THE

Pharmacologic Approach

TO THE

Critically Ill Patient

THIRD EDITION

THE

Pharmacologic Approach

TO THE

Critically Ill Patient

THIRD EDITION

EDITOR

Bart Chernow, M.D., F.A.C.P.

Professor of Medicine, Anesthesia, and Critical Care
The Johns Hopkins University School of Medicine
Physician-in-Chief
Sinai Hospital of Baltimore
Baltimore, Maryland
Editor-in-Chief
Critical Care Medicine

Associate Editors:
D. Craig Brater, M.D., Indianapolis, Indiana
John W. Holaday, Ph.D., F.C.C.M. Rockville Maryland
Gary P. Zaloga, M.D., F.A.C.P. Winston-Salem, North Carolina
Arno L. Zaritsky, M.D., Norfolk, Virginia

Editorial Assistant:
Lisa Daniel Sparks

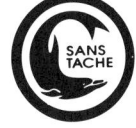

Williams & Wilkins

BALTIMORE • PHILADELPHIA • HONG KONG
LONDON • MUNICH • SYDNEY • TOKYO

A WAVERLY COMPANY

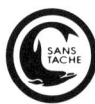

Editor: David C. Retford
Project Manager: Victoria Rybicki Vaughn, Kathleen Courtney Millet
Copy Editor: Stephen Siegforth, Dane Knighten
Designer: Norman W. Och
Illustration Planner: Lorraine Wrzosek

Copyright © 1994
Williams & Wilkins
428 East Preston Street
Baltimore, Maryland 21202, USA

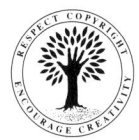

The authors, editor, and publisher have made every effort to provide accurate indications, adverse reactions, and dosage schedules for drugs discussed in this book, but it is possible that they may change. **The reader is urged to review the package information data of the manufacturers of the medications mentioned.**

Printed in the United States of America

Chapter reprints are available from the Publisher.

First Edition 1983
Second Edition 1988

Library of Congress Cataloging-in-Publication Data

The Pharmacologic approach to the critically ill patient/editor, Bart Chernow: associate editors, John W. Holaday, Gary P. Zaloga, Arno L. Zaritsky; editorial assistant, Lisa Daniel Sparks.—3rd ed.
   p. cm.
   Includes bibliographical references and index.
   ISBN 0-683-01524-9
   1. Pharmacology. 2. Critical care medicine. I. Chernow. Bart. [DNLM: 1. Pharmacology, Clinical. 2. Drug Therapy. 3. Critical Care. QV 38 P5355 1994]
RM301.P456 1994
615.5'8—dc20
DNLM/DLC
for Library of Congress
                             93-30220
                                 CIP

94 95 96 97 98
1 2 3 4 5 6 7 8 9 10

To my Parents, my Wife, and my Daughter

Preface

Critical care medicine has come into its own. The number of physicians, nurses, therapists, pharmacists, and other health professionals involved in the practice of critical care has increased dramatically over the last decade. The importance of clinical pharmacology in the care of the critically ill patient remains central to our therapeutic approach. The third edition of this textbook provides practitioners with an extended reference source in the arena of critical care pharmacology. This edition contains new chapters on drug monitoring, toxicology, muscle relaxants, sedation, immunotherapy, lazaroids, and mucolytic agents, with new attention focused on the pharmacologic approach to certain conditions, including stroke, muscle spasticity, burns, spinal cord injury, and even nerve gas poisoning. Nearly all of the other chapters have been completely rewritten.

Four associate editors have contributed their thoughts and assistance to this volume, and I owe each of them a debt of gratitude. Drs. Brater, Holaday, Zaloga, and Zaritsky have been important figures in the area of critical care pharmacology. Their insight and suggestions have been most helpful. The quality of our contributors is also impressive, and I hope that the reader appreciates the scholarly and thorough approach to the wide variety of subject matter presented. Unlike a number of reference sources, in this book I have permitted some degree of overlap, since several chapters would be incomplete if they did not contain certain information. However, the content varies so much from chapter to chapter, I am confident that the overlap will not be a distraction to readers. The index serves as a valuable adjunct to any clinical reference source. For that reason, numerous hours have been devoted to indexing this book.

It is inevitable that no reference source of this nature can be totally complete. Some would argue that we should extend this work to cover more specific clinical topics. However, as the editor, I found it necessary to consider page length, cost requirements, and the very favorable reviews of the first two editions of this book. It is a personal honor to have had the opportunity to edit the first three editions of this book, and I hope that in some way, the book's readers and their patients benefit from the contents.

Bart Chernow, M.D., F.A.C.P.

Contributors

David M. Angaran, M.S., F.C.C.P., F.A.S.H.P.
Professor of Pharmacy
Co-Director, Dubow Family Center for Research
    in Pharmaceutical Care
University of Florida College of Pharmacy
Gainesville, Florida

Allen I. Arieff, M.D., F.A.C.P.
Professor of Medicine
University of California, San Francisco
Chief, Geriatrics Research
Veterans Affairs Medical Center
San Francisco, California

Deborah K. Armstrong, Pharm.D., F.C.C.M.
Clinical Pharmacist
Mission Hospital Regional Medical Center
Mission Viejo, California

Patricia A. Arns, M.D.
Staff Physician in Internal Medicine
Baptist Hospital
Nashville, Tennessee

Frank J. Balestrieri, D.D.S., M.D., F.C.C.P.
Medical Director, Woodburn Surgery Center
Fairfax Hospital
Falls Church, Virginia
Assistant Clinical Professor
Department of Anesthesiology
George Washington University School of
    Medicine
Washington, DC
Assistant Clinical Professor
Department of Anesthesiology
Bowman Gray School of Medicine
Winston-Salem, North Carolina

Richard J. Battafarano, M.D.
Medical Fellow
Division of Surgical Infectious Diseases
Department of Surgery
University of Minnesota
Minneapolis, Minnesota

Luca M. Bigatello, M.D.
Instructor in Anaesthesia
Harvard Medical School
Assistant Anesthetist, Department of Anesthesia
Massachusetts General Hospital
Boston, Massachusetts

Lawrence Bortenschlager, M.D.
Staff Physician
Department of Critical Care Medicine
Methodist Hospital
Indianapolis, Indiana

William F. Boyer, M.D.
Assistant Professor
Department of Psychiatry
Emory University
Atlanta, Georgia

Robert A. Branch, M.D.
Professor of Medicine, Pharmacy,
    Pharmacology & Therapeutics
Director, Center for Clinical Pharmacology
University of Pittsburgh Medical Center
Pittsburgh, Pennsylvania

D. Craig Brater, M.D.
John B. Hickam Professor of Medicine
Chairman, Department of Medicine
Professor of Pharmacology and Toxicology
Chief, Division of Clinical Pharmacology
Indiana University Medical Center
Indianapolis, Indiana

Kenneth D. Burman, M.D., Col., M.C.
Professor of Medicine
Department of Medicine
The Uniformed Services University of the Health
    Sciences School of Medicine
Chief, Endocrine-Metabolism Service
Walter Reed Army Medical Center
Washington, DC

Hugh J. Carroll, M.D.
Professor of Medicine
Department of Medicine
State University of New York
Health Science Center at Brooklyn
Brooklyn, New York

Edwin H. Cassem, M.D.
Associate Professor of Psychiatry
Harvard University School of Medicine
Chief, Department of Psychiatry
Massachusetts General Hospital
Boston, Massachusetts

Robert Chasse, M.D.
Clinical Instructor
Section of Pulmonary/Critical Care Medicine
Department of Internal Medicine
Bowman Gray School of Medicine
Wake Forest University
Winston-Salem, North Carolina

Bart Chernow, M.D., F.A.C.P.
Professor of Medicine, Anesthesia, and Critical
  Care
The Johns Hopkins University School of
  Medicine
Physician-in-Chief
Sinai Hospital of Baltimore
Baltimore, Maryland
Editor-in-Chief
Critical Care Medicine

Robert Chin, Jr., M.D., F.C.C.P.
Assistant Professor of Medicine
Section of Pulmonary and Critical Care Medicine
Department of Medicine
Wake Forest University
Bowman Gray School of Medicine
Winston-Salem, North Carolina

Peter A. Chyka, Pharm.D., A.B.A.T.
Associate Professor of Clinical Pharmacology
University of Tennessee Center for the Health
  Sciences
Executive Director, Southern Poison Center, Inc.
Memphis, Tennessee

Robert D. Colucci, Pharm.D., F.C.P., F.C.C.M.
Assistant Director
Clinical Pharmacology, Clinical Research
Schering Plough Research Institute
Kenilworth, New Jersey

David J. Cullen, M.D., M.S.
Professor of Anaesthesia
Harvard Medical School
Anesthetist, Department of Anesthesia
Massachusetts General Hospital
Boston, Massachusetts

Joseph F. Dasta, M.Sc., F.C.C.M., F.C.C.P.
Associate Professor of Pharmacy and
  Anesthesiology
Division of Pharmacy Practice
The Ohio State University College of Pharmacy
Columbus, Ohio

Harold J. DeMonaco, M.S.
Assistant Professor
MGH Institute of Health Professions
Director, Pharmacy Department
Massachusetts General Hospital
Boston, Massachusetts

Louis DePalma, M.D.
Chief, Hematopathology
Associate Professor of Pathology and Anatomy
George Washington University Medical Center
Washington, DC

Douglas S. DeWitt, Ph.D.
Associate Professor
Department of Anesthesiology
University of Texas Medical Branch
Galveston, Texas

Michael N. Diringer, M.D.
Assistant Professor of Neurology, Neurosurgery,
  and Anesthesiology
Director, Neurology/Neurosurgery Intensive Care
  Unit
Washington University School of Medicine
St. Louis, Missouri

David L. Dunn, M.D., Ph.D.
Professor of Surgery
Head, Surgical Infectious Diseases
Division of Surgical Infectious Diseases
Department of Surgery
University of Minnesota
Minneapolis, Minnesota

Sudhir K. Dutta, M.D., F.A.C.P.
Professor of Medicine
University of Maryland School of Medicine
Director, Division of Gastroenterology
Sinai Hospital of Baltimore
Baltimore, Maryland

Donald Charles Eagerton, M.D.
Senior Fellow
Department of Endocrinology
Medical University of South Carolina
Charleston, South Carolina

Sergei Ermakov, M.D.
Clinical Research Fellow
Department of Critical Care Medicine
St. Francis Medical Center
Pittsburgh, Pennsylvania
Assistant Professor of Anesthesia
Medical Institute
Dnepropetrovsk, Russia

Mitchell P. Fink, M.D.
Associate Professor
Department of Surgery
Harvard Medical School
Chief, Division of Trauma and Critical Care
Beth Israel Hospital
Boston, Massachusetts

Sherry Fisher, R.N.
Pain Management Coordinator
Department of Anesthesiology
Fairfax Hospital
Falls Church, Virginia

Fun H. Fong, Jr., M.D., F.A.C.E.P.
Director, Radiation Medicine
Medical Sciences Division
Oak Ridge Institute for Science and Education
Oak Ridge, Tennessee

Robert M. Forstot, M.D.
Instructor of Anesthesiology
Division of Cardiothoracic Anesthesia
Department of Anesthesiology
Washington University School of Medicine
St. Louis, Missouri

Shirley A. Fry, M.B., B.Ch., M.P.H.
Associate Director
Medical Sciences Division
Oak Ridge Institute for Science and Education
Oak Ridge, Tennessee

David W. Fuhs, M.S., Pharm. D.
Assistant Director of Pharmacy
Clinical Services and Research
United and Children's Hospitals
St. Paul, Minnesota
Clinical Assistant Professor
University of Minnesota College of Pharmacy
Minneapolis, Minnesota

R. Brent Furbee, M.D., F.A.C.E.P., A.B.M.T.
Medical Director, Indiana Poison Center
Methodist Hospital of Indiana
Indianapolis, Indiana

Michael W. Gallagher, M.D.
Division of Obstetrics
Department of Obstetrics and Gynecology
Naval Medical Center
San Diego, California

Richard J. Galloway, M.D.
Department of Clinical Physiology
Walter Read Army Institute of Research
Washington, DC

Stephen A. Geraci, M.D., F.A.C.C., F.A.C.P., F.C.C.P.
Assistant Professor of Medicine and
    Pharmacology
Division of Cardiovascular Disease and Clinical
    Pharmacology
University of Tennessee College of Medicine
Memphis, Tennessee
Assistant Professor of Medicine and
    Pharmacology
Division of Cardiology
Uniformed Services of the Health Sciences
Bethesda, Maryland

Marye H. Godinez, M.D.
Research Associate
The Joseph Stokes Jr. Research Institute
The Children's Hospital of Philadelphia
Philadelphia, Pennsylvania

Rodolfo I. Godinez, M.D., Ph.D.
Associate Professor of Anesthesiology and
    Pediatrics
University of Pennsylvania School of Medicine
Associate Medical Director, Pediatric Intensive
    Care Unit
Medical Director, Respiratory Care Services
The Children's Hospital of Philadelphia
Philadelphia, Pennsylvania

Phillip J. Goldstein, M.D.
Chairman
Department of Obstetrics and Gynecology
Washington Hospital Center
Clinical Professor of Obstetrics and Gynecology
Georgetown University School of Medicine
Washington, DC

Steven A. Gould, M.D.
Chief of Service
Department of Surgery
Michael Reese Hospital and Medical Center
Professor of Surgery
University of Illinois College of Medicine
Chicago, Illinois

John P. Grant, M.D.
Associate Professor of Surgery
Duke University Medical Center
Durham, North Carolina

David J. Greenblatt, M.D.
Professor
Department of Pharmacology and Experimental
    Therapeutics
Tufts University School of Medicine
Division of Clinical Pharmacology
New England Medical Center Hospital
Boston, Massachusetts

Ake N.A. Grenvik, M.D., Ph.D., F.C.C.M.
Professor of Anesthesiology, Medicine, and
    Surgery
Director, Multidisciplinary Critical Care Training
    Program
University of Pittsburgh School of Medicine
Pittsburgh, Pennsylvania

Charles E. Halstenson, Pharm.D., F.C.C.P
Professor of Pharmacy
University of Minnesota College of Pharmacy
Co-Director, The Drug Evaluation Unit
Minneapolis Medical Research Foundation at
    Hennepin County Medical Center
Minneapolis, Minnesota

Paul M. Heerdt, M.D., Ph.D.
Associate Professor
Department of Anesthesiology
Assistant Professor
Department of Pharmacology
Cornell University Medical College
Assistant Member
Department of Anesthesiology and Critical Care
    Medicine
Memorial Sloan-Kettering Cancer Center
New York, New York

Mark A. Helfaer, M.D.
Associate Professor
Departments of Anesthesiology/Critical Care
    Medicine and Pediatrics
The Johns Hopkins University School of
    Medicine
Baltimore, Maryland

John W. Holaday, Ph.D., F.C.C.M.
Department of Medicine
The Johns Hopkins University School of
    Medicine
Baltimore, Maryland
President and Chief Executive Officer
EntreMed Inc.
Rockville, Maryland

John W. Hoyt, M.D., F.C.C.M., F.C.C.P.
Chairman
Department of Critical Care Medicine
St. Francis Medical Center
Clinical Professor of Anesthesiology/Critical Care
    Medicine
University of Pittsburgh School of Medicine
Pittsburgh, Pennsylvania

Judith Jacobi, Pharm.D., F.C.C.M.
Critical Care Pharmacist
Department of Pharmacy
St. Vincent Hospitals and Health Services
Indianapolis, Indiana

Allan S. Jaffe, M.D.
Professor of Medicine
Cardiovascular Division
Washington University School of Medicine
St. Louis, Missouri

Thomas C. Jannett, Ph.D.
Associate Professor
Department of Electrical and Computer
    Engineering
University of Alabama at Birmingham
Birmingham, Alabama

Jeffrey S. Kelly, M.D.
Assistant Professor of Anesthesia
Critical Care
Department of Anesthesia
Wake Forest University
Bowman Gray School of Medicine
Winston-Salem, North Carolina

Jeffrey R. Kirsch, M.D.
Associate Professor
Department of Anesthesiology/Critical Care
    Medicine
The Johns Hopkins University School of
    Medicine
Baltimore, Maryland

David J. Kramer, M.D.
Assistant Professor of Anesthesiology/Critical Care
    Medicine and Surgery
University of Pittsburgh School of Medicine
Co-Director, Liver Transplant ICU Services
Presbyterian-University Hospital
Pittsburgh, Pennsylvania

Gregory L. Krauss, M.D.
Assistant Professor
Department of Neurology
The Johns Hopkins University School of
    Medicine
Baltimore, Maryland

Edward P. Krenzelok, Pharm.D., A.B.A.T.
Professor
Department of Pharmacy and Therapeutics
School of Pharmacy
Department of Pediatrics
School of Medicine
University of Pittsburgh
Director, Pittsburgh Poison Center
Children's Hospital of Pittsburgh
Pittsburgh, Pennsylvania

Cheryl A. Kubisty, M.D.
Providence Everett Primary Care
Everett, Washington

Jane W. Kwan, B.S. Pharmacy, M.P.H.
Coordinator, Pharmacy Alternate Delivery
    Programs
Division of Pharmacy
The University of Texas
MD Anderson Cancer Center
Houston, Texas

C. Raymond Lake, M.D., Ph.D.
Professor and Chairperson
Department of Psychiatry
University of Kansas Medical Center
Kansas City, Kansas

Stanford I. Lamberg, M.D.
Associate Professor
Department of Dermatology
The Johns Hopkins University School of
    Medicine
Baltimore, Maryland

Daniel J. Lebovitz, M.D.
Instructor
Department of Pediatrics
Case Western Reserve University School of
    Medicine
Division of Pediatric Pharmacology and Critical
    Care
Rainbow Babies and Childrens Hospital
Cleveland, Ohio

Alex Lechleuthner, M.D., Ph.D.
Surgical Clinic
Department of Surgery
University of Cologne
Cologne, Germany

Brian Litt, M.D.
Instructor
Department of Neurology
The Johns Hopkins University School of
    Medicine
Division of Neurology
Department of Medicine
Sinai Hospital of Baltimore
Baltimore, Maryland

John D. Lockrem, M.D.
Department of Anesthesiology
Director, Surgical Intensive Care Unit
The Cleveland Clinic Foundation
Cleveland, Ohio

Naomi L.C. Luban, M.D.
Director, Blood Bank/Hematology
Department of Laboratory Medicine
Children's National Medical Center
Professor of Pediatrics and Pathology
George Washington University Medical Center
Washington, DC

Drew A. MacGregor, M.D.
Assistant Professor of Anesthesia (Critical Care)
    and Medicine (Pulmonary/Critical Care)
Department of Anesthesia
Wake Forest University
Bowman Gray School of Medicine
Winston-Salem, North Carolina

Diana S. Malcolm, Ph.D.
Research Associate Professor
Department of Surgery
F. Edward Hebert School of Medicine
Uniformed Services University of the Health
    Sciences
Bethesda, Maryland

J. A. Jeevendra Martyn, M.D., F.F.A.R.C.S.
Associate Professor of Anesthesia
Harvard Medical School
Anesthetist, Director, Clinical Pharmacology
Massachusetts General Hospital
Associate Director of Anesthesia,
Shriners Burn Institute
Boston, Massachusetts

Henry Masur, M.D.
Chief, Critical Care Medicine
Clinical Center, National Institutes of Health
Bethesda, Maryland
Professor of Clinical Medicine
George Washington University Medical Center
Washington, DC

Gerald S. Moss, M.D.
Dean
University of Illinois College of Medicine
Chicago, Illinois

James B. Mowry, Pharm.D., A.B.A.T.
Director, Indiana Poison Center
Methodist Hospital of Indiana
Indianapolis, Indiana

John J. Nanfro, M.D.
Rome, Georgia

Edmund Neugebauer, Ph.D.
Associate Professor of Theoretical Surgery
Head, Biochemical and Experimental Division
Department of Surgery
University of Cologne
Cologne, Germany

Daniel A. Notterman, M.D., F.A.A.P., F.C.C.M.
Associate Professor of Pediatrics, Clinical
    Pharmacology, and Pediatrics in Surgery
Director, Division of Pediatric Critical Care
    Medicine
New York Hospital-Cornell Medical Center
New York, New York

Man S. Oh, M.D.
Professor of Medicine
Department of Medicine
State University of New York
Health Science Center at Brooklyn
Brooklyn, New York

Joseph E. Parrillo, M.D.
James B. Herrick Professor of Medicine
Chief, Section of Cardiology
Chief, Section of Critical Care Medicine
Medical Director, Rush Heart Institute
Rush-Presbyterian-St. Luke's Medical Center
Chicago, Illinois

Donald S. Prough, M.D.
Professor and Chairman
Department of Anesthesiology
University of Texas Medical Branch
Galveston, Texas

Thomas G. Rainey, M.D., F.C.C.M.
Director, Critical Care
Fairfax Hospital
Falls Church, Virginia

Russell C. Raphaely, M.D.
Professor of Anesthesiology and Pediatrics
University of Pennsylvania School of Medicine
Medical Director, Pediatric Intensive Care Unit
Director, Division of Critical Care Medicine
The Children's Hospital of Philadelphia
Philadelphia, Pennsylvania

Charles A. Read, M.D., F.C.C.P.
Assistant Professor of Medicine
Division of Pulmonary and Critical Care
Georgetown University Medical Center
Washington, DC

Michael D. Reed, Pharm.D., F.C.C.P., F.C.P.
Associate Professor
Department of Pediatrics
Case Western Reserve University School of
    Medicine
Division of Pediatric Pharmacology and Critical
    Care
Rainbow Babies and Childrens Hospital
Cleveland, Ohio

John T. Repke, M.D.
Division of Maternal-Fetal Medicine
Department of Obstetrics, Gynecology, and
    Reproduction Biology
Harvard Medical School
Boston, Massachusetts

Dieter Rixen, M.D.
Surgical Clinic
Department of Surgery
University of Cologne
Cologne, Germany

Mark C. Rogers, M.D.
Vice Chancellor for Health Systems
Executive Director, Duke University Hospital
Distinguished Professor of Anesthesiology and
  Pediatrics
Duke University
Durham, North Carolina

Arthur L. Rosen, Ph.D.
Biophysicist, Surgical Research
Michael Reese Hospital and Medical Center
Chicago, Illinois

Alan J. Rosenbloom, M.D.
Assistant Professor of Anesthesiology/Critical Care
  Medicine
Division of Critical Care Medicine, Department
  of Anesthesiology
University of Pittsburgh School of Medicine
Pittsburgh, Pennsylvania

Laurence H. Ross, M.D.
Baltimore, Maryland

Anita C. Rudy, Ph.D.
Lecturer, Division of Clinical Pharmacology
Department of Medicine
Indiana University Medical Center
Wishard Memorial Hospital
Indianapolis, Indiana

Robert R. Ruffolo, Jr., Ph.D.
Vice President and Director
Pharmacological Sciences, U.S., U.K., Europe,
  and Australia
SmithKline Beecham Pharmaceuticals
King of Prussia, Pennsylvania

Pablo F. Ruiz-Ramon, M.D.
Nephrology and Hypertension
Santa Rosa, California

Colleen M. Ryan, M.D.
Assistant Professor of Surgery
Harvard Medical School
Massachusetts General Hospital
Boston, Massachusetts

Stefan Saad, M.D.
Surgical Clinic
Department of Surgery
University of Cologne
Cologne, Germany

Michael Salem, M.D.
Clinical and Research Fellow
Department of Anesthesiology/Critical Care
  Medicine
The Johns Hopkins University School of
  Medicine
Baltimore, Maryland

Joseph M. Scavone, M.S., Pharm.D.
Professor and Division Head
Clinical, Hospital, and Administrative Pharmacy
College of Pharmacy
University of Iowa
Assistant Clinical Professor of Psychiatry
Tufts University School of Medicine
Adjunct Assistant Professor of Community
  Medicine and Socio-Medical Sciences
Boston University School of Medicine
Boston, Massachusetts

Hansa L. Sehgal, B.S.
Supervisor, Surgical Research
Michael Reese Hospital and Medical Center
Chicago, Illinois

Lakshman R. Sehgal, Ph.D.
Director, Surgical Research
Michael Reese Hospital and Medical Center
Chicago, Illinois

Marissa Seligman, Pharm.D.
Vice President, Academic and Scientific Affairs
SCP Communications, Inc.
New York, New York

Louis C. Sheppard, Ph.D.
Associate Vice President for Bioengineering and
  Biotechnology
Director, Biomedical Engineering Center
Professor of Physiology and Biophysics
University of Texas Medical Branch
Galveston, Texas

Henry J. Silverman, M.D.
Associate Professor of Medicine
Director, Medical Intensive Care Unit
Pulmonary and Critical Care Medicine Division
University of Maryland School of Medicine
Baltimore, Maryland

Robert C. Smallridge, M.D.
Director
Division of Medicine
Walter Reed Army Institute of Research
Washington, DC

John C. Somberg, M.D., F.C.P.
Professor of Medicine and Pharmacology
University of Health Sciences
The Chicago Medical School
North Chicago, Illinois

Rajat Sood, M.D.
Fellow in Gastroenterology
Department of Medicine
Henry Ford Hospital
Detroit, Michigan

Wendy L. St. Peter, Pharm.D.
Assistant Professor of Pharmacy
University of Minneapolis College of Pharmacy
Clinical Scientist
The Drug Evaluation Unit
Hennepin County Medical Center
Minneapolis, Minnesota

Keith L. Stein, M.D.
Associate Professor of Anesthesiology/Critical
  Care Medicine and Surgery
University of Pittsburgh School of Medicine
Director, Cardiothoracic Surgical Intensive Care
  Unit
Presbyterian-University Hospital
Pittsburgh, Pennsylvania

Curt M. Steinhart, M.D.
Associate Professor of Pediatrics, Surgery, and
  Anesthesiology
Medical Director, Pediatric Intensive Care Unit
Medical College of Georgia
Augusta, Georgia

Barney J. Stern, M.D.
Associate Professor of Neurology
The Johns Hopkins University School of
  Medicine
Director, Division of Neurology
Sinai Hospital of Baltimore
Baltimore, Maryland

James K. Stoller, M.D.
Head, Section of Respiratory Therapy
Department of Pulmonary/Critical Care Medicine
The Cleveland Clinic Foundation
Cleveland, Ohio

Neelakantan Sunder, M.B.B.S.
Assistant Professor of Anesthesia
Harvard Medical School
Associate Anesthetist, Massachusetts General
  Hospital
Boston, Massachusetts

Richard J. Traystman, Ph.D.
Vice Chairman for Research
Distinguished Research Professor
Department of Anesthesiology/Critical Care
  Medicine
The Johns Hopkins University School of
  Medicine
Baltimore, Maryland

Ronald G. Tompkins, M.D., Sc.D.
Associate Professor of Surgery
Harvard Medical School
Chief, Trauma Service
Massachusetts General Hospital
Chief of Staff, Shriners Burns Institute
Boston, Massachusetts

Bertil K.J. Wagner, Pharm.D.
Assistant Professor
Department of Pharmacy Practice and
  Administration
Rutgers-The State University of New Jersey
College of Pharmacy
Piscataway, New Jersey

Peter J. Wedlund, Ph.D.
Associate Professor of Pharmacology
University of Kentucky College of Pharmacy
Lexington, Kentucky

Howard D. Weiss, M.D.
Division of Neurology
Sinai Hospital of Baltimore
Assistant Professor of Neurology
The Johns Hopkins University School of
  Medicine
Baltimore, Maryland

Wise Young, Ph.D., M.D.
Professor of Neurosurgery, Physiology, and
  Biophysics
Director of Neurosurgery Research
New York University Medical Center
New York, New York

Gary P. Zaloga, M.D., F.A.C.P.
Professor of Medicine and Anesthesia/Critical
  Care Medicine
Head, Section on Critical Care
Department of Anesthesia
Bowman Gray School of Medicine
Wake Forest University
Winston-Salem, North Carolina

Arno L. Zaritsky, M.D.
Associate Professor of Pediatrics
Eastern Virginia Medical School
Co-Director, Pediatric ICU
Children's Hospital of The King's Daughters
Norfolk, Virginia

Michael G. Ziegler, M.D.
Professor of Medicine
Director, Hypertension Services
Program Director, Clinical Research Center
University of California, San Diego Medical
  Center
San Diego, California

Jerry J. Zimmerman, Ph.D., M.D.
Associate Professor of Pediatrics
Director of Critical Care Fellowship and
  Research Programs
University of Wisconsin-Madison Medical School
Children's Hospital
Madison, Wisconsin

Contents

Section One *Clinical Pharmacology in the ICU*

Section Four   *Special Considerations in Critical Care Pharmacology*

SECTION ONE

Clinical Pharmacology in the ICU

CHAPTER 1

Pharmacokinetics

ANITA C. RUDY, Ph.D.
D. CRAIG BRATER, M.D.

When administering drugs to patients, one is concerned with the relationship between the dose of drug given and the response elicited. The obvious goal is to attain a therapeutic effect while minimizing toxicity. To attain this goal, clinicians need a working knowledge of the principles of drug absorption, distribution, and elimination and of how these processes are related to intensity and duration of drug action (pharmacokinetics). Using pharmacokinetic principles, therefore, can assist the clinician in determining the relationship between the dose administered and the concentration of drug achieved in the blood. There are several advantages to utilizing pharmacokinetic parameters, especially in the critically ill patient: (a) The proper use of kinetics can improve the overall care of the patient by more accurately attaining desired drug concentrations and response, as compared with the use of "hit-or-miss" therapy. (b) Utilizing pharmacokinetic parameters can decrease the incidence of toxicity from drugs having a narrow margin of safety. (c) Using kinetics properly can eliminate alterations in absorption, distribution, and elimination as causative factors in problem patients and thus allow the clinician to focus on pharmacodynamic efficacy (see below). (d) Finally, using pharmacokinetic parameters can help reduce the incidence of drug interactions that can complicate therapy (see Chapter 2).

When used properly, kinetic principles can be extremely helpful in the critical care setting; however, clinicians must also be aware of the limitations of applying pharmacokinetic principles. Clearly, the endpoint of drug therapy is clinical efficacy, not simply attaining a certain blood concentration of drug. Thus, to utilize blood concentrations without proper history, diagnosis, and clinical judgment would be a grave error. Indeed, the concentration of drug in the blood is only one tool to be used in assessing outcome. The relationship between the concentration of drug in blood and the clinical response (pharmacodynamics) is most critical (34). This relationship is a function of each patient's dose (concentration)-response curve and must be judged on an individual basis. In clinical practice we evaluate this parameter by clinical measures of response that can then be related to drug concentration and to dose in the individual patient. For example, in the use of quinidine to suppress ventricular ectopic beats, one can evaluate the decrease in ectopy as a measure of efficacy. Since widening of the QRS complex and prolongation of the Q-T interval are associated with quinidine toxicity, one can measure these as toxic endpoints in individual patients. Obviously, a dose of quinidine is sought that results in diminished ectopy (efficacy) without ECG changes of toxicity. This ratio of efficacy to toxicity (the therapeutic index) and the dose of drug that optimizes the ratio is highly individual. We know "average" doses of drugs that achieve "average" blood concentrations and "average" response in "average" patients. However, variability among patients is quite large, and disease states impact on both handling of and responses to drugs in patients. Therefore, to practice good therapeutics, we must attempt in each individual patient to define the optimal dose-response relationship.

The relationship between dose and response can be influenced by a variety of pharmacokinetic and pharmacodynamic parameters (Fig. 1.1). Using these parameters in concert with knowledge of how disease states influence absorption, distribution, and elimination of drugs and knowledge of the pharmacology of drugs, we can attempt to optimize drug therapy to the individual patient and measure clinical indices of response. In this chapter, principles of pharmacokinetics and pharmacodynamics are discussed in a general fashion, using specific, illustrative examples. The principles can then be applied in succeeding chapters. Rather than citing a voluminous literature, references are focused on timely reviews from which the interested reader can pursue more specific and detailed listings (10).

PHARMACOKINETIC PRINCIPLES (16, 22, 26, 27, 29, 43, 56, 66, 74)

In using and reading about drugs one encounters a variety of symbols and terminology (Table 1.1).

PHARMACOKINETICS

DOSING REGIMEN { DOSE / DOSING INTERVAL / ROUTE OF ADMINISTRATION

ABSORPTION

DISTRIBUTION

ELIMINATION { METABOLISM / EXCRETION / DIALYSIS

CONCENTRATION IN PLASMA

CONCENTRATION AT SITE OF ACTION

PHARMACODYNAMICS

EFFECT

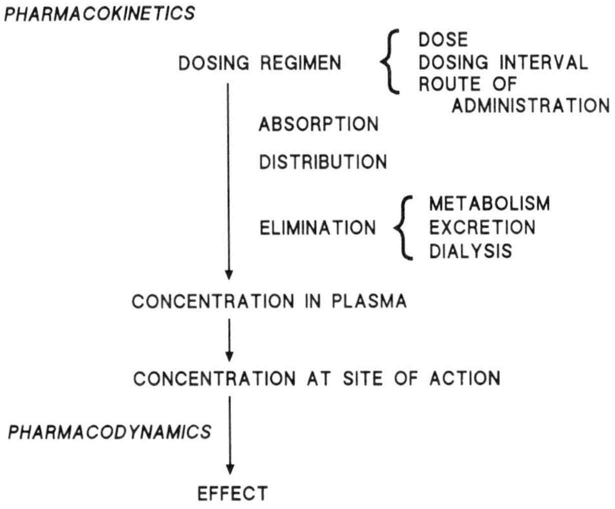

Figure 1.1. Schematic representation of the determinants of the relationship between the dose of a drug and the response it elicits.

DERIVATION OF PHARMACOKINETIC PARAMETERS

It is important to understand the symbols and terminology (Table 1.1) used in discussing pharmacokinetics and the derivation of some simple pharmacokinetic parameters. These pharmacokinetic calculations can be useful in determining drug dosing and, therefore, in the optimal care of the patient.

The majority of drugs used clinically obey first order or linear kinetics, as opposed to saturable kinetics, which may also be termed zero order, nonlinear, or Michaelis-Menten kinetics. With first order kinetics, a constant percentage of drug is removed per unit time; that is, as drug concentration increases, proportionally more drug is removed. The elimination half-life remains constant. With saturable kinetics, the percentage eliminated is different at different drug concentrations, usually resulting in long elimination half-lives with higher concentrations. The relevance of drugs obeying this latter type of elimination is discussed subsequently. Figure 1.2 shows an example of an orally administered drug obeying first order kinetics. A plot of the logarithm of the serum concentration vs. time allows derivation of a number of parameters. The straight, terminal segment of the curve, called the log-linear phase, can be extrapolated back to the Y axis. This component of the curve represents elimination, and from the slope of this line one can calculate k, the elimination rate constant (Fig. 1.2). For example,

$$Slope = \frac{\delta Y}{\delta X}$$

$$= \frac{\delta \, Concentration}{\delta \, time}$$

$$= \frac{ln \, 5.0 - ln \, 3.2}{4 - 5}$$

$$= \frac{1.61 - 1.16}{-1}$$

$$= -0.45$$

$$k = -slope = 0.45 \; (in \; units \; of \; reciprocal \; time)$$

The elimination half-life can then be calculated as $t_{1/2}$

Table 1.1.   Glossary of Pharmacokinetic Terms

$t_{1/2}$—half-life: The amount of time required for the concentration of drug to decrease by $\frac{1}{2}$.
k or ke—Elimination rate constant; determined by the slope of the terminal phase of a plot of the logarithm of the concentration of drug vs. time.
ka—Absorption rate constant.
kr—Elimination rate constant for the renal component of drug elimination.
knr—Elimination rate constant for the nonrenal component of drug elimination.
V_d—Volume of distribution that relates the concentration of drug in the plasma to the amount of drug in the body.
Cl—Clearance; the amount of blood, plasma, or serum from which all drug is removed per unit time.
Cl_r—The component of clearance accounted for by renal elimination.
Cl_{nr}—The component of clearance accounted for by nonrenal elimination.
f_e—Fraction of dose excreted unchanged in the urine.
F—Fraction of the dose that reaches the systemic circulation intact (bioavailability).
δ—Dosing interval; the time between doses.
Cp_{ss}—Average plasma concentration of drug at steady state.
Cp_{max}—The maximum or peak plasma concentration of drug at steady state.
Cp_{min}—The minimum or trough plasma concentration of drug at steady state.

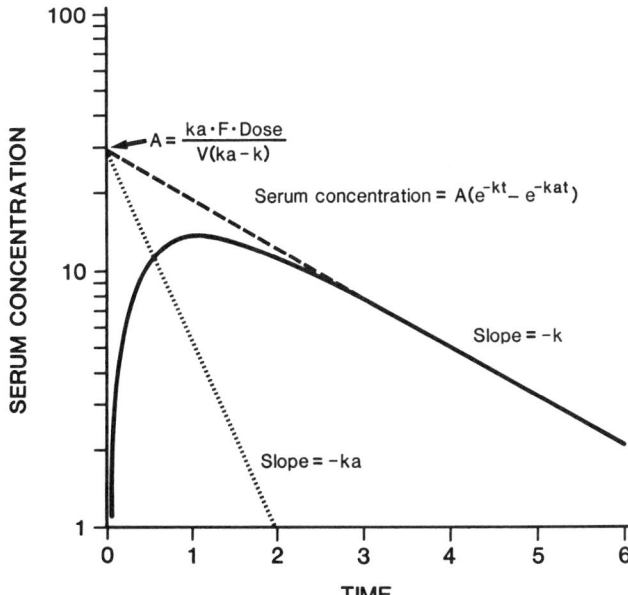

Figure 1.2. Semilogarithmic graph of serum concentration vs. time profile after oral administration of a drug. Pharmacokinetic parameters are shown. See text for explanation.

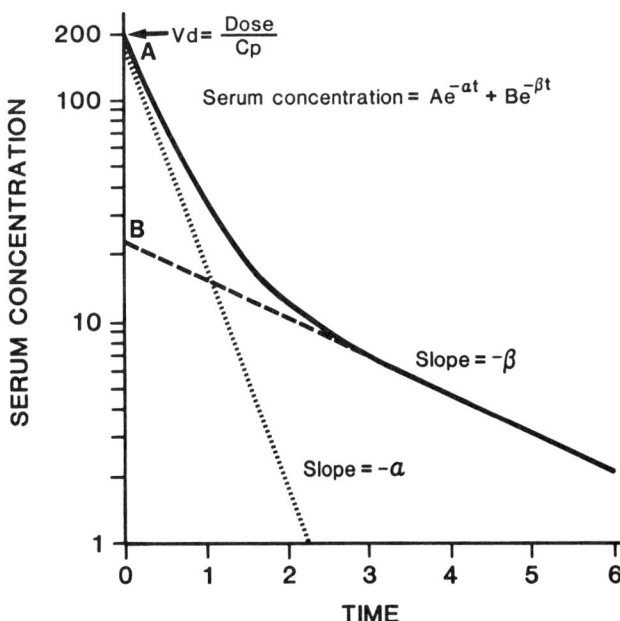

Figure 1.3. Semilogarithmic graph of serum concentration vs. time profile after intravenous administration of a drug with two compartment characteristics. Pharmacokinetic parameters are shown. See text for explanation.

elimination = $0.693/k$. Therefore, in Figure 1.2, $t_{1/2}$ elimination = $0.693/0.45 = 1.54$. (The units of time would be those used in the graph). The value in the numerator is the natural logarithm of 2. Alternatively, and probably more simply, any elimination half-life can be determined graphically by measuring the time interval for the serum concentration to decrease by one-half (for example, from 10 to 5)—in the case shown in Figure 1.2, approximately 1.5, i.e., the same as that calculated above.

Parameters for absorption can be calculated by using the method of residuals. By subtracting data points on the curve from the extrapolated log-linear phase (heavy dashed line), another straight line can be defined (small dashed line), the slope of which is a function of the absorption rate constant, k_a (Fig. 1.2). The half-life of absorption is then equal to $0.693/k_a$. The volume of distribution can also be calculated, using the intercept (A) of these straight lines with the Y axis, if one knows F, the fraction absorbed (bioavailability). This calculation is done using the equation:

$$A = k_a \cdot F \cdot Dose/V_d\,(k_a - k)$$

or

$$V_d = \frac{k_a \cdot F \cdot Dose}{A\,(k_a - k)}$$

A similar graph can be made for an intravenously administered drug. In this instance, the plasma decay curve has two components, the α phase (rapid or early phase), which usually represents a distribution phase, i.e., the drug is distributing into tissues, and the β phase, which represents elimination (Fig. 1.3). The terms α and β are both rate constants from which respective half-lives can be calculated; A and B are intercepts with the Y axis. The extrapolation of the β phase (heavy dashed line) defines B. Generation of another line

Table 1.2. Calculation of Pharmacokinetic Parameters after Intravenous Administration of a Drug

$$Cp = Ae^{-\alpha t} + Be^{-\beta t} \text{ (see Figure 1.3)}$$

$$V_{d_{area}} \text{ or } Vd_\beta = \frac{Dose}{\beta AUC} = \frac{Dose}{\beta\left(\dfrac{A}{\alpha} + \dfrac{B}{\beta}\right)}$$

$$Cl = \frac{Dose}{AUC} = \frac{Dose}{\dfrac{A}{\alpha} + \dfrac{B}{\beta}}$$

$$t_{1/2\alpha} = \frac{0.693}{\alpha} \text{ or measure directly}$$

$$t_{1/2\beta} = \frac{0.693}{\beta} \text{ or measure directly}$$

AUC refers to the *a*rea *u*nder the *c*urve relating plasma concentration to time.

(small dashed line) by subtracting the extrapolated β phase from the curve defines α and A. From A, B, α, and β, clearance and volume of distribution can be calculated (Table 1.2).

At clinically used doses, some drugs, particularly ethanol, phenytoin, salicylates, and mezlocillin, obey saturable or Michaelis-Menten kinetics. At usual therapeutic blood concentrations these drugs can saturate elimination pathways. Their handling, then, is best characterized by parameters for V_{max} and K_m, rather than by volume of distribution and clearance. For drugs such as these, clearance decreases and half-life increases with increasing doses of drug. Clinically, this characteristic means that at higher dosages a small increase in dose can result in a large increase in serum concentration of these drugs, with a longer half-life. For example, increasing a patient's phenytoin dose from 200 to 300 mg/day may result in a proportional increase in steady-state blood concentration from 10 to 15 μg/ml. However, as metabolizing enzymes become saturated, a further increase in dose from 300 to 400 mg/day may cause the blood concentration to rise from 15 to 30 μg/ml or more. The clinical lesson from this example is that dosage increments above the "usual normal dose" should be small with these drugs.

Disease states or drug interactions can adversely affect the elimination of drugs, which is of greatest concern for drugs that are cleared by saturable kinetics. A patient with hepatic disease, for example, may have a significantly lower V_{max} for a drug than a healthy individual. Consequently, lower concentrations could result in saturation of metabolizing enzymes. Thus, as discussed in the phenytoin example above, saturation may occur between 200- and 300-mg doses in the critically ill patient and cause unpredictably high drug concentrations at much lower dosages.

CLINICAL APPLICATION OF PHARMACOKINETIC PARAMETERS

In the clinical setting, the most important pharmacokinetic parameters are bioavailability (F), half-life ($t_{1/2}$), clearance (Cl), and volume of distribution (V_d). Proper knowledge of what these parameters represent and how they are used can assist in delivering proper dosing, in correctly utilizing therapeutic drug monitoring, and in optimizing drug therapy.

Bioavailability (F)

Bioavailability is defined as the percentage of an administered dose of drug that reaches the systemic circulation. If a drug is administered intravenously, for example, the bioavailability is obviously 100%, and F equals 1.0. When drugs are administered by other routes, however, the bioavailability in most instances is less than 100%. The degree of bioavailability is determined by the extent of drug absorption and degree of metabolism prior to the drug entering the systemic circulation. This subject is discussed in detail below under "Extent of Absorption." The clinician should have some quantitative estimate of bioavailability to correctly decide the dose of a drug the patient should receive. For example, morphine has an oral bioavailability of 20 to 30% due to rapid metabolism by the liver prior to entering the systemic circulation (first-pass effect). Consequently, the dose given orally is usually 3 to 5 times larger than the dose administered by means of parenteral routes.

Half-life (t₁/₂)

The most commonly used pharmacokinetic parameter is half-life, which is defined as the time it takes for the blood concentration of a drug to diminish by 50%. This term is often used inappropriately by clinicians as a term to define drug elimination. In contrast, half-life is a hybrid term, being a function of both clearance and volume of distribution. A change in half-life caused by a change in clearance has different therapeutic implications than does a change occurring because of an altered volume of distribution.

The most important use of half-life is to predict how long it takes for a dosing regimen to achieve steady-state concentrations of drug in blood. With initiation of therapy, if a loading dose is not administered—i.e., the patient is not "instantly" affixed at a desired serum drug concentration that is to be

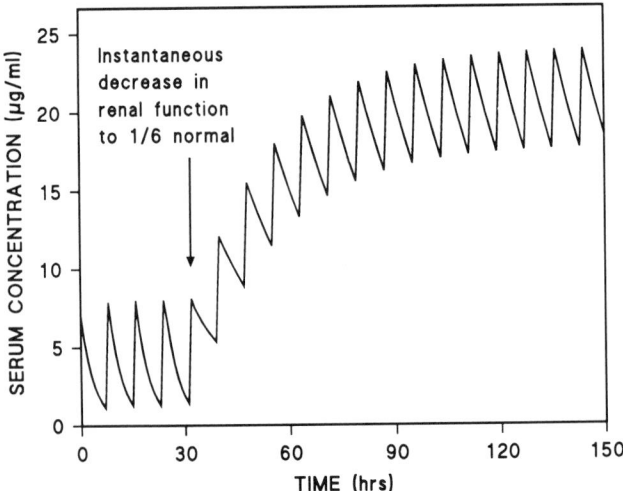

Figure 1.4. Schematic representing the effect of a 6-fold increase in half-life on the reattainment of steady-state blood concentrations of a drug. This schematic applies specifically to gentamicin or tobramycin if an instantaneous decrease of renal function to 1/6 of normal occurred.

maintained throughout therapy—four to five half-lives will elapse before the patient reaches steady-state drug concentrations. For a drug such as digoxin then, which has an average half-life of approximately 36 hours in patients with normal renal function, approximately 1 week must elapse before steady-state is achieved. If one evaluates such a patient clinically by obtaining a serum concentration of digoxin after only 2 days, and erroneously assumes that a steady-state has been reached, the drug concentration will be misinterpreted, and the clinician may have little, if any, insight into the patient's current status, as well as the patient's therapeutic or toxic state in the future.

Similarly, if the dose of a drug is either increased or decreased, 4 to 5 times the half-life must elapse to reattain steady state. Also, if drug half-life changes, such as may occur with a change in the patient's disease state, a new steady-state occurs after 4 to 5 times the new half-life (Fig. 1.4).

One must always try to maintain the perspective of whether or not the patient is at steady state. Interpreting blood drug concentration data is very difficult, if not impossible, unless one has some idea of the steady-state factor. Changing doses of a drug before the patient has reached steady state with one dose often becomes a confusing and potentially hazardous exercise. In the critically ill patient, this concept is exceedingly important, because the status of the patient's disease and of other coadministered drugs can change rapidly and dramatically with concomitant effects on drug handling and half-life.

Volume of Distribution

The volume of distribution is a proportionality constant that relates to concentration in the plasma and the amount of drug in the body. It is useful in estimating the concentration of drug attained in plasma by a given dose of drug or in estimating the dose required to achieve a desirable plasma drug concentration through the relationship concentration = amount in the body/V_d. After intravenous bolus administration of drug, one knows the amount in the body and the relationship becomes: concentration at time zero = Dose/V_d. Therefore, if one achieves an initial concentration of 10 μg/ml by administering a 1-g dose of a drug: by IV bolus, then

$$V_d = \frac{Dose}{Concentration\ at\ zero\ time}$$

$$= \frac{1\ g}{10\ g/liter}$$

$$= 100\ liter$$

This volume should not be ascribed physiologic meaning. It is a derived parameter. One might best think of the body as a bathtub; the volume of distribution simply describes the size of the bathtub for a given drug. Clinically, one may use the volume of distribution to calculate the loading dose of a drug required to reach an initial, target concentration of drug in blood. For example, if one wishes to achieve a drug concentration of 10 μg/ml and the volume of distribution is 100 liters, the loading dose would be 1000 mg from dose = V_d concentration at zero time. This calculation is independent of a drug's clearance or its half-life. Importantly, diseases can change a drug's volume of distribution, and the clinician who is not aware of this possibility can cause a serious disservice to patients. In the example just discussed, if the patient's disease caused the volume of distribution of the drug to decrease from 100 to 50 liters and this effect was not realized, resulting in the patient's being administered the same 1000-mg loading dose, the patient's serum concentration would predictably be 1000/50 = 20 μg/ml, as opposed to the desired concentration of 10 μg/ml. This type of mistake could result in toxicity.

Clearance (Cl)

Clearance is usually referred to as blood, plasma, or serum clearance, depending on whether concentrations of drug are measured in whole blood, plasma, or serum, respectively. With each use, clearance quantifies the amount of blood, or whatever variable, from which all drug is removed per unit time. Therefore, a plasma clearance of 100 ml/minute means that all drug can be removed from 100 ml of plasma in 1 minute. This removal can occur through distribution to tissues, metabolism, or excretion (see below).

Clinically, clearance is important for determining the amount of drug needed to maintain the concentration of drug at steady state. By definition, at steady state:

Rate of drug in = rate of drug out

The rate of drug entering is, in turn, a function of the dose administered, the fraction (*F*) of that dose absorbed if administered orally or intramuscularly, and the time interval over which it is administered (τ):

Rate in = F·dose/τ

The rate of drug leaving the body is a function of its steady-state concentration (Cp_{ss}) and its clearance:

Rate out = Cp_{ss}·Cl

Therefore, at steady-state

F·dose/τ = Cp_{ss}·Cl

or, rearranging the equation:

Cp_{ss} = F·dose/τ·Cl

It is obvious from this relationship that changes or individual differences in bioavailability, in dosing regimen (dose and dosing interval), and in clearance can influence the steady-state concentration of a drug (Fig. 1.4). Changes in clearance of a drug caused by disease must be compensated for by changes in dosing regimen.

Clinical Use of Pharmacokinetic Parameters

Table 1.3 summarizes the clinical importance of the various pharmacokinetic parameters discussed above. Briefly, *the volume of distribution is important for determining the loading dose, clearance for maintenance dose, and half-life for determining the time needed to reach steady state.* A change in half-life can occur by changes in volume of distribution and/or by changes in clearance. Therefore, for example, knowing only that the half-life of a drug is altered in a particular disease state does not allow one to decide appropriate adjustment of therapy. One must dissect this parameter into its component terms of volume of distribution and clearance and alter therapy accordingly.

These points can be illustrated with the drugs digoxin and lidocaine, showing how effects on volume of distribution and/or clearance affect therapeutic decisions (Table 1.4). As can be readily appreciated, the actual quantitative change in half-life is a function of the relative magnitude of change of each of its determinants. For example, assessing the effect of congestive heart failure only on the half-life of lidocaine would result in no dose adjustment while, clearly, V_d and *Cl* are both different, requiring changes in both loading and maintenance doses of this drug.

ABSORPTION (4, 7, 28, 30, 39, 47)

Drug absorption is influenced by a variety of factors, including site of absorption, ratio of ionized to nonionized drug, amount of drug metabolized before entry into the systemic circulation, and drug interactions. These factors can be highly variable among individuals and in different disease states. In fact, in many critical care situations, to circumvent these potential vagaries, one administers drugs intravenously if at all possible.

GENERAL PRINCIPLES OF ABSORPTION

Absorption can occur from many sites. Some drugs, such as dermatologics or nitroglycerin ointment, are absorbed through the skin. Others are injected intradermally, subcutaneously, or intramuscularly. Inherent variability in blood flow to these sites, disease-induced changes in perfusion, scarring from

Table 1.3. Pharmacokinetic Principles

$$\text{Initial concentration achieved after IV bolus} = C_0 = \frac{\text{Loading dose}}{\text{Volume of distribution}}$$

$$\text{Steady-state concentration maintained} = \frac{\text{Fraction absorbed} \cdot \text{maintenance dose}}{\text{Dosing interval} \cdot \text{clearance}}$$

$$\text{Half-life} = \frac{0.693 \cdot \text{Volume of distribution}}{\text{Clearance}}$$

Table 1.4. Clinical Illustration of Pharmacokinetic Principles

Clinical Setting	Kinetic Parameter			Dose		Time to Reach Steady State
	V_d	Cl	$t_{1/2}$	Loading	Maintenance	
Digoxin in mild-to-moderate renal failure	—	↓	↑	—	↓	↑
Digoxin in end stage renal failure	↓	↓↓	↑	↓	↓↓	↑
Lidocaine in liver disease	—	↓	↑	—	↓	↑
Lidocaine in CHF[a]	↓	↓	—	↓	↓	—

[a] CHF, congestive heart failure.

multiple injections, or injury can influence absorption characteristics from such sites. The nature of the drug and its formulation may also be important. For example, the injectable formulation of phenytoin is only soluble at a highly alkaline pH. When injected into muscle, the drug precipitates so that incomplete, erratic, and prolonged absorption occurs (60, 70). A similar phenomenon occurs with some of the benzodiazepines, emphasizing the inappropriateness of intramuscular administration of some of these tranquilizers (31, 37, 49). They are better and more predictably absorbed through the gastrointestinal tract.

Drugs can be absorbed throughout the length of the intestinal tract. Although most drug absorption occurs in the small intestine, in some instances it occurs through the oral mucosa. There are two important pharmacologic principles illustrated by absorption within the oropharynx. The general principle of passive, nonionic diffusion is well-illustrated here. Drugs that are nonionized more readily cross a lipid membrane than do ionized species. Therefore, an ambient pH favoring nonionized drug favors drug diffusion across membranes. In the gastrointestinal tract this characteristic favors absorption, whereas in the kidney it could favor elimination (see below). The degree to which absorption is modified is influenced by the pK_a of the drug, as well as by non-pH-dependent factors such as molecular size and lipid solubility. This principle and its application to absorption of drugs through the oral mucosa have been known by various cultures for centuries. For instance, cocaine and betel nut are both weak bases with pK_a values above 9. Local formulations of these drugs mix them with limestone to make the saliva more alkaline, thereby increasing the amount of nonionized drug and increasing absorption.

Another principle illustrated by absorption through the oral mucosa is the importance of the *first pass effect* or *presystemic elimination*. Drugs absorbed distal to the oropharynx enter the portal system and are delivered to the liver before reaching the systemic circulation. If the drug is rapidly metabolized in the liver, a substantial portion of the dose, although absorbed across the intestinal epithelium, may never reach circulating

levels in the body. A clue that the first pass effect is quantitatively important is that the dose of a drug given intravenously is considerably less than that administered by mouth. With propranolol, for example, a standard intravenous dose is 1 to 5 mg, whereas an oral dose needed to achieve similar serum concentrations is 40 to 80 mg. The difference is accounted for by the amount removed during the first pass through the liver after oral administration.

Drugs absorbed through the oral mucosa do not enter the portal circulation, and the first-pass effect is avoided. For example, nitroglycerin has sufficient first pass metabolism that very large doses must be given if it is swallowed. Consequently, patients place tablets under the tongue to achieve a rapid therapeutic effect. A direct analogy can be used to account for the similar efficacy of nitrates administered through the skin.

Gastric absorption is highly dependent on passive nonionic diffusion. Because of the acidic environment, appreciable absorption only occurs with weak acids such as salicylate and phenobarbital. Quantitatively, most absorption, even of weak acids, occurs in the proximal small intestine, which has a large surface area. Many drugs are also readily absorbed through the rectal mucosa, although the time course of absorption may differ, as compared to that with administration by mouth. Data assessing quantitative rectal absorption and its time course are scanty at best. The formulation administered rectally markedly influences absorption characteristics but not in a fashion that allows a priori predictions. This phenomenon is in need of further study (19).

In the gastrointestinal tract, a number of factors can influence drug absorption, and they are best considered in terms of three aspects: (*a*) the lag time for absorption to occur; (*b*) the extent of absorption; and (*c*) the rate of absorption.

LAG TIME FOR ABSORPTION

Lag time is defined as the time it takes for orally administered drug to enter the systemic circulation. It can vary from zero to many hours. For gastrointestinal absorption, the most important determinants of lag time are product formulation and gastric emptying time. For example, if a tablet is highly compressed, some time may be needed before dissolution occurs and drug becomes available for absorption. Since quantitatively most absorption occurs in the small bowel, the stomach must empty the drug to that site for the drug to enter the circulation. Disease states such as duodenal ulcer with gastric outlet obstruction, and drugs such as anticholinergics and narcotic analgesics, may delay gastric emptying, importantly affecting lag time. Similarly, a drug such as metoclopramide, which hastens gastric emptying, may diminish lag time (57, 58, 61).

Extent of Absorption (Bioavailability)

The extent of absorption (bioavailability) is obviously important, because it influences the total amount of drug entering the body, which in turn is directly related to the concentration of drug achieved in plasma at steady state, as shown in the equation

$$Concentration\ at\ steady\ state = F{\cdot}dose/\tau{\cdot}clearance$$

A representation of potential effects of changed bioavailability is shown in Figure 1.5. If one first considers the upper dashed horizontal line as representing the concentration of drug needed for efficacy, a decrease in bioavailability could result in lack of efficacy. If one then considers the lower horizontal line to be the effective blood concentration, a decrease in bioavailability results in still maintaining effective concentrations, but for a shorter time.

One must also consider the impact of changes in bioavailability in the opposite direction—namely, increases. If in Figure 1.5 the lower horizontal line represents an effective drug concentration and the upper horizontal line a toxic concentration, an increase in bioavailability could provide a longer time above the therapeutic concentration but at the expense of toxicity.

Product formulation and intestinal transit time may be important determinants of drug bioavailability. If a formulation dissolves very slowly and the patient has a shortened bowel or rapid intestinal transit because of disease or other

drugs, the medication may not spend sufficient time in the intestinal tract for "normal" absorption to occur. Physical complexing of drugs within the gastrointestinal tract may also occur, such as happens with milk products and tetracycline antibiotics, or cholestyramine or antacids with a number of drugs (see Chapter 2).

Finally, the magnitude of the first pass effect is an important determinant of overall bioavailability. If the liver's capacity to metabolize a drug changes, the total amount of drug reaching the systemic circulation can change. Changes in the liver's metabolic capacity can occur by several means:

1. Changed blood flow. For example, in cirrhosis or in treatment of patients with cimetidine or β-blockers, liver blood flow decreases.
2. Changed capacity of metabolizing enzymes, either (a) induced, such as with administration of rifampin (see Chapter 2), or (b) inhibited, such as occurs in cirrhosis or with enzyme-inhibiting drugs such as cimetidine (see below) (see Chapter 2).

A decrease in the liver's ability to metabolize drugs or a decrease in hepatic blood flow can increase bioavailability of drugs, having a substantial first-pass effect. This characteristic has been clearly demonstrated with propranolol, labetalol, and a few other drugs (37, 75). This effect can have a considerable impact on the circulating concentration of drugs.

Recall that concentration at steady state = $(F{\cdot}dose)/(\tau{\cdot}clearance)$. If bioavailability ($F$) is increased, and in addition the ability to metabolize the drug is also decreased (and clearance has decreased), then the overall effect on the serum concentration at steady state has undergone a "multiplier" effect and is disproportionate to the effect that would have occurred by changing bioavailability or clearance alone. Thus, critically ill patients may require substantial dosing modifications in order to avoid toxicity from some orally administered drugs.

RATE OF ABSORPTION

Changes in rate of drug absorption are also important. Figure 1.5 depicts serum concentration curves with different

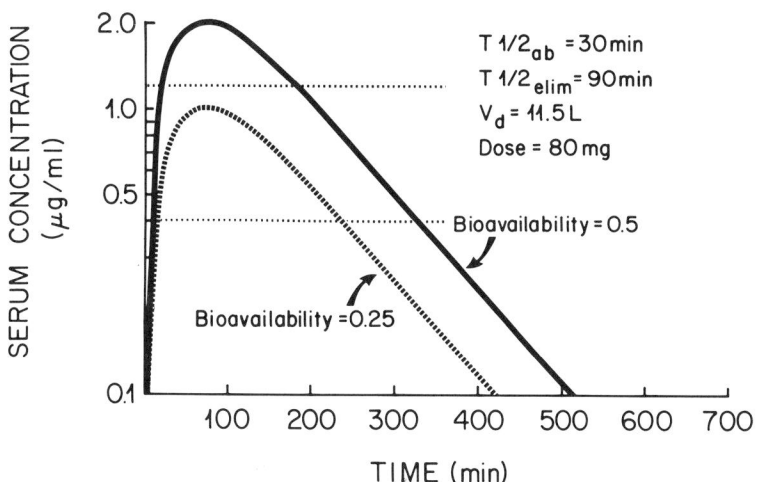

Figure 1.5. Schematic representation of the effect on serum concentration versus time curves of changes in bioavailability. Pharmacokinetic parameters in the figure are those of furosemide. See text for discussion.

Figure 1.6. Schematic representation of the effect on serum concentration versus time curves of changes in the rate of absorption with bioavailability remaining constant. See text for discussion.

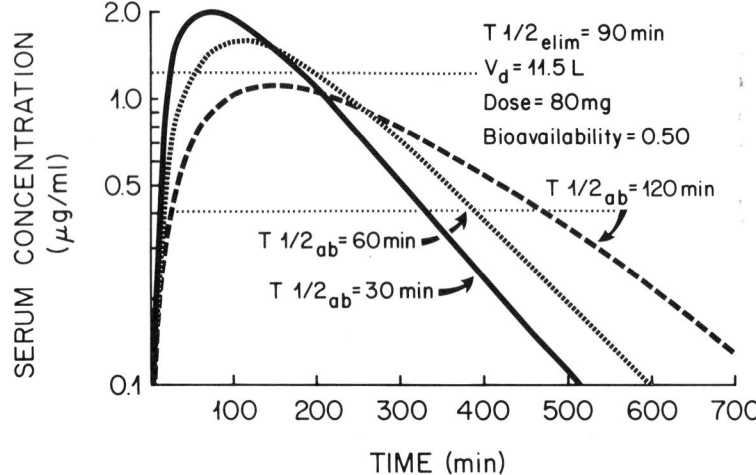

absorption half-lives, but which all have the same bioavailability.

If one first considers the lower horizontal line as the effective blood concentration, the curve with the slowest absorption half-life provides effective concentrations for the longest period of time. This phenomenon is the rationale for development of sustained-release preparations. However, such a phenomenon should not be expected necessarily to occur in all circumstances. For example, if the effective concentration were the upper horizontal line, the change to a slower absorption would result in lack of efficacy (Fig. 1.6). Assuming the lower horizontal line represents efficacy and the upper horizontal line represents toxicity (Fig. 1.6), changes in rate of absorption also influence whether toxicity occurs and its duration.

One cannot predict a priori which phenomenon will occur in individual patients or in the presence of significant disease. Consequently, it is a clinician's responsibility to obtain serum drug concentrations and to assess clinical endpoints in individual patients to discern the overall effect of a change in time course of absorption on response.

Rate of absorption is influenced by product formulation (as discussed with bioavailability), by drug interactions (see Chapter 2), and probably by gastrointestinal physiology-pathology, which has been little studied but likely occurs.

Any permutation and combination of all of the effects discussed can and will occur in individual patients.

DISTRIBUTION (9, 17, 25, 36, 38, 42, 63)

The determinants of distribution of drugs throughout the body are incompletely understood. Some drugs reach tissues by active transport, and their degree of distribution to a particular tissue may depend on their affinity for transport pumps, access to the pump(s), pump activity, distribution away from the tissue after reaching it, etc.

Lipid solubility and, in turn, ambient pH related to the drug's pK_a can influence distribution to certain tissues. For example, salicylate and phenobarbital have restricted access through the blood-brain barrier to the central nervous system (CNS). If the blood pH becomes more acidic, favoring the nonionized form of these weak acids, lipid permeability increases, and more drug distributes into the CNS (33). This

phenomenon explains the importance of reversing systemic acidemia in treating toxicity to facilitate exit of these agents from the CNS.

Binding of drugs to circulating proteins is an important determinant of distribution. Only unbound drug in blood can diffuse or be transported into tissues. Thus, the influence of protein binding is a limiting factor in drug distribution, especially with those drugs that are highly protein bound—in excess of 90 to 95%. Such drugs include penicillins, cephalosporins, sulfonamides, anticoagulants, nonsteroidal antiinflammatory drugs, propranolol, and others. The protein binding of these drugs can be affected by their relative concentrations in the blood (drug interactions), by changes in circulating protein concentration, and by diseases such as uremia that can result in accumulation of endogenous competitors for binding and/or alter the binding characteristics of protein (32).

In general, one must be concerned about changes in distribution with drugs that are highly protein-bound and/or drugs that have a small volume of distribution. Quantitatively important distribution-related effects have been described with phenytoin (52, 53), thiopental (14), valproic acid (13), warfarin (5), salicylates (33), and diazoxide (48).

In both hypoalbuminemia and uremia, phenytoin, valproic acid, and warfarin are displaced from albumin, increasing the amount of free drug in plasma. This displacement from binding in itself should cause an increased effect, inasmuch as the amount of drug accessible to its site of action is related to the amount of free drug in plasma. However, this free drug is also available for elimination and for distribution into tissues in which the drug is not active. The overall result is that a new steady state is reached in which the concentration of free drug in plasma is virtually the same as in the unperturbed condition; the pharmacologic effect is the same, but the total concentration of drug in blood (free plus bound) is less than that before displacement (42). This consequence is illustrated schematically for phenytoin in Figure 1.7.

The clinical importance of this phenomenon is that the amount of drug administered to the patient remains the same—i.e., for phenytoin approximately 300 mg/day. The "therapeutic" blood concentration of phenytoin in patients with the nephrotic syndrome or uremia, however, is one-half to one-third that in normal subjects. Consequently, the importance of this effect is in interpretation of measurements of phenytoin blood concentrations. "Low" total concentrations of phenytoin, thiopental, or valproic acid in a uremic or nephrotic patient should not be misinterpreted as subtherapeutic. This interpretive problem does not occur with warfarin, for one monitors the response to the anticoagulant, rather than its blood concentration.

Digoxin, although not highly protein-bound, can have clinically relevant changes in drug distribution. In end-stage renal failure, the volume of distribution of digoxin is decreased, and a smaller loading dose is needed to achieve a given blood concentration (Table 1.4) (3). The reduced maintenance dose of digoxin required in end-stage renal disease relates to decreased ability of the kidney to eliminate digoxin; additionally, the drug distributes into a smaller volume so that a diminished loading dose is also necessary.

Other influences on drug distribution might include factors such as overall tissue perfusion. For example, a diabetic who develops peripheral osteomyelitis often must undergo amputation because the disease has affected perfusion so severely that antibiotics never distribute to the site of infection. Patients with severe cirrhosis and portosystemic shunts do not distribute drug to the liver, where metabolism can occur.

It is important to reemphasize the difference between distribution to tissues and volume of distribution. They are undoubtedly related but not rigidly so. The latter should be thought of in the context discussed previously—namely, its therapeutic implications regarding loading dose and as one determinant of half-life. No physiologic implications should be attached to the magnitude of the volume of distribution, and disease-induced changes in volume of distribution do not warrant speculation as to actual effects on drug access to various tissues.

ELIMINATION

METABOLISM (6, 23, 24, 72, 73)

Most metabolism occurs in the liver, where drugs are converted to polar compounds that are then excreted by the kidney. Importantly, their metabolism does not necessarily imply that the metabolite is inactive. In fact, for some drugs such as chloral hydrate, encainide, and sulindac the parent drug is inactive, and metabolism to the active component must occur. For many other drugs, metabolites are also active and may cause pharmacologic effects, particularly in the setting of decreased renal function if their excretion is impaired

and they accumulate (11, 20, 43, 65). For example, procainamide is acetylated to *N*-acetylprocainamide (NAPA), which is itself an antiarrhythmic, eliminated by the kidney. Consequently, in renal failure NAPA accumulates in preference to procainamide and may do so in amounts that become toxic. Interpretation of serum concentrations of procainamide in a patient with azotemia becomes difficult, because both procainamide and NAPA contribute to the pharmacologic effect, but only the former is measured in many assays, and "therapeutic" concentrations for the latter have not been well-defined. Clinical assessment of pharmacologic effect is essential, rather than reliance on and possible misinterpretation of serum concentration measurements.

Some of the oral sulfonylureas are converted to active metabolites that accumulate in uremia, potentially causing prolonged and long-lasting hypoglycemia. Meperidine (pethidine) and propoxyphene are metabolized to normeperidine and norpropoxyphene, which depend on the kidney for elimination. Excess accumulation of these metabolites can result in seizures or cardiovascular collapse, respectively. These few examples illustrate the need for clinicians to understand the pharmacology of the drugs they use, including the pharmacology of metabolites.

The liver has a variety of pathways by which it can metabolize drugs, with the microsomal enzyme system with cytochrome P-450 playing a pivotal role. This system is important for oxidative reactions, such as dealkylation, hydroxylation, oxidation, sulfoxide formation, deamination, and desulfuration. Glucuronide synthesis and conjugation also occur in the microsomal system. Other metabolizing pathways also occur mainly in the liver but not via the microsomal enzyme system. These include reactions such as acetylation, methylation, and conjugation with glycine and sulfate, hydrolysis, and reduction reactions.

The microsomal enzyme system can be induced to greater activity or can be inhibited (see Chapter 2). The "classic" inducers of this system are the barbiturates; however, many agents can act as inducers. Inhibitors of the system include cimetidine and a variety of antituberculous drugs. These actions can affect the blood concentrations of drugs by impacting on bioavailability (for drugs with a substantial first-pass effect) and on clearance. Such changes, via effects on hepatic metabolism, whether caused by disease or other drugs, must be anticipated to select proper dosing regimens for individual patients.

EXCRETION (11, 12, 64)

By far the most important excretory route for both parent drug and metabolites is the kidney. It is easiest to consider renal modes of elimination in terms of the kidney's physiologic functions of filtration, active transport, and passive transport. In addition, the kidney metabolizes some drugs and conjugates others. These processes have been little explored, but there have been no reports of disease-induced changes or of drug interactions.

Filtration

The clinically relevant determinants of a drug's capacity to be filtered are molecular size and charge and the number of filtering ephrons.

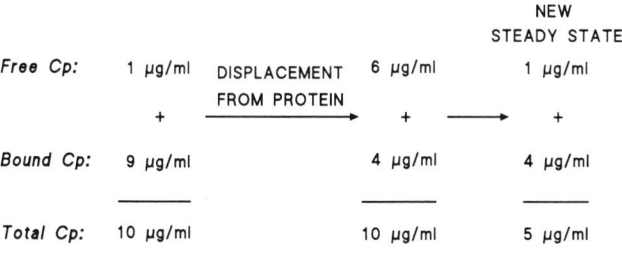

Free Cp:	1 µg/ml	DISPLACEMENT FROM PROTEIN	6 µg/ml	1 µg/ml
	+		+	+
Bound Cp:	9 µg/ml		4 µg/ml	4 µg/ml
Total Cp:	10 µg/ml		10 µg/ml	5 µg/ml

NEW STEADY STATE

Figure 1.7. Schematic representation of the effect of decreased protein binding on serum concentrations of phenytoin.

Effective molecular size is a limiting factor for excretion of mixed and high molecular weight dextrans. Dextran 40 used clinically is actually a mixture of different molecular weight species; the high molecular weight component (approximately 70,000) is selectively retained because it cannot be filtered (18, 67). Consequently, these preparations remain in patients for extended periods of time. Other drugs have sufficiently small molecular weights that there are essentially no size limitations to filtration.

Most studies and clinical attention are directed to influences of decreased numbers of functioning nephrons on the renal elimination of drugs. The effect of decreased creatinine clearance on the elimination of digoxin and aminoglycoside antibiotics is particularly well-known. In general, if 40% or more of the administered drug (or its active metabolites) is eliminated unchanged in the urine, decreased renal function will change handling of the drug and require dose adjustment (see Chapter 3).

Active Transport

The renal tubule can both actively secrete and actively reabsorb a variety of substrates. Active reabsorption appears to be inconsequential, except for iodipamide (a cholecystographic agent), which can induce marked uricosuria, presumably by decreasing the active reabsorption of uric acid in the proximal tubule (45). The uricosuria could cause the acute renal failure occasionally reported with this contrast agent. The same mechanism accounts for the uricosuria caused by probenecid. The uptake by pinocytosis from the proximal tubular lumen of gentamicin and other aminoglycoside antibiotics might be considered another example of active reabsorption (51). Sequestration of these drugs within tubular cells most likely contributes to nephrotoxicity, the mechanisms of which are being actively investigated.

The pars recta (straight segment) of the proximal tubule actively secretes into the tubular lumen a variety of organic acids (54, 69) and bases (50, 55). The pathways for acids and for bases appear to be separate, but within a group there is lack of specificity such that a variety of organic acids can compete with each other for transport, as can a variety of organic bases (see Chapter 2). If competing agents are coadministered, changes in clearance may occur, requiring a compensatory alteration of the dosing regimen.

A classic drug interaction of clinical consequence is the inhibition of the renal elimination of many acidic drugs by probenecid, a competitive inhibitor of renal secretion (67). Coadministration of probenecid with some acidic drugs results in an unexpected accumulation of drug and an increased possibility of toxic effects. Conversely, this interaction can be used on purpose to reduce the dose of drug needed to attain the same serum concentration.

A clinically important drug transport that is not of acids or bases is a secretory component of digoxin elimination, which can be competed for by spironolactone, quinidine, and verapamil (see Chapter 2). Patients to whom these drugs are coadministered develop higher serum concentrations of cardiac glycoside. The site of digitalis transport appears to be the distal nephron.

Table 1.5.   Drugs with Clinically Important Urine pH-dependent Elimination

Weak acids (alkaline urine increases excretion)
Phenobarbital
Salicylates
Sulfonamide derivatives
Weak bases (acid urine increases excretion)
Amphetamine
Ephedrine
Mexiletine
Pseudoephedrine
Quinine
Tocainide

Passive Transport

Passive transport of drugs is an important mechanism for both excretion and reabsorption of drugs in the kidney. Both weak acids and weak bases can be passively reabsorbed in the collecting duct (44, 46, 59), accounting for retention of many drugs. For this reabsorption to occur, these drugs must have gained entry into the tubular lumen at more proximal portions of the nephron by either glomerular filtration or active secretion. Even drugs with high rates of entry into the kidney can be almost completely reabsorbed in the collecting duct. This reabsorption is dependent mainly on two factors: urinary pH and flow rate through the lumen.

As discussed earlier, drugs in the nonionized state more readily pass through membranes, a fact that is important for drug absorption. The same principle applies for passive reabsorption in the collecting duct. Thus, if a large percentage of the drug is in the nonionized state, more drug is passively reabsorbed. For weak acids, as the pH decreases, the concentration of nonionized drug increases; for weak bases, an increase in pH results in more nonionized drug. Consequently, altering urinary pH can be a clinically important determinant of elimination for some drugs (Table 1.5).

Alkalinization of the urine, by favoring excretion of the ionized congener of phenobarbital or salicylate, is a mainstay of therapy for toxicity due to these agents. The small changes in urinary pH caused by modest doses of antacids can enhance the elimination of salicylate sufficiently to prevent attaining concentrations in blood necessary for an antiinflammatory effect.

The effect of urinary pH on the elimination of amphetamine may be better known to abusers of this drug than to clinicians. Since amphetamine is a weak base, alkalinizing the urine increases the amount of nonionized drug, favoring reabsorption. Amphetamine abusers regularly ingest baking soda to prolong the "high." Therapeutically, it would be important to acidify the urine of a patient with an overdose of amphetamine. The supposedly nontoxic pseudoephedrine accumulates to toxic levels in children with renal tubular acidosis in whom a persistently alkaline urine favors passive reabsorption of the drug. A similar phenomenon occurs with tocainide, an orally available lidocaine-like agent, for which the administration of bicarbonate decreases the elimination rate.

Not all weak acids and bases demonstrate urine pH-dependent elimination, however, and one cannot assume that these principles will apply to all weak acids and bases. Part of the lack of effect with some drugs probably relates to the drug's

pK_a and the lipid solubility of the congeners. For example, if even the nonionized species is poorly soluble in lipid, its ability to cross the tubular plasma membrane would not be enhanced. In this setting, changes in urinary pH would not cause changes in renal elimination.

Another modulator of the ability of the nonionized congener to pass across the lipid membrane may be antidiuretic hormone, which can increase by 50 to 100% the ability of lipophilic compounds to pass across the toad urinary bladder, a structure functionally analogous to the mammalian collecting duct (41). These findings have not been extrapolated to studies in humans. In many critical care settings, nonosmotic stimuli promote antidiuretic hormone release, which could conceivably affect renal drug handling. Other modulators of the effects of urinary pH on drug reabsorption are less well-defined.

Urinary flow rate can affect excretion of some drugs by decreasing the concentration gradient for reabsorption, because the urine is dilute, and by decreasing the time available for a drug to diffuse out of the urine. Urinary flow rate is an important determinant of elimination for chloramphenicol, ephedrine, phenobarbital, pseudoephedrine, and theophylline. This fact is probably clinically important only in patients with high urinary flow rates for prolonged periods of time.

Clinicians seem to pay little attention to the importance of urinary pH and flow rate, except in the case of salicylate or barbiturate overdose. As discussed above, more thought should be given to the importance of the urine pH for excretion of a broader gamut of drugs (Table 1.5).

DIALYSIS (11)

Elimination of drugs by dialysis is not discussed in great detail here and, in particular, dialysis techniques are not addressed. It is important, however, to review pharmacokinetic and pharmacologic aspects of some of the more pertinent determinants of a drug's dialyzability.

Determinants of Dialyzability

Molecular size influences a drug's dialyzability. In general, compounds of molecular weight less than 500 have flow-dependent dialyzability, while elimination of higher molecular weight drugs depends on dialyzer surface area. Vancomycin, with a molecular weight of 1800, has such a large molecular size that it is not dialyzable. Other drugs for which molecular size is clinically important are amphotericin B, erythromycin, morphine, and digoxin, all of which have poor dialyzability that is limited by membrane surface area. All other drugs have a sufficiently small molecular size for their dialysance to be determined by flow rate of blood and dialysate and by other factors to be discussed subsequently.

For a drug to be dialyzable, it must be water-soluble. (This rule does not apply to resin hemoperfusion.) Many of the sedative-hypnotics (such as glutethimide, methaqualone, meprobamate, ethchlorvynol, etc.) and the tricyclic antidepressants, although of small molecular weight, are relatively insoluble in water and are poorly dialyzable by conventional hemodialysis. Resin or charcoal hemoperfusion is not dependent on water solubility and therefore can remove these drugs effectively. In addition, drugs highly bound to serum proteins are, in general, poorly dialyzable. Protein binding is not a limiting factor with sorbent hemoperfusion.

Quantitative Aspects of Dialyzability

Whether dialysis can contribute to a drug's removal from the body relates to a drug's intrinsic plasma clearance—namely, how fast the body can eliminate the drug exclusive of dialysis. For dialysis to add a clinically important increment to overall drug elimination, clearance by dialysis should increase overall clearance by at least 30%. Some general principles can be appreciated by reconsidering the determinants of the clearance of a drug. Clearance can be expressed as a function of half-life and volume of distribution:

$$Cl = 0.693 \ V_d/t_{1/2}$$

From this relationship, it is clear that if the volume in which a drug distributes is large, clearance is large; for dialysis to add to clearance, dialyzability would have to be great. This observation seems to make sense intuitively in that a large volume of distribution means much of the body burden of the drug is in the peripheral tissues; dialysis can only remove the amount in the blood. Consequently, drug in the tissues is not accessible to the dialyzer, and the body burden of the drug is not significantly decreased by dialysis. The converse is true for a drug with a small volume of distribution unless it is highly protein bound and therefore does not cross the dialysis membrane.

Similarly, if the half-life is short (i.e., elimination is fast) the intrinsic clearance is great and dialysis would be less likely to have an effect. The converse is also true. The effect of dialysis on the clearance of aminoglycosides illustrates the validity of this concept. In a patient with normal renal function, the half-life of an aminoglycoside antibiotic is relatively short (2 to 3 hours). Therefore, clearance is large and dialysis in such a patient would not remove large amounts of the drug. However, aminoglycosides have long half-lives in patients with end-stage renal failure. Therefore, clearance is low and dialysis can eliminate enough of the antibiotic to require dosing after each dialysis.

In overdose settings, saturation of elimination pathways may occur (11, 12). If so, intrinsic clearance may be low at high blood concentrations of the drug and increase as concentrations decrease. In this situation, dialysis may contribute an important increment to elimination when drug concentrations are highest. This situation occurs with chloral hydrate and ethchlorvynol.

Hemodialysis

When to use hemodialysis or hemoperfusion (see below) for patients with drug overdoses is often debated and must be highly individualized to both patient status and the capacities of the hospital. For example, an identical patient might be treated differently depending on whether the local expertise is pulmonary care or technical skill in performing dialysis. A modification (11) of guidelines proposed by Schreiner is predicated on the ability of dialysis to contribute to elimination of the drug (Table 1.6).

Table 1.6. Guidelines for Dialysis of the Poisoned Patient

1. Severe clinical intoxication with life-threatening cardiovascular instability despite adequate volume replacement.
2. Ingestion and probable absorption of a potentially lethal dose.
3. A blood level of the drug that is in the range resulting in considerable mortality.
4. Impaired ability to eliminate the drug by endogenous routes either by disease itself, toxicity of the drug, or by saturation of pathways of elimination.
5. Prolonged coma in a setting in which expertise in hemodialysis exceeds expertise in respiratory care.
6. Methanol or ethylene glycol ingestion.

Table 1.7. Dose of Ethanol for Achieving a Target Concentration of 100 mg% in the Treatment of Methanol or Ethylene Glycol Ingestions

Loading dose[a]	0.6 g/kg
Maintenance dose	
Nondrinkers	66 mg/kg/hr
Chronic drinkers	154 mg/kg/hr
During hemodialysis	170 mg/kg/hr or 95% ethanol to achieve a dialysate concentration of 100 mg/ml

[a] Four and one-half 1-oz shots of 80 proof whiskey in a 70 kg patient.

Methanol and ethylene glycol ingestion warrant more detailed comments. Poisoning with either of these two agents is a clear indication for hemodialysis. Toxicity of massive doses can be completely prevented by appropriate treatment. Both methanol and ethylene glycol are benign and their toxicity is mediated by metabolic by-products. The first step in the metabolism of both of these compounds involves alcohol dehydrogenase for which ethanol is a preferred substrate. Consequently, adequate therapy entails not only hemodialysis to remove the parent methanol and ethylene glycol and any metabolites that may have formed, but also administration of sufficient ethanol to block formation of the toxic metabolites. The latter can be complicated, because ethanol itself is dialyzable and its infusion rate must be adjusted to maintain enzyme-blocking serum concentrations of ethanol (target concentration = 100 to 200 mg/100 ml). In addition, chronic (alcohol) drinkers have a higher capacity to metabolize ethanol and require higher maintenance infusion rates, unless, of course, they have liver disease. Clearly, the ethanol dose must be tailored to the individual patient and followed by determinations of serum concentrations if possible. Table 1.7 offers recommendations as a first approximation of the required ethanol dose. Hemodialysis for 4 to 6 hours appears sufficient for treatment of even massive overdoses. Ethanol infusion should probably be continued for up to 24 hours.

Many hospitals do not have the ability to measure serum concentrations of methanol or ethylene glycol. A reasonably accurate estimation of their concentrations can be obtained by measuring serum osmolality. The total number of osmoles in the sample includes the contribution of the agent in question, electrolytes, urea, and glucose. The last three can be calculated from their chemical measurement. The number of osmoles contributed by methanol or ethylene glycol can then be estimated by subtracting the osmolal contribution of normal blood constituents from total osmolality. Concentration of methanol or ethylene glycol can then be calculated based on

Table 1.8. Drugs for Which Resin Hemoperfusion Has Been Demonstrated to Remove Clinically Important Amounts

Barbiturates
Chloral hydrate (trichloroethanol)[a]
Chloroquine
Digitalis glycosides
Disopyramide
Ethchlorvynol
Glutethimide
Meprobamate
Methaqualone
N-Dexmethylmethsuximide
Phenylbutazone
Salicylate
Theophylline
Tricyclic antidepressants

[a] Trichloroethanol is the active metabolite; the parent, chloral hydrate, is rapidly converted to the metabolite.

its molecular weight (32 and 62, respectively). However, if ethanol is being administered, both ethanol and either methanol or ethylene glycol will contribute to the serum osmolality, with no means other than specific assay to ascertain the contribution of each.

Hemoperfusion

Recently, attempts have been made to increase the dialyzability of water-insoluble drugs that are severely toxic in overdose settings. Resins or activated charcoal have been used to bind these drugs and irreversibly extract them from the patient's blood. It is clear that these drugs can be removed efficiently by resin hemoperfusion. In fact, dialysis clearance for many of them is equal to blood flow through the dialyzer. Unfortunately, however, many of these drugs have large volumes of distribution so that the maximal reduction in blood concentrations is only short-lived, and the drug stores in peripheral tissues serve as a reservoir to refill the blood with drug as soon as hemoperfusion is stopped. In addition, the procedure itself can cause decrements in circulating formed elements in the blood. Clearer indications for use of resin hemoperfusion are likely to evolve. At present, the general indications for dialysis for poisoning (Table 1.6) would also apply for hemoperfusion, since hemoperfusion removes important amounts of a number of drugs in overdose settings (Table 1.8).

DOSING REGIMENS (6, 8, 15, 16, 26, 27, 29, 43, 56, 66, 74)

The aforementioned determinants of the relationship between the dose of drug administered to a patient and the concentration of that drug achieved in blood are a function of the individual characteristics of the patient, that patient's disease, and effects of coadministered drugs (see Chapter 2). On the other hand, dosing regimens are solely in the physician's control. Used wisely, they can mean the difference between success and failure; failure may result from allowing the disease to go untreated (lack of efficacy) or from drug-induced toxicity. A clinical example of this is the case of aminoglycoside antibiotics. Efficacy in Gram-negative bacteremia or pneumonia requires attainment of peak concentrations of tobramycin or gentamicin of more than 5 μg/ml (>20 μg/ml for amikacin). On the other hand, minimizing ototoxicity and/or nephrotoxicity from these drugs requires trough concentrations of less than 2 μg/ml (<5 μg/ml for amikacin). To achieve these goals the clinician must have a knowledge of dosing regimens, which in turn is a logical extrapolation of the pharmacokinetic principles discussed above.

The multiplicity of influences on the relationship between dose of a drug and its serum concentration (Fig. 1.1) emphasizes the importance of dosing regimens and use of assays of drug concentrations. Because so many factors affect this relationship, there is tremendous variability from patient to patient in handling of drugs and therefore in the concentration achieved by a dosing regimen. Tailoring the dosage regimen to the individual patient is the clinician's only tool to compensate for this variability and truly individualize therapy. To do so, the clinician must understand pharmacokinetic principles, know the medical literature on the handling of specific drugs in patients relative to their demographic characteristics and disease state, and use clinical endpoints of pharmacologic effect and measured drug concentrations to adjust therapy to the individual patient. These principles are illustrated schematically in Figure 1.8. For example, by knowing that a patient has congestive heart failure and that published data indicate that, on average, such patients have a decreased volume of distribution and clearance of lidocaine, an appropriate starting dosing regimen can be devised. Clearly, however, a patient may not be "average," which would be reflected by a measured lidocaine concentration that differed from the desired or predicted concentration. Presuming that clinical assessment corroborates conclusions based on the measured lidocaine concentration, an estimate of the individual patient's handling of lidocaine can be made with revision of the dosing regimen appropriate for the individual patient.

LOADING DOSE

A loading dose is administered to achieve therapeutic drug concentrations rapidly. Otherwise, one must wait 4 to 5 times the elimination half-life for steady state to occur. As discussed previously, the loading dose is determined by the volume of distribution of the drug; to reiterate:

Loading dose = desired concentration · volume of distribution

In emergent situations, loading doses are usually administered by vein. So doing ensures 100% bioavailability and a rapid attainment of desired serum drug concentrations. In less emergent situations, loading doses can be administered by other routes. When administered intravenously very high

serum concentrations may be achieved for transient periods of time. The height of concentrations achieved and their duration depends on the rate of administration and the rate at which drug distributes from blood into tissues. A loading dose given intravenously should be given over 3 to 5 minutes; to administer the drug faster is unnecessary and risky.

Studies with lidocaine demonstrate the types of problems that may occur when giving a loading dose (62). Considerable effort has been expended to develop a reasonable method for loading patients with lidocaine, minimizing excursions into the toxic range while achieving desired concentrations quickly. To date, the best method in patients with a normal volume of distribution is to administer 75 mg over 2 minutes followed by 150 mg by continuous intravenous infusion over 18 minutes (8.33 mg/min). This infusion is then followed by the maintenance infusion rate. A study comparing this rapid infusion method with three bolus injections of 50 mg over the same period found that all of 6 patients with bolus injections developed toxicity, compared with 1 of 12 after the infusion method (62).

No similar data exist for other drugs commonly used in emergent situations. Even with drugs in which bolus administration may pose no dangers, however, it seems logical to be conservative and administer the drug slowly. One may always increase the rate of infusion if deemed necessary; on the other hand, if too much drug has been administered too quickly, no recourse exists.

As was discussed in previous sections and as will be addressed in subsequent chapters for specific drugs and specific clinical conditions, a patient's disease state can influence the volume of distribution of a drug. The impact of such effects on dosing regimens is on loading rather than maintenance doses (Tables 1.3 and 1.4). The impact of disease on the volume of distribution of many drugs has not been explored. Consequently, it behooves the clinician to realize that changes from "normal" may exist in the individual patient. Consequently, one should err on the cautious side in estimating the needed loading dose. If an underestimate is made, it is easy to give more drug, in contrast to the potential consequences of having overestimated and administered too much.

MAINTENANCE DOSE

The maintenance dose determines the average concentration of drug at steady state. To reiterate:

$$Cp_{ss} = F \cdot dose/\tau \cdot clearance$$

Disease can influence both bioavailability of drugs (*F*) and their clearance. Such effects can be compensated for by

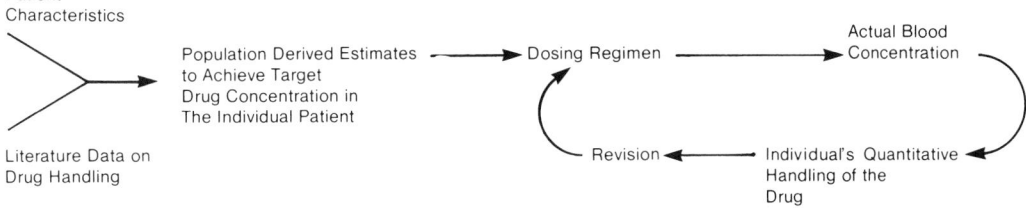

Figure 1.8. Steps for optimizing drug therapy to the individual patient.

changing the dose, the frequency with which it is administered, or both. The method selected for adjusting the dosing regimen influences the magnitude of difference between peak and trough concentrations of drug, i.e., the fluctuation above and below the average drug concentration. The more frequently a drug is administered, the less fluctuation, and the converse. One can estimate peak (Cp_{max}) and trough (Cp_{min}) concentrations of drug knowing pharmacokinetic parameters:

$$Cp_{max} = \frac{F \cdot dose/V_d}{1 - e^{-k\tau}}$$

and

$$Cp_{min} = Cp_{max} \, e^{-k\tau}$$

Such calculations might become important when using a drug with a narrow therapeutic range, when one is concerned about fluctuating from toxic to subtherapeutic concentrations of drug. For example, this phenomenon occurs in some patients when procainamide is administered in 750-mg doses every 6 hours as opposed to administering 375 mg every 3 hours. Because of variability among individuals, calculating estimated values for Cp_{max} and Cp_{min} is probably less informative than clinical evaluation of the patient at times of predicted peak and trough concentration of drug and obtaining measurements of actual drug concentration at these times.

No "best" method can be promulgated for adjusting the maintenance dose of a drug (16). Knowing the general relationship between dosing frequency and fluctuation of drug concentrations must be coupled with knowledge of the influence of specific disease states on the pharmacokinetics and dynamics of specific drugs. So doing allows approximation of a starting point for adjustment of dosing regimens, which must then be "fine tuned" to the individual patient by assessing clinical endpoints of response and measuring serum drug concentrations (Fig. 1.8).

DETERMINANTS OF THE RELATIONSHIP BETWEEN RESPONSE AND CONCENTRATIONS OF DRUG IN BLOOD

Understanding pharmacokinetics can help to clarify and compensate for the multitude of factors that influence the concentration of drug achieved in blood, relative to an administered dose. Many additional factors affect response. Their impact on the individual patient requires clinical assessment and cannot be quantified in pharmacokinetic terms. Optimal compensation for vagaries in response, however, then requires reapplication of pharmacokinetic principles to the modified goals derived from clinical assessment of pharmacodynamics.

Many clinical examples exist of changes in response to drugs; the increased toxicity of digitalis glycosides with hypokalemia, the decreased response to catecholamines in the acidemic patient, and the resistance to diuretics in severe congestive heart failure are all well known. Other examples must certainly exist. This entire area represents the "art" of therapeutics. Pharmacokinetics has evolved from a qualitative art to a quantitative science. Optimal therapeutics requires wedding the art of pharmacodynamic assessment to the science of pharmacokinetics.

Clearly, the use of therapeutic drug monitoring (TDM) has assisted clinicians' use of drugs. We now speak of therapeutic ranges, those serum concentrations at which the probability is high that the patient will receive optimal therapy and minimal toxicity. In critically ill patients especially, TDM has improved pharmacologic management.

It is important, however, for clinicians to utilize TDM correctly to optimize therapy and not overinterpret the serum drug concentration. Several confounding factors are important in interpreting serum drug concentrations, and many have been discussed in this chapter. For example, *if serum concentrations are measured during the distribution phase of drug dosing or prior to steady state, the use of the concentrations may lead to erroneous conclusions and inappropriate changes in therapy.* In addition, many drugs have active metabolites (23) and these are rarely measured. Lastly, the implications of free compared to protein-bound drug have been discussed.

Measurement of serum drug concentrations is useful if the clinician knows what information can be derived from the test and if the pharmacodynamic effect correlates with the serum concentration. Clearly, concentration can be critical in individualizing dosing, assuming that the true relationship between dose and sample collection is known. The concentration may not be useful if it does not correlate with therapeutic endpoints or if pharmacokinetic principles are ignored.

STEREOCHEMICAL CONSIDERATIONS (1, 2, 21, 40, 71)

The human body is a very chiral environment. It has the ability to differentiate between the optical isomers of endogenous substances as well as xenobiotics. In recent years, the role of stereochemistry in clinical pharmacology has been evolving. Continually improving technology has made possible the stereospecific evaluation of the pharmacokinetics and pharmacodynamics of therapeutic agents.

Approximately 20 to 25% of the therapeutic agents on the market are racemic mixtures. Racemates are 50:50 mixtures of optical isomers. Optical isomers that are nonsuperimposable mirror images of each other are known as enantiomers. Although closely related structurally, enantiomers usually differ in their pharmacokinetic and pharmacodynamic properties, both desirable as well as undesirable effects. This occurs because the human body often demonstrates preferential affinity for one enantiomer over another. One enantiomer may be active and the other inactive or, in some cases, have antagonist or undesirable side effects. In cases where the pharmacologic activity is associated with only one enantiomer, the pharmacokinetic profile of the racemate may or may not reflect the time course of the action of the single active enantiomer (e.g., warfarin). Despite common knowledge of the differences in the pharmacologic activity of enantiomers, much of the available pharmacokinetic information is based upon studies in which racemates rather than enantiomers were evaluated. Studies in which enantiomers were not resolved and quantitated are inaccurate and can be misleading. In the future, therapeutic drug monitoring will require stereospecific drug level determinations in order to yield information of value in the optimization of drug therapy in clinical practice.

REFERENCES

1. Ariens EJ: Stereochemistry, a basis for sophisticated nonsense in pharmacokinetics and clinical pharmacology. *Eur J Clin Pharmacol* 26:663–668, 1984.
2. Ariens EJ: Stereochemistry: a source of problems in medicinal chemistry. *Med Res Rev* 6:451–466, 1986.
3. Aronson JK: Clinical pharmacokinetics of digoxin 1980. *Clin Pharmacokinet* 5:137–149, 1980.
4. Azarnoff DL, Huffmann DH: Therapeutic implications of bioavailability. *Annu Rev Pharmacol Toxicol* 16:53–66, 1976.
5. Bachmann K, Shapiro R, Mackiewicz J: Influence of renal dysfunction on warfarin plasma protein binding. *J Clin Pharmacol* 16:468–472, 1976.
6. Bass NM, Williams RL: Guide to drug dosage in hepatic disease. *Clin Pharmacokinet* 15:396–420, 1988.
7. Benet LZ: Biopharmaceutics as a basis for the design of drug products. Ariens EJ (ed): *Drug Design.* Academic Press, New York, chapter I, pp 1–35. 1973.
8. Bennett WM: Guide to drug dosage in renal failure. *Clin Pharmacokinet* 15:326–354, 1988.
9. Blaschke TF: Protein binding and kinetics of drugs in liver diseases. *Clin Pharmacokinet* 2:32–44, 1977.
10. Bodenham A, Shelly MP, Park GR: The altered pharmacokinetics and pharmacodynamics of drugs commonly used in critically ill patients. *Clin Pharmacokinet* 14:347–373, 1988.
11. Brater DC: *Drug Use in Renal Disease.* ADIS, Sydney, 1983.
12. Brater DC: The pharmacological role of the kidney. *Drugs* 19:31–48, 1980.
13. Brewster D, Muir NC: Valproate plasma protein binding in the uremic condition. *Clin Pharmacol Ther* 27:76–82, 1980.
14. Burch PG, Stanski DR: Decreased protein binding and thiopental kinetics. *Clin Pharmacol Ther* 32:212–217, 1982.
15. Burton ME, Vasko MR, Brater DC: Comparison of drug dosing methods. *Clin Pharmacokinet* 10:1–37, 1985.
16. Chennavasin P, Brater DC: Nomograms for drug use in renal disease. *Clin Pharmacokinet* 6:193–214, 1981.
17. Craig WA, Kunin CM: Significance of serum protein and tissue binding of antimicrobial agents. *Annu Rev Med* 27:287–300, 1976.
18. Data JL, Nies AS: Dextran 40. *Ann Intern Med* 81:500–504, 1974.
19. deBoer AG, Moolenaar F, deLeede LGJ, Breimer DD: Rectal drug administration: clinical pharmacokinetic considerations. *Clin Pharmacokinet* 7:285–311, 1982.
20. Drayer DE: Pharmacologically active drug metabolites: therapeutic and toxic activities, plasma and urine data in man, accumulation in renal failure. *Clin Pharmacokinet* 1:426–443, 1976.
21. Drayer DE: Pharmacodynamic and pharmacokinetic differences between drug enantiomers in humans: an overview. *Clin Pharmacol Ther* 40:125–133, 1986.
22. Friedman H, Greenblatt DJ: Rational therapeutic drug monitoring. *JAMA* 256:2227–2233, 1986.
23. Garattini S: Active drug metabolites. An overview of their relevance in clinical pharmacokinetics. *Clin Pharmacokinet* 10:216–227, 1985.
24. George CF: Drug metabolism by the gastrointestinal mucosa. *Clin Pharmacokinet* 6:259–274, 1981.
25. Gibaldi M, Koup JR: Pharmacokinetic concepts—drug binding, apparent volume of distribution and clearance. *Eur J Clin Pharmacol* 20: 299–305, 1981.
26. Gibaldi M, Levy G: Pharmacokinetics in clinical practice. *JAMA* 235:1864–1867, 1987–1992, 1976.
27. Gibaldi M, Perrier D: *Pharmacokinetics.* Marcel Dekker, New York, 1975.
28. Goldman P: Rate-controlled drug delivery. *N Engl J Med* 307:286–290, 1982.
29. Greenblatt DJ, Koch-Weser J: Clinical pharmacokinetics. *N Engl J Med* 293:702–705, 964–969, 1975.
30. Greenblatt DJ, Koch-Weser J: Intramuscular injection of drugs. *N Engl J Med* 295:542–546, 1976.
31. Greenblatt DJ, Shader RI, MacLeod SM, Sellers EM, Franke K, Giles HG: Absorption of oral and intramuscular chlordiazepoxide. *Eur J Clin Pharmacol* 13:267–274, 1978.
32. Gugler R, Shoeman DW, Huffman DH, Cohlmia JB, Azarnoff DL: Pharmacokinetics of drugs in patients with the nephrotic syndrome. *J Clin Invest* 55:1182–189, 1975.
33. Hill JB: Salicylate intoxication. *N Engl J Med* 288:110–113, 1973.
34. Holford NHG, Sheiner LB: Understanding the dose-effect relationship: clinical application of pharmacokinetic-pharmacodynamic models. *Clin Pharmacokinet* 6:429–453, 1981.
35. Homeida M, Jackson L, Roberts CJC: Decreased first-pass metabolism of labetalol in chronic liver disease. *Br Med J* 2:1048–1050, 1978.
36. Jusko WJ, Gretch M: Plasma and tissue protein binding of drugs in pharmacokinetics. *Drug Metab Rev* 5:43–140, 1976.
37. Kanto J: Plasma concentrations of diazepam and its metabolites after peroral, intramuscular, and rectal administration: correlation between plasma concentration and sedatory effect of diazepam. *Int J Clin Pharmacol* 12:427–432, 1975.
38. Klotz U: Pathophysiological and disease-induced changes in drug distribution volume: pharmacokinetic implications. *Clin Pharmacokinet* 1:204–218, 1976.
39. Koch-Weser J: Bioavailability of drugs. *N Engl J Med* 291:233–236, 503–506, 1974.
40. Lam YW: Stereoselectivity: An issue of significant importance in clinical pharmacology. *Pharmacotherapy* 8:147–157, 1988.
41. Levine SD, Franki N, Einhorn R, Hays RM: Vasopressin-stimulated movement of drugs and uric acid across the toad urinary bladder. *Kidney Int* 9:30–35, 1976.
42. MacKichan JJ: Protein binding drug displacement interactions: fact or fiction? *Clin Pharmacokinet* 16:65–73, 1989.
43. Melmon KL, Morrelli HF: *Clinical Pharmacology—Basic Principles in Therapeutics.* Macmillan, New York, 1972.
44. Milne MD, Scribner BH, Crawford MA: Non-ionic diffusion and the excretion of weak acids and bases. *Am J Med* 24:709–729, 1958.
45. Mudge GH: Uricosuric action of cholecystographic agents. *N Engl J Med* 284:929–933, 1971.
46. Mudge GH, Silva P, Stibitz GR: Renal excretion by non-ionic diffusion. *Med Clin North Am* 59:681–698, 1975.
47. Parsons RL: Drug absorption in gastrointestinal disease with particular reference to malabsorption syndromes. *Clin Pharmacokinet* 2:45–60, 1977.
48. Pearson RM: Pharmacokinetics and response to diazoxide in renal failure. *Clin Pharmacokinet* 2:198–204, 1977.
49. Perry PJ, Wilding DC, Fowler RC, Hepler CD, Caputo JF: Absorption of oral and intramuscular chlordiazepoxide by alcoholics. *Clin Pharmacol Ther* 23:535–541, 1978.
50. Peters L: Renal tubular excretion of organic bases. *Pharmacol Rev* 12:1–35, 1960.
51. Porter GA, Bennett WM: Nephrotoxic acute renal failure due to common drugs. *Am J Physiol* 241:F1–F8, 1981.
52. Reidenberg MM: The binding of drugs to plasma proteins and the interpretation of measurements of plasma concentrations of drugs in patients with poor renal function. *Am J Med* 62:466–470, 1977.
53. Reidenberg MM, Affrime M: Influence of disease on binding of drugs to plasma proteins. *Ann NY Acad Sci* 226:115–126, 1973.
54. Rennick BR: Renal excretion of drugs: tubular transport and metabolism. *Annu Rev Pharmacol* 12:141–156, 1972.
55. Rennick BR: Renal tubule transport of organic cations. *Am J Physiol* 240:F83–F89, 1981.
56. Rowland M, Tozer TN: *Clinical Pharmacokinetics—Concepts and Applications,* ed 2. Philadelphia, Lea & Febiger, 1980.
57. Schulze-Delrieu K: Metoclopramide. *Gastroenterology* 77:768–779, 1979.
58. Schulze-Delrieu K: Metoclopramide. *N Engl J Med* 305:28–33, 1981.
59. Scribner BH, Crawford MA, Dempster WJ: Urinary excretion by nonionic diffusion. *Am J Physiol* 5:1135–1140, 1959.
60. Serrano EE, Roye DB, Hammer RH, Wilder BJ: Plasma diphenylhydantoin values after oral and intramuscular administration of diphenylhydantoin. *Neurology* 23:311–317, 1973.
61. Snape WJ, Battle WM, Schwartz SS, Braunstein SN, Goldstein HA, Alavi A: Metoclopramide to treat gastroparesis due to diabetes mellitus—double-blind, controlled trial. *Ann Intern Med* 96:444–446, 1982.
62. Stargel WW, Shand DG, Routledge PA, Barchowsky A, Wagner GS: Clinical comparison of rapid infusion and multiple injection methods for lidocaine loading. *Am Heart J* 102:872–876, 1981.
63. Vallner JJ: Binding of drugs by albumin and plasma protein. *J Pharm Sci* 66:447–465, 1977.
64. Van Ginneken CAM, Russel FGM: Saturable pharmacokinetics in the renal excretion of drugs. *Clin Pharmacokinet* 16:38–54, 1989.
65. Verbeck RK, Branch RA, Wilkinson GR: Drug metabolites in renal failure: pharmacokinetic and clinical implications. *Clin Pharmacokinet* 6:329–345, 1981.
66. Wagner JG: *Biopharmaceutics and Relevant Pharmacokinetics.* Drug Intelligence Publications, Chicago, 1971
67. Walkley JW, Tillman J, Bonnar J: The persistence of dextran 70 in blood plasma following its infusion, during surgery, for prophylaxis against thromboembolism. *J Pharm Pharmacol* 28:29–31, 1976.
68. Weiner IM: Inhibitors of tubular transport of organic compounds. In: Gilman AG, Rall TW, Nies AS, Taylor P, eds. *Goodman and Gilman's the Pharmacological Basis of Therapeutics.* Pergamon Press, New York, 1990.
69. Weiner IM, Mudge GH: Renal tubular mechanisms for excretion of organic acids and bases. *Am J Med* 36:743–762, 1964.
70. Wilensky AJ, Lowden JA: Inadequate serum levels after intramuscular administration of diphenylhydantoin. *Neurology* 23:318–324, 1973.
71. Williams K, Lee E: Importance of drug enantiomers in clinical pharmacology. *Drugs* 30:333–354, 1985.
72. Williams RL, Benet LZ: Drug pharmacokinetics in cardiac and hepatic disease. *Annu Rev Pharmacol Toxicol* 20:389–413, 1980.
73. Williams RL, Mamelok RD: Hepatic disease and drug pharmacokinetics. *Clin Pharmacokinet* 5:528–547, 1980.
74. Winter ME, *Basic Clinical Pharmacokinetics.* ed 2. Spokane WA, Applied Therapeutics, 1980.
75. Wood AJJ, Kornhauser DM, Wilkinson GR, Shand DG, Branch RA: The influence of cirrhosis on steady-state blood concentrations of unbound propranolol after oral administration. *Clin Pharmacokinet* 3:478–487, 1978.

CHAPTER 2

Drug Interactions

ANITA C. RUDY, Ph.D.
D. CRAIG BRATER, M.D.

In recent years, increasing emphasis has been placed on both the study and the clinical importance of drug interactions. Several books and reviews provide extensive listings of drug interactions, both observed and theoretical (128, 221, 272, 312, 328). These listings, although contributing valuable information, are often voluminous and include anecdotal case reports, extrapolations from animal data, and interactions of questionable clinical relevance. Literal use of these listings could, therefore, overcomplicate therapeutic decisions and hinder rather than assist the clinician. Since some drug interactions are critical for optimal patient care and since new interactions are routinely discovered, it is important for clinicians to be aware of various types of drug interactions and their mechanisms. This caveat is particularly true in critical care medicine in which multiple drugs with narrow therapeutic indices are frequently coadministered to severely ill patients. In such settings, the margin for error is small and a drug interaction can dictate the success or failure of therapy.

The purpose of this chapter is to illustrate pharmacologic principles that may be important in clinically relevant drug interactions. It is not the intent of this chapter to present comprehensive listings of drug interactions, but to use examples to illustrate the types of interactions that can occur. The reader should then be able to extrapolate these principles to individual patient situations (210).

GENERAL PRINCIPLES FOR DRUG INTERACTIONS

PHARMACOKINETIC INTERACTIONS

For the purposes of this chapter, pharmacokinetic drug interactions result from altered absorption, distribution, metabolism, or excretion of a drug (Table 2.1). Some of these interactions are beneficial to the patient, whereas most result in untoward effects.

Drug interactions at sites of absorption alter either the rate or extent of drug absorption. In general, the latter is more important clinically, since it can result in considerable reductions in steady-state plasma drug concentrations. Absorption of a drug has multiple determinants, including physicochemical properties of the drug, gastric pH, site of absorption in the gastrointestinal tract, rate of gastric emptying, intestinal motility, surface area for absorption, mucosal function, and blood flow to the absorption site. When two or more drugs are coadministered, interactions involving any of these factors may occur, particularly in critically ill patients whose condition may independently affect these same parameters.

Drug interactions can also occur by means of alterations in the tissue distribution of drugs. Many drugs bind reversibly to plasma proteins, and this binding limits the free drug concentration that is available to tissue sites of action. For example, a decrease from the normal 99% binding of coumarin to 96% may seem like a small decrement, but concurrently the concentration of free drug that is available to the site of action has quadrupled from 1 to 4%. In most instances, however, an increase in free drug concentration is transient and is rapidly compensated for by an increase in distribution of drug to nonpharmacologically active sites or an increase in metabolism and/or excretion of the free drug (207). If, however, the patient's disease or another drug interaction compromises drug elimination, the increased free concentration may be sustained, and serious consequences may result.

Table 2.1. Types of Drug Interactions

Pharmacokinetic
    Absorption
        Physicochemical complexing
        Changes in gastric pH
        Changes in gastrointestinal motility
        Effects on gastrointestinal mucosa
        Effects on gastrointestinal flora
        Changes in first pass effect
    Distribution
        Protein binding
    Elimination
        Metabolism
            Induction
            Inhibition
        Excretion
Pharmacodynamic
    Receptor (pharmacologic)
    Physiologic
    Modification of conditions at the site of action
    Physicochemical complexing

The majority of pharmacokinetic drug interactions involve elimination of drug by either metabolism or excretion. Metabolic drug interactions can result in an increase or decrease in the clearance of drugs and can occur by means of multiple mechanisms, including alterations in hepatic blood flow (affecting drugs for which the limiting step in metabolism is delivery to metabolic enzymes), competitive inhibition at sites of metabolism, or induction of liver microsomal enzymes. Because there are limited pathways for drug metabolism, many drugs are metabolized by means of similar pathways. Consequently, interactions involving competitive inhibition or induction of metabolic enzymes are common. It is important, therefore, for clinicians to be familiar with the metabolism of each drug administered to a patient to predict the possibility of an interaction.

Most drugs are metabolized by first order kinetics, i.e., the rate of metabolism is dependent on the drug concentration. Consequently, enzymatic sites of drug metabolism are not saturated, and an increase in drug concentration does not alter the rate of metabolism. In some instances, however, drugs are metabolized by zero-order kinetics, i.e., only a specific amount of drug is metabolized per unit time. In addition, drugs metabolized by first-order kinetics are capable of saturating their metabolic sites and shifting to zero-order kinetics. This phenomenon usually occurs only at high plasma concentrations. When two drugs are administered simultaneously, however, they may compete for the same metabolic sites, and lesser concentrations of each are needed to saturate the metabolic enzymes. Therefore, a drug interaction may result in a disproportional increase in the half-life and decreased clearance of drug if the interaction not only competes for metabolism but also causes a change from a nonsaturated to a saturated state. One could speculate that this phenomenon is more likely to occur in critically ill patients in whom diminished hepatic perfusion or metabolic function would readily occur because of their primary disease.

Finally, pharmacokinetic drug interactions can occur at sites of drug excretion, mainly the kidney, by affecting blood flow to the kidneys, glomerular filtration rate, urine pH, and secretion or reabsorption of the drug. Drug interactions can occur via any of these possible mechanisms or their combination.

PHARMACODYNAMIC DRUG INTERACTIONS

Pharmacodynamic drug interactions result in an alteration in the biochemical or physiologic effects of a drug (Table 2.1). In general, interactions of this type can be divided into four classes: *(a)* interactions at the drug receptor (pharmacologic); *(b)* interactions due to different cellular mechanisms acting in concert or in opposition (physiologic); *(c)* interactions by one drug changing the cellular environment and thereby altering the actions of a second drug; and *(d)* chemical neutralization of drugs.

A majority of pharmacodynamic drug interactions involve drugs binding to the same receptor. To exert the desired effect, most drugs bind to specific receptor sites (affinity), which activates a biochemical event or series of events that result in the pharmacologic action (intrinsic activity). *Drugs that have both high affinity for the receptor site and intrinsic activity are called agonists; drugs that have high affinity for binding sites but little or no intrinsic activity are called antagonists; drugs with varying degrees of affinity and intrinsic activity are termed mixed agonist-antagonists.* The overall outcome of drug interactions at receptor sites is dependent on the varying affinities and intrinsic activities of the different agents involved.

In many instances, drug interactions between agonists and antagonists are clinically useful. For example, the specific narcotic antagonist, naloxone, attenuates the undesirable actions of opioids. β-adrenergic antagonists are used extensively to block the effects of both endogenous and exogenous catecholamines. In some instances, however, receptor interactions are deleterious to the patient. For example, congestive heart failure or chronic obstructive pulmonary disease may worsen with β-adrenergic receptor antagonists by attenuating the beneficial effects of catecholamines.

Pharmacodynamic drug interactions of the physiologic type can also produce either an enhanced or attenuated response. The use of combinations of agents with different mechanisms of action to lower blood pressure is clearly beneficial to the patient. Conversely, indomethacin reduces the antihypertensive effects of captopril (221), β-adrenergic antagonists (86–88, 194), and hydralazine (65) and decreases the response to loop diuretics (42, 255), presumably by inhibiting prostaglandin synthesis.

The third type of pharmacodynamic interaction occurs when the action of one drug results in a change in the intracellular or extracellular environment that modifies the action of another drug. The best such example is the increased toxicity of cardiac glycosides when administered with drugs that cause potassium depletion (31, 48). Another example is the interaction between reserpine and indirectly acting agents (37, 50). Since reserpine depletes norepinephrine in nerve terminals (50), there is less response to drugs that act primarily by releasing the neurotransmitter.

The final type of interaction involves chemical neutralization of one drug by another. Several interactions of this type occur in the gastrointestinal tract and are discussed in detail below ("Interactions Affecting Drug Absorption"). This type

Table 2.2. Drug Interactions Affecting Absorption

Proposed Mechanism	Drug Affected	Drug Causing Effect	Results of Interaction	References
Physicochemical complexing	Atenolol	Antacids	Decreased absorption	121b
	Bishydroxycoumarin	Antacids	Increased absorption	8, 13
	Captopril	Antacids	Decreased absorption	85c, 121b
	Carbamazepine	Activated charcoal	Decreased absorption, increased elimination	229
	Cephalexin	Cholestyramine	Decreased absorption	254
	Chlorothiazide	Cholestyramine	Decreased absorption	154
	Chlorpromazine	Antacids, cimetidine	Decreased absorption	91, 267
	Diflunisal	Antacids	Decreased absorption	344
	Digitoxin	Cholestyramine	Decreased absorption, increased elimination	53, 56
	Digoxin	Activated charcoal	Decreased absorption	228
		Antacids	Decreased absorption	46, 158
		Cholestyramine	Decreased absorption	47
		Kaolin-pectin	Decreased absorption	9, 46
	Isoniazid	Antacids	Decreased absorption	141
	Levodopa	Iron	Decreased absorption	54b
	Methyldopa	Iron	Decreased absorption	54a
	Penicillamine	Antacids	Decreased absorption	251
	Phenobarbital	Activated charcoal	Decreased absorption, increased elimination	27, 187, 229
	Phenytoin	Activated charcoal	Decreased absorption	228
	Piroxicam	Activated charcoal	Increased elimination	121a
	Propranolol	Antacids	Decreased absorption	83
		Cholestyramine	Decreased absorption	136
	Quinine	Activated charcoal	Increased elimination	193a, 272a
	Quinolone antibiotics	Aluminum or magnesium containing antacids, sucralfate	Decreased absorption	103a, 121b, 238a, 253c, 267b
	Ranitidine	Antacids	Decreased absorption	211
	Tenoxicam	Activated charcoal	Increased elimination	121a
	Tetracyclines	Antacids	Decreased absorption	20, 105
	Theophylline	Activated charcoal	Decreased absorption, increased elimination	29
	Tolbutamide	Activated charcoal	Decreased absorption	230
	Valproate	Activated charcoal	Decreased absorption	230
	Warfarin	Cholestyramine	Decreased absorption, increased elimination	144, 284
Changes in gastric pH	Cimetidine	Antacids	Decreased absorption	122, 324
	Ketoconazole	Antacids, histamine H_2 antagonists, omeprazole	Decreased absorption	34a, 186
	Tetracyclines	Cimetidine	Decreased absorption	105
		Sodium bicarbonate	Decreased absorption	20
Changes in gastrointestinal motility				
Increase in motility	Acetaminophen	Metoclopramide	Increased rate of absorption	237
	Chlorothiazide	Metoclopramide	Increased rate of absorption	252
	Cimetidine	Metoclopramide	Decreased absorption	122, 152
	Digoxin	Metoclopramide	Decreased absorption	148
	Ethanol	Metoclopramide	Increased rate of absorption	108
	Lithium	Metoclopramide	Increased rate of absorption	69
Decrease in motility	Acetaminophen	Narcotic analgesics	Decreased rate of absorption	238
		Propantheline	Decreased rate of absorption	237
	Benzodiazepines	Antacids	Decreased rate of absorption	116, 118
	Bishydroxycoumarin	Amitriptyline	Increased absorption	269
	Chlorothiazide	Propantheline	Decreased rate of absorption	252
	Digoxin	Propantheline	Increased absorption	202
	Ethanol	Propantheline	Decreased rate of absorption	108
	Isoniazid	Antacids	Decreased rate of absorption	141
	Lithium	Propantheline	Decreased rate of absorption	69
	Phenytoin	Antacids	Decreased rate of absorption	103, 171
	Propranolol	Antacids	Decreased rate of absorption	83
Effects on gastrointestinal mucosa	Aminoglycoside antibiotics	Ethanol	Increased absorption due to mucosal damage	161
	Digoxin	Neomycin	Decreased absorption	191
		Sulfasalazine	Decreased absorption	149
	Furosemide	Phenytoin	Decreased absorption	96
Effects on gastrointestinal flora	Digoxin	Broad spectrum antibiotics	Increased absorption	192

Table 2.2. Drug Interactions Affecting Absorption (*Continued*)

Proposed Mechanism	Drug Affected	Drug Causing Effect	Results of Interaction	References
Changes in first-pass metabolism				
Induction	Cyclosporine	Anticonvulsants, rifampin	Decreased bioavailability	365a
	Felodipine	Anticonvulsants	Decreased bioavailability	54d
Inhibition	Bromocriptine	Erythromycin	Increased bioavailability	226c
	Cyclosporine	Erythromycin, ketoconazole	Increased bioavailability	122b, 365a
	Felodipine	Cimetidine	Increased bioavailability	99a, 312b, 341a
	Imipramine			
	Labetalol			
	Lidocaine			
	Metoprolol			
	Nisoldipine			
	Propranolol			
	Verapamil			
	Mercaptopurine	Allopurinol, methotrexate	Increased bioavailability	14a, 19a

of interaction also occurs within the circulation and may be desirable, as is the case with the use of protamine to neutralize heparin, or deleterious, as is illustrated by the inactivation of gentamicin by ureidopenicillins in patients with end-stage renal disease (266, 332, 355).

SPECIFIC TYPES OF DRUG INTERACTIONS

INTERACTIONS AFFECTING DRUG ABSORPTION

In this chapter, we are focusing on drug interactions affecting oral absorption since a large majority of documented drug interactions occur in the gastrointestinal (GI) tract. The principles applied here are also applicable, however, to other sites of drug absorption. In addition, the discussion does not include drug-food interactions. For these interactions and for a more extensive discussion of interactions of specific drugs affecting absorption, one should refer to reviews on the subject (129, 227, 356).

Drug interactions at sites of absorption can alter the rate and/or extent of drug absorption. The rate determines how rapidly the drug enters the blood and when the peak plasma concentration is achieved. The extent of absorption affects the total amount of the drug systemically available. In general, drug interactions altering the extent of absorption are of greater clinical importance than those affecting rate. If the patient requires a known concentration of drug in a short time, as often occurs in critical care settings, then intravenous administration can be used, thus obviating uncertainties about rate as well as extent of absorption. If one drug interferes with the total amount of another drug absorbed, then the relationship between dose and plasma concentrations achieved (and subsequently clinical effect) is altered, and dosing adjustments are required. For the most part, drug interactions of this type result in a decrease in circulating drug concentrations, and if this decrease is substantial, the interaction can compromise therapy. Less frequently, the interaction can result in increased absorption and can subject the patient to drug toxicity.

Since oral absorption of drugs is dependent on many factors involving both the properties of the drug and the characteristics of the GI tract, it is not surprising that interactions involve a number of mechanisms. In general, a majority of drug interactions affecting absorption involve (*a*) formation of drug complexes due to absorption, chelation, or binding; (*b*) alterations in gastric pH that change the ionization of drugs; and (*c*) changes in GI motility that affect the transit time of drugs. Other interactions, such as alterations in the GI mucosa (function, area, blood flow, or metabolism) also occur, but their clinical importance is yet to be determined. Some of these drug interactions involve only one mechanism while others are multifactorial. Table 2.2 summarizes some of the major drug interactions occurring at sites of drug absorption.

Several drugs can alter absorption by forming complexes with other agents. These drugs include antacids, activated charcoal, kaolin-pectin, and the hypocholesterolemic agents cholestyramine and colestipol (Table 2.2). In most instances, the complex formed between the drug and the ion is less soluble and thereby less absorbable, resulting in a decrease in the amount of drug absorbed. Compounds with reduced absorption include digoxin (46, 158), chlorpromazine (91), quinine (140), penicillamine (251), tetracyclines (20, 105), isoniazid (141), propranolol (83), ranitidine (211), and diflunisal (344). The resultant decrease in absorption can be 10 to 80%, depending on the drug involved; consequently, the interaction may be clinically important. Rarely, the drug complexes formed by interaction with antacids are more soluble, and thus increased absorption of drug occurs. For example, bishydroxycoumarin chelates with magnesium to form a more absorbable complex (8, 13). Thus, patients taking this anticoagulant with magnesium hydroxide antacids may develop higher serum drug concentrations and a greater anticoagulant effect. Interestingly, warfarin absorption does not appear to be affected by antacids (8, 284).

Both activated charcoal (227–229) and kaolin-pectin (9, 10, 46) adsorb many drugs in the GI tract. This adsorption can cause significant reductions in the amount of drug absorbed. For example, activated charcoal can reduce the bioavailability of tolbutamide and valproate by 90% and 65%, respectively (230). In addition, this adsorption can result in a significant increase in clearance of drug from the body. Many drugs are secreted into the gut, and then reabsorbed (so-called enterohepatic circulation). In the presence of charcoal, however, the secreted drugs are adsorbed, preventing their reabsorption into the body; thus, they are cleared more rapidly. This increased clearance of drugs has been observed for phenobarbital, carbamazepine, and theophylline (29, 229). This type of interaction could be of benefit in the acutely intoxicated patient, but it could prove harmful in therapeutic settings by reducing the steady-state plasma concentration of drugs below the therapeutic range. In a similar manner, cholestyramine and colestipol bind bile acids, cholesterol, and many other drugs in the GI tract (47, 53, 144, 186, 284). This binding results in the decreased absorption of many drugs, including chlorothiazide (154), propranolol (136), cephalexin (254), cardiac glycosides (47, 53), and anticoagulants (144, 284). To avoid the interaction rather than compensate for it, patients requiring these drug combinations should be administered drug (digoxin, digitoxin, or warfarin) 1 hour before or 4 hours after ingesting cholestyramine or colestipol.

The interaction between digitoxin or warfarin and cholestyramine is used to clinical advantage in patients who are toxic or poisoned with either of these agents. Both agents undergo enterohepatic circulation. Administration of cholestyramine sequesters drug in the gut, resulting in less reabsorption and decreasing serum concentrations (53, 56, 144, 284).

As mentioned above, some drugs affect the absorption of others by multiple mechanisms. For example, antacids not only form complexes with other drugs but also affect absorption by altering gastric pH. Drug absorption is dependent on both dissolution of drug and extent of ionization. In the acidic environment of the stomach, drugs that are weak acids are less ionized and more rapidly absorbed. The opposite is true for weak bases. Thus, alteration in gastric pH by antacids and/or histamine H_2-antagonists can affect drug absorption (34a, 186). (Table 2.2). Fortunately, this interaction is rarely of clinical importance since most drugs, whether weak acids or weak bases, are predominantly absorbed in the small intestine via pathways that are not pH-sensitive.

Since most drugs are absorbed in the small intestine, changes in gastric emptying can alter delivery to absorption sites and, thereby, alter the rate of drug absorption. Thus, antacids (356), narcotic analgesics (238), and drugs with anticholinergic properties that slow emptying decrease the rate of absorption of benzodiazepines (118), isoniazid (141), phenytoin (103, 171), and propranolol (83). In addition, the anticholinergic propantheline reduces gastric emptying and delays the absorption of acetaminophen (237), ethanol (108), and lithium (69).

Drugs that alter intestinal transit time can also affect the extent of drug absorption. Propantheline not only reduces gastric emptying but decreases GI motility. This slowed transit time increases the absorption of poorly soluble drugs such as chlorothiazide (252) and older preparations of digoxin (202). Presumably, amitriptyline increases the absorption of bishydroxycoumarin by the same mechanism (269). Many other drugs, including phenothiazines, other tricyclic antidepressants, antihistamines, and narcotic analgesics, may also reduce GI transit time, thereby altering either rate or extent of drug absorption.

In general, drugs that increase GI motility have the opposite effect on rate and extent of absorption (129). Thus, metoclopramide increases the rate of absorption of many drugs (69, 108, 237) and decreases quantitative absorption of cimetidine and of older preparations of digoxin (148, 152, 202).

Drug interactions affecting absorption also occur as a result of one drug affecting the intestinal metabolism and/or transport of another. Although there are only limited reports of these interactions, they are worth discussing since they involve drugs that may be used in critical care medicine. The antibiotics neomycin and sulfasalazine decrease the absorption and plasma concentrations of digoxin, presumably by affecting the integrity of the GI mucosa (149, 191). In contrast, erythromycin can increase digoxin absorption, the proposed mechanism being a decrease in flora that metabolize digoxin in the small intestine of approximately 10% of patients (192). The latter interaction can result in sufficient increases in serum digoxin concentrations to cause toxicity.

INTERACTIONS AFFECTING DRUG DISTRIBUTION

Once a drug is absorbed into the systemic circulation, it is distributed to various tissues, including the site of action. Many drugs bind extensively to plasma proteins, whereas only unbound drug is free to enter tissue storage sites or sites of action, or to be metabolized or excreted. The concentration of unbound drug in the circulation can be affected by competition of other drugs for binding sites. Consequently, displacement of one bound drug by another constitutes a major source of drug interaction. Recently, however, the relative clinical importance of displacement interactions has been questioned (195a, 207, 302), and it appears that these types of interactions are often misinterpreted.

The importance and occurrence of displacement interactions are dependent on three factors: the concentration of drug in the plasma; the relative binding affinity of the drug; and the volume of distribution (V_d). A high concentration of one drug relative to another will shift the binding equilibrium. Thus, assuming equal affinities, addition of large concentrations of one drug to the blood will rapidly decrease plasma protein binding of a second. Relative binding affinity is the second important factor. In general, only drugs with high binding affinity displace other drugs. These include digitoxin, bishydroxycoumarin, warfarin, diazoxide, phenytoin, clofibrate, valproic acid, hydralazine, quinidine, sulfonamides, tolbutamide, and most nonsteroidal antiinflammatory drugs, including salicylates. Finally, if a drug has a small V_d, more of the displaced drug can remain in the plasma and be delivered to sites of action with a concomitant increase in the pharmacologic effect.

The clinical relevance of displacement interactions is dependent on the therapeutic index of the drugs involved, the availability of other distribution sites, and the rate of elimination of the displaced drug. If a drug has a wide therapeutic index, then displacement from binding that results in higher free concentrations is of little concern. In addition, increasing the free drug concentration is less important clinically when the free drug can be distributed to other tissue storage sites. This is the reason that clinically important interactions are less likely with drugs that have a large V_d. Finally, for most drugs, elimination occurs by means of first-order kinetics. Thus, increasing the free concentration of drug is rapidly compensated for by an increase in metabolism or excretion

(207, 302). With increased elimination, a new steady-state is achieved with a free drug concentration similar to that existing before the interaction. However, if elimination is compromised by disease or other drug interactions, a higher concentration of free drug may be maintained, creating a greater risk of toxicity. This rule especially applies to drugs with a low V_d, since the increase in free drug does not redistribute to other tissue storage sites. Thus, in patients with compromised hepatic or renal function there is a greater potential that the displacement interaction will result in increased free drug concentration and increased pharmacologic effect.

Even though the effect of displacement interactions is usually transient, during the period of increased free drug concentration an increased pharmacologic response may occur. Consequently, clinicians should exercise caution in treating patients during this transitional period. For example, the most important drug interactions involving displacement from plasma protein-binding sites occur with coumarin anticoagulants (6, 33, 197). The transient period of increased unbound anticoagulant can result in bleeding. It is therefore important to determine successive prothrombin times when a potential interaction is suspected. The patient may remain relatively stable during the critical time of the interaction and return to the same baseline level of anticoagulation in a few days, but then again, he or she may not.

In drug displacement interactions, after a new steady state has been attained, the resulting *total* plasma concentration of drug may be below the "normal" therapeutic range. One should not misinterpret such "subtherapeutic" values, for they do not adequately reflect the concentration of free drug. The clinician must be aware of the potentially altered "therapeutic range" of that patient and also rely on clinical assessment of the drug effect.

In some instances, drug toxicity originally attributed to a displacement interaction is the result of multiple interactions, e.g., displacement plus impairment of metabolism. Phenylbutazone displaces warfarin from binding sites on serum proteins but also inhibits metabolism (6). Thus, the increased concentration of free anticoagulant is not compensated for by increased metabolism, increasing the likelihood of bleeding. A similar mechanism accounts for the increased incidence of phenytoin toxicity when tolbutamide is coadministered with the anticonvulsant (357). In contrast, lessening of potential toxicity can also occur with multiple drug interactions. Phenytoin displaces dicumarol from serum protein (126), but this has little importance in patients to whom phenytoin is chronically administered, because of induction of metabolism that increases elimination of the free dicumarol.

As mentioned above, displacement interactions with anticoagulants appear to be the most important clinically (Table 2.3). Several drugs can displace coumarin anticoagulants from plasma protein-binding sites, including the active metabolite of chloral hydrate (305, 399), clofibrate (33), phenylbutazone (6), salicylates (197), and phenytoin (126, 197). Displacement interactions with other drugs may also have clinical importance (Table 2.3). For example, patients taking tolbutamide may experience a hypoglycemic episode when started on high doses of salicylates (167, 362) or when administered phenylbutazone (268). In addition, the therapeutic range for total phenytoin in the plasma may be reduced in patients taking val-

Table 2.3. Drug Interactions due to Displacement from Protein-Binding Sites

Drug Displaced	Causative Agent	References
Coumarin anticoagulants	Chloral hydrate	305, 339
	Clofibrate	33
	Diazoxide	304
	Ethacrynic acid	304
	Mefenamic acid	304
	Nalidixic acid	304
	Phenylbutazone	6
	Phenytoin	126, 197
	Salicylates	197, 214a
Diazepam	Heparin	290
	Valproic acid	82
Phenytoin	Phenylbutazone	231
	Salicylates	98, 214a
	Tolbutamide	357
	Valproic acid	204, 262
Tolbutamide	Phenylbutazone	167, 268
	Salicylates	167, 362
Valproic acid	Salicylates	214a, 250

proic acid, salicylates, or tolbutamide since these drugs increase the free fraction of phenytoin (98, 204, 262, 357). In a similar manner, salicylates can transiently displace valproic acid from binding sites (250).

The clinical importance of many displacement interactions is currently being reassessed. Clinicians should, however, closely monitor patients given multiple drugs that exhibit plasma protein binding. This monitoring is especially important during the initial period after adding another drug to the patient's regimen or when the patient has compromised drug elimination, as may occur in critical care settings because of the influence of other drugs or the patient's primary disease.

INTERACTIONS DUE TO ALTERED DRUG METABOLISM

Drug interactions of metabolism are numerous and of varying clinical relevance. The vast majority of metabolic interactions occur with induction or inhibition of the hepatic microsomal P-450 system (51, 68, 107). Indeed, drugs as well as environmental chemicals that are metabolized by these mixed-function oxidases can induce their own metabolism (autoinduction) and also affect the metabolism of other agents (242b). In like manner, drugs that are metabolized by the same enzyme system can act as competitive inhibitors and decrease the biotransformation of other agents.

There is a great deal of individual variability in the metabolic capacity of the hepatic enzyme systems and the degree to which it may be induced or inhibited by drugs (51, 107). In addition, the time course of drug interaction varies with different drugs and with the patient's ability to metabolize them (i.e., disease, genetics, age, etc.). Thus it is difficult to predict a priori the extent of an interaction in an individual patient. Each patient must be followed closely with clinical evaluation of therapeutic and toxic endpoints and drug toxicity, and if possible, with measurement of serum drug concentrations to assess the clinical importance of a drug interaction.

Table 2.4. Examples of Drugs That Induce the Metabolism of Other Drugs

Drug Induced	Inducing Agent	References
Acetaminophen	Oral contraceptives	17a, 219
Carbamazepine	Phenytoin	62, 261, 263
Chloramphenicol	Phenobarbital	360
	Rifampin	274
Chlorpromazine	Phenobarbital	51
Cimetidine	Phenobarbital	320
Clofibrate	Oral contraceptives	17a
Clonazepam	Phenytoin	261, 262
Clozapine	Phenytoin	211b
Cyclosporin	Anticonvulsants, rifampin	99, 365b
Dapsone	Rifampin	367
Diazepam	Phenytoin, rifampin	242a, 261, 262
Diflunisal	Oral contraceptives	17a
Digoxin	Rifampin	106
Digitoxin	Phenobarbital	31, 316
	Phenytoin	31, 316
	Rifampin	31, 316
Disopyramide	Anticonvulsants	152a
Doxycycline	Phenytoin	259
Fluconazole	Rifampin	13b, 180a
Fludrocortisone	Phenytoin	156
Glucocorticoids	Phenytoin	102, 264
	Rifampin	28
Griseofulvin	Phenobarbital	51
Haloperidol	Anticonvulsants, rifampin	99b
Lovastatin	Propranolol	253a
Meprobamate	Chronic ethanol (prior to hepatic impairment)	193, 216, 301, 303
Methadone	Phenytoin	261, 263
Metoprolol	Rifampin	25
Mexiletine	Rifampin	258
Morphine	Oral contraceptives	17a
Oral anticoagulants	Carbamazepine	127, 168, 197
	Chronic ethanol	153, 309
	Gluthethimide	168, 197
	Griseofulvin	168, 197
	Phenobarbital	70, 168, 197, 309
	Phenytoin	126, 168, 197
	Rifampin	245, 247, 287
Oral contraceptives	Anticonvulsants, rifampin	17a
Pancuronium	Phenytoin	190a
Pefloxacin	Rifampin	139e
Pentobarbital	Chronic ethanol	193, 216, 301, 303
Phenylbutazone	Phenobarbital	51
Phenytoin	Carbamazepine	127, 261, 263
	Chronic ethanol	193, 296, 301
	Phenobarbital	49, 70, 173
	Rifampin	155
	Vigabatrin	283a
Pravastatin	Propranolol	253a
Quinidine	Phenytoin	72
	Rifampin	338
Salicylate	Oral contraceptives	17a
Temazepam	Oral contraceptives	17a
Theophylline	Cigarette smoking	120
	Moricizine	96a
	Phenobarbital	177
	Phenytoin	212
	Rifampin	38, 285
Tolbutamide	Chronic ethanol	153, 193, 301, 303
	Rifampin	51, 366
Valproic acid	Anticonvulsants	253b, 261, 263, 293
Verapamil	Phenobarbital	291a

Drug Interactions Resulting in Enhanced Metabolism

Although a number of agents induce the metabolism of other drugs (Table 2.4), emphasis is placed on a few drugs that induce the metabolism of many others, including the barbiturates (especially phenobarbital), ethanol, rifampin, and the anticonvulsants, phenytoin and carbamazepine. All of these agents induce the metabolism of oral anticoagulants, thereby increasing the dosage required to achieve therapeutic prolongation of the prothrombin time (70, 126, 127, 153, 168, 197, 309). For example, coadministration of rifampin with warfarin for 5 to 7 days doubles warfarin clearance, requiring an approximate 2-fold increase in dosing to maintain therapeutic plasma concentrations of the anticoagulant (16, 245, 247, 287). This type of interaction is important not only during the time of induced metabolism but also after the inducing agent is withdrawn (168). When the inducing stimulus is no longer present, the hepatic enzyme activity slowly decreases, increasing serum concentrations and resulting in increased anticoagulation with the possible consequence of disastrous bleeding. Consequently, after removal of an inducing agent, the dose of anticoagulant needs to be readjusted.

Phenobarbital is a potent inducer of hepatic microsomal enzymes (242b), resulting in reduced plasma concentrations and increased elimination of many drugs (Table 2.4), including chloramphenicol (360), cimetidine (320), phenytoin (49, 70, 173), dicumarol (70, 168, 197), nortriptyline (39), theophylline (177), and warfarin (168, 197). In a similar manner, phenytoin induces the metabolism of a large number of drugs (Table 2.4). Phenobarbital combined with phenytoin doubles the clearance of quinidine in humans, with a concomitant decrease in the elimination half-life of approximately 50% (73), presumably due to enzyme induction. Similarly, this anticonvulsant combination results in a significant increase in steroid clearance in transplant patients (102, 264). Since many epileptic patients receive long-term therapy with either phenytoin or phenobarbital or both, caution must be exercised when the patients receive additional medication.

Rifampin is one of the most potent inducers of metabolizing enzymes, increasing the clearance of warfarin (245, 247), glucocorticoids (28), digitoxin (31, 316), chloramphenicol (274), hexobarbital (366), metoprolol (25), and dapsone (367). Rifampin therapy also decreases the half-life of tolbutamide (51, 366), oral contraceptives (17), and theophylline (38, 285). Rifampin has a 2-fold effect on quinidine handling, decreasing quinidine's elimination half-life with no change in the volume of distribution (338). From the data, one would predict an approximate 3-fold increase in clearance with an identical decrement in the steady-state plasma concentration or area under the curve (AUC) of plasma concentration vs. time. The observed change in AUC of quinidine in these subjects, however, was a 6-fold decrease (338). The probable explanation for this discrepancy is a concomitant decrease in the bioavailability of quinidine due to an enhanced first-pass effect through an induced hepatic enzyme system. The net result is a "multiplier" effect on drug concentrations achieved in plasma.

Nonprescription drugs, ethanol, and cigarette smoking also induce the microsomal enzyme system. Indeed, the clinician is not always aware of the chronic use of ethanol or cigarettes and may initiate therapy with "normal doses" of drugs, which may not achieve therapeutic plasma concentrations. Consequently, it is important to be aware of possible drug interactions with "recreational" drugs. As is evident in Table 2.4, chronic ethanol use can result in increased metabolism of several drugs. However, the acute use of ethanol often has opposite effects on drug metabolism, as discussed in the next section. Thus, acute ethanol use appears to inhibit metabolism, while chronic use (prior to onset of liver disease) can result in enhanced metabolism due to enzyme induction (178). Finally, induction of the hepatic microsomal enzyme system by means of cigarette smoking may explain the increase in theophylline clearance in chronic smokers (120).

Several points regarding enzyme induction are important (Table 2.5). First, drug interactions involving induction are slow in onset and offset. It takes days or weeks before the enzymes are induced; consequently, patients need to be monitored for extended periods when clinically important interactions are predicted. For example, Romankiewicz and Ehrman (287) showed that the onset and offset of the increase in warfarin clearance produced by rifampin was maximal 5 to 7 days after starting and stopping rifampin therapy. Consequently, the critical period of this interaction occurs approximately 1 week after initiation of therapy and 1 week after discontinuing the inducing agent. Second, offset of the drug interaction is as clinically important as onset. If, for example, a dosage adjustment is made when a patient has been receiving rifampin and warfarin to compensate for the increased metabolism, then another adjustment is needed some days after the rifampin is discontinued to readjust for the decreased clearance and to prevent excessive bleeding. Third, the induction of the microsomal enzyme system may be specific for one isoenzyme (i.e., one pathway) or nonspecific. For example, rifampin administration appears to selectively induce certain pathways of antipyrine metabolism (337) but does not appear selective in theophylline metabolism (285). Another example of selective induction is seen with acetaminophen and oral contraceptives (219). Oral contraceptives appear to increase the clearance of acetaminophen by selectively increasing glucuronidation. Whether this selectivity can be exploited for clinical use in acetaminophen poisoning is yet to be determined. Finally, the overall clinical relevance of drug interactions involving induction is clearly dependent on the therapeutic index of the drug involved. Affected drugs with a narrow therapeutic range are more clinically important than those with a wide range.

Drug Interactions due to Inhibition of Metabolism

In general, drugs discussed above that are susceptible to induction of metabolism are also subject to inhibition (Table 2.6). Inhibitors are capable of decreasing the metabolism of any drug that is metabolized by the same enzyme system. As

Table 2.5. Important Considerations Concerning Enzyme Induction

1. Slow in onset and offset.
2. Dosage adjustment and clinical monitoring are as important during offset as during onset.
3. Induction may be specific or nonspecific.
4. Clinical relevance is a function of the therapeutic index of the interacting drugs.

with induction, the clinical importance of these interactions is largely a function of the therapeutic index of the drugs involved. Unlike induction interactions, however, the onset and offset of these interactions are fairly rapid.

Most drug interactions involving inhibition of metabolism occur in the liver and are due to competitive inhibition of enzymes involved in drug biotransformation. For example, cimetidine inhibits the metabolism of many drugs (Table 2.6), presumably by inhibiting the hepatic cytochrome P-450 mixed-function oxidases (164, 276, 322). This inhibition results in a decrease in elimination of many drugs and often requires a change in the dosing regimen (Table 2.6). Of most clinical importance, however, are interactions between cimetidine and theophylline, lidocaine, and oral anticoagulants, since these latter drugs have a narrow margin of safety and, thus, critical toxicity can occur. Cimetidine decreases theophylline clearance by approximately 50% with a corresponding doubling of the elimination half-life (54, 66, 143, 270, 278, 347). Volume of distribution does not change. The result, if a patient's dosing regimen were not modified, would be a doubling of the serum theophylline concentration. In a similar manner, cimetidine reduces the clearance of oral anticoagulants, potentiating their actions and requiring a decrease in dosage (168, 197, 244, 309, 318). Cimetidine also decreases the clearance of lidocaine by 25 to 42%, presumably because of a decrease in metabolism of the antiarrhythmic (22, 92, 361); however, this interaction increases the lidocaine serum concentration by 50%, indicating a concomitant decrease in volume of distribution (approximately 10 to 20%) (92, 361). Consequently, when coadministering lidocaine and cimetidine, one should decrease both the loading and maintenance lidocaine doses. Cimetidine may also decrease lidocaine clearance by reducing hepatic blood flow (92), thereby decreasing lidocaine access to the liver (327, 333), although the occurrence of this reduction in hepatic blood flow by means of cimetidine is controversial (134, 142, 361).

Other drugs clearly alter hepatic blood flow, resulting in a reduced elimination of drugs whose metabolism is limited by availability of drug to liver enzymes (drugs with a high extraction ratio). For example, the β-adrenergic blocking agents propranolol, nadolol, and metoprolol decrease lidocaine clearance by 20 to 50% (25, 297). In addition, hydralazine increases the peak concentration and AUC of metoprolol and propranolol after oral administration by diminishing hepatic blood flow (25, 298). Aspirin and indomethacin decrease clearance of indocyanine green without altering antipyrine clearance (94), suggesting that inhibition of prostaglandin synthesis may alter hepatic blood flow. These results imply that inhibitors of prostaglandin synthesis may have important interactions with drugs such as lidocaine and propranolol.

Many other drug interactions inhibiting metabolism are clinically relevant (Table 2.6). For example, acute administration of ethanol inhibits the metabolism of many drugs (178, 193, 301, 303), including chloral hydrate (306), some benzodiazepines (79, 307, 308), propranolol (85), tolbutamide (57), phenytoin (193, 301, 303), and warfarin (193, 301, 303). As discussed earlier, chronic ethanol has an opposite effect on the clearance of many of these drugs because of induction of drug metabolism (Table 2.4). Tolbutamide metabolism is reduced by the coadministration of several drugs (63, 301),

Table 2.6. Examples of Drugs That Inhibit the Metabolism of Other Drugs

Drug Causing Inhibition	Drugs Inhibited	References
Acetaminophen	Fenoldopam	367a
Allopurinol	6-Mercaptopurine	19, 19a, 226
	Flecainide	311
Amiodarone	Digoxin	185c
	Flecainide	185c
	Metoprolol	185b, 185c
	Phenytoin	114, 185c, 208, 239a
	Procainamide	185c, 292, 359a
	Quinidine	185c, 292
	Warfarin	157a, 185c, 249a, 350
Bishydroxycoumarin	Tolbutamide	168, 197
Calcium channel antagonists:	Antipyrine	23, 55
	Carbamazepine	45, 160a, 199, 299a
Verapamil > diltiazem ≫	Cyclosporine	44a, 160a, 200a, 299a, 365a
Dihydropyridine	Digitoxin	299a
(except nicardipine and	Digoxin	132a, 160a, 299a
nisoldipine)	Doxorubicin	299a
	Metoprolol	160a, 299a, 331a
	Prazosin	299a
	Propranolol	139a, 160a, 299a, 331a
	Quinidine	88c, 160a
	Theophylline	226a, 312a
Chloramphenicol	Carbamazepine	32, 63, 261
	Chlorpropamide	32, 63
	Oral anticoagulants	32, 63, 168, 197
	Phenobarbital	32, 63, 169
	Phenytoin	32, 63, 169, 261, 263
	Tolbutamide	32, 63, 272
Chlorpromazine	Phenytoin	261, 348
	Propranolol	346
Disulfiram	Benzodiazepines	198
	Phenytoin	159, 243
	Theophylline	193c
	Warfarin	168, 197, 246
Erythromycin	Alfentanil	21a
	Carbamazepine	211a, 363, 365
	Cyclosporine	203, 365a
	Felodipine	190b
	Theophylline	41, 206, 256a, 282, 283
Ethanol (acute)	Diazepam	196
	Meprobamate	193, 301, 303
	Pentobarbital	193, 301, 303
	Phenytoin	193, 261, 301, 303
	Tolbutamide	57, 193, 272
	Warfarin	168, 193, 197
Flecainide	Dextromethorphan	122c
	Propranolol	139a
Fluconazole	Chlorpropamide	114a
	Glyburide	114a
	Glipizide	114a
	Phenytoin	34b, 114a, 393
	Tolbutamide	114a, 393
	Warfarin	114a
Fluoxetine	Carbamazepine	119a
	Diazepam	185a
Histamine H₂-Antagonists:	Alprazolam	312b
Cimetidine = etintidine	Amitriptyline	71
≫ ranitidine, negligible	Benzodiazepines	79, 115, 162, 240a, 241, 291, 312b, 318
effect of famotidine,	Carbamazepine	200, 261
nizatidine, roxatidine	Chloroquine	88e
	Clozapine	330a, 176a
	Desipramine	324b
	Felodipine	85d, 88a, 294a
	5-Fluorouracil	19, 130
	Imipramine	4, 133, 312b
	Lidocaine	22, 92, 312b, 361

Table 2.6. Examples of Drugs That Inhibit the Metabolism of Other Drugs (*Continued*)

Drug Causing Inhibition	Drugs Inhibited	References
	Meperidine	121, 312b
	Metronidazole	312b
	Moricizine	96a
	Metoprolol	25, 334a
	Nifedipine	300a, 312b
	Pentoxifylline	204a
	Phenytoin	11, 135, 232, 294, 294b, 312b
	Piroxicam	344a
	Propranolol	93, 139c, 176a, 318
	Quinidine	312b
	Theophylline	35a, 54, 66, 143, 176a, 270, 278, 312b, 344c
	Tocainide	239b
	Tolbutamide	58
	Triamterene	222
	Warfarin	168, 244, 312b, 334c
	Urapadil	160b
Isoniazid	Acetaminophen	224a
	Carbamazepine	341, 364
	Haloperidol	180a
	Phenytoin	174, 225, 261
Ketoconazole	Cyclosporine	365a
	Methylprednisolone	151a
	Prednisolone	367a
	Terfenadine	220a
Methylphenidate	Phenobarbital	104, 261
	Phenytoin	104, 261
	Primidone	104, 261
Mexiletine	Theophylline	141a, 193d
Omeprazole	Diazepam	13a, 122a, 139b
	Nifedipine	139b
	Phenytoin	13a, 122a, 139b, 273a
	Warfarin	329a
Oral contraceptives	Chlordiazepoxide	17a
	Cyclosporine	17a
	Diazepam	2, 17a
	Imipramine	3
	Metoprolol	25
	Nitrazepam	17a
	Oral anticoagulants	80, 168, 197
	Prednisolone	17a, 184
	Theophylline	17a, 336
Oxyphenbutazone	Phenytoin	344a
	Tolbutamide	344a
	Warfarin	344a
Phenylbutazone	Phenytoin	344a
	Tolbutamide	344a
	Warfarin	344a
Probenecid	Carprofen	344a
	Indomethacin	344a
	Ketoprofen	344a
	Zidovudine	76a
Propafenone	Digoxin	136a
	Metoprolol	136a, 348a
	Propranolol	136a
	Warfarin	136a, 153a
Propoxyphene	Carbamazepine	73
	Doxepin	5
	Phenytoin	5, 261
Propranolol	Diazepam	242
	Flecainide	139a
	Lidocaine	40, 240
	Nifedipine	160a
	Nisoldipine	160a
Quinidine	Digitoxin	170
Via inhibition of cytochrome	Digoxin	132b
P450IID6	Desipramine	324a
	Imipramine	45a

Table 2.6.   Examples of Drugs That Inhibit the Metabolism of Other Drugs (*Continued*)

Drug Causing Inhibition	Drugs Inhibited	References
Quinolone Antibiotics: Enoxacin > ciprofloxacin = pefloxacin; negligible effect of norfloxacin and ofloxacin	Propafenone Propranolol Caffeine Theophylline Warfarin	101a 365c 54c, 88b, 134a, 341c 23a, 37a, 54c, 88b, 134a, 276a, 285b, 285c, 296a, 299b, 330b, 341c, 357a 88b, 134a, 334b
Sulfonamides	Carbamazepine Phenytoin Tolbutamide Warfarin	32, 150 32, 150, 195, 261 32, 195, 257, 272 32, 168, 195, 197
Sulfinpyrazone	Warfarin	335
Tamoxifen	Warfarin	193b
Thymidine	5-Fluorouracil	19
Ticlopidine	Theophylline	67a
Valproate	Carbamazepine	157b, 198a

which can result in long-lasting and profound hypoglycemia. Drug inhibition of phenytoin and carbamazepine metabolism has resulted in many incidences of toxicity with these agents (63, 125, 174, 195, 225, 261, 263). This toxicity, although usually not life-threatening, causes considerable trauma to the patient and often requires prolonged hospitalization. The potential consequences of drug interactions that inhibit metabolism of oral anticoagulants are obvious (80, 131, 166, 168, 195, 235, 246, 248, 249, 335), and to avoid potential toxicity, compensatory changes in dosing are necessary when therapy with an interacting drug is commenced or discontinued.

Interactions affecting drug metabolism can also occur with extrahepatic enzymes. As a major example, a number of drugs used clinically act by inhibiting monoamine oxidase (313). The significance of interactions with these drugs is only lessened by the appropriate infrequent use of these agents. However, procarbazine (81), a drug used in treating Hodgkin's disease, and isoniazid (185, 315) have monoamine oxidase inhibitory activity. Concomitant use of sympathomimetic agents with these drugs requires awareness of this potential effect. Monoamine oxidase metabolizes sympathetic neurotransmitters that are retaken up into the sympathetic nerve ending from the synaptic cleft. During inhibition of this enzyme, administration of catecholamines or agents that release catecholamines, such as tyramine, ephedrine, pseudoephedrine, and amphetamines, can cause potentially fatal hypertensive crisis since metabolism of these drugs and of endogenous catecholamine is inhibited. In addition, some antihypertensive agents such as reserpine, guanethidine, methyldopa, and clonidine may (rarely) acutely release endogenous catecholamine stores, paradoxically raising blood pressure to dangerous levels.

Several important points regarding drug interactions due to metabolic inhibition should be stressed (Table 2.7). First, as mentioned above, the onset of these interactions may be quite rapid. An effect can be seen with the first dose; the maximum effect is dependent on attainment of a new steady-state drug concentration and therefore requires 4 to 5 times the *new* half-life of the drug. Second, the interaction between two drugs may be dependent on the amount of the drug administered and the total duration of administration. For

Table 2.7.   Important Considerations Concerning Enzyme Inhibition

1. Onset can occur quickly.
2. Time to maximum effect depends on the new half-life of the affected drug.
3. Whether an interaction occurs may be dose-dependent.
4. The patient's primary disease may increase susceptibility.
5. The interaction may involve one, but not other, stereoisomers.

example, allopurinol at a dosage of 300 mg/day for 7 days does not alter the metabolism of theophylline in normal individuals, yet if the dosage is increased to 300 mg every 12 hours for 14 days, the clearance of theophylline is reduced 21% while the half-life and AUC are significantly increased (201). Thus, physicians must be cautious not only when adding a new drug to the therapeutic regimen but also when altering the dosage of a drug the patient is already taking. Third, other factors (i.e., liver function, genetics) affecting drug metabolism may influence the incidence of drug interactions. For example, Rollinghoff and Paumgartner (286) demonstrated that therapeutic doses of cimetidine reduced aminopyrine metabolism to a greater degree in patients with compromised liver function than in subjects with normal liver function. They concluded that patients with chronic liver disease may be at increased risk for drug interactions with drugs that compete for metabolism. Another factor involves the patient's inherited ability to metabolize drug. Genetic variability of drug metabolism is well-documented (65a, 143a, 150a, 176, 344b, 345, 353). The acetylation of isoniazid, for example, is rapid in approximately half the population and slow in the other half (89). Slow acetylation appears to predispose patients to increased toxicity from drugs metabolized by microsomal enzymes. This fact may explain the increased incidence of phenytoin toxicity in slow acetylators of isoniazid, as opposed to rapid acetylators (172). Phenytoin metabolism is also genetically controlled, certain individuals slowly metabolizing the drug (175, 343). This genetic variability may prove to be an additional, important determinant of susceptibility to drug interactions.

A fourth important point involves inhibition of drug metabolism that selectively affects one enantiomer of a racemic mixture of a drug. For example, warfarin used in therapy is a racemic mixture, with the S-enantiomer having the predominant anticoagulant effect. Several drugs, including metronidazole, (249), trimethoprim-sulfamethoxazole (248), and sulfinpyrazone (335), inhibit the metabolism of S-warfarin. When the interaction between these drugs and racemic warfarin is assessed, significant changes are observed in prothrombin time, yet no consistent or significant changes are observed in the pharmacokinetics of warfarin. The lack of a pharmacokinetic interaction is probably due to a masking of the inhibition of S-warfarin by R-warfarin. Consequently, clinicians should be aware that observed, yet unexplained, pharmacodynamic drug interactions may in fact have a pharmacokinetic component.

Finally, although this discussion has stressed drug interactions of metabolism that have deleterious consequences, some interactions of this type may be beneficial. For example, cimetidine selectively inhibits the oxidative metabolism of acetaminophen in the liver (1, 220). Since the oxidative metabolites of acetaminophen are more toxic than the conjugated metabolites, cimetidine-induced inhibition is potentially beneficial in treating acetaminophen overdose.

Ideally, the clinician should be aware of the metabolic pathways for various drugs, be able to predict potential drug interactions, and compensate for them. It is also possible, in some instances, for the clinician to substitute one drug for another if drug interactions are anticipated. For example, cimetidine inhibits the metabolism of several benzodiazepines, including diazepam and chlordiazepoxide, by inhibiting the mixed-function oxidases in the liver (78, 115, 162, 241, 291, 318). It does not, however, usually inhibit glucuronidation or sulfation. Consequently, if a benzodiazepine is needed in a patient receiving cimetidine, one can select oxazepam or lorazepam since cimetidine does not block glucuronidation of these drugs (256). If a drug is needed to decrease gastric acid secretion and the patient is receiving other drugs metabolized by the hepatic P-450 enzyme system, the clinician could select antacids, sucralfate, or ranitidine instead of cimetidine for therapy. Cimetidine (as discussed above) inhibits liver metabolism of many drugs, whereas ranitidine, a structurally different H_2-receptor blocker, does not appear to affect the metabolism of antipyrine, theophylline, warfarin, diazepam, tolbutamide, phenytoin, or β-adrenergic receptor blockers (43, 58, 132, 157, 163, 244, 270, 279, 310, 321, 351). Thus, ranitidine has the clinical advantage of limited potential for metabolic drug interactions.

INTERACTIONS AFFECTING DRUG EXCRETION

As noted previously, most drug excretion occurs in the kidney; consequently, emphasis is placed on drug interactions involving renal excretion of both parent drug and metabolites. Drugs can be excreted by filtration or active secretion and can be reabsorbed into the systemic circulation. Logically, all three functions are potential sites for drug interaction. The other major route of drug excretion involves biliary secretion into the intestinal tract. For such drugs, interactions can occur in the GI tract with other drugs that bind or adsorb the

secreted drugs (see "Interactions Affecting Drug Absorption"). This phenomenon is analogous to drug interactions decreasing the extent of absorption, as previously discussed.

Many drugs are eliminated by glomerular filtration; clinically important examples are the aminoglycoside antibiotics and digoxin. Theoretically, changes in glomerular filtration rate (GFR) affect handling of these and other drugs. Few studies, however, have addressed this potentially important area of drug interactions. Evidence suggests that furosemide causes a fall in GFR consequent to volume depletion (180). Presumably, by decreasing GFR, furosemide can reduce the clearance of digoxin and gentamicin (180, 334). Whether this interaction has clinical significance is yet to be determined. Furthermore, furosemide is a poor pharmacologic tool for assessing potential effects of GFR since the effect is most likely dependent on the degree of volume loss or replacement. Other pharmacologic agents can increase renal perfusion directly. For example, in dogs, dopamine increases GFR and the elimination of tobramycin (160). Such effects need further study in humans. However, many patients in critical care settings receive vasoactive drugs that can affect GFR. Similarly, many patients receive drugs dependent on glomerular filtration for excretion. It is important, therefore, for critical care physicians to consider the potential for these types of interactions, despite the paucity of available information.

A large number of drugs and metabolites are eliminated from the body by active secretion at the pars recta (straight segment) of the proximal tubule. This secretion occurs via two nonspecific transport systems, one for organic acids and one for bases. Since the transport is nonspecific, drugs can compete for transport with each other, and the resultant interactions can be clinically important (271, 280, 354). There is also a secretory pathway for digoxin, located in the distal tubule, which is a site for drug interactions affecting digoxin (109, 325).

Several drugs that are organic acids have clinically important renal secretion (Table 2.8). These include many diuretics, nonsteroidal antiinflammatory drugs (15), penicillins (151), cephalosporins (119), methotrexate (7, 19, 234), and sulfa compounds (260). Clearly, the different acids compete with each other for secretion; however, it is difficult to predict a priori the degree of competition.

Table 2.8. Organic Acids Actively Secreted by the Kidney[a]

Acetazolamide
p-Aminohippurate
Captopril
Cephalosporins (most)
Ciprofloxacin
Dapsone
Dyphylline
Heparin
Loop-acting diuretics
Methotrexate
Nonsteroidal antiinflammatory agents
Penicillins
Probenecid
Salicylates
Sulfonamides
Sulfonylureas
Thiazide diuretics

[a] Data taken from references 7, 15, 19, 54c, 119, 151, 183a, 205, 214a, 233a, 234, 260, 288, 289, 295, 330, 341c, 357.

Table 2.9. Organic Bases Actively Secreted by the Kidney[a]

Acecainide (*N*-acetylprocainamide)
Amantadine
Amiloride
Cimetidine
Ethambutol
Flecainide
Mecamylamine
Mepacrine (quinacrine)
Metformin
N-Methylnicotinamide
Procainamide
Pseudoephedrine
Ranitidine
Tetraethylammonium
Triamterene
Trimethoprim

[a] Data from references 64, 139d, 168a, 265, 281, 312b, 317, 319.

The interaction between methotrexate and probenecid illustrates the interaction between organic acids. When probenecid is administered to patients taking methotrexate, most clinicians decrease the dosage of the anticancer drug (7). Few physicians are aware, however, of a similar need to decrease the dose if other drugs secreted by the organic acid transport system are coadministered with methotrexate (19, 234). Indeed, the increased sensitivity to methotrexate seen in some patients may be due to coadministration of drugs that inhibit its active secretion.

In addition to exogenous organic acids, endogenous organic acids can also compete for the transport system. This mechanism may account for the large doses of organic acid diuretics, such as furosemide, that are required to cause diuresis in uremic patients (288, 289). The endogenous acids produced in uremia may compete with the diuretics for transport into the renal tubular lumen, i.e., to their site of action.

The active transport system for organic bases and its clinical importance are less well understood. Like organic acids, many bases undergo potentially important active secretion (Table 2.9). Of these, the only interactions studied clinically are those between the H$_2$-receptor antagonists cimetidine and ranitidine and the antiarrhythmic procainamide (64, 317, 319). Coadministration to healthy volunteers of cimetidine with procainamide results in a significant increase in AUC for procainamide and a significant decrease in the renal clearance of both procainamide and its major metabolite, *N*-acetylprocainamide (64, 319). Ranitidine produces similar effects, which are dependent on the plasma concentrations of the H$_2$-receptor antagonist (317). Whether other clinically significant interactions occur between organic bases is yet to be determined.

The decrease in secretion of digoxin caused by several drugs is one of the most important drug interactions affecting secretion (24, 30, 60, 84, 85a, 85e, 123, 139, 148a, 181–183, 223, 285a, 299, 326, 357b, 358). This phenomenon is reviewed in detail elsewhere (30). The interaction occurs in at least 90% of patients with coadministration of quinidine and digoxin, with, on the average, a doubling of the serum digoxin concentration. The magnitude of the effect appears to be dependent on the serum quinidine concentration. The predominant mechanism of the interaction is decreased tubular secretion of digoxin (109), resulting in decreased overall clearance and a need to halve the dose (on average) to maintain the same serum concentration of digoxin. In addition, approximately two-thirds of patients also demonstrate a 10% or more decrease in digoxin's volume of distribution. The mechanism of this effect is presumably the displacement of digoxin from muscle binding sites by quinidine (147, 299).

If displacement of digoxin from muscle occurs, does displacement occur from sites of action on cardiac muscle? If so, the increase in serum concentrations of digoxin would not result in an increased pharmacologic effect on the heart but may affect other systems. Data addressing this issue are inconsistent (24, 84, 138, 183, 299, 326, 357b, 358). Some studies report a decreased cardiac digoxin concentration with an increased concentration in the brain after quinidine administration (30). Although controversial, observations suggest enhanced electrophysiologic action on the heart (24, 183, 223) with a decrease in inotropism (81, 138, 299, 326, 358). The electrophysiologic actions may be due to enhanced central nervous system effects on atrioventricular nodal conduction. If these effects occur as a result of the interaction, one clearly needs to decrease the dosage of digoxin to maintain the "therapeutic range." This decrease may thereby compromise the inotropic actions of the drug. In fact, in those patients who do not require digoxin for effects on conduction, alternative therapy may be more appropriate.

This interaction with digoxin is not unique to quinidine. Amiodarone, quinine, spironolactone, verapamil, and flecainide also increase serum digoxin concentrations (85a, 85e, 95, 148a, 182, 189, 285a, 349, 352, 357b). Like quinidine, spironolactone affects both the volume of distribution and the clearance of digoxin (95, 349). On average, clearance decreases 26%; however, there is great variability among patients, with a range of 0 to 74%. Similarly, the effect on volume of distribution is highly variable. Therefore, some patients may require dose adjustment while others will not. In general, loading and maintenance doses of digoxin are decreased by one-third in patients receiving spironolactone; some patients may need subsequent upward titration.

Some drugs are reabsorbed in the nephron after having gained access to the tubular lumen by filtration or secretion. Reabsorption of drugs in the distal tubule and collecting duct is related to urinary flow rate and pH (214). High rates of urine flow induced by diuretics or fluid loading increase excretion of phenobarbital and theophylline, but these increased flow rates would have to be maintained for long periods of time before they became clinically important. In animal studies, digoxin clearly has a reabsorptive component, presumably in the proximal tubule (110). Consequently, renal excretion of digoxin involves filtration, proximal reabsorption, and secretion at more distal tubular sites. The mechanism of digoxin's reabsorption is unclear but appears to follow general reabsorptive activity of the proximal tubule. Administration of saline or mannitol decreases proximal tubular reabsorption of sodium and of digoxin, whereas agents acting more distally to increase sodium excretion and urinary volume do not affect digoxin excretion (110). Whether drug interactions occur in humans via this pathway is unclear. These interactions may, however, be particularly important in critical care settings in which fluctuations in volume status may have major effects on proximal tubule reabsorption. In such cases, digoxin handling should be followed closely.

Lithium is reabsorbed in the nephron in parallel with sodium, and changes in sodium homeostasis (particularly in the proximal tubule) can therefore alter renal excretion of lithium. The mild volume depletion attending chronic administration of thiazide diuretics causes increased proximal tubular reabsorption of sodium and concomitantly decreases lithium excretion (77, 137). Furosemide, on the other hand, appears to have little effect (146). Administration of indomethacin or diclofenac increases steady-state serum lithium concentrations by approximately 30%, presumably by facilitating the reabsorption of lithium in the proximal tubule (100, 277, 311a, 341b). Other agents affecting proximal reabsorption of sodium might also affect handling of lithium (18a, 85b, 118a, 226b).

Finally, altering the pH of the urine could alter passive transport of weak acids and bases. For example, administration of therapeutic doses of antacids may raise urinary pH sufficiently to change the excretion of some drugs in clinically important amounts (188).

PHARMACODYNAMIC DRUG INTERACTIONS

Many drug interactions do not involve changes in the absorption, distribution, or elimination of drugs but involve modification of the biologic effect of the drugs. These interactions may involve drug receptor interactions, may involve different cellular mechanisms, may be due to alterations in cellular environment, or may result from chemical neutralization.

Drug interactions at receptor sites are widely known and often used to clinical advantage. Clearly, drug antagonists are synthesized specifically for their effects on receptors, as is illustrated by the substantial number of β-adrenergic receptor blockers that are available. There are numerous examples of agonist/antagonist drug interactions. Often, however, antagonists lack specificity with regard to their receptor-blocking ability. For example, phenothiazines, tricyclic antidepressants, and butyrophenones have α-adrenergic antagonist properties, accounting for the enhanced activity of other α-adrenergic blockers used concomitantly. In addition, this antagonist activity accounts for the use of directly acting sympathomimetics to reverse toxic α-adrenergic blockade caused by these drugs.

In a similar manner, some tricyclic antidepressants have potent antimuscarinic effects (233, 239). Consequently, adverse drug interactions can occur when multiple drugs that block similar receptor sites are administered. The clinician, therefore, needs to be aware of possible multiple receptor effects of drugs, not just of the major classes of agonists or antagonists.

Unanticipated but predictable interactions may occur with use of agents that have multiple-receptor effects. For example, epinephrine is both an α- and α-adrenergic agonist; the α-effect predominates in most instances, causing arteriolar vasoconstriction. Concomitant use of an α-adrenergic antagonist not only attenuates the vasoconstriction but also may unveil the vasodilation caused by the β-effect. Similarly, the use of propranolol for the treatment of hypertension can, in rare instances, exacerbate the hypertension by blocking β-induced

vasodilation and potentiate preexisting α-mediated vasoconstriction, especially in patients with a pheochromocytoma (209, 236, 273). By means of a similar mechanism, in patients treated with clonidine, withdrawal of the drug during continued administration of propranolol can cause accentuation of the α-adrenergic effect of endogenous catecholamines (18).

Pharmacodynamic drug interactions also occur when two drugs administered together have different cellular mechanisms that either enhance or diminish the physiologic response. For example, indomethacin administration decreases the antihypertensive effects of captopril (101, 221), hydralazine (65), and propranolol (21, 86, 87, 194). The effect of indomethacin, although not known, may be due to inhibition of synthesis of prostaglandins responsible for vasodilation. This hypothesis is controversial, since the attenuation of the antihypertensive effects does not seem to occur with other inhibitors of prostaglandin synthesis (88).

In a similar manner, indomethacin decreases the acute response to furosemide, whereas aspirin has no effect in normal subjects (26, 42, 255, 340). The indomethacin effect is not a result of a change in the amount of furosemide reaching its intraluminal site of action (61). Whether this interaction is of clinical importance is unclear; patients chronically receiving both drugs show no effect on sodium excretion, although the antihypertensive effect of furosemide is blunted by indomethacin (255).

Tricyclic antidepressants and guanethidine block neuronal uptake of catecholamines at the synaptic cleft (36, 323). Because reuptake of catecholamines is the major mechanism of attenuation of their effect, the response to exogenously administered catecholamines may be increased if used with these agents (67). In studies of normal subjects given imipramine (25 mg 3 times daily) for 5 days, the pressor effect of phenylephrine was potentiated by 2 to 3 times, norepinephrine by 4 to 8 times, and epinephrine by 2 to 4 times (35). In a similar study in subjects given debrisoquine (a guanidinium antihypertensive agent that blocks the catecholamine reuptake system), the effects of phenylephrine were markedly potentiated and prolonged (12). Sympathomimetics that act indirectly would not be expected to have an enhanced effect with guanethidine-like drugs and would more likely have a decreased effect, since guanethidine, debrisoquine, and bethanidine deplete endogenous catecholamines.

Another set of important drug interactions involving the catecholamine reuptake mechanism is that occurring among the guanidinium antihypertensives, guanethidine, bethanidine, and debrisoquine, and a number of psychoactive agents. The former guanethidine antihypertensives are taken into the nerve ending by the catecholamine reuptake system, where they cause release and depletion of endogenous catecholamine stores. Tricyclic antidepressants reverse the antihypertensive effects of these agents by inhibiting their uptake to this site of action (36, 113, 124, 217, 218, 314, 329). Doxepin has less tendency to produce this effect than other antidepressants (90). A similar reversal of effect that probably results from inhibition of uptake or displacement from the site of action also occurs with amphetamine, ephedrine, methylphenidate, phenothiazines, butyrophenones, thiothixene, and possibly reserpine (59, 75, 76, 145, 329). A similar interaction has been reported with use of a nasal decongestant containing chlorpheniramine, isopropamide, and phenylpropanolamine (215). This last interaction is probably not clinically important in most patients, but use of over-the-counter "cold" remedies should be avoided in patients receiving guanethidine-like drugs.

Reversal of the antihypertensive effect of clonidine by desipramine is well documented (44, 49a, 342), implying that caution should be used when other tricyclic antidepressants and psychoactive drugs are administered to patients receiving clonidine.

There are several other examples of pharmacodynamic drug interactions resulting from different drug mechanisms. Phenothiazines and tricyclic antidepressants can produce a quinidine-like decrease in cardiac conduction time, resulting in a prolonged QRS complex and arrhythmias (14, 74, 97, 359). Concomitant use of quinidine, procainamide, or similar agents with these drugs could therefore have additive effects. Treatment of arrhythmias caused by phenothiazines or tricyclic antidepressants therefore requires agents that will not further depress conduction; these include lidocaine, tocainide, mexiletine, phenytoin, and β-adrenergic receptor blockers.

Verapamil, the slow calcium-channel antagonist, slows atrioventricular (A-V) nodal conduction by inhibition of calcium influx into the myocardial cells (190, 331). Both propranolol and digoxin can also slow A-V nodal conduction via other mechanisms. The concomitant administration of verapamil with either propranolol or digoxin could therefore result in additive suppression of A-V nodal conduction and cause bradycardia, A-V block, or ventricular asystole (253, 300). Thus although most patients can tolerate such combinations without difficulty, caution should be exercised when these drugs are given together.

The third type of pharmacodynamic drug interaction involves one drug changing the extracellular or cellular environment such that the action of a second drug is affected. Perhaps the best example of this is the changes in electrolyte status that affect the response to digitalis glycosides (31, 48). Many drugs, including diuretics (117, 165, 275), amphotericin B (213), ampicillin (111), carbenicillin (52), and lithium (224), can cause hypokalemia. Potassium depletion increases the risk of digoxin toxicity. This interaction is particularly easy to overlook because substantial decreases in intracellular potassium can occur with normokalemia. Hypercalcemia and hypomagnesemia similarly increase the sensitivity to digitalis.

Finally, drugs can neutralize each other by forming complexes either in solution or in situ. Perhaps the best example of this type of interaction in situ involves heparin and protamine. The administration of protamine to neutralize heparin is widely known and used to clinical advantage. Another important interaction of this type that can be critical to the patient's well-being is the neutralization of aminoglycoside antibiotics by certain penicillins in patients with renal disease (266, 332, 355). The penicillins: carbenicillin, ticarcillin, and piperacillin, complex with the aminoglycoside. The effect appears to be dependent on the patient's level of renal function (179) and is related to both concentration and time (34).

The preceding constitute but a few of the myriad pharmacodynamic drug interactions. It should be clear that anticipation of these interactions requires a collation of knowledge concerning the fundamental pharmacologic characteristics of the drugs administered to a patient and the pathophysiology of the patient's disease(s).

APPLICATIONS TO CRITICAL CARE PRACTITIONERS

Patients in critical care settings are particularly susceptible to drug interactions. They frequently receive multiple drugs that have narrow therapeutic indices and/or are frequently implicated in drug interactions. Antiarrhythmic agents, sympathomimetics, cardiac inotropes, and histamine H_2-receptor antagonists are but a few examples of drugs administered to many, if not most, patients in critical care medicine. To compound potential problems, the patient's primary disease can have great influence on drug disposition and response. For example, cardiovascular instability can affect hepatic and renal perfusion and thereby influence elimination of a number of drugs, especially those agents used in critical care settings. Examples include diminished hepatic elimination of lidocaine with congestive hepatopathy, diminished V_d of lidocaine in heart failure, and diminished renal excretion of digoxin or aminoglycoside antibiotics when renal perfusion is compromised. Not anticipating such effects can clearly lead to potentially disastrous drug-induced consequences. Unfortunately, critical care patients are often so sick that adverse drug effects can easily be misinterpreted as a manifestation of the patient's underlying condition. Because of this fact, and the great potential for drug interactions in this setting, the critical care practitioner must maintain a constant alert for drug interactions. So doing will allow one to avoid toxicity and maximize efficacy of the potent drugs at our disposal.

SUMMARY

In this chapter, drug interactions are discussed from a mechanistic point of view. We hope that the use of this approach provides a framework that assists clinicians in predicting potentially important drug interactions without memorizing extensive listings. Furthermore, as new drugs are introduced into clinical medicine, the principles discussed in this chapter can be applied to predict potential interactions prior to their documentation. For example, if aware that a new drug is metabolized by the liver microsomal enzyme system, the clinician is alerted to the potential for enzyme induction and/or inhibition by other agents handled in a similar manner. Conversely, knowing that a drug has a large V_d and is not extensively bound to plasma proteins, the clinician does not need to be concerned about displacement interactions.

With the increasing numbers of new drugs available to the clinician and with the use of multiple drugs in a given patient, it is essential to be aware of important drug interactions. By understanding basic pharmacokinetic principles and the characteristics of given drugs, the clinician can be alerted to potential drug interactions. The appropriate steps can then be taken: closely monitoring the patient; altering the dosing of one or both drugs; or changing one of the drugs to minimize the likelihood of an interaction.

REFERENCES

1. Abernethy DR, Greenblatt DJ, Divoll M, Ameer B, Shader RI: Differential effect of cimetidine on drug oxidation (antipyrine and diazepam) vs. conjugation (acetaminophen and lorazepam): prevention of acetaminophen toxicity by cimetidine. *J Pharmacol Exp Ther* 224:508–515, 1982.

2. Abernethy DR, Greenblatt DJ, Divoll M, Arendt R, Ochs HR, Shader RI: Impairment of diazepam metabolism by low-dose estrogen-containing oral-contraceptive steroids. *N Engl J Med* 306:791–792, 1982.

3. Abernethy DR, Greenblatt DJ, Shader RI: Imipramine disposition in users of oral contraceptive steroids. *Clin Pharmacol Ther* 35:792–797, 1984.

4. Abernethy DR, Greenblatt DJ, Shader RI: Imipramine-cimetidine interaction: impairment of clearance and enhanced absolute bioavailability. *J Pharmacol Exp Ther* 229:702–705, 1984.

5. Abernethy DR, Greenblatt DJ, Steel K, Shader RI: Impairment of hepatic drug oxidation by propoxyphene. *Ann Intern Med* 97:223–224, 1982.

6. Aggeler PM, O'Reilly RA, Leong L: Potentiation of anticoagulant effect of warfarin by phenylbutazone. *N Engl J Med* 276:496–501, 1967.

7. Aherne GW, Piall E, Marks V, Mould G, White WF: Prolongation and enhancement of serum methotrexate concentrations by probenecid. *Br Med J* 1:1097–1099, 1978.

8. Akers MA, Lach JL, Fischer LJ: Alterations in the absorption of bishydroxy-coumarin by various excipient materials. *J Pharm Sci* 62:391–395, 1973.

9. Albert KS, Ayres JW, DiSanto AR, Weidler DI, Sakmar E, Hallmark MR, Stoll RG, Desante KA, Wagner JG: Influence of kaolin-pectin suspension on digoxin bioavailability. *J Pharm Sci* 67:1582–1586, 1978.

10. Albert KS, DeSante KA, Welsh DD, DiSanto AR: Pharmacokinetic evaluation of a drug interaction between kaolin, pectin, and clindamycin. *J Pharm Sci* 67:1579–1582, 1978.

11. Algozzine GJ, Stewart RB, Springer PK: Decreased clearance of phenytoin with cimetidine (letter). *Ann Intern Med* 95:244–245, 1981.

12. Allum W, Aminu J, Bloomfield TH, Davies C, Scales AH, Vere DW: Interaction between debrisoquin and phenylephrine in man. *Br J Clin Pharmacol* 1:51–57, 1974.

13. Ambre JJ, Fisher LJ: Effect of coadministration of aluminum and magnesium hydroxides on absorption of anticoagulants in man. *Clin Pharmacol Ther* 14:231–238, 1973.

13a. Andersson T: Omeprazole drug interaction studies. *Clin Pharmacokinet* 21(3):195–212, 1991.

13b. Apseloff G, Hilligoss DM, Gardner MJ, Henry EB, Inskeep PB, Gerber N, Lazar JD: Induction of fluconazole metabolism by rifampin: *in vivo* study in humans. *J Clin Pharmacol* 31(4):358–361, 1991.

14. Arita M, Surawicz B: Electrophysiologic effects of phenothiazines on canine cardiac fibers. *J Pharmacol Exp Ther* 184:619–630, 1973.

14a. Arndt CAS, Balis FM, Lester McCully C, Jeffries SL, Doherty K, Murphy R, Poplack DG: Bioavailability of low-dose vs high-dose 6-mercaptopurine. *Clin Pharmacol Ther* 43:588–591, 1988.

15. Baber N, Halliday L, Sibeon R, Littler T, Orme ML'E: The interaction between indomethacin and probenecid. A clinical and pharmacokinetic study. *Clin Pharmacol Ther* 24:298–306, 1978.

16. Baciewicz AM, Self TH: Rifampin drug interactions. *Arch Intern Med* 144:1667–1671, 1984.

17. Back DJ, Breckenridge AM, Crawford FE: The effect of rifampin on the pharmacokinetics of ethynylestradiol in women. *Contraception* 21:135–143, 1980.

17a. Back DJ, Orme ML'E: Pharmacokinetic drug interactions with oral contraceptives. *Clin Pharmacokinet* 18(6):472–484, 1990.

18. Bailey RR, Neale TJ: Rapid clonidine withdrawal with blood pressure overshoot exaggerated by beta blockade. *Br Med J* 1:942–943, 1976.

18a. Baldwin CM, Safferman AZ: A case of lisinopril-induced lithium toxicity. *DICP Ann Pharmacother* 24:946–947, 1990.

19. Balis FM: Pharmacokinetic drug interactions of commonly used anticancer drugs. *Clin Pharmacokinet* 11:223–235, 1986.

19a. Balis FM, Holcenberg JS, Zimm S, Tubergen D, Collins JM, Murphy RF, Gilchrist GS, Hammond D, Poplack DG: The effect of methotrexate on the bioavailability of oral 6-mercaptopurine *Clin Pharmacol Ther* 41:384–387, 1987.

20. Barr WH, Adir J, Garrettson L: Decrease of tetracycline absorption in man by sodium bicarbonate. *Clin Pharmacol Ther* 12:779–784, 1971.

21. Barrientos A, Alcazar V, Ruilope L, Jarillo D, Rodio JL: Indomethacin and beta--blockers in hypertension. *Lancet* i:227, 1978.

21a. Bartkowski RR, Goldberg ME, Larijani GE, Boerner T: Inhibition of alfentanil metabolism by erythromycin. *Clin Pharmacol Ther* 46:99–102, 1989.

22. Bauer LA, Edwards AD, Randolph FP: Cimetidine-induced decrease in lidocaine metabolism. *Am Heart J* 108:413–414, 1984.

23. Bauer LA, Stenwall M, Horn JR, Davis R, Opheim K, Greene L: Changes in antipyrine and indocyanine green kinetics during nifedipine, verapamil, and diltiazem therapy. *Clin Pharmacol Ther* 40:239–242, 1986.

23a. Beckmann J, Elsaβer W, Gundert-Remy U, Hertrampf R: Enoxacin - a potent inhibitor of theophylline metabolism. *Eur J Clin Pharmacol* 33:227–230, 1987.

24. Belz GG, Doering W, Aust PE, Heinz M, Matthews J, Schneider B: Quinidine-digoxin interaction. Cardiac efficacy of elevated serum digoxin concentration. *Clin Pharmacol Ther* 31:548–554, 1982.

25. Benfield P, Clissold SP, Brogden RN: Metoprolol: an updated review of its pharmacodynamic and pharmacokinetic properties, and therapeutic efficacy, in hypertension, ischaemic heart disease and related cardiovascular disorders. *Drugs* 31:376–429, 1986.

26. Berg KJ: Acute effects of acetylsalicylic acid on renal function in normal man. *Eur J Clin Pharmacol* 11:117–123, 1977.

27. Berg MJ, Berlinger WG, Goldberg MJ, Spector R, Johnson GF: Acceleration of the body clearance of phenobarbital by oral activated charcoal. *N Engl J Med* 307:642–644, 1982.

28. Bergrem H, Refvem OK: Altered prednisolone pharmacokinetics in patients treated with rifampicin. *Acta Med Scand* 213:339–343, 1983.

29. Berlinger WG, Spector R, Goldberg MJ, Johnson GF, Quee CK, Berg MJ: Enhancement of theophylline clearance by oral activated charcoal. *Clin Pharmacol Ther* 33:351–354, 1983.

30. Bigger JT, Leahey EB: Quinidine and digoxin. An important interaction. *Drugs* 24:229–239, 1982.

31. Binnion PF: Drug interaction with digitalis glycosides. *Drugs* 15:369–380, 1978.

32. Bint AJ, Burtt I: Adverse antibiotic drug interaction. *Drugs* 20:57–68, 1980.

33. Bjornsson TD, Meffin PJ, Swezey S, Blaschke TF: Clofibrate displaces warfarin from plasma proteins in man: an example of a pure displacement interaction. *J Pharmacol Exp Ther* 210:316–321, 1979.

34. Blair DC, Duggan DO, Schroeder ET: Inactivation of amikacin and gentamicin by carbenicillin in patients with end-stage renal failure. *Antimicrob Agents Chemother* 22:376–379, 1982.

34a. Blum RA, D'Andrea DT, Florentino BM, Wilton JH, Hilligos DM, Gardner MJ, Henry EB, Goldstein H, Schentag JJ: Increased gastric pH and the bioavailability of fluconazole and ketoconazole. *Ann Intern Med* 114(9):755–757, 1991.

34b. Blum RA, Wilton JH, Hilligoss DM, Gardner MJ, Henry EB, Harrison NJ, Schentag JJ: Effect of fluconazole on the disposition of phenytoin. *Clin Pharmacol Ther* 49:420–425, 1991.

35. Boakes AJ, Laurence DR, Teoh PC, Barar FSK, Benedikter LT, Prichard BNC: Interactions between sympathomimetic amines and antidepressant agents in man. *Br Med J* 1:311–315, 1973.

35a. Boehningh W: Effect of cimetidine and ranitidine on plasma theophylline in patients with chronic obstructive airways disease treated with theophylline and corticosteroids. *Eur J Clin Pharmacol* 38:43–45, 1990.

36. Boulline DJ: The action of antidepressants on the effects of other drugs. *Primary Care* 2:669–688, 1975.

37. Boura ALA, Green AF: Adrenergic neurone blockade and other acute effects caused by N-benzyl-N-dimethylguanidine and its orthochloro derivative. *Br J Pharmacol* 20:36–55, 1963.

37a. Bowles SK, Popovski Z, Rybak MJ, Beckman HB, Edwards DJ: Effect of norfloxacin on theophylline pharmacokinetics at steady state. *Antimicrob Agents Chemother* 32(4):510–512, 1988.

38. Boyce EG, Dukes GE, Rollins DE, Sudds TW: The effect of rifampin on theophylline kinetics. *J Clin Pharmacol* 26:696–699, 1986.

39. Braitwaite RA, Flanagan RJ, Richens A: Steady state plasma nortriptyline concentrations in epileptic patients. *Br J Clin Pharmacol* 2:469–471, 1975.

40. Branch RA, Shand DG, Wilkinson GR, Nies AS: The reduction of lidocaine clearance by dl-propranolol: An example of hemodynamic drug interaction. *J Pharmacol Exp Ther* 184:515–519, 1973.

41. Branigan TA, Robbin RA, Cady WJ, Nickols JG, Ueda CT: The effects of erythromycin on the absorption and disposition kinetics of theophylline. *Eur J Clin Pharmacol* 21:115–120, 1981.

42. Brater DC: Analysis of the effect of indomethacin on the response to furosemide in man. Effect of dose of furosemide. *J Pharmacol Exp Ther* 210:386–390, 1979.

43. Breen KJ, Bury R, Desmond PV, Mashford ML, Morphett B, Westwood B, Shaw RG: Effects of cimetidine and ranitidine on hepatic drug metabolism. *Clin Pharmacol Ther* 31:297–300, 1982.

44. Briant RH, Reid JL, Dollery CT: Interaction between clonidine and desipramine in man. *Br Med J* 1:522–523, 1973.

44a. Brockmöller J, Neumayer HH, Wagner K, Weber W, Heinemeyer G, Kewitz H, Roots I: Pharmacokinetic interaction between cyclosporin and diltiazem. *Eur J Clin Pharmacol* 38:237–242, 1990.

45. Brodie MJ, MacPhee GJA: Carbamazepine neurotoxicity precipitated by diltiazem. *Br Med J* 292:1170–1171, 1986.

45a. Brosen K, Gram LF: Quinidine inhibits the 2-hydroxylation of imipramine and desipramine but not the demethylation of imipramine. *Eur J Clin Pharmacol* 37:155–160, 1989.

46. Brown DD, Juhl RP: Decreased bioavailability of digoxin due to antacids and kaolin pectin. *N Engl J Med* 295:1034–1037, 1976.

47. Brown DD, Juhl RP, Warner SL: Decreased bioavailability of digoxin due to hypocholesterolemia interventions. *Circulation* 58:164–172, 1978.

48. Brown DD, Spector R, Juhl RP: Drug interactions with digoxin. *Drugs* 20:198–206, 1980.

49. Buchanan RA, Heffelfinger JC, Weiss CF: The effect of phenobarbital on diphenylhydantoin metabolism in children. *Pediatrics* 43:114–116, 1969.

49a. Buckley M, Feely J: Antagonism of antihypertensive effect of guanfacine by tricyclic antidepressants. *Lancet* 337:1173–1174, 1991.

50. Burn JH, Rand MJ: The action of sympathomimetic amines in animals treated with reserpine. *J Physiol* 144:314–336, 1958.

51. Burns JJ, Conney AH: Enzyme stimulation and inhibition in the metabolism of drugs. *Proc R Soc Med* 58:955–960, 1965.

52. Cabizuca SV, Desser KB: Carbenicillin associated hypokalemic alkalosis. *JAMA* 236:956–957, 1976.

53. Caldwell JH, Greenberger NJ: Interruption of the enterohepatic circulation of digitoxin by cholestyramine. I. Protection against lethal digitoxin intoxication. *J Clin Invest* 50:2626–2637, 1971.

54. Campbell MA, Plachetka JR, Jackson JE, Moon JF, Finley PR: Cimetidine decreases theophylline clearance. *Ann Intern Med* 95:68–69, 1981.

54a. Campbell N, Paddock V, Sundaram R: Alteration of methyldopa absorption, metabolism, and blood pressure control caused by ferrous sulfate and ferrous gluconate. *Clin Pharmacol Ther* 43:381–386, 1988.

54b. Campbell NRC, Hasinoff B: Ferrous sulfate reduces levodopa bioavailability: Chelation as a possible mechanism. *Clin Pharmacol Ther* 45:220–225, 1989.

54c. Campoli-Richards DM, Monk JP, Price A, Benfield P, Todd PA, Ward A: Ciprofloxacin: A review of its antibacterial activity, pharmacokinetic properties and therapeutic use. *Drugs* 35:373–447, 1988.

54d. Capewell S, Freestone S, Critchley JAJH, Pottage A, Prescott LF: Reduced felodipine bioavailability in patients taking anticonvulsants. *Lancet* ii:480–482, 1988.

55. Carrum G, Egan JM, Abernethy DR: Diltiazem treatment impairs hepatic drug oxidation: studies of antipyrine. *Clin Pharmacol Ther* 40:140–143, 1986.

56. Carruthers SG, Dujovne CA: Cholestyramine and spironolactone and their combination in digitoxin elimination. *Clin Pharmacol Ther* 27:184–187, 1980.

57. Carulli N, Manenti F, Gallo M, Salvioli GF: Alcohol-drugs interaction in man: alcohol and tolbutamide. *Eur J Clin Invest* 1:421–424, 1971.

58. Cate EW, Rogers JF, Powell JR: Inhibition of tolbutamide elimination by cimetidine but not ranitidine. *J Clin Pharmacol* 26:372–377, 1986.

59. Chang CC, Costa E, Brodie BB: Reserpine-induced release of drugs from sympathetic nerve endings. *Life Sci* 3:839–844, 1964.

60. Chen T-S, Friedman HS: Alteration of digoxin pharmacokinetics by a single dose of quinidine. *JAMA* 244:669–672, 1980.

61. Chennavasin P, Seiwell R, Brater DC: Pharmacokinetic-dynamic analysis of the indomethacin-furosemide interaction in man. *J Pharmacol Exp Ther* 215:77–81, 1980.

62. Christiansen J, Dam M: Influence of phenobarbital and diphenylhydantoin on plasma carbamazepine levels in patients with epilepsy. *Acta Neurol Scand* 49:543–546, 1973.

63. Christensen LK, Skovested L: Inhibition of drug metabolism by chloramphenicol. *Lancet* 2:1397–1399, 1969.

64. Christian CD, Meredith CG, Speeg KV: Cimetidine inhibits renal procainamide clearance. *Clin Pharmacol Ther* 36:221–227, 1984.

65. Cinquegrani MP, Liang C-S: Indomethacin attenuates the hypotensive action of hydralazine. *Clin Pharmacol Ther* 39:564–570, 1986.

65a. Clark DWJ: Genetically determined variability in acetylation and oxidation. Therapeutic implications. *Drugs* 29:342–375, 1985.

66. Cluxton RJ, Rivera JO, Ritschel WA, Pesce AJ, Hanenson IB: Cimetidine-theophylline interaction (letter). *Ann Intern Med* 96:684, 1982.

67. Cocco G, Ague C: Interactions between cardioactive drugs and antidepressants. *Eur J Clin Pharmacol* 11:389–393, 1977.

67a. Colli A, Buccino G, Cocciolo M, Parravicini R, Elli GM, Scaltrini G: Ticlopidine-theophylline interaction. *Clin Pharmacol Ther* 41:358–362, 1987.

68. Conney AH: Pharmacological implications of microsomal enzyme induction. *Pharmacol Rev* 19:317–366, 1967.

69. Cramer JL, Rosser RM, Crane G: Blood levels and management of lithium treatment. *Br Med J* 3:650–654, 1974.

70. Cucinell SA, Conney AH, Sansur M, Burns JJ: Drug interaction in man. I. Lowering effect of phenobarbital on plasma levels of bishydroxycoumarin (Dicumarol) and diphenylhydantoin (Dilantin). *Clin Pharmacol Ther* 6:420–429, 1965.

71. Curry SH, DeVane CL, Wolfe MM: Cimetidine interaction with amitriptyline. *Eur J Clin Pharmacol* 29:429–433, 1985.

72. Data JL, Wilkinson GR, Nies AS: Interaction of quinidine with anticonvulsant drugs. *N Engl J Med* 294:699–702, 1976.

73. Dam M, Kristensen B, Hansen BS, Christiansen J: Interaction between carbamazepine and propoxyphene in man. *Acta Neurol Scand* 56:602–607, 1977.

74. Davis JM, Bartlett E, Termini BS: Overdosage of psychotropic drugs. A review. *Dis Nerv Syst* 29:157–164, 246–256, 1986.

75. Day MD: Effect of sympathomimetic amines on the blocking action of guanethidine, bretylium, xylocholine. *Br J Pharmacol* 18:421–439, 1962.

76. Day MD, Rand MJ: Antagonism of guanethidine by dexamphetamine and other related sympathomimetic amines. *J Pharm Sci* 14:541–549, 1962.

76a. de Miranda P, Good SS, Yarchoan R, Thomas RV, Blum MR, Myers CE, Broder S: Alteration of zidovudine pharmacokinetics by probenecid in patients with AIDS or AIDS-related complex. *Clin Pharmacol* 46:494–500, 1989.

77. Depaulo JR Jr, Correa EI, Sapir DG: Renal toxicity of lithium and its implications. *Johns Hopkins Med J* 149:15–21, 1981.

78. Desmond PV, Patwardhan RV, Schenker S, Speeg KV: Cimetidine impairs elimination of chlordiazepoxide (Librium) in man. *Ann Intern Med* 93:266–268, 1980.

79. Desmond PV, Patwardhan RV, Schenker S, Speeg KV: Short term ethanol administration impairs the elimination of chlordiazepoxide in man. *Eur J Clin Pharmacol* 18:275–278, 1980.

80. DeTeresa E, Vera A, Ortigosa J, Pulpon LA, Arus AP, DeArtaza M: Interaction between anticoagulants and contraceptives: an unsuspected finding. *Br Med J* 2:1260–1261, 1979.

81. DeVita VT, Hahn MA, Oliverio VT: Monoamine oxidase inhibition by a new carcinostatic agent, N-isopropyl(2-methyl-hydrazino)-p-toluamide (MIH). *Proc Soc Exp Biol Med* 120:561–565, 1965.

82. Dhillon S, Richens A: Serum protein binding of diazepam and its displacement by valproic acid in vitro. *Br J Clin Pharmacol* 12:591–592, 1981.

83. Dobbs JH, Skoutakis VA, Acchardio SR, Dobbs BR: Effects of aluminum hydroxide on the absorption of propranolol. *Curr Ther Res* 21:877–892, 1977.

84. Doering W: Quinidine-digoxin interaction. Pharmacokinetics, underlying mechanism and clinical implications. *N Engl J Med* 301:400–404, 1979.

85. Dorian P, Sellers EM, Carruthers G, Hamilton C, Fan T: Propranolol-ethanol pharmacokinetic interaction. *Clin Pharmacol Ther* 31:219, 1982.

85a. Dorian P, Strauss M, Cardella C, East DS, Ogilvie R: Digoxin-cyclosporine interaction: Severe digitalis toxicity after cyclosporine treatment. *Clin Invest Med* 11(2):108–112, 1988.

85b. Douste-Blazy PH, Rostin M, Livarek B, Tordjman E, Montastruc JL, Galinier F: Angiotensin converting enzyme inhibitors and lithium treatment. *Lancet* i:1448, 1986.

85c. Duchin KL, McKinstry DN, Cohen AI, Migdalof BH: Pharmacokinetics of captopril in healthy subjects and in patients with cardiovascular diseases. *Clin Pharmacokinet* 14:241–259, 1988.

85d. Dunselman PHJM, Edgar B: Felodipine clinical pharmacokinetics. *Clin Pharmacokinet* 21(6):418–430, 1991.

85e. Dunselman PHJM, Scaf AHJ, Kuntze CEE, Lie KI, Wesseling H: Digoxin-felodipine interaction in patients with congestive heart failure. *Eur J Clin Pharmacol* 35:461–465, 1988.

86. Durao B, Rico JMGT: Modification by indomethacin of the blood pressure lowering effect of pindolol and propranolol in conscious rabbits. *Eur J Pharmacol* 43:377–381, 1977.

87. Durao V, Prata MM, Gonclaves LMP: Modifications of antihypertensive effect of β-adrenoceptor-blocking agents by inhibition of endogenous prostaglandin synthesis. *Lancet* ii:1005–1007, 1977.

88. Easton PA, Koval A: Hypertensive reaction with sulindac. *Can Med Assoc J* 122:1273–1274, 1980.

88a. Edgar B, Lundborg P, Regårdh CG: Clinical pharmacokinetics of felodipine: A summary. *Drugs* 34(3):16–27, 1987.

88b. Edwards DJ, Bowles SK, Svensson CK, Rybak MJ: Inhibition of drug metabolism by quinolone antibiotics. *Clin Pharmacokinet* 15:194–204, 1988.

88c. Edwards DJ, Lavoie R, Beckman H, Blevins R, Rubenfire M: The effect of coadministration of verapamil on the pharmacokinetics and metabolism of quinidine. *Clin Pharmacol Ther* 41:68–73, 1987.

88d. Eichelbaum, M: Defective oxidation of drugs: pharmacokinetic and therapeutic implications. *Clin Pharmacokinet* 7:1–22, 1982.

88e. Ette EI, Brown-Awala EA, Essien EE: Chloroquine elimination in humans: Effect of low-dose cimetidine. *J Clin Pharmacol* 27:813–816, 1987.

89. Evans DAA, Mantey KA, McKusick VA: Genetic control of isoniazid metabolism in man. *Br Med J* 2:485–491, 1960.

90. Fann WE, Cavanaugh JH, Kaufmann JS: Doxepin: effects of transport of biogenic amines in man. *Psychopharmacologia* 22:111–125, 1972.

91. Fann WE, Davis JM, Janowsky DS, Sekerke WJ, Schmidt DM: Chlorpromazine: effects of antacids on its gastrointestinal absorption. *J Clin Pharmacol* 13:388–390, 1973.

92. Feely J, Wilkinson GR, McAllister CB, Wood AJJ: Increased toxicity and reduced clearance of lidocaine by cimetidine. *Ann Intern Med* 96:592–594, 1982.

93. Feely J, Wilkinson GR, Wood AJJ: Reduction of liver blood flow and propranolol metabolism by cimetidine. *N Engl J Med* 304:692–695, 1981.

94. Feely J, Wood AJJ: Effect of inhibitors of prostaglandin synthesis on hepatic drug clearance. *Br J Clin Pharmacol* 15:109–111, 1983.

95. Fenster PE, Hager WD, Goodman MM: Digoxin-quinidine-spironolactone interaction. *Clin Pharmacol Ther* 36:70–73, 1984.

96. Fine A, Henderson IS, Morgan DR, Wilstone WJ: Malabsorption of furosemide caused by phenytoin. *Br Med J* 2:1061–1062, 1977.

96a. Fitton A, Buckley MMT: Moricine; A review of its pharmacological properties, and therapeutic efficacy in cardiac arrhythmias. *Drugs* 40(1):138–167, 1990.

97. Fowler NO, McCall D, Chou T, Holmes JC, Hanenson IB: Electrocardiographic changes and cardiac arrhythmias in patients receiving psychotropic drugs. *Am J Cardiol* 37:223–230, 1976.

98. Fraser DG, Ludden TM, Evans RP, Sutherland EW: Displacement of phenytoin from plasma binding sites by salicylate. *Clin Pharmacol Ther* 27:165–169, 1980.

99. Freeman DJ, Laupacis A, Keown PA, Stiller CR, Carruthers SC: Evaluation of cyclosporin—phenytoin interaction with observations on cyclosporin metabolites. *Br J Clin Pharmacol* 18:887–893, 1984.

99a. Friedel HA, Sorkin EM: Nisoldipine; A preliminary review of its pharmacodynamic and pharmacokinetic properties, and therapeutic efficacy in the treatment of angina pectoris, hypertension and related cardiovascular disorders. *Drugs* 36:682–731, 1988.

99b. Froemming JS, Francis Lam YW, Jann MW, Davis CM: Pharmacokinetics of haloperidol. *Clin Pharmacokinet* 17(6):396–423, 1989.

100. Frolich JC, Leftwich R, Ragheb M, Oates JA, Reimann I, Buchanan D: Indomethacin increases plasma lithium. *Br Med J* 1:1115–1116, 1979.

101. Fujita T, Yamashita N, Yamashita K: Effect of indomethacin on antihypertensive action of captopril in hypertension patients. *Clin Exp Hypertension* 3:939–952, 1981.

101a. Funck-Brentano C, Kroemer HK, Pavlou H, Woosley RL, Roden DM: Genetically-determined interaction between propafenone and low dose quinidine: role of active metabolites in modulating net drug effect. *Br J Clin Pharmacol* 27:435–444, 1989.

102. Gambertoglio JH, Holford NHG, Kapusnik JE, Nishikawa R, Saltiel M, Stanik-Lizak P, Birnbaum JL, Hau T, Amend WJC Jr: Disposition of total and unbound prednisolone in renal transplant patients receiving anticonvulsants. *Kidney Int* 25:119–123, 1984.

103. Garnett WR, Carter BL, Bellock JM: Bioavailability of phenytoin administered with antacids. *Ther Drug Monitoring* 1:435–437, 1979.

103a. Garrelts JC, Godley PJ, Peteria JD, Gerlach EH, Yakshe CC: Sucralfate significantly reduces ciprofloxacin concentrations in serum. *Antimicrob Agents Chemother* 34(5):931–933, 1990.

104. Garrettson LK, Perel JM, Dayton PG: Methylphenidate interaction with both anticonvulsants and ethyl discoumacetate. *JAMA* 207:2053–2056, 1969.

105. Garty M, Hurwitz A: Effect of cimetidine and antacids on intestinal absorption of tetracycline. *Clin Pharmacol Ther* 28:203–207, 1980.

106. Gault H, Longerich L, Dawe M, Fine A: Digoxin-rifampin interaction. *Clin Pharmacol Ther* 35:750–754, 1984.

107. Geleherter TD: Enzyme induction. *N Engl J Med* 294:522–526, 589–595, 646–651, 1976.

108. Gibbons DO, Lant AF: Effects of intravenous and oral propantheline and metoclopramide on ethanol absorption. *Clin Pharmacol Ther* 17:578–584, 1975.

109. Gibson TP, Quintanilla AP: Effect of quinidine on the renal handling of digoxin. *J Lab Clin Med* 96:1062–1070, 1980.

110. Gibson TP, Quintanilla AP: Effect of volume expansion and furosemide diuresis on the renal clearance of digoxin. *J Pharmacol Exp Ther* 219:54–59, 1981.

111. Gill MA, DuBe JE, Young WW: Hypokalemic, metabolic alkalosis induced by high-dose ampicillin sodium. *Am J Hosp Pharm* 34:528–531, 1977.

112. Glynn AM, Slaughter RL, Brass C, D'Ambrosio R, Jusko WJ: Effects of ketoconazole on methylprednisolone pharmacokinetics and cortisol secretion. *Clin Pharmacol Ther* 39:654–659, 1986.

113. Gokhale SD, Gulati OD, Udwadia BP: Antagonism of the adrenergic neurone blocking action of guanethidine by certain antidepressant and antihistamine drugs. *Arch Int Pharmacodyn* 160:321–329, 1966.

114. Gore JM, Haffajee CI, Alpert JS: Interaction of amiodarone and diphenylhydantoin. *Am J Cardiol* 54:1145, 1984.

114a. Grant SM, Clissold SP: Fluconazole: A review of its pharmacodynamic and pharmacokinetic properties, and therapeutic potential in superficial and systemic mycoses. *Drugs* 39(6):877–916, 1990.

115. Greenblatt DJ, Abernethy DR, Morse DS, Harmatz JS, Shader RI: Clinical importance of the interaction of diazepam and cimetidine. *N Engl J Med* 310:1639–1643, 1984.

116. Greenblatt DH, Allen DA, Maclaughlin DS, Harmatz JS, Shader RJ: Diazepam absorption: effect of antacids and food. *Clin Pharmacol Ther* 24:600–609, 1978.

117. Greenblatt DJ, Duhme DW, Allen MD, Koch-Weser J: Clinical toxicity of furosemide in hospitalized patients. *Am Heart J* 94:6–13, 1977.

118. Greenblatt DJ, Shader RI, Harmatz JS, Franke K, Koch-Weser J: Influence of magnesium and aluminum hydroxide mixture on chlordiazepoxide absorption. *Clin Pharmacol Ther* 19:234–239, 1976.

118a. Griffin JH, Hahn SM: Lisinopril-induced lithium toxicity. *DICP Ann Pharmacother* 25:101, 1991.

119. Griffith RS, Black HR, Brier GL, Wolny JD: Effect of probenecid on the blood levels and urinary excretion of cefamandole. *Antimicrob Agents Chemother* 11:809–812, 1977.

119a. Grimsley SR, Jann MW, Carter JG, D'Mello AP, D'Souza MJ: Increased carbamazepine plasma concentrations after fluoxetine coadministration. *Clin Pharmacol Ther* 50:10–15, 1991.

120. Grygiel JJ, Brikett DJ: Cigarette smoking and theophylline clearance and metabolism. *Clin Pharmacol Ther* 30:491–496, 1981.

121. Guay DRP, Meatherall RC, Chalmers JL, Grahame GR: Cimetidine alters pethidine disposition in man. *Br J Clin Pharmacol* 18:907–914, 1984.

121a. Guenter TW, Defoin R, Mosberg H: The influence of cholestyramine on the elimination of tenoxicam and piroxicam. *Eur J Clin Pharmacol* 34:283–289, 1988.

121b. Gugler R, Allgayer H: Effects of antacids on the clinical pharmacokinetics of drugs; an update. *Clin Pharmacokinet* 18 (3):210–219, 1990.

122. Gugler R, Brand M, Somogyi A: Impaired cimetidine absorption by antacids and metoclopramide. *Eur J Clin Pharmacol* 20:225–228, 1981.

122a. Gugler R, Jensen JC: Omeprazole inhibits oxidative drug metabolism: Studies with diazepam and phenytoin *in vivo* and 7-ethoxycoumarin *in vitro*. Gastroenterol 89:1235–1241, 1985.

122b. Gupta SK, Bakran A, Johnson RWG, Rowland M. Cyclosporin-erythromycin interaction in renal transplant patients. *Br J Clin Pharmacol* 27:475–481, 1989.

122c. Haefeli WE, Bargetzi MJ, Follath F, Meyer UA: Potent inhibition of cytochrome P450IID₆ (Debrisoquin 4-hydroxylase) by flecainide *in vitro* and *in vivo*. *J Cardiovasc Pharmacol* 15:776–779, 1990.

123. Hager WD, Fenster P, Mayersohn M, Perrier D, Graves P, Marcus FI, Goldman S: Digoxin-quinidine interaction. Pharmacokinetic evaluation. *N Engl J Med* 300:1238–1241, 1979.

124. Hanahoe THP, Ireson JD, Large BJ: Interactions between guanethidine and inhibitors of noradrenaline uptake. *Arch Int Pharmacodyn* 182:349–353, 1969.

125. Hansen JM, Kristensen M, Skovsted L: Sulthiame (Opsollot^R) an inhibitor of diphenylhydantoin metabolism. *Epilepsia* 9:17–22, 1968.

126. Hansen JM, Siersbaek-Nielsen K, Kristensen M, Skovsted L, Christensen LK: Effects of diphenylhydantoin on the metabolism of dicoumarol in man. *Acta Med Scand* 189:15–19, 1971.

127. Hansen JM, Siersbaek-Nielsen K, Skovsted L: Carbamazepine-induced acceleration of diphenylhydantoin and warfarin metabolism in man. *Clin Pharmacol Ther* 12:539–543, 1971.

128. Hansen PD, Horn JR: *Drug Interactions and updates.* Malvern, PA, Lea & Febiger, 1990.

129. Harrington RA, Hamilton CW, Brogden RN, Linkewich JA, Romankiewicz JA, Heel RC: Metoclopramide: an updated review of its pharmacological properties and clinical use. *Drugs* 25:451–494, 1983.

130. Harvey VJ, Slevin ML, Dilloway MR, Clark PI, Johnston A, Lant AF: The influence of cimetidine on the pharmacokinetics of 5-fluorouracil. *Br J Clin Pharmacol* 18:421–430, 1984.

131. Haworth E, Burroughs AK: Disopyramide and warfarin interaction. *Br Med J* 2:866–867, 1977.

132. Heagerty AM, Castleden CM, Patel I: Failure of ranitidine to interact with propranolol. *Br Med J* 284:1304, 1982.

132a. Hedman A, Angelin B, Arvidsson A, Beck O, Dahlqvist R, Nilsson B, Olsson M, Schench-Gustafsson K: Digoxin-verapamil interaction: Reduction of biliary but not renal digoxin clearance in humans. *Clin Pharmacol Ther* 49:256–262, 1991.

132b. Hedman A, Angelin B, Arvidsson A, Dahlqvist R, Nilsson B: Interactions in the renal and biliary elimination of digoxin: Stereoselective difference between quinine and quinidine. *Clin Pharmacol Ther* 47:20–26, 1990.

133. Henaver SA, Hollister LE: Cimetidine interaction with imipramine and nortriptyline. *Clin Pharmacol Ther* 35:183–187, 1984.

134. Henderson JM, Ibrahim SZ, Millikan WJ Jr, Santi M, Warren WD: Cimetidine does not reduce liver blood flow in cirrhosis. *Hepatology* 3:919–922, 1983.

134a. Henwood JM, Monk JP: Enoxacin: A review of its antibacterial activity, pharmacokinetic properties and therapeutic use. *Drugs* 36:32–66, 1988.

135. Hetzel DJ, Bochner F, Hallpike F, Shearman DJC, Hann CS: Cimetidine interaction with phenytoin. *Br Med J* 282:1512, 1981.

136. Hibbard DM, Peters JR, Hunninghake DB: Effects of cholestyramine and colestipol on the plasma concentrations of propranolol. *Br J Clin Pharmacol* 18:337–342, 1984.

136a. Hii JTY, Duff HJ, Burgess ED: Clinical pharmacokinetics of propafenone. *Clin Pharmacokinet* 21(1):1–10, 1991.

137. Himmelhoch JM, Poust RI, Mallinger AG: Adjustment of lithium dose during lithium-chlorothiazide therapy. *Clin Pharmacol Ther* 22:225–227, 1977.

138. Hirsh PD, Weiner HJ, North RL: Further insights into digoxin-quinidine interaction: lack of correlation between serum digoxin concentration and inotropic state of the heart. *Am J Cardiol* 46:863–867, 1980.

138a. Ho G, Tierney MG, Dales RE: Evaluation of the effect of norfloxacin on the pharmacokinetics of theophylline. *Clin Pharmacol Ther* 44:35–38, 1988.

139. Holt DW, Hayler AM, Edmonds ME, Ashford RF: Clinically significant interaction between digoxin and quinidine. *Br Med J* 2:1401, 1979.

139a. Holtzman JL, Kvam DC, Berry DA, Mottonen L, Borrell G, Harrison LI, Conard GJ: The pharmacodynamic and pharmacokinetic interaction of flecainide acetate with propranolol: Effects on cardiac function and drug clearance. *Eur J Clin Pharmacol* 33:97–99, 1987.

139b. Howden CW: Clinical pharmacology of omeprazole. *Clin Pharmacokinet* 20(1):38–49, 1991.

139c. Huang SM, Weintraub HS, Marriott TB, Marinan B, Abels R: Etintidine-propranolol interaction study in humans. *J Pharmacokinet Biopharm* 15(6):557–568, 1987.

139d. Hughes B, Dyer JE, Schwartz AB: Increased procainamide plasma concentrations caused by quinidine: A new drug interaction. *Am Heart J* 114(4;1):908–909, 1987.

139e. Humbert G, Brumpt I, Montay G, Le Liboux A, Frydman A, Borsa-Lebas F, Moore N: Influence of rifampin on the pharmacokinetics of pefloxacin. *Clin Pharmacol Ther* 50:682–687, 1991.

139f. Hunt BA, Bottorff MB, Herring VL, Self TH, Lalonde RL: Effects of calcium channel blockers on the pharmacokinetics of propranolol stereoisomers. *Clin Pharmacol Ther* 47:584–591, 1990.

140. Hurwitz A: The effects of antacids on gastrointestinal drug absorption. II. Effect on sulfadiazine and quinine. *J Pharmacol Exp Ther* 179:485–490, 1971.

141. Hurwitz A, Schlozman DL: Effects of antacids on gastrointestinal absorption of isoniazid in rat and man. *Am Rev Respir Dis* 109:41–47, 1974.

141a. Hurwitz A, Vacek JL, Botteron GW, Sztern MI, Hughes EM, Jayaraj A: Mexiletine effects on theophylline disposition. *Clin Pharmacol Ther* 50:299–307, 1991.

142. Jackson JE: Reduction of liver blood flow by cimetidine (letter). *N Engl J Med* 305:99–100, 1981.

143. Jackson JE, Powell JR, Wandell M, Bentley J, Dorr R: Cimetidine decreases theophylline clearance. *Am Rev Respir Dis* 123:615–617, 1981.
143a. Jacqz E, Hall SD, Branch RA: Genetically determined polymorphisms in drug oxidation. *Hepatology* 6:1020–1032, 1986.
144. Jahnchen E, Meinertz T, Gilfrich H-J, Kersting F, Groth V: Enhanced elimination of warfarin during treatment with cholestyramine. *Br J Clin Pharmacol* 5:437–440, 1978.
145. Janowsky DS, El-Yousef MK, Davis JM, Fann WE: Antagonism of guanethidine by chlorpromazine. *Am J Psychiatry* 130:808–812, 1973.
146. Jefferson JW, Kalin NH: Serum lithium levels and long-term diuretic use. *JAMA* 241:1134–1136, 1979.
147. Jogestrand T, Schenck-Gustafsson K, Nordlander R, Dahlqvist R: Quinidine-induced changes in serum and skeletal muscle digoxin concentration; evidence of saturable binding of digoxin to skeletal muscle. *Eur J Clin Pharmacol* 27:571–575, 1984.
148. Johnson BF, Bustrack JA, Urbach DR, Hull JH, Marwaha R: Effect of metoclopramide on digoxin absorption from tablets and capsules. *Clin Pharmacol Ther* 36:724–730, 1984.
148a. Johnson BF, Wilson J, Marwaha R, Hoch K, Johnson J: The comparative effects of verapamil and a new dihydropyridine calcium channel blocker on digoxin pharmacokinetics. *Clin Pharmacol Ther* 42:66–71, 1987.
149. Juhl RP, Summers RW, Guillory JK, Blang SM, Cheng RH, Brown DD: Effect of sulfasalazine on digoxin bioavailability. *Clin Pharmacol Ther* 20:387–394, 1976.
150. Kabins SA: Interactions among antibiotics and other drugs. *JAMA* 219:206–212, 1972.
150a. Kalow W: Genetics of drug transformation. *Clin Biochem* 19:76–82, 1986.
151. Kampmann J, Hansen JM, Siersbaek-Nielsen K, Laursen H: Effect of some drugs on penicillin half–life in blood. *Clin Pharmacol Ther* 13:516–519, 1972.
151a. Kandrotas RJ, Slaughter RL, Brass C, Jusko WJ: Ketoconazole effects on methylprednisolone disposition and their joint suppression of endogenous cortisol. *Clin Pharmacol Ther* 42:465–470, 1987.
152. Kanto J, Allonen H, Jalonen H, Mantyla R: The effect of metoclopramide and propantheline on the gastrointestinal absorption of cimetidine. *Br J Pharmacol* 11:527–530, 1981.
152a. Kapil RP, Axelson JE, Mansfield IL, Edward DJ, McErlane B, Mason MA, Lalka D, Kerr CR: Disopyramid pharmacokinetics and metabolism: effect of inducers. *Br J Clin Pharmacol* 24:781–791, 1987.
153. Kater RMH, Roggin G, Tobon F, Zieve P, Iber FL: Increased rate of clearance of drugs from the circulation of alcoholics. *Am J Med Sci* 258:35–39, 1969.
153a. Kates RE, Yee YG, Kirsten EB: Interaction between warfarin and propafenone in healthy volunteer subjects. *Clin Pharmacol Ther* 42:305–311, 1987.
154. Kauffman RE, Azarnoff DL: Effect of colestipol on gastrointestinal absorption of chlorothiazide in man. *Clin Pharmacol Ther* 14:886–889, 1973.
155. Kay L, Kampmann JP, Svendsen TL, Vergman B, Hansen JE, Skovsted L, Kristensen M: Influence of rifampicin and isoniazid on the kinetics of phenytoin. *Br J Clin Pharmacol* 20:323–326, 1985.
156. Keilholz U, Guthrie GP Jr: Case Report: adverse effect of phenytoin on mineralocorticoid replacement with fludrocortisone in adrenal insufficiency. *Am J Med Sci* 291:280–283, 1986.
157. Kelly HW, Powell JR, Donohue JF: Ranitidine at very large doses does not inhibit theophylline elimination. *Clin Pharmacol Ther* 39:577–581, 1986.
157a. Kerin NZ, Blevins RD, Goldman L, Faitel K, Rubenfire, M: The incidence, magnitude, and time course of the amiodarone-warfarin interaction. *Arch Intern Med* 148:1779–1781, 1988.
157b. Kerr BM, Rettie AE, Eddy AC, Loiseau P, Guyot M, Wilensky AJ, Levy RH: Inhibition of human liver microsomal epoxide hydrolase by valproate and valpromide: *in vitro/in vivo* correlation. *Clin Pharmacol Ther* 46:82–93, 1989.
158. Khalil SAH: Bioavailability of digoxin in presence of antacids. *J Pharm Sci* 63:1641–1642, 1974 (letter).
159. Kiorboe E: Phenytoin intoxication during treatment with Antabuse (disulfiram). *Epilepsia* 7:246–249, 1966.
160. Kirby MG, Dasta JF, Armstrong DK, Tallman R Jr: Effect of low-dose dopamine on the pharmacokinetics of tobramycin in dogs. *Antimicrob Agents Chemother* 29:168–170, 1986.
160a. Kirch W, Kleinbloesem CH, Belz GG: Drug interactions with calcium antagonists. *Pharmacol Ther* 45:109–136, 1990.
160b. Kirsten R, Nelson K, Steinijans VW, Zech K, Haerlin R: Clinical pharmacokinetics of urapidil. *Clin Pharmacokinzn* 14:129–140, 1988.
161. Kitto R: Antibiotics and the ingestion of alcohol. *JAMA* 193:411, 1965.
162. Klotz U, Reimann IW: Delayed clearance of diazepam due to cimetidine. *N Engl J Med* 304:1012–1014, 1980.
163. Klotz V, Reimann IW, Ohnhaus EE: Effect of ranitidine on the steady state pharmacokinetics of diazepam. *Eur J Clin Pharmacol* 24:357–360, 1983.
164. Knodell RG, Holtzman JL, Crankshaw DL, Steele NM, Stanley LN: Drug metabolism by rat and human hepatic microsomes in response to interaction with H₂-receptor antagonist. *Gastroenterology* 82:84–88, 1982.
165. Kochar MS, Itskovitz HD: Effects of hydrochlorothiazide in hypertensive patients and the need for potassium supplementation. *Curr Ther Res* 15:298–304, 1973.
166. Koch-Weser J: Drug interactions in cardiovascular therapy. *Am Heart J* 90:93–116, 1975.

167. Koch-Weser J, Sellers EM: Binding of drugs to serum albumin. *N Engl J Med* 294:311–316, 526–531, 1976.
168. Koch-Weser J, Sellers EM: Drug interactions with coumarin anticoagulants. *N Engl J Med* 285:487–498, 547–558, 1971.
168a. Kosoglou T, Rocci ML, Vlasses PH: Trimethoprim alters the disposition of procainamide and N-acetylprocainamide. *Clin Pharmacol Ther* 44:467–477, 1988.
169. Koup JR, Gilbaldi M, McNamara P, Hilligoss DM, Colburn WA, Bruck E: Interaction of chloramphenicol with phenytoin and phenobarbital. *Clin Pharmacol Ther* 24:571–575, 1978.
170. Kuhlmann J, Dohrmann M, Marcin S: Effects of quinidine on pharmacokinetics and pharmacodynamics of digitoxin achieving steady-state conditions. *Clin Pharmacol Ther* 39:288–294, 1986.
171. Kulshrestha VK, Thomas M, Wadsworth J, Richens A: Interaction of phenytoin and antacids. *Br J Clin Pharmacol* 6:177–179, 1978.
172. Kutt H, Brennan R, Dehejia H, Verebely K: Diphenylhydantoin intoxication. A complication of isoniazid therapy. *Am Rev Resp Dis* 101:377–384, 1970.
173. Kutt H, Haynes J, Verebely K, McDowell F: The effect of phenobarbital on plasma diphenylhydantoin level and metabolism in man and in rat liver microsomes. *Neurology* 19:611–616, 1969.
174. Kutt H, Verebely K, McDowell F: Inhibition of diphenylhydantoin metabolism in rats and in rat liver microsomes by antitubercular drugs. *Neurology* 18:706–710, 1968.
175. Kutt H, Wolk M, Scherman R, McDowell F: Insufficient para-hydroxylation as a cause of diphenylhydantoin toxicity. *Neurology* 14:542–548, 1964.
176. Kronback T, Fisher V, Meyer UA: Cyclosporine metabolism in human liver: identification of a cytochrome P-450III gene family as the major cyclosporine-metabolizing enzyme explains interactions of cyclosporine with other drugs. *Clin Pharmacol Ther* 43:630–635, 1988.
176a. Labs RA: Interaction of roxatidine acetate with antacids, food and other drugs. *Drugs* 35(3):82–89, 1988.
177. Landay RA, Gonzalez MA, Taylor JC: Effect of phenobarbital on theophylline disposition. *J Allerg Clin Immunol* 62:27–29, 1978.
178. Lane EA, Guthrie S, Linnoila M: Effects of ethanol on drug and metabolite pharmacokinetics. *Clin Pharmacokinet* 10:228–247, 1985.
179. Lau A, Lee M, Flascha S, Prasad R, Sharifi R: Effect of piperacillin on tobramycin pharmacokinetics in patients with normal renal function. *Antimicrob Agents Chemother* 24:533–537, 1983.
180. Lawson DH, Tilstone WJ, Gray JMB, Srivastava PK: Effect of furosemide on the pharmacokinetics of gentamicin in patients. *J Clin Pharmacol* 22:254–258, 1982.
180a. Lazar JD, Wilner KD: Drug interactions with fluconazole. *Rev Inf Dis* 12(3):S327–S333, 1990.
181. Leahey EB, Rieffel JA, Drusin RE, Heissenbuttel RH, Lovejoy WP, Bigger JT: Interaction between quinidine and digoxin. *JAMA* 240:533–534, 1978.
182. Leahey EB, Reiffel JA, Giardina E-GV, Bigger JT: The effect of quinidine and other oral antiarrhythmic drugs on serum digoxin. *Ann Intern Med* 92:605–608, 1980.
183. Leahey EB, Reiffel JA, Heissenbuttel RH, Drusin RE, Lovejoy WP, Bigger JT: Enhanced cardiac effect of digoxin during quinidine treatment. *Arch Intern Med* 139:519–521, 1979.
183a. Lee BL, Medina I, Benowitz NL, Jacob P, Wofsy CB, Mills J: Dapsone, trimethoprim, and sulfamethoxazole plasma levels during treatment of pneumocystis pneumonia in patients with the acquired immunodeficiency syndrome (AIDS): Evidence of drug interactions. *Ann Intern Med* 110:606–611, 1989.
184. Legler UF, Benet LZ: Marked alterations in dose-dependent prednisolone kinetics in women taking oral contraceptives. *Clin Pharmacol Ther* 39:425–429, 1986.
185. Lejonc JL, Gusmini D, Brochard P: Isoniazid and reaction to cheese (letter). *Ann Intern Med* 91:793, 1979.
185a. Lemberger L, Rowe H, Bosomworth JC, Tenbarge JB, Bergstrom RF: The effect of fluoxetine on the pharmacokinetics and psychomotor responses of diazepam. *Clin Pharmacol Ther* 43:412–419, 1988.
185b. Leor J, Levartowsky D, Sharon C, Farfel Z: Amiodarone and β-adrenergic blockers: An interaction with metoprolol but not with atenolol. *Am Heart J* 116(1):206–207, 1988.
185c. Lesko LJ: Pharmacokinetic drug interactions with amiodarone. *Clin Pharmacokinet* 17(2):130–140, 1989.
186. Levine RR: Factors affecting gastrointestinal absorption of drugs. *Am J Digest Dis* 15:171–188, 1970.
187. Levy G: Gastrointestinal clearance of drugs with activated treated charcoal (editorial). *N Engl J Med* 307:676–678, 1982.
188. Levy G, Lampman T, Kamath BL, Garrettson LK: Decreased serum salicylate concentration in children with rheumatic fever treated with antacid. *N Engl J Med* 293:323–325, 1975.
189. Lewis GP, Holtzman JL: Interaction of flecainide with digoxin and propranolol. *Am J Cardiol* 53:52B–57B, 1984.
190. Lewis JG: Adverse reactions to calcium antagonists. *Drugs* 25:196–222, 1983.
190a. Liberman BA, Norman P, Hardy BG: Pancuronium-phenytoin interaction: a case of decreased duration of neuromuscular blockade. *Intern J Clin Pharmacol Ther Toxicol* 26(8):P371–374, 1988.

190b. Liedholm H, Nordin G: Erythromycin-felodipine interaction. *Ann Pharmacother* 25:1007–1008, 1991.

190c. Lin JH, Chremos AN, Chiou R, Yeh KC, Williams R: Comparative effect of famotidine and cimetidine on the pharmacokinetics of theophylline in normal volunteers. *Br J Clin Pharmacol* 24:669–672, 1987.

191. Lindenbaum J, Maulitz RM, Butler VP: Inhibition of digoxin absorption by neomycin. *Gastroenterology* 71:399–404, 1976.

192. Lindenbaum J, Rund DH, Butler VP, Tse-Eng D, Saha JR: Inactivation of digoxin by the gut flora: reversal by antibiotic therapy. *N Engl J Med* 305:789–794, 1981.

193. Linnoila M, Mattila MJ, Kitchell BS: Drug interactions with alcohol. *Drugs* 18:229–311, 1979.

193a. Lockey D, Bateman DN: Effect of oral activated charcoal on quinine elimination. *Br J Clin Pharmacol* 27:92–94, 1989.

193b. Lodwick R, McConkey B, Brown AM: Life threatening interaction between tamoxifen and warfarin. *Br Med J* 295:1141, 1987.

193c. Loi CM, Day JD, Jue SG, Bush ED, Costello P, Dewey LV, Vestal RE: Dose-dependent inhibition of theophylline metabolism by disulfiram in recovering alcoholics. *Clin Pharmacol Ther* 45:476–486, 1989.

193d. Loi CM, Wei X, Vestal RE: Inhibition of theophylline metabolism by mexiletine in young male and female nonsmokers. *Clin Pharmacol Ther* 49:571–580, 1991.

194. Lopez-Ovejero JA, Weber MA, Drayer JIM, Sealey JE, Laragh JH: Effects of indomethacin alone and during diuretic or β-adrenoreceptor-blockade therapy on blood pressure and the renin system in essential hypertension. *Clin Sci Mol Med* 55:203–205, 1978.

195. Lumholtz B, Siersbaek-Nielsen K, Skovsted L, Kampmann J, Hensen JM: Sulfamethizole-induced inhibition of diphenylhydantoin, tolbutamide, and warfarin metabolism. *Clin Pharmacol Ther* 17:731–734, 1975.

195a. MacKichan JJ: Protein binding drug displacement interactions: fact or fiction? *Clin Pharmacokinet* 16:65–73, 1989.

196. MacLeod SM, Giles HG, Patzalek G, Thiessen JJ, Sellers EM: Diazepam actions and plasma concentrations following ethanol ingestion. *Eur J Clin Pharmacol* 11:346–349, 1977.

197. MacLeod SM, Sellers EM: Pharmacodynamic and pharmacokinetic drug interactions with coumarin anticoagulants. *Drugs* 11:461–470, 1976.

198. MacLeod SM, Sellers EM, Giles HG, Billings BJ, Martin PR, Greenblatt DJ, Marshman JA: Interaction of disulfiram with benzodiazepines. *Clin Pharmacol Ther* 24:583–589, 1978.

198a. Macphee GJA, Mitchell JR, Wiseman L, McLellan AR, Park BK, McInnes GT, Brodie MJ: Effect of sodium valproate on carbamazepine disposition and psychomotor profile in man. *Br J Clin Pharmacol* 25:59–66, 1988.

199. Macphee GJA, Thompson GG, McInnes GT, Brodie MJ: Verapamil potentiates carbamazepine neurotoxicity: a clinically important inhibitory interaction. *Lancet* 1:700–703, 1986.

200. Macphee GJA, Thompson GG, Scobie G, Agnew E, Park BK, Murray T, McColl KEL, Brodie MJ: Effects of cimetidine on carbamazepine auto- and hetero-induction in man. *Br J Clin Pharmacol* 18:411–419, 1984.

200a. Maggio TG, Bartels DW: Increased cyclosporine blood concentrations due to verapamil administration. *Drug Intell Clin Pharmacol* 22:705–707, 1988.

201. Manfred RL, Vesell ES: Inhibition of theophylline metabolism by long-term allopurinol administration. *Clin Pharmacol Ther* 29:224–229, 1981.

202. Manninen V, Apajalahti A, Simonen H, Reissel P: Effect of propantheline and metoclopramide on absorption of digoxin. *Lancet* i:398, 1973.

203. Martell R, Heinrichs D, Stiller CR, Jenner M, Keown PA, Dupre J: The effects of erythromycin in patients treated with cyclosporine. *Ann Intern Med* 104:660–661, 1986.

204. Mattson RH, Cramer JA, Williamson PC, Novelly RA: Valproic acid in epilepsy: clinical and pharmacological effects. *Ann Neurol* 3:20–25, 1978.

204a. Mauro VF, Mauro LS, Hageman JH: Alteration of pentoxifylline pharmacokinetics by cimetidine. *J Clin Pharmacol* 28:649–654, 1988.

205. May CD, Jarboe CH: Inhibition of clearance of dyphylline by probenecid (letter). *N Engl J Med* 304:791, 1981.

206. May DC, Jarboe CH, Ellenburg DT, Roe EJ, Karibo J: The effects of erythromycin on theophylline elimination in normal males. *J Clin Pharmacol* 22:125–130, 1982.

207. McElnay JC, D'Arcy PF: Protein binding displacement interactions and their clinical importance. *Drugs* 25:495–513, 1983.

208. McGovern B, Geer VR, LaRaia PJ, Garan H, Ruskin JN: Possible interaction between amiodarone and phenytoin. *Ann Intern Med* 101:650–651, 1984.

209. McMurty RJ: Propranolol, hypoglycemia, and hypertensive crisis. *Ann Intern Med* 80:669–670, 1974.

210. Melmon KL, Nierenberg DW: Drug interactions and the prepared observer (editorial). *N Engl J Med* 304:723–724, 1981.

211. Mihaly GW, Marino AT, Webster LK, Jones DB, Louis WJ, Smallwood RA: High dose of antacid (Mylanta II) reduces bioavailability of ranitidine. *Br Med J* 285:998–999, 1982.

211a. Miles MV, Tennison MB: Erythromycin effects on multiple-dose carbamazepine kinetics. *Ther Drug Monit* 11:47–52, 1989.

211b. Miller DD: Effect of phenytoin on plasma clozapine concentrations in two patients. *J Clin Psychiatry* 52:23–25, 1991.

212. Miller M, Cosgriff J, Kwong T, Morken DA: Influence of phenytoin on theophylline clearance. *Clin Pharmacol Ther* 35:666–669, 1984.

213. Miller RP, Bates JH: Amphotericin B toxicity. A follow-up report of 53 patients. *Ann Intern Med* 71:1089–1095, 1969.

214. Milne MD, Scribner BH, Crawford MA: Non-ionic diffusion and the excretion of weak acids and bases. *Am J Med* 24:709–729, 1958.

214a. Miners JO: Drug interactions involving aspirin (acetylsalicylic acid) and salicylic acid. *Clin Pharmacokinet* 17(5):327–344, 1989.

215. Misage JR, McDonald RH: Antagonism of hypotensive action of bethanidine by "common cold" remedy. *Br Med J* 4:347, 1976.

216. Misra PS, Leferve A, Ishii H, Rubin E, Lieber CS: Increase of ethanol, meprobamate and pentobarbital metabolism after chronic ethanol administration in man and rats. *Am J Med* 51:346–351, 1971.

217. Mitchell JR, Arias L, Oates JA: Antagonism of the antihypertensive action of guanethidine sulfate by desipramine hydrochloride. *JAMA* 202:973–976, 1967.

218. Mitchell JR, Cavanaugh JH, Arias L, Oates JA: Guanethidine and related agents. III. Antagonism by drugs which inhibit the norepinephrine pump in man. *J Clin Invest* 49:1596–1604, 1970.

219. Mitchell MC, Hanew T, Meredith CG, Schenker S: Effects of oral contraceptive steroids on acetaminophen metabolism and elimination. *Clin Pharmacol Ther* 34:48–53, 1983.

220. Mitchell MC, Schnecker S, Speeg KV: Selective inhibition of acetaminophen oxidation and toxicity by cimetidine and other histamine H_2 receptor antagonists *in vivo* and *in vitro* in the rat and in man. *J Clin Invest* 73:383–391, 1984.

220a. Monahan BP, Ferguson CL, Killeavy ES, Lloyd BK, Troy J, Cantilena LR: Torsades de Pointes occurring in association with terfenadine use. *JAMA* 264(21):2788–27980, 1990.

221. Moore TJ, Crantz TR, Hollenberg NK, Koletsky RJ, Leboff MS, Swartz SL, Levine L, Podolsky S, Dluhy RG, Williams GH: Contribution of prostaglandins to the antihypertensive action of captopril in essential hypertension. *Hypertension* 3:168–173, 1981.

222. Muirhead MR, Somogyi AA, Rolan PE, Bochner F: Effect of cimetidine on renal and hepatic drug elimination: studies with triamterene. *Clin Pharmacol Ther* 40:400–407, 1986.

223. Mungall DR, Robichaux RP, Perry W, Scott JW, Robinson A, Burelle T, Hurst D: Effects of quinidine on serum digoxin concentration. *Ann Intern Med* 93:689–693, 1980.

224. Murphy DL, Bunney WE Jr: Total body potassium changes during lithium administration. *J Nerv Ment Dis* 152:381–389, 1971.

224a. Murphy R, Swartz R, Watkins PB: Severe acetaminophen toxicity in a patient receiving isoniazid. *Ann Intern Med* 113(10):799–800, 1990.

225. Murray FJ: Outbreak of unexpected reactions among epileptics taking isoniazid. *Am Rev Respir Dis* 86:729–732, 1962.

226. Murrell GAC, Rapeport WG: Clinical pharmacokinetics of allopurinol. *Clin Pharmacokinet* 11:343–353, 1986.

226a. Nafziger AN, May JJ, Bertino JS: Inhibition of theophylline elimination by diltiazem therapy. *J Clin Pharmacol* 27(11):862–865, 1987.

226b. Navis GJ, de Jong, PE, de Zeeuw D: Volume homeostasis, angiotensin converting enzyme inhibition, and lithium theraphy. *Am J Med* 86:621, 1989.

226c. Nelson MV, Berchou RC, Kareti D, LeWitt PA: Pharmacokinetic evaluation of erythromycin and caffeine administered with bromocriptine. *Clin Pharmacol Ther* 47:694–697, 1990.

227. Neuvonen PJ: Clinical pharmacokinetics of oral activated charcoal in acute intoxication. *Clin Pharmacokinet* 7:465–489, 1982.

228. Neuvonen PJ, Elfring SM, Elonen E: Reduction of absorption of digoxin, phenytoin and aspirin by activated charcoal in man. *Eur J Clin Pharmacol* 13:213–218, 1978.

229. Neuvonen PJ, Elonen E: Effect of activated charcoal on absorption and elimination of phenobarbitone, carbamazepine, and phenylbutazone in man. *Eur J Clin Pharmacol* 17:51–57, 1980.

230. Neuvonen PJ, Kannisto H, Hirvisalo EL: Effect of activated charcoal on absorption of tolbutamide and valproate in man. *Eur J Clin Pharmacol* 24:243–246, 1983.

231. Neuvonen PJ, Lehtovaara R, Bardy A, Elonen E: Antipyrine analgesics in patients on antiepileptic drug therapy. *Eur J Clin Pharmacol* 15:263–268, 1979.

232. Neuvonen PJ, Tokola RA, Kaste M: Cimetidine-phenytoin interactions: effect on serum phenytoin concentration and antipyrine test in man. *Eur J Clin Pharmacol* 21:215–220, 1981.

233. Newton RW: Physostigmine salicylate in the treatment of tricyclic antidepressant overdosage. *JAMA* 231:941–944, 1974.

233a. Ng HWK, Macfarlane AW, Graham RM, Verbov JL: Near fatal drug interactions with methotrexate given for psoriasis. *Br Med J* 295:752, 1987.

234. Nierenberg DW: Competitive inhibition of methotrexate in kidney slices by nonsteroidal anti-inflammatory drugs. *J Pharmacol Exp Ther* 226:1–6, 1983.

235. Nies AS: Adverse reactions and interactions limiting the use of antihypertensive drugs. *Am J Med* 58:495–503, 1975.

236. Nies AS, Shand DG: Hypertensive response to propranolol in a patient treated with methyl dopa—a proposed mechanism. *Clin Pharmacol Ther* 14:823–826, 1973.

237. Nimmo WS, Heading RC, Tothill P, Prescott LF: Pharmacological evaluation of gastric emptying: effect of propantheline and metoclopramide on paracetamol absorption. *Br Med J* 1:587–589, 1973.

238. Nimmo WS, Heading RC, Wilson J, Tothill P, Prescott LF: Inhibition of gastric emptying and drug absorption by narcotic analgesics. *Br J Clin Pharmacol* 2:502–513, 1975.

238a. Nix DE, Watson WA, Lener ME, Frost RW, Krol G, Goldstein H, Lettieri J, Schentag JJ: Effects of aluminum and magnesium antacids and ranitidine on the absorption of ciprofloxacin. *Clin Pharmacol Ther* 46:700–705, 1989.

239. Noble J, Matthew H: Acute poisoning by antidepressants: clinical features and management of 100 patients. *Clin Toxicol* 2:403–421, 1969.

239a. Nolan PE, Marcus FI, Hoyer GL, Bliss M, Gear K: Pharmacokinetic interaction between intravenous phenytoin and amiodarone in healthy volunteers. *Clin Pharmacol Ther* 46:43–50, 1989.

239b. North DS, Mattern AL, Kapil RP, Lalonde RL: The effect of histamine-2 receptor antagonists on tocainide pharmacokinetics. *J Clin Pharmacol* 28:640–643, 1988.

240. Ochs HR, Carstens G, Greenblatt DJ: Reduction in lidocaine clearance during continuous infusion and by coadministration of propranolol. *N Engl J Med* 303:373–377, 1980.

240a. Ochs HR, Greenblatt DJ, Friedman H, Burstein ES, Locniskar A, Harmatz JS, Shader RI: Bromazepam pharmacokinetics: Influence of age, gender, oral contraceptives, cimetidine, and propranol. *Clin Pharmacol Ther* 41:562–570, 1987.

241. Ochs HR, Greenblatt DJ, Gugler R: Cimetidine impairs nitrazepam clearance. *Clin Pharmacol Ther* 34:227–230, 1983.

242. Ochs HR, Greenblatt DJ, Verburg-Ochs B: Propranolol interactions with diazepam, lorazepam, and alprazolam. *Clin Pharmacol Ther* 36:451–455, 1984.

242a. Ohnhaus EE, Brockmeyer N, Dylewicz P, Habicht H: The effect of antipyrine and rifampin on the metabolism of diazepam. *Clin Pharmacol Ther* 42:148–156, 1987.

242b. Okey AB: Enzyme induction in the cytochrome P-450 system. *Pharmacol Ther* 45:241–298, 1990.

243. Olesen OV: Disulfiram (Antabuse[R]) as inhibitor of phenytoin metabolism. *Acta Pharmacol Toxicol* 24:317–322, 1966.

244. O'Reilly RA: Comparative interaction of cimetidine and ranitidine with racemic warfarin in man. *Arch Intern Med* 144:989–991, 1984.

245. O'Reilly RA: Interaction of chronic daily warfarin therapy and rifampin. *Ann Intern Med* 83:506–508, 1975.

246. O'Reilly RA: Interaction of sodium warfarin and disulfiram (Antabuse[R]) in man. *Ann Intern Med* 78:73–76, 1973.

247. O'Reilly RA: Interaction of sodium warfarin and rifampin. *Ann Intern Med* 81:337–340, 1974.

248. O'Reilly RA: Stereoselective interaction of trimethoprim-sulfamethoxazole with the separated enantiomers of racemic warfarin in man. *N Engl J Med* 302:33–35, 1980.

249. O'Reilly RA: The stereoselective interaction of warfarin and metronidazole in man. *N Engl J Med* 295:354–357, 1976.

249a. O'Reilly RA, Trager WF, Rettie AE, Goulart DA: Interaction of amiodarone with racemic warfarin and its separated enantiomorphs in humans. *Clin Pharmacol Ther* 42:290–294, 1987.

250. Orr JM, Abott FS, Farrell K, Ferguson S, Sheppard L, Godolphin W: Interaction between valproic acid and aspirin in epileptic children: serum protein binding and metabolic effects. *Clin Pharmacol Ther* 31:642–649, 1982.

251. Osman MA, Patel RB, Schuna A, Sundstrom WR, Welling PG: Reduction in oral penicillamine absorption by food, antacid and ferrous sulfate. *Clin Pharmacol Ther* 33:465–470, 1983.

252. Osman MA, Welling PG: Influence of propantheline and metaclopramide on the bioavailability of chlorothiazide. *Curr Ther Res* 34:404–408, 1983.

253. Packer M, Meller J, Medina N, Yushak M, Smith H, Holt J, Guererro J, Todd GD, McAllister RG, Gorlin R: Hemodynamic consequences of combined beta-adrenergic and slow calcium channel blockade in man. *Circulation* 65:660–668, 1982.

253a. Pan HY, Triscari J, DeVault AR, Smith SA, Wang-Iverson D, Swanson BN, Willard DA. Pharmacokinetic interaction between propranolol and the HMG-CoA reductase inhibitors pravastatin and lovastatin. *Br J Clin Pharmacol* 31:665–670, 1991.

253b. Panesar SK, Orr JM, Farrell K, Burton RW, Kassahun K, Abbott FS: The effect of carbamazepine on valproic acid disposition in adult volunteers. *Br J Clin Pharmacol* 27:323–328, 1989.

253c. Parpia SH, Nix DE, Hejmanowski LG, Goldstein HR, Wilton JH, Schentag JJ: Sucralfate reduces the gastrointestinal absorption of norfloxacin. *Antimicrob Agents Chemother* 33(1):99–102, 1989.

254. Parsons, RL, Paddock GM: Absorption of two antibacterial drugs, cephalexin and co-trimoxazole in malabsorption syndromes. *J Antimicrob Chemother* 1(suppl):59–67, 1975.

255. Patak RV, Mookerjee BK, Bentzel CJ, Hysert PE, Babej M, Lee JB: Antagonism of the effects of furosemide by indomethacin in normal and hypertensive man. *Prostaglandins* 10:649–659, 1980.

256. Patwardhan RV, Yarborough GW, Desmond PV, Johnson RF, Schenker S, Speeg KV: Cimetidine spares the glucuronidation of lorazepam and oxazepam. *Gastroenterology* 79:912–916, 1980.

256a. Paulsen O, Höglund P, Nilsson LG, Bengtsson HI: The interaction of erythromycin with theophylline. *Eur J Clin Pharmacol* 32:493–498, 1987.

257. Pedersen AK, Jackobsen P, Kampmann JP, Hansen JM: Clinical pharmacokinetics and potentially important drug interactions of sulphinpyrazone. *Clin Pharmacokinet* 7:42–56, 1982.

258. Pentikainen PJ, Koivula IH, Hiltunen HA: Effect of rifampicin treatment on the kinetics of mexiletine. *Eur J Clin Pharmacol* 23:261–266, 1982.

258a. Rodin SM, Johnson BF, Wilson J, Ritchie P, Johnson J: Comparative effects of verapamil and isradipine on steady-state digoxin kinetics. *Clin Pharmacol Ther* 43:668–672, 1988.

259. Penttila O, Neuvonen PJ, Aho K, Lehtovarra R: Interaction between doxycycline and some antiepileptic drugs. *Br Med J* 2:470–472, 1974.

260. Perel JM, Dayton PG, Snell MM, Yu TF, Gutman AB: Studies of interactions among drugs in man at the renal level: probenecid and sulfinpyrazone. *Clin Pharmacol Ther* 10:834–840, 1969.

261. Perucca E: Pharmacokinetic interactions with antiepileptic drugs. *Clin Pharmacokinet* 7:57–84, 1982.

262. Perucca E, Hebdige S, Gatti G, Leccini S, Frigo BM, Crema A: Interaction between phenytoin and valproic acid: plasma protein binding and metabolic effects. *Clin Pharmacol Ther* 28:779–789, 1980.

263. Perucca E, Richens A: Drug interactions with phenytoin. *Drugs* 21:120–137, 1981.

264. Petereit LB, Meikle AW: Effectiveness of prednisolone during phenytoin therapy. *Clin Pharmacol Ther* 22:912–916, 1977.

265. Peters L: Renal tubular excretion of organic bases. *Pharmacol Rev* 12:1–35, 1960.

266. Pickering IK, Rutherford I: Effect of concentration and time upon inactivation of tobramycin, gentamicin, netilmicin and amikacin by azlocillin, carbenicillin, mecillinam, mezlocillin and piperacillin. *J Pharmacol Exp Ther* 217:345–349, 1981.

266a. Pierce LR, Wysowski DK, Gross TP; Myopathy and rhabdomyolysis associated with lovastation—gemfibrozil combination therapy. *JAMA* 264(1):71–75, 1990.

267. Pinell OC, Fenimore DC, Davis GM, Fann WE: Drug-drug interactions of chlorpromazine and antacids (abstract). *Clin Pharmacol Ther* 23:125, 1978.

267a. Polk RE, Healy DP, Sahai J, Drwal L, Racht E: Effect of ferrous sulfate and multivitamins with zinc on absorption of ciprofloxacin in normal volunteers. *Antimicrob Agents Chemother* 33(11):1841–1844, 1989.

268. Pond SM, Birkett DJ, Wade DN: Mechanisms of inhibition of tolbutamide metabolism: phenylbutazone, oxyphenbutazone, sulfaphenazole. *Clin Pharmacol Ther* 22:573–579, 1978.

269. Pond SM, Graham GG, Birkett DJ, Wade DN: Effects of tricyclic antidepressants on drug metabolism. *Clin Pharmacol Ther* 18:191–199, 1975.

270. Powell JR, Rogers JF, Wargin WA, Cross RE, Eshelman FN: Inhibition of theophylline clearance by cimetidine but not ranitidine. *Arch Intern Med* 144:484–486, 1984.

271. Prescott LF: Mechanisms of renal excretion of drugs. *Br J Anaesth* 44:246–251, 1972.

272. Prescott LF: Pharmacokinetic drug interactions. *Lancet* 2:1239–1243, 1969.

272a. Prescott LF, Hamilton AR, Heyworth R: Treatment of quinine overdosage with repeated oral charcoal. *Br J Clin Pharmacol* 27:95–97, 1989.

273. Prichard BNC, Ross EJ: Use of propranolol in conjunction with alpha receptor blocking drugs in pheochromocytoma. *Am J Cardiol* 18:394–398, 1966.

273a. Prichard PJ, Walt RP, Kitchingman GK, Somerville KW, Langman MJS, Williams J, Richens A: Oral phenytoin pharmacokinetics during omeprazole therapy. *Br J Clin Pharmacol* 24:543–545, 1987.

274. Prober CG: Effect of rifampin on chloramphenicol levels. *N Engl J Med* 312:788–789, 1985.

275. Puschett JB, Rastegar A: Comparative study of the effects of metolazone and other diuretics on potassium excretion. *Clin Pharmacol Ther* 15:397–405, 1974.

276. Puurunen J, Solaniemi E, Pelkonen O: Effect of cimetidine on microsomal drug metabolism in man. *Eur J Clin Pharmacol* 18:185–187, 1980.

276a. Raoof S, Wollschlager C, Khan FA: Ciprofloxacin increases serum levels of theophylline. *Am J Med* 82(4A):115–118, 1987.

277. Reimann IW, Frolich JC: Effects of diclofenac on lithium kinetics. *Clin Pharmacol Ther* 30:348–352, 1981.

278. Reitberg DP, Bernhard H, Schentag JJ: Alteration of theophylline clearance and half-life by cimetidine in normal volunteers. *Ann Intern Med* 95:582–586, 1981.

279. Rendic S, Alebic-Kolbah T, Kajfez F: Interaction of ranitidine with liver microsomes. *Xenobiotica* 12:9–17, 1982.

280. Rennick BR: Renal excretion of drugs: tubular transport and metabolism. *Annu Rev Pharmacol* 12:141–156, 1972.

281. Rennick BR: Renal tubule transport of organic cations. *Am J Physiol* 240:F83–F89, 1981.

282. Renton KW, Gray JD, Hung OR: Depression of theophylline elimination by erythromycin. *Clin Pharmacol Ther* 30:422–426, 1981.

283. Richer C, Mathieu M, Bah H, Thuillex C, Duroux P, Giudicelli J-F: Theophylline kinetics and ventilatory flow in bronchial asthma and chronic airflow obstruction: influence of erythromycin. *Clin Pharmacol Ther* 31:579–586, 1982.

283a. Rimmer EM, Richens A: Interaction between vigabatrin and phenytoin. *Br J Clin Pharmacol* 27:27S–33S, 1989.

284. Robinson DS, Benjamin DM, McCormack JJ: Interaction of warfarin and nonsystemic gastrointestinal drugs. *Clin Pharmacol Ther* 12:491–495, 1971.

285. Robson RA, Miners JO, Wing LMH, Birkett DJ: Theophylline-rifampin interaction: non-selective induction of theophylline metabolic pathways. *Br J Clin Pharmacol* 18:445–448, 1984.

285a. Rogge MC, Solomon WR, Sedman AJ, Welling PG, Koup JR, Wagner JG: The theophylline-enoxacin interaction: II. Changes in the disposition of theophylline and its metabolites during intermittent administration of enoxacin. *Clin Pharmacol Ther* 46:420–428, 1989.

285b. Rogge MC, Solomon WR, Sedman AJ, Welling PG, Koup JR, Wagner JG: The theophylline-enoxacin interaction: II. Changes in the disposition of theophylline and its metabolites during intermittent administration of enoxacin. *Clin Pharmacol Ther* 46:420–428, 1989.

285c. Rogge MC, Solomon WR, Sedman AJ, Welling PG, Toothaker RD, Wagner JG: The theophylline-enoxacin interaction. I. Effect of enoxacin dose size on theophylline disposition. *Clin Pharmacol Ther* 44:579–587, 1988.

286. Rollinghoff W, Paumgartner G: Inhibition of drug metabolism by cimetidine in man: dependence on pretreatment microsomal liver function. *Eur J Clin Invest* 12:429–434, 1982.

287. Romankiewicz JA, Ehrman M: Rifampin and warfarin: a drug interaction. *Ann Intern Med* 82:224–225, 1975.

288. Rose HJ, Pruitt AW, Dayton PG, McNay JL: Relationship of urinary furosemide excretion rate to natriuretic effect in experimental azotemia. *J Pharmacol Exp Ther* 199:490–497, 1976.

289. Rose HJ, Pruitt AW, McNay J: Effect of experimental azotemia on renal clearance of furosemide in the dog. *J Pharmacol Exp Ther* 196:238–247, 1976.

290. Routledge PA, Kitchell BB, Bjornsson TD, Skinner T, Linnoila M, Shand DG: Diazepam and N-desmethyldiazepam redistribution after heparin. *Clin Pharmacol Ther* 27:528–532, 1980.

291. Ruffolo RL, Thompson JF, Segal JL: Diazepam-cimetidine drug interaction: a clinically significant effect. *South Med J* 74:1075–1078, 1981.

291a. Rutledge DR, Pieper JA, Mirvis DM: Effects of chronic phenobarbital on verapamil disposition in humans. *J Pharmacol Exper Ther* 246(1):7–13, 1988.

292. Saal AK, Werner JA, Greene HL, Sears GK, Graham EL: Effect of amiodarone on serum quinidine and procainamide levels. *Am J Cardiol* 53:1264–1267, 1984.

293. Sackellares JC, Sato S, Dreifuss FE, Penry JK: Reduction of steady state valproate levels by other antiepileptic drugs. *Epilepsia* 22:437–441, 1981.

294. Salem RB, Breland BD, Mishra SK, Jordan JE: Effect of cimetidine on phenytoin serum levels. *Epilepsia* 24:284–288, 1983.

294a. Saltiel E, Ellrodt AG, Monk JP, Langley MS: Felodipine: A review of its pharmacodynamic and pharmacokinetic properties, and therapeutic use in hypertension. *Drugs* 36:387–428, 1988.

294b. Sambol NC, Upton RA, Chremos AN, Lin ET, Williams RL: A comparison of the influence of famotidine and cimetidine on phenytoin elimination and hepatic blood flow. *Br J Clin Pharmacol* 27:83–87, 1989.

295. Sanchez G: Enhancement of heparin effect by probenecid (letter). *N Engl J Med* 292:48, 1975.

296. Sandor P, Sellers EM, Dumbrell M, Klouw V: Effect of short and long term alcohol use on phenytoin kinetics in chronic alcoholics. *Clin Pharmacol Ther* 30:390–397, 1981.

296a. Sano M, Kawakatus K, Ohkita C, Yamamoto I, Takeyama M, Yamashina H, Goto M: Effects of enoxacin, of loxacin and norfloxacin on theophylline disposition in humans. *Eur J Clin Pharmacol* 35:161–165, 1988.

297. Schneck DW, Luderer JR, Davis D, Vary JE: Effects of nadolol and propranolol on plasma lidocaine clearance. *Clin Pharmacol Ther* 36:584–587, 1984.

298. Schneck DW, Vary JE: Mechanism by which hydralazine increases propranolol bioavailability. *Clin Pharmacol Ther* 35:447–453, 1984.

299. Schenck-Gustafsson K, Jogestrand T, Nordlander R, Dahlqvist R: Effect of quinidine on digoxin concentration in skeletal muscle and serum in patients with atrial fibrillation. Evidence for reduced binding of digoxin in muscle. *N Engl J Med* 305:209–211, 1981.

299a. Schlanz KD, Myre SA, Bottorff MB: Pharmacokinetic interactions with calcium channel antagonists (Part I). *Clin Pharmacokinet* 21 (5):344–356, 1991.

299b. Schwartz J, Jauregui L, Lettieri J, Bachmann K: Impact of ciprofloxacin on theophylline clearance and steady-state concentrations in serum. *Antimicrob Agents Chemother* 32(1)75–77, 1988.

300. Schwartz JB, Keefe D, Kates RE, Kirsten E, Harrison DC: Acute and chronic pharmacodynamic interaction of verapamil and digoxin in atrial fibrillation. *Circulation* 65:1163–1170, 1982.

300a. Schwartz JB, Upton RA, Lin ET, Williams RL, Benet LZ: Effect of cimetidine or ranitidine administration on nifedipine pharmacokinetics and pharmacodynamics. *Clin Pharmacol Ther* 43:673–680, 1988.

301. Seixas FA: Alcohol and its drug interactions. *Ann Intern Med* 83:86–92, 1975.

302. Sellers EM: Plasma protein displacement interactions are rarely of clinical significance. *Pharmacology* 18:225–227, 1979.

303. Sellers EM, Holloway MR: Drug kinetics and alcohol ingestion. *Clin Pharmacokinet* 3:440–452, 1978.

304. Sellers EM, Koch-Weser J: Displacement of warfarin from human albumin by diazoxide and ethacrynic, mefenamic, and nalidixic acids. *Clin Pharmacol Ther* 11:524–529, 1970.

305. Sellers EM, Koch-Weser J: Potentiation of warfarin-induced hypoprothrombinemia by chloral hydrate. *N Engl J Med* 283:827–831, 1970.

306. Sellers EM, Lang M, Koch-Weser J, LeBlanc E, Kalant H: Interaction of chloral hydrate and ethanol in man. I. Metabolism. *Clin Pharmacol Ther* 13:37–49, 1972.

307. Sellers EM, Naranjo CA, Giles HG, Frecker RC, Beeching M: Intravenous diazepam and oral ethanol interaction. *Clin Pharmacol Ther* 28:638–645, 1980.

308. Sellman F, Kanto J, Raijola E, Pekkarinen A: Human and animal study on elimination from plasma and metabolism of diazepam after chronic alcohol intake. *Acta Pharmacol Toxicol* 36:33–38, 1975.

309. Serlin MJ, Breckenridge AM: Drug interactions with warfarin. *Drugs* 25:610–620, 1983.

310. Serlin MJ, Sibeon RG, Breckenridge AM: Lack of effect of ranitidine on warfarin action. *Br J Clin Pharmacol* 12:791–794, 1981.

311. Shea P, Lal R, Kim SS, Schechtman K, Ruffy R: Flecainide and amiodarone interaction. *J Am Coll Cardiol* 7:1127–1130, 1986.

311a. Shelley RK: Lithium toxicity and mefenamic acid: A possible interaction and the role of prostaglandin inhibition. *Br J Psych* 151:847–848, 1987.

312. Shinn AF, Shrewsbury RP: *Evaluation of Drug Interactions.* CV Mosby, St. Louis, 1985.

312a. Sirmans SM, Pieper JA, Lalonde RL, Smith DG, Self TH: Effect of calcium channel blockers on theophylline disposition. *Clin Pharmacol Ther* 44:29–34, 1988.

312b. Somogyi A, Muirhead M: Pharmacokinetic interactions of cimetidine 1987. *Clin Pharmacokinet* 12:321–366, 1987.

313. Sjoqvist F: Psychotropic drugs (2). Interaction between monoamine oxidase (MAO) inhibitors and other substances. *Proc R Soc Med* 58:967–977, 1965.

314. Skinner C, Coull DC, Johnston AW: Antagonism of the hypotensive action of bethanidine and debrisoquin by tricyclic antidepressants. *Lancet* ii:564–566, 1969.

315. Smith CK, Durack DT: Isoniazid and reaction to cheese. *Ann Intern Med* 88:520–521, 1978.

316. Solomon HM, Abrams WB: Interactions between digitoxin and other drugs in man. *Am Heart J* 83:277–280, 1972.

317. Somogyi A, Bochner F: Dose and concentration dependent effect of ranitidine on procainamide disposition and renal clearance in man. *Br J Clin Pharmacol* 18:175–181, 1984.

318. Somogyi A, Gugler R: Drug interactions with cimetidine. *Clin Pharmacokinet* 7:23–41, 1982.

319. Somogyi A, McLean A, Heinzow B: Cimetidine-procainamide pharmacokinetic interaction in man: evidence of competition for tubular secretion of basic drugs. *Eur J Clin Pharmacol* 25:339–345, 1983.

320. Somogyi A, Theilscher S, Gugler R: Influence of phenobarbital treatment on cimetidine kinetics. *Eur J Clin Pharmacol* 19:343–347, 1981.

321. Spahn H, Mutschler E, Kirch W, Ohnhaus EE, Janisch HD: Influence of ranitidine on plasma metoprolol and atenolol concentrations. *Br Med J* 286:1546–1547, 1983.

322. Speeg KV, Patwardham RV, Avant GR, Mitchell MC, Schenker S: Inhibition of microsomal drug metabolism by histamine H_2-receptor antagonist studied *in vivo* and *in vitro* in rodents. *Gastroenterology* 82:89–96, 1982.

323. Stafford JR, Fann WE: Drug interactions with guanidinium antihypertensives. *Drugs* 13:57–64, 1977.

323a. Staib AH, Stille W, Dietlein G, Shah PM, Harder S, Mieke S, Beer C: Interaction between quinolones and caffeine. *Drugs* 34(1):170-174, 1987.

324. Steinberg WM, Lewis JH, Katz DM: Antacids inhibit absorption of cimetidine. *N Engl J Med* 307:400–404, 1982.

324a. Steiner E, Dumont E, Spina E, Dahlqvist R: Inhibition of desipramine 2-hydroxylation by quinidine and quinine. *Clin Pharmacol Ther* 43:577–581, 1987.

324b. Steiner E, Spina E: Differences in the inhibitory effect of cimetidine on desipramine metabolism between rapid and slow debrisoquin hydroxylators. *Clin Pharmacol Ther* 42:278–282, 1987.

325. Steiness E: Renal tubular secretion of digoxin. *Circulation* 50:103–107, 1974.

326. Steiness E, Waldorff S, Hansen PB, Kjaergard H, Buch J, Egeblad H: Reduction of digoxin-induced inotropism during quinidine administration. *Clin Pharmacol Ther* 27:791–795, 1980.

327. Stenson RE, Constantino RT, Harrison DC: Interrelationships of hepatic blood flow, cardiac output, and blood levels of lidocaine in man. *Circulation* 43:205–211, 1971.

327a. Stille W, Harder S, Mieke S, Beer C, Shah PM, Frech K, Staib AH: Decrease of caffeine elimination in man during coadministration of 4-quinolones. *J Antimicrob Chemother* 20:729–734, 1987.

328. Stockley I: *Drug Interactions.* Blackwell Scientific Publications, Oxford, 1981.

329. Stone CA, Porter CC, Stavorski JM, Ludden CT, Totaro JA: Antagonism of catecholamine-depleting agents by antidepressant and related drugs. *J Pharmacol* 144:196–204, 1964.

329a. Sutfin T, Balmer K, Boström H, Eriksson S, Höglund P, Paulsen O: Stereoselective interaction of omeprazole with warfarin in healthy men. *Ther Drug Monit* 11:176–184, 1989.

330. Sweeney KR, Chapron DJ, Brandt JL, Gomolin IH, Feig PU, Kramer PA: Toxic interaction between acetazolamide and salicylate: case reports and a pharmacokinetic explanation. *Clin Pharmacol Ther* 40:518–524, 1986.

330a. Szymanski S, Lieberman JA, Picou D, Masiar S, Cooper T: A case report of cimetidine-induced clozapine toxicity. *J Clin Psychiatry* 52:21–22, 1991.

330b. Takagi K, Hasegawa T, Yamaki K, Suzuki R, Watanabe T, Satake T: Interaction between theophylline and enoxacin. *Intern J Clin Pharmacol Ther Toxicol* 26(6):288–292, 1988.

331. Talbert RL, Bussey HI: Update on calcium-channel blocking agents. *Clin Pharmacol* 2:403–416, 1983.

331a. Tateishi T, Nakashima H, Shitou T, Kumagai Y, Ohashi K, Hosoda S, Ebihara A: Effect of diltiazem on the pharmacokinetics of propranolol, metoprolol and atenolol. *Eur J Clin Pharmacol* 36:67–70, 1989.

332. Thompson MJB, Russo ME, Saxon BJ, Atkinthor E, Matsem JM: Gentamicin inactivation by piperacillin or carbenicillin in patients with end stage renal disease. *Antimicrob Agents Chemother* 21:268–273, 1982.

333. Thompson PD, Melmon KL, Richardson JA, Cohn K, Steinbrunn W, Cudihee R, Rowland M: Lidocaine pharmacokinetics in advanced heart failure, liver disease, and renal failure in humans. *Ann Intern Med* 78:499–508, 1973.

334. Tilstone WJ, Semple PF, Lawson DH, Boyle JA: Effects of furosemide on glomerular filtration rate and clearance of practolol, digoxin, cephaloridine, and gentamicin. *Clin Pharmacol Ther* 22:289–294, 1977.

334a. Toon S, Davidson EM, Garstang FM, Batra H, Bowes RJ, Rowland M: The racemic metoprolol H_2-antagonist interaction. *Clin Pharmacol Ther* 43:283–289, 1988.

334b. Toon S, Hopkins KJ, Garstang FM, Aarons L, Sedman A, Rowland M: Enoxacin-in-warfarin interaction: Pharmacokinetic and stereochemical aspects. *Clin Pharmacol Ther* 42:33–41, 1987.

334c. Toon S, Hopkins KJ, Garstang FM, Rowland M: Comparative effects of ranitidine and cimetidine on the pharmacokinetics and pharmacodynamics of warfarin in man. *Eur J Clin Pharmacol* 32:165–172, 1987.

335. Toon S, Low LK, Gibaldi M, Trager WF, O'Reilly RA, Motley CH, Goulart DA: The warfarin-sulfinpyrazone interaction: stereochemical considerations. *Clin Pharmacol Ther* 39:15–24, 1986.

336. Tornatore KM, Kanarkowski R, McCarthy TL, Gardner MJ, Yurchak AM, Jusko WJ: Effect of chronic oral contraceptive steroids on theophylline disposition. *Eur J Clin Pharmacol* 23:129–134, 1982.

337. Touerud EL, Boobis AR, Brodie MJ, Murray S, Bennett PN, Whitmarsh V, Davies DS: Differential induction of antipyrine metabolism by rifampicin. *Eur J Clin Pharmacol* 21:155–160, 1981.

338. Twun-Barima Y, Carruthers SG: Quinidine-rifampin interaction. *N Engl J Med* 304:1466–1469, 1981.

339. Udall JA: Warfarin-chloral hydrate interaction. Pharmacological activity and clinical significance. *Ann Intern Med* 81:341–344, 1974.

340. Valette H, Apoil E: Interaction between salicylate and two loop diuretics. *Br J Clin Pharmacol* 8:592–594, 1979.

341. Valsalan VC, Cooper GL: Carbamazepine intoxication caused by interaction with isoniazid. *Br Med J* 285:261–262, 1982.

341a. van Harten J, van Brummelen P, Lodewijks MTM, Danhof M, Breimer DD: Pharmacokinetics and hemodynamic effects of nisoldipine and its interaction with cimetidine. *Clin Pharmacol Ther* 43:332–341, 1988.

341b. Van Hecken A, Verbesselt R, Tjandra-Maga TB, De Schepper PJ: Pharmacokinetic interaction between indomethacin and diflunisal. *Eur J Clin Pharmacol* 36:507–512, 1989.

341c. Vance-Bryan K, Guay DRP, Rotschafer JC: Clinical pharmacokinetics of ciprofloxacin. *Clin Pharmacokinet* 19(6):434–461, 1990.

342. vanZwieten PA: The reversal of clonidine-induced hypotension by protryptyline and desipramine. *Pharmacology* 14:227–231, 1976.

343. Vasko MR, Bell RD, Daly DD, Pippenger CE: Inheritance of phenytoin hypometabolism: a kinetic study of one family. *Clin Pharmacol Ther* 27:96–103, 1980.

344. Verbeeck R, Tjandramaga TB, Mullie A: Effect of aluminum hydroxide on diflunisal absorption. *Br J Clin Pharmacol* 13:519–522, 1979.

344a. Verbeeck RK: Pharmacokinetic drug interactions with nonsteroidal anti-inflammatory drugs. *Clin Pharmacokinet* 19(1):44–66, 1990.

344b. Vesell ES: Pharmacogenetic perspectives: genes, drugs and disease. *Hepatology* 4:959–965, 1984.

344c. Vestal RE, Cusack BJ, Mercer GD, Dawson GW, Park BK: Aging and drug interactions.I. Effect of cimetidine and smoking on the oxidation of theophylline and cortisol in healthy men. *J Pharmacol Exp Ther* 241:488–499, 1987.

345. Otton SV, Inaba T, Kalow W: Competitive inhibition of sparteine oxidation in human liver by β-adrenoceptor antagonists and other cardiovascular drugs. *Life Sci* 34:73–80, 1984.

346. Vestal RE, Kornhauser DM, Hollifield JW, Shand DG: Inhibition of propranolol metabolism by chlorpromazine. *Clin Pharmacol Ther* 25:19–24, 1979.

347. Vestal RE, Thummel KE, Musser B, Mercer GD: Cimetidine inhibits theophylline clearance in patients with chronic obstructive pulmonary disease: a study using stable isotope methodology during multiple oral dose administration. *Br J Clin Pharmacol* 15:411–418, 1983.

348. Vincent FM: Phenothiazine-induced phenytoin intoxication (letter). *Ann Intern Med* 93:56–57, 1980.

348a. Wagner F, Kalusche D, Trenk D, Jähnchen E, Roskamm H: Drug interaction between propafenone and metoprolol. *Br J Clin Pharmacol* 24:213–220, 1987.

349. Waldorff S, Andersen JD, Heeboll-Nielson N, Nielsen OG, Moltke E, Sorensen U, Steiness E: Spironolactone-induced changes in digoxin kinetics. *Clin Pharmacol Ther* 24:162–167, 1978.

349a. Watkins PB, Murray SA, Winkelman LG, Heuman DM, Wrighton SA, Guzelian PS: Erithromycin breath test as an assay of glucocorticoid-inducible liver cytochromes P-450. *J Clin Invest* 83:688–97, 1989.

350. Watt AH, Stephens MR, Buss DC, Routledge PA: Amiodarone reduces plasma warfarin clearance in man. *Br J Clin Pharmacol* 20:707–709, 1985.

351. Watts RW, Hetzel DJ, Bochner F, Hallpike JF, Hann CS, Shearman DJC: Lack of interaction between ranitidine and phenytoin. *Br J Clin Pharmacol* 15:499–500, 1983.

352. Weeks CE, Conard GJ, Kvam DC, Fox JM, Chang SF, Paone RP, Lewis GP: The effect of flecainide acetate, a new antiarrhythmic, on plasma digoxin levels. *J Clin Pharmacol* 26:27–31, 1986.

353. Weber WW: The relationship of genetic factors to drug reactions. In Heyler L, Peck NM (eds): *Drug-Induced Diseases*. Excerpta Medica, Amsterdam, vol 4, 1972.

354. Weiner IM, Mudge GJ: Renal tubular mechanisms for excretion of organic acids and bases. *Am J Med* 36:743–762, 1964.

355. Weibert R, Keane W, Shapiro F: Carbenicillin inactivation of aminoglycosides in patients with severe renal failure. *Trans Am Soc Artif Intern Organs* 22:439–443, 1976.

356. Welling PG: Interactions affecting drug absorption. *Clin Pharmacokinet* 9:404–434, 1984.

357. Wesseling H, Mols-Thurkow I: Interaction of diphenylhydantoin (DPH) and tolbutamide in man. *Eur J Clin Pharmacol* 8:75–78, 1975.

357a. Wijnands WJA, Vree TB, Baars AM, van Herwaarden CLA: Steady-state kinetics of the quinolone derivatives ofloxacin, enoxacin, ciprofloxacin and pefloxacin during maintenance treatment with theophylline. *Drugs* 34(1):159–169, 1987.

357b. Wilerson RD, Beck BL: Increase in serum digoxin concentration produced by quinidine does not increase the potential for digoxin-induced ventricular arrhythmias in dogs. *J Pharmacol Exper Ther* 240(2):548–553, 1987.

358. Williams JF, Mathew B: Effect of quinidine on positive inotropic action of digoxin. *Am J Cardiol* 47:1052–1055, 1981.

359. Williams RB, Sherter C: Cardiac complications of tricyclic antidepressant therapy. *Ann Intern Med* 74:395–398, 1971.

359a. Windle J, Prystowsky EN, Miles WM, Heger JJ: Pharmacokinetic and electrophysiologic interactions of amiodarone and procainamide. *Clin Pharmacol Ther* 41:603–610, 1987.

360. Windorfer A Jr, Pringshein W: Studies on the concentration of chloramphenicol in the serum and cerebrospinal fluid of neonates, infants and small children. Reciprocal reactions between chloramphenicol, penicillin and phenobarbitone. *Eur J Pediatr* 124:129–138, 1977.

361. Wing LMH, Miners JO, Birkett DJ, Fornander T, Lillywhite K, Wanwimolruk S: Lidocaine disposition—sex differences and effects of cimetidine. *Clin Pharmacol Ther* 35:695–701, 1984.

362. Wishinsky N, Glasser EJ, Peakal S: Protein interactions of sulfonylurea compounds. *Diabetes* 2 (suppl):18–25, 1962.

363. Wong YY, Ludden TM, Bell RD: Effect of erythromycin on carbamazepine kinetics. *Clin Pharmacol Ther* 33:460–464, 1983.

364. Wright JM, Stokes EF, Sweeny VP: Isoniazid-induced carbamazepine toxicity and vice versa: a double drug interaction. *N Engl J Med* 307:1325–1327, 1982.

365. Wroblewski BA, Singer WD, Whyte J: Carbamazepine-erythromycin interaction. *JAMA* 255:1165–1167, 1986.

365a. Yee GC, McGuire TR: Pharmacokinetic drug interactions with cyclosporin (Part 1). *Clin Pharmacokinet* 19(4):319–332, 1990.

365b. Yee GC, McGuire TR: Pharmacokinetic drug interactions with cyclosporin (Part II). *Clin Pharmacokinet* 19(5):400–415, 1990.

365c. Zhou HH, Anthony LB, Roden DM, Wood AJJ: Quinidine reduces clearance of (+)-propranolol more than (−)-propranolol through marked reduction in 4-hydroxylation. *Clin Pharmacol Ther* 47:686–693, 1990.

365d. Ziemniak JA, Allison N, Boppana VK, Dubb J, Stote R: The effect of acetaminophen on the disposition of fenoldopam: Competition for sulfation. *Clin Pharmacol Ther* 41:275–281, 1987.

366. Zilly W, Breimer DD, Richter E: Induction of drug metabolism in man after rifampin treatment measured by increased hexobarbital and tolbutamide clearance. *Eur J Clin Pharmacol* 9:219–227, 1975.

367. Zuidema J, Hilbers-Modderman ESM, Merkus FWHM: Clinical pharmacokinetics of dapsone. *Clin Pharmacokinet* 11:299–315, 1986.

367a. Zürcher RM, Frey BM, Frey FJ: Impact of ketoconazole on the metabolism of prednisolone. *Clin Pharmacol Ther* 45:366–372, 1989.

CHAPTER 3

Pharmacologic Approach in Patients with Renal Failure

WENDY L. ST. PETER, Pharm.D.
CHARLES E. HALSTENSON, Pharm.D., F.C.C.P.

OVERVIEW

Altered drug disposition and the multiplicity of medications commonly required to treat critically ill patients with concomitant renal disease dictate that therapeutic regimens be individualized for this patient population. Without individualization of drug therapy, serious adverse events or suboptimal outcomes may occur. This chapter reviews the pharmacotherapy of acute and chronic renal failure. A basic overview of physiologic, pharmacokinetic, and pharmacodynamic alterations in renal failure and factors affecting the removal of drugs by various dialysis techniques is included. Recommendations on dosage adjustments of medications commonly used in intensive care unit settings is summarized for patients with various degrees of renal function. In addition, the effect of dialytic therapies on drug clearance is reviewed.

MEASUREMENT OF RENAL FUNCTION

Accurate assessment of renal function in critically ill patients is important in guiding individual adjustment of medication dosages but is often complicated by the presence of acute renal failure and/or multiple organ dysfunction. Unfortunately, there are very few well-controlled studies that compare renal assessment methods in critically ill populations.

Drug elimination by the kidneys depends on glomerular filtration, tubular secretion, and reabsorption. Any or all of these processes may be altered by type of renal disease and or concomitant organ dysfunction. Specifically, different types of renal disease result in different drug clearance rates among patients with the same degree of glomerular filtration (1, 2). Consequently, the nature of a patient's renal disease may be an important consideration when adjusting medication dosages in this population.

Traditionally, estimates of glomerular filtration rate (GFR) have been used to quantify the degree of renal insufficiency without regard to tubular secretion processes. Inulin clearance (CL_{IN}) remains the marker of choice for quantifying glomerular function (3). However, it must be administered intravenously with clearance calculated from multiple timed urine and blood samples, making this method impractical in an intensive care setting. Creatinine clearance (CL_{CR}) is widely used clinically to estimate GFR, but endogenous creatinine is not an ideal marker, as it is also eliminated by tubular secretion and by nonrenal mechanisms (3). In patients with renal insufficiency, the relative contribution of tubular secretion to overall creatinine elimination may increase. Therefore, as glomerular filtration declines, CL_{CR} progressively overestimates GFR (4, 5). Giovannetti and Barsotti (4) computed CL_{CR}/CL_{IN} ratios from a review of the literature in subjects with various degrees of renal dysfunction. They found that the ratio steadily increased to a peak of approximately 1.7 as renal function declined to a CL_{IN} of 30 ml/min. The ratio then decreased as CL_{IN} declined further. This interesting phenomenon may be due to accumulation of uremic inhibitors at low levels of renal function that compete with creatinine for tubular secretion (6). In addition, creatinine production and excretion may not be constant over

Table 3.1. Equations for Creatinine Clearance Estimation[a]

Cockcroft & Gault (17)

Male: $CL_{CR} = \dfrac{(140 - age)\ Wt}{72 \cdot Scr}$

Female: $CL_{CR} = CL_{CR}\ male \cdot 0.85$

Mawer et al. (16)

Male: $CL_{CR} = \dfrac{Wt\ [29.3 - (0.203 \cdot Age)]\ [1 - (0.03 \cdot Scr)]}{72 \cdot Scr}$

Female: $CL_{CR} = \dfrac{Wt\ [25.3 - (0.174 \cdot Age)]\ [1 - (0.03 \cdot Scr)]}{14.4 \cdot Scr}$

[a] Age is in years; Wt is actual body weight in kilograms; Scr is serum creatinine concentration.

time, particularly in acutely ill patients with a variety of disease states (3, 7, 8). In 1990 Freysz and colleagues (7) found a poor correlation between CL_{CR} and CL_{IN} in multiple trauma patients, demonstrating that absolute values of serum creatinine or CL_{CR} may not be particularly useful or representative of GFR in this population.

Several medications used in the ICU setting can create a pseudorenal failure scenario (9). Cimetidine, trimethoprim and, perhaps, salicylates interfere with the secretion of creatinine into the kidney tubules and increase serum creatinine concentrations without an attendant decrease in renal function. If any of these agents are instituted during hospitalization, the increase in serum creatinine may be erroneously interpreted as declining renal function. Interestingly, cimetidine may be useful in the clinical setting to improve the accuracy and precision of GFR estimation methods (10–12). Several cephalosporin antibiotics, methyldopa, high-dose furosemide, and lactose have been reported to interfere with creatinine measurement with analytical systems utilizing the Jaffe reaction (colorimetric method) (9). Although newer, more specific enzymatic methods are now available for creatinine determination (13), many hospitals continue to use colorimetric methods because they are less expensive (8).

The 24-hour urine collection for calculation of CL_{CR} remains the standard against which other methods of measuring or estimating CL_{CR} are compared. Accurate 24-hour collections are difficult to accomplish, and some investigators have evaluated shorter collection periods. Bauman and colleagues reported that CL_{CR} determined from an 8-hour urine collection were within 20% of the 24-hour value in 10 surgical intensive care unit (SICU) patients (14). A number of formulae have been developed for estimating CL_{CR} based on serum creatinine. Luke and associates (15) demonstrated that measured CL_{CR} by timed urine collections correlated well with CL_{CR} estimated by the methods of Mawer (16) and Cockcroft and Gault (17) (Table 3.1) in patients with stable renal function.

Some of these formulae may be less accurate in certain patient populations, particularly in acutely ill patients with unstable renal function. Large discrepancies between common methods used to measure or estimate CL_{CR} in ICU patients have been reported (8, 18, 19). Chow and Schweizer (20) compared several methods of CL_{CR} estimation, using simulated data for subjects with improving or declining renal function. They found that CL_{CR} calculated, using a 24-hour urine creatinine excretion along with a midpoint serum creatinine concentration, produced the lowest error. These data

were validated in seven postrenal transplant patients with improving renal function; therefore, it is difficult to extrapolate these data to patients with declining renal function and other patient populations.

Aminoglycoside clearance has been used clinically by pharmacists to estimate GFR and thus aid in the adjustment of other medications in various degrees of renal dysfunction. Aminoglycosides are primarily eliminated by renal mechanisms, and tubular secretion of aminoglycosides is limited (21). Recently, a well-designed trial evaluated several methods of estimating GFR and compared them to CL_{IN}, the gold standard method for evaluating GFR, in 10 critically ill patients (22). The GFR calculated from aminoglycoside serum concentration data showed a high correlation coefficient, as well as low absolute errors, when compared with CL_{IN}. The aminoglycoside method outperformed GFR estimates by the traditional 24-hour urine creatinine collection, as well as by the Cockcroft-Gault equation (16).

Methods for estimating GFR have not been rigorously compared to CL_{IN} in a large critically ill population (8). It is important for medical practitioners to be aware of the numerous limitations of using CL_{CR} to predict renal function in this patient population and to be familiar with the serum/urine creatinine assay that is being utilized at their institutions to ensure accurate creatinine concentrations. Estimating GFR using aminoglycoside clearance may be a practical method to use in ICU patients receiving aminoglycosides. Medical practitioners need to use sound clinical judgment in determining adequacy of renal function; multiple methods may be needed to predict renal function in individual cases.

ACUTE RENAL FAILURE

CRITICAL CARE IMPLICATIONS

Acute renal failure is a common disease occurring primarily in the hospital setting, and it is frequently iatrogenic. Acute renal failure is most often acquired in acute care facilities, reaching an incidence of 2 to 5% of hospitalized patients (23). Prerenal azotemia and acute tubular necrosis account for the majority of cases. Prerenal and postrenal failure not caused by malignant neoplasms carry an excellent prognosis when recognized early and treated appropriately. In contrast, acute tubular necrosis continues to be associated with high mortality. The risk of death in acute tubular necrosis correlates most closely with the underlying disease and its complications. Of those patients who survive acute tubular necrosis, renal function eventually improves enough in 99% to obviate the need for chronic dialysis (24).

The causes of acute renal failure may be divided into three broad categories: prerenal; intrinsic renal; and postrenal failure. Prerenal refers to a reduction in glomerular filtration rate that is secondary to diminished renal blood flow. Intrinsic renal causes are those that directly injure the renal parenchyma. This category encompasses a wide variety of systemic and primary renal diseases and includes acute tubular necrosis. Postrenal causes include obstruction of urine flow anywhere from the renal pelvis to the distal urethra.

Renal failure resulting from a wide variety of medications arises from either direct nephrotoxic damage (e.g., aminoglycoside nephrotoxicity), intrarenal and/or extrarenal hemodynamic effects (e.g., nonsteroidal antiinflammatory drugs and angiotensin-converting enzyme inhibitors), intrarenal tubular obstruction, renal inflammation (glomerular or interstitial), or a combination of the above mechanisms.

Acute renal failure is manifested by an increase in serum creatinine (S_{cr}) and blood urea nitrogen (BUN) and is frequently accompanied by diminished urine output. An increase in S_{cr} of 0.5 mg/dl or greater over 2 to 3 days when the baseline S_{cr} is less than 3.0 mg/dl is a commonly accepted guideline for the diagnosis of acute renal failure (25, 26).

A rapid deterioration of renal function is frequently accompanied by the development of acute fluid and electrolyte disturbances, severe azotemia, and various life-threatening complications. As a result, early and aggressive therapeutic intervention is extremely important in the management of acute renal failure. Principles of treatment include prevention of iatrogenic renal insults in patients with identified risks, an aggressive search for the etiology of renal dysfunction, and early diagnosis. The ability of diuretics, dopamine, and other agents to prevent or modify the course of acute renal failure remains unproven. Nutritional support, an aggressive search for and treatment of infection, as well as early dialysis may limit complications and alter the clinical course of acute renal failure.

THERAPEUTIC MANAGEMENT

Oliguria/Fluid Imbalance

Volume status must be assessed rapidly in patients with acute renal failure. Restoration of normal plasma volume is essential in patients who are volume-depleted to reverse prerenal acute renal failure (27). In contrast, patients who are volume-overloaded must be promptly treated to avoid complications such as pulmonary edema and respiratory arrest. Patients who are nonoliguric may respond to diuretics. However, patients with oliguria or anuria who do not respond to diuretics may need emergent dialysis to prevent life-threatening complications of volume overload.

The conversion of oliguria or anuria to nonoliguric acute renal failure has been associated with increased survival and reduced complications in patients with acute tubular necrosis (28). Therefore, several agents, including mannitol, furosemide, and dopamine, have been evaluated as potential modalities to alter the character and course of acute renal failure.

Studies of these pharmacologic agents have yielded controversial results that may be due to the uncontrolled design of the trials, small numbers of patients treated, variability in the patient populations, variable diagnostic criteria used, and markedly different therapeutic regimens utilized.

Mannitol protects the kidney from several types of nephrotoxic insults. The effect may be secondary to: (*a*) enhancement of solute excretion (29); (*b*) decreased cell swelling (30); (*c*) inhibition of tubular obstruction (31, 32); and (*d*) vasodilation (33, 34). It is often difficult to determine whether the effect of mannitol is direct, or whether it is secondary to the correction of volume status. Mannitol given at high doses has been reported to cause volume depletion and acute renal failure (35–37). Therefore, mannitol should be discontinued if initial doses are ineffective.

The protective effect of furosemide in acute renal failure may result from one or more of the following mechanisms: (*a*) decreased tubular obstruction; (*b*) suppressed tubuloglomerular feedback; and (*c*) renal vasodilatation (38). Although the intravenous administration of furosemide to patients with established acute renal failure increases urine flow (39–41), decreases the time of oliguria/anuria (41, 42), as well as reduces the need for dialysis (42–45), it does not appear to alter mortality (39, 40).

Despite the evidence that diuretics may have a minimal effect on the prevention of acute renal failure, they are commonly administered in this setting since the benefits potentially outweigh the risks. Mannitol is relatively nontoxic when administered appropriately. Complications of high-dose loop diuretics occur rarely and include permanent and severe deafness and volume depletion (39, 40). Therefore, mannitol, furosemide, or both may be used if blood pressure and volume status are adequate (Table 3.2). Although these treatment modalities may not improve the prognosis of acute renal failure, they may increase urine flow and thereby assist in nutritional and fluid management. Further discussion on diuretics can be found in Chapter 37.

Low-dose dopamine (1 to 5 µg/kg/min) may protect the kidney in acute renal failure by decreasing renal vascular resistance and increasing renal blood flow without altering peripheral vascular resistance and systemic arterial pressure (46–48). Although low-dose dopamine therapy has been used by several investigators to prevent or treat acute renal failure, its therapeutic efficacy remains unproved (49–51).

Table 3.2. Agents Used in the Treatment of Acute Renal Failure[a,b]

Agent	Dosage	Special Considerations
Mannitol (20%)	25 g i.v. (as a 15–25% solution) over 5–10 min. May repeat in 1 hr if no response. If urine output follows, mannitol can be continued as an intermittent infusion or as a continuous infusion. Maximum daily dosage: 100–200 g.	Monitor urine output and serum electrolytes to avoid fluid and electrolyte imbalances particularly fluid overload. Hemodialysis is indicated for fluid overload and hyperosmolality.
Furosemide	100 mg i.v.; if no response within 1 hr, 200 mg i.v.; if no response within 1 hr, 400 mg i.v.. Maximum suggested dose: 500–1000 mg	Monitor for fluid and electrolyte disturbances; rate should not exceed 4 mg/min as hearing loss may result if infused too rapidly.
Dopamine	1–5 µg/kg/min	Monitor urine output

[a] Adapted from 52 Heim-Duthoy KL, Kalil RSN, Kasiske BL: Acute renal failure. In DiPiro JT, Talbert RL, Hayes PE, Yee GC, Matzke GR, Posey LM (eds): Pharmacotherapy: a Pathophysiologic Approach. Appleton-Lange, Norwalk, CT, 1993, pp 660–672.
[b] Agents may expect beneficial effect when used within 24 hours following the onset of oliguria.

Table 3.3.   Agents Used in the Treatment of Hyperkalemia[a]

Agent	Mechanism	Dosage	Onset of Action	Special Considerations
Calcium Gluconate (10%)	Direct Antagonism	10–20 ml i.v. over 2–5 min	Immediate	Monitor with continuous ECG; calcium and sodium bicarbonate are incompatible.
Sodium bicarbonate (8.4%)	Redistribution	50 ml i.v. over 1–5 min; can be repeated	Minutes	Alkaline load.
Glucose/Insulin	Redistribution	2–3 g glucose/1 unit regular insulin; bolus: 50 ml D50W with 10 U regular insulin.	Minutes	Monitor blood sugar to prevent hypoglycemia.
Sodium polystyrene sulfonate (SPS, Kayexalate)	Increased elimination	15–60 g p.o. or rectally as retention enema up to 3 to 4 times/day; Sorbitol to be given concomitantly with SPS p.o.	2–12 hr	Approximately 1 mEq K+ adsorbed per gram of kayexalate administered. Monitor for fluid, electrolyte and GI disturbances; concomitant sorbitol to be administered for prevention of fecal impaction. Rectal route less effective.
B₂ agonists	Redistribution	Nebulized treatment of 20 mg albuterol in 4 ml normal saline inhaled over 10 minutes	30 min	Potassium-lowering effect extremely variable among patients. Combined therapy with insulin and glucose may be more effective than either therapy alone.
Dialysis	Increased elimination	—	2–4 hr	Feasibility includes appropriate access and availability.

[a] Compiled from references 52 and 203.

The primary method for preventing volume overload is fluid restriction. Fluid intake should approximate total fluid losses, including insensible losses, and, therefore, must be individualized. Body weight should be used as a guide for fluid replacement, but interpretation of body weight should take into account the fact that patients with acute renal failure may be extremely catabolic. Catabolic patients may be expected to lose up to ½ kg/day in fat and muscle mass (52). Serum sodium may be used as a gauge for water administration. A decreased serum sodium concentration results from water excess; therefore, more stringent water restriction is needed in this setting. If hyponatremia is severe and is associated with symptoms, hypertonic saline or dialysis may need to be used. An increased serum sodium concentration results from a loss of water that exceeds any loss of sodium and may be normalized by increasing the intake of free water.

Electrolyte and Acid-Base Disturbances

Hyperkalemia is a frequent problem in acute renal failure. Severe hyperkalemia (serum potassium concentration > 6 mEq/liter may be life-threatening. Therefore, the treatment of hyperkalemia should be given the highest priority when first evaluating a patient with acute renal failure. Although serum potassium concentrations may be used to monitor therapy, the best measure of severity is the ECG. A markedly increased serum potassium concentration in conjunction with ECG abnormalities (peaked T waves, prolonged QRS interval, etc.) is indicative of severe and urgent hyperkalemia, which must be treated emergently (Table 3.3). Calcium gluconate can be administered intravenously in conjunction with continuous ECG monitoring. Calcium gluconate directly antagonizes potassium cardiotoxicity and has an immediate onset of action.

The intravenous administration of glucose, insulin, and sodium bicarbonate is also effective in treating hyperkalemia. This combination shifts potassium intracellularly while sodium antagonizes the cardiotoxicity of potassium. Sodium bicarbonate should be administered slowly, since fluid overload may be exacerbated, and increases in plasma osmolality may actually shift intracellular potassium into the plasma.

Exogenous potassium administration, including potassium salts of other medications and potassium-sparing diuretics, should be avoided. The relatively slow-acting potassium-exchange resins may be used to treat hyperkalemia in patients with high serum potassium concentrations not associated with ECG changes. Sodium polystyrene sulfonate (Kayexalate, Winthrop-Breon) may be given orally or rectally as a retention enema. Sorbitol suspension is often administered concomitantly with oral exchange resins to prevent fecal impaction. Potassium-exchange resins will remove 1 mEq of potassium per gram when administered orally or ½ mEq/g when given as a retention enema. The onset of action after oral administration is approximately 2 hours and may be slower after rectal administration. Complications associated with the use of exchange resins include electrolyte imbalances, fluid overload secondary to the high sodium load (4.1 mEq/g), gastrointestinal upset, and fecal impaction.

The pharmacologic management of hyperkalemia discussed above is either slow, as in the case of polystyrene exchange resins, or temporary, as in the case with maneuvers that shift potassium into the cells. Hemodialysis is the most effective way to remove excess potassium from the body rapidly. Therefore, emergency hemodialysis should be considered in cases of severe hyperkalemia.

Severe metabolic acidosis (pH < 7.2) also requires prompt treatment. The correction of metabolic acidosis may help to prevent life-threatening hyperkalemia. Although sodium bicarbonate may be administered, dialysis is generally necessary because of the consequences of excessive sodium bicarbonate administration, i.e., fluid overload and pulmonary edema.

Calcium and phosphorus imbalances are also common in patients with acute renal failure. Twitching and convulsions may occur as a result of hypocalcemia, as well as from other electrolyte and fluid imbalances. Hyperphosphatemia may be prevented or treated by the administration of phosphate-binding antacids with meals. Antacids will chelate ingested phosphate in the intestine and prevent phosphorus absorption. However, magnesium antacids should be avoided since magnesium excretion is impaired in acute renal failure.

Treatment of hypocalcemia is generally reserved for patients in acute renal failure who are symptomatic, i.e., have tetany and cardiac arrhythmias. Symptomatic hypocalcemia is unusual in acute renal failure, except when acute renal failure is caused by rhabdomyolysis. Oral calcium, as well as parenteral, calcium may be administered in conjunction with appropriate cardiac monitoring.

Malnutrition

The caloric and protein requirements for acute renal failure patients are usually great but are highly variable and dependent on the underlying cause(s) of acute renal failure. Delivery of necessary nutrients often requires large volumes of intravenous fluids, which can exacerbate volume overload. Excessive exogenous protein supplementation may result in the accumulation of uremic waste products. On the other hand, an adequate supply of carbohydrates will minimize increases in nitrogenous waste products caused by endogenous protein catabolism.

The intake of calories, protein, and fluid may be more liberal for patients receiving dialysis. Excessive exogenous protein administration may exacerbate uremia, but protein is necessary to maintain a positive nitrogen balance and to decrease the hypercatabolic state frequently seen in acute renal failure patients (53–55). It is often a mistake to limit hyperalimentation in patients with acute renal failure in order to limit nitrogenous waste products, as hemodialysis therapy can be provided to correct nitrogenous waste product accumulation.

Unfortunately, the optimal amino acid/carbohydrate formula has not emerged from the multiple trials that have been conducted. Although existing data are conflicting, it appears that balanced solutions of amino acids may be beneficial for patients with acute renal failure and, ultimately, improve their clinical course (56).

Complications

Bacterial sepsis is a common cause of acute renal failure, and in acute renal failure from other causes, secondary infection is a frequent complication. Indeed, infection is the leading cause of death in patients with acute renal failure (57). The urinary tract and pulmonary system are the most common infection sites. Infectious complications of acute renal failure may result from, or be exacerbated by, abnormal host-defense mechanisms caused by impaired leukocyte function and depressed cell-mediated immunity. Uremia, acidosis, malnutrition, and various invasive procedures may predispose acute renal failure patients to infection, as well as increase severity of infection. Furthermore, the presence of an active infection may be masked due to an impaired immunologic response. Thus, the management of the patient with acute renal failure should include measures aimed at prevention of infection. If infection is suspected, an aggressive therapeutic regimen, including multiple bactericidal antibiotics, is often required.

Indwelling urinary catheters should not be used indefinitely, since the risk of urinary tract infections with their use increases over time. If urinary retention is present, intermittent catheterization may be used. Although hemodynamic monitoring with intravascular catheters may be necessary until the patient's cardiovascular status has stabilized, noninvasive clinical methods should be substituted as soon as possible. Patient mobilization and respiratory therapy should be initiated early to reduce the risk of pulmonary infection. Fungal infections may occur as a result of aggressive prophylactic antibiotic use in these patients. Oral antifungal agents may thus be indicated to prevent overgrowth of *Candida* species.

Nausea and vomiting are commonly encountered GI problems in acute renal failure patients and may be avoided by the early institution of dialysis. GI complications, including stress ulceration and GI bleeding, are not infrequent in these patients. The use of antacids may be effective in preventing these complications (58). H_2 blockers may be used alone or in combination with antacids for the prevention of GI bleeding (59, 60). Sucralfate has also been shown to be effective in preventing stress ulcers in critically ill patients (61) and may produce less incidence of nosocomial pneumonia (62). However, sucralfate acts as a phosphate-binding agent, and phosphorous concentrations should be monitored (63).

Cardiovascular complications that may occur with acute renal failure include hypertension, hypotension, cardiac failure, pulmonary edema, arrhythmias, and pericarditis. An increase in blood pressure may develop secondary to volume overload and may resolve with the initiation of dialysis. Cardiac failure and arrhythmias may result from volume overload, electrolyte imbalances, and/or hypertension. Correction of volume and electrolyte imbalances, as well as pharmacologic intervention, may be necessary in the management of cardiac failure and arrhythmias. On the other hand, volume depletion or sepsis may cause hypotension. Although pericarditis may occasionally complicate acute renal failure, it occurs less frequently than during chronic renal failure and may improve with frequent dialysis.

Neurologic manifestations of acute renal failure are variable and may be attributed to disorders of fluid and electrolytes, uremia, and/or drug toxicity. These abnormalities include lethargy, somnolence, coma, confusion, agitation, neuromuscular irritability, and seizures. These complications usually improve with dialysis therapy.

It is of critical importance that renally eliminated drugs be adjusted appropriately.

Current Research and Experimental Therapeutics

Various therapeutic modalities have been experimentally utilized to reverse acute renal failure by altering the resistance of renal vasculature or injury of epithelial cells (64). Renal hypoperfusion, secondary to renal vasoconstriction, has been proposed as a cause of renal failure. Therefore, the use of renal vasodilators may be beneficial in acute renal failure when renal blood flow is reduced. Investigators have explored the use of dopamine, calcium channel blockers (64–68), prostaglandin E_2, and prostacyclin (69–71). Furthermore, substances that block the effect of renal vasoconstrictors may ultimately produce the same result. Such inhibitors include adenosine (72, 73), thromboxane A_2, and angiotensin (64). Adjunctive therapy with intravenous human immunoglobulin G has been demonstrated to decrease mortality in a small number of patients with acute renal failure (74).

DIALYSIS

INDICATIONS

Hyperkalemia, volume overload, severe acidosis, pericarditis, and CNS symptoms are all indications for dialysis. In the setting of acute renal failure, it is better to initiate dialysis early to prevent uremic complications than to use dialysis later to treat complications. This practice is supported by data showing fewer complications when dialysis is initiated early (29, 75, 76).

METHOD OF DIALYSIS

Intermittent hemodialysis and continuous peritoneal dialysis remain the mainstays of dialytic therapy for acute renal failure. Slow continuous hemofiltration is a relatively new technique that employs a small hemofilter and uses the patient's arterial pressure as the driving force for the system (77). The filter can be hooked to wall suction if ultrafiltration is needed. This system eliminates the need for a sophisticated dialysis delivery system, blood pump, and air detectors. Slow continuous hemodialysis and continuous hemodiafiltration, a combination of hemodialysis and hemofiltration, have been described in the treatment of acute renal failure, but their role is yet to be defined (77). In a series of 49 patients with acute renal failure treated by spontaneous arteriovenous or pump-assisted venovenous hemofiltration, 37% survived. However, 63% of the patients died despite good control of uremia. Sepsis was the direct cause of death in 42% of the patients (78).

Hemodialysis is the most efficient of the above methods, being 10 to 20 times more efficient than peritoneal dialysis and slow continuous hemofiltration. This method allows prompt correction of life-threatening hyperkalemia and volume overload, as well as short treatment times. Its major disadvantages include a propensity to induce hypotension and arrhythmias.

Peritoneal dialysis offers the advantage of more gentle dialysis, less cardiovascular instability, and no anticoagulation. Its main disadvantages are its relative inefficiency, requiring long or continuous treatment, and the risk of peritoneal infection.

Although hemodynamic stability and simplicity make slow continuous hemofiltration attractive, it also requires continuous treatment and continuous systemic anticoagulation. Ultimately, the choice of the dialysis method for the individual patient will depend on the clinical situation and the technical expertise of the treatment center.

ALTERATIONS IN THE PHARMACOKINETICS OF MEDICATIONS USED IN THE PATIENTS WITH ACUTE RENAL FAILURE

Although the pharmacokinetic changes in patients with chronic renal failure have been well-described, little information is available on alterations in the pharmacokinetics of medications in patients with acute renal failure. There have been some recent investigations that have evaluated differences that may occur in the disposition of medications in patients with acute renal failure. In a small number of patients, the nonrenal clearance of vancomycin appears to be higher in the early phases of acute renal failure and appears to decrease with the duration of renal failure to that observed in chronic renal failure (79). Similarly, the nonrenal clearance of imipenem differs in patients with acute versus chronic renal failure (80). Hepatic function may be impaired secondary to decreases in systemic blood pressure or mean arterial pressure (81). Therefore, there may also be issues with medications that are eliminated by both renal and hepatic (biliary) excretion.

These findings suggest that application of dosing recommendations for other medications whose elimination are dependent on normal renal function may not be applicable to patients with acute renal failure. The majority of these recommendations were derived from pharmacokinetic studies performed in patients with stable renal insufficiency or failure and not in patients with acute renal dysfunction.

CHRONIC RENAL FAILURE

CRITICAL CARE IMPLICATIONS

End-stage renal disease patients are often admitted to the hospital with complex medical problems. In addition to renal disease, many dialysis patients have comorbid conditions, including diabetes, atherosclerotic cardiovascular disease, pulmonary disease, and hypertension (82). The presence of multiple medical problems often results in complex medication regimens, which may include antianginal therapy, antihypertensives, coumadin, aspirin, and insulin. Acutely ill dialysis patients present even greater medical complexities. Additional medications prescribed for treatment of acute illness have the potential for pharmacokinetic and pharmacodynamic interactions with chronic medication regimens.

PHYSIOLOGIC CHANGES IN RENAL FAILURE

The normal kidney serves both excretory and metabolic functions and is involved in the active production of various substances, including renin, erythropoietin, and 1,25-dihydroxyvitamin D_3 (calcitriol). Generally, a patient remains asymptomatic during initial loss of renal function. As GFR decreases to about 50% of normal, accumulation of creatinine and blood urea nitrogen (BUN) occurs. When CL_{CR} is reduced

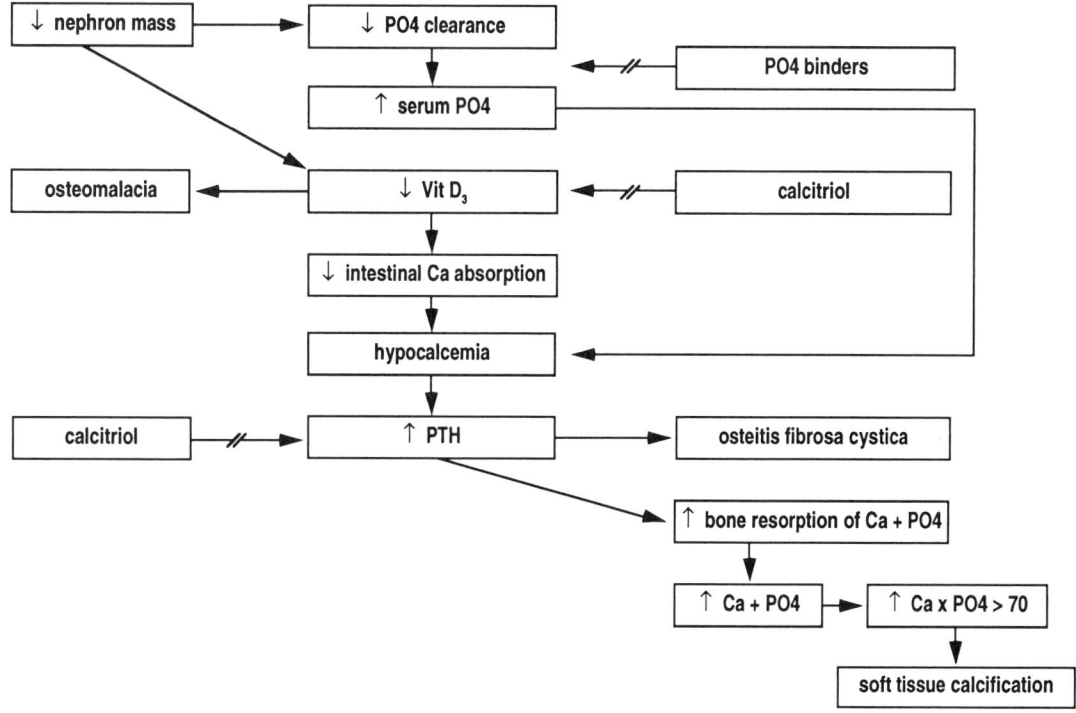

Figure 3.1. Pathophysiology of renal bone disease. (From Vargas-Ruiz M, St. Peter WL: Pharmacotherapeutic considerations in hemodialysis patients. *Wellcome Trends Hosp Pharm* 15(3):4, 5, and 7.)

to less than 30 ml/min, patients may become symptomatic with complaints of fatigue, decreased energy, cold intolerance, abnormal taste sensation, and decreased appetite. Metabolic and laboratory derangements, such as hyperphosphatemia, hypocalcemia, hyperkalemia, metabolic acidosis, and anemia, commonly occur. When end-stage renal disease (ESRD) is eminent (CL_{CR} of approximately 10 ml/min), patients may experience additional symptoms, including malaise, generalized pruritus, dyspnea, nausea and vomiting, and confusion. At this stage dialysis is indicated to remove uremic waste products, eliminate excess fluid, and correct laboratory abnormalities and metabolic acidosis (83).

Metabolic Acidosis

A clinically significant metabolic acidosis rarely develops until CL_{CR} drops below 20 ml/min. Until that point the kidney can produce enough ammonia to buffer excreted acid. Decreased urinary buffering capacity results in a positive hydrogen ion balance that exhibits systemically as a low plasma bicarbonate concentration (83).

Water Homeostasis

The kidney loses the ability to dilute or concentrate urine in chronic renal failure, and urine osmolality is fixed at approximately 300 mOsm/liter. Water balance is usually maintained, and urine volumes are fixed at approximately 2 liters/day. Fluid restrictions are usually unnecessary if the patient has an intact thirst mechanism and sodium intake is controlled, because he/she will drink enough fluids to maintain a normal serum osmolality. However, patients lack the ability to effectively handle larger volumes of oral or intravenous fluids.

Diuretic therapy may become necessary in some patients to maintain a normal water balance (83).

Sodium and Potassium Homeostasis

As nephron loss occurs, sodium balance is usually maintained by a progressive increase in the fractional excretion of sodium (FENa). Balance is maintained at the expense of volume expansion. Systemic vascular resistance increases by means of an unclear mechanism(s), and hypertension may result. The ability of the kidney to adjust to abrupt changes in sodium intake is impaired; therefore, sodium restriction is not generally recommended beyond a no-added-salt diet unless the patient is edematous or hypertensive (83).

Potassium balance is usually maintained until CL_{CR} is reduced to 10 ml/min because aldosterone-mediated increases in tubular secretion generally can keep pace with potassium intake. Potassium is also excreted through the colon by an aldosterone-mediated mechanism, which becomes important in patients with ESRD (83, 84).

Calcium and Phosphorous Homeostasis

In ESRD, phosphorous excretion is impaired, leading to an increase in serum phosphate. The normal physiological response to hyperphosphatemia is hypocalcemia (85). The kidney, gastrointestinal tract, and bone are the major organs involved in calcium balance. However, bone is quantitatively the body's primary source of calcium (86). Decreased serum calcium stimulates parathyroid hormone (PTH) release, which results in bone resorption through increased osteoclastic activity (87). Secondary hyperparathyroidism results and is manifested by a progressive increase in fibrous bone tissue that is referred to as osteitis fibrosa cystica (85). Bone resorption will result in increased serum concentrations of both phosphorus and calcium. If the serum calcium (mg/dl)-phosphorus (mg/dl) product exceeds 70 to 75, metastatic soft tissue calcification may occur (88). ESRD patients can not adequately synthesize calcitriol, the active form of vitamin D, from less-active precursors (vitamins D_2, D_3, or 25-hydroxyvitamin D). Osteomalacia occurs when bone mineralization is impaired from decreased serum calcitriol. Calcitriol deficiency also results in decreased calcium absorption from the gastrointestinal tract, leading to hypocalcemia that stimulates the release of PTH. Thus, altered synthesis of calcitriol by diseased kidneys also plays a role in the pathogenesis of secondary hyperparathyroidism and renal bone disease (85). Figure 3.1 summarizes the interrelationships of the two main pathways involved in the pathogenesis of renal osteodystrophy.

A rational pharmacotherapeutic approach helps dialysis patients maintain normal daily lives. Major therapeutic interventions in chronic renal failure and dialysis patients include: diuretics; systemic alkalinizing agents; phosphate-binding medications; erythropoietin; vitamin D analogues; vitamin and iron supplements; and antipruritic and muscle cramp medications.

MEDICATIONS COMMONLY USED IN CHRONIC RENAL FAILURE AND DIALYSIS PATIENTS

Diuretic Therapy

Diuretic therapy is commonly prescribed in patients approaching ESRD when moderate fluid restriction alone fails to control fluid balance. Loop or high-ceiling diuretics such as furosemide or bumetanide are the agents of choice, as thiazide diuretics generally lose their diuretic efficacy at CL_{CR} between 30 and 50 ml/min (89). Addition of a thiazide diuretic or metolazone may be indicated if the patient fails to respond to loop diuretics alone (90, 91). If combination therapy is initiated, frequent monitoring of urine output and serum electrolytes is necessary as a profound diuresis, natriuresis and kaliuresis may result (92). A further discussion on diuretics can be found under Acute Renal Failure in this chapter and in chapter 37.

Treatment of Metabolic Acidosis

Treatment of metabolic acidosis in ESRD patients is necessary to prevent bone demineralization, reduction in cardiac contractility, and cardiac irritability. Metabolic acidosis may also contribute to a decreased exercise tolerance, hyperkalemia, and fatigue (83). Patients who receive regular chronic dialysis treatments rarely require additional alkali therapy. Alkalinizing agents are indicated in predialysis patients who develop a metabolic acidosis. Usually, treatment is initiated when the serum bicarbonate concentration falls below 20 mEq/liter. Dosages of sodium citrate and citric acid solutions (Shohl's Solution or Bicitra) or sodium bicarbonate tablets are titrated to maintain a serum bicarbonate concentration above 20 mEq/liter.

Control of Hyperphosphatemia

Phosphate removal with hemodialysis is very poor (88). To achieve control of hyperphosphatemia, two modalities are used:

(1) dietary phosphorus restriction (800 to 1000 mg/day) and (2) use of phosphate-binding medications. The combination of both treatment modalities is almost always necessary to maintain serum phosphate homeostasis in ESRD patients. Currently, there are several aluminum- and calcium-containing phosphate-binding medications on the market. Hydroxy and carbonate salts of aluminum are the most potent phosphate-binding agents (93). Aluminum salts were the gold standard treatment for phosphorus control for many years. However, aluminum can accumulate in patients with renal disease during high-dose chronic use and has resulted in signs of aluminum toxicity (encephalopathy, aluminum bone disease, and anemia) (88). Therefore, it is important to avoid or minimize the use of aluminum-containing products whenever possible.

Calcium-containing salts used as phosphate binders include calcium acetate, calcium carbonate, and calcium citrate. Calcium carbonate is very inexpensive, contains a high amount of elemental calcium, and is generally well-tolerated (88). However, large quantities of calcium carbonate are usually needed to maintain adequate phosphorus control (94), and patients are at high risk of hypercalcemia unless low calcium dialysate baths are concurrently used (95). Calcium acetate is more effective in binding phosphate than either calcium carbonate or calcium citrate (88). Calcium acetate appears to bind twice the amount of phosphorus per amount of calcium ingested. However, the incidence of hypercalcemia appears to be the same, as compared to that of calcium carbonate, even though the amount of calcium absorbed is less with calcium acetate (96). In addition, gastrointestinal intolerance is higher than with calcium carbonate (96, 97). Calcium citrate has a binding capacity similar to that of calcium carbonate (98); however, calcium citrate increases the solubility and absorption of aluminum, and concurrent use should be avoided (99).

The therapeutic goal is to maintain a high normal serum phosphorus concentration while maintaining an adequate protein diet. Phosphate-binding medications should be given with meals for maximum efficacy. When dialysis patients are maintained on phosphate-binding medications, serum laboratory monitoring of phosphorus, calcium, albumin, and serum aluminum (if aluminum-containing phosphate binders are used) should be performed frequently.

Control of Calcium Balance

The therapeutic goal is to maintain a high normal serum calcium concentration to suppress PTH release. Serum calcium concentration is affected by the dialysate calcium concentration, calcium, and vitamin D supplements. Calcium carbonate contains more elemental calcium, mole per mole, than calcium acetate or calcium citrate and is the least expensive calcium supplement when a generic brand is used. When calcium carbonate is used as a calcium supplement, the tablets should be taken between meals, rather than with meals, for optimal absorption. Oral and intravenous calcitriol (or, occasionally, other vitamin D analogues) are also used to increase calcium absorption from the gastrointestinal tract.

Vitamin D Supplementation

Calcitriol (vitamin D_3) is necessary for calcium absorption from the gastrointestinal tract, for direct suppression of PTH release, and for normal bone mineralization (100). Pharmacologic doses of calcitriol are used in the treatment and prevention of renal osteodystrophy (93). Calcitriol is currently available in oral and parenteral forms. Oral calcitriol is more effective than parenteral calcitriol in enhancing calcium absorption from the gastrointestinal tract, but hypercalcemia is a common side effect (93). Parenteral calcitriol may be more effective than oral calcitriol in directly suppressing PTH release from the parathyroid gland. Chronic high-maintenance doses of intravenous calcitriol have been shown to effectively suppress PTH secretion in hemodialysis patients with secondary hyperparathyroidism refractory to conventional treatment, which included oral calcitriol (101). Interestingly, short-term studies evaluating large doses of oral calcitriol (1 to 3 times weekly) have been shown to favorably decrease PTH (102–104). These studies support the theory that obtaining high blood concentrations of calcitriol, rather than route of administration, appears to be the major factor in PTH suppression. Long-term studies are needed to evaluate the safety and continued efficacy of high-dose oral calcitriol.

Anemia of Chronic Renal Failure

The normochromic, normocytic anemia associated with chronic renal failure (CRF) has been attributed to multiple factors: inadequate erythropoietin production; blood loss through dialysis; decreased red blood cell survival time; aluminum intoxication; folic acid or iron deficiency; and inhibition of erythropoiesis by uremia (105, 106). Erythropoietin deficiency is the major mechanism for anemia of CRF (105). Blood transfusions and anabolic steroids were the traditional method of treatment for anemia in CRF patients. However, recombinant erythropoietin (epoetin) therapy has become the standard for treatment of anemia of chronic renal disease since its release in 1989. Epoetin stimulates the maturation and differentiation of red blood cells and produces a dose-dependent rise in hematocrit (107). The benefits of epoetin therapy in this population include increased exercise tolerance, improved quality of life (108, 109), and decreased need for red blood cell transfusions (110). Starting doses of epoetin range between 40 and 100 units/kg intravenously or subcutaneously, 1 to 3 times a week after each hemodialysis. Hematocrit values need to be monitored weekly until stabilized into the target range (30 to 33%) (111). Common side effects with epoetin therapy include hypertension and, less commonly, "flu-like" symptoms (110). When epoetin therapy is initiated, iron stores decrease secondary to increased erythropoietic response. The majority of dialysis patients given epoetin therapy should also receive iron supplements to prevent iron deficiency (112). The goal of iron therapy in dialysis patients is to maintain a serum ferritin greater than 100 ng/ml and transferrin saturation greater than 20%. For more information on erythropoietin, see Chapter 37.

ALTERATIONS IN PHARMACOKINETICS AND PHARMACODYNAMICS OF MEDICATIONS IN CHRONIC RENAL FAILURE

Bioavailability and Absorption

Bioavailability is a measure of the extent of drug appearance into the systemic circulation after extravascular adminis-

tration. There are only a few well-designed studies that specifically address the issue of drug bioavailability or absorption in patients with renal failure, using intravenous administration as a control (113–115). Instead, apparent bioavailability is often assessed by comparing peak plasma concentrations, time-to-peak concentrations and area under the plasma-concentration time curve, or fractional urine excretion (116). This makes it difficult to determine whether altered drug bioavailability in renal failure stems from changes in absorption or in first-pass metabolism.

Theoretically, drug bioavailability could be altered in renal failure due to multiple factors. Gastrointestinal symptoms such as nausea, vomiting, and diarrhea are common in uremia, and all may affect drug absorption. Gastric pH is increased in renal failure due to urea conversion to ammonia by gastric urease (117), use of orally administered alkalinizing agents such as sodium bicarbonate and citrate, and use of antacids for phosphate-binding effects. Therefore, those drugs that demonstrate pH-dependent absorption (ketoconazole, iron salts, tetracycline) may exhibit altered bioavailability (118). Bioavailability of fluoroquinolone antibiotics and isoniazid may be decreased by concomitant administration of antacids or phosphate-binding agents secondary to chelation (118–120).

Delayed gastric emptying with diabetic gastroparesis can alter drug absorption patterns. Kang (121) concluded that gastric emptying studies in uremic subjects have yielded conflicting results. In general, hemodialysis patients demonstrate normal gastric emptying of both solids and liquids, but uremic subjects not on dialysis can exhibit delayed gastric emptying. In addition, chronic ambulatory peritoneal dialysis patients may exhibit slowed gastric emptying of solids when dialysate is present in the peritoneal cavity (121).

Renal failure may affect the absorptive capacity of the small intestine. Craig and associates (122) showed that D-xylose absorption is reduced by one-third, and the time to appear in the systemic circulation is doubled in uremic patients.

Finally, the apparent bioavailability of some oral medications has been increased in uremic patients secondary to a decreased first-pass metabolism through the liver or gastrointestinal tract (123). Bianchetti and associates (124) observed that propranolol plasma concentrations were 2 to 3 times greater following a single oral dose in chronic renal failure patients, as opposed to those of hemodialysis patients or healthy volunteers. Interestingly, they also found that systemic bioavailability of propranolol was greater in hemodialysis patients on the day following hemodialysis than on the day of hemodialysis, which suggested that a dialyzable uremic substance was responsible for the change in bioavailability. The same effects have been observed with other β-blockers (123), dihydrocodeine (113), encainide (125), and propoxyphene (126).

Distribution

Apparent volume of distribution (V_d) depends on a number of factors, including plasma protein binding, tissue binding, and total body water. All of these factors may be altered in patients with renal insufficiency or failure. Hypermetabolic states (stress, trauma, sepsis, multiple-organ failure) contribute to decreases in binding proteins as protein degradation exceeds protein synthesis. It is unclear whether hemodialysis

Table 3.4. Effect of Renal Failure on Volume of Distribution (V_d) of Various Drugs[a]

Increased V_d	Decreased V_d
Amikacin	Chloramphenicol
Azlocillin	Digoxin
Bretyllium	Ethambutol
Cefazolin	Methicillin
Cefonicid	Pindolol
Cefoxitin	
Cefuroxime	
Clofibrate	
Cloxacillin	
Dicloxacillin	
Erythromycin	
Furosemide	
Gentamicin	
Isoniazid	
Moxalactam	
Naproxen	
Phenytoin	
Sulfamethopyrazine	
Trimethoprim	
Vancomycin	

[a] Adapted from Matzke GR, Frye RF: Drug dosing in patients with impaired renal function. In DiPiro JT, Talbert RL, Hayes PE, Yee GC, Matzke GR, Posey LM (eds): *Pharmacotherapy: A Pathophysiologic Approach.* Appleton & Lange, Norwalk, CT, 1993, pp 750–763.

changes V_d of drugs, since it is difficult to design a study to accurately assess the effects of dialysis on this parameter (127). Although commonly used dose adjustment methods oftentimes disregard V_d changes in their calculations, several drugs have been reported to have significant increases or decreases in distribution volumes in renal failure patients (Table 3.4).

Many drugs are bound to some extent to plasma proteins, including albumin (mainly, acidic drugs) and α-1-acid glycoprotein (AAG, primarily basic drugs). Binding alterations in patients with renal insufficiency can affect the V_d, the amount of free drug available for pharmacologic activity, and the rate and extent of elimination. Total drug concentrations are commonly used for therapeutic drug monitoring, although unbound (active) drug concentrations correlate more closely with drug efficacy. Monitoring total drug concentrations is adequate in the majority of patients, as the ratio between unbound to total drug concentrations remains constant between and within individuals (128). However, disease states such as renal failure can alter normal protein-binding ratios. Consequently, monitoring total drug concentrations may lead to misinterpretation of laboratory results and under- or overdosing of drugs.

There are limited data documenting changes in binding to AAG in renal failure. However, quantitative data suggest uremic patients and renal transplant patients exhibit serum levels of AAG up to three times those seen in normal human serum (129). These increases may result in significantly lower free fractions of agents bound primarily to AAG. Craig (130) has reported this effect with clindamycin. Increased lidocaine binding to AAG has been reported to be directly related to increased AAG plasma concentrations in uremic patients, but unbound (active) lidocaine concentrations remained unchanged (131). Increased binding of disopyramide to AAG has also been reported (129).

Conversely, the extent of binding of acidic drugs to albumin is generally decreased in ESRD patients (132). Mechanisms

for this reduction include a decrease in plasma albumin, displacement of drug by accumulated drug metabolites or uremic toxins, or configurational changes in albumin binding sites (132–134). Phenytoin is the classic example of a drug that exhibits binding alterations in renal failure secondary to decreases in serum albumin concentrations, as well as displacement by uremic metabolic products (132). Consequently, the free fraction of phenytoin increases from a normal value of approximately 10% up to 20 to 30% (116, unpublished data). Clinically, this results in decreased total phenytoin plasma concentrations, secondary to an increased V_d. It is critical that the medical practitioner understand that, although total phenytoin concentrations may be lower than the accepted therapeutic range of 10 to 20 μg/ml, the unbound (active) phenytoin concentration may be normal (1 to 2 μg/ml) because of the increased free fraction (135). Therefore, phenytoin-loading doses should not be altered in uremic patients, and it has been suggested that maintenance dosing be monitored by measurement of unbound (free) phenytoin concentrations.

If drugs are displaced by uremic toxins or accumulated metabolites, the degree of plasma protein binding immediately after hemodialysis might more closely approximate that of patients with normal renal function. Penicillin is one example of a drug that exhibits this type of binding pattern (136). However, Greene and Tice (137) have demonstrated that cefazolin exhibits a reduction in binding immediately after hemodialysis, perhaps due to drug displacement by free fatty acids generated by heparin activation of lipoprotein lipase (138).

Tissue binding changes occur with digoxin in patients with renal insufficiency or failure. Digoxin's V_d has been reported to decrease by 30 to 45% in renal failure secondary to displacement from tissue binding sites by endogenous uremic substances (139). As a result, reductions in digoxin-loading doses in patients with renal insufficiency have been advocated. However, it is unclear whether tissue binding alterations also affect digoxin pharmacodynamic effects on cardiac tissue (139). In addition, endogenous substances termed digoxin-like immunoreactive substance (DLIS) and digoxin metabolites that accumulate in renal failure can increase "apparent" digoxin concentrations measured by RIA, enzyme immunoassay, and fluorescence polarization immunoassay methods (139–142). Hemodialysis variably affects the DLIS concentrations (143). Clinicians need to be aware of the assay methodology utilized at their institution and understand the precision and sensitivity of the assay to digoxin and active metabolites in patients with renal failure.

It is difficult to predict the direction and/or absolute changes in protein binding that occur in patients with various degrees of renal function. Uremic patients may either experience increased or decreased protein binding of drugs, depending on the primary plasma or tissue protein that the drug binds to. Unfortunately, little information exists on alterations in dosing based on binding changes. For drugs such as antibiotics with wide therapeutic ranges, alterations in protein binding may be of more theoretical than practical importance. Clinically, unless free drug concentrations are altered with protein-binding changes, then dosing changes are probably not necessary. Practitioners need to appreciate that total phenytoin concentrations are decreased in renal failure and free (unbound) concentrations should be measured. In addition, digoxin loading doses should be more conservative in patients with renal insufficiency and failure.

Metabolism

Many drugs undergo hepatic biotransformation to water-soluble metabolites before renal excretion. There are several studies that demonstrate that renal failure may significantly affect both renal and nonrenal mechanisms of drug metabolism. Reviews of these alterations have been published (123, 144–147). Touchette and Slaughter (123) have pointed out the inherent difficulties of investigating the effects of renal failure on hepatic metabolism of drugs. Studies specifically addressing this phenomenon need to exclude other factors such as protein-binding changes and changes in hepatic blood flow for drugs with a high intrinsic clearance. Concurrent measurement of renal and hepatic clearance is necessary to detect effects of changes in either organ. Oral and intravenous dosing should be evaluated, when feasible, to demonstrate bioavailability changes in those drugs that exhibit high first-pass metabolism.

Proposed mechanisms for changes in hepatic metabolism secondary to renal failure include the accumulation of uremic inhibitory factors that compete for binding sites within the liver or affect the transport of organic anions into the liver (146). It has also been suggested that the accumulation of uremic end-metabolites may inhibit metabolism of drugs via feedback mechanisms or by product inhibition (146). Table 3.5 presents a list of drugs that have been shown to have a high, low, or unclear potential for inhibition of nonrenal clearance in renal failure.

The kidney itself contains many of the same metabolic enzymes found in the liver, and most are found within the renal cortex (146). There is a paucity of data on the effects of renal disease on these systems; however, Zenser et al (148) suggest that the presence of unilateral hydronephrosis reduces the function of these enzymatic pathways.

The formation of renally eliminated drug metabolites is also an important consideration when dosing patients with renal failure, because some metabolites are pharmacologically active (149). For example, acetylation metabolites of sulfonamides may retain the toxicities of the parent compounds (150). Norpropoxyphene and normeperidine, *N*-demethylated metabolites of propoxyphene, and meperidine, respectively, accumulate in renal failure (126, 151). Although these metabolites do not have opioid properties, norpropoxyphene can cause cardiac toxicity, and normeperidine can cause CNS excitation, culminating in seizures (126, 151). In addition, the metabolites of compounds such as cefotaxime and morphine retain some of the pharmacologic properties of the parent compound (152–154). *N*-acetyl-procainamide (NAPA), the main metabolic product of procainamide, displays antiarrhythmic properties distinct from those of procainamide (155).

Hemodialysis patients are regularly exposed to phthalate plasticizers leached from dialysis tubings (156). Long-term exposure to plasticizer metabolites has been shown to increase hepatic microsomal oxidative metabolism in rats, while acute exposure to both phthalate and its metabolites may produce inhibition of these enzyme systems (157). Consequently, when the nonrenal elimination of drugs is significantly changed by plasticizers or their metabolites, patients receiving chronic

Table 3.5. Drugs with High, Low, or Unclear Potential for Inhibition of Hepatic Metabolism in Renal Failure

High Potential	Low Potential	Unclear
Acyclovir	Cefamandol	Bisoprolol
Aztreonam	Cefoperazone	Cilazapril
Bufurolol	Cefpiramide	Flecainide
Captopril	Codeine	Oxazepam
Cefmenoxime	Cyclosporine	Propafenone
Cefmetazole	Isradipine	
Cefonicid	Lidocaine	
Cefotaxime	Metoprolol	
Cefotiam	Nifedipine	
Ceftizoxime	Nisoldipine	
Cefsulodin	Nitrendipine	
Cilastatin	Theophylline	
Desmethyldiazepam	Tocainide	
Encainide		
Erythromycin		
Imipenem		
Metoclopramide		
Moxalactam		
Nimodipine		
Nortriptyline		
Oxprenolol		
Propoxyphene		
Propranolol		
Verapamil		
Zidovudine		

a Compiled from Touchette MA, Slaughter RL: The effect of renal failure on hepatic drug clearance. *DICP* 25:1214–1224, 1991; Gibson TP: Renal disease and drug metabolism: an overview. *Am J Kidney Dis* 8:7–17, 1986.

hemodialysis may have increased clearance, compared with patients with significant renal dysfunction who are not yet on hemodialysis.

Pharmacodynamics of Drugs in Renal Failure

There is a paucity of literature evaluating drug response (pharmacodynamics) in renal failure patients and, therefore, medication dosage adjustments are often based on pharmacokinetic, rather than pharmacodynamic, data. Gladziwa and Klotz reviewed studies that evaluated the intragastric pH response following H_2 receptor antagonists in subjects with and without renal failure (158). One study compared famotidine effects on long-term intragastric pH monitoring in hemodialysis vs. healthy control subjects and found that in contrast to normal subjects, timing of intravenous famotidine doses did not affect the pH response in hemodialysis patients (159). Another study showed that one intravenous famotidine dose in renal failure patients sustained high gastric pH levels only two times longer than the same dose in normal subjects, although the half-life was prolonged approximately 5-fold (158). This shows that H_2 antagonist plasma concentrations do not correlate well with the pharmacodynamic actions of the drug and that dosing should be adjusted on pharmacodynamic response and not pharmacokinetic parameters alone.

Schmith and colleagues evaluated the pharmacokinetics and pharmacodynamics of alprazolam in a small group of hemodialysis and chronic ambulatory peritoneal dialysis patients, as compared to those in normal controls. Interestingly, they demonstrated that some psychomotor effects, corrected for the maximum free alprazolam concentration, were greater in the dialysis patients, indicating a greater sensitivity to the drug in this population (21).

Although morphine pharmacokinetics do not change in renal failure, there have been several reports in the literature suggesting that patients with renal failure have an increased sensitivity to morphine's effects (151). This finding has led to several investigations of morphine and metabolite pharmacokinetics and pharmacodynamics in normal and renal failure subjects (153, 160, 161). Based on these and other studies, it was found that a minor morphine metabolite, morphine 6-glucuronide, was pharmacologically active and many times more potent than morphine. Accumulation of this metabolite has been demonstrated in renal failure (154, 160, 162). Further investigations on the relationship between morphine-6-glucuronide plasma concentrations and pharmacodynamic effect in patients with various degrees of renal function are warranted.

EFFECTS OF DIALYSIS TECHNIQUES ON DRUG CLEARANCE

REMOVAL OF DRUGS BY DIALYSIS TECHNIQUES

Drug clearance by any dialysis technique is accomplished either through diffusion of the drug down a concentration gradient and/or by ultrafiltration of fluids containing the drug. Artificial membranes that are selectively permeable to various solutes are the mainstay of hemodialysis and hemofiltration techniques. The peritoneal membrane functions as a natural dialysis membrane during peritoneal dialysis. Levy suggested that clearance during dialysis must enhance total body clearance by at least 30% to be considered significant (163).

Hemodialysis

A number of factors affect the removal of drugs by hemodialysis. The physicochemical properties of the drug, such as molecular size, water solubility, extent of plasma protein binding, rate of equilibration between plasma and tissue, and apparent V_d all affect hemodialysis clearance (127). Removal of drug by dialysis depends on the concentration gradient of unbound, ultrafilterable solute between the plasma and the dialysate. Generally, drugs that have a molecular weight greater than 500 daltons (e.g., vancomycin) and/or are highly protein-bound (e.g., phenytoin), or are widely distributed to body tissues (e.g., digoxin, tricyclic antidepressants) are generally not effectively removed by hemodialysis (127).

Drug removal by hemodialysis also depends on a number of dialysis-specific factors, including blood flow to the dialyzer, dialysate flow rate, concentration gradient between plasma and dialysate, and intrinsic properties of the dialysis membrane itself. In general, the dialyzer clearance increases with membrane surface area and pore size (164). Standard dialysis membranes typically remove small molecules of less than 500 daltons. Most drugs have molecular weights less than 500 daltons. High-flux dialyzer membranes, which are becoming more popular, remove middle molecules up to 5000 daltons. Drugs such as vancomycin (MW 1486 daltons) are readily removed by these types of dialyzer membranes (165-167). Additional patient-specific factors, such as type of vascular access and degree of access recirculation, can affect the efficiency of drug clearance during hemodialysis (168). Therefore,

it is difficult to predict the exact amount of drug that will be removed during any particular dialysis session.

A rebound in plasma drug concentrations is common after hemodialysis. Rebound occurs when the hemodialysis process removes the drug from the blood more rapidly than the drug distributes from tissue compartments to the blood compartment. Significant rebound in aminoglycoside (conventional hemodialysis membranes) and in vancomycin concentrations (high-flux membranes) has been reported following hemodialysis (165, 169, 170). The time to maximal rebound occurs within 2 hours and from 1.7 to 12 hours with aminoglycosides and vancomycin, respectively (165, 170–172). Plasma concentrations should be drawn 2 hours (aminoglycosides) and 6–12 hours (vancomycin) following hemodialysis to avoid misinterpretation of posthemodialysis levels and potential antibiotic overdosing.

Hemodialysis clearance of drugs (CL_D) can be calculated by two general methods. Using the Fick principle (A-V pairs method), $CL_D = Q \cdot (A-V)/A$, where Q is blood flow through the dialyzer, A is drug concentration immediately before it enters the dialyzer, and V is drug concentration immediately after it comes out of the dialyzer. Generally, drug concentrations are determined in plasma; therefore, plasma flow rate, $Qp = (1-hematocrit) \cdot Q$, should be substituted for Q in the general equation above. Unfortunately, this method is fraught with problems because accuracy depends on a precise measurement of blood flow rate and a low rate of ultrafiltration during the procedure (173). The gold standard method to calculate CL_D is the amount recovered method (ARM): $CL_D = R/AUC_0^t$, where R is the total amount of drug recovered unchanged in the dialysate and AUC_0^t is the area under the curve of the plasma concentration-time curve during hemodialysis. Unlike the previous method, the ARM is independent of blood flow rate, the amount of ultrafiltrate, or the effects of plasma protein-binding. It is also a more difficult procedure, as it is necessary to collect the dialysate during the entire dialysis session, with aliquots taken for sample analysis.

Peritoneal Dialysis

Peritoneal dialysis (PD) is an accepted alternative to hemodialysis for the treatment of acute and chronic renal failure. The choice of modalities is dependent on vascular access, comorbid disease states, and availability (174). Unlike hemodialysis, where an artificial dialysis membrane is used to enhance solute and fluid clearance, the peritoneal membrane functions as a natural dialysis membrane. A peritoneal dialysate solution containing sodium, potassium, chloride, calcium, magnesium, and glucose is infused into the peritoneal cavity through a catheter that has been inserted through the abdominal wall. Waste products (solutes) and fluids pass from the blood into the dialysate within the peritoneal cavity. The dialysate, along with ultrafiltrate, is then drained from the peritoneal cavity. In continuous ambulatory peritoneal dialysis (CAPD), dialysate exchanges are usually performed by the patient about four times per day, three exchanges with a dialysate dwell time of about 4 to 6 hours and one overnight dwell time of 8 to 12 hours. In the critically ill hospitalized patient, automated forms of peritoneal dialysis are available. The patient is connected to an automatic cycling machine, which performs rapid exchanges; peritoneal dialysate is exchanged every 30 minutes to 2 hours for 10 to 12 hours.

Diffusion of drugs or solutes through the peritoneal membrane is dependent on the concentration gradient between the dialysate solution and blood; drug molecular weight and size, V_d, water solubility, ionic charge and protein binding; and peritoneal membrane resistance. The concentration gradient is best maintained by exchanging the dialysate within the peritoneal cavity frequently. Cycler-assisted PD provides more efficient waste and drug product removal because exchanges are performed more frequently. However, unlike CAPD, assisted PD is usually intermittent, and solute clearance decreases during the interdialytic period. Smaller weight substances, such as urea (MW 60), diffuse more rapidly across the peritoneal membrane than vitamin B_{12} (MW 1352). In contrast to hemodialysis artificial membranes, which have distinct molecular size and weight limitations in terms of solute clearance, the peritoneal membrane allows passage of large molecules, including proteins such as albumin (175). The V_d effects drug transfer across the peritoneal membrane. Drugs with a large V_d, such as digoxin or tricyclic antidepressants, have low plasma concentrations once equilibration takes place. Only small amounts will distribute into the peritoneal cavity, thus making PD an inefficient method for removing these drugs.

Calculation of the fraction of the dose removed by PD (f_{PD}) will determine whether supplemental dosing is necessary. Using the relationship $f_{PD} = CL_{PD}/CL$, one can estimate the fraction of the drug removed (f_{PD} is the fraction of the dose removed by PD, CL_{PD} is drug clearance via PD, and CL is total body clearance of the drug). As CL is difficult to determine in an individual patient, literature values for CL in ESRD patients can be used (176). If one assumes that an equilibrium has been reached between blood and dialysate by the end of the dwell period, and if the drug is not highly plasma protein bound, then the dialysate flow rate (usually 5 to 8 ml/min) can be used as a rough estimate of CL_{PD}. Using Levy's definition of significant clearance (30% enhancement of total body clearance), any drug having a total body clearance in ESRD greater than 27 ml/min would not be significantly removed by PD (163).

In general, the clearance of most drugs by peritoneal dialysis is quite low (177), and in most cases the dosage guidelines for patients with CL_{CR} less than 10 ml/minute can be applied to PD patients. Using the above criteria, drugs that have the potential to be significantly removed by PD include aminoglycosides, vancomycin, amoxicillin, ampicillin, ticarcillin, carbenicillin, cefadroxil, cefsulodin, ceftazidime, ceftizoxime, cefuroxime, cephalexin, amantadine, 5-fluorocytosine, phenobarbital, atenolol, sotalol, and lithium (177). Several investigators have confirmed that vancomycin and amikacin are significantly removed by CAPD (177); however, Bunke and colleagues (178) demonstrated that cephalexin, vancomycin, and tobramycin were not significantly removed by CAPD. For those patients receiving cyclic peritoneal dialysis on an intermittent basis, the total daily clearance of drugs should be comparable to that of CAPD, but doses of drugs should be administered after the procedure is finished, if feasible (179). Routine monitoring of aminoglycoside, vancomycin, 5-fluorocytosine, phenobarbital, and lithium plasma concentrations in PD patients is important to ensure efficacy while avoiding toxicity because of intersubject variability in pharmacokinetic parameters and the narrow therapeutic ranges of these agents. In general, plasma concentrations can be drawn anytime during CAPD, but in patients on intermittent cyclic PD, levels should be drawn following the procedure.

Administration of drugs by the intraperitoneal route may be desirable in cases where vascular access may be limited to administer insulin in diabetic patients and during episodes of peritonitis. In the former case, one needs to determine if drug absorption through the peritoneal cavity will be adequate to produce therapeutic systemic concentrations. Most drugs have significant absorption after intraperitoneal administration, and absorption is enhanced during peritonitis episodes (177). Drug distribution from the peritoneal space into the systemic circulation is promoted by a high concentration gradient between peritoneal dialysate and blood at the beginning of a dwell period. Table 3.6 shows several drugs and the fraction of the doses absorbed after various dwell times following intraperitoneal administration. These pharmacokinetic studies show that intraperitoneal administration of antimicrobials typically results in bioavailabilities exceeding 50% (177, 180). These pharmacokinetic studies were performed in healthy subjects or in patients with CAPD-related peritonitis. Efficacy studies that demonstrate the usefulness of intraperitoneal delivery of medications in critically ill patient populations are lacking. In addition, one needs to determine whether the drug has been shown to cause peritoneal irritation or it is chemically stable in dialysate fluid. Amphotericin B is very irritating to the peritoneal membrane (177), but many antibiotics have been successfully administered intraperitoneally in the treatment of CAPD peritonitis (181, 182). To ensure drug bioavailability, intravenous delivery of medications is preferable in critically ill patients, even in those with established intraperitoneal access. In patients in whom intravenous access is lacking, intraperitoneal administration is a consideration, but drug concentration monitoring should be performed to ensure therapeutic concentrations.

During peritonitis episodes, the treatment goal is to obtain high localized concentrations of antibacterial agents within the peritoneal cavity. Reviews on peritonitis treatment have been published elsewhere (181, 182).

Continuous Therapies

Continuous renal replacement therapies can be advantageous over conventional hemodialysis in critically ill patients with acute renal failure (183, 184). Intermittent hemodialysis sessions can result in large fluid and electrolyte shifts, leading to hemodynamic instability in predisposed patients. Continuous slow removal of fluids and solutes by either continuous hemofiltration or by continuous hemodialysis techniques may be tolerated better in some patients with cardiovascular instability, respiratory failure, acute renal failure, and multiple organ failure (183). In the past decade, a variety of continuous renal replacement techniques have been introduced into intensive care unit settings (185–187).

Two main types of slow hemofiltration and slow hemodialysis techniques are commonly used. Via continuous arteriovenous hemofiltration (CAVH) and continuous arteriovenous hemodialysis (CAVHD) one can take advantage of the patient's mean arterial blood pressure to drive blood through either a

Table 3.6. Reported Bioavailability of Various Antimicrobials after Intraperitoneal Administration in Subjects with or without Peritonitis[a]

Drug	Dose	Dwell Time (hr)	Bioavailability (%)
Aminoglycosides			
amikacin	7.5 mg/kg	5	53 ± 14
gentamicin	100 mg	6	49 ± 15
	1 mg/kg	6	84
	7.5 mg/kg	6	69
		6	85[b]
tobramycin	2 mg/kg	6	73 ± 10
	1.5 mg/kg	4	52
	100 mg	6	85
streptomycin	200 mg	6	75[b]
Cephalosporins			
cefamandol	1000 mg	6	72 ± 13
	1000 mg	6	71 ± 10
	1000 mg	6	71 ± 10
cefazolin	1000 mg	6	88[b]
	10 mg/kg	4	74
cefoperazone	1000 mg	10	95 ± 12
	2000 mg	6	61
cefotaxime	1000 mg	4	59 ± 6
	1000 mg	4	59 ± 5
	2000 mg	6	75 ± 21
	500 mg	5	61[c]
cefoxitin	50 mg/liter	6	71
ceftizoxime	500 mg	6	78 ± 4
ceftriaxone	2000 mg	5	74
	1000 mg	4	44 ± 13
cefuroxime	500 mg	5	70
moxalactam	1000 mg	4	57 ± 16
Miscellaneous			
acyclovir	1000 mg	4	61 ± 10
ampicillin/ sulbactam	2000 mg	6	60
	1000 mg	6	80
aztreonam	2000 mg	6	92[b]
	1000 mg	8	91
ciprofloxacin	5 mg/kg	4	84
	25 mg/liter	4	66
fluconazole	50 mg	6	87 ± 5
	150 mg	6	88 ± 4
impipenem/ cilastatin	500 mg	6	79 ± 8
piperacillin	1000 mg	6	83 ± 5[b]
	1000 mg	6	68 ± 9
trimethoprim-sulfamethoxazole	320 mg (trimethoprim)	4	84
	1600 mg (sulfamethoxazole)		66
vancomycin	30 mg/kg	6	52 ± 20
		?	91 ± 10[b]
	1000 mg	6	54 ± 17
	1000 mg	6	73 ± 11
	10 mg/kg	4	65
	37.5 mg/liter	3	70[a]
			39

[a] Compiled from references 177, 180, 204–209.
[b] With peritonitis.
[c] In pediatric patients.

hemofilter or a hemodialysis filter. A blood pump must be utilized if continuous venovenous hemofiltration (CVVH) or continuous venovenous hemodialysis (CVVHD) is chosen. Unlike hemodialysis techniques, hemofiltration does not involve a dialysate solution. As blood passes through the hemofilter an ultrafiltrate of blood is formed that contains dissolved solutes; thus, solute (and drug) removal during hemofiltration involves only convective forces. Fluid and electrolytes are then infused in amounts that restore the plasma to normal electrolyte balance. Slow hemodialysis techniques involve a countercurrent flow of dialysate through the outer compartment of the dialysis filter. Solute and drug elimination occurs mainly by diffusion down a concentration gradient into the dialysate. Convective forces play a lesser role in drug removal.

Drug removal via continuous hemofiltration and hemodialysis techniques is relatively inefficient when compared to intermittent hemodialysis, because blood flow rates are quite low. However, solute (drug) removal is continuous; thus over a period of time, drug loss can be significant by these slow, continuous dialysis methods. Unfortunately, data concerning the pharmacokinetics of medications during these procedures is sparse. Most articles address drug removal by hemofiltration techniques that are less efficient in drug removal than by continuous hemodialysis techniques. Aminoglycosides have been shown to adsorb to some hemofilter membranes in a concentration-dependent manner, which may lead to misinterpretation of the amounts removed (188, 189). Large molecular weight drugs, such as vancomycin, will be eliminated by different hemofilter and hemodialysis filters to variable extents, depending on the pore size of the particular membrane (190, 191). Mean vancomycin elimination half-lives of 24 to 56 hours have been reported during continuous hemofiltration or hemodialysis methods (192–194). Clearly, weekly vancomycin doses, which are typically administered to hemodialysis patients, would produce subtherapeutic concentrations in the majority of patients on slow continuous therapies. As many different filters are available for hemofiltration and hemodialysis, it is difficult to extrapolate information given in the literature to an individual patient.

Like the other extracorporeal methods outlined above, a drug is more likely to be significantly removed by continuous renal replacement therapies if it has a small V_d, a low molecular weight and size, and a low degree of protein binding. The extracorporeal clearance of a substance during continuous therapies can be calculated by determining the ratio of the amount of drug that is in the ultrafiltrate, compared to plasma (sieving), or in the combined ultrafiltrate plus dialysate to plasma (saturation). Saturation (Sa) or sieving (Si) is then multiplied by the flow rate of either the ultrafiltration (Q_{uf}-hemofiltration methods) or combined ultrafiltrate plus dialysate (Q_D-hemodialysis methods) to determine extracorporeal clearance (CL_{EX}) ($CL_{EX} = Si \cdot Q_{uf}$ or $CL_{EX} = Sa \cdot (Q_D + Q_{uf})$). Again, extracorporeal clearance can be considered clinically important if it enhances total body clearance by 30% or more. Reetze-Bonorden and colleagues (195) have determined that when typical saturation or sieving values are considered, any drug that has a total body clearance greater than 60 ml/min will not be significantly removed by slow continuous therapies. Thus supplemental dosing would be unnecessary with these drugs. Sieving or saturation becomes important with those drugs that have a total body clearance less than 60 ml/min. The smaller the total body clearance, the more important effect different ultrafiltration/dialysate flow rates and Si/Sa values have on CL_{EX} (195). Multiple variables, such as membrane filter type, ultrafiltration/dialysate flow rate, and protein binding changes in uremia, will all affect drug removal by continuous dialysis procedures. It is impossible to predict in an individual patient exactly how one procedure may affect drug clearance; therefore, plasma drug concentrations should be monitored when possible. Table 3.7 identifies those drugs that have the potential to be significantly removed by continuous hemofiltration or hemodialysis techniques, using typical flow rates and Si and Sa values (195).

DOSING IMPLICATIONS AND DRUG MONITORING

DOSAGE ADJUSTMENT IN RENAL FAILURE

The primary goal of dosage adjustment in renal insufficiency is to provide efficacious treatment of the medical problem without producing toxicity. Cost savings can be realized through appropriate dosing adjustment of medications by reducing drug and intravenous fluid costs, saving nursing and pharmacy time, and preventing iatrogenically induced disease.

One method of dosing adjustment is to administer a loading dose to reach a certain peak plasma concentration and then to administer subsequent usual maintenance doses at intervals determined by the elimination half-life of the antibiotic. Aminoglycoside dosing is adjusted in this manner, as aminoglycoside peak concentrations and area under the curve have been found to be important in determining clinical outcome in infected animals and patients (196). In addition, aminoglycosides, penem, and carbapenem antibiotics exhibit a postantibiotic effect (PAE); thus, it may not be necessary to maintain antibacterial concentrations above the minimum inhibitory concentration (MIC) for the entire dosing period with these antibiotics (196, 197).

Another method of adjustment is to reduce the medication dose and maintain the usual dosage interval, which results in more constant drug concentrations. This method is more acceptable with drugs with a narrow therapeutic range (digoxin, procainamide) and with β-lactam antibiotics. β-Lactam antibiotics, in general, do not produce a PAE, and antibacterial concentrations should be maintained above the MIC for the entire dosage interval (196). Both dosing methods will maintain the same average plasma concentrations; however, reduction of the medication dose, instead of lengthening of the interval, will result in less fluctuation between peak and trough plasma concentrations.

Standard medication loading doses should be administered with either dosing method to obtain therapeutic concentrations initially. One exception to this rule is digoxin. Digoxin's V_d is much lower in uremic patients secondary to decreased tissue binding and usual loading dose regimens may produce toxicity. In general, the initial digoxin loading regimen should be decreased to one-half or two-thirds of the normal loading regimen. If the patient does not respond, additional conservative digoxin doses can be administered based on the patient's clinical status.

Maintenance dosages should be adjusted based on the patient's level of renal function and drug characteristics. In individual cases, the dose and dosage interval may need adjustment for optimal patient management. Unfortunately, some oral medications come in specific dosage units that can not be divided. This restricts the practitioner to adjusting the medication dosing interval, which may result in suboptimal patient care. However, this is rarely a problem in the critical care setting, because most essential medications are available in an intravenous form.

Many pharmacokinetic articles include relationships between either drug clearance or elimination rate vs. CL_{CR}. These relationships can aid dosage adjustment in patients with various degrees of renal function. A compilation of antibiotic regression equations and correlation coefficients can be found in a recent review (176).

Many medications may be significantly removed by the various dialysis procedures (Table 3.7). Unfortunately, it is difficult to predict in an individual patient how much drug is actually removed unless plasma and/or dialysate concentrations can be measured. Drug removal by hemodialysis is influenced by dialysis membrane composition and surface area, blood flow rate, dialysate flow rate, type of hemodialysis access, amount of access recirculation, drug protein binding, and dialysis session length. Clearance of drugs during peritoneal dialysis is dependent on drug protein binding, on peritoneal membrane resistance and surface area, and on whether intermittent vs. continuous peritoneal dialysis is being performed. Ultrafiltrate and or ultrafiltrate plus dialysate flow rate, membrane composition and surface area, type of dialysis access and drug protein binding affect drug clearance during continuous dialysis techniques. Residue renal function also should be considered when one alters the dosage regimen in a patient. Since multiple variables affect drug clearance with each one of the dialysis techniques, it is easy to see why individual patient pharmacokinetic parameters may vary significantly from literature values. Maintenance or supplemental doses of medications that are significantly removed by hemodialysis or intermittent cyclic peritoneal dialysis should be administered after completion of the session on dialysis days. If the clinical condition of the patient dictates more aggressive dosing, maintenance doses may be given before hemodialysis with a supplemental dose after dialysis. Loading doses should be administered when appropriate.

Many review articles on medication dosage adjustment in patients with various degrees of renal function have been published (195, 198–201); however, information on drug removal by hemodialysis, peritoneal dialysis, and slow continuous dialysis procedures has not been included in one reference. Table 3.7 is a compilation of literature extracted from review articles and original publications regarding alterations in pharmacokinetic parameters in renal failure, suggested dosage adjustments in patients with various degrees of renal function and the effect of various dialysis techniques on drug removal. There are numerous issues encountered when analyzing and compiling data in this type of format. Early pharmacokinetic trials (before 1975) were generally less specific about study methodology, including sample collection, analytical techniques, and data analysis. Patient demographic information frequently was not reported, so pharmacokinetic parameters could not be normalized to total body weight.

Table 3.7. Drugs Commonly Used in Intensive Care Unit Patients: Dosage Adjustments in Various Degrees of Renal Function and with Dialytic Therapies[a]

THERAPEUTIC CATEGORY / Drug Class / Drug	V_d[b] (liter/kg) Normal	$t\frac{1}{2}\beta$ (h) CL_{CR} (ml/min) >50	<10	PPB (%) Normal	fe (%)	Dose for patients with CL_{CR} = >50 ml/min	Method	Adjustment for Renal Failure CL_{CR} = 10–50 ml/min	CL_{CR} = <10 ml/min	HD	PD	CAVH/ CVVH	CAVHD/ CVVHD
ANTIMICROBIAL AGENTS													
Aminoglycosides													
Dosage should be individualized using patient-specific parameters calculated from plasma concentrations. Initial dose should be based on population-based V_d; V_d is higher in edematous states, ESRD, ascites. Ototoxic, nephrotoxic potential.													
Amikacin	0.20	1.8	31.6	<5	87	Individualize	D or I	Individualize	Individualize	yes	yes	yes	yes
Gentamicin	0.27	2.7	41.8	0–25	81	Individualize	D or I	Individualize	Individualize	yes	yes	yes	yes
Concomitant penicillin therapy may decrease gentamicin levels.													
Netilmicin	0.22	3.3	37.6	<5	72	Individualize	D, I	Individualize	Individualize	yes	yes	yes	yes
May be less ototoxic.													
Streptomycin	0.24	2.6	61.9	34	67–91	Individualize	D, I	Individualize	Individualize	yes	yes	yes	yes
Tobramycin	0.25	2.1	58.1	<5	74–93	Individualize	D, I	Individualize	Individualize	yes	yes	yes	yes
Concomitant penicillin therapy may decrease tobramycin levels.													
Antitubercular agents													
Ethambutol	3.02	11.3	10.3	25	62–79	15 mg/kg q24h	D, I	75–100%	5%	no	no	no	no
Optic neuritis with decreased visual acuity.													
Isoniazid	0.71	2.3	4.3	4–30	3–11 h	5 mg/kg q24h	D	100%	100%	yes	no	no	?
Hepatotoxic; Dosages applicable to oral and IV dosing; isoniazid acetylator phenotype is major determinant of CL; absorption reduced with concomitant use of aluminum antacids; Maximum dose: 300 mg q 24h; usual dose should be given after HD.													
Pyrazinamide	0.74	9.5	25.6	<5	1–5	15–30 mg/kg q24h	I	Unknown	q48h	yes	ND	ND	ND
Hepatotoxic; Active metabolite with prolonged $t\frac{1}{2}$ in ESRD; Maximum dose: 2 grams; usual dose should be given after HD.													

Drug (notes)	V_d	$t_{1/2}$ (normal)	$t_{1/2}$ (ESRD)	% PB	% excreted	Dose	Method	GFR >50	GFR 10–50				
Rifampin — Hepatotoxic; Concomitant administration of aluminum antacids decreases absorption; PPB % affected by method of quantification; Maximum dose 600 mg.	0.96	3.3	11.0	57–90	9	10 mg/kg q24h	D	100%	100%	no	no	no	no
β-lactamase inhibitors — These agents are dosed in combination with beta-lactam antibiotics.													
Clavulanic acid	0.20	1.1	4.0	22	48	100 mg q4–6h	NA	NA	NA	yes	ND	ND	ND
Sulbactam	0.26	1.1	15.2	38	84	1g q6h	NA	NA	NA	yes	ND	ND	ND
Carbepenam and monobactam													
Aztreonam	0.25	1.8	7.5	56	64	1–2 g q6–8h	D, I	0.5–1 g q8h	0.5–1 g q12h	yes	no	ND	ND
Imipenem — Commercially available product contains equal amounts of cilastatin; post antibiotic effect exhibited.	0.28	1.0	3.4	20	49	0.25–1g q6h	D, I	0.25–0.5 g q6–8h	0.25–0.5 g q12h	yes	no	no	no
Cephalosporins													
Cefamandole — MTT side chain may prolong PT (INR); vitamin K reverses effect	0.20	0.9	9.5	70	54	1–2 g q6h	I	q8–12h	q24h	yes	no	no	yes
Cefazolin — HD: give 1–2g after HD.	0.11	2.2	32.5	84	75	1–2 g q6–8h	D, I	q12–24h	1 g q48h	yes	no	ND	ND
Cefmenoxime — Displays concentration dependent PPB.	0.30	1.4	10.6	43–75	74	1 g q4–6h	I	q6–12h	q24h	yes	no	ND	ND
Cefmetazole — MTT side chain may prolong PT (INR), vitamin K reverses effect.	0.18	1.4	20.8	85	85	2 g q6–8h	I	q12–24h	q48h	yes	no	ND	ND
Cefonicid — Displays concentration-dependent PPB.	0.14	4.9	62.3	97	88	1–2 g q24h	D, I	0.5–1 g q24–48h	0.25–0.5 g q48h	no	no	no	no
Cefoperazone — MTT side chain may prolong PT (INR), vitamin K reverses effect, some active metabolites.	0.22	1.8	3.7	89	27	1–2 g q12h	D	100%	100%	no	no	no	no
Cefotaxime — Active metabolite with prolonged $t_{1/2}$ in ESRD.	0.25	1.1	3.1	40	52	1–2 g q6–8h	I	q8–12h	q24h	yes	no	no	no
Cefotetan — MTT side chain may prolong PT (INR); vitamin K reverses effect.	0.15	3.7	16.5	90	72	1–2 g q12h	D, I	q12–24h	0.5–1 g q24h	?	ND	ND	ND

Table 3.7.   *(Continued)*

THERAPEUTIC CATEGORY Drug Class / Drug	$V_d{}^b$ (liter/kg) Normal	$t_{1/2}\beta$ (h) CL_{CR} (ml/min) >50	$t_{1/2}\beta$ (h) CL_{CR} (ml/min) <10	PPB (%) Normal	fe (%)	Dose for patients with CL_{CR} = >50 ml/min	Method	Adjustment for Renal Failure CL_{CR} = 10–50 ml/min	Adjustment for Renal Failure CL_{CR} = <10 ml/min	Removed Significantly by HD	Removed Significantly by PD	Removed Significantly by CAVH/ CVVH	Removed Significantly by CAVHD/ CVVHD
Cefoxitin Interferes with serum creatinine determination with Jaffé method.	0.13	0.6	11.6	73	80	1–2 g q6h	I	q8–12h	q24h	yes	no	no	yes
Ceftazidime 1 gm q24h in CAPD.	0.22	2.0	23.0	17	84	1–2 g q8h	I	q12–24h	q48h	yes	yes	yes	yes
Ceftizoxime	0.37	1.7	27.1	28	87	1–2 g q8h	I	q12–24h	q48h	yes	no	ND	ND
Ceftriaxone Displays concentration-dependent PPB.	0.11	6.1	14.7	83–95	46	1–2 g q24h	D	100%	100%	?	no	no	no
Cefuroxime (parenteral)	0.18	1.6	13.7	33	95	0.75–1.5 g q8h	D, I	q8–24h	1 g q24h	yes	yes	yes	yes
Cephalothin Active metabolite with prolonged t½ in ESRD.	0.23	0.4	3.1	65	52/6	0.5–2 g q4–6h	I	q6–8h	q12h	?	no	ND	ND
Moxolactam May inactivate gentamicin or tobramycin secondary to complexation. MTT side chain may prolong PT (INR); vitamin K reverses effect.	0.24	2.3	19.5	59	78	1–2 g q8h	D, I	1g q12–24h	1 g q24–48h	yes	no	yes	yes
Fluoroquinolones Aluminum, calcium and magnesium antacids, sucralfate, iron supplements have been shown to decrease bioavailability of oral quinolones by complexation reaction; quinolones are metabolized to active metabolites.													
Ciprofloxacin-parenteral	2.59	4.6	7.9	20–40	51	0.2–0.4 g q4–12h	D	75–100%	50%	no	no	no	no
Ofloxacin CAVHD/CVVHD: 0.1 g q8h.	1.55	5.6	32.5	30	71	0.4 g q12h	D, I	0.2–0.4 g q24h	0.1–0.2 g q24h	no	no	no	yes
Glycopeptides Dosage should be individualized using patient-specific parameters calculated from plasma concentrations. Initial dose should be based on population-based V_d.													

Drug	Vd	t½ normal	t½ ESRD	PB (%)	Excreted (%)	Dose for normal renal function	Method	GFR 10–50	GFR <10	HD	CAPD	CAVH
Vancomycin — Not removed significantly by conventional hemodialyzers; removed significantly with high flux hemodialyzer. Dosage should be individualized using patient-specific parameters calculated from plasma concentrations. Initial dose should be based on population-based V. CAPD: CL may be enhanced in peritonitis.	0.58	5.7	139.1	55	ND	Individualize	Individualize	Individualize	Individualize	no/yes	yes	yes
Macrolides												
Azithromycin — Displays concentration-dependent PPB.	ND	10–14	ND	12–50	5–12	0.25–0.5 g q24h	ND	ND	ND	?	ND	ND
Clarithromycin — Active metabolites; exhibits dose-dependent pharmacokinetics.	ND	4–11	ND	ND	ND	0.25–0.5 g q12h	ND	ND	ND	ND	ND	ND
Erythromycin (parenteral) — Ototoxicity associated with high doses in renal failure.	0.83	1.8	3.2	80–90	5–17	0.5–1 g q6h	D	100%	50%	no	no	no
Penicillins — Ureido penicillins (mezlocillin, piperacillin), and ticarcillin are associated with abnormal bleeding times which may be more pronounced in renal failure. HD: give dose for CL$_{CR}$ <10 after HD.												
Ampicillin-parenteral	0.29	1.2	19.0	18–28	81	1–2 g q6h	D, I	0.5 g q6-8h	0.5–1 g q12h	yes	yes	yes
Methicillin	0.36	0.3	4.0	40	80	1–2 g q4-6h	D, I	q6-8h	0.5–1 g q8-12h	no	ND	ND
Mezlocillin — Sodium 1.7 mEq/gm; exhibits dose-dependent pharmacokinetics.	0.23	1.1	2.6	16–40	49	2–4 g q4-6h	D, I	q4-6h	1–2 g q6h	no	no	no
Nafcillin	1.06	1.4	2.1	87	27/8	1–2 g q4-6h	D	100%	100%	no	ND	ND
Oxacillin (parenteral)	ND	0.4	0.8	93	39	1–2 g q4-6h	D	100%	50%	no	no	no
Penicillin G — HD: give dose for CL$_{CR}$ <10 after HD.	ND	0.6	4.1	52	ND	2–3 mU q4-6h	D, I	1–1.5 mU q4-6h	1 mU q8h	yes	ND	ND
Piperacillin — Sodium 1.9 mEq/g; may inactivate gentamicin or tobramycin secondary to complexation; displays dose-dependent pharmacokinetics. HD: give dose for CL$_{CR}$ <10 after HD.	0.23	1.0	2.8	16	45–80	3–4 g q6h	D, I	2–4 g q6h	2–3 q8h	yes	no	yes

Table 3.7.   *(Continued)*

THERAPEUTIC CATEGORY / Drug Class / Drug	V_d^b (liter/kg) Normal	$t\frac{1}{2}\beta$ (h) CL_{CR} (ml/min) >50	$t\frac{1}{2}\beta$ (h) CL_{CR} (ml/min) <10	PPB (%) Normal	fe (%)	Dose for patients with CL_{CR} = >50 ml/min	Method	Adjustment for Renal Failure CL_{CR} = 10–50 ml/min	Adjustment for Renal Failure CL_{CR} = <10 ml/min	Removed Significantly by HD	Removed Significantly by PD	Removed Significantly by CAVH/CVVH	Removed Significantly by CAVHD/CVVHD
Ticarcillin — Sodium 5.2 mEq/gm; May inactivate gentamicin or tobramycin secondary to complexation; HD: give dose for CL_{CR} <10 after HD.	0.16	1.2	8.9	35	81	3 g q6h	D, I	2 g q6–8h	2 g q12h	yes	yes	ND	ND
Tetracyclines													
Doxycycline	0.58	17.3	22.8	88	50/72	0.1 g q12h	D	100%	100%	no	no	no	no
Minocycline — May cause dose-related antianabolic effects	0.99	15.5	20.1	76	12/48	0.1 g q12h	D	100%	100%	no	ND	ND	ND
Tetracycline — Antianabolic effect with increase in BUN; avoid in CL_{CR} <30 ml/min; PPB derived from non-human data.	ND	6.2	63.4	56 y	70/96	0.25–0.5 g q12h	I	q12–24h	Avoid	no	ND	?	?
Miscellaneous													
Chloramphenicol succinate — Dosage should be individualized using patient-specific parameters calculated from plasma concentrations. Initial dose should be based on population-based V.	0.40	0.6	1.5	53	24	Individualize	D, I	Individualize 100%	Individualize 100%	?	no	ND	ND
Cilastatin — Renal dihydropeptidase inhibitor administered with imipenem; accumulates in renal failure; no apparent toxicity.	0.24	0.9	11.6	44	65	0.25–1 g q6h	NA	NA	NA	yes	no	ND	ND
Clindamycin (parenteral)	1.10	2.4	3.1	94	5	0.9 g q8h	D	100%	100%	no	no	no	no
Metronidazole — Active metabolite with prolonged $t\frac{1}{2}$ in renal failure	0.70	7.0	8.3	0–20	17	0.5 g q8h	D	100%	100%	yes	no	no	no
Pentamidine — Displays dose-dependent pharmacokinetics in both normal and renally-impaired patients.	55.70	29.0	73–118	69	4–29	3–4 mg/kg q24h	I	100%	100%	no	ND	ND	ND
Sulfamethoxazole (parenteral) — IV trimethoprim/sulfamethoxazole is available only as a combination product. Decreased PPB in renal failure; slightly active metabolites with prolonged $t\frac{1}{2}$ in renal insufficiency.	0.27	10.6	22.0	62	9	0.8 g q12h	I	q12–24h	q24h	yes	no	no	no

Drug / Notes	V_d (L/kg)	$t\frac{1}{2}$ Normal	$t\frac{1}{2}$ ESRD	Protein binding (%)	Excreted renal (%)	Dose	Method	Adj 1	Adj 2				
Trimethoprim (parenteral) — IV trimethoprim/sulfamethoxazole is available only as a combination product. Inhibits tubular secretion of creatinine; falsely high readings for serum creatinine may result but GFR not affected.	1.26	12.5	27.1	70	56	0.16 g q12h	I	q12–24h	q24h	yes	yes	no	no
ANTIFUNGAL AGENTS													
Amphotericin B — Nephrotoxic; renal tubular acidosis, magnesium and potassium wasting; initial $t\frac{1}{2}$ ~24–48 h; terminal $t\frac{1}{2}$ > 15 days.	4	24–48	24–48	90	<5	0.5–1 mg/kg q24h	D	100%	100%	no	no	no	no
Fluconazole — $t\frac{1}{2}$ 98–125 h in patients with mean CL_{CR} 13–14 ml/min; HD: 0.2 g after each HD	0.7	31.6	ND	12	73	0.100–0.400 g q24h	I	q24–48h	q48–72h	no	yes	yes	yes
Flucytosine (5-Fluorocytosine) — Dosage should be individualized using patient-specific parameters calculated from plasma concentrations. Bone marrow toxicity may be enhanced in renal failure.	0.6	3–6	75–200	<10	90	Individualize	D, I	Individualize	Individualize	yes	yes	yes	yes
Intraconazole	Large	21	25	99	Low	200 mg q12–24h	D	100%	50–100%	no	no	ND	no
Ketoconazole	1.9–3.6	2–3	2–3	84–99	13	200–400 mg q24h	D	100%	100%	no	ND	ND	ND
ANTIVIRAL AGENTS													
Acyclovir (parenteral) — ESRD patients more susceptible to neurotoxicity, rapid IV infusion can cause decreased CL_{CR} and acute renal failure.	0.7	2.1–3.8	20	15–30	40–70	5–10 mg/kg q8h	D, I	q12–24h	2.5–5.0 mg/kg q24h	yes	no	ND	ND
Ganciclovir — Neutropenia, HD: 1.25 mg/kg q24h, give after HD.	0.47	3–6	30–48.3	1–2	90–100	2.5–5 mg/kg q12h	D, I	1.25–2.5 mg/kg q24h	1.25 mg/kg q48h	yes	yes	ND	yes
ANTIHYPERTENSIVE AND CARDIOVASCULAR AGENTS — Antihypertensive agents: Blood pressure response best guide to dose and interval.													
Adrenergic modulators													
Clonidine — Transdermal system effective in ESRD up to dose of 0.12 mg/24 hr.	3–6	6–23	39–42	20–40	45	0.1–0.6 mg bid	D	100%	100%	no	no	no	no

Table 3.7.   *(Continued)*

THERAPEUTIC CATEGORY Drug Class Drug	V_d (liter/kg) Normal	$t\frac{1}{2}\beta$ (h) CL_{CR} (ml/min) >50	$t\frac{1}{2}\beta$ (h) CL_{CR} (ml/min) <10	PPB (%) Normal	fe (%)	Dose for patients with CL_{CR} = >50 ml/min	Method	Adjustment for Renal Failure CL_{CR} = 10-50 ml/min	Adjustment for Renal Failure CL_{CR} = <10 ml/min	Removed Significantly by HD	PD	CAVH/ CVVH	CAVHD/ CVVHD
Doxazosin Renal patients may be sensitive to small doses.	1–1.7	9.5–12.5	13	98	<5	1–15 mg/d	D	100%	100%	no	no	ND	ND
Guanabenz	10–12	12–14	ND	90	<5	8–16 mg bid	D	100%	100%	ND	ND	ND	ND
Methyldopa Active metabolites with long half-life.	0.5	1.5–6	6–16	<15	25–40	250–500 mg tid	I	q8–12h	q12–24h	yes	no	ND	ND
Prazosin Renal patients should be titrated starting with low doses.	0.6–0.8	2–3	2–3	97	<5	1–15 mg bid	D	100%	100%	no	no	no	no
Terazosin	0.2–0.4	9–12	8–12	90–94	10–15	1–20 mg/d	D	100%	100%	ND	ND	ND	ND
Angiotensin-converting enzyme inhibitors Hypotensive effects magnified by natriuretic agents or sodium depletion. Can cause hyperkalemia or metabolic acidosis. Acute renal dysfunction with bilateral renal artery stenosis, sodium depletion. Dry cough in 5 to 10%. Anaphylactoid reactions reported with concurrent angiotensin-converting enzyme inhibitors and polyacrylonitrile dialyzers.													
Captopril	0.7–0.8	1.9	21–32	25–30	30–40	25 mg q8–12h	D, I	50–75% q12h	50% q24h	yes	no	no	no
Enalapril Prodrug converted to active moiety.	ND	11–24	34–60	50–60	43	5–40 mg q24h	D	75–100%	50%	yes	no	no	no
Lisinopril	1.3–1.5	30	40–50	0–10	?	10–40 mg q24h	D	50–75%	25–50%	yes	no	ND	ND
Ramipril Prodrug converted to active moiety.	~1.3	5–8	15–35	55–70	20–50	2.5–20 mg q24h	D	50–75%	25–50%	yes	no	no	no
Benazepril Prodrug converted to active moiety.	0.2	25	>24	95	20	10–40 mg q24h	D	100%	50%	no	no	no	no
Fosinopril Prodrug converted to active moiety. Only ACE inhibitor with significant amount of hepatic elimination.	0.2	12	20	95	10–15	10–40 mg q24h	D	100%	100%	no	no	no	no

Drug / Notes													
Quinapril — Prodrug converted to active moiety; decreased conversion of quinapril to active moiety in renal failure.	ND	2.3	12.1	>90	37–50.9	10–80 mg q24h	D	50%	25%	no	no	no	no
β-Blockers — Hyperkalemia in ESRD.													
Acebutolol — Active metabolites with long half-life.	1.2	7–9	7	20	55	400–800 mg qd or bid	D	50%	30–50%	no	no	ND	ND
Atenolol — Accumulates in ESRD.	1.1	6.7	15–35	2	>90	50–100 mg qd	D, I	25–50 mg q48h	25 mg q48h	yes	no	yes	yes
Carteolol	3.5–4.5	5.7	30–40	15	55–65	2.5–10 mg/d	D	50%	25%	ND	no	ND	ND
Esmolol — Inactive metabolite accumulates. *See manufacturer's guidelines for titration regimen; stated dose is maintenance infusion.	1–1.5	7–15 min	7–15 min	55	<2	*50–200 µg/kg/min by infusion	D	100%	100%	no	no	ND	ND
Labetalol	5.6	3–9	3–9	50	<5	200–600 mg bid	D	100%	100%	no	no	no	no
Metoprolol	5.5	3.5	2.4–4.5	8	5	50–200 mg bid	D	100%	100%	yes	no	no	no
Nadolol	1.9	19	45	28	90	80–120 mg qd	D	50%	25%	yes	no	no	yes
Penbutolol	ND	22	24	>95	<10	10–40 mg qd	D	100%	100%	no	no	ND	ND
Pindolol	1.2	2.5–4	3–4	50	40	10–30 mg bid	D	100%	100%	no	no	no	no
Propranolol — Increased bioavailability in RF secondary to decreased first-pass metabolism.	2.8	2–6	1–6	93	<5	80–160 mg bid	D	100%	75–100%	no	no	no	yes
Sotalol	1.3	7.5–15	56	<1	60	160 mg qd	D	30%	15–30%	yes	ND	yes	yes
Timolol	1.7	2.7	4	60	15	10–20 mg bid	D	100%	100%	no	no	no	no
Vasodilators													
Diazoxide	0.2–0.3	17–31	30–60	>90	50	150–300 mg bolus	D	100%	100%	no	no	ND	ND
Hydralazine — Acetylator status determines rate of hepatic metabolism.	0.5–0.9	2–4.5	7–16	87	12–14	20–40 mg q6–8h	D	100%	100%	no	no	no	ND
Isosorbide — Active metabolites with long half-life; need nitrate-free interval of 10–12 h for continued effect.	1.5–4	0.15–0.5	4	72	10–20	10–40 mg tid	D	100%	100%	no	no	no	no
Minoxidil	2–3	2.8–4.2	2.8–4.2	0	15–20	5–30 mg bid	D	100%	100%	no	no	ND	ND
Nitroglycerin	2–3	2–4 min	2–4 min	ND	<1	Many methods and routes of dosing	D	100%	100%	no	no	no	no
Nitroprusside — Toxic metabolite, thiocyanate accumulates in RF and may cause seizures, coma. Thiocyanate is hemodialyzable. Measure thiocyanate levels after 48 h of high dose therapy.	0.2	<10 min	<10 min	0	<10	0.25–8 µg/kg/min by infusion, titrate	D	100%	100%	no	no	ND	ND

Table 3.7. (Continued)

64   *Section 1* / CLINICAL PHARMACOLOGY IN THE ICU

THERAPEUTIC CATEGORY Drug Class / Drug	V_d^b (liter/kg) Normal	$t_{1/2}\beta$ (h) CL_{CR} (ml/min) >50	<10	PPB (%) Normal	fe (%)	Dose for patients with CL_{CR} = >50 ml/min	Method	Adjustment for Renal Failure CL_{CR} = 10–50 ml/min	CL_{CR} = <10 ml/min	Removed Significantly by HD	PD	CAVH/ CVVH	CAVHD/ CVVHD
CARDIOVASCULAR DRUGS													
Antiarrhythmic agents Hepatic metabolism of encainide, flecainide, and propafene is genetically determined.													
Amiodarone Active metabolite.	70–140	14–120 d	14–120 d	96	<5	800–1600 mg load, 200–600 mg/dl	D	100%	100%	no	no	no	no
Bretylium	8.2	6–13.6	32–105	6	75	5–30 mg/kg load, 5–10 mg q6h or 1–2 mg/min infusion	D	25–50%	25%	no	no	no	no
Disopyramide Active metabolite; PPB dose-dependent. V_d decreased in ESRD.	0.8–2.6	5–8	10–18	54–81	35–65	100–200 mg q6h	I	q12–24h	q24h	?	no	ND	ND
Encainide Active metabolites which accumulate in RF.	2–2.7	3–9	1.5–9	75–81	5–60	25 mg q8h to 50 mg q6h	D	75–100%	50%	no	ND	ND	ND
Flecainide Excretion enhanced in acid urine.	8.4–9.5	12–19.5	19–26	52	10–40	100–200 mg q12h	D	100%	50–75%	no	no	no	no
Lidocaine	1.3–2.2	2–2.2	1.3–3	60–66	10	50 mg over 2 min, repeat q5 min × 3, then 1–4 mg/min	D	100%	100%	no	no	no	no
Mexiletine Increased renal excretion in acid urine.	5.5–6.6	8–13	16	70–75	10	100–300 mg q6–12h	D	100%	100%	no	no	no	no
N-Acetylprocainamide Redose by monitoring plasma levels. Hemofiltration useful in poisoning.	1.5–1.7	6–8	42–70	10–20	80	500 mg q6–8h	D, I	Individualize	Individualize	yes	no	?	no
Procainamide (parenteral) Redose by monitoring plasma level. Half-life and fe (%) acetylator phenotype-dependent. Active metabolite is N-acetylprocainamide. Hemofiltration useful in poisoning. V_d unchanged in RF.	2.2	2.5–4.9	5.3–14	15	50–60	Load: 12–17 mg/kg MD: Individualize	D, I	Load: 100% MD: Individualize	Load: 100% MD: Individualize	yes	no	no	no
Propafenone Half-life acetylator phenotype dependent.	3	2–3	2–3	>95	<1	150–300 mg q8h	D	100%	100%	no	no	no	no

Drug	t½ normal (h)	t½ ESRD (h)	Vd	PPB (%)	Excreted (%)	Dose	Method	GFR 10–50	GFR <10	Dial. 1	Dial. 2	Dial. 3	Dial. 4
Quinidine sulfate — Active metabolite. Excretion enhanced by acid urine. Hemodialysis useful in poisoning. Redose by monitoring plasma levels.	6	4–14	2–3.5	70–95	20	Initial: 10–15 mg/kg/d divided q6h	D	100% Individualize	100% Individualize	no	no	no	yes
Tocainide — Excretion decreased in alkaline urine.	14	22–27	3.2	10–20	10–40	400–600 mg q8h	D	100%	50%	yes	yes	no	yes
Calcium channel blockers													
Amlodipine	35–50	50	21	>95	<10	5–10 mg/d	D	100%	100%	ND	ND	no	no
Diltiazem (oral, parenteral) — Active metabolites. Continuous infusion can be used.	2–8	3.5	3–5	98	<10	60–120 mg q8h; 20–25 mg	D	100%	100%	no	no	no	no
Felodipine	10–14	21	9–7	99	<1	5–20 mg q24h	D	100%	100%	ND	ND	no	no
Isradipine	8–12	10–11	3–4	96	<5	2.5–5 mg bid	D	100%	100%	ND	ND	no	no
Nicardipine	5	5–7	1–1.5	98–99	<5	20–30 mg bid-tid	D	100%	100%	ND	ND	no	no
Nifedipine — PPB decreased in ESRD.	4–5.5	5–7	1.4	97	<5	10–30 mg q8h	D	100%	100%	no	no	no	no
Nimodipine — *Age-related hepatic impairment may be responsible for prolonged t½ reported in renal insufficiency patients.	1–2.8	22*	0.9–2.3	98	<1	60 mg q4h	D	100%	?	ND	ND	no	no
Nitrendipine	4.6	3.3–5.8	6.6	99	<1	20 mg bid	D	100%	100%	no	no	no	no
Verapamil (oral, parenteral) — Active metabolites.	3–7	2.4–4	3–6	83–93	<10	80–120 mg q8h; 5–10 mg	D	100%	100%	no	no	no	no
Cardiac glycosides													
Digitoxin — 8–10% converted to digoxin	144–200	210	0.6	94	20–25	0.1–0.2 mg/d	D	100%	100%	no	no	no	no
Digoxin — Vd and total body clearance decreased in ESRD. Decrease loading dose by 30–50% in ESRD. Various digoxin assays overestimate serum levels in uremia. Bioavailability of oral tablets only 65–75%.	36–44	80–120	5–8	20–30	76–85	10–15 μg/kg load, 0.25–0.5 mg/d	D, I	25–75% q24–48h	25% q48h	no	no	no	no
Diuretics — Thiazide diuretics generally ineffective alone in Cl_{CR} <30 ml/min but show synergism when administered with loop diuretics in renal failure.													
Amiloride — Increased risk of hyperkalemia in renal insufficiency and with concomitant ACE inhibitors.	6–8	10–144	5–5.2	30–40	50	5–10 mg q24h	D	50%	Avoid	NA	NA	NA	NA

Table 3.7. *(Continued)*

THERAPEUTIC CATEGORY / Drug Class / Drug	V_d^b (liter/kg) Normal	$t\frac{1}{2}\beta$ (h) CL_{CR} (ml/min) >50	$t\frac{1}{2}\beta$ (h) <10	PPB (%) Normal	fe (%)	Dose for patients with CL_{CR} = >50 ml/min	Method	Adjustment for Renal Failure CL_{CR} = 10–50 ml/min	CL_{CR} = <10 ml/min	Removed Significantly by HD	PD	CAVH/ CVVH	CAVHD/ CVVHD
Bumetanide Doses higher than 2 mg may be necessary in ESRD or ARF. Maximum daily dose: 20 mg; oral and iv dose identical.	0.2–0.5	1.2–1.5	1.5	96	33	1–2 mg q8–12h	D	100%	100%	no	no	no	no
Chlorothiazide (parenteral)	0.2	0.75–2	Increased	95	>95	0.5–1 g q12–24h	D	100%	Avoid	no	ND	no	no
Chlorthalidone	3.9	44–80	ND	76–90	50	25 mg/d	I	q24h	Avoid	ND	ND	ND	ND
Ethacrynic acid (parenteral) Higher incidence of ototoxicity than with furosemide or bumetanide; increased ototoxicity risk with low GFR.	0.1	2–4	ND	90	20	50 mg prn	I	100%	Avoid	no	ND	no	no
Furosemide (parenteral) Ototoxicity with rapid infusions; doses of 100 mg–1000 mg may be necessary in ESRD or ARF; oral bioavailability only 40–60%.	0.07–0.2	0.5–1.1	2–4	95	67	40–80 mg q12h	D	100%	100%	no	no	no	no
Hydrochlorothiazide	0.83	2.5	12–20	64	>95	25–50 mg qd	D	100%	Avoid	no	ND	no	no
Indapamide Ineffective in ESRD.	0.3–1.3	14–18	14–18	76–79	<5	2.5 mg/d	D	100%	Avoid	ND	ND	ND	ND
Metolazone High doses effective alone in ESRD; smaller doses synergistic with loop diuretics in ESRD.	1.6	4–20	ND	95	70	5–10 mg/d	D	100%	100%	no	no	no	no
Spironolactone Usually ineffective with GFR <30 ml/min. Active metabolite with long half-life; hyperkalemia.	ND	10–35	10–35	98	20–30	100–200 mg qd	D	50%	Avoid	no	ND	no	no
Triamterene Usually ineffective with GFR <30 ml/min; hyperkalemia.	2.2–3.7	2–12	10	40–70	4–10	50–100 mg q12h	D	100%	Avoid	ND	ND	ND	ND
Miscellaneous cardiac drugs													
Amrinone	1.3–1.6	2.6–8.3	ND	20–40	10–40	0.75 mg/kg load, 5–10 μg/kg/min, titrate daily dose <10 mg/kg	D	100%	?	ND	ND	yes	ND
Dobutamine	0.25	2 min	ND	ND	<10	2.5–15 μg/kg/min, titrate	D	100%	100%	no	no	no	no

Drug (comments)	Vd	t½ normal	t½ ESRD	Protein binding (%)	% excreted	Dose	Method	Adj A	Adj B	Dial 1	Dial 2	Dial 3	Dial 4
Dopamine — Increases renal blood flow at doses between 0.5 and 2 μg/kg/min.	ND	2 min	ND	ND	Small	0.5–20 μg/kg/min, titrate	D	100%	100%	no	no	no	no
Milrinone	0.25–0.35	1	1.5–3	70	80–85	15–75 μg/kg iv load, then 2.5–15 mg q6h po	D	100%	50–75%	no	ND	ND	ND
Norepinephrine	ND	min	ND	ND	Negligible	2–12 μg/min, titrate	D	100%	100%	no	no	no	no

SEDATIVES, HYPNOTICS, DRUGS USED IN PSYCHIATRY

Barbiturates
Charcoal hemoperfusion and hemodialysis more effective than peritoneal dialysis for overdose.

Drug (comments)	Vd	t½ normal	t½ ESRD	Protein binding (%)	% excreted	Dose	Method	Adj A	Adj B	Dial 1	Dial 2	Dial 3	Dial 4
Pentobarbital (parenteral) — PPB decreased in ESRD.	1	35–50	35–50	60–70	<1	100 mg prn	D	100%	100%	no	no	ND	no
Phenobarbital — PPB decreases in hypoalbuminemia. Monitor plasma levels; alkalinization of urine increases excretion.	0.6	60–150	117–160	40–60	25	1–3 mg/kg qd / Individualize	D	100% / Individualize	75–100% / Individualize	yes	yes	yes	yes
Secobarbital (parenteral)	1.5–2.5	20–35	ND	44	5	Anesthesia induction	D	100%	100%	no	ND	no	ND
Thiopental	1–1.5	4	6–18	72–86	<1	Anesthesia induction	D	100%	75%	ND	ND	ND	ND

Benzodiazepines

Drug (comments)	Vd	t½ normal	t½ ESRD	Protein binding (%)	% excreted	Dose	Method	Adj A	Adj B	Dial 1	Dial 2	Dial 3	Dial 4
Alprazolam — Active metabolite; does not accumulate in ESRD; PPB decreased in ESRD, HD, and CAPD—patients show enhanced sensitivity to some pharmacodynamic effects.	0.9–1.3	9.5–19	9.5–19	70–80	20	0.25–5 mg tid	D	100%	100%	ND	ND	ND	ND
Clonazepam	1.5–4.5	18–50	18–50	86	<1	0.5–5 mg tid	D	100%	100%	no	ND	no	no
Diazepam (parenteral) — Active metabolites; main metabolite does not appear to accumulate in RF; PPB decreased in ESRD; Vd increased in ESRD.	0.7–3.4	20–90	20–90	94–98	<1	5–20 mg prn	D	100%	100%	no	ND	no	ND
Flurazepam — Active metabolite.	3.4	47–100	47–100	96.6	<1	15–30 mg hs	D	100%	100%	no	ND	ND	ND
Lorazepam — Inactive metabolite.	0.9–1.3	10–20	32–70	87	<1	1–2 mg bid-tid	D	100%	100%	no	no	no	no
Midazolam — PPB decreased in ESRD; renal clearance of active metabolite decreased in ARF.	1–6.6	1.2–12.3	1.2–12.3	93–96	<1	titrate	D	100%	50–100%	no	no	ND	no

Table 3.7. (*Continued*)

THERAPEUTIC CATEGORY / Drug Class / Drug	V_d (liter/kg) Normal	$t\frac{1}{2}\beta$ (h) CL_{CR} (ml/min) >50	$t\frac{1}{2}\beta$ (h) CL_{CR} (ml/min) <10	PPB (%) Normal	fe (%)	Dose for patients with CL_{CR} = >50 ml/min	Method	CL_{CR} = 10–50 ml/min	CL_{CR} = <10 ml/min	HD	PD	CAVH/ CVVH	CAVHD/ CVVHD
								Adjustment for Renal Failure		*Removed Significantly by*			
Oxazepam — Inactive metabolite; PPB decreased and V_d increased in ESRD.	0.6–1.6	5–10	25–90	97	<1	10–30 mg tid, qid	D	100%	100%	no	ND	no	no
Temazepam — PPB decreased in renal disease.	1.3–1.5	4–10	ND	96	<1	15–30 mg hs	D	100%	100%	no	ND	no	no
Triazolam — PPB correlates with α-1 acid glycoprotein concentration.	1.1	2–4	2–4	85–95	2	0.125–0.25 mg hs	D	100%	100%	no	ND	no	no
Miscellaneous agents													
Buspirone — Active metabolite accumulates in ESRD, metabolite PPB 35–41%.	5	2–4	5.8	95	<1	5–10 mg tid	D	100%	50%	?	ND	ND	ND
Chloral hydrate — Active metabolite.	0.6	7–14	ND	70–80	<1	250 mg tid 500–1000 mg hs	D	ND	Avoid	?	ND	ND	ND
Haloperidol (parenteral)	14–21	10–36	ND	90–92	1	1–5 mg prn	D	100%	100%	no	no	no	no
Lithium carbonate — Dosage should be individualized using patient-specific parameters calculated from plasma concentrations. Plasma levels rebound after hemodialysis.	0.5–0.9	14–28	40	None	95	0.9–2.1 g qd in divided doses	D	Individualize 50–75%	Individualize 25–50%	yes	no	yes	yes
Phenothiazines													
Chlorpromazine (parenteral)	21	11–42	11–42	91–99	<1	25–50 mg q3–4h	D	100%	100%	no	no	no	no
Promethazine (parenteral) Excessive sedation	Large	9–12	ND	76–93	ND	12.5–50 mg q4h	D	100%	100%	ND	ND	ND	ND
Tricyclic antidepressants — Dosage reductions indicated for elderly and dehabilitated patients; daily doses should be divided initially and then consolidated in a single hs dose.													
Amitriptyline — Reduce dose in elderly.	6–36	24–40	24–40	96	<2	100–300 mg/d	D	100%	100%	no	no	no	no
Desipramine — Active metabolites.	28–60	12–54	ND	90	2	100–300 mg/d	D	100%	100%	no	no	no	no
Doxepin — PPB decreased in ESRD.	9–33	8–25	10–30	95	0	100–300 mg/d	D	100%	100%	no	no	no	no
Imipramine — Active metabolites.	9–15	6–20	ND	96	<2	100–300 mg/d	D	100%	100%	no	no	no	no
Nortriptyline	15–23	25–38	15–66	95	2	100–300 mg/d	D	100%	100%	no	no	no	no

Drug / Comments	Vd (L/kg)	t½ Normal	t½ ESRD	PPB (%)	Excreted (%)	Dose	Method	GFR 10–50	GFR <10	HD	CAPD	CAVH	
Protriptyline	15–31	54–98	ND	92	0	15–60 mg/d	D	100%	100%	no	no	no	no
Other antidepressants													
Fluoxetine — Active metabolite, which is hepatically metabolized with t½ 7–9 d.	35	2–3 d	2–3 d	95	<2.5	20–80 mg q am	D	100%	100%	no	no	no	no
Paroxetine — Dose-dependent pharmacokinetics.	ND	17.3	29.7 min CL_{CR} <30	95	2	20–50 mg q am	D	50–100%	50%	no	ND	ND	ND
Sertraline — Mildly active metabolite.	ND	26	NC	98	<1	50–200 mg q am	D	100%	100%	ND	ND	ND	ND
Narcotics and narcotic antagonists													
Alfentanil — Dosage ranges widely; PPB decreased in ESRD.	0.3–1	1–3	1–3	88–95	<1	Anesthetic induction	D	100%	100%	ND	ND	ND	ND
Butorphanol	9–11	2–4	ND	80	<5	2 mg q3–4h	D	ND	ND	ND	ND	ND	ND
Codeine — Active metabolites that accumulate in ESRD; narcosis reported in RF on standard doses.	3–4	4.4	13.0	7	0	30–60 mg q4–6h	D	75–100%	25–50%	no	no	no	
Fentanyl — Transdermal patch available for chronic pain control	2–4	2–7 min	NC	80–84	8	Anesthetic induction	D	100%	100%	NA	NA	NA	NA
Meperidine — Normeperidine, an active metabolite, accumulates in ESRD (t½–34h) and may cause seizures. CNS excitatory effects not reversed by naloxone. PPB reduced in ESRD. One-time doses OK in ESRD, but avoid chronic use.	4–5	2–7	2–7	70	1–25	50–100 mg q3–4h	D	50–100%	Avoid	no	no	ND	ND
Methadone — Fecal elimination is increased in ESRD. Acidic urine increases renal elimination.	3–6	13–58	ND	60–90	24	2.5–10 mg q6–8h	D	100%	100%	no	no	no	ND
Morphine (parenteral) — Active metabolite which accumulates in ESRD	3.5	1–4	1–4	20–30	6–10	2–10 mg q4h	D	75%	50%	ND	no	no	no
Naloxone	3	1–1.5	ND	54	0	0.4–2 mg	D	100%	100%	ND	ND	ND	ND
Propoxyphene — Active metabolite norpropoxyphene accumulates in ESRD and may cause cardiac toxicity. Cardiac toxicity not reversed by naloxone.	16	9–15	12–20	78	25	65 mg tid-qid	D	100%	Avoid	no	no	no	ND
Sufentanil — Dosage ranges widely.	2–3	2–5 min	2–5 min	92	6	Anesthetic induction	D	100%	100%	no	no	no	no

Table 3.7. *(Continued)*

THERAPEUTIC CATEGORY / Drug Class / Drug	V_d (liter/kg) Normal	$t\frac{1}{2}\beta$ (h) CL_{CR} (ml/min) >50	<10	PPB (%) Normal	fe (%)	Dose for patients with CL_{CR} = >50 ml/min	Adjustment for Renal Failure Method	CL_{CR} = 10–50 ml/min	CL_{CR} = <10 ml/min	Removed Significantly by HD	PD	CAVH/ CVVH	CAVHD/ CVVHD
Nonnarcotic analgesics													
Acetaminophen Metabolites may accumulate in ESRD.	1–2	2	2	20–30	3	650 mg q4h	I	q6h	q6h	no	no	no	no
Aspirin May decrease GFR when renal blood flow is prostaglandin-dependent. Excretion enhanced in alkaline urine. May add to uremic GI and hematologic symptoms. PPB reduced in ESRD. Low dose once-daily therapy for prophylaxis may be cautiously used in ESRD.	0.1–0.2	2–3	2–3	80–90	1.4	650 mg q4h	I	q4–6h	Avoid	yes	no	no	yes
Ketorolac May decrease GRF when renal blood flow is prostaglandin-dependent.	0.11–0.33	3.8–6.3	9–10	99	60	30–60 mg load 15–30 mg q6h	D	100%	15 mg q6h	ND	ND	ND	ND
MISCELLANEOUS AGENTS													
Antithrombotic agents													
Dipyridamole	2.4	12	ND	99	Small	75 mg tid	D	100%	100%	ND	ND	ND	ND
Heparin Half-life increases with dose, titrate dose to APTT.	0.06–0.1	0.3–2	0.3–2	>90	0	5000 U load 800–1500 U/hr	D	100%	100%	no	no	no	no
Streptokinase ESRD patients may be predisposed to bleeding complications; other dosage regimens have been used.	0.016	1–1.5	ND	ND	0	1.5 mU over 60 min or 250,000 U load, 100,000 U/h	D	100%	100%	ND	ND	ND	ND
Ticlopidine Neutropenia; active metabolite in rats, ? in humans; $t\frac{1}{2}$ increases after multiple doses.	ND	24–36	ND	98	<1	250 mg bid	D	100%	100%	ND	ND	ND	ND
Warfarin Titrate dose to INR or PT.	0.15	35–45	35–45	99	0	10 mg load × 2–3 d 2–10 mg/d	D	100%	100%	no	no	no	no
Anticonvulsants Monitor serum levels.													

Drug / remarks	V_d (L/kg)	$t_{1/2}$ Normal	$t_{1/2}$ ESRF	% PB	% Excr	Dose	Method	>50	10–50	<10	Hemo	CAPD	CAVH
Carbamazepine — Dosage should be individualized using patient-specific parameters calculated from plasma concentrations. Active metabolite with anticonvulsant and toxic effects, carbamazepine induces its own metabolism; other anticonvulsants induce metabolism; $t_{1/2}$ decreases with chronic therapy and with other concomitant anticonvulsant therapy.	0.8–1.8	24–40 h single dose; 6–25 h chronic dosing	NC	75	2–3	200 mg bid to 1200 mg/d in divided doses	D	100%	Individualize	100% Individualize	no	no	no
Ethosuximide	0.7	35–55	35–55	10	12–20	500–1500 mg/d	D	100%	100%	Individualize	yes	yes	ND
Phenytoin — Dosage should be individualized using patient-specific parameters calculated from plasma concentrations. Measure free levels in renal insufficiency or failure. PPB decreased and V_d increased in RF. Dose-dependent pharmacokinetics.	1	24	24	90	2	18 mg/kg load, 200–500 mg/d	D	100%	100% Individualize	100% Individualize	no	no	no
Primidone — Partially converted to phenobarbital and other metabolites with long half-life, monitor phenobarbital and primidone levels.	0.6	5–15	5–15	20	40	250–500 mg qid	D, I	Individualize	Individualize	Individualize	yes	ND	ND
Sodium valproate — Decreased PPB in uremia; $t_{1/2}$ decreases with polytherapy; monitoring total drug concentrations in ESRD may be misleading.	0.2	9–18	6–15	90	1–3	15–60 mg/kg qd divided bid-qid	D	100%	100%	100%	no	no	no
ANTIHISTAMINES													
H-1 antagonists													
Diphenhydramine	3.3–6.8	3.4–9.3	ND	80	2	25–50 mg q6–8h	D	100%	100%	100%	no	no	no
Hydroxyzine — Active metabolite excreted by the kidney.	19.5	14–20	ND	ND	0	25–100 mg q6h	D	?	?	?	no	no	ND
Antiulcer agents — Dosage of H_2 blockers (cimetidine, famotidine, ranitidine) should be guided by gastric pH monitoring in the acute care setting.													

Table 3.7. *(Continued)*

THERAPEUTIC CATEGORY / Drug Class / Drug	V_d (liter/kg) Normal	$t\frac{1}{2}\beta$ (h) CL_{CR} (ml/min) >50	$t\frac{1}{2}\beta$ (h) CL_{CR} (ml/min) <10	PPB (%) Normal	fe (%)	Dose for patients with CL_{CR} = >50 ml/min	Method	Adjustment for Renal Failure CL_{CR} = 10–50 ml/min	Adjustment for Renal Failure CL_{CR} = <10 ml/min	Removed Significantly by HD	Removed Significantly by PD	Removed Significantly by CAVH/ CVVH	Removed Significantly by CAVHD/ CVVHD
Cimetidine (parenteral) Inhibition of tubular secretion of creatinine. Mental confusion in patients with renal or hepatic disease.	0.8–1.3	1.5–2	5	20	50–70	300 mg q6h or 37.5–50 mg/h	D, I	q8–12h 25–37.5 mg/h	q12h 18–25 mg/h	yes	no	no	no
Famotidine (parenteral)	0.8–1.4	2.5–4	12–19	15–22	65–80	20–40 mg q12h	I	q12–24h	q24h	no	no	no	yes
Omeprazole	0.4–0.5	0.5–1	0.5–1	95	<1	20–40 mg qd	D	100%	100%	no	no	no	no
Ranitidine (parenteral)	1.1–1.9	1.5–3	6–9	15	80	50 mg q8h or 6.25 mg/h	I	q12h	q24h	yes	no	no	no
Arthritis and gout agents													
Allopurinol Renal excretion of active metabolite (oxypurinol) with half-life of 25 h.	0.5	2–8	2–8	<5	30	300 mg/d	D, I	150 mg qd	100 mg q24–72h	yes	ND	ND	ND
Colchicine (oral) Enterohepatic recycling of colchicine and metabolites. Acute: doses given until pain relief or GI symptoms appear. Avoid prolonged use in CL_{CR} <50 ml/min.	470–700	9–20	40	31	5–17	Acute: 0.5–1.3 mg, then 0.5–0.65 mg q 1–2 h prn Chronic: 0.5–0.65 mg qd or qod	I	?	?	no	ND	ND	ND
Bronchodilators													
Albuterol (oral) Aerosol available.	2–2.5	4	Increased	7	51–64	2–4 mg tid-qid	D	75%	50%	ND	ND	ND	ND
Diphylline	0.8	1.8–2.3	12	<3	85	15 mg/kg/d	D	50%	25%	yes	ND	ND	ND
Ipratropium	4.6	1.6	ND	ND	ND	2 inhalations qid	D	100%	100%	no	no	no	no
Terbutaline Large first-dose effect. Parenteral doses should be avoided in ESRD. Oral doses unchanged. Aerosol available.	0.94	14	ND	25	50	2.5–5 mg tid	D	50%	Avoid	ND	ND	ND	ND
Theophylline May exacerbate uremic gastrointestinal symptoms. Doses are expressed in terms of aminophylline. Monitor plasma levels of theophylline.	0.3–0.7	4–12	4–12	55	18	6 mg/kg load, 0.5–0.7 mg/kg/h	D	100%	100%	yes	ND	no	no
Corticosteroids													
Bethamethasone (parenteral)	1.4	5.5	ND	65	5	0.5–9 mg/d	D	100%	100%	ND	ND	ND	ND
Cortisone (oral)	ND	0.5–2	3.5	90	0	25–500 mg/d	D	100%	100%	no	no	no	no
Dexamethasone Oral and iv dose equivalent.	0.8–1	3–4	ND	70	2.6	0.75–9 mg/d	D	100%	100%	ND	ND	ND	ND

Drug	V_d	$t_{1/2}$ normal	$t_{1/2}$ ESRD	% Protein binding	% Excreted	Dose	Method	GFR 10–50	GFR <10	Hemo	CAPD	CAVH
Hydrocortisone — Oral and iv dose equivalent.	ND	1.5–2	1.5–2	ND	0	20–500 mg/d	D	100%	100%	ND	ND	ND
Methylprednisolone	1.2–1.5	2.3	2.3	78	4.9	10–150 mgqd	D	100%	100%	yes	ND	ND
Prednisolone — Oral and iv dose equivalent.	2.2	2.5–3.5	2.5–3.5	Saturable	26	5–60 mg/d	D	100%	100%	yes	no	ND
Prednisone	0.97	2.5–3.5	2.5–3.5	Saturable	3	5–60 mg/d	D	100%	100%	no	ND	ND
Triamcinolone (oral)	1.4–2.1	1.9–6	1.9–6	ND	ND	4–48 mg/d	D	100%	100%	ND	ND	ND
Hypoglycemic agents — Titrate insulin and oral hypoglycemic agents with blood glucose monitoring.												
Acetohexamide — May falsely elevate serum creatinine level. Active metabolite with half-life of 5–8 hours. Prolonged hypoglycemia in azotemic patients.	0.21	1–1.3	1–1.3	65–90	<1	250–1500 mg/d	I	Avoid	Avoid	ND	no	ND
Chlorpropamide — Prolonged hypoglycemia in azotemic patients.	0.09–0.27	24–42	50–200	88–96	20	100–500 mg/d	I	Avoid	Avoid	ND	no	ND
Glipizide — Inactive metabolites.	0.13–0.16	2–7	ND	97	4–5.7	2.5–15 mg/d	D	100%	100%	ND	ND	ND
Glyburide — Active metabolite prolongs hypoglycemic effect in rats.	0.16–0.3	7–10	ND	99	50	2.5–20 mg/d	D	Avoid	Avoid	no	no	no
Insulin — Renal metabolism of insulin decreases with azotemia.	0.15	2–4	13	5	0	Variable	D	75%	50%	no	no	no
Tolazamide — Weakly active metabolites.	ND	4–7	ND	94	7	100–500 mg/d	D	100%	100%	ND	ND	ND
Tolbutamide — Some patients may require divided doses.	0.1–0.15	4–6	4–6	95–97	0	1–2 g/d	D	100%	100%	no	no	no
Miscellaneous drugs												
Metoclopramide — Extrapyramidal side effects common in ESRD.	2–3.4	2.5–4	14–15	40	10–22	10–15 mg qid	D	75%	50%	no	ND	no
Cyclosporine	3.5–7.4	3–16	3–16	96–99	<1	3–10 mg/kg/d	D	100%	100%	no	no	ND
N-Acetylcysteine — Dosage indicated is for treatment of acetaminophen overdose.	0.34	2.3	ND	ND	30	140 mg/kg load, 70 mg/kg q4h for 17 doses	D	100%	100%	ND	ND	ND
Pentoxifylline	2.4	0.8	0.8	0	0	400 mg tid	D	100%	100%	ND	ND	ND
Neuromuscular agents												
Alfentanil	0.3–1	1.4–2	1.4–2	88–95	<1	8–245 µg/kg load, 0.5–3 µg/kg*min	D	100%	100%	ND	ND	ND

Table 3.7.   *(Continued)*

THERAPEUTIC CATEGORY Drug Class Drug	$V_d{}^b$ (liter/kg) Normal	$t^{1/2}\beta$ (h) CL_{CR} (ml/min) >50	$t^{1/2}\beta$ (h) CL_{CR} (ml/min) <10	PPB (%) Normal	fe (%)	Dose for patients with CL_{CR} = >50 ml/min	Adjustment for Renal Failure Method	CL_{CR} = 10–50 ml/min	CL_{CR} = <10 ml/min	Removed Significantly by HD	PD	CAVH/ CVVH	CAVHD/ CVVHD
Atracurium	0.15–0.18	0.3–0.4	0.3–0.4	82	0	0.4–0.5 mg/kg load, 0.08–0.1 mg/kg q15–25 min	D	100%	100%	ND	ND	ND	ND
Etomidate	2–4.5	4–5	4–5	75	0	0.2–0.6 mg/kg	D	100%	100%	ND	ND	ND	ND
Gallamine If blockade not responsive to neostigmine, dialysis may be useful.	0.21–0.24	2.3–2.7	6–20	30–70	85–100	0.5–1.5 mg/kg	D	Avoid	Avoid	NA	NA	NA	NA
Ketamine	1.8–3.1	2–3.5	2–3.5	ND	2–3	1–4.5 mg/kg	D	100%	100%	ND	ND	ND	ND
Metocurine	0.42–0.57	3.5–5.8	11.4	35	45–60	0.2–0.4 mg/kg	D	Avoid	Avoid	ND	ND	ND	ND
Neostigmine	0.5–1	1.3–3	3	0	67	15–375 mg/d	D	50%	25%	ND	ND	ND	ND
Pancuronium Active metabolite, which can accumulate in renal insufficiency.	0.15–0.38	2.3	4.3–8.2	70–85	30–40	0.04–0.1 mg/kg	D	50%	50%	ND	ND	ND	ND
Pyridostigmine Renal excretion decreased by basic drugs.	0.8–1.4	1.5–2	6	ND	80–90	60–1500 mg/d	D	35%	20%	ND	ND	ND	ND
Succinylcholine Hyperkalemia in ESRD.	ND	3	ND	ND	0	0.3–1.1 mg/kg load, 0.04–0.07 mg/kg prn	D	100%	100%	ND	ND	ND	ND
Sufentanil	1.7–5.2	2	2	92	1–2	1–30 µg/kg	D	100%	100%	ND	ND	ND	ND
Tubocurarine Prolonged neuromuscular blockade reported in ESRD.	0.22–0.39	2–4	5.5	30–50	40–60	0.1–0.2 mg/kg	D	50%	Avoid	ND	ND	ND	ND
Vecuronium Active metabolite, which can accumulate in renal insufficiency.	0.18–0.27	0.5–1.3	0.5–1.3	30	25	0.08–0.1 mg/kg load, 0.01–0.05 mg/kg	D	100%	Avoid	ND	ND	ND	ND

[a] Data compiled from references 151, 161, 176, 178, 210–263.
[b] APTT, activated partial thromboplastin time; CAVH/CAVHD, continuous arteriovenous hemofiltration or continuous arteriovenous hemofiltration or hemodialysis; CL, clearance; CVVH/CVVHD, continuous venovenous hemofiltration or hemodialysis; D, dose; ESRD, end-stage renal disease; GFR, glomerular filtration rate; HD, hemodialysis; I, interval; INR, international normalized ratio; LOAD, loading dose; MTT, methylthiotetrazole; NA, not applicable; NC, no change; ND, no data; PD, peritoneal dialysis; PT, prothrombin time; RF, renal failure; V_d, volume of distribution; ?, data equivocal or insufficient to make recommendations.

There are no established guidelines in the pharmacokinetic literature for the stratification of patients into categories of various degrees of renal function, using CL_{CR}. Investigators often report mean pharmacokinetic data from a selected range of CL_{CR} values that may or may not match those from other studies with the same drug. Furthermore, investigators from earlier clinical trials frequently neglected to mention whether CL_{CR} was estimated from an equation or whether a measured CL_{CR} had been performed.

Issues in trials in patients receiving intermittent or continuous hemodialysis or hemofiltration therapies included administering the particular drug immediately before or during the procedure and not allowing time for drug distribution to occur. Other common problems encountered included use of the arteriovenous method for calculation of hemodialysis clearance (202) and use of blood flow rate instead of plasma flow rate in calculations when plasma concentrations of the drug had been measured. Rebound of drug concentrations after hemodialysis have rarely been evaluated. Medical practitioners need to be cognizant of the numerous limitations of providing dosing information in a tabular review format.

A GUIDE TO INTERPRETING TABLE 3.7

Table 3.7 represents a list of those drugs more commonly used in an acute care environment and is not intended to be an exhaustive list of all medications.

CLASSIFICATION OF RENAL FUNCTION

Renal function in Table 3.7 was categorized according to measured or estimated CL_{CR}. The categories selected were: $CL_{CR} > 50$ ml/min, CL_{CR} 10 to 50 ml/min, and $CL_{CR} < 10$ ml/min. Although a $CL_{CR} > 50$ ml/min does not define normal renal function, dosage adjustment with medications is rarely advocated until CL_{CR} is less than 50 ml/min. Notable exceptions are aminoglycoside antibiotics, vancomycin, digoxin, procainamide, and 5-fluorocytosine (flucytosine) where dosing is usually individualized across the spectrum of renal function.

PHARMACOKINETIC PARAMETERS

V_d and plasma protein binding percent (PPB%) in subjects with normal renal function is supplied as a frame of reference. Clinically significant alterations that would result in dosage adjustment in renal failure are addressed under Comment. The terminal elimination half-life ($t^{1/2}\beta$) of each medication in patients with $CL_{CR} > 50$ ml/min and < 10 ml/min is presented to provide a comparison of patients with fairly normal renal function to those that have ESRD. The fraction of systemically available drug excreted unchanged in the urine (fe%) will indicate whether renal clearance is the major route of elimination of the drug.

DOSAGE ADJUSTMENT IN RENAL FAILURE

The dosage for patients with normal renal function reflects commonly administered dosages. This dosage should not be interpreted to be the only correct dosage for any indication in individual patients. After an appropriate loading dose, the maintenance dosage can be adjusted by lengthening the dosage interval (I) or by decreasing the dose (D), depending on the particular drug and clinical circumstance. See Dosing Implications and Drug Monitoring for further explanation. In Table 3.7, the preferred method of dosage alteration is indicated by an I or D. When "D" is displayed, then the dose should be reduced by the percentage indicated. Doses should be rounded off to practical units. If "I" is indicated, then the dose interval should be extended to the number of hours shown. Oftentimes, drug dosages can be altered using both methods simultaneously for optimal patient management; thus, "D or I" may be displayed.

SUPPLEMENTAL DOSING WITH DIALYTIC TECHNIQUES

For the purposes of Table 3.7, drugs that have been proven to be significantly removed (63) by dialytic methods or whose characteristics indicate the potential for significant removal are designated as "yes." Conversely, drugs that do not meet the criteria above are designated in the table as "no." Unfortunately, it is impossible to quantify the amount removed by a particular dialysis session in a given patient for reasons outlined in Effects of Dialysis Techniques on Drug Clearance. In the case of many drugs, such as most antibiotics, supplemental dosing may not be necessary after hemodialysis as long as the normal maintenance dose is scheduled for after hemodialysis. In other circumstances, supplemental doses may be required after hemodialysis. For instance, a patient receiving procainamide for control of atrial fibrillation may develop atrial fibrillation while on hemodialysis or after hemodialysis secondary to decreased procainamide and/or *n*-acetylprocainamide concentrations. In this case, additional doses should be given to supplement a regular maintenance dose. Hemodialysis provides a major route of elimination for aminoglycosides and vancomycin (high flux dialyzers) in ESRD. Thus, supplemental doses of aminoglycosides and vancomycin (high-flux dialyzers) should also be given after hemodialysis.

REFERENCES

1. Hori R, Okumura K, Kamiya A, Nihira H, Nakano H: Ampicillin and cephalexin in renal insufficiency. *Clin Pharmacol Ther* 34:792–798, 1983.
2. Kamiya A, Okumura K, Hori R: Quantitative investigation on renal handling of drugs in rabbits, dogs, and humans. *J Pharm Sci* 72:440–443, 1983.
3. Perrone RD, Madias NE, Levey AS: Serum creatinine as an index of renal function: new insights into old concepts. *Clin Chem* 38:1933–1953, 1992.
4. Giavannetti S, Barsotti G: In defense of creatinine clearance. *Nephron* 59:11–14, 1991.
5. Schuster VL, Seldin DW: Renal clearance. In: Seldin DW, Giebisch G (eds): *The Kidney: Physiology and Pathophysiology*. Raven Press, New York, pp 365–395, 1985.
6. Schück O, Taplan V, Nádvorníková H: The effect of haemodialysis on tubular secretion of creatinine in residual nephrons. *Nephrol Dial Transplant* 5:549–550, 1990.
7. Freysz M, Lafleur P, Dupont G, et al: Comparison of creatinine and inulin clearances in multiple trauma. *Biomed Pharmacother* 44:175–180, 1990.
8. Robert S, Zarowitz BJ: Is there a reliable index of glomerular filtration rate in critically ill patients? *DICP* 25:169–178, 1991.
9. Ducharme MP, Smythe M, Strohs G: Drug-induced alterations in serum creatinine concentrations. *Ann Pharmacother* 27:622–633, 1993.
10. Roubenoff R, Drew H, Moyer M, Petri M, Whiting-O'Keefe Q, Hellmann DB: Oral cimetidine improves the accuracy and precision of creatinine clearance in lupus nephritis. *Ann Intern Med* 113:501–506, 1990.

11. Hilbrands LB, Artz MA, Wetzels JFM, Koene RAP: Cimetidine improves the reliability of creatinine as a marker of glomerular filtration. *Kidney Int* 40:1171–1176, 1991.

12. Hirata-Dulas CAI, Kasiske BL, Halstenson CE: Improvement in the accuracy and precision of creatinine clearance as a measure of glomerular filtration rate with oral cimetidine in renal transplant recipients. *Clin Transplantation* in press, 1993.

13. Apple FS, Benson P, Abraham PA, Rosano TG, Halstenson CE: Assessment of renal function by inulin clearance: comparison with creatinine clearance as determined by enzymatic methods. *Clin Chem* 35:312–314, 1989.

14. Baumann TJ, Staddon JE, Horst HM, Bivins BA: Minimum urine collection periods for accurate determination of creatinine clearance in critically ill patients. *Clin Pharm* 6:393–398, 1987.

15. Luke DR, Halstenson CE, Opsahl JA, Matzke GR: Validity of creatinine clearance estimates in the assessment of renal function. *Clin Pharmacol Ther* 48:503–508, 1990.

16. Mawer CE, Knowles BR, Lucas SB, Stirland RA, Tooth JA: Computer-assisted prescribing of kanamycin for patients with renal insufficiency. *Lancet* i:12–15, 1972.

17. Cockcroft DW, Gault MH: Prediction of creatinine clearance from serum creatinine. *Nephron* 16:31–41, 1976.

18. Pesola GR, Akhavan I, Madu A, Shah NK, Carlon GC: Prediction equation estimates of creatinine clearance in the intensive care unit. *Intensive Care Med* 19:39–43, 1993.

19. Martin C, Alaya M, Bras J, Saux P, Gouin F: Assessment of creatinine clearance in intensive care patients. *Crit Care Med* 18:1224–1226, 1990.

20. Chow MSS, Schweizer R: Estimation of renal creatinine clearance in patients with unstable serum creatinine concentrations: comparison of multiple methods. *DICP* 19:385–390, 1985.

21. Schmith VD, Piraino B, Smith RB, Kroboth PD: Alprazolam in end-stage renal disease. II. Pharmacodynamics. *Clin Pharmacol Ther* 51:533–540, 1992.

22. Zarowitz BJ, Robert S, Peterson EL: Prediction of glomerular filtration rate using aminoglycoside clearance in critically ill medical patients. *Ann Pharmacother* 26:1205–1210, 1992.

23. Agmon Y, Brezis M: Acute renal failure: a multifactorial syndrome. Pathogenesis and prevention strategies. *Contrib Nephrol* 102:23–36, 1993.

24. Kjellstrand CM, Jacobson S, Lins L-E: Acute renal failure. In Maher JF (ed): *Replacement of Renal Function by Dialysis.* Kluwer Academic Publishers, Dordrecht, Holland, 616–649, 1993.

25. Acute renal failure: prerenal disease versus acute tubular necrosis. In Rose BD (ed): *Pathophysiology of Renal Disease.* McGraw-Hill, New York, pp 63–112, 1987.

26. Kahlmeter G, Dahlager JI: Aminoglycoside toxicity: a review of clinical studies published between 1975 and 1982. *J Antimicrob Chemother* 13:9–22, 1984.

27. Mandal AK, Visweswaran RK, Kaldas NR: Treatment considerations in acute renal failure. *Drugs* 44:567–577, 1992.

28. Dixon BS, Anderson RJ: Nonoliguric acute renal failure. *Am J Kidney Dis* 6:71–80, 1985.

29. Teschan PE, Lawson NL: Studies in acute renal failure. Prevention by osmotic diuresis and observations on the effect of plasma and extracellular volume expansion. *Nephron* 3:1–16, 1966.

30. Flores J, DiBona DR, Beck CH, Leaf A: The role of cell swelling in ischemic renal damage and the protective effect of hypertonic solute. *J Clin Invest* 51:118–126, 1972.

31. Burke TJ, Arnold PE, Schrier RW: Prevention of ischemic acute renal failure with impermeant solutes. *Am J Physiol* 244:F646–F649, 1983.

32. Hanley MJ, Davidson K: Prior mannitol and furosemide infusion in a model of ischemic acute renal failure. *AM J Physiol* 241:F556–F564, 1981.

33. Slekurt EE: Changes in renal clearance following complete ischemia of the kidney. *AM J Physiol* 144:395–403, 1945.

34. Morris CR, Alexander EA, Bruns FJ, Levinsky NG: Restoration and maintenance of glomerular filtration by mannitol during hypoperfusion of the kidney. *J Clin Invest* 51:1555–1564, 1972.

35. Gubern JM, Sancho JJ, Simo J, Sitges-Serra A: A randomized trial on the effect of mannitol on postoperative renal function in patients with obstructive jaundice. *Surgery* 103:39–44, 1988.

36. Dorman HR, Sondheimer JH, Cadnapaphornchai P: Mannitol-induced acute renal failure. *Medicine* 69:153–159, 1990.

37. Rabetoy GM, Fredericks MR, Hostettler CF: Where the kidney is concerned, how much mannitol is too much? *Ann Pharmacother* 27:25–28, 1993.

38. Brezis M, Rosen S, Epstein FH: Acute renal failure. In Brenner BM, Rector Jr FC (eds): *The Kidney.* WB Saunders, Philadelphia, pp 993–1061, 1991.

39. Brown CB, Ogg CS, Cameron JS, Bewick M: High dose frusemide in acute reversible intrinsic renal failure. A preliminary communication. *Scott Med J* 19(Suppl 1):35–39, 1974.

40. Brown CB, Ogg CS, Cameron JS: High dose frusemide in acute renal failure: a controlled trial. *Clin Nephrol* 15:90–96, 1981.

41. Krasna MJ, Scott GE, Scholz PM, Spotnitz AJ, Mackenzie JW, Penn F: Postoperative enhancement of urinary output in patients with acute renal failure using continuous furosemide therapy. *Chest* 89:294–295, 1986.

42. Cantarovich F, Galli C, Benedetti L, et al: High dose frusemide in established acute renal failure. *Br Med J* 4:449–450, 1973.

43. Minuth AN, Terrell JB, Suki WN: Acute renal failure: a study of the course of prognosis of 104 patients and of the role of furosemide. *Am J Med Sci* 271:317–324, 1976.

44. Fries D, Pozet N, Dubois N, Traeger J: The use of large doses of frusemide in acute renal failure. *Postgrad Med J* 47:Suppl:18–Suppl:20, 1971.

45. Karayannopoulos S: High-dose frusemide in renal failure. *BMJ* 2:278–279, 1974.

46. Riley AL: Effect of ischemia on renal blood flow in the rat: *Nephron* 21:107–113, 1978.

47. Schwartz LB, Gewertz BL: The renal response to low dose dopamine. *J Surg Res* 45:574–588, 1988.

48. Marik PE: Low-dose dopamine in critically ill oliguric patients: the influence of the renin-angiotensin system. *Heart Lung* 22:171–175, 1993.

49. Talley RC, Forland M, Beller B: Reversal of acute renal failure with a combination of intravenous dopamine and diuretics (abstract). *Clin Res* 18:518, 1970.

50. Lindner A: Synergism of dopamine and furosemide in diuretic-resistant, oliguric acute renal failure. *Nephron* 33:121–126, 1983.

51. Davis RF, Lappas DG, Kirklin JK, Buckley MJ, Lowenstein E: Acute oliguria after cardiopulmonary bypass: renal functional improvement with low-dose dopamine infusion. *Crit Care Med* 10:852–856, 1982.

52. Heim-Duthoy KL, Kalil RSN, Kasiske BL: Acute renal failure. In DiPiro JT, Talbert RL, Hayes PE, Yee GC, Matzke GR, Posey LM (eds): *Pharmacotherapy: a Pathophysiologic Approach.* Appleton & Lange, Norwalk, CT, pp 660–672, 1993.

53. Giordano C: Use of exogenous and endogenous urea for protein synthesis in normal and uremic patients. *J Lab Clin Med* 62:231–246, 1963.

54. Rose WC: The amino acid requirements of adult men. *Nutr Abstr Rev* 27:631–647, 1957.

55. Heidland A, Shaefer RM, Heidbreder E, Horl WH: Catabolic factors in renal failure: therapeutic approaches. *Nephrol Dial Transplant* 3:8–16, 1988.

56. Takala J: Nutrition in acute renal failure. *Crit Care Med* 3:155–166, 1987.

57. Woodrow G, Turney JH: Cause of death in acute renal failure. *Nephrol Dial Transplant* 7:230–234, 1992.

58. Priebe HJ, Skillman JJ: Methods of prophylaxis in stress ulcer disease. *World J Surg* 5:223–233, 1981.

59. Peterson WL, Richardson CT: Intravenous cimetidine or two regimens of ranitidine to reduce fasting gastric acidity. *Ann Intern Med* 104:505–507, 1986.

60. Peterson WL, Richardson CT: Sustained fasting achlorhydria: a comparison of medical regimens. *Gastroenterology* 88:666–669, 1985.

61. McCarthy DM: Drug therapy: sulcralfate. *N Engl J Med* 325:1017–1025, 1991.

62. Driks MR, Craven DE, Celli BR, et al: Nosocomial pneumonia in intubated patients given sulcralfate as compared with antacids or histamine type 2 blockers. *N Engl J Med* 317:1376–1382, 1987.

63. Sherman RA, Hwang ER, Walker JA, Eisinger RP: Reduction in serum phosphorus due to sucralfate. *Am J Gastroenterol* 78:210–211, 1983.

64. Burke TJ, Schrier RW: Acute renal failure. In Conick HC (ed) *Current Nephrology* Chicago: Year Book Medical Publishers, Inc., 245–261, 1990.

65. Russell JD, Churchill DN: Calcium antagonists and acute renal failure. *Am J Med* 87:306–315, 1989.

66. Schrier RW, Burke TJ: Calcium-channel blockers in experimental and human acute renal failure. *Adv Nephrol* 17:287–300, 1988.

67. Neumayer HH, Wagner K: Prevention of delayed graft function in cadaver kidney transplants by diltiazem: outcome of two prospective, randomized clinical trials. *J Cardiovasc Pharmacol* 10:S170–S177, 1987.

68. Shapiro JI, Cheung C, Itabashi A, Chan L, Schrier RW: The effect of verapamil on renal function after warm and cold ischemia in the isolated perfused rat kidney. *Transplantation* 40:596–600, 1985.

69. Neumayer HH, Wagner K, Preuschof L, Stanke H, Schultze G, Molzahn M: Amelioration of postischemic acute renal failure by prostacyclin analogue (iloprost): long-term studies with chronically instrumented conscious dogs. *J Cardiovasc Pharmacol* 8:785–790, 1986.

70. Kaufman Jr RP, Anner H, Kobzik L, Valeri CR, Shepro D, Hechtman HB: A high plasma prostaglandin to thromboxane ratio protects against renal ischemia. *Surg Gynecol Obstet* 165:404–409, 1987.

71. Higa EM, Schor N, Boim MA, Ajzen H, Ramos OL: Role of the prostaglandin and kallikrein-kinin systems in aminoglycoside-induced acute renal failure. *Braz J Med Biol Res* 18:355–365, 1985.

72. Lin JJ, Churchill PC, Bidani AK: Effect of theophylline on the initiation phase of postischemic acute renal failure in rats. *J Lab Clin Med* 108:150–154, 1986.

73. Lin JJ, Churchill PC, Bidani AK: Theophylline in rats during maintenance phase of post-ischemic acute renal failure. *Kidney Int* 33:24–48, 1988.

74. Keane WF, Hirata-Dulas CAI, Bullock ML, et al: Adjunctive therapy with intravenous human immunoglobulin G improves survival of patients with acute renal failure. *J Am Soc Nephrol* 2:841–847, 1991.

75. Conger JD: A controlled evaluation of prophylactic dialysis in post-traumatic acute renal failure. *J Trauma* 15:1056–1063, 1975.

76. Kleinknecht D, Jungers P, Chanard J, Barbanel C, Ganeval D: Uremic and non-uremic complications in acute renal failure: evaluation of early and frequent dialysis on prognosis. *Kidney Int* 1:190–196, 1972.

77. Kjellstrand CM, Berkseth RO, Klinkman H: Treatment of acute renal failure. In Schrier RW, Gottschalk CW (eds): *Disease of the Kidney.* Little, Brown, Boston, pp 1501–1540, 1988.

78. Keusch G, Schreier P, Binswanger U: Outcome in critically ill patients with acute renal failure treated by continuous hemofiltration. *Contrib Nephrol* 93:57–60, 1991.

79. Macias WL, Mueller BA, Scarim SK: Vancomycin pharmacokinetics in acute renal failure: preservation of nonrenal clearance. *Clin Pharmacol Ther* 50:688–694, 1991.

80. Mueller BA, Scarim SK, Macias WL: Comparison of imipenem pharmacokinetics in patients with acute or chronic renal failure treated with continuous hemofiltration. *Am J Kidney Dis* 21:172–179, 1993.

81. Heinmeyer G, Link J, Weber W, Meschede V, Roots I: Clearance of ceftriaxone in critical care patients with acute renal failure. *Intensive Care Med* 16:448–453, 1990.

82. Collins AJ, Hanson G, Umen A, Kjellstrand C, Keshaviah P: Changing risk factor demographics in end-stage renal disease patients entering hemodialysis and the impact on long-term mortality. *Am J Kidney Dis* 15:422–432, 1990.

83. Opsahl JA, Guay DRP, Ptachcinski RJ: Chronic renal failure and end-stage renal disease and renal transplantation. In DiPiro JT, Talbert RL, Hayes PE, Yee GC, Matzke GR, Posey LM (eds): *Pharmacotherapy: a Pathophysiologic Approach.* Appleton & Lange, Norwalk, CT, pp 673–700, 1993.

84. Salem MM, Rosa RM, Batlle DC: Extrarenal potassium tolerance in chronic renal failure: implications for the treatment of acute hyperkalemia. *Am J Kidney Dis* 18:421–440, 1991.

85. Sutton RAL, Cameron EC: Renal osteodystrophy: pathophysiology. *Semin Nephrol* 12:91–100, 1992.

86. Malluche H, Faugere M-C: Renal bone disease 1990: an unmet challenge for the nephrologist. *Kidney Int* 38:193–211, 1990.

87. Felsenfeld AJ, Llach F: Parathyroid gland function in chronic renal failure. *Kidney Int* 43:771–789, 1993.

88. Delmez JA, Slatopolsky E: Hyperphosphatemia: its consequences and treatment in patients with chronic renal disease. *Am J Kidney Dis* 19:303–317, 1992.

89. Brater DC: Use of diuretics in chronic renal insufficiency and nephrotic syndrome. *Semin Nephrol* 8:333–341, 1988.

90. Wollam GL, Tarazi RC, Bravo EL, Dustan HP: Diuretic potency of combined hydrochlorothiazide and furosemide therapy in patients with azotemia. *Am J Med* 72:929–938, 1982.

91. Brater DC, Pressley RH, Anderson SA: Mechanisms of the synergistic combination of metolazone and bumetanide. *J Pharmacol Exp Ther* 233:70–74, 1985.

92. Oster JR, Epstein M, Smaller S: Combined therapy with thiazide-type and loop diuretic agents for resistant sodium retention. *Ann Intern Med* 99:405–406, 1983.

93. Sakhaee K: Management of renal osteodystrophy. *Semin Nephrol* 12:101–108, 1992.

94. Slatopolsky E, Weerts C, Lopez-Hilker S, et al: Calcium carbonate as a phosphate binder in patients with chronic renal failure undergoing dialysis. *N Engl J Med* 315:157–161, 1986.

95. Slatopolsky E, Weerts C, Norwood K, et al: Long-term effects of calcium carbonate and 2.5 mEq/liter calcium dialysate on mineral metabolism. *Kidney Int* 36:897–903, 1989.

96. Hamida FB, Esper IE, Compagnon M, Morinière PH, Fournier A: Long-term (6 months) cross-over comparison of calcium acetate with calcium carbonate as phosphate binder. *Nephron* 63:258–262, 1993.

97. Caravaca F, Santos I, Cubero JJ, et al: Calcium acetate versus calcium carbonate as phosphate binders in hemodialysis patients. *Nephron* 60:423–427, 1992.

98. Sheikh MS, Maguire JA, Emmett M, et al: Reduction of dietary phosphorus absorption by phosphorus binders: a theoretical, in vitro and in vivo study. *J Clin Invest* 83:66–73, 1989.

99. Nolan CR, Califano JR, Butzin CA: Influence of calcium acetate or calcium citrate on intestinal aluminum absorption. *Kidney Int* 38:937–941, 1990.

100. Reichel H, Koeffler HP, Norman AW: The role of the vitamin D endocrine system in health and disease. *N Engl J Med* 320:980–991, 1989.

101. Malberti F, Surian M, Cosci P: Effect of chronic intravenous calcitriol on parathyroid function and set point of calcium in dialysis patients with refractory secondary hyperparathyroidism. *Nephrol Dial Transplant* 7:822–828, 1992.

102. Kwan JTC, Almond MK, Beer JC, Noonan K, Evans SJW, Cunningham J: 'Pulse' oral calcitriol in uraemic patients: rapid modification of parathyroid response to calcium. *Nephrol Dial Transplant* 7:829–834, 1992.

103. Tsukamoto Y, Nomura M, Takahashi Y, et al: The 'oral 1,25-dihydroxyvitamin D₃ pulse therapy' in hemodialysis patients with severe secondary hyperparathyroidism. *Nephron* 57:23–28, 1991.

104. Muramoto H, Haruki K, Yoshimura A, Mimo N, Oda K, Tofuku Y: Treatment of refractory hyperparathyroidism in patients on hemodialysis by intermittent oral administration of 1,25(OH)₂Vitamin D₃. *Nephron* 58:288–294, 1991.

105. Paganini EP: Overview of anemia associated with chronic renal disease: primary and secondary mechanisms. *Semin Nephrol* 9:3–8, 1989.

106. Schwenk MH, Halstenson CE: Recombinant human erythropoietin. *DICP* 23:528–536, 1989.

107. Eschbach JW, Egrie JC, Downing MR, Brown JK, Adamson JW: Correction of the anemia of end-stage renal disease with recombinant human erythropoietin. Results of a combined phase I and II clinical trial. *N Engl J Med* 316:73–78, 1987.

108. Levin NW: Quality of life and hemoatocrit level. *Am J Kidney Dis* 20:16–20, 1992.

109. McMahon LP, Dawborn JK: Subjective quality of life assessment in hemodialysis patients at different levels of hemoglobin following use of recombinant human erythropoietin. *Am J Nephrol* 12:162–169, 1992.

110. Eschbach JW, Abdulhadi MH, Browne JK, et al: Recombinant human erythropoietin in anemic patients with end-stage renal disease. *Ann Intern Med* 111:992–1000, 1989.

111. Ad Hoc Committee for the National Kidney Foundation: Statement on the clinical use of recombinant erythropoietin in anemia of end-stage renal disease. *Am J Kidney Dis* 14:163–169, 1989.

112. Van Wyck DB, Stivelman JC, Ruiz J, Kirlin LF, Katz MA, Ogden DA: Iron status in patients receiving erythropoietin for dialysis-associated anemia. *Kidney Int* 35:712–716, 1989.

113. Barnes JN, Williams AJ, Tomson MJF, Toseland PA, Goodwin FJ: Dihydrocodeine in renal failure: further evidence for an important role of the kidney in the handling of opioid drugs. *Br Med J* 290:740–742, 1985.

114. Plaisance KI, Drusano GL, Forrest A, Weir MR, Standiford HC: Effect of renal function on the bioavailability of ciprofloxacin. *Antimicrob Agents Chemother* 34:1031–1034, 1990.

115. Guay DRP, Matzke GR, Bockbrader HN, et al: Comparison of bioavailability and pharmacokinetics of cimetidine in subjects with normal and impaired renal function. *Clin Pharm* 2:157–162, 1983.

116. Matzke GR, Frye RF: Drug dosing in patients with impaired renal function. In DiPiro JT, Talbert RL, Hayes PE, Yee GC, Matzke GR, Posey LM (eds): *Pharmacotherapy: a Pathophysiologic Approach.* Appleton & Lange, Norwalk, CT, pp 750–763, 1993.

117. Aronoff GR: Antimicrobial therapy in patients with impaired renal function. *Am J Kidney Dis* 3:106–110, 1983.

118. *Drug Interaction Facts:* Facts and Comparisons, St. Louis, 1993.

119. Davies BI, Maesen FPV: Drug interactions with quinolones. *Rev Infect Dis* 11(Suppl 5):S1083–S1090, 1989.

120. Hurwitz A: Antacid therapy and drug kinetics. *Clin Pharmacokinet* 2:269–280, 1977.

121. Kang JY: The gastrointestinal tract in uremia. *Dig Dis Sci* 38:257–268, 1993.

122. Craig RM, Murphy P, Gibson TP, et al: Kinetic analysis of D-xylose absorption in normal subjects and in patients with chronic renal failure. *J Lab Clin Med* 101:496–506, 1983.

123. Touchette MA, Slaughter RL: The effect of renal failure on hepatic drug clearance. *DICP* 25:1214–1224, 1991.

124. Bianchetti G, Graziani G, Brancaccio D, et al: Pharmacokinetics and effects of propranolol in terminal uraemic patients and in patients undergoing regular dialysis treatment. *Clin Pharmacokinet* 1:373–384, 1976.

125. Bergstrand RH, Wang T, Roden DM, et al: Encainide disposition in patients with renal failure. *Clin Pharmacol Ther* 40:64–70, 1986.

126. Gibson TP, Giancomini KM, Briggs WA, Whitman W, Levy G: Propoxyphene and norproxyphene plasma concentrations in the anephric patient. *Clin Pharmacol Ther* 27:665–670, 1980.

127. Lee CS, Marbury TC: Drug therapy in patients undergoing haemodialysis. Clinical pharmacokinetic considerations. *Clin Pharmacokinet* 9:42–66, 1984.

128. MacKichan JJ: Influence of protein binding and use of unbound (free) drug concentrations. In Evans WE, Schentag JJ, Jusko WJ, Relling MV (eds): *Applied Pharmacokinetics.* Vancouver: Applied Therapeutics, pp 5.1–5.48, 1992.

129. Haughey DB, Kraft CJ, Matzke GR, Keane WF, Halstenson CE: Protein binding of disopyramide and elevated alpha-1-acid glycoprotein concentrations in serum obtained from dialysis patients and renal transplant recipients. *Am J Nephrol* 5:35–39, 1985.

130. Craig W: Enhanced protein binding of clindamycin in uremic sera—relationship to alpha-1-acid glycoprotein. 21st Interscience Conference on Antimicrobial Agents and Chemotherapy, Chicago, Nov. 4–6, 1981.

131. Grossman SH, Davis D, Kitchell BB, Shand DG, Routledge PA: Diazepam and lidocaine plasma protein binding in renal disease. *Clin Pharmacol Ther* 31:350–357, 1982.

132. Zini R, Riant P, Barré J, Tillement JP: Disease-induced variations in plasma protein levels. Implications for drug dosage regimens (Part I). *Clin Pharmacokinet* 19:147–159, 1990.

133. Boobis SW: Alteration of plasma albumin in relation to decreased drug binding in uremia. *Clin Pharmacol Ther* 22:147–153, 1978.

134. Craig WA: The effect of disease states on serum protein binding of antimicrobials. *Infection* 4(Suppl 2):S137–S141, 1976.

135. Tozer TN, Winter ME: Phenytoin. In Evans WE, Schentag JJ, Jusko WJ, Relling MV (eds): *Applied Pharmacokinetics.* Applied Therapeutics, Vancouver, 25.1–25.44, 1992.

136. Farrell PC, Grib NL, Fry DL, Popovich RP, Broviac JW, Babb AL: A comparison of in vitro and in vivo solute-protein binding interactions in normal and uremic subjects. *Trans Am Soc Artif Intern Organs* 18:268–276, 1972.

137. Greene DS, Tice AD: Effect of hemodialysis on cefazolin protein binding. *J Pharm Sci* 66:1508–1510, 1977.

138. Dromgoole SH: The effect of haemodialysis on the binding capacity of albumin. *Clin Chem Acta* 46:469–472, 1973.

139. Reuning RH, Geraets DR, Rocci Jr ML, Vlasses PH: Digoxin. In Evans WE, Schentag JJ, Jusko WJ, Relling MV (eds): *Applied Pharmacokinetics.* Applied Therapeutics, Vancouver, pp 20.1–20.48, 1992.

140. Graves SW, Brown B, Valdes R: An endogenous digoxin-like substance in patients with renal impairment. *Ann Intern Med* 99:604–608, 1983.

141. Pleasants RA, Gadsden RH, McCormack JP, Piveral K, Sawyer WT: Interference of digoxin-like immunoreactive substances with three digoxin immunoassays in patients with various degrees of renal function. *Clin Pharm* 5:810–816, 1986.

142. Fitzsimmons WE: Influence of assay methodologies and interferences on the interpretation of digoxin concentrations. *DICP* 20:538–542, 1986.

143. Madrenas J, Codina S, Monne J, et al: Digoxin-like immunoreacting activity in the serum of patients on regular hemodialysis. *Nephron* 43:303–304, 1986.

144. Anders MW: Metabolism of drugs by the kidney. *Kidney Int* 18:636–647, 1980.

145. Balant LP, Dayer P, Fabre J: Consequences of renal insufficiency on the hepatic clearance of some drugs. *Int J Clin Pharmacol Res* 3:459–474, 1983.

146. Gibson TP: Renal disease and drug metabolism: an overview. *Am J Kidney Dis* 8:7–17, 1986.

147. Reidenberg MM: The biotransformation of drugs in renal failure. *Am J Med* 62:482–485, 1977.

148. Zenser TV, Rapp NS, Mattammal MB, Davis BB: Renal cortical drug and xenobiotic metabolism following urinary tract obstruction. *Kidney Int* 25:747–752, 1984.

149. Drayer DE: Active drug metabolites and renal failure. *Am J Med* 62:486–489, 1977.

150. Adam WR, Henning M, Dawborn JK: Excretion of trimethoprim and sulphamethoxazole in patients with renal failure. *Aust NZ J Med* 3:383–387, 1973.

151. Chan GLC, Matzke GR: Effects of renal insufficiency on the pharmacokinetics and pharmacodynamics of opioid analgesics. *DICP* 21:773–783, 1987.

152. Doluisio JT: Clinical pharmacokinetics of cefotaxime in patients with normal and reduced renal function. *Rev Infect Dis* 4(Suppl):S333–S345, 1982.

153. Portenoy RK, Thaler HT, Inturrisi CE, Friedlander-Klar H, Foley KM: The metabolite morphine-6-glucuronide contributes to the analgesia produced by morphine infusion in patients with pain and normal renal function. *Clin Pharmacol Ther* 51:422–431, 1992.

154. Wolff J, Bigler D, Christensen CB, Rasmussen SN, Andersen HB, Tonnesen KH: Influence of renal function on the elimination of morphine and morphine glucuronides. *Eur J Clin Pharmacol* 34:353–357, 1988.

155. Coyle JD, Lima JJ: Procainamide. In Evans WE, Schentag JJ, Jusko WJ, Relling MV (eds): *Applied Pharmacokinetics—Principles of Therapeutic Drug Monitoring.* Applied Therapeutics, Vancouver, pp 22-1–22-33, 1992.

156. Gibson TP, Briggs WA, Boone BJ: Delivery of di-2-ethylhexyl phthalate to patients during hemodialysis. *J Lab Clin Med* 87:519–524, 1976.

157. Pollack GM, Shen DD, Door MB: Contribution of metabolites to the route- and time-dependent hepatic effects of di-(2-ethylhexyl)phthalate in the rat. *J Pharmacol Exp Ther* 248:176–181, 1989.

158. Gladziwa U, Klotz U: Pharmacokinetics and pharmacodynamics of H₂-receptor antagonists in patients with renal insufficiency. *Clin Pharmacokinet* 24:319–332, 1993.

159. Gladziwa U, Wagner S, Dakshinamurty KV, Bechtel B, Mann H, Sieberth H-G: Intragastric long-term pH-metry in hemodialysis patients. A study with famotidine. *Clin Nephrol* 36:97–102, 1991.

160. Osborne RJ, Joel SP, Slevin ML: Morphine intoxication in renal failure: the role of morphine-6-glucuronide. *BMJ* 292:1548–1549, 1986.

161. Glare PA, Walsh TD: Clinical pharmacokinetics of morphine. *Ther Drug Monit* 13:1–23, 1991.

162. Portenoy RK, Foley KM, Stulman J, et al: Plasma morphine and morphine-6-glucuronide during chronic morphine therapy for cancer pain: plasma profiles, steady-state concentrations and the consequences of renal failure. *Pain* 47:13–19, 1991.

163. Levy G: Pharmacokinetics in renal disease. *Am J Med* 62:461–465, 1977.

164. Lyman DJ: Membranes. In Drukker W, Parsons FM, Maher JF (eds): *Replacement of renal function by dialysis.* Martinus Nijhoff, Boston, pp 97–105, 1983.

165. DeSoi CA, Sahm DF, Umans JG: Vancomycin elimination during high-flux hemodialysis: kinetic model and comparison of four membranes. *Am J Kidney Dis* 20:354–360, 1992.

166. Quale JM, O'Halloran JJ, DeVincenzo N, Barth RH: Removal of vancomycin by high-flux hemodialysis membranes. *Antimicrob Agents Chemother* 36:1424–1426, 1992.

167. Torras J, Cao C, Rivas MC, Cano M, Fernandez E, Montoliu J: Pharmacokinetics of vancomycin in patients undergoing hemodialysis with polyacrylonitrile. *Clin Nephrol* 36:35–41, 1991.

168. Raja RM: Vascular access for hemodialysis. In Daugirdas JT, Ing TS (eds): Handbook of dialysis. Little, Brown, Boston, pp 40–58, 1988.

169. Catolico MM, Campbell S, Jones WM, Logan JL: Time course of gentamicin serum concentration rebound following hemodialysis. *DICP* 21:46–49, 1987.

170. Halstenson CE, Berkseth RO, Mann HJ, Matzke GR: Aminoglycoside redistribution phenomenon after hemodialysis: netilmicin and tobramycin. *Int J Clin Pharmacol Ther Toxicol* 25:50–55, 1987.

171. Pollard TA, Lampasona V, Mullins RE, Hooks MA, Wheaton R, Maroni BJ: Impact of vancomycin redistribution on dosing recommendations following high flux hemodialysis. (abstract) *J Am Soc Nephrol* 2:354, 1991.

172. Touchette MA, Patel RV, Anandan JV, Dumler F, Schmidt R, Zarowitz BJ: Vancomycin removal by F60 and F80 polysulfone hemodialysis filters in critically ill patients with end stage renal disease. (abstract). *Pharmacotherapy* 13:284, 1993.

173. Gibson TP: Problems in designing hemodialysis drug studies. *Pharmacotherapy* 5:23–29, 1985.

174. Bailie GR, Eisele G: Continuous ambulatory peritoneal dialysis: a review of its mechanics, advantages, complications, and areas of controversy. *Ann Pharmacother* 26:1409–1420, 1992.

175. Sorkin MI, Diaz-Buxo JA: Physiology of peritoneal dialysis. In *Handbook of Dialysis.* Little, Brown, Boston, pp 167–181, 1988.

176. St. Peter WL, Redic-Kill KA, Halstenson CE: Clinical pharmacokinetics of antibiotics in patients with impaired renal functions. *Clin Pharmacokinet* 22:169–210, 1992.

177. Keller E, Reetze P, Schollmeyer P: Drug therapy in patients undergoing continuous ambulatory peritoneal dialysis: clinical pharmacokinetic considerations. *Clin Pharmacokinet* 18:104–117, 1990.

178. Bunke CM, Aronoff GR, Luft FC: Pharmacokinetics of common antibiotics used in continuous ambulatory peritoneal dialysis. *Am J Kidney Dis* 3:114–117, 1983.

179. Maher JF: Influence of continuous ambulatory peritoneal dialysis on elimination of drugs. *Peritoneal Dialysis Bull* 7:159–167, 1987.

180. O'Brien MA, Mason NA: Systemic absorption of intraperitoneal antimicrobials in continuous ambulatory peritoneal dialysis. *Clin Pharm* 11:246–254, 1992.

181. Horton MW, Deeter RG, Sherman RA: Treatment of peritonitis in patients undergoing continuous ambulatory peritoneal dialysis. *Clin Pharm* 9:102–118, 1990.

182. The Ad Hoc Advisory Committee on Peritonitis Management: Peritoneal dialysis-related peritonitis treatment recommendations—1993 update. *Peritoneal Dialysis Int* 13:14–28, 1993.

183. Schäfer GE, Döring C, Sodemann K, Russ A, Schröder HM: Continuous arteriovenous and venovenous hemodialysis in critically ill patients. *Contrib Nephrol* 93:23–28, 1991.

184. McDonald BR, Mehta RL: Decreased mortality in patients with acute renal failure undergoing continuous arteriovenous hemodialysis. *Contrib Nephrol* 93:51–56, 1991.

185. Bellomo R, Parkin G, Love J, Boyce N: A prospective comparative study of continuous arteriovenous hemodiafiltration and continuous venovenous hemodiafiltration in critically ill patients. *Am J Kidney Dis* 21:400–404, 1993.

186. Golper TA: Continuous arteriovenous hemofiltration in acute renal failure. *Am J Kidney Dis* 6:373–386, 1985.

187. Alarabi A, Danielson BG, Wikström B: Continuous arteriovenous hemodialysis: outcome in intensive care acute renal failure patients. *Nephron* 64:58–62, 1993.

188. Cigarran-Guldris S, Brier ME, Golper TA: Tobramycin clearance during simulated continuous arteriovenous hemodialysis. *Contrib Nephrol* 93:120–123, 1991.

189. Kronfol NO, Lau AH, Barakat MM: Aminoglycoside binding to polyacrylonitrile hemofilter membranes during continuous hemofiltration. *Trans Am Soc Artif Intern Organs* 33:300–303, 1987.

190. Lau AH, Kronfol NO, John E: Increased vancomycin elimination with continuous hemofiltration. *Trans Am Soc Artif Intern Organs* 33:772–774, 1987.

191. Bellomo R, Ernest D, Parkin G, Boyce N: Clearance of vancomycin during continuous arteriovenous hemodiafiltration. *Crit Care Med* 18:181–183, 1990.

192. Reetze-Bonorden P, Böhler J, Kohler C, Schollmeyer P, Keller E: Elimination of vancomycin in patients on continuous arteriovenous hemodialysis. *Contrib Neprol* 93:135–139, 1991.

193. Thomson AH, Grant AC, Rodger RSC, Hughes RL: Gentamicin and vancomycin removal by continuous venovenous hemofiltration. *DICP* 25:127–129, 1991.

194. Davies SP, Azadian BS, Kox WJ, Brown EA: Pharmacokinetics of ciprofloxacin and vancomycin in patients with acute renal failure treated by continuous haemodialysis. *Nephrol Dial Transplant* 7:848–854, 1992.

195. Reetze-Bonorden P, Böhler J, Keller E: Drug dosage in patients during continuous renal replacement therapy: pharmacokinetic and therapeutic considerations. *Clin Pharmacokinet* 24:362–379, 1993.

196. Drusano GL: Role of pharmacokinetics in the outcome of infections. *Antimicrob Agents Chemother* 32:289–297, 1988.

197. Leitman PS: Pharmacokinetics of antimicrobial agents. In Mandell GL, Douglas Jr RG, Bennett JE (eds): *Principles and Practice of Infectious Diseases.* Churchill Livingstone, New York, pp 228–230, 1990.

198. Bennett WM, Aronoff GR, Morrison G (et al): Drug prescribing in renal failure: dosing guidelines for adults. *Am J Kidney Dis* 3:155–193, 1983.

199. Bernstein JM, Erk SD: Choice of antibiotics, pharmacokinetics, and dose adjustments in acute and chronic renal failure. *Med Clin North Am* 74:1059–1076, 1990.

200. Fillastre JP, Singlas E: Pharmacokinetics of newer drugs in patients with renal impairment (Part I). *Clin Pharmacokinet* 20:293–310, 1991.

201. Matzke GR, Keane WF: The use of antibiotics in patients with renal insufficiency. In Peterson PK, Verhoef J (eds): Antimicrobial agents annual I. Elsevier Science, Amsterdam, pp 472–488, 1986.

202. Gibson TP, Matusik E, Nelson LD, Briggs WA: Artificial kidneys and clearance calculations. *Clin Pharmacol Ther* 20:720–726, 1976.

203. Allon M, Copkney C: Albuterol and insulin for treatment of hyperkalemia in hemodialysis patients. *Kidney Int* 38:869–872, 1990.

204. Paap CM, Nahata MC, Mentser MA, Mahan JD, Puri SK, Hubbard JA: Cefotaxime and metabolite disposition in two pediatric continuous ambulatory peritoneal dialysis patients. *Ann Pharmacother* 26:341–343, 1992.

205. Rubin J: Vancomycin absorption from the peritoneal cavity during dialysis-related peritonitis. *Peritoneal Dialysis Intern* 10:283–285, 1990.

206. Sennesael JJ, Maes VA, Pierard D, Debeukelaer SH, Verbeelen DL: Streptomycin pharmacokinetics in relapsing mycobacterium xenopi peritonitis. *Am J Nephrol* 10:422–425, 1990.

207. Debruyne D, Ryckelynck J-P, Moulin M, Hurault de Ligny B, Levaltier B, Bigot M-C: Pharmacokinetics of fluconazole in patients undergoing continuous ambulatory peritoneal dialysis. *Clin Pharmacokinet* 18:491–498, 1990.

208. Dahl K, Walstad RA, Widerøe T-E: The effect of peritonitis on the transperitoneal transport of cefuroxime in patients of CAPD treatment. *Nephrol Dial Transplant* 5:275–281, 1990.

209. Burgess ED, Gill MJ: Intraperitoneal administration of acyclovir in patients receiving continuous ambulatory peritoneal dialysis. *J Clin Pharmacol* 30:997–1000, 1990.

210. AHFS Drug Information 93—American Hospital Formulary Service, Bethesda, American Society of Hospital Pharmacists, 1993.

211. Evans WE, Schentag JJ, Jusko WJ (eds): *Applied Pharmacokinetics—Principles of Therapeutic Drug Monitoring,* ed 3. Applied Therapeutics, Vancouver, 1992.

212. *Facts and Comparisons.* Facts and Comparisons, Inc., St. Louis, 1993.

213. Goodman GA, Rall TW, Nies AS, Taylor P (eds): *The Pharmacological Basis of Therapeutics,* ed 8. Pergamon Press, Elmsford, NY, 1990.

214. Achtert G, Scherrmann JM, Christen MO: Pharmacokinetics/bioavailability of colchicine in healthy male volunteers. *Eur J Drug Metab Pharmacokinet* 14:317–322, 1989.

215. Agoston S, Vandenbrom RHG, Wierda JMKH: Clinical pharmacokinetics of neuromuscular blocking drugs. *Clin Pharmacokinet* 22:94–115, 1992.

216. Barrie JR, Mousdale S: Ciprofloxacin levels in a patient undergoing venovenous haemodiafiltration. *Intensive Care Med* 18:437–438, 1992.

217. Blackwell BG, Leggett JE, Johnson CA, Zimmerman SW, Craig WA: Ampicillin and sulbactam pharmacokinetics and pharmacodynamics in continuous ambulatory peritoneal dialysis (CAPD). *Peritoneal Dialysis Intern* 10:221–226, 1990.

218. Boelaert J, Daneels R, Van Landuyt HW, Schurgers M: Multiple dose pharmacokinetics of acyclovir in patients on continuous ambulatory peritoneal dialysis (abstract). *Antimicrob Agents Chemother* 142, 1985.

219. Boulieu R, Bastien O, Bleyzac N: Pharmacokinetics of ganciclovir in heart transplant patients undergoing continuous venovenous hemodialysis. *Ther Drug Monit* 15:105–107, 1993.

220. Brass C, Galgiani JN, Blaschke TF, Defelice R, O'Reilly RA, Stevens DA: Disposition of ketoconazole, an oral antifungal, in humans. *Antimicrob Agents Chemother* 21:151–158, 1982.

221. Burgess ED, Blair AD: Pharmacokinetics of ceftizoxime in patients undergoing continuous ambulatory peritoneal dialysis. *Antimicrob Agents Chemother* 24:237–239, 1983.

222. Davenport A, Goel S, Mackenzie JC: Neurotoxicity of acyclovir in patients with end-stage renal failure treated with continuous ambulatory peritoneal dialysis. *Am J Kidney Dis* 20:647–649, 1992.

223. Debruyne D, Ryckelynck J-P: Clinical pharmacokinetics of fluconazole. *Clin Pharmacokinet* 24:10–27, 1993.

224. Debruyne D, Ryckelynck J-P, Hurault de Ligny B, Moulin M: Pharmacokinetics of piperacillin in patients on peritoneal dialysis with and without peritonitis. *J Pharm Sci* 79:99–102, 1990.

225. Doyle GD, Laher M, Kelly JG, Byrne MM, Clarkson A, Zussman BD: The pharmacokinetics of paroxetine in renal impairment. *Acta Psychiatr Scand* 80(Suppl 350):89–90, 1989.

226. Driessen JJ, Vree TB, Guelen PJM: The effects of acute changes in renal function on the pharmacokinetics of midazolam during long-term infusion in ICU patients. *Acta Anaesthesiol Belg* 42:149–155, 1991.

227. Fitzgerald J: Narcotic analgesics in renal failure. *Conn Med* 55:701–704, 1991.

228. Fletcher CV, Beatty C, Balfour Jr HH: Ganciclovir disposition in patients with renal insufficiency: implications for dose adjustment (abstract). *Pharmacotherapy* 11:277, 1991.

229. Gross ML, Somani P, Ribner BS, Raeader R, Freimer EH, Higgins Jr JT: Ceftizoxime elimination kinetics in continuous ambulatory peritoneal dialysis. *Clin Pharmacol Ther* 34:673–680, 1983.

230. Guay DRP, Awni WM, Findlay JWA, et al: Pharmacokinetics and pharmacodynamics of codeine in end-stage renal disease. *Clin Pharmacol Ther* 43:63–71, 1988.

231. Halvorsen MB, Whitmer JT, Halstenson CE: Hemodialysis clearance of encainide and metabolites. *Ther Drug Monit* 13:375–378, 1991.

232. Harford AM, Sica DA, Tartaglione T, Polk RE, Dalton HP, Poyner W: Vancomycin pharmacokinetics in continuous ambulatory peritoneal dialysis patients with peritonitis. *Nephron* 43:217–222, 1986.

233. Hoyer J, Schulte K-L, Lenz T: Clinical pharmacokinetics of angiotensin converting enzyme (ACE) inhibitors in renal failure. *Clin Pharmacokinet* 24:230–254, 1993.

234. Hui KK, Duchin KL, Kripalani KJ, Chan D, Kramer PK, Yanagawa N: Pharmacokinetics of fosinopril in patients with various degrees of renal function. *Clin Pharmacol Ther* 49:457–467, 1991.

235. Ito MK, Smith AR, Lee ML: Ticlopidine: a new platelet aggregation inhibitor. *Clin Pharm* 11:603–617, 1992.

236. Johnson C, Zimmerman S, Leggett J, et al: Pharmacokinetics and pharmacodynamics of ampicillin/sulbactam in CAPD patients (abstract). *Peritoneal Dialysis Intern* 7(Suppl):S40, 1987.

237. Johnson RJ, Blair AD, Ahmad S: Ketoconazole kinetics in chronic peritoneal dialysis. *Clin Pharmacol Ther* 37:325–329, 1985.

238. Josselson J, Narang PK, Adir J, Yacobi A, Sadler JH: Bretylium kinetics in renal insufficiency. *Clin Pharmacol Ther* 33:144–150, 1983.

239. Kaiser G, Ackermann R, Sioufi A: Pharmacokinetics of a new angiotensin-converting enzyme inhibitor, benazepril hydrochloride, in special populations. *Am Heart J* 117:746–751, 1989.

240. Keller E, Fecht H, Böhler J, Schollmeyer P: Single-dose kinetics of imipenem/cilastatin during continuous arteriovenous haemofiltration in intensive care patients. *Nephrol Dial Transplant* 4:640–645, 1989.

241. Kelly JG, O'Malley K: Clinical pharmacokinetics of the newer ACE inhibitors. *Clin Pharmacokinet* 19:177–196, 1990.

242. Kirch W, Ramsch KD, Duhrsen U, Ohnhaus EE: Clinical pharmacokinetics of nimodipine in normal and impaired renal function. *Int J Clin Pharmacol Res* 4:381–384, 1984.

243. Kowalsky SF, Echols M, Schwartz MT, Bailie GR, McCormick E: Pharmacokinetics of ciprofloxacin in subjects with varying degrees of renal function and undergoing hemodialysis or CAPD. *Clin Nephrol* 39:53–58, 1993.

244. Lawless ST, Restaino I, Azin S, Corddry D: Effect of continuous arteriovenous haemofiltration on pharmacokinetics of amrinone. *Clin Pharmacokinet* 25:80–82, 1993.

245. Lowenthal DT, Saris SD, Paran E, Cristal N: The use of transdermal clonidine in the hypertensive patient with chronic renal failure. *Clin Nephrol* 39:37–42, 1993.

246. Marquardt ED, Ishisaka DY, Batra KK, Chin B: Removal of ethosuximide and phenobarbital by peritoneal dialysis in a child. *Clin Pharm* 11:1030–1031, 1992.

247. Murdoch D, McTavish D: Sertraline. A review of its pharmacodynamic and pharmacokinetic properties, and therapeutic potential in depression and obsessive-compulsive disorder. *Drugs* 44:604–624, 1992.

248. Ochs HR, Rauh HW, Greenblatt DJ, Kaschell HJ: Clorzepate dipotassium and diazepam in renal insufficiency: serum concentrations and protein binding of diazepam and desmethyldiazepam. *Nephron* 37:100–104, 1984.

249. Parker CJR, Jones JE, Hunter JM: Disposition of infusions of atracurium and its metabolite, laudanosine, in patients in renal and respiratory failure in an ITU. *Br J Anaesth* 61:531–540, 1988.

250. Prendergast BD: Glyburide and glipisize, second-generation oral sulfonylurea hypoglycemic agents. *Clin Pharm* 3:473–485, 1984.

251. Przechera M, Bengel D, Risler T: Pharmacokinetics of imipenem/cilastatin during continuous arteriovenous hemofiltration. *Contrib Nephrol* 93:131–134, 1991.

252. Rello J, Roglan A, García-Cases C, Jané F, Net A: Effect of continuous arteriovenous hemodialysis on ganciclovir pharmacokinetics. *DICP* 24:544–545, 1990.

253. Rivey MP, Taylor JW, Mullenix TA: DIAS Rounds—Drug information analysis service. *DICP* 23:687–689, 1989.

254. Rosansky SJ, Johnson KL, McConnell J: Use of transdermal clonidine in chronic hemodialysis patients. *Clin Nephrol* 39:32–36, 1993.

255. Ruedy J: The effects of peritoneal dialysis on the physiological disposition of oxacillin, ampicillin and tetracycline in patients with renal disease. *Can Med Assoc J* 94:257–261, 1966.

256. Sabouraud A, Rochdi M, Urtizberea M, Christen MO, Achtert G, Scherrmann JM: Pharmacokinetics of colchicine: a review of experimental and clinical data. *Gastroenterology* 30(Suppl 1):35–39, 1992.

257. Schentag JJ: Cefmetazole sodium: pharmacology, pharmacokinetics, and clinical trials. *Pharmacotherapy* 11:2–19, 1991.

258. Schmith VD, Piraino B, Smith RB, Kroboth PD: Alprazolam in end-stage renal disease. I. Pharmacokinetics. *J Clin Pharmacol* 31:571–579, 1991.

259. Segredo V, Caldwell JE, Matthay MA, Sharma ML, Gruenke LD, Miller RD: Persistent paralysis in critically ill patients after long-term administration of vecuronium. *N Engl J Med* 327:524–528, 1992.

260. Sica DA: Kinetics of angiotensin-converting enzyme inhibitors in renal failure. *J Cardiovasc Pharmacol* 20(Suppl 10):S13–S20, 1992.

261. SmithKline Beecham Pharmaceuticals: *Package Insert for Paxil™ brand of paroxetine hydrochloride tablets,* (unpublished data), 1993.

262. Somani P, Freimer EH, Gross ML, Higgins Jr JT: Pharmacokinetics of imipenem-cilastatin in patients with renal insufficiency undergoing continuous ambulatory peritoneal dialysis. *Antimicrob Agents Chemother* 32:530–534, 1988.

263. Wallace SL, Singer JZ, Duncan GJ, Wigley FM, Kuncl RW: Renal function predicts colchicine toxicity: guidelines for the prophylactic use of colchicine in gout. *J Rheumatol* 18:264–269, 1991.

CHAPTER 4

Pharmacologic Approach in Patients with Heart Failure

STEPHEN A. GERACI, M.D.

INTRODUCTION

"Congestive heart failure" is a traditional term for the complex of signs and symptoms caused by chronic myocardial cell loss, secondary neurohumoral and vascular changes, and their consequences. This label is imprecise: abnormalities other than myocardial dysfunction can result in similar findings, while different myocardial insults, at various stages of progression, can display broad spectra of clinical findings. Precise physiologic diagnosis is important in the critical care setting, where multisystem disease, multiple drug therapy, and rapid clinical changes can mask, mimic, or produce myocardial dysfunction. Systolic failure is present when systemic blood flow is insufficient to meet the needs of peripheral tissues; neither arterial hypotension nor a low cardiac index per se is a prerequisite for diagnosis. Diastolic failure is present when ventricular filling pressure (and, therefore, pulmonary or systemic central venous pressure) exceeds tolerable levels, causing pathologic consequences (pulmonary edema, hepatic, or systemic congestion); similarly, this definition does not include a specific end-diastolic pressure, for many factors can influence a patient's tolerance of a given venous pressure. Both definitions should restrict the diagnosis of heart failure to abnormalities of myocardial performance.

In developing a pharmacologic approach to the patient with heart failure, we will first briefly review cardiovascular conditions that may produce low flow and congestive symptomatology. Principles of normal and abnormal cardiovascular physiology, including control and compensatory mechanisms, will be

discussed, emphasizing targets for pharmacologic modulation. On the basis of this background, an approach to setting therapeutic goals will be proposed. Finally, pharmacotherapeutic options to improve cardiovascular performance will be presented.

Space limitation precludes an in-depth discussion of this broad and multifaceted topic. Excellent reviews and research articles listed at the end of the chapter provide thorough discussions of the topics presented.

NORMAL AND ABNORMAL CARDIOVASCULAR PHYSIOLOGY

Before attempting to determine the physiologic aberrations producing heart failure in a patient, extramyocardial causes of low flow and congestive states must be excluded. Cardiovascular disorders can mimic systolic dysfunction, reducing cardiac output by inhibiting antegrade flow (valvular stenosis, thrombosis, embolus, pericardial disease, or arterial hypertension) or permitting retrograde ejection (valvular insufficiency or septal defects). Obstructing and regurgitant lesions can also imitate diastolic dysfunction, as can other disorders, such as intravascular hypervolemia and pulmonary injury (ARDS). Extramyocardial lesions may in fact produce their effects by altering cardiac performance or cause heart failure as a secondary phenomenon over time. It is crucial, however, to exclude or account for such diseases, even when true heart failure is also present, for incorrectly treating the former conditions (e.g., aortic stenosis) as the latter (e.g., with vasodilators) can have catastrophic results.

MECHANICAL ASPECTS OF CARDIOVASCULAR FUNCTION

Systolic Performance

Systolic performance is the ability of the heart to pump blood to peripheral tissues by developing and maintaining the pressure needed to eject an adequate stroke volume (SV) with sufficient frequency. Cardiac index (CI) reflects the sum product of four primary determinants: preload, afterload, contractility, and heart rate and rhythm.

Preload is the precontraction myocardial fiber length, best reflected clinically by ventricular end-diastolic volume (EDV); end-diastolic pressure (EDP) is a less precise estimate, as the diastolic pressure/volume (P/V) relationship is not linear (1). Increasing EDV through most of the normal physiologic range will increase the force and extent of contraction, if other factors are held constant (Starling effect). The dilated failing heart has exhausted much of this "preload reserve," while patients with noncompliant ventricles, increased pulmonary vascular permeability, and other disorders may not tolerate the EDP necessary to utilize this reserve fully (see below). Optimal preload for a given patient is one that maximally exploits the Starling effect without producing complications of elevated EDP.

Afterload is the active myocardial tension required to overcome all forces inhibiting ventricular ejection (2). The constituents of afterload are ventricular chamber radius, pressure and wall thickness (La Place relationship), ejection gradients, and aortic input impedance (including arteriolar or systemic vascular resistance (SVR), arterial stiffness, and reflected wave energy (3–5)). They interact throughout systole to determine inertial, force, and pressure loads faced by the contracting ventricle. Unlike the loss of preload effect, the decompensated ventricle is exquisitely sensitive to changes in afterload (6). Clinically, only some of the components (end-systolic volume (ESV), SVR) are easily measured. However, as different drugs may influence these factors to varying degrees, all should be considered when selecting optimal pharmacotherapy.

Contractility (inotropy) is the load-independent ability of a muscle fiber to generate force and shorten. Most clinical parameters used to estimate contractility (ejection fraction, dP/dt, and others) in fact vary greatly with loading conditions. Elastance, the relationship of ventricular pressure to volume throughout the cardiac cycle, is generally felt to be the most accurate assessment of inotropic state (7). Over physiologically obtainable ranges, the slope of the end-systolic pressure-volume relationship appears to be independent of both preload and afterload (8). Pressure/volume loops (9, 10), although not easily obtained at the bedside, permit detailed evaluation of inotropic and loading influences on stroke work (5, 11, 12). They comprise an important research tool in determining the results of pharmacologic intervention in heart failure.

Within limits, increasing heart rate proportionately increases cardiac output (CO) while independently augmenting contractility (7). Conversely, tachyarrhythmias may reduce forward flow by compromising diastolic filling time and atrioventricular (AV) synchrony. This latter factor, regardless of cause, impairs effective use of preload reserve (through loss of atrial systolic filling volume) and reduces the mechanical efficiency of contraction (1, 10).

Although they are distinct entities, these four factors interact intimately to determine overall systolic performance. For example, elevations in ventricular volume increase both preload (EDV) and afterload (chamber radius), while the reduction in SV caused by high aortic impedance (afterload) increases end-systolic—and subsequently, end-diastolic—volume (preload). When SV is reduced by contractile impairment, both preload and afterload rise with ventricular volume; the opposite effect occurs with inotropic stimulation. As previously noted, changes in heart rate may affect the other factors, while an alteration in CO or pressure will alter heart rate through neurohumoral reflexes (see below).

Diastolic Performance

Diastolic function or lusitropy, the ability of the ventricle to accept inflow volume, is determined by myocardial relaxation, passive stiffness, and filling dynamics. It is best (but incompletely) described with pressure/volume measurements (dV/dP or compliance; end-diastolic pressure-volume relationship) (1, 5, 9). Relaxation is largely an energy-dependent process (see below); although independent of preload (13), various afterloading factors can retard or accelerate the process (9, 13). Passive stiffness is determined by myocardial cell mass, interstitial structure, interventricular interactions, microvascular architecture, and pericardial influences (1, 14). Chamber geometry may effect both relaxation and stiffness, while influencing filling dynamics independently of ventricular compliance (14).

Although always assumed to accompany systolic failure (15), diastolic dysfunction (as an isolated phenomenon) is a well-recognized, distinct myocardial cause of central venous hypertension. It may occur acutely through ischemic or afterloading mechanisms or chronically via hypertrophy, fibrosis, or interstitial infiltration (13, 14). Active relaxation may be enhanced pharmacologically in the critical care setting through relief of precipitating events or improved diastolic reduction of cytosolic calcium (1, 5). Passive stiffness is not usually amenable to acute modulation.

Exclusive of obstructive and regurgitant lesions, hydrostatic pulmonary edema results from markedly elevated ventricular volume OR stiffness, or both. By definition, the noncompliant ventricle requires a higher EDP to achieve a given EDV (i.e., a steeper P/V curve). In this setting, simple reduction in inflow volume through venodilation or diuresis may relieve congestion but critically reduce effective preload, precipitating shock. Conversely, a positive lusitropic intervention may lower filling pressure while maintaining preload and systolic performance (9, 14, 16).

CELLULAR AND MOLECULAR ASPECTS OF CARDIOVASCULAR CONTROL

Cardiovascular mechanics are regulated through a complex system of autonomic and endocrine factors that attempt to maintain homeostasis. Their actions are, in turn, mediated through cellular and molecular pathways, many of which are potentially amenable to pharmacologic intervention.

Arterial baroreceptors respond to decreased distension (cardiac output and pressure) by disinhibiting central sympathetic outflow; this reflex arc is modulated by CNS inhibitory (adrenergic α_2) and excitatory (dopaminergic DA$_2$) receptors (17). Efferent sympathetic activity results in postganglionic neuronal release of norepinephrine (NE), which in turn is regulated by presynaptic inhibitory (α_2 and DA$_2$) and facilitory (angiotensin II (AT$_2$) and β_2) (18, 19) receptors. Postsynaptic neurotransmitter action is terminated largely through active neuronal reuptake and diffusion.

Myocardial surface adrenoreceptors (postsynaptic β_1 and extrasynaptic β_2) couple through a stimulatory guanine nucleotide (Gs) system to adenylate cyclase, enhancing synthesis of cyclic adenosine monophosphate (cAMP) from ATP. Adenylate cyclase activity is suppressed by activation of inhibitory (Gi)-coupled muscarinic and adenosine receptors (20, 21). Cyclic AMP promotes both contraction (by increasing systolic Ca^{2+} availability and actin-myosin cycling) and relaxation (through enhanced contractile protein Ca^{2+} release and cytosolic Ca^{2+} removal) (22). It is inactivated by cAMP-specific cytosolic phosphodiesterase (PDE) III. High cAMP concentrations have been linked to arrhythmogenesis (23, 24) and acceleration of myocyte damage (23, 25) in heart failure through their effects on energy consumption and Ca^{2+} handling.

Both contraction and relaxation are closely tied to myocardial Ca^{2+} flux. Extracellular Ca^{2+}, which enters the cell on depolarization through voltage-gated channels, activates the release of the larger sarcoplasmic reticular Ca^{2+} pool (20). Subsequent Ca^{2+} interaction with control and enzymatic elements of the contractile apparatus results in tension development (26). Relaxation occurs when cytosolic Ca^{2+} is removed by energy-dependent sarcoplasmic reuptake and sarcolemmal extrusion (22, 27) and through exchange for extracellular Na$^+$ by an energy-independent antiporter. The Na$^+$ gradient for antiporter function is maintained by Na$^+$/K$^+$ exchange, driven by a specific Na$^+$/K$^+$-dependent ATPase (22, 27).

Cardiovascular function is further modulated by neurohumoral factors that respond to reduced CO and blood pressure by increasing heart rate, ventricular contractility, vascular tone, and plasma volume. This is beneficial as short-term circulatory support in shock; however, neurohumoral activation in systolic failure also produces detrimental ventricular loading and energy consumption, central venous congestion, and redistribution of blood flow away from splanchnic and skeletal muscle beds. Chronic activation may also contribute to pathologic hypertrophy of ventricular and vascular smooth muscle (28, 29), hyponatremia (30), and impairment of acute control mechanisms (see below). Myocardial damage itself may be perpetuated by this process (25, 29).

Central sympathetic outflow results in β-receptor-mediated augmentation of inotropy, chronotropy, lusitropy, and oxygen consumption. Systemic release of epinephrine, renin (β_1-mediated), and arginine vasopressin (AVP) (also β_1-mediated) is enhanced. Stimulation of postsynaptic α-receptors causes arteriolar and venous constriction, increasing cardiac preload, and afterload (19).

Renin release is also stimulated when renal perfusion or Na$^+$ delivery fall (31). This enzyme catalyzes AT$_1$ synthesis, which is converted to AT$_2$ by angiotensin-converting enzyme (ACE). Systemically, AT$_2$ enhances NE activity through several pathways (32), while stimulating secretion of aldosterone

and AVP. Coronary and systemic vascular resistance, glomerular mesangial tone (32), and (perhaps) ventricular contractility (33) are acutely increased through AT$_2$ receptor-specific actions. (Chronic AT$_2$ and α-adrenergic action may also promote vascular smooth muscle and myocardial hypertrophy (32, 34).) Aldosterone leads to volume expansion by promoting renal Na$^+$ resorption (through K$^+$ and H$^+$ exchange) (35), while AVP enhances both free water resorption and systemic vasoconstriction (36).

Other modulators display contrasting actions. Atrial natriuretic peptide (ANP), released in response to atrial stretch and tachycardia (37), directly promotes renal Na$^+$ excretion, dilates most resistance and capacitance vessels, and counteracts AT$_2$ actions at many sites (38). Peripheral dopaminergic receptors inhibit NE and aldosterone release (DA$_2$); dilate splanchnic, coronary, and cerebral arteries (DA$_1$); and promote diuresis (39, 40). Extrasynaptic β_2-adrenoreceptors also promote vasodilation in skeletal muscle and mesenteric beds. A host of other factors contributes to organ-specific regulation of blood flow, including endothelium-derived relaxing factor (nitric oxide) (41), cyclooxygenase products (prostaglandins, thromboxanes) (42); tissue-limited renin-angiotensin (RA) systems (43, 44); neurogenic and paracrine mediators (19, 45); and metabolic factors (46).

Alterations in many segments of this intricate control system have been described in heart failure. Plasma levels of NE, renin, AT$_2$, AVP, aldosterone, and ANP are usually, but not invariably, elevated early in the clinical course (47, 48). Desensitization of aortic baroreceptors (49) may contribute to the excessive activation. Decreased myocardial NE concentration (50), reduced neuronal reuptake (34), β_2-receptor desensitization (via G protein uncoupling) (41), and β_1 downregulation (via internalization of the receptor complex) may occur acutely, while reduced β_1 turnover is seen in the chronically failing ventricle (51). Increased Gi/Gs activity ratio (52), reduced cAMP concentration (20, 23), impaired ATP production (25), and abnormal Ca^{2+} handling (53, 54) have also been described. Interestingly, the contractile response to Ca^{2+} is preserved (32). Many of these observations suggest an adaptive phenomenon, limiting the potentially toxic effects of ongoing hyperstimulation and energy depletion, and are reversible in experimental models. They may also partially explain the reduced myocardial responsiveness to inotropic stimulation by many drugs and the development of tachyphylaxis seen during therapy.

MYOCARDIAL ENERGY BALANCE

Just as ischemia can impair both systolic and diastolic performance, alterations in myocardial energy balance may contribute to heart failure and influence therapeutic outcome. Active tension development accounts for more than 90% of myocardial oxygen consumption (MVO$_2$). Oxygen consumption escalates with increases in contractility, systolic and diastolic wall stress (via increased ventricular radius or pressure), duration and rapidity of tension development, and heart rate. Determinants of oxygen delivery are more complex. Diastolic coronary perfusion will fall with decreased aortic pressure or increased intraventricular pressure (i.e., lowered coronary perfusion pressure), shortened perfusion time (tachycardia), and increased coronary resistance (via sympathetic outflow, postsynaptic α-stimulation, loss of dilatory β-agonism, atherosclerosis, or through actions of local modulators of autoregulation) (55). A given pharmacologic intervention may have conflicting effects on oxygen supply and demand or on different components of either factor.

Excellent discussions of mechanical, neurohumoral, and molecular pathophysiology in heart failure provide additional details on these and related topics. Identification of predominant pathophysiology in the patient is the first step in selecting optimal pharmacotherapy. Diagnostic modalities available to the intensivist are reviewed in the literature.

TREATMENT PLAN

The second step in heart failure pharmacotherapy is the selection of therapeutic goals, which should address immediate, intermediate, and long-term objectives. Although therapy directed toward these goals may be instituted simultaneously or sequentially, the treatment plan should be comprehensive, so that chosen measures are most consistent with the overall desired outcome.

Immediate therapeutic goals should seek to improve the acute hemodynamic abnormalities. Mechanical or pharmacologic modalities may be considered. Compromised organ perfusion may require augmentation of ventricular contractility, reduction in afterload components, volume loading or venoconstriction to increase preload, or a combination of these interventions. Pulmonary venous congestion could require improved ventricular relaxation and filling dynamics, redistribution of blood volume via venodilation, or salt and water removal. Acute ischemic dysfunction and sustained arrhythmias may cause both low output and venous hypertension; their specific therapies would be early priorities. Hemodynamic measures should be chosen to support optimal tissue oxygen delivery during the acute phase, while contributing to, or at least not compromising, definitive therapeutic efforts. Treatment for other acute precipitating or complicating events (severe anemia, electrolyte abnormalities, fever, hypoxia) is included with the immediate goals.

Intermediate goals should focus on definitive therapy for the underlying disease whenever possible, while limiting the potential for long-term damage from the acute insult. Definitive therapy may include mechanical or pharmacologic coronary reperfusion in acute heart failure from myocardial infarction, antibiotics for sepsis or infectious endocarditis, surgery for structural lesions, or enteric charcoal for certain cardiotoxic drug ingestions. As resuscitative efforts (e.g., catecholamine infusions) may place energy or load demands on a heart with limited reserves, secondary acute ischemic dysfunction may ensue. The intermediate objectives should include limitation of such secondary organ damage.

Intermediate goals can be the most difficult to set. Very often, several disease entities are contributing simultaneously to the presenting clinical picture, making choices for definitive therapy complex. Intermediate goals require frequent reevaluation, as ongoing interventions may alter the predominant findings. They are the most important goals, however, as the best resuscitative efforts will ultimately fail if reversible or treatable disease is addressed inadequately.

Evidence is growing that some drugs can improve long-term morbidity and mortality in chronic heart failure. Acute improvement of ventricular overload may reduce pathologic remodeling in certain conditions (56). In chronic heart failure, ACE inhibitors and combined vasodilator regimens can improve long-term survival (55, 57, 58). Such therapy is often instituted or continued in the critical care unit. Adjuvant treatments (e.g., anticoagulants, antiarrhythmics), that may influence outcome in some patients, are included here; these topics are debated in the literature (15, 59–61). Comprehensive therapeutic goals should therefore include elements of chronic drug therapy which, when begun prior to ICU discharge, might improve long-term functional capacity or reduce mortality.

PHARMACOTHERAPY

GENERAL APPROACH TO DRUG SELECTION

Drug therapy for the failing heart must match agent to patient. Both patient and drug factors (class actions and drug-specific characteristics) must be weighed in selecting pharmacotherapy. Note that division of patient-drug factors is somewhat arbitrary, as it is their dynamic interaction that determines final outcome.

Patient factors influencing drug selection are reflected in the pathophysiologic diagnosis (therapeutic goals), coexistent diseases influencing therapeutic or toxic responses, physiologic conditions affecting pharmacokinetics (PK) (drug absorption, distribution, metabolism, and elimination), concurrent drug therapy, pharmacogenetic considerations, and personal factors (age, sex, pregnancy, smoking, and alcohol history). Each may relatively preclude a specific agent or drug class, prohibit a given route of administration, or require dose or dosing frequency adjustment.

Drug factors are equally important in selecting a regimen. Pharmacodynamic (PD) action and mechanism are, of course, the primary concerns. Other important issues include dose, dosing frequency or rate, route of administration, specific formulation, time to onset of effect, time to steady state, maximal effect (if demonstrable), half-lives (distribution and elimination), production of active or toxic metabolites, and PK/PD susceptibility to individual patient factors and concurrently administered drugs. The incidence and frequency of adverse drug reactions, both predictable and idiosyncratic, must also be weighed in discerning the risk/benefit ratio of individual therapeutic options.

This multifaceted area of pharmacotherapy is discussed in classic references and elsewhere in this text. It is essential for the intensivist to be aware of relevant drug-drug and patient-drug interactions before starting therapy (62–64). Important new information on drug interactions and adverse reactions is reported frequently, and current literature should be followed to keep abreast of this dynamic field.

SPECIFIC PHARMACOLOGIC AGENTS

A detailed review of each drug used in heart failure therapy is beyond the scope of this chapter. Instead, we will briefly examine the effects of the major drug classes. Selected points regarding drug-specific pharmacokinetics or class interactions will be made, and potential alternatives for combination therapy presented. The reader is referred to the list of resources for detailed comprehensive discussions of individual agents and convenient handbooks for bedside use.

Sympathomimetic Agents

Catecholamines act by binding and activating adrenergic and dopaminergic membrane receptors, while some also influence the release of neurotransmitter from sympathetic nerve terminals. The drugs presently used in heart failure therapy are administered by intravenous infusion and are easily titrated by virtue of their short distribution and elimination half-lives.

Peripheral acting "pure" α-agonists (phenylephrine, mephenteramine, metaraminol) are rarely, if ever, indicated in heart failure, as they greatly increase preload, afterload, and MVO_2; they produce little, if any, inotropic action and reduce tissue perfusion in this condition. Similarly, agents that indiscriminately increase sympathetic neural outflow via CNS or peripheral actions (amphetamines, cocaine, tyramine, others) demonstrate PD/PK and side effect profiles that preclude their use in cardiovascular medicine. Selective β_2-agonists will be discussed briefly.

The pharmacodynamic actions of cardiotherapeutic sympathomimetic agents are predicted by their relative affinities for receptor subtypes (which may display dose dependency) and by their effect on NE turnover. All have been shown to have true positive inotropic action mediated through β-receptor-Gs-cAMP-Ca_{2+}-dependent pathways. They are less effective in failing ventricles due to β-receptor down-regulation and desensitization (65), while prolonged administration of some produces tachyphylaxis by means of these mechanisms (66). They are generally less effective in profoundly acidotic or hypoxemic patients and when coadministered with competitive β-receptor blockers (67). Although β-agonists can improve myocardial relaxation (68), these agents are not used in isolated diastolic dysfunction because of their other effects on chronotropy, inotropy, and the peripheral vasculature.

The toxic and adverse effects represent extensions of their pharmacodynamic actions. They tend to increase intrapulmonary shunt and raise pulmonary artery pressure in patients with parenchymal or vascular lung disease (67). They may precipitate arrhythmias and increase sinus rate and AV nodal conduction to a variable degree, an effect more pronounced in the presence of hyperthyroidism (69) or concurrently administered gaseous anesthetics (67). Extravascular actions that may contribute to adverse events include: altered insulin secretion (increased by β_2, decreased by α_2); increased hepatic glycogenolysis and gluconeogenesis (α and β_2); accelerated skeletal muscle glycogenolysis, potassium and phosphate uptake, and lactate production; and stimulation of lipolytic pathways (69).

These drugs are unstable in alkaline solutions, and most produce necrosis if extravasated into local tissues (63, 67). Their actions are terminated by neuronal uptake and enzymatic metabolism (catechol-O-methyltransferase, monoamine oxidase); they should be used with utmost caution if drugs that inhibit these processes have been recently administered

(67). In the presence of nonspecific β-blocking agents, sympathomimetics with combined α and β actions may precipitate diffuse arterial spasm from unopposed α_1-agonism (67).

Norepinephrine (NE) produces moderate β_1 activation at very low doses but shows virtually no β_2 activity at any concentration (69). In the pharmacologic doses usually used (0.01 to 0.03 μg/kg/min), α-stimulatory effects predominate. Direct postsynaptic actions far outweigh effects from presynaptic activity (α_2 and neuronal uptake/release). Infusions (which may be titrated every 3 to 5 minutes) result in marked increases in preload, inotropy, and all components of afterload; MVO_2 increases dramatically, although heart rate changes may be modest due to profound baroreceptor reflexes. The arrhythmogenic potential is somewhat less than that of epinephrine (69, 70).

This profile precludes the use of NE in most patients with systolic dysfunction. It is occasionally used in severe cardiogenic shock as part of a short-term regimen (including mechanical circulatory support), pending cardiac transplantation, or in combination with other agents.

Epinephrine (Epi) stimulates all adrenergic receptors with dose-dependent relative affinities. The plasma half-life of 2 minutes permits rapid titration. At low doses (<0.02 μg/kg/min), β effects predominate. Cardiac output, SV, and contractility increase, while vascular resistance in most beds declines or is unchanged. Electrophysiologic actions (sinus tachycardia, enhanced AV conduction and automaticity, and arrhythmogenicity) are pronounced. While coronary arterial resistance may decline, lowered diastolic blood pressure and increased MVO_2 usually produce a net negative effect on energy balance. At higher doses, the hemodynamic picture is dominated by vascular α effects. Arteriolar resistance increases, decreasing blood flow to renal, splanchnic, and coronary beds (65, 69).

The use of Epi in systolic failure is quite limited. As short-term support in selected patients (especially following cardioplegic arrest or anaphylactic shock with severe contractile impairment), its direct potent α- and β-effects will best support the circulation. Higher (α range) doses are otherwise reserved for profound cardiogenic shock.

Isoproterenol (Iso), a pure nonselective β-agonist, increases heart rate, contractility, AV conduction, and automaticity. Venous return and SVR decrease, resulting in significant falls in diastolic pressure, afterload, and preload in most patients. Cardiac output may increase or fall, depending on the actual loading responses (69). Because of unopposed β_2-effects, skeletal muscle blood flow may increase preferentially over splanchnic perfusion (65). Coronary resistance and ventricular diastolic pressure fall, but coronary blood flow decreases as diastolic aortic pressure and perfusion time decrease (65). The net effect on myocardial oxygen balance is almost always profoundly negative, however, due to excessively increased consumption (71).

With the advent of safer agents, Iso is rarely, if ever, used for inotropic support. In the ICU setting, it is used to accelerate sinus rate and AV conduction in life-threatening bradyarrhythmias (63) until a pacemaker is placed. This action may be particularly important in transplanted hearts, in which atropine is ineffective. Infusion is usually begun at 0.01 μg/kg/min and titrated every 3 to 5 minutes to effect. The terminal half-life is 2 to 3 minutes (69).

Dopamine (DA) displays (relative) dose-specific affinities for DA_1, DA_2, β- and α-receptors and facilitates NE release from presynaptic nerve terminals. Since a significant portion of the drug's action is due to this latter mechanism (50, 65), DA increases circulating NE (71) and is less effective in the NE-depleted state of chronic heart failure (50). Much of the tachyphylaxis observed during prolonged therapy may result from further neurotransmitter depletion. It does not readily cross the blood-brain barrier, but high doses will stimulate the area postrema, causing emesis (67). The drug's slightly longer terminal half-life (7 to 9 minutes) (69) suggests that it should be titrated at longer intervals (15 minutes), usually in increments of 2.5 to 5.0 μg/kg/min, if patient condition permits. When the infusion rate is increased more frequently, the patient should be observed for excessive vasoconstriction as steady state is reached.

During infusion of 2 to 3 μg/kg/min, DA_1-and DA_2-receptor-mediated actions predominate. Renal blood flow and sodium excretion increase; splanchnic arteriolar resistance declines; and aldosterone secretion is inhibited. Contractility may improve slightly via presynaptic effects. Both preload and afterload usually fall slightly, and pulmonary arterial resistance changes may be seen. Heart rate and MVO_2 are usually unchanged at this dose, especially in dilated ventricles. Infusions of 4 to 8 μg/kg/min result in predominant β ($β_1 > β_2$) actions, although α-stimulation is demonstrable. Both inotropy and lusitropy are augmented; CI and SV increase, as do heart rate and blood pressure. Venous return climbs as a result of increased forward flow. The effects on afterload and energy balance are variable and dependent upon the relative amount of α-stimulation and change in ventricular volume achieved. Although DA- and β-receptor agonism is maintained, doses in excess of 8 to 10 μg/kg/min result in hemodynamic changes dominated by peripheral $α_1$-stimulation. Aortic impedance increases as renal and splanchnic perfusion falls. Preload is increased by both venoconstrictive and afterload-mediated increases in ventricular volume. Pulmonary vasoconstriction and oxygen consumption increase markedly, while heart rate remains high (65, 72).

Doses in excess of 20 μg/kg/min are rarely used in treating heart failure (65), but infusions up to 50 μg/kg/min have been used in patients with shock of other etiologies and relatively intact baseline myocardial and coronary function (69). Dopamine's specific effects on splanchnic blood flow at low doses are especially useful and unique among drugs in this class.

Dobutamine (Dob) consists of stereoisomers with differing receptor affinities. The (+) isomer is a potent β-agonist ($β_1 > β_2$) but competitively blocks postsynaptic α-receptors. The (−) isomer, a less potent β stimulant, shows α-agonism (73). Neither molecule appears to bind DA receptors or directly influence neurotransmitter turnover (74). This profile provides for a relatively selective action in improving inotropy and lusitropy (via $β_1$ and $β_2$ activation) without elevating plasma NE concentration (75). Although tachycardia and arrhythmias are seen at higher doses, these effects are proportionately less, relative to inotropic effect, than with other agents in this class (76).

On initial administration to patients with systolic heart failure, Dob increases contractility, CI and SV with little effect on heart rate. Improved renal and splanchnic perfusion, natriuresis, and reductions in afterload and preload reflect the improved cardiac output, subsequent reduction of ventricular volume, and reduction in reflex-mediated sympathetic traffic. Myocardial oxygen balance generally improves in dilated hearts, although it may worsen in nondilated ventricles with associated coronary disease (67). Tachyphylaxis, demonstrable after 48 to 72 hours of continuous infusion, is felt to be caused by further receptor down-regulation and desensitization (77).

Dobutamine is usually begun at 2.5 μg/kg/min and titrated to the desired effect. Rapid distribution and a 3-minute terminal half-life permit dose adjustments at 10-minute intervals (63,69). In patients not receiving other β-agonists, a dose of 20 μg/kg/min usually produces the maximal inotropic effect; larger initial doses only increase adverse events (65), although higher doses may be of some additional benefit in patients treated for longer than 72 hours.

Intermittent Dob infusion as a regimen in chronic systolic failure has been abandoned, as treated patients showed poorer survival than controls (78, 79).

Other β-Agonists.   Attempts to treat chronic heart failure with $β_2$-selective agonists (albuterol, terbutaline, pirbuterol, and others) have been largely unsuccessful (79). Despite acute improvements in systolic performance and symptoms, their benefits are short lived (80). In some studies, mortality was increased by these agents (79). New partial selective agonists under investigation may display better efficacy and safety profiles.

Inodilators

These agents display both positive inotropic and vasodilatory properties. Their actions are partly explained by inhibition of cAMP-specific phosphodiesterase (PDE) III, the predominant isozyme in cardiovascular tissue. The bipyridines (amrinone and milrinone) may have additional actions, such as prolonging the release and/or delaying the reuptake of sarcoplasmic calcium (65, 81), but their actions are clearly independent of the β-receptor-Gs-adenylate cyclase and Na+/K+-dependent ATPase pathways. Their inotropic and lusitropic effects are less pronounced when intracellular cAMP levels are depressed, as in chronic systolic heart failure (75, 81, 82). Of this group, only intravenous amrinone and milrinone are marketed commercially in the U.S. Nonspecific PDE inhibitors, such as the methylxanthines, can lead to brief hemodynamic improvement in selected patients; however, rapid loss of efficacy, arrhythmogenicity, and pronounced side effects make them inappropriate for treating heart failure.

Inodilators produce load-independent improvement in systolic performance (contractility) (80, 81). Although most data suggest that this response is sustained (80), some studies have observed tachyphylaxis: the initial hemodynamic improvement and reduction in plasma NE concentration may be lost after 72 hours of continuous amrinone infusion (83). An improvement in myocardial lusitropy appears to be due to both cAMP-mediated enhancement of isovolumic relaxation and improved filling dynamics (81, 84).

Bipyridines are potent vasodilators, causing reductions in systemic and coronary arteriolar resistance. The effect is most pronounced in skeletal muscle beds, while no selective action on renal vascular resistance has been demonstrated. They also produce venodilation, through both direct vascular actions and reduction in reflex sympathetic tone (65, 80). Pulmonary vascular resistance may decline dramatically (65, 85). In patients with severely depressed systolic performance, low doses do not increase heart rate appreciably; higher doses may accelerate sinus rate and AV nodal conduction (66) but generally not to the degree seen with catecholamine inotropes. Similarly, aortic blood pressure is usually maintained in hypervolemic patients until higher doses are administered. Cardiac output and SV increase while atrial pressure declines. The reductions in preload, afterload, and coronary resistance, and improved diastolic relaxation usually offset the increased oxygen consumption accompanying inotropic augmentation and modest chronotropic stimulation to significantly improve energy balance in the dilated ventricle, unless diastolic hypotension is precipitated (80, 85, 86).

Amrinone's long-terminal half-life requires administration of an initial loading dose (0.75 mg/kg over 2 to 5 minutes) prior to constant infusion (5 to 10 μg/kg/min) (63) and subsequent boluses (30 to 50% of the initial loading dose) when the infusion rate is increased. An initial hemodynamic response is seen in about 7 minutes. The drug is metabolized by hepatic N-acetylation: in fast acetylators, the mean half-life is 1.5 to 2.0 hours, while in slow acetylators this value is 4.4 hours (67). Half-life increases to 6 to 8 hours in the presence of low output heart failure (87). Both parent drug and metabolite are excreted in the urine, although specific recommendations for dose reduction in renal failure are not available. The slow clearance will prolong complicating hypotension, but decreases in arterial pressure usually respond to volume administration.

During short-term infusion, unless hypotension develops, amrinone has relatively few side effects. As with all drugs that increase cAMP concentration, arrhythmias can occur more frequently during administration (66, 88). Consumptive thrombocytopenia, hypersensitivity reactions, fever, and hepatotoxicity (63, 67), which were common during trials of oral amrinone, are unusual (<3%) during short-term IV use if the total dose is held below 10 mg/kg/day (66, 87). Thrombocytopenia from this regimen is usually mild, rarely leads to hemorrhage, and may resolve even with continued administration. Platelet counts reliably return to normal several days after drug discontinuation (67).

Digoxin

Digitalis glycosides inhibit sarcolemmal Na+/K+-dependent ATPase, raising intracellular sodium and thus augmenting Na^+/Ca^{2+} exchange by the concentration-driven antiporter (87). Increased intracellular Ca^{2+} by this mechanism (89) (and perhaps by a direct effect on slow inward Ca^{2+} currents (87) increases myocardial contractility independent of cAMP concentration. Digoxin enhances vagal outflow, slowing sinus rate and AV nodal conduction (89). The drug may resensitize aortic baroreceptors in chronic heart failure (90) and, therefore, decrease sympathetic tone (89), although in some circumstances adrenergic tone may increase (87).

Although controversy continues, long-term digoxin therapy probably improves symptoms in at least some patients with chronic systolic heart failure and sinus rhythm (91, 92). In chronic atrial fibrillation, subtoxic levels partially control ventricular response (87, 93).

Acute initiation of intravenous digoxin therapy is no longer considered an appropriate inotropic intervention by most authors (76, 93, 94). The narrow toxic:therapeutic ratio, large number of interacting drugs and medical conditions that enhance toxicity and potential for undesirable neurologic and vascular events have contributed to this opinion (62, 67, 87, 95). The acute inotropic effects of this agent are minimal (66, 94). The long half-life (mean, 1.6 days (87) makes acute titration difficult and prolongs complications when they arise. Slow distribution (up to 4 to 6 hours following an IV dose (87) results in a considerable delay before peak inotropic effects are seen, while the times of peak effect and peak level do not correlate (87). In the early periinfarction period, digoxin has been shown to increase mortality (94, 96, 97) and to be less effective than other agents at improving systolic performance (98). More efficacious, titratable, short-acting inotropes have virtually replaced this drug in the acute treatment of systolic failure. Of course, there is no indication for digoxin in isolated diastolic dysfunction.

In the ICU, IV digoxin is still used commonly in two settings: for continuation of chronic therapy in patients who are unable to take oral medications due to intercurrent illness and to slow the ventricular response in some patients with rapid atrial fibrillation. Safety can be improved with attention to the well-described pharmacodynamics, pharmacokinetics, and toxicology of this drug. These have been reviewed extensively in the literature (64, 87).

Nitrovasodilators

These vasodilators (organic nitrates and nitroprusside), the most commonly used in the critical care setting, reduce vascular tone by reacting with sulfhydryl groups to form nitric oxide (NO). NO stimulates soluble guanylate cyclase to raise the cGMP concentration in vascular smooth muscle cells. Through a series of cGMP-dependent protein kinase phosphorylations, calcium efflux is enhanced, and myosin light chains are dephosphorylated (99, 100) reducing contractile protein cycling. Nitrovasodilators have no demonstrable direct myocardial actions but influence cardiac performance by altering loading conditions and coronary blood flow (99–101). Additional important effects may include activation of prostacyclin synthesis and inhibition of platelet aggregation (89, 99). Nitrovasodilators are metabolized to inactive or toxic metabolites in blood vessel walls, erythrocytes, and liver (99, 100). Class actions include worsening of ventilation-perfusion mismatching in patients with segmental lung disease (due to inhibition of hypoxic vasoconstriction) (102–104), excessive blood pressure effects when given with other hypotensive agents or in volume-depleted patients (99, 100), and rebound hemodynamic effects on acute discontinuation of high doses (105). Despite similarities in proposed molecular mechanisms, these agents show slightly different profiles of hemodynamic action.

Organic nitrates include nitroglycerin (intravenous, sublingual, and transdermal) and polyesterified polynitrates. They have a rapid onset of action (seconds) after introduction into the blood stream. Extensive first-pass hepatic metabolism is partially avoided with polyesterified formulations (isosorbide dinitrate, erythrityl tetranitrate, and pentaerythrital tetranitrate) (99). Oral bioavailability and longer half-lives constitute the only clinically important differences between these latter agents and nitroglycerin (NTG).

In the ICU, intravenous NTG is the preferred agent. The 60 to 180 second half-life allows establishment of steady-state levels within 5 to 10 minutes and, hence, rapid titration (99, 104). (Pharmacokinetic parameters of other nitrate preparations have been reviewed (99, 106).) Considerable variability in dose response is seen, especially in patients with systolic heart failure or nitrate tolerance (see below) (99, 107). As such, IV NTG is usually begun (with careful hemodynamic monitoring) as an infusion of 5 to 10 μg/min and titrated to effect or side effects every 3 to 10 minutes, in 5 to 10 μg/min increments (64, 104).

Although nitroglycerin shows relative dose-specific vascular actions, the actual doses at which these actions are seen vary widely among patients. At low doses, NTG dilates primarily capacitance vessels, reducing venous return and lowering ventricular EDP. This effect results in reduced pulmonary venous pressure and myocardial oxygen consumption, while arterial pressure, SVR, and heart rate remain unchanged; cardiac output is either unchanged (in decompensated failure) or reduced via Starling effect (89, 106). At moderate doses, large muscular arteries dilate, improving aortic distensibility and decreasing afterload (4). Dilation of large epicardial coronary arteries is seen, without impairment of coronary arteriolar autoregulation; combined with the improved perfusion pressure (from lowered intraventricular pressure), this action redistributes flow to subendocardial and regionally ischemic areas without altering total coronary blood flow (99). The resultant modulation of relative microcirculatory volume may partially explain the modest positive lusitropic action described with this agent (99, 101, 108). At higher doses, systemic arterioles also dilate, further reducing arterial impedance (99, 104). Pulmonary vascular impedance falls, but no appreciable change in renal or hepatic arteriolar resistance occurs (99). In volume-depleted patients or at a high-dose effect, arterial blood pressure may decrease. Unless diastolic hypotension or reflex tachycardia occurs, the result of titrated NTG is reduction in ventricular EDP (and perhaps preload in nondilated ventricles) and MVO_2, then reduction in most components of afterload; in the presence of coronary stenoses, oxygen delivery is also enhanced (89, 99).

The pharmacologic profile of intravenous NTG makes it an ideal drug for treating most patients with acute or chronic systolic failure, some patients with diastolic dysfunction, and those with coexistent coronary disease. Continuous administration by any route, however, leads to rapid vascular tolerance (107, 109). This may be due in part to depletion of reduced sulfhydryl groups in the vessel wall, but studies to restore sensitivity using –SH donors have had variable results (109–111). Diuretic administration may improve the drug's efficacy in a subgroup of edematous patients (106) or when fluid retention complicates therapy. Infusion rates must usually be increased frequently in patients treated for several days, although maximal effect will decline over time regardless of dose (107). With other nitrate preparations and in less critical patients, tolerance can be reduced with a daily 10- to 12-hour nitrate-free interval (112).

Most adverse events caused by nitrate therapy reflect exaggerated pharmacodynamic responses (hypotension, orthostasis, headache, edema). Other important but less common side effects include paradoxical vagotonia (causing hypotension and bradycardia) (113), worsened angina in patients with hypertrophic cardiomyopathy (63), prolonged bleeding time, and methemoglobinemia (113). A reduction in heparin's anticoagulant effect during IV nitrate therapy has been reported (63).

Sodium nitroprusside liberates NO when its ferrous ion reacts with a reduced sulfhydryl group in the blood vessel wall (100). With intravenous administration, initial response is seen in 30 seconds and peak response in 2 to 3 minutes; the effective half-life of 1 to 2 minutes allows for rapid dose titration (in increments of 0.10 to 0.25 μg/kg/min every 5 minutes) and prompt dissipation of effect on discontinuation (100, 104). The dose range depends upon indication, with lower doses (0.25 to 1.5 μg/kg/min) commonly effective in systolic failure; higher doses (up to 10 μg/kg/min) can often be required in hypertensive emergencies. As with nitroglycerin, significant interpatient variability has been described. Nitroprusside is metabolized to cyanide anion (and cyanomethemoglobin); through transulfuration reactions, thiocyanate is formed and excreted through the kidney. The drug is highly light- and pH-sensitive; it must be shielded with opaque materials and should be administered through a dedicated catheter (63, 100).

Nitroprusside produces balanced dilation of both capacitance and resistance vessels (89, 114). The reason for its somewhat different actions from those of NTG is not clear (115). At any given dose, arteriolar resistance decreases; medium and large artery compliance improves (4); and venous return falls (100). Afterload declines due to reductions in SVR, reflected wave components, and (often) ventricular volume. Ventricular EDP drops, and preload may decrease in nondilated hearts. No direct effect on active relaxation has been clearly demonstrated, although filling indices may improve by load-dependent changes in ventricular geometry. The effects on pulmonary and splanchnic vascular resistance are similar to those of nitroglycerin (116). In acute systolic failure, CI usually rises without significant hypotension unless the dose is excessive or preload is critically reduced; reflex neurohumoral activation (tachycardia, RA system stimulation) is more prominent in these latter instances (117). In decompensated chronic failure, when the heart is relatively preload-insensitive, forward flow increases in proportion to the degree of afterload reduction.

Nitroprusside's effect on myocardial oxygen balance is somewhat complex. The peripheral vascular actions and resultant reduction in intraventricular pressure lower oxygen demand and improve the coronary perfusion gradient. If neurohumoral activation ensues however, sympathetic outflow and AT_2 release may increase MVO_2. Concern regarding coronary steal was raised by demonstration of a worsened outcome in patients who received the drug less than 9 hours after symptom onset in acute infarction (89, 118). Subsequent trials have shown safety and efficacy when the drug is used carefully later in the periinfarction period (66, 119). Most authors now agree that nitroprusside has a net favorable effect on myocardial oxygen balance in the failing ventricle, unless diastolic hypotension or reflex tachycardia is precipitated (66, 94, 119).

Major adverse events during drug administration stem from its vascular actions and metabolism. Elevated intracranial pressure has been reported, while methemoglobinemia is exceedingly rare (113). Liberation of cyanide and formation of thiocyanate occur as part of nitroprusside's action and metabolism. Toxicity due to accumulation is very rare in the absence of renal failure (100), severe malnutrition (113), and with doses less than 2 μg/kg/min given for less than 3 days (63, 104, 113). Cyanide toxicity may be prevented and treated by infusion of sodium thiosulfate or hydroxycobalamin. Thiocyanate, which is normally cleared by the kidney, may be removed by dialysis. Curry and Arnold-Capell (113) have described these intoxications in detail.

"Direct" Arteriolar Dilators

Hydralazine, through poorly defined actions on vascular smooth muscle calcium flux (120), produces systemic arteriolar dilation in patients with heart failure. The acute hemodynamic response is a reduction in aortic impedance via decreased systemic vascular resistance (79). Pulmonary vascular resistance is lowered. Little direct effect on preload or inotropy is seen, although baroreceptor-mediated reflexes may increase sympathetic tone to the heart (100). The effect on myocardial energy supply-demand is variable. Reduction in afterload decreases, while reflex tachycardia increases, oxygen consumption. The coronary perfusion gradient benefits from lowered intraventricular pressure but falls if aortic diastolic hypotension ensues. Hence, the net effect will vary among patients.

The acute peak effect is seen 15 to 45 minutes following slow intravenous infusion, or 30 to 180 minutes after oral administration. It is about 90% protein bound and approximately 85% cleared by hepatic metabolism (to inactive products by N-acetylation and to active metabolites). The drug has an average excretion half-life of 2 to 4 hours and duration of action of 4 to 24 hours, largely influenced by acetylator status. Doses range from 5 to 20 mg IV and 25 to 150 mg orally every 6 to 12 hours. Dose reduction is necessary in either hepatic or renal dysfunction (63, 100).

The described acute hemodynamic improvements have failed to translate into long-term functional benefit or mortality reduction when hydralazine is used as the sole vasodilator in chronic heart failure. This may be due to secondary neurohumoral activation precipitated by reductions in blood pressure (79). However, improved survival has been demonstrated when oral hydralazine is combined with oral nitrates during long-term therapy (55).

Side effects have limited the drug's clinical utility in heart failure. After IV administration, profound and protracted hypotension may occur. At higher oral doses, chronic administration may cause significant GI upset, a lupus-like syndrome, pyridoxine-deficient neuropathy, and salt and water retention via RA system activation (60, 100, 121). Hydralazine is used infrequently in treating heart failure in the ICU, in favor of agents which are more easily titrated acutely (nitroprusside). or better tolerated chronically (ACE inhibitors) (122).

Minoxidil is a potent oral vasodilator with impressive side effects on chronic administration. It appears to have cardiovascular actions similar to those of hydralazine (15). Although short-term hemodynamic benefit has been demonstrated (15, 123), minoxidil administration in chronic heart failure may

cause clinical deterioration despite improved hemodynamics (123) through further neurohumoral activation (100). Diuretics must be coadministered to prevent excessive salt and water retention.

α-Adrenergic Blockers

Both nonselective (phentolamine, phenoxybenzamine) and α_1 selective (prazosin, terazosin, others) blockers have been studied in systolic heart failure. Acute vascular effects of decreased arteriolar resistance and venodilation (116) reduce ventricular afterload and preload and improve cardiac output, without appreciably influencing contractility (124). Reflex tachycardia (more pronounced with nonselective agents), orthostatic hypotension, and gastrointestinal side effects occur but are infrequent (63, 100). Although first-dose vascular effects are impressive (116), rapid development of tachyphylaxis (121, 125) has virtually excluded these agents from standard heart failure regimens. Indeed, the V-HeFT trial (55) showed prazosin to be indistinguishable from placebo in treating chronic heart failure. Additionally, the absence of parenteral availability and long half-lives of α_1-selective antagonists limit their utility in the critical care setting.

Angiotensin-converting Enzyme Inhibitors

The cardiovascular, endocrinologic and renal effects of AT_2 have been described above. Class actions of ACE inhibitors (captopril, enalapril, others) are largely explained by suppression of AT_2 production, although converting enzyme also has an important role in inactivating circulating bradykinin (113, 126). Other actions attributed to these agents in the heart failure patient include stimulation of prostacyclin synthesis (126), improved vascular responsiveness to ANP (127), resensitization of myocardial β-receptors (128), enhanced myocardial Gs activity (129), and reduction of postinfarction ventricular remodeling (130, 131). Whether these actions result from reduction in AT_2 effects alone or to other mechanisms is not clear. In addition to class actions, captopril's sulfhydryl group may permit this agent to scavenge free radicals as a means of cardioprotection (132) and to reduce nitrate tolerance.

Small doses of these drugs completely and reversibly inhibit systemic ACE activity (120, 133, 134). Saturation of available active sites limits the immediate effect in an individual patient and, hence, strict acute dose-response relationships have not been established (133, 135). (On chronic administration over weeks or months, additional hemodynamic effects are observed and have been attributed to drug action on vascular and tissue ACE (43, 44, 135).)

ACE inhibitors display a somewhat different pharmacodynamic profile in systolic failure patients than in those patients with uncomplicated hypertension. In heart failure, afterload decreases dramatically through reductions in systemic and pulmonary vascular resistance and ventricular volume; the latter effect accompanies a reduction in left and right heart filling pressures and systemic venodilation (136). Stroke volume increases significantly. Arterial blood pressure may remain constant or fall; a profound hypotensive response can be seen in patients who are intravascularly depleted, maintaining a marginal blood pressure with very high AT_2 activity, or are receiving concomitant therapy with other hypotensive agents (63, 113). Heart rate is usually unchanged or decreased. Although contractility may theoretically decline slightly as a result of reduced NE activity (33), overall systolic performance improves because of the more important alterations in loading. Circulating NE and AVP levels tend to decrease in patients with high baseline neurohumoral activation, though such observations are not invariable (31, 133, 137). Plasma renin activity increases dramatically following loss of feedback inhibition, while aldosterone levels fall more slowly due to the longer half-life of this hormone. Diuresis and natriuresis are observed as renal vascular resistance falls and hormonal influences on the distal nephron are lost (126). The net hemodynamic effects of ACE inhibitors are balanced reduction in preload and afterload, increased cardiac output, reduced venous congestion, and salt and water excretion. These actions appear sustained over long-term administration (130).

These agents also have complicated effects on myocardial energy balance. Reductions in afterload, especially in the absence of reflex tachycardia, reduce MVO_2. Decreased sympathetic stimulation and improved lusitropy (33, 43) may contribute to this effect. Reduced ventricular diastolic pressure and a sustained dilation of epicardial coronary arteries benefit coronary perfusion (136, 138, 139). However, vasorelaxation of the coronary arterioles may not be as pronounced or protracted (138, 140); if aortic hypotension develops, oxygen delivery may decrease (139).

Enalapril is available orally (a prodrug) and intravenously (as the active hydrolysis product, enalaprilat). The latter agent yields initial and peak responses in 15 and 30 minutes, respectively, while the peak effect from oral enalapril may not be seen for 3 to 4 hours (141). Approximately 40% of an oral dose eventually appears in the serum as enalaprilat (142). Serum half-life is approximately 11 hours, and both forms are excreted primarily through the kidneys. Minor differences in pharmacokinetic parameters have been noted in patients with systolic dysfunction (142), but dose reduction is generally advised only when creatinine clearance falls below 20 to 30 ml/min (63), and for patients receiving other hypotensive agents, such as diuretics (63, 113). The pharmacodynamic sensitivity displayed by patients with severely impaired systolic performance and marginal arterial pressure requires that initial doses be low, so that the acute "ceiling" effect of systemic ACE inhibition is not protracted; withholding diuretics and other hypotensive agents is advisable prior to initial administration (62, 126). Oral enalapril (2.5 to 20 mg) is usually administered every 12 to 24 hours, while IV enalaprilat (0.625 to 5 mg) may be given at 6- to 12-hour intervals. The higher doses are reserved for hypertensive patients or those on chronic enalapril therapy.

Oral captopril is about 65% bioavailable (fasting administration), showing a peak effect time of 30 to 90 minutes and a terminal half-life of 2 hours (113). This drug undergoes complex metabolism, forming disulfide bonds and dimeric compounds of unclear activity (141). It is dosed as 6.25 to 50 mg tablets every 6 to 12 hours, with precautions for concurrent drugs, renal function, and severity of heart failure similar to those described for enalapril (63). Newer agents (lisinopril, fosinopril, others) are longer-acting drugs that have not been studied as extensively in heart failure.

Most adverse hemodynamic events from ACE inhibition increase with dose, duration of drug action, and degree of intravascular depletion of the patient (126, 130, 143). Some side effects (potassium retention, azotemia, headache) are predictable from their known pharmacologic actions. Renal insufficiency is more likely in the presence of hyponatremia (113, 144). Allergic pneumonitis, angioedema, hypoproliferative hematologic disorders, and proteinuria are uncommon (113), while cough is seen more frequently. Some reactions (mucocutaneous lesions, immune complex glomerulopathy, altered taste sensation) appear more common with the sulfhydryl-containing captopril (113, 144). The class is generally considered contraindicated in patients with severe renal artery disease (113, 134). Other rare adverse effects have been reported (113).

Several important drug interactions have been described, in addition to those mentioned above. Potassium-sparing diuretics may precipitate severe hyperkalemia (63) and should be used carefully (if at all) with ACE inhibitors. Cyclooxygenase inhibitors decrease the magnitude of the hemodynamic effects (126). Lithium excretion is reduced by ACE inhibitors (63).

With chronic administration, captopril and enalapril have been shown to reduce mortality in chronic heart failure of many etiologies (130, 145). Symptomatic, hemodynamic, and myocardial structural benefits have been demonstrated in patients with mild or severe myocardial dysfunction (56, 130). These agents are better tolerated than the combination of hydralazine and isosorbide dinitrate (122); many of the adverse events reported during chronic ACE inhibitor trials may be attributed to the large fixed doses dictated by protocol (130, 143). To date, these agents appear to be the most important step toward mortality reduction in chronic heart failure.

Diuretics

Loop diuretics (furosemide, ethacrynic acid, bumetanide) and, occasionally, thiazide-type (metolazone, chlorthiazide) and potassium-sparing agents are employed in both acute and decompensated chronic heart failure in the critical care setting. The clinical pharmacology and application of this large group of drugs have been summarized in excellent reviews (146, 147).

Furosemide and bumetanide are potent sulfamoyl diuretics available both orally and intravenously. They are highly protein bound and act at the luminal surface of the thick ascending limb of Henle's loop to interfere with $Na^+/K^+/Cl^-$ exchange (146, 148). Primary delivery to the ultrafiltrate is by proximal tubular secretion, a process inhibited by organic anions, probenecid, penicillins, and cephalosporins (148). When renal plasma flow decreases, the drug is delivered mostly by glomerular filtration. Renal potency of these agents is reduced in low flow conditions, with normochloremic metabolic acidosis or concurrent drug therapy, and in hyperaldosteronemic states (148, 149). Diuretic resistance in these conditions can often be overcome with increased dose or by addition of chlorthiazide (available IV), metolazone, or agents that function on the distal nephron (amiloride, spironolactone, triamterene) (149).

Renal actions of loop diuretics include excretion of potassium, calcium, and magnesium. Sodium and water are excreted in a submaximally dilute urine; either hypernatremia or hyponatremia can occur, depending upon the patient's relative intake of salt and water. On repeated dosing, metabolic alkalosis may develop (149). These drugs increase renal blood flow, an effect mediated through local prostaglandin metabolism and sensitive to cyclooxygenase inhibition (150, 152). Via both renal and extrarenal actions, they stimulate renin release and elevate AT_2 and aldosterone levels (151, 153).

Nonrenal vascular actions of IV loop diuretics are of particular interest in the critical care unit and have been best described with furosemide. In pulmonary edema accompanying acute myocardial infarction, furosemide reduces filling pressure in minutes, an effect attributed to direct venodilation (153, 154). However, some studies (152), have shown acute vasoconstriction within 20 minutes of dosing in patients with decompensated chronic heart failure. This action may increase afterload and is most likely mediated by AT_2 (155). Vigorous diuresis or venodilation may critically reduce preload in the noncompliant ventricle, causing cardiac output to fall precipitously (64, 94). Conversely, many investigators have noted improved systolic function after effective diuresis has occurred (especially chronically) and attribute this to afterload reduction via decreased ventricular volume (wall stress), blood pressure, and SVR (aortic impedance) (48, 156). This complex hemodynamic profile dictates that intravenous loop diuretics be used cautiously in both acute and decompensated heart failure. The presence of ischemic heart disease requires additional consideration of potential load- and pressure-mediated effects on myocardial oxygen balance.

Furosemide is administered in multiples of 10 mg IV every 2 to 6 hours, to an average maximum dose of 6 mg/kg (157). Oral bioavailability is 50 to 60%. The time to onset of hemodynamic effect after IV administration is 5 to 15 minutes, while peak diuretic effect may not occur for 30 to 120 minutes. The terminal half-life of 0.5 to 2.0 hours may be markedly prolonged in cardiac, renal, or hepatic failure; at least 10% of the drug is excreted into the GI tract (63, 146, 157). Half-life may increase to 5.5 hours in severe systolic dysfunction and to 24 hours in chronic renal failure and severe multisystem organ failure (146, 157). Toxicity is generally a dose-related extension of its pharmacologic actions; other adverse events (hypoglycemia, blood dyscrasias, neuropathy, interstitial nephritis, and GI symptoms) are uncommon (64, 157). Ototoxicity is serious, very rare, and more common when furosemide is used concomitantly with other ototoxic drugs (157).

Bumetanide is approximately 40 times as potent and more lipid-soluble than furosemide. This latter feature makes it highly bioavailable on oral administration and less dependent upon proximal tubular secretion for efficacy (64, 157). Intravenous doses in increments of 0.5 mg may be given at 2- to 3-hour intervals, to an average maximum daily dose of 0.15 mg/kg (64, 157).

Narcotics

Morphine sulfate appears to act both via CNS μ-opioid receptors and by provoking release of histamine (158); newer selective μ-agonists (fentanyl, sufentanil) lack this latter property (158). The vascular actions of intravenous morphine (acute systemic venous and (mild) arteriolar dilation) reduce EDP, MVO_2, and stroke work (159). These, and perhaps secondary decreases in inotropy and lusitropy, occur with reduction in

central sympathetic efferent activity; no direct or significant myocardial effects have been demonstrated (158, 159). Cardiac output is either unchanged or mildly decreased. Bradycardia may occur and is more common with fentanyl than morphine (158).

Morphine is usually administered in 2 to 5 mg doses by slow IV injection, repeated at 15-minute intervals if needed. Its advantages include a rapid onset of action (3 to 5 minutes). and significant reversibility with naloxone (158). As it has little effect on myocardial relaxation, however, dangerous reductions in functional preload may occur in hypovolemic patients or those with chronically stiff ventricles. With a protean list of side effects (including respiratory depression, sedation, and emesis), its cardiovascular application in the ICU heart failure patient is usually limited to acute relief of hydrostatic pulmonary edema and treatment of acute myocardial infarction. The diverse systemic effects, side effects, contraindications, and drug interactions of narcotics have been well-described (158, 160).

Calcium Channel Antagonists

Three chemical classes of calcium channel blockers are now available in the U.S.: phenylalkylamines (verapamil), benzothiazepines (diltiazem), and 1,4-dihydropyridines (nifedipine and the newer agents nicardipine, nimodipine, isradipine, and felodipine). These agents have variably selective effects on the coronary and peripheral vasculature, myocardium, and nodal tissue. They are presently used to treat hypertension, angina, supraventricular tachyarrhythmias (verapamil and diltiazem), and posthemorrhagic cerebral vasospasm (nimodipine). At clinical doses, the dihydropyridines show somewhat greater vascular selectivity (161); the other groups have greater depressant effects on sinus node automaticity and AV conduction (162). All depress myocardial contractility, with nifedipine most potent on a molar basis and verapamil most often cited for clinical exacerbations of chronic heart failure (163, 164). Their potential utility in both systolic and diastolic heart failure has been of intense interest.

Many actions of these drugs are relevant to therapy of systolic heart failure. Potentially beneficial actions include relaxation of systemic arterioles and large muscular arteries (reducing aortic impedance) and reductions in coronary resistance (improving blood flow) and resting heart rate. Venous return is minimally altered (165). Calcium overload, which may perpetuate myocardial cell loss, might also be prevented by these drugs (166, 167). Possible detrimental effects include direct contractile depression, bradyarrhythmia-induced reduction in cardiac output, reflex neurohumoral activation, and direct stimulation of renin secretion (161, 167, 168).

Most studies of calcium blocker use in systolic heart failure have been deemed inconclusive or lent to differing interpretations (60, 165, 167, 169, 170). Most data suggest that both acute and chronic administration of phenylalkylamines and benzothiazepines are detrimental to patients with systolic heart failure (60, 167, 170); unless additional information is presented, they should probably be avoided in this setting. Nifedipine may also worsen systolic function (171, 172) and clinical symptoms in heart failure. While large controlled trials of newer agents are lacking, in the absence of evidence to the contrary, there is little justification for prescribing calcium channel antagonists to patients with systolic dysfunction who do not have an approved indication for their use (63).

The role of calcium blockers in diastolic failure is somewhat clearer. They are effective therapy for many disorders that lead to lusitropic abnormalities, including active ischemia and hypertension (99). Both symptomatic and hemodynamic improvement of patients with hypertrophic cardiomyopathy have been noted with these agents (most often, verapamil), although the incidence of serious adverse reactions is high in this population (1).

Verapamil and diltiazem appear to have a direct beneficial lusitropic effect in isolated diastolic dysfunction, as demonstrated by improved isovolumic and filling indices (1, 173). Less evidence is available on the effects of dihydropyridines in this regard. The benefits of improving diastolic performance in hydrostatic pulmonary edema of myocardial origin have been discussed above. While not presently approved by the FDA for this use, verapamil (and diltiazem) may offer a safer, effective treatment option for patients with pulmonary venous congestion caused by ventricular noncompliance.

Both intravenous verapamil and diltiazem are presently approved only as antiarrhythmic agents (63). Oral verapamil and diltiazem are available in short (6- to 8-hour) and long (12- to 24-hour)-acting formulations. They are cleared primarily by hepatic metabolism and have pharmacologically active metabolites (99). Excretion half-lives of these drugs are 3 to 5 hours but may be prolonged by fivefold in severe hepatic insufficiency. Dose-related toxicity may be seen in renal failure, probably due to retention of active metabolites (99). Important pharmacokinetic interactions may occur when these agents are coadministered with digoxin, rifampin, cyclosporine, lithium, histamine receptor (type 2) antagonists, muscle relaxants (including dantrolene), some anticonvulsant agents, and inhaled anesthetics (62, 63, 99).

Side effects and toxic manifestations are predominantly extensions of their effects on the heart (bradycardia, heart block, contractile depression) and smooth muscle (hypotension, edema, headache, constipation). Additive effects with any drug that has similar vascular, inotropic, or electrophysiologic actions can result in clinical toxicity. Inhibition of platelet aggregation, liver function abnormalities, and other infrequent side effects have been reported (63, 99).

Other Agents

β-adrenergic blockers, which relieve classical angina and reduce infarct size and sudden death in peri- and postinfarction patients (174, 175), are formally contraindicated in patients with overt heart failure. However, more than 16 trials have shown symptomatic and/or hemodynamic improvement in patients with idiopathic dilated cardiomyopathy treated chronically (>2 months) with oral β-blockers (176). Improved survival in these patients, and overall salutary responses in patients with heart failure from other causes (e.g., ischemic cardiomyopathy), have not yet been shown. Proposed beneficial actions in chronic systolic failure include β-receptor upregulation, reduced myocardial energy expenditure, and prevention of catecholamine-induced cardiotoxicity (174, 178, 177). Conversely, β-blockade may impair lusitropy (14, 174, 179).

In the critically ill patient with decompensated or acute nonischemic heart failure, β-blockers must still be considered contraindicated due to the risk of acute inotropic depression. Further investigation is required before such therapy can be considered an appropriate (chronic) treatment option (176).

Dopaminergic Agonists. The pharmacologic effects of dopamine and beneficial effects of DA receptor stimulation in heart failure have been discussed above. Levodopa (nonselective) and bromocriptine (DA_2-selective) are currently available oral dopaminergic agents. Trials in chronic heart failure thus far have been of short duration and complicated by high rates of CNS side effects (40). Neither drug has been evaluated in large controlled trials of chronic therapy and, hence, cannot be recommended as therapeutic options at this time. Newer selective agents with DA-receptor activity are under study (39, 180); though initial studies are promising, they presently remain investigational.

Combination Therapy

Often, drug combinations are employed in treating acute or decompensated chronic systolic failure in order to achieve a desired hemodynamic effect while limiting therapeutic complications. Although many different combinations are possible, they are usually chosen to exploit a dose-specific response, improve net myocardial energy balance, maintain splanchnic blood flow, or limit secondary neurohumoral reflexes. Only a few combinations will be described.

In acute heart failure management, the specific vascular effects of low dose dopamine may be combined with more specific inotropes (dobutamine) to improve contractility and renal perfusion while avoiding unwanted tachycardia. The addition of nitroglycerin (for preload, lusitropic, and coronary effects) to a combined α/β-agonist (high-dose dopamine) is often helpful in relieving pulmonary congestion and optimizing coronary perfusion while supporting blood pressure and improving contractility. The inotropic response to amrinone can be enhanced by increasing the intracellular concentration of conservable cAMP with β-agonists. If too pronounced, amrinone's vasodilatory action may be partially counteracted with moderate doses of dopamine, adding vasoconstriction (and $β_1$-agonism) to the final effect. A low dose of a balanced vasodilator (nitroprusside) may effectively lower preload and many components of afterload when short-term therapy with norepinephrine is required for profoundly reduced systolic performance. In general, diuretics must be added during prolonged infusions of nitrovasodilators to counteract unwanted salt and water retention. When diuretics are combined with ACE inhibitors, both balanced load reduction and limitation of potassium loss can be achieved. Indeed, if arterial pressure permits, addition of ACE inhibitors may afford some benefit to many patients when other agents (or the underlying disease) produce unwanted RA activation. Similar principles can be applied to multidrug combinations.

Several excellent reviews of drug groups and management strategies are listed for further reading (181–187).

CONCLUSION

This brief presentation of heart failure pharmacotherapy in the critically ill patient will hopefully stimulate the reader to pursue more detailed information on the topics presented. The need for precise pathophysiologic diagnosis translated into specific therapeutic goals, and selection of treatment based on sound pharmacologic principles, is paramount. The information provided above can only be viewed as a most general guideline. New pharmacologic agents, and new information on existing drugs, are being discovered at a breathtaking rate; yet, the ultimate therapeutic endpoint—improved patient survival with a good quality of life—has only been achieved recently for some patients. Constant vigilant study of the pharmacologic literature is the best prescription for the clinician responsible for critically ill patients with heart failure.

REFERENCES

1. Harizi RC, Bianco JA, Alpert JS: Diastolic function of the heart in clinical cardiology. *Arch Intern Med* 148:99–109, 1988.
2. Little RC, Little WC: Cardiac preload, afterload, and heart failure. *Arch Intern Med* 142:819–822, 1982.
3. Devereux RB: Toward a more complete understanding of left ventricular afterload. *J Am Coll Cardiol* 17:122–124, 1991.
4. Fitchett DH: Vascular reflections and the arterial load: their importance in the management of heart failure. *Congestive Heart Failure Index and Rev* 3:1, 24, 1990.
5. McElroy PA, Shroff SG, Weber KT: Pathophysiology of the failing heart. *Cardiol Clin* 7:25–37, 1989.
6. Kameyama T, Asanoi H, Ishizaka S, Sasayama S: Ventricular load optimization by unloading therapy in patients with heart failure. *J Am Coll Cardiol* 17:199–207, 1991.
7. Braunwald E, Sonnenblick EH, Ross J: Mechanisms of cardiac contraction and relaxation. In Braunwald E (ed): *Heart Disease: a Textbook of Cardiovascular Medicine*, ed 7. Philadelphia, WB Saunders Company, p. 383–425, 1988.
8. Suga H, Sagawa K, Shoukas AA: Load independence of the instantaneous pressure-volume ratio of the canine left ventricle and effects of epinephrine and heart rate on the ratio. *Cir Res* 32:314–322, 1973.
9. Katz AM: Influence of altered inotropy and lusitropy on ventricular pressure-volume loops. *J Am Coll Cardiol* 11:438–445, 1988.
10. Kass DA, Maughan WL: From 'Emax' to pressure-volume relations: a broader view. *Circulation* 77:1203–1211, 1988.
11. Elzinga G, Westerhof N: Pump function of the feline left heart: changes with heart rate and its bearing on the energy balance. *Cardiovasc Res* 14:81–92, 1980.
12. Mirsky I, Tajimi T, Peterson KL: The development of the entire end-systolic pressure-volume and ejection fraction-afterload relation: a new concept of systolic myocardial stiffness. *Circulation* 76:343–356, 1987.
13. Zile MR, Gaasch WH: Mechanical loads and the isovolumic and filling indices of left ventricular relaxation. *Prog Cardiovasc Dis* 32:333–346, 1990.
14. Stauffer JC, Gaasch WH: Recognition and treatment of left ventricular diastolic dysfunction. *Prog Cardiovasc Dis* 32:319–332, 1990.
15. Parmley WW: Pathophysiology and current therapy of congestive heart failure. *J Am Coll Cardiol* 13:771–785, 1989.
16. Dean JW, Poole-Wilson PA: Therapeutic implications of diastolic dysfunction in heart failure. *Postgrad Med J* 66:932–937, 1990.
17. Cohen JN: Abnormalities of peripheral sympathetic nervous system control in congestive heart failure. *Circulation* 82(suppl I):I59–I67, 1990.
18. Brodde O-E: Physiology and pharmacology of cardiovascular catecholamine receptors: implications for treatment of chronic heart failure. *Am Heart J* 120:1565–1572, 1990.
19. Francis GS: Modulation of peripheral sympathetic nerve transmission. *J Am Coll Cardiol* 12:250–254, 1988.
20. Morgan JP, Perreault CL, Morgan KG: The cellular basis of contraction and relaxation in cardiac and vascular smooth muscle. *Am Heart J* 121:961–968, 1991.
21. Bristow MR, Ginsberg R, Umans V, et al: β₁- and β₂-adrenergic receptor subpopulations in nonfailing and failing human ventricular myocardium: coupling of both receptor subtypes to muscle contraction and selective β₁-receptor down-regulation in heart failure. *Circ Res* 59:297–309, 1986.
22. Katz AM: Interplay between inotropic and lusitropic effects of cyclic adenosine monophosphate on the myocardial cell. *Circulation* 82 (suppl I):I17–I10, 1990.
23. Katz AM: Potential deleterious effects of inotropic agents in the therapy of chronic heart failure. *Circulation* 73 (suppl III):III184–III188, 1986.
24. Podrid PJ, Fuchs T, Candinas R: Role of the sympathetic nervous system in the genesis of ventricular arrhythmia. *Circulation* 82 (suppl I):I103–113, 1990.
25. Katz Am: Future perspectives in basic science understanding of congestive heart failure. *Am J Cardiol* 66:468–471, 1990.
26. Herzig JW, Ruegg JC, Solaro RJ: Myocardial excitation-contraction coupling as influenced through modulation of the calcium sensitivity of the contractile proteins. *Heart Failure* 6:244–250, 1990/1991.
27. Godfraind T: Comparative pharmacology of cardiac and vascular tissues in heart failure. *J Cardiovasc Pharmacol* 14 (suppl 8):S1–S20, 1989.
28. Francis GS, Cohn JN: Heart failure: mechanisms of cardiac and vascular dysfunction and the rationale for pharmacologic intervention. *FASEB J* 4:3068–3075, 1990.
29. Katz, AM: Cardiomyopathy of overload. *N Engl J Med* 322:100–110, 1990.
30. Goldsmith SR, Dodge-Brown DL, Katz A: Alpha₂-adrenergic stimulation and vasopressin in congestive heart failure. *J Cardiovasc Pharmacol* 14:425–429, 1989.

31. Kubo SH: Neurohormonal activity in congestive heart failure. *Crit Care Med* 18:S39–S44, 1990.
32. Francis GS: The relationship of the sympathetic nervous system and the renin-angiotensin system in congestive heart failure. *Am Heart J* 118:642–648, 1989.
33. Moravec CS, Schluchter MD, Paranandi L, et al: Inotropic effects of angiotensin II on human cardiac muscle in vitro. *Circulation* 82:1973–1984, 1990.
34. Francis GS: Neuroendocrine activity in congestive heart failure. *Am J Cardiol* (11):33D–39D, 1990.
35. Schulman M, Narins RG: Hypokalemia and cardiovascular disease. *Am J Cardiol* (10):4E–9E, 1990.
36. Cohen JN: Mechanisms in heart failure and the role of angiotensin-converting enzyme inhibition. *Am J Cardiol* Oct 2 66(11):2D–6D, 1990.
37. Raine AEG, Phil D, Erne P, et al: Atrial natriuretic peptide and atrial pressure in patients with congestive heart failure. *N Engl J Med* 315:533–537, 1986.
38. Cogan MG (principal discussant). Atrial natriuretic peptide. *Kidney Int* 37:1148–1160, 1990.
39. Murphy MB, Elliot WJ: Dopamine and dopamine receptor agonists in cardiovascular therapy. *Crit Care Med* 18:S14–S18, 1990.
40. Rajfer SI, Davis FR: Role of dopamine receptors and the utility of dopamine agonists in heart failure. *Circulation* 82(suppl I):I97–I102, 1990.
41. Hathaway DR, March KL: Molecular cardiology: new avenues for the diagnosis and treatment of cardiovascular disease. *J Am Coll Cardiol* 13:265–282, 1989.
42. Frelin C: Mechanisms of vasoconstriction. *Am Heart J* 121:958–960, 1991.
43. Dzau VJ, Hirsch AT: Emerging role of the tissue renin-angiotensin systems in congestive heart failure. *Eur Heart J* 11(suppl B):65–71, 1990.
44. Unger T, Gohlke P: Tissue renin-angiotensin systems in the heart and vasculature: possible involvement in the cardiovascular actions of converting enzyme inhibitors. *Am J Cardiol* 65:3I–10I, 1990.
45. Maisel AS, Scott NA, Motulsky HJ, et al: Elevation of plasma neuropeptide Y levels in congestive heart failure. *Am J Med* 86:43–48, 1989.
46. Wasserman K: The peripheral circulation and lactic acid metabolism in heart, or cardiovascular, failure. *Circulation* 80:1084–1086, 1989.
47. Rouleau JL, Kortas C, Bichet D, de Champlain J: Neurohumoral and hemodynamic changes in congestive heart failure: lack of correlation and evidence of compensatory mechanisms. *Am Heart J* 116:746–757, 1988.
48. Nishijima H, Yasuda H, Ito K, et al: Acute and chronic hemodynamic effects of the basic therapeutic regimen for congestive heart failure. *Jpn Heart J* 25:571–585, 1984.
49. Levine TB, Francis GS, Goldsmith ST, et al: Activity of the sympathetic nervous system and renin-angiotensin system assessed by plasma hormone levels and their relationship to hemodynamic abnormalities in congestive heart failure. *Am J Cardiol* 49:1659–1666, 1982.
50. Port JD, Gilbert EM, Larrabee P, et al: Neurotransmitter depletion compromises the ability of indirect-acting amines to provide inotropic support in the failing human heart. *Circulation* 81:929–938, 1990.
51. Bristow MR, Hershberger RE, Port JD, et al: Beta-adrenergic pathways in nonfailing and failing human ventricular myocardium. *Circulation* 82 (suppl I):I12–I25, 1990.
52. Horn EM, Bilezikian JP: Mechanisms of abnormal transmembrane signaling of the β-adrenergic receptor in congestive heart failure. *Circulation* 82 (suppl I):I26–I34, 1990.
53. Morgan JP: Abnormal intracellular modulation of calcium as a major cause of cardiac contractile dysfunction. *N Engl J Med* 325:625–631, 1991.
54. Morgan JP, Erny RE, Allen PD, Grossman W, Gwathmey JK: Abnormal intracellular calcium handling, a major cause of systolic and diastolic dysfunction in ventricular myocardium from patients with heart failure. *Circulation* 81 (suppl III):III21–III32, 1990.
55. Cohn JN, Archibald DG, Ziesche S, et al: Effect of vasodilator therapy on mortality in chronic congestive heart failure. Results of a Veterans Administration Cooperative Study (V-HeFT). *N Engl J Med* 314:1547–1552, 1986.
56. Pfeffer MA, Lamas GA, Vaughan DE, Parisi AF, Braunwald E: Effect of captopril on progressive ventricular dilatation after anterior myocardial infarction. *N Engl J Med* 319:80–86, 1988.
57. Mulrow CD, Mulrow JP, Linn WD, Aguilar C, Ramirez G: Relative efficacy of vasodilator therapy in chronic congestive heart failure. *JAMA* 259:3422–3426, 1988.
58. CONSENSUS Trial Study Group. Effects of enalapril on mortality in severe congestive heart failure: results of the Cooperative North Scandinavian Enalapril Survival Study (CONSENSUS). *N Engl J Med* 316:1429–1435, 1987.
59. Falk RH: A plea for a clinical trial of anticoagulation in dilated cardiomyopathy. *Am J Cardiol* 65:914–915, 1990.
60. Firth BG, Yancy CW: Survival in congestive heart failure: Have we made a difference? *Am J Med* 88:I3N–I8N, 1990.
61. Arnsdorf MF, Bump T: Management of arrhythmias in heart failure. *Cardiol Clin* 7:144–170, 1989.
62. Rudd C, Wilkman J, Plumb PD: Drug interactions in critical care. In Lumb PD, Bryan-Brown CW (eds): *Complications in Critical Care Medicine*. Chicago, Year Book Medical Publishers, pp. 262–279, 1988.
63. *Physicians' Desk Reference*. ed 46. Montvale, NJ, Medical Economics Data, 1992.
64. Purdy RE, Boucek RJ: *Handbook of Cardiac Drugs: Basic Science and Clinical Aspects of Cardiovascular Pharmacology*. Boston, Little, Brown, 1988.
65. Zaritsky AL, Chernow B. Catecholamines and other inotropes. In Chernow B (ed): *The Pharmacologic Approach to the Critically Ill Patient*, ed 2. Williams & Wilkins, Baltimore, pp. 584–602, 1988.
66. Passmore JM, Goldstein RA: Acute recognition and management of congestive heart failure. *Crit Care Clin* 5:497M–532, 1989.
67. Notterman DA: Inotropic agents—catecholamines, digoxin, amrinone. *Crit Care Clin* 7:583–613, 1991.
68. Katz AM: Changing strategies in the management of heart failure. *J Am Coll Cardiol* 13:513–523, 1989.

69. Hoffman BB, Lefkowitz RJ. Catecholamines and sympathomimetic drugs. In Gilman AG, Rall TW, Nies AS, Taylor P (eds): *The Pharmacologic Basis of Therapeutics,* ed 8. Pergamon Press, New York, pp 187–220, 1990.
70. Lollgen H, Drexler H: Use of inotropes in the critical care setting. *Crit Care Med* 18:S56–S60, 1990.
71. Maekawa K, Liang CS, Hood WB: Comparison of dobutamine and dopamine in acute myocardial infarction: effects of systemic hemodynamics, plasma catecholamines, blood flow, and infarct size. *Circulation* 67:750–759, 1983.
72. Wisenberg G, Zawadowski AG, Gebhardt VA, et al: Dopamine: its potential for inducing ischemic left ventricular dysfunction. *J Am Coll Cardiol* 6:84–92, 1985.
73. Ruffolo RR Jr, Spradlin TA, Pollock GD, Waddell JE, Murphy PJ: Alpha and beta adrenergic effects of the stereoisomers of dobutamine. *J Pharmacol Exp Ther* 219:447–452, 1981.
74. Leier CV, Unverferth DV: Dobutamine. *Ann Intern Med* 99:490–496, 1983.
75. Uretsky BF, Lawless CE, Verbalis JG, Valdes AM, Kolesar JA, Reddy PS: Combined therapy with dobutamine and amrinone in severe heart failure. *Chest* 92:657–662, 1987.
76. Roberts R: Inotropic therapy for cardiac failure associated with acute myocardial infarction. *Chest* 93(suppl):22S–24S, 1988.
77. Unverferth DV, Blandford M, Kates RE, Leier CV: Tolerance to dobutamine after a 72 hour continuous infusion. *Am J Med* 69:262–266, 1980.
78. Dies F, Krell MJ, Whitlow P, et al: Intermittent dobutamine in ambulatory outpatients with chronic cardiac failure (abstr.). *Circulation* 74(suppl 2):38, 1986.
79. Packer M: Vasodilator and inotropic drugs for the treatment of chronic heart failure: distinguishing hype from hope. *J Am Coll Cardiol* 12:1299–1317, 1988.
80. Colucci WS: Positive inotropic/vasodilator agents. *Cardiol Clin* 7:131–144, 1989.
81. Colucci WS, Wright RF, Braunwald E: New positive inotropic agents in the treatment of congestive heart failure: mechanisms of action and recent clinical developments (parts I and II). *N Engl J Med* 314:290–299, 349–358, 1986.
82. Bohm M, Diet F, Kemkes B, Erdmann E: Enhancement of the effectiveness of milrinone to increase force of contraction by stimulation of cardiac beta-adrenoceptors in the failing heart. *Klin Wochenschr* 66:957–962, 1988.
83. Maisel AS, Wright CM, Carter SM, Ziegler M, Motulsky HJ: Tachyphylaxis with amrinone therapy: association with sequestration and down-regulation of lymphocyte beta-adrenergic receptors. *Ann Intern Med* 110:195–201, 1989.
84. Monrad ES, McKay RG, Baim DS, et al: Improvement in indexes of diastolic performance in patients with congestive heart failure treated with milrinone. *Circulation* 70:1030–1037, 1984.
85. Monrad ES, Baim DS, Smith HS, et al: Effects of milrinone on coronary hemodynamics and myocardial energetics in patients with congestive heart failure. *Circulation* 71:972–979, 1985.
86. Baim DS: Effects of amrinone on myocardial energetics in severe congestive heart failure. *Am J Cardiol* 56:16B–18B, 1985.
87. Hoffman BF, Bigger JT: Digitalis and allied cardiac glycosides. In Gilman AG, Rall TW, Nies AS, Taylor P (eds): *The Pharmacologic Basis of Therapeutics,* ed 8. Pergamon Press, New York, pp 814–839, 1990.
88. DiBianco R, Shabetai R, Kostuk W, Moran J, Schlant RC, Wright R: A comparison of oral milrinone, digoxin, and their combination in the treatment of patients with chronic heart failure. *N Engl J Med* 320:677–683, 1989.
89. Chatterjee K: Digitalis and non-ACE inhibitor vasodilators in heart failure. *Cardiol Clin* 7:99–118, 1989.
90. Ferguson DW, Berg WJ, Sanders JS, Roach PJ, Kempf JS, Kienzle MG: Sympathoinhibitory responses to digitalis glycosides in heart failure patients: direct evidence from sympathetic neural readings. *Circulation* 80:65–77, 1989.
91. Guyatt GH, Sullivan MJ, Fallen EL, et al: A controlled trial of digoxin in congestive heart failure. *Am J Cardiol* 61:371–375, 1988.
92. Jaeschke R, Oxman AD, Guyatt GH: To what extent do congestive heart failure patients in sinus rhythm benefit from digoxin therapy? A systematic overview and meta-analysis. *Am J Med* 88:279–286, 1990.
93. Ewy GA: Urgent parenteral digoxin therapy: a requiem. *J Am Coll Cardiol* 15:1248–1249, 1990.
94. Cercek B, Shah PK: Complicated acute myocardial infarction: heart failure, shock, mechanical complications. *Cardiol Clin* 9:569–593, 1991.
95. Haustein KO, Assman I, Fiehring H: Problems of rapid digitalization in severe congestive heart failure. *Eur J Cardiol* 11:135–146, 1980.
96. Bigger JT, Fleiss JL, Rolnitzky IM, Merab JP, Ferrick KJ: Effect of digitalis treatment on survival after acute myocardial infarction. *Am J Cardiol* 55:623–630, 1985.
97. Moss AJ, Davis HT, Conard DL, DeCamilla JJ, Odoroff CH: Digitalis-associated cardiac mortality after myocardial infarction. *Circulation* 64:1150–1156, 1981.
98. Goldstein RA, Passamani ER, Roberts R: A comparison of digoxin and dobutamine in patients with acute infarction and cardiac failure. *N Engl J Med* 303:846–850, 1980.
99. Murad F. Drugs used for the treatment of angina: organic nitrates, calcium-channel blockers, and β-adrenergic antagonists. In Gilman AG, Rall TW, Nies AS, Taylor P (eds): *The Pharmacologic Basis of Therapeutics,* ed 8. Pergamon Press, New York, pp 764–783, 1990.
100. Gerber JG, Nies AS: Antihypertensive agents and the drug therapy of hypertension. In Gilman AG, Rall TW, Nies AS, Taylor P (eds): *The Pharmacologic Basis of Therapeutics,* ed 8. Pergamon Press, New York, pp 784–813, 1990.
101. Lavine SJ, Campbell CA, Held AC: Effect of nitroglycerin-induced reduction of left ventricular filling pressure on diastolic filling in acute dilated heart failure. *J Am Coll Cardiol* 14:233–241, 1989.
102. Bencowitz HZ, LeWinter MM, Wagner PD: Effect of sodium nitroprusside on ventilation-perfusion mismatching in heart failure. *J Am Coll Cardiol* 4:918–922, 1984.
103. Edwards JC, Ignarro LJ, Hyman AL, Kadowitz PJ: Relaxation of intrapulmonary artery and vein by nitrogen-oxide-containing vasodilators and cyclic GMP. *J Pharmacol Exp Ther* 228:33–42, 1984.
104. Parrillo JE. Vasodilator therapy. In Chernow B (ed): *The Pharmacologic Approach to the Critically Ill Patient,* ed 2. Williams & Wilkins, Baltimore, pp 346–364, 1988.
105. Packer M, Meller J, Medina N, Gorlin R, Herman M: Rebound hemodynamic events after the abrupt withdrawal of nitroprusside in patients with severe chronic heart failure. *N Engl J Med* 301:1193–1197, 1979.
106. Abrams J: Nitrates. *Med Clin North Am* 72:1–35, 1988.
107. Elkayam U, Kulick D, McIntosh N, Roth A, Hsueh W, Rahimtoola SH: Incidence of early tolerance to hemodynamic effects of continuous infusion of nitroglycerin in patients with coronary artery disease and heart failure. *Circulation* 76:577–584, 1987.
108. Hood WP, Amende I, Simon R, Lichten PR: The effects of intracoronary nitroglycerin on left ventricular systolic and diastolic function in man. *Circulation* 61:159–168, 1980.
109. Packer M, Lee WH, Kessler PD, Gottleib SS, Medina N, Yushak M: Prevention and reversal of nitrate tolerance in patients with congestive heart failure. *N Engl J Med* 317:799--804, 1987.
110. Levy WS, Katz RJ, Wasserman AG: Methionine restores venodilative response to nitroglycerin after the development of tolerance. *J Am Coll Cardiol* 17:474–479, 1991.
111. Munzel T, Holtz J, Mulsch A, Stewart DJ, Bassenge E: Nitrate tolerance in epicardial arteries or in the venous system is not reversed by N-acetylcysteine in vivo, but tolerance-independent interactions exist. *Circulation* 79:188–197, 1989.
112. Parker JO, Farrel B, Lahey KA, Moe G: Effect of intervals between doses on the development of tolerance to isosorbide dinitrate. *N Engl J Med* 316:1440–1444, 1987.
113. Curry SC, Arnold--Capell P: Nitroprusside, nitroglycerin, and angiotensin-converting enzyme inhibitors. *Crit Care Clin* 7:555–581, 1991.
114. Pouleur H, Covell JW, Ross J: Effects of nitroprusside on venous return and central blood volume in the absence and presence of acute heart failure. *Circulation* 61:328–337, 1980.
115. Miller RR, Vismara LA, Williams DO, Amsterdam EA, Mason DT: Pharmacological mechanisms for left ventricular unloading in clinical congestive heart failure: differential effects of nitroprusside, phentolamine, and nitroglycerin on cardiac function and peripheral circulation. *Circ Res* 39:127–133, 1976.
116. Leier CV: Regional blood flow responses to vasodilators and inotropes in congestive heart failure. *Am J Cardiol* 62:86E–93E, 1988.
117. Olivari MT, Levine TB, Cohn JN: Abnormal neurohumoral response to nitroprusside infusion in congestive heart failure. *J Am Coll Cardiol* 2:411–417, 1983.
118. Chiariello M, Gold HK, Leinbach RC, Davis MA, Maroko PR: Comparison between the effects of nitroprusside and nitroglycerin on ischemic injury during acute myocardial infarction. *Circulation* 54:766–773, 1976.
119. Perret C: Acute heart failure in myocardial infarction: principles of treatment. *Crit Care Med* 18:S26–S29, 1990.
120. Cohn JN: Future directions in vasodilator therapy for heart failure. *Am Heart J* 121:969–974, 1991.
121. Packer M: Therapeutic options in the management of chronic heart failure. *Circulation* 79:198–204, 1989.
122. Cohn JN, Johnson G, Ziesche S, et al: A comparison of enalapril with hydralazine-isosorbide dinitrate in the treatment of chronic congestive heart failure. *N Engl J Med* 325:303–310, 1991.
123. Franciosa JA, Jordan RA, Wilen MM, Leddy CL: Minoxidil in patients with left heart failure: contrasting hemodynamic and clinical effects in a controlled trial. *Circulation* 70:63–69, 1984.
124. Harper RW, Claxton H, Anderson S, Pitt A: The acute and chronic haemodynamic effects of prazosin in severe congestive heart failure. *Med J Aust* 2 (suppl):36–38, 1980.
125. Desch CE, Magorien RD, Triffon DW, Blanford MF, Unverferth DV, Leier CV: Development of pharmacodynamic tolerance to prazosin in congestive heart failure. *Am J Cardiol* 44:1178–1182, 1979.
126. Dzau VJ, Creager MA: Progress in angiotensin-converting enzyme inhibition in heart failure: rationale, mechanisms, and clinical response. *Cardiol Clin* 7:119–130, 1989.
127. Raya TE, Lee RW, Westhoff T, Goldman S: Captopril restores hemodynamic responsiveness to atrial natriuretic peptide in rats with heart failure. *Circulation* 80:1886–1892, 1989.
128. Maisel AS, Phillips C, Michel MC, Ziegler MG, Carter SM: Regulation of cardiac β-adrenergic receptors by captopril. Implications for congestive heart failure. *Circulation* 80:669–675, 1989.
129. Horn EM, Corwin SJ, Steinberg SF, et al: Reduced lymphocyte stimulatory guanine nucleotide regulatory protein and beta-adrenergic receptors in congestive heart failure and reversal with angiotensin converting enzyme inhibitor therapy. *Circulation* 78:1373–1379, 1988.
130. Deedwania P: Angiotensin-converting enzyme inhibitors in congestive heart failure. *Arch Intern Med* 150:1796–1805, 1990.
131. Pfeffer MA, Pfeffer JM, Steinberg C, Finn P: Survival after an experimental myocardial infarction: beneficial effects of long-term captopril. *Circulation* 72:406–412, 1985.
132. de Graeff PA, van Gilst WH, Bel K, De Langen CDJ, Kingma JH, Wesseling H: Concentration-dependent protection by captopril against myocardial damage after ischemia—reperfusion injury in a closed chest pig model. *J Cardiovasc Pharmacol* 9(suppl 2):S37–S42, 1987.
133. Kubo SH, Cody RJ, Laragh JH, et al: Immediate converting-enzyme inhibition with intravenous enalapril in chronic congestive heart failure. *Am J Cardiol* 55:122–126, 1985.
134. Packer M: Why do the kidneys release renin in patients with congestive heart failure? A nephrocentric view of converting-enzyme inhibition. *Eur Heart J* 11(suppl D):44–52, 1990.
135. Drexler H, Banhardt U, Meinertz T, Wollschlager H, Lehmann M, Just H: Contrasting peripheral short-term and long-term effects of converting enzyme inhibition in patients with congestive heart failure. *Circulation* 79:491–502, 1989.
136. Mancia G, Perondi R, Saino A, et al: Haemodynamic effects of ACE inhibitors. *Eur Heart J* 11(suppl D):27–32, 1990.

137. Swedberg K, Eneroth P, Kjekshus J, Wilhelmsen L, CONSENSUS Trial Study Group: Hormones regulating cardiovasular function in patients with severe congestive heart failure and their relation to mortality. *Circulation* 82:1730–1736, 1990.

138. Cleland JGF, Henderson E, McLenachan J, Findlay IN, Dargie HJ: Effect of captopril, an angiotensin-converting enzyme inhibitor, in patients with angina pectoris and heart failure. *J Am Coll Cardiol* 17:733–739, 1991.

139. Packer M, Kukin ML: Management of patients with heart failure and angina: do coexistent diseases alter the response to cardiovascular drugs? *J Am Coll Cardiol* 17:740–742, 1991.

140. Dargie HJ, Ray SG: The effects of angiotensin-converting enzyme inhibition on coronary blood flow and infarct size limitation. *J Hum Hypertens* 3(suppl I):I101–I106, 1989.

141. Garrison JC, Peach MJ. Renin and angiotensin. In Gilman AG, Rall TW, Nies AS, Taylor P (eds): *The Pharmacologic Basis of Therapeutics*, ed 8. Pergamon Press, New York, pp 749–763, 1990.

142. Dickstein K, Till AE, Aarsland T, et al: The pharmacokinetics of enalapril in hospitalized patients with congestive heart failure. *Br J Clin Pharmacol* 23:403–410, 1987.

143. Cody RJ: Pharmacology of angiotensin-converting enzyme inhibitors as a guide to their use in congestive heart failure. *Am J Cardiol* 66:7D–13D, 1990.

144. Borek M, Carlap S, Frishman WH: Angiotensin-converting enzyme inhibitors in heart failure. *Med Clin North Am* 73:315–338, 1989.

145. The SOLVD Investigators. Effect of enalapril on survival in patients with reduced left ventricular ejection fractions and congestive heart failure. *N Engl J Med* 325:293–302, 1991.

146. Boles-Ponto LL, Schoenwald RD. Furosemide (frusemide): a pharmacokinetic/pharmacodynamic review (part I). *Clin Pharmacokinet* 18:381–408, 1990.

147. Lant A. Diuretics: clinical pharmacology and therapeutic use (parts I and II). *Drugs* 29:57–87, 162–188, 1985.

148. Narins RG, Chusid P: Diuretic use in critical care. *Am J Cardiol* 57:26A–32A, 1986.

149. Puschett JB: Clinical pharmacologic implications in diuretic selection. *Am J Cardiol* 57:6A–13A, 1986.

150. Johnston GD, Hiatt WR, Nies AS, Payne NA, Murphy RC, Gerber JG: Factors modifying the early nondiuretic vascular effects of furosemide in man: the possible role of renal prostaglandins. *Circ Res* 53:630–635, 1983.

151. Francis GS, Benedict C, Johnstone DE, et al: Comparison of neuroendocrine activation in patients with left ventricular dysfunction with and without congestive heart failure. *Circulation* 82:1724–1729, 1990.

152. Francis GS, Siegel RM, Goldsmith SR, Olivari MT, Levine B, Cohn JN: Acute vasoconstrictor response to intravenous furosemide in patients with chronic congestive heart failure: activation of the neurohumoral axis. *Ann Intern Med* 103:1–6, 1985.

153. Sica DA, Gehr T: Diuretics in congestive heart failure. *Cardiol Clin* 7:87–97, 1989.

154. Dikshit K, Vyden JK, Forrester JS, Chatterjee K, Prakash R, Swan HJC: Renal and extrarenal hemodynamic effects of furosemide in congestive heart failure after acute myocardial infarction. *N Engl J Med* 228:1087–1090, 1973.

155. Goldsmith SR, Francis G, Cohn JN: Attenuation of the pressor response to intravenous furosemide by angiotensin converting enzyme inhibition in congestive heart failure. *Am J Cardiol* 64:1382–1385, 1989.

156. Wilson JR, Reichek N, Dunkman WB, Goldberg S: Effect of diuresis on the performance of the failing left ventricle in man. *Am J Med* 70:234–239, 1981.

157. Weiner IM. Diuretics and other agents employed in the mobilization of edema fluid. In Gilman AG, Rall TW, Nies AS, Taylor P (eds): *The Pharmacologic Basis of Therapeutics*, ed 8. New York, Pergamon Press, New York, pp 713–731, 1990.

158. Jaffe JH, Martin WR. Opioid analgesics and antagonists. In Gilman AG, Rall TW, Nies AS, Taylor P (eds): *The Pharmacologic Basis of Therapeutics*, ed 8. Pergamon Press, New York, pp 485–521, 1990.

159. Zelis R, Mansour EJ, Capone RJ, Mason DT: The cardiovascular effects of morphine: the peripheral capacitance and resistance vessels in human subjects. *J Clin Invest* 54:1247–1258, 1974.

160. Buck ML, Blumer JL: Opioids and other analgesics–adverse events in the intensive care unit. *Crit Care Clin* 7:615–637, 1991.

161. Packer M: Second generation calcium channel blockers in the treatment of chronic heart failure: Are they any better than their predecessors? *J Am Coll Cardiol* 14:1339–1342, 1989.

162. Piepho RW: Heterogeneity of calcium channel blockers. In *The Heterogeneity of Calcium Channel Blockers (Proceedings of a Symposium, Kansas City, MO, Fall 1989)*. McGraw-Hill, New York, pp 3–5, 1989.

163. Bohm M, Schwinger RHG, Erdmann E: Different cardiodepressant potency of various calcium antagonists in human myocardium. *Am J Cardiol* 65:1039–1041, 1990.

164. Henry PD: Comparative pharmacology of calcium antagonists: nifedipine, verapamil and diltiazem. *Am J Cardiol* 46:1047–1058, 1980.

165. Charlap S, Frishman WH: Calcium antagonists and heart failure. *Med Clin North Am* 73:339–359, 1989.

166. Kubo SH, Olivari MT, Cohn HN: Calcium antagonists in heart failure. *Ann NY Acad Sci* 522:553–564, 1988.

167. Packer M: Calcium channel blockers in chronic heart failure: the risks of "physiologically rational" therapy. *Circulation* 82:2254–2257, 1990.

168. Fakundig JL, Catt KJ: Dependence of aldosterone stimulation in adrenal glomerulosa cells on calcium uptake: effects of lanthanum and verapamil. *Endocrinology* 107:1345–1353, 1980.

169. Multicenter Diltiazem Postinfarction Trial Research Group. The effect of diltiazem on mortality and reinfarction after myocardial infarction. *N Engl J Med* 319:385–392, 1988.

170. Goldstein RE, Boccuzzi S, Cruess D, et al: Effects of diltiazem on occurance of heart failure after myocardial infarction (abstract). *Circulation* 80(suppl II):II–50, 1989.

171. Fifer MA, Colucci WS, Lorell BH, Jaski BE, Barry WH: Inotropic, vascular and neuroendocrine effects of nifedipine in heart failure: comparison with nitroprusside. *J Am Coll Cardiol* 5:731–737, 1985.

172. Elkayam U, Amin J, Mehra A, Vasquez J, Weber L, Rahimtoola SH: A prospective, randomized, double-blind, crossover study to compare the efficacy and safety of chronic nifedipine therapy with that of isosorbide dinitrate and their combination in the treatment of chronic congestive heart failure. *Circulation* 82:1954–1961, 1990.

173. Setaro JF, Zaret BL, Schulman DS, Black HR, Soufer R: Usefulness of verapamil for congestive heart failure associated with abnormal left ventricular diastolic filling and normal left ventricular systolic performance. *Am J Cardiol* 66:981–986, 1990.

174. Charlap S, Lichstein E, Frishman WH: Beta-adrenergic blocking drugs in the treatment of congestive heart failure. *Med Clin North Am* 73:373–385, 1989.

175. Chadda K, Goldstein S, Byington R, Curb JD: Effect of propranolol after acute myocardial infarction in patients with congestive heart failure. *Circulation* 73:503–510, 1986.

176. Krukemyer JJ: Use of β-adrenergic blocking agents in congestive heart failure. *Clin Pharm* 9:853–863, 1990.

177. Fowler MB, Bristow MR: Rationale for beta-adrenergic blocking drugs in cardiomyopathy. *Am J Cardiol* 55:120D–124D, 1985.

178. Rona G: Catecholamine cardiotoxicity. *J Mol Cell Cardiol* 17:291–306, 1985.

179. Colucci WS, Parker JD: Effects of β-adrenergic agents on systolic and diastolic myocardial function in patients with congestive heart failure. *J Cardiovasc Pharmacol* 14(suppl 5):S28–S37, 1989.

180. Carey RA, Jacob L: The role of dopaminergic agents and the dopamine receptor in treatment for CHF. *J Clin Pharmacol* 29:207–211, 1989.

181. Zaloga GP, Prielipp RC, Butterworth JF 4th, Royster RL: Pharmacologic cardiovascular support. *Crit Care Clin* 9(2):335–362, 1993.

182. Om A, Hess ML: Inotropic therapy of the failing myocardium. *Clin Cardiol* 16(1):5–14, 1993.

183. McGhie AL, Goldstein RA: Pathogenesis and management of acute heart failure and cardiopenic shock. *Chest* 102(5 Suppl 2): 6265–6325, 1992.

184. Ventura HO, Murgo JP, Smart FW, Stapleton DD, Arice HL: Current issues in advanced heart failure. *Med Clin North Am* 76(5):1057–82; Sep 1992.

185. Bonow RO, Udelson JE: Left ventricular diastolic dysfunction as a cause of congestive heart failure. Mechanism and management. *Ann Intern Med* 117(6): 502–10, 1992.

186. Cody RJ. Management of congestive heart failure. *Am J Cardiol* 69(18):141G–147G, 1992.

187. Pitt B. Congestive heart failure: new therapeutic strategies. *Clin Cardiol* 15 (Suppl) 1:12–4, 1992.

CHAPTER 5

Adjustment of Medications in Liver Failure

CHERYL A. KUBISTY, M.D.
PATRICIA A. ARNS, M.D.
PETER J. WEDLUND, PH.D.
ROBERT A. BRANCH, M.D.

Patients with liver disease are commonly treated with one or more different drugs in an effort to alleviate the numerous pathologic changes often associated with this and/or other concurrent disease processes. Commonly used drugs include diuretics, antibiotics, sedatives, and antiinflammatory, cardiovascular, and cancer chemotherapeutic agents. Of importance are the effects of liver disease on the absorption, distribution, elimination, and pharmacologic response to these drugs. Such changes may require reductions in drug dosage in order to avoid drug toxicity. The understanding of how liver disease can influence drug disposition and dosage requirements entails an appreciation for:

1. The various types of functions that the liver performs;
2. The pathologic changes produced by liver disease and how these changes alter hepatic function; and
3. The parameters that influence drug disposition and how they are affected by liver disease.

LIVER FUNCTION IN HEALTH AND DISEASE: IMPLICATIONS FOR DRUG DISPOSITION

HEPATIC FUNCTION

The liver plays an important role in the metabolism and elimination of drugs that may be too lipophilic to be removed efficiently by the kidneys. This function is carried out by a number of different enzymes located in liver cells. For example, one group of isoenzymes, referred to collectively as the cytochromes P-450, is important for carrying out many of the mixed function oxidative reactions that convert lipophilic compounds into more water-soluble products. Other enzymes in the liver may further transform these metabolites (or other drugs) by conjugating them with sugars, amino acids, sulfates, or acetate to form products that can be more readily eliminated in the bile or removed by the kidney. Still other liver enzymes (i.e., esterases, deaminases, hydrolases, and reductases) are important for the metabolic transformation and elimination of certain drugs and endogenous chemicals.

Many of these homeostatic and metabolic functions are compromised when the liver is damaged by different etiologic agents such as chemicals (including drugs) and diseases. The actual degree of damage to liver hemoperfusion, biliary excretion, and synthetic and metabolic functions in the liver can vary widely and therefore lead to variable changes in drug disposition within each disease entity (62, 102). Such changes in drug disposition reflect, to some extent, the degree to which the liver is impaired. For example, alcoholic liver disease can range from fatty liver, with little or no change in the disposition of most drugs, to severe cirrhosis, with major changes in the disposition of certain classes of drugs. Hepatic neoplasms also show great variability in the effect on drug disposition, depending on type (primary versus secondary), size, invasiveness, and vascularity of tumor mass. Moreover, certain acute injuries to the liver, as seen in viral hepatitis, may affect the disposition of some drugs, but this effect may be reversible as the injury subsides.

Hepatic reserves may help to maintain liver functions, and changes in drug metabolism may be slight since few, if any, liver functions are performed at 100% of their capacity (44). For example, under normal conditions, urea formation from ammonia and amino acids occurs at 60% of capacity. Glucose maintenance requires only 20% of liver function. Bilirubin elimination must fall below 10% of normal before jaundice develops, and albumin and clotting factors are synthesized by only a small percentage of the total liver cells at any one time. Furthermore, these and other liver processes may be increased when demand is increased. As a result, it is often difficult to determine the extent of liver damage caused by an agent because reserve and repair mechanisms tend to maintain hepatic function.

Such reserve and recuperative properties are obviously advantageous for the liver. This regenerative capability allows the liver to recover completely following acute liver insult. Even when the damage is extensive, if the causative agent is removed, the liver is capable of full recovery. However, if the etiologic agent is not removed so that the liver becomes exposed to chronic damage, then hepatic reserves may become seriously depleted. A limited repertoire of liver responses to such chronic damage will result in a characteristic pathophysiologic state of cirrhosis. Under such circumstances, significant changes in drug disposition may occur. The level of cytochrome P-450 enzymes in the liver, for example, may decline (37, 65, 143, 147, 159), and this change can seriously impair the liver's ability to metabolize endogenous products and drugs (32, 56, 112, 159, 160). Deterioration in other liver functions (i.e., the removal of bilirubin and fatty acids and the synthesis of plasma proteins) may lead to further alterations in drug disposition by influencing drug binding and distribution in the body (15, 167, 176).

ARCHITECTURE AND BLOOD FLOW IN CIRRHOSIS

The development of cirrhosis begins with initial hepatocellular damage producing inflammation, followed by phagocytic removal of dead or necrotic cells. This damage stimulates the secretion of collagen by fibroblasts, while the damaged and dead cells are repaired or replaced. As the damage continues, further collagen secretion is coupled with retraction of collagen fibrils. This leads to the formation of bands of connective scar tissue, inducing a deformation of normal architecture characteristic of cirrhosis. In compensation for hepatocellular damage, hepatocyte regeneration may lead to the clustered formation of new hepatocytes, which later form liver nodules. These nodules may increase in size and further distort the normal liver architecture.

As the liver architecture becomes distorted, the resistance to the flow of blood through the liver is increased. This increase, in turn, causes the portal venous pressure to increase. To alleviate an increased pressure, portal venous blood is shunted around the liver through collateral channels directly into the systemic circulation (43). The development of these collateral channels for shunting the portal venous blood occurs primarily where tributaries of the portal venous system lie in close proximity to those of the systemic circulation (i.e., submucosa of the esophagus, stomach, rectum, left renal vein, and abdomen).

The development of collateral channels for the shunting of portal venous blood around the liver can alter the effective hepatic blood flow and the amount of drug reaching the systemic circulation after oral administration (53, 127, 132, 155). These and other changes in drug disposition may require the dosage of some drugs to be reduced.

In addition, recent studies have shown that hepatic disease may also alter the microcirculation of the liver. Sinusoidal plasma in the healthy liver has direct access to the hepatocyte. Although the sinusoid is lined by endothelial cells, this is not a continuous layer; there is an incomplete basal lamina, and endothelial cells contain multiple fenestrations. Between the sinusoidal endothelium and the hepatocyte is the space of Disse, which contains the microvilli of hepatic cells, reticular fibers, and fat storage cells. Alcoholic liver disease is associated with an increase in type III collagen in the space of Disse, formation of a basal lamina, and a decrease in the number of fenestrations and porosity of the endothelial cell as seen with scanning electron microscopy (55, 87, 121, 158). This endothelialization transforms sinusoids into capillary-like channels and limits the access of the contents of sinusoidal blood to the hepatocyte. Studies using multiple indicator dilution techniques support the concept that conversion of loose interendothelial cell junctions to tight endothelial cell junctions may provide a barrier to the movement of molecules into the proximity of the hepatocyte (59–61). This intrahepatic shunting could be of importance in the diffusion of albumin and other large molecules, including protein-bound substances such as drugs, which may result in decreased ability for drug metabolism by the liver.

RENAL FUNCTION

Hemodynamic changes may also be present in the kidneys of patients with liver disease. Renal blood flow has been shown to be decreased in many patients with cirrhosis (137–139). Glomerular filtration rate is variable in cirrhosis, but may be decreased in patients with ascites (76). Moreover, the handling of electrolytes by the kidneys is disturbed in patients with cirrhosis. Renal sodium retention is a well-known phenomenon associated with this disease and contributes to the development of ascites. With progression of liver disease, a number of these factors will further depress kidney function to the point of renal failure (149). It follows that drugs having a major renal route of elimination may have an altered disposition in patients with liver disease, because of the secondary development of functional renal failure.

CHARACTERISTICS OF DRUG DISPOSITION

Whether pathologic changes associated with liver disease require an alteration in a normal drug regimen is determined by the dispositional characteristics of the drug and the biologic determinants of the system (12, 41, 180). Drug disposition, which includes both the distribution and elimination of drug, is determined in part by the physical properties of the drug. Important characteristics include molecular size, charge, pK_a, and lipid solubility. These factors will determine distribution as well as the route of elimination. In general, water-soluble drugs have a small volume of distribution and can be eliminated unchanged in urine, and lipid-soluble drugs have a large volume of distribution and require metabolism to more water-soluble moieties. Depending on the physical characteristics of any given drug, the balance of physiologic factors influencing that drug's disposition will vary. These physiologic factors have the potential to be altered by disease states. Thus, the influence of any one disease process can be complex; it can be mediated by a variety of factors and can influence the disposition of different drugs to a variable extent.

DISTRIBUTION

The major aspects of distribution affected by liver disease are volume of distribution (V_d) and plasma protein binding. Conceptually, the apparent volume of distribution is the volume into which a drug distributes in the body when it is at equilibrium and is related to the pool from which the drug concentration is measured. It is a theoretical concept and reflects the partitioning of drug between the fluid compartments in the body (e.g., plasma, interstitial fluid, and intracellular fluid). It is calculated by the equation:

$$V_d = D/Cp \tag{1}$$

where D represents the fraction of the dose absorbed and Cp is drug concentration at equilibrium. One way that liver disease can affect the V_d is by the production of ascites, which may produce an increase in the body's total fluid compartment. For example, propranolol has been shown to exhibit a 2-fold increase in V_d in patients with ascites, regardless of the extent of protein binding (18).

Most drugs in plasma are reversibly bound to proteins, such as albumin, globulin, α-1-acid glycoprotein, lipoproteins, ceruloplasmin, and transferrin. Acidic drugs commonly bind to albumin, whereas basic drugs more commonly bind to α-1-acid glycoprotein. Only unbound drug is available for distribution into tissues and capable of evoking a pharmacologic response (68, 82, 84, 126, 150). The extent of protein binding is therefore important in determining both pharmacologic response and drug disposition.

Cirrhosis causes a number of alterations that can also influence the binding of drugs within the blood, including (*a*) a decrease in serum albumin levels, (*b*) the appearance of altered or defective plasma proteins, and (*c*) the accumulation of endogenous and exogenous compounds that can displace drugs from protein binding sites. For example, acute viral hepatitis or primary biliary cirrhosis can lead to elevated serum bilirubin levels. The strong affinity of bilirubin for protein binding sites on albumin and the elevated levels are in part responsible for the displacement of some acidic drugs from the protein (15, 167, 182). Taken together, these factors can produce alterations in drug binding to proteins and in the unbound serum drug concentrations. As a result, changes may occur in drug distribution and elimination and pharmacologic response.

With a decrease in drug binding to plasma or blood proteins, more drug may become available for distribution into tissues, increasing the drug's apparent volume of distribution. This change can alter the drug's elimination half-life independently of any change in drug metabolism. The reason for this

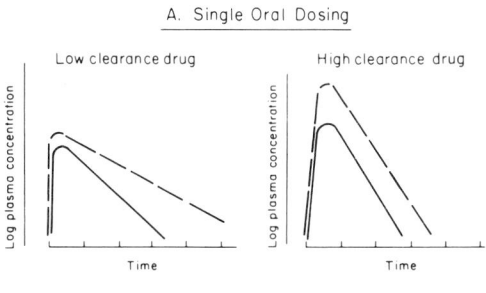

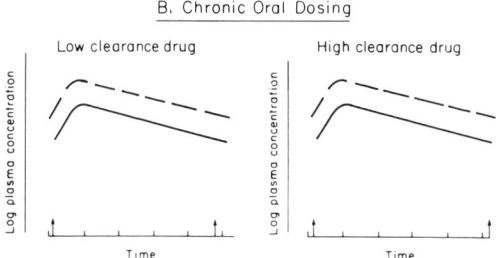

Figure 5.1. The effects of single (**A**) and chronic (**B**) oral dosing on low-clearance (enzyme-limited) and high-clearance (flow-limited) drugs in patients with cirrhosis (*dashed lines*) and in normal subjects (*solid lines*). *Arrows* indicate dosage interval for chronic dosing graphs.

change is apparent from the dependence of the half-life (*t*1/2) on both its total clearance from the blood (*Cl*) and its apparent volume of distribution (*V*d), according to the equation:

$$t1/2 = 0.693 \ V_d/Cl \tag{2}$$

As a result of this dependence, the half-life of a drug can be a misleading parameter when one is attempting to determine the effect(s) of liver disease on drug elimination. For example, an increase in the apparent volume of distribution of a drug may lead to a prolongation in its elimination half-life in the absence of any real change in metabolic drug elimination. An example of this phenomenon is the increase in the half-life of lorazepam (79) in patients with liver disease. This prolongation has been explained entirely by an increase in drug distribution secondary to decreased plasma binding, rather than by a reduction in clearance.

In addition to influencing drug distribution, changes in protein binding can influence drug elimination. A change in the free fraction of a drug in the blood can lead to an increase in the amount of drug available to the drug-metabolizing enzymes and therefore to an increase in the total clearance of some drugs. This increase can shorten the half-life of a drug in the absence of any change in the activity of drug-metabolizing enzymes. Indeed, the decrease in the half-life of tolbutamide (182) in acute viral hepatitis has been attributed solely to a decrease in its binding to plasma proteins, since it has been shown that even though total (free + bound) clearance of tolbutamide increases, protein binding decreases and free clearance remains unchanged.

The effect of protein binding on drug disposition is difficult to predict. At present, there are no guidelines for predicting the effect of liver disease on drug binding. However, two

Table 5.1. Drugs That Should be Used with Caution or Not at All in Liver Disease Patients

Group I: Drugs capable of causing hepatic damage
    Acetaminophen
    Acetylsalicylic acid
    Chlorpromazine
    Erythromycin estolate
    Methotrexate
    Methyldopa
Group II: Drugs that can compromise liver functions
    Anabolic and contraceptive steroids
    Prednisone (in acute viral hepatitis)
    Tetracycline
Group III: Drugs that may make complications of liver disease worse
    Cyclooxygenase inhibitors (indomethacin)
    Diuretics
    Meperidine and other CNS depressants
    Morphine
    Pentazocine
    Phenylbutazone

general rules may provide some insight into the more important factors influencing the extent of change: (*a*) If protein binding is altered by a particular liver disease, the degree of liver damage will influence the extent of change in drug binding to plasma proteins. (*b*) Changes in the extent of binding to plasma proteins will tend to be greater for extensively bound drugs (i.e., >60% bound) than for poorly bound drugs (i.e., <60% bound). Although these are general rules that have their exceptions, they should provide some appreciation for the effects of liver disease on plasma protein binding.

ELIMINATION

Elimination of drug is defined as the irreversible loss of drug from the site of measurement and includes both metabolism and excretion. Clearance is an important parameter that relates drug concentration to the rate of elimination, thereby providing a measure of efficiency of the elimination process. By definition, total or systemic clearance is a measure of the amount of plasma cleared of drug per unit time. This measure can be obtained from measurements of drug concentration in plasma after single doses (Equation 2) or at steady state:

$$Cl = \textit{rate of drug administration}/Cp_{ss} \qquad (3)$$

where Cp_{ss} is the steady-state plasma concentration. Clearance is independent of the mechanism of elimination involved, and if multiple routes of elimination occur concurrently, it provides an estimate of the sum of these processes.

When the rate of elimination is proportional to the amount of drug present, this is known as a first-order process. Clearance of drug is constant (linear) over a range of concentrations. Not all drugs undergo first-order kinetics; however, in some instances dose-dependent elimination occurs. Clearance in these cases is nonlinear and will vary depending on the achieved concentration of drug.

Clearance can also be described as the efficiency of removal of drug across an organ of elimination, the two major organs being liver and kidney. Hepatic clearance, (Cl_H), reflects the efficiency with which the liver irreversibly removes drug from

the blood. It is determined by both the fraction of drug removed or extracted (*E*) from the blood during passage through the liver and the liver blood flow (Q_H). The relationship between these parameters is given by the equation:

$$Cl_H = Q_H E \qquad (4)$$

Drugs that are given orally must first pass through the liver before reaching the systemic circulation. If hepatic enzymes extract drug from the blood as it passes through, then the fraction (*F*) of the total dose entering the general circulation is reduced. For drugs that are completely absorbed from the gastrointestinal tract, this fraction *F* (or bioavailability) is determined from the drug's extraction (*E*) by the liver according to the equation:

$$F = 1 - E \qquad (5)$$

The ability of the liver to extract a drug is, in turn, dependent on three separate factors: (*a*) the intrinsic activity of metabolic enzymes and transport processes within the liver that irreversibly remove drug from the blood, (*b*) the fraction of total drug in blood that is free to interact with enzymes responsible for its elimination, and (*c*) the rate at which drug passes or flows through the liver (129, 144, 179).

The irreversible removal of drug from the blood may be carried out by a number of separate enzymes in the liver. For simplicity, however, the elimination process is often considered as if it results only from a single enzyme system. Thus, metabolic and transport processes responsible for drug removal by the liver, defined as the free intrinsic drug clearance (Cl^u_{int}) can be described by a simple Michaelis-Menten equation as:

$$Cl^u_{int} = V_{max}/(K_m + C^u_L) \qquad (6)$$

where V_{max} represents the maximal rate of irreversible drug elimination by all liver enzymes, K_m is the Michaelis-Menten constant for the overall enzymatic removal process, and C^u_L is the concentration of unbound or free drug in liver.

The second factor that can contribute to the extraction of a drug by the liver is the free fraction of drug in blood (f_B). If the unbound fraction of total drug in the blood changes, then the free drug concentration at the site of elimination will also change. For some drugs, changes in binding can alter hepatic extraction by metabolic and transport enzymes in the liver.

Finally, the total amount of drug extracted by the liver is dependent on the rate at which the drug is delivered to the enzymes responsible for its elimination. This rate of delivery is determined by the liver blood flow (Q_H) perfusing functional hepatocytes. If intrinsic clearance is high, flow becomes the rate-limiting factor, and reductions in flow will not change hepatic extraction but rather will reduce hepatic clearance. If, on the other hand, intrinsic clearance is low, then as flow is decreased, hepatic extraction will increase and hepatic clearance will not be influenced by blood flow.

The relationship of the extraction (*E*) of a drug by the liver with its free intrinsic clearance (Cl^u_{int}), free fraction in the blood (f_B), and the total effective liver blood flow (Q_H) is given by the equation:

$$E = f_B Cl^u_{int}/(Q_H + f_B Cl^u_{int}) \qquad (7)$$

If Equation 7 is now substituted into Equation 4, which defines hepatic clearance, the expression obtained relates hepatic clearance with three variables: f_B, Q_H, and Cl^u_{int}. Thus, hepatic clearance may be written as:

$$Cl_H = Q_H E = Q_H f_B Cl^u_{int}/(Q_H + f_B Cl^u_{int}) \qquad (8)$$

Although these relationships may appear complex, it is important to recognize that hepatic clearance is determined by only these three physiologic variables, each of which can be changed independently by liver disease. The effect on drug disposition of any one of these variables can be anticipated by knowing the relative importance of each of these variables to that drug's disposition. This concept has been used to provide a framework for the classification of drugs into a system in which those drugs sharing a rate-limiting characteristic are grouped together.

DRUGS CLASSIFIED BY DISPOSITIONAL CHARACTERISTICS

Flow-limited Drugs

When the total intrinsic clearance $(f_B Cl^u_{int})$ of a drug is large relative to liver blood flow (Q_H), such that $E > 0.6$, hepatic clearance of the drug becomes dependent on liver blood flow (Equation 8). The rate at which the liver is able to remove these drugs from the blood is limited by their rate of presentation to the liver. Theoretically, metabolism and protein binding should not affect hepatic clearance of these drugs. Accordingly, this class of drugs is referred to as blood flow-limited and is sensitive to factors that can alter the effective liver blood flow. It should be noted that if the disease process reduces the intrinsic clearance so that it is less than the liver blood flow, the drug will lose its flow-sensitive characteristics.

Enzyme-limited Drugs

When the total intrinsic clearance of a drug is small relative to liver blood flow, such that $E < 0.2$, hepatic clearance becomes essentially dependent on the intrinsic activity of liver enzymes (Equation 8). Factors that influence the ability of the liver enzymes to remove drug become more important in altering drug elimination than changes in liver blood flow. Drugs with this characteristic belong to the class referred to as enzyme-limited. This class is further subdivided according to the extent of protein binding.

Enzyme-limited, Binding-insensitive Drugs. For enzyme-limited drugs with low binding to plasma or blood proteins (i.e., <50% bound), a change in plasma protein binding is not an important factor in altering hepatic drug elimination (Equation 8). This drug class is most affected by factors that change the level or activity of liver enzymes (Cl^u_{int}) responsible for their elimination. Drugs with these characteristics are referred to as enzyme-limited and binding-insensitive.

Enzyme-limited, Binding-sensitive Drugs. For enzyme-limited drugs that are extensively bound to plasma or blood proteins (i.e., >85% bound), hepatic clearance is sensitive to changes in protein binding in the blood (f_B) and/or liver enzyme activity (Cl^u_{int}). Drugs with these characteristics are referred to as enzyme-limited and binding-sensitive. Factors that may alter binding to proteins in the blood or the activity of liver enzymes responsible for drug elimination influence the hepatic clearance of these drugs.

Flow/Enzyme-sensitive Drugs

A drug may not be extensively bound or poorly extracted by the liver, but fall somewhere between the flow-limited and enzyme-limited classes. The clearance of these drugs from the blood may be sensitive to changes in liver blood flow, intrinsic clearance by the liver, and, in some cases, binding to plasma proteins (Equation 8). Drugs with these characteristics are referred to as flow- and enzyme-sensitive.

Drugs are classified according to this scheme to help provide a better appreciation of the importance of pathophysiologic changes produced by liver disease in altering drug disposition. Certain biologic determinants of metabolism (i.e., disease or genetic predisposition) may change the classification of a given drug for an individual.

It is now known that some people have genetic defects in the metabolism of certain drugs. Fast and slow acetylators of isoniazid have been recognized since the 1950s. More recently, independent genetic polymorphisms have been found for a number of other drugs metabolized by different oxidative enzymes. Poor and extensive metabolizers of debrisoquine, an antihypertensive agent (154), and mephenytoin, an anticonvulsant, are representative examples of two independent routes of oxidative metabolism mediated by cytochrome P-450 $2D_6$ and cytochrome P-450 $2C_{MP}$, respectively. Not only will the effect of liver disease have a greater effect on the clearance of this drug in extensive metabolizers than in poor metabolizers, but the effect of factors such as development of portal-systemic shunts will have a marked influence on systemic availability in extensive but not in poor metabolizer subjects.

INFLUENCE OF LIVER DISEASE ON DRUG DISPOSITION

As mentioned previously, both dispositional characteristics of a drug and biologic determinants of the system involved are important in determining the effects of liver disease on ultimate drug disposition. In the following sections, the effects of liver disease on each of these factors are discussed.

ROUTE OF ELIMINATION

Since there are multiple routes of elimination, only some of which involve the liver, it is important to determine which route is utilized for a given drug. For a drug that is excreted unchanged by the kidney, liver disease should have no effect on disposition, provided that there is no secondary or concomitant renal disease.

There is a strong relationship between the proportion of the drug that is eliminated following oxidative metabolism by the liver and the percentage of decrease in its free clearance caused by cirrhosis. Thus, liver disease has the greatest effect on those drugs that undergo extensive oxidative metabolism.

Table 5.2. The Dispositional Characteristics in Normal Subjects and in Patients with Liver Disease, Routes of Elimination, and Recommendations for Dose Adjustment for a Variety of Drugs[a]

Drug	Protein Binding (%)	Volume of Distribution (V_d) (liter/kg)	Half-life ($t_{1/2}$) (hr)	Clearance (Cl) (ml/min)	Class	Hepatic/Renal Elimination	Effect of Liver Disease on Drug Disposition	Adjustment of Dose	References
Antibiotic/Antiviral/Antifungal									
Amantadine	—	4.75	20.0	190	—	<10% Hepatic >90% Renal	Negligible unless renal function decreased	None	
Amikacin	5	0.26	2.5	85	—	<5% Hepatic >95% Renal	Negligible unless renal function decreased	None	
Ampicillin	30	0.28	1.0	340	—	<10% Hepatic >90% Renal	$t_{1/2}$ ↑; V_d ↑; Cl →; f_p ? →	None	83
Aztreonam	56	0.15	1.9	70	—	33% Hepatobiliary 66% Renal	$t_{1/2}$ ↑; V_d →; Cl →	Decrease if chronic, high-dosing	86
Carbenicillin	48	0.16	1.0	130	—	<10% Hepatic >90% Renal	Negligible unless renal function decreased	None	52
Cefaclor	24	0.35	1.0	280	—	<10% Hepatic >90% Renal	Negligible unless renal function decreased	None	
Cefamandole	74	0.16	1.0	130	—	<5% Hepatic >95% Renal	Negligible unless renal function decreased	None	
Cefazolin	84	0.15	1.8	68	—	<5% Hepatic >95% Renal	$t_{1/2}$ ↑; f_p ↑	None	113
Cefoperazone	90 nonlinear	0.20	1.7	80	Enzyme-limited, binding-sensitive	75% Hepatic 25% Renal	$t_{1/2}$ ↑; V_d →; Cl ↓ 60%; f_p ?	Decrease dose	16, 17
Cefotaxime	36	0.24	1.2	94	—	40% Hepatic 60% Renal	$t_{1/2}$ ↑; V_d ?; Cl ?	Unknown	98
Cefotetan	83	0.15	3.7	39.5	—	80% Renal 20% Biliary (unchanged)	Negligible unless renal function decreased	None	
Cefoxitin	73	0.12	1.0	98	—	15% Hepatic 85% Renal	Negligible unless renal function decreased	None	
Ceftazidime	17	0.2	1.7	75	—	10% Hepatic 90% Renal	$t_{1/2}$ ↑; V_d ?; Cl slight ↓	Negligible unless renal function decreased	123
Ceftriaxone	90	0.14	8.4	16	Enzyme-limited, binding-sensitive	60% Hepatobiliary 40% Renal	$t_{1/2}$ →; V_d ↑ if ascites present; Cl →; f_p ↑	None	162
Cefuroxime	30	0.33	1.2	210	—	<1% Hepatic >99% Renal	Negligible unless renal function decreased	None	117
Cephalothin	75	0.30	0.60	470	—	30–50% Hepatic 50–70% Renal	$t_{1/2}$ slight ↑; V_d →; Cl ↓	None	113
Chloramphenicol	70	1.0	3.0	170	Enzyme-limited, binding-sensitive	>90% Hepatic <10% Renal Glucuronidation of drug	$t_{1/2}$ ↑; V_d slight ↓; Cl ↓ 65%; f_p ? →; unknown if f_p changes	Decrease dose	101
Ciprofloxacin	30	2.3	4.0	350	—	40% Renal (unchanged) 15% Hepatic	Negligible unless renal function decreased	None	145, 97
Clindamycin	79	0.58	2.0	160	Enzyme-limited, binding-sensitive	90% Hepatic 10% Renal	$t_{1/2}$ slight ↑; V_d →; Cl ↓ 23%; f_p →	Decrease dose in severe cases	10, 51

Drug				Type	% Elimination	Pharmacokinetic changes	Dose adjustment	Ref.
Doxycycline	82	—	12.0	195	—	<10% Hepatic >90% Renal	Negligible unless renal function decreased	None	
Erythromycin	80	0.77	1.6	600	Enzyme-limited, binding-sensitive	>90% Hepatic <10% Renal	$t_{1/2}$ ↑; no other information	Decrease dose in moderate or severe disease	48, 81
Fluconazole	12	0.8	35	20	—	70% Renal (unchanged) 10% Hepatic	Negligible unless renal function decreased	None	63
Ganciclovir	2	0.5	3.0	185/1.73m²		>90% Renal (unchanged)	Negligible unless renal function decreased	None	
Gentamicin	<5	0.25	2.0	100		<5% Hepatic >95% Renal	Negligible unless renal function decreased	None	
Imipenem	25	0.33	1.1	186		70% Renal (unchanged) 25% Nonspecific hydrolysis	Negligible unless renal function decreased	None	
Isoniazid	<10	0.6	2.0 fast 6.0 slow	480 fast 170 slow	Enzyme-limited, binding-insensitive	85% Hepatic 15% Renal Drug acetylated	$t_{1/2}$ ↑; some assume Cl ↓; genetic differences more important than disease	Decrease dose in severe cases	3
Kanamycin	<10	0.20	3.0	55	—	<5% Hepatic >95% Renal	Negligible unless renal function decreased	None	
Metronidazole	10	0.75	8.0	85	—	>90% Hepatic <10% Renal	$t_{1/2}$ ↑; V_d ↓; Cl ↓	Decrease dose	29, 35
Nafcillin	90	0.4	1.0	580	Enzyme-limited, binding-sensitive	70% Hepatic 30% Renal	$t_{1/2}$ ↑ but little change; V_d ↓; Cl ↓ 50–60%; fp ? →	Decrease dose in moderate or severe disease	90
Neomycin	40	—	2.0	—		<5% Hepatic >95% Renal	Negligible unless renal function decreased	None	
Rifampin	85	0.4	2.5	180	Enzyme-limited, binding-sensitive	90% Hepatic 10% Renal	$t_{1/2}$ ↑; V_d ?; Cl ↓; f_p ?	Decrease in severe disease	72, 134
Streptomycin	35	0.26	2.5	85		<5% Hepatic >95% Renal	Negligible unless renal function decreased	None	
Sulfamethoxazole	66	0.17	9.0	15	Enzyme-limited, binding-sensitive	70% Hepatic 30% Renal Drug acetylated	Unknown, but probably little change unless there is severe liver disease	Slight decrease	
Tobramycin	<5	0.24	2.5	80		<5% Hepatic >95% Renal	Negligible unless renal function decreased	None	
Trimethoprim	45	1.5	12.0	96		30% Hepatic 70% Renal	Slight unless renal function decreased	None	
Vancomycin	55	0.4	5.0	80		<10% Hepatic >90% Renal	$t_{1/2}$ ↑; V_d →; Cl ↓	Decrease dose	21
Zidovudine	36	1.6	1.1	1900	Flow-limited	14% Renal (unchanged) 74% Hepatic	$t_{1/2}$, Cl, V_d	Decrease dose	165
Analgesic									
Acetaminophen	20	0.9	2.2	350	Flow/enzyme-sensitive	>95% Hepatic <5% Renal Mostly conjugated	$t_{1/2}$ ↑; V_d ?; Cl ↓ 54%; assume f_p →; little change in Cl if albumin >3.5 g/100 ml	Avoid chronic use; single dose—no change	9, 39, 153

Table 5.2. *Continued*

Drug	Protein Binding (%)	Volume of Distribution (V_d) (liter/kg)	Half-life ($t_{1/2}$) (hr)	Clearance (Cl) (ml/min)	Class	Hepatic/Renal Elimination	Effect of Liver Disease on Drug Disposition	Adjustment of Dose	References
Meperidine	65	4.5	4.5	900	Flow/enzyme-sensitive	>95% Hepatic <5% Renal	$t_{1/2}$↑; V_d →; Cl ↓ 50%; f_p →	Decrease oral dose by 50% in cirrhosis or acute viral hepatitis	105, 133
Methadone	80	4.0	28	150	Enzyme-limited, binding-sensitive	80% Hepatic 20% Renal	$t_{1/2}$↑ with severe liver disease; Cl →; V_d ↑ slightly	None or decrease	107, 108
Morphine	35	3.7	2.0	1200	Flow-limited	90% GI tract and liver, 10% renal Extensive glucuronidation	$t_{1/2}$→; V_d →; Cl →; f_p →, by some reports f_p ↑	None, but avoid in severe liver disease	119, 124, 125
Pentazocine	65	5.4	4.5	1000	Flow-limited	>95% Hepatic <5% Renal	$t_{1/2}$↑; V_d →; Cl ↓ 50%	Decrease oral dose by ⅔	105, 132
Propoxyphene	75	16	12	1200	Flow-limited	>95% GI tract and liver; <2% renal	$t_{1/2}$↑ slightly; V_d ?; Cl ↓ 25%; f_p →	Decrease oral dose by 50%	42
Anticancer									
Adriamycin	50	2.5	20	100	Enzyme-limited, binding-insensitive	>95% Hepatic <5% Renal Most biliary Active metabolite	$t_{1/2}$↑; V_d ?; Cl ?; f_p ?, assume f_p →	Unknown	13
Bleomycin	0	0.3	2.0	120	—	40% Hepatic 60% Renal	Unknown; probably not altered greatly	None ? Perhaps decrease	
Cyclophosphamide	14	0.6	5.0	120	Enzyme-limited, binding-insensitive	90% Hepatic 10% Renal Active metabolite	$t_{1/2}$↑; V_d ?→; Cl ↓ 43%; f_p ?→	Unknown	70, 175
Cytosine arabinoside	13	2.5	2.5	800	—	Extensive extrahepatic elimination; 40% renal	No data; probably little effect	None	
Etoposide	—	.28	5.6	39	—	65% Hepatic 35% Renal	$t_{1/2}$→; V_d →; Cl →	None	31, 49
5-Fluorouracil	—	0.5	0.1	—	Flow-limited	Hepatic and extrahepatic; <5% Renal	Some decrease in clearance expected	Probable slight decrease	
Methotrexate	50	0.5	9.0	80	—	15% Hepatic; mostly biliary; 85% Renal	No data; probably little effect. Drug is hepatotoxic and should be avoided if possible.	None	

Drug	% Bound				Classification	% Hepatic / % Renal	Effect of liver disease	Dose adjustment	References
Antiepileptic									
Carbamazepine	75	1.1	18.0 induced	—	Enzyme-limited, binding-sensitive	>98% Hepatic, <2% Renal	No data; expect a decrease in clearance and increase in $t_{1/2}$	Probably decrease dose	15, 119
Diphenylhydantoin	92	0.65	15.0 nonlinear	40	Enzyme-limited, binding-sensitive	>95% Hepatic, <5% Renal	AVH $t_{1/2} \to$; $Cl \to$; $f_p \uparrow$. Cirrhosis $f_p \uparrow$	Decrease dose in moderate to severe liver disease	7
Phenobarbital	50	0.8	100	8	Enzyme-limited, binding-insensitive	75% Hepatic, 25% Renal	$t_{1/2} \uparrow$; presumed $Cl \downarrow$	Decrease with severe liver disease	
Valproic acid	89 nonlinear	12	0.14	30	Enzyme-limited, binding-sensitive	>98% Hepatic, <25% Renal	$t_{1/2} \uparrow$; V_d slightly $\uparrow$; $Cl \downarrow$ 40%; $f_p \uparrow$	Decrease dose	88
Antipyretic/ Antiinflammatory									
Antipyrine	<10	0.58	12	50	Enzyme-limited, binding-insensitive	92% Hepatic, 8% Renal	$t_{1/2} \uparrow$; $V_d \uparrow$ or $\to$; $Cl \downarrow$ 60% or more, but actual decrease in Cl depends on disease	Not used clinically	23, 34, 54, 64, 80, 93, 96, 100, 130, 157, 159, 166
Dexamethasone	68	0.75	3.25	260	Flow/enzyme-sensitive	>97% Hepatic, <3% Renal	$f_p \downarrow$; $V_d \to$; $t_{1/2} \uparrow$; $Cl \downarrow$	Decrease dose	71
Fenprofen	>99	0.10	1.5	200	Enzyme-limited, binding-sensitive	>98% Hepatic, <2% Renal	No data; would expect $f_p \uparrow$; $Cl \uparrow$ or $\to$	Decrease dose	
Ibuprofen	>99	0.15 V area F	2.0	52	Enzyme-limited, binding-sensitive	>99% Hepatic, <1% Renal	$t_{1/2}$ slightly $\uparrow$ in severe LD; V_d ?; Cl ?	Decrease in severe liver disease if high doses	69
Indomethacin	90	0.17	8.0	125	Enzyme-limited, binding-sensitive	>98% Hepatic, <2% Renal	$t_{1/2} \uparrow$; no other information. Assume $Cl \downarrow$, $f_p \uparrow$	Decrease dose as required	50
Naproxen	99.6	0.10	14.0	5	Enzyme-limited, binding-sensitive	>90% Hepatic, <10% Renal	$t_{1/2} \uparrow$; $V_d \to$; $Cl \downarrow$ 28%; f_p ?	Decrease dose in moderate to severe disease	24, 184
Phenylbutazone	98.5	0.17	70	2	Enzyme-limited, binding-sensitive	>99% Hepatic, <1% Renal	$t_{1/2} \uparrow$ or $\to$; $f_p \uparrow$; V_d ?; Cl ? Assume $Cl \downarrow$ with liver disease	Decrease dose	20
Prednisolone	80	0.6	3.0	180	Enzyme-limited, binding-sensitive	>85% Hepatic, <15% Renal	$t_{1/2} \to$; $V_d \to$; $Cl \to$; $f_p \to$ or $\uparrow$. Drug little affected by liver disease.	None	71, 171
Salicylic acid	80–95 dose dependent	0.17 dose dependent	2.4–19	13 in therapeutic range	—	2–30% Renal; dose dependent	$t_{1/2} \to$; $V_d \to$; Cl ?; $f_p \uparrow$	None	141
Sulfinpyrazone	99	0.06	6.0	23	Enzyme-limited, binding-sensitive	65% Hepatic, 35% Renal	No data; would expect some decrease in Cl with liver disease	Slight decrease in dose	
Cardiovascular									
Atenolol	<5	0.55	6.5	55–130	—	10% Hepatic, 90% Renal	$t_{1/2} \to$; $V_d \to$; $Cl \to$	None	74
Captopril	27	0.7	1.9	13.3/kg	—	50% Hepatic, 40% Renal	Negligible unless renal function decreased	None	
Digitoxin	95	0.60	180	2.5	Enzyme-limited, binding-sensitive	70% Hepatic, 30% Renal	$t_{1/2} \to$ or $\downarrow$; $Cl \uparrow$ or $\to$; $f_p \uparrow$	None	73, 109

Table 5.2. *Continued*

Drug	Protein Binding (%)	Volume of Distribution (V_d) (liter/kg)	Half-life $(t_{1/2})$ (hr)	Clearance (Cl) (ml/min)	Class	Hepatic/Renal Elimination	Effect of Liver Disease on Drug Disposition	Adjustment of Dose	References
Digoxin	30	6.0	35	150	—	30% Heaptic 70% Renal	Appears negligible	None	88
Disopyramide	80 non-linear	1.0	8	100	—	45% Hepatic 55% Renal	No data; would not expect a tremendous change in liver disease	Probably slight decrease	—
Enalapril	50	1.0	4.0	125	Flow/enzyme-sensitive	Rapidly hydrolyzed to active enalaprilat in the liver, 60% excreted in the urine	$t_{1/2}$ enalaprilat C_{max} enalaprilat	None	11, 115
Esmolol	55	1.2	0.15	310/kg	—	80% Renal (rapidly hydrolyzed to inactive product in blood)	Negligible	None	22
Isradipine	95	3.0	8.0	1400	Flow-limited	<90% Hepatic >95% Hepatic <5% Renal	Cl, C_{max}, AUC, $t_{1/2}$, V_d $t_{1/2} \rightarrow$; $V_d \downarrow$; $Cl \rightarrow$ or $\downarrow$; f_p ?; assume $\uparrow$	Decrease dose Decrease oral dose; decrease i.v. dose to much smaller extent	1, 28 53
Labetalol	50	11.5	3.0	1600	Flow-limited				
Lidocaine	65 non-linear	1.1	2.0	1000	Flow-limited	97% Hepatic 3% Renal	$t_{1/2} \uparrow$; $V_d \uparrow$ or $\rightarrow$; $Cl \downarrow \sim 50\%$; f_p ? Low therapeutic ratio. Decrease in Cl depends on severity of disease	Decrease dose by 50% in severe liver disease	4, 39, 58, 168–170, 181
Lisinopril	<10	1.8	12	106	—	3% Hepatic 97% Unchanged 70% Fecal 30% Renal	Negligible unless renal function decreased	None	
Lorcainide	70	12.9	8.0	1700	Flow-limited	98% Hepatic 2% Renal	$t_{1/2} \uparrow$; $V_d \rightarrow$; $Cl \downarrow$ 29%; $f_p \uparrow$ slightly. Cl_{int} exhibits a very large decrease	Decrease dose	78
Metoprolol	10	3.2	4.0	800	Flow-limited	95% Hepatic 5% Renal	$t_{1/2} \uparrow$; $V_d \uparrow$ slightly; $Cl \downarrow$ 23%; f_p ?	Decrease dose slightly	135
N-Acetyl procainamide	10	1.4	8.0	210	—	20% Hepatic 80% Renal	No data; expect little change unless renal function altered assumed unaffected	None	
Nifedipine	98	1.0	3.0	600	Flow-limited, binding-sensitive	100% Hepatic	$t_{1/2} \uparrow$; $V_d \rightarrow$; $Cl \downarrow$; f_p	Decrease dose	75

Drug									Ref.
Pindolol	57	6.2	3.5	300	Enzyme-limited, binding-insensitive	70% Hepatic 30% Renal	Not affected by AVH. Cirrhosis Cl ↓ slightly and renal excretion of drug is increased	Some decrease in severe liver disease	114
Prazosin	97	1.3	3.0	450	Flow-limited	95% Hepatic 5% Renal	No data—would expect $t_{1/2}$ ↑; Cl ↓; f_p ↑	Decrease dose	33
Procainamide	15	2.2	3.0	600	—	45% Hepatic 55% Renal Drug acetylated	$t_{1/2}$ ↑; V_d ?; Cl ? probably decreased slightly	Some minor decrease in dose	
Propranolol	95	4.0	4.0	850	Flow-limited	>95% Hepatic <5% Renal	$t_{1/2}$ ↑; V_d ↑; Cl ~ 60%; f_p ↑.	Decrease dose depending on extent of damage	19, 129, 185
Quinidine	85	3.0	6.0	330	Flow/enzyme-sensitive	80% Hepatic 20% Renal	Tremendous decrease in Cl_{int}. Flow/enzyme-limited in cirrhosis $t_{1/2}$ ↑; V_d ↑; Cl →; f_p ↑; Cl_{int} decreased significantly	Decrease dose	5, 128
Tocainide	10	3.0	13	150	Enzyme-limited	60% Hepatic 40% Renal	$t_{1/2}$ ↑; V_d ?; Cl ↓	Decrease dose	120
Verapamil	92	6.7	3.5	1570	Flow-limited	95% Hepatic 5% Renal	$t_{1/2}$ ↑; V_d ↑; Cl ↓ 60%; f_p →; Cl_{int} decreases even more than 60%	Decrease dose by 50% in severe liver disease	155, 186
Diuretic									
Bumetanide	?	9.45	1.0	129		36% Hepatic 64% Renal	$t_{1/2}$ ↑; V_d ↓; Cl ↓	Minor decrease in dose	89
Furosemide	95	0.15	1.0	170		35% Hepatic 65% Renal	$t_{1/2}$ ↑ or →; V_d ↑ or →; Cl →; f_p ↑; the change in f_p compensates for decrease in Cl_{int} of liver	None or slight decrease in severe cases	40, 172, 174
Hydrochloro-thiazide	95	1.5	2.5	480		<10% Hepatic >90% Renal	No data; probably little affected unless renal function altered	None	
Spirono-lactone	98	—	20	—	Enzyme-limited, binding-sensitive, and extrahepatic metabolism	>85% Hepatic <15% Renal	No apparent change in drug disposition with liver disease; $t_{1/2}$ →	None	2, 146
Triamterene	50	2.5	2.0	1000	Flow-limited	95% Hepatic 5% Renal	Cl ↓; f_p →; expect $t_{1/2}$ ↑	Decrease dose	173
Sedative/Hypnotic									
Amylobarbital	60	1.2	21	35	Enzyme-limited, binding-insensitive	>95% Hepatic <5% Renal	$t_{1/2}$ ↑; V_d →; Cl ↓ 55%; f_p ↑. Little change if albumin >3.5 g/100 ml	Decrease dose	91
Chlordiaze-poxide	96	0.3	12 age-dependent	20	Enzyme-limited, binding-sensitive	>99% Hepatic <1% Renal	$t_{1/2}$ ↑; V_d ↑; Cl ↓ 60%; f_p ↑. Both AVH and cirrhosis affect drug	Decrease dose	141, 142

Table 5.2. *Continued*

Drug	Protein Binding (%)	Volume of Distribution (V_d) (liter/kg)	Half-life ($t_{1/2}$) (hr)	Clearance (Cl) (ml/min)	Class	Hepatic/Renal Elimination	Effect of Liver Disease on Drug Disposition	Adjustment of Dose	References
Diazepam	99	1.2	45	28	Enzyme-limited, binding-sensitive	>97% Hepatic <3% Renal	$t_{1/2}\uparrow$; $V_d\uparrow$; $Cl\downarrow$ 50%; $f_p\uparrow$. AVH and cirrhosis increase $t_{1/2}$. Large therapeutic index—safe	Single dose, no change; chronic, decrease dose	77, 92, 110
Flumazenil	40	0.85	0.8	1201	Flow-limited	>90% Hepatic	$t_{1/2}$, Cl, V_d	? Decrease dose	66
Hexobarbital	47	1.2	6.0	232	Enzyme-limited, binding-insensitive	>99% Hepatic <1% Renal	$t_{1/2}\uparrow$; $V_d\rightarrow$; $Cl\downarrow$ 62% (Cl decreased in AVH and cirrhosis, $Cl\rightarrow$ in cholestasis); $f_p\rightarrow$	Decrease during chronic dosing	136
Lorazepam	90	1.3	12.0	53	Enzyme-limited, binding-sensitive	>98% Hepatic <2% Renal Extensive glucuronidation	$t_{1/2}\uparrow$; $V_d\uparrow$; $Cl\rightarrow$; $f_p\uparrow$. Neither AVH nor cirrhosis affects drug dosing	None	79
Methohexital	—	61	2.0	829	Flow/enzyme-sensitive	>90% Hepatic <10% Renal	No data; assume $Cl\downarrow$, $t_{1/2}\uparrow$	Probably decrease dose	
Midazolam	—	1.3	1.6	624	Flow-limited	>95% Hepatic <5% Renal	$t_{1/2}\uparrow$; V_d slightly $\uparrow$; $Cl\downarrow$	Decrease dose	6, 85
Nitrazepam	87	1.9	26	63	Enzyme-limited	>99% Hepatic <1% Renal Mainly nitro-reduction	$t_{1/2}\rightarrow$; $V_d\rightarrow$; $Cl\rightarrow$; $f_p\uparrow$	None	67
Oxazepam	90	1.6	6.0	140	Enzyme-limited, binding-sensitive	>99% Hepatic <1% Renal Extensive glucuronidation	$t_{1/2}\rightarrow$; $V_d\rightarrow$; $Cl\rightarrow$; $f_p\rightarrow$. Neither AVH nor cirrhosis alters disposition significantly	None	152
Pentobarbital	65	1.0	30	30	Enzyme-limited, binding-sensitive	99% Hepatic <1% Renal	No data; expect $Cl\downarrow$, $t_{1/2}\uparrow$	Single dose, no change; chronic, lower dose	148
Primidone	19	0.86	17	41	—	60% Hepatic 40% Renal (in children)	$t_{1/2}\rightarrow$; V_d slight $\uparrow$; Cl slight $\uparrow$ in hepatitis	None	131
Temazepam	98	1.2	14	80	—	>98% Hepatic <2% Renal Mainly glucuronidation	$t_{1/2}\rightarrow$; $V_d\rightarrow$; $Cl\rightarrow$; $f_p\rightarrow$	None	111
Others									
Alfentanil	90	0.28	1.5	200	Flow/enzyme-sensitive	99% Hepatic 1% Renal	$t_{1/2}\uparrow$; $V_d\rightarrow$; $Cl\downarrow$; $f_p\uparrow$ (dose-dependent)	Decrease dose	38
Atracurium	—	0.16	0.33	385	—	Hofmann elimination; auto-metabolism	$t_{1/2}\rightarrow$; $V_d\uparrow$; $Cl\rightarrow$; long $t_{1/2}$ of metabolite	Decrease dose if long-term use	177

Drug									
Caffeine	31	0.54	6.0	63	Enzyme-limited, binding-insensitive	95% Hepatic, 5% Renal	$t_{1/2} \uparrow$ slightly; $V_d \to$; $Cl \downarrow 40\%$; $f_p \uparrow$; large therapeutic ratio	None	30
Chlormethiazole	64	0.12	7.0	1100	Flow-limited; vitamin B substitute	>99% Hepatic, <1% Renal	$t_{1/2} \uparrow$; $V_d \to$; $Cl \downarrow 28\%$; $f_p \uparrow$	Probably not necessary	127
Cimetidine	20	1.1	2.3	550	—	40% Hepatic, 60% Renal	$t_{1/2} \to$; $V_d \uparrow$ or $\downarrow$ or $\to$; $Cl \to$ or $\downarrow$; f_p changes assumed unimportant. Drug associated with increased incidence of mental confusion in cirrhotics	Decrease dose in severe liver disease	26, 45, 106
Clofibrate (CPIB)	95	0.15	18.0	8	Enzyme-limited, binding-sensitive	90% Hepatic, <10% Renal Glucuronidation of metabolite	$t_{1/2} \to$; $V_d \uparrow$ slightly; $Cl \to$; $f_p \uparrow$. AVH does not alter Cl; cirrhosis does have an effect on $Cl_{int} \downarrow 50\%$	Decrease dose in cirrhosis by 50%	46
Diphenhydramine	78	6.5	9.5	696	Flow-limited	>98% Hepatic, <2% Renal	$t_{1/2} \uparrow$; $V_d \to$; free $Cl \downarrow$; total $Cl \to$; $f_p \uparrow$	Decrease dose	94
Doxacurium	30	0.22	1.5	190	—	>90% Renal	Negligible unless renal function decreased	None	27
Famotidine	17	1.1	3.3	430	—	70% Renal (unchanged), 30% Hepatic	Negligible unless renal function decreased	None	116
Fentanyl	80	3.5	4.0	750	—	92% Hepatic, 8% Renal	$t_{1/2} \to$; $V_d \to$; $Cl \to$	None	47
Omeprazole	95	0.35	0.75	550	Flow-limited	>90% Hepatic	$t_{1/2}$ Cl, $V_d \to$; $Cl \to$	None	140
Ranitidine	15	1.5	2.3	600	—	30% Hepatic, 70% Renal	$t_{1/2} \to$; $V_d \to$ or $\downarrow$	None	99, 118
Sulfisoxazole	92	0.15	6.6	20	Enzyme-limited, binding-sensitive	50% Hepatic, 50% Renal Acetylation	$t_{1/2} \to$; $V_d \uparrow$; $Cl \uparrow$; $f_p \uparrow$	None	25
Theophylline	52	0.5	8.0	45	Enzyme-limited, binding-sensitive	91% Hepatic, 9% Renal	$t_{1/2} \uparrow$; $V_d \to$ cirrhosis, $\uparrow$ hepatitis and cholestasis; $Cl \downarrow 55\%$; $f_p \uparrow$. Low therapeutic index caution	Decrease dose by 50%	161
Thiopental	85	2.3	9.0	275	Enzyme-limited	>99% Hepatic, <1% Renal	$t_{1/2} \to$; $V_d \to$; $Cl \to$; $f_p \uparrow$	Uncertain; may need to decrease dose	122
Tolbutamide	98	0.15	5.0	20.0	Enzyme-limited, binding-sensitive	95% Hepatic, 5% Renal	$t_{1/2}$ slightly $\uparrow$ or $\to$; $V_d \to$; $Cl \uparrow$; $f_p \uparrow$. AVH has been reported to increase rate of elimination	None; probably not used in liver disease	167, 182
Warfarin	99	0.20	23	8.0	Enzyme-limited, binding-sensitive	99% Hepatic, 1% Renal	$t_{1/2} \to$; $V_d \to$; $Cl \to$; $f_p \to$ AVH no effect, but may be related to extent of liver damage	None; probably not used in liver disease	181

^a GI, gastrointestinal; AVH, acute viral hepatitis; LD, liver disease.

ROUTE OF METABOLISM

For drugs that are metabolized by the liver, the route of metabolism is also important in determining the effects of liver disease on drug disposition. All metabolic pathways are not affected equally by liver disease. For example, the elimination of lorazepam, morphine, and oxazepam, which are metabolized primarily by conjugation with glucuronic acid, is generally unaltered by liver disease, except in decompensated liver disease (57, 79, 124, 152, 156). The reason for this is unknown. It may reflect the sparing of conjugative pathways of drug metabolism in the liver during liver disease, and/or the importance of other organs to the elimination of drugs by this route. This preservation contrasts with reductions in clearance of drugs that are eliminated by oxidative metabolism.

ROUTES AND DURATION OF DRUG ADMINISTRATION

The effect of liver disease on drug disposition is determined by (a) the route of drug administration, (b) the class to which the drug belongs (i.e., flow-limited, flow/enzyme-sensitive, or enzyme-limited), and (c) duration of drug administration.

As noted previously, drugs that are taken orally, unlike those administered intravenously or intramuscularly, pass through the liver before reaching the systemic circulation and target tissues. This provides an opportunity for presystemic elimination, particularly for flow-limited drugs, with their high hepatic extractions, which normally have a low bioavailability. For flow-limited drugs, liver disease may increase their bioavailability. This increased bioavailability is partially explained by a decrease in the efficiency of drug extraction by liver enzymes. Another important factor contributing to this increase is the rerouting of blood from the portal vein through intrahepatic and extrahepatic portal-systemic shunts in response to portal hypertension caused by liver disease. In severely cirrhotic patients, this shunting may involve 60% or more of portal venous blood flow (46, 163, 164). This shunting allows a large amount of an orally administered drug to bypass the liver altogether and enter the systemic circulation directly. As a result of the changes in bioavailability of flow-limited drugs, peak blood concentrations following single oral dose administration are substantially higher in patients with cirrhosis than in normal subjects (Fig. 5.1). In contrast, the bioavailability of enzyme-limited drugs is high in normal subjects and remains unaffected in liver disease. Thus, peak concentrations following single oral dose administration are the same in cirrhotic and normal subjects (Fig. 5.1).

The case is somewhat different for chronic oral therapy: drug blood levels accumulate to an approximately steady-state situation that is dependent on drug clearance, the fraction of the dose that reaches the systemic circulation, and the dosage interval (Equation 3). Reductions in clearance resulting from liver disease create the potential for excessive drug accumulation during chronic therapy for both flow-limited and enzyme-limited drugs (Fig. 5.1). This may require dosage reduction in order to obtain the desired therapeutic objective.

In summary, the influence of liver disease on drug disposition is a function of how a drug is handled in healthy subjects. For flow-limited drugs, initial blood concentrations following intravenous or intramuscular administration can be expected to be similar in cirrhotic and normal subjects, whereas peak blood concentrations are higher in cirrhotic patients after single oral dose administration or at steady state during chronic therapy. In contrast, enzyme-limited drugs can be expected to have similar initial blood concentrations after both intravenous and single oral dose administration in cirrhotic and normal subjects, but increased blood concentrations at steady state during chronic therapy in cirrhotic subjects.

SEVERITY OF LIVER DISEASE

The type and severity of liver disease are variables that influence drug disposition. Not all drugs that undergo extensive oxidative metabolism are affected to an equal extent by all liver diseases. Acute viral hepatitis, for example, has no effect on the metabolic elimination (Cl^u_{int}) of tolbutamide, warfarin, diphenylhydantoin, or antipyrine (15, 36, 80, 182, 183), whereas it does produce changes in metabolic elimination of hexobarbital, meperidine, and chlordiazepoxide (178). These observations might reflect differences in the degree to which different oxidative pathways of drug elimination are affected by liver disease, but more likely reflect the differences in the severity of the disease process in patients used for the separate studies. Thus, it may not be possible to find any change in the metabolic elimination of drugs in patients with mild or moderate forms of hepatitis. Certainly, the levels of cytochrome P-450 drug-metabolizing enzymes are not altered in liver biopsies from such patients (37). With more extensive liver damage from viral hepatitis or other causes, the level of these enzymes declines (37, 147). This decline should cause a decrease in the free intrinsic clearance of those drugs that are oxidatively metabolized in the liver by this enzyme system (95).

DRUG INTERACTIONS IN LIVER DISEASE

Patients with liver disease are often on a multidrug regimen. Certain drugs are well-known to affect drug metabolism either by induction or inhibition of metabolic enzymes.

Phenobarbital, pentobarbital, tolbutamide, and phenytoin act as metabolic inducers, increasing the synthesis of metabolic enzymes. The administration of enzyme-inducing drugs to patients with moderate liver disease may offset the disease-induced decrease in cytochrome P-450 enzymes. This effect, however, is limited. With an increase in the severity of liver damage, liver reserves may become too depressed for drug administration to exert much of an effect on either the level or activity of these enzymes (37, 159).

Cimetidine, on the other hand, a drug commonly used in the treatment of patients with alcoholic liver disease, has been shown to decrease total plasma clearance of theophylline (161), chlordiazepoxide (106), as well as numerous other drugs, in both control and cirrhotic subjects. It is believed that cimetidine interferes with oxidative metabolism but does not alter hepatic blood flow (106). Consequently, patients with liver disease may have an additional risk of impaired drug metabolism. The study by Nelson and colleagues (106) showed the decrease in plasma clearance of chlordiazepoxide to be greater in the control group than in the cirrhotic group, suggesting that the greater the initial microsomal function, the greater the effect of an inhibitor. However, it should be emphasized that this further decrease in drug metabolism may still be of importance in a patient with liver disease who may already have decreased metabolic function.

RECOMMENDATIONS FOR DOSAGE ADJUSTMENTS

As seen from the discussion of pharmacokinetic considerations in liver disease, it is not easy to predict the effect of disease on drug disposition in individual patients. Although severity of disease seems to play a major role in distribution and elimination of a drug, there is no good predictor of hepatic function. Despite a considerable effort by a number of investigators (8, 14, 30, 130, 151), there is no useful noninvasive test of liver function to guide dosage adjustments (12, 180). The best that can be said for most of the so-called liver function tests (i.e., serum albumin, prothrombin time, bilirubin, serum glutamic-oxaloacetic and glutamic-pyruvic transaminases (SGOT and SGPT), alkaline phosphatase, etc.) is that they reflect but do not predict the extent of liver damage (44).

Measuring cytochrome P-450 enzyme levels from liver biopsies might be expected to provide a better measure of the degree to which oxidative drug metabolism in the liver has been damaged. The level of these enzymes, however, has not been found to be a useful predictor of the metabolic elimination of drugs by this organ (95, 159). One explanation for the poor predictive value is that this measure fails to account for total hepatic size (130).

Some measures do exist that correlate with drug clearance, such as tests of antipyrine (160), aminopyrine, and indocyanine green clearance; however, these studies are not usually conducted as part of a patient's routine clinical evaluation. Moreover, the correlation coefficients usually approximate only 0.6 in most studies, accounting for only 40% or less of variance. Therefore, a good predictor of hepatic function or drug clearance has not been found; and at the present time, there is not a good hepatic counterpart for glomerular filtration rate, which is a reliable indicator of renal function.

Before considering the influence of liver disease on drug dosage requirements, some mention must be made of the use of drugs in general. There are always risks associated with the use of any drugs, and these risks may become particularly pronounced in patients with liver disease. In a prospective drug-monitoring study of more than 2000 patients, Naranjo and colleagues (103, 104) found the frequency of adverse drug reactions (ADRs) to be higher in patients with cirrhosis than in those with renal disease, other liver diseases, or neither liver nor renal disease. In the group of cirrhotic patients, the frequency of ADRs was significantly correlated with the severity of liver dysfunction as measured by a composite clinical and laboratory index. Thus, consideration should be given to whether the drug is really needed and whether its benefits outweigh the risks. For example, the use of some drugs in patients with liver disease is associated with a particularly high risk, and they should be used with great caution or not at all in these patients (Table 5.1). In general, the drugs listed in Table 5.1 fall into three categories: (*a*) drugs capable of causing liver damage even in normal patients, (*b*) drugs that can further compromise depressed liver functions often found in liver disease patients, and (*c*) drugs that can make the complications of liver disease worse. In the above-cited study, diuretics were found to be the most common cause of ADRs and to cause the most severe reactions.

If drug treatment is required and alternatives are available, it is preferable to use a drug whose disposition is least affected by the liver disease (e.g., a drug that is excreted renally or metabolized by glucuronidation). If a drug must be prescribed that may be affected by the disease process, then a number of factors must be considered, including (*a*) the extent of liver damage, (*b*) the degree of hepatic elimination of the drug, (*c*) the degree of protein binding, (*d*) the class to which the drug belongs (i.e., enzyme-limited, flow/enzyme-sensitive, or flow-limited, (*e*) the route of administration, and (*f*) the duration of administration.

A considerable amount of information has been gathered over the years regarding disposition of specific drugs in liver disease. Most of this work has been done in cirrhosis, a lesser

Table 5.3. Considerations for Drug Dosage Adjustments in Liver Disease Patients

Extent of Change in Drug Dose	*Conditions or Requirements to Be Satisfied*
No change or minor change in dose	1. Mild liver disease 2. Extensive elimination of drug by kidneys and no renal dysfunction 3. Elimination by pathways of metabolism spared by liver disease 4. Drug is enzyme-limited and given acutely 5. Drug is flow/enzyme-sensitive and given acutely only by i.v. route 6. No alteration in drug sensitivity
Decrease in dose of >25%	1. Elimination by the liver does not exceed 40% of the dose; no renal dysfunction 2. Drug is flow-limited and given by i.v. route, with no large change in protein binding 3. Drug is flow/enzyme-limited and given acutely by oral route 4. Drug has a large therapeutic ratio
Decrease in dose of >25%	1. Drug metabolism is affected by liver disease; drug administered chronically 2. Drug has a narrow therapeutic range; protein binding altered significantly 3. Drug is flow-limited and given orally 4. Drug is eliminated by kidneys and renal function severely affected 5. Altered sensitivity to drug due to liver disease

amount in acute viral hepatitis, and very little in other types of liver disease. To help the clinician, Table 5.2 presents a compilation of the dispositional characteristics of a number of drugs in normal subjects, the route of elimination of these drugs, the effect of liver disease on their disposition, and recommendations for adjustment of dose.

For drugs not listed in Table 5.2, general guidelines for dosage adjustment are given in Table 5.3. Although these considerations may not be all-inclusive, they should provide some guidance as to the extent of dosage change required with liver disease.

ACKNOWLEDGMENT

This work was supported in part by U.S. Public Health Service Grant GM 31304.

REFERENCES

1. Abernethy D, Schwartz JB: Pharmacokinetics of calcium antagonists under development. *Clin Pharmacokinet* 15:1–14, 1988.
2. Abshagen U, Rennekamp H, Luszpinski G: Disposition kinetics of spironolactone in hepatic failure after single doses and prolonged treatment. *Eur J Clin Pharmacol* 11:169–176, 1977.
3. Acocella G, Bonollo L, Garimoldi M, Mainardi M, Tenconi LT, Hicolis FB: Kinetics of rifampin and isoniazid administered alone and in combination to normal subjects and patients with liver disease. *Gut* 13:47–53, 1972.
4. Adjepon-Yamoah KK, Himmo J, Prescott LF: Gross impairment of hepatic drug metabolism in a patient with chronic liver disease. *Br Med J* 4:387–388, 1974.
5. Affrime A, Reidenberg MM: The protein binding of some drugs in plasma from patients with alcoholic liver disease. *Eur J Clin Pharmacol* 8:267–269, 1975.
6. Allonen H, Zieglar G, Koltz U: Midazolam kinetics. *Clin Pharmacol Ther* 30:653–660, 1981.
7. Alvin J, Meltorse T, Hoyumpa A, Bush MT, Schenker S: The effect of liver disease in man on the disposition of phenobarbital. *J Pharmacol Exp Ther* 192:224–235, 1975.
8. Andreasen PB, Greisen G: Phenazone metabolism in patients with liver disease. *Eur J Clin Invest* 6:21–26, 1976.
9. Andreasen PB, Hutters L: Paracetamol (acetaminophen) clearance in patients with cirrhosis of the liver. *Acta Med Scand* [Suppl] 624:99–105, 1979.
10. Avant GR, Schenker S, Alford RH: The effect of cirrhosis on the disposition and elimination of clindamycin. *Am J Dig Dis* 20:223–230, 1975.
11. Baba T, Murabayashi S, Tomiyama T, Takebe K: The pharmacokinetics of enalapril in patients with compensated liver cirrhosis. *Br J Clin Pharmacol* 29:766–769, 1990.
12. Bass N, Williams R: Guide to drug dosage in hepatic disease. *Clin Pharmacokinet* 15:396–420, 1988.
13. Benjamin RS: Clinical pharmacology of adriamycin (NSC-123127). *Cancer Chemother Rep* 6:183–185, 1975.
14. Bircher J, Blankart R, Halpern A, Hacki W, Laissue J, Preisig R: Criteria for assessment of functional impairment in patients with cirrhosis of the liver. *Eur J Clin Invest* 3:72–85, 1973.
15. Blaschke TF, Meffin PJ, Melmon KL, Rowland M: Influence of acute viral hepatitis on phenytoin kinetics and protein binding. *Clin Pharmacol Ther* 17:685–691, 1975.
16. Boscia JA, Korzeniowski OM, Kobasa WD, Rocha H, Levison ME, Kaye D: Pharmacokinetics of cefoperazone in normal subjects and patients with hepatosplenic schistosomiasis. *J Antimicrob Chemother* 12:407–410, 1983.
17. Boscia JA, Korzeniowski OM, Snepar R, Kobasa WD, Levison ME, Kaye D: Cefoperazone pharmacokinetics in normal subjects and patients with cirrhosis. *Antimicrob Agents Chemother* 23:385–389, 1983.
18. Branch RA, James J, Read AE: A study of factors influencing drug disposition in chronic liver disease, using the model drug (+)-propranolol. *Br J Clin Pharmacol* 3:243–249, 1976.
19. Branch RA, Shand DG: Propranolol disposition in chronic liver disease: a physiological approach. *Clin Pharmacokinet* 1:264–279, 1976.
20. Brodie MJ, Boobis S: The effect of chronic alcoholic ingestion and alcoholic liver disease on binding of drugs to serum proteins. *Eur J Clin Pharmacol* 13:435–438, 1978.
21. Brown N, Ho DHW, Fong KL, Bogerd L, Maksymiuk A, Bolivar R, Fainstein V, Bodey GP: Effects of hepatic function on vancomycin clinical pharmacology. *Antimicrob Agents Chemother* 23:603–609, 1983.
22. Buchi KN, Rollins DE, Tolman KG, Achari R, Drissel D, Hulse JD: Pharmacokinetics of esmolol in hepatic disease. *J Clin Pharmacol* 27:880–884, 1987.
23. Burnett DA, Barak AJ, Tuma DJ, Sorrell MF: Altered elimination of antipyrine in patients with acute viral hepatitis. *Gut* 17:341–344, 1976.
24. Calvo MV, Dominguez-Gil A, Macias JG, Dietz JL: Naproxen disposition in hepatic and biliary disorders. *Int J Clin Pharmacol Ther Toxicol* 18:242–246, 1980.
25. Cello JP, Oie S: Binding and disposition of sulfisoxazole in alcoholic cirrhosis. *J Pharmacokinet Biopharm* 13:1–12, 1985.
26. Cello JP, Oie J: Cimetidine disposition in patients with Laennec's cirrhosis during multiple dosing therapy. *Eur J Clin Pharmacol* 25:223–229, 1983.
27. Cook DR, Freeman J, Lai A, Robertson K, Kang Y, Stiller R, Aggarwal S, Abou-Donia M, Welch R: Pharmacokinetics and pharmacodynamics of doxacurium in normal patients and in those with hepatic or renal failure. *Anesth Analg* 72:145–150, 1991.
28. Cotting J, Reichen J, Kutz K, Laplanche R, Nuesch E: Pharmacokinetics of isradipine in patients with chronic liver disease. *Eur J Clin Pharmacol* 38:599–603, 1990.
29. Daneshmend TK, Homeida M, Kaye CM, Elamin AA, Roberts CJC: Disposition of oral metronidazole in hepatic cirrhosis and in hepatosplenic schistosomiasis. *Gut* 23:807–813, 1982.
30. Desmond PV, Patwardhan RV, Johnson RF, Schenker S: Impaired elimination of caffeine in cirrhosis. *Dig Dis Sci* 25:193–197, 1980.
31. D'Incalci M, Rossi C, Zucchetti M, Urso R, Cavalli F, Mangioni C, Williams Y, Sessa C: Pharmacokinetics of etoposide in patients with abnormal renal and hepatic function. *Cancer Res* 46:2566–2571, 1986.
32. Doshi J, Luisada-Oppe A, Leevy CM: Microsomal pentobarbital hydroxylase activity in acute viral hepatitis. *Proc Soc Exp Biol Med* 140:492–495, 1975.
33. duSouich P, Erill S: Metabolism of procainamide and *p*-aminobenzoic acid in patients with chronic liver disease. *Clin Pharmacol Ther* 22:588–595, 1977.
34. El-Raghy I, Back DJ, Osman F, Nafeh MA, Orme M L'E: The pharmacokinetics of antipyrine in patients with graded severity of schistosomiasis. *Br J Clin Pharmacol* 20:313–316, 1985.
35. Farrell G, Baird-Lambert J, Cvejic J, Buchanan N: Disposition and metabolism of metronidazole in patients with liver failure. *Hepatology* 4:722–726, 1984.
36. Farrell GC, Cooksley WGE, Hart P, Powell LW: Drug metabolism in liver disease. Identification of patients with impaired hepatic drug metabolism. *Gastroenterology* 75:580–588, 1978.
37. Farrell GC, Cooksley WGE, Powell LW: Drug metabolism in liver disease: activity of hepatic microsomal metabolizing enzymes. *Clin Pharmacol Ther* 26:483–492, 1979.
38. Ferrier C, Marty J, Bouffard Y, Haberer JP, Levron JC, Duvaldestin P: Alfentanil pharmacokinetics in patients with cirrhosis. *Anesthesiology* 62:480–484, 1985.
39. Forrest JAH, Finlayson NDC, Adjepon-Yamoah KK, Prescott LF: Antipyrine, paracetamol, and lidocaine elimination in chronic liver disease. *Br Med J* 1:1384–1387, 1977.
40. Fuller R, Hoppel C, Ingalls ST: Furosemide kinetics in patients with hepatic cirrhosis with ascites. *Clin Pharmacol Ther* 30:461–467, 1981.
41. Gelman CR, Rumack BH: DRUGDEX® Information System. Micromedix, Inc., Denver, CO.
42. Giacomini KM, Giacomini JC, Gibson TP, Levy G: Propoxyphene and norpropoxyphene plasma concentrations after oral propoxyphene in cirrhotic patients with and without surgically constructed portacaval shunt. *Clin Pharmacol Ther* 28:417–424, 1980.
43. Giargcau AJ, Chalmers TC: The natural history of cirrhosis. I. Survival with esophageal varices. *N Engl J Med* 268:469–473, 1963.
44. Goldberg D, Brown D: Advances in the application of biochemical tests to diseases of the liver and biliary tract: their role in diagnosis, prognosis, and the elucidation of pathogenetic mechanisms. *Clin Biochem* 20:127–148, 1987.
45. Grahnen A, Jameson S, Lööf L, Tyllström J, Lindström B: Pharmacokinetics of cimetidine in advanced cirrhosis. *Eur J Clin Pharmacol* 26:347–355, 1984.
46. Groszman R, Kotelanski B, Khatri IM, Cohn JN: Quantitation of portasystemic shunting from the splenic and mesenteric beds in alcoholic liver disease. *Am J Med* 53:715–722, 1972.
47. Haberer JP, Schoeffler P, Couderc E, Duvaldestin P: Fentanyl pharmacokinetics in anaesthetized patients with cirrhosis. *Br J Anaesth* 54:1267–1270, 1982.
48. Hall KW, Nightingale CH, Gibaldi M, Nelson E, Bates TR, Disanto AR: Pharmacokinetics of erythromycin in normal and alcoholic liver disease subjects. *J Clin Pharmacol* 22:321–325, 1982.
49. Hande KR, Wedlund PJ, Noone RM, Wilkinson GR, Greco FA, Wolff SN: Pharmacokinetics of high-dose etoposide (VP-16-213) administered to cancer patients. *Cancer Res* 44:379–382, 1984.
50. Helleberg L: Clinical pharmacokinetics of indomethacin. *Clin Pharmacokinet* 6:245–258, 1981.
51. Hinthorn DR, Baker LH, Romig DR, Hassanien K, Liu C: Use of clindamycin in patients with liver disease. *Antimicrob Agents Chemother* 9:498–501, 1976.
52. Hoffman TA, Cestero R, Bullock WE: Pharmacodynamics of carbenicillin in hepatic and renal failure. *Ann Intern Med* 73:173–178, 1970.
53. Homeida M, Jackson L, Roberts CJC: Decreased first-pass metabolism of labetalol in chronic liver disease. *Br Med J* 2:1048–1050, 1978.

54. Homeida M, Roberts CJC, Halliwell M, Read AE, Branch RA: Antipyrine clearance per unit volume liver: an assessment of hepatic function in chronic liver disease. *Gut* 20:596–601, 1979.

55. Horn T, Christofferson P, Henriksen JH: Alcoholic liver injury: defenestration in noncirrhotic livers---a scanning electron microscopic study. *Hepatology* 7:77–82, 1987.

56. Howden C, Birnie G, Brodie M: Drug metabolism in liver disease. *Pharmacol Ther* 40:439–474, 1989.

57. Hoyumpa A, Schenker S: Is glucuronidation truly preserved in patients with liver disease? *Hepatology* 13(4):786–795, 1991.

58. Huet P, Lelorier J: Effects of smoking and chronic hepatitis B on lidocaine and indocyanine green kinetics. *Clin Pharmacol Ther* 28:208–215, 1980.

59. Huet P-M, Goresky CA, Villeneuve J-P, Marleau D, Lough JO: Assessment of liver microcirculation in human cirrhosis. *J Clin Invest* 70:1234–1244, 1982.

60. Huet P-M, Pomier-Layrargues G, Villeneuve J-P, Varin F, Viallet A: Intrahepatic circulation in liver disease. *Semin Liver Dis* 6:277–286, 1986.

61. Huet P-M, Villeneuve J-P, Pomier-Layrargues G, Marleau D: Hepatic circulation in cirrhosis. *Clin Gastroenterol* 14:155–168, 1985.

62. Huet P-M, Villeneuve J-P: Determinants of drug disposition in patients with cirrhosis. *Hepatology* 3(6):913–918, 1983.

63. Humphrey MJ, Jevons S, Tarbit MH: Pharmacokinetic evaluation of UK-49,858, a metabolically stable triazole antifungal drug, in animals and humans. *Antimicrob Agents Chemother* 28:648–653, 1985.

64. Ishizaki T, Chiba K, Sasaki T: Antipyrine clearance in patients with Gilbert's syndrome. *Eur J Clin Pharmacol* 27:297–302, 1984.

65. Iqbal S, Vickers C, Elias E: Drug metabolism in end-stage liver disease: in vitro activities of some phase I amd phase II enzymes. *J Hepatol* 11:37–42, 1990.

66. Janssen U, Walker S, Maier K, von Gaisberg U, Klotz U: Flumazenil disposition and elimination in cirrhosis. *Clin Pharmacol Ther* 46:317–323, 1989.

67. Jochemsen R, Van Beusekom BR, Spoelstra P, Janssens AR, Breimer DD: Effect of age and liver cirrhosis on the pharmacokinetics of nitrazepam. *Br J Clin Pharmacol* 15:295–302, 1983.

68. Johannessen SI, Gerna M, Bakke J, Strandjord RE, Morselli PL: CSF concentrations and serum protein binding of carbamazepine and carbamazepine-10gll-epoxide in epileptic patients. *Br J Clin Pharmacol* 3:575–582, 1976.

69. Juhl RP, VanThiel DH, Dittert LW, Albert KS, Smith RB: Ibuprofen and sulindac kinetics in alcoholic liver disease. *Clin Pharmacol Ther* 34:104–109, 1983.

70. Juma FD: Effect of liver failure on the pharmacokinetics of cyclophosphamide. *Eur J Clin Pharmacol* 26:591–593, 1984.

71. Kawai S, Ichikawa Y, Homma M: Differences in metabolic properties among cortisol, prednisolone, and dexamethasone in liver and renal diseases. Accelerated metabolism of dexamethasone in renal failure. *J Clin Endocrinol Metab* 60:848–854, 1985.

72. Kenny MT, Strates B: Metabolism and pharmacokinetics of the antibiotic rifampin. *Drug Metab Rev* 12:159–218, 1981.

73. Kirch W, Ohnhaus EE, Dylewicz P, Pabst J, Storstein L: Bioavailability and elimination of digitoxin in patients with hepatorenal insufficiency. *Am Heart J* 111:325–329, 1986.

74. Kirch W, Schafer-Korting M, Mutschler E, Ohnhaus EE, Braun W: Clinical experience with atenolol in patients with chronic liver disease. *J Clin Pharmacol* 23:171–177, 1983.

75. Kleinbloesem CH, van Harten J, Wilson JPH, Danhof M, van Brummelen P, Breimer DD: Nifedipine: kinetics and hemodynamic effects in patients with liver cirrhosis after intravenous and oral administration. *Clin Pharmacol Ther* 40:21–28, 1986.

76. Klinger EL, Vaamonde CA, Vaamonde LS, Lancestremere RG, Morosi HJ, Frisch E, Papper S: Renal function changes in cirrhosis of the liver. *Arch Intern Med* 125:1010–1015, 1970.

77. Klotz U, Antonin KH, Brugel H, Bieck PR: Disposition of diazepam and its major metabolite desmethyldiazepam in patients with liver disease. *Clin Pharmacol Ther* 21:430–436, 1977.

78. Klotz U, Fischer C, Muller-Seydlitz P, Schulz J, Mueller WA: Alterations in the disposition of differently cleared drugs in patients with cirrhosis. *Clin Pharmacol Ther* 26:221–227, 1979.

79. Kraus JW, Desmond PV, Marshall JP, Johnson RF, Schenker S, Wilkinson GR: Effects of aging and liver disease on disposition of lorazepam. *Clin Pharmacol Ther* 24:411–419, 1978.

80. Krausz Y, Zylber-Katz E, Levy M: Antipyrine clearance and its correlation to routine liver function tests in patients with liver disease. *Int J Clin Pharmacol Ther Toxicol* 18:253–257, 1980.

81. Kroboth PD, Brown A, Lyon JA, Kroboth FJ, Juhl RP: Pharmacokinetics of single-dose erythromycin in normal and alcohol liver disease subjects. *Antimicrob Agents Chemother* 21:135–140, 1982.

82. Levy G: Effect of plasma protein binding of drugs on duration and intensity of pharmacological activity. *J Pharm Sci* 65:1264–1265, 1976.

83. Lewis GP, Jusko WJ: Pharmacokinetics of ampicillin in cirrhosis. *Clin Pharmacol Ther* 18:475–484, 1975.

84. Lima JJ, Boudoulas H, Blanford M: Concentration-dependence of disopyramide binding to plasma protein and its influence on kinetics and dynamics. *J Pharmacol Exp Ther* 219:741–747, 1981.

85. MacGilchrist AJ, Birnie GG, Cook A, Scobie G, Murray T, Watkinson G, Brodie MJ: Pharmacokinetics and pharmacodynamics of intravenous midazolam in patients with severe alcoholic cirrhosis. *Gut* 27:190–195, 1986.

86. MacLeod CM, Bartley EA, Payne JA, Hudes E, Vernam K, Devlin RG: Effects of cirrhosis on kinetics of aztreonam. *Antimicrob Agents Chemother* 26:493–497, 1984.

87. Mak KM, Lieber CS: Alterations in endothelial fenestrations in liver sinusoids of baboons fed alcohol: a scanning electron microscopic study. *Hepatology* 4:386–391, 1984.

88. Malini PL, Sarti F, Dal Monte PR, Grepioni A, Boschi S, Ambrosioni E: Effect of chronic liver disease on plasma levels and metabolism of digoxin and betamethyl digoxin. *Int J Clin Pharmacol Res* 1:21–27, 1982.

89. Marcantonio LA, Auld WHR, Murdock WR, Purohit R, Skellern GG, Howes CA: The pharmacokinetics and pharmacodynamics of the diuretic bumetanide in hepatic and renal disease. *Br J Clin Pharmacol* 15:245–252, 1983.

90. Marshall JP, Salt WB, Elam RO, Wilkinson GR, Schenker S: Disposition of nafcillin inpatients with cirrhosis and extrahepatic biliary obstruction. *Gastroenterology* 73:1388–1392, 1977.

91. Mawer GE, Miller NE, Turnberg LA: Metabolism of amylobarbitone in patients with chronic liver disease. *Br J Pharmacol* 44:549–560, 1972.

92. McConnell JB, Curry SH, Davis M, Williams R: Clinical effects and metabolism of diazepam in patients with chronic liver disease. *Clin Sci* 63:75–80, 1982.

93. Mehta MU, Venkataramanan R, Burckart GJ, Ptachcinski RJ, Yang SL, Gray JA, Van Thiel DH, Starzl TE: Antipyrine kinetics in liver disease and liver transplantation. *Clin Pharmacol Ther* 39:372–377, 1986.

94. Meredith CG, Christian CD Jr, Johnson RF, Madhavan SV, Schenker S: Diphenhydramine disposition in chronic liver disease. *Clin Pharmacol Ther* 35:474–479, 1984.

95. Meyer B, Luo H, Bargetzi M, Renner E, Stalder G: Quantitation of intrinsic drug-metabolizing capacity in human liver biopsy specimens: support for the intact-hepatocyte theory. *Hepatology* 13(3):475–481, 1991.

96. Miguet J-P, Vuitton D, Deschamps J-P, Allemand H, Joanne C, Bechtel P, Carayon P: Cholestasis and hepatic drug metabolism: comparison of metabolic clearance rate of antipyrine in patients with intrahepatic or extrahepatic cholestasis. *Dig Dis Sci* 26:718–722, 1981.

97. Montay G, Gaillot J: Pharmacokinetics of fluoroquinolones in hepatic failure. *J Antimicrob Chemother* 26(suppl B):61–67, 1990.

98. Moreau L, Durand H, Biclet P: Cefotaxime concentrations in ascites. *J Antimicrob Chemother* 6(suppl A):121–122, 1980.

99. Morichau-Beauchant M, Houin G, Mavier P, Alexandre C, Dhumeaux D: Pharmacokinetics and bioavailability of ranitidine in normal subjects and cirrhotic patients. *Dig Dis Sci* 31:113–118, 1986.

100. Narang APS, Datta DV, Nath N, Mathur VS: Impairment of hepatic drug metabolism in patients with acute viral hepatitis. *Eur J Drug Metab Pharmacokinet* 7:255–258, 1982.

101. Narang APS, Datta DV, Nath N, Mathur VS: Pharmacokinetic study of chloramphenicol in patients with liver disease. *Eur J Clin Pharmacol* 20:479–483, 1981.

102. Narang APS, Kaur U, Bambery P: Drug metabolism and liver disease in India. *Drug Metab Rev* 23:65–81, 1991.

103. Naranjo CA, Busto U, Janecek E, Ruiz I, Roach CA, Kaplan K: An intensive drug monitoring study suggesting possible clinical irrelevance of impaired drug disposition in liver disease. *Br J Clin Pharmacol* 15:451–458, 1983.

104. Naranjo CA, Busto U, Mardones R: Adverse drug reactions in liver cirrhosis. *Eur J Clin Pharmacol* 13:429–434, 1978.

105. Neal EA, Meffin PJ, Gregory PB, Blaschke TF: Enhanced bioavailability and decreased clearance of analgesics in patients with cirrhosis. *Gastroenterology* 77:96–102, 1979.

106. Nelson DC, Avant GR, Speeg KV Jr, Hoyumpa AM Jr, Schenker S: The effect of cimetidine on hepatic drug elimination in cirrhosis. *Hepatology* 5:305–309, 1985.

107. Novick DM, Kreek MJ, Arns PA, Lau LL, Yancovitz SR, Gelb AM: Effect of severe alcoholic liver disease on the disposition of methadone in maintenance patients. *Alcoholism* 9:349–354, 1985.

108. Novick DM, Kreek MJ, Fanizza AM, Yancovitz SR, Gelb AM, Stenger RJ: Methadone disposition in patients with chronic liver disease. *Clin Pharmacol Ther* 30:353–362, 1981.

109. Ochs HR, Greenblatt DJ, Bodem G, Dengler HJ: Disease-related alterations in cardiac glycoside disposition. *Clin Pharmacokinet* 7:434–451, 1982.

110. Ochs HR, Greenblatt DJ, Eckardt B, Harmatz JS, Shader RI: Repeated diazepam dosing in cirrhotic patients: accumulation and sedation. *Clin Pharmacol Ther* 33:471–476, 1983.

111. Ochs HR, Greenblatt DJ, Verburg-Ochs B, Matlis R: Temazepam clearance is unaltered in cirrhosis. *Am J Gastroenterol* 81:80–84, 1986.

112. Oellerich M, Burdelski M, Lautz HU, Schulz M, Schmidt FW, Herrmann H: Lidocaine metabolite formation as a measure of liver function in patients with cirrhosis. *Ther Drug Monit* 12:219–226, 1990.

113. Ohashi K, Tsunoo M, Tsuneoka K: Pharmacokinetics and protein binding of cefazolin and cephalothin in patients with cirrhosis. *J Antimicrob Chemother* 17:347–351, 1986.

114. Ohnhaus EE, Münch U, Meier J: Elimination of pindolol in liver disease. *Eur J Clin Pharmacol* 22:247–251, 1982.

115. Ohnishi A, Tsuboi Y, Ishizaki T, Kubota K, Ohno T, Yoshida H, Kanezaki A, Tanaka T: Kinetics and dynamics of enalapril in patients with liver cirrhosis. *Clin Pharmacol Ther* 45:657–665, 1989.

116. Ohnishi K: Effects of hepatic disease on the pharmacokinetics of famotidine and effects of famotidine on hepatic hemodynamics and peptic ulcer. *Hepatogastroenterology* 37:6–10, 1990.

117. Okolicsanyi L, Venuti M, Orlando R, Xerri L, Pugina M: Pharmacokinetic studies of cefuroxime in patients with liver cirrhosis. *Arzneimittelforschung* 7:777–782, 1982.

118. Okolicsanyi L, Venuti M, Strazzabosco M, Orlando R, Nassuato G, Iemmolo RM, Lirussi R, Muraca M, Pastorino AM, Castelli G: Oral and intravenous pharmacokinetics of ranitidine in patients with liver cirrhosis. *Int J Clin Pharmacol Ther Toxicol* 22:329–332, 1984.

119. Olsen GD, Bennett WM, Potter GA: Morphine and phenytoin binding to plasma proteins in renal and hepatic failure. *Clin Pharmacol Ther* 17:677–684, 1976.

120. Oltmanns D, Pottage A, Endell W: Pharmacokinetics of tocainide in patients with combined hepatic and renal dysfunction. *Eur J Clin Pharmacol* 25:787–790, 1983.

121. Orrego H, Medline A, Blendis LM, Rankin JG, Kreaden DA: Collagenisation of the Disse space in alcoholic liver disease. *Gut* 20:673–679, 1979.

122. Pandele G, Chaux F, Salvadori C, Farinotti M, Duvaldestin P: Thiopental pharmacokinetics in patients with cirrhosis. *Anesthesiology* 59:123–126, 1983.

123. Pasko MT, Beam TR, Spooner JA, Camara DS: Safety and pharmacokinetics of ceftazidime in patients with chronic hepatic dysfunction. *J Antimicrob Chemother* 15:365–374, 1985.

124. Patwardhan R, Johnson R, Sheehan J, Desmond P, Wilkinson G, Hoyumpa A, Branch R, Schenker S: Morphine metabolism in cirrhosis. *Gastroenterology* 80:1344, 1981.

125. Patwardhan RV, Johnson RF, Hoyumpa A, Sheehan JJ, Desmond PV, Wilkinson GR, Branch RA, Schenker S: Normal metabolism of morphine in cirrhosis. *Gastroenterology* 81:1006–1011, 1981.

126. Pearson RM, Breckenridge AM: Renal function, protein binding and pharmacological response to diazoxide. *Br J Clin Pharmacol* 3:169–175, 1976.

127. Pentikainen PJ, Neuvonen PJ, Jostell K-G: Pharmacokinetics of chlormethiazole in healthy volunteers and patients with cirrhosis of the liver. *Eur J Clin Pharmacol* 17:275–284, 1980.

128. Perez-Mateo M, Erill S: Protein binding of salicylates and quinidine in plasma from patients with renal failure, chronic liver disease and chronic respiratory insufficiency. *Eur J Clin Pharmacol* 11:225–231, 1977.

129. Pessayre D, Lebrec D, Descatoire V, Peignoux M, Benhamou J-P: Mechanism for reduced drug clearance in patients with cirrhosis. *Gastroenterology* 74:566–571, 1978.

130. Pirttiaho HI, Sotaniemi EA, Ahlqvist J, Pitkanen U, Pelkonen RO: Liver size and indices of drug metabolism in alcoholics. *Eur J Clin Pharmacol* 13:61–67, 1978.

131. Pisani F, Perruca E, Primerano G, D'Agostino AA, Petrelli RM, Fazio A, Oteri G, Di Perri R: Single-dose kinetics of primidone in acute viral hepatitis. *Eur J Clin Pharmacol* 27:465–469, 1984.

132. Pond SM, Tong T, Benowitz NL, Jacob P: Enhanced bioavailability of pethidine and pentazocine in patients with cirrhosis of the liver. *Aust N Z J Med* 10:515–519, 1980.

133. Pond SM, Tong T, Benowitz NL, Jacob P, Rigod J: Presystemic metabolism of meperidine to normeperidine in normal and cirrhotic subjects. *Clin Pharmacol Ther* 30:183–188, 1981.

134. Pozzi E, Menghini P: Blood levels of rifampicin in liver diseases. *Int J Clin Pharmacol* 10:44–49, 1974.

135. Regardh G-G, Jordo L, Ervik M, Lundborg P, Olsson R, Ronn O: Pharmacokinetics of metoprolol in patients with hepatic cirrhosis. *Clin Pharmacokinet* 6:375–388, 1981.

136. Richter E, Breimer DD, Zilly W: Disposition of hexobarbital in intra- and extrahepatic cholestasis in man and the influence of drug metabolism-inducing agents. *Eur J Clin Pharmacol* 17:197–202, 1980.

137. Ring-Larsen H: Renal blood flow in cirrhosis: relation to systemic and portal haemodynamics and liver function. *Scand J Clin Lab Invest* 37:635–642, 1977.

138. Ring-Larsen H, Birger H, Henriksen JH, Christensen NJ: Sympathetic nervous activity and renal and systemic hemodynamics in cirrhosis: plasma norepinephrine concentration, hepatic extraction, and renal release. *Hepatology* 2:304–310, 1982.

139. Ring-Larsen H, Henriksen JH: Pathogenesis of ascites formation and hepatorenal syndrome: humoral and hemodynamic factors. *Semin Liver Dis* 6:341–352, 1986.

140. Rinetti M, Regazzi MB, Villani P, Tizzoni M, Sivelli R: Pharmacokinetics of omeprazole in cirrhotic patients. *Arzneimittelforschung* 41(I):420–422, 1991.

141. Roberts MS, Rumble RH, Wanwimolruk S, Thomas D, Brooks PM: Pharmacokinetics of aspirin and salicylate in elderly subjects and in patients with alcoholic liver disease. *Eur J Clin Pharmacol* 25:253–261, 1983.

142. Robinson JD, Whitney HAK Jr, Guisti DL, Morgan DD, Mendenhall CL: The absorption of intramuscular chlordiazepoxide (Librium) in patients with severe alcoholic liver disease. *Int J Clin Pharmacol Ther Toxicol* 21:433–438, 1983.

143. Roos F, Zysset T, Reichen J: Differential effect of biliary and micronodular cirrhosis on oxidative drug metabolism. *Biochem Pharmacol* 41(10):1513–1519, 1991.

144. Rowland M, Benet LZ, Graham GG: Clearance concepts in pharmacokinetics. *J Pharmacol Biopharm* 1:123–136, 1973.

145. Ruhnke M, Trautmann M, Borner K, Hopfenmuller W: Pharmacokinetics of ciprofloxacin in liver cirrhosis. *Chemotherapy* 36:385–391, 1990.

146. Sadee W, Schroder R, V Leitner E, Dagcioglu M: Multiple dose kinetics of spironolactone and canrenoate-potassium in cardiac and hepatic failure. *Eur J Clin Pharmacol* 7:195–200, 1974.

147. Schoene B, Fleischmann RA, Remmer H: Determination of drug metabolizing enzymes in needle biopsies of human liver. *Eur J Clin Pharmacol* 4:65–73, 1972.

148. Sessions JT, Minkel HP, Bullard JC, Ingelfinger FJ: The effect of barbiturates in patients with liver disease. *J Clin Invest* 33:1116–1127, 1954.

149. Shear L, Kleinerman J, Gabuzda GJ: Renal failure in patients with cirrhosis of the liver. *Am J Med* 39:184–198, 1965.

150. Shoeman DW, Azarnoff DL: Diphenylhydantoin potency and plasma protein binding. *J Pharmacol Exp Ther* 195:84–86, 1975.

151. Shreeve WW, Shoop JD, Ott DG, McInteer BB: Test for alcoholic cirrhosis by conversion of ^{14}C- or ^{13}C-galactose to expired CO_2. *Gastroenterology* 71:98–101, 1976.

152. Shull HJ, Wilkinson GR, Johnson R, Schenker S: Normal disposition of oxazepam in acute viral hepatitis and cirrhosis. *Ann Intern Med* 84:420–425, 1976.

153. Siegers C-P, Oltmanns D, Younes M: Effect of alcohol and chronic liver disease on the metabolic disposal of paracetamol in man. *Hepatogastroenterology* 28:304, 1981.

154. Sloan TP, Lancaster R, Shah RR, Idle JR, Smith RL: Genetically determined oxidation capacity and the disposition of debrisoquine. *Br J Clin Pharmacol* 15:443–450, 1983.

155. Somogyi A, Albrecht M, Kliens G, Schafer K, Eichelbaum M: Pharmacokinetics, bioavailability and ECG response of verapamil in patients with liver disease. *Br J Clin Pharmacol* 12:51–60, 1981.

156. Sonne J, Andreasen PB, Loft S, Dossing M, Andreasen F: Glucuronidation of oxazepam is not spared in patients with hepatic encephalopathy. *Hepatology* 11(6):951–956, 1990.

157. Sotaniemi EA, Luoma PV, Jarvensiva PM, Sotaniemi KA: Impairment of drug metabolism in polycystic non-parasitic liver disease. *Br J Clin Pharmacol* 8:331–335, 1979.

158. Sotaniemi EA, Niemala O, Risteli L, Stenback F, Pelkonen RO, Lahtela JT, Risteli J: Fibrotic process and drug metabolism in alcoholic liver disease. *Clin Pharmacol Ther* 40:46–55, 1986.

159. Sotaniemi EA, Pelkonen RO, Puukka M: Measurement of hepatic drug-metabolizing enzyme activity in man. *Eur J Clin Pharmacol* 17:267–274, 1980.

160. St. Peter J, Awni W: Quantifying hepatic function in the presence of liver disease with phenazone (antipyrine) and its metabolites. *Clin Pharmacokinet* 20(1):50–65, 1991.

161. Staib AH, Schuppan D, Lissner R, Zilly W, Bomhard GV, Richter E: Pharmacokinetics and metabolism of theophylline in patients with liver diseases. *Int J Clin Pharmacol Ther Toxicol* 18:500–502, 1980.

162. Stoeckel K, Tuerk H, Trueb V, McNamara PJ: Single-dose ceftriaxone kinetics in liver insufficiency. *Clin Pharmacol Ther* 36:500–509, 1984.

163. Syrota A, Paraf A, Gaudebout C, Desgrez A: Significance of intra- and extrahepatic portasystemic shunting in survival of cirrhotic patients. *Dig Dis Sci* 26:878–885, 1981.

164. Syrota A, Vinot J-M, Paraf A, Roucayrol JC: Scintillation splenoportography: hemodynamic and morphological study of the portal circulation. *Gastroenterology* 71:652–659, 1976.

165. Taburet A-M, Naveau S, Zorza G, Colin J-N, Delfraissy J-F, Chaput J-C, Singlas E: Pharmacokinetics of zidovudine in patients with liver cirrhosis. *Clin Pharmacol Ther* 47:731–739, 1990.

166. Teunissen MWE, Spoelstra P, Koch CW, Weeds B, Van Duyn W, Janssens AR, Breimer DD: Antipyrine clearance and metabolite formation in patients with alcoholic cirrhosis. *Br J Clin Pharmacol* 18:707–715, 1984.

167. Thiessen JJ, Sellers EM, Denbeigh P, Dolman L: Plasma protein binding of diazepam and tolbutamide in chronic alcoholics. *J Clin Pharmacol* 16:345–351, 1976.

168. Thomson PD, Melmon KL, Richardson JA, Cohn K, Steinbrunn W, Cudihee R, Rowland M: Lidocaine pharmacokinetics in advanced heart failure, liver disease, and renal failure in humans. *Ann Intern Med* 78:499–508, 1973.

169. Thomson PD, Rowland M, Melmon KL: The influence of heart failure, liver disease, and renal failure on the disposition of lidocaine in man. *Am Heart J* 82:417–421, 1971.

170. Tschang C, Steiner JA, Hignite CE, Huffman DH, Azarnoff DL: Systemic availability of lidocaine in patients with liver disease [Abstract]. *Clin Res* 25:609A, 1977.

171. Uribe M, Summerskill WHJ, Go VLW: Comparative serum prednisone and prednisolone concentrations following administration to patients with chronic active liver disease. *Clin Pharmacokinet* 7:452–459, 1982.

172. Verbeeck RK, Patwardhan RV, Villeneuve J-P, Wilkinson GR, Branch RA: Furosemide disposition in cirrhosis. *Clin Pharmacol Ther* 31:719–725, 1982.

173. Villeneuve J-P, Rocheleau F, Raymond G: Triamterene kinetics and dynamics in cirrhosis. *Clin Pharmacol Ther* 35:831–837, 1984.

174. Villeneuve J-P, Verbeeck RK, Wilkinson GR, Branch RA: Furosemide kinetics and dynamics in patients with cirrhosis. *Clin Pharmacol Ther* 40:14–20, 1986.

175. Wagner VT, Heydrich D, Bartels H, Hohorst HJ: The influence of damaged liver parenchyma, renal insufficiency and hemodialysis on the pharmacokinetics of cyclophosphamide and its activated metabolites. *Arzneimittelforschung* 30:1588–1592, 1980.

176. Wallace S, Brodie MJ: Decreased drug binding in serum from patients with chronic hepatic disease. *Eur J Clin Pharmacol* 9:429–432, 1976.

177. Ward S, Weatherley BC: Pharmacokinetics of atracurium and its metabolites. *Br J Anaesth* 58:6S–10S, 1986.

178. Wilkinson GR: The effects of liver disease and aging on the disposition of diazepam, chlordiazepoxide, oxazepam and lorazepam in man. *Acta Psychiatr Scand* 274:561–573, 1978.

179. Wilkinson GR, Shand DG: A physiological approach to hepatic drug clearance. *Clin Pharmacol Ther* 18:377–390, 1975.

180. Williams RL: Drug administration in hepatic disease. *N Engl J Med* 309(26):1616–1622, 1983.

181. Williams RL, Blaschke TF, Meffin PJ, Melman KL, Rowland M: Influence of viral hepatitis on the disposition of two compounds with high clearance: lidocaine and indocyanine green. *Clin Pharmacol Ther* 20:290–299, 1976.

182. Williams RL, Blaschke TF, Meffin PJ, Melmon KL, Rowland M: Influence of acute viral hepatitis on disposition and plasma binding of tolbutamide. *Clin Pharmacol Ther* 21:301–309, 1977.

183. Williams RL, Schary WL, Blaschke TF, Meffin PJ, Melmon KL, Rowland M: Influence of acute viral hepatitis on disposition and pharmacological effect of warfarin. *Clin Pharmacol Ther* 20:90–97, 1976.

184. Williams RL, Upton RA, Cello JP, Jones RM, Blitstein M, Kelly J, Nierenburg D: Naproxen disposition in patients with alcoholic cirrhosis. *Eur J Clin Pharmacol* 27:291–296, 1984.

185. Wood AJJ, Kornhauser DM, Wilkinson GR, Shand DG, Branch RA: The influence of cirrhosis on steady-state blood concentrations of unbound propranolol after oral administration. *Clin Pharmacokinet* 3:478–487, 1978.

186. Woodcock BG, Rietbrock I, Vohringer HF, Rietbrock N: Verapamil disposition in liver disease and intensive care patients: kinetics, clearance and apparent blood flow relationships. *Clin Pharmacol Ther* 29:27–34, 1981.

CHAPTER 6

Pharmacologic Approach in Patients with Pulmonary Failure

HENRY J. SILVERMAN, M.D.

BRONCHODILATORS

CONTROL OF AIRWAY TONE

Proper therapeutic use of bronchodilators requires an appreciation of the mechanism of action of the various agents available and, hence, an understanding of the anatomical and biochemical pathways involved in the control of airway tone.

Recent investigations have greatly expanded our knowledge of the neural control of human airways and have been the subject of extensive reviews (1–5). Autonomic control of the airway includes contributions from the sympathomimetic (adrenergic) and parasympathetic (cholinergic) nervous system and "third" nonadrenergic, noncholinergic nervous system (NANC), which includes several different neural mechanisms producing both bronchodilation and brochoconstriction (Fig. 6.1). Neural mechanisms also regulate mucous secretion from submucosal glands, permeability and blood flow in the bronchial circulation, fluid transport across airway epithelium, and release of mediators from mast cells and other inflammatory cells active in the response to injury and allergic reaction.

Parasympathetic innervation of the bronchi occurs via the vagus nerve as far down as the terminal bronchioles, whereas evidence for direct innervation by the sympathetic nervous system is sparse (1). Atropine produces bronchodilation from baseline, indicating the presence of resting airway

tone maintained by vagal motor activity, whereas administration of a β-antagonist does not result in bronchoconstriction in normal individuals, indicating the lack of tonic sympathetic influence. In asthmatics, however, β-antagonists cause bronchoconstriction, suggesting that adrenergic mechanisms are important in counteracting bronchospasm. NANC nerves were originally thought to be anatomically distinct from the autonomic nerves, but recent evidence suggests that NANC effects are mediated by the release of neurotransmitters from classic autonomic nerves (4, 5) and are, hence, thought to "fine tune" the autonomic system.

Hormones and neurotransmitters mediate airway tone by activating specific cell receptors. Acetylcholine released from parasympathetic postganglionic nerve endings stimulates muscarinic cholinergic receptors. These receptors are present in smooth muscle of large airways (6), the density of which decreases towards the terminal bronchioles (7). Hence, in humans, effects of anticholinergic drugs are more pronounced on larger airways, as compared with those on small airways (8).

Norepinephrine released by the sympathetic nerves and epinephrine released by the adrenal medulla mediate adrenergic mechanisms; these catecholamines activate α- and β-adrenoceptors on target cells (9, 10). β_2-receptors are present on airway smooth muscle, the density of which increases distally from the trachea to the smaller airways. β_1-receptors are absent and, hence, β_1 selective agonists exert no effect on the

114

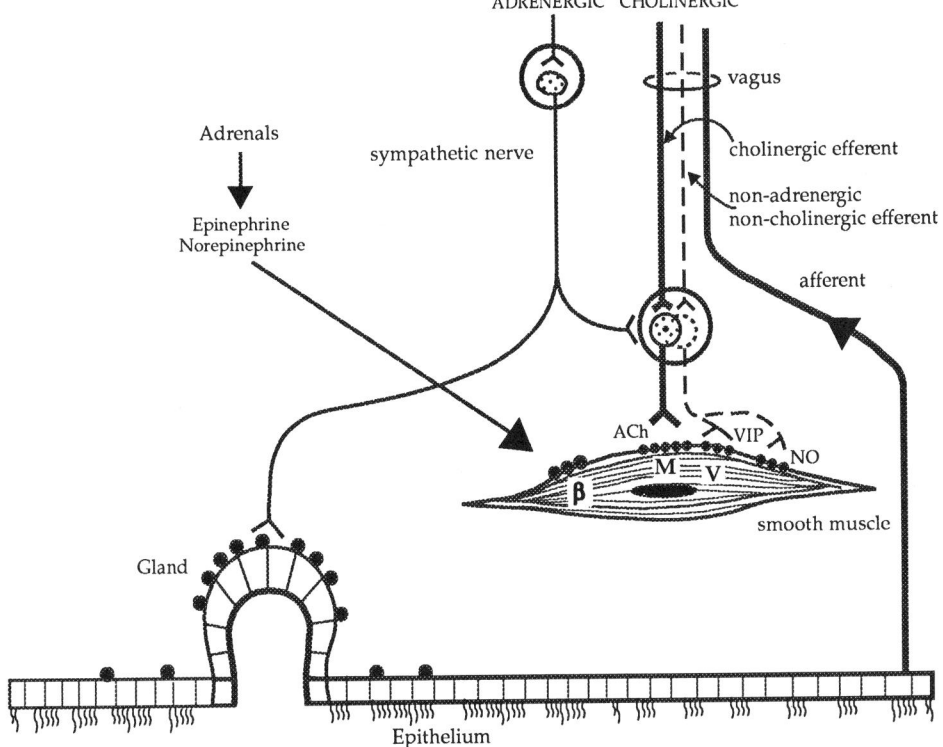

Figure 6.1. Innervation of human airway smooth muscle. The three components of the autonomic nervous system: adrenergic; cholinergic; and the noncholinergic, nonadrenergic pathway (*dashed lines*), which has both dilating and constricting effects on airway smooth muscle, the neurotransmitter of which is likely to be vasoactive intestinal peptide (*VIP*) and nitric oxide (*NO*). Specific receptors for these neurotransmitters present on airway smooth muscle cells: β, β-adrenergic; *M*, muscarinic cholinergic; *V*, VIP; and *Ach*, acetylcholine. (Modified from Barnes PJ: Neural control of airway smooth muscle. In Crystal RG, West JB (eds): *The Lung: Scientific Foundation*, vol 1. Raven Press, New York, 1991.)

human airway (9). Subtypes of α-receptors have been demonstrated in the human airway (11); α_1-receptors mediate contractile effects, and presynaptic α_2-receptors mediate negative feedback of norepinephrine release. Evidence exists for α-adrenergic hyperresponsiveness in the airways of asthmatics (12, 13), which may be "turned on" by inflammatory mediators (10, 14). However, α-blockers have not shown to be beneficial in asthma.

Although NANC nerves were originally thought of as an anatomically separate nervous system, the current thinking is that NANC effects are mediated by the release of several types of neurotransmitters from autonomic nerves (4). Release of vasoactive intestinal peptide and nitric oxide from cholinergic nerves mediates smooth muscle relaxation, whereas tachykinins released retrogradely from unmyelinated sensory nerves may facilitate cholinergic neurotransmission that produces bronchoconstriction. Specific clinical agents to manipulate this system are not yet available.

Airway patency normally depends on the balance between relaxant (via β-adrenergic receptors) and contractile (through α-adrenergic and cholinergic receptors) influences on bronchial smooth muscle cells. β-adrenergic receptor stimulation results in stimulation of adenylate cyclase, an enzyme that increases the production of cyclic AMP (cAMP). Conversely, cholinergic and α-receptor stimulation enhances cGMP production, while α-receptor stimulation can also reduce cAMP production by modulating phosphatidylinositol metabolism. Cyclic AMP apparently produces cell relaxation and is counteracted by cGMP, which tends to cause cell contraction.

β-ADRENERGIC AGENTS

Structure

Asthma treatment was initiated by the introduction of ephedrine more than 5000 years ago in China. Epinephrine appeared at the turn of the century, followed by the introduction of isoproterenol and ephedrine. Selective β_2 agonist agents were developed after investigations increased the understanding of the structure-function relation of the β-adrenergic drugs, which are discussed in several reviews (15–18).

Briefly, the β-adrenergic drugs are phenylethylamine derivatives containing two distinct regions: a benzene ring, which is important primarily for potency and secondarily for stability (duration of action) and selectivity to the β_1- and β_2-receptors, and an ethanolamine side chain, which confers selectivity and, to a lesser extent, potency (Fig. 6.2). For example, the most potent drugs (catecholamines) have hydroxyl groups substituted in the 3 and 4 positions of the benzene ring (known as catechol), a hydroxyl group at the β-carbon, a small group at the α-carbon (R_1) and a small N-substituted group (R_2). Selectivity is enhanced by increasing R_2 size, substitution of an ethyl group on the α-carbon (R_1), and a change of the catechol ring to resorcinol or saligenin. The resorcinols include metaproterenol, terbutaline, and fenoterol, whereas the only currently available saligenin is albuterol. A trade-off of potency for selectivity is necessary to diminish the unwanted cardiovascular side effects due to β_1 activation, provided that the decrease in potency is more than offset by the increase in selectivity.

Mode of Action

The β-adrenergic drugs act by stimulating β_2-adrenergic receptors, causing an increase in levels of cAMP, which produces bronchial smooth muscle relaxation (16).

Pharmacokinetics

The catecholamines are metabolized by monoamine oxidase (MAO) located in the presynaptic neurons and by catechol-*o*-methyltransferase (COMT) found in the liver, kidney, lung, erythrocytes, and the intestinal wall, which precludes the oral administration of these agents. However, the noncatecholamine β-adrenergic agonists metaproterenol, terbutaline (resorcinols), and albuterol (saligenin) are resistant to both MAO and COMT, prolonging their half-life and making them useful as oral agents.

The peak blood concentration of β-adrenergic agonists following oral administration and subcutaneous injection is 3 to 4 hours and 10 to 15 minutes, respectively (19). The peak blood concentration following inhalation of β-adrenergic agonists occurs earlier and is several times lower than that following oral or parenteral administration (20). The half-life of β-adrenergic drugs is quite variable: 3 minutes for epinephrine and isoproterenol; 1.5 hours for metaproterenol; 10 to 12 hours for terbutaline; and 3.5 to 4.6 hours for albuterol (21).

For oral or parenteral administration, the bronchodilation is closely related to blood levels, as are the systemic side effects. Following inhalation, the bronchodilating effect is independent of blood levels; consequently, the chance for systemic side effects is rarely observed.

Time Course of Bronchodilation

After oral administration, the β_2-agonists begin to dilate the bronchi after 30 minutes (22–24). A peak effect is reached after 1 to 2 hours and is maintained for 3 to 6 hours. The bronchodilating effects of subcutaneous administered epinephrine and terbutaline appear within a few minutes, peak in 15 to 20 minutes, and persist for 120 minutes for epinephrine and 180 to 240 minutes for terbutaline (25, 26). The intravenous administration of β-adrenergic agonists produces rapid, blood-related respiratory changes (27–30).

Depending on the drug used, the time course of bronchodilation produced by inhaled β-adrenergic agonists can follow two patterns (20, 22, 31, 32). The first pattern is a brisk, almost instantaneous onset of bronchodilation (within 1 to 3 minutes), reaching a peak at 5 to 15 minutes and progressively wearing off after 30 minutes to 1 hour. The drugs showing this pattern of response are all catecholamines. The second pattern, characteristic for inhaled resorcinols and saligenins, consists of a slower onset of bronchodilation (3 to 6 minutes), a delayed peak (20 to 60 minutes), and a sustained effect (4 to 6 hours).

Administration

The inhaled route is preferred for management of acute bronchoconstriction because (*a*) direct application of the drug

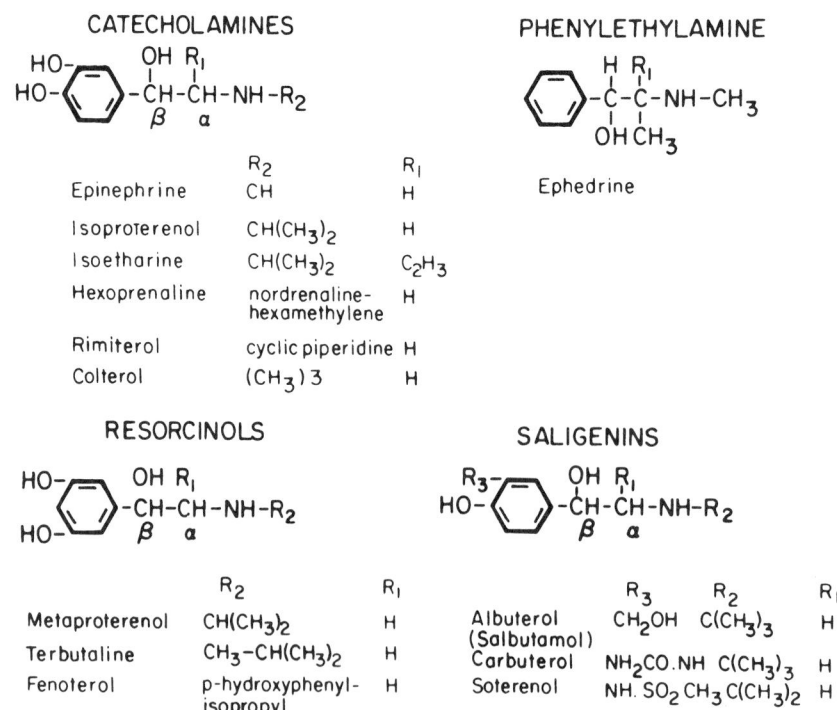

Figure 6.2. Chemical structures of β-adrenergic drugs. (Modified from Popa V: Beta-adrenergic drugs. In Ziment I, Popa V (eds): *Clinics in Chest Medicine: Respiratory Pharmacology,* vol 7. WB Saunders, Philadelphia, 1986.)

necessitates only a small quantity required for a therapeutic response, thereby minimizing side effects and (*b*) the onset of action is shorter than after oral administration and comparable with intravenous dosing. Additionally, several studies have shown that results with aerosol agents are equal to or better than those given parenterally (27–30, 33, 34).

Inhalation of drugs may be accomplished with a pressurized, fluorocarbon-powered, metered-dose inhaler (MDI) or a nebulizer driven by compressed air or ultrasound. MDIs and nebulizers deliver less than 10% of the administered dose to the small airways (35–37), and in intubated patients, less than 6% of the delivered dose is deposited in the lower respiratory tract for both modes of administration (38, 39). For MDIs, approximately 10% of the aerosol remains at the activator orifice; 80% impacts in the oropharynx; 9% is deposited in the lung; and only 1% is exhaled. Compared with MDIs, the nebulizers lead to a smaller deposition in the oropharynx (80% vs. 2%), but a larger proportion of the aerosol remains in the aerosolizer (about 10% vs. 70%) or is exhaled (about 1% vs. 10%).

Although the dose of β-adrenergic drugs currently prescribed for a nebulizer (e.g., 15 mg of metaproterenol) is 10 to 15 times higher than that delivered with an MDI (e.g., 0.065 mg of metaproterenol per puff), studies have shown comparable effects of repetitive MDI inhalations with nebulizer delivery (40–42), suggesting the inefficiency of nebulization. This observation, coupled with the decreased costs and ease of administration associated with MDIs compared with nebulizers suggest that MDIs should be used more frequently in intubated, mechanically ventilated adult patients (38, 39). Adapters are available to directly attach a MDI to a ventilator circuit. Nebulizers, however, may be preferred over MDIs in the nonintubated patient, because the acutely dyspneic patient may be unable to achieve proper hand-breath coordination. Spontaneously breathing patients may use a nebulizer with either a mouthpiece or a face mask.

Subcutaneous or intravenous β-agonist therapy may be considered in the face of refractory severe bronchoconstriction, based on the belief that the inhaled route may not deliver adequate drug because of severely obstructed airways (43). Agents available for subcutaneous use include epinephrine and terbutaline, whereas agents administered intravenously include isoproterenol and albuterol (34, 44, 44a). Intravenous administration, however, is associated with more cardiovascular side effects, compared with the inhalation route, and rebound bronchospasm may occur after discontinuation of the infusion.

Dosing

Table 6.1.

Side Effects

The most common adverse effects of β-adrenergic agents are skeletal muscle tremor, nervousness, tachycardia, and palpitations (45) and are due to stimulation of both $β_1$- and $β_2$-receptors. Tachycardia can represent either a direct $β_1$ effect or an indirect $β_2$ stimulation (reflex tachycardia secondary to marked peripheral vasodilation). Tachycardia is the dose-limiting side effect of nonselective β-agonists, whereas tremor limits the use of selective $β_2$-agonists. The side effects mediated via $β_1$-receptors are inevitable when $β_2$-agonists are administered intravenously, parenterally, or orally in large doses. The incidence of all side effects is very low following inhalation.

Other side effects occurring after relatively high subcutaneous, intravenous, or oral doses are headache, dizziness, nausea, weakness, sweating, mismatching of ventilation/perfusion (causing falls in PO_2), and paradoxical bronchoconstrictor response to inhaled catecholamines (observed particularly in status asthmaticus) (46–48). Significant hypokalemia following parenteral administration of β-adrenergic agonists has also been observed recently (49–51).

Tolerance

Diminished responsiveness, or tolerance, to bronchodilators may occur when receptors are repeatedly exposed to high concentrations of β-adrenergic agonist (52–56). The response to inhaled β-agonists, therefore, may be reduced considerably in patients with prolonged bronchospasm and may pertain to the β-adrenergic drugs with which the patient has been treated; hence, changing the β-agonist may overcome the tolerance.

Clinical Use

Bronchodilation represents the main therapeutic effect of β-adrenergic drugs in asthma. Other beneficial effects in asthma include an increase in ciliary movement (57a–c) and prevention of degranulation and release of mediators from sensitized mast cells challenged with the appropriate allergens (58–60).

ANTICHOLINERGIC AGENTS

This group of pharmacologic agents have a long and colorful history as medications, magic potions, and preferred poisons. Herbal preparations rich in belladonna and stramonium alkaloids were used by Indian and Middle Eastern civilizations for centuries for the treatment of asthma. These herbal formulations were introduced to Western medicine in the 19th century when British military physicians returned from India (61). Formulated as powders and dried leaves for inhalation or smoking, these "fuming asthma remedies" were the mainstay of bronchodilator therapy throughout Europe and North America in the 19th century. The popularity of these substances in the U.S. waned in the 1920s with the introduction of epinephrine as a pharmacologic preparation. Interest in this family of substances was rekindled in the 1970s, when a clear understanding of the parasympathetic nervous system in modulating airway tone was achieved and when the quaternary ammonium antimuscarinic drugs with favorable properties became available.

Structure

The alkaloid drugs obtained from the solanaceous plants contain tropine, a tertiary base that is esterified with 1-tropic acid to form tropine tropate, which upon racemization becomes atropine (Fig. 6.3). The atropinic compounds and acetylcholine contain three similar groups critical for activation of muscarinic receptors, the N-CH3 group, the ester O atom,

Table 6.1. β-Adrenergic Agonists

Drug	Preparation	Route of Administration	Dosage	
Epinephrine	1 mg/ml	Sub Q	Adult:	0.1–0.5 mg, repeated in 20–30 min
			Pediatric:	0.01 mg/kg
Epinephrine (racemic)	2.25% solution	Aerosol	Adult:	0.3–1.0 ml
			Pediatric:	0.3–0.6 ml
Isoproterenol	0.5% solution (5 mg/ml)	IV	Pediatric:	0.05–1.5 μg/kg/min
Metaproterenol	5% solution	Aerosol	Adult:	0.3 ml (15 mg) q2–4h
			Pediatric:	0.25–0.5 mg/kg q2–4h
	MDI (0.65 mg/puff)	Aerosol	Adult:	2–3 puffs q2–6h
			Pediatric:	1–3 puffs q4–6h
Terbutaline	0.1% solution	Sub Q	Adult:	0.2–0.4 ml (repeated in 15–30 min)
			Pediatric:	0.2 mg/kg, max = 6 mg
	MDI (0.2 mg/puff)	Aerosol	Adult:	1–2 puffs q4–6h
			Pediatric:	1–2 puffs q4–6h
Albuterol	5% solution	Aerosol	Adult:	2.5–5 mg q2–4h
			Pediatric:	0.05–0.15 mg q4–6h
	MDI (90 mg/puff)	Aerosol	Adult:	1–2 puffs q2–4h
			Pediatric:	1–2 puffs q4–6h
	5% solution	IV	Adult:	100 μg bolus followed by 300 μg in 15 min, 0.05–0.2 μg/kg/min
			Pediatric:	0.05–0.2 μg/kg/min

and the CO group but, the replacement of the acetyl group with a more bulky subunit in the atropinic compounds results in competitive blocking of the muscarinic receptor. Additions made to the nitrogen on the tropic acid subunit of the atropine molecule create charged derivatives (glycopyrrolate and ipratropium), which are poorly absorbed from the mucosal surfaces (62, 63).

Mode of Action

The atropinic compounds effectively compete with acetylcholine at the receptor site, causing inhibition of the generation of intracellular cGMP. The main effects are on the larger airways, with little action on small airways because muscarinic receptors occur mostly in the upper airway and are sparse in the terminal bronchi and bronchioles (64).

Pharmacokinetics

Atropine, the prototype antimuscarinic drug, is effective when given topically, orally, or by injection and is quickly and completely absorbed from mucosal surfaces and from the gastrointestinal tract. The serum half-life of absorbed medication is about 3 hours. After an aerosol dose, bronchodilation occurs in 15 minutes, peaks at approximately 1 hour, and persists for 4 to 6 hours (65, 66). Atropine disappears from the blood rapidly and is distributed throughout the body, including the central nervous system. Half of the drug is excreted unchanged in the urine and much of the rest as unknown metabolites.

The synthetic quaternary ammonium compounds are poorly absorbed from the mucosa and gut, which reduces major systemic side effects, and do not cross the blood-brain barrier, which minimizes central nervous system activity. Glycopyrrolate, used parenterally in the operating room to block vagal reflexes and to reduce gastric acid secretions, is widely used as an aerosol to produce bronchodilation that will begin in 15 minutes

and persist for 6 to 8 hours (67). Ipratropium bromide, available for administration as a metered-dose inhaler (MDI) (approved in the U.S.) and a solution (not approved in the U.S.), produces bronchodilation with 15 minutes, peaks at 1 hour, and persists for 4 to 6 hours. Higher doses increase the peak and extend the duration of action (68).

Dosing

Inhalation is the preferred mode for delivery of anticholinergic bronchodilators (Table 6.2).

Side Effects

The adverse effects associated with atropine include: palpitations; blurred vision; tachycardia; mydriasis; headache; weakness; speech disturbance; dysphagia; hot, dry, flushed skin; and urinary retention. These effects are dose-related and are greatly reduced when atropine is administered as an aerosol. The incidence of systemic side effects for the quaternary ammonium compounds is extremely low following inhalation. Atropine decreases mucous secretions, transmucosal electrolyte and water flux, ciliary motility, and mucous transport (69–71). Ipratropium bromide does not affect any of these functions, but data on whether inhalation of this agent decreases the volume of secretions in patients who have asthma or chronic bronchitis are conflicting (72–75).

Clinical Uses

Compared with β-adrenergic agonists, anticholinergic agents have a slower onset of action and, therefore, are not considered primary therapy for acute bronchospasm. However, the addition of an anticholinergic agent may enhance the bronchodilatory effects of a β-adrenergic agonist acting alone and extend the time course of bronchodilation (76, 77). Furthermore, these agents may be more effective than β-adrenergic agents for patients with chronic obstructive pulmonary disease (COPD), because their effects on larger airways may be more pronounced, compared with those of adrenergic aerosols, whose greatest effects are on the smaller airways (78–82).

THEOPHYLLINE

STRUCTURE

Theophylline (1,3-dimethylxanthine), together with caffeine (1,3,7-trimethylxanthine), are pharmacologically classified as methylxanthines. These compounds naturally occur in various plants and re found in tea, coffee, cola, chocolate, and cocoa. Theophylline was initially used for the treatment of

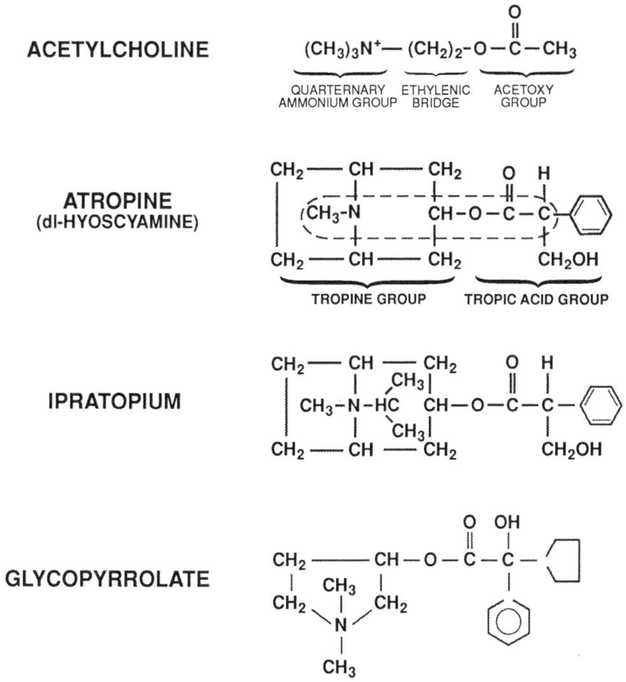

Figure 6.3. The stereochemical structure of acetylcholine that is responsible for receptor stimulation and shared by atropine (*dotted lines*) and other anticholinergic agents. Atropine is a tertiary ammonium compound, whereas glycopyrrolate and ipratropium are quaternary ammonium compounds. (Modified from Popa V: Anticholinergic Agents, In Ziment I, Popa V: *Clinics In Chest Medicine: Respiratory Pharmacology*, Vol 7. W.B. Saunders Company, Philadelphia, 1986.)

asthma more than 100 years ago (83), but its use did not become widespread until after 1936 (84).

Aminophylline, the "salt" form of theophylline, is a mixture of theophylline and the base ethylenediamine, which confers water solubility on the insoluble theophylline. By weight, aminophylline is 80% theophylline. The therapeutic activity of this salt form is attributed solely to theophylline. However, ethylenediamine can induce hypersensitivity reactions characterized by urticaria, generalized pruritus, angioedema, and bronchospasm (85).

MODE OF ACTION

For many years the pharmacologic action of theophylline in producing relaxation of bronchial smooth muscle had been attributed to an increase in intracellular cAMP levels via phosphodiesterase inhibition (86). Several observations, however, raise questions about the validity of this concept. First, the concentration of theophylline required to inhibit phosphodiesterase in vitro is higher than can be achieved therapeutically in humans (87, 88). Second, several chemically synthesized derivatives of theophylline that are extremely potent inhibitors of phosphodiesterase have been ineffective as bronchodilators (86, 89). Finally, theophylline-induced relaxation of contracted smooth muscle in isolated organ preparations does not correlate with significant changes in either cAMP or cGMP levels (89).

Alternatively, evidence suggests that theophylline may act as an adenosine antagonist (90, 91). Adenosine and theophylline are structurally similar, and theophylline competitively inhibits adenosine receptors in various tissues at concentrations well within its therapeutic range. Furthermore, adenosine-induced bronchoconstriction in asthmatic patients is reversed by inhaled theophylline, and the tracheorelaxant effect of theophylline is dose-dependently inhibited by adenosine (92, 93). However, enprofylline, a new xanthine that is more potent than theophylline as a bronchodilator, has little adenosine-blocking activity (94, 95). Other possible mechanisms of action include inhibition of intracellular calcium activity (96), prostaglandin antagonism (97), stimulation of endogenous catecholamines release (98), β-agonist activity (99), and inhibition of cGMP metabolism (100).

PHARMACOKINETICS

Many studies have been performed investigating the pharmacokinetics of theophylline (101–104). The volume of distribution of theophylline is between 0.3 and 0.7 liters/kg body

Table 6.2. Anticholinergic Drugs

Drug	Preparation	Route of Administration	Dosage	
Atropine	0.2 (0.5% solution)	Aerosol	Adult:	0.025–0.1 mg/kg q4–6h
			Pediatric:	0.025–0.1 mg/kg q4–6h
Glycopyrrolate	0.02% solution	IV	Adult:	0.1–0.2 mg
		Aerosol	Adult:	0.8–1.6 mg q6–8h
Ipratropium	MDI, 20 μg/puff	Aerosol	Adult:	2–4 puffs qid
			Pediatric:	1–2 puffs tid
	0.025% solution (Europe only)	Aerosol	Adult:	100–500 μg q6h

weight in adults and children and is not affected by sex, age, smoking, pulmonary edema, or asthma (104). It is increased in the presence of hepatic cirrhosis (105) and decreased in the presence of obesity (106).

Theophylline is about 90% metabolized by the liver microsomal system to inactive uric acid derivatives or to weakly active methylxanthine derivatives via oxidation and demethylation. The uric acid metabolites of theophylline have no known pharmacologic activity, whereas the metabolite, 3-methylxanthine, is characterized by a long biologic half-life and has pharmacologic and toxicologic actions similar to those of theophylline (107). This metabolite has the potential to produce theophylline toxicity in the presence of a therapeutic serum level of theophylline. The remaining 10% of theophylline is excreted unchanged through the kidneys.

Multiple factors affect the clearance of theophylline, and, therefore, the half-life of theophylline varies widely between individuals and even within individuals during changing conditions. For example, clearance of theophylline has been shown to vary with age (108, 109). In normal and asthmatic adults, the half-life ranges from 2.9 to 12.8 hours with a mean of approximately 5.8 hours (102, 103). In children, who metabolize theophylline faster than adults, the half-life varies from 1.4 to 7.9 hours with a mean of 3.7 hours (103, 110, 111). Theophylline clearance is reduced in infants and elderly patients. In infants, the decreased clearance is related to oxidative pathways that have not yet been established (112), whereas in elderly patients, the decrease in clearance is attributed to a relative loss in either functional activity or the amount of enzymes available (109).

Theophylline clearance is enhanced by polycyclic hydrocarbons in cigarette smoke (113–115), marijuana smoke (115), phenytoin (116), and phenobarbital (117, 118), whereas cimetidine (119, 120) and oral contraceptives (121) reduce cytochrome-related enzyme activity and decrease theophylline breakdown. Ranitidine, however, which is structurally dissimilar from cimetidine, has little effect on theophylline clearance (122). Hence, in situations where H_2-receptor blocking is required for a patient receiving theophylline, ranitidine should be the preferred drug.

Diets low in protein but high in carbohydrates give rise to lower rates of metabolism, whereas charcoal-broiled beef and a xanthine-free diet shorten theophylline half-life (123, 124).

The effects of erythromycin on theophylline clearance are unclear (125–130). No effects on theophylline kinetics were found when erythromycin was given for less than 5 days (125–127), whereas a decrease in elimination has been shown with longer duration (128–130). Alternatively, other studies have suggested that patients with chronic bronchitis or asthma may be more susceptible to interference of theophylline metabolism by erythromycin than normal healthy individuals (131, 132).

Since theophylline metabolism is dependent on the integrity of the liver and on hepatic blood flow, the half-life of theophylline is prolonged in patients with congestive heart failure, cor pulmonale, chronic obstructive pulmonary disease, or liver disease (105, 133–137). The half-life is also prolonged in patients with obesity (106) and viral upper respiratory infections (138).

The effect of acidemia on theophylline kinetics is controversial (139–142). Initially, investigators observed an inverse correlation between arterial pH and volume of distribution, but recent work has failed to substantiate these findings.

Few studies have investigated the pharmacokinetics of theophylline during pregnancy (143, 144). Clearance of theophylline in patients between 5 and 8 months of gestation has been reported to be unchanged, but volume of distribution, however, was increased. Hence, dosage adjustments appear to be prudent in pregnant patients, with increases adjusted to the patient's weight gain. Although theophylline crosses the placenta, there is no clear evidence for teratogenicity.

DOSING

Theophylline is manufactured as a variety of salts for oral, rectal, and parenteral administration, but it is the intravenous forms of theophylline that carry relevance for critically ill patients.

Several considerations warrant careful dosage titration when administering theophylline and for maintaining theophylline levels lower than the high end of the "therapeutic range." First, theophylline elimination has been shown to be dose-dependent at high plasma concentrations (zero-order kinetics) and, hence, a small change in dose can cause excessively high concentrations of theophylline (145). The concentration achieved may be well above that predicted from a previously determined rate of elimination in a given patient (146, 147).

Second, theophylline's effects on bronchodilation occur in proportion to the log of the serum or plasma concentration over the range of 5 to 25 μg/ml. The significance of this "log linear" relationship is that increases in indices of pulmonary function do not occur in proportion to the increase in the blood level of theophylline. Specifically, the increase in pulmonary function that occurs between a serum level of 15 and 20 μg/ml is not as great as that occurring between a serum level of 10 and 15 μg/ml. Hence as the theophylline level is increased in this former range, there is some increase in therapeutic effectiveness but with an increase in the likelihood of drug side effects (147).

Finally, because bronchodilation can be produced at the lower end of the therapeutic range (2 to 10 μg/ml) and because toxicity can occur in the high end of the therapeutic range (10 to 20 μg/ml), theophylline levels should be maintained between 5 and 10 μg/ml in those critically ill patients in whom theophylline's adverse side effects may not be well-tolerated.

Loading Dose

In clinical situations of acute bronchospasm, an intravenous loading dose of theophylline given over 30 minutes will rapidly establish a steady-state, therapeutic blood level of theophylline. The loading dose is given over 30 minutes to avoid the risk of inducing cardiac arrhythmia and blood pressure changes that can occur with rapid intravenous administration.

For the acutely ill patient who has not had any theophylline medications in the previous 24 hours, a loading dose of 5.6 mg/kg (calculated on the basis of the ideal body weight) of aminophylline will generate a mean serum level of theophylline of 10 μg/ml, with a range between 5 and 25 μg/ml. If

Table 6.3. Initial Intravenous Theophylline Maintenance Dosages

Patient Population	Theophylline Infusion Rate (mg/kg/hr)
Children 1 to 9 years old	0.8
Children over 9 years old	0.6
Healthy smokers (adult)	0.8
Healthy nonsmokers (adults)	0.5
Patient age > 60 years	0.3
Congestive heart failure or liver disease	0.2

the risk of toxicity is a concern, one-half the loading dose should be given instead. For patients taking oral theophylline compounds, one-half the calculated loading dose is administered intravenously if 12 hours or more have elapsed since ingestion of the last oral dose. An intravenous loading dose is not necessary if a long-acting oral dose of theophylline was taken within the preceding 12 hours.

If the patient has a known, subtherapeutic serum level of theophylline, the loading dose of theophylline to produce a higher serum concentration can be calculated as follows:

Loading dose (mg/kg) = [Desired serum level (μg/ml) − existing serum level (μg/ml)] × 0.5 liters/kg

Measurement of theophylline level should be performed within 1 hour after the completion of the intravenous loading dose, which allows for equilibrium distribution of theophylline from the central circulatory compartment into the peripheral tissue compartment.

Maintenance Therapy

The wide variability in theophylline metabolism among patients precludes the recommendation of one dosage for maintenance therapy for all patients. Instead, Table 6.3 may be used to estimate the initial maintenance dosage. Subsequently, the theophylline level should be determined approximately 12 to 18 hours after the institution of maintenance therapy and at intervals thereafter in order to achieve the proper individualization of the maintenance dosage rate to match the patient's rate of metabolism of theophylline.

SIDE EFFECTS

Toxicity due to theophylline is dose-related, but there is a wide variability among patients in the overlapping of the therapeutic and toxic serum ranges for theophylline. This overlapping of the therapeutic window with toxicity levels can occur even in the conventional range of 10 to 20 μg/ml.

Nonlife-threatening adverse effects of theophylline include gastrointestinal effects such as nausea, vomiting, and heartburn, which are both locally and centrally mediated. Central nervous system stimulation causes irritability, insomnia, and tremor (89).

Life-threatening adverse effects associated with theophylline administration are seizures and cardiac arrhythmias. Seizures occur with increasing frequency when serum theophylline concentrations are greater than 40 μg/ml and are particularly dangerous, because they may occur without warning signs of toxicity and are often refractory to usual anticonvulsant therapy (148). Mortality associated with theophylline-induced seizures has been reported to be about 50% (148).

A wide variety of cardiac rhythm disturbances can occur with theophylline administration. Theophylline enhances atrial automaticity (149) and accelerates intracardiac conduction (150). Sinus tachycardia is among the most common manifestations of theophylline toxicity, but its administration has also been associated with the development of supraventricular tacharrhythmias, such as multifocal atrial tachycardia, atrial fibrillation, and paroxysmal supraventricular tachycardia (151–154). Investigators have observed multifocal atrial tachycardia in elderly patients with therapeutic serum concentrations (154, 155).

Ventricular ectopy is rare in therapeutic doses, but during toxicity, frequent ventricular premature beats and, rarely, ventricular tachycardia may be present (156–159). Fortunately, these ventricular arrhythmias usually respond to lidocaine.

Metabolic disturbances associated with theophylline intoxication include hyperglycemia, hypophosphatemia, hypercalcemia, metabolic acidosis, and hypokalemia (160–163), with the latter being seen more frequently with acute, as opposed to chronic, overdose (163).

Other adverse reactions attributed to theophylline include incompetency of the lower esophageal sphincter (164), potentiation of sodium nitroprusside-induced hypotension (165), and suppression of pulmonary antibacterial defenses (166).

MANAGEMENT OF OVERDOSE

Methods that increase theophylline clearance include charcoal hemoperfusion (167) and administration of oral activated charcoal (168, 169). Prophylactic charcoal hemoperfusion has been recommended for patients with levels above 60 μg/ml resulting from an acute overdose (170–172). In contrast, in patients with a chronic overdose, life-threatening events are not predictable by using serum levels (173–176) and, therefore, initial treatment with oral charcoal therapy is recommended in these patients with non-life-threatening events, because hemoperfusion may be associated with adverse effects.

CURRENT ROLE IN BRONCHODILATOR THERAPY

Although once a mainstay in the treatment of bronchospasm, the importance of theophylline in the management of the critically ill patient with acute bronchospasm has been redefined during the past 10 years due to the emergence of more powerful aerosolized drugs, concerns with toxicity, and studies showing that theophylline administration does not add to the bronchodilating effects of β-agonist therapy (177–181). Hence, doses of aerosolized β-agonists, anticholinergics, and intravenous steroids should be maximized before therapy is begun with intravenous aminophylline.

In addition to airway smooth muscle bronchodilation, other effects of theophylline on the pulmonary system include acceleration of mucociliary clearance (182–184), stimulation of the respiratory center (185–187), and enhancement of diaphragmatic contractility (188–194), although the clinical significance of this latter effect remains to be elucidated. Nonpulmonary properties of theophylline include enhanced inotropy of both the right and left ventricles (195); dilation of the coronary, pulmonary, renal, and systemic arterioles and veins (196); diuresis (85, 86); relaxation of the smooth muscle of the gallbladder and gastrointestinal tract (85); suppression of responses to mast cell mediators (197, 198); and reduction in cerebral blood flow (199, 200).

CORTICOSTEROIDS

Glucocorticoids, rather than mineralocorticoids, are used to treat asthma and other pulmonary diseases. The standard oral agent is prednisone, which has a short plasma half-life of about 1 hour. It is relatively slow in onset of actions and is converted in the liver to its active congener, prednisolone; hence, it is less effective in patients with severe liver disease. For intravenous use, methylprednisolone is the standard agent, which has a plasma half-life of about 3 to 4 hours, but its physiological effects may persist for about 24 hours. Topical steroid preparations for inhalational use include beclomethasone, triamcinolone, and flunisolide.

Several mechanisms may be postulated to account for the bronchodilator actions of corticosteroids. Steroids may enhance the responsiveness of β_2 receptors to both endogenous catecholamines and administered sympathomimetic drugs (201, 202). This effect may be due to either an increase in the number of β-adrenergic receptors on smooth muscle cells or an increase in the proportion of receptors in the high-affinity state (203–205). The clinical relevance, however, of β-adrenergic receptor dysfunction in patients with bronchospasm remains controversial (206, 207).

Glucocorticoids also exert antiinflammatory actions via the inhibition of arachidonic acid metabolism, reduction in the release of inflammatory mediators, inhibition of interleukin-2 by lymphocytes, and suppression of immunoglobulin E (IgE) binding by receptors (208). Finally, corticosteroids may improve pulmonary function by enhancing mucociliary clearance, either by reducing mediator-induced mucous secretion or by their effects on epithelial inflammation (209–212).

INDICATIONS

Asthma

Although steroids are effective in chronic asthma, their use in treatment of acute exacerbations of asthma is less clear (213–216). Several studies have failed to document any early additive effect of steroids when administered with β-adrenergic agents (217, 218). Other investigations, however, have suggested an earlier onset for steroid action (219), and two recent studies showed a decreased hospital admission rate in those asthmatic patients who received an early dose of steroids (220, 221). Other studies (222–224) have demonstrated a delayed onset of steroid effects on pulmonary function, usually 6 to 12 hours after administration. Hence, the main value of corticosteroids in asthma is probably for hastening the resolution of attack, rather than treating the initial severity.

The appropriate dosage of steroids is still controversial. A study by Haskell and colleagues (224) showed that 125 mg of methylprednisolone every 6 hours produced slightly more rapid improvement than 40 mg every 6 hours; low-dose therapy (15 mg every 6 hours) was ineffective. Other studies (225–227), however, have failed to demonstrate an enhanced effect with high-dose steroid therapy, as compared to that with low-dose therapy. The current recommendation is to administer 40 mg of methylprednisolone every 6 hours intravenously for 36 to 48 hours (depending on the patient's condition), followed by a tapering regimen with oral prednisone (227a).

The major value of the aerosolized corticosteroid preparations in bronchospasm is to allow a substantial decrease in the oral steroid dose for the stable patient. There is no role for these agents in the treatment of the acute critically ill patient with bronchospasm.

Chronic Obstructive Pulmonary Disease

The value of corticosteroids in patients with chronic obstructive lung disease remains unclear (228). Albert and colleagues (229) showed an improvement in pulmonary function with the administration of steroids in acute exacerbation of COPD. However, these favorable results may have been due to a statistical artifact (230), and others have reported that steroid therapy has not been found to be useful in the emergency management of COPD (231). Steroid therapy may be useful in the subset of COPD patients who have a predominant asthmatic component and may enhance mucus secretion in selected cases (209–212).

Adult Respiratory Distress Syndrome

Although several authors (232–235) have suggested a role for steroids in the treatment of the adult respiratory disease syndrome (ARDS), large prospective clinical trials have failed to observe an effect of steroids in preventing ARDS in patients with the sepsis syndrome (236–240). Finally, when given to patients with established ARDS, corticosteroids do not alter outcome (241). Recent reports (242, 243), however, have documented a beneficial effect on the early fibrotic phase in ARDS, but these studies were not controlled.

Fat Emboli

Several reports, including a placebo-controlled trial, suggest a beneficial value of prophylactic administration of steroids in patients with a high risk of fat embolism syndrome (244–246).

Pneumonitis

No benefits have been observed with the administration of steroids for severe pulmonary infections or for direct irritative events, such as aspiration, near-drowning, smoke inhalation, or chemical exposure (247–250).

Pneumocystis carinii Pneumonia

Several studies (251–252b) have demonstrated that early adjunctive corticosteroid therapy can improve survival and decrease the likelihood of respiratory failure in patients with *Pneumocystis* pneumonia associated with moderate or severe pulmonary dysfunction as defined by an arterial oxygen pressure of less than 70 mm Hg (breathing room air) or an arterial-alveolar gradient of more than 35 mm Hg. The recommended dose is prednisone (40 mg bid) or methylprednisolone (40 mg every 6 hr, followed by a tapered regimen over a 3-week period) (253).

MAGNESIUM SULFATE

The bronchodilating effects of magnesium sulfate ($MgSO_4$) in bronchial asthma were first recognized more than 50 years ago (254). Recently, investigators have demonstrated (255–257) in patients with mild-to-severe asthma a rapid improvement in pulmonary functions with intravenously administered $MgSO_4$ (0.40 to 0.50 mmol/min). These effects, however, were temporary and significantly less than those observed with an aerosolized β_2 agonist. Administration of magnesium has been effective in severe acute cases of asthma that did not respond to β_2-agonist therapy (258–260) and, therefore, its use should be considered in this clinical situation.

The mechanism of action of magnesium may be due to an effect on calcium homeostasis (261–263). Results from a canine model (264) suggest that $MgSO_4$, like nifedipine, acts in the airway as a voltage-sensitive calcium channel blocker. Alternatively, magnesium may potentiate the effects of β-adrenergic agonists (265), inhibit histamine release from mast cells (266, 267), or inhibit acetylcholine release from cholinergic nerve terminals (268).

MUCOLYTICS

Although the use of physical methods to improve mucus clearance is well-known to the critical care physician, the use and efficacy of pharmacologic methods has been largely ignored due to the lack of well-designed clinical trials, the lack of objective measures of benefit, and uncertainty about the type of patients who are likely to benefit from this therapeutic modality.

Respiratory tract secretions in the tracheobronchial tree originate mainly from the submucosal bronchial glands and goblet cells. The submucosal glands are well-supplied by cholinergic fibers from the vagus nerve and, when stimulated, produce a fluid of relatively low viscosity. These glands are poorly supplied by sympathomimetic nerves. In contrast, the goblet cells are not controlled by the autonomic nervous system but respond to irritants by secreting a relatively viscous product (269).

Reduced mucociliary clearance may be due to an ineffective cough, abnormalities in ciliary function, enhanced epithelial permeability, or alterations in the viscoelasticity properties of the bronchial mucous (269–274). Mucous hypersecretion with retained secretions is seen in patients with asthma, chronic bronchitis, and heavy smokers.

Drugs that decrease mucous clearance include atropine, an anticholinergic agent, which acts by either reducing submucosal gland and epithelial secretions or by inhibiting ciliary activity (69–71). Ironically, atropine could have a beneficial effect on the low-viscosity secretions in the bronchorrhea that sometimes occurs in asthma (275). Results demonstrating the

effect of aerosolized ipratropium, a synthetic quaternary anticholinergic, on mucociliary function have been conflicting (72–75), but it is probably safe to administer it with careful monitoring.

Mucociliary clearance may be enhanced by the use of β_2-adrenergic agonists (57a–c) and theophyllines (182–184). Some of the improvement in clearance from bronchodilators may be due to enhanced cough based on bronchodilation and a higher peak flow rate. Corticosteroids may improve mucociliary clearance by reducing mediator-induced mucous secretion or by their effects on epithelial inflammation (209–212).

Mucoregulatory drugs have no effect on the mucus already formed but stimulate the activity of the secreting cells. These drugs include bromhexine, carbocysteine, sobrerol, letosteine, and strepronine. Studies with these agents, however, have shown conflicting results (276).

Mucolytics, in contrast, act by breaking up mucoprotein molecules in the mucus already formed in the air passages, promoting expectoration and resorption of the secretions, thus creating the conditions for rapid improvement in mucociliary transport. The best-studied mucolytic agent is *N*-acetylcysteine (283). This agent may be administered topically, orally, or intravenously. It possesses a free sulfhydryl group that can rupture disulphide chemical bonds. The aerosol can induce bronchospasm, which is prevented by concomitant bronchodilator therapy. The aerosol dose is 1 to 4 ml of a 10% solution of *N*-acetylcysteine, administered every 3 to 6 hours with a bronchodilator.

Iodide has had long-standing popularity as an oral or intravenous agent with both mucoregulatory and mucolytic effects (282–285). Iodide can be given as a saturated solution of potassium iodide (SSKI) (10 to 20 drops in a beverage 3 to 4 times/day). Side effects include an offensive taste and gastric irritation. A less toxic product is iodinated glycerol (Organidin), which has shown improvement in the clinical status of patients with chronic bronchitis and asthmatics (286). The oral dosage for adults is 60 to 120 mg 4 times/day.

OXYGEN

Oxygen is one of the most commonly used drugs administered by the critical care physician. This element was first discovered over 200 years ago and was soon recognized as having therapeutic value to patients with respiratory disorders (287). It was also found to be toxic to plants and animals if given in high concentrations for prolonged periods (288). Hence, the effects of this drug and its proper administration must be understood if it is to be used correctly.

ADMINISTRATION OF SUPPLEMENTAL OXYGEN

Oxygen is available from central sources, using either gaseous or liquid oxygen. The element can also be administered from portable oxygen cylinders, using compressed gas. Also available for domiciliary use are oxygen enrichers. These mechanisms utilize a molecular sieve to preferentially concentrate the oxygen present in room air.

Noninvasive oxygen therapy includes the use of nasal prongs, face tents, and face masks. The nasal cannula system is an example of a low-flow system, whereby the volume of fresh gas is inadequate to meet the inspiratory needs of the patient and, as a result, patients entrain variable quantities of room air with their inspiratory effort. Oxygen in higher flows can be delivered through a face mask with or without a reservoir bag to further increase the fractional inspired oxygen tension (FIO_2). Use of a "Venturi" face mask, which employs the Bernoulli principle, ensures delivery of an accurate FIO_2, and is most useful for patients with chronic COPD, in whom high concentrations of oxygen may cause excessive PCO_2 levels (see below). Noninvasive oxygen therapy is unlikely to deliver more than an FIO_2 of 0.60 to the lungs and, hence, is intended for the patient with a small-to-moderate amount of ventilation/perfusion ($\dot{V}/\dot{Q}$) disturbance.

Greater degrees of respiratory failure are usually accompanied by significant shunting requiring higher concentrations of inspired oxygen and positive end-expiratory pressure (PEEP), which are best delivered by a closed system through an endotracheal tube. A tight-fitting mask may also be used to deliver constant positive airway pressure (CPAP). The level of positive pressure maintained in the CPAP system is controlled by the exhalation valve and can be varied between 2 and 15 cm H_2O (289). The attractive features of CPAP by mask, which are the avoidance of intubation and high pleural pressures during inspiration, must be weighed against the possibility of gastric aspiration and the inability to suction and, hence, should only be used in conscious patients for only brief periods of time.

THERAPEUTIC USES

Tissue Hypoxia

Tissue hypoxia is due to an imbalance between the oxygen uptake and the oxygen demands of the tissues leading to an oxygen debt. An inadequate oxygen uptake may be due to failure of oxygen utilization by the cells (altered O_2 metabolism) or to an inadequate delivery of oxygen caused by arterial hypoxemia, circulatory failure, or an abnormal oxygen transport (anemia, abnormal hemoglobin, increased CO content).

The relationship between the determinants for delivery of oxygen to the peripheral tissues can be expressed by the following formula:

$$\dot{D}O_2 = CI \times (SAO_2 \times Hgb \times 1.34)$$

where $\dot{D}O_2$ is the oxygen delivery (ml/min/m^2), CI = cardiac index (L/min/m$_2$), SAO_2 = % saturation of hemoglobin, Hgb = hemoglobin concentration, and 1.34 is the amount of oxygen (ml) carried per gram of Hgb.

Of the variables important for oxygen delivery, therapeutic oxygen administration only corrects for arterial hypoxemia, and of the clinically important causes of arterial hypoxemia, oxygen primarily benefits those patients with low $\dot{V}/\dot{Q}$ defects. Oxygen administration fails to be beneficial when arterial hypoxemia is caused by a true shunt or by alveolar units acting like a shunt, because oxygen cannot reach the collapsed alveoli.

The oxygen consumption ($\dot{V}O_2$) of a normal human at rest is approximately 110 to 130 ml/m^2/min and can be measured directly by determining the difference between inspired and expired oxygen concentrations (290), by measuring the disappearance of oxygen from a closed system that contains a carbon dioxide absorber (291), or indirectly by use of the following Fick equation and calculating the arterial and mixed venous oxygen contents and measuring the cardiac output by thermodilution (292):

$$\dot{V}O_2 = CI \times (CAO_2 - C\bar{V}O_2) \times 10$$

where $\dot{V}O_2$ = the oxygen consumption (ml/min/m^2), CI = the cardiac index (L/min/m^2), CAO_2 = the arterial oxygen content (ml oxygen/100 ml blood), and $C\bar{V}O_2$ = the mixed venous oxygen content (ml oxygen/100 ml blood).

The advantages and disadvantages of the different ways of measuring or calculating $\dot{V}O_2$ have been reviewed recently (290).

Absolute measurements of systemic $\dot{D}O_2$ and systemic $\dot{V}O_2$ do not provide information about the adequacy of tissue oxygenation of either the whole organism or individual tissues. Since techniques for directly monitoring the adequacy of tissue oxygenation are not available in the clinical setting, much controversy surrounds the proper assessment of tissue oxygenation and is discussed in several reviews (293, 294).

Calculation of the alveolar-arterial oxygen gradient (A-aDO_2) can distinguish between hypoventilation or an abnormality in gas exchange as the cause of arterial hypoxemia. The arterial oxygen tension can be measured, whereas the actual alveolar concentration of oxygen can be calculated using the abbreviated form of the alveolar air equation:

$$PAO_2 = FIO_2 \times (P_{atm} - PH_2O) - PACO_2/R$$

where PAO_2 = alveolar O_2, FIO_2 = fractional inspired oxygen tension, P_{atm} = barometric pressure, P_{H2O} = water vapor pressure, $PACO_2$ = arterial CO_2, and R = respiratory exchange ratio assumed to be 0.8. However, A-aDO_2 varies with changes in FIO_2, which limits its usefulness for following the changes in gas exchange in a patient as the FIO_2 is altered. Alternatively, the a/APO_2 ratio is more stable than the A-aDO_2 with changing values of FIO_2 and, hence, can be used instead to monitor respiratory function (295, 296).

Chronic Obstructive Pulmonary Disease

Oxygen therapy is important for patients in acute respiratory failure to reverse life-threatening hypoxemia; however, its acute administration does little to the acute rise in pulmonary artery pressure observed in these patients (297). For patients with chronic COPD and arterial hypoxemia, several studies have shown that low flow domiciliary oxygen therapy prolongs survival (298, 299). The mechanisms by which oxygen therapy reduces mortality remain unclear and may be due to improvement in PO_2 providing enhanced oxygen delivery to the tissues or to a reduction in pulmonary artery resistance, leading to improved right ventricular function with consequent increase in oxygen delivery to the tissues (300–304).

Central Sleep Apnea

Oxygen administration may be a beneficial agent in treating central sleep apnea. Several investigators have reported either the complete abolition of or a reduction in the number of central apneic events in patients with central sleep apnea (305–307). The mechanism by which oxygen administration reduces central apneas has not yet been established.

Hyperbaric Oxygen Therapy

Hyperbaric oxygen therapy is useful for treatment of acute carbon monoxide poisoning and air embolism; its use in other clinical disorders remains problematic (308).

ADVERSE EFFECTS

Cell Toxicity

Several animal studies have documented the pulmonary pathological effects of hyperoxia (309–312), which appear related to the concentration of inspired oxygen and duration of exposure. Human studies have demonstrated clinical symptoms consisting of substernal discomfort, cough, and physiological changes, which include decreased tracheal mucus velocity, decreased lung volume, and diffusing capacity, and gas exchange abnormalities (313–318).

Morphologic changes occurring in humans exposed to hyperoxia include acute exudative changes involving congestion, edema, and hyaline membranes lining the alveolar septal spaces, whereas chronic exposure produces proliferative changes characterized by alveolar and septal edema along with fibrosis and hyperplasia of alveolar lining cells (319, 320).

The pathogenesis of O_2 toxicity involves the production of toxic oxygen radicals (superoxide, hydrogen peroxide, hydroxyl ions, and singlet oxygen). When generated in excess at elevated levels of intracellular PO_2, the normal antioxidant defenses, which include superoxide dismutases, catalase, and glutathione peroxidase, are overwhelmed (321–324).

Hypercapnia

Carbon dioxide retention is a serious effect of oxygen administration in patients with chronic obstructive pulmonary disease (COPD). The mechanism may be due to a depression of ventilation in those COPD patients who require arterial hypoxemia as a stimulus for breathing, as their ventilatory response to PCO_2 is depressed. A recent study, however, suggests that the increase in PCO_2 may be due to oxygen-induced increase in the inhomogeneity of ventilation-perfusion distribution (325). In practice, oxygen supplementation does not invariably lead to CO_2 retention, even in patients with preexisting CO_2 retention (326, 327).

Other Adverse Effects

Administration of 100% oxygen may cause alveoli distal to blocked airways to collapse due to complete absorption of oxygen and lack of inert nitrogen to act as a "splint." Absorption atelectasis decreases the vital capacity and increases shunting of blood through the lungs. Breathing 100% oxygen may also cause tracheobronchitis, which is manifested by substernal chest pain and continuous cough. This disorder is not known to cause any permanent pulmonary dysfunction. Chest pain due to tracheobronchitis may cause a decrease in inspiratory effort, resulting in further loss of vital capacity. Finally, chronic changes in the lung due to prolonged use of high concentrations of inspired oxygen can cause bronchopulmonary dysplasia, which is characterized by proliferation of lung fibroblasts, resulting in increased lung collagen synthesis (328).

SURFACTANT

Surfactant, a surface-active physiochemical agent that lines the alveolar surface of the lung (329), reduces surface tension (330) at the air-liquid interface at low end-expiratory volumes, increases lung compliance, and aids in keeping the alveoli dry as an "antiedema" factor (331). The importance of surfactant was recognized more than 50 years ago by Von Neergaard (332), who described how the lungs were more difficult to inflate with air than with fluid and by Avery and Mead (333), who demonstrated that the lungs of infants with hyaline membrane disease had a much higher surface tension than that found in normal lungs.

The components of natural pulmonary surfactant are lipids, proteins, and carbohydrates (334, 335). Phospholipids are the major components of surfactant, making up 80 to 90% of its weight. The two major classes of phospholipids are phosphatidylcholine and phosphatidylglycerol, with dipalmitoylphosphatidylcholine (DPPC) as the main surface active component. The functions of the other surfactant lipids are less well-defined. At least three lung-specific proteins (apoproteins) have been shown to be associated with pulmonary surfactant (336). Although still in dispute, it has become increasingly evident that these proteins aid in spreading surfactant on the alveolar surface, regulate surfactant phospholipid metabolism, and play a role in the immune defence system of the lung. The functional significance of the carbohydrate components remains to be established.

Pulmonary surfactant is secreted from the type II pneumocyte into the alveolar lumen. The surfactant is packaged and stored as lipid bilayers in lamellar bodies, which are exocytosed into the alveolar lumen. Ninety to ninety-five percent of secreted alveolar surfactant is recycled, reprocessed, refined, and repackaged for resecretion via the type II cells. A small fraction of surfactant undergoes macrophage degradation.

Clearance of surfactant material from the alveolar space of normal lungs appears to occur with a half-life of about 20 hours (335). There does not seem to be a large intracellular or extracellular reserve of alveolar surfactant. A number of studies have shown that a variety of agents can stimulate surfactant secretion, including adrenergic agonists, prostaglandins, and cholinergic agonists (336a).

Whereas a quantitative surfactant deficiency exists in neonatal respiratory distress syndrome (RDS), animal models of acute lung injury that simulate most of the pathophysiologic and morphologic features of ARDS (337–344), as well as studies in patients with ARDS (345, 346), have demonstrated biochemical and functional deficiencies of surfactant. Mechanisms of surfactant alterations include abnormalities in surfactant production by type II cells and biophysical inhibition of surfactant by constituents of permeability pulmonary edema (340, 341, 347–349). Other postulated mechanisms include attack by proteases present in epithelial lining fluid on surfactant apoproteins (350) and oxygen radical-induced oxidation of lung surfactant apoproteins or peroxidation of lung surfactant lipids (351).

Physiological effects of surfactant include increased pulmonary compliance and decreased shunt, leading to use of lower ventilating pressures and enhanced arterial oxygenation at lower FIO_2. These effects could theoretically reduce the risk of barotrauma and help the patient avoid toxic levels of oxygen, which may decrease the high morbidity and mortality associated with ARDS. Indeed, animal investigations studying the role of surfactant replacement therapy have demonstrated improved pulmonary function, as well as enhanced survival (351–354).

Subsequently, surfactant replacement has shown benefit in newborns at risk of developing or already having established respiratory distress syndrome (355–359). These studies have used natural human surfactant, an animal-based extracted surfactant, or a synthetic surfactant consisting of synthetic DPPC and an alcohol to help with spreading and adsorption (EXOSURF). Specifically, prophylaxis with these types of surfactant has reduced mortality by one-half, whereas surfactant treatment for established RDS has reduced mortality and morbidity due to pneumothorax, pulmonary interstitial emphysema, bronchopulmonary dysplasia, and intraventricular hemorrhage.

The dose of surfactant administered in these studies has varied from 50 to 200 mg of surfactant phospholipid per kg in a volume of 2 to 4 ml. This amount is roughly the size of the alveolar surfactant pool. The surfactant suspension was instilled via a fine-bore feeding tube into the trachea. The response was usually rapid, with an immediate increase in arterial oxygen tension and a decrease in oxygen requirements from around 80% to 50% or less within 30 minutes. Reductions in ventilatory settings occurred more slowly. In some babies, these improvements in pulmonary function were sustained after a single dose of surfactant, while in others multiple doses were required to maintain the improvement. Recently, the FDA granted approval for use of EXOSURF in newborns at risk of developing or having established RDS.

These encouraging results in RDS have led to investigations assessing the efficacy of surfactant replacement therapy in patients with ARDS. Replacement surfactant treatment in ARDS, compared to that in RDS, is probably more complex due to multiple and ongoing factors causing abnormalities in surfactant. Also to be considered is the delivery of adequate amounts of surface active material to the alveolar air-liquid interface due to the large absolute distances in the adult lung, compared to those in the neonate. Furthermore, injured lung units are closed, thus barring entry to the exogenous material. Techniques used have included selective endobronchial instillation under direct vision with the fiberoptic bronchoscope, as well as continuous nebulization.

Direct instillation of a porcine-derived surfactant have shown transient benefits in oxygenation in case reports (360, 361). Recently, aerosol delivery of EXOSURF in patients with septic-induced ARDS has shown improvement in pulmonary function and a trend towards improved survival (362, 363).

PROSTAGLANDINS

The intimate relationship between the pulmonary system and the prostaglandins is evidenced by the ability of the lungs to synthesize and catabolize many of the prostaglandins and by the potent vasoactive effects of several prostaglandins on the pulmonary system. Although the exact role of alterations in prostaglandin metabolism in acute lung injury remains undefined, recent research has focused on the therapeutic aspects of prostaglandins in lung diseases, especially the two prostaglandins known to vasodilate the pulmonary circulation, prostacyclin (PGI_2, epoprostenol) and PGE_1.

PGI_2 and PGE_1 are naturally occurring prostaglandins and are 20 carbon fatty acid products of the cyclooxygenase pathway of arachidonic acid. They have similar structures and are distinguished by the constituents of the cyclopentane ring and the number of double bonds in the attached 20-carbon unsaturated carboxylic acid side chain. These agents have short half-lives (2 to 3 minutes), and whereas PGI_2 is mainly metabolized by the liver (364), PGE_1 is rapidly degraded during a single passage through the lungs and, hence, its clearance is decreased with lung injury (365, 366).

In addition to being potent pulmonary vasodilators, properties shared by both agents include systemic vasodilation (367), enhancement of myocardial inotropy (368), inhibition of neutrophil activation (369), stabilization of cell membranes or cytoprotection (370–372), and inhibition of platelet aggregation, although PGI_2 is more powerful (373). One advantage, however, of PGI_2 over PGE_1 appears to be less intense and less prolonged platelet activation after discontinuation (374).

CLINICAL USES

Primary Pulmonary Hypertension

Patients in whom no cause can be found for elevated pulmonary pressures are diagnosed as having primary pulmonary hypertension (PPH) (375). Overall survival at 10 years is less than 10%, due predominantly to right ventricular failure. Several studies have demonstrated the safety and efficacy of PGI_2 in producing pulmonary vasodilatation, defined by a greater than 20% drop in pulmonary vascular resistance (375–383). The safety of PGI_2 is attributed to its short half-life, which minimizes the risk of sustained and catastrophic decreases in systemic arterial pressure (384–387). Studies have also shown that the acute response to PGI_2 has predictive value for subsequent oral vasodilator therapy (381, 382, 388, 389). The acutely favorable hemodynamic and symptomatic effects of this agent are maintained during prolonged infusions (379, 383), which makes this drug useful in patients awaiting heart-lung transplantation (379–387). The effect, however, of PGI_2 on long-term survival in PPH remains unknown (390, 391).

PGE_1 has reduced pulmonary vascular resistance in patients with PPH (392–394) and also has predictive value for the response to subsequent oral vasodilator therapy (395, 396). The number of studies evaluating the effects of PGE_1 on PPH are less than those with PGI_2. Furthermore, studies assessing prolonged infusions with PGE_1 have not been performed.

Chronic Obstructive Pulmonary Disease

Pulmonary hypertension complicating COPD is a poor prognostic sign (397) and, hence, an effort to lower pulmonary arterial pressure in order to reduce right ventricular afterload, improve cardiac output, and enhance oxygen delivery may be beneficial to survival. In COPD patients with acutely decompensated chronic lung disease, PGE_1 produced decreases in pulmonary vascular resistance and increases in cardiac output (398). In patients with stable COPD, both PGI_2 and a PGE_1 analog reduced pulmonary vascular resistance and increased oxygen delivery (399, 400). The clinical benefit, however, of pharmacologic reduction in right ventricular afterload in patients with pulmonary hypertension secondary to acute or chronic respiratory failure remains unknown.

Adult Respiratory Distress Syndrome

Therapy with prostaglandins has been suggested for the treatment of ARDS due to their antiinflammatory effect, as well as their vasodilator effect on the pulmonary circulation, because pulmonary hypertension is usually present in ARDS (401). Studies in animal models of ARDS have shown beneficial hemodynamic effects with prostaglandins (402–404). Several reports have documented beneficial effects of PGE_1 on pulmonary vascular resistance, cardiac output, and oxygen delivery in patients with ARDS (405–407). Although one small study demonstrated a trend toward improved survival in predominantly surgical patients with ARDS (408), a large multicenter placebo-controlled trial failed to show a survival benefit with PGE_1 administration (409).

STIMULANTS

Drugs with stimulant actions on the central respiratory system have been used to increase ventilation in patients with chronic COPD, primary alveolar hypoventilation syndrome, and the sleep apnea syndromes. Some respiratory stimulant drugs also appear to have a preferential effect on the activation of upper airway muscles to reverse sleep-related upper airway obstruction.

Doxapram, an analeptic agent, has been used in hastening arousal and reversing ventilatory depression following general anesthesia and to increase ventilation in patients with chronic COPD or with primary alveolar ventilation (410, 411), but its side effects, including hypertension, tachycardia, arrhythmias, and seizures, limit the use of this drug.

Theophylline increases respiratory activity by a direct effect on brainstem respiratory centers (185–187). This agent is effective in the management of idiopathic apnea of prematurity (412, 413) but has not been useful in adults with central sleep apnea (414).

Elevated levels of endogenous progesterone in pregnancy and during the progestational phase of the menstrual cycle lead to an increase in alveolar ventilation. Similarly, the administration of progestational agents has been shown to stimulate breathing in normal individuals and in patients with respiratory disorders (415–418). The oral form of medroxyprogesterone acetate (MPA) has been most widely evaluated for its respiratory stimulatory effects. Following oral administration, the drug is promptly absorbed from the intestinal tract. Metabolism takes place in the liver, but significant quantities are excreted in the urine. This agent has been used to increase alveolar ventilation in patients with COPD or with the obesity hypoventilation syndrome (419, 420). MPA in doses of 60 to 120 mg has had limited success in patients with obstructive sleep apnea (421).

Protriptyline, a tricyclic antidepressant, has been shown to relieve obstructive sleep apnea (422–424), which may be due to a selective activation of motor neurons to upper airway muscles to relieve the upper airway obstruction (425).

Acetazolamide, a reversible inhibitor of carbonic anhydrase, produces a metabolic acidosis and a parallel shift to the left of the ventilatory response to hypercapnia. With a left-shifted hypercapnic response, a smaller degree of hypoventilation is more likely to cause a respiratory stimulus. Acetazolamide has been used successfully to treat central sleep apneas (426), but recent reports have noted that central apneas may be replaced by obstructive apneas (427).

PHARMACOLOGIC APPROACH TO THE PATIENT WITH PULMONARY DISEASE

ASTHMA

Aerosolized β_2 agonists are the initial drugs of choice for management of acute bronchospasm. The high margin of safety for inhaled β_2 agonists allows these agents to be given as frequently as q20 minutes × the first 3 doses, then repeated q hour in severe cases (180). Sequential inhalation may maximize the therapeutic effects of β-adrenergic agonists by allowing better penetration of the bronchodilator aerosol after some bronchodilation has been achieved (428). Continuous nebulization has also been used (429), but the efficacy of this mode of delivery has yet to be shown.

In most patients with an attack of bronchospasm, especially if airway narrowing is predominantly due to spasm and not to mucosal edema, control can be achieved with aerosolized β_2 agonists within the first hour (429a). Intravenous aminophylline should not be part of the initial management of acute severe bronchospasm, because this agent in combination with a sympathomimetic is neither additive nor synergistic and may increase the toxicity of inhaled β-adrenergic agonists (179–181). Intravenous steroids may be administered as part of initial treatment in patients who present with severe bronchospasm (peak expiratory flow rate (PEFR) < 100 L/min).

Status asthmaticus is present when there is no improvement or further deterioration occurs after initial treatment. At this time, concern with the inability of an aerosol dose to penetrate the lower airways due to mucus plugs and/or airway edema may warrant the use of SC or IV preparations. Corticosteroids should also be administered, if not already given, and intravenous aminophylline should be started at this time. Magnesium sulfate may also be administered as a 1.2-g bolus in 50 ml of saline over 20 minutes.

Although anticholinergic agonists should not be used as primary therapy because of their slow time course of action and medium potency, their administration may help prolong the duration of bronchodilation. Aerosolized corticosteroids have no role during the acute exacerbation of asthma, because they can cause bronchial irritation and potentially worsen the attack. Antibiotics should not be administered unless there is a strong suspicion of pneumonia based on clinical and radiographic findings and the Gram stain (430).

Oxygen therapy should be given to all patients with bronchospasm to mitigate paradoxical bronchodilator-induced hypoxemia and reverse hypoxic pulmonary vasoconstriction. If mechanical ventilation is instituted, sedatives may be useful to minimize peak airway pressure due to agitation; paralyzing agents (vecuronium bromide or pancuronium bromide) may also be beneficial in reducing airway pressures by decreasing chest wall compliance. The anesthetic gases halothane and ether may also cause further bronchodilation. The mucolytic agent *N*-acetylcysteine may be useful when combined with therapeutic bronchoscopy for bronchial lavage to remove tenacious mucus (431).

CHRONIC OBSTRUCTIVE PULMONARY DISEASE

The administration of supplemental, low-flow oxygen is probably the single most useful treatment in most cases of acute exacerbations of COPD (432). Although COPD is characterized by irreversible airflow obstruction, there may be a reversible component in the setting of an acute exacerbation (433–435) and, therefore, aerosolized β_2 agonists should initially be administered in conjunction with oxygen. If no response occurs, then an aerosolized anticholinergic agent may be helpful. Intravenous aminophylline has not been shown to be helpful in acute exacerbations of COPD (177). The benefit of corticosteroids in the treatment of an acute exacerbation is controversial, but a short-term administration may be warranted in those refractory to initial treatment. Mucolytics agents may be beneficial in the presence of tenacious sputum. *N*-acetylcysteine (1 to 4 ml of a 10% solution) can be aerosolized with a bronchodilator.

Diuretics are helpful when increased extravascular lung water is present. Antibiotics are useful only when there is evidence for bronchitis or pneumonia (436). Respiratory stimulants may prevent intubation and mechanical ventilation by allowing time for the beneficial actions of bronchodilators, corticosteroids, and oxygen to take effect, but the high incidence of side effects associated with these agents cause their administration to be controversial (451).

ADULT RESPIRATORY DISTRESS SYNDROME

The overall mortality rate of 50 to 70% associated with ARDS has remained unchanged during the past 10 to 20 years, not only due to the increased prevalence of sicker patients presenting with this syndrome but also to the lack of therapy aimed at treating the underlying pathogenesis.

Recent advances, however, made in elucidating the pathophysiology of this syndrome have started to influence the pharmacologic approach to patients with this syndrome. Briefly, investigators have emphasized the importance of sepsis as a cause of ARDS and have focused on the relationships between endotoxin, macrophages, and circulating cytokines in mediating the manifestations of this syndrome (438–443). Consequently, ARDS is considered as simply the pulmonary component of a generalized panendothelial inflammation affecting multiple organs and caused by circulating mediators released in response to systemic sepsis, trauma, or another major insult.

The appreciation that nosocomial infections, especially pneumonia, enhance the mortality rate in patients with ARDS (444–447), has led to strategies aimed at preventing these infections. One strategy involves selective decontamination of the digestive tract (SDD) with the use of oral and systemic antibiotics. The rationale for this therapy is to suppress the growth of potentially pathogenic aerobic Gram-negative gut bacteria that may aspirate directly into the lungs or invade the systemic circulation via bacterial translocation (448–451). Although several studies have reported a decrease in the incidence of nosocomial pneumonias in patients treated with a SDD protocol, compared to that of control patients, only two studies have shown a significant decrease in mortality (452).

Gastric acid neutralization with H_2-receptor antagonists or antacids with subsequent gastric microbial growth may increase the incidence of aspiration pneumonia. Studies comparing sucralfate, a cytoprotective agent that has in vitro antibacterial properties, with pH-altering agents have suggested a decreased incidence of nosocomial pneumonias with this agent (453–455) and, therefore, its use should be considered in patients tolerating enteral feedings.

The demonstration of pathological oxygen supply dependency in ARDS leading to tissue hypoxia and subsequent multiple organ failure has led several investigators to suggest therapy aimed at maximizing oxygen delivery (455a–c). Methods to minimize oxygen demand may also be beneficial in restoring the balance between oxygen demand and uptake. Fever, increased work of breathing, anxiety, and the metabolic stresses of sepsis, trauma, and the associated tissue repair processes all increase the metabolic demand for oxygen. Hence, antipyretics to correct hyperthermia, as well as agents to induce sedation and muscular paralysis, may be beneficial. No study, however, has yet demonstrated that optimizing DO_2 and VO_2 enhances survival.

The central role that endotoxin may play in initiating the immunoinflammatory cascade has led to investigations on the efficacy of antibodies to endotoxin in sepsis. Initial studies with antiendotoxin antibodies were optimistic (456, 457), but recent studies employing monoclonal antibodies have been less impressive (458, 459).

Tumor necrosis factor (TNF), a mediator released by macrophages in response to endotoxin, may play a role in promoting lung injury (460–462). Recent animal studies have demonstrated the efficacy of antibodies to TNF in endotoxin shock (463, 464) and, currently, phase I as well as phase III clinical trials are underway to determine the safety and efficacy of such antibodies in humans with the sepsis syndrome.

Therapeutic strategies have also focused on modulating the inflammatory response in ARDS. Nonsteroidal antiinflammatory drugs that inhibit cyclooxygenase products have reduced the extent of pulmonary injury in animal models of sepsis and ARDS (465–467). Promising results have been observed in initial clinical trials, using ibuprofen (468–479). Corticosteroids and PGE_1 have not been shown to benefit patients with ARDS (238–241, 409).

Survival statistics demonstrating that approximately only 10% of patients die from respiratory failure (445) suggest that therapeutic strategies focused on alleviating pulmonary injury may not be rewarding. Indeed, newer ventilatory strategies, including extracorporeal techniques, have not enhanced survival in patients with ARDS (471). However, hyperoxia lung damage is a concern, because elevated concentrations of oxygen must be given to patients due to increased pulmonary shunting. Some pulmonary oxygen toxicity could be avoided if intracellular PO_2 monitoring indicated adequate cellular oxygenation at lower FIO_2 levels. Unfortunately, current therapeutic prescription of oxygen is based empirically on arterial PO_2, which does not reflect the adequacy of cellular oxygen utilization. Hence, the lowest possible concentration of oxygen that maintains tissue oxygenation should be administered in order to avoid further pulmonary injury from hyperoxia. At the present time, it is recommended that PEEP be employed to maintain the $PAO_2 > 60$ mm Hg at an FIO_2 at or below 0.6. Surfactant may help with limiting the use of high concentrations of oxygen, but it awaits further clinical trials before its safety and efficacy can be assessed.

PULMONARY EMBOLISM

Treatment of pulmonary embolism begins with a high level of suspicion, followed by appropriate diagnostic studies, which has been the focus of several reviews (472–475). When pulmonary embolism is initially suspected and there are no contraindications to its use, heparin therapy should begin with a loading dose of 5000 to 10,000 units, followed by a maintenance infusion of 1000 to 2000 units/h, which is continued for 7 to 10 days if a pulmonary embolism is confirmed. Therapy is monitored by the partial thromboplastin time (PTT) and a therapeutic effect is achieved when the baseline PTT is 1.5 to 2.0 times that of the control. The PTT is checked q12h for 2 days, then daily if the patient remains stable. Oral anticoagulation with warfarin is begun 1 or 2 days after heparin therapy has been initiated and is monitored by the prothrombin time (PT), with the dose titrated to maintain the PT $1\frac{1}{2}$ to 2 times above the control value.

Thrombolytic therapy should probably be reserved for those patients with hemodynamic compromise; although studies have shown more rapid resolution of pulmonary emboli with thrombolytic agents (476, 477), the 8% overall mortality rate of treated pulmonary embolism has not been improved with thrombolytic therapy (478). Streptokinase is given intravenously as a 250,000-unit bolus over 30 minutes, followed by a maintenance infusion of 100,000 units/h for 24 hours. If after 2 to 3 hours the thrombin time cannot be prolonged despite an infusion rate in excess of 200,000 units/h, the patient is probably resistant to streptokinase due to circulating antistreptococcal antibodies in high titer. Consequently, urokinase should be administered. After 24 hours, thrombolytic therapy is discontinued, and the patient is started on heparin in a full anticoagulant dose as soon as the thrombin time, followed serially every few hours after discontinuation of streptokinase, falls to within $2\frac{1}{2}$ times the control value.

Tissue plasminogen activator is also effective for thrombolytic therapy in patients with pulmonary emboli and is administered intravenously as an initial bolus of 20 mg over 1 hour, followed by an infusion of 10 mg/h for a total dose of 40 to 100 mg (479, 480).

In addition to lytic therapy, pulmonary embolism associated with hemodynamic compromise should be supported with fluids to elevate right ventricular preload and to permit more effective right ventricular emptying against the acute increase in afterload and, if necessary, sympathomimetic agents should be given to improve right ventricular function (481).

PULMONARY HYPERTENSION

Pulmonary hypertension is most amenable to pharmacologic therapy in disorders in which active vasoconstriction plays a major pathogenic role and includes patients with COPD or primary pulmonary hypertension.

Chronic Obstructive Pulmonary Disease

In patients with COPD, reversible pulmonary hypertension is due to hypoxic vasoconstriction, which occurs from alterations in pulmonary gas exchange. Several efforts can be used that are directed towards this pathophysiologic mechanism. One, inhaled bronchodilators (β_2 agonists and/or anticholinergic agents) can improve alveolar ventilation and alleviate alveolar hypoxia by producing bronchodilation and enhanced mucociliary clearance. Subcutaneous administration of terbutaline (0.25 mg) can also effect pulmonary vasodilation and provide inotropic support for the right side of the heart (482, 483). Theophylline, in addition to its bronchodilator effects, may also improve right ventricular function and cause pulmonary vasodilation.

Supplemental oxygen should be administered chronically only when the initial hypoxemia has failed to respond to intensive pharmacotherapy, which may take up to 3 months. Presently, oxygen is recommended for patients with either a $PO_2 < 55$ mm Hg while breathing room air or a PO_2 of 55 to 65 mm Hg in the presence of secondary erythrocytosis, mental dysfunction responsive to oxygen, or cor pulmonale.

The treatment of right heart failure in cor pulmonale is guided by the presence of the patient's symptoms. Diuretics can treat systemic venous congestion and peripheral edema and relieve dyspnea by reducing pulmonary capillary congestion and extravascular lung water. Diuretics may also enhance left ventricular function by reducing the size of the right ventricle, which can impair left ventricular (LV) filling when dilated (484). Diuretics must be given cautiously, because excessive reduction in right ventricular end-diastolic volume may cause cardiac output to decrease, and excessive use may generate a metabolic alkalosis, which can depress ventilation and thereby elicit alveolar and arterial hypoxemia.

Digitalis has only been shown to be useful in patients with both right and left ventricular function (485–487). Although this agent increases right ventricular contractility, it can also cause pulmonary vasoconstriction (488). This effect, coupled with the enhanced risk of digitalis toxicity in the presence of hypoxemia, acidosis, catecholamine excess, and hypokalemia, has led to the disuse of digitalis in most patients with pulmonary hypertension (489).

Vasodilators should be considered only when conventional therapy and oxygen have failed to ameliorate signs of right ventricular failure in view of the potential adverse consequences of these agents. Hence, careful assessment of their effects on hemodynamics and oxygenation must be undertaken, which usually requires invasive right-sided catheterization.

If vasodilators are used, a beneficial hemodynamic response to a vasodilator is considered when (*a*) pulmonary vascular resistance is reduced by more than 20% and cardiac output is increased or unchanged and (*b*) pulmonary arterial pressure is decreased or unchanged, and systemic blood pressure is not significantly reduced (490).

Vasodilator therapy in COPD patients includes the use of hydralazine, nitrates, or calcium channel blockers. Results with hydralazine have been mixed, with some studies showing beneficial hemodynamic effects (491–496), while others indicate limited or detrimental effects, such as excessive ventilation causing increased dyspnea (497–499). Nitrates have produced significant reductions in pulmonary arterial pressure and pulmonary vascular resistance, but due to their vasodilating effects, cardiac output usually falls (491).

Nifedipine often produces an acute decrease in pulmonary vascular resistance, an increase in cardiac output and, in many cases, decreases in pulmonary artery pressure (500–505). A decrease in PAO_2 may occur in some patients as a result of an unfavorable influence on pulmonary ventilation-perfusion relationships caused by reversal of hypoxic vasoconstriction, but this effect is usually mild, and oxygen delivery still may be increased because of the favorable effect of nifedipine on cardiac output. Use of nifedipine should probably be limited to the short-term management of acute decompensations of cor pulmonale, because one study showed lack of long-term hemodynamic effects with this agent, as well as a paradoxical detrimental interaction with concurrent oxygen use (500). Diltiazem and verapamil have not been shown to have an effect on pulmonary hemodynamics in COPD patients (506, 507). PGE_1 has demonstrated favorable hemodynamic effects in acutely decompensated chronic lung disease (398).

Primary Pulmonary Hypertension

Vasodilator therapy remains the mainstay of therapy for patients with PPH. A short-acting intravenous vasodilator, either PGE_1 or PGI_2, should be administered to assess acute pulmonary vasodilator responsiveness. A wide range of different oral pharmacologic agents can then be given and includes α-adrenergic antagonists, β-adrenergic agonists, calcium channel-blocking agents, inhibitors of angiotensin-converting enzyme, and nitrates (508–513). Trials with multiple agents of different pharmacologic classes may be necessary, because marked variability in responses to different agents is a common finding. Calcium channel-blocking agents are usually well-tolerated by patients and, hence, may be chronically administered.

New therapeutic approaches have included the use of high-dose calcium channel-blocking agents in patients who do not respond to conventional test doses of calcium channel-blocking agents (514). continuous intravenous PGI_2 have been used for those patients who are not responsive to, or are intolerant of, oral vasodilator therapy, or are severely ill and awaiting heart-lung or lung transplantation.

In addition to vasodilator therapy, other options include administration of diuretics for symptoms of right heart failure and oxygen for evidence of arterial hypoxemia, either at rest or during exercise. The occurrence of in situ thrombosis in patients with PPH has led to the use of anticoagulants or treatment with antiplatelet agents; aspirin, possibly in combination with dipyridamole (515, 516).

REFERENCES

1. Nadel JA, Barnes PJ: Autonomic regulation of the airways. *Annu Rev Med* 35:451–467, 1984.
2. Barnes PJ: Neural control of human airways in health and disease. State of the art. *Am Rev Respir Dis* 134:1289–1314, 1986.
3. Richardson JB: Nonadrenergic inhibitory innervation of the lung. *Lung* 159:315–322, 1981.
4. Barnes PJ, Baraniuk JN, Belvisi MG: Neuropeptides in the respiratory tract. Part I. *Am Rev Respir Dis* 144:1181–1198, 1991.
5. Barnes PJ, Baraniuk JN, Belvisi MG: Neuropeptides in the respiratory tract. Part II. *Am Rev Respir Dis.* 144:1391–1399, 1991.
6. Murlas C, Nadel JA, Roberts JM: The muscarinic receptors of airway smooth muscle: their characterization in vitro. *J Appl Physiol* 52:1084–1091, 1982.
7. Barnes PJ, Basbaum CB, Nadel JA: Autoradiographic localization of autonomic receptors in airway smooth muscle: marked differences between large and small airways. *Am Rev Respir Dis* 127:758–762, 1983.
8. Ingram RH Jr, Wellman JJ, McFadden ER Jr, Mead J: Relative contribution of large and small airways to flow limitation in normal subjects before and after atropine and isoproterenol. *J Clin Invest* 59:696–703, 1977.
9. Carstairs JR, Nimmo A, Barnes PJ: Autoradiographic visualization of beta-adrenoceptor subtypes in human lung. *Am Rev Respir Dis* 132:541–547, 1985.
10. Kneussl MP, Richardson JB: Alpha-adrenergic receptors in human and canine tracheal and bronchial smooth muscle. *J Appl Physiol* 45:307–311, 1978.
11. Hoffman BB, Lefkowitz RJ: Alpha-adrenergic receptor subtypes. *N Engl J Med* 302:375–392, 1980.
12. Black JL, Salome CM, Yan K, Shaw J: Comparison between airways response to an α-adrenoceptor agonist and histamine in asthmatic and non-asthmatic subjects. *Br J Clin Pharmacol* 14:464–465, 1982.
13. Henderson WR, Shelhamer JH, Reingold DB, Smith LJ, Evans III R, Kaliner M: Alpha-adrenergic hyper-responsiveness in asthma. Analysis of vascular and pupillary responses. *N Engl J Med* 300:642–647, 1979.
14. Barnes PJ, Skoogh B-E, Brown JK, Nadel JA: Activation of alpha-adrenergic responses in tracheal smooth muscle: a post-receptor mechanism. *J Appl Physiol* 54:1469–1476, 1983.
15. Popa V: Clinical pharmacology of adrenergic drugs. *J Asthma* 78:442–744, 1984.
16. Skidmore IF: Drugs acting at adreno-receptors. In Buckle DR and Smith H (eds): *Development of Anti-Asthma Drugs*. London, Butterworths, pp 185–204, 1984.
17. Tashkin DP, Jenne JW: Alpha and beta adrenergic agents. In Weiss EB, Segal MS, Stein, M. (eds): *Bronchial Asthma Mechanisms and Therapeutics*. Little, Brown, Boston, pp 604–645, 1985.
18. Ziment I: *Respiratory Pharmacology and Therapeutics*. WB Saunders, Philadelphia, 1978.
19. Van den Berger W, Lefrink JG, Maes RAA, et al: The effects of oral and subcutaneous administration of terbutaline in asthmatic patients. *Eur J Respir Dis* 65(Suppl 134):181–193, 1984.
20. Walker SR, Evans ME, Richards AJ, et al: The clinical pharmacology of oral and inhaled salbutamol. *Clin Pharmacol Ther* 13:861–867, 1972.
21. Popa V: Beta-adrenergic drugs: In Zimet I, Popa V, (eds): *Respiratory Pharmacology, Clinics in Chest Medicine*, vol 7. WB Saunders, Philadelphia, p 313–329, 1986.
22. Webb J, Rees J, Clark TJH: A comparison of the effects of different methods of administration of beta₂ sympathomimetics in patients with asthma. *Br J Dis Chest* 76:341–359, 1982.
23. Larsson S, Svedmyr N: A comparison of two modes of administering beta₂ adrenoreceptor stimulants in asthmatics: tablets and metered aerosol. *Scand J Respir Dis* 101(suppl):79–85, 1977.
24. Tabachnick IIA: A summary of the pharmacology and toxicology of albuterol (Proventil). *Ann Allergy* 47:379–383, 1981.
25. Smith PA, Henrich AE, Leffler CT, et al: A comparative study of subcutaneously administered terbutaline and epinephrine in the treatment of acute bronchial asthma. *Chest* 71:129–135, 1977.
26. Da Costa JL, Goth BK: A comparative trial of subcutaneous terbutaline: the 1165a and adrenaline in bronchial asthma. *Med J Aust* 2:588–592, 1973.
27. Fagerstrom PO: Pharmacokinetics of terbutaline after parenteral administration. *Eur J Respir Dis* 65(suppl 134):101–110, 1984.
28. Lawford P, Jones BJM, Milledge JS: Comparison of intravenous and nebulized salbutamol in initial treatment of severe asthma. *Br Med J* 1:84–86, 1978.
29. Thiringer G, Svedmyr N: Comparison of infused and inhaled terbutaline in patients with asthma. *Scand J Respir Dis* 101(suppl):95–99, 1977.
30. Williams SJ, Winner SJ, Clark TJH: Comparison of inhaled and intravenous terbutaline in acute severe asthma. *Thorax* 36:629–631, 1981.
31. Benjamin C: A comparative study of the bronchodilator effect of five beta-adrenoreceptor drugs in patients with reversible bronchoobstruction. *Med Proc* 18:35–43, 1972.
32. Watanabe S, Renzetti AD, Bergin R, et al: Airway responsiveness to a bronchodilator aerosol. I. Normal subjects. *Am Rev Respir Dis* 109:530–537, 1974.
33. Hetzel MR, Clark IJH: Comparison of intravenous and aerosol salbutamol. *Br Med J* 1:919, 1976.

34. Spiro SG, Johnson AJ, May CS, et al: Effect of intravenous injection of salbutamol in asthma. *Br J Clin Pharmacol* 2:484, 1975.

35. Newman SP: Therapeutic aerosols. In Clarke SW, Pavia, D. (eds): *Aerosols and the Lung: Clinical and Experimental Aspects.* London, Butterworths, pp 197–224, 1984.

36. Kradjan WA, Lakshminarayan S: Efficiency of air compressor-driven nebulizers. *Chest* 87:512–516, 1985.

37. Christensson P, Arborelius M Jr, Lilja B: Salbutamol inhalation in chronic asthma bronchiale: dose aerosol vs. jet nebulizer. *Chest* 79:416–419, 1981.

38. Hess D: Aerosol bronchodilator delivery during mechanical ventilation. Nebulizer or inhaler? *Chest* 100:1103–1104, 1991.

39. Hess D: How should bronchodilators be administered to patients on ventilators? *Respir Care* 36:377–394, 1991.

40. Shim CS, Williams MH: Effect of bronchodilator therapy administered by cannister versus jet nebulizer. *J Allergy Clin Immunol* 73:387–390, 1984.

41. Newhouse M, Dolovich M: Aerosol therapy: nebulizer vs metered dose inhaler. *Chest* 91:799, 1987.

42. Morley TF, Marozsan E, Zapposodi SJ, et al: Comparison of beta-adrenergic agents delivered by nebulizer vs metered dose inhaler with InspirEase in hospitalized asthmatic patients. *Chest* 94:1205–1210, 1988.

43. Appel D, Karpel JP, Sherman M: Epinephrine improves expiratory flow rates in patients with asthma who do not respond to inhaled metaproterenol sulfate. *J Allergy Clin Immunol* 84:90, 1989.

44. Parry WH, Martorano F, Colton EK: Management of life-threatening asthma with intravenous isoproterenol infusion. *Am J Dis Child* 130:39, 1976.

44a. Herman JJ, Noah ZL, Moody RR: Use of intravenous isoproterenol for status asthmaticus in children. *Crit Care Med* 11:716, 1983.

45. Sly RM, Anderson JA, Bierman CW, et al: Adverse effects and complications of treatment of beta-adrenergic agonist drugs. *J Allergy Clin Immunol* 75:443–449, 1985.

46. Keighley JF: Iatrogenic asthma associated with adrenergic aerosols. *Ann Intern Med* 65:985–990, 1966.

47. Stanescu DS, Van de Woestinje KP: Asthma attack induced by isoprenaline aerosols. *Respiration* 29:532–536, 1972.

48. Van Metre Jr TE: Adverse effects of inhalation of excessive amounts of nebulized isoproterenol in status asthmaticus. *J Allergy* 43:101–113, 1969.

49. Clifton GD, Hunt BA, Patel RC, Burki NK: Effects of sequential doses of parenteral terbutaline on plasma levels of potassium and related cardiopulmonary responses. *Am Rev Respir Dis* 141:575–579, 1990.

50. DaCruz D, Holburn C: Serum potassium responses to nebulized salbutamol administered during an acute asthmatic attack. *Arch Emerg Med* 6:22–26, 1989.

51. Spector SL: Adverse reactions associated with parenteral beta agonists: serum potassium changes. *N Engl Reg Allergy Proc* 8:317–321, 1987.

52. Bhatia SP, Davies HJ: Evaluation of tolerance after continuous and prolonged oral administration of salbutamol to asthmatic patients. *Br J Clin Pharmacol* 2:463–469, 1975.

53. Chervinsky P: The development of drug tolerance during long-term beta₂-agonist bronchodilator therapy. *Chest* 73:1001–1009, 1978.

54. Jenne JW, Strickland RD, Chick TW, et al: Induction of β receptor tolerance by terbutaline. *J Allergy Clin Immunol* 55:96–104, 1975.

55. Larsson S, Svedmyr N, Thiringer G: Lack of bronchial β adrenoreceptor tolerance in asthmatics during long term treatment with terbutaline. *J Allergy Clin Immunol* 59:93–99, 1977.

56. Nelson HS, Raine D, Brandi B, et al: Adrenergic subsensitivity induced by chronic administration of terbutaline and albuterol. *J Allergy Clin Immunol* 57:259–265, 1976.

57a. Sackner MA, Epstein S, Wanner A: Effects of beta adrenergic agonists aerosolized by freon propellant on tracheal mucous velocity and cardiac output. *Chest* 69:593–598, 1976.

57b. Foster WM, Bergofsky EH, Bohning DE, Lippman M: Effect of adrenergic agents and their mode of action on mucociliary clearance. *J Appl Physiol* 41:146–152, 1976.

57c. Clarke SW, Lopez-Vidriero MT: The effect of beta-2 agonist on the activity of human bronchial cilia in vitro. *J Physiol* 336:40–41, 1982.

58. Basran GS, Paul W, Morely J, et al: Evidence in man of synergistic interaction between putative mediators of acute inflammation and asthma. *Lancet* i:935–936, 1982.

59. Gronneberg R, Strandberg K, Stahlenheim G, et al: Effect in man of antiallergic drugs on the immediate and late phase cutaneous allergic reactions induced by anti-IgE. *Allergy* 36:201–208, 1981.

60. Orange RP, Austen WG, Austen KF: Immunological release of histamine and slow reacting substance of anaphylaxis from human lung. I. Modulation by agents influencing cellular levels of cyclic 3′,5″-adenosine monophosphate. *J Exp Med* 134:136s–141s, 1971.

61. Gandevia B: Historical review of the use of parasympatholytic agents in the treatment of respiratory disorders. *Postgrad Med J* 51(suppl 7): 13–20, 1975.

62. Cullumbine H: Cholinergic blocking drugs. In DiPalma JR (ed): *Drill's Pharmacology in Medicine*, 4. McGraw-Hill, New York, 1971.

63. Weiner N: Atropine, scopolamine, and related anti-muscarinic drugs. In Gilman AG, Goodman LS, Rall TW, et al. (eds): *Goodman and Gilman's The Pharmacognosy*, 7. Macmillan, New York, 1985.

64. Nadel JA, Barnes PJ: Autonomic regulation of the airways. *Annu Rev Med* 35:451–467, 1984.

65. Gross NJ, Skorodin MS: The place of anticholinergic agents in the treatment of airways obstruction. *Immunol Allergy Pract* 7:224–231, 1986.

66. Ziment I, Au JP: Anticholinergic agents. *Clin Chest Med* 7:355–366, 1986.

67. Gal TJ, Suratt PM, Lu J-Y: Glycopyrrolate and atropine inhalation: comparative effects on normal airway function. *Am Rev Respir Dis* 129:871–873, 1984.

68. Massey KL, Gotz VP: Ipratropium bromide. *Drug Intelligence Clin Pharm* 19:5–12, 1985.

69. Annis P, Landa J, Lichtiger M: Effects of atropine on velocity of tracheal mucus in anesthetized patients. *Anesthesiology* 44:74–77, 1976.

70. Corssen G, Allen CR: Acetylcholine: its significance in controlling ciliary activity of human respiratory epithelium in vitro. *J Appl Physiol* 14:901–904, 1959.

71. Groth ML, Langenback EG, Foster WM: Influence of inhaled atropine on lung mucociliary function in humans. *Am Rev Respir Dis* 144:1042–1047, 1991.

72. Pavia D, Batement JRM, Sheahan NF, et al: Effect of ipratropium bromide on mucociliary clearance and pulmonary function in reversible airways obstruction. *Thorax* 34:501–507, 1979.

73. Matthys H, Hundenborn J, Daikeler G, Kohler D: Influence of 0.2 mg ipratropium bromide on mucociliary clearance in patients with chronic bronchitis. *Respiration* 48:329–339, 1985.

74. Foster WM, Langenback EG, Bergofsky EH: Acute effect of ipratropium bromide at therapeutic dose on mucus transport of adult asthmatics. *Eur J Resp Dis* 64(Suppl 128):554–557, 1983.

75. Ruffine RE, Wolff RK, Dolorich MB, Rossman CR, Fitzgerald JD, Newhouse MT: Aerosol therapy with Sch 1000. Short-term mucociliary clearance in normal and bronchitic subjects and toxicology in normal subjects. *Chest* 73:501–506, 1978.

76. Higgins RM, Stradling JR, Lane DJ: Should ipratropium bromide be added to beta-agonists in treatment of acute severe asthma? *Chest* 94:718–722, 1988.

77. Rebuck AS, Chapman KR, Abboud R, et al: Nebulized anticholinergic and sympathomimetic treatment of asthma and chronic obstructive airways disease in the emergency room. *Am J Med* 82:59–64, 1987.

78. Mann JS, George CF: Anticholinergic drugs in the treatment of airway disease. *Br J Dis Chest* 79:209–228, 1985.

79. Marini JJ, Lakshminarayan S: The effect of atropine inhalation in "irreversible" chronic bronchitis. *Chest* 77:591–596, 1980.

80. Braun SR, McKenzie WN, Copeland C, et al: A comparison of the effect of ipratropium and albuterol in the treatment of chronic airway disease. *Arch Intern Med* 149:544–547, 1989.

81. Gross NJ, Petty TL, Friedman M, et al: Dose response to ipratropium as a nebulized solution in patients with chronic obstructive pulmonary disease. *Am Rev Respir Dis* 139:1185–1191, 1989.

82. Gross NJ, Skorodin MS: Anticholinergic, antimuscarinic bronchodilators. *Am Rev Respir Dis* 128:856–970, 1984.

83. Salter H: On some points in the treatment and clinical history of asthma. *Edinburgh Med J* 4:1109–1115, 1958.

84. May CD: History of the introduction of theophylline into the treatment of asthma. *Clin Allergy* 4:211–217, 1974.

85. McEvoy GK: Theophylline. In McEvoy GK (ed): *AHFS Drug Information 1987.* American Society of Hospital Pharmacists, Bethesda, MD, pp 1952–1959, 1987.

86. Kelly HW: Controversies in asthma therapy with theophylline and the beta-2-adrenergic agonist aerosols. *Clin Pharm* 3:386–395, 1984.

87. Bergstrand H: Phosphodiesterase inhibition and theophylline. *Eur J Respir Dis* 61(S109):37–44, 1980.

88. Lohman SM, Miech RP, Butcher FR: Effects of isoproterenol, theophylline and carbachol on cyclic nucleotide levels and relaxation of bovine tracheal smooth muscle. *Biochim Biophys Acta* 499:238–250, 1977.

89. Miech RP, Stein M: Methylxanthines. *Clin Chest Med* 7:331–340, 1986.

90. Holgate ST, Mann JS, Cushey MJ: Adenosine as a bronchoconstriction mediator in asthma and its antagonism by methylxanthines. *J Allergy Clin Immunol* 74:302–306, 1984.

91. Winn HR: Methylxanthines, adenosine, and the pulmonary system. *Chest* 91:800–801, 1987.

92. Cushley MJ, Tattersfield AE, Holgate ST: Inhaled adenosine and guanosine on airway resistance in normal and asthmatic subjects. *Br J Clin Pharmacol* 15:161–165, 1983.

93. Fredholm BB: Theophylline actions on adenosine receptors. *Eur J Respir Dis* (suppl) 109:29–36, 1980.

94. Pauwels R, Van Renterghem DV, Van Der Straeten M, Johannesson N, Persson CG: The effect of theophylline and enprofylline on allergen-induced bronchoconstriction. *J Allergy Clin Immunol* 76:583–590, 1985.

95. Lunell E, Anderson KE, Persson CG, Svedmyr N: Intravenous enprofylline in asthma patients. *Eur J Respir Dis* 65:28–34, 1984.

96. Iafrate RP, Massey KL, Hendeles L: Current concepts in clinical therapeutics: asthma. *Clin Pharm* 5:206–227, 1986.

97. Horrobin DF, Manku MS, Franks DJ, Hamet P: Methylxanthine phosphodiesterase inhibitors behave as prostaglandin antagonists in a perfused rat mesenteric artery preparation. *Prostaglandins* 13:33–40, 1977.

98. Higbee MD, Kumar M, Glant SP: Stimulation of endogenous catecholamine release by theophylline: a proposed additional mechanism of action for theophylline effects. *J Allergy Clin Immunol* 70; 377–382, 1982.

99. Mackay AD, Baldwin CJ, Tattersfield AE: Action of intravenously administered aminophylline on normal airways. *Am Rev Respir Dis* 127:609–613, 1983.

100. Fenger M, Eriksen PB, Andersen O, Nielsen MK, Knudsen PJ: Plasma concentrations of the cyclic nucleotides, adenosine 3',5'-mono-phosphate and guanosine 3',5'-monophosphate, in healthy adults treated with theophylline. *Pharmacology* 24:215–221, 1982.

101. Hendeles L, Weinberger M: Theophylline: a state of the art review. *Pharmacotherapy* 3:2–44, 1983.

102. Mitenko PA, Ogilvie RI: Rational intravenous doses of theophylline. *N Engl J Med* 289:600–603, 1973.

103. Ogilvie RI: Clinical pharmacokinetics of theophylline. *Clin Pharmacokinet* 3:267–293, 1978.

104. McFadden ER: Introduction: methylxanthine therapy and reversible airway obstruction. *Am J Med* 79(S6A):1–4, 1985.

105. Piafsky KM, Sitar DS, Rangno RE, Ogilvie RI: Theophylline disposition in patients with hepatic cirrhosis. *N Engl J Med* 296:1495–1497, 1977.

106. Gal P, Jusko WJ, Yurchak AM, Franklin BA: Theophylline disposition in obesity. *Clin Pharmacol Ther* 23:438–444, 1978.

107. Persson CG, Andersson KE: Respiratory and cardiovascular effects of 3-methylxanthine, a metabolite of theophylline. *Acta Pharmacol Toxicol* 40:529–536, 1977.

108. Nassif EG, Weinberger MM, Shannon D, et al: Theophylline disposition in infancy. *J Pediatr* 98:158–161, 1981.

109. Nielsen-Kudsk F, Magnussen I, Jakobsen P: Pharmacokinetics of theophylline in ten elderly patients. *Acta Pharmacol Toxicol* 42:226–234, 1978.

110. Ellis EF, Koysooko R, Levy G: Pharmacokinetics of theophylline in children with asthma. *Pediatrics* 1976; 58:542–547.

111. Longhuan PM, Siar DS, Ogilvie RI, Eisen A, Fox Z, Neims AH: Pharmacokinetic analysis of the disposition of intravenous theophylline in young children. *J Pediatr* 88:874–879, 1976.

112. Tserng K-Y, King KC, Takieddine FN: Theophylline metabolism in premature infants. *Clin Pharmacol Ther* 29:594–600, 1981.

113. Hunt SN, Jusko WJ, Yurchal AM: Effect of smoking on theophylline disposition. *Clin Pharmacol Ther* 24:405–410, 1978.

114. Grygiel JJ, Birkett DJ: Cigarette smoking and theophylline clearance and metabolism. *Clin Pharmacol Ther* 30:491–496, 1981.

115. Jusko WJ, Schentag JJ, Clark JH, Gardner MS, Yurchak AM: Enhanced biotransformation of theophylline in marijuana and tobacco smokers. *Clin Pharmacol Ther* 24:405–410, 1978.

116. Marquis J-F, Caruthers SG, Spence JD, Brownstone YS, Toogood JH: Phenytoin-theophylline interaction. *N Engl J Med* 30:1189–1190, 1982.

117. Lohman SM, Miech RP: Theophylline metabolism by the rat liver microsomal system. *J Pharmacol Exp Ther* 196:213–225, 1976.

118. Landay RA, Gonzalez MA, Taylor JC: Effect of phenobarbital on theophylline disposition. *J Allergy Clin Immunol* 62:27–29, 1978.

119. Reitberg DP, Bernhard H, Schentag JJ: Alteration of theophylline clearance and half-life by cimetidine in normal volunteers. *Ann Intern Med* 95:582–585, 1981.

120. Jackson JE, Powell JR, Wandell M, Bentley J, Door R: Cimetidine decreases theophylline clearance. *Am Rev Respir Dis* 123:615–617, 1981.

121. Jusko WJ, Gardner MJ, Mangione A, Shentag JJ, Doup JR, Vance JW: Factors affecting theophylline clearances: age, tobacco, marijuana, cirrhosis, congestive heart failure, obesity, oral contraceptives, benzodiazepines, barbiturates, and ethanol. *J Pharm Sci* 68:1358–1366, 1979.

122. Breen KJ, Burry R, Desmond PV, et al: Effects of cimetidine and ranitidine on hepatic drug metabolism. *Clin Pharmacol Ther* 31:297–300, 1982.

123. Kappas A, Anderson KE, Conney AH, Alvares AP: Influence of dietary protein and carbohydrate on antipyrine and theophylline metabolism in man. *Clin Pharmacol Ther* 20:643–653, 1976.

124. Kappas A, Alvares AP, Anderson KE, et al: Effect of charcoal-broiled beef on antipyrine and theophylline metabolism. *Clin Pharmacol Ther* 23:445–450, 1978.

125. Pfeifer HJ, Greenblatt DJ, Friedman P: Effect of three antibiotics on theophylline kinetics. *Clin Pharmacol Ther* 26:36–40, 1979.

126. Maddux MS, Leeds NH, Organek HW, Hasegawa GR, Bauman JL: The effect of erythromycin on theophylline pharmacokinetics at steady state. *Chest* 81:563–565, 1982.

127. Iliopoulou A, Aldhous ME, Johnston A, Turner P: Pharmacokinetic interaction between theophylline and erythromycin. *Br J Clin Pharmacol* 14:495–499, 1982.

128. May DC, Jarboe CH, Ellenburg CJ, Roe EJ, Karibo J: The effects of erythromycin on theophylline elimination in normal males. *J Clin Pharmacol* 22:125–130, 1982.

129. Prince RA, Wing DS, Weinberger MM, Hendeles LS, Riegelman S: Effect of erythromycin on theophylline kinetics. *J Allergy Clin Immunol* 68:427–431, 1981.

130. Renton KW, Gray JD, Hung OR: Depression of theophylline elimination by erythromycin. *Clin Pharmacol Ther* 30:422–426, 1981.

131. Reisz G, Pingelton SK, Melethil S, Ryan PB: The effect of erythromycin on theophylline pharmacokinetics in chronic bronchitis. *Am Rev Respir Dis* 127:581–584, 1983.

132. Richer C, Mathieu M, Bah H, Thuillez C, Duroux P, Giudicelli J-F: Theophylline kinetics and ventilatory flow in bronchial asthma and chronic airflow obstruction: influence of erythromycin. *Clin Pharmacol Ther* 31:579–586, 1981.

133. Piafsky KM, Sitar DS, Rangno RE, Ogilvie RI: Theophylline kinetics in acute pulmonary edema. *Clin Pharmacol Ther* 21:310–316, 1977.

134. Powell JR, Vozeh S, Hopewell P, Costello J, Sheiner LB, Reigelman S: Theophylline disposition in acutely ill hospitalized patients: the effect of smoking, heart failure, severe airway obstruction, and pneumonia. *Am Rev Respir Dis* 118:229–238, 1978.

135. Vicuna N, McNay JL, Ludden TM, Schwertner H: Impaired theophylline clearance in patients with cor pulmonale. *Br J Clin Pharmacol* 7:33–37, 1979.

136. Mangione A, Imhoff TE, Lee RV, Shum LY, Jusko WJ: Pharmacokinetics of theophylline in hepatic disease. *Chest* 73:616–622, 1978.

137. Staib AH, Schuppan D, Lissner R, Zilly W, von Bonmhard G, Richter E: Pharmacokinetics and metabolism of theophylline in patients with liver diseases. *Int J Clin Pharmacol Ther Toxicol* 18:500–502, 1980.

138. Chang KC, Lauer BA, Bell TD, Chai H: Altered theophylline pharmacokinetics during acute respiratory viral illness. *Lancet* i:1132–1133, 1978.

139. Resar RK, Walson PD, Fritz WL, Perry DF, Barbee RA: Kinetics of theophylline: variability and effect of arterial pH in chronic obstructive lung disease. *Chest* 76:11–16, 1979.

140. Vallner JJ, Speir Jr WA, Kolbeck RC, Harrison GN, Brandsome Jr ED: Effect of pH on the binding of theophylline to serum proteins. *Am Rev Respir Dis* 120:83–86, 1979.

141. Clozel J-P, Saunier C, Royer-Morot M-J, Royer RJ, Sadoul P: Respiratory acidemia and theophylline pharmacokinetics in the awake dog. *Chest* 80:631–633, 1981.

142. Westerfield BT, Carder AJ, Light RW: The relationship between arterial blood gases and serum theophylline clearance in critically ill patients. *Am Rev Respir Dis* 124:17–20, 1981.

143. Sutton PL, Koup JR, Rose JQ, Middleton E: The pharmacokinetics of theophylline in pregnancy (abstr). *J Allergy Clin Immunol* 61:174, 1978.

144. Lobovitz E, Spector S: Placental theophylline transfer in pregnant asthmatics. *JAMA* 247:786–788, 1982.

145. Weinberger MW, Ginchanski EJ: Dose-dependent kinetics of theophylline disposition in asthmatic children. *J Pediatr* 91:820–924, 1977.

146. Tang-Liu DD, Williams RL, Riegelman S: Nonlinear theophylline elimination. *Clin Pharmacol Ther* 31:358–369, 1982.

147. Rogers RM, Owens GR, Pennock BE: The pendulum swings again toward a rational use of theophylline. *Chest* 87:280–282, 1985.

148. Zwillich CW, Sutton TD, Neft TA, et al: Theophylline-induced seizures in adults: correlations with serum concentration. *Ann Intern Med* 81:784–787, 1975.

149. Lin C, Chuang I, Cheng K, Chiang BN: Arrhythmogenic effects of theophylline in human arterial tissue. *Int J Cardiol* 17:289–297, 1987.

150. Eiriksson CE, Writer SL, Vestal RE: Theophylline-induced alterations in cardiac electrophysiology in patients with chronic obstructive pulmonary disease. *Am Rev Respir Dis* 135:322–326, 1987.

151. Paloucek FP, Rodvold KA: Evaluation of theophylline overdoses and toxicities. *Ann Emerg Med* 17:135–144, 1988.

152. Sessler CN, Cohen M, Garnett AR: Cardiac arrhythmias during theophylline toxicity. *Chest* 94:8S, 1988.

153. Marchlinski FE, Miller JM: Atrial arrhythmias exacerbated by theophylline: response to verapamil and evidence for triggered activity in man. *Chest* 88:931–934, 1985.

154. Levine JH, Michael JR, Guarnieri T: Multifocal atrial tachycardia: a toxic effect of theophylline. *Lancet* i:12–14, 1985.

155. Bittar G, Friedman H: The arrhythmogenicity of theophylline: a multivariate analysis of clinical determinants. *Chest* 99:1415–1420, 1991.

156. Dutt AK, de Soyza ND, Au WY, Hargis JL, Tuck RL: The effect of aminophylline on cardiac rhythm in advance chronic obstructive pulmonary disease: correlation with serum theophylline levels. *Eur J Respir Dis* 64:264–270, 1983.

157. Banner AS, Sunderrajan EV, Agarwal MK, Addington WW: Arrhythmogenic effects of orally administered bronchodilators. *Arch Intern Med* 139:434–437, 1979.

158. Hendeles L, Bighley L, Richardson RH, Hepler CD, Carmichael J: Frequent toxicity from IV aminophylline infusion in critically ill patients. *Drug Intelligence Clin Pharm* 11:12–18, 1977.

159. Sessler CN, Cohen MD: Cardiac arrhythmias during theophylline toxicity: a prospective continuous electrocardiographic study. *Chest* 98:672–678, 1990.

160. Parr MJ, Anaes FC, Day AC, Kletchko SL, Crone PK, Rankin APN: Theophylline poisoning—a review of 64 cases. *Intensive Care Med* 16:394–398, 1990.

161. Sessler CN: Theophylline toxicity: clinical features of 116 consecutive cases. *Am J Med* 88:567–576, 1990.

162. McPherson ML, Prince SR, Atamer ER, Maxwell DB, Ross-Clunis H, Estep HL: Theophylline-induced hypercalcemia. *Ann Intern Med* 105:52–54, 1986.

163. Shannon M, Lovejoy FH: Hypokalemia after theophylline intoxication: the effects of acute vs chronic poisoning. *Arch Intern Med* 149:2725–2729, 1989.

164. Johannesson B, Andersson KE, Joelsson B, et al: Relaxation of lower esophageal sphincter and stimulation of gastric secretion and diuresis by antiasthmatic xanthines. Role of adenosine antagonism. *Am Rev Respir Dis* 131:26, 1985.

165. Pearl RG, Rosenthal MH, Murad F, et al: Aminophylline potentiates sodium nitroprusside-induced hypotension in the dog. *Anesthesiology* 61:712, 1984.

166. Nelson S, Summer WR, Jakab GJ: Aminophylline-induced suppression of pulmonary antibacterial defenses. *Am Rev Respir Dis* 131:923, 1985.

167. Fleetham JA, Ginsburg JC, Nakatsu K, Wigle RD, Munt PW: Resin hemoperfusion as treatment of theophylline-induced seizures. *Chest* 75:741–742, 1979.

168. Berlinger WG, Spector R, Goldberg MJ, Johnson GF, Quee CK, Berg MJ: Enhancement of theophylline clearance by oral activated charcoal. *Clin Pharmacol Ther* 33:351–354, 1983.

169. Mahutte CK, True RJ, Michiels TM, Berman JM, Light RW: Increased serum theophylline clearance with orally administered activated charcoal. *Am Rev Respir Dis* 128:820–822, 1983.

170. Ehlers SM, Zaske DE, Sawchuk RJ: Massive theophylline overdose: rapid elimination by charcoal hemoperfusion. *JAMA* 240:474, 1978.

171. Weinberger MM, Hendeles L: Role of dialysis in the management and prevention of theophylline toxicity. *Dev Pharmacol Ther* 1:26–30, 1980.

172. Park GD, Spector R, Roberts RJ, Goldberg MJ, Weismann D, Shillerman A, et al: Use of hemoperfusion for treatment of theophylline intoxication. *Am J Med* 74:961–966, 1983.

173. Aitken ML, Martin TR: Life-threatening theophylline toxicity is not predictable by serum levels. *Chest* 91:10–14, 1987.

174. Bertino JS, Walker JW: Reassessment of theophylline toxicity. *Arch Intern Med* 147:757–760, 1987.

175. Parr MJ, Anaes FC, Day AC, Kletchko SL, Crone PD, Rankin APN: Theophylline poisoning—a review of 64 cases. *Intensive Care Med* 16:394–398, 1990.

176. Sessler CN: Theophylline toxicity: clinical features of 116 consecutive cases. *Am J Med* 88:567–576, 1990.

177. Rice KL, Leatherman JW, Duane PG, Snyder LS, Harmon KR, Abel J, Niewoehner DE: Aminophylline for acute exacerbations of chronic obstructive pulmonary disease. *Ann Intern Med* 107:305–309, 1987.

178. Littenberg B: Aminophylline treatment in severe, acute asthma: a meta-analysis. *JAMA* 259:1678–1684, 1988.

179. Fanta CH, Rossing TH, McFadden ER Jr: Treatment of acute asthma. Is combination therapy with sympathomimetics and methylxanthines indicated? *Am J Med* 80:5–10, 1986.

180. Rossing TH, Fanta CH, Goldstein DH, Snapper JR, McFadden ER Jr: Emergency therapy of asthma: comparison of the acute effects of parenteral and inhaled sympathomimetics and infused aminophylline. *Am Rev Res Dis* 122:365–371, 1980.

181. Siegel D, Sheppard D, Gelb A, Weinberg PF: Aminophylline increases the toxicity but not the efficacy of an inhaled beta-adrenergic agonist in the treatment of acute exacerbations of asthma. *Am Rev Respir Dis* 132:283–286, 1985.

182. Welsh MJ, Widdicombe JH, Nadel JA: Fluid transport across the canine tracheal epithelium. *J Appl Physiol* 49:905–909, 1980.

183. Serafini SM, Wanner A, Michaelson ED: Mucociliary transport in central and intermediate size airways: effect of aminophylline. *Bull Eur Physiopathol Respir* 12:415–422, 1976.

184. Sutton PP, Pavia D, Bateman JRM, et al: The effect of oral aminophylline on lung mucociliary clearance in man. *Chest* 80S:889–891, 1981.

185. Dowell AR, Heyman A, Sieker HO, Tripathy K: Effect of aminophylline on respiratory center sensitivity in Cheyne-Stokes respiration and in pulmonary emphysema. *N Engl J Med* 273:1447–1453, 1965.

186. Eldridge FL, Millhorn DE, Waldrop TG, et al: Mechanism of respiratory effects of methylxanthines. *Respir Physiol* 53:239–261, 1983.

187. Sanders JS, Berman TM, Bartlett MM, et al: Increased hypoxic ventilatory drive due to administration of aminophylline in normal men. *Chest* 78:279–282, 1980.

188. Aubier M, DeTroyer A, Sampson M, Macklem PT, Roussos C: Aminophylline improves diaphragmatic contractility. *N Engl J Med* 305:249–252, 1981.

189. Aubier M, Murciano D, Vires N, Lecocguic Y, Palacois S, Pariente R: Increased ventilation caused by improved diaphragmatic efficiency during aminophylline infusion. *Am Rev Respir Dis* 127:148–154, 1983.

190. Murciano D, Aubier M, Lecocguic Y, Pariente R: Effects of theophylline on diaphragmatic strength and fatigue in patients with chronic obstructive pulmonary disease. *N Engl J Med* 311:349–353, 1984.

191. Dureuil B, Besmonts JM, Mankikian B, et al: Effects of aminophylline on diaphragmatic dysfunction after upper abdominal surgery. *Anesthesiology* 62:242–246, 1985.

192. Supinski GS, Seal EC, Kelsen SG: The effects of caffeine and theophylline on diaphragm contractility. *Am Rev Respir Dis* 130:429–433, 1984.

193. Murciano D, Aubier M, Viires N, Mal R, Pariente R: Effects of theophylline and enprofylline on diaphragm contractility. *J Appl Physiol* 63:51–57, 1987.

194. Janssens S, Derom E, Reid MB, Tjandramaga TB, Decramer M: Effects of theophylline on canine diaphragmatic contractility and fatigue. *Am Rev Resp Dis* 144:1250–1255, 1991.

195. Matthay RA, Berger JH, Loke J, Gottschal A, Zarat BL: Effects of aminophylline upon right and left ventricular performance in chronic obstructive pulmonary disease. *Am J Med* 65:903–910, 1978.

196. Andersson KE, Persson CG: Extra-pulmonary effects of theophylline. *Eur J Respir Dis* 62(S109):17–28, 1980.

197. McWilliams BC, Menendez R, Kelly HW, Howick J: Effects of theophylline on inhaled methacholine and histamine in asthmatic children. *Am Rev Respir Dis*. 130:193–197, 1984.

198. Cartier A, Lemire I, L'Archeveque J, Ghezzo H, Martin RR, Malo JL: Theophylline partially inhibits bronchoconstriction caused by inhaled histamine in subjects with asthma. *J Allergy Clin Immunol* 77:570–575, 1986.

199. Magnaussen I, Hoedt-Rasmussen K: The effects of intraarterial administered aminophylline on cerebral hemodynamics in man. *Acta Neurol Scand* 55:131–136, 1977.

200. Bowton DL, Alford PT, McLees BD, Prough DS, Stump DA: The effect of aminophylline on cerebral blood flow in patients with chronic obstructive pulmonary disease. *Chest* 91:874–877, 1987.

201. Ellul-Micallef R, Fench FF: Effect of intravenous prednisolone in asthmatics with diminished adrenergic responsiveness. *Lancet* ii:1269–1270, 1975.

202. Holgate ST, Baldwin CJ, Tattersfield AE: Beta-adrenergic agonists resistance in normal airways. *Lancet* ii:375–377, 1977.

203. Paterson JW, Lulich KM, Goldie RG: Drug effects on beta-adrenoreceptor function in asthma. In Morley, J (ed): *Beta-Adrenoceptors in Asthma.* Academic Press, London, 1984.

204. Fraser CM, Benter JC: The synthesis of β-adrenergic receptors in cultural human lung cells: induction by glucocorticoids. *Biochem Biophys Res Commun* 94:390–397, 1980.

205. Mano K, Akbarzadek A, Townley RG: Effect of hydrocortisone on β-adrenergic receptors in lung membranes. *Life Sci* 25:1925–1930, 1979.

206. Tashkin OP, Connally ME, Deutsch RI, et al: Subsensitization of β-adrenoceptors in airways and lymphocytes of healthy and asthmatic subjects. *Am Rev Respir Dis* 125:185–193, 1982.

207. Holgate ST, Baldwin CJ, Tattersfield AE: β-adrenergic agonist resistance in normal human airways. *Lancet* ii:375–377, 1977.

208. Morris HG: Mechanisms of action and therapeutic role of corticosteroids in asthma. *J Allergy Clin Immunol* 75:1–13, 1985.

209. Agnew JE, Bateman JRM, Sheahan NF, et al: Effect of oral corticosteroids in mucus clearance by cough and mucociliary transport in stable asthma. *Bull Eur Physiopathol Respir* 19:37–41, 1983.

210. Lundgren JD, Kaliner MA, Shelhamer JH: Mechanisms by which glucocorticosteroids inhibit secretion of mucus in asthmatic airways. *Am Rev Respir Dis* 141 (suppl): S52–S58, 1990.

211. Wiggins J, Elliott JA, Stevenson RD, Stockley RA: Effect of corticosteroids on sputum sol-phase protease inhibitors in chronic obstructive pulmonary disease. *Thorax* 37:652–656, 1982.

212. Marom Z, Shelhammer J, Alling D, et al: The effects of corticosteroids on mucous glycoprotein secretion from human airways in vitro. *Am Rev Respir Dis* 129:62–65, 1984.

213. Pierson WE, Bierman CW, Kelley VC: A double-blind trial of corticosteroid therapy in status asthmaticus. *Pediatrics* 54:282–288, 1974.

214. Shapiro GG, Furukawa CT, Pierson WE, Gardinier R, Bierman CW: Double-blind evaluation of methylprednisolone versus placebo for acute asthma. *Pediatrics* 71:510–514, 1983.

215. Fanta CH, Rossing TH, McFadden Jr ER: Glucocorticoids in acute asthma: a critical controlled trial. *Am J Med* 74:845–851, 1983.

216. Harkell RJ, Wong BM, Mansen JE: A double-blind, randomized clinical trial of methylprednisolone in status asthmaticus. *Arch Intern Med* 143:1324–1327, 1983.

217. Pinkerton Jr HH, Metre Jr TR: Immediate therapy for acute attack of asthma. *N Engl J Med* 258:363–366, 1958.

218. Kattan M, Gurwitz D, Levinson H: Corticosteroids in status asthmaticus. *J Pediatr* 96:596–599, 1980.

219. Ellul-Micallef R, Fench FF: Intravenous prednisolone in chronic bronchial asthma. *Thorax* 30:312–315, 1975.

220. Littenberg B, Gluck EH: A controlled trial of methylprednisolone in the emergency treatment of acute asthma. *N Engl J Med* 314:150–152, 1986.

221. Schneider SM, Pipher A, Britton HL, Borok Z, Harcup CH: High dose methylprednisolone as initial therapy in patients with acute bronchospasm. *J Asthma* 25:189–193, 1988.

222. McFadden ER Jr, Kiser R, deGroot WJ, Holmes B, Kiker R, Viser G: A controlled study of the effects of single doses of hydrocortisone on the resolution of acute attacks of asthma. *Am J Med* 74:845–851, 1983.

223. Collins JV, Clark TJ, Brown D, Townsend J: The use of corticosteroids in the treatment of acute asthma. *Q J Med* 44:259–273, 1975.

224. Haskell RJ, Wong BM, Hansen JE: A double-blind, randomized clinical trial of methylprednisolone in status asthmaticus. *Arch Intern Med* 143:1324–1327, 1983.

225. Tanaka RM, Santiago SM, Kuhn GJ, et al: Intravenous methylprednisolone in adults in status asthmaticus. Comparison of two dosages. *Chest* 82:438–440, 1982.

226. Britton MG, Collins JV, Brown D, et al: High-dose corticosteroids in severe acute asthma. *Br Med J* 2:73–74, 1976.

227. Harfi H, Hanissian AS, Crawford LV: Treatment of status asthmaticus in children with high doses and conventional doses of methylprednisolone. *Pediatrics* 61:829–831, 1978.

227a. McFadden ER Jr: Dosages of cortiscosteroids in asthma. *Am Rev Respir Dis* 147:1306–1310, 1993.
228. Sahn SA: Corticosteroids in chronic bronchitis and pulmonary emphysema. *Chest* 73:389–396, 1978.
229. Albert RK, Martin TR, Lewis SW. Controlled clinical trial of methylprednisolone in patients with chronic bronchitis and acute respiratory insufficiency. *Ann Intern Med* 92:753–758, 1980.
230. Glenny RW: Steroids in COPD. The scripture according to Albert. *Chest* 91:289–290, 1987.
231. Emerman CL, Connors AF, Lukens RTW, et al: A randomized controlled trial of methylprednisolone in the emergency treatment of acute exacerbations of COPD. *Chest* 95:563–567, 1989.
232. Nicholson DP: Glucocorticoids in the treatment of shock and the adult respiratory distress syndrome. *Clin Chest Med* 3:121–132, 1982.
233. Sibbald WJ, Anderson RR, Reid B, et al: Alveolo-capillary permeability in human septic ARDS: effect of high-dose corticosteroid therapy. *Chest* 79:133–142, 1981.
234. Brigham KL, Bowers RE, McKeen CR: Methylprednisolone prevention of increased lung vascular permeability following endotoxemia in sheep. *J Clin Invest* 67:1103–1110, 1981.
235. Schumer W: Steroids in the treatment of clinical septic shock. *Ann Surg* 184:333–341, 1976.
236. Weigelt JA, Norcross JF, Borman KR, et al: Early steroid therapy for respiratory failure. *Arch Surg* 120:536–540, 1985.
237. Schein RM, Bergman R, Marcial EH, et al: Complement activation and corticosteroid therapy in the development of the adult respiratory distress syndrome. *Chest* 91:850–854, 1987.
238. Sprung CL, Caralis PV, Marcial EH, et al: The effects of high-dose corticosteroids in patients with septic shock: a prospective controlled study. *N Engl J Med* 311:1137–1143, 1984.
239. Veterans Administration Systems Sepsis Cooperative Study Group: Effect of high dose glucocorticoid therapy on mortality in patients with clinical signs of systemic sepsis. *N Engl J Med* 317:659–665, 1987.
240. Luce JM, Montgomery AB, Marks JD, et al: Ineffectiveness of high-dose methylprednisolone in preventing parenchymal lung injury and improving mortality in patients with septic shock. *Am Rev Respir Dis* 138:62–68, 1988.
241. Bernard GR, Luce JM, Sprung CL, et al: High-dose corticosteroids in patients with the adult respiratory distress syndrome. *N Engl J Med* 317:1565–1570, 1987.
242. Hooper RG, Kearl RA: Established ARDS treated with a sustained course of adrenocortical steroids. *Chest* 97:138–143, 1990.
243. Meduri GU, Bolenchia JM, Estes RJ, Wanderink RG, El Torky M, Leeper KV: Fibroproliferative phase of ARDS: clinical findings and effects of corticosteroids. *Chest* 100:943–952, 1991.
244. Alho A, Saikku K, Eerola P, Koskinen M, Hamalainen M: Corticosteroids in patients with a high risk of fat embolism syndrome. *Surg Gynecol Obstet* 147:358–362, 1978.
245. Stoltenberg JJ, Gustilo RB: The use of methylprednisolone and hypertonic glucose in the prophylaxis of fat embolism syndrome. *Clin Orthop* 143:211–212, 1979.
246. Schonfeld SA, Ploysongsang Y, Dilisio R, et al: Fat embolism prophylaxis with corticosteroids: a prospective study in high-risk patients. *Ann Intern Med* 99:438–443, 1983.
247. Wolfe JE, Bone RC, Ruth WE: Effects of corticosteroids in the treatment of patients with gastric aspiration. *Am J Med* 63:719–722, 1977.
248. Zorab JSM: Pulmonary aspiration. *Br Med J* 288:1631–1632, 1984.
249. Wynne JW, Reynolds JC, Hood JI, et al: Steroid therapy for pneumonitis induced in rabbits by aspiration of foodstuff. *Anesthesiology* 51:11–19,1979.
250. Glauser FL, Millen JE, Falls R: Increased alveolar epithelial permeability with acid aspiration: the effect of high-dose steroids. *Am Rev Respir Dis* 120:1119–1123, 1979.
251. Montaner JSG, Lawson LM, Levitt N, Belzberg A, Schechter MT, Ruedy J: Corticosteroids prevent early deterioration in patients with moderately severe *Pneumocystis carinii* pneumonia and the acquired immunodeficiency syndrome (AIDS). *Ann Intern Med* 113:14–20, 1990.
252a. Gagnon S, Boota AM, Fischal MA, Baier H, Kirksey OW, La Vaie L: Corticosteroids as adjunctive therapy for severe *Pneumocystis carinii* pneumonia in the acquired immunodeficiency syndrome: a double-blind, placebo-controlled trial. *N Engl J Med* 1990; 323:1444–1450.
252b. Bozzette SA, Sattler FR, Chiu J, et al: A controlled trial of early adjunctive treatment with corticosteroids for *Pneumocystis carinii* pneumonia in the acquired immunodeficiency syndrome. *N Engl J Med* 323:1451–1457, 1990.
253. The National Institutes of Health-University of California Expert Panel for Corticosteroids as Adjunctive Therapy for Pneumocystis Pneumonia: Consensus statement on the use of corticosteroids as adjunctive therapy for *Pneumocystis* pneumonia in the acquired immunodeficiency syndrome. *N Engl J Med* 323:1500–1504, 1990.
254. Haury VG: The broncho-dilator action of magnesium and its antagonistic action (dilator action) against pilocarpine, histamine and barium chloride. *J Pharmacol Exp Ther* 64:58–64, 1938.
255. Okayama H, Aikawa T, Okayama M, et al: Bronchodilatory effect of intravenous magnesium sulfate in bronchial asthma. *JAMA* 257:1076–1078, 1987.
256. Rolla G, Bucca C, Caria E, Arossa W, Bugiani M, Cesano L, Caropreso A: Acute effect of intravenous magnesium sulfate on airway obstruction of asthmatic patients. *Ann Allergy* 61:388–391, 1988.
257. Noppen M, Vanmaele L, Impens N, Schandevyl W: Bronchodilating effect of intravenous magnesium sulfate in acute severe bronchial asthma. *Chest* 97:373–376, 1990.
258. Okayama H, Okayama M, Aikawa T, Sasaki M, Takishima T: Treatment of status asthmaticus with intravenous magnesium sulfate. *J Asthma* 28:11–17, 1991.
259. McNamara RM, Spivey WH, Skobeloff EM, Jacubowitz S: Intravenous magnesium sulfate in the management of acute respiratory failure complicating asthma. *Ann Emerg Med* 18:197–199, 1989.
260. Spivey WH, McNamara RM, Skobeloff EA: Intravenous magnesium sulfate for the treatment of acute asthma in the emergency department. *JAMA* 262:1210–1213, 1989.
261. Turlapaty PDMV, Carrier O: Influence of magnesium on calcium-induced responses of atrial and vascular muscle. *J Pharmacol Exp Ther* 187:86–98, 1973.
262. Dunnett J, Nayler WG: Calcium efflux from cardiac sarcoplasmic reticulum: effect of calcium and magnesium. *J Mol Cell Cardiol* 10:487–498, 1978.
263. Levine BS, Coburn JW: Magnesium, the mimic/antagonist of calcium. *N Engl J Med* 310:1253–1255, 1984.
264. Lindeman KS, Hirshman CA, Freed AN: Effect of magnesium sulfate on bronchoconstriction in the lung periphery. *J Appl Physiol* 66:2527–2532, 1989.
265. Rolla G, Bucca C, Bugiani M. Arossa W, Spinaci S: Reduction of histamine-induced bronchoconstriction by magnesium in asthmatic subjects. *Allergy* 42:186–188, 1987.
266. Bois P: Effect of magnesium deficiency on mast cells and urinary histamine in rats. *Br J Exp Pathol* 44:151–155, 1963.
267. Del Castillo J, Engbaek L: The nature of the neuromuscular block produced by magnesium. *J Physiol* 124:370–384, 1954.
268. Rolla G, Bucca C, Bugiani M, et al: Effect of magnesium in salbutamol-induced bronchodilation in asthmatics. *Am Rev Respir Dis* 139(suppl):A431, 1989.
269. Ziment I: Mucus in Bronchial Asthma. In Allergra L, Bragu PC (eds): *Bronchial Mucology and Related Disease.* Raven Press, New York, pp 127–140, 1990.
270. Clarke SW: Rationale of airway clearance. *Eur Respir J* 2:599–604, 1989.
271. Puchelle E, Zahm JM, Girard D, et al: Mucociliary transport in vivo and in vitro. Relations to sputum properties in chronic bronchitis. *Eur J Respir Dis* 61:254–264, 1980.
272. Lundgren JD, Shelhamer JH: Pathogenesis of airway mucus hypersecretion. *J Allergy Clin Immunol* 85:399–417, 1990.
273. Wanner A: Clinical aspects of mucociliary transport. *Am Rev Respir Dis* 115:73–125, 1977.
274. Sleigh MA, Blake JR, Liron N: The propulsion of mucus by cilia. *Am Rev Respir Dis* 137:726–741, 1988.
275. Wick MM, Ingram RH: Bronchorrhea responsive to aerosolized atropine. *JAMA* 235:1356–1357, 1976.
276. Ziment I: Mucokinetic agents. In Ziment I (ed): *Respiratory pharmacology and therapeutics.* WB Saunders, Philadelphia, pp 60–104, 1978.
277. Holdiness MR: Clinical pharmacokinetics of N-acetylcysteine. *Clin Pharmacokinet* 20:123–134, 1991.
278. Olivieri D, Marsico SA, Del Donno M: Improvement of mucociliary transport in smokers by mucolytics. *Eur J Respir Dis* 66(Suppl 139):142–145, 1985.
279. Rasmussen JB, Glennow C: Reduction in days of illness after long-term treatment with N-acetylcysteine controlled-release tablets in patients with chronic bronchitis. *Eur Resp J* 1:351–355, 1988.
280. Bowman G, Backer U, Larsson S, Melander B, Whalander L: Oral acetylcysteine reduces exacerbation rate in chronic bronchitis: report of a trial organized by the Swedish Society for Pulmonary Diseases. *Eur J Respir Dis* 64:405–415, 1983.
281. Multicenter Study Group: Long-term oral acetylcysteine in chronic bronchitis: a double-blind controlled study. *Eur J Respir Dis.* 61(Suppl 111):93–108, 1980.
282. Ziment I: Inorganic and organic iodides. In Braga PC, Allegra L (eds): *Drugs in Bronchial Mycology.* Raven Press, New York, 1989.
283. Pavia D, Agnew JE, Glassman JM, Sutton PP, Lopez-Vidriero MT, Soyka JP, et al: Effects of iodopropylidene glycerol on tracheobronchial clearance in stable, chronic bronchitic patients. *Eur J Respir Dis* 67:177–184, 1985.
284. Repsher LM, Glassman JM, Soyka JP: Evaluation of iodopropylidene glycerol as adjunctive therapy in stable, chronic asthmatic patients on theophylline maintenance. *Today's Ther Trends* 1:77–89, 1983.
285. Prenner BM: Chronic respiratory disease complicated by mucus: results of a clinical evaluation of the mucolytic agent iodinated glycerol in a four-week, open trial of adult asthmatics. *Immunol Allergy Pract* 10:17–20, 1988.
286. Petty TL: The National Mucolytic Study. Results of a randomized, double-blind placebo-controlled, study of iodinated glycerol in chronic obstructive bronchitis. *Chest* 97:75–83, 1990.
287. Leigh JM: Early treatment with oxygen. *Anaesthesia* 29:194–208, 1974.
288. Deneke SM, Fanburg BL: Normobaric oxygen toxicity of the lung. *N Engl J Med* 303:76–86, 1980.

289. Civetta JM, Brons R, Gabel JC: A simple and effective method of employing spontaneous positive-pressure ventilation. *J Thorac Cardiovasc Surg* 62:312–317, 1972.

290. Snyder JV, Pinsky MR, Buran MJ (eds): *Oxygen Consumption. Transport in the Critically Ill.* Year Book, Chicago, pp 16–21, 1987.

291. Bartlett RH, Dechert RE, Mault JR, et al: Measurement of metabolism in multiple organ failure. *Surgery* 92:771–779, 1982.

292. Weissman C, Kemper M, Askanazi J, et al: Resting metabolic rate of the critically ill patient: measured versus predicted. *Anesthesiology* 64:673–679, 1986.

293. Reinhart K: Clinical assessment of tissue oxygenation: value of hemodynamic and oxygen transport related variables. In Gutierrez G, Vincent JL (eds): *Update in Intensive Care and Emergency Medicine*, vol 12. Springer-Verlag, New York, pp 269–285, 1991.

294. Synder JV: Assessment of systemic oxygen transport. In Snyder JV, Pinsky MR (eds): *Oxygen Transport in the Critically Ill.* Year Book, Chicago, pp 179–198, 1987.

295. Gilbert R, Auchincloss JH, Kuppinger M, Thomas MV: Stability of the arterial/alveolar oxygen partial pressure ratio: effects of low ventilation/perfusion regions. *Crit Care Med* 7:267–272, 1979.

296. Gilbert R, Keighley JF: The arterial/alveolar oxygen tension ratio. An index of gas exchange applicable to varying inspired oxygen concentrations. *Am Rev Resp Dis* 109:142–145, 1974.

297. Abraham AS, Cole RB, Green ID, et al: Factors contributing to the reversible pulmonary hypertension of patients with acute respiratory failure studied by serial observations during recovery. *Circ Res* 24:54–60, 1969.

298. Medical Research Council Working Party: Long-term domiciliary oxygen therapy in chronic hypoxic cor pulmonale complicating chronic bronchitis and emphysema. *Lancet* i:681–686, 1981.

299. Nocturnal Oxygen Therapy Trial Group: Continuous or nocturnal oxygen therapy in hypoxemic chronic obstructive lung disease: a clinical trial. *Ann Intern Med* 93:391–398, 1980.

300. Ashutosh K, Mead G, Dunksy M: Early effects of oxygen administration and prognosis in chronic obstructive pulmonary disease and cor pulmonale. *Am Rev Respir Dis* 127:399–404, 1983.

301. Weitzenblum E, Sautegeau A, Ehrhart M, et al: Long-term oxygen therapy can reverse the progression of pulmonary hypertension in patients with chronic obstructive pulmonary disease. *Am Rev Respir Dis* 131:493–498, 1985.

302. France AJ, Prescott RJ, Biernacki W, et al: Does right ventricular function predict survival in patients with chronic obstructive pulmonary disease? *Thorax* 43:621–626, 1988.

303. Morrison DA, Henry R, Goldman S: Preliminary study for the effects of low flow oxygen on oxygen delivery and right ventricular function in chronic obstructive lung disease. *Am Rev Respir Dis* 133:390–395, 1986.

304. Wiedemann HP, Matthay RA: Cor pulmonale in pathophysiology and new concepts of therapy. In Simmons DH (ed): *Current Pulmonology*, vol 8. Year Book, Chicago, pp 127–162, 1987.

305. Martin R, Saunders M, Gray B, et al: Acute and long-term ventilatory effects of hyperoxia in the adult sleep apnea syndrome. *Am Rev Resp Dis* 125:175–180, 1982.

306. McNicholas W, Carter J, Rutherford R, et al: Beneficial effect of oxygen in primary alveolar hypoventilation with central sleep apnea. *Am Rev Respir Dis* 125:772–775, 1982.

307. Gold A, Smith P, Haponik E, et al: Effects of low flow oxygen on central sleep apnea. *Am Rev Respir Dis* 129:A274, 1984.

308. NHLBI Workshop Summary: Hyperbaric oxygenation therapy. *Am Rev Respir Dis* 144:1414–1421, 1991.

309. Adamason I, Bowden D, Wyatt J: Oxygen poisoning in mice. Ultrastructural and surfactant studies during exposure and recovery. *Arch Pathol* 90:463–472, 1970.

310. Barry BE, Crapo JD: Patterns of accumulation of platelets and neutrophils in rat lungs during exposure to 100% and 85% oxygen. *Am Rev Respir Dis* 132:548–555, 1985.

311. Berend N: The effect of bleomycin and oxygen on rat lung. *Pathology* 16:136–139, 1984.

312. Holm B, Notter R, Leary J, et al: Alveolar epithelial changes in rabbits after a 21-day exposure to 60% O_2. *J Appl Physiol* 62:2230–2236, 1987.

313. Comroe J, Dripps R, Dimke P, et al: Oxygen toxicity. The effect of inhalation of high concentrations of oxygen of twenty-four hours on normal men. *JAMA* 128:710–717, 1945.

314. Caldwell P, Lee W, Schildkraut H, et al: Changes in lung volume, diffusing capacity, and blood gases in men breathing oxygen. *J Appl Physiol* 21:1477–1483, 1966.

315. Burger E, Mead J: Static properties of lungs after oxygen exposure. *J Appl Physiol* 27:191–197, 1969.

316. Barber R, Lee J, Hamilton W: Oxygen toxicity in man: a prospective study in patients with irreversible brain damage. *N Engl J Med* 283:1478–1484, 1970.

317. Singer MM, Wright F, Stanley L, et al: Oxygen toxicity in man: a prospective study in patients after open heart surgery. *N Engl J Med* 283:1473–1478, 1970.

318. Sackner M, Landa J, Hirsch J, et al: Pulmonary effects of oxygen breathing. A six-hour study in normal men. *Ann Intern Med* 82:40–43, 1975.

319. Gould V, Tosco R, Wheelis R, et al: Oxygen pneumonitis in man. Ultrastructural observations on the development of alveolar lesions. *Lab Invest* 26:499–508, 1972.

320. Nash G, Blennerhassett JB, Pontoppidan H: Pulmonary lesions associated with oxygen therapy and artificial ventilation. *N Engl J Med* 276:368–374, 1967.

321. Jenkinson SG: Pulmonary oxygen toxicity. *Clin Chest Med* 3:109, 1982.

322. Clark J, Lambertsen C: Pulmonary oxygen toxicity: a review. *Pharmacol Rev* 23:37–133, 1971.

323. Haugaard N: Cellular mechanisms of oxygen toxicity. *Physiol Rev* 48:311–373, 1968.

324. Travis J: Oxidants and antioxidants in the lung. *Am Rev Respir Dis* 135:773–774, 1987.

325. Aubier M, Murciano D, Milic-Emili J, et al: Effects of the administration of O_2 on ventilation and blood gases in patients with chronic obstructive pulmonary disease during acute respiratory failure. *Am Rev Respir Dis* 122:747–754, 1980.

326. Warren PM, Jeffrey A, Haslett C, et al: Controlled oxygen therapy in acute exacerbations of chronic bronchitis and emphysema. Clin Sci 63:53P, 1982.

327. Warren PM, Flenley DC, Millar JS, Avery A: Respiratory failure revisited: acute exacerbations of chronic bronchitis between 1961–68 and 1970–76. *Lancet* i:467–471, 1980.

328. Tierney DF, Ayers L, Kasuyama RS: Altered sensitivity to oxygen toxicity. *Am Rev Respir Dis* 114:59, 1977.

329. Sanders RL. The composition of pulmonary surfactant. In Farrell PM (ed): *Lung Development: Biological and Clinical Perspectives.* Academic Press, New York, p 183, 1982.

330. Clements JA: Dependence of pressure-volume characteristics of lungs on intrinsic surface active material. *Am J Physiol* 187:592, 1956.

331. Pattle RE: Surface lining of the lung alveoli. *Physiol Rev* 45:48–79, 1965.

332. Von Neergaard K: New notions on a fundamental principle of respiratory mechanisms. The retractile force of the lungs, dependent on the surface tension in the alveoli (translated by Arnold R, Hahn H). In Comroe JH (ed). *Pulmonary and Respiratory Physiology.* Dowden, Hutchison, and Ross, Stroudsburg, PA, 214–234, 1976.

333. Avery ME, Mead J: Surface properties in relation to atelectasis and hyaline membrane disease. *Am J Dis Child* 97:517–523,1959.

334. Wright JR, Clements JA: Metabolism and turnover of lung surfactant. *Am Rev Respir Dis* 135:426–444, 1987.

335. Holm BA, Matalon S: Role of pulmonary surfactant in the development and treatment of adult respiratory distress syndrome. *Anesth Analg* 69:805–818, 1989.

336. Weaver TE: Surfactant proteins and SP-D. *Am J Respir Cell Mol Biol* 5:4–5, 1991.

336a. Hollingsworth M, Gilfillan AM: The pharmacology of lung surfactant secretion. *Pharmacol Rev* 36:69–90, 1984.

337. Lachmann B, Hallman M, Bergmann KC: Respiratory failure following anti-lung serum: study on mechanisms associated with surfactant system damage. *Exp Lung Res* 12:163–180, 1987.

338. Berry D, Ikegami M, Jobe A: Respiratory distress and surfactant inhibition following vagotomy in rabbits. *J Appl Physiol* 61:1741–1748, 1986.

339. Holm BA, Notter RH, Seigle J, Matalon S: Pulmonary physiological and surfactant changes during injury and recovery from hyperoxia. *J Appl Physiol* 59:1402–1409, 1985.

340. Ikegami M, Jobe A, Jacobs H: A protein from airways of premature lambs that inhibits surfactant function. *J Appl Physiol* 57:1134–1142, 1984.

341. Seeger W, Stohr G, Wolf HRD: Alteration of surfactant function due to protein leakage: special interaction with fibrin monomer. *J Appl Physiol* 58:326–338, 1985.

342. Fuchimukai T, Fujiwara T, Takahashi A, Enhorning G: Artificial pulmonary surfactant inhibited by proteins. *J Appl Physiol* 62:429–437, 1987.

343. Ryan SF, Lian DF, Loomis-Bell AL, et al: Correlation of lung compliance and quantities of surfactant phospholipids after acute alveolar injury from N-nitroso-N-methylurethane in the dog. *Am Rev Resp Dis* 123:200–204, 1981.

344. Pison U, Oberatacke U, Brand M, Seeger W, Joka T, Bruch J, Schmit-Neuerburg KP: Altered pulmonary surfactant in uncomplicated and septicemia-complicated courses of acute respiratory failure. *J Trauma* 30:19–26, 1990.

345. Petty TL, Silvers GW, Paul GW, et al: Abnormalities in lung elastic properties and surfactant function in adult respiratory distress syndrome. *Chest* 75:571–574, 1979.

346. Hallman M, Spragg R, Harrell JH, et al: Evidence of lung surfactant abnormality in respiratory failure. *J Clin Invest* 70:673–683, 1982.

347. Holm BA, Notter RH, Finkelstein JN: Surface property changes from interactions of albumin with natural lung surfactant and extracted lung lipids. *Chem Phys Lipids* 38:287–298, 1985.

348. Holm BA, Notter RH: Effects of hemoglobin and cell membrane lipids on pulmonary surfactant activity. *J Appl Physiol* 63:1434–1442, 1987.

349. Holm BA, Enhorning GE, Notter RH: A biophysical mechanism by which plasma proteins inhibit surfactant activity. *Chem Phys Lipids* 49:49–55, 1988.

350. Merritt TA, Hallman M, Spragg R, Heldt GP, Gilliard N: Exogenous surfactant treatments for neonatal respiratory distress syndrome and their potential role in the adult respiratory distress syndrome. *Drugs* 38:591–611, 1989.

351. Matalon S, Holm BA, Notter RH: Mitigation of pulmonary hyperoxic injury by administration of exogenous surfactant. *J Appl Physiol* 62:756–761, 1987.

352. Loewen GM, Holm BA, Milanowski I, Wild LM, Matalon S: Alveolar hyperoxic injury in rabbit receiving exogenous surfactant. *J Appl Physiol* 66:1087–1092, 1988.

353. Kobayashi T, Kataoka H, Ueda T, Murakami S, Takada Y, Kokubo M: Effects of surfactant supplement and end-expiratory pressure in lung-lavaged rabbits. *J Appl Physiol* 57:995–1001, 1984.

354. Berggren P, Lachmann B, Curstedt T, Grossman G, Robertson B: Gas exchange and lung morphology after surfactant replacement in experimental adult respiratory distress syndrome induced by repeated lung lavage. *Acta Anaesthesiol Scand* 30:321–328, 1986.

355. Merit TA, Hallman M, Bloom BT: Prophylactic treatment of very premature infants with human surfactant. *N Engl J Med* 315:785–790, 1986.

356. Collaborative European Multicenter Study Group: Surfactant replacement therapy for severe neonatal respiratory distress syndrome: an international randomized clinical trial. *Pediatrics* 82:683–691, 1988.

357. Horbar JD, Soll SF, Sutherland JM et al: A multicenter, randomized, placebo-controlled trial of surfactant therapy for respiratory distress syndrome. *N Engl J Med* 320:959–965, 1989.

358. Corbet AJ, Goldman SA, Lombrady L, Mammel MA, Long WA: Decreased mortality in small premature infants treated at birth with a single dose of synthetic surfactant: a multicenter trial. *J Pediatr* 118:277–284,1991.

359. Long WA, Thompson T, Sundell H, Schumacher R, Volberg F, Guthrie R: Effects of two rescue doses of synthetic surfactant on mortality in 700-1300 gram infants with RDS. *J Pediatr* 118:595–605, 1991.

360. Richmann PS, Spragg RG, Merritt TA, Curstedt T: The adult respiratory distress syndrome: first trials with surfactant replacement. *Eur Respir J* 2(suppl):109–111, 1989.

361. Lachmann B: Animal models and clinical pilot studies of surfactant replacement in adult respiratory distress syndrome. *Eur Respir J* 2(suppl):98:103, 1989.

362. Weg J, Reines H, Balk R, et al: Safety and efficacy of an aerosolized surfactant (EXOSURF) in human sepsis-induced ARDS. *Chest* 100:137S, 1991.

363. Reines HD, Silverman H, Hurst J: Effects of two concentrations of nebulized surfactant (EXOSURF) in sepsis-induced adult respiratory distress syndrome (ARDS). *Crit Care Med* 20:S61, 1992.

364. Dusting GJ, Moneada S, Vane JR: Recirculation of prostacyclin in the dog. *Br J Pharmacol* 64:315–320, 1978.

365. Gillis CN, Pitt BR, Wiedemann HP, Hammond GL: Depressed prostaglandin E₁ and 5-hydroxytryptamine removal in patients with adult respiratory distress syndrome. *Am Rev Respir Dis* 134:739–744, 1986.

366. Cox JW, Andreadis NA, Bone RC, Maunder RJ, Pullen RH, Ursprung JJ, Vassar MJ: Pulmonary extraction and pharmacokinetics of prostaglandin E₁ during continuous intravenous infusion in patients with adult respiratory distress syndrome. *Am Rev Respir Dis* 137:5–12, 1988.

367. Dusting JD, Moncada S, Van J: Prostaglandins, their intermediates and precursors: cardiovascular actions and regulatory roles in normal and abnormal circulatory systems. *Prog Cardiovasc Dis* 21:405–430, 1979.

368. Metsa-Ketela T: Cyclic AMP-dependent and -independent effects of prostaglandins on the contraction-relaxation cycle of spontaneously beating isolated rat atria. *Acta Physiol Scand* 112:481–485, 1981.

369. Goldstein I, Malmsten C, Samuelsson B, Weissman G: Prostaglandins, thromboxanes and polymorphonuclear leukocytes. *Inflammation* 2:309, 1977.

370. Robert A: Cytoprotection by prostaglandins. *Gastroenterology* 77:761, 1979.

371. Araki H, Lefer A: Cytoprotective actions of prostacyclin during hypoxia in the isolated perfused cat liver. *Am J Physiol* 238:H176, 1980.

372. Sikujara O, Monden M, Toyoshima K, Okamura J, Kosaki G: Cytoprotective effect of prostaglandin I2 (prostacyclin) on ischaemia induced hepatic cell injury. *Transplantation* 36:238, 1983.

373. Whittle BJ, Moncada S, Vane JR: Comparison of the effects of prostacyclin, prostaglandin E1 and D2 on platelet aggregation of different species. *Prostaglandins* 16:373–388, 1978.

374. Sinzinger H, Reiter R: The intrafusion platelet rebound during and following PGE-infusion is faster and more intensive than that with PGI2. *Prostaglandins Leukat Med* 13:281–288, 1984.

375. Rich S: Primary pulmonary hypertension. *Prog Cardiovasc Dis* 31:205–238, 1988.

376. Szczeklik J, Szczeklik A, Nizankowski R: Hemodynamic effects produced by prostacyclin in man. *Br Heart J* 44:254–258, 1980.

377. Guadagni DN, Ikram H, Maslowski AH: Haemodynamic effects of prostacyclin (PGI₂) in pulmonary hypertension. *Br Heart J* 45:385–388, 1981.

378. Rubin LJ, Groves BM, Reeves JT, Frosolono M, Handel F, Cata AE: Prostacyclin-induced acute pulmonary vasodilation in primary pulmonary hypertension. *Circulation.* 66:334–338, 1982.

379. Higenbottam T, Wells F, Wheeldon D, Wallwork J: Long-term treatment of primary pulmonary hypertension with continuous intravenous epoprostenol (prostacyclin). *Lancet* ii:1046–1047, 1984.

380. Kaapa P, Koivisto M, Ylikorkala O, Kouvalainen K: Prostacyclin in the treatment of neonatal pulmonary hypertension. *J Pediatr* 107:951–953, 1985.

381. Groves BM, Rubin LJ, Frosolono MF, Cato AE, Reeves JT: A comparison of the acute hemodynamic effects of prostacyclin and hydralazine in primary pulmonary hypertension. *Am Heart J* 110:1200–1204, 1985.

382. Barst RJ: Pharmacologically induced pulmonary vasodilation in children and young adults with primary pulmonary hypertension. *Chest* 89:497–503, 1986.

383. Rubin LJ, Mendoza J, Hood M, McGoon M, Barst R, Williams WB, Diehl JH, Crow J, Long W: Treatment of primary pulmonary hypertension with continuous intravenous prostacyclin (epoprostenol). *Ann Intern Med* 112:485–491, 1990.

384. Packer M: Vasodilator therapy for primary pulmonary hypertension: limitations and hazards. *Ann Intern Med* 103:258–270, 1985.

385. Packer M: Is it ethical to administer vasodilator drugs to patients with primary pulmonary hypertension? *Chest* 95:1173–1175, 1989.

386. Long W, Barst R, Fishman AP, et al: Acute hemodynamic effects of prostacyclin in 65 primary pulmonary hypertension patients. *J Crit Care* 1:127–128, 1986.

387. Long WA, Rubin LJ: Prostacyclin and PGE₁ treatment of pulmonary hyeprtension. *Am Rev Respir Dis* 136:773–776, 1987.

388. Palevsky HI, Long W, Crow J, Fishman AP: Prostacyclin and acetylcholine as screening agents. *Circulation* 82:2018–2026, 1990.

389. Reeves JT, Groves BM, Turkevich D: The case for treatment of selected patients with primary pulmonary hypertension. *Am Rev Respir Dis* 134:342–346, 1986.

390. Rich S, Brundage BH, Levy PS: The effect of vasodilator therapy on the clinical outcome of patients with primary pulmonary hypertension. *Circulation* 71:1191–1196, 1985.

391. Rozkovec A, Stradling JR, Shepherd G, MacDermot J, Oakley CM, Dollery CT: Prediction of favourable responses to long term vasodilator treatment of pulmonary hypertension by short term administration of epoprostenol (prostacyclin) or nifedipine. *Br Heart J* 59:696–705, 1988.

392. Watkins WD, Peterson MB, Crone RK, Shannon DC, Levine L: Prostacyclin and prostaglandin E₁ for severe idiopathic pulmonary artery hypertension (letter).*Lancet* 2:1083, 1980.

393. Swan PK, Tibballs J, Duncan AW: Prostaglandin E₁ in primary pulmonary hypertension. *Crit Care Med* 14:72–73, 1986.

394. Vandenbossche JL, Melot C, Naeije R: Prostaglandin E₁ in primary pulmonary hypertension. Acta Ther 6:44, 1980.

395. Lambert RJ, Corrigan PE, Caldwell EJ: The use of PGE₁ to improve the safety of vasodilators in pulmonary hypertension.*Chest* 89:459S, 1986.

396. Halpern SM, Shah PK, Lehrman S, Goldberg HS, Jasper AC, Koerner SK: Prostaglandin E₁ as a screening vasodilator in priamry pulmonary hypertension. *Chest* 92:686–691, 1987.

397. Burrows B, Earle RH: Course and prognosis of chronic obstructive lung disease: a prospective study of 200 patients. *N Engl J Med* 280:397–404, 1969.

398. Naeije R, Melot C, Mols P, Hallemans R: Reduction in pulmonary hypertension by prostaglandin E₁ in decompensated chronic obstructive pulmonary disease. *Acta Ther* 6:29, 1980.

399. Ishizaki T, Miyabo S, Mifune J, et al: OP-1206, a prostaglandin E₁ derivative: effects of oral administration to patients with chronic lung disease. *Chest* 85:383–386, 1984.

400. Jones K, Higenbottam TW, Wallwork J: Pulmonary vasodilation with prostacyclin in primary and secondary pulmonary hypertension. *Chest* 96:784–88, 1989.

401. Zapol WMC, Snider MT: Pulmonary hypertension in severe acute respiratory failure. *N Engl J Med.* 296:476–480, 1977.

402. Smith ME, Gunther R, Zaiss C, et al: Prostaglandin infusion and endotoxin-induced lung injury. *Arch Surg* 117:175–180, 1982.

403. Slotman GJ, Machiedo GW, Casey KF, Lyons MJ: Histologic and hemodynamic effects of prostacyclin and prostaglandin E1 following oleic acid infusion. *Surgery* 92:93–100, 1982.

404. Radermacher P, Santak B, Wust HJ, Tarnow J, Falke KJ: Prostacyclin for the treatment of pulmonary hypertension in the adult respiratory distress syndrome: effects on pulmonary capillary pressure and ventilation—perfusion distributions. *Anesthesiology* 72:238–244, 1990.

405. Appel PL, Shoemaker WC: Hemodynamic; and oxygen transport effects of prostaglandin E₁ in patients with adult respiratory distress syndrome. *Crit Care Med* 12:528–529, 1984.

406. Tokioka H, Kobayashi O, Ohta Y, Wakabayashi T, Kosaka F: The acute effects of prostaglandin E₁ on the pulmonary circulation and oxygen delivery in patients with adult respiratory distress syndrome. *Intensive Care Med* 11:61–64, 1985.

407. Shoemaker WC, Appel PL: Effects of prostaglandin E₁ in adult respiratory distress syndrome. *Surgery* 99:275–283, 1986.

408. Holcroft JW, Vassar MJ, Weber CJ: Prostaglandin E₁ and survival in patients with the adult respiratory distress syndrome. *Ann Surg* 203:371–378, 1986.

409. Bone RC, Slotman G, Maunder R, et al: Randomized double-blind, multicenter study of prostaglandin E₁ in patients with the adult respiratory distress syndrome. *Chest* 96:114–119, 1989.

410. Lugliani R, Whipp BJ, Wasserman K: Doxapram hydrochloride: a respiratory stimulant for patients with primary alveolar hypoventilation. *Chest* 76:414–419, 1979.

411. Moser KM, Luchsinger PC, Adamason JS, et al: Respiratory stimulation with intravenous doxapram in respiratory failure. *N Engl J Med* 288:427–431, 1973.
412. Gerhardt T, McCarthy J, Bancalari E: Effects of aminophylline on respiratory center and reflex activity in premature infants with apneas. *Pediatr Res* 17:188–191, 1983.
413. Aranda JV, Turman T: Methylxanthines in apnea of prematurity. *Clin Perinatol* 6:87–108, 1979.
414. Guilleminault C, Vanden Hoed J, Mitler: Clinical overview of the sleep apnea syndrome. In Guilleminault C, Dement WC (eds): *Sleep Apnea Syndromes*. Alan R. Liss, New York, pp 1–11, 1978.
415. Delaunois L, Delwiche JP, Lulling J: Effect of medroxyprogesterone on ventilatory control and pulmonary gas exchange in chronic obstructive patients. *Respiration* 47:107–113, 1985.
416. Schoene RB, Pierson DJ, Lakshminarayan S, et al: Effect of medroxyprogesterone acetate on respiratory drives and occlusion pressure. *Bull Eur Physiopathol Respir* 16:645–653, 1980.
417. Skatrud JB, Dempsey JA, Bhansali P, et al: Determinants of chronic carbon dioxide retention and its correction in humans. *J Clin Invest* 65:813–821, 1980.
418. Skatrud JB, Dempsey JA, Kaiser DG: Ventilatory response to medroxyprogesterone acetate in normal subjects: time course and mechanism *J Appl Physiol* 44:939–944, 1978.
419. Sutton FD Jr, Zwillich CW, Creagh CE, et al: Progesterone for outpatient treatment of Pickwickian syndrome. *Ann Intern Med* 83:476–479, 1975.
420. Tyler JM: The effect of progesterone on the respiration of patients with emphysema and hypercapnea. *J Clin Invest* 39:34–41, 1960.
421. Strohl KP, Hensley MJ, saunders NA, et al: Progesterone administration and progressive sleep apneas. *JAMA* 245:1230–1232, 1981.
422. Bromnell LG, West P, Sweatman P, et al: Protriptyline in obstructive sleep apnea. *N Engl J Med* 307:1037–1042, 1982.
423. Conway WA, Zorick F, Piccione P, et al: Protriptyline in the treatment of sleep apnea. *Thorax* 37:49–53, 1982.
424. Smith PL, Haponik EF, Allen RM, et al: The effects of protriptyline in sleep-disordered breathing. *Am Rev Resp Dis* 127:8–13, 1983.
425. Bonora M, St. John WM, Bledsoe TA: Differential elevation by protriptyline and depression by diazepam of upper airway respiratory motor activity. *Am Rev Respir Dis* 131:41–45, 1985.
426. White DP, Zwillich CW, Pickett CK, et al: Central sleep apnea: improvement with acetazolamide therapy. *Arch Intern Med* 142:1816–1819, 1982.
427. Sharp J, Druz W, D'Souza V, et al: Effect of metabolic acidosis and alkalosis upon sleep apnea. *Am Rev Respir Dis* 125(suppl):233, 1982.
428. Heimer D, Shim C, Williams Jr MH: The effects of sequential inhalations of metaproterenol in asthma. *J Allergy Clin Immunol* 66:75–77, 1980.
429. Colacone A, Wolkone N, Stern E, et al: Continuous nebulization of albuterol (salbutamol) in acute asthma. *Chest* 97:693, 1990.
429a. Fanta CH, Rossing TH, McFadden Jr ER: Emergency room treatment of asthma: relationships among therapeutic combinations, severity of obstruction and time course of response. *Am J Med* 72:416–422, 1982.
430. Graham VAL, Milton AF, Knowles GK, et al: Routine antibiotics in hospital management of acute asthma. *Lancet* ii:418, 1982.
431. Millman M, Good AH, Goldstein IM, et al: Status asthmaticus: use of acetylcysteine during bronchoscopy and lavage to remove mucus plug. *Ann Allergy* 50:85, 1963.
432. Degaute JP, Domenighetti G, Naeije R, et al: Oxygen delivery in acute exacerbation of chronic obstructive lung disease. Effects of controlled oxygen therapy. *Am Rev Respir Dis* 124:26, 1981.
433. Irwin RS, Corraro WM, Erickson AD, et al: A true exacerbation of chronic obstructive bronchitis can be objectively defined. *Am Rev Respir Dis* 123(suppl):57, 1981.
434. Schmidt GA, Hall JB: Acute or chronic respiratory failure: assessment and management of patients with COPD in the emergency setting. *JAMA* 261:3444, 1989.
435. Dull WL, Alexander MR, Sadoul P, et al: The efficacy is isoproterenol inhalation for predicting the response to orally administered theophylline in chronic obstructive pulmonary disease. *Am Rev Respir Dis* 126:656, 1982.
436. Anthonisen NR, Monfreda J, Warren CPW, Hershfeld ES, Harding GKM, Nelson NA: Antibiotic therapy in exacerbations of chronic obstructive pulmonary disease. *Ann Intern Med* 106:196, 1987.
437. Derenne J-P, Fleury B, Pariente R: Acute respiratory failure of chronic obstructive pulmonary disease. *Am Rev Respir Dis* 138:1006–1033, 1988.
438. Fein A, Lippmann M, Holtzman H, et al: The risk factors, incidence and prognosis of the adult respiratory distress syndrome following septicemia. *Chest* 83:40–42, 1983.
439. Fowler AA, Hamman RF, Good JT, et al: Adult respiratory distress syndrome: risk with common predisposition. *Ann Intern Med* 98:593–597, 1983.
440. Brigham KL, Meyrick B, Berry LC, et al: Antioxidants protect cultured bovine lung endothelial cells from injury by endotoxin. *J Appl Physiol* 63:840–850, 1987.
441. Parsons PE, Worthen GS, Moore EE, et al: The association of circulating endotoxin with the development of the adult respiratory distress syndrome. *Am Rev Respir Dis* 140:294–301, 1989.
442. Border JR: Hypothesis: sepsis, multiple systems organ failure and the macrophage. *Arch Surg* 123:285–286, 1988.
443. Said SI, Foda HD: Pharmacologic modulation of lung injury. *Am Rev Respir Dis* 139:1553–1564, 1989.
444. Seidenfeld JJ, Pohl DF, Bell RD, et al: Incidence, site, and outcome of infections in patients with the adult respiratory distress syndrome. *Am Rev Respir Dis* 134:12–16, 1986.
445. Montgomery AB, Stager MA, Carrico C, et al: Causes of mortality in patients with the adult respiratory distress syndrome. *Am Rev Respir Dis* 132:485–489, 1985.
446. Hyers TM, Fowler AA: Adult respiratory distress syndrome: causes, morbidity, and mortality. *Fed Proc* 45:25–29,1986.
447. Bell RC, Coalson JJ, Smith JD, et al: Multi-organ system failure and infection in adult respiratory distress syndrome. *Ann Intern Med* 99:293–298, 1983.
448. Van Deventer SJH, ten Cate JW, Tytgat GNJ: Intestinal endotoxemia: clinical significance. *Gastroenterology* 94:825, 1988.
449. Deitch EA, Berg R, Specian R: Endotoxin promotes in the translocation of bacteria from the gut. *Arch Surg* 122:185, 1986.
450. Van Saene HKF, Stoutenbeek CP, Zandstra DF: Concept of selective decontamination of the digestive tract in the critically ill. In van Seane HKF, Stoutenbeek CP, Lawin P, et al (eds). *Infection Control by Selective Decontamination*. Springer-Verlag, Berlin, pp 88–94, 1989.
451. Redl H, Schlag G: Pathophysiology of multi-organ failure (MOF)—Proposed mechanisms. *Clin Intensive Care* 1:66, 1990.
452. Vandenbroucke-Grands CM, Vandenbroucke JP: Effect of selective decontamination of the digestive tract on respiratory tract infections and mortality in the intensive care unit. *Lancet* ii:859–862, 1991.
453. Cook DJ, Laine LA, Guyalt GH, Raffin TA: Nosocomial pneumonia and the role of gastric pH: a meta-analysis. *Chest* 100:7–13, 1991.
454. Heyland D, Mandell ZA: Gastric colonization by gram-negative bacilli and nosocomial pneumonia in the intensive care unit patient evidence for causation. *Chest* 101:187–193, 1992.
455. Eddlestone JM, Vohra A, Scott P, et al: A comparison of the frequency of stress ulceration and secondary pneumonia in sucralfate—or ranitidine—treated intensive care unit patients. *Crit Care Med* 19:1491–1496, 1991.
455a. Vincent LJ, Roman A, de Backer D, Kahn RJ: Oxygen uptake/supply dependency: effects of a short-term dobutamine infusion. *Am Rev Respir Dis* 142:2–7, 1990.
455b. Bihari D, Smithies M, Gimson A, Tinker J: The effects of vasodilation with prostacyclin on oxygen delivery and uptake in critically ill patients. *N Engl J Med* 317:397–404,1987.
455c. Shoemaker WC, Appel PL, Kram HB, Waxman K, Lee TS: Prospective trial of supranormal values of survivors as therapeutic goals in high risk surgical patients. *Chest* 94:1176–1186, 1988.
456. Ziegler EJ, McCutchan AM, Fiererr J, et al: Treatment of gram-negative bacteremia and shock with human antiserum to a mutant *Escherichia coli*. *N Engl J Med* 307:1225–1230, 1982.
457. Baumgartner JD, Glauser MP, McCutchan JA, et al: Prevention of gram negative shock and death in surgical patients by antibody to endotoxin. *Lancet* ii:59–63, 1985.
458. Greenman RL, Schein RMH, Martin MA, et al: A controlled clinical trial of E5 murine monoclonal IgM antibody to endotoxin in the treatment of gram-negative sepsis. *JAMA* 266:1097–1102, 1991.
459. Ziegler EJ, Fisher CJ Jr, Sprung CL, et al: Treatment of gram-negative bacteremia and septic shock with HA-1A human monoclonal antibody against endotoxin—a randomized double blind, placebo-controlled trial. *N Engl J Med* 324:429–436, 1991.
460. Mathison JC, Wolfson D, Ulevith RJ: Participation of tumor necrosis factor in the mediation of gram negative bacterial lipopolysaccharide-induced injury in rabbits. *J Clin Invest* 81:1925–1937, 1988.
461. Tracey KJ, Lowry SF, Cerami A: Cachetin/TNF-α in septic shock and septic adult respiratory distress sydrome. *Am Rev Respir Dis* 138:1377–1379, 1988.
462. Stephens KE, Ishizaka A, Larrick JW, et al: Tumor necrosis factor causes increased pulmonary permeability and edema. *Am Rev Respir Dis* 147:1364–1370, 1988.
463. Beutler B, Milsark IW, Cerami AC: Passive immunization against cachectic tumor necrosis factor protects mice from lethal effects of endotoxin. *Science* 229:869–871, 1985.
464. Tracey KJ, Fong Y, Wesse DG, et al: Anti-cathectin/TNF monoclonal antibodies prevent septic shock during lethal bacteremia. *Nature* 330:662–664, 1987.
465. Metz CA, Sheagren JN: Ibuprofen in animal models of septic shock. *J Crit Care* 5:206, 1990.
466. Snapper JR, Hutchison AA, Ogletree ML, et al: Effects of cyclooxygenase inhibitors on the alterations in lung mechanics caused by endotoxemia in the unanesthetized sheep. *J Clin Invest* 72:63, 1983.
467. Balk RA, Jacobs RF, Tryka AF, et al: Effects of ibuprofen on neutrophil function and acute lung injury in canine endotoxin shock. *Crit Care Med* 16:1121, 1988.
468. Bernard GR, Reines HD, Metz CA, et al: Effects of a short course of ibuprofen in patients with severe sepsis. *Am Rev Respir Dis* 137:138, 1988.
469. Haupt MT, Justremski MS, Clemmer TP, Metz CA, Goris GB: Effect of ibuprofen in patients with severe sepsis: a randomized, double-blind, multicenter study. *Crit Care Med* 19:1339–1347, 1991.

470. Bernard GR, Reines HD, Halushka PV, et al: Prostacyclin and thromboxane A₂ formation is increased in human sepsis syndrome. Effect of cyclooxygenase inhibition. *Am Rev Respir Dis* 144:1095–1101, 1991.

471. Zopol WM, Snider MT, Hill JD, et al: Extracorporeal membrane oxygenation in severe acute respiratory failure. *JAMA,* 242:2193–2196, 1979.

472. Hull RD, Hirsh J, Carter CJ, et al: Pulmonary angiography, ventilation lung scanning, and venography for clinically suspected pulmonary embolism with abnormal perfusion lung scan. *Ann Intern Med* 98:891–899, 1983.

473. The PIOPED Investigators: Value of the ventilation/perfusion scan in acute pulmonary embolism. Results of the prospective investigation of pulmonary embolism diagnosis (PIOPED). *JAMA* 263:2753–2759, 1990.

474. Kelley MA, Carson JL, Palevsky HI, Schwartz S: Diagnosing pulmonary embolism: new facts and strategies. *Ann Intern Med* 114:300–306, 1991.

475. Hull RD, Raskob GE: Low-probability lung scan findings: a need for change. *Ann Intern Med* 114:142–144, 1991.

476. Bell WR, Meek AG: Guidelines for the use of thrombolytic agents. *N Engl J Med* 301:1266, 1979.

477. Genton E: Thrombolytic therapy of pulmonary thromboembolism. *Prog Cardiovasc Dis* 21:333, 1979.

478. Dalen JE: The case against fibrinolytic therapy. *J Cardiovasc Med* 5:798, 1980.

479. Gore JM, Thompson MJ, Becker RC: Rapid resolution of acute core pulmonale with recombinant tissue plasminogen activator. *Chest* 96:939, 1989.

480. PIOPED Investigators: Tissue plasminogen activator for the treatment of acute pulmonary embolism. *Chest* 97:528, 1990.

481. Molloy WD, Leeky, Girling L, Schick U, Prewitt RM: Treatment of shock in a canine model of pulmonary embolism. *Am Rev Respir Dis* 130:870–874, 1984.

482. Brent BN, Mahler D, Verger HJ, et al: Augmentation of right ventricular performance in chronic obstructive pulmonary disease by terbutaline: a combined radionuclide and hemodynamic study. *Am J Cardiol* 50:313–319, 1982.

483. Ringsted CV, Eliasen K, Andersen JB, et al: Ventilation-perfusion distributions and central hemodynamics in chronic obstructive pulmonary disease: effects of terbutaline administration. *Chest* 96:976–983, 1989.

484. Fishman AP: Chronic cor pulmonale. *Am Rev Respir Dis* 114:775–794, 1976.

485. Mathur PN, Powles ACP, Pugsley SO, et al: Effect of digoxin on right ventricular function in severe chronic airflow obstruction. *Ann Intern Med* 95:283–288, 1981.

486. Brown SE, Pakron FJ, Milne N, et al: Effects of digoxin on exercise capacity and right ventricular function during exercise in chronic airflow obstruction. *Chest* 85:187–191, 1984.

487. Mathur PN, Powles ACP, Pubsley SO, et al: Effect of long-term administration of digoxin on exercise performance in chronic airflow obstruction. *Eur J Respir Dis* 66:273–283, 1985.

488. Kim YS, Aviado DM: Digitalis and the pulmonary circulation. *Am Heart J* 62:680–686, 1961.

489. Green LH, Smith TW: The use of digitalis in patients with pulmonary disease. *Ann Intern Med.* 87:459–465, 1977.

490. Rubin LJ: Vasodilators and pulmonary hypertension: where do we go from here? *Am Rev Respir Dis* 135:288–293, 1987.

491. Brent BN, Berger HJ, Matthay RA, et al: Contrasting acute effects of vasodilators (nitroglycerin, nitroprusside, and hydralazine) on right ventricular performance in patients with chronic obstructive pulmonary disease and pulmonary hypertension: a combined radionuclide-hemodynamic study. *Am J Cardiol* 51:1682–1689, 1983.

492. Corriveau ML, Minh V-D, Dolan GF: Long-term effects of hydralazine on ventilation and blood gas values in patients with chronic obstructive pulmonary disease and pulmonary hypertension. *Am J Med* 83:886–892, 1987.

493. Corriveau ML, Rosen BJ, Keller CA, et al: Effect of posture, hydralazine, and nifedipine on hemodynamics, ventilation, and gas exchange in patients with chronic obstructive pulmonary disease. *Am Rev Respir Dis* 138:1494–1498, 1988.

494. Dal Nogare AR, Rubin LJ: The effects of hydralazine on exercise capacity in pulmonary hypertension secondary to chronic obstructive pulmonary disease. *Am Rev Respir Dis* 133:385–389, 1986.

495. Keller CA, Shepard JW, Chun DS, et al: Effects of hydralazine in hemodynamics, ventilation and gas exchange in patients with chronic obstructive pulmonary disease and pulmonary hypertension. *Am Rev Respir Dis* 130:606–611, 1984.

496. Rubin LJ, Peter RH: Hemodynamics at rest and during exercise after oral hydralazine in patients with cor pulmonale. *Am J Cardiol* 47:116–122, 1981.

497. Lupi-Herrera E, Seoane M, Verdejo J: Hemodynamic effect of hydralazine in advanced, stable chronic obstructive pulmonary disease with cor pulmonale: immediate and short-term evaluation at rest and during exercise. *Chest* 85:156–163, 1984.

498. McGoon MD, Seward JB, Vlietstra RE, et al: Hemodynamic response to intravenous hydralazine in patients with pulmonary hypertension. *Br Heart J* 50:579–585, 1983.

499. Packer M, Greenberg B, Massie B, et al: Deleterious effects of hydralazine in patients with pulmonary hypertension. *N Engl J Med* 1306:1326–1331, 1982.

500. Agostoni P, Doria E, Galli C, et al: Nifedipine reduces pulmonary pressure and vascular tone during short—but not long—term treatment of pulmonary hypertension in patients with chronic obstructive pulmonary disease. *Am Rev Respir Dis* 139:120–125, 1989.

501. Kennedy TP, Michael JR, Huang C-K, et al: Nifedipine inhibits hypoxic pulmonary vasoconstriction during rest and exercise in patients with chronic obstructive pulmonary disease. *Am Rev Respir Dis* 129:544–551, 1984.

502. Melot C, Hallemans R, Naeije R, et al: Deleterious effect of nifedipine on pulmonary gas exchange in chronic obstructive pulmonary disease. *Am Rev Respir Dis* 130:612–616, 1984.

503. Morley TF, Zappasodi SJ, Belli A, et al: Pulmonary vasodilator therapy for chronic obstructive pulmonary disease and cor pulmonale: treatment with nifedipine, nitroglycerin, and oxygen. *Chest* 92:71–76, 1987.

504. Simonneau G, Escourrou P, Duroux P, et al: Inhibition of hypoxic pulmonary vasoconstriction by nifedipine. *N Engl J Med* 304:1582–1585, 1981.

505. Sturani C, Bassein L, Schiavina M, et al: Oral nifedipine in chronic cor pulmonale secondary to severe chronic obstructive pulmonary disease (COPD): short- and long-term hemodynamic effects. *Chest* 84:135–142, 1983.

506. Brown ES, Linden GS, King RR, et al: Effects of verapamil on pulmonary hemodynamics during hypoxemia, at rest, and during exercise in patients with chronic obstructive pulmonary disease. *Thorax* 38:840–844, 1983.

507. Clozel JP, Delorme N, Battistella P, et al: Hemodynamic effects of intravenous diltiazem in hypoxic pulmonary hypertension. *Chest* 91:171–175, 1987.

508. Hughes JD, Rubin LJ: Primary pulmonary hypertension: an analysis of 28 cases and a review of the literature. *Medicine* 65:56–72, 1986.

509. Rich S: Primary pulmonary hypertension. *Prog Cardiovasc Dis* 65:205–238, 1988.

510. Palevsky HI, Schloo BL, Pietra GG, et al: Primary pulmonary hypertension: vascular structure, morphometry and responsiveness to vasodilator agents. *Circulation* 80:1207–1221, 1989.

511. Rubin LJ, Peter RH: Therapy of pulmonary heart disease. In Rubin LJ (ed): *Pulmonary Heart Disease.* Martinus Nijhoff, Boston, pp 325–353, 1984.

512. Weir EK, Rubin LJ, Ayres SM, et al: The acute administration of vasodilators in primary pulmonary hypertension: experience from the National Institutes of Health Registry on Primary Pulmonary Hypertension. *Am Rev Respir Dis* 140:1623–1630, 1989.

513. McGoon MD, Vliestra RE: Vasodilator therapy for primary pulmonary hypertension. *Mayo Clin Proc* 59:672–677, 1984.

514. Rich S, Brundage BH: High-dose calcium channel-blocking therapy for primary pulmonary hypertension: evidence for long-term reduction in pulmonary arterial pressure and regression of right ventricular hypertrophy. *Circulation* 76:134–141, 1987.

515. Fuster V, Steele PM, Edwards WD, Gersh BJ, McGoon MD, Frye RL: Primary pulmonary hypertension: natural history and the importance of thrombosis. *Circulation* 70:580–587, 1984.

516. Cohen M, Fuster V, Edwards WD: Anticoagulation in the treatment of pulmonary hypertension. In Fishman AP (ed): *The Pulmonary Circulation: Normal and Abnormal: Mechanisms, Management and the National Registry.* University of Pennsylvania Press, Philadelphia, pp 501–510, 1990.

CHAPTER 7

Pediatric Pharmacotherapy

DANIEL A. NOTTERMAN, M.D., F.A.A.P., F.C.C.M.

Children develop and grow, and their response to drug therapy is conditioned by age, size, and stage of development. It is axiomatic that the change in body size associated with growth is a factor in determining dosage and response. However, even when the effect of size is accommodated, age and level of maturity exert a profound effect on response to pharmacotherapy. The influence of developmental factors is modulated, and usually amplified, by the imposition of critical illness, multiple organ system failure, heredity, and coadministration of other drugs. In infants and small children, vagaries of drug delivery systems and administration techniques assume significance (48, 60, 81, 102, 132, 133). This chapter provides a review of selected aspects of pediatric clinical pharmacology. The pharmacology of individual agents is reviewed in greater detail in other chapters. The purpose here is to describe specific features that distinguish pharmacologic responses of children from those of adults, and to indicate, when possible, which observed pharmacologic differences are likely to result in important clinical differences.

Age-related differences in response are both pharmacokinetic and pharmacodynamic in origin (6, 16, 137, 139). The pharmacokinetic description concerns the relationship, over time, between drug *dosage* and drug concentration. The pharmacodynamic description concerns the relationship between this concentration and the resulting *response*. Narrowly construed, "pharmacodynamics" means "sensitivity," and applies to the relationship between unbound drug concentration (theoretically at the site of action; in practice, in the plasma) and magnitude of effect. Broadly conceived, pharmacodynamics comprises all of the biochemical and physiologic effects of a substance (137). Sensitivity is graphically represented in several ways (137); most often as a plot of the log of drug concentration versus intensity of pharmacologic response. Figure 7.1, described in more detail in a subsequent section, is from a study by Driscoll and associates (35) and displays the pharmacodynamic relationship between dopamine concentration and the resulting inotropic effect in puppy ventricles from animals of different ages. In some instances, immaturity is associated with enhanced sensitivity to a pharmacologic effect. For example, as indicated in Figure 7.2, the concentration of vecuronium necessary to induce a 50% depression of twitch tension is less in infants (mean age 6.6 months) than it is in children (mean age 41.4 months) or adults.

A fundamental requirement for pharmacodynamic analysis is that there be precise pharmacokinetic information regarding the drug of interest *in the population in question*. Such is gradually becoming available in the pediatric age group.

PHARMACODYNAMIC VARIATION

Pharmacodynamic differences between the responses of pediatric patients and adult patients will be considered in the context of (*a*) effects that are unique in children, (*b*) adverse effects, and (*c*) therapeutically desired effects. This last category will focus on the catecholamines.

139

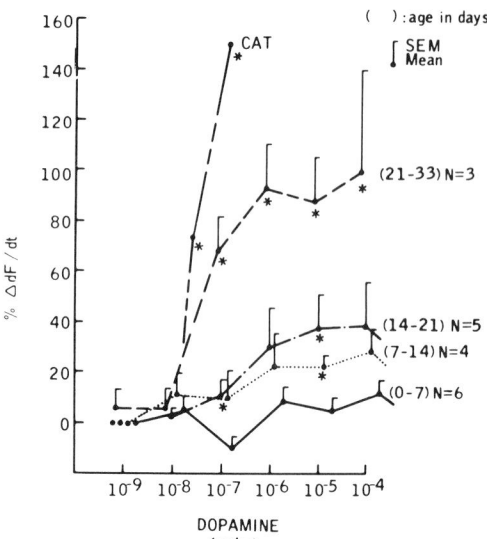

Figure 7.1. Inotropic (%ΔdF/dt) dose-response curves of puppy ventricles and adult cat ventricle treated with dopamine. There is an increasing inotropic responsiveness with age of isolated puppy ventricle to dopamine * P<0.05 using puppies 0 to 7 days old as control. (From Driscoll DJ, Gillette PC, Ezrailson EG, et al: Inotropic response of the neonatal canine myocardium to dopamine. *Pediatr Res* 12:42, 1978.)

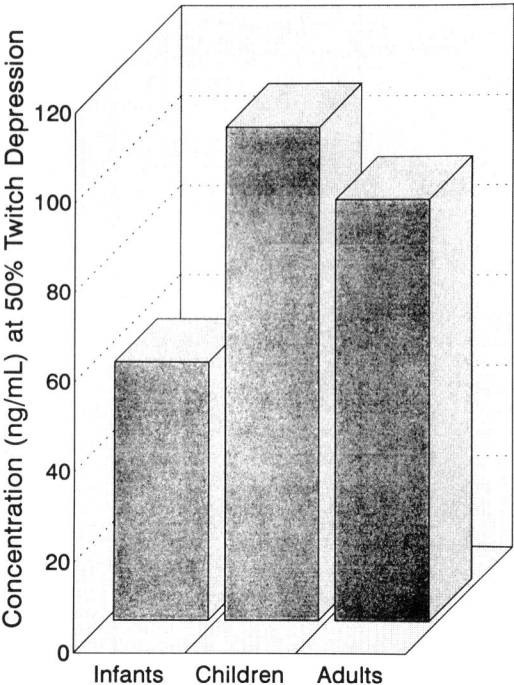

Figure 7.2. Effect of age upon pharmacodynamic response to vecuronium. The concentration of vecuronium needed to achieve 50% depression of twitch tension is lower in the infant than in older children or adults. This implies a pharmacodynamic increase in sensitivity to the drug. (Adapted from data in Fisher DM, Castagnoli K, Miller RD: Vecuronium kinetics and dynamics in anesthetized infants and children. *Clin Pharmacol Ther* 37:402, 1985.)

UNIQUE EFFECTS

Drugs may have unique effects in children. Examples include substances that disturb patterns of growth and differentiation that occur only during particular phases of life (87a). Notable in this regard are teratogens, which have unique adverse effects on the fetus (16, 87a, 90, 132, 151). To a certain extent, children share this special vulnerability with the fetus until growth and development cease at maturity. Thus, the tetracyclines affect bone growth in the fetus and newborn infant (25), as well as development of the teeth in children less than 6 years of age (62, 182). Corticosteroids, among their other adverse effects, suppress the linear growth of children (87), an effect that cannot occur in adults.

Cartilage toxicity is a concern with nalidixic acid (158) and related fluoroquinoline antibiotics such as ciprofloxacin and norfloxacin (69, 105). These newly developed quinoline derivatives should be avoided in children until age 17, when skeletal growth is presumed complete (69, 105).

ADVERSE EFFECTS

Increased Occurrence or Sensitivity

Metoclopramide and other dopamine antagonists such as prochlorperazine (Compazine), haloperidol, and chlorpromazine, have a variety of potential critical care indications (77, 93, 129, 171). These drugs produce acute dystonic reactions much more frequently in children and adolescents than in adults (7, 9, 160). A pharmacokinetic basis for this increase in dystonic reactions has been examined and rejected (7). The increase in CNS sensitivity to a variety of dopamine antagonists might be caused by the greater concentration of dopamine-2 receptors in the brains of young subjects (178).

Verapamil, a calcium entry blocking agent, is used to treat supraventricular tachycardia and other atrial dysrhythmias in children (61, 122, 154). There are clinical reports of infants developing acute severe cardiorespiratory failure following administration of the drug (40, 53, 124). For this reason, verapamil should not be administered to individuals less than 1 year of age (46, 53, 124). Fortunately, adenosine, which has been recently introduced for treatment of supraventricular tachycardia, has been shown to be safe and effective in infants and children. The initial dosage employed is 50 μg/kg. The dosage is increased by 50 μg/kg and the dose repeated in 30 seconds until the dysrhythmia resolves (185b and c).

In infants, elastic and resistive properties of the lung entail optimal efficiency at high respiratory rates with low tidal volumes (121). Thus, the resting respiratory rate is higher, and the infant responds to the need for hyperventilation by increasing rate in preference to tidal volume (121). The need to maintain rapid respiratory rates implies greater sensitivity to respiratory depressants. Indeed, some years ago, Way and associates (169) demonstrated that compared with adults, infants required one-third the dose of morphine (on a weight-normalized basis) for comparable depression in CO_2 sensitivity. Pharmacokinetic factors were not excluded, and further work on the effect of depressant drugs on the immature respiratory system would be useful.

Valproic acid is a broad spectrum anticonvulsant, but its use is limited by concern regarding hepatic toxicity. There is evidence that the incidence of toxicity is increased in children younger than 2 years of age and is rare over the age of 10 years (185d). Paradoxical excitement and hyperactivity very frequently complicate therapy with barbiturates (185e and f). This problem often requires termination of therapy and is more frequent in young children. Of greater concern are reports that indicate that long-term treatment of children with phenobarbital may adversely affect intelligence (185g). While the potential effects of phenobarbital upon behavior and intelligence are of concern during chronic management, they are not relevant during acute therapy and do not contraindicate treatment with these drugs in the critical care unit.

Continuous intravenous infusion of sedative-hypnotics and analgesics is employed in critically ill children for control of movement, pain, and anxiety. Midazolam, a benzodiazepine with a short half-life, and fentanyl, an opioid, have been extensively employed for this purpose in pediatric intensive care units (185h). Recently, reports of serious movement and cognitive disorders following cessation of infusions with these compounds have been of concern (185i). It is likely that these abnormalities represent an abstinence syndrome. It is not known whether induction of such a syndrome occurs with greater facility in children than adults. However, these reports indicate a need for caution before adopting into pediatric practice new therapeutic strategies, such as long-term, continuous intravenous infusion of drugs of this type (185j).

Decreased Occurrence or Sensitivity

Children enjoy relative protection from the adverse effects of several drugs. In most cases, the mechanism responsible for the relative immunity of youth has not been determined.

Several drugs cause hepatic injury less frequently in children than in adults. These include isoniazid (5, 38, 46, 108, 155), halothane (18, 21, 42, 89, 92, 168), and acetaminophen (3, 45, 103, 140, 141, 159).

Therapy with isoniazid (INH) is associated with asymptomatic increases in hepatic enzymes in 10 to 20% of adults (5, 38). In children 9 to 14 years of age, 17% had elevations of serum glutamic-oxaloacetic transaminase (SGOT) or glutamic-pyruvic transaminase (SGPT), similar to the proportion in adults (155). INH hepatitis, a potentially fatal disorder, develops in some individuals receiving the drug. The risk of developing INH hepatitis increases with age: 0 per 1000 in patients less than 20 years of age; 3 per 1000 for those 20 to 34 years of age; 12 per 1000 for those 35 to 49 years old; 23 per 1000 for those 50 to 65 years of age; and 8 per 1000 for those older than 65 years (46). Despite occasional reports of INH hepatitis in children (155), usually when INH and rifampin are coadministered (108), the incidence is still extremely low, and measurement of SGOT is not routinely performed in children receiving INH alone. Neither the mechanism of INH hepatitis, nor the reason for the relative protection of youth, has been elucidated.

Although there are isolated case reports to the contrary (21, 168), halothane hepatotoxicity appears to be extremely rare in children, even following multiple exposures to the drug, which increases risk in adults (168). Again, the mechanism of protection is unknown.

Acetaminophen produces marked elevation (>1000 IU/liter) of SGOT following ingestion of a substantial overdose (>150 mg/kg) (140). Without administration of an antidote, such as N-acetylcysteine (141), severe hepatitis occurs in 10%

of adults, with an associated mortality of 10 to 20% (45). Of individuals with potentially toxic acetaminophen levels, 5.5% of those less than 12 years of age had SGOT levels above 1000 IU/liter, while 29% of those older than 12 years had an increase of this magnitude (140). The protection conferred by young age has been related to ingestion of relatively small quantities of drug and to early emesis (140, 141). This fact is not the only explanation, since severe hepatotoxicity in children is rare even in the presence of levels associated with severe injury to adults (140). Children younger than about 9 years of age conjugate acetaminophen with sulfate as well as glucuronate (159). It is suggested that this additional pathway of detoxification reduces flux through the mixed-function oxidase pathway implicated in acetaminophen hepatotoxicity (140, 159), or that children have increased availability of glutathione, used to detoxify acetaminophen metabolites (140). These explanations remain speculative. Cases of severe acetaminophen toxicity and death have occurred in children (3, 103). Thus, children who ingest a potentially toxic quantity should be fully evaluated and treated with N-acetylcysteine if the concentration of acetaminophen exceeds the "probable risk" line of the Rumack nomogram (141) or if more than 150 mg/kg has been ingested and a serum level cannot be determined within 16 hours of ingestion (140).

Aminoglycoside ototoxicity and nephrotoxicity are probably less common in infants and children than in adults (28, 68, 91, 125). There is experimental and clinical evidence that the kidney of the infant or child is more tolerant of aminoglycoside exposure (28, 68). Enzymuria, a marker of renal tubular injury, is less in infants and children following treatment with an aminoglycoside, and there is less renal accumulation of these drugs in infants (68). In an analysis of controlled studies, the incidence of cochlear and vestibular toxicity was not found to be greater in infants receiving aminoglycosides than in control subjects (91). The relatively low incidence of aminoglycoside toxicity in infants and children should not be taken as evidence that these drugs are innocuous (91). The usual precautions for minimizing aminoglycoside toxicity, including therapeutic drug monitoring when appropriate, are indicated.

Infants tolerate higher serum concentrations of digoxin than do older children or adults 57, 110, 113), although some investigators dispute this observation (66). Lessened susceptibility to glycoside-induced arrhythmias may be a result of decreased norepinephrine content and sympathetic innervation of ventricular myocardium (51, 66, 75, 113), increased vagal tone (117), and/or a healthier myocardium without superimposed coronary artery disease (113).

Three other points should be mentioned regarding digoxin. *First,* the observation that infants tolerate higher concentrations of digoxin without manifesting toxicity does not mean that they require higher concentrations in order to achieve therapeutic benefit. In fact, no therapeutic advantage accrues to maintaining serum digoxin levels greater than those also associated with therapeutic efficacy (1 to 2 ng/ml) in adults (98, 113, 114, 120). Infants with relatively high and relatively low digoxin levels have comparable shortening of systolic time intervals (120, 142). An average level of 1.3 ng/ml provides adequate cardiac functional improvement in infants with congestive heart failure (113, 114). *Second,* when normalized by weight, the dose of digoxin needed to achieve a particular digoxin concentration is larger in infants than adults (98, 113, 114). This fact represents a true pharmacokinetic difference between the two populations and is reflected in different dosage requirements (98, 113). As discussed, this pharmacokinetic observation does not mean that infants are less sensitive to the drug. *Third*, the discovery of an endogenous digoxinlike substance that interacts with digoxin assays employing antibody systems (161, 162) means that older information concerning digoxin pharmacokinetics and dosage in infants and patients with hepatic or renal failure may need revision.

THERAPEUTICALLY DESIRED EFFECTS

Cardiac Glycosides

An earlier incorrect belief that infants require higher serum concentrations of digoxin to achieve comparable pharmacologic effect is discussed above.

Neuromuscular Blocking Agents

Newborns and infants respond differently from older children and adults to neuromuscular blocking agents. For example, they require smaller dosages of the competitive (nondepolarizing) agents pancuronium and *d*-tubocurarine (9, 10, 26, 176, 180). This finding probably represents a pharmacodynamic increase in sensitivity. The dose of *d*-tubocurarine or pancuronium needed to induce paralysis is much lower in young infants: Bennett and associates (10) found that 40 μg/kg of pancuronium produced apnea in the 1-day-old infant, whereas 92 μg/kg was required at 1 month. Similar results have been reported with *d*-tubocurarine (9, 176). This difference persists even when *d*-tubocurarine is prescribed on the basis of surface area (neonate: 4.1 mg/m^2 adult: 7.0 mg/m^2) (26). The reduced dosage requirement of infants cannot be explained on a pharmacokinetic basis, since clearance is *greater* (109) or the same (185k) in infants as in adults. In contrast, equal doses of succinylcholine, per unit weight, yield a shorter duration of apnea in infants than in adults (26, 27, 176). On the basis of body weight, infants require twice the adult dose to produce equivalent degrees of blockade (107). The discrepancy is attenuated when dose is normalized to body surface area rather than mass, and a uniform dose of 40 mg/m^2 produces equivalent duration of effect in infants and adults (26, 176). This finding suggests a pharmacokinetic, rather than true pharmacodynamic, basis for the apparent decrease in sensitivity of infants to succinylcholine. In line with this conclusion, the elimination half-life of succinylcholine is shorter in infants than in older children and adults (176).

Vecuronium and atracurium are nondepolarizing muscle relaxants that have recently been introduced into pediatric critical care practice. As described previously, the sensitivity to vecuronium varies with age (Fig. 7.2). This observation of altered pharmacodynamics must be distinguished from the pharmacokinetic observation that the volume of distribution (V_D) of vecuronium is greater in infants than in older children; clearance is similar in infants and adults. A consequence of the greater volume of distribution is a longer half-life $t_{1/2}$ and, consequently, a longer duration of action (185l). The net effect

Table 7.1.   Dosage of Neuromuscular Blocking Drugs in Children

Drug	Dosage (mg/kg)
Succinylcholine	
Newborns, infants	2
Children to adults	0.6–1
Pancuronium	
Newborn	0.02–0.04
2–4 weeks	0.06–0.08
>4 weeks	0.1
Continuous infusion[a]	0.1 mg/kg/hr
Atricurium[b]	
All ages	0.4–0.5 mg/kg
Vecuronium[b]	
All ages[c]	0.08–1.0 mg/kg
Continuous infusion[a]	0.1 mg/kg/hr

[a] Titrate.
[b] Not examined in neonates.
[c] Duration of action prolonged in infants.

is that similar dosages of vecuronium produce a lower concentration in infants. However, the drug lingers for a longer duration. The clinical outcome is that infants have similar dosage requirements for single doses of the drug but a longer duration of paralysis. The dosage requirements during continuous infusion of vecuronium in children have not been systematically explored. Data in children indicate that an average hourly dosage of 0.11 mg/kg/hr will completely abolish the Train of Four (185m). As predicted, in adults a similar infusion rate of 0.103 mg/kg/hr was effective in abolishing three responses to the Train of Four (about a 90% block of the neuromuscular junction) (185n). Additional work, incorporating measurement of vecuronium plasma concentration, is needed in critically ill children receiving vecuronium by continuous infusion. This need is highlighted by recent reports that document prolonged neuromuscular paralysis following vecuronium infusion (185o).

The clinical pharmacology of atracurium also differs from that of other nondepolarizing agents. For example, in one study, infants were not found to be pharmacodynamically more sensitive to atracurium, as they are for vecuronium and pancuronium. In this study, both the volume of distribution and the clearance of atracurium were greater in infants and children than in adults. However neither elimination half-life nor $t_{1/2}$ nor time to recovery varied with age for this agent (185p). Although the higher clearance in infants and children would lead one to predict a higher dosage requirement in these populations, in fact, steady state infusion requirements for atracurium are similar for infants and children (185o and q). This finding suggests the need for further study in the critical care environment.

Dosage guidelines incorporate these observations, and are summarized in Table 7.1.

Sympathomimetic Agents

The clinical use of sympathomimetic agents, particularly the catecholamines, is reviewed in Chapter 31. The following discussion summarizes recent information concerning the clinical pharmacology of the catecholamines in children.

It has been suggested that the immature cardiovascular system responds differently to inotropic agents, including exogenously administered catecholamines. For example, Driscoll and coworkers (35) examined the inotropic response of isolated, perfused ventricles from puppies of different ages as the preparations were exposed to perfusate containing varying concentrations of dopamine and isoproterenol. Figure 7.1 displays the data obtained when dopamine was in the perfusate. Sensitivity increased with increasing puppy age from 0 to 7 days to 21 to 33 days. This relationship was ablated by pretreatment with reserpine. These observations suggested that the blunted inotropic response to dopamine of preparations from younger animals resulted from incomplete sympathetic innervation and reduced norepinephrine stores. Relative deficiencies of sympathetic innervation have been demonstrated in newborn animals (49, 51, 54, 117) but have not been evaluated in human infants, and the timing of complete myocardial innervation has not been elucidated (51). Others have also observed cardiac subsensitivity to exogenous catecholamines in newborn animals (35, 36, 134). However, results have varied between laboratories, even when the same species was examined. For example, Rockson and associates (134) administered bolus injections of isoproterenol to intact puppies and, unlike Driscoll and associates, found that there was a close relationship between age and inotropic response to isoproterenol. Geis and coworkers (54) reported that compared with adult dogs, puppies responded equally well to isoproterenol and exhibited a greater chronotropic response to norepinephrine. Methodologic rather than physiologic differences may play a role in the diversity of these observations. Structural and physiologic cardiovascular differences between the fetus, infant, child, and adult have been recently examined and are only summarized here (4, 22, 49, 50, 117, 183).

The immature heart has a greater proportion of noncontractile relative to contractile tissue (49, 50) and has a lower compliance (50, 117, 135, 136). Stroke volume is smaller when normalized to weight (127). Decreased compliance and stroke volume imply that the immature heart has a limited "preload reserve" (50, 117). The increase in stroke volume that follows volume loading is smaller than expected (135, 136). Newborn ventricles exhibit greater interdependence than those from adult animals (135), which is also expected to limit the efficacy of volume loading. A high baseline heart rate (117), coupled with limited ability to augment stroke volume, impairs the ability of the heart to increase cardiac output. Stroke volume may not be augmented by the usual inotropic agents; increases in cardiac output may depend on drug-induced acceleration of heart rate (50, 117). It is in this context that Friedman and George (50) have referred to the limited "total functional reserve" of the infant heart.

The cardiovascular response to catecholamines may also be limited by differences in the number and function of adrenergic receptors. Binding studies of peripheral white blood cells indicate that β-adrenergic receptor number may be reduced in infants and children (128, 131). It is not certain that the number of β-receptors on peripheral white cells reflects the number in the myocardium. Work in the elderly (166) and in patients with heart failure (59) suggests that this fact may be so. Evidence against a role for the adrenergic receptor in neonatal cardiac subsensitization was provided by Rockson

and associates (134), who observed that the density of β-adrenergic binding sites was *increased* in immature animals, and that these receptors generated cyclic AMP appropriately, even though the inotropic response to isoproterenol and norepinephrine was reduced. This finding was thought to represent an adaptive response to decreased myocardial innervation but suggests that diminished number and function of receptors does not play a major role in the limited response of immature animals to catecholamines.

Studies in nonhuman neonates have shown age-related or maturational-related differences in α- and β-adrenergic receptor content of lung, brain, liver, platelets, and fat cells (172). It would not be surprising if these differences produced qualitative and quantitative alterations in noncardiovascular pharmacologic effects of catecholamine infusions. Postnatal changes in vascular responsiveness to adrenergic agents have been extensively explored. Decreased vascular sensitivity to a variety of catecholamines has been a fairly constant (4, 19, 39) but not invariant (39) finding in immature animals. The newborn pig requires a higher dose of isoproterenol than does the adult to reduce vascular resistance (20), and sheep display greater sensitivity to both norepinephrine and isoproterenol with increasing fetal and postnatal age (4). Interestingly, the authors of this study related increasing sensitivity to closure of vascular shunts rather than to maturation of the neuroeffector system. These in vivo experiments are supported by in vitro work with isolated vascular muscle strips and rings and by experiments in which the microvasculature is directly observed. This work has been reviewed recently (39).

In human infants and children, several published clinical studies have evaluated the use of dopamine or dobutamine. More recent work includes measurement of plasma catecholamine levels. Surprisingly, these studies do not provide unambiguous evidence that pediatric patients display a diminished or different response to catecholamines (185r).

Lang and coworkers (86) treated five children (ages, 1 to 24 months; mean age, 8 months) with dopamine following cardiovascular surgery. For the group as a whole, neither heart rate, blood pressure, nor cardiac output increased significantly at infusion rates less than 15 μg/kg/min. Increases in cardiac output were related to higher heart rate rather than to greater stroke volume. Adults display increases in blood pressure and cardiac output at infusion rates below 5 to 10 μg/kg/min and increases in heart rate below 10 μg/kg/min (11, 24, 56, 156, 175). Lang's study has been taken to support the view that the cardiovascular system of infants and children is less sensitive to dopamine (50). However, the study was uncontrolled and included a heterogeneous group of patients. Driscoll and associates (37) evaluated dopamine in 24 children (ages, 2 days to 18 years; mean age, 39 months) with shock of disparate medical and surgical causes (20 of 24 had congenital heart disease). The infusion was started at 2 to 10 μg/kg/min and titrated to desired response. More than half of the subjects responded favorably to the infusion (≥15% increase in systolic blood pressure), at a mean dosage in responders of 8.3 ± 1.5 μg/kg/min. In this group, blood pressure increased significantly, but heart rate did not. The study design did not permit evaluation of a dose-response relationship. Perez and colleagues (115) observed that a group of five hypotensive newborn infants studied prospectively required a dopamine infusion rate of greater than 20 μg/kg/min to achieve adequate blood pressure, capillary refill, and urine output. The average infusion rate of dopamine required to increase mean arterial pressure from 27 to 54 mm Hg was 25 ±10 μg/kg/min, and the highest dosage was 50 μg/kg/min. At this dosage, urine output increased and there was no clinical evidence of cutaneous vasoconstriction. Since infusion rates of this magnitude in adults are often associated with marked peripheral vasoconstriction, Perez and associates interpreted their findings to support the concept of cardiac and peripheral vascular subsensitization to catecholamines during infancy. In contrast, in a placebo-controlled study of infants, DiSessa and associates (32) observed that relatively modest (2.5 μg/kg/min) dosages of dopamine were associated with improvement in blood pressure and myocardial performance, evaluated by echocardiogram; Seri and coworkers (149) made similar observations.

These clinical studies do not permit firm conclusions. The subjects had diverse underlying and coexisting conditions, including structural cardiac disease, recent cardiac operation, asphyxia, pulmonary hypertension, and septicemia. Indications for pressor therapy, volume status, and measure of pharmacologic response were not standardized. A large variety of factors other than age and development, reviewed elsewhere in this text, are known to affect adrenergic receptor function and cardiovascular response to catecholamine infusion (24, 183, 184). These factors were not controlled, and plasma dopamine levels were not measured. Padbury and colleagues (112) incorporated measurement of dopamine concentration with assessment of cardiovascular response in newborn infants. Infusion rates as low as 0.5 to 1.0 μg/kg/min were associated with important effects on blood pressure and cardiac output. Heart rate increased at infusion rates of 2 to 3 μg/kg/min. The calculated thresholds for changes in selected hemodynamic functions were in the range of 14 to 35 ng/ml. Of importance is that, when compared with experience in older subjects, the newborns seemed at least as sensitive to equivalent plasma concentrations of dopamine. The dopamine clearance reported by Padbury and associates was 48 to 60 ml/kg/min and did not correlate with age or birth weight. In critically ill neonates, Zaritsky observed an average clearance of 96.2 ml/kg/min, which was lower (although not with statistical significance) than the average clearance in older children: 58.8 ml/kg/min (185s). Values recorded in adults have also been within this range (664, 72). However, our group found that dopamine clearance varied substantially with age. In this study, children younger than 2 years of age had a clearance that was nearly twofold greater than that observed in older children (82 vs 46 ml/kg/min) (185t). This difference in clearance could account for the clinical observation, described earlier, that infants display a requirement for higher dosages of dopamine.

The hemodynamic effects of dobutamine in children have been examined in several studies (13, 34, 116, 144, 157). Detailed pharmacodynamic and kinetic information is available for healthy and acutely ill adults (74, 83, 84), and it is becoming available in children.

Age-related differences in response to dobutamine have not been consistently observed. In addition to the anticipated increase in cardiac output and stroke volume, Driscoll and Gillette (34) found a fairly consistent increase in systemic vascular resistance, contrary to the behavior of adults with congestive heart failure (76, 83). Driscoll's subjects had structural congenital heart disease, and most were not in heart failure—these differences, rather than age, probably account for the disparity. Perkin and Levin (116) found dobutamine to be effective in augmenting cardiac output and stroke volume in a variety of conditions associated with shock. Subjects younger than 12 months old displayed a trend (not statistically significant) toward an attenuated response to the inotropic effect of the drug. In newborn infants with "heart failure" of diverse etiology, Stopfkuchen and associates (157) found that abnormal left ventricular systolic time intervals changed significantly during infusion of dobutamine. This change was associated with a significant chronotropic effect. Schranz and coworkers (144) documented a substantial positive inotropic effect with little acceleration of heart rate in 12 children with shock of various etiologies.

In children emerging from cardiopulmonary bypass, dobutamine may not be a desirable agent because of undesirable chronotropy and slight improvement in stroke volume (15). A small left ventricle is thought to limit the inotropic effect of dobutamine in children who are recovering from repair of tetralogy of Fallot (13). In these children, increases in cardiac output depend on dobutamine-associated increases in heart rate. This effect illustrates that differences that appear to be developmental may actually reflect structural peculiarities of congenital heart disease, as well as the fact that myocardial dysfunction and CHF may not be characteristic of the circulatory status of many children undergoing cardiac surgery. More work will be needed to clarify the relative importance of development, type of structural lesion, and cardiopulmonary bypass in producing these differences.

One group recently provided pharmacokinetic and pharmacodynamic information regarding dobutamine infusion in critically ill neonates (185u). Infusion of 2.5 to 5.0 μg/kg/min was associated with a stepwise increase in cardiac output. The mean increase was 25% of baseline (range, 6% to 63%). The threshold dobutamine concentration associated with an increase in output was 39 ng/ml, and the mean total body clearance was 90 ml/kg/min. The data fit a first-order kinetic model. These values are consistent with work in adults: in one study involving adults, there was a progressive increase in cardiac function as dobutamine concentration rose from 40 to 190 ng/ml (83).

In a different study involving older children (0.13 to 17 years), somewhat more complex pharmacokinetics were observed (185v), providing evidence that a simple, single-compartment first-order kinetic model may not adequately describe the compound's behavior. Sensitivity was not directly examined in this study, but the average dobutamine concentration (in patients receiving dobutamine alone) was 94 ng/ml, suggesting that the therapeutic range for dobutamine is similar in children, neonates, and adults. Nonlinear (i.e., dose-dependent) kinetics have been observed for dobutamine (185w and u) and dopamine (185x), although this finding has not been observed by all groups.

Thus, work in infants and adults has not as yet documented systematic age-related differences in catecholamine pharmacodynamics. Pharmacokinetic differences in the disposition of catecholamines between adults, children, and infants probably exist but require more study. The extent of our knowledge in humans, however, is limited by methodologic problems and by limited pharmacokinetic data in infants and children. There is detailed pharmacokinetic and pharmacodynamic information concerning each of the clinically employed catecholamines in healthy and, to a limited extent, critically ill adults (29, 30, 44, 58, 82, 83, 153). As more information becomes available in children, the relationship between age, maturity, and response to catecholamine infusion will become more definite.

PHARMACOKINETIC VARIATION

The weight of the average 18-year-old male (63 kg) exceeds that of the average term newborn infant (3.4 kg) (87a), by a factor of 19. Expressed in terms of surface area, this factor becomes 8.5. Thus, it is not surprising that infants and children require smaller dosages than adults. In this section, the effect of changing size and function on pharmacokinetics will be examined. Such alterations affect each of the major aspects of drug disposition: absorption, distribution (including protein binding), biotransformation, and excretion of changed and unchanged drug (16, 98, 130, 1391). Lack of awareness of the need to account for altered function as well as altered size has been responsible for serious therapeutic misadventures, such as the "gray syndrome" (170) of the 1960s (neonatal chloramphenicol toxicity) and the "gasping syndrome" (47, 55) of the 1980s (neonatal benzyl alcohol toxicity).

SPECIAL PROBLEMS IN DRUG DELIVERY TO CHILDREN

Children require and tolerate smaller volumes of intravenous fluid than do adults. This fact limits the volume of intravenously administered fluid in which a drug can be diluted and the maximum rate at which the drug can be infused. These problems are magnified by the imposition of fluid limits associated with critical cardiac, respiratory, or renal disease.

Dilution volumes of intravenous medications can be adjusted, but physical properties of many drugs, as well as concern for safety, place a limit on maximum drug concentration. Current recommendations for dilution of several drugs employed in pediatric critical care are listed in Table 7.2. These recommendations (48, 102) are based on both clinical observation and pharmaceutical information concerning solubility and stability but may not have been subjected to experimental testing. Stock drug solutions are often too concentrated for appropriate pediatric dosages. Errors during dilution may result in over- or underdosage.

Low intravenous flow rates result in a substantial delay before delivery of drug actually starts or is completed. The magnitude of this delay depends on the rate of infusion, the drug dosage volume, and the site of introduction of the drug into the intravenous tubing. The length of delay can be surprising. For example, when drug is added to the fluid reservoir of a system in which the rate of flow is 25 ml/hr, delivery of drug does not begin for nearly 2 hours and is not complete for 4 hours (133). Delayed drug delivery has several untoward consequences, which were recently summarized by Roberts (115). (a) In one study, 36% of the total daily dose of certain intravenous medications was inadvertently discarded when

Table 7.2. Maximum Drug Concentration for Intravenous Infusions in Infants and Children[a]

Drug	Concentration
Antibiotics	
Acyclovir	7 mg/ml
Amikacin	6 mg/ml
Amphotericin B	0.1 mg/ml
β-Lactams[b]	50–100 mg/ml
Chloramphenicol	100 mg/ml
Clindamycin	12 mg/ml
Co-Trimoxazole[c]	1 mg/15 ml
Erythromycin lactobionate	5 mg/ml
Gentamicin	2 mg/ml
Imipenem/Cilastatin	5 mg/ml
Kanamycin	6 mg/ml
Metronidazole	8 mg/ml
Penicillin G	50,000–100,000 units/ml
Tobramycin	2 mg/ml
Vancomycin	5 mg/ml
Vidarabine	0.7 mg/ml
Neuromuscular Blocking Agents	
Atracurium	10 mg/ml
Pancuronium	1–2 mg/ml
Vecuronium	1 mg/ml
Inotropes and Pressors	
Dobutamine	5 mg/ml
Dopamine	3.2 mg/ml
Epinephrine	100 mg/ml
Norepinephrine	4 mg/ml
Other Cardiovascular Drugs	
Bretylium Tosylate	10 mg/ml
Lidocaine	0.2–1.2 mg/ml
Methyldopate	10 mg/ml
Nitroprusside	100–200 μg/ml
Procainamide	2-4 mg/ml
Miscellaneous	
Aminophylline	25 mg/ml
Cimetidine	6 mg/ml
Diphenhydramine	50 mg/ml
Ethacrynate	2 mg/ml
Magnesium	200 mg/ml
Ranitidine	2 mg/ml

[a] From Ford DC, Leist ER, Phelkps SJ: *Guidelines for Administration of Intravenous Medications to Pediatric Patients*, ed 3. Bethesda, MD, American Society of Hospital Pharmacists, 1988; Lipkin F: Personal communication, 1992.
[b] β-Lactams, penicillin derivatives and cephalosporins.
[c] Co-trimoxazole is trimethoprim/sulfamethoxazole.

intravenous sets were routinely changed. (b) Therapeutic drug monitoring becomes inaccurate when the precise time of delivery of drug cannot be determined. (c) When the rate of infusion is less than or equal to the drug's elimination rate, plasma drug levels will be negligible. Clearly, precise knowledge of the characteristics of drug delivery systems must be an important consideration in devising treatment plans.

Gould, Roberts, and Leff (60, 81, 133) evaluated several methods of intravenous drug delivery as alternatives to the standard, anterograde injection technique. These methods include retrograde injection and syringe pump infusion (Fig. 7.3). Syringe pump infusion is generally preferred, because it permits controlled drug delivery at a rate that is not dependent upon the primary infusion rate. The reader is referred to the original publications for details (60, 81, 133).

ABSORPTION

Absorption of drug occurs from the gastrointestinal tract (mouth, stomach, small intestine, rectum), from intramuscular or subcutaneous sites of injection, from the skin, and from lung. Agents that are administered by vein or artery bypass the process of absorption.

The effect of age on enteral absorption is not uniform and is difficult to predict. Newborns absorb drugs more slowly but not necessarily less completely than older children and adults (16, 97, 98, 132). Drugs known to be well-absorbed when given orally to adults may not be available in a form suitable for administration to young children. For example, when isoniazid tablets are crushed and administered with applesauce, as some researchers recommend, the INH is poorly absorbed. This practice has led to failed treatment of tuberculous meningitis (106). Untested, extemporaneous forms of medication should not be administered to children.

Absorption from intramuscular sites may be quite variable in critically ill patients and, so is not generally recommended in this population. Occasionally this route may be appropriate. Considerable information is now available concerning absorption following intramuscular administration to neonates and has been summarized recently (185y).

In the past, rectal suppository administration was frequently prescribed for drugs such as phenobarbital, aspirin, acetaminophen, aminophylline, belladonna, opium, and others. Rectal suppository administration is generally not desirable in the critical care setting, and many substances are slowly and unpredictably absorbed by this route (16). Therapeutic failure and severe intoxication have occurred with rectal administration of aminophylline (16, 104). However, the rectal route has been effective for administration of diazepam and valproic acid to control and prevent recurrences of febrile seizures (96, 164, 185z and aa). Midazolam, diazepam, and morphine have each been effectively employed in children when administered rectally for analgesia or pre-anesthetic sedation (185bb).

Transdermal drug delivery has not been exploited in therapy of children. Since percutaneous absorption is facilitated by the relatively thin stratum corneum of the infant and child (98) and the high surface area-to-weight ratio, both therapeutic and toxic effects of topically applied substances will be greater than in adults. Numerous examples of inadvertent systemic absorption and toxicity in infants have been recorded (23, 43, 57, 71, 99, 138, 143, 150, 177). The pediatric intensive care physician should be cautious about application of presumably innocuous substances to the integument of these patients. Viscous lidocaine has produced seizures following topical application to the oral mucosa (138), and delirium has been reported after administration of aerosolized tripelennamine, an antihistamine (143).

Intraosseous administration of emergency medications has been reintroduced (12, 70, 111, 152) and is now a standard of emergency care. The relevant anatomy, indications and contraindications, and technique have been recently reviewed (185cc). The technique is simple, rapid, and rarely associated with major complications. Following intraosseous administration, brisk appearance in the bloodstream has been documented for several emergency drugs: catecholamines; calcium; bicarbonate; blood; colloid; and saline (111, 152).

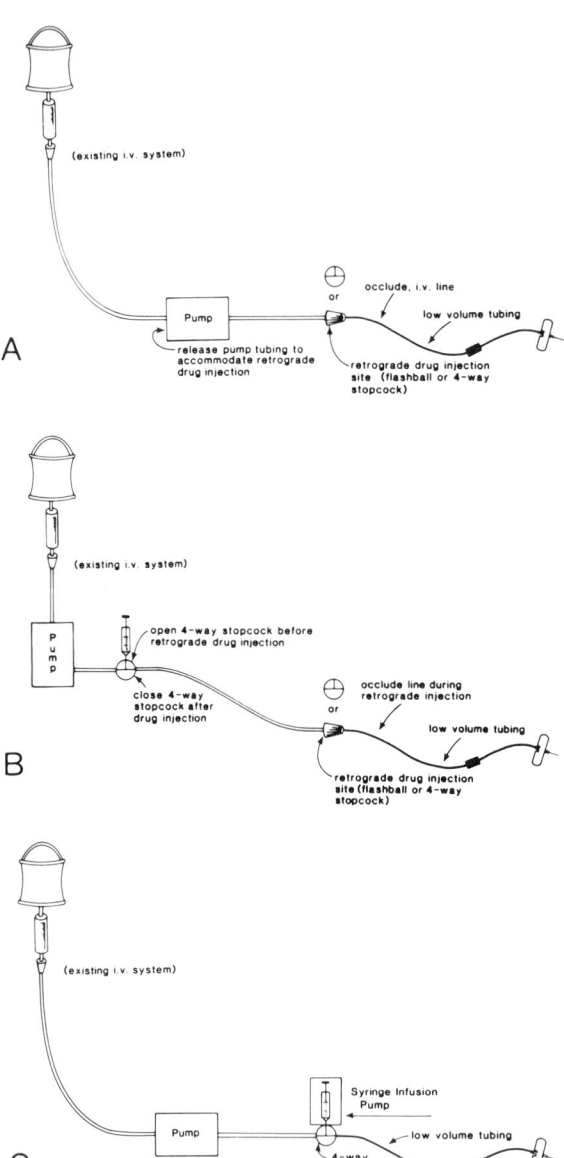

Figure 7.3. **A,** Construction of an intravenous system for manual retrograde injection. An injection site (flashball or stopcock) and low-volume extension tubing are located at the distal end of the existing intravenous setup. **B,** Construction of intravenous system for retrograde injection modified for a volume infusion pump device unable to accept retrograde injection. System consists of existing intravenous setup to which is attached an extension set with a proximal 4-way stopcock and distal flashball injection site. A large-volume syringe is attached to the 4-way stopcock and acts as an overflow reservoir for the intravenous fluid displaced by the dose volume. **C,** Construction of mechanical (syringe) infusion system. A 4-way stopcock and low-volume extension tubing are attached distal to the existing intravenous system. The dosing syringe is attached directly to the 4-way stopcock before placement on the syringe infusion device. For details see original sources. (Adapted from Leff RD, Roberts RJ: Methods of intravenous drug administration in the pediatric patient. *J Pediatr* 98:681, 1981; and Roberts RJ: Intravenous administration of medications in pediatric patients: problems and solutions. *Pediatr Clin North Am* 28:23, 1986.)

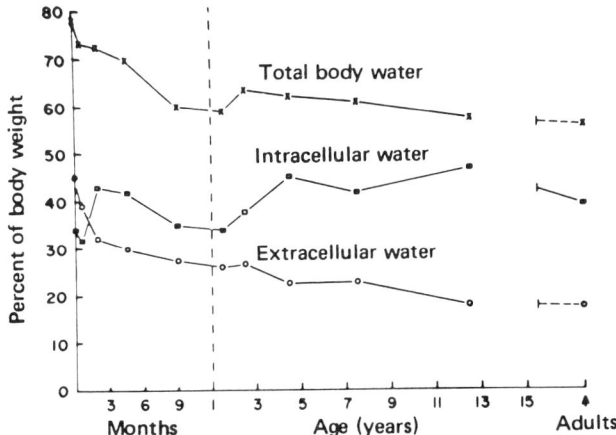

Figure 7.4. Developmental changes in total body, intracellular, and extracellular water in infants and children. The changes are expressed as percentages of body weight. (From Rane A, Wilson JT: Clinical pharmacokinetics in infants and children. In Gibaldi M, Prescott L (eds): *Handbook of Clinical Pharmacokinetics.* ADIS Health Science Press, New York, 1983. Data from Friis-Hansens B: *Pediatrics* 28:169, 1961.)

Intraosseous administration permits continuous infusion of catecholamines and resuscitation fluid and permits bolus injection of most standard emergency medications. This technique is an important advantage over the intratracheal route (167). Considering the difficulty in securing vascular access during a cardiorespiratory or hemodynamic emergency, intraosseous administration is the method of choice for administration of emergency drugs and fluids when intravenous access cannot be secured within a few minutes. This method is preferred over intracardiac administration (111) or the intratracheal route.

DISTRIBUTION

Distribution refers to the movement of drug from the central compartment to peripheral compartments and, ultimately, to the site of action and elimination. Changes in volume of distribution (V_d) result in reciprocal changes in the drug concentration (C) following a single drug dose or during repetitive drug dosing (see Chapter 1).

Distribution is affected by several parameters, including the cardiac output, individual organ blood flow, composition and relative size of body compartments, pH of body fluids, and extent of drug binding to plasma proteins and peripheral tissues (74, 78, 98, 139). Important age-related changes include differences in body composition and protein binding.

Body Composition

In the neonate, infant, and child, the various body compartments have a different absolute and relative size than in adults. The size and composition of these compartments vary continuously. As indicated in Figure 7.4, total body water (expressed as percentage of body weight) decreases from about 80% in the newborn infant to 60% in the adult, whereas extracellular

water (ECW) decreases from 45% to 20% during the same interval (127). Conversely, expressed as a function of body surface area, ECW is relatively constant (6, 16). As a percentage of body mass, adipose tissue doubles during the first year of life. In the infant, skeletal muscle mass is reduced, and the brain and liver are much larger in relation to body weight than they are in the adult (98).

Protein Binding

Many drugs are less avidly bound to plasma proteins in the neonate and infant than they are in the older patient (16, 98, 132, 179). Decreased binding affects acidic drugs (e.g., phenytoin), which are bound to albumin (163), as well as basic drugs (e.g., lidocaine), which are bound to 1-glycoprotein (14, 118, 179). Reduced binding to plasma proteins is associated with at least three potentially important effects: (*a*) increase in apparent volume of distribution (V_d) (132); (*b*) decrease in the total plasma drug concentration following a standard dosage (139, 173); and (*c*) decrease in the range of total plasma drug concentrations associated with both therapeutic efficacy and toxicity. These effects are important for extensively protein-bound drugs that have a low hepatic extraction ratio (139, 173).

Although the protein binding of many drugs is reduced in the newborn, these observations have not been extended into later infancy (97, 98, 132). Reduced binding is of definite clinical importance for drugs that are both extensively bound and subject to therapeutic drug monitoring. Phenytoin (85, 163) is the usual example. When an infant is treated with this anticonvulsant, the free rather than the total phenytoin concentration should be monitored. Other extensively bound drugs with reduced binding in early infancy include quinidine (119), diazepam (100), furosemide (100), some antibiotics (16, 98), propranolol, and thiopental (16). However, the effect on therapy has not been delineated, and it would be incorrect to assume that these alterations in protein binding must be clinically important. Further investigation is warranted. Protein binding of certain neuromuscular blocking agents is reduced in infancy (176, 180), but the substances are so weakly bound in adults (180) that this observation is not likely to have clinical significance.

Changes in protein binding affect other kinetic functions and calculations, including clearance and volume of distribution. These are reviewed in Chapter 1 and in several publications (98, 132, 139, 163, 165, 173), which include a discussion of the manner in which efficiency of hepatic extraction interacts with the extent of protein binding to affect total and unbound drug clearance. The net effect of greater ECW, diminished protein binding, and the relatively large brain and liver in the infant is to increase, on a weight-normalized basis, the V_d of most drugs (98, 139). This change in V_d may entail a larger dosage of these drugs, but this is not necessarily the case because of the potential countervailing influence of reduced elimination or altered sensitivity.

Binding of unconjugated bilirubin to plasma proteins is affected by drug therapy (16). This subject has been extensively reviewed, and is not considered in this chapter.

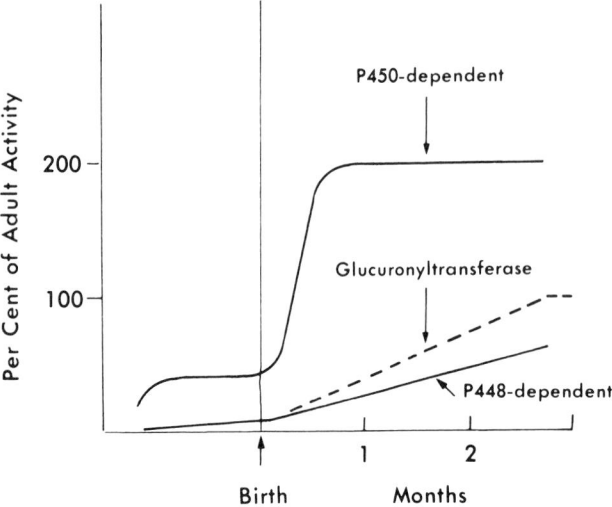

Figure 7.5. Developmental pattern of cytochrome P-450- and P-448-dependent reactions and of UDP-glucuronyltransferase in human liver. (From Vessey DA: Hepatic metabolism of drugs and toxins. In Zakim D, Boyer TD (eds): *Hepatology*. WB Saunders, Philadelphia, 1982.)

Table 7.3. Selected Drugs That Undergo Oxidation: Plasma Half-lives in Full-term Newborns and Adults[a]

| | *Elimination Half-life (hr)* | |
Drug	*Newborns*	*Adults*
Aminopyrine	30–40	2–4
Bupivacaine	25	1.3
Caffeine	95	4
Carbamazepine	8–28	21–36
Diazepam	25–100	15–25
Indomethacin	14–20	2–11
Lidocaine	2.9–3.3	1.0–2.2
Meperidine	22	3–4
Mepivacaine	8.7	3.2
Nortriptyline	56	18–22
Phenobarbital	28–43	36–38
Phenylbutazone	21–34	12–30
Phenyltoin	21	11–29
Theophylline	24–36	3–9
Tolbutamide	10–40	4.4–9

[a] Adapted from Rane A: Basic principle of drug disposition and action. In Yaffe SJ (ed): *Pediatric Pharmacology*. Grune & Stratton, New York, 1980; and Morselli PL, Franco-Morselli R, Bossi L: Clinical pharmacokinetics in newborns and infants. *Clin Pharmacokinet* 5:485, 1980.

ELIMINATION

Elimination of drug from the body occurs by two processes, biotransformation (metabolism) and excretion (85, 139). Age-related differences in both processes are well-described and are of clinical importance.

Biotransformation

Drug biotransformation is divided into two phases, phase 1 and phase 2 (174). Phase 1 reactions are catalyzed by oxidoreductases and hydroxylases, which produce carboxyl, epoxide, hydroxyl, amino, and sulfur groups (33, 88). These reactive groups promote elimination and permit phase 2 conjugation reactions with moieties, such as acetate, amino acids, glucuronic acid, sulfate, and glutathione. Conjugation leads to more polar products that are readily eliminated via the kidney or gastrointestinal tract. The hepatic contribution to biotransformation is the largest and best-characterized (165). Hepatic phase 1 and phase 2 reactions are both depressed in the neonate but increase during later infancy and childhood, often to rates much greater than those seen in the adult (98).

Phase 1 Reactions. Phase 1 biotransformation of many drugs is slow in newborn infants (97, 98, 132). At birth, the cytochrome P-450 content of the liver is only 28% of the adult level. Activity of a variety of monooxygenases is depressed to less than 50% of adult activity (165). Depressed rates of metabolism persist for a variable but substantial period of time. Table 7.3 indicates selected compounds that may display different rates of oxidation in newborn infants. This category of reaction is most consistently impaired in the newborn period (88, 126), although even here exceptions are important. Thus, the elimination rate of phenytoin is similar in newborns and adults (185dd). In contrast, demethylation reactions, as illustrated by diazepam, are relatively intact (16, 98), indicating that each class of compound must be individually evaluated.

As expected, the newborn and young infant display reduced oxidative activity toward theophylline and caffeine.

Instead of undergoing *N*-demethylation, as in adults, theophylline is *N*-methylated to caffeine (65), a compound with similar biological activity. By 7 to 9 months of age, the adult metabolic pattern is attained (65). This fact illustrates that not only is biotransformation slower as a rule, in early infancy, but also the end products may be different.

Deficient phase 1 activity is not limited to the mixed-function oxidase system. Other enzymes known to be deficient in the newborn are reviewed elsewhere (88, 98, 99), and include (with their substrates in parentheses) alcohol dehydrogenase (ethyl alcohol, methyl alcohol, chloral hydrate), plasma esterase (local anesthetics), and *N*-acetyltransferase (INH, hydralazine) (94).

Phase 2 Reactions. Conjugation reactions are also limited at birth. Glucuronic acid conjugation is severely impaired for some (not all) compounds; this is implicated in intoxication with chloramphenicol (170). Sulfate and glycine conjugation are well-preserved in the neonate, and sulfonation of steroids occurs at near adult rates (88). Thus, as with phase 1 reactions, generalization regarding the effect of immaturity on phase 2 reactions can be misleading. Each reaction must be individually evaluated.

Maturation of Biotransformation. Concurrent with the maturation of hepatic biotransformation (Fig. 7.5), there is a dramatic acceleration of the elimination rates of many compounds (98, 139). Beyond early infancy, children clear many substances more rapidly than do adults. In part, these increased clearance rates reflect the large volumes of distribution that characterize infancy, but to a considerable extent they reflect a true augmentation of rates of hepatic biotransformation. As Morselli and associates (98) indicate, disposition rates that are less than 30% of adult values in the newborn become severalfold greater than adult values by the end of the first year of life. The intensive care physician caring for infants and children thus encounters a heterogeneous population of subjects with regard to drug elimination. Figure 7.6 illustrates the effect of age on elimination half-life ($t_{1/2}$) of diazepam. Detailed information about maturation of hepatic biotransformation is available (16, 88, 98, 132, 139, 165, 185cc).

Renal Elimination

At birth, many aspects of renal function are reduced, even when normalized to body weight or to surface area. In full-term neonates, the glomerular filtration rate (GFR) is 2 to 4 ml/min (15 ml/min/1.73 m²) (2, 63). It doubles during the first 2 weeks of life. When normalized to surface area, adult rates of filtration (90 to 130 ml/min/1.73 m²) are achieved by 6 months of age (2). Thereafter, there is a linear relation between GFR and body surface area (Fig. 7.7). Tubular function is also reduced in the newborn, and maturation of tubular function is slower than maturation of glomerular filtration (16). Neonates display decreased transport capacity for a variety of substances, including acids, bases, glucose, protein, and bicarbonate (2, 63, 98).

Many substances are eliminated by the kidney in unchanged form. Whether it be due to immaturity or to disease, reduced renal function decreases clearance and prolongs elimination half-life. This result may entail a reduction in dosage. Rane and Wilson (127) have elegantly shown how reduced glomerular filtration or tubular secretion in the infant can affect drug $t_{1/2}$. They examined two drugs—*p*-aminohippurate, assumed to be eliminated exclusively by tubular secretion, and inulin, assumed to be eliminated exclusively by glomerular

filtration. Based on age-appropriate V_d and measured total body clearances (*Cl*) for these substances, it is simple to calculate resulting elimination half-life, since:

$$t_{1/2} = \frac{0.693 \times V_d}{Cl} \tag{1}$$

The calculations are shown in Table 7.4. Inulin, representing drugs that are cleared by filtration (e.g., aminoglycosides), displays a 50% increase in its $t_{1/2}$ in the infant, as compared with that in the adult. *p*-Aminohippurate, representing drugs cleared by tubular secretion (e.g., penicillin), displays a 3-fold increase in its $t_{1/2}$. These theoretic calculations conform reasonably well to measured values (123). Thus, kinetic studies with ampicillin, penicillin G, and methicillin indicate that *t* decreases progressively after birth. This finding is also true for furosemide, accounting for the prolonged diuretic effect with this drug that is observed in neonates (185x and ee). As renal function matures (Fig. 7.7), these values approach those seen in adults.

Generalization is problematic, since renal elimination of some drugs is either unchanged in infancy (e.g., colistin) (123) or actually greater than in adults. The latter is the case for lidocaine (95) and digoxin (113) and may represent maturation of filtration prior to tubular reabsorptive function (114).

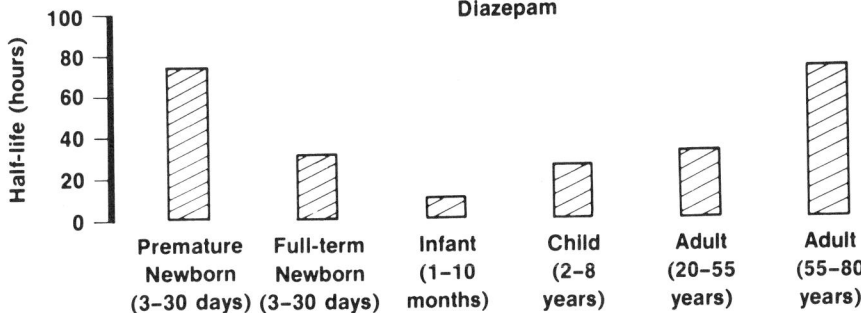

Figure 7.6. The elimination half-life of diazepam is shortest in the infant and longest in the newborn and the elderly. (Adapted from Rowland M, Tozer TN: *Clinical Pharmacokinetics.* Lea & Febiger, Philadelphia, 1980. Adapted from the data of Morselli PL: *Drug Disposition During Development.* Spectrum Publications, New York, 1977; and Klotz U, Avant GR, Hoyumpa A, et al: The effect of age and liver disease on the disposition and elimination of diazepam in adult man. *J Clin Invest* 55:347, 1975.)

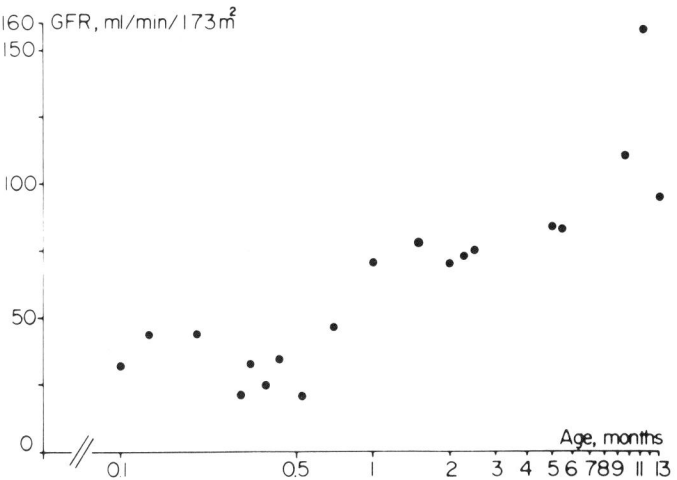

Figure 7.7. Glomerular filtration rate (*GFR*) during the first year of life, related to the logarithm of age. Determined by inulin disappearance curve. (From Aperia A, Broberger O, Thodenius K, et al: Development of renal control of salt and fluid homeostasis during the first year of life. *Acta Paediatr Scand* 64:393, 1975.)

Table 7.4. Calculation of Half-life for a Proposed Drug with the Same Clearance as Inulin (Glomerular Filtration) or *p*-Aminohippuric Acid (PAH) (Tubular Secretion) in an Infant (1.5 months old) and Adult[a,b]

Weight (kg)	ECW			Inulin		PAH	
	% of Weight	Total Volume (ml)		Clearance (ml/min)	$t_{1/2}$ (min)	Clearance (ml/min)	$t_{1/2}$ (min)
4.5	32	1,440		10	100	25	40
70.0	18	12,600		130	67	650	13

[a] From Rane A, Wilson JT: Clinical pharmacokinetics in infants and children. In Gibaldi M, Prescott L (eds): *Handbook of Clinical Pharmacokinetics*. ADIS Health Science Press, New York, 1983.
[b] The drug distributes in the extracellular water space (ECW). Calculation is based on $t_{1/2} = 0.693 \times V_d \times Cl^{-1}$.

Digoxin elimination provides an interesting example of maturation of renal function. In neonates, clearance of this drug is lower than in older infants and children, reflecting immature rates of filtration and elimination (98, 113). Clearance of digoxin increases between the 2nd and 3rd months of life, to the extent that it is greater in children than in adults (86, 98, 113). A portion of this increase in clearance can be attributed to the fact that the V_d of digoxin is 1.5 to 2 times greater in the child than in the adult ($Cl = K_e \times V_d$, where K_e is elimination rate constant). An additional factor is that in children, but not adults, glomerular filtration of digoxin is augmented by secretion (86). During adolescence, net tubular secretion and total renal clearance of digoxin decrease toward adult values. This decrease is correlated with sexual maturity stage (Tanner stages 4 and 5) rather than chronological age (86). A relationship between sexual maturity (rather than size or age) and drug elimination rate may also have significance for drugs other than digoxin.

IMPAIRMENT OF RENAL DRUG ELIMINATION BY DISEASE

Serum creatinine is lower in the pediatric age group than in healthy adults. By the 5th day of life, the plasma creatinine is 0.40 ± 0.02 mg/dl (63). During the balance of childhood (up to 18 years of age), creatinine values are lower than 0.8 mg/dl in healthy individuals (148), reflecting lesser muscle mass. Creatinine values that would be considered normal in young and middle-aged adults can represent significant degrees of renal dysfunction in the child.

Modifying drug dosage to account for impaired renal function depends on an estimate of the extent of impairment. This estimate usually involves measurement or estimation of creatinine clearance. Timed urine collection is difficult in the child and may not be complete before therapeutic decisions are necessary. However, unless age is taken into account, an isolated serum creatinine measurement does not provide an accurate estimate of renal function. For example, at 6 months of age, a serum creatinine value of 1.0 mg/dl is associated with a clearance of approximately 30 ml/min/1.73 m2. At 20 years, the same creatinine level indicates a clearance of approximately 115 ml/min/1.73 m2. In relatively healthy children, it is possible to accurately estimate creatinine clearance from knowledge of the patient's age, sex, length, and plasma creatinine (145–147). The equation and appropriate constants are indicated in Table 7.5.

Table 7.5. Method for Calculating Cl_{cr} in Children Aged 1 Week to 21 Years[a,b]

Cl_{cr} (ml/min/1.73 m²) = length (cm) × k/P_{cr} (mg dl)	
Age	k
Infant (1–52 weeks)	0.45
Child (1–13 years)	0.55
Adolescent (14–21 years)	
Male	0.7
Female	0.55

[a] Based on Schwartz and associates (145–147).
[b] This method is valid for individuals without severe muscle wasting and with stable plasma creatinine (P_{cr}) values.

Adjustment of dosage in renal failure is discussed in detail in Chapter 3. A method that is satisfactory in relatively healthy children is presented here. First, the creatinine clearance is estimated using the method indicated in Table 7.5. The following equation is used to estimate corrected dosage:

$$D_r = D_n \times [1 - f(1 - R)] \tag{2}$$

where R, the fraction of remaining renal function, is given by

$$R = \frac{estimated\ Cl_{cr}\ of\ patient\ (per\ 1.73\ m^2)}{normal\ Cl_{cr}\ for\ age\ (per\ 1.73\ m^2)} \tag{3}$$

During the first year of life, normal Cl_{cr} for age is estimated as shown in Figure 7.7. Subsequently, it is assumed to be 100 ml/min/1.73 m². Other terms in Equation 2 are as follows: f, fraction of drug excreted unchanged by the kidney in a normal subject (Table 7.6); D_r, daily dose during renal failure; and D_n, daily dose in a normal subject (of the same age). D_r, the total daily dose during renal failure, can be delivered by administering the usual dose at an extended interval or by offering a reduced dose at the usual interval. It may be most appropriate both to reduce individual dose and to extend dosing interval. Further details are available in a number of publications (1, 31, 41, 130, 139).

EXAMPLE: A 3-year-old child (weight, 15 kg; length, 96 cm) with a serum creatinine of 1.2 mg/dl requires gentamicin ($f = 1.0$). The usual dosage for this age is 5 mg/kg/day (75 mg), divided into three 8-hourly doses. The corrected dosage for this child is calculated as follows:

1. Creatinine clearance of patient:

$$Cl_{cr} = \frac{0.55 \cdot 96 \; cm}{1.2 \; mg/dl}$$

$$= 44 \; ml/min/m^2$$

2. Calculation of dosage

$$R = \frac{44 \; ml/min/m^2}{100 \; ml/min/m^2}$$

$$= 0.44$$

$$D_r = 75 \; mg/day \cdot [1-1.0 \; (1-0.44)]$$

$$= 33 \; mg/day$$

This dosage can be given at the usual (8-hour interval, 11 mg every 8 hours, or at an extended interval, 33 mg every 24 hours. The 8-hourly schedule prevents prolonged subtherapeutic concentrations, whereas the 24-hourly schedule permits the usual peak, trough, and mean drug concentrations. A reasonable compromise would be to administer 22 mg every 16 hours.

Unfortunately, predicting creatinine clearance is not as straightforward in critically ill children as the preceding example suggests. For example, in a recent study in critically ill children (185ff), there was a marked discrepancy between estimated and measured creatinine clearance, with the estimated clearance usually too high. Indeed, in 37 of 100 of the patients studied, the discrepancy was greater than 50%. Thus, there is an important possibility of overdosage when an estimated creatinine clearance is employed in critically ill children to establish a drug regimen. Therefore, when employing an estimate of renal function based on serum creatinine measurement to prescribe the dosage of potentially toxic drugs, it is essential to very carefully monitor the serum drug concentration. This monitoring may require the precaution of drug concentration measurement following the first dose. Although this drug level information will be preliminary, not reflecting the effect of drug accumulation, early measurement will avoid drug concentrations that are grossly high or low.

This presentation does not take into account excretion of products of hepatic drug metabolism by the kidney or the effect of altered renal function on drug metabolism in the liver and other organs. These subjects are reviewed in Chapters 1 to 6 and elsewhere (1, 132, 139). In addition, while dosage adjustment for renal failure is *relatively* simple because the reduction in clearance is proportionate to an easily measured term Cl_{cr}, this is not the case for functional alterations in renal drug elimination that are due to changes in renal blood flow (i.e., digoxin), state of hydration (i.e., lithium), coadministration of other drugs (i.e., probenecid), or urine pH (i.e., phenobarbital). Such changes are frequent and should be anticipated in appropriate contexts.

EXCHANGE TRANSFUSION

Exchange transfusion is performed in neonates for control of hyperbilirubinemia. In older infants and children, this procedure is occasionally advocated for therapy of diverse hematological and metabolic conditions. Usually, a double volume

exchange is performed, although "partial" exchange transfusions employing lesser volumes are occasionally employed. Exchange of the blood volume represents an additional mode of elimination and perturbs distribution of drugs. Lackner (79) presented the following equation for estimating the fraction of drug removed (f_x) as a result of an exchange transfusion of volume (v), when the drug has a volume of distribution,

$$f_x = 1 - e^{-V/V_d} \tag{4}$$

In most instances, the amount of drug loss is trivial (<20%). With the possible exception of theophylline (f_x=32.4%), specific drug replacement is not necessary unless exchanges are numerous or greater than two blood volumes.

ADJUSTMENT FOR SIZE

Adjusting dosage to body size can be complex: Ritschel (130) was able to count no less than 23 separate approaches,

Table 7.6. Fraction of Dose Excreted Unchanged in Urine (f) with normal renal function[a]

Antibiotics	f
Acyclovir[b]	0.8
Aminoglycosides[b]	1.0
Ampicillin[b]	0.8
Amphotericin	0
Erythromycin	0.1
[b]Cefazolin	0.8
Cefoperazone	0.3
Cefotaxime	0.5
[b]Cefoxitin	0.9
[b]Ceftazidime	0.9
Ceftriaxone	0.5
[b]Cefuroxime	0.9
Chloramphenicol	0
Clindamycin	0.1
[b]Ganciclovir	1.0
[b]Imipenem/Cilastin	0.7
[b]Methicillin	0.9
Metronidazole	0.1
Nafcillin	<0.2
[b]Oxacillin	0.8
[b]Penicillin	0.9
Rifampin	0
[b]Sulfamethoxazole	0.9
[b]Trimethoprim	0.7
[b]Vancomycin	1.0

Miscellaneous	f
Acetaminophen	0
[b]Atenolol	0.9
Atricurium	0
[b]Cimetidine	0.6
[b]Digoxin	0.7
[b]Lithium	1.0
Lorazepam	0
Midazolam	0
[b]Pancuronium	0.7
[b]Ranitidine	0.7
Vecuronium	0.2

[a] Adapted from Rowland M, Tozer TN: Clinical Pharmacokinetics. Lea & Febiger, 1980 Philadelphia.
[b] Indicates that dosage reduction may be necessary with clinically significant renal dysfunction. Individual product information should be consulted.

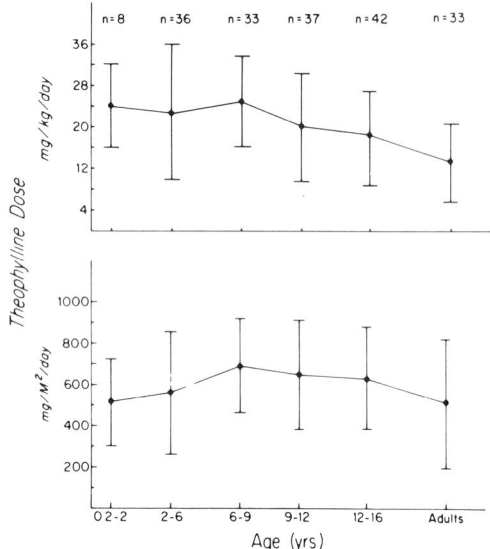

Figure 7.8. Weight-adjusted (*upper*) and body surface area-adjusted (*lower*) theophylline dose requirements (mean ±2 SD). Dosage was adjusted to maintain peak serum theophylline concentrations between 10 and 20 μg/ml during chronic therapy. (From Wyatt R, Weinberger M, Hendeles L: Oral theophylline dosage for the management of chronic asthma. *J Pediatr* 92:125, 1978.)

employing a total of 52 different equations! Most methods involve adjustment for body weight or adjustment for body surface area.

Adjustments for body weight have the advantage of simplicity and familiarity. In most reference sources, pediatric dosages are presented in terms of body weight. The theoretic and practical objection to this method is that the weight-normalized dosage of many drugs increases as weight decreases. If a constant per unitweight dosage is employed, small individuals (children) will receive too small a dose.

Basing dosage on surface area has the apparent advantage of *approximating* constant dosage over a wide range of body size and age. This supposition is illustrated in Figure 7.8 for theophylline (181) and was discussed earlier in connection with succinylcholine. It is true of a variety of drugs used in critical care (16, 52).

The relative linearity between surface area and dosage is not easily explained. In part, it reflects that for many drugs, V_d is related to the volume of the extracellular water (ECW). ECW increases relative to mass as size decreases (Fig. 7.4). However, ECW remains nearly constant relative to surface area as size decreases. Thus, relative to mass, V_d increases with decreasing size; relative to surface area, V_d tends to remain constant. This cannot be the entire reason, since the increase in V_d alone would shorten t but not affect drug clearance or the relationship between drug dosage and mean drug concentration. Probably, it is also important that the magnitude or velocity of other physiological processes that affect drug disposition is also directly related to surface area rather than mass. These include cardiac output, GFR, intestinal surface area, and hepatic blood flow (16, 52).

The apparently constant relationship between surface area and dosage leads many to advocate this method of normalization. While there are compelling reasons to employ surface area normalization—(a) during new drug development trials (55); (b) for extrapolation from dosages in adults; and (c) at extremes of weight (obesity, malnutrition) (130)—there appears to be no intrinsic advantage in routine clinical practice. Calculation of surface area is laborious, and many nomograms are inaccurate (7). For theophylline, use of surface area-normalized dosages does not reduce interpatient variability (181). Thus, it makes sense to employ a weight-based method for drug dosing, but to recognize that the dosage may be higher, on a weight basis, in infants than in adults.

CONCLUSION

The axiom that children are not merely small adults is manifest nowhere more than in the consideration of pediatric pharmacotherapy. Pharmacodynamic and pharmacokinetic differences between children and adults are common and important; these differences are derived from the significant changes in human physiology that attend growth and development. Knowledge of basic pharmacological principles guides the clinician in adapting information derived from experience in adults to children, but these basic (and general) principles must be supplemented by rigorous and detailed knowledge of specific drugs and their application to children.

REFERENCES

1. Anderson RJ: Drug prescribing for patients in renal failure. *Hosp Pract* 18(2):145, 1983.
2. Aperia A, Broberger O, Thodenius K, et al: Development of renal control of salt and fluid homeostasis during the first year of life. *Acta Paediatr Scand* 64:393, 1975.
3. Arena JM, Rourk MH Jr, Sibrack CD: Acetaminophen: report of an unusual poisoning. *Pediatrics* 61:68, 1978.
4. Assali NS, Brinkman CR, Woods JR, et al: Development of neurohumoral control of fetal, neonatal, and adult cardiovascular functions. *Am J Obstet Gynecol* 129:748, 1977.
5. Bailey WC, Weill H, DeRoven, et al: The effect of isoniazid on transaminase levels. *Ann Intern Med* 81:200, 1974.
6. Barthels H: Drug therapy in childhood: what has been done and what has to be done. *Pediatr Pharmacol* 3:31, 1983.
7. Bateman DN, Croft AW, Nicholson E, et al: Dystonic reactions and the pharmacokinetics of metoclopramide in children. *Br J Clin Pharmacol* 15:557, 1983.
8. Bateman DN, Rawlins MD, Simpson JM: Extrapyramidal reactions to prochlorperazine and haloperidol in the United Kingdom. *Q J Med* 59:549, 1986.
9. Bennett EJ, Ignacio A, Patel K, et al: Tubocurarine and the neonate. *Br J Anaesthesiol* 48:687, 1976.
10. Bennett EJ, Ramamurthy S, Dalal FY, et al: Pancuronium and the neonate. *Br J Anaesthesiol* 47:75, 1975.
11. Beregovich J, Bianchi C, Rubler S: Dose-related hemodynamic and renal effects of dopamine in congestive heart failure. *Am Heart J* 87:550, 1974.
12. Berg RA: Emergency infusion of catecholamines into bone marrow. *Am J Dis Child* 138:810, 1984.
13. Berner M, Rouge JC, Friedli B: The hemodynamic effect of phentolamine and dobutamine after open heart operations in children: influence of the underlying heart defect. *Ann Thorac Surg* 35:643, 1983.
14. Bienvenu J, Sann L, Bienvenu F, et al: Laser nephelometry of orosomucoid in serum of newborns: reference intervals and relation to bacterial infections. *Clin Chem* 27:721, 1981.
15. Bohn DJ, Poirier CS, Edmonds JF, et al: Hemodynamic effects of dobutamine after cardiopulmonary bypass in children. *Crit Care Med* 8:367, 1980.
16. Boreus LO: *Principles of Pediatric Pharmacology.* New York, Churchill Livingstone, 1982.
17. Brion L, Fleischman AR, Schwartz GJ: Evaluation of four length-weight formulas for estimating body surface area in newborn infants. *J Pediatr* 107:801, 1985.

18. Brown BR Jr: Halothane hepatitis revisited. *N Engl J Med* 313:1347, 1985.
19. Buckley NM, Brazeau P, Gootman P: Maturation of circulatory responses to adrenergic stimuli. *Fed Proc* 42:1643, 1983.
20. Buckley NM, Gootman PM, Yellin EL, et al: Age-related cardiovascular effects of catecholamines in anesthetized piglets. *Circ Res* 45:282, 1979.
21. Carney FT, Van Dyke RA: Halothane hepatitis: a critical review. *Anesth Analg* 51:135, 1972.
22. Casella ES, Rogers MC, Zahka KG: Developmental physiology of the cardiovascular system. In Rogers MC (ed): *Textbook of Pediatric Intensive Care*. Baltimore, Williams & Wilkins, 1987.
23. Chabrolle JP, Rossier A: Goitre and hypothyroidism in the newborn after cutaneous absorption of iodine. *Arch Dis Child* 53:495, 1978.
24. Chernow B, Rainey TG, Lake CR: Endogenous and exogenous catecholamines in critical care medicine. *Crit Care Med* 10:409, 1982.
25. Cohlan SQ, Bevelander G, Tiamsic T: Growth inhibition of prematures receiving tetracycline: clinical and laboratory investigation. *Am J Dis Child* 105:453, 1963.
26. Cook DR: Muscle relaxants in infants and children. *Anesth Analg* 60:335, 1981.
27. Cook DR, Fischer CG: Neuromuscular blocking effects of succinylcholine in infants and children. *Anesthesiology* 42:662, 1975.
28. Cowan RH, Jukkola AF, Arant BS: Pathophysiologic evidence of gentamicin nephrotoxicity in neonatal puppies. *Pediatr Res* 14:1204, 1980.
29. Cryer PE: Physiology and pathophysiology of the human sympathoadrenal neuroendocrine system. *N Engl J Med* 303:436, 1980.
30. Cryer PE, Rizza RA, Haymond MW, et al: Epinephrine and norepinephrine are cleared through betaadrenergic, but not alpha-adrenergic, mechanisms in man. *Metabolism* 29:1114, 1980.
31. Dettli L: Drug dosage in renal disease. In Gibaldi M, Prescott L (eds): *Handbook of Clinical Pharmacokinetics*. New York, ADIS Health Science Press, 1983.
32. DiSessa TG, Leitner M, Ching CT, et al: The cardiovascular effects of dopamine in the severely asphyxiated neonate. *J Pediatr* 99:772, 1981.
33. Drayer DE: Pathways of drug metabolism in man. *Med Clin North Am* 58:927, 1974.
34. Driscoll DJ, Gillette PC: Hemodynamic effects of dobutamine in children. *Am J Cardiol* 43:581, 1979.
35. Driscoll DJ, Gillette PC, Ezrailson EG, et al: Inotropic response of the neonatal canine myocardium to dopamine. *Pediatr Res* 12:42, 1978.
36. Driscoll DJ, Gillette PC, Lewis RM, et al: Comparative hemodynamic effects of isoproterenol, dopamine, and dobutamine in the newborn dog. *Pediatr Res* 13:1006, 1979.
37. Driscoll DJ, Gillette PC, McNamara DG: The use of dopamine in children. *J Pediatr* 92:309, 1978.
38. Drugs for tuberculosis. *Med Lett Drugs Ther* 24:17, 1982.
39. Duckles SP, Banner W Jr: Changes in vascular smooth muscle reactivity during development. *Annu Rev Pharmacol Toxicol* 24:65, 1984.
40. Epstein ML, Kiel EA, Victorica BE: Cardiac decompensation following verapamil therapy in infants with supraventricular tachycardia. *Pediatrics* 75:737, 1983.
41. Fabre J, Balant L: Renal failure. In Gibaldi M, Prescott L (eds): *Handbook of Clinical Pharmacokinetics*. New York, ADIS Health Science Press, 1983.
42. Farrell G, Prendergast D, Murray M: Halothane hepatitis. Detection of a constitutional susceptibility factor. *N Engl J Med* 313;1310, 1985.
43. Filloux F: Toxic encephalopathy caused by topically applied diphenhydramine. *J Pediatr* 108:1018, 1986.
44. Fitzgerald GA, Barnes P, Hamilton CA, et al: Circulating adrenaline and blood pressure: the metabolic effects and kinetics of infused adrenaline in man. *Eur J Clin Invest* 10:401, 1980.
45. Flower RJ, Moncada S, Vane JR: Analgesic-antipyretics and anti-inflammatory agents; drugs used in the treatment of gout. In Gilman AG, Goodman LS, Roll TW, Murad F (eds): *The Pharmacological Basis of Therapeutics*, ed 7. New York, Macmillan, 1985.
46. Food and Drug Administration: FDA Drug Bull 8:11, 1978.
47. Food and Drug Administration: FDA Drug Bull 12:10, 1982. 48. Ford DC, Leist ER, Algren JT: *Guidelines for Administration of Intravenous Medications to Pediatric Patients*, ed 2. Bethesda, American Society of Hospital Pharmacists, 1984.
49. Friedman WF: The intrinsic physiologic properties of the developing heart. *Prog Cardiovasc Dis* 15:87, 1972.
50. Friedman WF, George BL: New concepts and drugs in the treatment of congestive heart failure. *Pediatr Clin North Am* 31:1197, 1984.
51. Friedman WF, Pool PE, Jacobiwitz D, et al: Sympathetic innervation of the developing rabbit heart. Biochemical and histochemical comparisons of fetal, neonatal, and adult myocardium. *Circ Res* 23:25, 1968.
52. Garson A: Dosing the newer antiarrhythmic drugs in children: considerations in pediatric pharmacology. *Am J Cardiol* 57:1405, 1986.
53. Garson A: Medicolegal problems in the management of cardiac arrhythmias in children. *Pediatrics* 79:84, 1987.
54. Geis WP, Tatooles CJ, Priola DV: Factors influencing neurohumoral control of the heart in the newborn dog. *Am J Physiol* 228:1685, 1975.
55. Gershanik J, Boecler B, Ensley H, et al: The gasping syndrome and benzyl alcohol poisoning. *N Engl J Med* 307:1384, 1982.

56. Goldberg LI: Dopamine—clinical use of an endogenous catecholamine. *N Engl J Med* 291:707, 1974.
57. Goldbloom RB, Goldbloom A: Boric acid poisoning, *J Pediatr* 43:631, 1953.
58. Goldstein DS, Zimlichman R, Stull R, et al: Plasma catecholamine and hemodynamic responses during isoproterenol infusions in humans. *Clin Pharmacol Ther* 40:233, 1986.
59. Gordon EP, Bristow MR, Laser JA, et al: Correlation between beta-adrenergic receptors in human lymphocytes and heart. *Circulation* 68:99, 1983.
60. Gould T, Roberts RJ: Therapeutic problems arising from the intravenous route for drug administration. *J Pediatr* 95:465, 1979.
61. Greco R, Musto B, Arienzo V: Treatment of paroxysmal supraventricular tachycardia in infancy with digitalis, adenosine-5-triphosphate, and verapamil: a comparative study. *Circulation* 66:504, 1982.
62. Grossman ER, Walchek A, Freedman H, et al: Tetracycline and permanent teeth: the relation between dose and tooth color. *Pediatrics* 47:567, 1971.
63. Guignard JP: Renal function in the newborn infant. *Pediatr Clin North Am* 29:777, 1982.
64. Gundert-Remy U, Penzien J, Hildebrandt R, et al: Correlation between the pharmacokinetics and pharmacodynamics of dopamine in healthy subjects. *Eur J Clin Pharmacol* 26:163, 1984.
65. Haley TJ: Metabolism and pharmacokinetics of theophylline in human neonates, children, and adults. *Drug Metab Rev* 14:295, 1983.
66. Halkin H, Radomsky M, Blieden L, et al: Steady state serum digoxin concentration in relation to digitalis toxicity in neonates and infants. *Pediatrics* 61:184, 1978.
67. Hayes GJ, Butler VP Jr, Gersony WM: Serum digoxin studies in infants and children. *Pediatrics* 52:561, 1973.
68. Heimann G: Renal toxicity of aminoglycosides in the neonatal period. *Pediatr Pharmacol* 3:251, 1983.
69. Hooper DC, Wolfson JS: The fluoroquinolones: pharmacology, clinical uses and toxicities in humans. *Antimicrob Agents Chemother* 28:716, 1985.
70. Iserson KV, Criss E: Intraosseous infusions: a usable technique. *Am J Emerg Med* 4:540, 1986.
71. James LS: Hexachlorophene. *Pediatrics* 49:492, 1972.
72. Jarnberg PO, Bengesson L, Erstrand J, et al: Dopamine infusion in man. Plasma catecholamine levels and pharmacokinetics. *Acta Anaesthesiol Scand* 25:334, 1981.
73. Kaplan JM, McCracken GH Jr, Horton CJ, et al: Pharmacologic studies in neonates given large dosages of ampicillin. *J Pediatr* 84:571, 1974.
74. Kates RE, Leier CV: Dobutamine pharmacokinetics in severe heart failure. *Clin Pharmacol Exp Ther* 24:537, 1978.
75. Kelliher GJ, Roberts J: Effect of age on the cardiotoxic action of digitalis. *J Pharmacol Exp Ther* 197:10, 1976.
76. Kho TL, Henquet JW, Punt R, et al: Influence of dobutamine and dopamine on hemodynamics and plasma concentrations of noradrenaline and renin in patients with low cardiac output following acute myocardial infarction. *Eur J Clin Pharmacol* 18:213, 1980.
77. Kittinger JW, Sandler RS, Heizer WD: Efficacy of metoclopramide as an adjunct to duodenal placement of small bore feeding tubes: a randomized, placebo-controlled, double-blind study. *J Parenter Enteral Nutr* 11:33, 1987.
78. Klotz U: Pathophysiology and disease-induced changes in drug distribution volume. In Gibaldi M, Prescott L (eds): *Handbook of Clinical Pharmacokinetics*. New York, ADIS Health Science Press, 1983.
79. Lackner TE: Drug replacement following exchange transfusion. *J Pediatr* 100:811, 1982.
80. Lang P, Williams RG, Norwood WI, et al: Hemodynamic effects of dopamine in infants after corrective cardiac surgery. *J Pediatr* 96:630, 1980.
81. Leff RD, Roberts RJ: Methods of intravenous drug administration in the pediatric patient. *J Pediatr* 98:631, 1981.
82. Legan E, Chernow B: Catecholamine response to acute illness. *Semin Respir Med* 7:88, 1985.
83. Leier CV, Unverferth DV, Kates RE: The relationship between plasma dobutamine concentrations and cardiovascular responses in cardiac failure. *Am J Med* 66:238, 1979.
84. Leier CV, Unverferth DV: Dobutamine. *Ann Intern Med* 99:490, 1983.
85. Levy RH, Bauer LA: Basic pharmacokinetics. *Ther Drug Monit* 8:47, 1986.
86. Linday LA, Drayer DE, Kahn MAA, et al: Pubertal changes in net renal tubular secretion of digoxin. *Clin Pharmacol Ther* 35:438, 1984.
87. Leob JN: Corticosteroids and growth. *N Engl J Med* 295:547, 1976.
87a. Lowrey GH: *Growth and Development of Children*, ed 7. Chicago, Year Book, 1978.
88. Mannering GJ: Drug metabolism in the newborn. *Fed Proc* 44:2302, 1985.
89. Marshall BE, Wollman H: General anesthetics. In Gilman AG, Goodman LS, Roll TW, Murad F (eds): *The Pharmacological Basis of Therapeutics*, ed 7. New York, Macmillan, 1985.
90. McBride WG: Thalidomide and congenital abnormalities. *Lancet* 2:1358, 1961.
91. McCracken GH Jr: Aminoglycoside toxicity in infants and children. *Am J Med* 80:172, 1986.
92. McLain GE, Sipes IG, Brown BR Jr: An animal model of halothane hepatotoxicity: roles of enzyme induction and hypoxia. *Anesthesiology* 91:321, 1979.

93. Metoclopramide for gastroesophageal reflux. *Med Lett Drugs Ther* 27:21, 1985.

94. Miceli JN, Olson, WA, Cohen SN: Elimination kinetics of isoniazid in the newborn infant. *Dev Pharmacol Ther* 2:225, 1981.

95. Mihaly GW, Moore RG, Thomas JW, et al: The pharmacokinetics and metabolism of the anilide local anesthetics in neonates. *Eur J Clin Pharmacol* 13:143, 1978.

96. Milligan N, Dhillon S, Richens A, et al: Rectal diazepam in the treatment of absence status: a pharmacodynamic study. *J Neurol Neurosurg Psychiatry* 44:914, 1981.

97. Morselli PL: Clinical pharmacokinetics in neonates. *Clin Pharmacokinet* 1:81, 1976.

98. Morselli PL, Franco-Morselli R, Bossi L: Clinical pharmacokinetics in newborns and infants. *Clin Pharmacokinet* 5:485, 1980.

99. Mullick FC: Hexachlorophene toxicity. Human experience at the Armed Forces Institute of Pathology. *Pediatrics* 51:395, 1973.

100. Nau H, Luck W, Kuhnz W, et al: Serum protein binding of diazepam, desmethyldiazepam, furosemide, indomethacin, warfarin, and phenobarbital in human fetus, mother, and newborn infant. *Pediatr Pharmacol* 3:219, 1983.

101. Nelson JD: Antimicrobial drugs. In Yaffe SJ (ed): *Pediatric Pharmacology*. New York, Grune & Stratton, 1980.

102. Nelson JD: *Pocketbook of Pediatric Antimicrobial Therapy*, ed 7. Baltimore, Williams & Wilkins, 1987.

103. Nogen AG, Bremner JE: Acetaminophen overdosage in a young child. *J Pediatr* 92:832, 1978.

104. Nolke AC: Severe toxic effects from aminophylline and theophylline suppositories in children. *JAMA* 161:693, 1956.

105. Norfloxacin. *Med Lett Drugs Ther* 29:25, 1987.

106. Notterman DA, Nardi M, Saslow JG: Effects of dose formulation on isoniazid absorption in two young children. *Pediatrics* 77:850, 1986.

107. Nugent SK, Laravuso R, Rogers MC: Pharmacology and use of muscle relaxants in infants and children. *J Pediatr* 94:481, 1979.

108. O'Brien RJ, Long MW, Cross FS, et al: Hepatotoxicity from isoniazid and rifampin among children treated for tuberculosis. *Pediatrics* 72:491, 1983.

109. O'Keefe, Gregory GA, Stanski DR, et al: *d*-Tubocurarine: pharmacodynamics and kinetics in children. *Anesthesiology* 51:S270, 1979.

110. O'Mally K, Coleman EN, Doig WB, et al: Plasma digoxin levels in infants. *Arch Dis Child* 48:99, 1973.

111. Orlowski JP: My kingdom for an intravenous line. *Am J Dis Child* 138:803, 1984. 112. Padbury JF, Agata Y, Baylen BG, et al: Dopamine pharmacokinetics in critically ill newborn infants. *J Pediatr* 110:293, 1987.

113. Park MK: Use of digoxin in infants and children with specific emphasis on dosage. *J Pediatr* 108:871, 1986.

114. Park MK, Ludden T, Arom KV, et al: Myocardial vs serum digoxin concentrations in infants and adults. *Am J Dis Child* 136:418, 1982.

115. Perez CA, Reimer JM, Schreiber MD, et al: Effect of high dose dopamine on urine output in newborn infants. *Crit Care Med* 14:1045, 1986.

116. Perkin RM, Levin DL: Dobutamine: a hemodynamic evaluation in children with shock. *J Pediatr* 100:97, 1982.

117. Perloff WH: Physiology of the heart and circulation. In Swedlow DB, Raphaely RC (eds): *Cardiovascular Problems in Pediatric Critical Care*. New York, Churchill Livingstone, 1986.

118. Piafsky, KM: Disease induced changes in the plasma binding of basic drugs. *Clin Pharmacokinet* 5:246, 1980.

119. Pikoff AS, Kessler KM, Singh S, et al: Age related differences in the protein binding of quinidine. *Dev Pharmacol Ther* 3:108, 1981.

120. Pinsky WW, Jacobsen JR, Gillette PC, et al: Dosage of digoxin in premature infants. *J Pediatr* 96:639, 1976.

121. Polgar G, Weng TR: The functional development of the respiratory system. *Am Rev Respir Dis* 120:625, 1979.

122. Porter CJ, Garson A, Gillette PC: Verapamil: an effective calcium blocking agent for pediatric patients. *Pediatrics* 71:748, 1983.

123. Prandota J: Clinical pharmacokinetics of changes in drug elimination in children. *Dev Pharmacol Ther* 8:311, 1985.

124. Radford D: Side effects of verapamil in infants. *Arch Dis Child* 58:465, 1983.

125. Rajchgot P, Prosber CG, Soldins S, et al: Aminoglycoside related nephrotoxicity in the premature newborn. *Clin Pharmacol Ther* 35:394, 1984.

126. Rane A: Basic principle of drug disposition and action. In Yaffe SJ (ed): *Pediatric Pharmacology*. New York, Grune & Stratton, 1980.

127. Rane A, Wilson JT: Clinical pharmacokinetics in infants and children. In Gibaldi M, Prescott L (eds): *Handbook of Clinical Pharmacokinetics*. New York, ADIS Health Science Press, 1983.

128. Reinhardt D, Zehmisch T, Becker B, et al: Age dependency of alpha and beta-adrenoreceptor on thrombocytes and lymphocytes of asthmatic and nonasthmatic children. *Eur J Pediatr* 142:111, 1984.

129. Ricci DA, Saltzman MB, Meyer C, et al: Effect of metoclopramide in diabetic gastroparesis. *J Clin Gastroenterol* 7:25, 1985.

130. Ritschel WA: *Handbook of Basic Pharmacokinetics*, ed 2. Hamilton, IL, Drug Intelligence Publications, 1980.

131. Roan Y, Galant SP: Decreased neutrophil beta adrenergic receptors in the neonate. *Pediatr Res* 16:591, 1982.

132. Roberts RJ: *Drug Therapy in Infants*. Philadelphia, WB Saunders, 1984.

133. Roberts RJ: Intravenous administration of medications in pediatric patients: problems and solutions. *Pediatr Clin North Am* 28:23, 1986.

134. Rockson SG, Homcy CJ, Quinn P, et al: Cellular mechanisms of impaired adrenergic responsiveness in neonatal dogs. *J Clin Invest* 67:319, 1981.

135. Romero T, Covell J, Freidman WF: A comparison of pressure volume relations of the fetal, newborn and adult heart. *Am J Physiol* 222:1285, 1972.

136. Romero T, Friedman WF: Limited left ventricular response to volume overload in the neonatal period: a comparative study with the adult animal. *Pediatr Res* 13:910, 1979.

137. Ross EM, Gilman AG: Pharmacodynamics: mechanisms of drug action and the relationship between drug concentration and effect. In Gilman AG, Goodman LS, Roll TW, Murad F (eds): *The Pharmacological Basis of Therapeutics*, ed 7. New York, Macmillan, 1985.

138. Rothstein P, Dornbusch J, Shaywitz BA: Prolonged seizures associated with the use of viscous lidocaine. *J Pediatr* 101:461, 1982.

139. Rowland M, Tozer TN: *Clinical Pharmacokinetics*. Philadelphia, Lea & Febiger, 1980.

140. Rumack BH: Acetaminophen overdose in young children. *Am J Dis Child* 138:428, 1984.

141. Rumack BH, Peterson RC, Koch G, et al: Acetaminophen overdose. *Arch Intern Med* 141:380, 1981.

142. Sandor GGS, Bloom KR, Izukawa T, et al: Noninvasive assessment of left ventricular function related to serum digoxin levels in neonates. *Pediatrics* 65:541, 1980.

143. Schipioe PG: An unusual case of antihistamine poisoning. *J Pediatr* 71:589, 1967.

144. Schranz D, Stopfkuchen H, Jungst BK, et al: Hemodynamic effects of dobutamine in children with cardiovascular failure. *Eur J Pediatr* 139:4, 1982.

145. Schwartz GJ, Feld LG, Langford DJ: A simple estimate of glomerular filtration rate in full term infants during the first year of life. *J Pediatr* 104:849, 1984.

146. Schwartz GJ, Haycock GB, Edelmann CM Jr, et al: A simple estimate of glomerular filtration rate in children derived from body length and plasma creatinine. *Pediatrics* 58:259, 1976.

147. Schwartz GJ, Haycock GB, Gauthier B: A simple estimate of glomerular filtration rate in adolescent boys. *J Pediatr* 106:522, 1985.

148. Schwartz GJ, Haycock GB, Spitzer A: Plasma creatinine and urea concentration in children: normal values for age and sex. *J Pediatr* 88:828, 1976.

149. Seri I, Tulassay T, Kiszel J, et al: Cardiovascular response to dopamine in hypotensive preterm neonates with severe hyaline membrane disease. *Eur J Pediatr* 142:3, 1984.

150. Shawn DH, McGuigan MA: Poisoning from dermal absorption of promethazine. *Can Med Assoc J* 130:1460, 1984.

151. Shaywitz SE, Caparulo BK, Hodgson ES: Developmental language disability as a consequence of prenatal exposure to ethanol. *Pediatrics* 68:850, 1981.

152. Shoor PM, Berryhill RE, Benumof JL: Intraosseous infusion: pressure-flow relationship and pharmacokinetics. *J Trauma* 19:772, 1979.

153. Silverberg AB, Shah SD, Haymond MW, et al: Norepinephrine: hormone and neurotransmitter in man. *Am J Physiol* 234:E252, 1978.

154. Singh BN, Nademanee K, Baky SH: Calcium antagonists. Clinical use in the treatment of arrhythmias. *Drugs* 25:125, 1983.

155. Spyridis P, Sinaniotis C, Papadea I, et al: Isoniazid liver injury during chemoprophylaxis in children. *Arch Dis Child* 94:65, 1979.

156. Stoner JD, Bolen JL, Harrison DC: Comparison of dobutamine and dopamine in treatment of severe heart failure. *Br Heart J* 39:536, 1977.

157. Stopfkuchen H, Schranz R, Huth R, et al: Effects of dobutamine on left ventricular performance in newborns as determined by systolic time intervals. *Eur J Pediatr* 146:135, 1987.

158. Tatsumi H, Senda H, Yatera S, et al: Toxicological studies on pipemidic acid. V. Effect on diarthrodial joints of experimental animals. *J Toxicol Sci* 3:357, 1978.

159. Tenenbein M: Pediatric toxicology: current controversies and recent advances related to nephrotoxicity in the premature newborn. Clinical and recent advances. *Curr Probl Pediatr* 16:185, 1986.

160. Terrin BN, McWilliams NB, Maurer HM: Side effects of metoclopramide as an antiemetic in childhood cancer chemotherapy. *J Pediatr* 104:138, 1984.

161. Valdes R Jr: Endogenous digoxin-like immunoreactive factors: impact on digoxin measurement and potential physiological implications. *Clin Chem* 31:1985, 1985.

162. Valdes R Jr, Graves SW, Brown BA: Endogenous substance in newborn infants causing false-positive digoxin measurements. *J Pediatr* 152:947, 1983.

163. Vallner JJ: Binding of drugs by albumin and plasma protein. *J Pharm Sci* 66:447, 1977.

164. van-der-Kleijn E, Baars AM, Vree TB, et al: Clinical pharmacokinetics of drugs used in the treatment of status epilepticus. *Adv Neurol* 34:421, 1983.

165. Vessey DA: Hepatic metabolism of drugs and toxins. In Zakim D, Boyer TD (eds): *Hepatology*. Philadelphia, WB Saunders, 1982.

166. Vestal RE, Wood AJJ, Shand DG: Reduced beta-adrenoreceptor sensitivity in the elderly. *Clin Pharmacol Ther* 26:181, 1979.

167. Ward JT: Endotracheal drug therapy. *Am J Emerg Med* 1:71, 1983.

168. Warner LO, Beach TP, Garvin JP: Halothane and children. The first quarter century. *Anesth Analg* 63:838, 1984.

169. Way WL, Costley EC, Way EL: Respiratory sensitivity of the newborn infant to meperidine and morphine. *Clin Pharmacol Ther* 6:454, 1962.

170. Weiss CF, Glazko AJ, Weston JK: Chloramphenicol in the newborn infant. *N Engl J Med* 262:787, 1960.

171. Whately K, Turner WW Jr, Dey M, et al: When does metoclopramide facilitate transpyloric intubation? *J Parenter Enteral Nutr* 8:679, 1984.

172. Whitsett JA, Noguchi A, Moore JJ: Developmental aspects of alpha and beta-adrenergic receptors. *Semin Perinatol* 6:125, 1982.

173. Wilkinson GR, Shand DC: A physiologic approach to hepatic drug clearance. *Clin Pharmacol Ther* 7:377, 1975.

174. Williams RT: *Detoxification Mechanisms*. New York, John Wiley & Sons, 1959.

175. Wilson RF, Sibbald WJ, Jaanimagi JL: Hemodynamic effects of dopamine in critically ill septic patients. *J Surg Res* 20:163, 1976.

176. Wingard LB, Cook DR: Clinical pharmacokinetics of muscle relaxants. *Clin Pharmacokinet* 2:330, 1977.

177. Wolff JA: Methemoglobinemia due to benzocaine. *Pediatrics* 20:915, 1957.

178. Wong DF, Wagner HN, Dannals RF, et al: Effects of age on dopamine and serotonin receptors measured by positron tomography of the living human brain. *Science* 226:1393, 1984.

179. Wood M, Wood AJJ: Changes in plasma drug binding and alpha₁-acid glycoprotein in mother and newborn infant. *Clin Pharmacol Ther* 4:522, 1981.

180. Wood M, Wood AJJ: Neuromuscular blocking agents. In Wood M, Wood AJJ (eds): *Drugs and Anesthesia*. Baltimore, Williams & Wilkins, 1982.

181. Wyatt R, Weinberger M, Hendeles L: Oral theophylline dosage for the management of chronic asthma. *J Pediatr* 92:125, 1978.

182. Yaffe SJ, Bierman CW, Cann HM, et al: Requiem for tetracyclines. *Pediatrics* 55:142, 1975.

183. Zaritsky A, Chernow B: Use of catecholamines in pediatrics. *J Pediatr* 105:341, 1984.

184. Zaritsky A, Eisenberg MG: Ontogenetic considerations in the pharmacotherapy of shock. In Chernow B, Shoemaker W (eds): *Critical Care—State of the Art*. vol 7. Fullerton, CA, Society of Critical Care Medicine, 1986, vol 7.

185a. Ciprofloxacin: *Med Let Drugs Ther* 30: 11, 1989.

185b. Till J, Shinebourne EA, Rigby ML, et al: Efficacy and safety of adenosine in the treatment of supraventricular tachycardia in infants and children. *Br Heart J* 62: 204, 1989.

185c. Overholt ED, Rheuban KS, Gutgesell HP, et al: Usefulness of adenosine for arrhythmias in infants and children. *Am J Cardiol* 61: 336, 1988.

185d. Dreifuss FE, Langer DH, Molinbe KA, Maxwell JE: Valproic acid hepatic fatalities. *Neurology* 39:201, 1989.

185e. American Academy of Pediatrics. Behavioral and cognitive effects of anticonvulsant therapy. Committee on Drugs. *Pediatrics* 76:644, 1985.

185f. Herranz JL, Armijo JA, Arteaga-R: Clinical side effects of phenobarbital, primidone, phenytoin, carbamazepine, and valproate during monotherapy in children. *Epilepsia* 29:794, 1988.

185g. Farwell JR, Lee YJ, Hirtz, DG, et al: Phenobarbital for febrile seizures — effects on intelligence and on seizure recurrence. *N Engl J Med* 322:364, 1990.

185h. Hartwig S, Roth B, Theisohn M: Clinical experience with continuous intravenous sedation using midazolam and fentanyl in the paediatric intensive care unit. *Eur J Pediatr* 150: 784, 1991.

185i. Bergman I, Steeves M, Burckart G, Thompson-A: Reversible neurologic abnormalities associated with prolonged intravenous midazolam and fentanyl administration. *J Pediatr* 119: 644, 1991.

185j. Kauffman RE: Fentanyl, fads, and folly: who will adopt the therapeutic orphans?. *J Pediatr* 119: 588, 1991.

185k. Fisher DM, O'Keeffe C, Stanski DR, et al: Pharmacokinetics and pharmacodynamics of d-tubocurarine in infants, children, and adults. *Anesthesiology* 57:203, 1982.

185l. Fisher DM, Castagnoli K, Miller RD: Vecuronium kinetics and dynamics in anesthetized infants and children. *Clin Pharmacol Ther* 37:402, 1985.

185m. Eldadah MK, Newth CJ: Vecuronium by continuous infusion for neuromuscular blockade in infants and children. *Crit Care Med* 7:989, 1989.

185n. Darrah WC, Johnston JR, Mirakhur RK: Vecuronium infusions for prolonged muscle relaxation in the intensive care unit. *Crit Care Med* 17:1297, 1989.

185o. Vanderheyden BA, Reynolds HN, Gerold KB, et al: Prolonged paralysis after long-term vecuronium infusion. *Crit Care Med* 20:304, 1992.

185p. Fisher DM, Canfell PC, Spellmann MJ: Pharmacokinetics and pharmacodynamics of atracurium in infants and children. *Anesthesiology* 73:33, 1990.

185q. Kalli, Meretoja OA: Infusion of atracurium in neonates, infants and children. *Br J Anaesth* 60:651, 1988.

185r. Notterman DA: Pharmacology of the cardiovascular system. In Fuhrman B, Zimmerman J (eds): *Pediatric Critical Care*. St Louis, Mosby Year Book, 1992, p 323.

185s. Zaritsky, A, Lotze A, Stull R: Steady state dopamine clearance in critically ill infants and children. *Crit Care Med* 16:3, 1988.

185t. Notterman DA, Greenwald BM, Moran, F, et al: Dopamine clearance in critically ill children: effect of age and organ system dysfunction. *Clin Pharm Ther* 48:138, 1990.

185u. Martinez AM, Padbury JF, Thio S: Dobutamine pharmacokinetics and cardiovascular response in critically ill neonates. *Pediatrics* 89:47, 1992.

185v. Schwartz PH, Eldadah MK, Newth CJL: The pharmacokinetics of dobutamine in pediatric intensive care unit patients. *Crit Care Med* 19:614, 1991.

185w. Banner W, Vernon DD, Minton, SD, Dean JM: Nonlinear dobutamine pharmacokinetics in a pediatric population. *Crit Care Med* 19:871, 1991.

185x. Banner W, Vernon DD, Dean, JM, Swenson: Nonlinear dopamine pharmacokinetics in pediatric patients. *J Pharmacol Exp Ther* 249:131, 1989.

185y. Blumer JL and Reed MD: Principles of neonatal pharmacology, in Yaffe SJ and Aranda JV (eds): *Pediatric Pharmacology*, ed 2. Philadelphia, WB Saunders, 1992, p 167.

185z. Daugbjerg P, Brems M, Mai J, et al: Intermittent prophylaxis in febrile convulsions: diazepam or valproic acid. *Acta Neurol Scand* 82: 17, 1990.

185aa. Van Hoogdalem E, de Boer AG, Breimer DD: Pharmacokinetics of rectal drug administration (part I). *Clin Pharmacokinet* 21:11, 1991.

185bb. Holm Knudsen, Clausen TG, Eno D: Rectal administration of midazolam versus diazepam for preanesthetic sedation in children. *Anesth Prog* 37:29, 1990.

185cc. Fiser DH: Intraosseous infusion. *N Engl J Med* 322:1579, 1990.

185dd. Rane A: Drug disposition and action in infants and children. In Yaffe SJ and Aranda JV (eds): *Pediatric Pharmacology*, ed 2. Philadelphia, WB Saunders, 1992, p 10.

185ee. Aranda JV, Perez J, Sitar DS, et al: Pharmacokinetic disposition and protein binding of furosemide in newborn infants. *J Pediatr* 93: 407, 1978.

185ff. Fong J, Notterman D, Valentino T: Calculated creatinine clearance fails to predict creatinine cleareance in critically ill children. *Crit Care Med* 19:S37, 1991.

CHAPTER 8

Role of the Pharmacist in Caring for the Critically Ill Patient

JOSEPH F. DASTA, M.Sc., F.C.C.M., F.C.C.P.

JUDITH JACOBI, Pharm.D., F.C.C.M.

DEBORAH K. ARMSTRONG, Pharm.D., F.C.C.M.

Critical care medicine has undergone considerable change in the past decade and has evolved into a multidisciplinary specialty with highly trained practitioners. Likewise, the profession of pharmacy is undergoing change as pharmacists become further integrated into the complex health care environment. One of the newest specialty practice areas within pharmacy is critical care pharmacy practice. Many pharmacists currently practice in intensive care units (ICUs). However, wide variations in pharmacy practice exist. Some pharmacists perform primarily dispensing functions, while others, with significant clinical expertise, actively participate in drug therapy decision-making (1, 2). Despite an increased involvement in direct patient care, pharmacists' potential contributions may not be universally recognized. For example, a recent task force on recommendations (3) for services and personnel delivering care to critically ill patients indicated the necessity of 24-hour pharmacy services but listed pharmacy in the "other" category, along with housekeeping and the unit clerk.

The purpose of this chapter is to provide an overview of pharmaceutical services, to introduce the concept of "pharmaceutical care," and to describe and quantify activities of pharmacists practicing in ICUs. It is hoped that readers will gain a better appreciation of the role pharmacists can play in the multidisciplinary pharmacologic management of the critically ill patient.

INTRODUCTION TO PHARMACEUTICAL SERVICES

From the early 20th century, pharmacists procured, prepared, and sold medications (4). A primary obligation was the dispensing of drugs in proper dosage forms, since many drugs were available only in bulk form.

The 1960s and 1970s heralded significant changes as pharmacy began to shift its focus from the drug product to the patient. Studies conducted during this time reported that medication errors were common in hospitals using traditional methods of drug control, such as the ward-stock system (5). In response to these problems, hospitals developed unit-dose and intravenous admixture services, in an attempt to reduce errors and improve drug use control. Having drugs prepared by pharmacists in patient-labeled, ready-to-administer forms relieved the nurse of compounding duties, reduced medication-related errors, and increased the sterility of intravenous dosage forms. Currently, 89% of hospitals have complete unit-dose systems and 70% have complete intravenous admixture programs; 77% of hospitals with more than 400 beds have both types of services (6).

Disturbing reports of prescribing errors began to appear in the 1970s. A 1972 article, for example, reported that 65% of antibiotics were prescribed inappropriately (7). Improvements in drug distribution systems alone could not solve these problems. Involvement of pharmacists in medical education and in the decision-making process was a logical means of improving the documented problems of drug therapy prescribing.

The clinical pharmacy movement, which began in the mid 1960s, applies specialized drug therapy knowledge to patient-specific problems and requires a close association of the pharmacist with the patient, physician, nurse, and other health care personnel (8). The Study Commission on Pharmacy concluded

Table 8.1. Events in the Drug Use Process[a]

Identifying the patient's problems (diagnosis)
Determining the patient's history of drug use
Prescribing medications
Selecting the drug product
Dispensing the drug
Educating and counseling the patient
Administering the drug
Monitoring drug therapy
Reviewing drug usage
Educating professionals on pharmacology and therapeutics

[a] Reproduced with permission from McLeod DC: Philosophy of pharmacy practice. In McLeod DC, Miller WA (eds): *The Practice of Pharmacy.* Cincinnati, OH,
Harvey Whitney Books, 1981, pp 1–10.

that, although pharmacy should still be concerned with compounding and dispensing drugs, it should now be defined as a system rendering a service grounded in knowledge about drugs and their effects on humans and animals (9). Recent writings corroborate that pharmacy is a system of concepts dealing with the acquisition, translation, transmission, and utilization of drug knowledge (10). The concept of clinical pharmacy does not imply the abdication of drug distribution responsibilities, but rather expands the role of the pharmacist to ensure optimal safety in both the distribution and use of medications (11). Table 8.1 lists the complex series of events surrounding "drug use control," where the goal is to cure the patient and improve his or her quality of life.

The modern pharmacy curriculum contains information from the basic behavioral and social sciences and the preclinical biomedical sciences of physiology, pathophysiology, physical assessment, anatomy, and statistics. Pharmaceutical science courses include medicinal chemistry, pharmacology (generally 1 year), pharmacotherapeutics, pharmaceutics, pharmacokinetics, and pharmacy administration. Clinical science training provides the opportunity for students to apply this knowledge, under the supervision of preceptors, in structured clinical clerkships in inpatient and outpatient environments. Beginning in the mid-1960s, schools of pharmacy began to offer advanced clinical work leading to the Doctor of Pharmacy (Pharm.D.) degree (12). This degree may be obtained as a first professional degree (entry level) or as a post-baccalaureate program. The Pharm.D. curriculum generally provides more in-depth coverage of material and experiences than do baccalaureate degree programs. However, much debate exists on the optimal approach to educating pharmacists.

Pharm.D. graduates may pursue additional clinical and/or research training. Residencies or research fellowships, from 1 to 3 years in duration, are available in areas including pharmacokinetics, pediatrics, nutrition support, cardiology, drug information, critical care, and other specialty areas of internal medicine (2). Besides obtaining the State Board of Pharmacy-issued license to practice pharmacy, it is now possible for pharmacists to become board certified in pharmacotherapy, nutrition support, or nuclear pharmacy.

Clinical pharmacists are sometimes incorrectly called clinical pharmacologists, who are usually physicians with specialty training in drug action. Pharmacists apply their unique knowledge of basic, pharmaceutical, and clinical sciences to drug therapy optimization (13). As with any profession, the sophistication of these services varies with the education and experience of the pharmacist and the practice environment.

Many institutions currently employ highly trained pharmacists whose primary responsibility is to ensure rational drug therapy. At present, nearly 80% of hospitals have pharmacists actively monitoring drug therapy, more than 90% have programs in adverse drug reaction monitoring and drug use evaluation, 34% report drug management of medical emergencies by pharmacists, and 28% have nutritional support consultations involving pharmacists (6). Clinical pharmacokinetics has been a major area of contribution, since pharmacists receive extensive training in this area. Currently, 42% of hospitals have formal pharmacokinetic consultation programs, with more than 82% of pharmacists' recommendations being adopted by the medical staff (6). Pharmacists also collaborate with physicians in drug-related research and publish their findings in pharmacy and medical journals. A review of 65 medical journals from 1977 to 1986 revealed 854 articles written by individuals with a Pharm.D. degree (14). A review of *Critical Care Medicine* from 1989 to 1992 revealed 50 articles (excluding letters to the editor) with pharmacist authors; in 24 of those articles, a pharmacist was the primary author. The training, experience, and performance of modern pharmacists have prompted Dr. George Lundberg, editor of *JAMA*, to conclude that clinical pharmacy has emerged from a need for an interface between drugs and people, and that the most qualified individual at this interface is the pharmacist (15).

PHARMACEUTICAL CARE

To consolidate the many facets of pharmacy practice and to align the profession with current trends in health care, a new paradigm called *pharmaceutical care* has been developed (4, 16). This philosophy highlights pharmacy's responsibility to provide optimal drug therapy with the intent of improving the patient's quality of life. It is centered on the individual *patient* as the ultimate receiver of care. The pharmaceutical care concept is consistent with the evolving health care standard that requires providers of services to assess and document the risk versus the benefit of their services to both patients and populations (17). Relman (18) points out that the era of assessment and accountability is upon us. It is possible that reimbursement for pharmaceutical services may be determined by the relative impact of these services on patient outcome (19).

Pharmaceutical care places an increased responsibility for drug therapy success and failure on the pharmacist (16). It is essentially a component of care that can be best accomplished by a competent pharmacist through application of pharmaceutical knowledge (16). In this scheme, the pharmacist must be an active participant in health care delivery and not just a conduit through which information on drugs flows.

IMPACT OF PHARMACEUTICAL CARE

Adverse drug reactions, drug interactions, and drug errors (sometimes called drug misadventures) continue to occur. A recent study of a tertiary care teaching hospital revealed 3.13 prescribing errors per 1000 orders written (20). Three to eight percent of patients are admitted to hospitals because of an adverse drug reaction, and 3 to 43% of hospitalized patients experience an adverse drug reaction (21). In a 1991 study of adverse events in 30,195 hospitalized patients, drug complications were the most common single type of adverse event, accounting for 19% of all events (22). The annual cost of drug-related morbidity in the United States is estimated at $7 billion (4).

Pharmacists have instituted programs and services to improve patient care. From 1974 to 1984, 305 studies (classified in Table 8.2) were published documenting pharmacists' activities in institutional settings (23). These and other investigations (24) reported a widespread acceptance of clinical pharmacy services by physicians that resulted in more appropriate use of drugs and serum drug concentrations, cost-effective drug therapy, and improved quality of care. One study, for example, examined the effects of 1027 interactions with physicians by clinical pharmacists on drug therapy problems at a 530-bed tertiary care teaching hospital (25). Physicians fully accepted 90% of the recommendations of pharmacists, while 6% were partially followed. A multidisciplinary peer review committee judged that 96% of recommendations were appropriate, and that these recommendations also resulted in an annual cost saving of nearly $900,000.

CRITICAL CARE PHARMACEUTICAL SERVICES

EVOLUTION OF CRITICAL CARE PHARMACY

The involvement of pharmacists in critical care has been relatively slow to develop (26). A 1984 survey of critical care personnel and services in the United States, for example, did not reveal participation by pharmacists (27).

Historical reasons for this slow growth include a lack of formalized training programs in critical care pharmacy, exclusion of ICUs from early unit-dose and intravenous admixture programs, and the significant allocation of time needed to practice in critical care units (26, 28).

One of the earliest reports of pharmacy involvement in critical care appeared in 1972, as a letter to the editor in the *New England Journal of Medicine*, in which a pharmacist was

Table 8.2.   Documented Clinical Pharmacy Services[a]

Monitoring drug therapy
   Provision of written consultations
   Participation in drug utilization review
   Conducting patient care audits
   General monitoring of drug therapy
   Preparation of patient medication histories
Drug information and education
Participation in management of medical emergency and chronic
   diseases
Detection and reporting of adverse drug reactions
Control of medication administration
Computer applications
Financial and personnel management
General clinical pharmacy
Clinical drug investigations

[a] Reproduced with permission from Hatoum HT, Catizone C, Hutchinson RA, Purohit A: An
eleven-year review of the pharmacy literature: documentation of the value and acceptance of clinical pharmacy. *Drug Intell Clin Pharm* 20:33–48, 1986.

mentioned as a member of the cardiac arrest team (29). Notable pharmacy practitioners with established practices in the 1970s were David Angaran, M.S., at the University of Wisconsin Trauma and Life Support Center (28), Thomas Majerus, Pharm.D., at the Maryland Shock Trauma Center (30), and Robert Elenbaas, Pharm.D., at the University of Missouri-Kansas City Emergency Department (31). Pharmacy services have expanded to various ICUs (adult and pediatric), the operating room, and the emergency department, where pharmacists have established drug therapy monitoring programs and efficient drug delivery systems (1, 32–40).

FORMALIZED TRAINING AND ORGANIZATIONAL EFFORTS OF CRITICAL CARE PHARMACISTS

Considerable attention has been given recently to education and organizational participation of critical care pharmacists (41). Approximately a dozen postdoctoral critical care pharmacy residencies or fellowships, of 1 or 2 years, currently exist. Standards for a critical care pharmacy residency have recently been published (42).

Several professional organizations now have formal programs for critical care pharmacists. Pharmacists practicing in operating room (OR) satellite pharmacies, for example, have recently formed an OR Satellite Pharmacy Association (43). The American Society of Hospital Pharmacists (ASHP) has implemented a Specialty Practice Group in Critical Care Pharmacy practice, and the American College of Clinical Pharmacy (ACCP) has formed a Practice Research Network in critical care. Each has approximately 60-90 members. In 1989, a Clinical Pharmacology and Pharmacy Section was formed in the Society of Critical Care Medicine (SCCM) (44). In 1993, there are over 200 members (mostly pharmacists), and six pharmacists are Fellows of the Society. The goals of the Section are to promote activities of section members and to encourage and support research, practice, and teaching in multidisciplinary clinical pharmacology and pharmacy.

NATIONAL SURVEY OF CRITICAL CARE PHARMACEUTICAL SERVICES

A recent national survey of 613 hospitals with more than 100 beds identified 764 ICU pharmacists, with an additional 301 full-time equivalent (FTE) ICU pharmacists and 34 more ICU satellite pharmacies anticipated in the next 2 years (45, 46). One hundred twenty-four hospitals had ICU satellite pharmacies that usually provided services for 8 to 16 hours per day and were staffed, on average, by three FTE pharmacists and two FTE pharmacy technicians. Unit-dose services were available to more than 85% of ICU patients; however, only 48 to 63% of hospitals reported complete intravenous admixture services to ICU patients, depending on the presence of an ICU satellite pharmacy. Also, nurses were reported to prepare most of the intravenous products in 13% of hospitals with an ICU satellite and in 20% of those without an ICU satellite pharmacy.

Table 8.3 revealed that pharmacists actively monitor many drugs prescribed for ICU patients. As expected, most monitoring involves antimicrobials, total parenteral nutrient solutions, vasoactive agents or inotropes, and antiarrhythmics. ICU

Table 8.3. Level of Pharmacist Involvement with Critically Ill Patients[a]

Type of Activity	Mean Level of Involvement[b]
Drug selection or monitoring	
Antimicrobial agents	4.0
Total parenteral nutrient solutions	3.8
Vasoactive agents or inotropes	3.5
Antiarrhythmics	3.3
Stress ulcer prophylaxis drugs	3.3
Antihypertensives	3.1
Colloids	2.9
Analgesics	2.7
Diuretics	2.5
Review of drug orders for ICU patients	
Concurrent review (e.g., during rounds)	3.2
Retrospective review in ICU	3.9
Retrospective review in pharmacy	2.3
Pharmacokinetic consultation	3.6
Hemodynamic monitoring	2.7
Participation in cardiopulmonary resuscitation attempts	2.7
Calculation of infusion rates	3.7
Cost containment programs	3.6
Participation in research	2.5
Nursing inservice education programs	3.5
Physician inservice education programs	2.8
Preceptorship for baccalaureate students	3.1
Preceptorship for Pharm.D. or M.S. students	2.2

[a] Reproduction with permission from Dasta JF, Segal R, Cunningham A: National survey of critical care pharmaceutical services. *Am J Hosp Pharm* 46:2308–2312, 1989.

[b] Key to scale: 1 = not involved, 2 = minimally involved, 3 = moderately involved, 4 = involved, and 5 = very involved. From ICU pharmacists not affiliated with a satellite pharmacy.

Table 8.4. Percentage of Patients Receiving Drugs in Intensive Care Units

Drug Class	SICU[a] (48)	TICU[b] (49)	BT/SICU[c] (50)
Antibiotics	92.6	70.5	86.7
Analgesics	90.3	88.4	70.5
Antacids	55.1	60.1[d]	42.6
Antiarrhythmics	54.5	11.5[e]	41.9
Antianginal	50.0	NL[f]	53.6[g]
H$_2$ blocker	49.4	NL	44.1
Diuretic	39.2	NL	27.9
Psychotropic/sedative	33.5	48.9[h]	47.0
Antihypertensive	30.1	16.9[i]	20.5
Antifungal	33[j]	NL	9.5
Colloids	24.4	NL	NL
Bronchodilators	23.9	41[k]	19.8
Vitamins	21.6	NL	NL
Catecholamines	20.5	11.5[e]	19.8[l]
Insulin	19.3	NL	12.5
Corticosteroids	18.7	NL	8.1
Acetaminophen	15.9	40.6	36
Antiplatelet	12.5	NL	NL
Anticoagulant	10.8	11.5[m]	9.5
Laxative	9.1	17.6	NL
Aspirin	9.1	NL	NL
Anticonvulsant	6.2	6.8	9.5
Neuromuscular blocker	2.8	48.9[h]	NL
Antiemetics	NL	49.6	NL

[a] Surgical Intensive Care Unit.
[b] Trauma Intensive Care Unit.
[c] Burn-trauma Intensive Care Unit.
[d] H$_2$ blockers, antacids, and sucralfate.
[e] Inotropes, pressors, and antiarrhythmics.
[f] Not listed.
[g] Nitrates and calcium channel antagonists.
[h] Sedatives and muscle relaxants.
[i] Antihypertensives and vasodilators.
[j] Topical and systemic.
[k] Bronchodilators and mucolytics.
[l] Vasoactive and inotropes.
[m] Heparin.

pharmacists were involved with concurrent review of drug orders, pharmacokinetic consultations, cardiopulmonary resuscitation attempts, calculation of infusion rates, cost containment programs, provision of nursing inservices, and preceptorship of pharmacy students. These data suggest that pharmacy services to critically ill patients are diverse and that an increasing number of pharmacists are caring for critically ill patients.

PATTERNS OF DRUG USE IN THE ICU

Several studies have begun to characterize drug use patterns in modern ICUs (47–51). Table 8.4 compares the percentages of patients receiving different drug therapies in various types of ICUs. Drugs used in at least 50% of patients include antibiotics, analgesics, drugs for stress ulcer prophylaxis, antiarrhythmics, and antianginal drugs. The mean number of drugs prescribed per day varied from 5.6 to 8.6 (range 1 to 18), and the mean total number of drugs ordered was between 7.6 and 12.1 (range 1 to 44). Drug therapy is not only complex in these patients but also expensive, accounting for nearly 14% of total hospital charges (48). ICU patients are often diagnostic-related group (DRG) outliers, with revenue losses, under a prospective payment system, averaging nearly $18,000 per patient. In surgical ICU patients receiving catecholamines, triple antibiotics, or total parenteral nutrient solutions, revenue losses averaged more than $40,000 during their ICU stay, with pharmacy charges from the ICU averaging 27 to 47% of their total pharmacy bill (48). Reimbursement of ICU patients' bills by nonprivate carriers, at one hospital, ranged from only 30 to 55% (51).

ADVERSE EFFECTS OF DRUGS

Critically ill patients are susceptible to drug interactions and adverse drug reactions, since they are often elderly, have multiple drugs prescribed, and are hemodynamically unstable with multiple organ system dysfunction (52, 53). One study reported that 47% of visits to an emergency department resulted in the addition of medications to a patient's concurrent drug regimen, with a potential adverse interaction introduced by this therapy in about 10% of visits (54). Another study revealed that medications were responsible for 54% of the iatrogenic cardiac arrests, with most events considered preventable (55). Furthermore, 37% of patients remaining in ICUs longer than 72 hours experience iatrogenic complications; 38% of these are related to problems of drug administration (55a). In addition, about 6-20% of ICU admissions result from drug reactions, and many of these drug-induced problems may be preventable (56, 56a). In one pediatric ICU, 32% of the iatrogenic causes of admission resulted from drug-induced events (57). Finally, a computer-based system of adverse drug reaction reporting detected 648 patients hospital-wide who experienced 701 adverse drug events in an 18-month period (58). About one-third of patients experienced their first adverse drug event while in an ICU. Drugs therefore result in and complicate the ICU admission.

THE PHARMACIST'S ROLE IN ASSESSING PHARMACOKINETICS OF CRITICALLY ILL PATIENTS

ICU patients have altered drug disposition and require frequent monitoring and dosage adjustments to achieve and maintain therapeutic drug concentrations (59–62). Altered organ blood flow, dysfunction of drug eliminating organs, and changes in fluid compartment volumes may account for variability in volume of distribution, elimination half-life, and clearance. Standard doses of drugs used in stable ward patients therefore cannot be applied universally to the critically ill patient.

Information on pharmacokinetics in critically ill patients has become available only relatively recently. More than 30 articles have been published between 1989 and 1991 on pharmacokinetic considerations in critically ill patients, focusing on drugs such as the aminoglycosides, vancomycin, penicillins, phenytoin, theophylline, and dopamine. Clinical pharmacists specializing in critical care can have an impact on patient care by optimizing drug therapy through knowledge and application of pharmacokinetics and disease state influences in critically ill patients.

Critical care pharmacists can assist physicians, for example, by calculating aminoglycoside dosages to achieve optimal serum concentrations during the first 24 hours of therapy. Standard loading doses of aminoglycosides are often too low to achieve therapeutic serum concentrations, as a result of an increased volume of distribution of these drugs (63). Kreger et al have demonstrated that 50% of deaths secondary to Gram-negative bacteremia occur in the initial 24 to 48 hours (64). Achieving early, therapeutic aminoglycoside concentrations in patients with Gram-negative infections has been shown to influence outcomes positively (65, 66). Although the volume of distribution is increased during the septic process, pharmacokinetic parameters change as the patient improves, and therefore frequent modification of the dosing regimen is often necessary (60).

Pharmacists can also coordinate timing of serum drug concentration samples and interpretation of results. Although it may seem simple to document the time of blood drawing in relation to the dose for serum concentration determination, errors in sampling can produce erroneous values and hence incorrect interpretations for subsequent dosage adjustments.

A 1-month audit of 167 serum drug concentrations ordered for surgical ICU patients revealed 42% inappropriate samples, 83% inappropriate requests, and 17% of samples drawn at incorrect times (67). Forty-seven percent of serum drug concentrations were outside the therapeutic ranges for the drugs involved.

Several studies have evaluated the effects of individualized pharmacokinetic dosing of the aminoglycosides on outcome. Unfortunately, the ideal study has not been conducted, and studies often possess methodologic inadequacies (66). Studies comparing outcomes of pharmacist versus physician drug dosing reveal that pharmacist-managed dosing of aminoglycosides results in more serum concentrations within the therapeutic range. These studies further demonstrated reduced mortality, fewer hospital days, shorter febrile periods, and associated reductions in hospital costs with pharmacokinetic dosing (68–71). A recent prospective, randomized clinical trial examined the outcomes of physician-managed versus pharmacist-managed aminoglycoside dosing in patients with ultimately fatal underlying diseases (72). Patients with pharmacist-managed drug therapy received more aggressive drug dosing and experienced a significantly lower mortality rate. Although this paper has been criticized because of small sample size (73), a more global evaluation of the literature reveals a consistent pattern of documented effectiveness of pharmacokinetic dosing of aminoglycosides. Using solely empirical dosing techniques in seriously ill patients with changing hemodynamics is inconsistent with the current understanding of modern pharmacotherapeutics.

Thus, the ICU patient represents a significant challenge to the clinician in selecting, dosing, and monitoring drugs to optimize drug therapy and control unnecessary drug costs. Together with physicians, pharmacists need to document further the impact of therapeutic drug monitoring programs on outcome and costs.

PEDIATRIC CRITICAL CARE PHARMACY

Pediatric considerations in drug therapy and specialized pharmaceutical services are important roles for critical care pharmacists specializing in pediatrics or neonatology (1, 74, 75). Pediatrics is considered a therapeutic orphan, since there are often few data on drug therapy in this population when new drugs are released. Few companies seek Food and Drug Administration (FDA) indications for pediatrics and often leave it to practitioners to document indications, dosage, and side effects in the pediatric population. Some new drugs such as flumazenil and HA-1A may be particularly useful in pediatric pharmacotherapy; however, studies in this patient population are needed. There is an analogy to the paucity of data in pediatric patients with adult critically ill patients, since most adult drug studies are not conducted in critically ill patients.

Specific areas in which pharmacists can provide guidance include pharmacokinetic dosing and optimization of drug therapy in pediatric ICU patients. The Department of Pharmacy at Children's Hospital Los Angeles, for example, publishes a manual (*Housestaff Manual*) that provides drug dosages, indications, pharmacokinetics, and nursing considerations for drugs used in pediatrics. The need to document pharmacists' drug therapy interventions in pediatric intensive care parallels that in adult intensive care. By attending physician rounds, the pharmacist can intervene before the order is written and provide information on controversies in the literature or cost-related issues. An average of 33 therapeutic interventions per month were documented at Children's Hospital Los Angeles by one critical care pharmacist during an 11-month period from March 1991 through February 1992. In contrast, approximately 25 interventions per month were performed by pharmacists monitoring noncritical care patients at that same institution, perhaps reflecting the more drug-intensive nature of the critically ill pediatric patient (Taketomo C, unpublished data).

Other areas in which pharmacists are routinely sought for advice include the management of fluid therapy and intravenous compatibility. Although references exist (76, 77), new drugs have not been well-studied and little information exists to make an educated judgment for the pediatric patient. Because fluid is often limited in the critically ill child, common questions asked of the pharmacist often pertain to intravenous compatibility, maximum drug concentrations, and infusion rates. In addition, the pharmacist should understand the use of retrograde infusion techniques and how this method can affect aminoglycoside or vancomycin serum concentrations (78). Residents are often not educated about the significance of retrograde infusion technique and how different administration procedures affect serum drug concentrations.

Evidence of the impact that the critical care pharmacist can make in regard to physician education and patient care is seen, for example, with theophylline. The drug has a narrow therapeutic range, and close monitoring is essential. In the year before a pharmacist-directed educational effort was begun, approximately 4.6% of theophylline concentrations were above the therapeutic range at Children's Hospital Los Angeles. This value fell to 2.2% following the educational program (Taketomo C, unpublished data).

Potential areas of research by pharmacists include quantification of the pharmacologic response to drugs in children, intravenous compatibility of new drugs in parenteral nutrient solutions, and determination of maximum allowable drug concentrations for specific pediatric indications.

ASSESSING CRITICAL CARE PHARMACY SERVICES

Factors such as polypharmacy and altered drug disposition in ICU patients illustrate the need for a pharmacotherapy specialist to evaluate and monitor drug therapy. Quantifying the impact of critical care pharmacists is difficult, since studies often use historical controls and make assumptions about drug therapy outcomes in the absence of pharmacist interventions. Although the pharmaceutical care concept dictates performing pharmacy services for optimal outcome or improved quality of life, quantifying the effect of these interventions is hampered by the myriad of factors that influence mortality and quality of life. The presence of a physician with formal training in critical care medicine, however, has been shown to decrease mortality in septic shock patients (79). More indirect methods, such as cost avoidance, are often used to assess critical care pharmaceutical services.

Close monitoring of drug therapy is particularly important during critical care nursing shortages that lead to inadequate staffing and overworked nurses (80). Medication administration studies in ICUs reveal error rates as high as 38% (81, 82). A 1-year study of critical incidents in one ICU showed that drug administration-related errors accounted for 17% of the 110 critical incidents involving human error (83).

Although several hundred publications have evaluated the impact of clinical pharmacy services in hospitalized patients (23, 24), only a few studies have been conducted in critically ill patients. Physician acceptance of clinical pharmacist recommendations and cost savings from changing to optimal drug therapy are often used as endpoints. For example, albumin, a high-cost drug used for critically ill patients, was used suboptimally 74% of the time (84). A pharmacist intervention program increased the percentage of albumin prescribed appropriately and resulted in annualized cost savings of more than $83,000 (85). As members of the cardiopulmonary resuscitation team, pharmacists have been evaluated by physicians and nurses and defined as important contributors and necessary members of this team (86). Physician acceptance of pharmacists providing on-call clinical pharmacy services was evaluated in an emergency department setting (87). Of more than 2000 drug-related recommendations by pharmacists over a 2-year period, 91% were accepted unchanged by physicians. Pharmacists also prevented medication prescribing errors at two children's hospitals, at a rate of about five errors per 1000 medication orders (88). The greatest number of errors occurred in children under 2 years of age and in pediatric ICU patients. Pharmacists have also developed effective drug education programs for critical care nurses (89).

Six (90–95) pharmacist-intervention studies have been conducted in ICU patients. These studies document the delivery of pharmaceutical care and evaluate the potential impact of this care on the cost of drug therapy.

Examples of pharmacist interventions include discontinuation of unnecessary drug therapy, changes in drug therapy to more cost-effective regimens, prevention of unnecessary laboratory tests, and detection and minimization of problems relating to drug therapy. Cost savings in these studies are substantial, with annualized values ranging from $18,000 to more than $500,000 (85–89). A wide variety of drugs have been the focus of these intervention studies, including albumin, various antibiotics, and sedatives. Although health care providers are operating in a cost-constrained environment, the drug regimen that costs the least is not necessarily the best when evaluating outcome and cost of hospitalization. Canafax et al calculated that the cost of one drug regimen for a renal transplant patient was $3987 higher than that for a standard regimen (96). However, the new regimen resulted in an average of $9543 per patient less in total hospitalization charges, as a result of the shorter initial hospitalization, decreased rate of rehospitalization, lower frequency of acute rejection, and lower infection rates. The effect of pharmacist management of fluid therapy in fluid-restricted ICU patients receiving parenteral nutrition was compared with that in a group of patients not managed by the pharmacist (95). The fluid intake of patients receiving pharmacist monitoring was significantly less than that of control patients with similar fluid output values in both groups. The result was better fluid balance secondary to pharmacist involvement.

RECOMMENDATIONS FOR DELIVERING PHARMACEUTICAL CARE

Twenty-four hour pharmacy services are listed as an essential service in the SCCM Guidelines for services and personnel (3). However, the scope of those services was not delineated. In order to provide direction for the profession and care of the critically ill patient, a detailed description of services consistent with current trends in health care and pharmaceutical care is proposed. Essential services are those most hospitals should be able to provide. Pharmacies should strive to deliver services listed in the "optimum" category to maximize the role of the pharmacist. All services are suggested in the context of multidisciplinary critical care.

Essential Pharmaceutical Services

Essential pharmaceutical care services encompass efficient and prompt dispensing of the drug product as well as pharmacist evaluation and optimization of drug therapy. Rapid availability of drug products is a vital component of pharmacy services, especially with the tenuous status of many ICU patients. This goal may be best accomplished with a satellite pharmacy located in close proximity to the critical care unit (39). Critical care satellites can be more flexible to meet the needs of priority patients and can provide greater continuity of care than can centralized dispensing areas (97). An efficient pharmacy system will minimize turn-around time, maximize capture of appropriate charges, and ensure prompt availability of needed products. Detailed descriptions of satellite pharmacy services to medical (37, 98), surgical (67, 90, 99–102), and medical/surgical (39, 91, 93, 103) critical care units have been published. However, the importance of the physical location of a pharmacy is minimized if an effective communication and delivery system exists. A pharmacist should be at the bedside evaluating patient needs, anticipating orders, making drug therapy recommendations, and communicating with the dispensing area (97). Whatever dispensing system is utilized, the medication handling requirements of the nursing staff should be minimized.

For most efficient administration by the nurses, all medications should be dispensed 24 hours a day in a ready-to-use unit-dose form. Use of a system with both pharmacy and nursing double-checking of the medication should minimize errors. Floor drug stock should be minimized to prevent errors related to dose or item selection. Drugs should be prepared under the supervision of a pharmacist. Intravenous products prepared aseptically in a laminar air-flow hood, for example, are less prone to contamination than those compounded at bedside (104). The use of various prepackaged products (Add-Vantage Intravenous Piggy Back (IVPBs), premixed IVs, frozen IVPBs, etc.) may simplify the dispensing process, decrease waste, and decrease nursing time. Standardizing IV concentrations may also decrease waste by allowing unused products to be relabeled for another patient (105). Standard preparation and drug dilution techniques will also produce a more consistent product (106–108). However, pharmacists should consider

Table 8.5. Category of References for a Critical Care Pharmacy Satellite[a]

IV compatibility
Drug interactions
Pharmacology
Critical care
Toxicology
Drug dosing in organ system failure
Emergency drug therapy
Pharmacokinetics
Neonatal/pediatric pharmacotherapy

[a] Selections from references 114–141.

individualized dilutions, when indicated, to minimize fluid overload that may result from multiple intravenous drug and nutritional therapies (95, 109, 110).

Pharmacists must be prepared to provide intravenous compatibility information. The need to administer multiple drugs through a limited number of access sites challenges the pharmacist to extrapolate the limited intravenous compatibility data. Multiple lumen catheters have simplified the problem somewhat, but y-site administration is still common. The type of multilumen catheter used, however, may influence the possibility of precipitate formation when two incompatible drugs are infused through separate lumens (111). Unfortunately, most of the compatibility studies have tested drug concentrations that are not used clinically, and they report results over long periods (112). These data do not relate to the questions that arise from short-term mixing in the line or at the y-site. Published compatibility charts may assist nurses but are difficult to keep current (113).

A critical care pharmacy should have the necessary equipment and personnel to allow rapid preparation of IV solutions, refrigeration, adequate supplies of unit-specific drugs, and appropriate space for work areas and references. The reference area should include one source from each category listed in Table 8.5 to facilitate responses to individual drug information questions (114–140).

Additional support from a drug information center or medical library with current critical care journals and other standard references, computerized literature search capabilities, and access to a poison information center are also desirable. Other useful services include drug information, assistance in screening/enrollment of patients, and participation in ongoing pharmacotherapeutic research through maintenance of investigational drug inventories.

Some medications will be needed too rapidly to permit distribution from the pharmacy. Emergency medications should be available in an emergency cart on the unit for rapid resuscitation of patients. A pharmacist should participate in these resuscitations, to evaluate the impact of the patient's medication history and concurrent therapy, and to assist with rapid preparation, administration, and documentation of life-saving therapies (86).

The pharmacist at the bedside should be a contributing member of the critical care team and be responsible for all aspects of drug therapy, including the evaluation of the need for expensive and potentially toxic therapeutic agents. The critical care pharmacist should work with the critical care team to develop therapeutic protocols and guidelines for use of critical care drug therapies and to evaluate the effect on patient outcome. The drug product, however, is only one part of the medication use system. Multidisciplinary problem-solving, using total quality management tools, should address issues more globally than does traditional drug use evaluation. Outcome of a critically ill patient depends on many factors in addition to drug therapy. The critical care team can assess the entire process required to ensure optimal pharmacotherapy and patient outcome (141, 142).

Pharmacist input into pharmacotherapy at the time orders are written is preferred in order to adequately evaluate and optimize therapy for the disease state and related co-morbidities. Other essential activities for the critical care pharmacist include pharmacokinetics and therapeutic drug monitoring (scheduling and interpreting serum concentration results), individualization of nutritional support, regular review of the medication profile, and adverse drug reaction identification, prevention, and reporting. The pharmacist should participate in programs to facilitate optimal drug therapy usage, such as teaching and inservice education for the nursing staff and other critical care personnel. Other essential services for pharmacists include obtaining drug therapy histories and preventing drug interactions (2, 37). Ideally, the critical care pharmacist should be able to spend more than 50% of the day in these patient-focused activities (46). However, projections for clinical services in a 20-bed surgical ICU estimate that 12.7 hours per day will be required (100). Productivity standards can be used to estimate and evaluate pharmacist and technician staffing requirements for the provision of pharmaceutical care services.

Critical care pharmacists must document their contributions to patient care. The record of pharmacist drug therapy interventions should be a part of the medical record, just as is standard for other personnel such as nurses and physical, occupational, or respiratory therapists (141, 143).

Optimal Pharmaceutical Services

Optimal critical care pharmaceutical services include all of the aforementioned services, plus continuous provision of pharmaceutical care services, 24 hours a day, 7 days a week from a pharmacy satellite in the critical care area staffed with specialized practitioners. The critical care pharmacy team should consist of pharmacy technicians and pharmacists, and a highly trained critical care pharmacy specialist. A pharmacist should participate in daily patient rounds and be involved whenever therapy decisions are made. The role of the specialist will depend on the needs of the area. In smaller facilities, the critical care specialist may be the primary pharmaceutical care provider. In larger critical care units, the specialist may serve more as a resource to the satellite pharmacists by problem-solving with the most complicated patients, while participating in daily pharmaceutical care services. In addition, the critical care specialist should be responsible for the continuing education of the critical care pharmacy team, through formal education, daily discussion of patient care goals, and effective role modeling.

Optimally, pharmaceutical care plans will be developed and used, much as nursing has used a problem-oriented approach to patient care. An example of a systematic guideline for the documentation of drug therapy evaluation is provided in Table 8.6 (144). The pharmaceutical care plan can be used

Table 8.6. Pharmacist Workup of Drug Therapy[a]

I. Identifying issues associated with the patient's drug therapy
  A. Patient description
    1. Age, sex, and race
      a. Increased risk of side effects because of age, sex, or race?
      b. Metabolism and elimination of certain drugs likely to be affected because of age, sex, or race?
    2. Height: Lean body weight calculations dependent on height
    3. Weight: How does patient's weight affect dosage calculations?
    4. Lean body weight: Kinetic parameters and dosage recommendations calculated by lean body weight.
  B. Medical problem list/diagnosis
  C. History of present illness and medical history
  D. Present medications
  E. Medication history
  F. Allergies
  G. Smoking/alcohol/recreational drug use history
  H. Compliance
  I. Systems review
    1. Vital signs: temperature, heart rate, blood pressure, respiration.
    2. Renal
      a. Is patient receiving a drug that can alter renal function?
      b. Is the patient's renal function affecting the elimination of certain drugs?
  J. Pertinent laboratory values
    1. What tests are needed to determine efficacy of present drug therapy?
    2. What tests are needed to determine whether present drug therapy is causing toxicity?
    3. What baseline laboratory values are needed in anticipation of therapeutic effectiveness and toxicity monitoring of drugs?
II. Patient-specific, drug-related problem list
  A. What problems are you (as a clinical pharmacist) going to solve for this patient?
  B. What problems are you (as a clinical pharmacist) going to assume responsibility for?
III. Desired therapeutic outcomes
IV. Therapeutic alternatives
V. Pharmacist's drug recommendation and individualization
VI. Therapeutic drug monitoring
  A. What information do I need to ensure that the recommended drug therapy is producing the desired effect?
  B. With what frequency and for what duration do I need to collect the relevant information?

[a] Reproduction with permission from Strand LM, Cipolle RJ, Morley PC: Documenting the clinical pharmacist's activities: back to basics. *Drug Intell Clin Pharm* 22:63–67, 1988.

to train new practitioners and facilitate standardization of services. This approach is not unique to pharmacy, but the care plans should reflect the emphasis on drug therapy selection, dosing, monitoring, and follow-up evaluation. In complicated cases, an organ system approach helps the pharmacist evaluate the large amount of patient data more effectively. The pharmacist should identify and evaluate possible drug-induced problems.

Evaluation of pharmaceutical care services for effects on patient outcome and assessment of the quality of these services are important. The specialist should participate as a member of hospital committees such as a critical care committee, infection control committee, pharmacy and therapeutics committee, and quality review committee. The specialist should also provide regular educational programs, participate in ongoing research activities, and contribute to the literature of critical care by collaborative research and projects. Pharmacists have been approved as primary investigators by the FDA (145). The specialist should also have expertise in research design and statistical analysis.

New technology will allow optimal use of the expertise of critical care pharmacists and minimize time spent in technical activities. Devices such as the Pyxis, Meditrol, and Sure-Med will dispense to nurses and automatically record use of floor-stock items and narcotics (146, 147). With the support of technicians and the evolution of cart-filling devices such as the ATC 212, Medispence, and other automated/robotic systems, the pharmacist will have more time to practice at the bedside as an information resource (146). High-technology infusion devices will allow more control over the rate of infusion of intermittent and continuous infusions. (148) Closed-loop infusion systems allow computerized titration of rate according to the programmed criteria. With more predictable drug delivery, especially with drugs dosed intermittently, the critical care pharmacist will have more opportunity to characterize the pharmacokinetic parameters of critical care patients.

Computerized patient data management systems will allow evaluation of current multidisciplinary patient data (hemodynamics, ventilation, medication administration, laboratory data, etc.) from a single terminal (149). The computer systems are designed to increase the productivity of critical care staff, lower the cost of ICU care, and enhance the quality of care by improving the flow and quality of information. Pharmacist input into the development and application of these systems is essential.

SUMMARY

The pharmacist's role in ICUs has evolved over the last 10 years. Pharmacists are currently an important component of many ICUs as they provide supervision for drug distribution and advice on pharmacotherapy issues. Further documentation of the impact of pharmaceutical services on mortality and quality of life is needed. The pharmacist, working in concert with physicians, nurses, and other health care personnel, can provide optimal pharmaceutical care in the pharmacologic management of critically ill patients.

REFERENCES

1. Majerus TC, Dasta JF (eds): Practice of critical care pharmacy. Rockville, MD, Aspen Systems, 1985.
2. Dasta JF, Angaran DM: Evolving role of the pharmacist in critical care. *Crit Care Med* 20:563–565, 1992.
3. Task Force on Guidelines: Recommendations for services and personnel for delivery of care in a critical care setting. *Crit Care Med* 16:809–811, 1988.
4. Hepler CD, Strand LM: Opportunities and responsibilities in pharmaceutical care. *Am J Hosp Pharm* 47:533–543, 1990.
5. Allan EL, Barker KN: Fundamentals of medication error research. *Am J Hosp Pharm* 47:555–571, 1990.
6. Crawford SY: ASHP national survey of hospital-based pharmaceutical services—1990. *Am J Hosp Pharm* 47:2665–2695, 1990.
7. Roberts AW, Visconti JA: The rational and irrational use of systemic antimicrobial drugs. *Am J Hosp Pharm* 29:828–834, 1972.
8. McLeod DC: Philosophy of pharmacy practice. In McLeod DC, Miller WA (eds): *The Practice of Pharmacy.* Cincinnati, OH, Harvey Whitney Books, pp 1–10, 1981.
9. Millis JS: *Pharmacists for the Future.* Ann Arbor, MI, Health Administration Press, p 161, 1975.
10. Brodie DC, McGhan WF, Lindon J. The theoretical base of pharmacy. *Am J Hosp Pharm* 48:536–540, 1991.
11. Brodie DC: Drug-use control—keystone to pharmaceutical services. *Drug Intell Clin Pharm* 1:63–65, 1967.
12. Biles JA: The doctor of pharmacy. *JAMA* 249:1157–1160, 1983.
13. Smith WE, Benderev K: Levels of pharmaceutical care: a theoretical model. *Am J Hosp Pharm* 48:540–546, 1991.
14. Visconti JA, Benson HB: PharmD authored publications in the medical literature: a review of two decades (1967–1986). *Am J Pharm Ed* 53:370–375, 1989.
15. Lundberg GD: The clinical pharmacist. *JAMA* 249:1193, 1983.
16. Strand LM, Cipolle RJ, Morley PC, Perrier DG: Levels of pharmaceutical care: a needs-based approach. *Am J Hosp Pharm* 48:547–550, 1991.
17. Angaran DM: Measuring and monitoring health care. *Top Hosp Pharm Manage* 10:1–11, 1990.
18. Relman AS: Assessment and accountability—the third revolution in medical care. *N Engl J Med* 319:1220–1222, 1988.
19. Hatoum HT, Vlasses PH: Patient outcome and the future practice of pharmacy. *DICP Ann Pharmacother* 25:208–210, 1991.
20. Lesar TS, Briceland LL, Delcoure K, Parmalee JC, Masta-Gornic V, Pohl H: Medication prescribing errors in a teaching hospital. *JAMA* 263:2329–2334, 1990.
21. Manasee HR: Medication use in an imperfect world: drug misadventuring as an issue of public policy, part 1. *Am J Hosp Pharm* 46:929–944, 1989.
22. Leape LL, Brennan TA, Laird N, et al: The nature of adverse events in hospitalized patients: results of the Harvard medical practice study II. *N Engl J Med* 324:377–384, 1991.
23. Hatoum HT, Catizone C, Hutchinson RA, Purohit A: An eleven-year review of the pharmacy literature: documentation of the value and acceptance of clinical pharmacy. *Drug Intell Clin Pharm* 20:33–48, 1986.
24. Willett MS, Bertch KE, Rich DS, Ereshefsky L: Prospectus on the economic value of clinical pharmacy services—a position statement of the American College of Clinical Pharmacy. *Pharmacotherapy* 9:45–56, 1989.
25. Hatoum HT, Hutchinson RA, Witte KW, Newby GP: Evaluation of the contribution of clinical pharmacists: inpatient care and cost reduction. *Drug Intell Clin Pharm* 22:252–259, 1988.
26. Dasta JF: Critical care therapeutics: a frontier for clinical pharmacy. *Drug Intell Clin Pharm* 16:398–399, 1982.
27. Greenbaum DM: Availability of critical care personnel, facilities, and services in the United States. *Crit Care Med* 12:1073–1077, 1984.
28. Angaran DM: Critical care clinical pharmacy services. In McLeod DC, Miller WA (eds): *The Practice of Pharmacy.* Cincinnati, OH, Harvey Whitney Books, pp 171–181, 1981.
29. Elenbaas RM: Pharmacist on resuscitation team [Letter]. *N Engl J Med* 287:151, 1972.
30. Majerus TC: Shock-trauma: clinical pharmacy in emergency medicine. *Top Hosp Pharm Manage* 2:87–93, 1982.
31. Elenbaas RM, Waeckerle JF, McNabney WK: The clinical pharmacist in emergency medicine. *Am J Hosp Pharm* 34:843–846, 1977.
32. Crisp CB: The pharmacist's role on the critical care team. *Calif J Hosp Pharm* 2:33–34, 1990.
33. Schwerman E, Schwartau N, Thompson CO, Didier EP: The pharmacist as a member of the cardiopulmonary resuscitation team. *Drug Intell Clin Pharm* 7:298–308, 1973.
34. Kasuya A, Bauman JL, Curtis RA, Duarte B, Hutchinson RA: Clinical pharmacy on-call program in the emergency department. *Am J Emerg Med* 4:464–467, 1986.
35. Hall K, Guay M: The implementation of comprehensive critical care pharmacy services through the development of a 24-hour satellite pharmacy. *Can J Hosp Pharm* 35:184–188, 1982.
36. Keicher PA, Mcallister JC: Comprehensive pharmaceutical services in the surgical suite and recovery room. *Am J Hosp Pharm* 42:2454–2462, 1985.
37. Ellinoy BR, Clarke JE, Wagers PW, Swinney RS: Comprehensive pharmaceutical services in a medical intensive care unit. *Am J Hosp Pharm* 41:2335–2342, 1984.
38. Chin Y, Vogel DP: A team approach to patient care in the medical intensive care units at Robert Wood Johnson University Hospital. *Top Hosp Pharm Manage* 10:83–89, 1991.
39. Armitstead JA, Lobas NH, Ivey MF: Planning and operation of a critical care pharmacy satellite. *Crit Care Nurs Q* 14:39–50, 1991.
40. Moleski RJ, Easley S, Barash PG, Shier NQ, Schrier RI: Control and accountability of controlled substance administration in the operating room. *Anesth Analg* 64:989–995, 1985.
41. Dasta JF: Progress in critical care pharmacy. *Drug Intell Clin Pharm* 18:156–157, 1984.
42. Anonymous: ASHP supplemental standard and learning objectives for residency training in critical care pharmacy practice. *Am J Hosp Pharm* 47:609–612, 1990.
43. Rodriguiz AM, Overeem AC: Operating room satellite pharmacies: demographics services and implementation. *Hosp Pharm* 26:1026–1034, 1991.
44. Dasta JF, Jacobi JJ: Pharmacist involvement in the Society of Critical Care Medicine. *DICP Ann Pharmacother* 25:1398–1399, 1991.
45. Dasta JF: Assessment of critical care pharmacy practice. *Calif J Hosp Pharm* 2:30–32, 1990.
46. Dasta JF, Segal R, Cunningham A: National survey of critical care pharmaceutical services. *Am J Hosp Pharm* 46:2308–2312, 1989.

47. Dasta JF: Drug use in a surgical intensive care unit. *Drug Intell Clin Pharm* 20:752–756, 1986.
48. Dasta JF, Armstrong DK: Pharmacoeconomic impact of critically ill surgical patients. *Drug Intell Clin Pharm* 22:994–998, 1988.
49. Boucher BA, Kuhl DA, Coffey BC, Fabian TC: Drug use in a trauma intensive care unit. *Am J Hosp Pharm* 47:805–810, 1990.
50. Gundlach CA, Faulkner TP, Souney PF: Drug usage patterns in the ICU: profile of a major metropolitan hospital and comparison with other ICUs. *Hosp Formul* 26:132–136, 1991.
51. Gundlach CA, Faulkner TP: Charge and reimbursement analysis for intensive care unit patients in a large tertiary teaching hospital. *DICP Ann Pharmacother* 25:1231–1235, 1991.
52. Brodie MJ, Feely J: Adverse drug interactions. *BMJ* 296:845–849, 1988.
53. Dasta JF: Drug interactions in the ICU. In Cerra F (ed): *Perspectives in Critical Care.* St. Louis, MO, Quality Medical Publishing, pp 61–85, 1989.
54. Beers MH, Storrie M, Lee G: Potential adverse drug interactions in the emergency room. *Ann Intern Med* 112:61–64, 1990.
55. Bedell SE, Dietz DC, Leeman D, Delbanco TL: Incidence and characteristics of preventable iatrogenic cardiac arrests. *JAMA* 265:2815–2820, 1991.
55a. Ferraros VA, Propp ME: Outcome in critical care patients: a multivariate study. *Crit Care Med* 20:967–976, 1992.
56. Trunet P, Borda IT, Rouget AV, Rapin M, Lhoste F: The role of drug-induced illness in admissions to an intensive care unit. *Intens Care Med* 12:43–46, 1986.
56a. Tietze KJ, Wittbrodt ET, Lanken PN: The frequency of drug-related MICU/IMCU admissions. *Clin Pharmacol Ther* 53:214, 1993 (Abstract).
57. Stambouly JJ, Pollack MM: Iatrogenic illness in pediatric critical care. *Crit Care Med* 18:1248–1251, 1990.
58. Classen DC, Pestotnik SL, Evans RS, Burke JP: Computerized surveillance of adverse drug events in hospital patients. *JAMA* 266:2847–2851, 1991.
59. Boucher BA, Kuhl DA, Fabian TC, Robertson JT: Effect of neurotrauma on hepatic drug clearance. *Clin Pharmacol Ther* 50:487–497, 1991.
60. Dasta JF, Armstrong DK: Variability in aminoglycoside pharmacokinetics in critically ill surgical patients. *Crit Care Med* 16:327–330, 1988.
61. Bodenham A, Shelly MP, Park GR: The altered pharmacokinetics and pharmacodynamics of drugs commonly used in critically ill patients. *Clin Pharmacokinet* 14:347–373, 1988.
62. van Dalen R, Vree TB: Pharmacokinetics of antibiotics in critically ill patients. *Intens Care Med* 16(suppl 3):S235–S238, 1990.
63. Watling SM, Dasta JF: Aminoglycoside dosing considerations in intensive care unit patients. *Ann Pharmacother* 27:351–357, 1993.
64. Kreger BE, Craven DE, McCabe WR: Gram-negative bacteremia: IV reevaluation of clinical features in 612 patients. *Am J Med* 68:344–355, 1980.
65. Moore RD, Smith CR, Lietman PS: The association of aminoglycoside plasma levels with mortality in patients with gram-negative bacteremia. *J Infect Dis* 149:443–448, 1984.
66. Rodvold KA, Zokufa H, Rotschafer JC: Aminoglycoside pharmacokinetic monitoring: an integral part of patient care. *Clin Pharm* 7:608–613, 1988.
67. Crisp CB, Lane JR, Murray W: Audit of serum drug concentration analysis for patients in the surgical intensive care unit. *Crit Care Med* 18:734–737, 1990.
68. Bootman JL, Wertheimer AI, Zaske D, Rowland C: Individualizing gentamicin dosage regimens in burn patients with gram-negative septicemia: a cost-benefit analysis. *J Pharm Sci* 68:267–272, 1976.
69. Dillon KR, Dougherty SH, Casner P, Polly S: Individualized pharmacokinetic versus standard dosing of amikacin: a comparison of therapeutic outcomes. *J Antimicrob Chemother* 24:581–589, 1989.
70. Destache CJ, Meyer SK, Bittner MJ, Hermann KG: Impact of a clinical pharmacokinetic service on patients treated with aminoglycosides: a cost-benefit analysis. *Ther Drug Monit* 12:419–426, 1990.
71. Burton ME, Ash CL, Hill DP, Handy T, Shepherd MD, Vasco MR: A controlled trial of the cost benefit of computerized bayesian aminoglycoside administration. *Clin Pharmacol Ther* 49:685–694, 1991.
72. Whipple JK, Ausman RK, Franson R, Quebbeman EJ: Effect of individualized pharmacokinetic dosing on patient outcome. *Crit Care Med* 19:1480–1485, 1991.
73. DeMonaco HJ: Pharmacokinetics—the emperor's new clothes. *Crit Care Med* 19:1462–1463, 1991.
74. Lobas NH, Armitstead JA, Ivey MF: Expanding staff pharmacists' responsibilities to maintain pharmacy services in a neonatal intensive care unit. *Am J Hosp Pharm* 48:1708–1711, 1991.
75. Zenk KE: The pharmacist—a member of the neonatal interdisciplinary team. *J Calif Perinatal Assoc* 1:54–59, 1983.
76. Trissel LA: Handbook on injectable drugs. Bethesda, MD, American Society of Hospital Pharmacists, 1992.
77. Ford DC, Leist ER, Phelps SJ: Guidelines for administration of intravenous medications to pediatric patients. Bethesda, MD, American Society of Hospital Pharmacists, 1988.
78. Nahata MC: Influence of infusion methods on therapeutic drug monitoring in pediatric patients. *Drug Intell Clin Pharm* 20:367–369, 1986.
79. Reynolds HN, Haupt MT, Thil-Baharozian MC, Carlson RW: Impact of critical care physician staffing on patients with septic shock in a university hospital medical intensive care unit. *JAMA* 260:3446–3450, 1988.
80. Searle LD: The extent of the nursing shortage in critical care. *Heart Lung* 17:25A–29A, 1988.
81. Tisdale JE: Justifying a pediatric critical care pharmacy by medication error reporting. *Am J Hosp Pharm* 43:368–371, 1986.
82. Girotti MJ, Garrick C, Tierney MG, Chesnick K, Brown SJL: Medication administration errors in an adult intensive care unit. *Heart Lung* 16:449–453, 1987.
83. Wright D, Mackenzie SJ, Buchan I, Cairns CS, Price LE: Critical incidents in the intensive therapy unit. *Lancet* 338:676–678, 1991.
84. Alexander MR, Stumpf JL, Nostrant TT, Khanderia U, Eckhauser FE, Colvin CL: Albumin utilization in a university hospital. *DICP Ann Pharmacother* 23:214–217, 1989.
85. Stumpf JL, Lechner JL, Ryan ML: Use of albumin in a university hospital: the value of targeted physician intervention. *DICP Ann Pharmacother* 25:239–243, 1991.
86. Ludwig DJ, Abramowitz PW: The pharmacist as a member of the CPR team: evaluation by other health professionals. *Drug Intell Clin Pharm* 17:463–465, 1983.
87. Kasuya A, Bauman JL, Curtis RA, Duarte B, Hutchinson RA: Clinical pharmacy on-call program in the emergency department. *Am J Emerg Med* 4:464–467, 1986.
88. Folli HL, Poole RL, Benitz WE, Russo JC: Medication error prevention by clinical pharmacists in two children's hospitals. *Pediatrics* 79:718–722, 1987.
89. Hassan E: Pharmacy-based drug education program for critical care nurses. *Am J Hosp Pharm* 44:1629–1631, 1987.
90. Miyagawa CI, Rivera JO: Effect of pharmacist interventions on drug therapy costs in a surgical intensive care unit. *Am J Hosp Pharm* 43:3008–3013, 1986.
91. Bearce WC, Wiley GA, Fox RL, Coleman LT: Documentation of clinical interactions: quality of care issues and economic considerations in critical care pharmacy. *Hosp Pharm* 23:883–890, 1988.
92. Katona BG, Ayd PR, Walters JK, Caspi M, Finkelstein BW: Effect of a pharmacist's and nurse's interventions on cost of drug therapy in a medical intensive care unit. *Am J Hosp Pharm* 46:1179–1182, 1989.
93. Rosenbaum CL, Fant WK, Miyagawa CI, Armitstead JA: Inability to justify a part-time clinical pharmacist in a community hospital intensive care unit. *Am J Hosp Pharm* 48:2154–2157, 1991.
94. Hadbavny AM, Hoyt JW: Promotion of cost-effective benzodiazepine sedation. *Am J Hosp Pharm* 50:660–661, 1993.
95. Broyles JE, Brown RO, Vehe KL, Nolly RJ, Luther RW: Pharmacist interventions improve fluid balance in fluid-restricted patients requiring parenteral nutrition. *DICP Ann Pharmacother* 25:119–122, 1991.
96. Canafax D, Gruber SA, Chang L, et al: The pharmacoeconomics of renal transplantation: increased drug costs with decreased hospitalization costs. *Pharmacotherapy* 10:205–210, 1990.
97. Task force on guidelines for the Society of Critical Care Medicine: recommendations for critical care unit design. *Crit Care Med* 16:796–806, 1988.
98. Caldwell RD, Tuck B: Justification and operation of a critical care satellite pharmacy. *Am J Hosp Pharm* 40:2141–2145, 1983.
99. Ferris NH: Justification of a critical care satellite pharmacy. *Calif J Hosp Pharm* 2:35–37, 1990.
100. Ferris NH, Crisp CB, Hoyt DB, et al: Analysis of workload and staffing requirements for a critical care satellite pharmacy. *Am J Hosp Pharm* 47:2473–2478, 1990.
101. Kelly WN, Meyer JD, Flatley CJ: Cost analysis of a satellite pharmacy. *Am J Hosp Pharm* 43:1927–1930, 1986.
102. Armstrong DK, Dasta JF, Schobelock M, Schneider PJ: The pharmacist in surgical intensive care and anesthesiology. In Majerus TC, Dasta JF (eds): *Practice of Critical Care Pharmacy.* Rockville, MD, Aspen Systems Corp., 1985, pp 127–161.
103. Dobson K, Holt P, Falkowski M, et al: The establishment of a critical care pharmacy: a nursing perspective. *Crit Care Nurs* 4:20–22, 1984.
104. Quercia RA, Hills SW, Klimek JJ, et al: Bacteriologic contamination of intravenous infusion delivery systems in an intensive care unit. *Am J Med* 80:364–367, 1986.
105. Gonzalez ER, Sojka PA, Clapham CE, et al: Cost containment in the intensive care unit: standardized regimens of dopamine and dobutamine. *Parenterals* 6:1–8, 1988.
106. Sulzbach LM, Munro BH: Survey of nursing practice related to decanting intravenous solutions. *Heart Lung* 20:624–630, 1991.
107. Hall K, Guay M, Armstrong G, Nazeravich, D: Development of an intravenous drug manual for a critical care satellite pharmacy. *Can J Hosp Pharm* 35:189–191, 1982.
108. Dasta JF, Bonfiglio MF, Rague NG, Shields BJ: Accuracy and variability of intravenous theophylline preparations. *Ther Drug Monitor* 12:554–557, 1990.
109. Robinson DC, Cookson TL, Grisafe JA: Concentration guidelines for parenteral antibiotics in fluid-restricted patients. *Drug Intell Clin Pharm* 21:985–989, 1987.
110. Quandt CM: The pharmacist in neurosurgery intensive care. In Majerus TC, Dasta JF (eds): *Practice of Critical Care Pharmacy.* Rockville, MD, Aspen Systems Corp., 1985, pp 163–185.
111. Collins JL, Lutz RJ: In vitro study of simultaneous infusion of incompatible drugs in multilumen catheters. *Heart Lung* 20:271–277, 1991.

112. Dasta JF, Hale KN, Stauffer GL, Tschampel MM: Comparison of visual and turbidimetric methods for determining short-term compatibility of intravenous critical care drugs. *Am J Hosp Pharm* 45:2361–2366, 1988.

113. Zeller FP, Anders RJ: Compatibility of intravenous drugs in a coronary intensive care unit. *Drug Intell Clin Pharm* 20:349–352, 1986.

114. King JC: *Guide to Parenteral Admixtures*. St. Louis, MO, Kabivitrum, Inc., 1992.

115. Tatro DS, Olin BR, Hebel SK (eds): *Drug Interaction Facts*. St. Louis, MO, JB Co., 1992.

116. Hansten PD, Horn JR (eds): *Drug Interactions and Updates*. Vancouver, WA, Applied Therapeutics, Inc., 1992.

117. Zucchero FJ, Hogan MJ (eds): *Evaluations of Drug Interactions*. St. Louis, MO, Professional Drug Systems, Inc., 1992.

118. McEvoy GK, Litvak K (eds): *AHFS Drug Information*. Bethesda, MD, American Society of Hospital Pharmacists, 1992.

119. Olin BR, Hebel SK, Dombeck CE (eds): *Drug Facts and Comparisons*. St. Louis, MO, JB Lippincott, 1992.

120. Chernow B: *The Pharmacologic Approach to the Critically Ill Patient*. Baltimore, MD, Williams & Wilkins, 1988.

121. Ornato JR, Gonzalez ER: *Drug Treatment in Emergency Medicine*. New York, Churchill Livingstone, 1990.

122. DiPiro JT, Talbert RL, Hayes PE, et al (eds): *Pharmacotherapy, A Pathophysiologic Approach*. New York, Elsevier, 1989.

123. Young LY, Koda-Kimble MA: *Applied Therapeutics, the Clinical Use of Drugs*, ed 5. Vancouver, WA, Applied Therapeutics, Inc., 1992.

124. Shoemaker WC, Grenvik A, Holbrook PR, Thompson WL (eds): *Textbook of Critical Care*. Philadelphia, PA, WB Saunders, 1989.

125. Civetta JM, Taylor RW, Kirby RR (eds): *Critical Care*. Philadelphia, JB Lippincott, 1988.

126. Rippe JM, Irwin RS, Alpert JS, Fink MP (eds): *Intensive Care Medicine*. Boston, MA, Little, Brown, 1991.

127. Parrillo JE (ed): *Current Therapy in Critical Care Medicine*. Philadelphia, BC Decker, 1991.

128. Cerra FB: *Manual of Critical Care*. St, Louis, MO, CV Mosby, 1987.

129. Rumack BH (ed): *Poisindex*. Denver, CO, Micromedex, 1992.

130. Ellenhorn MJ (ed): *Medical Toxicology, Diagnosis and Treatment of Human Poisoning*. New York, Elsevier, 1988.

131. Haddad LM (ed): *Clinical Management of Poisoning and Drug Overdose*. Philadelphia, WB Saunders, 1990.

132. Bennett WM, Aronoff GR, Golper TA, et al: *Drug Prescribing in Renal Failure*. Philadelphia, American College of Physicians, 1987.

133. Fillastre JP, Singlas E: Pharmacokinetics of newer drugs in patients with renal impairment (part I). *Clin Pharmacokinet* 20:293–310, 1991.

134. Singlas E, Fillastre JP. Pharmacokinetics of newer drugs in patients with renal impairment (part II). *Clin Pharmacokinet* 20:389–410, 1991.

135. Bickley SK: Drug dosing during continuous arteriovenous hemofiltration. *Clin Pharm* 7:198–206, 1988.

136. Eisenberg MS, Cummins RO, Ho MT: Code blue: cardiac arrest and resuscitation. Philadelphia, WB Saunders, 1987.

137. Jaffe AS: Textbook of advanced cardiac life support. Dallas, TX, American Heart Association, 1987.

138. Evans WE, Schentag JJ, Jusko WJ (eds): *Applied Pharmacokinetics, Principles of Therapeutic Drug Monitoring*. Spokane, WA, Applied Therapeutics, Inc., 1986.

139. Winter ME: *Basic Clinical Pharmacokinetics*. Spokane, WA, Applied Therapeutics, Inc., 1988.

140. Bennett WM, Tatro S (eds): *Pediatric Drug Handbook*. Chicago, Yearbook Medical Publishers, 1988.

141. Rogove HJ, Moore KA (eds): Critical care medicines. Columbus, OH, Contemporary Critical Care Resources, Inc., 1993.

142. Angaran DM: Quality assurance to quality improvement: measuring and monitoring pharmaceutical care. *Am J Hosp Pharm* 48:1901–1907, 1991.

143. Enright SM, Flagstad MS: Quality and outcome: pharmacy's professional imperative. *Am J Hosp Pharm* 48:1908–1911, 1991.

144. Blissenbach H: The justification of critical care pharmacy positions in hospitals. In Majerus TC, Dasta JF (eds): *Practice of Critical Care Pharmacy*. Rockville, MD, Aspen Systems Corp., pp 13–27, 1985.

145. Strand LM, Cipolle RJ, Morley PC: Documenting the clinical pharmacist's activities: back to basics. *Drug Intell Clin Pharm* 22:63–67, 1988.

146. Anonymous: FDA again states PharmD appropriate as P.I. *ACCP Report* 9:1, 1990.

147. Hynniman CE: Drug product distribution systems and departmental operations. *Am J Hosp Pharm* 48:S24–S35, 1991.

148. Sham SM, Hollis RC: A cooperative approach to implementing automated medication distribution. *Top Hosp Pharm Manage* 10:59–66, 1991.

149. Kwan JW: High-technology i.v. infusion devices. *Am J Hosp Pharm* 48:S36–S51, 1991.

150. Dasta JF: Computers in critical care: opportunities and challenges. *DICP Ann Pharmacother* 24:1084–1092, 1990.

CHAPTER 9

Cardiovascular Adrenoceptors: Physiology and Critical Care Implications

ROBERT R. RUFFOLO, JR., PH.D.

The cardiovascular system is regulated by α- and β-adrenoceptors. The neurotransmitter norepinephrine influences cardiovascular function under normal homeostatic conditions and in a variety of pathophysiologic conditions. In addition, the actions of the circulating bloodborne hormone epinephrine and exogenously administered catecholamines are largely mediated through interaction with α- and β-adrenoceptors in the major effector organs of the cardiovascular system, such as the heart, vasculature, and kidney. An understanding of these receptors, in terms of their function, location, and distribution, is of primary importance in treating the critically ill patient, inasmuch as the best available pharmacologic treatments for these patients involve the stimulation or blockage of α- and β-adrenoceptors in the cardiovascular system.

There have been many recent developments in our understanding of α- and β-adrenoceptors and the functions they subserve in the regulation of the cardiovascular system. This chapter is a review of these major recent developments, with emphasis on the clinical setting and the use of drugs currently available or being developed that perturb the cardiovascular system through stimulation or blockade of α- and β-adrenoceptors.

CONTROL OF THE CARDIOVASCULAR SYSTEM

ORGANIZATION OF THE AUTONOMIC NERVOUS SYSTEM

The cardiovascular system is under the control and regulation of the autonomic nervous system. Although effector organs of the cardiovascular system (heart, vasculature, kidneys) function in the absence of autonomic nerves, the sympathetic and parasympathetic divisions of the autonomic nervous system provide a delicate balance involving closed reflex loops to maintain these organs in an optimal functional state.

The autonomic nervous system is composed of the parasympathetic division, in which the neurotransmitter at the effector organ is acetylcholine, and the sympathetic division, in which the neurotransmitter is norepinephrine. The parasympathetic division exits the central nervous system from the brainstem (vagus) and the sacral region of the spinal cord. These nerves are characterized by long preganglionic neurons and short postganglionic neurons, the latter innervating the effector organs. The neurotransmitter in the parasympathetic ganglia is acetylcholine. The heart receives a dense cholinergic innervation from the vagus, and cholinergic "tone" in the heart predominates over adrenergic tone. In general, there is no significant parasympathetic innervation to the vasculature, although blood vessels nonetheless contain muscarinic cholinergic receptors that are stimulated by acetylcholine and mediate vasodilation through release of an endothelial derived relaxant factor (43).

The sympathetic division of the autonomic nervous system originates from the intermediolateral cell column of the thoracic and lumbar portions of the spinal cord. The relatively short preganglionic fibers characteristic of sympathetic nerves terminate in the sympathetic ganglia chain, where the neurotransmitter is acetylcholine. The postganglionic sympathetic neurons are long and liberate norepinephrine, which interacts postsynaptically with adrenoceptors in the heart, vasculature, and kidney. The innervation to the vasculature is almost exclusively adrenergic, where the end-organ response is vasoconstriction.

Although the sympathetic and parasympathetic components of the autonomic nervous system originate in the spinal cord and are considered peripheral nerves, both divisions are under the control of nuclei located in the brainstem, which in turn receive input from higher centers in the brain. Most of the cardiovascular reflex loops consist of afferent nerves from various peripheral chemoreceptors and baroreceptors, which travel to the regulatory nuclei in the brainstem, where the information is integrated. The efferent component of the reflex loop involves descending pathways originating from the brainstem nuclei that ultimately recruit the sympathetic and parasympathetic divisions of the autonomic nervous system to make the necessary alterations in the functional state of the various effector organs of the cardiovascular system.

CARDIOVASCULAR REFLEXES

Cardiovascular reflexes maintain cardiovascular function, in particular blood pressure, within a relatively narrow optimal range. A sensitive and highly efficient series of positive and negative feedback loops detects deviations from normal cardiovascular function and then "up-regulates" or "down-regulates" the function of peripheral organs of the cardiovascular system after integration in the central nervous system. Pressure receptors in the carotid sinus and aortic arch sense changes in peripheral arterial blood pressure and initiate the cardiovascular reflex. Afferents from the carotid sinus and aortic arch enter the central nervous system through cranial nerves IX (glossopharyngeal) and X (vagus), respectively, and form, in part, the solitary tract in the medulla. The first synapse in the cardiovascular reflex loop occurs in the nucleus tractus solitarii, where the neurotransmitter appears to be l-glutamate (109). Synapses are made within the nucleus tractus solitarii, both with inhibitory neurons that course to the ventrolateral medulla, which ultimately regulates sympathetic outflow, and with excitatory neurons that send connections to the dorsal motor nucleus of the vagus, which in turn, regulates parasympathetic outflow.

Increases in systemic arterial blood pressure activate the afferent component of the cardiovascular reflex loop. As a result, the inhibitory neurons originating in the nucleus tractus solitarii and terminating in the ventrolateral medulla are activated, reducing sympathetic outflow to the heart, vasculature, and kidney. As a direct consequence, heart rate, stroke volume (and, therefore, cardiac output), and total peripheral vascular resistance are reduced, and blood pressure is reduced to within normal limits. In addition, the excitatory neurons that originate from the nucleus tractus solitarii and terminate in the dorsal motor nucleus of the vagus are activated, and cholinergic outflow is increased, further decreasing heart rate and cardiac output (74) and thus augmenting the reduction in arterial blood pressure. This reduction restores the afferent input to a near-normal level such that the "error signal" becomes small, and the system achieves a new steady state.

α-ADRENOCEPTORS

Adrenoceptors may be subdivided into the α- and β-type (114). β-Adrenoceptors are selectively activated by epinephrine, norepinephrine, and isoproterenol. α-Adrenoceptors are also stimulated by epinephrine and norepinephrine but are resistant to isoproterenol. β-Adrenoceptors may be subdivided further into the β_1- and β_2-subtypes; isoproterenol and epinephrine stimulate both subtypes, and norepinephrine stimulates only the β_1-subtype. Likewise, α-adrenoceptors have been subdivided into the α_1- and α_2-subtypes, and epinephrine and norepinephrine stimulate both. Although the naturally occurring catecholamines cannot distinguish between α_1- and α_2-adrenoceptors, many synthetic drugs do. Thus, phenylephrine and methoxamine are potent and highly selective α_1-adrenoceptor agonists, whereas clonidine and α-methylnorepinephrine (the latter being the active metabolite of α-methyldopa) are potent and selective -$\alpha_2$adrenoceptor agonists (116).

CENTRAL α-ADRENOCEPTORS

Stimulation of central α_2-adrenoceptors in the ventrolateral medulla induces a reduction in sympathetic outflow to the periphery, manifested as a reduction in arterial blood pressure accompanied by bradycardia. This response has been studied extensively over the past 2 decades, and several comprehensive reviews are available (74, 112, 122, 143). Quantitative structure-activity studies have shown excellent correlation between the α_2-adrenoceptor agonist potency of a series of clonidine analogs and blood pressure reduction, provided a lipophilicity term is included to correct for penetration through the blood-brain barrier, which is required in order to gain access to the site of action within the central nervous system (119).

The characteristic response to intravenous administration of an α_2-adrenoceptor agonist in a normotensive or hypertensive animal is an immediate pressor response, due to stimulation of peripheral arterial postjunctional α_1- and α_2-adrenoceptors (119). This response is also seen in human subjects following intravenous administration of clonidine (100). This pressor response is relatively short-lived and is followed by a slow decline in arterial blood pressure to levels lower than those observed prior to drug administration. This long-lasting depressor/antihypertensive response is a result of central α_2-adrenoceptor stimulation. Heart rate declines immediately following administration and continues to be reduced for the duration of drug action. If the α_2-adrenoceptor agonist is administered directly into the central nervous system, or via the vertebral artery, which allows for easy access to the central nervous system, the initial pressor response is not observed (140). High oral doses of centrally acting α-adrenoceptor agonists, such as clonidine or guanfacine, can also transiently increase blood pressure via peripheral arterial α-adrenoceptor stimulation (29), and this increase may provide an explanation for the "therapeutic window" seen with clonidine in antihypertensive therapy (42).

The antihypertensive action of α_2-adrenoceptor agonists results from stimulation of postsynaptic α_2-adrenoceptors in the brainstem. A brainstem site appears likely, based on the inability of transection at the intercollicular level or at the pontomedullary junction to attenuate the antihypertensive activity of clonidine (123). Many experiments have been performed in an attempt to locate more precisely the site of action of α_2-adrenoceptor agonists within the brainstem. Although the nucleus tractus solitarius has often been considered as the principal site of action of central α_2-adrenoceptor agonists (122), recent studies using microinjections of clonidine suggest the lateral reticular nucleus in the ventrolateral medulla as a more likely candidate (46). This nucleus is readily accessible from the ventral surface of the medulla, where α_2-adrenoceptor agonists have been shown to be effective following local application (13, 46).

In addition to a reduction in sympathetic outflow, central α_2-adrenoceptor stimulation can enhance parasympathetic outflow. This action has usually been demonstrated as a potentiation of the reflex bradycardia induced by intravenous injection of a pressor agent such as angiotensin II (74). This action also requires penetration of the α_2-adrenoceptor agonist into the central nervous system (74), but the precise site of action has not yet been determined (46).

Central α_2-adrenoceptor stimulation is utilized clinically for antihypertensive therapy. In addition to the directly acting central α_2-adrenoceptor agonists discussed above, α-methyldopa, which has been extensively employed for nearly 2 decades, is now known to stimulate central α_2-adrenoceptors following metabolic conversion to α-methylnorepinephrine (142), which has much greater α_2-adrenoceptor selectivity than norepinephrine (115). Following chronic treatment with α-methyldopa in rats, medullary norepinephrine stores are almost completely replaced by α-methylnorepinephrine (25), which is available for interaction with medullary α_2-adrenoceptors to inhibit sympathetic outflow. The therapeutic and side effect profile of α-methyldopa is similar to that observed with the directly acting central α_2-adrenoceptor agonists (143).

In addition to clonidine and α-methyldopa, guanfacine is now in general use as an antihypertensive drug. This compound has an in vitro pharmacologic profile similar to that of clonidine (125) but appears to have a longer duration of action (108). Clinical trials have been conducted with several other α_2-adrenoceptor agonists, including St 600 (73), tiamenidine (22), monoxidine, lofexidine (126), and B-HT 933 (azapexole) (108). The latter compound is more selective than clonidine for α_2- vis-à-vis α_1-adrenoceptors (141), and its antihypertensive activity confirms an α_2-adrenoceptor-mediated mechanism. As in animal studies, the clinical cardiovascular profiles of the various α_2-adrenoceptor agonists are relatively similar (107). Besides their antihypertensive indication, the sympatholytic action of the centrally active α_2-adrenoceptor agonists may offer clinical benefit in congestive heart failure and angina pectoris, again through a centrally mediated reduction in sympathetic outflow. Although extensive evaluation for efficacy in these conditions has not yet been performed, preliminary trials in patients are encouraging (46).

One important issue associated with antihypertensive therapy with centrally acting α_2-adrenoceptor agonists is the "rebound hypertension" or "withdrawal" phenomenon that often occurs when treatment is abruptly terminated (55). This phenomenon is characterized by tachycardia and abrupt rises in blood pressure, sometimes to levels greater than those observed before initiation of therapy (54). Studies in animals have confirmed the presence of a hyperadrenergic state following abrupt termination of chronic clonidine therapy (54). Administration of an α_2-adrenoceptor antagonist, such as yohimbine, can also precipitate this withdrawal phenomenon (54).

The withdrawal phenomenon observed following abrupt cessation of α_2-adrenoceptor agonist therapy bears some similarity to opiate withdrawal (55) and appears to involve overactivity of locus ceruleus neurons (37). This effect may represent a rebound phenomenon following chronic suppression of the firing rate of these neurons during chronic antihypertensive treatment. In view of the similarities and possible receptor interactions between α_2-adrenoceptors and opiate receptors, it is not surprising that morphine can suppress, via a naloxone-sensitive mechanism, some of the cardiovascular rebound effects observed following termination of clonidine infusion in rats (139).

PERIPHERAL ARTERIAL α-ADRENOCEPTORS

SYSTEMIC CIRCULATION

It is now widely accepted that arterial vasoconstriction may be mediated by a mixed population of postjunctional vascular α_1- and α_2-adrenoceptors. We are now beginning to understand the physiologic function and/or distribution of these receptors. It appears that in the arterial circulation, postjunctional vascular α-adrenoceptors located at the neuroeffector junction (i.e., extrajunctional receptors) are of the α_2-subtype. Support for this concept of junctional α_1- and extrajunctional α_2-adrenoceptors in the arterial circulation has been obtained in many arterial test systems (20, 80, 81, 144, 145).

The physiologic role of the postsynaptic junctional arterial α_1- and α_2-adrenoceptors appears to be in maintaining resting vascular tone. Presumably, these receptors, which are located in the vicinity of the neurovascular junction, interact with endogenous norepinephrine liberated from sympathetic nerves. The physiologic role of the extrajunctional α_1- and α_2-adrenoceptors is not fully understood, but a number of proposals have been made. The extrajunctional α_1- and α_2-adrenoceptors would not normally interact with liberated norepinephrine since they are located at some distance from the adrenergic nerve terminal, and the highly efficient neuronal uptake pump keeps synaptic levels of norepinephrine sufficiently low, preventing diffusion of the neurotransmitter to the extrajunctional sites (80). The extrajunctional α_1- and α_2-adrenoceptors may respond to circulating epinephrine liberated from the adrenal gland and acting as a bloodborne hormone (81). Although circulating catecholamines may be below the levels required to exert a physiologic effect, in times of stress these levels may be elevated to threshold levels at which postsynaptic vascular α_2-adrenoceptors are activated (27). The contribution made by arterial extrajunctional α_2-adrenoceptors to total peripheral vascular resistance may be greater in certain hypertensive states than in normotensive patients (11, 69), implying that postjunctional vascular α_2-adrenoceptors may play an important role in pathophysiologic states such as hypertension and possibly congestive heart failure, in which circulating catecholamine levels are high (24, 84). It is unclear at the present time whether epinephrine is in fact responsible for stimulating the extrajunctional α_2-adrenoceptors in these states since circulating levels of norepinephrine are also particularly high and could account, at least in part, for α_2-adrenoceptor activation in disease states such as hypertension and congestive heart failure.

CORONARY CIRCULATION

Although the precise role of α-adrenoceptor stimulation in the dynamic regulation of coronary blood flow is still unclear, it has been known for some time that following β-adrenoceptor blockade, α-adrenoceptor agonists or cardiac sympathetic nerve stimulation can produce coronary artery vasoconstriction, leading to an increase in coronary arterial resistance and a decrease in coronary artery blood flow. α-Adrenoceptor agonists, such as phenylephrine (105), methoxamine (56), and norepinephrine (56), produce coronary artery vasoconstriction in the dog, as well as in other species. In animals pretreated with β-adrenoceptor blocking agents, cardiac sympathetic nerve stimulation produces a decrease in coronary artery blood flow that can be blocked by α-adrenoceptor antagonists, demonstrating that α-adrenoceptors can mediate vasoconstrictive response to endogenous as well as exogenous norepinephrine in the coronary circulation (38).

It has recently been suggested that α_2-adrenoceptors may play a role in the α-adrenoceptor-mediated regulation of coronary artery blood flow. In the presence of β-adrenoceptor blockade, intracoronary administration of the selective α_1-adrenoceptor agonist phenylephrine and the selective α_2-adrenoceptor agonist B-HT 933 produces a rapid decrease in coronary artery blood flow, and these effects are blocked by the α_1- and α_2-adrenoceptor antagonists, prazosin and rauwolscine, respectively (63). These same investigators have demonstrated that the reduction in coronary artery blood flow elicited by exogenously administered norepinephrine is antagonized to a greater degree by rauwolscine than by prazosin, thus suggesting a more prominent role of α_2-adrenoceptors in the regulation of coronary artery blood flow. The presence of α_1-adrenoceptors on the large epicardial coronary arteries has recently been demonstrated (60), whereas α_2-adrenoceptors appear to be located primarily on the smaller subendocardial resistance vessels of the coronary vascular bed (75). In addition, it has been found that the pressure of a flow-limiting coronary artery stenosis can unmask a vasoconstrictor response mediated by sympathetic nerve stimulation, and that this response can be antagonized by the nonselective α-adrenoceptor antagonist phentolamine, as well as by the selective α_2-adrenoceptor antagonist rauwolscine but not by the selective α_1-adrenoceptor antagonist prazosin (59). These results suggest that α_2-adrenoceptor-mediated coronary artery vasoconstriction may occur in the coronary circulation under pathologic conditions (i.e., coronary artery disease, angina, or coronary artery vasospasm), and that α_2-adrenoceptors might, therefore, represent a novel therapeutic target.

The selective α_2-adrenoceptor antagonist, idazoxan, has recently been shown to produce a greater degree of blockade of the coronary vasoconstrictor response to sympathetic nerve stimulation than does the selective α_1-adrenoceptor antagonist

prazosin. It thus appears that α_1- and α_2-adrenoceptors coexist in the coronary circulation, and that both α-adrenoceptor subtypes mediate coronary artery vasoconstriction. Furthermore, the data suggest that postjunctional vascular α_2-adrenoceptors may play a more important functional role than postjunctional vascular α_1-adrenoceptors in the coronary circulation, and that α_2-adrenoceptors may be preferentially innervated (i.e., junctional), since they may be selectively activated by endogenous norepinephrine liberated from sympathetic nerves on electrical stimulation.

PULMONARY CIRCULATION

Postjunctional vascular α_1- and α_2-adrenoceptors mediate vasoconstriction in the pulmonary circulation of the dog (129). This fact is evidenced by the dose-related increase in pulmonary perfusion pressure produced by the selective α_1-adrenoceptor agonist methoxamine, which is highly sensitive to blockade by the α_1-adrenoceptor antagonist prazosin, and resistant to blockade by the α_2-adrenoceptor antagonist rauwolscine. Accordingly, the pulmonary pressor effects mediated by the selective α_2-adrenoceptor agonist B-HT 933 are sensitive to blockade by rauwolscine and are resistant to prazosin. The results indicate that postjunctional vascular α_1- and α_2-adrenoceptors coexist in the pulmonary circulation, and that both α-adrenoceptor subtypes mediate vasoconstriction (65, 129).

Prazosin and rauwolscine both antagonize the increases in pulmonary perfusion pressure elicited by exogenously administered norepinephrine, indicating that norepinephrine has the capacity to stimulate both postjunctional α_1- and α_2-adrenoceptors in the pulmonary circulation (129). Pulmonary pressor responses to endogenous norepinephrine released from sympathetic nerves are antagonized primarily by prazosin, with little or no effect of rauwolscine. It appears, therefore, that endogenous norepinephrine acts primarily on α_1-adrenoceptors in the pulmonary vascular bed of the dog (130), and that endogenously released norepinephrine stimulates predominantly junctional α_1-adrenoceptors, whereas exogenously administered norepinephrine stimulates both junctional α_1- and extrajunctional α_2-adrenoceptors in the canine pulmonary vascular bed. Similar conclusions have been made regarding the peripheral arterial circulation of the dog, in which preferential innervation of postjunctional vascular α_1-adrenoceptors has been demonstrated (82).

The ability of selective α_2-adrenoceptor agonists and exogenously administered norepinephrine to elicit increases in pulmonary perfusion pressure may indicate that under some conditions, circulating catecholamines play a role in maintaining or elevating pulmonary vascular tone by a mechanism involving, at least in part, postsynaptic vascular α_2-adrenoceptors. Hyman and associates (66) have infused epinephrine into the perfused pulmonary circulation of the cat (after propranolol treatment) to elicit a large increase in pulmonary perfusion pressure (10 to 20 mm Hg). Recently, Sawyer and colleagues (121) demonstrated that circulating catecholamines are responsible for α_2-adrenoceptor-mediated pressor effects in the spontaneously hypertensive rat. Therefore, in certain disease states, such as congestive heart failure, in which pulmonary pressure is increased and circulating catecholamine levels are high (24), α_2-adrenoceptor-mediated increases in pulmonary vascular resistance may possibly be secondary to the increased circulating catecholamines.

When pulmonary vascular tone is elevated even slightly with a vasoconstrictor agent, responses to the selective α_2-adrenoceptor agonist B-HT 933 are markedly potentiated (130). Furthermore, the enhanced responsiveness of α_2-adrenoceptors is tone-dependent and highly selective for α_2-adrenoceptors, since responses to the α_1-adrenoceptor agonist methoxamine or to angiotensin II are not potentiated by increasing pulmonary vascular tone (130). The nature of the vasoconstrictor agent used to increase pulmonary vascular tone does not influence the enhanced α_2-adrenoceptor responsiveness, although the manner in which pulmonary vascular pressure is increased is critically important. When pulmonary perfusion pressure is increased by increased pulmonary blood flow, as opposed to pulmonary vasoconstriction, responses to α_2-adrenoceptor agonists are not potentiated as they are when vasoconstrictor agents are utilized to elevate pulmonary pressure (130). This observation indicates that pulmonary vascular smooth muscle tone, and not pulmonary pressure per se, is the major determinant of the potentiation in α_2-adrenoceptor responsiveness in the pulmonary vasculature. The selective potentiation of α_2-adrenoceptor-mediated vasoconstriction in the pulmonary circulation under conditions of high pulmonary vascular tone may be relevant to certain pathophysiologic conditions, such as congestive heart failure, in which pulmonary vascular resistance is increased and circulating catecholamine levels are high. Both of these factors may predispose the patient to a further exacerbation of the increase in pulmonary vascular resistance by this selective potentiation mechanism.

RENAL CIRCULATION

The kidneys receive approximately 20% of the cardiac output and provide a significant contribution to total systemic vascular resistance. Their dense adrenergic innervation extends to both the afferent and efferent arterioles (7, 26). Stimulation of the renal nerves and administration of α-adrenoceptor agonists produce an increase in renal vascular resistance with redistribution of blood flow from the cortical to the medullary areas. This response is blocked by phenoxybenzamine or phentolamine (26, 101), indicating the activation of α-adrenoceptors. Initial in vivo studies of the α-adrenoceptor subtype mediating renal vascular responses to exogenously administered agonists suggested an almost exclusive role of α_1-adrenoceptors in the renal vasculature of the rat (124), cat (34), and dog (64). More recent studies show that α_2-adrenoceptor activation may also produce an increase in renal vascular resistance (58). However, despite evidence demonstrating the presence of postjunctional α_2-adrenoceptors in the renal arterial vasculature, it does appear that postjunctional α_1-adrenoceptors predominate.

MESENTERIC CIRCULATION

The splanchnic circulation receives approximately 20 to 25% of the cardiac output and contains a similar proportion of the blood volume. The major part of the splanchnic blood supply is received by the mesenteric circulation, which supplies the small intestine and the upper two-thirds of the large intestine via the superior mesenteric artery. Consequently, the mesenteric circulation has the potential to play a major role in the determination of total systemic vascular resistance. Sympathetic nerve stimulation and exogenous administration of norepinephrine produce mesenteric arteriolar vasoconstriction by activation of α-adrenoceptors (52). Studies using the in situ autoperfused superior mesenteric arterial bed of the rat suggest that only α_1-adrenoceptors are present in the mesenteric vasculature, since vasoconstrictor responses to norepinephrine are blocked exclusively by low doses of prazosin and are relatively unaffected by yohimbine (97). However, Hiley and Thomas (62) have recently shown that the mesenteric vasculature of the rat does indeed possess postjunctional vascular α_2-adrenoceptors in addition to the previously identified α_1-subtype, with an apparent greater density of α_1-adrenoceptors relative to that of α_2-adrenoceptors. Similarly, studies in the cat (34) and the dog (131) have demonstrated a significant population of postjunctional vascular α_2-adrenoceptors in the superior mesenteric arterial bed. Neuronally released norepinephrine, which presumably acts exclusively on α_1-adrenoceptors in the resistance vessels, does not produce a significant redistribution of blood flow within the intestinal wall. Thus, α_1-adrenoceptors appear to be relatively uniformly distributed throughout the arterial circulation in the gut wall.

CEREBRAL CIRCULATION

The arteries supplying blood to the brain clearly have different pharmacologic characteristics from those of peripheral arteries. A marked decrease in sensitivity to norepinephrine is seen just prior to the entry of the vessel into the subarachnoid space (10). This point of transition corresponds to the change in embryologic origin of the proximal and distal portions of each of these blood vessels.

Although cerebral blood vessels have extensive and active sympathetic innervation (35), the α-adrenoceptor-mediated responses of these vessels to sympathetic nerve stimulation are small, compared with those of peripheral vessels (92). This difference may be related either to insensitivity of the α-adrenoceptor or to reduced α-adrenoceptor number (9). Nevertheless, there is evidence that the sympathetic nervous system can modulate cerebral blood flow in the conscious animal thorough an α-adrenoceptor-mediated effect, as measured by hypothalamic washout of radioactive xenon in the rabbit (110).

In vitro characterization of α-adrenoceptors on cerebral blood vessels has not yet yielded a uniform picture. Radioligand binding studies show the presence of both α_1- and α_2-adrenoceptors in membranes from human and monkey cerebral arteries.

Much information on the role of the α-adrenoceptor subtypes in mediating vasoconstriction of cerebral arteries still remains to be elucidated. Nevertheless, in certain species, including humans, both α_1- and α_2-adrenoceptors can be demonstrated in radioligand binding studies; by vasoconstriction induced by α_1- and α_2-adrenoceptor agonists; and by blockade of the response to the physiologic neurotransmitter norepinephrine by selective α_1- and α_2-adrenoceptor antagonists.

ENDOTHELIUM

It has recently been demonstrated that vascular endothelial cells mediate relaxation of arterial smooth muscle in response to certain vasodilators, such as acetylcholine, bradykinin, and substance P, by the release of the so-called endothelial derived relaxing factor (EDRF) (43). Activation of α_2-adrenoceptors on endothelial cells is thought to stimulate the release of EDRF (23, 36, 91), an action that would tend to antagonize vasoconstriction produced by activation of postjunctional vascular α-adrenoceptors. Thus, removal of endothelial cells from arteries produces an increase in responsiveness to α-adrenoceptor agonists (36). Removal of endothelium enhances the vasoconstrictor response produced by norepinephrine in canine and porcine circumflex coronary artery; and after blockade of α_1-adrenoceptors, norepinephrine can produce yohimbine-sensitive and idazoxan-sensitive relaxation of precontracted arteries only in the presence of an intact endothelium (23). Additional studies have shown that α_2-adrenoceptors mediate the release of EDRF from carotid, mesenteric, renal, and femoral arteries of dogs and pigs, although there do appear to be species differences in the magnitude of this response (3). Furthermore, endothelial α_2-adrenoceptors may mediate release of EDRF in coronary microvessels (3). Thus, α_2-adrenoceptor agonists do, indeed, appear to have the capability of modulating vascular responsiveness via stimulation of EDRF release in large arteries and the microcirculation, but this effect does not occur uniformly in all blood vessels. Recent evidence suggests that EDRF may be chemically identical to nitric oxide (102).

PERIPHERAL VENOUS α-ADRENOCEPTORS

SAPHENOUS VEIN

The most commonly studied vein is the canine saphenous vein. DeMey and Vanhoutte (31, 41) first reported the potent vasoconstrictor activity of clonidine in this tissue. Additional studies have shown that highly selective α_2-adrenoceptor agonists, such as B-HT 920, B-HT 933, and UK 14,304, produce a vasoconstrictor response that is resistant to antagonism by prazosin and sensitive to blockade by rauwolscine (120). In the canine saphenous vein, norepinephrine, which can activate both α_1- and α_2-adrenoceptors, appears to activate preferentially the α_2-subtype.

Experiments in isolated human saphenous vein (96) show results similar to those reported for the canine saphenous vein. The response to low concentrations of norepinephrine is essentially unaffected by prazosin but potently antagonized by yohimbine, suggesting that α_2-adrenoceptors may be more important than α_1-adrenoceptors.

The venous circulation resembles the arterial circulation in that postjunctional vascular α_1- and α_2-adrenoceptors coexist, with each α-adrenoceptor subtype mediating vasoconstriction (32, 39). However, in contrast to the arterial circulation, postjunctional vascular α_2-adrenoceptors in veins appear to be preferentially innervated, and postjunctional vascular α_1-adrenoceptors are innervated to a lesser degree and are possibly located predominantly extrajunctionally (39).

PULMONARY VEIN

Assessment of postjunctional α-adrenoceptor activity in the pulmonary vasculature in vitro provides some interesting correlates to what is observed in canine and human saphenous veins. Intralobar pulmonary veins have been reported to contract in response to the selective α_2-adrenoceptor agonist B-HT 933, and this response is sensitive to inhibition by the selective α_2-adrenoceptor antagonist rauwolscine (99, 130). In contrast, intralobar pulmonary arteries are relatively unresponsive to B-HT 933 in vitro. These results indicate that postjunctional vascular α_2-adrenoceptors may be preferentially located on the venous side of the pulmonary circulation, as also appears to be the case in the peripheral circulation (113).

HEPATIC PORTAL SYSTEM

A situation similar to that described in the saphenous vein also exists in vivo in the intestinal venous circulation (103). In addition, in the hepatic venous circulation of the cat in vivo, blood volume responses to norepinephrine are mediated by postjunctional vascular α_2-adrenoceptors, as is the hepatic venous response to sympathetic nerve stimulation (128). These results are suggestive of a dominance of α_2- over α_1-adrenoceptors in the hepatic venous circulation, as well as a preferential, if not exclusive, junctional location of vascular α_2-adrenoceptors (128). Furthermore, α_2-adrenoceptor-mediated responses in the venous circulation appear to be more marked than those in the arterial circulation, consistent with the notion that postjunctional vascular α_2-adrenoceptors may play a more important functional role in venous than in arterial blood vessels (113).

OTHER VEINS

Most other veins have less of an α_2-adrenoceptor contribution relative to that observed in the saphenous vein. Shoji and associates (132) compared the responsiveness of many canine veins to norepinephrine, phenylephrine and clonidine. The saphenous and cephalic veins have the greatest response to the α_2-adrenoceptor agonist clonidine, followed by the femoral vein. Interestingly, longitudinal but not helical strips of portal vein, mesenteric vein, and vena cava readily respond to clonidine. Evidence for postjunctional α_2-adrenoceptors in human femoral vein has been provided by the failure of prazosin to antagonize the response to low concentrations of norepinephrine in this tissue, and by the potent contractile effect observed with guanfacine, a moderately selective α_2-adrenoceptor agonist (47).

In a quantitative analysis of α_1- and α_2-adrenoceptor characteristics in femoral and saphenous veins, the selective α_2-adrenoceptor agonist UK 14,304 was much less effective in inducing contraction in the femoral vein (22% of norepinephrine maximum) than in the saphenous vein (86% of norepinephrine maximum) (40). As seen in some arteries, the response to norepinephrine in certain veins, such as the canine splenic vein, may be sensitive to blockade by both rauwolscine and prazosin, even though the tissue is unresponsive to highly selective α_2-adrenoceptor agonists (61).

PHYSIOLOGIC SIGNIFICANCE OF VENOUS α_2-ADRENOCEPTORS

The physiologic significance of venous α_2-adrenoceptors is unclear. In vivo studies with α_2-adrenoceptor agonists in the rat (45) or dog (146) cannot demonstrate a significant hemodynamic effect, clearly attributable to effects on venous capacitance vessels (96). Since venous α_2-adrenoceptors are most prominent in the cutaneous veins (39), the venous α_2-adrenoceptor may be involved in blood flow redistribution to optimize the thermoregulatory process. It has recently been reported that α_2-adrenoceptor-mediated vasoconstriction can significantly reduce venous capacitance and thereby increase venous return to the heart, resulting in an increase in cardiac output (70).

MYOCARDIAL α-ADRENOCEPTORS

The predominant postsynaptic adrenoceptor in the heart is the α_1-adrenoceptor, which mediates a positive inotropic and chronotropic response (16). However, in the hearts of most mammalian species, including humans, there are postsynaptic α_1-adrenoceptors that mediate a positive inotropic response without notably changing heart rate (127). The mechanism by which cardiac α_1-adrenoceptors increase force of contraction has not been established, but it appears not to be associated with accumulation of cyclic AMP (cAMP) or stimulation of adenylate cyclase (17). In this respect, α_1-adrenoceptors differ from α_1-adrenoceptors in the myocardium. Other differences between myocardial α_1- and α_1-adrenoceptors are the longer rate of onset and longer duration of action of α_1-adrenoceptor-mediated inotropic responses (127). Differences among electrophysiologic actions mediated by α_1- and α_1-adrenoceptors have also been observed (50). α_1-Adrenoceptor-mediated inotropic responses occur at all rates of contraction, but the effect mediated by α_1-adrenoceptors is most prominent at lower rates (16).

RENAL α-ADRENOCEPTORS

The presence of α-adrenoceptors in the kidney has been known for many years, and α-adrenergic drugs produce a variety of renal effects. Only now are we beginning to understand the functions and locations of the renal α-adrenoceptors (137). Radioligand binding studies indicate that α_1- and α_2-adrenoceptors coexist in the kidneys of a variety of mammalian species; however, the number, proportion, and distribution of each α-adrenoceptor subtype may vary from one species to another (137).

α_1-Adrenoceptors are believed to predominate in the human renal vasculature and to mediate a vasoconstrictor response, thereby modulating renal blood flow (57). α_2-Adrenoceptors have been identified in the juxtaglomerular apparatus and appear to inhibit renin release (137). Recently, it has been demonstrated that stimulation of renal α_2-adrenoceptors can inhibit the effects of vasopressin on water and sodium excretion (133). This effect mediated by α_2-adrenoceptors appears to involve inhibition of adenylate cyclase and reductions in cellular cAMP and may occur at the level of the cortical collecting tubule (78). The α_2-adrenoceptor-mediated enhancement in sodium and water excretion occurs simultaneously with a decrease in potassium secretion (44). α-Adrenoceptors, possibly of the α_1-subtype, may enhance sodium and water reabsorption in the proximal convoluted tubules. Gluconeogenesis in the proximal convoluted tubule has been shown to be under α_1-adrenoceptor control (72).

The density of renal α_2-adrenoceptors is higher in spontaneously hypertensive and Dahl salt-sensitive hypertensive rats than in normotensive controls, and high-sodium diets may increase α_2-adrenoceptor number even further (51, 104). Thus, renal α_2-adrenoceptors may be involved in certain forms of genetic hypertension.

PLATELETS

Adrenaline has long been known to induce aggregation of human platelets and to potentiate aggregation induced by other agents, such as ADP and thrombin. The response is normally biphasic, consisting of a reversible, partial aggregation followed by a rapid, irreversible aggregation. α_2-Adrenoceptor antagonists, such as yohimbine, block the effect of adrenaline, suggesting an α_2-adrenoceptor-mediated mechanism. However, many synthetic α_2-adrenoceptor agonists, such as clonidine, do not usually induce human platelet aggregation. The failure of most α_2-adrenoceptor agonists to induce platelet aggregation likely results from their low efficacy combined with low α_2-adrenoceptor density in platelets. In most experiments, clonidine will block adrenaline-induced platelet aggregation, a typical finding for a partial agonist, and a few investigators have observed a small aggregatory response to clonidine, usually corresponding in magnitude to the initial phase of adrenaline-induced aggregation. UK-14,304, a highly potent and selective α_2-adrenoceptor agonist, produces an effect comparable with that produced by adrenaline. Consistent with this observation is the fact that UK-14,304 has a higher efficacy than clonidine and most other imidazolines at the α_2-adrenoceptor. Several close analogs of UK-14,304 are also capable of inducing aggregation of human platelets.

α_2-Adrenoceptor-mediated platelet aggregation is not as prominent in animal platelets. This finding seems to be related both to low α_2-adrenoceptor density and the poor coupling between α_2-adrenoceptor occupancy and the triggering of the aggregation response. Typical biphasic platelet aggregation is observed only in primates and, occasionally, in cats. This potentiating action can be blocked by α_2-adrenoceptor antagonists. Addition of subthreshold concentrations of a calcium ionophore will also follow a full aggregatory response to occur to adrenaline and UK-14,304 in rabbit platelets. Platelets from the rat and guinea pig are unresponsive to adrenaline, both for induction of aggregation and for potentiation of ADP-induced aggregation. This lack of activation correlates with the failure to demonstrate specific [^{3}H] yohimbine-binding sites in platelets from these species (47).

The functional role of α_2-adrenoceptor-mediated platelet aggregation is not clearly understood. Many substances normally present in blood can induce aggregation, and the in vitro concentrations of adrenaline required to induce platelet aggregation are generally higher than those found in vivo. The most likely situation is that the physiologic control of platelet aggregation involves the action of multiple aggregatory hormones, each present at levels below those necessary for induction of platelet aggregation individually. It is possible that increased levels of catecholamines in the systemic circulation during stress, and in the coronary circulation during myocardial ischemia, may produce platelet aggregation and/or platelet hyperaggregability. This possibility is supported by observations in a canine model of platelet-dependent coronary artery thrombosis in which stenosis of an endothelial-damaged coronary artery produces platelet-dependent cyclic flow reductions. In this model, the α_2-adrenoceptor antagonist yohimbine, but not the α_1-adrenoceptor antagonist prazosin, reduces the frequency of cyclic flow reductions. Thus, it would appear that adrenaline can act to potentiate the actions of aggregating agents in vivo, such that inhibition of this effect, presumably produced by circulating epinephrine, produces an inhibition, albeit incomplete, of platelet aggregation.

CARDIOVASCULAR EFFECTS OF α-ADRENERGIC DRUGS

PERIPHERAL α-ADRENOCEPTOR BLOCKING AGENTS AS ANTIHYPERTENSIVES

Since vascular tone is mediated predominantly by α-adrenoceptors, it is logical to assume that pharmacologic antagonists of α-adrenoceptors abate hypertension. Indeed, the α-adrenoceptor antagonists tolazole (Priscoline) and phentolamine (Regitine) were introduced as clinical antihypertensive agents many years ago. These competitive α-adrenoceptor antagonists do, in fact, lower blood pressure, but their clinical efficacy has been unaccountably low. One explanation for their ineffectiveness is their ability to potentiate neuronal norepinephrine release (136). Both tolazoline and phentolamine are nonselective α-adrenoceptor antagonists and, therefore, have potent antagonist activity at prejunctional α_2-adrenoceptors, in addition to their postjunctional α-adrenolytic effects. Their prejunctional α_2-adrenoceptor antagonist activity appears to interrupt the inhibitory negative feedback loop that regulates neurotransmitter release, increasing synaptic levels of norepinephrine. The increased levels of norepinephrine in the synaptic cleft may partially overcome the postjunctional α_1-adrenoceptor antagonist effects and, thus, limit antihypertensive efficacy. This hypothesis has been widely accepted, primarily in light of the high antihypertensive efficacy observed with prazosin (Minipress), a selective α_1-adrenoceptor antagonist (28). Since prazosin possesses only weak antagonist activity at presynaptic α_2-adrenoceptors, the neuronal negative feedback loop remains intact to prevent elevation of synaptic concentrations of norepinephrine (28).

In human forearm, yohimbine, a selective α_2-adrenoceptor antagonist, produces arterial vasodilation and increases blood flow (12). This finding suggests that, at least in this vascular bed, the postsynaptic extrajunctional α_2-adrenoceptor may also play an important role, along with the junctional α_1-adrenoceptor, in maintaining vascular tone. Vasoconstrictor activity mediated by postsynaptic extra junctional α_2-adrenoceptors may play more of a role in the hypertensive state, as shown both in animal studies (90, 93) and in clinical studies in which increased vasodilatory activity of yohimbine has been observed in patients with essential hypertension (12).

Circulating catecholamines are known to be increased in a major subpopulation of patients with essential hypertension (49), and these high plasma catecholamine levels have been suggested as contributors to the increased vascular resistance characteristic of essential hypertension (2). Since circulating catecholamines appear to be the endogenous agonists for the extrajunctional vascular α_2-adrenoceptors, in this subgroup of patients, postjunctional α_2-adrenoceptors may, in fact, contribute to the increased peripheral vascular resistance. As such, α_2-adrenoceptor blockade may prove to be beneficial in some forms of hypertension.

α_1-ADRENOCEPTOR ANTAGONISTS IN CONGESTIVE HEART FAILURE

Vasodilators have assumed a more prominent role in the treatment of congestive heart failure during the past decade. In most patients with congestive heart failure, the optimal vasodilator is one that acts relatively equally on the arterial and venous beds. Sodium nitroprusside acts in this way but must be administered intravenously. Prazosin, an orally active selective α_1-adrenoceptor antagonist, has been shown to mimic the hemodynamic effects of nitroprusside in congestive heart failure, increasing cardiac output, decreasing left ventricular filling pressure and system and pulmonary vascular resistance, and maintaining heart rate (6). Although acute tolerance has been observed after multiple doses of prazosin over a period of 24 to 72 hours (5), the beneficial effect often returns with continued therapy, and long-term clinical trials with prazosin show chronic efficacy in patients with congestive heart failure (135). Prazosin improves symptoms most during exercise (111).

Since there is evidence that the degree of sympathetic tone is proportional to the severity of heart failure (98, 138), and the level of plasma cathecholamines has been implicated as a primary risk factor in patients with congestive heart failure (24), the use of α-adrenoceptor antagonists in low-output cardiac failure may have a rational advantage over other vasodilators. An additional benefit may be that anginal frequency decreases with reduced afterload, and cardiac oxygen needs may be diminished (8).

The factor that best correlates with mortality in patients with heart failure is a high level of circulating catecholamines (24). Because, as discussed earlier, circulating catecholamines may be the natural substrates for postsynaptic extrajunctional α_2-adrenoceptors in the arterial circulation, and because high plasma catecholamine levels may contribute to the increased total peripheral vascular resistance characteristic of congestive heart failure (14, 98), the evaluation of an α_2-adrenoceptor antagonist in low-output cardiac failure is indicated.

α-ADRENOCEPTOR ANTAGONISTS IN MYOCARDIAL ISCHEMIA

There is evidence to suggest that α-adrenoceptor blockade may be effective in the treatment of angina pectoris. In a trial of prazosin in congestive heart failure, two patients with severe resting angina obtained a beneficial effect that persisted throughout the 6-month treatment period (8). This antianginal effect is probably the result of a reduction in cardiac oxygen requirements caused by the reduction in afterload produced by prazosin. In vasospastic angina, the localized constriction of an apparently normal coronary artery may be mediated, at least in part, by activation of coronary vascular α_1-adrenoceptors. In clinical practice, α-adrenoceptor antagonists, such as phentolamine, phenoxybenzamine, and prazosin, are sometimes used in angina if primary therapy with nitrates and calcium channel blockers is ineffective.

Prazosin has been shown to have nitroprusside-like effects in patients with acute myocardial infarction, reducing both pre- and afterload and increasing cardiac output (135). Prazosin may be useful as a second-line drug in acute myocardial infarction, following intravenous nitroprusside and nitroglycerin.

α-ADRENOCEPTOR ANTAGONISTS IN CARDIAC ARRHYTHMIAS

Despite the unquestionable beneficial effects of α_1-adrenoceptor antagonists in experimental models of arrhythmia (see above), the α-adrenoceptor antagonists have not been used clinically to a significant extent, perhaps as a result of their hypotensive activity. Recently, a prazosin analog, UK 52046, has been postulated as having selectivity for cardiac vs. vascular α_1-adrenoceptors. No in vitro data have been reported to support this selectivity or, indeed, to demonstrate α_1-adrenoceptor blockade by UK 52046, although studies in normal volunteers showed blockade of phenylephrine-induced increases in systolic and diastolic blood pressure.

UK 52046 has been shown to be an effective antiarrhythmic agent in a variety of animal models, including the ischemic isolated guinea pig heart and conscious dogs 24 hours following coronary artery ligation. UK 52046 had no hemodynamic or electrophysiologic effects in nonischemic cardiac patients. In another group of patients with stable coronary artery disease, UK 52046 produced a slight decrease in blood pressure, accompanied by a slight increase in heart rate and cardiac index. Hence, this compound appears to be well-tolerated in humans and should allow a test of whether an α_1-adrenoceptor antagonist will show clinically useful antiarrhythmic activity in humans.

α₂-ADRENOCEPTOR AGONISTS IN HYPERTENSION

Central α_2-adrenoceptor stimulation has been utilized clinically for many years in the treatment of hypertension. The most commonly used drugs are clonidine, a moderately selective α_2-adrenoceptor agonist that can readily cross the blood-brain barrier, and α-methyldopa, which is actively transported into the brain, then metabolized to α-methylnoradrenaline, which preferentially activates the α_2-adrenoceptor (142). The therapeutic and side effect profiles of these two agents are quite similar (143).

In addition to clonidine and α-methyldopa, guanabenz and guanfacine are now in general use as antihypertensive drugs. Clinical trials have been conducted with many other α_2-adrenoceptor agonists, including St 600, tiamenidine, monoxidine, lofexidine, rilmenidine (S-3341), and B-HT 933 (azepexole) (73, 108, 126).

Both animal and clinical studies are consistent with the hypothesis that α_2-adrenoceptor agonists can lower blood pressure and heart rate by an action on central postsynaptic α_2-adrenoceptors to inhibit sympathetic outflow to the periphery (140). Although there is a large body of experimental evidence in support of this hypothesis, controversy remains with respect to the exact site of action within the brain, and the potential involvement of nonadrenergic "imidazoline" receptors has been proposed. Many of the divergent results have been obtained when drugs are locally administered to various central sites. Thus, the blood pressure reduction induced by local administration of clonidine to the rostral ventrolateral medulla is insensitive to blockade by SK&F 86466, a nonimidazoline α_a-adrenoceptor antagonist. However, the hypotensive effect of clonidine in the anesthetized normotensive rat is sensitive to blockade by SK&F 86466 (J. P. Hieble, personal communication). This disparity suggests that α_2-adrenoceptor agonists may act *via* a different mechanism upon local microinjection in the brain than when systemically administered to an intact animal or to human subjects.

Clonidine and guanfacine are effective antihypertensive drugs, with a desirable clinical profile. Reflex tachycardia has not been observed, and orthostatic hypotension has not been a common side effect. However, the use of α_2-adrenoceptor agonists has been limited by the prevalence of sedation. This side effect results from stimulation of a different population of central α_2-adrenoceptors, probably located at prejunctional sites. No pharmacologic difference has been shown between the α_2-adrenoceptors mediating central inhibition of sympathetic outflow and those mediating sedation, and studies of agents purported to show less sedation ultimately produced equivalent sedation as clonidine when administered by the same route in the same species. All of the α_2-adrenoceptor agonists claimed to be less sedative than clonidine are also less potent antihypertensive agents, compared to clonidine, and the lower incidence of sedation observed in clinical trials may be a consequence of differing positions of the administered dose on the concentration-response curve for blood pressure reduction.

β-ADRENOCEPTORS

CENTRAL β-ADRENOCEPTORS

β-Adrenoceptors have been identified on many neurons of the central nervous system (67), but their role in cardiovascular regulation is unclear. Activating central β-adrenoceptors has been shown to elevate blood pressure and heart rate (30). This observation is supported by the finding that injecting β-adrenoceptor antagonists into the central nervous system decreases blood pressure and heart rate (30). In addition, systemically administering β-adrenoceptor antagonists produces decreases in resting splanchnic sympathetic nerve discharges that correlate with reductions in arterial blood pressure (85). Intravenously administered propranolol has been reported to interrupt the cardiovascular reflex loop in the central nervous system and inhibit sympathetic outflow (33). Increases in blood pressure and heart rate evoked by sinoaortic denervation may be attenuated by injecting small doses of propranolol into the central nervous system (95). These results are highly suggestive of a centrally mediated tonic β-adrenoceptor influence to increase blood pressure and of a possible central mechanism for the antihypertensive effects of β-blockers (77). However, β-adrenoceptor antagonists that do not penetrate the blood-brain barrier, such as atenolol, are also highly effective antihypertensive agents, suggesting that the peripheral antihypertensive effects of β-adrenoceptor antagonists are also significant.

PERIPHERAL β-ADRENOCEPTORS

PRESYNAPTIC β-ADRENOCEPTORS

The best understood presynaptic adrenoceptor is the α_2-adrenoceptor that inhibits neurotransmitter liberation. More recently, presynaptic α_2-adrenoceptors have been identified and shown to facilitate neurotransmitter release. It has been shown that presynaptic α_2-adrenoceptors enhance stimulus-evoked norepinephrine release, suggesting that prejunctional α_2-adrenoceptors mediate a positive feedback effect on sympathetic neurotransmission. The prejunctional α_2-adrenoceptor has been found in a variety of species, including humans (20, 87, 89).

Most experiments characterizing the prejunctional α_2-adrenoceptor have used either epinephrine or isoproterenol as agonists. Norepinephrine is not a potent presynaptic α_2-adrenoceptor agonist (88), acting instead on the presynaptic α_2-adrenoceptor to inhibit neurotransmitter release. It is, therefore, logical to assume that epinephrine is the physiologic ligand for the presynaptic α_2-adrenoceptor. This assumption has led to the "epinephrine hypothesis" of essential hypertension, which suggests that activation of prejunctional α_2-adrenoceptors by neuronally released epinephrine may initiate the disease process.

EPINEPHRINE HYPOTHESIS OF ESSENTIAL HYPERTENSION

Epinephrine, synthesized and released by the adrenal gland, has a short half-life in the systemic circulation. Although circulating epinephrine levels during stress are equivalent to the threshold concentration for in vitro activation of prejunctional α_2-adrenoceptors (79), any α_2-adrenoceptor-mediated effect of circulating epinephrine on neuronal norepinephrine release should be transient. However, circulating epinephrine is readily accumulated by sympathetic nerve terminals via the neuronal uptake pump for sympathomimetic amines (uptake$_1$). In the sympathetic nerve terminal, epinephrine can be costored and coreleased with norepinephrine (88). Increases in the epinephrine content of tissues with dense sympathetic innervation are observed after stimulation-induced adrenal epinephrine secretion (106). Since epinephrine, but not norepinephrine, will activate the prejunctional α_2-adrenoceptor, epinephrine coreleased with norepinephrine will shift the balance toward increased α_2- relative to α_2-adrenoceptor-mediated prejunctional effects, thus increasing the net efficiency of sympathetic neurotransmission. Increased norepinephrine release in response to neuronally released epinephrine has been demonstrated in vitro in guinea pig and rat atrial tissue (89) and in vivo in humans (18).

Continuous infusion of low doses of epinephrine induces hypertension in rats (89). This effect is not mimicked by norepinephrine infusion and can be blocked by propranolol, suggesting an action on prejunctional α_2-adrenoceptors. Tachycardia is often an additional consequence of epinephrine infusion; this tachycardia is attenuated by neuronal uptake blockade and is much more persistent after epinephrine infusion than after isoproterenol, the latter not being a substrate for neuronal uptake (19).

The results of a large-scale clinical study in Great Britain correlating blood pressure and plasma catecholamines in hypertensive and prehypertensive subjects support the role of epinephrine in the development of the hypertensive state (18). Although the mechanism(s) of the antihypertensive activity of β-adrenoceptor blocking agents has not been established, the blockade of presynaptic facilitative β-adrenoceptors and the resulting inhibition of neurotransmitter liberation must be considered.

MYOCARDIAL β-ADRENOCEPTORS

The postsynaptic β-adrenoceptor of the heart that mediates an increase in both the rate and force of contraction is predominantly the β_1-subtype (16). Biochemical studies indicate that the positive inotropic and chronotropic responses to catecholamines are mediated by β_1-adrenoceptor activation of adenylate cyclase, with the ultimate generation and accumulation of cAMP (16).

Recent studies have shown that myocardial β_2-adrenoceptors may be present in the sinoatrial node in some mammalian species, including humans. The functional significance of these β_2-adrenoceptors is not known, and they appear to be noninnervated (16). It has been proposed that noninnervated extrajunctional β_2-adrenoceptors in the heart may represent "hormonal" adrenoceptors that are responsive to circulating blood-borne epinephrine (4).

Available data indicate that in congestive heart failure, myocardial β-adrenoceptors undergo "down-regulation," a cellularly mediated decrease in surface receptor number (15). This decrease in β-adrenoceptor number is proportional to the degree of myocardial dysfunction and the loss of contractility that occurs in congestive heart failure. Myocardial β-adrenoceptor down-regulation is chamber-specific, occurring to the greatest degree in the most severely affected ventricular chamber, and is specific to the β_1-adrenoceptor subtype. β-adrenoceptor down-regulation may be the result of the excessively high levels of plasma catecholamines seen in congestive heart failure, inasmuch as a similar phenomenon of β-adrenoceptor down-regulation is seen in animals treated with high doses of catecholamines. The specific down-regulation in cardiac β-adrenoceptors may be, in part, the cause of the decrease in myocardial function observed during long-term β-adrenoceptor stimulation, and an actual decrease in β-adrenoceptor number has been observed in myocardial tissue from patients with congestive heart failure (117). Down-regulation of β-adrenoceptors in congestive heart failure results in a decrease or loss of efficacy of β-adrenoceptor agonists on long-term administration. Although β-adrenoceptors are down-regulated in congestive heart failure, myocardial β_1-adrenoceptors and histamine H_2-receptors do not appear to be subject to this same regulatory process.

VASCULAR β-ADRENOCEPTORS

Postsynaptic vascular $β_2$-adrenoceptors mediate vasodilation. The vascular $β_2$-adrenoceptors, like the vascular $α_2$-adrenoceptors, appear to be noninnervated (i.e., are located extrajunctionally) (4). It has been proposed, therefore, that extrajunctional vascular $β_2$-adrenoceptors are "hormonal" receptors that mediate vasodilation in response to circulating epinephrine in certain vascular beds at times of stress, when plasma levels of epinephrine are increased. As recently shown, the vasodilatory response mediated by vascular $β_2$-adrenoceptors after ganglionic stimulation is abolished by bilateral adrenalectomy, indicating that this response results from the action of circulating epinephrine liberated by the adrenal glands (4).

RENAL β-ADRENOCEPTORS

The kidney is also heavily under adrenergic control. Probably the most important adrenergic effect in the kidney is the regulation of renin release from the juxtaglomerular apparatus (71). Renin release from the juxtaglomerular cells is enhanced by $β_1$-adrenoceptor stimulation and/or stimulation of renal adrenergic nerves (71). The increase in renin release evoked by the exogenous administration of β-adrenoceptor agonists or by adrenergic nerve stimulation is antagonized by β-adrenoceptor blocking agents such as propranolol. The juxtaglomerular cells appear to be under a constant adrenergic tone since β-adrenoceptor blocking agents also inhibit basal renin release (71). It has been suggested that the magnitude of the antihypertensive response to β-adrenoceptor antagonists depends on the initial plasma renin activity and the degree of its suppression by β-adrenoceptor blockade (21). However, the relevance of the decrease in renin release mediated by β-adrenoceptor antagonists to the antihypertensive effects of these compounds has been questioned, since the reduction in blood pressure does not always parallel the reduction in renin release. In addition, some β-adrenoceptor blockers with intrinsic sympathomimetic activity may themselves promote renin release by their inherent β-adrenoceptor agonist properties (71), yet these compounds nonetheless are effective antihypertensive agents in humans.

Renal β-adrenoceptors also appear to regulate renal blood flow at the vascular level. $β_2$-Adrenoceptors in the vasculature have been identified pharmacologically and mediate the expected vasodilatory response, resulting in an increase in renal blood flow.

β-Adrenoceptors may also affect renal salt and water metabolism, but these effects are controversial, and the results are often contradictory (71).

CARDIOVASCULAR EFFECTS OF β-ADRENERGIC DRUGS

β-ADRENOCEPTOR ANTAGONISTS USED IN THE MANAGEMENT OF HYPERTENSION

β-Adrenoceptor blocking agents are commonly used to treat hypertension. Several β-adrenoceptor antagonists are available and differ significantly. Certain β-adrenoceptor antagonists, such as propranolol, are nonselective in that they antagonize both $β_1$- and B_2-adrenoceptors. Other β-adrenoceptor antagonists, such as atenolol, are termed "cardioselective," preferentially antagonizing myocardial $β_1$-adrenoceptors. Finally, a class of β-adrenoceptor antagonists with intrinsic sympathomimetic activity is now available; the prototype is pindolol. These different classes of β-adrenoceptor antagonists produce qualitatively and quantitatively distinct hemodynamic responses in humans and, therefore, should not be considered as one homogenous class of drugs possessing similar pharmacologic activities.

As indicated earlier, the mechanism of action of β-adrenoceptor antagonists in hypertension is still a matter of controversy. From the previously discussed effects that may be attributed to central β-adrenoceptors and peripheral presynaptic and postsynaptic β-adrenoceptors in the heart, vasculature, and kidneys, four logical mechanisms for the antihypertensive activity of β-blocking agents may be postulated: (*a*) an action within the central nervous system that antagonizes the central β-adrenoceptor-mediated increases in blood pressure and heart rate; (*b*) presynaptic β-adrenoceptor blockade that inhibits the β-adrenoceptor-mediated positive feedback effect on neurotransmitter (norepinephrine) liberation in the heart, vasculature, and kidneys; (*c*) blockade of postsynaptic cardiac $β_1$-adrenoceptors that decreases the rate and force of myocardial contraction and thereby decreases cardiac output; and (*d*) inhibition of renin release, which is stimulated by $β_1$-adrenoceptor activation.

All classes of β-adrenoceptor antagonists lower blood pressure, regardless of β-adrenoceptor subtype selectivity or the presence of intrinsic sympathomimetic activity. Furthermore, no one mechanism will adequately account for the antihypertensive activity of β-adrenoceptor antagonists in general. Thus, some β-adrenoceptor blockers do not penetrate the blood-brain barrier, whereas others with intrinsic sympathomimetic activity may enhance renin release. In addition, β-adrenoceptor antagonists decrease heart rate and cardiac output acutely, yet the antihypertensive effect of β-adrenoceptor blockers may take days to develop. Thus, several of these mechanisms may contribute to the antihypertensive activity of any one β-adrenoceptor blocker.

When β-adrenoceptor antagonists (without intrinsic sympathomimetic activity) are first administered, there is an acute decrease in heart rate and cardiac output and a reflex increase in total peripheral vascular resistance, such that no net change in blood pressure results. After a period of latency, total peripheral vascular resistance begins to decrease toward initial values in the face of continued reduced cardiac output, and the net effect is a decrease in blood pressure (76). At times, total peripheral resistance may only return to normal levels, but cardiac output remains low, and the net effect is still a reduction in blood pressure (94).

In spite of the initial increase in total peripheral vascular resistance, the antihypertensive effect of propranolol follows closely the secondary decrease in peripheral vascular resistance that occurs with time, even when there is some restoration in cardiac output.

β-ADRENOCEPTOR BLOCKING AGENTS IN ANGINA

The β-adrenoceptor blocking agents are useful in angina pectoris because they decrease three aspects of myocardial oxygen demand: (*a*) myocardial wall tension, which is a function of ventricular pressure and the radius of the left ventricle; (*b*) heart rate; and (*c*) contractility. β-adrenoceptor antagonists produce a decrease in heart rate and contractile force, simply by β-adrenoceptor blockade. The chronic antihypertensive effect of β-adrenoceptor blockers also serves to reduce myocardial wall tension by decreasing ventricular systolic developed pressure. Therefore, the utility of β-adrenoceptor antagonists in treating angina results from the ability of these compounds to decrease the myocardial oxygen demand by affecting each of the three factors known to determine oxygen demand (53).

β-ADRENOCEPTOR AGONISTS IN CONGESTIVE HEART FAILURE

In heart failure, the goal of therapy is usually to increase cardiac output, and this is often done by increasing the contractile state of the myocardium. One mechanism that may be used to augment cardiac function is activation of myocardial β_1-adrenoceptors, which increases heart rate and contractility and, therefore, increases cardiac output. The increase in heart rate that occurs with isoproterenol may be undesirable since it increases myocardial work and oxygen demand. With certain inotropic agents, myocardial contractility can be selectively increased with little or no increase in heart rate.

Intravenous infusion of dobutamine generally increases cardiac output by augmenting stroke volume (1) through enhanced left ventricular contractility (dp/dt) (68). Total peripheral vascular resistance (afterload) is reduced in part by reflex withdrawal of sympathetic tone (86) and in part by direct arterial vasodilation (118). The reduction in afterload produced by dobutamine further increases left ventricular stroke volume by reducing the impedance to left ventricular ejection. Furthermore, the decrease in total peripheral vascular resistance offsets the contribution made by cardiac output to blood pressure, such that mean arterial pressure is only minimally affected while cardiac output is significantly increased (83).

Dobutamine infusion is generally associated with decreases in central venous pressure, right and left atrial pressures, pulmonary artery pressure and resistance, and pulmonary capillary wedge pressure (83). Consequently, left ventricular end-diastolic volume (preload, represented by left ventricular end-diastolic pressure) is lowered, allowing the enlarged myocardium characteristic of congestive heart failure to reduce to a more efficient size (134). The decrease in left ventricular end-systolic volume also decreases myocardial wall tension, an important determinant of myocardial oxygen consumption (53).

For doses of isoproterenol and dobutamine that produce comparable increases in cardiac output, larger decreases in total peripheral vascular resistance and, hence, greater reductions in blood pressure are observed with isoproterenol (134). In addition, tachycardia is more pronounced with isoprotere-

nol (5), resulting from a greater direct positive chronotropic effect and an additional reflex increase in cardiac rate secondary to the greater reduction in vascular tone. The more profound increase in cardiac rate observed with isoproterenol than with dobutamine, at doses that produce equivalent increases in cardiac output, indicates that a smaller contribution to cardiac output is derived from augmentation of stroke volume with isoproterenol than with dobutamine.

When dopamine and dobutamine are infused at doses that produce equivalent increases in cardiac output, dobutamine is generally associated with greater reductions in left ventricular filling pressure and pulmonary capillary wedge pressure (83). Quite commonly, dopamine is associated with no change or even an increase in pulmonary artery pressure, pulmonary capillary wedge pressure, and left ventricular end-diastolic pressure. Whereas dobutamine tends to have minimal effects on blood pressure, dopamine is more likely to produce an increase in total peripheral vascular resistance and mean arterial blood pressure (83). At low doses, dopamine has been shown to produce a selective increase in renal blood flow, secondary to a decrease in renal vascular resistance (48). This action of dopamine, which is lacking with dobutamine, has been ascribed to selective renal vasodilation resulting from activation of renal DA_1-dopamine receptors. In contrast, the improvement in renal function observed with dobutamine appears to be secondary to an increase in cardiac output and a reflex decrease in total peripheral vascular resistance (83).

At doses that produce comparable increases in cardiac output, epinephrine and norepinephrine cause more tachycardia and greater increases in total peripheral vascular resistance than dobutamine. Consequently, dobutamine tends to increase stroke volume while not greatly affecting blood pressure or heart rate, whereas epinephrine and norepinephrine may cause a smaller increase in stroke volume because of the increased impedance to left ventricular ejection resulting from elevation of afterload, the latter serving to limit increases in stroke volume elicited by improved myocardial contractility.

ACKNOWLEDGMENT

I would like to thank Sue Tirri for expert secretarial assistance.

REFERENCES

1. Akhtar N, Mikulik E, Cohn JN, Chaudhry MH: Hemodynamic effect of dobutamine in patients with severe heart failure. *Am J Cardiol* 36:202, 1975.
2. Amann FW, Bolli P, Kiowski W, Buhler FR: Enhanced α-adrenoceptor-mediated vasoconstriction in essential hypertension. *Hypertension* 3(Suppl 1):I119, 1981.
3. Angus JA, Cocks TM, Satoh K: The α-adrenoceptors on endothelial cells. *Fed Proc* 45:2355–2359, 1986.
4. Ariens EJ: The classification of α-adrenoceptors. *Trends Pharmacol Sci* 2:170, 1981.
5. Arnold SB, Williams RL, Ports TA, Benet LZ, Parmley WW, Chatterjee K: Attenuation of prazosin effect on cardiac output in chronic heart failure. *Ann Intern Med* 91:345, 1979.
6. Awan NA, Miller RR, Maxwell KS, Mason DJ: Effects of prazosin on forearm resistance and capacitance vessels. *Pharmacol Ther* 22:79, 1977.
7. Barajas L, Wang P: Localization of tritiated norepinephrine in the renal arteriolar nerves. *Anat Rec* 195:525, 1979.
8. Bertel O, Burkart R, Buhler FR: Sustained effectiveness of chronic prazosin therapy in severe chronic congestive heart failure. *Am Heart J* 5:529, 1981.
9. Bevan JA: Autonomic pharmacologist's guide to the cerebral circulation. *Trends Pharmacol Sci* 5:234–236, 1986.

10. Bevan JA: Sites of transition between functional systemic and cerebral arteries of rabbits occur at embryological junctional sites. *Science* 204:635–637, 1979.

11. Bolli P, Erne P, Ji BH, Block LH, Kiowski W, Buhler FR: Adrenaline induces vasoconstriction through postjunctional alpha₂-adrenoceptors and this response is enhanced in patients with essential hypertension. *J Hypertens* 2(Suppl 3):115–118, 1984.

12. Bolli P, Erne P, Kiowski W, Ji BH, Amann FW, Buhler FR: Important contribution of post-junctional α₂-adrenoceptor-mediated vasoconstriction to arteriolar tone in man. *J Hypertens* 1(Suppl 2):257, 1983.

13. Bousquet P, Guertzenstein PG: Localization of the central cardiovascular action of clonidine. *Br J Pharmacol* 49: 573–579, 1973.

14. Bristow MR: The adrenergic nervous system in heart failure. *N Engl J Med* 311:850, 1984.

15. Bristow MR, Ginsberg R, Minobe WA, Harrison DC, Reitz BA, Stinson EB: β-Adrenergic receptor measurements in normal and failing human right and left ventricle. *Circulation* 66(Suppl II):II207, 1982.

16. Broadley KJ: Cardiac adrenoceptors. *J Auton Pharmacol* 2:119–145, 1982.

17. Brodde O-E, Motomura S, Endoh M, Schumann HJ: Lack of correlation between the positive inotropic effect evoked by α-adrenoceptor stimulation and the levels of cyclic AMP and/or cyclic GMP in the isolated ventricle strip of the rabbit. *J Mol Cell Cardiol* 10:207–219, 1978.

18. Brown MJ: The role of adrenaline in essential hypertension in man. In Bevan JA, Godfraind T, Maxwell RA, Worcel M (eds): *Proceedings of the Vascular Neuroeffector Symposium*, IRL Press, Oxford, 1985.

19. Brown MJ, Brown DC, Murphy MB: Hypokalemia from β₂-adrenoceptor stimulation by circulating epinephrine. *N Engl J Med* 309:1414, 1983.

20. Brown MJ, Macquin I: Is adrenaline the cause of essential hypertension? *Lancet* ii:1079, 1981.

21. Buhler FR, Laragh JH, Baer JH, Vaughn ED, Brunner HR: Propranolol inhibition of renin secretion. A specific approach to the diagnosis and treatment of renin-dependent hypertensive disease. *N Engl J Med* 287:1209, 1972.

22. Clifton CG, O'Neill WM, Wallin JD: Tiamenidine, a new antihypertensive agent: efficacy, safety and rebound hypertension. *Curr Ther Res* 30:397–404, 1981.

23. Cocks TM, Angus JA: Endothelium-dependent relaxation of coronary arteries by noradrenaline and serotonin. *Nature* 305:627–630, 1983.

24. Cohn JN, Levine TB, Olivari MM, Garberg V, Luva D, Francis GS, Simon AB, Rector T: Plasma norepinephrine as a guide to prognosis in patients with chronic congestive heart failure. *N Engl J Med* 311:819, 1984.

25. Conway EL, Louis WJ, Jarrott B: The effect of acute α-methyldopa administration on catecholamine levels in anterior hypothalamic and medullary nuclei in rat brain. *Neuropharmacology* 18:279–286, 1979.

26. Cooke JH, Johns EJ, MacLeod JH, Singer B: Effect of renal nerve stimulation, renal blood flow and adrenergic blockade on plasma renin activity in the cat. *J Physiol* 226:15–36, 1972.

27. Cutter WE, Bier DM, Shah SD, Cryer PE: Epinephrine plasma clearance rates and physiologic thresholds for metabolic and hemodynamic actions in man *J Clin Invest* 66:94–101, 1980.

28. Davey MJ: Relevant features of the pharmacology of prazosin. *J Cardiovasc Pharmacol* 2(Suppl 3):S287, 1980.

29. Davis DS, Wingl LMH, Reid JL, Neill E, Tippett P, Dollery CT: Pharmacokinetics and concentration-effect relationships of intravenous and oral clonidine. *Clin Pharmacol Ther* 21:593–600, 1977.

30. Day MD, Roach AG: Cardiovascular effects of dopamine after central administration into conscious cats. *Br J Pharmacol* 58:505, 1976.

31. DeMey J, Vanhoutte PM: Uneven distribution of postjunctional α₁- and α₂-like adrenoceptors in canine arterial and venous smooth muscle. *Circ Res* 48:875–884, 1981.

32. Docherty JR, Hyland L: Neuro-effector transmission through postsynaptic α₂-adrenoceptors in human saphenous vein. *Br J Pharmacol* 83:362P, 1984.

33. Dorward PK, Korner PI: Effect of propranolol on renal sympathetic baroreflex properties and aortic baroreceptor activity. *Eur J Pharmacol* 52:61, 1978.

34. Drew GM, Whiting SB: Evidence for two distinct types of postsynaptic α-adrenoceptor in vascular smooth muscle in vivo. *Br J Pharmacol* 67:207–215, 1979.

35. Duckles SP: Functional activity of the noradrenergic innervation of large cerebral arteries. *Br J Pharmacol* 69:193–199, 1980.

36. Egleme C, Godfraind T, Miller RC: Enhanced responsiveness of isolated rat aorta to clonidine after removal of the endothelial cells. *Br J Pharmacol* 81:16–18, 1984.

37. Engberg G, Elam M, Svensson TH: Clonidine withdrawal: activation of brain noradrenergic neurons with specifically reduced α₂-receptor sensitivity. *Life Sci* 30:235–243, 1982.

38. Feigl EO: Sympathetic control of coronary circulation. *Circ Res* 20:262–270, 1967.

39. Flavahan NA, Rimele TJ, Cooke JP, Vanhoutte PM: Characterization of post-junctional α₁- and α₂-adrenoceptors activated by exogenous or nerve-released norepinephrine in the canine saphenous vein. *J Pharmacol Exp Ther* 230:699–705, 1984.

40. Flavahan NA, Vanhoutte PM: Alpha₁ and α₂-adrenoceptor: response coupling in canine saphenous and femoral veins. *J Pharmacol Exp Ther* 238:131–138, 1986.

41. Flavahan NA, Vanhoutte PM: The effect of cooling on α₁- and α₂-adrenergic responses in canine saphenous and femoral veins. *J Pharmacol Exp Ther* 238:139–147, 1986.

42. Frisk-Holmberg M, Paalzow L, Wibell L: Relationship between the cardiovascular effects and steady-state kinetics of clonidine in hypertension. *Eur J Clin Pharmacol* 26:309–313, 1984.

43. Furchgott RF, Zawadzki JV: The obligatory role of endothelial cells in the relaxation of arterial smooth muscle by acetylcholine. *Nature* 288:373, 1980.

44. Gellai M, Ruffolo RR Jr: Renal effects of selective α₁- and α₂-adrenoceptor agonists in conscious, normotensive rats. *J Pharmacol Exp Ther* 240:723–728, 1987.

45. Gerold M, Haesler G: Alpha₂-adrenoceptors in rat resistance vessels. *Naunyn-Schmiedebergs Arch Pharmacol* 322:29–33, 1983.

46. Giles TD, Thomas MG, Sander GE, Quiroz AC: Central α-adrenergic agonists in chronic heart failure and ischemic heart disease. *J Cardiovasc Pharmacol* 7(Suppl 8):S51–S55, 1985.

47. Glusa E, Markwardt F: Characterization of α₂-adrenoceptors on blood platelets from various species using [³H]-yohimbine. *Haemostasis* 13:96–101, 1983.

48. Goldberg LI, Hsieh YY, Resnekov L: Newer catecholamines for treatment of heart failure and shock: an update on dopamine and a first look at dobutamine. *Prog Cardiovasc Dis* 19:327, 1977.

49. Goldstein DS: Plasma catecholamines and essential hypertension: an analytical review. *Hypertension* 5:86, 1983.

50. Govier WC: A positive inotropic effect of phenylephrine mediated through α-adrenergic receptors. *Life Sci* 6:1361–1365, 1967.

51. Graham RM, Pettinger WA, Sagalowsky A, et al: Renal α-adrenergic receptor abnormality in the spontaneously hypertensive rat. *Hypertension* 4:881, 1982.

52. Granger DN, Richardson PDI, Kvietys PR, Mortillaro NA: Intestinal blood flow. *Gastroenterology* 78:837–863, 1980.

53. Gross GJ, Urquilla PR: Antianginal drugs. In Craig CR, Stitzel RE (eds): *Modern Pharmacology*. Boston, Little, Brown, 1982, pp 283–294.

54. Hansson L: Clinical aspects of blood pressure crisis due to withdrawal of centrally acting antihypertensive drugs. *Br J Clin Pharmacol* 15:485S–489S, 1973.

55. Hansson L, Hunyor SN, Julius S, Hoobler SW: Blood pressure crisis following withdrawal of clonidine, with special reference to arterial and urinary catecholamine levels and suggestions for acute management. *Am Heart J* 85:605–610, 1973.

56. Hashimoto K, Shigel T, Imai S, Saito Y, Yago N, Uei I, Clark RE: Oxygen consumption and coronary vascular tone in the isolated fibrillating dog heart. *Am J Physiol* 198:965–970, 1960.

57. Hepburn ER, Bentley GA: The effects of α-agonists on various vascular beds. In Bevan JA, Godfraind T, Maxwell RA, Vanhoutte PM (eds): *Vascular Neuroeffector Mechanisms*. Raven Press, New York, 1980, pp 249–251.

58. Hesse IFA, Johns EJ: An in vivo study of the α-adrenoceptor subtypes on the renal vasculature of the anaesthetized rabbit. *J Auton Pharmacol* 4:145–152, 1984.

59. Heusch G, Duessen A: The effects of cardiac sympathetic nerve stimulation on perfusion of stenotic coronary arteries in the dog. *Circ Res* 53.8–15, 1983.

60. Heusch G, Deussen A, Schipke J, Thamer V: Alpha₁- and alpha₂-adrenoceptor-mediated vasoconstriction of large and small canine coronary arteries in vivo. *J Cardiovasc Pharmacol* 6:961–968, 1984.

61. Hieble JP, Woodward DF: Different characteristics of postjunctional α-adrenoceptors on arterial and venous smooth muscle. *Naunyn-Schmiedebergs Arch Pharmacol* 328:44–50, 1984.

62. Hiley CR, Thomas GR: Effects of alpha-adrenoceptor agonists on cardiac output and its regional distribution in the pithed rat. *Br J Pharmacol* 90:61–70, 1987.

63. Holtz J, Saeed M, Sommer O, Bassenge E: Norepinephrine constricts the canine coronary bed via postsynaptic α₂-adrenoceptors. *Eur J Pharmacol* 82:199–202, 1982.

64. Horn PT, Kohli JD, Listinsky JJ, Goldberg LI: Regional variation in the α-adrenergic receptors in the canine resistance vessels. *Naunyn-Schmiedebergs Arch Pharmacol* 318:166–172, 1982.

65. Hyman AL, Kadowitz PJ: Evidence for existence of postjunctional α₁- and α₂-adrenoceptors in cat pulmonary vascular bed. *Am J Physiol* 249:H891–H898, 1985.

66. Hyman AL, Lippton HL, Kadowitz PJ: Autonomic regulation of the pulmonary circulation. *J Cardiovasc Pharmacol* 7:S80–S95, 1985.

67. Iversen LL: Catecholamine-sensitive adenylate cyclases in nervous tissue. *J Neurochem* 29:5, 1977.

68. Jewitt D, Mitchell A, Birkhead J, Dollery C: Clinical cardiovascular pharmacology of dobutamine. *Lancet* ii:363, 1974.

69. Jie K, van Brummelen P, Vermey P, Timmermans PBMWM, van Zwieten PA: Alpha₁- and alpha₂-adrenoceptor-mediated vasoconstriction in the forearm of normotensive and hypertensive subjects. *J Cardiovasc Pharmacol* 8:190–196, 1986.

70. Kalkman HO, Thoolen MJMC, Timmermans PBMWM, van Zwieten PA: The influence of α₁- and α₂-adrenoceptor agonists on cardiac output in rats and cats. *J Pharm Pharmacol* 36:265–268, 1984.

71. Keeton TK, Campbell WB: The pharmacologic alteration of renin release. *Pharmacol Rev* 32:81, 1980.

72. Kessar P, Saggerson ED: Evidence that catecholamines stimulate renal gluconeogenesis through an α_1-type of adrenoceptor. *Biochem J* 190:119, 1980.

73. Kho TL, Schalekamp MADH, Zaal GA, Wester A, Birkenhager WH: Comparison between the effects of St 600 and clonidine. *Arch Intern Pharmacodyn* 217:162–169, 1975.

74. Kobinger W: Central α-adrenergic system as targets for hypotensive drugs. *Rev Physiol Biochem Pharmacol* 81:39, 1978.

75. Kopia GA, Kopaciewicz LJ, Ruffolo RR Jr: α-Adrenoceptor regulation of coronary artery blood flow in normal and stenotic canine coronary arteries. *J Pharmacol Exp Ther* 239:641–647, 1986.

76. Korner PI: Discussion to: systemic hemodynamic effects of centrally acting antihypertensive agents. In Onesti G, Fernandes M, Kim E (eds): *Regulation of Blood Pressure by the Central Nervous System*. Grune & Stratton, New York, p 412, 1976.

77. Korner PI, Angus JA: Central nervous control of blood pressure in relation to antihypertensive drug treatment. *Pharmacol Ther* 13:321, 1981.

78. Krothapalli RK, Suki W: Functional characterization of the α-adrenergic receptor modulating the hydroosmotic effect of vasopressin on the rabbit cortical collecting tubule. *J Clin Invest* 73:740, 1984.

79. Langer SZ: Presynaptic receptors and their role in the regulation of transmitter release. *Br J Pharmacol* 60:481, 1977.

80. Langer SZ, Shepperson NB: Postjunctional α_1- and α_2-adrenoceptors: preferential innervation of α_1-adrenoceptors and the role of neuronal uptake. *J Cardiovasc Pharmacol* 4:S8–S13, 1982.

81. Langer SZ, Shepperson BN: Recent developments in vascular smooth muscle pharmacology: the postsynaptic α_2-adrenoceptor. *Trends Pharmacol Sci* 3:440–444, 1982.

82. Langer SZ, Shepperson NB, Massingham R: Preferential noradrenergic innervation of α_1-adrenergic receptors in vascular smooth muscle. *Hypertension* 3(Suppl I):I112–I118, 1981.

83. Leier CV, Unverferth DV: Dobutamine. *Ann Intern Med* 99:490, 1983.

84. Levine TB, Francis GS, Goldsmith SR: Activity of the sympathetic nervous system assessed by plasma hormone levels and their relation to hemodynamic abnormalities in congestive heart failure. *Am J Cardiol* 49:1659–1666, 1982.

85. Lewis PJ, Haeusler G: Reduction in sympathetic nervous activity as a mechanism for hypotensive effect of propranolol. *Nature* 256:440, 1975.

86. Liang CS, Hood WB: Dobutamine infusion in conscious dogs with and without autonomic nervous system inhibition: effects of systemic hemodynamics, regional blood flows and cardiac metabolism. *J Pharmacol Exp Ther* 211:698, 1979.

87. Majewski H, Hedler L, Starke K: The noradrenaline release rate in the anesthetized rabbit: facilitation by adrenaline. *Naunyn-Schmiedebergs Arch Pharmacol* 321:20, 1982.

88. Majewski H, Rand MJ, Tung LH: Activation of prejunctional β-adrenoceptors in rat atria by adrenaline applied exogenously or released as a co-transmitter. *Br J Pharmacol* 73:669, 1981.

89. Majewski H, Tung LH, Rand MJ: Adrenaline activation of prejunctional β-adrenoceptors and hypertension. *J Cardiovasc Pharmacol* 4:99, 1982.

90. Majewski H, Tung LH, Rand MJ: Adrenaline-induced hypertension in rats. J Cardiovasc Pharmacol 3:179, 1981.

91. Matsuda H, Kuon E, Holtz J, Busse R: Endothelium-mediated dilations contribute to the polarity of the arterial wall in vasomotion induced by α_2-adrenergic agonists. *J Cardiovasc Pharmacol* 7:680–688, 1985.

92. McCalden TA: Sympathetic control of the cerebral circulation. *J Auton Pharmacol* 1:421–431, 1981.

93. Medgett IC, Hicks PE, Langer SZ: Smooth muscle α_2-adrenoceptors mediate vasoconstrictor responses to exogenous norepinephrine and to sympathetic stimulation to a greater extent in spontaneously hypertensive than in Wistar Kyoto rat tail arteries. *J Pharmacol Exp Ther* 231:159, 1984.

94. Meier M, Orwin J, Rogg H, Brunner H: β-Adrenoceptor antagonists in hypertension. In Scriabine A (ed): *Pharmacology of Antihypertensive Drugs*. Raven Press, New York, pp 179–194, 1980.

95. Montastruc J-L, Montastruc P: Effect of intracisternal application of 6-hydroxydopamine on the antihypertensive action of propranolol in the dog. *Eur J Pharmacol* 63:103, 1980.

96. Muller-Schweinitzer E: Alpha-adrenoceptors, 5-hydroxytryptamine receptors and the action of dihydroergotamine in human venous preparations obtained during saphenectomy procedures for varicose veins. *Naunyn-Schmiedeberg's Arch Pharmacol* 327:299–303, 1984.

97. Nichols AJ, Hiley CR: Identification of adrenoceptors and dopamine receptors mediating vascular responses in the superior mesenteric arterial bed of the rat. *J Pharm Pharmacol* 37:110–115, 1985.

98. Ogasawara B, Ogawa K, Hayashi H, Sassa H: Plasma renin activity and plasma concentration of norepinephrine and cyclic nucleotides in heart failure after prazosin. *Clin Pharmacol Ther* 29:464, 1981.

99. Ohlstein EH, Shebuski RJ, Ruffolo RR Jr: Localization of α_2-adrenoceptors in the canine pulmonary vasculature. *Pharmacologist* 28:141, 1986.

100. Onesti G, Schwartz AB, Kim KE: Antihypertensive effect of clonidine. *Circ Res* 28(Suppl 2):53–69, 1971.

101. Oswald H, Greven J: Effects of adrenergic activators and inhibitors on kidney function. In Syekeres L (ed): *Handbook of Experimental Pharmacology*. Springer-Verlag, Berlin, vol 54, pp 241–288, 1981.

102. Palmer RMJ, Ferrige AG, Moncade S: Nitric oxide release accounts for the biological activity of endothelium derived relaxing factor. *Nature* 327:524–526, 1987.

103. Patel P, Bose D, Greenway C: Effects of prazosin and phenoxybenzamine on α- and β-receptor mediated responses in intestinal resistance and capacitance vessels. *J Cardiovasc Pharmacol* 3:1050–1059, 1981.

104. Pettinger WA, Gandler T, Sanchez A, et al: Dietary sodium and renal α-adrenoceptors in Dahl hypertensive rats. *Clin Exp Hypertension* A4(4 and 5):819, 1982.

105. Pitt B, Elliot EC, Gregg DE: Adrenergic receptor activity in the coronary arteries of the unanesthetized dog. *Circ Res* 21:75–84, 1967.

106. Raab W, Gigee W: Die katecholamine des herzens. *Naunyn-Schmiedeberg's Arch Pharmacol* 219:248, 1953.

107. Reid JL: Central α_2-receptors and the regulation of blood pressure in humans. *J Cardiovasc Pharmacol* 7(Suppl 8):S45–S50, 1985.

108. Reid JL, Rubin PC, Howden CW: Central α_2-adrenoceptors and blood pressure regulation in man: studies with guanfacine (BS 100–141) and azapexole (B-HT 933). *Br J Clin Pharmacol* 15(Suppl 4):463–469, 1983.

109. Reis DJ: The brain and hypertension: reflections on 35 years of inquiry into the neurobiology of the circulation. *Circulation* 70:III31, 1984.

110. Rosendorff C, Mitchell G, Scriven DR, Shapiro C: Evidence for a dual innervation affecting local blood flow in the hypothalamus of the conscious rabbit. *Circ Res* 38:140–145, 1976.

111. Rubin SA, Chatterjee K, Gelberg HJ, Ports TA, Brundage BH, Parmley WW: Paradox of improved exercise but not resting hemodynamics with short term prazosin in chronic heart failure. *Am J Cardiol* 43:810, 1979.

112. Ruffolo RR Jr: α-Adrenoceptors. *Monogr Neural Sci* 10:224–253, 1984.

113. Ruffolo RR Jr: Distribution and function of peripheral α-adrenoceptors in the cardiovascular system. *Pharmacol Biochem Behav* 22:827–833, 1985.

114. Ruffolo RR Jr: Relative agonist potency as a means of differentiating α-adrenoceptors and α-adrenergic mechanisms. *Clin Sci* 68(Suppl 10):9S–14S, 1985.

115. Ruffolo RR Jr: Stereochemical requirements for activation and blockade of α_1- and α_2-adrenoceptors. *Trends Pharmacol Sci* 5:160–164, 1984.

116. Ruffolo RR Jr: Structure-activity relationships of α-adrenoceptor agonists. In Kunos G (ed): *Adrenoceptors and Catecholamine Action, Part B*. John Wiley & Sons, New York, pp 1–50, 1983.

117. Ruffolo RR Jr, Kopia GA: The importance of receptor regulation in the pathophysiology and therapy of congestive heart failure. *Am J Med* 80(Suppl 2B):67–72, 1986.

118. Ruffolo RR Jr, Morgan EL: Interaction of novel inotropic agent, ASL-7022, with α- and β-adrenoceptors in the cardiovascular system of the pithed rat: comparison with dobutamine and dopamine. *J Pharmacol Exp Ther* 229:364, 1984.

119. Ruffolo RR Jr, Nichols AJ, Hieble JP: Functions mediated by α_2-adrenergic receptors. In Limbird L (ed): *The α-Adrenergic Receptors*. Clifton, NJ, Humana Press, pp 187–280, 1988.

120. Ruffolo RR Jr, Zeid RL: Relationship between α-adrenoceptors occupancy and response for the α-adrenoceptor agonist, cirazoline, and the α_2-adrenoceptor agonist, B-HT 933, in canine saphenous vein. *J Pharmacol Exp Ther* 235:636–643, 1985.

121. Sawyer R, Warnock P, Docherty JR: Role of vascular α_2-adrenoceptors as targets for circulating catecholamines in the maintenance of blood pressure in anesthetized spontaneously hypertensive rats. *J Cardiovasc Pharmacol* 7:809–812, 1985.

122. Schmitt H: Action des α-sympathomimetiques sur les structures nerveuses. *Actual Pharmacol* 24:93–131, 1971.

123. Schmitt H, Schmitt H: Localization of the hypotensive effect of 2-(2,6-dichlorophenylamino)-2-imidazoline hydrochloride. *Eur J Pharmacol* 6:8–12, 1969.

124. Schmitz JM, Graham KM, Saglowsky A, Pettinger WA: Renal α_1- and α_2-adrenergic receptors: biochemical and pharmacological correlations. *J Pharmacol Exp Ther* 219:400–406, 1981.

125. Scholtysik G: Pharmacology of guanfacine. *Br J Clin Pharmacol* 10:21S–24S, 1980.

126. Schultz HS, Chertien SD, Brewer DD, Eltorai MT, Weber MA: Centrally acting antihypertensive agents: a comparison of lofexidine with clonidine. *J Clin Pharmacol* 21:65–71, 1981.

127. Schumann HJ, Endoh M, Brodde O-E: The time course of the effects of β- and α-adrenoceptor stimulation by isoprenaline and methoxamine on the contractile force and cAMP level of the isolated rabbit papillary muscle. *Arch Pharmacol* 289:291–302, 1975.

128. Segstro R, Greenway C: α-Receptor subtype mediating sympathetic mobilization of blood from the hepatic venous system in anesthetized cats. *J Pharmacol Exp Ther* 236:224, 1986.

129. Shebuski RJ, Fujita T, Ruffolo RR Jr: Evaluation of α_1- and α_2-adrenoceptor-mediated vasoconstriction in the in situ, autoperfused, pulmonary circulation of the anesthetized dog. *J Pharmacol Exp Ther* 238:217–223, 1986.

130. Shebuski RJ, Ohlstein EH, Smith JM Jr, Ruffolo RR Jr: Enhanced pulmonary α_2-adrenoceptor responsiveness under conditions of elevated pulmonary vascular tone. *J Pharmacol Exp Ther* 242:158–165, 1987.

131. Shepperson NB, Langer SZ: The effects of the 2-amino-tetrahydronaphthalene derivative, M7, a selective α_2-adrenoceptor agonist in vitro. *Naunyn-Schmiedeberg's Arch Pharmacol* 318:10–13, 1981.

132. Shoji T, Tsuru H, Shigei T: A regional difference in the distribution of postsynaptic α_2-adrenoceptor subtypes in canine veins. *Nuanyn-Schmiedeberg's Arch Pharmacol* 324:246–255, 1983.

133. Smyth DD, Umemura S, Pettinger WA: α_2-Adrenoceptors and sodium reabsorption in the isolated perfused rat kidney. *Am J Physiol* 247:F680–F685, 1985.

134. Sonnenblick EH, Frishman WH, LeJemtel TH: Dobutamine: a new synthetic cardioactive sympathetic amine. *N Engl J Med* 300:17, 1979.

135. Stanaszek WF, Kellerman D, Brogden RN, Romankiewicz JA: Prazosin update—a review of its pharmacological properties and therapeutic use in hypertension and congestive heart failure. *Drugs* 25:339, 1983.

136. Stokes GS, Marwood JF: Review of the use of α-adrenoceptor antagonists in hypertension. *Methods Find Exp Clin Pharmacol* 6:197, 1984.

137. Summers RJ, McPherson GA: Radioligand studies of α-adrenoceptors in the kidney. *Trends Pharmacol Sci* 3:291, 1982.

138. Thomas JA, Marks BH: Plasma norepinephrine in congestive heart failure. *Am J Cardiol* 41:233, 1978.

139. Thoolen JMC, Timmermans PBMWM, van Zwieten PA: Cardiovascular effects of withdrawal of some centrally acting antihypertensive drugs in the rat. *Br J Clin Pharmacol* 15:491S–505S, 1983.

140. Timmermans PBMWM, Hoefke W, Stahle H, van Zwieten PA: Structure-activity relationships in clonidine-like imidazolidines and related compounds. *Prog Pharmacol* 3:1–104, 1980.

141. van Meel JCA, deJonge A, Timmermans PBMWM, van Zwieten PA: Selectivity of some alpha-adrenoceptor agonists for peripheral alpha-1 and alpha-2 adrenoceptors in the normative pithed rat. *J Pharmacol Exp Ther* 219:760–767, 1981.

142. van Zwieten PA: Pharmacology of centrally acting hypotensive drugs. *Br J Clin Pharmacol* 10:13S–20S, 1980.

143. van Zwieten PA, Thoolen MJMC, Timmermans PBMWM: The pharmacology of centrally acting antihypertensive drugs. *Br J Clin Pharmacol* 15:455S–462S, 1983.

144. Wilffert B, Timmermans PBMWM, van Zwieten PA: Extrasynaptic location of α_2- and noninnervation β_2-adrenoceptors in the vascular system of the pithed normotensive rat. *J Pharmacol Exp Ther* 221:762–768, 1982.

145. Yamaguchi I, Kopin IJ: Differential inhibition of α_1- and α_2-adrenoceptor-mediated pressor responses in pithed rats. *J Pharmacol Exp Ther* 214:275–281, 1980.

146. Zandberg P, Timmermans PBMWM, van Zwieten PA: Hemodynamic profiles of methoxamine and B-HT 933 in spinalized ganglion-blocked dogs. *J Cardiovasc Pharmacol* 6:256–262, 1984.

CHAPTER 10

Therapeutic Drug Monitoring

BERTIL K.J. WAGNER, Pharm.D.
DAVID M. ANGARAN, M.S., F.C.C.P., F.A.S.H.P.
DAVID W. FUHS, M.S., Pharm.D.

INTRODUCTION

Critically ill patients often present with varying degrees of organ dysfunction and with metabolic abnormalities that alter drug pharmacokinetics and pharmacodynamics. These changes need to be considered when administering drugs to critically ill patients. Individualized dosing of drugs can improve patient survival and decrease cost of therapy and length of intensive care unit (ICU) stay for critically ill patients (1, 2). In addition, the patient's changing condition requires constant monitoring and adjustment of medications. The drugs used to treat diseases in critically ill patients often have narrow or undefined therapeutic ranges. Drug toxicity may also be exacerbated in these patients due to underlying organ dysfunction. The clinician must have a working knowledge of the pharmacokinetic and pharmacodynamic properties of drugs used in the ICU in order to determine a rational loading dose and maintenance dosing regimen to achieve the desired therapeutic endpoint. The goals of this chapter are to describe changes in drug pharmacokinetic and pharmacodynamic parameters commonly observed in the critically ill patient population, to provide a discussion of pharmacokinetic laboratory considerations, and to elaborate on therapeutic drug monitoring in the ICU.

PHARMACOKINETIC CONCEPTS

Pharmacokinetics defines the movement of drugs within the body and can be subdivided into four categories:

absorption; distribution; metabolism; and excretion. Absorption is the process by which the drug is taken into the body and is dependent both on the agent's physiochemic properties and the route of administration. Bioavailability is defined as the rate and extent of drug absorption into the systemic circulation. Drug distribution describes the movement of the drug within the body following absorption and is influenced primarily by drug molecular size, degree of ionization, tissue perfusion, and plasma and tissue drug-protein binding. The term "apparent volume of distribution" (V_d) defines the relationship between blood or plasma drug concentrations (C) and the total amount of drug in the body (A). This relationship is expressed as $A = C/V_d$. Drugs with a small V_d (<0.6 liters/kg) are distributed primarily into body water (3). The elimination of drug from the body may occur through metabolism, excretion, or both. Hepatic biotransformation, the major route of drug metabolism, is primarily dependent on liver blood flow, drug plasma protein binding, and the hepatocytes' ability to clear drug, i.e., the intrinsic clearance. The kidney represents the major route of elimination of drugs and drug metabolites. A number of drugs are also metabolized by the lungs or plasma enzymes. Some drugs also undergo biliary elimination to be excreted in the feces or reabsorbed at a later stage in the small intestine, i.e., enterohepatic recycling. Drug clearance is defined in terms of the rate of the blood or plasma volume that can be cleared of drug per unit time. The elimination rate (k_e) constant describes the rate of disappearance of drug from the blood and is dependent on total body clearance (Cl_{TB}) and the volume of distribution (V_d). This relationship can be expressed as $k_e = Cl/V_d$. The drug's half-life ($t_{1/2}$) describes the time it takes for a drug's concentration to decrease by 50% and is related to the elimination rate as follows: $t_{1/2} = 0.693/k_e$.

The pharmacokinetic parameters—half-life, clearance, and volume of distribution—are very useful in therapeutic drug monitoring. Most pharmacokinetic formulas are useful only when steady-state or near steady-state conditions are present. The half-life can be used to determine the time until steady-state drug concentrations have been achieved, when the rate of drug input is equal to the rate of drug elimination. Given constant dosing, it takes four to five half-lives until 90 to 95% steady-state has been achieved (3). For example, in a healthy adult, plasma concentrations of theophylline or digoxin following constant dosing, will plateau after a period of 1 to 2 or 6 to 8 days, respectively (4, 5).

An estimate of the volume of distribution can be used to determine drug loading doses. Loading doses do not alter the time until achievement of steady-state conditions (Fig. 10.1) but are often used to provide concentrations in the therapeutic range from the onset with drugs that have long half-lives. Half-lives can also be used to determine the time course of drug toxicity for drugs with a clear concentration-effect relationship, e.g., theophylline, and when drug dosing should be reinstated following toxicity. Clearance (*Cl*) can be used to predict average drug concentrations (*Cave*$_{ss}$) during steady-state drug administration, where the dose (*D*) and dosing interval (τ) are constant. This relationship can be expressed as Dose/τ = *Cl* x *Cave*$_{ss}$ and is often used for quick determination of a new dosing regimen given steady-state conditions (3).

EFFECT OF CRITICAL ILLNESS ON DRUG PHARMACOKINETICS

CIRCULATORY FAILURE

Circulatory failure occurs when there is insufficient blood flow to meet tissue oxygen demand. Causes of circulatory failure include trauma, hypertension, surgery, infection, myocardial infarction resulting in arrhythmias, hemorrhage, and organ failure. The body acutely responds to circulatory failure with increased sympathetic tone and local autoregulation of blood flow. Attempts to increase myocardial contractility, by the use of inotropic agents, may or may not be adequate to meet tissue oxygen demand. In addition, vasoconstriction in muscle, skin, and splanchnic organs decreases the amount of blood flow to these areas, and vasodilation of vascular beds in the brain and heart maintains blood flow to these vital organs (6). Critically ill patients often require drug therapy, surgery, mechanical ventilation, nutrition, pacemakers, or circulatory assist devices. These therapies and the body's responses to circulatory failure also affect the pharmacokinetics of the drugs used in the ICU (Fig. 10.2) (6).

DRUG ABSORPTION

Critically ill patients are often unable to take medication by mouth because of slow or incomplete absorption, an inability to swallow due to altered consciousness, intubation, frequent nasogastric suctioning, or an ileus. Likewise, topical,

subcutaneous, and intramuscular administration may produce delayed or variable serum concentrations (6). Therefore, the intravenous route is most commonly used in the ICU, resulting in immediate and complete drug absorption. During cardiac arrest, when an intravenous route may not be available, the endotracheal route can be effectively used for lidocaine, epinephrine, naloxone, and atropine (7). In fact, the endotracheal administration of β-agonists results in enhanced therapeutic effect and less systemic side effects (8).

The oral absorption of drugs in patients with end-stage renal disease may be markedly decreased due to a higher gastric pH, binding to antacids, and decreased gastrointestinal motility. The absorption of ranitidine following an oral dose was shown to be delayed in renal failure (9). The rate and extent of drug absorption are decreased in patients with congestive heart failure due to poor gut perfusion (10). Liver disease and portal hypertension may decrease first-pass metabolism of drugs, resulting in enhanced bioavailability (11). The absorption of drugs administered by subcutaneous injection is delayed if the injection site is edematous, or if there are alterations in circulation (12).

The intravenous administration of drugs by use of continuous infusions can result in error. Most automatic infusion pumps are very accurate, within 5 to 10% (13). In addition, they alert the user in cases of sudden changes in flow and allow for preset volumes to be infused. These safeguards decrease the risk for inadvertent, gravity-fed, excessive infusion rates and subcutaneous extravasation. However, infusion pump failure and line obstructions can occur and may result in sudden changes in patient status. The use of nonautomatic infusion devices may result in significant changes in flow rates (14) and cannot be recommended for infusion of vasoactive medications.

DRUG DISTRIBUTION

Changes in the drug distribution and V_d have been demonstrated in renal disease, hepatic disease, and in the elderly (15). Concentrations of drugs that have a slow distribution phase, such as digoxin, are probably not affected by acute cardiac failure. However, decreased perfusion decreases tissue penetration of drugs with a rapid distribution phase (16). Conversely, the amount of drug that is presented to the brain and heart is higher than normal due to preferential blood flow to these areas. Lidocaine is an example of a rapidly distributing drug that exhibits a smaller volume of distribution in heart failure with elevated concentrations and slower initial tissue distribution, which also explains the central nervous system toxicity seen following single rapid injections of normal doses (17). With chronic circulatory failure and third-spacing of fluids, the V_d of water-soluble drugs increases. This increase may be due to vasodilation, an expanded extracellular fluid volume, or changes in the concentrations and characteristics of the various plasma or tissue binding proteins. Unfortunately, using the aminoglycosides as an example, the magnitude of the increase in V_d in the critically ill is unpredictable but, in general, ICU patients have an increased volume of distribution of 0.3 to 0.35 liters/kg (18). Similar pharmacokinetic changes have been observed with piperacillin in critically ill patients (19).

Figure 10.1. Plasma drug concentrations resulting from an intravenous bolus dose and infusion.

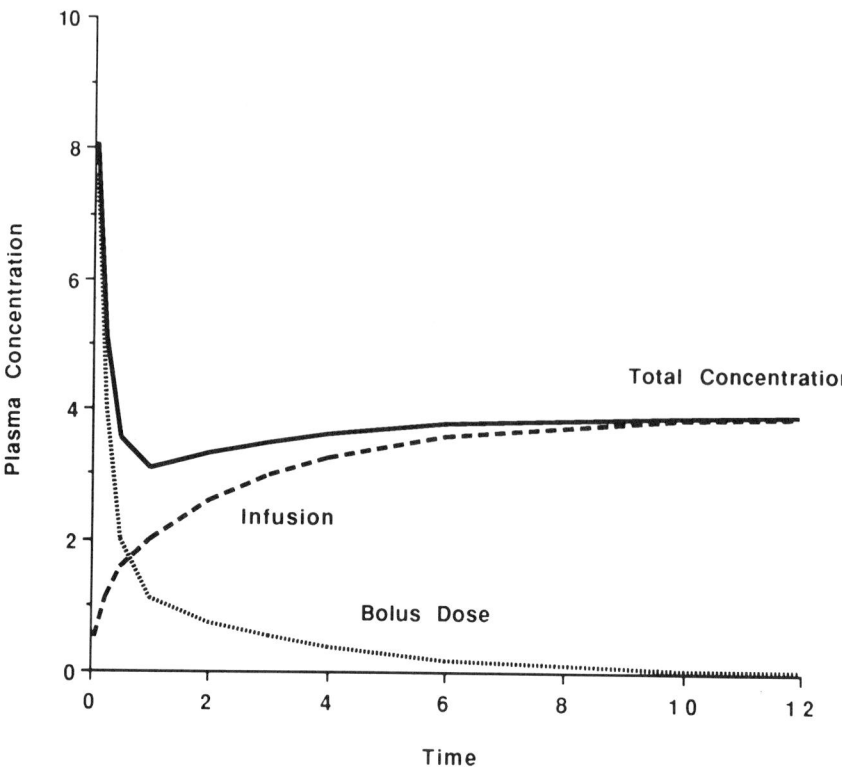

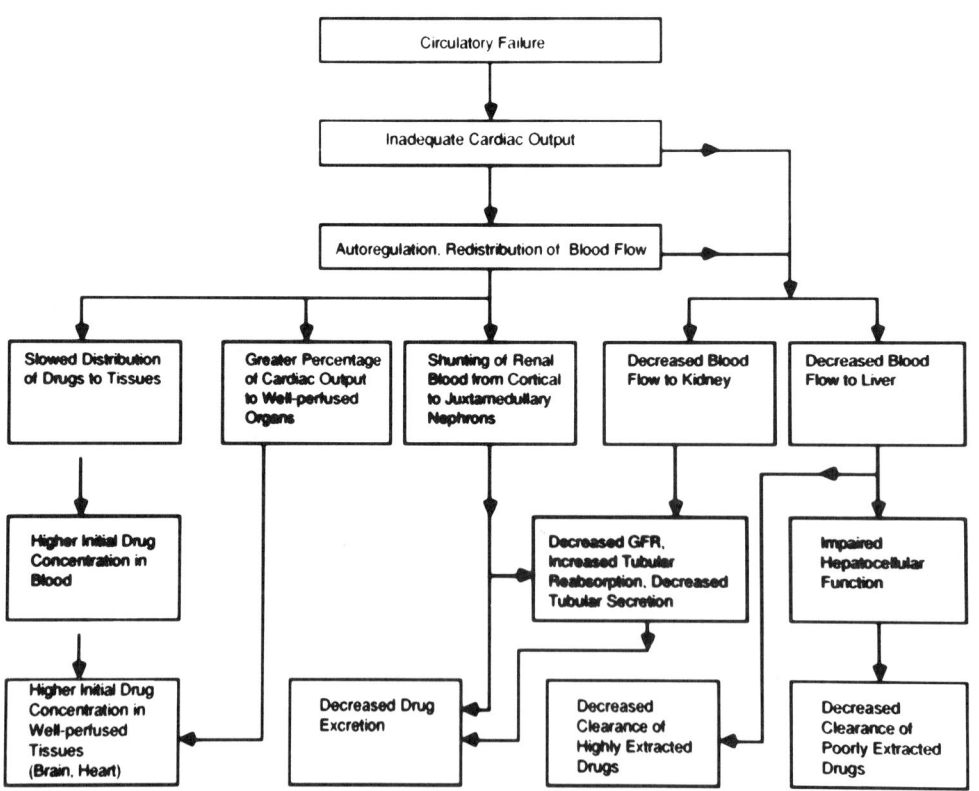

Figure 10.2. Pharmacokinetic consequences of circulatory failure. *GFR*, glomerular filtration rate. (From Pentel P, Benowitz N: Pharmacokinetic and pharmacodynamic considerations in drug therapy of cardiac emergencies. *Clin Pharmacokinet* 9:273–308, 1984. Used with permission of the publisher.)

Table 10.1. Drug Dosage Adjustment in Hepatic Failure

Drug	% Protein Bound	Mechanism	Method of Adjustment
Cefoperazone	90	EL, BS[a]	Decrease dose
Chloramphenicol	70	EL, BS	Decrease dose
Cimetidine	20	FL	Decrease dose if severe
Clindamycin	79	EL, BS	Decrease dose if severe
Diazepam	97	EL, BS	Decrease dose
Erythromycin	80	EL, BS	Decrease dose
Labetalol	50	FL	Decrease dose
Lidocaine	65	FL	Decrease dose
Lorazepam	90	EL, BS	None
Meperidine	65	FL and EL	Decrease dose, avoid if severe
Morphine	35	FL	Decrease dose, avoid if severe
Phenobarbital	50	EL, BI	Decrease dose
Phenytoin	92	EL, BS	Decrease dose
Propranolol	95	FL	Decrease dose
Quinidine	85	FL and EL	Decrease dose
Ranitidine	15	FL	Decrease dose (oral), intravenous (none)
Theophylline	52	EL, BI	Decrease dose
Verapamil	92	FL	Decrease dose

[a] From Mann HJ, Fuhs DW, Cerra FB: Pharmacokinetics and pharmacodynamics in critically ill patients. *World J Surg* 11:210–217, 1987. Used with permission of the publisher.

[b] FL, flow limited; EL, enzyme limited; BI, binding insensitive; BS, binding sensitive.

DRUG METABOLISM

The liver is the major organ responsible for drug metabolism. The kidneys and lungs also metabolize some drugs, while others (adenosine, esmolol, and atracurium) are degraded by enzymes in the blood or the reticuloendothelial system. Hepatocellular function is primarily affected in acute liver disease, while in mild-to-moderate cirrhosis, shunting and alterations in hepatic blood flow predominate (20, 21). Attempts to correlate endogenous substances such as bilirubin with the hepatic clearance of drugs have not been successful. The exogenous substances, antipyrine and indocyanine green, have been used with mixed results but are often not practical at the bedside. Serum drug concentrations and pharmacodynamic effects are used to estimate liver function in the absence of good indicators of hepatic clearance. Some of the hepatically cleared drugs for which serum concentrations are routinely available include theophylline, procainamide, quinidine, phenobarbital, phenytoin, and valproic acid. Drugs cleared by the liver for which serum concentrations are not generally available include β-blockers, verapamil, antipsychotics, benzodiazepines, and narcotics. Therefore, the clinical responses and data from pharmacokinetic studies must be used as dosing guidelines.

Drugs metabolized by the liver are classified as having either a high or low extraction ratio. Drugs with a high extraction ratio are usually not affected by hepatocellular damage because the metabolic capacity is much greater than the rate at which the drug is presented to the liver. The clearance of high extraction drugs is dependent on hepatic blood flow and is also not affected by protein binding. Cirrhotic liver disease can cause a shunting of blood away from the liver, resulting in a decreased clearance of flow-dependent high extraction ratio drugs. Some examples of flow-dependent drugs are lidocaine, meperidine, morphine, metoprolol, midazolam, propranolol, and verapamil (Table 10.1) (22). Liver blood flow is decreased during hypotension, anesthesia, surgery (23), sepsis,

hypoxia, and mechanical ventilation with positive end expiratory pressure (PEEP) (23, 24). Increased catecholamine secretion in the early posttrauma period reduces hepatic blood flow, but after several days, flow is often increased (25, 26). Drugs that improve cardiac output may increase hepatic blood flow, causing an increased clearance of flow-dependent drugs, while vasopressors may decrease the clearance of flow-dependent drugs.

The clearance of low extraction ratio drugs is not dependent on hepatic blood flow but is, instead, highly dependent on protein binding and the intrinsic clearance of the liver (21, 27). Drugs dependent on hepatic enzyme activity for clearance may accumulate due to hypoxia, trauma, hepatocellular damage, or drug-induced depression of enzyme activity. A change in hepatic clearance in liver disease may be seen earlier for drugs with a low intrinsic clearance than for drugs with a high intrinsic clearance (21). Ampicillin, barbiturates, chloramphenicol, diazepam, furosemide, phenytoin, procainamide, theophylline, and warfarin are examples of low extraction ratio drugs. For example, the pharmacokinetics of theophylline were studied in 26 acutely ill patients and compared with those of 31 normal volunteers. The clearance of theophylline was decreased to 43% of normal in patients with congestive heart failure, 37% of normal in patients with pneumonia, and 84% in patients with severe bronchial obstruction (25). The difference in clearance would result in markedly elevated serum theophylline concentrations if dosed according to the standard nomograms based on age and body weight. The pharmacokinetics of theophylline in acutely ill patients are unpredictable and can vary greatly.

Liver disease has also been shown to significantly decrease the hepatic clearance of barbiturates and narcotic analgesics. The half-lives of these drugs are prolonged, and accumulation may occur with continued dosing, so a dose reduction of 50% is recommended (22). The hepatic clearance of diazepam may decrease by 50% in acute viral hepatitis or cirrhosis. Diazepam has active metabolites, but in hepatic failure, the half-life of the parent drug and metabolites is extended. Lorazepam and oxazepam are not affected by acute viral hepatitis or cirrhosis because they do not require oxidative metabolism since the primary metabolic pathway is glucuronidation (22).

The potential problems of racemic mixtures of drugs should be considered. A number of agents (verapamil, bupivacaine, barbiturates, propranolol) are racemic mixtures of enantiomers. These enantiomers have similar physical and chemical properties but may have dissimilar pharmacokinetic and pharmacodynamic properties. The differences stem largely from the ability of the enantiomer to bind to sites of action or metabolizing enzymes. For instance, verapamil is less potent when it is given orally due to stereoselective first-pass metabolism of the more active enantiomer. Oral verapamil will, therefore, exert greater activity in patients with liver cirrhosis. The reverse is observed with propranolol (28). Labetalol is a mixture of four stereoisomers with different α- and β-adrenergic activities. Dilevalol, the R,R-isomer, is responsible for most of the β-blockade whereas the S,R-isomer produces predominantly α-blockade (29). The shift towards β-blocking activity of labetalol following oral administration (30) may be due to enhanced first-pass metabolism of the S,R-isomer.

Critically ill patients receive a large number of medications, and the potential for drug interactions is great. Equimolar amounts of cimetidine and ranitidine, but not famotidine, have been shown to significantly decrease hepatic cytochrome P-450 activity (31). However, the potential drug interactions with ranitidine are less than for cimetidine since lower doses are needed to suppress gastric hydrogen ion secretion. Cimetidine will not affect glucuronidation and will, therefore, not alter the metabolism of drugs such as oxazepam or lorazepam which are eliminated this way (32). Phenobarbital, phenytoin, and carbamazepine stimulate cytochrome P-450 activity and usually lower serum concentrations of drugs that undergo hepatic oxidative metabolism (33). A more complete list of drug interactions can be found elsewhere (34).

PROTEIN BINDING

Albumin and other plasma proteins maintain colloid osmotic pressure and act as carriers for both endogenous and exogenous substances. As a rule, basic drugs bind to α-1-acid glycoprotein and lipoproteins while acidic drugs often bind to albumin (35). Serum concentrations of the acute phase proteins, α-1-acid glycoprotein, haptoglobulin, and C-reactive protein, increase following trauma, surgery, or severe illness, while albumin, prealbumin, and transferrin decrease (36–38). A decrease in the serum concentration of albumin, due to increased capillary permeability, decreased hepatic synthesis, or hemodilution may increase the concentration of unbound drug. The hypoalbuminemia of the nephrotic syndrome or liver disease results in decreased protein binding of drugs. Fatty acidemia and hyperlipidemia can also cause competition for binding sites on the albumin molecule, leading to a higher unbound fraction of various drugs (39). In addition, changes in the binding characteristics of albumin have been demonstrated in hepatic (20) and renal failure (40), perhaps due to competition for binding sites during accumulation of endogenous metabolites. The larger free fraction is then available

for hepatic extraction and renal excretion that may diminish any increased pharmacodynamic effects (35, 40). Changes in protein binding may affect the volume of distribution and the clearance of drugs. Changes in the pH of blood can also affect the protein binding of drugs, but the clinical significance of this is unclear. The serum concentration and pharmacodynamic effect of drugs such as lidocaine, quinidine, propranolol, and verapamil, which bind to the acute-phase proteins, may be altered. For example, the increase in α-1-acid glycoprotein concentrations following myocardial infarction can cause an apparent accumulation of lidocaine during its infusion (41). Despite high measured concentrations of total lidocaine (bound and unbound) in these patients, the lack of toxicity suggests that the unbound active drug concentration is unchanged, or even lower than that in normal patients. However, the decreased plasma protein binding during and after cardiopulmonary bypass surgery may lead to clinically important drug toxicity (42). Phenytoin is another example of a drug exhibiting an increased free fraction in critically ill patients. The total drug concentration may be decreased, but the concentration of free phenytoin may be increased due to hypoalbuminemia and/or uremia (43). Normally, 90% of phenytoin is bound to serum albumin, and 10% is free. The normal therapeutic range for total phenytoin concentrations is 10 to 25 μg/ml and, correspondingly, 1.0 to 2.5 μg/ml for free phenytoin. However, when hypoalbuminemia or uremia is present, the free fraction can increase to 20 or 30%. For instance, if the total phenytoin concentration is only 12 μg/ml, the corresponding free concentration could be as high as 2.4 to 3.6 μg/ml. Because both efficacy and toxicity are related to the free, rather than the total, drug concentration, it would be best to measure the free drug concentration. Technical difficulties have prevented the routine use of free drug concentrations in clinical practice for most drugs other than phenytoin. Table 10.2 lists highly protein-bound drugs that are commonly used in the ICU.

DRUG EXCRETION

Most drugs are excreted by the kidney, either unchanged or following one or more metabolic processes. The lung is another organ responsible for drug elimination, especially for the clearance of anesthetic agents. The lungs also play a significant role in the metabolism of endogenous hormones such as norepinephrine, angiotensin and serotonin (44). In addition, fentanyl, meperidine (45), morphine (46), and lidocaine (47) are taken up by the lungs and may be later released. The clinical significance of pulmonary extraction or metabolism of other drugs and their alteration in disease states is unknown. Drugs that enter the biliary system may be excreted in the feces or undergo reabsorption (enterohepatic recycling). This route of drug excretion is important for neuromuscular blocking agents (48), some antibiotics, digoxin, and imipramine (49). The management of digoxin and antidepressant overdoses by multiple-dose charcoal administration is based on the concept of removing active and metabolite drugs that are eliminated in the bile.

Renal drug excretion is affected by cardiac failure and mechanical ventilation with PEEP when renal blood flow is

Table 10.2. Pharmacokinetic Parameters of and Monitoring Guidelines for Drugs Commonly Used in the Intensive Care Unit 117

Drug	PPB (%)[a]	Active Metabolites	Elimination	Monitoring Guidelines
Antiarrhythmics				
Lidocaine	70	MEGX	Hepatic, metabolite renal	Therapeutic serum concentration 3–6 mg/ml. Initial toxicity with muscle twitching and CNS excitation. Toxicity most common in patients with CHF.
Digoxin	25	None	Renal (60%), hepatic and biliary	Therapeutic serum concentration 0.8–2.5 ng/ml. Monitor ECG (PR prolongation, T wave flattening, ST sloping). DLIS is a problem.
Procainamide	16	NAPA	Hepatic, metabolite renal	Therapeutic serum concentration 4–12 mg/ml. Monitor ECG (QRS prolongation, QT prolongation).
Anticonvulsants				
Phenytoin	90	None	Hepatic	Therapeutic serum concentration 10–20 mg/ml. Monitor free concentration (1–2 mg/ml) if uremic or hypoalbuminemic.
Valproic acid	93	None	Hepatic	Therapeutic serum concentration 30–100 mg/ml
Phenobarbital	51	None	Hepatic	Therapeutic serum concentration 10–25 mg/ml
Antihypertensives				
Nitroprusside		Cyanate thiocyanate	Hepatic, metabolite (T) renal	Maintain serum thiocyanate concentration <10 mg/ml. Monitor if patient has renal insufficiency and is receiving the drug for more than 3 days.
Analgesics and sedatives				
Morphine	35	Morphine-6-glucuronide	Hepatic, metabolite renal	Monitor CNS status. Patients with CHF, cirrhosis, and renal failure are at increased risk for toxicity.
Meperidine	58	Desmethyl-meperidine	Hepatic, metabolite renal	Monitor CNS status. Patients with renal insufficiency are at increased risk for seizures.
Diazepam	>95	Desmethyl-diazepam	Hepatic	Avoid large doses and continuous infusions in patients with liver disease. Rapid injections will produce apnea and hypotension.
Midazolam	>95	α-hydroxy-midazolam	Hepatic	Same as for diazepam. Tolerance is a major problem. Metabolite may accumulate during long-term infusions.
Lorazepam	93	None	Hepatic	Rapid injection will produce apnea and hypotension
Haloperidol	92	Reduced haloperidol	Hepatic	Rapid injection will produce hypotension. Metabolite accumulation is not a problem with short-term use.
Antiasthmatics				
Theophylline	56	None	Hepatic	Therapeutic serum concentration 5–15 mg/ml. Signs of toxicity include tachycardia and hypertension
Antimicrobials				
Aminoglycosides	<10	None	Renal	Renal and ototoxicity. Therapeutic peak serum concentration 4–8 mg/ml. Amikacin (8–16 mg/ml). Avoid trough concentration above 2 and 4 mg/ml, respectively.
Vancomycin	30	None	Renal	Therapeutic peak and trough serum concentration 20–40 and <10 mg/ml, respectively.
Neuromuscular agents[48]				
Pancuronium	30	3-hydroxy-pancuronium	Renal (35%), Metabolite renal and bile	Avoid high doses and prolonged infusions in patients with renal insufficiency. Monitor twitch response, "train of four."
Vecuronium	30–90	3-hydroxy-vecuronium, 3-desacetyl-vecuronium	Mostly bile. Renal (20%)	Same as for pancuronium.
Antiulcer agents				
H$_2$-receptor blockers	20	None	Renal (65%)	Monitor CNS status. Avoid high doses and prolonged infusions with renal insufficiency. Drug interactions (see text)

[a] PPB, plasma protein binding; MEGX, monoethylglycylxylidine; DLIS, digoxin-like immunoreactive substance; NAPA, *n*-acetylprocainamide.

decreased by more than 20%. There is a decrease in glomerular filtration rate and secretion due to decreased blood flow, and an increase in tubular reabsorption may occur. In critically ill patients, these effects may be masked by concomitant failure of the liver or kidneys. Acute renal failure is common in the ICU setting due to sepsis, major surgery (especially cardiovascular), trauma, and nephrotoxins, such as drugs or contrast dye. Renal failure alters pharmacokinetic parameters, and

patients are, therefore, prone to the adverse effects of drugs that accumulate. This increased sensitivity may be due to functional or morphologic modifications of the receptor sites, electrolyte abnormalities, or metabolite accumulation. Acidosis secondary to renal disease can decrease renal tubular reabsorption and slow the degradation of curare-like drugs (50). Meningeal and cerebral permeability are often increased, and there is an increased incidence of clinically significant neurotoxicity in patients with decreased renal function (16). Decreased tissue uptake may also occur in end-stage renal disease (ESRD), as seen with digoxin, in which the myocardial-to-serum digoxin ratio decreases as the glomerular filtration rate (GFR) declines (51). The symptoms of azotemia may be controlled by hemodialysis, peritoneal dialysis, or continuous arteriovenous hemofiltration (52). These methods may be used to clear small molecular weight and water-soluble substances that have a small volume of distribution (53). Continuous arteriovenous hemofiltration clears drugs less efficiently than conventional hemodialysis because of the limited volume of hemofiltrate removed and the lack of a concentration gradient. Hemofiltration clearance is restricted by the free plasma drug concentration and the volume filtered.

DOSE ADJUSTMENT IN RENAL FAILURE

There are two main methods of dosage regimen adjustment in renal failure. Since the drug half-life is increased in renal failure, decreasing the dose and keeping the dosing interval the same should maintain the concentration of the drug in the body. This method is ideal for digoxin since a relatively constant serum concentration is desired. The other method of dosage adjustment is to keep the dose the same but change the dosage interval, which maintains peak and trough concentrations similar to those achieved in normal patients. This method is preferred for aminoglycosides because peak concentrations have been correlated with enhanced bacterial kill power (54), and these drugs also exhibit a significant postantibiotic effect (55). In addition, drug toxicity can be minimized if the trough concentrations are kept at levels less than 2 μg/ml.

Estimates and measurements of the creatinine clearance (CrCl) are often used to approximate the GFR and serve as a guide in dosing patients with varying degrees of renal function. As renal function declines, the kidney secretes creatinine in order to maintain homeostasis, until the GFR reaches 50 ml/min, and the serum creatinine concentration begins to rise. Calculated CrCls are less accurate than measured CrCls in changing renal function, and both methods significantly overestimate the GFR as renal function decreases (56). Clearance measurements may also be unreliable in the cachectic patient with long-standing illness. It is important to recognize the limitations of the CrCl since it is still the most commonly used indicator of renal function for drug dosage adjustment.

The same loading dose is usually given, regardless of the patient's renal function. In fact, it may be more important to give a loading dose to patients with renal failure because the longer half-life prolongs the time to reach an effective steady-state concentration; however, the loading dose should be reduced for anesthetics, sedatives, and hypnotics that are known to cause adverse reactions in patients with renal disease (51). Nomograms have been constructed, suggesting dosage adjustments in patients with varying degrees of renal failure. One of the most comprehensive compilations was published by Bennett (57). Table 10.3 provides the half-life of some common drugs in normal renal function and in patients with ESRD, the suggested method of dosage adjustment, and specific suggestions based on the GFR, which can be approximated by

the CrCl. Several formulas based on age, weight, height, sex, and serum creatinine have been devised to calculate the CrCl (58). These formulas are very easy to use and usually provide a relatively accurate estimate of the patient's renal function. However, these formulas do not accurately predict the CrCl in patients with very poor renal function (CrCl < 10 ml/min) (59). For those patients, a measured 24-hour CrCl is preferable. Shorter collection periods (8 hours) have been shown to be acceptable (60).

The half-life of most drugs that are excreted primarily by the kidney increases slowly until the GFR decreases to less than 30 ml/min when marked increases in half-life and rapid accumulation occur. The metabolites of drugs that are hepatically eliminated will also accumulate in renal failure if they are excreted by the kidney. For example, the accumulation of the normeperidine metabolite of meperidine in renal failure can result in tremor, myoclonus, and seizures (61). Morphine has an active metabolite, morphine-6-glucuronide, which accumulates in renal failure (62). This polar metabolite penetrates the blood-brain barrier and may be a more potent analgesic than the parent compound (63, 64). Pancuronium and vecuronium are metabolized to several active and renally eliminated metabolites that can cause prolonged neuromuscular blockade in patients with renal insufficiency (48). Other drugs commonly used in the ICU that are subject to metabolite accumulation are procainamide (N-acetyl procainamide metabolite), nitroprusside (thiocyanate metabolite), and sulfonamides (N-acetyl metabolites).

Many of the antibiotics used in the ICU are excreted by the kidney and require dosage adjustment in renal failure and a supplemental dose following dialysis. Aminoglycosides, vancomycin, and the semisynthetic penicillins require extra attention. The aminoglycosides are primarily excreted unchanged by the kidney. As renal function declines, the serum aminoglycoside concentrations rise because of decreased renal clearance. The renal tubular damage and subsequent decrease in GFR that can occur with aminoglycoside therapy occurs after several days of treatment. The toxicity is presumably due to high aminoglycoside trough concentrations and the long-term treatment frequently seen in the ICU setting (65). The tissue accumulation of gentamicin and amikacin was studied in 27 critically ill patients, using a 2-compartment pharmacokinetic model to describe the rate and extent of the accumulation. In this matched population, nephrotoxicity was observed in 16% of the patients treated with gentamicin and 20% of the patients who received amikacin (66). In the ICU setting, where rapid swings in renal function, fluid status, and hemodynamic parameters can occur, even the same patient may exhibit very different pharmacokinetic parameters from one day to the next. The most reliable way to adjust the dosage regimen is to measure serum concentrations and individualize the dose (67). In patients with renal failure, the prolonged half-life of the semisynthetic penicillins results in accumulation, which can cause an increased bleeding time (68). The importance of individualized dosing has also been examined for vancomycin. In a study of 37 critically ill patients who were administered vancomycin using a common nomogram for varying renal function, vancomycin serum concentrations were found to be higher than expected (69). The mean peak and trough concentrations observed were 61.2 μg/ml and 22.6

μg/ml. The elimination of half-life was markedly prolonged in patients with a decreased CrCl, and the correlation coefficient between the CrCl and vancomycin clearance was 0.78. There were large interpatient variations in volume of distribution and total body clearance. Individualized vancomycin dosing based on serum concentrations is, therefore, recommended in critically ill patients.

The histamine receptor antagonists are commonly used in the ICU setting for stress ulcer prophylaxis and to treat acute gastrointestinal bleeding. Cimetidine, ranitidine, and famotidine are all filtered at the glomerulus and secreted in the proximal tubules. Concentrations in patients with severe renal impairment are approximately twice as high as in patients with normal renal function, and the elimination half-lives drugs are increased. The adverse effects associated with cimetidine, such as mental confusion and arrhythmias, are much more common in patients with renal impairment (70, 71). The effect of renal failure on drugs that are highly protein-bound is usually a decrease in protein binding. Hypoproteinemia and the elevated blood urea nitrogen level of renal failure result in an elevated free fraction of phenytoin, which can lead to increased toxicity. The increased volume of distribution seen with phenytoin is probably due to the decrease in protein binding. Phenytoin metabolism may also be increased in renal failure due to decreased protein binding and the increased free fraction. While the binding of acidic drugs is usually decreased in renal failure, that of basic drugs may be either decreased or unchanged. Hemodialysis has also shown a variable effect on protein binding, causing an increase (penicillins), a decrease (sulfonamides and phenytoin), or no effect (carbamazepine). If dialysis becomes necessary, the amount of drug lost during the procedure must be considered. Dialyzability is a function of the V_d, molecular weight, lipophilicity, and electric charge. The V_d of a drug may be used as an indicator of how well it will be dialyzed (72): $V_d > 2$ liters/kg = not well dialyzed, V_d 1 to 2 liters/kg = marginally dialyzed, $V_d < 1$ liter/kg = well dialyzed.

Some general recommendations for the dosing of drugs in renal failure are (*a*) use drugs not affected by renal disease or with a wide margin of safety when possible, (*b*) adjust dose based on the best estimate of GFR available, (*c*) measure serum levels and alter dosage using individualized pharmacokinetic parameters, and (*d*) use clinical judgment to evaluate the pharmacodynamic response.

PHARMACODYNAMICS

Pharmacokinetics is defined as the process controlling drug concentrations, at any time, after one or more doses of a drug. It is a function described by both drug concentration and time. Pharmacodynamics is independent of time and describes an equilibrium (time-independent relationship between concentration and effect). A simpler way to differentiate between these two concepts is: pharmacokinetics is what the body does to drugs, and pharmacodynamics is what drugs do to the body (73).

PHARMACODYNAMIC MODELING

The traditional models used to relate drug serum concentrations (SC) to pharmacologic effect are used to define potency (sensitivity of an organ to a drug) and efficacy (the maximum achievable response) during steady-state conditions (74).

One of the classic pharmacodynamic models is the E_{max} model, where $E = E_{max}(C)/(EC_{50} + C)$. The variables are defined as follows: E = effect; C = concentration; E_{max} = maximal effect attributable to the drug; EC_{50} = drug serum concentration producing 50% of E_{max}. This pharmacodynamic model displays a dose-response curve that is hyperbolic in shape and demonstrates the law of diminishing returns. The greatest pharmacologic effects occur at lower drug concentrations, and even greater increases in concentrations are needed to produce comparable changes in effect (Fig. 10.3).

Table 10.3. Drug Dosage Adjustment in Renal Failure[a]

Drug	Half-life Normal	Half-life ESRD	Method of Adjustment	Adjustment Based on Creatinine Clearance >50	10–50	<10	Supplement for Dialysis[b]
Acyclovir	2.5	20	I (D)[c]	8	24	24 (50%)	Yes (H)
Aminoglycosides	2	30	I	8–12	12–18	24–48	Yes (H, P)
Cimetidine	1.8	3.5	I	6	8	12	No
Digoxin	24–36	72–96	D	100%	25–75%	10–25%	No (H, P)
Cephalosporins[d]	1–2	18–36	I	6–8	8–12	24–48	Yes (H, P)
Cefoperazone	1.8	2.1	I		None		Yes (H)
Ceftriaxone	7	12	I		None		No (H)
Cephalosporins[e]	1–2	2–20	I	6–8	8–12	24–48	Yes (H)
Flucytosine	4	75–200	I (D)	6	12–24	24 (50%)	Yes (H)
Nafcillin	0.5	1.2			None		No (H)
Penicillin G	0.5	6–20	I	6–8	8–12	12	Yes (H), no (P)
Piperacillin	1	3–5	I	4–6	6–8	8	Yes (H)
Procainamide	3.5	11–20	I	4	6–12	12–24	Yes (H)
Ranitidine	2.2	8.7	I		12	24	Yes (H)
Ticarcillin	1	16	I	8–12	12–24	24–48	Yes (H, P)
Vancomycin	6	240	I	24–72	72–240	240	No (H, P)

[a] From Mann HJ, Fuhs DW, Cerra FB: Pharmacokinetics and pharmacodynamics in critically ill patients. *World J Surg* 11:210–217, 1987. Used with permission of the publisher.
[b] H, hemodialysis; P, peritoneal dialysis.
[c] I, interval extension; D, dose reduction.
[d] First and second generation cephalosporins.
[e] Other third generation cephalosporins.

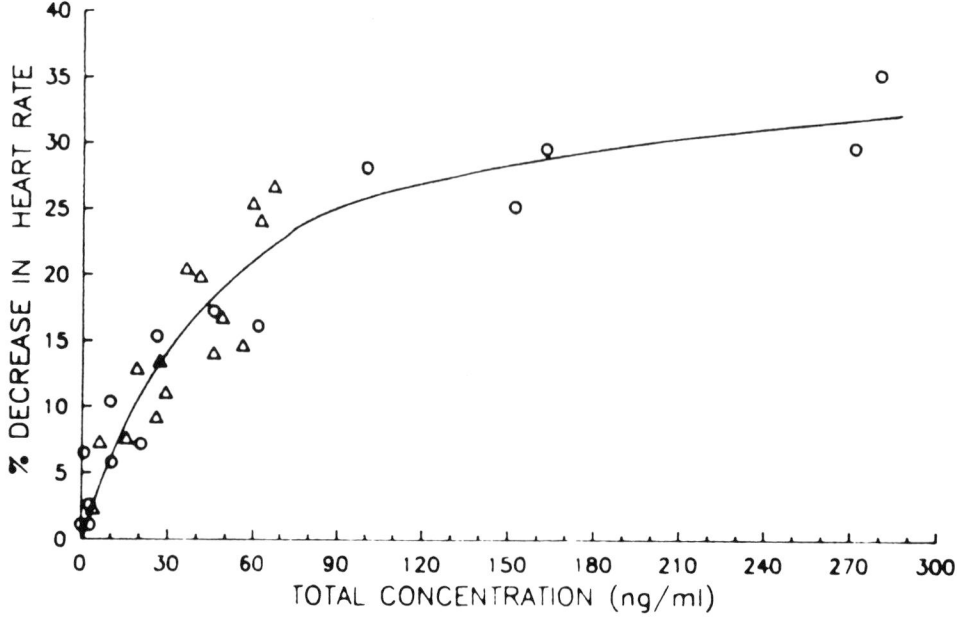

Figure 10.3. Propranolol serum concentration-effect relationship. The solid line was obtained by nonlinear least-squares regression using the E_{max} model. (From Lalonde RL, Straka RJ, Pieper JA, Bottorf MB, Mirvis DM: Propranolol pharmacodynamic modeling using unbound and total concentrations in healthy volunteers. *J Pharmacokinet Biopharm* 15:569–582, 1987. Used with permission of publishers.)

Table 10.4. Relationship between Increase in Concentration (C) and Increase in Effect as Predicted by the E_{MAX} Model[a]

Function E = $\dfrac{E_{max}\ C}{EC_{50} + C}$

C	Effect
	$(\%E_{max})$
(Multiples of EC_{50})	
0.5	33
1	50
2	66.6
3	75
4	80
9	90
99	99

[a] Holford NHG, Sheiner LB: Understanding the dose-effect relationship: clinical application of pharmacokinetic-pharmacodynamic models. *Clin Pharmacokinet* 6:429–453, 1981. Used with permission of the publisher.

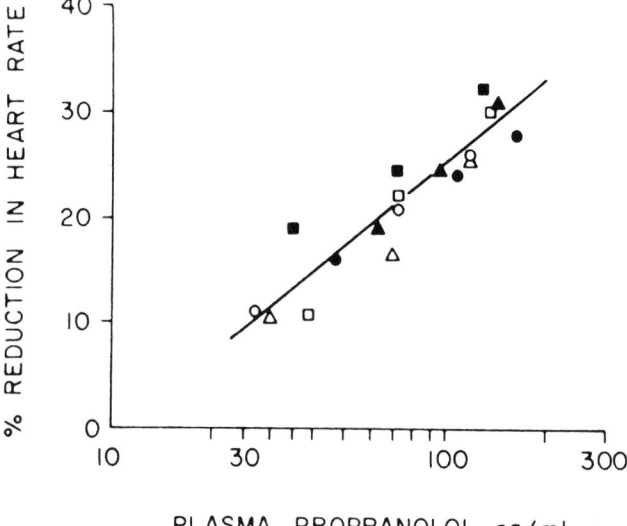

Figure 10.4. Relationship between percent reduction in exercise tachycardia and log plasma propranolol concentration. The line of best fit is shown. (From McDevitt DG, Shand DG: Plasma concentrations and the time course of β-blockade due to propranolol. *Clin Pharmacol Ther* 18:708–713, 1975. Used with permission of the publishers.)

Table 10.4 enumerates the multiples by which one has to increase drug SC to achieve a certain percentage increase in pharmacologic effect. For example, theophylline has an EC_{50} of 10 μg/ml and an increase to the upper limit of the therapeutic range (20 μg/ml) only increases the pharmacologic effect by 17% (74).

Some concentration-effect relationships are portrayed using a log-linear model (Fig. 10.4). This transformation is empiric but has useful properties. A logarithmic transformation expands the initial portion of the concentration scale, where the greatest pharmacologic effect is occurring, while compressing the end concentration portion. The log-linear E_{max} model, which is linear between EC_{20} and EC_{80} of the maximum effect, was particularly useful before nonlinear regression **techniques** were commonly available for statistical analysis of

sigmoidal or hyperbolic curves. However, the log-linear model is unable to predict an effect associated with the absence of the drug or the maximum effect (74).

The establishment of a relationship between serum drug concentrations and pharmacologic effect at nonsteady-state conditions is a relatively recent phenomenon. The concurrent modeling of kinetic and dynamic processes is described as a kinetic-effect model (KEM). The complex mathematical models necessary to accomplish KEM are beyond the scope of this chapter but hold much promise (Table 10.5) (75). KEM may be used to test bioequivalence, therapeutic equivalence, and onset and duration of action; to devise dosage regimens; and to investigate kinetic and dynamic instability. KEM can also be useful as described above in explaining a number of observed relationships between SC and pharmacodynamic effects.

ONSET OF DRUG ACTION

The onset of action for a drug is influenced by the route of administration, drug dosage form, dose, serum concentration response relationship, the EC_{50}, and slope of the response curve (76). A KEM can be useful in understanding the relationship between SCs and response to a drug when the response compartment is outside the vascular system. Verapamil, when given intravenously as a single dose, acts within 1 to 5 minutes to control the heart rate in supraventricular arrhythmias, with a maximum effect in 10 to 20 minutes. The SC profile in relationship to the PR interval shows the characteristic counterclockwise hysteresis (Fig. 10.5). The increasing PR interval with declining SCs is explained by the initial diffusion from

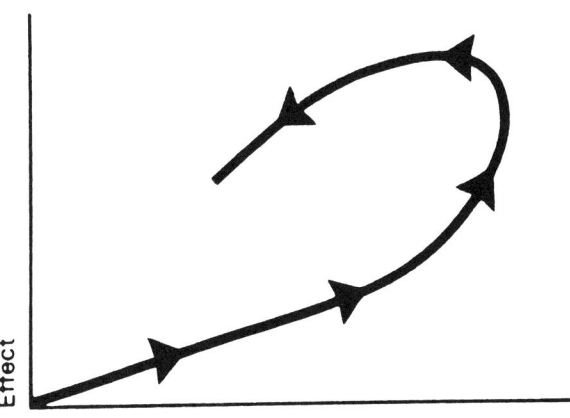

Effect

Plasma concentration

Figure 10.5. Anticlockwise hysteresis loop indicating equilibration delay between plasma concentration and the effect site producing the effect. (From Holford NHG, Sheiner LB: Understanding the dose-effect relationship: clinical application of pharmacokinetic-pharmacodynamic models. *Clin Pharmacokinet* 6:429–453, 1981. Used with permission of the publishers.)

the vascular system into the atrioventricular (AV) node, followed by redistribution from the AV node to the vascular system, terminating the effect. A KEM model with an AV node compartment would establish a relationship between SC, AV node concentration, and the PR interval. The equilibration half-time may range from 2 minutes for disopyramide, to 30 minutes for cimetidine, and to 200 minutes for digoxin (74).

INTENSITY AND DURATION/DOSAGE REGIMEN DESIGN

The relationship between declining SC and pharmacodynamic effect can be broken into three phases (Fig. 10.6). Phase I exists when the SC is greater than the EC_{80}, and the relationship between concentration and effect is shallow. A 9% change in effect, from 90 to 99%, requires a 90-fold change in SC (Table 10.4). In this range, SCs appear to have little influence on drug effect. Phase II occurs when the SC is between the EC_{20} and the EC_{80} of the maximum response. The exponential decay of SCs is accompanied by a linear decrease in effect. Phase III exists when the effect is less than 20% of maximum. During this phase, the effect is proportional to the SC and declines exponentially with time parallel to the plasma level (76).

These concepts can be applied to the design of dosage regimens. Propranolol has a pharmacokinetic half life of 2 to 5 hours, yet it can be dosed on a once- or twice-daily basis. The reason for this dosing regimen is that the SCs achieved with common oral dosing (100 to 250 ng/ml) can greatly exceed the EC_{50} for β-blockade (0.5 to 20 ng/ml) and give it an effective therapeutic duration of 12 hours or more. If the EC_{50} were much higher, e.g., ventricular arrhythmia suppression at 200 ng/ml, larger and/or more frequent doses would be needed (77).

The duration of the pharmacodynamic effect is a function of SC, therapeutic index, EC_{50}, and the elimination rate from the effect compartment. The previously cited verapamil example demonstrates a duration of action influenced primarily by equilibration. Repeated doses of IV verapamil within a short interval will increase the postdistribution SCs and maintain a therapeutic level at the AV node. Its duration and intensity will depend on the EC_{50} and verapamil metabolic elimination. The EC_{50} of the AV node may be altered by endogenous or exogenous catecholamine stimulation.

Table 10.5. Comparison of Methods Related to Clinical Pharmacokinetics and to KEM[a]

| | Methods and Criteria | |
Problem	Clinical Pharmacokinetics	KEM
Design of a dosing regimen	Proof of linear PK[b]	Proof of stability of PD
	Clearance, C_p at steady state	E(t) at steady-state
	Elimination half-life	Duration of effect
	Optimal range of C_p	Therapeutically desired effect
Design of controlled-release formulations	Optimal Cp(t) profile	Optimal E(t) profile
Test of bioequivalence between different formulations	Comparison of AUCs and absorption kinetics	Comparison of E(t) profiles
Individualization of drug therapy	Therapeutic drug monitoring	Control system with effect as feedback

[a] From Grevel J: Kinetic-effect models and their applications. *Pharm Res* 4:86–91, 1987. Used with permission of Plenum Publishing Corp.
[b] PK, pharmacokinetics; PD, pharmacodynamics.

At steady-state pharmacokinetic and pharmacodynamic conditions, the duration of effect increases by one half-life with each doubling of the dose and is proportional to the logarithm of the dose (76). (see Fig. 10.5). The clinician uses this information in two ways:

1. The pharmacodynamic duration of action can be lengthened by increasing the dose, rather than the frequency, or by using a continuous infusion. The rate-limiting step for narrow therapeutic index drugs, e.g., theophylline, is the increasing probability of toxicity as peak concentrations increase,
2. The time to offset can be predicted for a drug that's been discontinued to allow for patient evaluation. An example would be a patient confined to the coronary care unit following a myocardial infarction, with PVCs that have been suppressed by intravenous lidocaine. The lidocaine infusion is discontinued, and transfer is planned if the patient is no longer dysrhythmic. The question arises as to when the lidocaine SC will become subtherapeutic to allow patient evaluation. In Table 10.6, lidocaine SC at the time of discontinuance, drug half-life, and minimum effective lidocaine SC, are altered to indicate when the patient's underlying dysrhythmia status can be evaluated without the influence of a therapeutic lidocaine SC.

PHARMACODYNAMIC STEADY-STATE

The difference between pharmacokinetic steady-state and pharmacodynamic plateau can be a point of confusion. Drug

action is dependent on the pharmacokinetic properties of drugs but also on drug-receptor interaction, receptor distribution and sensitivity, and postreceptor changes. It is necessary to differentiate between the immediate dynamic effects of an agent and the ultimate expression of change in the disease state being treated. The initial hemodynamic effects of oral captopril, measured by cardiac index or pulmonary artery wedge pressure, have an onset of 20 to 30 minutes with a peak response at 1 to 2 hours. Captopril has a pharmacokinetic half-life of 2 to 3 hours in patients with normal renal function. Yet, the patient being treated for congestive heart failure may not achieve the ultimate therapeutic benefit, as measured by exercise tolerance or a change in NYHA classification, until after 2 to 3 months of treatment. This example serves to highlight both the pharmacodynamic steady-state concept and the complex interaction between physiologic adaptation and the therapeutic index. Dosage regimen design must consider the parameters of drug distribution, the concentration and

Table 10.6. Duration of Lidocaine Therapeutic Effectiveness

SC[a]	$t_{1/2}$	EC	WAIT
4.0	4.0	2.1	4.0
4.0	2.0	2.1	2.0
4.0	2.0	1.1	4.0
2.0	4.0	1.1	4.0
2.1	4.0	2.0	0.1

[a] SC, serum concentration (μg/ml) at time of discontinuance; $t_{1/2}$, drug elimination half-life (hours); EC, minimum effective antiarrhythmic serum concentration (μg/ml); WAIT, time until lidocaine is no longer therapeutically effective (hours).

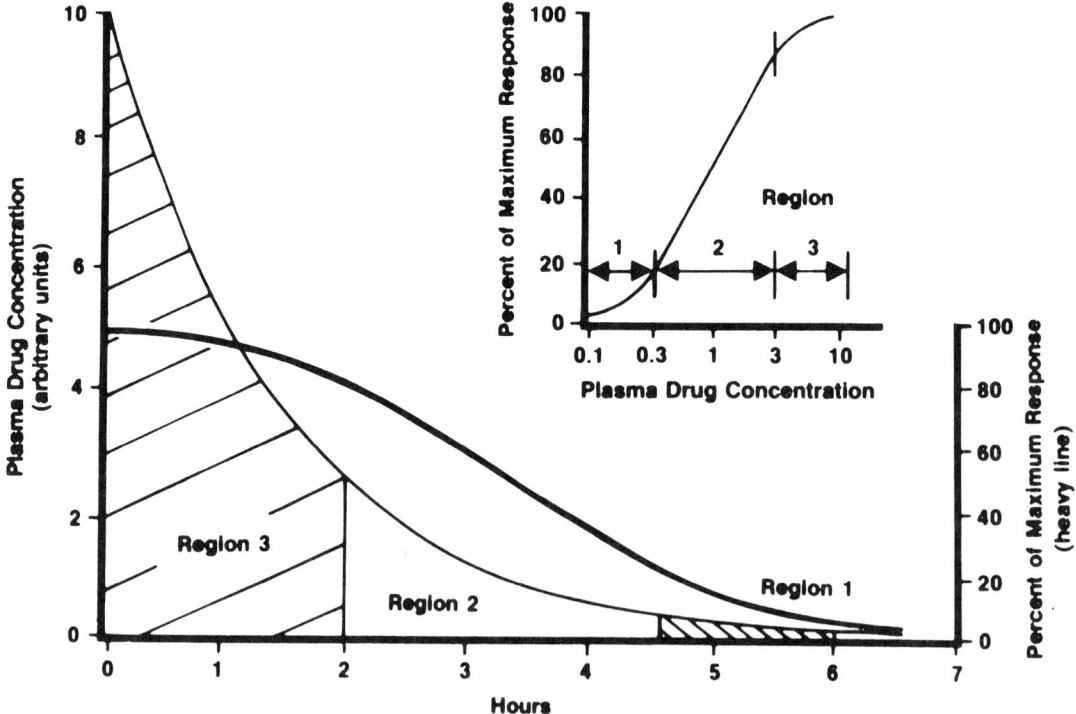

Figure 10.6. The decline in the intensity of pharmacologic effect with time, following a single large dose, has three parts corresponding to the regions of the concentration-response curve (*inset*). Initially, in region 3, the response remains almost maximal despite a 75% fall in the concentration. Thereafter, as long as the concentration is within region 2, the intensity of response approximately declines linearly with time. Only when the concentration falls into region 1 does the decline in response parallel that of drug in the body. (From Rowland M, Tozer TN: *Clinical Pharmacokinetics: Concepts and Applications.* ed 2. Lea & Febiger, Philadelphia, PA, 1989. Reprinted with permission.)

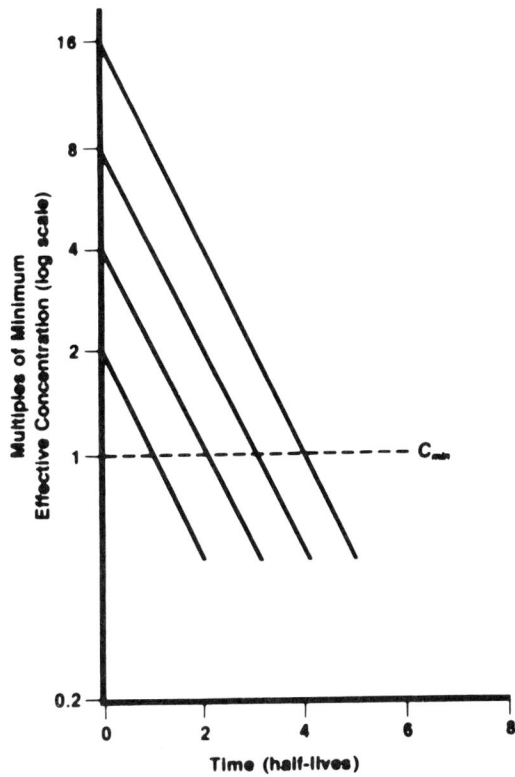
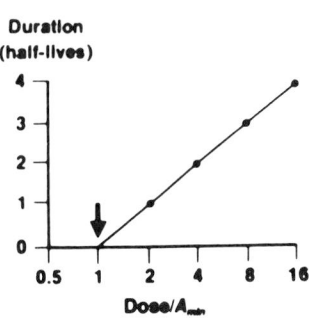

Figure 10.7. The duration of effect increases by one half-life with each doubling of the dose. Duration is proportional to the logarithm of the dose (*inset*). (From Rowland M, Tozer RN: *Clinical Pharmacokinetics: Concepts and Applications.* ed 2. Lea & Febiger, Philadelphia, PA, 1989. Reprinted with permission.)

effect relationship, and the desired therapeutic response. The dosages of drugs used in the ICU vary greatly from patient to patient, and clinical endpoints should be used to guide therapy. The patient care implications of this background information will be discussed in the next part of this chapter, dealing with the serum concentration and pharmacodynamic interface in critical care practice.

THERAPEUTIC INDEX/THERAPEUTIC RANGE

The therapeutic index is the ratio between the median toxic dose and the median effective dose. The therapeutic range is defined as the lowest effective SC and the maximum tolerable effective SC. Often, there is not a clear separation between maximum efficacy and the risk of SC-related toxicity (82). Designation of the upper therapeutic limit is a process of weighing the probability of therapeutic benefit against the probability of toxicity. Drugs with a wide therapeutic index include the penicillin and cephalosporin antibiotics, in contrast to drugs with a narrow therapeutic index, such as digoxin or the aminoglycosides.

The therapeutic index is not absolute for all patients and may change in an individual patient over time due to concurrent disease and/or drug therapy. The therapeutic index for digoxin is considered to be 0.9 to 2 ng/ml. At SCs above 2 ng/ml, there is a 50% chance of toxicity, and above 4 ng/ml, a 90% chance of toxicity. These probabilities of toxicity are increased and occur at lower digoxin SCs if the patient is hypokalemic (78). Table 10.7 provides a summary of five major

studies investigating the relationship between digoxin SC and toxicity. This summary illustrates the interpatient and intrastudy variation that is present for many drugs.

Establishing the probability of toxicity given a certain SC can be expressed as the likelihood ratio (LR). The LR is the relative likelihood that a certain result will occur within a given range of SCs. In therapeutic drug monitoring, the LR of toxicity is defined as the [(number of toxic patients having SCs within the specified SC range/total number of toxic patients)] / [(number of nontoxic patients having SCs within the same SC range / total number of nontoxic patients)]. The greater the LR, the stronger the association between the drug and the toxicity.

The therapeutic index is commonly presented in terms of a stated range without comment on the intensity of the therapeutic response or probability of toxicity. The practitioner needs to know both for clinical decision making. Toxicity must also be defined in discreet terms to allow proper use of the therapeutic index for patient care. Theophylline-induced nausea is one magnitude of importance, compared to cardiac arrhythmias or seizures. Table 10.8 provides a dual therapeutic index describing both therapeutic benefit and type of toxicity (79).

The clinician is still faced with the difficult task of using the therapeutic index. Decision analysis was developed as a structured approach to making choices in the clinical arena. Weinstein et al (80) have provided a detailed description of decision analysis, and the idea and general concepts are presented here. Decision analysis is based on the assumption of assigning the prior probability that a certain sign or symptom indicates drug-induced toxicity. This prior probability is then modified by obtaining a SC and determining its relationship to the therapeutic range. In general, the higher the SC, the greater the probability that the patient is truly toxic from the drug.

Schumacher and Barr (81) provide an example using theophylline. Serum theophylline concentrations (STCs) were obtained and associated with toxicity in a population of 1087 hospitalized patients. The authors used this data to calculate the family of LR curves depicted in Figure 10.8. This figure is used in the following way. A clinician estimates the prior probability of theophylline-induced toxicity in a selected patient to be 0.33. Subsequently, the patient's STC is found to be 23 μg/ml, and inspection of the 23 to 24.9 μg/ml LR curve in Figure 10.8 allows the clinician to revise the estimate upward to a 0.63 posterior probability of toxicity, nearly twice the initial estimate. If the STC reported were 11 μg/ml, the posterior probability of toxicity would be approximately 0.1.

The probability of a patient being toxic can thus be calculated but is only part of the therapeutic decision making process. All toxicities are not the same and, therefore, they have different levels of importance. The results of nontreatment or therapeutic failure are different for each disease state and even within patients having the same condition. Decision analysis combines the probability of each of the above events and assigns a utility (relative value) for each outcome, e.g., discontinue the drug in a nontoxic patient vs. continue the drug in a toxic patient. The assignment of utilities can be difficult and varies greatly between clinicians and the specific patients involved. An expected utility (EU) can be computed once a decision analysis table has been completed, and Table 10.9 provides an example. The greater EU represents the best choice, and even though the differences between numbers do not seem large, it is a function of the calculations.

PHARMACODYNAMIC EXAMPLES IN THE CRITICALLY ILL PATIENT

The pharmacokinetics and pharmacodynamics of new drugs are often not studied in complex critically ill patients during the pre-FDA approval process. It is only after the drugs are in common use that this information is slowly accumulated. This process is not surprising considering the number of drugs

Table 10.7.   Comparative Values of Likelihood Ratio Obtained for Serum Digoxin Concentration (SDC) Test Outcomes[a]

SDC Outcome (ng/ml)	Study	Probability of SDC in Toxic Patients	Probability of SDC in Patients without Toxicity	Likelihood Ratio for Toxicity Given SDC
0.0–0.99	Evered and Chapman	0	0.41	
	Carruthers et al	0	0.50	
	Park et al	0	0.63	
	Waldorff and Buch	0	0.54	
	Eraker and Sasse	0.35	0.61	
	Weighted Mean Values	**0.075**	**0.54**	**0.14**
1.0–1.99	Evered and Chapman	0.090	0.41	
	Carruthers et al	0	0.35	
	Park et al	0.14	0.27	
	Waldorff and Buch	0.29	0.42	
	Eraker and Sasse	0.18	0.35	0.51
	Weighted Mean Values	**0.125**	**0.353**	**0.35**
2.0–2.99	Evered and Chapman	0.27	0.13	
	Carruthers et al	0.77	0.091	
	Park et al	0.29	0.083	
	Waldorff and Buch	0.57	0.012	
	Eraker and Sasse	0.24	0.020	
	Weighted Mean Values	**0.375**	**0.072**	**5.18**
≥3.0	Evered and Chapman	0.64	0.058	
	Carruthers et al	0.23	0.057	
	Park et al	0.57	0.019	
	Waldorff and Buch	0.14	0.024	
	Eraker and Sasse	0.24	0.020	
	Weighted Mean Values	**0.425**	**0.036**	**11.73**
>2.0	Evered and Chapman	0.91	0.19	4.89
	Carruthers et al	1.00	0.15	6.77
	Park et al	0.86	0.10	8.42
	Waldorff and Buch	0.71	0.036	19.76
	Eraker and Sasse	0.47	0.040	11.53
	Beller et al	0.71	0.15	4.84
	Huffman et al	0.84	0.036	23.63
	Weighted Mean Values	**0.788**	**0.104**	**7.55**

[a] From Eraker SA, Sasse L: The serum digoxin test and digoxin toxicity: a Bayesian approach to decision making. Circulation 64:409–420, 1981. Used with permission of the American Heart Association.

Table 10.8. Adverse Effects of Theophylline[a]

Serum Concentration	Symptoms	Frequency	Duration	Comments
5–20 μg/ml	Nausea, cramps, insomnia headache	Rare—if dose is slowly titrated over 1–2 weeks	Transient	
		Common—if therapeutic serum concentrations are rapidly attained	Transient	Avoided by dose titration
	Tremor	Rare—with concurrent administration of oral β₂-adrenergic	Unknown	Avoided if β₂-agonist is administered by inhalation
	Excessive gastric acid secretion	Rare		
15–35 μg/ml	Nausea, vomiting, diarrhea, stomach ache, headache, irritability, nervousness, insomnia, sinus tachycardia	Common—at serum concentrations >20 μg/ml	Persistent	Decrease dose
	Hyperglycemia	Rare—may occur in neonates	Persistent	
>35 μg/ml	Seizures, cerebral hypoxia, arrhythmias, cardiorespiratory arrest, death	Common	Persistent	Minor adverse effects often do not precede life-threatening toxicity

[a] Adapted from Hendeles L, Weinberger M: Theophylline: therapeutic use of serum concentration monitoring. In Taylor WJ, Finn AL (eds): *Individual Drug Therapy: Practical Applications of Drug Monitoring*. Gross, Townsend, Frank, Hoffman, New York, 1981, vol 1, pp 32–65. Used with permission of the publishers.

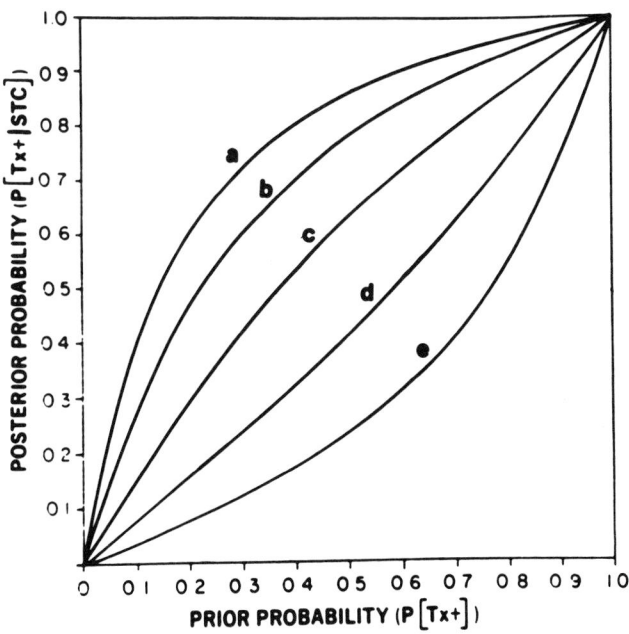

Figure 10.8. Conditional probability curves relating prior probability of toxicity and STC to posterior probability of toxicity. STC ranges and LRs corresponding to curves are as follows: *a*, STC = 27 to 28.9 mg/ml; *LR*, 6.38; *b*, STC = 23 to 24.9 mg/ml, *LR* = 3.55; *c*, STC, 19 to 20.9; *LR*, 1.67; *d*, STC = 15 to 16.9 mg/ml, *LR*, 0.71; *e*, STC, 11 to 12.9 mg/ml, *LR* = 0.31. (Originally published in Schumacher GE, Barr JT: Applying decision analysis in therapeutic drug monitoring: using decision trees to interpret serum theophylline concentrations. *Clin Pharm* 5:325–333, 1986. © 1986, American Society of Hospital Pharmacists, Inc. All rights reserves. Reprinted with permission (R9326).)

and the many disease states associated with the critically ill patient. Table 10.10 is a nonexhaustive list of the information known about the alterations of pharmacodynamics in critically ill patients. Only those drugs for which there is some evidence for a change in potency or efficacy are included. A change in pharmacodynamic response secondary to the accumulation of drug due to hepatic or renal failure or an associated change in binding was not considered a reason to be included in this table.

DRUG CONCENTRATION MONITORING

Optimization of drug therapy often involves serum drug concentration (SC) monitoring and maintenance of SC in the therapeutic range. The therapeutic range is the range of drug concentrations with a high probability of desired clinical response and a relatively low probability of unacceptable drug toxicity (82). Today's intensive care practitioner is confronted with an increasing number of drugs with previously undefined therapeutic ranges. Recent research has also questioned previously established therapeutic ranges for commonly monitored medications, such as theophylline, the aminoglycosides, digoxin, and phenytoin (83, 84).

Therapeutic drug monitoring commonly includes patient-specific factors (age, weight, height, sex, history of drug exposure, concurrent disease states), along with drug pharmacology, dose, pharmacokinetic model, route of administration, potential drug interactions, sample processing and analysis, and therapeutic endpoint. Much emphasis is usually placed on SCs since they provide very useful information. However, frequent sampling of blood may be detrimental to the patient's condition. The usefulness SCs should, therefore, always be assessed prior to sampling since other patient data may provide information of equal importance. SCs should generally be obtained when therapy is initiated to document concentration/therapeutic response relationship or when dosing changes are planned due to inadequate therapeutic results or toxicity. Other situations when SCs are helpful include therapeutic evaluations of drugs with a poor relationship between dose and serum concentrations that lack specific/sensitive measures to detect therapeutic failure and/or adverse reactions (phenytoin), determination of compliance, and establishment of a diagnosis following overdoses. The proper timing of drug concentration samples is crucial. Samples for serum drug concentrations should be obtained 2 to 4 hours after the administration of rapid-release medications, immediately before the next dose for slow-release medications, and at any time after steady-state has been attained during a constant-rate intravenous infusion. Serum samples for concentrations of anticonvulsant and antiarrhythmic medications should always be obtained immediately prior to the next dose. Serum samples for digoxin, which has an exceptionally long distribution half-life, should be obtained at least 8 hours after the dose. The Sawchuk-Zaske method (85) is useful for sampling of aminoglycoside serum concentrations and can also be applied to vancomycin therapeutic drug monitoring (86). The Chiou method (87) is used frequently for determination of theophylline pharmacokinetics during constant-rate infusions.

The location of the sampling port may be important. Due to regional uptake of drug and increased drug elimination in the lower portion of the body, samples obtained from the superior vena cava may have a greater drug concentration than samples from the inferior vena cava or peripheral sites (88, 89). The drug sample should ideally not be obtained from the same port through which the drug was infused. If the same port has to be used, the port should be flushed thoroughly with saline prior to sampling.

LABORATORY CONSIDERATIONS

Rapid and automated enzyme multiplied immunoassay techniques (EMIT) and fluorescence immunoassays (FIA or FPIA) have replaced many of the older and more time-consuming methods, such as gas-liquid chromatography (GLC), high-performance liquid chromatography (HPLC), radioimmunoassay (RIA), and bioassays, and are now the primary assay methods used in the clinical laboratory for therapeutic drug monitoring. Radioimmunoassays were developed in the 1950s and use ^{57}Co-, ^{3}H-, or ^{125}I-tagged drugs. These drugs

are displaced from antibodies by free drug in serum samples, and the amount of displaced radioactive drug can be counted by γ-counters and is proportional to the amount of drug in the sample. Although RIA techniques are extremely sensitive, they are used primarily for research since their clinical usefulness is limited by poor specificity and precision, expensive equipment, and concerns over the disposal of radioactive wastes.

The very high specificity of the HPLC assay makes this technique useful in therapeutic drug monitoring of drugs with active metabolites, such as quinidine (90), cyclosporine (91), chloramphenicol (92), carbamazepine (93), digoxin (94), and tricyclic antidepressants (95), which may cross-react with the parent compound if other assays are used. However, the HPLC assay is time-consuming, requires significant operator expertise, and is used primarily in research or commercial laboratories.

Fluorescence immunoassays (FIA) (Syva Advance) and fluorescence immunopolarization assays (FPIA) (Abbott TDx) use fluorescein-labeled drug that competes with unlabeled drug for antibody binding sites. The EMIT assay involves displacement of a drug-enzyme complex from an antibody by free drug in a sample. When the drug-enzyme complex is displaced from the antibody, it can use substrate (NAD) that, when catalyzed, can be detected spectrophotometrically. These newer and simpler assay methods are used in hospital, commercial, and office laboratories to assay aminoglycosides, anticonvulsants, chloramphenicol, digoxin, tricyclic antidepressants, antiarrythmics, and theophylline serum concentrations. Table 10.11 compares several assay procedures. More recently, rapid, disposable enzyme immunochromatography methods that use fingerstick blood samples have become popular for theophylline (96), phenytoin, phenobarbital, and carbamazepine (97) therapeutic drug monitoring.

Several factors may adversely affect drug assay results. Active metabolites and endogenous substances may cross-react with the parent compound, producing falsely elevated measured concentrations. The clinician may, therefore, lower the dose when, in reality, no change in volume of distribution or drug clearance exists. Resultant inadequate therapy may, therefore, ensue. Digoxin-like immunoreactive substance (DLIS) is an endogenous compound that cross-reacts with digoxin when the RIA analytic method is used. DLIS produces falsely increased serum digoxin concentrations in neonates (98) and patients with liver (99) or renal impairment (94). Elevated serum digoxin concentrations in these patient populations should, therefore, always be viewed in light of subjective patient complaints, concurrent disease states, vital signs,

Table 10.9. Expected Utilities for Possible Decisions in Three Prototype Cases

Case	Prior Probability of Toxicity	Serum Theophylline Concentration (µg/ml)	Posterior Probability of Toxicity	Continue the Same Dosage	Discontinue the Drug	Lower the Dosage
				Expected Utility for Decision		
1	0.25	20	0.36	**0.71**	0.60	0.67
2	0.5	20	0.63	0.50	**0.75**	0.73
3	0.5	16	0.42	0.66	0.63	**0.68**

[a] Adapted from and originally published in Schumacher GE, Barr JT: Applying decision analysis in therapeutic drug monitoring: using decision trees to interpret serum theophylline concentrations. *Clin Pharm* 5:325–333, 1986. © 1986, American Society of Hospital Pharmacists, Inc. All rights reserved. Reprinted with permission. (R9326).

and ECG findings. The FPIA assay is less influenced by DLIS and is preferred when the presence of DLIS is suspected (100). The in vitro inactivation of aminoglycosides by semisynthetic penicillins presents a special problem. The issue is especially of concern in patients with poor renal function. Samples that contain these drugs should be placed on ice and analyzed immediately or frozen prior to analysis (101).

EVALUATION OF DRUG MONITORING DATA

Pharmacokinetic forecasting is an important part of therapeutic drug monitoring. Various approaches have been used to predict drug concentrations in patients. These approaches can generally be grouped into three different categories: individualized forecasting; nomograms; and Bayesian forecasting. Individualized forecasting uses patient-specific data only. The data are generally fitted to some basic pharmacokinetic model, and predictions are made based on this model and the patient's medical condition and concurrent medications. Most commonly, monitored drugs, such as the aminoglycosides and vancomycin, are usually monitored by individualized forecasting methods (85). Nomograms are based on specific patient population pharmacokinetic estimates and usually prompt the user for some patient-specific factors, such as age, weight, and/or the CrCl. This approach is used in the therapeutic drug monitoring of digoxin (102), phenytoin (103–105), aminoglycosides (106) and vancomycin (107, 108). Advances in microcomputerization have allowed the widespread use of Bayesian forecasting methods. Most commercially available pharmacokinetic software packages give the user the option of using either individualized or Bayesian (pseudoindividualized) forecasting. Bayesian methods use both population and patient-specific pharmacokinetic parameters. Initial Bayesian pharmacokinetic estimates are based solely on population pharmacokinetic parameters. With additional patient-specific drug concentration data, subsequent Bayesian pharmacokinetic estimates are based to a greater degree on the patient's own data, and less weight is given to the population parameters. Theophylline (109) and phenytoin (110) are often dosed by using a Bayesian forecasting approach but can also be monitored by using individualized methods (87, 111). Yuen et al (110) evaluated the predictive power of Bayesian forecasting, individual forecasting, and nomograms on phenytoin dosing. For single data points, the Bayesian method was equivalent to published nomograms. With multiple doses, the Bayesian approach demonstrated better accuracy and fewer toxic doses (110). The Bayesian method yields superior results compared to the individualized approach (109, 110). Bayesian forecasting in critical care therapeutic drug monitoring does have a major drawback: the initial estimates used for the computer programs are generally derived from other patient populations and may provide erroneous initial dosing estimates. The clinician should, therefore, use data from the critical care patient population whenever possible. Computerized therapeutic drug monitoring in the ICU can provide accurate dose predictions and can also be used to build a patient data base that can be used for patient- and unit-specific data analysis.

A multidisciplinary approach, involving a variety of health care professionals, including physicians, pharmacists, nurses, and medical technologists (112), to therapeutic drug monitoring service (TDMS) also improves professional communication, team spirit, data gathering and analysis, and implementation of recommendations. Pharmacokinetic dosing services involving pharmacists are available in approximately half of all the hospitals in the U.S. (113). A TDMS can also provide opportunities for education and research if reports and feedback are presented on a regular basis to the professional staff. Studies have shown that TDMS can have a positive impact on toxic drug reactions, drug dosing, and appropriate serum sample collection (114). Critically ill patients often represent a "loss" in hospital revenues, and the number of patients is increasing with time. Approximately 25% of total pharmacy charges may be generated during the time when the patient is in the ICU. Catecholamines, antibiotics, total parenteral nutrition, systemic antifungals, and colloids contribute most to the cost of ICU drug therapy (115). Many of these products are not yet available in generic form and are therefore quite expensive. The search for alternative inexpensive medications, deletion of unnecessary duplication of therapy, and use of enteral feeding where possible may decrease the cost of intensive care therapy.

The effectiveness of a TDMS is difficult to judge. The process-outcome relationship of TDMS is often difficult to ascertain, and confounding variables should be evaluated. A TDMS process strictly adhered to (i.e., elimination of trough serum phenytoin concentrations less than than 10 μg/ml) may not always result in improved patient therapy. Serum drug concentrations should not be considered as being "supratherapeutic," "therapeutic," or "subtherapeutic," but rather "appropriate" or "inappropriate" in reference to the patient's condition (a "subtherapeutic" total serum phenytoin concentration of 8 μg/ml may be "appropriate" in a uremic patient due to decreased plasma protein binding of the drug). Other outcome parameters, such as the length of stay and readmission frequency, may be affected by concurrent disease states or unforeseen complications. A reduction in the number of SDC measurements may not be related to patient outcome but could result in substantial cost savings if inappropriate SDC measurements are minimized. Although patient care cost analysis is important, it should not be used alone since fiscal outcome may be unrelated to clinical patient outcome. TDMS is an important part of improving patient outcome, but further research in defining the exact effects of TDMS is needed (116).

CONCLUSIONS

Therapeutic drug monitoring is an essential part of modern health care and should be conducted by a multidisciplinary team for maximum use of resource personnel. Critically ill patients require special monitoring due to the pharmacokinetic and pharmacodynamic changes observed in this patient population. These patients are also rarely at steady-state, and therapeutic outcomes must constantly be reassessed. The clinician needs to recognize that critically ill patients respond differently to drugs, as compared to other patient populations, and should tailor drug therapy to accommodate changes in drug distribution and elimination pathways. The use of drugs with ultrashort half-lives that are eliminated by blood esterases

Table 10.10. Alteration of Drug Pharmacodynamics in Critically Ill Patients

Drugs	Dynamics	Disease State	Reason	Therapeutic Alternative
Antiarrhythmics	Proarrhythmias Death (?) CHF	CHF^a, ISHD, MI, Malignant arrhythmias CHF, MI	Increased sensitivity, CC-hypoxia, K$^+$, Mg^{2+}	Use with caution. Monitor serum levels
Dopamine/dobutamine	Worsen DD, Wall motion, ABN, increased PCWP, angina, ST changes	CHF, ISHD	DD MVO$_2$ balance, LV compliance	DOP > DOB use vasodilators. Avoid HR + SBP > 12,000
	Arrhythmogenic	CHF, ISHD Cardiomyopathy	Increased sensitivity, CC-hypoxia, ISHD, K$^+$, Mg^{2+}	Avoid or use at lowest possible doses
	Decreased myocardial contractile response, Tolerance within 48–72 hours	CHF, ISHD Cardiomyopathy	Down-regulation of β-receptors, DD	Intermittent therapy, use vasodilators
Digoxin	Toxicity, death (?)	CHF, ISHD	Direct toxicity, indirect sympathetic stimulation, CC-ISHD, CC-hypoxia, K$^+$, Ca^{2+}, Mg^{2+}	Use vasodilators first. Monitor other conditions closely.
	PCWP	CHF, ISHD	Activates sympathetic nervous system. Direct action, vasoconstriction.	Avoid rapid (<10 min) IV administration
β-blockers	Increased CO or SV	CHF-associated DD, ISHD	Reverses DD, ISHD-induced LV compliance	Unpredictable—use cautiously
	Decreased CO	CHF, ISHD	Decreased contractility, β-blockade	Use cautiously and observe
Calcium channel blockers	Decreased CO	Severe CHF	Decreased contractility	Caution with all, including nifedipine. Monitor carefully.
	Increased CO	ISHD	Improves DD	All agents are capable.
Vasopressors Dopamine Norepinephrine	Decreased BP response	Sepsis	α-receptor desensitization	Monitor, increase doses.
Fluids Preload challenge	Blunted CO response	Sepsis/shock, ARDS	LV dysfunction, RVF with PAP	Monitor
	Noncardiogenic pulmonary edema	ARDS	Increased capillary permeability	Use lowest PCWP compatible with best DO$_2$
Diuretics Furosemide	Slow onset, decreased diuresis	Shock, ARF, CHF	Decreased renal blood flow	Use higher doses cautiously and mannitol and/or dopamine (low doses)
Warfarin	Increased PT response	CHF	Decreased metabolism	Use lower doses. Monitor carefully.
Nutrition	Increased VO$_2$, worsening of DO$_2$/VO$_2$ match, hypercarbia	Shock, CHF COPD, ARDS	Overfeeding, VO$_2$ Excess carbohydrate calories, RQ > 1	Moderate caloric input Decrease carbohydrate, increase fat input
	Fat intolerance	Severe sepsis	Metabolic intolerance	Decrease or discontinue fat input
Insulin	Hyperglycemia, insulin resistance	DM, stress-induced, sepsis/shock	Insulin receptor changes, CC-stress steroids, glucagon, GH, catecholamines	Minimize exogenous glucose
Vasodilators Nitroprusside	Worsening myocardial ischemia	MI, angina, ISHD	Coronary steal, dilates capacitance and resistance vessels, MVO$_2$ imbalance	Use nitroglycerin
	Arterial hypoxemia	ARDS/shock	Increased pulmonary shunting, dilates pulmonary blood vessels	Monitor. Increase FIO$_2$.
Nitroglycerin	Increased EF and CO	ISHD, MI	Reverses ISHD and DD asynergy, LV compliance	
H$_2$ Blockers Cimetidine	Confusion, disorientation	Hepatic/renal failure	? increased penetration CSF/CNS blockade	Decrease dose or switch to other agents.
	Hypotension/cardiac arrest/bradyarrhythmias	MI, COPD	H$_2$ myocardial blockade with high concentrations	Slow (>15 minutes IV)

Table 10.10. *continued*

Drugs	Dynamics	Disease State	Reason	Therapeutic Alternative
ACE inhibitors	*First-dose hypotension*	*CHF*	*Increased with hyponatremia, high ACE*	*Start with small dose, e.g., Captopril 6.25 mg po.*

[a] ACE, angiotensin-converting enzyme; ARDS, adult respiratory distress syndrome; ARF, acute renal failure; BP, blood pressure; CC, concurrent; CHF, congestive heart failure; CO, cardiac output; COPD, chronic obstructive pulmonary disease; DD, diastolic dysfunction; DM, diabetes mellitus; DOB, dobutamine; DOP, dopamine; DO_2, oxygen delivery; EF, ejection fraction; GH, growth hormone; HR, heart rate; ISHD, ischemic heart disease; LV, left ventricular; MI, myocardial infarction; MVO_2, myocardial oxygen consumption; RQ, respiratory quotient; PT, prothrombin time; SV, stroke volume; VO_2, total body oxygen consumption.

Table 10.11. Comparison of Analytical Techniques[a]

	Analytical Method[a]				
	HPLC	GLC	RIA	EI	FPIA
Sample					
Size (µl)	100–500	100–500	100	50	50
Type[b]	P, S, U, SI	P, S, U, SI	P, S, U, SI	P, S, U	P, S
Analysis time (hr)	0.5	0.5	0.25	0.1–0.3	0.1–0.2
Sensitivity[c]	1	1	2	3	2
Specificity[c]	1	1	4	4	3
Accuracy[c]	2	2	2	2	2
Precision[c]	3	3	2	1	1
Specialized Training[c]	5	5	3	3	2
Cost[c]					
Equipment	4	4	5	3	4
Reagent	3	2	2	3	2
Preference[c]					
Clinical	4	5	4	2	1
Research	1	2	3	3	3
Usefulness					
Aminoglycosides	•		•	•	•
Anticonvulsants	•	•		•	•
Chloramphenicol	•	•		•	•
Digoxin		•	•	•	•
Imipramine	•	•	•	•	•
Lidocaine	•	•		•	•
Methotrexate	•		•	•	•
Procainamide	•	•		•	•
Quinidine	•	•	•	•	•
Theophylline	•	•		•	•

[a] Adapted from Pieper JA, Rutledge DR: *Current Concepts: Laboratory Techniques for Pharmacists.* Upjohn Corp, Kalamazoo, MI, 1989. Used with permission of the publisher.
[b] EI, enzyme immunoassay. B, whole blood; P, plasma; S, serum; U, urine; SI, saliva.
[c] Arbitrary ranking scale of 1 (excellent) to 5 (poor).

can be useful in patients with multisystem organ failure. Therapeutic drug monitoring in the ICU has in the past been complicated by a lack of reliable pharmacokinetic and pharmacodynamic drug data. The advent of ICU computerization will facilitate therapeutic drug monitoring since patient data can be more easily accessed and specific critical care databases can be assembled easily.

REFERENCES
1. Zaske DE, Bootman JL, Solem LB, Strate RG: Increased burn patient survival with individualized dosages of gentamicin. *Surgery* 91:142–149, 1982.
2. Bootman JL, Wertheimer AI, Zaske D, Rowland C: Individualizing gentamicin dosage regimens in burn patients with gram-negative septicemia: A cost-benefit analysis. *J Pharm Sci* 68:267–272, 1979.
3. Gibaldi M, Perrier D: Pharmacokinetics. ed 2. Marcel Dekker, New York, 1982.
4. Hendeles L, Mannsanari M, Weinberger M. Theophylline. In Evans WE, Schentag JJ, Jusko WG (eds): *Applied Pharmacokinetics, Principles of Therapeutic Drug Monitoring*, ed 2. Applied Therapeutics, Spokane, WA, 1986, pp 1105–1188.
5. Aronson JK: Clinical pharmacokinetics of digoxin 1980. *Clin Pharmacokinet* 5:137–149, 1980.
6. Pentel P, Benowitz N: Pharmacokinetic and pharmacodynamic considerations in drug therapy of cardiac emergencies. *Clin Pharmacokinet* 9:273–308, 1984.
7. Raehl CA: Endotracheal drug therapy in cardiopulmonary resuscitation. *Clin Pharm* 5:572–579, 1986.
8. Salmeron S, Brochard L, Mal H, et al: Intravenous or inhaled salbutamol in status asthmaticus? A multicenter double blind study. *Chest* 96 (Suppl):136S, 1989.
9. Roberts CJC: Clinical pharmacokinetics of ranitidine. *Clin Pharmacokinet* 9:211–221, 1984.
10. Rodighiero V: Effects of cardiovascular disease on pharmacokinetics. *Cardiovasc Drugs Ther* 3:711–730, 1989.
11. Colli A, Buccino G, Cocciolo M, Parravicini R, Scaltrini G: Disposition of a flow-limited drug (lidocaine) and a metabolic capacity-limited drug (theophylline) in liver cirrhosis. *Clin Pharmacol Ther* 44:642–649, 1988.
12. Maher JF: Pharmacokinetics in patients with renal failure. *Clin Nephrol* 21:39–46, 1984.
13. Runciman WB, Ilsley AH, Rutten AJ, Baker D, Fronsko RL: An evaluation of intravenous infusion pumps and controllers. *Anaesth Intens Care* 15:217–228, 1987.
14. Carlton BC, Cipolle RJ, Larson SD, Canafax DM: Method for evaluating drip-rate accuracy of intravenous flow-regulating devices. *Am J Hosp Pharm* 48:2422–2426, 1991.
15. Klotz U: Pathophysiological and disease induced changes in drug distribution volumes: Pharmacokinetic implications. *Clin Pharmacokinet* 1:204–218, 1976.

16. Fabre J, Balant L: Renal failure, drug pharmacokinetics, and drug action. *Clin Pharmacokinet* 1:99–120, 1976.

17. Benowitz N, Forsyth RP, Melmon KL, Rowland M: Lidocaine disposition kinetics in monkey and man. I. Prediction by a perfusion model. *Clin Pharmacol Ther* 16:87–98, 1974.

18. Fuhs DW, Mann HJ, Kubajak CAM, Cerra FB: Intrapatient variation of aminoglycoside pharmacokinetics in critically ill surgery patients. *Clin Pharm* 7:207–213, 1988.

19. Shikuma LR, Ackerman BH, Weaver RH, et al: Effects of treatment and the metabolic response to injury on drug clearance: a prospective study with piperacillin. *Crit Care Med* 18:37–41, 1990.

20. Blaschke TF: Protein binding and kinetics of drugs in liver diseases. *Clin Pharmacokinet* 2:32–44, 1977.

21. Barre J, Houin G, Brunner F, Bree F, Tillement JP: Disease-induced modifications of drug pharmacokinetics. *Int J Clin Pharmacol Res* 3:215–226, 1983.

22. Williams RL: Drug administration in hepatic disease. *N Engl J Med* 309:1616–1622, 1983.

23. Gelman SI: Disturbances in hepatic blood flow during anesthesia and surgery. *Arch Surg* 111:881–883, 1976.

24. Perkins MW, Dasta JF, DeHaven B: Physiologic implications of mechanical ventilation on pharmacokinetics. *DICP Ann Pharmacother* 23:316–323, 1989.

25. Powell JR, Vozeh S, Hopewell P, Costello J, Sheiner LB, Riegelman S: Theophylline disposition in acutely ill hospitalized patients. The effect of smoking, heart failure, severe airway obstruction, and pneumonia. *Am Rev Respir Dis* 118:229–238, 1978.

26. Gottlieb ME, Stratton HH, Newell JC, Shah DM: Indocyanine green. Its use as an early indicator of hepatic dysfunction following injury in man. *Arch Surg* 119:264–268, 1984.

27. Wilkinson GR, Shand DG: Commentary: a physiological approach to hepatic drug clearance. *Clin Pharmacol Ther* 18:377–390, 1975.

28. Tucker GT, Lennard MS: Enantiomer specific pharmacokinetics. *Pharmacol Ther* 45:309–329, 1990.

29. Baum T, Sybertz EJ: Pharmacology of labetalol in experimental animals. *Am J Med* 75(4A):15–23, 1983.

30. Richards DA, Prichard NC, Boakes AJ, Tuckman J, Knight EJ: Pharmacological basis for antihypertensive effects of intravenous labetalol. *Br Heart J* 39:99–106, 1977.

31. Klotz U, Arvela P, Pasanen M, et al: Comparative effects of H2-receptor antagonists on drug metabolism in vitro and in vivo. *Pharmacol Ther* 33:157–161, 1987.

32. Greenblatt DJ, Abernethy DR, Koepke HH, Shader RI: Interaction of cimetidine with oxazepam, lorazepam, and flurazepam. *J Clin Pharmacol* 24:187–193, 1984.

33. Levy RH, Wilensky AJ, Friel PN: Other antiepileptic drugs. In Evans WE, Schentag JJ, Jusko WG (eds): *Applied Pharmacokinetics, Principles of Therapeutic Drug Monitoring*, ed 2. Applied Therapeutics, Spokane, WA, 1986, pp 540–569.

34. Hansten PD, Horn JR (eds): *Drug Interactions*. ed 6. Lea & Febiger, 1989.

35. Piafsky KM: Disease-induced changes in the plasma binding of basic drugs. *Clin Pharmacokinet* 5:246–262, 1980.

36. West JG, Trunkey DD, Lim RC: Systems of trauma care. A study of two countries. *Arch Surg* 114:455–460, 1979.

37. Hasselgren PO, Jagenburg R, Karlström L, Pedersen P, Seeman T: Changes of protein metabolism in liver and skeletal muscle following trauma complicated by sepsis. *J Trauma* 24:224–228, 1984.

38. Border JR, Chenier R, McMenamy RH, et al: Multiple systems organ failure: muscle fuel deficit with visceral protein malnutrition. *Surg Clin North Am* 56:1147–1167, 1976.

39. Gugler R, Azarnoff DL: Drug protein binding and the nephrotic syndrome. *Clin Pharmacokinet* 1:25–35, 1976.

40. Koch-Weser J, Sellers EM: Binding of drugs to serum albumin. *N Engl J Med* 294:311–316, 526–531, 1976.

41. Routledge PA, Bartlowsky A, Bjornsson TD, Kitchall BB, Shand DG: Lidocaine plasma protein binding. *Clin Pharmacol Ther* 27:347–354, 1980.

42. Davies RF, Dubé, Mousseau N, McGilveray I, Beanlands DS: Perioperative variability of binding of lidocaine, quinidine, and propranolol after cardiac operations. *J Thorac Cardiovasc Surg* 96:643–641, 1988.

43. Bauer LA, Edwards WAD, Dellinger EP, Raisys VA, Brennan C: Importance of unbound phenytoin serum levels in head trauma patients. *J Trauma* 23:1058–1060, 1983.

44. Hook GER: The metabolic potential of the lungs. In George CF, Shand DG, Renwick AG (eds): *Presystemic Drug Elimination*. Butterworth Scientific, London, 1982, pp 117–146.

45. Roerig DL, Kortly KJ, Vucins EJ, et al: First pass uptake of fentanyl, meperidine, and morphine in the human lung. *Anesthesiology* 67:466–472, 1987.

46. Persson MP, Wiklund L, Hartvig P, Paalzow L: Potential pulmonary uptake and clearance of morphine in postoperative patients. *Eur J Clin Pharmacol* 1986;30:567–574

47. Jorfeldt L, Lewis DH, Lofstrom B, Post C: Lung uptake of lidocaine in healthy volunteers. *Acta Anesth Scand* 23:567–574, 1979.

48. Buck ML, Reed MD: Use of nondepolarizing neuromuscular blocking agents in mechanically ventilated patients. *Clin Pharm* 10:32–48, 1991.

49. Dobrinska MR: Enterohepatic circulation of drugs. *J Clin Pharmacol* 29:577–580, 1989.

50. Gibaldi M, Levy G, Hayton WL: Tubocurarine and renal failure. *Br J Anesth* 44:163–165, 1972.

51. Jusko WJ, Weintraub M: Myocardial distribution of digoxin and renal function. *Clin Pharmacol Ther* 16:449–454, 1974.

52. Dodd MJ, O'Donovan RM, Bennett-Jones PN, et al: Arteriovenous haemofiltration: a recent advance in the management of renal failure. *Br Med J* 287:1008–1010, 1983.

53. Gibson TP, Nelson HA: Drug kinetics and artificial kidneys. *Clin Pharmacokinet* 2:403–426, 1977.

54. Moore RD, Lietman PS, Smith CR: Clinical response to aminoglycoside therapy: importance of the ratio of peak concentration to minimal inhibitory concentration. *J Infect Dis* 155:93–99, 1987.

55. Zhanel GG, Hoban DJ, Harding GKM: The postantibiotic effect: a review of in vitro and in vivo data. *DICP Ann Pharmacother* 25;153–163, 1991.

56. Bauer JH, Brooks CS, Burch RN: Clinical appraisal of creatinine clearance as a measurement of glomerular filtration rate. *Am J Kidney Dis* 2:337–346, 1982.

57. Bennett WM: Guide to drug dosage in renal failure. *Clin Pharmacokinet* 15:326–354, 1988.

58. Robert S, Zarowitz BJ: Is there a reliable index of glomerular filtration rate in critically ill patients? *DICP Ann Pharmacother* 25:169–178, 1991.

59. Hull JH, Hak LJ, Koch GG, Wargin WA, Chi SL, Mattocks AM: Influence of renal function and liver disease on predictability of creatinine clearance. *Clin Pharmacol Ther* 29:516–521, 1981.

60. Baumann TJ, Staddon JE, Horst HM, Bivins BA: Minimum urine collection periods for accurate determination of creatinine clearance in critically ill patients. *Clin Pharm* 6:393–398, 1987.

61. Szeto HH, Inturrisi CE, Houde R, Saal S, Cheigh J, Reidenberg MM: Accumulation of normeperidine, an active metabolite of meperidine, in patients with renal failure or cancer. *Ann Intern Med* 86:738–741, 1977.

62. Osborne RJ, Joel SP, Slevin ML: Morphine intoxication in renal failure: the role of morphine-6-glucuronide. *Br Med J* 292:1548–1549, 1986.

63. Yoshimura H, Ida S, Ogurik K, Tsukamoto H: Biochemical basis for analgesic activity of morphine-6-glucuronide. I. Penetration of morphine-6-glucuronide in the brain of rats. *Biochem Pharmacol* 22:1423–1430, 1972.

64. Yoshimura H, Natsuki R, Ida S, Ogurik K: Chemical reactivity of morphine and morphine-6-conjugates and their binding to rat brain. *Chem Pharm Bull* 24:901–906, 1976.

65. Dahlgren JG, Anderson ET, Hewitt WL: Gentamicin blood levels: a guide to nephrotoxicity. *Antimicrob Agent Chemother* 8:58–62, 1975.

66. French MA, Cerra FB, Plaut ME, Schentag JJ: Amikacin and gentamicin accumulation pharmacokinetics and nephrotoxicity in critically ill patients. *Antimicrob Agents Chemother* 19:147–152, 1981.

67. Lesar TS, Rotschafer JC, Strand LM, Solem LD, Zaske DE: Gentamicin dosing errors with four commonly used nomograms. *JAMA* 248:1190–1193, 1982.

68. Johnson GJ, Rao GHR, White JG: Platelet dysfunction induced by parenteral carbenicillin and ticarcillin. *Am J Pathol* 91:85–106, 1978.

69. Garaud JJ, Regnier B, Inglebert F, Faurisson F, Bauchet J, Vachon F: Vancomycin pharmacokinetics in critically ill patients. *J Antimicrob Chemother* 14(Suppl. D):53–57, 1984.

70. Schentag JJ, Cerra FB, Calleri G, DeGlopper E, Rose JQ, Bernhard H: Pharmacokinetic and clinical studies in patients with cimetidine-associated mental confusion. *Lancet* i:177–181, 1979.

71. MacMahon B, Bakshi M, Walsh MJ:. Cardiac arrhythmias after intravenous cimetidine. *N Engl J Med* 305:832–833, 1981.

72. Lee CS, Marbury TC: Drug therapy in patients undergoing haemodialysis: clinical pharmacokinetic considerations. *Clin Pharmacokinet* 9:42–66, 1984.

73. Holford NHG, Sheiner LB: Kinetics of pharmacologic response. *Pharmacol Ther* 16:143–166, 1982.

74. Holford NHG, Sheiner LB: Understanding the dose-effect relationship: clinical application of pharmacokinetic-pharmacodynamic models. *Clin Pharmacokinet* 6:429–453, 1981.

75. Grevel J: Kinetic-effect models and their applications. *Pharm Res* 4:86–91, 1987.

76. Rowland M, Tozer TN (eds): *Clinical Pharmacokinetics, Concepts and Applications*. ed 2. Lea & Febiger, Philadelphia, PA, 1989, pp 323–346.

77. Gengo F, Green JA: Beta blockers. In Evans WE, Schentag JJ, Jusko WG (eds): *Applied Pharmacokinetics, Principles of Therapeutic Drug Monitoring*, ed 2. Applied Therapeutics, Spokane, WA, 1986, pp 735–781.

78. Eraker SA, Sasse L: The serum digoxin test and digoxin toxicity: a Bayesian approach to decision making. *Circulation* 64:409–420, 1981.

79. Seligman M: Bronchodilators. In Chernow B (ed): *The Pharmacologic Approach to the Critically Ill Patient*. ed 2. Williams & Wilkins, Baltimore, MD, 1988, p 441.

80. Weinstein MC, Fineberg AV: *Clinical Decision Analysis*. WB Saunders, Philadelphia, PA, 1980.

81. Schumacher GE, Barr JT: Applying decision analysis in therapeutic drug monitoring: using decision trees to interpret serum theophylline concentrations. *Clin Pharm* 5:325–333, 1986.

82. Ross EM, Gilman AG: Pharmacodynamics: mechanisms of drug action and the relationship between drug concentration and effect. In Goodman LS,

Gilman A (eds): *The Pharmacological Basis of Therapeutics*. ed 8. MacMillan, New York, NY, 1990, pp 35–48.

83. Schumacher GE, Barr JT: Using population-based serum drug concentration cutoff values to predict toxicity: test performance and limitations compared with Bayesian interpretation. *Clin Pharm* 9:788–796, 1990.

84. Schumacher GE, Barr JT, Browne TR, Collins JF: Test performance characteristics of the serum phenytoin concentration (SPC): the relationship between SPC and patient response. *Ther Drug Monit* 13:318–324, 1991.

85. Sawchuk RJ, Zaske DE, Cipolle RJ, Wargin WA, Strate RG: Kinetic model for gentamicin dosing with the use of individual patient parameters. *Clin Pharmacol Ther* 21:362–369, 1977.

86. Rybak MJ, Boike SC: Individualized adjustment of vancomycin dosage: comparison with two dosage nomograms. *DICP Ann Pharmacother* 20:64–68, 1986.

87. Chiou WL, Gadalla MAF, Peng GW: Method for the rapid estimation of the total body drug clearance and adjustment of dosage regimens in patients during a constant rate intravenous infusion. *J Pharmacokinet Biopharm* 6:135–151, 1977.

88. Major E, Aun C, Yate PM, et al: Influence of sample site on blood concentrations of ICI 35 868. *Br J Anaesth* 55:371–375, 1983.

89. Upton RN, Runciman WB, Mather AL, McLean CF, Ilsley AH: The uptake and elution of lignocaine and procainamide in the hindquarters of the sheep described using mass balance principles. *J Pharmacokinet Biopharm* 16:31–40, 1988.

90. Ueda CT. Quinidine: In Evans WE, Schentag JJ, Jusko WG (eds): *Applied Pharmacokinetics, Principles of Therapeutic Drug Monitoring*, ed 2. Applied Therapeutics, Spokane, WA, 1986, pp 735–781.

91. Yee GC, Kennedy MS: Cyclosporine. In Evans WE, Schentag JJ, Jusko WG (eds): *Applied Pharmacokinetics, Principles of Therapeutic Drug Monitoring*, ed 2. Applied Therapeutics, Spokane, WA, 1986, pp 826–851.

92. Nahata MC: Chloramphenicol. In Evans WE, Schentag JJ, Jusko WG (eds): *Applied Pharmacokinetics, Principles of Therapeutic Drug Monitoring*, ed 2. Applied Therapeutics, Spokane, WA, 1986, pp 437–462.

93. Monaco F, Piredda S: Carbamazepine-10-11-epoxide determined by EMIT carbamazepine reagent. *Epilepsia* 21:475–477, 1980.

94. Graves SW, Brown B, Valdes R: An endogenous digoxin-like substance in patients with renal impairment. *Ann Int Med* 99:604–608, 1983.

95. DeVane CL: Cyclic antidepressants. In Evans WE, Schentag JJ, Jusko WG (eds): *Applied Pharmacokinetics, Principles of Therapeutic Drug Monitoring*, ed 2. Applied Therapeutics, Spokane, WA, 1986, pp 852–907.

96. Vaughan LM, Milavetz G, Ellis E, et al: Multicentre evaluation of disposable visual measuring device to assay theophylline from capillary blood sample. *Lancet* i:184–186, 1986.

97. Monaco F, Gianelli M, Dimanico U, Mutani R: A simple and disposable visual measuring device to assay antiepileptic drugs from whole blood samples. *Ther Drug Monit* 12:359–361, 1990.

98. Pudek MR, Seccombe DW, Whitfield MF: Digoxin-like immunoreactivity in premature and full-term infants not receiving digoxin therapy. *N Engl J Med* 308;904–905, 1983.

99. Nanji AA, Greenway DC: Falsely raised plasma digoxin concentrations in liver disease. *Br J Med* 290:432–433, 1985.

100. Pleasants RA, Gadsden RH, McCormack JP, Piveral K, Sawyer WT: Interference of digoxin-like immunoreactive substances with three digoxin immunoassays in patients with various degrees of renal function. *Clin Pharm* 5:810–816, 1986.

101. Pickering LK, Rutherford I: Effect of concentration and time upon inactivation of tobramycin, gentamicin, netilmicin, and amikacin by azlocillin, carbenicillin, mecillinam, mezlocillin, and piperacillin. *J Pharmacol Exp Ther* 217:345–349, 1981.

102. Hyneck ML, Johnson MH, Wagner JG, Williams GW: Comparison of methods for estimating digoxin dosing regimens. *Am J Hosp Pharm* 38:69–73, 1981.

103. Richens A, Dunlop A: Phenytoin dosage nomogram. *Lancet* ii:1305–1306, 1975.

104. Winter ME, Tozer TN: Phenytoin. In Evans WE, Schentag JJ, Jusko WG (eds): *Applied Pharmacokinetics, Principles of Therapeutic Drug Monitoring*, ed 2. Applied Therapeutics, Spokane, WA, 1986, pp 493–539.

105. Rambeck B, Boenigk HE, Dunlop A, Mullen PW, Wadsworth J, Richens A: Predicting phenytoin dose—a revised nomogram. *Ther Drug Monit* 1:325–333, 1979.

106. Hull JH, Sarubbi FA: Gentamicin serum concentrations: pharmacokinetic predictions. *Ann Intern Med* 85:183–189, 1976.

107. Moellering RC, Krogstad DJ, Greenblatt DJ: Vancomycin therapy in patients with impaired renal function: a nomogram for dosage. *Ann Intern Med* 94:343–346, 1981.

108. Matzke GR, McGory RW, Halstenson CE, et al: Pharmacokinetics of vancomycin in patients with various degrees of renal function. *Antimicrob Agents Chemother* 25:433–437, 1984.

109. Sheiner LB, Beal SL: Bayesian individualization of pharmacokinetics: simple implementation and comparison with non-Bayesian methods. *J Pharm Sci* 71:1344–1348, 1982.

110. Yuen GJ, Taylor JW, Ludden TM, Murphy MJ: Predicting phenytoin dosages using Bayesian feedback: a comparison with other methods. *Ther Drug Monit* 5:437–441, 1983.

111. Ludden TM, Allen JP, Valutsky WA, Vicuna AV, Nappi JM, Hoffman SF, et al: Individualization of phenytoin dosage regimens. *Clin Pharmacol Ther* 21:287–293, 1977.

112. Cox S, Walson PD: Providing effective therapeutic drug monitoring services. *Ther Drug Monit* 11:310–322, 1989.

113. Crawford SY: ASHP national survey of hospital-based pharmaceutical services-1990. *Am J Hosp Pharm* 47:2665–2695, 1990.

114. Ried LD, McKenna DA, Horn JR: Meta-analysis of research on the effect of clinical pharmacokinetics services on therapeutic drug monitoring. *Am J Hosp Pharm* 46:945–951, 1989.

115. Dasta JF, Armstrong DK: Pharmacoeconomic impact of critically ill surgical patients. *DICP Ann Pharmacother* 22:994–998, 1988.

116. Reents S, Hatton RC: Influence of methods on the evaluation of therapeutic drug-monitoring services. *Am J Hosp Pharm* 48:1553–1559, 1991.

117. Gilman AG, Goodman LS, Gilman A: *The Pharmacological Basis of Therapeutics*. ed 6. MacMillan, New York, NY, 1990.

CHAPTER 11

Pharmacotherapy in the Elderly

JOSEPH M. SCAVONE, M.S., Pharm.D.

The proper use of drugs in the elderly patient is an issue of social and medical concern. Problems associated with optimal drug selection—the patient's ability and desire to take medications as prescribed, the effects of aging on drug therapy, and the misunderstandings about the goal(s) of drug therapy—have led to many discussions about the use of drugs in elderly patients. It is extremely important for clinicians to be well-informed about the effects of aging on all drugs. Many elderly patients are taking a number of medications that may interact with drugs prescribed by the clinician. Patients may also be taking over-the-counter drugs that could affect a treatment plan. Thus, whenever a patient's clinical status is evaluated, both prescription and nonprescription drugs must be reviewed with the patient. Appropriate choice of drug therapy, dose selection, duration of therapy and potential interactions with a patient's coexistent disease states, other drug therapies, cigarette smoking, ethanol use, and life style requirements must all be delicately balanced in an elderly patient.

Evaluating drug therapy in the elderly is difficult because both the frequency of drug therapy and the number of drugs taken progressively increases with age. It has been estimated that two-thirds of all Americans over the age of 65 years take at least one prescription drug. At hospital discharge, 25% of elderly patients receive prescriptions for 6 or more drugs. In nursing homes it is not uncommon for some patients to be receiving 12 to 15 drugs.

Almost 70% of elderly patients regularly use over-the-counter medications, as compared to about 10% of the general adult population. It is estimated that over-the-counter preparations account for at least 40% of all drugs used by the elderly. Since the incidence of adverse drug effects increases with age and number of medications used, the elderly may suffer adverse drug reactions $1\frac{1}{2}$ to 3 times more than the younger and middle-age adult population (1).

This chapter will review information about the use of drugs in the elderly. It will also describe the elements of drug therapy that are affected by the aging process. It is necessary to explain factors such as physiologic changes, mechanisms of drug interactions, and adverse effects, that govern drug disposition and response. It is imperative that all clinicians have a working knowledge of these concepts, so that they can better understand the clinical importance of the effects of aging on pharmacotherapy.

THE EFFECTS OF AGING ON DRUG THERAPY

It is well-known that the elderly may exhibit an exaggerated pharmacologic response to medications. A therapeutic response may develop in elderly patients at doses far below what is recommended for younger adults. Elderly patients may also experience drug toxicity at doses that are within the usual therapeutic range.

Studies of drug response in the elderly have suggested that at least two types of phenomena may explain these changes in sensitivity. The first explanation is based on pharmacokinetics. The ability to biotransform and/or eliminate drugs from the

Table 11.1. Factors That Can Affect the Pharmacokinetics of Drugs

Patient Variables
    Age
    Gender
    Body composition
    Body weight
    Drugs
    Nutritional status
    Ethanol use
    Cigarette smoking
Medical Conditions
    Congestive heart failure
    Kidney disease
    Cirrhosis
    Hepatitis
    Fever
    Sepsis
    Burns (severe)
    Anemia
    Shock

body declines with age. If the total elimination (clearance) of drug is reduced, then chronic therapy at any given dose will lead to higher steady-state drug concentrations in systemic circulation, and the likelihood of toxicity is increased. The second explanation is a pharmacodynamic one. Receptor site sensitivity to pharmacologic actions of drugs may increase with age. Thus, at any given drug concentration, the presence of the drug at the receptor site may lead to a greater response. Such an increase in drug sensitivity may be evident clinically as a greater likelihood of excessive drug effect(s) or toxicity at what are usually regarded as safe therapeutic doses. Reduced drug sensitivity in the aged can also occur, but it has only been described in a few cases.

PHARMACOKINETICS AND PHARMACODYNAMICS

When studying the effects of drugs in the elderly, one is quickly introduced to many terms that are used to describe the consequences of drug therapy. The term "pharmacokinetics" is often encountered and usually causes a fair amount of apprehension to those who are not familiar with the basic concepts. Pharmacokinetics is the mathematical analysis of the time course of drug concentration in a body fluid or tissue. It describes the amount of drug in the body over time and includes factors that control the time course of drug absorption, distribution, and biotransformation and elimination, parameters collectively referred to as drug disposition.

The pharmacokinetic profile of a drug is based on several interrelated factors, which include the relationship of plasma or serum drug concentrations to the size and frequency of dose, the relationship of free or unbound drug concentration to the amount that is bound to proteins or other blood components, the equilibrium of ionized and un-ionized bound and unbound drug with receptors, and the dissipation of drug effects in relation to the elimination of the drug from the receptor site (2). Other factors that can influence the pharmacokinetics of drugs are listed in Table 11.1.

It is important to realize that absorption, distribution, biotransformation (often referred to as metabolism), and elimination occur simultaneously at rates that change over time. The

process is complex, but the essentials of pharmacokinetics should be understood by all persons involved in prescribing and monitoring the effects of pharmacologic agents. Since the goal of drug therapy is to treat a patient in such a way that a drug provides a therapeutic, yet nontoxic, way to manage various conditions, an understanding and cautious application of pharmacokinetic principles can assist the clinician in making correct decisions when choosing or evaluating an elderly patient's drug therapy (3). It can also allow for more educated decisions about drug selection, dose, frequency of administration, route of administration and monitoring therapeutic response, ineffectiveness, or toxicity. The application of the principles of pharmacokinetics is extremely important for safe and effective drug therapy in the elderly, but it should never replace clinical judgment. Pharmacokinetics provides the framework for understanding drug behavior, but it oversimplifies the complicated physiologic events that govern drug disposition.

The other term that often appears in discussions about drug therapy in the elderly is "pharmacodynamics." Pharmacodynamics refers to the interaction of the drug molecule with its target receptor site. The interaction of drug and receptor is analogous to an enzyme-substrate or lock-and-key type of interaction. In order to fully understand how and why a drug causes a particular effect or the mechanism of drug interactions, its pharmacodynamics must be defined. The effects of aging on receptor sensitivity, specificity, number, and affinity are now being studied. When the pharmacodynamic effects of aging are correlated with pharmacokinetic changes, it will enable the clinician to more accurately predict the effects of drugs in the elderly patient (4).

ABSORPTION

The oral route is the safest, most convenient, and most economical delivery route for drugs intended to have a systemic effect. Orally administered drugs are absorbed from the gastrointestinal tract into systemic circulation and distributed to the site of action. Numerous factors govern the absorption process. In discussions of drug absorption three variables that describe the bioavailability (systemic availability in terms of rate and extent) of a drug should be identified: time of peak plasma drug concentration (T_{max}); peak plasma drug concentration (C_{max}); and the area under the plasma drug concentration-time curve (AUC). Knowledge of the bioavailability of a drug is important because it can be used as a guide when choosing between a "brand name" and generic form of a drug, or when changing from one dosage form or product to another. The intention of drug therapy is also an important factor. Drugs can be administered as a single dose for a specific time-limited situation or in multiple doses for chronic therapy. For example, if the patient is taking a medication as a single dose for the treatment of acute pain or as a sedative/hypnotic, it is important that the drug is absorbed quickly and that it produces a high enough blood level for a long enough time to be clinically effective. However, if a medication, such as an antibiotic, is needed for a long period of time, it is more important that the drug provides an average or steady-state (constant) concentration in the blood.

After a tablet or capsule is swallowed, it must disintegrate before the active drug can dissolve and become absorbed into systemic circulation. If a drug does not get absorbed from the stomach, it will pass into the small intestine, where most drugs are actually absorbed. Factors that govern the absorption of drugs from the gut include the amount of fluid that is coingested with the dosage form, pharmaceutical aspects of the dosage form (such as tablet coatings, formulation, and hardness), the presence of other substances (other drugs, antacids, food, ethanol) in the stomach, gastric emptying time, and intestinal transit time. All of these variables influence the bioavailability profile of a drug. Other considerations include medications that can delay gastric emptying (anticholinergics or opiates) and slow gastrointestinal transit time, drugs that accelerate gastric emptying (metoclopramide), and drugs that can bind other drugs (antihypercholesterolemic resins, kaopectate, psyllium-type laxatives).

Another concern is that some drugs, such as nonsteroidal antiinflammatory agents (including salicylates), potassium tablets and capsules, and iron supplements, can be extremely irritating to the gut mucosa. Gastrointestinal bleeding, ulceration, and perforation have all been reported with the aforementioned drugs.

The presence of food in the gut may cause a delay in drug absorption, but it should not be a clinically important problem if the drugs are taken as chronic multiple-dose therapy.

Other routes of administration that involve drug absorption include the oral route, in which a drug can be used sublingually, buccally, or as a perioral spray; the intramuscular route; the subcutaneous route (including injection and implantation); the intranasal route; the ophthalmic route; and the transdermal route. There is not much information about the effects of aging on the absorption of drugs from these routes of administration. However, based on clinical experience it is assumed that aging does not significantly affect the absorption of drugs from these routes. Anecdotal information suggests that if an aging person has diminished salivary production and if they are taking an anticholinergic drug, such as an antihistamine, tricyclic antidepressant, or antipsychotic medication, these drugs may sufficiently dry the mouth so that it takes longer for the tablet to dissolve. Although this effect has not yet been studied in a controlled fashion, it may explain why some elderly patients have difficulty with sublingual dosage forms. The sublingual route of drug administration is becoming more popular because in some patients, oral administration may be undesirable because of nausea, vomiting, or other situations in which the use of the gastrointestinal tract needs to be avoided. Drugs such as triazolam, alprazolam, captopril, opiate analgesics, antiarrhythmics, nitroglycerin, and others are administered by this route (5, 6).

The coingestion of food and other drugs can significantly affect the bioavailability of a drug. Certain drugs, such as propranolol, griseofulvin, and others, actually have an increased bioavailability when taken with food, whereas the coingestion of food can delay absorption of analgesics, hypnotics, and other drugs so dramatically, the desired clinical effect following a single dose will not occur.

When drugs are given in multiple doses as chronic therapy, the extent of drug absorption (AUC) is more important than either T_{max} or C_{max}. Since the object of drug therapy is to maintain a certain average blood level of the drug, the time course of absorption is less important than the actual amount of drug that replaces that which has been cleared by the body.

Numerous studies performed on the effects of aging on the gastrointestinal tract suggest the possibility of altered drug absorption in the elderly gut (7, 8). Reasons for this suggestion include increased gastric pH because of a reduction in gastric parietal cell function, resulting in decreased gastric acid output (9); decreased splanchnic blood flow, resulting from a decrease in cardiac output (10); a reduction in gastric emptying time; and a decrease in gastrointestinal motility (11). In addition, altered active transport processes of some nutrients in the elderly have led to the belief that drug absorption may be similarly impaired (12). However, for most drugs used in clinical practice, the rate and extent of absorption are determined by passive diffusion during contact with the surface of the proximal small intestine (7). Despite speculation to the contrary, there is essentially no evidence that drug absorption is impaired in the elderly (13–15). Any changes, if they actually do occur, are often small and are unlikely to be of any clinical importance, especially during chronic therapy (16, 17). In summary, changes in drug absorption appear to be the least important of the age-related pharmacokinetic changes. Knowledge of how drug absorption affects the onset and duration of clinical effects for drugs that are given as single doses can assist the clinician in targeting the desired therapeutic effects of a drug for a specific situation.

DISTRIBUTION

Once it is in the body, a drug will distribute to various body fluids and tissues. Fat-soluble drugs such as digoxin, diazepam, and imipramine distribute readily and have relatively large distribution volumes, whereas water-soluble drugs such as cephalosporins, penicillins, and aminoglycosides are considered to have small volumes of distribution. Understanding drug distribution is sometimes difficult because the distribution volumes or compartments are actually derived from mathematics, rather than from anatomy and physiology. Thus, pharmacokinetic compartments are imaginary mathematical spaces and do not correspond to actual anatomic entities, even though the compartments are assigned numeric dimensions of volume (milliliters, liters) (3).

After a drug reaches systemic circulation its passage into body tissue and fluids depends on the drug's molecular size, degree of ionization, solubility, and ability to cross biologic membranes. The goal is to have the drug reach the receptor at the intended site of activity and to cause the desired effect. If too much reaches the receptor site, toxicity could result, and if not enough drug reaches the target, a subtherapeutic response can result. Furthermore, if the drug is available to reach other sites, adverse effects may occur. For example, an antihistamine may be prescribed for the treatment of an allergy, cough, or colds, but in addition to alleviating the symptoms, it can act in the central nervous system and cause drowsiness and confusion; in the eyes it can cause a mydriasis and a blurring of vision; in the gastrointestinal tract it can cause a decrease in gut motility, resulting in constipation; and in many other areas, resulting in urinary retention, diminished salivary flow, and various other effects.

If the drug is able to penetrate many areas in the body, the range of adverse effects can be dramatic. Certain drugs are specifically designed to have different lipid and water-solubility characteristics so that the intended action is more predictable based on its distribution profile. Since many drugs need to be present at the site of activity at a certain minimum effective concentration, the distribution profile of a drug can be used clinically to actually plan a desirable duration of effect. For example, benzodiazepines such as midazolam and diazepam are administered intravenously as a preanesthetic/induction agent for surgery, or orally (diazepam, alprazolam) for conscious sedation or as anxiolytics (18). They are extremely fat-soluble substances that readily distribute throughout the body following the administration of the dose. Because of their extensive distribution, the central nervous system concentrations diminish to a level where the drug is not active any longer. Thus, the termination of clinical effect is governed by the distribution of the drug throughout the body, causing a dilution of the amount available to the receptors located in the brain, and not by the biotransformation or excretion of drug from the body. If a lipid-soluble drug with a large volume of distribution is given chronically, as is oftentimes the case with diazepam, the compartments will sequester drug, and the result will be the accumulation of drug in various tissues. This accumulation can lead to residual effects secondary to increased total body levels of drug. Benzodiazepines, which are relatively more hydrophilic, will exhibit longer durations of clinical effect than their more lipophilic counterparts following single doses but will accumulate to a lesser extent after chronic dosing. The level of response to a medication may increase over time independent of an increase in dose to the patient. Although this concept is extremely important, many clinicians forget that drug accumulation can occur. Some reasons for this accumulation include that the body maintains homeostasis through adaptive mechanisms at the receptor site. It is a rather complicated process, but the message is that despite the protective mechanisms, the body's homeostatic mechanisms can be overridden after a period of time due to changes in reserve capacity.

Several factors, such as decreased cardiac output, increased peripheral vascular resistance, decreased blood flow to the liver and kidney, and increased fraction of cardiac output to cerebral, coronary, and skeletal muscle circulations, affect the distribution of drugs in the elderly person (8, 19). In addition, age-related changes in body habitus (composition) can affect drug distribution. The elderly generally experience a decrease in total body water, extracellular fluid, muscle, and lean body mass and a relative doubling in the proportion of adipose tissue. For example, the fat content in the body of young adult males is approximately 18% and can increase to approximately 36% in elderly males. The percentage of fat in young adult females is approximately 33% and can increase to approximately 48% in elderly females (7). These changes in body habitus can affect the volume of drug distribution, depending on the drug's fat and water solubility. Thus, it appears that there is a gender-related difference in the elderly regarding the volume of distribution of drugs. Women will have a larger distribution of fat-soluble drugs (20–22) and a smaller distribution volume for relatively water-soluble drugs (23, 24). Various fat-soluble drugs, such as diazepam and lidocaine, are more extensively distributed in the elderly, whereas various relatively water-soluble drugs (less lipid-soluble), such as ethanol, antipyrine, and acetaminophen, have a decreased volume of distribution in elderly individuals (7, 25–27).

After drugs enter the systemic circulation they become bound to circulating plasma proteins. Albumin and α_1-acid glycoprotein (AAG), an acute-phase reactant, are the two most important proteins to which drugs can bind. The attachment of drugs to a protein involves a reversible bonding of ionic, hydrogen, or van der Vaal type, which is relatively weak and loose (28). Acidic drugs preferentially bind to albumin (for example, nonsteroidal antiinflammatory agents, salicylates, benzodiazepines, warfarin, phenytoin), whereas basic drugs (tricyclic antidepressants, β-adrenergic antagonists, lidocaine, and other drugs) bind to α_1-acid glycoprotein. Not all drugs are equally bound, and the actual binding of drugs is a dynamic process. In any given situation there is an equilibrium that is established between the amount of drug that is bound and the amount of drug that is unbound or free. The percentage of free drug is known as the free fraction and represents a ratio between the free drug concentration and the total (free plus bound) drug concentration. The distribution of drug to plasma proteins contributes to the actual volume of distribution because only the unbound drug is available to leave the systemic circulation and travel to the receptor site. Additionally, it is the free drug that is available for elimination from the body and to other body tissues and fluids. Although some controversy exists, an age-related reduction in plasma albumin concentrations and age-related increases in α_1-acid glycoprotein have been consistently reported (29, 30). Elderly patients who are undernourished, are severely debilitated, or have advanced disease especially have a substantial decrease in plasma albumin concentrations (31). Healthy, well-nourished elderly persons have lower albumin concentrations than young persons, even though they may not fall below the usual normal range (7). The degree of drug binding to plasma proteins may be reduced in the elderly because of the decrease in the amount of albumin and because of suspected alterations in the affinity of albumin for drugs (8, 28).

The clinical implications of protein binding have often been overestimated. Plasma protein binding, or changes in binding that may occur as a result of drug interactions or disease, seldom have any direct clinical importance. It is neither a benefit nor a disadvantage for a drug to be extensively bound to plasma protein because the free drug concentration is that which is available for pharmacologic activity, distribution, and clearance. The free concentration depends only on the drug dosing rate and the clearance of free drug, not on the actual extent of protein binding (32). Drugs that are considered highly protein-bound are generally greater than 80% bound (Table 11.2). Changes in free fraction could be important for drugs that are 80 to 90% bound but much more important for those which are greater than 90% bound. When the free fraction is small, slight variations can have important consequences. Drugs that are less than 80% bound generally imply that the consequences of protein binding are relatively unimportant (3).

While protein binding interactions do not directly influence clinical activity, alterations in binding can have an enormous effect on the interpretation of total serum or plasma

Table 11.2. Examples of Protein-Bound Drugs

Greater than 90% Bound
   Warfarin
   Ibuprofen
   Phenylbutazone
   Indomethacin
   Diazepam
   Chlordiazepoxide
   Temazepam
   Oxazepam
   Furosemide
   Thiazide diuretics
   Oral hypoglycemics (first generation)
   Propranolol[a]
   Chlorpromazine[a]
80% to 90% Bound
   Lorazepam
   Sulfisoxazole
   Salicylates
   Phenytoin
   Oxazepam
   Clofibrate
   Haloperidol[a]
   Methadone[a]
   Quinidine[a]
   Tricyclic antidepressants[a]

[a] Bound to α_1 acid glycoprotein. All other drugs listed are bound to albumin.

drug concentrations. When drug levels in the serum, plasma, or whole blood are monitored, the laboratory usually reports the total (free plus bound) amount of drug, even though it is only the free drug that is available to cross cell membranes and interact with the receptor. Luckily, the free concentration remains stable over the course of a patient's therapy, and the variability between and within patients is relatively small (33).

When more than one highly protein-bound drug is given to a patient, drug binding to serum protein may be substantially altered. A "new" drug added to a therapeutic regimen can displace the present drug(s) from their protein binding site(s), resulting in a reduction in binding accompanied by an increase in free fraction (10, 34). Such interactions have been misinterpreted. In reality these interactions are unlikely to be clinically important because the transient increase in free concentrations will equilibrate rapidly and will be available for clearance (7, 10, 34, 35). The total drug concentration will be reduced as a result of redistribution and may result in a lowering of the therapeutic and toxic ranges for the total serum or plasma drug level (33).

For example, if a patient who was taking phenytoin (Dilantin) for the treatment of a seizure disorder and routinely had steady-state plasma concentrations averaging about 15 µg/ml and was well-controlled (seizure- and side effect-free) received a prescription for aspirin, a drug interaction will most likely occur because of the displacement of phenytoin from protein-binding sites by the salicylate. However, this drug interaction would not likely be of clinical importance since only the total blood level of phenytoin would decrease (36). Protein-binding interactions are complex, yet transient, and the net result is usually harmless to the patient. The misinterpretation of what actually occurs is the main problem and could result in an inappropriate and potentially hazardous intervention. Since the elderly take more medications, the frequency, as well as

the confusion of such interactions, is much greater than in younger patients.

In summary, a change in drug binding to plasma proteins does not itself alter clinical drug effects. However, alterations in binding may influence the interpretation of plasma or serum drug concentrations (blood levels) used to monitor therapy (7). For highly protein-bound drugs whose binding is decreased and resulting free fraction is increased, clinicians should anticipate lower ranges of both toxic and therapeutic plasma or serum concentrations of total (free plus bound) drug. Regarding drug distribution, altered drug distribution itself in the elderly will not alter steady-state plasma concentrations during chronic drug administration because the maintenance of steady-state plasma concentrations depends only on the dosing rate and the total clearance of the drug.

CLEARANCE

In order to understand how the body eliminates drugs, it is important to be familiar with terms such as clearance and elimination half-life.

The concept of total clearance is extremely important when evaluating the pharmacokinetic properties of all drugs. Clearance is expressed in units of volume divided by time (such as milliliters per minute (ml/min) or liters per hour (liters/hr) and is the single most reliable index of an organism's capacity to biotransform (metabolize) or excrete a given drug (32). Most clinicians are familiar with the concept of clearance in the context of renal function, for which the clearance of creatinine is used as an index of kidney function. Creatinine clearance schematically represents the total volume of blood from which creatinine is completely removed per unit of time. The clearance of drugs is conceptually similar. Most drugs are primarily cleared by either the liver or the kidney. A given drug's clearance numerically describes the capacity of a given individual to remove that drug from the body. A drug's clearance cannot exceed the rate of drug delivery or blood flow to the clearing organ.

Clearance is important in clinical practice because it is a major determinant of steady-state plasma or serum concentration during multiple dosage. In fact, the total clearance of a drug will influence a patient's therapeutic outcome. When a medication has been administered as a multiple dose long enough for steady state to occur, the general equation describing the steady-state concentration in blood, plasma, or serum (C_{ss}) is as follows:

$$C_{ss} = \frac{Dosing\ rate}{Clearance}$$

It is important for clinicians to appreciate this equation because dosing rate is the variable over which they have control (assuming a patient cooperates with the therapeutic plan and is compliant); it is the rate of drug administration, expressed in units of amount of drug divided by time (such as milligrams per hour (mg/hr) or grams per day (g/d)). By varying the size of each dose or the interval between doses (dosage schedule), the clinician can directly control the dosing rate and, ultimately, the steady-state concentration. Clearance appears in the denominator of this equation as the biologic variable describing the individual's capacity to remove the drug from the body. However, in a medically stable patient the clearance of a drug is assumed to be constant. Variables that can dramatically alter the rate of drug clearance in humans include: changes in hepatic or renal status secondary to aging or disease; the addition or deletion of drugs or substances that affect hepatic drug biotransformation processes, such as cigarette smoking, ethanol consumption, and other drugs that are hepatic microsomal enzyme inducers or inhibitors; and drugs that affect kidney function, such as those that compete for tubular absorption or secretion and those that change the pH of the urine. Thus, at any given rate, C_{ss} will increase as clearance decreases (7). If aging is associated with the reduction in total clearance of a given drug, C_{ss} will increase accordingly, and the clinician can either extend the dosing interval or give a lower maintenance dose to the elderly patient for a desired steady-state concentration.

Knowledge of a drug's pathway of biotransformation and of factors that could influence its clearance can help clinicians to anticipate how patient characteristics, drug interactions, or disease states might alter clearance. Many drugs yield active metabolites upon biotransformation that contribute to the therapeutic or toxic effect of the parent compound. The ultimate goal of multiple-dose drug administration is to achieve a steady-state plasma concentration that lies within a "therapeutic" range and to avoid toxic or clinically ineffective blood levels (32).

ELIMINATION HALF-LIFE

Elimination half-life is probably the most commonly discussed and most misinterpreted pharmacokinetic variable for drugs used in clinical practice. Most drugs are eliminated by a characteristic kinetic behavior known as a first-order process. In order for a drug to fit this first-order model, the rate of change of drug concentrations over time must vary continuously in relation to the concentration (3). Drug concentration in body fluids usually declines with time, and when the concentrations are high (i.e., following drug administration), the rate of decline is also high; when concentrations are low, the rate of decline is smaller. Since the rate of drug disappearance varies continuously as a function of time as the concentration changes, an exponential function is used to describe this behavior. Fortunately, first-order exponential processes can be described using the concept of half-life. The elimination half-life of a drug is the time necessary for the drug concentration in blood, serum, plasma, or any other body fluid or tissue to fall by one-half, or 50%. Each time an interval equal to a half-life elapses, the concentration falls to one-half the value at the beginning of that interval. The amount of drug that has been eliminated from the system decreases with the passing of each half-life, but the percentage or ratio of change (50%) is always constant. The important facts (3) to remember about the clinical use of half-lives are as follows:

1. All first-order processes are more than 90% complete after four half-life intervals have elapsed.

2. First-order processes are never 100% complete, no matter how much time elapses.

3. It takes approximately four to five half-lives to elapse before a drug is considered to be in the steady-state condition.

4. It takes approximately four to five half-lives to elapse before a drug is considered to be virtually eliminated from the system, even though first-order processes are considered to be essentially complete after approximately eight half-life intervals.

It is also important that clinicians understand that the elimination half-life is a dependent biologic variable related to a drug's volume of distribution (V_d) and inversely related to its total clearance as follows:

$$Elimination\ half\text{-}life = \frac{0.693 \times V_d}{Clearance}$$

If the volume of distribution is relatively constant, then the elimination half-life will be inversely related to total clearance. Therefore, when clearance is low, half-life is long and, conversely, when clearance is high, half-life is short. However, when the volume of distribution is not constant, changes in volume of distribution may influence elimination half-life without a change in clearance (37). The potential pitfalls of elimination half-life must always be recognized.

Elimination half-life is a clinically important variable because it is related to the rate and extent of drug accumulation during multiple dosage. When a drug is administered at dosing intervals that are shorter than its elimination half-life, a large fraction of each prior dose will remain in the body when the next dose is administered. This result leads to drug accumulation, which continues until the steady-state condition is reached, at which point there is no further accumulation. Likewise, the time necessary to reach steady-state following the start of multiple-dose therapy is also related to the drug's elimination half-life. This concept is used clinically in situations in which a loading dose is administered to a patient in order to quickly initiate a therapeutic response.

Many categories of drugs contain representatives in their class that vary widely in their elimination half-life. This characteristic raises questions about which type of drug is more appropriate for an elderly patient. There are benefits, as well as disadvantages, for both long half-life and short half-life compounds. Drugs with relatively short values of elimination half-life (such as ibuprofen, triazolam, temazepam, lorazepam, and alprazolam) are usually termed "nonaccumulating." For these drugs, the steady-state condition is reached rapidly after the start of therapy. This fact may provide some therapeutic benefit in terms of ease of dosage titration because little delay occurs between initiation of treatment and the attainment of steady state. Short half-life compounds also have some potential disadvantages since multiple daily doses are usually required to maintain adequate plasma levels throughout the day. Furthermore, when treatment is discontinued, or if doses are inadvertently or deliberately missed, serum concentrations will decrease rapidly, which may lead to rapid recurrence of symptoms, withdrawal, or rebound effects. For long half-life compounds (such as piroxicam, digoxin, diazepam, chlordiazepoxide, and desmethyldiazepam), a theoretic disadvantage is that attainment of steady state may be delayed. There is also a delay in the achievement of a new steady-state condition if the dosage must be increased or decreased. There is also a long elimination (wash-out) phase upon discontinuation of the drug, which must be accounted for when a patient's treatment response is reevaluated after starting a different drug therapy. On the other hand, a potential advantage is that the number of doses that the patient takes per day is decreased, which could possibly translate into enhanced patient compliance. Furthermore, when treatment is discontinued, or when doses are missed, plasma levels will not decrease promptly, thereby minimizing the likelihood of a rapid recurrence of symptoms.

In general, many clinicians prefer to use drugs with a shorter half-life in elderly patients because of tighter control when adjusting or individualizing doses and because of the decreased likelihood of accumulation occurring.

BIOTRANSFORMATION

Biotransformation, commonly referred to as drug metabolism, is a considerably complex process that primarily occurs in the liver. Liver cells carry out many biotransformation reactions that contribute to the removal of drugs from the body. Oxidation and conjugation are the two most important subdivisions of hepatic clearance. These reactions can be categorized into either phase I, also referred to as preparative reactions, or phase II, also known as synthetic reactions. Phase I biotransformation includes the oxidation reactions, such as hydroxylation, dealkylation, sulfoxidation, nitroreduction, and hydrolysis. These reactions generally constitute minor molecular modifications, usually resulting in a more water-soluble (polar) metabolite. The product of these reactions also retains part or all of the pharmacologic activity of the parent compound (7). Examples of drugs that undergo phase I biotransformation reactions that yield active metabolites include (parent drug to active metabolite): diazepam to desmethyldiazepam; flurazepam to desalkylflurazepam; imipramine to desipramine; and amitriptyline to nortriptyline. Hepatic microsomal oxidation is often termed a "susceptible" metabolic pathway, in that its activity can be impaired by numerous factors, such as old age, hepatitis, cirrhosis, severe debilitation, or the coadministration of many agents known to impair oxidizing capacity (38, 39). The hepatic microsomal enzymes that are responsible for phase I reactions appear to be significantly impaired in the elderly. The result is a reduction in total drug clearance, higher steady-state plasma drug concentrations during multiple dosage, and an increase in elimination half-life. Phase II reactions involve the attachment or conjugation of the drug molecule to a glucuronide, sulfate, or acetate moiety. The resulting conjugates are generally pharmacologically inactive (except for some acetylated metabolites), are much more polar than the parent molecule, and are usually excreted in the urine (7). Hepatic conjugation is considered to be a "nonsusceptible" pathway and is relatively uninfluenced by old age, disease states, or drug interactions (22, 32). Thus, a prior knowledge of a drug's major metabolic pathway (oxidation vs. conjugation) may be of help to the clinician in predicting whether clearance is susceptible to change in a specific clinical situation (Tables 11.3 and 11.4). In addition, it can be helpful in drug selection for the elderly patient. For example, the benzodiazepines diazepam, chlordiazepoxide, desalkylflurazepam and desmethyldiazepam are all subject to oxidation reactions during clearance from the body. The clearance of many drugs is reduced in elderly patients, and the likelihood for increased accumulation is a concern in that patient population. Since

Table 11.3. Examples of Drugs That Are Biotransformed by Phase I (Preparative) Reactions

Alprazolam
Amitriptyline
Antipyrine
Barbiturates
Carbamazepine
Chloramphenicol
Chlorpromazine
Clonazepam
Codeine
Desipramine
Desmethyldiazepam
Diazepam
Dimenhydrinate
Doxylamine
Flurazepam
Glutethimide
Ibuprofen
Imipramine
Lidocaine
Meperidine
Methamphetamine
Nortriptyline
Midazolam
Phenacetin
Phenylbutazone
Phenytoin
Prazepam
Quinidine
Trazodone
Triazolam
Warfarin

Table 11.4. Examples of Drugs That Are Biotransformed by Phase II (Synthetic) Reactions

Acetaminophen
Acetylsalicylic acid (aspirin)
Clonazepam
Hydralazine
Lorazepam
Nitrazepam
Oxazepam
Phenelzine
Procainamide
Sulfanilamide
Temazepam

the metabolism of the parent drug yields metabolites that are also clinically active, there is a concern about the accumulation not only of the parent drug but also of the active metabolites as well. The accumulation of metabolites could theoretically contribute to the development of adverse or increased effects. On the other hand, the benzodiazepines oxazepam, temazepam, and lorazepam undergo conjugation reactions, have no active metabolites, and are relatively unaffected by old age. Thus, drug selection for the elderly patient can essentially make more sense if the prescribing clinician considers the drug's metabolic fate.

Hepatic blood flow can be more important for some drugs than is microsomal enzyme activity as a major determinant of total drug clearance (40). Partially as a result of an age-related reduction in cardiac output, liver blood flow declines an estimated 40 to 45% in elderly persons, as compared to that in young adults (9). Hepatic size, both in absolute terms and as a percentage of total body weight, decreases with age.

One would expect that the clearance of high liver blood flow-dependent drugs would be uniformly affected, but the data are conflicting. For example, a reduction in the total clearance occurs for propranolol but not for lidocaine (26, 41, 42). Theoretically, the bioavailability of drugs that have a high first-pass hepatic extraction (following drug absorption from the gastrointestinal tract before reaching the general systemic circulation) may also be affected by aging, but there is no conclusive evidence available at this time.

It is difficult to predict the influence of age on biotransformation since hepatic drug-metabolizing capacity may not be uniformly affected. Changes in total clearance of hepatic microsomal enzyme-mediated drug oxidation reactions can be impaired in an elderly individual, even though the patient has normal liver function tests. Thus, normal values on liver function tests do not imply normal drug metabolism. In addition, the effect of age on hepatic drug clearance depends on the metabolic pathway of the drug, in addition to the influence of liver blood flow, size, and other coingested substances and drugs. It appears that aging affects drug clearance in elderly males to a greater extent than in elderly females.

ELIMINATION (RENAL CLEARANCE)

The effect of age on renal drug clearance is more straightforward and predictable. Glomerular filtration rate decreases by about 35% over a person's lifetime, so that drugs excreted mainly by the kidney can be expected to have reduced total clearance (7, 8, 41, 43). In order to adequately predict the effect of the aging kidney on total drug clearance, it is necessary to know the status of a patient's level of renal function. This status is usually determined by evaluating a serum creatinine level or estimating a glomerular filtration rate (GFR), using creatinine clearance as an indicator. Serum creatinine concentration depends on endogenous creatinine production, as well as on renal creatinine clearance. Evaluating renal function based on serum creatinine is oftentimes misleading, because the age-related decrease in lean body (muscle) mass results in a decrease in daily endogenous creatinine production. As a result, in the elderly, creatinine clearance must decrease to a greater extent than in a younger person before the serum creatinine increases (43). Thus, the use of serum creatinine concentration as the only indicator of renal function may actually overestimate renal function. In an elderly patient, serum creatinine may be in the normal range while renal function is substantially reduced (7, 8). Ideally, creatinine clearance determinations based on 24-hour urinary excretion should be used along with serum creatinine to evaluate renal function. In reality this is not always feasible, so clinicians must rely only on serum creatinine concentrations. However, there are various nomograms and formulas available to estimate creatinine clearance from serum creatinine. One formula (44) that is considered useful is the following:

Creatinine clearance in males =
$$\frac{(140 - age) \times body\ weight\ (kg)}{72 \times serum\ creatinine\ level}$$

Creatinine clearance in females = 0.85 × above value

where creatinine clearance is in milliliters per minute (ml/min), serum creatinine is in milligrams per deciliter (mg/dl), age is in years, and weight is in kilograms (kg).

In general, the dosage of a drug that is excreted principally by the kidney must be reduced in order to prevent excessive accumulation of the drug (Table 11.5). Following reduction in the initial doses of drugs excreted by the kidney, the clinical status of the patient can be reviewed, and dosage adjustments can be made.

PHARMACODYNAMICS: THE EFFECTS OF AGING ON DRUG SENSITIVITY

It is generally believed that the elderly are more sensitive to drug effects than the young and, consequently, experience more adverse reactions (8, 23). These observations have stimulated much speculation about the cause of these clinical impressions, but conclusive evidence is still lacking about the reasons and mechanisms for altered responsiveness. Since it is not possible in many cases to measure in humans the true in vivo receptor sensitivity, many of these questions will go unanswered (45). Data from experiments using animal models, tissue, and/or cell cultures and studies in humans correlating serum, plasma, or tissue level to a resulting pharmacodynamic response are the basis for evaluating the effects of aging on drug response.

There are conflicting data and considerable debate about the mechanisms underlying the altered sensitivity to drugs in elderly humans. There are basically two interrelated hypotheses that are used to explain the differences. The pharmacodynamic hypothesis suggests that receptors change in their sensitivity to certain drugs, such that a given drug concentration at the receptor site leads to a greater effect in an elderly individual than in a young individual. The age-related changes appear to occur at the level of either the affinity of the receptor for a drug, the number of functioning receptors, the concentration or density of receptors in a given area, the sensitivity of the receptor, the presence or absence of second or subsequent messengers, or the cellular responsiveness to these messengers (8). The second possible mechanism for altered drug sensitivity is a pharmacokinetic one. Previously

Table 11.5. Examples of Drugs That Are Excreted by the Kidney

Amantadine
Amikacin
Cephalosporins
Cimetidine
Digoxin
Erythromycin
Furosemide
Gentamicin
Lithium
Methanamic acid
Nitrofurantoin
Penicillins
Phenobarbital
Procainamide
Quinidine
Sulfonamides
Tetracycline
Tobramycin
Vancomycin

in this chapter, age-related changes in pharmacokinetics were discussed. Information about a decrease in total metabolic clearance and changes in volume of distribution raised the issue that, at any given dosing rate, steady-state concentrations will be higher in the elderly than in young individuals. Since the effects of many drugs parallel receptor occupancy, the more drug available to the receptor at a given dose results in increased pharmacodynamic (therapeutic or toxic) activity.

Studies in humans documenting a change in pharmacodynamic sensitivity to drugs among the elderly are less numerous than those describing pharmacokinetic changes. This fact is because it is often difficult to isolate aging from confounding variables such as coexistent medical or psychiatric disease, other drug therapies, and altered nutritional status and body habitus. No consistent generalizations can be made about drug effects in the elderly because intrinsic changes in drug sensitivity are difficult to quantitate in well-controlled studies. Drug responses in the elderly may be increased, decreased, or unchanged, depending on the nature of the study population and the particular variable evaluated. Thus, the interpretation of altered drug sensitivity in the elderly has to be described for each drug category.

SELECTED DRUG CATEGORIES

SLEEP DISORDERS AND THE USE OF HYPNOTICS

Sleep disorders are extremely common in the elderly. Each year, approximately 10 million Americans consult a physician about their sleep problems, and about half of these receive prescriptions for hypnotic medications (46). Insomnia is the second most common indication requiring drug therapy. More than 50 million prescriptions are dispensed annually for hypnotic drugs and countless more over-the-counter hypnotics are sold (47).

Insomnia is the major complaint among elderly patients seeking help for a sleep disorder. Insomnia is sometimes used as a catch-all term for different types of sleep disturbances. Therefore, it is necessary for the clinician who is evaluating the patient to obtain a thorough history and description of the condition causing the complaint. Sleep disturbances are oftentimes clinical manifestations of other diseases or problems such as psychiatric illness, incontinence, cardiac conditions, pain, and others. Thus, the complaint of insomnia may be secondary to a problem that can be readily treated. If a patient with a sleep problem, which is secondary to another condition, is treated with a hypnotic agent, aggravation of the preexisting condition and/or worsening of the primary disorder could ensue. The presence of other disturbances that may be associated with symptoms of sleep disturbance must be ruled out before hypnotics are prescribed for the patient.

The complaint of insomnia may be further clarified into either one or a combination of the following: difficulty in falling asleep (increased sleep latency); frequent nocturnal awakenings; and/or early morning awakenings with the inability to fall back to sleep. Each problem may have to be treated differently because of the characteristics of the available drug therapies.

HYPNOTICS

Formal clinical studies evaluating the effects of aging on the pharmacokinetics and pharmacodynamics of various hypnotics such as chloral hydrate, barbiturates, glutethimide, ethchlorvynol, methyprylon, and most antihistamines have not been done. With the exception of low doses of chloral hydrate (e.g., 0.25 to 0.5 g) and diphenhydramine (e.g., 25 mg) administered occasionally, the other drugs listed are not considered to be reasonable choices for the elderly.

Data on the safety, efficacy, and toxicity of benzodiazepine hypnotics following single dosage and during chronic use are available from sleep laboratory studies and from controlled clinical trials. In general, benzodiazepines are safe and effective for the treatment of insomnia when used in the lowest effective dose for the shortest time. However, some patients do suffer from chronic insomnia and have to take hypnotics for long periods of time.

BENZODIAZEPINES

Data on the efficacy and toxicity of benzodiazepine hypnotics following single dosage and during chronic use are available from sleep laboratory studies and from controlled clinical trials. Results from these two research settings do not always agree, but some generalizations have been made. The clinical efficacy of benzodiazepines used in the short-term or intermediate-term treatment of insomnia that is unrelated to identifiable medical or psychiatric disease is well-known. The use of hypnotic agents to treat insomnia constitutes only one management option in the overall clinical approach to patients with insomnia. Individualized clinical judgment must be used when deciding which patients are candidates for hypnotic medications. Most patients with insomnia do not require long-term treatment, and the hazards of well-monitored therapy of limited duration with hypnotic drugs appear to be small. Currently, there are five benzodiazepine derivatives that are indicated specifically for the treatment of sleep disorders in the U.S. A number of other benzodiazepines are equally useful as hypnotics, although they do not carry specific labeling for the insomnia indication (48). It would be incorrect to state that hypnotic benzodiazepines have important neuropharmacologic differences from anxiolytic benzodiazepines. In fact, all of these drugs act as antianxiety agents at low doses and sedative/hypnotics at higher doses. The primary approved therapeutic indication reflects a combination of research direction taken during clinical development and testing, together with specific pharmacokinetic properties that might make a particular drug suitable as a hypnotic.

A clear relationship between plasma benzodiazepine concentrations and clinical sedative and/or anxiolytic effects has not yet been demonstrated. Therefore, it cannot be stated with certainty that the pharmacokinetic profile of a particular benzodiazepine derivative explains its clinical properties. Observations during clinical and sleep laboratory studies of the various benzodiazepine hypnotics are highly consistent with the pharmacokinetic properties of these drugs.

The principal determinant of the onset of action of hypnotic drugs is the rate of absorption. The faster the rate of absorption, the quicker and more intense is the onset of action.

The duration of clinical effect following a single dose is governed mainly by distribution and not by the elimination half-life. However, for a drug with an extremely short elimination half-life, such as triazolam, elimination does contribute to the termination of action.

Multiple-dose effects are a combination of the effect of any given dose together with residual effects from prior doses (48). Elimination is a major determinant of accumulation. Accumulation of compounds with long elimination half-lives increases the likelihood of continued efficacy during repeated dosage and minimizes the probability that rebound insomnia will occur upon discontinuation of the drug. The chance of the occurrence of residual effects such as daytime drowsiness and impairment of performance is also increased but is partly offset by adaptation and/or tolerance. Nonaccumulating hypnotics with short elimination half-lives have a reduced likelihood of adverse daytime sequelae. Although previously disputed, evidence now indicates that there is an increased probability of transient rebound-insomnia following the discontinuation of hypnotics with short elimination half-lives.

The relevance of these pharmacokinetic principles becomes evident when the properties of the benzodiazepine hypnotics are considered individually.

FLURAZEPAM

Flurazepam hydrochloride was the first benzodiazepine to become available in the U.S. for specific use as a hypnotic agent. Flurazepam has been extensively used since its introduction in 1970. As a result, most other hypnotic agents are compared to flurazepam in clinical trials.

The pharmacokinetic profile of flurazepam in humans is extremely complex. Flurazepam appears to act as a mixture of short- and long-acting hypnotics. When the blood or serum from a patient taking flurazepam is evaluated, a number of active substances are found to be present. Flurazepam has at least three metabolites that are pharmacologically active. Hydroxyethyl flurazepam and flurazepam aldehyde appear and disappear rapidly, so they are termed "short-acting substances." These two metabolites are likely to contribute to the induction of sleep. There is desalkylflurazepam, the principal metabolite, which both appears and is eliminated slowly. Flurazepam is a complicated compound with respect to what is actually inducing sleep, what is maintaining sleep, what is causing residual effects, and what is accumulating following multiple dosage.

The metabolic pathway of desalkylflurazepam involves hepatic hydroxylation, which is an oxidative reaction. It is influenced by aging (especially in males), liver disease, and microsomal enzyme inducers and inhibitors. The elimination half-life of desalkylflurazepam in healthy, normal adults ranges from 40 to 200 hours and may be as long as 300 hours in the elderly. Accumulation of desalkylflurazepam during multiple dosage with flurazepam occurs and is directly related to its long elimination half-life and clearance.

Elderly males accumulate desalkylflurazepam to a greater degree than do young males. However, values for elderly females are no different than those for young females (49).

Clinical ratings of sleep patterns and daytime sedation have also been correlated with pharmacokinetic data. Results indicate an increase over time in daytime sedation, in addition to improvement in sleep parameters, which are generally consistent with the profile of desalkylflurazepam accumulation. The changes over time in clinical effects did not occur in parallel with the increases in desalkylflurazepam plasma concentration, probably due to the capacity of benzodiazepines to produce clinical tolerance and adaptation to their effect.

As a result of the long elimination half-life of desalkylflurazepam in the elderly due to a reduction in clearance, many clinicians avoid its use in patients over 60 years old. Short-term occasional doses of flurazepam (15 mg) have been shown clinically to be "safe" for the elderly. Issues dealing with carryover, residual or hangover effects compared with tolerance, and adaptation are still unclear at this time, so definitive recommendations cannot be made. Flurazepam at a dosage of 15 mg appears to be safe in most patients younger than 60 years old, but caution must be emphasized with its use in elderly patients who may receive chronic therapy.

QUAZEPAM

Quazepam is available as a product named Doral (formerly Dormalin). Claims that quazepam is selective for the BZ-1 receptor, which affects the neural pathways involved in the generation of natural sleep, remain to be proved. Quazepam is a precursor of desalkylflurazepam and as such can be expected to be an accumulating hypnotic agent, especially in the elderly. The same cautions for flurazepam apply to quazepam.

TEMAZEPAM

Temazepam was introduced as an hypnotic agent in 1981 as Restoril. It is a 3-hydroxybenzodiazepine derivative and is biotransformed in the liver by conjugation rather than oxidation. The major metabolite is glucuronide conjugate. Temazepam glucuronide has no pharmacologic activity and is excreted in the urine. Smaller amounts of temazepam are metabolized by *N*-demethylation to yield oxazepam, which then appears in the urine as oxazepam glucuronide.

Following administration of the hard-gelatin capsule preparation of temazepam that is currently available in the U.S., the appearance rate of temazepam in plasma is slow. Peak concentrations are reached in an average of 2.5 hours after administration (50). Part of this slow rate of appearance is the result of the formulation of the hard-gelatin capsule and part is due to temazepam's intrinsic physicochemical properties. Clearly, temazepam is not ideal for patients with insomnia characterized primarily by difficulty in falling asleep (increased sleep latency), particularly when the drug is taken directly at bedtime. This finding is consistent with clinical studies showing its minimal efficacy in sleep latency insomnia (49). The slow absorption of temazepam may be partly offset by ingestion of the dose 1 to 2 hours before bedtime rather than immediately at the time of retiring. However, if the dose is coingested with food, there may be a further delay in the time to reach peak plasma concentrations and the onset of clinical effect.

Clinical studies of temazepam performed in the United Kingdom and Europe are not applicable to the use of temazepam in the U.S. The soft-gelatin capsule preparation of temazepam that is available in Europe provides a much more rapid rate of absorption than does the hard-gelatin capsule. Thus, it is impossible to extrapolate or compare clinical trials using one or the other preparation.

The mean elimination half-life of temazepam is approximately 13 to 14 hours, with a range of 10 to 20 hours. In some individuals it can be longer than 30 hours. Therefore, temazepam is characterized as having an intermediate rather than a short half-life. As a result, an intermediate degree of accumulation will occur, with the accumulation profile falling between the extremes of benzodiazepines with long, as opposed to short, elimination half-life values (50). The clinical consequence of the temazepam accumulation profile is not clearly established.

Because temazepam is biotransformed by conjugation rather than oxidation, its metabolic pathway is less likely to be influenced by factors such as aging. It has been speculated that despite its absorption problems, temazepam may be more appropriate for the treatment of frequent nocturnal awakenings and/or early morning awakenings, especially in the elderly.

In summary, temazepam is an intermediate-acting benzodiazepine with no long-acting metabolites. Doses of 15 to 30 mg increase total sleep time and decrease the frequency of duration of nocturnal awakenings in insomniac patients. Temazepam does not appear to decrease the latency to sleep onset and, therefore, would not be appropriate for a patient whose only complaint was difficulty in falling asleep. In the elderly, a dose of 15 mg daily should be used initially, and the patient should be reevaluated before it is increased to 30 mg.

TRIAZOLAM

Triazolam (Halcion) is a triazolobenzodiazepine hypnotic with a short elimination half-life. In the majority of individuals, the elimination half-life falls between 1.5 and 5 hours. A typical dose is almost completely eliminated 12 to 15 hours after ingestion. Therefore, triazolam is an essentially nonaccumulating hypnotic. This lack of accumulation probably minimizes the likelihood of residual daytime effects.

The absorption rate of triazolam is in the intermediate range, with peak concentrations occurring between 1 and 2 hours after dosage. Triazolam can also be administered sublingually. Following sublingual administration, there is approximately a 28% increase in bioavailability, presumably due to avoidance in first-pass hepatic extraction (51). Triazolam is metabolized principally by hepatic microsomal oxidation. The effects of age, liver disease, or metabolic inhibitors or enhancers on its pharmacokinetic profile cannot yet be generalized. Factors influencing the pharmacokinetic profile of triazolam may differ from those of other oxidized benzodiazepines (49).

The current recommended initial starting dose of triazolam in adults is 0.125 to 0.25 mg unless the patient is unresponsive. In the elderly, dosages greater than 0.25 mg are not recommended. Elderly patients should initially be started at a dose of 0.125 mg. If this appears to be too much, then one-half of a 0.125-mg tablet (0.0625 mg) can be given. The use of triazolam for several consecutive nights may lead to a transient period of "rebound-insomnia" that usually lasts for one to two nights following the abrupt discontinuation of the drug. This effect should be anticipated and can be minimized by tapering treatment over time.

Triazolam, in addition to other benzodiazepines, can also cause "anterograde-amnesia." The intensity and duration of this effect appears to increase with dosage. It is not clearly established at this time whether the amnestic effects are any more frequent or severe than those that occur during treatment with other benzodiazepine derivatives. Various psychologic disturbances have been anecdotally associated with triazolam, but controlled clinical trials suggest that this is not a substantial concern (49).

In summary, triazolam is a short-acting benzodiazepine. In doses of 0.125 to 0.25 mg it increases sleep duration and decreases nocturnal awakening in latency to sleep onset. Triazolam alters the distribution of REM sleep during the night but has little, if any, effect on the total amount of REM sleep. Triazolam also appears to have no effect on delta sleep, which distinguishes it from chlordiazepoxide, diazepam, flurazepam, and temazepam. In comparative studies, triazolam is subjectively judged to be equal to, or better than, flurazepam, diazepam, or oxazepam (48). Clearly, this appears to be the benzodiazepine hypnotic of choice in an elderly patient who has trouble falling asleep.

ESTAZOLAM

Estazolam is a triazolobenzodiazepine derivative. The mean elimination half-life in elderly subjects ranges from 13.5 to 34.6 hours, as compared to 10 to 24 hours in young subjects. The recommended initial dose for elderly patients is 0.5 mg at bedtime; however, 1 mg may be necessary. Estazolam is biotransformed in the liver to 4-hydroxyestazolam and 1-oxoestazolam. These metabolites have some pharmacologic activity but because of their low potencies and low concentrations, they are not thought to significantly contribute to the hypnotic effect of estazolam. Estazolam is relatively new to the U.S. market, so clinical experience in the elderly is limited.

OTHER BENZODIAZEPINES

Other benzodiazepines may also serve as hypnotics. The lack of a Food and Drug Administration-approved specific indication for sleep disorders by no means precludes the use of a benzodiazepine as a hypnotic agent. Many benzodiazepines indicated primarily for anxiety can serve equally well as sleep-inducing agents, provided that the clinical approach is adapted for this objective and the drug's kinetic properties are well-understood. Both diazepam and clorazepate are rapidly absorbed from the gastrointestinal tract and can be very useful in the treatment of sleep disorders characterized by difficulty in falling asleep. Furthermore, their extensive volume of distribution tends to minimize residual hangover effects. However, the cumulative profile of desmethyldiazepam during multiple dosage closely resembles that of flurazepam, with the associated risks and benefits. Lorazepam and oxazepam may also be used as hypnotics. The rate of lorazepam and oxazepam absorption and elimination half-life is intermediate. Therefore, it is best taken approximately 1 hour before bedtime if it is used in patients with increased sleep latency. During multiple dosage, an intermediate degree of accumulation can be anticipated.

Benzodiazepines are clearly superior to other classes of hypnotic agents in safety and, possibly, in efficacy. Clinically meaningful differences among the various benzodiazepines are often subtle but could result in a significant alteration in clinical response. Therefore, understanding the pharmacokinetic similarities and differences among the various benzodiazepine sedative-hypnotics is extremely important and should help the health care practitioner to make a more informed judgment as to the appropriateness of a choice of a particular agent for his/her patient.

ANTIANXIETY AGENTS

Benzodiazepines are the most frequently prescribed anxiolytic agents. They are usually recommended for the short-term relief of anxiety, whereas psychotherapy or counseling is chosen for long-term management (52). In general, the aging process does not result in any change in the absorption rate of benzodiazepines. Age-related changes in body habitus can result in accumulation of the more lipophilic and so-called "long-acting" benzodiazepines (diazepam, desmethyldiazepam, flurazepam, desalkylflurazepam, quazepam, prazepam, clorazepate, and chlordiazepoxide) and their metabolites due to a larger volume of distribution. These long-acting benzodiazepines are cleared via the hepatic microsomal mixed-function oxidase system and will be metabolized at a slower rate in the elderly. Age-related changes in clearance and volume of distribution result in a prolongation in the elimination half-life. These pharmacokinetic changes coupled with increased sensitivity in pharmacodynamic effects in the elderly explain why this group experiences a more profound drug effect at any given dose (52–54). The benzodiazepines lorazepam and oxazepam are less lipid-soluble than the others and undergo conjugation in the liver as their means of clearance. This biotransformation pathway is relatively unaffected by aging, so these drugs are better choices for the elderly. Alprazolam is a comparatively intermediate-acting drug that is primarily cleared by phase I biotransformation. However, alprazolam does not yield any clinically important metabolites. In lower doses it is also a reasonable choice for the elderly.

All benzodiazepines can produce lethargy, sedation, cognitive impairment, and central nervous system depression that can lead to ataxia and motor incoordination (48, 55, 56). They can also interact synergistically or additively with other central nervous system depressants. They are contraindicated in patients with sleep apnea and respiratory depression because of their respiratory depressant effects.

In summary, for the elderly patient short- to intermediate-acting benzodiazepines (short to intermediate elimination half-life) are preferred to long-acting agents (long elimination half-life) and hydrophilic alternatives that are metabolized via conjugation reactions are preferred to those that are oxidized and yield active metabolites. Drug interactions with benzodiazepines and the potential aggravation of underlying medical or psychiatric conditions must be considered before these drugs are prescribed for the elderly.

Buspirone is a nonbenzodiazepine anxiolytic that is classified as an azapirone. Its exact mechanism of action is not known, but it appears to involve complex interactions among central nervous system neurotransmitters, especially serotonin (57–59). Buspirone is metabolized to active and inactive metabolites, but aging does not appear to affect its clearance. It is an appealing drug for treating the elderly because of its lack of serious side effects. Buspirone lacks sedative, muscle relaxant, and anticonvulsant effects of benzodiazepines (59). The most common adverse effects are dizziness, nervousness, and headaches, which are dose-related. Buspirone does not cause cognitive or psychomotor impairment; does not interact with alcohol or other central nervous system depressants; does not decrease respiratory function or impair driving skills (57, 59). It has also been shown to be as effective as other benzodiazepines in the treatment of anxiety (60). The major drawback with buspirone is the lag-time of approximately 1 to 2 weeks before its anxiolytic effect occurs. This drawback should not preclude its use, but patients should be counseled about therapeutic expectations. It also seems to work better in benzodiazepine-naive patients because many patients who have taken benzodiazepines miss the characteristic "buzz," which does not occur following the ingestion of buspirone.

Antihistamines, β-adrenergic blockers, antidepressants, and neuroleptics are also used to treat anxiety. β-blockers are useful when patients have somatic components to anxiety, such as palpitations, diaphoresis, tremulousness, urinary frequency, and tachycardia (56). Antihistamines may be useful in patients with depressed respiratory function, such as those with chronic obstructive pulmonary disease. Neuroleptics are useful in patients who suffer from severe anxiety and agitation, and antidepressants are useful in anxious patients with coexisting depression. These drugs are discussed elsewhere in this chapter.

ANTIDEPRESSANTS

Antidepressants can be safely prescribed for the elderly if underlying medical conditions and concurrent drug therapy are carefully evaluated. It is important to consider the many drugs that a patient is taking that cause or contribute to depression. Various medical conditions may also aggravate or contribute to depression, and other medical conditions could be adversely affected by drug therapy. The choice of which antidepressant is most appropriate for a given patient is determined largely by its adverse effect profile (i.e., sedative, cardiovascular, and anticholinergic), the patient's ability to tolerate its side effects, prior patient response to the drug or other antidepressants, the patient's medical and psychiatric status, and age-related changes in the pharmacokinetics of a drug and its metabolites (55, 61–63). Generally, antidepressant drug doses for the elderly should be 30 to 50% of those used in younger patients, and the dosage should be gradually increased until the desired therapeutic effect is achieved or until intolerable or potentially dangerous adverse effects develop. If side effects occur, the drug should be substituted for another, usually from the same class, with a lower incidence of the adverse effect that occurred (52). The elderly patient must be closely monitored for both side effects and response. Antidepressants should be continued for a minimum of 4 weeks before a decision is made that they are not effective (61). The elderly may take longer to respond to therapy than do younger patients (64). It should be noted that electroconvulsive therapy and psychotherapy are safe and effective treatments for depression in the elderly, but they will not be addressed in this chapter.

Tricyclic antidepressants are considered the drugs of choice in treating depression in the elderly (56, 61, 63). The mechanisms of action of tricyclic antidepressants include inhibition of the reuptake of biogenic amines (especially norepinephrine and serotonin), muscarinic acetylcholine receptor antagonism, and histamine (H_1 and H_2) receptor antagonism (61). The tricyclics differ from each other by their relative anticholinergic and sedative effects (65). The elderly are especially sensitive to the anticholinergic effects of tricyclics, which include blurred vision, urinary retention, tachycardia, dry mouth, mild memory loss, orientation difficulties, confusional reactions, constipation, and precipitation of narrow-angle glaucoma. Elderly patients may not differ from younger patients in the likelihood of becoming hypotensive on tricyclics, but they are more likely to experience serious complications after falls (61). Of these agents amitriptyline and doxepin are the most sedative; protriptyline is the least sedative; amitriptyline, trimipramine, doxepin, and protriptyline have the highest anticholinergic activity; desipramine has the weakest anticholinergic effects; and nortriptyline may cause less orthostatic hypotension than the other tricyclics (55, 61).

Tricyclics can also be categorized by chemical structure and biotransformation. The tertiary amines (amitriptyline, doxepin, imipramine, and trimipramine) are metabolized in the liver by demethylation to yield active metabolites that are secondary amines. The age-related decrease in the rate of hepatic biotransformation has been previously discussed. Thus, there tends to be a higher ratio of tertiary to secondary amines. Generally, the tertiary amines produce greater anticholinergic, hypotensive, and cardiac effects than the secondary amines, so it appears to be more reasonable that the secondary amines (desipramine, nortriptyline, and protriptyline) are used initially in the elderly patient (55).

The tricyclic antidepressants are especially useful and effective in the elderly patient. When the patient is properly diagnosed and concomitant medications, and coexisting medical and psychiatric problems have been evaluated in terms of their effect on depression and potential interaction with tricyclic antidepressants, appropriate drug and dose selection will often result in safe and effective therapy.

Fluoxetine is a bicyclic antidepressant that inhibits the presynaptic reuptake of serotonin with an apparent impressive side effect profile. It is biotransformed in the liver to its demethylated metabolite norfluoxetine. One study evaluating the effect of aging on the pharmacokinetics of fluoxetine found no difference between young and elderly subjects (66). The frequency of side effects is low and dose-related, with the most common being nausea, anxiety, insomnia, anorexia, diarrhea, and nervousness (67).

MONOAMINE OXIDASE INHIBITORS

Monoamine oxidase (MAO) inhibitors are not used as frequently as the tricyclics in the elderly. Reasons for this include severe orthostatic hypotension and interactions with tyramine-containing foods and sympathomimetic drugs, resulting in hypertensive crisis (61, 68, 69). MAO inhibitors still need to be further evaluated in the elderly because monoamine oxidase increases with age, whereas the synthesis of biogenic amines decreases (70); they do not produce cardiac arrhythmias; they have few anticholinergic effects; and they do not adversely affect cognitive function (61).

OTHER DRUGS

Trazodone is a phenylpiperazine derivative that selectively inhibits the uptake of serotonin (71). The major side effect of trazodone is sedation, which is found less with chronic dosing than acute dosing; it most likely does not impair psychomotor function or memory in elderly patients; it has few anticholinergic effects, a low incidence of cardiovascular toxicity, and a good safety profile in overdosage. Dry mouth and constipation do occur, but it is thought to be a result of α-adrenergic blocking activity. Major cardiovascular side effects include a mild reduction of heart rate and blood pressure, and the possibility of exacerbating preexisting arrhythmias (61). The worst adverse effect is priapism. Trazodone offers many advantages over tricyclic antidepressants and MAO inhibitors in the management of depression in the elderly.

Maprotiline is a tetracyclic antidepressant that blocks the reuptake of norepinephrine and has antihistaminic and peripheral anticholinergic effects (72). Unfortunately, maprotiline is associated with a high incidence of seizures at therapeutic levels; has cardiovascular side effects that are similar to those of the tricyclics; and is considered to be extremely toxic in overdosage. Its use is not favored in any age group (73, 74).

Amoxapine is a demethylated metabolite of loxapine, a neuroleptic, and belongs to the dibenzoxapine class of tricyclics. It is a dopamine antagonist and a potent inhibitor of norepinephrine uptake. It has a relatively benign cardiac toxicity profile, but it has been associated with atrial arrhythmias and conduction abnormalities at therapeutic doses in the elderly (61).

Amoxapine can also cause tardive dyskinesia, dystonias, parkinsonism, akinesias, and neuroleptic malignant syndrome, which makes it a poor choice for elderly patients.

Bupropion is a phenylaminoketone that has dopaminergic properties but no significant effect on norepinephrine or serotonin (75). It has no cardiovascular effects, minimal anticholinergic effects, a mild anxiolytic effect, and no sedative effects. Dry mouth is the major side effect. Dose-related seizures have been reported, but its implication to elderly patients is not known at this time (61).

ANTIPSYCHOTIC AGENTS

Antipsychotic drugs or neuroleptics are used for treating chronic schizophrenia, psychotic paranoid states, bipolar disorders, agitated depression, and agitation and confusion of delirium and dementia (52). Chlorpromazine, thioridazine, thiothixene, haloperidol, perphenazine, trifluoperazine, and fluphenazine are of equal therapeutic efficacy when prescribed in equipotent dosages. Haloperidol and fluphenazine are considered to be high-potency antipsychotics and have the greatest incidence of extrapyramidal effects, pseudo-parkinsonism, akathesias, and dystonias (52). However, they are associated with a lower incidence of sedation, hypotension, and anticholinergic effects. Due to age-related changes in the central nervous system, the elderly are more likely to have side effects of the pseudo-parkinsonian type and tardive dyskinesia but less likely to have dystonias than younger patients (76). Chlorpromazine and thioridazine are classified as low-potency drugs. They are associated with a higher incidence of sedation and anticholinergic effects. Side effects related to α-adrenergic antagonism, such as orthostatic hypotension, myocardial infarction, cerebrovascular accidents, and hypersensitivity reactions, are more common with chlorpromazine and thioridazine (52, 55). Higher plasma levels of chlorpromazine occur in the elderly following similar doses to younger patients (77). In summary, age-related increases in sensitivity to antipsychotic drugs appear to be explained by a combination of pharmacokinetic changes involving decreased clearance and pharmacodynamic alterations related to changes in receptor sites (number and density) and receptor sensitivity. It is presumed that elderly patients require reduced doses of antipsychotic drugs, but interpatient variability is high. As with most other drugs, antipsychotic drug doses should start out low and be gradually increased until the desired clinical response is reached with minimal side effects.

LITHIUM

Lithium is primarily excreted via the kidneys. Since renal function declines secondary to aging, a predictable decrease in lithium clearance occurs. Therefore, serum lithium levels should be closely monitored in elderly patients. Many drugs can also affect lithium clearance. Diuretics may cause sodium depletion, resulting in lithium retention and methyldopa, and nonsteroidal antiinflammatory drugs can decrease the renal clearance of lithium (52). It has been suggested that red blood cell lithium binding decreases in the elderly, but this is unconfirmed. The major age-related change in lithium disposition is related to decreased renal function.

ANTIHYPERTENSIVE AGENTS

Most elderly people are hypertensive (both combined diastolic and systolic, >140/90 mm Hg; or isolated systolic >160 mm Hg) and, if diagnosed, are receiving antihypertensive therapy. Epidemiologic studies have demonstrated the increased risk of cardiovascular morbidity and mortality associated with untreated hypertension in the elderly (78, 79). Nonpharmacologic therapies, such as weight reduction in the obese, moderated sodium restriction (2 g of sodium or 5 g of sodium chloride), moderation of alcohol intake, and exercise are just as effective in the elderly as they are in younger patients and usually result in decreases of about 9 mm Hg for both diastolic and systolic pressures. If drug therapy is chosen, an equal hypotensive effect can be expected in both younger and elderly patients. In general, there are no risk-free or universally effective drugs, and no single drug or combination of drugs is regarded as best for the elderly (78). As with younger patients, African-Americans respond less well to angiotensin-converting enzyme inhibitors and β-adrenergic antagonists. As with other drugs, specific therapy should be tailored to each patient. It is wiser to initiate antihypertensive drug therapy with a reduced dose (approximately one-half of the normal) and to titrate slowly and gradually.

DIURETICS

Diuretics are commonly used as monotherapy in the elderly. When given at reduced dosage (12.5 mg/day of hydrochlorothiazide or its equivalent), diuretics are well-tolerated (78, 80, 81). Adverse effects are dose-related, and doses greater than 25 to 50 mg daily of hydrochlorothiazide are of little therapeutic benefit (82). Advantages of diuretics over other antihypertensives include usefulness in patients with heart failure, peripheral edema, proven efficacy, low cost, and convenient dosing (78). Adverse effects include hypokalemia, hyponatremia, hyperuricemia, hyperglycemia, azotemia, and hypercholesterolemia. Furosemide and metolazone are useful in patients with renal insufficiency. In the elderly, the volume of distribution of furosemide is increased; renal clearance is decreased; and elimination half-life is prolonged (83).

β-ADRENERGIC RECEPTION ANTAGONISTS

β-blockers are effective antihypertensive agents in the elderly despite theoretical concerns about the elderly having decreased β-receptor response and low renin state. They are especially useful in patients with angina pectoris and tachyarrhythmias. Both hydrophilic and lipophilic β-blockers cause central nervous system effects such as depression, sleep disturbance, and lethargy but, anecdotally, many elderly patients tolerate the water-soluble drugs better than the lipophilic versions. Adverse effects to β-blockers include atrioventricular conduction delay or block, increased peripheral vascular resistance, negative inotropy, hypertriglyceridemia, lowered high-density lipoprotein cholesterol, bradycardia, and bronchospasm in asthmatics.

ANGIOTENSIN-CONVERTING ENZYME INHIBITORS

Angiotensin-converting enzyme (ACE) inhibitors act as peripheral vasodilators by blocking the effect of the renin-angiotensin-aldosterone system. They appear to work equally well in young and elderly patients (78). The advantages of ACE inhibitors are their ability to reverse left ventricular hypertrophy, their usefulness in the treatment of congestive heart failure, and their lack of peripheral vascular symptoms, orthostatic hypotension, and central nervous system effects. However, ACE inhibitors can worsen renal function in patients with congestive heart failure. Other adverse effects include a nonproductive cough and hyperkalemia, especially in patients taking potassium supplements or potassium-sparing diuretics.

CALCIUM CHANNEL ANTAGONISTS

Calcium channel blockers may be slightly more effective in elderly than in young individuals (79). As a class of drugs, calcium channel blockers do not affect electrolyte, lipid, or hormonal levels; they have few contraindications; and they rarely cause orthostatic hypotension or central nervous system side effects (78). The most common problems associated with calcium channel blockers are abdominal discomfort and constipation, but these problems are managed with the use of smaller doses and by increasing the patient's intake of dietary fiber.

Age-related decreases in clearance resulting in increased plasma concentrations have been shown for verapamil and sustained-release nifedipine (84, 85). No differences in the clearance and elimination half-life of diltiazem were found following the administration of a single intravenous dose and chronic oral doses to elderly and young hypertensive patients (86).

α_1-ANTAGONISTS

Prazosin and terazosin are selective α_1-antagonists that reduce blood pressure by decreasing peripheral resistance. These drugs can cause orthostatic hypotension, which is enhanced in the elderly patient secondary to impaired baroreceptor reflex (78). Orthostasis is usually avoided if an initial dose not greater than 1 mg is taken at bedtime following abstinence from diuretics for 2 to 3 days. Little reflex tachycardia or tachyphylaxis and no compromise in cerebral blood flow have been observed in the elderly (78, 87).

CENTRALLY- ACTING α_2-AGONISTS AND DIRECT-ACTING VASODILATORS

Clonidine, guanabenz, guanfacine, and methyldopa reduce blood pressure by decreasing central sympathetic outflow. They are associated with many central nervous system side effects, such as dry mouth, sedation, and orthostatic hypotension. Although effective, they are not used in the elderly because of their adverse effects and the availability of safer agents (78).

Hydralazine, a direct-acting vasodilator, is generally well-tolerated and does not cause orthostasis. In the elderly it may reduce blood pressure and cause less reflex tachycardia than in younger patients, so that concomitant β-adrenergic blockers or other sympatholytic agents may not be necessary (78). However, hydralazine is not used frequently because of its inability to cause a regression in left ventricular hypertrophy and its association with increased adverse effects in African-Americans and patients with renal insufficiency.

In summary, diuretics, β-adrenergic blockers, calcium channel blockers, and ACE inhibitors are all useful in treating the elderly hypertensive patient. Calcium channel blockers and ACE inhibitors are appealing because of the relatively low incidence of hemodynamic, electrolyte, central nervous system, and metabolic adverse effects. As with the treatment of many disease states, low doses, careful titration, and the use of nondrug therapies result in safe and effective management of hypertension in the elderly.

DIGOXIN

The extensive use of digoxin in the elderly may not be clinically justified because the frequency of digitalis toxicity may outweigh the therapeutic benefit (88). Digoxin is used in the treatment of left ventricular failure, in chronic atrial fibrillation with a rapid ventricular response rate, and in the prevention of some atrial tachyarrhythmias. The peak age of onset of chronic atrial fibrillation is between 65 and 70 years of age (89).

Digoxin is a drug with a narrow therapeutic margin. Age-related changes in digoxin disposition do occur. As a result, steady-state serum digoxin concentrations resulting from a given maintenance dose are on the average twice the level in patients older than 80 years of age (average elimination half-life is 70 hours) as in patients between the ages of 30 and 50 (average elimination half-life is 30 to 40 hours) (88, 90).

Digoxin is primarily (approximately 75%) eliminated from the body by the kidney. Thus, the age-related decline in glomerular filtration rate results in accumulation of digoxin. In addition, digoxin is distributed primarily to lean body mass, which is diminished in the elderly. These changes result in higher serum digoxin concentrations for any given dose. In the elderly population, the range in magnitude of the changes in digoxin pharmacokinetics is variable and unpredictable. Therefore, digoxin dosage must be carefully tailored to the individual patient, using a combination of clinical judgment, estimates of renal function (calculated creatinine clearance), and serum digoxin concentrations (88). Adverse effects resulting from digoxin toxicity include anorexia, nausea, vomiting, bradycardia, bigeminy, delirium, delusions, confusional states, visual and auditory hallucinations, and disturbances in color vision and visual acuity. Potassium depletion secondary to diuretic therapy can predispose patients to digoxin toxicity.

In summary, digoxin use in the elderly is a controversial subject. However, it appears to be safe when close patient monitoring accompanies its use. Digoxin doses should be calculated for elderly patients based on creatinine clearance, lean body weight, and steady-state serum concentrations.

ANTIARRHYTHMICS

In the elderly the incidence of lidocaine toxicity was found to be twice that of young patients (91). The volume of distribution of lidocaine is also greater in the elderly, which may account for a significant increase in elimination half-life without a change in plasma clearance in elderly compared to young patients (26, 90). Additionally, variables such as congestive heart failure, hepatic disease, and decreased hepatic blood flow are associated with increased lidocaine toxicity (92).

Steady-state serum concentrations of procainamide and its active metabolite *N*-acetylprocainamide have been found to increase in the elderly (93). This change is associated with the age-related decrease in renal function and a decrease in renal tubular secretion. Both in hepatic and renal clearance of quinidine decrease with age and, therefore, lower initial doses and gradual increases should be used in the elderly (94–96). Disopyramide has potent anticholinergic effects that account for a majority of side effects in the elderly. It is especially not tolerated well by males with benign prostatic hypertrophy and urinary retention (97). The effects of aging on β-adrenergic blockers and calcium ion antagonists have already been addressed in this chapter. In summary, the effects of aging on antiarrhythmics mostly result in an increase in elimination half-life, which results in higher steady-state blood levels. Dosage reduction and careful monitoring of serum or plasma drug concentrations are necessary when these drugs are used in aged patients.

ANTICOAGULANTS

Anticoagulant use in the elderly is associated with higher risks of complications. Although the pharmacokinetic parameters of heparin are poorly understood, patients older than 60 years of age (particularly females) experience an increased incidence of bleeding (98–100).

Warfarin is highly plasma protein-bound. Since aging is associated with a decrease in plasma albumin concentrations, the elderly have less circulating albumin, which results in a decrease in bound warfarin and an increase in free (unbound) warfarin (98). Thus, at any given dose, elderly patients effectively have a higher free warfarin concentration, are at an increased risk for dose-related complications, are more likely to experience bleeding and are less likely to achieve a desired therapeutic outcome. When the pharmacokinetics of warfarin were evaluated in young vs. elderly patients, no differences were found in elimination half-life, volume of distribution, or clearance (101, 102).

Other factors that may contribute to the development of problems associated with anticoagulant therapy in the elderly include a decrease in hematostatic response, resulting from a 33 to 50% decrease in the synthesis of clotting factors in the elderly as opposed to the young; the increased potential for drug interactions with warfarin; age-related reductions in receptor sensitivity to vitamin K; increased clearance of vitamin K; and age-related increases in the active metabolite of warfarin, vitamin K oxide, in the elderly (98). Thus, when elderly patients receive anticoagulant therapy, they should be very closely monitored for signs of bleeding. When warfarin is used, a dose reduction for elderly patients is in order, and cautious titration of dose should be accompanied by frequent monitoring of prothrombin times.

GASTROINTESTINAL DRUGS

Drugs used to treat peptic ulcer disease are frequently prescribed for the elderly. Options for treatment include the use of histamine$_2$, (H$_2$) receptor antagonists, sucralfate, antacids, omeprazole, and misoprostil; pirenzepine, colloidal bismuth, carbenoxolone, and antibiotics are still under investigation at this time. Of these, H$_2$ antagonists and sucralfate are considered to be the safest and most efficient choices for the treatment of peptic ulcer disease. Four H$_2$ antagonists have been approved in the U.S.: cimetidine; ranitidine; famotidine; and nizatidine. The major difference between these drugs is their advance effect and drug interaction profiles. Cimetidine, the first available H$_2$ antagonist, is associated with the most problems. Cimetidine binds to hepatic cytochrome P-450 microsomal mixed-function oxidase enzymes and inhibits their function. As a result, clinically important decreases in clearance, resulting in an increase in elimination half-life of drugs such as phenytoin, warfarin, theophylline and others, can

occur (103–106). Since elderly patients may take many medications, alterations in the clearance of drugs, especially those with a narrow therapeutic margin, can result in increased adverse effects and/or toxicity. In addition to drug interactions, cimetidine use is associated with mental confusion, elevations of creatinine, increased values for liver function tests, and antiandrogenic effects (107–109). Ranitidine, nizatidine, and famotidine are not associated with clinically significant changes in drug clearance (110, 111). Thus, it is reasonable to recommend that if H$_2$ receptor antagonists are to be used in elderly patients who are taking other drugs that are hepatically metabolized by oxidative biotransformation, ranitidine, famotidine, or nizatidine should be used instead of cimetidine.

Sucralfate is an interesting alternative to the H$_2$ antagonists. It is not absorbed systemically and has few side effects. If patients experience problems with the H$_2$ antagonists or if systemic therapy is not desired, sucralfate can be used. The only clinically important problems associated with the use of sucralfate are constipation, the potential for sucralfate to bind to other drugs and interfere with their absorption, and the tablet being so large that some patients have trouble swallowing it.

Antacids can be useful in some situations, but because of their bad taste, patient compliance is the biggest problem. Aluminum-containing antacids can cause constipation, and magnesium- and calcium-containing products can cause diarrhea. The sugar content of antacid products is especially important for diabetic patients (55).

Other gastrointestinal drugs, such as hypocholesterolemics, prokinetics (e.g., metoclopramide), antiinflammatory agents, hydrogen ion pump inhibitors (e.g., omeprazole), antibacterial agents, and antidiarrheal drugs have not been sufficiently studied in the elderly, so recommendations about their use in this population cannot be made. The use of laxatives in the elderly should be avoided if possible. Nonpharmacologic measures, such as increasing fluid intake, exercise, and dietary fiber, should be used before drugs are prescribed. Evaluation of the drugs a patient is taking, such as anticholinergics and iron salts, should be performed, and alternate agents should be substituted if possible. Stool softeners, such as dioctyl sodium sulfosuccinate or dioctyl calcium sulfosuccinate, should be considered when diet and exercise are ineffective.

ANTIBACTERIAL AGENTS

A review of the effects of aging on antibiotics reveals that for most agents, the age-related decrease in renal clearance results in predictable prolongation in elimination half-life (112). Therefore, dose reductions for most antibacterial agents are indicated for the elderly patient. The reduction of dose should be carefully managed so that the blood level or tissue concentration necessary for bacteriocidal or bacteriostatic activity is achieved. β-Lactam drugs, such as the penicillins and cephalosporins, tetracyclines, and sulfonamides, have an extremely good safety profile in the elderly. Aminoglycosides, quinolones, vancomycin, and β-lactams, all excreted by the kidney, may require dose adjustments based on creatinine clearance. The toxicity of aminoglycosides (ototoxicity and renal toxicity) cannot be overstated, and dose reductions for elderly patients are almost always required.

Antibacterials that are primarily cleared by the liver may also require dosage reduction. These drugs include isoniazid, metronidazole, quinolones, rifampin, and the macrolides (i.e., erythromycin). Thus, when antibacterial agents are used in the elderly patient the clinician should anticipate decreased clearance and an increase in elimination half-life.

Most of the agents are inherently safe, so changes in pharmacokinetics could present as an increased likelihood of adverse effects. On the other hand, aminoglycosides and vancomycin should be monitored and used with extreme caution since their toxicities are dose-related and usually avoidable.

MISCELLANEOUS DRUGS

Studies evaluating the effects of aging on the pharmacokinetics and pharmacodynamics of other drugs exist, but oftentimes they raise more questions about the clinical relevance of their results. Reasons for this include the study of drugs in normal healthy (disease-free) elderly volunteers, the study of pharmacokinetics without pharmacodynamic evaluation and, likewise, the evaluation of clinical response or toxicity in the absence of pharmacokinetic determinations. Other problems include the study of patients with concomitant disease states who may be taking other medications. Predictable age-related changes in clearance, plasma protein binding, and volume of distribution occur for many drugs, and the necessity for starting therapy in elderly patients with smaller doses than those used in young adults and with adjusting therapy gradually cannot be overstated.

The anticonvulsant phenytoin has been reported to be susceptible to age-related changes in protein binding and clearance. However, studies have shown that plasma phenytoin level may either increase or decrease as a function of aging (113–115). However, reports of the increased incidence of neurologic and hematologic toxicity in elderly patients is often dose-related, so if patients are maintained at lower steady-state plasma phenytoin concentrations, these complications can be avoided.

Narcotic analgesic use in the elderly is often associated with increased incidence of adverse effects such as nausea, hypotension, and excess respiratory depression. In addition, increased pain relief from normal adult doses occurs in elderly patients. The pharmacokinetic and pharmacodynamic reasons for these effects are not completely understood, but lower initial doses and cautious titration are usually adequate to solve these problems. However, care must be taken to avoid the undertreatment of pain (116). No significant age-related effects have been reported for either aspirin or acetaminophen.

There is no evidence that the elderly respond any differently to theophylline than the young do. However, theophylline is mainly biotransformed in the liver, and the clearance may be decreased in the elderly. Monitoring serum theophylline concentrations will adequately protect patients from overdosage.

The delivery of insulin to systemic circulation, the metabolic clearance, and the sensitivity of insulin do not change with age (98, 117). The clearance and volume of distribution of oral hypoglycemic agents may be affected by aging, but lower doses and monitoring of serum glucose levels result in the selection of appropriate doses for the patient.

DRUG SELECTION

Generally, the fewer drugs the elderly patient takes, the better. There are no specific rules about which drugs should only be used in the elderly patient, because many factors contribute to drug and dose selection. Some variables include a patient's medical status, other drugs the patient is taking, and specific pharmacokinetic and pharmacodynamic aspects of individual drugs and combinations. From the information presented earlier in this chapter, some helpful guidelines can be suggested about how certain drugs are selected over others.

The design of a dosage form (tablet, capsule, liquid) and the size and taste of the medication can all be used to guide drug selection. The choice of a sustained-release drug product instead of a single-release dosage form may make more sense in certain patients, because the patient does not have to take the drug as frequently. However, if the patient has had a prior history of problems with sustained-release products, e.g., dose-dumping or short duration of clinical effect, avoidance of time-release drug formulations makes sense. There have been some anecdotal claims that dose-dumping from sustained-release dosage forms occurs more frequently in the elderly, but no data are available to support them. If a patient is already in the habit of taking other prescription medications at certain times, the choice of a drug with an overlapping administration schedule makes the most sense.

Another important selection variable for drugs used in the elderly is the elimination half-life of a drug. In general, the shorter the half-life, the less likelihood that the drug will cause problems secondary to accumulation. Likewise, if an adverse reaction or side effect occurs, abatement of the problem is sooner for a drug with a short elimination half-life vs. a long half-life. Classes of drugs that are assumed to be therapeutically equivalent can be categorized based on elimination half-lives. Depending upon the treatment objective, those with a shorter half-life should be tried first for the elderly patient.

The route of clearance of a drug can also be used to guide drug selection. For drugs that are predominantly cleared by the liver, a drug that undergoes conjugation (phase II biotransformation) is more desirable than one that is metabolized via oxidation (phase I) pathways. If the choice is among drugs that are oxidized, the drug with the least number of active metabolites should be chosen. In this situation, further assessment of the lipophilicity and elimination half-life of the metabolites will help to select the most appropriate agent. An example would be the choice of alprazolam, lorazepam, or oxazepam over diazepam, clorazepate, or chlordiazepoxide.

The volume of distribution of a drug should also be considered when selecting or reevaluating a patient's medications. The relative fat vs. water solubility of a drug may predict or explain the clinical effects of a medication. For example, if a β-adrenergic antagonist, i.e., if propranolol (lipophilic) is prescribed for a hypertensive patient and the patient complains of nightmares and/or daytime somnolence but is otherwise experiencing an acceptable therapeutic response, the clinician can simply switch to atenolol (hydrophilic). Atenolol is a less fat-soluble β-blocker that has fewer central nervous system effects than propranolol. Alternatively, if a β-blocker is being prescribed for the management of physical symptoms of anxiety, i.e., palpitations, nervousness, or tremor, a more lipophilic version may be more desirable than a hydrophilic one. Volume of distribution concerns related to body habitus and accumulation are important determinants in drug selection in the elderly.

The route of excretion is also a factor that must be considered. For drugs that are primarily excreted via the kidney, an appropriate evaluation of renal function is essential. In a patient who has compromised renal function, adjustments in dose and/or dosing interval will have to be made. However, if an alternate drug that is biotransformed by the liver, rather than excreted by the kidney exists, selection of this agent would be prudent. Likewise, if a patient's liver function is compromised or if he/she is taking drugs that may affect hepatic microsomal mixed-function oxidase enzymes, it would make more sense to select a drug that is excreted by the kidney.

The drug interaction profile of a drug can also guide the selection process. Potential drug-drug, drug-disease state, and drug-food/nutrition interactions should be considered before a certain drug is used in a patient. The adverse effect (side effect) profile can also be used as selection criteria. Avoidance of drugs with overlapping side effect profiles, i.e., anticholinergics, central nervous system depressants, gastrointestinal tract irritation, and others, should be avoided if possible because of synergistic or additive effects. Likewise, if patients are experiencing side effects from their medications, an assessment of all the prescription and nonprescription medications in terms of their adverse effect profile should be performed. Simply changing one or more of the medications may be all that is necessary.

The cost of medications is another important factor. Various therapeutic alternatives can be more or less expensive for the patient. Certain generic forms of drugs may be available, and consideration of less expensive alternatives may be more reasonable for elderly patients on fixed incomes. For example, it is less expensive for the patient if ampicillin or a sulfa drug is chosen, instead of a cephalosporin or quinolone, for the treatment of an uncomplicated urinary tract infection. Aspirin could be used before more expensive nonsteroidal antiinflammatory drugs for the management of rheumatoid arthritis.

There are many variables that can contribute to the appropriate selection of drugs for the elderly patient. Factors such as the clinical pharmacology of a drug and socioeconomic and psychosocial factors all have to be balanced in order to ensure that the patient is receiving optimal therapy.

REFERENCES

1. Picozzi, A, and Neidle EA: Geriatric pharmacology for the dentist: an overview. *Dent Clin North Am* 28:581–593, 1984.
2. Ogilvie RI: An introduction to pharmacokinetics. *J Chron Dis* 36:121–127, 1983.
3. Greenblatt DJ, Shader RI: *Pharmacokinetics in Clinical Practice*. WB Saunders, Philadelphia. 1985.
4. Dorris RL, Taylor SE: Significant adverse interactions of drugs in dentistry. *Dent Clin North Am* 28:555–562, 1984.
5. Scavone JM, Greenblatt DJ, Friedman H: Enhanced bioavailability of triazolam following sublingual versus oral administration. *J Clin Pharmacol* 26:208–210, 1986.
6. Scavone JM, Greenblatt DJ, Goddard JE, et al: Alprazolam kinetics following sublingual and oral administration. *J Clin Psychopharmacol* 7:332–334, 1987.
7. Greenblatt DJ, Sellers EM, Shader RI: Drug disposition in old age. *N Engl J Med* 306:1081–1088, 1982.
8. Ouslander JG: Drug therapy in the elderly. *Ann Intern Med* 95:711–722, 1981.
9. Geokas MC, Haverback BJ: The aging gastrointestinal tract. *Am J Surg* 117:881–892, 1969.
10. Sellers EM: Plasma protein displacement interactions are rarely of clinical significance. *Pharmacology* 18:225–227, 1979.
11. Evans MA, Triggs EJ, Cheung M, et al: Gastric emptying rate in the elderly: implications for drug therapy. *J Am Geriatr Soc* 29:201–205, 1981.
12. Montgomery R, Haeney MR, Ross IN, et al: The ageing gut: a study of intestinal absorption in relation to nutrition in the elderly. *Q J Med* 47:197–211, 1978.
13. Kramer PA, Chapron DJ, Benson J, et al: Tetracycline absorption in elderly patients with achlorhydria. *Clin Pharmacol Ther* 23:467–472, 1978.
14. Ochs HR, Greenblatt DJ, Allen MD, et al: Effect of age and Billroth gastrectomy on absorption of desmethyldiazepam from clorazepate. *Clin Pharmacol Ther* 26:449–456, 1979.
15. Ochs HR, Otten H, Greenblatt DJ, et al: Diazepam absorption: effects of age, sex, and Billroth gastrectomy. *Dig Dis Sci* 27:225–230, 1982.
16. Divoll M, Ameer B, Abernethy DR: Age does not alter acetaminophen absorption. *J Am Geriatr Soc* 30:240–244, 1982.
17. Greenblatt DJ, Shader RI, Franke K, et al: Pharmacokinetics and bioavailability of intravenous, intramuscular, and oral lorazepam in humans. *J Pharm Sci* 68:57–63, 1979.
18. Terezhalmy GT, Bowen LL, Rye LA, et al: Pharmacotherapeutics in urgent dental care. *Dent Clin North Am* 30:399–420, 1986.
19. Bender AD: The effect of increasing age on the disturbances of peripheral blood flow in man. *J Am Geriatr Soc* 13:192–198, 1965.
20. Greenblatt DJ, Allen MD, Harmatz JS, et al: Diazepam disposition determinants. *Clin Pharmacol Ther* 27:301–312, 1980.
21. Allen MD, Greenblatt DJ, Harmatz JS, et al: Desmethyldiazepam kinetics in the elderly after oral prazepam. *Clin Pharmacol Ther* 28:196–202, 1980.
22. Greenblatt DJ, Divoll M, Puri SK, et al: Clobazam kinetics in the elderly. *Br J Clin Pharmacol* 12:631–636, 1981.
23. Greenblatt DJ, Divoll M, Abernethy DR, et al: Antipyrine kinetics in the elderly: prediction of age-related changes in benzodiazepine oxidizing capacity. *J Pharmacol Exp Ther* 220:120–126, 1982.
24. Divoll M, Abernethy DR, Ameer B, et al: Acetaminophen kinetics in the elderly. *Clin Pharmacol Ther* 31:151–156, 1982.
25. Vestal RE, McGuire EA, Tobin JD, et al: Aging and ethanol metabolism. *Clin Pharmacol Ther* 21:343–354, 1977.
26. Nation RL, Triggs EJ, Selig M: Lignocaine kinetics in cardiac patients and aged subjects. *Br J Clin Pharmacol* 4:439–448, 1977.
27. Klotz U, Avant GR, Hoyumpa A, et al: The effects of age and liver disease on the disposition and elimination of diazepam in adult man. *J Clin Invest* 55:347–359, 1975.
28. Richey DP, Bender AD: Pharmacokinetic consequences of aging. *Annu Rev Pharmacol Toxicol* 17:49–65, 1977.
29. Dybkaer R, Lauritzen M, Krakauer R: Relative reference values for clinical chemical and haematological quantities in 'healthy' elderly people. *Acta Med Scand* 209:1–9, 1981.
30. Greenblatt DJ: Reduced serum albumin concentration in the elderly: a report from the Boston Collaborative Drug Surveillance Program. *J Am Geriatr Soc* 27:20–22, 1979.
31. MacLennan WJ, Martin P, Mason BJ: Protein intake and serum albumin levels in the elderly. *Gerontology* 23:360–367, 1977.
32. Greenblatt DJ, Scavone JM: Pharmacokinetics of oxaprozin and other nonsteroidal antiinflammatory agents. *Semin Arth Rheum* 15(Suppl 2):18–26, 1986.
33. Friedman H, Greenblatt DJ: Rational therapeutic drug monitoring. *JAMA* 256:2227–2233, 1986.
34. Koch-Weser J, Sellers EM: Binding of drugs to serum albumin. *N Engl J Med* 294:311–316, 526–531, 1976.
35. McElnay JC, D'Arcy PF: Protein binding displacement interactions and their clinical importance. *Drugs* 25:495–513, 1983.
36. Fraser DG, Ludden TM, Evens RP, et al: Displacement of phenytoin from plasma binding sites by salicylate. *Clin Pharmacol Ther* 27:165–169, 1980.
37. Abernethy DR, Greenblatt DJ, Harmatz JS, et al: Alterations in drug distribution and clearance due to obesity. *J Pharmacol Exp Ther* 217:681–685, 1981.
38. Williams RL: Drug administration in hepatic disease. *N Engl J Med* 309:1616–1622, 1983.
39. Gibaldi M, Perrier D: Clinical pharmacokinetics. *N Engl J Med* 293:702–705, 964–970, 1975.
40. Wilkinson GR, Shand DG: A physiological approach to hepatic drug clearance. *Clin Pharmacol Ther* 18:377–390, 1975.
41. Vestal RE: Drug use in the elderly. *Clin Pharmacokinet* 1:280–296, 1978.
42. Casteleden CM, George CF: The effect of age on the hepatic clearance of propranolol. *Br J Clin Pharmacol* 7:49–54, 1979.
43. Rowe JW, Andres R, Tobin JD, et al: The effect of age on creatinine clearance in man: a cross-sectional and longitudinal study. *J Gerontol* 31:155–163, 1976.
44. Cockroft DW, Gault MH: Prediction of creatinine clearance from serum creatinine. *Nephron* 16:31–41, 1976.

45. Stevenson IH: Drugs for the elderly. In Lemberger L, Reidenberg MM (eds): *Proceedings of the Second World Conference on Clinical Pharmacology and Therapeutics.* Bethesda, MD. *Am Soc Pharmacol Exp Ther* pp 64–73, 1984.
46. Dement WC, Miles LE, Carskadon MA, et al: "White Paper" on sleep and aging. *J Am Geriatr Soc* 30:25–35, 1982.
47. Lasagna L: Hypnotic drugs. *N Engl J Med* 287:1182–1184, 1972.
48. Greenblatt DJ, Abernethy DR, Divoll M, et al: Pharmacokinetic properties of benzodiazepine hypnotics. *J Clin Psychopharmacol* 3:129–132, 1983.
49. Greenblatt DJ, Divoll M, Abernethy DR, et al: Benzodiazepine hypnotics: kinetic and therapeutic options. *Sleep* 5:18–27, 1982.
50. Ochs HR, Greenblatt DJ, Heur HI: Is temazepam an accumulation hypnotic? *J Clin Pharmacol* 24:58–64, 1984.
51. Scavone JM, Greenblatt DJ, Friedman H: Enhanced bioavailability of triazolam following sublingual versus oral administration. *J Clin Pharmacol* 26:208–210, 1986.
52. Thompson TL, Moran MG, Nies AS: Psychotropic drug use in the elderly. *N Engl J Med* 308:134–138, 194–199, 1983.
53. Pomara N, Stanley B, Block R, et al: Increased sensitivity of the elderly to the central depressant effects of diazepam. *J Clin Psychiatry* 46:185–187, 1985.
54. Greenblatt DJ: Disposition of cardiovascular drugs in the elderly. *Med Clin North Am* 73:487–494, 1989.
55. Lamy PP, Love RC: Psychotropic agents. *Elder Care News* 4:9–15, 1988.
56. Jenike MA: Handbook of geriatric psychopharmacology. PSG Publishing, Littleton, MA, 1985.
57. Goa KC, Ward A: Buspirone: a preliminary review of its pharmacological properties and therapeutic efficacy as an anxiolytic. *Drugs* 32:114–129, 1986.
58. Eison AS, Temple DL: Buspirone: review of its pharmacology and current perspectives on its mechanism of action. *Am J Med* 80(Suppl 3B):1–9, 1986.
59. Kastenholz KV, Crimson ML: Buspirone, a novel nonbenzodiazepine anxiolytic. *Clin Pharm* 3:600–607, 1984.
60. Rickels K, Weisman K, Norstad N, et al: Buspirone and diazepam in anxiety. *J Clin Psychiatry* 43:81–86, 1982.
61. Peabody CA, Whiteford HA, Hollister LE: Antidepressants and the elderly. *J Am Geriatr Soc* 34:869–874, 1986.
62. Baldessarini RJ: Current status of antidepressants: clinical pharmacology and therapy. *J Clin Psychiatry* 50:117–126, 1989.
63. Blazer D: Depression in the elderly. *N Engl J Med* 320:164–166, 1989.
64. Lazarus LW, Davis JM, Dysken MW: Geriatric depression: a guide to successful therapy. *Geriatrics* 40:43–53, 1985.
65. Hollister LE: Tricyclic antidepressants. *N Engl J Med* 2:1106–1109, 1978.
66. Bergstrom RF: The pharmacokinetics of fluoxetine in elderly subjects. In *Abstracts of the Second World Conference on Clinical Pharmacology and Therapeutics.* Washington, DC, Vol 2, p 120, 1983.
67. Sommi RW, Crimson ML, Bowden CL: Fluoxetine: a serotonin-specific, second generation antidepressant. *Pharmacotherapy* 7:1–15, 1987.
68. Rabkin JG, Quitkin FM, McGrath P, et al: Adverse monoamine oxidase inhibitors. Part II. Treatment correlates with clinical management. *J Clin Psychopharmacol* 5:2–9, 1985.
69. Scavone JM, Marx CM: Drug-food and drug nutrition interactions. *NARD J* 5:55–59, 1983.
70. Robinson DS: Relation of sex and aging to monoamine oxidase activity of human brain, plasma, and platelets. *Arch Gen Psychiatry* 24:536–539, 1971.
71. Riblet LA, Taylor DP: Pharmacology and neurochemistry of trazodone. *J Clin Psychopharmacol* 1(Suppl):17S–22S, 1981.
72. Richelson E: The newer antidepressants: structures, pharmacokinetics and proposed mechanisms of action. *Psychopharmacol Bull* 20:213–223, 1984.
73. Gruter W, Poldinger W: Maprotiline. *Mod Probl Pharmacopsychiatry* 18:17–48, 1982.
74. Burckhardt D, Müller V, Imhoff P, et al: Cardiovascular effects of tricyclic and tetracyclic antidepressants. *JAMA* 239:213–216, 1978.
75. Dufresne RL, Weber SS, Becker RE, et al: Bupropion hydrochloride. *Drug Intell Clin Pharm* 18:957–964, 1984.
76. Hamilton LD: Aged brain and the phenothiazines. *Geriatrics* 21:131–138, 1966.
77. Rivera-Calimlim L, Nasrallah H, Gift T, et al: Plasma levels of chlorpromazine: effect of age, chronicity of disease, and duration of treatment. *Clin Pharmacol Ther* 21:115–116, 1977.
78. Tjoa HI, Kaplan NM: Treatment of hypertension in the elderly. *JAMA* 264:1015–1018, 1990.
79. Kaplan NM: Calcium entry blockers in the treatment of hypertension: current status and future prospects. *JAMA* 262:817–823, 1989.
80. Hulley SB, Furberg CD, Gurland B, et al: Systolic Hypertension in the Elderly Program (SHEP): antihypertensive efficacy of chlorthalidone. *Am J Cardiol* 56:913–920, 1985.
81. Goldstein G, Materson BJ, Cushman WC, et al: Treatment of hypertension in the elderly. II. Cognitive and behavioral function: results of a Department of Veterans Affairs cooperative study. *Hypertension* 15:361–369, 1990.
82. Materson BJ, Cushman WC, Goldstein G, et al: Treatment of hypertension in the elderly. I. Blood pressure and clinical changes: results of a Department of Veterans Affairs cooperative study. *Hypertension* 15:348–360, 1990.
83. Fujimura A, Ohira H, Shiga T, et al: Chronopharmacology of furosemide in the elderly. *J Clin Pharmacol* 32:838–842, 1992.
84. Abernethy DR, Schwartz JB, Todd EL, et al: Verapamil pharmacodynamics and disposition in young and elderly hypertensive patients. *Ann Intern Med* 105:329–336, 1986.
85. Chase SL (ed): Calcium antagonists and cardiovascular diseases of the elderly. *Phila Coll Pharm Sci* 1:1–31, 1989.
86. Abernethy DR, Montamat SC: Acute and chronic studies of diltiazem in elderly versus young hypertensive patients. *Am J Cardiol* 60(Suppl I):116I–120I, 1987.
87. Ram CVS, Meese R, Kaplan NM, et al: Antihypertensive therapy in the elderly: effects on blood pressure and cerebral blood flow. *Am J Med* 82(Suppl 1A):53–57, 1987.
88. Stults BM: Digoxin use in the elderly. *J Am Geriatr Soc* 30:158–164, 1982.
89. Morris DC, Hurst JW: Atrial fibrillation. *Curr Probl Cardiol* 5:1–12, 1980.
90. Cusack B, Kelly J, O'Malley K, et al: Digoxin in the elderly: pharmacokinetic consequences of old age. *Clin Pharmacol Ther* 25:772–776, 1979.
91. Pfeifer HJ, Greenblatt DJ, Koch-Weser J: Clinical use and toxicity of intravenous lidocaine. *Am Heart J* 92:168–173, 1976.
92. Thomson PD, Richardson JH, Melmon KL, et al: Lidocaine pharmacokinetics in advanced heart failure, liver disease, and renal failure in humans. *Ann Intern Med* 78:499–508, 1973.
93. Reidenberg MM, Comacho MC, Kluger J, et al: Aging and renal clearance of procainamide and acetylprocainamide. *Clin Pharmacol Ther* 28:732–735, 1980.
94. Ochs HR, Greenblatt DJ, Woo E, et al: Reduced clearance of quinidine in elderly humans. *Clin Res* 25:513A, 1977.
95. Ochs HR, Greenblatt DJ, Woo E, et al: Reduced quinidine clearance in elderly persons. *Am J Cardiol* 42:481–485, 1978.
96. Drayer DE, Hughes M, Lorenzo B, et al: Prevalence of high (3S)-3-hydroxyquinidine/quinidine ratios in serum, and clearance of quinidine in cardiac patients with age. *Clin Pharmacol Ther* 27:72–75, 1980.
97. Baines MW, Davies JE, Kellett DW, et al: Some pharmacologic effects of disopyramide and a metabolite. *J Int Med Res* 4(Suppl 1):5–7, 1976.
98. Garnett WR, Barr WH: Geriatric pharmacokinetics. The Upjohn Company, Kalamazoo, MI. pp 1–27, 1984.
99. Jick HD, Slone D, Borda IT, et al: Efficacy and toxicity of heparin in relation to age and sex. *N Engl J Med* 279:284–286, 1968.
100. Vieweg WVR, Piscatelli RL, Houser JJ, et al: Complication of intravenous administration of heparin in elderly women. *JAMA* 213:1303–1306, 1970.
101. Hayes MJ, Langman MJ, Short AH, et al: Changes in drug metabolism with increasing age. I. Warfarin binding and plasma proteins. *Br J Clin Pharmacol* 2:69–72, 1975.
102. Hewick DS, Moreland TA, Shepherd AMM, Stevenson IH: The effect of age on the sensitivity to warfarin sodium. *Br J Clin Pharmacol* 2:189P–190P, 1975.
103. Somogyi A, Muirhead M: Pharmacokinetic interactions of cimetidine. *Clin Pharmacokinet* 12:321–366, 1987.
104. Gerber MC, Tejwani GA, Gerber N, et al: Drug interactions with cimetidine: an update. *Pharmacol Ther* 27:353–370, 1985.
105. McInnes GT, Brodie MJ: Drug interactions that matter: a critical re-appraisal. *Drugs* 36:83–110, 1988.
106. Griffin JW, May JR, DiPiro JT: Drug interactions: theory versus practice. *Am J Med* 77(Suppl 5B):85–89, 1984.
107. Gordon C: Differential diagnosis of cimetidine-induced delirium. *Psychosomatics* 22(3):251–252, 1981.
108. Brier KL, Dasta JF, Kidwell GA, et al: Cimetidine and mental confusion. *Crit Care Med* 8(12):760–761, 1980.
109. Jenike MA: Cimetidine in elderly patients: review of uses and risks. *J Am Geriatr Soc* 30:170–173, 1982.
110. Mitchard M, Harris A, Mullinger BM: Ranitidine drug interactions—a literature review. *Pharmacol Ther* 32:293–325, 1987.
111. Krishna DR, Klotz U: Newer H₂-receptor antagonists: clinical pharmacokinetics and drug interaction potential. *Clin Pharmacokinet* 15:205–215, 1988.
112. Meyers BR, Wilkinson P: Clinical pharmacokinetics of antibacterial drugs in the elderly: implications for selection and dosage. *Clin Pharmacokinet* 17:385–395, 1989.
113. Patterson M, Heazelwood R, Smithhurst B, et al: Plasma protein binding of phenytoin in the aged: in vivo. *Br J Clin Pharmacol* 13:423–425, 1982.
114. Hayes MJ, Langman MJS, Short AH: Changes in drug metabolism with increasing age. II. Phenytoin clearance and protein binding. *Br J Clin Pharmacol* 2:73–79, 1975.
115. Houghton GW, Richens A, Leighton M, et al: Effect of age, height, weight and sex on serum phenytoin concentration in epileptic patients. *Br J Clin Pharmacol* 2:251–256, 1975.
116. Wallace DE, Watanabe AS: Drug effects in geriatric patients. *Drug Intelligence in Clinical Pharmacy* 11:597–603, 1977.
117. Barbagallo-Sangiorgi G: The pancreatic beta cell response to intravenous administration of glucose in elderly subjects. *J Am Geriatr Soc* 18:529–538, 1970.

Principles of Toxicology and Therapeutics

EDWARD P. KRENZELOK, Pharm.D., A.B.A.T.

INTRODUCTION

In 1991 approximately 1.84 million poisoning cases were reported by poison information centers to the American Association of Poison Control Centers (AAPCC) (1). Since all toxicologic exposures are not reported to poison centers, conservative estimates suggest that the actual annual number of exposures exceeds 4.4 million cases (1). The magnitude of this volume of cases dictates that the physician who cares for the critically ill patient will encounter a significant number of toxicologically compromised patients in his or her practice.

The majority of toxicology cases are relatively insignificant and are responded to with intervention and observation at home under the direction of a poison information center since they do not necessitate referral to a health care facility. Sixty percent of the exposures involve children less than 6 years of age, and 83% of all exposures have a medical outcome that results in no adverse effect or only minor toxic manifestations (1). However, these statistics are skewed by the inordinate number of pediatric exposures that are generally associated with low morbidity and mortality, and they therefore fail to represent the nearly 5-fold increase in serious morbidity and mortality that accompanies adult toxic exposures (1).

Pediatric exposures frequently are limited in regard to both the toxic substance and the extent of the exposure. Children may swallow small amounts of medications, cosmetics, plants, or household cleaning products, but the extent of the exposure is often only incidental as a result of adult supervision. Furthermore, the majority of these exposures are accidental, whereas the adult may ingest extraordinary quantities of a toxin with the sole intent of drug abuse or self-harm. There is actually an inverse relationship between the number of poisoning exposures and fatalities in children versus adults (1). The nature of the substance with intentional overdoses is far different than in the pediatric overdose. It is often a medication with a narrow therapeutic index, such as psychotropic or cardiovascular medications.

The majority of reported toxicology-related fatalities involve pharmacologic agents rather than hydrocarbons and gases such as carbon monoxide (1). During the last 5 years cyclic antidepressants have been responsible for more fatalities than any other category (1–5). In 1991, 0.525% of all antidepressant-related overdoses that were managed by poison information centers resulted in death, as compared with analgesic-related overdoses, which resulted in a similar number of fatalities but had a mortality index of only 0.104% (1). Street drug overdoses (0.434%) and cardiovascular medication overdoses (0.348%) had significant mortality indexes but slightly lower than those associated with antidepressants (1). There is also an inherent bias in these data, since they represent outcomes from poison information centers and do not take into consideration overdoses or successful suicide patients who died before entering the health care system. These overdoses require a significant amount of supportive pharmacotherapy and gastric decontamination intervention as well as the use of a limited number of antidotes and occasional aggressive use of extracorporeal means of enhancing their elimination. This chapter focuses on the pharmacotherapeutic aspects of the management of acute poisoning emergencies.

INITIAL BASIC MANAGEMENT

There are few specific pharmacologic antagonists or antidotes, so good supportive care is inherent in the management of all poisoned patients. Immediate and appropriate medical intervention cannot be overlooked in pursuit of antidotal therapy. Aggressive medical intervention will limit adverse outcomes. Stabilization of the patient and adherence to the ABC's of life support are essential to good patient management. Securing a patent airway takes priority over any pharmacologic intervention.

AIRWAY

The indications for endotracheal intubation in the poisoned patient usually are consistent with the general medical indications for intubation. Many pharmacologic toxins such as opioids produce respiratory depression, and intubation is necessary to maintain adequate ventilation. Overdose patients with a decreased level of consciousness are at a greater risk of vomiting; therefore, airway protection may be necessary to prevent subsequent aspiration. Intubation may also be necessary in the combative patient whose behavior precludes normal therapeutic intervention such as fluid management, administration of antagonists or pressors, or gastric decontamination. Finally, endotracheal intubation is indicated in patients who have ingested medications that may produce a rapid loss of consciousness and deterioration. Most notably, those drugs include tricyclic antidepressants, calcium channel blockers, and clonidine.

INTRAVENOUS ACCESS

During patient stabilization, intravenous access should be established with at least one large-bore intravenous line. The appropriate solution should be administered as determined by the patient's cardiovascular status, fluid and electrolyte needs, and compatibility with pharmacotherapeutic agents such as pressors and antidotes. Ultimately, the placement of a central venous or Swan-Ganz catheter may be necessary to assess fluid status accurately.

COMA DRUGS

Few pharmacologic antagonists readily reverse a decreased level of consciousness or overt coma. In the past, analeptic agents such as nikethamide and picrotoxin were administered to reverse the central nervous system depression associated with sedative-hypnotic overdoses. The indiscriminate use of those agents actually increased morbidity and mortality, and basic life support alone is superior to that type of therapeutic intervention. Contemporary management of the patient with a decreased level of consciousness includes the use of a triad of agents commonly referred to as coma drugs—glucose, thiamine, and naloxone (6).

Glucose

Glucose 50% (1 to 2 ml/kg) should be administered intravenously to all patients with a decreased level of consciousness if a rapid determination of the patient's blood glucose cannot be made (6). Patients suffering from insulin-induced hypoglycemia or an overdose of oral hypoglycemic medications such as chlorpropamide or glyburide will respond to the glucose if hypoglycemic-induced brain damage has not occurred. Oral hypoglycemic agents may produce protracted hypoglycemia in acute overdose and need not be used for 24 hours, requiring prolonged administration of a glucose-containing solution such as dextrose 10%. If intravenous access cannot be attained, glucagon 1 mg intramuscularly may reverse the hypoglycemia. Parenteral glucose is preferred to the administration of oral glucose in the comatose patient because of the risk of aspiration.

Thiamine

If glucose is administered to the adult patient, thiamine 100 mg either intravenously or intramuscularly should be administered simultaneously to prevent Wernicke's encephalopathy (6). Glucose administration may further deplete thiamine stores, which are already diminished in the nutritionally compromised alcoholic patient.

Naloxone

Naloxone (Narcan), the opioid antagonist, is customarily administered to all unconscious patients (6). This is considered to represent the standard of care in all patients with a decreased level of consciousness. However, at least one study has questioned the utility of administering it as a diagnostic agent unless the patient is comatose with decreased respirations—a common presentation of opioid overdose. The standard dosage recommendation is to administer 0.4 to 2.0 mg intravenously every 2 to 3 minutes until the desired level of consciousness is achieved or a maximum of 10 mg is administered (7). If intravenous access cannot be established, naloxone can be administered via intralingual or sublingual injection or via the endotracheal tube. The failure to respond to naloxone 10 mg suggests that the patient's decreased level of consciousness is not the result of an opioid overdose or that there may be a mixed overdose and the other agent (e.g., ethanol or a benzodiazepine) may be contributing to the coma. Other explanations for the failure to respond to naloxone include medical conditions or trauma that contributes to the central nervous system depression and the use of an insufficient quantity of naloxone. Some synthetic opioids such as propoxyphene and illicit drugs of abuse such as fentanyl derivatives may require substantial amounts of naloxone, even exceeding 10 mg.

OTHER ANTIDOTES

Very few effective antidotes are used to reverse the adverse sequelae associated with acute poisoning emergencies. Naloxone was used in only 7136 of the 1.84 million poisoning cases reported to the AAPCC in 1991 (1). This was followed by *N*-acetylcysteine, which was used to treat 7075 patients suffering from acetaminophen poisoning (1). The remainder of the common pharmacologic antagonists were each used in fewer than 1000 reported cases (1). Although these agents can reduce morbidity and mortality, they are utilized only infrequently. The most common and important antidotes for acute poisoning problems are discussed briefly below.

N-acetylcysteine

Acetaminophen is partially metabolized via the p-450 system to a toxic metabolite (*N*-acetyl-*p*-benzoquinonimine) that is detoxified by endogenous glutathione (8). After glutathione has been substantially depleted, the metabolite selectively binds to and destroys hepatocytes, producing centrilobular necrosis. *N*-acetylcysteine serves as a glutathione surrogate and prevents hepatotoxicity. It is most effective if it is administered within the first 8 hours after ingestion of the acetaminophen (9). The Rumack-Matthew nomogram is used to plot serum acetaminophen levels and to determine the risk of hepatotoxicity and the need to administer *N*-acetylcysteine. In the United States it is approved only for oral use. The dosing regimen consists of a loading dose of 140 mg/kg followed by 17 maintenance doses of 70 mg/kg at 4-hour intervals (9). Intravenous *N*-acetylcysteine use is not approved in the United States. Dosing protocols differ from those for the oral route, in that the length of therapy is reduced from 72 hours to 24 to 48 hours (10, 11).

Flumazenil

Only acetaminophen and antibiotics are responsible for more accidental and intentional poisonings than are the benzodiazepines (1). Although it is rare for benzodiazepines to be solely responsible for fatalities, their synergistic central nervous system depressant effects often complicate otherwise only minor to moderate exposures to ethanol, sedatives, and other agents with central nervous system depressant properties. Flumazenil, a specific benzodiazepine antagonist, may rectify those problems by producing partial to complete reversal of the sedative effects and psychomotor impairment consistent with benzodiazepine overdose (12). Much like naloxone, flumazenil has a rapid onset of action and a short half-life (40 to 80 minutes), which may necessitate repeated administration to continuously reverse the effects of benzodiazepines such as diazepam (13). In suspected benzodiazepine overdoses, 0.2 mg should be administered intravenously over 30 seconds. If no response is apparent after an additional 30 seconds, a subsequent dose of 0.3 mg is recommended. Additional doses in 0.5 mg increments may be administered at 1-minute intervals until the desired response is achieved or a total of 3.0 mg is administered (13). The drug should be used with great caution in patients who are suspected to be physiologically dependent upon benzodiazepines, since flumazenil may precipitate withdrawal, which has life-threatening potential. Flumazenil is contraindicated in patients suffering from mixed ingestions involving both a cyclic antidepressant and a benzodiazepine. Flumazenil may unmask the seizure potential of cyclic antidepressants by antagonizing the antiseizure effect of benzodiazepines. Because of this potential, the indiscriminate use of flumazenil as a coma drug with glucose, thiamine, and naloxone is not advised.

Atropine

Atropine exerts its primary effect by blocking muscarinic receptors and, therefore, finds extensive use in the treatment of poisonings resulting from cholinesterase inhibitors such as carbamate and organophosphate insecticides. It is also occasionally used to reverse the cholinergic effects associated with the excessive use of the cholinesterase inhibitor physostigmine. Cholinergic crisis from pesticide poisoning may require the administration of 2 to 4 mg per dose, which may need to be repeated at intervals of 2 to 5 minutes until muscarinic signs abate (14). Since organophosphates irreversibly render red blood cell cholinesterase ineffective, if pralidoxime is not used, atropine administration may have to be administered for several weeks in severe cases.

Pralidoxime

Pralidoxime, also known as 2-PAM, is used to permanently restore cholinesterase activity in patients who are suffering from organophosphate toxicity. If pralidoxime is administered within the first 24 hours after an organophosphate exposure, the pesticide-cholinesterase bond is severed and activity returns (14). Unlike atropine, which is a temporizing measure and blocks the muscarinic receptors, pralidoxime opposes the nicotinic effects of organophosphate insecticides (15). Pralidoxime generally is not indicated in carbamate insecticide poisoning, since the cholinesterase inhibition is more transient in nature and responds to atropine administration (15). The customary adult dose is 1 to 2 g infused in 100 ml of saline over 15 to 30 minutes.

Deferoxamine

Iron poisoning is one of the most common pediatric poisonings and in 1991 accounted for more pediatric fatalities than any other agent (1). Most iron overexposures necessitate only very conservative therapy, which may include some form of gastrointestinal decontamination (16). However, patients who experience moderate to serious iron poisoning, which is often characterized by gastrointestinal bleeding, hypotension, and shock, are candidates for deferoxamine therapy (17). Serum levels should be used adjunctively to confirm significant overexposure to iron but should not be used as the sole indication for deferoxamine therapy unless the levels are inordinately high, since there is not a good correlation between toxicity and total iron binding capacity at moderate serum levels. Deferoxamine chelates iron to form a water-soluble complex, ferrioxamine, which is excreted in the urine. Ferrioxamine usually imparts a pink to orange hue to the urine, and in the absence of serum iron levels the disappearance of this color is an excellent indicator that deferoxamine therapy can be terminated. Since iron toxicity is often associated with hypotension, intravenous administration of deferoxamine is preferred over the intramuscular route. The initial dose is 1 g followed by subsequent doses of 500 mg at 4-hour intervals as necessary and as dictated by the clinical response and serum iron levels (18). The rate of administration should not exceed 15 mg/kg/hr, and the maximum daily dose is 6 g.

Ethanol

Ethanol is specifically used to treat ethylene glycol and methanol toxicity. Following the concurrent administration of ethanol in either an ethylene glycol or methanol poisoning incident, ethanol is preferentially metabolized by alcohol dehydrogenase. This prevents the metabolic conversion of ethylene glycol and methanol to toxic metabolites, thus allowing the parent compounds to be renally eliminated or removed via extracorporeal techniques. The oral loading dose of ethanol is 600 to 700 mg/kg followed by hourly maintenance doses of approximately 125 mg/hr (19, 20). Ethanol can be administered orally as a 20 to 25% solution or intravenously as a 5 to 10% solution. Ethanol maintenance doses must be doubled during hemodialysis to maintain serum levels of at least 100 mg/dl to effectively inhibit the metabolism of ethylene glycol and methanol (19, 20).

Digoxin Immune Fab

Digoxin immune Fab fragments are specific antidigoxin antibodies that are harvested from sheep. They are effective in the treatment of digitalis glycoside overdoses that include both digoxin and digitoxin (21). They have some cross-reactivity with similar glycosides such as those found in the very poisonous botanical oleander. Their high affinity for digoxin significantly reduces the morbidity and mortality associated with both intentional and nosocomial digitalis glycoside overdoses. The indications for use include life-threatening digitalis glycoside overdose, which may manifest as arrhythmias unresponsive to conventional therapy, the acute ingestion of 10 mg of digoxin (in previously healthy adults), steady-state serum levels in excess of 10 ng/ml, and/or hyperkalemia (22, 23). Dosage recommendations are specified in the product literature. If the amount of digitalis glycoside ingested is unknown, the administration of 10 to 20 vials is recommended (23). Caution should be exercised against indiscriminate use of digoxin immune Fab in patients dependent upon the inotropic effects of digitalis glycosides.

Pyridoxine

Tuberculosis is becoming more common in the United States as a consequence of foreign immigration patterns and restricted public health funds. Isoniazid is commonly used in the treatment and prophylaxis of this ailment and overdoses are prevalent among people who are being treated with it. Isoniazid overdoses produce metabolic acidosis as well as pronounced and often recalcitrant seizure activity as a result of the decrease in endogenous γ-aminobutyric acid concentrations in the brain (24). This results from isoniazid-induced inhibition of pyridoxal-5'-phosphate activity, which is countered by the expeditious administration of pyridoxine. Pyridoxine is administered intravenously in a gram-for-gram dosage based upon the amount of isoniazid ingested (25). If the amount of isoniazid cannot be verified, a 5-g dose of pyridoxine is administered.

Physostigmine

Physostigmine is a cholinesterase inhibitor that has a limited role in the treatment of acute poisoning emergencies. It rose to prominence as a specific antagonist for tricyclic antidepressant overdoses. However, the life-threatening effects associated with tricyclic antidepressant overdose are not anticholinergically mediated—physostigmine is not indicated in those overdoses. It finds its only indications in the treatment of anticholinergic effects from *Datura* species (jimson weed) poisoning, since these agents contain inordinate amounts of belladonna alkaloids, and a limited number of other overdoses such as severe antihistamine poisoning. Physostigmine should be administered intravenously in small dosage increments of 0.5 mg with administration rates of not less than 2 to 3 minutes (26). Rapid intravenous administration may produce seizures and a cholinergic crisis.

Antidotes are important adjuncts in the management of acute toxicologic emergencies. In conjunction with aggressive life support measures they can substantially reduce the morbidity and mortality associated with a limited number of poisoning emergencies. However, gastric decontamination of the patient is more important than antidotes and utilized in nearly every poisoning emergency, since 80% of all poisonings are ingestions. These procedures can prevent further absorption of the toxin and, perhaps, eliminate the need for more aggressive therapeutic intervention.

GASTROINTESTINAL DECONTAMINATION

Following the implementation of life support measures, if such measures are necessary, the traditional management of poisoning emergencies has dictated some type of gastrointestinal decontamination to prevent further absorption if the toxin was ingested. Conventional clinical practice standards have recommended the induction of emesis for alert patients and the use of gastric lavage for patients with a decreased level of consciousness. Activated charcoal was administered as an adsorbent and followed by cathartic use, and both were considered more as adjunctive than mandatory therapy. However, choosing the optimal type of gastrointestinal decontamination is not so straightforward, and a number of factors must be considered, such as the temporal separation between the ingestion and treatment, the substance ingested, the level of consciousness or potential for rapid deterioration, the amount of toxin, and efficacy and risks of each gastrointestinal technique. Furthermore, the validity of all gastrointestinal decontamination techniques has been challenged, and some authorities recommend the elimination of gastric emptying in favor of using only activated charcoal as the sole means of gastrointestinal decontamination. Others advocate whole-bowel irrigation as the most efficacious procedure. The section that follows examines the risks, benefits, and limitations of these procedures in the acutely poisoned patient.

SYRUP OF IPECAC-INDUCED EMESIS

Overview

The standard approach to gastric emptying has been the induction of emesis. A variety of agents, both with and without a pharmacologic basis, have been used. Home remedies such as egg whites and mustard water are ineffective. Salt water has been advocated as an emetic for decades. Although a concentrated sodium chloride solution may be irritating, it is not an effective emetic and the dangers of hypernatremia, especially in the pediatric patient, far outweigh the benefits of its use. Copper sulfate is an effective emetic that was popular as recently as the early 1970s. However, the acute toxicity associated with the absorption of copper, particularly if emesis is unsuccessful, does not justify its use. Apomorphine is an effective emetic that is no longer used in humans but finds extensive use in veterinary medicine. It is a very effective emetic but suffers from the fact that it is an opioid and may complicate poisonings and overdoses from agents that have synergistic central nervous system effects. There is no role for this agent in the contemporary management of acute poisoning emergencies. Mild liquid dishwashing detergents contain surfactants that produce an emetic response, but their palatability restricts their general use. Syrup of ipecac is the emetic of choice, and it enjoys widespread popularity as a convenient, safe, and effective emetic that can be used at home.

Critical Care Implications

Syrup of ipecac was the time-honored means of gastric decontamination in all alert patients, even those who had taken overdoses of drugs associated with high morbidity and mortality, such as tricyclic antidepressants. The early literature clearly demonstrated it to be more effective than gastric lavage (27–29). Until the last decade there were no studies that compared it with current lavage techniques or activated charcoal, and it was widely used in most overdoses. Although ipecac will effectively produce emesis, its use has never been validated in regard to its ability to reduce morbidity and mortality among poisoned patients. Furthermore, contemporary studies have clearly demonstrated that properly performed gastric lavage is superior to ipecac-induced emesis in the removal of marker drugs (30, 31). Activated charcoal alone has been demonstrated to be more effective than ipecac in preventing the absorption of medications. This effect is especially true when there is a delay of 30 to 60 minutes after toxin ingestion (32–33).

Ipecac has very limited use in the critical care patient. Many critical care patients present with a decreased level of consciousness and hemodynamic compromise. There is generally at least a 3-hour delay between exposure and presentation for treatment (32). Therefore, substantial toxin absorption has already occurred, and ipecac-induced emesis is contraindicated in patients with a decreased level of consciousness and in those who have taken agents that may cause an impending loss of consciousness. Its application may be limited to patients who have recently ingested agents that do not lend themselves to gastric lavage (e.g., poisonous mushrooms) and in children.

Indications

Syrup of ipecac is a viable agent to induce vomiting in the home setting in the pediatric or adult patient who has accidentally ingested a potentially toxic agent (and in whom emesis is not contraindicated) that can be at least partially removed via emesis (34). It has limited usefulness in the emergency department because of the delays between ingestion and treatment.

Mechanism of Action

Emetine and cephaline are the primary alkaloidal ingredients in syrup of ipecac (35). The primary mechanism of action functions via peripheral gastrointestinal irritation and secondarily through absorption of the alkaloids and subsequent direct stimulation of the vomiting center in the chemoreceptor trigger zone (35). Emesis begins in 16 to 26 minutes, and the time to onset appears to be dose dependent (36). A dose of 30 ml will produce emesis approximately 10 minutes faster than a conventional pediatric dose of 15 ml. Emesis occurs successfully in more than 99% of patients following the use of 30 ml and in 92% of patients following the use of 15 ml (36).

Pharmacokinetics

The pharmacokinetics of syrup of ipecac have not been fully elucidated. The absorption of the alkaloids is minimal in most patients as a result of the rapid onset of emesis. Emetine is metabolized hepatically, and the process is very slow. The half-life of emetine is long and may be detected in urine for up to 60 days (37). Therefore, it will accumulate with repetitive use, as may be the case in bulimic patients.

Dosage and Route of Administration

Syrup of ipecac is always administered orally. The dose for children younger than 1 year of age is 5 to 10 ml. Children ages 1 to 12 years of age receive 15 ml, and in adolescents and adults the recommended dosage is 30 ml (38). A popular alternative is to administer 30 ml to all individuals older than 1 year of age (36). This method eliminates the problems of underdosing caused by using kitchen flatware spoons and improves compliance. The ipecac is followed by the administration of a minimum of 120 to 240 ml of water or other suitable clear liquid such as juice or soda. Contrary to popular opinion, milk will not interfere with the action of ipecac; however, it is less desirable than clear fluids, since the milk may obscure remnants of medications in the emesis (39, 40). If the initial dose of ipecac does not successfully induce vomiting within 20 to 30 minutes, an additional dose and more fluid are indicated. The label on ipecac bottles warns against the concurrent use of activated charcoal, as the charcoal allegedly prevents the emetic effects of ipecac. This allegation is not valid, and since the primary mechanism of action of ipecac is to produce vomiting via peripheral irritation, the two may be used together. Otherwise, the administration of activated charcoal will need to be delayed until the emetic process has ceased.

Adverse Effects and Contraindications

Ipecac-induced emesis is generally well-tolerated. Emesis usually ceases within 15 to 30 minutes, and only occasionally do patients have protracted courses of vomiting that exceed 1 hour. Consistent with the therapeutic use of ipecac is occasional diarrhea, cramping, and even drowsiness. The use of even multiple doses of ipecac in the management of acute poisonings is not associated with systemic toxicity. Rare but reported consequences of ipecac use include Mallory-Weiss tears of the esophagus, aspiration pneumonitis, pneumomediastinum, retropneumoperitoneum, one case of intracranial bleeding in an elderly individual, and death of a child from herniation of the stomach through a preexisting diaphragmatic hernia (41–46).

Chronic abuse of ipecac in individuals with eating disorders can lead to a variety of complications as a consequence of the accumulation of emetine (47). Cardiomyopathy and cardiac arrhythmias have been reported. Emetine is also directly myotoxic (48, 49). Laboratory analysis for the alkaloids generally is unavailable on an acute basis, and pathognomonic of chronic ipecac toxicity are electrocardiogram (EKG) abnormalities and, especially, inverted T waves (35).

Contraindications to emesis include a decreased or impending loss of consciousness and the ingestion of corrosive agents. Generally, emesis is contraindicated in patients who have ingested hydrocarbons because of the risk of aspiration. The use of ipecac in children younger than 1 year of age and during pregnancy is not contraindicated, but its use is advised only in a health care facility.

GASTRIC LAVAGE

Overview

Until the last decade, gastric lavage was reserved solely for use in the patient with a decreased level of consciousness. Early research comparing lavage with emesis used small-bore nasogastric tubes, inadequate fluid volumes, and poor technique. Contemporary studies that incorporated the use of larger-bore tubes and voluminous amounts of lavage fluid demonstrated the superiority of lavage over ipecac-induced emesis (30, 31). However, as with ipecac, the impact on morbidity and mortality has never been validated. Yet, gastric lavage is an important technique in the management of acute poisoning emergencies.

Critical Care Implications

Only two practical means of gastrointestinal decontamination are available to the physician who is treating the critically ill patient: activated charcoal and gastric lavage. The intentional overdose or drug abuse victim is frequently comatose or disoriented and cannot be relied upon for an accurate history. It is therefore prudent to gastrically evacuate the patient. Gastric lavage is the only realistic means of removing toxins from the stomach. Although activated charcoal may adsorb those same toxins, it can be administered only via a large-bore orogastric tube in patients with a decreased level of consciousness. Furthermore, toxins can desorb from activated charcoal as the toxin:charcoal complex traverses the bowel. The removal of toxins remaining in the stomach ensures that they are not bioavailable to produce systemic effects. This is an important procedure from both a medical and legal perspective.

Indications

Gastric lavage is indicated whenever a rapidly acting toxin associated with high morbidity and mortality, such as a tricyclic antidepressant or cyanide, has been ingested (41). It is generally indicated in the comatose overdose or poisoned patient who is a candidate for gastrointestinal decontamination. Overdoses involving agents that are not adsorbed effectively by activated charcoal, such as iron, alcohols, and lithium, are good indications for gastric lavage.

Procedure

Gastric lavage is accomplished by introducing a large-bore orogastric lavage tube (24 to 28 French in children and 34 to 40 French in adults) orally down the esophagus and into the stomach (6). Large-bore tubes are essential both to maximize the introduction of lavage fluid and to facilitate removal of toxin and other gastric debris. Small-bore tubes with small and a limited number of orifices are of little value unless the toxin is a liquid. Gastric lavage is performed most effectively by using a technique referred to as gravity flow lavage. A receptacle containing the lavage fluid is elevated on an IV pole over the patient, and fluid is introduced into the lavage tube. The lavage instillation tube is then clamped to restrict further flow, a tube leading from the lavage tube into a closed collection receptacle near the floor is opened, and the lavage fluid is removed via gravity from the patient who is lying on his or her left side in Trendelenburg's position. The process is repeated continuously. Lukewarm tap water may be used in the adult patient and instilled in 300-ml increments until the lavage returns are clear of macroscopic debris and a total of 10 to 20 liters of lavage fluid has been instilled (6, 41). Comatose patients should always be intubated with a cuffed endotracheal tube prior to performing gastric lavage.

Adverse Effects and Contraindications

Gastric lavage is relatively safe, but there are some attendant risks associated with the procedure. Trauma and esophageal perforation secondary to the rigid nature and size of the tubes is an ever-present risk. Aspiration may occur while the tube is being inserted. This can be eliminated for the most part if the patient is endotracheally intubated prior to tube insertion. Children are at risk of developing fluid and electrolyte derangement if tap water is used (41). Normal or half-normal saline warmed to body temperature is advised in the pediatric patient.

There are few absolute contraindications to gastric lavage. Most notably, lavage should not be implemented if a strong corrosive agent has been ingested, since the risk of perforation is very high. Lavage should not be used if the patient cannot protect his or her airway or unless the patient is intubated. Lavage may be performed without prior intubation on fully alert patients with an intact gag reflex.

Other Considerations

The typical candidate for gastric lavage has a decreased level of consciousness. This also complicates the administration of activated charcoal, which requires the patient's cooperation or the placement of a large-bore orogastric tube for administration. Although to do so is not conventional, activated charcoal should be administered to the patient at the beginning of the lavage process to adsorb toxin that may not be removed during lavage and that is subsequently gastrically emptied into the small intestine (50). Furthermore, the presence of activated charcoal in the lavage fluid can serve as a marker to signal when lavage is complete. In other words, the gross macroscopic absence of activated charcoal in the lavage returns is an accurate signal that the stomach has been thoroughly evacuated.

ACTIVATED CHARCOAL

Overview

Activated charcoal has been used as a poison "antidote" for centuries. During the 20th century it became popular as a component of the fabled but ineffective universal antidote, which also contained tannic acid and magnesium oxide. Prior to the 1980s, the use of activated charcoal was relegated to that of an adjunct that was used when it was convenient to do so following gastric emptying with either ipecac or gastric lavage. However, its undisputed value became apparent in a large number of studies that revealed that activated charcoal alone was as effective as either lavage or emesis, and in many cases even superior, in preventing the absorption of the study toxin (32, 33, 51–53). As with the other procedures, there is a lack of adequate validation that the use of activated charcoal reduces morbidity and mortality from poisonings, but it is abundantly clear that it does enhance toxin elimination via several mechanisms. Single doses of activated charcoal prevent the absorption of toxin that has not been absorbed, and multiple doses can actually enhance the elimination of agents that are already absorbed or given parenterally and then resecreted into the gut. The use of activated charcoal will continue to grow, and in 1990 it surpassed both ipecac and lavage as the primary means of gastric decontamination in the poisoned patient (2). However, the sole use of activated charcoal has yet to be accepted totally as the standard of care, and it is prudent also to lavage patients who have ingested agents that are associated with high morbidity and mortality (54).

Critical Care Implications

The use of activated charcoal offers distinct advantages in the critically ill patient. Most notable is the ability of activated charcoal to adsorb toxins that have traversed the stomach and now reside in the small intestine. These toxins are nonretrievable with conventional gastric emptying, and, at least in theory, activated charcoal can "catch up" with those toxins. This effect may be especially relevant following the ingestion of agents that reduce gastrointestinal motility, such as anticholinergics and opioids (55). Profound hypotension often accompanies serious overdoses and thereby reduces splanchnic circulation and subsequent absorption of the toxin. When hemodynamic balance is restored, the presence of activated charcoal in the bowel may minimize the absorption of unabsorbed toxins. The critically ill patient may require extensive stabilization, making lavage both inappropriate and impractical. The administration of activated charcoal can prevent toxin absorption and delay gastric lavage until the patient is stable. Extracorporeal elimination of drugs is not without complications. Multiple doses of activated charcoal may be efficacious in enhancing the elimination of selected drugs such as theophylline and phenobarbital, thereby eliminating the need for more

invasive procedures such as hemodialysis and hemoperfusion, which are not universally available.

Indications

Activated charcoal is indicated in nearly all poisoning emergencies that result from the ingestion of a toxin. Only a limited number of agents are not adsorbed effectively by activated charcoal: heavy metals, iron, lithium, alcohols, and a few others (37). Many intentional overdoses involve co-ingestants that may be adsorbed by charcoal. Therefore, charcoal is not contraindicated even when one or more of the toxins may not be adsorbed effectively. Multiple-dose activated charcoal therapy is effective in adsorbing agents that are secreted into the gut (e.g., theophylline, phenobarbital, etc.) or enterohepatically circulated (digitoxin) (41). Unlike gastric lavage and emesis, the administration of activated charcoal is still indicated several hours after the ingestion of agents that may have undergone complete gastric emptying, such as liquid preparations.

Mechanism of Action

Activated charcoal is refined carbonaceous material that is produced from the combustion of either organic matter such as wood pulp or petroleum. The activation process removes debris from the charcoal and creates a network of pores, which results in extensive surface area and the resultant adsorptive properties. Activated charcoal USP has a minimum surface area of 950 m². Commercially available activated charcoal products have surface areas of up to 2000 m². Activated charcoal will adsorb but not irreversibly bind inorganic and organic substances with a molecular weight range of 100 to 1000 daltons (33). The charcoal:toxin complex will then be eliminated via the gastrointestinal tract. Multiple-dose activated charcoal therapy is based upon the enteroenteric or enterohepatic secretion of toxins into the gastrointestinal tract (56). The multiple pulses of activated charcoal coming through the gastrointestinal tract will bind toxin that is being secreted constantly or intermittently and prevent the reabsorption of the agent, therefore enhancing elimination.

Pharmacokinetics

Activated charcoal is pharmacologically inert and it is not absorbed. Its elimination is via the gastrointestinal tract and cathartics are sometimes used to hasten its elimination.

Dosage, Route of Administration, and Frequency

Activated charcoal is administered orally. Commercial products are slurries and not true suspensions. Therefore, they must be agitated vigorously prior to administration. A minimum of 30 seconds of agitation is advised, and the container should be rinsed thoroughly to ensure that all of the charcoal has been administered to the patient (57). For either single- or multiple-dose therapy, the dose for infants is 1 to 2 g/kg, for children, 25 to 50 g, and for adults, 50 to 100 g (58). During multiple-dose therapy the charcoal is usually administered at intervals of 4 to 6 hours. However, that interval can be shortened to accommodate a variety of needs. For example, theophylline lends itself to enhanced elimination by multiple-dose charcoal, but a common side effect of theophylline toxicity is vomiting. A 50-g dose of activated charcoal in a minimum of 240 ml of fluid may be difficult for a patient to retain if he or she is already afflicted with repetitive vomiting. The use of smaller amounts (e.g., 12.5 g every hour or 25 g every 2 hours) over shorter intervals is equally effective and may reduce the incidence of emesis (59). Cathartics are often administered with activated charcoal to hasten the elimination of the charcoal:toxin complex. Caution must be exercised when using cathartics during multiple-dose therapy—the cathartics should not be used with each dose of charcoal.

Adverse Effects and Contraindications

Activated charcoal is inert and will not cause systemic toxicity. Although the risks associated with its use are limited, they must not be overlooked. Vomiting is a common side effect and is most prevalent when activated charcoal is combined with the cathartic sorbitol (41). Diarrhea is also a complication of using a charcoal:sorbitol mixture (60). If excessive sorbitol is administered, the patient may become dehydrated (61). Patients should be warned that their stools will turn black. Pulmonary aspiration of activated charcoal is generally not a serious event. However, a limited number of reports describe bronchiolitis obliterans and airway obstruction as a result of the physical presence of lumps of charcoal (62, 63). Some agents such as tricyclic antidepressants and opioids may decrease bowel motility or even produce an ileus. Activated charcoal should not be administered in the absence of bowel sounds (41). Activated charcoal in sorbitol should not be given to infants, since the cathartic dose of sorbitol is fixed and may produce severe dehydration (61). Contrary to popular opinion, activated charcoal will not interfere with the emetic effects of syrup of ipecac and is not contraindicated. In addition, N-acetylcysteine is not adsorbed significantly by activated charcoal, and the use of charcoal in acetaminophen overdose is not contraindicated.

Special Considerations: Cathartics

Activated charcoal will bind toxins spontaneously, but the binding process is not irreversible. Cathartics traditionally have been used to hasten the elimination of the charcoal:toxin complex through the bowel to decrease the risk of reabsorption of desorbed toxin. The saline cathartics magnesium sulfate and sodium sulfate enjoyed wide popularity until magnesium citrate and sorbitol were clearly demonstrated to be superior (60). Although there is no documented evidence that cathartics reduce morbidity and mortality, when used in conjunction with activated charcoal they have been documented to be superior to the use of activated charcoal alone (64). This effectiveness is most prominent when the charcoal and cathartic are ingested within 1 hour of the ingestion of a marker drug. The customary cathartic dose of magnesium citrate is 4 to 5 ml/kg. Sorbitol is the superior cathartic in a dose of 1.0 to 1.5 g/kg (65). In volunteer studies, catharsis of activated charcoal was evident in less than 1 hour. However, in overdoses of agents that reduce bowel motility, the time to catharsis was several hours. Cathartics are effective only if peristalsis is not compromised. Cathartics should be used cautiously because they produce third-spacing of fluid in the gastrointestinal tract,

which may result in fluid and electrolyte derangement (61). Hypermagnesemia may result from overly aggressive use of magnesium citrate (66). Magnesium citrate should also be avoided in patients with compromised renal function.

WHOLE-BOWEL IRRIGATION

Overview

Whole-bowel irrigation has long been used as a means of preoperative bowel preparation, and only recently has its utility in the management of poisoning emergencies been realized. It has very limited application, but it provides a means of cleansing the bowel of foreign material without the risks of impending fluid and electrolyte problems. Since voluminous amounts of fluid are introduced orally, its use is limited to noncomatose patients (41). It is of little value in the treatment of conventional overdoses in which gastric emptying and activated charcoal therapy may suffice.

Critical Care Implications

Whole-bowel irrigation finds its greatest application in the treatment of the patient who will have impending critical care needs. The patient who has ingested a large amount of an iron-containing preparation, which is easily visualized on a radiograph, is an excellent candidate for whole-bowel irrigation. The iron tablets can be purged before they have a chance to produce local corrosive effects or be absorbed. Cocaine "stuffers," who swallow crack cocaine rocks or small bags of cocaine to eliminate evidence and avoid arrest, and "body packers," who smuggle scores of cocaine packets in their bowel, are at a high risk of developing intestinal ischemia and systemic effects if the container breaks or leaks (41). Expeditiously performed whole-bowel irrigation can prevent these patients from developing severe toxicity. The nature of whole-bowel irrigation does not lend itself to use in comatose and critically ill patients.

Indications

Whole-bowel irrigation may be indicated in patients who have ingested iron salts or heavy metals such as lead that can be visualized on a radiograph. Its use in the treatment of body packers and stuffers is well-established. It may also have some utility in the treatment of patients who have ingested sustained-release medications or who have medication bezoars.

Mechanism of Action

Polyethylene glycol electrolyte solution, which is isoosmotic, is consumed or instilled via a nasogastric tube, and the entire gastrointestinal tract is flushed. The process is continued until the rectal effluent has the same clarity and consistency as the infusate fluid. This endpoint does not guarantee that all of the toxic agent has been eliminated. That can be ascertained only through collaborating histories, radiographs, laboratory values, and clinical manifestations.

Dosage, Routes of Administration, and Frequency

Polyethylene glycol electrolyte solution is administered orally in compliant patients or via a nasogastric tube at the rate of approximately 1 to 2 liters/hr (41). This rate is continued to the endpoint as described in the preceding section; typically, 10 liters are used.

Adverse Effects and Contraindications

The voluminous amount of fluid that is administered often produces bloating, vomiting, and abdominal cramping. It should not be used in patients with an ileus or who are at risk of gastrointestinal perforation. Its use is restricted to noncomatose, medically stable patients. It should not be used in comatose patients because of the risk of vomiting and aspiration. The combative or noncompliant patient is not a good candidate for this procedure, since it may require several hours to complete.

ENHANCING TOXIN ELIMINATION

The majority of poisoned patients will be managed adequately with conservative therapy and gastrointestinal decontamination. A limited number of patients will require pharmacologic intervention and the use of antidotal agents. An even more limited number of patients will require the use of extracorporeal means to eliminate the toxin. In 1991, only 865 of the reported 1.84 million poisoning cases were treated by hemoperfusion, hemodialysis, or peritoneal dialysis (1).

Extracorporeal elimination has limited application. Many of the very toxic agents such as tricyclic antidepressants have pharmacokinetic profiles that do not lend themselves to removal. For a drug to be removed effectively, it should have a low molecular weight, low volume of distribution, high water solubility, and low protein binding. Most of the agents that produce severe toxicity do not match this profile. A limited number of agents are hemodialyzable: ethanol, ethylene glycol, methanol, lithium, phenobarbital, salicylates, theophylline, and the like. The indications for hemodialysis are stringent, and rarely do patients require such extraordinary therapy.

Charcoal hemoperfusion differs from hemodialysis in that blood is filtered through a charcoal filter. It has the advantage of being able to adsorb more lipid-soluble and protein-bound drugs. It is not universally available, and it has limited application despite its advantages over hemodialysis with some agents.

Ion-trapping, or manipulation of urinary pH to ionize and trap a drug, has academic merit but little application in the management of poisoning emergencies.

REFERENCES

1. Litovitz TL, Bailey KM, Holm KC, et al: 1991 annual report of the American Association of Poison Control Centers National Data Collection System, Washington, DC. *Am J Emerg Med* 10:452–505, 1992.
2. Litovitz TL, Bailey KM, Schmitz BF, et al: 1990 annual report of the American Association of Poison Control Centers National Data Collection System. *Am J Emerg Med* 9:461–509, 1991.
3. Litovitz TL, Schmitz BF, Bailey KM: 1989 annual report of the American Association of Poison Control Centers National Data Collection System. *Am J Emerg Med* 8:394–442, 1990.
4. Litovitz TL, Schmitz BF, Holm KC: 1988 annual report of the American Association of Poison Control Centers National Data Collection System. *Am J Emerg Med* 7:495–545, 1989.
5. Litovitz TL, Schmitz BF, Matyunas N, et al: 1989 annual report of the American Association of Poison Control Centers National Data Collection System. *Am J Emerg Med* 6:479–515, 1988.
6. Krenzelok EP, Dunmire SM: Acute poisoning emergencies—resolving the gastric decontamination controversy. *Postgrad Med* 91:179–186, 1992.
7. Anon: Naloxone. In: *American Hospital Formulary Service*. Bethesda, MD, American Society of Hospital Pharmacists, 1992, pp 1178–1181.
8. Corcoran GB, Mitchell JR, Vaishnav YN, et al: Evidence that acetaminophen and N-hydroxyacetaminophen form a common arylating intermediate, N-acetyl-p-benzoquinoneimine. *Mol Pharmacol* 18:536–542, 1980.
9. Smilkstein MJ, Knapp GL, Kulig KW, et al: Efficacy of oral N-acetylcysteine in the treatment of acetaminophen overdose: analysis of the national multicenter study (1976–1985). *N Engl J Med* 319:1557–1562, 1988.
10. Keays R, Harrison PM, Wendon JA, et al: Intravenous acetylcysteine in paracetamol induced fulminant hepatic failure: a prospective controlled trial. *BMJ* 303:1026–1029, 1991.
11. Smilkstein MJ, Bronstein AC, Linden C, et al: Acetaminophen overdose: a 48-hour intravenous N-acetylcysteine treatment protocol. *Ann Emerg Med* 20:1058–1063, 1991.
12. Votey SR, Bosse GM, Bayer MJ, et al: Flumazenil: a new benzodiazepine antagonist. *Ann Emerg Med* 20:181–188, 1991.
13. Anon: Benzodiazepine antagonist approved by the FDA. *Clin Pharm* 11:287–288, 1992.
14. Bryson PD: *Comprehensive Review in Toxicology*. Rockville, MD, Aspen Publications, pp 533–545, 1989.
15. Ellenhorn MJ, Barceloux DG: *Medical Toxicology—Diagnosis and Treatment of Human Poisoning*. New York, Elsevier, pp 1069–1078, 1988.
16. Klein-Schwartz W, Oderda GM, Gorman RL, et al: Assessment of management guidelines. *Clin Pediatr* 29:316–321, 1990.
17. Engle JP, Polin KS, Stile IL: Acute iron intoxication: treatment controversies. *Drug Intell Clin Pharm* 21:153–159, 1987.
18. Anon: Deferoxamine. In: *American Hospital Formulary Service*. Bethesda, MD, American Society of Hospital Pharmacists, pp 1800–1801, 1992.
19. McCoy HG, Cipolle RJ, Ehlers SM, et al: Severe methanol poisoning: application of a pharmacokinetic model for ethanol. *Am J Med* 67:804–807, 1979.
20. Ekins BR, Rollins DE, Duffy DP, et al: Standardized treatment of severe methanol poisoning with ethanol and hemodialysis. *West J Med* 142:337–340, 1985.
21. Smith TW: Review of clinical experience with digoxin immune Fab (ovine). *Am J Emerg Med* 9(suppl 1):1–6, 1991.
22. Bayer MJ: Recognition and management of digitalis intoxication: implications for emergency medicine. *Am J Emerg Med* 9(suppl 1):29–32, 1991.
23. Ellenhorn MJ, Barceloux DG: *Medical Toxicology—Diagnosis and Treatment of Human Poisoning*. New York, Elsevier, pp 200–207, 1988.
24. Orlowski JP, Paganini EP, Pippenger CE: Treatment of a potentially lethal dose isoniazid ingestion. *Ann Emerg Med* 17:73–76, 1988.
25. Shannon MW, Lovejoy FH: Isoniazid. In Haddad LM, Winchester JF (eds): *Clinical Management of Poisoning and Drug Overdose*. Philadelphia, WB Saunders, pp 970–976, 1990.
26. Anon: Physostigmine salicylate. In: *American Hospital Formulary Service*. Bethesda, MD, American Society of Hospital Pharmacists, 1992, pp 628–630.
27. Arnold FJ, Hodges JB, Barta RA, et al: Evaluation of the efficacy of lavage and induced emesis in treatment of salicylate poisoning. *Pediatrics* 23:286–301, 1959.
28. Boxer L, Anderson FP, Rowe DS: Comparison of ipecac-induced emesis with gastric lavage in the treatment of acute salicylate ingestion. *J Pediatr* 74:800–803, 1969.
29. Abdallah AH, Tye A: A comparison of the efficacy of emetic drugs and stomach lavage. *Am J Dis Child* 113:571–575, 1967.
30. Auerbach PS, Osterloh J, Braun O, et al: Efficacy of gastric emptying: gastric lavage versus emesis induced with ipecac. *Ann Emerg Med* 15:692–698, 1986.
31. Tandberg D, Diven BG, McLeod JW: Ipecac-induced emesis versus gastric lavage: a controlled study in normal adults. *Am J Emerg Med* 4:205–209, 1986.
32. Kulig K, Bar-Or D, Cantrill SV, et al: Management of acutely poisoned patients without gastric emptying. *Ann Emerg Med* 14:562–567, 1985.
33. Neuvonen PJ, Vartiainen M, Olkkola KT: Comparison of activated charcoal and ipecac syrup in prevention of drug absorption. *Eur J Clin Pharmacol* 24:557–562, 1983.
34. Krenzelok EP: Is it time to abandon ipecac in the treatment of overdoses and poisonings? *ACCP Report* 10:3, 1990.
35. Manno BR, Manno JE: Toxicology of ipecac: a review. *Clin Toxicol* 10:221–242, 1977.
36. Krenzelok EP, Dean BS: Effectiveness of 15 ml versus 30 ml doses of syrup of ipecac in children. *Clin Pharm* 6:715–717, 1987.
37. Ellenhorn MJ, Barceloux DG: *Medical Toxicology—Diagnosis and Treatment of Human Poisoning*. New York, Elsevier, pp 54–63, 1988.
38. Anon: Ipecac. *Drug Information for the Health Care Professional*. USP DI, Rockville, MD, United States Pharmacopeial Convention, Inc, pp 1640–1641, 1992.
39. Grbcich PA, Lacouture PG, Lewander WJ, et al: Effect of milk on ipecac-induced emesis. *J Pediatr* 110:973–975, 1987.
40. Klein-Schwartz W, Litovitz T, Oderda GM, et al: The effect of milk on ipecac-induced emesis. *J Toxicol Clin Toxicol* 29:505–511, 1991.

41. Hall AH, Krenzelok EP: Gastrointestinal decontamination: sifting through supportive therapeutic options. In Krenzelok EP (ed): *Updates in Toxicology II.* Atlanta, GA, American Health Consultants, pp 1–8, 1992.

42. Robertson WO: Syrup of ipecac associated fatality: a case report. *Vet Hum Toxicol* 21:87–89, 1979.

43. Knight KM, Doucet HJ: Gastric rupture and death caused by ipecac syrup. *South Med J* 80:786–787, 1987.

44. Timberlake GA: Ipecac as a cause of the Mallory-Weiss syndrome. *South Med J* 77:804–805, 1984.

45. Wolowodink DJ, McMicken DB, O'Brien P: Pneumomediastinum and retropneumomediastinum: an unusual complication of syrup of ipecac induced emesis. *Ann Emerg Med* 13:1148–1151, 1984.

46. Klein-Schwartz W, Gorman RL, Oderda GM, et al: Ipecac use in the elderly: the unanswered question. *Ann Emerg Med* 13:1152–1154, 1984.

47. Friedman EJ: Death from ipecac intoxication in a patient with anorexia nervosa. *Am J Psychiatry* 141:702–703, 1984.

48. Mateer JE, Farrell BJ, Chou SS, et al: Reversible ipecac myopathy. *Arch Neurol* 42:188–190, 1985.

49. Sugie H, Russin R, Verity MA: Emetine myopathy: two case reports with pathobiochemical analysis. *Muscle Nerve* 7:54–59, 1984.

50. Burton BT, Bayer MJ, Barron L, et al: Comparison of activated charcoal and gastric lavage in the prevention of aspirin absorption. *J Emerg Med* 1:411–416, 1984.

51. Tenenbein M, Cohen S, Sitar DS: Efficacy of ipecac-induced emesis, orogastric lavage, and activated charcoal for acute drug overdose. *Ann Emerg Med* 16:838–841, 1987.

52. Albertson TE, Derlet RW, Foulke GE, et al: Superiority of activated charcoal alone compared with ipecac and activated charcoal in the treatment of acute toxic ingestions. *Ann Emerg Med* 18:56–59, 1989.

53. Kornberg AE, Dolgin J: Pediatric ingestions: charcoal alone versus ipecac and charcoal. *Ann Emerg Med* 20:648–651, 1991.

54. Olson KR: Is gut emptying all washed up? *Am J Emerg Med* 8:560–561, 1990.

55. Harchelroad F, Cottington E, Krenzelok EP: Gastrointestinal transit times of a charcoal/sorbitol slurry in overdose patients. *J Toxicol Clin Toxicol* 27:91–99, 1989.

56. Neuvonen PJ, Olkkola KT: Oral activated charcoal in the treatment of intoxications: role of single and repeated doses. *Med Toxicol Adverse Drug Exp* 3:33–58, 1988.

57. Krenzelok EP, Lush RM: Container residue after the administration of aqueous activated charcoal products. *Am J Emerg Med* 9:445–448, 1991.

58. Anon: Activated charcoal. In: *Drug Information for the Health Care Professional.* USP DI, Rockville, MD, United States Pharmacopeial Convention, Inc, pp 875–876, 1992.

59. Ilkhanipour K, Yealy DM, Krenzelok EP: The comparative efficacy of various multiple dose activated charcoal regimens. *Am J Emerg Med* 10:298–300, 1992.

60. Krenzelok EP, Keller R, Stewart RD: Gastrointestinal transit times of cathartics combined with charcoal. *Ann Emerg Med* 14:1152–1155, 1985.

61. Farley TA: Severe hypernatremic dehydration after use of an activated charcoal-sorbitol suspension. *J Pediatr* 109:719–722, 1986.

62. Elliott CG, Colby TV, Kelly TM, et al: Charcoal lung: bronchiolitis obliterans after aspiration of activated charcoal. *Chest* 96:672–674, 1989.

63. Menzies DG, Busuttil A, Prescott LF: Fatal pulmonary aspiration of oral activated charcoal. *Br Med J* 297:459–460, 1988.

64. Keller RE, Schwab RA, Krenzelok EP: Contribution of sorbitol combined with activated charcoal in prevention of salicylate absorption. *Ann Emerg Med* 19:654–656, 1990.

65. Minocha A, Krenzelok EP, Spyker DA: Dosage recommendations for activated charcoal-sorbitol treatment. *Clin Toxicol* 23:579–583, 1986.

66. Garrelts JC, Watson WA, Holloway KD, et al: Magnesium toxicity secondary to catharsis during management of theophylline toxicity. *Am J Emerg Med* 7:34–37, 1989.

SECTION TWO

Resuscitation Pharmacology

CHAPTER 13

Resuscitation Pharmacology

ARNO L. ZARITSKY, M.D.

The goals of cardiopulmonary resuscitation (CPR) are (*a*) to restore stable circulatory and ventilatory function, and (*b*) to maintain vital critical organ function until such stabilization can be achieved. Early definitive care (usually defibrillation in adults and ventilatory support in infants) is the first priority. Thereafter, the maintenance of circulatory and ventilatory function (with chest compression and assisted ventilation using supplemental oxygen) and pharmacologic interventions aimed at reestablishing more normal cardiopulmonary functioning may improve the success of subsequent efforts. Treatment with pharmacologic agents has the potential to:

1. Suppress or reverse ventricular tachycardia and/or fibrillation;
2. Maintain coronary and cerebral perfusion until the restoration of more normal cardiopulmonary function;
3. Evoke a rhythm more likely to be associated with an adequate perfusion pressure in patients with asystole or electromechanical dissociation;
4. Correct hypoxemia and acidosis;
5. Improve hemodynamics and organ perfusion.

These goals are similar in all arrest situations, although there may be some unique circumstances (e.g., trauma) in which additional therapies also may be required. This chapter provides a review of the pharmacology, indications, dosages, and potential complications of each agent used during resuscitation. Indications and dosage recommendations have undergone revision following the 1992 National Conference on Cardiopulmonary Resuscitation. This chapter contains recommendations from that conference (1).

GENERAL GUIDELINES FOR ADMINISTERING MEDICATIONS

During cardiac arrest, intravenous drug administration is preferred. Central venous drug administration produces higher and more rapid peak drug concentrations than do peripheral injections during resuscitation (2). Since drugs administered into the venous circulation must be distributed to organs via arterial blood flow, achieving higher central venous drug concentrations is an important determinant of drug effectiveness. Drugs such as epinephrine exert their beneficial effects on the arterial rather than the venous circulation (3).

The placement of a central "line" is time consuming, requires the discontinuation of compressions and ventilations, usually for a potentially deleterious duration, and is associated with substantial morbidity to adjacent structures. In the past, an advocacy for the placement of central lines via the femoral vein obviated some of these considerations. However, unless a long catheter can be advanced into the chest, this route should not be used since compression-induced blood return to the heart from below the diaphragm is much lower than blood flow above the diaphragm (4). Thus, in adults the brachial vein is the site of choice for the placement of an intravenous line (1). Peripheral venous drug administration followed by a fluid bolus effectively increases drug delivery into the

233

central circulation (5), although the onset of drug effect is not as rapid as after central venous administration (6). Therefore, to enhance delivery to the central circulation, each peripheral venous injection should be followed by a bolus of 10 to 20 ml of normal saline.

In pediatric patients, rapid intravenous access can be difficult in general (7), and cannulation of the superior vena caval system is particularly difficult. It has not been established that the difference in blood flow between the upper and lower parts of the body during chest compression in adults also occurs in infants. Furthermore, it is likely that higher cardiac and cerebral blood flow and perfusion pressure are produced in children by direct cardiac compression (8, 9). Therefore, in children any venous access site, including the intraosseous route, is acceptable. The administration of intravenous drugs should be followed, as in the adult, with an injection of saline (5 to 10 ml). Intraosseous injection (usually via the proximal tibia) also can be used to provide an access site for the administration of fluids and drugs, (10) including potent catecholamines (11). Although intraosseous infusions are considered safe, fat and bone marrow pulmonary emboli (12), tibial fractures (13), and bilateral lower extremity compartment syndromes (14) have been reported.

If intravenous access is not readily available, endotracheal administration of certain lipid-soluble drugs (i.e., epinephrine, atropine, lidocaine, and naloxone) can be utilized (15, 16). Optimal endotracheal doses have not been defined. In some animal studies as much as 10 times the intravenous dose of epinephrine is required to produce the same hemodynamic effects (17, 18). A similar finding was noted in a clinical study comparing the administration of epinephrine by the i.v. vs. the endotracheal route in adults with out-of-hospital asystolic arrest. There was no change in measured epinephrine levels following 1 mg by the endotracheal route; a 3- to 4-fold increase was seen after the same dose was given intravenously (19). Based on these observations, a larger dose should be used by the endotracheal route compared with the i.v. route. In children, an initial dose of 0.1 mg/kg of 1:1000 epinephrine (10 times the current dose) is recommended in the treatment of asystolic arrest (1).

Using a larger endotracheal epinephrine dose may improve its effectiveness, but the lungs may subsequently act as a depot, sometimes producing profound hypertension for up to 30 minutes after administration (18, 20). In addition, the reliability of endotracheal epinephrine has been questioned in a number of studies (21, 22). Even using a dose of 0.1 mg/kg may not produce changes in perfusion pressure despite increasing the plasma epinephrine concentration (22).

Other agents may be given endotracheally, such as lidocaine, bretylium, isoproterenol, and propranolol (23–25), but these usually are not required as emergently as epinephrine and may be given after intravenous access has been obtained. Moreover, there are few data on the pharmacokinetics of endotracheal administration of these agents. Data suggest that endotracheal atropine in the same dose as used intravenously is effective (16). Based on measurements of blood lidocaine concentrations following endotracheal administration in adult prehospital arrest patients, a lidocaine dose of 3 mg/kg is recommended (26).

In addition, lidocaine is better absorbed when diluted in sterile water rather than normal saline (15); this absorption results from the tonicity of lidocaine whereby dilution in water produces a more nearly isotonic solution.

Drug absorption occurs in the distal airways, but the best method of drug delivery is not certain. When the endotracheal route is used, medications should be instilled deeply into the trachea either using a catheter positioned beyond the end of the endotracheal tube or by discontinuing compressions and ventilations during the instillation and hyperventilating the patient thereafter (24). Improved drug absorption may be achieved by dilution; saline is the preferred diluent since it causes the least adverse effect on blood gases. A comparison of lidocaine administration by various techniques showed that dilution of the drug in saline was most effective, with flushing of the endotracheal tube with saline being the next most efficacious (27).

Although drug dilution can improve drug absorption, the optimal quantity of diluent is uncertain. In a canine arrest model comparing 6, 12, and 25 ml of diluent, lidocaine concentrations were highest when diluted with 6 ml of saline (25), whereas in a clinical study the highest plasma lidocaine concentrations in adults were obtained with 10 ml of saline flush compared with 5 and 3 ml (28). In the latter study, however, the larger volume of flush results in prolonged hypoxemia. In the absence of clinical data, it seems reasonable to use 5 to 10 ml of saline to flush the drug into the distal airways.

Once a stable rhythm is restored and vascular access is obtained, vasopressors are often used to support the circulation. Catecholamines are compatible with many intravenous solutions (normal saline, 0.45N saline, Ringer's lactate, and 10% dextrose and water), but 5% dextrose and water usually is preferred in adults. In children, D5 0.9N saline, 0.9N saline, or Ringer's lactate are usually used. Postarrest, catecholamine infusions should be initiated at a sufficiently rapid rate to clear the intravenous tubing of other solutions; otherwise, a substantial delay may occur before a drug effect is observed, particularly in pediatric patients in whom lower infusion rates are typical. Toxicity is avoided by using the lowest possible dose that achieves the desired effect and rapidly decreasing the infusion rate when a toxic effect is seen. Catecholamines should not be mixed in the same intravenous solution bag with alkaline solutions (e.g., bicarbonate, phenytoin, or aminophylline) because catecholamines are autooxidized by basic solutions (29).

ESSENTIAL RESUSCITATION MEDICATIONS

OXYGEN

Pharmacology

Many factors contribute to severely impaired oxygenation during cardiac arrest. Exhaled gas delivered during mouth-to-mouth rescue breathing provides only 16 to 17% oxygen, which at best produces an alveolar oxygen tension of 80 mm Hg (normal arterial oxygen tension in room air is approximately 104 mm Hg, depending in part on altitude). Cardiopulmonary resuscitation is accompanied by right-to-left intrapulmonary shunting, by impairment of oxygen delivery by mismatches between ventilation and perfusion (30), and often by the inhibition of oxygen transport across the alveolus by aspiration and/or pulmonary edema. Because properly performed chest compression delivers only 25 to 35% of a normal cardiac output (31), oxygen delivery to the tissues is additionally impaired. To compensate, tissue extraction increases, and mixed venous oxygen tension is low. The admixture of this highly desaturated venous blood with poorly oxygenated "arterial" blood further decreases arterial oxygen tension. The net result is that oxygen delivery is compromised markedly during cardiac arrest and resuscitation.

Hypoxemia at the tissue level leads to anaerobic metabolism, lactic acid production, and local acidosis, augmenting intracellular acidosis and cellular dysfunction and eventually leading to cell death. Although the effectiveness of oxygen administration is not certain, aggressive attempts to maximize tissue oxygenation are worthwhile, as long as the clinician recognizes that even a supranormal arterial oxygen concentration does not ensure adequate tissue oxygen delivery since the latter results from the product of cardiac output and arterial oxygen content. Certainly, if the baseline oxygen tension is on the steep portion of the oxyhemoglobin saturation curve, even small increments in oxygen tension may markedly improve the delivery of oxygen to the tissues.

Indications and Dose

Oxygen should be provided in the highest concentration possible (usually 100%) during cardiopulmonary resuscitation; there should be no concern about the development of oxygen toxicity with short exposure. Oxygen should not be withheld in any patient with hypoxemia, even if chronic lung disease and carbon dioxide retention are present. By increasing arterial oxygen tension, oxygen content in blood and therefore tissue oxygen delivery may be enhanced.

Although the administration of oxygen improves arterial oxygen tension and content, it does not guarantee adequate oxygen delivery to the tissues. Animal (32) and clinical (33) studies show that during cardiopulmonary resuscitation there is a progressive decrease in mixed venous oxygen tension, probably the best indicator of the adequacy of tissue oxygen delivery, even when arterial oxygen tension is well-maintained. Accordingly, additional therapy is needed to improve tissue oxygen delivery.

EPINEPHRINE

Pharmacology

The pharmacologic actions of epinephrine are complex and dose-related (see Chapter 24). The large doses used during cardiopulmonary resuscitation produce both α-adrenergic and β-adrenergic effects. During cardiopulmonary resuscitation, epinephrine's α-adrenergic effects on vascular tone are of primary importance because aortic diastolic pressure is the critical determinant of the success or failure of resuscitative efforts in both animals (34, 35) and humans (36). During chest compression, aortic and right atrial pressure are equal and there is little or no coronary blood flow. During diastole, there is a small gradient favoring flow. By increasing arterial vasoconstriction and preventing arterial

collapse of intrathoracic arteries via its effects on α-adrenergic tone, epinephrine elevates aortic diastolic pressure and therefore coronary perfusion pressure, increasing coronary blood flow (3, 8). The potent peripheral vasoconstrictive action redirects blood flow from the much larger splanchnic and skeletal muscle vascular beds to the heart and brain (8, 37). Thus, overall cardiac output often falls despite an increase in coronary perfusion pressure and flow following epinephrine administration (37, 38).

In animals, epinephrine also augments cerebral perfusion. Cerebral blood flow can be maintained at approximately 70% of normal levels with a continuous infusion of epinephrine combined with simultaneous ventilation and compression cardiopulmonary resuscitation in some experimental models (37). Similar results with epinephrine infusion were observed in an infant piglet model (8).

The impact of the β-adrenergic effects of epinephrine is more controversial. Epinephrine's inotropic and chronotropic effects increase myocardial oxygen demand, and many have argued that the increased demand may obviate the benefits of increased coronary flow (39). A recent study using open chest CPR showed a worse outcome following fibrillation arrest treated with higher epinephrine doses as a result of an adverse effect on the myocardium, presumably from β-adrenergic stimulation (40). Furthermore, data suggest that it is the α-adrenergic rather than the β-adrenergic effects of epinephrine that enhance the susceptibility of ventricular fibrillation to electrical defibrillation (41).

These contentions, along with the possible adverse effects of hypertension and/or arrhythmias that may be induced synergistically by the β- plus α-adrenergic effects of epinephrine following restoration of spontaneous circulation, have led some investigators to advocate the replacement of epinephrine with a more selective α-adrenergic agent such as phenylephrine or methoxamine. Despite methoxamine's theoretic advantage of increasing coronary perfusion pressure without stimulating increased myocardial oxygen demand through β-adrenergic stimulation, two double-blind comparisons of epinephrine vs. methoxamine in the treatment of a total of 80 adults with electromechanical dissociation failed to show any benefit from methoxamine (42, 43), although relatively small doses of methoxamine were used (5 mg and 10 mg, respectively). In a swine fibrillation model, epinephrine produced significantly better myocardial blood flow, myocardial oxygen utilization, and defibrillation success rates than did methoxamine in a wide range of doses (0.1, 1.0, and 10 mg/kg), and epinephrine was significantly better at maintaining cerebral blood flow (44). Conversely, a possible role for a pure α-adrenergic agonist like methoxamine has been suggested in prolonged arrest, based upon a swine ventricular fibrillation study (45).

Phenylephrine is another α-adrenergic agent having no advantage over epinephrine in animal studies (46). Norepinephrine is also considered to have more selective α-adrenergic effects, although it also stimulates β1-adrenergic receptors. Norepinephrine may be superior to epinephrine in ventricular fibrillation, but not in asphyxial arrest (47). Large doses of norepinephrine increase coronary perfusion pressure and regional cerebral blood flow as effectively as do high doses of epinephrine (48). Furthermore, a preliminary study comparing epinephrine with norepinephrine in adults with ventricular fibrillation suggests that norepinephrine more effectively restores a stable circulation (49). Additional clinical data are needed before any change in drug recommendations is indicated.

Indications and Dose

Despite experimental data suggesting that a more selective α-adrenergic agent may be superior in certain arrest settings, epinephrine remains the most effective drug in the clinical treatment of cardiac arrest, regardless of mechanism, in infants, children, and adults (1). The optimal dose, however, is controversial. In animals, doses in the range of those recommended during resuscitation in humans (7.5 to 15 μg/kg) do not increase diastolic blood pressure. Doses of 45, 75, and 150 μg/kg must be used to induce a diastolic pressure of 30 mm Hg or more for up to 5 minutes (50). Additional animal studies in various arrest models also showed that epinephrine doses ranging from 10 to 20 times higher than those currently used more effectively increase brain and heart blood flow (51). These studies utilized models simulating out-of-hospital arrest where coronary perfusion pressure is low secondary to prolonged ischemia. In this setting, higher doses of epinephrine are more effective, but this regimen may not apply to settings with short arrest times.

Clinical reports also suggested that higher doses of epinephrine are more effective. Higher coronary perfusion pressures were measured in adults following prolonged arrest using higher epinephrine doses (52), and improved rates of survival have been reported in children failing to respond to two standard doses of epinephrine (53). Counterbalancing these animal and clinical reports, two multicenter, randomized blinded studies in adults failed to show a beneficial effect of high-dose (10 to 15 mg) epinephrine (54, 55). Furthermore, some animal data suggest a worse outcome in ventricular fibrillation with high-dose epinephrine (40, 56), which may result from excessive β-adrenergic stimulation since treatment with a β-blocker postarrest decreases the risk of early death (57). It should be noted that these studies used a brief arrest time (40) or CPR with high perfusion pressures (56). In these settings, higher myocardial epinephrine delivery and less acidosis to impair adrenergic receptor responsiveness may have increased myocardial epinephrine-induced contractility and oxygen demand. This result would explain the failure of high-dose epinephrine in adult cardiac arrest, which is often secondary to ventricular fibrillation complicating poor myocardial perfusion secondary to coronary artery disease.

Until better data are available, epinephrine in a dose of 1 mg in an adult and 10 μg/kg in a child is recommended in the initial treatment of cardiac arrest. Subsequent doses of epinephrine in adult arrest may be increased to 10 to 15 mg, as long as the potential adverse effects of these larger doses are recognized. In children, in whom the coronary circulation is usually normal, cardiac arrest typically is characterized by asystole or wide-complex bradycardia. Therefore, if the child fails to respond to the initial dose of epinephrine, subsequent doses of 0.1 to 0.2 mg/kg should be used every 3 to 5 minutes of continued cardiac arrest. The shorter interval between epinephrine doses is based

on human data showing that the peak effect following intravenous epinephrine is achieved in 3 to 4 minutes (58). Epinephrine, like other catecholamines, should not be mixed with bicarbonate, since alkaline solutions autooxidize the drug (29).

ATROPINE

Pharmacology

Atropine has predominant parasympatholytic effects at clinically relevant doses. It accelerates sinus or atrial pacemakers and enhances atrioventricular conduction (59) by competitively antagonizing muscarinic receptors and therefore inhibiting vagal tone. Its use in cardiac arrest is based on its cardiac vagolytic actions. Extensive cholinergic innervation of the ventricular conducting system (60) suggests that parasympathetic stimulation may be important in cardiac arrest. Since high ventricular vagal tone may suppress automaticity, atropine has been recommended in ventricular asystole and slow idioventricular rhythms.

At low doses, atropine has central and peripheral parasympathomimetic actions that may induce paradoxic vagotonic effects (61, 62). Atropine is excreted renally and hepatically, each accounting for about 50% of drug elimination. The half-life in normal individuals is about 2.5 hours (63). Prolonged elimination should be expected during arrest and the postresuscitation period. Although the amount needed for complete parasympathetic blockade may range from 2 to 6 mg (64), doses of more than 2 mg of atropine, which is a totally vagolytic dose for most individuals (65), are usually adequate during cardiopulmonary arrest.

Indications and Dose

Atropine is the drug of choice for the treatment of bradycardia, particularly when it results from sinus bradycardia or heart block at the nodal level accompanied by hemodynamic compromise or ventricular ectopy. When bradycardia complicates a severe hypoxic-ischemic insult to the myocardium, it is unlikely that this insult represents excess vagal tone responsive to atropine. Its benefit in ventricular asystole is based on the supposition that asystole is the end stage of a spectrum of bradycardias, and on the apparent benefit observed in small numbers of patients (66), especially those in a hospital setting in which there is a very rapid initiation of resuscitation. The benefit of atropine in asystole occurring in the outpatient setting is doubtful (67). Atropine should be used cautiously in the presence of myocardial ischemia or infarction since excessive increases in heart rate may increase the extent of infarction (65) and can, on occasion, induce ventricular tachycardia or fibrillation (68, 69). Bradycardia in most pediatric cardiac arrest patients, and in many adult patients with severe pulmonary disease, results most often from hypoxemia and shock; therefore, it is best treated by improving ventilation and circulation.

The recommended doses of atropine are 1.0 mg for asystole and 0.5 mg for symptomatic bradycardia (1), with a minimal dose of 0.5 mg. A total dose of 2.0 mg generally results in full vagal blockage (65). In pediatric patients, the dose is 0.02 mg/kg intravenously or endotracheally, with a minimum dose of

0.1 mg. The dose may be repeated in 5 minutes, up to 1.0 mg in a child and 2.0 mg in an adolescent. As noted earlier, smaller doses of atropine, less than 0.5 mg in adults and less than 0.1 mg in pediatric patients, can induce paradoxic vagotonic effects (61, 62). Although atropine dilates the pupils, data in children show that its administration should not be used as an explanation of fixed, dilated pupils in a postarrest patient (70).

LIDOCAINE

Pharmacology

Lidocaine is a membrane anesthetic of the amide type that is also a class 1 antiarrhythmic agent. Its primary mode of action is via its membrane-stabilizing effects, mediated predominantly by blockade of sodium channels (71). It decreases automaticity by slowing the slope of phase 4 depolarization (72). Lidocaine has differential effects on the duration of the action potential and the effective refractory period in normal and ischemic tissue. In normal tissue lidocaine tends to shorten these intervals slightly, whereas in ischemic tissue it prolongs them. By narrowing the differences in these intervals between normal and ischemic myocardium, lidocaine may inhibit the propagation of reentrant arrhythmias (73).

Lidocaine also increases the amount of energy required to induce ventricular fibrillation (the ventricular fibrillation threshold) (74, 75), but high plasma levels appear to be required (76, 77). However, lidocaine does not reduce the energy required to terminate ventricular fibrillation (the ventricular defibrillation threshold). Indeed, data suggest that it increases the energy needed, though only modestly (78, 79).

Although lidocaine has long been recommended in the treatment of both ventricular tachycardia and ventricular fibrillation, recent data suggest that it may be ineffective at best, and detrimental at worst (80). Metaanalysis of clinical studies have suggested only a mild protective effect on subsequent development of ventricular fibrillation in patients having a myocardial infarction (81). In addition, this analysis suggested an increased risk of asystole associated with the use of lidocaine, although the difference was not significant (95% confidence interval showing a 2% reduction of risk to a 95% increase in risk) (81). In a recent study, Weaver and associates (82) found a 25% occurrence rate of asystole with repeated lidocaine administration for ventricular fibrillation after the first countershock. This represents a 3-fold greater rate compared with epinephrine administration alone. Furthermore, giving lidocaine before the second shock was associated with a significantly reduced survival. The mechanism of this adverse effect of lidocaine is uncertain but may be related to lidocaine-induced attenuation of sympathetic nervous system activity.

In patients with ventricular dysrhythmias but no ischemia, lidocaine appears to have limited effectiveness (80). For example, in 31 episodes of sustained wide-complex tachycardia, lidocaine was effective in terminating the tachycardia in not more than six episodes (83). All but three of the 25 patients in this study had coronary artery disease, but none had acute ischemia. These findings are consistent with experimental data showing a lack of lidocaine's effectiveness in suppression of reentry tachycardias under nonischemic conditions (84).

About 70% of plasma lidocaine is protein bound (85), and it is cleared by the liver at a rate close to that of hepatic blood flow (86). Thus, changes in hepatic blood flow have important effects on lidocaine plasma concentrations. In normal subjects, lidocaine's volume of distribution is about 1 liter/kg, although this volume is substantially reduced in patients with heart failure. Its elimination has both an α-distributive and a β-half-life. In normal subjects, the half-life of lidocaine after a bolus injection (its α-distributive half-life) is 8.3 minutes, and its half-life after achieving a steady state with a constant infusion (the β-half-life) is 86 to 108 minutes. Thus, bolus doses of lidocaine are required to obtain therapeutic blood levels until a steady state concentration (reached after five half-lives) is achieved with a constant infusion. One-half of the steady-state concentration is reached at one half-life. For example, a 4 mg/min infusion will achieve a therapeutic concentration of approximately 2 μg/ml in 86 to 108 minutes, assuming normal pharmacokinetics and a therapeutic range of 2 to 5 μg/ml.

Clinical conditions in which hepatic blood flow or cardiac output is reduced and those in which the volume of distribution is altered (older patients, heart failure) will lead to increased levels of lidocaine for any given dose (86). Accordingly, dose adjustments are required in patients with reduced cardiac output to the liver (e.g., those patients with shock), in those patients with congestive heart failure or hepatic dysfunction in which hepatic metabolism is reduced, and in those patients over the age of 70 in whom the volume of distribution and clearance is decreased. In addition, after a 24-hour infusion, the ability of the liver to clear lidocaine appears to decrease, mandating a reduced infusion rate if toxicity is to be avoided (87). Although renal disease does not affect the clearance of lidocaine or its volume of distribution, metabolites of lidocaine will accumulate after prolonged infusions (88). There is little information concerning lidocaine pharmacokinetics or pharmacodynamics during cardiopulmonary resuscitation. However, probably as a consequence of the marked reduction in cardiac output, levels after conventional bolus doses are above or within the therapeutic range for at least 20 minutes (77, 89). Lidocaine levels should be monitored in patients on a lidocaine infusion to avoid toxicity.

Toxic effects of lidocaine usually occur when levels are above the therapeutic range or when the drug is infused very rapidly (89, 90). These effects include central nervous system manifestations such as drowsiness, confusion, numbness and tingling, muscle twitching, and (predominantly) agitation. Seizures requiring treatment can occur. At high concentrations, lidocaine can decrease myocardial contractility (91), induce hypotension by peripheral vasodilation, decrease sinus node function, and worsen high-grade atrioventricular block (92).

Indications and Dose

The prophylactic use of lidocaine to prevent ventricular fibrillation in patients highly suspected of having acute myocardial infarction has been widely recommended (1, 93) because of data suggesting that it reduces the incidence of ventricular fibrillation (74, 75). However, the risk-benefit ratio on which this recommendation is based has been questioned (80), in part because few data have suggested that primary ventricular fibrillation itself is associated with an adverse prognosis (81, 94). If therapy is not initiated prophylactically, traditional indications for the use of lidocaine in suspected acute myocardial infarction include ventricular premature complexes that are more frequent than 6/min, are multiform, encroach on the T wave of the QRS complex, or occur in bursts of two or more in succession (1). In this circumstance, a loading dose of lidocaine can be administered as multiple, slow boluses of 50 mg every 5 minutes to a total dose of 200 to 300 mg, or at a rate of 20 mg/min to a total dose of 3 to 5 mg/kg followed by a continuous infusion of 2 to 4 mg/min for 24 hours (93). If the infusion is continued for more than 24 hours, the rate should be reduced by one-half (95). The initial doses and the infusion rate should be decreased (many clinicians empirically reduce them by 50%) in the presence of congestive heart failure, hepatic dysfunction, patient age above 70 years, or hypotension (88).

A similar regimen can also be used in more emergent situations (e.g., when rapid ventricular tachycardia is present) to achieve and maintain therapeutic levels as quickly as possible. In general, lidocaine is the drug of choice for most malignant ventricular arrhythmias associated with myocardial ischemia or those arrhythmias induced by digitalis toxicity. Patients with wide-complex tachycardia may respond better to other agents such as procainamide (83). Patients with ventricular tachycardia who fail to respond to lidocaine and those with compromised perfusion require cardioversion.

When an antiarrhythmic agent is required during cardiopulmonary resuscitation (i.e., ventricular tachycardia or ventricular fibrillation that fails to reverse following defibrillation or cardioversion, respectively), a bolus of 1 mg/kg of lidocaine will provide levels in or above the therapeutic range for at least 20 minutes (77), during which time defibrillation should be reattempted. Since levels remain high for a prolonged period, only one dose is generally required, although some may prefer to use repetitive doses of 0.5 mg/kg every 8 to 10 minutes before changing to bretylium (1).

Similar doses of lidocaine (1 mg/kg) followed by repeat defibrillation attempts are appropriate for pediatric patients with ventricular tachycardia and ventricular fibrillation, although these rhythm disturbances occur in less than 10% of pediatric cardiac arrests (96). If ventricular tachycardia/fibrillation is not reversed, a second 1 mg/kg bolus of lidocaine is recommended, followed by an infusion of 20 to 50 μg/kg/min and repeated attempts at defibrillation or cardioversion. The infusion rate of lidocaine for children who have received loading doses of lidocaine and require maintenance infusions should be reduced by at least 50% if shock, congestive heart failure, or hepatic dysfunction is present (1).

BRETYLIUM TOSYLATE

Pharmacology

Bretylium is a quaternary ammonium compound with both adrenergic and direct myocardial effects (97, 98). It is classified as a type III antiarrhythmic agent. Although class III antiarrhythmics have diverse pharmacologic actions, they all share the ability to prolong the duration of the action potential and the refractory period in Purkinje and ventricular muscle fibers by increasing repolarization time (71). They have little effect on the rate of rise of phase zero or on the resting membrane potential, but they substantially increase the ventricular fibrillation threshold (99). Bretylium is thought to terminate reentrant arrhythmias by markedly prolonging refractoriness without affecting propagation of the cardiac impulse (100).

Additional acute effects of bretylium in vivo are complex and probably partly a result of adrenergic stimulation, which will cause repolarization and increased rate of conduction in abnormal depolarized regions (71). Bretylium's adrenergic effects are biphasic. It initially causes the release of norepinephrine from adrenergic nerve terminals, inducing transient (approximately 20 minutes) hypertension, tachycardia, and, in some patients, increases in cardiac output (71). Once norepinephrine is depleted, release is inhibited, and by 45 to 60 minutes hypotension (especially orthostatic) may be present (98, 101). Since bretylium blocks the uptake of norepinephrine, it may potentiate the effects of exogenously administered catecholamines (97). For some time it was thought that the adrenergic effects of bretylium had little to do with its effects on ventricular fibrillation, since neither reserpine nor sympathectomy changed the ventricular fibrillation threshold (102). However, more recent data support the hypothesis that bretylium's pharmacologic action may be critically dependent on its adrenergic effects (103). Initial catecholamine-stimulated increase in the upstroke velocity of phase zero of the action potential in infarcted regions (104), in concert with direct myocardial effects of lengthening of the effective refractory period, is essential to the antiarrhythmic mechanism of the agent (105). Bretylium reduces disparities in refractory periods and conduction velocities between ischemic and normal tissues, and delays the conduction of premature impulses into normal tissue contiguous with ischemic zones ("border zones") (106).

Despite more than 25 years of study, the relative importance of bretylium's direct electrophysiologic effects vs. the release of catecholamines or adrenergic neuronal blockade remains uncertain (97, 103, 107). Bretylium's antifibrillatory onset of action following i.v. administration is delayed for 10 to 15 minutes (77). This delayed onset of action is related to the slow uptake of the drug into the myocardium; myocardial concentrations correlate with its antifibrillatory effect (108). Peak effect may not be achieved for 3 to 6 hours following a dose (108), but bretylium's duration of action is much longer than that observed with lidocaine (77, 109).

In experimental animals and in anecdotal reports in patients, bretylium is capable of terminating ventricular fibrillation (110, 111). Bretylium also has been reported to increase markedly the fibrillation threshold, even when ischemia or reperfusion is present (103, 108, 112). Bretylium either does not change or lowers *de*fibrillation threshold (the energy required to terminate ventricular fibrillation) (79, 113). Despite a pharmacologic profile suggesting that bretylium should be more effective than lidocaine in the treatment of ventricular fibrillation, controlled clinical trials have shown only a small benefit (114, 115) or no difference in efficacy of these drugs in treating ventricular fibrillation (95, 116). Possibly, the late administration of antiarrhythmic agents during cardiac arrest therapy is responsible for the lack of difference. Since lidocaine has a rapid onset of action and the effect of bretylium is delayed, more prolonged, combined therapy may be most efficacious (109).

Bretylium is utilized only intravenously. Its effects generally are delayed for 10 to 15 minutes when used in conventional doses for ventricular tachyarrhythmias (108). In this setting, doses often are diluted and administered slowly or via an infusion to reduce adverse adrenergic and gastrointestinal effects. A delay in onset also likely results from the need to concentrate the drug in the myocardium (106, 108, 111). Higher doses administered as a bolus without dilution are warranted during cardiac arrest and have more immediate effects. Bretylium is excreted unchanged in the urine and has a half-life of about 9 hours that increases to 15 to 30 hours with renal insufficiency (98). Accordingly, dosage adjustments are required for patients with renal failure. When renal function is normal, 72% is excreted within the first 24 hours and 100% by 72 hours (98, 117). Elimination from myocardium and plasma is similar, with an elimination half-life in humans of 4 to 17 hours (98, 108).

The principal side effect of bretylium is delayed hypotension, especially orthostatic hypotension, and nausea and vomiting. Hypotension occurs in 50 to 75% of patients, depending on the dose and rapidity of administration (97). Because bretylium impairs the reuptake of catecholamines, it can potentiate the effects of exogenously administered pressors and/or inotropes (97). Other side effects include negative synergism with other antiarrhythmic agents, but the clinical importance of these interactions in critically ill patients is unclear (110). There is also the possibility that digitalis toxicity could be exacerbated by adrenergic stimulation (97). The treatment for severe hypotension caused by bretylium relies on tricyclic antidepressants, which block the access of bretylium to sympathetic neurons but do not affect its antiarrhythmic effects (71).

Indications and Dose

Bretylium is indicated for the treatment of ventricular arrhythmias that are resistant to other treatments, or when other treatments are for some reason contraindicated. For ventricular tachycardia with a pulse, bretylium is usually used after lidocaine and, in most instances, procainamide, in a dose of 5 to 10 mg/kg diluted 1:4. Good results have been obtained even in patients with digitalis toxicity, despite concerns about catecholamine stimulation (98). Bretylium is administered slowly, over 8 to 10 minutes, and the dose can be repeated once or twice, followed by intermittent bolus doses every 6 to 8 hours or a continuous infusion of 1 to 2 mg/min (97). For ventricular tachycardia without a pulse or ventricular fibrillation, bretylium is recommended if lidocaine was ineffective or was contraindicated. The required dose of bretylium is 5 mg/kg given as a bolus, followed by 10 mg/kg if ventricular fibrillation does not respond to defibrillation. Repeated doses of 10 mg/kg can be given every 15 to 30 minutes, to a maximum dose of 30 mg/kg (97). The indications and doses for pediatric arrests are identical to those for adults. It is noted, however,

that the pharmacologic basis for this recommendation in children is lacking; there are only anecdotal reports of successful use of bretylium in children (118, 119).

INTRAVENOUS PROCAINAMIDE

Pharmacology

Procainamide is a type IA antiarrhythmic agent. It reduces the rate of phase 4 depolarization in isolated ventricular muscle and Purkinje fibers (71), slows ventricular conduction by reducing the slope of phase 0 of the action potential (120), and increases the refractory period of ventricular tissue (121). If conduction is already slowed, as seen in ischemic myocardium, further slowing may produce a bidirectional block, preventing or terminating reentrant arrhythmias (122, 123).

The clearance of procainamide depends on both hepatic and renal function. Approximately 60% of any given dose is excreted unchanged in the urine (72) if normal renal function is present, and the remainder undergoes N-acetylation in the liver (124). Thus, elimination is reduced during renal failure or in congestive heart failure if renal and/or hepatic perfusion is impaired, requiring a reduction in dose (125). In addition, patients may be fast or slow hepatic acetylators of the agent, which can have clinically important effects on plasma levels (124). In fast acetylators or in those patients with renal insufficiency, 40% or more of the administered procainamide may be excreted as N-acetylprocainamide (NAPA); concentrations of NAPA in plasma may equal or exceed those of the parent drug (71). The NAPA derivative has antiarrhythmic properties that are somewhat different from those of the parent compound (126), and it is also excreted renally (71).

Although the metabolism of procainamide is complex, the measurement of both the parent compound and the N-acetyl derivative is routinely available, facilitating more chronic treatment. Difficulties in rapidly obtaining therapeutic blood levels make the agent difficult to use in the emergency setting. Procainamide is a ganglionic blocker with significant vasodilating effects and, at high doses, some negative inotropic effects (127). These effects limit the rapidity with which procainamide can be administered (127). Accordingly, the agent must be administered cautiously to patients with hypotension and heart failure or to those whose clearance of procainamide may be impaired (those with hepatic and/or renal dysfunction). Since procainamide slows conduction and increases the refractory period, it can induce heart block, widening of the QRS complex, and Q-T$_c$ prolongation and associated arrhythmias (128).

Indications and Dose

Procainamide is indicated for the treatment of malignant ventricular arrhythmias, particularly refractory ventricular tachycardia that does not respond to lidocaine, or when treatment with lidocaine is contraindicated (129). It also may be used intravenously to treat supraventricular arrhythmias (129), but it is rarely used to treat ventricular fibrillation because it takes too long to achieve therapeutic levels.

The intravenous loading dose is 50 mg every 5 minutes unless hypotension occurs, the QRS complex has widened by more than 50%, 1 g has been administered, or the arrhythmia has been suppressed. In urgent circumstances, an infusion of

20 mg/min has been given, titrated to the same endpoints (129). The maintenance infusion is 1 to 4 mg/min to achieve therapeutic blood levels of 4 to 10 μg/ml (125). An alternative regimen utilizes a loading dose of 17 mg/kg given over 1 hour, followed by a maintenance infusion of 2.8 mg/kg/hr. In patients who might clear the agent slowly, the loading dose is reduced to 12 mg/kg and the infusion rate to 1.4 mg/kg/hr (125). With this regimen, some patients have therapeutic levels by 15 minutes (122). There are no unique considerations concerning the use of procainamide in children other than to appreciate the fact that ventricular arrhythmia is a rare cause of cardiac arrest, which more commonly develops secondary to acute respiratory failure (96).

OTHER MEDICATIONS OF POTENTIAL USE

SODIUM BICARBONATE

Pharmacology

During cardiopulmonary arrest, metabolic and respiratory acidosis are inevitable. Acidosis results in vasodilation locally, which may compromise further vital organ perfusion by leading to peripheral blood pooling and by lowering central aortic pressures and thus diastolic coronary perfusion pressure (see the section entitled "Epinephrine" above). Acidosis may antagonize the action of catecholamines (130, 131); however, the applicability of this concept to the cardiac arrest setting and the doses of epinephrine utilized is unclear (132, 133). As reviewed elsewhere (133), even severe acidosis (pH <7.0) in an intact animal may not produce negative inotropic effects secondary to endogenous sympathetic nervous system activity. Acidosis increases pulmonary vascular resistance, vasodilates systemic vascular beds, and decreases glycolytic pathway activity, thus impairing ATP synthesis (132, 134).

Respiratory acidosis results from inadequate ventilation and is partly antagonized by providing assisted ventilation. As discussed in greater detail below, respiratory tissue acidosis may persist despite having normalized arterial PCO_2. Metabolic acidosis results from inadequate tissue perfusion and oxygenation, which lead to anaerobic metabolism and the production of lactic acid (135). Acute respiratory and acute metabolic acidosis have very different effects on intracellular pH. Acute increases in PCO_2 acutely decrease intracellular pH because carbon dioxide diffuses rapidly into cells, whereas acute increases in the extracellular hydrogen ion concentration decrease intracellular pH less rapidly because both H^+ and HCO_3^- diffuse across cell membranes relatively slowly.

The adverse effects of acidosis appear to be related to changes in the intracellular and extracellular pH and carbon dioxide concentration. Ischemia during cardiopulmonary resuscitation induces increased myocardial intracellular PCO_2 to 300 mm Hg (40 kPa) or greater, and a decrease in intracellular pH to below 6.5 (136, 137). Intracellular acidosis and hypercarbia have been related to diminished contractile performance and an elevated end-diastolic pressure (138, 139). This effect is accentuated by increases in PCO_2 even when extracellular pH is held constant (140). Thus, severe respiratory acidosis may preclude successful resuscitation (139).

There also is concern that a high PCO_2 will reduce diaphragmatic function and exacerbate respiratory distress, especially in infants (141).

During cardiac arrest, substantial gradients between central venous and arterial pH and PCO_2 exist (33). The pH gradients are largely explained by the differences in PCO_2 between central venous and arterial blood (33), and do not result from the administration of bicarbonate. Once spontaneous circulation returns, the pH gradient between central venous and arterial blood rapidly disappears. Similarly, when artificial perfusion during arrest is achieved by open-chest cardiac compression, which maintains a higher cardiac output, the mixed venous-arterial gradient is much less (142). The occurrence of a marked arterial-venous pH gradient is at least partly explained by examining the Fick equation, using carbon dioxide content (CCO_2) rather than oxygen content:

$$Q = VCO_2/(CVCO_2 - CACO_2)$$

where Q is cardiac output and VCO_2 is carbon dioxide production from the lungs. $CVCO_2$ and $CACO_2$ are the mixed venous and arterial carbon dioxide contents, respectively. On rearrangement:

$$CVCO_2 - CACO_2 = VCO_2/Q$$

Thus, a wide arterial-venous gradient occurs when cardiac output is low, as in cardiac arrest. After intubation and ventilation, the small amount of blood flow through the pulmonary circulation is usually well-oxygenated and ventilated, as reflected in arterial blood gases, although epinephrine administration during an arrest appears to increase dead-space ventilation and ventilation/perfusion mismatch (143).

An appreciation of the marked venous and myocardial acidosis, the effects of intracellular acidosis on cardiovascular function, and the differences in diffusion among CO_2 and H^+ and HCO_3^- ions has led to a substantial rethinking of the use of buffers during cardiopulmonary resuscitation. Originally, sodium bicarbonate in combination with epinephrine was reported to improve the success of defibrillation and survival during resuscitation; sodium bicarbonate alone was no better than placebo (144). When coronary perfusion pressure is maintained near the critical level between poor and good outcome, sodium bicarbonate (1 mEq/kg) failed to affect the success of defibrillation or improve the chances for return of spontaneous circulation or survival (145). Likewise, even when cardiac output is well-maintained using open-chest CPR, bicarbonate administration (2 mEq/kg) was not better than an equimolar amount of NaCl (142). A comparison of 2.5 mEq/kg of sodium bicarbonate to Carbicarb (an equimolar mixture of $NaHCO_3$ and Na_2CO_3 that does not generate CO_2) (146) again showed no benefit from $NaHCO_3$ (147). Other studies also have failed to observe a beneficial effect from sodium bicarbonate administration (148), although a recent study evaluating neurologic outcome following resuscitation in a canine model shows a beneficial effect from $NaHCO_3$ (149).

Why should bicarbonate have an adverse effect during CPR? Sodium bicarbonate buffers excess protons through the reaction: $HCO_3^- + H^+ \Leftrightarrow H_2CO_3 \Leftrightarrow H_2O + CO_2$. Thus, in the presence of H^+ ion, more carbon dioxide is formed. The combination of the intrinsic CO_2 concentration plus that formed by the aforementioned reaction will diminish both extracellular and intracellular pH (150). Thus, it should not be surprising that rapid administration of bicarbonate transiently increases PCO_2 and diminishes left ventricular performance even in the absence of cardiac arrest (151). In critically ill patients with metabolic acidosis, bicarbonate did not improve cardiac output compared with an equimolar amount of NaCl, despite an increase in pH (152). Furthermore, bicarbonate may compromise cardiac resuscitation by reducing coronary perfusion pressure (153), and by failing to improve intramyocardial acidosis (136).

Adverse effects of bicarbonate have also been observed in the presence of lactic acidosis with hypoxemia. In this setting, sodium bicarbonate (2.5 mEq/kg administered over 1 hour) diminished blood pressure, impaired splanchnic blood flow, and markedly decreased liver intracellular pH compared with animals who received an equimolar amount of saline alone (154). Blood lactate and lactic acid production were substantially augmented in animals treated with bicarbonate. In a model of cardiac arrest, administration of bicarbonate increased arterial pH but decreased cerebrospinal fluid pH, because CO_2 diffuses into the central nervous system more rapidly than does H^+ or HCO_3^- ions (155). When metabolic acidosis is produced by administration of acid (HCl) or by experimental diabetic ketoacidosis, bicarbonate impairs cerebral oxygen availability, probably by decreasing cerebral blood oxygen content and/or tissue oxygen release from hemoglobin (156). The latter appears to result from a shift in the oxyhemoglobin dissociation curve to the left as a result of arterial alkalosis, which impairs tissue oxygen delivery. The effects of excess CO_2 cannot be overcome by hyperventilation alone because of the limited pulmonary blood flow induced during chest compression and ventilation, as noted previously.

In addition to the adverse effects that result from a high venous PCO_2, administration of sodium bicarbonate during cardiac arrest may cause hyperosmolarity and hypernatremia (157) and extracellular alkalosis (147). Alkalosis induced by excessive bicarbonate administration may reduce the concentration of ionized calcium (152), decrease plasma potassium concentration, shift the oxyhemoglobin dissociation curve to the left (inhibiting the release of oxygen), and induce malignant arrhythmias (79). Precipitation of calcium carbonate occurs when bicarbonate is mixed with calcium.

Indications and Dose

The American Heart Association guidelines deemphasized the role of sodium bicarbonate in both pediatric and adult resuscitation (1), since adverse effects have been noted in experimental models and few data document a benefit of bicarbonate during cardiopulmonary resuscitation. Bicarbonate should not be used until the airway is secured, adequate ventilation and chest compressions have been administered, and the patient fails to respond to defibrillation, antiarrhythmic therapy, and epinephrine. Acidosis, if present, should be treated with judicious hyperventilation and attempts to increase tissue perfusion. Attention to airway management is particularly important in pediatric patients, since respiratory failure is a major cause of cardiopulmonary arrest (96).

Monitoring blood gases during cardiac arrest to determine the degree of acidosis, and subsequently to guide alkali therapy, can be misleading. As noted, a large gradient between arterial and mixed venous pH exists during CPR (33). The presence of a normal arterial pH and hypocarbia is consistent with little cardiac output and thus little pulmonary blood flow participating in gas exchange. Indeed, improved cardiac output results in arterial respiratory and metabolic acidosis during resuscitation (38). Furthermore, intramyocardial pH is poorly reflected by arterial pH. During ventricular fibrillation, intramyocardial pH decreased from a mean of 7.24 to 6.88, whereas arterial pH remained above 7.30 (137). Severe myocardial hypercarbia may then preclude successful resuscitation (139).

Following the restoration of spontaneous circulation, the role of bicarbonate is more controversial. Lactate may be "washed out" of reperfused tissue beds with an acute exacerbation of central metabolic acidosis. Bicarbonate should be administered only if an adequate pH cannot be achieved with hyperventilation. It is probably unnecessary to treat mild-to-moderate metabolic acidosis (pH >7.20), especially when it results from correctable hemodynamic causes. Bicarbonate is still useful to help antagonize the adverse electrophysiologic effects of hyperkalemia.

When bicarbonate is used, the dose is 1 mEq/kg by slow intravenous infusion for both adult and pediatric patients. Subsequent doses of 0.5 mEq/kg may be given every 10 minutes as needed. In infants, it is preferable to dilute the bicarbonate 1:1 with sterile water to decrease the hyperosmolarity of the 8.4% solution (1).

CALCIUM

Pharmacology

Calcium is essential to the process of excitation-contraction coupling. It enters the myocardial cell through voltage-dependent channels, stimulating the intracellular release of calcium from the sarcoplasmic reticulum. The transient increase in intracellular calcium concentration activates actin-myosin coupling through interaction with regulatory proteins. Contraction terminates when calcium is pumped out of the cell or back into the sarcoplasmic reticulum. Normally, there is approximately a 10,000-fold concentration gradient between extracellular and intracellular calcium concentration, which is maintained by energy-requiring mechanisms. Although calcium has a positive inotropic effect, it may also impair cardiac relaxation (158). Furthermore, if the intracellular calcium concentration becomes increased, such as following ischemic insults, cell death results, in part through calcium-mediated mechanisms (159, 160).

Calcium has variable effects on peripheral vascular tone, although most clinical studies suggest that it increases systemic vascular resistance and blood pressure (161, 162). Recently, calcium administration producing increases in the ionized concentration within the normal range has been reported to attenuate the peripheral vascular and inotropic effects of catecholamines, such as epinephrine (163). Excessive calcium doses producing hypercalcemia may precipitate or exacerbate digitalis toxicity, leading to severe arrhythmias, including life-threatening bradycardias (164). Calcium forms an insoluble precipitate (calcium carbonate) if mixed with bicarbonate, is sclerosing to peripheral veins, and, if it infiltrates into the subcutaneous tissues, can produce a severe chemical burn.

Indications and Dose

Advocacy of the use of calcium in cardiopulmonary arrest was stimulated by the observation that calcium administration resulted in positive inotropic effects in patients after cardiopulmonary bypass (165) and during hemodialysis (166). Despite these beneficial effects, clinical studies show that calcium is ineffective in the treatment of refractory electromechanical dissociation (167) and/or asystole (168), although an increased rate of restoration of spontaneous circulation in patients with out-of-hospital arrest and electromechanical dissociation has been reported (169).

In addition to the lack of data concerning the efficacy of calcium in cardiac arrest, there is also concern that postischemic cell injury (so-called reperfusion injury) is exacerbated by the excessive plasma calcium concentrations known to occur when calcium is administered during critical illness or cardiopulmonary resuscitation (170, 171).

Balancing calcium's lack of effectiveness are data showing that ionized hypocalcemia is common in out-of-hospital cardiac arrest (172) and in animal models of prolonged cardiac arrest (173). These studies do not provide an explanation for the decrease in ionized calcium concentration, but there is an inverse relationship between lactate concentration and ionized calcium concentration (173); lactate can bind calcium. It remains to be seen whether calcium is beneficial in patients with prolonged arrest.

Thus, calcium should be used during cardiopulmonary resuscitation only to correct suspected or documented ionized hypocalcemia, to reverse the adverse effects of hyperkalemia and/or hypermagnesemia, or to treat calcium channel blocker toxicity (1). Although animal and in vitro data suggest that calcium chloride and gluconate are equivalent (174), clinical response in critically ill patients shows increased bioavailability of the chloride salt (175). There is little information as to the optimal dose. A dose of 2 ml of 10% calcium chloride (elemental calcium, 2 to 4 mg/kg) is recommended in adults (1). In pediatric patients, a larger dose (10% calcium chloride, 20 mg/kg; elemental calcium, 5 to 7 mg/kg) is recommended. The dose should be infused slowly and may be repeated after 10 minutes if required, based on measured ionized hypocalcemia.

ISOPROTERENOL

Pharmacology

Isoproterenol is a potent, very-short-acting synthetic catecholamine with nearly pure β-adrenergic stimulating properties. As such, isoproterenol induces marked increases in heart rate and contractility and potent peripheral and coronary vasodilation. It also markedly increases myocardial work (176).

By increasing myocardial oxygen demand, isoproterenol may induce or exacerbate ischemia in patients with coronary artery disease (176, 177). Because it decreases coronary perfusion pressure, it increases mortality during experimental resuscitation (178) and may cause myocardial ischemia in children with normal coronary vessels (179). Isoproterenol can induce ventricular arrhythmias, especially in patients with digitalis toxicity (180).

Indications and Dose

Isoproterenol is not indicated during the management of cardiac arrest, since it appears to increase mortality (178) and has been supplanted as a pressor/inotrope by dopamine and dobutamine. Its only role at present is in the temporary treatment of life-threatening bradycardia resulting from heart block or sinus arrest until a pacemaker can be inserted. When bradycardia is the end result of a severe hypoxic-ischemic insult, it is less likely that isoproterenol will be effective. Furthermore, the availability of reliable external pacemakers (181) makes the use of isoproterenol less important. When isoproterenol is used to treat bradycardia, the dose required usually is quite low because it has such potent chronotropic effects. Accordingly, the initial dose should be 2 μg/min. Doses as high as 10 μg/min may be needed to maintain an adequate heart rate (usually approximately 60 beats/min).

In pediatric patients, bradycardia usually results from hypoxia. Therefore, attention to ventilation should precede isoproterenol administration. Epinephrine is preferable to isoproterenol in pediatric patients since it does not induce vasodilation and thus should better maintain coronary perfusion pressure (182). The infusion dose of isoproterenol is 0.1 to 1.0 μg/kg/min.

MAGNESIUM

Pharmacology

Magnesium is an important cofactor for a number of enzymes. Its deficiency leads to inadequate sodium-potassium ATPase activity and thus to alterations in the intracellular to extracellular concentrations of potassium and sodium (183). Subsequent abnormalities of potassium homeostasis affect depolarization, repolarization, and pacemaker activity (184). The exact role of intracellular and extracellular magnesium on modulating normal and abnormal cardiac electrophysiology, either directly or indirectly through its effects on potassium homeostasis, is not clear. Increased extracellular magnesium concentrations can reverse the effects of hyperkalemia (185). Furthermore, increasing the intracellular magnesium concentration inhibits slow inward calcium current, whereas depleted intracellular magnesium has the opposite action (186). Magnesium also can affect the sodium flux across the cell membrane (184). Finally, magnesium can affect endothelial cell function, which may have an important effect on vascular tone (187, 188).

Based on its electrophysiologic effects, it should not be surprising that magnesium deficiency is associated with cardiac arrhythmias (189, 190). Magnesium deficiency states are common in critically ill patients (191). It is seen with the use of loop and thiazide diuretics, inadequate magnesium intake, digitalis toxicity, acute myocardial infarction, alcoholism, gastrointestinal losses, diabetes, and congestive heart failure (192–194). A high percentage (38 to 42%) of patients receiving diuretic therapy and having hypokalemia also have hypomagnesemia (194, 195). Recognition of magnesium deficiency is complicated by the fact that it is largely intracellular; extracellular (i.e., serum) concentrations may not reflect total body magnesium content (196).

Torsade de pointes is a life-threatening form of ventricular tachycardia characterized by a wandering vector of cardiac depolarization. It occurs in conditions producing prolongation of the Q-T interval, most frequently secondary to toxicity from the type IA antiarrhythmic drugs, such as quinidine or disopyramide (197, 198). Bradycardia, hypokalemia, and hypomagnesemia can increase the likelihood of developing torsade de pointes and may be the only cause in unusual circumstances (199, 200). Intravenous magnesium sulfate has been shown to be very effective in the treatment of torsade de pointes (198). Of interest, it was even effective in patients who had normal serum magnesium concentrations but low potassium concentrations.

Several large placebo-controlled, double-blind trials have examined the effects of magnesium administration in patients with known or suspected acute myocardial infarction (201, 202). Although the studies were limited by lack of rigorous arrhythmia quantification and outcome assessment, they showed an approximately 50% reduction of arrhythmias in the treated patients, and a reduction of early and late mortality. The precise role of magnesium therapy is not clear, but it is suggested that magnesium levels should be checked in all patients with an acute infarct, and that patients requiring potassium supplementation should be assumed to have magnesium deficiency as well (198).

Ventricular arrhythmias resulting from digitalis toxicity are often very sensitive to magnesium therapy; magnesium can suppress digoxin-induced ventricular arrhythmias in patients with either normal or low magnesium serum concentrations (203, 204). Indeed, when magnesium serum concentrations are normal, the intracellular level is frequently low in digitalis-intoxicated patients (204). Magnesium probably exerts its beneficial effect by counteracting the inhibitory effect of digoxin on sodium-potassium ATPase.

Indications and Dose

There are several well-accepted indications for the use of magnesium sulfate in the treatment of life-threatening arrhythmias. These are torsade de pointes, ventricular arrhythmias complicating acute myocardial infarction and failing to respond to standard therapy, and digoxin overdose (184, 193, 198). Other less well-accepted indications include the treatment of multifocal atrial tachycardia and atrial fibrillation (193). Certainly, magnesium therapy is indicated in patients with documented hypomagnesemia and arrhythmias, but magnesium levels may be difficult to obtain rapidly and may correlate poorly with the intracellular concentration, as previously discussed.

Magnesium administration is safe as long as the patient does not have impaired renal function. The recommended dose is 20% magnesium sulfate, 10 to 15 ml infused over 1 minute (2 to 3 gm), followed by 500 ml of 2% solution (10 gm) over 5 hours (193). Potassium chloride, 20 to 40 mEq, should be added to the magnesium solution if the serum potassium concentration is ≤4 mEq/liter. In patients with documented hypomagnesemia, an additional 500 ml of 2% magnesium sulfate may be given over the next 10 hours. Dosage information for pediatric patients is not certain. Recommended doses for the treatment of hypomagnesemia range from 25 to 50 mg/kg of magnesium sulfate given i.m. or slowly i.v. In the acute care setting the i.v. route is preferred, using

an infusion concentration of 10 mg/ml given over 15 to 20 minutes.

Manifestations of magnesium intoxication include hypotension, bradycardia, hypotonia with possible respiratory failure, and hypocalcemia secondary to suppressed parathyroid gland action. The neuromuscular and cardiac toxicities related to hypermagnesemia may be antagonized by the administration of calcium.

REFERENCES

1. Emergency Cardiac Care Committee and Subcommittees, American Heart Association: Guidelines for cardiopulmonary resuscitation and emergency cardiac care. *JAMA* 268:2171–2295, 1992.
2. Doan LA: Peripheral vs. central delivery of medications during CPR. *Ann Emerg Med* 13(2):784–786, 1984.
3. Otto C, Yakaitis R, Blitt C: Mechanism of action of epinephrine in resuscitation from asphyxial arrest. *Crit Care Med* 9:321–324, 1981.
4. Dalsey W, Barsan W, Joyce S, Hedges J, Lukes S, Doan L: Comparison of superior vena caval and inferior vena caval access using a radioisotope technique during normal perfusion and cardiopulmonary resuscitation. *Ann Emerg Med* 13:881–884, 1984.
5. Emerman CL, Pinchak AC, Hancock D, Hagen JF: The effect of bolus injection on circulation times during cardiac arrest. *Am J Emerg Med* 8:190–193, 1990.
6. Keats S, Jackson RE, Kosnik JW, Tworek RM, Zwanger M: Effect of peripheral vs. central injection of epinephrine on changes in aortic diastolic pressure during closed chest massage in dogs. *Ann Emerg Med* 14:495, 1985.
7. Rosetti V, Thompson B, Aprahamian C, Darin J, Mateer J: Difficulty and delay in intravascular access in pediatric arrests. *Ann Emerg Med* 13:406, 1984.
8. Schleien CL, Dean JM, Koehler RC, et al: Effect of epinephrine on cerebral and myocardial perfusion in an infant animal preparation of cardiopulmonary resuscitation. *Circulation* 73:809–817, 1986.
9. Orlowski JP: Optimum position for external cardiac compression in infants and young children. *Ann Emerg Med* 15:667–673, 1986.
10. Fiser D: Intraosseous infusion. *N Engl J Med* 322:1579–1581, 1990.
11. Berg R: Emergency infusion of catecholamines into bone marrow. *Am J Dis Child* 138:810–811, 1984.
12. Orlowski JP, Julius CJ, Petras RE, Porembka DT, Gallagher JM: The safety of intraosseous infusions: risks of fat and bone marrow emboli to the lungs. *Ann Emerg Med* 18:1062–1067, 1989.
13. La Fleche FR, Slepin MJ, Vargas J, Milzman DP: Iatrogenic bilateral tibial fractures after intraosseous infusion attempts in a 3 month old infant. *Ann Emerg Med* 18:1099–1101, 1989.
14. Galpin RD, Kronick JB, Willis RB, Frewen TC: Bilateral lower extremity compartment syndromes secondary to intraosseous fluid resuscitation. *J Pediatr Orthop* 11:773–776, 1991.
15. Hähnel J, Lindner K, Schürmann C, Prengel A, Ahnefeld F: Plasma lidocaine levels and PaO₂ with endobronchial administration: Dilution with normal saline or distilled water? *Ann Emerg Med* 19:1314–1317, 1990.
16. Johnston C: Endotracheal drug delivery. *Pediatr Emerg Care* 8:94–97, 1992.
17. Roberts JR, Greenberg MI, Knaub MA, Kendrick ZV, Baskin SI: Blood levels following intravenous and endotracheal epinephrine administration. *J Am Coll Emerg Phys* 8:53–56, 1979.
18. Ralston S, Tacher W, Showen L, Carter A, Babbs C: Endotracheal vs. intravenous epinephrine during electromechanical dissociation with CPR in dogs. *Ann Emerg Med* 14:1044–1048, 1985.
19. Quinton DN, O'Byrne G, Aitkenhead AR: Comparison of endotracheal and peripheral intravenous adrenaline in cardiac arrest. Is the endotracheal route reliable? *Lancet* i:828–829, 1987.
20. Hörnchen U, Schüttler J, Stoeckel H, Eichelkraut W, Hahn N: Endobronchial instillation of epinephrine during cardiopulmonary resuscitation. *Crit Care Med* 15:1037–1039, 1987.
21. Orlowski JP, Gallagher JM, Porembka DT: Endotracheal epinephrine is unreliable. *Resuscitation* 19:103–113, 1990.
22. Crespo SG, Schoffstall JM, Fuhs LR, Spivey WH: Comparison of two doses of endotracheal epinephrine in a cardiac arrest model. *Ann Emerg Med* 20:230–234, 1991.
23. Scott B, Martin F, Matchett J, White S: Canine cardiovascular responses to endotracheally and intravenously administered atropine, isoproterenol and propranolol. *Ann Emerg Med* 16:1–10, 1987.
24. Raehl C: Endotracheal drug therapy in cardiopulmonary resuscitation. *Clin Pharm* 5:572–579, 1986.
25. Mace SE: Differences in plasma lidocaine levels with endotracheal drug therapy secondary to total volume of diluent administered. *Resuscitation* 20:185–191, 1990.
26. McDonald J: Serum lidocaine levels during cardiopulmonary resuscitation after endotracheal and intravenous administration. *Crit Care Med* 13:914–915, 1985.

27. Mace SE: Effect of technique of administration on plasma lidocaine levels. *Ann Emerg Med* 15:552–556, 1986.
28. Hähnel JH, Lindner KH, Schürmann C, Prengel A, Ahnefeld FW: What is the optimal volume of administration for endobronchial drugs? *Am J Emerg Med* 8:504–508, 1990.
29. Newton DW, Fung EF, Williams DA: Stability of five catecholamines and terbutaline sulfate in 5% dextrose in the absence and presence of aminophylline. *Am J Hosp Pharm* 38:1314–1319, 1981.
30. Ornato JP, Bryson BL, Donovan PJ, Farqualharson RR, Jaeger C: Measurement of ventilation during cardiopulmonary resuscitation. *Crit Care Med* 11:79–82, 1983.
31. Voorhees WD, Jaeger CS, Babbs CR, et al: Regional blood flow during cardiopulmonary resuscitation in dogs. *Crit Care Med* 8:134–136, 1980.
32. Ralston S, Voorhees W, Showen L, Schmitz P, Kougias C, Tacker WA: Venous and arterial blood gases during and after cardiopulmonary resuscitation in dogs. *Am J Emerg Med* 3:132–136, 1985.
33. Weil M, Rackow E, Trevino R, Grundler W, Falk J, Griffel M: Difference in acid-base state between venous and arterial blood during cardiopulmonary resuscitation. *N Engl J Med* 315:153–156, 1986.
34. Niemann JT, Criley JM, Rosborough JP, Niskanen RA, Alferness C: Predictive indices of successful cardiac resuscitation after prolonged arrest and experimental cardiopulmonary resuscitation. *Ann Emerg Med* 14:521–528, 1985.
35. Sanders A, Ewy G, Taft T: Prognostic and therapeutic importance of the aortic diastolic pressure in resuscitation from cardiac arrest. *Crit Care Med* 12:871–878, 1984.
36. Paradis NA, Martin GB, Rivers EP, et al: Coronary perfusion pressure and the return of spontaneous circulation in human cardiopulmonary resuscitation. *JAMA* 263:1106–1113, 1990.
37. Michael J, Guerci A, Koehler R, et al: Mechanisms by which epinephrine augments cerebral and myocardial perfusion during cardiopulmonary resuscitation in dogs. *Circulation* 69:822–835, 1984.
38. Angelos MG, DeBehnke DJ, Leasure JE: Arterial blood gases during cardiac arrest: markers of blood flow in a canine model. *Resuscitation* 23:101–111, 1992.
39. Ditchey R: High dose epinephrine does not improve the balance between myocardial oxygen supply and demand during cardiopulmonary resuscitation in dogs. *J Am Coll Cardiol* 3:596, 1984.
40. Hörnchen U, Schüttler J, Berg P: Potential risks of high doses of epinephrine during CPR after short term cardiac arrest in a porcine CPR model. *Anesthesiology* 75:A1116, 1991.
41. Otto CW, Yakaitis RW: The role of epinephrine in CPR: a reappraisal. *Ann Emerg Med* 13(2):840–843, 1984.
42. Olson DW, Thakur R, Stueven HA, et al: Randomized study of epinephrine vs. methoxamine in prehospital ventricular fibrillation. *Ann Emerg Med* 18:250–253, 1989.
43. Turner LM, Parsons M, Luetkemeyer RC, Ruthman JC, Anderson RJ, Aldag JC: A comparison of epinephrine and methoxamine for resuscitation from electromechanical dissociation in human beings. *Ann Emerg Med* 17:443–449, 1988.
44. Brown CG, Davis EA, Werman HA, Hamlin RL: Methoxamine vs. epinephrine on regional cerebral blood flow during cardiopulmonary resuscitation. *Crit Care Med* 15:682–686, 1987.
45. Roberts D, Landolfo K, Dobson K, Light RB: The effects of methoxamine and epinephrine on survival and regional distribution of cardiac output in dogs with prolonged ventricular fibrillation. *Chest* 98:999–1005, 1990.
46. Brillman J, Sanders A, Ottow C, Fahmy H, Bragg S, Ewy G: Comparison of epinephrine and phenylephrine for resuscitation and neurologic outcome of cardiac arrest in dogs. *Ann Emerg Med* 16:11–17, 1987.
47. Lindner KH, Ahnefeld FW: Comparison of epinephrine and norepinephrine in the treatment of asphyxial or fibrillatory cardiac arrest in a porcine model. *Crit Care Med* 17:437–441, 1989.
48. Brown C, Robinson L, Jenkins J, et al: The effect of norepinephrine vs. epinephrine on regional cerebral blood flow during cardiopulmonary resuscitation. *Am J Emerg Med* 7:278–282, 1989.
49. Lindner KH, Ahnefeld FW, Grünert A: Epinephrine vs. norepinephrine in prehospital ventricular fibrillation. *Am J Cardiol* 67:427–428, 1991.
50. Kosnik JW, Jackson RE, Keats S, Tworek RM, Freeman SB: Dose-related response of centrally administered epinephrine on the change in aortic diastolic pressure during closed chest massage in dogs. *Ann Emerg Med* 14:204–208, 1985.
51. Brown C, Werman H: Adrenergic agonists during cardiopulmonary resuscitation. *Resuscitation* 19:1–16, 1990.
52. Gonzales E, Ornato J, Garnett A, Levine R, Young D, Racht E: Dose-dependent vasopressor responses to epinephrine during CPR in human beings. *Ann Emerg Med* 18:920–926, 1989.
53. Goetting MG, Paradis NA: High-dose epinephrine improves outcome from pediatric cardiac arrest. *Ann Emerg Med* 20:22–26, 1991.
54. Stiell IG, Hebert PC, Weitzman BN, et al: High-dose epinephrine in adult cardiac arrest. *N Engl J Med* 327:1045–1050, 1992.
55. Callaham M, Madsen CD, Barton CW, Saunders CE, Daley M, Pointer J: A randomized trial of high-dose epinephrine and norepinephrine vs. standard dose epinephrine in prehospital cardiac arrest. *JAMA* 268:2667–2672, 1992.
56. Berg R, Otto C, Kern K, Sanders A, Ewy G: High dose epinephrine does not improve survival from prolonged cardiac arrest. *Crit Care Med* 20:S10, 1992.
57. Otto C, Berg R, Milander M, Kern K, Sanders A, Ewy G: Beta blockade attenuates tachycardia and early death after resuscitation from prolonged cardiac arrest with high dose epinephrine. *Crit Care Med* 20:S74, 1992.
58. Paradis N, Martin G, Rosenberg J, et al: The effect of standard- and high-dose epinephrine on coronary perfusion pressure during prolonged cardiopulmonary resuscitation. *JAMA* 265:1139–1144, 1991.
59. Dhingra RC, Amat-y-Leon F, Wyndham C, et al: Electrophysiologic effects of atropine on human sinus node and atrium. *Am J Cardiol* 38:429–434, 1976.
60. Kent KM, Epstein SE, Cooper T, Jacobowitz DM, et al: Cholinergic innervation of the canine and human ventricular conducting system: an anatomic and electrophysiologic correlation. *Circulation* 50:948–955, 1974.
61. Koltmeier C, Gravenstein J: The parasympathomimetic activity of atropine and atropine methylbromide. *Anesthesiology* 29:1125–1133, 1968.
62. Dauchot P, Gravenstein JS: Effects of atropine on the electrocardiogram in different age groups. *Clin Pharmacol Ther* 12:274–280, 1971.
63. Prete M, Hanan C, Burkle F: Plasma atropine concentrations via intravenous, endotracheal, and intraosseous administration. *Em J Emerg Med* 5:101–104, 1987.
64. Schweitzer P, Mark H: The effect of atropine on cardiac rhythm and conduction. Part 1. *Am Heart J* 100:119–127, 1980.
65. O'Rourke G, Greene N: Autonomic blockade and the resting heart rate in man. *Am Heart J* 80:469–474, 1970.
66. Brown D, Lewis A, Criley J: Asystole and its treatment: the possible role of the parasympathomimetic system in cardiac arrest. *J Am Coll Emerg Phys* 8:448–453, 1979.
67. Stueven HA, Tonsfeldt DJ, Thompson BM, Whitcomb J, Kastenson E, Aprahamian C: Atropine in asystole: human studies. *Ann Emerg Med* 13(2):815–817, 1984.
68. Cooper M, Abinader E: Atropine-induced ventricular fibrillation: case report and review of the literature. *Am Heart J* 97:225–228, 1979.
69. Scheinman MM, Thorburn D, Abbott JA: Use of atropine in patients with acute myocardial infarction and bradycardia. *Circulation* 52:627–633, 1975.
70. Goetting M, Contereas E: Systemic atropine administration during cardiac arrest does not cause fixed and dilated pupils. *Ann Emerg Med* 20:55–57, 1991.
71. Bigger JT Jr, Hoffman BF: Antiarrhythmic drugs. In Gilman AG, Rall TW, Nies AS, Taylor P (eds): *Goodman and Gilman's The Pharmacological Basis of Therapeutics*, ed 8. Pergamon Press, New York, 1990, pp 840–873.
72. Bigger JT Jr, Mandel WJ: Effect of lidocaine on the electrophysiologic properties of ventricular muscle and Purkinje fibers. *J Clin Invest* 49:63–77, 1970.
73. Kupersmith J: Electrophysiological and antiarrhythmic effects of lidocaine in canine acute myocardial ischemia. *Am Heart J* 97:360–366, 1979.
74. Borer J, Harrison LA, Kent KM, Levy R, Goldstein RE, Epstein SE: Beneficial effects of lidocaine on ventricular electrical stability and spontaneous ventricular fibrillation during experimental myocardial infarction. *Am J Cardiol* 37:860–863, 1976.
75. Spear JF, Moore EN, Gerstenblith G: Effect of lidocaine on the ventricular fibrillation threshold in the dog during acute ischemia and premature ventricular contractions. *Circulation* 46:65–73, 1972.
76. Anderson JL: Antifibrillatory vs. antiectopic therapy. *Am J Cardiol* 54:7A-12A, 1984.
77. Chow MSS, Kluger J, DiPersio DM, Lawrence R, Fieldman A: Antifibrillatory effects of lidocaine and bretylium immediately post-CPR. *Am Heart J* 110:938–943, 1985.
78. Babbs CF, Yim GKW, Whistler SJ, Tacker WA, Geddes LA: Elevation of ventricular defibrillation threshold in dogs by antiarrhythmic drugs. *Am Heart J* 98:345–350, 1979.
79. Kerber RE, Pandian NG, Jensen SR, et al: Effect of lidocaine and bretylium on energy requirements for transthoracic defibrillation: Experimental studies. *J Am Coll Cardiol* 7:397–405, 1986.
80. Wesley RC Jr, Resh W, Zimmerman D: Reconsiderations of the routine and preferential use of lidocaine in the emergent treatment of ventricular arrhythmias. *Crit Care Med* 19:1439–1444, 1991.
81. MacMahon S, Collins R, Peto R, Koster RW, Yusuf S: Effects of prophylactic lidocaine in suspected acute myocardial infarction. An overview of results from the randomized, controlled trials. *JAMA* 260:1910–1916, 1988.
82. Weaver WD, Fahrenbruch CE, Johnson DD, Hallstrom AP, Cobb LA, Compass MK: Effect of epinephrine and lidocaine therapy on outcome after cardiac arrest due to ventricular fibrillation. *Circulation* 82:2027–2034, 1990.
83. Armengol RE, Graff J, Baerman JM, Swiryn S: Lack of effectiveness of lidocaine for sustained, wide complex QRS complex tachycardia. *Ann Emerg Med* 18:254–257, 1989.
84. Kirby DA, Hottinger S, Ravid S, Lown B: Inducible monomorphic sustained ventricular tachycardia in the conscious pig. *Am Heart J* 119:1042–1049, 1990.
85. Boynes RN, Scott DB, Jebson PJ, Goodman MJ, Julian DG: Pharmacokinetics of lidocaine in man. *Clin Pharmacol Ther* 12:105–116, 1971.
86. Nies AS, Shand DG, Wilkinson GR: Altered hepatic blood flow and drug disposition. *Clin Pharmacokinet* 1:135–155, 1976.
87. LeLorier J, Moisan R, Gagne J, Caille G: Effect of the duration of infusion on the disposition of lidocaine in dogs. *J Pharmacol Exp Ther* 203:507–511, 1977.

88. Thompson PD, Melmon KL, Richardson JA, et al: Lidocaine pharmacokinetics in advanced heart failure, liver disease, and renal failure in humans. *Ann Intern Med* 78:499–508, 1973.

89. Chow MMS, Ronfeld RA, Hamilton RA, Helmink R, Fieldman A: Effect of external cardiopulmonary resuscitation on lidocaine pharmacokinetics in dogs. *J Pharmacol Exp Ther* 224:531–537, 1983.

90. Lie KI, Wellens HJ, van Capelle FJ, Durrer D: Lidocaine in the prevention of primary ventricular fibrillation. *N Engl J Med* 291:1324–1326, 1974.

91. Lown B, Vassaux C: Lidocaine in acute myocardial infarction. *Am Heart J* 76:685–690, 1968.

92. Collingsworth KA, Kalman SM, Harrison DC: The clinical pharmacology of lidocaine as an antiarrhythmic drug. *Circulation* 50:1217–1230, 1974.

93. Bethesda Conference Report: Thirteenth Bethesda conference: emergency cardiac care. *Am J Cardiol* 50:365–420, 1982.

94. Carruth JE, Silverman ME: Ventricular fibrillation complicating acute myocardial infarction: reasons against the routine use of lidocaine. *Am Heart J* 104:545–550, 1985.

95. Haynes RE, Chinn TL, Copass MK, Cobb LA: Comparison of bretylium tosylate and lidocaine in management of out-of-hospital ventricular fibrillation. A randomized clinical trial. *Am J Cardiol* 48:353–356, 1981.

96. Eisenberg M, Bergner L, Hallstrom A: Epidemiology of cardiac arrest and resuscitation in children. *Ann Emerg Med* 12:672–674, 1983.

97. Koch-Weser J: Drug therapy: bretylium. *N Engl J Med* 300:473–477, 1979.

98. Heissenbuttel RH, Bigger JT Jr: Bretylium tosylate: a newly available antiarrhythmic drug for ventricular arrhythmias. *Ann Intern Med* 90:229–238, 1979.

99. Kniffen FJ, Lomas TE, Counsell RE, Lucchesi BR: The antiarrhythmic and antifibrillatory actions of bretylium and its o-iodobenzyl trimethylammonium analog, UM-360. *J Pharmacol Exp Ther* 192:120–128, 1975.

100. Singh BN, Nademanee K: Control of cardiac arrhythmias by selective lengthening of the repolarization: theoretic considerations and clinical observations. *Am Heart J* 109:421–430, 1985.

101. Chatterjee K, Mandel WJ, Vyden JK, Parmley WW, Forrester JS: Cardiovascular effects of bretylium tosylate in acute myocardial infarction. *JAMA* 223:757–760, 1973.

102. Cervoni P, Ellis CH, Maxwell RA: The antiarrhythmic action of bretylium in normal reserpine-pretreated and chronically denervated dog hearts. *Arch Int Pharmacodyn Ther* 190:91–102, 1971.

103. Euler D, Scanlon PJ: Mechanism of the effect of bretylium on the ventricular fibrillation threshold in dogs. *Am J Cardiol* 55:1396–1401, 1985.

104. Cardinal R, Sasyniuk BI: Electrophysiologic effects of bretylium tosylate on subendocardial Purkinje fibers from infarcted canine hearts. *J Pharmacol Exp Ther* 204:159–174, 1978.

105. Nishimura M, Watanabe Y: Membrane action and catecholamine release action of bretylium tosylate in normoxic and hypoxic canine Purkinje fibers. *J Am Coll Cardiol* 2:287–295, 1983.

106. Fujimoto T, Hamamoto H, Peter T, et al: Electrophysiologic effects of bretylium on canine ventricular muscle during acute ischemia and reperfusion. *Am Heart J* 105:966–972, 1983.

107. Peterson E, Luccheri BR: Bretylium: a prototype for future development of antidysrhythmic agents. *Am Heart J* 106:426–431, 1983.

108. Anderson JL, Patterson E, Conlon M, Pasyk S, Pitt B, Lucchesi BR: Kinetics of antifibrillatory effects of bretylium: correlation with myocardial drug concentrations. *Am J Cardiol* 46:583–592, 1980.

109. Hanyok JJ, Chow MSS, Kluger J, Fieldman A: Antifibrillatory effects of high dose bretylium and a lidocaine-bretylium combination during cardiopulmonary resuscitation. *Crit Care Med* 16:691–694, 1988.

110. Bacaner MB: Quantitative comparison of bretylium with other antifibrillatory drugs. *Am J Cardiol* 21:504–512, 1968.

111. Sanna G, Arcidiacono R: Chemical defibrillation of the human heart with bretylium tosylate. *Am J Cardiol* 32:982–987, 1973.

112. Vachiery J-L, Reuse C, Blecic S, Contempre B, Vincent J-L: Bretylium tosylate vs. lidocaine in experimental cardiac arrest. *Em J Emerg Med* 8:492–495, 1990.

113. Koo CC, Allen JD, Pantridge JF: Lack of effect of bretylium tosylate on electrical ventricular defibrillation in a controlled study. *Cardiovasc Res* 18:762–767, 1984.

114. Holder DA, Sniderman AD, Fraser G, Fallen EL: Experience with bretylium tosylate by a hospital cardiac arrest team. *Circulation* 55:541–544, 1977.

115. Harrison EE, Amey BD: The use of bretylium in prehospital ventricular fibrillation. *Em J Emerg Med* 1:1–6, 1983.

116. Olson DW, Thompson BM, Darin JC, Milbrath MH: A randomized comparison study of bretylium tosylate and lidocaine in resuscitation of patients from out-of-hospital ventricular fibrillation in a paramedic system. *Ann Emerg Med* 13(2):807–810, 1984.

117. Narang PK, Adir J, Josselson J, Yacobi A, Sadler J: Pharmacokinetics of bretylium in man after intravenous administration. *J Pharmacokinet Biopharm* 8:363–372, 1980.

118. Castaneda A, Bacaner M: Effect of bretylium tosylate on the prevention and treatment of postoperative arrhythmias. *Am J Cardiol* 25:461–466, 1970.

119. Mongkolsmai C, Dove J, Kyrouac J: Bretylium tosylate for ventricular fibrillation in a child. *Clin Pediatr* 23:696–698, 1984.

120. Shenasa TM, Gilbert CJ, Schmidt DH, Akhtar M: Procainamide and retrograde atrioventricular nodal conduction in man. *Circulation* 65:355–362, 1982.

121. Shechter JA, Caine R, Friehling T, Kowey PR, Engel TR: Effect of procainamide on dispersion of ventricular refractoriness. *Am J Cardiol* 52:279–282, 1983.

122. Kastor JA, Josephson ME, Guss SB, Horowitz LN: Human ventricular refractoriness. II. Effects of procainamide. *Circulation* 56:462–467, 1977.

123. Arnsdorf MF: Electrophysiologic properties of antidysrhythmic drugs as a rational basis for therapy. Med Clin North Am 60:213–232, 1976.

124. Reidenberg MM, Drayer DE, Levy M, Warner H: Polymorphic acetylation of procainamide in man. *Clin Pharmacol Ther* 17:722–730, 1975.

125. Lima JJ, Goldfarb AL, Conti DR, et al: Safety and efficacy of procainamide infusions. *Am J Cardiol* 43:98–105, 1979.

126. Jaillon P, Winkle RA: Electrophysiologic comparative study of procainamide and N-acetyl-procainamide in anesthetized dogs: concentration response relationships. *Circulation* 60:1385–1394, 1979.

127. Harrison D, Sprouse JH, Morrow AG: The antiarrhythmic properties of lidocaine and procainamide. *Circulation* 28:486–491, 1963.

128. Boccardo D, Pitchon R, Weiner I: Adverse reactions and efficacy of high-dose procainamide therapy in resistant tachyarrhythmias. *Am Heart J* 102:797–798, 1981.

129. Giardina EGV, Heissenbuttel RH, Bigger JT Jr: Intermittent intravenous procainamide to treat ventricular arrhythmias: correlation of plasma concentration with effect on arrhythmia, electrocardiogram, and blood pressure. *Ann Intern Med* 78:183–193, 1973.

130. Mitchell JH, Wildenthal K, Johnson RL Jr: The effects of acid-base disturbance on cardiovascular and pulmonary function. *Kidney Int* 1:375–389, 1972.

131. Korstanje C, Mathy MJ, van Charldorp K, de Jonge A, van Zwieten PA: Influence of respiratory acidosis or alkalosis on pressor responses mediated by alpha-1- and alpha-2-adrenoceptors in pithed normotensive rats. *Naunyn Schmiedebergs Arch Pharmacol* 330:187–192, 1985.

132. Anderson MN, Borden JR, Mouritzen CV: Acidosis, catecholamines, and cardiovascular dynamics: when does acidosis require correction? *Ann Surg* 166:344–356, 1967.

133. Mehta P, Kloner R: Effects of acid base disturbance, septic shock, and calcium and phosphorus abnormalities on cardiovascular function. *Crit Care Clin* 3:747–758, 1987.

134. Roos A, Boron WF: Intracellular pH. *Physiol Rev* 61:296–434, 1981.

135. Weil MH, Affifi AA: Experimental and clinical studies on lactate and pyruvate as indicators of the severity of acute circulatory failure (shock). *Circulation* 41:989–1001, 1970.

136. Kette F, Weil MH, Von Planta M, Gazmuri RJ, Rackow EC: Buffer agents do not reverse intramyocardial acidosis during cardiac resuscitation. *Circulation* 81:1660–1666, 1990.

137. von Planta M, Weil MH, Gazmuri RJ, Bisear J, Rackow EC: Myocardial acidosis associated with CO$_2$ production during cardiac arrest and resuscitation. *Circulation* 80:684–692, 1989.

138. Tang W, Weil M, Gazmuri R, Bisera J, Rackow E: Reversible impairment of myocardial contractility due to hypercarbic acidosis in isolated perfused rat heart. *Crit Care Med* 19:218–224, 1991.

139. von Planta I, Weil MH, von Planta M, Gazmuri RJ, Duggal C: Hypercarbic acidosis reduces cardiac resuscitability. *Crit Care Med* 19:1177–1182, 1991.

140. Cingolani HE, Mattiazzi AR, Blesa ES, Gonzalez NC: Contractility in isolated mammalian heart muscle after acid base changes. *Circ Res* 26:269–278, 1970.

141. Juan G, Calverley P, Talamo C, Schnader J, Roussos C: Effect of carbon dioxide on diaphragmatic function in human beings. *N Engl J Med* 310:874–879, 1984.

142. Federiuk C, Sanders A, Kern K, Nelson J, Ewy G: The effect of bicarbonate on resuscitation from cardiac arrest. *Ann Emerg Med* 20:1173–1177, 1991.

143. Tang W, Weil MH, Gazmur RJ, Sun S, Duggal C, Bisera J: Pulmonary ventilation/perfusion defects induced by epinephrine during cardiopulmonary resuscitation. *Circulation* 84:2101–2107, 1991.

144. Redding J, Pearson J: Resuscitation from ventricular fibrillation: drug therapy. *JAMA* 203:255–260, 1968.

145. Guerci A, Chandra N, Johnson E, et al: Failure of sodium bicarbonate to improve resuscitation from ventricular fibrillation in dogs. *Circulation* 74(suppl IV):IV75–IV79, 1986.

146. Filley G, Kindig N: Carbicarb, an alkalinizing ion-generating agent of possible clinical usefulness. *Trans Am Clin Climatol Assoc* 96:141–153, 1984.

147. Gazmuri RJ, von Planta M, Weil MH, Rackow EC: Cardiac effects of carbon dioxide-consuming and carbon dioxide-generating buffers during cardiopulmonary resuscitation. *J Am Coll Cardiol* 15:482–490, 1990.

148. Minuck M, Sharma GP: Comparison of THAM and sodium bicarbonate in resuscitation of the heart after ventricular fibrillation in dogs. *Anesth Analg* 56:38–45, 1977.

149. Bircher NB: Sodium bicarbonate improves cardiac resuscitability, 24 hour survival and neurologic outcome after 10 minutes of cardiac arrest in dogs. *Anesthesiology* 75:A246, 1991.

150. Ostrea E, Odell G: The influence of bicarbonate administration on blood pH in a "closed system": clinical implications. *J Pediatr* 80:671–680, 1972.

151. Kindig NB, Filley GF: Intravenous bicarbonate may cause transient intracellular acidosis (letter). *Chest* 83:712, 1983.

152. Cooper D, Walley K, Wiggs B, Russell J: Bicarbonate does not improve hemodynamics in critically ill patients who have a lactic acidosis. A prospective, controlled clinical study. *Ann Intern Med* 112:492–498, 1990.

153. Kette F, Weil MH, Gazmuri RJ: Buffer solutions may compromise cardiac resuscitation by reducing coronary perfusion pressure. *JAMA* 266:2121–2126, 1991.

154. Graf H, Leach W, Arieff A: Metabolic effects of sodium bicarbonate in hypoxic lactic acidosis in dogs. *Am J Physiol* 249:F630–F635, 1985.

155. Berenyi K, Wolk M, Killip T: Cerebrospinal fluid acidosis complicating therapy of experimental cardiopulmonary arrest. *Circulation* 52:319–324, 1975.

156. Bureau M, Begin R, Berthiaume Y, Shapcott D, Khoury K, Gagnon N: Cerebral hypoxia from bicarbonate infusion in diabetic ketoacidosis. *J Pediatr* 96:968–973, 1980.

157. Mattar JA, Neil MH, Shubin H, Stein L: Cardiac arrest in the critically ill. II. Hyperosmolal states following cardiac arrest. *Am J Med* 56:162–168, 1974.

158. Katz AM: Potential deleterious effects of inotropic agents in the therapy of heart failure. *Circulation* 73 (Suppl III):III184–III190, 1986.

159. Katz A, Reuter H: Cellular calcium and cardiac cell death. *Am J Cardiol* 44:188–190, 1979.

160. Cheung J, Bonventre J, Malis C, Leaf A: Calcium and ischemic injury. *N Engl J Med* 314:1670–1676, 1986.

161. Maynard J, Cruz C, Kleerekoper M, Levin N: Blood pressure response to changes in serum ionized calcium during hemodialysis. *Ann Intern Med* 104:358–361, 1986.

162. Drop L: Ionized calcium, the heart, and hemodynamic function. *Anesth Analg* 64:432–451, 1985.

163. Zaloga GP, Strickland RA, Butterworth JF IV, Mark JL, Mills SA, Lake CR: Calcium attenuates epinephrine's β-adrenergic effects in postoperative heart surgery patients. *Circulation* 81:196–200, 1990.

164. Smith TW, Antman EM, Friedman PL, Blatt CM, Marsh JD: Digitalis glycosides: mechanisms and manifestations of toxicity. *Prog Cardiovasc Dis* 26:413–445, 1984.

165. Stulz PM, Scheidegger D, Drop LJ, Lowenstein E, Laver MB: Ventricular pump performance during hypocalcemia. *J Thorac Cardiovasc Surg* 78:185–194, 1979.

166. Henrich W, Hunt J, Nixon J: Increased ionized calcium and left ventricular contractility during hemodialysis. *N Engl J Med* 310:19–23, 1984.

167. Stueven H, Thompson B, Aprahamian C, Tonsfeldt D, Kastenson E: The effectiveness of calcium chloride in refractory electromechanical dissociation. *Ann Emerg Med* 14:626–629, 1985.

168. Stueven H, Thompson B, Aprahamian C, Tonsfeldt D, Kastenson E: Lack of effectiveness of calcium chloride in refractory asystole. *Ann Emerg Med* 14:630–632, 1985.

169. Harrison E, Amey B: The use of calcium in cardiac resuscitation. *Em J Emerg Med* 3:267–273, 1983.

170. Carlon G, Howland W, Kahn R, Schweizer O: Calcium chloride administration in normocalcemic critically ill patients. *Crit Care Med* 8:209–212, 1980.

171. Dembo D: Calcium in advanced life support. *Crit Care Med* 9:358–359, 1981.

172. Urban P, Scheidegger D, Buchmann B, Barth B: Cardiac arrest and blood ionized calcium levels. *Ann Intern Med* 109:110–113, 1988.

173. Cairns C, Niemann J, Pelikan P, Sharma J: Ionized hypocalcemia during prolonged cardiac arrest and closed-chest CPR in a canine model. *Ann Emerg Med* 20:1178–1182, 1991.

174. Heining M, Band D, Linton R: Choice of calcium salt. *Anaesthesia* 39:1079–1082, 1984.

175. Broner C, Stidham G, Westenkirchner D, Watson D: A prospective, randomized, double-blind comparison of calcium chloride and calcium gluconate therapies for hypocalcemia in critically ill children. *J Pediatr* 117:986–989, 1990.

176. Mueller H, Ayres SM, Gregory JJ, Gianelli S Jr, Grace WR: Hemodynamics, coronary blood flow and myocardial metabolism in coronary shock; response to *l*-norepinephrine and isoproterenol. *J Clin Invest* 49:1885–1902, 1970.

177. Vatner SF, Baig H: Comparison of the effects of ouabain and isoproterenol on ischemic myocardium of conscious dogs. *Circulation* 58:654–662, 1978.

178. Niemann JT, Haynes KS, Garner D, Rennie CJ III, Jagels G, Stormo O: Post countershock pulseless rhythms: response to CPR, artificial cardiac pacing and adrenergic agonists. *Ann Emerg Med* 15:112–120, 1985.

179. Matson J, Loughlin G, Struck R: Myocardial ischemia complicating the use of isoproterenol in asthmatic children. *J Pediatr* 5:776–778, 1978.

180. Becker DJ, Nonkin PM, Bennett LD, Kimball SG, Sternberg MS, Wasserman F: Effect of isoproterenol in digitalis cardiotoxicity. *Am J Cardiol* 10:242–247, 1962.

181. Zoll PM, Zoll RH, Falk RH, Clinton JE, Eitel DR, Antman EM: External noninvasive temporary cardiac pacing: clinical trials. *Circulation* 71:937–944, 1985.

182. Anonymous: Fluid therapy and medications. In Chameides L (ed): *Textbook of Pediatric Advanced Life Support*. American Heart Association, Dallas, 1988, pp 47–59.

183. Dubey A, Solomon R: Magnesium, myocardial ischemia and arrhythmias: the role of magnesium in myocardial infarction. *Drugs* 37:1–7, 1989.

184. Roden DM: Magnesium treatment of ventricular arrhythmias. *Am J Cardiol* 63:43G–46G, 1989.

185. Kraft LF, Katholi RE, Woods WT, James TN: Attenuation by magnesium of the electrophysiologic effects of hyperkalemia on human and canine heart cells. *Am J Cardiol* 45:1189–1195, 1980.

186. White RE, Hartzell HC: Effects of intracellular free magnesium on calcium current in isolated cardiac myocytes. *Science* 239:778–780, 1988.

187. Shattock MJ, Hearse DJ, Fry CH: The ionic basis of the anti-ischemic and anti-arrhythmic properties of magnesium in the heart. *J Am Coll Nutr* 6:27–33, 1987.

188. Altura BT, Altura BM: Endothelium-dependent relaxation in coronary arteries requires magnesium ions. *Br J Pharmacol* 91:449–451, 1987.

189. Roden DM, Iansmith DHS: Effects of low potassium or magnesium concentrations on isolated cardiac tissue. *Am J Med* 82 (Suppl 3A):18–23, 1987.

190. Dyckner T: Serum magnesium in acute myocardial infarction. *Acta Med Scand* 207:59–66, 1980.

191. Ryzen E, Wagers PW, Singer FR, Rude RK: Magnesium deficiency in a medical ICU population. *Crit Care Med* 13:19–21, 1985.

192. Whang R: Magnesium deficiency: pathogenesis, prevalence, and clinical implication. *Am J Med* 82(suppl 3A):24–29, 1987.

193. Iseri LT: Role of magnesium in cardiac tachyarrhythmias. *Am J Cardiol* 65:47K–50K, 1990.

194. Boyd JC, Bruns DED, Wills MR: Frequency of hypomagnesemia in hypokalemic states. *Clin Chem* 29:178–179, 1983.

195. Whang R, Oei TO, Aikawa JK, et al: Predictors of clinical hypomagnesemia: hypokalemia, hypophosphatemia, hyponatremia, and hypocalcemia. *Arch Intern Med* 144:1794–1796, 1984.

196. Reinhart RA: Magnesium metabolism. A review with special reference to the relationship between intracellular content and serum levels. *Arch Intern Med* 148:2415–2420, 1988.

197. Tzivoni D, Keren A, Stern S: Torsade de pointes vs. polymorphous ventricular tachycardia. *Am J Cardiol* 52:639–640, 1983.

198. Tzivoni D, Keren A: Suppression of ventricular arrhythmias by magnesium. *Am J Cardiol* 65:1397–1399, 1990.

199. Keren A, Tzivoni D, Gavish A, et al: Etiology, warning signs and therapy of torsade de pointes: a study of 10 patients. *Circulation* 64:1167–1174, 1981.

200. Curry P, Fitchett D, Stubbs W, Krikler D: Ventricular arrhythmias and hypokalemia. *Lancet* ii:231–233, 1976.

201. Abraham AS, Rosenmann D, Kramer M, et al: Magnesium in the prevention of lethal arrhythmias in acute myocardial infarction. *Arch Intern Med* 147:753–755, 1987.

202. Rasmussen AS, McNair P, Norregard P, Backer V, Lindenberg O, Balsen T: Intravenous magnesium in acute myocardial infarction. *Lancet* i:234–236, 1986.

203. Whang R, Oei T, Watanabe A: Frequency of hypomagnesemia in hospitalized patients receiving digitalis. *Arch Intern Med* 145:655–656, 1985.

204. Cohen L, Kitzes R: Magnesium sulfate and digitalis-toxic arrhythmias. *JAMA* 249:2808–2810, 1983.

CHAPTER 14

Cerebral Protection

DONALD S. PROUGH, M.D.
DOUGLAS S. DeWITT, Ph.D.

Cerebral ischemia causes neurologic injury in such diverse diseases as stroke, subarachnoid hemorrhage, and cardiac arrest, and after surgical procedures on the brain or the cerebral vasculature. Less obviously, important deterioration in neurologic and cognitive function after head trauma or cardiac surgery may result from cerebral ischemia. However, despite major advances that have occurred during the past decades in the understanding of the pathogenesis of cerebral ischemia, few clinically applicable treatment strategies have evolved. Treatments that are effective in experimental models often are associated with apparently favorable physiologic or pharmacologic effects when used in uncontrolled clinical practice but fail to improve outcome when investigated in properly designed clinical trials. Clinical trials may fail because of differences in the timing of interventions between the precise experimental sequences possible in animals and the heterogeneous presentation of patients. Clinical failure may also reflect differences in tolerance for therapeutic interventions between healthy animals and aging patients with systemic diseases.

Effective treatment of ischemic injury must decrease the magnitude or duration of ischemia, or must increase the ability of neural tissue to withstand ischemic insults. Although studies of tissue responses to injury usually must involve animal experiments, some evidence is available regarding the tolerance of the human brain for ischemia. Finnerty et al, using the Kety-Schmidt technique, studied global cerebral blood flow (CBF) and cerebral metabolism associated with the onset of symptoms of cerebral hypoperfusion in volunteers subjected to orthostatic stress (74). The critical CBF value was determined to be 31 ml·100 g^{-1}·min^{-1}. Sundt et al, in patients undergoing carotid cross-clamping during carotid endarterectomy under general anesthesia, found that the electroencephalogram showed ischemic changes if CBF was less than 15 ml·100 g^{-1}·min^{-1} (282). Rossen et al, using neck-tourniquet compression in volunteers and schizophrenics, demonstrated that unconsciousness followed approximately 6 to 6.5 seconds of nearly complete ischemia (244). The duration of total cerebral ischemia that would be tolerated in normothermic humans without irreversible injury is unknown; however, data in nonhuman primates suggest that intervals of 15 minutes or more may be compatible with good recovery (151, 274).

The development of a comprehensive pathophysiologic understanding of cerebral edema and brain ischemia promises rapid evolution of novel treatment strategies (76, 261, 306). However, because clinical trials usually attempt to apply basic information accumulated 5 or more years ago, neurologic intensive care has focused on the application of the potential neuroprotective effects of interventions such as barbiturates, calcium entry blockers, and glucocorticoids. In some instances the results have been gratifying, as in the demonstration by Nussmeier and colleagues (203) that sodium thiopental could, under carefully defined conditions, limit focal neurologic injury during valvular heart surgery. However, the theory that barbiturates might protect against the neurologic injury that commonly follows cardiac arrest has finally and conclusively been disproved (28). Calcium entry blockers have proved effective in preventing and treating delayed ischemic neurologic deficits caused by vasospasm in patients after

247

subarachnoid hemorrhage, have proved equivocally effective in stroke (87, 88, 286), and have failed to improve survival or neurologic salvage after cardiac arrest (29, 80, 239). Corticosteroids have proved useless in the management of closed head injury (249) and after cardiac arrest (127).

Our understanding of cerebral ischemia is now expanding rapidly. Experimental data emphasize the role of excitatory amino acids (22, 42, 199) and oxygen free radicals (101, 265) in the pathogenesis of ischemic neural damage. Nitric oxide (NO), one candidate for the role of the endothelium-derived relaxant factor (EDRF) (123), appears to play an important part in the responses of the cerebral vasculature. Although each new insight into the pathophysiology of cerebral ischemia raises the possibility of new therapeutic approaches, it is important to remember that many steps lie between demonstration of efficacy in experimental animals and the application of a new treatment modality in humans.

Among the many hurdles that must be overcome, perhaps the most formidable is timing. Clinical management of ischemia can be divided into *preischemic* treatment, which encompasses both prevention of ischemia and preservation of brain during ischemia, and *postischemic* treatment, after restoration of cerebral perfusion. Most therapeutic interventions in the laboratory work best when administered *before* an ischemic insult. Unfortunately, only a few clinical situations (e.g., carotid endarterectomy) permit pretreatment. Most patients require intervention either during an ongoing ischemic insult, such as a stroke, or after the termination of an ischemic insult, such as cardiac arrest.

This chapter reviews the normal physiologic regulation of CBF and intracranial pressure, the pathophysiology of cerebral injury, and the pharmacologic basis of experimental and clinical cerebral protective therapy.

REGULATION AND MONITORING OF CEREBRAL HEMODYNAMICS

PHYSIOLOGIC REGULATION AND MONITORING OF CEREBRAL BLOOD FLOW

Cerebral perfusion is tightly regulated in normal physiologic states. The major determinants of CBF include cerebral metabolic demand, arterial O_2 tension, arterial CO_2 tension, and cerebral perfusion pressure (CPP), as defined by the following equation:

$$CPP = MAP - ICP \qquad (1)$$

where "MAP" denotes mean arterial pressure and "ICP" denotes intracranial pressure. The outflow pressure of the cerebral circulation is either ICP or jugular venous pressure, whichever is greater. The influence of CPP on CBF is influenced by the autoregulatory capacity of the cerebral circulation (see below).

Physiologic Regulation

Metabolic Activity. More than a century ago, Roy and Sherrington (246) suggested that the brain possesses "an automatic mechanism . . . well fitted to provide for a local variation of the blood-supply in accordance with local variations of the

functional activity." Thus, the concept of coupling between functional and metabolic activity and CBF is far older than most of the techniques currently used to investigate this important relationship. Techniques such as double-label autoradiography, [133]Xenon (^{133}Xe) clearance, and positron emission tomography have left little question that CBF and metabolism are tightly coupled in both experimental animals (90) and normal humans (240). Although seizures most dramatically illustrate the effects of an increase in the cerebral metabolic rate for oxygen ($CMRO_2$) on CBF, CBF also increases measurably in appropriate brain regions in response to simple motor activity, sensory stimulation, eye movement, reading, and thinking (172, 241, 242). Flow-metabolism coupling is variably preserved in patients who have neurologic injury (Fig. 14.1). However, there is some uncertainty about the nature of the mechanism(s) that link CBF to the functional activity of the neuroaxis. Changes in extracellular H^+ and K^+ concentrations, which will affect CBF levels, are no longer believed to be important in normal coupling between CBF and metabolism (148). Adenosine, which is involved in the maintenance of resting cerebral vascular tone and in vasodilatory responses to hypoxia (195, 217), is likely to be an important mediator of cerebral vascular responses to certain stimuli.

More recent evidence suggests that the cerebral vascular endothelium plays an important role in vascular responses and, perhaps, in the coupling of CBF and metabolism. In 1980, Furchgott and Zawadzki (84) reported that an intact

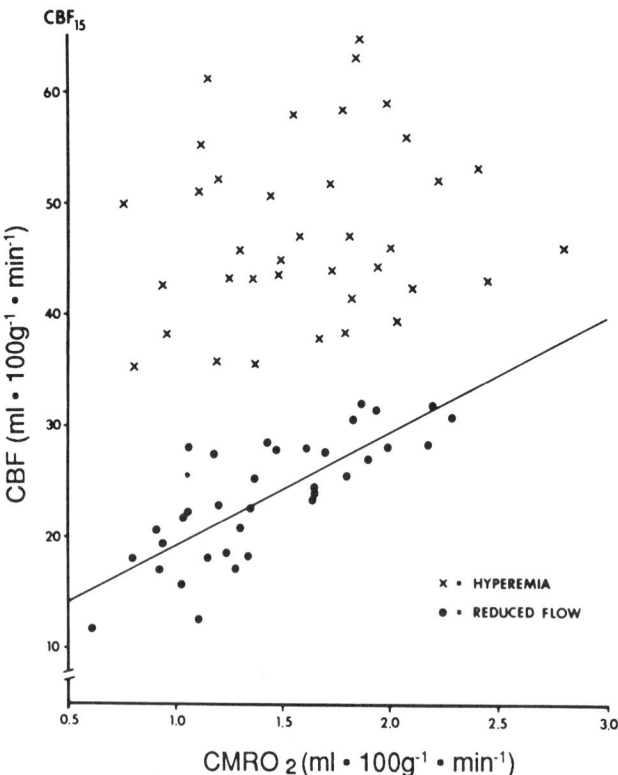

Figure 14.1. Flow-metabolism coupling in patients who have acute head injury. The solid circles and the regression line demonstrate normal coupling of cerebral blood flow (*CBF*) and the cerebral metabolic rate for oxygen (*CMRO₂*), albeit at values lower than normal (CBF 50 ml·100 g⁻¹·min⁻¹ and CMRO₂ 3.5 ml·100 g⁻¹·min⁻¹). The x characters represent values of CBF that exceed metabolic need (i.e., uncoupled values).

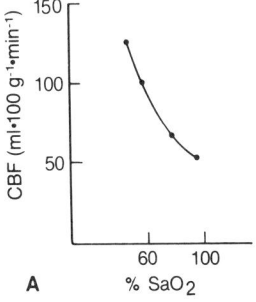
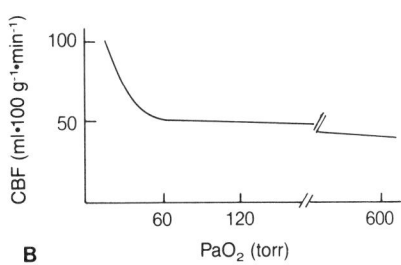

Figure 14.2. Response of cerebral blood flow (*CBF*) to changes: **A**, in arterial oxygen saturation (*SAO₂*), and **B**, in PAO₂. Cerebral blood flow is inversely related to oxygen content. Therefore, CBF increases rapidly when SAO₂ is decreased below 90% (**A**) or as PAO₂ is decreased below 60 mm Hg (**B**). (Reprinted with permission, Prough DS, Michenfelder JD: Cerebral blood flow. In Cerra FB, Shoemake WC (eds): *Critical Care State of the Art.* Baltimore, Williams & Wilkins, 1987, p 54.)

vascular endothelium was required for acetylcholine-induced vasodilation in vitro. Subsequent studies suggested that one EDRF responsible for acetylcholine-induced vasodilation is NO, an oxygen radical (123), although the cerebral vascular EDRF may not be NO in all species (169). Wei and Kontos (300) reported that EDRF is a nitrosothiol metabolite of NO such as S-nitroso-L-cysteine. EDRF, whether NO or a related compound, is involved in the regulation of resting cerebral vascular tone (72, 284). In addition, NO is now believed to be important in intercellular signalling processes (86), especially in glutamatergic neurons (33), suggesting that it may couple CBF and functional neuronal activity. Although it is likely that NO or other endothelium-derived mediators will prove to play an important role in the control of the cerebral circulation, available experimental data remain controversial. Conflicting results are likely the result, in part, of physiologic differences between in vivo and in vitro models (see reference 168).

Arterial Oxygen Tension (PAO₂). Decreases in arterial oxygen saturation (SAO₂) and PAO₂ cause reciprocal changes in CBF. CBF increases rapidly as SAO₂ is decreased below 90% (Fig. 14.2) or as PAO₂ is decreased below 60 mm Hg (8.0 kPa) (Fig. 14.2). The mechanism by which decreased oxygen availability increases CBF may be the same as that by which neural activation increases CBF, specifically, the local release of adenosine (118, 219). Adenosine antagonism by caffeine and theophylline decreases CBF and perhaps limits the ability of the cerebral vasculature to respond to lack of oxygen (27, 171). Recent evidence that low oxygen tension increases (and high oxygen tension decreases) the half-life of EDRF suggests that EDRF may mediate the CBF to changes in PAO₂ (82). However, NO synthetase inhibitors did not block increases in CBF during hypoxia (215). Increases in PAO₂ produce modest decreases in CBF (about 15% below normal at a PAO₂ of 600 mm Hg [80 kPa]).

Arterial Carbon Dioxide Tension (PACO₂). Changes in PACO₂ influence CBF through alterations of the brain extracellular H^+ concentration (143). As PACO₂ is acutely decreased from 40 to 20 mm Hg (5.3 to 2.7 kPa), CBF is halved (98) (Fig. 14.3). As PACO₂ increases from 40 to 80 mm Hg (5.3 to 10.7 kPa), CBF doubles (98). On the average, CBF increases 4% for every 1.0 mm Hg (0.13 kPa) increase in PACO₂ (98). Because rapid changes in PACO₂ produce rapid changes in both CBF and cerebral blood volume, acute hypercapnia may precipitate intracranial hypertension in patients with decreased intracranial compliance. If PACO₂ is changed

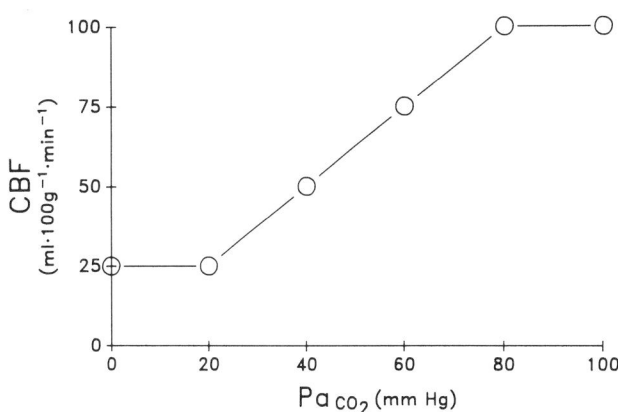

Figure 14.3. Response of cerebral blood flow (*CBF*) to changes in PACO₂. As PACO₂ is acutely decreased from 40 to 20 mm Hg, CBF is halved.

acutely and then maintained at a new level for 24 to 36 hours, CBF returns toward normal values as the brain extracellular H^+ concentration returns to normal (255).

Pressure Autoregulation. *Autoregulation* is the term applied to the process by which cerebral vascular resistance varies directly with changes in CPP (or MAP) to maintain a constant CBF. Under normal circumstances, autoregulation results in a nearly constant CBF over a CPP range from 60 to at least 150 mm Hg (see reference 213 for review) (Fig. 14.4). The myogenic theory, the most widely accepted mechanism of autoregulation, states that an increase in wall tension within a cerebral arteriole produces a reflex increase in smooth muscle tone, perhaps by changing smooth muscle cell membrane permeability to Ca^{2+} and other ions (32). Decreases in transmural pressure may lead to the release of EDRF and, therefore, autoregulatory vasodilation to hypotension (213). However, recent evidence that NO synthetase inhibitors do not block vasodilatory responses to hypotension argue against a role of EDRF in the autoregulatory responses to decreased MAP (59).

In contrast to the myogenic hypothesis, the metabolic hypothesis suggests that changes in perfusion pressure result in transient changes in local blood flow that alter the release of a vasodilator substance. Kontos et al (147) observed that vasodilation in pial vessels during hypotension could be prevented by local hyperoxia, suggesting an oxygen-sensitive mechanism. Reports that caffeine, an adenosine antagonist,

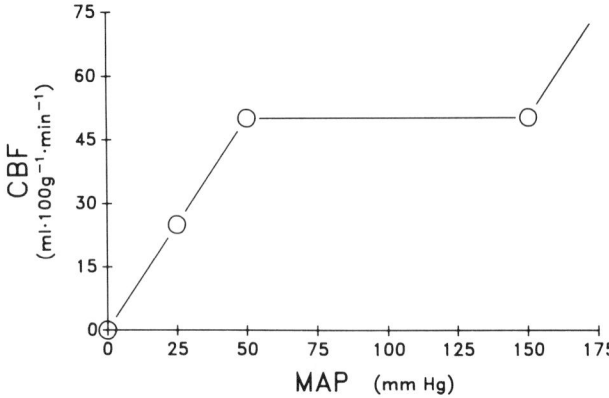

Figure 14.4. Response of cerebral blood flow (*CBF*) to changes in mean arterial pressure (MAP). Under normal circumstances, pressure autoregulation results in a nearly constant CBF over a MAP range from 60 to approximately 150 mm Hg.

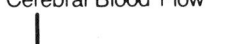
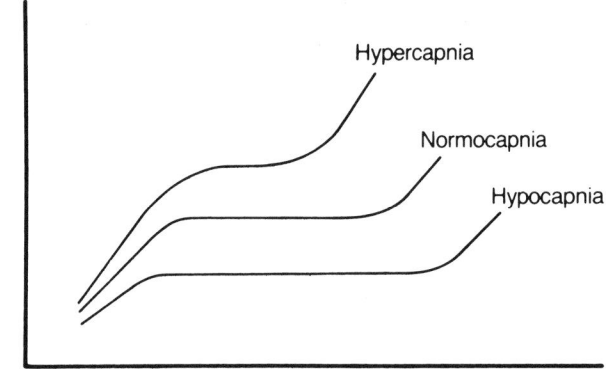

Figure 14.5. Cerebral autoregulation is impaired by coexistent cerebral vasodilatory stimuli. In the presence of hypercapnia, cerebral blood flow is higher and the upper limit of autoregulation is shifted to a lower mean blood pressure.

does not affect autoregulation argue against adenosine as the metabolic mechanism of autoregulation (218).

The lower limit of autoregulation is, in part, determined by the type of physiologic or pharmacologic change that produces the reduction in CPP. In hemorrhagic shock, for instance, the lower limit of autoregulation is shifted toward higher pressure, an effect that is abolished by cervical sympathectomy (77). In addition, the response to regulatory stimuli such as changes in $PACO_2$ may be blunted or abolished when CPP is near the lower threshold for autoregulation (10).

Cerebral autoregulation is impaired by coexistent cerebral vasodilatory stimuli. Hypercapnia severely impairs autoregulation (63, 106) (Fig. 14.5), an effect that diminishes as hypercapnia becomes more chronic (234). Cerebral vasodilators may impair autoregulation.

Cerebral Blood Flow Monitoring

The first quantitative method for the measurement of human CBF was the Kety-Schmidt technique (139), in which global CBF was calculated from the difference between the arterial and jugular bulb saturation curves of an inhaled, inert gas. Shortly thereafter, techniques were developed that were based upon the clearance from the brain of an intraarterially injected radioisotope such as ^{133}Xenon (^{133}Xe) as detected by scintillation counters positioned over the scalp (207). Subsequently, mathematical techniques were devised to correct clearance curves for recirculation of ^{133}Xe, thereby permitting measurement of CBF after inhaled (205) or intravenous administration of ^{133}Xe.

^{133}Xe clearance estimates of regional cortical CBF represent a powerful research technique. Nevertheless, despite the prognostic value of CBF measurements in patients who have suffered closed head injury, ^{133}Xe clearance has not been generally useful for primary diagnosis, surveillance, or goal-directed management. Among the obstacles to wider use are the cumbersome regulations governing the administration of radionuclides, the technically demanding nature of the measurements, and the sustained stable conditions (5 to 15 minutes) required to perform a single measurement.

Arterial flow velocity can be readily measured in intracranial vessels, especially the middle cerebral artery (MCA), in most patients using commercially available transcranial Doppler (TCD) equipment. TCD measurements offer useful diagnostic information in "detecting severe stenosis (>65%) in the major basal intracranial arteries; assessing patterns and extent of collateral circulation . . . evaluating and following vasoconstriction . . . especially after subarachnoid hemorrhage (SAH); detecting arteriovenous malformations . . . and assessing patients with suspected brain death" (7).

TCD assesses blood flow *velocity* rather than blood flow *per se*. Velocity is a function not only of blood flow rate but also of vessel diameter. Therefore, when CBF declines as a consequence of cerebral vasospasm after SAH, flow velocity in the MCA first increases, then decreases as vasospasm resolves (253). If the diameter of the MCA remains constant, changes in velocity are proportional to changes in CBF measured using ^{133}Xe clearance; however, intersubject differences in flow velocity correlate poorly with intersubject differences in CBF measured using ^{133}Xe clearance (25).

As a monitor for patients who are at risk for ischemic cerebral complications, TCD appears promising. Entirely noninvasive, TCD measurements can be repeated at frequent intervals or even applied continuously. However, further work is necessary to define those situations in which the excellent capacity for rapid trend monitoring can be exploited.

PHYSIOLOGIC REGULATION AND MONITORING OF INTRACRANIAL PRESSURE

Physiologic Regulation

ICP, normally less than 15 mm Hg (200 mm H_2O), reflects the volume of the three compartments—tissue, blood, and cerebrospinal fluid (CSF)—within the noncompliant skull. A small, gradual increase in any one of these compartments is partially compensated for by modest decreases in the volume of one or both of the other components (Fig. 14.6), and ICP remains within normal limits. Once a critical volume is reached, however, any further increments in intracranial volume produce large increments in ICP. Common causes of intracranial hypertension include intracranial neoplasms, subdural and epidural hematomas, intracerebral hemorrhage, acute hydrocephalus, and cerebral edema.

Intracranial Pressure Monitoring

Increased ICP may produce cerebral ischemia by reducing CPP. A sufficient reduction in CPP produces global cerebral ischemia, whereas herniation produces localized ischemic brain damage. Neurologic disease may increase intracranial volume and ICP via the mechanisms listed in Table 14.1. Although CBF cannot be inferred directly from knowledge of MAP and ICP, severe increases in ICP will reduce both CPP and CBF. In head-injured patients and children with Reye's syndrome, ICP monitoring is an accepted part of management (191, 248, 258). In other clinical situations, including severe central nervous system infections (14), anoxic cerebral insults, SAH (11), and hepatic failure, ICP monitoring has provided interesting descriptive information but has not been widely employed.

Clinicians have applied systematic, though institutionally specific, protocols for avoidance of intracranial hypertension and for reduction of ICP exceeding a therapeutic threshold of 15 or 20 mm Hg. Decisions about diuretics, hyperventilation, position changes, and additional diagnostic procedures may be influenced by ICP information. Although ICP monitoring has been credited by some investigators with an improving prognosis from acute closed head injury (191, 248), others question whether concurrent improvements in management, rather than ICP monitoring, explain the improvement (49). In patients who have nontraumatic coma, data defining the impact of ICP monitoring on outcome are more fragmentary and less convincing.

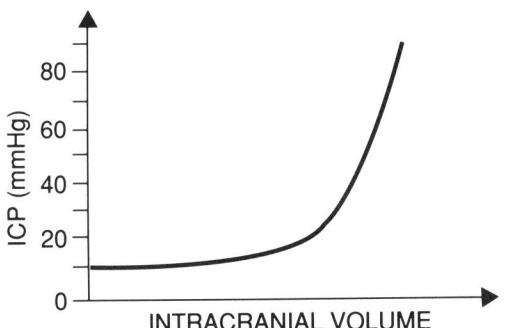

Figure 14.6. Relationship between intracranial volume and intracranial pressure (*ICP*). As the volume of one compartment (tissue, cerebrospinal fluid, or blood) increases, compensation initially is adequate; however, once a critical volume is obtained, intracranial pressure rapidly increases.

The equipment used for ICP monitoring has evolved progressively. The introduction of the subarachnoid screw facilitated effective, safe monitoring (297), despite occasional errors in measurement (190). Recently, many centers have begun to use fiberoptic catheters, which are less susceptible to short-term malfunction than the previous generation of fluid-filled, subdural catheters (53). Whenever ICP monitoring is employed, the potential complications, the most important of which is infection, must be considered (46). Intraventricular catheters carry a greater risk of infection than do subdural monitors.

Many investigators have attempted to enhance the clinical value of ICP monitoring. The pressure volume index (PVI) is calculated by removing or adding volume to cerebrospinal fluid through a ventricular cannula according to the following equation:

$$PVI = V/\log P_0 / P_m \text{ or } p \qquad (2)$$

where "V" denotes the volume withdrawn or injected; "P_0" denotes the pressure before withdrawing or injecting fluid; "P_m" denotes the minimum pressure following fluid withdrawal; and "P_p" denotes the peak pressure following volume addition. A lower PVI, implying reduced brain compliance, is associated with the subsequent development of intracranial hypertension and with poorer neurologic outcome (170). The critical value for PVI appears to be approximately 13 ml, below which level treatment is likely to be necessary either to reduce ventricular fluid pressure or to improve compliance (285). If the PVI is <10 ml, reduction of ICP is nearly always required. Robertson et al correlated the PVI with a computerized frequency analysis of the ICP waveform in 55 severely head-injured patients and determined that this continuous technique provided information that correlated very highly with the PVI, provided earlier evidence of changes in intracranial compliance than ICP alone, and did not require manipulation of intracranial fluid volume (237).

PATHOPHYSIOLOGY OF CEREBRAL INJURY

PATHOPHYSIOLOGY OF CEREBRAL ISCHEMIA

Overview

Cerebral ischemia refers to the inadequate delivery of oxygen to brain tissue, whether caused by inadequate oxygen supply, increased cerebral metabolic demand, or impaired tissue uptake. Cerebral ischemia can result from a critical reduction of any of the components of cerebral oxygen delivery

Table 14.1. Causes of Intracranial Hypertension

Cause	Mechanism
Intracranial mass lesions	Local expansion
Brain edema	Increased brain volume
Cellular (cytotoxic)	Cellular swelling secondary to hypoxia or ischemia
Vasogenic	Breakdown of blood-brain barrier with interstitial protein accumulation
Interstitial (hydrocephalic)	Block of CSF (reabsorption)
Brain engorgement (hyperemia)	Increased cerebral blood volume
Hypercarbia	Increased extracellular [H^+]
Hypoxia	Mechanism undetermined (adenosine?)
Hypertension	Impaired autoregulation
Improper head positioning	Obstruction of cerebral venous drainage

(CDO$_2$), including CBF, hemoglobin (Hgb) concentration, and arterial Hgb saturation (SAO$_2$). A fundamental mechanism of injury in many neurologic insults, cerebral ischemia even contributes to morbidity and mortality after closed head trauma. Although mechanical injury adequately explains most traumatic neurologic damage, histopathologic changes from cerebral ischemia frequently can be demonstrated postmortem (4).

Insufficient delivery of oxygen to the brain must be viewed in comparison with normal values for cerebral oxygen supply and demand (Table 14.2). The normal brain, representing about 2% of body mass, receives 15% of the cardiac output, and a greater amount of oxygen is extracted from blood perfusing the brain than from blood perfusing most other tissues. Consequently, jugular venous (JV) oxygen content (CJVO$_2$), tension (PJVO$_2$), and saturation (SJVO$_2$) are lower than systemic mixed venous oxygen content (CVO$_2$), tension (PVO$_2$), and saturation (SVO$_2$).

The brain is highly sensitive to oxygen deprivation for several reasons, including a high resting energy requirement, the absence of oxygen stores, and the absence of unperfused "reserve" capillaries. Brain tissue is not homogeneously vulnerable to ischemic damage. Certain regions, especially the arterial boundary zones, the cerebellum, the basal ganglia, and parts of the hippocampus, are especially prone to damage (93). Table 14.3 displays experimental thresholds at which ischemic dysfunction and injury occur. Below a CBF level of 8 to 10 ml·100 g^{-1}·min^{-1}, cell death becomes imminent unless flow is restored promptly. Clinical thresholds have been less well-established because clinical techniques lack the resolution of experimental techniques. However, the thresholds

based on data acquired during carotid endarterectomy appear to be similar to those observed in animals (Table 14.4) (256).

The deficit produced by an ischemic insult is dependent not only on the magnitude of flow reduction but also on the regionality and the duration of the event. Magnitude refers to whether the ischemia is complete, as in cardiac arrest, or partial, as in shock states or intracranial hypertension. Regionality describes whether the insult is focal, as in stroke, or global, as in cardiac arrest (Table 14.5). Describing ischemia in these terms helps to predict the likely response to therapeutic interventions. For instance, focal cerebral ischemia often involves an area of cell death surrounded by an ischemic penumbra of viable but nonfunctional tissue, much of which may be salvageable by appropriate treatment (263, 264). In experimental focal ischemia, hyperventilation increases cerebral vascular resistance in noninvolved areas, thereby redirecting flow to areas of viable but nonfunctioning tissue, a process termed an "inverse steal." Conversely, hypercapnia may "steal" flow from ischemic tissue to well-perfused tissue.

The duration of cerebral ischemia exerts an important effect on outcome. When CBF declines abruptly and severely, reversible neurologic dysfunction develops within seconds, and the insult becomes irreversible after a critical threshold of duration. In monkeys, paralysis develops if regional CBF declines below about 23 ml·100 g^{-1}·min^{-1} (194). Infarction of brain tissue, however, requires that CBF remain below 18 ml·100 g^{-1}·min^{-1} (194). Therefore, prolonged paralysis is potentially reversible if the paralysis is associated with CBF values of 18 to 23 ml·100g^{-1}·min^{-1}. The tolerable duration of more profound ischemia is inversely proportional to the severity of CBF reduction (i.e., CBF <10 ml·100 g^{-1}·min^{-1} for 2 hours results in infarction). Although conventional wisdom states that the human brain is irreversibly damaged if flow is completely interrupted for more than 4 minutes, recent studies in primates suggest that the brain can recover function after complete ischemia of 17 minutes or longer (151, 274).

Even if flow is restored to neural tissue after a period of ischemia, prolonged postischemic hypoperfusion typically follows (Fig. 14.7). This state, which is associated with a profound increase in cerebral vascular resistance, was first described by Ames and associates, who coined the term "no-reflow phenomenon" (8). The profound vasoconstriction is

Table 14.2. Normal Cerebral Oxygen Supply and Utilization[a]

Cerebral blood flow (CBF)	50 ml·100g^{-1}·min^{-1}
CMRO$_2$ = CBF × C(A-JV)O$_2$	3.5 ml·100g^{-1}·min^{-1}
C(A-JV)O$_2$	7.0 ml·100ml^{-1}
CAO$_2$	20 ml·100ml^{-1}
CJVO$_2$	13 ml·100ml^{-1}
SJVO$_2$	65%
PJVO$_2$	35 mm Hg
CDO$_2$ = CBF × CAO$_2$	10 ml·100g^{-1}·min^{-1}

[a] CMRO$_2$, metabolic consumption of oxygen; CAO$_2$, arterial oxygen content; CJVO$_2$, jugular bulb oxygen content; C(a-jv)O$_2$, cerebral arteriovenous oxygen content difference; SJVO$_2$, jugular bulb oxygen saturation; CDO$_2$, cerebral oxygen delivery.

Table 14.3. Cerebral Blood Flow (CBF) Thresholds During Cerebral Ischemia in Experimental Animals

CBF (ml·100g^{-1}·min^{-1})	Endpoint	Species	Reference
28	EEG slowing, reduced SEP amplitude	Cat	Gregory et al (96)
25	Histologic damage	Rat	Tyson et al (294)
23	Increased extracellular K$^+$	Gerbil	Mies et al (189)
20	Motor paralysis	Primate	Morawetz et al (194)
20	ATP levels decrease by 30%	Gerbil	Crockard et al (52)
20	Increased brain edema	Gerbil	Crockard et al (51)
20–10	Infarction in boundary zones	Cat	Graham et al (94)
15	Loss of spontaneous EEG activity	Primate	Morawetz et al (194)
15–12	SEP amplitude reduced or abolished	Primate	Branston et al (30)
15–10	Increased brain edema	Cat	Hossmann and Schuler (120)
12	Infarction if prolonged 1–2 hrs.	Primate	Morawetz et al (194)
10	Increased extracellular K$^+$ Decreased extracellular Ca^{2+}	Primate	Harris et al (107)
6	Increased extracellular K$^+$	Primate	Morawetz et al (194)

Table 14.4. Cerebral Blood Flow (CBF) Thresholds During Cerebral Ischemia in Humans

CBF (ml·100g⁻¹·min⁻¹)	Endpoint	Reference
35–29	Confusion, staring, yawning	Finnerty et al (74)
22–16	Significant EEG slowing	Sundt et al (281)
14	EEG flattening	Trojaborg and Boysen (293)

Table 14.5. Examples of Types of Cerebral Ischemia

Clinical Situation	Characteristics
Hypotension	Global, incomplete
Hypoxemia	Global, incomplete
Cardiac arrest	Global, complete
Stroke	Focal, incomplete
Subarachnoid hemorrhage with vasospasm	Focal, incomplete
Head trauma	Focal, incomplete

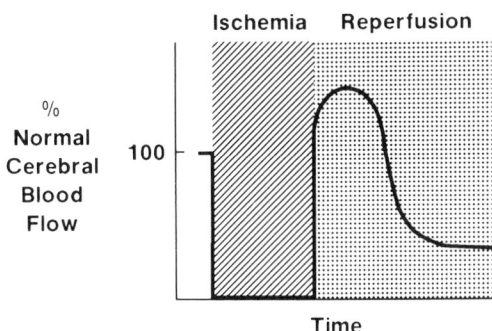

Figure 14.7. Following relief of global cerebral ischemia (represented by termination of a period of vascular occlusion), blood flow typically increases, then declines to a fraction of its preischemic value. Similar events occur following regional ischemia. (Reprinted with permission from Ref. 226.)

Table 14.6. Pathogenesis of Ischemic Injury

Neuronal Injury	Vascular Injury
Intracellular acidosis	Platelet aggregation
Membrane injury	Vasospasm
Release of excitatory neurotransmitters	Vasogenic edema
Intracellular calcium overload	
Intracellular (cytotoxic) edema	

associated with edema of surrounding tissue, increased intracellular Ca^{2+}, and evidence of increased tissue and intravascular levels of thromboxane A_2 (138, 228). Both the severity of postischemic vasoconstriction and the severity of cerebral edema are directly related to the duration of ischemia (289, 290).

Biochemical Consequences of Cerebral Ischemia

Metabolic Failure. Even a transient reduction in cerebral oxygenation rapidly depletes high-energy phosphate stores, thereby setting in motion a cascade of events that leads to neuronal and vascular injury (Table 14.6). Neuronal injury is characterized by intracellular acidosis, cell membrane dysfunction, release of excitatory neurotransmitters, intracellular calcium overload, and cytotoxic edema. Vascular injury, which is associated with an increase in vascular resistance resulting from platelet aggregation or vasospasm, and with disruption

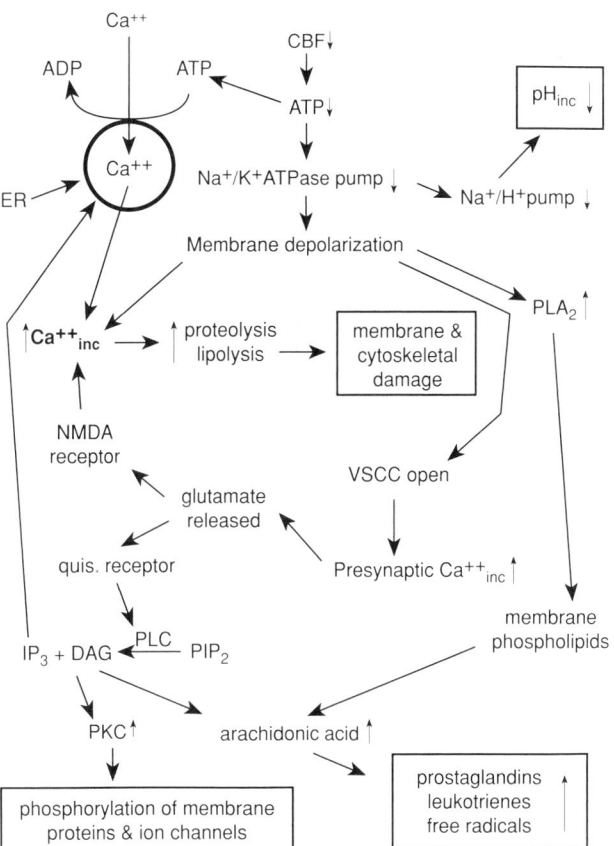

Figure 14.8. Biochemical events associated with ischemic injury to neural cells and the cerebral vasculature. A reduction in oxygen availability results in a decline in high-energy phosphate metabolites, ATP, and phosphocreatine and a shift to anaerobic metabolism. Cell membrane dysfunction results in ionic shifts, intracellular calcium overload, the release of excitatory neurotransmitters, and the production of oxygen free radicals and free fatty acids.

of the blood-brain barrier, causes plasma extravasation (vasogenic edema). All of the aforementioned are major features of ischemic injury to which many biochemical events contribute (Fig. 14.8). The failure of ATP and phosphocreatine production occurs quickly after tissue oxygen tension declines; rapid consumption leads to depletion of high-energy substrates (260). The failure of aerobic ATP production leads to an increase in anaerobic glycolysis. Although insufficient to maintain cell energy needs, anaerobic glycolysis nevertheless results in a rapid accumulation of lactic acid and a precipitous decline in intracellular pH (182). Acidosis further enhances free radical formation (261). Hyperglycemia, if present, may worsen intracellular acidosis and neurologic outcome by providing additional substrate for anaerobic glycolysis (91).

Subsequently, because of dysfunction of the ATP-dependent Na^+/K^+ transport system, extracellular Na^+ enters and intracellular K$^+$ leaks from the cell (93, 263, 264, 283). At a critical level of extracellular K$^+$, Ca^{2+} floods the cell (93, 263, 264, 283). Increasing concentrations of intracellular Ca^{2+} activate phospholipase A$_2$, which subsequently releases free fatty acids, including arachidonic acid, from cell membranes (260). The release of free fatty acids increases intracellular acidosis. If oxygen is available (as in incomplete ischemia or after reperfusion of ischemic tissue), arachidonate is metabolized, producing thromboxane A$_2$, leukotrienes, and free radicals (138, 140, 228, 309) (Fig. 14.9).

Glutamate, Calcium, and Excitotoxicity. The toxic effects of glutamate in the retina and brain were first established in 1957 and 1969, respectively (164, 208). Since then, considerable evidence has accumulated, indicating that glutamate-mediated, "excitotoxic" mechanisms contribute to ischemic damage to the central nervous system (for review see references 21 and 37). After ischemia, extracellular glutamate concentrations increase markedly in the hippocampus, a brain region that is particularly vulnerable to ischemic injury (21). Ischemia-induced glutamate release is believed to be from transmitter pools (calcium-dependent) as well as from cytosolic sources (calcium-independent) (199). Glutamate application in cell cultures produces morphologic damage (42) similar to that observed after cerebral ischemia (233). Although excessive swelling secondary to Na$^+$ and Cl$^-$ influx may contribute to glutamate-mediated cell death (245), increases in intracellular Ca^{2+} concentrations are more likely to play a central role (21, 266).

An understanding of the excitotoxic effects of glutamate requires a brief review of the different types of receptors at which glutamate acts. To date, at least five separate glutamate receptors, named for their specific agonists, have been identified (193) (Table 14.7). The most widely studied, the *N*-methyl-*D*-aspartate (NMDA) receptor, is connected to a Ca^{2+} channel that is normally blocked by Mg^{2+} ions. The kainate and α-amino-3-hydroxy-5-methylisoxazole-4-propionate (AMPA) (formerly quisqualate) receptors act as gates for channels for monovalent cations (i.e., K$^+$, Na$^+$). L-AP4-amino-4-phosphonobutyrate (L-AP4) and trans-1-aminocyclopentyl-1,3-dicarboxylate (ACPD) receptors, the least understood of the glutamate receptors, are believed to mediate presynaptic inhibition and phosphatidylinositol metabolism, respectively.

Briefly, Ca^{2+}-mediated excitotoxicity begins when glutamate, released as a consequence of ischemia, acts at kainate and AMPA receptors to allow Na$^+$ and K$^+$ influx and depolarization. Membrane depolarization releases Mg^{2+} ions, which normally block the NMDA channel. Glutamate then opens the NMDA-gated channel, allowing Ca^{2+} influx. It appears that glutamate also acts at the ACPD receptors to trigger the formation of inositol triphosphate (IP$_3$) from phosphatidylinositol (PI) (see below). IP$_3$ causes the release of intracellular Ca^{2+} stores from the endoplasmic reticulum, which increases cytoplasmic free Ca^{2+} without requiring the influx of extracellular Ca^{2+} (193).

However, glutamate is released not only by ischemia, a cell-damaging process, but also by nondestructive processes such as cortical spreading depression and long-term potentiation. Although cortical spreading depression and long-term potentiation also markedly increase cytosolic Ca^{2+} levels, cell death does not occur as it does after cerebral ischemia (266). Siesjo and Bengtsson (266) suggest that ischemia-induced, glutamate-mediated Ca^{2+} influx is deleterious because the absence of ATP prevents cells from using energy requiring membrane pumps to reestablish Ca^{2+} homeostasis. In addition, the lack of ATP prevents glutamate reuptake, thereby increasing extracellular glutamate levels (21). Thus, it appears that glutamate acts at multiple receptors to alter intracellular ion concentrations in a manner that leads to irreversible cell loss if depleted energy stores prevent active restoration of ionic homeostasis.

Phosphoinositide Metabolism. Considerable evidence suggests that many neurotransmitters (i.e., glutamate and acetylcholine) act through GTP-binding proteins (G-proteins) to activate several phospholipase C isozymes, which cleave phosphatidylinositol bisphosphate (PIP$_2$) to IP$_3$ and diacylglycerol (DAG) (23, 44, 75, 201). As described above, IP$_3$ increases cytosolic Ca^{2+} levels by releasing stored Ca^{2+}. IP$_3$ also causes protein kinase C (PKC) to translocate to cell membranes, where it is activated by DAG. Although the importance of PI hydrolysis in the pathophysiology of cerebral ischemia remains unclear, Lin et al (158) reported that PI metabolism increased in brain regions that sustained severe ischemic damage following experimental MCA occlusion.

Protein Kinase. PKC, an enzyme with a variety of substrates within the central nervous system and the cerebral vasculature, requires calcium, phospholipids (i.e., phosphatidylserine), and DAG to be fully activated (132). Within the central nervous system, PKC influences neuronal conductances to Ca^{2+}, Cl$^-$, and K$^+$, and increases neurotransmitter release (132). Although the relative contributions of these effects of PKC to the pathophysiology of cerebral ischemia are unknown, inhibition of PKC prevents postischemic neuronal damage in rodents (105). In addition to its action on neurons, PKC affects smooth muscle contraction. Rasmussen et al (235) suggested that prolonged vasoconstriction during cerebral vasospasm may result from phosphorylation of smooth muscle contractile proteins by PKC, based upon the evidence that

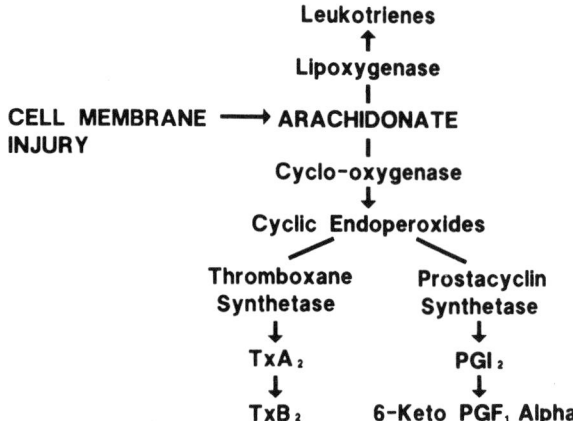

Figure 14.9. If oxygen is available (as in incomplete ischemia or following reperfusion of ischemic tissue), arachidonate is metabolized by cyclooxygenase and lipoxygenase, producing prostaglandins, thromboxane A$_2$, leukotrienes, and oxygen free radicals. The cyclic endoperoxides, substrate for thromboxane A$_2$ production, also constrict the cerebral vasculature and promote platelet aggregation.

Table 14.7. Glutamate Receptor Subtypes[a]

Receptor Type[b]	*Ion Channel*	*Putative Function*	*Agonist(s)*	*Antagonist(s)*
NMDA[c]	Na^{2+}, Ca^{2+}	LTP	NDMA	MK-801, PCP, ketamine, dextrophan, APV
Kainate	Na^{2+}	LTP	Kainic acid	DNQX, CNQX
AMPA	Na^{2+}	LTP	AMPA, quis.	DNQX, CNQX
APB	K^+	Presynaptic inhibition	APB	?
ACPD (metabotropic)	None	PI metabolism, neuronal NO synthesis	ACPD, quis.	AP3

[a] (Modified from Monaghan DT, Bridges RJ, Cotman CW: The excitatory amino acid receptors: their classes, pharmacology, and distinct properties in the function of the central nervous system. *Annu Rev Pharmacol Toxicol* 29:365–402, 1989.) (See also references 13 and 319.)

[b] Each receptor type represents a family rather than a single receptor. Therefore, the functions, agonists, or antagonists listed may pertain to individual receptors within of the family.

[c] NMDA = *N*-methyl-*D*-aspartate; LTP = long-term potentiation; ACPD = *trans*-1-amino-1,3-cyclopentane decarboxylate; PI = phosphoinositol; PCP = phencyclidine; AMPA = α-amino-3-hydroxy-5-methyl-4-isoxazolepropionic acid; DNQX = 6, 7-dinitroquinoxaline-2,3-dione; CNQX = 6-cyano-7-nitroquinoxaline-2,3-dione; quis. = quisqualate; APV = amino-phosphonovaleric acid; APB = L-2-amino-4-phosphonobutyrate; NO = nitric oxide.

PKC inhibitors reduced vascular spasm in isolated segments of canine basilar artery. Thus, it appears that activation of PKC may contribute to brain injury by affecting neuronal ion conductances as well as by directly influencing the cerebral vasculature.

Arachidonic Acid Metabolites and Free Radicals. Various agonist-receptor interactions result in the activation of phospholipases A_2 and C and the subsequent release of arachidonic acid. Arachidonate is converted to prostaglandins and thromboxanes by cyclooxygenase, to leukotrienes by lipoxygenases, to epoxyeicosatrienoic acid by cytochrome P-450, and to several hydroperoxy acids (i.e., HPETE) by autohoxidation (259). Arachidonate metabolites have a wide variety of functions in many organ systems (259). Of particular interest to central nervous system injury are thromboxane A_2 (TxA_2), a potent vasoconstrictor (309), and the leukotrienes C_4, D_4, and E_4, which together make up the slow-reacting substances of anaphylaxis (122). Leukotrienes, which increase after cerebral ischemia (309), stimulate contraction of vascular smooth muscle and increase vascular permeability. Most attempts to regulate arachidonate metabolism to reduce ischemic neuronal loss or changes in CBF have focused on the cyclooxygenase pathways. Inhibition of cyclooxygenase with ibuprofen improves postischemic CBF in dogs (97). Indomethacin, a cyclooxygenase inhibitor, reduces neuronal damage in the hippocampal CA_1 layer after ischemia in gerbils (247). Recent evidence that arachidonate and many of its metabolites affect ion channels in neurons and vascular smooth muscle (210, 259) and that arachidonate metabolites may serve as intracellular messengers (259) suggests that these agents may play a more complex role in the pathophysiology of cerebral ischemia than has previously been realized.

In addition to the products of arachidonate metabolism described earlier, the actions of cyclooxygenase and lipoxygenase on arachidonate produce oxygen free radicals, primarily the superoxide anion radical ($\cdot O_2^-$)(142). The superoxide radical dismutes spontaneously, or in the presence of superoxide dismutase, to form hydrogen peroxide (H_2O_2) and oxygen (265). In the presence of Fe^{2+}, H_2O_2 can combine with additional superoxide to form OH⁻, oxygen, and a hydroxyl radical ($\cdot OH^-$) (101). The unstable hydroxyl radical is extremely reactive and attacks membranes, DNA, and various proteins that may be bound to receptors and ion channels (265). Radical attacks on neuronal membrane polyunsaturated fatty acids

produce hydroperoxides which, in the presence of certain metals (i.e., iron), decompose to additional radicals. Lipid hydroperoxides can also produce other reactive agents that cross-link proteins and inactivate receptors and enzymes (252).

An additional target of the superoxide anion radical is NO, itself an oxygen radical, which combines with O_2^- to form the peroxynitrite anion, which rapidly decomposes into a highly reactive oxidant (18). Therefore, in addition to producing reactive species such as the hydroxyl radical, superoxide anion may inactivate NO, an important cerebral vasodilator. Although oxygen radicals have a short half-life and are difficult to detect (see references 19, 265, and 292), their role in the pathophysiology of cerebral ischemia has been investigated using agents that eliminate free radicals or reduce radical damage (292). Superoxide dismutase and catalase, which together convert superoxide anion radicals to O_2 and water, reduced infarct size in focal ischemia (160). U74006F, an experimental 21-aminosteroid believed to inhibit lipid peroxidation, reduced neuronal loss in a gerbil ischemia model (103).

Cerebral Acidosis. Brain intracellular acidosis, produced by cerebral ischemia, may lead to protein denaturation and enzymatic dysfunction. Recent evidence suggests that acidosis may impair ion homeostasis, thereby enhancing ischemia-induced increases in cytosolic Ca^{2+} levels (102). There is also evidence that acidosis decreases the binding capacity of iron-binding proteins, thereby increasing free iron concentrations and encouraging the production of hydroxyl radicals (165). Finally, it appears that acidosis impairs synaptic function and that lactic acidosis may do so irreversibly (298).

PATHOPHYSIOLOGY OF TRAUMATIC BRAIN INJURY

Overview

Secondary insults complicate the course of 48% of comatose head-injured patients (Table 14.8) (191). After cerebral trauma, hypoxia or hypotension that would normally be well tolerated may produce cerebral ischemia. After experimental brain injury, moderate hypoxemia (PAO_2 = 40 mm Hg [5.3 kPa]) or hypotension worsens neurologic deficits, disrupts cerebral high-energy phosphate stores, and generates intracerebral lactic acidosis (124, 125). In cats subjected to head injury, autoregulation was impaired (i.e., hemorrhagic hypotension reduced CBF more than in uninjured animals) (157).

Compensatory increases in CBF also failed to occur in response to hemodilution after hemorrhage in head-injured animals (58).

Severely head-injured patients usually demonstrate depressed $CMRO_2$, less markedly decreased CBF, and highly variable pressure autoregulation and carbon dioxide reactivity. In some patients, the decline in CBF appears to occur secondary to the reduction in $CMRO_2$ (i.e., CBF and $CMRO_2$ are coupled; in others, CBF may be less depressed than $CMRO_2$) (204) (see Fig. 14.1). Despite impaired autoregulation, CBF may not increase to normal levels even at high levels of CPP (198). Patients with coupled but reduced CBF and $CMRO_2$ may be vulnerable to excessive vasoconstriction during acute hyperventilation. Nearly 20% of patients develop a wide cerebral arteriovenous oxygen content difference ($A-VDO_2$) during hyperventilation, suggesting that hyperventilation therapy perhaps should be accompanied by an estimate of the adequacy of cerebral perfusion (204).

Because of the vulnerability of the acutely injured brain to hypotension, prompt reversal of hypovolemic shock accompanying acute head injury is essential. The selection of resuscitation fluid requires an understanding of the relationship between intravenous fluids and brain water and ICP. The blood-brain barrier, because of its relative impermeability to sodium, enhances the importance of changes in osmolality and reduces the importance of alterations in oncotic pressure (318). Hypotonic solutions (including lactated Ringer's solution) increase brain water and ICP. Lactated Ringer's solution is more likely to increase brain water content than are fluids such as 0.9% saline, 6.0% hydroxyethyl starch in 0.9% saline, or 5.0% albumin in 0.9% saline, all of which have higher osmolality (291). Accordingly, rapid resuscitation with 6.0% hydroxyethyl starch in 0.9% saline increased ICP less than did hemodynamically comparable resuscitation using hypotonic lactated Ringer's solution (222). In experimental animals, resuscitation with hypertonic (3.0 to 7.5%) saline solutions was associated with lower ICP than was resuscitation with isotonic or slightly hypotonic fluids (99, 227). Less hypertonic solutions (250 mEq/liter Na^+), infused at a rate sufficient to maintain stable cardiac output after resuscitation in dogs, were not appreciably superior to slightly hypotonic solutions (305). Glucose-containing solutions generally should be avoided. Hyperglycemia has been associated with poorer neurologic outcome in head-injured patients (149, 225).

The development of sound animal models of closed head injury should facilitate the development of more effective clinical strategies. The feline fluid-percussion model developed at the Medical College of Virginia is a well-characterized model that duplicates many of the electrophysiologic (95), vascular (157), and systemic physiologic features of human closed head injury. Fluid-percussion injury produces transient increases in CBF that return to control levels within 30 minutes without evidence of posttraumatic ischemia (56). This finding is consistent with reports that CBF is reduced in some head-injured patients, but seldom to ischemic levels in the absence of extensive mass lesions (150). However, the normally tight coupling between CBF and metabolism may be impaired after injury. Changes in the relationship between CBF and metabolism in discrete brain regions (hippocampus) occur after low-level fluid-percussion injury in cats, and these changes may affect regional energy metabolism (314). Thus, animal models can provide important information contributing to a better understanding of the mechanisms underlying human brain injury. Other studies of the effects of fluid-percussion injury on cerebral metabolic activity using the autoradiographic 2-deoxyglucose technique (270) led Hayes and coworkers (112) to the hypothesis that a cholinergic site in the feline brainstem, when activated by fluid-percussion injury, produces transient posttraumatic unconsciousness. This region was subsequently shown to be a complex group of nuclei that may also mediate spinal motor and sensory function (137).

The fluid-percussion injury model has recently been adapted for use in rats (60), allowing metabolic and physiologic effects to be correlated with behavioral effects of closed concussive brain injury. Fluid-percussion injury has been found to suppress reflexes and to impair motor activity (e.g., balancing and walking on a narrow wooden beam) (113). The cholinergic antagonist scopolamine, whether administered before or after injury, reverses these traumatic effects on reflexes and motor activity (111, 166).

Biochemical Effects of Traumatic Brain Injury

Excitatory Amino Acids in Trauma. In 1989, Jenkins et al (128) suggested that excitotoxicity may play an important role in central nervous systemic damage after traumatic brain injury (TBI), especially if TBI is followed by even mild cerebral ischemia (130). There is now considerable evidence that the release of abnormal levels of excitatory amino acids (i.e., glutamate) contributes to the pathophysiology of TBI (70, 129, 136, 175). In rodents, extracellular glutamate levels increase markedly after TBI (70, 136). Glutamate receptor antagonists such as phencyclidine (129), dextrorphan (70), or MK-801 (175) reduce brain edema and improve neurologic scores after TBI. Glutamate-mediated excitotoxicity in ischemia is believed to involve increases in intracellular Ca^{2+} concentrations

Table 14.8. Influence of Remediable Causes of Secondary Injury on Outcome after Head Injury

Secondary Insult	Definition	Poor outcome (%)[a,b]
Hypoxemia	$PAO_2 < 60$ mm Hg	59
Hypotension	SBP < 90 mm Hg	65
Anemia	Hct < 30%	62
Hypercarbia	$PACO_2 > 45$ mm Hg	78
Intracranial hypertension	ICP > 20, reducible	45
	ICP > 20, not reducible	95

[a] (Modified from Miller JD, Butterworth JF, Gudeman SK, et al: Further experience in the management of severe head injury. J Neurosurg 54:289, 1981, with permission.)

[b] Poor outcome = severe disability, persistent vegetative state, or death. SBP = systolic blood pressure; Hct = hematocrit; ICP = intracranial pressure.

Table 14.9. Experimental Strategies for Reduction of Ischemic Injury

Increase cerebral blood flow
  Hemodilution—dextran, albumin
  Alter blood rheology—pentoxifylline
  Decrease cerebral vascular tone—calcium entry blockers
  Inhibit thromboxane production
    Thromboxane synthetase inhibitors
    Cyclooxygenase inhibitors
Decrease CMRO$_2$
  Seizure control
    Barbiturates
    Phenytoin
    Hypothermia
  Electrophysiologic suppression—barbiturates
Decrease cerebral edema; decrease ICP
  Vasogenic edema—glucocorticoids
  Decrease water in normal brain—mannitol
  Decrease CSF production—furosemide

Decrease cell membrane injury
  Inhibit phospholipase—glucocorticoids
  Inhibit free radical production—superoxide dismutase
Antagonize intracellular calcium overload—calcium
  entry blockers
Decrease intracellular acidosis
  THAM
  Dextrose-free fluids
Antagonize excitatory amino acids
Reverse effects of endogenous opioids
Influence cell recovery—gangliosides

---

(266) (see above), but the effects of increases of extracellular glutamate concentrations on intracellular Ca^{2+} after TBI are less clear. TBI reduces brain tissue Mg^{2+} concentrations (295), and the decline in intracellular Mg^{2+} levels correlates with severity of neuronal injury. McIntosh et al (174) reported that Mg^{2+} deficiency exacerbates and Mg^{2+} supplementation reduces behavioral deficits after TBI. Mg^{2+} ions are important for a number of critical cellular processes (see reference 174), including a voltage-dependent blockade of agonist-operated Ca^{2+} channels (i.e., NMDA receptors) (202). The absence of Mg^{2+} potentiates the activity of glutamate and aspartate on NMDA and kainate receptors (200), suggesting that trauma-induced decreases in intracellular Mg^{2+} concentrations may exacerbate the effects of glutamate released after TBI.

Arachidonic Acid Metabolites and Free Radicals. Experimental TBI increases phospholipase C activity (302), resulting in increases in brain tissue prostaglandin levels in cats (67) and rats (57). 12-HETE, a lipoxygenase product, also increases after TBI in cats (66). Increased cyclooxygenase and lipoxygenase activity is associated with generation of oxygen free radicals (see above and reference 144), with impaired cerebral vascular reactivity (301) and damage to the cerebral vascular endothelium (145). Kontos et al (146) reported that arachidonate interferes with the generation or release of EDRF, probably caused by endothelial damage by the hydroxyl radical. Endothelial damage and impaired vascular reactivity can be restored after TBI using free radical scavengers and cyclooxygenase inhibitors (65, 301). These data indicate that oxygen free radicals play an important role in the pathophysiology of TBI as well as cerebral ischemia.

PHARMACOLOGY OF CEREBRAL PROTECTION

EXPERIMENTAL APPROACHES

Many drugs and strategies are used clinically or are under investigation for the treatment of cerebral ischemia, cerebral trauma, and intracranial hypertension. Table 14.9 summarizes the potential abilities of a variety of drugs and physiologic interventions to limit the severity of ischemia by increasing CBF or decreasing CMRO$_2$, decrease cerebral edema, reduce

cell membrane injury, antagonize intracellular calcium overload, decrease intracellular acidosis, limit the toxicity of excitatory amino acids, antagonize the effects of endogenous opioids, and influence neural cell recovery using gangliosides.

Increase Cerebral Oxygen Delivery

CDO$_2$, the product of CBF and CAO$_2$, can be increased by increasing any of its components, assuming that the other components do not decrease simultaneously. CBF can be increased by physiologic interventions, such as hypercapnia, or by cerebral vasodilators. Until recently, no clinically available cerebral vasodilator demonstrated a beneficial effect in the acute or chronic management of reduced flow in the diseased cerebral circulation. However, the advent of the calcium entry blockers, such as nimodipine, suggests the possibility of effective therapy. Nimodipine appears to dilate preferentially the cerebral vasculature in intact animals and in animals with focally ischemic brain regions (109, 173, 184), thereby providing the rationale for its use in stroke and in clinical states, such as vasospasm after SAH, associated with pathologic cerebral vasoconstriction.

Cerebral perfusion also can be improved by changing blood rheology, either by inducing hemodilution or by the use of drugs. In brain tissue distal to an experimental MCA occlusion, hypervolemic hemodilution with dextran significantly improves CBF (312, 313). If CDO$_2$ increases, tissue with borderline viability may be preserved. Pentoxifylline, which alters blood rheology and improves flow in tissue perfused by partially occluded vessels, recently became the first drug to receive approval from the Food and Drug Administration for the symptomatic treatment of intermittent claudication resulting from peripheral arterial occlusive disease (273). An oral dose of 400 mg three times daily appears to limit the incidence of recurrent transient ischemic attacks (116). Chronic oral administration of pentoxifylline improves CBF in patients with chronic cerebrovascular disease (108), but as yet no data document clinical neurologic or neuropsychologic improvement associated with increased CBF.

Cerebral Metabolic Depression

In diseases such as stroke and postischemic hypoperfusion in which CDO$_2$ may be inadequate to meet oxygen demand, depression of metabolic demand theoretically should limit the extent of brain injury. Therefore, control of seizures, which markedly increase $CMRO_2$, and fever, which increases $CMRO_2$ approximately 7.0% per degree Celsius, should preserve ischemically threatened brain. Some of the therapeutic effect of barbiturates and phenytoin in experimental ischemia may be attributable to seizure prevention. Barbiturates, in large intravenous doses (sodium thiopental, 20 to 30 mg/kg; sodium pentobarbital, 30 mg/kg; phenobarbital, 60 mg/kg), by profoundly suppressing the electrical activity of the brain, reduce both $CMRO_2$ and CBF by approximately 50% (187). Depression of $CMRO_2$ by barbiturates provides protection in animal models of incomplete focal cerebral ischemia (188, 267). Because barbiturates also improve intracranial hypertension, they have been widely used as therapy for intracranial hypertension associated with closed head trauma, Reye's syndrome, and near-drowning. At the present time, however, despite the unequivocal observation that barbiturate loading reduces ICP, there is little evidence that barbiturates materially affect survival in any of those disorders.

Another conventional means of decreasing cerebral metabolism is through reduction of body temperature. Moderate decreases in brain and body temperature have been reported to be protective in cerebral ischemia (43, 304), trauma (47), and cardiac arrest (155). In both rats (192) and gerbils (304), hypothermia to 35°C (cranial and rectal temperatures) during ischemia reduces, and hypothermia to 33°C prevents, hippocampal neuronal damage. Clifton et al (47) reported that brain temperatures of 30°C but not 36°C or 33°C significantly reduced mortality and behavioral deficits in rats after experimental TBI. Mild hypothermia (34 to 36°C) during and after cardiac arrest in dogs improves neurologic outcome (155).

Hypothermia is not uniformly effective under all circumstances. Chopp et al (43) reported that postischemic hypothermia (rectal temperature 34°C) reduced hippocampal neuron loss after 8 minutes but not after 12 minutes of forebrain ischemia. In contrast, Welsh and Harris (303) observed that postischemic hypothermia (33°C and 23°C, rectally and cranially) did not protect gerbils from hippocampal cell loss after 5 minutes of forebrain ischemia.

The mechanisms underlying the protective effects of hypothermia are likely related, in part, to decreased metabolic requirements. However, there is now evidence that hypothermia decreases tissue glycine concentrations and decreases release of excitatory neurotransmitters after cerebral ischemia (12, 39). Glycine facilitates the activity of glutamate at agonist operated Ca^{2+} channels (266), and reductions in both tissue glycine and excitatory amino acid levels would serve to reduce neuronal damage resulting from ischemia-induced Ca^{2+} influx.

Decrease Cerebral Edema

If sufficiently severe, brain injury resulting from ischemia, tumor, trauma, inflammation, or metabolic causes may produce cerebral edema. Three types of cerebral edema have been described experimentally (76), although in individual patients more than one type of edema may be present. Interstitial edema occurs with hydrocephalus. Vasogenic edema, which accompanies intracranial tumors, is associated with increased permeability of the blood-brain barrier to protein.

The most clearly established use of glucocorticoids in neurologic intensive care is to treat the vasogenic edema associated with brain tumors and brain abscesses (236). Cytotoxic edema, which accompanies hypoxic or traumatic injury, is characterized by cellular swelling and is not responsive to glucocorticoids (76). Therefore, glucocorticoids appear to be ineffective in closed head injury (249) and in focal and global cerebral ischemia (117, 153).

Diuretics are commonly used to reduce the intracranial hypertension associated with cerebral edema. Osmotic diuretics acutely reduce brain volume, primarily by removing water osmotically from uninjured brain in which the blood-brain barrier is intact. Mannitol and other osmotic diuretics also reduce blood viscosity and may improve microcirculatory flow (117, 198). This effect, in conjunction with the reduction in ICP produced by osmotic diuretics, limits the extent of infarction in animal models of focal ischemia (117, 159). Furosemide, 20 to 40 mg intravenously, reduces ICP acutely in animal models and in patients (50, 236). Although the initial effect is to reduce brain water, furosemide also inhibits the elaboration of CSF, thereby reducing another of the three components of intracranial volume.

Decrease Cell Membrane Injury

Glucocorticoids commonly are given in an attempt to decrease cell membrane injury or to stabilize ischemic cell membranes. The proposed mechanisms of action of glucocorticoids include facilitated clearance of vasogenic edema, stabilization of cellular membranes, and inhibition of the release of arachidonate from cell membranes.

Research into antiinflammatory drugs has produced a variety of agents that limit the production of the by-products of arachidonic acid metabolism. In vitro, glucocorticoids inhibit phospholipase A_2. Cyclooxygenase inhibitors, such as indomethacin and ibuprofen, can virtually eliminate the production of the cyclic endoperoxides, the precursor molecules from which many endogenous prostaglandins are synthesized. Recent data suggest that, after experimental ischemic injury, ibuprofen, 12.5 mg/kg administered intravenously, suppresses the release of thromboxane A_2 in the cerebral vasculature, an effect that is associated with increased postischemic blood flow (97). In rats subjected to four-vessel occlusion, the cyclooxygenase inhibitor zomepirac sodium, 5 mg/kg intravenously, improved postischemic CBF and electroencephalographic (EEG) recovery (277). Since cyclooxygenase inhibitors also inhibit the production of prostacyclin, an extremely potent cerebral vasodilator, Hallenbeck and Furlow (104) combined indomethacin with prostacyclin and heparin and markedly improved regional CBF after an experimental ischemic insult. In theory, specific thromboxane synthetase inhibitors should prevent the production of thromboxane A_2, while permitting continued production of vasodilator prostaglandins such as prostacyclin. However, thromboxane synthetase inhibitors have failed to improve CBF after either global or regional ischemic insults (196, 228), possibly because the cyclic endoperoxides, which also exert cerebral vasoconstrictive and platelet aggregatory effects, accumulate if the more distal enzymatic pathway is blocked (Fig. 14.9) (78, 250). Finally, investigators have speculated that nimodipine or other calcium entry blockers might act, in part, by inhibiting calcium-mediated activation of phospholipase A_2.

Antagonism of Intracellular Calcium Overload

The cerebral effects of calcium entry blockers are undergoing extensive investigation, suggesting that this promising class of drugs may ultimately be widely employed in neurologic disease. The calcium entry blockers are a diverse group of drugs, the potential therapeutic effects of which may be related to nonspecific cerebral vasodilation, blockade of the cellular toxicity of calcium (such as activation of phospholipase A_2), or antagonism of the vascular effects of increased calcium release (postischemic hypoperfusion). Consequently, nimodipine has therapeutic potential for managing focal stroke, cerebral vasospasm associated with SAH, and the reduction in CBF that occurs after cardiac arrest.

Reversal of Intracellular Acidosis

Bicarbonate, the buffer most commonly employed to increase systemic pH, crosses the intact blood-brain barrier to a minimal extent and is therefore ineffective for the management of brain intracellular acidosis. In addition, exogenous bicarbonate increases $PACO_2$ if minute ventilation remains constant; because carbon dioxide does cross the blood-brain barrier, intracellular acidosis may be aggravated. The buffer trishydroxymethylamino methane (THAM) penetrates the blood-brain barrier and may produce intracellular alkalinization after neural injury (243). Further studies are needed to characterize the potential efficacy of THAM in a variety of neurologic insults. In areas of low flow resulting from either pathologic vasoconstriction or obstructive vascular lesions, adequate delivery of the intracellular buffer might require combination with cerebral vasodilator therapy.

Limit the Toxicity of Excitatory Amino Acids

Considerable evidence suggests that one critical mechanism of ischemic and traumatic brain injury is the release of excitatory amino acids (152, 263, 264). Consequently, drugs that effectively block the adverse effects of excitatory amino acids might improve outcome in patients with cerebral ischemia or brain trauma. The effects of experimentally available NMDA and non-NMDA receptor antagonists recently have been reviewed (176). One of the more extensively studied NMDA antagonists, MK-801, provided protection against cerebral hypoperfusion after incomplete focal cerebral ischemia (181). However, such compounds must be screened carefully to exclude toxic effects from the drugs themselves (209). Some less severe side effects, such as sedation from MK-801, may also reduce the utility of some of these agents. Despite these concerns, sufficient experience exists with several NMDA antagonists, including MK-801, dextrorphan, dextromethorphan, and ketamine, that preliminary clinical trials appear to be warranted (5, 36) and have been initiated.

Antagonize Endogenous Opioids

A full review of the extensive literature regarding the role of endogenous opioids in the pathogenesis of ischemia and trauma exceeds the scope of this chapter. However, conventional opiate antagonists have yet to find a significant role in clinical management of cerebral ischemia or trauma, despite experimental data suggesting that they should be effective (71, 110, 119). Perhaps more promising are thyrotropin releasing hormone (TRH) and TRH analogues, which once were thought to function as opiate antagonists but now are known to exert a variety of physiologic effects independent of endogenous opioids (69, 71, 119).

Preserve Neural Cells and Cell Function Using Gangliosides

Various monosialoganglioside derivatives appear to protect ischemic brain against injury. Although the mechanisms of protection remain controversial, nonspecific membrane protection and reduction of brain edema appear to be involved (212). In experimental animals, cellular survival, electrophysiologic function, and cognitive function appear to be better preserved if gangliosides or their derivatives are given (154, 211, 254). Preliminary clinical trials appear to confirm the animal data (41, 212).

CLINICAL APPLICATIONS

Many neurologic diseases, particularly those involving cerebral ischemia, have resisted attempts at therapy. Today, there is reason for cautious optimism that the extent of neurologic injury produced by a given insult ultimately may be reduced. Much of that optimism is based on the introduction of new drugs, such as the calcium entry blockers, and on increasing research into the biochemical basis of neural injury produced by ischemia and reperfusion. Intracranial hypertension, a problem contributing to adverse outcome in several neurologic diseases, usually can be controlled using established protocols. Encouraging progress has been accomplished in the management of stroke. Intense interest has been focused on the neurologic sequelae of cardiac arrest, the management of cerebral vasospasm after SAH, and the mechanisms of permanent neurologic dysfunction occurring after closed head injury. The effects of hemorrhagic shock and resuscitation on CBF and cerebral metabolism have received attention, at least in part, because of the common association between closed head injury and hypovolemia in patients who have sustained vehicular trauma. Recently, investigators have directed attention at the high incidence of cognitive deficits after cardiac surgery.

Control of Intracranial Hypertension

Control of increased ICP depends on effective control of cerebral tissue volume, cerebral blood volume, and CSF volume (Table 14.10). The therapy of intracranial hypertension must either decrease the volume of the component that caused the original problem (e.g., tumor or hematoma removal) or decrease the volume of one of the other components (Fig. 14.10). On an emergent basis, intracranial hypertension is most quickly treated by reducing cerebral blood volume, usually by intentionally using acute hyperventilation to decrease CBF.

Table 14.10. Strategies for Controlling ICP [a]

Strategy	Mechanism
Endotracheal intubation	Prevention of hypoxia and hypercarbia
Neuromuscular blockade[b]	Prevention of coughing and straining
Passive hyperventilation[b]	Reduction of CBF[a] and cerebral blood volume
Fluid restriction[b]	Limitation of cerebral edema
Head positioning[b]	Facilitation of cerebral venous drainage
Osmotic diuresis	Reduction of brain water
Sedation/narcosis[b]	Reduction of CMRO$_2$[a], limitation of CBF response to noxious stimuli
Fever control	Limitation of CMRO$_2$
Barbiturates[c]	Reduction of CMRO$_2$, CBF, ICP [a]
Glucocorticoids[c]	Limitation of cerebral edema
Decompressive craniectomy[b]	Increase space for brain expansion

[a] ICP = intracranial pressure; CBF = cerebral blood flow; CMRO$_2$ = cerebral metabolic rate for oxygen.
[b] Controversial.
[c] Little or no demonstrable benefit.

Reduction of Cerebral Tissue Volume. Brain tissue volume can be reduced medically or surgically. Medical control conventionally is based on glucocorticoid administration, fluid restriction, and the use of osmotic diuretics. Glucocorticoids appear to be ineffective in reducing cerebral edema in patients with closed head injury (249) and after cardiac arrest (127), and they are of questionable value after stroke. Chronic fluid restriction does not effectively reduce brain tissue volume. Osmotic diuretics, on the other hand, effectively reduce brain tissue volume by dehydrating normal brain tissue. Mannitol reduces ICP for 3 to 4 hours. An i.v. bolus of 1.0 to 1.5 g/kg provides brain decompression in anticipation of surgical mass removal (i.e., tumor removal or hematoma drainage). Smaller doses (0.25 to 0.5 g/kg) have been used effectively for maintenance reduction of ICP in patients with closed head trauma. Because its effects depend on the integrity of the blood-brain barrier, mannitol may be less effective in patients with severe, diffuse brain injury.

Reduction of Cerebral Blood Volume. Cerebral blood volume may be reduced by reducing CBF or by facilitating cerebral venous drainage. Endotracheal intubation and mechanical ventilation facilitate maintenance of adequate gas exchange, thereby limiting the likelihood of inadvertent increases in CBF resulting from hypoxemia or hypercarbia. Adequate sedation and analgesia, by limiting the effects of brain stimulation on CMRO$_2$ and CBF, are useful in the control of ICP. Patients with multiple injuries, including closed head trauma, may require potent narcotic analgesic agents in sufficient doses to control pain if intracranial hypertension is to be managed effectively. In such narcotized patients, control of ventilation is essential. Passive hyperventilation is commonly used to reduce CBF, both as a sustained therapeutic measure and as an acute response to sudden increases in ICP. Hyperventilation, which reduces ICP by reducing cerebral blood volume, is most commonly used; however, limited attention has been paid to the maintenance of adequate CBF during therapeutic hyperventilation. Mechanical hyperventilation frequently reduces SJVO$_2$ below acceptable average levels (204), perhaps explaining the adverse effects of hyperventilation on outcome in patients with head trauma (see below).

Blood pressure represents a particularly difficult problem in patients with intracranial hypertension. Autoregulation is attenuated or abolished in areas of injured brain. Consequently, decreased systemic blood pressure may reduce CBF and worsen cerebral ischemia. Increased blood pressure may, in some patients, increase CBF and cerebral blood volume, thereby increasing ICP. Pharmacologic reduction of systemic blood pressure may have adverse effects on intracranial hemodynamics. Nitroprusside has been associated both with cerebral ischemia resulting from rapid blood pressure reduction (100) and with intracranial hypertension (40, 167). In awake individuals, sodium nitroprusside reduces MAP, CBF, and PJVO$_2$ (114, 115). Although sodium nitroprusside may decrease CBF, it increases ICP, apparently by increasing cerebral blood volume. Rapid administration of nitroprusside is likely to cause an untoward increase in ICP when intracranial compliance is reduced (40, 167). Nitroglycerin, like nitroprusside, may increase ICP (38). When nitroprusside or nitroglycerin is used to reduce blood pressure in patients with intracranial lesions, the net effect on ICP is the result of reduced cerebral blood volume in injured areas that do not autoregulate and increased cerebral blood volume in intact regions where the drug therapy itself inhibits autoregulation. Other antihypertensive drugs also influence CBF. The calcium entry blocker nifedipine maintains or increases CBF (24). Labetalol, a combination β- and α-antagonist, causes little change in blood flow in hypertensive patients (214).

Reduction of Cerebrospinal Fluid Volume. CSF volume can be reduced mechanically, through dehydration, or by pharmacologic intervention. CSF can be withdrawn through intraventricular catheters, which are placed more commonly in patients who have intraventricular hemorrhage and less commonly in other situations involving intracranial hypertension. Dehydration decreases the production of CSF. Drugs such as furosemide; acetazolamide, 250 mg orally or intravenously; and digoxin also reduce CSF production, although they are uncommonly used in acute situations.

Stroke

Recent advances suggest that the neurologic morbidity produced by stroke may be modified effectively. Theoretically, clinical stroke is the expression of brain ischemia that does not uniformly involve threatened tissue. In the center, or focus, of the ischemic zone, regional CBF is so severely reduced that cells cannot recover viability. In penumbral tissue surrounding the central focus, regional perfusion is reduced, but cell viability potentially can be preserved if perfusion is increased, if metabolism is reduced, or if cell-damaging processes can be slowed or stopped (262). Regional perfusion theoretically could be increased by increasing perfusion pressure, by reducing blood viscosity (to increase flow through partially obstructed or collateral vessels), or by vasodilating or otherwise relieving obstruction of constricted segments.

Induced hypertension potentially can increase CBF in areas of focal ischemia distal to partially obstructed cerebral arteries. Since ischemia abolishes autoregulation in the involved areas, flow may be increased by an increase in MAP. Administration of vasopressor drugs has improved neurologic status in some anecdotal reports of patients after ischemic events (308). However, conclusive evidence of the clinical efficacy of induced hypertension requires additional study.

Hemodilution, particularly if combined with hypervolemia, has been studied extensively in patients with stroke. However, clinical application has been impeded by concern regarding two physiologic risks. First, hypervolemia may produce cardiac failure or myocardial ischemia in patients who have coexisting cerebrovascular and coronary occlusive disease. Second, although flow may be improved slightly by moderate hemodilution, the reduction in oxygen-carrying capacity may prevent any improvement in local oxygen delivery.

In patients with acute stroke, normovolemic hemodilution increases CBF and improves EEG activity (311). However, the effectiveness of hemodilution in clinical stroke remains somewhat controversial, in part because of the risk associated with aggressive volume expansion of patients who often are elderly and have associated cardiovascular disease. The Scandinavian Stroke Study Group, which randomized 373 patients to receive either conventional therapy or normovolemic hemodilution after stroke, demonstrated an increased incidence of cardiovascular complications and an increased early mortality among hemodiluted patients (251). The Italian Acute Stroke Study Group randomized 1267 patients to receive conventional therapy or normovolemic hemodilution and found no difference in outcome (126). However, both studies were constrained by the cardiovascular risk of volume expansion. In contrast, the Hemodilution in Stroke Study Group used invasive cardiovascular monitoring to guide hypervolemic hemodilution and increase cardiac output with pentastarch in patients with acute ischemic stroke (287). Although overall mortality and neurologic outcome were not superior in the hemodilution group, neurologic outcome apparently was improved in patients who were entered into the trial within 12 hours of the onset of stroke and those who had an increase of cardiac output ≥10% of baseline.

Calcium entry blockers appear to improve CBF and exert a protective effect on focally ischemic brain distal to mechanically occluded blood vessels (183, 184). Both CBF and intracellular pH are improved by nimodipine, suggesting a possible therapeutic role in human stroke. Several major clinical trials (87, 88, 286) appear to demonstrate that nimodipine produces a slight but measurable improvement in outcome. The major potential drawbacks of nimodipine relate to its systemic hypotensive effects and its tendency to increase ICP. Theoretically, titration of nimodipine, coupled with support of blood volume and blood pressure, should maximally improve regional CBF in patients at minimal risk for intracranial hypertension.

Because extensive experimental results suggest that prostaglandin I_2 antagonizes the adverse effects of thromboxane A_2 on cerebral vascular tone and platelet aggregation, an extensive study was performed to determine whether the infusion of prostacyclin would ameliorate acute stroke (121). The data suggest that prostacyclin is not effective, a finding in concert with the lack of efficacy of prostacyclin alone in experimental cerebral ischemia.

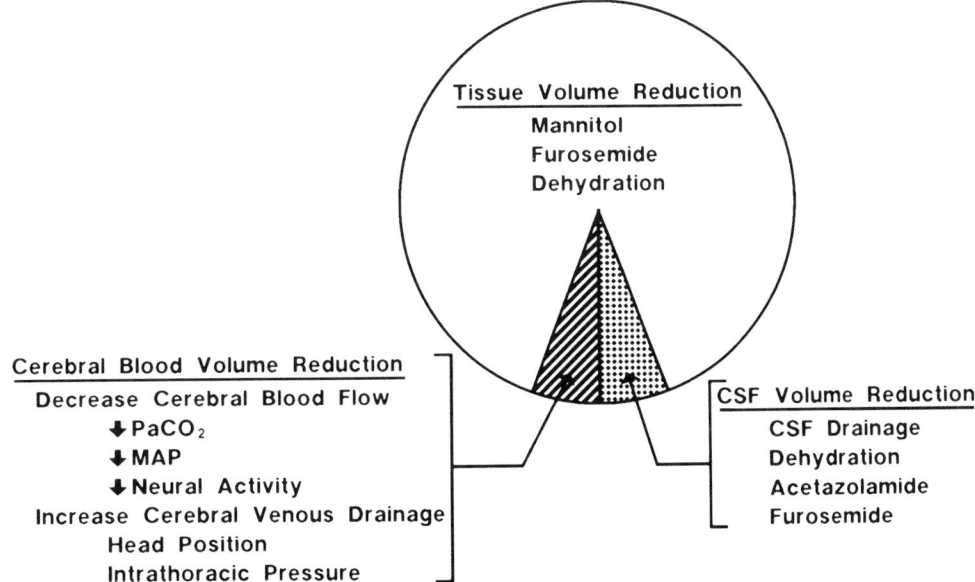

Figure 14.10.   Strategies for reducing intracranial pressure based on the intracranial compartments: tissue volume, cerebrospinal fluid (*CSF*) volume, or cerebral blood volume (*MAP*, mean arterial pressure). The therapy of intracranial hypertension must either decrease the volume of the component that caused the original increase in ICP or decrease the volume of one of the other components.

Osmotic brain dehydration may become a useful component of stroke therapy, if combined with other interventions. Bayer and associates recently reported a double-blind randomized clinical trial in which 173 patients received either 500 ml of 10% glycerol in normal saline or 500 ml of normal saline daily for 6 days after acute stroke (17). Treatment with glycerol reduced acute mortality but did not significantly change the degree of neurologic disability in survivors. Since potentially useful treatments such as nimodipine or hypervolemic hemodilution may increase ICP, the reduction in ICP produced by osmotherapy could permit more aggressive use of other treatments.

Cerebral metabolic considerations may become important in the management of acute stroke. Hyperglycemia has been associated with worse neurologic outcome in patients after stroke (232), probably because more severe neurologic injury is associated with stress-induced hyperglycemia rather than that hyperglycemia *per se* aggravates injury (162). Nevertheless, because hyperglycemia worsens outcome after ischemia in experimental animals, control of blood glucose may be prudent in patients with stroke.

Theoretically, general depression of cerebral metabolism should preserve marginally perfused brain tissue. However, barbiturate therapy has not been subjected to a definitive clinical trial in human stroke because of the poor tolerance of elderly patients with cardiovascular disease to the hemodynamic depression produced by high doses of barbiturates and because of the necessity for prolonged ventilatory support.

Perhaps, ultimately, therapy designed to interrupt the biochemical cascade of ischemic events may be combined with medical thrombolysis or surgical revascularization. Thrombolysis using tissue plasminogen activator has been effective in experimental studies of stroke (317) and in preliminary clinical studies (316). Emergency surgical revascularization, if performed sufficiently soon after the onset of ischemia, could result in reperfusion of still viable brain tissue. Antiischemic medical therapy could stabilize injured neurons until surgical therapy could be performed, perhaps for as long as 6 hours or more. Both emergency carotid endarterectomy (185) and middle cerebral embolectomy (186) have been performed with promising results, suggesting the clinical evidence of a penumbral zone of electrophysiologically dysfunctional but viable tissue.

Cardiac Arrest

After the global cerebral ischemic insult that occurs during cardiac arrest, many patients recover adequate cardiovascular, pulmonary, and renal function but are left with profound neurologic deficits (28, 156). Recent experimental work has emphasized the likely occurrence of reperfusion injury, damage that occurs after restoration of flow in neural tissue or in the cerebral vasculature (Fig. 14.11). The therapeutic implications of progressive injury during reperfusion are obvious. Therapeutic interventions could perhaps decrease the neurologic morbidity that follows cardiac arrest if the mechanisms underlying progressive injury could be identified. Preservation of brain viability during cardiopulmonary resuscitation is the most important consideration other than restoration of effective cardiac activity. Although many experimental models address issues related to brain perfusion, only the issue of

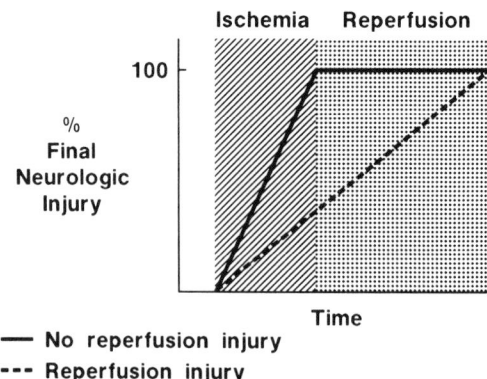

Figure 14.11. Experimental work has emphasized the likely occurrence of reperfusion injury in the cerebral circulation. Reperfusion injury is damage that occurs in neural tissue or in the cerebral vasculature after cerebral blood flow is restored. A central part of the hypothesis is that ischemic injury is not maximal at the time that ischemia resolves.

high-dose epinephrine has been addressed definitively in randomized clinical trials. High-dose epinephrine potentially could improve outcome either by improving cerebral perfusion during cardiopulmonary resuscitation or by more rapidly restoring effective cardiac function and CBF. In two trials, patients undergoing cardiopulmonary resuscitation were randomized to receive either conventional doses (0.02 mg/kg) or high doses (0.2 mg/kg) of epinephrine (35, 278). In neither trial was there evidence of improved outcome.

Postischemic treatment is most often applied in situations in which the cerebral circulation has been interrupted and then restored. Such circumstances include patients who have undergone successful resuscitation from cardiac arrest and patients who have a temporary interruption of focal or global cerebral circulation as part of surgical management (i.e., carotid cross-clamping during carotid endarterectomy, temporary occlusion of major vessels while approaching an intracranial aneurysm, or temporary circulatory arrest). One central assumption regarding postischemic treatment is that neurologic injury not only results from the ischemic episode per se but also continues during reperfusion.

Figure 14.7 schematically depicts the typical sequence of transient hyperemia followed by profound oligemia that occurs after complete experimental cerebral ischemia. After restoration of cerebral perfusion, animals typically develop a transient hyperemia, after which CBF decreases to a fraction of preischemic values (269, 275). Early work, using Kety-Schmidt estimates of global CBF, suggested that humans also developed postischemic hypoperfusion and that $CMRO_2$ was less suppressed than CBF, suggesting the possibility of potentially reversible cerebral ischemia (20). Later work, using ^{133}Xe clearance to estimate cortical blood flow, suggested that cerebral hyperemia, rather than hypoperfusion, is commonly associated with adverse outcome (48). Regardless, it seems unlikely that simple interventions designed to increase postischemic CBF will improve outcome.

As discussed earlier, hyperglycemia in patients initially resuscitated from cardiac arrest is associated with worse neurologic outcome (161–163); however, hyperglycemia appears to be an effect of more protracted and difficult resuscitation rather than an independent cause of worse neurologic injury

(162). Control of postischemic blood glucose is prudent but unproved as a therapeutic intervention.

When global cerebral hypoperfusion was believed to be a major contributing factor to poor neurologic outcome after cardiac arrest, many clinicians and investigators believed that postischemic administration of barbiturates would improve outcome. The Brain Resuscitation Clinical Trial I effectively terminated that belief by demonstrating no difference in outcome between patients who were provided good intensive care after arrest versus those randomized to receive large doses of thiopental (28).

As enthusiasm regarding barbiturate treatment was waning, experimental data suggested that calcium entry blockers might offer effective postischemic treatment. Forsman et al randomized patients to receive intravenous nimodipine or placebo while in transit from out-of-hospital cardiac arrest to the hospital (80). A low dose of nimodipine was used because of concern regarding drug-associated hypotension. Although patients who ultimately awakened did so more quickly if they received nimodipine, the percentage of patients who regained consciousness was not significantly greater (80). The high percentage of patients who had poor prearrest physical status, coupled with the small numbers entered into the trial, virtually assured a negative result (226). Roine et al also failed to find any improvement in neurologic outcome in patients given nimodipine (239). The Brain Resuscitation Clinical Trial II, which randomized 520 patients to receive lidoflazine or placebo, also failed to demonstrate clinical efficacy (29).

Although glucocorticoids are relatively ineffective against cytotoxic cerebral edema (76), many clinicians still tend to use dexamethasone or methylprednisolone in patients who have been resuscitated from cardiac arrest. Although no large-scale trial has specifically randomized patients to receive glucocorticoids or placebo, Jastremski et al, in an analysis of outcome in patients who had been entered into the Brain Resuscitation Clinical Trial I, failed to find any evidence of efficacy (127).

Subarachnoid Hemorrhage

Each year, 19,000 patients in the U.S. die or are disabled as a consequence of SAH (133, 134). Among patients who acutely survive the initial insult, rebleeding and vasospasm constitute the primary sources of morbidity and mortality. Neurologic deficits following SAH frequently are secondary to reversible cerebral ischemia resulting from cerebral vasospasm (45, 288, 307). The more severe the reduction in CBF, the worse the neurologic outcome (89, 288). Older patients are particularly likely to develop cerebral ischemia after SAH (180).

The mechanism of vasospasm occurring from SAH is unclear (135). Considerable experimental evidence suggests that some of the reduction in vessel caliber is caused by active smooth muscle contraction in response to spasmogenic substances released from blood in the CSF. A related hypothesis is that vascular relaxation is impaired by abnormalities of vessel wall metabolism or substances present in bloody CSF. The involved vessels ultimately undergo structural changes, such as smooth muscle hypertrophy, inflammation, and fibroblastic infiltration (135).

To reduce the incidence of rebleeding, many neurosurgeons now prefer to operate within the first 24 to 48 hours after the event. To control the neurologic complications of vasospasm, clinical investigators have used hypervolemic hemodilution to improve blood flow through spastic vessels and calcium entry blockers to prevent or antagonize vasospasm. Therapeutic attempts to improve CBF in patients with cerebral vasospasm have been partially successful. Intravascular volume expansion and induced systemic hypertension return CBF toward normal values (197, 223). Finn et al devised a strategy in which two factors (unoperated vs. operated and vasospastic vs. nonvasospastic) are used to divide patients into four categories (73). Hemodynamic support can be applied most aggressively in those patients who have surgically eradicated aneurysms and evidence of vasospasm. In such patients, both hypervolemic hemodilution and induced hypertension can be employed. Hemodynamic support is least aggressive in those patients who have not been surgically repaired and who have no neurologic deficits. The use of hypervolemic hemodilution is often combined with early operation because of the inherent risk of increasing systemic blood pressure in patients who have a recently ruptured intracranial aneurysm. Clinical investigators have offered uncontrolled data supporting this approach (271).

Certain calcium entry blockers antagonize the cerebral vasospasm associated with experimental SAH. An extensive multicenter study has demonstrated a prophylactic effect of nimodipine (0.35 mg/kg orally every 4 hours) on the subsequent development of vasospasm in patients entering the hospital with acute SAH but with minimal neurologic deficits (6). Nimodipine also improves the proportion of patients with good outcome from approximately 9.8% to 29.2% among those who have severe neurologic deficits secondary to vasospasm (216). The intraoperative course of patients who undergo aneurysm clipping while under treatment with calcium entry blockers appears to be minimally affected (280). Consequently, there currently is little controversy about the routine use of nimodipine in patients who have suffered SAH (177). However, as in the management of stroke, there is little objective evidence to guide the titration of therapy with the combination of nimodipine and hemodilution. Other calcium entry blocking agents such as nicardipine (79) may ultimately supplant nimodipine in the management of SAH.

Closed-Head Injury

Closed-head injury occurs frequently in young, productive, and otherwise healthy people who, because of their residual disability, may require years of custodial care. The clinical concept that governs the present management of closed-head injury is that the ultimate extent of disability results from the cumulative effects of both the primary mechanical injury and the secondary injuries produced by associated physiologic derangements. Secondary injury refers to the effects of subsequent events, such as hypoxemia or hypotension, that may compound the injury. The histopathologic evidence of cerebral ischemia frequently seen in fatal closed-head injury illustrates the potential importance of recognizing and limiting secondary injury (4).

Much of the current clinical strategy for the management of acute closed-head injury is directed toward a reduction in ICP, since the control of intracranial hypertension appears to improve outcome (248). Intracranial hypertension is a particularly important cause of secondary neural injury, because it is possible to monitor and reduce ICP effectively in most patients. However, very aggressive control of ICP does not reverse the effects of the primary injury. Severe, irreversible primary insults usually result in an unfavorable neurologic outcome, regardless of how well ICP has been controlled.

Therapeutic reduction of both CBF and $CMRO_2$, which can be accomplished with barbiturates, appears to be a physiologically sound strategy for the reduction of ICP without adversely affecting brain oxygenation. Marshall and associates have reported good results in a pilot study in which sodium pentobarbital, 3 to 5 mg/kg followed by an infusion of 100 to 200 mg every 30 to 60 minutes, was given to patients with severe closed-head injury (169a). Nevertheless, the overall response to barbiturate therapy after closed head trauma has been disappointing (299), perhaps reflecting the variability in CBF responsiveness to barbiturates in this heterogeneous population, as well as variability in the extent of primary injury. Recently, Eisenberg et al have defined a limited role for barbiturates in closed-head injury associated with refractory intracranial hypertension (62).

Hemorrhagic Shock

CBF is reduced during hemorrhagic shock, an effect that apparently results in part from massive sympathetic nervous system activation by the hemorrhage (77). The ultimate extent of central nervous system damage caused by the shock-induced partial cerebral ischemia depends on the magnitude and duration of the hypotensive insult. The effects of hypotension may be most critical in patients with coexisting traumatic neurologic injury, since in these patients morbidity from partial cerebral ischemia may be added to the primary insult.

Recent studies have focused not only on the effects of shock on CBF, but also on the effects of resuscitation on CBF and ICP. The evidence to date suggests that volume resuscitation from shock, if it does not include red blood cells, may actually result in a reduction of CDO_2 below the levels associated with shock (221, 222, 227). This results from two factors. First, during volume resuscitation from experimental hemorrhage, CBF increases transiently as MAP improves during expansion of intravascular volume, but then quickly decreases to levels no greater than those present during the shock state. These hemorrhage-related changes in CBF are strikingly different from the predictable increase in CBF that accompanies blood-free volume infusion in the absence of shock. Second, the concentration of hemoglobin is reduced if major blood loss is replaced with crystalloid or colloid. Further studies are necessary to determine the implications of reduced CDO_2 after volume expansion in cases of craniocerebral trauma or intracranial mass lesions.

Catecholamines are often administered with fluid resuscitation for the clinical treatment of circulatory shock. The effects of α-, β-, and dopaminergic receptor agonists consist both of their direct pharmacologic actions and the indirect effects of drug-induced increases in blood pressure, cardiac output, or both. Pure β-agonists, such as isoproterenol, cause no change in CBF (55, 206). Epinephrine and norepinephrine increase both $CMRO_2$ and CBF under specific conditions. CBF is increased only if blood pressure is increased beyond the upper limit of autoregulation, and only if the blood-brain barrier is disrupted (1, 54, 61). Dopamine dilates cerebral vessels independently of changes in blood pressure (296), but increases $CMRO_2$ only if the blood-brain barrier is disrupted (64). The effects on coexisting injury of catecholamines used during resuscitation from shock require further study.

Cardiopulmonary Bypass

The neurologic sequelae of cardiopulmonary bypass and open heart surgery represent an iatrogenic problem of considerable magnitude, primarily because of the 300,000 coronary revascularization procedures that are performed in the U.S. each year. Clinically demonstrable neurologic insults can be divided into permanent deficits, and transient focal and diffuse deficits. Although their cause remains unclear, the percentage of these complications is increasing, probably as a consequence of an aging cardiac surgical population, after more than a decade of progressive improvement in the incidence of postoperative stroke (2, 31, 34, 85). The current incidence of discrete, permanent stroke following coronary artery bypass surgery is 1 to 2% (34), but cognitive dysfunction occurs with alarming frequency (257, 268, 272). Studies of subclinical neurologic injury, as manifested by release of adenylate kinase into the CSF, suggest that it is 50% or greater (3). Clearly, further investigations of these subtle but potentially disabling effects of cardiopulmonary bypass on memory, learning, and emotional stability are required.

Because of the high incidence of neurologic and neuropsychologic dysfunction after cardiac surgery (257), many investigators have attempted to define the physiology of cardiopulmonary bypass and to identify interventions that might reduce injury. Implicit in these efforts is the assumption that neurologic dysfunction after cardiac surgery is secondary to ischemic injury, whether caused by macroembolism, microembolism, or global hypoperfusion. Early experience with cardiac surgery suggested that aggressive efforts to limit macroembolism could reduce the incidence of postoperative deficits (2). More recently, membrane oxygenation has been shown to produce fewer intraoperative occlusions of the retinal microvasculature than bubble oxygenation, implying a potential advantage (26).

Control of physiologic variables during cardiopulmonary bypass offers a potential method of controlling the incidence of postoperative sequelae. Hotly debated issues include the control of $PACO_2$, the management of blood pressure and blood glucose, and the use of hypothermia. During hypothermic cardiopulmonary bypass, $PACO_2$ can be managed either to maintain a level of 40 mm Hg (5.3 kPa) when measured in the blood gas analyzer at 37°C, or of 40 mm Hg (5.3 kPa) when the measured value is corrected to the patient's actual temperature. For example, the former (α-stat) method of management would result in a $PACO_2$ of 27 mm Hg (3.6 kPa) at a body temperature of 27°C; the latter (pH-stat) method would require a $PACO_2$ of 60 mm Hg (8 kPa) in the blood gas analyzer if the temperature-corrected $PACO_2$ were 40 mm Hg (5.3 kPa) at 27°C. $PACO_2$ exerts powerful control over the cerebral circulation during cardiopulmonary bypass (230, 231), as it does under other circumstances. Two randomized clinical trials have investigated the influence of $PACO_2$ management on postoperative outcome and have reached different conclusions. Bashein et al concluded that outcome, measured using neuropsychologic testing, was unaffected (16), whereas Stephan et al found that the pH-stat method was associated with a significantly higher incidence of neurologic deficits (276).

Whether hypotension during cardiopulmonary bypass contributes to postoperative deficits has been argued for many years (279). Cerebral pressure autoregulation appears to be intact during cardiopulmonary bypass (92, 238). However, both retrospective analyses (68, 141) and prospectively collected data (16) have failed to demonstrate a convincing relationship. Too few data are available to permit conclusions regarding the risk of hypotension in elderly patients or those with cerebrovascular disease.

Hyperglycemia has been associated with worse neurologic outcome in patients after stroke (232), cardiac arrest (161–163), and closed-head injury (149). Hyperglycemia, commonly occurring during cardiopulmonary bypass, theoretically should aggravate ischemic neurologic injury; prevention of hyperglycemia should lessen the incidence or reduce the severity of injury. However, the use of a glucose-containing solution to prime the bypass circuit, while further increasing blood sugar during cardiopulmonary bypass, did not result in an increased incidence of gross neurologic deficits (178). Frasco et al were also unable to demonstrate an association between intraoperative hyperglycemia and cognitive dysfunction after cardiac surgery (83). Conclusive resolution of the debate, however, awaits the demonstration that tight control of blood glucose during cardiopulmonary bypass does or does not influence the incidence and severity of deficits, especially since there are apparent nonneurologic advantages of a glucose-containing priming solution (178).

Hypothermia, routinely employed during cardiopulmonary bypass in many centers, theoretically should also protect the brain from ischemic insults by reducing cerebral metabolism. Certainly, profound hypothermia greatly increases the duration of neurologic tolerance for complete circulatory arrest. The resurgent use of "warm bypass" that has accompanied improvements in intraoperative cardiac protection greatly increases the clinical importance of the question regarding hypothermic brain protection. Thus far, the evidence is inconclusive. Wong et al found improved performance on neuropsychologic tests by patients who had been managed with "warm bypass" in contrast to those managed at a mean temperature of 27.8°C (310).

In addition to mechanical and physiologic strategies, clinicians have attempted a variety of pharmacologic interventions to reduce neurologic injury after cardiac surgery. Most prominent have been the barbiturates and calcium entry blockers. Barbiturates have produced mixed results. Doses of thiopental sufficient to suppress the EEG reduce the total incidence of gross neurologic and psychiatric changes after valvular heart surgery conducted using a glucose-containing priming solution and slightly hypothermic perfusion, but at the price of prolonged requirements for postoperative ventilation and an increased need for inotropic support (203). Smaller doses of thiopental, timed to provide protection during the intervals of greatest risk, did not result in an increased incidence in comparison with a group

of valvular surgery patients randomized to receive larger doses throughout bypass (179), but that study is difficult to interpret because it did not include an untreated control group (229). In clear contrast to the experience with valvular heart surgery patients, administration of EEG-suppressing doses of thiopental to patients undergoing coronary bypass grafting did not produce a decrease in the incidence of stroke, although hemodynamic depression and prolonged need for ventilatory support were evident (315). To date, no published study has thoroughly evaluated the influence of barbiturates on postoperative cognitive function.

Because of the likelihood that deficits after cardiac surgery represent focal cerebral ischemic insults, nimodipine is a logical prophylactic intervention to study in patients undergoing cardiac surgery. To date, the only major study is that of Forsman et al, who randomized cardiac surgical patients to receive nimodipine or placebo and demonstrated that nimodipine conferred no benefit with regard to neurologic status (81).

Recently, there has been considerable interest in the concept that brain monitoring could be used to detect and reverse cerebral ischemia during cardiopulmonary bypass. The question is whether focal ischemia secondary to embolic phenomena or regional cerebrovascular disease, or global ischemia secondary to excessive vasoconstriction or hypotension, can be identified and reversed, thereby reducing the neurologic and cognitive sequelae of cardiac surgery. An uncontrolled clinical series, using a historical comparison group, suggested improved neurologic outcome using interventions based upon EEG monitoring (9). However, a randomized clinical trial failed to demonstrate any practical value of EEG monitoring during cardiopulmonary bypass (15).

INTEGRATION OF BRAIN MONITORING AND PHARMACOLOGIC THERAPY

In many critically ill patients, long-term neurologic outcome may depend on the adequacy of regional or global CBF as well as specific etiologic treatment of the primary process. Despite this possibility, useful clinical algorithms regarding appropriate physiologic and pharmacologic management of the cerebral circulation have developed slowly. Although protocols for the management of stroke, SAH, cardiac arrest, head injury, and cardiopulmonary bypass are based in part on cerebral circulatory considerations, they are derived more from physiologic inference rather than data obtained by monitoring.

Although CBF has been measured and to some extent manipulated in patients with intracranial hypertension, the only commonly monitored variable in such patients is ICP. ICP is the outflow pressure for the cerebral circulation in the presence of intracranial hypertension. However, ICP measurements alone, in the absence of measurements of CBF or $CMRO_2$, provide the same potential for erroneous interpretation of the adequacy of cerebral circulation that one would expect if pulmonary capillary wedge pressure were used as the sole measure of the adequacy of systemic circulation.

Two recent developments suggest that cerebral circulatory monitoring might soon become feasible on a wider scale.

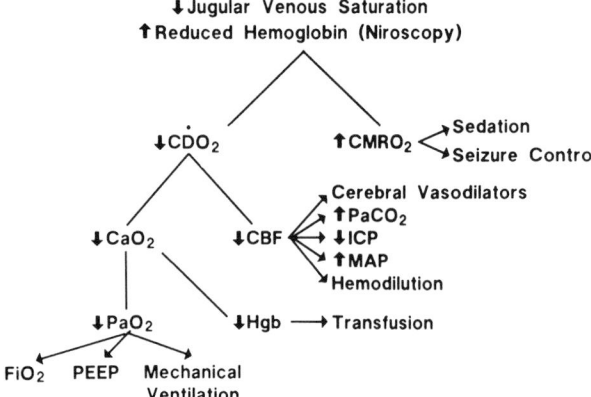

Figure 14.12. Schematic depiction of possible factors contributing to a decrease in jugular venous saturation. *Hgb*, hemoglobin; *FiO₂*, fractional inspired oxygen concentration; *PEEP*, positive end-expiratory pressure. Other abbreviations are explained in the text. Since blood in either jugular bulb represents a "mixed" sample from the entire brain, a reduction in $SJVO_2$ can result only from a reduction in $C\dot{D}O_2$ or an increase in $CMRO_2$.

First, the introduction of continuous monitoring of $SJVO_2$ as a research tool suggests that this parameter might be used clinically to monitor the net balance of cerebral oxygen supply and demand for the whole brain. Since blood in either jugular bulb represents a "mixed" sample from the entire brain, a reduction in $SJVO_2$ can result only from a reduction in CDO_2 or an increase in $CMRO_2$ (Fig. 14.12). In turn, a reduction in CDO_2 can result only from a reduction in either CAO_2 or CBF, and a reduction in CAO_2 can be caused only by a reduction in SAO_2 or hemoglobin. Consequently, continuous monitoring of $SJVO_2$ in patients at risk for global cerebral ischemia may provide a mechanism for early detection of insufficient oxygen availability, after which a rapid, sequential analysis can be made of possible contributing factors. Alternatively, near-infrared spectroscopy, a technique that detects changes in cerebral arteriovenous hemoglobin saturation differences by transcranial penetration of near-infrared light, might noninvasively provide qualitative evidence that CBF is insufficient to meet metabolic demand (131, 220, 224).

The second major development that promises to improve the monitoring of cerebral circulation is the use of portable systems for measuring CBF based on the clearance of ^{133}Xe or the inferring of data regarding CBF from the measurement of MCA flow velocity. Regional CBF measurements provide discrete focal information about cortical flow and, in combination with CAO_2 and $CJVO_2$ values, allow a rough approximation of $CMRO_2$. Consequently, in the near future perhaps all of the factors that contribute to cerebral oxygen balance can be estimated quickly at the bedside of the critically ill patient. Rapid evaluation of CAO_2 may be performed with arterial blood gas analysis and CO-Oximetry or may be monitored on-line with pulse oximetry. Together, CBF and CAO_2 constitute CDO_2. Continuous monitoring of the processed EEG may permit detection and management of increased electrophysiologic activity (suggesting seizures) or decreased activity (suggesting ischemia). Prompt, effective recognition and management of hypoxemia, cerebral hypoperfusion, and increased metabolic demand should improve the rate of favorable neurologic recovery.

REFERENCES

1. Abdul-Rahman A, Dahlgren N, Johansson BB, Siesjö BK: Increase in local cerebral blood flow induced by circulating adrenaline: involvement of blood-brain barrier dysfunction. *Acta Neurol Scand* 107:227–232, 1979.
2. Aberg T, Kihlgren M: Cerebral protection during open-heart surgery. *Thorax* 32:525–533, 1977.
3. Aberg T, Ronquist G, Tydén H, Brunnkvist S, Hultman J, Bergström K, Lilja A: Adverse effects on the brain in cardiac operations as assessed by biochemical, psychometric, and radiologic methods. *J Thorac Cardiovasc Surg* 87:99–105, 1984.
4. Adams JH, Graham DI, Gennarelli TA: Contemporary neuropathological considerations regarding brain damage in head injury. In Becker DP, Povlishock JT (eds): *Central Nervous System Trauma Status Report*. Bethesda, MD, National Institutes of Health, 1985, pp 65–77.
5. Albers GW, Goldberg MP, Choi DW: N-methyl-D-aspartate antagonists: ready for clinical trial in brain ischemia? *Ann Neurol* 25:398–403, 1989.
6. Allen GS, Ahn HS, Preziosi TJ, et al: Cerebral arterial spasm—a controlled trial of nimodipine in patients with subarachnoid hemorrage. *N Engl J Med* 308:619–624, 1983.
7. American Academy of Neurology: Assessment: transcranial Doppler. *Neurology* 40:680, 1990.
8. Ames A, Wright RL, Kowada M, Thurston JM, Majno G: Cerebral ischemia. II. The no-reflow phenomenon. *Am J Pathol* 52:437–453, 1968.
9. Arom KV, Cohen DE, Strobl FT: Effect of intraoperative intervention on neurologic outcome based on electroencephalographic monitoring during cardiopulmonary bypass. *Ann Thorac Surg* 48:476–483, 1989.
10. Artru AA, Colley PS: Cerebral blood flow responses to hypocapnia during hypotension. *Stroke* 15:878–883, 1984.
11. Bailes JE, Spetzler RF, Hadley MN, et al: Management of morbidity and mortality of poor-grade aneurysm patients. *J Neurosurg* 72:559, 1990.
12. Baker AJ, Zornow MH, Grafe MR, Scheller MS, Skilling SR, Smullin DH, Larson AA: Hypothermia prevents ischemia-induced increases in hippocampal glycine concentrations in rabbits. *Stroke* 22:666–673, 1991.
13. Barnes JM, Henley JM: Molecular characteristics of excitatory amino acid receptors. *Prog Neurobiol* 39:113–133, 1992.
14. Barnett GH, Ropper AH, Romeo J: Intracranial pressure and outcome in adult encephalitis. *J Neurosurg* 68:585–588, 1988.
15. Basheir G, Nessly ML, Bledsoe SW, Townes BD, Davis KB, Coppel DB, Hornbein TF: Electroencephalography during surgery with cardiopulmonary bypass and hypothermia. *Anesthesiology* 76:878–891, 1992.
16. Basheir G, Townes BD, Nessly ML, Bledsoe SW, Hornbein TF, Davis KB, Goldstein DE, Coppel DB: A randomized study of carbon dioxide management during hypothermic cardiopulmonary bypass. *Anesthesiology* 72:7–15, 1990.
17. Bayer AJ, Pathy MSJ, Newcombe R: Double-blind randomised trial of intravenous glycerol in acute stroke. *Lancet* 1:405–407, 1987.
18. Beckman JS, Beckman TW, Chen J, Marshall PA, Freeman BA: Apparent hydroxyl radical production by peroxynitrite: implications for endothelial injury from nitric oxide and superoxide. *Proc Natl Acad Sci USA* 87:1620–1624, 1990.
19. Beckman JS, Freeman BA: Antioxidant enzymes as mechanistic probes of oxygen-dependent toxicity. In *Physiology of Oxygen Radicals*. American Physiological Society, Bethesda, MD 1986, pp 39–53.
20. Beckstead JE, Tweed WA, Lee J, MacKeen WL: Cerebral blood flow and metabolism in man following cardiac arrest. *Stroke* 9:569–573, 1978.
21. Benveniste H: The excitotoxin hypothesis in relation to cerebral ischemia. *Cerebrovasc Brain Metab Rev* 3:213–245, 1991.
22. Benveniste H, Drejer J, Schousboe A, Diemer NH: Elevation of the extracellular concentrations of glutamate and aspartate in rat hippocampus during transient cerebral ischemia monitored by intracerebral microdialysis. *J Neurochem* 43:1369–1374, 1984.
23. Berridge MJ, Irvine RF: Inositol trisphosphate, a novel second messenger in cellular signal transduction. *Nature* 312:315–321, 1984.
24. Bertel O, Conen D, Radu EW, Muller J, Lang C, Dubach UC: Nifedipine in hypertensive emergencies. *Br Med J* 286:19–21, 1983.
25. Bishop CCR, Powell S, Rutt D, Browse NL: Transcranial Doppler measurement of middle cerebral artery blood flow velocity: a validation study. *Stroke* 17:913–915, 1986.
26. Blauth CI, Smith PL, Arnold JV, Jagoe JR, Wootton R, Taylor KM: Influence of oxygenator type on the prevalence and extent of microembolic retinal ischemia during cardiopulmonary bypass. Assessment by digital image analysis. *J Thorac Cardiovasc Surg* 99:61–69, 1990.
27. Bowton DL, Alford PT, McLees BD, Prough DS, Stump DA: The effect of aminophylline on cerebral blood flow in patients with chronic obstructive pulmonary disease. *Chest* 91:874–877, 1987.
28. Brain Resuscitation Clinical Trial I Study Group: Randomized clinical study of thiopental loading in comatose survivors of cardiac arrest. *N Engl J Med* 31:397–403, 1986.
29. Brain Resuscitation Clinical Trial II Study Group: A randomized clinical study of a calcium-entry blocker (lidoflazine) in the treatment of comatose survivors of cardiac arrest. *N Engl J Med* 324:1225–1231, 1991.

30. Branston NM, Symon L, Crockard HA, Pasztor E: Relationship between the cortical evoked potential and local cortical blood flow following acute middle cerebral artery occlusion in the baboon. *Exp Neurol* 45:195–208, 1974.

31. Branthwaite MA: Prevention of neurological damage during open-heart surgery. *Thorax* 30:258–261, 1975.

32. Brayden JE, Nelson MT: Regulation of arterial tone by activation of calcium-dependent potassium channels. *Science* 256:532–535, 1992.

33. Bredt DS, Snyder SH: Nitric oxide mediates glutamate-linked enhancement of cGMP levels in the cerebellum. *Proc Natl Acad Sci USA* 86:9030–9033, 1989.

34. Breuer AC, Furlan AJ, Hanson MR, Lederman RJ, Loop FD, Cosgrove DM, Greenstreet RL, Estafanous FG: Central nervous system complications of coronary artery bypass graft surgery: prospective analysis of 421 patients. *Stroke* 14:682–687, 1983.

35. Brown CG, Martin DR, Pepe PE, Stueven H, Cummins RO, Gonzalez E, Jastremski M, The Multicenter High-Dose Epinephrine Study Group: A comparison of standard-dose and high-dose epinephrine in cardiac arrest outside the hospital. *N Engl J Med* 327:1051–1055, 1992.

36. Buchan AM: Do NMDA antagonists protect against cerebral ischemia: are clinical trials warranted? *Cerebrovasc Brain Metab Rev* 2:1–26, 1990.

37. Buchan AM: Do NMDA antagonists protect against cerebral ischemia: are clinical trials warranted? *Cerebrovasc Brain Metab Rev* 2:1–26, 1991.

38. Burt DER, Verniquet AJW, Homi J: The response of canine intracranial pressure to systemic hypotension induced with nitroglycerine. *Br J Anaesth* 54:665–671, 1982.

39. Busto R, Globus MY, Dietrich WD, Martinez E, Valdes I, Ginsberg MD: Effect of mild hypothermia on ischemic-induced release of neurotransmitters and free fatty acids in rat brain. *Stroke* 20:904–910, 1989.

40. Candia GJ, Heros RC, Lavyne MH, Zervas NT, Nelson CN: Effect of intravenous sodium nitroprusside on cerebral blood flow and intracranial pressure. *Neurosurgery* 3:50–53, 1978.

41. Carolei A, Fieschi C, Bruno R, Toffano G: Monosialoganglioside GM1 in cerebral ischemia. *Cerebrovasc Brain Metab Rev* 3:134–157, 1991.

42. Choi DW, Maulucci-Gedde M, Kriegstein AR: Glutamate neurotoxicity in cortical cell culture. *J Neurosci* 7:357–368, 1987.

43. Chopp M, Chen H, Dereski MO, Garcia JH: Mild hypothermic intervention after graded ischemic stress in rats. *Stroke* 22:37–43, 1991.

44. Chuang D-M: Neurotransmitter receptors and phosphoinositide turnover. *Annu Rev Pharmacol Toxicol* 29:71–110, 1989.

45. Chyatte D, Sundt TM Jr: Cerebral vasospasm after subarachnoid hemorrhage. *Mayo Clin Proc* 59:498–505, 1984.

46. Clark WC, Muhlbauer MS, Lowrey R, et al: Complications of intracranial pressure monitoring in trauma patients. *Neurosurgery* 25:20, 1989.

47. Clifton GL, Jiang JY, Lyeth BG, Jenkins LW, Hayes RL: Marked protection by moderate hypothermia in experimental traumatic brain injury. *J Cereb Blood Flow Metab* 11:114–121, 1991.

48. Cohan SL, Mun SK, Petite J, Correia J, Tavelra da Silva AT, Waldhorn RE: Cerebral blood flow in humans following resuscitation from cardiac arrest. *Stroke* 20:761–765, 1989.

49. Colohan ART, Alves WM, Gross CR, Torner JC, Mehta VS, Tandon PN, Jane JA: Head injury mortality in two centers with different emergency medical services and intensive care. *J Neurosurg* 71:202–207, 1989.

50. Cottrell JE, Robustelli A, Post K, Turndorf H: Furosemide- and mannitol-induced changes in intracranial pressure and serum osmolality and electrolytes. *Anesthesiology* 47:28–30, 1977.

51. Crockard A, Iannotti F, Hunstock AT, Smith RD, Harris RJ, Simon L: Cerebral blood flow and edema following carotid occlusion in the gerbil. *Stroke* 11:494–498, 1980.

52. Crockard HA, Gadian DG, Frackowiak RSJ, Proctor E, Allen K, Williams SR, Russell RWR: Acute cerebral ischemia: concurrent changes in cerebral blood flow, energy metabolites, pH, and lactate measured with hydrogen clearance and ^{31}P and ^1H nuclear magnetic resonance spectroscopy. II. Changes during ischemia. *J Cereb Blood Flow Metab* 7:394–402, 1987.

53. Crutchfield JS, Narayan RK, Robertson CS, Michael LH: Evaluation of a fiberoptic intracranial pressure monitor. *J Neurosurg* 72:482–487, 1990.

54. Dahlgren N, Rosen I, Sakabe T, Siesjo BK: Cerebral functional, metabolic and circulatory effects of intravenous infusion of adrenaline in the rat. *Brain Res* 184:143–152, 1980.

55. Davis DH, Sundt TM Jr: Relationship of cerebral blood flow to cardiac output, mean arterial pressure, blood volume, and alpha and beta blockade in cats. *J Neurosurg* 52:745–754, 1980.

56. DeWitt DS, Jenkins LW, Wei EP, Lutz H, Becker DP, Kontos HA: Effects of fluid percussion brain injury on regional cerebral blood flow and pial vessel diameter. *J Neurosurg* 64:787–794, 1986.

57. DeWitt DS, Kong DL, Lyeth BG, Jenkins LW, Hayes RL, Wooten ED, Prough DS: Experimental traumatic brain injury elevates brain prostaglandin E_2 and thromboxane B_2 levels in rats. *J Neurotrauma* 5:303, 1988.

58. DeWitt DS, Prough DS, Taylor CL, Whitley JM, Deal DD, Vines SM: Regional cerebrovascular responses to progressive hypotension after traumatic brain injury in cats. *Am J Physiol Heart Circ Physiol* 32:H1276–H1284, 1992.

59. DeWitt DS, Prough DS, Colonna DM, Deal DD, Vines SM: Effects of nitric oxide synthase inhibitors on cerebral blood flow and autoregulation in rats [Abstract]. *Anesthesiology* 77(Suppl 3A):A689, 1992.

60. Dixon CE, Lyeth BG, Povlishock JT, Findling RL, Hamm RJ, Marmarou A, Young HF, Hayes RL: A fluid percussion model of experimental brain injury in the rat. *J Neurosurg* 67:110–119, 1987.

61. Edvinsson L, Lancombe P, Owman C, Reynier-Rebuttel AM, Seylaz J: Quantitative changes in regional cerebral blood flow of rats induced by alpha- and beta-adrenergic stimulants. *Acta Neurol Scand* 107:289–296, 1979.

62. Eisenberg HM, Frankowski RF, Contant CF, Marshall LF, Walker MD: High-dose barbiturate control of elevated intracranial pressure in patients with severe head injury. *J Neurosurg* 69:15–23, 1988.

63. Ekstrom-Jodal B, Haggendal E, Linder L-E, Nilsson NJ: Cerebral blood flow autoregulation at high arterial pressures and different levels of carbon dioxide tension in dogs. *Eur Neurol* 6:6–10, 1971.

64. Ekstrom-Jodal B, Larsson LE: Effects of dopamine on cerebral circulation and oxygen metabolism in endotoxic shock: an experimental study in dogs. *Crit Care Med* 10:375–377, 1982.

65. Ellis EF, Dodson LY, Police RJ: Restoration of cerebrovascular responsiveness to hyperventilation by the oxygen radical scavenger *n*-acetylcysteine following experimental traumatic brain injury. *J Neurosurg* 75:774–779, 1991.

66. Ellis EF, Police RJ, Rice LY, Grabeel M, Holt S: Increased plasma PGE$_2$ 6-keto-PGF$_{1\alpha}$, and 12-HETE levels following experimental concussive brain injury. *J Neurotrauma* 6:31, 1989.

67. Ellis EF, Wright KF, Wei EP, Kontos HA: Cyclooxygenase products of arachidonic acid metabolism in cat cerebral cortex after experimental concussive brain injury. *J Neurochem* 37:892–896, 1981.

68. Ellis RJ, Wisniewski A, Potts R, Calhoun C, Loucks P, Wells MR: Reduction of flow rate and arterial pressure at moderate hypothermia does not result in cerebral dysfunction. *J Thorac Cardiovasc Surg* 79:173–180, 1980.

69. Faden AI: TRH analog YM-14673 improves outcome following traumatic brain and spinal cord injury in rats: dose-response studies. *Brain Res* 486:228–235, 1989.

70. Faden AI, Demediuk P, Panter SS, Vink R: The role of excitatory amino acids and NMDA receptors in traumatic brain injury. *Science* 244:798–800, 1989.

71. Faden AI, Vink R, McIntosh TK: Thyrotropin-releasing hormone and central nervous system trauma. *Ann NY Acad Sci* 553:380–384, 1989.

72. Faraci FM: Role of endothelium-derived relaxing factor in cerebral circulation: large arteries vs. microcirculation. *Am J Physiol* 261:H1038–H1042, 1991.

73. Finn SS, Stephensen SA, Miller CA, Drobnich L, Hunt WE: Observations on the perioperative management of aneurysmal subarachnoid hemorrhage. *J Neurosurg* 65:48–62, 1986.

74. Finnerty FA Jr, Guillaudeu RL, Fazekas JF: Cardiac and cerebral hemodynamics in drug induced postural collapse. *Circ Res* 5:34–39, 1957.

75. Fisher SK, Heacock AM, Agranoff BW: Inositol lipids and signal transduction in the nervous system: an update. *J Neurochem* 58:18, 1992.

76. Fishman RA: Brain edema. *N Engl J Med* 293:706–711, 1975.

77. Fitch W, MacKenzie ET, Harper AM: Effects of decreasing arterial blood pressure on cerebral blood flow in the baboon. Influence of the sympathetic nervous system. *Circ Res* 37:550–557, 1975.

78. FitzGerald GA, Reilly IAG, Pedersen AK: The biochemical pharmacology of thromboxane synthetase inhibition in man. *Circulation* 72:1194–1201, 1985.

79. Flamm ES: The potential use of nicardipine in cerebrovascular disease. *Am Heart J* 117:236–242, 1989.

80. Forsman M, Aarseth HP, Nordby HK, Skulberg A, Steen PA: Cerebral blood flow, intracranial pressure and neurologic outcome after cardiac arrest: effects of nimodipine. *Anesth Analg* 68:436–443, 1989.

81. Forsman M, Olsnes BT, Semb G, Steen PA: Effects of nimodipine on cerebral blood flow and neuropsychological outcome after cardiac surgery. *Br J Anaesth* 65:514–520, 1990.

82. Förstermann U, Neufang B: The endothelium-dependent vasodilator effect of acetylcholine: characterization of the endothelial relaxing factor with inhibitors of arachidonic acid metabolism. *Eur J Pharmacol* 103:65–70, 1984.

83. Frasco P, Croughwell N, Blumenthal J, Will C, Leone B, White W, Goodman D, Reves JG: Association between blood glucose level during cardiopulmonary bypass and neuropsychiatric outcome [Abstract]. *Anesthesiology* 75(3A):A55, 1991.

84. Furchgott RF, Zawadzki JV: The obligatory role of endothelial cells in the relaxation of arterial smooth muscle by acetylcholine. *Nature* 288:373–376, 1980.

85. Gardner TJ, Horneffer PJ, Manolio TA, Pearson TA, Gott VL, Baumgartner WA, Borkon AM, Watkins L Jr, Reitz BA: Stroke following coronary artery bypass grafting: a ten-year study. *Ann Thorac Surg* 40:574–581, 1985.

86. Garthwaite J: Glutamate, nitric oxide and cell-cell signalling in the nervous system. *Trends Neurosci* 14:60–67, 1991.

87. Gelmers HJ, Gorter K, de Weerdt CJ, Wiezer HJA: A controlled trial of nimodipine in acute ischemic stroke. *N Engl J Med* 318:203–207, 1988.

88. Gelmers HJ, Hennerici M: Effect of nimodipine on acute ischemic stroke. Pooled results from five randomized trials. *Stroke* 21(Suppl IV):IV-81–IV-84, 1990.

89. Geraud G, Tremoulet M, Guell A, Bes A: The prognostic value of noninvasive CBF measurement in subarachnoid hemorrhage. *Stroke* 15:301–305, 1984.

90. Ginsberg MD, Dietrich WD, Busto R: Coupled forebrain increases of local cerebral glucose utilization and blood flow during physiologic stimulation of a somatosensory pathway in the rat: demonstration by double-label autoradiography. *Neurology* 37:11–19, 1987.

91. Ginsberg MD, Welsh FA, Budd WW: Deleterious effect of glucose pretreatment on recovery from diffuse cerebral ischemia in the cat. I. Local cerebral blood flow and glucose utilization. *Stroke* 11:347–354, 1980.

92. Govier AV, Reves JG: Cerebral blood flow: autoregulation during cardiopulmonary bypass. In Hilberman M (ed): *Brain Injury and Protection during Heart Surgery.* Martinus Nijhoff, Boston, 1988, pp 27–45.

93. Graham DI: The pathology of brain ischaemia and possibilities for therapeutic intervention. *Br J Anaesth* 57:3–17, 1985.

94. Graham DI, Fitch W, MacKenzie ET, Harper AM: Effects of hemorrhagic hypotension on the cerebral circulation. III. Neuropathology. *Stroke* 10:724–727, 1979.

95. Greenberg RP, Hyatt MS, Becker DP: Transient electrical dysfunction in head-injured cats: a mechanism for loss of consciousness. *Surg Forum* 32:492–494, 1981.

96. Gregory PC, McGeorge AP, Fitch W, Graham DI, MacKenzie ET, Harper EM: Effects of hemorrhagic hypotension on the cerebral circulation. *Stroke* 10:719–723, 1979.

97. Grice SC, Chappell ET, Prough DS, Whitley JM, Su M, Watkins WD: Ibuprofen improves cerebral blood flow after global cerebral ischemia in dogs. *Stroke* 18:787–791, 1987.

98. Grubb RL Jr, Raichle ME, Eichling JO, Ter-Pogossian MM: The effects of changes in PACO₂ on cerebral blood volume, blood flow, and vascular mean transit time. *Stroke* 5:630–639, 1974.

99. Gunnar W, Jonasson O, Merlotti G, Stone J, Barrett J: Head injury and hemorrhagic shock: studies of the blood-brain barrier and intracranial pressure after resuscitation with normal saline solution, 3% saline solution, and dextran-40. *Surgery* 103:398–407, 1988.

100. Haas DC, Streeten DHP, Kim RC, Naalbandian AN, Obeid AI: Death from cerebral hypoperfusion during nitroprusside treatment of acute angiotensin-dependent hypertension. *Am J Med* 75:1071–1076, 1983.

101. Haber F, Weiss J: The catalytic decomposition of hydrogen peroxide by iron salts. *Proc R Soc Med* 147:332–351, 1934.

102. Hakim AM, Shoubridge EA: Cerebral acidosis in focal ischemia. *Cerebrovasc Brain Metab Rev* 1:115–132, 1989.

103. Hall ED, Yonkers PA: Attenuation of postischemic cerebral hypoperfusion by the 21-aminosteroid U74006F. *Stroke* 19:340–344, 1988.

104. Hallenbeck JM, Furlow Jr TW: Prostaglandin I₂ and indomethacin prevent impairment of post-ischemic brain reperfusion in the dog. *Stroke* 10:629–637, 1979.

105. Hara H, Onodera H, Yoshidomi M, Matsuda Y, Kogure K: Staurosporine, a novel protein kinase C inhibitor, prevents postischemic neuronal damage in the gerbil and rat. *J Cereb Blood Flow Metab* 10:646–653, 1990.

106. Harper AM: The inter-relationship between PACO₂ and blood pressure in the regulation of blood flow through the cerebral cortex. *Acta Neurol* 41(Suppl 41):94–103, 1965.

107. Harris RJ, Symon L, Branston NM, Bayhan M: Changes in extracellular calcium activity in cerebral ischaemia. *J Cereb Blood Flow Metab* 1:203–209, 1981.

108. Hartmann A: Effect of pentoxifylline on regional cerebral blood flow in patients with cerebral vascular disorders. *Eur Neurol* 22(Suppl 1):108–115, 1983.

109. Haws CW, Heistad DD: Effects of nimodipine on cerebral vasoconstrictor responses. *Am J Physiol* 247:H170–H176, 1984.

110. Hayes RL, Kulkarni P, Galinat BJ, Becker DP: Evidence for the release of endogenous opiate substances after experimental closed-head injury in the cat. *Science* 179–188, 1982.

111. Hayes RL, Lyeth BG: Neurochemical mechanisms of mild and moderate head injury: implications for treatment. In Levin HS, Eisenberg HM, Benton AL (eds): *Mild Head Injury.* Oxford University Press, Oxford, England, 1989, pp 54–79.

112. Hayes RL, Pechura CM, Katayama Y, Povlishock JT, Giebel ML, Becker DP: Activation of pontine cholinergic sites implicated in unconsciousness following cerebral concussion in the cat. *Science* 223:301–303, 1984.

113. Hayes RL, Stonnington HH, Lyeth BG, Dixon CE, Yamamoto T: Metabolic and neurophysiologic sequelae of brain injury: a cholinergic hypothesis. *CNS Trauma* 3:163–173, 1986.

114. Henriksen L, Paulson OB: The effects of sodium nitroprusside on cerebral blood flow and cerebral venous blood gases. II. Observations in awake man during successive blood pressure reduction. *Eur J Clin Invest* 12:389–393, 1982.

115. Henriksen L, Paulson OB, Lauritzen M: The effects of sodium nitroprusside on cerebral blood flow and cerebral venous blood gases. I. Observations in awake man during and following moderate blood pressure reduction. *Eur J Clin Invest* 12:383–387, 1982.

116. Herskovits E, Famulari A, Tamaroff L, Gonzalez AM, Vazquez A, Dominguez R, Fraiman H, Vila J: Preventive treatment of cerebral transient ischemia: comparative randomized trial of pentoxifylline versus conventional antiaggregants. *Eur Neurol* 24:73–81, 1985.

117. Hoff JT: Cerebral protection. *J Neurosurg* 65:579–591, 1986.

118. Hoffman WE, Albrecht RF, Miletich DJ: The role of adenosine in CBF increases during hypoxia in young vs aged rats. *Stroke* 15:124–129, 1984.

119. Holaday JW, Long JB, Martinez-Arizala A, Chen H-S, Reynolds DG, Gurll NJ: Effects of TRH in circulatory shock and central nervous system ischemia. *Ann NY Acad Sci* 553:370–379, 1989.

120. Hossmann K-A, Schuler FJ: Experimental brain infarcts in cats. I. Pathological observations. *Stroke* 11:583–592, 1980.

121. Hsu CY, Faught Jr RE, Furlan AJ, Coull BM, Huang DC, Hogan EL, Linet OI, Yatsu FM: Intravenous prostacyclin in acute nonhemorrhagic stroke: a placebo-controlled double-blind trial. *Stroke* 18:352–358, 1987.

122. Hsu CY, Liu TH, Hogan EL, Chao J, Sun G, Tai HH, Beckman JS, Freeman BA: Arachidonic acid and its metabolites in cerebral ischemia. *Ann NY Acad Sci* 559:282–295, 1989.

123. Ignarro LJ, Buga GM, Wood KS, Byrns RE, Chaudhuri G: Endothelium-derived relaxing factor produced and released from artery and vein is nitric oxide. *Proc Natl Acad Sci USA* 84:9265–9269, 1987.

124. Ishige N, Pitts LH, Berry I, Nishimura MC, James TL: The effects of hypovolemic hypotension on high-energy phosphate metabolism of traumatized brain in rats. *J Neurosurg* 68:129–136, 1988.

125. Ishige N, Pitts LH, Pogliani L, Hashimoto T, Nishimura MC, Bartkowski HM, James TL: Effect of hypoxia on traumatic brain injury in rats. Part 2: changes in high energy phosphate metabolism. *Neurosurgery* 20:854–858, 1987.

126. Italian Acute Stroke Study Group: Haemodilution in acute stroke: results of the Italian Haemodilution Trial. *Lancet* i:318–323, 1988.

127. Jastremski M, Sutton-Tyrell K, Vaagenes P, Abramson N, Heiselman D, Safar P, Brain Resuscitation Clinical Trial I Study Group: Glucocorticoid treatment does not improve neurological recovery following cardiac arrest. *JAMA* 262:3427–3430, 1989.

128. Jenkins LW, Lyeth BG, Hayes RL: The role of agonist-receptor interactions in the pathophysiology of mild and moderate head injury. In Hoff JT, Anderson PE, Cole T (eds): *Contemporary Issues in Neurological Surgery.* 1. Mild to Moderate Brain Injury. Blackwell Scientific Publications, Boston, 1989, pp 47–61.

129. Jenkins LW, Lyeth BG, Lewelt W, Moszynski K, DeWitt DS, Balster RL, Miller LP, Clifton GL, Young HF, Hayes RL: Combined pretrauma scopolamine and phencyclidine attenuate posttraumatic increased sensitivity to delayed secondary ischemia. *J Neurotrauma* 5:275–287, 1988.

130. Jenkins LW, Moszynski K, Lyeth BG, et al: Increased vulnerability of the mildly traumatized rat brain to cerebral ischemia: the use of controlled secondary ischemia as a research tool to identify common or different mechanisms contributing to mechanical and ischemic brain injury. *Brain Res* 477:211–224, 1989.

131. Jobsis FF: Noninvasive, infrared monitoring of cerebral and myocardial oxygen sufficiency and circulatory parameters. *Science* 198:1264–1267, 1977.

132. Kaczmarek LK: The role of protein kinase C in the regulation of ion channels and neurotransmitter release. *Trends Neurosci* 10:30, 1987.

133. Kassell NF, Drake CG: Timing of aneurysm surgery. *Neurosurgery* 10:514–519, 1982.

134. Kassell NF, Drake CG: Review of the management of saccular aneurysms. *Neurol Clin* 1:73–86, 1983.

135. Kassell NF, Sasaki T, Colohan ART, Nazar G: Cerebral vasospasm following aneurysmal subarachnoid hemorrhage. *Stroke* 16:562–572, 1985.

136. Katayama Y, Becker DP, Tamura T, Hovda DA: Massive increases in extracellular potassium and the indiscriminate release of glutamate following concussive brain injury. *J Neurosurg* 73:889–900, 1990.

137. Katayama Y, DeWitt DS, Becker DP, Hayes RL: Behavioral evidence for a cholinoceptive pontine inhibitory area: descending control of spinal motor output and sensory input. *Brain Res* 296:241–262, 1984.

138. Kempski O, Shohami E, von Lubitz D, Hallenbeck JM, Feuerstein G: Postischemic production of eicosanoids in gerbil brain. *Stroke* 18:111–119, 1987.

139. Kety SS, Schmidt CF: The nitrous oxide method for the quantitative determination of cerebral blood flow in man: theory, procedure and normal values. *J Clin Invest* 27:476–483, 1948.

140. Kiwak KJ, Moskowitz MA, Levine L: Leukotriene production in gerbil brain after ischemic insult, subarachnoid hemorrhage, and concussive injury. *J Neurosurg* 62:865–869, 1985.

141. Kolkka R, Hilberman M: Neurologic dysfunction following cardiac operation with low-flow, low-pressure cardiopulmonary bypass. *J Thorac Cardiovasc Surg* 79:432–437, 1980.

142. Kontos HA: Oxygen radicals in cerebral vascular injury. *Circ Res* 57:508–516, 1985.

143. Kontos HA, Raper AJ, Patterson JL: Analysis of vasoactivity of local pH, PCO₂, and bicarbonate on pial vessels. *Stroke* 8:358–360, 1977.

144. Kontos HA, Wei EP, Ellis EF, Jenkins LW, Povlishock JT, Rowe GT, Hess ML: Appearance of superoxide anion radical in cerebral extracellular space during increased prostaglandin synthesis in cats. *Circ Res* 57:142–151, 1985.

145. Kontos HA, Wei EP, Povlishock JT, Dietrich WD, Magiera CJ, Ellis EF: Cerebral arteriolar damage by arachidonic acid and prostaglandin G₂. *Science* 209:1242–1245, 1980.

146. Kontos HA, Wei EP, Povlishock JT, Kukreja RC, Hess ML: Inhibition by arachidonate of cerebral arteriolar dilation from acetylcholine. *Am J Physiol* 256:H665–H671, 1989.

147. Kontos HA, Wei EP, Raper AJ, Rosenblum WI, Navari RM, Patterson JL: Role of tissue hypoxia in local regulation of cerebral microcirculation. *Am J Physiol* 234:H582–H591, 1978.

148. Kuschinsky W: Coupling between functional activity, metabolism and blood flow in the brain: state of the art. *Microcirculation* 2:357–378, 1983.

149. Lam AM, Winn HR, Cullen BF, Sundling N: Hyperglycemia and neurological outcome in patients with head injury. *J Neurosurg* 75:545–551, 1991.

150. Langfitt TW, Obrist WD: Cerebral blood flow and metabolism after intracranial trauma. *Prog Neurol Surg* 10:14–48, 1981.

151. Lanier WL, Stangland KJ, Scheithauer BW, Milde JH, Michenfelder JD: The effects of dextrose infusion and head position on neurologic outcome after complete cerebral ischemia in primates: examination of a model. *Anesthesiology* 66:39–48, 1987.

152. Lee KS: Selective neuronal vulnerability and the distribution of N-methyl-D-aspartate (NMDA) receptors. *Neurobiol Aging* 10:611–613, 1989.

153. Lee MC, Mastri AR, Waltz AG, Loewenson RB: Ineffectiveness of dexamethasone for treatment of experimental cerebral infarction. *Stroke* 5:216–218, 1974.

154. Leon A, Lipartiti M, Seren MS, Lazzaro A, Massari S, Koga T, Toffano G, Skaper SD: Hypoxic-ischemic damage and the neuroprotective effects of GM$_1$ ganglioside. *Stroke* 21(Suppl III):III-95–III-97, 1990.

155. Leonov Y, Sterz F, Safar P, Radovsky A, Oku K-I, Tisherman S, Stezoski SW: Mild cerebral hypothermia during and after cardiac arrest improves neurologic outcome in dogs. *J Cereb Blood Flow Metab* 10:57–70, 1990.

156. Levy DE, Caronna JJ, Singer BH, Lapinski RH, Frydman H, Plum F: Predicting outcome from hypoxic-ischemic coma. *JAMA* 253:1420–1426, 1985.

157. Lewelt W, Jenkins LW, Miller JD: Autoregulation of cerebral blood flow after experimental fluid percussion injury of the brain. *J Neurosurg* 53:500–511, 1980.

158. Lin T-N, Liu TH, Xu J, Hsu CY, Sun GY: Brain polyphosphoinositide metabolism during focal ischemia in rat cortex. *Stroke* 22:495–498, 1991.

159. Little JR: Modification of acute focal ischemia by treatment with mannitol and high-dose dexamethasone. *J Neurosurg* 49:517–524, 1978.

160. Liu TH, Beckman JS, Freeman BA, Hogan EL, Hsu CY: Polyethylene glycol-conjugated superoxide dismutase and catalase reduce ischemic brain injury. *Am J Physiol* 256:H589-93, 1989.

161. Longstreth WT, Diehr P, Inui TS: Prediction of awakening after out-of-hospital cardiac arrest. *N Engl J Med* 308:1378–1382, 1983.

162. Longstreth WT Jr, Diehr P, Cobb LA, Hanson RW, Blair AD: Neurologic outcome and blood glucose levels during out-of-hospital cardiopulmonary resuscitation. *Neurology* 36:1186–1191, 1986.

163. Longstreth WT Jr, Inui TS: High blood glucose level on hospital admission and poor neurological recovery after cardiac arrest. *Ann Neurol* 15:59–63, 1984.

164. Lucas DR, Newhouse JP: The toxic effect of sodium L-glutamate on the inner layers of the retina. *Arch Ophthalmol* 58:193–201, 1957.

165. Lundgren J, Zhang H, Agardh C-D, Smith M-L, Evans PJ, Halliwell B, Siesjö BK: Acidosis-induced ischemic brain damage: are free radicals involved? *J Cereb Blood Flow Metab* 11:587–596, 1991.

166. Lyeth BG, Dixon CE, Giebel ML, Robinson SE, Hamm RJ, Stonnington HH, Young HF, Hayes RL: The effects of scopolamine pre- and post-treatment on the responses to concussive brain injury in the rat. *Soc Neurosci* 12:967, 1986.

167. Marsh ML, Aidinis SJ, Naughton KVH, Marshall LF, Shapiro HM: The technique of nitroprusside administration modifies the intracranial pressure response. *Anesthesiology* 51:538–541, 1979.

168. Marshall JJ, Kontos HA: Endothelium-derived relaxing factors. A perspective from in vivo data. *Hypertension* 16:371–386, 1990.

169. Marshall JJ, Wei EP, Kontos HA: Independent blockade of cerebral vasodilation from acetylcholine and nitric oxide. *Am J Physiol* 255:H847–H854, 1988.

169a. Marshall LF, Smith RW, Shapiro HM: The outcome with aggressive treatment in severe head injuries. Part II: acute and chronic barbiturate administration in the management of head injury. *J Neurosurg* 50(1):26–30, 1979.

170. Maset AL, Marmarou A, Ward JD, Choi S, Lutz HA, Brooks D, Moulton RJ, DeSalles A, Muizelaar JP, Turner H, Young HF: Pressure-volume index in head injury. *J Neurosurg* 67:832–840, 1987.

171. Mathew RJ, Wilson WH: Caffeine induced changes in cerebral circulation. *Stroke* 16:814–817, 1985.

172. Maximilian VA, Prohovnik I, Risberg J: Cerebral hemodynamic response to mental activation in normo- and hypercapnia. *Stroke* 11:342–347, 1980.

173. McCalden TA, Nath RG, Thiele K: The effects of a calcium antagonist (nimodipine) on basal cerebral blood flow and reactivity to various agonists. *Stroke* 15:527–530, 1984.

174. McIntosh TK, Faden AI, Yamakami I, Vink R: Magnesium deficiency exacerbates and pretreatment improves outcome following traumatic brain injury in rats: ^{31}P magnetic resonance spectroscopy and behavioral studies. *J Neurotrauma* 5:17, 1988.

175. McIntosh TK, Vink R, Soares H, Simon R: Possible role of excitatory amino acid neurotransmitters in pathophysiology of experimental brain injury [Abstract]. *J Cereb Blood Flow Metab* 9:S77, 1989.

176. Meldrum B: Protection against ischaemic neuronal damage by drugs acting on excitatory neurotransmission. *Cerebrovasc Brain Metab Rev* 2:27–57, 1990.

177. Messeter K, Brandt L, Ljunggren B, Svendgaard NA, Algotsson L, Romner B, Ryding E: Prediction and prevention of delayed ischemic dysfunction after aneurysmal subarachnoid hemorrhage and early operation. *Neurosurgery* 20:548–553, 1987.

178. Metz S, Keats AS: Benefits of a glucose-containing priming solution for cardiopulmonary bypass. *Anesth Analg* 72:428–434, 1991.

179. Metz S, Slogoff S: Thiopental sodium by single bolus dose compared to infusion for cerebral protection during cardiopulmonary bypass. *J Clin Anesth* 2:226–231, 1990.

180. Meyer CHA, Lowe D, Meyer M, Richardson PL, Neil-Dwyer G: Subarachnoid haemorrhage: older patients have low cerebral blood flow. *Br Med J* 285:1149–1153, 1982.

181. Meyer FB, Anderson RE, Friedrich PF: MK-801 attenuates capillary bed compression and hypoperfusion following incomplete focal cerebral ischemia. *J Cereb Blood Flow Metab* 10:895–902, 1990.

182. Meyer FB, Anderson RE, Sundt Jr TM, Yaksh TL: Intracellular brain pH, indicator tissue perfusion, electroencephalography, and histology in severe and moderate focal cortical ischemia in the rabbit. *J Cereb Blood Flow Metab* 6:71–78, 1986.

183. Meyer FB, Anderson RE, Sundt TM, Sharbrough FW: Selective central nervous system calcium channel blockers—a new class of anticonvulsant agents. *Mayo Clin Proc* 61:239–247, 1986.

184. Meyer FB, Anderson RE, Yaksh TL, Sundt TM Jr: Effect of nimodipine on intracellular brain pH, cortical blood flow, and EEG in experimental focal cerebral ischemia. *J Neurosurg* 64:617–626, 1986.

185. Meyer FB, Piepgras DG, Sandok BA, Sundt Jr TM, Forbes G: Emergency carotid endarterectomy for patients with acute carotid occlusion and profound neurological deficits. *Ann Surg* 203:82–89, 1986.

186. Meyer FB, Piepgras DG, Sundt Jr TM, Yanagihara T: Emergency embolectomy for acute occlusion of the middle cerebral artery. *J Neurosurg* 62:639–647, 1985.

187. Michenfelder JD: The interdependency of cerebral functional and metabolic effects following massive doses of thiopental in the dog. *Anesthesiology* 41:231–236, 1974.

188. Michenfelder JD, Milde JH: Influence of anesthetics on metabolic, functional and pathological responses to regional cerebral ischemia. *Stroke* 6:405–410, 1975.

189. Mies G, Kloiber O, Drewes LR, Hossman K-A: Cerebral blood flow and regional potassium distribution during focal ischemia of gerbil brain. *Ann Neurol* 16:232–237, 1984.

190. Miller JD, Bobo H, Kapp JP: Inaccurate pressure readings for subarachnoid bolts. *Neurosurgery* 19:253–255, 1986.

191. Miller JD, Butterworth JF, Gudeman SK, Faulkner JE, Choi SC, Selhorst JB, Harbison JW, Lutz HA, Young HF, Becker DP: Further experience in the management of severe head injury. *J Neurosurg* 54:289–299, 1981.

192. Minamisawa H, Nordström C-H, Smith M-L, Siesjo BK: The influence of mild body and brain hypothermia on ischemic brain damage. *J Cereb Blood Flow Metab* 10:365–374, 1990.

193. Monaghan DT, Bridges RJ, Cotman CW: The excitatory amino acid receptors: their classes, pharmacology, and distinct properties in the function of the central nervous system. *Annu Rev Pharmacol Toxicol* 29:365–402, 1989.

194. Morawetz RB, Crowell RH, DeGirolami U, Marcoux FW, Jones TH, Halsey JH: Regional cerebral blood flow thresholds during cerebral ischemia. *Fed Proc* 38:2493–2494, 1979.

195. Morii S, Ngai AC, Ko KR, Winn HR: Role of adenosine in regulation of cerebral blood flow: effects of theophylline during normoxia and hypoxia. *Am J Physiol* 253:H165–H175, 1987.

196. Moufarrij NA, Little JR, Skrinska V, Lucas FV, Latchaw JP, Slugg RM, Lesser RP: Thromboxane synthetase inhibition in acute focal cerebral ischemia in cats. *J Neurosurg* 61:1107–1112, 1984.

197. Muizelaar JP, Becker DP: Induced hypertension for the treatment of cerebral ischemia after subarachnoid hemorrhage. Direct effect on cerebral blood flow. *Surg Neurol* 25:317–325, 1986.

198. Muizelaar JP, Lutz HA III, Becker DP: Effect of mannitol on ICP and CBF and correlation with pressure autoregulation in severely head-injured patients. *J Neurosurg* 61:700–706, 1984.

199. Nicholls DG: Release of glutamate, aspartate and gamma-aminobutyric acid from isolated nerve terminals. *J Neurochem* 52:331–341, 1989.

200. Nicoletti F, Wroblewski JT, Costa E: Magnesium ions inhibit the stimulation of inositol phospholipid hydrolysis by endogenous excitatory amino acids in primary cultures of cerebellar granule cells. *J Neurochem* 48:967–973, 1987.

201. Nicoll RA: The coupling of neurotransmitter receptors to ion channels in the brain. *Science* 241:545, 1988.

202. Nowak L, Bregestovski P, Ascher P, Herbelt A, Prochiantz A: Magnesium gates glutamate-activated channels in mouse central neurons. *Nature* 307:462–465, 1984.

203. Nussmeier NA, Arlund C, Slogoff S: Neuropsychiatric complications after cardiopulmonary bypass: cerebral protection by a barbiturate. *Anesthesiology* 64:165–170, 1986.

204. Obrist WD, Langfitt TW, Jaggi JL, Cruz J, Gennarelli TA: Cerebral blood flow and metabolism in comatose patients with acute head injury. Relationship to intracranial hypertension. *J Neurosurg* 61:241–253, 1984.

205. Obrist WD, Thompson HK Jr, Wang HS, Wilkinson WE: Regional cerebral blood flow estimated by ^{133}Xenon inhalation. *Stroke* 6:245–256, 1975.

206. Olesen J, Hougard K, Hertz M: Isoproterenol and propranolol: ability to cross the blood-brain barrier and effects on cerebral circulation in man. *Stroke* 9:344–349, 1978.

207. Olesen J, Paulson OB, Lassen NA: Regional cerebral blood flow in man determined by the initial slope of the clearance of intra-arterially injected ^{133}Xe. Theory of the method, normal values, error of measurement, correction for remaining radioactivity, relation to other flow parameters and response to PACO$_2$ changes. *Stroke* 2:519–540, 1971.

208. Olney JW: Brain lesions, obesity, and other disturbances in mice treated with monosodium glutamate. *Science* 164:719–721, 1969.

209. Olney JW, Labruyere J, Price MT: Pathological changes induced in cerebro-cortical neurons by phencyclidine and related drugs. *Science* 244:1360–1362, 1989.

210. Ordway RW, Singer JJ, Walsh Jr JV: Direct regulation of ion channels by fatty acids. *Trends Neurosci* 14:96, 1991.

211. Ortiz A, MacDonall JS, Wakade CG, Karpiak SE: GM1 ganglioside reduces cognitive dysfunction after focal cortical ischemia. *Pharmacol Biochem Behav* 37:679–684, 1990.

212. Papo I, Benedetti A, Carteri A, Merli GA, Mingrino S, Bruno R: Monosialo-ganglioside in subarachnoid hemorrhage. *Stroke* 22:22–26, 1991.

213. Paulson OB, Strandgaard S, Edvinsson L: Cerebral autoregulation. *Cerebro-vasc Brain Metab Rev* 2:161–192, 1990.

214. Pearson RM, Griffith DNW, Woollard M, James IM: Comparison of effects on cerebral blood flow of rapid reduction in systemic arterial pressure by diazoxide and labetalol in hypertensive patients: preliminary findings. *Br J Clin Pharmacol* 8:195S–198S, 1979.

215. Pellegrino DA, Koenig HM, Albrecht RF: Nitric oxide synthesis and regional cerebral blood flow responses to hypercapnia and hypoxia in the rat. *J Cereb Blood Flow Metab* 13:80–87, 1993.

216. Petruk KC, West M, Mohr G, et al: Nimodipine treatment in poor-grade aneurysm patients: results of a multicenter double-blind placebo-controlled trial. *J Neurosurg* 68:505–517, 1988.

217. Phillis JW: Adenosine in the control of the cerebral circulation. *Cerebrovasc Brain Metab Rev* 1:26–54, 1989.

218. Phillis JW, DeLong RE: The role of adenosine in cerebral vascular regulation during reductions in perfusion pressure. *J Pharm Pharmacol* 38:460–462, 1986.

219. Phillis JW, Preston G, DeLong RE: Effects of anoxia on cerebral blood flow in the rat brain: evidence for a role of adenosine in autoregulation. *J Cereb Blood Flow Metab* 4:586–592, 1984.

220. Piantadosi CA, Hemstreet TM, Jobis-Vandervliet FF: Near-infrared spectro-photometric monitoring of oxygen distribution to intact brain and skeletal muscle tissues. *Crit Care Med* 14:698–706, 1986.

221. Poole GV Jr, Johnson JC, Prough DS, Stump DA, Stullken EH: Cerebral hemodynamics after hemorrhagic shock: effects of the type of resuscitation fluid. *Crit Care Med* 14:629–633, 1986.

222. Poole Jr GV, Prough DS, Johnson JC, Stullken EH, Stump DA, Howard G: Effects of resuscitation from hemorrhagic shock on cerebral hemodynamics in the presence of an intracranial mass. *J Trauma* 27:18–23, 1987.

223. Pritz MB, Giannotta SL, Kindt GW, McGillicuddy JE, Prager RL: Treatment of patients with neurological deficits associated with cerebral vasospasm by intravascular volume expansion. *Neurosurgery* 3:364–368, 1978.

224. Proctor HJ, Cairns C, Fillipo D, Palladino GW, Rosner MJ: Brain metabolism during increased intracranial pressure as assessed by niroscopy. *Surgery* 96:273–279, 1984.

225. Prough DS, Coker LH, Lee S, Yates F, McWhorter JM: Hyperglycemia and neurologic outcome in patients with closed-head injury [abstr]. *Anesthesiology* 69(Suppl 3a):A584, 1988.

226. Prough DS, Furberg CD: Nimodipine and the "no-reflow phenomenon"—experimental triumph, clinical failure? *Anesth Analg* 68:431–435, 1989.

227. Prough DS, Johnson JC, Stump DA, Stullken EH, Poole GV Jr, Howard G: Effects of hypertonic saline versus lactated Ringer's solution on cerebral oxygen transport during resuscitation from hemorrhagic shock. *J Neurosurg* 64:627–632, 1986.

228. Prough DS, Kong D, Watkins WD, Stout R, Stump DA, Beamer WC: Inhibition of thromboxane A2 production does not improve post-ischemic brain hypoperfusion in the dog. *Stroke* 17:1272–1276, 1986.

229. Prough DS, Mills SA: Should thiopental sodium administration be a standard of care for open cardiac procedures? *J Clin Anesth* 2:221–225, 1990.

230. Prough DS, Rogers AT, Stump DA, Mills SA, Gravlee GP, Taylor C: Hyper-carbia depresses cerebral oxygen consumption during cardiopulmonary bypass. *Stroke* 21:1162–1166, 1990.

231. Prough DS, Stump DA, Roy RC, Gravlee GP, Williams T, Mills SA, Hinshel-wood L, Howard G: Response of cerebral blood flow to changes in carbon dioxide tension during hypothermic cardiopulmonary bypass. *Anesthesiology* 64:576–581, 1986.

232. Pulsinelli WA, Levy DE, Sigsbee B, Scherer P, Plum F: Increased damage after ischemic stroke in patients with hyperglycemia with or without estab-lished diabetes mellitus. *Am J Med* 74:540–544, 1983.

233. Pulsinelli WA, Waldman S, Rawlinson D, Plum F: Moderate hyperglycemia augments ischemic brain damage: a neuropathologic study in the rat. *Neurol-ogy* 32:1239–1246, 1982.

234. Raichle ME, Stone HL: Cerebral blood flow autoregulation and graded hyper-capnia. *Eur Neurol* 6:1–5, 1971.

235. Rasmussen H, Takuwa Y, Park S: Protein kinase C in the regulation of smooth muscle contraction. *FASEB J* 1:177–185, 1987.

236. Reulen HJ: Vasogenic brain oedema. New aspects in its formation, resolution and therapy. *Br J Anaesth* 48:741–752, 1976.

237. Robertson CS, Narayan RK, Contant CF, Grossman RG, Gokaslan ZL, Pahwa R, Sherwood AM: Clinical experience with a continuous monitor of intracran-ial compliance. *J Neurosurg* 71:673–680, 1989.

238. Rogers AT, Stump DA, Gravlee GP, Prough DS, Angert KC, Wallenhaupt SL, Roy RC, Phipps J: Response of cerebral blood flow to phenylephrine infusion during hypothermic cardiopulmonary bypass: influence of PACO$_2$ management. *Anesthesiology* 69:547–551, 1988.

239. Roine RO, Kaste M, Kinnunen A, Nikki P, Sarna S, Kajaste S: Nimodipine after resuscitation from out-of-hospital ventricular fibrillation. A placebo-controlled, double-blind, randomized trial. *JAMA* 264:3171–3177, 1990.

240. Roland PE: Changes in brain blood flow and oxidative metabolism during mental activity. *NIPS* 2:120, 1987.

241. Roland PE, Friberg L: Localization of cortical areas activated by thinking. *J Neurophysiol* 53:1219–1243, 1985.

242. Rosenfeld D, Wolfson LI: The effects of activation procedures on regional cerebral blood flow in humans. *Semin Nucl Med* 11:172–185, 1981.

243. Rosner MJ, Becker DP: Experimental brain injury: successful therapy with the weak base, tromethamine. *J Neurosurg* 60:961–971, 1984.

244. Rossen R, Kabat H, Anderson JP: Acute arrest of cerebral circulation in man. *Arch Neurol Psychiatr* 50:510–528, 1943.

245. Rothman SM, Olney JW: Excitotoxicity and the NMDA receptor. *Trends Neurosci* 10:299–302, 1987.

246. Roy CS, Sherrington MB: On the regulation of the blood-supply of the brain. *J Physiol (Lond)* 11:85–108, 1890.

247. Sasaki T, Nakagomi T, Kirino T, Tamura A, Noguchi M, Saito I, Takakura K: Indomethacin ameliorates ischemic neuronal damage in the gerbil hippo-campal CA$_1$ sector. *Stroke* 19:1399, 1988.

248. Saul TG, Ducker TB: Effect of intracranial pressure monitoring and aggressive treatment on mortality in severe head injury. *J Neurosurg* 56:498–503, 1982.

249. Saul TG, Ducker TB, Saloman M, Carro E: Steroids in severe head injury. A prospective randomized clinical trial. *J Neurosurg* 54:596–600, 1981.

250. Saussy Jr DL, Mais DE, Knapp DR, Halushka PV: Thromboxane A$_2$ and prostaglandin endoperoxide receptors in platelets and vascular smooth mus-cle. *Circulation* 72:1202–1207, 1985.

251. Scandinavian Stroke Study Group: Multicenter trial of hemodilution in acute ischemic stroke. I. Results in the total patient population. *Stroke* 18:691–699, 1987.

252. Schmidley JW: Free radicals in central nervous system ischemia. *Stroke* 21:1086–1090, 1990.

253. Sekhar LN, Wechsler LR, Yonas H, Luyckx K, Obrist W: Value of transcranial Doppler examination in the diagnosis of cerebral vasospasm after subarach-noid hemorrhage. *Neurosurgery* 22:813–821, 1988.

254. Seren MS, Rubini R, Lazzaro A, Zanoni R, Fiori MG, Leon A: Protective effects of a monosialoganglioside derivative following transitory forebrain ischemia in rats. *Stroke* 21:1607–1612, 1990.

255. Severinghaus JW, Chiodi H, Eger EIII, Brandstater B, Hornbein TF: Cere-bral blood flow in man at high altitude. Role of cerebrospinal fluid pH in normalization of flow in chronic hypocapnia. *Circ Res* 19:274–282, 1966.

256. Sharbrough FW, Messick Jr JM, Sundt Jr TM: Correlation of continuous electroencephalograms with cerebral blood flow measurements during carotid endarterectomy. *Stroke* 4:674–683, 1973.

257. Shaw PJ, Batens D, Cartlidge NEF, French JM, Heaviside D, Julian DG, Shaw DA: Neurologic and neuropsychological morbidity following major surgery: comparison of coronary artery bypass and peripheral vascular sur-gery. *Stroke* 18:700–707, 1987.

258. Shaywitz BA, Rothstein P, Venes JL: Monitoring and management of in-creased intracranial pressure in Reye syndrome: results in 29 children. *Pediat-rics* 66:198–204, 1980.

259. Shimizu T, Wolfe LS: Arachidonic acid cascade and signal transduction. *J Neurochem* 55:1, 1990.

260. Siesjö BK: Cell damage in the brain: a speculative synthesis. *J Cereb Blood Flow Metab* 1:155–185, 1981.

261. Siesjö BK, Bendek G, Koide T, Westerberg E, Wieloch T: Influence of acidosis on liquid peroxidation in brain tissues in vitro. *J Cereb Blood Flow Metab* 5:253–258, 1985.

262. Siesjö BK, Wieloch T: Cerebral metabolism in ischaemia: neurochemical basis for therapy. *Br J Anaesth* 57:47–62, 1985.

263. Siesjö BK: Pathophysiology and treatment of focal cerebral ischemia. Part I: Pathophysiology. *J Neurosurg* 77:169–184, 1992.

264. Siesjö BK: Pathophysiology and treatment of focal cerebral ischemia. Part II: Mechanisms of damage and treatment. *J Neurosurg* 77:337–354, 1992.

265. Siesjo BK, Agardh C-D, Bengtsson F: Free radicals and brain damage. *Cerebrovasc Brain Metab Rev* 1:165–211, 1989.

266. Siesjo BK, Bengtsson F: Calcium fluxes, calcium antagonists, and calcium-related pathology in brain ischemia, hypoglycemia, and spreading depression: a unifying hypothesis. *J Cereb Blood Flow Metab* 9:127–140, 1989.

267. Smith AL, Hoff JT, Nielsen SL, Larson CP: Barbiturate protection in acute focal cerebral ischemia. *Stroke* 5:1–7, 1974.

268. Smith PLC, Treasure T, Newman SP, Joseph P, Ell PJ, Schneidau A, Harrison MJG: Cerebral consequences of cardiopulmonary bypass. *Lancet* 2:823–825, 1986.

269. Snyder JV, Nemoto EM, Carroll RG, Safar P: Global ischemia in dogs: intracranial pressures, brain blood flow and metabolism. *Stroke* 6:21–27, 1975.

270. Sokoloff L, Reivich M, Kennedy C, Des Rosiers MH, Patlak CS, Pettigrew KD, Sakurada O, Shinohara M: The ^{14}C deoxyglucose method for the measurement of local cerebral glucose utilization: theory, procedure, and normal values in the conscious and anesthetized albino rat. *J Neurochem* 28:897–916, 1977.

271. Solomon RA, Fink ME, Lennihan L: Early aneurysm surgery and prophylactic hypervolemic hypertensive therapy for the treatment of aneurysmal subarachnoid hemorrhage. *Neurosurgery* 23:699–704, 1988.

272. Sotaniemi KA, Mononen H, Hokkanen TE: Long-term cerebral outcome after open-heart surgery. A five-year neuropsychological follow-up study. *Stroke* 17:410–416, 1986.

273. Spittell Jr JA: Pentoxifylline and intermittent claudication. *Ann Intern Med* 102:126–127, 1985.

274. Steen PA, Gisvold SE, Milde JH, Newberg LA, Scheithauer BW, Lanier WL, Michenfelder JD: Nimodipine improves outcome when given after complete cerebral ischemia in primates. *Anesthesiology* 62:406–414, 1985.

275. Steen PA, Michenfelder JD, Milde JH: Incomplete versus complete cerebral ischemia: improved outcome with a minimal blood flow. *Ann Neurol* 6:389–398, 1979.

276. Stephan H, Weyland A, Kazmaier S, Henze T, Menck S, Sonntag H: Acid-base management during hypothermic cardiopulmonary bypass does not affect cerebral metabolism but does affect blood flow and neurological outcome. *Br J Anaesth* 69:51–57, 1992.

277. Stevens MK, Yaksh TL, Hansen II RB, Anderson RE: Effect of preischemia cyclooxygenase inhibition by zomepirac sodium on reflow, cerebral autoregulation, and EEG recovery in the cat after global ischemia. *J Cereb Blood Flow Metab* 6:691–702, 1986.

278. Steill IG, Hebert PC, Weitzman BN, Wells GA, Raman S, Stark RM, Higginson LAJ, Ahuja J, Dickinson GE: High-dose epinephrine in adult cardiac arrest. *N Engl J Med* 327:1045–1050, 1992.

279. Stockard JJ, Bickford RG, Chir B, Schauble JF: Pressure-dependent cerebral ischemia during cardiopulmonary bypass. *Neurology* 23:521–529, 1973.

280. Stullken EH, Balestrieri FJ, Prough DS, McWhorter JM: The hemodynamic effects of nimodipine in patients anesthetized for cerebral aneurysm clipping. *Anesthesiology* 62:346–348, 1985.

281. Sundt TM, Sharbrough FW, Anderson RF, Michenfelder JD: Cerebral blood flow measurements and electroencephalography during carotid endarterectomy. *J Neurosurg* 41:310–320, 1974.

282. Sundt TM Jr, Sharbrough FW, Piepgras DG: Correlation of cerebral blood flow and electroencephalographic changes during carotid endarterectomy. *Mayo Clin Proc* 56:533–543, 1981.

283. Symon L: Flow thresholds in brain ischaemia and the effects of drugs. *Br J Anaesth* 57:34–43, 1985.

284. Tanaka K, Gotoh F, Gomi S, Takashima S, Mihara B, Shirai T, Nogawa S, Nagata E: Inhibition of nitric oxide synthesis induces a significant reduction in local cerebral blood flow in the rat. *Neurosci Lett* 127:129–132, 1991.

285. Tans JTJ, Poortvliet DCJ: Intracranial volume-pressure relationship in man. Part 2: Clinical significance of the pressure-volume index. *J Neurosurg* 59:810–816, 1983.

286. The American Nimodipine Study Group: Clinical trial of nimodipine in acute ischemic stroke. *Stroke* 23:3–8, 1992.

287. The Hemodilution in Stroke Study Group: Hypervolemic hemodilution treatment of acute stroke. Results of a randomized multicenter trial using pentastarch. *Stroke* 20:317–323, 1989.

288. Thie A, Spitzer K, Kunze K: Spontaneous subarachnoid hemorrhage: assessment of prognosis and initial management in the intensive care unit. *J Intensive Care Med* 2:103–115, 1987.

289. Todd NV, Picozzi P, Crockard HA, Russell RR: Reperfusion after cerebral ischemia: influence of duration of ischemia. *Stroke* 17:460–466, 1986.

290. Todd NV, Picozzi P, Crockard HA, Russell RWR: Duration of ischemia influences the development and resolution of ischemic brain edema. *Stroke* 17:466–471, 1986.

291. Tommasino C, Moore S, Todd MM: Cerebral effects of isovolemic hemodilution with crystalloid or colloid solutions. *Crit Care Med* 16:862–868, 1988.

292. Traystman RJ, Kirsch JR, Koehler RC: Oxygen radical mechanisms of brain injury following ischemia and reperfusion. *Am J Physiol* 1185, 1991.

293. Trojaborg W, Boysen G: Relationship between EEG, regional cerebral blood flow and internal carotid artery pressure during carotid endarterectomy. *Electroencephalogr Clin Neurophysiol* 34:61–69, 1973.

294. Tyson GW, Teasdale GM, Graham DI, McCulloch J: Focal cerebral ischemia in the rat: topography of hemodynamic and histopathological changes. *Ann Neurol* 15:559–567, 1984.

295. Vink R, McIntosh TK, Demediuk P, Weiner MW, Faden AI: Decline in intracellular free Mg^{2+} is associated with irreversible tissue injury after brain trauma. *J Biol Chem* 263:757–761, 1988.

296. von Essen C: Effects of dopamine on the cerebral blood flow in the dog. *Acta Neurol Scand* 50:39–52, 1974.

297. Vries JK, Becker DP, Young HF: A subarachnoid screw for monitoring intracranial pressure. *J Neurosurg* 39:416–419, 1973.

298. Walz W, Harold DE: Brain lactic acidosis and synaptic function. *Can J Physiol Pharmacol* 68:164–169, 1990.

299. Ward JD, Becker DP, Miller DJ: Failure of prophylactic barbiturate coma in the treatment of severe head injury. *J Neurosurg* 62:383–388, 1985.

300. Wei EP, Kontos HA: H$_2$O$_2$ and endothelium-dependent cerebral arteriolar dilation. Implications for the identity of endothelium-derived relaxing factor generated by acetylcholine. *Hypertension* 16:162–169, 1990.

301. Wei EP, Kontos HA, Dietrich WD, Povlishock JT, Ellis EF: Inhibition by free radical scavengers and by cyclooxygenase inhibitors of pial arteriolar abnormalities from concussive brain injury in cats. *Circ Res* 48:95–103, 1981.

302. Wei EP, Lamb RG, Kontos HA: Increased phospholipase C activity after experimental brain injury. *J Neurosurg* 56:695–698, 1982.

303. Welsh FA, Harris VA: Postischemic hypothermia fails to reduce ischemic injury in gerbil hippocampus. *J Cereb Blood Flow Metab* 11:617–620, 1991.

304. Welsh FA, Sims RE, Harris VA: Mild hypothermia prevents ischemic injury in gerbil hippocampus. *J Cereb Blood Flow Metab* 10:557–563, 1990.

305. Whitley JM, Prough DS, Brockschmidt JK, Vines SM, DeWitt DS: Cerebral hemodynamic effects of fluid resuscitation in the presence of an experimental intracranial mass. *Surgery* 110:514–522, 1991.

306. Wieloch T, Siesjo BK: Ischemic brain injury: the importance of calcium, lipolytic activities, and free fatty acids. *Pathol Biol* 30:269–277, 1982.

307. Wilkins RH: Attempts at prevention or treatment of intracranial arterial spasm: an update. *Neurosurgery* 18:808–825, 1986.

308. Wise G, Sutter R, Burkholder J: The treatment of brain ischemia with vasopressor drugs. *Stroke* 3:135–140, 1972.

309. Wolfe LS: Eicosanoids: prostaglandins, thromboxanes, leukotrienes, and other derivatives of carbon-20 unsaturated fatty acids. *J Neurochem* 38:1–14, 1982.

310. Wong BI, McLean RF, Naylor CD, Snow WG, Harrington EM, Gawel MJ, Woods RB, Fremes SE: Central-nervous-system dysfunction after warm or hypothermic cardiopulmonary bypass. *Lancet* 339:1383–1384, 1992.

311. Wood JH, Polyzoidis KS, Epstein CM, Gibby GL, Tindall GT: Quantitative EEG alterations after isovolemic-hemodilutional augmentation of cerebral perfusion in stroke patients. *Neurology* 34:764–768, 1984.

312. Wood JH, Simeone FA, Fink EA, Golden MA: Hypervolemic hemodilution in experimental focal cerebral ischemia. Elevation of cardiac output, regional cortical blood flow, and ICP after intravascular volume expansion with low molecular weight dextran. *J Neurosurg* 59:500–509, 1983.

313. Wood JH, Snyder LL, Simeone FA: Failure of intravascular volume expansion without hemodilution to elevate cortical blood flow in region of experimental focal ischemia. *J Neurosurg* 56:80–91, 1982.

314. Yang MS, DeWitt DS, Becker DP, Hayes RL: Regional brain metabolite levels following mild experimental head injury in the cat. *J Neurosurg* 63:617–621, 1985.

315. Zaidan JR, Klochany A, Martin WM, Ziegler JS, Harless DM, Andrews RB: Effect of thiopental on neurologic outcome following coronary artery bypass grafting. *Anesthesiology* 74:406–411, 1991.

316. Zeumer H, Hacke W, Ringelstein EB: Local intraarterial thrombolysis in vertebrobasilar thromboembolic disease. *AJNR* 4:401–404, 1983.

317. Zivin JA, Fisher M, DeGirolami U, Hemenway CC, Stashak JS: Tissue plasminogen activator reduces neurological damage after cerebral embolism. *Science* 230:1289–1292, 1985.

318. Zornow MH, Todd MM, Moore SS: The acute cerebral effects of changes in plasma osmolality and oncotic pressure. *Anesthesiology* 67:936–941, 1987.

319. Zorumski CF, Thio LL: Properties of vertebrate glutamate receptors: calcium mobilization and desensitization. *Prog Neurobiol* 39:295–336, 1992.

CHAPTER 15

Pharmacology of Colloids and Crystalloids

THOMAS G. RAINEY, M.D., F.C.C.M.
CHARLES A. READ, M.D., F.C.C.P.

This chapter reviews the use of colloids and crystalloids in the therapy of shock. Controversy exists as to the changes in body compartment composition in critical illness. Some investigations show depletion of extracellular fluid in shock from hemorrhage (with intravascular and interstitial fluid volumes both depleted) and an increase in intracellular water secondary to cell membrane and sodium-potassium pump dysfunction (25, 163–165). On the other hand, in surgical patients posttrauma, extracellular fluid is found not to be decreased but actually increased, whereas intravascular volume is depleted (44, 156). Despite this controversy, one thing is agreed upon—intravascular volume is depleted in many types of critical illness. Prompt restoration of intravascular volume depletion is essential to reestablish cellular perfusion and accomplish successful resuscitation.

A thorough knowledge of the distribution and pharmacokinetics of plasma expanders allows the clinician to promptly and efficiently resuscitate patients in shock from various causes, including trauma, sepsis, hemodilution, and burns. An understanding of this pharmacologic subject helps the physician to minimize side effects associated with overaggressive volume resuscitation (respiratory failure, peripheral edema) or inadequate resuscitation (renal failure, refractory shock). The chapter begins with a discussion of the general principles of fluid distribution within the body, and then reviews the pharmacology of common plasma volume-expanding agents and their application in various clinical situations.

BODY FLUID DISTRIBUTION BY COMPARTMENTS

The total body water (TBW) ranges from 45 to 65% of total body weight in the human adult. The average adult man's TBW equals 60% of total body weight (38, 57, 124), or 48 liters for an 80-kg man (147) (Table 15.1). Body water is distributed into two main compartments, the intracellular fluid (ICF) space, and the extracellular fluid (ECF) space. Two-thirds (32 liters) of the TBW resides in the ICF space and one-third (16 liters) in the ECF space (Fig. 15.1). The ECF space is further subdivided into the intravascular space and the interstitial space. Normally, approximately one-fourth of ECF resides in the intravascular compartment (4 liters) and three-fourths in the interstitial compartment (12 liters). The membranes separating these compartments are freely permeable to water, which moves under the force of osmotic drive until the osmolality in each compartment is equivalent.

When water is added into one compartment it distributes evenly throughout the TBW, and the amount of volume added to any given compartment is proportional to its fractional representation of TBW. As an example, if 3 liters of "free" water (no osmotically active particles) is added to the intravascular space (assuming none of that water exists in the body), the compartment volumes change from 16 to 17 liters in the ECF space and 32 to 34 liters in the ICF space (Fig. 15.2). Note that the placement of 3 liters of free water in the intravascular space results in a net increase of only 250 ml in the

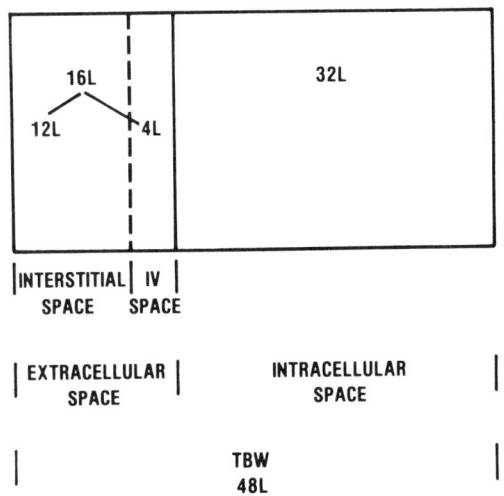

Figure 15.1. Distribution of total body water (TBW) in an 80-kg man (*IV*, intravascular).

Table 15.1. Total Body Water as Percentage of Body Weight[a]

Build	Total Body Water (% of Body Weight)	
	Male	*Female*
Thin	65	55
Average	60	50
Obese	55	45

[a] Modified from Scribner BH (ed): University of Washington Teaching Syllabus for the Course on Fluid and Electrolyte Balance. University of Washington Press, Seattle, 1969.

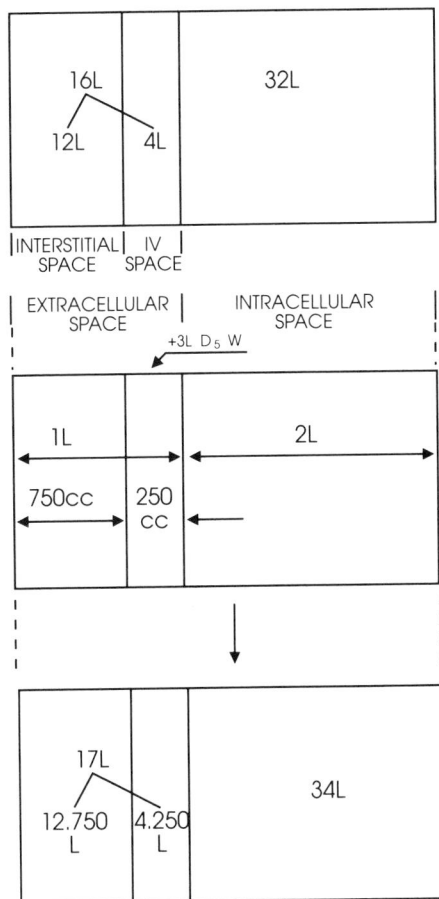

Figure 15.2. Distribution of 3 liters of free water (5% dextrose in water, D5W) in an 80-kg man with total body water of 48 liters (*IV*, intravascular).

intravascular volume after equilibration takes place. Approximately 30 minutes after a rapid volume infusion, less than one-tenth of the volume infused remains in the intravascular space (180)! If the 3 liters of infused solution are isotonic with plasma (Ringer's lactate, normal saline), a different fluid distribution occurs (Fig. 15.3). Since there is no difference in osmolality between the infused fluid and the body fluids, there is no driving force to cause water to diffuse into the intracellular compartment. The intact membrane between the interstitial space and the intravascular space is permeable to ions and small particles, whereas the membrane surrounding the ICF space functionally is not. Consequently, the ECF space is the distribution space for isotonic fluids such as normal saline and Ringer's lactate. It also should be noted that knowledge of the distribution space for isotonic fluid has important practical applications for resuscitation. Only one-fourth of the volume of isotonic fluid infused remains in the intravascular space after 30 minutes.

Application of these basic concepts allows one to predict the space of distribution for any standard intravenous solution, since these solutions are all some combination of free water and isotonic fluid. For example, 1000 ml of 0.45% saline can be thought of as 500 ml of normal (0.9%) saline plus 500 ml of free water. The portion that is isotonic (saline) distributes through the ECF space, and the portion that is water distributes through the TBW. If one tries to expand the intravascular volume of a hypotensive patient by giving 1000 ml of 0.45% saline over 1 hour, the resultant increase in intravascular

volume is only 165 ml! After distribution, the 500 ml of free water adds only 40 ml, and the 500 ml of normal saline adds approximately 125 ml to the intravascular volume. What initially appears to be a large volume of fluid adds very little to the intravascular volume of 4 to 5 liters. Writing intravenous fluid prescriptions and predicting the outcome of therapy becomes simple when fluid balance and distribution are thought of in these terms.

CRYSTALLOIDS

The term *crystalloid* as used here refers to solutions that contain sodium as their major osmotically active particle. Ringer's lactate and normal saline are the first solutions considered. A subsequent section addresses hypertonic saline.

ISOTONIC CRYSTALLOIDS: PHYSIOLOGY AND PHARMACOKINETICS

As described in the previous section, isotonic fluids such as Ringer's lactate and normal saline distribute evenly throughout the extracellular space. In normal healthy adults, approximately one-fourth of the volume infused remains in the intravascular space after 1 hour. Equilibration with the extracellular space occurs within 20 to 30 minutes after infusion. In the critically ill or injured patient, only one-fifth of the volume (56) or less (23) may remain in the circulation 1 to 2 hours after infusion. The "dwell time" in the circulation is the same in shock as in nonshock states (56).

In experimental acute blood loss leading to circulatory collapse, plasma volume becomes reduced and returns to normal over 3 to 4 days. As this equilibration occurs, hematocrit progressively decreases. It takes 24 hours or longer for the hematocrit to stabilize as intravascular volume is restored at the expense of interstitial and ICF volume. By 2 hours, 14 to 36% of the ultimate change in hematocrit occurs; 36 to 50% occurs in 8 hours and 63 to 77% in 24 hours (41). When any plasma expander, including crystalloid, is infused (exogenous fluid), a more immediate decrease in hematocrit occurs. However, as redistribution of resuscitation fluid out of the intravascular space occurs, the hematocrit again increases. The apparently erratic changes in serial hematocrit values seen during large volume crystalloid resuscitations are often the result of these fluid shifts rather than repeated episodes of bleeding.

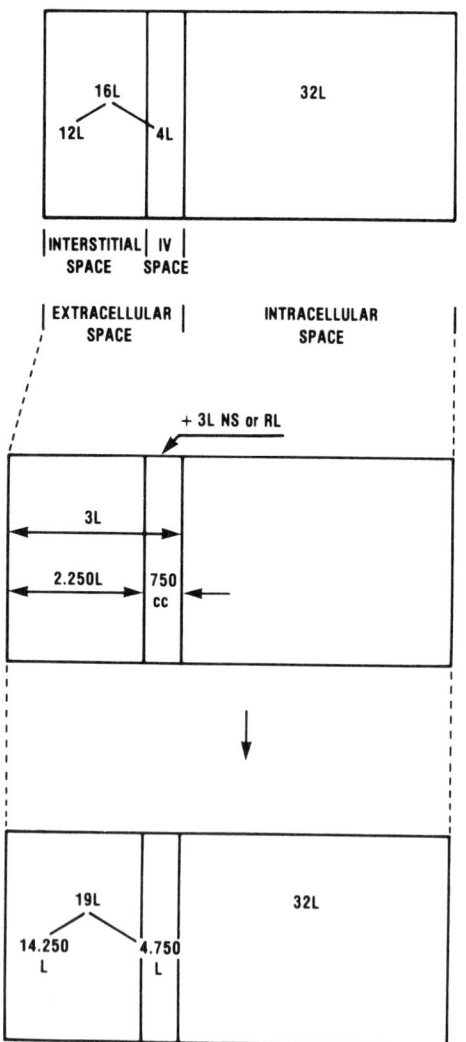

Figure 15.3. Distribution of 3 liters of normal saline (*NS*) or Ringer's lactate (*RL*) in an 80-kg man with total body water of 48 liters (*IV*, intravascular).

The total serum protein levels show similar changes. Endogenous restoration of depleted intravascular volume occurs through movement of interstitial fluid into the intravascular space. Catecholamines mediate arteriolar vasoconstriction, which diminishes capillary bed hydrostatic pressure favoring influx of interstitial fluid into the vascular tree distal to the arteriolar constriction. Subsequently, lymphatic flow returns plasma proteins to the intravascular space. Increases in interstitial pressure caused by crystalloid distribution into the interstitial space may augment lymphatic flow and thus the "protein-refill" mechanism (91). This process, combined with increased albumin synthesis and spontaneous diuresis secondary to volume repletion, explains the return of serum protein levels to normal within days after crystalloid resuscitation (164, 192).

Normal saline and Ringer's lactate can be used interchangeably (see the section of this chapter entitled "Prescribing Information"). The lactate load in Ringer's lactate solution does not potentiate the lactic acidemia associated with shock (187). Rather, as circulating blood volume is restored, diminished lactic acid production and decreased serum lactate levels are found (22, 137, 187). The use of Ringer's lactate does not alter the reliability of blood lactate measurements (96).

The theoretic concern that large volumes of normal saline produce a "dilution acidosis" is not a problem clinically. Normal saline, like Ringer's lactate, causes no acidosis when studied in traumatic shock for which large volumes are administered (96). Saline resuscitation provides an excess of circulating chloride ion, which normally is excreted by the kidney without problem. In patients with acidosis caused by an organic acid (ketoacidosis or lactic acidosis), hyperchloremic acidosis may be seen during the postresuscitation period (121). However, this acidosis results from loss of the bicarbonate substrate (ketones) in the urine rather than occurring secondary to the administered chloride load.

INDICATIONS

Isotonic crystalloid solutions are indicated for plasma volume expansion (95, 113). They are inexpensive (Table 15.2), readily available, easily stored, and reaction free, and they help to correct extracellular electrolyte and volume deficits. In hemorrhagic shock, crystalloids can be used to replace plasma volume immediately (while blood is being crossmatched) and can limit the total amount of blood required for resuscitation (153). Crystalloids decrease blood viscosity as the blood volume is expanded. In the oliguric patient, a diagnostic "volume challenge" with crystalloid may safely help to distinguish between intravascular volume depletion and acute renal failure.

SIDE EFFECTS

Crystalloid solutions are nontoxic and free from side effects if used appropriately. Excessive crystalloid administration may cause peripheral and pulmonary edema.

Peripheral Edema

Edema is expected from isotonic crystalloid use, since three-quarters or more of the volume administered distributes

Table 15.2.   Comparative Prices of Volume-Expanding Agents

Agent	Amount (ml)	Average Cost ($)	Cost per 400–500 ml IV Expansion ($)[a]
Albumin 5%	500	105.50	105.50
Albumin 25%	100	100.00	100.00
Hydroxyethyl starch (Hetastarch)	500	63.18	64.00
Dextran-40	500	85.69	45.00–85.00
Dextran-70	500	52.91	25.00–52.00
Pentastarch	500	66.00	47.15
Ringer's lactate	1000	7.90[b]	10.50–21.07
Normal saline	1000	6.31[b]	8.30–1660
Hypertonic (3%) saline	500	5.19[b]	5.19[b]

[a] Cost based on AWP as listed in Cardinale VA (ed): Drug Topics Redbook 1991. Economics, 1991. Copyright © *Drug Topics Red Book 1991* edition, published by Medical Economics Data, Montvale, NJ.
[b] Cost based on average list price as quoted by major manufacturers.

in the interstitial compartment of the extracellular space. Edema can be limited by appropriate monitoring of the adequacy of resuscitation to prevent volume overload.

Pulmonary Edema

Isotonic crystalloid resuscitation lowers colloid oncotic pressure by reducing the serum protein concentrations (55, 196). Whether the reduction in plasma proteins and consequent lowering of plasma colloid oncotic pressure decreases lung function is a controversial issue (56, 61, 132, 145, 157, 163, 193). "Edema safety factors," such as increased lymphatic flow, diminished pulmonary interstitial oncotic pressure, and increased interstitial hydrostatic pressure, limit the effect of lowered colloid oncotic pressure to increase fluid transudation from the vascular space (91). When the total crystalloid volume administered is controlled to prevent volume overload, there is no difference in lung function in resuscitation of shock using crystalloid or colloid solutions (59, 95, 113, 115, 192). The development of the adult respiratory distress syndrome (ARDS) is associated more closely with the presence of sepsis than with the type of fluid used in shock resuscitation.

RECOMMENDATIONS FOR USE

Shock

Crystalloid solutions are used in shock of various etiologies for the restoration of intravascular volume and repletion of interstitial water and electrolyte deficits (115, 152, 156, 176, 193). The volume of isotonic crystalloid required to attain adequate volume repletion varies from three (38, 56, 115, 165) to 12 (35) times the volume of colloid solution required to reach the same hemodynamic endpoint. The patient who is in shock, whether from trauma, hemorrhage, or sepsis, should receive immediate volume replacement with crystalloid solutions during evaluation of the clinical situation. Two to three liters administered promptly may restore blood pressure and peripheral perfusion. If the hematocrit is greater than 30% and hemodynamic stability remains, further aggressive fluid resuscitation may be unnecessary. Acute blood loss of 10 to 20% of the blood volume may be replaced adequately with crystalloid if given in a quantity of three to four times the volume of blood lost (12, 161, 191, 196). If continued fluid resuscitation is required and the hematocrit remains above

30%, the authors recommend the use of crystalloid in conjunction with 5 to 10% colloid solutions in a ratio of 4:1 (crystalloid:colloid by volume). If the hematocrit falls below 30%, packed red blood cells should be transfused. If the serum albumin level decreases below 2 to 2.5 g/dl, albumin or another colloid should be added to maintain the colloid oncotic pressure. Other blood components should be administered as necessitated by serial measurement of platelet count, prothrombin time, and partial thromboplastin time.

The major pitfall to avoid in isotonic crystalloid resuscitation is inadequate fluid administration. Five liters of isotonic crystalloid may be needed to replenish a 1-liter blood loss (160). Edema is to be expected and should not be interpreted as intravascular volume overload. Adequacy of intravascular volume repletion must be assessed by the usual parameters that indicate adequacy of peripheral perfusion—stable mean arterial pressure of 70 to 80 mm Hg, heart rate less than 100 beats/min, warm extremities with good capillary refill, adequate CNS function, urine volume of 0.5 to 1 ml/kg/hr, and absence of advancing acidosis. In massive resuscitation or other critical situations, pulmonary artery occlusion pressure, cardiac output, mixed venous oxygen content, and arteriovenous oxygen concentration difference ($AVDO_2$) must supplement these other parameters in guiding fluid administration. A more detailed discussion of hemodynamic monitoring in resuscitation of shock may be found elsewhere (155).

Diagnosis of Oliguria

Oliguria (urine output <0.5 ml/kg/hr) may indicate prerenal hypoperfusion resulting from intravascular volume depletion or congestive heart failure (CHF). In the critically ill patient (who often has underlying chronic obstructive pulmonary disease, ARDS, edema resulting from large volume resuscitation, hypoproteinemia, or sepsis with capillary leak) it may be impossible to distinguish volume depletion from CHF by physical examination. A volume challenge (500 ml over 5 minutes) with isotonic crystalloid solution can be helpful. If after an adequate volume challenge the patient's urine output increases, the diagnosis of intravascular volume depletion is confirmed, and subsequent fluid management can be altered appropriately. If the oliguria is not a result of intravascular volume depletion, no increase in urine output occurs with volume challenge. Since crystalloid fluids distribute out of the intravascular space rapidly, only a transient increase in intravascular volume results from a fluid challenge, and the patient with CHF does not experience a prolonged increase in vascular volume.

An adequate fluid challenge consists of no less than 500 ml of crystalloid Ringer's lactate or normal saline given over 5 minutes. A smaller volume or a longer time for infusion will not expand the intravascular volume significantly. Only 100 to 150 ml of the 500 ml administered will remain in the intravascular space after 30 minutes. If the volume challenge is given over 30 minutes, the intravascular volume (5 liters for a 70-kg man) would be expanded by a trivial 100 to 150 ml, thereby providing no information on the etiology of the oliguria since the intravascular volume was never expanded. Similarly, increasing the infusion rate of an oliguric patient from 100 ml/hr to 200 or 300 ml/hr provides no answer to the question of etiology of the oliguria, nor does it adequately treat volume depletion.

Prolonged prerenal hypoperfusion can lead to renal failure. The timely diagnosis and treatment of oliguria secondary to volume depletion is essential to avoid this disastrous consequence. If crystalloid volume challenge does not provide the answer, invasive diagnosis with a pulmonary artery catheter may be required. Colloid solutions should not be used to differentiate between intravascular volume depletion and CHF, since their dwell time in the intravascular space is much longer and osmotic diuresis occurs immediately with some preparations (dextran, hydroxyethyl starch).

PRESCRIBING INFORMATION

The contents of normal saline and Ringer's lactate solutions are shown in Table 15.3, and their costs in relation to other volume-expanding agents are listed in Table 15.2 (74).

Ringer's lactate contains 28 mEq of lactate, which must undergo hepatic metabolism to bicarbonate to release 28 mEq of free base per liter of solution. In patients with renal failure, this bicarbonate source may be useful as an acid buffer; however, when hyperkalemia is a problem, use of normal saline avoids the 4 mEq/liter potassium content of Ringer's lactate. Similarly, normal saline is preferred in hypercalcemic or hyponatremic states. In the presence of established hyperchloremic metabolic acidosis, Ringer's lactate is preferred to provide a

bicarbonate source and to diminish the administered chloride load.

HYPERTONIC SALINE

PHYSIOLOGY AND PHARMACOKINETICS

Hypertonic saline (7.5%) is advocated as an effective resuscitation fluid for hypovolemic shock and burns (63, 64, 110).

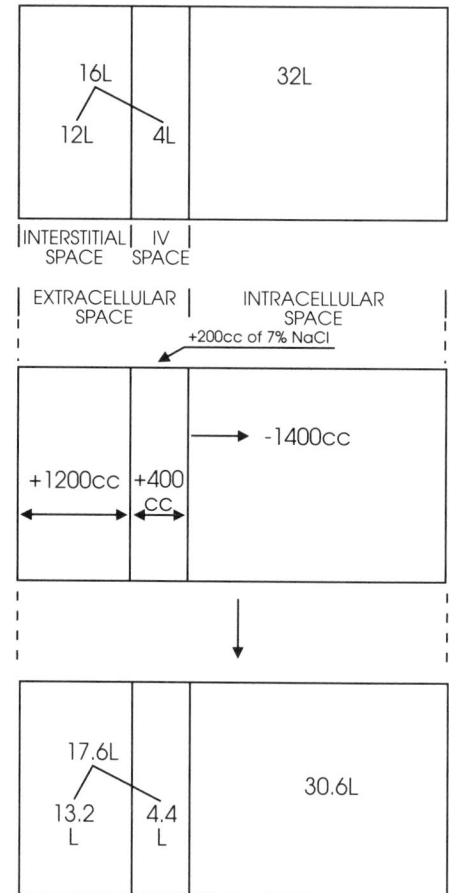

Figure 15.4. Distribution of 200 cc of 7% NaCl in an 80-kg man with total body water of 48 liters.

Table 15.3. Ionic Composition of Various Volume-Expanding Agents

Agent	Component (mEq/liter)				
	Na⁺	Cl⁻	K⁺	Ca²⁺	Lactate
Ringer's lactate	130	109	4	3	28
Normal saline	154	154	—	—	—
Albumin 5%	130–160	130–160	<1	—	—
Albumin 25%	130–160	130–160	<1	—	—
Dextran-40					
10% in normal saline	154	154	—	—	—
10% in water	0	0	—	—	—
Dextran-70					
6% in normal saline	154	154	—	—	—
6% in water	0	0	—	—	—
Hydroxyethyl starch (hetastarch)	154	154	—	—	—

Because of its hypertonicity, it provides more rapid resuscitation to normal hemodynamic parameters with less total volume infused than do standard crystalloids (122). In addition to the volume infused, hypertonic saline can increase extracellular volume by recruiting intracellular fluid into the extracellular space. Upon immediate infusion of 7.5% NaCl, there is fluid movement from the intracellular space into the extracellular space secondary to the increased tonicity. This action provides approximately 7 ml of free water for every 1 ml of hypertonic saline infused (112). Therefore, resuscitation with 200 ml of hypertonic saline results in a net extracellular volume increase of 1600 ml (200 ml infused and 1400 ml recruited) (Fig. 15.4). The intravascular hypertonic benefit dissipates within 15 minutes as a result of the redistribution between intravascular and interstitial space. This problem is solved with the addition of a hyperoncotic agent such as 6% dextran. The majority of clinical trials utilize the combination of 7% NaCl and 6% dextran-70. (The effects of dextran care are discussed in the section of this chapter entitled "Colloids.")

In addition to the direct volume expanding effects of hypertonic saline, there are indirect reflex mediated positive hemodynamic responses. Hypertonic saline evokes a vagal pulmonary reflex that leads to selective blood flow restriction to the skeletal muscles and causes visceral and pulmonary precapillary dilation (117, 134, 139). The combined effects result in restoration of normal blood flow to the vital organs and shunting from skeletal muscles. The reflex is thought to be dependent on the presence of high concentrations of sodium ions in the interstitium (48). Hypertonic saline has also been reported to increase cardiac output, which appears to be separate from the improvement of preload itself. This increase in cardiac output may be secondary to a positive inotropic effect or to the decreased afterload secondary to the visceral capillary dilation (117, 178). Another theory is that hypertonic saline improves cardiac compliance when compared with isotonic saline resuscitation, as the latter leads to increased muscle water, which decreases the muscle compliance (32). The improvement in cardiac output offsets the dilution effect that hypertonic saline resuscitation has on the oxygen carrying capacity so that there is no significant deterioration of systemic oxygen delivery or uptake (32). In resuscitation of hypovolemic dogs to identical hemodynamic endpoints, hypertonic saline provided a better oxygen supply/delivery balance during the first hour than isotonic saline (185).

Finally, hypertonic saline, by improving systemic blood pressure, improves cerebral blood flow in the head injury patient. Unlike other crystalloids, however, the hypertonicity prevents development of cerebral edema and consequent increases of intracranial pressures. Therefore, the overall effect is improvement in the cerebral perfusion pressure (195).

INDICATIONS

Use of 7.5% NaCl and 6% dextran-70 for resuscitation is still pending approval by the Food and Drug Administration (FDA); however, numerous studies have advocated its use in hemorrhagic shock and burn victims (14, 63, 64, 110, 117, 118). In trauma patients, when hypertonic saline is compared with Ringer's lactate as the initial 250-ml volume expander, it is both safe and, when compared to historical controls,

decreases mortality rates (64, 103, 190, 202). Hypertonic saline has also been shown to be effective in resuscitation for various types of head injury models, as it rapidly expands the intravascular volume and therefore improves the cerebral perfusion pressure without a concomitant increase in the intracranial pressure (195). Finally, hypertonic saline/dextran in small volumes has been effective as a volume expander in animal models of endotoxic shock (80). It may have a future role in the management of septic shock.

SIDE EFFECTS

Electrolyte Abnormalities

The use of hypertonic saline has the potential for causing hypernatremia, hyperchloremia, and hypokalemia. In one clinical trial, the use of 250 ml of 7.5% NaCl and 6% dextran-70 led to a mean increase in patients' serum sodium to 151 mEq/liter and in serum chloride to 118 mEq/liter, and to a serum potassium decrease to 3.8 mEq/liter (103). In addition, serum osmolarity increased to a mean of 340 mOsm/kg H_2O. These effects corrected within 24 hours and no arrhythmias, neurologic sequelae, or other adverse effects were noted. Therefore, with the amounts of hypertonic saline used clinically, these side effects had no clinical significance.

Pulmonary Edema

As with all other fluids, there is potential for the development of pulmonary edema if volume resuscitation is overvigorous, resulting in marked increase in pulmonary vascular hydrostatic pressures. Excluding this complication of management, there seems to be no added risk for the development of pulmonary edema with hypertonic saline compared with standard crystalloids. When the amount of lung lymphatic drainage is used as a measurement of the development of pulmonary edema, there is no added increase when hypertonic saline is used compared with Ringer's lactate (118). In addition, intravascular hydrostatic pressure may be reduced slightly as a result of the pulmonary precapillary dilation induced by the hypertonic saline. With the addition of dextran to the hypertonic saline, there is less potential for decreasing the intravascular oncotic pressure by dilution than with standard crystalloids.

Coagulation

Hypertonic saline will increase the ionic strength of the plasma. As ionic strength increases, it affects enzyme function and cellular metabolism, leading to a deterioration of clotting mechanisms. Hypertonic saline in amounts sufficient to cause a 10% dilution of plasma volume produces a clinically significant prolongation of the partial prothromboplastin time and interferes with platelet aggregation (130). These problems are not of clinical significance, as the amounts of hypertonic saline normally used are much smaller (58). Theoretically, because hypertonic saline restores circulating volume rapidly, perfusion pressure may be restored before adequate hemostasis is achieved, resulting in significant blood loss in trauma patients. This effect is not directly related to the hypertonic saline *per se* but rather to the early restoration of perfusion pressure (79).

Finally, dextran has been associated with coagulopathy (see below), so its use in conjunction with hypertonic saline may compound bleeding problems.

RECOMMENDATIONS FOR USE

The role of 7.5% NaCl/6% dextran-70 in resuscitation of circulatory shock is still undergoing trials and awaiting approval by the FDA. In the previously published trials (64, 103, 110), it is limited to an initial infusion of 4 ml/kg or 250 ml total given as an intravenous bolus. Subsequently, usual crystalloid/colloid infusions may be used according to the recommendations made in other sections of this chapter.

PRESCRIBING INFORMATION

A 7.5% NaCl/6% dextran-70 solution has a calculated osmolality of 2400 mOsm/kg, with the dextran adding only 1 mOsm/kg to the tonicity. It may be prepared by adding 75 ml of 23.4% NaCl to 175 ml of 6% dextran in 0.9% NaCl (64). It is currently awaiting approval by the FDA as a prepackaged mixture.

COLLOID

The term *colloid* refers to large molecular weight substances that do not pass readily across capillary walls.

ALBUMIN

Human serum albumin is effective in restoring blood volume in intravascular volume depletion (168). Its clinical indications are controversial, and it costs more than other plasma volume-expanding agents.

PHARMACOLOGY AND PHARMACOKINETICS

Endogenous Albumin

Albumin is produced in the liver and represents 50% of hepatic protein production (141). Its molecular weight ranges from 66,300 to 69,000 daltons (188). In a healthy person, approximately 12 to 14 g/day, or 130 to 200 mg/kg/day, are produced by the body (91, 141, 189). Albumin is the major oncotically active plasma protein, contributing about 80% of the plasma colloid oncotic pressure (91, 180). A 50% reduction of the serum albumin concentration decreases the colloid oncotic pressure to one-third of normal (180). Albumin binds cations and anions despite its strong negative charge and is a major transport protein for metals, drugs, fatty acids, hormones, and enzymes (188).

In the adult, 4 to 5 grams of albumin per kilogram of body weight are available in the extracellular space, and 30 to 40% is present in the intravascular compartment. Albumin is secreted directly from the hepatocyte into the sinusoidal plasma. The final serum concentration of 3.5 to 5.0 g/dl results

Table 15.4. Potential Albumin Losses in Pathologic States

Fluid	Albumin
Edema	
Congestive heart failure	1 g/dl
Renal disease	
Cirrhosis	
Lymphedema	>2 g/dl
Ascites	1–2 g/dl
Urine—nephrosis[a]	Usually 100–400 mg/kg/day, but may be more or less

[a] Requires proteinuria of ≥3 g/24 hr.

from the combination of albumin secretion, volume of distribution, rate of loss from the intravascular space, and ultimate degradation. In cirrhosis with portal hypertension, a large portion of the albumin produced enters directly into the peritoneal space (ascites) rather than the intravascular space, contributing to hypoproteinemia despite a normal or even increased synthetic rate.

Approximately 50 to 60% of endogenous albumin is in the interstitial space. Some is tissue-bound and unavailable to the circulation. Free interstitial space albumin returns to the intravascular compartment by lymphatic drainage. This return of non-tissue-bound albumin increases during intravascular volume depletion, as do the synthesis and secretion of new albumin (92, 163). Interstitial space albumin that is tissue-bound is subsequently incorporated into the intracellular space, where it is metabolized to amino acids, which return to the liver in a cycle similar to the Cori cycle (157). Catabolism increases albumin metabolism, perhaps accounting for part of stress-induced hypoalbuminemia. Decreases in the degradation of albumin and increases in its distribution in the interstitial space help to compensate for hypoalbuminemia resulting from protein loss (nephrotic syndrome, hemorrhage, bowel obstruction) or diminished production (starvation) (138, 141). In injury or stress, albumin synthesis decreases acutely, whereas the production and serum levels of acute phase reactants (such as globulins, fibrinogen, and haptoglobin) increase. In such situations, a 50% depletion of albumin can be corrected by translocation of interstitial albumin into the intravascular space (114). Subsequently, albumin synthesis can increase if hepatic function and the supply of nutrients are adequate (138). For instance, albumin synthesis increases after hemorrhage and burns, although acutely, serum levels and synthesis decrease (141). When appropriate nutrients are provided, albumin synthesis increases in the critically ill patient (138, 165). Albumin synthesis is increased by thyroid hormone and cortisone (91, 139, 142) through stimulation of RNA production, is decreased by malnutrition, and is finely regulated by the oncotic environment of the hepatocytes (141). The serum albumin level exerts no feedback control on albumin synthesis except through albumin's contribution to colloid oncotic pressure (141).

Albumin loss can occur through various body fluids (Table 15.4).

Exogenous Albumin

The major clinical use of albumin is as a plasma volume expander, and there are 50 years of experimental evidence to document its effectiveness (59). The reader is referred elsewhere for specific data concerning albumin use in human shock, trauma, or major surgery (7, 19, 33, 56, 78, 81–84, 123, 149, 154, 162, 164, 192) and animal shock (20, 35, 37, 38, 61, 62, 114, 125, 126). The increase in plasma volume resulting from infusion of albumin solutions is associated with hemodynamic improvement (154) (Figs. 15.5 and 15.6).

Administered albumin distributes itself throughout the extracellular space. It is a commonly held, but false, assumption that albumin distributes solely in the intravascular space. It is only a transient passenger in this compartment, although its length of stay is long compared with that of crystalloid fluids. The plasma half-life of albumin is 16 hours, the same as that of endogenously produced albumin. After 2 hours, 90% remains in the intravascular space. In a healthy person, the half-life of albumin in the body is approximately 20 days (91). One gram of intravascular albumin binds 18 ml of water by its oncotic activity (52, 61, 91, 145).

Albumin is clinically available as a 5% or 25% solution in isotonic saline. When 100 ml of 25% albumin solution (25 g albumin) are infused, an increase in the intravascular volume

occurs over 30 to 60 minutes to a final volume of 450 ml (56). The intravascular volume is expanded by the translocation of 350 ml of interstitial fluid into the intravascular space (Fig. 15.7). In the face of extracellular volume depletion, this equilibration is not sufficiently brisk or complete unless supplemental isotonic fluid is provided as part of the resuscitation regimen (91, 201). A 500-ml solution of 5% albumin contains 25 g of albumin and increases the intravascular space by 450 to 500 ml; however, in this instance the albumin is administered in conjunction with the fluid to be retained.

INDICATIONS

Albumin is most widely used for its oncotic properties in the resuscitation of patients with an acutely diminished intravascular volume. It has beneficial effects on viscosity and is used for pump priming in cardiopulmonary bypass and hemodialysis. Its properties as a transport protein have been

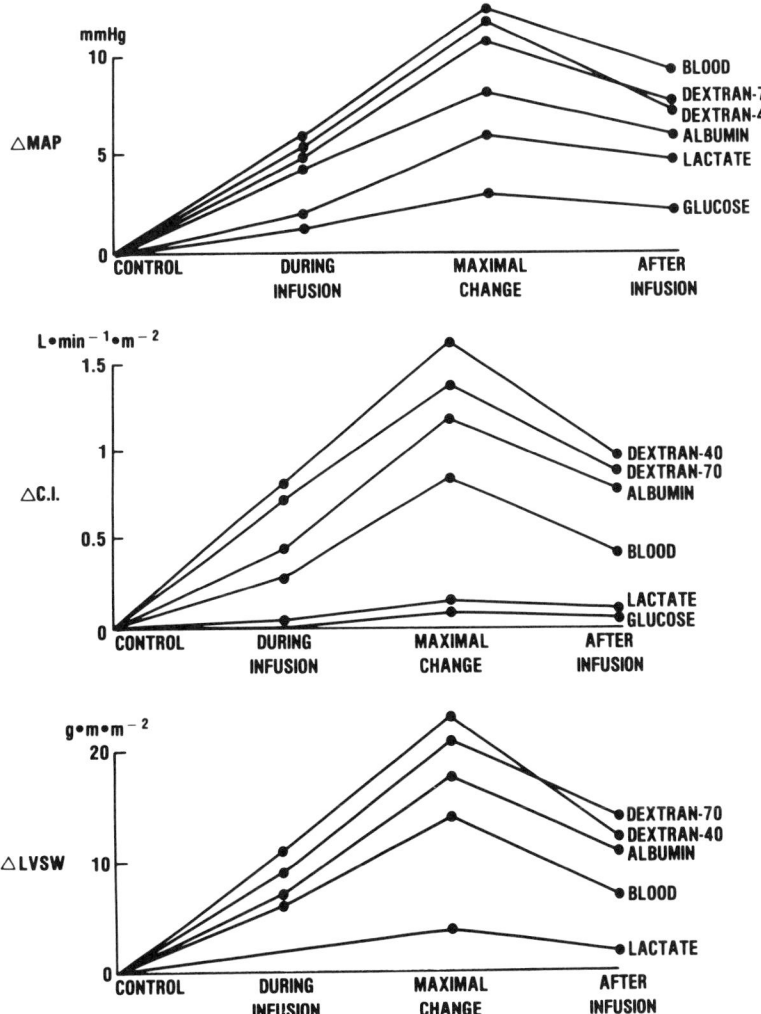

Figure 15.5. Hemodynamic effects of 500 ml of whole blood, 5% albumin, 10% dextran-40, dextran-70, and 1000 ml of 5% glucose or Ringer's lactate all infused over 1 hour. (*MAP*, mean arterial pressure; *C.I.*, cardiac index; *LVSW*, left ventricular stroke work). (Modified from Shoemaker WC: Comparison of the relative effectiveness of whole blood transfusions and various types of fluid therapy in resuscitation. *Crit Care Med* 4:71–78, copyright Williams & Wilkins 1976.)

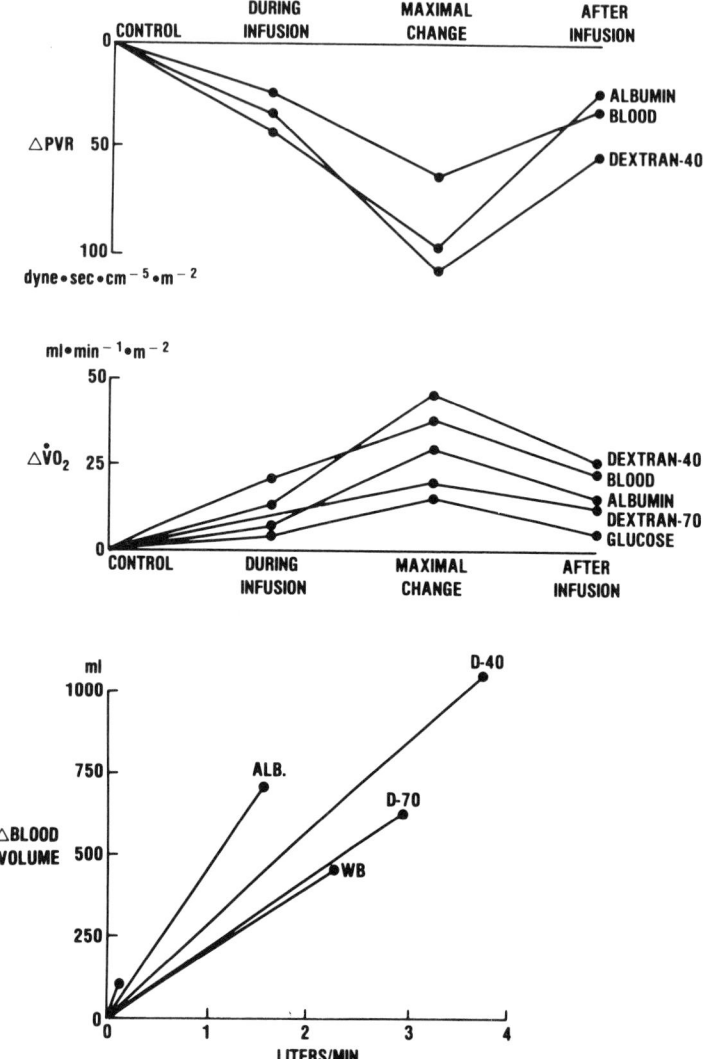

Figure 15.6. Hemodynamic effects of 500 ml of whole blood, 10% dextran-40, dextran 70, and 1000 ml of 5% glucose or Ringer's lactate all infused over 1 hour. (*PVR*, pulmonary vascular resistance; $\dot{V}O_2$ oxygen consumption. (Modified from Shoemaker WC: Comparison of the relative effectiveness of whole blood transfusions and various types of fluid therapy in resuscitation. *Crit Care Med* 4:71–78, copyright Williams & Wilkins, 1976.)

used advantageously in binding bilirubin during therapy of hemolytic disease of the newborn.

SIDE EFFECTS

Pulmonary Edema

The "colloid-crystalloid debate" has produced conflicting animal and human studies, some showing adverse effects (33, 67, 78, 97, 99, 160, 198) and others showing beneficial effects of albumin (19, 24, 49, 81–84, 95, 113, 114, 125, 149, 164, 192). The method of resuscitation, overall volume used, and presence or absence of sepsis affect pulmonary function to a far greater extent than does the type of resuscitation fluid used (44, 125, 158, 191, 194).

Decreased Ionized Calcium Levels

Albumin may lower the serum ionized calcium concentration, producing a negative inotropic effect on the myocardium

(33, 78, 97, 99, 198) and coagulopathy (28); however, these data are controversial.

Anaphylaxis

The occurrence rate of albumin-induced anaphylaxis is between 0.47 and 1.53% (141). Such reactions are short-lived and include urticaria, chills, fever, and, very rarely, hypotension. Purified protein fraction has an increased frequency of associated hypotension (compared with albumin), perhaps secondary to the presence of kinins or prekallikrein activator (3, 15, 30, 54).

Hepatitis Risk

There is no hepatitis risk with albumin. The preparations are heated during processing to 60°C for 10 hours—sufficient time to inactivate the hepatitis virus.

Acquired Immune Deficiency Syndrome Risk

There is no known risk of acquired immune deficiency syndrome (AIDS) with albumin.

Cost

Albumin is expensive. Hospital units have shown that albumin accounts for 10 to 30% of pharmacy budgets (189). The cost per liter of albumin is more than that of other colloid solutions and 30 times the cost of the intravascular volume-equivalent amount of crystalloid solution (Table 15.2).

RECOMMENDATIONS FOR USE

In 1975, a National Institutes of Health task force examined the appropriate use of albumin in light of increasing cost and apparent indiscriminate use (188). The authors' recommendations for albumin use are similar to the guidelines of the task force (Table 15.5). Albumin is used for its oncotic activity in the resuscitation of shock. In shock therapy, a major goal is prompt repletion of the intravascular volume in order to restore tissue perfusion. For major volume resuscitation (replacement of more than 30% of the blood volume), colloids such as albumin or hydroxyethyl starch should be used as part of the resuscitation regimen. If colloids are used early, peripheral perfusion may be restored more promptly than with crystalloid alone. Blood component therapy is dictated by the coagulation profile, hemoglobin concentration, and platelet count. The total volume of crystalloid administered, and thus the potential interstitial space fluid distribution, can be limited by using 5% albumin solution as part of the resuscitation treatment. If the patient is edematous, 25% albumin should be used to mobilize the patient's own interstitial volume. A solution of 100 ml of 25% albumin becomes 400 to 500 ml of intravascular volume over the course of 30 to 60 minutes. The greatest problem with its use is avoiding unintentional volume overload and pulmonary edema. Because of albumin's long "dwell time" in the intravascular space, volume overload persists unless diuresis or preload reduction is instituted.

A colloid oncotic pressure (COP) of ≥ 20 mm Hg, a serum albumin of ≥ 2.5 g/dl, or a total serum protein of ≥ 5 g/dl indicates adequate plasma oncotic activity in most situations. Large volumes of crystalloid fluids decrease COP, whereas colloids (including albumin) increase COP (55). "Edema safety factors" limit the effect of decreased COP on the development of pulmonary edema; these factors include decreased interstitial oncotic pressure, increased lymphatic flow, and increased interstitial tissue pressure. The importance of decreased COP in pulmonary edema development remains unsettled (46, 98, 143, 157, 193).

Shock is associated with loss of capillary wall integrity ("capillary leak"), especially in the lung, with subsequent development of ARDS. The use of albumin in the presence of capillary leak (ARDS, sepsis, intestinal obstruction) must be limited, since albumin crosses the capillary wall and exerts its oncotic influence in the interstitial rather than the intravascular space. The authors recommend that colloid use during capillary leak be minimized. Crystalloid fluids should be used until the capillary leak has resolved. Colloids, including albumin, may then be useful in supporting plasma volume during spontaneous or forced diuresis. Unfortunately, determining when capillary leak is present or has resolved is difficult. In burns (141) and intestinal obstruction (143), capillary integrity is restored after approximately 24 hours. In sepsis or ARDS, the "leak" may persist.

In ARDS, as in shock, it is skillful fluid management rather than the type of fluid used that is important. In the complicated care of the postshock patient with ARDS, the goal of supportive therapy is to minimize further fluid accumulation in the lung while perfusing body tissues. To achieve this goal requires adequate monitoring with the use of pulmonary artery, arterial, and bladder catheters. A cardiac output adequate to support tissue perfusion must be obtained, but at the lowest possible capillary hydrostatic pressure to minimize fluid extravasation into the lung. In the presence of a capillary leak, the higher the capillary hydrostatic pressure, the greater the loss of fluid from the intravascular space into the interstitium of the lung.

There are a few clinical situations in which albumin is commonly but inappropriately used (72, 119, 120). Infusion of albumin to normalize a marginally lowered serum albumin concentration in the face of chronic disease such as malnutrition, cirrhosis, or nephrotic syndrome is unjustified. The serum albumin level is simply an indicator of some more basic underlying problems, and infusing albumin does not solve the problem. Rosenoer and associates (138) make this analogy: "If one's gas gauge points to empty, one simply need smash the glass and move the indicator up to full." Appropriate nutrition, even in cirrhosis, replenishes albumin stores more efficiently than does albumin infusion. Using albumin as a protein nutrient source is inefficient and more expensive than other forms of parenteral nutrition. Albumin does not contain all the essential amino acids (140, 165), and those amino acids it does have are unavailable for immediate protein synthesis because of albumin's long half-life (91).

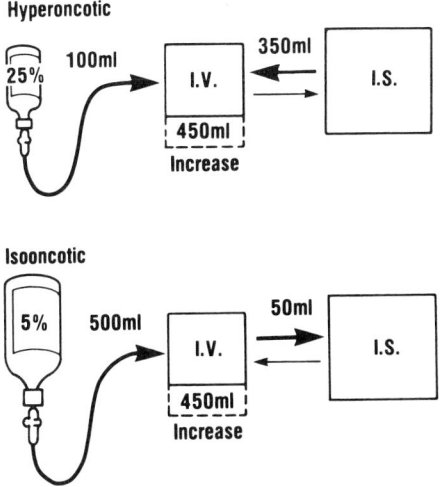

Figure 15.7. Schematic drawing of the influence of albumin solutions on the distribution of water to the intravascular (*I.V.*) and interstitial (*I.S.*) fluid compartments of the body. (Modified from Lamke LO, Liljedahl SO: Plasma volume expansion after infusion of 5%, 20%, and 25% albumin solutions in patients. *Resuscitation* 5:85–92, 1976.)

In cirrhosis, infused albumin equilibrates with ascites and may decrease endogenous albumin synthesis (91, 202). In nephrosis, endogenous albumin synthesis is increased, and there is no evidence that chronic edema or the underlying disease is improved by albumin infusion. Rather, infused albumin is lost in the urine. Although inappropriate for chronic use in each of these situations, the use of albumin for plasma volume support is appropriate (e.g., after paracentesis, dialysis, acute blood loss, and diuretic-induced hypotension).

PRESCRIBING INFORMATION

Albumin is provided as three distinct preparations (Table 15.6) (11): normal serum albumin, 5% and 25%, and purified protein fraction. None of these products contains coagulation components, and hemodilution of the cellular and protein components of blood occurs with albumin use in large volume. Red blood cells and fresh frozen plasma should be added as appropriate to the resuscitation fluids. Normal serum albumin has a shelf life of 3 to 5 years, depending on the storage conditions. A 25% solution of normal serum albumin is hypertonic, with an osmolarity of 1500 mosm/liter, resulting in its expansion to four to five times the administered volume (1 g of albumin binds 18 ml of H_2O in the intravascular space). A 5% solution of normal serum albumin is isotonic with plasma. The protein content of normal serum albumin preparations is 96% albumin. Purified protein fraction preparations contain only 83% albumin, with the remainder being α- and β-globulins. Purified protein fraction is associated with an increased incidence of hypotension, thought to be secondary to kinins or the presence of prekallikrein activator activity among these other proteins (13, 15, 30, 54).

A 25% albumin solution is often referred to as "salt-poor" albumin. This terminology dates from World War II, when albumin preparations had to be stabilized with a "salt-rich"

Na^+ content of 300 mEq/liter. Improved stabilization methods have now reduced the Na^+ content of all albumin preparations to 145 ± 15 mEq/liter (11). The "salt-poor" label has persisted, although "salt-rich" solutions are no longer made (54). Selection among the albumin solutions can alter the amount of Na^+ a patient receives. Expansion of the intravascular space by 500 ml can be accomplished by using 100 ml of 25% albumin, adding 14.5 mEq of Na^+ (100 ml of a solution with 145 mEq/liter), or 500 ml of 5% albumin, adding 72.5 mEq of Na^+ (500 ml of a solution with 145 mEq/liter).

DEXTRAN

Dextran is a large glucose polymer, isolated originally from sugar beets contaminated with bacteria. In its native form it is a branched polysaccharide of 200,000 glucose units (Fig. 15.8). Partial hydrolysis produces polysaccharides of smaller size, which are available commercially as preparations having average molecular weights of 40,000 daltons (dextran-40; D-40) or 70,000 daltons (dextran-70; D-70). Dextran is used clinically as a volume-expanding agent; however, it is also used to prevent thromboembolism and to increase peripheral blood flow.

PHARMACOLOGY AND PHARMACOKINETICS

Dextran molecules distribute in the extracellular space, mainly in the intravascular compartment. The particle size of the various dextrans affects the "dwell time" in the intravascular space and the duration of volume expansion accomplished. The major route of loss of dextran from the intravascular space is through the kidney. Smaller particles (<15,000 daltons molecular weight) are rapidly filtered, not reabsorbed, and lost in the urine; however, while in the circulation, they exert

Table 15.5.   Appropriate Use of Albumin

Clinical Situations	*Guidelines for Use (See Text)*
1. Acute intravascular volume depletion, including hemorrhage, trauma, acute hemodilution, acute vasodilation	In conjunction with crystalloid to limit edema from massive crystalloid volume resuscitation in the elderly or in patients with cardiopulmonary impairment or acute blood loss of >30% blood volume
	To keep serum albumin >2.5 g/dl in acute resuscitation
	Albumin 5% if patient is not edematous
	Albumin 25% if patient is edematous
2. "Third space" fluid loss, including acute peritonitis, mediastinitis, postoperative radical surgery	Same guidelines as above
3. Burns	Greater than 50% surface area burn
	Use after first 24 hours when capillary leak has diminished
	Maintain serum albumin >2.5 g/dl
	Use in conjunction with hyperalimentation
4. Chronic disease (cirrhosis, nephrotic syndrome) associated with acute volume depletion (post paracentesis, dialysis, or overaggressive diuresis)	For acute intravascular volume resuscitation
	Same guidelines as #1 above
5. Post cardiopulmonary bypass with hemodilution	Albumin ≥2.5 g/dl
6. Adult respiratory distress syndrome	Maintain lowest PAW that provides a CO adequate for tissue perfusion
	Use only after capillary leak has resolved
	Albumin >2.5 g/dl
	T protein ≥5 g/dl
	Colloid osmotic pressure >20 mm Hg
	To correct intravascular volume depletion associated with diuretic use

Table 15.6.   Human Serum Albumin Products for Clinical Use[a]

Normal serum albumin (human)(NSA)
   25 ± 1.5% protein
     or
   5 ± 0.3% protein

Purity:	At least 96% of the total protein in the final product must be albumin
pH:	6.9 ± 0.5
Sodium:	25% NSA: not more than 160 mEq/liter
	5% NSA: 130–160 mEq/liter
Dating:	When stored at 2–10°C: 5 years
	When stored at room temperature, no warmer than 37°C: 3 years

Plasma protein fraction (human) (PPF)
   5 ± 0.3% protein

Purity:	At least 83% of the total protein in the final product must be albumin; no more than 17% shall be globulins; no more than 1% of globulins shall be γ-globulin
pH:	7.0 ± 0.3
Sodium:	100–160 mEq/liter
Potassium:	No more than 2 mEq/liter
Dating:	When stored at 2–8°C: 5 years
	When stored at no warmer than 30°C: 3 years

Applicable to NSA and PPF
   Heated at 60°C ± 0.5°C for 10 hours
   No preservatives
   Pass standard tests for sterility and for pyrogenic substances

Stabilizers:	0.16 mmol sodium acetyltryptophanate
	or 0.08 mmol sodium acetyltryptophanate and
	0.08 mmol sodium caprylate

[a] From Barker LF: *Proceedings of the Workshop on Albumin,* February 12–13, 1975. Department of Health, Education and Welfare, Washington, DC, DHEW Publication No. (NIH) 76-925, 1976.

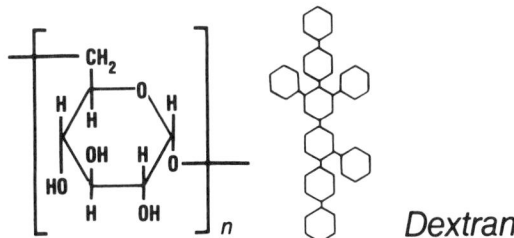

Figure 15.8.   Dextran: glucose subunit and polymer.

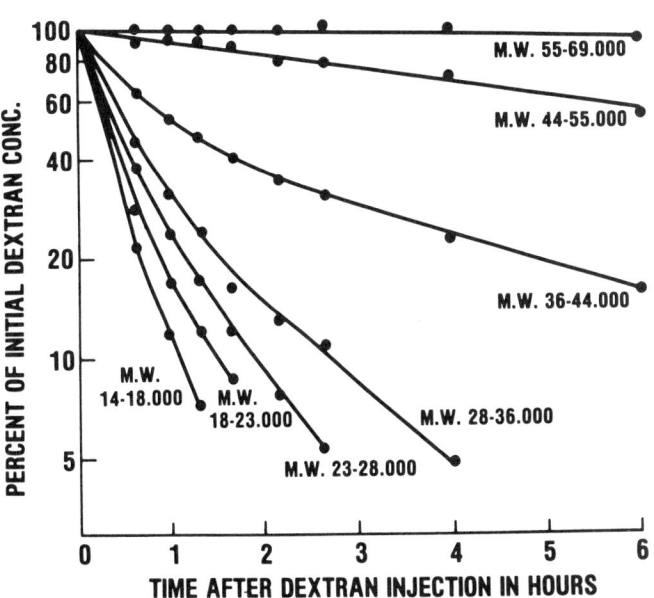

Figure 15.9.   The disappearance rate of dextrans of different molecular weights from plasma. (From Arthurson G: The intravascular persistence of Dextran of different molecular sizes in normal humans. *Scand J Clin Lab Invest* 16:76–80, 1964.)

osmotic activity. Larger particles remain in the circulation longer but exert less osmotic activity. D-40 and D-70 contain particles with molecular weights ranging from 10,000 to 80,000 (34) and 40,000 to 100,000 daltons, respectively. The circulating half-life of dextran varies with its particle size (38). The half-life for particles with molecular weights of 14,000 to 18,000 daltons is 15 minutes, whereas for those particles greater than 55,000 daltons it is several days (Fig. 15.9). Sixty to seventy percent of D-40 and 30 to 40% of D-70 is cleared in 12 hours (6, 8, 184). Since smaller particles are cleared more rapidly than larger ones, and D-40 contains smaller particles than does D-70, D-40 is lost from the circulation faster than D-70. As a general rule, only 20% of a D-40 dose and 30% of a D-70 dose remains in the circulation after 24 hours, and accumulation of large particles occurs over days of administration. For each preparation, after 24 hours the particles that accumulate have an average molecular weight of more than 80,000 daltons. With renal impairment small species accumulate. The larger particles are taken up by the reticuloendothelial system and eventually are metabolized to

carbon dioxide and water. Other particles cross into the interstitial space and are recirculated through the lymphatic system.

INDICATIONS

Volume Expansion

Dextran has ideal properties as a plasma volume expander: a long dwell time and ultimate biodegradability. In shock, dextran increases survival (35, 37, 38, 154, 163, 176) and improves hemodynamic parameters (29, 36, 51, 85, 133, 154). Dextran infusion is associated with increased renal plasma flow and a decrease in plasma antidiuretic hormone levels when used in hypovolemia (184). It has favorable hemodynamic effects in restoring intravascular volume in shock when compared with other volume expanders (109, 154) (Figs. 15.5 and 15.6).

The reported degree of dextran-induced volume expansion varies, based on the type and concentration of solution used and the experimental setting. Dextran infusion increases the intravascular volume by an amount greater than or equal to that infused; however, the subsequent osmotic diuresis limits the duration of the volume expansion. One gram of dextran obligates 20 to 30 ml of water to the intravascular space (38, 53, 184). A 500-ml bolus of D-40 produces a 750-ml expansion of intravascular volume at 1 hour and 1050 ml at 2 hours (154). Some volume expansion may persist up to 8 hours in hypovolemic patients. (77). Studies of shock in dogs show similar volume expansion, with 47% of the bolus infused remaining in the intravascular space after 4 hours (38). Four to six hours after the infusion of either D-40 or D-70, the degree of intravascular volume expansion is similar and approximately equal to the amount infused (184).

Promotion of Peripheral Blood Flow

In addition to increasing plasma volume, dextran has other effects on blood flow that potentiate flow in the microvasculature (4). By coating endothelial surfaces, dextran reduces interaction with the cellular elements in blood (184). The sludging and cellular aggregation seen in shock are reduced by reduction of blood viscosity (29) and coating of cellular elements. Altered platelet function, including diminished adherence and degranulation, limits thrombus formation and activation of the clotting cascade mechanism (1, 90, 199). Dextran is also reported to copolymerize with fibrin monomer, resulting in a less stable clot that is more susceptible to endogenous lysis (1).

Prevention of Thromboembolism

Dextran is effective in reducing the incidence of thromboembolic disease (9, 21, 137, 144). It is beneficial, compared with controls, in the prevention of deep venous thrombosis in general surgery patients and following total hip replacement. However, data for the use of heparin in this same group are as good or better (50, 68), without the attendant risks of dextran.

Other Uses

Isovolemic hemodilution is a common preoperative procedure to obtain autologous blood and an accepted therapy for microcirculatory disorders in ischemic diseases. In a Phase I trial, isovolemic hemodilution with D-60 was proven to be beneficial in treatment of pancreatitis (73). Dextran has been used in the therapy of ischemic ulceration of the skin, arterial occlusion, frostbite, and stroke, and in cell harvest in plasmapheresis and priming for extracorporeal circulation.

SIDE EFFECTS

Renal Failure

Dextran-induced renal failure may occur (27, 40, 47, 101, 102), especially in the presence of unrecognized hypovolemia. The mechanism for the renal failure is tubular obstruction secondary to concentration and precipitation of dextran in the tubules with cast formation (26). Three conditions are necessary to cause this side effect: (*a*) decreased renal perfusion pressure, (*b*) dextran in the tubule, and (*c*) a continued stimulus for water reabsorption. Unfortunately, these conditions exist in intravascular volume depletion and its resuscitation with dextran, especially if the intravascular volume repletion is inadequate.

Anaphylaxis

The incidence of anaphylactic reactions to dextran is between 1% (131) and 5.3% (180). Reactions occur early, within one-half hour after the infusion is begun, and may include urticaria, rash, nausea, bronchospasm, shock, and death. Dextran is a potent antigen and has cross-reactivity with bacterial polysaccharide antigens. Patients with *Streptococcus pneumoniae* or *Salmonella* infections may therefore be more prone to dextran reactions. Gut flora make endogenous dextran from dextrose, and a small portion of the patient population has never received dextran yet has circulating precipitins to the dextran molecule.

Osmotic Diuresis

As previously noted, osmotic diuresis occurs almost immediately upon infusion of any dextran preparation, as smaller species are filtered and not reabsorbed. The effect is greater with D-40 than with D-70 because of the prevalence of small species in D-40. In the presence of this obligate osmotic diuresis, urine volume cannot serve as a guide to the adequacy of intravascular volume repletion. If blood volume is restored inadequately in the patient who is receiving dextran, the stage is set for all the conditions to be met to produce renal failure.

Biochemical Alterations

Blood glucose levels can be increased falsely in patients who are receiving dextran if the glucose measurement is done by analysis using acid, which converts dextran to dextrose. Dextran may also cause false increases of the total protein concentration. Total protein measurements can be checked using a refractometer. The refractometer reading is within 1 g/dl of the true value.

Dextran can interfere with the cross-matching of blood. The coating action of dextran on red blood cells causes cells to aggregate, mimicking a (nonexistent) cross-match problem. This effect is a problem especially when blood is drawn from a site proximal to the dextran intravenous infusion site, and is handled simply by drawing blood prior to dextran infusion or notifying the blood bank that the patient is receiving dextran. Other biochemical alterations include false increases in the serum bilirubin level and alteration of colloid oncotic pressure measurements (54).

Bleeding Diathesis

Dextran inhibits erythrocyte aggregation in vivo (29). It adheres to vessel walls and cellular elements of the blood (16, 90); decreases platelet adhesiveness (90, 200), serum fibrinogen, and other factor levels (34); and increases Ivy bleeding time and incisional bleeding (180). In dogs, clinical bleeding is not observed until 80% replacement of plasma volume has been achieved (177). At doses less than 1.5 g/kg/day, clinical bleeding is not encountered (184).

Reticuloendothelial Blockade

Dextran temporarily impairs reticuloendothelial system function (86, 146), and by so doing may diminish immune competence.

RECOMMENDATIONS FOR USE

Dextran is an effective agent for intravascular volume expansion and has some specific beneficial effects on blood flow through the microvasculature that make its use in shock very attractive. In addition, it is ultimately biodegradable. Its side effects, as described above, are noteworthy in the critically ill population. Dextran can cause a bleeding diathesis and interfere with blood cross-matching in a patient who is suffering from hemorrhagic shock. Its use can produce renal failure whenever renal perfusion is impaired (i.e., in any shock situation). Dextran causes an immediate osmotic diuresis, which, if misinterpreted, may potentiate volume depletion and ultimately renal failure, especially in critically ill patients with underlying diseases such as diabetes mellitus.

PRESCRIBING INFORMATION

Preparations

Dextran-40 is commercially available as a 10% solution in normal saline or 5% dextrose in water. Dextran-70 is commercially available as a 6% solution in normal saline or 5% dextrose in water or in 10% invert sugar. These preparations require no mixing and can be "hung" just as supplied.

Dosage

To avoid bleeding diathesis, the total administered dosage should remain less than 1.5 g/kg/day of D-40 and 2 g/kg/day of D-70. For restoration of blood volume in shock, this amount (approximately 1000 ml of 10% D-40 for a 70-kg man) may be given acutely in conjunction with crystalloid, packed red blood cells, and plasma as necessary. The *Medical Letter on Drugs and Therapeutics* recommends using less than 1000 ml/day of D-40 (2). For use in prophylaxis of thromboembolic disease or peripheral vascular disease, the dosage should be increased to 50 ml/hr in 5 ml increments of D-40, with monitoring of urine output and specific gravity. Infusion should be discontinued for specific gravity greater than 1.030 and urine volume less than 0.5 ml/kg/hr (179).

HYDROXYETHYL STARCH

HETASTARCH AND PENTASTARCH

Hetastarch is a synthetic starch molecule that closely resembles glycogen. Its development is the result of a concerted effort to find a colloidal volume-expanding agent that is free from the toxicities of previously developed plasma expanders. Its similarity to glycogen may account for its relative freedom from immune reactions (Fig. 15.10).

Pentastarch is another synthetic starch molecule that is an analog of hetastarch. It possesses a lower average molecular weight than hetastarch (264,000 daltons for pentastarch versus 450,000 daltons for hetastarch) and has fewer hydroxyethyl groups added per molecule (Fig. 15.11). Originally used in leukopheresis (169), pentastarch is now being investigated as a colloid volume expander with qualities similar to those of hetastarch yet fewer potential side effects (65, 93, 129, 171, 199).

PHYSIOLOGY AND PHARMACOKINETICS

Hetastarch is available for clinical use as a 6% solution in normal saline. The average molecular weight of the particles is 450,000 daltons, with a range of 400,000 to 550,000 daltons. Glucose subunits are linked in α-1,4 and α-1,6 linkages to form a polymer that is more branched than dextran and is globular rather than linear. In addition, hydroxyethyl groups are substituted on the glucose subunits, which slows degradation in vivo (Figs. 15.10 and 15.11).

After intravenous infusion there is an almost immediate appearance of smaller particles in the urine (molecular weight, 50,000 daltons) (106). Studies in normal human volunteers show that 46% of an administered dose is excreted in the urine by 2 days and 64% by 8 days (128, 203). Larger particles remain in the circulation longer. Their rate of disappearance depends on their absorption by tissues (notably liver and spleen), gradual return to the circulation, uptake by the reticuloendothelial system, and subsequent degradation to smaller particles cleared through urine and bile. Blood α-amylase also degrades larger particles to smaller starch polymers and free

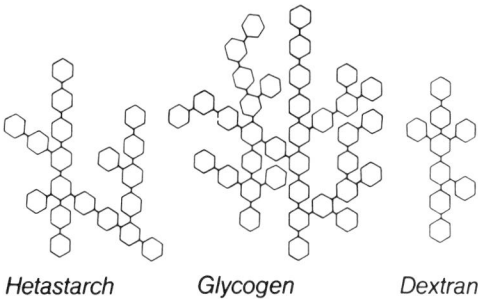

Hetastarch   Glycogen   Dextran

Figure 15.10. Two-dimensional representations of hydroxyethyl starch (hetastarch), glycogen, and dextran molecules. (Modified from Thompson WL: *Proceedings from a Symposium: Hespan (Hetastarch): Historical Perspective and Development.* Toronto, February 1982.)

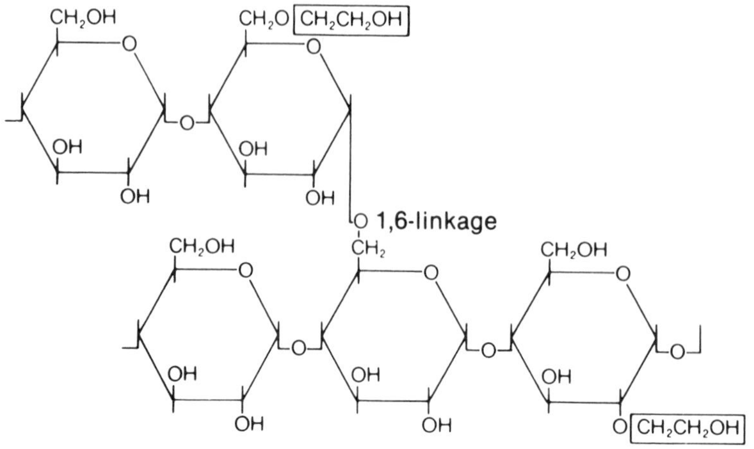

Figure 15.11.   The hydroxyethyl starch molecule. Note the α-1,6-linkage and hydroxyethyl groups in boxes. (Modified from *Answers to Frequently Asked Questions about Hespan (Hetastarch)*. American Critical Care Publications, McGraw Park, IL, p 111, 1981.

glucose. However, the amount of glucose produced does not cause clinically significant hyperglycemia even in the diabetic model (60). The rate of amylase degradation of hetastarch is slow compared with the rate for naturally occurring starches, probably because of the presence of hydroxyethyl groups substituted on 70% of the glucose subunits. Less than 1% of infused hetastarch can be recovered as exhaled carbon dioxide.

As with dextran, the half-life of hetastarch represents a composite of the half-lives of various-sized particles. Sixty-four percent of the dose is eliminated in the urine within 8 days. Ninety percent of a single infusion of hetastarch leaves the circulation in 42 days, with a terminal half-life of 17 days (203). The remaining 10% has a half-life of 48 days. Small amounts of hetastarch have been measured in the circulation as long as 17 weeks after a single infusion (18). The uptake of hetastarch molecules by the cells of the reticuloendothelial system has caused concern that the immune function of the patient could be compromised. However, clinically significant reticuloendothelial system dysfunction has not been demonstrated (89, 150, 172).

Plasma volume expansion after infusion of hetastarch is equal to or greater than that produced by dextran-70 (88, 105, 167, 177, 181, 182) or 5% albumin. Studies in humans show an increase in blood volume from 2.3 liters/m² to 2.9 liters/m², with a duration of at least 3 hours (87). Although there is some variability, infusions of hetastarch increase intravascular volume by an amount equal to or greater than the volume infused (10, 70, 85, 87, 105, 167, 183). The increase in intravascular volume is associated with improvement in hemodynamic parameters in critically ill patients (39, 71, 87, 100, 128, 151). The increase in colloid pressure is similar to that seen with albumin (55, 71).

Pentastarch is available as a 10% solution in normal saline. The average molecular weight is 264,000 daltons, with a range of 150,000 to 350,000 daltons. When compared with hetastarch, pentastarch has a lower average molecular weight as well as fewer moles of hydroxyethyl starch per mole of glucose, resulting in a shorter tissue retention time. Pentastarch is both hydrolyzed and excreted by the kidney more rapidly, resulting in an average half-life of only 2.5 hours (107). Studies in normal human volunteers have demonstrated that within 24 hours of an infusion of pentastarch, 66% of the total dose has been excreted in the urine, 4% remains in the intravascular space, and the remaining 30% is unaccounted for (108).

The higher concentration formulation of pentastarch (10%) results in an increased volume expansion per volume infused and is slightly greater than that of hetastarch. A 700-ml increase in plasma volume results within 30 minutes of infusion of 500 ml of pentastarch (69). The increase in colloid oncotic pressure as well as the augmentation of mean arterial pressure, cardiac index, and cardiac filling pressures seen with pentastarch are similar to that with albumin infusion (93).

INDICATIONS

Hetastarch is indicated for use as a plasma volume-expanding agent in shock from hemorrhage, trauma, sepsis, or burns. It has adjunctive application in leukopheresis and as a pump prime and volume expander in cardiopulmonary bypass.

Currently, the only FDA approval for pentastarch is as an adjunctive to leukopheresis. However, several case clinical trials have demonstrated use in sepsis and burns and as a volume expander in cardiac surgery (93, 129, 196). In addition, pentastarch has recently been investigated for inducing hypervolemia in hemodilution treatment of acute stroke (65).

SIDE EFFECTS

Coagulopathy

Hetastarch is associated with minor alterations in laboratory measurements, but not with clinical bleeding when used in doses below 1500 ml/day (88, 116, 162); doses greater than 1500 ml/day have been administered without bleeding complications (151). Dilutional effects on cellular and protein elements of the blood clotting cascade are produced secondary to the blood volume-expanding effect. However, the laboratory abnormalities are not explained by dilution alone. Coagulation profile discrepancies include a transient decrease in platelet count, prolonged prothrombin and partial thrombo-plastin times, and a decrease in the tensile clot strength (136, 166, 173–175, 197). In clinical series bleeding is a problem in only a small minority of cases (88, 166). Experience with hetastarch in leukopheresis is extensive, with bleeding compli-cations occurring only rarely (45, 170).

In patients undergoing leukopheresis with pentastarch, there was a prolongation of the partial thromboplastin time, a decrease in concentration of fibrinogen and factor VIII, and a decrease of the thrombin time, but these effects are less extensive than those seen with hetastarch. In addition, there was no effect on the urokinase-activated clot lysis time (171). The aforementioned effects are caused primarily by hemodilu-tion, without any direct effect on the coagulation system as found with hetastarch. When compared with albumin as a volume expander in cardiac surgery patients, pentastarch in doses up to 2000 ml produces no significant difference in clotting time, coagulation factor levels, or bleeding time and no increase in clinical parameters of bleeding or hemostasis at 1 to 7 days (93).

Pulmonary Edema

Hetastarch has been used successfully in critically ill pa-tients with various forms of shock without producing pulmo-nary edema or change in pulmonary function (87, 128).

Anaphylaxis

The incidence of anaphylactic reactions to hetastarch (mo-lecular weights >16,000 daltons) infusions is less than 0.085%. The incidence of severe reactions, including shock or cardio-pulmonary arrest, is 0.008% (131). Hetastarch is not immuno-genic (104, 132) and does not induce histamine release (94). There have been no reported cases of anaphylactic reactions to pentastarch.

Hyperamylasemia

Serum amylase levels are increased following hetastarch administration (75). Complexes of amylase and hetastarch mol-ecules create macroamylase particles, which undergo urinary excretion at a much slower rate than the solitary amylase molecule. Serum amylase levels commonly are twice as high as normal after hetastarch infusion. There is no alteration of normal pancreatic function. A similar effect can be seen with pentastarch.

RECOMMENDATIONS FOR USE

Hetastarch may be used whenever colloid is required to restore plasma volume. Its properties as a volume-expanding agent are similar to those of 5% albumin solutions (127). At doses of 1500 ml/day or less, bleeding complications are avoided; doses greater than 1500 ml/day have been adminis-tered without bleeding complications (151). Hetastarch, like other colloid solutions, does not carry oxygen and must be administered in conjunction with packed red blood cells to maintain adequate oxygen content of the blood. Although rare, clinical bleeding has been associated with its use. Fresh frozen plasma and platelets should be replaced as indicated by clini-cal bleeding and the results of serial coagulation profiles. Hetastarch should be used with extreme caution in the pres-ence of a known bleeding diathesis.

Adequate monitoring for detection of volume overload is as crucial for hetastarch as it is for infusion of all other volume expanders. Volume overload pulmonary edema may be pro-duced unwittingly despite careful monitoring of left heart filling pressures, as the osmotic action of the infused hetastarch draws interstitial space water into the circulation. The imme-diate osmotic diuresis associated with its use offers some protection from this phenomenon. Urine volume must be expected to increase acutely secondary to the osmotic diuresis, and must not be misinterpreted as a sign of adequate periph-eral perfusion. Patients with renal impairment are particularly subject to initial volume overload and to accumulation of hetastarch in the circulation and tissues with repeated admin-istration (76). In these patients, initial volume resuscitation accomplished with hetastarch should be maintained with an-other plasma volume expander, such as albumin or crystalloid.

Serum amylase values will be approximately twice normal levels after hetastarch infusion and are *not* indicative of pan-creatitis. When serum amylase measurements are important (as in pancreatitis, bowel obstruction, and parotitis), serum levels should be measured prior to infusion of hetastarch. Increases in serum amylase values may persist for 5 days postinfusion.

Hetastarch costs about two-thirds as much as an equivalent amount of 5% albumin (Table 15.2). Although dextran prepara-tions cost even less than hetastarch, their use is associated with more side effects, such as anaphylactoid reactions, inter-ference with blood typing and cross-matching, antigenicity, coagulopathy, and renal failure.

The guidelines for the use of pentastarch are similar to those for hetastarch, with the exception that the intravascular volume expands to a greater degree with similar amounts of pentastarch than with hetastarch. In doses up to 2000 ml of pentastarch, clinically significant effects on coagulation have not been observed.

PRESCRIBING INFORMATION

Hetastarch Preparations

Hetastarch is available as a 6% solution of 0.9% sodium chloride. The pH is 5.5 and the osmolarity 310 mOsm/liter. It is bottled ready for infusion in 500-ml bottles.

Dosage

Usual total dosage is 20 ml/kg/day, but this is not an abso-lute upper limit. The total volume may be administered over 1 hour if the clinical situation demands adequate volume resuscitation.

For leukopheresis, 250 to 700 ml may be infused in the ratio of 1:8 with venous blood. Ten repetitions over the course of 5 weeks have been reported to be safe; however, hetastarch accumulation in the tissues will occur. Safety beyond this duration and frequency of administration is not known.

Pentastarch Preparations

Pentastarch is available at 10% solution in 0.9% sodium chloride. The pH is 5.0 and the osmolarity 326 mOsm/liter. It is supplied in 500-ml bottles.

Dosage

In studies using pentastarch as a volume expander, it is given as a 500-ml bolus infusion with a limit of 2000 ml total.

REFERENCES

1. Aberg M, Hedner V, Bergentz S: Effect of dextran on factor VIII and platelet function. *Ann Surg* 189:243–247, 1979.
2. Abramowicz M (ed): *Med Lett Drugs Ther* 10(1):3, 1968.
3. Alving BM, Hojima Y, Pisano JJ: Hypotension associated with prekallikrein activator (Hageman-factor fragments) in plasma protein fraction. *N Engl J Med* 299:66–70, 1978.
4. Amundson B, Jennische E, Haljamae H: Skeletal muscle microcirculatory and cellular metabolic effects of whole blood. Ringer's acetate and dextran-70 infusions in hemorrhagic shock. *Circ Shock* 7:111–120, 1980.
5. Appel PL, Shoemaker WC: Evaluation of fluid therapy in adult respiratory failure. *Crit Care Med* 9:862–869, 1981.
6. Arthurson G, Granath K, Thoren L, Wallenius G: The renal excretion of LMW dextran. *Acta Clin Scand* 127:543–551, 1964.
7. Arthurson G, Wallenius G: The renal clearance of dextran of different molecular sizes in normal humans. *Scand J Clin Lab Invest* 16:81–86, 1964.
8. Atik M: Dextran-40 and dextran-70, a review. *Arch Surg* 94:664–672, 1967.
9. Atik M: The uses of dextran in surgery: a current evaluation. *Surgery* 65:548–562, 1969.
10. Ballinger WF: Preliminary report on the use of hydroxyethyl starch solution in man. *J Surg Res* 6:180–183, 1966.
11. Barker LF: Albumin products and the Bureau of Biologics. In Proceedings of the Workshop on Albumin, February 12–13, 1975. Washington, DC, Department of Health, Education and Welfare, DHEW Publication No. (NIH) 76–925, pp 22–27, 1976.
12. Baue AE, Tragus ET, Wolfson SK: Hemodynamic and metabolic effects of Ringer's lactate solution in hemorrhagic shock. *Ann Surg* 166:29–38, 1697.
13. Bergentz SE: Dextran prophylaxis of pulmonary embolism. *World J Surg* 2:19–24, 1978.
14. Bitterman H, Triolo J, Lefer AM. Use of hypertonic saline in the treatment of hemorrhagic shock. *Circ Shock* 21:271–283, 1987.
15. Bland JHL, Laver MB, Lowenstein E: Vasodilation effect of commercial 5% plasma protein fraction solutions. *JAMA* 224:1721–1724, 1973.
16. Bloom WL, Harmer J, Bryant MF: Coating of blood vessel surfaces and blood cells: a new concept in the prevention of intravascular thrombosis. *Proc Soc Exp Biol Med* 115:384–386, 1964.
17. Bogan RK, Gale GR, Walton RP: Fate of 14C labelled hydroxyethyl starch in animals. *Toxicol Appl Pharmacol* 15:206–211, 1969.
18. Boon JC, Jesch F, Ring J, Messmer K: Intravascular persistence of hydroxyethyl starch in man. *Eur Surg Res* 8:497–503, 1976.
19. Boutros AR, Ruess R, Olson L: Comparison of hemodynamic, pulmonary and renal effects of use of 3 types of fluid after major surgical procedures on abdominal aorta. *Crit Care Med* 7:9–13, 1979.
20. Brinkmeyer DO, Safar P, Motoyama E: Superiority of colloid over electrolyte solution for fluid resuscitation (severe normovolemic hemodilution). *Crit Care Med* 9:369–371, 1981.
21. Browse NL, Clemeson G, Bateman NT: Effect of IV dextran-70 and pneumatic leg compression on incidence of post-op pulmonary embolism. *Br Med J* 2:1281–1284, 1976.
22. Canizaro PC, Prager MC, Shires GT: The influence of Ringer's lactate solution during shock: changes in lactate, excess lactate and pH. *Am J Surg* 122:494–501, 1971.
23. Carey JS, Scharschmidt BF, Culliford AT: Hemodynamic effectiveness of colloid and electrolyte solutions for replacement of simulated operative blood loss. *Surg Gynecol Obstet* 131:679–686, 1970.
24. Carey LC, Lowery BD, Cloutier CT: Hemorrhagic shock. *Curr Probl Surg* 1:3–48, 1971.
25. Carrico CJ, Canizaro PC, Shires GT: Fluid resuscitation following injury; rationale for the use of balanced salt solutions. *Crit Care Med* 4:46–54, 1976.
26. Chinitz JL: Pathophysiology and prevention of dextran-40 induced anuria. *J Lab Clin Med* 77:76–87, 1971.
27. Christensen EI, Moundsback AB: Effects of dextran on lysosomal ultrastructure and protein digestion in renal proximal tubule. *Kidney Int* 16:301–311, 1979.
28. Coghill TH, Moore EE, Dunn EI: Coagulation changes after albumin resuscitation. *Crit Care Med* 9:22–26, 1981.
29. Cohn JN, Luria MH, Daddario RC: Studies in clinical shock and hypotension. V. Hemodynamic effects of dextran. *Circulation* 35:316–326, 1967.
30. Coleman RW: Paradoxical hypotension after volume expansion with plasma protein fraction. *N Engl J Med* 299:97–98, 1978.
31. Croft D, Dion YM, Dumont M, Langlois D: Cardiac compliance and effects of hypertonic saline. *Can J Surg* 35:139–144, 1992.
32. Curtis SE, Cain SM: Systemic and regional O₂ delivery and uptake in bled dogs given hypertonic saline, whole blood, or dextran. *Am J Physiol* 262(3):H778–H786, 1992.
33. Dahn MS, Lucas CE, Ledgerwood AM: Negative inotropic effect of albumin resuscitation for shock. *Surgery* 86:235–241, 1979.
34. Data JL, Nies AS: Dextran 40. *Ann Intern Med* 81:500–504, 1974.
35. Dawidson I, Eriksson B: Statistical evaluations of plasma substitutes based on 10 variables. *Crit Care Med* 10:653–657, 1982.
36. Dawidson I, Eriksson B, Gelin LE: Oxygen consumption and recovery from surgical shock in rats: a comparison on the efficacy of different plasma substitutes. *Crit Care Med* 7:460–465, 1979.
37. Dawidson I, Gelin LE, Haglind E: Plasma volume, intravascular protein content, hemodynamic and oxygen transport changes during intestinal shock in dogs. Comparison of relative effectiveness of various plasma expanders. *Crit Care Med* 8:73–80, 1980.
38. Dawidson I, Gelin LE, Hedman L: Hemodilution and recovery from experimental intestinal shock in rats: a comparison of the efficacy of three colloids and one electrolyte solution. *Crit Care Med* 9:42–46, 1981.
39. Diehl JT, Lester JL, Cosgrove DM: Clinical comparison of hetastarch and albumin in postoperative cardiac patients. *Ann Thorac Surg* 34:674–679, 1982.
40. Diomi P: Studies on renal tubular morphology and toxicity after large doses of dextran-40 in the rabbit. *Lab Invest* 22:355–360, 1970.
41. Ebert RV, Stead EA Jr, Gibson JG: Response of normal subjects to acute blood loss with special reference to the mechanism of restoration of blood volume. *Arch Intern Med* 68:578–590, 1941.
42. Elkington JR, Danowski TS: The Body Fluids: Basic Physiology and Practical Therapeutics. Baltimore, Williams and Wilkins, 1955.
43. Elwyn DH, Bryan-Brown CW, Shoemaker WC: Nutritional aspects of body water dissociations in postoperative and depleted patients. *Ann Surg* 182:76–85, 1975.
44. Esrig BC, Fulton RL: Sepsis, resuscitated hemorrhagic shock and "shock lung." An experimental correlation. *Ann Surg* 182:218–227, 1975.
45. Farrales FB, Belcher C, Summers T, Bayer WL: Effect of hydroxyethyl starch on platelet function following granulocyte collection using the continuous flow cell separator. *Transfusion* 17:635–647, 1977.
46. Feeley TW, Mihm FG, Halperin BD, Rosenthal MH: Failure of the colloid oncotic-pulmonary artery wedge pressure gradient to predict changes in extravascular lung water. *Crit Care Med* 13:1025–1028, 1985.
47. Feest TG: Low molecular weight dextran: a continuing cause of acute renal failure. *Br Med J* 2:1300, 1976.
48. Fulton RL. The absorption of sodium and water by collagen during hemorrhagic shock. *Ann Surg* 172:861–869, 1975.
49. Gaisford WD, Pandey D, Jensen CG: Pulmonary changes in hemorrhagic shock. II. Ringer's solution vs. colloid infusion. *Am J Surg* 124:738–743, 1972.
50. Gallus AS, Hirsch J, O'Brien SE: Prevention of venous thrombosis with small, subcutaneous doses of heparin. *JAMA* 235:1980–1984, 1976.
51. Gelin LE, Solvell L, Zederfeldt B: Plasma volume expanding effect of low viscous dextran and macrodex. *Acta Chir Scand* 122:309–322, 1961.
52. Granger DN, Gabel JC, Drahe RE, Taylor AD: Physiologic basis for the clinical use of albumin solutions. *Surg Gynecol Obstet* 146:97–104, 1978.
53. Gruber VF, Messmer K: Colloids for blood volume support. *Prog Surg* 15:49–76, 1977.
54. Guyton AC: Textbook of Medical Physiology, ed 4. Philadelphia, WB Saunders, 1971.
55. Haupt MT, Rackow EC: Colloid osmotic pressure and fluid resuscitation with hetastarch, albumin and saline solutions. *Crit Care Med* 10:159–162, 1982.
56. Hauser CJ, Shoemaker WC, Turpin I: Oxygen transport responses to colloids and crystalloids in critically ill surgical patients. *Surg Gynecol Obstet* 150:811–816, 1980.
57. Hays RM: Dynamics of body water and electrolytes. In Maxwell MH, Kleeman CR (eds): Clinical Disorders of Fluid and Electrolyte Metabolism. New York, McGraw-Hill, 1972.
58. Hess J, Dubick MA, Summary JJ, Bangal NR, Wade CE: The effects of 7.5% NaCl/6% dextran-70 on coagulation and platelet aggregation in humans. *J Trauma* 32(1):40–44, 1992.
59. Heye JT, Janeway CA: The use of human albumin in military practice. *US Navy Med Bull* 40:785–791, 1942.
60. Hofer RE, Lanier WL: Effect of hydroxyethyl starch solutions on blood glucose concentrations in diabetic and non-diabetic rats. *Crit Care Med* 20:211–215, 1992.
61. Holcroft JW, Trunkey DD: Extravascular lung water following hemorrhagic shock in the baboon: comparison between resuscitation with Ringer's lactate and plasmanate. *Ann Surg* 180:408–417, 1974.
62. Holcroft JW, Trunkey DD: Pulmonary extravasation of albumin during and after hemorrhagic shock in baboons. *J Surg Res* 18:91–97, 1979.
63. Holcroft JW, Vassar MT, Perry CA, et al: Use of 7.5% NaCl/6% dextran-70 solution in the resuscitation of injured patients in the emergency room. *Prog Clin Biol Res* 299:331–338, 1989.
64. Holcroft JW, Vassar MT, Turner JE, Derlet RW, Kramer GC: 3% NaCl and 7.5% NaCl/dextran-70 in the resuscitation of severely injured patients. *Ann Surg* 206:279–288, 1987.
65. Hemodilution in Stroke Study Group: Hypervolemic hemodilution treatment of acute stroke. Results of a randomized trial using pentastarch. *Stroke* 20(3):317–323, 1989.
66. Janeway CA, Gibson ST, Woodruff LM: Albumin in the treatment of shock. *J Clin Invest* 23:465–475, 1944.
67. Johnson D, Lucan CE, Gerrick SJ: Altered coagulation after albumin supplements for treatment of oligemic shock. *Ann Surg* 114:379–383, 1979.
68. Kakkar VV: International multicenter trial: prevention of fatal postoperative pulmonary embolism by low doses of heparin. *Lancet* 2:45–51, 1975.

69. Khosropour R, Lackner F, Steinbereithnerk, et al: Comparison of the effect of pre- and intraoperative administration of medium molecular weight hydroxyethyl starch (HES 200/0.5) and dextran 40(60) in vascular surgery. *Anaesthesist* 29:616–622, 1980.
70. Kilian J, Spilker D, Borst R: Effect of 6% hydroxyethyl starch, 4.5% dextran 60 and 5.5% oxypolygelatine on blood volume and circulation in human volunteers. *Anaethesist* 24:193–197, 1975.
71. Kirklin JK, Lell WA, Kouchoukos NT: Hydroxyethyl starch vs. albumin for colloid infusion following cardiopulmonary bypass in patients undergoing myocardial revascularization. *Ann Thorac Surg* 37:40–46, 1984.
72. Klapp D, Harrison WL: Evaluation of albumin use by medical audit. *Am J Hosp Pharm* 36:1205–1209, 1979.
73. Kohler H, Kirch W, Klein H: The effect of 6% hydroxyethyl starch-induced macroamylasemia. *Int J Clin Pharmacol* 15:428–431, 1977.
74. Knipping WJ (ed): Drug Topics Redbook, ed 90. Oradell, NJ, Medical Economics, 1986.
75. Kohler H, Kirch W, Horstmann HJ: Hydroxyethyl starch-induced macroamylasemia. *Int J Clin Pharmacol* 15:428–431, 1977.
76. Kohler H, Kirch W, Klein H: The effect of 6% hydroxyethyl starch 450/0.7, 10% dextran 40 and 3.5% gelatin on plasma volume in patients with terminal renal failure. *Anaesthesist* 24:193–197, 1975.
77. Kohler H, Zschiedrich H, Clasen R: Blutvolumen, kolloidosmotischer Druck un Nierenfunktion von Probanden nach Infusion Mittelmolekularer 10% Hydroxyethylstarke 200/0.5 and 10% dextran 40. *Anaesthesist* 31:61–67, 1982.
78. Kovalik SG, Ledgerwood AM, Lucas CE: The cardiac effect of altered calcium homeostasis after albumin resuscitation. *J Trauma* 21:275–279, 1981.
79. Krausz MM, Landau EH, Klin B, Gross D: Hypertonic saline treatment of uncontrolled hemorrhagic shock at different periods from bleeding. *Arch Surg* 127:93–96, 1992.
80. Kreimeier U, Frey L, Dentz J, Herbel T, Messmer K. Hypertonic saline dextran resuscitation during the initial phase of acute endotoxemia: effect on regional blood flow. *Crit Care Med* 19(6): 801–809, 1991.
81. Laks H, O'Connor NE, Anderson W, et al: Crystalloid versus colloid hemodilution in man. *Surg Gynecol Obstet* 142:506–512, 1976.
82. Laks H, Pilon RN, Anderson W: Intraoperative prebleeding in man: effect of colloid hemodilution on blood volume, lung water, hemodynamics and oxygen transport. *Surgery* 78:130–137, 1975.
83. Laks H, Pilon RN, Anderson W, et al: Acute normovolemic hemodilution with crystalloid vs colloid replacement. *Surg Forum* 25:21–22, 1974.
84. Laks H, Pilon RN, Klovekorn WP: Acute hemodilution: its effects on hemodynamics and oxygen transport in anesthetized man. *Ann Surg* 180:103–109, 1974.
85. Lamke LO, Liljedahl SO: Plasma volume changes after infusion of various plasma expanders. *Resuscitation* 5:93–102, 1976.
86. Lamke LO, Liljedahl SO: Plasma volume expansion after infusion of 5%, 20%, and 25% albumin solutions in patients. *Resuscitation* 5:85–92, 1976.
87. Lazrove S, Waxman K, Shippy C: Hemodynamic blood volume and oxygen transport responses to albumin and hydroxyethyl starch infusions in critically ill post operative patients. *Crit Care Med* 8:302–306, 1980.
88. Lee WH, Cooper N, Weidner MG: Clinical evaluation of a new plasma expander: hydroxyethyl starch. *J Trauma* 8:381–393, 1968.
89. Lenz G, Hempel V, Jurger H, Worle H: Effect of hydroxyethyl starch, oxypolygelatin and human albumin on the phagocytic function of the reticuloendothelial system in healthy subjects. *Anaesthesist* 35:423–428, 1986.
90. Lewis JH, Szetol LF, Beyer WL: Severe hemodilution with hydroxyethyl starch and dextrans. *Arch Surg* 93:941–950, 1966.
91. Lewis RT: Albumin: role and discriminative use in surgery. *Can J Surg* 23:322–328, 1980.
92. Liljedahl JO, Rieger A: Blood volume and plasma protein. IV. Importance of thoracic duct lymph in restitution of plasma volume and plasma proteins after bleeding and immediate substitution in splenectomized dogs. *Acta Chir Scand* Suppl 379:39–51, 1967.
93. London MJ, Ho JS, Triedman JK, et al: A randomized clinical trial of 10% pentastarch (low molecular weight hydroxyethyl starch) versus 5% albumin for plasma volume expansion after cardiac operations. *J Thorac Cardiovasc Surg* 97(5):785–797, 1989.
94. Lorenz W, Dolniche A, Freund M: Plasma histamine levels in man following infusion of hydroxyethyl starch: a contribution to the question of allergic or anaphylactoid reactions following administration of a new plasma substitute. *Anaesthesist* 24:228–230, 1975.
95. Lowe RJ, Moss GS, Jilek J, et al: Crystalloid vs. colloid in the etiology of pulmonary failure after trauma: a randomized trial in man. *Surgery* 81:676–683, 1977.
96. Lowery BD, Cloutier CT, Carey LC: Electrolyte solutions in resuscitation in human hemorrhagic shock. *Surg Gynecol Obstet* 133:273–284, 1971.
97. Lucas CE, Ledgerwood AM, Higgins RF: Impaired pulmonary function after albumin resuscitation from shock. *J Trauma* 20:446–451, 1980.
98. Lucas CE, Ledgerwood AM, Rachwel WJ, Grabow D, Saxe JM: Colloid oncotic pressure and body water dynamics on septic and injured patients. *J Trauma* 31(7):927–933, 1991.
99. Lucas CE, Weaver D, Higgins RF: Effects of albumin vs. nonalbumin resuscitation on plasma volume and renal excretory function. *J Trauma* 18:564–570, 1978.
100. Maggio RA, Rha CC, Somberry ED, Praeger PI, Pasley RW, Reed GE: Hemodynamic comparison of albumin and hydroxyethyl starch in postoperative cardiac surgery patients. *Crit Care Med* 11:943–945, 1983.
101. Mailoux L, Swartz CD, Capizzi R, et al: Acute renal failure after administration of LMW dextran. *N Engl J Med* 277:1113–1118, 1967.
102. Matheson NA, Diomi P: Renal failure after the administration of dextran-40. *Surg Gynecol Obstet* 131:661–668, 1970.
103. Mattox KL, Maningas PA, Moore EE, et al: Prehospital hypertonic saline/dextran infusion for post-traumatic hypotension. *Ann Surg* 213(5):482–491, 1991.
104. Maurer PH, Berardinelli B: Immunologic studies with hydroxyethyl starch (HES). *Transfusion* 8:265–268, 1968.
105. Metcaff W, Papadopoulos A, Talano R: Clinical physiologic study of hydroxyethyl starch. *Surg Gynecol Obstet* 131:255–267, 1970.
106. Mishler JM, Borberg H, Emerson PM: Hydroxyethyl starch, an agent for hypovolemic shock treatment. II. Urinary excretion in normal volunteers following three consecutive daily infusions. *Br J Pharmacol* 4:591–595, 1977.
107. Mishler JM, Hester JP, Heustis DW, Rock GA, Strauss RG: Dosage and scheduling regimens for erythrocyte-sedimenting molecules. *J Clin Apheresis* 1:130–143, 1983.
108. Mishler JM, Parry ES, Sutherland BA, Bushrod JR: A clinical study of low molecular weight hydroxyethyl starch, a new plasma expander. *Br J Clin Pharm* 7:619–622, 1979.
109. Modig J: Effectiveness of dextran 70 vs. Ringer's acetate in traumatic shock and adult respiratory distress syndrome. *Crit Care Med* 14:454–457, 1986.
110. Monaof WW, Chuntrasakul C, Aywazian VH. Hypertonic sodium solutions in the treatment of burn shock. *Am J Surg* 126:778–783, 1973.
111. Moore FD, Daher FJ, Boyden CM: Hemorrhage in normal man. I. Distribution and dispersal of saline infusions following acute blood loss: clinical kinetics of blood volume support. *Ann Surg* 163:485–504, 1966.
112. Moss GS, Gould SA: Hypertonic saline. *Prog Clin Biol Res* 299:293–302, 1989.
113. Moss GS, Lower RJ, Jilek J, et al: Colloid of crystalloid in the resuscitation of hemorrhagic shock. A controlled clinical trial. *Surgery* 89:434–438, 1981.
114. Moss GS, Proctor JH, Homer LD: A comparison of asanguinous fluids and whole blood in the treatment of hemorrhagic shock. *Surg Gynecol Obstet* 129:1247–1257, 1969.
115. Moss GS, Siegel DC, Cochin A, et al: Effects of saline and colloid solutions on pulmonary function in hemorrhagic shock. *Surg Gynecol Obstet* 133:53–58, 1971.
116. Muller N, Popov-Cenic S, Kladetzky RG: The effect of hydroxyethyl starch on the intra- and postoperative behavior of haemostasis. *Bibl Anat* 16:460–462, 1977.
117. Nakayama S, Sibley C, Gunther RA, et al: Small volume resuscitation and hypertonic saline (2400 mOsm/liter) during hemorrhagic shock. *Circ Shock* 13:149–159, 1984.
118. Nerlich M, Gunther R, Demling RH: Resuscitation from hemorrhagic shock with hypertonic saline or lactated ringer's (effect on the pulmonary and systemic microcirculation). *Circ Shock* 10:179–188, 1983.
119. Nilsson E, Lamke LO, Liljedahl SO: Is albumin therapy worthwhile in surgery for colorectal cancer? *Acta Chir Scand* 146:619–622, 1980.
120. O'Riordan JP: Current concepts in utilization and provision of human albumin. *Haematologia* 13:175–184, 1980.
121. Oh MS, Carroll HT, Goldstein DA: Hyperchloremic acidosis during the recovery phase of diabetic ketosis. *Ann Intern Med* 89:925–927, 1978.
122. Pascual JMS, Watson JC, Runyon AE, Wade CE, Kramer GC: Resuscitation of intraoperative hypovolemia: a comparison of normal saline and hyperosmotic/hyperoncotic solutions in swine. *Crit Care Med* 20:200–210, 1992.
123. Paul K, Schlesinger RG, Schanfield MS: Reaction to albumin (letter to the editor). *JAMA* 245:234–235, 1981.
124. Pitts RF: Volume and composition of the body fluids. In Physiology of the Kidney and Body Fluids. Year Book, Chicago, 1974.
125. Poole GV, Meredity JW, Pernell T, et al: Comparison of colloids and crystalloids in resuscitation from hemorrhagic shock. *Surg Gynecol Obstet* 154:577–586, 1982.
126. Proctor HJ, Moss GS, Homer LD, et al: Changes in lung compliance in experimental shock and resuscitation. *Ann Surg* 169:82–92, 1969.
127. Puri VK, Howard M, Paidipaty B: Comparative studies of hydroxyethyl starch and albumin in hypovolemia (abstr.) *Crit Care Med* 10:230, 1982.
128. Puri VK, Paidipaty B, White L: Hydroxyethyl starch for resuscitation of patients with hypovolemia in shock. *Crit Care Med* 9:833–837, 1981.
129. Rackow EC, Mecher C, Astiz ME, Griffel M, Falk JL, Weil H: Effects of pentastarch and albumin infusion on cardiorespiratory function and coagulation in patients with severe sepsis and systemic hypoperfusion. *Crit Care Med* 17(5):394–398, 1989.
130. Reed RL, Johnston TD, Chen Y, Fischer RP: Hypertonic saline alters plasma clotting times and platelet aggregation. *J Trauma* 31(1):8–14, 1991.
131. Ring J, Messmer K: Incidence and severity of anaphylactoid reactions to colloid volume substitutes. *Lancet* 1:466–469, 1977.
132. Ring J, Siefert J, Messmer K: Anaphylactoid reactions due to hydroxyethyl starch infusion. *Eur Surg Res* 8:389–399, 1976.
133. Risberg B, Miller E, Hughes J: Comparison of the pulmonary effects of rapid infusion of a crystalloid and a colloid solution. *Acta Chir Scand* 147:613–618, 1981.
134. Rocha-Silva M, Negraes GA, Soares AM, Pontieri V, Loppnow L: Hypertonic resuscitations from severe hemorrhagic shock: patterns of regional circulation. *Circ Shock* 19:165–175, 1986.
135. Rocha-e-Silva M, Vleasco IT, Nogueira da Silva RI, Negraes GA, Oliveira MA: Hyperosmotic sodium salts reverse severe hemorrhagic shock; other solutes do not. *Am J Physiol* H751–H762, 1987.
136. Rock G, Wise P: Plasma expansion during granulocyte procurement. Cumulative effects of hydroxyethyl starch. *Blood* 53:1156–1163, 1979.
137. Rose SD: Prophylaxis of thromboembolic disease. *Med Clin North Am* 63:1205–1224, 1979.
138. Rosenoer VM, Skillman JJ, Hastings PR: Albumin synthesis and nitrogen balance in postoperative patients. *Surgery* 87:305–312, 1980.
139. Rothschild MA, Bauman A, Yalow RS: The effect of large doses of desiccated thyroid on the distribution and metabolism of albumin in euthyroid subjects. *J Clin Invest* 36:422–428, 1957.
140. Rothschild MA, Oratz M, Schreiber SS: Albumin metabolism. *Gastroenterology* 64:324–337, 1973.
141. Rothschild MA, Oratz M, Schreiber SS: Albumin synthesis. *N Engl J Med* 286:748–756, 816–820, 1972.
142. Rothschild MA, Schreiber SS, Oratz M: The effects of adrenocortical hormones on albumin metabolism studies with albumin. *J Clin Invest* 37:1229–1235, 1958.
143. Rowe MI, Arango A: Colloid vs. crystalloid resuscitation in experimental bowel obstruction. *J Pediatr Surg* 11:635–643, 1976.
144. Sasahara AA, Sharma GV, Parisi AF: New developments in the detection and prevention of venous thromboembolism. *Am J Cardiol* 43:1214–1224, 1979.

145. Scattchard G, Batchelder AC, Brown A: Chemical, clinical and immunological studies on the products of human plasma fraction. VI. The osmotic pressure of plasma and serum albumin. *J Clin Invest* 23:458–464, 1944.

146. Schildt B, Bouvang RM, Sollenberg M: Plasma substitute induced impairment of the reticuloendothelial system function. *Acta Chir Scand* 141:7–13, 1975.

147. Scribner BH (ed): University of Washington Teaching Syllabus for the Course of Fluid and Electrolyte Balance. Seattle, University of Washington Press, 1969.

148. Sgouris JT, Rene A (eds): Proceedings of the Workshop on Albumin, February 12–13, 1975. Washington, DC, Department of Health, Education and Welfare, DHEW Publication No. (NIH) 76–925, 1976.

149. Shah DM, Browner BD, Dutten RE: Cardiac output and pulmonary wedge pressure, use for evaluation of fluid replacement in trauma patients. *Arch Surg* 112:1161–1164, 1977.

150. Shatney CH, Chaudry IH: Hydroxyethyl starch administration does not depress reticuloendothelial function of increase mortality from sepsis. *Circ Shock* 13:21–26, 1984.

151. Shatney CH, Deapiha K, Militello PR. Majerus TC, Dawson RB: Efficacy of hetastarch in the resuscitation of patients with multisystem trauma and shock. *Arch Surg* 118:804–809, 1983.

152. Shires GT, Canizaro PC: Fluid resuscitation in the severely injured. *Surg Clin North Am* 53:1341–1366, 1973.

153. Shires CT, Cohn D, Carrico J: Fluid therapy in hemorrhagic shock. *Arch Surg* 88:688–693, 1964.

154. Shoemaker WC: Comparison of the relative effectiveness of whole blood transfusions and various types of fluid therapy in resuscitation. *Crit Care Med* 4:71–78, 1976.

155. Shoemaker WC: Fluids and electrolyte problems in the adult. In Shoemaker WC, Thompson WL (eds): Critical Care State of the Art. Fullerton, CA, Society of Critical Care Medicine, 1982.

156. Shoemaker WC, Bryan-Brown CW, Quigley L: Body fluids shifts in depletion and post-stress states and their correction with adequate nutrition. *Surg Gynecol Obstet* 136:371–374, 1973.

157. Shoemaker WC, Hauser CJ: Critique of crystalloid vs colloid therapy in shock and shock lung. *Crit Care Med* 7:117–124, 1979.

158. Shoemaker WC, Schluchter M, Hopkins JA: Comparison of the relative effectiveness of colloids and crystalloids in emergency resuscitation. *Am J Cardiol* 142:73–84, 1981.

159. Shoemaker WC, Schluchter M, Hopkins JA: Fluid therapy in emergency resuscitation: clinical evaluation of colloid and crystalloid regimens. *Crit Care Med* 9:367–368, 1981.

160. Siegel SC, Moss GS, Cochin A: Pulmonary changes following treatment for hemorrhagic shock: saline vs. colloid infusion. *Surg Forum* 921:17–19, 1970.

161. Singh G, Chaudry KI, Chaudry IH: Crystalloid is as effective as blood in resuscitation of hemorrhagic shock. *Ann Surg* 215(4):377–382, 1992.

162. Skillman JJ: The role of albumin and oncotically active fluids in shock. *Crit Care Med* 4:55–61, 1976.

163. Skillman JJ, Hassan AK, Moore FD: Plasma protein kinetics of the early transcapillary refill after hemorrhage in man. *Surg Gynecol Obstet* 125:983–996, 1967.

164. Skillman JJ, Restall DS, Salzman EW: Randomized trial of albumin vs. electrolyte solutions during abdominal aortic operations. *Surgery* 78:291–303, 1975.

165. Skillman JJ, Rosenoer VM, Smith PC: Improved albumin synthesis in postoperative patients by amino acid infusion. *N Engl J Med* 295:1037–1040, 1976.

166. Solanke TF: Clinical trial of 6% hydroxyethyl starch (a new plasma expander). *Br Med J* 3:783–785, 1968.

167. Solanke TF, Khwaja MS, Madojemu EI: Plasma volume studies with four different plasma volume expanders. *J Surg Res* 11:140–143, 1971.

168. Stead EA Jr, Ebert RV: Studies on human albumin. In Mudd S, Thaliver W (eds): Blood Substitutes and Blood Transfusion. Springfield, IL, Charles C Thomas, 1942.

169. Strauss RG, Hester JP, Volger WR, et al: A multicenter trial to document the efficacy and safety of a rapidly excreted analog of hydroxyethyl starch for leukopheresis with a note on steroid stimulation of granulocyte donors. *Transfusion* 26:258–264, 1986.

170. Strauss RG, Koepke JA, McGuire LC, et al: Clinical and laboratory effects on donors in intermittent flow centrifugation platelet-leukopheresis performed with hydroxyethyl starch and citrate. *Clin Lab Haematol* 2:1–11, 1980.

171. Strauss RG, Stansfield C, Henriksen RA, Villahaauer PJ: Pentastarch may cause fewer effects on coagulation than hetastarch. *Transfusion* 28:257–260, 1988.

172. Strauss RG, Snyder EL, Stuber J, Fick RB: Ingestion of hydroxyethyl starch by human leukocytes. *Transfusion* 26:88–90, 1986.

173. Strauss RG, Stump DC, Henrikson RA: Hydroxyethyl starch accentuates von Willenbrand's disease. *Transfusion* 25:235–237, 1985.

174. Strauss RG, Stump DC, Henrikson RA, Saunders R: Effects of hydroxyethyl starch on fibrinogen, fibrin clot formation and fibrinolysis. *Transfusion* 25:230–234, 1985.

175. Stump DC, Strauss RG, Henrikson RA, Peterson RE, Saunders R: Effects of hydroxyethyl starch on blood coagulation, particularly factor VIII. *Transfusion* 25:349–354, 1985.

176. Takaori M, Safar P: Acute severe hemodilution with lactated Ringer's solution. *Arch Surg* 94:67–73, 1967.

177. Takaori M, Safar P: Treatment of massive hemorrhage with colloid and crystalloid solutions. *JAMA* 199:297–302, 1967.

178. Templeton GH, Mitchell JH, Wildenthal K: Influence of hyperosmolarity on left ventricular stiffness. *Am J Physiol* 222:1406–1411, 1972.

179. Thomas JM, Silva JR: Dextran 40 in the treatment of peripheral vascular disease. *Arch Surg* 106:138–141, 1973.

180. Thompson WL: Rational use of albumin and plasma substitutes. *Johns Hopkins Med J* 136:220–225, 1975.

181. Thompson WL, Britton JJ, Walton RP: Persistence of starch derivatives and dextran when infused after hemorrhage. *J Pharmacol Exp Ther* 136:125–132, 1962.

182. Thompson WL, Fukushima T, Rutherford RB, et al: Intravascular persistence, tissue shortage and excretion of hydroxyyethyl starch. *Surg Gynecol Obstet* 131:965–972, 1970.

183. Thompson WL, Walton RP: Circulatory responses to intravenous infusions of hydroxyethyl starch solutions. *J Pharmacol Exp Ther* 146:359–364, 1964.

184. Thoren L: The dextrans—clinical data. Joint WHO/IABS symposium on the standardization of albumin plasma substitutes and plasmapheresis, Geneva 1980. *Dev Biol Stand* 48:157–167, 1981.

185. Tobias TA, Schertel ER, Schmell LM, Wilber N, Muir WW: Comparative effects of 7.5% NaCl in 6% Dextran-70 and .09% NaCl on cardiorespiratory parameters after cardiac output controlled resuscitation from canine hemorrhage shock. *Circ Shock* 398:139–146, 1993.

186. Trinkle JK, Rush BF, Eiseman B: Metabolism of lactate following major blood loss. *Surgery* 63:782–787, 1968.

187. Trudnowski RJ, Goel SB, Lam FT, Evers JT: Effect of Ringer's lactate solution and sodium bicarbonate on surgical acidosis. *Surg Gynecol Obstet* 125:807–814, 1967.

188. Tullis JL: Albumin. I. Background and use. *JAMA* 237:355–360, 1977.

189. Tullis JL: Albumin. 2. Guidelines for clinical uses. *JAMA* 237:460–463, 1977.

190. Vassar MJ, Perry CA, HolCroft JW: Prehospital resuscitation of hypotensive trauma patients with 7.5% NaCl versus 7.5% NaCl with added Dextran. A controlled trial. *J Trauma* 34:622–633, 1993.

191. Virgilio RW: Crystalloid vs. colloid resuscitation (reply to letter to editor). *Surgery* 86:515, 1979.

192. Virgilio RW, Rice CL, Smith DE: Crystalloid vs colloid resuscitation: is one better? A randomized clinical study. *Surgery* 85:129–139, 1979.

193. Virgilio RW, Smith DE, Zarino DK: Balanced electrolyte solutions: experimental and clinical studies. *Crit Care Med* 7:98–106, 1979.

194. Vito L, Dennis RC, Weisel RD: Sepsis presenting as acute respiratory insufficiency. *Surg Gynecol Obstet* 138:896–900, 1974.

195. Walsh JC, Zhuamg J, Shackford SR. A comparison of hypertonic to isotonic fluid in the resuscitation of brain injury and hemorrhagic shock. *J Surg Res* 50(3):284–292, 1991.

196. Waxman K, Holness R, Tominaga G, Chela P, Grimes J: Hemodynamic and oxygen transport effects of pentastarch in burn resuscitation. *Ann Surg* 209(3):341–345, 1989.

197. Weatherbee L, Spencer HH, Knopp CT: Coagulation studies after the transfusion of hydroxyethyl starch protected frozen blood in primates. *Transfusion* 14:109–115, 1974.

198. Weaver DW, Ledgerwood AM, Lucas CE: Pulmonary effects of albumin resuscitation for severe hypovolemic shock. *Arch Surg* 113:387–392, 1978.

199. Weil MH, Henning RJ, Puri VK: Colloid oncotic pressure: clinical significance. *Crit Care Med* 7:113–116, 1979.

200. Weiss HJ: The effect of clinical dextran on platelet aggregation, adhesion and ADP release in man: in vivo and in vitro studies. *J Lab Clin Med* 69:37–46, 1967.

201. Woodruff LM, Gobsin ST: Use of human albumin in military medicine. Clinical evaluation of human albumin. *US Navy Med Bull* 40:791–796, 1942.

202. Wong PY, Carroll RE, Lipinski TL: Studies on the renin-angiotension-aldosterone system in patients with cirrhosis and ascites: effect of saline and albumin infusion. *Gastroenterology* 77:1171–1176, 1979.

203. Yacobi A, Stoll RG, Sum CY: Pharmacokinetics of hydroxyethyl starch in normal subjects. *J Clin Pharmacol* 22:206–212, 1982.

204. Younes RN, Aun F, Accioly CQ, Casale LPL, Szanjnbok I, Birolini D: Hypertonic solutions in the treatment of hypovolemic shock: a prospective, randomized study in patients admitted to the emergency room. *Surgery* 111(4):380–385, 1992.

CHAPTER 16

Anesthetic Pharmacology and Critical Care

DAVID J. CULLEN, M.D., M.S.
LUCA M. BIGATELLO, M.D.
HAROLD J. DeMONACO, M.S.

INTRODUCTION

Anesthetic pharmacology is an integral part of intensive care therapeutics for two major reasons. *First*, many patients enter the intensive care unit (ICU) following either elective or emergency surgical procedures performed under a variety of anesthetics whose effects persist for varying lengths of time. The kinetics, pharmacologic actions, and potential toxicities of anesthetic drugs during the recovery period are important. *Second*, anesthetic drugs possess attributes that are useful and often essential in the ICU management of postoperative patients. Concerns over premedication and anesthetic administration must be appreciated both by the intensivist and the anesthesiologist. Problems involved in using common anesthetics to manage the critically ill, and drug interactions that apply to this unique and susceptible group of patients are discussed.

PREMEDICATION

The main purpose of premedication is to reduce fear and anxiety, enabling the patient to anticipate surgery calmly and confidently. Premedicants may also potentiate anesthesia, diminish anesthetic side effects, enhance gastric emptying, and dry the mouth when oral instrumentation is anticipated. The effects of premedication for most patients entering the ICU from the operating room (OR) will have been dissipated and, therefore, are of little or no concern to the ICU staff. Barbiturates are rarely used for premedication and have no important

role in medicating the ICU patient about to undergo a surgical procedure.

Opioids (Table 16.1). Opioids are often used for premedication, and residual effects may persist into the recovery period, particularly with longer-acting drugs such as morphine. When morphine is used for premedication by the i.m. route, its onset of action occurs within 15 to 30 min and peaks at 45 to 90 min. Opioids obtund the response to painful stimuli at several loci in the central nervous system (CNS). They may act by decreasing conduction of impulses of primarily afferent fibers when they enter the spinal cord and decrease activity in other sensory nerve endings. There are numerous opioid binding sites, μ-receptors, in the spinal cord. Morphine-like drugs acting at this site are thought to decrease the release of neurotransmitters, such as substance P, that mediate transmission of pain impulses. Opioids, especially morphine, may sedate and ultimately induce sleep in large doses. The sedative effect of morphine make it particularly suitable for premedication. Opioids lack a reliable amnestic action: small doses of barbiturates or a benzodiazepine may be added for this purpose; in patients who are deemed too unstable to tolerate these drugs, scopolamine (0.2 to 0.4 mg) provides reliable amnesia. Morphine has little effect on cardiovascular function unless the patient is tilted head-up, in which case morphine-induced venous pooling may cause hypotension. The respiratory effects of intramuscular morphine, however, are substantial, especially in critically ill patients. It will significantly decrease the sensitivity of the respiratory center to carbon

Table 16.1. Use of Opioids in Adult ICU Patients

	Premedication	Induction of Anesthesia	
		Opioid alone	With thiopental
Morphine	5–10 mg i.m.	0.5–1 mg/kg	5–15 mg
Meperidine	50–75 mg i.m.	Not recommended: histamine release, negative inotrope	75–150 mg
Fentanyl	Too potent agents; not ideal for premedication.	10–50 μg/kg	3–10 μg/kg
Alfentanil		50–125 μg/kg	20–50 μg/kg
Sufentanil		3–30 μg/kg	1–10 μg/kg
Comments:	Pleasant sedative effect. Stable hemodynamics in the recumbent position. All inhibit gastric emptying.	Large doses of opioids induce general anesthesia. A few patients (10–20%) may not be amnestic or may show a hemodynamic response if used alone. Chest wall rigidity.	

dioxide or other stimuli. Airway reflexes may become diminished, which is an advantage to intubated and ventilated patients but a potential risk to those patients whose airway is unprotected. Even small (7.5 mg) subcutaneous doses of morphine significantly decrease the hypoxic ventilatory response (1), and it is likely that this action occurs with other opiates as well. Morphine is particularly useful in patients undergoing extensive and invasive monitoring procedures before induction of anesthesia or in patients about to undergo nerve blocks.

Although meperidine is a synthetic opioid, its effects in equianalgesic doses are very similar to those actions of morphine. Its onset of action is more rapid, and its duration of effect is approximately one-half that of morphine. Patients receiving monoamine oxidase inhibitors may experience a serious drug interaction with meperidine, consisting of fever, delirium, respiratory depression, and cyanosis (2).

The agonist/antagonist opioids were developed to produce less respiratory depression than the pure agonists. Butorphanol tartrate (10 mg)(3) and nalbuphine hydrochloride (2 mg)(4) have respiratory effects similar to those of 10 mg of morphine; however, no further depression occurs with higher doses, nor does analgesia improve either.

When ICU patients are being premedicated, respiratory depressants such as opioids should be avoided until endotracheal intubation and access to controlled ventilation is immediately available. Often, however, the medications previously used to control pain within the ICU can be continued and even considered as premedicants when such critically ill patients must return for additional surgical procedures. The anesthesiologist should accompany ICU patients to the OR when possible to ensure that the patient is adequately monitored and ventilated during transport.

Tranquilizers. Oral tranquilizers have little use in ICU patients, except for premedicating surgical patients. Oral benzodiazepines have both a calming and amnesic effect; however, their effects on postoperative patients arriving in the ICU are minimal. Intravenous diazepam (1 to 5 mg) or midazolam (0.5 to 2 mg) may be very effective before ICU patients are transported to the OR. Except in hypovolemic situations, the benzodiazepines have little cardiovascular effect.

The benzodiazepines are particularly useful in reinforcing the sedative effects of opioids while permitting smaller doses of opioids to provide analgesia. They also have a powerful

anticonvulsant action. Diazepam and midazolam are not commonly used for induction of anesthesia because of slow onset of action and burning pain (diazepam) when given i.v. Occasionally, severe cardiorespiratory depression may occur with large anesthetic doses.

Diazepam is very lipid-soluble, accounting for its rapid onset of action, though its onset is not as rapid as that of thiopental. The effect of redistribution and protein binding accounts for its prolonged duration of action. Diazepam's half-life is 20 to 40 hours in most subjects. After repeated doses, blood levels of diazepam accumulate, and prolonged effects may be seen. Diazepam is primarily metabolized by the microsomal enzyme system of the liver and prolonged effects are possible in patients with liver dysfunction. When i.v. diazepam is used in critically ill adult patients, a test dose of 1 to 2.5 mg i.v. should be given before larger doses are administered.

Midazolam (5) is a water-soluble benzodiazepine with a shorter onset of action and duration of action than diazepam. Being water-soluble, midazolam can be injected i.v. pain-free and can be used i.m. without concern. The incidence of thrombophlebitis at the site of injection is extremely low, compared to that of diazepam. Because it is very lipophilic and has a high degree of affinity for benzodiazepine receptors, its onset of action is faster than that of diazepam (usually, about 1 minute). It is probably three to four times as potent as diazepam, and the dose should be reduced accordingly. Midazolam is an effective premedicant, with significant anterograde amnesia of relatively short duration. Premedication doses i.m. range from 0.07 to 0.1 mg/kg. In the less-healthy patients, iv doses should range from 0.5 to 1 mg. Midazolam has significant respiratory depressant effects and reduces the ventilatory response to hypercarbia and hypoxia. Of major concern is the interaction with opioids to produce profound respiratory depression. Lorazepam is also a useful oral premedicant in doses ranging from 0.5 to 2 mg p.o. A specific benzodiazepine antagonist, flumazenil, has been available in Europe and Israel and has just been released for clinical use in the USA. Flumazenil antagonizes the central effects of benzodiazepines and other hypnotics that interact with benzodiazepine receptors. In clinical trials, flumazenil caused reversal of postoperative sedation associated with the administration of midazolam (6–8) and of coma secondary to benzodiazepine intoxication.

Phenothiazines and the butyrophenones, haloperidol and droperidol, are usually avoided as premedicants in critically ill patients because their cardiovascular side effects are unpredictable.

Anticholinergics. Autonomic nervous system activity should be minimized during anesthesia and surgery. Cholinergic effects, such as bronchial and salivary secretions, and bradycardia may be alleviated by anticholinergic premedication. Preoperative i.m. administration of atropine, scopolamine, or glycopyrrolate will inhibit secretions, which is especially useful in patients undergoing upper airway procedures such as bronchoscopy or esophagoscopy.

Scopolamine is often used for its amnestic properties and lack of hemodynamic effects in hemodynamically unstable patients. Occasionally, however, patients returning from the OR who have been premedicated with scopolamine will become delirious, disoriented, and uncooperative. The central anticholinergic effects of scopolamine may be antagonized with physostigmine (1 to 2 mg i.v.), rapidly converting the patient into a conscious, cooperative individual (9). Physostigmine is a tertiary ammonium compound that is lipid-soluble, thus rapidly crossing the blood-brain barrier to antagonize acetylcholinesterase, the enzyme responsible for hydrolyzing acetylcholine. Therefore, more acetylcholine is available to compete with scopolamine at the CNS cholinergic receptor. Physostigmine may also reverse the central effects of benzodiazepines, phenothiazines, and the butyrophenones.

The patient at risk from excessive sympathetic nervous system activity, e.g., one with myocardial ischemia, usually requires continuation of β-adrenergic receptor blockade therapy, particularly if that patient had received propranolol preoperatively. This approach will minimize hypertension and tachycardia during laryngoscopy and intubation.

Prophylaxis against Aspiration of Gastric Contents. Pulmonary aspiration of gastric contents is one of the most common causes of severe morbidity related to anesthesia. Although many ICU patients scheduled for surgery are already endotracheally intubated, they may, during the OR course, undergo additional procedures such as change of the endotracheal tube or institution of a tracheostomy, during which the airway remains unprotected for variable periods of time. Furthermore, they almost invariably receive opioids, which significantly delay gastric emptying. Patients receiving enteral nutrition should have their feeding stopped for 6 to 8 hours before surgery. Pharmacologic prophylaxis of aspiration has two main objectives: inhibition of gastric acid secretion and stimulation of gastric peristalsis. The first objective is accomplished most effectively with histamine 2 (H_2) receptor antagonists. Cimetidine and ranitidine have both been effective in increasing gastric pH preoperatively; neither drug, however, completely eliminates the risk of aspiration in all patients (10). Omeprazole (11) is a recently introduced drug available only for oral administration that blocks the H^+ - K^+ ATPase of the gastric parietal cells. Unlike H_2-antagonists, omeprazole completely abolishes acid production for up to 48 hours; however, as the drug is destroyed in an acid environment, peak effect is delayed. The effect of omeprazole before anesthesia has not been evaluated as yet. The second objective may be best attempted with the administration of metoclopramide: 10 to 20 mg i.v. results in gastric emptying in 20 to 30 minutes. The clinical efficacy of metoclopramide is not uniform, and its effects are completely abolished by opioids.

INDUCTION OF ANESTHESIA

Induction of general anesthesia is accomplished with potent, short-acting hypnotics; occasionally, repeated dosage or continuous infusions are used, and residual pharmacologic effects may persist at the time of admission to the ICU. Also, induction of anesthesia may be needed in ICU patients for procedures such as direct laryngoscopy, gastrointestinal endoscopies, special radiologic tests, and minor surgical procedures in patients deemed too unstable to be transferred to the operating room. Among the drugs of importance in anesthetic induction for critically ill patients are the barbiturates, benzodiazepines, ketamine, propofol, and etomidate.

Barbiturates. Ultrashort-acting barbiturates used for induction of general anesthesia include thiopental, thiamylal, and methohexital. Their pharmacologic profile is quite similar, and thiopental, the most widely used, may be considered the prototype of this class. Sodium thiopental is provided as a 2.5% solution that is strongly basic (pH 10.6). The usual dosage for induction of anesthesia is 3 to 5 mg/kg, though less drug may be needed in sicker patients and in the elderly. At usual dosages, loss of consciousness occurs within one or two circulation times and lasts 10 to 30 minutes. The rapid decay in blood and brain concentrations of thiopental is a result of rapid redistribution to muscle and fat (12). The elimination of thiopental is slow, with an elimination half-life of about 5 hours (13). Elimination occurs almost entirely via hepatic metabolism. A large fraction of circulating thiopental is bound to serum proteins (60 to 96%). In patients who are depleted of serum proteins, more free thiopental is available for diffusion into brain and heart, thus prolonging sleep times and enhancing cardiovascular depression (14).

The cardiovascular effects of thiopental include a dose-dependent decrease of myocardial contractility, venous pooling, and decreasing preload (15). Patients with low cardiac output, circulatory shock, or congestive heart failure whose cerebral and coronary blood flows are preserved at the expense of other organ blood flows are vulnerable to drugs such as thiopental because the amount of thiopental circulating to the brain and heart will be proportionally greater. Hence, the initial dose of thiopental must be carefully reduced in abnormal circulatory states. Furthermore, thiopental is a dose-dependent direct myocardial depressant and peripheral vasodilator. Thus, hypotension and respiratory depression, which often occur transiently following thiopental administration, may further decrease venous return, cardiac output, and coronary blood flow, leading to myocardial ischemia.

Apnea, usually lasting less than one minute, occurs after a single injection of thiopental, but this transient effect is reversed once CO_2 increases spontaneously to stimulate respiration. Although the CNS effects of thiopental dissipate rapidly after the first dose, multiple doses of thiobarbiturates may prolong respiratory depression, particularly if supplemented by opioids which, of course, greatly potentiate respiratory depression.

Thiopental decreases cerebral metabolism and oxygen consumption and causes a decrease in cerebral blood flow (16) that makes thiopental particularly useful in managing patients with increased intracranial pressure and in patients at risk for regional cerebral ischemia.

Hepatic metabolism accounts for about 50% of the thiopental removed from the circulation. Patients with severe liver dysfunction will not metabolize thiopental effectively, and its action will be prolonged. Thiopental-induced EEG changes may persist hours after the clinical effects have disappeared. If additional drugs, such as opioids or benzodiazepines, are given while this residual barbiturate effect is present, potentiation may occur.

Contraindications to the use of thiopental include severe cardiac decompensation or peripheral circulatory failure, porphyria, and known allergic reactions to previous administration of barbiturates. Thiobarbiturates are especially useful for anesthetic induction in patients with increased intracranial pressure to avoid airway irritability, particularly in patients with asthma, to aid endotracheal intubation within the ICU, and to facilitate a rapid induction for patients with a full stomach.

Benzodiazepines.   When administered in doses five to ten times larger than those dosages used for mild sedation, benzodiazepines reliably induce general anesthesia. Their hemodynamic and respiratory effects at these high doses are similar to those actions of sodium thiopental. Their slower onset of action, however, has limited the use of benzodiazepines for induction of anesthesia. Compared to diazepam, midazolam (5, 17) has the advantage of a relatively faster onset and, being water-soluble, of not causing pain at the site of injection; in very fragile patients it can be a safe induction agent.

Opioids (Table 16.1).   Large doses of opioids are often employed to induce and maintain general anesthesia in patients with limited cardiovascular reserve. Since the report by Lowenstein et al in 1969 (18) on the safety and efficacy of morphine (1 mg/kg) in patients undergoing coronary artery bypass surgery, high doses of opioids (e.g., fentanyl 10 to 25 μg/kg, sufentanil 3 to 10 μg/kg) have been widely employed for induction of general anesthesia in critically ill patients. However, the hemodynamic response to endotracheal intubation is not uniformly blunted (19), amnesia is not ensured, and hypotension may still occur, particularly in hypovolemic patients.

Ketamine (20).   Ketamine is used to induce anesthesia in those awake but unstable patients who may be disturbed by laryngoscopy, yet at risk of profound cardiovascular decompensation from thiopental or midazolam. Its onset of action is between 30 and 60 seconds, only slightly slower than that of thiopental. The usual adult induction dose is approximately 1 to 2 mg/kg i.v., but this must be adjusted according to the severity of illness. Intramuscular administration, often used in children, is inappropriate in the adult ICU patient. Ketamine is a cataleptic analgesic and anesthetic agent without hypnotic properties whose mechanism of action differs greatly from that of thiopental. It has been called a dissociative anesthetic characterized by complete analgesia with only superficial sleep.

In healthy patients, ketamine raises the blood pressure by 20% to 40%. However, with smaller doses and in critically ill patients, blood pressure usually does not increase. Its cardiovascular effects include hypertension, tachycardia, and increased cardiac output probably mediated by increased central sympathetic outflow. Baroreflexes may be impaired, and norepinephrine is potentiated by a cocaine-like action on adrenergic nerve terminals, which prevents reuptake and inactivation of catecholamines. Although ketamine is a direct myocardial depressant, this effect is usually overcome by sympathetic activation. Because of its substantial increase in myocardial oxygen consumption, ketamine is relatively contraindicated in patients with coronary artery disease. Its routine use is not warranted particularly because it is a potent hallucinogen. Awakening is slow, even after a single dose that further limits its usefulness for short procedures where immediate arousal is important. The drug is specifically contraindicated in patients with increased intracranial or intraocular pressure because these pressures increase dramatically after a single dose of ketamine. Upper airway procedures cannot be safely carried out using ketamine alone, but it may be useful for induction of anesthesia in patients requiring such operations.

Etomidate.   Etomidate (21) is a short-acting benzylimidazole that rapidly induces apnea and unconsciousness, but little analgesia, in doses of 0.3 to 0.4 mg/kg. Etomidate shares with sodium thiopental the ability of decreasing cerebral blood flow and metabolism, which makes it suitable for induction of general anesthesia in patients with increased intracranial pressure. Etomidate causes minimal cardiovascular depression and, possibly, less hypotension when compared with equipotent doses of thiopental. Its short duration of action (3 to 5 minutes) is determined both by redistribution and by rapid hepatic metabolism. Unpleasant side effects are pain at the site of injection, a high (30 to 50%) incidence of myoclonus, and the frequent occurrence of nausea and vomiting on emergence. The main untoward effect is the inhibition of adrenal steroidal biosynthesis, which contraindicates the continuous infusion of etomidate for long-term sedation in the ICU. Inhibition of steroidogenesis is measurable following a single injection, although this problem has not been associated with perioperative complications (22).

Propofol.   Propofol (23) is an alkylphenol, unrelated to any other currently used intravenous anesthetic. Propofol is presently available as a 1% solution in soybean oil, glycerol, and egg phosphatide; previously reported anaphylactoid and anaphylactic reactions were attributed to the solubilizing agent Cromophor EL, which is no longer part of the formulation. Propofol produces rapid onset of unconsciousness in doses of 1.5 to 3 mg/kg; its effects on the cerebral circulation, as well as on the cardiovascular system, are quite similar to those actions of sodium thiopental and etomidate (24). The reports of a lower incidence of postoperative nausea and vomiting have not been substantiated on a large scale. The main pharmacodynamic difference between propofol and all the other intravenous and inhalational anesthetics seems to be a more rapid emergence with minimal confusion. The duration of action of a single dose is very short (2 to 3 minutes) due to rapid hepatic and extrahepatic clearance. No significant prolongation of its hypnotic effect has been reported in patients with hepatic or renal disease; in elderly patients, however, the clearance is significantly lower than in young patients, suggesting that propofol should be used in reduced doses in the elderly population. The pharmacokinetic profile of propofol, as well as the particularly rapid recovery that follows its administration, make it a very attractive drug for administration in continuous infusion.

MAINTENANCE OF ANESTHESIA

Anesthetic maintenance of critically ill patients undergoing surgery is accomplished with inhalation anesthetics, with intravenous drugs or, most commonly, with combinations of smaller doses of several drugs utilizing the best properties of each.

Opioids (Table 16.1). Opioids are often used in large doses for anesthetic management of critically ill patients because they maintain cardiovascular stability. Morphine releases histamine, depresses sympathetic activity, resulting in venous pooling and reduced ventricular filling pressures, and induces bradycardia. In the supine patient, however, morphine is unlikely to produce hypotension unless the patient's blood pressure has been maintained by increased central sympathetic activity. Hypotension that may occur is the result of sedation and analgesia, rather than a direct vascular effect of morphine. Direct myocardial depression is not seen in clinical doses.

Meperidine decreases central sympathetic output and has a negative inotropic effect (25), which results in decreased blood pressure. Meperidine can increase heart rate (26) probably due to an anticholinergic effect, as it is structurally similar to atropine.

Fentanyl is approximately 100 times as potent as morphine and has a shorter duration of action than either meperidine or morphine (27). Because it is so lipid-soluble, large doses of fentanyl accumulate and prolong its duration of action for many hours. Even massive doses of fentanyl (50 to 100 μg/kg) do not impair myocardial contractility; reduction in cardiac output is usually the result of bradycardia.

Sufentanil is a potent analogue of fentanyl and is useful in producing anesthesia in patients who require high-dose narcotic techniques to maintain cardiovascular stability (28). It is five to ten times as potent as fentanyl, and doses should be scaled accordingly. Sufentanil is a pure opioid agonist, highly selective for μ-receptors. When used in high-dose techniques, prolonged respiratory depression and the need for ventilatory support are expected. Like fentanyl, hemodynamic stability is its major advantage over other drugs, though bradycardia usually occurs after larger doses of either drug. Like fentanyl, sufentanil attenuates the hemodynamic response to many surgical stimuli, including surgical incision and endotracheal intubation, though some patients with good ventricular function may "break through" and become hypertensive (18). Both fentanyl and sufentanil reduce the endocrine and metabolic responses to surgical stress, one of the major reasons for their use in critically ill patients. Since rapid injection of either drug can produce truncal rigidity, sometimes before loss of consciousness the use of muscle relaxants must be anticipated, and the operator must be ready to intubate and ventilate such patients immediately. The only important advantage of sufentanil over fentanyl appears to be a shorter duration of action, though this characteristic often depends on clinical factors more than on the pharmacokinetics of the drug.

Alfentanil has entirely different pharmacokinetic and pharmacodynamic effects, compared to fentanyl and sufentanil. Alfentanil is also a pure opioid agonist, whose effects are mediated through opioid μ-receptors in the central nervous system. Onset of action is extremely rapid, and duration of analgesia is short. Alfentanil has a much smaller volume of distribution than fentanyl, especially in muscle and fat, and thus, because plasma concentration is higher, it is more easily eliminated from the body (29). Alfentanil is approximately one-fifth as potent as fentanyl, but its blood concentration decreases below threshold levels for surgical anesthesia within 30 to 60 minutes after bolus injection. Because it equilibrates across the brain more rapidly than does fentanyl, its narcotic effect peaks within 1 or 2 minutes. Its small volume of distribution (both initial and steady-state), ensures that alfentanil is rapidly eliminated from the body with an elimination half-life of 1 to 1.5 hours.

Alfentanil has been useful in attenuating the hemodyanmic response to endotracheal intubation (30). Extrapolating from these data, the authors occasionally use a bolus of alfentanil (10 to 20 μg/kg) in intubated, ventilated patients, just prior to chest physiotherapy or other airway stimulating procedures that might be detrimental to those patients with severe coronary artery disease, increased intracranial pressure, or bronchospastic disease.

The postoperative result of narcotic anesthesia is usually prolonged respiratory depression, regardless of which narcotic was used. However, this effect may be beneficial in critically ill patients for whom postoperative ventilation is anticipated.

Reversing narcotic effects in critically ill patients with naloxone is usually unsatisfactory because of unwanted drug side effects. Naloxone is a pure narcotic antagonist that causes no paradoxical respiratory depression even when administered in large doses. Its mechanism of action is competitive inhibition; naloxone prevents opioids from occupying their central nervous system receptors by binding to these sites itself. It promptly reverses respiratory depression associated with residual narcotic drugs by increasing respiratory rate and tidal volume. Of great importance is naloxone's short duration of action (31). It rapidly penetrates the brain because it is very lipid-soluble. Brain-naloxone concentrations decline quickly, compared to morphine or other residual opioids because, like thiopental, it rapidly redistributes to other lipid-soluble tissues. Thus, respiratory depression may recur when the naloxone antagonism subsides. The side effects of naloxone, which may be important in the ICU, include nausea, vomiting, hypertension, tachycardia, and acute pain manifested by the patient pulling out tubes, intravenous catheters, and dressings. If one administers naloxone in the narcotized, extubated patient, it is useful to titrate 0.04- to 0.1-mg doses until the patient is awake enough to maintain adequate ventilation and airway protection. If, however, the patient is intubated, having received large doses of opioids for anesthesia, and is still drowsy or somnolent, controlled ventilation is safest until the narcotic effect disappears, permitting the patient to breathe spontaneously at normal levels of $PACO_2$.

Inhalation Anesthesia. Inhalation anesthesia results when an appropriate brain anesthetic partial pressure is achieved. Therefore, recovery from inhalation anesthesia requires that the brain anesthetic partial pressure decrease to levels which permit awakening and depends on the rate of decrease of the alveolar anesthetic concentration. The rate of anesthetic "wash-out" from the brain depends on cerebral blood flow and the relative solubility of the anesthetic in the tissue and blood, as well as the difference in partial pressure of the drug from tissue to blood. When cerebral blood flow is decreased, less anesthetic is washed out of the central nervous system and emergence is slowed. Anesthetics with higher-lipid solubility (halothane, enflurane, and isoflurane) have more drug in the brain and require more time to move from the brain to the blood. Anesthetics with lower solubility (nitrous oxide) have less of a reservoir in the brain and move more readily to the blood. The partial pressure difference of anesthetic from tissue to blood is the gradient along which the drug moves. If the partial pressure gradient is small, little anesthetic is transferred from brain to blood, and emergence is slowed. This situation arises if the arterial blood is saturated with anesthetic because the lungs fail to eliminate the drug.

Elimination of inhaled anesthetic from the lungs is governed to a large extent by the same factors that govern uptake during induction of anesthesia (32). These factors include cardiac output, blood/gas solubility, and alveolar ventilation. The alveolar partial pressure of anesthetic determines the amount of anesthetic in the arterial blood perfusing the brain. A lower alveolar partial pressure produces lower arterial saturation and speeds wash-out from the brain. The more soluble an anesthetic is in the blood, the longer it takes for emergence (Fig 16.1)(33). This phenomenon occurs because larger amounts of a more soluble drug are in the tissues and the drug has less tendency to move from the blood to gas phase. Isoflurane has a lower blood-gas solubility coefficient than halothane or enflurane, thus allowing for more rapid emergence. The less soluble anesthetics, such as nitrous oxide and desflurane, have less of a reservoir in the tissues and move readily from the blood to the alveoli, hence, emergence is

rapid. Finally, the amount of alveolar ventilation is very important in determining the rate of emergence from inhalation anesthesia. The effect of ventilation is more marked for more soluble agents (Fig 16.2)(32). If the patient hypoventilates while recovering from halothane, as might occur when given a narcotic for pain, emergence is slowed.

Several other factors can affect a patient's rate of recovery from inhalational anesthesia, including: (*a*) duration of anesthesia; (*b*) ventilation/perfusion abnormalities; (*c*) changes in solubility; (*d*) hypothermia; (*e*) metabolism; and (*f*) presence of other drugs.

The longer a patient has been anesthetized, the longer the time for recovery because, as the anesthetic proceeds, more anesthetic accumulates in muscle and fat. This fact is particularly true for the more soluble anesthetics.

Alterations of solubility change the rate of emergence. The clearest example of this problem is hypothermia in which solubility is increased and emergence is slowed. In addition, during hypothermia, anesthetic potency is increased, and a lower partial pressure of anesthetic is required for awakening (34). Anesthetics that undergo hepatic metabolism, such as halothane and methoxyflurane, have a rate of clearance from the circulation that is affected by the rate of metabolism.

All of the above factors affect the rate of change of alveolar partial pressure which, in turn, determines anesthetic pressure in the brain. Some factors, such as hypothermia, can affect the potency of anesthetics and thus delay emergence because a lower partial pressure of anesthetic in the alveoli must be achieved. Sedative/hypnotic drugs, opioids, lidocaine, and certain antihypertensives, such as α-methyldopa and clonidine, increase the potency of inhalation anesthetics. In addition, less anesthetic is required in pregnant women and the elderly, and these patients may take longer to recover from anesthesia (35). In summary, emergence from general inhalation anesthesia is a complex process whose rate is determined by the many variables, including factors that affect wash-out of the drug, concomitant medications, and the preexisting condition of the patient.

Nitrous Oxide. Nitrous oxide (N_2O) is the anesthetic gas with the lowest solubility in use today. Nitrous oxide is nonflammable, has a molecular weight of 44, and is supplied in

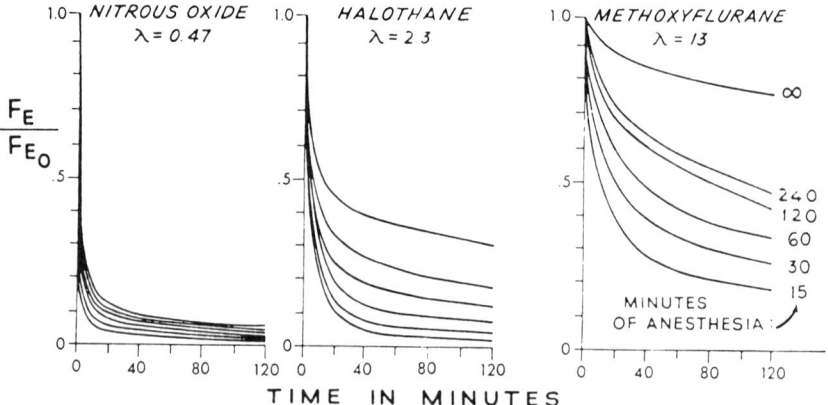

Figure 16.1. Analog recovery curves illustrating the effects of duration of anesthesia (equilibrium 15, 30, 60, 120 and 240 minutes) and solubility on the rate of recovery at a constant alveolar ventilation (4 liters/min). F_E/F_{EO} is the ratio of alveolar gas tension at each time in the recovery divided by the alveolar gas tension at the start of recovery. (From Stoelting RK, Eger II ET: Ventilation and anesthetic solubility on recovery from anesthesia: an in vivo and analog analysis before and after equilibration. *Anesthesiology* 30:296, 1969, with permission of Stoelting RK and JB Lippincott.)

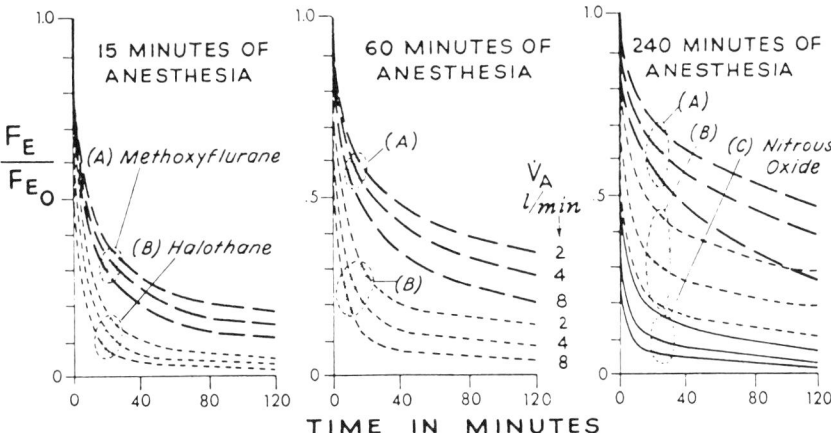

Figure 16.2. In vivo alveolar recovery curve (dashed lines) following equilibrium at ventilations controlled to maintain alveolar PCO_2 values at 20, 40 and 80 mm Hg, are plotted during 30 minutes of recovery. The solid lines represent the corresponding analog recovery curves at alveolar ventilations of 2, 4 and 8 liters/min. The in vivo F_E/F_{EO} ratios for nitrous oxide and halothane were derived from alveolar gas values, while arterial concentrations were used for methoxyflurane ratios. F_E/F_{EO} is the ratio of alveolar gas tension at each time in recovery divided by the alveolar gas tension at the start of recovery. (From Stoelting RK, Eger III ET: Ventilation and anesthetic solubility on recovery from anesthesia: an in vivo and analog analysis before and after equilibration. *Anesthesiology* 30:296, 1969, with permission of Stoelting RK and JB Lippincott.)

blue cylinders that contain the vapor over liquid. It has a blood-gas solubility coefficient of 0.47, about one-fifth that of halothane. Because of the low solubility of nitrous oxide, a higher alveolar partial pressure is quickly achieved, as little is taken up by the blood. For this reason, induction and recovery from anesthesia are rapid.

Nitrous oxide is much less potent than other anesthetics. Anesthetic potency is described in terms of minimal alveolar concentration (MAC) required to prevent movement to incision in 50% of patients. The MAC for nitrous oxide is about 105%, (36) a figure that can only be achieved in a hyperbaric chamber. Although it can be used alone as an analgesic, nitrous oxide must be supplemented with other volatile anesthetic or intravenous drugs when used for OR anesthesia.

The cardiovascular effects of nitrous oxide are variable. When used alone, there is an apparent sympathomimetic effect (36, 37) that is associated with increased circulating catecholamine concentrations and results in increased cardiac output and mean arterial and pulmonary artery pressures. When combined with potent inhalational anesthetics or opioids, nitrous oxide produces moderate decreases in cardiac output and elevates systemic vascular resistance (38). There is little effect of administered nitrous oxide on respiration, although when added to halothane, tidal volume decreases, and respiratory rate increases (39).

The overall toxicity of nitrous oxide is very low, but complications with its use may arise. Diffusion hypoxia can occur during the first few minutes of emergence from nitrous oxide (40). Nitrous oxide moves rapidly from the blood to the alveoli during emergence and dilutes alveolar oxygen, and arterial oxygen tension decreases sharply (41). Carbon dioxide is also diluted during this period, and ventilation may be depressed. Supplemental oxygen is appropriate during this time. Another consequence of the low solubility of nitrous oxide is its tendency to move from the blood into body air cavities (42). For this reason, nitrous oxide is relatively contraindicated in patients with bowel obstruction or pneumothorax and in situations where air embolism is a risk. Finally, prolonged administration (days) of nitrous oxide results in leukopenia

and megaloblastic anemia, possibly by binding to vitamin B_{12}-inhibiting methionine and DNA synthesis (43).

Potent Inhalation Anesthetics. Halothane is a myocardial depressant, the primary cause of hypotension and decreased blood flow, since peripheral vascular resistance is usually unchanged. Enflurane, like halothane, is a potent myocardial depressant, producing hypotension in dose-dependent fashion, but it also has peripheral vasodilating effects. Isoflurane produces hypotension primarily because of decreased peripheral vascular resistance. Cardiac output remains fairly constant because tachycardia usually compensates for decreased vascular tone. Anesthetic concentrations of halothane sensitize the myocardium to catecholamines, increasing the risk of ventricular arrhythmias, whereas enflurane and isoflurane do not sensitize the heart.

Recently, isoflurane has been shown to reduce coronary vascular resistance by dilating small coronary vessels, leading to the potential for myocardial ischemia in patients with coronary artery disease (44–46). Reiz et al have demonstrated electrocardiographic and metabolic evidence of ischemia at 1% isoflurane in patients (47). Restoration of aortic pressure did not relieve ischemia in three of their patients. Recent studies involving large numbers of patients undergoing cardiac surgery have failed to demonstrate any difference in outcome when isoflurane is compared to other inhalation or narcotic analgesic techniques (48, 49). The issue of isoflurane and coronary steal has been exhaustively debated and reviewed (50). While the evidence that isoflurane may be able to induce coronary steal certainly exists, its clinical significance has not been demonstrated: in patients with a "steal-prone" anatomy, isoflurane is potentially dangerous under hemodynamic conditions that may favor steal. This characteristic may, however, be true for all anesthetics, as well as for many other therapeutically efficacious drugs.

All potent inhalation anesthetics are respiratory depressants, halothane less so than enflurane or isoflurane. Halothane irritates the respiratory tract least, and intubation may often be performed without muscle relaxation. There is little increase in salivary or bronchial secretions, even in subjects who have not received atropine. Clinical concentrations of all three inhalation anesthetics produce bronchodilation and can be used in patients suffering from chronic bronchitis, emphysema, or bronchospasm. Induction with enflurane or isoflurane is more difficult because they irritate airway reflexes more than halothane, particularly in the presence of an endotracheal tube.

All inhalation anesthetics dilate the cerebral vasculature to increase cerebral blood flow and, possibly, intracranial pressure while concomitantly reducing cerebral metabolism. Thus, for ICU patients in whom increasing intracranial pressure is a concern, the inhalation anesthetics are contraindicated until control of intracranial pressure has been initiated and maintained.

Newer inhalational anesthetics are currently under clinical investigation, and two of these anesthetics may soon be approved for clinical use in the U.S. Sevoflurane (51) is a fluorinated ether with a very low solubility in blood (half that of isoflurane, almost twice that of nitrous oxide). Induction and recovery are more rapid than with the presently available potent agents. Sevoflurane seems to decrease myocardial contractility less than halothane and to decrease vascular tone less than isoflurane, features that make its use potentially attractive in patients with cardiac disease. This anesthetic, however, is not stable, and contact with soda lime leads to the formation of decomposition products that are still under investigation. Desflurane (52) is also a fluorinated ether similar in structure to isoflurane, with a solubility in blood equivalent to that of nitrous oxide. Induction and recovery are, therefore, extremely rapid. Cardiovascular effects are similar to those of isoflurane. Since its potency is much higher than that of nitrous oxide (MAC in humans is 6 to 7%), desflurane might combine the characteristics of an insoluble agent with those of a potent anesthetic and be used as a single agent with rapid induction and emergence; however, its pungency and tendency to provoke coughing and breathholding make induction of anesthesia clearly more difficult than with halothane and may limit its use for this purpose.

Interaction of Anesthetics with Hypoxia.   Essentially, all patients requiring ICU admission from the operating room will have residual anesthesia, usually with inhalation anesthetics or narcotic analgesics. Studies in dogs and man have demonstrated profound interference with the normally vigorous ventilatory response to hypoxia when inhalation anesthesia is present. With severe hypoxia (PAO_2 = 30 mm Hg; 4.1 kPa), light halothane anesthesia resulted in almost immediate respiratory arrest in spontaneously breathing dogs and cardiac arrest in dogs whose ventilation was controlled (53). Halothane (1.1%) reduced the ventilatory response to moderate hypoxia by 50% of the awake, control response in dogs and, as arterial PO_2 decreased to 40 mm Hg (5.4 kPa), the hypoxic ventilatory response during 1.1% halothane almost disappeared (54). An equivalent response occurred in man, even at subanesthetic concentrations as low as one-tenth that required for clinical anesthesia (55). Although subclinical doses of halothane had no discernible effect on resting ventilation and end-tidal PCO_2 or the ventilatory response to CO_2, the ventilatory response to hypoxia was greatly diminished.

An extreme example of not responding to hypoxia occurred in patients who underwent bilateral carotid thromboendarterectomy, in whom the hypoxic ventilatory response was lost completely (56). These experimental results in healthy animals, human volunteers, and healthy patients must be extrapolated to debilitated, medicated, systemically ill postsurgical patients requiring intensive care. Thus, a less vigorous response will occur at far lower residual anesthetic concentrations in patients. Instead of the normal physiologic responses to hypoxia, such as agitation, hypertension, tachycardia, hyperventilation, etc., the hypoxic patient with residual anesthesia is likely to develop respiratory and circulatory depression, leading to cardiorespiratory arrest.

Residual narcotic analgesia may be no safer than halothane. Morphine (7.5 mg sc) decreased the hypoxic ventilatory response by 60% (1). ICU patients, who receive large doses of potent narcotic for anesthesia or analgesia will be depressed by hypoxia and subject to the same risk of cardiorespiratory arrest as patients receiving inhalation anesthetics. Thus, patients admitted to the ICU from the operating room may require ventilation with high concentrations of oxygen until they are able to maintain an acceptable baseline steady-state level of oxygenation.

Combined General and Epidural Anesthesia.   In recent years the focus has been on regional anesthesia techniques to reduce perioperative morbidity in high-risk surgical patients, specifically in those patients with limited cardiovascular reserve or with preexisting respiratory dysfunction. Regional anesthesia, in particular epidural anesthesia and postoperative analgesia, has shown favorable effects in selected circumstances (57–59). Regional anesthesia allows the patient to remain awake or lightly sedated, without endotracheal intubation; this approach avoids irritating the tracheobronchial tree and interfering with ciliary clearance of secretions, yet retains spontaneous respiration. However, such patients may hypoventilate, not receive adequate tracheobronchial toilet, or lose their respiratory drive entirely. A second approach now commonly employed utilizes epidural anesthesia in combination with light, general endotracheal anesthesia. Epidural anesthesia may be carried out with a combination of opioids and a local anesthetic in low concentration, e.g., 3 to 5 ml/hour of a mixture of fentanyl (10 μg/ml) and 0.1 % bupivacaine; light general anesthesia may be provided with nitrous oxide and oxygen alone or in combination with a low concentration of a potent anesthetic, e.g., 0.5% isoflurane or enflurane. This approach minimizes pharmacologic interference with cardiovascular performance and with respiration, so that most patients are able to maintain hemodynamic stability and regain respiratory control upon emergence, even after major operations such as aortic surgery, prolonged intraabdominal procedures, and lung resections. The added advantage of administration of opioids via the epidural catheter for postoperative pain relief is also an important consideration. Clinical experience with these techniques has been extremely satisfactory at the Massachusetts General Hospital, where they are now employed routinely for major vascular, thoracic, and gastrointestinal surgery, allowing early extubation and shorter ICU stay in most cases. Although several studies have looked at the effect of these anesthetic techniques on outcome (57–59), they all have limitations in their design, and definite evidence of the superiority of the combined technique over the traditional modalities of general anesthesia is not presently available.

SEDATION AND PAIN MANAGEMENT IN THE ICU

Adequate analgesia and sedation are an essential part of the management of all ICU patients. Even when the surgical wound has healed and incisional pain has subsided, anxiety, fear, and pain from multiple sources (dressing changes, endotracheal suction, invasive procedures, indwelling catheters, and tubes) are still part of the stressful routine of the ICU.

Sedation. Appropriate sedation may result in a more cooperative patient, assure amnesia and facilitate sleep, which is essential for physical and mental recovery. Sedation may be accomplished with a variety of hypnotics and sedatives: while many different commercially available drugs may be safely used, the benzodiazepines are often preferred for their reliable amnestic action, cardiovascular stability, and minor ventilatory depression. In patients requiring very large doses of sedatives bacause of excessive agitation and confusion, a continuous infusion of a sedative-hypnotic may be very effective. Drugs suitable for continuous infusion should have a short duration of action, fast recovery, minimal hemodynamic effect, and should exhibit a flexibility in their pharmacodynamic action, so that changes in the rate of infusion will result in different levels of sedation. The introduction in recent years of shorter-acting opioids (alfentanil, sufentanil) and hypnotics (midazolam, propofol) has stimulated the use of continuous intravenous infusion of these drugs for maintenance of general anesthesia. Potential advantages offer better hemodynamic stability when compared to inhalation anesthesia, more uniform blood levels and pharmacodynamic effect when compared to repeated administration, and a faster recovery. Continuous intravenous infusion of sedative-hypnotics may be particularly appropriate in the ICU setting, where prolonged and yet easily reversible sedation is often required. Midazolam in doses ranging from 0.4 to 5 mg/kg/hour and propofol (0.01 to 0.25 mg/kg/hour) were compared in 101 ICU patients (60). Both regimens provided satisfactory sedation without untoward hemodynamic or respiratory effects; recovery after discontinuation of the infusion was almost immediate in the majority of patients, but more patients in the midazolam group required a longer period of time (20 or more minutes) to fully recover. Continuous infusion of propofol (2 to 4 mg/kg/hour) for 24 hours provided excellent sedation and rapid recovery for neurologic evaluation in ICU patients with head injury (61). The growing clinical experience with propofol seems to indicate an extreme versatility of this drug in providing a wide range of effects according to the dose employed, from very mild sedation without respiratory depression to full anesthesia; rapid recovery seems to occur even at the higher doses.

Pain Management. Short-term administration of pain medication anticipating rapid return to floor care is not a therapeutic goal. Thus, intravenous opioids in sufficient amounts to control pain are appropriate. For long-term pain relief and sedation, intravenous morphine, potentiated if necessary by haloperidol, usually provided 4 to 8 hours of analgesia, sedation, and tranquilization. Diazepam, lorazepam, or midazolam may be substituted for haloperidol, but their tranquilizing effects are more variable. Short-acting barbiturates such as pentobarbital are also effective when combined with opioids to relieve pain and induce sleep in the ICU environment.

Nonsteroidal antiinflammatory drugs (NSAIDs) may be a useful alternative or adjunct to opiates. Indomethacin (25 to 50 mg per rectum every 6 to 8 hours) may provide satisfactory analgesia, although it often requires supplementation with opioids initially. Ketorolac (62) is a recently introduced NSAID with powerful analgesic properties, possibly comparable in efficacy to morphine and meperidine, and yet devoid of any respiratory depression. The potential for coagulopathy and gastrointestinal bleeding has to be assessed in a large trial, but from the available experience it does not seem to be a more frequent occurrence than with any other NSAID. Ketorolac is presently approved in the U.S. only for intramuscular use (15 to 60 mg loading dose followed by half the amount every 6 hours), although it has been safely used intravenously in Europe.

Local anesthetics for nerve blockade may relieve postoperative pain. Intercostal nerve block is often used to relieve the pain of thoracoabdominal incisions and rib fractures. Several intercostal levels are blocked, usually two or three above and below the incision using 3 ml of 0.25 to 0.5% bupivacaine with epinephrine (to prolong the duration of a bupivacaine block, as well as decrease the rate of intravascular absorption). Eight to ten hours of pain relief may be expected for each series of injections. This procedure is safest when the patient has a chest tube in place, as pneumothorax is a potential complication of intercostal block. These blocks are practical when patients are weaning from controlled ventilation over short time periods. However, in patients in whom early weaning is not advisable, different modalities of analgesia should be considered.

Attention has been directed to epidural administration of opioids in order to provide postoperative analgesia (63–64) (Table 16.2). This technique has advantages over systemic narcotic use because much less drug is required and the cardiovascular and respiratory effects are minimal. The resulting analgesia is profound and can last for more than 24 hours with one dose of intrathecal morphine or as long as necessary with continuous infusion techniques. Unlike local anesthetics, there is no loss of motor function with epidural opioids, nor is there sympathetic blockade. Spinal opiates are thought to act on specific opiate receptors in the dorsal horn of the spinal cord, since little narcotic reaches the systemic circulation.

For postoperative pain relief, the usual route of administration is an epidural catheter in the lumbar or thoracic region. Preservative-free morphine (PFM, 0.01 mg/kg in the CSF or 5 to 10 mg epidurally) has a slow onset and a long duration of action, usually lasting more than 24 hours; as the benefit of analgesia is long-lasting, so is the potential for respiratory depression, which has been observed for up to 18 to 24 hours following central administration of PFM. Respiratory depression results from rostral spread of the drug in the cerebrospinal fluid reaching the respiratory center (65). This fact mandates prolonged observation in a closely monitored environment, which may be undesirable in busy surgical ICUs, where bed availability for more unstable patients might potentially be jeopardized. Fentanyl, a more lipophilic opioid, has a faster onset than PFM when injected into the epidural space (15 to 20 minutes, as compared to 1 hour or more for PFM) and a shorter duration of action (65). Attendant to this pharmacokinetic profile, the potential for respiratory depression is limited, and cases of delayed respiratory arrest following epidural administration of fentanyl have not yet been reported. Its pharmacokinetic profile also makes it particularly suitable for continuous infusions. A concentration of 10 μg/ml at rates varying from 3 to 8 ml/hour provides adequate pain relief in most patients; for catheters placed in the thoracic spine, rates in the lower range are generally adequate. The high lipophilicity of fentanyl causes a faster reabsorption into the bloodstream, and plasma levels are detectable soon after institution of an epidural infusion; at high rates of infusion (70 to 100 μg/hour), plasma levels have been found to be adequate to cause systemic analgesia, and it is possible that at these rates the analgesic effect may be secondary to systemic narcosis. The addition of a local anesthetic in low concentrations (e.g., bupivacaine 0.075% to 0.125%) seems to act synergistically with fentanyl, improving analgesia and decreasing the requirement of the opioid. The synergism between opioids and local anesthetics has been attributed to the existence of nociceptors in the substantia gelatinosa of the spinal cord that are blocked by local anesthetics and not by narcotics. Many different mixtures of fentanyl and local anesthetics have been successfully employed. At the Massachusetts General Hospital, two standard mixtures are provided from the hospital pharmacy: fentanyl (10 μg/ml with 0.1% bupivacaine) and fentanyl (3 μg/ml with 0.1% bupivacaine). The latter is used routinely in pediatric patients and occasionally in adults who seem particularly sensitive to the side effects of the opioid. Although in most circumstances hypotension attributable to the local anesthetic is not observed, this effect may occur at times, even at these low concentrations, in which case a straight opioid infusion is used. Besides acute and delayed respiratory depression, complications of epidural opioids include pruritus, urinary retention, and nausea. These side effects are reversed by

naloxone titrated to effect either by bolus or continuous infusion. The goal of naloxone administration is to suppress the side effect without reversing analgesia. Treatment of respiratory depression with naloxone includes an initial bolus (100 to 400 μg), followed by an infusion of 40 to 80 μg/hr. Lower doses are required to counteract pruritus or nausea, e.g., 10 to 20 μg/hr. The impact of postoperative epidural analgesia on the outcome of critically ill patients is as yet unknown and is likely to remain as such, since so many uncontrollable variables are present in this patient population that a reliable comparison seems extremely difficult to design. At present, clinical experience and overwhelming patient acceptance clearly justify their use.

Patient-controlled analgesia (PCA) (66) is another newer modality that has reached widespread use (Table 16.2). With this technique, the patient self-administers small amounts of opioid in response to pain; a preset lockout interval avoids overdosing. Although somewhat less efficacious than epidural administration, this technique is certainly superior to intermittent intramuscular administration because it allows a more constant blood level of opioids to be maintained. PCA is less frequently utilized in ICUs, since in this environment the closer observation by the nursing staff allows for effective IV administration of opioids in boluses or by continuous infusion. Even in the ICU, however, PCA may be useful in selected cases, such as in alert patients who cannot receive or benefit from epidural analgesia because of coagulopathy, spinal surgery, or surgical wounds in sites inaccessible to epidural blockade.

MUSCLE RELAXANTS

Succinylcholine. Knowledge of the basic mechanisms of action and the side effects of neuromuscular blocking agents is required prior to their use in critically ill patients. There are two important types of neuromuscular blockade. The first, a depolarizing block, follows the intravenous administration of succinylcholine and is characterized by muscle fasciculations approximately 60 seconds after injection, because succinylcholine initially depolarizes the postjunctional membrane. A few minutes of blockade follow due to reduced membrane potential at the motor end-plate, and the membrane remains

Table 16.2.   Use of Opioids in Adult ICU Patients

| | Postoperative Analgesia | | |
	Continuous Infusion	*PCA*	*Epidural*
Morphine	5 mg/hr, up to 20–30 mg/hr	e.g., boluses of 1–2 mg at lockout intervals of 6–10 min	Preservative-free: 0.25–1 mg/hr
Meperidine	Not reported	Equivalent doses, no advantage over morphine	Preservative-free form not available in U.S.
Fentanyl	50–100 μg/hr		3–10 μg/ml at 5–10 ml/hr
Alfentanil	500–1500 μg/hr	Too potent not ideal for PCA	Not frequently used in U.S.
Sufentanil	Not reported	Too potent not ideal for PCA	Not frequently used in U.S.
Comments	Very large individual variations Tachyphylaxis Respiratory depression Most patients are intubated	Very large individual variations	In most instances epidural opioids are more effective when mixed with local anesthetics: 0.075% to 0.125% bupivacaine

Table 16.3. Succinylcholine-induced Hyperkalemia and Ventricular Fibrillation

1. After the first several days of:
   (*a*) massive trauma
   (*b*) extensive burns
   (*c*) lower motor neuron paralysis
   (*d*) denervation and spinal cord transection
2. During generalized illness with:
   (*a*) muscle-wasting diseases
   (*b*) muscular dystrophy
   (*c*) multiple sclerosis
   (*d*) uremia

Table 16.4. Muscle Relaxants

Relaxant	Intubating Dose (mg/kg)	Duration of Clinical Effect (min)
1. Depolarizing		
Succinylcholine	1–2	10–20
2. Nondepolarizing		
d-tubocurarine	0.6	60–90
Metocurine	0.4	60–90
Pancuronium	0.1	60–90
Atracurium	0.4	30–60
Vecuronium	0.08	30–60
Mivacurium	0.15	15–20

depolarized. The duration of depolarization block depends on redistribution of succinylcholine occupying the receptor site and metabolism of succinylcholine by plasma or pseudocholinesterase. Thus, a profound neuromuscular paralysis is produced, lasting 5 to 10 minutes in normal patients. Other characteristics of a depolarizing block include absence of fade at slow and fast rates of stimulation; absence of posttetanic potentiation; antagonism of the block by *d*-tubocurarine (a nondepolarizing neuromuscular blocking drug); and potentiation of the block by anticholinesterase drugs such as neostigmine. Inhalation anesthetics do not potentiate the effects of succinylcholine. Succinylcholine is rapidly metabolized by plasma cholinesterase unless the patient has a genetic variant of the enzyme that fails to metabolize succinylcholine, or the patient has severe liver disease that limits adequate production of plasma cholinesterase. In patients with disorders often seen in the ICU (Table 16.3), a massive efflux of intracellular potassium occurs when succinylcholine depolarizes skeletal muscle. Acute hyperkalemia and ventricular fibrillation may occur. When muscle relaxation is required to intubate patients suffering from these disorders, a large dose of nondepolarizing muscle relaxant, such as 0.15 to 0.2 mg/kg pancuronium, vecuronium, or mivacurium, may be substituted for succinylcholine (67). However, controlled ventilation must be anticipated until the nondepolarizing relaxant wears off. Other side effects of succinylcholine administration include increased intraocular and intragastric pressure. If succinylcholine is administered to children, bradycardia may occur, particularly after a second dose. If succinylcholine is administered to adults, this problem occurs less commonly but may develop with repeated doses of succinylcholine. Pretreatment with atropine usually prevents succinylcholine-induced bradycardia. Succinylcholine is extremely useful to facilitate intubation in difficult situations, provided the operator is skilled with laryngoscopy and intubation. It allows an entirely quiet field of vision, open vocal cords, and absence of vomiting, bucking, and coughing when the endotracheal tube is inserted. Of course, when possible, anesthesia is administered before succinylcholine is given, usually with thiopental, midazolam, or ketamine.

Side effects from succinylcholine may occur, because it is structurally similar to acetylcholine and, therefore, may stimulate both nicotinic and muscarinic cholinergic receptors. The net effects of succinylcholine vary individually, but tachycardia or bradycardia may be seen. Succinylcholine may decrease ventricular threshold to catecholamine-induced arrhythmias in man, which is one reason why ventricular irritability associated with endotracheal intubation is not surprising. Succinylcholine also increases serum potassium by

0.5 to 1 mEq/liter after intravenous injection of 1 mg/kg in normal patients. Although uremic patients do not have a hyperkalemic response to succinylcholine, they may be hyperkalemic initially

Nondepolarizing Neuromuscular Blockade. Nondepolarizing muscle relaxants are used much more frequently in the ICU both because patients come from the operating room with residual neuromuscular blockade and because these muscle relaxants are used to aid optimal ventilatory management of critically ill patients with severe respiratory dysfunction. A nondepolarizing block is produced when the postjunctional membrane receptors are occupied by drugs such as *d*-tubocurarine, metocurine, or pancuronium. These drugs combine reversibly with the receptor but do not change the receptor's membrane permeability. The duration of block depends on the rate at which the relaxant is redistributed. A nondepolarizing block is characterized by lack of fasciculation, a fading response to twitch or tetanus, posttetanic potentiation, and antagonism of the drug by anticholinesterase-blocking drugs such as neostigmine.

The long-acting relaxants (Table 16.4) include *d*-tubocurarine (curare), metocurine (Metubine) and pancuronium (Pavulon), and the newer drugs doxacurium (68) and pipecuronium (69). These long-acting relaxants peak 2 to 5 minutes after an intubating dose, with additional doses required every 45 to 90 minutes. The intermediate-acting relaxants, atracurium and vecuronium, generally require redosing every 20 to 40 minutes and are therefore usually given by continuous infusion when used for long-term paralysis. All of these drugs are highly ionized with low lipid solubility, having a volume of distribution roughly equivalent to the extracellular fluid space. The relative potencies of the relaxants are reflected in the doses needed to produce intubating conditions (Table 16.4). Sensitivity to muscle relaxants varies greatly among patients, and for that reason, it is best to titrate relaxants to effect.

Inhalation anesthetics potentiate the muscle relaxation of nondepolarizing drugs, with isoflurane and enflurane showing a greater effect than halothane. Patients with myasthenia gravis and myasthenic syndrome are exquisitely sensitive to nondepolarizing muscle relaxants and require careful neuromuscular monitoring when they are used. Other types of neuromuscular disease result in unpredictable responses to the nondepolarizing muscle relaxants (70)(Table 16.5). The dose of muscle relaxants varies widely in man. Since complete twitch inhibition is unnecessary in the ICU, small doses are sufficient to paralyze respiratory efforts and improve chest wall compliance. In general, *d*-tubocurarine, in initial doses of 9 to 18 mg and maintenance doses of approximately 3 to

Table 16.5. Disease-Muscle Relaxant Interactions (46)

Disease	*Types of Relaxant Interactions and Clinical Implications*
Myasthenia gravis	(1) Resistance to depolarizing drugs. (2) Extreme sensitivity to nondepolarizers (*d*-tubocurarine test). The weakness responds to anticholinesterase.
Myasthenic syndrome (Eaton-Lambert syndrome)	(1) Marked sensitivity to nondepolarizing relaxants. Block not readily reversed with neostigmine. In contrast to myasthenia gravis, the response to fast rates of stimulation is a progressive increase in twitch amplitude to as much as six times the initial height. (2) Release sensitivity to an average clinical dose of depolarizing relaxant.
Thyrotoxic myopathy	(1) Decreased response to succinylcholine (pseudocholinesterase levels are at the upper limit of normal or increased). (2) Increased sensitivity to decamethonium. (3) Normal *d*-tubocurarine requirement.
Amyotropic lateral sclerosis, syringomyelia, and poliomyelitis	(1) Defective neuromuscular transmission and nerve conduction. (2) Exaggerated response to nondepolarizers.
von Recklinghausen's disease	Variable response. Some subjects show prolonged responses to both nondepolarizing and depolarizing relaxants. Others, like myasthenics, are sensitive to *d*-tubocurarine and resistant to succinylcholine.
Myotonic syndrome (*a*) Myotonia dystrophica (*b*) Myotonia congenita (*c*) Paramyotonia	Generalized muscle spasm (myotonic response) occurs after depolarizing agents. Myotonia is alleviated by quinine and procainamide.
Muscular dystrophy Obscure congenital myopathies Familial periodic paralysis Steroid myopathy Myxedemia myopathy Alcoholic myopathy Diabetic myopathy	Unpredicatable response to relaxants, their use is better avoided. Unpredictable response to relaxants.
Polymyositis Dermatomyositis Systemic lupus erythmatosus Polyarteritis nodosa	Muscle weakness and fatigability. Respond to neostigmine, hence the term "myasthenic state."
Hypokalemia Hyperkalemia (1) Traumatized patients (2) Burn patients (3) Muscle-wasting disease Lower motor neuron lesions with hemiplegia Muscular dystrophy Denervation and spinal cord transection Multiple sclerosis Tetanus Denervation	Theoretically increased sensitivity to nondepolarizing relaxants Theoretically increased sensitivity to depolarizing relaxants and decreased sensitivity to nondepolarizing relaxants.
Primary muscle disease or myopathy	High incidence of malignant hyperpyrexia in these patients and susceptible relatives. Usually, the myopathy is mild or subclinical. Squints, hernias, and minor orthopaedic problems are often found in affected families. Malignant hyperpyrexia muscle is more sensitive to caffeine-induced rigor than normal muscle.

a From Ali HH, Savarese JJ: Monitoring of neuromuscular function. *Anesthesiology* 45:216–249, 1976.

6 mg/hr, will prevent respiratory activity in most patients. However, this dose schedule must be individualized, depending on the clinical situation and the patient's response. Pancuronium is five to six times as potent as *d*-tubocurarine and approximately two to three times as potent as metocurine, so doses for these drugs must be reduced accordingly.

The route of elimination of the commonly used, nondepolarizing relaxants varies and may be important in selecting a drug for use in the ICU. Metocurine and gallamine rely entirely on renal excretion, resulting in prolonged paralysis in

renal failure (71). Partial hepatic clearance of curare makes it a useful drug in renal failure patients (72). Although pancuronium is 80% eliminated in the urine, the remaining 20% is metabolized in the liver, and its duration of action is prolonged in hepatic failure (73). Up to 80% of a dose of vecuronium can be recovered in the bile, both metabolized and unchanged, therefore leading to a prolonged effect in cirrhotic patients. Atracurium is unique among the nondepolarizing relaxants in that its clearance is independent of hepatic and renal function with breakdown of the drug occurring by Hoffman elimination and ester hydrolysis (74). Hoffman elimination can be impaired in severe hypothermia and acidosis, prolonging atracurium's effect in those conditions.

Clinical doses of nondepolarizing neuromuscular blocking drugs affect cardiovascular function in two ways: (*a*) stimulation or inhibition of peripheral autonomic sites and (*b*) release of histamine and possibly other vasoactive substances. Thus, *d*-tubocurarine is a weak ganglionic blocker and a potent histamine-releasing drug that may cause hypotension following intravenous administration. Bronchospasm fortunately is exceedingly rare, though it has been reported. Metocurine, structurally very similar to *d*-tubocurarine, does not have similar autonomic effects until massive doses are given and, hence, it usually offers extreme cardiovascular stability (75). Pancuronium and gallamine block cardiac muscarinic receptors, leading to tachycardia. With gallamine, tachycardia may occur even before neuromuscular blockade begins. These two drugs, however, do not block ganglia or release histamine. Thus, gallamine and pancuronium should be avoided in patients at risk from myocardial ischemia.

Atracurium can cause some histamine release, resulting in hypotension when given rapidly in large boluses (76). Vecuronium has no hemodynamic side effects when used in clinical doses.

New Neuromuscular Agents. Three nondepolarizing muscle relaxants have recently become available in the U.S. Doxacurium chloride (68) is a benzylisoquinolone devoid of clinically important autonomic effects and histamine release. Its duration of action is longer, compared to that of an equipotent dose of pancuronium, but both drugs have a similar onset of action. Because it lacks hemodynamic side effects, doxacurium could be indicated in the management of critically ill patients during prolonged surgical procedures or in the ICU. Pipecuronium bromide (69) is structurally similar to pancuronium and vecuronium and also has minimal cardiovascular effects. Its onset of action is shorter than pancuronium, and its duration of action is midway between vecuronium and pancuronium. Both doxacurium and pipecuronium undergo little or no metabolism and are eliminated primarily by the kidney. Mivacurium chloride is a short-acting benzylisoquinolone, with minimal cardiovascular effects, secondary to histamine release. Mivacurium (77) was synthesized in an attempt to create a nondepolarizing muscle relaxant pharmacokinetically similar to succinylcholine. Like succinylcholine, mivacurium is metabolized by plasma cholinesterase, but at a somewhat slower rate. Clinical studies show that mivacurium has the fastest onset and shortest duration of action among the currently available nondepolarizing relaxants. However, both onset and duration are still significantly longer than succinylcholine.

Reversal of Neuromuscular Blockade. Many factors affect the degree of neuromuscular blockade. In terms of acid-base balance, both respiratory acidosis and metabolic alkalosis augment nondepolarizing blockade (78). In a patient recovering from anesthesia with residual neuromuscular blockade, hypoventilation leads to greater neuromuscular blockade, and a downhill spiral can ensue, leading to respiratory failure. Electrolyte imbalances, such as hypokalemia, hyponatremia, hypocalcemia, and hypermagnesemia, each potentiate neuromuscular blockers (70). Several types of antibiotics, including aminoglycosides, polymyxins, neomycin, streptomycin, tetracycline, and clindamycin, accentuate relaxant-induced blockade (70). Patients with major burns require larger doses of nondepolarizing relaxants to achieve paralysis (79), as do many patients who have been immobile for prolonged periods.

A major concern in critically ill patients receiving muscle relaxants is reversal of neuromuscular blockade. The ability to consistently reverse the effects of nondepolarizing muscle relaxants with neostigmine, edrophonium, or pyridostigmine depends first on redistribution and elimination of most of the relaxant before pharmacologic reversal is attempted.

The neuromuscular junction has a large margin of safety because more than 80% of the receptors must be occluded by nondepolarizing drug before twitch response is depressed. The twitch response is completely obliterated when more than 95% of the receptors are occupied. Thus, extensive receptor occlusion may persist, even though the twitch response returns to normal (80). Measurement of tidal volume does not adequately indicate the degree of reversal of neuromuscular blockade. It is possible to assess neuromuscular blockade at the bedside by clinical tests if the patient is cooperative. Bedside tests used to determine the degree of residual nondepolarizing neuromuscular blockade include 5 seconds of sustained head lift, eye opening, hand grasping, and tongue protrusion. A vital capacity maneuver of 10 to 15 ml/kg with an inspiratory force of at least -25 cm H_2O quantitates adequate respiratory effort. These clinical tests have been correlated with a quantitative measurement of the exact degree and rate of change of neuromuscular blockade called the train-of-four method (70). In addition to studies in healthy volunteers and patients, studies were conducted in moderately sick patients whose muscle relaxants were allowed to wear off spontaneously (81). In cooperative patients, clinical testing of neuromuscular and respiratory function reliably assessed reversal of neuromuscular blockade, eliminating the need for sophisticated mon-itoring of neuromuscular function. Conversely, in patients unable to cooperate because of residual anesthesia or inherent disease process, the train-of-four method offered a sensitive, quantitative and reliable approach to assess the degree of neuromuscular blockade. Another important lesson gleaned from this study was that when muscle relaxants were allowed to wear off spontaneously, a range of 2 to 10 hours was needed for complete reversal to occur after the last dose of muscle relaxant administered in the operating room. This finding demonstrates the variable, but prolonged, effect of nondepolarizing neuromuscular blockade in sick patients, many of whom are hypothermic and have abnormal binding, distribution, and elimination of drugs.

When a nondepolarizing muscle relaxant has been used in fully paralyzing doses, reversal with an anticholinesterase drug accompanied by an anticholinergic drug should always be given unless there are specific contraindications or unless control of ventilation in the ICU is anticipated for several hours. Some anesthesiologists believe that all patients should be reversed to provide a safety margin in the ICU if the ventilator disconnects. Others feel that the completely reversed patient is far more difficult to manage when controlled ventilation is necessary. Neostigmine reverses nondepolarizing neuromuscular blockade by binding to acetylcholinesterase at the neuromuscular junction, thus preventing enzymatic hydrolysis of acetylcholine. Thus, acetylcholine accumulates and competitively overcomes the block. However, it is not always possible to completely reverse a nondepolarizing block with 0.07 mg/kg neostigmine iv within a short period of time in adults. This fact is particularly true if twitch is completely inhibited before reversal is attempted. If reversal is incomplete after neostigmine, the patient should be ventilated until the block diminishes spontaneously through redistribution, metabolism, and elimination of the muscle relaxant. Otherwise, respiratory acidosis, which limits neostigmine's ability to antagonize a nondepolarizing neuromuscular block, may occur, leading to a vicious cycle of more hypercapnia and more interference with neostigmine (82). Atropine (0.4 mg) or glycopyrrolate (0.2 mg) should be administered intravenously for each 1 mg of neostigmine to prevent the undesirable muscarinic side effects of bradycardia and excessive salivation.

RENAL DYSFUNCTION

ICU patients with renal dysfunction present difficult anesthetic challenges. In general, anesthesia reduces renal blood flow and glomerular filtration, depending on depth of anesthesia, effects on blood pressure, and alterations in sympathetic tone. Important considerations for patients with renal failure undergoing anesthesia and surgery are strict attention to fluid administration, sodium intake, and potassium balance. Since hypercapnia increases serum potassium as a result of decreasing pH, respiratory depression must be avoided in patients already hyperkalemic. Most general anesthetics cause a slight metabolic acidosis that will be added to the persistent metabolic acidosis common in uremia. Since hemoglobin concentrations are chronically reduced, the margin of safety for hemorrhage is limited. However, blood transfusion is more problematic, and patients are often transfused with frozen, washed cells. Renal failure patients are usually hypertensive and receive antihypertensive medications, including α-methyldopa, a drug that reduces the anesthetic requirement in man (83), and β-blocking drugs. Hypertension should be controlled as much as possible before induction of anesthesia to lessen the wide swings in blood pressure associated with anesthesia and surgery. Thus, antihypertensive medications should be continued into the intraoperative period.

Anesthesia for patients with severe renal dysfunction is best accomplished with inhalation anesthetics since their elimination occurs via the lung. Fixed drugs behave quite unpredictably in patients with renal failure, and prolonged effects may result. Hypotension is uncommon since these patients usually have excess blood volume; therefore, thiopental is a useful induction drug. Nitrous oxide and isoflurane are appropriate to maintain anesthesia in most cases. A major advantage of the inhalation anesthetics is that by potentiating neuromuscular blockade, smaller doses of nondepolarizing muscle relaxants are needed, as compared to anesthetic techniques using opioids or other fixed drugs that do not potentiate the muscle relaxant effect (84). Thus, reversal of neuromuscular blockade is more easily accomplished, and reparalyzation is less likely.

EFFECTS OF LIVER DYSFUNCTION ON DRUG METABOLISM AND ELIMINATION

Most drugs used in the perioperative period are metabolized or excreted partially or completely in the liver. Therefore, the presence of hepatic dysfunction, common in critically ill patients, may greatly modify the actions of these drugs. Low serum albumin concentrations, a result of liver disease, may prolong the effects of protein-bound drugs such as thiopental and digoxin.

Local anesthetic drugs of the amide class, such as lidocaine, are metabolized in the liver. Hence, their effects may also be prolonged in patients with hepatic dysfunction. Ester-type local anesthetics, such as procaine, are hydrolyzed by plasma cholinesterase and theoretically should follow normal pharmacokinetics. However, severe liver dysfunction also reduces plasma cholinesterase, prolonging the effects of these drugs as well. Since trimethaphan (Arfonad), procainamide (Pronestyl), and mivacurium are also metabolized by plasma cholinesterase, administration of these drugs must be carefully titrated. Patients with severe liver dysfunction may require postoperative mechanical ventilation to ensure that all drug effects have worn off before allowing them to resume spontaneous ventilation, weaning, and extubation.

SPECIAL INDICATIONS FOR CONTINUOUS INFUSIONS OF SEDATIVES, OPIOIDS, AND MUSCLE RELAXANTS

Most patients admitted to intensive care require analgesia, sedation and, in rare instances, neuromuscular paralysis at some time during their stay. ICU patients are subjected to a nearly continuous array of stimuli as a result of both their underlying disease and its therapy. Pain related to trauma or surgery and discomfort related to the endotracheal tube, nasogastric tube, and mechanical ventilation are but two of the continuous noxious stimuli. In addition, patients are subjected to intermittent stimuli such as chest physiotherapy, dressing changes, tracheal suctioning, and repositioning.

An individual's requirement for analgesia, sedation, and paralysis depends on the patient's presenting condition, severity of illness, and the intensity of treatment (85). Analgesia would be necessary in patients who have suffered recent trauma or undergone major surgery. Sedation may be required in patients to allay fear and anxiety. Neuromuscular blocking

Table 16.6. Most Commonly Used Drugs and Method of Administration for Sedation during Mechanical Ventilation[a]

Drug	Method of Administration	Frequency of Reported Use (%)
Morphine	Intermittent IV	95
Lorazepam	Intermittent IV	86
Midazolam	Intermittent IV	81
Diazepam	Intermittent IV	78
Pancuronium	Intermittent IV	82
Vecuronium	Intermittent IV	60
Atracurium	Continuous infusion	17

[a] Adapted from Hansen-Flaschen JH, Brazxinsky S, Basile C, et al: Use of sedating and neuromuscular blocking agents in patients requiring mechanical ventilation for respiratory failure: a national survey. *JAMA* 266:2870–2875, 1991.

Table 16.7. Dose and Cost of Most Commonly Used Neuromuscular Blocking Drugs in Mechanically Ventilated Patients

Drug	Maintenance Dose[a]	Cost/Day[b] ($)
SEDATIVE/HYPNOTIC		
Phenobarbital	15–90 mg every 6–8 hours	3.25
Pentobarbital	100–200 mg every 6–8 hours	12.50
Thiopental	25–200 mg/hr	15.00
Propofol	50–300 mg/hr	300.00
ANXIOLYTICS		
Diazepam	5–10 mg IV every 6 hours	1.50
Lorazepam	2–4 mg IV every 6 hours	70.00
Midazolam	2.5–25 mg/hr	550.00
NARCOTICS		
Morphine	5–50 mg/hr	17.00
Fentanyl	50–500 μg/hr	17.25
Alfentanil	250–2500 μg/hr	210.00
Sufentanil	10–100 μg/hr	430.00
NEUROMUSCULAR BLOCKERS		
d-Tubocurarine	2–10 mg/hr	19.00
Pancuronium	1–3 mg/hr	38.00
Metocurine	1–5 mg/hr	56.00
Vecuronium	2–4 mg/hr	170.00
Atracurium	20–30 mg/hr	293.00

[a] The maintenance dose listed is the usual dose range for a 70-kg patient.
[b] Institutional costs are approximated and represent the acquisition cost for a 24-hour supply of the maximum dose listed.

drugs are frequently used in the management of patients with respiratory failure who require positive pressure mechanical ventilation. A published survey of 265 U.S. hospitals noted widespread use of sedatives and neuromuscular blocking drugs in critically ill patients (86)(Tables 16.6 and 16.7). Yet, surveys of discharged ICU patients suggest that despite an adequate armamentarium of drugs, many patients suffer from inadequate pain relief, anxiety, and unpleasant recollections while paralyzed (87–89).

Neuromuscular blocking drugs are used occasionally in approximately 70% of the ICUs surveyed and frequently in 26% of ICUs surveyed. Yet, peripheral nerve stimulators are rarely used to monitor the level of paralysis induced by neuromuscular blocking drugs, with only 4% of responders reporting routine use. There is considerable variation in the choice of drugs used, the frequency, and the method of administration. Tables 16.6 and 16.7 list the drugs most commonly administered to patients and their reportedly preferred method of administration (86).

Several factors may alter the requirement for sedation of critically ill patients. The severity of illness has been demonstrated to lower analgesic requirements. Thus, patients with high APACHE II scores require lower serum levels of morphine to achieve deeper levels of sedation than patients with less severe illness (90). Frequent reassurance and communication by the patient's direct caregivers can also lower the level of anxiety. Strict attention to a day-night cycle and the presence of windows in the room dramatically reduce the incidence of delirium in critically ill patients (91).

A critical factor in designing a rational therapeutic plan is clarifying the patient's expected course. Short-term interventions (less than 72 hours) require the use of drugs with short durations of action and ease of adjustment. Conversely, long-term problems (greater than 72 to 96 hours) are best managed using drugs with prolonged durations of action, where ease of titration is not necessary or desirable. This stratification of patients by long- and short-term goals allows for a reasonable

Table 16.8. Scoring System for Assessment of Sedation in ICU Patients

Level	Response
1	Anxious and agitated or restless
2	Cooperative, oriented, tranquil
3	Responds to commands only
4	Asleep but brisk response to glabellar tap or loud auditory stimulus
5	Asleep, sluggish response to glabellar tap or loud auditory stimulus
6	No response

and cost-effective choice of drug therapy (Table 16.7). No data support the contention that shorter-acting sedatives or neuromuscular blocking drugs are safer, reduce length of stay, or alter outcome. Shelly et al reported that the metabolism of midazolam is reduced in critically ill patients when given by continuous infusion for several days, resulting in delayed recovery of sensorium (92). In children, midazolam infusion may cause prolonged neurologic dysfunction after long-term continuous administration in combination with fentanyl (93). For patients requiring short-term sedation, especially those weaning from mechanical ventilation, infusions of short-acting drugs, such as midazolam, are effective and without important side effects. If the infusion is maintained for longer than 72 to 96 hours, the patient should be slowly weaned from midazolam, and a low dose of a long-acting benzodiazepine, such as diazepam, may be added during the weaning process.

Before using sedatives in the critically ill patient, the desired clinical endpoints should be defined. Ramsay has suggested a useful scoring system to define objective clincal endpoints (94)(Table 16.8). Most patients require a moderate level of sedation. However, patients who become agitated due to intermittent procedures such as deep endotracheal suctioning or repositioning will require a deeper level of sedation or will require supplemental administration of short-acting drugs such as midazolam or fentanyl/alfentanil.

For critically ill patients subjected to mechanical ventilation for a prolonged (greater than 72 to 96 hours) period of time, long-acting drugs are very useful. Continuous infusions of morphine or fentanyl is titratable to effect. The addition of a benzodiazepine (diazepam 5 to 10 mg every 6 hours) helps reduce the hemodynamic response to a variety of stimuli. As tolerance develops, patients may require relatively large doses of morphine. Morphine metabolites (3- and 6-glucuronide) are active and excreted renally and thus may contribute to prolonged narcosis in patients with renal failure (90). It is important to reassess patients daily and to adjust therapy based on the anticipated patient status 48 hours after assessment. Narcotics should always be weaned over several days if they have been administered to patients for more than 3 to 4 days. Occasional patients require additional therapy beyond simple sedation. Neuromuscular blocking drugs are often used in the ICU for the following reasons unrelated to their use during surgery and anesthesia:

a. To induce respiratory paralysis in intubated and fully ventilated patients who cough or buck excessively or when previous attempts to match the ventilatory pattern with the patient's needs have failed.
b. As an adjunct to reduce oxygen requirements of an intubated ventilated patient. Neuromuscular blockers also prevent the normal physiologic response of shivering to hypothermia.
c. To reduce peak airway pressures in intubated, fully ventilated patients, helping to reduce the risk of barotrauma.
d. To ease the management of status epilepticus, tetanus, and botulism resistant to more conventional methods of treatment in intubated and fully ventilated patients.
e. To intubate patients when other more conventional methods to secure the airway have failed or are not possible.

Patients requiring neuromuscular blocking drugs should always be adequately sedated prior to initiation of paralysis. Adequate sedation using a narcotic/anxiolytic combination will ensure a lack of recall or awareness by the patient. Many drugs other than inhalation anesthetics reduce the required dose of muscle relaxants to produce a given level of paralysis, including midazolam and diazepam (95, 96).

Although only a small number of ICUs routinely use peripheral nerve stimulators to assess paralysis, their use should be encouraged. Ideally, maintaining one twitch using the "train of four" testing method is the desired endpoint. The presence of at least one twitch indicates that 90 to 95% of all receptors are blocked. The absence of any twitch response indicates all of the receptors are blocked. The administered dose may be well above the ED_{100}; hence, paralysis may persist long after discontinuing the drug.

The elimination of nondepolarizing drugs is varied and will impact on the choice of drug to be used for long-term muscle relaxation. Metocurine is eliminated solely by renal excretion; therefore, in patients with abnormal renal function, the duration of paralysis may be prolonged, an effect that may be of benefit in patients needing prolonged paralysis and a very stable level of neuromuscular blockade. *d*-Tubocurarine is eliminated by both renal and hepatic pathways, making accumulation and prolonged duration of action somewhat less likely. Pancuronium is excreted renally, although about 20%

of the administered dose is excreted hepatically. Up to 80% of the administered dose of vecuronium is excreted hepatically, resulting in accumulation and prolonged duration of action in patients with hepatic dysfunction. Segredo et al. reported several patients with renal dysfunction in whom paralysis was prolonged, presumably due to accumulation of active renally excreted vecuronium metabolites (97). Atracurium is metabolized through a nonenzymatic process called Hoffman degradation. Metabolites of atracurium (which are active on the central nervous system) are excreted renally. Hoffman degradation can be altered by severe acidosis and hypothermia. *In general, the differences in side effects are attenuated when continuous infusion is employed, as compared to bolus injection.*

Neuromuscular blockade and muscle paralysis should only be initiated after adequate methods of ensuring sedation and analgesia have been taken. Therapeutic endpoints should be defined prior to drug administration, and clear, objective criteria should be established with regard to both level of sedation and paralysis. Bolus dosing techniques should not be used in critically ill patients since this technique will enhance the side effects of each of the drugs. Morphine sulfate by continuous infusion is the sedative drug of choice during neuromuscular blockade unless specifically contraindicated. Morphine sulfate is readily available, inexpensive, and easily reversed. Additional drugs such as a benzodiazepine may be added, especially in younger patients. We routinely administer diazepam by intermittent intravenous injection as an adjunct.

Unless rapid paralysis is required, muscle relaxants should be continuously infused, avoiding bolus or loading doses (Table 16.7). Although any of the available neuromuscular blocking drugs can be used, we routinely use *d*-tubocurarine. Adequate attention should be given to eye care (ocular lubricants and taping of eyelids), as well as to skin care for the sedated and paralyzed patient. Tachycardia and/or hypertension during normal care may indicate inadequate sedation or analgesia. The decision to continue paralysis should be reconsidered at least daily. Reversal of neuromuscular blockade is not recommended, and paralysis should be allowed to resolve with the patient under adequate sedation.

CONCLUSION

Knowledge of anesthetic pharmacology is essential to critical care patient management. Specific information regarding the patient's disease process will help the physician choose the most appropriate anesthetic technique to safely return the patient to the intensive care unit. The intensivist must be aware of the residual effects of anesthetic drugs that may affect the awakening process and the ability to maintain homeostasis within the intensive care unit.

REFERENCES

1. Weil JV, McCullough RE, Kline JS, et al: Diminished ventilatory response to hypoxia and hypercapnia after morphine in normal man. *N Engl J Med* 292:1103–1106, 1975.
2. Brownlee G, Williams GW: Potentiation of amphetamine and pethidine by monoamineoxidase inhibitors. *Lancet* i:669, 1963.
3. Nagashima H, Karamanian A, Malovany R, et al: Respiratory and circulatory effects of intravenous butorphanol and morphine. *Clin Pharmacol Ther* 19:738–745, 1976.

4. Romagnoli A, Keats AS: Ceiling effect for respiratory depression by nalbuphine. *Clin Pharmacol Ther* 27:478–485, 1980.
5. Brown CR, Sarnquist FH, Canup CA, et al: Clinical, electroencephalographic, and pharmacokinetic studies of a water-soluble benzodiazepine, midazolam maleate. *Anesthesiology* 50:467–470, 1979.
6. Alon A, Baitella L, Hossli G: Double-blind study of the reversal of midazolam-supplemented general anesthesia with RO 15–1788. *Br J Anaesth* 59:455–548, 1987.
7. Ricou B, Forster A, Bruckner A, et al.: Clinical evaluation of a specific benzodiazepine antagonist (RO 15-1788). *Br J Anesth* 67:A659, 1986.
8. Hojer J, Baehrendtz S, Magnusson A, Gustaffson LL: A placebo-controlled trial of flumazenil given by continuous infusion in severe benzodiazepine overdosage. *Acta Anesthesiol Scand* 35:584–590, 1991.
9. Holzgrafe RE, Vondrell JJ, Mintz SM: Reversal of postoperative reactions to scopolamine with physostigmine. *Anesth Analg* 52:921–925, 1973.
10. Morgan M: Control of intragastric pH and volume. *Br J Anesth* 56:47–57, 1984.
11. Maton PN: Omeprazole. *N Engl J Med* 324:965–975, 1991.
12. Saidman LJ, Eger EI II: The effect of thiopental metabolism on duration of anesthesia. *Anesthesiology* 27:118–126, 1966.
13. Morgan DJ, Blackman GL, Paull JD, et al: Pharmacokinetics and plasma binding of thiopental. I. Studies in surgical patients. *Anesthesiology* 54:468–473, 1981.
14. Ghoneim MM, Pandya HB, Kelley SE, et al: Binding of thiopental to plasma proteins: effects on distribution in the brain and heart. *Anesthesiology* 45:635–639, 1976.
15. Etsten B, Li TH: Hemodynamic changes during thiopental anesthesia in humans: cardiac output, stroke volume, total peripheral resistance, and intrathoracic blood volume. *J Clin Invest* 34:500–510, 1955.
16. Pierce EC Jr, Lambertsen CJ, Deutsch S, et al: Cerebral circulation and metabolism during thiopental anesthesia and hyperventilation in man. *J Clin Invest* 41:1664–1671, 1962.
17. Reves JG, Fragen RJ, Vinik R, Greenblatt DJ: Midazolam: pharmacology and uses. *Anesthesiology* 62:310–324, 1985.
18. Lowenstein E, Hallowell P, Levine FH, et al.: Cardiovascular response to large doses of intravenous morphine in man. *N Engl J Med* 281:1389–1393, 1969.
19. Philbin DM, Rosow CE, Schnider RC, et al: Fentanyl and sufentanil anesthesia revisited: how much is enough? *Anesthesiology* 73:5–11, 1990.
20. White PF, Way WL, Trevor AJ: Ketamine—its pharmacology and therapeutic uses. *Anesthesiology* 56:119–136, 1982.
21. Van Hamme MJ, Ghoneim NM, Amber JJ: Pharmacokinetics of etomidate, a new intravenous anesthetic. *Anesthesiology* 49:274, 1978.
22. Wagner RL, White PF: Etomidate inhibits adrenocortical function in surgical patients. *Anesthesiology* 60:647, 1984.
23. Sebel PS, Lowdon JD: Propofol: a new intravenous anesthetic. *Anesthesiology* 71:260–277, 1989.
24. Edelist G: A comparison of propofol and thiopentone as induction agents in outpatients surgery. *Can J Anaesth* 34:110–116, 1987.
25. Strauer BE. Contractile responses to morphine, piritramide, meperidine, and fentanyl: a comparative study of effects on the isolated ventricular myocardium. *Anesthesiology* 37:304–310, 1972.
26. King BD, Elder JD, Dripps RD: The effect of the intravenous administration of meperidine upon the circulation of man and upon the circulatory response to tilt. *Surg Gynecol Obstet* 94:591–597, 1952.
27. Sanford TJ, Smith NT, Dec-Silver H, et al: A comparison of morphine, fentanyl, and sufentanil anesthesia for cardiac surgery: induction, emergence, and extubation. *Anesth Analg* 65:259–266, 1986.
28. Rosow CE: Sufentanil citrate: a new opioid analgesic for use in anesthesia. *Pharmacotherapy* 4:11–19, 1984.
29. Bovill JG, Sebel PS, Blackburn CL, et al: The pharmacokinetics of alfentanil (R39209): a new opioid analgesic. *Anesthesiology* 57:439–443, 1982.
30. Crawford DC, Fell D, Achola KJ, et al: Effects of alfentanil on the pressor and catecholamine responses to tracheal intubation. *Br J Anaesth* 59:707–712, 1987.
31. Longnecker DE, Grazis PA, Eggers Jr. GWN: Naloxone for antagonism of morphine-induced respiratory depression. *Anesth Analg* 52:447–453, 1973.
32. Eger II EI: *Anesthetic Uptake and Action.* Williams & Wilkins, Baltimore, 1974.
33. Stoelting RK, Eger II EI: The effects of ventilation and anesthetic solubility on recovery from anesthesia: an in vivo and analog analysis before and after equilibration. *Anesthesiology* 30:290–296, 1969.
34. Regan MJ, Eger II EI: Effect of hypothermia in dogs on anesthetizing and apneic doses of inhalation agents. Determination of the anesthetic index (apnea/MAC). *Anesthesiology* 28:689–700, 1967.
35. Gregory GA, Eger II EI, Munson ES: The relationship between age and halothane requirement in man. *Anesthesiology* 30:488–491, 1969.
36. Leighton KM, Koth B: Some aspects of the clinical pharmacology of nitrous oxide. *Can Anaesth Soc J* 20:94–103, 1973.
37. Lunn JK, Liu W-S, Stanley TH, et al: Peripheral vascular and cardiac effects of nitrous oxide in the bovine. *Can Anaesth Soc J* 24:571–585, 1977.
38. Eisele Jr. JH: Cardiovascular effects of nitrous oxide. In: Eger II EI, Ed. *Nitrous oxide.* New York: Elsevier, 125–156, 1985.
39. Hornbein TF, Martin WE, Bonica JJ, et al: Nitrous oxide effects on the circulatory and ventilatory responses to halothane. *Anesthesiology* 31:250–260, 1969.
40. Fink BR: Diffusion anoxia. *Anesthesiology* 16:511–519, 1955.
41. Sheffer L, Steffenson JL, Birch AA: Nitrous-oxide-induced diffusion hypoxia in patients breathing spontaneously. *Anesthesiology* 37:436–493, 1972.
42. Munson ES: Transfer of nitrous oxide into body air cavities. *Br J Anaesth* 46:202–209, 1974.
43. Nunn JF, Chanarin I: Nitrous oxide and vitamin B_{12}. *Br J Anaesth* 50:1089–1090, 1978.
44. Becker LC: Is isoflurane dangerous for the patient with coronary artery disease? *Anesthesiology* 66:259–261, 1987.
45. Buffington CW, Romson JL, Levine A, et al: Isoflurane induces coronary steal in a canine model of chronic coronary occlusion. *Anesthesiology* 66:280–292, 1987.
46. Priebe H-J, Foex P: Isoflurane causes regional myocardial dysfunction in dogs with critical coronary artery stenoses. *Anesthesiology* 66:293–300, 1987.
47. Reiz S, Balfors E, Sorensen MB, et al: Isoflurane—a powerful coronary vasodilator in patients with coronary artery disease. *Anesthesiology* 59:91–97, 1983.
48. Slogoff S, Keats AS: Randomized trial of primary anesthetic agents on outcome of coronary artery bypass operations. *Anesthesiology* 70:179–188, 1989.
49. Tuman KJ, McCarthy RJ, Spiess BD, et al: Does choice of anesthetic agents significantly affect outcome after coronary artery surgery? *Anesthesiology* 70:189–198, 1989.
50. Priebe H-J: Isoflurane and coronary hemodynamics. *Anesthesiology* 71:960–976, 1989.
51. Weiskopk RB, New inhaled anesthetics. *Curr Opin Anesth* 2:421–424, 1989.
52. Jones RM: Desflurane and Sevoflurane. Inhalation anesthetics for this decade? *Br J Anaesth* 65:527–536, 1990.
53. Cullen DJ, Eger II EI. The effects of halothane on respiratory and cardiovascular responses to hypoxia in dogs: a dose-response study. *Anesthesiology* 33:487–496, 1970.
54. Weiskopf RB, Raymond LW, Severinghaus JW: Effects of halothane on canine respiratory responses to hypoxia with and without hypercarbia. *Anesthesiology* 41:350–360, 1974.
55. Knill RL, Gelb AW: Ventilatory responses to hypoxia and hypercapnia during halothane sedation and anesthesia in man. *Anesthesiology* 49:244–251, 1978.
56. Wade JG, Larson Jr CP, Hickey RF, et al: Effect of carotid endarterectomy on carotid chemoreceptor and baroreceptor function in man. *N Engl J Med* 282:823–829, 1970.
57. Yeager MP, Glass DD, Neff RK, Brink-Johnsen T: Epidural anesthesia and analgesia in high-risk surgical patients. *Anesthesiology* 66:729–736, 1987.
58. Baron J-F, Bertrand M, Barre E, et al: Combined epidural and general anesthesia versus general anesthesia for abdominal aortic surgery. *Anesthesiology* 75:611–618, 1991.
59. Temec BK, Schafer PW, Park WY, Harmon JW: Epidural anesthesia in patients undergoing thoracic surgery. *Arch Surg* 124:415–418, 1989.
60. Aitkenhead AR, Pepperman ML, Willats SM, et al.: Comparison of propofol and midazolam for sedation in critically ill patients. *Lancet* 8665;704–708, 1989.
61. Farling PA, Johnston JR, Coppel DL: Propofol infusion for sedation of patients with head injury in intensive care. *Anaesthesia* 44:222–226, 1989.
62. Kenny GNC: Ketorolac trometamol—a new non-opioid analgesic. *Br J Anaesth* 65:445–447, 1990.
63. Bromage PR, Camporesi E, Chestnut D: Epidural opioids for postoperative analgesia. *Anesth Analg* 59:473–480, 1980.
64. Martin R, Salbaing J, Blaise G, et al: Epidural morphine for postoperative pain relief: a dose-response curve. *Anesthesiology* 56:423–426, 1982.
65. Cousins MJ, Mather LE: Intrathecal and epidural administration of opioids. *Anesthesiology* 61:276–310, 1984.
66. Ferrante FM, Ostheimer G, Covino BG: Patient-controlled analgesia. Blackwell Scientific Publications, London, 1990.
67. Brown EM, Krishnaprasad D, Smiler BG: Pancuronium for rapid induction technique for tracheal intubation. *Can Anaesth Soc J* 26:489–491, 1979.
68. Basta SJ, Savarese JJ, Ali HH, et al: Clinical pharmacology of doxacurium chloride. *Anesthesiology* 69:478–486, 1988.
69. Larijani GE, Bartkowski RR, Azad SS, et al: Clinical pharmacology of pipecuronium bromide. *Anesth Analg* 68:734–739, 1989.
70. Ali HH, Savarese JJ: Monitoring of neuromuscular function. *Anesthesiology* 45:216–249, 1976.
71. Meijer DKF, Weitering JG, Vermeer GA, et al: Comparative pharmacokinetics of *d*-tubocurarine and metocurine in man. *Anesthesiology* 51:402–407, 1979.
72. Cohen EN, Brewer HW, Smith D: The metabolism and elimination of *d*-tubocurarine-H^3. *Anesthesiology* 28:309–317, 1967.
73. Duvaldestein P, Agoston S, Henzel D, et al: Pancuronium pharmacokinetics in patients with liver cirrhosis. *Br J Anaesth* 50:1131–1136, 1978.
74. Miller RD, Rupp SM, Fisher DM, et al: Clinical pharmacology of vecuronium and atracurium. *Anesthesiology* 61:444–453, 1984.
75. Savarese JJ: The autonomic margin of safety of metocurine and *d*-tubocurarine in the cat. *Anesthesiology* 50:40–46, 1979.
76. Scott RPF, Savarese JJ, Basta S, et al: Atracurium: clinical strategies for the prevention of histamine release. *Br J Anaesth* 57:550–553, 1985.
77. Savarese JJ, Ali HH, Basta SJ, et al: The clinical neuromuscular pharmacology of mivacurium chloride (BW B1090U): a short-acting nondepolarizing ester neuromuscular blocking drug. *Anesthesiology* 68:723–732, 1988.
78. Miller RD, Roderick LL: Acid-base balance and neostigmine antagonism of pancuronium neuromuscular blockade. *Br J Anaesth* 50:317–324, 1978.

79. Martyn JA: The use of neuromuscular relaxants in burn patients. *Problems in Anesth* 3:478–488, 1989.
80. Paton WDM, Waud DR. The margin of safety of neuromuscular transmission. *J Physiol (Lond)* 191:59–90, 1967.
81. Brand JB, Cullen DJ, Wilson NE, et al: Spontaneous recovery from nondepolarizing neuromuscular blockade: correlation between clinical and evoked responses. *Anesth Analg* 56:55–58, 1977.
82. Miller RD, Van Nyhuis LS, Eger II EI, et al: The effect of acid-base balance on neostigmine antagonism of *d*-tubocurarine-induced neuromuscular blockade. *Anesthesiology* 42:377–383, 1975.
83. Miller RD, Way WL, Eger II EI: The effects of alpha-methyldopa, reserpine, guanethidine, and iproniazid on minimum alveolar anesthetic requirement (MAC). *Anesthesiology* 29:1153–1158, 1968.
84. Miller RD, Eger II EI., Way WL, et al: Comparative neuromuscular effects of Forane and halothane alone and in combination with *d*-tubocurarine in man. *Anesthesiology* 35:38–42, 1971.
85. Aitkenhead AR: Analgesia and sedation in intensive care. *Br J Anaesth* 63:196–206, 1989.
86. Hansen-Flaschen JH, Brazxinsky S, Basile C, et al: Use of sedating and neuromuscular blocking agents in patients requiring mechanical ventilation for respiratory failure: a national survey. *JAMA* 266:2870–2875, 1991.
87. Bion JF: Sedation and analgesia in the intensive care unit. *Hosp Update* 14:1272–1286, 1988.
88. Hewitt PB: Subjective follow-up of patients from a surgical intensive therapy ward. *Br Med J* 4:669–673, 1970.
89. Jones J, Hoggart B, Withey J, et al: What the patients say: a study of reactions to an intensive care unit. *Intensive Care Med* 5:89–92, 1979.
90. Bion JF, Logan BK, Newman PM, et al: Sedation in intensive care: morphine and renal function. *Intensive Care Med* 12:359–365, 1986.
91. Wilson LM: Intensive care delirium. The effect of outside deprivation in a windowless unit. *Arch Intern Med* 130:225–226, 1972.
92. Shelley MP, Mendell L, Park GR: Failure of critically ill patients to metabolize midazolam. *Anaesthesia* 42:619–626, 1987.
93. Bergman I, Steeves M, Burckart G, Thompson A: Reversible neurologic abnormalities associated with prolonged intravenous midazolam and fentanyl administration. *J Pediatr* 119:644–649, 1991.
94. Ramsay MA, Savege TM, Simpson BR, Goodwin R: Controlled sedation with alphaxalone-alphadolone. *Br Med J* 2:656–659, 1974.
95. Feldman SA, Crawley BE: Interaction of diazepam with the muscle relaxant drugs. *Br Med J* 2:336–338, 1970.
96. Driessen JJ, Van Egmond J, van der Pol F, Crul JF: Effects of two benzodiazepines and a benzodiazepine antagonist on muscle blockade in the anesthetized cat. *Arch Int Pharmacodyn Ther* 286(1):58–70, 1987.
97. Segredo V, Matthay MA, Sharma ML, et al: Prolonged neuromuscular blockade after long term administration of vecuronium in two critically ill patients. *Anesthesiology* 72:566–570, 1990.

CHAPTER 17

Muscle Relaxants

NEELAKANTAN SUNDER, M.B.B.S.
J. A. JEEVENDRA MARTYN, M.D., F.F.A.R.C.S.

INTRODUCTION

Mechanical ventilation is required in approximately 80% of critically ill intensive care patients (1), and muscle relaxants (MR) have become an integral part of the pharmacologic armamentarium during mechanical ventilation (2, 3). These drugs, by occupying the acetylcholine receptors in the postjunctional membrane, prevent the transmission of neural impulses mediated by acetylcholine. The muscle relaxation or paralysis that results from this effect not only facilitates endotracheal intubation but also, and more importantly, results in more effective synchronization and control of mechanical ventilation (4, 5). This result is particularly advantageous when patients receive high positive end-expiratory pressure. It has been suggested that the negative pleural pressure during spontaneous respiration and the ventilator-delivered breath are additive to transpulmonary pressure (6, 7). The decrease in chest wall compliance from relaxation may contribute to decreased transpulmonary pressure and decreased barotrauma (7). The work of breathing, consisting of only 1 to 2% of total oxygen consumption in normal patients, can be as high as 15 to 20% during pathologic states of the lung (8, 9). Effective muscle paralysis and mechanical ventilation will, therefore, decrease oxygen consumption (8). The decreased oxygen consumption will become important in the presence of hypoxia and/or pathological states of the lung where total oxygen delivery may be decreased (9, 10). Although MR should never be used without sedation, the coadministration of MR may also decrease the requirement for centrally acting drugs (11, 12).

Another use of MR is to prevent shivering in hypothermic patients (13, 14); shivering, particularly in a hypoxic or hypercatabolic patient, may have deleterious effects, as shivering increases metabolic heat production by 200% (15). Finally, an important advantage of MR that is increasingly evident is their ability to prevent coughing response during endotracheal suctioning. Coughing and "bucking" increase pulmonary vascular (16), as well as intracranial, pressures (17, 18). Thus, MR are indicated for a variety of reasons and are a useful pharmacologic adjunct during mechanical ventilation of critically ill patients.

DEPOLARIZING MUSCLE RELAXANTS

MR, based on pharmacologic characteristics, can be classified into depolarizing and nondepolarizing muscle relaxants (NDMR). Depolarizing relaxants replicate the effects of acetylcholine at the neuromuscular junction and initially depolarize the muscle membrane. In contrast to acetylcholine, whose effects dissipate quickly because of its rapid breakdown, these drugs prevent repolarization of the muscle membrane and, hence, produce for a period of time a nonexcitable zone that results in muscle paralysis. Succinylcholine and decamethonium belong to this class of drugs in which only succinylcholine is used clinically.

SUCCINYLCHOLINE

Succinylcholine is structurally similar to acetylcholine. It is, in fact, a *bis*-acetylcholine, two acetylcholine molecules

309

held together by ester linkage. It is very short-acting due to its rapid hydrolysis by the enzyme plasma cholinesterase. A prolonged neuromuscular effect of succinylcholine may be due to (a) decreased synthesis of the enzyme, as in severe liver disease or malnutrition; (b) drug-induced decreased cholinesterase enzyme activity (e.g., anticholinesterases, pancuronium, chlorpromazine, organophosphorous compounds, echothiophate eyedrops); and/or (c) presence of genetically determined atypical enzyme variants that do not adequately metabolize succinylcholine (19). Plasma cholinesterase activity should be determined in cases where there has been prolonged apnea after succinylcholine, and there is strong suspicion of abnormal enzyme activity. There are four main genetic variants of the enzyme: normal; atypical; fluoride-resistant; and silent. The presence or absence of a genetic cause of decreased metabolism of succinylcholine can be determined by the "dibucaine number." For details of genetic variants, refer to reviews by Robertson or Kalow (19, 20).

When prolonged apnea due to succinylcholine is encountered, one can continue to ventilate the patient until spontaneous recovery occurs. Spontaneous recovery will occur when the succinylcholine is eliminated by the kidneys, after approximately 3 to 5 hours. In the ICU patient, the morbidity associated with mechanical ventilation for an additional 3 to 5 hours may be minimal. Alternately, a highly purified cholinesterase is available to enhance the metabolism of succinylcholine and to restore neurotransmission (21–23). With increased awareness of even the remote possibility of blood-borne transmission of diseases, including AIDS, one should resort to purified cholinesterase therapy only when there is a definite indication.

The inhibition of neuromuscular transmission produced by succinylcholine is recognized by the (a) depression of the nerve-stimulated contractile response of muscle (twitch paralysis), which is preceded by fasciculation; (b) absence of fade or decrease in muscle tension, with repetitive (tetanic high frequency) stimulation; (c) absence of posttetanic potentiation of the paralysis; (d) lack of fade on train of four; and (e) absence of reversal of the paralysis by anticholinesterase drugs (e.g. neostigmine). Prolonged or repeated use of succinylcholine produces a different kind of block than that described above and is referred to as phase-II block or desensitization block. Characteristic features of this type of block include tetanic fade, posttetanic potentiation, and reversibility with anticholinesterase drugs. In other words, the distinguishing features of a depolarizing block are not present, but there is similarity to NDMR-type block (see below) (24). Although anticholinesterase drugs reverse a phase-II block, it is not common practice to use these drugs for reversal.

Unwanted Effects of Succinylcholine

—Hyperkalemia (see under Critical Care Implications)
—Increased intraocular pressure. Succinylcholine can cause increased intraocular pressure as a result of sustained contracture of the extraocular muscles.
—Hypersensitivity reactions. Anaphylatic reactions to succinylcholine have been reported (25, 26). One survey found hypersensitivity reactions to succinylcholine the most common compared to other muscle relaxants (27).

—Muscle pains are common after its use and may be ameliorated by the prior administration of small doses of d-tubocurarine (3 mg) or pancuronium (0.05 mg).
—Rhabdomyolysis and myoglobinemia are of concern in select cases (28). Myoglobinuria, when it occurs, should be treated to prevent renal damage.
—Malignant hyperthermia. Succinylcholine has been shown to be a triggering agent of the development of malignant hyperthermia. It is absolutely contraindicated in patients with a history of this syndrome.

NONDEPOLARIZING MUSCLE RELAXANTS

NDMRs produce muscle relaxation or paralysis by inhibiting the binding of the neurotransmitter acetylcholine to its receptor. They are, therefore, described as competitive inhibitors or antagonists of the acetylcholine receptor. At high concentrations of NDMR, an additional noncompetitive mechanism (i.e., channel block) may become operative, which may explain the difficulty in reversing a NDMR-induced profound paralysis. The inhibition of neuromuscular transmission produced by NDMRs is characterized by (a) depression of twitch height, (b) fade on tetanic stimulation; (c) presence of posttetanic facilitation; and (d) reversibility of the paralysis by anticholinesterase drugs.

A brief review of the NDMRs approved by the Food and Drug Administration is discussed below. Refer to Table 17.1 for clinical pharmacology and pharmacodynamics.

D-TUBOCURARINE

D-tubocurarine, also known as curare, was obtained from the extract of the vine *Chondrodendron tomentosum*, found in Ecuador. This was the first muscle relaxant used clinically approximately 50 years ago (29). The neuromuscular paralysis produced by curare is of long duration (90 to 120 minutes) and is readily reversed by anticholinesterases. Increasing the dose increases the duration of action, an effect that may be due, in part, to occupation of the acetylcholine receptor channel by the drug (channel blockade) (30). Tubocurarine administered as a bolus lowers blood pressure because of histamine release (31) and inhibition of transmission through autonomic ganglia (32). Approximately 30 to 40% of the administered dose is eliminated by the kidney, and the remainder is eliminated through bile (33). Thus, prolonged duration of action may be seen when repeated doses are administered to patients with renal failure. Although it has been used in patients with renal failure, the potential for recurarization is ever present.

METOCURINE

Metocurine (trimethylated derivative of tubocurarine) is a semisynthetic drug first studied in man in 1948. It is twice as potent as d-tubocurarine but releases much less histamine and has fewer cardiovascular side effects (34). Metocurine is primarily eliminated by the kidneys and, hence, it should be avoided in patients with renal failure (35).

Table 17.1. Clinical Pharmacology of Neuromuscular Blockers

Drug	ED_{95} (mg/kg)	Intubating Dose (mg/kg)	Time to Recovery (min)	Route of Elimination
Succinylcholine	0.2	1	10–15	Plasma cholinesterase
d-Tubocurarine	0.5	0.5–0.6	80–100	Kidney; liver
Metocurine	0.28	0.3	80–100	Kidney
Gallamine	3	3–4	100–180	Kidney
Pancuronium	0.07	0.1	80–100	Kidney
Pipecuronium	0.05	0.05–0.1	80–100	Kidney
Atracurium	0.3	0.05–0.6	30–60	Hofman elimination
Vecuronium	0.07	0.1	30–60	Liver; kidney
Doxacurium	0.03	0.03–0.04	80–100	Kidney
Mivacurium	0.08	0.15–0.2	15–20	Plasma cholinesterase

GALLAMINE

Gallamine was first synthesized in 1947 and was introduced to clinical practice in 1950. It has a more potent vagolytic effect than any other neuromuscular blocking drug, which results in significant tachycardia even from small doses (36). This effect may be useful in children, whose cardiac output can be enhanced by increasing heart rate. The neuromuscular block of gallamine is difficult to reverse with anticholinesterases, which is probably due to its channel-blocking property (37). Its elimination is entirely dependent on the kidneys, and its neuromuscular effect can be prolonged in patients with renal failure. The elimination of gallamine in patients with renal failure can be enhanced by hemodialysis and peritoneal dialysis (38). Currently, gallamine is very rarely used in clinical practice.

PANCURONIUM

The concept of fusing acetylcholine-like fragments with a steroidal skeleton to produce neuromuscular block evolved from the discovery of malouetine, a naturally occurring extract of a plant used as an arrow poison by the natives in Zaire. With the steroidal structure of malouetine in mind, a series of compounds was designed by manipulating its molecular structure (39). Pancuronium was the first of these compounds to be introduced into clinical practice (39). Although pancuronium does not produce histamine release or ganglionic blockade, it does cause tachycardia. The latter effect may be due to several mechanisms: (*a*) blocking of muscarinic cholinergic receptors in the heart (40); (*b*) postganglionic cardiac vagal inhibitory action causing norepinephrine release (40); (*c*) blocking of dopaminergic interneurons (SIF cells) on sympathetic ganglia, thereby facilitating ganglionic transmission; and (*d*) inhibition of neuronal reuptake of norepinephrine (uptake 1) (41).

Approximately 60 to 80% of pancuronium is eliminated by the kidney. The elimination half-life of pancuronium and, therefore, the duration of neuromuscular block are prolonged in renal failure (42). A small fraction of pancuronium is deacetylated to 3-OH and 17-OH metabolites, which are half as potent as the parent compound. The 3-17 dihydroxy metabolite is essentially inactive (43). Although only 10% of pancuronium is eliminated by the liver, prolonged duration of action has been seen in patients with liver disease (44, 45). Renal failure or hepatic failure is not an absolute contraindication to the use of pancuronium,

but careful monitoring of the neuromuscular function is necessary when repeated doses are given.

VECURONIUM

Vecuronium is the monoquarternary analogue of the steroidal relaxant pancuronium. Despite a very minor change in its structure, its pharmacologic properties are somewhat different from those of pancuronium. It produces no cardiovascular side effects (46). Its relatively short duration of action may be due to rapid redistribution of the drug to the liver with little tendency to produce cumulative effect. Repetitive large doses or prolonged infusions, however, can saturate the hepatic tissue stores, resulting in cumulative effects. In contrast to pancuronium, 40 to 60% of vecuronium is eliminated by the liver (47). Prolonged duration of the action of vecuronium can be expected in hepatic cirrhosis or cholestasis (48, 49). Long-term infusions in patients with renal failure will also result in prolongation of effect due to accumulation of parent drug and its active metabolites (50).

PIPECURONIUM

Pipecuronium synthesized and evaluated in 1980 in Hungary is now approved for use in the U.S. It is slightly more potent than pancuronium and has remarkably similar pharmacodynamic and pharmacokinetic profile, but it produces no cardiovascular side effects (51). As in pancuronium and vecuronium, its deacetylated metabolites can be detected in plasma. Increased elimination half-life and slower clearance are found in patients with renal failure (52).

ATRACURIUM

Atracurium is a potent NDMR with intermediate duration of action, which is easily reversed with anticholinesterase agents (46). At doses higher than 0.5 mg/kg (twice the effective dose), atracurium releases histamine, which causes decreased blood pressure and increased heart rate (53). The hemodynamic effects of histamine release can be prevented or attenuated by prior treatment with H_1 and H_2-receptor antagonists or by injecting the drug over several seconds (54).

Atracurium undergoes a unique self-destructing process called "Hofman elimination," a mechanism dependent on temperature and pH. The by-products of this process are laudanosine and acrylates, both of which are inactive at the neuromuscular junction. Laudanosine in very high concentrations has been shown to cause seizures in animals and increase the anesthetic requirement (55, 56). Although laudanosine can accumulate in patients with renal failure, clinical doses of atracurium are unlikely to cause elevated laudanosine levels, which can produce clinically important central effects (46). Atracurium also undergoes ester hydrolysis independent of plasma cholinesterase. Normal neuromuscular response to atracurium was seen in a patient with no plasma cholinesterase activity (57). Thus, the breakdown of atracurium by Hofman elimination and ester hydrolysis is not dependent on the kidney, liver, or any other organ function, but occurs spontaneously throughout its volume of distribution. Consequently, it is a very useful drug in patients with renal or hepatic failure. It can be used as an infusion drug at the rate of 6 to 10 μg/kg/min, which provides a 90 to 95% block during balanced anesthesia. This infusion rate may have to be increased or decreased in ICU patients, depending on the neuromuscular response.

DOXACURIUM

Doxacurium (BW 938u) is a very potent new, nondepolarizing neuromuscular blocking agent. It has a duration of action somewhat similar to that of pancuronium and, in clinically effective doses, is free of hemodynamic effects (58). It is excreted unchanged by the kidney. In patients with renal failure, normal onset times and duration of action were found in one study (59), while only a marginal increase in elimination half-life and slower clearance were observed in another (60). Liver disease appears to have no significant effect on the pharmacokinetics of doxacurium (60).

MIVACURIUM

Mivacurium (BW 1090u) is a short-acting nondepolarizing ester neuromuscular blocking drug. It undergoes hydrolysis by human plasma cholinesterase, although no correlation can be found to plasma cholinesterase activity and neuromuscular recovery of individual patients (61). The neuromuscular block produced by mivacurium lasts approximately 20 to 25 minutes and is also easily reversible (61). There are no significant hemodynamic changes when twice the effective doses are administered. When higher doses are administered, histamine release and cardiovascular side effects may become evident (62). Elevations of plasma histamine levels correlate well with decreased blood pressure, which is very transient. The incidence and magnitude of histamine release can be reduced by injecting the drug over 60 seconds (62).

Mivacurium is ideal for use as a continuous infusion. The neuromuscular block recovers spontaneously within 15 minutes of termination of infusion or its effects can be easily reversed by anticholinesterase drugs. No cumulative effects are seen, and the recovery of the block is independent of the duration of infusion (62). The recovery of neuromuscular paralysis is slightly faster than that of succinylcholine infused

for a similar length of time (62). The pharmacokinetics and pharmacodynamics of mivacurium during long-term infusions in ICU patients are unknown.

MONITORING OF NEUROMUSCULAR BLOCK

If a muscle relaxant is used, the depth of the neuromuscular block or recovery should be monitored whenever possible. In an awake and cooperative patient, the recovery of muscle power can be determined by various objective tests like handgrip strength, sustained head lift, and vital capacity. Quantitative information in an unconscious or sedated patient can be obtained by stimulating a peripheral nerve and observing or recording the evoked response in a muscle supplied by that nerve. Stimulation of the ulnar nerve and observing the evoked response at the adductor pollicis is the most common practice. If the ulnar nerve is not available or easily accessible, the facial nerve can be used, and the response at the orbicularis occuli be easily observed. Care must be taken that the observed response (contraction) is not due to direct stimulation of the muscle. Whenever necessary, the posterior tibial nerve can be stimulated behind the medial malleus and plantar flexion of the great toe can be observed, or the peroneal nerve can be stimulated around the fibular head, and dorsiflexion of the foot can be recorded. The evoked response observed in the muscle will depend on the pattern of nerve stimulation, which may be a single twitch, tetanic, or train-of-four stimulation. The evoked responses can be painful and, therefore, are not always practical in patients who are conscious.

SINGLE TWITCH

Stimulus frequency of 0.1 Hz (i.e., one stimulus every 10 seconds) is usually employed. The degree of suppression of twitch at this frequency correlates to clinical relaxation (63). One major drawback of this method of monitoring in the ICU is that a baseline twitch height needs to be established prior to administration of the muscle relaxant since the twitch suppression or recovery is expressed as a percentage of the initial twitch height. Also, patients can have a significant degree of residual paralysis (presence of fade) despite the twitch height recovering to 95% of baseline twitch height.

TRAIN OF FOUR

This approach uses a train (series) of four stimuli at a frequency of 2 Hz for 2 seconds. These stimuli can be repeated every 10 to 20 seconds or at longer intervals. The ratio of the fourth to the first evoked response in the train (T_4 ratio) is a very useful and practical index of neuromuscular recovery. Several portable models of nerve stimulators that give single as well as multiple stimuli are commercially available.

TETANUS

Other modes of stimulation, including tetanic stimulation, posttetanic count (PTC), posttetanic single twitch stimulation, and double-burst stimulation (DBS) have been recommended (64). The utility of these methods over the train of four is unclear. Most importantly, these modes of stimulation are all extremely painful and their use in awake patients may elicit an unwanted stress response.

INTEGRATED EMG

Where available, EMG can be a very useful monitor. The raw EMG signal from the recorded muscle is integrated and presented in graphic and digital form. The information from recording the first dorsal interosseus correlates well to ulnar nerve stimulated thumb adduction measured mechanically (64).

REVERSAL OF NEUROMUSCULAR EFFECTS OF NDMR

When the decision to terminate the administration of muscle relaxant is made, the effects of the drug will dissipate over time due to metabolism and/or elimination of the drug. Alternately, reversal drugs can be used. Anticholinesterases are the drugs of choice for reversal of neuromuscular paralysis induced by NDMRs. The anticholinesterases, by inhibiting the breakdown of acetylcholine and increasing its concentration at the neuromuscular junction, reverse the effects of NDMR. The efficacy and adequacy of the reversal of NDMR will depend on several factors, including depth of block, type and amount of relaxant used, method of administration (single-bolus or infusion), type and dose of reversal agent, and the temperature of the patient.

DEPTH OF BLOCK

Profound neuromuscular paralysis evidenced by complete suppression of evoked twitch response is difficult to reverse, especially when long-acting drugs such as *d*-tubocurarine, metocurine, and pancuronium have been used (65, 66). Reversal of deep paralysis may be difficult, even with intermediate-duration relaxants such as atracurium and vecuronium (67, 68). It is, therefore, important to recognize this phenomenon and to avoid reversal of the neuromuscular block when twitch response is completely suppressed. Overdosing can be avoided by careful monitoring of the nerve-stimulated evoked response described previously.

Neostigmine (0.04 to 0.06 mg/kg), pyridostigmine (0.2 to 0.3 mg/kg), and edrophonium (0.5 to 1 mg/kg) are the most commonly used anticholinesterase drugs for reversal of neuromuscular block. Anticholinergics need to be coadministered to prevent such unpleasant muscarinic side effects as bradycardia and increased secretion. Atropine (20 to 30 μg/kg) and glycopyrrolate (10 μg/kg) are the most commonly used anticholinergic drugs. Initial tachycardia and late bradycardia are seen frequently during reversal. These effects may be of great concern in critically ill patients with ischemic heart disease. When atropine and neostigmine are used together, it is common to see initial tachycardia and late bradycardia. The changes in heart rate can be minimized by giving the injection slowly (69). Glycopyrrolate (10 μg/kg) and neostigmine (50 μg/kg) administered together produce a stable heart rate (70). Atropine may be the preferred drug when used in combination with edrophonium, however, since the onset of their effects on the heart (tachycardia and bradycardia, respectively) is similar (71).

Anticholinesterase agents themselves can cause muscle weakness. This effect may be due to an increased concentration of acetylcholine in the synaptic cleft, which causes negative feedback and decreases in transmitter release (72). A single effective dose of reversal drug is unlikely to produce clinically important anticholinesterase-induced muscle weakness (73).

ASSESSMENT OF RECOVERY FROM NEUROMUSCULAR PARALYSIS

Adequacy of recovery of neuromuscular function can be assessed clinically by the ability of the patient on command to open the eyes wide, to sustain protrusion of the tongue, to lift the head for 5 seconds, to maintain an effective handgrip, or to produce an effective cough (63, 64). Maximum peak negative inspiratory pressure of -10 to -16 cm H_2O was found to correlate to breathing capability of maintaining a normal $PACO_2$ (74). Doubling this pressure to -20 to -30 cmH_2O to increase the margin of safety became the standard for patients recovering from respiratory failure in the ICU (75). When the train of four ratio (TOF) of >0.7, that is, when the intensity of all four nerve-stimulated muscle contractions is almost equal, normal vital capacity, sustained head lift over 5 seconds, and maximum inspiratory pressure of -20 to -25 cm H_2O can be generated (64). Thus, a TOF of >0.7 and maximum inspiratory pressure of -25 cm H_2O are useful objective indicators of muscle strength. Several reports suggest that residual paralysis may still be present in upper airway muscles (masseter, geniohyoid) despite complete recovery of the adductor pollicis (76, 77). Some authors have suggested, therefore, that since muscles of deglutition are necessary for protection and maintenance of the airway, a higher level of muscle function (e.g., -50 cm H_2O maximum inspiratory pressure) may be required (78).

CRITICAL CARE IMPLICATIONS

As indicated previously, MR used in the critically ill ICU patients have a number of advantages (see Introduction). Depolarizing relaxants and nondepolarizing relaxants, however, have several unwanted effects. The presence of concurrent disease states and/or the coadministration of other drugs can alter the response to these drugs. These aberrant responses to MR may be due to neuromuscular-junctional (pharmacodynamic) factors, such as qualitative and quantitative changes in acetylcholine receptors or to (pharmacokinetic) changes in the body's ability to distribute and eliminate the drug or its metabolite. Since several confounding components can affect both the pharmacodynamics and pharmacokinetics of the MR in ICU patients, these components should be taken into consideration prior to and during administration of MR (79).

ACETYLCHOLINE RECEPTORS AND SENSITIVITY TO MUSCLE RELAXANTS

An important factor affecting the sensitivity of MR is the acetylcholine receptors' (AChR) quality and quantity. The terms up-regulation and down-regulation generally refer to increased and decreased numbers of AChRs, respectively. The typical condition where up-regulation of AChR occurs is following upper or lower motor neuron denervation (80). In this condition not only is there an increase in receptor number but also qualitative changes occur in the receptor, altering its functional and pharmacologic characteristics (80). Multiple factors are present in the critically ill patient that seem to induce or contribute to denervation-like changes in muscle, including up-regulation of AChR. These factors include immobilization, malnutrition, infection (toxins), and coadministration of many drugs that affect the prejunctional or postjunctional membrane. Immobilization of skeletal muscle causes nerve sprouting and the spread of AChR beyond the junctional area (81). Chronic protein-calorie malnutrition in the absence of any other pathology prolongs nerve conduction-velocity and produces neuromuscular changes (82). Toxins released by organisms, probably by inhibiting the acetylcholine release, can up-regulate AChR number (82, 83). Chronic use of the NDMR alone can produce denervation-like changes in the skeletal muscle membrane (84). This effect of NDMRs and toxins can be further compounded by chronic use of drugs such as antibiotics and antiepileptics, which inhibit the release of acetylcholine and may upregulate AChR (85). It is not surprising, therefore, that electromyographic evidence of polyneuropathy or denervation is present in many critically ill patients in the ICU (86, 87).

An increase in AChR number is usually associated with resistance to competitive antagonists (NDMRs) and increased sensitivity to depolarizing relaxants such as succinylcholine (80, 88, 89). Increased sensitivity to succinylcholine in the extreme form can result in a lethal hyperkalemic response (80, 88). Sensitivity to succinylcholine and resistance to NDMR can generally be seen as early as 3 to 7 days after the insult or injury. The duration of these responses in not known.

MECHANISMS OF HYPERKALEMIA WITH SUCCINYLCHOLINE

Succinylcholine consists of two acetylcholine molecules joined together by an ester bond and, therefore, it replicates the depolarization caused by acetylcholine at the postsynaptic membrane. In the normal neuromuscular junction, the opening of the AChR channel occurring with depolarization allows the efflux of potassium from the cell into extracellular fluid through receptors that are present only in the end-plate area. This causes serum potassium in the extracellular fluid or plasma to rise about 0.5 mEq/L with no cardiovascular consequences. With up-regulation of AChRs to the extrajunctional regions, the area of chemosensitivity expands, and depolarization and chemical transmission can occur through junctional (end-plate) as well as extrajunctional AChRs. With up-regulation, therefore, more ion channels are available to release potassium during depolarization. When many muscles are involved, this flooding of the extracellular fluid with potassium can result in hyperkalemia and, sometimes, lethal cardiovascular consequences (80).

The conditions under which hyperkalemia, following the administration of succinylcholine, leads to cardiac arrest have been observed to include burns (80); spinal cord injury (90); tetanus (91); severe intraabdominal infections (92); encephalopathy (93); chronically ill patients in the ICU (94–96); polyneuropathy, including Guillaine-Barré syndrome (97, 98); and metastic disease with and without radiation (80, 99). Succincylcholine was used in all these patients primarily for intubation or for change of tracheostomy tube. Although hyperkalemia was not documented in all of these instances, cardiac arrest following succinylcholine was the common denominator. As indicated previously, the hyperkalemia to succinylcholine in ICU patients may be related to up-regulation of AChR due to critical illness polyneuropathy (86, 87), immobilization (81), bacterial toxins (82, 83), and prolonged use of NDMR and other drugs (84, 85).

MECHANISMS OF RESISTANCE (INSENSITIVITY) TO NDMR

Numerous authors have reported tolerance to the effects of NDMRs in ICU patients (50, 100–102). The up-regulation of AChR caused by immobilization, sepsis, and polyneuropathy may play a significant role in the resistance to NDMR (80, 84, 89, 103). It is now clear that the chronic administration of NDMR itself can be a significant factor in the development of tolerance to these drugs and the development of extrajunctional receptors (84). This increased dose requirement for an antagonist (NDMR) of the AChR during up-regulation of that receptor is consistent with classical receptor dogma that an increase in receptor is associated with tolerance to antagonists and increased sensitivity to agonists (80). An additional factor that may induce tolerance can be the qualitative change occurring in the AChR, which alters its affinity for NDMRs (80).

Despite the pharmacologic basis explaining the need for increased amounts of NDMRs, their continued use might cause residual paralysis for days to months after termination of use (104–108). Polyneuropathy of critical illness, immobilization atrophy, and concurrent use of drugs that affect neuromuscular transmission (see Drug Interactions) may all contribute to this prolonged weakness. It is of interest that all reports of prolonged muscle weakness in ICU patients have followed the use of vecuronium or pancuronium. Whether this apparently high incidence is due to their more popular use is unclear. A recent survey indicates that pancuronium is used in 21% of the ICUs vs. 17% for atracurium (3), yet there are no reports of prolonged muscle weakness following atracurium. Prolonged weakness following pancuronium and vecuronium may be related to their unique chemical (steroidal) nature, both of which have pharmacologically active metabolites (50).

DRUG INTERACTIONS

Anticonvulsants

Several studies have demonstrated resistance to NDMR after prolonged therapy with phenytoin or carbamazepine (109–111). Additionally, studies in humans have confirmed varying forms of sensory, motor, and neuromuscular junction disorders in patients on long-term anticonvulsant therapy (112). Whether these neuromuscular disorders (?denervation syndrome) contribute to the resistance is unknown. Anticonvulsants are also potent inducers of liver metabolizing enzymes (113) and may enhance metabolic clearance of NDMRs.

Table 17.2. Commonly Used Antibiotics and Their Interactions with NDMR

—Polymyxin:	Most potent of the antibiotics to have an effect on the neuromuscular junction. Blocks AChR ion channel.	
—Aminoglycosides:	Neomycin	—Decreases acetylcholine release
	Gentamicin Kanamycin Amikacin	—Lowers sensitivity of the postjunctional membrane to acetylcholine
—Tobramycin:	May also have a direct effect on the muscle.	
—Lincomycin:	Blocks ion channels and also has a direct depressant action on contractility of the muscle.	
—Clindamycin:	Direct action on the muscle and may also block acetylcholine receptor ion channel.	

The acute-phase reactant proteins released by the liver as a result of enzyme induction, particularly α_1-acid glycoprotein, can cause increased protein binding of many drugs, including MR (Table 17.2). The increased protein binding (decreased free fraction) that leaves less free drug available for action at the neuromuscular junction may play a role in decreased sensitivity to NDMRs following chronic anticonvulsant therapy (85). The administration of NDMR following acute phenytoin therapy, however, will result in potentiation of neuromuscular effects (114).

Antibiotics

Antibiotics are the drugs most commonly used in the ICU that can have an interaction with MR. They can potentiate the neuromuscular effects of MR, in the intraoperative and postoperative periods (115). Antibiotic-induced inhibition of neurotransmission can occur even in the absence of the concomitant administration of muscle relaxants (e.g., myasthenia gravis). The etiology of the reduced neurotransmission varies with the antibiotic and can affect acetylcholine release, acetylcholine receptor ion channel activity, and postjunctional sensitivity to acetylcholine. Some antibiotics (e.g., clindamycin) exert a direct action on the muscle itself (115). As a rule, the inhibition of neurotransmission produced by antibiotics is not easily reversed by reversal agents, such as neostigmine. Although 4-aminopyridine and Ca^{2+} salts are effective reversal drugs for some antibiotic-induced muscle paralysis, their clinical use is not recommended.

Steroids

Interaction of steroids and NDMRs may have clinical implications. A few case reports have been made of antagonism of neuromuscular blockade after glucocorticoids (116), after testosterone (117), and after betamethasone therapy (118, 119). The mechanism for this interaction is not clear, although both prejunctional and postjunctional effects have been proposed.

Phosphodiesterase Inhibitors

Drugs like theophylline (120), furosemide (121), and azathioprine (122) that have an inhibitory action on phosphodiesterase enzyme have been found to antagonize pancuronium-induced neuromuscular blockade. Aminophylline also increases the contractility of the diaphragm (123), an effect that

may be due to increased levels of cyclic AMP causing an enhanced release of acetylcholine. Although theophylline alone has no effect on neuromuscular transmission, concomitant administration of *d*-tubocurarine has distinct effects on the neuromuscular junction dependent on the plasma concentration of theophylline (124).

Dantrolene

Dantrolene is the drug of choice for treatment of malignant hyperthermia. It is also used therapeutically to control various forms of muscle spasticity. Dantrolene is known to produce weakness in healthy volunteers and this effect may be of significance, especially if dantrolene is given prophylactically to patients with neuromuscular disease (125). Whenever dantrolene is used in the presence of a neuromuscular disease or with NDMR, a more profound weakness should be anticipated and the patient carefully monitored.

Dantrolene has been shown to produce clinical improvement in experimental autoimmune myasthenia gravis (EAMG) (126). This effect may be due to an increased release of acetylcholine due to changes in intracellular calcium at the nerve terminal. Resistance to the relaxant effect of dantrolene quantitated by evoked twitch response has been reported in a patient with myasthenia gravis (127).

POTASSIUM, CALCIUM, AND MAGNESIUM

Electrolyte disturbances are commonly seen in the ICU. Changes in potassium, calcium, and magnesium have definite effects on the neuromuscular junction. Hypokalemia increases the potency of NDMR and also increases the amount of anticholinesterase required for reversal (128, 129). Hyperkalemia or hypercalcemia decreases the sensitivity of the neuromuscular junction to *d*-tubocurarine or pancuronium (130). Increased magnesium levels in plasma enhance the neuromuscular block produced by both succinylcholine and NDMRs (131, 132). Changes in magnesium levels may become important in the parturient and the fetus when magnesium sulfate is administered for eclampsia (132). Although Ca^{2+} increases (and Mg^{2+} decreases) enhance the release of acetylcholine, the interaction of calcium channel blockers with neuromuscular blockers in unclear.

RENAL FAILURE

Renal failure increases elimination half-life and thereby prolongs the duration of action of all commonly used NDMRs, with the exception of atracurium. The intensity of this effect will depend on the importance of the renal route for the elimination of the drug.

d-Tubocurarine has been safely used in patients with renal failure for many years. Prolonged duration of action due to increased elimination half-life results, however (33).

Metocurine is primarily eliminated by the kidneys and, hence, it should be avoided in patients with renal failure (35).

Gallamine is almost exclusively eliminated by the kidneys, and its duration of action can be prolonged for days in patients with renal failure. It is readily reversed with hemodialysis and peritoneal dialysis (38).

Pancuronium should be used with caution in patients with renal failure, as prolonged duration of action occurs due to decreased clearance of the drug (43).

Vecuronium-induced neuromuscular paralysis can be prolonged in patients with renal failure due to increased elimination half-life (46, 47). The delayed recovery from paralysis following chronic rise of vecuronium may be related to decreased elimination of vecuronium metabolites (50).

Atracurium may be the drug of choice in patients with renal failure, since no significant changes in both duration of action and elimination half-life occur. (133).

Pipecuronium clearance may be decreased and the elimination half-life increased in patients with renal failure (52).

Doxacurium's duration of action was prolonged and more variable in patients with renal failure than in normal controls (60).

LIVER DISEASE/FAILURE

Patients with liver disease may show altered responses to NDMRs due to the pharmacodynamic and pharmacokinetic changes associated with the disease, including protein binding, volume of distribution, associated renal dysfunction, and nutritional status (133, 134). Liver is less important than the kidney in the elimination of most MR. The hepatic route of elimination accounts for about 10% of pancuronium and *d*-tubocurarine. Although only 10% of pancuronium is eliminated by the liver, prolonged duration of action has been seen in patients with liver disease (44, 45) . Metocurine and gallamine are not dependant on the liver for clearance. Slower clearance and increased elimination half-life, however, have been shown in patients with cirrhosis and cholestasis (48, 49).

Atracurium is not dependent on any organ function for its elimination. Its metabolism is unique in that it is degraded by "Hofman elimination" and ester hydrolysis (134). It can be very safely administered to patients with hepatic failure (135).

HYPOTHERMIA

Temperature plays a complex role in the function of the neuromuscular junction. Hypothermia is seen often in ICU patients, especially after major surgery, multiple trauma, and massive fluid resuscitation. Decreases in body temperature alter acetylcholine receptor functions, nerve conduction, the contractile mechanisms of the muscle, and the pharmacokinetics and metabolism of the drug.

A fall in temperature, for example, reduces the sensitivity to *d*-tubocurarine. This effect seen during hypothermia may be due to (*a*) direct membrane depolarization and slowing of repolarization, both of which augment the effect of acetylcholine; (*b*) more acetylcholine available at the junction because of reduced activity of acetylcholine-esterase enzyme and increased transmitter release; and (*c*) reduced affinity of the receptors to tubocurarine (136). Decreased temperature also affects the metabolism of all NDMRs, and their actions may, therefore, be prolonged (137, 138).

MYASTHENIA GRAVIS

Myasthenia gravis is a disorder causing muscle weakness that becomes worse on repeated voluntary effort but that can be improved by rest or anticholinesterase drugs (139, 140). Antibodies to acetylcholine receptor protein are detected in the serum of patients with myasthenia gravis, although the antibody titers may not correlate to the severity of the disease. These antibodies combine with the α-subunits of the acetylcholine receptors and lead to destruction of a large percentage of receptors. Histological abnormalities of the thymus are found in a large percentage of myasthenic patients and surgical removal produces clinical remission in about 80% of patients. Thymus contains muscle-like cells that have acetylcholine receptors, and these cells may be the source of antigen in the development of antibodies (141). The reduced number of acetylcholine receptors available decreases the margin of safety for neurotransmission. Fade of the evoked twitch response on tetanic and train-of-four stimulation is seen. A typical myasthenic patient shows resistance to the neuromuscular effects of succinylcholine (142) and is extremely sensitive to NDMRs (143). Patients with myasthenia gravis may, however, present at various stages of the disease process; the response to MR will depend on the effectiveness of the current therapy the patient is receiving and the severity of the disease.

MYASTHENIC SYNDROME (LAMBERT-EATON SYNDROME)

This syndrome, originally reported in association with bronchogenic carcinoma, is also characterized by muscular weakness (144). Other studies have confirmed the association of this disease with small cell carcinoma of multiple-tissue origins (141). Myasthenic syndrome is a prejunctional phenomenon affecting the release of acetylcholine from the nerve endings due to autoimmune antibodies directed against the voltage-gated calcium channels. In contrast to myasthenia gravis, the postjunctional acetylcholine receptors are normal, and antibodies to acetylcholine receptors are absent. Increased sensitivity to depolarizing and nondepolarizing muscle relaxants is seen in myasthenic syndrome.

CHRONIC CHOLINESTERASE INHIBITORS

Pathological elevations of acetylcholine activity can be seen in overdose of cholinesterase inhibitors in the treatment of myasthenia gravis (139), in the chronic administration of reversible cholinesterase inhibitors as prophylaxis during the threat of chemical (nerve gas) warfare (145), and in acute and chronic exposure to organophosphorous insecticides compounds (146). In myasthenia gravis, effectiveness of anticholinesterase drug treatment may be diminished by its chronic use. This effect may be due to further down regulation of the number of AChR as a result of excessive amounts of acetylcholine at the neuromuscular junction (147). Acute organophosphorous pesticide poisoning is seen around the world from absorption through the skin or deliberate or accidental ingestion (146). The potential for organophosphates (nerve gas) to be used during war is ever present.

Clinically, organophosphorous compound poisoning presents in three different phases. In the acute stage the inhibition of acetylcholinesterase results in acute elevations of acetylcholine. The metabolism of succinylcholine will be impaired due to inhibition of all esterase enzymes (148). Resistance to NDMRs may be present due to increased levels of acetylcholine. After the first 24 hours, in the intermediate phase, electromyographic features resemble those of myasthenia gravis, or a postsynaptic defect (149). The continued presence of high concentrations of acetylcholine during this time results in a decreased number of receptors (147). One might anticipate increased sensitivity to NDMRs, though this has never been quantitated. In the late stages a neurotoxic polyneuropathy occurs during which neural (denervation-like) and myopathic changes occur together (150). The response to neuromuscular blockers at this stage is not known.

THERAPEUTIC CONSIDERATIONS FOR ADMINISTRATION OF MUSCLE RELAXANTS

Although MR facilitate mechanical ventilation, it is important to stress that every patient who requires ventilation does not necessarily require MR. Recent surveys of U.S. hospitals that participate in training pulmonary fellows indicated that mechanical ventilation was required in approximately 80% of ICU patients, yet only 20% of medical intensive care unit patients required MR (3). This number may be higher in surgical intensive care units run by anesthesiologists. Despite their many advantages, MR are not devoid of side effects. Numerous reports indicate the presence of prolonged muscle weakness following critical illness (50, 102, 106, 107). These reports have implicated MR and/or their pharmacologically active metabolites in the muscle weakness, and in all of these reports steroidal relaxants, pancuronium or vecuronium were the drugs involved. None of these reports, however, has characterized the confounding effects of organ failure, concomitant sepsis, disuse atrophy, and coadministered drugs. Concurrent disease, including release of certain hormones (e.g., steroids) may have aggravated the muscle weakness.

Another fact requiring emphasis is that MR are not effective narcotics, sedatives, or anxiolytics. Although sleep can be induced by local instillation of MR into cerebral ventricles (11), the utility of these drugs for central nervous system inhibition is controversial. The stress of pain and anxiety has multiple effects, including those on immune response and wound healing (151–153). The afferent responses that increase the hypermetabolic (stress) response to trauma, injury, and sepsis can be accentuated by the brain, particularly in the presence of pain and anxiety (154). In a preliminary study, it has been reported that patients with persistently high endorphins and, possibly, catecholamines developed sepsis (154). The question has been raised as to whether these substances will decrease oxygen delivery, alter immune response, and make them more prone to sepsis. The administration of sedatives and opiates has been shown to decrease endogenous endorphin levels and improve morbidity and mortality (154). Psychosis is another side effect of a paralyzed but "awake" patient (155). Being paralyzed, but helpless and unable to express one's feelings, including pain, can be terrifying.

Evaluation of depth of sedation and pain control, although difficult in paralyzed patients, is important to prevent excessive or undertreatment. Contrary to popular belief, pain and episodes of fear and anxiety cannot be reliably detected by changes in heart rate and blood pressure (156). Other measures of depth of analgesia and sedation, such as lower esophageal sphincter activity or frontalis muscle tone, also fail to predict awareness. At present, the most promising measure of consciousness or awareness appears to be oscillatory electrical activity recorded in response to auditory and visual stimuli (156). The utility of auditory evoked responses for evaluation of sedation in ICU patients has been tested (157). The sedative drugs used included fentanyl and propofol. This study documented the feasibility of its use in critically ill patients, although guidelines for its use were not outlined. Further work should investigate the sensitivity and specificity of these monitors. In spite of these difficulties in assessing adequacy of sedation and pain relief, the importance of adequate control of pain and anxiety cannot be overemphasized. With increased availability of opiate and benzodiazepine antagonists (e.g., narcan, flumanezil), the reluctance to appropriately medicate critically ill patients with central depressants may be less of a problem in the future. Thus, drugs such as the benzodiazepines, narcotics and, occasionally, neuroleptics such as haloperidol should always be coadministered with MR.

CONCLUSION

Muscle relaxants are useful adjuncts for facilitating mechanical ventilation. Used in conjunction with sedatives and narcotics, MR can reduce barotrauma, decrease oxygen consumption, improve pulmonary compliance, and improve arterial oxygenation and oxygen delivery in the critically ill patient (4–10). Increases in central vascular and intracranial pressures during coughing and "bucking" can also be attenuated by the use of sedation and/or MR (16–18). There are, however, a number of side effects of MR. The most important is the potentially lethal hyperkalemic response to the depolarizing relaxant succinylcholine (80). Persistent muscle weakness for days to months after critical care illness has been attributed to prolonged use of NDMRs (104–108). There is no conclusive evidence for implicating NDMR, since malnutrition, sepsis, coadministration of other drugs, and polyneuropathy of critical illness confound the picture. Nevertheless, since the prolonged muscle weakness of ICU patients has long-term effects on the rehabilitation of these patients, it may seem prudent to limit the dosage of MR by monitoring the depth of neuromuscular paralysis and allowing patients to emerge intermittently from paralysis during its administration.

Prolonged muscle paralysis due to MR can be anticipated if normal doses are administered in the presence of renal and hepatic failure. Atracurium has advantages in this respect. Although atracurium was used for long periods in approximately 20% of patients requiring MR (3), no long-term side effects have been reported (3, 158). Short-acting muscle relaxants (atracurium, vecuronium, and mivacurium) have theoretical advantages over the long-acting muscle relaxants (e.g., *d*-tubocurarine, pancuronium, and metocurine). In this day of cost containment in medical practice, the cost of drugs should also be considered. The cost of short-acting drugs (e.g., midazolam with atracurium or vecuronium) for 24 hours is approximately $1000 per patient, as compared to $50 per patient for long-acting drugs (e.g., pancuronium with diazepam) that are no longer under patent.

Continued use of MR results in tolerance to their effectiveness. Whenever neuromuscular blockers are administered, evoked responses such as train-of-four monitoring should be performed in order to avoid relative overdosing or underdosing. Succinylcholine may be a relative contraindication for reintubation in critically ill patients, particularly after long-term immobilization and/or prolonged use of NDMR.

REFERENCES

1. Klessig HT, Geiger HJ, Murray MJ, Cousin DB. A national survey on the practice patterns of anesthesiologist intensivists in the use of muscle relaxants. *Crit Care Med* 20:1341–1345, 1992.
2. Hansen-Flaschen J, Cowen J, Raps EC: Neuromuscular blockade in the intensive care unit. *Am Rev Respir Dis* 147:234–236, 1993.
3. Hansen-Flaschen JH, Brazinsky S, Basile C, Lanken PN: Use of sedating drugs and neuromuscular blocking agents in patients requiring mechanical ventilation. *JAMA* 266:2870–2875, 1991.
4. Miller-Jones CMH, Williams JH: Sedation for ventilation: a retrospective study of 50 patients. *Anaesthesia* 35:1104–1106, 1981.
5. Bishop JM: Hemodynamic and gas exchange effects on pancuronium bromide in sedated patients with respiratory failure. *Anesthesiology* 60:396–371, 1984.
6. Pollitzer MJ, Reynolds EO, Shaw DG, Thomas RG: Pancuronium during mechanical ventilation speeds recovery of lungs of infants with hyaline membrane disease. *Lancet* i:346–348, 1981.
7. Greenough A, Wood S, Morley CJ, Davis JA: Pancuronium prevents pneumothoracies in ventilated premature babies who actively expire against positive pressure inflation. *Lancet* i:1–3, 1984.
8. Wilson RS, Sullivan SF, Malm JR, Bowman FO: The oxygen cost of breathing following anesthesia and cardiac surgery. *Anesthesiology* 39:387–393, 1973.
9. Thung N, Herzog P, Ignacies II, Thompson WM, Dammann JF: The cost of respiratory effort in postoperative cardiac patients. *Circulation* 28:552–559, 1963.
10. Cameron CB, Gregory GA, Rudolph AM, Heymann MA: Cardiovascular effects of *d*-tubocurarine and pancuronium in newborn lambs during normoxia and hypoxia. *Pediatr Res* 20:246–252, 1986.
11. Haranath PSRK, Venkata-Bhatt H: Sleep induced by drugs injected into inferior horn of lateral cerebral ventricles in dogs. *Br J Pharmacol* 59:231–236, 1977.
12. Forbes AR, Cohen NH, Eger EI: Pancuronium reduces halothane requirement in man. *Anesth Analg* 58:497–501, 1979.
13. Liem ST, Aldrete JA: Control of post anesthetic shivering. *Can Anaesth Soc J* 21:506–510, 1974.
14. Domino SF: Sites of action of some central nervous system depressants. *Annu Rev Pharmacol* 2:215–236, 1962.
15. Sessler DI: *Temperature Monitoring in Anesthesia*, ed 3. Miller RD (ed.) Churchill-Livingstone, New York, 1991, pp. 1227–1242.
16. Hickey PF, Hausen DD, Wessel DL, Lang P, Jonas RA, Elixson EM: Blunting of stress responses in the pulmonary circulation of infants by fentanyl. *Anesth Analg* 64:1137–1142, 1985.
17. Klezi M, Wesba A, Illevich U, Schramm W, Spiss CK: Effects of atracurium on elevated intracranial pressure during routine endotracheal suctioning. *Anesthesiology* 75:1211, 1991.
18. Fanconi S, Duc G: Intratracheal suctioning in sick preterm infants: prevention of intracranial hypertension and cerebral hypoperfusion by muscle paralysis. *Pediatrics* 79:538–543, 1987.
19. Robertson GS: Serum cholinesterase deficiency. I. Disease and inheritance. *Br J Anaesth* 38:355–360, 1966.
20. Kalow W: Pharmacogenetics and anesthesia. *Anesthesiology* 25:377–387, 1964.
21. Goedde HW, Held KR, Altlan DK: Hydrolysis of succinylcholine and succinylcholine in human serum. *Mol Pharmacol* 4:274–287, 1968.
22. Goedde HW, Altlan DK, Schloot W: Therapy of prolonged apnea after suxamethonium with purified pseudocholinesterase. New data on kinetics of the hydrolysis of succinylcholine and succinylmonocholine and further data on N-acetyltransferase polymorphism. *Ann NY Acad Sci* 151:742–751, 1968.
23. Benzer A, Luz G, Oswald E, Schmoigl C, Menardi G: Succinylcholine-induced prolonged apnea in a week old newborn: treatment with human plasma cholinesterase. *Anesth Analg* 74:137–138, 1992.
24. Ramsey FM, Lebowitz PW, Savarese JJ, Ali HH: Clinical characteristics of a long-term succinylcholine neuromuscular blockade during balanced anesthesia. *Anesth Analg* 59:110–116, 1980.
25. Moss J, Fahmy N, Sunder N, Beaven MA: Hormonal and hemodynamic profile of an anaphylactic reaction in man. *Circulation* 63:210–213, 1981.
26. Mathews MD, Ceglarski JZ, Pabari M: Anaphylaxis to suxamethonium. A case report. *Anaesth Intensive Care* 5:235, 1977.
27. Watkins J. Anaphylactoid response to neuromuscular blockers (atracurium in perspective). In *Recent Developments in Muscle Relaxation: Atracurium in Perspective*. Royal Society of Medicine Services International Congress and Symposium Series 131. RM Jones and JP Payne (eds). Royal Society of Medicine Services, London, pp. 13–20, 1988.
28. Miller RD, Sanders DB, Rowlington FG, et al: Anesthesia induced rhabdomyolysis in a patient with Duchenne-muscular dystrophy. *Anesthesiology* 48:146–148, 1978.
29. Griffith HR, Johnson GE: The use of curare in general anesthesia. *Anesthesiology* 3:418–420, 1942.
30. Colquhoun D, Dryer F, Sheriden RE: The action of tubocurarine at the frog neuromuscular junction. *J Physiol (Lond)* 293:247–284, 1979.
31. Moss J, Roscow CE, Savarese JJ, Philbin D, Kniffen KJ: Role of histamine in the hypotensive action of *d*-tubocurarine in humans. *Anesthesiology* 55:19–25, 1981.
32. Bermingham AT, Hussein SZ: A comparison of skeletal neuromuscular and autonomic ganglion blocking potencies of five non-depolarizing relaxants. *Br J Pharmacol* 70:501–506, 1980.
33. Miller RD, Matteo RS, Benet LZ, et al: The pharmacokinetics of d-tubocurarine in man with and without renal failure. *J Pharmacol Exp Ther* 202:1–7, 1977.
34. Savarese JJ, Ali HH, Antonio RP: The clinical pharmacology of metocurine: dimethyl tubocurarine revisited. *Anesthesiology* 47:277–284.
35. Brotherton WP, Matteo RS: Pharmacokinetics of metocurine in man with renal failure. *Anesthesiology* 53:S268, 1980.
36. Bowman WC: Nonrelaxant properties of neuromuscular blocking drugs. *Br J Anaesth* 54:147–160, 1982.
37. Colquhoun D, Sheriden RE. The modes of action of gallamine. *Proc R Soc Lond (Series B)* 211:181–203, 1981.
38. Lowenstein E, Goldfine C, Flache WE: Administration of gallamine in the presence of renal failure-reversal of neuromuscular blockade by peritoneal dialysis. *Anesthesiology* 33:556–558, 1970.
39. Buckett WR, Hewett CL, Savage DS: Pancuronium, bromide and other steroidal neuromuscular blocking agents containing acetylcholine fragments. *J Med Chem* 16:1116–1124, 1973.
40. Bowman WC: *Pharmacology of Neuromuscular Function*, ed 2. Butterworth, London, 1990, pp. 181–189.
41. Ivankovich AD, Miletich DJ, Albrecht RT, et al: The effect of pancuronium on myocardial contraction and catecholamine metabolism. *J Pharm Pharmacol* 27:837–841, 1975.
42. Miller RD, Agoston S, et al: The comparative potency and pharmacokinetics of pancuronium and its metabolites in anesthetized man. *J Pharmacol Exp Ther* 207:539–543, 1978.
43. McLeod K, Watson MJ, Rawlins MD: Pharmacokinetics of pancuronium in patients with normal and impaired renal function. *Br J Anaesth* 48:341–345, 1978.
44. Westra P, Vermeer GA, DeLange AR, et al: Hepatic and renal disposition of pancuronium and gallamine in patients with extra-hepatic cholestasis. *Br J Anaesth* 51:331–338, 1981.
45. Somogyi AA, Shanks CA, Triggs EJ: Disposition kinetics of pancuronium bromide in patients with total biliary obstruction. *Br J Anaesth* 49:1103–1108, 1977.
46. Miller RD, Rupp SM, Fisher DM, et al: Clinical pharmacology of vecuronium and atracurium. *Anesthesiology* 61:443–453, 1984.
47. Bencini AF, Scaf AHJ, Sohn YJ, et al: Hepatobiliary disposition of vecuronium bromide in man. *Br J Anaesth* 58:988–995, 1986.
48. Lebrault C, Berger JL, D'Hollander, Gomeni R, Henzel D, Duvaldestin P: Pharmacokinetics and pharmacodynamics of vecuronium (ORG NC 45) in patients with cirrhosis. *Anesthesiology* 62:601–605, 1985.
49. Lebrault C, Duvaldestin P, Henzel D, Chauvin M, Guesnon P: Pharmacokinetics and pharmacodynamics of vecuronium in patients with cholestasis. *Br J Anaesth* 58:983–987, 1986.
50. Segredo V, Matthay MA, Sharma ML, Gruenke LD, Caldwell JE, Miller RD: Prolonged neuromuscular blockade after long-term administration of vecuronium in two critically ill patients *Anesthesiology* 72:566–570, 1990.
51. Larijani GE, Bartkowski RR, Azad S, et al: Clinical pharmacology of pipecuronium bromide. *Anesth Analg* 68:734–739, 1989.
52. Caldwell JE, Canfell PC, Castagnoli KP, et al: The influence of renal failure on the pharmacokinetics and duration of action of pipecuronium bromide in patients anesthetized with halothane and nitrous oxide. *Anesthesiology* 70:7–12, 1989.
53. Basta SJ, Ali HH, Savarese JJ, Sunder N, et al: Clinical pharmacology of atracurium besylate (BW 33A): a new neuromuscular blocking agent. *Anesth Analg* 61:723–729, 1982.
54. Scott RPF, Savarese JJ, Ali HH, Basta SJ, Sunder N: Atracurium: clinical strategies for preventing and alternating the hemodynamic response. *Br J Anaesth* 57:550–553, 1985.
55. Shi WZ, Fahey MR, Fisher DM, et al: Laudanosine (a metabolite of atracurium) increases the minimum alveolar concentration of halothane in rabbits. *Anesthesiology* 63:584–588, 1985.

56. Fahey MR, Shi WZ, Miller RD: Inhaled anesthetics alter the seizure threshold of laudanosine in rabbits (abstr), *Anesthesiology* 65:A115, 1986.

57. Baraka A: Neuromuscular blockade of atracurium versus succinylcholine in a patient with complete absence of plasma cholinesterase activity. *Anesthesiology* 66:80–81, 1987.

58. Basta SJ, Savarese JJ, Ali HH, et al: Clinical pharmacology of doxacurium chloride. A new long-acting non-depolarizing muscle relaxant. *Anesthesiology* 69:478–486, 1988.

59. Cashman JN, Luke JJ, Jones RM: Neuromuscular block with doxacurium (BW 938u) in patients with normal and absent renal function. *Br J Anaesth* 64:186–192, 1990.

60. Cook RD, Freeman JA, Lai AA, Robertson KA, et al: Pharmacokinetics and pharmacodynamics of doxacurium in normal patients and in those with hepatic or renal failure. *Anesth Analg* 72:145–150, 1991.

61. Savarese JJ, Ali HH, Basta SJ, et al: The clinical neuromuscular pharmacology of mivacurium chloride (BW 1090u)—A short-acting nondepolarizing ester neuromuscular blocking drug. *Anesthesiology* 68:723–732, 1988.

62. Savarese JJ, Ali HH, Basta SJ, Scott RPF, et al: The cardiovascular effects of mivacurium chloride (BW 1090u) in patients receiving nitrous oxide-opiate-barbiturate anesthesia. *Anesthesiology* 70:3:8–16, 1989.

63. Ali HH, Savarese JJ, Lebowitz PW, et al: Twitch, tetanus and train of four as indices of recovery from non-depolarizing neuromuscular blockade. *Anesthesiology* 54:294–297, 1981.

64. Ali HH: Monitoring neuromuscular function. *Semin Anesthesia* 8:158–168, 1989.

65. Katz RL: Clinical neuromuscular pharmacology of pancuronium. *Anesthesiology* 34:550–556, 1971.

66. Baraka A: Irreversible curarization. *Anaesth Intensive Care* 5:244–246, 1977.

67. Caldwell JE, Robertson EN, Baird WLM: Antagonism of profound neuromuscular blockade induced by vecuronium or atracurium. Comparison of neostigmine with edrophonium. *Br J Anaesth* 58:1285–1289, 1986.

68. Smith CE, Donati F, Bevan DR: Dose-response relationship for edrophonium and neostigmine as antagonists of atracurium and vecuronium neuromuscular blockade. *Anesthesiology* 71:37–43, 1989.

69. Harper KW, Bali IM, Gibson FM, et al: Reversal of neuromuscular block: heart rate changes with slow injection of neostigmine and atropine mixtures. *Anaesthesia* 39:772–775, 1984.

70. Mirakhur R, Dundee JW, Jones CJ, et al: Combination of glycopyrrolate (10 μg/kg) and neostigmine (50 μgm/kg) administered together produces a stable heart rate. *Anesth Analg* 60:557–562, 1981.

71. Mirakhur RK: Antagonism of the muscarinic effects of edrophonium with atropine or glycopyrrolate: a comparative study. *Br J Anaesth* 57:1213–1216, 1985.

72. Chang CC, Chen SM, Hong SJ: Reversal of neostigmine induced tetanic fade and endplate potential rundown with respect to the autoregulation of transmitter release. *Br J Pharmacol* 95:1255–1261, 1988.

73. Goldhill DR, Wainwright AP, Stuart CS, Flynn PJ: Neostigmine after spontaneous recovery from neuromuscular blockade. Effect on depth of blockade monitored with train of four and tetanic stimuli. *Anaesthesia* 44:293–299, 1989.

74. Westcott DA, Bendixen HH: Neostigmine on a curare antagonist—A clinical study. *Anesthesiology* 23:324–332, 1962.

75. Sahn S, Lakshminarayan S: Bedside criteria for discontinuation of mechanical ventilation. *Chest* 63:1002–1007, 1973.

76. Donati F, Bevan DR: Not all muscles are the same. *Br J Anaesth* 68:235–236, 1992.

77. Isono S, Kochi T, Mizuguchi T, Nishino T: Differential effects of vecuronium on diaphragm and geniohyoid in anaesthetized dogs. *Br J Anaesth* 68:239–243, 1992.

78. Pavlin EG, Holle RH, Schoene RB: Recovery of airway protection compared with ventilation in humans after paralysis with curare. *Anesthesiology* 70:381–385, 1989.

79. Fiamengo S, Savarese J: Use of muscle relaxants in intensive care units. *Crit Care Med* 19:12:1457–1458, 1991.

80. Martyn JAJ, White DA, Gronert GA, Jaffe RS, Ward JM: Up and down regulation of acetylcholine receptors: effect on neuromuscular blockers. *Anesthesiology* 76:822–843, 1992.

81. Fambrough DM: Control of acetylcholine receptors in skeletal muscle. *Physiol Rev* 59:165–227, 1979.

82. Tomera JF, Martyn JAJ: Intraperitoneal endotoxin, but not protein malnutrition shifts d-tubocurarine dose-response curves in mouse gastrocnemius. *J Pharmacol Exp Ther* 250:921–926, 1989.

83. Simpson LL: Molecular pharmacology of botulinum toxin and tetanus toxin. *Annu Rev Pharmacol Toxicol* 26:427–453, 1986.

84. Hogue CW, Ward JM, Itani MS, Martyn JAJ: Tolerance and upregulation of acetylcholine receptor follows chronic infusion of d-tubocurarine. *J Appl Physiol* 72:1326–1331, 1992.

85. Kim CS, Arnold FJ, Martyn JAJ: Decreased sensitivity to metocurine during chronic phenytoin may be due to protein binding and acetylcholine receptor changes. *Anesthesiology* 77:500–506, 1992.

86. Witt NJ, Zochodne DW, et al: Peripheral nerve function in sepsis and multiple organ failure. *Chest* 99:176–184, 1991.

87. Mezza JBL, Garcia A: Acute polyneuropathy in critically ill patients. *Intensive Care Med* 16:159–162, 1990.

88. Goldhill GA, Martyn JAJ: Succinylcholine induced hyperkalemia. Muscle relaxants. Azar I (ed): Marcel Dekker, New York, 1987, pp. 93–113.

89. Hogue CW Jr, Itani MS, Martyn JAJ: Resistence to *d*-tubocurarine in lower motor neuron injury is related to increased acetylcholine receptors at the neuromuscular junction. *Anesthesiology* 73:703–709, 1990.

90. Tobey RE. Paraplegia, succinylcholine and cardiac arrest. *Anesthesiology* 32:359–364, 1970.

91. Roth F, Wuthrich H: The clinical importance of hyperkalemia following suxamethonium administration. *Br J Anaesth* 41:311–316, 1969.

92. Kohlschutter B, Baur H, Roth F: Suxamethonium induced hyperkalemia in patients with severe intra-abdominal infections. *Br J Anaesth* 48:557–561, 1976.

93. Tong TK: Succinylcholine induced hyperkalemia in near drowning. *Anesthesiology* 66:5:720, 1987.

94. Horton WA, Fergusson NV: Hyperkalemia and cardiac arrest after the use of suxamethonium in intensive care. *Anaesthesia* 43:890–891, 1988.

95. Hemming AE, Charleton S, Kelly P: Hyperkalemia, cardiac arrest, suxamethonium and intensive care. *Anaesthesia* 45:990–991, 1990.

96. Sarubin J, Gebert E: Serumkaliumanstieg nach depolarisierenden muskelrelaxantien. I. Abhangigkeit von der immobilisationsdauer. *Anaesthetist* 30:246–250, 1981.

97. Feldman JM: Cardiac arrest after succinylcholine administration in a pregnant patient recovered from Guillain-Barré Syndrome. *Anesthesiology* 72:942–944, 1990.

98. Fergusson RJ, Wright DJ, Willey RF, Compton GK, Grant IWB: Suxamethonium is dangerous in polyneuropathy. *Br Med J* 18:1990–2001, 1981.

99. Krikken-Hogenberk LG, DeJong JR, Bovill JG: Succinylcholine induced hyperkalemia in a patient with metastatic rhabdomyosarcoma. *Anesthesiology* 70:3:553–555, 1989.

100. Callahan DL: Development of resistance to pancuronium in adult respiratory distress syndrome. *Anesth Analg* 64:1126–1128, 1985.

101. Coursin DB, Klasek G, Goelzer SL: Increased requirements for continuously infused vecuronium in critically ill patients. *Anesth Analg* 69:518–521, 1989.

102. Vanderheyden BA, Reynolds HN, Gerald KB, Emanuele T: Prolonged paralysis after long-term vecuronium infusion. *Crit Care Med* 20:304–307, 1992.

103. Gronet GA: Disuse atrophy with resistance to pancuronium. *Anesthesiology* 55:547–549, 1981.

104. Subramony SH, Carpenter DE, Raju S, Pride M, Evans OB: Myopathy and prolonged neuromuscular blockade after lung transplant. *Crit Care Med* 19:1580–1582, 1991.

105. Gooch JL, Suchyta MR, Balbierz JM, Petajan JH, Clemmer TP: Prolonged paralysis after treatment with neuromuscular junction blocking agents. *Crit Care Med* 19:1125–1131, 1991.

106. Rossiter A, Souney PF, McGowan S, et al: Pancuronium induced prolonged neuromuscular blockade. *Crit Care Med* 19:1583–1587, 1991.

107. Partridge BL, Abrams JH, Bazemore C, Rubin R: Prolonged neuromuscular blockade after long-term infusion of vecuronium bromide in the intensive care unit. *Crit Care Med* 18:1177–1179, 1990.

108. Op de coul AAW, Lambregts PCLA, Koeman J, Van Puynbroek MJE, Terlaak HJ, Gabreels-Festen AAWN: Neuromuscular complications in patients given pavulon (pancuronium bromide) during artificial ventilation. *Clin Neurol Neurosurg* 87:17–22, 1985.

109. Tempelhoff R, Modica P, Jellish WS, Spitznrgel EL: Resistance to atracurium induced neuromuscular blockade in patients with intractable seizure disorders treated with anti-convulsants. *Anesth Analg* 71:665–669, 1990.

110. Ornstein E, Matteo RS, Schwartz AE, Silverberg PA, Young WL, Diaz J: The effect of phenytoin on the magnitude and duration of neuromuscular block following atracurium or vecuronium. *Anesthesiology* 67:191–196, 1987.

111. Roth S, Ebrahim ZY: Resistance to pancuronium in patients receiving carbamazepine. *Anesthesiology* 66:691–693, 1987.

112. Argov Z, Mastaglia FL: Drug induced peripheral neuropathies. *Br Med J* 1:663–666, 1979.

113. Nation RL, Evans AM, Milne RW: Pharmacokinetic drug interactions with phenytoin. *Clin Pharmacokinet* 18:1312–1350, 1980.

114. Gray HS, Slater RM, Pollard BJ: The effect of acutely administered phenytoin on vecuronium induced neuromuscular blockade. *Anaesthesia* 44:379–381, 1989.

115. Sokoll MD, Gergis SD: Antibiotics and neuromuscular function. *Anesthesiology* 55:148–161, 1981.

116. Meyers EF: Partial recovery from pancuronium neuromuscular blockade following hydrocortisone administration. *Anesthesiology* 46:148–150, 1977.

117. Reddy P, Guzman A, Robalino J, Shevde K: Resistance to muscle relaxants in a patient receiving prolonged testosterone therapy. *Anesthesiology* 70:871–873, 1989.

118. Parr SM, Galletly DC, Robinson BJ: Betamethasone induced resistance to vecuronium: A potential problem in neurosurgery. *Anaesth Intens Care* 19:103–105, 1991.

119. Parr SM, Robinson BJ, Rees D, Galletly DC: Interaction between betamethasone and vecuronium. *Br J Anaesth* 67:447–451, 1991.

120. Doll DC, Rosenberg H: Antagonism of neuromuscular blockade by theophylline. *Anesth Analg* 58:139–140, 1979.

121. Azar I, Cottrell J, Gupta B, Turndorf H: Furosemide facilitates recovery of evoked twitch response after pancuronium. *Anesth Analg* 59:55–57, 1980.

122. Glidden RS, Martyn JAJ, Tomera JF: Azathioprine fails to alter dose-response curves of *d*-tubocurarine. *Anesthesiology* 68:595–598, 1988.

123. Aubier M, deTroyer A, Sampson M, Macklum PT, Roussos C: Aminophylline improves diaphragmatic contractility. *N Engl J Med* 305:249–252, 1981.

124. Fuke N, Martyn JAJ, Kim CS, Basta S: Concentration dependent interaction of theophylline with *d*-tubocurarine. *J Appl Physiol* 62:1970–1974, 1987.

125. Flewellen EH, Nelson TE, Jones WP, Arens JF, Wagner DL: Dantrolene dose response in awake man: implications for management of malignant hyperthermia. *Anesthesiology* 59:275–280, 1983.

126. Takamori M, Sakato S, Matsubara S, Okumura S: Therapeutic approach to experimental autoimmune myasthenia gravis by dantrolene sodium. *J Neurol Sci* 58:17–24, 1983.

127. Mora CT, Eisenkraft JB, Papatesta S: Intravenous dantrolene in a patient with myasthenia gravis. *Anesthesiology* 64:371–373, 1986.

128. Feldman SA: Effect of changes in electrolytes, hydration and pH upon the reactions to muscle relaxants. *Br J Anaesth* 35:546–551, 1963.

129. Miller RD, Roderick LL: Diuretic induced hypokalemia, pancuronium, neuromuscular blockade and its antagonism by neostigmine. *Br J Anaesth* 50:541–544, 1978.

130. Waud BE, Waud DR: Interaction of calcium and potassium with neuromuscular blocking agents. *Br J Anaesth* 52:863–866, 1980.

131. DeSilva AJC: Magnesium intoxication: an uncommon cause of prolonged curarization. Case report. *Br J Anaesth* 45:1228–1229, 1973.

132. James MFM: Clinical use of magnesium infusions in anesthesia. *Anesth Analg* 74:129–136, 1992.

133. deBros F, Lai A, Scott R, et al: Pharmacokinetics and pharmacodynamics of atracurium during isoflurane anesthesia in normal and anephric patients. *Anesth Analg* 65:743–746, 1986.

134. Fisher DM, Canfell PC, Fahey MR, et al: Elimination of atracurium in humans: contribution of Hofman elimination and ester hydrolysis versus organ based elimination. *Anesthesiology* 65:6–12, 1986.

135. Ward S, Neill EAM: Pharmacokinetics of atracurium in acute hepatic failure (with acute renal failure). *Br J Anaesth* 55:1169–1172, 1983.

136. Bowman WC: Pharmacology of neuromuscular function. WC Bowman (ed): Wright, Butterworth, pp. 192–193, 1990.

137. Ham J, Miller RD, Benet LZ, et al: The effect of temperature on the pharmacokinetics and pharmacodynamics of d-tubocurarine. *Anesthesiology* 49:324–328, 1978.

138. Miller RD, Agoston S, van der Pol F, et al: Hypothermia and pharmacokinetics and pharmacodynamics of pancuronium in the cat. *J Pharmacol Exp Ther* 207:532–538, 1978b.

139. Engel AG: Myasthenia gravis and myaesthenic syndromes. *Ann Neurol* 16:519–534, 1984.

140. Drachman DB: Myaesthenia gravis (Medical Progress). *N Engl J Med* 298:136–142, 186–193, 1978.

141. Zweiman B, Arnason BG: Immunologic aspects of neurological and neuromuscular diseases. *JAMA* 258:2970–2973, 1987.

142. Eisenkraft JB, Book WJ, Mann SM, Papatestas AE, Hubbard M: Resistance to succinylcholine in myasthenia gravis: a dose response study. *Anesthesiology* 69:760–763, 1988.

143. Nilsson E, Merotoja OA: Vecuronium dose-response and maintenance requirements in patients with myasthenia gravis. *Anesthesiology* 73:28–32, 1990.

144. Vincent A, Lang B, Newsom-Davis J: Autoimmunity to the voltage gated calcium channel underlies the Lambert-Eaton myasthenic syndrome, a paraneoplastic disorder. *Trends Neurosci* 12:496–502, 1989.

145. Keeler JR, Hurst CG, Dunn MA: Pyridostigmine used as a nerve agent pretreatment under wartime conditions. *JAMA* 266:693–695, 1991.

146. Karralliedde J, Senanayake N: Organophosphorous insecticide poisoning. *Br J Anaesth* 63:736–750, 1989.

147. Fambrough DM, Drachman DB, Satyamurti S: Neuromuscular junction in myasthenia gravis: decreased acetylcholine receptors. *Science* 182:293–295, 1973.

148. Selden BS, Curry SC: Prolonged succinylcholine induced paralysis in organophosphate insecticide poisoning. *Ann Emerg Med* 16:215–217, 1987.

149. Davies JE: Changing profiles of pesticide poisoning. *N Engl J Med* 316:807–808, 1987.

150. Rosenstock L, Keifer M, Daniel WE, McConnell R, Claypole K: Chronic nervous system effects of acute organophosphate pesticide intoxication. *Lancet* 2:338:223–227, 1991.

151. Fauman MA: The central nervous system and immune system. *Biol Psychiatry* 17:1459–1482, 1982.

152. Riley V: Psychoneuroendocrine influences on immunocompetence and neoplasia. *Science* 212:1100–1109, 1981.

153. Watkins J, Glynn LE: Symposium on trauma, stress and immunity at Bath. *Anaesthesia* 36:647–653, 1981.

154. Demling RH: What are the functions of endorphins following thermal injury (discussion)? *J Trauma* 24:S172–176, 1984.

155. Evan JM: Consciousness, awareness, and pain in general anesthesia. Rosen M, Lunn JN (eds). Butterworths, London, pp. 184–192, 1987.

156. Kulli J, Koch C: Does anesthesia cause loss of consciousness? *Trends Neurol Sci* 14:6–10, 1991.

157. Sneyd JR, Wang DY, Edward D, et al: Effect of physiotherapy on auditory evoked response of paralysed, sedated patients in the intensive care unit. *Br J Anaesth* 68:349–351, 1992.

158. Dulin PG, Gillard L, Williams CJ: Sedating drugs and neuromuscular blockade during mechanical ventilation (letter to the editor). *JAMA* 267:1775, 1992.

CHAPTER 18

Sedation: Intravenous Benzodiazepines in Critical Care Medicine

DAVID J. GREENBLATT, M.D.

The clinical term "sedation" refers to nonspecific CNS depression associated with a number of drug classes, including benzodiazepines, barbiturates, and ethanol. Sedation is also produced as a secondary pharmacologic effect by other drug classes having different primary actions. Most notable are the opiates, whose secondary sedative effects are often used in critical care medicine.

Of drug classes whose primary pharmacologic action is sedation, benzodiazepines are by far the most widely used in critical care medicine. Some barbiturates, such as the "short-acting" derivative thiopental, continue to be used to some degree, particularly in the context of preanesthetic induction. However, the benzodiazepine derivatives have the advantage of producing relatively less cardiovascular and respiratory depression than clinically equivalent doses of barbiturates (1–3). Furthermore, the capacity of benzodiazepines to produce physical dependence is considerably less than that of barbiturates (4), and the benzodiazepines do not produce hepatic microsomal enzyme induction during long-term use (5).

This chapter reviews the pharmacologic and pharmacokinetic properties of benzodiazepines used intravenously in the context of critical care medicine.

HISTORY OF BENZODIAZEPINES

Chlordiazepoxide (Librium) was the first benzodiazepine introduced into clinical practice in the year 1960 (2). Since that time, numerous derivatives have become available and are now widely used. Because benzodiazepines as a class are lipophilic (lipid-soluble) agents, the development of formulations suitable for parenteral administration has been a difficult problem. A parenteral formulation of chlordiazepoxide is available and can be administered intravenously (6, 7). However, intravenous chlordiazepoxide has never gained wide acceptance. The three parenterally available benzodiazepines now in common clinical use are: diazepam, lorazepam, and midazolam. Each has relative benefits and disadvantages.

MECHANISM OF ACTION

All benzodiazepine derivatives are presumed to exert their primary pharmacologic actin via interaction with a specific binding site termed the benzodiazepine receptor (8-10). This receptor is a high-affinity binding site found in human brain and in all mammalian systems studied to date. Receptor binding of "benzodiazepine-positive" agents (compounds having primary sedative, anxiolytic, and anticonvulsant effects) is closely linked with the binding to the same receptor complex of the endogenous neurotransmitter γ-aminobutyric acid (GABA). That is, benzodiazepine binding facilitates GABA binding, and vice versa. Receptor binding of benzodiazepines and/or GABA to this complex causes an opening of a chloride channel in the cell membrane. Chloride ions enter the cell and cause cell hyperpolarization. A more polarized cell is more difficult to depolarize, and the clinical result is the benzodiazepine agonist effect of sedation and the associated

Table 18.1. Characteristics of Benzodiazepines Used Intravenously in Critical Care Medicine[a]

Parent Drug	Metabolite of Potential Importance	Benzodiazepine Receptor K_i (nM)	Lipid Solubility Index (vs. Diazepam)	Usual Range of Elimination $t_{1/2}$ (hr)
Diazepam		9.57	1.00	20–70
	Desmethyldiazepam	5.58	0.79	36–90
Lorazepam		1.64	0.48	10–20
Midazolam		0.44	1.54	1–4
	1-Hydroxymidazolam	2.23	0.71	

[a] See refs. 11 and 14.

Table 18.2. Composition of Solvents Used for Parenteral Preparations of Benzodiazepines

Drug	Solvent Composition
Diazepam (5 mg/ml)	40% propylene glycol 10% ethyl alcohol 5% sodium benzoate/benzoic acid 1.5% benzyl alcohol
Midazolam (5 mg/ml, 1 mg/ml)	0.8% sodium chloride 0.1% disodium EDTA 1% benzyl alcohol pH adjusted to 3
Lorazepam (2 mg/ml, 4 mg/ml)	2.0% benzyl alcohol 0.18 ml polyethylene glycol-400 in propylene glycol per ml of injectable preparation.

events, including reduction of anxiety, anticonvulsant effects, transient amnesia, slowing of reaction time, slowed psychomotor performance, difficulty with visual accommodation, and ataxia.

When the intrinsic affinity of various benzodiazepines for the specific receptor site is measured using brain homogenates in vitro, very different quantitative results are obtained (Table 18.1). Of the three benzodiazepines used in critical care medicine, midazolam has the smallest affinity constant. This constant indicates that midazolam has high intrinsic affinity, since small molar amounts are needed to produce a given degree of receptor occupancy. Diazepam, in contrast, has a higher affinity constant, indicating lower intrinsic potency. Lorazepam falls in between. These differences in intrinsic potency do not indicate a difference in the qualitative character of the drug-receptor interaction. At a given degree of receptor occupancy, the character of the "benzodiazepine agonist" effects produced by all benzodiazepines is essentially identical. Quantitative differences in milligram potency are adjusted for in clinical practice by appropriate adjustments in total amount of drug administered. For example, higher absolute doses of diazepam, compared to those for midazolam or lorazepam, are needed to produce a given degree of clinical sedation.

Metabolic products of benzodiazepines, formed by hepatic biotransformation in vivo, must also be considered in evaluating overall clinical effects (11). Midazolam has two human metabolites, one of which may be of clinical importance (12, 13). However, the intrinsic receptor affinities of both metabolites are lower than the parent drug, and their uptake into brain tissue is relatively low (14). The principal metabolite of lorazepam (lorazepam glucuronide) appears to have essentially

no pharmacologic activity (15). Desmethyldiazepam, the major metabolite of diazepam, has intrinsic affinity higher than that of the parent drug (14). However, desmethyldiazepam is generated relatively slowly and acquires clinical importance only during multiple dosage with diazepam.

PHARMACOKINETIC PROPERTIES

Experimental studies indicate that the "driving force" for the interaction of a benzodiazepine with its receptor site is simply the amount of drug available to bind to the receptor (16). The extent of receptor occupancy is predictably related to the amount of drug present in brain. As whole brain concentrations increase or decrease, the degree of receptor occupancy and, subsequently, the degree of sedation change correspondingly. Brain concentrations of drug, in turn, depend on plasma concentrations, since uptake of drug from plasma into brain is a process determined largely by passive diffusion. For these reasons, pharmacokinetic differences among benzodiazepines are a major determinant of apparent differences in clinical action, even though intrinsic drug effects on the receptor site are similar or identical among the drugs.

IMPLICATIONS OF LIPID SOLUBILITY

All benzodiazepines are relatively lipid-soluble substances (11). One major consequence of this physicochemical property is the inherent difficulty in preparing a solution suitable for intravenous administration. Diazepam and lorazepam are available only in free base form, as opposed to a salt form. The parenteral preparation of both of these drugs contains a high concentration of the "oily" substance propylene glycol (Table 18.2). The diazepam solvent also contains ethyl alcohol, benzyl alcohol, and sodium benzoate/benzoic acid. This combination of solvents renders diazepam very irritating at local intravenous injection sites, causing local discomfort on injection and, sometimes, subsequent phlebitis. For this reason diazepam is recommended for intravenous injection into a large vein, and slow injection may be necessary to avoid local discomfort. The parenteral preparation of lorazepam has a lower fraction of lipoidal material but still can cause local pain and irritation after intravenous injection. Midazolam has the advantage of being available as a water-soluble salt, provided the pH of the injection solution is buffered to the acidic range. Since the injection solvent for midazolam is aqueous, local reactions at the injection site are relatively unusual. The characterization of midazolam as being "water-soluble" applies only to this injection preparation. Once buffered to physiologic pH in vivo, midazolam is a very lipid-soluble substance.

Although all benzodiazepines are lipophilic, there are considerable differences among the individual derivatives in relative lipid solubility (11). Diazepam and midazolam (in free base form) are highly lipid-soluble, whereas lorazepam has low or intermediate lipid solubility. These differences have important implications for in vivo intravenous administration.

ONSET OF ACTION: UPTAKE INTO BRAIN

After rapid intravenous injection of a benzodiazepine, the time of onset of activity, as well as the time to maximal activity, will depend on the rate of drug uptake into brain tissue. Because the blood-brain barrier is a lipoidal membrane system, drug diffusion across this barrier is facilitated by lipid solubility. Differences among benzodiazepines in lipid solubility have direct clinical implications in this context.

The time-course of benzodiazepine agonist effects after rapid intravenous injection has been compared under identical experimental conditions for diazepam, midazolam, and lorazepam (17, 18). CNS effects of all three drugs after 1-minute intravenous injections were quantitated by computer analysis of the EEG to determine the density of activity in the "benzodiazepine-responsive" frequency range of 13 to 30 cycles/sec. Lorazepam contrasted sharply with the other two drugs (Fig. 18.1). Even after rapid intravenous injection, the onset of action of lorazepam was relatively slow, with peak effects not attained until approximately 30 minutes after injection. The onset of activity of the other two drugs was much more rapid. Maximal effects of diazepam were reached almost immediately after the end of the injection. Midazolam also had a fast onset of action, but peak effects did not occur until approximately 5 minutes after the injection. Experimental studies strongly suggest that these differences correspond almost exactly to rates of drug entry into brain. In an animal model, actual measurement of diazepam and lorazepam concentrations in brain after intravenous injection showed differences closely corresponding to the time-course of clinical activity in humans (18–21).

These differences in onset of clinical activity indicate that intravenously administered benzodiazepines are not interchangeable. Diazepam is highly suited for clinical situations in which second-to-second titration of dosage and response is necessary. These situations might include intravenous administration for sedation prior to endoscopy or cardioversion, or for induction prior to general anesthesia. Lorazepam is not suited for these purposes but would be more useful for situations requiring longer duration of action, as opposed to immediate onset (22) (see below). Midazolam more closely resembles diazepam in its onset properties, but second-to-second titratability should not be anticipated. Several minutes should elapse to assess the effect of one dose of midazolam before the next dose is given.

DURATION OF ACTION: PERIPHERAL DISTRIBUTION

Lipid solubility also influences the duration of action of benzodiazepines after single intravenous doses. Disappearance of benzodiazepines from plasma following rapid intravenous injection generally follows a biphasic pattern (11). The initial rapid phase of drug disappearance corresponds to the process of drug distribution out of central compartment

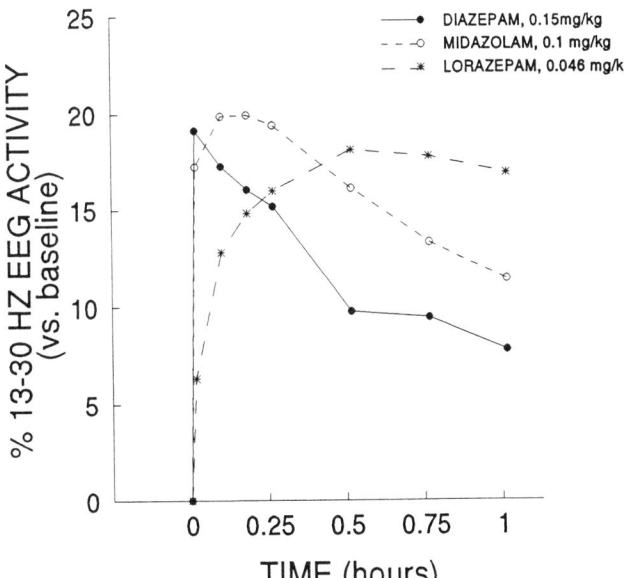

Figure 18.1. CNS effects of three different benzodiazepines as measured by the increase over predrug baseline in the percent of EEG amplitude falling in the frequency range of 13 to 30 cycles/sec. Medications were administered to healthy volunteer subjects by intravenous infusion into a peripheral vein over a period of 1 minute, beginning at time zero. For diazepam, effects were maximum at the end of the infusion. For midazolam, maximum effects were delayed until 5 minutes postinfusion. In the case of lorazepam, there was a 30- to 45-minute delay until CNS effects were maximal. (See references 17 and 18.)

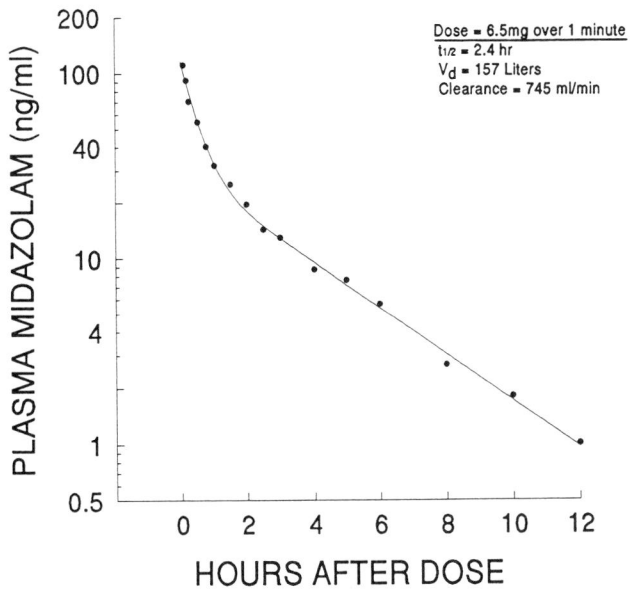

Figure 18.2. Plasma midazolam concentrations in a healthy male volunteer who received a 6.5-mg intravenous dose over a period of 1 minute. The *solid line* represents the fitted pharmacokinetic function. Based on this function, values of elimination half-life ($t^{1/2}$), volume of distribution (V_d), and clearance are shown.

tissues (including circulating blood and brain) into peripheral sites of distribution (including adipose tissue and muscle). The process of attainment of distribution equilibrium generally requires anywhere from 30 minutes to 4 hours. After distribution is complete, drug disappearance from plasma proceeds at a slower rate (Fig. 18.2) During this phase, irreversible hepatic biotransformation generally accounts for drug removal. Values for elimination half-life cited in the pharmacologic literature almost always refer to the half-life of drug disappearance in the postdistributive phase, after distribution equilibrium is complete. As such, elimination half-life may bear little relationship to the duration of drug action after single doses. The extensive decline in plasma concentrations due to distribution, on the other hand, often is the major determinant of the duration of action (23, 24) (Fig. 18.3).

In general, more lipid-soluble drugs have a greater extent of peripheral distribution than do drugs of lower lipid solubility. Diazepam has a much larger volume of distribution (after correction for protein binding) than does lorazepam, and the extent of distribution-related plasma level decline for diazepam is much greater than for lorazepam (18, 23).

CONTINUOUS INFUSION

A constant level of clinical sedation can theoretically be attained by continuous intravenous infusion of a benzodiazepine at a constant rate, termed a "zero-order" infusion. In practice, diazepam is not well-suited for this purpose, because of the long elimination half-life of diazepam and its major metabolite desmethyldiazepam. After initiation of a zero-order infusion of diazepam, attainment of the steady-state condition would require several days. Administration of a loading dose at the start of the infusion could reduce the time necessary to attain steady-state. However, drug elimination after the termination of the infusion, or attainment of a new steady-state after reduction of the infusion rate, would still require a number of days.

Because of its short elimination half-life, midazolam is well-suited to use by continuous infusion in critical care medicine (25–30). Loading doses are generally administered at the start of infusions to accelerate the attainment of steady-state (Fig. 18.4). Computer-controlled infusion pumps have been used to deliver the loading dose via continuously changing infusion rates rather than single rapid injections, thereby attaining steady-state more rapidly and directly.

An "effective" steady-state plasma concentration range for midazolam has not been established. As a general principle, steady-state plasma levels within a given individual will increase in direct proportion to the final infusion rate. However, at any given infusion rate, steady-state levels will change inversely with metabolic clearance, which is variable among individuals (Fig. 18.5). Unfortunately, midazolam clearance for a given patient cannot be accurately determined without a study of midazolam pharmacokinetics in that particular patient. In actual practice, some estimation and titration is needed. An initial "target" steady-state plasma level is chosen, and midazolam clearance is then estimated from published averages based on the patient's age, gender, weight, and degree of debility. The infusion rate is calculated as the product

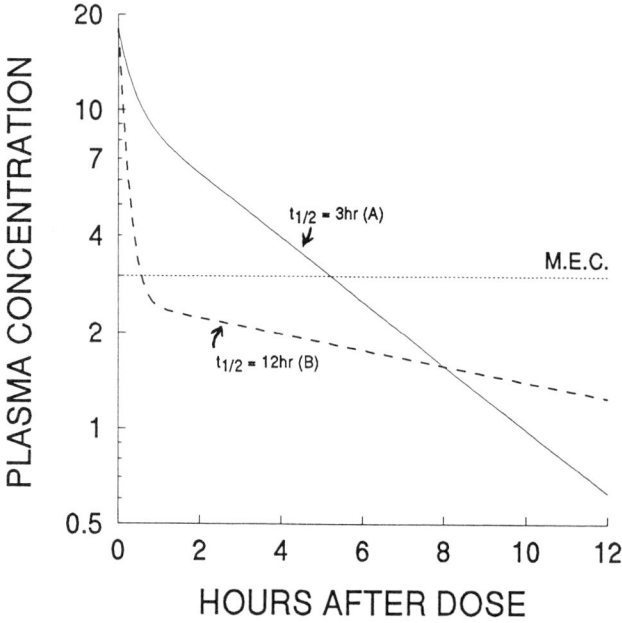

Figure 18.3. Computer-simulated pharmacokinetic functions for two drugs given by rapid intravenous injection. It is assumed that the dose of both drugs is the same and that both drugs have the same clearance. The only difference is that Drug B is more lipid-soluble than Drug A, such that the volume of distribution of Drug B is 4 times that of Drug A. This difference causes the elimination half-life of Drug B to be 4 times that of Drug A (12 hr vs. 3 hr). If the *horizontal dotted line* represents the minimum effective concentration (*M.E.C.*), then Drug B, despite its longer half-life, will have a shorter duration of clinical action than Drug A.

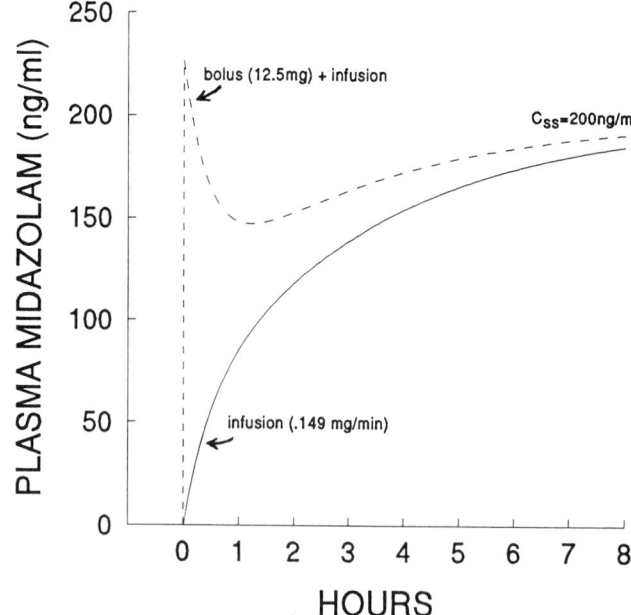

Figure 18.4. Plasma midazolam concentrations predicted by computer if the same volunteer as in Figure 18.2 were to receive a constant-rate infusion of midazolam, at a rate of 0.149 mg/min, starting at time zero. The predicted steady-state concentration (C_{ss}) is 200 ng/ml. If the infusion is started without a loading dose (*solid line*), there is a delay in attainment of steady-state. Administration of a loading dose coincident with the start of the infusion (*dashed line*) allows more rapid attainment of steady-state.

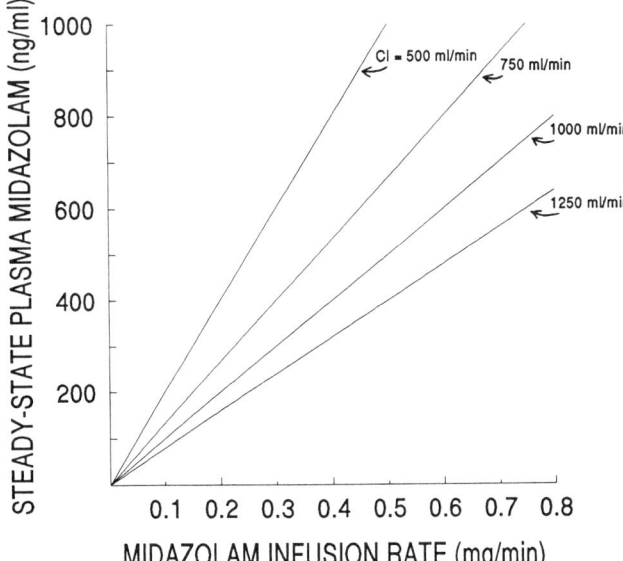

Figure 18.5. Nomogram showing the relation of midazolam infusion rate (*X* axis) to steady-state plasma midazolam concentration (*Y* axis) for various values of midazolam clearance (*Cl*).

of clearance and target steady-state plasma level. Infusion rates are subsequently adjusted after observation of clinical response.

HAZARDS AND ADVERSE REACTIONS

Adverse effects of benzodiazepines are attributable to their primary pharmacologic actions (1–3). Excessive plasma and brain concentrations of any benzodiazepine will produce excessive generalized CNS depression. The time-course and intensity of such effects depend on dosage, infusion rate, and the pharmacokinetic properties discussed above. As a class, benzodiazepines are among the safest of CNS-active medications with respect to their propensity to produce clinically important respiratory and cardiovascular dysfunction. Nonetheless, excessive CNS depression due to high plasma and brain concentrations of benzodiazepines can be accompanied by respiratory and cardiovascular depression in susceptible individuals.

Use of pharmacokinetic principles to guide administration of parenteral benzodiazepines can reduce the likelihood of excessive or prolonged CNS depression. For example, upward titration of midazolam dosage should be done with the knowledge that the maximum sedative effect of a given intravenous bolus dose will be delayed from 5 to 10 minutes after the injection is complete. In the case of lorazepam, maximum effects of an intravenous dose can be delayed up to 30 minutes after dosage. In the phase of recovery from intravenous sedation, recovery from midazolam-induced sedation should be relatively rapid due to its high clearance and large volume of distribution. The reverse is true for lorazepam-sedative effects of intravenous administration may persist for many hours after dosage.

Treatment of excessive CNS depression due to benzodiazepines is conservative and supportive. All manifestations should be completely reversible, as the active compounds are removed from the central receptor site by distribution and clearance. The benzodiazepine receptor "antagonist" flumazenil can be administered in unusual clinical situations in which CNS effects of benzodiazepines need to be reversed on an urgent basis (31–33). However, it should be cautioned that flumazenil has a high clearance and short half-life in humans. The effects of a single dose of flumazenil are likely to be of short duration, and CNS depression may recur as the antagonist is cleared.

COMMENT

Intravenously administered benzodiazepines are highly useful sedative/amnestic agents in critical care medicine, whether administered by discrete injection, continuous infusion, or a combination of the two. Understanding of dose-concentration-response relationships, and the use of objective numerical response measures (such as the computer-analyzed EEG) (13, 17, 18, 26, 30, 34–38), has increased substantially during the last decade and should enhance the ability of clinicians to utilize these drugs for maximum clinical benefit.

ACKNOWLEDGMENT

Supported, in part, by Grant MH-34223 from the Department of Health and Human Services.

REFERENCES

1. Kanto J, Klotz U: Intravenous benzodiazepines as anaesthetic agents: pharmacokinetics and clinical consequences. *Acta Anaesth Scand* 26:554–569, 1982.
2. Greenblatt DJ, Shader RI: *Benzodiazepines in Clinical Practice*. Raven Press, New York, 1974.
3. Greenblatt DJ, Shader RI, Abernethy DR: Current status of benzodiazepines. *N Engl J Med* 309:354–358, 410–416, 1983.
4. Woods JH, Katz JL, Winger G: Abuse liability of benzodiazepines. *Pharmacol Rev* 39:251–419, 1987.
5. Greenblatt DJ, Shader RI: Long-term administration of benzodiazepines: pharmacokinetic versus pharmacodynamic tolerance. *Psychopharmacol Bull* 22:416–423, 1986.
6. Greenblatt DJ, Shader RI, Franke K, MacLaughlin DS, Ransil BJ, Koch-Weser J: Kinetics of intravenous chlordiazepoxide: sex differences in drug distribution. *Clin Pharmacol Ther* 22:893–903, 1977.
7. Greenblatt DJ, Shader RI, MacLeod SM, Sellers EM: Clinical pharmacokinetics of chlordiazepoxide. *Clin Pharmacokinet* 3:381–394, 1978.
8. Haefely WE: The GABA$_A$-benzodiazepine receptor: biology and pharmacology. In *Handbook of Anxiety, Vol. 3: The Neurobiology of Anxiety.* Burrows GD, Roth M, and Noyes Jr. R, (eds): Elsevier Science Publishers B.V. (Biomedical Division), Amsterdam, 1990, pp. 165–188.
9. Zorumski CF, Isenberg KE: Insights into the structure and function of GABA-benzodiazepine receptors: ion channels and psychiatry. *Am J Psychiatry* 148:162–173, 1991.
10. Miller LG, Greenblatt DJ: Neurochemistry of the benzodiazepines. In Watson RR, (ed): *Drugs of Abuse and Neurobiology.* CRC Press, Boca Raton, FL, 1992, pp. 182.
11. Greenblatt DJ, Shader RI: Pharmacokinetics of antianxiety agents. In Meltzer HY (ed): *Psychopharmacology: The Third Generation of Progress.* Raven Press, New York, 1987, pp. 1377–1386.
12. Reves JG, Fragen RJ, Vinik HR, Greenblatt DJ: Midazolam: pharmacology and uses. *Anesthesiology* 62:310–324, 1985.
13. Mandema JW, Tuk B, van Steveninck AL, Breimer DD, Cohen AF, Danhof M: Pharmacokinetic-pharmacodynamic modeling of the central nervous system effects of midazolam and its main metabolite α-hydroxymidazolam in healthy volunteers. Clin Pharmacol Ther 51:715–728, 1992.
14. Arendt RM, Greenblatt DJ, Liebisch DC, Luu MD, Paul SM: Determinants of benzodiazepine brain uptake: lipophilicity versus binding affinity. Psychopharmacology 93:72–76, 1987.
15. Greenblatt DJ: Clinical pharmacokinetics of oxazepam and lorazepam. *Clin Pharmacokin* 6:88–105, 1981.

16. Miller LG, Greenblatt DJ, Paul SM, Shader RI: Benzodiazepine receptor occupancy in vivo: correlation with brain concentrations and pharmacodynamic actions. J Pharmacol Exp Ther 240:516–522, 1987.

17. Greenblatt DJ, Ehrenberg BL, Gunderman J, Locniskar A, Scavone JM, Harmatz JS, Shader RI: Pharmacokinetic and electroencephalographic study of intravenous diazepam, midazolam, and placebo. *Clin Pharmacol Ther* 45:356–365, 1989.

18. Greenblatt DJ, Ehrenberg BL, Gunderman J, Scavone JM, Tai NT, Harmatz JS, Shader RI: Kinetic and dynamic study of intravenous lorazepam: comparison with intravenous diazepam. *J Pharmacol Exp Ther* 250:134–140, 1989.

19. Jack ML, Colburn WA, Spirt NM, Bautz G, Zanko M, Horst WD, O'Brien RA: A pharmacokinetic/pharmacodynamic/receptor binding model to predict the onset and duration of pharmacological activity of the benzodiazepines. *Prog Neuro-Psychopharmacol Biol Psychiatry* 7:629–635, 1983.

20. Greenblatt DJ, Sethy VH: Benzodiazepine concentrations in brain directly reflect receptor occupancy: studies of diazepam, lorazepam, and oxazepam. *Psychopharmacology* 102:373–378, 1990.

21. Walton NY, Treiman DM: Lorazepam treatment of experimental status epilepticus in the rat: relevance to clinical practice. *Neurology* 40:990–994, 1990.

22. Ameer B, Greenblatt DJ: Lorazepam: a review of its clinical pharmacological properties and therapeutic uses. *Drugs* 21:161–200, 1981.

23. Greenblatt DJ, Divoll M: Diazepam versus lorazepam: relationship of drug distribution to duration of clinical action. In *Status Epilepticus: Mechanisms of Brain Damage and Treatment* (Advances in Neurology, Volume 34) Delgado-Escueta AV, Wasterlain CG, Treman DM, Porter RI, (eds): Raven Press, New York, 1983, pp. 487–491.

24. Arendt RM, Greenblatt DJ, deJong RH, Bonin JD, Abernethy DR, Ehrenberg BL, Giles HG, Sellers EM, Shader RI: In vitro correlates of benzodiazepine cerebrospinal fluid uptake, pharmacodynamic action, and peripheral distribution. *J Pharmacol Exp Ther* 227:95–106, 1983.

25. Lauven PM, Schwilden H, Stoeckel H, Greenblatt DJ: The effects of a benzodiazepine antagonist Ro15-1788 in the presence of stable concentrations of midazolam. *Anesthesiology* 63:61–64, 1985.

26. Lauven PM, Stoeckel H, Schwilden H: A pharmacokinetically-based infusion model for midazolam. *Anaesthetist* 31:15–20, 1982.

27. Persson MP, Nilsson A, Hartvig P: Relation of sedation and amnesia to plasma concentrations of midazolam in surgical patients. *Clin Pharmacol Ther* 43:324–331, 1988.

28. Allonen H, Ziegler G, Klotz U: Midazolam kinetics. *Clin Pharmacol Ther* 30:653–661, 1981.

29. Persson P, Nilsson A, Hartvig P, Tamsen A: Pharmacokinetics of midazolam in total I.V. anaesthesia. *Br J Anaesth* 59:548–556, 1987.

30. Klotz U, Ziegler G, Ludwig L, Reimann IW: Pharmacodynamic interaction between midazolam and a specific benzodiazepine antagonist in humans. *J Clin Pharmacol* 25:400–406, 1985.

31. Brogden RN, Goa KL: Flumazenil. A preliminary review of its benzodiazepine antagonist properties, intrinsic activity and therapeutic use. *Drugs* 35:448–467, 1988.

32. Nilsson A, Persson MP, Hartvig P: Effects of the benzodiazepine antagonist flumazenil on postoperative performance following total intravenous anaesthesia with midazolam and alfentanil. *Acta Anaesthesiol Scand* 32:441–446, 1988.

33. Riishede L, Krogh B, Nielsen JL, Freuchen I, Mikkelsen BO: Reversal of flunitrazepam sedation with flumazenil. A randomized clinical trial. *Acta Anaesthesiol Scand* 32:433–436, 1988.

34. Breimer LTM, Hennis PJ, Burm AGL, Danhof M, Bovill JG, Spierdijk J, Vletter AA: Quantification of the EEG effect of midazolam by aperiodic analysis in volunteers. Pharmacokinetic/pharmacodynamic modelling. *Clin Pharmacokinet* 18:245–253, 1990.

35. Veselis RA, Reinsel R, Alagesan R, Heino R, Bedford RF: The EEG as a monitor of midazolam amnesia: changes in power and topography as a function of amnesic state. *Anesthesiology* 74:866–874, 1991.

36. Bührer M, Maitre PO, Hung O, Stanski DR: Electroencephalographic effects of benzodiazepines. I. Choosing an electroencephalographic parameter to measure the effect of midazolam on the central nervous system. *Clin Pharmacol Ther* 48:544–554, 1990.

37. Bührer M, Maitre PO, Crevoisier C, Stanski DR: Electroencephalographic effects of benzodiazepines. II. Pharmacodynamic modeling of the electroencephalographic effects of midazolam and diazepam. *Clin Pharmacol Ther* 48:555–567, 1990.

38. Herkes GK, Wszolek ZK, Westmoreland BF, Klass DW: Effects of midazolam on electroencephalograms of seriously ill patients. *Mayo Clin Proc* 67:334–338, 1992.

CHAPTER 19

Use and Administration of Blood and Components

NAOMI L.C. LUBAN, M.D.
LOUIS DePALMA, M.D.

Modern transfusion therapy entails the process of fractionation of whole blood into various blood components to give patients the specific part of blood that they need most. The appropriate use of blood and its components is essential to the management of the critically ill patient. The composition of various blood components (Table 19.1), indications and contraindications for their use, potential adverse effects, and appropriate administration and dosage are delineated. In addition, alternatives to blood transfusion, as well as the utilization of autologous blood transfusion, are described.

BLOOD COMPONENTS AND DERIVATIVES

WHOLE BLOOD

A unit of whole blood has an approximate volume of 500 ml. It is composed of red blood cells, nonviable leukocytes and platelets, plasma, and an anticoagulant-preservative. Whole blood has a hematocrit ranging between 35 and 40% and must be stored between 1°C and 6°C in a monitored refrigerator. The shelf-life of the unit of whole blood is dependent on the anticoagulant used. Blood collected in citrate-phosphate-dextrose (CPD) can be stored for up to 21 days, while the preservative CPD adenine-1 (CPDA-1) allows storage for 35 days.

Whole blood serves both as a volume expander and as a source of red blood cells. Whole blood should be reserved for briskly bleeding patients who require both volume expansion, as well as oxygen-carrying capacity (1). It is also indicated

in the rare circumstances where one or more blood volumes are to be exchanged and in selected cases of cardiovascular bypass pump priming, particularly in neonates. It is contraindicated in patients with chronic anemia who are normovolemic; while whole blood contains plasma coagulation proteins, it is deficient in labile coagulation factors V and VIII (2). Adverse reactions that may occur following the transfusion of whole blood are similar to those adverse reactions that occur with other blood components (Table 19.2). These transfusion-related problems include hemolytic, allergic, and febrile reactions, as well as circulatory overload and transfusion-transmitted infectious diseases (Table 19.3).

Whole blood must be ABO identical with the recipient and must be administered through a blood filter. The infusion time should not exceed 4 hours. Each unit of whole blood should increase the hemoglobin concentration of a 70-kg adult by 1 g/dl or the hematocrit by 3%.

RED BLOOD CELL PRODUCTS

Red Blood cells, also referred to as packed red blood cells (PRBC), are prepared from whole blood following centrifugation or sedimentation. PRBC units have a volume of 250 ml, a hematocrit of 70 to 80%, and consist of 120 to 180 ml of PRBCs in 70 to 100 ml of plasma. Removal of most of the plasma during preparation reduces the amount of anticoagulant solution, lactic acid, and other plasma analytes and also reduces the isoagglutinins anti-A and/or anti-B present in

327

Table 19.1. Blood Components and Indications

Components	Major Indications	Precautions
Whole blood	Symptomatic anemia and hypovolemia	Must be ABO-identical
Red blood cells	Symptomatic anemia	Must be ABO-compatible
Red blood cells Leukocytes removed (centrifugation or filtration)	Symptomatic anemia, febrile reactions from leukocyte antibodies, prevention of CMV[a] (?)	Must be ABO-compatible
Red blood cells, washed	Symptomatic anemia, febrile and/or allergic reactions, prevention of CMV (?)	Must be ABO-compatible, component expires 24 hours after washing procedure
Fresh frozen plasma	Deficit of labile and stable plasma coagulation factors	Should be ABO-compatible
Platelets, random	Bleeding of thrombocytopenia or platelet function abnormality	Should be ABO-compatible
Platelets, pheresis (HLA-matched)	Same as above, plus presence of anti-HLA or platelet-specific antibodies	Should be ABO-compatible
Granulocytes	Neutropenia with infection	Must be ABO-compatible
Cryoprecipitate	von Willebrand's disease, Hemophilia A, Hypofibrogenemia, Factor XIII deficiency	Close laboratory monitoring of Factor VIII, VWF, as well as fibrinogen, is necessary

[a] CMV, cytomegalovirus; HLA, human leukocyte antigen; VWF, von Willebrand factor.

Table 19.2. Adverse Reactions to Blood Components and Derivatives

Type	Cause	Prevention
Acute hemolytic	Immunologic (ABO, alloantibody) or nonimmunologic (mechanical, overheating of blood, use of hypotonic solutions)	Appropriate patient identification, use of monitored blood warmers, use of 0.9% sodium chloride only, appropriate storage conditions
Acute febrile nonhemolytic	Antibody to leukocyte or platelet antigens	Premedication with antipyretics, slow rate of infusion. In repetitive or severe cases; use of filtered components
Pulmonary hypersensitivity (noncardiogenic pulmonary edema)	HLA or antileukocyte or platelet antibodies	Washed or filtered cells
Allergic	IgE- and IgG-mediated sensitivity to plasma proteins	Premedicate with diphenhydramine
Anaphylaxis	IgA deficiency with presence of IgG, anti-IgA antibody	Washed cells or use of IgA deficient plasma
Bacterial contamination	Improper collection or storage of blood or components	Use of proper techniques of storage
Viral	Hepatitis B, C, HIV, CMV, EBV,[a] HTLV-1, others	Decreased use of unnecessary blood components, appropriate use of screening donors and serologic testing
Graft-versus-host disease	Transfusion of viable immunocompetent lymphocytes into an immunoincompetent host	Irradiation of blood components

[a] EBV, Epstein-Barr virus; HTLV-1, human T cell lymphotropic virus-1, HIV, human immunodeficiency virus.

the donor plasma. When additive solutions such as Adsol, Nutricel, or Optisol are used as the anticoagulant, the hematocrit is reduced to 50 to 60%. The viscosity of these red blood cells is reduced; hence, their flow rate is more rapid than that of standard PRBCs. It is important to know what type of anticoagulant has been used in order to assess the adequacy of the posttransfusion hematocrit increment; if additive anticoagulants are used, the posttransfusion hematocrit increment will be less than when packed red blood cells without an additive anticoagulant are used.

Other red blood cell preparations include leukopoor, washed, and frozen deglycerolized red blood cells. Leukopoor PRBCs are prepared by a number of different techniques. Leukopoor products have been modified to remove at least 70% of the original leukocytes, although most of the currently used techniques remove more. The use of so-called third generation in-line and bedside filters to produce leukopoor red cells has been recently reviewed (3); such filters remove as much as 95% of leukocytes. These filters should not be confused with either standard 170 μm filters or the so-called microaggregate blood filters.

Cells may be washed in either automated cell washers (Cobe 2991, Haemonetics V50) or by using manual techniques. Washing removes 70 to 90% of leukocytes, as well as much of the original plasma, platelets, anticoagulant, and microaggregates. Red blood cells may be cryopreserved using one of two methods that employ glycerol as a cryoprotectant. Deglycerolization requires thawing and washing, employing automated cell washers. Frozen, deglycerolized red cells are virtually free of white blood cells, platelets, plasma, anticoagulant solution, microaggregates, and, if frozen within hours of collection, have high levels of 2,3-diphosphoglycerate (DPG) and adenosine triphosphate (ATP). As with washed red blood cells, deglycerolized cells have the disadvantage of a 24-hour expiration interval once they have been manipulated by washing. Deglycerolized, washed cells of rare blood cell phenotype can be refrozen for future use but with loss of red blood cell number and decreased in vivo survival.

PRBCs are indicated to restore red blood cell mass and to prevent or to treat shock. They are particularly useful when it is difficult to assess the rate of volume depletion, demands on oxygen delivery, and cardiopulmonary reserve of the patient. Their use is contraindicated in compensated anemias and when the anemia can be treated with hematinics like iron, folic acid, and vitamin B_{12}. PRBCs are also indicated in patients with symptomatic anemia to increase oxygen delivery. They can be used with crystalloid solutions in surgical patients to replace operative losses of five to six units of blood. Specialized leukopoor PRBCs are indicated in patients who have recurrent or severe febrile transfusion reactions not prevented by pretransfusion antipyretics. These reactions develop secondary to the development of antileukocyte antibodies; these antibodies may be antineutrophil-specific but are most often anti-HLA specific and usually occur in previously pregnant females or in individuals who have had repeated transfusions. These specially prepared red blood cell products have several characteristics in common: they require more time to prepare; they are more costly; they must be transfused within 24 hours of preparation; and they result in some red blood cell loss. Frozen deglycerolized PRBCs are indicated in those patients with high-incidence red blood cell alloantibodies requiring blood of rare phenotype available from rare donor registries, in those patients who have IgA deficiency to avoid anaphylaxis

secondary to recipient anti-IgA antibodies, and in those patients with recurrent febrile reactions to transfusion despite pretransfusion medication with antipyretics or leukoreduction by more common methods.

Several formulas can be used to predict hemoglobin increments in transfused patients. In the setting of the ICU, hemoglobin and hematocrit determinations frequently do not adequately reflect ongoing losses. On the other hand, the ICU setting permits close observation and quantitation of those physiologic mechanisms that compensate for blood loss, result in increased oxygen demands, and reflect oxygen delivery.

Red Blood Cell Transfusion Formulas

(1) 6 ml of whole blood/kg of body weight increases the hemoglobin by 1 g/dl.
(2) 3 ml of packed red blood cells/kg of body weight increases the hemoglobin by 1g/dl.
(3) *ml of blood to be transfused =*

$$\frac{(wt\ in\ kg)(blood\ volume\ in\ ml/kg)(desired\ Hb - actual\ Hb)}{22\ g/dl}$$

where by 3 months of age an infant's blood volume is 70 to 75 ml/kg and where 22 g/dl is the average hemoglobin of a PRBC unit.

PLATELETS

A unit of random donor platelets is prepared by centrifugation of a whole blood unit within 8 hours of collection. The supernatant platelet-rich plasma undergoes a second centrifugation step at higher centrifugal force, resulting in a cell-free plasma component used in the manufacturing of plasma by products. When the platelet pellet is resuspended in 50 to 75 ml of residual plasma, it is called a platelet concentrate. Each platelet concentrate contains 0.7 to 0.9×10^{11} platelets (minimum 5.5×10^{10}) in 50 to 75 ml of plasma. The volume of plasma is critical to maintenance of a pH of 6.0 and greater in the platelet container. Platelets are stored at 22°C on a mechanical rotator to ensure their viability and may be stored for up to 5 days. Single-donor platelets are obtained by plateletpheresis, using any one of several automated blood cell processors. Depending upon the number of blood volumes cycled through the apheresis machine, 6 to 12 units of platelet concentrate in 200 to 300 ml of plasma may be collected. Each plateletpheresis component contains at least 3×10^{11} platelets. They are collected in sterile systems that permit 5-day storage, although occasionally plateletpheresis components with a 24-hour outdate may be provided; they are also stored at 22°C on a mechanical rotator. For selected pediatric patients, a plateletpheresis unit can be sterilely separated into three or more bags, providing a single-donor product for the 5-day life of the product; a sterile connecting device is needed to ensure sterility. The degree of red blood cell and white blood cell contamination varies according to the technique and the machine used. Platelets have an in vivo survival of 9 to 10 days and are hemostatically effective for 3 to 5 days.

Platelets are indicated for quantitative and qualitative platelet disorders. They are used to prevent hemorrhage and

Table 19.3. Transfusion-Transmitted Infectious Diseases

Disease	Cause
AIDS	HIV-1, HIV-2
Tropical spastic paraparesis/ HTLV-associated myelopathy	HTLV-1, HTLV-II
HTLV-associated adult T-cell leukemia/lymphoma?	HTLV-I
Hepatitis A	HAV[a]
Hepatitis B	HBV
Non A-, non-B hepatitis (hepatitis C)	HCV
Cytomegalovirus infection	CMV
Epstein-Barr virus infection	EBV
Syphilis	*Treponema pallidum*
Malaria	*Plasmodium malariae, P. ovale, P. vivax, P. falciparum*
Lyme disease (?)	*Borrelia burgdorferi*
Babesiosis	*Babesia microti*
Trypanosomiasis	*Trypanosoma cruzi*
Toxoplasmosis	*Toxoplasma gondii*
Filariasis	Various species
Various bacterial diseases	*Pseudomonas aeruginosa, Yersinia enterocolitica, Escherichia coli, etc.*

[a] HAV, hepatitis A virus; HBV, hepatitis B virus; HCV, hepatitis C virus; EBV, Epstein-Barr virus.

to stop or attenuate ongoing bleeding. Clinical factors to be considered prior to platelet transfusion include the primary diagnosis of the patient; the chance for marrow recovery and adequate platelet production; presence of fever; splenomegaly; sepsis; ongoing oozing or bleeding, which would increase consumption of platelets; and use of antibiotics or drugs, which might induce platelet dysfunction. The decision to use platelets must be based on an assessment of these factors, as there are no prospective studies to guide the intensivist. Single-donor platelets are used when alloantigen exposure needs to be kept at a minimum (e.g., aplastic anemia patients prior to bone marrow transplantation) or when platelets with a known HLA antigen phenotype are required (e.g., patients with anti-HLA antibodies).

A platelet count of 50,000/mm³ appears to be adequate for hemostasis, as has been supported by the adult oncologic literature (4). Even major abdominal surgery can be performed with platelet counts in this range, if there is no other coagulopathy (5). Platelet counts between 20,000 and 30,000/mm³ are usually an indication for platelet transfusion, although many patients with platelets in this range will not bleed, especially if the marrow is recovering and producing young, large, sticky platelets (6). However, clinical judgment must be used, especially in the patient with additional factors that might predispose to hemorrhage, in those patients undergoing invasive neurosurgical or general surgical procedures such as liver biopsy, and in those patients who are septic or who have rapidly falling counts. Such individuals may or may not require transfusion to bring their platelet count to above 50,000/mm³. Similarly, there are no guidelines that help establish platelet counts above which it is safe to perform less invasive procedures like bone marrow aspiration, lumbar puncture, venous or arterial catheterization, or endotracheal intubation.

Clinical judgment and knowledge of the cause for both the thrombocytopenia and the bleeding is essential. For example, antibody-mediated idiopathic thrombocytopenic purpura (ITP) is frequently associated with profound thrombocytopenia (platelets < 10,000/mm³). Patients having this diagnosis will not benefit from platelet transfusions because the transfused platelets are complexed with antibody and rapidly removed from the circulation by the reticuloendothelial system, sometimes within minutes of transfusion (6). Platelet transfusion in this circumstance should be reserved only for life-threatening hemorrhage along with other therapeutic modalities.

The use of prophylactic platelet transfusions is very controversial, and few studies have been performed in children (7, 8). Their use is limited to otherwise stable patients with leukemia, with solid tumors, or bone marrow transplant recipients with severe thrombocytopenia (< 15,000 to 20,000/mm³), who are expected not to make platelets because of their therapy. If platelet counts are dropping rapidly, or if there is an increased risk of hemorrhage from concomitant illness, prophylactic transfusions might be indicated for a specific period of time (9, 10).

Patients who have been massively transfused (i.e., who receive more than one blood volume in 24 hours) and in whom more than one blood volume has been replaced in a relatively short time may suffer from thrombocytopenia. In these patients, there is a combination of loss of endogenous platelets and dilution from use of both banked blood devoid of functioning platelets, as well as crystalloid or colloid solutions. Studies in both adults (11) and children (12) demonstrate an inverse relationship between platelet counts and blood volume transfused, but the decrease in platelet count is less than predicted from published wash-out formulae. These studies suggest that there is mobilization of platelets from endogenous sources, most likely, the spleen. In one study of massive trauma in children, the initial platelet count was a predictor of the need for platelet transfusion; only 3 of 26 patients had excessive bleeding requiring platelet transfusion, and each patient had an initial platelet count of less than 50,000/mm³. Some trauma transfusion algorithms recommend routine prophylactic use of platelets. One should not transfuse platelet concentrates based on number of units of red blood cells transfused, as many patients will not bleed despite low counts. Use of formulae may be helpful, however, in determining when platelet transfusion will be necessary based on the initial platelet count of the patient who has been massively transfused (13).

Cardiopulmonary bypass induces platelet dysfunction and is associated with thrombocytopenia. The thrombocytopenia may develop because of platelet adhesion to the cardiotomy reservoir and bypass circuitry and because of consumption at the surgical site. Platelet counts rarely fall below the number considered hemostatic, so that bleeding not considered to be "surgical" bleeding is more likely related to a functional defect or to fibrinolysis. Following bypass, the relationship between platelet count and bleeding time has been shown to be disparate, with prolonged bleeding times at platelet counts of greater than 100,000/mm³; this finding is likely due to release of α-granules and dense bodies from the platelet (14, 15). Platelet transfusions would be indicated in such circumstances where platelet dysfunction was proven or suspected following the bypass procedure.

PLATELET TRANSFUSION FORMULAE

Most formulae have been developed for adults. The effective posttransfusion platelet count will depend upon the size of the patient, number of platelets per unit, and complicating clinical factors. For these reasons, the corrected count increment (CCI) is more helpful in assessing posttransfusion effectiveness than the platelet count alone (10).

$$CCI = \frac{\text{Post-transfusion platelet count} - \text{Pretransfusion platelet count} \times BSA}{\text{No. of platelets in units} \times 10^{11}}$$

The CCI should be measured 1 hour after a platelet transfusion. Clinically stable patients have CCIs of 20,000 to 32,000/mm³ 1 hour after transfusion. Other formulae which may be useful are listed below:

$$\text{Expected increment} = \frac{2}{3} \frac{([0.7 \times 10^{11}] \times n)}{BV}$$

where 2/3 = corrects for splenic sequestration; n = number of platelet units; BSA = body surface area (in m²); and BV = blood volume in microliters. One unit of platelet concentrate per 10 kilograms body weight should increase the platelet count by 10,000/mm³, and one unit of platelet concentrate per m² should raise the platelet count by 5,000 to 8,000/mm³.

Poor CCIs may indicate the presence of anti-HLA, as well as antiplatelet specific antibodies. Platelets from an HLA-matched donor (plateletpheresis) are indicated when anti-HLA antibodies are documented. Platelet counts obtained 12 to 24 hours following platelet transfusion reflect platelet survival rather than adequacy of the platelet transfusion.

ABO antigens are present on platelets and may have relevance to the effectiveness of platelet transfusion. There are conflicting data concerning the survival of ABO incompatible platelets. ABO matching can improve the response to platelet transfusions (16, 17). Another concern in infants and young children is the transfusion of isoagglutinins A and B present in the plasma of the platelet concentrate. Sufficient anti-A and/or anti-B may be present in plasma to produce a positive direct Coombs test or hemolysis of recipient RBCs (18). Rh antigens are not present on the platelet membrane, so anti-Rh antibody should not affect platelet survival. However, red blood cells are present in platelet concentrates as a "contaminant" of the preparation of platelets and have caused Rh sensitization.

Whenever possible, ABO-compatible platelets should be administered. If ABO-incompatible platelets are to be administered and the blood group and transfusion needs of the patient are such that large volumes of incompatible plasma will be transfused, the platelets should be pooled, volume reduced, and platelets resuspended in a reduced volume (19). Following plasma reduction, the component must not be stored long-term, as platelet viability deteriorates due to high platelet counts and the limited amount of buffering capacity of the residual plasma.

If Rh-positive platelet components are to be administered to Rh-negative females, Rh immunoglobulin should be used to prevent alloimmunization, secondary to the pressure of Rh-positive red cells. The dose necessary can be calculated as follows:

Quantity of red blood cells in platelet concentrate = Volume(ml) × hematocrit of platelet concentrate = Volume RBC (in ml) per concentrate

Usual hematocrit of one platelet concentrate is 0.25%

Two other formulae that may be useful are:

No. of platelet concentrates transfused × 0.5 ml = RBC transfused per transfusion episode

No. of vials needed =
$$\frac{Volume\ of\ blood\ component \times Hct\ of\ infused\ product}{15}$$

A standard dose (300 μg) vial is protective for up to 15 ml of red blood cells, while a microdose vial (50 μg) can be used for 2.5 ml of red blood cells.

PLASMA AND PLASMA PRODUCTS

Plasma is prepared from whole blood during the preparation of either red blood cells or platelet concentrates. To be labelled as fresh frozen plasma (FFP), plasma must be separated from the red blood cells and stored at −18°C within 8 hours of collection. It may be stored frozen for 1 year, and once thawed it must be transfused within 24 hours. Single-donor plasma is plasma that has been separated on or before the fifth day after the expiration date of a unit of whole blood. Alternately, some blood banks stock frozen plasma that has been frozen up to 24 hours after collection; preliminary studies indicate that there is no appreciable difference in coagulation factors in plasma held before freezing for either 8 or 24 hours (2).

Cryoprecipitated antihemophiliac factor (AHF) is the cold-insoluble portion of plasma remaining after FFP has been thawed between 1 and 6° and then refrozen. It is most commonly known as cryoprecipitate. Each bag of 20 to 40 ml contains 80 units of Factor VIII and between 100 and 350 mg of fibrinogen; these bags are frequently referred to as "units" of cryoprecipitate, confusing those individuals trying to order units of Factor VIII activity. Cryoprecipitate also contains Factor VIII: vWF (von Willebrand factor) and fibronectin, an opsonic protein that aids in phagocytosis of particulate debris. There are no standards for the quantity of either of these two proteins in the manufacture of cryoprecipitate. Once thawed, cryoprecipitate should be transfused within 4 hours.

An NIH consensus conference has evaluated the indications for use of fresh frozen plasma (20). FFP is one of the most inappropriately used blood components. FFP is indicated for deficiency of plasma proteins when no other more specific factor concentrates are available. Examples include congenital deficiencies of Factors II, V, VII, X, and XI; antithrombin III; Protein C; and Protein S. Adequate replacement of Factor II and XI may be difficult with the volumes of plasma necessary to achieve greater than 50% concentration in homozygous deficiencies. FFP is most commonly used to treat multiple coagulation deficiencies, such as might occur in patients with liver disease, fat-soluble vitamin K deficiency due to malabsorption, biliary disease, starvation (when coumarin anticoagulants are used), or when disseminated intravascular coagulation has developed. Other less common indications include provision of C1 esterase inhibitor in patients with hereditary angioedema and in patients with hemolytic uremic syndrome, and thrombotic thrombocytopenic purpura as a simple transfusion or as part of plasma exchange (21). FFP should not be used as a volume expander or to replace trace minerals, as the risk from transfusion-transmitted diseases is as great as with cellular products; use of albumin or plasma protein fractions, which are pasteurized, or crystalloid, which has no viral transmission risk, are preferable.

The appropriate volumes or FFP in milliliters for treatment of single-coagulation deficiencies are easy to calculate. Calculations are based on the assumption that there is 1 ml of factor activity for each milliliter of FFP. For most factor deficiencies, 30% of factor activity is sufficient for hemostasis, but a higher percentage of factor activity would be required for invasive surgical procedures and major hemorrhage, such as central nervous system hemorrhage. Factor VIII and IX deficiencies are most often treated with lyophilized factor concentrates that are heat-treated, solvent-detergent treated, or monoclonally prepared. Because the risk of viral transmission is reduced through these processes, even mild deficiencies of Factors VIII and IX requiring treatment might benefit from commercial concentrates instead of multiple plasma infusions.

The amount of Factor V required for replacement in a Factor V-deficient patient with 5% Factor V who requires surgery at 30% Factor V can be calculated as follows:

(a) *Weight in kilograms* × *70 ml/kg = blood volume in ml*
(b) *Blood volume in ml* × *(1.0 − hematocrit) = plasma volume in ml*
(c) *Plasma volume (ml)* × *(desired Factor V μm/ml − initial Factor V Um/ml) = units Factor V*

Specifics: 35 kilogram child × *70 ml/kg = 2450 ml blood volume*
2450 × *(1.0 − 0.4) = 1470 ml plasma volume*
1470 × *(0.3 − 0.05) = 370 units of Factor V*
1 unit factor activity per milliliter of plasma means that 370 ml of plasma would need to be infused.

One also needs to know the half-life of transfused factor to plan the next infusion dose (see reference 22). Measurement of the specific factor is helpful in monitoring transfusion frequency, as active consumption or ongoing blood loss will decrease the expected increment.

CRYOPRECIPITATE

Cryoprecipitate is indicated in the treatment of von Willebrand's disease, and for quantitative or qualitative deficiency of fibrinogen and of Factor XIII, either congenital or acquired. The most likely causes of acquired deficiencies are disseminated intravascular coagulation (DIC), severe liver disease, and dilutional hypofibrinogenemia.

Quantitative deficiencies of fibronectin are associated with massive trauma, and fibronectin replacement in the form of cryoprecipitate has been recommended by some intensivists, although randomized, controlled therapeutic trials are lacking as of this writing (23, 24). Fibronectin depletion may develop during starvation, sepsis, with burn injuries, and in fulminant hepatic failure (25–27), but few studies have correlated administration of fibronectin in these settings with survival advantage (25, 28).

For quantitative fibrinogen deficiency, the same formulae can be applied as for any factor deficiency, except that the normal circulating fibrinogen concentration should be estimated at 250 mg/dl in the adult and child, with quantitatively lower estimates in premature infants (150 to 200 mg/dl). The quantity of fibrinogen per milliliter of cryoprecipitate is approximately 2 mg/ml, with one bag of cryoprecipitate containing approximately 25 to 50 ml. For von Willebrand's disease, one usually does not employ formulae, as von Willebrand's factor is not quantitated. Replacement for major hemorrhage is usually based on increasing Factor VIII coagulant activity to between 80 and 100% and the bleeding time to normal. In practice, 1 to 2 bags of cryoprecipitate per 10 kg body weight are administered with additional doses at 8- or 12-hour intervals based on quantitative Factor VIII coagulant levels and the clinical status of the patient. There are approximately 55 mg of fibronectin per ml of cryoprecipitate. Fibronectin is rarely quantitated, and there are no formulae to replace it.

FFP and cryoprecipitate should be ABO-compatible with the recipient's red blood cells. Because there are no red blood cells in FFP or cryoprecipitate, the Rh type is not considered.

Compatibility testing (cross-match) is not required. When large volumes of FFP or cryoprecipitate are administered, the isoagglutinins A and B in the product may produce a positive antiglobulin test and, rarely, hemolysis (18). Adverse reactions to plasma are similar to those from cellular components, but there are disproportionately more anaphylactic and allergic reactions, as well as cases of fluid overload (Table 19.2). Large doses of cryoprecipitate given to patients with normal circulating fibrinogen concentrations may increase the fibrinogen level and precipitate acute thrombosis and DIC.

For complex coagulation factor deficiencies, FFP may be administered in combination with cryoprecipitate. No controlled studies support these practices. Therapy in DIC should be directed at correcting the underlying disease, using antibiotics, volume expansion or, if applicable, the surgical removal of whatever precipitated the episode (e.g., infarcted bowel). In the face of clinically apparent bleeding, 10 to 15 ml/kg of FFP may be administered every 12 to 24 hours with 1 bag of cryoprecipitate per 10 kg of body weight if the fibrinogen concentrate is reduced. If the platelet count is <20,000/mm³, platelet concentrates are also indicated. Coagulation tests need to be repeated frequently to make sure component therapy is appropriate. Component therapy should not be used prophylactically or empirically. Other conditions where the use of FFP is questionable include treatment of capillary leak syndromes, massive loss of lymph fluid, and in nonbleeding patients with prolonged coagulation times (1.5 times normal) who are not candidates for invasive procedures (20, 29).

GRANULOCYTE CONCENTRATES

Granulocyte concentrates are obtained by cytapheresis and contain 1×10^{10} cells in 200 to 400 ml. They are indicated in severely neutropenic patients who have a chance of marrow recovery and who have not responded to antibiotic therapy. They are usually administered for 4 to 6 days. Because granulocyte concentrates have a hematocrit of 0.15%, they should be ABO and, if possible, Rh-compatible with the recipient. Many adverse reactions to granulocyte transfusion have been reported, including fever, rigors, and pulmonary reactions, including respiratory distress syndrome and deoxygenation. In infants, their use has been advocated at 1×10^{9} PMN per kg per transfusion. Products should be cytomegalovirus (CMV)-negative and irradiated to prevent posttransfusion CMV and graft vs. host disease (GVHD). A recent review of collection, storage, and indications for granulocyte concentrates can be found in Reference 30. Their use is limited due to their lack of availability and, more importantly, to the new bacteriocidal antibiotics and the use of IV IgG.

SPECIALIZED BLOOD PRODUCTS

Occasionally, specialized blood products may be indicated for patients in the ICU. Such components should be used only after consultation with a transfusion medicine physician and with the patient's primary care physician.

BLOOD PRODUCTS PREPARED TO REDUCE THE RISK OF CYTOMEGALOVIRUS

CMV is an ubiquitous virus of the herpes family that is harbored in white blood cells. A significant proportion of blood donors (30 to 70%) are CMV-seropositive, although there are regional differences; older age, female sex, and lower socioeconomic strata predispose to higher seroprevalence rates (31). Despite studies that confirm that seropositive donors can transmit CMV to seronegative recipients, only one study has been able to document viremia in blood donors (32). This finding has led to the concept that both actively and latently infected donors can transmit CMV.

There are three types of CMV infections seen in the transfusion recipient. These infections include primary infection, and two kinds of secondary infections: reactivation and reinfection. Primary infection occurs in a seronegative recipient of blood from a donor who is actively or latently infected. It is frequently symptomatic with a mononucleosis-like syndrome that is heterophile-negative. Viremia, viruria, an IgM-specific, and then IgG-specific anti-CMV antibody response can be demonstrated. Reactivation occurs when a CMV-seropositive recipient is transfused with blood from either a CMV-seropositive or seronegative donor. The donor leukocytes trigger an allograft reaction that reactivates the recipient's latent CMV (33). An increase in antibody titer and viral shedding may be found. Infections are usually asymptomatic, unless the patient is immunocompromised (31). Reinfection or coinfection occurs in a CMV-seropositive recipient of blood with a strain of CMV that differs from the strain that initially infected the recipient. IgM and IgG responses, as well as viral shedding, may be seen. The only way to distinguish reinfection is to use molecular markers specific for different strains of virus.

There is a wide clinical spectrum associated with posttransfusion CMV infection. CMV infection may be asymptomatic and only discovered because of serial serological tests, or it may produce clinically important morbidity and mortality. The intensivist must be cognizant of certain select patient groups at risk for pneumonia, cytopenias, hepatopathy, graft rejection, unexplained fever, and increased risk of bacterial and fungal infections associated with posttransfusion CMV. These groups include low birth-weight neonates, specifically those neonates less than 1250 g who are seronegative and who required large amounts of blood. Bone marrow and solid organ transplant recipients and infants who receive intrauterine transfusions are other patients at risk. Other immunocompromised patients, whether seronegative or seropositive, do not appear to be at increased risk for increased morbidity from CMV. As of this writing, no studies have addressed the need for specialized CMV attenuated components for either seronegative or seropositive patients with HIV infection.

There are a number of different methods that can be used to prevent or decrease the chance of developing posttransfusion CMV. Because the virus is likely harbored in the white blood cells (34), manipulations that can reduce or decrease leukocyte cell number should reduce the risk of transmission. These methods include washing and freezing, followed by washing and filtration. Lower rates of CMV infection have been seen in open heart and neonatal patients receiving washed red blood cells (35, 36). The use of frozen deglycerolized red blood cells, regardless of the serostatus of the product, is effective in preventing CMV in neonates (37, 38) and patients on dialysis (39). Recently, third generation leukocyte depletion filters have been developed for both platelets and red cell products and have been shown to be highly effective in preventing primary CMV infection in neonates (40) and in adult patients with hematologic malignancies (41). Standard leukodepletion filters do not remove a sufficient leukocyte number to be as effective; the exact number of leukocytes that need to be removed is not known.

Some oncologists would argue that patients who *may* undergo bone marrow transplantation, regardless of marrow donor serology, should have blood and blood products manipulated to prevent reactivation of CMV or reinfection. There have been no studies that support this practice, although theoretically, infection with CMV may be as high as 51% in these patients, and clinical manifestations of newly acquired CMV diseases are significant. CMV pneumonia may develop in 10% of transplant patients, and 60 to 80% of these infections may be fatal (42–44). More routine use of the third generation filters may well be able to provide an acceptable product that does not depend on donor serostatus.

Both prospective and retrospective studies have demonstrated that IgG-seronegative blood and blood products have a low-to-nonexistent risk of transmitting CMV. Donors with IgM-specific CMV antibody may be more able to transmit CMV, as those donors are more likely to have acute viral infection and replication (45). IgM antibody assays, however, are not yet well-standardized. Hence, use of IgG-seronegative blood is considered to be "gold standard," despite the fact that most IgG-seropositive units are not infectious.

γ- or cesium irradiation of blood to inhibit DNA replication (vide infra) will not prevent CMV infection (46). Many patients undergoing chemotherapy with or without transplantation receive irradiated blood for prevention of postgraft graft-versus-host disease. Similarly, many patients who receive blood that is CMV-seronegative or leukodepleted receive CMV hyperimmune globulin or intravenous immunoglobulin with variable titers to CMV antibody and, in addition, may be receiving fresh frozen plasma for coagulopathy. They receive these plasma products to attenuate the development of graft-induced CMV or nosocomial acquisition of CMV (47, 48). It may be very difficult to assess the serostatus of these individuals because of passive acquisition of CMV antibody. Tests for CMV early antigen or molecular markers will be necessary to establish posttransfusion CMV in these individuals, but these tests are not yet routinely available.

IRRADIATED BLOOD

Posttransfusion graft-versus-host disease occurs when an immunosuppressed or immunodeficient transfusion recipient receives immunologically competent donor lymphocytes through transfused blood products. The transfused histincompatible T-lymphocytes proliferate and engraft in the immunocompromised host, who is incapable of rejecting foreign cells. The degree of similarity between the HLA antigens of the blood donor and the recipient enhances the potential for engraftment. Once engraftment occurs, donor lymphocyte proliferation occurs and clinical symptoms begin, usually 4 to 30 days following transfusion. Clinical manifestations include fever, erythematous rash, anorexia, nausea, vomiting, and profuse watery diarrhea. The rash may progress to bullae and to desquamation. Liver dysfunction, from increases in liver enzyme values in blood to fulminant hepatic coma can occur. The bone marrow hematopoietic progenitors are particularly affected and produce severe cytopenias. Posttransfusion graft-versus-host disease is fatal in 90% of reported cases in children (49). Diagnosis is usually made post-mortem but can be made premortem with biopsy of the skin or GI tract, by looking for chimerism, using DNA analysis (restriction fragment length polymorphisms) tissue (50).

Patient groups at risk for posttransfusion graft-versus-host disease include bone marrow transplant recipients of any age, infants with congenital immunodeficiency, and those patients who received exchange or simple transfusion following intrauterine transfusion. Infants with unsuspected congenital immuno-deficiency disease may also develop posttransfusion graft-versus-host disease, as well as older children with immunodeficiency acquired congenitally or through chemotherapy. In addition, patients receiving ablative chemotherapy for diverse forms of malignancy, as well as patients with lymphoma, are also at increased risk.

The incidence of posttransfusion graft-versus-host disease is not known. Estimates for patients with leukemia range from 0.1 to 1%(49) and 2% for lymphoma (51), but such rates are impossible to verify. Most oncology units caring for children are part of large cooperative groups or specialized cancer hospitals and have been using irradiated products for several years. There are several reports of premature infants and one full-term infant developing posttransfusion graft-versus-host disease following exchange transfusion (reviewed in Ref. 52). Some neonatal centers use irradiated blood for all premature infants on the basis of the known cellular and humoral immune dysfunction in these infants, but this practice is not agreed upon by all (53). It is likely that only the most severe cases of posttransfusion graft-versus-host disease are reported or, alternately, that many are missed because of the similarities between the clinical manifestations of posttransfusion graft-versus-host disease and chemotherapy and radiation-induced toxicities.

The incidence of posttransfusion graft-versus-host disease is further attenuated by its pathobiology. A certain number of viable lymphocytes, likely 1×10^7/kg, must be transfused to the recipient at a point at which the recipient is maximally immunosuppressed. Therefore, certain malignancies or stages of a given malignancy are not associated with posttransfusion graft-versus-host disease, because the immunosuppression may be less intense at one point in the care of the same patient (54). Other factors that may attenuate posttransfusion graft-versus-host disease are kind of chemotherapy used, concomitant use of radiotherapy, or other immunosuppressive regimens. The kind of product used is also critical. Although posttransfusion graft-versus-host disease has been associated with whole blood, PRBC, frozen deglycerolized red blood cells, white blood cells, platelets, and fresh plasma, it has not been associated with frozen-thawed plasma or frozen-thawed cryoprecipitate.

Because the lymphocyte is the most likely initiator of graft-versus-host disease, the disease can be prevented by reducing the number of lymphocytes, or by rendering them mitotically inactive. Since posttransfusion graft-versus-host disease has been reported following use of leukodepleted blood products, γ-irradiation is currently the only adequate method of preventing posttransfusion graft-versus-host disease. The dose to be used should abrogate mixed lymphocyte culture response while producing no harm to the cellular components. Doses between 1500 and 5000 rads (15 to 50 Gy) have been used, with either cesium or cobalt source irradiators. Recent studies suggest 2500 rads to the midplane of the bag is necessary. Cesium 137 blood irradiators are designed to hold blood bags and rotate during the process ensuring adequate radiation exposure (55) while cobalt 60 sources, available in radiotherapy departments, have not been as standardized for blood bags (56). Irradiation of platelet bags at 3000 rads followed by storage does not alter platelet function (57). The lack of adverse effect of irradiation of red blood cells (58) has recently come into question; several investigators have found that irradiation produces increases in plasma potassium and plasma hemoglobin concentrations when irradiated units are stored for periods of time that are still within their shelf-life (59, 60). Red blood cell products transfused to fetuses, to neonates, or to children unable to tolerate potassium loads should be irradiated immediately prior to use and not stored (60) until additional data are available. Studies on the effect of irradiation of granulocyte products have produced variable results. While chemotaxis (61) and bactericidal killing (62) remain intact at 5000 rads, superoxide production was adversely affected at 2500 and 5000 rads (63, 64).

PARENTS AS DONORS

Fear over transfusion-transmitted viruses has caused many parents to demand that their blood be used for their children. This practice has produced a new series of potential and real immunologic concerns. Although well-recognized in Japan as postoperative erythroderma, there are now several reports of posttransfusion graft-versus-host disease occurring in nonimmunocompromised individuals following transfusion of blood donated by family members (65–69). In these cases, the first-degree relatives' donors are homozygous for two HLA haplotypes and share one HLA haplotype with the recipient. The recipient is incapable of eliminating the donor's lymphocytes because of the shared HLA haplotype. However, the donor recognizes the unshared recipient haplotype as "non-self" and may attack the host with a graft-versus-host disease type of reaction. U.S. blood collection agencies have recommended careful identification of units of blood and blood products obtained from first degree relatives followed by irradiation of such units (70, 71). This practice has many implications for small hospitals, where irradiation facilities may not be readily available. If blood centers irradiate for small hospitals, there are issues of storage and transportation. Serum potassium concentrations of 53 to 67 mmol/l have been reported in irradiated packed cells that were then stored for 7 days or more (59), which might well cause clinically important increases in patient potassium levels if blood is used for exchange transfusion or during cardiopulmonary bypass.

When parents are donors, there are other concerns that are serological in nature. Maternal plasma may contain alloantibodies directed toward paternal antigens; these may be red cell-, granulocyte-, or platelet-specific or have HLA specificities. Transfusion of a maternal blood component containing plasma exposes the infant to these antibodies directed against paternally derived blood cell antigens. In utero, the placenta protects against passage of these antibodies to the fetus. In a recent study of 25 healthy women tested at time of delivery, 16% had lymphocytotoxic and granulocytotoxic antibodies (72). Although the clinical significance of these antibodies is as yet unknown, they are known to produce noncardiogenic pulmonary edema and purpura in adults (73).

Use of the biologic father's blood also has possible consequences. Most maternal alloantibodies are directed toward paternally derived antigens. An infant may have passively acquired maternal alloantibody, which will be missed by standard pretransfusion testing. This fact is because the antibody may be directed toward a low incidence or "private" red cell antigen not present on the cells used for pretransfusion testing. In addition, most infants are not routinely cross-matched against donor units; the cross-match would provide a mechanism to pick up these alloantibodies; thus, an incompatibility might be easily missed. Therefore, in cases where a parent is to serve as a donor, a full major (parent cells and infant serum) and minor cross-match (parent serum and infant red cells) should be performed to prevent a possible hemolytic transfusion episode. Products screened for and found to be positive for HLA-, platelet-, and granulocyte-specific antibodies or plasma-containing components from mothers should be excluded (74).

TRANSFUSION PRACTICES

CHOICE OF RESUSCITATION FLUIDS AND THE MASSIVELY TRANSFUSED PATIENT

The primary treatment for a hemorrhaging patient who has lost 20 to 25% or less of his or her blood volume should be nonsanguinous fluids, such as crystalloids and colloids; such solutions are readily available, are rapidly administered, and are effective even at low hematocrits at improving microvascular flow (75). As volume is restored, an assessment of extent of red blood cell loss can be made and red blood cells requested, if clinically indicated. In the emergency situation, O-positive or O-negative packed cells may be provided without compatibility testing, which must be completed at a later time. Type-specific blood can be available in 5 to 10 minutes, while full compatibility testing of donor and recipient requires 45 minutes to 1 hour. Only normal saline (0.9% sodium chloride) should be used in their same "line" as blood. Ringer's lactate solution contains calcium, which chelates with the citrate anticoagulant and causes blood to clot in the bag while 5% dextrose in water is hypotonic and causes red blood cells to lyse.

When red blood cells are transfused rapidly to a bleeding patient, several adverse reactions may occur. These reactions include hypothermia, secondary to the cold blood, and metabolic adverse effects, including hypocalcemia, hyper- and hypokalemia, hypernatremia, and hypo- and hyperglycemia. Hypertension secondary to rapid expansion of the intravascular space may also occur.

Hypothermia can produce a left shift of the oxygen dissociation curve, and increase oxygen affinity while decreasing peripheral oxygen offloading, arrhythmia, low cardiac output, and DIC (76). Hypothermia can be avoided by using commercially available blood warmers. They should have automatic audible and visible alarms for temperature control; transfusion of heat-hemolyzed blood products may produce anaphylaxis, DIC, and death. Many warmers are designed to pass blood across warming plates; these warmers restrict flow rate, limiting their usefulness. Modified warmers have been developed for red blood cells (77) and for FFP, using a modified microwave (78). Blood and blood products should never be heated in uncontrolled water baths, or other warming devices, including standard microwave heaters. Electromechanical devices may be used for infusion of blood, platelets, plasma, and cryoprecipitate. They vary from syringe infusion to volume displacement devices and may require specific cassettes that increase the dead volume of the transfusion. High-viscosity, high-hematocrit-packed red blood cells may hemolyze when some of these devices are used. Their use should be restricted to controlled infusion of small volumes in patients with specific needs for such slow infusion, such as cardiovascular instability. Transfusion of large volumes rapidly using these devices is contraindicated.

Hypocalcemia is one of the most critical metabolic abnormalities to occur posttransfusion because of its association with depressed myocardial contractility. Studies on the extent of this problem are contradictory, but the liver transplant patient serves as the best model. Most transplant patients are anhepatic for a part of the procedure and, therefore, cannot metabolize citrate; they also receive large volumes of blood over a relatively short time. In such patients, rapid infusion of blood is associated with decreased cardiac index, decreased ventricular function, and hypotension, and calcium infusion is indicated (79, 80). Other massively transfused patients should be monitored but need not receive prophylactic calcium infusions. Hyperkalemia secondary to massive transfusion may also decrease myocardial contractility and should also be monitored (81). Because banked blood is acidic due to the initial anticoagulant and the production of lactic acid during storage, a metabolic acidosis is expected in the massively transfused recipient. It is more likely, however, that the acidosis is the result of hypoxemia and poor tissue perfusion (82). Prophylactic administration of bicarbonate is not indicated, but arterial blood pH should be monitored, and metabolic defects treated as they are discovered.

BLOOD SALVAGE AND AUTOLOGOUS TRANSFUSION

The collection and reinfusion of a patient's own blood can decrease the need for homologous blood transfusion. This goal may be accomplished by one or a combination of the following modalities: (*a*) preoperative blood donation with subsequent blood bank storage and reinfusion during or following surgery; (*b*) acute normovolemic hemodilution, whereby blood is collected immediately preceding or following anesthetic induction and reinfused at the end of the surgical procedure; and (*c*) intraoperative and postoperative blood salvage, whereby blood shed into the operative field or enclosed space is collected, washed, and reinfused during or after surgery. These procedures have been used frequently in adults and are gaining acceptance in the pediatric population (83).

The pediatric patient admitted to the intensive care unit following a surgical procedure in which any combination of the above methods may have been employed may be at risk for the development of dilutional coagulopathy. Because these patients are receiving salvaged, washed packed red cells, coagulation factors, as well as platelets, may decrease to levels that place the patient at risk for hemorrhage. Laboratory monitoring of the platelet count, as well as screening coagulation assays, should be used to gauge the need for replacement therapy. Although some investigators advocate resuspension of the washed salvaged red cells with fresh frozen plasma, this approach may be unnecessary (84). Only careful monitoring of both the clinical and laboratory data should dictate the need for additional blood components.

Special care should be taken to ensure appropriate labelling of the salvaged product; the products should always be used within the outdate on the bag and never more than 4 hours. It should never be transfused to any person other than the autologous patient. In some postoperative collection systems, the blood is not washed prior to reinfusion. No data are currently available on the use of these products in pediatric patients.

REFERENCES

1. Counts RB, Haisch C, Simon TL et al: Hemostatis in massively transfused trauma patients. *Ann Surg* 190:91–98, 1979.
2. Nilsson L, Hedner U, Nilsson IM, Robertson B: Shelf-life of bank blood and stored plasma with special reference to coagulation factors. *Transfusion* 23:377–381, 1983.
3. Wenz B: Leukocyte-free red cells: The evoluton of a safer blood product. I. In McCarthy LJ and Baldwin ML (eds): *Controversies of Leukocyte-Poor Blood and Components* AABB, Arlington, VA, 1989.
4. Dutcher JP, Schiffer CA, Aisner J, et al: Incidence of thrombocytopenia and serious hemorrhage among patients with solid tumors. *Cancer* 53:557–562, 1983.
5. Simpson MB: Platelet fuction and transfusion therapy in the surgical patient. In Smith DM and Summers SH (eds): *Platelets*. AABB, Arlington VA, p 129–166, 1988.
6. Aster RH, Jandle JH: Platelet sequestration in man. II. Immunological and clinial studies. *J Clin Invest* 43:856–869, 1964.
7. Ilett SJ, Lilleyman JS: Platelet transfusion requirements of children with newly diagnosed lymphoblastic leukemia. *Acta Haemat* 62:86–89, 1979, (Basel).
8. van Eyes J, Thomas D, Olivos B: Platelet use in pediatric oncology: a review of 393 transfusions. *Transfusion* 18:169–173, 1978.
9. Schiffer CA, Aisner J: Platelet and granulocyte transfusion therapy for patients with cancer. In Petz LD and Swisher SN (eds): *Clinical Practice of Blood Transfusion*. Churchill Livingstone, New York, 1981.
10. Schiffer CA (ed): *Platelet Physiology and Transfusion*. AABB, Washington, DC, 1978.
11. Reed RL, Ciavarella D, Heimbach DM, et al: Prophylactic platelet administration during massive transfusion. *Ann Surg* 203:40–48, 1986.
12. Cote CJ, Liau LMP, Szyfelbein SK, Goudsouzian NG, Daniels AL: Changes in serial platelet counts following massive blood transfusion in pediatric pateints. *Anesthesiology* 62:197–201, 1985.
13. Noe DA, Graham SM, Luff R, et al: Platelet counts during rapid massive transfusion. *Transfusion* 22:392–395, 1982.
14. Bick RL: Hemostasis defects associated with cardiac surgery, prosthetic devices and other extracorporeal circuits. *Semin Thromb Hemost* 2:249–280, 1985.
15. Harker LA, Malpass TW, Branson HE, et al: Mechanisms of abnormal bleeding in patients undergoing cardiopulmonary bypass: acquired dysfunction associated with α granule release. *Blood* 56:824–834, 1980.
16. Murphy S: ABO blood groups and platelet transfusion. *Transfusion* 28:401–402, 1988.
17. Skogen B, Rossebo-Hansen B, Husebekk A, et al: Minimal expression of blood group A antigen on thrombocytes from A2 individuals. *Transfusion* 28:456–459, 1988.
18. Pierce RN, Reich LM, Mayer K: Hemolysis following platelet transfusions from ABO incompatible donors. *Transfusion* 25:60–62, 1985.
19. Moroff G, Friedman A, Robkin-Kline L, et al: Reduction of the volume of stored platelet concentrations for neonatal use. *Transfusion* 24:144–146, 1984.
20. Consensus Conference: Fresh frozen plasma: indications and risks. *JAMA* 253:551–553, 1985.
21. Shepard KV, Bukowski RM: The treatment of thrombotic thrombocytopenic purpura with exchange transfusion, plasma infusions and plasma exchange. *Semin Hematol* 24:178–193, 1987.
22. Goldsmith JC: Plasma component therapy. In Luban NLC (ed): *Pediatric Transfusion Medicine*, Johns Hopkins University Press, Baltimore, 1990.
23. Saba TM, Jaffe E: Plasma fibronectin: its synthesis by vascular endothelial cells and its role in cardiopulmonary integrity following trauma as related to reticuloendothelial function. *Am J Med* 68:577–594, 1980.
24. Scovill WA, Saba TM, Blumenstock FA, et al: Opsonic alpha-2 surface binding glycoprotein therapy during sepsis. *Ann Surg* 188:521–529, 1978.
25. Hesselvic JF: Plasma fibronectin levels in sepsis: influencing factors. *Crit Care Med* 15:1092–1097, 1987.
26. Schena FP, Pertosa G: Fibronectin and the kidney. *Nephron* 48:177–182, 1988.
27. Yoder MC, Douglas SD, Gerdes J, Kline J, Polin RA: Plasma fibronection in healthy newborn infants: respiratory distress syndrome and perinatal asphyxia. *J Pediatr* 102:777–780, 1983.
28. Fredell J, Takyi Y, Gwenigale W, et al: Fibronectin as a possible adjunct in the treatment of severe malnutrition. *Lancet* ii:962, 1987.
29. Snyder AJ, Gottschall JL, Menitove JE: Why is fresh frozen plasma transfused? *Transfusion* 26:107–112, 1986.
30. Blajchman MA: Granulocyte transfusions. *Tranfusion Med Rev* 4:1–23, 1990.
31. Tegtmeier GE: Posttransfusion cytomegalovirus infections. *Arch Pathol Lab Med* 113:236–246, 1989.
32. Diosi P, Moldovan E, Tomescu N: Latent cytomegalovirus infection in blood donors. *Br Med J* 4:660–662, 1969.
33. Lang DJ: Cytomegalovirus infectins in organ transplantation and posttransfusion: an hypothesis. *Arch Gesamte Virusforsch* 37:365–377, 1972.
34. Winston SJ, Ho WG, Howell CL, et al: Cytomegalovirus infections associated with leukocyte transfusions. *Ann Intern Med* 102:16–20, 1985.
35. Lang DJ, Ebert PA, Rogers BM, et al: Reduction of postperfusion cytomegalovirus infections following the use of leukocyte depleted blood. *Transfusion* 17:391–395, 1977.
36. Luban NLC, Williams AE, MacDonald MG, et al: Low indicence of acquired cytomegalovirus infections transfused with washed red blood cells. *Am J Dis Child* 141:416–419, 1987.
37. Brady MT, Milam JD, Anderson DC, et al: Use of deglycerolized red blood cells to prevent posttransfusion infection with cytomegalovirus in neonates. *J Infect Dis* 150:334–339, 1984.
38. Taylor BJ, Jacovs RF, Baker RL, et al: Frozen deglycerolized blood prevents transfusion acquired cytomegalovirus infection in neonates. *Pediatr Infect Dis J* 5:188–191, 1986.
39. Tolkoff-Rubin NE, Ruben RH, Keller EE, et al: Cytomegalovirus infection in dialysis patients and personnel. *Ann Intern Med* 89:625–628, 1978.
40. Gilbert GL, Hayes K, Hudson IL, et al: Prevention of transfusion-acquired cytomegalovirus infection in infants by blood filtration to remove leukocytes. *Lancet* ii:1228–1231, 1989.
41. DeGraan-Hentzen YCE, Gratama JW, Mudde GC, et al: Prevention of primary cytomegalovirus infection in patients with hematologic malignancy by intensive white cell depletion of blood products. *Transfusion* 29:757–760, 1989.
42. Bowden RA, Sayers M, Flournoy N, et al: Cytomegalovirus immune globulin and seronegative blood products to prevent primary cytomegalovirus infection after marrow transplantation. *N Engl J Med* 314:1004–1010, 1986.
43. Meyers JD, Flournoy N, Thomas ED: Risk factors for cytomegalovirus infection after human marrow transplant. *J Infect Dis* 153:478–488, 1986.
44. Pecago R, Hill R, Applebaum FR, et al: Interstitial pneumonitis following autologous bone marrow transplant. *Transplantation* 42:515–517, 1986.
45. Lamberson HV, McMillan JA, Weiner LB, et al: Prevention of transfusion-associated cytomegalovirus (CMV) infection in neonates by screening donors for IgM for CMV. *J Infect Dis* 157:820–823, 1988.
46. Chou S, Kim DY, Norman DJ: Transmission of cytomegalovirus by pretransplant leukocyte transfusions in renal transplant candidates. *J Infect Dis* 155:565–567, 1987.
47. Slichter SJ: Transfusin and bone marrow transplantation. *Trans Med Rev* 2:1–17, 1988.
48. Winston DJ, Ho WG, Lin C, et al: Intravenous immune globulin for prevention of cytomegalovirus infection and interstitial pneumonia after bone marrow transplantation. *Ann Intern Med* 106:12–18, 1987.
49. Von Fliedner V, Higby DJ, Kim U: Graft-versus-host reaction following blood transfusion. *Am J Med* 72:951–961, 1982.
50. Dinsmore RE, Straus DJ, Pollack MS: Fatal graft-versus-host disease following blood transfusion in Hodgkin's disease documented by HLA typing. *Blood* 55:831–834, 1980.
51. Stutzman L, Nisce L, Friedman M, et al: Increased toxicity of total nodal irradiation following combination chemotherapy. *ASCO Abst* C411:391, 1979.
52. Holland P: Prevention of transfusion-associated graft-versus-host disease. *Arch Pathol Lab Med* 113:285–291, 1989.

53. Sacher RA, Luban NLC, Strauss RG: Current practice and guidelines for the transfusion of cellular blood components in the newborn. *Trans Med Rev* 3:39–54, 1989.

54. Holohan TV, Terasaki PI, Deisseroth AB: Suppression of transfusion-related alloimmunization in intensively treated cancer patient. *Blood* 58:122–128, 1981.

55. Fearon TC, Luban NLC: Practical dosimetric aspects of blood and blood product irradiation. *Transfusion* 26:457–459, 1986.

56. McMican A, Luban NLC, Sacher RA et al: Practical aspects of blood irradiatin. *Lab Med* 18:299–303, 1987.

57. Read EJ, Kodis C, Carter CS, et al: Viability of platelets following storage in the irradiated state. *Transfusion* 28:446–450, 1988.

58. Moore GL, Ledford ME: Effects of 4000 rad irradiation on the in vitro storage properties of packed cells. *Transfusion* 25:583–585, 1985.

59. Ramirez AM, Woodfield DG, Scott R, et al: High potassium levels in stored irradiated blood. *Transfusion* 27:444, 1987.

60. Rivet C, Baxter A, Rock G: Potassium levels in irradiation blood. *Transfusion* 29:185, 1989.

61. Valerius NH, Johansen KS, Nielson OS, et al: Effect of in vitro x-irradiation on lymphocyte and granulocyte function. *Scand J Haematol* 27:9–18, 1981.

62. Holley TR, Van Epps DE, Harvey RL: Effect of high doses of radiation of human neutrophil chemotaxis, phagocytosis and morphology. *Am J Pathol* 75:61–68, 1974.

63. Buescher ES, Gallin JI: Radiation effects on cultured human monocytes and on monocyte-derived macrophages. *Blood* 63:1402–1407, 1984.

64. Eastlund DT, Charbonneau TT: Superoxide generation and cytotaxic response of irradiated neutrophils. *Transfusion* 28:368–370, 1988.

65. Arsura EL, Bartelle A, Minkowitz S, et al: Transfusion-associated graft-versus-host disease in a presumed immunocompetent patient. *Arch Intern Med* 148:1941–1944, 1988.

66. Juji T, Shibata Y, Ide H, et al: Host-transfusion graft-versus-host disease in immunocompetent patients after cardiac surgery in Japan. *N Engl J* 321:56, 1989.

67. Sakakibara T, Juji T: Post transfusion graft-versus-host disease after open heart surgery. *Lancet* ii:1099, 1986.

68. Sheehan T, McLaren KM, Brettle R, et al: Transfusion-induced graft-versus-host disease in pregnancy. *Clin Lab Haematol* 9:205–207, 1987.

69. Thaler M, Shamiss A, Orgad S, et al: The role of blood from HLA homozygous donors in fatal transfusion-associated graft-versus-host disease affect open heart surgery. *N Engl J Med* 321:25–28, 1989.

70. American Association of Blood Banks Memorandum to AABB Institution Members, November 6, 1989.

71. American Red Cross, Blood Services Letter #89–91, November 29, 1989.

72. Elbert C, Strauss RG, Barrett F, et al: Biological mothers may be dangerous blood donors for their neonates. *Acta Haematol* 85:189–191, 1991.

73. Yomtovian R, Kline W, Press C, et al: Severe pulmonary hypersensitivity associated with passive transfusion of a neutrophil-specific antibody. *Lancet* i:244–246, 1984.

74. Strauss RG, Sacher RA: Directed donations for pediatric patients. *Transfusion Med Rev* 2:58–64, 1988.

75. Isley MR, Kaley ER, Lucas WJ, et al: The hemodynamic and oxygen transport responses to automated acute normovolemic hemodilution. *Anesth Analg* 66:587, 1987.

76. Rueler JB: Hypothermia: pathophysiology, clinical settings and management. *Ann Intern Med* 89:519–527, 1978.

77. Kruskall MS, Racini DG, Malynn ER, et al: Evaluation of a blood warmer that utiizes a 40°C heat exchanger. *Transfusion* 30:7–11, 1990.

78. Sohngen D, Kretschmer V, Franke K, et al: Thawing of fresh-frozen plasma with a new microwave oven. *Transfusion* 28:576–580, 1988.

79. Gray TA, Buckley BM, Sealey MM, et al: Plasma ionized calcium monitoring during liver transplantation. *Transplantation* 41:335–339, 1986.

80. Marquez J, Martin D, Virji MA, et al: Cardiovascular depression secondary to ionic hypocalcemia during hepatic transplantation in humans. *Anesthesiology* 65:457–461, 1986.

81. Linko K, Tigerstedt I: Hyperpotassemia during massive blood transfusion. *Acta Anesthesiol Scand* 28:220–221, 1984.

82. Collins JA, Simmons RL, James PM, et al: Acid-base status of seriously wounded combat casualties: resuscitation with stored blood. *Ann Surg* 173:6–18, 1971.

83. DePalma L, Luban NLC: Autologous blood transfusion in pediatrics. *Pediatrics* 85:125–128, 1990.

84. Estrin JA, Belani KG, Karnavas AG, et al: A new approach to massive blood transfusion during pediatric liver resection. *Surgery* 99:6–8, 1986.

Red Cell Substitutes: A Current Appraisal

STEVEN A. GOULD, M.D.

LAKSHMAN R. SEHGAL, PH.D.

ARTHUR L. ROSEN, PH.D.

HANSA L. SEHGAL, B.S.

GERALD S. MOSS, M.D.

The two acellular oxygen carriers currently being evaluated as red cell substitutes are hemoglobin solutions and fluorocarbon emulsions. The primary indication for such a product would be the unavailability of blood. The most important properties of a suitable red cell substitute should be the ability to effectively transport oxygen and carbon dioxide and to support circulatory dynamics. In addition, the preparation should be nontoxic and temperature-stable; should have a long shelf storage time and a suitable intravascular persistence; should require no cross-match before administration; and should be effective when the recipient is on room air.

We have shown that both hemoglobin solutions and fluorocarbon emulsions can maintain normal levels of oxygen consumption, carbon dioxide production, and circulatory dynamics in primates in the virtual absence of red blood cells (16). Although each solution, therefore, satisfies the most important criteria for a red cell substitute, certain problems exist with both that must be resolved prior to their clinical application. This chapter will assess the current status of both products.

HEMOGLOBIN SOLUTIONS

For the last 15 years we have pursued the possibility that a hemoglobin solution prepared from outdated blood could serve as a temporary substitute for the red blood cell (17, 25, 26). This interest is based on several remarkable characteristics of the hemoglobin molecule. First, hemoglobin has the capacity to chemically bind oxygen: 1 g of hemoglobin binds 1.34 ml of oxygen. Second, the hemoglobin molecule has the ability to become fully oxygen-saturated at ambient oxygen pressures. Few, if any, biologically acceptable substances have a greater oxygen capacity at physiologic pressures. Thus, hemoglobin is a fully effective oxygen carrier without the addition of supplemental oxygen to the inspired air. Third, oxygen is normally unloaded from hemoglobin in the capillary at oxygen pressures of approximately 40 torr. This unloading characteristic allows for oxygen molecules to flow from hemoglobin to the intracellular mitochondria without producing interstitial hypoxia. Despite these features, an acceptable hemoglobin solution has not yet been used in the clinical setting.

UNMODIFIED HEMOGLOBIN

The basic unmodified hemoglobin solution is currently prepared from outdated blood. The red cells are first washed and lysed with pyrogen-free water (Fig. 20.1). A series of filtration steps permits the complete separation of the red cell membrane debris ("stroma") from the hemoglobin molecules. The resultant hemoglobin solution is essentially free of these contaminants and is commonly referred to as "stroma-free hemoglobin," or SFH. Since the blood type characteristics are located on the cell membrane, SFH is universally compatible and can be infused without regard to specific blood type. The properties of this unmodified tetrameric or "stripped" hemoglobin solution are shown in Table 20.1. The P_{50} of 12 to 14 torr compares with a normal value of 26 torr (25).

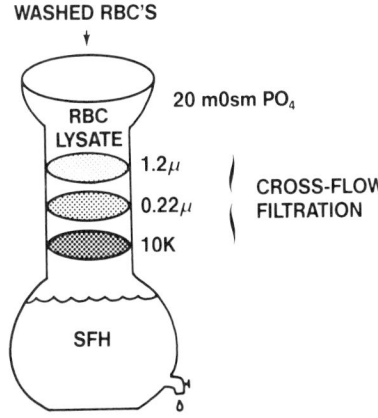

Figure 20.1. Schematic drawing of preparation process for stroma-free hemoglobin (SFH). *RBC*, red blood cell.

Table 20.1[a]. Properties of Stroma-free Hemoglobin (SFH)

Hemoglobin content	6–8 g/dl
P_{50}	12–14 torr
Colloid osmotic pressure	20–25 torr
Half-life	2–4 hr

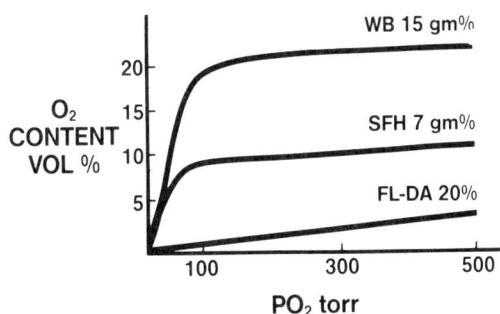

Figure 20.2. Oxygen content curves for 15 g/dl *(gm%)* of whole blood *(WB)*, 7 g/dl *(gm%)* of stroma-free hemoglobin *(SFH)*, and 20% Fluosol-DA *(FL-DA)*.

Although SFH can be prepared with a [Hb] of 14 g/dl, the solution would have a colloid osmotic pressure (COP) of greater than 60 torr (17). This hyperoncotic solution would not be acceptable for clinical use. The [Hb] of 7 g/dl is, therefore, required to maintain an isoncotic product. The low P_{50} is due to the loss of 2,3-diphosphoglycerate (2,3-DPG) during the preparation. The O_2 content curve of SFH is thus both anemic ($\downarrow$[Hb]) and leftward-shifted ($\downarrow P_{50}$). A comparison with a 15 g/dl whole blood product and Fluosol-DA, 20%, is shown in Figure 20.2.

Despite these limitations, SFH will support life in primates in the absence of red cells, documenting effective O_2 transport (25). Animals survive a total exchange transfusion with SFH to zero hematocrit with maintenance of normal O_2 consumption (VO_2), cardiac output (CO), and arteriovenous O_2 content difference (AVDO2). Although still normal, there is a decline in some of these parameters from the baseline values. In addition, a considerable decrease occurs in the mixed venous oxygen tension (PMVO$_2$) from roughly 50 to 20 torr.

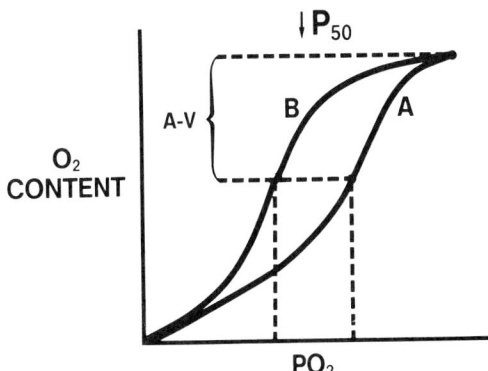

Figure 20.3. Oxygen content curves showing how a leftward shift *(P$_{50}$)* with a constant AVDO$_2$ leads to a lower PMVO$_2$.

The PMVO$_2$ is the tension at which oxygen unloads from the hemoglobin molecule and is in equilibrium with the tissue PO$_2$. This decline indicates a marked increase in O_2 extraction and is the mechanism used to compensate for the fall in [Hb] and P_{50}. Such a low PMVO$_2$ caused us concern and led us to attempt to restore a more normal value.

ANALYSIS OF MIXED VENOUS OXYGEN TENSION

The factors that lower PMVO$_2$ include a decrease in cardiac output, hemoglobin mass, P_{50} ($\uparrow$ affinity state), arterial saturation, and an increase in O_2 consumption (12). In reviewing the data we could eliminate changes in O_2 consumption, arterial saturation, and cardiac output as explanations for the decline in PMVO$_2$. The major changes were the fall in [Hb] and P_{50} that occurred during the exchange transfusion. We believed that the low [Hb] and P_{50} of the infused SFH were responsible for these results (18). Our subsequent efforts have focused on normalizing these values and obtaining a product with a normal O_2-carrying capacity.

PYRIDOXYLATED HEMOGLOBIN

Our initial efforts were focused on improving the oxygen affinity state of SFH. The increase in affinity state ($\downarrow P_{50}$) in SFH is related to the loss of the organic ligand, 2,3-DPG, normally found in the red blood cell. Figure 20.3 demonstrates how a leftward shift in the O_2 content curve with no change in VO$_2$, CO, or AVDO$_2$ produces a decrease in the oxygen tension at which unloading occurs—the PMVO$_2$ (15). Attempts to normalize P_{50} by the simple addition of 2,3-DPG to the hemoglobin solution were unsuccessful because the DPG disappears rapidly from the circulation after infusion (38). Benesch (1), Greenburgh (21), Sehgal (36), and their coworkers have described a modification of the hemoglobin molecule by the addition of pyridoxal phosphate. The resulting pyridoxylated hemoglobin (SFH-P) has a P_{50} of 20 to 22 torr, considerably higher than the P_{50} of the unmodified SFH.

The SFH-P was evaluated in eight baboons (9). Four received SFH (P_{50}, 12 torr) and four received SFH-P (P_{50}, 22 torr). The hemoglobin concentration of both solutions was approximately 7 g/dl. The exchange transfusion again was carried out until zero hematocrit was achieved. The PMVO$_2$

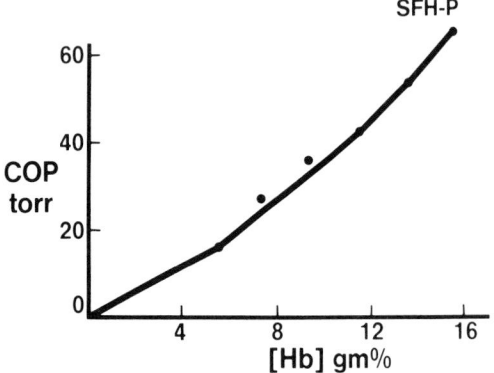

Figure 20.4. Relationship between *[Hb]* and colloid osmotic pressure *(COP)* for tetrameric *SFH-P.*

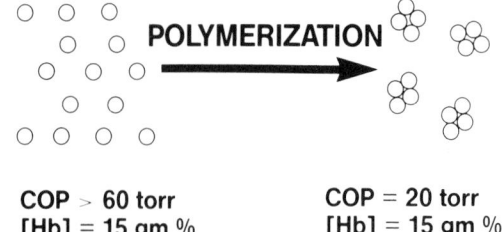

Figure 20.5. Schematic explanation of polymerization of 15 g/dl *(gm%)* tetrameric to 15 g/dl *(gm%)* polymerized hemoglobin. *COP,* colloid osmotic pressure.

Table 20.2. Properties of Polymerized, Pyridoxylated Stroma-free Hemoglobin (Poly SFH-P)

Hemoglobin content	14–16 g/dl
P_{50}	16–20 torr
Colloid osmotic pressure	20–25 torr
Half-life	24–48 hr

levels were significantly higher at the end of the exchange in the animals receiving SFH-P. Although the hemodynamics were maintained in a normal range, there was once again a decline from the baseline values in both groups.

These results illustrate three points. First, they confirm that rightward shifts in the dissociation curve ($\uparrow P_{50}$) result in an increased PMVO$_2$ as long as the other determinants of PMVO$_2$ remain constant (9). This fact is physiologically important because it allows O$_2$ unloading to occur at a higher tissue PO$_2$. Second, although increased, the PMVO$_2$ level (near 25 torr) in the animals treated with SFH-P still was substantially lower than the normal value of 40 to 50 torr found in control animals. Third, the hemodynamics still showed a reduction from the baseline values. Thus, we began to search for other means to normalize the PMVO$_2$ and the hemodynamics. The remaining option was to raise the hemoglobin concentration of the SFH (18).

POLYMERIZED HEMOGLOBIN

Preparation

It is possible to prepare a hemoglobin solution with a normal hemoglobin concentration. However, the COP of such a product will be in excess of 60 torr (Fig. 20.4) (17, 26). Such a solution might produce large fluid shifts from the extravascular to the intravascular space following infusion and, therefore, is not a suitable product. An alternate approach to developing a product with a normal O$_2$ capacity and a normal COP value is polymerization of the hemoglobin molecule. The COP of any solution is proportional to the number of colloidal particles in the solution. If a 15 g/dl solution of hemoglobin is polymerized, the number of molecules is reduced along with the COP, whereas no change occurs in hemoglobin concentration (Fig. 20.5). We have successfully prepared such a product in large volumes (33–35). The characteristics of such a polymerized, pyridoxylated hemoglobin solution (Poly SFH-P) are shown in Table 20.2.

PRELIMINARY STUDIES

Two kinds of preliminary studies have been completed. The first documented the efficacy of the polyhemoglobin in

rats at otherwise lethal hematocrits (34), and the second investigated polyhemoglobin half-life in the baboon (33). Much of the tetramer is cleared by the kidneys following dissociation into dimers, with a resultant half-life of 2 to 4 hours. The polyhemoglobin shows a striking increase in half-life to 38 hours, compared with about 4 hours for pyridoxylated hemoglobin (33). Thus, at the same COP, the O$_2$ capacity is greater, and the intravascular persistence is much longer for Poly SFH-P than for any unpolymerized product.

EFFICACY

We recently completed two studies to evaluate the efficacy of Poly SFH-P in baboons. The first examined the effects on P_{50} (11). Although the [Hb] of 14 g/dl of Poly SFH-P is a significant improvement over the [Hb] of the unpolymerized tetramer, the polymerization process results in a modest decrease in the P_{50}, from 22 to 24 torr for SFH-P to 16 to 20 torr for Poly SFH-P. Because O$_2$ unloading may decrease as P_{50} falls (18), there is concern about the ability of Poly SFH-P to transport O$_2$ effectively in the presence of red cells with their normal P_{50} of 26 torr. This issue is relevant because the clinical use of Poly SFH-P is likely to be in the presence of a reduced, but significant, red cell mass. In this setting, O$_2$ is carried in three separate compartments: RBCs; the plasma; and the Poly SFH-P, as shown:

$$[O_2]\ total = [O_2]\ RBC + [O_2]\ plasma + [O_2]\ Poly\ SFH\text{-}P$$

We previously reported that the efficacy of any O$_2$ carrier can be assessed quantitatively by determining its individual contribution to total O$_2$ delivery and O$_2$ consumption (11, 29). Using this methodology we evaluated the efficacy of Poly SFH-P as an O$_2$ carrier in a clinically relevant range of hematocrits and have shown that SFH-P effectively transports O$_2$ in the presence of red cells.

Seven adult baboons underwent a total exchange transfusion with Poly SFH-P with a [Hb] of 14.3 ± 2 g/dl and a P_{50} of 19.6 ± 0.4 torr. The data were compared with previously reported data using unpolymerized SFH-P with a [Hb] of 7.3 ± 0.2 g/dl and a P_{50} of 22.1 ± 1 torr. All animals receiving Poly SFH-P survived. The results show that Poly SFH-P supports life at zero hematocrit and that it makes significant contributions to both total O_2 delivery and O_2 consumption in the presence of red cells. Poly SFH-P permits a higher plasma [Hb] (Fig. 20.6) and has a longer intravascular persistence than any unpolymerized hemoglobin solution. Poly SFH-P, thus, is an effective O_2 carrier (13).

The second study focused on the hemodynamics (19). As stated above, although animals survive exchange transfusion with SFH-P, there is a decrease from baseline values in VO₂, mean arterial pressure (MAP), and CO and an increase in heart rate (HR) at zero hematocrit. It is possible that these changes are due to the low [Hb] of SFH-P, because the final plasma [Hb] in these animals is only 4 g/dl. Our hypothesis was that Poly SFH-P might normalize the final [Hb] and, thus, maintain baseline hemodynamics in the absence of red cells.

Six adult baboons were anesthetized, paralyzed, intubated, and mechanically ventilated on room air. Arterial, venous, and pulmonary artery catheters were inserted. A total exchange transfusion was performed with Poly SFH-P (Hb, 14.2 g/dl; P_{50}, 19.2 torr). The exchange volumes were adjusted to maintain the pulmonary capillary wedge pressure at baseline values. Cardiac output, O_2 consumption, MAP, and HR were measured. All baboons survived the exchange to a hematocrit (Hct) below 1%. The mean ± SEM for VO₂, MAP, HR, and CO at baseline (before exchange) and Hct below 1% (after exchange) are shown in Table 20.3. The results are compared with our prior data from six animals receiving the unpolymerized SFH-P ([Hb], 6.6 g/dl; P_{50}, 18.3 torr). The final plasma [Hb] at Hct below 1% was 9.7 g/dl for Poly SFH-P and 3.7 g/dl for the unpolymerized SFH-P. The hemodynamics and

O_2 consumption were well-maintained throughout with Poly SFH-P (19).

Poly SFH-P and SFH-P both support life in the absence of red cells. In contrast to SFH-P, Poly SFH-P achieves a near-normal plasma [Hb] and maintains baseline hemodynamics and O_2 consumption at zero hematocrit. Its intravascular persistence is prolonged significantly. These observations suggest that Poly SFH-P is an improved red cell substitute for use in the clinical setting.

SAFETY

The limiting factor prior to clinical testing is the concern about the safety of Poly SFH-P. The main uncertainty is the effect of this product on renal function. Nephrotoxicity was reported in early studies following the infusion of hemoglobin solution (22). Further investigations suggested that the stroma was the toxic factor, probably because of thrombosis of the small renal vasculature (27). In 1967 Rabiner and associates (28) reported that hemoglobin solution, relatively free of stroma, produced no deterioration in renal function following infusion in dogs. These findings were subsequently confirmed in monkeys, even in the stressful circumstances of dehydration and shock (2). The key observation was made in 1978 when Savitsky and coworkers (32) reported the results of a clinical safety trial in humans, using stroma-free hemoglobin. Eight healthy male volunteers received a 250-ml infusion of stroma-free hemoglobin at a rate of 2 to 4 ml/min. The hemoglobin concentration of this solution was 6.4 g/dl. The P_{50} was not reported. Two control patients received similar infusions at 5% albumin.

The most striking finding of this study was a decline in creatinine clearance in the hemoglobin solution recipients from a baseline value of 148 ml/min to 73 ml/min, 1 hour after infusion. This value returned to normal in the second hour following infusion. This alteration in kidney function was accompanied by a sharp decline in urine volume in these patients. In the albumin control patients, no changes were seen in urine volume or creatinine clearance. The authors stressed that this deterioration in kidney function was transient and not associated with permanent renal damage. Nevertheless, these results had a chilling effect on further clinical research.

As Savitsky and coworkers (32) pointed out, there are several possible explanations for the observed nephrotoxicity. The first is stromal toxicity—the authors did report a stroma lipid level of 1.6 mg/dl. However, since this represents only 1% of the original level of phospholipid, and since the infusion

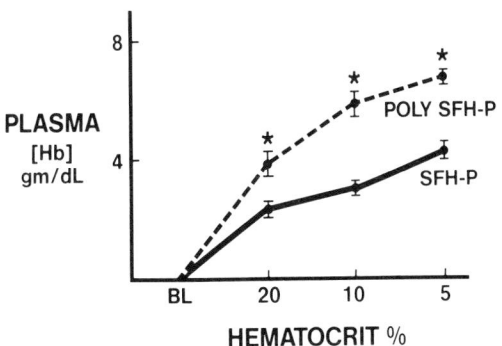

Figure 20.6. Plasma *[Hb]* (mean ± SEM) at intermediate hematocrits with Poly *SFH-P* or *SFH-P*. *BL*, baseline.

Table 20.3. Hemodynamics and Oxygen Consumption Before and After Exchange Transfusion

	Poly SFH-P		SFH-P	
	Baseline	*Hct < 1%*	*Baseline*	*Hct < 1%*
Oxygen consumption (ml/min)	60.1 ± 8.5	58.0 ± 4.8	85 ± 10	50 ± 10[a]
Mean arterial pressure (torr)	138 ± 8	140 ± 8	128 ± 7	95 ± 7[a]
Heart rate (beats/min)	114 ± 3	117 ± 10	108 ± 8	138 ± 11[a]
Cardiac output (liters/min)	1.63 ± 0.26	1.30 ± 0.2	2.72 ± 0.32	2.0 6 ± 0.46[a]

[a] Significant difference from baseline ($P < 0.05$).

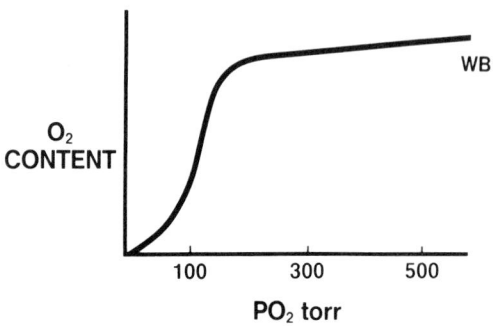

Figure 20.7. Oxygen content curve for whole blood *(WB)*. (From Civetta, Taylor, Kirby (eds): Fluorocarbons as oxygen carriers in surgical patients. *Surg Rounds 3(11):37–46, 1988.)*

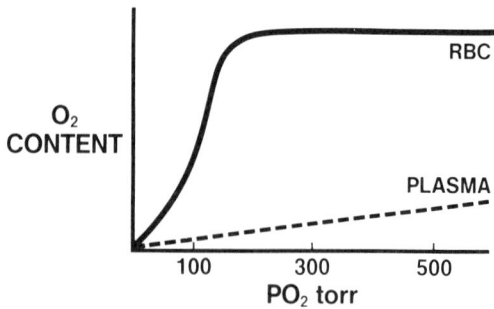

Figure 20.8. Oxygen content curves for red blood cells *(RBC)* and plasma. (From Civetta, Taylor, Kirby (eds): Fluorocarbons as oxygen carriers in surgical patients. *Surg Rounds 3(11):37–46, 1988.)*

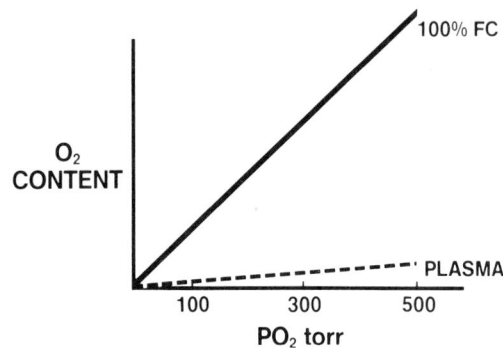

Figure 20.9. Oxygen content curves for 100% fluorocarbon *(FC)* and plasma. (From Civetta, Taylor, Kirby (eds): Fluorocarbons as oxygen carriers in surgical patients. *Surg Rounds 3(11):37–46, 1988.)*

of hemoglobin solution did not produce detectable disseminated intravascular coagulation in the recipients, stromal toxicity is an unlikely explanation. A second possibility is that the changes in renal function were simply related to the filtration of free hemoglobin through the kidneys. Perhaps hemoglobin filtration in some way interferes with normal kidney function. Once the hemoglobinemia disappears, renal function returns to normal. This is an interesting argument, since the highest level of plasma hemoglobin in the human volunteers was only 57 mg/dl. In actual clinical practice, we expect plasma hemoglobin levels to rise to 6 to 8 g/dl, a 1000-fold increase over the levels seen in the clinical safety trials. Elevations of plasma hemoglobin of such a magnitude would probably produce even greater changes in renal function, especially in a setting of hemorrhagic shock.

A significant problem has been the absence of a reliable animal model to assess the safety of each product. We have recently developed a sensitive and reproducible animal model that virtually duplicates these findings (31). Infusion of tetrameric hemoglobin solution in the unanesthetized primate produces the same changes in hemodynamics and renal function that were observed in the human volunteers. It is our hypothesis that since the large polymerized hemoglobin molecule will not traverse the renal tubules, it may not produce these same effects. We have completed the evaluation of Poly SFH-P, essentially free of unmodified tetrameric hemoglobin in this same model and shown it to be safe. We have confirmed this finding in human volunteers. There was no evidence of vasoconstriction or renal dysfunction in this group. Expanded safety and efficacy studies in patients are in progress.

PERFLUOROCHEMICAL EMULSIONS

Perfluorochemicals have potential as oxygen carriers because of their relatively high solubility for oxygen when compared with blood or plasma (3). However, this high solubility exists only for pure perfluorochemicals. Since perfluorochemicals are not miscible with water (i.e., plasma), current products are prepared as an emulsion, which lowers the concentration of fluorocarbon. The properties of the currently available perfluorochemical emulsions can best be understood by looking at several oxygen content curves. The oxygen content curve for whole blood is shown in Figure 20.7 and is the composite of the oxygen content curves for red cell hemoglobin and

plasma, as shown in Figure 20.8 (7). The curve illustrates that the majority of oxygen in whole blood is chemically bound to the hemoglobin molecule. The hemoglobin becomes fully saturated at a PO_2 of 150 torr (20 kPa). As the PO_2 increases beyond 150 torr (20 kPa), however, there is still an increase in the amount of oxygen in whole blood (Fig. 20.7), which reflects the dissolved O_2 in the aqueous phase of plasma (Fig. 20.8). Thus, as the oxygen tension in the blood is increased, the oxygen content will similarly increase despite the complete saturation of the hemoglobin molecule. Since the dissolved oxygen content of blood at the ambient PO_2 of 100 torr (13 kPa) is only 0.3 ml/dl, it is generally ignored when discussing oxygen content.

The potential value of perfluorochemicals as oxygen carriers is shown in Figure 20.9 (20). The curve illustrates that pure fluorocarbons have a solubility coefficient approximately 10 to 20 times that of plasma. In a sense, the fluorocarbons are functioning as a "super water." Unfortunately, however, pure fluorocarbons cannot be administered. A major development in perfluorochemical research was the ability to make a stable emulsion using pluronic F-68 as the emulsifying agent. By creating this emulsion, the concentration of fluorocarbon is lowered dramatically. Figure 20.10 shows oxygen content curves for 20% and 40% fluorocarbon emulsions, as compared to those of plasma. Clearly, the lower the concentration of fluorocarbon, the lower the oxygen content. The oxygen content of the perfluorochemical depends on both the PO_2 and the volume concentration of fluorocarbon (fluorocrit). For any given fluorocrit, the higher the PO_2, the higher the concentration of dissolved oxygen. Similarly, for any given PO_2, the higher the amount of fluorocarbon, the higher the oxygen content (Fig. 20.10).

The commercially prepared perfluorochemical emulsion is Fluosol-DA, 20%. This product has been evaluated extensively in animals and humans in Japan and in several series in the U.S. A comparison of whole blood with a hemoglobin of 15 g/dl and Fluosol-DA, 20%, is shown in Figure 20.11 (20). Although the Fluosol-DA does offer some value as an oxygen carrier, there are several limiting factors. First, the patient must breathe a high concentration of inspired oxygen in order to maximize the O_2 content of the Fluosol-DA. Second, even at a PO_2 of 500 torr (67 kPa) (fractional inspired O_2 concentration (FIO_2), 1.0), with the maximum achievable fluorocrit, the O_2 content is still less than 5 ml/dl, as compared to 20 ml/dl in whole blood. The infusion of Fluosol-DA would, therefore, add very little to the total O_2 content unless the [Hb] were considerably reduced from normal levels. The point of this observation is that although a potential benefit of Fluosol-DA does exist, there are significant limitations. Furthermore, the restrictions on the amount of Fluosol-DA that can be administered to any patient (40 ml/kg) limits the achievable fluorocrit, which will further decrease the amount of oxygen that can be carried by the Fluosol-DA.

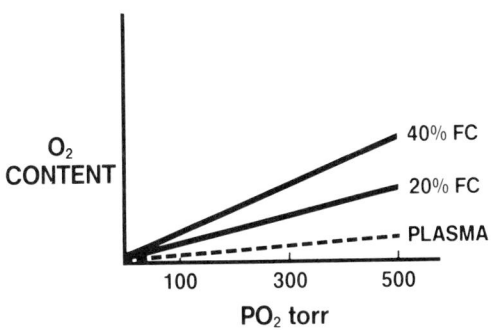

Figure 20.10. Oxygen content curves for plasma; also, 20% and 40% fluorocarbons *(FC)*. (From Civetta, Taylor, Kirby (eds): Fluorocarbons as oxygen carriers in surgical patients. *Surg Rounds 3(11):37–46, 1988.*)

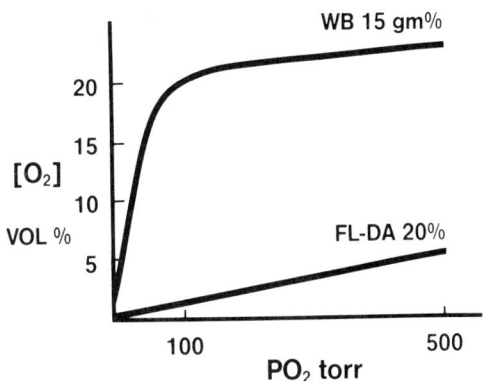

Figure 20.11. Oxygen content curves for 15 g/dl *(gm%)* of whole blood *(WB)* and 20% Fluosol-DA *(FL-DA)*. (From Civetta, Taylor, Kirby (eds): Fluorocarbons as oxygen carriers in surgical patients. *Surg Rounds 3(11):37–46, 1988.*)

LABORATORY STUDIES

Our initial effort was to answer the question: How good are fluorocarbon emulsions as oxygen carriers? Because the principal requirement of any O_2 carrier is the ability to load and unload oxygen, these functions must be accurately evaluated. We have shown that adult baboons can survive a total exchange transfusion with Fluosol-DA to zero hematocrit if they are ventilated at an FIO_2 of 1.0 (11). The animals maintain normal hemodynamics and oxygen transport in the virtual absence of red blood cells. Although these data suggest that Fluosol-DA is an effective oxygen carrier, we also demonstrated that control animals survive at zero hematocrit on an FIO_2 of 1.0 without Fluosol-DA (13). This remarkable observation leads to the conclusion that Fluosol-DA is not necessary at an FIO_2 of 1.0, at least in this acute setting.

These results can be explained by an understanding of the way in which the fluorocarbons carry oxygen. In the presence of red blood cells and fluorocarbon (FC), the total oxygen content in the blood can be considered as the sum of three separate oxygen carriers:

$$[O_2] \; total = [O_2] \; RBC + [O_2] \; plasma + [O_2] \; FC \qquad (2)$$

Survival depends on total oxygen content but does not distinguish between each of the oxygen carriers (14, 30). Thus, at a PO_2 of 500 torr (67 kPa) the plasma becomes a very significant carrier of oxygen and is capable of supporting oxygen consumption, even in the complete absence of both red cells and fluorocarbon. Because the plasma oxygen content will always be increased at an FIO_2 of 1.0, the actual need for the Fluosol-DA is unclear.

Although this study documents the efficacy of plasma as an oxygen carrier at an FIO_2 of 1.0, we are concerned about the potential risk of oxygen toxicity to the lungs in the clinical setting (5). A safe level of prolonged supplemental oxygen is thought to be an FIO_2 below 0.6. Our data suggest that the Fluosol-DA might not be necessary at an FIO_2 of 1.0, but we cannot assume the same to be true at lower levels of supplemental oxygen.

CLINICAL TRIAL

The results of the animal study led us to design a clinical trial to evaluate the safety and efficacy of Fluosol-DA as an oxygen carrier (7, 10). We sought to distinguish between the contribution of the dissolved oxygen in the plasma and the dissolved oxygen in the Fluosol-DA compartment and to minimize the risk of toxicity from breathing 100% oxygen. The objective, therefore, was to provide sufficient O_2 delivery with Fluosol-DA at a FIO_2 below 0.6. Unlike most clinical trials, the protocol for Fluosol-DA was nonblinded and had a crossover design, with each patient serving as his or her own control for each O_2 carrier. Such a design let us define the physiologic need for, and evaluate the efficacy of, Fluosol-DA in acute anemia.

Patients had to be at least 18 years old in order to be admitted into the study. Furthermore, the patient's arterial blood PO_2 (PAO_2) had to reach 300 torr (40 kPa) or greater when receiving supplemental oxygen, and the patient had to be normovolemic. The physiologic criteria of need for supplementing oxygen content were derived from our control studies in baboons: [Hb] below 3.5 g/dl; PMVO$_2$ below 25 torr; and O$_2$ extraction ratio above 50% (6, 14).

A patient who met one of the inclusion criteria was first treated with 100% oxygen. An attempt was made to stabilize the patient's condition at the clinically safe inspired oxygen level of 60% by a gradual tapering process. If successful, the patient was considered to have no physiologic need for an increased O$_2$ content and did not receive Fluosol-DA. If unsuccessful, the patient was crossed over to the Fluosol-DA, and received up to a maximum permissible dose of 40 ml/kg of body weight. Once again, an attempt was made to stabilize the patient's condition at 60% oxygen with Fluosol-DA.

GOALS

The study had three goals: (*a*) to identify a physiologic need for an additional oxygen carrier when the red cell compartment became inadequate, as defined by the physiologic criteria; (*b*) to attempt an increase in the oxygen content, using only the plasma as an oxygen carrier at a safe FIO$_2$; and (*c*) to evaluate Fluosol-DA as an oxygen carrier if the physiologic criteria of need still existed at an unsafe FIO$_2$.

RESULTS

Twenty-three surgical patients with blood loss and having religious objections to receiving blood transfusions were evaluated. Fifteen moderately anemic patients with a mean hemoglobin level (±SE) of 7.2 ± 0.5 g/dl had no evidence of a physiologic need for increased arterial oxygen content and did not receive Fluosol-DA. Eight severely anemic patients with a mean hemoglobin level of 3.0 ± 0.4 g/dl met the criteria of need and received the drug until the physiologic need disappeared or a maximal dose of 40 ml/kg of body weight was reached. All patients breathed supplemental O$_2$. We observed no adverse reactions to Fluosol-DA.

The volume of Fluosol-DA infused ranged from 2 to 10 units. Six of the eight patients received the maximum allowable dose. One patient survived after receiving only 2 units. Another died before his total dosage had been infused.

The maximal arterial oxygen content added by Fluosol-DA in the eight patients ranged from 0.3 to 1.2 ml/dl, with a mean increment of 0.7 ± 0.1 ml/dl. The data for FIO$_2$, fluorocrit, and partial pressure of arterial oxygen at the time of this peak in arterial oxygen content are shown in Table

Table 20.4. Arterial Oxygen Content at Peak Effect of Fluosol-DA[a]

	Mean ± SE
Partial pressure of arterial O$_2$ (torr)	430 ± 19
Fluorocrit (%)	5 ± 1
Fractional inspired O$_2$ concentration	1.0 ± 0.0
Arterial O$_2$ content (ml/dl)	
In Fluosol-DA phase	0.7 ± 0.1
In plasma phase	1.3 ± 0.1
Of red cells	2.8 ± 0.6

[a] Civetta, Taylor, Kirby (eds): Fluorocarbons as oxygen carriers in surgical patients. *Surg Rounds* 3(11): 37–46, 1988.

20.4. The simultaneous level of arterial oxygen carried by the plasma was 1.3 ± 0.1 ml/dl, and the level of oxygen carried by the red cells was 2.8 ± 0.6 ml/dl.

Table 20.5 shows the extent of oxygen unloading from the three phases. Eighty-two percent of the oxygen carried by the plasma and Fluosol-DA phases was unloaded. In contrast, only 19% was unloaded from the red cell phase. The relative contribution to total oxygen consumption for each of the three phases is also shown in Table 20.5. The plasma contributes the most (50%), whereas Fluosol-DA contributes 28% and the red cells only 22%.

The hemodynamic and oxygen transport values before and after Fluosol-DA are shown in Table 20.6. The only statistically significant differences were a minor reduction in heart rate and an increase in partial pressure of arterial oxygen (following an increased FIO$_2$ in one patient).

The intravascular persistence of the Fluosol-DA was determined in five patients. The mean half-life was 24.3 ± 4.3 hours, with a range of 12 to 37 hours.

SURVIVAL

Six of the eight patients receiving Fluosol-DA died. One of the surviving patients received red cell transfusions against his wishes, under a court order, after receiving his maximal allowable dose of Fluosol-DA (7). He probably would have died in the absence of red cell therapy. The minimal hemoglobin level observed in these eight patients was 1.8 ± 0.4 g/dl.

The 15 patients not receiving Fluosol-DA had a minimal hemoglobin level of 7.2 ± 0.5 g/dl during their hospital stay. Fourteen of these patients survived.

IMPLICATIONS OF THE CLINICAL STUDY

The principal requirement of any oxygen carrier is the ability to load and unload oxygen effectively. The product must remain in the intravascular space long enough to satisfy the need for which it was administered, and it must be free from any undesirable side effects.

The data illustrate that Fluosol-DA provides poor arterial oxygen content supplementation. This study shows that the fluorocrit achieved clinically with the currently available product is only about 5%. As shown in Table 20.4, a 5% concentration of Fluosol-DA at a PO$_2$ of 430 torr (57 kPa) has an oxygen content of 0.7 ml/dl, or approximately half the oxygen carried by plasma (1.3 ml/dl). This value is equivalent to an increase in hemoglobin concentration of only 0.5 g/dl. This relation between the amount of oxygen carried by Fluosol-DA at this fluorocrit and the amount carried by plasma is valid, regardless of PO$_2$, since the oxygen content curves for both carriers are straight lines (Fig. 20.12). The potential benefit of the Fluosol-DA is that even this small amount of oxygen is additive to the amount carried by plasma (Equation 2). However, the observed increase in total oxygen content of 0.7 ml/dl was not clinically important in our eight patients, as evidenced by the absence of any discernible physiologic benefit after the Fluosol-DA infusion.

In contrast, Fluosol-DA unloads oxygen very effectively. The AVDO$_2$ of the Fluosol-DA phase is 0.5 ml/dl (Table 20.5).

Table 20.5. Oxygen Dynamics of Three Phases at Peak Effect of Fluosol-DA[a]

| | Mean ± SE | | |
	Fluosol-DA	Plasma	Red Cells
Arterial O$_2$ content (ml/dl)	0.7 ± 0.1	1.3 ± 0.1	2.8 ± 0.6
Venous O$_2$ content (ml/dl)	0.2 ± 0.1	0.2 ± 0.1	2.2 ± 0.4
Oxygen unloaded (%)	82 ± 5	82 ± 5	19 ± 5
Contribution to O$_2$ consumption (%)	28 ± 5	50 ± 5	22 ± 7

[a] From Civetta, Taylor, Kirby (eds): Fluorocarbons as oxygen carriers in surgical patients. *Surg Rounds* 3(11): 37–46, 1988.

Table 20.6. Hemodynamics and Oxygen Transport Before and After Fluosol-DA Administration[a]

| | Mean ± SE | |
	Before Fluosol-DA	After Fluosol-DA[b]
Heart rate beats/min	117 ± 5	106 ± 4[c]
Mean arterial pressure (torr)	74 ± 6	78 ± 5
Cardiac index (liters/min/m²)	4.5 ± 0.7	4.2 ± 0.7
Hemoglobin (g/dl)	3.0 ± 0.4	2.0 ± 0.4
Total arterial O$_2$ content (ml/dl)	5.3 ± 0.5	4.8 ± 0.6
O$_2$ delivery (ml/min/m²)	235 ± 27	197 ± 32
O$_2$ consumption (ml/min//m²)	109 ± 13	88 ± 11
Partial pressure of arterial O$_2$ (torr)	356 ± 24	430 ± 19[c]
Partial pressure of mixed venous O$_2$ (torr)	40.0 ± 3.9	78.2 ± 23.3
O$_2$ extraction ratio (%)	46.0 ± 2.5	47.6 ± 3.8

[a] From Civetta, Taylor, Kirby (eds): Fluoro-carbons as oxygen carriers in surgical patients. *Surg Rounds* 3(11): 37–46, 1988.
[b] Data were obtained at peak arterial oxygen content after Fluosol-DA.
[c] The difference between values before and after Fluosol-DA is statistically significant ($P < 0.05$).

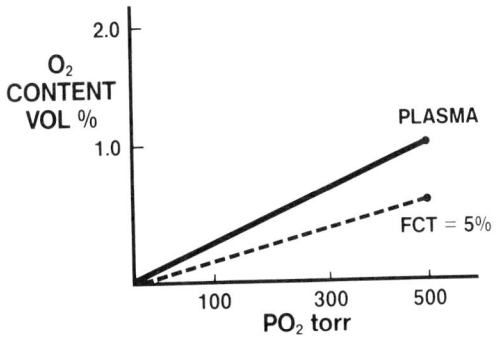

Figure 20.12. Oxygen content curves for plasma and Fluosol at a fluorocrit *(FCT)* of 5%.

Most of the oxygen carried by the Fluosol-DA is thus unloaded. The data also confirm previous reports that Fluosol-DA makes an important contribution to total oxygen consumption (39–41). However, the lack of any apparent physiologic effect despite this efficient oxygen unloading again suggests that this contribution is inadequate.

The intravascular persistence of Fluosol-DA is also insufficient, at least when red cells cannot be subsequently used. The half-life of 24 hours and the maximal allowable dose of 40 ml/kg led to a loss of the Fluosol-DA from the circulation before the patients were able to regenerate an adequate red cell mass to recover from their severe anemia (8). The mean hemoglobin level in the eight patients fell from an initial level of 3.0 to a low of 1.8 g/dl. This hemoglobin level is not compatible with survival, and six of the eight patients died of progressive anemia. The combination of too small an increment in arterial oxygen content and an inadequate duration of Fluosol-DA probably contributed to this unsatisfactory outcome. One of the survivors did require and eventually received red cells (against his wishes) after his total Fluosol-DA dose. It is thus possible that an evaluation of Fluosol-DA in a setting of short-term unavailability of red cells might result in a better outcome.

The mortality results should be compared with those of previous studies (23, 24, 39, 41). In the four earlier reports, representing a total of 200 patients, only three patients had a hemoglobin level of less than 3 g/dl. Two of these three patients died. In contrast, the less severely anemic patients receiving Fluosol-DA had satisfactory outcomes. This is consistent with our experience. Fifteen of the 23 patients evaluated had no physiologic evidence of a need for increased arterial oxygen content, despite their minimal hemoglobin level of 7.2 g/dl. They appeared to do as well as the comparable patients who received Fluosol-DA or those who would have received red cells if they were willing, because their hemoglobin level was below 10 g/dl. Fourteen of these moderately anemic patients not receiving Fluosol-DA survived. This good outcome justifies our physiologic assessment of when supplementation of oxygen content is needed and raises some questions about the manner in which decisions about transfusions are made. The mortality rate is high among severely anemic patients refusing red cells, despite Fluosol-DA therapy. Patients with less extreme blood loss who refuse red cells do well, with or without Fluosol-DA.

In conclusion, the results suggest that in acute blood loss, Fluosol-DA is unnecessary when anemia is moderate and ineffective when it is severe. Fluosol-DA is, therefore, an inadequate red cell substitute. New formulations of perfluorochemicals that correct the observed shortcomings of Fluosol-DA may be more effective (4, 37), such as achieving higher fluorocarbon concentrations and a longer intravascular persistence. In the near future, however, there is no likely perfluorochemical that will be an effective red cell substitute.

SUMMARY

The possibilities for the use of these oxygen carriers in the future are rather exciting. Both products meet some of the criteria of an ideal red cell substitute; both have shortcomings that will influence their clinical utility. The fluorocarbons appear to be quite safe. Their major current deficiency is that they are not likely to be useful in the clinical setting because of the requirement for supplemental O_2. The fluorocarbons are ineffective O_2 carriers when patients are breathing room air. In contrast, Poly SFH-P has been shown to be highly effective and has an O_2-carrying capacity equivalent to that of red blood cells. The unknown factor at this time is the safety of this hemoglobin solution. However, we are hopeful that Poly SFH-P will eliminate the undesirable effects of prior products. Clinical trials with Poly SFH-P are now in progress. Other areas of use for these O_2 carriers are being explored, such as use in coronary angioplasty, myocardial and cerebral ischemia, and radiation and chemotherapy. In addition, both products may be useful in cardioplegia and organ preservation. Once the safety and efficacy issues are resolved, other innovative uses may be identified. The development of both products remains active.

REFERENCES

1. Benesch RE, Benesch R, Renthal RD, et al: Affinity labeling of the polyphosphate binding site of hemoglobin. *Biochemistry* 11:3576, 1972.
2. Birndorf NI, Lopas H: Effects of red cell stroma-free hemoglobin solution on renal function in monkeys. *J Appl Physiol* 29:573, 1970.
3. Biro GP, Blais P: Perfluorocarbon blood substitutes. *CRC Crit Rev Oncol Hematol* 6(4):311, 1987.
4. Clark LC Jr, Clark EW, Moore RE, et al: Room temperature-stable biocompatible fluorocarbon emulsions. In Bolin RB, Geyer RP, Nemo GJ (eds): *Advances in Blood Substitute Research*. Alan R. Liss, New York, p 169, 1983.
5. Davis WB, Rennard SI, Bitterman PB, Crystal RG: Pulmonary oxygen toxicity: early reversible changes in human alveolar structure induced by hyperoxia. *N Engl J Med* 309:878, 1983.
6. Gould SA, Rice CL, Moss GS: The physiologic basis of the use of blood and blood products. *Surg Annu* 16:13, 1984.
7. Gould SA, Rosen AL, Sehgal LR, et al: Clinical experience with Fluosol-DA. In Bolin RB, Geyer RP (eds): *Advances in Blood Substitute Research*. Alan R. Liss, New York, p 331, 1983.
8. Gould SA, Rosen AL, Sehgal LR, et al: Depressed red cell recovery following acute blood loss (abstract). *Fed Proc* 44:1265, 1985.
9. Gould SA, Rosen AL, Sehgal L, et al: The effect of altered hemoglobin-oxygen affinity on oxygen transport by hemoglobin solution. *J Surg Res* 28:246, 1980.
10. Gould SA, Rosen AL, Sehgal LR, et al: Fluosol-DA as a red cell substitute in acute anemia. *N Engl J Med* 315:1653, 1986.
11. Gould SA, Rosen AL, Sehgal LR, et al: How good are fluorocarbon emulsions as O_2 carriers? *Surg Forum* 32:299, 1981.
12. Gould SA, Rosen AL, Sehgal LR, et al: Is cardiac output the principal determinant of Pmvo$_2$? *Crit Care Med* 9:273, 1981.
13. Gould SA, Rosen AL, Sehgal LR, et al: Is polyhemoglobin an effective O_2 carrier? *J Trauma* 26:903, 1986.
14. Gould SA, Rosen AL, Sehgal, LR, et al: O_2 extraction ratio: a physiologic indicator of transfusion need (abstract). *Transfusion* 23:416, 1983.
15. Gould SA, Rosen AL, Sehgal LR, et al: Plasma: an alternative oxygen carrier (abstract 7864)? *Fed Proc* 41:1615, 1982.
16. Gould SA, Rosen AL, Sehgal LR, et al: Red cell substitutes: hemoglobin solution or fluorocarbon? *J Trauma* 22:736, 1982.
17. Gould SA, Sehgal LR, Rosen AL, et al: The development of polymerized pyridoxylated hemoglobin solution as a red cell substitute. *Ann Emerg Med* 15:1416, 1986.
18. Gould SA, Sehgal LR, Rosen AL, et al: Hemoglobin solution: is a normal [Hb] or P$_{50}$ more important? *J Surg Res* 33:189, 1982.
19. Gould SA, Sehgal LR, Rosen AL, et al: Polyhemoglobin: an improved red cell substitute. *Surg Forum* 36:30, 1985.
20. Gould SA, Sehgal LR, Rosen AL, et al: Red cell substitutes: an update. *Ann Emerg Med* 14:798, 1985.
21. Greenburg AG, Hayashi R, Siefert I, et al: Intravascular persistence and oxygen delivery of pyridoxylated, stroma-free hemoglobin during gradations of hypotension. *Surgery* 86:13, 1979.
22. Hamilton PB, Hiller A, Van Slyke DD: Renal effects of hemoglobin infusions in dogs in hemorrhagic shock. *J Exp Med* 85:477, 1948.
23. Karn KE, Ogburn PL Jr, Julian T, et al: Use of a whole blood substitute, Fluosol-DA 20%, after massive postpartum hemorrhage. *Surg Obstet Gynecol* 65:127, 1985.
24. Mitsuno T, Ohyanagi H, Naito R: Clinical studies of a perfluorochemical whole blood substitute (Fluosol-DA): summary of 186 cases. *Ann Surg* 195:60, 1982.
25. Moss GS, DeWoskin R, Rosen AL, et al: Transport of oxygen and carbon dioxide by hemoglobin-saline solution in the red cell-free primate. *Surg Gynecol Obstet* 142:357, 1976.
26. Moss GS, Gould SA, Sehgal LR, et al: Hemoglobin solution—from tetramer to polymer. *Surgery* 95:249, 1984.
27. Rabiner SF, Friedman, LH: The role of intravascular hemolysis and the reticuloendothelial system in the production of hypercoagulable state. *Br J Haematol* 14:105, 1968.
28. Rabiner SF, Helbert JR, Lopas H, Friedman LH: Evaluation of a stroma-free hemoglobin solution for use as a plasma expander. *J Exp Med* 126:1127, 1967.
29. Rosen AL, Gould SA, Sehgal LR, et al: Evaluation of efficacy of stroma free hemoglobin solutions. In Bolin RB, Geyer RP (eds): *Advances in Blood Substitutes*. Alan R. Liss, New York, p 79, 1983.
30. Rosen AL, Sehgal LR, Gould SA, et al: Fluorocarbon emulsions: methodology to assess efficacy. *Crit Care Med* 10:149, 1982.
31. Rosen AL, Sehgal LR, Gould SA, et al: Renal response to hemoglobin solutions. *Physiologist* 29:4, 1986.
32. Savitsky JP, Doczi J, Black J, Arnold JD: A clinical safety trial of stroma-free hemoglobin. *Clin Pharmacol Ther* 23:73, 1978.
33. Sehgal LR, Gould SA, Rosen AL, et al: Polymerized pyridoxylated hemoglobin: a red cell substitute with normal O_2 capacity. *Surgery* 95:433, 1984.
34. Sehgal L, Rosen AL, Gould SA, et al: In vitro and in vivo characteristics of polymerized pyrodoxylated hemoglobin solution (abstract 2383). *Fed Proc* 39:718, 1980.
35. Sehgal LR, Rosen AL, Gould SA, et al: Preparation and in vitro characteristics of polymerized pyridoxylated hemoglobin. *Transfusion* 23:148, 1983.
36. Sehgal LR, Rosen AL, Noud G, et al: Large volume preparation of pyridoxylated hemoglobin with high in vivo P$_{50}$. *J Surg Res* 30:14, 1981.
36a. Sehgal LR, Sehgal HL, Gould DA, et al: Characteristics of polymerized pyridoxylated hemoglobin solution under clinical investigation. Vth ISBS, San Diego, March 17–20, H104, 1993.
37. Sloviter HA, Mukherji B: Prolonged retention in the circulation of emulsified lipid-coated perfluorochemicals. In Bolin RB, Geyer RP (eds): *Advances in Blood Substitute Research*. Alan R. Liss, New York, p 181, 1983.
38. Sunder-Plassman L, Dieterle R, Seifert J, et al: Stroma free haemoglobin solution as a blood replacement fluid: actual state and problems. *Eur J Intensive Care Med* 1:37, 1975.
39. Tremper KK, Friedman AE, Levine EM, et al: The preoperative treatment of severely anemic patients with a perfluorochemical oxygen-transport fluid, Fluosol-DA. *N Eng J Med* 307:277, 1982.
40. Tremper KK, Lapin R, Levine E, et al: Hemodynamic and oxygen transport effects of a perfluorochemical blood substitute. Fluosol-DA (20%). *Crit Care Med* 8:738, 1980.
41. Waxman K, Tremper KK, Cullen BF, Mason GR: Perfluorocarbon infusion in bleeding patients refusing blood transfusion. *Arch Surg* 119:721, 1984.

CHAPTER 21

Thrombolytic Therapy

ALLAN S. JAFFE, M.D.

The use of thrombolytic agents for the treatment of thrombotic disorders has been investigated extensively since the initial observations by Tillet and Garner in 1933 (265) that filtrates of β-hemolytic streptococci had fibrinolytic activity. Initially, because of the potential for bleeding and the lack of adequate documentation of benefit, the indications for the use of thrombolytic agents were limited. During the 1980s, enthusiasm for thrombolytic therapy increased because of the development of agents with greater clot specificity and the demonstration that prompt reperfusion of coronary arteries occluded by thrombi in patients with acute myocardial infarction led to a reduction in mortality (104, 142, 242) and preservation of ventricular function (215, 240, 241). These phenomena stimulated new research to define the optimum means for inducing fibrinolysis and to redefine the indications and contraindications for the use of these agents. Presently, four preparations of plasminogen activators are available for clinical use: streptokinase (SK); urokinase (UK); tissue plasminogen activator (t-PA); and acylated streptokinase/plasminogen complexes (APSAC).

OVERVIEW OF THE FIBRINOLYTIC SYSTEM

The fibrinolytic system is an enzymatic system present in blood that induces clot dissolution via the formation of the enzyme plasmin. Plasmin is derived from the circulating zymogen, plasminogen, by the action of agents known as plasminogen activators. Once generated, plasmin degrades fibrin,

as well as fibrinogen, prothrombin, factor V, factor VIII, prekallikrein, several components of the complement system, and other circulating proteins (6). The proteolytic activity of plasmin is controlled by rapid interactions with several circulating inhibitors in blood (51).

Plasminogen is a single-chain glycoprotein that exists in several forms. Native plasminogen has a glutamic acid at the amino terminus, and is referred to as "glu-plasminogen" (290). Limited plasmin digestion of plasminogen during activation results in a modified glycoprotein with lysine, alanine, or methionine at the amino terminus, referred to collectively as "lys-plasminogen." Within the plasminogen molecule are sites referred to as the lysine-binding sites, which serve as the points of interaction for the binding of plasminogen to fibrin or to its inhibitor, α-2-antiplasmin (51, 301). Lys-plasminogen has a higher affinity for fibrin than does glu-plasminogen and is also more rapidly converted to plasmin by the plasminogen activator, UK (49, 211).

MECHANISM OF ACTION OF PLASMINOGEN ACTIVATORS

Plasminogen can be activated by a number of mechanisms. It is activated by factor XII, prekallikrein, high molecular weight kininogen, and possibly other plasm constituents of the kallikrein system (140). The physiologic importance of this type of activation (intrinsic) is undetermined. The significance of activation due to the secretion of plasminogen activators from tissue or endothelium is better understood (extrinsic activation). t-PA has been extensively studied and is probably identical to blood plasminogen activator and vascular plasminogen activator (219). It has very little plasminogen activator activity in isolation; however, in the presence of fibrin, activation of plasminogen increases markedly (122). Thus, in physiologic systems, t-PA converts only fibrin-bound plasminogen to plasmin, providing a localized mechanism for clot dissolution (54). Activation of t-PA is modulated by a variety of inhibitors. The rapidly acting inhibitor, plasminogen activator inhibitor-1 (PAI-1), is the most common and binds to t-PA, inactivating it. PAI-1 also inhibits urokinase but not single-chain urokinase-like plasminogen activator (scu-PA) or streptokinase (154). PAI-1 increases in response to administration and/or elaboration of t-PA (169).

UK is a two-chain serum protease that has been isolated from human urine and cultured kidney cells (202, 305). It exists in both a high and low molecular weight form (299). Two-chain UK activates plasminogen by lysis of a single arginine-valine bond (221). A single-chain proenzyme form of UK (scu-PA) also has been isolated and has plasminogen activator activity, even without conversion to the two-chain form (55, 109).

SK, in contrast, activates plasminogen indirectly. It first forms an equimolar complex with plasminogen, which exposes an active site on plasminogen and transforms it into an activator complex (43, 178). SK-plasminogen complexes (APSAC) have been modified by the synthesis of derivatives containing acyl groups at the active site (246). In the circulation, acylation prevents plasminogen activation. These derivatives are deacylated slowly, and active SK-plasmin(ogen) activator complexes result. It was thought that this strategy would lead to less systemic plasminogen activation, greater clot specificity, and greater efficacy (7). However, at the doses required for rapid fibrinolysis, fibrin specificity is lost (50). The major advantage of APSAC is that it can be administered as a one-time bolus (173).

Once generated, plasmin is rapidly inhibited by the formation of an equimolar complex with α-2-antiplasmin (300). Plasmin interacts with fibrin at the enzyme's lysine-binding site. Plasmin that is bound to fibrin is protected from rapid inhibition by α-2-antiplasmin since the lysine-binding site is occupied by fibrin. α-2-macroglobulin also inhibits plasmin, although more slowly (51).

CLINICAL PHARMACOLOGY OF FIBRINOLYTIC AGENTS

STREPTOKINASE (Streptase; Hoechst Celanse, Inc., Somerville, NJ, and Kabikinase, Kabi Vitrum AB, Stockholm, Sweden)

Because streptokinase (SK) is derived from a common bacterial species, antibodies to it are present in most patients. Although allergic reactions can occur, a well-documented case of anaphylaxis with currently available preparations has not been reported. When SK is administered systemically, an initial large dose is used to overcome the inhibitory effect of high-antibody titers. The administration of 250,000 units overcomes antibody resistance and induces a systemic lytic state in more than 90% of patients (118). The maintenance dose used subsequently varies but in theory must be sufficient to generate enough plasmin to overcome circulating inhibitors. An excessive dose of SK could in theory consume or complex all of the available plasminogen, leaving none for further activation. Thus, both insufficient and/or excessive doses could result in less effective therapy.

After injection of radiolabeled SK, an initial α-distributive half-life of 18 minutes has been observed, followed by a β-distributive half-life of 83 minutes (84). However, the clearance of functionally active SK-plasminogen complexes has been estimated to be only 23 minutes (182). Nonetheless, fibrinolytic activity can be demonstrated for as long as 4 hours after administration of SK, despite clearance of active complexes from plasma (79). A rate of administration of 750,000 units over 30 minutes induces a mean decrease in systolic blood pressure of 35 ± 19 mm Hg and in diastolic blood pressure of 20 ± 14 mm Hg. More severe and symptomatic hypotension also can occur in patients with poor left ventricular function (167).

Since SK activates both circulating plasminogen and plasminogen bound to fibrin, both local and systemic effects are observed after its administration. Degradation of circulating fibrinogen, plasminogen, and coagulation factors is the most significant hemostatic alteration (239). Formation of fibrinogen degradation products may exacerbate the tendency toward bleeding induced by the low levels of circulating fibrinogen and other coagulation factors by inhibiting thrombin and fibrin polymerization (158, 174, 212). Low-dose local infusions of SK have been used to limit these adverse systemic effects.

SK induces a procoagulant response when administered (75). Increases in thrombin activity occur with all activators but, judging from in vitro studies, the extent of this effect appears greater with SK (73, 74). In addition to increases in thrombin activity, enhanced platelet activation is also observed (83). Activation may be secondary to increases in thrombin activity or due to an independent process. Some of the increases in thrombin activity may be derived from preformed thrombin in the clot itself (88) or reflect the influence of the endothelium reexposed after clot dissolution. However, judging from the results of in vivo and in vitro studies, new thrombin is generated by activation of prothrombin by plasmin (74, 81). The fact that SK elaborates more plasmin systemically than more fibrin-specific activators may explain why the extent of procoagulation appears greater. Procoagulation may retard the rapidity of lysis. This fact may be the reason for the lower patency rate at 90 minutes observed with SK, compared to that observed with agents such as t-PA in patients with acute myocardial infarction (48, 282, 286).

UROKINASE (Abbokinase; Abbott Laboratories, North Chicago, IL).

Urokinase (UK) has also been used extensively as a fibrinolytic agent. Since UK is not antigenic in humans and is a direct activator of plasminogen, the dose-response relationships of this activator are less complex. After administration, UK is cleared with a half-life of 14 ± 6 minutes. Since UK activates both circulating plasminogen and plasminogen bound to fibrin, intravenous administration of UK results in systemic effects similar to those observed after SK (85). Local infusions of UK have also been used to minimize these effects. In general, the effects of UK and the actions of SK are similar. In the past, UK has been considerably more expensive than SK.

TISSUE PLASMINOGEN ACTIVATOR (Alteplase; Boehringer Ingelheim, activase; Genentech, Inc., South San Francisco, CA)

Human recombinant tissue-type plasminogen activator (t-PA) is the first of the so-called fibrin-specific agents. Initial studies used product isolated from a human melanoma cell (24, 277) until a recombinant product could be made (58, 276). t-PA exists in one- and two-chain forms (289) that have similar fibrinolytic activity in purified systems. However, in plasma, one-chain t-PA is converted to the two-chain form during fibrinolysis (218). After a bolus injection, predominantly two-chain t-PA is cleared from plasma with a half-life of approximately 4.1 to 6.3 minutes (91, 190). With longer infusions, a β-distributive half-life of 41 to 50 minutes is evident (91, 283). Predominantly single-chain preparations have a slightly shorter initial half-life of 3.6 to 4.6 minutes and a β-distributive half-life of 39 to 53 minutes (91). Thus, plasma levels will vary, depending on the preparation used. After administration of t-PA, lytic activity persists for many hours after clearance of activator (79). There are preparations other than the one available for routine clinical use in the U.S. that have been used for research purposes (13, 52). The extent of single-, compared to two-chain material, the clearance of the agents (related to the extent of glycosylation), and the potency of each on a milligram basis may vary and must be assessed individually for each preparation (13, 52).

Unlike UK or SK, t-PA has little systemic effect at low doses (57, 277). The markedly enhanced activation of plasminogen by t-PA in the presence of fibrin should result in clot lysis without significant systemic plasminogen activation. However, the selectivity for plasminogen bound to fibrin is only relative, and in the presence of very high concentrations of t-PA, circulating plasminogen is degraded as well (248, 263). Thus, in clinical trials in patients with acute myocardial infarction, higher doses (100 to 150 mg) of t-PA produce some systemic plasminogen activation and fibrinogen breakdown (53, 80). Data also exist to suggest that excessive breakdown of plasminogen can occur and lead to a loss of plasminogen within the clot itself, retarding lysis (249). Nonetheless, these systemic effects are less with t-PA than with other activators.

Trials of recombinant t-PA in patients with acute myocardial infarction generally have used intravenous preparations to permit treatment as early as possible. However, infusions into the coronary artery and peripheral arteries have also been employed and offer the advantage of allowing administration of a significantly lower dose with similar beneficial effects (58, 101) when rapid treatment is less critical. Increases in thrombin activity and enhanced platelet activation also occur in response to t-PA (145, 209, 210). The extent of these increases is a predictor of the success or failure of treatment (108, 145). Judging from in vitro studies, changes in thrombin activation with t-PA appear to be less than those changes observed with activators that are less fibrin-specific (73, 74). Because t-PA does not markedly degrade fibrinogen, it does not generate fibrinogen degradation products to antagonize thrombin activity or deplete fibrinogen to the same extent as nonfibrin-specific activators (53). This fact may make t-PA more prone to reocclusion in the absence of antithrombotic treatment. The maintenance of the high degree of early coronary patency induced by t-PA is critically dependent on the early and effective administration of heparin (26, 123).

As is the case for all plasminogen activators, the fibrinolytic activity of t-PA in plasma is modulated by circulating plasmin inhibitors to some extent. Studies have shown t-PA is protected from inhibition once bound to fibrin (51, 300) but is rapidly inhibited by plasminogen inhibitor-1 (154), which is known to be elevated in patients with ischemic heart disease (112, 179, 198) and to increase in response to administration and/or elaboration of t-PA (169).

ACYLATED STREPTOKINASE/PLASMINOGEN COMPLEX DERIVATIVES (APSAC, Eminase; SmithKline Beecham Pharmaceuticals, Philadelphia, PA, and Upjohn Co., Kalamazoo, MI).

It had been hypothesized that acylated SK-plasminogen complexes would induce clot lysis, while inducing less systemic lytic activity than SK (245). However, deacylation is slow (half-life = 40 minutes), mandating the use of doses for rapid thrombolysis that induce significant systemic plasminogen activation (22, 119, 141, 173, 252, 287). Thus the primary benefit of this approach has been to permit administration as a one-time bolus dose (173). Other biochemical and pharmacologic effects appear similar to the actions of SK, except that APSAC in the dose used clinically (30 mg is equivalent to 1,100,000 units of SK) appears to induce hypotension less frequently than SK in its most commonly used dose (1,500,000 units) (10). About 5% of patients develop possible allergic reactions; in 0.2 to 0.4% they are classified as severe (3, 134). A purpuric rash can also occur and at times may be severe (3, 37, 134). In direct comparative trials, APSAC results in a greater frequency of coronary patency than does SK by 90 minutes after treatment of patients with acute myocardial infarction (45), but this advantage is no longer present at 24 hours. The patency rate associated with APSAC at 90 minutes after treatment appears comparable to that induced with intracoronary SK (10, 32). In the only available direct comparative trial reported thus far, t-PA induced a greater patency rate at 90 minutes than does APSAC (186). By 24 hours, patency with APSAC and t-PA is equivalent (11, 286). There were no differences in mortality rates between patients receiving APSAC, SK, or t-PA in the only comparative clinical trial reported thus far (244).

ACTIVATORS NOT AVAILABLE FOR ROUTINE CLINICAL USE

There are several plasminogen activators under development that may with time provide for more fibrin specificity. They have been called by some "second generation fibrin-specific agents" and include single-chain UK plasminogen activators (scu-PA) (60, 168), a variety of activators that are linked to fibrin-specific monoclonal antibodies (27, 28, 110) and an activator isolated from vampire bat salivary gland known as Bat-PA (92).

Scu-PA is the only one of these agents that has been investigated in a systematic way in patients (69, 139, 278, 279). scu-PA is thought to be able to activate some plasminogen to plasmin directly. Plasmin then converts scu-PA into the two-chain form of UK, resulting in still further plasminogen activation (60, 168). In plasma, activation of plasminogen by scu-PA is limited by inhibitors (168) that appear to be inactivated in the presence of fibrin. The half-life of scu-PA in experimental models is similar to that of UK. Preliminary trials with scu-PA demonstrate greater clot selectivity in humans than with UK (278), but less than with t-PA. Synergism with t-PA and UK has been demonstrated (29, 30, 56, 59).

MONITORING OF THE COAGULATION SYSTEM

Ideally, laboratory monitoring of coagulation during treatment with fibrinolytic agents should provide precise information regarding the effect of the activator on coagulation and, hence, the intensity of fibrinolytic activity, the extent of clot dissolution, and the potential for bleeding. Conventional assays of coagulation can only document the presence of a systemic lytic state when it is induced and do not distinguish between the effects of the activators and those of heparin (239). With the newer, more clot-selective plasminogen activators, monitoring has focused primarily on detection of systemic lytic activity as an index of excessive dosage. Once the lytic state has waned, assays of coagulation are used to titrate the dose of heparin.

Conventional laboratory monitoring of the effects of thrombolytic therapy may include assays of thrombin time, activated partial thromboplastin time, prothrombin time, fibrinogen, fibrinogen degradation products, and euglobulin lysis time. An understanding of each test and how it is affected by plasminogen activation is essential to proper interpretation of results (239).

The thrombin time depends on the concentration of fibrinogen in plasma and is extremely sensitive to heparin and fibrinogen degradation products in the sample (133). It is prolonged after administration of fibrinolytic agents, if fibrinogen is depleted, and if fibrin(ogen) degradation products are formed. When heparin has been administered, the addition of protamine sulfate to the plasma sample reverses the effects of heparin, allowing for detection of the consequences of systemic lytic activity alone.

The activated partial thromboplastin time (aPTT) assesses the activity of the coagulation factors other than factors VII and XIII and is used primarily to monitor the effects of heparin (206). It is affected by decreased fibrinogen and increases in fibrinogen degradation products but to a lesser extent than is the thrombin time. Once the systemic lytic state has resolved, the aPTT is the best presently available coagulation test for monitoring and titrating the dose of heparin. However, values do not reflect thrombin activity as measured with more precise but less clinically available assays (77).

The prothrombin time measures the activity of factors V, VII, and X; prothrombin; and fibrinogen. It is affected to an even lesser extent than the aPTT by low levels of fibrinogen and/or fibrin(ogen) degradation products.

Determination of fibrinogen degradation is one of the most common criteria for documenting systemic plasminogen activation. Several methods are available for measurement of fibrinogen. The Clauss procedure measures the kinetics of clot formation and, hence, clottable fibrinogen. This assay is sensitive to the presence of fibrin(ogen) degradation products that are not clottable or inhibit polymerization of fibrin and is inaccurate when fibrinogen levels are extremely low (generally less than 55 mg/dl), as is frequently the case after intravenous administration of nonfibrin-specific activators. The Ellis method of measuring fibrinogen is an endpoint assay that measures the total amount of fibrinogen clotted after prolonged incubation. This assay is less affected by fibrin(ogen) degradation products and generally yields higher values for fibrinogen than those obtained from the Clauss method, particularly when the fibrinogen level is very low. Large amounts of heparin in the sample can lead to spuriously low values. Reversal of the effects of heparin with protamine sulfate corrects for this effect. Precipitation procedures and most immunologic methods generally do not differentiate fibrinogen from large clottable fibrinogen degradation products.

The most commonly used procedure for measurement of fibrin(ogen) degradation products utilizes antifibrinogen antibody-coated latex particles. This method and most others detect products of both fibrinogen and fibrinolysis (259).

The euglobulin lysis time measures the functional activity of plasminogen activators in plasma in the absence of inhibitors that are not contained in the fraction (153). Enhanced lytic activity in the euglobulin fraction on plasma clots or fibrin plates or on clots in other systems is evidence of the presence of functional plasmin activity in vivo.

Monitoring generally includes baseline measurements of the aPTT, thrombin time, fibrinogen, and/or fibrin(ogen) degradation products. With nonfibrin-specific activators, a repeat fibrinogen is often useful to document induction of the lytic state (239). Reduction of fibrinogen to 50% of baseline values or less has been suggested as a criterion. When very low levels of fibrinogen are present, the Ellis assay is more likely to be accurate. Subsequently, a normal protamine-corrected thrombin time can be used to document the absence of residual effects of plasminogen activation. Once the systemic lytic state has resolved, the aPTT may be used to titrate the dose of heparin. With more clot-specific activators, such as t-PA, that may not induce systemic plasminogen activation, a shortened euglobulin lysis time may be the only evidence of circulating plasminogen activator, since fibrinogen degradation and other alterations of coagulation may only be present after large doses.

Fibrinopeptide A (FPA) is a 16-amino acid peptide cleaved from fibrinogen by thrombin as part of the formation of fibrin. Thus, with rare exception (295), it is a measure of thrombin activity (191). Other measures, such as the prothrombin fragment F1.2 (81) and thrombin-antithrombin 3 complexes, can also be used to assess thrombin activity (108). Several assays have been developed recently to distinguish fibrin from fibrinogen degradation products (89, 229, 298). These assays have been used to show that fibrin dissolution after t-PA and SK persists for many hours after these activators are cleared from the circulation (79), to detect fibrinolysis when fibrin-specific

Table 21.1. Results of Trials Comparing Thrombolysis and Heparin for the Acute Treatment of Deep Venous Thrombosis

Study	Agent	Venographic Improvement (% Patients)[a]		Bleeding (% Patients)[a,b]	
		Thrombolysis	Heparin	Thrombolysis	Heparin
Arneson (15)	SK[c]	71 (15/21)	14 (3/21)	14 (3/21)	14 (3/21)
Elliot (82)	SK	65 (17/26)	0 (0/25)	12 (3/26)	0 (0/25)
Goldhaber (98)	t-PA	41 (20/49)	18 (2/11)	24 (12/49)	0 (0/12)
Kakkar (137)	SK	78 (8/9)	22 (2/9)	40 (4/10)	22 (2/9)
Marder (175)	SK	58 (7/12)	25 (3/12)	58 (7/12)	8 (1/12)
Robertson (223)	SK	66 (6/9)	29 (2/7)	35 (6/17)	29 (2/7)
Rosch (226)	SK	45 (10/22)	27 (7/26)	NA	NA
Tsapogas (273)	SK	53 (10/19)	7 (1/15)	NA	NA
Watz (291)	SK	67 (12/18)	36 (6/17)	17 (3/18)	12 (2/17)

[a] Number of patients is in parentheses.
[b] Includes all bleeding.
[c] SK, streptokinase; t-PA, tissue plasminogen activator.

activators are used, and to quantitate the relative amount of fibrin vs. fibrinogen degradation (80).

Assays that directly measure t-PA and PAI-1 antigen and activity have recently been developed; these assays permit distinction of free from bound activator (170). Increases in PAI-1 have been observed in response to administration of t-PA and may be responsible for reocclusion in some patients (169).

CLINICAL APPLICATIONS OF THROMBOLYSIS

DEEP VENOUS THROMBOSIS

The traditional objective of therapy for lower extremity venous thrombosis has been to prevent pulmonary embolism and its often-catastrophic complications (62, 136, 146). Although this goal can be accomplished by heparin, heparin alone usually does not result in dissolution of the thrombus. As a consequence of residual thrombosis, morbidity due to venous valvular insufficiency with lower extremity edema, aching, stasis dermatitis, and ulceration (postphlebitic syndrome) may occur, especially after extensive proximal venous thrombosis (35, 304). As many as 80% of patients treated with heparin for venous thrombosis ultimately develop signs and/or symptoms of the postphlebitic syndrome (193). Fibrinolytic agents have the potential to more thoroughly dissolve occlusive thrombi. Since residual clot is considered the etiology of the "postphlebitic syndrome," this therapy should reduce its incidence.

RANDOMIZED TRIALS COMPARING STREPTOKINASE WITH HEPARIN

Nine randomized trials performed in the 1960s and 1970s have compared the efficacy of clot lysis induced by SK with that induced by heparin, as assessed by venography (14, 23, 82, 137, 175, 223, 226, 273, 291). In six, long-term endpoints were also assessed (15, 61, 82, 137, 138, 273). In response to SK, generally administered as a bolus of 250,000 units followed by an intravenous infusion of 100,000 units/hr for 24 to 72 hours, improved venous patency was observed in 62% of patients treated with SK (Table 21.1). Only 20% of patients treated with heparin demonstrated similar improvement. However, bleeding complications were much greater after

SK. Despite the improved efficiency of clot lysis with SK, the short-term clinical response was similar with either regimen in most series.

Long-term clinical benefit was more evident in patients treated with SK (Table 21.2). Approximately 60% of the patients who received this thrombolytic had normal or only minor abnormalities on follow-up venography at intervals from 2 to 6½ years; 74% were asymptomatic. In contrast, only 20% of the patients treated with heparin alone demonstrated similar findings by venography, and more than 70% had symptomatic postphlebitic syndrome. Thus, fibrinolytic therapy results in more rapid and more complete resolution of deep venous thrombosis acutely and less morbidity over the long term.

Several clinical factors may modulate the response to SK. Fresher clots are lysed more readily than older clots. The response to treatment is excellent for up to 3 days after the onset of symptoms (257), and the response appears less favorable after 7 days (175). Between 4 and 7 days, the chances of success decrease (16, 237), but in some series good late results have been obtained (71, 234). In addition, both the extent and location of the deep vein thrombosis affect the results of treatment. Incompletely occlusive thrombi seem to respond more favorably than completely occlusive clots in some series (36, 46, 82, 177), perhaps due to better access of the activator to the clot itself. However, the presence of a total occlusion does not preclude total resolution of thrombus (46, 137). In addition, proximal venous thrombi seem to respond better than distal thrombi (71, 132).

Recently, what has been termed ultrahigh-dose SK treatment (1,500,000 units/hr for 6 hours) has been advocated (176). With this massive dose regimen, there was "total clearance" in 42% of 176 cases and partial clearance (some areas of occlusion remaining) in another 36.4%. Patients with subclavian thrombi and those patients who had more recently formed clots responded better. Bleeding was infrequent and only four patients developed pulmonary emboli (176), a known complication with the use of lytic therapy for deep venous thrombosis (31, 121).

APSAC also is effective (246); however, at doses higher than 5 mg/day, significant fibrinogen degradation occurs (141). Whether it will have advantages over SK other than the convenience of bolus dosing is unclear at present. Recently, a comparative analysis by Graor et al (102) has suggested that prolonged intravenous infusions of UK and SK have comparable

Table 21.2. Results of Trials Comparing Thrombolysis and Heparin for the Treatment of Deep Venous Thrombosis (Late Results)

Study	Agent	Normal Venogram (% Patients)[a]		Asymptomatic (% Patients)[a]	
		Thrombolysis	*Heparin*	*Thrombolysis*	*Heparin*
Arneson (15)	SK[b]	44 (7/16)	0 (0/18)	77 (13/17)	33 (6/18)
Beiger (23)	SK	100 (5/5)	20 (1/5)	60 (3/5)	40 (2/5)
Elliot (82)	SK	55 (11/20)	0 (0/25)	62 (16/26)	10 (2/21)
Kakkar (137)	SK	57 (4/7)	14 (1/7)	NA	NA
Rosch (226)	SK	40 (6/15)	8 (1/12)	NA	NA
Watz (291)	SK	92 (11/12)	13 (1/8)	NA	NA

[a] Number of patients is in parentheses.
[b] SK, streptokinase.

efficacy for the treatment of deep venous disease, but that the incidence of significant bleeding was substantially less with UK. If the cost of treating the complications of SK treatment is factored in, UK is no longer appreciably more expensive. However, increased bleeding with SK has not been documented in all studies.

t-PA induces complete lysis in some patients without evidence of systemic plasminogen activation (293). A recent large study comparing t-PA with and without the adjunctive use of heparin to treatment with heparin alone found more complete clot dissolution with little morbidity in patients given t-PA in a dose of 0.05 mg/kg/hr for 24 hours to a maximum dose of 150 mg (98). Complete or more than 50% lysis occurred in 28% of patients, whether heparin was used adjunctively or not. This degree of lysis was not observed in any patient receiving heparin alone. In fact, 83% of patients receiving heparin alone demonstrated no lysis at all (Table 21.1). One patient developed nonfatal intracranial bleeding. Comparative trials of plasminogen activators for the treatment of deep venous thrombosis have not been accomplished.

SUMMARY

Thrombolytic therapy of deep venous thrombosis results in more complete dissolution of thrombi, which prevents venous valvular damage and venous hypertension and reduces the incidence of postphlebitic syndrome. Thrombolytic therapy should be considered in well-selected younger patients with extensive proximal venous thrombosis, who are free of contraindications to treatment (Table 21.3); the bleeding risks in such patients appear reasonable. However, the risk-to-benefit relationship in patients with relative contraindications and the agent of choice and its dose have not been established. After treatment, patients should receive heparin titrated to maintain the aPTT at approximately twice normal, followed by long-term treatment with coumadin.

PULMONARY EMBOLISM

The use of heparin for the treatment of pulmonary embolism markedly reduces the mortality rate from recurrent emboli (18). Once treatment has been initiated, the mortality rate is approximately 8% and often is secondary to associated illness (64). Nonetheless, patients with severe reduction in the cross-sectional area of the pulmonary artery (greater than 50%) frequently have right ventricular failure and shock and have a poor prognosis despite treatment with heparin.

Table 21.3. Contraindications to Thrombolytic Therapy

Absolute contraindications
  Active bleeding
  Cerebrovascular accident within 2 months or active
    intracerebral process
Major relative contraindications
  Major recent surgery, organ biopsy, or invasive vascular
    procedure within 10 days
  Active malignancy
  Recent serious trauma, including prolonged cardiopulmonary
    resuscitation
  Severe hypertension (systolic $\geq$ 180 mm Hg or diastolic $\geq$ 110
    mm Hg)
Other relative contraindications
  Chronic or acute renal failure
  Endocarditis
  Pregnancy or immediate postpartum state
  Age (75 yr or older)
  Diabetic hemorrhagic retinopathy
  Chronic therapeutic anticoagulation
  Inflammatory bowel disease
  Cutaneous ulcerations
  Chronic liver disease
  Disorders of hemostasis
  History of cerebrovascular accident

Several controlled trials in the 1970s demonstrated convincingly that there is more rapid clot dissolution with fibrinolytic agents than with heparin alone (171, 262, 268, 274). However, it was unclear that the more rapid clot dissolution improved prognosis. The largest trial had two phases. In the first, the effects of a 12-hour infusion of UK were compared with the effects of infusion of heparin alone [Urokinase Pulmonary Embolism Trial or UPET (268)] and in the second, 12- and 24-hour infusions of UK and a 24-hour infusion of SK were compared (Urokinase-Streptokinase Pulmonary Embolism Trial or USPET) (274). In both phases, patients received heparin for 5 days, then coumadin for 14 days. In these reports and several smaller series, fibrinolytic therapy accelerated the dissolution of pulmonary emboli (Table 21.4), led to a more rapid decrease of mean pulmonary artery pressure and pulmonary vascular resistance, and was associated with improvements in cardiac index (Table 21.5). However, after 5 days or more of treatment, the degree of lung scan resolution was similar, regardless of treatment received (UPET). Mortality rate was similar in patients who presented in shock (5 to 6%), whether or not they received thrombolytic agents. Bleeding was more common after thrombolytic therapy: 45% of patients given UK and 27% of patients given heparin. However, invasive procedures to permit intrapulmonary infusion of drug or to document the effects of the agents were used, and most of the bleeding in both groups was at catheterization sites.

Two smaller randomized controlled trials also compared the effects of SK with the actions of heparin in patients with massive pulmonary emboli (171, 262). In both trials, SK was administered for 72 hours at a rate of 100,000 units/hr and resulted in more rapid and complete dissolution of emboli than heparin alone. Bleeding complications occurred in 30% of the patients who received SK and 18% of those patients who received heparin alone. The more rapid dissolution of emboli appeared to be associated with an improved clinical course in patients with massive insults. It is possible that trials of this group of patients would find a beneficial effect on mortality as well, and reports of the success of intrapulmonary treatment with thrombolytic agents continue (106, 161). However, enthusiasm for fibrinolytic therapy in most patients with pulmonary emboli has been blunted in the past by the high incidence of bleeding.

The evolution of high-dose intravenous bolus regimens with or without subsequent infusions has led to new interest in the use of thrombolytic agents in patients with acute pulmonary embolism. The concept, developed in part from the positive experiences observed in patients with acute myocardial infarction, avoids invasive procedures and thus markedly reduces risks of bleeding. Since the early resolution of emboli is most important in individuals who have massive or submassive emboli, most trials have focused on this group. Both SK in doses as high as 3 million units given acutely (157, 196) and APSAC given generally in 5 mg boluses up to a dose of 30 mg as needed (25, 230) have been used. In general, rapid resolution of emboli have been documented by angiography or ventilation perfusion imaging in association with clinical improvement, with very few instances of severe bleeding in the absence of invasive procedures. Similar studies have been done with UK. A bolus dose of 15,000 IU/kg administered into the right atrium was associated with marked reduction in the extent of perfusion defects, improved right heart and pulmonary arterial hemodynamics, and clinical improvement, especially during the initial 3 hours after treatment (199).

Most recent studies have used t-PA that, in an animal model of pulmonary embolism, appeared superior to UK (205). In addition, efficacy of intravenous and intrapulmonary administration was comparable (284). Clinical studies also suggest that t-PA is more effective than UK (97). When a dose of 100 mg of t-PA given over 2 hours was compared with the dose of UK used in UPET, clot dissolution was far more rapid with t-PA. Hemostatic measurements and bleeding complications were similar. After an initial positive experience with t-PA (33, 99), several recent trials have used t-PA to treat patients with pulmonary emboli with disparate results (156, 165, 201, 284). A variety of dosing regimens have been employed. The Pioped Investigators used a dose of between 40 and 80 mg administered over 40 to 90 minutes and found little evidence of clot dissolution after 2 hours, despite modest reductions in pulmonary resistance. After 24 hours, these was not a statistically significant difference between those patients receiving t-PA and those patients receiving heparin alone. Massive bleeding occurred in one patient (201). Other groups have had a more positive experience (156, 284). In response to 100 mg of t-PA given over a 7-hour period, with a variable initial bolus, and in the presence of adjunctive treatment with heparin, t-PA induced substantial amounts of clot lysis and rapid improvement in hemodynamics. However, bleeding complications were frequent, likely because of the need for

Table 21.4. Resolution of Lung Scan Defects in the National Institutes of Health Trials with Thrombolytic Agents

Protocol	Lung Scan Resolutions (%)				
	1 Day	*2 Days*	*5 Days*	*14 Days*	*3 Mos.*
UPET[a]					
Urokinase (12 hr)[a]	6.2	8.0	11.3	14.9	
Heparin only	2.7	4.9	9.3	14.7	
USPET					
Urokinase (12 hr)[a]	9.0				28.6
Urokinase (24 hr)[a]	11.6				26.0
Streptokinase (24 hr)[a]	7.0				21.6

[a] UPET, Urokinase Pulmonary Embolism Trial; USPET, Urokinase-Streptokinase Pulmonary Embolism Trial.
[b] All patients received heparin after infusion of the fibrinolytic agent.

Table 21.5. Hemodynamic Response to Thrombolysis in the National Institutes of Health Trials[a]

Protocol	PA[b] Mean (mm Hg)		Cardiac Index (liters/min/m^2)		Total Pulmonary Resistance (dyne/sec/cm^{-5})	
	Pre	*Post*	*Pre*	*Post*	*Pre*	*Post*
UPET						
Urokinase (12 hr)	26.3	20.7	3.2	3.3	330.3	244.7
Heparin only	26.0	24.8	3.1	3.0	365.0	395.7
USPET						
Urokinase (12 hr)	27.4	20.1	2.9	3.0	403.4	298.9
Urokinase (24 hr)	27.5	20.0	2.6	2.9	365.0	244.7
Streptokinase (24 hr)	26.2	20.9	2.8	3.6	181.3	121.5

[a] Measurements made before (pre) and 24 hours after (post) start of infusion of the fibrinolytic agent. Urokinase 12-hour group had been on heparin for 12 hours at time of posttreatment measurements.
[b] PA, pulmonary artery pressure; UPET, Urokinase Pulmonary Embolism Trial; USPET, Urokinase-Streptokinase Pulmonary Embolism Trial.

invasive procedures to assess the results of treatment. Levine et al used a 2-minute infusion of t-PA in a dose of 0.6 mg/kg in 33 patients and compared the results with those results in patients who received a saline placebo. All patients received heparin (165). They took this approach because in experimental studies it was found that high-dose boluses of t-PA given over a short period of time (15 minutes) induced a greater degree of thrombolysis than administration of the same dose over 90 minutes (204). Perfusion defects were found to be reduced by more than 50% at 24 hours in 34% of the patients receiving t-PA and in only 12% of those treated with placebo. Overall, the mean reduction in the perfusion defect at 24 hours was 37% in patients treated with t-PA, compared with 18.8% in those receiving heparin alone. After 7 days, there were no differences. Other reports have suggested that the increased rapidity of thrombolysis observed can be of great benefit in patients with pulmonary embolism and shock (100, 126, 184, 200). Thus, the best results have been documented with large initial bolus doses. If future studies substantiate this approach and the optimal dose of activator can be determined and the need for invasive procedures reduced, clot-selective activators may become the preferred treatment for patients with pulmonary emboli.

SUMMARY

At present, thrombolytic therapy should be used if contraindications to treatment are not present when pulmonary embolism is massive and complicated by right ventricular failure or hypotension, or when obstruction of 50% or more of a major pulmonary artery is documented. Therapy with SK or UK should be given for 24 hours or less. SK is generally given as an intravenous bolus of 250,000 units over 15 to 30 minutes, followed by infusion of 100,000 units/hr. For UK, a bolus of 300,000 units, followed by infusion of 2000 units/kg/hr, is as efficacious as higher doses (4400 units/kg/hr) (103). An initial bolus of 0.6 mg/kg of t-PA should be used. In most patients who manifest shock, additional drug has been administered (100, 126, 184, 200). Some also advocate the use of t-PA if there is hemodynamic compromise or obstruction of blood flow to a lobe or to multiple pulmonary segments (96). Before and during therapy, meticulous management to avoid bleeding due to vascular trauma is essential. Pulmonary artery catheters for monitoring or angiography should be placed through antecubital fossa venous cut-downs, rather than percutaneously in noncompressible vessels (i.e., large central veins) whenever possible. Arterial blood gases should be obtained only if essential with a 23-gauge needle from the radial artery. The artery should then be compressed for a minimum of 15 minutes. Whenever possible, noninvasive monitoring of oxygen saturation is preferred.

ACUTE MYOCARDIAL INFARCTION

The use of thrombolytic therapy for acute myocardial infarction was first reported in 1958 (86, 87). However, until the 1980s, data demonstrating benefit were not sufficiently persuasive to justify its use in view of the potential for serious hemorrhage. In addition, during the 1970s, skepticism regarding the role of coronary thrombosis in acute myocardial infarction further discouraged the use of antithrombotic and fibrinolytic agents. The rediscovery of the importance of coronary thrombosis in transmural infarction can be attributed to DeWood and associates (67), who demonstrated total coronary occlusion in 87% of 126 patients studied within the first 4 hours of the onset of infarction and nearly total obstruction in an additional 10%. In patients studied later (12 to 24 hours), the incidence of total occlusion decreased to 65%. These data, coupled with the retrieval of thrombus during subsequent emergent coronary revascularization in a subset of 51 patients, conclusively established the presence of coronary thrombosis early during the evolution of acute myocardial infarction. Although Chazov and coworkers (47) were the first to report pharmacologic coronary fibrinolysis, Rentrop et al (216) popularized the concept that coronary reperfusion could be achieved by guidewire fragmentation, followed by intracoronary SK. Subsequently it was demonstrated that intracoronary administration of SK elicits recanalization in approximately 70% of cases.

Patients with acute transmural myocardial infarction have increased levels of thrombin activity early after the onset of symptoms (78) and little evidence of spontaneous fibrinolysis (76). Both fibrinolysis (79) and thrombin activity increase after treatment with plasminogen activators (77, 108, 209, 210). Thrombin activity subsequently decreases markedly when recanalization occurs (77, 108). In patients in whom recanalization does not occur, markers of thrombin activity increase, suggesting that continued clot formation competes with dissolution. Thus, the failure of recanalization is not due to inadequate fibrinolysis but to more intense thrombus formation (77, 108). These data emphasize the importance of antithrombotic treatment in the success or failure of thrombolysis. They suggest that either the frequency of coronary recanalization or its rapidity will be enhanced by the use of antithrombotic interventions. Since nonfibrin-specific activators induce greater increases in thrombin activity, judging from in vitro experiments (73, 74), aggressive interventions to inhibit thrombin activity may be of more benefit in regard to initial recanalization with these activators than with more fibrin-specific agents. The early administration of heparin increases the rapidity of recanalization after administration of SK (166) and may reduce mortality rates (231). Over time, the initial procoagulant stimulus wanes, and the generation of fibrin(ogen) degradation products with their antithrombin effects and the depletion of fibrinogen induced by nonfibrin-specific activators may protect against reocclusion. With fibrin-specific activators, it is clear that antithrombotic treatments are essential to maintain coronary artery patency (26, 123).

Initially, patients with acute myocardial infarction were treated with intracoronary fibrinolytics because lower doses could be administered; systemic lytic effects were thought to be minimal; and the results of therapy could be immediately appreciated. However, rapid mixing of the activator in the systemic circulation occurred after intracoronary administration and resulted in systemic activation of plasminogen and induction of a systemic lytic state (63, 227). In addition, coronary angiography may delay the initiation of treatment by as much as 90 minutes, during which time the magnitude of

Table 21.6. Mortality-based Trials of Intravenous Thrombolysis and Conventional Management in Patients with Acute Myocardial Infarction (264)

Trial	Thrombolytic Agent	Mortality (%) Control	Mortality (%) Thrombolysis
AIMS	APSAC	12.2	6.4
ECSG (1979)	SK	30.6	15.6
GISSI I	SK	13.0	10.7
ISAM	SK	7.1	6.3
ISIS II	SK	12.2	9.2
New Zealand I	SK	12.9	2.5
ASSET	t-PA	9.8	7.9
NHF Australian	t-PA	2.8	9.6
TICO	t-PA	5.6	5.4
ECSG II	t-PA	6.2	1.6
ECSG V	t-PA	5.7	2.8

Table 21.7. Mortality-based Comparative Trials of Intravenous Thrombolytic Agents (264)

Study	Mortality (%) by Thrombolytic Agent SK	APSAC	t-PA	UK	scu-PA
ECSG I	4.6		4.7		
GAUS			4.8	4.1	
New Zealand II	7.4		3.7		
PAIMS	8.2		4.7		
PRIMI	4.9				3.5
TIMI I	8.2		4.9		
GISSI II International	8.5		8.9		
ISIS III	10.5	10.6	10.3[a]		
GUSTO	7.3		6.3[b]		

[a] A different preparation of t-PA ("duteplase") was used in this study.
[b] Statistically different.

potential benefit from reperfusion is diminishing. It is for this reason as well that treatment with thrombolytic agents is preferred over direct angioplasty, except in those rare centers where angioplasty can be accomplished with little if any delay.

All thrombolytic agents substantially reduce mortality rates when administered to patients early after the onset of acute myocardial infarction (264) (Table 21.6). Most experimental and clinical data suggest that the mechanism of benefit is predominantly, if not exclusively, reduction in the extent of myocardial injury related to the prompt restoration of coronary perfusion (149, 150). When coronary reperfusion occurs within 2 hours after the onset of acute transmural myocardial infarction, regional left ventricular wall motion often improves, and mortality rates (both short-term and long-term) are reduced, particularly in patients with anterior infarction (4, 104, 152, 215, 228, 240–242). When treatment is started later, benefit is of lesser magnitude and less consistent (8, 9, 142, 143, 147, 217, 225, 236). At present, the conventional time window during which thrombolysis is considered effective is up to 6 hours from the onset of infarction. However, at least one trial has shown a benefit of treatment up to 24 hours after the onset of infarction (128). This may be due to the effects of an open infarct-related coronary artery on ventricular remodeling (159) or to a decrease in the propensity to the development of life-threatening arrhythmias (281). Two current trials that have attempted to document the benefit of treatment after 6 hours have thus far been unable to do so (68, 269). Accordingly, the initiation of treatment at the earliest possible time in patients who are appropriate candidates for treatment should be of the highest priority. To this end, every possible effort should be made to decrease the time for triage of patients who are candidates. It appears that the median time to treatment (the so-called "door-to-needle" time) at this time in the U.S. is roughly 90 minutes (144). This time lag is too long and could be reduced in most patients by more expeditious triage, more rapid collection of electrocardiograms [by, for example, obtaining such studies before the patient's arrival in the emergency department (144, 292)], minimizing administrative procedures and ancillary diagnostic tests, and maximizing the availability of the fibrinolytic agents in the treatment area. The feasibility of early administration

in the out-of-hospital setting by physicians has been demonstrated (294), and the possibility of administration by nonphysicians has been considered. It is unclear as to whether this approach will be a cost-effective one (292).

Recently, the issue of the mechanism of benefit from treatment with thrombolytic agents has been challenged by the results of several large clinical trials (105, 129, 244). It has been established that intravenous t-PA elicits a higher incidence of coronary patency by 90 minutes after treatment than does intravenous SK (48, 282) or APSAC (286). By 24 hours, however, the incidence of coronary patency is high with all activators (11, 45). If the predominant mechanism of benefit is the early induction of coronary patency, t-PA should reduce mortality rates to a greater extent than SK. This contention was supported by several smaller trials (264). However, in direct large comparative trials, this finding has not been the case; both agents result in similar reductions in mortality rates (105, 129, 244) (Table 21.7). These findings could be interpreted as indicating that early coronary patency is not the only mechanism of benefit. It could be that effects on ventricular remodeling (159) or the propensity to malignant arrhythmias (163, 281) may be more important than reduction in the extent of infarction. Alternatively, it might be that it is coronary patency, regardless of when it is achieved, that is of importance. It is also possible and perhaps likely that the lack of appropriate antithrombotic treatment in these trials led to an excessive number of reocclusions, and, therefore, masked differences in early patency. The essentiality of such treatment, especially with fibrin specific activators, has been shown in several studies (26, 123) (Table 21.8). Thus, the effects of early coronary opening may not have been tested due to a high incidence of reocclusion. Ongoing trials have been designed to address this issue more definitively.[a]

Regardless of mechanism, a reduced mortality rate in patients with acute myocardial infarction has been shown to occur whether thrombolytics are administered via the intracoronary or intravenous route (264). To date, differences in mortality rate between activators has not been documented. Patients with ST segment elevation and perhaps those patients with left bundle branch block (128) who can be treated within 6 hours of the onset of infarction clearly benefit from treatment. Patients with anterior wall infarction who have a higher mortality rate than those with inferior wall infarction benefit more (104). Treatment with intravenous heparin, regardless

Table 21.8.   Effects of Heparin on Coronary Patency in Patients Treated with Fibrin Specific Activators[a]

Study	Time of Angiography after Treatment (hr)			Patency of the Infarct-related Artery		
	Number	Mean	Range	With Heparin	Without Heparin	
HART	205	18	(7–24)	82% (−ASA)[b]	48% (+ASA)	Alteplase
Bleich et al	83	57	(48–72)	71% (−ASA)	44% (−ASA)	Alteplase
ECSG-6	609	81	(48–120)	84% (+ASA)	75% (+ASA)	Alteplase
Tebbe	118	8	(6–12)	81%	60%	Saruplase

[a] From Sobel BE: Thrombolysis in the treatment of acute myocardial infarction. *Thromb Cardiol Disord*:289–326, 1992.
[b] ASA refers to the use (+) or lack (−) of protocol-mandated aspirin.

Table 21.9.   Effects of Heparin on Early Mortality (42 Days)[a]

	Placebo Group		Treatment Group		% Reduction in Mortality (Treatment vs. Placebo)
	No.	Mortality (%) (No.)	No.	Mortality (%) (No.)	
With intravenous heparin	3090	9.2 (294)	9,298	5.5 (514)	39
Without intravenous heparin	16,331	13,1 (2,144)	34,581	9.3 (3,226)	29

[a] From Tiefenbrunn AJ, Sobel BE: Thrombolysis and myocardial infarction. *Fibrinolysis* 5:1–15, 1991.

of the plasminogen activator used, also improves survival (264) (Table 21.9). Improvement in patients treated after 6 hours of the onset of infarction (68, 269), in those patients with normal ECGs, or in those with ST segment depression has not yet been proven (128).[b] Although the complications of treatment increase as age increases, so does the mortality rate associated with infarction (45, 186). Thus, treatment should not be withheld on the basis of age alone.

Although preservation of myocardium is thought to be the predominant mechanism of benefit in patients receiving thrombolysis and should result in improved left ventricular performance, this mechanism has been difficult to prove, especially in groups of patients (40). This difficulty is likely due to selection bias, the use of global measurements of left ventricular performance, and the differential death rates between treated and control patients (275). This hypothesis is supported by improvements in sequential measurements in patients who have recanalized, compared to improvements in those who have remained totally occluded (213, 235, 240, 241). Improvement is greater in those patients treated earlier and in patients with anterior infarction (220, 240, 241). Benefit in patients with inferior infarction has been documented only with t-PA (20, 195).

USE OF SPECIFIC ACTIVATORS   (Table 21.10).

When used for coronary thrombolysis, the conventional dose of SK is 1,500,000 units given over 1 hour intravenously (104, 105, 244). Infusion rates ≥750,000 units/min are associated with hypotension (167). Allergic reactions are sufficiently rare that pretreatment is no longer employed routinely. SK cannot be given a second time for up to 6 months due to the development of antibodies (118). Although in many major trials, heparin has not been given or its administration has been delayed (104, 105, 244), in vitro and clinical data indicate that the rapidity of lysis is increased (164), and the mortality rate is decreased (231, 264) by the concomitant use of heparin. Heparin is usually given intravenously before treatment or at the end of the infusion, and the dose is titrated to maintain the aPTT at greater than 1.5 to 2 times normal.

The use of acylated SK plasminogen complexes (BRL-26921, ASPAC) to treat patients with acute myocardial infarction also has been studied extensively (22, 104, 109, 173,

---

[a] After submission of this chapter, the results of the Global Utilization of Streptokinase (SK) and tissue plasminogen activator (t-PA) for Occluded Coronary Arteries (GUSTO) were reported (1). This study compared t-PA and streptokinase under conditions that minimized reocclusion rates by administering (in most but not all arms of the study) intravenous heparin at the same time as the thrombolytic agents. It was documented that t-PA (given as a front-loaded regimen) opened vessels more rapidly than did streptokinase, so that by 90 minutes after treatment, the use of t-PA was associated with a patency rate of roughly 81%, as compared to 61% for streptokinase (also with concomitant intravenous heparin). The improved patency rate represented a difference predominantly in TIMI grade 3 flow (normal flow of angiographic dye), which has recently been found to translate into much greater benefits in preventing mortality (2, 3). By 180 minutes, patency with the two regimens were comparable. Thus, GUSTO tested whether the increased rapidity of patency (in this instance, induced by t-PA) was of benefit and found that it was. Mortality was reduced in the t-PA group by 1% in absolute terms, which represents roughly a 14% reduction in the risk of death from acute infarction. In addition to benefits in mortality, there was less congestive heart failure in patients who received t-PA. There was a slight excess of intracranial bleeding in patients who received t-PA, but the difference was small and thus did not alter the conclusions of the study. Thus, the results of the GUSTO study strongly support the concept that the primary mode of benefit in patients treated with thrombolytic agents is the early induction of coronary recanalization. Because t-PA is more efficient in this regard, it is a more effective agent. Issues related to the costs for any given increment of benefit will continue to be controversial.
1. The GUSTO Investigators: An International randomized trial comparing four thrombolytic strategies for acute myocardial infarction. *N Eng J Med* 329:673, 1993.
2. Vogt A, von Essen R, Tebbe U, Feuerer W, Appel K-F, Neuhaus K-L: Impact of early perfusion status of the infarct-related artery on short-term mortality after thrombolysis for acute myocardial infarction: retrospective analysis of four German multicenter trials. *J Am Coll Cardiol* 21:1391, 1993.
3. Lincoff A, Ellis S, Galeana A, Sigmon K, Lee K, Rosenschein U (for the TAMI Study Group): Is a coronary artery with TIMI grade 2 flow "patent"? Outcome in the thrombolysis and angioplasty in myocardial infarction (TAMI) trial. *Circulation* 86:I–268, 1993.

[b] Since the initial writing of this chapter, new data has been reported, indicating that the treatment of patients who present with ST segment elevation between 6 and 12 hours after the onset of infarction reduces in-hospital mortality. The nature of the patients benefitted and the details of the trial are not yet available for scrutiny (1).
1. Wilcox R, Late Assessment of Thrombolytic Efficacy (the LATE trial), presented at the *14th Annual Congress of the European Society of Cardiology*, September 1992.

252). Because deacylation to the active streptokinase plasminogen activator complex is relatively slow, the agent can be administered as an intravenous bolus. Optimal rates of recanalization appear to require a dose of at least 30 mg, which results in significant systemic lytic activity (173). Treatment with ASPAC has been shown to induce a greater incidence of coronary patency at 90 minutes than SK in some trials (45) but is not as effective as t-PA (286). ASPAC and SK result in similar degrees of systemic fibrinogen depletion (45). Hypotension and allergic reactions similar to those observed with SK can occur with APSAC (3, 10, 134). Issues related to the proper administration of heparin with APSAC are similar to those outlined for SK.

The intravenous dose for UK is 2,000,000 units/hr (285). Allergic reactions do not occur. In the only comparative trial completed to date, intravenous UK induced a 90-minute patency rate equivalent to that induced by t-PA (189). A conjunctive heparin regimen similar to that used with SK is recommended.

t-PA has been the most extensively studied of the more fibrin-specific activators. Initial data demonstrated the ability of very low doses of intravenous t-PA to induce coronary thrombolysis in patients with acute myocardial infarction (58, 277). However larger doses induce lysis more rapidly (185). At present, the recommended dose is 100 mg over 3 hours. In general, 10% of the dose is given as an initial bolus (34). Front-loaded regimens in which t-PA is administered over 90 minutes have been developed in the hope of achieving coronary patency earlier, but a direct comparison of the relative safety and efficacy of the two approaches is lacking. The most commonly used front-loaded regimen consists of 15 mg as a bolus, followed by 50 mg over the initial 30 minutes, then 35 mg over the remaining 60 minutes (188). Individuals weighing less than 65 kg may benefit from weight-adjusted dosing (1 mg/kg) since high doses that induce significant fibrinogenolysis are associated with bleeding (80). The concomitant use of intravenous heparin for at least 24 hours after treatment is recommended. After 1 day of heparin, aspirin alone appears adequate to maintain coronary patency (260). Coadministration of heparin with t-PA does not improve initial patency rates but may speed lysis (270). However, in the absence of

Table 21.10. Conventional Doses of Plasminogen Activators for Patients with Acute Myocardial Infarction

Agent	Dosing
t-PA[a]	
"Conventional"	100 mg or 1 mg/kg for those ≤65 kg, over 3 hr with 10% of the dose given as an initial bolus
"Front-loaded"	100 mg over 1.5 hr with a 15 mg initial bolus
SK	1,500,000 units over 1 hr
APSAC	30 mg over 2 to 5 min
UK	2,000,000 units over 1 hr
scu-PA	80 mg over 1 hr with 20 mg given as an initial bolus

[a] t-PA, tissue-plasminogen activator; SK, streptokinase; APSAC, acylated streptokinase/plasminogen complexes; UK, urokinase; scu-PA, single-chain urokinase-like plasminogen activator.

intravenous heparin administered either with or immediately after the infusion, coronary patency is decreased by approximately 30% during the first 24 hours (26, 123).

Scu-PA is also highly effective in inducing recanalization in patients with acute myocardial infarction (278, 279). In general, coronary reperfusion has been induced at a rate similar to that observed for t-PA. However, rapid thrombolysis requires a dose that is associated with a more marked degree of systemic lytic activity than is usually induced by t-PA (278). Since the half-life of scu-PA is relatively short (approximately 8 minutes), a continuous infusion is required. At the present time, the therapeutic-toxic ratio seems to be less favorable than that demonstrated for t-PA. Low doses of t-PA and scu-PA may be synergistic (56).

ADDITIONAL CONSIDERATIONS

Aspirin has become standard adjunctive treatment with thrombolytic agents. The rationale for such treatment is that clotting and platelet activation are ongoing and, to some extent, are exacerbated by the use of plasminogen activators (83, 145). Aspirin has been shown to inhibit some of these platelet effects (83). In addition, aspirin is known to reduce the mortality rate in patients with unstable angina (258), and in one trial of patients with acute infarction, the effects of aspirin alone were equivalent to those effects of SK alone and synergistic with those actions of the thrombolytic agent (128). Based on these data, aspirin in a dose of 60 to 325 mg is generally given concomitantly with thrombolytic treatment for acute myocardial infarction. Recent data suggest aspirin may also augment fibrinolysis (256).

After successful coronary thrombolysis, a high-grade residual stenosis generally persists. Since this stenosis is a potential site of reocclusion and reinfarction, it was initially assumed that aggressive management was essential. It is now clear that routine catheterization and angioplasty do not improve prognosis (243, 266, 268) but are associated with increased complications during the acute phase. Clinically important bleeding occurs in 20 to 25% (243, 266, 268). In most studies, groups of patients treated conservatively fare equally well or better than those who undergo routine intervention (17, 224). However, there are subsets of patients that may benefit, including those in whom thrombolysis does not induce coronary recanalization. These patients are known to have increased mortality and morbidity rates (65, 251) that appear to be lessened by angioplasty (1). Unfortunately, these patients are hard to identify. Clinical indicators of successful coronary recanalization include a rapid rise and early peaking of MB creatine kinase, evidence of reperfusion arrhythmias, and rapid resolution of ST segment elevation and chest discomfort after administration of plasminogen activators. When all of these indicators are concordant, the ability to predict the success or failure of recanalization is excellent. Unfortunately, concordance occurs in only about 10% of patients (41). Newer techniques employing continuous monitoring of the ECG (66) or the rate of rise of markers of myocardial injury (2) are promising but not yet refined for routine clinical use. Patients with continuing chest discomfort and ECG changes, especially if hemodynamically unstable, are good candidates for catheterization to assess the appropriateness of additional intervention.

In addition, patients at high risk (i.e., those patients with extensive anterior infarction, previous infarction, recurrent pain or arrhythmia, congestive heart failure, or hypotension (with or without shock) who cannot tolerate further loss of viable myocardium and do not appear to have responded to treatment, should be considered for intervention, which may include emergency bypass surgery or angioplasty. Other patients may not require catheterization unless they have recurrent symptoms or positive stress results.

Angioplasty is preferred to treatment with thrombolytic agents under some circumstances. It is generally accepted that patients with cardiogenic shock and acute infarction are best served by prompt emergency angioplasty (50). In addition, in a few institutions, angioplasty can be accomplished with such a high level of expertise and so rapidly that it competes with thrombolysis as the approach of choice. This technique also can be applied to the group of patients who have contraindications to the use of thrombolytic agents.

β-adrenergic blockers (117, 127) and, to a lesser extent, intravenous nitroglycerin (39, 130) have been reported to reduce infarct size and improve survival in patients with acute myocardial infarction. There is little direct information to support the benefit of nitroglycerin in conjunction with thrombolysis. In theory, nitroglycerin may reduce thrombosis via its effects on endothelium-derived relaxing factor (125, 254), but there is evidence suggesting that nitroglycerin may antagonize the effects of heparin (21, 164) and reduce the efficacy of t-PA (85b). There are experimental and clinical data to support the use of β-blockers adjunctively with thrombolytic agents (222, 280), but the results have not been sufficiently impressive to support a recommendation for their routine use. For example, in a recently reported study, metoprolol given at the time of administration of thrombolytic agent (t-PA) reduced the incidence of recurrent infarction, compared with the incidence in patients given the agent later during hospitalization for secondary prevention. However, this effect was only observed in patients treated within 2 hours of the onset of symptoms and only in those patients in the low-risk group; it did not have an impact on mortality rate (222). Unfortunately, the suggestion from that study that β-blockers may reduce the incidence of intracranial bleeding has not been supported by results in other trials (105).

Ongoing research suggests that calcium channel blockers (116, 148, 151), α-adrenergic blockers (302), β-adrenergic blockers (111), and oxygen free-radical scavengers (38, 135, 187, 208) may enhance the salvage of myocardium after thrombolysis. However until the results of ongoing clinical trials are available, these agents should not be used because of the potential for deleterious effects.

Heparin has been used almost universally after administration of fibrinolytic agents to prevent recurrent coronary thrombosis. Reocclusion after coronary recanalization with all activators is common (194). It is prudent to administer heparin for at least 24 hours after initiation of thrombolysis, although this approach may be less essential with SK and APSAC than with more fibrin-specific activators (192) (Table 21.10). The intravenous route in preferred since the attainment of consistent and stable anticoagulation with subcutaneous administration is difficult (124). In addition, the risk of reocclusion is greatest immediately after recanalization, and it is during this early period that subcutaneous administration is particularly unreliable. If bleeding develops, heparin should be discontinued, and angiography should be performed if symptoms recur. It is now clear that heparin is not an ideal agent for inhibiting thrombin. The heparin-antithrombin 3 complex is too large to inhibit thrombin bound to clot (297). Agents such as hirudin will likely be more potent and are under investigation at this time (114, 183). Their increased effectiveness may be manifested not only by the increased efficacy of thrombolysis but also by increases in bleeding. Other approaches to inhibit coagulation also are being developed. Agents that inhibit platelet function by blocking platelet receptors with either monoclonal antibodies (93) or small peptides (114) are being tested, as are approaches that inhibit the initiators of clotting, such as tissue factor (115). In each case of use of these agents, the benefit will have to be weighed against the increased propensity to bleeding. An alternative strategy has been to use a fibrin- and a nonfibrin-selective activator concomitantly (42, 107) or to use prolonged infusions of thrombolytic agents (94). Both approaches appear promising.

The data concerning whether anticoagulants are essential to the maintenance of long-term patency are contradictory. One small randomized trial found that the frequency of reinfarction, unstable angina, pulmonary edema, and/or death by 30 months after infarction was 16% in patients treated with coumadin and 37% in those who received aspirin (232). Another study found no differences between patients treated with coumadin and those patients given aspirin (181).

Lidocaine often is administered concomitantly with thrombolytic agents because of concern that, in addition to the significant incidence of malignant arrhythmias associated with infarction, recanalization itself may further exacerbate these arrhythmias. However, the data suggest that thrombolysis reduces the incidence of malignant arrhythmias (281, 285). Furthermore, experimental evidence suggests that reperfusion arrhythmias should not respond to lidocaine (203). One nonrandomized study has claimed to show the benefit of prophylactic lidocaine (172), but the only randomized study has not (131). Thus, although commonly advocated, the use of lidocaine cannot be said to be well-supported scientifically.

The major complication associated with the use of plasminogen activators for the treatment of patients with acute myocardial infarction is bleeding. Bleeding is related to the dissolution of hemostatic plugs, the degree to which clotting is inhibited by fibrinogen depletion, and other manifestations of the systemic lytic state (212), as well as to the use of antithrombotic agents (e.g., heparin, aspirin, etc.). All activators can cause both local and systemic bleeding. Despite controversy, in general it appears that there is little difference in the incidence of overall or intracranial bleeding in association with the various activators (105, 244). Excessive doses of t-PA may exacerbate bleeding (180), and for that reason dose adjustment for smaller individuals (≤65 kg) is advised. Prevention of bleeding is an important component of safe treatment. Only essential venous and/or arterial punctures should be undertaken, and then only with the understanding that their performance is a relative contraindication to the use of thrombolytic agents. Noncompressible vessels should not be punctured at all.

SUMMARY

When coronary reperfusion is accomplished within 1 to 2 hours after the onset of symptoms, patients benefit, especially those patients with anterior wall myocardial infarction. When treatment is initiated later, improvement is less consistent. Whether treatment occurs at all after 6 hours after the onset of infarction is controversial. Thus, the decision to administer thrombolytic therapy more than 6 hours after the onset of infarction depends on the risk vs. the potential benefit for each individual patient. Since rapid initiation of therapy is essential, intravenous fibrinolytic agents are the treatment of choice. The challenge of the 90s will be to administer treatment sooner after the onset of symptoms.

UNSTABLE ANGINA PECTORIS

There has been considerable enthusiasm for the use of thrombolytic agents for the treatment of patients with unstable angina pectoris because of the known association of thrombi with the lesions observed on invasive study of their coronary arteries and because of the absence of evidence of spontaneous fibrinolysis (72). To date, the results of clinical trials have yielded conflicting results (233), perhaps because patients with unstable angina are a heterogeneous group or because the intensity of thrombosis is less in this group (72).

ACKNOWLEDGMENT

The author appreciates the editorial assistance of Ms. Beth Engeszer.

REFERENCES

1. Abbotsmith CW, Topol EJ, George BS, et al: Fate of patients with acute myocardial infarction with patency of the infarct-related vessel achieved with successful thrombolysis versus rescue angioplasty. *J Am Coll Cardiol* 16:770–778, 1990.
2. Abendschein DR, Ellis AK, Eisenberg PR, et al: Prompt detection of coronary recanalization by analysis of rates of change of concentrations of macromolecular markers in plasma. *Coronary Artery Dis* 2:201–212, 1991.
3. AIMS Trial Study Group: Effect of intravenous APSAC on mortality after acute myocardial infarction: preliminary report of a placebo-controlled clinical trial. *Lancet* I:545, 1988.
4. AIMS Trial Study Group. Long-term effects of intravenous anistreplase in acute myocardial infarction: final report of the AIMS study. *Lancet* 335(8687):427–431, 1990.
5. Alderman EL, Jutzky KR, Berte LE, et al: Randomized comparison of intravenous versus intracoronary streptokinase for myocardial infarction. *Am J Cardiol* 54:14, 1984.
6. Alkjaersig N, Fletcher AP, Sherry S: The mechanism of clot dissolution by plasmin. *J Clin Invest* 38:1086, 1959.
7. Anderson JL: Development and evaluation of anisoylated plasminogen streptokinase activator complex (APSAC) as a second generation thrombolytic agent. *J Am Coll Cardiol* 10:22B–27B, 1987.
8. Anderson JL, Marshall HW, Askens JC, et al: A randomized trial of intravenous and intracoronary streptokinase in patients with acute myocardial infarction. *Circulation* 70:606, 1983.
9. Anderson JL, Marshall HW, Bray BE, et al: A randomized trial of intracoronary streptokinase in treatment of acute myocardial infarction. *N Engl J Med* 308:1312, 1983.
10. Anderson JL, Rothbard RL, Hackworthy RA, et al: Multicenter reperfusion trial of intravenous anisoylated plasminogen streptokinase activator complex (LAPSAC) in acute myocardial infarction: controlled comparison with intracoronary streptokinase. *J Am Coll Cardiol* 11(6):1153–1163, 1988.
11. Anderson JL, Sorensen SG, Moreno FL, et al: Multicenter patency trial of intravenous anistreplase compared with streptokinase in acute myocardial infarction. The TEAM-2 Study Investigators. *Circulation* 83(1):126–140, 1991.
12. Andrade-Gordon P, Strickland S: Interaction of heparin with plasminogen activators and plasminogen: effects on the activation of plasminogen. *Biochemistry* 25:403, 1986.
13. Armstrong PW, Baigrie S, Daly, PA, et al: Tissue plasminogen activator: Toronto (TPAT) placebo-controlled randomized trial in acute myocardial infarction. *J Am Coll Cardiol* 13:1469–1476, 1989.
14. Arneson H, Heilo A, Jakobsen E, et al: A prospective study of streptokinase and heparin in the treatment of deep vein thrombosis. *Acta Med Scand* 203:457–463, 1978.
15. Arneson H, Hoiseth A, Ly B: Streptokinase or heparin in the treatment of deep venous thrombosis. *Acta Med Scand* 21:65, 1982.
16. Astedt B, Robertson B, Haeger K: Experience with standardized streptokinase therapy of deep venous thrombosis. *Surg Gynecol Obstet* 139:387–388, 1974.
17. Barbash GI, Roth A, Hod H, et al: Randomized controlled trial of late in-hospital angiography and angioplasty versus conservative management after treatment with recombinant tissue-type plasminogen activator in acute myocardial infarction. *Am. J. Cardiol* 66(5):538–545, 1990.
18. Barritt DW, Jordan SC: Anticoagulant drugs in the treatment of pulmonary embolism. A controlled trial. *Lancet* 1:1309, 1960.
19. Bates ER, Topol EJ: Limitations of thrombolytic therapy for acute myocardial infarction complicated by congestive heart failure and cardiogenic shock. *J Am Coll Cardiol* 18(4):1077–1084, 1991.
20. Bates ER, Topol EJ, Kline EM, et al: Early reperfusion therapy improves left ventricular function after acute myocardial infarction associated with right coronary artery disease. *Am Heart J.* 114:261–267, 1987.
21. Becker RC, Corrao JM, Bovill EG, et al: Intravenous nitroglycerin-induced heparin resistance: a qualitative antithrombin III abnormality. *Am Heart J* 119(6):1254–1261, 1990.
22. Been M, de Bona DP, Muir AL, et al: Coronary thrombolysis with intravenous anisoylated plasminogen streptokinase complex BRL26921. *Br Heart J* 53:253, 1985.
23. Beiger R, Boehout-Mussert RJ, Hohmann F: Is streptokinase useful in the treatment of deep venous thrombosis? *Acta Med Scand* 199:81, 1976.
24. Bergmann SR, Fox KAA, Ter-Pogossian MM, et al: Clot selective coronary thrombolysis with tissue-type plasminogen activator. *Science* 220:1181, 1983.
25. Bett JHN, Bunce IH, Cade JF, et al: Initial experience with a new fibrinolytic agent (APSAC) in patients with major pulmonary embolism. *Aust NZ J Med* 17:77–79, 1987.
26. Bleich SD, Nichols TC, Schumacher RR, et al: Effect of heparin on coronary arterial patency after thrombolysis with tissue plasminogen activator in acute myocardial infarction. *Am J Cardiol* 66(20):1412–1417, 1990.
27. Bode C, Runge M, Eberle T, et al: Enhanced thrombolysis in plasma and in vivo by single-chain urokinase-type plasminogen activator (scuPA) conjugated to an antifibrin antibody. *Trans Assoc Am Physicians* 102:7–12, 1989.
28. Bode C, Runge MS, Newell JB, et al: Thrombolysis by a fibrin-specific antibody Fab'-urokinase conjugate. *J Mol Cell Cardiol* 19(4):335–341, 1987.
29. Bode C, Schoenermark S, Schuler G, et al: Efficacy of intravenous prourokinase and a combination of prourokinase and urokinase in acute myocardial infarction. *Am J Cardiol* 61(13):971–974, 1988.
30. Bode C, Schuler G, Nordt T, et al: Intravenous thrombolytic therapy with a combination of single-chain urokinase-type plasminogen activator and recombinant tissue-type plasminogen activator in acute myocardial infarction. *Circulation* 81(3):907–913, 1990.
31. Bolgiano EB, Foxwell MM, Brown BJ, et al: Deep venous thrombosis of the upper extremity: diagnosis and treatment. *J Emerg Med* 8(1):85–91, 1990.
32. Bonnier HJ, Visser RF, Klomps HC, et al: Comparison of intravenous anisoylated plasminogen streptokinase activator complex and intracoronary streptokinase in acute myocardial infarction. *Am J Cardiol* 62(1):25–30, 1988.
33. Bounameaux HM, Vermylen J, Collen D: Thrombolytic treatment with recombinant tissue-type plasminogen activator in a patient with massive pulmonary embolism. *Ann Intern Med* 103:64, 1985.
34. Braunwald E, Knatterud GL, Passamani E: Update from the thrombolysis in myocardial infarction trial. *J Am Coll Cardiol* 10:970, 1987.
35. Browse NL, Clemenson G, Lea Thomas ML: Is the postphlebitic leg always postphlebitic? Relationship between phlebographic appearances of deep-vein thrombosis and late sequelae. *Br Med J* 281:1167, 1980.
36. Browse NL, Thomas ML, Pim HP: Streptokinase and deep vein thrombosis. *Br Med J* 3:717–720, 1968.
37. Burrows N, Jones RR: Rash after treatment with anistreplase *Br Heart J* 65(4):289–290, 1990.
38. Burton KP: Superoxide dismutase enhances recovery following myocardial ischemia. *Am J Physiol* 248:H637, 1985.
39. Bussman W, Passek D, Seidel E: Reduction of CK and CK-MB indices of infarct size by intravenous nitroglycerine. *Circulation* 63:615, 1981.
40. Califf RM, Harrelson-Woodlief L, Topol EJ: Left ventricular ejection fraction may not be useful as an end point of thrombolytic therapy comparative trials. *Circulation* 82:1847–1853, 1990.
41. Califf RM, O'Neil W, Stack RS, et al: Failure of simple clinical measurements to predict perfusion status after intravenous thrombolysis. *Ann Intern Med* 108:658–662, 1988.
42. Califf RM, Topol EJ, Stack RS, et al: Evaluation of combination thrombolytic therapy and timing of cardiac catheterization in acute myocardial infarction.

Results of thrombolysis and angioplasty in myocardial infarction—phase 5 randomized trial. TAMI Study Group. *Circulation* 83(5):1543–1556, 1991.

43. Castellino FJ: A unique enzyme-protein substrate modifier reaction: plasmin/streptokinase interaction. *Trends Biochem Sci* 4:1, 1979.

44. Chaitman BR, Thompson B, Wittry MD, et al: The use of tissue-type plasminogen activator for acute myocardial infarction in the elderly: results from thrombolysis in myocardial infarction Phase I, open label studies and the Thrombolysis in Myocardial Infarction Phase II pilot study. The TIMI Investigators. *J Am Coll Cardiol* 14(5):1159–1165, 1989.

45. Charbonnier B, Cribier A, Monassier JP, et al: A European multicenter and randomized study of APSAC versus streptokinase in myocardial infarction. *Arch Mal Coeur* 82(9):1565–1571, 1989.

46. Chavatzas D, Martin P: A study of streptokinase in deep vein thrombosis of the lower extremities. *Vasa* 4:68–72, 1975.

47. Chazov EL, Mateeva LS, Mazaev AV, et al: Intracoronary administration of fibrinolysis in acute myocardial infarction. *Ter Arkh* 48:8–19, 1976.

48. Chesbro JH, Knatterud G, Roberts R, et al: Thrombolysis in myocardial infarction (TIMI) trial phase 1. A comparison between intravenous tissue plasminogen activator and intravenous streptokinase. *Circulation* 76:142, 1987.

49. Claeys H, Vermylen J: Physico-chemical and proenzyme properties of NH2-terminal lysine human plasminogen. Influence of 6-aminohexanoic acid. *Biochim Biophys Acta* 342:351, 1974.

50. Col JJ, Col-De Beys CM, Renkin JP, et al: Pharmacokinetics, thrombolytic efficacy and hemorrhagic risk of different streptokinase regimens in heparin-treated acute myocardial infarction. *Am J Cardiol* 63(17):1187–1192, 1989.

51. Collen D: On the regulation and control of fibrinolysis. *Thromb Haemost* 45:77, 1981.

52. Collen D, Lu H-R, Lijnen HR, Nelles L, Stassen JM: Thrombolytic and pharmacokinetic properties of chimeric tissue-type and urokinase-type plasminogen activators. *Circulation* 84(3):1216–1234, 1991 Sep.

53. Collen D, Bounameaux H, De Cock F, et al: Analysis of coagulation and fibrinolysis during intravenous infusion of recombinant human tissue-type plasminogen activator in patients with acute myocardial infarction. *Circulation* 73:511, 1986.

54. Collen D, Lijnen HR: The fibrinolytic system in man. An overview. In Collen D, Lijnen HR, Verstraete M (eds): *Thrombolysis; Biological and Therapeutic Properties of New Thrombolytic Agents.* Churchill Livingstone, Edinburgh 1985.

55. Collen D, Stassen JM, Blaber M, et al: Biological and thrombolytic properties of the proenzyme and active forms of human urokinase. III. Thrombolytic properties of natural and recombinant urokinase in rabbits with experimental jugular vein thrombosis. *Thromb Haemost* 52:26, 1984.

56. Collen D, Stassen J, Stump DC, et al: Synergism of thrombolytic agents in vivo. *Circulation* 74:838, 1986.

57. Collen D, Stassen JM, Verstraete M: Thrombolysis with human extrinsic (tissue-type) plasminogen activator in rabbits with experimental jugular vein thrombosis. Effect of molecular form and dose of activator, age of thrombus, and route of administration. *J Clin Invest* 71:1012, 1984.

58. Collen D, Topol EJ, Tiefenbrunn AJ, et al: Coronary thrombolysis with recombinant human tissue-type plasminogen activator: a prospective, randomized, placebo-controlled trial. *Circulation* 70:1012, 1984.

59. Collen D, Van de Werf F: Coronary arterial thrombolysis with low-dose synergistic combinations of recombinant tissue-type plasminogen activator (rt-PA) and recombinant single-chain urokinase-type plasminogen activator (rscu-PA) for acute myocardial infarction. *Am J Cardiol* 60(7):431–434, 1987.

60. Collen D, Zamarron C, Lijnen HR, et al: Activation of plasminogen by pro-urokinase. 2. Kinetics. *J Biol Chem* 261:1259, 1986.

61. Common HH, Seaman AJ, Rosch J, et al: Deep vein thrombosis treated with streptokinase or heparin. *Angiology* 27:645, 1976.

62. Coon WW, Willis PW, Symons MJ: Assessment of anticoagulant treatment of venous thromboembolism. *Ann Surg* 170:559, 1969.

63. Cowley MJ, Hastillo A, Vetrovec GW: Effects of intracoronary streptokinase in acute myocardial infarction. *Am Heart J* 102:1149, 1981.

64. Dalen JE, Alpert JS: Natural history of pulmonary embolism. *Prog Cardiovasc Dis* 17:259, 1975.

65. Dalen JE, Gore JM, Braunwald E, et al: Six and twelve month follow-up on the Phase I thrombolysis in myocardial infarction (TIMI) trial. *Am J Cardiol* 62:179–185, 1988.

66. Dellborg M, Topol EJ, Swedberg K: Dynamic QRS complex and ST segment vectorcardiographic monitoring can identify vessel patency in patients with acute myocardial infarction treated with reperfusion therapy. *Amer Heart J* 122(4, Part I)943–948:1991.

67. DeWood MA, Spores J, Notske RN, et al: Prevalence of total coronary occlusion during the early hours of transmural myocardial infarction. *N Engl J Med* 303:897, 1980.

68. Rapaport E: Early versus late opening of coronary arteries: the effect of timing. *Clin Cardiol* 13(8 Suppl 8):VIII18–VIII22, 1990.

69. Diefenbach C, Erbel R, Pop T, et al: Recombinant single-chain urokinase-type plasminogen activator during acute myocardial infarction. *Am J Cardiol* 61(13):966–970, 1988.

70. Dodge HT, Sheehan FH, Mathey DG, et al: Usefulness of coronary artery bypass graft surgery or percutaneous transluminal angioplasty after thrombolytic therapy. *Circulation* 72(part 2):39, 1984.

71. Ducker F, Muller G, Nyman E, et al: Treatment of deep vein thrombosis with streptokinase. *Br Med J* 1:479–481, 1975.

72. Eisenberg PR, Kenzore JL, Sobel BE, et al: Relation between ST segment shifts during ischemia and thrombin activity in patients with unstable angina. *J Am Coll Cardiol* 18:898–903, 1991.

73. Eisenberg PR, Miletich JP: Induction of marked thrombin activity by pharmacologic concentrations of plasminogen activators in nonanticoagulated whole blood. *Thromb Res* 55:635, 1989.

74. Eisenberg PR, Miletich JP, Sobel BE, et al: Differential effects of activation of prothrombin by streptokinase compared with urokinase and tissue-type plasminogen activator (t-PA). *Thromb Res* 50:707, 1988.

75. Eisenberg PR, Sherman LA, Jaffe AS: Differential effects of activation of prothrombin by streptokinase compared with urokinase and tissue-type plasminogen activator (t-PA). *Thromb Res* 50:707, 1988.

76. Eisenberg PR, Sherman LA, Perez J, et al: Relationship between elevated plasma levels of crosslinked fibrin degradation products (SL-FDP) and the clinical presentation of patients with myocardial infarction. *Thromb Res* 46:109–120, 1987.

77. Eisenberg PR, Sherman LA, Rich M, et al: Importance of continued activation of thrombin reflected by fibrinopeptide A to the efficacy of thrombolysis. *J Am Coll Cardiol* 7:1255, 1986.

78. Eisenberg PR, Sherman LA, Schechtman K, et al: Fibrinopeptide A: a marker of acute coronary thrombosis. *Circulation* 71:912, 1985.

79. Eisenberg PR, Sherman LA, Tiefenbrunn AJ, et al: Sustained fibrinolysis after t-PA in man. *Thromb Haemost* 57:35, 1987.

80. Eisenberg PR, Sobel BE, Jaffe AS: Characterization *in vivo* of the fibrin specificity of activators of the fibrinolytic system. *Circulation* 78:592–597, 1988.

81. Eisenberg PR, Sobel BE, Jaffe AS: Activation of prothrombin accompanying thrombolysis with rt-PA. *J Am Coll Cardiol* 19:1065–1069, 1992.

82. Elliot MS, Immelman EJ, Jeffrey P, et al: A comparative randomized trial of heparin versus streptokinase in the treatment of acute proximal venous thrombosis: an interim report of a prospective trial. *Br J Surg* 66:838, 1979.

83. Fitzgerald DJ, Catella F, Roy L, et al: Marked platelet activation in vivo after intravenous streptokinase in patients with acute myocardial infarction. *Circulation* 77:142, 1988.

84. Fletcher AP, Alkjaersig N, Sherry S: The clearance of heterologous protein from the circulation of normal and immunized man. *J Clin Invest* 37:1306, 1959.

85. Fletcher AP, Alkjaersig N, Sherry S, et al: The development of urokinase as a thrombolytic agent. Maintenance of a sustained thrombolytic state in man by its intravenous infusion. *J Lab Clin Med* 65:713, 1965.

86. Fletcher AP, Alkjaersig N, Smyrniotis FE, et al: The treatment of patients suffering from early myocardial infarction with massive and prolonged streptokinase therapy. *Trans Assoc Am Physicians* 71:287, 1958.

87. Fletcher AP, Sherry S, Alkjaersig N, et al: The maintenance of a sustained thrombolytic state in man. II. Clinical observations on patients with myocardial infarction and other thromboembolic disorders. *J Clin Invest* 38:111, 1959.

88. Frances CW, Markham RE Jr, Barlow GH, et al: Thrombin activity of fibrin thrombi and soluble plasmic derivatives. *J Lab Clin Med* 102:220–230, 1983.

89. Gaffney PJ, Perry MJ: Unreliability of current serum fibrin degradation product (FDP) assays. *Thromb Haemost* 53:310, 1984.

90. Ganz W, Geft I, Lew AS, et al: Intravenous streptokinase in evolving acute myocardial infarction. *Am J Cardiol* 53:1209, 1984.

91. Garabedian HD, Gold HK, Leinbach RC, et al: Comparative properties of two clinical preparations of recombinant human tissue-type plasminogen activator in patients with acute myocardial infarction. *J Am Coll Cardiol* 9:599, 1987.

92. Gardell SJ, Ramjit DR, Stabilito II, et al: Effective thrombolysis without marked plasminemia after bolus intravenous administration of vampire bat salivary plasminogen activator in rabbits. *Circulation* 84:244–253, 1991.

93. Gold HK, Coller BS, Yasuda T, et al: Rapid and sustained coronary artery recanalization with combined bolus injection of recombinant tissue-type plasminogen activator and monoclonal antiplatelet GPIIb/IIIa antibody in a canine preparation. *Circulation* 77(3):670–677, 1988.

94. Gold HK, Leinbach RC, Garabedian HD, et al: Acute coronary reocclusion after thrombolysis with recombinant human tissue-type plasminogen activator: prevention by a maintenance infusion. *Circulation* 73:347, 1986.

95. Goldberg S, Urban PL, Greenspon A, et al: Combination therapy for evolving myocardial infarction: intracoronary thrombolysis and percutaneous transluminal angioplasty. *Am J Med* 72:994, 1982.

96. Goldhaber SZ: Thrombolysis for pulmonary embolism. *Prog Card Dis* (2):113–134, 1991.

97. Goldhaber SZ, Kessler CM, Heit J, Markis J, Sharma GVRK, Dawley D, Nagel JS, Meyerovitz M, Kim D, Vaughan DE, Parker JA, Tumeh SS, Drum D, Loscalzo J, Reagan K, Selwyn AP, Anderson J, Braunwald E: Randomized controlled trial of recombinant tissue plasminogen activator versus urokinase in the treatment of acute pulmonary embolism. *Lancet* ii(8606):293–298, 1988.

98. Goldhaber SZ, Meyerovitz MF, Green D, et al: Randomized controlled trial of tissue plasminogen activator in proximal deep venous thrombosis. *Am J Med* 88:235, 1990.

99. Goldhaber SZ, Vaughn DE, Markis JE, et al: Acute pulmonary embolism treated with tissue plasminogen activator. *Lancet* ii:886, 1986.

100. Gore JM, Thompson MJ, Becker RC: Rapid resolution of acute cor pulmonale with recombinant tissue plasminogen activator. *Chest* 96:939–941, 1989.

101. Graor RA, Risius B, Young JR, et al: Peripheral artery and bypass graft thrombolysis with recombinant human tissue-type plasminogen activator. *J Vasc Surg* 3:115, 1985.

102. Graor RA, Young JR, Risius B, et al: Comparison of cost effectiveness of streptokinase and urokinase in the treatment of deep vein thrombosis. *Ann Vasc Surg* 1:524–528, 1987.

103. Groupe de Recherche Urokinase-Embolie Pulmonaire: Rapport prepare par B. Charbonnie, Tours. Etude Multicentrique sur seux protocoles d'urokinase dans l'embolie pulmonaire grave. *Arch Mal Coeur* 7:773, 1984.

104. Gruppo Italiano per lo Studio della Sreptochinasi nell'Infarcto Miocardio (GISSI): Effectiveness of intravenous thrombolytic treatment in acute myocardial infarction. *Lancet* i:398, 1986.

105. Gruppo Italiano per lo Studio della Sreptochinasi nell'Infarcto Miocardio (GISSI). 2: A factorial randomised trial of alteplase versus streptokinase and heparin versus no heparin among 12,490 patients with acute myocardial infarction. *Lancet* 336(8707):65–71, 1990.

106. Grau E, Fontcuberta J, Pages MA, et al: Massive pulmonary embolism: short-term effects of thrombolytic treatment. *Angiology* 37:832–839, 1986.

107. Grines CL, Nissen SE, Booth DC, et al: A prospective, randomized trial comparing combination half-dose tissue-type plasminogen activator and streptokinase with full-dose tissue-type plasminogen activator. Kentucky Acute Myocardial Infarction Trial (KAMIT) Group. *Circulation* 84(2):540–549, 1991.

108. Gulba DC, Barthels M, Westhoff-Bleck M, et al: Increased thrombin levels during thrombolytic therapy in acute myocardial infarction. Relevance for the success of therapy. *Circulation* 83(3):937–944, 1991.

109. Gurewich V, Pannell R, Louie S, et al: Effective and fibrin-specific clot lysis by a zymogen precursor form of urokinase (prourokinase). A study in vitro and in two animal species. *J Clin Invest* 73:1731, 1984.

110. Haber E: Antibody-directed fibrinolysis. An antibody specific for both fibrin and tissue plasminogen activator. *J Biol Chem* 264(2) 944–948, 1980.

111. Hammerman H, Kloner RA, Briggs LL, et al: Enhancement of salvage of reperfused myocardium by early beta-adrenergic blockade (timolol). *J Am Coll Cardiol* 3:1438, 1984.

112. Hamsten A, Wiman B, De Faire U, Blomback M: Increased plasma levels of a rapid inhibitor of tissue plasminogen activator in young survivors of myocardial infarction. *N Engl J Med* 313:1557, 1985.

113. Harrison DC, Ferguson DW, Collin SM, et al: Rethrombosis after reperfusion with streptokinase: importance of geometry of residual lesions. *Circulation* 69:991, 1984.

114. Haskel EJ, Prager NA, Sobel BD, et al: Relative efficacy of antithrombin compared with antiplatelet agents in accelerating coronary thrombolysis and preventing early agents in accelerating coronary thrombolysis and preventing early reocclusion. *Circulation* 83(3):1048–1056, 1991.

115. Haskel EJ, Torr SR, Day KC, et al: Prevention of arterial reocclusion after thrombolysis with recombinant lipoprotein-associated coagulation inhibitor. *Circulation* 84(2):821–827, 1991.

116. Henry PD, Schuchleib R, Davis J, et al: Myocardial contracture and accumulation of mitochondrial calcium in ischemic rabbit heart. *Am J Physiol* 233:H677, 1977.

117. Herltiz J, Elmfeldt D, Holmberg S, et al: Goteberg Metoprolol Trial: Mortality and causes of death. *Am J Cardiol* 53:9D, 1984.

118. Hirsch J, O'Sullivan EF, Martin M: Evaluation of a standard dosage schedule with streptokinase. *Blood* 35:341, 1970.

119. Hoffman JJML, van Rey FJW, Bonnier JJRM: Systemic effects of BRL 26921 during thrombolytic treatment of acute myocardial infarction. *Thromb Res* 37:567, 1985.

120. Holmes DR Jr, Smith HC, Vlietstra RE, et al: Percutaneous transluminal coronary angioplasty, alone or in combination with streptokinase therapy, during acute myocardial infarction. *Mayo Clin Proc* 60:449, 1985.

121. Holmstrom M, Bratt G, Tornebohm E: Fatal pulmonary embolism caused by streptokinase treatment of deep venous thrombosis of the leg? *J Intern Med* 228(6):647–649, 1990.

122. Hoylaerts M, Rijken DC, Lijnen HR, et al: Kinetics of the activation of plasminogen by human tissue-type plasminogen activator. Role of fibrin. *J Biol Chem* 257:2912, 1982.

123. Hsia J, Hamilton WP, Kleinman N, et al: A comparison between heparin and low-dose aspirin as adjunctive therapy with tissue plasminogen activator for acute myocardial infarction. Heparin-Aspirin Reperfusion Trial (HART) Investigators *N Engl J Med* 323(21):1433–1437, 1990.

124. Hull, RD, Raskob GE, Hirsh J, et al: Continuous intravenous heparin compared with intermittent subcutaneous heparin in the initial treatment of proximal-vein thrombosis. *N Engl J Med* 315(18):1109–1114, 1986.

125. Ignarro LJ: Endothelium-derived nitric oxide: pharmacology and relationship to the actions of organic nitrate esters. *Pharm Res* 6(8):651–659, 1989.

126. Intenzo CM, Park CH, Kim SM: Rapid resolution of pulmonary embolism by tissue plasminogen activator. *Clin Nucl Med* 14:800, 1989.

127. ISIS Group: Vascular mortality after early IV beta blockade in acute myocardial infarction (MI). *Circulation* 72:111, 1985.

128. ISIS-2 (Second International Study of Infarct Survival) Collaborative Group: Randomised trial of intravenous streptokinase, oral aspirin, both, or neither among 17,187 cases of suspected acute myocardial infarction. *Lancet* ii(8607):349–360, 1988.

129. International Study Group: In-hospital mortality and clinical course of 20,891 patients with suspected acute myocardial infarction randomised between alteplase and streptokinase with or without heparin. *Lancet* 336(8707):71–75, 1990.

130. Jaffe AS, Geltman EM, Teifenbrunn AJ, et al: Reduction of infarct size in patients with inferior infarction with intravenous glyceryl trinitrate. A randomized study. *Br Heart J* 49:452, 1982.

131. Jannasch B, Schluter M, Schofer J, et al: Ineffective use of lidocaine in preventing reperfusion arrhythmias in patients with acute myocardial infarct. *Z Kardiol* 74(3):185–190, 1985.

132. Jarvinen P, Aromaa U, Roiha M: Streptokinase and concomitant oral anticoagulants in the treatment of deep venous thrombosis. *Klin Wochenschr* 58:801–804, 1978.

133. Jim RTS: A study of plasma prothrombin time. *J Lab Clin Med* 50:45, 1957.

134. Johnson ES, Cregeen RJ: An interim report of the efficacy and safety of anisoylated plasminogen streptokinase activator complex (APSAC). *Drugs* 33(Suppl 3):298, 1987.

135. Jolly SR, Kane WJ, Bailie MB, et al: Canine myocardium reperfusion injury, its reduction by the combined administration of superoxide dismutase and catalase. *Circ Res* 54:277, 1984.

136. Kakkar VV, Flanc C, Howe CT, et al: Natural history of post-operative deep vein thrombosis. *Lancet* ii:230, 1969.

137. Kakkar VV, Flanc C, Howe CT, et al: Treatment of deep venous thrombosis. A trial of heparin, streptokinase, and Arvin. *Br Med J* 1:806–810, 1969.

138. Kakkar VV, Howe CT, Laws JW, et al: Late results of treatment of deep venous thrombosis. *Br Med J* 1:810, 1969.

139. Kambara H, Kawai C, Kajiwara N, et al: Randomized, double-blinded multicenter study. Comparison of intracoronary single-chain urokinase-type plasminogen activator, pro-urokinase (GE-0943), and intracoronary urokinase in patients with acute myocardial infarction. *Circulation* 78(4):899–905, 1988.

140. Kaplan AP: Initiation of the intrinsic coagulation and fibrinolytic pathways of man: the role of surfaces, Hagemann factor, prekallikrein, HMW kininogen, and factor XI. *Prog Hemost Thromb* 4:127, 1978.

141. Kasper W, Erbel R, Meinertz T: Intracoronary thrombolysis with an acylated streptokinase plasminogen activator (BRL 26921) in patients with acute myocardial infarction. *J Am Coll Cardiol* 4:357, 1984.

142. Kennedy JW, Ritchie RL, Davis KB, et al: Western Washington randomized trial of intracoronary streptokinase in acute myocardial infarction. *N Engl J Med* 309:1477, 1983.

143. Kennedy JW, Ritchie RL, Davis KB, et al: The Western Washington randomized trial of intracoronary streptokinase: a 12 month follow up. *N Engl J Med* 312:1073, 1985.

144. Kereiakes DJ, Weaver WD, Anderson JL, et al: Time delays in the diagnosis and treatment of acute myocardial infarction: a tale of eight cities. *Am Heart J* 120 (4):773–780, 1990.

145. Kerins DM, Roy L, FitzGerald DJ: Platelet and vascular function during coronary thrombolysis with tissue-type plasminogen activator. *Circulation* 80(5):1718–1725, 1989.

146. Kernogan RJ, Todd C: Heparin therapy in thromboembolic disease. *Lancet* i:621, 1966.

147. Khaja F, Walton JA, Brymer JF, et al: Intracoronary fibrinolytic therapy in acute myocardial infarction: report of a prospective randomized trial. *N Engl J Med* 308:756, 1983.

148. Klein HH, Schobothe M, Nebendahl K, et al: The effects of two different diltiazem treatments on infarct size in ischemic reperfused porcine hearts. *Circulation* 69:1000, 1984.

149. Kloner RA, Alker KJ: Effect of streptokinase on intramyocardial hemorrhage, infarct size, and the no-reflow phenomenon during coronary reperfusion. *Circulation* 70:513–521, 1984

150. Kloner RA, Alker K, Campbell C, et al: Does tissue-type plasminogen activator have direct beneficial effects on the myocardium independent of its ability to lyse intracoronary thrombi? *Circulation* 79:1125–1136, 1989.

151. Knabb RM, Rosamond TI, Fox KAA, et al: Enhanced salvage of reperfused ischemic myocardium by diltiazem. *J Am Coll Cardiol* 8:861, 1986.

152. Koren G, Weiss AT, Hasin Y, et al: Prevention of myocardial damage in acute myocardial ischemia by early treatment with intravenous streptokinase. *N Engl J Med* 313:1384, 1985.

153. Kowalski E, Kopec M, Niewiarowski S: An evaluation of the euglobulin method for determination of fibrinolysis. *J Clin Pathol* 12:215, 1959.

154. Kruithof EKO: Plasminogen activator inhibitors—a review. *Enzyme* 40:113, 1988.

155. Kwon K, Freedman B, Wilcox I, et al: The unstable ST segment early after thrombolysis for acute infarction and its usefulness as a marker of recurrent coronary occlusion. *Am J Cardiol* 67:109–115, 1991.

156. Lang M, Charbonnier B, Quilliet L, et al: Activateur tissul du plasminogene (alteplase) dans l'embolie pulmonaire aigue massive. *Arch Mal Coeur* 82:1803–1811, 1989.

157. Langer JE, Velchik MG: Rapid resolution of massive pulmonary embolism due to streptokinase therapy: documented by ventilation/perfusion imaging *Clin Nucl Med* 13:874–877, 1988.

158. Larrieu MJ, Rigollot C, Marder VJ: Comparative effects of fibrinogen degradation products D and E on coagulation. *Br J Haematol* 72:719, 1973.

159. Lavie CJ, O'Keefe JH, Chesebro JH, et al: Prevention of late ventricular dilatation after acute myocardial infarction by successful thrombolytic reperfusion. *Am J Cardiol* 66:31–36, 1990.

160. Lee G, Low RI, Takeda P, et al: Importance of follow-up medical and surgical approaches to prevent reinfarction, reocclusion, and recurrent angina following intracoronary thrombolysis with streptokinase in acute myocardial infarction. *Am Heart J* 104:921, 1982.

161. Leeper KV, Popovich J, Lesser BA, et al: Treatment of massive acute pulmonary embolism. The use of low doses of intrapulmonary arterial streptokinase combined with full doses of systemic heparin. *Chest* 93(2):234–240, 1988.

162. Leibhoff RH, Katz RJ, Wasserman AG, et al: A randomized angiographically controlled trial of intracoronary streptokinase in acute myocardial infarction. *Am J Cardiol* 53:404, 1984.

163. Leor J, Hod H, Rotstein Z, et al: Effects of thrombolysis on the 12-lead signal-averaged ECG in the early postinfarction period. *Am. Heart J* 120(3):1990.

164. Lepor NE, Amin DK, Berberian L, et al: Does nitroglycerin induce heparin resistance? *Clin Cardiol* 12(8)432–434, 1989.

165. Levine M, Hirsh MD, Weitz J, et al: A randomized trial of a single bolus dosage regimen of recombinant tissue plasminogen activator in patients with acute pulmonary embolism. *Chest* 98:1473–1479, 1990.

166. Lew AS, Cercek B, Hod H, et al: Usefulness of residual plasma fibrinogen after intravenous streptokinase for predicting delay or failure of reperfusion in acute myocardial infarction. *Am J Cardiol* 58(9):680–685, 1986.

167. Lew AS, Laramee P, Cercek B, et al: The hypotensive effect of intravenous streptokinase in patients with myocardial infarction. *Circulation* 72:1321, 1985.

168. Lijnen HR, Zamarron C, Blaber M, et al: Activation of plasminogen by pro-urokinase. 1. Mechanism. *J Biol Chem* 261:1253, 1986.

169. Lucore CL, Fujii S, Sobel BE: Dependence of fibrinolytic activity on the concentration of free rather than total tissue-type plasminogen activator in plasma after pharmacologic administration. *Circulation* 79:1204–1213, 1989.

170. Lucore CL, Hagan RR, Sobel BE: Disparate changes in free and total t-PA quantified with a novel, rapid, immunoassay during and after coronary thrombolysis. *Circulation* 84(Suppl 11):11–290, 1991.

171. Ly B, Anreson H, Eie H, et al: A controlled trial of streptokinase and heparin in the treatment of major pulmonary embolism. *Acta Med Scand* 1203:465, 1978.

172. Marco MR, Moya VL, Pardo JG, et al: Lignocaine prophylaxis for reperfusion arrhythmias during treatment with streptokinase in acute myocardial infarction. *Lancet* Oct. 7, 1989.

173. Marder VJ, Rothbard RL, Fitzpatrick PG, et al: Rapid lysis of coronary artery thrombi with anisoylated plasminogen:streptokinase activator complexes. *Ann Intern Med* 104:304, 1986.

174. Marder VJ, Shulman NR: High molecular weight derivatives of human fibrinogen produced by plasmin. *J Biol Chem* 244:2120, 1969.

175. Marder VJ, Soulen RL, Atichartakarn V, et al: Quantitative venographic assessment of deep vein thrombosis in the evaluation of streptokinase and heparin therapy. *J Lab Clin Med* 89:1018–1029, 1977.

176. Martin M, Othmar Fieback BJ: Short-term ultrahigh streptokinase treatment of chronic arterial occlusions and acute deep vein thromboses. *Semin Thromb and Hemost* 17(1):21–38, 1991.

177. Mayor GE, Bennett B, Galloway JMD, et al: Streptokinase in iliofemoral venous thrombosis. *Br J Surg* 56:5764–5790, 1969.

178. McKlintock DK, Bell PH: The mechanism of activation of human plasminogen by streptokinase. *Biochem Biophys Res Commun* 43:694, 1971.

179. Mehta J, Mehta P, Lawson D, et al: Plasma tissue plasminogen activator inhibitor levels in coronary artery disease: correlation with age and serum triglyceride concentrations. *J Am Coll Cardiol* 9:263, 1987.

180. Mehta JL, Nicolini FA, Nichols WW, et al: Concurrent nitroglycerin administration decreases thrombolytic potential of tissue-type plasminogen activator. *J Am Coll Cardiol* 17:805–811, 1991.

181. Meijer A, Werter CJ, Freek WA: The apricot study: coumadin versus aspirin in the prevention of reocclusion after successful thrombolysis, a prospective placebo-controlled angiographic study. *Circulation* 84 (4):II–571, 1991.

182. Mentzer RL, Budynski AZ, Sherry S: High-dose, brief duration intravenous infusion of streptokinase in acute myocardial infarction: description of effects on the circulation. *Am J Cardiol* 57:1220, 1986.

183. Mirshahi M, Soria J, Soria C, et al: Evaluation of the inhibition of heparin and hirudin of coagulation activation during r-tPA-included thrombolysis. *Blood* 74(3):1025–1039, 1989.

184. Mitchell JP, Trulock EP: Tissue-plasminogen activator for pulmonary embolism resulting in shock: two case reports and discussion of the literature. *Am J Med* 90:255, 1991.

185. Mueller HS, Rao AK, Forman SA, et al: Thrombolysis in myocardial infarction (TIMI): comparative studies of coronary reperfusion and systemic fibrinogenolysis with two forms of recombinant tissue-type plasminogen activator. *J Am Coll Cardiol* 10:479, 1987.

186. Muller DW, Topol EJ: Selection of patients with acute myocardial infarction for thrombolytic therapy. *Ann Intern Med* 113(2):949–960, 1990.

187. Myers ML, Bolli R, Lekich RF, et al: Enhancement of recovery of myocardial function by oxygen free-radical scavengers after reversible regional ischemia. *Circulation* 72:915, 1985.

188. Neuhaus KL, Feuerer W, Jeep-Tebbe S, et al: Improved thrombolysis with a modified dose regimen of recombinant tissue-type plasminogen activator. *J Am Coll Cardiol* 14:1566–1569, 1989.

189. Neuhaus KL, Tebbe U, Gottwik M, et al: Intravenous infusion of recombinant tissue-type plasminogen activator (rt-PA) and urokinase in acute myocardial infarct: intermediate results of the G.A.U.S. study (German Activator Urokinase Study). *Klin-Wochenschr* 66(Suppl 12):102–108, 1988.

190. Nilsson T, Wallen P, Mellbring G: Turnover of human extrinsic (tissue-type) plasminogen activator in man. *Haemostasis* 14:90, 1984.

191. Nossel HL, Yudelman I, Caufield RE, et al: Measurement of fibrinopeptide A in human blood. *J Clin Invest* 54:43, 1974.

192. O'Connor CM, Meese R, Navetta F, et al: A randomized trial of heparin in conjunction with anistreplase (APSAC) in acute myocardial infarction. *Circulation* 85(4):II–571, 1991.

193. O'Donnell TF, Browse NL, Burnand KG, et al: The socioeconomic effects of an iliofemoral venous thrombosis. *J Surg Res* 22:483, 1977.

194. Ohman EM, Califf RM, Topol EJ, et al: Consequences of reocclusion after successful reperfusion therapy in acute myocardial infarction. TAMI Study Group. *Circulation* 82(3):781–791, 1990.

195. O'Rourke M, Baron D, Keogh A, et al: Limitations of myocardial infarction by early infusion of recombinant tissue-type plasminogen activator. *Circulation* 77:1311–1315, 1988.

196. Ozbek C, Sen S, Frank S, et al: Rapid high dose streptokinase in severe pulmonary embolism. *Lancet* 2:229–230, 1989.

197. Paques EP, Stohr HA, Heimburger N: Study on the mechanism of action of heparin and related substances on the fibrinolytic systems: relationship between plasminogen activator and heparin. *Thromb Res* 42:797, 1986.

198. Paramo JA, Colucci M, Van De Werf CD: Plasminogen activator inhibitors in the blood of patients with coronary artery disease. *Br Med J* 291:573, 1985.

199. Petitpretz P, Simmoneau G, Cerrina J, et al: Effects of a single bolus of urokinase in patients with life-threatening pulmonary emboli: a descriptive trial. *Circulation* 70(5)861–866, 1984.

200. Petronis J: Sequential ventilation/perfusion imaging of massive pulmonary embolism treated with recombinant tissue plasminogen activator. *Clin Nucl Med* 15:150–153, 1990.

201. A collaborative study by the PIOPED investigators: Tissue plasminogen activator for the treatment of acute pulmonary embolism. *Chest* 97:528–533, 1990.

202. Ploug J, Kheldgaard NO: Urokinase: an activator of plasminogen from urine. 1. Isolation and properties. *Biochim Biophys Acta* 24:282, 1957.

203. Pogwizd SM, Corr PB: Electrophysiologic mechanisms underlying arrhythmias due to reperfusion of ischemic myocardium. *Circulation* 76(2):404–426, 1987.

204. Prewitt RM: Principles of thrombolysis in pulmonary embolism. *Chest* 99:4, 1991.

205. Prewitt RM, Hoy C, Kong A, et al: Thrombolytic therapy in canine pulmonary embolism. Comparative effects of urokinase and recombinant tissue plasminogen activator. *Am Rev Respir Dis* 141:290–295, 1990.

206. Proctor RR, Rapaport SI: The partial thromboplastin time with kaolin. *Am J Clin Pathol* 6:212, 1963.

207. Prowse CV, Dawes J, Lane DA, Ireland H, Knight I: Proteolysis of fibrinogen in healthy volunteers following major and minor vivo plasminogen activation. *Thromb Res* 27(1):91–97, 1982.

208. Przyklenk K, Kloner RA: Superoxide dismutase plus catalase improve contractile function in the canine model of "stunned myocardium." *Circ Res* 58:148, 1986.

209. Rapold HJ: Promotion of thrombin activity by thrombolytic therapy without simultaneous anticoagulation. *Lancet* i:481–482, 1990.

210. Rapold HJ, Weiss M, Baur H, et al: Monitoring of fibrin generation during thrombolytic therapy of acute myocardial infarction with recombinant tissue-type plasminogen activator. *Circulation* 79:980–989, 1989.

211. Rakoczi I, Wiman B, Collen D: On the biological significance of the specific interaction between fibrin, plasminogen, and antiplasmin. *Biochim Biophys Acta* 1540:295, 1978.

212. Rao AK, Pratt C, Berke A, et al: The thrombolysis in myocardial infarction trial-Phase 1: hemorrhagic manifestations and changes in plasma fibrinogen and the fibrinolytic system in patients treated with recombinant tissue plasminogen activator and streptokinase. *J Am Coll Cardiol* 11:1–11, 1988.

213. Reduto LA, Smalling RW, Freund CG, et al: Intracoronary infusion of streptokinase in patients with acute myocardial infarctions: effects of reperfusion on left ventricular performance. *Am J Cardiol* 48:403–409, 1981.

214. Rentrop KP: Thrombolytic therapy in patients with acute myocardial infarction. *Circulation* 71:627, 1985.

215. Rentrop P, Blanke H, Karsch KR, et al: Changes in left ventricular function after intracoronary streptokinase infusion in clinical evolving myocardial infarction. *Am Heart J* 102:1188, 1981.

216. Rentrop P, Blanke H, Karsch KR, et al: Selective intracoronary thrombolysis in acute myocardial infarction and unstable angina pectoris. *Circulation* 63:307, 1981.

217. Rentrop KP, Feit F, Blanke H, et al: Effects of intracoronary streptokinase and intracoronary nitroglycerine infusion on coronary angiographic patterns and mortality in patients with acute myocardial infarction. *N Engl J Med* 311:1457, 1984.

218. Rijken DC, Hoylaerts M, Collen D: Fibrinolytic properties of one-chain and two chain human extrinsic (tissue-type) plasminogen activator. *J Biol Chem* 257:2920, 1982.

219. Rijken DC, Wijngaards G, Collen D: Tissue-type plasminogen activator from human tissue and cell cultures and its occurrence in plasma. In Collen D, Lijnen HR, Verstraete M (eds): *Thrombolysis: Biological and Therapeutic Properties of New Thrombolytic Agents.* Churchill Livingstone, Edinburgh, 1985.

220. Ritchie JL, Cerqueria M, Maynard C, et al: Ventricular function and infarction size: the Western Washington Intravenous Streptokinase in Myocardial Infarction Trial. *J Am Coll Cardiol* 11:689–697, 1988.

221. Robbins KC: The human plasma fibrinolytic system: regulation and control. *Mol Cell Biochem* 20:149, 1978.

222. Roberts R, Rogers WJ, Mueller HS, et al: Immediate versus deferred B-blockade following thrombolytic therapy in patients with acute myocardial infarction. Results of the thrombolysis in myocardial infarction (TIMI) 11-B study. *Circulation* 83:422–437, 1991.

223. Robertson BR, Nilsson IM, Nylander G: Thrombolytic effect of streptokinase as evaluated by phlebography of deep venous thrombi of the leg. *Acta Chir Scand* 136:173, 1970.

224. Rogers WJ, Baim DS, Gore JM, et al: Comparison of immediate invasive, delayed invasive, and conservative strategies after tissue-type plasminogen activator. Results of the thrombolysis in myocardial infarction (TIMI) phase 11-A trial. *Circulation* 81:1457–1476, 1990.

225. Rogers WJ, Mantle JA, Hood WP: Prospective randomized trial of intravenous and intracoronary streptokinase in acute myocardial infarction. *Circulation* 68:1051, 1983.

226. Rosch J, Dotter CT, Seaman AJ, Porter JM, et al: Healing of deep venous thrombosis: venographic findings in a randomized study comparing streptokinase and heparin. *AJR* 127:553, 1976.

227. Rothbard RL, Fitzpatrick PG, Francis CW, et al: Relationship of the lytic state to successful reperfusion with standard and low dose intracoronary streptokinase. *Circulation* 71:562, 1985.

228. Rovelli F, De-Vita C, Feruglio GA, et al: Gruppo italiano per la sperimentazione della streptochinasi nell'infarto miocardico. *J Am Coll Cardiol* 10(5 Suppl B):33B–39B, 1987.

229. Rylatt DB, Blake AS, Cottis LE, et al: An immunoassay for human D dimer using monoclonal antibodies. *Thromb Res* 31:767, 1983.

230. Sande JV, Bossaert L, Brochier M, et al: Thrombolytic treatment of pulmonary embolism with APSAC. *Eur Respir J* 1:721–725, 1988.

231. Scati (Studio sulla calciparina nell'angina e nella trombosi ventricolare nell'infarto) group: Randomised controlled trial of subcutaneous calcium-heparin in acute myocardial infarction. *Lancet* ii(8656):182–186, 1989.

232. Schrieber TL, Miller DH, Silvasi D, et al: Superiority of warfarin over aspirin long term after thrombolytic therapy for acute myocardial infarction. *Am Heart J* 119:1238, 1990.

233. Scrutinio D, Biasco MG, Rizzon P: Thrombolysis in unstable angina: results of clinial studies. *Am J Cardiol* 68:99B–104B, 1991.

234. Serradimigni A, Bory M, Djiane P, et al: Treatment of venous thrombosis and pulmonary embolism by streptokinase. *Angiology* 29:825–831, 1978.

235. Schroeder R, Biamino G, Von Leitner ER, et al: Intravenous short-term infusion of streptokinase in acute myocardial infarction. *Circulation* 67:536, 1983.

236. Schroeder R, Neuhaus KL, Leizorovicz A, et al: A prospective placebo-controlled double-blind multicenter trial of intravenous streptokinase in acute myocardial infarction (ISAM): long-term mortality and morbidity. *J Am Coll Cardiol* 9:197, 1987.

237. Seaman AJ, Common HH, Rosch J, et al: Deep vein thrombosis treated with streptokinase or heparin. *Angiology* 27:549–556, 1976.

238. Serruys PW, Wijns W, van den Brand M, et al: Is transluminal coronary angioplasty mandatory after successful thrombolysis? Quantitative coronary angiographic study. *Br Heart J* 50:257, 1983.

239. Shafer KE, Santoro SA, Sobel BE, et al: Monitoring of fibrinolytic agents. A therapeutic challenge. *Am J Med* 76:879, 1984.

240. Sheehan FH, Detley GM, Schofer J, et al: Effect of interventions in salvaging left ventricular function in acute myocardial infarction: a study of intracoronary streptokinase. *Am J Cardiol* 52:431, 1983.

241. Sheehan FH, Mathey DS, Schofer J, et al: Factors that determine recovery of left ventricular function after thrombolysis in patients with acute myocardial infarction. *Circulation* 71:1121, 1985.

242. Simoons ML, Brand M, de Zwaan C, et al: Improved survival after early thrombolysis in acute myocardial infarction. *Lancet* ii:578, 1985.

243. Simoons ML, Arnold AER, Betriu A, et al: Thrombolysis with tissue plasminogen activator in acute myocardial infarction: no additional benefit from immediate percutaneous coronary angioplasty. *Lancet* i:197–202, 1988.

244. ISIS-3: a randomised comparison of streptokinase vs tissue plasminogen activator vs anistreplase and of aspirin plus heparin vs aspirin alone among 41,299 cases of suspected acute myocardial infarction. ISIS-3 (Third International Study of Infarct Survival) Collaborative Group. *Lancet* 339(8796):753–770, 1992.

245. Smith RAG, Dupe RJ, English PD, et al: Acyl-enzymes as thrombolytic agents in a rabbit model of venous thrombosis. *Thromb Haemost* 47:269, 1982.

246. Smith RAG, Dupe RJ, English PD, et al: Fibrinolysis with acyl enzymes: a new approach to thrombolytic therapy. *Nature* 290:505, 1981.

247. Sobel BE: Thrombolysis in the treatment of acute myocardial infarction. In Foster and Verstralte (eds): *Thrombosis in Cardiovascular Disorders.* WB Saunders, Philadelphia, pp 289–326, 1992.

248. Sobel BE, Gross RW, Robison AK: Thrombolysis, clot selectivity, and kinetics. *Circulation* 70:160, 1984.

249. Sobel BE, Nachowiak DA, Fry ETA, et al: Paradoxical attenuation of fibrinolysis attributable to "plasminogen steal" and its implications for coronary thrombolysis. *Coronary Artery Dis* 1:111–119, 1990.

250. Spann JF, Sherry S, Carabello BA, et al: Coronary thrombolysis by intravenous streptokinase in acute myocardial infarction: acute and follow-up studies. *Am J Cardiol* 53:655, 1984.

251. Stadius ML, Davis K, Maynard C, et al: Risk stratification for one year survival based on characteristics identified in the early hours of acute myocardial infarction. *Circulation* 74:703–711, 1986.

252. Stainforth DH, Smith RAG, Hibbs M: Streptokinase and anisoylated streptokinase plasminogen complex. Their action on haemostasis in human volunteers. *Eur J Pharmacol* 24:751, 1983.

253. Stampfer MJ, Goldhaber SZ, Yusef S, et al: Effect of intravenous streptokinase on acute myocardial infarction. Pooled results from randomized trials. *N Engl J Med* 307:1180, 1982.

254. Stamler JS, Vaughan DE, Loscalzo J: Synergistic disaggregation of platelets by tissue-type plasminogen activator, prostaglandin E1, and nitroglycerin. *Circ Res* 65(3):796–804, 1989.

255. Taylor GJ, Mikell SL, Moses HW, et al: Intravenous versus intracoronary streptokinase therapy for acute myocardial infarction in community hospitals. *Am J Cardiol* 54:256, 1984.

256. Terres W, Beythien C, Kupper W, et al: Effects of aspirin and prostaglandin E on in vitro thrombolysis with urokinase. *Circulation* 79:1309–1314, 1989.

257. Theiss W, Wirtzield A, Fink J, et al: The success rate of fibrinolytic therapy in fresh and old thrombosis of the iliac and femoral veins. *Angiology* 34:61–69, 1983.

258. Theroux P: Antiplatelet and antithrombotic therapy in unstable angina. *Am J Cardiol* 68:92B–98B, 1991.

259. Thomas D, Niewiarowski S, Meyers AR, et al: A comparative study of four methods for detecting fibrinogen degradation products in patients with various diseases. *N Engl J Med* 283:663, 1970.

260. Thompson PL, Aylward PE, Federman J, et al: A randomized comparison of intravenous heparin with oral aspirin and dipyridamole 24 hours after recombinant tissue-type plasminogen activator for acute myocardial infarction. *Circulation* 83:1534–1542, 1991.

261. The Thrombolysis Myocardial Infarction (TIMI) Trial: phase 1 findings. *N Engl J Med* 312:932, 1985.

262. Tibbutt DA, Davies JA, Anderson JA, et al: Comparison by controlled clinical trial of streptokinase and heparin in treatment of life-threatening pulmonary embolism. *Br Med J* 1:343, 1974.

263. Tiefenbrunn AJ, Robison AK, Kurnik PB, et al: Clinical pharmacology in patients with evolving myocardial infarction of tissue-type plasminogen activator produced by recombinant DNA technology. *Circulation* 71:110, 1985.

264. Tiefenbrunn AJ, Sobel BE: Thrombolysis and myocardial infarction. *Fibrinolysis* 5:1–15, 1991.

265. Tillet WS, Garner RL: The fibrinolytic activity of hemolytic streptococci. *J Exp Med* 58:485, 1933.

266. TIMI Research Group: Immediate vs delayed catheterization and angioplasty following thrombolytic therapy for acute myocardial infarction. TIMI 11 A results. *JAMA* 260:2849–2858, 1988.

267. Topol EJ, Califf RM, George BS, et al: A multicentered randomized trial of intravenous recombinant tissue plasminogen activator and emergency coronary angioplasty for acute myocardial infarction: preliminary report from the TAMI study. *Circulation* 74:11–74, 1986.

268. Topol EJ, Califf RM, George BS, et al: A randomised trial of immediate versus delayed elective angioplasty after intravenous tissue plasminogen activator in acute myocardial infarction. *N Engl J Med* 317:581–588, 1987.

269. Topol EJ, Ellis SG, Wall TC, et al: A randomised controlled trial of late (6–24 hour) reperfusion for acute myocardial infarction. *Circulation* 83(4):539, 1990.

270. Topol EJ, George BS, Kereiakes DJ, et al: A randomized controlled trial of intravenous tissue plasminogen activator and early intravenous heparin in acute myocardial infarction. *Circulation* 79:281–286, 1989.

271. Topol EJ, O'Neill WW, Langburd AB, et al: A randomized, placebo-controlled trial of intravenous recombinant tissue-type plasminogen activator and emergency coronary angioplasty in patients with acute myocardial infarction. *Circulation* 75:420, 1987.

272. Topol EJ, Weiss JL, Brinker JA, et al: Regional wall motion improvement after coronary thrombolysis with recombinant tissue plasminogen activator: importance of coronary angioplasty. *J Am Coll Cardiol* 6:426, 1985.

273. Tsapogas MJ, Peabody RA, Wu KT, et al: Controlled trial of thrombolytic therapy in deep vein thrombosis. *Surgery* 74:973, 1973.

274. Urokinase-Streptokinase Pulmonary Embolism Trial, phase 2 results. *JAMA* 229:1606, 1974.

275. Van de Werf F: Discrepancies between the effects of coronary reperfusion on survival and left ventricular function. *Lancet* i:1367–1369, 1989.

276. Van de Werf F, Bergmann SR, Fox KAA, et al: Coronary thrombolysis with intravenously administered human tissue-type plasminogen activator produced by recombinant DNA technology. *Circulation* 69:605, 1984.

277. Van de Werf F, Ludbrook PA, Bergmann SR, et al: Coronary thrombolysis with intravenously administered human tissue-type plasminogen activator in patients with acute myocardial infarction. *N Engl J Med* 311:609, 1984.

278. Van de Werf F, Nobuhara M, Collen D: Coronary thrombolysis with human single-chain urokinase-type plasminogen activator (prourokinase) in patients with acute myocardial infarction. *Ann Intern Med* 104:345, 1984.

279. Van de Werf F, Vanhaecke J, de Geest H, et al: Coronary thrombolysis with recombinant single-chain urokinase type plasminogen activator in patients with acute MI. *Circulation* 74:1066, 1986.

280. Van de Werf F, Vanhaecke J, Jang IK, et al: Reduction in infarct size and enhanced recovery of systolic function after coronary thrombolysis with tissue-type plasminogen activator combined with beta-adrenergic blockade with metoprolol. *Circulation* 75:830–836, 1987.

281. Vermeer F, Simmons ML, Lubsen J: Reduced frequency of ventricular fibrillation after early thrombolysis in myocardial infarction. *Lancet* i:1147–1148, 1986.

282. Verstraete M, Bory M, Collen D, et al: Randomized trial of intravenous recombinant tissue-type plasminogen activator versus intravenous streptokinase in acute myocardial infarction. *Lancet* i:842, 1985.

283. Verstraete M, Bounameoux H, De Cock F, et al: Pharmacokinetics and systemic fibrinogenolytic effects of recombinant human tissue-type plasminogen activator (rt-PA) in humans. *J Pharmacol Exp Ther* 235:506, 1985.

284. Verstraete M, Miller GAH, Boundameaux H, et al: Intravenous and intrapulmonary recombinant tissue-type plasminogen activator in the treatment of acute massive pulmonary embolism. *Circulation* 77:353–360, 1988.

285. Volpi A, Cavalli A, Santoro E, et al: Incidence and prognosis of secondary ventricular fibrillation in acute myocardial infarction. Evidence for a protective effect of thrombolytic therapy. *GISSI Investigators Circulation* 82(4):1279–1288, 1990.

286. Neuhaus KL, von Essen R, Tebbe U, Vogt A, Roth M, Riess M, Niederer W, Forycki F, Wirtzfeld A, Maeurer W, et al: Improved thrombolysis in acute myocardial infarction with front-loaded administration of alteplase: results of the rt-PA-APSAC patency study (TAPS). *J Am Coll Cardiol* 19(5):885–891, 1992.

287. Walker ID, Davidson JR, Rae AP, et al: Acylated streptokinase-plasminogen complex in patients with acute myocardial infarction. *Thromb Haemost* 51:204, 1984.

288. Wall TC, Phillips III HR, Stack RS, et al: Results of high dose intravenous urokinase for acute myocardial infarction. *Am J Cardiol* 65(3):124–131, 1990.

289. Wallen P, Bergsdorf N, Ranby M: Purification and identification of two structural variants of porcine tissue plasminogen activator by affinity adsorption of fibrin. *Biochim Biophys Acta* 719:318, 1982.

290. Wallen P, Wiman B: Characterization of human plasminogen. II. Separation and partial characterization of different molecular forms of human plasminogen. *Biochim Biophys Acta* 257:122.

291. Watz R, Savidge GF: Rapid thrombolysis and preservation of valvular function in high deep venous thrombosis. *Acta Med Scand* 205:293, 1979.

292. Weaver WD, Eisenberg MS, Martin JS, et al: Myocardial infarction triage and intervention project—Phase I: Patient characteristics and feasibility of prehospital initiation of thrombolytic therapy. *J Am Coll Cardiol* 15:925–931, 1990.

293. Weimar W, Stibbe AJ, van Seyen AJ, et al: Specific lysis of an iliofemoral thrombus by administration of extrinsic (tissue type) plasminogen activator. *Lancet* ii:1018, 1980.

294. Weiss AT, Fine DG, Applebaum D, et al: Prehospital coronary thrombolysis. A new strategy in acute myocardial infarction. 92(1):124–128, 1987.

295. Weitz JI, Cruickshank MK, Thong B, et al: Human tissue-type plasminogen activator releases fibrinopeptides A and B from fibrinogen. 82(5):1700–1707, 1988.

296. Weiss AT, Fine DG, Applebaum D, et al: Prehospital coronary thrombolysis. A new strategy in acute myocardial infarction. 92(1):124–128, 1987.

297. Weitz JI, Hudoba M, Massel D, et al: Clot-bound thrombin is protected from inhibition by heparin-antithrombin III but is susceptible to inactivation by antithrombin III-dependent inhibitors. *J Clin Invest* 85:385–391, 1990.

298. Whitaker AN, Elms NJ, Masci PP: Measurement of crosslinked fibrin derivatives in plasma: an immunoassay using monoclonal antibodies. *J Clin Pathol* 37:882, 1984.

299. White WF, Barlow GH, Mozen MN: The isolation and characterization of plasminogen activators (urokinase) from human urine. *Biochemistry* 5:2160, 1966.

300. Wiman B, Collen D: On the kinetics of the reaction between human antiplasmin and plasmin. *Eur J Biochem* 84:573, 1978.

301. Wiman B, Collen D: Purification and characterization of human antiplasmin, the fast-acting plasmin inhibitor in plasma. *Eur J Biochem* 78:19, 1977.

302. Yamada K, Saffitz JE, Sobel BE, et al: Enhanced salvage of reperfused ischemic myocardium by alpha-adrenergic blockade. *J Am Coll Cardiol* 7:54, 1986.

303. Yasuno M, Saito Y, Ishida M, et al: Effects of percutaneous transluminal coronary angioplasty: intracoronary thrombolysis with urokinase in acute myocardial infarction. *Am J Cardiol* 53:1217, 1984.

304. Young AE, Lea Thomas M, Browse NL: Comparison between sequelae of surgical and medical treatment of venous thromboembolism. *Br Med J* 4:127, 1974.

305. Zammarron C, Lijnen HR, Van Hoef B, et al: Biological and thrombolytic properties of proenzyme and active forms of human urokinase. 1. Fibrinolytic and fibrinogenolytic properties in human plasma in vitro of urokinases obtained from human urine or by recombinant DNA technology. *Thromb Haemost* 52:19, 1984.

CHAPTER 22

Immunotherapy in Critically Ill Patients

RICHARD J. BATTAFARANO, M.D.
DAVID L. DUNN, M.D., Ph.D.

INTRODUCTION

The incidence of significant nosocomial infections in the U.S. continues to increase each year. Approximately 400,000 cases occur per year, of which at least 30% are caused by Gram-negative bacterial organisms (1–3). Despite improvements in antimicrobial therapy, intensive care (e.g., aggressive fluid resuscitation hemodynamic monitoring and metabolic support), survival subsequent to Gram-negative bacterial sepsis has improved only modestly during the last 30 years. Gram-negative bacteremia and its attendant sequelae are a frequent cause of multisystem organ failure and death in surgical intensive care units, contributing to or directly causing over 40,000 deaths per year in the U.S. (4).

Although virtually every Gram-negative bacterial pathogen has been identified as being capable of causing bacteremia, enteric organisms, such as *Escherichia coli* and isolates of *Klebsiella, Enterobacter, Serratia,* and *Pseudomonas,* predominate in overall frequency. Bacteremias due to *Pseudomonas* species and polymicrobial bacteremias are associated with a higher lethality than those caused by other single pathogens, probably as a result of both the virulence of the organism and because this type of bacteremia occurs with higher frequency in immunosuppressed hosts with concurrent serious underlying illness.

Although many disease processes may predispose patients to develop Gram-negative bacterial infection, the precise sequence of events that culminates in bacteremia has not been clearly defined. Systemic spread of microorganisms from a focus of infection may be responsible in many cases, while translocation of enteric organisms across the gut barrier may be etiologic in other individuals, particularly neutropenic patients. The presence of indwelling catheters in the urinary or respiratory tracts or the bloodstream provides additional potential sources of infection in critically ill patients (5–7).

Patient susceptibility to Gram-negative bacteremia is greatly increased by disease processes and treatments that depress the host immune system or modify the host microflora. Examples of agents or disease states that lead to this type of immunologic alteration consist of cancer chemotherapy, administration of immunosuppressive agents to patients undergoing organ transplantation, malnutrition, a major operative event, polytrauma, diabetes mellitus, congestive heart failure, and uremia.

The overall mortality attributable to this disease process is substantial (10–20%) and is >30% in immunodeficient patient populations (3, 5, 6, 8–17). The continued high mortality of Gram-negative bacterial infections, sepsis, and septic shock, despite standard treatment with currently available measures, has provided an impetus for the development of new adjuvant forms of therapy. Because the Gram-negative bacterial cell wall component lipopolysaccharide (endotoxin, LPS) appears to be causally related to the high morbidity and mortality associated with serious Gram-negative bacterial infections, the concept that it may be possible to target therapy directly against this toxic compound has been studied intensively.

Current evidence suggests that endotoxin may exert deleterious effects upon the host by directly affecting host tissues, by provoking the production of secondary monokine mediators that affect host tissues, or both. Host monokines, such as tumor

Table 22.1.   Potential Immunotherapeutic Agents for the Treatment of Sepsis

Biologic Response Modifiers	Lipid A Analogs	Antibody Immunotherapy	Monokine Abrogation
Muramyl dipeptide	Lipid X	Normal polyclonal antibody preparations	Anti-TNF mAb
Thymopentin	SDZ MRL 953	Anti-*E. coli* J5 polyclonal antibody preparations	CB0006
Tuftsin	Monophosphoryl lipid A	Anti-Lipid A mAbs	IL-1 receptor antagonist
Levamisole		E5	Soluble IL-1 receptor
GM-CSF		HA-1A	
G-CSF		T-88	

necrosis factor (TNF) interleukin-1 (IL-1), and interleukin-6 (IL-6), are secreted by host macrophages during Gram-negative bacterial infections and following endotoxin challenge and are integral components of the host response to such infections (18). Unfortunately, endotoxin may not only initiate but also is capable of perpetuating the release of these monokines, and it has become obvious that excessive monokine production may, in and of itself, produce end-organ damage, organ failure, and death.

Thus, the overall host response to a septic insult may represent a composite of host mediator-related events and the direct toxicity caused by the infecting pathogen. More effective therapy for Gram-negative bacterial sepsis most likely will require elimination of microbial growth, neutralization of microbial virulence factors, and abrogation of the effects of the secondary host mediators that are released during infection (19). This concept constitutes the conceptual basis for the use of agents directed against endotoxin and endotoxin-induced monokines as adjuvant treatment of Gram-negative bacterial infections. These new therapies will hopefully serve to reduce the high mortality associated with clinical Gram-negative bacterial sepsis and shock.

PATHOPHYSIOLOGY OF GRAM-NEGATIVE BACTERIAL INFECTION

The host physiologic response to Gram-negative bacterial infection consists of fever, systemic acidosis, arterial hypoxemia, disordered substrate metabolism and oxygen utilization, hyperglycemia, decreased systemic vascular resistance, elevated cardiac output, hypotension, and failure of organ systems distant from the site of local infection. Although blood-borne bacteria or bacterial toxins play an important role in mediating the toxicity of Gram-negative bacterial infection, more complex interactions certainly occur.

The amplification of several host mediator systems plays an important role in the response to Gram-negative bacterial sepsis. Activation of the complement and coagulation cascades has been associated with macrophage activation, polymorphonuclear leukocyte aggregation, and thrombocytopenia. Cellular release of cytokines, prostaglandins, superoxide radicals, and lysosomal enzymes accompanies the initial activation steps, and increasing evidence suggests that organ failure and death may occur secondary to an exaggerated host response (20–22).

Bacteria, bacterial toxins, or host-mediated events individually cannot account for all of the alterations that occur in host physiology, suggesting that a composite effect may be responsible. Specifically, results obtained from both experimental and clinical studies demonstrate that cellular mediators are released in response to a variety of stimuli, including bacterial products, and that excessive mediator secretion causes target organ damage and failure (23, 24). However, the exact series of events that culminates in lethality remains unknown.

Gram-negative bacterial LPS is that portion of the Gram-negative bacterial cell membrane responsible for many, if not all, of the toxic effects that occur during Gram-negative bacterial sepsis (25–27). The biochemical structure of LPS has been determined for many species of Gram-negative microorganisms, and this molecule is comprised of 3 regions: (*a*) lipid A, the toxic moiety of LPS; (*b*) the core region, a series of 10 to 11 saccharide residues, common to many Gram-negative bacteria; and (*c*) O-antigen, a series of 30 to 100 repeating polysaccharide residues, an antigen unique to each bacterial strain (28–35). Because of the central role of LPS in mediating the toxicities associated with Gram-negative bacterial sepsis, the immunologic and physiologic effects of this substance have been extensively studied.

The host response to LPS includes macrophage activation, nonspecific polyclonal B lymphocyte proliferation, monokine secretion, and production of antibody directed against various portions of the LPS molecule following repeated challenge with either LPS or intact bacteria. Direct administration of LPS induces responses similar to those observed during Gram-negative bacterial sepsis, including hypoxemia, hypotension, acidosis, white blood cell and platelet margination, bacterial translocation across the gut, complement and coagulation cascade activation, and death (36–38).

The septic response almost assuredly is a result of both the direct and indirect effects of LPS. Indirect effects arise from LPS stimulation of host macrophages. Activated macrophages secrete a wide array of monokines that includes TNF, IL-1, IL-6, and interferon-α. Although the paracrine effects of these monokines probably act to bolster local host defenses, systemic dissemination of these monokines results in host morbidity. Investigation of the effects of TNF has provided the most compelling demonstration that this monokine may, in and of itself, be directly responsible for many of the deleterious effects of endotoxin. Four lines of reasoning provide support for this contention: (*a*) Patients who develop Gram-negative bacterial sepsis exhibit increased serum levels of TNF. (*b*) Administration of endotoxin to humans and nonhuman primates leads to increased levels of TNF. (*c*) Administration of purified TNF induces a clinical response similar to that of endotoxic shock with characteristic end-organ dysfunction and high mortality. (*d*) Administration of anti-TNF antibodies has been shown to improve survival after experimental endotoxin and Gram-negative bacterial challenge (39–47).

Other macrophage-derived cytokines, such as IL-1 and IL-6, may also play an important role in the septic host response. Serum IL-1 levels are increased in humans after exogenous administration of endotoxin and are elevated after Gram-negative bacterial challenge in nonhuman primates (44, 48–51). Protective doses of anti-TNF antibody abrogate this increase in IL-1 (52). IL-6 levels are also elevated systemically and at the infected site in animal and clinical studies, and anti-TNF antibodies also abrogate this increase in IL-6 (52–54). Interestingly, although IL-6 administration does not lead to increased mortality, anti-IL-6 antibodies have been shown to improve survival after experimental Gram-negative bacterial challenge (55).

Two problems arise in treating patients with serious Gram-negative bacterial infections: (*a*) Patients frequently present with evidence of systemic sepsis and shock prior to a specific site of infection or organism being identified. (*b*) Antimicrobial therapy is incapable of counteracting the toxicity associated with LPS after release from the Gram-negative bacterial outer membrane occurs. In an attempt to reduce the high mortality associated with Gram-negative bacterial sepsis, potentially additive forms of therapy, therefore, have been developed and examined. The principal areas of investigation include: (*a*) administration of immunostimulatory agents that may serve to enhance either phagocytic (polymorphonuclear or macrophage) or lymphocytic cellular defense mechanisms; (*b*) blockade of various deleterious aspects of host mediator systems; and (*c*) immunorepletion in the form of either nonspecific or specific antibody preparations directed against bacterial pathogens or specific toxic bacterial compounds, such as Gram-negative bacterial LPS (Table 22.1).

There is renewed interest in developing and testing immunopharmacologic agents that directly augment immune responses and host defenses. Patients who have undergone surgery have been found to exhibit altered host defenses, including a reduced ability of B and T lymphocytes to respond to mitogens, diminished antimicrobial and chemotactic activity of polymorphonuclear leukocytes, suppression of natural killer cell cytotoxicity, and impaired macrophage function (56–60).

Agents that act as nonspecific immunostimulants and augment host defenses include muramyl dipeptide (MDP), thymopentin (TP-5), tuftsin, and levamisole. Granulocyte-macrophage colony-stimulating factor (GM-CSF) specifically stimulates maturation of cells of the granulocyte and monocyte lineage, thereby replenishing these important components of host defenses. Lipid A analogs [monophosphoryl lipid A (MPL), SDZ MRL 953, and lipid X] appear to provide protection during Gram-negative bacterial sepsis by competitively inhibiting the toxic interaction of lipid A with mammalian cells. However, MPL and SDZ MRL 953 also possess immunostimulatory properties, increasing the therapeutic potential of these two agents in the treatment of Gram-negative bacterial sepsis. Herein, the mechanism of action and the results of experimental use of these agents will be individually reviewed.

IMMUNOSTIMULANTS

MURAMYL DIPEPTIDE

Whole cells or cell wall fractions of the mycobacterium *bacillus Calmette-Guérin* (BCG) are capable of nonspecifically stimulating host immune systems. This augmentation of host defenses has been shown to enhance resistance to experimental infection due to Gram-positive and Gram-negative bacteria and yeast (61–66). The minimum portion necessary to mediate the immunostimulatory activity of BCG is muramyl dipeptide (MDP).

MDP consists of a hexamino acid water-soluble peptidoglycan. In vitro, MDP appears to stimulate macrophage phagocytic acticity and augment proliferation and cytotoxicity of T lymphocytes (67–74). T lymphocyte stimulation probably is not caused by a direct effect of MDP but occurs via MDP-induced macrophage producton of soluble factors, such as IL-1.

A great number of in vivo studies have examined the immunostimulatory effects of MDP. For example, administration of MDP plus low-dose chloramphenicol significantly enhanced the survival of mice infected with *Klebsiella pneumoniae*, as compared to that of mice treated with chloramphenicol alone (75, 76). MDP and various MDP analogs exerted a protective effect during either *Pseudomonas aeruginosa* or *Candida albicans* infection in a murine sepsis model (61, 77). Murabutide, an MDP analog, is perhaps one of the most promising agents. Currently, it is being tested in phase II clinical trials as an antiinfective immunostimulant in leukemia patients (70, 78).

THYMOPENTIN

Thymopentin (TP-5) is a pentapeptide corresponding to amino acid residues 32 to 36 of the thymic hormone thymopoietin, and both possess the same biological properties in vitro and in vivo (60, 70, 79). A large number of studies have been performed, using animal models of thermal injury to examine the ability of this compound to reverse the attendant severe immunosuppression and infectious complications that occur subsequent to a major burn. TP-5 has been observed to reverse the in vitro B lymphocyte mitogenic response to sheep red blood cells in splenocytes harvested from guinea pigs after burn injury (80). Thymopentin also has been shown to enhance macrophage and neutrophil bactericidal function in burned guinea pigs (81).

Stinnett et al demonstrated improved survival in burned guinea pigs that were given TP-5 and then challenged with a subeschar inoculum of *P. aeruginosa* (82). In addition, Waymack et al demonstrated that burned guinea pigs that received TP-5 and were subjected to bacterial peritonitis with *E. coli* and *Bacteroides fragilis* exhibited an improved survival when compared with controls (83). A multicenter study of the impact of TP-5 on septic complications in burn patients is currently being conducted.

TUFTSIN

Tuftsin is a naturally occurring tetrapeptide generated in the serum by two enzymatic cleavages of the parent molecule, a cytophilic immunoglobulin. It represents amino acid residues 289 to 292 of the constant region of the IgG heavy chain and is only active in the free state apart from the parent molecule. It augments a wide variety of macrophage, monocyte, and granulocyte functions that include chemotaxis, phagocytosis, bactericidal activity, and increased antibody secretion (70, 84–88).

Tuftsin has been shown to augment host defenses when tested in animal models of bacterial infection. Hisatsune and Nozaki showed that treatment of immunosuppressed mice with tuftsin prior to *C. albicans* infection resulted in increased survival (89). Martinez and Winternitz showed an increased rate of bacterial clearance from the blood of tuftsin-pretreated mice infected with *E. coli, Listeria monocytogenes,* or *Staphylococcus aureus,* and the survival rate of mice infected with a standard inoculum of *Streptococcus pneumoniae* increased from 15 to 50% by prior administration of tuftsin (60, 90). Chu et al studied the effects of tuftsin on splenectomized mice that were subsequently challenged with *S. pneumoniae* and observed that treatment with tuftsin provided a statistically significant increase in survival that approached that of nonsplenectomized control animals (91).

LEVAMISOLE

Levamisole is a synthetic antihelminthic agent that also has been noted to possess immunostimulatory properties. Treatment of mice with tetramisole (the levoisomer of levamisole) 2 days prior to administration of a *Brucella* vaccine led to enhanced protection of these animals from subsequent challenge with *Brucella abortus* (92, 93). Subsequent to this report, the immune-enhancing properties of this compound have been extensively studied. In vitro, levamisole restores polymorphonuclear leukocyte (PMN) macrophage phagocytosis, opsonization, and chemotaxis. In addition, levamisole appears to augment many T lymphocyte functions, such as cell-mediated cytotoxicity and lymphokine production (92–94).

In the clinical setting, anergic patients appear to benefit from levamisole administration. Meakins et al studied the effects of levamisole administration in 39 preoperative anergic patients in a prospective, randomized, double-blind trial. The occurrence of major sepsis (defined by a positive blood culture or an intraabdominal abscess) was significantly increased in the placebo group, as compared to the rate of major infection in the levamisole-treated group (45 vs. 16%; *P* < 0.05). While the incidence of mortality and minor sepsis (urinary tract infections, or infiltrate on chest x-ray) was lower in the levamisole treatment group, and the reversal of anergic skin tests also was more common in the treatment group, they did not reach statistical significance (95). Other investigators have shown that levamisole administration to anergic patients with cancer restores responsiveness to skin testing with dinitrochlorobenzene and tuberculin PPD (96, 97). Although levamisole administration has been shown to reverse anergy, it has not been shown to alter the outcome of patients with life-threatening infections. Incidentally, this agent is being used primarily as an adjuvant form of therapy in the treatment of colon carcinoma.

GRANULOCYTE-MACROPHAGE COLONY-STIMULATING FACTOR

GM-CSF is a cytokine that was initially isolated from activated T lymphocytes and that acts to induce maturation and development of granulocyte and macrophage bone marrow

colonies in vitro. It is one member of a family of cytokines that stimulate and support the development of hematopoietic progenitor cells. Other members of this family of cytokines include interleukin-3 (IL-3), granulocyte colony-stimulating factor (G-CSF), and macrophage colony-stimulating factor (M-CSF). Recently, the gene encoding GM-CSF has been identified and cloned, providing large amounts of recombinant human GM-CSF for therapeutic purposes (98, 99).

In vitro, GM-CSF augments macrophage tumoricidal activity (100) and enhances macrophage-mediated elimination of intracellular parasitic infection (101). GM-CSF is also a potent activator of neutrophils (102, 103). Because GM-CSF has been shown in vitro to augment these important host defense functions, it also has been extensively studied in vivo as an immunostimulant.

Administration of recombinant human GM-CSF in vivo produces an increase in monocytes, PMNs, and eosinophils in the systemic circulation. Use of GM-CSF in patients with myelodysplastic syndromes led to increased granulocyte counts, and administration to patients with delayed engraftment following bone marrow transplantation resulted in decreased bacterial and fungal infections, as compared to similar historical controls (104–106). Patients suffering chemotherapy-induced myelosuppression have also benefited from GM-CSF administration that resulted in normalization of granulocyte counts and decreased incidence of infection (107). It is clear that GM-CSF will be an important adjunctive treatment in those patients with underlying neutropenia who are critically ill.

LIPID A ANALOGS

Although Gram-negative bacterial LPS induces multiple toxic effects on mammalian cells in vitro and in vivo, it has also been found to possess immunostimulatory properties consisting of B lymphocyte mitogenicity, increased immunoglobulin synthesis, and increased natural killer cell activity (35). Both the immunostimulatory and toxic effects of LPS are mediated by the lipid A portion of the LPS molecule. The nonspecific immunostimulatory effects that are associated with LPS administration have been shown to augment host resistance in animals to a subsequent challenge with either microbial pathogens or tumor cells (108). Systemic toxicity (e.g., hypotension and fever) associated with LPS and lipid A administration in humans, however, has limited its clinical use as an immunostimulant. In an effort to circumvent the inherent toxicity of LPS while retaining its immunostimulatory properties, investigators have studied the protective capacity of the truncated lipid A molecules lipid X, SDZ MRL 953, and monophosphoryl lipid A (MPL) in animal models of sepsis.

LIPID X

Lipid X is a monosaccharide precursor of lipid A that accumulates in certain mutants of *E. coli* that are deficient in phospholipid synthesis. This compound was originally thought to possess immunostimulatory activities similar to those of LPS, but these properties were found to be caused by contamination with *N,O*-acylated disaccharide-1-phosphate (109). In vitro studies have demonstrated that lipid X can competitively inhibit the priming of human neutrophils by endotoxin in a dose-dependent manner (109, 110).

In a murine model of overwhelming Gram-negative bacterial sepsis, lipid X was unable to protect when administered alone, but if injected with ticarcillin provided survival benefit (111). In addition, lipid X administration is able to reverse the lethal effects of LPS even if it is administered 6 hours after the induction of Gram-negative bacterial infection in animal sepsis models (111, 113). Overall, it appears that lipid X acts as a potent competitive inhibitor of LPS, acting to inhibit LPS-induced toxicity.

SDZ MRL 953

SDZ MRL 953 is a synthetic monosaccharide lipid A analog that was developed in the hope of mimicking the immunostimulatory activities of endotoxin without provoking toxicity. It is chemically related to lipid X, possessing an additional 3(R)-hydroxy-myristic acid moiety attached to the hydroxy group at C-4 that appears to impart immunostimulatory properties not observed with lipid X. In vitro, SDZ MRL 953 causes mouse macrophages to release cytokines IL-6 and TNF and to induce colony-stimulating activity (114).

Prophylactic administration of SDZ MRL 953 to myelosuppressed or immunocompetent mice that were subsequently challenged with a lethal dose of either *E. coli*, *P. aeruginosa*, or *S. aureus* provided significant protective capacity (114). In a murine model of severe sepsis in which antibiotic treatment was withheld until the animals appeared moribund, animals pretreated with SDZ MRL 953 were protected against a subsequent challenge of either *E. coli* or *S. aureus*, that otherwise caused lethality in those animals solely treated with antibiotics (115). The possible mechanisms by which SDZ MRL 953 provides protection against bacterial challenge in vivo include both immunostimulation and competitive inhibition of lipid A toxicity, but the relative contribution of each mechanism to protective capacity is unknown.

MONOPHOSPHORYL LIPID A

Chemical treatment of lipid A by acid hydrolysis results in the loss of the phosphate group at the 1-position of the reducing sugar and yields a relatively nontoxic compound termed monophosphoryl lipid A (MPL) (116). Although MPL has been shown to be nontoxic and nonpyrogenic, compared to the parent endotoxin, it retains the ability to induce cytokine production, splenocyte mitogenesis, macrophage activation, and a variety of other effects on immune reactivity (117–119). Pretreatment with MPL has been shown to be protective in animal models of both Gram-positive and Gram-negative bacterial sepsis. For example, Chase et al pretreated animals with MPL that were subsequently challenged with an intraperitoneal inoculum of either *Staphylococcus epidermidis* or *E. coli*, and noted that survival was statistically increased in the MPL treatment group (119). In addition, Rackow et al demonstrated that pretreatment of rats with MPL 15 minutes prior to the administration of LPS prevented the decrease in

cardiac output, central venous oxygen saturation, and arterial pressure observed in untreated animals (120).

The mechanism by which MPL provides protection in these animal models of sepsis is unclear. Although MPL has been shown to act as an immunostimulant in vitro, its structural similarity to lipid A may allow it to also function as a competitive inhibitor of LPS in vivo. In support of this contention, Heiman et al have shown that MPL inhibits neutrophil priming by LPS in a dose-dependent manner (121). In addition, although MPL appeared to provide protection against both Gram-positive and Gram-negative organisms in the study cited above, 10-fold less MPL was required to protect against Gram-negative bacterial organisms (119). A phase I drug trial has already shown that MPL can be safely administered to patients, thus facilitating further large scale testing of this potentially important drug during the treatment of sepsis (122).

Immunostimulants as a class may also play an important role in the treatment of Gram-negative bacterial sepsis since they appear to directly augment host defenses. This effect is especially marked in animals with preexisting immune defects such as severe burns (TP-5), chemotherapy-induced immunosupression (tuftsin), neutropenia (GM-CSF), and anergy (levamisole). The lipid A analogs (lipid X, SDZ MRL 953, and MPL) represent potentially powerful adjuvants in the treatment of critically ill patients with Gram-negative bacterial sepsis since they appear to be able to directly counteract the toxic effects of LPS both in vitro and in vivo. The ability of lipid X to provide protective capacity even when administered 6 hours after the onset of Gram-negative bacterial sepsis in animal models makes the use of this compound especially attractive. Most likely, more effective treatment in these patients will require both appropriate antimicrobial agents and therapy targeted directly against LPS-mediated toxicity. In addition to their adjunctive use during active infection, the immunostimulants and lipid A analogs also might be used prophylactically in patients in whom the risk of occurrence of Gram-negative bacterial infections is especially high.

ANTIBODY IMMUNOTHERAPY OF GRAM-NEGATIVE BACTERIAL SEPSIS

Antibodies directed against all three regions of the LPS molecule, (O-antigen, core, and lipid A) have been generated and studied with regard to their ability to provide protection during LPS or Gram-negative bacterial challenges. Antibody preparations directed against the O-antigen provide protection only against bacterial or LPS challenge from organisms of the same bacterial serotype against which the antibodies were generated. Although an antibody preparation consisting of multiple protective anti-O antigen monoclonal antibodies (mAbs) directed against a panel of the most common serotypes of Gram-negative bacterial pathogens, such as *E. coli*, *K. pneumoniae*, *P. aeruginosa*, and *Enterobacter cloacae*, might circumvent this problem, the extreme diversity in Gram-negative bacterial serotypes probably would still limit the reliability and effectiveness of such an antibody preparation.

For this reason, most investigators have concentrated their efforts on developing and characterizing cross-reactive antiendotoxin antibody preparations. These antibody preparations take advantage of the fact that many different types of LPS possess a relatively homogeneous common antigenic core/lipid A region. Antibodies directed against this region of LPS have the dual conceptual advantage of binding to both a common region and to the toxic moiety of the LPS molecule, thereby increasing the ability of these antibodies to afford protection during Gram-negative bacterial sepsis and shock.

Polyclonal immunoglobulin preparations directed against the core region of LPS have been prepared by immunizing animals or humans with LPS obtained from *E. coli* J5, which lacks the enzyme uridine diphosphate galactose-4-epimerase. Mutants lacking this enzyme are unable to incorporate galactose residues into LPS during its synthesis and exhibit rough colonial morphology, as compared to the smooth appearance of organisms that possess an intact core LPS and O-antigen structure. *E. coli* J5 bacteria lack the entire O-antigen side chain, possess only the intermediate but not the outer portion of core LPS, and thus are similar to the Rc chemotype of *Salmonella minnesota*. The Re chemotype of *S. minnesota* exhibits a defect in the synthesis of core LPS at a more proximal step, exposing the deep core/lipid A region extensively upon the bacterial cell surface. Immunoglobulins isolated from the serum of humans or animals immunized with the LPS obtained from these rough mutant bacteria have been isolated, yielding antibody preparations that exhibit high titers directed against the deep/core lipid A region of LPS. More recently, murine and human monoclonal antibodies directed against core and lipid A epitopes also have been developed (123–134).

There is some controversy concerning the extent of expression of the core LPS and lipid A epitopes on either the intact Gram-negative bacterial outer membrane or smooth LPS isolated from wild type Gram-negative bacterial pathogens. Evidence has accumulated, however, showing that even smooth strains may express substantial amounts of unmodified core LPS upon their cell surface, as well as O-antigen residues of various chain lengths (135). In addition, some evidence exists to support the presence of host serum enzymes, which serve to cleave O-antigens exposing core determinants in vivo (136).

Using polyclonal antibody, Young and Stevens demonstrated that the Re chemotype determinant (presumably a deep core epitope) was available on smooth bacteria but that the lipid A determinant was not. In addition, they showed that smooth organisms with intact O-antigen side chains possess core antigens that will precipitate antibody directed against LPS cleaved from the *S. minnesota* Re 595 deep core chemotype (137). Ito et al demonstrated that anti-*E. coli* J5 antiserum reacted in an enzyme-linked immunoabsorbant assay (ELISA) with *E. coli* O111:B4 and also concluded that core LPS was accessible on wild-type organisms (138). Further support was provided by Eskenazy et al, who demonstrated that acid hydrolysis of whole bacterial cells exposed core LPS determinants to a greater extent (139). Subsequently, Dunn et al provided evidence that anti-*E. coli* J5 polyclonal antibody reacts extensively against a wide array of Gram-negative bacteria or their derived outer membrane LPS, and both Dunn et al and Bogard et al noted extensive binding of mAbs (the primary specificity of which was directed against deep core/lipid A and isolated lipid A epitopes) to both the heat-killed

wild-type whole organisms and to the LPS derived from these organisms (124, 132, 140, 141).

Many studies using anti-core /lipid A mAbs have been performed that provide cogent data in support of the contention that both core and lipid A epitopes are, indeed, expressed upon the outer membrane of smooth Gram-negative bacteria and are available for binding in vitro and in vivo. Dunn et al demonstrated that murine mAbs raised against *E. coli* J5 LPS bound to whole bacteria and LPS isolated from *E. coli* J5, *E. coli* O111:B4, *K. pneumoniae*, *P. aeruginosa*, and *S. minnesota* Re when tested by ELISA (124). Nelles and Niswander described cross-reactive anticore mAbs that bound to *E. coli* O111:B4, *S. typhimurium*, and *K. pneumoniae* (127). Mutharia et al demonstrated that a murine anti-core/ lipid A mAb bound to the bacterial membrane or purified LPS from 34 of 35 Gram-negative bacterial strains tested. Analyzed by Western immunotransblots, this mAb bound to the lipid A band of 14 clinical isolates of *P. aeruginosa*, and of purified LPS isolated from *K. pneumoniae*, *S. marcescens*, and *E. coli* O55:B5 (126).

Although anticore/lipid A antibody binding to smooth bacteria and LPS has been observed by many investigators, this has not been a universal finding. For example, Pollack et al demonstrated that although an antilipid A mAb bound to free lipid A and to the lipid A region of *S. minnesota* Re lipid A, it did not bind to LPS derived from rough mutant bacteria derived from other genera that exhibit slightly different core LPS structures (142). Gigliotti and Schenep isolated murine mAbs that bound to both isolated *E. coli* J5 LPS and intact J5 bacterial cells but found that none of the mAbs bound to intact cells of *E. coli* O111:B4 or unrelated *E. coli* strains (143).

Using panels of anti-LPS mAbs, both Priest et al and Pollack et al were able to demonstrate that small differences in the structure of the core and deep core/lipid A regions of LPS create unique epitopes that may be recognized because of the fine specificity of the antibody response, allowing the isolation of mAbs that are not cross-reactive (142, 144). These findings may help to explain some of the discrepancies in the results reported by different investigators. In addition, the assay used to determine mAb binding specificity may create differences in epitope availability that affect mAb binding. In the ELISA assay, lipid A or LPS is associated with the polystyrene matrix through electrostatic interactions, while in the passive hemolysis assay (PHA), lipid A-associated fatty acids are intercalated into the red cell membrane through hydrophobic forces. LPS is likely displayed differently in the two assays, and these differences in antigen presentation may account for differences observed in antibody binding (125–130, 141, 142, 145).

In summary, the majority of studies provide firm evidence that antibodies directed against the deep core/lipid A region of LPS are capable of binding to rough and smooth Gram-negative bacteria and their derived LPS. Overall, the data can be interpreted to support the hypothesis that binding of these mAbs to the genus of rough mutant against which the antibody initially was generated is a necessary but not sufficient condition for cross-reactivity. Determination of cross-reactive capacity, therefore, requires extensive in vitro testing of an antibody against many different smooth and rough bacteria and their derived LPS and lipid A.

ANIMAL PROTECTION STUDIES

Because antisera and mAbs obtained after immunization with rough mutants exhibited cross-reactive binding to many different types of Gram-negative bacteria, the protective capacity of these antibody preparations was studied in animal models of sepsis. Initially, Ziegler et al demonstrated that the administration of anti-*E. coli* J5 antisera provided protection against subsequent bacteremia from two smooth strains of *E. coli*, or *K. pneumoniae* in neutropenic rabbits (146). In an endotoxin model, passive immunization with antilipid A antiserum provided protection against subsequent administration of a lethal challenge of LPS from multiple gram-negative bacterial sources (147). Subsequently, Dunn and Ferguson demonstrated that pretreatment of animals with anti-*E. coli* J5 antiserum enhanced survival in animals challenged with *E. coli* O111:B4 or *P. aeruginosa* (148).

The administration of antisera directed against the core/lipid A region of LPS has not invariably been associated with protection. In an endotoxin model, Greisman et al found that pretreatment of animals with antisera possessing high titers to *E. coli* J5 and *S. minnesota* Re did not provide protection from a subsequent injection of endotoxin isolated from a variety of smooth bacteria, including *E. coli* O111:B4, *S. typhimurium*, *S. minnesota*, and *Citrobacter freundii* (149, 150). In addition, Sakulramrung and Domingue found that antisera directed against *E. coli* J5 did not provide protection against subsequent bacterial or endotoxin challenge with *S. typhimurium* but did provide protection against a bacterial challenge of *E. coli* J5 in a murine sepsis model (151).

Experiments utilizing murine mAbs also have been performed to study the ability of purified homogeneous anticore/lipid A mAb preparations to provide protection against bacterial or endotoxin challenges. Priest et al were able to show that a panel of mAbs that exhibited cross-reactive binding in vitro also provided protection in vivo against a large number of various species of Gram-negative bacteria or their derived outer membrane LPS (129). Other investigators have provided similar data (18, 124, 132, 152). Human monoclonal anticore/lipid A antibodies have also been isolated that provide protection in experimental models of Gram-negative bacterial infection (3, 128, 133, 134). Teng et al developed a human monoclonal IgM antibody that bound to the lipid A moiety of LPS. The extensive cross-reactive and cross-protective capacities of this mAb were demonstrated by: (*a*) broad cross-reactivity of mAbs to a variety of Gram-negative bacterial species isolated from the blood of patients, (*b*) abrogation of the dermal Shwartzman reaction in mice, and (*c*) protection of mice against lethal bacteremia induced by a broad range of Gram-negative bacterial organisms (133). Because this mAb was shown to be cross-protective in animal studies, it was subsequently studied as adjuvant treatment for critically ill patients with sepsis in a phase II clinical trial. The results of this trial will be discussed later in this section.

Although large numbers of cross-reactive mAbs have been generated, protective capacity of these mAbs has not been a consistent finding in studies using lethal endotoxin or bacterial challenges. For example, Miner et al found that although binding to whole heat-killed bacteria in vitro was observed in an ELISA assay, these cross-reactive mAbs failed to protect in animal models (131). However, in a metaanalysis of the protective capacity of antiendotoxin antibodies performed by Cody and Dunn, the weight of the published data suggested that anticore/lipid A mAbs provide protection in experimental models of Gram-negative bacterial sepsis (18).

While these animal studies reveal that anticore/lipid A mAbs provide protection in models of Gram-negative bacterial sepsis, the mechanisms by which these antibodies provide protection has not been elucidated. Current evidence, however, supports the hypothesis that neutralization of endotoxin coupled with the inhibition of host cytokine release may be key factors. Primarily, the observation that these mAbs protect in endotoxin models of Gram-negative bacterial infection suggests that the neutralization of endotoxin is a critical mechanism of protection. In addition, polyclonal horse anti-*E. coli* J5 F(ab')₂ antibody fragments provide protection against lethal Gram-negative bacteremia (153). Priest et al and Mayoral et al demonstrated that both anti-O-antigen and anticore/lipid A mAbs inhibited TNF production by macrophages in vitro (144, 154). In addition, Mayoral et al demonstrated in a murine sepsis model that pretreatment of animals with this same anti-O-antigen mAb resulted in decreased serum TNF levels at 1.5 and 3 hours after bacterial challenge, a finding that correlated with survival (155).

In contrast, although Silva et al demonstrated that pretreatment of animals with an anticore/lipid A mAb provided protection against an *E. coli* O111:B4 challenge, no differences in serum TNF levels were observed during the initial 5 hours after bacterial challenge (156). Baumgartner et al directly compared the ability of anti-O-antigen, anticore/lipid A antibodies to inhibit the production of TNF in mice challenged with either LPS or Gram-negative bacteria. In this study, serum TNF levels were decreased only in animals pretreated with anti-O-antigen antisera and subsequently challenged with homologous LPS or bacteria. The anticore/lipid A antibodies tested neither provided protection nor did they alter serum TNF levels in this model (157). Lastly, Chia et al studied a panel of anti-O-antigen, anticore/lipid A mAbs with regard to their ability to inhibit LPS-induced TNF production by macrophages in vitro and noted that none of the mAbs tested decreased TNF production (158).

In summary, neutralization of endotoxin appears to be an important mechanism by which anticore/lipid A antibodies provide protective capacity during experimental Gram-negative bacterial sepsis. Although the protective capacity of anti-O-antigen antibodies has been shown to correlate with a decrease in TNF levels after LPS or bacterial challenge, similar data concerning anticore/lipid A antibodies has not been forthcoming. Because LPS and TNF probably act synergistically to induce toxicity during Gram-negative bacterial infections (159), effective binding to LPS and abrogation of cytokine release by both of these agents may well be required for protection. Further studies assuredly must be performed to clarify the importance of cytokine inhibition produced by protective anti-LPS mAbs to optimize their clinical application as adjuvant therapy in the treatment of patients with life-threatening Gram-negative bacterial infections.

CLINICAL TRIALS OF ANTIENDOTOXIN ANTIBODIES

NORMAL POLYCLONAL ANTIBODY PREPARATIONS

Naturally occurring antiendotoxin antibodies in human sera have been identified, and their presence appears to impart some survival benefit during Gram-negative bacterial infection. This benefit has led investigators to study the effects of administration of commercially available immunoglobulin preparations (which are derived from the plasma or sera of healthy individuals) as adjuvant treatment in the treatment of Gram-negative bacterial sepsis.

In a prospective, randomized, double-blind, controlled study, Dominioni et al studied the effect of administering polyclonal IgG antibody to 62 consecutive surgical patients admitted to the intensive care unit with sepsis scores ≥20. Patients in the treatment group received 0.4 g/kg polyclonal IgG (Sandoglobulin) on days 0 and 1 and received 0.2 g/kg on day 5. Patients were included in the study only if they survived to day 2 and had received at least two doses of IgG or placebo. The mortality was substantially reduced in the treatment group, as compared to that of the placebo group (38 vs. 67%; $P < 0.05$). The difference in mortality observed in the treatment group appeared to result from a decrease in the rate of death from septic shock (7 vs. 33%; $P < 0.05$), whereas death from multiple-organ failure was not altered (31 vs. 33%) (160).

Recently, the use of normal polyclonal immunoglobulin preparations was studied in a subset of 74 postoperative critically ill patients who exhibited measurable serum endotoxin levels (determined by the limulus lysate assay). Those patients whose serum contained endotoxin on 2 consecutive days and whose temperature was greater than 38.5°C were randomized to treatment and nontreatment groups. The treatment group received standard immunoglobulin (0.25 g/kg IV) for 2 days, and the control group received no additional treatment. A total of 46 patients were enrolled in the study. Sixty-three percent (15 of 24) of the patients died in the treatment group, as compared to 86% (19 of 22) in the control group. Due to the small numbers of patients in each group, however, these differences did not achieve statistical significance (161).

The effectiveness of commercially prepared immunoglobulin in the treatment of Gram-negative bacterial sepsis was evaluated in a second study by Schedel et al. Fifty-five patients who met stringent criteria for septic shock (fever, hypotension, thrombocytopenia, etc.), had detectable levels of endotoxemia, and whose symptoms of septic shock had appeared within 24 hours prior to enrollment in the study were randomized over a 3-year period. Those patients in the treatment group received a standard human immunoglobulin preparation (38 g/liter IgG, 6 g/liter IgM, and 6 g/liter IgA) containing anti-LPS antibody binding titers that were 4 to 8 times higher, compared to those from normal human donor serum. This preparation was administered on 3 successive days (600 ml day 1; 300 ml days 2 and 3) after enrollment in the study. Only one patient died in the treatment group (caused by pulmonary embolism in an individual who had responded to therapy and had no signs of sepsis at the time of death), as compared to nine patients who died in the placebo group (4 vs. 32%; $P = 0.008$) (162).

It is unclear whether patients who exhibited measurable endotoxemia represent an important subgroup in which these standard immunoglobulin preparations are efficacious. The role of endotoxemia in the clinical course of patients in shock was prospectively studied by Danner et al, who identified measurable serum endotoxin levels in 43 of 100 patients with septic shock (T > 38°C, mean arterial pressure < 60), but in only 1 of 10 patients in a control group with shock from nonseptic causes (hemorrhage, myocardial infarction, or adrenal insufficiency). The rates of multiple-organ system failure and depression of left ventricular ejection fraction were significantly higher in septic patients with endotoxemia when compared with nonendotoxemic septic patients. However, there was no statistical difference in mortality between these two groups (163). Other investigators previously also have observed this limitation in predicting clinical outcome in patients who exhibit endotoxemia (164, 165).

Thus, although the results of the aforementioned studies utilizing standard immunoglobulin preparations as adjunctive treatment in patients with measurable endotoxemia are very encouraging, other studies using polyclonal immunoglobulin preparations have shown no survival benefit (169, 170). Further studies are required before the routine use of normal nonspecific immunoglobulin preparations in critically ill patients for the treatment of Gram-negative bacterial sepsis can be recommended.

ANTISERA DIRECTED AGAINST CORE ENDOTOXIN

Because many investigators had shown that antisera directed against the core/lipid A region of the LPS molecule (anti-*E. coli* J5, anti-*S. minnesota* Re) provided protection during Gram-negative bacterial sepsis in animal models, clinical studies utilizing these reagents were undertaken. Ziegler et al reported the results of a randomized, double-blind study in which a single unit of human antisera directed against *E. coli* J5 or preimmune control serum was administered to critically ill patients with a presumptive diagnosis of Gram-negative bacterial sepsis. There was a fivefold difference in the mean titers of antibody to *E. coli* J5 LPS between the control and immune sera, although there was considerable variability in antibody titers among individual lots of immune sera administered in this study. Three hundred-four patients were enrolled in the study, 191 of whom had Gram-negative bacteremia. Mortality associated with Gram-negative bacteremia occurred less frequently in those patients given human anti-*E coli* J5 antiserum than in those given preimmune serum (24 vs. 38%; $P = 0.04$), and the survival benefit was greater in a subgroup of patients with clinical evidence of shock, with or without positive blood cultures compared to similar patients who received placebo (46 vs. 76%; $P = 0.009$). Although the results of this study suggested that anticore antibodies provided protection during Gram-negative bacteremia, survival benefit in the entire study population did not correlate well with the titer of administered J5 antibody. Analysis of a subgroup of 80 patients in profound shock revealed that mortality in a further subgroup of 53 bacteremic patients who received serum with anti-*E. coli* J5 antibody titers of >1:8 was significantly lower than the mortality in 27 bacteremic

Table 22.2. Comparison of Mortality (%) Using E5 and HA-1A in Treating Critically Ill Patients with Sepsis

	E5	Placebo	HA-1A	Placebo
Overall mortality	40	41	39	43
Mortality due to Gram-negative bacterial sepsis	38	41		
Shock present	45	40		
Shock absent	30	43[a]		
Mortality due to Gram-negative bacteremia			30	49[a]
Shock present			33	57[a]
Shock absent	27	37	27	40

[a] $P < 0.05$.

patients who received serum with antibody titers <1:8 (53 vs. 74%; $P = 0.07$) (166).

In an attempt to extend the benefits of protection afforded by anti-*E. coli* J5 antisera, Baumgartner et al performed a randomized, double-blind trial in which control or immune serum was administered prophylactically to surgical patients who were at high risk for Gram-negative bacterial infection. On admission to the intensive care unit, patients in the treatment group received anti-*E. coli* J5 serum, while those in the control group received preimmune serum from the same donors. The incidence of septic shock (5 vs. 11%; $P = 0.05$) and death from this process (2 vs. 7%; $P = 0.03$) were significantly lower in patients who received anti-*E. coli* J5 antisera. Survival, however, correlated solely with administration of immune sera and was not correlated with regard to anti-*E. coli* J5 titers (167).

McCutchan et al also studied the effects of anti-*E. coli* J5 antiserum in a patient population at high risk for Gram-negative bacterial infection. In this study of anti-*E. coli* J5 antiserum prophylaxis, the administration of pre-and postimmune anti-*E. coli* J5 antisera to neutropenic patients resulted in no reduction in bacteremia, febrile episodes, or mortality. One possible explanation for the failure of anti-*E coli* J5 antiserum to provide protection in this study was the small number of cases of Gram-negative bacteremia observed (168).

Overall, these studies utilizing anti-*E. coli* J5 antiserum in the treatment or prophylaxis of Gram-negative bacterial sepsis suggested that immune sera does seem to provide protection. The difficulty in characterizing polyclonal anti-LPS antibody preparations, however, and establishing precise correlation with regard to antibody binding capacity and survival benefit led to the performance of several clinical trials using anti-LPS mAbs.

ANTILIPID A MONOCLONAL ANTIBODIES

E5 is a murine antilipid A IgM mAb that has been shown to bind to Gram-negative bacteria and LPS of many different genera and species. This IgM mAb initially was determined to be safe and without significant side effects or allergic reactions in a Phase I clinical study (134). Subsequently, a randomized, double-blind, controlled trial using E5 was performed in a group of 468 patients with presumed Gram-negative bacterial infection. The treatment group (242 patients) received two intravenous doses of E5 (2 mg/kg) 24 hours apart, and a control group (226 patients) received placebo. Overall, there was no demonstrable difference in 30-day mortality between treatment and placebo groups (40 vs. 41%). However,

the 30-day mortality was significantly decreased in the E5-treated subgroup of patients with Gram-negative bacterial sepsis who did not have refractory shock (29% of all study patients), compared to that of control patients (30 vs. 43%; $P = 0.01$). Additional analysis of this subgroup of patients without shock revealed that treatment with E5 produced a trend toward decreased mortality in both the 71 patients with bacteremia and the 66 nonbacteremic patients, although the differences between treatment and placebo groups did not reach statistical significance. E5 administration also was found to statistically improve the rate of recovery from organ failure in treatment patients who did not have refractory shock (54 vs. 30%; $P = 0.05$). Importantly, 179 patients with refractory shock associated with Gram-negative bacterial infection received no benefit from E5 therapy, and as would be expected, 152 patients who developed sepsis that was not of Gram-negative bacterial origin did not benefit from E5 therapy (17).

A second antilipid A mAb, HA-1A, has also been studied for its ability to provide protection in patients with Gram-negative bacterial sepsis. This mAb is a human monoclonal antilipid A IgM antibody. In a double-blind, randomized, multicenter trial, patients with sepsis and suspected Gram-negative bacterial infection and bacteremia were randomly assigned to receive HA-1A (100 mg IV) or placebo upon entry into the study. Within the entire study population there was no difference in mortality observed between the treatment and placebo groups (39 vs. 43%; $P = 0.24$). However, upon subgroup analysis of the 196 patients with Gram-negative bacteremia, a statistically significant difference in 28-day mortality was observed between the treatment and control groups (49 vs. 30%; $P = 0.014$). A difference in mortality among patients who developed septic shock due to Gram-negative bacteremia was also noted between patients receiving HA-1A and placebo (33 vs. 57%; $P = 0.017$). There was no survival benefit observed in 201 patients with nonbacteremic Gram-negative bacterial infections and in 142 patients with sepsis not caused by Gram-negative bacteria (51 Gram-positive bacterial infections, 7 fungal infections, and 84 patients with no infection identified) (3).

The E5 and HA-1A mAbs both appear to provide varying degrees of benefit in patients who develop Gram-negative bacterial infection. E5 appears to provide protection in patients with Gram-negative bacterial infections who are not in shock, regardless of whether they are bacteremic. In contrast, HA-1A appears to provide protection only in patients with Gram-negative bacteremia, regardless of whether shock is present (Table 22.2). Because these two studies differed in the design (patients received two doses of E5 vs. one dose of HA-1A), entrance criteria (patients enrolled in the E5 had lower mean APACHE II scores than those patients in the HA-1A study), and methods of subgroup analysis (HA-1A study only analyzed patients with Gram-negative bacteremia), it is not clear what real differences in protective capacity exist between E5 and HA-1A (3, 17, 171).

One would not expect mAbs directed against the same portion of the endotoxin molecule to result in such different patterns of protection. The importance of anti-LPS antibody binding specificity in providing protection against various Gram-negative pathogens has been addressed above, and yet, very little published data on the LPS binding specificities of either E5 or HA-1A is available (133, 134). Antibody binding specificity may be an important reason for the observed differences in protection between E5 and HA-1A. A caveat arises from the interpretation of data provided by Baumgartner et al, who studied HA-1A and found that this mAb was incapable of providing protection against LPS or Gram-negative bacterial challenge in an animal model (157, 172). Thus, there is still considerable debate in the literature concerning the effectiveness of anticore/lipid A antibody preparations in the treatment of patients with Gram-negative bacterial infections. Additional studies using E5 and HA-1A mAbs and the results from a current study with a new cross-reactive antilipid A mAb (T-88), may provide further information concerning their efficacy.

ABROGATION OF THE CYTOKINE RESPONSE

Anti-LPS antibodies are likely to be a useful adjunct to standard treatment modalities; however, their usefulness will be limited to treating patients with Gram-negative bacterial infections. Since a number of microorganisms initiate the cytokine cascade associated with sepsis, new therapies directed at the host response to microbial products may prove effective in patients with polymicrobial infections and in those patients without a particular infectious source identified. The best characterized of these approaches consists of the use of antibodies to abrogate the biologic activity of TNF.

Based on substantial animal data demonstrating the protective effect of polyclonal and monoclonal antibodies directed against TNF, one study has been performed using a murine anti-TNF mAb (CB0006) in the treatment of septic patients. This mAb is of the IgG$_1$ subclass and is directed against recombinant human TNF. Severe septic shock was defined as systolic BP <90 and at least one of the following: oliguria; fever or hypothermia; hypoxia; acidosis; thrombocytopenia; increased fibrin degradation products; or respiratory alkalosis. Fourteen patients with severe septic shock received CB0006, three of whom were alive at 28 days. In this phase I study, no acute toxicity attributable to the antibody was reported (47).

IL-1 receptor antagonists (IL-1ra) and soluble IL-1 receptors have also shown promise in animal models of Gram-negative bacterial infections (173). A phase I multicenter clinical trial utilizing IL-1ra is currently in progress. As with other immunomodulatory therapies, however, a cautious approach toward therapies that abrogate the cytokine response is warranted. Although substantial evidence implicates TNF, IL-1, and IL-6 as critical mediators of the toxicity associated with Gram-negative bacterial infections, each has been shown to

have significant beneficial immunostimulatory functions. Inhibition of beneficial effects such as local recruitment of host defenses potentially could have untoward and unexpected consequences.

CONCLUSION

The future use of immunotherapeutic agents in the treatment of critically ill patients is very promising. Although the administration of many of the agents discussed above remains investigational, GM-CSF is currently approved for clinical use and provides an important adjunctive therapy in the care of neutropenic bone marrow transplant patients. The administration of the antilipid A mAbs to critically ill septic patients has resulted in a decrease in mortality within certain subgroups of patients, but problems exist regarding how best to target these expensive reagents in order solely to treat patients with Gram-negative bacterial sepsis and not other types of infection. Continued research is necessary to determine the optimal binding specificity, to identify the mechanisms by which these anti-LPS mAbs provide protection, and to establish means of early rapid diagnosis of these infections in order to optimize this form of therapy. Critically ill patients continue to receive these mAbs under compassionate use protocols, and analysis of the results of these ongoing studies may help to identify those patients most likely to benefit from this adjunctive treatment and provide valuable information that can be used to better implement the testing of newer forms of immunotherapy.

REFERENCES

1. Increase in national hospital discharge survey rates for septicemia-United States, 1979–1987. *MMWR* 39:31–34, 1990.
2. Bone RC, Fisher CJ Jr, Clemmer TP, et al: A controlled clinical trial of high dose methylprednisolone in the treatment of severe sepsis and septic shock. *N Engl J Med* 317:653–658, 1987.
3. Ziegler EJ, Fisher CJ Jr, Sprung Cl, et al: Treatment of gram-negative bacteremia and septic shock with HA-1A human monoclonal antibody against endotoxin. *N Engl J Med* 324:429–436, 1991.
4. Brown JM, Grosso MA, and Harken AH: Cytokines, sepsis and the surgeon. *Surg Gynecol Obstet* 169:568–675, 1989.
5. Dunn DL: Immunotherapeutic advances in the treatment of gram-negative bacterial sepsis. *World J Surg* 11:233–240, 1987.
6. Dunn DL: Antibody immunotherapy of gram-negative bacterial sepsis. *Pharmacotherapy* 7:S31–35, 1987.
7. Dunn DL: Development and potential use of antibody directed against lipopolysaccharide for the treatment of gram negative bacterial sepsis. *J Trauma* 30:S100-106,1990.
8. McCabe W, Kreger B, Johns M: Type-specific and cross-reactive antibodies in gram-negative bacteria. *N Engl J Med* 287:261–267,1972.
9. Ledingham IM, McCardle CS: Prospective study of the treatment of shock. *Lancet* i:1194–1197, 1978.
10. Kreger BE, Craven DE, McCabe WR: Gram-negative bacteremia. IV. Reevaluation of clinical features and treatment in 612 patients. *Am J Med* 68:344–355, 1980.
11. Bryan CS, Reynolds KL, Brenner ER: Analysis of 1,186 episodes of gramnegative bacteremia in non-university hospitals. The effects of antimicrobial therapy. *Rev Infect Dis* 5:629–638, 1983.
12. Klastersky J, Glauser M, Schimpff S, Zinner SH, Gaya H: The European Organization for Research on treatment of Cancer Antimicrobial Therapy Project Group. Prospective randomized comparison of three antibiotic regimens for empiric therapy of suspected bacteremic infection in febrile granulocytopenic patients. *Antimicrob Agents Chemother* 29:263–270, 1986.
13. The EORTC International Antimicrobial Therapy Cooperative Group: Ceftazidime combined with a short or long course of amikacin for empiric therapy of gram-negative bacteremia in cancer patients with granulocytopenia. *N Engl J Med* 317:1692–1698, 1987.
14. Ispahani P, Pearson N, Greenwood D: An analysis of community and hospital-acquired bacteraemia in a large teaching hospital in the United Kingdom. *Q J Med* 63:427–440, 1987.

15. Dunn DL: Vaccines and antibody immunotherapy in surgical patients. *Am J Surg* 153:409–416, 1987.

16. Leroy O, Beuscart C, Mouton Y: Gram-negative nosocomial infection: incidence, pathogens, compromised host. *Br J Clin Pract* 57:27–35, 1988.

17. Greenman RL, Schein RMH, Martin MA, et al: A controlled clinical trial of E5 murine monoclonal IgM antibody to endotoxin in the treatment of gram-negative sepsis. *JAMA* 266:1097–1102, 1991.

18. Cody C, Dunn DL: Endotoxins in septic shock. In Neugebauer E, Holaday J (eds): *Handbook of Mediators in Septic Shock*. CRC Press Inc, Boca Raton, FL, 1993, App 1–37.

19. Michie H, Wilmore D: Sepsis, signals, and surgical sequelae (a hypothesis). *Arch Surg* 125:531–536, 1990.

20. Pruitt BA. The pathogenesis of multiple organ failure. *Arch Surg* 123:1518, 1988.

21. Nuytinck KS, Offermans XJ, Kubat K, Goris JA: Whole body inflammation in trauma patients: an autopsy study. *Arch Surg* 123:1519–1524, 1988.

22. Cerra FB, West M, Keller G, et al: Hypermetabolism/organ failure: the role of the activated macrophage as a metabolic regulator. *Prog Clin Biol Res* 264:27– 42, 1988.

23. Trunkey DD: Inflammation and trauma. *Arch Surg* 123:1517, 1988.

24. Watters JM, Bessey PQ, Dinarello CA, et al: Both inflammatory and endocrine mediators stimulate host responses to sepsis. *Arch Surg* 121:179–190, 1986.

25. Hinshaw LB, Solomon LA, Holmes DD, Greenfield LJ: Comparison of canine responses to *Escherichia coli* organisms and endotoxin. *Surg Gynecol Obstet* 23:981–988, 1968.

26. Morrison DC: Endotoxins and disease mechanisms. *Annu Rev Med* 38:417–432, 1987.

27. Suffredini A, Fromm R, Parker M, et al: The cardiovascular response of normal humans to the administration of endotoxin. *N Engl J Med* 321:280–287, 1989.

28. Luderitz O, Staub AM, Westphal O: Immunochemistry of O and R antigens of *Salmonella* and related *Enterobacteriaceae*. *Bacteriol Rev* 30:192–225, 1966.

29. Gmeiner J, Luderitz O, Westphal O: Biochemical studies on lipopolysaccharides of *Salmonella* R mutants VI: investigations on the structure of the lipid A component. *Eur J Biochem* 7:370–379, 1969.

30. Costerton JW, Ingram JM, Cheng KJ: Structure and function of the cell envelope of gram-negative bacteria. *Bacteriol Rev* 38:87–110, 1974.

31. Schmidt G, Fromme I, Mayer H: Immunochemical studies on core lipopolysaccharides of *Enterobacteriaceae* of different genera. *Eur J Biochem* 14:357–366, 1970.

32. Kim YB, Watson DW: Biologically active endotoxins from *Salmonella* mutants deficient in O- and R-polysaccharides and heptose. *J Bacteriol* 94:1320– 1326, 1967.

33. Schmidt G, Jann B, Jann K: Immunochemistry of R lipopolysaccharides of *Escherichia coli*: studies of R mutants with an incomplete core derived from *E. coli* 08:K27. *Eur J Biochem* 16:382–392, 1970.

34. Galanos C, Rietschel ET, Luderitz O, et al: Biological activities of lipid A complexed with bovine serum albumin. *Eur J Biochem* 31:230–233, 1972.

35. Morrison DC, Ryan JL: Bacterial endotoxins and host immune responses. *Adv Immunol* 28:298–450, 1979.

36. Morrison DC, Ulevitch R: The effects of bacterial endotoxins on host mediator systems. *Am J Pathol* 93:527–617, 1978.

37. Solomkin JS, Cotta LA, Satoh PS, et al: Complement activation and clearance in acute illness and injury: evidence for C5a as a cell directed mediator of the adult respiratory distress syndrome in man. *Surgery* 97:668–678, 1985.

38. Deitch EA, Berg R, Specian R: Endotoxin promotes the translocation of bacteria from the gut. *Arch J Surg* 122:185–190, 1987.

39. Tracey KJ, Beutler B, Lowery SF, et al: Shock and tissue injury induced by recombinant human cachectin. *Science* 234:470–474, 1986.

40. Tracey KJ, Lowry SF, Fahey TJ III, et al: Cachectin/tumor necrosis factor induces lethal shock and stress hormone responses in the dog. *Surg Gynecol Obstet* 164:415–422, 1987.

41. Beutler B, Cerami A: Cachectin: more than a tumor necrosis factor. *N Engl J Med* 316:379–385, 1987.

42. Olds LJ: Tumour necrosis factor: another chapter in the long history of endotoxin. *Nature* 330:602–603, 1987.

43. Waage A, Halstensen A, Espevik T: Association between tumor necrosis factor in serum and fatal outcome in patients with meningococcal disease. *Lancet* i:355–357, 1987.

44. Hesse DG, Tracey KJ, Fong Y, et al: Cytokine appearance in human endotoxemia and other non-human primate bacteremia. *Surg Gynecol Obstet* 166:147–153, 1988.

45. Michie HR, Manogue KR, Spriggs DR, et al: Detection of circulating tumor necrosis factor after endotoxin administration. *N Engl J Med* 318:1481– 1486, 1988.

46. Tracey KJ, Fong Y, Hesse DG, et al: Anti-cachectin/TNF monoclonal antibodies prevent septic shock during lethal bacteremia. *Nature* 330:662–664, 1987.

47. Exley AR, Cohen J, Burman B, et al: Monoclonal antibody to TNF in severe septic shock. *Lancet* 335:1275–1276, 1990.

48. Dinarello CA: Interleukin-1. *Rev Infect Dis* 6:51–95, 1984.

49. Dinarello CA, Wolf SM: Molecular basis of fever in humans. *Am J Med* 72:799–819, 1982.

50. Dinarello CA, Clowes GHA Jr, Gordon AH, et al: Cleavage of human interleukin-1:isolation of a peptide fragment from plasma of febrile humans and activated monocytes. *J Immunol* 133:1332–1338, 1984.

51. Cannon JG, Tompkins RG, Gelfand JA, et al: Circulating interleukin-1 and tumor necrosis factor in septic shock and experimental endotoxin fever. *J Infect Dis* 161:79–84, 1990.

52. Fong Y, Tracey KJ, Moldawer LL, et al: Antibodies to cachectin/TNF reduces interleukin-1-β and interleukin-6 appearance during lethal bacteremia. *J Exp Med* 170:1627–1633, 1989.

53. Fong Y, Moldawer LL, Marano M, et al: Endotoxemia elicits increased circulating beta 2-IFN/IL-6 in man. *J Immunol* 142:2321–2324, 1989.

54. Hack CE, de Groot ER, Felt-Bersma RJ, et al: Increased plasma levels of interleukin-6 in sepsis. *Blood* 74:1704–1710, 1989.

55. Yim JH, Tewari A, Pearce MK, et al: Monoclonal antibody against murine interleukin-6 prevents the lethal effects of *Escherichia coli* sepsis and tumor necrosis factor challenge in mice. *Surg Forum* 41:114–117, 1990.

56. Riddle P: Disturbed immune reactions following surgery. *Br J Surg* 54:882–886, 1967.

57. Jubert A, Lee E, Hersh F, McBride C: Effects of surgery anesthesia and intraoperative blood loss on immunocompetence. *J Surg Res* 15:339–403, 1973.

58. Saba TM, Antikatzides TG: Decreased resistance to intravenous tumor cell challenge during reticuloendothelial depression following surgery. *Br J Cancer* 34:381–389, 1976.

59. Pollack RE, Babcock GF, Romsdahl M, Nishioka K: Surgical stress-mediated suppression of natural killer cell cytotoxicity. *Cancer Res* 44:3888, 1984.

60. Alexander JW, Babcock GF, Waymack JP: Immunotherapeutic approaches to the prevention and treatment of infection in the surgical patient. In Simmons RL, Howard RJ (eds): *Surgical Infectious Diseases*, ed 2. Appleton & Lange, East Norwalk, CT, 1988, pp.307–317.

61. Fraser-Smith E, Mathers T: Protective effect of MDP analogs against infection of *Pseudomonas aeruginosa* or *Candida albicans* in mice. *Infect Immun* 34:676–683, 1981.

62. Weiss DW: Nonspecific stimulation and modulation of the immune response and states of resistance by the methanol-extraction residue fraction of tubercle bacilli. *Natl Cancer Inst Monogr* 35:157–171, 1972.

63. Sher NA, Chaparas SD, Greenberg LE, Bernard S: Effects of BCG, *Corynebacterium parvum*, and methanol-extraction residue in the reduction and mortality from *Staphylococcus* and *Candida albicans* infections in immunosuppressed mice. *Infect Immun* 12:1325–1330, 1975.

64. Howard JG, Biozzi G, Halpern BN, Stiffel C, Mouton D: The effect of *Mycobacterium tuberculosis* (BCG) infection on the resistance of mice to bacterial endotoxin and *Salmonella enteritidis* infection. *Br J Pathol* 40:281–290, 1959.

65. Senterfitt VC, Shands JW Jr: Salmonellosis in mice infected with *Mycobacterium bovis* BCG. II. Resistance to infection. *Infect Immun* 1:583–586, 1970.

66. Weiss DW: Enhanced resistance of mice to infection with *Pasteurella pestis* following vaccination with fractions of phenol-killed tubercle bacilli. *Nature* 186:1060–1061, 1960.

67. McCoy DM, Brown GL, Ausobsky JR, Polk HC: Muramyl dipeptide enhances in vitro peritoneal macrophage phagocytic activity. *Am Surg* 11:634–636, 1985.

68. Azuma I, Sugimura K, Taniyama T, et al: Adjuvant activity of mycobacterial fractions: adjuvant activity of synthetic N-acetylmuramyl-dipeptide and the related compounds. *Infect Immun* 14:18–27, 1976.

69. Igarashi T, Okada M, Azuma I, et al: Adjuvant activity of synthetic N-acetylmuramyl-L-alanyl-D-isoglutamine and related compounds on cell mediated cytotoxity in syngeneic mice. *Cell Immunol* 34:270–278, 1977.

70. Ruszala-Mallon V, Lin YI, Durr FE, et al: Low molecular weight immunopotentiators. *Int J Immunopharmacol* 10:497–510, 1988.

71. Fraser-Smith EB, Waters RV, Matthews TR: Correlation between in vivo anti-*Pseudomonas* and anti-*Candida* activities and clearance of carbon by the reticuloendothelial system for various muramyl dipeptide analogs using normal and immunosuppressed mice. *Infect Immun* 35:105–110, 1982.

72. Wuest B, Wachsmuth ED: Stimulatory effect of N-acetyl muramyl dipeptide in vivo: proliferation of bone marrow progenitor cells in mice. *Infect Immun* 37:452–462, 1982.

73. Tanaka A, Nagao S, Nagoa R, et al: Stimulation of the reticuloendothelial system of mice by muramyl dipeptide. *Infect Immun* 24:302–317, 1979.

74. Waters RV, Ferraresi RW: Muramyl dipeptide stimulation of particle clearance in several animal species. *J Reticuloendothel Soc* 28:457–471, 1980.

75. Polk HC, Galland JC, Ausobsky J: Nonspecific enhancement of resistance to bacterial infections. *Ann Surg* 196:436–441, 1982.

76. Galland R, Trachtenberg L, Rynerson N, Polk HC: Nonspecific enhancement of resistance to local bacterial infection in starved mice. *Arch Surg* 117:161–164, 1982.

77. Ausobsky JR, Cheadle WG, Broskey BG, Polk HC: Muramyl dipeptide increases tolerance to shock and bacterial challenge in mice. *Br J Surg* 71:151–153, 1984.

78. Oberling F, Morin A, Duclos B, et al: Enhancement of antibody response to a natural fragment of Streptococcal M protein by murabutide administered to healthy volunteers (abstract). *Int J Immunopharmacol* 7:398, 1985.

79. Schlesinger DH, Goldstein G, Scheid MP, et al: Chemical synthesis of a peptide fragment of thymopoietin II that induces selective T-cell differentiation. *Cell* 5:367–370, 1975.

80. Maghsudi M, Miller CL: The immunomodulating effect of TP-5 and indomethacin in burn induced hypoimmunity. *J Surg Res* 37:133–138, 1984.

81. Waymack J, Miskell P, Gonce S, Alexander JW: Mechanisms of action of two new immunomodulators. *Arch Surg* 120:43–48, 1985.

82. Stinnett JD, Loose LD, Miskell P, et al: Synthetic immunomodulators for prevention of fatal infections in a burned guinea pig model. *Ann Surg* 198:53–57, 1983.

83. Waymack JP, Miskell P, Gonce SJ, et al: Immunomodulators in the treatment of peritonitis in burned and malnourished animals. *Surgery* 96:308–314, 1984.

84. Najjar VA: The physiologic role of gamma-globulin. *Methods Enzymol* 41:129–178, 1974.

85. Edelman GM, Cunningham BA, Gall WE, et al: The covalent structure of an entire gamma-globulin immunoglobulin molecule. *Proc Natl Acad Sci USA* 63:78–85, 1969.

86. Nishioka K, Amoscato AA, Babcock GF: Tuftsin: a hormone-like tetrapeptide with antimicrobial and antitumor activities. *Life Sci* 28:1081–1090, 1981.

87. Najjar VA, Bump NJ: Tuftsin (THR-LYS-PRO-ARG). A stimulator of all known functions of the macrophage. In Fenichel RL, Chirigos MA (eds): *Immune Modulation Agents and Their Mechanisms*. Marcel Dekker, New York, 1984,pp.229–242.

88. Florentin I, Bruley-Rosset M, Kiger N, et al: In vivo immunostimulation by tuftsin. *Cancer Immun Immunother* 5:211–216, 1978.

89. Hisatsune K, Nozaki S: A biochemical study of the phagocytic activities of tuftsin and its analogues. *Ann NY Acad Sci* 419:205–213, 1983.

90. Martinez J, Winternitz F: New synthetic and natural tuftsin-related compounds and evaluation of their phagocytosis-stimulating activity. *Ann NY Acad Sci* 419:23–34, 1983.

91. Chu DZJ, Nishioka K, El-Hagin T, et al: Effects of tuftsin on postsplenectomy sepsis. *Surgery* 97:701–706, 1985.

92. Symoens J, Rosenthal M: Levamisole in the modulation of the immune response: the current experimental and clinical state. *J Reticuloendothel Soc* 21:175–221, 1977.

93. Drews J: The experimental and clinical use of immune-modulating drugs in the prophylaxis and treatment of infections. *Infection* 13(suppl 2):S241–250, 1985.

94. Amery WK: The mechanism of action of levamisole: immune restoration through enhanced cell maturation. *J Reticuloendothel Soc* 24:187–193, 1978.

95. Meakins JL, Christou NV, Shizgal HM, MacLean LD: Therapeutic approaches to anergy in surgical patients: surgery and levamisole. *Ann Surg* 190:286–296, 1979.

96. Tripodi D, Parks LC, Brugmans J: Drug-induced restoration of cutaneous delayed hypersensitivity in anergic patients with cancer. *N Engl J Med* 289:354–357, 1973.

97. Flanery GR, Rolland JM, Nairn RC: Levamisole (letter to editor). Lancet i:750–751, 1975.

98. Wong GG, Witek JS, Temple PA, et al: Human GM-CSF: molecular cloning of the complimentary DNA and purification of the natural and recombinant proteins. *Science* 228:810–815, 1985.

99. Gillis S: T-cell-derived lymphokines. In Paul WE (ed): *Fundamental Immunology*, ed 2. Raven Press, New York, 1989, pp.628–629.

100. Grabstein KH, Urdal DL, Tushinski RJ, et al: Induction of macrophage tumoricidal activity by granulocyte-macrophage colony-stimulating factor. *Science* 232:506–508, 1986.

101. Weiser WY, van Niel A, Clark SC, David JR, Remold HG: Recombinant human granulocyte/macrophage colony-stimulating factor activates intracellular killing of *Leishmania donovani* by human monocyte-derived macrophages. *J Exp Med* 166:1436–1446, 1987.

102. Weisbart RH, Kwan L, Golde JDW, Gasson JC: Human GM-CSF primes neutrophils for enhanced oxidative metabolism in response to the major physiologic chemoattractants. *Blood* 69:18–21, 1987.

103. Lopez AF, Williamson DJ, Gamble JR, et al: Recombinant human granulocyte-macrophage colony-stimulating factor stimulates in vitro mature human neutrophil and eosinophil function, surface receptor expression, and survival. *J Clin Invest* 78:1220–1228, 1986.

104. Vadhan-Raj S, Keating M, LeMaistra A, et al: Effects of recombinant human granulocyte-macrophage colony-stimulating factor in patients with myelodysplastic syndromes. *N Engl J Med* 317:1545–1552, 1987.

105. Vandhan-Raj S, Buescher B, Broxmeyer HE, et al: Stimulation of myelopoiesis in patients with aplastic anemia by recombinant human granulocyte-macrophage colony-stimulating factor. *N Engl J Med* 319:1628–1634, 1988.

106. Vose JM, Bierman PJ, Kessinger A, Coccia PF, Anderson J, Oldham FB, et al: The use of recombinant human granulocyte-macrophage colony-stimulating factor for the treatment of delayed engraftment following high dose therapy and autologous hematopoietic stem cell transplantation for lymphoid malignancies. *Bone Marrow Transplant* 7:139–143, 1991.

107. Antman KS, Griffin JD, Elias A, et al: Effect of granulocyte-macrophage colony-stimulating factor on chemotherapy-induced myelosuppression. *N Engl J Med* 319:593–598, 1988.

108. Ribi E, Cantrell JL, Takayama K, Qureshi N, Peterson J, Ribi HO: Lipid A and immunotherapy. *Rev Infect Dis* 6:567–572, 1984.

109. Lam C, Hildebrandt J, Schutze E, et al: Immunostimulatory, but not antiendotoxin, activity of lipid X is due to small amounts of contaminating *N,O*-acylated disaccharide-1 phosphate: in vitro and in vivo reevaluation of the biolgocial activity of synthetic lipid X. *Infect Immun* 59:2351–2358, 1991.

110. Danner RL, Joiner KA, Parrillo EJ: Inhibition of endotoxin-induced priming of human neutrophils by lipid X and 3-Aza-lipid X. *J Clin Invest* 80:605–612, 1987.

111. Golenbock DT, Leggett JE, Rasmussen P, et al: Lipid X protects mice against fatal *Escherichia coli* infection. *Infect Immun* 56:779–784, 1988.

112. Proctor RA, Will JA, Burhop KE, Raetz CRH: Protection of mice against lethal endotoxemia by a lipid A precursor. *Infect Immun* 52:905–907, 1986.

113. Golenbock DT, Will JA, Raetz CRH, Proctor RA: Lipid X ameliorates pulmonary hypertension and protects sheep from death due to endotoxin. *Infect Immun* 55:2471–2476, 1987.

114. Lam C, Schutze E, Hildebrandt J, et al: SDZ MRL 953, a novel immunostimulatory monosaccharidic lipid A analog with an improved therapeutic window in experimental sepsis. *Antimicrob Agents Chemother* 35:500–505, 1991.

115. Lam C, Schutze E, Liehl E, Stutz P: Effect of SDZ MRL 953 on the survival of mice with advanced sepsis that cannot be cured by antibiotics alone. *Antimicrob Agents Chemother* 35:506–511, 1991.

116. Takayama K, Qureshi N, Ribi E: Separation and characterization of toxic and nontoxic forms of lipid A. *Rev Infect Dis* 6:439–443, 1984.

117. Ribi E: Beneficial modification of the endotoxin molecule. *J Biol Response Modif* 3:1–9, 1984.

118. Johnson AG, Tomai M, Solem L, Beck L, Ribi E: Characterization of a nontoxic monophosphoryl lipid A. *Rev Infect Dis* 9:S512–516, 1987.

119. Chase JJ, Kubey W, Dulek MH, et al: Effect of monophosphoryl lipid A on host resistance to bacterial infection. *Infect Immun* 53:711–712, 1986.

120. Rackow EC, Astiz ME, Kim YB, Weil MH: Monophosphoryl lipid A blocks the hemodynamic effects of lethal endotoxemia. *J Lab Clin Med* 113:112–117, 1989.

121. Heiman DF, Astiz ME, Rackow EC, et al: Monophosphoryl lipid A inhibits neutrophil priming by lipopolysaccharide. *J Lab Clin Med* 116:237–241, 1990.

122. Vosika GJ, Barr C, Gilbertson D: Phase 1 study of intravenous modified lipid A. *Cancer Immunol Immunother* 18:107–112, 1984.

123. Dunn DL, Mach PA, Dalmnasso AP, et al: Protection from the metabolic derangements of gram-negative bacterial sepsis by use of *E. coli* J5 antiserum. *J Surg Res* 38:298–304, 1985.

124. Dunn DL, Ewald D, Chandan N, Cerra FB: Immunotherapy of gram-negative bacterial sepsis: a single murine monoclonal antibody provides cross-genera protection. *Arch Surg* 121:58–62, 1986.

125. Kirkland TN, Colwell DE, Michalek SM, et al: Analysis of the fine specificity and cross-reactivity of monoclonal anti-lipid A antibodies. *J Immunol* 137:3614–3619, 1986.

126. Mutharia LM, Crockford G, Bogard WC, et al: Monoclonal antibodies specific for *Escherichia coli* J5 lipopolysaccharide: cross-reaction with other gram-negative species. *Infect Immuno* 45:631–636, 1984.

127. Nelles MJ, Niswander CA: Mouse monoclonal antibodies reactive with J5 lipopolysaccharide exhibit extensive serologic cross-reactivity with a variety of gram-negative bacteria. *Infect Immun* 46:677–681, 1984.

128. Pollack M, Raubitschek A, Larrick J: Human monoclonal antibodies that recognize conserved epitopes in the core-lipid A region of lipopolysaccharides. *J Clin Invest* 7:1421–1430, 1987.

129. Priest BP, Brinson DN, Schroeder DA, Schroeder DA, et al: Treatment of experimental gram-negative bacterial sepsis with murine monoclonal antibodies against LPS. *Surgery* 106:147–155, 1989.

130. Young LS, Alam S, Gascon R: Monoclonal antibody directed against the core glycolipid of endobacterial endotoxin (abstract). *Clin Res* 30:552a, 1982.

131. Miner K, Manyak C, Williams E, et al: Characterization of murine monoclonal antibodies to *Escherichia coli* J5. *Infect Immun* 52:56–62, 1986.

132. Dunn DL, Bogard W, Cerra F: Efficacy of type-specific and cross-reactive murine monoclonal antibodies directed against endotoxin during experimental sepsis. *Surgery* 98:283–289, 1985.

133. Teng N, Kaplan H, Herbert J, et al: Protection against gram-negative bacteremia and endotoxemia with human monoclonal IgM antibodies. *Proc Natl Acad Sci USA* 82:1790–1794, 1985.

134. Harkonen S, Scannon P, Mischak R, et al: Phase I study of a murine monoclonal anti-lipid A antibody in bacteremic and non-bacteremic patients. *Antimicrob Agents Chemother* 32:710–716, 1988.

135. Schneider H, Hale TL, Zollinger WD, et al: Heterogeneity of molecular size and antigenic expression within lipopolysaccharides of individual strains of *Neisseria gonorrhoeae* and *Neisseria meningitidis*. *Infect Immun* 45:544–549, 1984.

136. Chedid L, Parant M, Boyer F: A proposed mechanism for natural immunity to enterobacterial pathogens. *J Immunol* 100:292–301, 1968.

137. Young LS, Stevens PR: Precipitating antibody against core glycolipid of *Enterobacteriaceae*. *Experientia* 30:192–193, 1973.

138. Ito JI, Lyons WJ, Davis CE, et al: Role of magnesium in the enzyme-linked immunosorbent assay for lipopolysaccharides of rough *Escherichia coli* strain J5 and *Neisseria gonorrhoeae*. *J Infect Dis* 142:532–537, 1980.

139. Eskenazy M, Konstantinov G, Ivanova R: Detection by immunofluorescence of common antigenic determinants in unrelated gram-negative bacteria and their lipopolysaccharides. *J Infect Dis* 135:965–969, 1977.

140. Dunn DL, Bogard W, Cerra F: Enhanced survival during murine gram-negative sepsis by use of a murine monoclonal antibody. *Arch Surg* 120:50–53, 1985.

141. Bogard W, Dunn DL, Abernathy K, et al: Isolation and characterization of murine monoclonal antibodies specific for gram-negative bacterial lipopolysaccharide: Association of cross-genus reactivity with lipid A specificity. *Infect Immun* 55:899–908, 1987.

142. Pollack M, Chia JK, Koles NL, et al: Specificity and cross-reactivity of monoclonal antibodies reactive with the core and lipid A regions of bacterial lipopolysaccharide. *J Infect Dis* 159:168–188, 1989.

143. Gigliotti F, Schenep JL: Failure of monoclonal antibodies to core glycolipid to bind intact smooth strains of *Escherichia coli*. *J Infect Dis* 151:1005–1011, 1985.

144. Priest B, Bankey P, Cerra F, Dunn D: An immunoprotective antibody directed against lipopolysaccharide inhibits tumor necrosis factor production in vitro. *Surg Forum* 39:29–30, 1988.

145. Brade L, Kosma P, Appelmelk BJ, et al: Use of synthetic antigens to determine the epitope specificities of monoclonal antibodies against the 3-deoxy-D-manno-Octulosonate region of bacterial lipopolysaccharide. *Infect Immun* 55:462–466, 1987.

146. Ziegler E, Douglas H, Sherman J, Davis C, Braude A: Treatment of *E. coli* and *Klebsiella* bacteremia in agranulocytic animals with antiserum to a UDP-gal epimerase-deficient mutant. *J Immunol* 11:433–438, 1973.

147. Mullan NA, Newsome PM, Cunnington PG, et al: Protection against gram-negative infections with antisera to lipid A from *Salmonella minnesota* Re 595. *Infect Immun* 10:1195–1201, 1974.

148. Dunn DL, Ferguson R: Immunotherapy of gram-negative bacterial sepsis: enhanced survival in guinea pig model by use of rabbit antiserum to *Escherichia coli* J5. *Surgery* 92:212–219, 1982.

149. Greisman S, Johnston C: Failure of antisera to J5 and R595 rough mutants to reduce endotoxic lethality. *J Infect Dis* 157:54–64, 1988.

150. Greisman S, DuBuy B, Woodward C: Experimental gram-negative bacterial sepsis: re-evaluation of the ability of rough mutant antisera to protect mice. *Proc Soc Exp Biol* 15:482–490, 1978.

151. Sakulramrung R, Domingue G: Cross-reactive immunoprotective antibodies to *Escherichia coli* O111 rough mutant J5. *J Infect Dis* 151:995–1004, 1985.

152. Dunn DL, Priest B, Condie R: Protective capacity of polyclonal and monoclonal antibodies directed against endotoxin during experimental sepsis. *Arch Surg* 123:1389–1393, 1988.

153. Dunn DL, Mach PA, Condie RM, et al: Anti-core endotoxin F(ab')$_2$ equine immunoglobulin fragments protect against lethal effects of gram-negative bacterial sepsis. *Surgery* 96:440–446, 1984.

154. Mayoral J, Dunn D: Cross-reactive murine monoclonal antibodies directed against the core/lipid A region of endotoxin inhibit production of tumor necrosis factor. *J Surg Res* 49:287–292, 1990.

155. Mayoral J, Schweich C, Dunn D: Decreased tumor necrosis factor production during the initial stages of infection correlates with survival during murine gram-negative bacterial sepsis. *Arch Surg* 125:24–28, 1990.

156. Silva A, Appelmelk B, Buurman W, Bayston K, Cohen J: Monoclonal antibody to endotoxin core protects mice from *Escherichia coli* sepsis by a mechanism independent of tumor necrosis factor and interleukin 6. *J Infect Dis* 162:454–459, 1990.

157. Baumgartner J, Heumann JD, Gerain J, Weinbreck P, Grau G, Glauser M: Association between protective efficacy of anti-lipopolysaccharide (LPS) antibodies and suppression of LPS-induced tumor necrosis factor and interleukin 6. Comparison of O side chain-specific antibodies with core LPS antibodies. *J Exp Med* 171:889–896, 1990.

158. Chia J, Pollack M, Guelde G, Koles N, Miller M, Evans M: Lipopolysaccharide (LPS)-reactive monoclonal antibodies fail to inhibit LPS-induced tumor necrosis factor secretion by mouse-derived macrophages. *J Infect Dis* 159:872–880, 1989.

159. Rothstein JL, Schreiber H: Synergy between tumor necrosis factor and bacterial products causes hemorrhagic necrosis and lethal shock in normal mice. *Proc Natl Acad Sci USA* 85:607–611, 1988.

160. Dominioni I, Dionigi R, Zanello M, et al: Effects of high-dose IgG on survival of surgical patients with sepsis scores of 20 or greater. *Arch Surg* 126:236–240, 1991.

161. Grungman R, Hornung M: Immunoglobulin therapy in patients with endotoxemia and postoperative sepsis—a prospective randomized study. In *Bacterial Endotoxins: Pathophysiological Effects, Clinical Significance, and Pharmacologic Control*. Alan R. Liss, New York, pp. 339–349, 1988.

162. Schedel I, Dreikhausen U, Nentwig B, et al: Treatment of gram-negative septic shock with an immunoglobulin preparation: a prospective, randomized clinical trial. *Crit Care Med* 19:1104–1113, 1991.

163. Danner RL, Elin RJ, Hosseini JM, Wesley RA, Reilley JM, Parillo JE: Endotoxemia in human shock. *Chest* 90:169–175, 1991.

164. Stumacher RJ, Kovnat MJ, McCabe WR: Limitations of the usefulness of the limulus assay for endotoxin. *N Engl J Med* 283:1261–1264, 1973.

165. Elin RJ, Robinson RA, Levine AS, Wolff SM: Lack of clinical usefulness of the limulus test in the dignosis of endotoxemia. *N Engl J Med* 293:521–524, 1975.

166. Ziegler E, McCutchan J, Fierer J, et al: Treatment of gram-negative bacteremia and shock with human antisera to a mutant *Escherichia coli*. *N Engl J Med* 307:1225–1230, 1982.

167. Baumgartner J, Glauser M, McCutchan J, et al., Prevention of gram-negative shock and death in surgical patients by antibody to endotoxin core glycolipid. *Lancet* 8446:59–63, 1985.

168. McCutchan J, Wolf J, Ziegler E, Braude A: Ineffectiveness of single-dose human antiserum to core glycolipid (*E. coli* J5) for prophylaxis of bacteremic, gram-negative infections in patients with prolonged neutropenia. *Schweiz Med Wochenschr* 113(suppl):40–45, 1983.

169. Just HM, Vogel W, Metzger M, Pelka RD, Daschner FD: Treatment of intensive care unit patients with severe nosocomial infections. *Intensive Care Med* 345–352, 1986.

170. Jesdinsky HJ, Tenpel JG, Castrup HJ, Seifert J: Cooperative group of additional immunoglobulin therapy in severe bacterial infections: results of a multicenter randomized controlled trial in cases of diffuse fibrinopurulent peritonitis. *Klin Wochenschr* 65:1132–1138, 1987.

171. Bone R: A critical evaluation of new agents for the treatment of sepsis. *JAMA* 266:1686–1691, 1991.

172. Baumgartner J, Heuman D, Glauser M: Letter to the Editor. *N Engl J Med* 325:282, 1991.

173. Ohlsson K, Björk P. Bergenfelft M, Hageman R, Thompson RC: Interleukin-1 receptor antagonist reduces mortality from endotoxic shock. *Nature* 348:550–552, 1990.

CHAPTER 23

Lazaroids: The Potential Role of 21-Aminosteroids in Treating Critically Injured Patients

MARK A. HELFAER, M.D.

JEFFREY R. KIRSCH, M.D.

RICHARD J. TRAYSTMAN, Ph.D.

MARK C. ROGERS, M.D.

INTRODUCTION

Patients admitted to critical care units have suffered severe insults. The role of the caregivers in this setting is to preserve the physiologic functions that will reverse the deleterious effects of injuries and to prevent ongoing damage. This ongoing damage may be caused by a compromise in perfusion due to diminished upstream pressure (i.e., blood pressure) as occurs, for example, with heart failure, or by an elevation of downstream pressure (e.g., venous capillary pressure), as occurs with edema formation. Although these latter goals are vital, critical care in the 1990s has extended beyond the maintenance of perfusion pressure and oxygen delivery into the biochemical realm of the interruption of the production and consequences of chemical mediators. One of the most exciting areas in this regard is the pharmacologic approach to the inhibition of lipid peroxidation. Since the majority of work with 21-aminosteroids has been done in relationship to prevention of brain injury, it is the main focus of this chapter. However, we will also review the potential therapeutic efficacy of these drugs for prevention of tissue injury from myocardial ischemia, shock, multiple sclerosis, and renal ischemia.

PATHOPHYSIOLOGY LEADING TO LIPID PEROXIDATION IN BRAIN FOLLOWING ISCHEMIA AND REPERFUSION

Neurologic injury may occur in a 2-step process. The primary injury is the immediate one and, in the case of trauma or ischemia, it results in immediate and irreversible damage. After the insult, other pathophysiologic processes may take place that will result in secondary injury. Oxygen radical mechanisms have been hypothesized to be important mediators of brain injury from ischemia and reperfusion in brain (1) and in the case of neurotrauma (2). In brief, oxygen radical production may result from an overreduced electron transport chain during ischemia (3), or may occur during reperfusion via pathways that involve breakdown of arachidonic acid (4), or adenosine (5), or a mechanism involving leukocytes (6, 7). Radical species can be released when leukocytes migrate to injured tissue and degranulate as part of the inflammatory process (7, 8). Another mediator of neurologic injury is calcium (9, 10). Free intracellular calcium concentrations increase during ischemia. Calcium increases the release of superoxide by endothelial cells (11) and plays an important role in stimulating oxygen radical production via the arachidonic acid (12), adenosine (13, 14), or leukocyte pathways (15). Calcium also enhances free radical damage in vitro (9).

Superoxide is one oxygen radical which, although not as reactive as other radical species, can be produced by these processes and result in either direct injury (16, 17) or can react with other species to produce more injury. In the presence of a metal catalyst (e.g., iron, ferrous ion but not ferric), superoxide can be converted to the more reactive hydroxyl radical by Fenton chemistry. The source for iron is not completely understood but may involve transferrin and ferritin. Release of iron from transferrin may be stimulated by acidosis and released from ferritin by superoxide anions (18, 19). Once formed, hydroxyl radicals react with almost every type of molecule found in living cells (20).

Recently, a nitric oxide mechanism has been proposed to explain the sequence of events leading to radical mediated brain injury. Nitric oxide is produced during conversion of arginine to citrulline by nitric oxide synthase in endothelium, astrocytes, and neurons (21). Increased nitric oxide production presumably occurs during ischemia via a mechanism that involves release of excitatory amino acids and stimulation of N-methyl-D-aspartate (NMDA) receptors (22). Although nitric oxide itself does not appear to be toxic to brain, reaction with superoxide produced during ischemia and reperfusion may result in formation of a hydroxyl radical-like species (23).

Regardless of the source, these species (hydroxyl radical or related species) may provoke a process of lipid peroxidation that is an iron-dependent process where the unpaired electron of a radical attacks unsaturated fatty acids within the cell membrane (20). In short, a hydroxyl-like radical is able to remove hydrogen from polyunsaturated fatty acids, creating a carbon-centered radical that quickly reacts with oxygen to produce a peroxy radical (24). Peroxy radical can perpetuate the chain and convert itself into a lipid hydroperoxide. Lipid hydroperoxides can produce alkoxy and peroxy radicals in the presence of transition metal ions (e.g., iron) to yield carbonyl products. These radicals are highly reactive and may rapidly induce formation of conjugated dienes (25, 26). Lipid peroxidation is enhanced in in vitro systems by lactic acidosis (27); however, that has not been substantiated in in vivo systems (28). Evidence for lipid peroxidation can be obtained by measuring tissue levels of conjugated dienes or malonaldehyde (29, 30). More indirect evidence for lipid peroxidation in brain following ischemia and reperfusion comes from detecting a change in endogenous levels of naturally occurring antioxidants (31, 32).

In brain, lipid peroxidation has been demonstrated in in vitro preparations of anoxia and reoxygenation (33, 34) and in some (35–37) in vivo models of ischemia and reperfusion. There is a correlation of increased lipid peroxidation in regions with increased vulnerability to ischemia and reperfusion (37). Thus, secondary injury can be ongoing long after the primary insult has been completed, and it explains the sometimes delayed deterioration that can occur following the insult. The importance of lipid peroxidation in the pathophysiology of brain injury from ischemia and reperfusion remains controversial. Information available to delineate the potential importance of lipid peroxidation comes from studies that have administered inhibitors of oxygen radical pathways or, specifically, of lipid peroxidation, and determined whether these agents prevent neurologic injury following transient cerebral ischemia.

Inhibitors of oxygen radicals have limited success as therapeutic agents. For example, exogenously administered superoxide dismutase alone does not diminish hyperemia (38) or delayed hypoperfusion (39) or improve neurologic outcome (40) following global ischemia and reperfusion. In the setting of focal cerebral ischemia, however, administration of superoxide dismutase has been associated with improved neurologic outcome (16, 17, 41). Likewise, superoxide dismutase decreases the amount of delayed development of vasogenic brain edema following brain injury (42). Some of the limitation of the therapeutic efficacy of superoxide dismutase may be due to its poor ability to penetrate the blood-brain barrier (43, 44).

Several antioxidants have also been tested for therapeutic efficacy in the setting of ischemia and reperfusion. For example, α-tocopherol is a nonenzymatic inhibitor of oxygen toxicity (45) that has been demonstrated to inhibit lipid peroxidation in brain taken from animals exposed to ischemia and reperfusion (46). Likewise, α-tocopherol administration is associated with decreased lipid peroxidation in vivo, improved recovery of electrical function, decreased brain edema, and improved neurologic outcome (47–50). A new inhibitor of lipid peroxidation, LY178002 (5-[[3,5-bis(1,1-dimethyl-ethyl)-4-hydroxyphenyl]methylene]-4-thiazolidinone) prevents brain injury when administered prior to and following transient global cerebral ischemia (51).

Corticosteroids have been used in a variety of clinical situations, including cases of neurologic injury. Promising anecdotal evidence prompted many physicians to investigate the efficacy of steroids in cases of neurologic injury including stroke, and traumatic brain and spinal cord injury. In severe nonmissile-related head injury, high-dose dexamethasone does not ameliorate intracranial hypertension (52) or improve overall morbidity or mortality (53). In some models of cerebral ischemia, steroids have been demonstrated to decrease the flux of ions and fluid, which leads to cerebral edema (54). However, in other models steroids do not treat edema caused by ischemia (55–57). Steroids are also not effective in decreasing brain injury from focal (58) or global (59) ischemia in patients.

Steroids have also been evaluated in the setting of spinal cord trauma. With the failure of the first trial of steroids in the National Acute Spinal Cord Injury Study (NASCIS 1), enthusiasm was diminished for the use of steroids in spinal cord injury. The first systematic improvement in neurologic function following injury came with NASCIS 2, which evaluated a higher dose of methylprednisolone (initially 30 mg/kg) and demonstrated that methylprednisolone reduced the morbidity associated with spinal cord injury (60). Steroid therapy, however, has always been associated with problematic side effects, such as hyperglycemia, catabolic states, and increased incidence of serious infections (61–63). These confounding metabolic effects of the glucocorticoids could have minimized the otherwise salutary effects of the drugs (64). Bolstered by the modest successes of high-dose methylprednisolone studies, development of related drugs continued. The focus was to develop compounds with a similar structure-function relationship that would preserve the therapeutic effects of the steroids without the confounding metabolic effects.

The modest efficacy of steroid therapy in neurologic injury was demonstrated at doses that were far in excess of those used clinically, which led to the speculation that the mechanism of action was one different from the antiinflammatory actions attributed to steroids. The group of drugs that has shown the most promise is those with the steroid moiety backbone but substituted in the 21 position.

GENERAL CHARACTERISTICS OF 21-AMINOSTEROIDS

The best-studied of the 21-aminosteroids is tirilazad mesylate (U74006F;21-[4-2(2,6-di-1-pyrrolidinyl-4-pyrimidinyl)-1-piperazinyl]-16α-pregna-1,4,9(11)-triene-3,20-dione, monomethane sulfonate). In in vitro systems, tirilazad mesylate inhibits ACTH secretion in cultured pituitary cells (65). In in vivo systems, tirilazad mesylate stimulates release of ACTH in adrenalectomized rats (65); however, it has no effect on the pituitary-adrenal axis in normal rats. Chronic tirilazad mesylate administration is also not associated with hyperglycemia, alteration in electrolytes, or loss of body weight due to hormonally mediated myopathic effects (66, 67). Tirilazad mesylate administration has no effect on thymus weight and no reduction in phytohemagglutinin-stimulated T cell proliferation, which has been interpreted to indicate that the drug does not cause significant immunosuppression (66). Although 21-aminosteroids are not potent oxygen radical scavengers, one 21-aminosteroid, U74500A, decreases oxygen radical production by monocytes in normal patients and patients with multiple sclerosis (68) and from polymorphonuclear leukocytes in normal patients (69). Whereas decreased oxygen radical production by leukocytes may be beneficial for several pathologic states caused by excessive leukocyte activity, it may have negative implications for infectious disease problems. The effects of tirilazad mesylate on oxygen radical production have not been investigated.

21-AMINOSTEROIDS AND NEUROLOGIC ISCHEMIA

The 21-aminosteroids tirilazad mesylate (70) and U78517F (71) have been shown to reverse the tendency toward intracellular accumulation of calcium following cerebral ischemia. By the above synthesis, the last common pathway of neurologic injury, regardless of the initiating event, is by lipid peroxidation; therefore, inhibition of lipid peroxidation should be an efficacious way to ameliorate the damage in neurologic injury. Tirilazad mesylate inhibits lipid peroxidation in vitro by a mechanism relatively independent of iron, in much the same way as α-tocopherol inhibits lipid peroxidation. In contrast, U74500A also acts as an iron chelator. Endogenous substances within brain that prevent lipid peroxidation, such as α-tocopherol, are consumed in the face of ischemia, but when treated with 21-aminosteroids, α-tocopherol levels are preserved (72). In vitro, tirilazad mesylate and U74500A also demonstrate a protective effect in the face of glucose deprivation. With an in vitro analog to ischemia (i.e., combined oxygen-glucose deprivation), U74500A affords protection against cell death. This effect was less than the effect of NMDA antagonists but was additive with the latter, suggesting that the mechanism afforded by 21-aminosteroids is not related to the NMDA receptor (73).

Results of studies evaluating the therapeutic efficacy of tirilazad mesylate are consistent with what would be expected from its actions to prevent lipid peroxidation through some mechanism involving membrane function. We have discussed potential therapeutic effects of tirilazad based on the characteristics of the ischemic paradigm. For example, it may be expected that the salutary effects of tirilazad mesylate may be greater in paradigms with accentuated lipid peroxidation and in models that allow sufficient time during reperfusion for lipid peroxidation to occur.

When tirilazad mesylate is administered after 12.5 minutes of cardiac arrest (74), there is no effect on delayed hypoperfusion or return of CMRO$_2$ 4 hours following the insult. However, the investigators indicate that the cardiac resuscitation efforts in the drug-treated animals were conducted with greater ease. In spite of demonstrating no immediate short-term therapeutic efficacy of tirilazad mesylate in terms of blood flow and metabolism, other investigators have demonstrated improved neurological outcome following transient global ischemia. Following 10 minutes of normothermic ventricular fibrillation, dogs treated during resuscitation with tirilazad mesylate demonstrated an improved neurologic status and decreased mortality 24 hours after ischemia. However, this improvement could not be demonstrated until 10 hours after the insult (67). It is not clear that diminished mortality in tirilazad mesylate treated animals (83% vs. 33%) may be partially attributed to a neuroprotective effect of the drug, rather than to a nonneurological effect on the cardiovascular or the renal system (75). Pretreatment prior to reperfusion with tirilazad mesylate also improved neurologic outcome following 12 minutes of complete cerebral ischemia produced by elevation of intracranial pressure (72). Forty-eight hours following this injury, all tirilazad mesylate-treated animals had a normal neurologic outcome, in contrast to the placebo-treated animals, who had significant neurologic impairments.

The neuroprotective effects are somewhat different in the setting of incomplete ischemia. For example, early reports (76) demonstrated attenuation of hypoperfusion 3 hours following 5 minutes of near complete cerebral ischemia induced by neck tourniquet inflation in cats. However, arterial blood pressure and cerebral blood flow (CBF), were better maintained in drug-treated animals. Associated with this improved maintenance of CBF was an improved recovery of somatosensory-evoked potential amplitude in drug-treated animals. Pretreatment with tirilazad mesylate 30 minutes prior to 10 minutes of bilateral carotid occlusion with hemorrhagic hypotension (50 mm Hg) in rats afforded benefits at 24 and 72 hours. The parameters demonstrating an improvement were magnetic resonance imaging in neocortex (but not hippocampus) on each day after the insult, which correlated with histopathologic findings on day 3 (77). These findings might be due in part to the fact that tirilazad mesylate attenuates the cardiovascular deterioration that follows 2 hours of hemorrhagic hypotension (78).

In rats, however, treatment with tirilazad mesylate prior to and following transient forebrain ischemia did not result in improved histopathologic outcome (79). Following transient forebrain ischemia we (80) and others (81) demonstrated improved rate of recovery of high-energy phosphates with no affect of drug treatment on ultimate metabolic, blood flow, or electrical recovery. On the contrary, in the setting of hyperglycemia, when accentuated lipid peroxidation would be anticipated, treatment with tirilazad mesylate improves both the rate, as well as the ultimate metabolic recovery, of dogs subjected to incomplete global ischemia (80).

Testing of 21-aminosteroids in the setting of focal cerebral ischemia has resulted in mixed results. Following 3 hours of unilateral carotid artery occlusion, gerbils have improved survival 24 and 48 hours after ischemia when treated with 10 mg/kg of tirilazad mesylate. Other animals that survived this insult had histologic evidence of protection with drug administration (82) after 24 hours. Hall et al demonstrated that tirilazad mesylate inhibits brain edema (83). However, Young et al (84) found that tirilazad mesylate can inhibit postischemic edema formation only if collateral flow is present. Utilizing a middle cerebral artery occlusion model in rats, treatment after the occlusion resulted in less ionic flux and edema formation 24 hours after the occlusion (84). On the contrary, Hoffman and colleagues reported no improvement in neurologic outcome score or histopathology for 3 days following unilateral carotid occlusion with hemorrhagic hypotension (30 mm Hg) for 30 minutes (85) in rat. The lack of delivery of the drug during ischemia would explain the negative results of Hoffman et al (85), in which the ischemic insult (30 minutes of unilateral carotid occlusion coupled with hypotension to 35 mm Hg) could prevent sufficient quantities of drug in the tissue during ischemia. Likewise, we have found that treatment with tirilazad mesylate either before or following 90 minutes of focal ischemia did not improve recovery of blood flow or electrical function.

Some encouraging results examining the effects upon spinal cord ischemia have been reported, using a model of 25 minutes of infrarenal aortic clamping in rabbits. Pretreatment with 10 mg/kg of tirilazad mesylate 10 minutes prior to ischemia and 0.75 mg/kg every hour for 6 hours following release of the cross-clamp conferred significant neurologic protection. Specifically, 5 out of 9 tirilazad mesylate-treated animals were neurologically normal, whereas only 1 out of 10 of the vehicle treated animals was normal (86).

The results of these studies evaluating the efficacy of 21-aminosteroids in models of ischemic nervous tissue are enticing, yet conflicting. On the basis of these animal experiments, we have more to investigate before we understand what, if any role, 21-aminosteroids may play in clinical practice.

THE ROLE OF 21-AMINOSTEROIDS IN NEUROTRAUMA

The cascade of events following neurotrauma has been hypothesized to be similar to that described for cerebral ischemia. In particular, oxygen radical production with subsequent lipid peroxidation has been demonstrated to occur following traumatic brain injury. It is, therefore, not surprising that 21-aminosteroids have also been tested for therapeutic efficacy in the setting of head trauma.

When mice are subjected to 900 gm-cm closed-head trauma by dropping a 50-g weight from a height of 18 cm, all lose their righting reflex, and 30% die. In survivors of this injury, treatment within 5 minutes following this injury with tirilazad mesylate (1 mg/kg), followed by a repeat dose 1.5 hours later, changes the 1 week survival from 27.3% in vehicle-treated animals to 78.6%. Tirilazad mesylate also improved the 1-hour postinjury neurologic status of these mice (87). The mechanism by which this protective effect is conferred may be due to inhibition of cerebral edema. When rats are

subjected to 2.5 to 2.6 atmospheres delivered by a fluid percussion model into a craniotomy site, the time of maximum cerebral edema occurs at 48 hours after injury. In the cortex, thalamus, and hippocampus on the ipsilateral side of the injury, water content (brain edema) is diminished significantly when the animals are treated with two doses of 3 mg/kg 15 minutes and 3 hours following the injury (88).

Tirilazad mesylate has also been evaluated as a neuroprotective agent in the setting of spinal cord trauma. Tirilazad mesylate treatment improved neurologic outcome 3 to 4 weeks following spinal cord injury in cats. In this study, a dose-response study demonstrated that greater than 1.6 mg/kg 48 hr was required to achieve an advantage over control animals (89). In a similar model, 10 mg/kg of tirilazad mesylate administered after the injury prevented the fall in spinal cord blood flow, which normally occurs following trauma (90). This partial reversal of posttraumatic spinal cord ischemia, occurring within the first 4 hours following the trauma, may be the mechanism by which improvement of neurologic outcome is conferred.

THE ROLE OF 21-AMINOSTEROIDS IN SUBARACHNOID HEMORRHAGE

Since vasospasm is thought to be the cause of delayed ischemia and neurologic deficits following aneurysmal subarachnoid hemorrhage, much effort has been expended to understand its etiology and potential therapies. Following aneurysmal subarachnoid hemorrhage, a cascade of events is postulated to occur that results in formation of radical species and lipid peroxidation within the blood vessel wall. Some investigators have hypothesized that this production of vascular oxygen radicals and lipid peroxides may be important in the mechanism of vasospasm. Cerebral vasospasm can be inhibited by pretreatment with 1 mg/kg of tirilazad mesylate prior to experimental subarachnoid hemorrhage induced by injection of 4.5 ml of autologous blood into the cisterna magna of rabbits (91). Likewise, in primate studies, tirilazad mesylate has been shown to decrease the angiographic evidence of vasospasm, as well as to improve the cerebral energy profile (ATP/[ADP + AMP]) of ischemic tissue (92). The blood-brain barrier is disrupted following subarachnoid hemorrhage, as demonstrated by Evans Blue extravasation. This increased permeability can be prevented by tirilazad mesylate and may be a mechanism by which the drug prevents edema formation (93).

AMINOSTEROIDS AND THE HEART

Tirilazad administered to dogs 1 hour after initiation of left descending coronary artery occlusion (lasting a total of 2 hours) reduces the typical increase in plasma-conjugated dienes for up to 6 hours. This effect implies that tirilazad treatment inhibits lipid peroxidation in the injured myocardium. In this setting, however, there was no improvement in regional myocardial blood flow or infarct size conferred by tirilazad (94). In a different model of myocardial injury, the left circumflex artery is occluded for 10 minutes followed by a period of limited reperfusion in dogs. In this model, myocardial function can be preserved by pretreatment with tirilazad mesylate (95). Similarly, when the left circumflex artery is occluded for 40 minutes, followed by 60 minutes of reperfusion, mitochondrial ATPase is better preserved in tirilazad-treated animals. Other parameters measured in this model, such as depletion of glutathione, tissue ATP levels, and thiobarbituric acid-reactive substances were unaffected by the therapy (96). The models differ most importantly in that acute occlusions (analogous to embolic events) have a different time course and pattern of ongoing injury, as compared to acute occlusions associated with limited reperfusion (analogous to thrombotic events). Although somewhat conflicting, these findings suggest that limitation of lipid peroxidation associated with myocardial ischemia and infarction may offer a therapeutic approach to patients with this disease. Adding 21-aminosteroids to the existing therapies for myocardial ischemia, such as thrombolytic therapy, prevention of dysrhythmias, and vasodilating coronary collaterals may well contribute to improved morbidity and mortality in these patients.

21-AMINOSTEROIDS AND MULTIPLE SCLEROSIS

Monocytes are recruited to active sites in multiple sclerosis demyelination. Macrophages (from which these monocytes are derived) are producers of toxic oxygen metabolites which, when released into tissues, produce damage. In this way, some of the exacerbations of multiple sclerosis may in part be due to a white cell mechanism. In vitro, the 21-aminosteroid U74500A reduces hydrogen peroxide generation and decreases chemiluminescence of stimulated human leukocytes. If toxic oxygen radicals contribute to the pathophysiology in multiple sclerosis, and if a 21-aminosteroid inhibits the production of these radicals, then there may be a role for the latter to play in the future treatment of multiple sclerosis patients suffering neurologic deterioration (68, 69).

THE ROLE OF 21-AMINOSTEROIDS IN SHOCK

21-Aminosteroids have been tested for efficacy in several models of shock. When 2 hours of hemorrhagic shock (mean arterial pressure to 45 to 50 mm Hg) is induced in cats, mean arterial pressure is better maintained during the subsequent resuscitation in tirilazad mesylate-treated animals, as compared to vehicle- or methylprednisolone-treated animals (78). Likewise, when shock is induced by occluding the celiac and superior mesenteric arteries for 40 minutes in rats, tirilazad mesylate treatment maintained blood pressure greater during the reperfusion period, maintained a lower hematocrit (implying less third space losses), and improved survival (97). In a model of nonhemorrhagic shock, mice subjected to trauma have a dose-dependent improved survival when treated with tirilazad mesylate. These studies offer some mechanistic insights into better understanding observed beneficial effects. The chemical mediators that reflect or confer the damage in these models can be modified by treatment with the 21-aminosteroids. Specifically, there is a dose-dependent decrease in plasma concentration of cathepsin D activity, free amino-nitrogen, and myocardial depressant factor following traumatic insult (98).

The mechanism for ameliorating the injury in these models is somewhat obscure. It seems reasonable that these drugs may inhibit edema formation in the damaged tissue and, thereby, improve microvascular circulation. In so doing the tissues would be better perfused with substrate, causing less ischemic injury. If these animal experiments are repeated with the same compelling results, then clinically, along with our present approach, 21-aminosteroids may someday play a role in the early resuscitation of patients presenting in shock from any number of causes.

21-AMINOSTEROIDS AND RENAL ISCHEMIA

Tirilazad mesylate has been evaluated for therapeutic efficacy in transient renal ischemia. Rats subjected to a right nephrectomy and 45 minutes of left renal artery occlusion followed by reperfusion have a better recovery of renal function when pretreated with tirilazad. This better recovery is documented by a lower serum creatinine concentration, as well as by evidence of less severe histologic damage (75). Once again, these drugs may act by inhibiting edema formation and, consequently, improve substrate delivery to otherwise ischemic tissue. This evidence would suggest that future use of 21-aminosteroids may play a role during reconstructive aortic surgery, kidney transplantation, or resuscitation from shock or trauma.

CONCLUSIONS

The protective effect of the 21-aminosteroids in a variety of different models of tissue injury may be based on antiinflammatory properties or ability to inhibit lipid peroxidation. The antiinflammatory properties are similar to those of the glucocorticoid steroids but without the hyperglycemic effects. These antiinflammatory effects may be most clear in cases in which the drug inhibits edema formation and deleterious ion fluxes. The mechanism by which swelling and edema formation are inhibited may be due to the property of the drug to inhibit lipid peroxidation. Regardless of the mechanism, 21-aminosteroid administration does not ameliorate all injury from ischemia or trauma.

The natural next step, then, is to evaluate an approach in preventing tissue injury that attacks more than just one pathway of injury. This multifaceted approach, advocated by Safar and colleagues (99), seems to hold the most promise to finding a successful regimen to take advantage of the understanding we have of the pathophysiology leading to ongoing injury following the primary insult. 21-Aminosteroids may play an important role, along with many of the other modalities available, in optimizing outcome following serious injuries. Initiation of some of these modalities could begin preceding the anticipated insult, such as in cases of aortic reconstructive surgery, cardiopulmonary bypass surgery, transplantation, or intracranial operations. Treatment after the insult to prevent secondary injury holds promise for interrupting ongoing processes, as long as there is sufficient blood flow to the injured area, such as in the case of acute stroke, myocardial ischemia, cardiac arrest, shock, neurotrauma, and subarachnoid hemorrhage. In the future, 21-aminosteroids are likely to be evaluated in many other conditions where lipid peroxidation has been implicated, such as in crush injuries (100). Once more is known about these agents, we will likely see more clinical studies evaluating their efficacy. If they clinically demonstrate some of the promising properties that have been seen in the laboratories, they will likely offer an additional pharmacologic agent for the critically ill patient.

REFERENCES

1. Traystman RJ, Kirsch JR, Koehler RC: Oxygen radical mechanisms of brain injury following ischemia and reperfusion. *J Appl Physiol* 71:1185–1195, 1991.
2. Kontos HA, Wei EP. Superoxide production in experimental brain injury. *J Neurosurg* 64:803–807, 1986.
3. Cino M, Del Maestro RF: Generation of hydrogen peroxide by brain mitochondria: the effect of reoxygenation following postdecapitative ischemia. *Arch Biochem Biophys* 269:623–638, 1989.
4. Armstead WM, Mirro R, Busija DW, Leffler CW: Postischemic generation of superoxide anion by newborn pig brain. *Am J Physiol* 255:H401–H403, 1988.
5. Patt A, Harken AH, Burton LK, et al: Xanthine oxidase-derived hydrogen peroxide contributes to ischemia reperfusion-induced edema in gerbil brains. *J Clin Invest* 81:1556–1562, 1988.
6. Kochanek PM, Dutka AJ, Hallenbeck JM: Indomethacin, prostacyclin, and heparin improve postischemic cerebral blood flow without affecting early postischemic granulocyte accumulation. *Stroke* 18:634–637, 1987.
7. Hallenbeck JM, Dutka AJ, Tanishima T, et al: Polymorphonuclear leukocyte accumulation in brain regions with low blood flow during the early postischemic period. *Stroke* 17:246–253, 1986.
8. Giulian D, Robertson C: Inhibition of mononuclear phagocytes reduces ischemic injury in the spinal cord. *Ann Neurol* 27:33–42, 1990.
9. Braughler JM, Duncan LA, Goodman T: Calcium enhances in vitro free radical-induced damage to brain synaptosomes, mitochondria, and cultured spinal cord neurons. *J Neurochem* 45:1288–1293, 1985.
10. Siesjo BK: Cell damage in the brain: a speculative synthesis. *J Cereb Blood Flow Metab* 1:155–185, 1981.
11. Matsubara T, Ziff M: Superoxide anion release by human endothelial cells: synergism between a phorbol ester and a calcium ionophore. *J Cell Physiol* 127:207–210, 1986.
12. Wieloch T, Siesjo BK: Ischemic brain injury: the importance of calcium, lipolytic activities, and free fatty acids. *Pathol Biol* 30:269–277, 1982.
13. Kinuta Y, Kimura M, Itokawa Y, Ishikawa M, Kikuchi H: Changes in xanthine oxidase in ischemic rat brain. *J Neurosurg* 71:417–420, 1989.
14. McCord JM: Oxygen-derived free radicals in postischemic tissue injury. *N Engl J Med* 312:159–163, 1985.
15. Robinson JM, Badwey JA, Karnovsky ML, Karnovsky MJ: Superoxide release by neutrophils: synergistic effects of a phorbol ester and a calcium ionophore. *Biochem Biophys Res Comm* 122:734–739, 1984.
16. Imaizumi S, Woolworth V, Fishman RA, Chan PH: Liposome-entrapped superoxide dismutase reduces cerebral infarction in cerebral ischemia in rats. *Stroke* 21:1312–1317, 1990.
17. Matsumiya N, Koehler RC, Kirsch JR, Traystman RJ. Conjugated superoxide dismutase reduces extent of caudate injury after transient focal ischemia in cats. *Stroke* 22:1193–1200, 1991.
18. Aust SD, Morehouse LA, Thomas CE: Role of metals in oxygen radical reactions. *J Free Radical Biol Med* 1:3–25, 1985.
19. Miller JP, Perkins DJ: Model experiments for the study of iron transfer from transferrin to ferritin. *Eur J Biochem* 10:146–151, 1969.
20. Halliwell B, Gutteridge JM: Oxygen toxicity, oxygen radicals, transition metals and disease. *Biochem J* 219:1–14, 1984.
21. Palmer RM, Moncada S: A novel citrulline-forming enzyme implicated in the formation of nitric oxide by vascular endothelial cells. *Biochem Biophys Res Commun* 158:348–352, 1989.
22. Garthwaite J, Garthwaite G, Palmer RM, Moncada S: NMDA receptor activation induces nitric oxide synthesis from arginine in rat brain slices. *Eur J Pharmacol* 172:413–416, 1989.
23. Beckman JS, Beckman TW, Chen J, Marshall PA, Freeman BA: Apparent hydroxyl radical production by peroxynitrite: implications for endothelial injury from nitric oxide and superoxide. *Proc Natl Acad Sci USA* 87:1620–1624, 1990.
24. Bielski BH, Arudi RL, Sutherland MW: A study of the reactivity of HO2/O2- with unsaturated fatty acids. *J Biol Chem* 258:4759–4761, 1983.
25. Hasegawa K, Patterson LK: Pulse radiolysis studies in model lipid systems: formation and behavior of peroxy radicals in fats. *Photochem Photobiol* 28:817–823, 1978.
26. Small RD, Scaiano JC, Patterson LK: Radical processes in lipids. A laser photolysis study of t-butoxy radical reactivity toward fatty acids. *Photochem Photobiol* 29:49–51, 1979.
27. Rehncrona S, Hauge HN, Siesjo BK: Enhancement of iron-catalyzed free radical formation by acidosis in brain homogenates: differences in effect by lactic acid and CO2. *J Cereb Blood Flow Metab* 9:65–70, 1989.
28. Lundgren J, Zhang H, Agardh C-D, et al: Acidosis-induced ischemic brain damage: Are free radicals involved? *J Cereb Blood Flow Metab* 11:587–596, 1991.
29. Pryor WA, Stanley JP, Blair E: Autoxidation of polyunsaturated fatty acids. II. A suggested mechanism for the formation of TBA-reactive materials from prostaglandin-like endoperoxides. *Lipids* 11:370–379, 1976.
30. Dahle LK, Hill EG, Holman RT: The thiobarbituric acid reaction and the autoxidations of polyunsaturated fatty acid methyl esters. *Arch Biochem Biophys* 98:253–261, 1962.
31. Rehncrona S, Smith DS, Akesson B, Esterberg E, Siesjo BK: Peroxidative changes in brain cortical fatty acids and phospholipids, as characterized during Fe²⁺- and ascorbic acid-stimulated lipid peroxidation in vitro. *J Neurochem* 34:1630–1638, 1980.
32. Siesjo BK, Bendek G, Koide T, Westerberg E, Wieloch T: Influence of acidosis on lipid peroxidation in brain tissues in vitro. *J Cereb Blood Flow Metab* 5:253–258, 1985.
33. Kogure K, Watson BD, Busto R, Abe K: Potentiation of lipid peroxides by ischemia in rat brain. *Neurochem Res* 7:437–454, 1982.
34. Yoshida S, Abe K, Busto R, Watson BD, Kogure K, Ginsberg MD: Influence of transient ischemia on lipid-soluble antioxidants, free fatty acids and energy metabolites in rat brain. *Brain Res* 245:307–316, 1982.
35. Watson BD, Busto R, Goldberg WJ, Santiso M, Yoshida S, Ginsberg MD: Lipid peroxidation in vivo induced by reversible global ischemia in rat brain. *J Neurochem* 42:268–274, 1984.
36. Yoshida S, Abe K, Busto R, Watson BD, Kogure K, Ginsberg MD: Influence of transient ischemia on lipid-soluble antioxidants, free fatty acids and energy metabolites in rat brain. *Brain Res* 245:307–316, 1982.
37. Bromont C, Marie C, Bralet J: Increased lipid peroxidation in vulnerable brain regions after transient forebrain ischemia in rats. *Stroke* 20:918–924, 1989.
38. Helfaer MA, Kirsch JR, Haun SE, Moore LE, Traystman RJ: Polyethylene glycol conjugated superoxide dismutase fails to blunt post-ischemic reactive hyperemia. *Am J Physiol* 261:H548–H553, 1991.
39. Schurer L, Grogaard B, Gerdin B, Arfors KE: Superoxide dismutase does not prevent delayed hypoperfusion after incomplete cerebral ischemia in the rat. *Acta Neurochir* 103:163–170, 1990.
40. Forsman M, Fleischer JE, Milde JH, Steen PA, Michenfelder JD: Superoxide dismutase and catalase failed to improve neurologic outcome after complete cerebral ischemia in the dog. *Acta Anaesthesiol Scand* 32:152–155, 1988.
41. Liu TH, Beckman JS, Freeman BA, Hogan EL, Hsu CY: Polyethylene glycol-conjugated superoxide dismutase and catalase reduce ischemic brain injury. *Am J Physiol* 256:H589–H593, 1989.
42. Chan PH, Longar S, Fishman RA: Protective effects of liposome-entrapped superoxide dismutase on posttraumatic brain edema. *Ann Neurol* 21:540–547, 1987.
43. Petkau A, Chelack WS, Kelly K, Barefoot C, Monasterski L: Tissue distribution of bovine 125-I-superoxide dismutase in mice. *Res Commun Chem Pathol Pharmacol* 15:641–654, 1976.
44. Haun SE, Kirsch JR, Helfaer MA, Kubos KL, Traystman RJ: Polyethylene glycol-conjugated superoxide dismutase fails to augment brain superoxide dismutase activity in piglets. *Stroke* 22:655–659, 1991.
45. Tappel AL: Vitamin E and free radical peroxidation of lipids. *Ann NY Acad Sci* 203:12–28, 1972.
46. Yoshida S, Busto R, Santiso M, Ginsberg MD: Brain lipid peroxidation induced by postischemic reoxygenation in vitro: effect of vitamin E. *J Cereb Blood Flow Metab* 4:466–469, 1984.
47. Yamamoto M, Shima T, Uozumi T, Sogabe T, Yamade K, Kawasaki T: A possible role of lipid peroxidation in cellular damages caused by cerebral ischemia and the protective effect of alpha-tocopherol administration. *Stroke* 14:977–982, 1983.
48. Suzuki J, Abiko H, Mizoi K, Oba M, Yoshimoto T: Protective effect of phenytoin and its enhanced action by combined administration with mannitol and vitamin E in cerebral ischaemia. *Acta Neurochir (Wien)* 88:56–64, 1987.
49. Yoshida S, Busto R, Santiso M, Ginsberg MD: Brain lipid peroxidation induced by postischemic reoxygenation in vitro: effect of vitamin E. *J Cereb Blood Flow Metab* 4:466–469, 1984.
50. Fleischer JE, Lanier WL, Milde JH, Michenfelder JD: Failure of deferoxamine, an iron chelator, to improve neurologic outcome following complete cerebral ischemia in dogs. *Stroke* 18:124–127, 1987.
51. Panetta JA, Phillips ML, Wolski K, Clemens JA: Effects of two inhibitors of lipid peroxidation on ischemic brain damage. In Krieglestein J, Oberpichler H (eds). *Pharmacology of Cerebral Ischemia*, Wissenschaftliche Verlagsgesellschaft mbH, Stuttgart, pp. 351–356, 1990.
52. Dearden NM, Gibson JS, McDowall DG, Gibson RM, Cameron MM: Effect of high-dose dexamethasone on outcome from severe head injury. *J Neurosurg* 64:81–88, 1986.
53. Braakman R, Schouten HJA, Blaauw-Van Dishoeck M, Minderhoud JM: Megadose steroid in severe head injury. *J Neurosurg* 58:326–330, 1983.
54. Betz AL, Coester HC: Effect of steroids on edema and sodium uptake of the brain during focal ischemia in rats. *Stroke* 21:1199–1204, 1990.
55. Plum F: Effects of steroids on experimental cerebral infarction. *Arch Neurol* 9:571–573, 1963.
56. Ito U, Ohno K, Suganuma Y, Suzuki K, Inaba Y: Effect of steroid on ischemic brain edema. Analysis of cytotoxic and vasogenic edema occurring during ischemia and after restoration of blood flow. *Stroke* 11:166–172, 1980.

57. Siegel BA, Studer RK, Potchen EJ: Steroid therapy of brain edema. Ineffectiveness in experimental cerebral microembolism. *Arch Neurol* 27:209–212, 1972.

58. Patten BM, Mendell J, Bruun B, Curtin W, Carter S: Double-blind study of the effects of dexamethasone on acute stroke. *Neurology* 22:377–383, 1972.

59. Jastremski M, Sutton Tyrrell K, Vaagenes P, Abramson N, Heiselman D, Safar P: Glucocorticoid treatment does not improve neurological recovery following cardiac arrest. Brain Resuscitation Clinical Trial I Study Group. *JAMA* 262:3427–3430, 1989.

60. Bracken MB, Shepard MJ, Collins WF, et al: A randomized, controlled trial of methylprednisolone or naloxone in the treatment of acute spinal-cord injury. Results of the second national acute spinal cord injury study. *N Eng J Med* 322:1405–1411, 1990.

61. DeMaria EJ, Reichman W, Kenney PR, Armitage JM, Gann DS: Septic complications of corticosteroid administration after central nervous system trauma. *Ann Surg* 202:248–252, 1985.

62. Deutschman CS, Konstantinides FN, Raup S, Cerra FB: Physiological and metabolic response to isolated closed-head injury. Part 2. Effects of steroids on metabolism. Potentiation of protein wasting and abnormalities of substrate utilization. *J Neurosurg* 66:388–395, 1987.

63. Robertson CS, Clifton GL, Goodman JC: Steroid administration and nitrogen excretion in the head-injured patient. *J Neurosurg* 63:714–718, 1985.

64. Sapolsky RM, Pulsinelli WA: Glucocorticoids potentiate ischemic injury to neurons: therapeutic implications. *Science* 229:1397–1400, 1985.

65. Burrin JM, Hart GR: Effects of a novel 21-amino steroid, U74006F, on the rat pituitary-adrenocortical axis. *J Endocrinol* 126:203–209, 1990.

66. Braughler JM, Chase RL, Neff GL, et al. A new 21-aminosteroid antioxidant lacking glucocorticoid activity stimulates adrenocorticotropin secretion and blocks arachidonic acid release from mouse pituitary tumor (AtT-20) cells. *J Pharmacol Exp Ther* 244:423–427, 1988.

67. Natale JE, Schott RJ, Hall ED, Braughler JM, D'Alecy, LG: Effect of the aminosteroid U74006F after cardiopulmonary arrest in dogs. *Stroke* 19:1371–1378, 1988.

68. Fisher M, Levine PH, Doyle EM, et al: A 21-aminosteroid inhibits stimulated monocyte hydrogen peroxide and chemiluminescence measurements from MS patients and controls. *Neurology* 41:297–299, 1991.

69. Fisher M, Levine PH, Cohen RA: A 21-aminosteroid reduces hydrogen peroxide generation by and chemiluminescence of stimulated human leukocytes. *Stroke* 21:1435–1438, 1990.

70. Hall ED, Pazara KE, Braughler JM: Effects of tirilazad mesylate on postischemic brain lipid peroxidation and recovery of extracellular calcium in gerbils. *Stroke* 22:361–366, 1991.

71. Hall ED, Pazara KE, Braughler JM, Linesman KL, Jacobsen EJ: Nonsteroidal lazaroid U78517F in models of focal and global ischemia. *Stroke* 21:III83–III87, 1990.

72. Perkins WJ, Milde LN, Milde JH, Michenfelder JD: Pretreatment with U74006F improves neurologic outcome following complete cerebral ischemia in dogs. *Stroke* 22:902–909, 1991.

73. Monyer H, Hartley DM, Choi DW: 21-Aminosteroids attenuate excitotoxic neuronal injury in cortical cell cultures. *Neuron* 5:121–126, 1990.

74. Sterz F, Safar P, Johnson DW, Oku K-I, Tisherman SA: Effects of U74006F on multifocal cerebral blood flow and metabolism after cardiac arrest in dogs. *Stroke* 22:889–895, 1991.

75. Podrazik RM, Obedian RS, Remick DG, Zelenock GB, D'Alecy, LG: Attenuation of structural and functional damage from acute renal ischemia by the 21-amino steroid U74006F in rats. *Curr Surg* 46:287–292, 1989.

76. Hall ED, Yonkers PA: Attenuation of postischemic cerebral hypoperfusion by the 21-aminosteroid U74006F. *Stroke* 19:340–344, 1988.

77. Lesiuk H, Sutherland G, Peeling J, Butler K, Saunders J: Effects of U74006F on forebrain ischemia in rats. *Stroke* 22:896–901, 1991.

78. Hall ED, Yonkers, PA, McCall JM: Attenuation of hemorrhagic shock by the non-glucocorticoid 21-aminosteroid U74006F. *Eur J Pharmacol* 147:299–303, 1988.

79. Beck T, Bielenberg GW: Failure of the lipid peroxidation inhibitor U74006F to improve neurological outcome after transient forebrain ischemia in the rat. *Brain Res* 532:336–338, 1990.

80. Maruki Y, Koehler RC, Kirsch JR, Traystman RJ: Improved metabolic, pH and evoked potential recovery after normoglycemic and hyperglycemic incomplete ischemia with 21-aminosteroid (U74006F) pretreatment. *J Cereb Blood Flow Metab* 11:S141, 1991.

81. Haraldseth O, Gronas T, Unsgard G: Quicker metabolic recovery after forebrain ischemia in rats treated with the antioxidant U74006F. *Stroke* 22:1188–1192, 1991.

82. Linberg JV: Orbital compartment syndromes following trauma. *Adv Ophthalmic Plast Reconstr Surg* 6:51–62, 1987.

83. Hall ED, Travis MA: Inhibition of arachidonic acid-induced vasogenic brain edema by the non-glucocorticoid 21-aminosteroid U74006F. *Brain Res* 451:350–352, 1988.

84. Young W, Wojak JC, DeCrescito V: 21-Aminosteroid reduces ion shifts and edema in the rat middle cerebral artery occlusion model of regional ischemia. *Stroke* 19:1013–1019, 1988.

85. Hoffman WE, Baughman VL, Polek W, Thomas C: The 21-aminosteroid U74006F does not markedly improve outcome from incomplete ischemia in the rat. *J Neurosurg Anesthesiol* 3:96–102, 1991.

86. Fowl RJ, Patterson RB, Gewirtz RJ, Anderson DK: Protection against postischemic spinal cord injury using a new 21-aminosteroid. *J Surg Res* 48:597–600, 1990.

87. Hall Ed, Yonkers PA, McCall JM, Braughler JM: Effects of the 21-aminosteroid U74006F on experimental head injury in mice. *J Neurosurg* 68:456–461, 1988.

88. McIntosh TK, Banbury M, Smith D, Thomas M: The novel 21-aminosteroid U-74006F attenuates cerebral oedema and improves survival after brain injury in the rat. *Acta Neurochir Suppl* 51:329–330, 1990.

89. Anderson DK, Braughler JM, Hall ED, Waters TR, McCall JM, Means ED: Effects of treatment with U-74006F on neurological outcome following experimental spinal cord injury. *J Neurosurg* 69:562–567, 1988.

90. Hall ED: Effects of the 21-aminosteroid U74006F on posttraumatic spinal cord ischemia in cats. *J Neurosurg* 68:462–465, 1988.

91. Vollmer DG, Kassell NF, Hongo K, Ogawa H, Tsukahara T: Effect of the nonglucocorticoid 21-aminosteroid U74006F experimental cerebral vasospasm. *Surg Neurol* 31:190–194, 1989.

92. Steinke DE, Weir BK, Findlay JM, Tanabe T, Grace M, Krushelnycky BW: A trial of the 21-aminosteroid U74006F in a primate model of chronic cerebral vasospasm. *Neurosurgery* 24:179–186, 1989.

93. Zuccarello M, Anderson DK: Protective effect of a 21-aminosteroid on the blood-brain barrier following subarachnoid hemorrhage in rats. *Stroke* 20:367–371, 1989.

94. Ovize M, de Lorgeril M, Ovize A, Ciavatti M, Delaye J, Renaud S: U74006F, a novel 21-aminosteroid, inhibits in vivo lipid peroxidation but fails to limit infarct size in a canine model of myocardial ischemia reperfusion. *Am Heart J* 122:681–689, 1991.

95. Holzgrefe HH, Buchanan LV, Gibson JK: Effects of U74006F, a novel inhibitor of lipid peroxidation, in stunned reperfused canine myocardium. *J Cardiovasc Pharmacol* 15:239–248, 1990.

96. Godin DV, Garnett ME, Ko KM: Effects of a steroidal antioxidant (U74006F) in an acute model of myocardial ischemia/reperfusion injury. *Proc West Pharmacol Soc* 33:189–192, 1990.

97. Johnson G, III, Lefer AM: Protective effects of a novel 21-aminosteroid during splanchnic artery occlusion shock. *Circ Shock* 30:155–164, 1990.

98. Aoki N, Lefer AM: Protective effects of a novel nonglucocorticoid 21-amino steroid (U74006F) during traumatic shock in rats. *J Cardiovasc Pharmacol* 15:205–210, 1990.

99. Gisvold SE, Safar P, Rao G, Moossy J, Kelsey S, Alexander H: Multifaceted therapy after global brain ischemia in monkeys. *Stroke* 15:803–812, 1984.

100. Odeh M: The role of reperfusion-induced injury in the pathogenesis of the crush syndrome. *N Eng J Med* 324:1417–1422, 1991.

Medication Groups

CHAPTER 24

Catecholamines, Inotropic Medications, and Vasopressor Agents

ARNO L. ZARITSKY, M.D.

Management of the critically ill patient often necessitates the use of one or more inotropic agents to maintain adequate tissue perfusion. Catecholamines and other sympathomimetics are the most important group of inotropic agents currently available; however, a number of new, noncatecholamine agents are used increasingly in critically ill patients. This chapter reviews the pharmacology, cardiovascular actions, and clinical indications of catecholamines, the new bipyridine inotropes, such as amrinone, and selected other inotropes undergoing active clinical investigation. In addition, adrenergic receptor physiology and endogenous catecholamine responses in the critically ill patient are discussed, particularly with reference to how they influence the patient's response to vasoactive agents.

CATECHOLAMINE PHARMACODYNAMICS

Clinical use of inotropes requires an understanding of several important pharmacologic principles. These are discussed in detail in Chapter 1 but are reviewed briefly here. Whenever a drug is administered to a patient, its clinical actions result from a complex interaction between the concentration of drug in the plasma, its elimination rate from the body, diffusion to its site of action, and response of the target tissue to the drug. For inotropic agents, plasma drug concentration is modified by changes in the rate of drug infusion (i.e., drug dose), distribution, and changes in the organ(s) responsible for its elimination. The tissue response is influenced by changes in receptor and tissue responsiveness.

Pharmacokinetics is the mathematical expression of the time course of all processes leading to drug distribution and elimination. This time course typically is determined by quantifying drug concentration in the plasma compartment. In the critical care setting, most inotropic agents are administered by continuous intravenous infusion, making the kinetics relatively simple. Although a close relationship between plasma drug concentration and drug effect is assumed, this relationship may not be true, particularly for the catecholamines. As shown in Figure 24.1, drug administered into the blood must diffuse across the endothelium to reach its receptor. During distribution, a portion of the catecholamine will be removed by nonspecific tissue uptake, termed uptake (1). An additional quantity is removed by uptake into local sympathetic nerves, termed $uptake_1$ (2). The remaining drug is then available to act at accessible adrenergic receptors.

Pharmacodynamics is the relationship between drug concentration, usually measured in plasma samples, and drug effect. In the case of inotropic agents, measurable drug-induced physiologic actions include a change in cardiac output, blood pressure, and heart rate. When inotropes are used clinically, their pharmacodynamic effects are not related to the drug plasma concentration in a simple manner, since the patient's illness may influence the net hemodynamic effect observed.

In patients with circulatory shock, for example, drug within the plasma compartment may not be distributed to the active site because of poor organ perfusion. As the patient's clinical

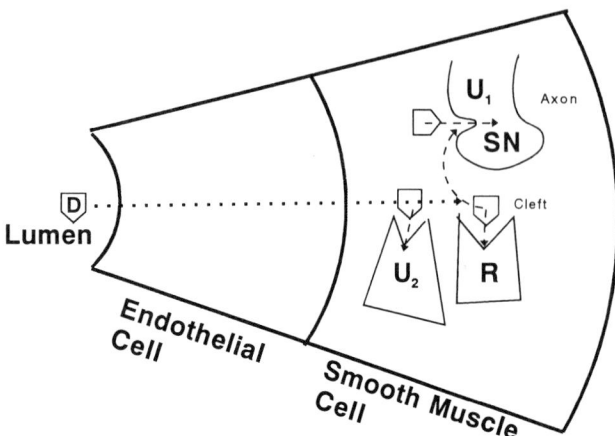

Figure 24.1. Administered catecholamine drug (*D*) diffuses from the capillary lumen through the endothelial cell to act subsequently at the adrenergic receptor (*R*). Diffused catecholamine is metabolized by uptake$_2$ (*U$_2$*), a low-affinity, high-capacity system that degrades catecholamines via the enzyme catechol-*O*-methyltransferase (COMT) and uptake$_1$ (*U$_1$*). The latter system is located on sympathetic nerve (*SN*) axons and is stereoselective. Catecholamines removed by U$_1$ are either stored in vesicles for later release or catabolized by monoamine oxidase.

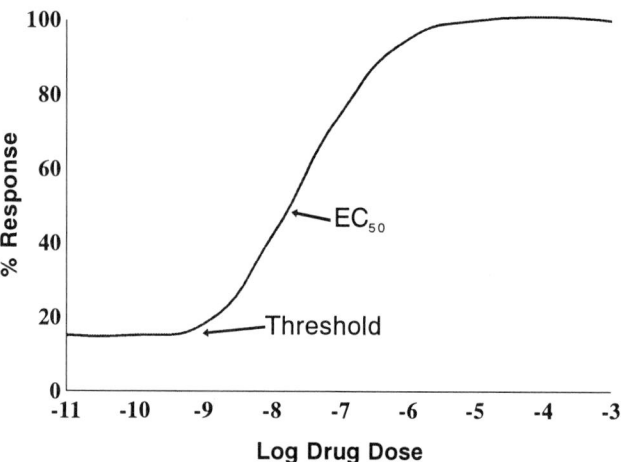

Figure 24.2. Typical relationship between log [catecholamine concentration] and effect. *EC$_{50}$*, drug concentration associated with 50% maximal drug response. *Threshold*, the concentration that produces a noticeable effect.

condition changes, the pharmacokinetics and pharmacodynamics of administered inotropes may also change, necessitating frequent reassessment of the patient and adjustment of the infusion rate. The clinical application of the dose-response relationship of inotropes is further complicated by the kinetics of drug-receptor interactions. A typical catecholamine concentration-response curve obtained in animal studies is seen in Figure 24.2. Note that the concentration range from the threshold to maximal drug response often spans a 2- to 3-fold logarithmic change in the drug concentration. This variation in concentration is much larger than that used clinically, in part because a vasoactive agent rarely is infused to achieve maximal drug effect because of its undesirable side effects. Understanding the threshold effect and the logarithmic concentration-response relationship has therapeutic implications.

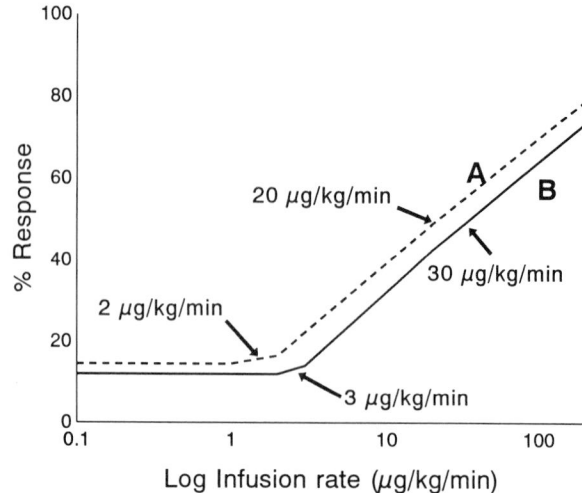

Figure 24.3. The relationship between log [infusion dose] and peak response is seen for two patients (*A* and *B*). Both patients have similar total body clearance rates and slopes of the concentration-response relationship, but the threshold responses are different. The infusion rate needed to achieve 50% of peak response is seen to differ by 10 μg/kg/min despite a minor difference in threshold infusion rate (see text).

Recent studies document that a threshold concentration associated with a given physiologic endpoint can be determined for an individual patient (3, 4). Subsequent logarithmic increases in the plasma concentration produce linear increases in drug effect. Since all of the clinically used inotropes are cleared by first-order kinetics, changes in infusion rate are linearly related to changes in plasma concentration (5–7). Thus, as seen in Figure 24.3, logarithmic changes in the infusion rate are associated with approximately linear changes in response. The clinical implications are seen by comparing the concentration-response relationship for two patients, as shown in Figure 24.3. For illustrative purposes, they have different threshold concentrations, producing an increase in heart rate, but similar plasma drug clearance rates and similar slopes of the concentration-effect curve. The threshold concentration is 10,000 pg/ml in patient A, which was achieved at an infusion rate of 2 μg/kg/min. If the desired endpoint is a heart rate equal to 50% of maximal response, this goal is achieved with a one-logarithm increase in concentration. Thus, an infusion rate of 20 μg/kg/min is needed, based on linear kinetics. Patient B's threshold plasma concentration is 15,000 pg/ml, achieved at an infusion rate of 3 μg/kg/min. To achieve the same pharmacologic effect as in patient A will require an infusion of 30 μg/kg/min.

Stated differently, it is important to recognize that linear changes in drug infusion rate are not associated with linear changes in drug effect, since the latter is logarithmically related to changes in plasma drug concentration. A 2-fold increase in dobutamine infusion rate from 5 to 10 μg/kg/min should produce a change in hemodynamic effect similar in magnitude to a doubling of the infusion rate from 2.5 to 5, or 10 to 20, μg/kg/min. In the discussion of individual inotropes that follows, statements regarding hemodynamic effects observed with specific infusion doses should be recognized as approximations; individual adjustment is essential for each patient.

ADRENERGIC RECEPTORS

ADRENERGIC RECEPTOR SUBTYPES

Adrenergic receptors constitute a complex group of glycoproteins responsible for the transduction of a signal from a circulating hormone (e.g., epinephrine) or neurotransmitter (e.g., norepinephrine) into altered cellular function. The actions of catecholamines are determined by their binding at three major classes of receptors: α-adrenergic, β-adrenergic, and dopaminergic (DA) receptors. Molecular biology has revealed a greater degree of complexity among these receptors than was initially appreciated by studies examining different pharmacologic agonists and antagonists. There are at least eight subtypes of adrenergic receptors identified by gene cloning (8). For practical purposes, there are two functional subtypes of each of these receptors, termed α_1 and α_2; β_1 and β_2; and DA_1 and DA_2.

β-Adrenoceptors initially were classified as cardiac (β_1), and vascular and bronchial smooth muscle (β_2) (9). Subsequently, the existence of both β_1- and β_2-myocardial adrenoceptors was confirmed by radioligand binding (10). The percentage of myocardial β_2-adrenoceptors approximates 14 to 40% of the total β-adrenoceptors in human ventricular myocardium and 20 to 55% in human atrial tissue (10, 11). Both receptor subtypes mediate positive inotropic and chronotropic actions in response to β-agonists (12). Furthermore, β_2-adrenoceptors are found prejunctionally on sympathetic nerves, and activation of these receptors stimulates neurotransmitter release (13).

α-Adrenoceptors initially were classified with respect to their relationship with sympathetic nerve endings. The postsynaptic, "innervated" receptor was α_1 and the presynaptic receptor on the sympathetic nerve was α_2 (14, 15). Stimulation of the α_1-adrenoceptor produced smooth muscle contraction, whereas excitation of the presynaptic α_2-adrenoceptor inhibited norepinephrine release, producing local feedback regulation of activity at the sympathetic nerve terminus. Subsequently, α_2-adrenoceptors located on postsynaptic smooth muscle were identified; activation of these receptors produced smooth muscle contraction (16). These postsynaptic α_2-adrenoceptors are considered to be "hormonal" receptors since they are not associated with sympathetic nerves and instead are likely activated by circulating epinephrine.

Besides increasing smooth muscle tone, α_1-adrenoceptors are also located on myocardial muscle cells, although in relatively low concentration compared with β-adrenoceptors in the human heart (17). Stimulation of cardiac α_1-adrenoceptors produces a slow-onset, prolonged increase in the inotropic state of the heart (18). The role of these α-adrenoceptors in patients with heart failure is uncertain. Clinical studies variously report either no change in α_1-adrenoceptor density or response (17), or a depressed inotropic response of both α_1- and β_1-adrenoceptors that is proportional to the severity of heart failure (19).

In a manner analogous to that of the α-adrenoceptors, DA receptors initially were classified as innervated, postsynaptic

DA_1 receptors and presynaptic DA_2 receptors (20, 21). DA_1 receptors are located on smooth muscle within the renal, splanchnic, coronary, and cerebral vascular beds; their activation results in vasodilation mediated by increased intracellular cyclic AMP (cAMP) production (20, 22). When stimulated, DA_2 receptors, like α_2-adrenoceptors, inhibit norepinephrine release from sympathetic nerve terminals.

More recently, DA_1 receptors have been identified on proximal renal tubular cells where their stimulation produces inhibition of Na^+ reabsorption from the tubular fluid (23, 24). DA_2 receptors are located within autonomic ganglia as well as sympathetic nerve endings; in both locations they inhibit sympathetic nerve activity (25). Activation of DA_2 receptors in the adrenal cortex inhibits aldosterone synthesis and release (26). DA_2 receptors are also located in the anterior pituitary gland, where they modulate thyroid and prolactin hormone release (27), and in the carotid body, where their activation inhibits the ventilatory response to hypoxia (28, 29).

RECEPTOR REGULATION

All of the adrenergic receptors mediate their actions through interaction with a group of intracellular proteins known as "G proteins," since they bind guanine triphosphate and diphosphate. This G protein-coupled receptor system is widely distributed; approximately 80% of known hormones and neurotransmitters activate cellular signal transduction mechanisms by activating G protein-coupled receptors (30). The ubiquitous distribution of this coupling system has important implications in modulating the cellular response to divergent stimuli, as discussed below.

Signal transduction of the β-adrenoceptor has been best studied (31). As seen in Figure 24.4, this comprises a complex series of events between the heterotrimeric G protein and adenylate cyclase (30, 32). Six classes of G proteins have been identified as having different actions (30). The β-adrenoceptors and DA_1 receptor stimulate adenyl cyclase activity by activation of Gs, whereas α_2 and DA_2 adrenoceptors are associated with an inhibitory G protein (Gi) that decreases activity of adenyl cyclase (33). The α_1-adrenoceptor transduces the signal from an agonist, presumably through an unidentified G protein that stimulates phospholipase C activity, increasing the production of inositol triphosphate and diacylglycerol (32, 34). These actions result in an increase in intracellular calcium concentration, which mediates the effects of receptor stimulation by facilitating smooth muscle contraction.

Note that adrenergic receptors function as an amplification system: agonist binding of a single β-adrenoceptor, for example, results in the potential activation of multiple G proteins. Each active G protein can then interact with an adenyl cyclase enzyme, thus stimulating the synthesis of multiple cAMP molecules. This amplification system provides intermediary steps that may be modulated by competing cellular systems. Thus, receptor-agonist binding does not produce a consistent change in cell activity.

The complex regulation of adrenergic receptors that modulate the clinical and pharmacologic response to vasoactive drugs has important implications in the therapy of critically

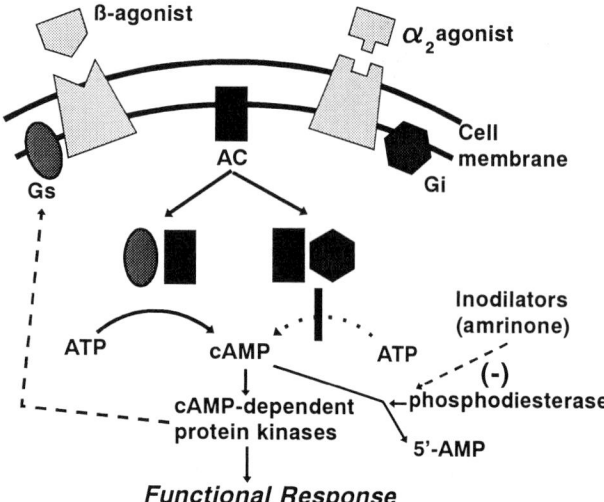

Figure 24.4. Adrenoceptor-G protein interaction is represented. β- and DA$_1$-adrenoceptors activate the stimulatory G protein, Gs, which then dissociates from the receptor and activates membrane-bound adenyl cyclase (*AC*). α$_2$- and DA$_2$- adrenoceptors activate the inhibitory G protein (*Gi*), which dissociates from the receptor and blocks adenyl cyclase activity. The effect of both G proteins is terminated when bound GTP is hydrolyzed to GDP (not shown). Adenyl cyclase catalyzes the conversion of ATP to cAMP; the latter stimulates protein kinases, which results in changed cellular functions. cAMP-dependent protein kinase also phosphorylates the β-adrenoceptor, leading to desensitization (see text). Inodilators, such as amrinone, inhibit phosphodiesterase III, resulting in an increase in cAMP concentration for any level of cAMP production.

ill patients. For example, diminished receptor function (desensitization) following prolonged exposure to an agonist is well-characterized for the β-adrenoceptor and probably occurs for other G protein-coupled receptors (35). Receptor desensitization is defined by the need for an increase in the agonist concentration to produce half-maximal stimulation of activity, such as cAMP production. Cellular processes that contribute to desensitization include phosphorylation of the receptor, physical removal of the receptor from the cell surface, and phosphorylation of the G proteins (8, 35). β-Adrenoceptors may be phosphorylated either by protein kinase A (36), whose activity is increased by an increase in cAMP production, or by a β-adrenoceptor protein kinase (37). The latter enzyme requires agonist binding by the receptor, whereas the former does not (36, 37). Phosphorylation by protein kinase A provides a mechanism whereby the β-adrenoceptor may be regulated by other adenyl cyclase-coupled receptors.

β-Adrenergic receptor redistribution from the cell surface is further divided into two processes: (*a*) sequestration, the rapid (within 5 minutes), reversible removal of functional receptors from the cell surface following agonist exposure, and (*b*) down-regulation, the internalization and subsequent destruction of receptors (8). Down-regulation occurs more slowly than sequestration, needing several hours, and it requires phosphorylation of the receptor, which is not required for sequestration (38).

Besides the changes in receptor density induced by agonist exposure, other conditions modulate the density of adrenoceptors on the cell surface (Table 24.1). These alterations may mediate important differences in adrenergic responsiveness. For example, the number and functional responsiveness of

β$_1$-adrenoceptors is reduced in the hearts of patients with severe congestive heart failure (39, 40). This down-regulation presumably results from the increased sympathetic nervous system activity characteristically observed in heart failure (41, 42), although the pattern of receptor alteration is not consistent. β$_1$-Adrenoceptors are selectively reduced in patients with idiopathic dilated cardiomyopathy (39, 40), but both β$_1$- and β$_2$-adrenoceptors are reduced in patients with end-stage ischemic cardiomyopathy, tetralogy of Fallot (43), and mitral valve disease (44). Further complicating the adrenergic response in patients with congestive heart failure is the observation that both β-adrenoceptors and stimulatory G proteins (Gs) are down-regulated in patients with congestive heart failure; Gs was reduced to 20% of normal (45).

In septic shock, diminished responsiveness to adrenergic vasoconstrictor stimulation characteristically is observed (46). This altered responsiveness probably reflects a complex mechanism, but a portion of the diminished responsiveness likely results from decreased α$_1$-adrenoceptor density in the peripheral vasculature (46, 47). Similarly, adrenergic receptor density may be altered by ontogenetic influences (48). Infants have diminished responsiveness to vasoactive agents such as epinephrine and isoproterenol compared with adults (48); a portion of this phenomenon is probably related to diminished receptor density. In summary, adrenergic agonist-induced effects reflect an intricate interplay among cellular regulatory mechanisms. Simple agonist-receptor binding is insufficient to explain the observed differences in response in different clinical states. Finally, these cellular interactions reflect a dynamic process that requires careful reassessment of the patient's response over time.

ENDOGENOUS CATECHOLAMINE RESPONSE

The sympathetic nervous system renders an important homeostatic function to maintain blood pressure and vital organ perfusion in response to shock and other stresses. Conversely, activation of the sympathetic nervous system may have adverse effects by increasing afterload in the patient with congestive heart failure (49), or by producing arrhythmias in the patient with myocardial ischemia (50).

Likewise, the neurohumoral response to critical illness has important effects on the pharmacodynamics of inotropes. Besides altering adrenergic receptor affinity state and cell density as outlined above, endogenous catecholamines exert vasoactive effects: stimulating heart rate and cardiac contractility, modulating peripheral vascular tone, and partly mediating the metabolic changes characteristic of critical illness (51). When an inotrope is administered to a critically ill patient, the net hemodynamic effect reflects the pharmacodynamic action of the drug and the modifying influence of the patient's endogenous catecholamine response.

The majority of plasma norepinephrine is derived from synaptic nerve clefts. Norepinephrine is the neurotransmitter of the sympathetic nervous system; it is released from sympathetic nerves and acts locally. The plasma norepinephrine concentration serves as a marker of sympathetic nerve activity (52), although it is influenced by the rate of norepinephrine release, the rate of norepinephrine reuptake by the sympathetic nerve, the rate of metabolic degradation at the effector site, and the rate of metabolic clearance from the plasma. For example, Esler et al. (53) showed that a normal plasma norepinephrine concentration may be associated with an increased rate of norepinephrine release balanced by an increased rate of metabolic clearance. Therefore, caution should be exercised when interpreting plasma norepinephrine concentrations as a reflection of sympathetic nervous system activity. Plasma norepinephrine (and epinephrine) concentrations are also influenced by the site of sampling; epinephrine is increased and norepinephrine decreased in forearm arterial versus venous blood (54). Finally, increases in plasma norepinephrine concentration reflect neuronal activity; endogenous plasma concentrations are usually well below the threshold concentration of 1800 pg/ml needed to produce a clinically measurable hemodynamic effect (55).

The release of norepinephrine from sympathetic nerves is controlled by a complex interplay between presynaptic receptors (for catecholamines, acetylcholine, angiotensin, and other mediators) (56) and modulation by such other factors as pH, adenosine concentration, and prostaglandin E_2 that can either increase or decrease norepinephrine release (56, 57). Many of these hormonal or metabolic systems are abnormal in critical illness and may modulate the local release and action of catecholamines.

Circulating epinephrine is derived largely from the adrenal gland, with a small contribution from other chromaffin tissue. Unlike norepinephrine, epinephrine functions as a circulating hormone; small changes in plasma concentration produce significant alterations in hemodynamic effects (58). Normal plasma epinephrine concentrations are in the range of 24 to 74 pg/ml; a small increase to 75 to 125 pg/ml elevates heart rate and systolic blood pressure (58).

The increase in plasma catecholamines in critical illness may function in concert with other counterregulatory hormones to mediate some of the hemodynamic and metabolic alterations characteristic of stress (59), although the degree of correlation between plasma catecholamine concentrations and cardiac effects is unclear since the circulating norepinephrine concentration reflects a variable organ-specific increase in norepinephrine release combined with diminished clearance (42). The extent of plasma catecholamine increase has been correlated with the severity of congestive heart failure (60) and the severity of injury early after trauma (61). Myocardial

infarction (62), hemorrhagic hypotension (63), and cardiopulmonary arrest (64), to name a few disorders, are also associated with substantial increases in circulating norepinephrine and/or epinephrine concentrations. Based on these observations, endogenous catecholamine responses to critical illness undoubtedly influence the net hemodynamic response (pharmacodynamics) of exogenously administered inotropes.

SPECIFIC INOTROPIC AGENTS

EPINEPHRINE

Pharmacology

As noted previously, epinephrine is an important endogenous hormone synthesized from norepinephrine (Fig. 24.5) that is produced and released primarily from the adrenal gland in response to stress. The direct cardiac effects of epinephrine are mediated through β_1- and β_2-adrenoceptors. Epinephrine shortens systole more than diastole, in part by increasing conduction through the atrioventricular (AV) node and Purkinje system. It accelerates the spontaneous depolarization rate of the SA node directly, and accelerates ectopic foci. In addition, it decreases the refractory period of ventricular muscle, predisposing the myocardium to arrhythmias. Although epinephrine therapy may increase coronary blood flow, particularly in patients with coronary artery disease, epinephrine often increases myocardial oxygen demand more than oxygen delivery so that a mismatch occurs (65).

When epinephrine is infused, its hemodynamic actions are determined by the infusion rate: at low rates (0.005 to 0.02 μg/kg/min in adults) epinephrine principally stimulates β-adrenoceptors, resulting in peripheral vasodilation and increased heart rate and contractility. The net hemodynamic effects are to widen the pulse pressure, decrease systemic and pulmonary vascular resistance, and increase stroke volume, left ventricular stroke work, and cardiac output, provided that the patient's circulating blood volume is adequate. As the infusion rate is increased, more α-adrenergic-mediated effects are seen, resulting in increased systemic vascular resistance, increase of blood pressure, and variable effects on cardiac output (the latter action depends on the myocardium's ability to maintain stroke volume as afterload is increased).

Table 24.1.   Disease and Conditions That Alter Receptor Density on Effector Cells[a]

Disease or Condition	Receptor Altered	Change
Congestive heart failure	β (heart)	Increased[b]
Sepsis	α (liver, vasculature)	Decreased
Myocardial ischemia	β (heart)	Decreased
Myocardial ischemia	α (heart)	Increased
Asthma[c]	β (lung, leukocytes)	Decreased
Cystic fibrosis	β (leukocytes)	Decreased
Fetal and neonatal life	α, β (heart, platelets, leukocytes)	Decreased
Agonist administration	α, β (heart, platelets, leukocytes)	Decreased
Antagonist administration	α, β (heart, platelets, leukocytes)	Increased
Hyperthyroidism	β (heart)	Increased
Hypothyroidism	β (heart)	Decreased
Glucocorticoids	β (heart, leukocytes)	Increased

[a] From Zaritsky A, Eisenberg, MG: Ontogenetic considerations in the pharmaco-therapy of shock. In Chernow B, Shoemaker WC (eds): Critical Care: State of the Art, vol 7. Society of Critical Care Medicine, Fullerton, CA, 1986, pp 485–534.
[b] β-Adrenergic receptors are decreased in severe heart failure.
[c] If on β-agonist therapy for asthma.

Figure 24.5. Chemical structure of the catecholamines. (From Chernow B, Rainey TG, Lake CR: Endogenous and exogenous catecholamines in critical care medicine. Crit Care Med 10:409–416, 1982.)

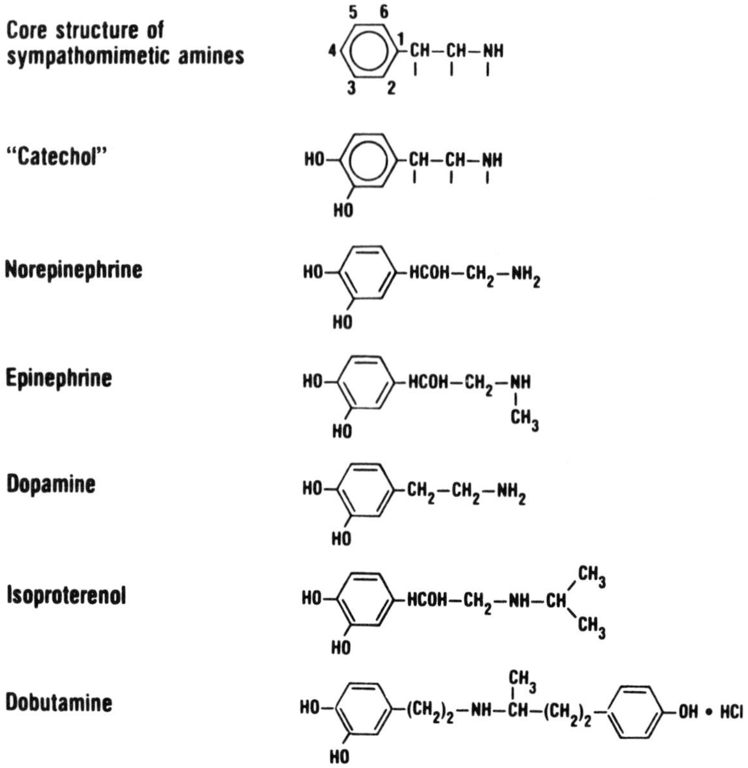

Similar epinephrine-induced actions are seen in pediatric patients, although the dosage ranges are substantially different (based on infusion rate/weight). Thus, infusions up to 0.3 μg/kg/min in infants and children often produce a predominant β-adrenergic effect with little evidence of increased systemic vascular resistance.

Epinephrine has important effects on the respiratory system since the airways are poorly innervated by sympathetic nerves (66), suggesting a key role for circulating epinephrine (67, 68). Activation of β$_2$-adrenoceptors in bronchial smooth muscle results in bronchodilation, whereas stimulation of β$_2$-adrenoceptors on cholinergic nerves inhibits acetylcholine release and bronchoconstriction (66). Furthermore, beneficial effects in asthma result from the inhibition of mast cell degranulation mediated through β$_2$-adrenergic stimulation (69).

Epinephrine is a potent renal artery vasoconstrictor, which limits its usefulness in patients with shock. Infusions as low as 0.035 μg/kg/min induce a 10% decrease in renal plasma flow in humans (70). A portion of epinephrine's vasoconstrictive effect probably is also mediated by increased renin activity following direct stimulation of β-adrenoceptors of the juxtaglomerular apparatus (71). The net effect is to reduce renal blood flow and urine output. Despite these limitations, in patients with low cardiac output epinephrine may increase urine output by increasing cardiac output and therefore renal blood flow (72).

Infusion of epinephrine to achieve plasma concentrations seen with exercise or stress causes plasma glucose, lactate, β-hydroxybutyrate, and free fatty acid concentrations to increase (58, 73), and serum potassium (74, 75) and phosphorus (76) concentrations to decrease. The former effects are mediated by increased gluconeogenesis from the liver (73), skeletal muscle insulin resistance (77), and inhibition of insulin release

(58). Epinephrine-induced hypokalemia occurs through a β$_2$-adrenergic mechanism; mean plasma potassium concentration decreases 0.8 mEq/liter in response to epinephrine concentrations achieved during myocardial infarction (74, 75). Coincident with the decline in potassium, T-wave flattening and QTc prolongation were observed (75). These electrophysiologic effects in combination with epinephrine-induced hypokalemia may predispose the critically ill patient to serious dysrhythmias. Similar decreases in plasma potassium are seen with the use of other β$_2$-agonists, such as agents used in asthma or to inhibit labor (78).

Indications and Dose

Epinephrine infusions are most frequently used in pediatric patients; in adults, their potential toxicity in patients with coronary artery disease limits their utility (Table 24.2). The recommended infusion rate in adults to produce principally a β-adrenergic effect is 0.005 to 0.02 μg/kg/min (51). In pediatric patients, initial infusion rates of 0.05 to 0.3 μg/kg/min are recommended in the treatment of cardiogenic or septic shock (79). Although norepinephrine is frequently used in the treatment of septic shock that is unresponsive to fluid resuscitation and dopamine (see the section of this chapter entitled "Norepinephrine"), epinephrine is also useful in adults with septic shock (80). Epinephrine may be particularly useful when combined with afterload reduction in cardiogenic shock (81) and is preferable to dopamine in pediatric patients with cardiogenic shock in whom catecholamine stores may be depleted (see the section of this chapter entitled "Dopamine").

In the treatment of acute asthma, epinephrine may be administered subcutaneously in a dose of 0.01 mg/kg, up to 0.3 mg every 15 to 20 minutes, although its use has been

Table 24.2. Suggested Uses of Inotropes by Age[a]

Condition	Infant	Child	Adult
Cardiogenic, hypotensive shock	EPI[a] or NE DA[b], Dobut	EPI or NE DA[b], Dobut	NE, EPI DA[b]
Cardiac failure, normotensive	Dobut, amrinone DA, EPI	Dobut, amrinone DA, EPI	Dobut, amrinone DA, EPI
Septic shock, hypotensive	EPI or NE DA[b]	EPI or NE DA[b]	NE or EPI DA[b]
Septic shock, normotensive	DA, EPI Dobut, amrinone	DA[b], EPI Dobut, amrinone	DA or Dobut Amrinone
Hypovolemic shock	Not indicated	Not indicated	Not indicated
Shock from bradycardia	EPI Iso	EPI Iso	Iso or EPI
Anaphylactic shock	EPI	EPI	EPI
Decreased renal blood flow or urine output	DA[c]	DA[c]	DA[c]

[a] Listed in order of preference. DA, dopamine; EPI, epinephrine; NE, norepinephrine; Dobut, dobutamine; Iso, isoproterenol.
[b] High-dose dopamine (typically >10 µg/kg/min).
[c] Low-dose dopamine, 1–3 µg/kg/min; may also combine with other vasopressors to maintain splanchnic blood flow.

Table 24.3. Prescribing Infusions of Inotropic Agents: Deriving Concentrations[a]

Inotrope	How Supplied	Diluent	Concentration
Epinephrine (adrenaline chloride)	1-mg (1 ml) dosette ampules of 1:1000 epi; also in 30-ml vial of 1 mg/ml[b,c]	250 ml of either D₅W or 0.9% NaCl	4 µg/ml
Norepinephrine (noradrenaline)	4-mg ampule of NE bitartrate; each ampule has 4 ml of fluid with 1 mg NE/ml[b,c]	500 ml of either D₅W, or NaCl or 0.45% NaCl	8 µg/ml
Dopamine	200-mg ampules (5 ml) of dopamine HCl (40 mg/ml); also available in 400 mg and 800 mg, 5 ml vials[b,c]	250 ml of D₅W or 0.9% NaCl	800 µg/ml
Dobutamine	250 mg in 20-ml vials of dobutamine HCl[b,c]	250 ml of either D₅W or 0.9% NaCl	1000 µg/ml
Isoproterenol	1-mg ampule of 1:5000 isoproterenol HCl; each ampule has 1 mg/5 ml of fluid[b]	250 ml of either D₅W or 0.9% NaCl	4 µg/ml
Amrinone (Inocor)	100 mg in 20-ml ampules[d]	20 ml of 0.9% NaCl or 0.45% NaCl	2.5 mg/ml

[a] EPI, epinephrine; NE, norepinephrine.
[b] Protect ampules from light.
[c] Avoid use with alkaline solutions.
[d] Do not mix in dextrose-containing solutions.

replaced largely by inhaled β-agonists. It is also administered subcutaneously in the treatment of acute allergic, local reactions (e.g., bee stings), and it may be administered intravenously (5 to 10 ml of the 1:10,000 solution) in the treatment of anaphylaxis. In cardiac arrest, epinephrine is the most effective pharmacologic agent, although the optimal dose is uncertain (see Chapter 13).

Administration and Toxicity

Epinephrine (adrenaline) is available in several forms: prediluted in syringes (1:10,000 concentration; 0.1 mg/ml) for use in cardiac arrest and anaphylaxis, and in vials for subcutaneous administration (1-ml vials) and the preparation of intravenous infusions (30-ml vials) (Tables 24.3 and 24.4).

Epinephrine pharmacokinetics have been examined in a number of studies, but always in normal adult volunteers (54, 58). Epinephrine is cleared rapidly from the plasma at mean rates of 35 to 89 ml/kg/min, depending on the site of sampling and the rate of epinephrine infusion (54, 58). Clearance is accomplished largely by the liver and kidney, which contain substantial concentrations of the enzymes catechol-*O*-methyltransferase and monoamine oxidase (82). Rapid clearance

(half-life about 2 minutes) requires a continuous infusion to maintain hemodynamic effects. Since substantial interindividual variation in epinephrine clearance is reported in normal adults, during critical illness greater variation in clearance would be expected, emphasizing the importance of individual titration of the infusion rate.

Epinephrine is absorbed from the tracheobronchial tree, although the plasma concentration and hemodynamic effects are only about 1/10 those seen with a similar dose given intravenously (83). Endotracheal administration is reserved for patients in cardiac arrest or severe anaphylaxis in whom vascular access is not readily available (see Chapter 13).

Preferably, epinephrine should be administered through a central venous line, since infiltration from peripheral venous administration can result in local ulceration. If infiltration occurs and is recognized early, local injection of the site with 5 to 10 mg of phentolamine in 10 to 15 ml of saline may be effective. The epinephrine infusion rate should be controlled by a constant infusion pump to avoid inadvertent boluses. Epinephrine is compatible with a number of intravenous solutions (Table 24.3); alkaline solutions, particularly when exposed to bright fluorescent light, should be avoided as diluents

Table 24.4.   Preparation of Inotrope Infusions in Children

Inotrope	Preparation	Dose
Epinephrine Norepinephrine Isoproterenol	$0.6 \times$ body weight (kg) is the number of milligrams added to diluent to make final volume of 100 ml	1 ml/hr delivers 0.1 μg/kg/min
Dopamine Dobutamine Amrinone[a]	$6 \times$ body weight (kg) is the number of milligrams added to diluent to make final volume of 100 ml	1 ml/hr delivers 1 μg/kg/min

[a] A loading dose of 3–4.5 mg/kg should precede the continuous infusion; the loading dose should be given as repeated 1–1.5 mg/kg infusions over several minutes with careful monitoring of blood pressure.

for epinephrine and other catecholamines that are inactivated at the higher pH (84).

Epinephrine-induced toxicities include restlessness, fear, throbbing headache, tachycardia, tachydysrhythmias (PVCs, ventricular tachycardia, and ventricular fibrillation), severe hypertension with secondary cerebral hemorrhage, and anginal pain resulting from an increase in myocardial oxygen demand relative to myocardial oxygen delivery.

NOREPINEPHRINE

Pharmacology

Norepinephrine is the neurotransmitter of the sympathetic nervous system and is the biosynthetic precursor of epinephrine, differing only by a methyl group on its amino terminus (Fig. 24.5). It possesses both α- and β-adrenergic receptor activity; low-infusion doses produce mainly β-adrenergic effects: cardiac contractility, conduction velocity, and chronotropy increase, with little change in peripheral vascular resistance. More commonly, in the doses used during hypotensive shock, mixed α- and β-adrenergic effects occur. Peripheral vascular resistance is increased by α_1- and α_2-adrenergic-mediated vasoconstriction. Cardiac contractility, cardiac work, and stroke volume all increase if the augmentation in afterload is tolerated by the ventricle. Chronotropy generally is blunted by baroreceptor-mediated vagal effects to slow the heart rate in response to the norepinephrine-induced increase in blood pressure.

Like epinephrine, norepinephrine is a potent renal and splanchnic vasoconstrictor, which limits its clinical usefulness (71, 85). It vasoconstricts the pulmonary as well as the systemic vascular bed and should be used with caution in patients with pulmonary artery hypertension. Norepinephrine infusion at 5.0 μg/min in normal adults increases blood glucose, glycerol, β-hydroxybutyrate, and acetoacetate, although not as potently as does epinephrine (55). The metabolic effects of infusions in critical illness have not been reported.

Indications and Dose

Norepinephrine's major indication is to increase blood pressure in hypotensive patients who failed to respond to adequate volume resuscitation and other, less potent, inotropes. The most frequent clinical condition that generates this state is septic shock, since profound abnormalities in vascular tone and adrenergic responsiveness characterize this condition (46, 86). In septic patients, norepinephrine increases blood pressure and systemic vascular resistance, often without

altering cardiac output (87). Furthermore, norepinephrine often improves renal blood flow and urine output in these patients by increasing splanchnic perfusion pressure (88, 89), without compromising cardiac index, oxygen delivery, and oxygen consumption by the increase in systemic vascular resistance (90).

Norepinephrine may be useful in myocardial infarction shock, since the major determinant of myocardial oxygen delivery is the diastolic blood pressure-left ventricular end-diastolic pressure gradient (91). The goal is to increase coronary perfusion pressure to 50 to 60 torr by increasing mean arterial pressure to 70 to 80 torr, at which time coronary blood flow improves (92). Use of a potent vasoconstrictor must be balanced against the increase in ventricular afterload, which heightens myocardial oxygen demand; therefore, norepinephrine should be considered only a temporizing measure until intraaortic balloon counterpulsation is initiated. Finally, norepinephrine may be added to gastric lavage solutions used in the treatment of acute gastrointestinal bleeding, with 16 mg of norepinephrine added to 200 ml of iced saline (93).

In nonseptic patients, norepinephrine is a renal vasoconstrictor that compromises renal function. Low-dose dopamine, however, ameliorates the vasoconstrictive action of norepinephrine in dogs (94). The clinical combination of dopamine and norepinephrine therefore may provide both the desired increase in coronary perfusion pressure and the maintenance of adequate renal function.

Administration and Toxicity

Norepinephrine bitartrate (Levophed bitartrate) is available in 4-ml ampules of 1 mg/ml (Table 24.3). Norepinephrine is cleared rapidly from the plasma following intravenous administration; its average half-life is 2 to 2.5 minutes, although substantial interindividual variation has been noted (95). Norepinephrine is cleared by enzymatic degradation in the liver and kidney and by uptake and degradation in neuronal and nonneuronal effector organ sites.

An initial norepinephrine infusion rate of 2 to 4 μg/min is typical and subsequently is increased until the desired change in blood pressure is achieved. In septic adults, remarkably high infusion rates (up to 1.5 μg/kg/min) have been used safely, producing beneficial effects on renal function (88, 90). In pediatric patients, norepinephrine infusions may be prepared as shown in Table 24.4; initial infusion rates are 0.05 to 0.1 μg/kg/min and subsequently are titrated up to 1.5 μg/kg/min.

Preferably, norepinephrine infusions should be given through a central vein. Careful monitoring of arterial pressure, perfusion, and renal function is necessary during norepinephrine infusions to prevent organ ischemia and excessive increases in ventricular afterload. Inadvertent boluses may precipitate profound hypertension resulting in myocardial infarction or cerebral hemorrhage (96). Infiltrated infusions may produce local skin necrosis and ulceration; if recognized early, these conditions should be treated with local phentolamine injection (see the section of this chapter entitled "Toxicity," under "Epinephrine"). Anxiety, respiratory difficulty, palpitations, angina, and transient headaches also occur.

ISOPROTERENOL

Pharmacology

Isoproterenol is a synthetic *N*-alkylated catecholamine similar in structure to epinephrine (Fig. 24.5). As a potent β-adrenergic agonist it increases cardiac contractility, heart rate, and conduction velocity. It also shortens atrioventricular nodal conduction and may incite either ventricular or atrial dysrhythmias. Stimulation of peripheral $β_2$-adrenoceptors results in vascular smooth muscle relaxation, reducing systemic vascular resistance and diastolic blood pressure. Since $β_2$-adrenergic vascular receptors are most prevalent in the skeletal muscle vascular bed, isoproterenol may redirect cardiac output from the splanchnic bed to the skeletal muscle bed, producing a "splanchnic steal" (97).

The net hemodynamic effect produced by isoproterenol infusion is an increase in cardiac output, provided circulating blood volume is adequate. When circulating blood volume is low, vasodilation may impair venous return and, therefore, cardiac output. Pulse pressure widens secondary to the increase in systolic pressure generated by enhanced cardiac contractility and the decrease in diastolic blood pressure mediated by peripheral vasodilation. Although isoproterenol has positive inotropic effects, much of the increase in cardiac output is often related to the change in heart rate, rather than an increase in stroke volume, particularly in pediatric patients (97, 98).

Isoproterenol also relaxes pulmonary vascular and bronchial airway smooth muscle; pulmonary vascular resistance decreases and bronchospasm may be reversed. By overcoming hypoxic pulmonary vasoconstriction, isoproterenol can increase intrapulmonary shunt and lower arterial oxygen tension when used in patients with parenchymal lung disease (99, 100).

Since heart rate and contractility are increased, myocardial oxygen demand is enhanced. At the same time, isoproterenol-induced decreases in diastolic filling time and diastolic coronary perfusion pressure may impair myocardial oxygen supply, which results in myocardial ischemia (91), particularly in the presence of coronary artery stenosis (101).

Isoproterenol does not produce the same degree of hyperglycemia as epinephrine, probably because β-adrenergic stimulation enhances insulin release, whereas epinephrine-mediated $α_2$-adrenergic stimulation inhibits insulin release (102).

Indications and Dose

Once a popular inotrope, isoproterenol has fallen out of favor because of its propensity to produce myocardial ischemia and excessive tachycardia and because more selective inotropes are available (Table 24.2). Isoproterenol may be used to treat hemodynamically significant bradycardia, particularly in the setting of heart block, but should be considered only as a temporizing measure until more definitive therapy, such as cardiac pacing, is obtained (103). In bradycardic pediatric patients, low-dose epinephrine infusion may be more useful since it maintains diastolic coronary perfusion pressure better than does isoproterenol (104).

Isoproterenol is effective in pediatric patients with status asthmaticus (105) and those patients with pulmonary artery hypertension (106). Isoproterenol also may be used as an inotrope in postoperative cardiac surgery patients, particularly with right heart dysfunction (107), although other agents that have fewer side effects are available. In adults with coronary artery disease, isoproterenol should be avoided, since myocardial ischemia is likely (91).

Infusions are usually begun at 0.01 µg/kg/min and are adjusted to produce the desired hemodynamic effect. As with other catecholamines, isoproterenol should be infused through a secure intravenous line using a calibrated infusion pump. Isoproterenol may be given through a secure peripheral i.v., since it lacks vasoconstrictive actions. The patient's heart rate and blood pressure must be monitored carefully during the infusion.

Administration and Toxicity

The parenteral form of isoproterenol (Isuprel HCl) is available in 5-ml vials containing 1 mg (1:5000 solution; Table 24.3). For adults, one vial (1 mg) is added to 250 ml of saline or D_5W, giving a concentration of 4 µg/ml.

After intravenous administration, isoproterenol is cleared rapidly from the plasma; it has a half-life of about 2 minutes (108). It is cleared largely in the liver, and to a lesser extent it is taken up by effector organs throughout the body. It is also well-absorbed from the tracheobronchial tree and is thus available in an aerosol form for treatment of asthma, although more selective $β_2$-adrenergic agonists, such as albuterol, have largely replaced aerosolized isoproterenol.

The major side effects of isoproterenol are tachycardia and tachydysrhythmias, particularly ventricular tachycardia. Angina and myocardial infarction may result from the unfavorable action of isoproterenol on myocardial oxygen demand relative to oxygen delivery (91, 101), even in pediatric patients with normal coronary circulation treated for status asthmaticus (109, 110). Palpitation, headache, and flushing of the skin are common, whereas nausea, tremor, dizziness, and weakness are less common side effects.

DOPAMINE

Pharmacology

Dopamine is the immediate precursor of norepinephrine in the endogenous catecholamine biosynthetic pathway and differs from norepinephrine by the absence of a β-hydroxyl group (Fig. 24.5). Dopamine also serves as a neurotransmitter in both the central and peripheral nervous systems (111, 112). In the latter, it modulates autonomic activity at sympathetic ganglia, decreases gastrointestinal activity, decreases aldosterone synthesis and release (113), and increases renal blood flow (111, 112) and renal sodium excretion (23, 114). When infused in pharmacologic concentrations, dopamine has complex actions because of its mixed direct and indirect sympathomimetic effects.

Unlike the other catecholamines, dopamine's hemodynamic effects are attributed to release of norepinephrine from sympathetic nerves (indirect effect), as well as direct stimulation of α-, β- and DA-receptors (115, 116). Pretreatment of dogs with reserpine to deplete endogenous norepinephrine stores suggests that as much as 50% of dopamine's hemodynamic action may be produced by norepinephrine release (117). In clinical studies, dopamine infusions increase plasma norepinephrine in a dose-dependent manner (118, 119), reflecting its indirect action. Dopamine's hemodynamic effect is less pronounced than that observed with a direct-acting catecholamine, such as dobutamine, in clinical conditions characterized by myocardial norepinephrine depletion (120, 121).

When infused at 2 to 5 μg/kg/min in normal subjects, dopamine increases cardiac contractility and cardiac output, with little change in heart rate, blood pressure, or systemic vascular resistance (25, 115). Doses up to 10 μg/kg/min in normal subjects further increase cardiac output, with small increases in heart rate and blood pressure (115). Renal blood flow and urine output increase at doses of 0.5 to 2.0 μg/kg/min secondary to selective action at both DA$_1$-vascular and renal receptors, and DA$_2$-adrenoceptors (23, 114). Sodium excretion is enhanced by the increase in renal flow and dopamine-mediated inhibition of proximal tubular sodium reabsorption (23, 114). Further improvement in renal function may occur at higher infusion rates related to an improved global cardiac output. At infusion rates in excess of 10 μg/kg/min an increasing α-adrenergic effect may be seen, with increases in systemic vascular resistance and subsequently in mean arterial pressure (122). The salutary effect of dopamine on renal blood flow may be lost at higher doses as a result of predominant α-adrenergic effects (115, 123).

In patients with pulmonary hypertension, dopamine infusions may lead to further increases in mean pulmonary artery pressure (124, 125), and dopamine enhances hypoxic pulmonary vasoconstriction (100, 126). In the absence of pulmonary hypertension, dopamine increases pulmonary blood flow, with little change in mean pulmonary artery pressure or pulmonary capillary wedge pressure (115). Dopamine constricts capacitance veins that may increase central venous and pulmonary capillary wedge pressure (127, 128); serious consequences may then result by means of the increase in myocardial wall tension, and therefore myocardial oxygen demand, and by means of the worsening of hydrostatic pulmonary edema (120). Furthermore, dopamine may limit the expected increase in coronary blood flow associated with catecholamine-induced increased metabolic demand (129).

Dopamine has several potentially important metabolic effects in the critically ill patient. Stimulation of dopamine receptors in the zona glomerulosa of the adrenal cortex decreases aldosterone secretion (130). Conversely, dopamine receptor blockade (e.g., following the administration of metoclopramide) increases plasma aldosterone concentration (26). Dopamine inhibits thyroid-stimulating hormone (TSH) and prolactin release (27, 131); the former blunts the TSH response to thyrotropin-releasing hormone (TRH), making discrimination between the patient with hypothyroidism and the one with the euthyroid-sick syndrome more difficult. Insulin secretion is also inhibited by a direct action of dopamine on pancreatic islet cell α$_2$-adrenoceptors (132), although the clinical importance of this effect during dopamine infusion is unclear.

Indications and Dose

Dopamine is commonly used in the intensive care unit (ICU) to manage patients with shock and congestive heart failure. It is also used to maintain or enhance renal and splanchnic perfusion, and to enhance urine output and sodium excretion. Of the currently available inotropes, dopamine is the only one that selectively increases renal and splanchnic flow.

In myocardial infarction-induced cardiogenic shock, a mean dopamine infusion rate of 17.2 μg/kg/min was required to raise mean arterial pressure to 65 to 70 torr (133); dopamine also increased heart rate, mean arterial pressure, and cardiac index, and decreased pulmonary capillary wedge pressure (PCWP), central venous pressure (CVP), and systemic vascular resistance (SVR). Myocardial oxygen extraction significantly increased along with lactate production, indicating that the improvement in cardiac performance occurred at the expense of an increase in myocardial oxygen demand. This result is similar to observations on dopamine's effects on coronary perfusion and myocardial oxygen extraction following coronary artery surgery (129). Furthermore, dopamine did not influence experimental infarct size (134, 135), whereas dobutamine decreased the area of ischemic infarction (134). Dopamine-responsiveness in cardiogenic shock may discriminate survivors from nonsurvivors, since survivors had improved cardiac output, urinary flow, PCWP, and heart rate at mean infusions of 9.1 μg/kg/min, whereas nonsurvivors failed to show beneficial effects at mean infusion rates of 17.1 μg/kg/min (136).

Combined administration of dopamine and dobutamine may have advantages over the administration of either agent alone in cardiogenic shock (137). Dopamine alone (15 μg/kg/min) consistently increased mean arterial pressure, but also increased PCWP, had variable effects on stroke index, and reduced PaO$_2$. Dobutamine alone (15 μg/kg/min) failed to increase mean arterial pressure but more consistently improved stroke volume. The combination of dopamine and dobutamine (7.5 μg/kg/min each) had the most beneficial effects: mean arterial pressure, cardiac index, and stroke volume index all increased, with no change in PCWP, mean pulmonary artery pressure, or PaO$_2$ (137). All three infusion combinations increased intrapulmonary shunt. This effect is common to inotropes that increase cardiac output and results from improved perfusion of poorly ventilated lung segments (138). Typically, inotrope-mediated increases in oxygen delivery balance the increase in shunt, and PaO$_2$ is unchanged; dopamine, however, caused hypoxemia in this (137) and other studies (139), probably because of an increase in PCWP.

As in cardiogenic shock, dobutamine is superior to dopamine in chronic heart failure (120). Based on animal studies, dopamine's inotropic response is attenuated in chronic heart failure because myocardial norepinephrine stores are depleted (117, 121). In addition, dopamine loses its inotropic effect after 24 hours of infusion in experimental myocardial infarction, possibly as a result of dopamine-mediated stimulation of myocardial norepinephrine release, which rapidly depletes stores (134).

After coronary artery bypass grafting, dopamine frequently is used to support the circulation. Dopamine had increasing inotropic action during a 24-hour observation period after bypass graft (140), unlike the response seen in experimental myocardial infarction (134). Despite this beneficial effect, when compared with dobutamine, dopamine produces a relatively smaller enhancement of left ventricular contractility (141). Differences in the hemodynamic response to dopamine and dobutamine in the postoperative period may be related to the state of the ventricle (142). In normal ventricles, dobutamine had a greater chronotropic response; in volume-loaded ventricles, both drugs had similar effects on heart rate and cardiac output, but dobutamine caused a greater reduction in systemic vascular resistance and pulmonary vascular resistance (142). Neither agent (at 5 µg/kg/min) produces a change in hemodynamics in the pressure-loaded ventricle.

In septic shock, dopamine is effective in improving cardiac output, although intrapulmonary shunt may increase (143, 144). The latter can be prevented by the application of positive end-expiratory pressure (144). Since many septic patients are hypotensive, dopamine has the advantage of increasing systemic vascular resistance, and therefore blood pressure, and may be preferable over dobutamine in this clinical setting (145). An additional advantage of dopamine is its beneficial effect on urine output (146) and lack of adverse effects on splanchnic flow, even when used at high infusion rates during sepsis (147). Despite these advantages, dopamine may increase PCWP and pulmonary artery pressure in septic patients (144, 146), requiring invasive hemodynamic monitoring for optimal therapy.

Dopamine's major clinical benefit is that it causes a selective increase in renal and splanchnic blood flow. A low-dose infusion (1 to 3 µg/kg/min) augments urine output following cardiopulmonary bypass (148), and in patients with oliguria and critical illness (114). Low-dose dopamine may also antagonize the vasoconstrictive action of norepinephrine and other adrenergic vasoconstrictors (94). In experimental studies, it improves blood flow and protein synthesis in the postischemic liver (149) and protects renal function in patients undergoing orthotopic liver transplantation (150). Despite its beneficial effects on renal blood flow, however, it is not certain that dopamine has a beneficial effect in patients with acute renal failure (123).

Infusion rates of 0.5 to 2 µg/kg/min result in selective dopaminergic actions on the renal and splanchnic vasculature. With infusion rates between 5 and 10 µg/kg/min, β-adrenergic effects usually dominate; infusions between 10 and 20 µg/kg/min have mixed α- and β-adrenergic effects, whereas infusions in excess of 20 µg/kg/min usually have predominant α-adrenergic effects.

Administration and Toxicity

Dopamine is available in a number of commercial formulations (Table 24.3). In adults, 200 mg may be diluted in 250 ml of diluent (e.g., D₅W), producing a final dopamine concentration of 800 µg/ml. As with other catecholamines, dopamine should not be mixed in an alkaline solution.

After intravenous administration, dopamine is cleared rapidly from the plasma, although the kinetics of elimination are variably reported as representing first-order (5, 6, 151), or nonlinear, clearance (152). Most studies report a terminal elimination half-life of 6 to 9 minutes (5, 6, 153). Mean steady-state plasma clearance of dopamine (50 to 70 ml/kg/min) is similar in both adults and infants (6, 7, 153), although substantial interindividual variation is noted in all studies. A portion of the interindividual variation may result from abnormal organ function, since alterations of renal and/or liver function are associated with diminished dopamine clearance (7, 151).

Nausea, emesis, and tachyarrhythmias are the most frequent side effects associated with dopamine (154). Anginal pain, myocardial ischemia (134), serious hypertension, and profound vasoconstriction may occur (155, 156). Local infiltration may be treated successfully with local injection of phentolamine up to 12 hours after dopamine infiltration (156). In patients who are dependent on hypoxic ventilatory drive, dopamine may depress ventilation and worsen hypoxemia (28, 29).

DOBUTAMINE

Pharmacology

Dobutamine was developed by systematic modification of the catecholamine molecule in the search for an agent that would have selective inotropic activity with little peripheral vascular effect (157). Dobutamine has a large substitution on the amino terminus of the catecholamine molecule (Fig. 24.5), and, like isoproterenol, it is administered as a racemic mixture of the (+) and (−) isomers. This racemic mixture provides dobutamine with its characteristic β₁-adrenergic selectivity: the (−)-isomer is a potent, selective α₁-adrenergic agonist, and the (+)-isomer potently stimulates both β-adrenoceptors (158, 159). Dobutamine's net hemodynamic effect is determined by its direct action at these receptors, combined with a decrease in sympathetic nervous system tone associated with a dobutamine-induced increase in cardiac output (160). Further confusing its pharmacodynamic action is the possibility that dobutamine's major metabolite, 3-O-methyldobutamine (161), is a potent inhibitor of α-adrenoceptors (162).

At usual infusion rates (5 to 15 µg/kg/min), dobutamine's predominant effect is on the heart, with an increase in contractility and a relatively smaller increase in heart rate. Dobutamine typically decreases or has little effect on systemic and peripheral vascular resistance (120, 163), probably because of the balanced activation of α₁- and β₂-adrenergic receptors (158). Dobutamine generally decreases central venous and pulmonary wedge pressure and has little effect on pulmonary vascular resistance (120, 163). Like other inotropes, dobutamine can increase intrapulmonary shunt by augmenting cardiac output and thus perfusion of poorly ventilated lung regions (164).

Although it lacks a selective renal vascular effect, dobutamine often enhances urine output by improving cardiac output and thus renal perfusion (165). Despite dobutamine's action at multiple adrenoceptors, no significant metabolic side effects are reported.

Unlike dopamine, dobutamine's pharmacologic action does not depend upon releasable stores of norepinephrine (115). Its clearance appears to be complex, with wide interpatient variability (3, 166, 167). In a small group of adults, clearance was 2.35 liters/min/m^2 (168), whereas reported clearance ranges from 32 to 1300 ml/kg/min in pediatric patients (3, 166, 167). It is uncertain whether dobutamine follows first-order kinetics (3) or nonlinear kinetics (166). Furthermore, co-infusion of other inotropes such as dopamine has been variously reported to affect (166) or not affect (167) dobutamine clearance. The clinical implication of these data is that variable kinetics should be expected, requiring careful titration of drug infusion rate to effect.

Dobutamine loses its hemodynamic effect during prolonged infusion (169), presumably because of down-regulation of receptors. However, dobutamine maintains its hemodynamic effect much better than does dopamine during continuous infusion, since the latter depletes myocardial norepinephrine stores (170).

Indications and Dose

Dobutamine is indicated in clinical conditions that require increased contractility with little effect on peripheral vascular resistance. This setting most often occurs in normotensive patients with congestive heart failure (163). In patients with congestive heart failure, including neonates and children (171, 172), dobutamine increases stroke volume and cardiac output while reducing the elevated filling pressure accompanying this clinical state (165, 173). When dobutamine is used in lower dosages (2 to 10 μg/kg/min), little change in heart rate is seen (163, 171). In patients with very poor myocardial function and higher baseline plasma norepinephrine concentrations, however, dobutamine's effect on cardiac index is attenuated (174).

In patients with myocardial failure and nonobstructed coronary arteries, dobutamine improves coronary blood flow and myocardial oxygen supply equal to, or in excess of, the increase in myocardial oxygen demand elicited by its positive inotropic action (129, 175). Supplementation of myocardial perfusion may partly explain dobutamine's ability to produce sustained improvement of cardiac function in patients with congestive heart failure following short-term infusions (176, 177). In one study, a 72-hour dobutamine infusion improved endomyocardial ATP/creatinine ratio and the ultrastructural appearance of mitochondria (178).

Patients with myocardial infarction benefit from dobutamine infusion, even those who have hypotension prior to therapy (179, 180). Patients with hypotensive cardiogenic shock, however, may fail to improve with dobutamine, since it has relatively less peripheral vascular action; dopamine may be superior in this setting (163, 181).

In postoperative cardiovascular surgical patients, dobutamine improves stroke volume and decreases ventricular filling pressures with less positive chronotropy than observed with dopamine (182). In addition, dobutamine enhances myocardial blood flow more than does dopamine (129). In patients after heart transplant, myocardial sympathetic innervation is destroyed. Since dobutamine's inotropic action does not depend on myocardial stores of norepinephrine, it is a better inotrope in the transplant recipient than dopamine (183). In a mixed population of critically ill surgical postoperative patients, dobutamine produced greater increases in oxygen delivery and consumption with less adverse effect on intrapulmonary shunt and filling pressures than produced by dopamine (139, 184).

Because dobutamine lacks clinically important vasoconstrictive effects, it may be disadvantageous in the patient with septic shock and hypotension. Dobutamine will often increase cardiac output, oxygen delivery, and oxygen consumption in volume-resuscitated septic patients, while having variable effects on blood pressure (185). Unfortunately, the increase in oxygen delivery does not necessarily mean that splanchnic organ flow improves (186). Although dobutamine-induced increases in cardiac output and peripheral tissue flow theoretically could increase pulmonary and tissue edema in septic patients, this effect has not been observed in an animal model (187). Dobutamine is ideally employed for septic patients with combined ventricular dysfunction and increased filling pressures who have received adequate fluid resuscitation (139, 164).

Administration and Toxicity

Dobutamine (Dobutrex) is supplied in 250-mg, 20-ml vials (Table 24.3). One vial is usually diluted into 250 ml of an appropriate diluent, achieving a final drug concentration of 1000 μg/ml. In stable adults with congestive heart failure, a good correlation exists between dobutamine dose, plasma concentration, and hemodynamic effects (188). Unfortunately, the variable clearance observed in more recent studies (3, 166, 167) suggests that such good correlation between infusion rate and effect is unlikely in the ICU. Dobutamine is cleared rapidly by catechol-O-methyltransferase and rapid redistribution from the plasma compartment (161, 168). As with the other catecholamines, dobutamine preferably should be administered into a central venous site using a continuous infusion pump.

Dysrhythmias are the most frequent toxic side effect, although they are less frequent than with dopamine or isoproterenol (189). Other side effects include excessive tachycardia, headaches, anxiety, tremors, and excessive increases or decreases in blood pressure (163).

AMRINONE AND OTHER INODILATORS

Pharmacology

The bipyridine amrinone was discovered in the search for positive inotropic drugs with a better therapeutic : toxic ratio than digoxin. Amrinone possesses positive inotropic and, to a lesser extent, chronotropic actions on the heart and has potent vasodilator properties (190). These properties are shared by other drugs in this group, leading to their classification as "inodilators." Amrinone is effective following intravenous administration but is not useful orally. Milrinone is a methyl carbonitrile derivative of amrinone that is orally effective, but it was removed from the market because of its side effects (191). Intravenous milrinone is under investigation and may prove beneficial since its half-life is shorter than that of amrinone (192). A number of new inodilators are also under

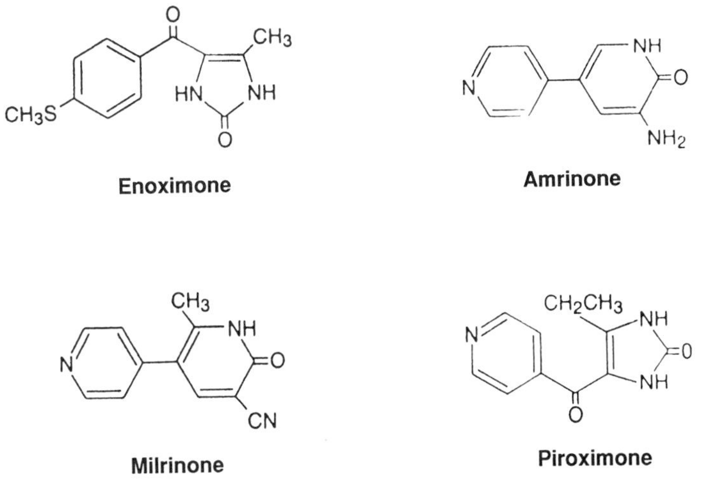

Figure 24.6. Chemical structures of enoximone, amrinone, milrinone, and piroximone.

active development, including enoximone and piroximone (193, 194).

Pharmacologically, these compounds differ from catecholamines and cardiac glycosides. They possess a unique structure, unlike that of any of the other inotropic agents (Fig. 24.6). Although their mechanism of action is still not completely understood, they share a similar pharmacologic action with methylxanthines (190, 195); both inhibit phosphodiesterase, resulting in an increase in intracellular cAMP. Amrinone and other inodilators selectively inhibit phosphodiesterase type III, which is in high concentrations in the heart and vascular smooth muscle. Increased cAMP activates protein kinase, which phosphorylates a sarcolemmal calcium channel and activates the calcium pump (192). The latter produces a lusitropic effect, enhancing ventricular relaxation and diastolic compliance (194). Thus, like most other inotropic agents, the inodilator's inotropic action is characterized by an increase in intracellular calcium concentration (196), which can be attenuated by pretreatment with calcium channel blockers (190). Unlike catecholamines and other drugs whose inotropic effect is mediated only by increasing cAMP concentration, amrinone also appears to prolong the release and/or delay the reuptake of calcium by the sarcoplasmic reticulum (196). Furthermore, amrinone and other inodilators may increase the sensitivity of the contractile elements to calcium, and may directly activate a sodium-dependent calcium channel (197).

Amrinone increases cAMP concentrations in vascular smooth muscle, relaxing tone (198) and thus decreasing peripheral and pulmonary vascular resistance, and dilating coronary vessels (194, 199). Based on studies in isolated tissue, the potency of these drugs in vascular tissue is 10 to 100 times greater than their inotropic action (196), suggesting that a large part of their action in heart failure is related to afterload reduction.

In intact animals and humans, the bipyridines increase cardiac contractility, stroke volume, cardiac output, and, to a lesser extent, heart rate. Although the bipyridines decrease systemic vascular resistance, systemic blood pressure is unchanged with low doses because the drug-induced increase in stroke volume compensates for the decrease in resistance (190, 200). In the pulmonary vascular bed, pulmonary systolic and diastolic blood pressures usually decline (190, 200), but intrapulmonary shunt may worsen (201). The bipyridines are

particularly beneficial in cardiac failure since they reduce afterload by peripheral vasodilation and increase cardiac contractility, often without an increase in myocardial oxygen consumption (194, 202, 203). The net hemodynamic effect is dose related: increasing doses produce greater afterload reduction and increased contractility.

Complicating the pharmacology of amrinone and milrinone is the observation of species-dependent and age-dependent differences in their inotropic effects (204, 205). In newborn puppies and piglets, amrinone administration induces a significant decrease in both peak myocardial tension developed and the rate of myocardial tension development (204, 205); in puppies, this result changed to a positive inotropic effect by 3 days of age and increased in magnitude thereafter (206). These effects are not a result of developmental changes in the effects of amrinone on phosphodiesterase (204). It is speculated that the observed ontogenetic differences are related to inadequate development of the T-tubule-sarcoplasmic reticulum system in the newborn (190, 207). Supporting this theory is the observation that amrinone has negative inotropic effects in adult Purkinje fibers, another tissue that lacks a T-tubular system (208).

Amrinone is eliminated largely by glucuronidation and acetylation; 10 to 40% is excreted unchanged in the urine (209). Studies with amrinone reveal a mean half-life of 3.6 hours, with slower elimination seen in patients with congestive heart failure (half-life, 5 to 8 hours) (210, 211), and in patients who are slow acetylators (209). The relatively slow elimination observed in sicker patients has potential therapeutic implications, since a continuous infusion of amrinone may result in progressive increase in drug plasma concentrations over several hours. Furthermore, critically ill patients often have changing hepatic and renal function complicating the maintenance of a steady-state plasma concentration.

The elimination kinetics in pediatric patients is age-dependent; neonates (<4 weeks) have prolonged half-lives (212). The mean half-life in infants was 6.8 hours, compared with 22.2 hours in neonates (212). The clearance in older children appears to be similar to that observed in infants (213). The pharmacodynamic response in infants and children is not known, but negative inotropic responses have not been observed despite the animal data noted previously (212, 213).

Indications and Dose

Most of the clinical data on these drugs are derived from studies in either normal populations or patients with chronic congestive heart failure; few data are available in patients with acute, critical illness. In patients with heart failure, amrinone augments dP/dt without significant changes in heart rate or blood pressure (214, 215). Amrinone also reduces left ventricular filling pressure, mean pulmonary artery pressure, right atrial pressure, and pulmonary and systemic vascular resistances (201, 214). In perioperative patients with low cardiac output, amrinone had similar beneficial effects on resistance, filling pressures, and cardiac output (216). The magnitude of these changes varies depending on the underlying clinical state of the patient and the dosage regimen employed. Indeed, in patients with end-stage heart failure, inodilators had greatly reduced inotropic effect, probably reflecting diminished cAMP production secondary to reduced β-adrenoceptor density and responsiveness (217). In general, phosphodiesterase inhibitors appear to have ideal hemodynamic properties in patients with severe heart failure: cardiac index is enhanced and filling pressure is reduced, with minimal effect on myocardial oxygen demand.

Despite having vasodilating properties that may worsen hypotension in septic shock, amrinone has potential utility in these patients since it is a potent pulmonary vasodilator and may unload the right ventricle. Amrinone potently increased cardiac output in dogs with endotoxic shock, although mean arterial pressure remained low (218). More intriguing are data showing that pharmacologic concentrations of amrinone potently inhibit lipopolysaccharide-induced tumor necrosis factor production (219). This effect was additive to the inhibitory action of dexamethasone on tumor necrosis factor production. In the author's experience, amrinone has been useful in septic shock patients, as long as adequate volume resuscitation is provided.

Individual variation in the peripheral vascular and myocardial response makes it difficult to select the correct infusion rate in critically ill patients. Since the half-life of amrinone is substantially longer than that of either catecholamines or intravenous vasodilators used in cardiogenic shock, it is probably preferable to individually titrate an inotrope and vasodilator in the unstable patient, rather than use an agent such as amrinone that possesses both activities. By virtue of its vasodilator action, amrinone may also result in clinically important hypotension (220), which could compromise diastolic coronary filling in the patient with cardiogenic shock. Conversely, in more stable patients, amrinone is often quite effective. Unlike catecholamines, cardiac output is often increased without significant tachycardia or increased myocardial metabolic demand.

The manufacturer's recommended dosage for amrinone is an initial intravenous loading dose of 0.75 mg/kg over 3 to 5 minutes, followed by a second equal bolus 30 minutes later if required. Data in pediatric patients reveal a larger volume of distribution, requiring a total load of 3 to 4.5 mg/kg (212, 213). Anecdotal (221) and kinetic (222) data in adults also suggest that a larger bolus dose is required to provide therapeutic concentrations and acute effectiveness. The bolus should be given in divided infusions of 1 to 1.5 mg/kg over several minutes, with close observation of blood pressure; more rapid infusions may result in hypotension (212). Subsequent bolus doses are given every 10 minutes. The bolus should be followed by a continuous intravenous infusion of 5 to 10 μg/kg/min, with the total daily dose not exceeding 10 mg/kg (214). In neonates, the infusion should not exceed 5 μg/kg/min, since their clearance is much lower than that of older children (212). After an intravenous bolus, peak effects are seen in several minutes; with an intravenous infusion alone, peak effects will not occur until 7 or more hours (214).

Administration and Toxicity

Amrinone lactate (Inocor) is available as a solution of 100 mg in 20-ml vials. The drug generally is diluted in normal or half-normal saline to a concentration of 1 to 3 mg/ml. Glucose-containing solutions should not be used, since a slow chemical interaction causes the loss of 11 to 13% of amrinone's activity over 24 hours when it is mixed with dextrose (223). This interaction does not preclude the co-infusion of amrinone with dextrose-containing solutions using a Y-connector. Furosemide precipitates when mixed with amrinone, so the two cannot be co-administered (223).

Intravenous amrinone produces reversible thrombocytopenia in approximately 2 to 4% of patients (223, 224); the frequency increases with total daily doses in excess of 24 mg/kg. Increase of liver enzymes has been reported with long-term, but not short-term, use (224). No increased risk of arrhythmias has been documented with amrinone (223).

The relatively long half-life and the resultant slow attainment of a new steady state with changes in continuous infusion rate of amrinone make it less attractive in the critical care setting. There is no information about drug excretion in patients with hepatic or renal failure; therefore, amrinone should be used cautiously, if at all, in this population.

SUMMARY

The pharmacology of catecholamines, bipyridines, and other selected inotropes is reviewed in this chapter. These compounds possess potent myocardial and peripheral vascular actions when used in critically ill patients to maintain cardiac function and manipulate peripheral and pulmonary vascular tone. Optimal use of these valuable drugs requires an understanding of their pharmacology and the influence of critical illness on the hemodynamic actions resulting from their administration. In pediatric applications, age-related changes in drug kinetics or dynamics may occur, further complicating these drugs' administration to infants and children and emphasizing the need to titrate the infusion rate individually to observed hemodynamic changes.

REFERENCES

1. Trendelenburg U: Extraneuronal uptake and metabolism of catecholamines as a site of loss. *Life Sci* 22:1217–1222, 1978.
2. Bevan JA, Bevan RD, Kuckles SP: Adrenergic regulation of vascular smooth muscle. *Handbook Physiol* 2:515–566, 1980.
3. Martinez AM, Padbury JF, Thio S: Dobutamine pharmacokinetics and cardiovascular responses in critically ill neonates. *Pediatrics* 89:47–51, 1992.
4. Padbury JF, Habib DM, Martinez AM: Thresholds for the physiologic effects of adrenergic agents: a methodologic appraisal. *Dev Pharmacol Ther* 14:115–124, 1990.

5. Bhatt MV, Nahata MC, McClead RE, Menke JA: Dopamine pharmacokinetics in critically ill newborn infants. *Eur J Clin Pharmacol* 40:593–597, 1991.

6. Padbury JF, Agata Y, Baylen BG, et al: Pharmacokinetics of dopamine in critically ill newborn infants. *J Pediatr* 117:472–476, 1990.

7. Zaritsky A, Lotze A, Stull R, Goldstein D: Steady-state dopamine clearance in critically ill infants and children. *Crit Care Med* 16:217–220, 1988.

8. Kobilka B: Adrenergic receptors as models for G protein-coupled receptors. *Annu Rev Neurosci* 15:87–114, 1992.

9. Lands AM, Arnold A, McAuliff JP, Ludicna FP, Frown G: Differentiation of receptor systems activated by sympathomimetic amines. *Nature* 214:597–598, 1967.

10. Brodde O-E, Karad K, Zerkowski HR, Rohm N, Reidemeister JC: Coexistence of β_1- and β_2-adrenoceptors in human right atrium. *Circ Res* 53:752–758, 1983.

11. Heitz A, Schwartz J, Velly J: β-Adrenoceptors of the human myocardium: determination of β_1- and β_2-subtypes by radioligand binding. *Br J Pharmacol* 80:711–717, 1983.

12. Kauman AJ, Hall JA, Murray KJ, Wells FC, Brown MJ: A comparison of the effects of adrenaline and noradrenaline on human heart: the role of β_1- and β_2-adrenoceptors in the stimulation of adenylate cyclase and contractile force. *Eur Heart J* 10(suppl B):29–37, 1989.

13. Majowki H: Modulation of noradrenaline release through activation of presynaptic β-adrenoceptors. *J Auton Pharmacol* 3:47–60, 1983.

14. Langer SZ: Presynaptic regulation of catecholamine release. *Biochem Pharmacol* 23:1793–1800, 1974.

15. Starke K: α-Adrenoceptor subclassification. *Rev Physiol Biochem Pharmacol* 88:199–236, 1981.

16. van Zwieten PA, Timmermans PBMWM: Cardiovascular α_2-receptors. *J Mol Cell Cardiol* 15:717–733, 1983.

17. Böhm M, Diet F, Feiler G, Kemkes B, Erdmann E: α-Adrenoceptors and α-adrenoceptor-mediated positive inotropic effects in failing human myocardium. *J Cardiovasc Pharmacol* 12:357–364, 1988.

18. Govier WC: Myocardial alpha-adrenergic receptors and their role in the production of a positive inotropic effect by sympathomimetic agents. *J Pharmacol Exp Ther* 159:82–90, 1968.

19. Schmitz W, Kohl C, Neumann J, Scholz H, Scholz J: On the mechanism of positive inotropic effects of alpha-adrenoceptor agonists. *Basic Res Cardiol* 84(suppl 1):23–33, 1989.

20. Goldberg LI, Volkman PH, Kohli JD: A comparison of the vascular dopamine receptor with other dopamine receptors. *Annu Rev Pharmacol Toxicol* 18:57–79, 1978.

21. Willems JL, Buylaert WA, Lefebvre RA, Bogaert MG: Neuronal dopamine receptors on autonomic ganglia and sympathetic nerves and dopamine receptors in the gastrointestinal system. *Pharmacol Rev* 37:165–217, 1985.

22. Goldberg LI, Kohli JD: Peripheral dopamine receptors: a classification based on potency series and specific antagonism. *Trends Pharmacol Sci* 4:64–66, 1983.

23. Hegde SS, Ricci A, Amenta F, Lokhandwala MF: Evidence from functional and autoradiographic studies for the presence of tubular dopamine-1 receptors and their involvement in the renal effects of fenoldopam. *J Pharmacol Exp Ther* 251:1237–1245, 1989.

24. Felder RA, Blecher M, Eisner GM, Jose PA: Cortical tubular and glomerular dopamine receptors in the rat kidney. *Am J Physiol* 246:F557–F568, 1984.

25. Goldberg LI: The role of dopamine receptors in the treatment of congestive heart failure. *J Cardiovasc Pharmacol* 14(suppl 5):S19–S27, 1989.

26. Carey RM, Thorner MO, Ortt EM: Dopaminergic inhibition of metoclopramide-induced aldosterone secretion in man. *J Clin Invest* 66:10–18, 1980.

27. Levinson PD, Goldstein DS, Munson PJ, Gill JR Jr, Keiser HR: Endocrine, renal, and hemodynamic responses to graded dopamine infusions in normal men. *J Clin Endocrinol Metab* 60:821–826, 1985.

28. Olson LG, Hensley MJ, Saunders NA: Ventilatory responsiveness to hypercapnic hypoxia during dopamine infusion in humans. *Am Rev Respir Dis* 126:783–787, 1982.

29. Ward DS, Bellville JW: Reduction of hypoxic ventilatory drive by dopamine. *Anesth Analg* 61:333–337, 1982.

30. Birnbaumer L, Abramowitz J, Brown AM: Receptor-effector coupling by G proteins. *Biochem Biophys Acta* 1031:163–224, 1990.

31. Stiles GL, Caron MG, Lefkowitz RJ: β-adrenergic receptors: biochemical mechanisms of physiological regulation. *Physiol Rev* 64:661–743, 1984.

32. Cotecchia S, Kobilka BK, Daniel KW, et al: Multiple second messenger pathways of α-adrenergic receptor subtypes expressed in eukaryotic cells. *J Biol Chem* 265:63–69, 1990.

33. Gilman AG: G proteins: transducers of receptor-generated signals. *Annu Rev Biochem* 56:615–649, 1987.

34. Minneman KP: α_1-Adrenergic receptor subtypes, inositol phosphates, and sources of cell Ca^{2+}. *Pharmacol Rev* 40:87–119, 1988.

35. Lefkowitz RJ, Hausdorff WP, Caron MG: Role of phosphorlyation in desensitization of the β-adrenoceptor. *Trends Pharmacol Sci* 11:190–194, 1990.

36. Benovic JL, Pike LJ, Cerione RA, et al: Phosphorlation of the mammalian β-adrenergic receptor by cyclic AMP-dependent protein kinase. *J Biol Chem* 260:7094–7101, 1985.

37. Benovic JL, Mayor F, Staniszewski E, Lefkowitz RJ, Caron MG: Purification and characterization of beta-adrenergic receptor kinase. *J Biol Chem* 262:9026–9032, 1987.

38. Hausdorff WP, Caron MG, Lefkowitz RJ: Turning off the signal: desensitization of β-adrenergic receptor function. *FASEB J* 4:2881–2889, 1990.

39. Brodde O-E, Schuler S, Kretsch R, et al: Regional distribution of β-adrenoceptors in the human heart: coexistence of functional β_1- and β_2-adrenoceptors in both atria and ventricles in severe congestive cardiomyopathy. *J Cardiovas Pharmacol* 8:1235–1242, 1986.

40. Bristow MR, Ginsburg R, Umasns V, et al: β_1- and β_2-adrenergic-receptor subpopulations in nonfailing and failing human ventricular myocardium: coupling of both receptor subtypes to muscle contraction and selective β_1-receptor down-regulation in heart failure. *Circ Res* 59:297–309, 1986.

41. Francis GS, Cohn JN: The autonomic nervous system in congestive heart failure. *Annu Rev Med* 37:235–247, 1986.

42. Hasking GJ, Esler MD, Jennings GL, Burton D, Johns JA, Korner PI: Norepinephrine spillover to plasma in patients with congestive heart failure: evidence of increased overall and cardiorenal sympathetic nervous activity. *Circulation* 73:615–621, 1986.

43. Brodde O-E, Zerkowski H-R, Borst MG, Maier W, Michel MC: Drug- and disease-induced changes of human cardiac β_1- and β_2-adrenoceptors. *Eur Heart J* 10(suppl B):38–44, 1989.

44. Brodde O-E, Zerkowski H-R, Doetsch N, Motomura S, Khamssi M, Michel MC: Myocardial beta-adrenoceptor changes in heart failure: concomitant reduction in beta$_1$- and beta$_2$-adrenoceptor function related to the degree of heart failure in patients with mitral valve disease. *J Am Coll Cardiol* 14:323–331, 1989.

45. Horn EM, Corwin SJ, Steinberg SF, et al: Reduced lymphocyte stimulatory guanine nucleotide regulatory protein and β-adrenergic receptors in congestive heart failure and reversal with angiotensin converting enzyme inhibitor therapy. *Circulation* 78:1373–1379, 1988.

46. Sibbald WJ, Fox G, Martin C: Abnormalities of vascular reactivity in the sepsis syndrome. *Chest* 100(suppl):155S–159S, 1991.

47. McKenna TM, Martin FM, Chernow B, Briglia FA: Vascular endothelium contributes to decreased aortic contractility in experimental sepsis. *Circ Shock* 19:267–273, 1986.

48. Zaritsky AL, Eisenberg MG: Ontogenetic considerations in the pharmacotherapy of shock. In: Chernow B, Shoemaker W (eds): *Critical Care State of the Art.* Fullerton, CA, Society of Critical Care Medicine, 1986, pp 485–534.

49. Levine TB, Francis GS, Goldsmith SR, Simon AB, Cohn JN: Activity of the sympathetic nervous system and renin-angiotensin system assessed by plasma hormone levels and their relation to hemodynamic alterations in congestive heart failure. *Am J Cardiol* 49:1659–1666, 1982.

50. Verrier RL, Lown B: Behavioral stress and cardiac arrhythmias. *Annu Rev Physiol* 46:155–176, 1984.

51. Chernow B, Rainey T, Lake C: Endogenous and exogenous catecholamines in critical care medicine. *Crit Care Med* 10:409–416, 1982.

52. Goldstein D: Plasma norepinephrine as an indicator of sympathetic neural activity in clinical cardiology. *Am J Cardiol* 48:1147–1154, 1981.

53. Esler M, Leonard P, O'Dea K, Jackman G, Jennings G, Korner P: Biochemical quantification of sympathetic nervous activity in humans using radiotracer methodology: fallibility of plasma noradrenaline measurements. *J Cardiovasc Pharmacol* 4:S152–S157, 1982.

54. Best JD, Halter JB: Release and clearance rates of epinephrine in man: importance of arterial measurements. *J Clin Endocrinol Metab* 55:263–268, 1982.

55. Silverberg AB, Shah SD, Haymond MW, Cryer PE: Norepinephrine: hormone and neurotransmitter in man. *Am J Physiol* 234:E252–E256, 1978.

56. Shepherd JT, Vanhoutte PM: Local modulation of adrenergic neurotransmission. *Circulation* 64:655–660, 1981.

57. Stjärne L, Brundin J: Frequency dependence of ^{3}H-noradrenaline secretion from human vasoconstrictor nerves; modification by factors intering with alpha- or beta-adrenoceptor or prostaglandin E$_2$-mediated control. *Acta Physiol Scand* 101:199–210, 1977.

58. Clutter WE, Bier DM, Shah SD, Cryer PE: Epinephrine plasma metabolic clearance rates and physiologic thresholds for metabolic and hemodynamic actions in man. *J Clin Invest* 66:94–101, 1980.

59. Gelfand RA, Matthews DE, Bier DM, Sherwin RS: Role of counterregulatory hormones in the catabolic response to stress. *J Clin Invest* 74:2238–2248, 1984.

60. Cohn JN, Levine TB, Olivari MT, et al: Plasma norepinephrine as a guide to prognosis in patients with chronic congestive heart failure. *N Engl J Med* 311:819–823, 1984.

61. Davies CL, Newman RJ, Molyneux SG, Grahame-Smith DG: The relationship between plasma catecholamines and severity of injury in man. *J Trauma* 24:99–105, 1984.

62. Bertel O, Bühler FR, Baitsch G, Ritz R, Burkart F: Plasma adrenaline and noradrenaline in patients with acute myocardial infarction. *Chest* 82:64–68, 1982.

63. Chernow B, Lake CR, Barton M, et al: Sympathetic nervous system sensitivity to hemorrhagic hypotension in the subhuman primate. *J Trauma* 24:229–232, 1984.

64. Wortsman J, Frank S, Cryer PE: Adrenomedullary response to maximal stress in humans. *Am J Med* 77:779–784, 1984.

65. Schechter E, Wilson MF, Yin-Suen K: Physiologic responses to epinephrine infusion: the basis for a new stress for coronary artery disease. *Am Heart J* 105:554–560, 1983.

66. Barnes PJ: Modulation of neurotransmission in airways. *Physiol Rev* 72:699–729, 1992.

67. Barnes PJ: Endogenous catecholamines and asthma. *J Allergy Clin Immunol* 77:791–795, 1986.

68. Warren JB, Dalton N: A comparison of the bronchodilator and vasopressor effects of exercise levels of adrenaline in man. *Clin Sci* 64:475–479, 1983.

69. Assem ESK, Schild HO: Inhibition by sympathomimetic amines of histamine release induced by antigen in passively sensitized human lung. *Nature* 224:1028–1029, 1969.

70. Gombos EA, Hulet WH, Bopp P, Goldring W, Baldwin DS, Chasis H: Reactivity of renal and systemic circulations to vasoconstrictor agents in normotensive and hypertensive subjects. *J Clin Invest* 41:203–217, 1962.

71. Insel PA, Snavely MD: Catecholamines and the kidney: receptors and renal function. *Annu Rev Physiol* 43:625–636, 1981.

72. Coffin LH Jr, Ankeney JL, Beheler EM: Experimental study and clinical use of epinephrine for treatment of low cardiac output syndrome. *Circulation* 33(Suppl 1):I78–I85, 1965.

73. Soman VR, Shamoon H, Sherwin RS: Effects of physiologic infusion of epinephrine in normal humans: relationship between the metabolic response and β-adrenergic binding. *J Clin Endocrinol Metab* 50:294–297, 1980.

74. Brown MJ: Hypokalemia from beta$_2$-receptor stimulation by circulating epinephrine. *Am J Cardiol* 56:3D–9D, 1985.

75. Struthers AD, Whitesmith R, Reid JL: Metabolic and haemodynamic effects of increased circulating adrenaline in man. *Br Heart J* 50:277–281, 1983.

76. Body J-J, Cryer PE, Offord KP, Heath H III: Epinephrine is a hypophosphatemic hormone in man. *J Clin Invest* 71:572–578, 1983.

77. Bessey PQ, Brooks DC, Black PR, Aoki TT, Wilmore DW: Epinephrine acutely mediates skeletal muscle insulin resistance. *Surgery* 94:172–178, 1983.

78. Küng M, White JR, Burki NK: The effect of subcutaneously administered terbutaline on serum potassium in asymptomatic adult asthmatics. *Am Rev Respir Dis* 129:329–332, 1984.

79. Zaritsky A, Chernow B: Use of catecholamines in pediatrics. *J Pediatr* 105:341–350, 1984.

80. Bollaert PE, Bauer P, Audibert G, Lambert H, Larcan A: Effects of epinephrine on hemodynamics and oxygen metabolism in dopamine-resistant septic shock. *Chest* 98:949–953, 1990.

81. Benzing G III, Helmsworth JA, Schreiber JT, Kaplan S: Nitroprusside and epinephrine for treatment of low output in children after open-heart surgery. *Ann Thorac Surg* 27:523–528, 1979.

82. Kopin I: Catecholamine metabolism: basic aspects and clinical significance. *Pharmacol Rev* 37:333–364, 1985.

83. Chernow B, Holbrook P, D'Angona DS Jr, et al: Epinephrine absorption after intratracheal administration. *Anesth Analg* 63:829–832, 1984.

84. Newton DW, Fung EYY, Williams DA: Stability of five catecholamines and terbutaline sulfate in 5% dextrose injection in the absence and presence of aminophylline. *Am J Hosp Pharm* 38:1314–1319, 1981.

85. Greenway CV, Stark RD: Hepatic vascular bed. *Physiol Rev* 51:23–65, 1971.

86. Astiz M, Tilly E, Rackow E, Weil M: Peripheral vascular tone in sepsis. *Chest* 99:1072–1075, 1991.

87. Dasta JF: Norepinephrine in septic shock: renewed interest in an old drug. *DICP* 24:153–156, 1990.

88. Desjars P, Pinaud M, Bugnon D, Tasseau F: Norepinephrine therapy has no deleterious renal effects in human septic shock. *Crit Care Med* 17:426–429, 1989.

89. Fukuoka T, Nishimura M, Imanaka H, Taenaka N, Yoshiya I, Takezawa J: Effects of norepinephrine on renal function in septic patients with normal and elevated serum lactate levels. *Crit Care Med* 17:1104–1107, 1989.

90. Saux MP, Eon B, Aknin P, Gouin F: Septic shock: a goal-directed therapy using volume loading, dobutamine and/or norepinephrine. *Acta Anaesth Scand* 34:413–417, 1990.

91. Mueller H, Ayres SM, Gregory JJ, et al: Hemodynamics, coronary blood flow and myocardial metabolism in coronary shock: response to *l*-norepinephrine and isoproterenol. *J Clin Invest* 49:1885–1902, 1970.

92. Passmore JM, Goldstein RA: Acute recognition and management of congestive heart failure. *Crit Care Clin* 5:497–532, 1989.

93. Douglas HO Jr: Levarterenol irrigation: control of massive gastrointestinal bleeding in poor risk patients. *JAMA* 230:1653–1657, 1974.

94. Schaer GL, Fink MP, Parillo JE: Norepinephrine alone versus norepinephrine plus low-dose dopamine: enhanced renal blood flow with combination pressor therapy. *Crit Care Med* 13:492–496, 1985.

95. FitzGerald GA, Hossmann V, Hamilton CA, Reid JL, Davies DS, Dollery CT: Interindividual variation in kinetics of infused norepinephrine. *Clin Pharmacol Ther* 26:669–675, 1979.

96. Hoffman BB, Lefkowitz RJ: Catecholamines and sympathomimetics. In: Gilman AG, et al (eds): *Goodman and Gilman's The Pharmacologic Basis of Therapeutics.* New York, Pergamon Press, 1990, pp 187–220.

97. Halloway EL, Stinson EB, Derby GC, Harrison DC: Action of drugs in patients early after cardiac surgery. I. Comparison of isoproterenol and dopamine. *Am J Cardiol* 35:656–659, 1975.

98. Driscoll DJ, Gillette PC, Fukushige J, et al: Comparison of the cardiovascular action of isoproterenol, dopamine and dobutamine in the neonatal and mature dog. *Pediatr Cardiol* 1:307–312, 1980.

99. Gazioglu K, Condemi JJ, Hyde RW, Kaltreider NL: Effect of isoproterenol on gas exchange during air and oxygen breathing in patients with asthma. *Am J Med* 50:185–190, 1971.

100. Furman WR, Summer WR, Kennedy TP, Sylvester JT: Comparison of the effects of dobutamine, dopamine, and isoproterenol on hypoxic pulmonary vasoconstriction in the pig. *Crit Care Med* 10:371–374, 1982.

101. Lekven J, Kjekshun JK, Mjös OD: Cardiac effects of isoproterenol during graded myocardial ischemia. *J Clin Lab Invest* 33:161–171, 1974.

102. Porte D Jr: Sympathetic regulation of insulin secretion. *Arch Intern Med* 123:252–260, 1969.

103. Anonymous: Standards and guidelines for cardiopulmonary resuscitation and emergency cardiac care. *JAMA* 255:2841–2989, 1986.

104. Anonymous: Fluid therapy and medications. In: Chameides L (ed): *Textbook of Pediatric Advanced Life Support.* Dallas, TX, American Heart Association, 1988, pp 47–59.

105. Herman JJ, Noah ZL, Moody RR: Use of intravenous isoproterenol for status asthmaticus in children. *Crit Care Med* 11:716–720, 1983.

106. Lupi-Herrera E, Sandoval J, Seonane M, Bialostozky K, Attie F: The role of isoproterenol in the preoperative evaluation of high-pressure, high-resistance ventricular septal defect. *Chest* 81:42–46, 1982.

107. Kirklin JK, Kirklin JW: Management of the cardiovascular subsystem after cardiac surgery. *Ann Thorac Surg* 32:311–319, 1980.

108. Goldstein DS, Simlichman R, Stull R, Keiser HR: Plasma catecholamine and hemodynamic response during isoproterenol infusions in humans. *Clin Pharmacol Ther* 40:233–238, 1986.

109. Raper R, Fisher M, Bihari D: Profound, reversible myocardial depression in acute asthma treated with high-dose catecholamines. *Crit Care Med* 20:710–712, 1992.

110. Maguire JF, O'Rourke PP, Colan SD, Geha RS, Crone R: Cardiotoxicity during treatment of severe childhood asthma. *Pediatrics* 88:1180–1186, 1991.

111. Lackovic A, Relja M: Evidence for a widely distributed peripheral dopaminergic system. *Fed Proc* 42:3000–3004, 1983.

112. Dinerstein RJ, Jones RT, Goldberg LI: Evidence for dopamine-containing renal nerves. *Fed Proc* 42:3005–3008, 1983.

113. Sowers JR, Brickman AS, Sowers DK, Berg G: Dopaminergic modulation of aldosterone secretion in man is unaffected by glucocorticoids and angiotensin blockage. *J Clin Endocrinol Metab* 52:1078–1083, 1981.

114. Schwartz LB, Gewertz BL: The renal response to low dose dopamine. *J Surg Res* 45:574–588, 1988.

115. Goldberg LI, Hsieh Y-Y, Resnekov L: Newer catecholamines for treatment of heart failure and shock: an update on dopamine and a first look at dobutamine. *Prog Cardiovasc Dis* 19:327–340, 1977.

116. Brodde O-E: Vascular dopamine receptors: demonstration and characterization by in vitro studies. *Life Sci* 31:289–306, 1982.

117. Driscoll DJ, Gillette PC, Ezrailson EG: Inotropic responses of the neonatal canine myocardium to dopamine. *Pediatr Res* 12:42–45, 1978.

118. Kho TL, Henquet JW, Punt R, Birkenhäger WH, Rahn KH: Influence of dobutamine and dopamine on hemodynamics and plasma concentrations of noradrenaline and renin in patients with low cardiac output following acute myocardial infarction. *Eur J Clin Pharmacol* 18:213–217, 1980.

119. Stopfkuchen H, Rackë K, Schwörer H, Queisser-Luft A, Vogel K: Effects of dopamine infusion on plasma catecholamines in preterm and term newborn infants. *Eur J Pediatr* 150:503–506, 1991.

120. Loeb HS, Bredakis J, Gunnar RM: Superiority of dobutamine over dopamine for augmentation of cardiac output in patients with chronic low output cardiac failure. *Circulation* 55:375–381, 1977.

121. Chidsey CA, Braunwald E, Morrow AG, Mason DT: Myocardial norepinephrine concentration in man. Effects of reserpine and of congestive heart failure. *N Engl J Med* 269:653–658, 1963.

122. Robie NW, Goldberg LI: Comparative systemic and regional hemodynamic effects of dopamine and dobutamine. *Am Heart J* 90:340–345, 1975.

123. Vincent JL: Do we need a dopaminergic agent in the management of the critically ill? *J Auton Pharmacol* 10(suppl 1):S123–S127, 1990.

124. Holloway EL, Palumbo RA, Harrison DC: Acute circulatory effects of dopamine in patients with pulmonary hypertension. *Br Heart J* 37:482–485, 1975.

125. Stephenson LW, Edmunds LH Jr, Raphaely R, Morrison DF, Hoffman WS, Rubis LJ: Effects of nitroprusside and dopamine on pulmonary arterial vasculature in children after cardiac surgery. *Circulation* 60(suppl I):I104–I110, 1979.

126. Mentzer RM Jr, Alegre CA, Nolan SP: The effects of dopamine and isoproterenol on the pulmonary circulation. *J Thorac Cardiovasc Surg* 71:807–814, 1976.

127. Lang P, Williams RG, Norwood WI, Castaneda AR: The hemodynamic effects of dopamine in infants after corrective cardiac surgery. *J Pediatr* 96:630–644, 1980.

128. Marino RJ, Romagnoli A, Keats AS: Selective venoconstriction by dopamine in comparison with isoproterenol and phenylephrine. *Anesthesiology* 43:570–572, 1975.

129. Fowler MB, Alderman EL, Oesterle SN, et al: Dobutamine and dopamine after cardiac surgery: greater augmentation of myocardial blood flow with dobutamine. *Circulation* 70(suppl I):I103–I111, 1984.

130. Whitfield L, Sowers JR, Tuck ML, Golub MS: Dopaminergic control of plasma catecholamine and aldosterone response to acute stimuli in normal man. *J Clin Endocrinol Metab* 51:724–729, 1980.

131. Leebaw W, Lee L, Woolf P: Dopamine affects basal and augmented pituitary hormone secretion. *J Clin Endocrinol Metab* 47:480–486, 1978.

132. Zern RT, Foster LB, Blalock JA, et al: Characteristics of the dopaminergic and noradrenergic systems of the pancreatic islets. *Diabetes* 28:185–189, 1979.

133. Mueller HS, Evans DR, Ayres SM: Effect of dopamine on hemodynamics and myocardial metabolism in shock following acute myocardial infarction in man. *Circulation* 57:361–365, 1978.

134. Maekawa K, Liang C-S, Hood WB Jr: Comparison of dobutamine and dopamine in acute myocardial infarction. *Circulation* 67:750–759, 1983.

135. Arnold JMO, Braunwald E, Sandor T, Kloner RA: Inotropic stimulation of reperfused myocardium with dopamine: effects on infarct size and myocardial function. *J Am Coll Cardiol* 6:1026–1034, 1985.

136. Holzer J, Karliner JS, O'Rourke RA, Pitt W, Ross J Jr: Effectiveness of dopamine in patients with cardiogenic shock. *Am J Cardiol* 32:79–84, 1973.

137. Richard C, Ricome JL, Rimailho A, Bottineau G, Auzepy P: Combined hemodynamic effects of dopamine and dobutamine in cardiogenic shock. *Circulation* 67:620–626, 1983.

138. Jardin F, Eveleigh MC, Gurdjian F, Margairaz A: Venous admixture in human septic shock. *Circulation* 60:155–159, 1978.

139. Shoemaker WC, Appel PL, Kram HB: Oxygen transport measurements to evaluate tissue perfusion and titrate therapy: dobutamine and dopamine effects. *Crit Care Med* 19:672–688, 1991.

140. Trigt PV, Spray TL, Pasque MK, et al: The influence of time on the response to dopamine after coronary artery bypass grafting: assessment of left ventricular performance and contractility using pressure/dimension analyses. *Ann Thorac Surg* 35:3–13, 1983.

141. Trigt PV, Spray TL, Pasque MK, Peyton RB, Pellom GL, Wechsler AS: The comparative effects of dopamine and dobutamine on ventricular mechanics after coronary artery bypass grafting: a pressure dimension analysis. *Circulation* 70(suppl I):I112–I117, 1984.

142. DiSesa VJ, Brown E, Mudge GH Jr, Collins JJ Jr, Cohn LH: Hemodynamic comparison of dopamine and dobutamine in the postoperative volume-loaded, pressure-loaded, and normal ventricle. *Thorac Cardiovasc Surg* 83:256–263, 1982.

143. Schreuder WO, Schneider AJ, Groeneveld AB, Thijs LG: Effect of dopamine vs norepinephrine on hemodynamics in septic shock. Emphasis on right ventricular performance. *Chest* 95:1282–1288, 1989.

144. Regnier B, Kapin M, Gory G, Lemaire F, Teisseire B, Harari A: Hemodynamic effects of dopamine in septic shock. *Intensive Care Med* 3:47–53, 1977.

145. Wilson RF, Sibbald WJ, Jaanimagi JL: Hemodynamic effects of dopamine in critically ill septic patients. *J Surg Res* 20:163–172, 1976.

146. De La Cal MA, Miravalles E, Pascual T, Esteban A, Ruiz-Santana S: Dose-related hemodynamic and renal effects of dopamine in septic shock. *Crit Care Med* 12:22–25, 1984.

147. Ruokonen E, Takala J, Usaro A: Effect of vasoactive treatment on the relationship between mixed venous and regional oxygen saturation. *Crit Care Med* 19:1365–1369, 1991.

148. Davis RF, Lappas DG, Kirklin JK, Buckley MJ: Acute oliguria after cardiopulmonary bypass: renal functional improvement with low-dose dopamine infusion. *Crit Care Med* 10:852–856, 1982.

149. Hasselgren P-O, Biber B, Fornander J: Improved blood flow and protein synthesis in the postischemic liver following infusion of dopamine. *J Surg Res* 34:44–52, 1983.

150. Polson RJ, Park GR, Lindop MJ, Farman JV, Calne RY, Williams R: The prevention of renal impairment in patients undergoing orthotopic liver grafting by infusion of low dose dopamine. *Anaesthesia* 42:15–19, 1987.

151. Notterman DA, Greenwald BM, Moran F, DiMaio HA, Metakis L, Reidenberg MM: Dopamine clearance in critically ill infants and children: effect of age and organ system dysfunction. *Clin Pharmacol Ther* 48:138–147, 1990.

152. Banner W Jr, Vernon DD, Dean JM, Swenson E: Nonlinear dopamine pharmacokinetics in pediatric patients. *J Pharmacol Exp Ther* 249:131–133, 1989.

153. Jarnberg PO, Bengtsson L, Edstrand J, Hamberger B: Dopamine infusion in man. Plasma catecholamine levels and pharmacokinetics. *Acta Anaesth Scand* 25:328–331, 1981.

154. Guller B, Fields AI, Coleman MG, Holbrook PR: Changes in cardiac rhythm in children treated with dopamine. *Crit Care Med* 6:151–154, 1978.

155. Golbranson FL, Lurie L, Vance RM, Vandell RF: Multiple extremity amputations in hypotensive patients with dopamine. *JAMA* 243:1145–1146, 1980.

156. Siwy BK, Sadove AM: Acute management of dopamine infiltration injury with regitine. *Plast Reconstr Surg* 80:610–612, 1987.

157. Tuttle RR, Mills J: Dobutamine: Development of a new catecholamine to selectively increase cardiac contractility. *Circ Res* 36:185–196, 1975.

158. Ruffolo RR Jr: Review: the pharmacology of dobutamine. *Am J Med Sci* 294:244–248, 1987.

159. Ruffolo RR Jr, Yaden EL: Vascular effects of the stereoisomers of dobutamine. *J Pharmacol Exp Ther* 224:46–50, 1983.

160. Liang CS, Hood WB: Dobutamine infusion in conscious dogs with and without autonomic nervous system inhibition: effects of systemic hemodynamics, regional blood flows and cardiac metabolism. *J Pharmacol Exp Ther* 211:698–705, 1979.

161. Murphy PJ, Williams GL, Kau DLK: Disposition of dobutamine in the dog. *J Pharmacol Exp Ther* 199:423–431, 1976.

162. Ruffolo RR Jr, Messick K, Horng JS: Interactions of the enantiomers of 3-O-methyldobutamine with α- and β-adrenoceptors in vitro. *Nauyn Schmeidebergs Arch Pharmacol* 329:244–252, 1985.

163. Leier CV, Unverferth DV: Dobutamine. *Ann Intern Med* 99:490–496, 1983.

164. Jardin F, Sportiche M, Bazin M, Bourokba A, Margairaz A: Dobutamine: a hemodynamic evaluation in human septic shock. *Crit Care Med* 9:329–332, 1981.

165. Leier CV, Hebran PT, Huss P, Bush CA, Lewis RP: Comparative systemic and regional hemodynamic effects of dopamine and dobutamine in patients with cardiomyopathic heart failure. *Circulation* 58:466–475, 1978.

166. Banner W Jr, Vernon DD, Minton SD, Dean JM: Nonlinear dobutamine pharmacokinetics in a pediatric population. *Crit Care Med* 19:871–873, 1991.

167. Schwartz PH, Eldadah MK, Newth CJ: The pharmacokinetics of dobutamine in pediatric intensive care unit patients. *Drug Metab Dispos* 19:614–619, 1991.

168. Kates RE, Leier CV: Dobutamine pharmacokinetics in severe heart failure. *Clin Pharmacol Ther* 24:537–541, 1978.

169. Unverferth DV, Blanford M, Kates RE, Leier CV: Tolerance to dobutamine after a 72 hour continuous infusion. *Am J Med* 69:262–266, 1980.

170. MacCannell KL, Giraud GD, Hamilton PL, Groves G: Haemodynamic responses to dopamine and dobutamine infusions as a function of duration of infusion. *Pharmacology* 26:26–39, 1983.

171. Bhatt-Mehta V, Nahata MC: Dopamine and dobutamine in pediatric therapy. *Pharmacotherapy* 9:303–314, 1989.

172. Stopfkuchen H, Schranz D, Huth R, Jüngst B-K: Effects of dobutamine on left ventricular performance in newborns as determined by systolic time intervals. *Eur J Pediatr* 146:135–139, 1987.

173. Andy JJ, Curry CL, Ali N, Mehratra PP: Cardiovascular effects of dobutamine in severe congestive heart failure. *Am Heart J* 94:175–182, 1977.

174. Colucci WS, Wright RF, Jaski BE, Fifer MA, Braunwald E: Milrinone and dobutamine in severe heart failure: differing hemodynamic effects and individual patient responsivenes. *Circulation* 73(suppl III):III175–III183, 1986.

175. Magorien RD, Unverferth DV, Brown GP, Leier CV: Dobutamine and hydralazine: comparative influences on positive inotropy and vasodilation on coronary blood flow and myocardial energetics in nonischemic congestive heart failure. *J Am Coll Cardiol* 1:499–505, 1983.

176. Liang C-S, Sherman LG, Doherty JU, Wellington K, Lee VW, Hood WB Jr: Sustained improvement in patients with congestive heart failure after short-term infusion of dobutamine. *Circulation* 69:113–119, 1984.

177. Applefeld MM, Newman KA, Grove WR, et al: Intermittent, continuous outpatient dobutamine infusion in the management of congestive heart failure. *Am J Cardiol* 51:455–458, 1983.

178. Unverferth DV, Magorien RD, Altschuld R, Kolibash AJ, Lewis RP, Leier CV: The hemodynamic and metabolic advantages gained by a three-day infusion of dobutamine in patients with congestive cardiomyopathy. *Am Heart J* 106:29–34, 1983.

179. Renard M, Bernard R: Clinical and hemodynamic effects of dobutamine in acute myocardial infarction with left heart failure. *J Cardiovasc Pharmacol* 2:543–552, 1980.

180. Keung ECH, Siskind SJ, Sonnenblick EH, Ribner HS, Schwartz WJ, LeJemtel TH: Dobutamine therapy in acute myocardial infarction. *JAMA* 245:144–146, 1981.

181. Francis GS, Sharma B, Hodges M: Comparative hemodynamic effects of dopamine and dobutamine in patients with acute cardiogenic circulatory collapse. *Am Heart J* 103:995–1000, 1982.

182. Gray R, Shah PK, Sing B, Conklin C, Matloff JM: Low cardiac output states after open heart surgery. Comparative hemodynamic effects of dobutamine, dopamine and norepinephrine plus phentolamine. *Chest* 80:16–22, 1981.

183. Edwards H, Olafsson O, Hyman AI, Drusin RE, Reemtsma K: Dobutamine in the rejecting transplanted heart. *Crit Care Med* 9:498–499, 1981.

184. Shoemaker WC, Appel PL, Kram HB, Duarte D, Harrier HD, Ocampo HA: Comparison of hemodynamic and oxygen transport effects of dobutamine and dopamine in critically ill surgical patients. *Chest* 96:120–126, 1989.

185. Haywood GA, Tighe D, Moss R, et al: Goal directed therapy with dobutamine in a porcine model of septic shock: effects on systemic and renal oxygen transport. *Postgrad Med J* 67(suppl 1):S36–S41, 1991.

186. Vincent JL, Roman A, Kahn RJ: Dobutamine administration in septic shock: addition to a standard protocol. *Crit Care Med* 18:689–693, 1990.

187. Knox J, Youn Y-K, Lalonde C, Demling R: Effect of dobutamine on oxygen consumption after fluid and protein losses after endotoxemia. *Crit Care Med* 19:525–531, 1991.

188. Leier CV, Unverferth DV, Kates RE: The relationship between plasma dobutamine concentrations and cardiovascular responses in cardiac failure. *Am J Med* 66:238–242, 1979.

189. Sonnenblick EH, Frishman WH, LeJental TH: Dobutamine. A new synthetic cardioactive sympathetic amine. *N Engl J Med* 300:17–22, 1979.

190. Alousi AA, Johnson DC: Pharmacology of the bipyridines: amrinone and milrinone. *Circulation* 73(suppl 3):3–10, 1986.

191. DiBianco R, Shabetai R, Kostuk W, et al: A comparison of oral milrinone, digoxin, and their combination in the treatment of patients with chronic heart failure. *N Engl J Med* 320:677–683, 1989.

192. Honerjäger P: Pharmacology of bipyridine phosphodiesterase III inhibitors. *Am Heart J* 121(part 2):1939–1944, 1991.

193. Vernon MW, Heel RC, Brogden RN: Enoximone. A review of its pharmacologic properties and therapeutic potential. *Drugs* 42:997–1017, 1991.
194. Chatterjee K: Phosphodiesterase inhibitors: alterations in systemic and coronary hemodynamics. *Basic Res Cardiol* 84(suppl 1):213–224, 1989.
195. Thompson WJ: Cyclic nucleotide phosphodiesterases: pharmacology, biochemistry and function. *Pharmacol Ther* 51:13–33, 1991.
196. Morgan JP, Gwathmey JK, DeFeo TT, Morgan KG: The effects of amrinone and related drugs on intracellular calcium in isolated mammalian cardiac and vascular smooth muscle. *Circulation* 73(suppl III):III65–III77, 1986.
197. Hayes J, Bowling N, Boden G, Kauffman R: Molecular basis for the cardiovascular activities of amrinone and AR-L57. *J Pharmacol Exp Ther* 230:124–132, 1984.
198. Meisheri KD, Plamer RF, van Breemen C: The effects of amrinone on contractility, Ca² uptake ←and cAMP in smooth muscle. *Eur J Pharmacol* 61:159–165, 1980.
199. Zannad F, Juillere Y, Royer RF: The effects of amrinone on cardiac function, oxygen consumption and lactate production of an isolated, perfused, working guinea-pig heart. *Arch Int Pharmacodyn Ther* 263:264–271, 1983.
200. Benotti JR, Grossman W, Braunwald E, Davolos DD: Hemodynamic assessment of a new inotropic agent. *N Engl J Med* 299:1373–1377, 1978.
201. Prielipp RC, Butterworth JF IV, Zaloga GP, Robertie PG, Royster RL: Effects of amrinone on cardiac index, venous oxygen saturation and venous admixture in patients recovering from cardiac surgery. *Chest* 99:820–825, 1991.
202. Benotti JR, Grossman W, Braunwald E, Carabello BL: Effects of amrinone on myocardial energy metabolism and hemodynamics in patients with severe congestive heart failure due to coronary disease. *Circulation* 62:28–34, 1980.
203. Baim D: Effects of amrinone on myocardial energetics in severe congestive heart failure. *Am J Cardiol* 56:16B–18B, 1985.
204. Binah O, Sodowick B, Vulliemoz Y, Danilo P Jr, Rosen M: The inotropic effects of amrinone and milrinone on neonatal and young canine cardiac muscle. *Circulation* 73(suppl III):III46–III51, 1986.
205. Ross-Ascuitto N, Ascuitto R, Chen V, Downing SE: Negative inotropic effects of amrinone in the neonatal piglet heart. *Circ Res* 61:847–852, 1987.
206. Binah O, Legato MJ, Danilo P Jr, Rosen MR: Developmental changes in the cardiac effects of amrinone in the dog. *Circ Res* 52:747–752, 1983.
207. Legato MJ: Cellular mechanisms of normal growth in the mammalian heart. II. A quantitative and qualitative comparison between the right and left ventricular myocytes in the dog from birth to five months of life. *Circ Res* 44:263–279, 1979.
208. Rosenthal JE, Ferrier GR: Inotropic and electrophysiologic effects of amrinone on untreated and digitalized ventricular tissues. *J Pharmacol Exp Ther* 221:188–196, 1982.
209. Ward A, Brogden RN, Heel RC, Speight TM, Avery GS: Amrinone: a preliminary review of its pharmacological properties and therapeutic use. *Drugs* 26:468–502, 1983.
210. Edelson J, LeJemtel TH, Alousi AA, Biddlecome CE, Maskin CS, Sonneblick EH: Relationship between amrinone plasma concentration and cardiac index. *Clin Pharmacol Ther* 29:723–728, 1981.
211. Edelson J, Stroshane R, Benziger DP, et al: Pharmacokinetics of the bipyridines amrinone and milrinone. *Circulation* 73(suppl III):III145–III152, 1986.
212. Lawless S, Burckart G, Diven W, Thompson A, Siewers R: Amrinone in neonates and infants after cardiac surgery. *Crit Care Med* 17:751–754, 1989.
213. Lawless ST, Zaritsky A, Miles M: The acute pharmacokinetics and pharmacodynamics of amrinone in pediatric patients. *J Clin Pharmacol* 31:800–803, 1991.
214. Goldstein RA: Clinical effects of intravenous amrinone in patients with congestive heart failure. *Circulation* 73(suppl III):III191–III195, 1986.
215. Evans DB: Overview of cardiovascular physiologic and pharmacologic aspects of selective phosphodiesterase peak III inhibitors. *Am J Cardiol* 63:9A–11A, 1989.
216. Gunnicker M, Hess W: Preliminary results with amrinone in perioperative low cardiac output syndrome. *Thorac Cardiovasc Surg* 35:219–225, 1987.
217. Schmitz W, von der Leyen H, Meyer W, Neumann J, Scholz H: Phosphodiesterase inhibition and positive inotropic effects. *J Cardiovasc Pharmacol* 14(suppl 3):S11–S14, 1989.
218. Vincent J-L, Domb M, Van der Linden P, et al: Amrinone administration in endotoxic shock. *Circ Shock* 25:75–83, 1988.
219. Giroir BP, Beutler B: Effect of amrinone on tumor necrosis factor production in endotoxic shock. *Circ Shock* 36:200–207, 1992.
220. Jaski BE, Fifer MA, Wright RF, Braunwald E, Colucci WS: Positive inotropic and vasodilator actions of milrinone in patients with severe congestive heart failure. Dose-response relationship and comparison to nitroprusside. *J Clin Invest* 75:643–649, 1985.
221. Olsen KH, Kluger J, Fieldman A: Combination high dose amrinone and dopamine in the management of moribund cardiogenic shock after open heart surgery. *Chest* 94:503–506, 1988.
222. Bailey JM, Levy J, Rogers G, Szlam F, Hug CC Jr: Pharmacokinetics of amrinone during cardiac surgery. *Anesthesiology* 75:961–968, 1991.
223. Treadway G: Clinical safety of intravenous amrinone-A review. *Am J Cardiol* 56:39B–40B, 1985.
224. Kullberg MP, Freeman GB, Biddlecome C, Alousi AA, Edelson J: Amrinone metabolism. *Clin Pharmacol Ther* 29:394–401, 1981.

CHAPTER 25

Antihypertensive Therapy

MICHAEL G. ZIEGLER, M.D.
PABLO F. RUIZ-RAMON, M.D.

Hypertension is the most common chronic illness of industrialized societies. Hypertensives develop critical cerebrovascular and cardiovascular disease at a much higher rate than normal subjects, thus, patients arriving at intensive care units frequently have received antihypertensive drugs (Table 25.1). These drugs alter cardiovascular responses to severe illness and may diminish the ability to maintain the circulation during shock. Many other common drugs, such as caffeine, ethanol, nicotine, over-the-counter decongestants, diet pills, and recreational drugs, alter blood pressure and are considered in this chapter. Food is also an important determinant of blood pressure, especially in patients dependent on intravenous nutrition. The interaction of all of these chemicals is a complex but important facet of the regulation of the cardiovascular system.

NUTRITIONAL PHARMACOLOGY OF HYPERTENSION

Diet is not an alternative usually considered in the drug therapy of hypertension, but dietary factors have potent effects on blood pressure and interact with antihypertensive drugs. Dietary manipulations alone can often provide effective therapy of hypertension and may be prescribed in place of antihypertensive medication. The most important dietary factors are caloric intake, ethanol, sodium, potassium, calcium, and tyrosine.

CALORIC INTAKE

Carbohydrate ingestion increases sympathetic nervous system activity, whereas consumption of protein or fat has little acute effect (1). When obese adults are switched from a 2600-kcal/day diet to a 600-kcal/day diet, they have a 40% decrease in the urinary excretion of 3-methoxy-4-hydroxymandelic acid, a metabolite of norepinephrine (2). The acute effects of carbohydrate ingestion on sympathetic nervous activity may be mediated by insulin, since maintenance of a constant serum insulin level prevents the carbohydrate-associated increase in circulating norepinephrine (3). All antihypertensive drugs have direct or indirect influences onthe sympathetic nervous system, and carbohydrate ingestion can alter the effect of these drugs.

Obesity has chronic effects on the sympathetic and cardiovascular systems (4). Obesity augments cardiac output, stroke volume, left ventricular filling pressure, and intravascular volume, and lowers total peripheral resistance. Obesity is strongly associated with hypertension. Sixty-two percent of hypertensive subjects are more than 20% overweight. Weight loss can decrease or cure hypertension (5). The effect of weight reduction on blood pressure reduction can be greater than the effect of drug therapy (6). The hyperinsulinemia of obesity promotes sodium retention (7) and sympathetic neuronal overactivity.

Fasting lowers blood pressure by decreasing sympathetic nervous activity and by activating an opiate-mediated vasodepressor response (8). After 8 to 12 weeks of a low calorie diet,

Table 25.1. Antihypertensive Therapies

Nutritional
    Weight loss
    Sodium restriction
    Ethanol restriction
    Potassium
    Calcium
Diuretics
    Thiazides
    Loop diuretics
    Potassium-sparing diuretics
Sympatholytics
    α-Adrenergic Receptor Blockers
        Phenoxybenzamine
        Phentolamine
        Prazosin
        Terazosin
        Doxazosin
    β-Adrenergic Receptor Blockers
        Atenolol
        Metoprolol
        Nadolol
        Propranolol
        Timolol
        Acebutolol
        Labetalol
        Penbutolol
        Betaxolol
        Dilevalol
        Carteolol
        Esmolol
    α_2-Adrenergic receptor agonists
        Clonidine
        Guanabenz
        Methyldopa
        Guanfacine
Vasodilators
    Diazoxide
    Hydralazine
    Minoxidil
    Nitroprusside
    Nitroglycerin
Calcium channel blockers
    Nifedipine
    Diltiazem
    Verapamil
    Nicardipine
    Felodipine
Converting-enzyme inhibitors
    Captopril
    Enalapril
    Lisinopril
    Fosinopril
    Benazapril
    Ramipril

plasma renin activity and aldosterone levels both decrease, irrespective of sodium intake (9). Thus, weight loss reduces plasma insulin, norepinephrine, renin, and aldosterone levels, and cardiac output, all of which lower blood pressure.

The average hypertensive can expect to decrease systolic blood pressure by 1 mm Hg and diastolic pressure by 3/4 mm Hg for every pound lost. As long as the weight is not gained back, there is no evidence of any rebound in blood pressure; thus, the cure of a patient's obesity may simultaneously cure hypertension.

Diet has short-term effects on blood pressure as well. If dietary intake is less than 600 kcal/day, starvation ketosis causes natriuresis and hypotension. Carbohydrate consumption increases sympathetic nervous activity, but foods rich in the amino acid tyrosine may increase central norepinephrine release and, thereby, act to decrease peripheral sympathetic tone (10).

ETHANOL

The consumption of more than three alcoholic drinks daily is associated with an increase in mean blood pressure and in the incidence of hypertension. Approximately 5% of the hypertension encountered in the U.S. may be attributed to alcohol consumption. Surprisingly, the incidence of myocardial infarction decreases with increasing alcohol ingestion, even in the face of increased blood pressure; however, stroke is more common in alcoholics. Moderate doses of ethanol increase plasma renin activity, plasma aldosterone, and cortisol (11). Extremely high doses of ethanol may acutely activate central enkephalin neurons and lower blood pressure (12). The acutely ill patient in an alcoholic coma is usually hypotensive while intoxicated. As time progresses, blood pressure in this intoxicated patient can be expected to increase, frequently into the hypertensive range, as the patient undergoes alcohol withdrawal.

SODIUM

Patients with malignant hypertension reduce their blood pressure dramatically by eating a 10-mEq/day sodium diet (13). However, an increase in sodium from 10 to 35 mEq/day increases the blood pressure almost to pretreatment levels (14). The value of moderate sodium restriction has been contested, but controlled studies of moderate sodium restriction in hypertension show a decrease in mean blood pressure of about 7 mm Hg (15) and a marked decrease in the requirement for antihypertensive medications (16). A similar decrement in blood pressure occurs in hospitalized patients who receive a 35-mEq/day sodium diet (17). Moderate sodium restriction can control mild hypertension, but severe hypertension requires severe sodium restriction for blood pressure control. The change in blood pressure that occurs with sodium restriction is acutely related to a change in plasma volume (17).

DIURETICS

THIAZIDES

Thiazide diuretics are first-line drugs for some subgroups of patients with essential hypertension. Thiazides are also used in edematous states, idiopathic hypercalciuria, and diabetes insipidus. Initially, thiazide therapy decreases blood volume and cardiac output. During chronic treatment these parameters return to normal, however, and blood pressure falls as peripheral vascular resistance decreases (18). The antihypertensive effects of thiazide diuretics can be negated by a large salt intake or infusion of saline, although a similar increase in blood volume via a dextran infusion fails to increase blood pressure (19). Thiazides cause an increase in renin, aldosterone, and sympathetic nervous system activity (20), which may prevent a decrease in blood pressure. Patients who fail to respond to thiazides because of compensatory homeostatic mechanisms are especially prone to the antihypertensive effect of sympatholytic drugs (21). Other patients do not respond to thiazides because they eat or retain too much salt. Obese, African-American, and elderly hypertensives respond favorably to thiazides.

Thiazide diuretics are similar, except for their varying duration of action. Current doses of diuretics used to treat hypertension are excessive. Treatment with 12.5 mg of hydrochlorothiazide (22) and 25 mg of chlorthalidone (23) lowers blood pressure maximally in patients with normal renal function. The thiazides are not very effective at glomerular filtration rates less than 35 ml/min, and patients with a glomerular filtration rate between 35 and 70 ml/min often require higher doses of diuretic. Metolazone is the only exception, having activity at glomerular filtration rates as low as 10 ml/min. It is best to use the lowest effective dose to treat hypertension because deleterious side effects multiply with increasing dose.

Thiazide therapy can cause a decrease in serum potassium and magnesium concentrations and an increase in serum glucose, triglyceride, uric acid, and calcium concentrations. Hypokalemic alkalosis may develop with chronic therapy. Thiazides increase serum cholesterol values by increasing low-density lipoprotein levels without causing a similar increase in high-density lipoproteins. The hypercholesterolemia is most prominent in men and postmenopausal women, and it is feared that these changes might underlie an increased mortality rate in patients receiving thiazides (24). The hypokalemia seen after high doses of thiazides can induce ventricular arrhythmias. Hypersensitivity reactions to thiazides are similar to those reactions secondary to the sulfonamides and include photosensitivity rash, thrombocytopenia, leukopenia, interstitial nephritis, and pancreatitis. The effects of thiazides on calcium are beneficial in the elderly, where the rate of bone loss and fractures is decreased (25).

Since the antihypertensive actions of thiazide diuretics take up to 3 weeks to fully manifest, they are not useful as single agents in the acute care of hypertension. The lack of initial antihypertensive efficacy is due to homeostatic mechanisms, such as an increase in norepinephrine and renin release. These mechanisms can be blocked by sympatholytic drugs, so that acute therapy with a diuretic and sympatholytic drugs or angiotensin converting enzyme (ACE) inhibitors can rapidly lower blood pressure.

Thiazides are effective as monotherapy and in combined therapy of hypertension in many patients; however, high doses worsen gout, diabetes mellitus, and hypercholesterolemia.

LOOP DIURETICS

Loop diuretics, such as furosemide, bumetanide, and ethacrynic acid, are more potent natriuretic agents than the thiazides. Furosemide decreases blood volume but not peripheral vascular resistance. Rather, it elicits a reflex increase in sympathetic nervous activity and in renin release (26, 27), which may increase peripheral vascular resistance. Renovascular resistance, however, is decreased as a result of increased local production of vasodilatory prostaglandins. If a vasodilator or

sympatholytic is given to diminish peripheral vascular resistance, then the combined effects may adequately decrease blood pressure. Loop diuretics are useful for hypertensive patients with a creatinine clearance less than 35 ml/min or in those patients who have fluid retention. Patients with malignant hypertension are often volume-depleted, so loop diuretics may impair tissue perfusion and worsen vasospasm. Nonsteroidal antiinflammatory agents decrease the natriuretic response of loop diuretics.

Unlike thiazides, loop diuretics increase calcium excretion. Hypomagnesemia and hyponatremia can occur. The same sulfa related hypersensitivity reactions seen with thiazides can occur with furosemide. Permanent or reversible ototoxicity is dose-related and can occur with the use of loop diuretics, particularly in patients with renal disease and those patients treated with other ototoxic drugs.

POTASSIUM-SPARING DIURETICS

Spironolactone, triamterene, and amiloride inhibit sodium reabsorption at the distal nephron. They inhibit potassium excretion and are often combined with thiazide diuretics to counteract hypokalemia. They have little antihypertensive effect, but they can cause hyperkalemia. Spironolactone causes gynecomastia and impotence in men and dysmenorrhea in women (28). Triamterene can cause nephrolithiasis, and when combined with indomethacin, can cause acute renal failure due to a reduction of renal vasodilatory protaglandins caused by both triamterene and indomethacin. Amiloride, however, causes an increase in renal vasodilatory prostaglandins (29).

β-ADRENERGIC RECEPTOR ANTAGONISTS

β-adrenergic receptor antagonists (β-blockers) lower blood pressure by means of several mechanisms. Cardiac output is promptly reduced, but increased peripheral vascular resistance compensates for this action. Days to weeks later, peripheral vascular resistance diminishes, almost reaching pretreatment values, and blood pressure decreases. The β-blockers inhibit renin secretion and lower blood pressure more in high-renin patients than in those patients with low renin values (30), but these agents still have some hypotensive effect in low-renin patients. The β-blockers may alter prostaglandin levels in vascular tissue, and indomethacin can diminish some of their hypotensive effects (31). Atrial natriuretic peptide increases in animals and humans given β-blockers, thereby influencing renal excretion of sodium (32, 33). In animals, the β-blockers enhance the central release of norepinephrine, which diminishes peripheral sympathetic tone. They also increase baroreflex sensitivity (34). Some β-blockers cause renal vasoconstriction, while others cause renal vasodilation (35). β-blockers lower blood pressure by causing a reduction in cardiac output and renin release. It is unclear how important prostaglandins, the central nervous system, and intrarenal effects are in lowering blood pressure.

The effectiveness of β-blocker therapy depends on the patient's age, race, renin status, and duration of hypertension. Patients with high plasma renin levels have the greatest hypotensive response to β-blocker therapy. Although this effect is statistically significant, it is not sufficiently striking to justify the use of renin-sodium classification in individual hypertensives (36). Both cardiac chronotropic and inotropic responsiveness to β-stimulation diminishes with age (37), and β-blockade has less of a cardiac effect in the elderly than in the young. The net effect is that β-blockers work less well to lower blood pressure in the elderly than in the young but can be more dangerous in the elderly since they may accentuate heart block and bronchospasm. In contrast, young patients with recent onset of hypertension tend to have a hyperdynamic cardiac output and have hypertension based more on increased cardiac output than on increased peripheral vascular resistance. These young hypertensives respond very well to β-blockade (38).

African-American hypertensives respond poorly to β-blockade. A group of African-American patients who had a decrease in mean blood pressure of 14 mm Hg with diuretic therapy had only a 5 mm Hg blood pressure decrease in response to β-blockade (39). Combination therapy with a β-blocker and low-dose diuretic, however, is still more efficacious than high-dose diuretic therapy alone in this group of patients (40). Hollifield and associates (41) reported that when *low-dose* propranolol fails to work, propranolol doses in the range of 320 to 960 mg/day diminish blood pressure. However, other investigators found that 80 mg of propranolol per day was as effective as 480 mg/day. It is not clear whether extremely high doses of β-blockers provide any additional hypotensive effect, but they do increase side effects and cost.

β-blocking drugs differ in their receptor affinity and pharmacokinetic properties (Table 20.2). Propranolol has a half-life of only 3 to 6 hours, but its effect persists with once-daily dosing (42), with fewer nighttime side effects. Propranolol blocks both $β_1$- and $β_2$-adrenergic receptors. The $β_1$-receptors mediate cardiac effects (Table 20.3), and $β_2$-receptors mediate bronchodilation and arteriolar dilation. A variety of other effects, including renin release, are influenced by both types of receptors (Table 20.4). Atenolol, metoprolol, acebutolol, and betaxolol are $β_1$-selective and thus are less likely to block β-adrenergic bronchodilation or vasodilation. Their cardioselectivity is not absolute, however, and in the higher dose range these agents can cause broncho-constriction. When a β-blocking agent is necessary in the treatment of a patient with bronchospasm or an insulin-dependent diabetic (43), $β_1$-selective agents are safer than nonselective agents. However, β-blockers should not be used at all in these patients unless absolutely necessary. Atenolol and metoprolol can be successfully used with $β_2$-agonist agents, and newly developed β-blockers that possess $β_2$-agonist properties may be useful in patients with bronchoconstriction.

β-blockers also differ in their fat solubility and rate of elimination (Table 20.2). Atenolol, nadolol, and carteolol are not soluble in fat and are not extensively metabolized by the liver. They do not undergo a "first pass" metabolism by the liver as rapidly as more lipophilic agents. Their longer half-lives allow once-daily dosing, but the dose needs to be adjusted in renal failure because these drugs are excreted by the kidneys. Nonlipophilic agents do not penetrate the brain very effectively. People metabolize β-blockers at very different rates, and dosage must be adjusted by clinical response. When heart rate slows and the increment in heart rate on standing decreases, β-blockade is effective. As shown in Table 20.2,

the variation in plasma levels with the same dose of drug is greatest with propranolol and tends to be less with agents that are excreted by the kidney than those medications metabolized by the liver.

The first β-blocker synthesized was dichloroisoproterenol. It was a partial β-agonist and was not used in humans because of its β-receptor stimulant activity. Pindolol, acebutolol, penbutolol, and carteolol have sympathomimetic activity since they are partial agonists as well. Dilevalol has $β_2$-selective agonist activity. These agents do not decrease resting heart rate but antagonize the increase in heart rate with exercise. Pindolol has the most intrinsic sympathomimetic activity (ISA) and is the least likely to cause heart block and bradycardia. Angina may occur in a patient abruptly changed from another β-blocker to pindolol because of its stimulant activity. Acebutolol has less intrinsic sympathomimetic activity and usually does not change heart rate (44). β-blockers with intrinsic sympathomimetic activity are less likely to increase airways resistance in patients with reactive airways disease (45).

The available β-blocking agents differ in their pharmacokinetic profile and in their $β_1$ selectivity. There is no convincing evidence that any of these agents is either more effective or associated with fewer side effects in the average hypertensive patient. However, in particular patients there are some clear advantages to specific agents. Cardioselectivity is an advantage for patients with bronchospasm or those patients who tend to develop cold hands or Raynaud's phenomenon. These drugs can also be used with $β_2$-agonist bronchodilators and are the drugs of choice when a β-blocker must be used in a patient with impaired respiratory function. The β-blockers with longer half-lives may be more useful when treating angina pectoris, but shorter-acting drugs, such as propranolol, seem equally effective for the treatment of hypertension when given once daily.

Propranolol, when given acutely or chronically, lowers both renal plasma flow and glomerular filtration rate. Nadolol, β-blockers with intrinsic sympathomimetic activity, and those drugs with vasodilating properties such as labetalol and dilevalol do not alter renal hemodynamics significantly (35). The decrease in renal blood flow with most β-blocking agents is too small to increase serum creatine and blood urea nitrogen levels and, in most cases, is of little clinical importance. β-blockers may induce hyperkalemia in patients with poor renal function. Most side effects of the different β-blocking agents are similar. In a study of 10,000 patients, propranolol worsened exercise tolerance-associated dyspnea. It tended to cause nausea and rhinorrhea early in therapy and cold hands later in therapy (46). Rhinorrhea and Raynaud's phenomenon may be less of a problem with cardioselective β-blocking drugs. Although more fat soluble drugs have easier access to the brain, lipophilicity is not clearly associated with an increase in CNS side effects (47). β-blockers may cause congestive heart failure in situations where increased sympathetic drive or tachycardia associated with restricted stroke volume compensate underlying impaired myocardial function. Although studies in animals have shown that agents with intrinsic sympathomimetic activity may be more favorable in cases of impaired cardiac function, there are few human studies (48). Bradyarrhythmias or impaired atrioventricular conduction defects may occur in patients with sick sinus syndrome or partial

Table 25.2. Properties of Oral β-Adrenergic Receptor-Blocking Drugs

Generic name: Brand name:	Propranolol Inderal	Atenolol Tenormin	Metoprolol Lopressor	Nadolol Corgard	Pindolol Visken	Timolol Blocardren	Acebutolol Sectral	Labetalol Trandate	Carteolol Cartrol	Betaxolol Kerlone	Penbutolol Levatol	Dilevalol Unicard
Oral bioavailability (%)	30	40	50	30	90	75	40	25	85	90	>95	30
Dose in hypertension (mg)	80–640	50–100	100–450	80–320	15–60	20–60	200–1200	200–2400	2.5–10	5–40	10–80	200–800
Variation in plasma levels between patients	20X[a]	4X	10X	7X	4X	7X	7X	7X	3X	2X	5X	2X
Protein-bound (%)	93	<5	12	30	60	10	25	50	25	50	95	75
Half-life (hr)	3–6	6–9	3–4	14–24	3–4	3–4	3–13	6–8	6	14–22	26	8–12
Fat solubility	+	0	+	0	+	0	0	+	0	+	+	+
Eliminated by	Liver	Kidney	Liver	Kidney	Kidney and liver	Liver	Kidney and liver	Kidney and liver	Kidney	Liver and kidney	Kidney	Kidney and liver
Membrane-stabilizing effect	++	0	±	0	+	0	+	+	0	±	±	0
Cardioselectivity	0	+	+	0	0	0	+	0	0	+	0	0
Intrinsic sympathomimetic activity	0	0	0	0	++	±	+	0	+	0	+	+(β_2)
Active metabolites	+	0	0	0	0	0	+	0	+	0	0	0
Potency (relative)	10	10	10	10	60	60	5	2	100	90	50	10

[a] x, fold increase; +, increased or present; ++, markedly increased; ±, little to none; 0, none or absent.

Table 25.3. Clinical Settings That Influence the Use of β-Adrenergic Receptor Blockers (β-Blockers)

Clinical Setting	Consideration in β-Blocker use.
Bronchospasm	Avoid β-blockers. Drugs with intrinsic sympathomimetic activity (ISA) such as pindolol and dilevalol or drugs with β₁ selectivity can be used in low doses with close monitoring.
Angina pectoris	Drugs with ISA are usually contraindicated. Labetalol may be useful in variant angina. Use other β-blockers with caution. Drugs with a short half-life need to be given frequently.
Heart failure	β-blockers are usually contraindicated.
Cardiac conduction defects	β-blockers are usually contraindicated; however, those with intrinsic sympathomimetic activity can be tried with close monitoring.
Bradycardia	β-blockers with ISA affect heart rate to a lesser extent.
Raynaud's phenomenon and peripheral vascular disease	Avoid β-blockers if possible. Drugs with ISA and β₁ selectivity better.
Insulin-dependent diabetes mellitus	β₁-selective drugs and those with ISA favored.
Pheochromocytoma	Avoid all β-blockers, except with concurrent α-blocker use.
Renal insufficiency	Use lower doses of renally excreted agents. Drugs with active metabolites may accumulate.
Depression	Avoid β-blockers if possible.
Clonidine	Enhanced rebound phenomenon with clonidine withdrawal.

Table 25.4. α-Adrenergic and β-Adrenergic Responses

Organ	Function[a]	Effect of Receptor Stimulation				
		α₁	α₂	β₁	β₁ & β₂	β₂
Blood vessels	Arteriolar tone	↑	↑	-		↓
	Venous tone	↑	↑	-		-
Heart	SA node discharge (rate)	-	-	↑		-
	Contractility	↑	-	↑		-
	Conduction velocity	-	-	↑		-
Lung	Bronchial muscle tone	-	-	-		↓
	Bronchial gland secretion	-	-	-		↑
GI tract	Peristalsis	↓	-		↓	
	Sphincter tone	↑	-		-	
	Jejunal secretion	-	↓		-	
Uterus	Muscle contraction	↑	-	-		↓
Central nervous system	Neurotransmission	↑	↓	-		-
	Pituitary ADH release	-	-	↑		-
Salivary gland	Secretion	↑	-	-		↑
Endocrine	Lipolysis	-	↓		↑	
	Insulin release	-	↓		↑	
	cAMP formation	-	-		↑	
	Fasting blood sugar	↑	-		↑	
	Renin secretion	-	↓		↑	

[a] S-A, sinoatrial; cAMP, cyclic AMP; ADH, antidiuretic hormone; ↑, increases; ↓, decreases; -, no effect.

or complete atrioventricular conduction defects. Finally, except for β-blockers with intrinsic sympathomimetic activity, most β-blockers cause an increase in blood triglyceride and a decrease in HDL-cholesterol concentrations. Table 20.3 outlines clinical situations that can influence the proper choice of a β-blocker.

β-blocking drugs should not be withdrawn abruptly in patients with angina pectoris or in those patients at risk of ventricular arrhythmias. Patients treated with β-blockers for hypertension can develop a reproducible hyperadrenergic withdrawal syndrome when abruptly withdrawn from treatment (49). Twenty-four hours after drug withdrawal, blood pressure and heart rate may increase, although hypertensive crises have not been observed. These symptoms increase to a maximum at 48 hours and disappear by 7 days. This syndrome is mediated by an increased density or sensitivity of β-receptors. Patients abruptly withdrawn from propranolol

had the highest incidence of intraoperative ischemia and arrhythmias in a large prospective study (50). When treatment was maintained until just before surgery, there was a lower incidence of these findings. In some cases, it may be necessary to continue intravenous β-blocker therapy during the immediate postoperative period. Longer-acting agents, such as atenolol, nadolol, and betaxolol, or agents with intrinsic sympathomimetic activity, such as pindolol, acebutolol, and carteolol, may be less likely to cause this syndrome. Another possible cause of the increased incidence of myocardial ischemia in this syndrome is increased platelet aggregation (50).

There are five β-blockers available for use in intravenous form: esmolol; propranolol; atenolol; metoprolol; and labetalol. Esmolol is an ultrashort-acting (half-life 9 minutes) cardioselective β-blocker without intrinsic sympathomimetic activity used primarily for control of supraventricular arrhythmias and symptomatic sinus tachycardia. It has, however, been used effectively to control postoperative hypertension (51). Labetalol is a nonselective β-blocking drug that also possesses some α-blocking activity. Dilevalol has less α-blocking effect and manifests β$_2$-selective agonist activity. Other β-blocking drugs initially increase peripheral vascular resistance, but this increased resistance is prevented by the α-blocking activity of labetalol and β$_2$-agonist properties of dilevalol (52). Labetalol is useful for the acute therapy of severe hypertension. After intravenous injection of labetalol, symptomatic postural hypotension is common. During chronic use, the drug possesses the side effects of β- and α-blockers and may cause nausea. However, labetalol is more effective than other β-blockers in lowering blood pressure, and its effects are potentiated by diuretics (53).

α-ADRENERGIC CONTROL OF BLOOD PRESSURE

The antihypertensive drugs methyldopa, clonidine, guanabenz, prazosin, terazosin, doxazosin, phenoxybenzamine, and phentolamine all act on α-adrenergic receptors. Their hypotensive effect is most easily understood in terms of their effects on various types of α-receptors with differing anatomic distribution. α$_1$ and α$_2$-receptors (previously referred to as postsynaptic and presynaptic receptors) can be distinguished by their affinity for various drugs (Table 20.5). Epinephrine and norepinephrine stimulate, while phentolamine and phenoxybenzamine block, both types of receptors. However, newer drugs such as prazosin or clonidine can selectively block α$_1$-receptors or stimulate α$_2$-receptors, respectively. Because of their specificity, these agents cause fewer side effects than nonspecific drugs. The drugs can be classified by receptor-binding affinities or physiologic effect, and these classifications agree with one another.

In the vasculature, α-receptors near noradrenergic nerve terminals are usually of the α$_1$ type, while receptors away from these terminals, but accessible to circulating catecholamines, are more often of the α$_2$ type. α-Receptors in the brain are predominantly of the α$_2$ type, although all adrenergically innervated organs have both types of receptors present.

Presynaptic α$_2$-adrenergic receptors on sympathetic nerve terminals inhibit the release of norepinephrine (54). When α$_2$- receptors on the nerves are stimulated, they antagonize calcium influx and enhance calcium efflux, thereby inhibiting further release of norepinephrine. These presynaptic α$_2$-receptors inhibit norepinephrine release from nerves in the periphery and in the brain. α$_2$-receptors in the brain are also located postsynaptically, and postsynaptic α-receptors mediate the central antihypertensive actions of clonidine and methyldopa (55).

There are two ways that α$_2$-receptors lower blood pressure. The stimulation of peripheral α$_2$-receptors inhibits norepinephrine release from sympathetic nerves (54), and stimulation of central α$_2$-receptors diminishes sympathetic activity. The central action is by far the more important, so all clonidine-like drugs have central side effects, such as sedation.

In general, peripheral α$_1$-receptors mediate vasoconstriction, and peripheral α$_2$-receptors inhibit norepinephrine release. Central α$_2$-receptors decrease sympathetic nervous system activity and enhance vagal activity (see Table 20.4). Drugs that stimulate α$_2$-receptors or block α$_1$-receptors lower blood pressure and can do so with fewer side effects than nonspecific agents.

α$_1$-ADRENERGIC RECEPTOR BLOCKERS

Prazosin is structurally related to papaverine and was first thought to act as a vasodilator. However, it fails to vasodilate vasculature that is not stimulated by α-agonists, such as norepinephrine. Prazosin, terazosin, and doxazosin block α$_1$-receptors, and this blockade is responsible for their antihypertensive efficacy. The α-blocking agents phenoxybenzamine and phentolamine have more side effects because they nonselectively block both α$_1$- and α$_2$-receptors. The nonselective blockade of α$_2$-receptors enhances norepinephrine release, which causes tachycardia and increases renin release. In contrast, selective α$_1$-blockers have little effect on heart rate or renin levels. They do not affect presynaptic α$_2$-receptors and allow them to inhibit norepinephrine release normally. α$_1$-blockers tend to improve cardiac output during exercise. They lower blood pressure by reducing systemic vascular resistance. They are relatively weak antihypertensives, and prazosin and clonidine are no more effective in combination than is clonidine alone (56).

α$_1$-Blockers preserve renal blood flow and glomerular filtration (57) and are effective in low doses in patients with renal disease. They slightly reduce total cholesterol and total triglyceride values and increase HDL-cholesterol levels and are particularly useful in treating hypertensives with lipid abnormalities (58). These agents do not affect glucose metabolism, respiratory function, or electrolytes and are safe for diabetics, asthmatics, and persons with renal insufficiency. These effects

Table 25.5. Relative Binding Affinity of Drugs for α$_1$ and α$_2$ Receptors

	Agonists	*Antagonists*	
α$_2$ ↑ ↑ ↑ ↑	Guanfacine Guanabenz Clonidine α-Methylnorepinephrine Epinephrine	Yohimbine	α$_2$ ↑ ↑ ↑ ↑
α$_1$ and α$_2$ ↓	Norepinephrine	Phentolamine Phenoxybenzamine	α$_1$ and α$_2$ ↓
α$_1$	Phenylephrine Methoxamine	Labetalol Prazosin Doxazosin Terazosin	α$_1$

Table 25.6.   Properties of Oral α₁-Adrenergic Receptor Blockers

Generic Name Brand Name	Prazosin Minipress	Terazosin Hytrin	Doxazosin Cardura
Dose (mg)	1–20 mg	1–20 mg	1–16 mg
Oral bioavailability	55%	70%	65%
Half-life, (hr)	2–3	12	22
Major route of elimination	Liver	Liver	Liver
Dosing	2–3 x/day	1–2 x/day	Daily

contrast with those properties of propranolol that include decreased renal blood flow, bronchoconstriction, and hyperlipidemia. The combination of prazosin and propranolol results in a partial amelioration of propranolol's effects on cholesterol and triglyceride levels. Unlike β-blockers, α₁-blockers are effective in all age groups and races (59).

The three currently available α₁-blockers differ in their bioavailability and half-lives, but otherwise have similar hemodynamic effects and side effect profiles (Table 20.6). Prazosin undergoes extensive hepatic inactivation such that a "first pass" effect clears almost 50% of the drug. This first pass clearance is markedly diminished in uremic patients (60), thus very small doses of prazosin (approximately one-third the usual dose) are effective in renal failure. Terazosin is more water-soluble, undergoes little first-pass effect, and has a longer half-life. Doxazosin's longer half-life is related to the slower rate of elimination by liver metabolism. The characteristics of the latter two agents allow once daily dosing.

α₁-Blockers are effective antihypertensives alone or in combination with diuretics. Their antihypertensive efficacy may diminish because of salt and water retention (61). These drugs have a pronounced effect after the first dose, but there may be a 6- to 8-week delay before prazosin affects diastolic pressure demonstrably (62). The combination of these α₁-blockers with α₂-agonists such as methyldopa or clonidine is not effective (63). A combination of α₁-blockers with β-blockers is generally effective (64).

As might be expected, prazosin is extremely effective in the treatment of hypertension due to pheochromocytoma (65). A prolonged profound response to α₁-blockers should make one suspicious of the presence of this tumor. The "first-dose effect" is the major side effect of α₁-blockers. After abrupt α-blockade, massive blood pooling in the capacitance veins leads to postural hypotension (66). This complication is dose-related. Among 74 hypertensives initially treated with a 2-mg dose of prazosin, 2 experienced syncope, and 10 others had symptoms of postural hypotension (67). First-dose syncope can be avoided by withholding diuretics the day before the first dose and administering a 1-mg capsule at bedtime (68). The first-dose effect may be slightly less dramatic with terazosin and doxazosin. The postural hypotension persists during chronic therapy but usually does not cause symptoms.

PHENOXYBENZAMINE

Phenoxybenzamine irreversibly blocks α₁- and α₂-adrenergic receptors. It is also a potent antihistamine and has a fairly weak effect on serotonin and acetylcholine receptors. Its important clinical effects are almost all related to its α-blocking activity. It is clinically related to nitrogen mustards and has a tertiary amine that forms a reactive intermediate molecule. This reactive intermediate binds with α-adrenergic receptors. Phenoxybenzamine has a relatively slow onset of action, and peak effect is not attained until an hour after IV administration due to the time required for the formation of the reactive intermediate. Weak α-adrenergic blockade may be observed for a week after the drug is discontinued. This prolonged duration of action is most likely due to the requirement for synthesis of new α-receptors to replace those receptors covalently bound to the drug. Phenoxybenzamine also inhibits the uptake of catecholamines into nerves and extraneuronal tissue.

Phenoxybenzamine blocks feedback mechanisms, increases the rate of turnover of norepinephrine, and increases the amount of norepinephrine released by each nerve impulse by blocking presynaptic α₂-receptors (69). The most striking physiologic effect is a reflex tachycardia, the result of lower blood pressure, enhanced release of norepinephrine, and decreased inactivation of norepinephrine. Impaired vasoconstriction causes postural hypotension, which becomes more pronounced during exercise or other vasodilating activities. Although phenoxybenzamine effectively lowers blood pressure, reflex responses to hypotension limit its usefulness in man. The drug can reverse the pressor effects of epinephrine by blocking its α-adrenergic effects, leaving β effects unopposed. Because of this phenomenon, phenoxybenzamine can cause hypotension during stress. The drug exaggerates the vasodepressor effects of opiates and vasodilators by preventing compensatory vasoconstriction. The α-blockade also leads to miosis, nasal stuffiness, and inhibition of ejaculation. It has CNS effects that include a characteristic loss of time perception and, in high doses, cause nausea, vomiting, hyperventilation, and even convulsions. Lower doses cause sedation and fatigue, but it is not clear if α-blocking activity induces these CNS effects since they develop and terminate more rapidly than does the peripheral α-blockade.

The major use of phenoxybenzamine is for treating hypertension caused by pheochromocytoma. Prazosin may be an equally useful α-blocker in this setting, but there is less clinical experience with prazosin. Phenoxybenzamine is available for oral use in 10-mg capsules; the IV form is available only by special arrangement with the manufacturer.

PHENTOLAMINE AND TOLAZOLINE

Phentolamine competitively blocks both α₁ and α₂-receptors. Its effects are most dramatic in patients with a pheochromocytoma. However, adequate doses of the drug have hemodynamic effects in almost all people. The blockade of vascular receptors causes vasodilation of both arterioles and veins with a prompt decrease in peripheral resistance and a decrease in blood pressure. The blockade of α_2-receptors on adrenergic nerve terminals disinhibits norepinephrine release, which stimulates β-adrenergic receptors. This β stimulation can cause tachycardia, arrhythmias, and angina. The drug probably also has nonspecific effects on serotonin, histamine, and acetylcholine receptors, which frequently lead to GI stimulation and, occasionally, stimulate salivary, lachrymal, respiratory tract, and pancreatic secretions.

Phentolamine is available in 50-mg oral tablets but is most frequently used in parenteral form, supplied in 5-mg ampules. An injected 5-mg dose dramatically decreases blood pressure in patients with pheochromocytoma or clonidine withdrawal.

Tolazoline is chemically and pharmacologically related to phentolamine. It is used in the treatment of clonidine overdose, since it blocks the α-receptors that are stimulated by clonidine and penetrates the central nervous system more easily than does phentolamine. The side effects of tolazoline are similar to those of phentolamine but tend to be more severe, since tolazoline is less specific for α-receptors than phentolamine.

CENTRALLY ACTING SYMPATHOLYTICS

This important class of antihypertensive agents includes clonidine, guanabenz, guanfacine, and α-methyldopa. Their net effect is to reduce activity of the sympathetic nervous system via stimulation of α_2-receptors. Their principal site of action is the α_2-receptors in the vasomotor centers of the medulla oblongata, particularly at the nucleus tractus solitarius. This α_2-stimulation decreases sympathetic activity, increases vagal stimulation, and lowers plasma norepinephrine, epinephrine, and renin release (70). As a result, peripheral vascular resistance at rest and with exercise is reduced. These drugs are efficacious in lowering blood pressure in all age groups and races and have little effect on lipid levels, electrolytes, or renal function. Methyldopa and clonidine may cause salt and water retention, particularly at higher doses (71). Sedation and dry mouth occur as a direct result of central α_2-stimulation and are dose-dependent. After acute withdrawal, sympathetic nervous activity increases, and plasma norepinephrine levels and blood pressure increase to pretreatment levels. Abrupt withdrawal can cause insomnia, headache, flushing, sweating, apprehension, tremulousness and, rarely, ventricular arrhythmias (72). The longer half-life of methyldopa and guanfacine diminish the severity of withdrawal. Central α-agonists have antihypertensive effects when used in combination with diuretics or vasodilators. They also appear to be effective when combined with ACE inhibitors or calcium channel blockers. In contrast, combinations with selective α_1-blockers and central sympatholytics are not as useful. There is evidence that β-blockers that penetrate the CNS, such as propranolol, may interfere with the antihypertensive effects of clonidine (73). β-blockers may also be dangerous during withdrawal of a central sympatholytic, when β-blockade allows unopposed vasoconstriction (74).

To produce hypotensive effects, clonidine must penetrate the CNS. Intravenously administered clonidine transiently increases blood pressure by stimulating peripheral α_1-receptors but subsequently causes a decrease in blood pressure that is maximal at 20 minutes and persists for many hours. The pressor phase is not seen when clonidine is given orally since peak blood levels are not reached until 90 minutes after ingestion. The drug is about 75% bioavailable with a half-life of 8 hours. Sixty percent of the drug is cleared unchanged by the kidney. The hypotensive effects of clonidine and its side effects of sedation and dry mouth follow plasma levels very closely (75). Some of clonidine's central effects may occur via release of β-endorphin (76). Naloxone reverses the antihypertensive effect of clonidine in laboratory animals and in some, but not all, human subjects. Although many people find that the sedative effects of a nighttime dose of these agents aids sleep, they produce a dose-dependent inhibition of paradoxical sleep, which may be related to nighttime hallucinations and dementia when clonidine is given to the elderly (77). Sympathetic nervous activity and blood pressure normally decrease during sleep, and clonidine further lowers sympathetic nervous system activity and blood pressure at night (78).

Clonidine is available in a transdermal formulation that has a 7-day duration of action and provides constant plasma concentrations of the drug so that side effects are less noticeable. It is also useful for treatment of hypertension in patients who cannot swallow, but there is a 2-day lag before onset of action. Withdrawal effects are virtually eliminated since it takes 3 to 4 days to clear the drug after the patch is removed. Steady-state drug concentrations are achieved after 2 days and remain constant when new patches are replaced each 7 days. Dermatologic reactions occur in about 20% of patients, ranging from skin irritation with erythema to an allergic contact dermatitis.

Clonidine progressively lowers blood pressure with increasing doses up to 0.8 mg daily, but beyond this dose range it has a U-shaped dose-response curve. In the range of 1.2 to 1.6 mg daily, clonidine begins to increase blood pressure as its peripheral vasoconstrictor effects override its central hypotensive effects (79). The withdrawal syndrome is most severe in patients taking more than 1.2 mg of oral clonidine daily (80) and seems particularly likely to occur postoperatively (80, 81). Symptoms are most marked at 24 to 72 hours after clonidine is withdrawn but then subside spontaneously (79). The clonidine withdrawal syndrome rarely occurs at doses less than 0.3 mg daily, but patients receiving doses higher than this amount should be cautioned not to stop the drug abruptly.

Oral clonidine has been recommended for treating severe hypertension (82) in a dose of 0.2 mg initially followed by 0.1 mg hourly. Since clonidine acutely decreases cardiac output and cerebral blood flow (83), there are some theoretical objections to the safety of this procedure, but clinical experience has been favorable.

Guanabenz, like clonidine, stimulates α_2-receptors and has similar blood pressure-lowering effects and side effects. Guanabenz's half-life of 6 hours is short and it can cause a withdrawal syndrome similar to that of clonidine. Guanabenz is given in a dose of 4 to 32 mg twice daily, but the highest doses may cause a pressor response and severe side effects, as with high doses of clonidine.

Guanfacine has a long half-life of 16 hours, which permits once-daily dosing of 1 to 3 mg with effective control of blood pressure. It is readily absorbed and about 30% is excreted in the urine; the rest is hepatically metabolized. Withdrawal effects are infrequent due to the longer half-life (84).

α-Methyldopa is metabolized to an α_2-agonist that has actions similar to those of clonidine. Only about one-fourth of methyldopa is absorbed unchanged, since it is metabolized in the gut wall and in the liver before gaining access to the systemic circulation. The drug is enzymatically converted to active metabolites and inhibitors of the enzymes dopa-decarboxylase and dopamine-β-hydroxylase prevent its hypotensive effects. Methyldopa is converted to α-methyldopamine, then to α-methylnorepinephrine, a potent agonist of α_2-receptors. α-Methylnorepinephrine is stored in nerve endings and released by nerve stimulation. Several hours may elapse after methyldopa is given before enough metabolite is formed to lower blood pressure. Since the body stores this active metabolite, the effect persists for as long as 24 hours, even though the half-time of elimination for plasma α-methyldopa is about 2 hours. The *O*-methylated metabolites of methyldopa may also contribute to its hypotensive action. The usual starting dose of methyldopa is 250 mg once or twice daily. This dosage can be increased to a maximum of 2.0 g/day, but most patients respond at 500 to 1000 mg daily.

Methyldopa metabolites stimulate α_2-receptors, causing side effects similar to those adverse actions of clonidine. Acute doses of methyldopa impair judgment (85) and depress behavior. The drug causes hypothermia and prolactin secretion, which may cause gynecomastia in men. It can also cause fever with or without associated transient hepatocellular dysfunction (86). In contrast to clonidine, it increases rapid eye movement sleep in humans and causes less dry mouth and bradycardia than clonidine. It is more likely than the other central sympatholytics to cause sexual dysfunction and an adverse lipid profile (87). Methyldopa also has important immunologic side effects. Twenty-five percent of patients taking 1 g of methyldopa daily for 6 months develop a positive direct Coomb's test. The drug stimulates production of IgG antibody directed at the Rh locus of the red blood cell membrane (88). The positive Coomb's test is not a contraindication to continuation of therapy; however, in somewhat less than 25% of individuals with a positive Coomb's test, a hemolytic anemia occurs. Rebound hypertension can occur after abrupt withdrawal of methyldopa (89), but this rebound is much rarer than with clonidine.

The α_2-agonists can increase blood pressure when given in doses high enough to stimulate peripheral vasoconstriction. They should not be given in higher-than-recommended doses. Methyldopa, clonidine, guanabenz, and guanfacine should not be given in combination since their α_2-stimulating activities may be addictive.

VASODILATORS

Vasodilators increase blood flow to vital organs, such as the brain and kidney; their peripheral mode of action avoids CNS side effects. When used properly, vasodilators are potent hypotensive agents. Some of these drugs can lower blood pressure to normal, even in patients with hypertension that is resistant to all other modes of therapy.

The vasodilating activity of these drugs leads to predictable side effects. Hydralazine, minoxidil, and diazoxide dilate the precapillary arterioles with little effect on postcapillary circulation or capacitance vessels. Nitroprusside has a balanced effect to dilate both arterioles and veins; whereas the nitrates, such as nitroglycerin, are primarily venodilators. The arterial vasodilators lower blood pressure by allowing a relatively unimpeded flow of blood through the arterial circulation. Since capacitance vessels are not dilated, this blood returns promptly to the heart. The lower blood pressure reflexly increases sympathetic tone to the heart. Increased blood return to the heart and increased sympathetic stimulation cause tachycardia and a greater cardiac output. The patient may experience these combined effects as a racing heart beat with palpitations, a pounding headache, and rushing vascular noises in the head. All of these cardiac manifestations of unopposed arterial vasodilation can be blocked by the β-blocking drugs or central sympatholytics.

Although the vasodilators tend to increase renal blood flow, with the exception of calcium antagonists, they cause sodium retention. This problem is particularly prominent with diazoxide, which has an intrinsic antinatriuretic effect, and with minoxidil. In contrast, calcium antagonists induce a mild natriuresis. The vasodilators cause a redistribution in renal blood flow, a decrease in perfusion pressure to the kidney, and an increase in renal renin output. Diuretics can counteract fluid retention, and sympatholytic agents lower renin output.

Blood pressure lowering with vasodilators has several major advantages. These agents counteract hypertensive vasoconstriction, preserve renal and cerebral blood flow, and are effective anti-hypertensives. However, the side effects of the arterial vasodilators prevent them from being used alone, and they should be combined with a sympatholytic and a diuretic.

HYDRALAZINE

Hydralazine is available for both parenteral and oral administration. The drug is extensively metabolized by the liver. After oral administration there may be low bioavailability due to first pass metabolism in the liver. Hepatic acetylation is a major route of metabolism, and rapid acetylators have about 30% bioavailability of the drug, as compared to the 50% bioavailability in slow acetylators. The plasma elimination half-time of hydralazine is about 4 hours, but plasma hydralazine levels correlate poorly with antihypertensive efficacy, probably because the agent is directly bound to arterioles at its site of action. Although the drug's circulating half-life is about 3 hours, the half-time of its effect on blood pressure is about 100 hours (90). As a result, the drug is equally as effective when given twice per day as when given 4 times a day (90).

Hydralazine acts by causing vasodilation, which is most marked in the splanchnic, coronary, cerebral, and renal vasculature. Blood flow does not increase in skin or muscle, however. The antihypertensive potency of hydralazine is severely limited by a reflex increase in cardiac output and fluid retention. β-blocking drugs that diminish the reflex increase in plasma renin activity are synergistic with hydralazine, and it is possible to carefully devise a regimen of diuretic, β-blocker, and hydralazine that can markedly lower blood pressure with minimal side effects (91).

Although symptomatic side effects elicited by vasodilation from hydralazine can be combated with the addition of a diuretic and a β-blocker, other side effects idiosyncratic to the drug cannot be blocked. A drug-induced lupus-like syndrome occurs in 10 to 20% of patients who receive prolonged therapy in doses exceeding 400 mg daily. This syndrome occurs more rarely at doses in the range of 200 mg/day and manifests primarily in caucasians who eliminate the drug slowly because of their acetylation phenotype. This lupus-like syndrome is reversible when the drug is withdrawn and is characterized by joint pain and skin rash. Renal toxicity is infrequent. Hydralazine can also cause drug fever. A peripheral neuropathy may occur, which can be corrected with pyridoxine, probably because the drug binds with this vitamin (92).

The drug is available for intravenous or intramuscular injection. The usual parenteral dose is 10 to 40 mg, but response is quite variable, and its effects develop gradually over 15 to 20 minutes after IV administration. Hydralazine is available for oral use in 10-, 25-, 50-, and 100-mg tablets. It is usually started in low doses so that the side effects of tachycardia and fluid retention can be combated with sympatholytics and diuretics before they become severe.

MINOXIDIL

Minoxidil is an extremely effective vasodilator, with actions similar to those of hydralazine. However, the agent is more efficacious and more potent than hydralazine and causes different side effects.

Ninety percent of an orally administered dose of minoxidil is absorbed; 85% of the drug is metabolized by the liver; and 15% is excreted unchanged in the kidney. The plasma half-life of minoxidil is approximately 4 hours, but it is effective for over 24 hours, probably because it is retained by vascular smooth muscle (93). The maximum effect of the drug is apparent 6 hours after an oral dose.

The ultimate dose of minoxidil required to control hypertension is extremely varied, and therapy should be begun with a small dose, such as 2.5 or 5 mg. This dose may then be doubled every 6 hours when the maximum effect of the prior dose becomes apparent, until blood pressure control is obtained. The effective dose can then be administered every 12 to 24 hours. As with hydralazine, minoxidil must always be administered with a diuretic and a sympatholytic agent, such as a β-blocker or clonidine. The drug is presently approved only for therapy of hypertension resistant to other avenues of treatment. Minoxidil is effective in renal failure and has successfully controlled blood pressure in patients with severe hypertension and end-stage renal disease.

Minoxidil's potent vasodilating effects can elicit marked hemodynamic responses. The sympathetic nervous system is activated to such a degree that plasma catecholamine levels may mimic those levels seen in patients with a pheochromocytoma (94). This sympathetic nervous activation stimulates renin secretion, and the vasoconstrictor effects of norepinephrine and angiotensin II diminish the hypotensive effects of minoxidil unless they are blocked with a sympatholytic. The renal tubules avidly retain sodium in the patient treated with minoxidil, although glomerular filtration is not changed. Early in the course of therapy, even patients given large doses of furosemide may retain sodium. The unopposed cardiac stimulation of minoxidil is associated with absence of regression or even progression of cardiac hypertrophy (95). The fluid retention may be overcome by combining furosemide with a thiazide diuretic or metolazone, and with subsequent therapy fluid retention is less avid. It is sometimes necessary to lower the dose of minoxidil to effect a diuresis in patients who have some degree of renal insufficiency.

Minoxidil causes hypertrichosis (excessive hair growth involving the face, arms and legs), which occurs in most patients several weeks to months after the drug is instituted and sometimes takes up to 6 months to disappear after the drug is stopped. Many women find this side effect intolerable. Minoxidil is available for topical use for the treatment of male pattern baldness, and although this route of administration does not affect blood pressure, changes in cardiac output and left ventricular mass have been noted (96). Pathologic lesions of the heart have been reported in two animal studies using minoxidil, but no such lesions have been reported in man (97). Pulmonary hypertension has been reported during treatment with minoxidil, but there have also been reports of decreased pulmonary vascular resistance during therapy. Pericardial effusion occasionally progressing to pericardial tamponade has been described in patients receiving minoxidil, but these problems usually occur in those patients who have congestive heart failure or renal failure. Approximately 2% of patients treated with this drug show no response, even to a large dose (98). In 98% of hypertensives, minoxidil is one of the most effective drugs available.

DIAZOXIDE

Diazoxide is chemically related to the thiazide diuretics, but it causes fluid retention, rather than a natriuresis. Thiazide diuretics have a minor vasodilating effect, but diazoxide is a very effective vasodilator. Diazoxide directly dilates arterioles but has little effect on large veins, although it can dilate the small postcapillary resistance vessels. Diazoxide is usually given by rapid intravenous injection for the treatment of hypertension, and when given by this route, 90% of the drug is eventually bound to albumin, and about one-third of the drug is cleared through the kidneys. The serum half-life of diazoxide is about 30 hours, and in patients with impaired renal function, the half-life increases proportionally. Diazoxide tends to accumulate with repeated administration, but there is no correlation between the total serum concentration and the intensity of its hypotensive action, because the hypotensive effects of diazoxide depend on the concentration of drug in the arterioles. Since the drug binds to both albumin and the arterioles, there is competition between these sites, and only the drug in the arterioles has a hypotensive effect. As a result, if a bolus of the drug is injected rapidly, it can reach arteriolar sites more effectively than when given slowly, and its hypotensive usefulness is more beneficial and dramatic. When given this way, maximum hypotensive effect is attained in 3 to 5 minutes. Fifty to 150 mg of the drug can be given as a bolus, injected over 30 seconds or less. If the patient has already received a diuretic and a β-blocker, the drug may be given by slow intravenous infusion.

Diazoxide increases cardiac output and causes sympathetic stimulation and fluid retention. Its effects can be greatly potentiated by sympatholytic agents or diuretics. If the patient is volume-depleted or receiving a sympatholytic agent, the dose of diazoxide needs to be reduced in order to avoid hypotension. There are other side effects characteristic of this agent; cerebral blood flow is diminished (99), and the drug may cause extrapyramidal symptoms with prolonged use (100). It inhibits release of insulin from the pancreas, thereby increasing blood glucose levels. In patients with diabetes mellitus or renal failure, treatment of the hyperglycemia may become necessary in a few days. It suppresses tubular transport of uric acid and leads to hyperuricemia, as do the other thiazides. Since the drug binds strongly to albumin, it displaces warfarin anticoagulants.

In clinical practice, the side effects of diazoxide are usually relatively minor, and its ease of use is one of its major advantages. In contrast to nitroprusside, diazoxide can be given in hypertensive emergencies to a patient who is not on continuous blood pressure monitoring because its maximum effect is reached in 5 minutes, and blood pressure gradually returns to pretreatment level within 5 to 12 hours. This duration of action allows time to introduce other antihypertensive therapies. The drug should not be used alone in patients in whom cardiac stimulation may be deleterious, such as those patients with severe coronary artery disease or aortic dissection. In most patients with severe hypertension, diazoxide can successfully lower blood pressure without the need for continuous monitoring.

SODIUM NITROPRUSSIDE

Sodium nitroprusside's hypotensive capability has been recognized for 50 years, but it was little used until it was commercially marketed and promoted as Nipride. Its hypotensive effect is probably due to the iron-nitroso (Fe-NO) grouping in the intact nitroprusside molecule, and the drug causes both venous and arterial vasodilation, as do the nitrates. This balanced vascular dilation, which includes venous capacitance vessels, gives nitroprusside a slightly different spectrum of effect than the other vasodilators. The venodilation results in a decreased cardiac preload, instead of the increased preload seen with the "pure" arterial vasodilators. In the absence of heart failure, cardiac output either decreases or does not change in response to nitroprusside. However, if myocardial disease has diminished cardiac output, nitroprusside may increase output as a result of diminished afterload. Nitroprusside usually causes a 20 to 30% increase in heart rate, but if there is a preexisting tachycardia due to heart failure, heart rate may actually decrease slightly. The decreased preload may diminish cardiac work, and angina often improves when nitroprusside is given, in contrast to the "pure" arterial vasodilators that may cause myocardial ischemia.

Since nitroprusside causes venous pooling, it can induce a profound postural hypotension, unlike the pure arterial vasodilators. If a critically ill patient receives nitroprusside and becomes acutely hypotensive, he is usually intravascularly depleted and requires fluid replacement. In the upright posture, nitroprusside causes a decrease in cardiac output, which may have a major effect on the drug's hypotensive impact.

In supine patients, the decrease in cardiac output is responsible for about one-fourth of its hypotensive activity. Nitroprusside-induced hypotension activates the sympathetic nervous system, which increases cardiac output and heart rate. Renal blood flow and glomerular filtration rate do not change. Since nitroprusside does not increase cardiac preload, it is a good drug for treating patients with congestive heart failure, myocardial dysfunction, or aortic dissection, where hyperkinetic cardiac output would be harmful. It is also useful in treating hypertension associated with myocardial infarction and an unstable blood pressure since its effects can be rapidly terminated by stopping its infusion.

Sodium nitroprusside given by intravenous infusion (0.25 to 2.5 μg/kg/min, advancing to a maximum of 10 μg/kg/min) lowers blood pressure within seconds, and the hypotensive effect dissipates within 1 to 2 minutes after stopping the infusion. The drug is extremely effective and can lower blood pressure markedly in any person. Because of its rapid action and potency, nitroprusside should be administered with an infusion pump while blood pressure is continually monitored. After the first 2 hours of administration, the rate of drug infusion frequently needs to be increased to maintain an equivalent hypotensive effect, because nitroprusside causes an increase in cardiac index without inducing tachycardia (101). The increased cardiac index is due to fluid accumulation and sympathetic nervous stimulation and can be effectively counteracted with a diuretic or β-blocking agent. The drug can increase or maintain cerebral blood flow, and this response can lead to increased intracranial pressure, which might be deleterious in patients with head injury.

Nitroprusside is broken down to cyanide, which is rapidly converted in the body to thiocyanate. Cyanide toxicity from the drug is uncommon, but thiocyanate is handled by the body in essentially the same manner as chloride and bromide. The thiocyanate may thus be retained by patients with renal failure or by those patients receiving low-sodium diets; its half-life is normally 4 days. If the concentration of thiocyanate exceeds 10 mg/dl, weakness, hypoxia, nausea, tinnitus, muscle spasm, disorientation and psychosis may occur. Thiocyanate interferes with transport of iodide by the thyroid gland and may cause hypothyroidism. If nitroprusside is infused for a long time and in high doses, blood levels of thiocyanate need to be monitored. Nitroprusside-treated patients who stand may experience postural hypotension, and some may encounter nasal stuffiness and increased body warmth, dizziness, weakness, muscle twitching, and nausea.

Sodium nitroprusside (Nipride) is supplied as a powder (50 mg vials) for reconstitution in 250 ml of 5% dextrose (yielding a concentration of 200 μg/ml). This solution may be used for 24 hours after reconstitution but should be protected from light. Deeply colored solutions should be discarded because development of a visible color indicates loss of potency.

Patients given sodium nitroprusside must have their blood pressure continuously measured. Although nitroprusside is not necessary for treating most cases of severe hypertension, it is one of the better agents available for treating hypertensive emergencies. Since the drug becomes less effective and leads to accumulation of thiocyanate with prolonged infusion, patients should be given other antihypertensive drugs soon after the initiation of therapy. Diuretics and sympatholytics markedly potentiate the effects of this vasodilator and decrease the dose of drug required.

NITROGLYCERIN

Nitroglycerin was initially used as a sublingual antianginal agent in the late 1800s. This organic nitrate has been widely used in its intravenous form in the intensive care setting for the treatment of coronary insufficiency, due to its ability to cause coronary artery vasodilation and thus improve myocardial oxygenation. However, nitroglycerin also relaxes smooth muscles in veins, arterioles, bronchioles, the biliary tract, the gastrointestinal tract, and the uterus. The smooth muscle relaxant effect of nitrates is mediated by the production of nitric oxide which in turn stimulates guanylate cyclase, the enzyme responsible for producing cyclic guanosine monophosphate (102). In lower dosages, venous capacitance vessels are more sensitive to nitroglycerin, while at higher doses one observes additional arterial vasodilation. This combined action on venous and arterial systems leads to a reduction in left ventricular filling pressure, right atrial pressure, central venous pressure, mean arterial pressure, and systemic vascular resistance. The reduction of systolic blood pressure is greater than that of diastolic blood pressure (103). At high doses, a large drop in blood pressure may induce a reflex tachycardia, which may antagonize the favorable effects of the drug on cardiac workload.

Nitroglycerin has a rapid onset of action and has an elimination half-life of minutes, allowing for return of baseline blood pressure approximately 10 minutes following cessation of intravenous infusion. Due to nitroglycerin's hepatic metabolism and degradation, impaired liver function may decrease clearance. Renal failure does not alter nitrate clearance. Nitroglycerin may be absorbed and adsorbed by polyvinylchloride (PVC) plastics, leading to decreases in desired concentrations when nitroglycerin is mixed in PVC (104). Nitroglycerin is well-tolerated. The most common side effect is hypotension, which is easily reversed by decreasing the rate of infusion. Other side effects include headache, bradycardia, and tachycardia. Nitroglycerin given as an intravenous infusion is begun at 5 μg/min and titrated in 5 μg/min increments to the desired effect.

Nitroglycerin is useful for the treatment of congestive heart failure, since its venodilating action will reduce cardiac preload. The coronary vasodilating properties of nitroglycerin make it ideal in treating unstable angina, vasospastic angina, and acute myocardial infarction. Nitroglycerin is widely used in the surgical setting to provide controlled hypotension or to treat postoperative hypertension. Patients with hypertension in association with ischemic heart disease or left ventricular failure respond to nitroglycerin by lowering systemic blood pressure and reducing myocardial oxygen demand.

CALCIUM ANTAGONISTS

The myocardium and smooth muscle cells have slow calcium channels in their cell membranes that regulate the influx of calcium into the cytoplasm. Increased free intracellular calcium increases smooth muscle contractility, peripheral resistance, and blood pressure. Various vasoactive systems, such as the renin-angiotensin-aldosterone system and sympathetic nervous system, may be involved in the regulation of intracellular calcium levels. Calcium-blocking drugs (also known as calcium entry blockers, calcium antagonists, and calcium channel blockers) lower intracellular calcium levels and cause vasodilation. Large arteries are less sensitive to the vasodilating effects of calcium blockers than peripheral resistance vessels, cerebral arteries, coronary arteries, and mesenteric arteries. α_2-Receptor stimulation by endogenous catecholamines is mediated by an influx of calcium ions and may be inhibited by calcium antagonists. Although most vasodilators cause fluid retention, some calcium channel blockers induce a mild natriuresis (105). These drugs have varying effects on myocardial contractility, sinus and atrioventricular node function, and regional vascular beds (Table 20.7). All of these drugs are effective in treating essential hypertension (106, 107). The coronary vasodilating properties of the drugs make them useful in the treatment of angina pectoris (108). Diltiazem and verapamil depress sinoatrial node automaticity; slow AV node conduction; and are, therefore, useful in treating supraventricular arrhythmias. There are three chemical classes of calcium channel blockers: phenylalkylamines, benzothiazepines, and dihydropyridines (Table 20.7). All of these agents are well-absorbed from the gastrointestinal tract; however, they undergo extensive first-pass metabolism, so their bioavailabilities range from 10 to 50%. Calcium channel blockers are highly protein-bound, and their main route of elimination is the liver. Most calcium channel blockers are rapidly metabolized and have short half-lives. Slow release preparations are available for nifedipine, verapamil, diltiazem, and felodipine.

Nifedipine, the prototypical dihydropyridine, decreases blood pressure more in elderly and low-renin hypertensives than in high renin hypertensives (109). It can rapidly lower blood pressure when given sublingually (110) or orally (111). Acutely, nifedipine reflexly increases cardiac output. With chronic use, however, nifedipine's direct cardiodepressant activity counteracts its reflex stimulant effects so that heart rate and contractility do not change much (112). After several months, the hypotensive effect of nifedipine tends to diminish when the drug is given alone but is maintained when the drug is administered with propranolol or clonidine (111).

Calcium channel blockers are effective in lowering blood pressure when used alone or in conjunction with β-blocking drugs, angiotensin-converting enzyme inhibitors, and central sympatholytics. Their efficacy in controlling blood pressure appears to be similar. Verapamil, however, is usually not used in combination with β-blockers, as both agents decrease AV node conduction and myocardial contractility (113). Although these effects are not as pronounced with diltiazem, β-blockers should be administered cautiously with diltiazem.

Oral and sublingual nifedipine has been used to treat hypertensive crisis and severe hypertension (114). Its quick onset of action and preservation of both cardiac output and cerebral perfusion (114) make it useful in this setting. Intravenous diltiazem and verapamil have also been used effectively in acute situations (115), and intravenous nicardipine is under study for control of accelerated hypertension.

Calcium channel blockers have no effects on electrolytes, lipids, glucose, or respiratory function. There is evidence that they may have antiatherogenic properties (116). They improve

Table 25.7. Properties of Oral Calcium Channel Blockers Used in Treating Hypertension

Generic Name *Brand Name*	*Verapamil* *Calan, Isoptin*	*Diltiazem* *Cardizem*	*Nifedipine* *Adalat, Procardia*	*Nicardipine* *Cardene*	*Isradipine* *Dynacirc*	*Felodipine* *Plendil*
Chemical Class	P[a]	B	D	D	D	D
Daily dose (mg)	120–480	120–360	30–180	60–120	5–20	5–20
Bioavailability	20–25%	40%	45–70%	10–30%	15–20%	20%
Half-life (hr)	5–18	3–4.5	2–5	8.6	8	11–16
Protein binding	85%	80%	95%	98%	95%	>99%
Elimination	Hepatic	Renal & hepatic	Hepatic	Hepatic	Hepatic	Hepatic
Active metabolites	+	+	0	0	0	0
Peripheral vasodilation	↑↑	↑↑	↑↑↑	↑↑↑	↑↑↑	↑↑↑
Heart rate	↔	↔	↑*/↔[+a]	↑*/↔[+]	↔	↑*/↔[+]
Myocardial contractility	↓	↓	↔	↔	↔	↔
Coronary vasodilation	↑	↑	↑↑	↑↑	↑↑	↑↑
AV conduction	↓↓	↓	↔	↔	↔	↔
Cardiac output	↔	↔	↑*/↔[+]	↑*	↔	↔
Myocardial O$_2$ demand	↓	↓	↓	↓	↓	↓

[a] +, chronic use; *, acute use; P, phenylalkylamine; B, Benzothiazepine; D, Dihydropyridine.

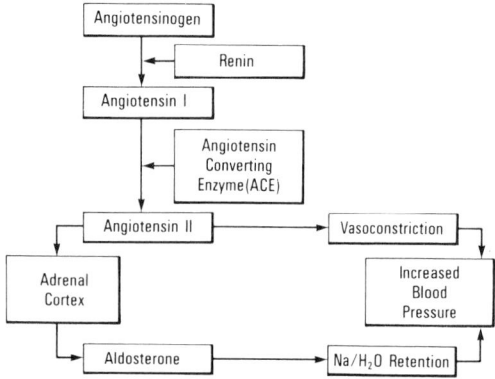

Figure 25.1. The renin-angiotensin-aldosterone system.

renal perfusion by causing glomerular afferent arteriolar dilation (117) and are safe to use in patients with renal dysfunction. Calcium channel blockers are effective in lowering blood pressure in African-Americans and whites, and in young and old patients but may be most effective in African-Americans and the elderly. Unlike β-blockers, they are useful in treating Raynaud's phenomenon. Adverse effects of calcium channel blockers include those consequences associated with vasodilation such as flushing, headache, and dizziness, which are more frequent with the dihydropyridines. Ankle edema develops in some people; is dose-related; and again is more common with the dihydropyridines. Ankle edema is usually the result of vasodilation and does not always indicate fluid retention. Underlying sinus node or AV node conduction abnormalities or concomitant use of β-blockers may cause severe sinus bradycardia or AV block when verapamil or diltiazem are used. Verapamil commonly causes constipation. Cutaneous adverse reactions to calcium channel blockers occur rarely (118).

ANGIOTENSIN-CONVERTING ENZYME INHIBITORS (ACE INHIBITORS)

Renin is released from the kidney and enzymatically converts circulating angiotensinogen to angiotensin I. Angiotensin I is then rapidly converted to angiotensin II by angiotensin-converting enzyme, which is present in blood vessel walls and in the lung (Fig. 20.1). Angiotensin II is a very potent vasoconstrictor that also stimulates aldosterone release. Renin levels are markedly increased in renovascular hypertension and malignant hypertension and are above normal in about one-fourth of patients with essential hypertension. The pressor effects of renin can be blocked by inhibition of angiotensin-converting enzyme. The first inhibitor of this enzyme, teprotide, was derived from snake venom. Captopril was specifically designed to interfere with the active site of angiotensin-converting enzyme, and enalapril, lisinopril, fosinopril, benazapril, and ramipril have similar modes of action. ACE inhibitors are potent antihypertensive agents that act primarily by preventing the production of angiotensin II. As a result, aldosterone levels are reduced, and renin levels increase. ACE inhibitors also mediate their effect on tissue-specific renin-angiotensin systems, as well as on the circulating renin-angiotensin system (119). Angiotensin-converting enzyme also causes the breakdown of circulating bradykinin, a potent vasodilator (120). Bradykinin acts locally in tissues to release vasodilatory prostaglandins; treatment with indomethacin diminishes the hypotensive activity of infused bradykinin and the hypotensive activity of captopril. Angiotensin II potentiates both the release and the pressor responses to norepinephrine. ACE inhibitors lower blood pressure by lowering levels of angiotensin II, by enhancing bradykinin levels, and by inhibiting the effects of angiotensin II on sympathetic nerves (121).

The hemodynamic actions of ACE inhibitors differ from those of other antihypertensive agents and may be beneficial in patients with hypertensive damage to the kidneys and heart (122). After an acute dose of captopril, blood pressure reduction is related to the initial plasma renin activity (123). Patients with high renin levels have a rapid captopril-induced decrease in blood pressure, which then rebounds nearly to pretreatment levels. Over subsequent days, blood pressure slowly decreases but not to as low a level as encountered during the initiation of therapy. Patients with normal or low renin levels have a more prolonged and gentler decrease in blood pressure. The initial hypotensive response is exaggerated in patients who are volume depleted, and this excessive hypotension can be treated with intravenous saline.

ACE inhibitors lower total peripheral resistance and cause little change in cardiac output, heart rate, or pulmonary artery occlusion pressure in most hypertensives. However, in patients with congestive heart failure, they can increase cardiac output by diminishing afterload (124). Prolonged ACE inhibition reduces left ventricular hypertrophy in hypertensives (125). ACE inhibitors decrease renal vascular resistance enough to increase renal blood flow, even while decreasing blood pressure. Glomerular filtration rate is usually unchanged, and intraglomerular pressure decreases due to a greater vasodilation of efferent glomerular arterioles. Renal hemodynamic abnormalities found in the hypertensive kidney may be reversed by ACE inhibitors (126). Proteinuria is sometimes reduced by ACE inhibitors, and it has been suggested that progression of glomerular injury may be slowed (127). Reversible oliguric renal failure or increases in the serum creatinine concentration may occur during therapy, particularly if there is bilateral renal artery stenosis, a solitary kidney with renal artery stenosis (such as a transplanted kidney), severe bilateral hypertensive nephrosclerosis (128), or low cardiac output. ACE inhibitors do not cause postural hypotension and lower blood pressure without a reflex increase in sympathetic nervous system activity. Norepinephrine levels remain unchanged during therapy and respond to stress normally (129).

ACE inhibitors are effective as monotherapy, particularly in young white hypertensives who usually have high renin levels. African-American and elderly patients respond less often to ACE inhibition monotherapy, but a combination of an ACE inhibitor and a diuretic will control blood pressure in 85% of subjects (130). Combinations with an ACE inhibitor and other drugs that increase renin levels, such as calcium antagonists (131) and minoxidil, are also very effective (132). ACE inhibitors are particularly effective in renovascular hypertension not amenable to surgery and in patients with congestive heart failure. They correct both the hypertension and hypokalemia caused by markedly increased renin levels. Angiotensin II stimulates release of aldosterone and potassium excretion. Potassium supplementation, potassium-sparing diuretics, and combination diuretics, such as triamterene-hydrochlorothiazide combinations, should usually be avoided during ACE inhibitor therapy. Patients with renal insufficiency and elderly diabetics may develop severe hyperkalemia with ACE inhibitors.

Of the more than 50 ACE inhibitors developed, six are available for clinical use: captopril; enalapril; lisinopril; fosinopril; benazapril; and ramipril. Their chemical classification is based on the ligand that binds the zinc ion in angiotensin-converting enzyme (133). The characteristics of these drugs are listed in Table 20.8. Captopril has a sulfhydryl group as a ligand that can, rarely, cause dose-related immunologic side effects, such as a rash, fever, eosinophilia, proteinuria, and neutropenia. These side effects are related to captopril blood levels and are most common in patients with renal insufficiency who are given high doses. Blood levels peak in 30 to 90 minutes after oral administration and even more rapidly when captopril is given sublingually.

The other ACE inhibitors lack a sulfhydryl group and may have fewer immunologic side effects. They have a slower onset of action than captopril. Some are pro-drugs, which are converted to active metabolites in the gut wall and liver (Table 20.8). The pro-drug enalapril is converted to enalaprilat, which is available for intravenous administration.

Lisinopril is not a pro-drug and does not have a sulfhydryl group. It has a prolonged half-life that allows once-daily dosing. Fosinopril, benazapril, and ramipril are all pro-drugs that are converted to their active forms by the liver. They have long terminal half-lives, which allow for once-daily dosing. Although ramipril has a primary half-life of 4 hours, it has a terminal half-life of 110 hours, indicating prolonged binding and inhibition of angiotensin-converting enzyme. Fosinopril is the only ACE inhibitor that is partially eliminated in the bile, thus allowing for fixed-dosing regimens in patients with renal impairment. The other ACE inhibitors must be given in smaller doses to these patients.

Captopril can be successfully employed in hypertensive emergencies (134). It is usually a very potent agent in malignant hypertension, but its effects are difficult to control in this setting. Enalaprilat, the active diacid metabolite of enalapril, is available for use in intravenous form. It has been used successfully in the treatment of hypertensive crisis (135) and moderate or severe systemic hypertension (136).

All of the ACE inhibitors impair the breakdown of bradykinin. This action may cause a persistent dry cough at times associated with wheezing or life-threatening angioedema. ACE inhibitors should not be used in pregnancy, as they reduce placental blood flow and cause acute renal failure and hypotension in newborns (137).

COMBINED DRUG THERAPY OF HYPERTENSION

The critically ill patient with severe hypertension often cannot attain normal blood pressure in response to a single drug. Large doses of an individual drug are more likely to cause a number of side effects than smaller doses of drugs that potentiate one another. It is often possible to take advantage of drug combinations to attain an adequate hypotensive effect with minimal side effects by using more than one drug. However, some drug combinations are ineffective or toxic. Many drugs lower blood pressure as a side effect of their primary use (Table 20.9), and some are potent antihypertensive agents when used with a diuretic.

One can take advantage of the increase in renin, aldosterone, and sympathetic nervous system activity that occurs during diuretic or vasodilator treatment by blocking these effects with other antihypertensives and attaining a synergistic blood pressure response (Table 20.10). This approach explains the high success rate in lowering blood pressure when an ACE inhibitor, which lowers angiotensin-II, is combined with a thiazide, which increases renin and angiotensin-II. Sympatholytic drugs block the increase in sympathetic nervous system activity that results from volume depletion or vasodilation, again achieving a synergistic effect on blood pressure. The combination of a diuretic and a central sympatholytic agent is particularly effective in elderly patients with systolic hypertension.

The β-blocking drugs are all quite similar in their antihypertensive efficacy and should not be combined with one another. Clonidine acts to diminish the sympathetic nervous

Table 25.8.   Properties of Oral ACE Inhibitors Used in Treating Hypertension

Generic Name	Captopril	Enalapril	Lisinopril Zestril, Prinivil	Fosinopril	Ramipril	Benazapril
Brand Name	Capoten	Vasotec	Prinivil	Monopril	Altace	Lotensin
Zinc ligand	Sulfhydryl	Carboxyl	Carboxyl	Phosphinyl	Carboxyl	Carboxyl
Prodrug	No	Yes	No	Yes	Yes	Yes
Daily dose (mg)	25–150	5–20	20–40	10–40	2.5–20	5–40
Bioavailability (%)	70	40	25	30	60	28
Route of elimination	Kidney	Kidney	Kidney	Kidney and liver	Kidney	Kidney
Terminal half-life (hr)	2	11	12	12	110	21
Onset of action (hr)	0.5–1	1–2	2–4	2–6	1–2	1–2

Table 25.9.   Drugs That Lower Blood Pressure

Drug	Action	Drug Interactions
Neuroleptics, especially chlorpromazine	α-Blockade	Potentiated by diuretics
Dopamine agonists L-dopa Bromocriptine Dopamine Pimozide	Stimulate dopamine receptors, inhibit NE[a] release	
Fenfluramine	Inhibits NE release	Potentiated by diuretics
Tricyclic antidepressants	Myocardial depression	Inhibits clonidine effect
MAO[a] inhibitors	?	Hypertension with tyramine, reserpine
Marijuana	Inhibits NE effects	
Opiates	Vasodilation, inhibits norepinephrine release	
Antiarrhythmics Disopyramide	Myocardial depression, vasodilation	

[a] NE, norepinephrine; MAO, monoamine oxidase.

Table 25.10.   Effects of Combination Antihypertensive Therapy[a]

	Salt Restriction	Thiazides	α-Blockers	β-Blockers	α₂-Agonists	Vasodilators	Calcium Channel Blockers	ACE Inhibitor
Salt restriction	0	+	+	+	+	+	0	+
Thiazides	+	0	+	+	+	+	0	++
α-Blockers	+	+	0	+/0	0	?	+	+
β-Blockers	+	+	+/0	0	-	+	+/-*	0
α₂-Agonists	+	+	0	-	0	+	+	+
Vasodilators	+	+	?	+	+	0	0	++
Calcium channel blockers	0	0	+	+/-*	+	0	0	+
ACE inhibitors	+	++	+	0	+	++	+	0

[a] +, additive effect; 0, no additive effect; ++, strong additive effect; -, adverse effect; *, do not combine two drugs that depress AV node conduction/myocardial contractility.

system release of norepinephrine, and the β-blockers antagonize the effects of norepinephrine. In experimental animals, β-blockers such as propranolol that penetrate the central nervous system inhibit the antihypertensive efficacy of clonidine. In humans, the combination of clonidine and propranolol has been reported as both effective and ineffective (138, 139). Clonidine may exacerbate hypertension in some patients receiving a β-blocker (63), and β-blockers worsen the hypertension found during clonidine withdrawal (74).

The combination of the α-blocking agent prazosin with a β-blocking drug seems to be a reasonable approach to the control of hypertension. Labetalol, a drug with both peripheral α- and β-blocking activity, is an effective antihypertensive agent. However, according to some reports, the antihypertensive efficacy of prazosin combined with propranolol is not more effective than either agent used alone (63, 140). Prazosin also does not enhance the antihypertensive efficacy of clonidine (141).

It has not proven clearly beneficial to combine sympatholytic drugs in the treatment of hypertension, except for the combination of α- and β-blocking agents in a patient with pheochromocytoma. On the other hand, there are numerous reports of unexpected pressor responses and a predictable increase in the number of side effects occurs as more sympatholytic drugs are added. In general, patients should be treated with a single sympatholytic agent.

The arterial vasodilators reflexly increase sympathetic nervous system activity and cardiac output. The vasodilators also increase renin and aldosterone production and cause fluid retention. Consequently, vasodilators are not very effective in lowering blood pressure by themselves; they need to be combined with a diuretic and a sympatholytic for maximal hypotensive effect and to avoid the side effects of edema and palpitations. Minoxidil and diazoxide cause such avid fluid retention that a loop diuretic, such as furosemide, is often necessary.

Most sympatholytic drugs potentiate the antihypertensive effects of the vasodilators. β-Blocking drugs block the increased cardiac output and renin secretion engendered by the vasodilators. In fact, when β-blockers are used in appropriate doses, they can eliminate the palpitations, headaches, and vascular noises that may be caused by the vasodilators. β-Blockers diminish β-adrenergic effects engendered by vasodilators, but they do not block α-adrenergic effects. If β-blockers do not lower blood pressure adequately, it is reasonable to change to an α$_2$-agonist such as clonidine. Clonidine should be substituted for the β-blocker, not added to the previous drug regimen, since clonidine can increase blood pressure in a patient treated with the combination of a diuretic, hydralazine, and a β-blocker (63). Combining a vasodilator with an ACE inhibitor, which decreases renin effects, is also very effective. Many hypertensive patients develop coronary insufficiency and angina pectoris. A vasodilator used alone can worsen the angina, but a vasodilator can safely be used if the patient is already on adequate doses of a diuretic and a β-blocker.

The ACE inhibitors work well in patients with high renin levels. The diuretics and vasodilators cause high renin levels, so patients receiving these drugs usually have a good hypotensive response to ACE inhibitors (142). This synergism can be so dramatic that it is often advisable to withhold diuretic drugs for 3 days prior to initiation of ACE inhibition to avoid hypotension.

The calcium channel blockers have vasodilating and diuretic effects. They increase renin and norepinephrine levels, so they act synergistically with ACE inhibitors and some sympatholytics. The combination of a calcium channel blocker with an ACE inhibitor is expensive but very effective antihypertensive therapy. Verapamil and diltiazem prolong cardiac conduction time, so heart block is a potential complication when they are combined with β-blockers. On the other hand, the dihydropyridine calcium channel blockers do not affect AV node conduction and may be safely and effectively combined with β-blockers.

EVALUATION OF THE SEVERELY HYPERTENSIVE PATIENT

Essential hypertension is a lifelong disease, and therapy ideally should be initiated slowly with the drugs least likely to cause side effects. However, patients presenting with severe hypertension may have a poor prognosis unless they receive prompt, effective treatment. The most common cause of a markedly increased blood pressure is a stress reaction (143). Some patients who are only slightly hypertensive in their normal environment respond to the stress of a medical examination with severe hypertension, which subsides when they return to their usual surroundings. Ganglion-blocking drugs, such as guanethedine, can block stress-induced hypertension, but clonidine or methyldopa do not. The effects of clonidine or methyldopa can be overridden during severe stress, allowing normal discharge from the sympathetic nervous system.

On physical examination, the patient with stress-induced hypertension lacks the stigmata of hypertensive disease, and funduscopic exam shows a relatively undamaged retinal vasculature. Examination of the urine will be normal, in contrast to the proteinuria which may be seen in a chronically hypertensive patient. Administering potent antihypertensive agents to these patients leaves them hypotensive when they return to a less stressful environment.

DRUG-INDUCED HYPERTENSION

Many drugs used in clinical practice or present in over-the-counter preparations can produce hypertension, at times mimicking the pressor response to a pheochromocytoma (Table 20.11). Phenylpropanolamine is a popular over-the-counter anorectic agent, frequently combined with ephedrine or caffeine and marketed for the treatment of obesity, drowsiness, and nasal congestion. This drug causes α-adrenergic-mediated vasoconstriction and increases blood pressure even when given in normal doses, and can cause marked hypertension resulting in cerebral hemorrhage when taken in excessive doses (144). Over-the-counter asthma preparations may contain epinephrine, racinepherine, and ephedrine. Phenylephrine, present in nasal sprays, cough drops, and cold tablets, may raise blood pressure by α-stimulation.

Monoamine oxidase inhibitors have had a resurgence in popularity for the treatment of depression. They ordinarily lower blood pressure, but when taken with a food containing tyramine, such as cheese or wine, they can cause severe hypertension. They can also worsen the hypertension caused by drugs such as ephedrine and phenylpropanolamine, which are degraded by monoamine oxidase.

Several recreational drugs transiently increase blood pressure. Cocaine inhibits norepinephrine reuptake and stimulates norepinephrine release. Acute hypertension, cardiac arrhythmias, and cerebrovascular events may develop (145). Phencyclidine (PCP) causes sympathetic activation and hypertension in over 50% of users (146). Other drugs that may cause hypertension are listed in Table 20.11.

Abrupt withdrawal of clonidine in doses greater than 0.2 mg/day can cause a rebound increase in sympathetic nervous system release of norepinephrine and an overshoot hypertension. All of the above mentioned drug reactions increase blood pressure through α-adrenergic stimulation, and they are best treated acutely with α-blocking drugs. Although patients with a pheochromocytoma or with one of these drug reactions are usually tachycardic and tremulous, they should not initially receive β-blocking drugs, which may worsen the patient's hypertension. However, abrupt withdrawal of β-blocking drugs produces a syndrome of hypertension, tachycardia, and tremulousness mediated by supersensitive β-adrenergic receptors. The best therapy for this syndrome is small doses of β-blockers.

Table 25.11. Drugs That Increase Blood Pressure

Drug	Action	Drug Interactions
Ethanol	↓ Aldosterone metabolism	Enhances diuretic K⁺ loss; enhances sedation with methyldopa & clonidine
Nicotin	Vasoconstriction	
Caffeine	Sympathetic stimulation	Synergystic with nicotine and α-stimulants, mild diuresis
Stimulants		
Phencyclidine		
Amphetamine	Norepinephrine release, blockage of reuptake	Paradoxical hypertension with β-blockers
Methylphenidate		
Methamphetamine		
Phenmetrazine		
Cocaine		
Racinephrine		
Pseudoephedrine	α- and β-stimulation	Inhibited by α- and β-blockers
Epinephrine		
Isoproterenol		
Isoetharine	β-stimulation	Inhibited by β-blockers
Terbutaline		
Phenylephrine		
Phenylpropanolamine	α-stimulation	Inhibited by α₁-blockers
Ephedrine		
MAO inhibitor and tyramine	Enhanced tryamine effect	
Mineralocorticoids	Sodium retention	Enhance K⁺ loss with diuretics
Glucocorticoids	?	
Glycyrrhizic acid (licorice)	Altered steroid metabolism	
Carbenoxalone	↓ Cortisol metabolism	
Estrogens, oral contraceptives	↑ Angiotensinogen	
Nonsteroidal antiinflammatory drugs	Blocks prostaglandin vasodilation	↓ Diuretic effects
Cyclosporine A	?	Improved by diuretics and calcium antagonists

HYPERTENSIVE CRISIS

Severe asymptomatic hypertension with a diastolic blood pressure above 120 mm Hg is often called a hypertensive urgency. It is not clear whether urgent treatment of the hypertensive urgency is beneficial, but lowering blood pressure too rapidly can be harmful. Severe hypertension with end organ damage is a hypertensive emergency that calls for an immediate reduction in blood pressure, often with parenteral agents given in a monitored hospital setting. Malignant hypertension is a hypertensive emergency where one observes grade IV Keith Wagener retinopathy, increased intracranial pressure, and rapid vascular deterioration (147). It has a mortality rate of 50% in 6 months.

Vasospasm, renin release, and increased sympathetic tone can all initiate a hypertensive crisis (Table 20.12). If blood pressure remains high enough, diffuse vascular damage causes the release of angiotensin II, norepinephrine, and vasopressin, which further intensify vasoconstriction. This action induces platelet and fibrin deposition, causing the pathologically observed entity of fibrinoid necrosis of the arterioles. These damaged arterioles lose their ability to autoregulate and become narrowed and cause ischemia. Tissue ischemia then causes further release of pressor hormones. Most organs autoregulate blood flow, so that tissue perfusion remains constant over a 25% or larger change in blood pressure. Patients with chronic hypertension reset their autoregulatory range around their chronic blood pressure. Thus, a patient who has had a diastolic blood pressure of 120 mm Hg for weeks is likely to develop ischemia if blood pressure is abruptly lowered to the normal range. During episodes of malignant hypertension, tissue ischemia can occur in the presence of markedly increased pressures due to increased peripheral vascular resistance. In order to prevent ischemia during therapy of malignant hypertension it is necessary to lower blood pressure slowly, treat with vasodilating drugs, avoid vasoconstricting drugs, and monitor heart, kidney, and cerebral function for signs of ischemia.

End-organ consequences of malignant hypertension include CNS manifestations such as encephalopathy, intracranial bleeding, and retinal changes, including hemorrhages, exudates, and papilledema. Increased myocardial oxygen demand may cause angina and congestive heart failure. The shearing forces of severe hypertension on the aorta may cause aortic dissection, particularly in patients with preexisting atherosclerosis or Marfan's syndrome. Vascular injury in the kidney may lead to oliguria, azotemia, proteinuria, and hematuria. Diffuse endothelial damage with platelet deposition and arteriolar narrowing in the setting of high pressures can lead to microangiopathic hemolytic anemia. Therefore, an evaluation of a patient with a severe increase in blood pressure should include a medical history directed at determining a possible cause (Table 20.12), a careful physical exam looking for signs of end-organ damage, and a laboratory evaluation looking for abnormalities in the various organ systems possibly affected by the severe hypertension. These include a chest radiograph, electrocardiogram, urinalysis, electrolytes, blood urea nitrogen, creatinine, and a complete blood count.

When the cause of a hypertensive crisis is known (Table 20.12), then a drug to counteract that cause is best. Usually, hypertensive crises are an exacerbation of long-standing hypertension with worsening vasospasm. Initial therapy should reverse the vasospasm to preserve organ perfusion. Diuretics and β-blockers cause an initial increase in peripheral vascular resistance and can lower renal blood flow and are not first-line therapy for vasospastic hypertension. Furthermore, the high pressures induce a sodium-water pressure diuresis in these patients. A number of drugs that relieve vasospasm are effective agents that can lower blood pressure while maintaining tissue perfusion. Direct vasodilators, such as nitroprusside and diazoxide, and the calcium channel blockers directly relax vascular smooth muscle. ACE inhibitors block formation of angiotensin II and cause vasodilation. Sympatholytics, such as clonidine and the α-blockers, prevent norepinephrine mediated vasoconstriction. The initial choice among these agents depends on how soon blood pressure must be controlled; nitroprusside is very rapid; clonidine may require 3 hours to attain full effect. Once an initial agent is begun, further therapy must be directed at control of angiotensin II and norepinephrine pressor effects, cardiac output, and blood volume.

SPECIFIC CONDITIONS ASSOCIATED WITH HYPERTENSIVE CRISIS

The choice of antihypertensive therapy will depend on the clinical situation being considered. Table 20.13 lists the parenteral antihypertensive drugs and specific hypertensive emergencies for which they are useful. Oral agents should be used after initial control of blood pressure.

Table 25.12. Causes of Hypertensive Crisis

1. Vasospasm
   —Exacerbation of essential hypertension
   —Scleroderma
   —Vasculitis
   —Preeclampsia and eclampsia
2. ↑ Renin release
   —Renal artery stenosis
   —Acute glomerulonephritis
   —Renal parenchymal diseases
   —Cholesterol embolization syndrome
   —Renin-secreting tumors
3. ↑ Central sympathetic activity
   —Stroke
   —Head trauma
   —Clonidine withdrawal
   —Spinal cord dysreflexia
   —CNS Drugs
4. ↑ Peripheral sympathetic activity
   —Pheochromocytoma
   —Monoamine oxidase inhibitor and tyramine ingestion
   —Sympathomimetic drugs
   —Extensive burns, trauma, and pain

INTRACRANIAL PROCESSES

Two-thirds of patients develop hypertension after a stroke, and one-half of patients with acute strokes have a history of hypertension. Many of these patients require parenteral therapy to control blood pressure, but the degree to which blood pressure should be reduced must be balanced against the risk of cerebral hypoperfusion brought about by the loss of cerebral blood flow autoregulation. Autoregulation is lost with cerebral infarction and intracranial bleeding, and subarachnoid hemorrhage causes cerebral vascular spasm. Treatment of extreme increases in blood pressure (diastolic blood pressure above 120 mm Hg) is generally recommended (148), and blood pressure should be gradually reduced by 20 to 25% in the first 24 hours. There are no controlled trials to address whether treatment is beneficial for smaller increases in blood pressure, but it is generally agreed that diastolic blood pressure should not drop below 100 mm Hg (147). Sodium nitroprusside is a useful agent in these conditions due to its short half-life, which allows for rapid dose adjustment guided by changes in neurologic status. Nitroprusside increases intracranial pressure due to venodilation and increased cerebral blood flow (149), and specific treatment for this circumstance may be necessary.

Labetalol, diazoxide, and nifedipine are alternative treatments, especially in settings where intensive monitoring is not available. The calcium channel blocker nimodipine is useful in subarachnoid hemorrhage (150). Sedating drugs, such as clonidine, and drugs that reduce cardiac output and cerebral perfusion, such as β-blockers, should be avoided.

HYPERTENSIVE ENCEPHALOPATHY

The patient with hypertensive encephalopathy has a severe headache and frequently has visual disturbances, paralysis, convulsions, vomiting, stupor, and coma. Other intracranial processes also associated with hypertension must be excluded. The onset of encephalopathy occurs over 12 to 48 hours, and diastolic blood pressure is usually above 140 mm Hg, although patients with no preexisting hypertension may present with lower diastolic blood pressures. At these high pressures it is believed that cerebral autoregulation fails, and this failure results in diffuse cerebral edema, petechial hemorrhages, and microinfarctions. Because of the rapid onset, patients may not have developed papilledema, but arteriolar spasm and a retinal sheen are always present. There may be evidence of pulmonary edema and renal failure and, if untreated, the patient will die in several hours or days. This condition needs to be treated immediately, and intravenous nitroprusside or ganglionic blockers are the agents of choice. Intravenous diazoxide and labetalol can be used in hypertensive encephalopathy if the patient cannot be continuously monitored in an intensive care unit. Rapid institution of therapy in hypertensive encephalopathy is lifesaving. Blood pressure should be reduced by 25% over several hours.

AORTIC DISSECTION

Patients with aortic dissection present with severe tearing or ripping chest pain of sudden onset that radiates to the back

Table 25.13.   Parenteral Drugs for Hypertensive Emergencies

Drug	Dose	Onset	Duration	Recommended for	Avoid In
Sodium nitroprusside	0.25 μg/kg/min–8 μg/kg/min intravenous infusion	Seconds	3–5 minutes	Hypertensive encephalopathy, cerebral infarction, cerbral hemorrhage, left ventricular failure, aortic dissection, eclampsia, burns	Renal failure
Nitroglycerin	5–100 μg/min IV infusion	1–2 min	5–10 min	Myocardial ischemia, postcoronary bypass surgery.	
Diazoxide	50–150 mg IV bolus, may repeat every 5–10 min up to 600 mg *or* 15–30 mg/min infusion	1–2 min	10 hours	Substitute when nitroprusside not available	Myocardial ischemia and infarction, aortic dissection, pregnancy
Trimethaphan	0.5–5 mg/min IV infusion	1–5 min	10 min	Aortic dissection	Myocardial ischemia, renal insufficiency, pregnancy
Hydralazine	10–20 mg IV 10–50 mg IM	10–30 min	2–4 hours	Eclampsia, post-op hypertension	Left ventricular failure, myocardial ischemica, mycocardial infarction, aortic dissection, intracranial processes
Phentolamine	5–15 mg IV every 5–15 min	1–2 min	3–10 min	Pheochromocytoma, recreational drugs, MAO inhibitors and tyramine, spinal cord dysreflexia	
Labetalol	2 mg/min IV or 20 mg IV bolus, then 20–80 mg at 10 min (300 mg/max)	5–10 min	3–6 hours	Eclampsia, spinal cord dysreflexia, intracranial process when nitroprusside not available	Heart failure
Methyldopa	250–500 mg IV	30–60 min	6–12 hours	Eclampsia, perioperative hypertension	Myocardial ischemia, myocardial infarction, aortic dissection
Enalaprilat	1.25–5 mg every 6 hours	15 min	12–24 hours	Scleroderma crisis, left ventricular failure, renovascular hypertension, acute glomerulonephritis	Pregnancy
Nicardipine	5 mg/hr increase by 1–2 mg/hr every 15 min up to 15 mg/hr	5–15 min	4–6 hours	(Still being evaluated)	

and abdomen. It may be associated with a murmur of aortic insufficiency, disparate pulses between upper and lower extremities, neurologic abnormalities, and acute renal failure. A widened mediastinum may be seen on chest radiograph; however, angiography is diagnostic. Blood pressure must be immediately reduced to prevent extension of the dissection. The ganglionic blocker trimethaphan reduces blood pressure and diminishes aortic shear forces via its negative inotropic effect. It is a good agent in this setting but may cause ileus, neurogenic bladder, respiratory muscle paralysis, orthostatic hypotension, and tachyphylaxis at 24 to 48 hours. Labetalol or nitroprusside in combination with a β-blocker are alternative choices. Drugs that cause tachycardia or increased cardiac contractility should be avoided. Systolic blood pressure should be quickly reduced to 100 to 120 mm Hg or as low as can be tolerated.

CORONARY INSUFFICIENCY

Drugs that improve coronary perfusion and reduce left ventricular wall tension by reducing systemic vascular resistance are preferred in the treatment of hypertension associated with myocardial infarction and ischemia. The venodilatory effects of nitroglycerin accomplish these desired effects (151). Drugs that induce tachycardia such as hydralazine and diazoxide should be avoided. Labetalol and calcium channel blockers are useful alternatives or adjuncts, as they both improve myocardial oxygenation. Sodium nitroprusside may "steal" blood supply from the poststenotic circulation by virtue of its arteriolar vasodilation (152), although a reduction of preload may reduce cardiac work and thus reduce angina.

ACUTE CONGESTIVE HEART FAILURE

Hypertensive emergencies are often associated with left ventricular failure and acute pulmonary edema. Reduction in preload and afterload are beneficial, and this goal can be accomplished with nitroprusside. Morphine sulfate and diuretics are useful adjuncts. Negative inotropic agents and drugs that cause tachycardia should be avoided. The afterload-reducing qualities of an ACE inhibitor such as enalaprilat can be useful in this setting.

PREECLAMPSIA/ECLAMPSIA

Preeclampsia is defined as hypertension, proteinuria, and edema seen after the 20th week of gestation. Eclampsia demonstrates the additional finding of convulsions. Vasoconstriction is a usual association and, thus, diuretics are not useful. If delivery is not feasible and blood pressure is greater than 160/110 mm Hg, antihypertensive therapy should be started (153). Intravenous hydralazine has been the agent of choice due to extensive experience and lack of fetal side effects. Intravenous labetalol has also been used effectively (154). Diazoxide and calcium channel blockers may inhibit uterine contractions, and trimethaphan increases the risk of meconium ileus. There have been concerns about cyanide accumulation in the fetus with the use of nitroprusside, but there is little evidence to support this finding in humans, and this agent can be safely used with close monitoring (153).

CATECHOLAMINE EXCESS STATES

Pheochromocytoma can produce episodic severe hypertension in response to circulating norepinephrine. A hypertensive crisis may ensue with induction of anesthesia, during surgery, or with the use of certain drugs (e.g., metoclopramide) (155). Patients with pheochromocytoma are usually volume-depleted from the pressor effects of norepinephrine, so treatment with diuretic may cause circulatory compromise to vital organs. β-Blocking drugs should not be given to the patient with a pheochromocytoma until adequate α-adrenergic receptor blockade has been achieved, since blockade of β-adrenergic-mediated vasodilation allows unopposed α-vasoconstriction and may worsen the hypertension. On the other hand, treatment with α-blocking drugs, such as prazosin and phenoxybenzamine, may be strikingly effective in lowering blood pressure, and a prolonged hypotensive response to a low dose of prazosin should make one suspect the presence of pheochromocytoma. Calcium-channel blockers are also very effective in pheochromocytoma, as they impair catecholamine release from the tumor. If parenteral therapy is needed, phentolamine and sodium nitroprusside are good choices.

Drug and food interactions with monoamine oxidase (MAO) inhibitors, ingestion of sympathomimetic drugs, and clonidine withdrawal are also associated with increased levels of circulating catecholamines. These problems should be treated with the agents used to treat pheochromocytoma and patients in clonidine withdrawal should receive clonidine.

RENAL CAUSES OF HYPERTENSIVE CRISIS

Acute glomerulonephritis, renal artery stenosis, and the postrenal transplant state may be associated with hypertensive crisis. In situations where total renal perfusion is compromised, such as bilateral renal artery stenosis or a single kidney with renal artery stenosis. ACE inhibitors may decrease renal clearance and may, rarely, precipitate renal failure. ACE-inhibitors such as enalaprilat are very effective in treating hypertension associated with high renin levels. Calcium-channel blockers and sodium nitroprusside are effective in these disorders, although thiocyanate levels should be followed closely when sodium nitroprusside is used in patients with renal insufficiency.

HYPERTENSIVE URGENCIES

A hypertensive urgency represents a situation where one observes a marked increase in blood pressure in the absence of end-organ damage. Rapid blood pressure reduction is often necessary in situations such as perioperative hypertension. In an outpatient, the risk of a negative outcome within 24 hours of presentation is unknown and likely to be small. Although the rapid reduction of blood pressure in such situations is a common practice in emergency rooms, simple initiation of therapy with assurance of close follow-up is likely to be adequate (156).

Table 25.14 lists oral agents that have been used to rapidly lower blood pressure. It is important to lower blood pressure gently; captopril and prazosin sometimes cause an abrupt drop in blood pressure. Sublingual nifedipine is popular in the treatment of hypertensive urgencies. Although generally safe, there are several case reports of myocardial ischemia following its use.

REFERENCES

1. Joossens JV, Geboers J. Nutrition and essential hypertension. *Biblthca Nutr Dieta* 1986;37:104-118.
2. Young JR, Landsberg L. Suppression of sympathetic nervous system during fasting. *Science* 1977;190:1473-1475.
3. Landsberg L, Young JB. Fasting, feeding and regulation of the sympathetic nervous system. *N Eng J Med* 1978;298:1295-1302.

Table 25.14. Oral Drugs for Hypertensive Urgencies

Drug	Dose	Onset	Duration	Comments
Nifedipine	10–20 mg	5–15 min	3–5 hr	Oral, buccal, or sublingual administration have similar effects. Causes tachycardia.
Clonidine	0.2 mg, then 0.1 mg/hr (max 0.8 mg)	0.5–2 hr	6–8 hr	Sedating.
Captopril	6.5–25 mg	15 min	4–6 hr	Avoid in pregnancy and compromised renal perfusion. May abruptly decrease blood pressure.
Prazosin	1–2 mg, repeat after 1 hr	15–30 min	8 hr	Useful in catecholamine excess states. Watch for orthostatic hypotension.
Minoxidil	2.5–10 mg every 4–6 hrs	0.5–1 hr	12–16 hr	Causes tachycardia.

4. Lavie CJ, Messerli FH. Cardiovascular adaptation to obesity and hypertension. *Chest* 1986;90:275-279.
5. Dustan HP. Obesity and hypertension. *Ann Int Med* 1985;103:1047-1049.
6. MacMahon SW, MacDonald GJ, Berstein I, Andrews G, Blacket RB. Comparison of weight reduction with metoprolol in treatment of hypertension in young overweight patients. *Lancet I* 1985;1223-1236.
7. Sims EAH, Berchtold P. Obesity and hypertension. Mechanisms and implications for management. *JAMA* 1982;247:49-52.
8. Einhorne D, Young JB, Landsberg L. Hypotensive effect of fasting: Possible involvement of the sympathetic nervous system and endogenous opiates. *Science* 1982;217:727-729.
9. Tuck ML, Sowers J, Dornfeld L, Kledzik G. Maxwell M. The effect of weight reduction on blood pressure, plasma renin activity, and plasma aldosterone levels in obese patients. *N Eng J Med* 1981;304:930-933.
10. Agharanya JC, Alonso R. Wurtman RJ. Changes in catecholamine excretion after short-term tyrosine ingestion in normally fed human subjects. *Am J Clin Nutr* 1981;34:82-87.
11. Jenkins JS, Conolly J. Adrenocortical response to ethanol in man. *Br Med J* 1968;5607:804-805.
12. Jeffreys DB, Flanagan RJ, Volans GN. Reversal of ethanol-induced coma with naloxone. *Lancet* 1980;(Feb 9):308-309.
13. Kempner W. Treatment of hypertensive vascular disease with rice diet. *Am J Med* 1948;4:545-577.
14. Watkin DM, Frobe HF, Hatch TF, Gutman AB. Effects of diet in essential hypertension II. Results with unmodified Kempner rice diet in 50 hospitalized patients. *Am J Med* 1950;9:441-493.
15. MacGregor GA, Best FA, Cam JM, et al. Double-blind randomized crossover trial of moderate sodium restriction in essential hypertension. *Lancet* 1982;(Feb 13):351-354.
16. Beard TC, Gray WR, Cooke HM, Barge R. Randomized controlled trial of a no-added sodium diet for mild hypertension. *Lancet* 1982;(Aug 28):455-458.
17. Warren SE, O'Connor DT. The antihypertensive mechanism of sodium restriction. *J Cardiovasc Pharmacol* 1981;3:781-790.
18. Dustan HP, Bravo EL, Tarazi RC. Volume dependent, essential and steroid hypertension. *Am J Cardiol* 1973;32:606.
19. Winer BM. The antihypertensive actions of benzothiadiazenes. *Circulation* 1961;23:211-218.
20. Lake CR, Ziegler MG, Coleman MD, Kopin IJ. Hydrochlorothiazide-induced sympathetic hyperactivity in hypertensive patients. *Clin Pharmacol Ther* 1979;26:428-432.
21. Lake CR, Ziegler MG, Coleman MD, Kopin IJ. Fenfluramine potentiation of antihypertensive effects of thiazides. *Clin Pharmacol Ther* 1980;28:22-27.
22. Berglund G, Andersson O. Low doses of hydrochlorothiazide in hypertension: Antihypertensive and metabolic effects. *Eur J Clin Pharmacol* 1976;10:177-182.
23. Materson BJ, Oster JR, Michael UF, et al. Dose responses to chlorthalidone in patients with mild hypertension. *Clin Pharmacol Ther* 1978;24:192-198.
24. Kolata G. Heart study produces a surprise result. *Science* 1982;218:31.
25. Felson DT, Sloutkis D, Anderson JJ, Anthony JM, Kiel OP. Thiazide diuretics and the risk of hip fracture: Results from the Framingham study. *JAMA* 1991;265:370-373.
26. Lake CR, Ziegler MG. Effect of acute volume alterations on norepinephrine and dopamine-beta hydroxylase in normotensive and hypertensive subjects. *Circulation* 1978;57:774-778.
27. Taylor AA, Pool JL, Lake CR, et al. Plasma norepinephrine concentrations: No differences among normal volunteers and low, high or normal renin hypertensive patients. *Life Sci* 1978;22:1499-1510.
28. Skluth HA, Gums JG. Spironolactone: A re-examination. *DIEP* 1990;24:52-59.
29. Fawada ET. Antihypertensive therapy with trimtrene-hydrochlorothiazide VS amiloride-hydrochlorothiazide: Comparison of effects on urinary prostaglandin E_2 excretion. *Arch Intern Med* 1986;146:1312-1314.
30. Buhler FR, Laragh JH, Baer L, Vaughan ED, Brunner HR. Propranolol inhibition of renin secretion. *N Engl J Med* 1972;287:1209-1214.
31. Jackson EK, Campbell WB. A possible antihypertensive mechanism of propranolol: Antagonism of angiotensin II enhancement of sympathetic nerve transmission through prostaglandins. *Hypertension* 1981;3:23-33.
32. Nakaoka H, Kitahara Y, Amano M, et al. Effect of β-adrenergic receptor blockade on atrial natriuretic peptide in essential hypertension. *Hypertension* 1987;10:221-225.
33. Struyker-Boudier HA, Smits JF. Antihypertensive action of beta-adrenoreceptor blocking drugs. The role of intrarenal mechanisms. *Am J Hypertens* 1989;2:237S-240S.
34. O'Connor DT, Preston RA. Propranolol effects on autonomic function in hypertensive men. *Clin Cardiol* 1982;5:340-346.
35. Beaufils M. Alterations in renal hemodynamics during chronic and acute beta-blockade in humans. *Am J Hypertens* 1989;2:233S-236S.
36. Woods JW, Pittman AW, Pulliam CC, Werk EE, Waider W, Allen CA. Renin profiling in hypertension and its use in treatment with propranolol and chlorthalidone. *N Eng J Med* 1976;294:1137-1143.
37. Weisfeldt ML. Aging of the cardiovascular system. *N Eng J Med* 1980;303:1172-1173.
38. Frolich ED, Dustan HP, Page IH. Hyperdynamic beta-adrenergic circulatory state. *Arch Intern Med* 1966;117:614-619.
39. Holland OB, Fairchild C. Renin classification for diuretic and beta blocker treatment of black hypertensive patients. *J Chron Dis* 1982;35:179-182.
40. Hawkins DW, Diekmann MR, Horner RD. Diuretics and hypertension in black adults. *Arch Intern Med* 1988;148:803-805.
41. Hollifield JW, Sherman K, Zwagg RV, Shand DG. Proposed mechanisms of propranolol's antihypertensive effect in essential hypertension. *N Eng J Med* 1976;295:68-73.
42. van de Brink G, Boer P, van Asten P, Mees EJD, Geyskes GG. One and three doses of propranolol a day in hypertension. *Clin Pharmacol Ther.* 1980;27:9-15.
43. Dornhurst A, Powell SH, Pensy J. Aggravation by propranolol of hyperglycaemic effect of hydrochlorothiazide in type II diabetics without alteration of insulin secretion. *Lancet* 1985;(Jan):123-126.
44. Vandongen R, Margetts B, Deklerk N, Beilin LJ, Rogers P. Plasma catecholamines following exercise in hypertensives treated with pindolol: Comparison with placebo and metoprolol. *Br J Clin Pharmacol* 1986;21:627-632.
45. Ruffin RE, McIntyre ELM, Latimer KM, et al. Assessment of β-adrenoceptor antagonists in asthmatic patients. *Br J Clin Pharmacol* 1982;13(Suppl 2):325S-335S.
46. Medical Research Council. Adverse reactions to bendrofluazide and propranolol for the treatment of mild hypertension. *Lancet* 1981;(Sept 12):539-542.
47. Gengo FM, Gabos C. Central nervous system considerations in the use of β-Blockers, ACE-inhibitors, and thiazide diuretics in managing essential hypertension. *Am Heart J* 1988;116:305-310.
48. Frishman WH. β-Adrenergic receptor blockers. Adverse effects and drug interactions. *Hypertension II* 1988;(Suppl. II):II21-II29.
49. Pederson OL, Mikkelsen E, Nielsen JL, Christensen NJ. Abrupt withdrawal of beta-blocking agents in patients with arterial hypertension. Effect on blood pressure, heart rate and plasma catecholamines and prolactin. *Eur J Clin Pharmacol* 1979;15:215-217.
50. Frishman WH. Beta adrenergic blocker withdrawal. *Am J Cardiol* 1987;59:26F-32F.
51. Gibson BE, Black S, Maas L, Eucchiara RF. Esmolol for the control of hypertension after neurologic surgery. *Clin Pharmacol Ther* 1988;44:650-653.
52. Frohlich E. Vasodilatory β-blockers: Systemic and regional hemodynamic effects. *Am Heart J* 1991;121:1012-1017.
53. Michelson E, Frishman WH, Lewis JE, et al. Multicenter clinical evaluation of long-term efficacy and safety of labetalol in treatment of hypertension. *Am J Med* 1983;(October):68-80.
54. Langer SZ. The role of alpha and beta-presynaptic receptors in the regulation of noradrenaline release elicited by nerve stimulation. *Clin Sci Mol Med* 1976;51:423s-426s.
55. Kobinger W. Alpha-adrenoceptors in cardiovascular regulation. In: Ziegler MG, Lake CR, eds. Frontiers of Clinical Neuroscience, Vol. 4: Norepinephrine. Baltimore: Williams & Wilkins, 1984.
56. Oates HF, Stoker LM, Stokes GS. Interactions between prazosin, clonidine, and direct vasodilators in the anaesthetized rat. *Clin Exp Pharmacol Physiol* 1978;5:85-89.
57. O'Connor DT, Preston RA, Sasso EH. Renal perfusion changes during treatment of essential hypertension: Prazosin versus propranolol. *J Cardiovasc Pharmacol* 1979;1(Suppl 1):S38-S42.
58. Nash DT. Alpha-adrenergic blockers: Mechanism of action, blood pressure control, and effects on lipoprotein metabolism. *Clin Cardiol* 1990;13:764-772.
59. Luther RR. New perspectives on selective alpha$_1$ blockade. *Am J Hypertens* 1989;2:729-735.
60. Graham RM, Thornell G, Gain IR. Prazosin: The first dose phenomenon. *Br Med J* 1976;2:1293.
61. Baner JH, Jones LB, Gaddy P. Effects of prazosin therapy on blood pressure, renal function, and fluid composition. *Arch Intern Med* 1984;144:1196-1200.
62. Mroczek WJ, Finnerty FA. A double-blind evaluation of a new antihypertensive agent. In: Cotton, ed. Prazosin. Amsterdam: Excerpta Medica, 1974.
63. Kuokkanen K, Mattila MJ. Antihypertensive effect of prazosin in combination with methyldopa, clonidine or propranolol. *Ann Clin Res* 1979;11:18-24.
64. Holtzman JL, Kaihlanen PM, Rider A, et al. Concomitant administration of terazosin and atenolol for the treatment of essential hypertension. *Arch Intern Med* 1988;148:539-543.
65. Wallace JM, Gill DP. Prazosin in the diagnosis and treatment of pheochromocytoma. *JAMA* 1978;240:2752-2753.
66. Cavero I, Roach AG. The pharmacology of prazosin, a novel antihypertensive agent. *Life Sci* 1980;27:1525-1540.
67. Semplicini A, Pessina AC, Pallatini P, et al. Orthostatic hypotension after the first administration of prazosin in hypertensive patients. *Clin Exp Pharmacol Physiol* 1981;8:1-10.
68. Stokes GS, Braham RM, Gain JM, Davis PR. Influence of dosage and dietary sodium on the first-dose effects of prazosin. *Br Med J* 1977;1:1507.
69. Starke K. Regulation of noradrenaline release by presynaptic receptor systems. *Rev Physiol Biochem Pharmacol* 1977;77:1-124.
70. Mitchell HC, Pettinger WA. Dose-response of clonidine on plasma catecholamines in the hypernoradrenergic state associated with vasodilator beta-blocker therapy. *J Cardiovasc Pharmacol* 1981;3:647-654.

71. Campese VM, Romanoff M, Telfer N, Weidman P, Massry SG. Role of sympathetic nerve inhibition and body sodium volume state in the antihypertensive action of clonidine in essential hypertension. *Kidney Int* 1980;18:351-357.

72. Peters RW, Hamilton BP, Hamilton J, Kuzbida B, Pavlis R. Cardiac arrhythmias after clonidine withdrawal. *Clin Pharmacol Ther* 1983;34:435-439.

73. Garvey HL, Ram N. Centrally induced hypotensive effects of beta adrenergic blocking drugs. *Eur J Pharmacol* 1975;33:283-294.

74. Mehta JL, Lopez LM. Rebound hypertension following abrupt cessation of clonidine and metoprolol. *Arch Intern Med* 1987;147:389-390.

75. Dollery CT, Davies DS, Draffan GH, et al. Clinical pharmacology and pharmacokinetics of clonidine. *Clin Pharmacol Ther* 1975;19:11-17.

76. Kunos G, Farsand C. Beta endorphin: Possible involvement in the antihypertensive effect of central alpha-receptor activation. *Science* 1981;211:82-84.

77. Brown MJ, Salmon D, Rendell M. Clonidine hallucinations. *Ann Int Med* 1980;93:456-457.

78. Maling TJB, Dollery CT, Hamilton CA. Clonidine and sympathetic activity during sleep. *Clin Sci* 1979;57:509-514.

79. Reid JL, Dargie HJ, Davies DS, Wing LMH, Hamilton CA, Dollery CT. Clonidine withdrawal in hypertension. *Lancet* 1977;(June 4):1171-1174.

80. Brodsky JB, Bravo JJ. Acute postoperative clonidine withdrawal syndrome. *Anesthesiology* 1976;44:519-521.

81. Brenner WI, Lieberman AN: Acute clonidine withdrawal syndrome following open-heart operation. *Ann Thoracic Surg* 1977;24:80-82.

82. Anderson RJ, Hat GR, Crumpler CP, Reed WG, Matthews CA. Oral clonidine loading in hypertensive emergencies. *JAMA* 1981;246:848-850.

83. Larbi JI, Zaimise E. Effect of acute intravenous administration of clonidine on cerebral blood flow in man. *Br J Pharmacol* 1970;39:198P-199P.

84. Jerie P. Clinical experience with guanfacine in long-term treatment of hypertension; adverse reactions to guanfacine. *Br J Clin Pharmacol* 1980;10(Suppl 1):157-164.

85. Beal D, Dujovne C, Gillis JA. The effect of methyldopa on human judgment in hypertensive patients and normal volunteers. *Res Comm Psychol Psychiatry Behav* 1980;5:205-217.

86. Stanley P, Mijch A. Methyldopa: An often overlooked cause of fever and transient hepatocellular dysfunction. *Med J Aust* 1986;144:603-604.

87. Oster JR, Epstein M. Use of centrally acting sympatholytic agents in the management of hypertension. *Arch Intern Med* 1991;151:1638-1644.

88. LoBuglio AF, Jandl JH, The nature of the α-methyldopa red-cell antibody. *N Engl J Med* 1967;276:658-665.

89. Burden AC, Alexander CPT. Rebound hypertension after acute methyldopa withdrawal. *Br Med J* 1976;(May):1055-1057.

90. O'Malley K, Segal JL, Israili ZH, Boles M, McNay JL, Dayton PG. Duration of hydralazine action in hypertension. *Clin Pharmacol Ther* 1975;18:581-586.

91. Zacest R, Gilmore E, Koch-Weser J. Treatment of essential hypertension with combined vasodilation and beta-adrenergic blockade. *N Eng J Med* 1972;286:617-622.

92. Koch-Weser J. Vasodilator drugs in the treatment of hypertension. *Arch Int Med* 1974;133:1017-1025.

93. Linas SL, Nies AS. Minoxidil. *Ann Int Med* 1981;94:61-65.

94. Meier A, Weidmann P, Ziegler WH. Catecholamine, renin, aldosterone, and blood volume during chronic minoxidil therapy. *Klin Wochenschr* 1981;59:1231-1236.

95. Leenen FHH, Smith DL, Farkas RM, Reeves RA, Marquez-Julio A. Vasodilators and regression of left ventricular hypertrophy. *Am J Med* (1987);82:969-978.

96. Leenen FHH, Smith DL, Unger NP. Topical minoxidil: Cardiac effects in bald man. *Br J Clin Pharmac* 1988;26:481-485.

97. Sobota JT. Review of cardiovascular findings in humans treated with minoxidil. *Toxicol Path* 1989;17:193-202.

98. Wells, JD. Unusual cases of resistance to minoxidil therapy. *J Cardiovascular Pharmacol* 1980;(Suppl 2):S228-S235.

99. Pearson RM, Griffith DNW, Wollard M, James IM. Comparison of effects on cerebral blood flow of rapid reduction in systemic arterial pressure by diazoxide and labetalol in hypertensive patients: Preliminary findings. *Br J Clin Pharmacol* 1979;8:155S-198S.

100. Neary D, Thurston H, Pohl JEF. Development of extrapyramidal symptoms in hypertensive patients treated with diazoxide. *Br Med JP* 1973;(Sept 1):474-475.

101. Rouby JJ, Gory G, Bourrelli B, Glaser P, Viars P. Resistance to sodium nitroprusside in hypertensive patients. *Crit Care Med* 1982;10:301-304.

102. Abrams SA, A Reappraisal of nitrate therapy. *JAMA* 1988;259:396-401.

103. Sorkin EM, Brogden RN, Romankiewicz JA. Intravenous glyceryl trinitrate. *Drugs* 1984;27:45-80.

104. Cote DD, Torchia MG. Nitroglycerin absorption to polyvinylchloride seriously interferes with its clinical use. *Anesth Analg* 1982;61:541-543.

105. Ruilope LM, Miranda B, Oliet A, Alcazar JM, Bigorra J, Rodicio JL. Persistence of the natriuretic effect of calcium entry blockers. *J Cardiovasc Pharm* 1988;12:S136-S139.

106. Pool PE, Massie BM, Venkataraman K, Hirsch AT, Samant DR, Seagren SC, Gaw J, Salel AF, Tubau JF. Diltiazem as monotherapy for systemic hypertension: A multicenter, randomized placebo-controlled trial. *Amer J Cardiol* 1986;57:212-217.

107. Cummings DM, Amadio P, Nelson L, Fitzgerald JM. The role of calcium channel blockers in the treatment of essential hypertension. *Arch Intern Med* 1991;151:250-259.

108. Frischman W, Charlap S, Kimmel B, et al. Diltiazem, nifedipine, and their combination in patients with stable angina pectoris: Effects on angina, exercise tolerance, and the ambulatory electrocardiographic ST segment. *Circulation* 1988;77:774-786.

109. Resnick KLM, Nicholson JP, Laragh JH. Calcium, the renin-aldosterone system, and the hypertensive response to nifedipine. *Hypertens* 1987;10:254-258.

110. Corea L, Miele N, Bentivoglio M, Boschetti E, Abagiti-Rosei E, Muiesan G. Acute and chronic effects of nifedipine on plasma renin actvity and plasma adrenaline and noradrenaline in controls and hypertensive patients. *Clin Sci* 1979;57:115s-117s.

111. Imai Y, Abe K, Otsuke Y, et al. Management of severe hypertension with nifedipine in combination with clonidine or propranolol. *Arzneim.-Firsch/Drug Res* 1980;30:674-678.

112. Stern HC, Matthews JH, Belz, GG. Intrinsic and reflex actions of verapamil and nifedipine: Assessment in normal subjects by noninvasive techniques and autonomic blockade. *Eur J Clin Pharmacol* 1986;29:541-547.

113. Caruthers SG, Freeman DJ, Bailey DG. Synergistic adverse hemodynamic interaction between oral verapamil and propranolol. *Clin Pharmacol Ther* 1989;46:469-477.

114. Bertel O, Conen D, Rader EW, Muller J, Land C, Cubrich UC. Nifedipine in hypertensive emergencies. *Br Med J* 1983;283:19-21.

115. Bauer JH, Reams GP. The role of calcium entry blockers in hypertensive emergencies. *Circulation* 1987;75:(Suppl V):V174-V180.

116. Weinstein DB, Heider JG. Antiatherogenic properties of calcium antagonists. *Am J Med* 1989;86(Suppl 4A):27-32.

117. Benstein JA, Dworkin LO. Renal vascular effects of calcium channel blockers in hypertension. *Am J Hypertens* 1990;3:3055-3125.

118. Stern R, Khalsa JH. Cutaneous adverse reactions associated with calcium channel blockers. *Arch Intern Med* 1989;149:829-832.

119. Dzau VJ. Implications of local angiotensin production in cardiovascular physiology and pharmacology. *Am J Cardiovasc* 1987;59:59A-65A.

120. Edwards CR, Padfield PL. Angiotensin-converting enzyme inhibitors: Past, present, and bright future. *Lancet* 1985;(January 5):30-34.

121. Katzman PL, Hulthen UL, Hokfelt B. The effect of 8 weeks treatment with the calcium antagonist felodipine on blood pressure, heart rate, working capacity, plasma renin activity, plasma angiotensin II, urinary catecholamines and aldosterone in patients with essential hypertension. *Br J Clin Pharmac* 1986; 21:633-640.

122. Helgeland A, Strommen R, Hagelund CH, Tretli S: Enalapril, atenolol and hydrochlorothiazide in mild to moderate hypertension. *Lancet* 1986; (April 19):872-875.

123. Brunner HR, Gavras H, Waeber B, et al. Oral angiotensin-converting enzyme inhibitor in long-term treatment of hypertensive patients. *Ann Int Med* 1979;90:19-23.

124. Turini GA, Bribic M, Brunner HR, Waeber B, Gavras H. Improvement of chronic congestive heart-failure by oral captopril. *Lancet* 1979;(June 9):1213-1215.

125. Nakashima Y, Foudd F, Tarazi RC. Regression of left ventricular hypertrophy from systemic hypertension by enalapril. *Am J Cardiol* 1984;53:1044-1049.

126. Bauer JH, Reamy GP, Lal SM. Renal protective effect of strict blood pressure control with enalapril therapy. *Arch Intern Med* 1987;147:1397-1400.

127. Keane WF, Anderson S, Anvell M, de Zeeuw D, Narins RG, Povarg G. Angiotensin converting enzyme inhibitors and progressive renal insufficiency. *Ann Intern Med* 1989;111:503-516.

128. Toto RD, Mitchell HC, Lee HC, Milam C, Pettinger WA. Reversible renal insufficiency due to angiotensin converting enzyme inhibitors in hypertensive nephrosclerosis. *Ann Intern Med* 1991;115(7):513-519.

129. Manhem P, Bramnert M, Hulthen UL, Hokfelt B. The effect of captopril on catecholamines, renin activity, angiotensin II and aldosterone in plasma during physical exercise in hypertensive patients. *Eur J Clin Invest* 1981;11:389-395.

130. Townsend RR, Holland B. Combination of converting enzyme inhibitor with diuretic for the treatment of hypertension. *Arch Intern Med* 1990;150:1175-1183.

131. Singer DRJ, Markandu ND, Shore AC, MacGregor GA. Captopril and nifedipine in combination for moderate and severe essential hypertension. *Hypertens* 1987;9:629-633.

132. Matson JR, Norby LH, Robillard JE. Interaction of minoxidil and captopril in the treatment of refractory hypertension. *Am J Dis Child* 1981;135:256-258.

133. Kostis JB. Angiotensin converting enzyme inhibitors: Emerging differences and new compounds. *Am J Hypertens* 1989;2:57-64.

134. Sakano T, Okuda N, Sakura N. Yahata H, Tabe Y, Eno S, Kurogane H, Usui T. Captopril in hypertensive emergencies. *Hiroshima J Med* 1981;30:30-45.

135. Strauss R, Garvas I, Vlahakos D, Garvas H. Enalaprilat in hypertensive emergencies. *J Clin Pharmacol* 1986;26:39-43.

136. Rutledge J, Ayers C, Davidson R, et al. Effect of intravenous enalaprilat in moderate and severe systemic hypertension. *Am J Cardiol* 1988;62:1062-1067.

137. Scott A, Scott AA, Purohit DM, et al. Neonatal renal failure: A complication of maternal antihypertensive therapy. *Am J Ob Gyn* 1989;160:1223-1224.

138. Weber MA, Drayer JIM, Laragh JH. The effects of clonidine and propranolol separately and in combination on blood pressure and plasma renin activity in essential hypertension. *J Clin Pharmacol* 1978;18:233.

139. Wilja M, Jonnela AJ, Juustila H, Mattila MJ. Interaction of clonidine and beta blockers. *Acta Med Scand* 1980;207:173.

140. Mattila MG. Antihypertensive effect of prazosin in combination with methyldopa. Clonidine or Propranolol? *Ann Clin Res* 1979;11:18.

141. Hubbell FA, Weber MA, Drayer JM, Rose DE. Central alpha-adrenergic stimulation by clonidine overrides the antihyper-tensive effect of peripheral alpha adrenergic blockade induced by prazosin. 8th Mtg Intl Soc Hypertension 1081;Milan, Italy.

142. MacGregor GA, Markandu ND, Smith SJ, Sagnella GA. Captopril: Contrasting effects of adding hydrochlorothiazide, propranolol, or nifedipine. *J Cardiovasc Pharmacol* 1985;7:S82-S87.

143. Mancia G, Grassi G, Pomdiossi G, et al. Effects of blood- pressure measurements by the doctor on patient's blood pressure and heart rate. *Lancet* 1983;(Sept 24):695-697.

144. Bravo EL. Phenylpropanolamine and other over-the-counter vasoactive compounds. *Hypertension* 1988;11(Suppl II):II7-II10.

145. Levine SR, Braust JCM, Futrell N, et al. Cerebrovascular complications of the use of the "crack" form of alkaloidal cocaine. *N Engl J Med* 1990;323:699-704.

146. McCarron MM, Schulze BW, Thompson GA, et al. Acute phencyclidine intoxication: Incidence of clinical findings in 1,000 cases. *Ann Emerg Med* 1981;10:237-242.

147. Houston MC. Pathophysiology, clinical aspects, and treatment of hypertensive crisis. *Prog Cardiovasc Dis* 1989;32(2):99-148.

148. Brett T, Reed RL. Intensive care for acute stroke in the Community Hospital setting. *Stroke* 1989;20(5):694-697.

149. Van Aken H, Cottrell JE, Angler G, Puchstein C. Treatment of intraoperative hypertensive emergencies in patients with intracranial disease. *Am J Cardiol* 1989;53:43C-47C.

150. Tattenborn D, Dycka J. Prevention and treatment of delayed ischemic dysfunction in patients with aneurysmal subarachnoid hemorrhage. *Stroke* 1990;21(Suppl IV):IV83-IV89.

151. Flaherty JT. Comparison of intravenous nitroglycerin and sodium nitroprusside in acute myocardial infarction. *Am J Med* 1983;74(6B):53-60.

152. Mann T, Cohn PF, Holman L, Green L, Markis JE, Phillipi DA. Effect of nitroprusside on regional myocardial blood flow in coronary artery disease. *Circulation* 1978;57:732-737.

153. Silver HM. Acute hypertensive crisis in pregnancy. *Med Clin NA* 1989;73:623-638.

154. Jouppila P, Kirkinen P, Koivula A, et al. Labetalol does not alter the placental and fetal blood flow or maternal prostanoids in pre-eclampsia. *Br J Obstet Gynaecol* 1986;93:543-547.

155. Abe M, Orita Y, Nakashima Y, et al. Hypertensive crisis induced by metoclopramide in a patient with pheochromocytoma. *Angiology* 1984;35:122-128.

156. Zeller KR, Von Kuhnert L, Matthews C. Rapid reduction of severe asymptomatic hypertension. A prospective, controlled trial. *Arch Intern Med* 1989;149:2186-2189.

CHAPTER 26

Heart Rate Control

PAUL M. HEERDT, M.D., Ph.D.

ROBERT M. FORSTOT, M.D.

Few hemodynamic variables routinely monitored in critically ill patients can change as quickly, and sometimes disastrously, as heart rate. Reflecting an intrinsic rate of contraction that, in turn, is modified by extrinsic control mechanisms, the heart rate has a profound influence on cardiac output and myocardial oxygen consumption. The discussion that follows focuses on mechanisms for initiation, conduction, and regulation of heart rate, and then outlines how these mechanisms can be pharmacologically altered in the treatment of bradycardia and supraventricular tachyarrhythmias. Information regarding drugs used specifically to halt atrial ectopy arising from nonnodal tissue, or primary ventricular tachycardia, can be found in other chapters.

INTRINSIC CONTROL OF HEART RATE

It appears that all chambers of the heart have cells that are capable of spontaneously depolarizing and producing a generalized cardiac contraction. Under most circumstances, cells in the sinoatrial (SA) node display the fastest rate of spontaneous depolarization (automaticity), followed by those in the atrioventricular (AV) node and some ventricular Purkinje fibers. This "chain of command" is physiologically significant in that if a more rapid pacemaker shuts down—or if impulses from the atria to ventricles are completely blocked—then a slower pacemaker predominates to avoid asystole. However, pathologic or pharmacologic influences on the heart may: (a) cause the AV node, a subsidiary atrial pacemaker, or even atrial or ventricular muscle, to depolarize (either via enhanced automaticity or reentry) at a rate exceeding the normal SA node rate, resulting in a nonsinus tachycardia; (b) allow rapid or chaotic atrial impulses to be conducted to the ventricles; or (c) block transmission of impulses through the AV node and/or suppress normal and ectopic pacemakers enough to allow cardiac standstill.

Located in the posterior right atrium near the entrance of the superior vena cava (sulcus terminalis), the SA node is composed of three cell types: (a) P cells—small, round cells that appear pale on both light and electron-microscopy and are primarily involved in impulse generation; (b) transitional cells—elongated cells primarily involved in impulse conduction that display characteristics of both P cells and atrial myocytes; and (c) true atrial myocytes incorporated within nodal tissue (1). In humans, blood to the SA node is supplied by a sinus node artery originating from either the right coronary (55%) or left circumflex artery (45%). A characteristic SA node action potential is shown in Figure 26.1. In comparison to the membrane potential characteristics of atrial myocytes, SA node cells display a less negative resting membrane (or diastolic) potential, spontaneous depolarization during phase 4, a lower depolarization threshold, a slower phase 0, no plateau, and a gradual rate of repolarization. The frequency of SA nodal rhythmicity is thus influenced by the slope of phase 4, as well as diastolic and threshold potentials, which in turn can be modified by extrinsic factors such as autonomic tone (Fig. 26.2).

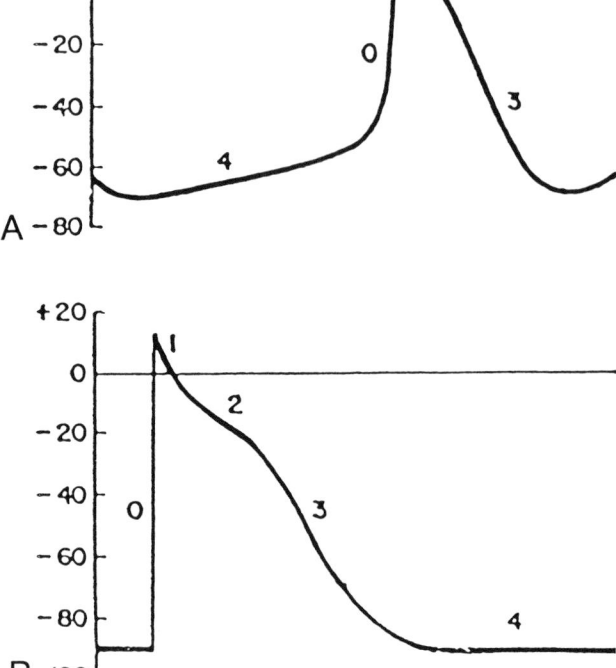

Figure 26.1. Representative action potentials recorded from cells in the SA node (**A**) and atrium (**B**); sweep speed in **A** is one-half that in **B**. (Redrawn from Berne RM, Levy MN: Cardiac physiology. St. Louis, CV Mosby, 1981.)

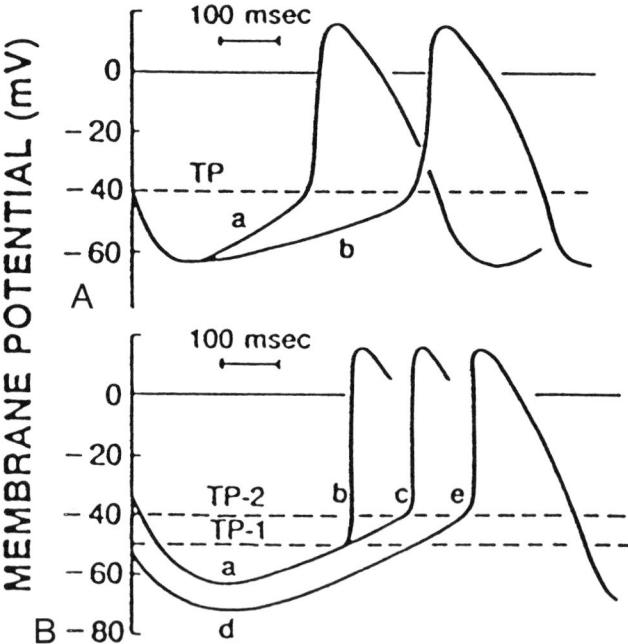

Figure 26.2. Action potential tracings representing mechanisms for changing automaticity of nodal cells. In **A**, an increase in the slope of phase 4 from *b* to *a* will increase the frequency of pacemaker firing. In **B**, an increase in the magnitude of the diastolic potential from *a* to *d* will reduce automaticity, as will an increase in threshold potential (*TP*) from *b* to *c*. (Redrawn from Atlee JL: Perioperative cardiac dysrhythmias. Chicago, Year Book Medical Publishers, 1990.)

Impulses generated in the SA node are conducted to the left atrium by specialized conducting fibers (Bachmann's bundle) and to the AV node via the anterior, middle, and posterior internodal pathways. The true physiologic significance of these pathways, however, remains controversial (2). Multiple atrial regions with "subsidiary" atrial pacemaker activity have been defined, including the coronary sinus, inferior sulcus terminalis, Bachmann's bundle, and atrial "plateau" fibers (3). These areas, which appear to have less vagal innervation than the SA node, may be responsible for some supraventricular arrhythmias, and for the appearance of a nonsinus atrial rate faster than AV node rhythmicity that occurs from minutes to days after SA arrest.

Located near the ostium of the coronary sinus on the right side of the interatrial septum, the AV node is a long (22 mm), thin (3 mm) structure on which the internodal pathways converge. The AV node contains P cells and transitional cells (many of which display histological variation from those in the SA node) that are arranged into anatomically and functionally discrete areas. Connection of the AV node to the ventricular His bundle appears to occur in some of these specialized regions (4). Blood is supplied to the AV node via a branch of the right coronary artery in nearly 90% of humans, with the remaining 10% receiving blood from the circumflex branch of the left coronary artery.

The nature of phase 4 depolarization in pacemaker tissue has been studied extensively and appears to vary between nodal cells and Purkinje fibers. In general, automaticity of SA and AV nodal cells depends upon a slow inward current of calcium to produce depolarization during phase 4, and is independent of inward sodium ion movement (i.e., it is not altered by sodium channel blockade with tetrodotoxin) (5). It is important to note that in the AV node, the chronotropic role provided by automatic properties is secondary to the primary role of impulse conduction (dromotropy). Pharmacologic manipulation of the rate of rise and amplitude of action potentials in some AV nodal cells influences the time it takes for an impulse to be conducted, while alterations in the recovery of cell excitability influence effective refractory period. AV nodal cells display the intrinsic property of prolonged conduction time in response to increased heart rate (6). This phenomenon has been termed "AV nodal accommodation," and, under normal circumstances, protects the ventricle from many supraventricular tachycardias.

Drugs are now available that influence both chronotropy and dromotropy, primarily through intrinsic mechanisms. Interference with the slow inward movement of calcium, for example, reduces the rate of spontaneous depolarization (slope of phase 4), thus decreasing automaticity of both the SA and AV nodes. Furthermore, direct, acute changes in AV node conduction time and refractory period are often beneficial in curtailing reentrant arrhythmias and controlling the ventricular response to supraventricular tachycardia.

EXTRINSIC CONTROL OF HEART RATE

At any point in time, heart rate reflects complex, second-to-second variations in cardiac autonomic tone that, in turn, are modified by factors such as age, homeostatic reflexes, disease, drugs, and emotion. In the absence of any autonomic influence (e.g., denervation), the intrinsic adult heart rate is estimated to be 105 beats per minute (7). Given that the rate of a normal, innervated heart is about 70 beats per minute, it appears that the human SA node is predominantly under parasympathetic control at rest.

Anatomic studies have demonstrated extensive, discrete autonomic innervation of the SA node, while terminal autonomic fibers in the AV node have not been as clearly defined (8). Cardiac sympathetic fibers originate in the upper thoracic, and probably lower cervical, spinal cord with preganglionic fibers in white rami, and synapses primarily in caudal cervical and stellate ganglia. Postganglionic fibers reach the cardiac plexus via superior, middle, and inferior cardiac nerves. Parasympathetic innervation of the heart arises in the medulla oblongata, courses through the vagus nerve, and enters the heart along with sympathetic fibers in the cardiac plexus to synapse within the heart itself. Modulation of autonomic input to the heart has been reviewed extensively (9, 10) and is extraordinarily complex, with multiple cerebral cortical influences (i.e., anxiety) and hypothalamic factors (i.e., temperature regulation) meshed with medullary and local preganglionic, ganglionic, postganglionic, and end-organ influences.

SYMPATHETIC EFFECTS

In normal humans, sympathetic blockade of the heart produces only a slight reduction in heart rate, consistent with the contention that the predominant autonomic input at rest is parasympathetic. However, when sympathetic tone is high—as during congestive heart failure or sepsis—the negative chronotropic response to cardiac sympathetic blockade may be profound. It has long been known that the predominant adrenergic receptor found in SA and AV nodal tissue is of the β_1 variety, although recent evidence has suggested the possibility of α-adrenergic influence as well (11). At the end-organ level, norepinephrine released by adrenergic nerve terminals binds to β-receptors, which are coupled to membrane-bound adenylate cyclase by a guanine nucleotide-binding protein (12). Activation of adenylate cyclase ensues, leading to generation of intracellular adenosine 3':5'-cyclic phosphate (cAMP) and a cascade of events culminating in the phosphorylation of proteins either within, or in close proximity to, calcium channels. Individual channels then exhibit prolonged "open time"—and reduced "closed time"—thus increasing the probability that the channel will be open. The resultant increase in whole-cell calcium current is responsible for the physiologic responses of enhanced automaticity and decreased conduction time (13, 14). It has been clearly demonstrated that, in comparison with vagally mediated effects, the cardiac response to sympathetic stimulation both arises and dissipates relatively slowly (10). The current rationale for this latency includes the nature of norepinephrine dispersion (reuptake) at the nerve terminal, and dependence on a second messenger for end-organ effect.

PARASYMPATHETIC EFFECTS

In contrast to sympathetic stimulation, the cardiac response to parasympathetic stimulation occurs almost immediately (i.e., within 100 msec) and dissipates nearly as quickly as a result of the extremely rapid hydrolysis of acetylcholine by acetylcholinesterase. Mediated by the binding of acetylcholine to muscarinic receptors linked directly to sarcolemmal potassium channels by a guanine nucleotide-binding protein, parasympathetic stimulation produces membrane hyperpolarization (Fig. 26.2) along with inhibition of the hyperpolarization-activated pacemaker current (15). Furthermore, stimulation of muscarinic receptors coupled via another guanine nucleotide-binding protein to adenylate cyclase leads to inhibition of the enzyme, thus opposing the effects of adrenergic stimulation (16). Thus, enhanced vagal tone decreases pacemaker automaticity while increasing AV node conduction time and increasing refractory period.

It is extremely important to understand that changes in cardiac chronotropy or dromotropy are not merely the result of unidirectional changes in either sympathetic or parasympathetic tone, but stem from concomitant opposing fluctuations in the cardiac input of both autonomic components. The moment-to-moment magnitude of cardiac tone provided by one division of the autonomic nervous system is profoundly influenced by the simultaneous level of input from the other component; when autonomic activity is altered by disease or pharmacologic manipulation, these interactions become even more complex. For example, although the cardiac response to sympathetic stimulation is generally opposite that of vagal stimulation, under some circumstances simultaneous stimulation of sympathetic nerve fibers may actually exaggerate parasympathetic responses (10). This finely tuned interaction between both branches of the autonomic nervous system has been shown to occur at both prejunctional and postjunctional locations, with much of the interaction dependent upon interneuronal and intracellular mechanisms. Thus, when treating disturbances in heart rate, clinicians should consider underlying causes of autonomic disturbance.

DRUGS USED IN THE TREATMENT OF SUPRAVENTRICULAR TACHYCARDIA

Acute pharmacologic control of heart rate in critically ill patients is directed toward slowing sinus tachycardia, producing abrupt cessation of enhanced automaticity in the AV node or subsidiary pacemakers, and depressing AV node conduction to break reentrant junctional tachycardia or prevent ventricular tachycardia during atrial fibrillation or flutter. Clinicians should at all times consider factors that may promote autonomic contribution to the rhythm (Table 26.1).

CALCIUM CHANNEL BLOCKERS

Clinical Use

The calcium channel blockers are a chemically diverse group of compounds that produce varying degrees of negative chronotropy, dromotropy, and inotropy, coupled with arterial vasodilation. This diversity permits a wide range of therapeutic uses in the critical care setting (17). In the control of heart rate, negative dromotropic effects at the AV node make calcium channel blockers extremely valuable in the treatment of supraventricular arrhythmias; these drugs do not have a role in the treatment of ventricular arrhythmias except those

Table 26.1.   Dose, Kinetics, and Side Effects of Drugs Used to Treat Supraventricular Tachycardia

	Dosage (Adult)	*Elimination*	*Side Effects*
Intrinsic action			
Calcium channel blockers			
Verapamil	*Bolus:* 2.5 mg to 10 mg i.v. over 2 min; may repeat in 30 min *Infusion (short-term):* 0.005 mg/kg/min, up to total of 1 mg/min	Hepatic $t^{\frac{1}{2}} = 4$ hr	Hypotension, AV block, myocardial depression, constipation
Diltiazem	*Bolus:* 0.25 mg/kg over 2 min; may repeat in 15 min: 0.35 mg/kg over 2 min. *Infusion:* 5 to 15 mg/hr	Hepatic $t^{\frac{1}{2}} = 4$ to 6 hr	Hypotension, flushing, AV block, constipation, pruritus
Adenosine	Rapid i.v. bolus 6 mg; repeat 12 mg in 1 to 2 min	Plasma/endothelial cells $t^{\frac{1}{2}}$ 1-3 seconds	Dyspnea, flushing, chest pain, transient AV block/asystole, bronchospasm
Sympatholytic action			
β-blockers			
Esmolol	*Loading:* 500 μg/kg over 4 min *Infusion:* 50 to 300 μg/kg/min	Plasma hydrolysis $t^{\frac{1}{2}} = 9$ min	Bradycardia, hypotension, myocardial depression, bronchospasm
Propranolol	*Bolus:* 15 to 45 μg/kg (1 to 3 mg) slowly (1 mg/min); may repeat in 3 min	Hepatic $t^{\frac{1}{2}} = 4$ hr	See the section entitled Esmolol
Vagotonic action			
Digoxin	*Loading:* 0.75 to 1.0 mg i.v. in 3 divided doses over 12 to 24 hr	Renal $t^{\frac{1}{2}} = 36$ to 48 hr	Nausea, arrhythmias, AV block
Anticholinesterase			
Edrophonium	10 to 20 mg i.v. bolus (single dose) for heart rate control	66% renal 33% hepatic $t^{\frac{1}{2}} = 110$ min	Cholinergic crisis, bronchoconstriction, bradycardia, AV block, muscle weakness
α$_1$-agonist			
Phenylephrine	*Bolus:* 50 to 100 μg i.v. *Infusion:* 50 μg/min titrated to effect	Hepatic $t^{\frac{1}{2}} = 2$ to 3 hr (although clinical duration of action is short)	Bradycardia, hypertension, cardiac failure

secondary to coronary vasospasm-induced myocardial ischemia.

Verapamil was the first calcium channel blocker approved for use as an antiarrhythmic, where it is indicated in the treatment of paroxysmal supraventricular tachycardia (PSVT), reentrant arrhythmias, and control of ventricular rate during atrial fibrillation or flutter. Composed of a racemic mixture in which the (−) enantiomer is more active, verapamil has a gastrointestinal (GI) absorption of nearly 100%, but marked first-pass hepatic metabolism decreases bioavailability to about 20% in patients with normal hepatic function. Peak effect of verapamil is reached 30 to 60 minutes after oral administration, and 15 minutes after i.v. injection. The effect on AV conduction begins within 1 to 2 minutes, with a duration of effect of up to 6 hours. Plasma protein binding of verapamil is nearly 90%, with a volume of distribution of approximately 5 liters/kg; clearance is 15 ml/min/kg, and the elimination half-life is 4 hours. Protein binding and clearance are decreased, and volume of distribution and elimination half-life increased, by hepatic dysfunction. Verapamil elimination is not appreciably altered by renal failure, since less than 3% of verapamil undergoes urinary excretion unchanged. Hepatic demethylation of verapamil results in norverapamil, a weakly active metabolite with a half-life of 10 hours. Chronic administration of calcium channel blockers has been reported to increase bioavailability and prolong half-life as a result of saturation of hepatic metabolism (17).

Intravenous verapamil is supplied in a dose of 2.5 mg/ml, with a usual dose of 5 to 10 mg (75 to 150 μg/kg) given over 2 minutes, which may be repeated in 30 minutes. Continuous infusions of verapamil have been used for short-term maintenance of heart rate control at doses of 0.005 mg/kg/min up to a total dose of 1 mg/min. Verapamil is available in p.o. form in doses of 40, 80, or 120 mg, as well as 180 mg or 240 mg SR (sustained release). The usual dose is 80 to 120 mg p.o. three times daily, to a daily maximum of 480 mg.

Intravenous diltiazem has recently become available for heart rate control during atrial fibrillation and flutter. The bolus dose is 0.25 mg/kg over 2 minutes, which can be repeated in 15 minutes at 0.35 mg/kg. This administration may be followed by an infusion of 5 to 15 mg/hr. The elimination of diltiazem is primarily hepatic, with a half-life of 4 to 6 hours.

Mechanism of Action

There are four chemical classes of calcium channel blockers: (*a*) phenylalkylamines (verapamil, a derivative of papaverine); (*b*) dihydropyridines (nicardipine, nifedipine, and nimodipine); (*c*) benzothiazepines (diltiazem); and (*d*) diphenylpiperazines (none currently approved for clinical use). These compounds vary in their relative cardiovascular effects, but all act through the blockade of the slow inward current or calcium channel (18). This slow influx of calcium ions is responsible for automaticity in pacemaker cells and maintains the plateau phase (phase 2) of the action potential in myocytes. The voltage-sensitive calcium channels located on the extracellular membrane have been divided into three subtypes, designated L, N, and T (19). Currently available calcium channel blockers bind only to the L subtype calcium channel. The relative pharmacodynamic selectivity of calcium channel blockers is secondary to the abundance of L calcium channels in cardiac and vascular smooth muscle. Furthermore, the calcium channel blockers of each chemical class bind to different sites on the L channel. The extent of calcium channel opening is further modulated by a phosphorylation-dependent gate located on the intracellular membrane. The dihydropyridines such as nifedipine may also inhibit cyclic nucleotide phosphodiesterases, thereby increasing cAMP and decreasing cytosolic calcium levels, further relaxing vascular smooth muscle (20). Additionally, verapamil and the benzothiazepine diltiazem possess some local anesthetic properties in their ability to partially block the fast-current sodium channels responsible for phase 0 of the action potential (21).

Depolarization of vascular smooth muscle is caused primarily by an influx of calcium, which results in an increase in cytosolic free calcium. This increase allows calcium binding to calmodulin, thereby activating myosin light chain kinase, which, in turn, phosphorylates the myosin light chain and promotes smooth muscle contraction (22). Blockade of voltage-dependent calcium channels, and thus of Ca^{2+} influx, results in arterial vasodilation with little change in venous capacitance (23).

In cardiac myocytes, depolarization occurs secondary to inward current through both fast sodium channels and slow calcium channels. Alternatively, cardiac pacemaker cell depolarization results primarily from the slow calcium current. The negative inotropic effect of calcium channel blockers thus reflects inhibition of the slow inward calcium current. However, the negative chronotropic and dromotropic effects of calcium channel blockers also depend, in part, on inhibition of the calcium channel rate of recovery from the inactivated state. For example, verapamil decreases both the slow inward calcium current and the rate of channel recovery from the inactivated to the resting state (24). Also, verapamil and diltiazem share with local anesthetic antiarrhythmic drugs such as lidocaine and procainamide the property of use-dependent blockade: as frequency of stimulation increases in cardiac pacemaker cells, channels accumulate in the inactive state until a steady state is reached (25). Verapamil and diltiazem thereby are able to decrease SA node automaticity and AV node conduction, the basis for their antitachyarrhythmic effects. In contrast, nifedipine exhibits neither use-dependent blockade nor the ability to slow transition from the inactivated channel to the resting state (26). Thus, nifedipine does not result in the negative chronotropic and dromotropic effects seen with verapamil or, to a lesser extent, diltiazem.

Side Effects/Toxicity

The primary adverse effects of verapamil are gastrointestinal (constipation) and cardiovascular; serum levels are not useful clinically to predict drug side effects. Arterial vasodilation secondary to calcium channel blockade resulting in unwanted hypotension usually starts within 3 to 5 minutes of i.v. administration and lasts 10 to 20 minutes. Some clinicians advocate calcium pretreatment to avoid this hypotensive effect, while preserving the antiarrhythmic properties of verapamil (27). The negative inotropic effect of verapamil is usually offset by a reflex increase in sympathetic autonomic outflow

secondary to arterial vasodilation. However, verapamil is relatively contraindicated in patients with severe left ventricular dysfunction. In patients treated simultaneously with the antiarrhythmic disopyramide or β-adrenergic receptor antagonists, bradycardia, AV block, asystole, and ventricular fibrillation in response to verapamil have been reported (28). The concurrent use of verapamil with β-adrenergic blockers or digoxin should be undertaken cautiously, since an additive effect on the sinus or AV nodes often results. Verapamil may also interact with digoxin kinetically to increase digoxin levels (29). Conversely, agents that increase intracellular cAMP, such as β-agonists or the phosphodiesterase inhibitors, will oppose the effects of verapamil. Adverse effects can be reversed by various agents, including i.v. calcium, glucagon, isoproterenol, or atropine. Paradoxically, verapamil can increase the ventricular response rate to atrial fibrillation in patients with Wolff-Parkinson-White syndrome by allowing increased AV conduction through the bypass tract. Verapamil is contraindicated in patients with malfunctioning pacemakers, AV conduction abnormalities, or sick sinus syndrome.

Side effects of diltiazem are similar to those of verapamil, with hypotension and junctional rhythm/AV block the most common. Flushing and pruritus may occur, and constipation can also be a problem.

β-ADRENERGIC BLOCKERS

Clinical Use

The β-adrenergic receptor antagonists have been found to be effective in the treatment of hypertension, acute myocardial infarction, hypertrophic cardiomyopathy, angina pectoris, and both supraventricular and ventricular arrhythmias (30). Structurally, β-blockers are derivatives of the β-agonist isoproterenol, consisting of an aromatic moiety and a substituted alkylamine. The levoisomer of the racemic mixture is primarily responsible for the β-antagonist effects.

The β-blockers can be distinguished functionally by their relative affinity for β₁- and β₂-receptors (nonselective vs. β₁-selective), intrinsic sympathomimetic activity (ISA), blockade of α-adrenergic receptors, lipid solubility, and pharmacokinetics. The β₁-selective blockers, such as metoprolol, esmolol, and atenolol, offer the advantage of less bronchoconstriction and vasoconstriction secondary to β₂-receptor antagonism (31, 32). However, this selectivity is lost at higher doses. Intrinsic sympathomimetic activity—slight residual agonist effect at β-receptors in the absence of catecholamines—is characteristic of the β-blockers pindolol and acebutolol (33). In theory, less resting bradycardia and negative inotropy result from these drugs than from β-blockers without ISA properties. Labetalol is the only currently available β-blocker that also acts as a competitive antagonist at α₁-receptors. The hydrophilic β-antagonists nadolol and atenolol tend to be excreted renally and have the longest elimination half-lives, permitting once-daily dosing. Their reduced penetration of the blood-brain barrier may lead to a lower incidence of CNS side effects, such as lethargy or depression (34). Finally, high doses of β-blockers may produce quinidine-like membrane stabilizing effects, but this is not believed to be clinically significant (35).

Specific Compounds. As the first β-blocker introduced into clinical use, **propranolol** is considered the prototype to which other β-receptor antagonists can be compared. Propranolol is a nonselective lipophilic β-blocker without ISA or α-blocking properties. Propranolol blocks β$_1$- and β$_2$-receptors equally, although the negative chronotropic effects appear to outlast negative inotropy (36). Propranolol undergoes extensive hepatic first-pass metabolism, resulting in the active metabolite 4-hydroxy propranolol, which is less potent than the parent compound and has a shorter half-life. Alterations in hepatic enzyme activity or decreases in hepatic blood flow will affect propranolol clearance. Propranolol's lipophilicity results in a large volume of distribution and allows it to cross the blood-brain barrier readily. Propranolol is extensively protein bound, and thus drugs such as heparin that activate lipoprotein lipase and increase plasma free fatty acids will increase the amount of free drug in the plasma (37). The relationship between plasma concentration of propranolol and hemodynamic effects is unclear. The half-life of propranolol is only 4 hours, yet its pharmacodynamic effects permit once- or twice-daily oral dosing. Oral dosing of propranolol for the treatment of hypertension or angina usually starts at 40 to 80 mg/day. The dosage of intravenous propranolol for treatment of arrhythmias is usually 15 to 45 μg/kg (a total dose of 1 to 3 mg) administered as a slow i.v. bolus (less than 1 mg/min), which may be repeated after several minutes.

Other β-blockers commonly used in the intensive care setting to achieve rapid heart rate control include the β$_1$-selective compounds metoprolol and esmolol, and the combined α/β-blocker labetalol.

Metoprolol is a β$_1$-selective blocker without ISA. It undergoes extensive first-pass hepatic metabolism without production of active metabolites. Protein binding is low at 10%. Plasma concentration is unrelated to therapeutic effects, and half-life is 3 to 4 hours. The oral dosage is 100 to 200 mg/day. The usual intravenous dose is 5 mg every 2 minutes to a maximum of 15 mg.

Esmolol is a β$_1$-selective blocker without appreciable ISA that has the advantage of rapid onset with a short duration of action (38). Esmolol's ester linkage is rapidly hydrolyzed by plasma and erythrocyte esterases (distinct from the plasma pseudocholinesterase that metabolizes succinylcholine), resulting in a half-life of 9 minutes. The resulting carboxylic acid metabolite has only 1/500 the potency of the parent compound but does have a prolonged half-life of 4 hours and is renally excreted. The peak effect of esmolol occurs within 6 minutes of the loading dose, and appreciable effects dissipate within 15 to 20 minutes after stopping the drug. Esmolol is extremely effective in attenuating heart rate responses to noxious stimuli, although concomitant hypotension may result (39). For the treatment of SVT, an esmolol loading dose of 500 μg/kg over 4 minutes has been suggested, followed by an infusion of 50 μg/kg/min. If the desired effect is not achieved, the loading dose is repeated and the infusion is increased to 100 μg/kg/min. This process may be repeated up to a maximum infusion rate of 300 μg/kg/min (40). Caution and clinical judgment must be exercised with this loading dose. Many clinicians find gentle titration of the loading dose in 10-mg bolus increments to be desirable. The safety of prolonged infusion of esmolol over 48 hours has not been established.

Labetalol exerts competitive antagonist effects at α$_1$-, β$_1$-, and β$_2$-receptors, along with cocaine-like inhibition of neuronal uptake of norepinephrine, and perhaps some direct vasodilating capacity (41). The drug contains two chiral centers, resulting in equal concentrations of four diastereoisomers with different pharmacologic properties that account for the drug's myriad effects. Overall, the potency for β-receptor antagonism by labetalol is 5- to 10-fold greater than for α-blockade; the drug also exhibits some ISA at the β$_2$-receptor (42). It is this combination of α$_1$-blockade and partial β$_2$-agonism that results in arterial smooth muscle vasodilation, while β$_1$-blockade blunts reflex tachycardia. Labetalol undergoes extensive first-pass hepatic metabolism, undergoing oxidation and glucuronidation with less than 5% appearing unchanged in the urine (43). The elimination half-life is 4 to 6 hours, with prolongation in the setting of hepatic dysfunction. Oral dosing starts at 100 mg twice daily up to 800 mg maximum. Intravenous labetalol may be titrated in boluses (anywhere from 5 mg to 80 mg at a time) at 10-minute intervals to 300 mg maximum. Infusions of 2 mg/min may also be used, titrated to effect. Labetalol is particularly useful in the intensive care setting when both tachycardia and hypertension are encountered, and sympatholysis with an opioid or sedative is undesirable.

Mechanism of Action

The effects of β-adrenergic receptor antagonism can be predicted from a knowledge of Ahlquist's original hypothesis that catecholamine effects are mediated through distinct α- and β-subsets of end-organ receptors (44). Clinically available β-blockers act by competitive inhibition; binding to adrenergic receptors is reversible, and thus these compounds can be displaced from the receptors by increasing amounts of agonist. Chronic administration of β-blockers leads to up-regulation of β-adrenergic receptors, thereby producing increased sensitivity to endogenous and exogenous catecholamines if these drugs are discontinued abruptly (45).

The net effect of β-blockade on the cardiovascular system depends not only on β$_1$- and β$_2$-receptor location and density, but also on the corresponding level of sympathetic activity. For example, β-blockade has little effect on a normal resting heart. However, the positive chronotropic and inotropic effects of elevated cardiac sympathetic tone or infused catecholamines are blunted by blockade of β-receptors, resulting in a slowing of the heart rate and a decrease in myocardial contractility (33). Blockade of β$_2$-receptors produces increased peripheral vascular resistance, reduced coronary and renal blood flow, and preserved cerebral blood flow (46). The decrease in renal blood flow is not clinically significant in patients with normal kidneys (47). With time, total peripheral resistance returns to normal. Both the β-blocker-induced reduction in coronary blood flow and the increased end-diastolic pressure and systolic ejection period would predict a decrease in myocardial oxygen supply and an increase in oxygen demand, aggravating myocardial ischemia. However, β-blockers exert the opposite effect clinically by blunting catecholamine-induced increases in myocardial oxygen demand, thus favorably improving the balance of myocardial supply and demand, and actually improving exercise tolerance in patients limited by angina pectoris (48, 49).

The effect of β-blockade on chronotropy may result from β₂- as well as β₁-receptor inhibition (50). The β-blockers decrease the rate of spontaneous phase 4 depolarization in pacemaker cells, both sinus and ectopic. They also slow conduction (increase conduction time) through the AV node, thereby decreasing ventricular response to atrial fibrillation and terminating reentrant arrhythmias.

The mechanism by which β-blockade reduces blood pressure in hypertensive patients is not entirely clear. Possible explanations include inhibition of sympathetically mediated renin release from the renal juxtaglomerular apparatus, although these agents are effective without decreasing plasma renin activity. Another possibility is that blockade of presynaptic β-receptors reduces release of norepinephrine from nerve terminals. This as yet unexplained primary antihypertensive effect of β-blockade appears to result from a delayed-onset fall in peripheral vascular resistance that persists despite reduced cardiac output (51). It is interesting to note that β-receptor antagonism paradoxically may augment the vasopressor response to endogenous or exogenously administered catecholamines by unmasking α-agonism, a feature particularly relevant in patients with pheochromocytoma.

Side Effects/Toxicity

The most common adverse effects of β-blockers are cardiovascular, including precipitation of congestive heart failure and bradyarrhythmias such as junctional escape rhythms, particularly with concomitant use of verapamil or digitalis. Treatment of profound bradycardia may be difficult, and atropine (70 μg/kg) or high concentrations of isoproterenol (2 to 25 μg/min) may be required. A transvenous temporary pacemaker can be lifesaving if pharmacologic therapy is unsuccessful. Myocardial depression can be reversed by high doses of β-receptor agonists such as isoproterenol or dobutamine, as well as by drugs that act independently of the adrenergic receptors, such as calcium chloride (250 to 1000 mg) or glucagon (1 to 5 mg). Patients with peripheral vascular disease and intermittent claudication, or those with Raynaud's phenomenon, may experience exacerbation of these symptoms with β-blockade. Abrupt discontinuation of chronically administered β-receptor antagonists is dangerous and may result in rebound hypertension, worsening of angina, and increased risk of sudden death (52). In the lung, blockade of β-receptors in bronchial smooth muscle has little effect on normal individuals but may precipitate life-threatening bronchospasm in patients with obstructive or reactive airway disease.

The metabolic effects of β-receptor antagonism include a reduction in catecholamine-induced glycogenolysis (thus delaying recovery from hypoglycemia in critically ill patients receiving exogenous insulin), along with attenuated mobilization of free fatty acids (53, 54). Central nervous system side effects include fatigue, depression, and sleep disturbances (34).

Finally, catecholamines induce intracellular uptake of potassium ion, primarily into skeletal muscle, counteracting K⁺ ion efflux from skeletal muscle during exercise or stress (55).

This catecholamine buffer to K⁺ efflux is ablated by β-blockade, resulting in a relative hyperkalemia with stress.

ADENOSINE

Clinical Use

Adenosine is indicated for the termination of PSVT, including AV node reentrant tachycardia, AV reciprocating tachycardia, and Wolff-Parkinson-White syndrome. The drug is not effective in terminating atrial flutter, atrial fibrillation, or ventricular tachycardias. Adenosine may also be useful in the differential diagnosis of narrow- and wide-complex tachycardia (56). Additionally, adenosine has been used as a coronary vasodilator during thallium radionuclide imaging for cardiac stress tests, and to induce deliberate hypotension.

Endogenous adenosine is formed from two sources: (a) extra- and intracellular dephosphorylation of AMP by 5'-nucleotidase; and (b) S-adenosyl-homocysteine (SAH) catalyzed formation of adenosine and homocysteine via a methionine-dependent reaction. Cardiac myocytes appear to be the major source of adenosine (57).

When released into cardiac tissue, adenosine is removed both by simple washout and cytosolic degradation involving adenosine kinase (which phosphorylates adenosine to AMP), and adenosine deaminase (which forms vasoinactive inosine, which can be degraded further to hypoxanthine by nucleoside phosphorylase). The primary site of adenosine metabolism appears to be endothelial cells, which possess an efficient nucleoside transport system. It is by blockade of this system that dipyridamole retards adenosine degradation, thereby potentiating its effects.

Therapeutically, exogenous adenosine is administered initially as a rapid i.v. bolus of 6 mg. If this is ineffective, a second bolus of 12 mg may be tried in 1 to 2 minutes and then repeated once. Doses of 1 to 6 mg (37.5 μg/kg) have been used successfully and safely in infants and children (58).

Mechanism of Action

Adenosine has multiple electrophysiologic effects on the heart, including negative chronotropy at the SA node, negative dromotropy at the AV node, and decreased ventricular automaticity. The compound also acts as a negative atrial inotrope, attenuates catecholamine-induced ventricular inotropy, and produces coronary vasodilation (57). The mechanism of adenosine action is somewhat controversial. Both adenosine and ATP interact with two cell membrane purine receptors, P₁ and P₂, which produce inhibition of adenylate cyclase (59). Adenosine and adenosine analogs modified on the ribose (R) ring can also bind to membrane receptors, designated A₁ and A₂, which are competitively inhibited by methylxanthines. The A₁- and A₂-receptors are currently believed to be the primary site of the physiologic action of adenosine.

Adenosine is a negative chronotrope at the SA node, causing sinus bradycardia or sinus arrest after an i.v. bolus. The drug also shifts the site of earliest pacemaker cell activation from the SA node to subsidiary pacemaker cells in the crista terminalis (60). Dipyridamole potentiates this effect, while methylxanthines, but not atropine, antagonize it. Depression of cardiac automaticity may be mediated by increased inward

K^+ current and hyperpolarization of the pacemaker cells in a manner similar to the actions of acetylcholine (61). Adenosine also attenuates catecholamine-induced increases in calcium current in SA node cells.

The negative dromotropic action of the adenine nucleotides ATP, ADP, and AMP are likely a result of their degradation to adenosine, although the response to ATP may in part be vagally mediated. In the proximal AV node, adenosine increases the A-H interval in a dose-dependent manner without affecting the H-V interval. This increase in A-H interval is primarily a result of increasing K^+ conductance of the nodal cells with a subsequent increase in the N-H interval (62). The negative dromotropic actions of adenosine are also competitively antagonized by the methylxanthines, but not by atropine, in a manner that is specific for adenosine and independent of phosphodiesterase inhibition (63). The mechanism by which adenosine can terminate reentrant tachycardias involving the AV node is thus clear. Furthermore, adenosine may inhibit catecholamine-dependent ventricular arrhythmias mediated by elevated cAMP levels, including delayed afterdepolarizations and triggered automaticity. However, under certain electrophysiologic conditions adenosine may be proarrhythmic, facilitating intraatrial reentry and leading to atrial fibrillation (57).

Clinically, the electrophysiologic effects of adenosine seem to depend on whether the compound is administered as a bolus or as an infusion. A single bolus injection of adenosine to patients in sinus rhythm results in a sinus bradycardia within 10 to 20 seconds after injection. The sinus bradycardia lasts less than 10 seconds and is followed by reflex (autonomic-mediated) sinus tachycardia. AV block follows a similar time course. Continuous infusion of adenosine results in a dose-dependent sinus tachycardia and no effect on AV conduction, possibly because sympathetic reflex activation overrides direct effects of the drug. Thus, adenosine should not be administered as a maintenance infusion after termination of an SVT. Bolus adenosine also produces a chemoreceptor-mediated pressor response—with elevated blood pressure coincident with the onset of bradycardia and AV block—followed by a decrease in blood pressure with the development of the sinus tachycardia. Continuous infusion of adenosine results in a decrease in pulmonary and systemic vascular resistance secondary to direct vasodilation, with a simultaneous increase in pulse pressure and minimal change in mean arterial pressure, as cardiac output increases in compensation.

Adenosine may have a diagnostic as well as therapeutic role. Although adenosine will terminate the majority of narrow-complex tachycardias whose underlying mechanism is AV nodal and atrioventricular reentry, it will not affect supraventricular tachycardias that do not involve the AV node, such as intraatrial reentrant tachycardia, atrial flutter, atrial fibrillation, and sinoatrial reentrant tachycardia. However, during these arrhythmias, the junctional block produced by adenosine may unmask unrecognized flutter waves (64). Interestingly, adenosine has been reported to terminate sinus node reentrant tachycardia and automatic intraatrial tachycardia, two rare forms of supraventricular tachycardia not involving the AV node (65, 66). Adenosine may also have a diagnostic role in patients with paroxysmal SVT by unmasking lateral preexcitation accessory pathways (67).

The differential diagnosis of a regular wide-complex tachycardia includes ventricular tachycardia, a preexcited atrial arrhythmia, or an SVT with aberrant conduction. Verapamil is relatively contraindicated in two of these situations (ventricular tachycardia and preexcited rhythm), because of profound hemodynamic deterioration. This is in contrast to the apparently benign effects of adenosine in patients with ventricular tachycardia (68). In a study of patients with atrial arrhythmias and WPW, adenosine produced no clinically significant hemodynamic deterioration, although ventricular rate did increase transiently in some patients (69). Adenosine will terminate a rare form of ventricular tachycardia, right ventricular outflow-tract tachycardia (70), which is also responsive to verapamil.

In addition to its electrophysiologic effects, adenosine acts as a direct negative atrial inotrope via a cAMP-independent mechanism, and although it exhibits no direct suppression of ventricular myocardium, adenosine mediates an indirect, cAMP-dependent attenuation of catecholamine-induced inotropy (71, 72). Adenosine produces coronary vasodilation via stimulation of endothelial cell A_2-receptors (73). Postreceptor events remain unclear but may involve increases in intracellular cAMP that are then coupled to vascular smooth muscle cell relaxation by an undetermined pathway involving the cell surface A_1-receptor (74). Coronary vasodilation produced by exogenously administered adenosine is blocked by the methylxanthines. Conversely, dipyridamole potentiates the vascular action of adenosine by preventing nucleoside uptake and intracellular degradation. It should be noted that, in comparison with effects on exogenous adenosine, antagonism of endogenous cardiac adenosine by methylxanthines is slower in onset, although the ultimate degree of blockade is equivalent. This response possibly results from the primarily interstitial location of endogenous adenosine, thus requiring extravascular diffusion of the methylxanthine.

Side Effects/Toxicity

Bolus administration of adenosine can result in dose-related dyspnea, flushing, or chest pain that may mimic that of angina or peptic ulcers and that is possibly myocardial in origin. Adenosine-induced dyspnea and hyperventilation are believed to be chemoreceptor-mediated, whereas the flushing most likely results from cutaneous vasodilation. These effects show large interpatient variability, and although they usually are transient, they can be treated with aminophylline. Bronchoconstriction is also a potential adverse reaction to adenosine that, unlike other adverse effects, may be prolonged in duration. Thus, reactive airway disease is a relative contraindication to adenosine use.

DIGITALIS

Clinical Use

Although relatively toxic, the cardiac glycosides—known generically as "digitalis"—remain widely used to slow transmission of cardiac impulses through the AV node when atrial contractions are aberrant or abnormally rapid, and to enhance the contractility of failing myocardium (75). Structurally, these compounds are composed of a steroid moiety (a cyclopentanoperhydrophenanthrene nucleus with an unsaturated lactone ring attached to the C-17 position) with one to four sugar molecules bound to the C-3 position. In general, the sugar moiety dictates kinetic properties and potency of the drug, and the steroid (or aglycone) component contributes pharmacologic activity, with a double bond at the C-14 position of the lactone ring an essential feature.

In critically ill patients, digitalis compounds are often beneficial in the treatment of atrial flutter or fibrillation with rapid ventricular response, and recurrent paroxysmal atrial tachycardia. The only absolute contraindication to digitalis administration is digitalis toxicity. Relative contraindications include idiopathic hypertrophic subaortic stenosis, heart block, and severe hypokalemia.

Dosages of digitalis compounds should be "titrated" to the patient's cardiovascular pathology, concomitant noncardiac disease, and age. In general, larger initial doses are required to slow ventricular response in supraventricular tachydysrhythmias than to treat congestive heart failure. Additionally, renal failure lowers the maintenance dose, and elderly patients tend to require less drug (29). By far the most commonly used digitalis compound in the critical care setting is digoxin. Derived from the leaves of *Digitalis lanata*, digoxin may be given orally or intravenously, has a relatively long duration of action (plasma half-life of 36 to 48 hours in patients with normal renal function), and can be readily assayed in the serum. The drug exhibits only modest (25%) protein binding, is extensively bound in peripheral tissues, and displays a volume of distribution of about 7.3 liters/kg. The primary route of elimination is via the kidney, where unchanged digoxin is both filtered and secreted (29).

The benefit of serum digoxin levels as a guide to therapeutic response is limited. There is wide variability among patients in the serum concentration of drug required to achieve a desired response. Also, a number of other frequently used drugs raise serum digoxin levels. Quinidine, amiodarone, verapamil, diltiazem, spironolactone, triamterine, and indomethacin have all been shown to increase serum digoxin levels (29, 76). Furthermore, falsely elevated serum digoxin levels (either from an endogenous digitalis-like factor or altered biotransformation) have been reported in neonates and in the setting of hypertension, renal and hepatic disease, and pregnancy (77). Serum digoxin levels are of most benefit in ensuring that the dose given is sufficient to achieve measurable blood concentrations and in confirming a clinical suspicion of overdose or toxicity.

Mechanism of Action

The cardiovascular response to digitalis reflects both direct and indirect actions and is profoundly influenced by cardiac disease and basal sympathetic nervous tone. Substantial evidence suggests that direct cardiac actions of digitalis result from inhibition of membrane-bound sodium, potassium-activated adenosine triphosphatase (Na K-ATPase), the biochemical correlate of the "sodium pump" (78, 79). In contrast, the ability of digitalis to stimulate autonomic nervous activity accounts for the vast majority of indirect actions (80).

At therapeutic concentrations, the predominant electrical effects of digitalis are the result of increased parasympathetic input to the heart, as well as enhanced sensitivity of SA and AV node tissue to acetylcholine and reduced sensitivity to norepinephrine (81). Cardiac glycosides stimulate or facilitate vagal activity at central nuclei and the nodose ganglion, at peripheral autonomic ganglia, and in vagal efferents (80). Additional evidence suggests that digitalis sensitizes baroreceptors to produce a greater increase in vagal tone for a given elevation in pressure (82, 83) and is capable of directly stimulating cardiac receptors involved with the bradycardic Bezold-Jarisch reflex (80).

Side Effects/Toxicity

A major limitation of digitalis use is an exceptionally low therapeutic index. Many side effects of digitalis are well-known and relatively common in outpatients, but particular attention should be paid to assessing possible adverse effects in debilitated patients with multisystem disease.

Cardiotoxicity. Although nausea is perhaps the most common side effect of digitalis treatment, the most serious is development of cardiac arrhythmias. Digitalis cardiotoxicity has been widely investigated and the literature extensively reviewed (84–86). The diagnosis of digitalis toxicity is a clinical one and should not be based entirely on elevated digoxin levels or electrocardiogram (ECG) alterations. Factors frequently encountered in the critical care setting, such as old age, myocardial ischemia or acute infarction, hypokalemia, hypomagnesemia, renal insufficiency, hepatic dysfunction, carotid sinus massage, electrical cardioversion, hypothyroidism, and concomitant drug therapy, all have been shown to influence digitalis kinetics or dynamics in such a way as to enhance cardiotoxicity. Mechanistically, digitalis arrhythmogenesis can be regarded as having two components: (*a*) a direct effect on cardiac tissue secondary, perhaps, to excessive inhibition of the sodium pump and overaccumulation of intracellular calcium, and (*b*) an indirect component resulting from activation of the autonomic nervous system. Both components serve to alter the automaticity, conduction, and excitability of cardiac tissue.

When toxic drug levels are achieved, digitalis compounds are capable of producing virtually every ECG abnormality known. Relatively frequent disturbances include atrial tachycardia with or without block, AV conduction delay more pronounced than simple lengthening of the P-R interval, AV dissociation, junctional escape rhythms, and ventricular dysrhythmias, particularly premature ventricular contractions. Digitalis-induced arrhythmias may be life-threatening, particularly in critically ill patients with underlying multisystem disease. Initial intervention should include discontinuation of the drug; ECG monitoring, since arrhythmias may be intermittent or progressively malignant; and assessment of the patient for predisposing factors (e.g., hypokalemia, renal compromise, catecholamine infusion). Administration of potassium chloride is often beneficial in the treatment of ventricular or supraventricular ectopy even if the patient is normokalemic. A solution of 60 mEq of potassium per liter in normal or half-normal saline infused through a large vein at the rate of 0.5 mEq/min may be used. Potassium may not be advantageous when the primary toxicity is a conduction disturbance, since potassium has been shown to further depress conduction. Diuretics should not be administered, nor should glucose solutions without potassium. High-degree AV block and bradydysrhythmia may require temporary pacing. Supraventricular and ventricular tachyarrhythmias are frequently responsive to diphenylhydantoin or lidocaine, although additional therapy with propranolol, procainamide, or verapamil may be required. Direct current countershock should be avoided because of the potential for worsening arrhythmias. Hemodialysis is of no benefit for drug removal because of extensive tissue binding. Severe digoxin toxicity with malignant arrhythmias refractory to antiarrhythmic agents and producing hemodynamic compromise may require administration of digoxin-specific Fab fragments (Digibind, Burroughs Wellcome) (87). This fragment of antidigoxin antibody binds serum digoxin, rendering it pharmacologically inactive. The fragment-digoxin complex is then excreted renally.

Nontherapeutic Effects.   Digitalis causes constriction of isolated arteries (88), and studies in humans and animals have demonstrated a rise in arterial pressure and systemic vascular resistance following digitalis administration (89–91). However, the magnitude of increases in vascular resistance are profoundly influenced by basal sympathetic activity; if "tone" is high (as during low flow states), then increased cardiac output brought about by digitalis leads to a withdrawal of vascular tone, which counterbalances direct vasoconstriction by the drug, and vasodilation occurs (80). Specific investigation of regional systemic and pulmonary circulations have further demonstrated the vasoconstrictor actions of digitalis (92, 93), which appear to be mediated both by direct vascular and adrenergically mediated effects. Vasoconstriction in response to digoxin is most pronounced when the drug is administered rapidly. Thus, in critically ill patients—who may require rapid parenteral digitalization for heart rate control—vascular actions of digitalis are worthy of consideration. Vasoconstriction of coronary, mesenteric, and renal circulation in response to digoxin infusion has been reported (91, 92), as has potentiation of the pressor actions of norepinephrine and angiotensin (94).

Digoxin administration may potentially exacerbate myocardial ischemia by causing both increased oxygen demand and coronary vasoconstriction. Since digitalis compounds are expected to produce ST segment changes on the ECG, alterations resulting from ischemia may well be missed. There is also good evidence that ischemic myocardium is much more susceptible to cardiotoxicity (95, 96).

Although the effects of cardiac glycosides on pulmonary function vary widely and are difficult to interpret (80), cardiotoxicity is apparently increased in patients with pulmonary disease (97). Additionally, digoxin-induced pulmonary vasoconstriction may potentially exacerbate underlying pulmonary hypertension, although this has not been confirmed in animal models (98).

In the kidney, cardiac glycosides produce a diuresis by inhibiting intrarenal Na K-ATPase, and a natriuresis most probably by inhibiting sodium reabsorption in the distal nephron (99). As noted above, digitalis compounds can produce relatively intense renal vasoconstriction, an action that may be detrimental in patients with compromised renal perfusion.

Inhibition of Na K-ATPase increases smooth muscle tone in a variety of organ systems, the most evident of which is the gastrointestinal tract, with resultant diarrhea. Nausea probably results from stimulation of the medullary vomiting center. Mesenteric vasoconstriction in response to digoxin

appears to be potentiated by nonsteroidal antiinflammatory agents (100) and has been implicated in bowel ischemia (101).

Central nervous system manifestations of digitalis treatment are common and should be considered in debilitated patients who may be confused or disoriented; nightmares, hallucinations, mania, and depression have been reported. Visual symptoms are frequent, especially halos and yellow discoloration (xanthopsia), and appear to reflect stimulation of visual pathways by the glycoside (80).

Electrocardiographic Changes.   The multiple influences of digitalis on cardiac muscle and conducting system electrophysiology are manifest, in part, as alterations in the ECG. At nontoxic doses, relatively consistent changes include lengthening of the P-R interval, ST segment depression and shortening (often described as "sagging"), and reduction of T-wave amplitude. In the His-Purkinje system at least, these changes appear to reflect changes in the duration and slope of phases 2 and 3 of the action potential (84). Less frequently, U-waves appear, and symmetrical T-wave inversion similar to that seen during ischemia or pericarditis may occasionally occur. Electrocardiographic alterations, particularly ST segment changes, may become magnified by underlying myocardial disease, concomitant tachycardia, and high-amplitude QRS complexes.

Potassium, Calcium, and Magnesium Homeostasis.   Hypokalemia predisposes the patient to digitalis cardiotoxicity under both clinical and experimental conditions. Mechanistically, low potassium augments inhibition of Na K-ATPase and development of afterdepolarizations (84). Administration of potassium chloride can effectively oppose early manifestations of digitalis cardiotoxicity but should be undertaken carefully, since hyperkalemia may enhance cardiac glycoside-induced slowing of AV nodal conduction velocity (102). Particular attention should be paid to assessing potassium homeostasis during the initiation of digitalis therapy in patients who are dependent on parenteral nutrition, as well as those who are receiving diuretic therapy or carbohydrate and insulin infusion (103).

Calcium influences both the therapeutic and direct toxic effects of digitalis and thus should be considered during both the initiation and maintenance of therapy. Inhibition of Na K-ATPase by the cardiac glycosides leads to an accumulation of intracellular calcium and enhanced inotropy. Not surprisingly, insensitivity to digitalis has been reported in the setting of hypocalcemia (104). Alternatively, overaccumulation of calcium predisposes the patient to afterdepolarization development and cardiac ectopy. Hypercalcemia has been demonstrated to exacerbate virtually all forms of cardiotoxicity, a phenomenon that is opposed by calcium channel blockade (105).

Magnesium is required for the appropriate functioning of Na K-ATPase. The amount required, however, is minuscule, and thus magnesium infusion will not overcome inhibition of the sodium pump (106). Clinical hypomagnesemia probably has minimal influence on the inotropic response to cardiac glycosides, but there is evidence that it nearly doubles the amount of digoxin required to acutely control ventricular rate in patients with atrial fibrillation (107). Animal studies have shown a reduction in the arrhythmogenic dose of digitalis during concomitant hypomagnesemia (108), and magnesium sulfate infusion has been effective in the treatment of various digitalis-induced arrhythmias, including some that are resistant to lidocaine (102). As with replacement of potassium or calcium, magnesium should be administered judiciously, since hypermagnesemia can produce AV block and slowing of intraventricular conduction.

ANTICHOLINESTERASE DRUGS

Clinical Use

Anticholinesterase drugs are indicated primarily for reversal of nondepolarizing neuromuscular blockade, reduction of intraocular pressure, diagnosis and treatment of myasthenia gravis, treatment of nonobstructive paralytic ileus and atony of the bladder, and adverse reactions to anticholinergic drugs. A secondary role for anticholinesterase drugs is in the treatment of SVT. Because of a rapid onset (1 to 2 minutes) and limited duration of action (5 to 10 minutes) in low doses, edrophonium is the anticholinesterase primarily used to treat SVT. Usual doses are 10 to 20 mg administered as an i.v. bolus. The anticholinesterases have an elimination half-life of 80 to 100 minutes, with primarily renal excretion of 50 to 75%. Half-lives are correspondingly prolonged with renal dysfunction (109–111).

Mechanism of Action

Acetylcholine (Ach) released into a synaptic cleft is hydrolyzed by acetylcholinesterase to choline and acetic acid in a manner so efficient that up to 3×10^5 Ach molecules per molecule of enzyme are degraded per minute (112). In the heart, this rapidity of action is necessary to allow the myocyte refractory period to be longer than the residence time of free Ach in the synapse. Thus, a single impulse results in only a single action potential. Anticholinesterase drugs inhibit the enzyme by one of three mechanisms: (a) reversible competitive inhibition (edrophonium); (b) reversible inhibition by competitive substrate (physostigmine, neostigmine, and pyridostigmine); and (c) irreversible inhibition (organophosphates) (113, 114).

Edrophonium, the most frequently used anticholinesterase in the critical care setting, is a quaternary amine-substituted phenol that blocks Ach substrate binding to the enzyme by electrostatic attachment to the anionic site and hydrogen bonding to the esteratic site of the enzyme. This reversible binding, in combination with rapid renal elimination, accounts for its brief duration of action. An additional presynaptic release of Ach by edrophonium may contribute to the rapid onset of action (115).

The cardiovascular actions of anticholinesterase drugs are complicated by the fact that the accumulated Ach affects both preganglionic nicotinic receptors and postganglionic muscarinic receptors. High doses of anticholinesterases give unpredictable hemodynamic effects as a result of their ability first to excite and then to inhibit autonomic ganglia as well as medullary vasomotor and cardiac regulatory centers (112). The small doses of edrophonium (10 to 20 mg) typically used to counteract a tachycardia usually have minimal side effects. Therapeutically, enhanced muscarinic agonism following anticholinesterase administration reduces nodal automaticity while it increases nodal refractory period and conduction time. The onset of action is usually rapid and may be abrupt, occasionally precipitating profound bradycardia or asystole; temporary AV sequential or ventricular pacing may be required. Peripherally, accumulated Ach may produce systemic vasodilation via a second messenger such as endothelium-derived relaxing factor (116). In the central circulation, the reactions of the coronary and pulmonary vasculature to accumulated Ach are less predictable (117) and generally are overridden by local autoregulation.

Side Effects/Toxicity

Overdose of anticholinesterase can precipitate a cholinergic crisis characterized by excessive secretory gland activity, bronchoconstriction, muscular weakness from unsynchronized fasciculations similar to the depolarizing action of succinylcholine, and CNS depression. Treatment is with atropine and supportive measures.

ADRENERGIC AGONISTS

Clinical Use

Prior to the advent of specific AV node blocking agents, bolus administration of a vasopressor was frequently the first-line treatment for SVT with hypotension. Mediated by a reflex increase in vagal tone following abrupt systemic vasoconstriction, this treatment is often sufficient to break a reentrant tachycardia. Furthermore, increased coronary perfusion pressure may be beneficial if ischemia contributes to the arrhythmia. The drug most commonly used for this purpose is phenylephrine, although methoxamine, metaraminol, and mephenteramine have also been used (33).

Structurally similar to epinephrine, phenylephrine has only one hydroxyl group on the benzene ring and is thus a noncatecholamine refractory to degradation by catechol-o-methyltransferase (COMT). The drug is metabolized by monoamine oxidase (MAO), accounting for its brief duration of action. The usual dose of phenylephrine for the treatment of tachycardia and hypotension is an i.v. bolus of 50 to 100 μg followed by repeated boluses or an i.v. infusion of approximately 50 μg/min titrated to effect.

The α_2-agonists (e.g., clonidine, guanfacine, and guanabenz) also reduce heart rate but are not primarily indicated for treatment of tachycardia. It is believed that central stimulation of presynaptic α_2-receptors in the nucleus tractus solitarius of the medullary vasomotor center produces a decrease in central sympathetic outflow, subsequently reducing blood pressure and heart rate (118, 119). These compounds may also centrally increase vagal tone, contributing to the resultant bradycardia.

Mechanism of Action

Phenylephrine is a direct α_1-adrenergic agonist (some β-agonism is also apparent at high doses) that produces marked arterial and venous vasoconstriction. The rapid increase in systolic and diastolic blood pressure following bolus administration leads to an equally rapid baroreceptor-mediated increase in cardiac parasympathetic tone. This reflex bradycardic effect may be exaggerated by simultaneous administration of β-adrenergic antagonists or drugs that sensitize baroreceptors such as digoxin (80). Alternatively, baroreceptor desensitization, as occurs with chronic hypertension or advanced age, may diminish the response (120).

Side Effects/Toxicity

Phenylephrine should be used carefully in patients with left ventricular dysfunction, aortic insufficiency, or mitral regurgitation, since rapid changes in ventricular afterload occur; the drug usually decreases cardiac output as well as renal and splanchnic blood flow. Alternatively, coronary blood flow is often increased because elevated perfusion pressure more than offsets moderate direct vasoconstriction. Pulmonary vasoconstriction may also occur, although data suggest that in the setting of preexisting pulmonary hypertension, phenylephrine may actually produce dilation (121).

DRUGS USED IN THE TREATMENT OF BRADYCARDIA

ANTICHOLINERGICS

Clinical Use

Clinically used anticholinergic drugs include the tertiary amine belladonna alkaloids atropine and scopolamine, and the quaternary amine synthetic derivative glycopyrrolate. Producing antagonism primarily of muscarinic cholinergic receptors, these compounds display a wide range of uses and side effects. In the intensive care unit (ICU), the major indication for anticholinergic drugs is the acute treatment of hemodynamically significant bradyarrhythmias. In general, atropine has the greatest efficacy for increasing heart rate (followed by glycopyrrolate) and is thus the anticholinergic most frequently used in emergency situations. Given as an intravenous bolus of 0.4 to 1.0 mg, atropine generally increases heart rate within seconds. The magnitude of the chronotropic response, however, is variable. It has been estimated that in adults, complete blockade of cardiac muscarinic receptors is achieved by a total atropine dose of 2.0 mg (122), thus larger doses usually will not increase heart rate further. In nonemergency situations when modest chronotropy of long duration (2 to 3 hours) is desired, glycopyrrolate (0.2 to 0.4 mg) is often effective. Other actions of anticholinergic drugs that potentially are beneficial in critically ill patients include sedation, mucosal drying, bronchodilation, smooth muscle relaxation (biliary, ureteral, and bladder), mydriasis and cycloplegia, and decreased gastric acid secretion. Additionally, transdermal scopolamine has become widely used as an antiemetic, and other centrally acting anticholinergics are routinely administered to treat extrapyramidal symptoms in patients with Parkinson's disease or mental illness who require protracted treatment with phenothiazines (Table 26.2).

A racemic mixture of *d*- and *l*-hyoscyamine (the active form), atropine is lipid soluble and readily absorbed by respiratory mucosa, thus allowing for intratracheal administration during emergency situations. Both atropine and scopolamine cross the blood-brain barrier to produce central effects. In contrast, the quaternary amine glycopyrrolate does not enter the CNS and exhibits only peripheral effects. Atropine has a half-life of about 4 hours, with approximately 50% undergoing hepatic degradation (ester hydrolysis to form tropic acid), and the other 50% eliminated unchanged in the urine. Glycopyrrolate also undergoes hepatic degradation.

Mechanism of Action

These compounds competitively inhibit muscarinic cholinergic receptors at postganglionic parasympathetic neuroeffector junctions, neurons, and ganglia (123). Interestingly, although vascular smooth muscle cells lack cholinergic innervation, they do possess muscarinic receptors, accounting for the systemic vasodilation induced by exogenous acetylcholine (116). Antimuscarinic drugs also exhibit nicotinic receptor blockade at high doses and may interfere with ganglionic and neuromuscular cholinergic actions (122). This effect is most pronounced with synthetic quaternary amines, such as glycopyrrolate. At least three subclasses of muscarinic receptors exist (M_1, M_2, and M_3), and although currently available antimuscarinic compounds are nonselective with regard to these subclasses, newer selective antagonists, such as pirenzepine, are being developed (124).

The predominant cardiovascular effect of muscarinic receptor antagonism in normal patients is an increase in resting heart rate; blockade of M_2-receptors in the SA node increases automaticity. In the AV node, muscarinic blockade decreases conduction time (shortens the PR interval irrespective of rate), decreases functional refractory period, and also increases automaticity (125). Thus, in some patients with slow junctional rhythm, atropine may not restore sinus rhythm but rather may accelerate the nodal beats. The chronotropic response to a given dose of antimuscarinic depends on the patient's intrinsic rhythm and the degree of baseline cardiac parasympathetic tone. Young adults have the greatest level of resting vagal tone compared with infants and the elderly, and thus exhibit the largest increase in heart rate (126). It is interesting to note that low doses of atropine may produce a transient paradoxical slowing of the heart rate (reduced by 4 to 8 beats per minute), followed thereafter by the expected tachycardia. Originally believed to reflect central vagal stimulation, the same transient decrease in heart rate has been observed after administration of glycopyrrolate, whose actions are limited to the periphery. It is now thought that an initial blockade of M_1-receptors on postganglionic parasympathetic neurons results in a decrease in the negative feedback presynaptic inhibition of acetylcholine release, similar to the role of presynaptic α_2-receptors in the adrenergic system (127).

It is important to note that not all parasympathetically innervated organs are equally sensitive to the effects of antimuscarinic drugs. This spectrum of sensitivities most likely reflects that fact that the various end-organs are controlled by differing degrees of parasympathetic tone, rather than by varying receptor affinities to the same compound. Thus, a chronotropic response usually cannot be achieved without anhydrosis, mydriasis, cycloplegia, and the drying of secretions. Doses higher than those routinely used in the treatment of bradycardia are required to achieve bladder, ureteral, and gastrointestinal atony and to inhibit gastric acid secretion (128, 129).

Table 26.2. Dose, Kinetics, and Side Effects of Drugs Used to Treat Bradycardia

	Dosage (Adult)	*Elimination*	*Side Effects*
Vagolytic			
Antimuscarinic			
Atropine	*Bolus:* 0.4 to 1.0 mg i.v.	50% hepatic 50% renal $t\frac{1}{2}$ = 4 hr	Paradoxical bradycardia (with low doses), drying of secretions, mental status changes/sedation, central anticholinergic syndrome, mydriasis/cycloplegia
Sympathomimetic			
Direct			
Isoproterenol	*Infusion:* 1 to 5 μg/min i.v.	Hepatic (COMT) $t\frac{1}{2}$ = 2 min	Tachycardia, tachyarrhythmia, flushing, myocardial ischemia
Indirect			
Ephedrine	*Bolus:* 5 to 25 mg i.v.	60% hepatic—MAO 40% renal unchanged $t\frac{1}{2}$ = 3 to 6 hr	Tachycardia, hypertension, tachyphylaxis

Side Effects/Toxicity

Adverse effects of antimuscarinics depend on the initial indication for their use. Atropine treatment of bradycardia, for example, will produce a dry mouth, while glycopyrrolate administered as an antisialagogue will increase heart rate.

It is important to note that large doses of atropine or scopolamine (as may be used during cardiopulmonary resuscitation) can enter the CNS in sufficient quantity to precipitate the central anticholinergic syndrome, characterized first by restlessness, hallucinations, and delirium, followed by seizures, medullary respiratory center paralysis, CNS depression, coma, and death. Since mental status changes are not uncommon in ICU patients, recent treatment with an anticholinergic should be considered in the differential diagnosis. Furthermore, nicotinic cholinergic blockade at high doses may result in skeletal muscle weakness and orthostatic hypotension. In addition to supportive measures, specific treatment for central anticholinergic syndrome is the tertiary amine acetylcholinesterase inhibitor physostigmine in doses of 15 to 60 μg/kg (1 to 4 mg i.v., 0.5 mg i.v. for children). It should be noted that the rapid metabolism of physostigmine may necessitate redosing every 1 to 2 hours to prevent a relapse of symptoms. Overdose by quaternary amine antimuscarinics does not cause significant CNS toxicity but may possibly produce ganglionic and neuromuscular blockade. It is also important to consider that patients with narrow-angle glaucoma may display acutely elevated intraocular pressure—with the ensuing danger of blindness—following treatment with an antimuscarinic. Should such a patient require atropine to treat a life-threatening bradyarrhythmia, prompt treatment with a topical cholinomimetic alkaloid such as pilocarpine can substantially reduce the risk of blindness. However, if patients are already being treated with topical anticholinesterases or cholinomimetics, deleterious effects of emergency antimuscarinic treatment are minimal.

β-ADRENERGIC AGONISTS

Clinical Use

The naturally occurring catecholamines and their synthetic sympathomimetic derivatives comprise a diverse class of compounds with multiple clinical uses. All catecholamines are derived from substituted phenylethylamines, with relative selectivity of individual drugs for α- or β-receptors dictated by the hydroxyl and alkyl moieties attached to the parent compound. In critically ill patients, these agents are most frequently employed as positive inotropes, chronotropes, and vasopressors; other uses include bronchodilation, pulmonary vascular dilation, treatment of anaphylactoid reactions, and resuscitation following cardiopulmonary arrest. The overall systemic response to catecholamine infusion, however, is complicated by several factors: (*a*) affinities of specific compounds for adrenergic receptor subtypes vary (i.e., at low doses β$_2$-mediated vasodilation may occur, but at high doses α-mediated constriction predominates); (*b*) various organs differ in the predominant type and density of adrenergic receptors; and (*c*) homeostatic reflexes tend to counterbalance some direct effects of the drug.

Isoproterenol, a potent β$_1$- and β$_2$-agonist, is the catecholamine most often selected when positive chronotropy is the goal. In patients with profound sinus bradycardia or high-degree heart block, isoproterenol is administered as an i.v. infusion of 1 to 5 μg/min (0.01 to 0.1 μg/kg/min). The drug is rapidly metabolized by COMT in the liver and other tissues and has a half-life of 2 minutes. Unlike endogenous catecholamines, isoproterenol does not undergo significant reuptake into postganglionic adrenergic nerve terminals and thus is not significantly metabolized by MAO.

Mechanism of Action

In the heart, β$_1$-receptor stimulation increases automaticity of the SA node and decreases conduction time through the AV node, thus making isoproterenol useful in sinus bradycardia and heart block. However, β$_1$-adrenergic agonism may also enhance conduction through anomalous pathways and promote ectopic automaticity in both the atria and ventricles. Isoproterenol infusion produces significant β$_2$-mediated vasodilation in skeletal muscle and renal and splanchnic beds, with a fall in systemic vascular resistance. In some patients, reduced arterial pressure coupled with tachycardia may result in a deleterious effect on myocardial oxygen supply-demand balance that leads to ischemia (33).

Not all sympathomimetics act directly on adrenergic receptors. The so-called "indirect-acting" sympathomimetics enter the postganglionic adrenergic nerve terminal and displace norepinephrine from storage vesicles into the synaptic cleft (130). Presynaptic catecholamine reuptake-blockers such as cocaine—which potentiate the effects of direct-acting sympathomimetics (131)—prevent access of indirect-acting agents to their site of action, thus dramatically decreasing their efficacy. The most commonly used indirect sympathomimetic, ephedrine, also displays direct effects on α- and β-adrenergic receptors. The drug predictably increases heart rate, systolic and diastolic blood pressure, and myocardial contractility when administered in 5- to 25-mg boluses, and it is often beneficial in the acute treatment of bradycardia and hypotension. However, although the response to a single ephedrine dose may last 5 to 10 minutes, tachyphylaxis to repeated doses often develops, possibly as a result of depletion of presynaptic catecholamine stores (132). Forty percent of ephedrine is excreted unchanged in the urine, with the remainder slowly deaminated by MAO and conjugated in the liver, thus accounting for the relatively prolonged duration of action.

Side Effects/Toxicity

Prominent side effects of isoproterenol include skin flushing, sinus tachycardia, atrial and ventricular tachydysrhythmias, and myocardial ischemia. Although catecholamines in general tend to produce hyperglycemia (via increased hepatic gluconeogenesis coupled with insulin resistance and impaired release), this effect is less prominent with isoproterenol (133).

REFERENCES

1. James TN, Sherf L, Schlant RC, et al: Anatomy of the heart. In Hurst JW (ed): *The Heart*, ed 5. New York, McGraw-Hill, pp 22–74, 1982.
2. Sommer JR, Jennings RB: Ultrastructure of cardiac muscle. In Fozzard HA, Haber E, Jennings RB, et al (eds): *The Heart and Cardiovascular System*. New York, Raven Press, pp 61–100, 1986.
3. Jones SB, Euler DE, Hardie E, et al: Comparison of SA nodal and subsidiary atrial pacemaker function and location in the dog. *Am J Physiol* 234:H471–H476, 1978.
4. Hecht HH, Kossmann CE, Childers RW, et al: Atrioventricular and intraventricular conduction: revised nomenclature and concepts. *Am J Cardiol* 31:232–244, 1973.
5. Irisawa H, Giles WR: Sinus and atrioventricular node cells: cellular electrophysiology. In Zipes DP, Jalife J (eds): *Cardiac Electrophysiology*. Philadelphia, WB Saunders, pp 95–102, 1990.
6. Tuna IC, Barragry TP, Walker M, et al: Effects of transplantation on atrioventricular nodal accommodation and hysteresis. *Am J Physiol* 253:H1514–H1522, 1987.
7. Berne RM, Levy MN: Control of the heart. In *Cardiovascular Physiology*. St. Louis, CV Mosby, p 145, 1981.
8. Anderson RH, Ho SY, Becker AE: Gross anatomy and microscopy of the conducting system. In Mandel JW (ed): *Cardiac Arrhythmias: Their Mechanism, Diagnosis, and Management*, ed 2. Philadelphia, JB Lippincott, pp 13–52, 1987.
9. Zipes DP, Miyazaki T: The autonomic nervous system and the heart: basis for understanding interactions and effects on arrhythmia development. In Zipes DP, Jalife J (eds): *Cardiac Electrophysiology*. Philadelphia, WB Saunders, pp 312–329, 1990.
10. Salata JJ, Zipes DP: Autonomic nervous system control of heart rate and atrioventricular nodal conduction. In Zucker IH, Gilmore JP (eds): *Reflex Control of the Circulation*. Boston, CRC, pp 67–101, 1991.
11. Rosen MR, Bilezikian JP, Cohen IS, Robinson RB: α-adrenergic modulation of cardiac rhythm. In Zipes DP, Jalife J (eds): *Cardiac Electrophysiology*. Philadelphia, WB Saunders, pp 300–304, 1990.
12. Gilman AG: G proteins and dual control of adenylate cyclase. *Cell* 36:577–579, 1984.
13. Rasmussen H: The calcium messenger system. Part 1. *N Engl J Med* 314:1094–1101, 1986.
14. Rasmussen H: The calcium messenger system. Part 2. *N Engl J Med* 314:1164–1170, 1986.
15. DiFrancesco D, Ducouret P, Robinson RB: Muscarinic modulation of cardiac rate at low acetylcholine concentrations. *Science* 243:669–671, 1989.
16. Sorota S, Tsugi Y, Tajima T, Pappano AJ: Pertussis toxin treatment blocks hyperpolarization by muscarinic agonists in chick atrium. *Circ Res* 57:748–758, 1985.
17. Murad F: Drugs used for the treatment of angina: organic nitrates, calcium-channel blockers, and α-adrenergic antagonists. In Gilman AG, Rall TW, Nies AS, Taylor P (eds): *Goodman and Gilman's The Pharmacological Basis of Therapeutics*, 8th ed. New York, Pergamon Press, pp 774–780, 1990.
18. Kohlhardt M, Bauer B, Krause H, Fleckenstein A: Differentiation of the transmembrane Na and Ca channels in mammalian cardiac fibres by the use of specific inhibitors. *Pflugers Arch* 335:309–322, 1972.
19. Schwartz A, McKenna E, Vaghy PL: Receptors for calcium antagonists. *Am J Cardiol* 62:3G–6G, 1988.
20. Antman EM, Stone PH, Muller JE, Braunwald E: Calcium channel blocking agents in the treatment of cardiovascular disorders. Part I. Basic and clinical electrophysiology effects. *Ann Intern Med* 93:875–885, 1980.
21. Kraynack BJ, Lawson NW, Gintautas J: Local anesthetic effect of verapamil in vitro. *Reg Anaesth* 7:114–117, 1982.
22. Bolton TB: Mechanism of action of transmitters and other substances on smooth muscle. *Physiol Rev* 59:606–718, 1979.
23. Robinson BF, Dobbs RJ, Kelsey CR: Effects of nifedipine on resistance vessels, arteries, and veins in man. *Br J Clin Pharmacol* 10:433–438, 1980.
24. Ehara T, Daufmann R: The voltage- and time-dependent effects of (–)-verapamil on the slow inward current in isolated cat ventricular myocardium. *J Pharmacol Exp Ther* 207:49–55, 1978.
25. Hondegheim LM: Antiarrhythmic agents: modulated receptor applications. *Circulation* 75:514–520, 1987.
26. Kohlhardt M, Fleckenstein A: Inhibition of the slow inward current by nifedipine in mammalian ventricular myocardium. *Naunyn Schmiedebergs Arch Pharmcol* 298:267–272, 1977.
27. Barnett JC, Touchon RC: Short-term control of supraventricular tachycardia with verapamil infusion and calcium pretreatment. *Chest* 97:1106–1109, 1990.
28. Verapamil for arrhythmias. *Med Lett Drugs Ther* 23(6):29–30, 1981.
29. Rodin SM, Johnson BF: Pharmacokinetic interactions with digoxin. *Clin Pharmacokinet* 15:227–244, 1988.
30. Choice of a beta-blocker. *Med Lett Drugs Ther* 28(707):20–22, 1986.
31. Shand DG: State of the art: comparative pharmacology of the α-adrenoceptor blocking drugs. *Drugs* 25(suppl 2):92–99, 1983.
32. Sheppard D, DiStefano S, Byrd RC, Eschenbacher WL, Bell V, Steck J, Laddu A: Effects of esmolol on airway function in patients with asthma. *J Clin Pharmacol* 26:169–174, 1986.
33. Hoffman BB, Lefkowitz RJ: Adrenergic receptor antagonists. In Gilman AG, Rall TW, Nies AS, Taylor P (eds): *Goodman and Gilman's The Pharmacological Basis of Therapeutics*, 8th ed. New York, Pergamon Press, pp 221–243, 1990.
34. Betts TA, Alford C: β blocking drugs and sleep. A controlled trial. *Drugs* 25(suppl 2):268–272, 1983.
35. Shand DG: Propranolol. *N Engl J Med* 293:280–284, 1975.
36. Boudoulas H: Differential time course of inotropic and chronotropic blockade after oral propranolol. *Cardiovasc Med* 2:511–518, 1977.
37. Wood M, Shand DG, Wood AJJ: Propranolol binding in plasma during cardiopulmonary bypass. *Anesthesiology* 51:512–516, 1979.
38. Esmolol—a short-acting IV beta-blocker. *Med Lett Drugs Ther* 29(742):57–58, 1987.
39. Menkhaus PG, Reves JG, Kisson I, et al: Cardiovascular effects of esmolol in anesthetized humans. *Anesth Analg* 64:327–334, 1985.
40. The Esmolol Research Group: Intravenous esmolol for the treatment of supraventricular tachyarrhythmia: results of a multicenter, baseline-controlled safety and efficacy study in 160 patients. *Am Heart J* 112:498–505, 1986.
41. Gold EH, Chang W, Cohen M, Baum T, Ehrreich S, Johnson G, Prioli N, Sybertz EJ: Synthesis and comparison of some cardiovascular properties of the stereoisomers of labetalol. *J Med Chem* 25:1363–1370, 1982.
42. Baum T, Watkins RW, Sybertz EJ, Vemulapalli S, Pula KK, Eynon E, Nelson S, Vlict GV, Glennon J, Moran RM: Antihypertensive and hemodynamic actions of SCH 19927, the R,R-isomer and labetalol. *J Pharmacol Exp Ther* 218:444–452, 1981.
43. Labetalol for hypertension. *Med Lett Drugs Ther* 26(670):83–85, 1984.
44. Ahlquist RP: A study of the adrenotropic receptors. *Am J Physiol* 153:586–600, 1948.
45. Roth J, Lesniak MA, Bar RS, Muggeo M, Megyesi K, Harrison LC, Flier JS, Wachslicht-Rodbard H, Gorden P: An introduction to receptors and receptor disorders. *Proc Soc Exp Biol Med* 162:3–12, 1979.
46. Nies AS, Evans GH, Shand DG: Regional hemodynamic effects of beta-adrenergic blockade with propranolol in the unanesthetized primate. *Am Heart J* 85:97–102, 1973.
47. Epstein M, Oster JR: Beta-blockers and the kidney. *Miner Electrolyte Metab* 8:237–254, 1982.
48. Yusuf S, Peto R, Lewis J, Collins R, Sleight P: Beta blockade during and after myocardial infarction: an overview of the randomized trials. *Prog Cardiovasc Dis* 27(5):335–371, 1985.
49. Thadani U, Davidson C, Singleton W, Taylor SH: Comparison of five beta-adrenoreceptor antagonists with different ancillary properties during sustained twice daily therapy in angina pectoris. *Am J Med* 68:243–250, 1980.
50. Brodde OE: The functional importance of beta₁ and beta₂ adrenoceptors in the human heart. *Am J Cardiol* 62:24C–29C, 1988.

51. Man in't Veld AJ, Van den Meiracker AH, Schalekamp MA: Do beta-blockers really increase peripheral vascular resistance? Review of the literature and new observations under basal conditions. *Am J Hypertens* 1:91–96, 1988.

52. Houston MC, Hodge R: Beta adrenergic blocker withdrawal syndromes in hypertension and other cardiovascular diseases. *Am Heart J* 116:515–523, 1988.

53. Deacon SP, Karunanuyake A, Barnett D: Acebutolol, atenolol, and propranolol and metabolic responses to acute hypoglycemia in man. *Br Med J* 2:1255–1257, 1977.

54. Miller NE: Effects of adrenoceptor-blocking drugs on plasma lipoprotein concentrations. *Am J Cardiol* 60:17E–23E, 1987.

55. Brown MJ, Brown DC, Murphy MB: Hypokalemia from beta$_2$-receptor stimulation by circulating epinephrine. *N Engl J Med* 309:1414–1419, 1983.

56. Adenosine. *Med Lett Drugs Ther* 32(821):63, 1990.

57. Belardinelli L, Linden J, Berne RM: The cardiac effects of adenosine. *Prog Cardiovasc Dis* 32(1):73–97, 1989.

58. Overholt ED, Rheuban KS, Gutgesell HP, Lerman BB, DiMarco JP: Usefulness of adenosine for arrhythmias in infants and children. *Am J Cardiol* 61:336–340, 1988.

59. Londos C, Wolff J: Two distinct adenosine-sensitive sites on adenylate cyclase. *Proc Natl Acad Sci USA* 74:5482–5486, 1977.

60. West GA, Belardinelli L: Sinus slowing and pacemaker shift caused by adenosine in rabbit SA node. *Pflugers Arch* 403:66–74, 1985.

61. Camm AJ, Garratt CJ. Adenosine and supraventricular tachycardia. *N Engl J Med* 325(23):1621–1629, 1991.

62. Belardinelli L, West GA, Clemo SHF: Regulation of atrioventricular node function by adenosine. In Gerlach E, Becker B (eds): *Topics and Perspectives of Adenosine Research*. Berlin, Springer-Verlag, pp 344–355, 1987.

63. Belardinelli L, Fenton RA, West A, et al: Extracellular action of adenosine and the antagonism by aminophylline on the atrioventricular conduction of isolated perfused guinea pig and rat hearts. *Circ Res* 51:569–579, 1982.

64. Brugada P, Brugada J, Mont L, Smeets J, Andries EW: A new approach to the differential diagnosis of a regular tachycardia with a wide QRS complex. *Circulation* 83:1649–1659, 1991.

65. Griffith MJ, Garratt CJ, Ward DE, Camm AJ: The effects of adenosine on sinus node reentrant tachycardia. *Clin Cardiol* 12:409–411, 1989.

66. Perelman KS, Krikler DM: Termination of focal atrial tachycardia by adenosine triphosphate. *Br Heart J* 58:528–530, 1987.

67. Belhassen B, Shoshani D, Laniado S: Unmasking of ventricular preexcitation by adenosine triphosphate: its usefulness in the assessment of the ajmaline test. *Am Heart J* 118:634–636, 1989.

68. Sharma AO, Klein GJ, Yee R: Intravenous adenosine triphosphate during wide QRS complex tachycardia: safety, therapeutic efficacy, and diagnostic utility. *Am J Med* 88:337–343, 1990.

69. Garratt CJ, Griffith MJ, O'Nunain S, Ward DE, Camm AJ: Effects of intravenous adenosine on antegrade refractoriness of accessory atrioventricular connections. *Circulation* 84(5):1962–1968, 1991.

70. Lerman BB, Belardinelli L, West GA, Berne RM, DiMarco JP: Adenosine-sensitive ventricular tachycardia: evidence suggesting cyclic AMP-mediated triggered activity. *Circulation* 74:270–280, 1986.

71. Dobson JG: Adenosine reduces catecholamine contractile responses in oxygenated and hypoxic atria. *Am J Physiol* 245:H468–H474, 1983.

72. Schrader J, Baumann G, Gerlach E: Adenosine as inhibitor of myocardial effects of catecholamines. *Pflugers Arch* 372:29–35, 1977.

73. Kusachi S, Thompson RD, Olsson RA: Ligand selectivity of dog coronary adenosine receptor resembles that of adenylate cyclase stimulating (Ra) receptors. *J Pharmacol Exp Ther* 227:316–321, 1983.

74. Kurtz A: Adenosine stimulates guanylate cyclase activity in vascular smooth muscle cells. *J Biol Chem* 262:6296–6300, 1987.

75. Duca P, Brest AW: Indications, contraindications, and nonindications for digitalis therapy. *Cardiovasc Clin* 4:131–139, 1974.

76. Marcus FI: Pharmacokinetic interaction between digoxin and other drugs. *J Am Coll Cardiol* 5:82A–90A, 1985.

77. Gault H, Vusdev S, Vlusses P, et al: Interpretation of serum digoxin levels in renal failure. *Clin Pharmacol Ther* 39:530–536, 1986.

78. Allen JC, Entman ML, Schwartz A: The nature of the transport ATPase-digitalis complex. VIII. The relationship between in vivo bound ^{3}H-ouabain-Na, K-ATPase complex and ouabain-induced positive inotropism. *J Pharmacol Exp Ther* 192:105–112, 1975.

79. Schwartz A, Lindenmayer GE, Allen JC: The sodium-potassium adenosine triphosphatase: pharmacological, physiological and biochemical aspects. *Pharmacol Rev* 27:1–134, 1975.

80. Gillis RA, Quest JA: The role of the nervous system in the cardiovascular effects of digitalis. *Pharmacol Rev* 31:19–97, 1980.

81. Nadeau RA, Amir-Jahad AK, Gauther P, Porlier GA: Effects of cardiac glycosides injected into the atrioventricular node artery of the dog. *Can J Physiol Pharmacol* 49:113–126, 1971.

82. Ferrari A, Gregorini L, Ferrari MC, Prete L, Mancia G: Digitalis and baroreceptor reflexes in man. *Circulation* 63:279–285, 1981.

83. Thames MD: Acetylstrophanthidin-induced reflex inhibition of canine renal sympathetic nerve activity mediated by cardiac receptors with vagal afferents. *Circ Res* 44:8–15, 1979.

84. Akera T, Brown BS: Cardiovascular toxicity of cardiotonic drugs and chemicals. In Van Stee EW (ed): *Cardiovascular Toxicology*. New York, Raven Press, 1982, pp 109–134.

85. Smith TW, Autman EM, Freidman PL, et al: Digitalis glycosides: mechanisms and manifestations of toxicity. Parts I, II, and III. *Prog Cardiovasc Dis* 26:413, 495, 1984; 27:21, 1984.

86. Haustein KO: Cardiotoxicity of digitalis. *Arch Toxicol Suppl* 9:197–204, 1986.

87. Smith TW, Butler VP Jr, Haber L, Fozzard H, Marcus FI, Bremner WF, Schulman IC, Phillips A: Treatment of life-threatening digitalis intoxication with digoxin-specific Fab fragments: experience in 24 cases. *N Engl J Med* 307:1357–1362, 1982.

88. Mikkelson E: Effects of digoxin on isolated human pulmonary vessels. *Acta Pharmacol Toxicol* 45:139–144, 1979.

89. Mason DT, Braunwald E: Studies on digitalis. X. Effects of ouabain on forearm vascular resistance and venous tone in normal subjects and patients in heart failure. *J Clin Invest* 43:532–543, 1964.

90. Schinz A, Schnelle K, Klein G, Blomer H: Time sequence of direct vascular and inotropic effects following intravenous administration of digoxin in normal man. *Int J Clin Pharmacol* 15(4):189–193, 1977.

91. Vatner SF, Higgins CB, Franklin D, Braunwald E: Effects of a digitalis glycoside on coronary and systemic hemodynamics in conscious dogs. *Circ Res* 28:470–479, 1971.

92. Higgins CB, Vatner SF, Braunwald E: Regional hemodynamic effects of a digitalis glycoside in the conscious dog with and without experimental heart failure. *Circ Res* 30:406–417, 1972.

93. Mecca TE, Elam JT, Caldwell RW: Mechanism of the pulmonary vasoconstrictor action of digoxin in the dog. *J Cardiovasc Pharmacol* 7:833–840, 1985.

94. Guthrie GP: Effects of digoxin on responsiveness to the pressor actions of angiotensin and norepinephrine in man. *J Clin Endocrinol Metab* 58:76–80, 1984.

95. Harriman RJ, Zeiler RH, Gough WB, El-Sherif N: Enhancement of triggered activity in ischemic Purkinje fibers by ouabain: a mechanism of increased susceptibility to digitalis toxicity in myocardial infarction. *J Am Coll Cardiol* 5:672–679, 1985.

96. Kim DH, Akera T, Kennedy RH: Ischemia-induced enhancement of digitalis sensitivity in isolated guinea pig heart. *J Pharmacol Exp Ther* 226:335–342, 1983.

97. Green LH, Smith TW: The use of digitalis in patients with pulmonary disease. *Ann Intern Med* 87:459–465, 1977.

98. Heerdt PM, Caldwell RW: The cardiovascular response to digoxin in conscious dogs with left atrial obstruction. *J Cardiothoracic Anesth* 4:687–694, 1990.

99. Brady JM, Nechay BR: Maximal effects of ouabain on renal sodium reabsorption and ouabain-sensitive adenosine triphosphatase activity in the dog. *J Pharmacol Exp Ther* 190:346–357, 1974.

100. Nies AS, Gerber JG: Non-steroidal anti-inflammatory drugs potentiate the vasoconstrictor effects of ouabain in the dog. *Circ Res* 48(6):844–849, 1981.

101. Levinsky RA, Lewis RM, Bynum TE, Hanley HG: Digoxin induced intestinal vasoconstriction. *Circulation* 52:130–136, 1975.

102. Kleeman K, Singh BN: Serum electrolytes and the heart. In Maxwell MH, Kleeman CR (eds): *Clinical Disorders of Fluid and Electrolyte Metabolism*. New York, McGraw-Hill, 1980, pp 169–173.

103. Hall RJ, Gellbart A, Silverman M, Goldman RH: Studies on digitalis-induced arrhythmias in glucose- and insulin-induced hypokalemia. *J Pharmacol Exp Ther* 201:711, 1977.

104. Chopra D, Janson R, Sawin CT: Insensitivity to digoxin associated with hypocalcemia. *N Engl J Med* 296:917, 1977.

105. Jonkman FAM, Boddeke HWGM, van Zweiten PA: Protective activity of calcium entry blockers against ouabain intoxication in anesthetized guinea pigs. *J Cardiovasc Pharmacol* 8:1009–1013, 1986.

106. Specter MJ, Schweizer E, Goldman RH: Studies on magnesium's mechanism of action in digitalis-induced arrhythmias. *Circulation* 52:1001, 1975.

107. DiCarli C, Sprouse G, LaRosa JC: Arrhythmias and conduction disturbances: serum magnesium levels in symptomatic atrial fibrillation and their relation to rhythm control by intravenous digoxin. *Am J Cardiol* 57:956–959, 1986.

108. Kleiger RE, Katsutaka S: Effects of chronic depletion of potassium and magnesium on the action of acetylstrophanthidin. *Am J Cardiol* 17:520, 1966.

109. Cronnelly R, Stanski DR, Miller RD, Shenner LB, Sohn YJ: Renal function and the pharmacokinetics of neostigmine in anesthetized patients. *Anesthesiology* 51:222–226, 1979.

110. Cronnelly R, Morris RB: Antagonism of neuromuscular blockade. *Br J Anaesth* 54:183–193, 1982.

111. Morris RB, Cronnelly R, Miller RD, Stanski DR, Fahey MR: Pharmacokinetics of edrophonium and neostigmine when antagonizing d-tubocurarine neuromuscular blockade in man. *Anesthesiology* 54:399–402, 1981.

112. Taylor P: Anticholinesterase agents. In Gilman AG, Rall TW, Nies AS, Taylor P (eds): *Goodman and Gilman's The Pharmacological Basis of Therapeutics*, 8th ed. New York, Pergamon Press, pp 131–149, 1990.

113. Holmstedt B: Structure-activity relationships of the organophosphorus anticholinesterase agents. In Cholinesterases and Anticholinesterase Agents. Koelle GB (ed): *Handbuch der Experimentellen Pharmakologie*, vol 15. Berlin, Springer-Verlag, pp 428–485, 1963.

114. Usdin E: Reactions of cholinesterases with substrate inhibitors and reactivators. In Karczmar AG (ed): *Anticholinesterase Agents. International Encyclopedia of Pharmacology and Therapeutics*, vol 1, sect 13. Oxford, Pergamon Press, pp 47–354, 1970.

115. Cronnelly R, Morris RB, Miller RD: Edrophonium: duration of action and atropine requirements in humans during halothane anesthesia. *Anesthesiology* 57:261–266, 1982.

116. Vanhoutte PM: Endothelium and control of vascular function. *Hypertension* 13:658–667, 1989.

117. Feigl EO: Reflex parasympathetic coronary vasodilation elicited from cardiac receptors in the dog. *Circ Res* 37:175–182, 1975.

118. Langer SZ, Cavero I, Massingham R: Recent developments in noradrenergic neurotransmission and its relevance to the mechanism of action of certain antihypertensive agents. *Hypertension* 2:372–382, 1980.

119. Kobinger W: Central alpha-adrenergic systems as targets for hypotensive drugs. *Rev Physiol Biochem* 81:39–100, 1978.

120. Sleight P: Reflex control of the heart. *Am J Cardiol* 44:889–894, 1979.

121. Hyman AL, Lippton HL, Dempsey CW, et al: Autonomic control of the pulmonary circulation. In Weir EK, Reeves JT (eds): *Pulmonary Vascular Physiology and Pathophysiology*. New York, Marcel Dekker, pp 291–324, 1989.

122. Brown JH: Atropine, scopolamine and related antimuscarinic drugs. In Gilman AG, Rall TW, Nies AS, Taylor P (eds): *Goodman and Gilman's The Pharmacological Basis of Therapeutics*, 8th ed. New York, Pergamon Press, pp 150–165, 1990.

123. Yamamura HI, Snyder SH: Muscarinic cholinergic receptor binding in the longitudinal muscle of the guinea pig ileum with [³H] quinuclidinyl benzilate. *Mol Pharmacol* 10:861–867, 1974.

124. Bonner TI: The molecular basis of muscarinic receptor diversity. *Trends Neurosci* 12:148–151, 1989.

125. Gravenstein JS, Andersen TW, DePadua CB: Effects of atropine and scopolamine on the cardiovascular system in man. *Anesthesiology* 25:123–130, 1964.

126. Dauchot P, Gravenstein JS: Effects of atropine on the electrocardiogram in different age groups. *Clin Pharmacol Ther* 12:274–280, 1971.

127. Wellstein A, Pitschner HF: Complex dose-response curves of atropine in man explained by different functions of M₁ and M₂-cholinoceptors. *Naunyn Schmiedebergs Arch Pharmacol* 338:19–27, 1988.

128. Bolton TB: Mechanisms of action of transmitters and other substances on smooth muscle. *Physiol Rev* 59:606–718, 1979.

129. North RA, Slack BE, Surprenant A: Muscarinic M₁ and M₂ receptors mediate depolarization and presynaptic inhibition in guinea pig enteric nervous system. *J Physiol (Lond)* 368:435–452, 1985.

130. Bönisch H, Trendelenburg U: The mechanism of action of indirectly acting sympathomimetic amines. In Trendelenburg U, Weiner N (eds): *Catecholamines I. Handbook of Experimental Pharmacology*, vol 90. Berlin, Springer-Verlag, pp 247–278, 1988.

131. Iversen LL: Uptake processes for biogenic amines. In Iversen LL, Iversen SD, Snyder SH (eds): *Handbook of Psychopharmacology*, vol 3. New York, Plenum Press, pp 381–442, 1975.

132. Lefkowitz RJ, Hoffmann BB, Taylor P: Neurohumoral transmission: The autonomic and somatic motor nervous systems. In Gilman AG, Rall TW, Nies AS, Taylor P (eds): *Goodman and Gilman's The Pharmacological Basis of Therapeutics*, 8th ed. New York, Pergamon Press, pp 84–121, 1990.

133. Somar VR, Shamoon H, Sherwin RS: Effects of physiologic infusion of epinephrine in normal man: relationship between metabolic response and β adrenergic binding. *J Clin Endocrinol Metab* 50:294, 1980.

CHAPTER 27

Treatment of Cardiac Arrhythmias

ROBERT D. COLUCCI, PHARM.D., F.C.P., F.C.C.M.
JOHN C. SOMBERG, M.D., F.C.P.

The treatment of cardiac arrhythmic emergencies has undergone considerable change. Our approach to the treatment of supraventricular arrhythmias has changed considerably, as well as the modalities to treat life threatening ventricular arrhythmias. However, it remains the cornerstone of diagnosis and therapy to search for reversible etiologies of the culprit arrhythmia: hypoxia, myocardial ischemia; heart failure; acid-base or electrolyte imbalances. Treating an arrhythmia that has a reversible etiology is often ineffective and inappropriate since the risks associated with antiarrhythmic therapy could have been avoided. However, antiarrhythmic therapy will be needed for patient stabilization, arrhythmia termination, and then the chronic prophylaxis of arrhythmia reoccurrences. An understanding of antiarrhythmic pharmacology is needed to effectively utilize current therapy. To understand and effectively use antiarrhythmic therapy a basic knowledge of cellular electrophysiology will give order to an otherwise bewildering array of agents.

CELLULAR ELECTROPHYSIOLOGY

The cardiac action potential is comprised of 5 stages (Fig. 27.1). These stages represent the movement of ions across the cardiac cell membrane. The interior of the cardiac cell is electrically negative, compared to the extracellular space. This electrostatic potential is due to the preponderance of Na outside the cell and K+ primarily inside the cell. This ionic concentration gradient is maintained by the energy-dependent Na^+K^+ ATP ase ion pump. The intracellular K concentration is approximately 150 mM, while the extracellular K^+ is approximately 3 mM. The cell is somewhat permeable to K^+, so K^+ leaks out of the cell into the intracellular space, leaving negative charges on intracellular protein to predominate, making the cell electronegative inside to outside. This equilibrium between the chemical and electrostatic forces creates a resting potential that can be described by the Nernst equation:

$$E_K = -61.5 \log (K+ \; interval/K+ \; external)$$

When an applied stimulus is of sufficient amplitude to cause an inward current that is greater than the K+ outward current, ion channels open, permitting Na^+ to rush into the cell, depolarizing it. A rapid depolarization changes the resting membrane potential to a more positive one, about +25 to +35 mV, approaching the Na^+ equilibrium potential. Following this rapid depolarization there is a change in K^+ channel conductance that leads to K^+ being less permeable, sustaining phase 0 depolarization. In addition, a second K channel is activated, causing a small repolarization current (Phase 1). Then there occur further changes in ion channels, permitting a slow inward current of Ca^{2+} that prolongs repolarization. This slow channel opens when the membrane channel reaches -60 mV from the resting -90 mV, permitting the inward movement of Ca^{2+} that contributes to the continued inward depolarizing current, forming a "plateau" phase. The Ca^{2+} slow inward channel begins to close, and a second K^+ channel

445

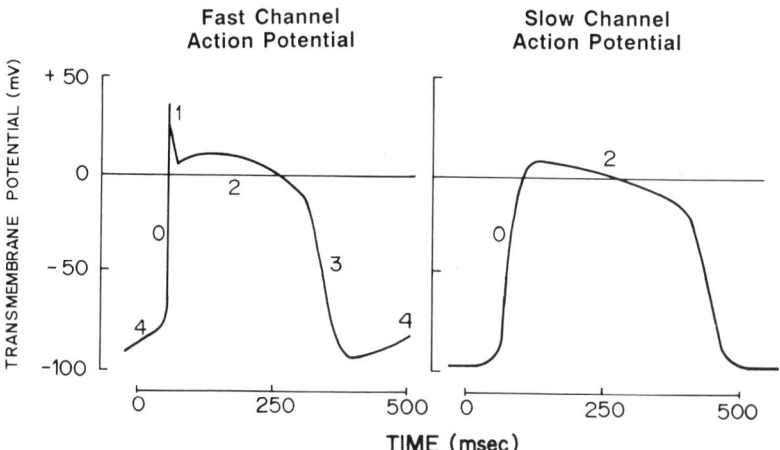

Figure 27.1.   Representative cardiac action potentials from tissues dependent on either fast response (Na^+ channels) or slow response (CA^{2+} channels) for action potential generations.

opens and allows the outward movement of K^+, permitting membrane repolarization (phase 3) to the resting potential.

The pacemaker cells in the heart, the sinoatrial node (SA node) behaves somewhat differently. There occurs in the SA node a spontaneous decline in K^+ conductance. Thus the outward K^+ flux is stopped. An inward current due to the Ca^{2+} remains with the cell depolarizing. The SA node has the highest degree of this spontaneous depolarization, called automaticity, and thus the SA node is the dominant cardiac pacemaker. The rate of the automaticity of the SA node is modulated by the activity of both divisions of the autonomic nervous system. The release of acetylcholine from cholinergic vagal fibers increases potassium conductance in the SA node; more K^+ moving outward gives the cell a greater negative potential, thus hyperpolarizing the cell, making it less likely to depolarize. On the other hand, sympathetic stimulation decreases membrane permeability to K^+, leading to early cell depolarization and, thus, to enhanced automaticity. Other cells in the atrium, atrioventricular (AV node), His-Purkinje system, and working ventricular myocardia can manifest automaticity, but this effect usually occurs due to cell injury (ischemia), electrolyte imbalance (hypokalemia), or catecholamine excess.

The movement of the electrical force, cardiac conduction, is essential for the effective contraction of the heart. While the impulse originates at the SA node initiating atrial contraction, the ventricle needs to contract from apex to base. This contraction is accomplished by a delay at the AV junction, followed by rapid conduction through specialized fibers (Purkinje fibers) to the working myocardium, initiating contraction at the apex and then running up to the base pushing blood out of the heart through the aorta. One can readily see why a ventricular tachycardia originating the His-Purkinje system would be tolerated well, while one originating in the high left ventricular free wall would lead to outflow obstruction (base contracting before apex), hemodynamic collapse, and arrest in rapid sequence.

The major determinants of conduction velocity include the rate of depolarization and the resting membrane potential. Conduction velocity is proportional to the rate of rise of phase 0; in other words, the rate of Na^+ ions influx into the cell, through the fast sodium channel. During the depolarization

period and the early part of repolarization the heart cannot be depolarized by an extra stimulus, and this is termed the refractory period. The effective refractory period is the interval between the preceding spontaneous depolarization to the point at which an extra premature stimulus is just able to produce a depolarization (minimal internal).

THE GENESIS OF ARRHYTHMIAS

Cardiac arrhythmias may be due to disorders of impulse formation or disorders of conduction. Sinus tachycardia is the simplest and most common example of enhanced impulse formation due to release of circulating catecholamines or β-adrenergic stimulation. With hypoxia, hypokalemia, hypomagnesium, and myocardial stretch, as well as other conditions, permeability to K^+ and Na^+ is changed, which can lead to spontaneous cellular depolarization. The increase in intracellular Ca^{2+} concentrations may lead to oscillation in the resting membrane potential. When the oscillations are of sufficient magnitude, cell depolarization will occur. These oscillations may be termed afterdepolarization. Afterdepolarization may occur early in the electrical cycle, termed early afterdepolarization, or late in the cycle, termed delayed afterdepolarization, and may occur in response to hypothermia, electrolyte imbalance, catecholamine excess, or myocardial distention. Digitalis excess in the laboratory may give rise to late afterdepolarization (see Fig. 27.2).

Cardiac conduction disorders are common causes of clinical arrhythmias. A simple construct of an impulse reaching two tissues, each with different states of refractoriness and, thus, different abilities to conduct an impulse exemplifies the condition of reentry. The impulse may be conducted down one pathway while the other is not able to conduct. However, the second pathway may be able to conduct in a retrograde fashion, thus turning the impulse to its origin and reexciting the antegrade pathway such that a circular or reentry circuit of depolarization wavefront develops. This is classical reentry, as shown in diagrammatic form in Figure 27.3. The impulse initializing the arrhythmia may originate from a sinus beat that is held up in a diseased area, then reenters and forms a

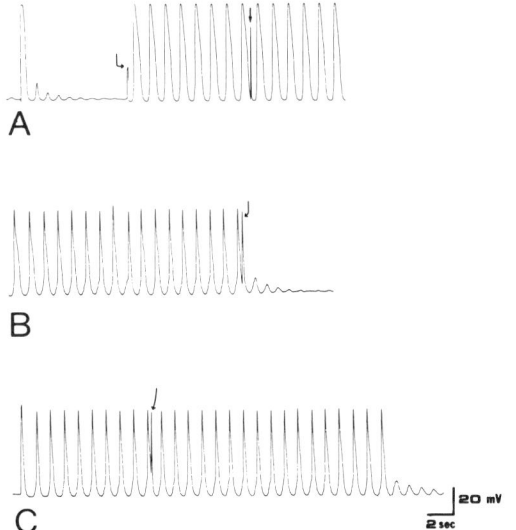

Figure 27.2. Triggered automaticity in an isolated superfused guinea pig myocyte. **A, B,** and **C** depict action potential recordings obtained from an impaled myocyte in the presence of isoproterenol, 10 μM. **A,** The first action potential is followed by several delayed afterpolarizations that fail to achieve threshold. At the *arrow,* an applied stimulus initiates sustained rhythmic activity. **B.** A single extrastimulus terminates the arrhythmia. Subthreshold delayed afterepolarizations are again observed. As shown in **C,** triggered activity may also terminate spontaneously. (Courtesy of Dr. L. Belardinelli, University of Virginia.)

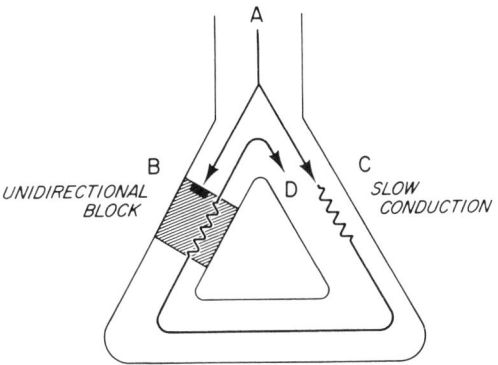

Figure 27.3. Diagram of the requirements for reentry. A premature impulse from some proximal point arrives at a branch point *(A)* with unequal conduction in the two branches. On side *B,* the tissue is still refractory and anterograde conduction block occurs. On side *C,* the impulse is slowed but traverses the area. It can then conduct around to point *B,* which has sufficiently recovered to permit retrograde conduction. If the tissue at *D* has recovered excitability, the reentry loop is completed and may continue.

cirrus movement tachycardia. Arrhythmia initiation may also be from a depolarization due to abnormal automaticity being premature or late in the cardiac cycle reentering a pathway, catching the dispersion of refractoriness in such a way as to perpetuate a reentry tachycardia. The state of the autonomic nervous system as it modifies refractoriness and depolarization may greatly influence the reentry circuit. Reentry is dependent on a heterogeneity of refractoriness. Heterogeneity is dependent on diseased tissue and the differential effect of disease on cardiac actions and repolarization to result in reentry. The reentry may be macro, involving the AV node specialized conducting system, or it may be micro, involving an

isolated segment of the heart that is heterogenous due to myocardial injury most likely secondary to a myocardial infarction. An anatomical anomaly with atrial tissue connecting the atrium to the ventricle may also give rise to a macro reentry in the Wolff-Parkinson-White preexcitation syndromes. The conduction may be down the normal pathway (anterograde conduction), then up the bypass connection between the atrium and ventricle, or it can be down the bypass tract and up the His-Purkinje AV node pathway (retrograde tachycardia). Once again, the state of the autonomic nervous system can greatly influence the tachyarrhythmia by changing refractoriness in the various components of the anatomical structures that make up the pathway. A hallmark of reentry tachycardia is that a carefully timed stimulus may initiate, as well as terminate, the tachyarrhythmia. While this is a hallmark of reentry, afterdepolarization in tissue bath preparations caused by excessive amounts of digitalis may trigger afterdepolarization combined with pacing, and pacing may, indeed, terminate afterdepolarization as well. Thus, the extra stimulus techniques of arrhythmia initiation and termination are not foolproof in differentiating a tachycardia due to reentry vs. abnormal automaticity.

Pharmacodynamic agents have markedly different effects on the tachycardias due to differences in their mechanism. A reentry supraventricular tachycardia involving the AV node could be terminated by a drug that increases AV node refractoriness. Vagal stimulation increased by pharmacologic means or endogenous pureness, such as ATP or adenosine, increases outward K$^+$ currents, hyperpolarizing the cell, inhibiting depolarization. Calcium channel blockers of the verapamil or diltiazem grouping may prolong AV node refractoriness, terminating the tachycardia. Membrane active drugs may increase refractoriness at the AV node or in other components of the reentry circuit also terminating the tachycardia. Tachycardias involving the ventricular myocardium need to have the balance in refractoriness and conduction modified in the limbs of the reentry circuit. A large number of agents can change the balance of refractoriness and repolarization. A description of the agents available, how they work and are classified, follows below.

One can see how the β-blockers, by attenuating the effects of catecholamine, decrease automaticity and can slow conduction. The calcium channel blockers, by affecting the voltage-dependent slow Ca^{2+} channels involved in AV node refractoriness and conduction, may be effective in terminating arrhythmias that involve the SA and AV nodes. Membrane-active agents, the prototypic one being quinidine, work on the sodium channel by inhibiting depolarization. One can see how this could effect automaticity, as well as influencing conduction and refractoriness, thus affecting a reentrant rhythm. The drugs of this class have been termed class I agents by Vaughan Williams. Interestingly, there are three major groupings of agents of this class, and these groupings can be based on the Na$^+$ channel kinetics, with agents that demonstrate rapid "on-off" kinetics to the Na channel being Class Ib and those with very slow "on-off" kinetics being of the Ic grouping. Another grouping of drugs may influence arrhythmias by prolonging repolarization by delaying the inward K$^+$ flux that drives repolarization. Amiodarone, *N*-acetyl procainamide (NAPA), and sotalol are agents that fit into this class III category. Thus, an understanding of the molecular mechanism that underlies arrhythmias and that is effected by antiarrhythmic agents may, indeed, help in the therapeutic approach to arrhythmias.

ANTIARRHYTHMIC DRUG CLASSIFICATION

The development of an antiarrhythmic drug classification was first proposed and utilized over 20 years ago (1, 2). A variety of classifications have emerged as a result of increasing research with newer antiarrhythmic compounds, as well as the advancement in technology that allows one to specifically record electrophysiologic properties (2, 3). Although each of these classifications possesses limitations, they each assist in the development of a framework for antiarrhythmics, based on the drugs mechanism of actions. Vaughan Williams proposed the first antiarrhythmic classification. Today, his classification system is utilized most frequently, both in clinical practice and research.

Antiarrhythmic drugs are classified into four major groups. Class I antiarrhythmic drugs affect the fast sodium channels by inhibiting the conduction through excitable tissue. This effect is achieved principally through decreasing phase 0 of the action potential. Class I antiarrhythmic drugs also affect the refractory period and depress automaticity by lowering phase 4 potential.

Class I antiarrhythmics demonstrate various degrees of effect on conduction, refractoriness, and on the action potential. As a result they are further subdivided into Ia, Ib and Ic. Class Ia agents have a moderate effect on phase 0 depression, slow conduction, and prolong repolarization. Class Ib antiarrhythmics are characterized by having little effect on phase 0 depolarization, slowing conduction while shortening repolarization. Class Ic antiarrhythmics are characterized by producing a marked effect on sodium conductance, prolonging conduction but with no effect on repolarization.

Class II antiarrhythmics are classically the β-adrenergic blockers. These drugs depress automaticity and increase the effective refractory period of the AV node. This group of antiarrhythmic agents may exert a membrane-stabilizing effect at pharmacologic and suprapharmacologic serum concentrations; however, this is of little clinical significance.

Class III antiarrhythmics are characterized by significantly prolonging the action potential. As a result, the repolarization period and refractoriness are prolonged without an appreciable effect on excitability. These agents also have important antifibrillatory effects.

Class IV antiarrhythmics consist of the calcium channel blockers. Their electrophysiologic effects are primarily due to prolonging of the AV nodal conduction and prolongation of the functional refractory period.

The Vaughan Williams classification system has proven to be an effective way of grouping antiarrhythmic drugs. The initial intent of this grouping was to classify the antiarrhythmic action, not the specific action of individual agents. Each of the antiarrhythmic agents and their metabolites possesses a multitude of electrophysiologic properties that may vary in different patient populations. Therefore, the response of an individual antiarrhythmic agent should not be interpreted as the response of an entire class.

INDIVIDUAL ANTIARRHYTHMIC AGENTS

The following is an overview of the individual antiarrhythmic agents within the Vaughan Williams classification system. Table 27.1 lists the individual agents and general recommendations for their use.

CLASS IA ANTIARRHYTHMICS

Quinidine

Quinidine is one of the oldest antiarrhythmics available. Quinidine was first developed in the 18th century (4). It continues to be used frequently and has been shown to be effective for both supraventricular and ventricular arrhythmias.

Pharmacology/Electrophysiology. Quinidine is derived from the bark of the cinchona tree. Quinidine is a weak base and, depending on its salt formulation, the percent of quinidine may vary from 60 to 83%. Quinidine is considered to be the prototype of class Ia antiarrhythmics. Its electrophysiologic effects include prolongation of the action potential and effective refractory period in atrial, ventricular, and Purkinje fibers. Quinidine additionally demonstrates a decrease in the action potential and rate of rise of Phase O (5, 6). In electrophysiology studies, quinidine prolongs the AV interval, refractory period, and AV nodal conduction. On the ECG, quinidine significantly prolongs the QRS and QT intervals.

Quinidine possesses α-adrenergic blocking activity. This activity can result in a reflex activation that may increase the sinus node rate and sinus node conduction (7). Rapid intravenous administration is generally not recommended, other than in acute testing procedures and in emergency situations. Rather, a slow intravenous administration has been used safely (8).

Pharmacokinetics. The bioavailability of quinidine may vary from 43 to 93%, depending on the salt formulation (9). Since quinidine is a weak base, the primary area of absorption is in the small intestine. The peak plasma concentration is achieved 2 to 4 hours following administration of quinidine sulfate. The volume of distribution of quinidine is 3 liters/kg and follows a 2-compartment kinetic model (10). Approximately 70 to 90% of quinidine is bound to glycoprotein (pharmacologically inactive). Quinidine protein binding has been shown to decrease in patients following a myocardial infarction, trauma, or surgery (11, 13).

Quinidine undergoes both hepatic and renal elimination. The half-life of quinidine is 6 to 8 hours in patients receiving quinidine gluconate. Several metabolites have been identified following liver metabolism. The principle metabolites are 3-hydroxyquinidine and 2-oxoquinidine. The effects of renal or hepatic dysfunction on the pharmacokinetics of quinidine have not been clearly defined, although the liver appears to play a more important role in quinidine's elimination. Marked adjustments in dosage for moderate-to-severe renal or hepatic disease have not been uniformly required, although higher levels have been noted in cirrhotics and following propranolol administration (14).

The plasma concentration of quinidine is 2 to 4 μg/ml. Patients whose concentrations were >8 μg/ml may present with clinically significant ECG changes and signs of toxicity.

Table 27.1. Antiarrhythmic Agents[a,b]

Drug	Indication	Route	Dosing[c] (mg/day)	Adverse Effects
Class Ia				
Quinidine	AF, PSVT VT, WPW	IV	6–10 mg/kg (infusion)	Hypotension, GI, thrombocytopenia, cinchonism
		Oral	(QG) 648–972	
			(QP) 550–825	
			(QS) 600–1200 (RR)	
			(QS) 1200–1800 (SR)	
Procainamide	AF, VT, WPW	IV	5–15 mg/kg, LD	GI, CNS, lupus fever, hematological, anticholinergic effects
			2–6 mg/min, MD	
		Oral	2000–5000 (SR)	
Disopyramide	AF, VT	Oral	400–800 (RR)	Anticholinergic effects, CHF
			400–800 (SR)	
Class Ib				
Lidocaine	VT, VF, PVC	IV	1–2 mg/kg, LD (may repeat × 1)	CNS, GI
			1–4 mg/min, MD	CNS, blood dyscrasia
Mexilitene	VT	Oral	600–1200	GI, CNS
Tocainide	VT	Oral	1200–1800	GI, CNS, pulmonary aggranulocytosis
Class Ic				
Encainide	VT	Oral	75–200	GI, CNS,
Flecainide	VT	Oral	200–400	CHF, GI, CNS, blurred vision
Propafenone	VT	Oral	450–900	GI, blurred vision, dizziness
Moricizine	VT	Oral	600–900	Dizziness, nausea, rash, seizures
Class II				
Propranolol	SVT, VT, PVC, digoxin toxicity	IV	1–3 mg (may repeat × 1)	CHF, bradycardia, hypotension, CNS, fatigue
			30–120 (RR)	
		Oral	120–160 (SR)	
Esmolol	ST, SVT	IV	500 µg/kg/min for 1 min, followed by 50 µg/kg/min for 4 min, then titrate with repeat LD 50–300 µg/kg/min MD	CHF, CNS, lupus-like syndrome, hypotension, bradycardia bronchospasm
Class III				
Amiodarone	VT	Oral	800–1600 (21 days LD)	CNS, GI, thyroid, pulmonary fibrosis, liver, corneal deposits
			600–800 MD (30 days, LD) 400 MD	
Bretylium	VT, VF	IV	5–10 mg/kg, LD may repeat as needed 5–10 mg/kg q6–8 hr or 1–2 mg/min MD	GI, orthostatic hypotension, CNS
Sotalol	VT	PO	320–640	Bradycardia, hypotension, CHF, CNS, fatigue
Class IV				
Verapamil	AF, PSVT	IV	5–10 mg (may repeat after 15–30 min)	Hypotension, CHF, bradycardia, vertigo, constipation
		Oral	240–480 (RR)	
			120–480 (SR)	
Diltiazem	AF, PSVT	IV	0.25 mg/kg × 2 min LD	Hypotension, GI, liver
			0.35 mg/kg × 2 min (2nd LD optional)	
			5–15 mg/hr, MD	
			120–360 (RR)	
		Oral		
Miscellaneous				
Adenosine	SVT, PSVT,	IV	6 mg (may repeat up to 12 mgs)	Flushing, dizziness, bradycardia, syncope
Digoxin	AF, PSVT	IV	0.4–1 LD	GI, CNS, arrhythmias
			0.125–0.375 MD	
		PO	0.750–1.25 LD	
			0.125–0.375 MD	
Magnesium	VT, VF	IV	1–2 gm LD	Hypotension, CNS hypothermia, myocardial depression
			0.5–1. gm/hr MD	

[a] All doses and indications are based on current standards of practice that are subject to change, and all recommendations should be verified before being clinically implemented.

[b] LD, loading dose; MD, maintenance dose; WPW, Wolff-Parkinson-White; ST; Sinus Tachycardia, RR; regular release, SR; sustained release, QG; quinidine gluconate, QP; quinidine polygalactoronate.

[c] Total dosing for one day, unless otherwise noted.

Clinical Use.   Quinidine has been demonstrated to be effective in a variety of atrial and ventricular arrhythmias. Similar to other class I antiarrhythmics, quinidine suppresses premature ventricular contractions (PVCs) and ventricular arrhythmias in approximately 60 to 80% of patients by Holter monitoring. However, following programmed electrical stimulation (PES) testing, overall efficacy decreases to 30% (15).

Quinidine is effective in treating supraventricular tachycardia, including Wolff-Parkinson-White syndrome, by prolonging the effective refractory period of the accessory pathway in the anterograde direction. Its efficacy in converting atrial fibrillation or atrial tachycardia to normal sinus rhythm is 10 to 20% (16).

Adverse Effects.   Quinidine causes mild depression in myocardial contractility and automaticity. Dose-related prolongation of the QRS interval has been demonstrated, and AV block can develop with severe quinidine toxicity. Increased ventricular response in atrial fibrillation or flutter may be more likely with quinidine than procainamide because of quinidine's anticholinergic action. A syndrome of quinidine syncope characterized by the development of ventricular tachycardia or fibrillation has been described and estimated to occur in up to 3% of the patients receiving quinidine for atrial fibrillation (17). The mechanism of this syndrome is unknown but may be related to the development of prolonged Q-T interval and enhanced myocardial instability.

The most common adverse effects following chronic therapy are gastrointestinal, including nausea, diarrhea, abdominal pain, vomiting, and anorexia. Central nervous system toxicity of quinidine (cinchonism) includes tinnitus, hearing loss, visual disturbances, confusion, delirium, and coma. Allergic reactions may manifest as rashes, fever, immune-mediated thrombocytopenia, hemolytic anemia and, rarely, anaphylaxis. Quinidine is highly protein bound (about 80%) and may cause bleeding in patients receiving the oral anticoagulant coumadin by displacement of coumadin from its protein binding. Cimetidine has been reported to cause a rise in plasma quinidine concentration (18), and rifampin lowers quinidine concentrations by inducing hepatic enzymes (19). Quinidine has also been shown to raise serum digoxin levels (20) which, if not dealt with, may lead to a significant incidence of digitalis toxicity.

Dosage and Administration.   Depending on the oral formulation used (sulfate, gluconate, or polygalacturonate) various amounts of quinidine ares found in the base formulation. The gluconate and polygalacturonate salts are the slow-release preparations. The immediate-release preparation is usually given every 6 hours, and the slow-release preparation is given every 8 to 12 hours. Quinidine is orally administered with an initial dose of 600 to 1200 mgs daily in divided doses. The use of intravenous administration has been shown to be safe and effective (21). The usual dose of 6 to 10 mg/kg is infused at a rate of 0.4 to 0.5 mg/kg/min (equivalent to 0.25 to 0.31 mg/kg/min of quinidine base). The infusion rate may be decreased or terminated due to decreased blood pressure.

Procainamide

In the 1930s, procainamide was identified as having antiarrhythmic activity. However, it took nearly 20 years before a more stable formulation was introduced.

Pharmacology Electrophysiology.   Procainamide is an analogue of procaine hydrochloride. The cardiac and electrophysiology activities are similar to other class Ia antiarrhythmics. However, unlike quinidine, procainamide has no α-blocking properties and much weaker vagolytic effects (22).

Procainamide slows conduction, also prolonging the effective refractory period and action potential duration. Procainamide demonstrates dose-related changes on the surface ECG, which includes a widening of the QRS and QT intervals (less pronounced than with quinidine).

Pharmacokinetics.   The bioavailability of oral procainamide is 75% to 95% in most patients. Peak plasma concentration following the immediate-release preparation occurs 1 to 2 hours postadministration. The volume of distribution of procainamide is 2 liters/kg. The volume of distribution decreases approximately 25% in patients with congestive heart failure (CHF). Contrary to quinidine, procainamide is minimally protein bound. The elimination half life of procainamide is 3 to 4 hours; however, this half-life may be significantly prolonged (up to 20 hours) in patients with renal dysfunction. The sustained release formulation was developed to increase the half-life (5 to 7 hours), which minimizes the dosing regimen and plasma concentration fluctuations.

Procainamide undergoes metabolism by the liver and is eliminated via the kidneys. Procainamide undergoes first order pharmacokinetics and acetylation in the liver. The acetylation phenotype, genetically determined, controls the rate of metabolism of procainamide. Approximately 40% of patients are fast and 40% slow acetylators, respectively. The remaining 20% of patients is intermediate. The major metabolite of procainamide following acetylation is *N*-acetyl procainamide (NAPA) (23, 24). This metabolite occurs in 16–21% of slow acetylators and 24 to 33% of fast acetylators. NAPA is excreted via the kidneys and undergoes minimal metabolism. NAPA has different electrophysiologic properties than the parent compound, behaving like a class III drug, prolonging the action potential duration. The contribution of NAPA to antiarrhythmic activity is small, given its low concentrations. However, in patients with renal dysfunction and who are rapid acetylators, NAPA accumulates. The recommended therapeutic plasma concentration of procainamide is 4 to 8 µg/ml, and for NAPA it is 10 to 24 µg/ml, respectively. It is incorrect to add the NAPA and procainamide levels together since each has a distinctly different therapeutic range. Cimetidine has been observed to reduce procainamide elimination.

Clinical Use.   Procainamide is an effective agent in the management of both ventricular and supraventricular arrhythmias. Although lidocaine has been preferred for the emergency intravenous therapy of life-threatening ventricular arrhythmias, some patients who fail to respond to lidocaine may be treated safely and successfully with procainamide. Procainamide therapy for patients with the Wolff-Parkinson-White syndrome has produced variable results. Reduction in the number of premature atrial complexes (which often initiate tachycardia) and production of retrograde block in the accessory pathway during atrial fibrillation or flutter are potentially beneficial effects of procainamide. However, procainamide may also have deleterious effects in this syndrome, causing an increase in the anterograde refractory period of the accessory pathway and a lesser effect on the shorter refractory period of the AV node. Procainamide may, rarely, facilitate AV nodal reentry and development of paroxysmal tachycardia in patients with the Wolff-Parkinson-White syndrome (25). However, procainamide is still the agent of choice in patients with rapid atrial arrhythmias who could possibly have preexcitation syndrome.

Adverse Effects. Adverse cardiovascular effects of procainamide include prolonged conduction, negative inotropy, and decreased automaticity. Severe cardiovascular toxicity may manifest as high-grade AV block or intraventricular block with prolongation of the QRS complex (a potential life-threatening toxicity terminating in asystole due to procainamide-induced suppression of automaticity in subsidiary pacemakers). Ventricular tachyarrhythmias and shock may develop from toxic doses of procainamide (26). Excessively rapid administration may produce hypotension that is partially due to a ganglionic blocking action that produces peripheral vasodilation.

Adverse effects following chronic oral use of procainamide include gastrointestinal intolerance (nausea, vomiting, and diarrhea) and skin rash. In addition, up to 40% of patients on long-term procainamide may develop a syndrome resembling systemic lupus erythematosus, with arthralgias, myalgias, fever, pleuropericarditis, and circulating antinuclear antibodies. Virtually all patients eventually develop a positive antinuclear antibody test; however, antinuclear antibodies and the clinical syndrome occur sooner among slow acetylators of the drug (24).

Dosage and Administration. In the emergency setting, procainamide is administered intravenously. An initial 5 to 15 mg/kg loading dose is given as a continuous infusion or small boluses (100 mg every 5 minutes to a dose of 1000 mg), followed by a maintenance infusion of 2 to 6 mg/min. It is generally recommended that the intravenous loading infusion should not exceed 25 to 50 mg/min. Throughout the intravenous administration, careful monitoring of the blood pressure and ECG must be performed.

Conversion to oral therapy is based on the total daily dose divided by the appropriate intervals. One half-life (3 to 4 hours on average) should elapse before introducing the oral therapy following cessation of infusion. The introduction of the sustained-release formulation of procainamide has greatly facilitated patient compliance by lengthening the dosing interval to 6 hours.

Disopyramide

In 1962 disopyramide was first demonstrated to have antiarrhythmic properties in an animal model. By 1977 disopyramide was approved for ventricular arrhythmias.

Pharmacology/Electrophysiology. Disopyramide is a synthetic antiarrhythmic that is chemically unlike quinidine or procainamide, although its electrophysiologic properties resemble class Ia antiarrhythmic agents. The effect on the myocardium and conduction are mediated in part through muscarinic blockade. In animals and humans, the direct depressant effect is offset in partly an increase in heart rate (27). In patients with SA node dysfunction, disopyramide may cause clinically important conduction disturbance (28).

In atrial and ventricular muscle, both the action potential duration and effective refractory period are increased in a concentration-dependent manner. The electrocardiographic changes observed with disopyramide include widening of the QRS and QT intervals and prolongation of the PR interval.

Pharmacokinetics. Disopyramide is rapidly and almost completely absorbed from the gastrointestinal tract. Peak absorption is achieved within 2 hours, using the immediate-release formulation. In the liver, approximately 25% of the dose of disopyramide is metabolized to a mono-*N*-dealkyl disopyramide (29). It possesses mild antiarrhythmic activity and may slowly accumulate following chronic use. Disopyramide is principally cleared via the kidneys through glomerular filtration and active tubule secretion. A reduced dose is required in patients with renal dysfunction. The elimination half-life varies from 4 to 10 hours in patients with normal renal function. Protein binding ranges from 5 to 50% to the α-1-acid glycoprotein following nonlinear (zero-order) pharmacokinetics (30, 31). Therefore, even with a small increase in dose, a significant increase in unbound drug may occur.

The effective therapeutic plasma concentration of disopyramide is 2 to 4 μg/ml. However, in the treatment of ventricular arrhythmias, a plasma concentration of 4 to 8 μg/ml may be required (32).

Clinical Use. Similar to quinidine and procainamide, disopyramide is effective in suppressing premature ventricular contractions and ventricular arrhythmias. Controlled trials have demonstrated the efficacy of oral disopyramide in preventing ventricular arrhythmias following an acute myocardial infarction and in preventing recurrent atrial fibrillation after direct-current cardioversion (33, 34). Disopyramide has been reported to be effective in the treatment of some patients with refractory ventricular tachycardia.

Additionally, since disopyramide slows conduction and prolongs refractoriness in accessory pathways, it has been demonstrated to be effective in the treatment of the Wolff-Parkinson-White syndrome (35). Since the drug markedly decreases left ventricular function, due both to a direct as well as an indirect effect, it has found utility in treating patients with idiopathic hypertrophic subaortic stenosis (IHSS) who also manifest arrhythmias. The drug is to be avoided in patients with left ventricular ejection fraction (LVEF) of less than 30%.

Adverse Effects. The adverse effects of disopyramide are most commonly related to its anticholinergic properties; dry mouth, blurred vision (impaired visual accommodation), constipation, and urinary retention. The latter may be particularly prominent in elderly males. Potential adverse cardiovascular effects are similar to those of quinidine, including AV block, increased ventricular response to atrial flutter or fibrillation, hypotension, and idiosyncratic paroxysmal ventricular arrhythmias resembling quinidine syncope (36). The negative inotropic potential of disopyramide is considerable and substantially exceeds that of quinidine and procainamide, with a significant occurrence of severe cardiac failure in association with its use (37). Precautions should be taken among patients receiving both disopyramide and other negative inotropic agents, such as propranolol and verapamil, since the additive cardiac depressant actions may be deleterious.

Dosage and Administration. Disopyramide is available in immediate release and controlled release formulations. Standard dosing includes a loading dose of 300 mg, followed by a maintenance dose of 100 to 200 mg every 6 hours.

Controlled-released preparation allows for a convenient 12-hour dosing interval. Patients with renal insufficiency will require a longer dosing interval.

CLASS Ib ANTIARRHYTHMICS

Lidocaine

Lidocaine was first introduced as a local anesthetic in the 1940s. Further research has documented its antiarrhythmic properties, and now it is considered a standard therapy of choice in the treatment of most acute ventricular arrhythmias.

Pharmacology/Electrophysiology. Lidocaine is classified as a class Ib antiarrhythmic. It possesses unique electrophysiologic properties that make it valuable for acute therapy.

In isolated tissue lidocaine exerts its major electrophysiologic effect by depressing the action potential amplitude. Purkinje fiber action potential amplitude and conduction velocity are reduced, and membrane responsiveness is suppressed (38). Lidocaine has minimal or no effect on the SA node or AV node conduction velocity or refractory period (39).

In general, lidocaine does not significantly demonstrate changes in the surface ECG, although at times the PR and QRS durations may decrease. Furthermore, lidocaine shortens the QT interval in some patients by shortening repolarization.

Pharmacokinetics. Due to lidocaine's poor absorption properties and extensive first-pass hepatic metabolism, intravenous administration is the preferred route of administration. Lidocaine undergoes liver metabolism to form two principle metabolites. Each of these metabolites has antiarrhythmic properties and is found in significant concentrations. The first metabolite is monoethylglycine xylidide, which is formed by *N*-deethylation of lidocaine. It has a half-life of 120 minutes and is eliminated by the plasma. Following further metabolism, the second metabolite glycine xylidide is formed. It has a half-life of 10 hours and is excreted principally by the kidneys (90%).

Lidocaine follows a 2-compartment model and has a β-half-life of approximately 100 minutes. Lidocaine equilibrates into various compartments of the body having high blood flow (e.g., liver, kidneys, brain). Conditions such as liver failure, CHF, and renal failure have shown to alter the disposition of lidocaine and, thus, require dosage adjustment. The therapeutic plasma concentration of lidocaine is between 2 and 5 μg/ml. Patients with plasma concentrations >6 μg/ml may manifest signs of toxicity. Cimetidine causes a significant increase in serum lidocaine concentration (40).

Clinical Use. Lidocaine is uniquely useful in ischemic situations where it may convert a unidirectional block into a bidirectional block, thus preventing a reentrant ventricular tachycardia. Lidocaine also appears to normalize conduction in the ischemic zone while prolonging it in normal tissue, decreasing the dispersion of refractoriness and the propensity to sustain a ventricular tachycardia.

The utility of lidocaine is that one can achieve therapeutic concentrations rapidly (intravenously or intramuscularly) to control ventricular arrhythmias, especially in the ischemic milieux. In patients resuscitated from out-of-hospital ventricular tachycardia or fibrillation, lidocaine is as effective as bretylium in preventing recurrent episodes of ventricular arrhythmias (41). In patients with a myocardial infarction (MI) within

6 hours, lidocaine prophylaxis reduced episodes of ventricular fibrillation, compared to the performance of placebo (42). Other investigators have not reported advantages of prophylactic lidocaine (43), and some have argued for prophylactic lidocaine in only selected patients (44). A recent review by Yusuf et al discussed an adverse effect of lidocaine when data from multiple trials are pooled (45).

Lidocaine has little effect on atrial tissue and has minimal myocardial depressant properties. Thus, lidocaine can be used more easily than class Ia or Ic antiarrhythmics in patients with sinus node disease or AV conduction disturbance. However, in patients with a severely compromised conduction system, lidocaine must be used with great caution.

The use of lidocaine in the treatment of atrial flutter must be used with caution since lidocaine may lead to an acceleration of the ventricular response. In the Wolff-Parkinson-White preexcitation syndrome, the response to lidocaine may be unpredictable, and in patients with a known short effective refractory period of the accessory pathway, lidocaine may accelerate the ventricular response during atrial fibrillation (46). In a macroreentry tachycardia involving the bypass tract in an anterograde fashion (atrium to ventricle), then up the His-Purkinje system and AV node to the atrium (retrograde), lidocaine may terminate the arrhythmia in the retrograde component of the circuit.

Adverse Effects. The most common adverse effects observed with lidocaine are those associated with the central nervous system. These include dizziness, drowsiness, tinnitus, paresthesias, and visual disturbance. These effects can be more often observed in geriatric patients and are concentration-dependent. Reversal of these effects are often seen following decreased dosing. More severe CNS effects can be seen at higher doses, including seizures or coma. Other effects include a mild peripheral vasodilation, resulting in a decrease in the blood pressure. AV block or sinus node dysfunction is very rare.

Dosing and Administration. Lidocaine is administered intravenously by bolus, followed by a maintenance infusion. Usually, the therapeutic plasma concentration can be achieved by a 1 to 2 mg/kg loading dose (administered as a 50- or 100-mg bolus), followed by a 1 to 4 mg/min continuous infusion. If the arrhythmia is not suppressed a second bolus of 50 to 75 mg may be required, and the continuous infusion should also be increased, to a maximum of 4 mg/min. Patients who are small (under 50 kg) or who are hemodynamically compromised require a lower bolus and maintenance dose. Monitoring of plasma concentrations may be helpful in avoiding toxicity with prolonged administration.

Mexiletine

Mexiletine is an oral analogue of lidocaine. It was approved by the FDA in 1986.

Pharmacology/Electrophysiology. Mexiletine is a class Ib antiarrhythmic. The cardiac electrophysiology effects are similar to those of lidocaine. Mexiletine depresses the rate of rise of the action potential without prolonging action potential duration. Mexiletine has no effect on the atrial refractory period, sinus node function, or refractory period (47, 48). In the His-Purkinje system, both the effective and relative refractory periods are prolonged. As with lidocaine, the electrocardiogram is often unchanged.

Pharmacokinetics. Mexiletine is rapidly absorbed following oral administration and peak absorption is achieved in 4 hours. Mexiletine has a markedly reduced first-pass metabolism. The mean elimination half-life of mexiletine following chronic therapy ranges between 11 and 15 hours in patients with coronary artery disease (49).

Mexiletine is primarily eliminated by hepatic metabolism. Approximately 85% of mexiletine is metabolized to inactive metabolites; parahydroxy mexiletine and hydroxymethyl mexiletine. The remainder is excreted via the kidneys.

Mexiletine does not significantly accumulate in patients with renal insufficiency (50). Alkalinization of the urine results in an increase in the plasma concentration, increasing reabsorption in the distal tubule. The normal therapeutic plasma concentration is relatively narrow, 0.7 to 1.6 μg/ml; thus, monitoring of the serum concentration may be useful to prevent adverse side effects.

Clinical Use. Mexiletine is indicated in the treatment of ventricular arrhythmias. It has been shown to be effective in suppression of PVCs following chronic dosing (51) and drug-resistant ventricular tachycardia (52). The effectiveness of mexiletine alone evaluated by PES techniques shows efficacy comparable to lidocaine, about 10% on average. While some studies find mexiletine effective alone in the electrophysiologic laboratory (53), several recent reports have found limited efficacy of the drug, except when combined with quinidine or other class I antiarrhythmic agents (54).

Adverse Effects. The most frequent adverse effects of mexiletine involve the central nervous system and gastrointestinal tract. These effects are often dose-related. They include tremors, nystagmus, blurred vision, dizziness, drowsiness, confusion, ataxia, paresthesia, dysarthria, insomnia, tinnitus, nausea, vomiting, and convulsions. Often, the gastrointestinal disturbance can be decreased when mexiletine is taken with food.

Dosage and Administration. Mexiletine is usually administered at 8-hour intervals at dosages of between 200 and 400 mg. Patients begin at 200 mg administered every 8 hours, and the dosage is increased every 3 to 5 days until very early toxic signs develop, or until the arrhythmia is controlled.

Tocainide

Tocainide is the second oral class Ib antiarrhythmic to become available. It was approved by the Food and Drug Administration for ventricular arrhythmias.

Pharmacology/Electrophysiology. Tocainide is a primary amine analogue of lidocaine. The electrophysiologic properties of tocainide are similar to those of both lidocaine and mexiletine. Tocainide shortens the action potential and effective refractory period in the atrial, AV node, and ventricle and has minimal effect on the Purkinje fibers (55). Due to its minimal effect on SA and AV nodal conductions, tocainide has been reported as safe in patients with abnormal conduction (56). Tocainide does not significantly alter ECG intervals.

Pharmacokinetics. Tocainide is nearly 100% bioavailable following oral administration. Tocainide undergoes little presystemic elimination; therefore, peak plasma concentration is achieved within 4 hours. Although food has been shown to delay the rate of absorption, the extent of absorption is unchanged. The mean elimination half-life of tocainide is 11 hours (57). Higher elimination half-lives have been observed

in patients with CHF and renal dysfunction. They may range from 13 to 22 hours. Tocainide undergoes partial hepatic metabolism to lactylxylidide and tocainide carbamoyl glucuronide. Each of these metabolites are inactive and are excreted renally, and 35% of tocainide is excreted unchanged. Dosage adjustments are usually required in patients with renal dysfunction. The recommended effectilasma concentration is 3 to 7 μg/ml.

Clinical Use. Tocainide is effective in the suppression of ventricular ectopy after a single oral dose and after chronic oral dosing of 400 to 600 mg every 12 hours (58). A number of studies have suggested that in patients with drug-resistant arrhythmias, efficacy of tocainide may be predicted by response to lidocaine (59). In patients with recurrent ventricular tachycardia it was shown that 11 of 15 patients favorably responded to the therapy (60). It is possible that tocainide, by shortening the refractory period (61), like lidocaine may prevent a reentrant tachycardia from being induced by PES techniques. Since tocainide is similar to lidocaine in pharmacodynamic properties, it is not surprising that the drug has been studied extensively in the postmyocardial infarction period, in which it has been effective in reducing ventricular ectopy (62, 63). It is also effective in prophylaxis against postinfarction arrhythmias (64), as well as in a postsurgical population (65).

Adverse Effects. Tocainide causes side effects, resulting in 10 to 20% of patients discontinuing therapy (66). The side effects are largely neurologic and include tremors, hot and cold flashes, nausea, dizziness, anxiety, vertigo, diplopia, emesis, paresthesia, and coma. Rash, constipation, and fever have also been reported. Most side effects can be reduced by decreasing the drug dose, but doing so may reduce antiarrhythmic efficacy. A small but significant incidence of neutropenia and agranulocytosis has been reported. Because of this possible effect, the drug has been recommended for patients unresponsive to other therapy who possess life-threatening arrhythmias and demonstrable lidocaine responsive arrhythmias.

Dosage and Administration. Tocainide is available in 400 to 600-mg tablets. The recommended initial dose is 1200 mg divided in 3 equal doses.

CLASS Ic ANTIARRHYTHMICS

Encainide

Encainide is a class Ic antiarrhythmic. It was approved by the Food and Drug Administration for the treatment of life-threatening ventricular arrhythmias in 1987 and withdrawn by the proposing drug company in 1990, except for those patients with a life-threatening event who were responsive only to encainide therapy.

Pharmacology/Electrophysiology. Encainide is a benzanilide derivative possessing local anesthetic activity. Its chemical structure is similar to procainamide; however, its electrophysiologic properties are different. It prolongs conduction markedly in atrial, AV node, and myocardial tissue (67). The drug has less negative inotropic action than other Class IC agents. The ECG effects observed with encainide include prolongation of the PR and QRS intervals.

Pharmacokinetics. The extent by which encainide is metabolized is dependent on the patients' genetic phenotype.

Two patient populations have been identified, extensive metabolizers and poor metabolizers, each possessing different pharmacokinetic profiles. Approximately 93% of patients are extensive metabolizers. The two major metabolites, which are formed following this pathway, are O-dimethyl encainide (ODE) and 3-methoxy-O-dimethyl (MODE) encainide, which have greater potency and contribute to the therapeutic, as well as to the adverse effects of encainide (68). Peak plasma concentrations following oral administration occur at 1.5 hours for encainide, 1.4 hours for ODE, and 5.7 hours for MODE. The systemic bioavailability is variable, ranging from 14 to 38% due to the significant first pass effects. The volume of distribution is 27 L, and protein binding at steady state is 70%. The elimination half-life of encainide and ODE range from 30 min to 4 hours and 5 to 37 hours, respectively. Both ODE and MODE accumulate significantly following encainide metabolism and are renally eliminated, accounting for 40% of the urinary excretion products. Encainide clearance is decreased in extensive metabolizers with renal dysfunction, and both ODE and MODE concentrations may increase (80 and 15%, respectively) following long-term dosing. Therefore, dosage adjustment may be required.

Seven percent of patients receiving encainide are poor metabolizers and form minimal amounts of ODE and MODE. In this patient population, encainide is primarily metabolized to N-desmethyl encainide, which has equal antiarrhythmic potency as encainide and is observed in both plasma and urine. The elimination half-life for encainide is much longer, ranging from 8 to 22 hours. In contrast to extensive metabolizers, there is an increase in the bioavailability (approximately 85%) and protein binding (78%).

Due to the complex metabolism of encainide and the activity of the parent compound and metabolites, monitoring of the plasma concentration of both encainide and its metabolites offers minimal advantage. The drug's prolongation of the QRS is a good way to assess increased or possibly excessive drug concentrations.

Clinical Use.   Encainide is effective in the treatment of supraventricular and ventricular arrhythmias (69). Studies have demonstrated nearly complete suppression of ventricular ectopy in patients with significant arrhythmias (70).

The occurrence of proarrhythmia of encainide varies from 2.8 to 16.0%, depending on the severity of the arrhythmia and concurrent risk factors. Recent results from the cardiac arrhythmia suppression trial (CAST) study (71) reported an increase in sudden death with encainide and flecainide, as compared to that in patients treated with a placebo postmyocardial infarction when their PVC's were suppressed on Holter. Encainide should not be used in patients postmyocardial infarction but only in those patients with a life-threatening arrhythmia who have undergone electrophysiologic testing.

Adverse Effects.   The most common side effects of encainide are dizziness (26%) and visual disturbances (19%) (72). Other common adverse effects include nausea (11%), headaches (15%), taste disturbances (4%), and tremors (3%). These side effects are responsible for discontinuation of therapy in approximately 5 to 10% of patients.

Dosage and Administration.   The initial dose of encainide in patients with normal renal function is initiated at 25 mg administered every 8 hours. The dosage may then be subsequently increased to 35 mg every 8 hours, then 50 mg every 8 hrs with 3 days or more between increments. This time period is needed since the enzyme system metabolizing encainide to active metabolites takes days to be fully expressed. Due to the increased risk of proarrhythmic events at higher doses, it is generally recommended that the lowest dose that suppresses the arrhythmia should be used.

Flecainide

Flecainide was the first Class Ic antiarrhythmic available in the U.S. It was synthesized in 1972 and approved in 1986. The drug is indicated for the treatment of life-threatening ventricular arrhythmias, as well as for the treatment of supraventricular arrhythmias (an indication granted in 1991).

Pharmacology/Electrophysiology.   Flecainide is a fluorinated aromatic hydrocarbon. It is distinctly different from quinidine and procainide. The drug has prolonged binding kinetics to the sodium channel, decreases the rate of rise of the action potential, and markedly prolongs conduction in the atrial, AV nodal, and ventricular myocardial tissues (73).

The electrophysiographic effects of flecainide include significant increases in PR and QRS duration. The repolarization component of the QT interval remains unchanged.

Pharmacokinetics.   The pharmacokinetics of flecainide have been evaluated following oral and intravenous administration. The oral bioavailability of flecainide is approximately 95%. Peak serum concentrations are rapidly achieved within 90 minutes. Approximately 40% of flecainide is protein bound. Flecainide undergoes hepatic metabolism to form meta-O-dealkylated flecainide and the meta-O-dealkylated lactam of flecainide (74). Each of these metabolites are found in the plasma and excreted in the urine. They possess no clinically significant electrophysiologic or antiarrhythmic properties at normal therapeutic doses.

Following chronic dosing, flecainide's half-life ranges from 9 to 23 hours. Approximately 25% of flecainide is principally cleared via the kidneys unchanged. Renal dysfunction and heart failure have been reported to prolong flecainide's half-life (75, 76). A correlation has been reported between the plasma concentration of flecainide and suppression of premature ventricular contractions. The recommended plasma concentrations are between 200 and 1000 ng/ml, while plasma concentration >1000 ng/ml may be associated with toxicity.

Clinical Use.   Flecainide has been shown to be effective in both atrial and ventricular arrhythmias (77, 78). Patients undergoing electrophysiologic evaluation for ventricular arrhythmias have reported a greater overall efficacy with flecainide than with either class Ia or Ib antiarrhythmics (79). Flecainide is approved for the treatment of atrial arrhythmias and has been found effective in suppressing ectopic and reentrant atrial arrhythmias, AV nodal reentrant atrial arrhythmias, and AV reciprocating tachycardia (80, 81). It should be used for patients without structural heart disease, since those patients with structural heart disease may be subject to the proarrhythmic effects of the drug.

Adverse Effects.   Flecainide passes negative inotropic activity, and it lengthens ventricular refractoriness. Thus, patients with significant congestive heart failure and severe conduction disturbances have relative contraindications to flecainide administration. We have noticed that patients with a history of sick sinus syndrome often require implantation of a permanent pacemaker (79).

Perhaps the main consideration in the use of flecainide is the potential proarrhythmic effects of the drug. Increased potency seems to also involve an increased proarrhythmic potential. Patients with low ejection fraction and a history of sustained ventricular tachycardia or cardiac arrest seem especially prone to the proarrhythmic effects of the drug. The proarrhythmic effects of the drug may be manifested by the development of a wide complex ventricular tachycardia that may be unresponsive to electroshock. This arrhythmia may accelerate and become incessant leading to the patient's death. We have observed that patients who are unresponsive to electroshock and suffering from flecainide toxicity may respond to lidocaine boluses followed by an infusion (82).

The recent report of the Cardiac Arrhythmia Suppression Trial (CAST) showed that flecainide can be well-tolerated and suppress VPCs in post MI patients. However, patients receiving flecainide are at a greater risk of dying than those taking placebo (71). One can hypothesize that the proarrhythmia potential is greater than the arrhythmia risk for this population and the benefit offered by flecainide.

Other adverse reactions of flecainide include CNS and GI toxicity, with headache, drowsiness, dry mouth, nausea, and vomiting reported.

Dosage and Administration. The dosage of flecainide is initiated at 100 mg twice daily. After the patient is on 100 mg twice daily and is loaded over 3 or 4 days, obtaining an appropriate trough serum level can be helpful in guiding therapy. For patients with cardiac dysfunction, a starting dose of 50 mg twice daily is recommended.

Propafenone

Propafenone is a recently approved antiarrhythmic that was developed in Europe. It is classified as a class Ic antiarrhythmic. At doses often higher than those used clinically, propafenone demonstrates mild β-adrenergic and calcium channel-blocking properties. The drug is indicated only for the treatment of life-threatening ventricular arrhythmias.

Pharmacology/Electrophysiology. Propafenone has a variety of antiarrhythmic characteristics that are concentration-dependent. The principle electrophysiologic activity is depression of the action potential in the atrium, ventricles, and Purkinje fibers (83, 84). Propafenone has no effect on the action potential duration and a minor effect on the effective refractory period. The drug markedly prolongs conduction. Propafenone also decreases automaticity in the SA node, atrial, and Purkinje fibers. In patients with AV node accessory pathways, propafenone prolongs the conduction in both the anterograde and retrograde direction, making it effective in treating preexcitation-mediated arrhythmias (85).

Following chronic oral therapy in patients with left ventricular dysfunction, propafenone has been reported to further impair LV function, with reductions up to 20% (86).

The ECG effects of propafenone are dose-dependent. Propafenone prolongs PR and QRS intervals but does not effect the QT, JT, and QTC intervals. Placement of intracardiac catheters during electrophysiology studies has shown prolongation of the AH and HV intervals and refractory period of the right atrium, ventricle, and AV node.

Pharmacokinetics. Propafenone is completely absorbed following oral administration. Peak plasma concentration is achieved within 2 to 3 hours. Due to first-pass metabolism, bioavailability is low; however, this increases with high doses. The volume of distribution of propafenone is 1.9 to 3.6 liters/kg and is 95% protein-bound. In the liver, propafenone undergoes oxidative metabolism to form metabolic products of glucuronide and sulfate conjugates. Elimination is primarily observed in the feces and urine. The principle metabolites are 5-hydroxypropafenone and N-depropylpropafenone (87). The 5-hydroxypropafenone has been reported to have significant electrophysiologic activity. Slow and fast metabolizers have been identified that are genetically determined. Approximately 90% of patients receiving propafenone are fast metabolizers, and 10% of patients are slow metabolizers (88). The mean elimination half-life for fast metabolizers is 5.5 hours, and for slow metabolizers it is 17.2 hours.

Clinical Use. Propafenone has shown to be effective in the treatment of supraventricular and ventricular arrhythmias. In supraventricular arrhythmias propafenone has been reported to be effective in AV nodal reentry, Wolff-Parkinson-White syndrome (89), and atrial flutter and fibrillation (90). The drug is currently not approved for the treatment of supraventricular arrhythmias.

In the treatment of ventricular arrhythmias, propafenone is effective in suppressing ventricular ectopy and nonsustained ventricular tachycardia (VT). In suppressing chronic stable ventricular arrhythmias, propafenone has been reported to be more effective and better tolerated than disopyramide, although it shows efficacy similar to that of quinidine. In the treatment of more severe arrhythmias propafenone has been reported to be less effective. In studies in patients with sustained ventricular tachycardia induced by programmed electrical stimulation, propafenone has a high proarrhythmic incidence (91).

Adverse Effects. Propafenone possesses myocardial depressant properties similar to those of flecainide. Propafenone may precipitate or exacerbate congestive heart failure, conduction disturbances, and aggravation of arrhythmias. Additional adverse effects include a bitter or metallic taste, constipation, nausea, dizziness, diplopia, paresthesia fatigue, and headache. These effects may occur in as many as 20% of patients, although the incidence can be reduced by decreasing dosage. Propafenone, as an Ic antiarrhythmic, probably should be used with the same caution as flecainide, given the CAST results with the Ic agents.

Dosage and Administration. Propafenone is available in 150- to 300-mg tablets. The initial dose is 150 mg every 8 hours. The maximum chronic dosing is 900 mg/day in divided doses.

Moricizine

Moricizine is a class Ic antiarrhythmic. It was initially developed in the Soviet Union in 1964. By 1976, clinical studies were initiated in the U.S. which led to its approval by the FDA in 1990 for the treatment of life-threatening ventricular arrhythmias.

Pharmacology/Electrophysiology. Moricizine is a phenothiazine derivative. Its principle electrophysiologic effects are caused by a concentration-dependent blockade of the sodium channels, and electrophysiologically it acts like a Class Ic antiarrhythmic (92). Moricizine decreases the maximum upstroke velocity of the action potential, along with increasing the rate of membrane repolarization. In addition, both the action potential duration and effective refractory period are decreased. In electrophysiologic testing, moricizine markedly slows intraatrial, AV nodal, and intraventricular conduction (93). The electrocardiographic changes observed include prolongation of the PR and QRS intervals, placing it in the Class Ic category.

Pharmacokinetics.   The pharmacokinetics of moricizine has been described with the oral formulations. Following oral administration, moricizine undergoes rapid absorption and first pass metabolism (94). Peak plasma concentrations are achieved within 1 to 2 hours following administration. Approximately 38% of the total moricizine dose is absorbed. In healthy volunteers the volume of distribution ranges from 8.3 to 11.1 liters/kg. Moricizine is significantly bound to 2- glycoprotein, albumin, and peripheral tissue in the range of 95%.

In the liver, moricizine undergoes significant metabolism (95). In animals 30 to 40 metabolites have been reported, and in humans a minimum of 9 metabolites have been identified in urine and feces. Two metabolites have been shown to possess significant antiarrhythmic activity; these include moricizine sulfoxide and phenothiazine 2- carbon-acid-ethyl-ester-sulfoxide. Moricizine and its metabolites are cleared, 56% in the feces and 39% in the urine (96). The plasma clearance ranges from 2.2 to 2.6 liters/min in healthy volunteers. The mean elimination half life of moricizine following chronic dosing is 19.2 hours. Decreases in hepatic blood flow and hepatic dysfunction alter the pharmacokinetics of moricizine, while congestive heart failure does not.

Due to the complex hepatic metabolism and significant number of metabolites, plasma concentration of moricizine has not yet demonstrated a strong correlation with antiarrhythmic efficacy.

Clinical Use.   Moricizine has been evaluated for treatment in a variety of ventricular arrhythmias. It has been shown to be effective in suppressing VPCs and nonsustained ventricular tachycardia (97, 99). The response to symptomatic nonsustained ventricular tachycardia, sustained ventricular tachycardia, and ventricular fibrillation has been variable. The overall response of these arrhythmias in patients undergoing PES is approximately 20%. The CAST study (CAST II) has reported an initial higher mortality in the moricizine treatment group than in the placebo treated group, causing the study to be stopped (100).

Adverse Effects.   Moricizine is well-tolerated in the recommended doses. The adverse effects that have been observed are attributed to its phenothiazine structure. The noncardiac adverse effects include dizziness, nausea, headaches, hypothesis, elevation of liver enzymes, and abdominal pain. Cardiac adverse effects include congestive heart failure, chest pain, and asymptomatic arrhythmias. The occurrence of proarrhythmic events is 3.2% without relationship to dose. The malignant neuroleptic syndrome has been reported with moricizine (101).

Dosage and Administration.   Moricizine is available in 200-, 250-, and 300-mg tablets. The recommended dosage ranges from 600 to 900 mg/day. Higher doses have been used. However, they have been associated with adverse events.

CLASS II ANTI-ARRHYTHMIC AGENTS

β-*Adrenergic Blocking Agents*

Numerous β-blockers are presently available. Their clinical utility have been shown to be effective in a variety of cardiovascular, as well as non cardiovascular, conditions (102).

Pharmacology/Electrophysiology.   The antiarrhythmic effects of the β-adrenergic receptor blocking drugs are chiefly related to their capacity to inhibit the β-receptor (103). Most of our information on the antiarrhythmic actions of β-blockers comes from studies with propranolol. To the extent they have been evaluated, other β-blockers have produced similar results on the heart. Propranolol and some of the other β-blockers have "quinidine-like" membrane-stabilizing effects that may play a small part in the antiarrhythmic effects of these drugs. However, in clinically relevant doses of β-blockers, these membrane-active effects are minimal. Additional antiarrhythmic properties include slow conduction and increasing AV nodal refractoriness.

Pharmacokinetics.   Many β-adrenergic blocking agents exist, and the pharmacokinetics may favor one over another agent. Table 27.2 describes the pharmacokinetic properties of the most common β-blockers available. Propranolol is frequently used and is considered to be the prototype of other β-blockers. However, in the ICU setting, where acute therapy is required, esmolol has been reported to be effective due to attractive pharmacokinetic properties (104) (i.e., rapid onset of action and a short half-life). However, the volume in which the drug needs to be administered often severely limits its utilization.

Due to the wide variability in concentration among the β-blockers, monitoring of serum concentration is usually not warranted. Rather, monitoring of heart rate and blood pressure are used to evaluate the degree of β-blockade.

Clinical Use.   The β-blockers have been reported to be useful in the prevention and treatment of supraventricular arrhythmias, especially those due to the Wolff-Parkinson-White syndrome. These drugs are also effective in arrhythmias related to excessive cardiac adrenergic stimulation, such as those associated with thyrotoxicosis, pheochromocytoma, exercise, emotion, and anesthesia with cyclopentane and halothane. The β-blockers appear to be the drugs of choice for treating patients with ventricular arrhythmias associated with the prolonged QT interval syndrome (105). They are also effective in preventing exercise-induced augmented ventricular ectopy in patients with coronary disease, in treating arrhythmias associated with mitral valve prolapse syndrome, and in reducing the number and complexity of premature ventricular complexes after myocardial infarction, the significance of which is unknown. Several studies have demonstrated a reduction in the incidence of sudden death following myocardial infarction in patients chronically treated with β-adrenergic blockers, such as practolol, propranolol, timolol, metoprolol, and atenolol. The reduction in sudden death is on the average of 25% in relative risk. This reduction translates into a significant reduction in sudden death after myocardial infarction. This reduction is related to the attenuation of sympathetic stimulation by the β-blocking agents. β-blockers with intrinsic sympathomimetic activity, except the small study

Table 27.2. Selected Properties of β-Adrenergic-Blocking Drugs

Drug	Relative β₁ Selectivity	ISA[a]	MSA	Absorption (%)	Bio availability (%)	Elimination Half-Life	Major Route Elimination
Acebutolol	+	+	+	70	50	3–4 hr	Renal
Atenolol	+	−	−	50	40	6–9 hr	Renal
Esmolol	+	−	−	—	—	9–10 min	Hepatic
Metoprolol	+	−	−	90	50	3–4 hr	Hepatic
Nadolol	−	−	−	30	30	14–24 hr	Renal
Pinadolol	−	+ +	+	90	90	3–4 hr	Renal, hepatic
Propranolol	−	−	+ +	90	30	3–4 hr	Hepatic
Sotalol	−	−	−	70	60	8–10 hr	Renal
Timolol	−	−	−	90	75	4–5 hr	Renal, hepatic

[a] ISA, intrinsic sympathomimetic activity; MSA, membrane-stabilizing activity.

with practolol, have not shown a reduction in sudden death in the postinfarction patient.

Adverse Effects. The most common adverse effects seen with β-blockers are not cardiovascular (103). These include exacerbation of asthma, chronic obstructive pulmonary disease, fatigue, insomnia, impotence, and depression. Cardiac effects may include worsening of LV function with the development of congestive heart failure, sinus node dysfunction, AV block, claudication and Raynaud's phenomenon.

CLASS III ANTIARRHYTHMIC AGENTS

Amiodarone

Initially introduced as an antianginal drug, amiodarone is a benzofuran derivative that has had considerable application as an antiarrhythmic agent for over 20 years worldwide. It is highly effective, but because of significant toxicity, is reserved for patients unresponsive to other antiarrhythmic agents. It was approved in 1988 for the treatment of life-threatening ventricular arrhythmias when other modalities of therapy failed.

Pharmacology/Electrophysiology. Amiodarone possesses a variety of pharmacologic and electrophysiologic effects on the myocardium. Its principal effects include prolongation of the action potential duration in the atrium and ventricles and prolongation of the effective refractory period in the atrium, ventricles, AV node, and His Purkinje system (106). Amiodarone has been shown to increase the refractoriness of the accessory pathways both in the anterograde and retrograde direction.

α- and β-antagonist properties for amiodarone have been identified. These effects are partially responsible for the slowing of the SA rate. Other effects include a calcium channel blocking action that may inhibit depolarization-induced automaticity and delayed afterdepolarization.

The ECG effects observed with amiodarone are prolongation of the PR and QT intervals. The most prominent and pharmacodynamically important action is QT prolongation. This action has corresponded with amiodarone's antiarrhythmic efficacy (107). Measurement made by intracardiac catheters demonstrates prolongation in the AH and AV intervals.

Pharmacokinetics. Absorption of oral amiodarone is slow and variable. Peak concentrations are usually achieved 6.5 hours postingestion. The drug is widely distributed into body compartments including fat, muscle, liver, lung, and spleen. Amiodarone is 96% protein bound, primarily to albumin. The half-life of amiodarone has been estimated at 55 days while the elimination half-life of amiodarone may be as long as 100 days following chronic dosing (108). Plasma concentrations required for a pharmacologic action take a minimum of 1 to 3 weeks in the absence of a loading dose (109).

Amiodarone undergoes hepatic metabolism. The principle metabolite that has been identified in humans is desmethylamiodarone. It possesses antiarrhythmic activity and has a longer half-life than amiodarone. Hepatic excretion in the bile is the principle route of elimination for both amiodarone and demethylamiodarone. Correlations between the plasma concentration of amiodarone and dose have been evaluated, and plasma levels correlate with an effective range of drug action (110).

Clinical Use. Amiodarone has been reported effective in treating a wide variety of supraventricular (111) and ventricular arrhythmias (112, 113). It is particularly effective in arrhythmias associated with the Wolff-Parkinson-White syndrome (114) and in the prevention of recurrent ventricular tachycardia and ventricular fibrillation. In many such cases, amiodarone is the sole agent to which patients with these difficult arrhythmias have responded (115).

Amiodarone is effective when administered intravenously in a loading dose. If oral loading is not employed, oral administration may take months to reach an effective steady-state level sufficient to provide antiarrhythmic action. Amiodarone's effects against atrial arrhythmias and those of the Wolff-Parkinson-White syndrome may require a lower dose than what is needed in the treatment of the most severe ventricular arrhythmias. A recent report by Horowitz and colleagues has shown amiodarone to be guided effectively by electrophysiologic testing (116). Additionally, in a randomized study comparing amiodarone therapy to the success of the implantable defibrillator, Horowitz and colleagues found them to be equally effective (117).

The intravenous preparation, while experimental, has been reported in many antidotal reports and in a few consecutive series to be very effective in patients with unresponsive ventricular tachycardia (118). While amiodarone itself has limited negative inotropic action, the diluent used to solubilize the amiodarone, Tween-80, causes hypotension and negative inotropy. An IV amiodarone without Tween 80 is currently in clinical trials in the U.S.

Adverse Effects. In antiarrhythmic doses, amiodarone has little effect on myocardial contractility. However, there have been cases of LV depression associated with amiodarone. Corneal microdeposits are reported in most patients following chronic administration. Rash, skin discoloration, photosensitivity, thyroid dysfunction, serious neurologic side effects, including peripheral neuropathy, constipation, and gastrointestinal symptoms, are but a few of the side effects of this agent. The most serious adverse actions are hepatic, renal, and pulmonary. Pulmonary fibrosis, which can be severe and cause death, occurs in about 15% of patients receiving very high chronic oral doses of amiodarone (119, 120).

Dosage and Administration. To avoid gastrointestinal side effects, the drug is usually administered in 2 or 3 doses daily. One dosing regimen used is 800 to 1600 mg daily for 2 to 3 weeks, followed by a maintenance dose of 600 to 800 mg/day for 4 weeks, then 400 mg/day thereafter. Many physicians experienced in the use of amiodarone are turning to low dose approaches. The European experience has been that lower doses may be associated with a lower complication rate and an adequate efficacy profile. Studies are needed to confirm that the doses of 100 to 200 mg/day may be as effective as higher doses. Further reduction in amiodarone doses is needed in patients on amiodarone for 1 year or more when the drug concentration accumulates. Monitoring drug levels and keeping the amiodarone and its metabolites desethyl amiodarone between 1.5 and 2 ng/ml may avoid toxicity. Additionally, monitoring the QT or JT prolongation may be a physiologic indicator of drug effect.

Bretylium

Bretylium was first introduced in the 1950s as an antihypertensive agent, but it was subsequently discontinued due to orthostatic hypotension and other adverse effects. Further work subsequently revealed significant antifibrillatory and antiarrhythmic activity. It was reintroduced for this use in 1978 and was approved for intravenous administration in the treatment of life-threatening ventricular arrhythmias.

Pharmacology/Electrophysiology. Bretylium is a bromobenzyl quaternary ammonium structure. The antiarrhythmic actions of bretylium is a result of its indirect stimulation of the adrenergic nervous system and direct stimulation of the cardiac membrane (121). The acute electrophysiologic changes of bretylium as a result of its adrenergic effects include increased automaticity of the sinus node, Purkinje fibers, conduction velocity, and V_{max}. The action potential amplitude is also increased while the action potential duration and effective refractory period are reduced.

Direct effects, after prolonged administration, seen on the myocardium include an increase in action potential duration and the effective refractory period in the Purkinje fibers and ventricular muscle. Bretylium possesses significant antifibrillatory properties. The drug may also spontaneously terminate ventricular fibrillation through catecholamine release and blockade of reuptake. Bretylium may also reduce energy requirements for cardiac defibrillation.

Pharmacokinetics. Bretylium is available in a parenteral formulation. The intramuscular administration of bretylium has been used, although its onset is somewhat slower and its absorption erratic. Bretylium is extensively distributed into adrenergic nerves. The volume of distribution of bretylium ranges from 3 to 5 liters/kg. Bretylium is not significantly protein bound and is primarily cleared via the kidneys. The terminal half life is long and ranges from 7 to 13 hours after loading and prolonged administration (122). The clearance of bretylium has been correlated with creatinine clearance in patients with renal dysfunction. The utility of therapeutic plasma monitoring offers little value in predicting therapeutic efficacy or toxicity (123).

Clinical Use. Bretylium is indicated for the treatment of sustained ventricular tachycardias and/or ventricular fibrillation. Its use in the drug selection process has primarily been when lidocaine fails. In the setting of a ventricular fibrillation arrest, there appears to be no greater efficacy with bretylium than that compared to lidocaine (124). Additionally, bretylium may impair hemodynamic recovery following ventricular arrest, as demonstrated in animals (125). Peak antiarrhythmic effects (class III action) are commonly observed several hours following administration, contrary to its antifibrillatory effects, which are seen within minutes.

Adverse Effects. Initial observations seen with bretylium are an increase in blood pressure and heart rate, followed by hypotension, as a result of its released of norepinephrine from nerve endings and the blockade of reuptake. Hypotension causes discontinuation of therapy in approximately 10% of patients. The use of protriptyline, a tricyclic antidepressant 5 to 10 mg every 6 to 8 hours, has been found effective in preventing the orthostatic hypotension, observed following bretylium administration (126).

Nausea, vomiting, and retching have been reported with rapid intravenous administration. The use of intramuscular bretylium causes irritation at the site of injection; thus, it is recommended that the sites of injection be rotated. Additional adverse reactions include diarrhea, flushing, anxiety, dyspnea, diaphranesis, and nasal stuffiness.

Dosing and Administration. Bretylium is administered as a 5 to 10 mg/kg bolus injection for the treatment of unstable ventricular tachycardia or ventricular fibrillation. Maintenance therapy may be continued, using bolus dosing of 5 to 10 mg/kg every 6 to 8 hours or as a continuous infusion of 1.0 to 2.0 mg/min.

SOTALOL

Sotalol is a β-adrenergic blocking agent that has been available in Europe for the treatment of hypertension. Sotalol possesses both class II and class III antiarrhythmic properties. It was recently approved by the Food and Drug Administration for the treatment of life-threatening ventricular arrhythmias (1992).

Pharmacology/Electrophysiology. Sotalol is a nonselective β-adrenergic blocking agent. Contrary to other β-blockers, its chemical structure is a methanesufulonamide-substituted phentolamine. It is devoid of both intrinsic sympathomimetic activity and local anesthetic activity. Sotalol has approximately one-third the β-blocking activity of propranolol.

Sotalol possesses potent electrophysiologic effects not observed with conventional β-blockers. These effects include prolongation of the effective refractory period in both the atria ventricles, atrioventricular node, and by-pass tracts (127). Sotalol decreases the resting heart rate and, hemodynamically, the cardiac output is decreased without changing stroke volume in hypertensive patients with CHF. However, in the normotensive patient without CHF, cardiac output is not altered.

Electrocardiographically, sotalol increases the QTC and JT intervals. Sotalol does not affect the PR or QRS intervals.

Pharmacokinetics. Sotalol approaches nearly 100% absorption. Following oral administration, peak plasma concentration is achieved within 3 hours. Sotalol undergoes no hepatic metabolism and is principally excreted by the kidneys through glomerular filtration. Both plasma clearance and renal clearance have correlated with creatine clearance (128). The elimination half-life ranges from 7 to 18 hours in patients with normal renal function and increases with renal dysfunction.

Clinical Efficacy. Sotalol has been evaluated in a variety of supraventricular arrhythmias. Sotalol has been shown to be effective in terminating proximal supraventricular tachycardia. In a series of studies, IV sotalol converted atrial flutter and atrial fibrillation in 62% and 27%, respectively. Sotalol prevented inducible supraventricular tachycardia in 59% of patients compared with 28% with metoprolol (129).

In the treatment of ventricular arrhythmias sotalol appears to be effective in suppressing premature ventricular contractions (primarily, higher grades of ventricular ectopy). In two separate electrophysiology studies, IV sotalol prevented ventricular tachycardia and ventricular fibrillation (VT/VF) reinducibility in 45.5% and 67%, respectively (130, 131). Sotalol prevents ventricular tachycardia induction in 33% of patients, as contrasted to procainamide with an efficacy rate of 22% (132).

Adverse Effects. As with the other β-blocking agents, sotalol has similar cardiac and noncardiac side effects. These effects include bradycardia, hypotension, dyspnea, dizziness, worsening CHF, fatigue, and impotence. Sotalol causes marked QT (JT) prolongation and, thus, close monitoring is needed for torsade de pointe arrhythmia that can be worsened by hypokalemia or hypomagnesemia. The occurrence of proarrhythmia ranges between 5 and 20%.

Dosage/Administration. Sotalol is available in 50-, 100-, and 200-mg tablets. The daily dose ranges from 320 to 640 mg/day.

MISCELLANEOUS

Verapamil

Verapamil was the first agent to be identified to selectively inhibit the transmembrane flux of calcium ions in excitable tissue. Following 20 years of worldwide research, it gained FDA approval in 1980. Its use is recommended in the treatment of angina, hypertrophic cardiomyopathy, hypertension, and supraventricular arrhythmias.

Pharmacology/Electrophysiology. Verapamil is a dephenylalkamine, which is structurally different from other calcium channel-blocking agents. It exerts its antiarrhythmic effect by blocking the transmembrane movement of calcium ions within the myocardium (133). Electrophysiologically, its greatest effects are observed in the SA and AV nodes by inhibiting depolarization. Verapamil slows conduction and has peripheral vasodilatory actions. Verapamil has lesser effects on the atrial tissue and minimal effects on ventricular and Purkinje fibers. Electrocardiographically, verapamil prolongs the AH interval and the effective refractory period of the AV node. On the surface ECG, verapamil prolongs the PR interval.

Pharmacokinetics. Following oral administration, verapamil is rapidly absorbed. Peak serum concentrations are usually achieved within 90 minutes (134). Verapamil undergoes significant first pass metabolism and, thus, only 10 to 20% of the drug is bioavailable. In patients with liver cirrhosis or hepatic dysfunction, bioavailability approaches 100%. The volume of distribution ranges from 3 to 6 liters/kg, and the protein binding is approximately 90%. Verapamil undergoes extensive hepatic metabolism. The principle metabolite is norverapamil; it possesses approximately 20% of the antiarrhythmic activity of verapamil. The elimination half-life of verapamil is 4 to 5 hours following acute dosing. However, following chronic administration, nonlinear accumulation occurs, and the half-life increases to 8 to 12 hours. Plasma concentrations are not routinely used; however, concentrations range from 80 to 300ng/ml.

Clinical Use. Intravenous verapamil is very effective in the treatment of supraventricular arrhythmias (135, 136). This agent results in a clinically significant reduction of the ventricular response in atrial fibrillation or flutter and can convert paroxysmal supraventricular tachycardia to sinus rhythm (137). Verapamil has not been effective in reducing the frequency of ventricular ectopic beats or in immediately terminating ventricular arrhythmias (138), although some authors have reported variable degrees of success (139, 140). Verapamil is not effective in preventing ventricular tachycardia induction in the PES laboratory. In patients with normal LV function with "verapamil-responsive" ventricular tachycardia, the drug is effective in therapy. The efficacy of verapamil in preventing induction of ventricular tachycardia, using electrophysiology techniques, has been observed to be considerably less than that seen with procainamide (141). The lack of ectopy suppression, combined with the prevention of ventricular tachycardia induction, demonstrates that triggering mechanism and threshold for inducibility may be affected differently by the same drug. The long-term clinical efficacy of verapamil in preventing recurrence of ventricular tachycardia and ventricular fibrillation remains to be determined. Certainly, the antiischemic action of the drug may be a contributing factor to its antiarrhythmic effects, and this attribute will have to be taken into consideration while the drug is used in clinical practice. Verapamil may be especially effective in the control of the ventricular response in atrial fibrillation in the ambulatory patient. While digoxin may slow the ventricular response at rest, it is not effective during exercise while verapamil is effective.

Adverse Effects. The most commonly observed adverse effect with verapamil is transient lowering of the blood pressure. This effect occurs following intravenous administration.

Preadministration of calcium salts has been shown to be beneficial in preventing hypotension and may not alter the antiarrhythmic activity (142).

Bradycardia, or AV block, has occurred primarily in patients concomitantly receiving β-blocker therapy. Verapamil is not recommended in patients with sick sinus syndrome, with 2nd or 3rd degree AV block, or with left ventricular ejection fraction less than 30%.

Other adverse effects that may occur following chronic dosing include constipation, headache, dizziness, and peripheral edema. Verapamil should not be used in patients with a possible preexcitation syndrome since the AV node may be blocked, permitting rapid conduction of the atrial depolarization (especially when the patient is in atrial fibrillation) to the ventricle by way of the accessory pathway, causing hemodynamic collapse.

Dosage and Administration.   Verapamil is available both in oral and intravenous formulations. The recommended oral dose ranges from 240 to 480 mg/day. A sustained release formulation is available in 120-mg, 180-mg, 240-mg, and 300-mg doses. The recommended intravenous dose is 0.075 to 0.15 mg/kg or 5 to 10 mg over 1 to 3 minutes. If optimal response is not achieved, a second bolus may be administered after 5 to 10 minutes. Alternately, a continuous infusion of 5 mg/hour has been demonstrated to be effective in preventing the hemodynamic fluctuations seen with repeated boluses (143).

Diltiazem

Diltiazem is a calcium channel blocking agent that has been extensively used in the treatment of angina and hypertension. Although it has been known to demonstrate antiarrhythmic activity, its use has been limited. The recent development of the intravenous formulation has allowed it to be used in the acute setting for the treatment of supraventricular tachycardia (SVT). The drug was approved for SVT therapy by the FDA in 1991.

Pharmacology/Electrophysiology.   Diltiazem is a benzothiazepine derivative. Its mechanism of action is comparable to other calcium channel blocking agents through inhibition of slow inward current of calcium in voltage-dependent channels. Electrophysiologic studies have shown that diltiazem slows AV nodal conduction and prolongs AV nodal refractoriness (144). Diltiazem has no significant effect on refractory periods of the atrial, ventricular, or Purkinje fibers. In comparison to verapamil, diltiazem has less of an affect on the AV node but with greater vasodilatory properties. Diltiazem has less of an effect on left ventricular function than verapamil. Thus, diltiazem may have an advantage in preserving left ventricular function in patients with SVT and impaired LV function. On the surface ECG, diltiazem prolongs the PR interval.

Pharmacokinetics.   Diltiazem is 90% absorbed following oral administration. It undergoes rapid first-pass metabolism to form several metabolites. *N*-monodesmethyl diltiazem is the principle metabolite and possess 20% of diltiazem activity. The mean oral bioavailability is 30 to 40% Diltiazem is 80 to 90% protein bound to albumin. The elimination half-life of diltiazem ranges from 2 to 11 hours following oral administration and 2 to 5 hours following intravenous administration.

The pharmacokinetics of diltiazem are not altered in patients with renal dysfunction. However, the pharmacokinetics of diltiazem are altered in patients with hepatic dysfunction or impaired hepatic clearance.

Clinical Efficacy.   Diltiazem has been shown to be effective clinically in the treatment of supraventricular tachycardia (145). Oral diltiazem has been shown to be effective in the treatment of paroxysmal supraventricular tachycardia (PSVT) caused by assessory pathway (i.e., Wolff-Parkinson-White syndrome), however, it should be used cautiously (146). Recently, with the availability of the intravenous formulation, diltiazem has been demonstrated to be safe and effective in the acute treatment of atrial fibrillation/flutter, administered as a bolus or as a continuous infusion (147).

Adverse Effects.   Diltiazem is well-tolerated by patients receiving the oral and the intravenous formulations. Adverse effects that may be observed include headache, flushing, hypotension, nausea, dryness of the mouth, and constipation. Significant AV block may occur, although it is principally seen in patients receiving concomitant medication (i.e., β-blockers).

Dosage and Administration.   Oral dosing of diltiazem ranges from 120 to 360 mg/day. The recommended dose of the intravenous formulation that is approved for supraventricular tachycardia is 0.25 mg/kg over 2 minutes. If the response is inadequate the patients may be rebolused with 0.35 mg/kg over 2 minutes followed by a maintenance infusion 5 to 15 mg/hr.

Adenosine

Adenosine is a naturally occurring compound that has been recently approved for the acute treatment of supraventricular arrhythmias.

Pharmacology/Electrophysiology.   Adenosine is an endogenous purine nucleoside that has been described as having a variety of physiologic effects. Its activity on the myocardium is through stimulation of cyclic AMP and the adenosine receptor. Two adenosine receptors (A_1 and A_2) have been identified. Adenosine has many physiologic actions. Adenosine causes both arterial vasodilation and coronary vasodilation (148). The principle electrophysiologic effect of adenosine is prolongation of AV refractoriness and conduction. Adenosine also causes a slowing of the heart rate. In electrophysiologic studies, adenosine demonstrates a dose-dependent increase in AH conduction with AV block.

Pharmacokinetics.   Adenosine is administered intravenously. In plasma, adenosine is rapidly taken up by the erythrocytes in the endothelial system. The drug is rapidly metabolized in the circulation, resulting in an ultrashort-acting half-life, ranging from 0.6 to 1.5 seconds, and a duration of effect lasting approximately 1 to 2 minutes.

Clinical Efficacy.   Adenosine has been shown to be effective in the termination of proximal supraventricular tachycardia. Rarely, it may terminate an adenosine-responsive ventricular tachycardia. Adenosine IV has been used with success in the treatment of AV nodal tachycardia and Wolff-Parkinson-White syndrome tachycardias, using the AV node as part of the reentry circuit. It yields additional benefits in the diagnosis of wide complex tachycardia vs. supraventricular tachycardia. However, the use of adenosine with ventricular tachycardia has resulted in profound hypotension, causing cardiac collapse and arrest. The sensitivity and specificity of adenosine in diagnosing a wide complex tachycardia vs. supraventricular tachycardia is high (149). The great advantage of adenosine is its rapid onset of action, as well as the drug's brief duration of action, enabling rapid termination of effect. While it may cause ventricular standstill in patients with atrial flutter, the effect is momentary, to the physician's and patient's relief.

Adverse Effects. The most frequently adverse effects observed by intravenous adenosine include "facial flushing," dyspnea, nausea, light-headedness, dizziness, and syncope (148). Hypotension and bradycardia may occur transiently. Acute treatment with aminophylline has been shown to block these effects. Conversely, dipyridamole has been demonstrated to potentiate adenosine's action, and their combined use is to be avoided.

Dosage and Administration. The recommended dose for treatment of SVT is 6 mg over 1 to 2 minutes. A second dose may be administered if the desired affect has not been achieved. Alternately, an incremental dosing regimen has also been suggested. This regimen includes the administration of 1 to 3 mg initially, followed by 2.5 to 3.0 mg, until a maximum dose of 20 mg is administered.

Digoxin

The digitalis glycosides have been around for over 200 years and are one of the oldest cardiovascular agents. Digoxin is one of the most frequently prescribed medications in the treatment of CHF and atrial arrhythmias.

Pharmacology/Electrophysiology. Digoxin exerts its cardiovascular effects in part through cholinergic stimulation and directly on cardiac cells (150). Digoxin's principal electrophysiologic effect is slowing of the AV node conduction and prolongation of the AV node refractory period. Sinus node automaticity is also slowed. This slowing is mediated principally through the vagus nerve. The ECG effect seen is PR prolongation and, possibly, ST and T wave changes.

Pharmacokinetics. The absorption of digoxin varies, depending on the formulation (151). The biovailability for the tablets is 60 to 80%; for capsules, 70 to 80%; and for the elixir, 90 to 100%. The VD of digoxin is 7 l/kg and follows a 2-compartment distribution model. Approximately 20 to 25% of digoxin is protein-bound. Partial breakdown of digoxin occurs in the gut in approximately 10% of patients. Digoxin is cleared principally by the kidneys. The elimination half-life of digoxin is 20 to 30 hours in healthy volunteers. In patients with renal dysfunction (and as patients age), the elimination half-life increases; thus, a dosage adjustment is required. Therapeutic serum concentration of digoxin ranges from 0.9 to 2.0 ng/ml. Patients with a serum concentration > 2 ng/ml usually present with signs of toxicity.

Clinical Use. Digoxin is primarily used in the treatment of atrial fibrillation and paroxysmal supraventricular tachycardia. Digoxin has been demonstrated to be as effective as the β-blockers or calcium channel blocking agents in the treatment of these arrhythmias, although the agent does not convert AF to normal sinus rhythm (NSR). Digoxin is ineffective in the treatment of Wolff-Parkinson-White syndrome, since it primarily alters anterograde conduction at the AV node. Patients who are undergoing concurrent electrical cardioversion while receiving digoxin are not subject to ventricular arrhythmias. However, patients who present with elevated serum digoxin concentrations are advised to delay electrical conversion, since their risk for ventricular arrhythmias may be greater.

Adverse Effects. Acute adverse effects that are often seen with digoxin are often early signs of toxicity. Adverse effects include a wide variety of cardiac and noncardiac manifestations. Cardiac effects include ventricular premature beats, atrial premature beats, ventricular tachycardia, ventricular bigeminy and trigeminy, junctional rhythm, and 2nd or 3rd degree AV block. Noncardiac effects include nausea and vomiting, anorexia, malaise, fatigue, delirium, and seizures.

Digoxin toxicity is occasionally encountered, especially in the elderly. Treatment of toxicity is supportive; activated charcoal may be employed for acute overdose. Arrhythmias commonly encountered include ventricular tachycardia, ventricular fibrillation, complete AV block with slow ventricular escape rhythm, and asystole. Lidocaine and phenytoin are commonly used to treat the arrhythmias. Other agents used to correct specific rhythms include β-blockers, magnesium sulfate, procainamide, and atropine. Rapid and successful reversal of acute toxicity can be accomplished with the use of digoxin-specific antibodies (Fab fragments) (152, 153).

Dosage and Administration. Digoxin is available both orally and intravenously. In the ICU setting, the IV formulation may be initially used for rapid digitalization, though this is rarely indicated at present. The suggested IV dose is 8 to 12 µg/kg over 24 hours, administered in 3 equally divided doses. This regimen is then followed by an oral maintenance dose of 0.125 to 0.25 mg/daily. With difficult-to-control atrial fibrillation and with the exclusion of thyrotoxicosis as an etiology, patients may receive up to 0.5 mg/day with monitoring of serum digoxin levels. When one is treating atrial flutter or fibrillation, the ventricular response is often adequate to gauge digoxin administration. Still, one must be cautious to not overdigitalize. It is still possible to make the patient digitalis-toxic when the patient is in AF. In sinus rhythm, no guide exists to establish adequate digitalization. In sinus rhythm, measurement of the serum digoxin levels at least 4 hours from the last digoxin dose is effective in guiding therapy and avoiding toxicity.

Magnesium

Magnesium has been known to possess antiarrhythmic properties (154). Its use as an antiarrhythmic, with its success in reducing sudden death in patients following a myocardial infarction, has been reported (155, 156). Acute administration in cardiac arrest patients reduced the incidence of arrhythmias (157).

Pharmacology/Electrophysiology. Magnesium is an intracellular cation that is distributed in both muscle and bone. Magnesium is involved in a variety of physiologic actions providing maintenance of electrical homeostasis (158). Alteration in the magnesium serum concentration has been demonstrated to affect the electrical field strength and to change membrane excitability. Magnesium has electrophysiologic effects similar to those of class III agents and, in fact, has been compared to amiodarone.

Magnesium slows the conduction through the AV node and prolongs the refractory period in the atria and ventricles (154). Magnesium does not alter the sinus node function or ventricular refractory period.

Pharmacokinetics. Magnesium may be administered orally, intramuscularly, or intravenously. Intravenous administration achieves the most rapid onset of action. Magnesium is principally eliminated via the kidneys (158). Due to significant reabsorption in the kidney, only 2 to 3% of magnesium is eliminated in the urine.

Clinical Use. The administration of magnesium to patients has been reported to be effective in supraventricular (159), as well as ventricular, arrhythmias (157). There exist many case reports that magnesium may be effective in patients with life-threatening ventricular tachycardia unresponsive to other antiarrhythmic agents. Magnesium has been likened to the "poor man's" IV amiodarone and, in some ways, considered to behave electrophysiologically like amiodarone, prolonging repolarization. Magnesium administration has been found effective in reducing sudden death post MI (156) in patients with polymorphic VT, in patients with the long QT syndrome (160), and in cases of digitalis toxicity (161). While magnesium would not be considered a first-line therapy and not a chronic therapy, the acute administration of magnesium in patients unresponsive to other therapeutic modalities may be beneficial.

Adverse Effects. The major complications associated with magnesium and the most frequent adverse one following bolus or continuous infusion is hypotension. Often, this complication can be rapidly reversed by decreasing the infusion rate. Hypotension in patients minimally compensated may lead to hemodynamic collapse, ischemia, ventricular fibrillation, and death, if electroshock is not immediately applied. Other adverse effects include myocardial depression, hypothermia, and coma.

Dosage and Administration. Both the sulfate and chloride salt formulations of magnesium have been used successfully. The total dose of magnesium has varied among studies. The mean amount reportedly administered varies considerably. In general, doses of 1 to 2 g are administered initially, followed by a continuous infusion of 0.5 to 1 g/hour.

Treatment of Arrhythmias

Arrhythmias can be fast tachycardias, or they can be slow bradycardias; each grouping is of consequence, demanding attention and appropriate therapy.

Tachycardias may be supraventricular, or they may be ventricular in origin. The supraventricular arrhythmias are often not life-threatening but can be quite bothersome and cause hemodynamic compromise. The goal in treating supraventricular arrhythmias needs to be clearly determined. If symptoms are to be alleviated, clearly, the arrhythmia must be identified, and a treatment or therapy must be shown to reduce arrhythmia symptoms. Often, the arrhythmias are intermittent, and obtaining a 24-hour recording of the electrocardiogram, a Holter monitor does not catch the offending arrhythmia. The transtelephonic systems that are now available with immediate memory loops and the ability to transmit the arrhythmia transtelephonically at a later date may be optimal for arrhythmia detection and subsequent follow-up.

While the majority of atrial arrhythmias are benign, some prove more problematic to patients. Atrial fibrillation may suggest underlying disease, be it cardiac enlargement, valvular disease, atherosclerosis, or hyperthyroidism. These conditions should be identified and treated. Still, atrial fibrillation often persists and is associated with an increased incidence of stroke due to embolization (162, 163). Appropriate conversion to sinus rhythm should usually be attempted if the atria are of reasonable size, with antiarrhythmic therapy as prophylaxis against arrhythmia reoccurrence. If the AF cannot be converted to sinus rhythm, then rate control is mandatory. While digitalis is effective at rest, on exercise digitalis is poor at rate control (ventricular response), and verapamil or diltiazem or the β-blockers are more effective in controlling rate.

Supraventricular arrhythmias are especially important when associated with the preexcitation syndromes. Rapid SVTs may be conducted to the ventricle at such high rates as to cause hemodynamic compromise. AF can activate the ventricle at rates between 200 and 400 beats/min, leading to ventricular fibrillation. Thus, therapy of SVT in conjunction with an underlying preexcitation system needs to take into account the effects of the drug both on the AV node and on the preexcitation pathway. An acute presentation of a patient with possible preexcitation in an SVT usually demands an electrical intervention or the administration of a class Ia antiarrhythmic, usually procainamide. Procainamide slows conduction in the AV node and by-pass tract while verapamil, for instance, slows the AV node more than the by-pass tract, permitting an acceleration of the arrhythmia down the by-pass tract which, combined with the hypotensive effects of verapamil, can lead to hemodynamic deterioration. Patients who have electrocardiographic evidence of preexcitation and are symptomatic with an SVT episode should be studied at an electrophysiologic laboratory to determine the potential for rapid atrial fibrillation. There have been significant advances in mapping the anatomical location of the pathway and preparing the patient for a surgical or more recently available electrical catheter ablation. These techniques are safe, definitive, readily available, and can permit the patient to avoid a lifetime of pharmacologic therapy.

The treatment of ventricular arrhythmias has undergone tremendous change. Our understanding of the problem has evolved, as well as our appreciation of the risk of therapy. The problem is perhaps best analyzed from the vantage point of assessing the trigger and the substrate. Arrhythmias can be triggered, and then they need to be sustained by substrate. If the mechanism is reentry the substrate is a heterogeneity of refractoriness in a diseased heart. Heightened automaticity may be due to substrate modification, the excess of sympathetic tone, electrolyte imbalance, or drug toxicity, such as an excess of digitalis. When evaluating a patient with a ventricular arrhythmia, clearly the potential risk the arrhythmia poses to the patient and the mechanism of its initiation and propagation need to be assessed. Trigger mechanism can be looked upon as VPC frequency. This frequency can be assessed by Holter monitoring. The frequency of VPCs, more complex forms, and runs of nonsustained ventricular tachycardia can be identified and quantified by Holter monitoring or telemetry. However, there is no evidence to support the theories that suppression of the arrhythmias reduce risk. In fact, in the CAST (164),

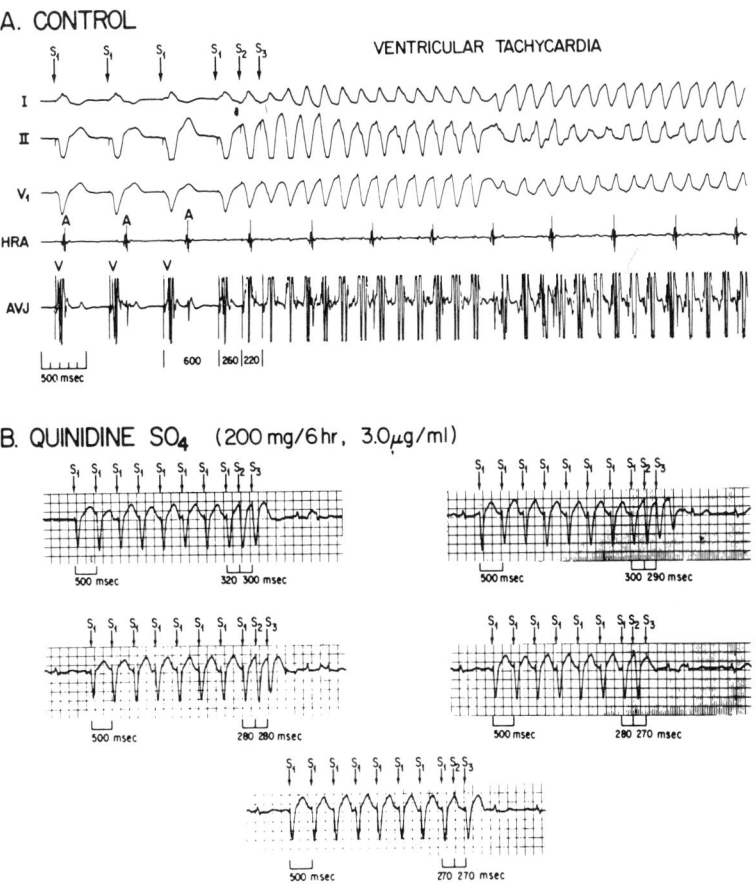

Figure 27.4. Electrophysiologic testing in a patient with cardiac arrest. **A,** Surface ECG leads I, II, and V, and intracardiac recordings from the high right atrium *(HRA)* and the AV junction *(AVJ)*. Two extrastimuli with coupling intervals of 260 and 220 msec initiated a rapid ventricular tachycardia that required countershock for termination. **B,** Repeat testing on quinidine shows that no arrhythmia is inducible. (From DiMarco JP, Garan H, Ruskin JN: Quinidine for ventricular arrhythmias: value of electrophysiologic testing. *Am J Cardiol* 51:90–95, 1983.)

effective suppression of VPCs in a post-MI patient population with a Ic antiarrhythmic was not an effective treatment. In fact, the group receiving antiarrhythmic therapy that effectively suppressed VPC group frequency did worse than the group on placebo (71). The antiarrhythmic drugs flecainide and encainide in CAST I and moricizine in CAST II (100) clearly made the situation worse. This may be a proarrhythmic effect of those drugs, but the VPC suppression hypothesis must be critically questioned in light of these results. We know that post-MI patients who have frequent VPCs are at greater risk for sudden death. The VPCs were suppressed, but mortality of these post-MI patients was adversely affected.

In addition to these problems with the suppression hypotheses, patients at highest risk for sudden death are those who had a sustained ventricular tachycardia or an episode already of sudden death (cardiac arrest). Nearly 50% of these high-risk patients do not have frequent arrhythmias on Holter monitoring, making risk detection using Holter techniques questionable in those patients. Electrophysiologic testing has developed because of the problem of not having identifiable arrhythmia markers in many patients at risk. Electrophysiology techniques have also developed because of an understanding of reentry arrhythmias, the ability to initiate and terminate ventricular tachycardia. The paradigm of electrophysiologic testing is described in Figure 27.4, utilizing the introduction

of one, two, or three extra stimuli to provoke ventricular tachycardia. Provocation of the tachycardia identifies patients at risk for sudden death. Administration of antiarrhythmic agents and then retesting using PES techniques can identify patients who, on antiarrhythmic drugs, cannot be induced into ventricular tachycardia. These patients have a lower rate of arrhythmia recurrence if on effective therapy (165–169). Thus, in patients with life-threatening arrhythmias, electrophysiologic testing appears to be a safe and effective way of assessing risk, then selecting appropriate antiarrhythmic therapy. However, only 20 to 40% of patients can have an effective drug selected at testing. Large numbers of patients need alternative therapy, and empiric amiodarone was employed for a number of years. Recently, the development of the implantable defibrillator has revolutionized arrhythmia management. While the procedure is costly, currently requires a thoracotomy, and may require frequent battery unit replacement, its efficiency rate has been found to be superior to antiarrhythmic therapy in some situations or comparable in others (117).

While antiarrhythmic agents may be needed in up to half the patients with the defibrillator device, still many of the side effects of drugs can be avoided with very minimal adverse effects from the device. β-blockers are often used to control heart rate, since increments in heart rate can cause the device to be triggered. The implantable device can now be inserted without a thoracotomy, which will further increase its utilization in patients with very poor heart function.

Many, if not most, of the arrhythmias of ventricular origin are due to reentry. A new technique that may identify patients with possible reentry pathways that could put them at risk for life-threatening arrhythmias is the signal-averaged ECG. The premise of this system is that the slow part of the reentry pathway may give rise to delayed activation, even when not actively involved in an arrhythmia. By amplifying the ECG signal, filtering out the high amplitude signals, and focusing in on the terminal part of depolarization, the late activation of the QRS can be detected. The presence of these delayed pathways in patients with coronary artery disease post MI correlates with a significantly increased risk for sudden death. Currently, the effects of antiarrhythmic agents are not readily discerned by the signal-averaged ECG. Patients with a prior MI history who have a positive signal-averaged ECG should be evaluated with electrophysiologic techniques to determine the need for antiarrhythmic therapy.

The decision to use noninvasive or invasive electrophysiologic techniques to determine therapy is still not clear (as to optimum approach). In patients thought to be at high risk but not demonstrating arrhythmias, invasive techniques are required. Results were reported for a recent comparison of invasive vs. noninvasive arrhythmic assessment techniques in patients with frequent VPCs called the ESVEM Trial (Electrophysiologic Study Versus Electrocardiographic Monitoring for Selection of Antiarrhythmic Therapy of Ventricular Tachyarrhythmias) (170, 171). The results showed no appreciable difference in outcome between the two groups. However, the electrophysiologic study methods used only two extra stimuli in many cases and analyzed the results based on the intention to treat. A more definitive trial is needed, but until additional results are available, the predominant evidence suggests the utility of invasive electrophysiology testing to guide antiarrhythmic therapy in patients with life-threatening arrhythmias (165–169).

Not all patients who are to receive antiarrhythmic therapy have life-threatening arrhythmias. Given the possibility of creating life-threatening arrhythmias due to the proarrhythmic action of antiarrhythmic therapy, clear goals need to be established for treating patients. Incessant palpitations that disrupt a patient's life may be a reason for therapy. One must be cautious as to which drugs are chosen, since underlying heart disease may change the equation from benefit to the side of risk. While, for example, flecainide may be useful for patients with SVT or for bothersome PVCs in patients with normal hearts, those with structural heart disease are at risk from the changes in refractoriness and conduction that can increase the electrical dispersion of the heart to favor sustaining a ventricular tachycardia. The risk of worsening arrhythmias is termed proarrhythmia, and this is a serious risk with antiarrhythmic drugs. Thus, the selection of agents like β-blockers and Ca^{2+} channel blockers that are associated with less proarrhythmia are favored before one turns to class Ia and Ic agents. Class III drugs are disparate regarding proarrhythmia. Amiodarone has a very low proarrhythmic potential but causes protein-adverse side effect. Sotalol is tolerated well but is associated with a significant incidence of proarrhythmia sometimes manifested as torsade de pointe ventricular tachycardia.

Acute Arrhythmic Therapy

The acute treatment for arrhythmias differs considerably from chronic arrythmic therapy. Often the arrhythmia that is being observed, by its nature, is not always clear. One should strive to identify the rhythm, using standard electrocardiographic techniques, double-paper speed, double standard, Lewis leads, esophageal leads if needed and, if all else fails, diagnostic electrophysiology techniques if available. Therapy is dependent upon the specific arrhythmia; PSVT, AV nodal reentrant tachycardias are now treated with adenosine as first line therapy followed by verapamil or diltiazem, selection of which may be based on the patient's cardiac function. SVT in the postsurgical patient is in the setting of a hyperadrenergic state with possible ischemia, and here the ultrashort-acting β-blocker esmolol may be the first choice. Patients who are young, have a fast tachycardia, and possibly have a suggestion of preexcitation on the ECG receive procainamide as first-line therapy. All SVTs that are associated with hemodynamic compromise require immediate cardioversion. Cardioversion is R wave-synchronized direct current shock. As with pharmacology a dose-effect curve exists with energy strength and arrhythmic termination. High-current strengths may cause myocardial injury and, thus, the lowest current to terminate the arrhythmia is optimum. Atrial flutter requires 25 to 50 joules; atrial fibrillation may require 150 to 380 joules.

Ventricular tachycardia that is hemodynamically unstable can be treated with low-voltage cardioversion; energies as low as 5 joules may be effective. Ventricular fibrillation (VF) needs defibrillation to terminate the arrhythmia, since there is no R wave to synchronize on for cardioversion discharge. The longer the VF the greater the energy requirement to terminate, with 200 to 380 joules required. Placement of the paddles is different for cardioversion of SVT and VT since the atria and the ventricle lie on different planes. VF is best approached with front to back placement of the paddles for discharge. Some defibrillators go beyond the standard 380-joule limits, and this can be useful in the large patient or the one with an incessant arrhythmia unresponsive to lower voltages. In patients in whom defibrillation fails or who are initially stable, lidocaine may be first-line therapy, with bretylium next. IV amiodarone, while experimental, is uniquely effective and may prove to be first-line therapy in the future. Intravenous procainamide is an alternative, but it may take up to an hour to administer, making its use problematic. A bolus of magnesium in patients not otherwise responsive may be useful in terminating ventricular tachycardia. Clearly, acute success requires follow-up with an infusion, usually lidocaine, followed by evaluation for definitive therapy.

Bradyarrhythmias

As with tachyarrhythmias, determining underlying cause is essential. A patient on β-blocker therapy who has symptomatic bradycardia does not need permanent pacing. Patients with ischemia and syncope need the ischemic problem addressed, with possibly an interventional procedure, before consideration for pacing. Clearly, temporary and permanent pacing has

Table 27.3. Guidelines for Implantation of Cardiac Pacemakers (Permanent)

Class I (agreement exists for permanent pacemaker insertion)
  AV block
    Complete with symptoms
    2nd degree type II (Mobitz)—symptomatic
    Pauses greater than 3 sec
  Periinfarction period
    Complete heart block
    New bifascicular block (RBBB & LAH)[a] with Mobitz II Sick sinus syndrome
    SSS and syncope
Class II (experts disagree on pacemaker indication)
  AV block
    Complete heart block asymptomatic or HR > 40/min
      Mobitz II asymptomatic
  Periinfarction period
    AV node block (complete without symptoms)
    Isolated bifascicular block (RBBB and LAH, LBBB)
Class III (agreement against pacemaker implantation)
  AV Block
    1st degree
    2nd degree AV block Type I (supra His)
  Periinfarction Period:
    Isolated left anterior hemiblock
    1st degree AV block
  Sick sinus syndrome
    Asymptomatic

[a] RBBB, right bundle branch block; LBBB, left bundle branch block; LAH, left anterior hemiblock; HR, heart rate; SSS, sick sinus syndrome.

Table 27.4. Indications for Temporary Pacing

SA node dysfunction
  Sick sinus syndrome—symptomatic with syncope
AV node disease
  Acute complete heart block
  Type II (Mobitz II) with symptoms
  Symptomatic pauses greater than 3 sec
Periinfarction period
  Acute Mobitz II
  Acute RBBB and LAH[a]
  Acute trifascicular block (1st degree AV block with RBBB and LAH or 1st degree and LBBB)
  Isolated acute LBBB

[a] RBBB, right bundle branch block; LBBB, left bundle branch block. LAH, left anterior hemiblock.
[b] Disagreement exists among experts.

greatly improved, replacing the need for alternative therapy. Rarely does one turn to an isoproterenol infusion to maintain cardiac rate; temporary pacing is a safer and more reliable method. The indication for pacing has been reviewed and is the subject of a report of a special committee on pacemaker implantation from the American Heart Association Task Force on Assessment of Diagnostic and Therapeutic Cardiovascular Procedure and the American College of Cardiology (172). These recommendations are well thought out and need review by all those involved in emergency cardiac care. Table 27.3 summarizes the indications for pacing as recommended by the committee on pacemaker implantation. Table 27.4 summarizes the indications for temporary pacing.

THE MANAGEMENT OF SPECIFIC ARRHYTHMIAS

Proximal Atrial Tachycardia

Proximal atrial tachycardia (PAT) may involve the sinoatrial node, ectopic atrial sites, or the AV node. By increasing vagal tone one is often able to terminate the arrhythmia or slow rate to make an appropriate diagnosis. Carotid massage can cause increased vagal tone but the presence of carotid artery disease, a carotid bruie, the presence of diffuse atherosclerosis, or a prior neurologic event are relative contradictions to carotid massage. Once diagnosis is made, the preferred pharmacologic therapy is administration of adenosine intravenously. If adenosine fails, alternative therapies are verapamil and diltiazem administered intravenously. The old-line forms of therapy—the cardiac glycosides, the β-blockers, edrophonium, intravenous procainamide—are rarely ever used due to the safety and success with the newer armamentarium.

Proximal Supraventricular Tachycardia

PSVT may be due to several mechanisms—atrial ventricular reentry tachycardia, AV nodal reentry tachycardia, automatic atrial tachycardia, or ectopic atrial tachycardia. These tachycardias are normally handled as a PAT is except when the possibility of the preexcitation is suggested by the patient's age or is based on evidence from a prior ECG of preexcitation. When preexcitation is suspected, the use of intravenous procainamide is preferred over that of verapamil or diltiazem. While some may argue that adenosine has such a short half-life and is a good way to identify the problem and will rapidly dissipate, if there are adverse electrophysiologic effects, still the hypotension that adenosine could cause may destabilize the patient, causing the need for immediate cardioversion or defibrillation. The reason for caution when one is using adenosine or the calcium channel blockers is that they have a differential effect on cardiac conduction. These agents slow the AV node but not the by-pass pathway, thus permitting a rapid conduction down the by-pass tract and accelerating the ventricular response. This response may possibly lead to ventricular fibrillation. This effect is especially true if the atrial arrhythmia is flutter or fibrillation. This reason is also why the digitalis glycosides that increase atrial excitability and conduction in atrial tissue while prolonging conduction at the AV node may preferentially favor development of a fast ventricular response and hemodynamic collapse in some patients with preexcitation.

Atrial Flutter

Atrial flutter is characterized by rapid atrial activity at a rate of between 200 and 350 beats/min. Atrial flutter may be treated by slowing the ventricular response using digitalis, the calcium channel blockers (verapamil & diltiazem), β-blockers, or a class I antiarrhythmic agent. Only the class I (A or C) antiarrhythmic agent will favor conversion from atrial flutter to fibrillation. Some agents, such as flecainide or amiodarone, may cause conversion in up to 40 to 50% of patients, while procainamide and quinidine may be effective in 20 to 35% of patients treated. An effective therapy is cardioversion for those patients who do not convert on a class I antiarrhythmic agent. An alternative approach in skilled hands is the technique of pacing termination. One type of atrial flutter is quite amendable to entrainment.

Atrial Fibrillation

Atrial fibrillation's treatment may be aimed at controlling the ventricular response or in terminating the arrhythmia. Conversion of the first episode of atrial fibrillation should always be attempted if the rhythm persists after treatment of reversible causes and if the atria are only modestly enlarged. Twenty to thirty-five percent of patients undergo successful cardioversion by pharmacologic therapy with a class Ia or Ic antiarrhythmic agent with a flecainide more potent in some studies than quinidine or procainamide. Sotalol and amiodarone have been reported to be more effective in converting atrial fibrillation to sinus rhythm. In addition, patients following cardioversion have a greater likelihood of staying in sinus rhythm on a class III antiarrhythmic than the class Ic and a greater likelihood of remaining in sinus rhythm on a Ic than a class Ia. The risk of underlying heart disease influences the potential for proarrhythmia from the Ics. The adverse side effect profile of the class III agents make selection of therapy dependent on each individual patient to assess the risk benefit ratio. Patients who do not respond to medications alone should undergo transthoracic cardioversion 2 to 3 weeks after effective anticoagulation to prevent the risk of thromboembolism from occurring following the return to sinus rhythm. In patients with new-onset atrial fibrillation, and those who are hemodynamically symptomatic, atrial fibrillation may need to be cardioverted on an emergent basis without anticoagulation. In these cases, transesophageal echocardiography to identify left atrial thrombus is useful for the stable patient. Those patients failing cardioversion or whose left atrial size precludes conversion need adequate rate control. Digitalis glycosides have been the mainstay of therapy, although they are not very effective against the enhanced ventricular response secondary to catecholamine stimulation. Here β-blockers and calcium channel blockers (diltiazem or verapamil) are most useful.

Nonproximal Junctional Tachycardia

Nonproximal junctional tachycardia is a type of tachycardia arising from the AV junction. The rate is between 60 and 150 beats/min. AV dissociation or one-to-one AV conduction may be observed. The causes may be catecholamine stimulation, sinus node depression due to drugs, such as lithium or digoxin, or following cardiac surgery. These arrhythmias are difficult to treat, and reversing the underlying ideologies may be most useful. Some have tried lidocaine if the toxicity is due to digitalis or verapamil, but pharmacologic therapy is often unsuccessful. Overdrive pacing may provide some hemodynamic benefit.

Multifocal Atrial Tachycardia

Multifocal atrial tachycardia due to enhanced automaticity of multiple ectopic atrial sites shows multiple p wave morphologies and a rapid tachycardia, 120 to 200 beats/min with 1:1 AV conduction. This arrhythmia is most commonly seen in patients who have severe obstructive pulmonary disease and hypoxia. Excess catecholamine may also initiate multifocal atrial tachycardia. Treatment requires treating the underlying etiologies—hypoxia, catecholamine excess. Verapamil may be useful, but the negative inotropic effects may limit its use in patients with poor ventricular function.

Ventricular Tachycardia

Ventricular tachycardia might present in a patient appearing stable or with a patient in cardiovascular collapse. Treatment should be directed at remedying these underlying problems. Lidocaine administered by bolus followed by infusion might be useful. If the needed expertise exists, inserting a pacing catheter into the right ventricle and pacing termination of the tachycardia is an alternative modality to be considered. Cardioversion may be a superior approach to the use of intravenous bretylium, which may cause hypotension, leading to hemodynamic instability in a previously stable patient.

Ventricular Fibrillation

Ventricular fibrillation is a premorbid arrhythmia needing immediate intervention. Defibrillation is indicated; if that fails, lidocaine, bretylium and, if available, IV amiodarone, may be effective. The appropriate use of the defibrillator, gels to improve conductivity, the proper selection of voltage (joules), and the appropriate positioning of the paddles (front-to-back optimum) are requisite for effective results. Clearly, the sooner the arrhythmia is terminated, the greater the potential for success.

REFERENCES

1. Vaughan Williams EM: A classification of antiarrhythmic actions reassessed after a decade of new drugs. *J Clin Pharmacol* 24:129–147, 1984.
2. Natel S: Antiarrhythmic drug classifications. A critical appraisal of their history, present status and clinical reference. *Drugs* 41:(5)672–701, 1991.
3. Ling GN, Gerald RW: The normal membrane potential of frog sartorius fibers. *Journal of Cellular and Comparative Physiology* 34:383–396, 1949.
4. Willus FA, Keys TE: Cardiac clinics. XCIV. A remarkable easy reference to the use of cinchona in cardiac arrhythmia. *Mayo Clin Proc* 17:249–258, 1942.
5. Mason JW, Hondeghem LM: Quinidine. *Ann NY Acad Sci* 432:162–176, 1984.
6. Mason JW, Winkle RA, Rider AK, et al: The electrophysiologic effects of quinidine in the transplanted human heart. *J Clin Invest* 59:481–489, 1977.
7. Mirro MJ, Watanabe AM, and Baily JC: Electrophysiologic effects of the optical isomer of disopyramide and quinidine in the dog: dependence on stereochemistry. *Circ Res* 48:867-876, 1981.
8. Torres V, Flowers D, Miura D, et al: Intravenous quinidine by intermittent bolus for electrophysiologic studies in patients with ventricular tachycardia. *Am Heart J* 108:1437–1442, 1984.
9. Riggen JT: Management of arrhythmias. In Braunwald E (ed): *Heart Disease: a Textbook of Cardiovascular Medicine*. Philadelphia, WB Saunders, pp. 743–791, 1980.
10. Ueda CT, Hirschfeld DS, Scheinman MM, et al: Disposition kinetics of quinidine. *Clin Pharmacol Ther* 19:30–36, 1976.
11. Fremstad D, Bergerud K, Haffner JF, et al: Increased plasma binding of quinidine after surgery: a preliminary report. *Eur J Clin Pharmacol* 10:441, 1976.
12. Kessler KM, Lisker B, Conde C, et al: Abnormal quinidine binding in survivors of prehospital cardiac arrest. *Am Heart J* 107:665–669, 1984.
13. Garfinkel D, Mameluk RD, Blascke TF: Altered therapeutic range for quinidine after myocardial infarction and cardiac surgery. *Ann Intern Med* 107:48–50, 1987.
14. Kessler KM, Humphries WC, Black M, et al: Quinidine pharmacokinetics in patients with cirrhosis or receiving propranolol. *Am Heart J* 96:627–636, 1978.
15. Ruskin JN, Dimarco JP, Garan H: Out of hospital cardiac arrest: electrophysiological observations and selection of long term therapy. *N Engl J Med* 303;607–613, 1980.
16. Rossi M, Lown B: The use of quinidine in cardio version. *Am J Med* 19:234–238, 1967.
17. Reynolds EW, Vander Ark CR: Quinidine syncope and the delayed repolarization syndromes. *Mod Concepts Cardiovasc Dis* 45:117–122, 1976.
18. Hardy B, Zador IT, Golden L, et al: Effect of cimetidine on the pharmacodynamics of quinidine. *Am J Cardiol* 52:172-175, 1983.
19. Twum-Barima Y, Carruthers SG: Quinidine-rifampin interaction. *N Engl J Med* 304:1466–1469, 1981.
20. Leahe EB Jr, Reiffel JA, Drusin RE, et al: Interaction between digoxin and quinidine. *JAMA* 240:533–534, 1978.
21. Swerdlow CD, Yu Jo, Jacobson E, et al: Safety and efficacy of intravenous quinidine. *Am J Med* 75:36–42, 1983.

22. Josephson ME, Caracta AR, Ricciotti MA, et al: Electro-physiologic properties of procainamide in man. *Am J Cardiol* 33:596–603, 1974.

23. Ridenberg MM, Drayer DE, Levy M: Polymorphic acetylation of procainamide in man. *Clin Pharmol Ther* 17:722–730, 1975.

24. Woosley RL, Drayer DE, Reidenberg MM, et al: Effect of acetylation phenotype on the rate at which procainamide induces antinuclear antibodies and lupus syndrome. *N Engl J Med* 298:1157–1159, 1978.

25. Wu D, Denes P, Bauernfiend R, et al: Effects of procainamide on atrial ventricular nodal re-entrant paroxysmal tachycardia. *Circulation* 57:1171–1179, 1978.

26. Strasbert B, Sclarovsky S, Erdberg A, et al: Procainamide induced polymorphous ventricular tachycardia. *Am J Cardiol* 47:1309–1313, 1981.

27. Josephson ME, Caract AR, Lau SH, et al: Electrophysiological evaluation of disopyramide in man. *Am Heart J* 86:771–8, 1973.

28. LaBarre A, Strauss HC, Scheinman MM, et al: Electro-physiologic effects of disopyramide phosphate on sinus node function in patients with sinus node dysfunction. *Circulation* 59:226–235, 1979.

29. Kates RE: Metabolites of cardiac antiarrhythmic drugs: their clinical roles. *Ann NY Acad Sci* 432:75, 1984.

30. Bredesen JE, Kierulf P: Relationship between alpha 1-acid glycoprotein and plasma binding of disopyramide and mono-N-dealkyldiospyramide. *Br J Clin Pharmacol* 18:779–784, 1984.

31. Haughey DB, Lima JJ: Influence of concentration dependent protein binding on serum concentrations and urinary excretion of disopyramide and its metabolite following oral administration. *Biopharm Drug Dispos* 4:103–112, 1983.

32. Josephson ME, Horowitz LN: Electrophysiologic approach to therapy of recurrent sustained ventricular tachycardia. *Am J Cardiol* 43:631–642, 1979.

33. Zainal N, Carmichael DJS, Griffiths JW, et al: Oral disopyramide for the prevention of arrhythmias in patients with acute myocardial infarction admitted to open wards. *Lancet* 1977;ii:887–889.

34. Hartel G, Louhija A, Konttinen A. Disopyramide in the prevention of recurrence of atrial fibrillation after electroconversion. *Clin Pharmacol Ther* 15:551–555, 1974.

35. Spurrell RAJ, Thorburn CW, Camm J, et al: Effects of disopyramide on electrophysiologic properties of specialized conduction system in man and on accessory atrio-ventricular pathway in the Wolff-Parkinson-White syndrome. *Br Heart J* 37:861–867, 1975.

36. Riccioni N, Castiglioni M, Bartolomei C: Disopyramide induced QT prolongation and ventricular tachyarrhythmias. *Am Heart J* 105:870–871, 1983.

37. Podrid PG, Schoeneberger A, Lown B: Congestive heart failure caused by oral disopyramide. *N Engl J Med* 302:614–617, 1980.

38. Davis LD, Temte JV: Electrophysiologic actions of lidocaine on canine ventricular muscle and Purkinje fibers. *Circ Res* 24:639–655, 1969.

39. Josephson ME, Caracta AR, Lau SH, et al: Effects of lidocaine on refractory period of man. *Am Heart J* 84:778–786, 1972.

40. Knapp AB, Maguire W, Keren, et al: The cimetidine-lidocaine interaction. *Ann Intern Med* 98(2):174–177, 1983.

41. Haynes R, Chinn T, Copass M, Cobb L: Comparison of bretylium tosylate and lidocaine in management of out-of-hospital ventricular fibrillation: a randomized clinical trial. *Am J Cardiol* 48:353, 1981.

42. Lie K, Wellen H, VanCapelle F, Durrer D: Lidocaine in the prevention of primary ventricular fibrillation. A double-blind randomized study of 212 consecutive patients. *N Engl J Med* 291:1324–1326, 1974.

43. MacMahon S, Collins R, Peto R, et al: Effects of prophylactic lidocaine in suspected acute myocardial infarction. *JAMA* 260:1910–1916, 1988.

44. Wyse EDG, Kellen J, Rademaker A: Prophylactic versus selective lidocaine for early ventricular arrhythmias of myocardial infarction. *J Am Coll Cardiol* 12:507–513, 1988.

45. Yusuf S, Sleight P, Held P, et al: Routine medical management of myocardial infarction. *Circulation* 82:117–134, 1990.

46. Akhtan M, Gilbert CJ, Shenasa M: Effect of lidocaine on atrioventricular response via the accessory pathway in patients with Wolff-Parkinson-White syndrome. *Circulation* 63:435–441, 1981.

47. McComish M, Robinson C, Kitson D, et al: Clinical electrophysiological effects of mexilitene. *Postgrad Med J* 53:85–91, 1977.

48. Roos JC, Paalman DCA, Dunning AJ: Electrophysiological effects of mexiletine in man. *Postgrad Med J* 53:92–94, 1977.

49. Campbell NPS, Kell JG, Adgey AAJ, et al: The clinical pharmacology of mexilitene. *Br J Clin Pharmacol* 6:103, 1978.

50. Monk JP, Brogden RN: Mexilitene. A review of its pharmacodynamic and pharmacokinetic properties, and therapeutic use in the treatment of arrhythmias. *Drugs* 40:374–411, 1990.

51. Talbot RG, Julian DG, Prescott LF: Long term treatment of ventricular arrhythmias with oral mexiletine. *Am Heart J* 91:58–65, 1976.

52. Lange R, Lee T, Wong K, et al: Mexiletine in the treatment of recurrent ventricular tachycardia. Prediction of long term arrhythmia suppression from acute and short term response. *J Clin Pharm* 23:89–92, 1983.

53. DiMarco JP, Garan H, Ruskin GN: Mexiletine for refractory ventricular arrhythmias: results using serial electrophysiologic testing. *Am J Cardiol* 47:131–137, 1981.

54. Duff HJ, Rosen D, Drimm K, et al: Mexiletine in the treatment of resistant ventricular arrhythmias, enhancement of efficacy in reduction of dose related side effects in combination with quinidine. *Circulation* 67:1124–1128, 1983.

55. Anderson JL, Mason JW, Winkle RA, et al: Clinical electrophysiology of tocainide. *Circulation* 57:685–691, 1978.

56. Horowitz LN, Josephson ME, Farshidi A: Human electro-physiology of tocainide, a lidocaine congener. *Am J Cardiol* 42:276–280, 1978.

57. Lalka D, Meyer M, Duce B, et al: Kinetics of the oral antiarrhythmic, lidocaine, congener tocainide. *Clin Pharmacol Ther* 19:757–766, 1976.

58. Woosley RL, McDermott DG, Nies AS, et al: Suppression of ventricular ectopic depolarization by tocainide. *Circulation* 56:980–984, 1977.

59. Winkle R, Mason JW, Harrison DC: Tocainide for drug resistant ventricular arrhythmias: efficacy, side effects and lidocaine responsiveness for predicting tocainide success. *Am Heart J* 100:1041–1045, 1980.

60. Maloney JD, Nissen RG, McColgan GM: Open clinical studies at a referral center: chronic maintenance tocainide therapy in patients with current sustained ventricular tachycardia refractory to conventional antiarrhythmic agents. *Am Heart J* 100:1023–1030, 1980.

61. Ikram H: Hemodynamic and electrophysiological interaction between antiarrhythmic drugs and beta blockers with special reference to tocainide. *Am Heart J* 100:1076–1080, 1980.

62. Haffajee CI, Alpert JS, Dalen GE: Tocainide for refractory ventricular arrhythmias of myocardial infarction. *Am Heart J* 100:1013–1016, 1980.

63. Bastian BC, Macfarlane PW, McLaughlan JH, et al: A prospective randomized trial of tocainide in patients following myocardial infarction. *Am Heart J* 100:1017–1022, 1980.

64. Ryden L, Arnman K, Conradson T, et al: Prophylaxis of ventricular tachyarrhythmias with intravenous and oral tocainide in patients with and recovering from acute myocardial infarction. *Am Heart J* 100:1006–1012, 1980.

65. Morganroth J, Harlen S, MacVargh H, et al: Lidocaine in the treatment of ventricular arrhythmias after open heart surgery. *J Am Coll Cardiol* 1:700(A), 1983.

66. Horn H, Haddian Z, Johnson J, et al: Safety evaluation of tocainide in the American emergency use program. *Am Heart J* 100:1037–1040, 1980.

67. Jackman WM, Zipes DP, Naccarelli GU, et al: Electrophysiology of oral encainide. *Am J Cardiol* 49:1270–1278, 1982.

68. Winkle RA, Peters F, Kates RE, et al: Possible contribution of encainide metabolites to the long term antiarrhythmic efficacy of encainide. *Am J Cardiol* 51:1182–1188, 1983.

69. Winkle R, Peters F, Kates R, et al: Clinical pharmacology and antiarrhythmic efficacy of encainide in patients with chronic ventricular arrhythmias. *Circulation* 64:290–296, 1981.

70. Roden D, Reele S, Higgens S, et al: Total suppression of ventricular arrhythmias by encainide. *N Engl J Med* 302:877–882, 1980.

71. Echt DS, Liebson PR, Mitchell B, et al. Mortality and morbidity in patients receiving encainide, flecainide, or placebo. *N Engl J Med* 324:781–788, 1991.

72. Soyka LF: Safety of encainide for the treatment of ventricular arrhythmias. *Am J Cardiol* 58:96C–103C, 1986.

73. Hellestrand KJ, Bexton RS, Nathan AW, et al: Acute electrophysiological effects of flecainide acetate on conduction and refractoriness in man. *Br Heart J* 48:140–148, 1982.

74. Conrad GJ, Ober RE: Metabolism of flecainide. *Am J Cardiol* 53:418, 1984.

75. Franciosa JA, Wilen M, Weeks CE, et al: Pharmacokinetics and hemodynamic effects of flecainide in patients with chronic low output heart failure. *J Am Coll Cardiol* 1:669A, 1983.

76. Conrad GJ, Ober RE: Metabolism of flecainide. *Am J Cardiol* 53:41B–51B, 1984.

77. Banitt EF, Bronn WR, Coyne WE, et al: Antiarrhythmia synthesis and antiarrhythmic N-(piperidylalkyl) trifluoroethoxybenzamides. *J Med Chem* 20:821–826, 1977.

78. Anderson JL, Stewart JR, Perry BA, et al: Oral flecainide acetates for the treatment of ventricular arrhythmias. *N Engl J Med* 305:473–477, 1981.

79. Flowers D, O'Gallagher D, Torres V, et al: Flecainide: long term treatment using a reduced dosing schedule. *Am J Cardiol* 55:79–83, 1985.

80. Hellestrand KJ, Nathan AW, Bexton RS, et al: Electro-physiologic effects of flecainide acetate on sinus node function, anomalous atrioventricular connections and pacemaker thresholds. *Am J Cardiol* 53:30B–38B, 1984.

81. Hellestrand KJ: Intravenous flecainide acetate for supraventricular tachycardias. *Am J Cardiol* 62:16D, 1988.

82. Schwartz J, Crocker K, Somberg J: Refractoriness as a determinant of right ventricular inducibility. *Clin Res* 35:325A, 1987.

83. Ledda I, Mantelli L, Manzini S, et al: Electrophysiologic and antiarrhythmic properties of propafenone in isolated cardiac preparations. *J Cardiovasc Pharmacol* 3:1162–1173, 1981.

84. Karaqueuzian HS, Kato T, Sugi K, et al: Electrophysiologic effects of propafenone, a new antiarrhythmic drug, on isolated cardiac tissue. *Circulation* 66:375(A), 1982.

85. Breithardt G, Burggrefe M, Wiebringhaus E, et al: Effect of propafenone in the Wolff-Parkinson-White syndrome. Electrophysiologic findings and long term follow-up. *Am J Cardiol* 54:29D, 1984.

86. Baker BJ, Desoyza N, Boyd CM, et al: Effects of propafenone on left ventricular function (abstr.). *Circulation* 67:II–267, 1982.

87. Somberg JC, Tepper D, Landau S: Propafenone: a new antiarrhythmic agent. *Am Heart J* 115:1274–1279, 1988.

88. Siddoway LA, McAllister CB, Want T, et al: Polymorphic oxidative metabolism of propafenone in man. *Circulation* 68:64(A), 1983.

89. Frank R, Tonet JL, Lacroix H, et al: Electrophysiological effects and efficacy of oral propafenone in the Wolff-Parkinson White-syndrome. *Circulation* 70:442(A), 1984.

90. Shen EN, Keung E, Huyeke E, et al: Intravenous propafenone for the termination of re-entrant supraventricular tachycardia: a placebo-controlled, randomized, double blind, crossover study. *Ann Intern Med* 105:655–661, 1986.

91. Doherty JU, Waxman HL, Kienzle MG, et al: Limited role of intravenous propafenone hydrochloride in the treatment of sustained ventricular tachycardia: electrophysiological effects and results of programmed ventricular stimulation. *J Am Coll Cardiol* 4:378–381, 1984.

92. Vaughan Williams EM: Classification of the antiarrhythmic action of moricizine. *J Clin Pharm* 31:216–221, 1991.

93. Wyndham CRC, Pratt CM, Mann D, et al: Electrophysiology of ethmozine (moricizine HCL) for ventricular tachycardia. *Am J Cardiol* 60:67F–72F, 1987.

94. Woosely RL, Morganroth J, Fogoros RN, et al: Pharmacokinetics of moricizine. *Am J Cardiol* 35F–39F, 1987.

95. Siddoway LA, Schwartz SL, Barbey JT, et al: Clinical pharmacokinetics of moricizine. *Am J Cardiol* 65:21D–25D, 1990.

96. Howrie DL, Pieniaszek HJ, Fogoros RN, et al: Disposition of moricizine (ethmozine) in healthy subjects after oral administration of radiolabelled drug. *Eur J Clin Pharmacol* 32:607–610, 1987.

97. Podrid PJ, Lyakisheu A, Lown B, et al: Ethmozine, a new antiarrhythmic drug for suppressing ventricular premature complexes. *Circulation* 61:450–457, 1980.

98. Pratt CM, Yepsen SC, Taylor AA, et al: Ethmozine suppression of single and repetitive ventricular premature depolarization during therapy: documentation of efficacy and long-term safety. *Am Heart J* 106:85–91, 1983.

99. Morganroth J, Pratt CM, Kennedy HL, et al: Efficacy and tolerance of ethmozine(moricizine HCl) in placebo controlled trials. *Am J Cardiology* 60:48F–51F, 1987.

100. Cardiac Arrhythmias Suppression Trial II Investigators: Effect of the antiarrhythmic agent moricizine on survival after myocardial infarction. *N Engl J Med* 327:227–233, 1992.

101. Miura D, Wynn J, Torres V, et al: Antiarrhythmic efficacy of ethmozine in patients with ventricular tachycardia as determined by programmed electrical stimulation. *Am Heart J* 111:661–666, 1985.

102. Molinoff PB: Evolving properties of B-Adrenergic receptor antagonists. *Pharmacotherapy* 12:144–153, 1992.

103. Upward JW, Waller DG, George CF: Class II antiarrhythmic agents. *Pharmacol Therapy* 37:81–109, 1988.

104. Gray RJ, Bateman TM, Czer LSC, et al: Esmolol: a new ultrashort-acting beta-adrenergic blocking agent for rapid control of heart rate in postoperative supraventricular tachyarrhythmias. *J Am Coll Cardiol* 5:1451–1456, 1985.

105. Olley PM, Fowler RS: The pseudo-cardiac syndrome and therapeutic observations. *Br Heart J* 32:467–471, 1970.

106. Sloskey GE: Amiodarone: a unique antiarrhythmic agent. *Clin Pharm* 2:330–340, 1983.

107. Torres V, Flowers D, Wynn J, et al: QT prolongation and the antiarrhythmic efficacy of amiodarone. *J Am Coll Cardiol* 7:142–147, 1986.

108. Riva E, Gerna M, Latini R, et al: Pharmacokinetics of amiodarone in man. *J Cardiovasc Pharmacol* 4:264–269, 1982.

109. Puech P: Practical aspects of the use of amiodarone. *Drugs* 41:67–73, 1991.

110. Mostow N, Rakita L, Blumer J: Amiodarone: correlation of serum concentration with clinical efficacy. *Circulation* 66:223A, 1982.

111. Rosenbaum MB, Chiale PA, Halpern MS: Clinical efficacy of amiodarone as an antiarrhythmic agent. *Am J Cardiol* 38:934–944, 1976.

112. Kaski JC, Girotti LA, Mesuti H: Long-term management of sustained, recurrent, symptomatic ventricular tachycardia with amiodarone. *Circulation* 64:273–279, 1981.

113. Nademanee K, Hendrixing JA, Cannom DS, et al: Control of refractory life threatening ventricular tachycardias by amiodarone. *Am Heart J* 101:759–768, 1981.

114. Ward DE, Camm AJ, Spurrell RA: Clinical antiarrhythmic effects of amiodarone in patients with resistant paroxysmal tachycardia. *Br Heart J* 44:91–95, 1980.

115. Fogoros RN, Anderson KP, Winkle RA, et al: Amiodarone, clinical efficacy and toxicity in 96 patients with recurrent drug refractory arrhythmias. *Circulation* 68:88–94, 1983.

116. Horowitz LN, Greenspan AM, Spielman SR, et al: Usefulness of electrophysiologic testing in evaluation of amiodarone therapy for sustained ventricular tachyarrhythmias associated with coronary heart disease. *Am J Cardiol* 55:367–371, 1985.

117. Gottlieb CD, Slivka T, Langan MN, et al: Do implantable defibrillators prolong survival compared to electrophysiologic guided therapy. *Circulation* 86:655A, 1982.

118. Somberg JC: Intravenous amiodarone. *Clin Prog Pacing Electrophysiol* 4:430–435, 1986.

119. Marchlinski FE, Gansler TS, Waxman HL, et al: Amiodarone pulmonary toxicity. *Ann Intern Med* 97:839–845, 1982.

120. Fogoros RN, Anderson KP, Winkle RA, et al: Amiodarone, clinical efficacy and toxicity in 96 patients with recurrent drug refractory arrhythmias. *Circulation* 68:88–94, 1983.

121. Koch-Wesner J: Bretylium. *N Engl J Med* 300:473–477, 1979.

122. Rapaport WG: Clinical pharmacokinetics of bretylium. *Clin Pharmacokinet* 10:248–256, 1985.

123. Anderson JL, Patterson E, Conlon M, et al: Kinetics and antifibrillatory effects of bretylium: correlation with myocardial drug concentrations. *Am J Cardiol* 46:583–590, 1980(A).

124. Hayes RE, Chinn TL, Cupass MK, et al: Comparison of bretylium tosylate and lidocaine in management of out of hospital ventricular fibrillation. A randomized clinical trial. *Am J Cardiol* 48:353–356, 1981.

125. Euler DE, Zeman TW, Wallock ME, et al: Deleterious effects of bretylium on hemodynamic recovery from ventricular fibrillation. *Am Heart J* 112:25–31, 1986.

126. Woosely RL, Reele SB, Roden DM, et al: Pharmacological reversal of the hypotensive effect that complicates antiarrhythmic therapy with bretylium. *Clin Pharmacol Ther* 32:313–321, 1982.

127. Touboul P, Atallah G, Kirkorian G, et al: Clinical electrophysiology of intravenous sotalol, a beta blocking drug with Class III antiarrhythmic properties. *Am Heart J* 107(5):888–895, 1984.

128. Blair AD, Burgess ED, Maxwell BM, et al: Sotalol kinetics in renal insufficiency. *Clin Pharmacol Ther* 29(4):457–463, 1981.

129. Rizos I, Senges J, Jauernig R, et al: Differential effects of sotalol and metoprolol on induction of paroxysmal supraventricular tachycardia. *Am J Cardiol* 53:1022–1027, 1984.

130. Senges J, Lengfelder W, Javernig R, et al: Electrophysiologic testing of therapy with sotalol for sustained ventricular tachycardia. *Circulation* 72:577–583, 1985.

131. Nademanee K, Feld G, Hendrickson JA, et al: Electrophysiologic and antiarrhythmic effects of sotalol in patients with life-threatening ventricular tachyarrhythmias. *Circulation* 72(3):555–564, 1985.

132. Nademanee K, Lee IK, Singh BN: Sotalol versus procainamide in the prevention of ventricular tachycardia induction: a double blind parallel multicenter study. *Circulation* 74:1242A, 1986.

133. Mitchell LB, Schroeder JS, Mason JW: Comparative clinical electrophysiologic effects of diltiazem, verapamil and nifedipine: a review. *Am J Cardiol* 49:629–635, 1982.

134. Kates RE: Calcium antagonists: pharmacokinetic properties. *Drugs* 28:405, 1985.

135. Schamroth L, Krikler DM, Garrett C: Immediate effects of intravenous verapamil in cardiac arrhythmias. *Br Heart J* 1:660–662, 1972.

136. Schamroth L: Immediate effects of intravenous verapamil on atrial fibrillation. *Cardiovasc Res* 5:419–424, 1971.

137. Waxman HL, Meyerberg RJ, Apple R, et al: Verapamil for control of ventricular rate in paroxysmal supraventricular tachycardia and atrial fibrillation or flutter. *Ann Intern Med* 94:1–6, 1981.

138. Heng MK, Singh BN, Roche AH, et al: Effects of intravenous verapamil on cardiac arrhythmias and on the electrocardiogram. *Am Heart J* 90:487–498, 1975.

139. Bender F, Reploh HD: Treatment of ventricular tachycardia with Isoptin. *Medinische Klin* 63:715–717, 1968.

140. Wellens HJ, Farre J, Bar FW: The role of the slow inward current in the genesis of ventricular tachyarrhythmias in man. The slow inward current and cardiac arrhythmias. *Dev Cardiovasc Med* 7:507–514, 1980.

141. Siegel L, Keren G, Torres V, et al: Antiarrhythmic action of verapamil in preventing programmed stimulation induced ventricular tachycardia. *Clin Res* 31:633A, 1983.

142. Weiss AT, Lewis BS, Halon DA, et al: The use of calcium with verapamil in the management of supraventricular tachyarrhythmias. *Int J Cardiol* 4:275–280, 1983.

143. Iberti TJ, Benjamin E, Paluch TA, et al: Use of constant- infusion verapamil for the treatment of postoperative supraventricular tachycardia. *Crit Care Med* 14:283–284, 1986.

144. Kawai C, Konishi T, Matsuyama E, et al: Comparative effects of three calcium antagonists, diltiazem, verapamil, and nifedipine on the sinoatrial and atrioventricular nodes: experimental and clinical studies. *Circulation* 63:1035–1042, 1981.

145. Huycke E, Sung R, Dias V, et al: Intravenous diltiazem for termination of re-entrant supraventricular tachycardia: a placebo-controlled, randomized double-blind multicenter study. *J Am Coll Cardiol* 13:538–544, 1989.

146. Salerna D, Dias V, Kleiger R, et al: Efficacy and safety of intravenous diltiazem for treatment of atrial fibrillation and atrial flutter. *Am J Cardiol* 63:1046–1051, 1989.

147. Ellenbogen KA, Dias VC, Plumb VJ, et al: A placebo-controlled trial of continuous intravenous diltiazem infusion for 24 hour heart rate control during atrial fibrillation and atrial flutter: a multicenter study. *J Am Col Cardiol* 18:891–897, 1991.

148. Faulds D, Crisp P, Buckley MT: Adenosine: an evaluation of its use in cardiac diagnostic procedures, and in the treatment of paroxysmal supraventricular tachycardia. *Drugs* 41:596–624, 1991.

149. Sharma A, Klein GJ, Yee R: Intravenous adenosine triphosphate during wide QRS complex tachycardia: safety, therapeutic efficacy and diagnostic utility. *Am J Med* 88:337–343, 1990.

150. Smith TW, Braunwald E, Kelley R: The management of heart failure. In *Braunwald Heart Disease: A Textbook of Cardiovascular Medicine*, ed 4. Philadelphia, WB Saunders 464–519, 1992.

151. Smith TW: Pharmacokinetics, bioavailability and serum levels of cardiac glycosides. *J Am Coll Cardiol* 5:43A–50A, 1985.

152. Wenger TL, Butler VP, Haber E, et al: Treatment of 63 severely digitalis-toxic patients with digoxin-specific antibody fragments. *J Am Coll Cardiol* 5:118A–123A, 1985.

153. Ujheiyi MR, Colucci RD, Cummings DM, et al: Monitoring serum digoxin concentrations during digoxin immune lab therapy. *DICP Ann Pharmacother* 25:1047–1049, 1991.

154. Rasmussen HS, Thomsen PEB: The electrophysiological effects of intravenous magnesium on human sinus node, atrioventricular node, atrium, and ventricle. *Clin Cardiol* 12:85–90, 1989.

155. Rasmussen HS, Norregard P, Lindeneg O, et al: Intravenous magnesium in acute myocardial infarction. *Lancet* i:234–236, 1986.

156. Rasmussen HS, Gronbaet M, Cirrtin C, et al: One year death rate in 270 patients with suspected acute myocardial infarction initially treated with intravenous magnesium or placebo. *Clin Cardiol* 11:377–381, 1988.

157. Smith LF, Heagerty AM, Bing RF, et al: Intravenous infusion of magnesium sulfate after acute MI: effects on arrhythmias and mortality. *Int J Cardiol* 12:175–180, 1986.

158. Wacker WEC, Parisi AF: Magnesium metabolism. *N Engl J Med* 278:658–662, 1968.

159. Wesley R, Haines D, Lerman B, et al: Effect of intravenous magnesium sulfate on supraventricular tachycardia. *Am J Cardiol* 63:1129–1131, 1989.

160. Peticone F, Adinolfi L, Bonduce D: Efficacy of magnesium sulfate in the treatment of torsade de pointes with magnesium sulfate. *Circulation* 77:392–397, 1988.

161. Seller R: The role of magnesium in digitalis toxicity. *Am Heart J* 82:551–556, 1971.

162. Kannel WB, Abbott RD, Savage DD, et al: Epidemiologic features of chronic atrial fibrillation: the Framingham study. *N Engl J Med* 306:1018–1022, 1982.

163. Wolf PA, Dawber TR, Thomas HE Jr, et al: Epidemiologic assessment of chronic atrial fibrillation and risk of stroke: the Framingham study. *Neurology* 28:973–977, 1978.

164. The Cardiac Arrhythmia Suppression Trial (CAST) Investigators. Preliminary report: effect of encainide and flecainide on mortality in a randomized trial of arrhythmia suppression after myocardial infarction. *N Engl J Med* 321:406–412, 1988.

165. Ruskin JN, DiMarco JP, Garan H: Out-of-hospital cardiac arrest: electrophysiologic observations and selection of long-term antiarrhythmic therapy. *N Engl J Med* 303:607, 1980.

166. Josephson ME, Horowitz LN, Spielman SR, et al: Electro-physiologic and hemodynamic studies in patients resuscitated from cardiac arrest. *Am J Cardiol* 46:948, 1980.

167. Morady F, Scheiman MM, Hess DS, et al: Electrophysiologic testing in the management of survivors of out-of-hospital cardiac arrest. *Am J Cardiol* 51:85–95, 1983.

168. Swerdlow CD, Winkle RA, Mason JW: Determinants of survival in patients with ventricular tachyarrhythmias. *N Engl J Med* 308:1436, 1983.

169. Wilber DJ, Garan H, Firkelstein D, et al: Out-of-hospital cardiac arrest—Use of electrophysiologic testing in the prediction of long-term outcome. *N Engl J Med* 318:19–24, 1988.

170. The Electrophysiologic Study Versus Electrocardiographic Monitoring Investigators. Electrophysiologic study versus electrocardiographic monitoring for selection of antiarrhythmic therapy of ventricular tachyarrhythmias. *Circulation* (79)6:1354–1360, 1989.

171. The ESVEM Investigators: Incidence of drug efficacy predictions in the electrophysiologic study versus electrocardiographic monitoring trial (ESVEM). *J Am Coll Cardiol* 19:387A, 1992.

172. A Report of the American College of Cardiology/American Heart Association Task Force on Assessment of Diagnostic and Therapeutic Cardiovascular Procedures (Committee on Pacemaker Implantation): Guidelines for implantation of cardiac pacemakers and antiarrhythmia devices. *Circulation* (1)84:455–467, 1991.

---

* All doses and indications are based on current standards of practice that are subject to change and all recommendations should be verified before being clinically implemented.

CHAPTER 28

Vasodilator Therapy

JOSEPH E. PARRILLO, M.D.

Although the principles of afterload reduction with vasodilator therapy were enumerated almost 50 years ago (113), it is only in the past 20 years that clinical applications of vasodilator therapy in the treatment of moderate to severe cardiac failure have gained relatively widespread acceptance (17, 30). As early as 1944, spinal anesthesia-induced vasodilation was employed successfully to reverse cardiogenic pulmonary edema (113). In the early 1960s, the principles of afterload reduction as a method to improve cardiac performance were confirmed and extended (12, 112). However, frequent clinical use of vasodilators required the ability to document a salutary hemodynamic response and the capability of closely monitoring adverse consequences of this therapy. In the 1970s, the development of the Swan-Ganz balloon flotation catheter (117) allowed hemodynamic monitoring at the bedside, which was previously available only in the cardiac catheterization laboratory. Today, the physician can serially measure cardiac outputs and calculate systemic vascular resistance to document a salutary or adverse response to therapy. Further, routine use of arterial pressure catheters allows a beat-to-beat measure of the major adverse consequence of vasodilators, namely, hypotension.

In 1971, phentolamine, an α-adrenergic receptor antagonist, was reported to be effective in relieving symptoms and improving the hemodynamics of patients with severe heart failure secondary to ischemic heart disease (81). One year later, nitroprusside-induced vasodilation was shown to increase cardiac output, reduce ventricular filling pressures, and relieve symptoms in postmyocardial infarction patients with severe heart failure, or even cardiogenic shock (49).

Subsequent studies have documented the usefulness of vasodilation therapy in subsets of patients with severe intractable heart failure (61), cardiogenic shock (33), and severe mitral (21) or aortic (9) regurgitation.

The purpose of this chapter is to review the physiologic mechanisms underlying vasodilator therapy, the appropriate indications for use of vasodilators, and the usefulness of specific vasodilator agents. The practical considerations of vasodilator therapy in the management of critically ill patients are reviewed. Emphasis is placed on the physiology and pathogenic mechanisms that provide a foundation for proper patient care. Reviews of more specific aspects of vasodilator therapy are available (6, 7, 25, 42, 44, 53, 82, 86, 92, 95, 106, 122, 123, 128).

PHYSIOLOGIC MECHANISMS OF ACTION OF VASODILATORS

FACTORS DETERMINING VENTRICULAR FUNCTION

The heart's major function is to supply blood flow to the tissues to satisfy the metabolic requirements of the body. There are four major determinants of cardiac function: preload, afterload, contractility, and heart rate (12, 26). These factors can be manipulated clinically to produce optimal ventricular function in any given patient. Depending on the patient's physiology, pathology, and clinical status, the physician

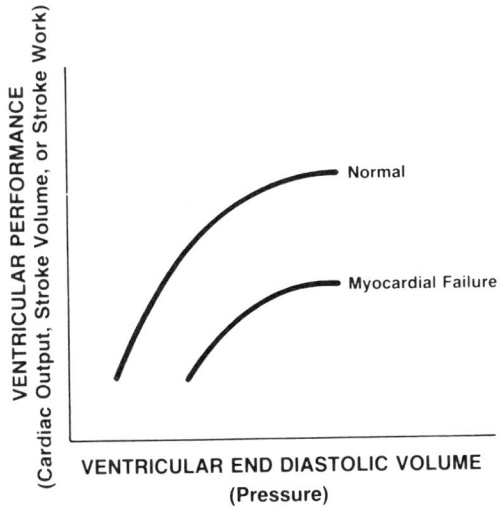

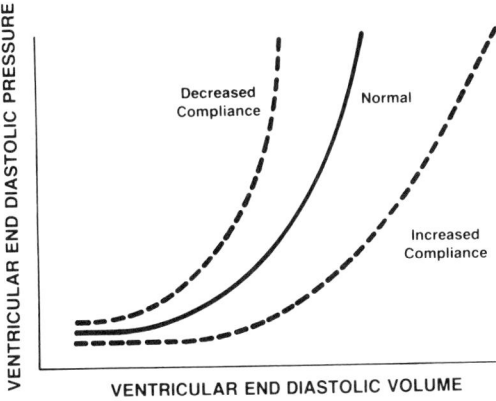

Figure 28.1. Frank-Starling ventricular performance curves. In the normal ventricle, as ventricular end-diastolic volume is increased, there is a concomitant increase in ventricular performance until a plateau is reached. Patients with myocardial dysfunction and heart failure demonstrate a shift of this curve downward and to the right. In heart failure, an increase in end-diastolic volume produces less of an increase in ventricular performance, and a "plateau" is reached at a much lower level of ventricular performance.

Figure 28.2. Diastolic pressure-volume relationship of the left ventricle. At low ventricular volumes, substantial changes in volume produce little change in ventricular pressure. At higher ventricular volumes, small changes produce exponentially greater increases in pressure. Increasing ventricular compliance with vasodilator therapy shifts the curve to the right, allowing a greater end-diastolic volume at a lower pressure. See text for details.

can choose from a wide variety of methods to augment cardiovascular function.

Preload

Preload is defined as the amount the myocardium is stretched prior to the onset of contraction. Isolated papillary muscle experiments originally demonstrated an increase in myocardial tension development with an increase in the resting length of the cardiac muscles (13), with maximal tension development occurring when there was the most overlap of actin and myosin filaments. In the intact ventricle, this Frank-Starling relationship is manifested by enhanced ventricular performance as the end-diastolic volume of the left or right ventricle is increased (13) (Fig. 28.1). In the normal heart, at low end-diastolic volumes, small increases in preload cause a substantial increase in stroke volume and cardiac output; as one increases end-diastolic volume further, similar increases in end-diastolic volume produce progressively less of an increase in stroke volume, finally reaching a plateau beyond which increases in diastolic volume do not increase stroke volume (or other measures of ventricular performance) (116).

Clinically, measuring end-diastolic ventricular volumes is difficult, whereas end-diastolic pressure can be obtained relatively easily from intracardiac catheter readings. When plotting the relationship between end-diastolic pressure and ventricular performance, one sees a relationship similar to that shown in Figure 28.1: on increasing end-diastolic pressure, ventricular performance increases substantially, then more modestly, finally plateauing. It is clinically useful to recognize that the relationship between end-diastolic pressure and volume is not linear (Fig. 28.2). Thus, at low volumes, a substantial increase in end-diastolic volume (producing an increase in stroke volume) can cause little or no change in end-diastolic pressure. At higher volumes, the relationship between volume

and pressure becomes more linear, and changes in volume will be associated with increases in the end-diastolic ventricular pressure. Therefore, when dealing with low end-diastolic volumes, increasing the end-diastolic volume with fluid administration can produce considerable increases in stroke volume with little or no change in ventricular filling pressures.

The ventricle's intrinsic ability to increase its volume and pressure in response to an increase (or decrease) in intravascular volume is termed compliance, a measure of the ventricle's distensibility. Ischemia, fibrosis, hypertrophy, and certain pharmacologic agents such as vasodilators (see below) can profoundly influence ventricular compliance (11). Several studies suggest that left ventricular compliance is altered by high right ventricular diastolic pressures (8), which presumably alter left ventricular geometry with a displaced septum. Other studies suggest that an intact pericardium is important in right ventricular induced decreases in left ventricular compliance (99), arguing that changes in the right side of the heart affect the left side because of the pericardial "closed space."

In a more compliant ventricle, for any ventricular end-diastolic volume the ventricular pressure will be lower. This is a practical clinical concern since pulmonary edema occurs when left ventricular end-diastolic pressure rises above approximately 20 mm Hg. Thus, a more compliant ventricle allows for a greater increase in end-diastolic volume (enhancing systolic ventricular performance) than does a noncompliant ventricle, which will develop a high pressure at a lower ventricular volume.

Afterload

Afterload is defined as the sum of the factors that oppose the shortening of muscle fibers—a definition derived from isolated papillary muscle experiments (89). In the intact cardiovascular system, afterload refers to the impedance against which the ventricle must eject during systole. Precise determination of aortic impedance to ventricular ejection requires sophisticated analysis of a series of harmonics, each of which depends on amplitude, phase angle, and frequency. These harmonics describe a spectrum of instantaneous relationships between pressure and flow (89, 107). Because of its complexity and the difficulty of its determination, afterload is usually defined clinically as vascular resistance, a value that defines the steady state (frequency-independent) characteristics of impedance to aortic flow.

Systemic vascular resistance (SVR) is defined by the following equation:

$$\frac{MAP - mean\ right\ atrial\ pressure}{CO}$$

where MAP is mean arterial blood pressure and CO is cardiac output (60). This equation demonstrates why afterload cannot be derived from blood pressure measurements alone: an arterial dilator can reduce SVR and cause an increase in CO resulting in no change in blood pressure, though the afterload confronting the ventricle is substantially reduced. Thus, SVR has become the most commonly used clinical parameter to reflect afterload or outflow impedance.

The nature of the relationship between afterload and stroke volume is important to an understanding of changes in cardiac function when SVR varies. Stroke volume varies as the function of increasing SVR (Fig. 28.3). In the normally functioning ventricle (*upper curve*), mild to moderate increases in SVR do not decrease stroke volume, although the blood pressure increases modestly. Severe increases in SVR (e.g., malignant hypertension) may decrease stroke volume (17, 30, 112). One of the major reasons that the normal ventricle's stroke volume does not become decreased with increasing afterload is the ventricle's ability to increase preload by rising on the steep portion of the Starling curve (Fig. 28.1) (24, 32, 112). Thus, in an experimental setting in which preload and contractility are kept constant, an increase in afterload decreases stroke volume secondary to a reduction in the extent and velocity of myocardial wall shortening (15, 124). Analogously, a ventricle with myocardial dysfunction operates on the plateau of the Starling function (Fig. 28.1) and is unable to increase stroke volume by increasing end-diastolic volume. Therefore, in a dysfunctional ventricle, increases in SVR decrease stroke volume. These physiologic principles provide the basis for effective vasodilator therapy: in a moderately or severely dysfunctional ventricle, a decrease in SVR commonly causes an increase in stroke volume, therefore augmenting CO (Fig. 28.3, *lower curve*).

Contractility

Contractility refers to the inherent ability of the ventricle to increase the velocity and/or extent of contraction. Studies have defined contractility as changes in ventricular performance that cannot be ascribed to preload or afterload. Another useful operational definition is that an increase in contractility (holding afterload constant) produces a shift in the Starling preload curve upward and to the left (Fig. 28.4). A negative inotropic effect shifts the Starling curve downward and to the right. Positive inotropic agents that augment the contractility of the ventricle include the catecholamines, digitalis, glucagon, and thyroxine. Negative inotropic agents include phenobarbital, most general anesthetics, and propranolol.

The relationship of intrinsic myocardial contractility to afterload is also important in optimal vasodilator therapy. In the normal ventricle, increases in afterload are well-tolerated with no decrease in stroke volume; however, in a depressed, poorly contractile ventricle, increases in afterload result in decreased stroke volume and CO (Fig. 28.3, *lower curve*). Thus, in many patients with heart failure and an increased SVR, reduction of SVR results in an augmented stroke volume and CO (Fig. 28.3).

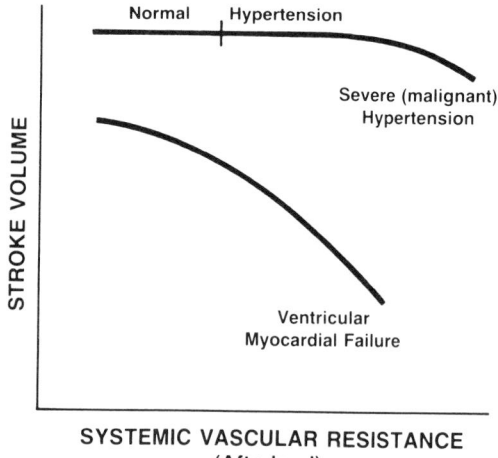

Figure 28.3.   Relationship of systemic vascular resistance to stroke volume in a normal and dysfunctional ventricle. Increases in afterload do not cause a decrease in stroke volume in a normal ventricle (*upper curve*), except at very high levels of afterload when severe hypertension causes ventricular decompensation. In a failing ventricle (*lower curve*), however, an increase in afterload causes a progressive depression of stroke volume and cardiac output. Thus, vasodilator-induced reductions in afterload enhance stroke volume in patients with severe ventricular dysfunction.

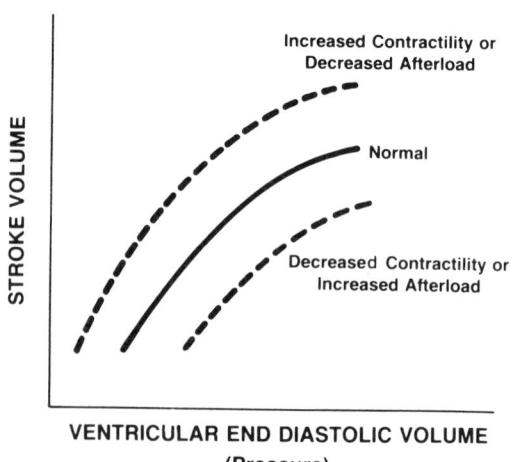

Figure 28.4.   Ventricular function curves demonstrating the effects of changes in contractility or afterload. If afterload is held constant, an increase in contractility of the ventricle will shift the functional curve upward and to the left, demonstrating improved ventricular performance at any given level of end-diastolic volume. If ventricular contractility is left unchanged, a decrease in afterload will produce a similar shift in the ventricular function curve.

Heart Rate

If stroke volume is held constant, CO increases linearly with increases in heart rate, since CO is equal to the product of heart rate and stroke volume. However, faster heart rates allow less time for diastolic filling and may decrease preload; the ultimate CO depends on the extent of the increase in heart rate versus the decrease in preload. In addition, increases in heart rate cause an increase in ventricular contractility; this augmented contractility with increased heart rate occurs in ventricles with myocardial dysfunction and in normal ventricles (66, 76).

Many pharmacologic interventions have important effects on several of the aforementioned parameters affecting CO. The ultimate pharmacologic effect on cardiac performance depends on the magnitude and direction of the changes produced in each individual parameter, and also on the baseline hemodynamics of the treated patient. Further, one must consider reflex responses (autonomic or renin-angiotensin system) activated by the pharmacologic intervention; these reflexes tend to counteract many of the therapeutic effects. Thus, in order to predict the ultimate outcome of any particular pharmacologic intervention on cardiac performance, one must know the pharmacologic effect on each individual parameter (preload, afterload, contractility, and heart rate) and the patient's hemodynamic status (76, 112). Even with this knowledge, one cannot always accurately predict the ultimate outcome of certain interventions; in such cases, a therapeutic trial following objective hemodynamic parameters is required.

PATHOPHYSIOLOGIC ABNORMALITIES IN CONGESTIVE HEART FAILURE

When myocardial function is decreased, the body activates a number of compensatory mechanisms designed to maintain CO and systemic blood pressure (11–13, 17, 30). The possible etiologies of the cardiac dysfunction and failure include ischemic heart disease, primary cardiomyopathy, infiltrative cardiomyopathies, chronic pressure overload (e.g., aortic stenosis), chronic volume overload (e.g., mitral regurgitation, aortic regurgitation, ventricular septal defect), and direct myocardial depression by drugs or disease states (e.g., septic shock or myocarditis). Regardless of the underlying causes of heart failure, the compensatory mechanisms are similar and include the following: First, dilation of the left ventricle (i.e., increasing the left ventricular end-diastolic volume) optimizes preload. Patients with heart failure are operating on the plateau portion of a depressed left ventricular function curve (Fig. 28.1). Once the end-diastolic volume reaches the plateau, further increases of preload do not improve stroke volume or ventricular performance and have an undesirable effect, namely, increase of left ventricular end-diastolic pressure, increased pulmonary capillary wedge pressure, and pulmonary edema (11, 13, 15). Further increases in end-diastolic volume increase left ventricular wall stress (La Place relationship) and in turn increase myocardial oxygen consumption, potentially precipitating acute ischemic events in patients with coronary artery disease (17). In some patients with heart failure, left ventricular dilation causes mitral regurgitation, adding a regurgitant volume load to an already compromised ventricle (112). Although elevation of end-diastolic volume is a useful mechanism in increasing cardiac performance, it can have deleterious effects on cardiac function once preload increases past the plateau of the Starling curve. In some patients, reduction of this inappropriately elevated preload (especially the pressure component) to prevent pulmonary congestion becomes important. This reduction can be performed clinically with diuretics, but vasodilators, with the ability to venodilate and increase the capacitance of the venous system, are also highly effective in reducing even severe elevations of ventricular end-diastolic pressure and volume (17, 30, 82).

A secondary compensatory mechanism in many patients with congestive heart failure is an increase in adrenergic stimulation of the heart, enhancing cardiac contractility and increasing heart rate and subsequently CO (130).

A third mechanism that serves to maintain blood pressure, presumably a response to depressed stroke volume, is elevated SVR (30, 126). This mechanism is mediated at least partially via baroreceptor activation of the sympathetic nervous system, increased activation of the renin-angiotensin system, accumulation of salt and water in blood vessel walls, and some other mechanisms (50, 126–129). Importantly, in many patients with heart failure, the SVR becomes inappropriately increased (i.e., the resistance is higher than that needed to maintain an adequate blood pressure) and is high enough actually to decrease stroke volume because of the effect of an increased afterload on a dysfunctional ventricle (30). If this inappropriately high SVR is lowered with a vasodilator agent, stroke volume and CO may improve with little change in blood pressure. It is important to realize that this reflex increase in afterload does not reduce stroke volume in a normal ventricle (Fig. 28.3) (116) but does reduce stroke volume in a dysfunctional and failing ventricle. Thus, paradoxically, one of the compensatory mechanisms (increased afterload) in the clinical syndrome of heart failure, in which a depression of stroke volume is likely to occur, may actually worsen overall cardiac performance.

MECHANISM OF VASODILATOR ACTION

The major mechanism by which vasodilators increase CO and reduce ventricular filling pressures is by decreasing arterial and venous vasoconstriction. Vasodilators that cause predominantly arterial dilation reduce afterload or outflow impedance, and those that produce predominantly venodilation decrease preload (ventricular end-diastolic volume and/or pressure). Most vasodilators produce their effect by relaxing vascular smooth muscle in resistance and capacitance vessels. Some agents produce this relaxation via a direct smooth muscle effect, whereas other agents stimulate or inhibit mechanisms that regulate smooth muscle tone.

The relationship of vascular resistance to the size of the vascular bed is expressed in Poiseuille's law:

$$Resistance\ to\ flow = \frac{viscosity \times vessel\ length \times 8}{(vessel\ radius)^4}$$

Resistance varies inversely with the vessel radius to the fourth power. The arterial vascular radius (or cross-sectional area) is determined largely by the smooth muscle tone in the arterioles, and this smooth muscle tone is the direct or indirect site of vasodilator action. Changes in smooth muscle tone

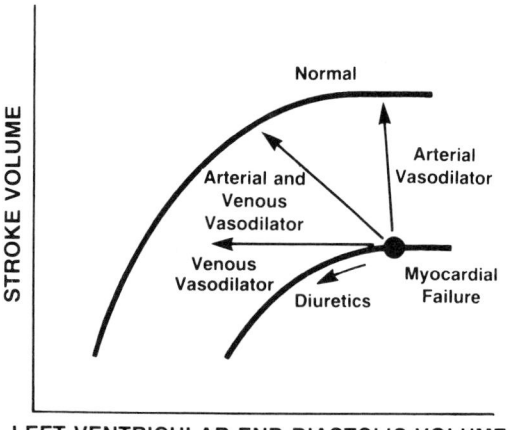

Figure 28.5.. Ability of different types of vasodilators to shift depressed ventricular function curve toward normal. Arterial vasodilators produce an increase in stroke volume with few or no changes in preload. Venous vasodilators produce a reduction in end-diastolic volume with little or no change in stroke volume. Vasodilators with both arterial and venous effects improve stroke volume and reduce filling pressures. An inotropic agent, along with a vasodilator, would shift the depressed curve even closer toward normal. At low levels of end-diastolic volume (on the slope rather than the plateau of the ventricular function curve), vasodilators may cause decreases in stroke volume and/or end-diastolic volume, resulting in decreased cardiac performance and hypotension. See text for details.

have a different effect on the arterial and venous circulations. Increases in arteriolar vessel tone increase resistance to blood flow in the arterial circuit (i.e., increased afterload). Increases in venular and venous vessel tone decrease the amount of blood stored in the venous system. Since the venous system and venules have approximately 70 to 80% of the body's blood volume, venous vasoconstriction decreases the amount of blood returned to the heart (59, 86). When one is conceptualizing the circulatory system and comparing it with electrical systems, the arterial circuit is best considered as a resistor and the venous system as a capacitor circuit.

Different vasodilator agents may have effects on arteriolar vessel tone, venous vessel tone, or a combination of arteriolar and venous tone. Further, vasodilators can have different effects on the systemic versus the pulmonary circulation (59). Depending on these effects and the baseline clinical hemodynamics, the ultimate effect or the general direction of hemodynamic change of a vasodilator agent can be predicted (Fig. 28.5). Although specific vasodilators are classified as venous or arterial in their action, none has "pure" effects on one circuit; nonetheless, the major effect is commonly regarded as predominantly arterial or venous.

In general, the goal of vasodilator therapy in heart failure is to improve CO by reducing unnecessary increases in afterload and to improve elevated ventricular filling pressures by reducing preload. On the arterial side, a decrease in outflow impedance increases stroke volume and thus CO. In most patients with heart failure treated with vasodilators, the heart rate does not increase and the blood pressure decreases slightly or not at all. The lack of change in blood pressure results from a proportional increase in stroke volume enhancing CO in response to the vasodilator-induced decrease in SVR (17, 30).

Thus, the vasodilator reverses an inappropriate increased vascular resistance and induces an increase in CO. When this reaction occurs, most patients report symptomatic improvement, with decreased dyspnea and fatigue. Patients commonly demonstrate reversal of signs of poor organ perfusion such as mental obtundation, cool, clammy skin, and elevations of blood urea nitrogen secondary to depressed renal perfusion. Better renal perfusion increases the excretion of salt and water, which tends to decrease vascular filling pressures (17, 30, 59, 112). Decreased sodium concentrations in vessel walls further decrease vessel tone. If mitral or aortic regurgitation is a part of the cardiovascular pathophysiology, the regurgitant fraction is reduced, with an increase in forward stroke volume.

Vasodilators become more effective as ventricular function worsens, and these agents can dramatically improve severe heart failure. Several studies have found a correlation between baseline CO and the vasodilator-induced increase in CO (i.e., the patients with the lowest resting CO have the best response to vasodilators) (19, 45, 46, 48, 49, 79, 80, 88, 90). One study shows a strong positive correlation between the initial SVR and the ability of the vasodilators to reduce SVR (i.e., the highest impedance has the greatest chance of response) (52). Most patients with severe myocardial dysfunction and failure have a steep impedance-to-stroke-volume relationship (Fig. 28.3, *lower curve*), and decreasing impedance raises stroke volume. In contrast, patients with normal or near-normal cardiac function have no change in stroke volume with decreased impedance (Fig. 28.3, *upper curve*); the preload reduction decreases stroke volume because these patients are operating on the steep portion of the Starling curve, and the reduced stroke volume and CO may result in substantial decreases in blood pressure. The hypotensive effect is desirable in hypertensive patients, and vasodilator therapy is an effective antihypertensive regimen (97); however, in patients with severe heart failure, blood pressure usually changes minimally for the reasons enumerated previously.

With venodilation, ventricular filling pressures decrease. Since most patients with heart failure are operating on the plateau portion of a depressed Starling curve (Fig. 28.1), reductions in preload generally do not reduce ventricular performance. However, reductions of filling pressures below a certain level reduce the stroke volume and can result in serious hypotension and/or a low output syndrome. The pulmonary capillary wedge pressure or left ventricular end-diastolic pressures can be reduced to approximately 15 mm Hg without affecting stroke volume in most patients; reductions below this level should be avoided because they depress stroke volume and CO (17, 30).

Despite many studies suggesting that vasodilator therapy in moderate to severe heart failure is not associated with an important blood pressure reduction, an occasional patient does develop symptomatic hypotension with vasodilator administration. If this occurs, one should suspect that the filling pressures are not elevated and that preload has been reduced too low, or that ventricle function is only mildly impaired. Patients with obstructive cardiac lesions in whom forward output cannot be increased (e.g., aortic stenosis, mitral stenosis, or obstructive hypertrophic cardiomyopathy) also may have a hypotensive response to vasodilators. Patients with restrictive cardiomyopathy from amyloidosis or endomyocardial fibrosis are also prone to hypotensive responses to vasodilators, in the author's experience. After the aforementioned possible causes of a hypotensive reaction to vasodilators are considered, an occasional patient with proven high filling pressures and poor CO, in severe heart failure, does not tolerate vasodilator therapy because of hypotension. It is assumed that this patient has not developed the usual inappropriate elevation of SVR seen in most patients with severe heart failure, though the reasons for this fact remain obscure.

CELLULAR AND BIOCHEMICAL MECHANISMS INVOLVED IN VASODILATOR ACTIONS

The final common pathway of vasodilator effect is to relax vascular smooth muscle tone. At the cellular and biochemical level, three major classes of vasodilators are at present recognized to produce this vasodilation: (*a*) inhibitors of the renin-angiotensin system, such as saralasin, captopril, enalapril, or lisinopril; (*b*) sympathetic nervous system blocking agents that negate α-adrenergic stimulation, such as phentolamine, prazosin, and trimethaphan; and (*c*) direct smooth muscle relaxers, as exemplified by nitroprusside, nitrates, hydralazine, and minoxidil. The effects of some direct-acting vasodilators may result from release of endothelial-derived relaxing factor (EDRF) from endothelial cells. However, these agents work at the vascular level and not via sympathetic or renin-angiotensin blockade. The specific mechanisms of action of the individual vasodilator agents are considered below (see the section entitled "Specific Vasodilator Agents").

EFFECTS OF VASODILATORS ON MYOCARDIAL ISCHEMIA

An area of myocardial ischemia represents an imbalance between myocardial oxygen demand and supply. In patients with coronary artery disease, blood supply is limited by coronary artery narrowing and, in some patients, by coronary spasm (10, 65, 114). When myocardial oxygen demand increases, blood cannot reach certain areas of myocardium, which then become segmentally ischemic and dysfunctional. The major determinants of myocardial oxygen consumption are arterial (or ventricular) systolic pressure, heart rate, heart size, and the ventricular contractile state. Arterial systolic pressure and heart size are the major determinants of wall stress, according to the La Place relationship (11–13). Vasodilators have a number of mechanisms for favorably altering the balance between myocardial oxygen demand by decreasing preload and reducing ventricular size; the ventricular pressure also reduces myocardial oxygen needs.

Vasodilators can increase blood flow to an ischemic area by reducing vasoconstrictor influences in the collateral flow to ischemic zones. Vasodilators reduce end-diastolic pressures, favoring subendocardial flow. Several studies have shown that segmental wall motion abnormalities are improved following nitroglycerin administration (64), providing evidence that certain vasodilators can influence the myocardial oxygen supply/demand balance favorably. The ultimate effect of a vasodilator on ischemic myocardium in a particular patient depends on a number of factors: the baseline hemodynamic state of the ventricle, the coronary anatomy and collateral flow, and the type of vasodilator employed. Conflicting and contradictory results are common in this field. Some have reported that nitroglycerin decreases, whereas nitroprusside increases, evidence of myocardial ischemia (23). Others have reported that nitroprusside can decrease the S-T segment evidence of ischemia (5).

Two large, controlled studies investigated the effects of nitroprusside infusion in patients with acute myocardial infarction (31, 40). One study found a statistically significant reduction in mortality in the nitroprusside group, along with a nitroprusside-induced reduction in the incidence of cardiogenic shock, clinical signs of heart failure, and levels of creatine kinase isoenzymes (40). In a second multicenter trial, nitroprusside was not associated with any change in overall mortality when given to patients with myocardial infarction and a pulmonary capillary wedge pressure greater than 12 mm Hg (31). In this latter study, patients whose nitroprusside infusions were begun within 9 hours of chest pain had an increased mortality, whereas infusions begun later were associated with a decreased mortality. These two studies do not lend themselves to a simple interpretation of the effect of this vasodilator agent on myocardial ischemia in the postinfarction phase of acute myocardial infarction. Nonetheless, the two studies were well-controlled and properly performed, and the contradictory results argue for the complexity of predicting the response of vasodilators in patients with myocardial ischemia.

Controlled trials have also evaluated nitroglycerin in the treatment of acute myocardial infarction (69, 16, 67, 43, 70). The most recent trials suggest that intravenous nitroglycerin can reduce infarct size, improve ejection fraction, reduce left ventricular asynergy, and improve Killip class score. Nitroglycerin treatment was associated with a decreased incidence of cardiogenic shock and infarct extension. Nitroglycerin produced a reduced in-hospital and 1-year mortality, although this survival advantage was limited to the anterior infarction subgroup. Treatment was most effective when mean blood pressure was kept greater than 80 mm Hg. It is important to note that this study was completed prior to the use of thrombolytic therapy for acute myocardial infarction, and that the value of nitroglycerin with thrombolysis has not been evaluated. However, this study suggests that intravenous nitroglycerin reduces morbidity and mortality in acute myocardial infarction.

Vasodilator therapy has also been shown to be effective in preventing the ventricular remodeling (increased cavity size and alteration in ventricular shape) following myocardial infarction (109). Remodeling has been associated with reduced ventricular performance and a higher mortality, and therapy with angiotensin-converting enzyme inhibitors or nitroglycerin has been shown to reduce this remodeling process. Effects on remodeling may be linked to vasodilator influence on ventricular compliance (see below). Large clinical trials are being conducted to define the influence of vasodilator treatment on the remodeling process.

EFFECT OF VASODILATORS ON VENTRICULAR COMPLIANCE

Another possible mechanism by which vasodilators improve ventricular function is induction of an increase in ventricular compliance (18, 104). The volume-pressure relationship of the ventricle is curvilinear (Fig. 28.2). At small end-diastolic volumes, ventricular size can change with little change in pressure; at higher ventricular volumes, a small change in volume produces a much greater pressure increase. If a pharmacologic agent shifts the volume-pressure curve to the right, there is a greater increase in end-diastolic volume without reaching a ventricular pressure that induces pulmonary edema. Assuming one has not reached the plateau portion of the Starling curve (Fig. 28.1), this increased volume at lower pressure produces better ventricular performance.

Studies suggest that vasodilators improve ventricular compliance (11, 78, 79, 105, 108), though further investigation is necessary to decide whether this is an important mechanism of vasodilator-induced improvement in ventricular performance. The mechanism of this improvement in compliance is not clear. Some investigators postulate a reduction in ischemia; others argue for an intrinsic increase in ventricular relaxation (14, 18), or right ventricular relaxation causing increased left ventricular compliance within a confined pericardial space (33, 78). Vasodilators are capable of preventing ventricular remodeling following myocardial infarction (see above), which may represent an influence of these agents on ventricular compliance.

VASODILATOR-INDUCED REDISTRIBUTION EFFECTS

Most of the literature on vasodilators focuses on their ability to reduce afterload and/or preload and improve ventricular performance. Another potentially important capability of vasodilators in critical care medicine is reduction or redistribution of blood flow away from certain nonessential vascular beds and toward vital areas. For example, patients with septic shock commonly have a high CO, low filling pressures, and a low overall peripheral vascular resistance; however, many organs in the body are not receiving appropriate blood supply, as evidenced by lactic acidosis and progressive organ system dysfunction (e.g., rising blood urea nitrogen with renal dysfunction). In this setting, the appropriate vasodilator could potentially redirect blood flow toward the vital organs. Many forms of shock are postulated to have inappropriate sympathetic outflow causing arteriolar vasoconstriction; some investigators advocate the use of vasodilators in the treatment of shock (108). However, in shock, where one is faced with hypotension that is commonly difficult to control, vasodilators may further decrease blood pressure. In the absence of clear efficacy and with the potential of worsening already existing hypotension, vasodilators are not widely accepted in the treatment of noncardiogenic shock.

In cardiogenic shock and severe intractable heart failure (33, 61), vasodilator therapy increases stroke volume and CO, and in some cases reverses cardiogenic shock. Commonly, vasodilator therapy in cardiogenic shock is used in conjunction with an inotropic agent such as dopamine (85, 94) or with intraaortic balloon counterpulsation (62). In severe heart failure, the body's compensatory mechanisms (sympathetic outflow, the renin-angiotensin system, and the organ's autoregulatory capacity) redistribute blood flow to preferentially maintain cerebral and coronary perfusion. In this setting, renal

perfusion does not change or decrease, and flow to the mesenteric and limb circulations is considerably diminished (131). If vasodilator therapy increases CO, flow to these vascular beds increases. In cardiogenic shock, the body's compensatory mechanisms are redistributing a very reduced CO to those organs of vital importance to survival. In other forms of shock (e.g., septic shock), CO is adequate or increased, but the distribution of flow is commonly inappropriate, resulting in lactic acidosis and vital organ dysfunction. The cause of this inappropriate redistribution of flow in septic shock, and whether vasodilators can redirect the flow, are questions that are unanswered and will require further study.

VASODILATOR THERAPY IN MECHANICAL DEFECTS

Patients with mitral regurgitation, aortic regurgitation, or a ventricular septal defect frequently respond to vasodilator therapy with an improvement in their hemodynamics and clinical symptoms of heart failure (9, 21). Although the definitive treatment for these mechanical lesions is corrective cardiac surgery, vasodilator therapy can be employed when surgery is not possible or when it is wise to defer surgery.

In mitral regurgitation, the severity of the regurgitation is dependent on the degree of anatomic derangement of the mitral apparatus as well as aortic outflow impedance (21, 104). Increasing afterload increases the regurgitant fraction (11, 12); vasodilator-induced reduction of aortic impedance should decrease regurgitation through the mitral valve. A number of clinical studies have documented that vasodilator-induced reductions in SVR produce marked hemodynamic improvements in patients with mitral regurgitations (21, 55, 59, 63, 125). Nitroprusside increases forward stroke volume and CO (mean increase, approximately 50%), decreases regurgitant volumes, decreases pulmonary artery and capillary wedge pressures, and causes large V-waves in the pulmonary capillary wedge tracing to decrease markedly or disappear. These effects are a result of vasodilator-induced redistribution of the left ventricular stroke volume, causing more blood to be ejected into the aorta than into the left atrium. The major mechanism for this effect is a reduction of aortic impedance; however, a reduction in ventricular size with closer approximation of mitral leaflets and, in some cases, a reduction of papillary muscle ischemia may also contribute to the vasodilator-induced improvement in regurgitation.

In severe aortic regurgitation, the body may reflexively increase SVR to maintain blood pressure and thereby initiate a vicious cycle that increases regurgitation further. Nitroprusside is capable of reducing the aortic regurgitant fraction and increasing the forward stroke volume in chronic aortic regurgitation (9, 14, 87, 121). Vasodilators also produce increases in forward CO in acute aortic regurgitation (104).

In a large ventricular septal defect, the magnitude of the left-to-right shunt is determined largely by the ratio of the vascular resistances in the pulmonary versus systemic circuits. A reduction in SVR decreases the left-to-right shunt and favors flow from the left ventricle to the aorta (i.e., it increases systemic CO). Nitroprusside induces a favorable hemodynamic response in patients with acute ventricular septal defects complicating myocardial infarction (119). It should be recognized that if vasodilator therapy reduces pulmonary resistance more than systemic, the left-to-right shunt increases and systemic flow decreases. One must repeatedly measure flows and shunts to be sure that a sustained beneficial effect is resulting from such therapy.

EFFECT OF VASODILATOR THERAPY ON MORTALITY IN PATIENTS WITH MODERATE TO SEVERE CONGESTIVE HEART FAILURE

Vasodilators have been shown to produce profound changes in cardiovascular physiology, especially in patients with moderate to severe congestive heart failure. There is no question that vasodilator therapy can decrease elevated filling pressures and increase cardiac output and stroke volume in many patients with significant heart failure. Concomitant with these improved hemodynamics, many patients note a decrease in symptomatology and improvement in signs of heart failure: decreased dyspnea, improved energy, and improved organ blood flow and function. However, one of the most important questions regarding vasodilator therapy is its effect on survival of patients with severe heart failure. Several recent trials have addressed this question.

The first Veterans Administration (VA) Cooperative Study assigned 642 men with moderate to severe heart failure already receiving digitalis and diuretics to receive additional double-blind treatment with (*a*) placebo, (*b*) prazosin (20 mg/day), or (*c*) a combination of hydralazine (300 mg/day) and isosorbide dinitrate (160 mg/day) (27, 28). The mortality in the hydralazine/isosorbide dinitrate group was lower than that in the placebo group throughout the entire follow-up period (average, 2.3 years). The mortality risk reduction in the group treated with hydralazine/isosorbide dinitrate was 36% by 3 years. The mortality in the prazosin group was similar to that in the placebo group. Further, the serially determined left ventricular ejection fraction increased in the hydralazine/isosorbide dinitrate group but not in the placebo or prazosin groups. Thus, this study demonstrates that addition of hydralazine/isosorbide dinitrate to digitalis/diuretic therapy can result in improved left ventricular function and decreased mortality.

Another prospective, double-blind analysis evaluated the effect of an angiotensin-converting enzyme inhibitor, enalapril, in 253 patients under treatment for severe heart failure (35). The enalapril group had a highly significant 27% decrease in mortality compared with the placebo group. Interestingly, the entire reduction in total mortality was found to be among patients with progressive heart failure, and no reduction was seen in the incidence of sudden cardiac death.

The recently reported Study Of Left Ventricular Dysfunction (SOLVD) trial (93) has extended these findings to patients with mild to moderate heart failure. Enalapril therapy again resulted in a significant mortality reduction (risk reduction averaged 16% at 41 months of follow-up). A second VA Cooperative Trial (34) compared the efficacy of hydralazine-isordil with that of enalapril. At 2 years of follow-up, mortality was significantly lower in the enalapril group, although hydralazine-isosorbide produced a greater initial improvement in left ventricular ejection fraction and oxygen consumption at peak

Table 28.1. Vasodilators Classified by Their Principal Site of Action

Arterial and venous vasodilators—"balanced vasodilators"
Nitroprusside
Phentolamine
Prazosin
Captopril
Enalapril
Lisinopril
Nifedipine
Verapamil
Diltiazem
Arterial vasodilators
Hydralazine
Minoxidil
Venous vasodilators
Nitrates (nitroglycerin, isosorbide dinitrate)

exercise. These multicenter trials have demonstrated the survival advantage of both hydralazine-isosorbide and enalapril, with enalapril showing a greater survival improvement. Future studies will address whether a combination of both regimens should be employed in severe heart failure patients.

SPECIFIC VASODILATOR AGENTS

Clinically, the most useful method of classifying vasodilator agents is based on their major peripheral vascular actions (Fig. 28.5; Table 28.1) (130). One group of vasodilators is considered to have its major effect by dilating arterioles, a second group dilates predominantly veins and venules, and a third group has relatively equal effects dilating arterioles and veins ("balanced" vasodilation). In general, vasodilators that affect arterioles increase CO through an enhanced stroke volume but have little or no effect on pulmonary or systemic venous pressures. Agents that dilate veins and venules reduce pulmonary and systemic venous pressures with little or no change in CO. Vasodilators with effects on both the arterial and venous circuits reduce pulmonary and systemic venous hypertension and increase CO (Fig. 28.5).

Although this classification is clinically useful, it has several limitations. Of the currently available vasodilator agents, none has pure arteriolar or venodilator properties; all have some effect on both circuits, though certain agents have such a predominant effect on the arteriolar or venous side that they are best regarded as arteriolar or venous vasodilators. Perhaps the most accurate representation of these vasodilator properties would be as a spectrum of effects ranging from pure venodilation, to balanced venous and arteriolar effects, to pure arteriolar dilation. A second limitation is that the hemodynamic response to any vasodilator depends on the baseline hemodynamic status of the patient (see the section of this chapter entitled "Mechanism of Vasodilator Action"). Patients' responses to the same vasodilator agent are usually variable, and one must consider this fact when instituting therapy. Despite these limitations, the classification proposed (Table 28.1) is highly useful, both conceptually and clinically, and allows prediction of a vasodilator's probable site of action and probable hemodynamic outcome.

In the critical care setting, use of rapidly acting parenteral vasodilator agents predominates, and therefore the emphasis is on parenteral (usually intravenous) vasodilator agents. However, some mention is also made of nonparenteral agents that are of use in the intensive care unit.

ARTERIAL AND VENOUS VASODILATORS

Nitroprusside

Because of its rapid onset of action, rapid reversibility when discontinued, relatively specific effect on vascular smooth muscle, balanced effect on the arteriolar and venous systems, and lack of tachyphylaxis, nitroprusside is the vasodilator of choice for many situations in the critical care unit.

Nitroprusside has both an interesting history and chemistry. Its original use in the 1850s was as a chemical color indicator. Its hypotensive properties were not described until 1929 (68). The chemical structure of nitroprusside contains five cyanide groups per molecule (29, 103), and concern about cyanide toxicity delayed development of the agent as a pharmaceutical until 1955, when its safety and potent hypotensive effects were demonstrated in a group of hypertensive patients (102). In 1972, nitroprusside was shown to improve left ventricular function in patients with acute myocardial infarction (49), and subsequent studies have shown the drug's ability to improve left ventricular function in severe heart failure resulting from ischemic heart disease, cardiomyopathy, or cardiac regurgitant lesions (9, 14, 21, 33, 61).

Nitroprusside causes direct relaxation of arterial and venous smooth muscle. At therapeutic doses, it has no effect on uterine or duodenal smooth muscle and no direct effect on myocardial contractility (29). Nitroprusside relaxes the lower esophageal sphincter (38); however, in general the drug affects vascular smooth muscle in a relatively specific manner. Nitroprusside-induced vascular smooth muscle relaxation is not dependent on the sympathetic nervous system or adrenergic receptors. Its cellular mechanism of action is unknown, though possible mechanisms include interaction with intracellular sulfhydryl groups, inhibition of calcium transport, or changes in intracellular cyclic nucleotides (112).

Nitroprusside is useful for all of the clinical indications outlined below in the section entitled "Clinical Indications for Vasodilator Therapy." It is the classic example of a balanced vasodilator with capability to reduce both pulmonary venous and systemic venous pressures as well as to increase stroke volume and CO in patients with severe heart failure. Heart rate usually decreases slightly or remains unchanged, and blood pressure may fall slightly or remain unchanged. Concomitant with this salutary hemodynamic effect, most patients have symptomatic improvement, with relief of dyspnea, lessened fatigue, warming of the skin, and diuresis (17, 30, 49, 61).

In patients with severe heart failure requiring intensive care, nitroprusside therapy should be initiated and continued using constant arterial pressure monitoring and employing a Swan-Ganz pulmonary artery catheter to determine serial pulmonary artery pressures, pulmonary capillary wedge pressures, and thermodilution COs. Nitroprusside has an onset of action within seconds of initiating the drug, and its duration of effect is only 1 to 3 minutes, allowing slow increase of the dose every few minutes while the arterial pressure is watched carefully. Serial determinations of hemodynamic values allow

correlation of clinical with hemodynamic improvement. Once an optimal pulmonary capillary wedge pressure (usually 14 to 18 mm Hg) and maximal CO are achieved, oral vasodilator agents can be started and nitroprusside tapered. Serial hemodynamics can again help determine the optimal dose and combination of vasodilator agents for a particular patient.

The major complication of nitroprusside therapy is hypotension. Most patients with severe heart failure respond to relatively low doses of nitroprusside with an increase in CO and only minimal decreases in pressure; however, patients with low filling pressures commonly respond to nitroprusside with a reduced CO and hypotension resulting from inadequate preload (Fig. 28.1). Some authors recommend that vasodilators not be used with a diastolic pressure of less than 60 mm Hg (17, 104), but others state that nitroprusside therapy can be used in most patients with systolic pressures between 90 and 105 mm Hg without precipitating hypotension (29). Most patients whose blood pressure decreases with nitroprusside respond to discontinuation of the drug, and the nitroprusside usually can then be restarted at a lower dosage. A hypotensive response to nitroprusside should always cause the physician to consider whether the filling pressures are lower than suspected. Profound hypotension with nitroprusside that does not respond to discontinuation of infusion and fluid administration within a few minutes should be treated with an inotropic agent such as dopamine; this therapy usually restores blood pressure promptly.

For patients with severe heart failure, a nitroprusside infusion is started at 10 μg/min and may be increased by 10-μg/min increments every 5 to 15 minutes. There is great variability in individual responses to nitroprusside, but most patients with heart failure show a positive response to 1 to 2 μg/kg/min (approximately 70 to 140 μg/min) with a drop in the pulmonary capillary wedge pressure and/or an increase in CO. Although hemodynamic responses are highly variable, a decrease of 20 to 50% in wedge pressure and an increase of 20 to 40% in CO are considered positive responses to nitroprusside. In patients with pulmonary edema with hypertension, nitroprusside is started at 10 μg/min but is increased by 20-μg/min increments every 3 to 5 minutes in order to rapidly reduce filling pressures and relieve symptoms. When nitroprusside is used for hypertension, usually the doses required to decrease blood pressure are considerably higher than those required to treat heart failure.

Besides hypotension, the other major side effects of nitroprusside are thiocyanate/cyanide toxicity and mild reductions in arterial oxygen tension resulting from nitroprusside-induced inhibition of the pulmonary vasoconstrictor response (91, 110). Thiocyanate toxicity is manifested by confusion, hyperreflexia, and convulsions; cyanide toxicity is first manifested by a metabolic acidosis resulting from cyanide's combining with cytochromes and inhibiting aerobic cellular metabolism. Thiocyanate or cyanide toxicity occurs almost exclusively in patients receiving high doses of nitroprusside for a prolonged period. Infusion rates of less than 3 μg/kg/min for less than 72 hours are not associated with toxicity.

Deaths during long infusions of high doses of nitroprusside have been ascribed to cyanide toxicity. Cyanide conversion to thiocyanate is facilitated by thiosulfate, sodium nitrate, or hydroxocobalamin (26, 36), and these three agents should be considered as therapy in patients demonstrating toxicity from nitroprusside with metabolic acidosis and confusion when discontinuation of the nitroprusside does not reverse the toxicity. Monitoring blood thiocyanate levels is useful to follow toxicity in patients requiring infusions for longer than 2 to 3 days. Levels of thiocyanate below 10 mg/dl are considered safe.

On rapid discontinuation of a nitroprusside infusion, a rebound beyond the prenitroprusside baseline occurs, with an increase in SVR, increase in pulmonary capillary wedge pressure, and decrease in CO (99). This phenomenon probably results from vasodilator-induced activation of the sympathetic and renin-angiotensin systems. A slow nitroprusside taper while oral vasodilator therapy is instituted usually avoids this rebound depression of cardiac performance.

Phentolamine

Phentolamine was the first vasodilator used clinically to improve cardiovascular performance in heart failure (81). It is considered one of the classical α-adrenergic blocking agents and causes blockade at both the postsynaptic (α-1) and presynaptic (α-2) receptors. Its potent vasodilator capabilities are secondary to both α-blockade (56, 112) and a direct vasodilator effect on vascular smooth muscle (118). Norepinephrine release may actually increase reflexively because of baroreceptor activation caused by the fall in blood pressure and the blockade of the presynaptic α-2-receptors, the inhibition promoting further release. This circulating norepinephrine frequently results in a tachycardia and positive cardiac inotropic stimulation.

Phentolamine can relax arteriolar as well as venous vascular smooth muscle and thus can increase CO and reduce pulmonary and systemic venous pressures in patients with moderate to severe heart failure of all etiologies. The ability of phentolamine to increase CO is comparable with that of nitroprusside; however, it produces less of a decrease in filling pressures. The ability of phentolamine to increase CO and its less-than-expected decreases in venous tone may be caused by the enhanced release of norepinephrine, which increases cardiac contractility and heightens venous vasoconstriction. Although phentolamine is generally well-tolerated in ischemic cardiac failure, the tachycardia and norepinephrine release can worsen ischemia in patients with coronary artery disease.

Phentolamine is given as an intravenous infusion starting at 0.1 mg/min and increasing slowly up to 2 mg/min in increments of 0.2 to 0.4 mg/min every 10 to 30 minutes. Hemodynamic effects occur at 15 minutes, usually peak by 30 minutes, and persist up to 60 minutes after the drug is stopped. The drug can be given orally in doses of 50 to 150 mg every 4 to 6 hours.

In addition to the tachycardia, the major side effects of phentolamine are gastrointestinal: vomiting, abdominal pain, diarrhea, and hypermotility. Because tolerance to the drug develops rapidly, phentolamine is used only on an acute basis.

Prazosin

Prazosin is a selective α-1 (postsynaptic) adrenergic receptor antagonist that causes arteriolar and venous vasodilation exclusively by its receptor-blocking effects (57, 115). Since it is available only in oral form, its use in the intensive care environment is as a subacute or chronic agent after therapy is initiated with a parenteral vasodilator. In patients with heart failure, prazosin has balanced hemodynamic actions similar to those of nitroprusside, with elevation in CO and reductions in systemic and pulmonary venous pressures (58).

Prazosin is well-absorbed from the gastrointestinal tract and is given in doses of 1 to 10 mg every 6 to 8 hours. Its onset of action is 30 to 60 minutes, with maximal hemodynamic effect at 2 to 6 hours postdose. In many patients, the first dose of drug will produce orthostatic syncope, so patients should be warned to rise slowly from the supine position.

A subset of patients develop tachyphylaxis to the beneficial hemodynamic effect of this drug after several days of therapy (4, 39, 96). The mechanism is unknown, but increasing the drug dose or adding diuretics does not help. If tachyphylaxis occurs, prazosin should be discontinued and another vasodilator used. This tachyphylaxis may account for prazosin's failure to improve survival in heart failure patients (see above).

Captopril

With the onset of moderate to severe heart failure, the renin-angiotensin-aldosterone system is activated and serves as an important compensatory mechanism to maintain blood pressure and cause volume retention. In advanced heart failure, some of the "inappropriate" increase in afterload may be maintained by the vasoconstrictor substance angiotensin II. Inhibition of the renin-angiotensin system reduces afterload or impedance and enhances cardiac performance. A number of inhibitors of the renin-angiotensin system are being tested, and captopril is a prototype of the angiotensin converting enzyme (ACE) inhibitors commercially available.

In patients with heart failure, captopril produces a hemodynamic pattern similar to that seen with nitroprusside (75) or prazosin (71). From what is known of angiotensin II physiology, one would predict that a pure inhibitor of angiotensin II production would cause a reduction in afterload with little effect on preload. Yet, captopril does reduce preload, prompting some to argue that captopril has an additional mechanism of action causing vasodilation. The mechanism of captopril-induced vasodilation is unknown, but it is postulated to result from inhibition of the enzyme that degrades bradykinin, leading to an increase in the circulating level of this potent vasodilator (41).

Captopril is available only in an oral preparation, and therapy is started with 6.125 mg every 6 hours and increased to a maximum daily dosage of 450 mg. Onset of a hemodynamic change is within 30 minutes, with peak effect at 1 to 3 hours and disappearance by 4 to 8 hours. The duration of the hemodynamic effect is dose-dependent, but the magnitude is not. Tolerance to the drug does not develop in patients treated for as long as 6 to 12 months.

Enalapril and lisinopril are somewhat longer-acting ACE inhibitors. Enalapril is also available for intravenous administration as enalaprilat, a product of particular use in the critically ill. The usual dose is 1.25 mg every 6 hours i.v. over 5 minutes. A clinical response is usually seen within 15 minutes, although peak effects may not occur until 4 hours following the dose.

Nifedipine

Calcium channel blockers inhibit the contraction of vascular smooth muscle and therefore have vasodilator properties; however, few studies are available to evaluate the efficacy of these agents in heart failure. In one study, patients in cardiogenic pulmonary edema were treated with nifedipine (10 mg sublingually), causing reduction in symptoms of dyspnea, decreases in systemic and pulmonary venous pressures, and a rise in CO (111). Nifedipine also produces a sustained hemodynamic improvement in patients with chronic heart failure (7). Many clinicians are reluctant to use calcium channel blockers in heart failure because these agents have a direct depressant effect on the myocardium. With nifedipine, the decrease in afterload is more profound than the myocardial depressant effect, resulting in overall enhanced hemodynamics. Heart failure is a relative contraindication to calcium channel blocker therapy.

Verapamil, another calcium channel blocker, has vasodilator properties but its direct myocardial depressant effect is more profound, and this may seriously aggravate heart failure in patients with severe myocardial dysfunction. Diltiazem also has vasodilator and myocardial depressant properties.

ARTERIAL VASODILATORS

Hydralazine

Hydralazine has been used in the treatment of hypertension for 30 years. It is a potent direct dilator of vascular smooth muscle and mostly affects arterioles. In patients with heart failure, hydralazine produces impressive increases in stroke volume by reducing arteriolar resistance and has no effect or only a modest lowering effect on systemic or pulmonary venous pressures (9, 22). For a given change in blood pressure, hydralazine increases CO more than does nitroprusside or nitrates. There is conflicting evidence as to whether hydralazine has a reflex or direct cardiac inotropic effect as an explanation for its potent ability to increase CO (98, 112). Hydralazine can also increase limb and renal blood flow, thus promoting diuresis.

When hydralazine is used in a critical care setting, intravenous administration is the most reliable route, but it must be given slowly and with constant hemodynamic monitoring to avoid hypotension. Administration should begin with 5 to 10 mg given as a slow intravenous drip over 20 minutes. Maximal effect occurs 15 to 45 minutes after injection, and the effect can last 4 to 24 hours. One can administer up to 20 mg intravenously every 6 hours. Given orally, the dosage is usually 25 to 100 mg every 6 hours, with onset of action at 60 minutes and peak effect at 2 to 3 hours. Some studies suggest that high doses of hydralazine (150 to 200 mg) are necessary in some patients to produce a beneficial effect on cardiac performance (20, 97); the need for this high oral dose in some patients may result from mesenteric venous hypertension's causing malabsorption of the drug.

A small number of patients with heart failure develop tachycardia with hydralazine administration. Exacerbation of angina pectoris can occur with hydralazine, especially (but not exclusively) in patients with ischemic heart disease who develop a tachycardia during therapy (72). Prolonged administration of hydralazine is associated with a lupus-like syndrome in 10 to 20% of patients, especially in those taking more than 400 mg daily (2).

Minoxidil

Minoxidil is a potent, direct-acting, vascular smooth muscle relaxant that acts largely on the arterial bed (51). In doses of 5 to 20 mg orally, the drug produces hemodynamic effects similar to those of hydralazine in patients with heart failure (i.e., a rise in CO, decrease in SVR, and no change in pulmonary venous, or arterial, pressure) (47). Side effects include hirsutism and pericardial effusion.

VENOUS VASODILATORS

Organic esters of nitric acid have been established therapy for angina pectoris for more than 100 years. Only in the past 10 years have they been used to treat congestive heart failure. Nitrates have a direct smooth-muscle-relaxing capability, especially on vascular smooth muscle. Recent evidence suggests that nitrates may act on smooth muscle by releasing prostacyclin (a potent vasodilator) from vessel endothelial cells (74).

In patients with heart failure, the most prominent action of nitrates is to lower ventricular filling pressures by dilation of pulmonary and systemic veins (54). The volume of the left and right ventricles decreases and the compliance of the left ventricle increases (37, 77, 78). The mechanism of this improved compliance is unclear; however, it may result from altered constraints on the left ventricle caused by a decrease in right ventricle size.

Nitrates also decrease arterial vascular resistance, but CO may increase, remain unchanged, or decrease in response to nitrates (112). In some patients treated with nitrates, the CO does not increase because a concomitant fall in preload causes a depression in stroke volume (18, 104). Other patients not showing an increase in CO in response to nitrates have received a dose that is insufficient to produce a significant fall in impedance. At lower doses of nitrate, the vasodilatory effect is largely on the venous system, with decreases in filling pressures. At higher nitrate doses, impedance falls and CO rises. As with nitroprusside, the increase in CO with nitrates is proportional to the reduction in SVR (45, 100) and is correlated inversely with the patient's baseline CO (45, 80, 100). Some authors note a positive correlation between baseline SVR and the nitrate-induced rise in CO (52), although others do not support this finding (3, 100).

The effects of nitrates and nitroprussides on ischemic heart disease were considered previously in the section entitled "Effects of Vasodilators on Myocardial Ischemia."

In an intensive care environment, the optimal nitrate preparation is intravenous nitroglycerin because it allows exact titration of dose and the ability to quickly terminate drug infusion. It is important to be certain that the left ventricular filling pressures are high or optimal because even low doses of nitroglycerin can precipitously decrease filling pressures. Intravenous infusions should begin at 10 μg/min, and one can increase the dosage in increments of 10 μg/min every 5 to 10 minutes to a dose of 50 to 100 μg/min. Most patients demonstrate a vasodilator effect at this dose, but up to 400 μg/min can be given if clinically indicated. High doses of nitroglycerin are well-tolerated for several days. Treatment can then be changed to oral isosorbide dinitrate, 20 to 100 mg every 4 hours, nitroglycerin ointment, ½ to 1½ inches every 4 hours, or a transdermal delivery system for nitroglycerin (1, 120).

In recent years a nitrate tolerance syndrome has been clearly described. If administered continuously for more than 24 to 48 hours, many patients develop a tolerance to the hemodynamic and/or antianginal effects of nitroglycerin and other nitrates (101). To prevent this tolerance when therapy is initiated, patients should be given a nitrate-free period of 6 to 8 hours during a 24-hour period.

Nitrates and hydralazine are used together to combine nitrate-induced reductions in filling pressures with hydralazine's ability to increase CO, producing an oral regimen comparable with that of nitroprusside (72, 73, 83, 84). The hemodynamic changes seen with the combination are roughly additive (72, 83, 84), and are similar to those produced by nitroprusside. This combination produced improved survival in heart failure patients. As with all vasodilator regimens, hypotension can complicate this therapy and necessitate alteration in dosage or discontinuation of one of the drugs.

CLINICAL INDICATIONS FOR VASODILATOR THERAPY

The following are the clinical situations in which vasodilator therapy is beneficial:

1. In acute heart failure, in combination with diuretics and digitalis, vasodilator therapy will reduce filling pressures and usually improve cardiac output. In chronic heart failure, enalapril and (to a somewhat lesser degree) hydralazine/isosorbide dinitrate have been shown to improve long-term mortality.
2. In acute cardiogenic pulmonary edema, vasodilator therapy with acute vasodilation can rapidly reduce high filling pressures and reverse symptoms. Vasodilators can be used in conjunction with supplemental oxygen, rotating tourniquets, morphine, and intravenous diuretics.
3. In acute or chronic mitral regurgitation, aortic regurgitation, or ventricular septal defect, vasodilator-induced decreases in SVR increase forward (systemic) CO. Vasodilators are usually employed in these situations as a temporizing measure to allow time to prepare the patient for cardiac surgery.
4. Intravenous nitroglycerin has been shown to reduce infarct size and improve mortality in acute myocardial infarction. Nitrate therapy is useful in treating stable and unstable angina. Vasodilators such as nitroprusside can reduce myocardial oxygen consumption in patients with persistent chest pain who are hypertensive.
5. In patients with cardiogenic shock, vasodilator therapy combined with inotropic drugs (e.g., dopamine or dobutamine) or intraaortic balloon counterpulsation can produce substantial hemodynamic improvement. Once stabilized, such patients can be considered for revascularization.
6. As reviewed in other chapters of this book, vasodilators are highly useful to treat hypertension, malignant hypertension, and dissecting aortic aneurysms (in conjunction with β-blockade) and possibly may be useful in some patients with primary pulmonary hypertension.

ACKNOWLEDGMENTS

The author thanks Ms. Veronica Powell for her excellent secretarial assistance and Ms. Geri Byrd for her superb administrative and editorial assistance.

REFERENCES

1. Abrams JA: Nitroglycerin and long-acting nitrates. *N Engl J Med* 302:1234–1237, 1980.
2. Alarcon-Segovia D: Drug-induced antinuclear antibodies and lupus syndromes. *Drugs* 12:69–77, 1976.
3. Armstrong PW, Armstrong JA, Markes CS: Pharmacokinetic hemodynamic studies of intravenous nitroglycerin in congestive heart failure. *Circulation* 62:160–166, 1980.
4. Arnold SB, Williams RL, Ports TA, Baughman RA, Benet LZ, Parmley WW, Chatterjee K: Attenuation of prazosin effect on cardiac output in chronic heart failure. *Ann Intern Med* 91:345–349, 1979.
5. Awan NA, Miller RR, Zakanddin V, DeMaria AN, Amsterdam EA, Mason DT: Reduction of ST segment elevation with infusion of nitroprusside in patients with acute myocardial infarction. *Am J Cardiol* 38:425–439, 1976.
6. Bache RJ, Dymek DJ: Local and regional regulation of coronary vascular tone. *Prog Cardiovasc Dis* 24:191–212, 1981.
7. Bellocui F, Ansalone G, Scabia E, Viencenzo A, Peitro S, Laperfido F, Paolo Z: Sustained beneficial effect of nifedipine in chronic refractory heart failure. *Am J Cardiol* 47:407, 1981.
8. Bemis CF, Serue JR, Borkenhagen D, Sonnenblick EH, Urschel CW: Influence of right ventricular filling pressure on left ventricular pressure and dimension. *Circ Res* 34:498–504, 1974.
9. Bolen JL, Alderman EL: Hemodynamic consequence of afterload reduction in patients with chronic aortic regurgitation. *Circulation* 53:879–883, 1976.
10. Braunwald E: Control of myocardial oxygen consumption. *Am J Cardiol* 27:416–432, 1971.
11. Braunwald E: Pathophysiology of heart failure. In Braunwald E (ed): *Heart Disease: A Textbook of Cardiovascular Medicine*, ed 3. Philadelphia, WB Saunders, pp 426–448, 1988.
12. Braunwald E, Ross J, Sonneblick EH: *Mechanisms of Contraction of the Normal and Failing Heart*. Boston, Little, Brown & Co, 1976.
13. Braunwald E, Sonnenblick EH, Ross J: *Contraction of the normal heart*. In Braunwald E (ed): Heart Disease: A Textbook of Cardiovascular Medicine. Philadelphia, WB Saunders, 1980.
14. Brodie BR, Grossman W, Mann T, McLaurin LP: Effects of sodium nitroprusside on left ventricular diastolic pressure/volume relations. *J Clin Invest* 59:59–68, 1977.
15. Burns JW, Covell JW, Ross J: Mechanics of isotonic left ventricular contractions. *Am J Physiol* 224:725–732, 1973.
16. Bussmann WD, Passek D, Seidel W, Kaltenbach M: Reduction of CK and CK-MB indexes of infarct size by intravenous nitroglycerin. *Circulation* 63:615–622, 1981.
17. Chatterjee K, Parmley WW: The role of vasodilator therapy in heart failure. *Prog Cardiovasc Dis* 19:301–325, 1977.
18. Chatterjee K, Parmley WW: Vasodilator therapy for chronic heart failure. *Annu Rev Pharmacol Toxicol* 20:475–512, 1980.
19. Chatterjee K, Parmley WW, Ganz W, Forrester J, Walinsky P, Crexells C: Hemodynamic and metabolic responses to vasodilator therapy in the acute myocardial infarction. *Circulation* 48:1183–1193, 1973.
20. Chatterjee K, Parmley WW, Massie B: Oral hydralazine therapy for chronic refractory heart failure. *Circulation* 54:879–883, 1976.
21. Chatterjee K, Parmley WW, Swan HJ, Berman G, Forrester J: Beneficial effects of vasodilator agents in severe mitral regurgitation due to dysfunction of subvalvular apparatus. *Circulation* 48:684–690, 1973.
22. Chatterjee K, Ports TA, Brundage BH, Massie B, Holly AN, Parmley WW: Oral hydralazine in chronic heart failure: sustained beneficial hemodynamic effects. *Ann Intern Med* 92:600–604, 1980.
23. Chiariello M, Gold HK, Leinbach RC, Davis MA, Maroko PR: Comparison between the effects of nitroprusside and nitroglycerin on ischemic injury during acute myocardial infarction. *Circulation* 54:766–773, 1976.
24. Clancy RI, Graham TP, Ross J, Sonnenblick EH, Braunwald E: Influence of aortic pressure induced homeometric autoregulation on myocardial performance. *Am J Physiol* 214:1186–1192, 1968.

25. Cohn JN: Marriage of the heart and the peripheral circulation. *Prog Cardiovasc Dis* 24:189–190, 1981.
26. Cohn JN: Vasodilator therapy for heart failure. *Circulation* 48:5–8, 1973.
27. Cohn JN, Archibald DG, Ziesche S, et al: Effects of vasodilator therapy on mortality in chronic congestive heart failure. Results of a Veterans Administration Cooperative Study. *N Engl J Med* 314:1547–1552, 1986.
28. Cohn JN, Archibald DG, Francis GS, et al: Veterans Administration Cooperative Study on vasodilator therapy of heart failure: influence of prerandomization variables on the reduction of mortality by treatment with hydralazine and isosorbide dinitrate. *Circulation* 75(suppl IV):IV-49, 1987.
29. Cohn JN, Burke LP: Nitroprusside. *Ann Intern Med* 91:752–757, 1979.
30. Cohn JN, Franciosa JA: Vasodilator therapy of cardiac failure. *N Engl J Med* 297:254–258, 1977.
31. Cohn J, Franciosa JA, Francis GS, et al: Effect of short term infusion of sodium nitroprusside on mortality rate in acute myocardial infarction complicated by left ventricular failure. Results of a Veterans Administration Cooperative Study. *N Engl J Med* 306:1129–1135, 1982.
32. Cohn JN, Masniro I, Levine TB, Mehta J: Role of vasoconstrictor mechanisms in the control of left ventricular performance of the normal and damaged heart. *Am J Cardiol* 44:1019–1022, 1979.
33. Cohn JN, Mathew KJ, Franciosa JA, Snow JA: Chronic vasodilator therapy in the management of cardiogenic shock and intractable left vasodilator failure. *Ann Intern Med* 81:777–790, 1974.
34. Cohn JN, Johnson G, Ziescher S, et al: A comparison of enalapril with hydralazine-isosorbide dinitrate in the treatment of chronic congestive heart failure. *N Engl J Med* 325:303–310, 1991.
35. CONSENSUS Trial Study Group: Effects of enalapril on mortality in severe congestive heart failure. Results of the Cooperative North Scandinavian Enalapril Survival Study (CONSENSUS). *N Engl J Med* 316:1429–1435, 1987.
36. Cottrell JE, Casthely P, Brodie JO, Patel K, Klein A, Turndorf H: Prevention of nitroprusside-induced cyanide toxicity and hydroxocobalamin. *N Engl J Med* 298:808–811, 1978.
37. DeMaria AN, Vismara LA, Auditore K, Amsterdam EA, Aelis R, Mason DT: Effects of nitroglycerine on left ventricular cavity size and cardiac performance determined by ultrasound in man. *Am J Med* 57:754–760, 1974.
38. Dent J, Dodds WJ, Arndorfer RC: Effect of nitroprusside and verapamil on esophageal smooth muscle contractility in the opposum. *Gastroenterology* 74:1119, 1978.
39. Desch CE, Magorien RD, Triffon DW, Blanford MF, Unverferth DV, Leier CV: Development of pharmacodynamic tolerance to prazosin in congestive heart failure. *Am J Cardiol* 44:1178–1182, 1979.
40. Durrer JD, Lie KI, Van Capelle FJL, Durrer D: Effect of sodium nitroprusside on mortality in acute myocardial infarction. *N Engl J Med* 306:1121–1128, 1982.
41. Dzau VJ, Colucci WS, Williams GH, Curfoman G, Meggs L, Hollenberg NK: Sustained effectiveness of converting-enzyme inhibition in patients with severe congestive heart failure. *N Engl J Med* 302:1373–1379, 1980.
42. Finkelstein SM, Collins VR: Vascular hemodynamic impedance measurement. *Prog Cardiovasc Dis* 24:401–418, 1982.
43. Flaherty JT, Becker LC, Bulkley BH, Weiss JL, Gersten-Weisfeldt ML: A randomized prospective trial of intravenous nitroglycerin in patients with acute myocardial infarction. *Circulation* 68:576–588, 1983.
44. Franciosa JA: Effectiveness of long-term vasodilator administration in the treatment of chronic left ventricular failure. *Prog Cardiovasc Dis* 24:319–330, 1982.
45. Franciosa JA, Blank RC, Cohn JN, Miculec E: Hemodynamic effects of topical, oral and sublingual nitroglycerin in left ventricular failure. *Curr Ther Res* 22:231–245, 1977.
46. Franciosa JA, Blank RC, Cohn JN: Nitrate effects on cardiac output and left ventricular outflow resistance in chronic congestive heart failure. *Am J Med* 64:207–213, 1978.
47. Franciosa JA, Cohn JN: Effects of minoxidil on hemodynamics in patients with congestive heart failure. *Circulation* 63:652–657, 1981.
48. Franciosa JA, Cohn JN: Sustained hemodynamic effects without tolerance during long-term isosorbide dinitrate treatment of chronic left ventricular failure. *Am J Cardiol* 45:648–654, 1980.
49. Franciosa JA, Cuiha NH, Limas CJ, Rodriguera E, Cohn JN: Improved left ventricular function during nitroprusside infusion in acute myocardial infarction. *Lancet* 1:650–654, 1972.
50. Gaffney TF, Braunwald E: Importance of the adrenergic nervous system in the support of circulatory function in patients with congestive heart failure. *Am J Med* 34:320–324, 1963.
51. Gilmore E, Weil J, Chidsey C: Treatment of essential hypertension with a new vasodilator in combination with beta-adrenergic blockade. *N Engl J Med* 282:521–531, 1970.
52. Goldberg S, Mann T, Grossman W: Nitrate therapy of heart failure in valvular heart disease. Importance of resting level of peripheral vascular resistance in determining cardiac output response. *Am J Med* 65:161–166, 1978.
53. Goldstein RE: Coronary vascular responses to vasodilator drugs. *Prog Cardiovasc Dis* 24:419–436, 1982.
54. Gomes JAC, Carambas CR, Moran HE: The effect of isosorbide dinitrate on left ventricular size, wall stress and left ventricular function in the chronic refractory heart failure. *Am J Med* 65:794–801, 1978.
55. Goodman DJ, Rossen RM, Holloway FL, Alderman EF, Harrison DC: Effect of nitroprusside on left ventricular dynamics in mitral regurgitation. *Circulation* 50:1025–1032, 1974.
56. Gould L, Zahir M, Ettinger S: Phentolamine and cardiovascular performance. *Br Heart J* 31:154–162, 1969.
57. Graham RM, Oats HF, Stoker LM, Stokes GS: Alpha blocking action of the antihypertensive agent, prazosin. *J Pharmacol Exp Ther* 201:747–762, 1977.
58. Graham RM, Pettinger WA: Prazosin. *N Engl J Med* 300:232–236, 1979.
59. Grossman W, Harshaw CW, Munro AB, Becker L, McLaurin LP: Lowered aortic impedance as therapy for severe mitral regurgitation. *JAMA* 230:1011–1013, 1974.
60. Grossman W, McLaurin LP: Clinical measurement of vascular resistance and assessment of vasodilator drugs. In Grossman W (ed): *Cardiac Catheterization and Angiography*, ed 2. Philadelphia, Lea & Febiger, 1980.
61. Guiha NH, Cohn JN, Mikulic E: Treatment of refractory heart failure with infusion of nitroprusside. *N Engl J Med* 291:587–592, 1974.
62. Harper RW, Gold HK, Leinbach RC: Acute myocardial infarction. In Harper E, Austen WC (eds): *The Practice of Cardiology*. Boston, Little, Brown & Co, 1980.
63. Harshaw CW, Grossman W, Munro AB, McLaurin LP: Reduced systemic vascular resistance as therapy for severe mitral regurgitation of valvular origin. *Ann Intern Med* 83:312–316, 1975.
64. Helfant RH, Banka VS, Bodenheimer MM: Left ventricular dysfunction in coronary heart disease: a dynamic problem. *Cardiovasc Med* 2:557–571, 1977.
65. Herman MV, Heinle RA, Klein MD, Gorlin R: Localized disorders in myocardial contraction. *N Engl J Med* 277:222–232, 1967.
66. Higgins CB, Vatner SF, Franklin D, Braunwald E: Extent of regulation of the heart's contractile state in the conscious dog by alteration in the frequency of contraction. *J Clin Invest* 52:1187–1194, 1973.
67. Jaffe AS, Geltman EM, Tiefenbrunn AJ, Ambos HD, Strauss HD, Sobel BE, Roberts R: Reduction of infarct size in patients with inferior infarction with intravenous glycerol trinitrate. A randomized study. *Br Heart J* 49:452–460, 1983.
68. Johnson CC: The actions and toxicity of sodium nitroprusside. *Arch Int Pharmacodyn Ther* 35:481–482, 1929.
69. Jugdutt BI, Warnica JW: Intravenous nitroglycerin therapy to limit myocardial infarct size, expansion, and complications. Effect of timing, dosage, and infarct location. *Circulation* 78:906–917, 1988.
70. Jugdutt BI, Sussex BA, Warnica JW, Rossall RE: Persistent reduction in left ventricular asynergy in patients with acute myocardial infarction by intravenous infusion of nitroglycerin. *Circulation* 68:1264–1273, 1983.
71. Kluger J, Cody RF, Smith V, Laragh JH: Comparative hemodynamic effects and humoral correlations of prazosin and captopril in heart failure. *Clin Res* 29:215A, 1981.
72. Koch-Weser J: Hydralazine. *N Engl J Med* 295:320–323, 1976.
73. Leier CV, Magorien RD, Desch CE, Thompson MJ, Unverferth DV: Hydralazine and isosorbide dinitrate: comparative central and regional hemodynamic effects when administered alone or in combination. *Circulation* 63:102–107, 1981.
74. Levin RI, Weksler BB, Jaffe EA: Nitroglycerin induces production of prostacyclin by human endothelial cells. *Clin Res* 28:471A, 1980.
75. Levine TB, Franciosa JA, Cohn JN: Acute and long-term response to an oral converting-enzyme inhibitor, captopril, in congestive heart failure. *Circulation* 62:35–41, 1980.
76. Liedtke AJ, Buoncristiani JF, Kirk ES, Sonnenblick EH, Urschel CW: Regulation of cardiac output after administration of isoproterenol and ouabain: interactions of systolic impedance and contractility. *Cardiovasc Res* 56:325–332, 1972.
77. Ludbrook PA, Byrne JD, Kurnik PB, McKnight RC: Influence of reduction of preload and afterload by nitroglycerin on left ventricular diastolic pressure-volume relations and relaxation in man. *Circulation* 56:937–943, 1977.
78. Ludbrook PA, Byrne JD, McKnight RC: Influence of right ventricular diastolic pressure-volume relations in man. *Circulation* 59:21–31, 1979.
79. Lukes SA, Romero CA, Resnekov L: Hemodynamic effects of sodium nitroprusside in 21 subjects with congestive heart failure. *Br Heart J* 41:187–191, 1979.
80. Magrini F, Niarchos AP: Ineffectiveness of sublingual nitroglycerin in acute left ventricular failure in the presence of massive peripheral edema. *Am J Cardiol* 45:841–847, 1980.
81. Majid PA, Sharma B, Taylor SH: Phentolamine for vasodilator treatment of severe heart-failure. *Lancet* 22:719–726, 1971.
82. Mason DT: Afterload reduction and cardiac performance. *Am J Med* 65:106–107, 1978.
83. Massie B, Chatterjee K, Werner J, Greenberg B, Hart R, Parmley WW: Hemodynamic advantage of combined administration of hydralazine orally and nitrates nonparenterally in the vasodilator therapy of chronic heart failure. *Am J Cardiol* 40:794–801, 1977.
84. Massie BM, Kramer B, Shen E, Haughloom F: Vasodilator treatment with isosorbide dinitrate and hydralazine in chronic heart failure. *Br Heart J* 45:376, 1981.
85. Miller RR, Awan NA, Joyce JA: Combined dopamine and nitroprusside therapy in congestive heart failure. Greater augmentation of cardiac performance by addition of inotropic stimulation to afterload reduction. *Circulation* 55:881–884, 1977.

86. Miller RR, Fennell WH, Young JB, Palomo AR, Quinones MA: Differential systemic arterial and venous actions and consequent cardiac effects of vasodilator drugs. *Prog Cardiovasc Dis* 24:353–374, 1982.

87. Miller RR, Vismara LA, DeMaria AN, Salel AF, Mason DT: Afterload reduction therapy with nitroprusside in severe aortic regurgitation: improved cardiac performance and reduced regurgitant volume. *Am J Cardiol* 38:564–567, 1976.

88. Miller RR, Vismara LA, Zelis R, Amsterdam EA, Mason DT: Clinical use of sodium nitroprusside in chronic ischemic heart disease. *Circulation* 51:328–336, 1975.

89. Milnor WR: Arterial impedance as ventricular afterload. *Circ Res* 36:565–570, 1975.

90. Mookherjee S, Henion W, Warner R, Erch RH, Smulyan H, Obeid AI: Sodium nitroprusside therapy in congestive cardiomyopathy: variability in hemodynamic response. *J Clin Pharmacol* 18:67–75, 1978.

91. Mookherjee S, Keighley JFH, Warner RA, Bowser MA, Obeid AI: Hemodynamic, ventriculatory and blood gas changes during infusion of sodium nitroferricyanide (nitroprusside). *Chest* 72:273–278, 1977.

92. Nichols WW, Pepine CJ: Left ventricular afterload and aortic input impedance: implications of pulsatile blood flow. *Prog Cardiovasc Dis* 24:293–306, 1982.

93. The SOLVD Investigators: Effect of enalapril on survival in patients with reduced left ventricular ejection fractions and congestive heart failure. *N Engl J Med* 325:293–302, 1991.

94. Packer M, Leier CV: Survival in congestive heart failure during treatment with drugs with positive inotropic actions. *Circulation* 75(suppl IV):IV-55, 1987.

95. Packer M, LeJemtel TH: Physiologic and pharmacologic determinants of vasodilator response: a conceptual framework for rational drug therapy for chronic heart failure. *Prog Cardiovasc Dis* 24:275–292, 1982.

96. Packer M, Meller J, Gorlin R, Herman MV: Hemodynamic and clinical tachyphylaxis to prazosin mediated afterload reduction in severe chronic congestive heart failure. *Circulation* 59:531–539, 1979.

97. Packer M, Meller J, Medine N, Gorlin R, Herman MV: Dose requirements of hydralazine in patients with severe chronic congestive heart failure. *Am J Cardiol* 45:655–660, 1980.

98. Packer M, Meller J, Medina N, Gorlin R, Herman MV: Hemodynamic evaluation of hydralazine dosage in refractory heart failure. *Clin Pharmacol Ther* 27:337–346, 1980.

99. Packer M, Meller J, Medina N, Gorlin R, Herman MV: Rebound hemodynamic events after the abrupt withdrawal of nitroprusside in patients with severe chronic heart failure. *N Engl J Med* 301:1193–1197, 1979.

100. Packer M, Meller J, Medine N, Yushak M, Gorlin R: Determinants of drug response in severe chronic heart failure. I. Activation of vasoconstrictor forces during vasodilator therapy. *Circulation* 64:506–514, 1981.

101. Packer M, Lee WH, Kessler PD, et al: Prevention and reversal of nitrate tolerance in patients with congestive heart failure. *N Engl J Med* 317:799–804, 1987.

102. Page IH, Corcoran AC, Dustan HP, Kuppanyi T: Cardiovascular actions of sodium nitroprusside in animals and hypertensive patients. *Circulation* 11:188–198, 1955.

103. Palmer RF, Lasseter KC: Sodium nitroprusside. *N Engl J Med* 292:294–497, 1975.

104. Parmley WW, Chatterjee K: Vasodilator therapy. In Harvey P (ed): *Current Problems in Cardiology.* Chicago, Year Book, 1978.

105. Parmley WW, Chuck L, Chatterjee K, Swan HJC, Klausner SC, Glantz SA, Ratshin RA: Acute changes in the diastolic pressure volume relationship of the left ventricle. *Eur J Cardiol* 4:105–120, 1976.

106. Pepine CJ, Nichols WW: Aortic input impedance in cardiovascular disease. *Prog Cardiovasc Dis* 24:307–318, 1982.

107. Pepine CJ, Nichols WW, Conti CR: Aortic input impedance in heart failure. *Circulation* 58:460–465, 1978.

108. Petersdorf RG, Dale DC: Gram negative bacteremia and septic shock. In Petersdorf RG, Wilson J. (eds): *Harrison's Textbook of Medicine.* New York, McGraw-Hill, 1980.

109. Pfeffer MA, Braunwald E: Ventricular remodeling after myocardial infarction. Experimental observations and clinical implication. *Circulation* 81:1161–1172, 1990.

110. Pierpont G, Hale KA, Franciosa JA, Cohen JN: Effects of vasodilators on pulmonary hemodynamics in gas exchange in left ventricular failure. *Am Heart J* 99:208–216, 1980.

111. Polese A, Fiorentine C, Olivari MT, Guazzi MD: Clinical use of a calcium antagonistic agent (nifedipine) in acute pulmonary edema. *Am J Med* 66:825–830, 1979.

112. Ribner HS, Breshnan D, Hsieh A, Silverman R, Tommaso C, Coath A, Askenazi J: Acute hemodynamic responses to vasodilator therapy in congestive heart failure. *Prog Cardiovasc Dis* 25:1–45, 1982.

113. Sarnoff SJ, Farr HW: Spinal anesthesia in the therapy of pulmonary edema: a preliminary report. *Anesthesiology* 5:69–76, 1944.

114. Schlant RC: Altered cardiovascular physiology of coronary atherosclerotic disease. In Hurst JW, Logue RB, Schlant RC (eds): *The Heart.* New York, McGraw-Hill, 1978.

115. Scivolett R, Toledo AJO, Gomes Da Silva AC, Nigro D: Mechanism of the hypotensive effect of prazosin. *Arch Int Pharmacodyn Ther* 223:333–338, 1976.

116. Sonnenblick EH: Force velocity relations in mammalian heart muscle. *Am J Physiol* 202:931–936, 1962.

117. Swan HJ, Ganz W, Forrester JS, Marcus H, Diamond G, Chonette D: Catheterization of the heart in man with the use of a flow-directed balloon tip catheter. *N Engl J Med* 283:444–451, 1970.

118. Taylor SH, Sutherland GR, MacKenzie CJ, Staunton HP, Donald KW: The circulatory effects of intravenous phentolamine in man. *Circulation* 31:741–754, 1965.

119. Teckleberg PL, Fitzgerald J, Allaire BI, Alderman EL, Harrison DC: Afterload reduction in the management of post-infarction ventricular septal defect. *Am J Cardiol* 38:956–958, 1976.

120. Transdermal delivery systems for nitroglycerin. *Med Lett Drugs Ther* 24:35, 1982.

121. Warner RA, Bowser M, Zuehlke A, Mookherjee S, Obeid AI: Treatment of acute aortic insufficiency with sodium nitroferricyanide. *Chest* 72:375–379, 1977.

122. Webb RC, Bohr DF: Regulation of vascular tone, molecular mechanisms. *Prog Cardiovasc Dis* 24:213–242, 1981.

123. Weber KT, Janicki JS, Hunter WC, Shroff S, Perlman ES, Fishman AP: The contractile behavior of the heart and its functional coupling of the circulation. *Prog Cardiovasc Dis* 24:375–400, 1982.

124. Weber KT, Janicki JS, Reeves RC: Determinants of stroke volume in the isolated canine heart. *J Appl Physiol* 37:742–746, 1974.

125. Yoran C, Yellin EL, Becker RM, Gabbay S, Frater R, Sonnenblick EH: Mechanism of reduction of mitral regurgitation with vasodilator therapy. *Am J Cardiol* 43:773–777, 1979.

126. Zelis R: The contribution of local factors to the elevated venous tone of congestive heart failure. *J Clin Invest* 54:219–224, 1974.

127. Zelis R, Delea CS, Coleman HN, Mason DT: Arterial sodium content in experimental congestive heart failure. *Circulation* 41:213–224, 1970.

128. Zelis R, Flaim SF: Alterations in vasomotor tone in congestive heart failure. *Prog Cardiovasc Dis* 24:437–459, 1982.

129. Zelis R, Lee G, Mason DT: Influence of experimental edema on metabolically determined blood flow. *Circ Res* 34:482–490, 1974.

130. Zelis R, Mason DT, Braunwald E: A comparison of the effects of vasodilator stimuli on peripheral resistance vessels in normal subjects and in patients with congestive heart failure. *J Clin Invest* 47:960–970, 1968.

131. Zelis R, Nellis SH, Longhurst J: Abnormalities in the regional circulations accompanying congestive heart failure. *Prog Cardiovasc Dis* 18:181–197, 1975.

CHAPTER 29

Pharmacologic Approach to Acute Seizures and Antiepileptic Drugs

BRIAN LITT, M.D.
GREGORY L. KRAUSS, M.D.

OVERVIEW

In this chapter we present pharmacologic principles and practical guidelines for managing acute seizures in the critical care setting. We will focus on:

(1) The major types of seizures encountered in the ICU, their pathophysiology, clinical manifestations, treatment, and how seizure type affects prognosis and choice of antiepileptic drugs;

(2) Antiepileptic drugs (AEDs) that are useful in critical care management, their properties, interactions, and practical suggestions for their effective use;

(3) An introduction to the pathophysiology and classification of types of acute seizures and status epilepticus;

(4) Medical conditions frequently encountered in critical care units that require special consideration with regard to management and AED treatment.

CLINICAL DIAGNOSIS AND THE BASIS OF EPILEPSY

Seizures are a frequent problem in critically ill patients, both as a reason for hospital admission and as a complication of underlying brain or systemic pathology. In one study of 1850 patients admitted to the medical intensive care unit at Rush-Presbyterian-St. Luke's Medical Center in Chicago, over 28% of the patients who had neurologic complications of primarily nonneurologic disease had seizures (1). The most common mechanisms involved in epileptogenesis in the critical care setting are outlined in Table 29.1 below.

Other factors that may promote seizures, particularly in those patients with known seizure disorders, are fever, stress, sleep deprivation, exercise, and being in the perimenstrual period. In the critical care setting epileptogenesis is often multifactorial. The contribution of multiple factors to causing seizures is expressed as the notion of a seizure threshold.

> *Seizure threshold:* A limit beyond which anyone can be made to seize, when subjected to a sufficient number of epileptogenic factors.

Normal individuals have a higher seizure threshold, that is, they require more or stronger epileptogenic factors to make them seize than do people predisposed toward seizures, such as those with a history of CNS infection, brain injury, or epilepsy. All of the processes listed in Table 29.1 can lower the seizure threshold. This list is not exhaustive, and there are other precipitants, such as hyperventilation and photic stimulation, that may be related to seizure type.

> A guiding principle of seizure prophylaxis and treatment is to minimize the number of factors that lower the seizure threshold.

BACKGROUND AND TERMINOLOGY

Focal seizures begin in a region of brain, usually cortical, in which the usual balance between excitatory and inhibitory

Table 29.1. Common Causes of Seizures in Critically Ill Patients

Condition	Examples
Mechanical brain injury	Trauma, neurosurgery, SAH/ICH[a]
Hypoxic/ischemic insult	Stroke, hemorrhage, shock, cardiac arrest, cerebral edema
CNS infection	Meningitis, encephalitis, (especially herpes simplex), abscess, sepsis
Metabolic disorders	Electrolyte abnormalities (low Na, low Mg, high Ca), hepatic failure, renal failure, hypo- or hyperglycemia, very rare genetic disorders
Drug sensitivity/toxicity	Theophylline, phenothiazines, alcohol, cocaine
Idiopathic epilepsy	Absence, complex partial
Seizure prone states	Alcohol abuse, eclampsia, drug withdrawal
Electric shock	Lightning, electroconvulsive therapy (ECT)
Tumor	Primary brain, metastases, other

[a] SAH, subarachnoid hemorrhage; ICH, intracranial hemorrhage; CNS, central nervous system.

influences has been disturbed. This type of seizure may be triggered by a number of stimuli, such as trauma, infection, or toxins (see Table 29.1). The area of brain generating epileptiform activity is called the **epileptic focus,** a volume of tissue thought to contain thousands of cells, though its actual size remains in debate. Under normal conditions focal seizure activity is limited to this volume, though circumstances that diminish seizure threshold may propagate activity to other regions of brain. Seizures may then *generalize,* or spread throughout the entire cortical mantle.

Focal seizure activity is frequently asymptomatic, depending upon its site of origin and upon its duration. For example, clinical observations indicate that focal seizure activity must be, depending upon its location, sustained for seconds (often between 10 and 30 seconds) before it becomes symptomatic. Clinical manifestations of seizures vary greatly and may present with any movement or sensation that normal brain can generate. For example, focal activity in the hand area of the precentral gyrus may present with uncontrolled contralateral hand movements; laughing, crying, anger, or fear may emanate from limbic foci; sensations of amorphous flashes of light (phosphenes) may emanate from occipital foci; and medial temporal foci may generate impairment of consciousness with or without mechanical-like movements, such as eye blinking, picking movements, lip smacking, or meaningless repetitive movements (automatisms). Widespread seizure activity may present with generalized tonic-clonic (GTC) activity, subtle confusion, automatisms, or no clinical activity at all (generalized nonconvulsive seizures) (2).

In addition to the clinical manifestations of seizures, EEG findings vary according to seizure type, in both the location and form of epileptiform activity. Classifying seizures according to their clinical manifestations and EEG findings is useful, as treatment and prognosis are often a function of seizure type. The most commonly used classification, at present, is the scheme put forth in 1981 by the International League against Epilepsy and revised in 1985 (3, 4). This scheme is based primarily upon the clinical manifestations of seizures and separates seizure types according to the following questions:

Is consciousness impaired?

Simple seizures: Consciousness is not impaired.
Complex seizures: Consciousness is impaired (though patients may still respond).

Are the seizures focal or generalized in origin?

Partial (focal) seizures: Focal in origin, may spread after a time, sometimes throughout the entire brain (called secondary generalization).

Generalized seizures: Erupt over the entire brain at once. Have many different forms (e.g., absence, tonic-clonic, tonic, clonic, atonic, myoclonic, etc.).

Unclassified seizures: Not easily separable into the above categories.

Seizures are usually short-lived and limited to several minutes of clinical electrical activity (the ictal period). Seizures that are prolonged, or come in rapid succession without the patient regaining consciousness, may present a life-threatening emergency called *status epilepticus.*

Status Epilepticus

Status epilepticus (SE) has been defined by prolonged or repeated seizures leading to a "fixed and lasting epileptic condition" (3). The condition is practically defined as sustained seizure activity, or repeated seizures without the patient regaining consciousness, for 15 to 30 minutes or longer. The exact time at which status begins is in debate, and is based upon animal data that suggest 30 minutes of sustained seizure activity as the time beyond which irreversible neuronal injury takes place (5, 6). Any seizure type may give rise to status epilepticus. Some specific types of SE that are of particular importance in critical care are described later in this chapter.

Postictal Phenomena

Prolonged seizure (ictal) activity may be followed by a period of decreased function in the distribution of seizing neurons, usually lasting up to 48 hours, though after bouts of status epilepticus deficits may take several days to resolve. A transient deficit resulting from seizure activity is usually called a postictal state. "Todd's paralysis" is an example of a postictal state characterized by a motor weakness in the distribution of muscles innervated by seizing motor neurons (7). Other examples of postictal phenomena include transient blindness after an occipital seizure and loss of memory after a complex partial seizure originating in the temporal lobe. Generalized seizures may be followed by minutes to hours of sleep, confusion, or unresponsiveness.

One dilemma in acute seizure management is determining whether or not a neurologic deficit after a seizure is due to a postictal state, which will resolve on its own, or another process that may require immediate treatment. This task is complicated by the fact that fever, headache, and disorientation may be normal sequela of seizures. Three rules of thumb for approaching this question are: (*a*) In the critically ill patient, a postictal state is a diagnosis of exclusion; other causes of postictal deficits must be investigated. (*b*) Any postictal state lasting more than 24 hours must be investigated aggressively for other causes. (*c*) Any postictal fever in a critically ill patient must be investigated as a new, unexplained fever. Postictal fever is a diagnosis of exclusion.

COMMON SEIZURE TYPES ENCOUNTERED IN THE CRITICALLY ILL PATIENT

Simple Partial (Focal) Seizures

These seizures usually result from focal cerebral injury but may also be triggered by systemic processes, such as hypoglycemia. They may present with any signs or symptoms that normal brain can generate, such as simple motor, sensory or special sensory phenomena (olfactory, visual, etc.). Simple partial seizures are a common manifestation of focal cortical injury, such as that caused by tumor, trauma, infection, or stroke. EEG may or may not show focal epileptiform discharges (spikes or sharp waves) during and between seizures (interictal). When prolonged or repeated, they give rise to simple partial status epilepticus. Simple partial status, also called *epilepsy partialis continua*, can be difficult to control in some patients, sometimes requiring multiple AEDs or surgical excision of a focal lesion (2).

Complex Partial Seizures (CPS)

This is the most common seizure type in adults. They are manifested by a disturbance of consciousness often accompanied by staring and mechanical behaviors called automatisms, such as lip smacking, picking at clothing or bed clothes, and eye blinking. CPS usually originate from temporal more frequently than frontal lobe foci, areas that are especially vulnerable to trauma and ischemic injury (8, 9). EEGs often show focal interictal discharges over the affected region, but deep temporal or frontal foci may be electrically silent on scalp EEG. Seizures often begin with a warning, or aura, consisting of a strange smell or taste, sense of fear, falling, ringing in the ears (tinnitus), movement in space or, most commonly, as a strange feeling in the abdomen. Auras are actually focal seizure activity in regions that control the sensations that they produce. Recent experience with intracranial recording has demonstrated that focal seizure activity must be, depending on its location, sustained for seconds (often 10–30 seconds) before it is perceived as an aura by patients. Complex partial seizures may be prolonged, giving rise to complex partial status epilepticus. If left untreated, complex partial status may result in cognitive impairment, memory loss, personality changes, and behavioral disturbances (10, 11).

Generalized Tonic-Clonic (GTC) Seizures

Generalized tonic-clonic seizures are common in the intensive care setting and may have many potential etiologies. These seizures usually result from regions of focal cortical injury, which trigger partial seizures that then secondary generalize. GTC seizures may also *begin* as generalized events, emanating from as yet undefined subcortical structures. Patients may or may not report an aura (usually with secondarily generalized partial seizures). Loss of consciousness occurs early, followed by a variable tonic phase, characterized by global rigidity. This phase is followed by synchronous, repeated clonic movements. There is usually a postictal period of sleep, confusion, and amnesia for the event. Tongue biting and urinary incontinence are common. Generalized tonic-clonic seizures form the most common type of status epilepticus (12), a life-threatening emergency, which may result in neuronal injury and death (13).

Absence Seizures (a Type of Generalized Seizure)

These seizures are of two types. Childhood absence, the most common form in the community, usually begins in the first or second decade of life and is marked by multiple brief episodes of staring, up to hundreds of times per day, without loss of body tone. Spells are sometimes accompanied by automatisms. EEGs show a classical generalized 3/second spike and slow wave pattern, with frontocentral maximum (14). Absence seizures commonly resolve with age but may persist into adulthood. When they progress to status epilepticus, they usually respond to treatment with low-dose benzodiazepines. Patients with a history of childhood absence epilepsy form a small minority of patients in the critical care setting with absence status epilepticus (15).

In critical care units, absence status epilepticus occurs most often in elderly patients with no prior seizure history (16, 17). It is most commonly caused by toxic or metabolic processes and has a characteristic EEG, which shows a slow 1.5 to 2.5/sec spike and wave pattern that may be irregular and demonstrate some focality (14, 18, 19). Patients with this condition appear confused, are variably responsive, and may or may not display automatisms. This state may persist for long periods of time, (up to months in one report) before it is detected (18, 20).

Myoclonic Seizures (a Type of Generalized Seizure)

These seizures occur primarily in two settings: (*a*) in patients with a history of myoclonic epilepsy and (*b*) in ICU patients with toxic/metabolic disorders or after anoxic-ischemic injury, such as cardiac arrest. In patients with a history of myoclonic epilepsy, seizures consist of focal or generalized rapid, uncontrolled muscle movements, which are usually synchronous. Consciousness may or may not be impaired. EEGs show irregular spikes and polyspikes that may be focal, multifocal, or generalized (21). When these patients present with uncontrolled seizures, prognosis for full recovery is good with proper treatment (22).

Approximately 17% of patients who experience anoxic-ischemic injury that results in coma develop focal, multifocal, or generalized periodic myoclonic movements, often eye blinking, chewing movements, or multifocal twitching (10). The EEG shows one of several characteristic patterns: burst-suppression; suppression; or periodic generalized discharges (22). Prognosis for meaningful recovery is poor. Postanoxic myoclonus is notoriously difficult to control and may be continuous, giving rise to myoclonic status epilepticus. This problem will be discussed in more detail below.

Pseudoseizures

These are episodes of clinical seizure-like activity that do not result from abnormal electrochemical activity in the brain. The most common forms in the ICU are psychogenic seizures and decerebrate or decorticate posturing. Posturing can usually be distinguished from seizure activity by history and careful neurologic examination. Psychogenic seizures are a potentially life-threatening condition, due to iatrogenic morbidity from attempts to control seizures. Psychogenic seizures may progress to psychogenic status epilepticus, resulting in ICU admission, intubation, and treatment with high-dose AEDs.

Patients with psychogenic seizures may sometimes be distinguished by a history of psychiatric disease, an unusual medical history, or an atypical response to antiepileptic drugs. Clinically, they present most commonly with unresponsiveness and minor movements, though sometimes they may present with generalized tonic-clonic movements. Features that are sometimes reliable are side-to-side head movements, asynchronous motor movements, pelvic thrusting, forced eye closure, guarding of the face when presumed unresponsive, and alerting to stimuli during generalized tonic-clonic activity. A further challenge to the clinician results from the fact that up to 20% or more of patients with psychogenic seizures may also have real seizures (23–25).

SECOND INTERNATIONAL CLASSIFICATION SCHEME

Another classification scheme that has become more popular among epileptologists over the past several years arises from our growing experience with intracranial recordings of seizures and localization of sources of epileptiform activity. This system was first proposed by the ILAE Commission on Classification and Terminology in 1985 and was revised in 1989 (2, 4). This system divides the major epilepsies as follows.

Localization-related Epilepsies and Syndromes

These are seizure types that occur in cortical regions whose function is known and easily recognized. For example, as above, seizures arising from the visual cortex begin with disturbances of vision; temporal lobe seizures may begin with olfactory auras, déja vu, or auditory symptoms.

Generalized Epilepsies and Syndromes

These also have many different forms, such as the staring spells characteristic of absence seizures, primary generalized tonic-clonic seizures, myoclonic seizures, etc.

Epilepsies and Syndromes, Determined Whether Focal or Generalized

This is an area currently under intense investigation.

Special Syndromes (e.g., Lennox-Gastaut, Hypsarrhythmia)

With this basic background, we will now briefly review some basic neurobiology before approaching the management of seizures in critically ill patients. This information will be useful when discussing the mechanisms of action of many clinically important antiepileptic drugs (AEDs).

BACK TO BASICS (THE CELLULAR STORY)

Normal brain function requires a balance of excitatory and inhibitory processes. The major excitatory neurotransmitter in the brain is glutamate; the major inhibitory neurotransmitter is gamma-aminobutyric acid (GABA). There are a large number of active peptides in the CNS, mostly inhibitory, many of which work through membrane-bound second messenger systems (26).

Seizures can result from increasing or deregulating excitatory function or decreasing or deregulating inhibitory function. Some ways in which this can occur are through alterations in:

1. Neuronal structure (e.g., trauma);
2. Electrolyte flux;
3. Ion channel function;
4. Neurotransmitters and/or their receptors;
5. Second messenger systems (e.g., membrane-bound enzyme systems acting through cyclic AMP or GMP).

The major ions involved in epileptic phenomena are sodium and calcium (mostly extracellular), potassium (mostly intracellular), chloride (equally distributed), and magnesium (acting primarily at the channel and enzyme level). Neurons communicate electrochemically, among other ways, via action potentials, which can be triggered by mechanical, electrical, or chemical stimuli. Action potentials are asynchronous and integrated at target neurons into postsynaptic potentials (PSPs). Seizure activity results from synchronous volleys of excitatory postsynaptic potentials (EPSPs) and disruption of the normal pattern of inhibitory postsynaptic potentials (IPSPs). Lowering membrane potential (hyperpolarization) makes action potentials less likely. Increasing membrane potential (depolarization) triggers action potentials when the membrane potential surpasses a threshold value.

Ion channels are **glycoproteins** imbedded in the cell membrane that, when activated, can change their configuration to create pores through which ions flow. Ion channels usually fall into four categories, depending upon what stimulus triggers them: mechanically sensitive; voltage-sensitive; chemically (e.g. neurotransmitter) activated; and those activated by changes in the intracellular milieu (usually direct channels between adjacent cells, called gap junctions). Chemically sensitive channels usually exist as part of receptor-channel complexes. Two important examples of receptor-channel complexes relevant to our discussion of epileptogenesis are the glutamate-sensitive sodium channel and the GABA-activated chloride channel (5, 27).

Channels tied to the GABA receptor also contain receptors for benzodiazepines and barbiturates, two potent classes of AEDs. When GABA, or a compound in one of these AED classes, binds to this receptor-channel complex, the channel opens and allows an influx of chloride ions, lowering the membrane potential.

Channels tied to the glutamate receptor have multiple subtypes, some of which also contain receptors for N-methyl-D-aspartate (NMDA) or kainic acid, both potent epileptogenic agents. Stimulation of this receptor-channel complex triggers a rapid influx of sodium and calcium and generation of excitatory postsynaptic potentials. Calcium influx activates a number of intracellular pathways, triggering proteases, lipases, mitochondrial enzymes, and further NMDA receptor activation, all of which can result in excitotoxic cell injury when stimulated excessively (28). Many of these channels also contain receptors for the agents PCP, ketamine, or MK-801, which block channel function and may be protective to the cell (5, 28, 29). These agents have been the target of research into a number of new agents to prevent the excitotoxic cell injury that results from prolonged seizure activity or ischemia.

KINETICS: A FEW PERTINENT PRINCIPLES

Below are a few key concepts directly relevant to acute seizure therapy. In the drug section below, specific aspects of each drug described will be outlined. Good references for reviewing these concepts are Goodman and Gilman's *The Pharmacological Basis of Therapeutics* and the article, Pharmacokinetics of Antiepileptic Drugs, by Scheyer and Cramer, referenced at the end of this chapter (30, 31).

BLOOD-BRAIN BARRIER

Tight junctions between endothelial cells in brain capillaries and between glial cell membranes surrounding these capillaries restrict the passage of organic acids and bases into the cerebrospinal fluid (CSF) and extracellular fluid of the brain parenchyma. Lipid-soluble compounds pass through the blood-brain barrier with relative ease, their diffusion limited primarily by brain blood flow. The blood-brain barrier and its permeability to lipid-soluble compounds accounts for the slow onset of action of many AEDs, such as phenytoin and carbamazepine, and the rapid onset of lipid-soluble agents, such as benzodiazepines and barbiturates (30).

BIOAVAILABILITY

Bioavailability is loosely defined as the amount of therapeutically effective (active) drug delivered to the target tissue, in this case the brain, for a particular dose of drug. Bioavailability varies, depending upon drug preparation, route of administration, and the specific biochemical milieu at the time of administration. In the acute seizure patient it is important that the bioavailability of a specific AED be known and reliable. Bioavailability in acute seizure therapy is usually guaranteed by administering standard preparations of medications intravenously, or intramuscularly in rare cases, and restricting conditions that may inhibit systemic drug absorption, penetration into, or action in the brain. Examples of situations that may alter bioavailability in the acute care setting are the decreased bioavailability of oral phenytoin in the presence of continuous enteral feedings and the increased bioavailability of benzodiazepines in the presence of alcohol or metoclopramide (30).

ENZYME INDUCTION AND INCREASED METABOLISM

A number of AEDs that are metabolized by the liver increase the production of microsomal enzymes that metabolize them. This increase can occur as rapidly as over several days with some medications. Increased metabolism causes a gradual decline in serum and brain levels of AEDs and necessitates frequent monitoring of AED drug levels during treatment. For example, the metabolism of pentobarbital increases over several days when it is administered in high doses for refractory status epilepticus (32). Some drugs may compete for or inhibit metabolic enzymes that act on other agents, resulting in decreased metabolism and, therefore, increased serum levels of the initial agent. An example of this interaction is the inhibited metabolism of phenobarbital by valproic acid (2, 33).

PROTEIN BINDING AND DISPLACEMENT

Most AEDs are at least partially protein-bound, usually to albumin and other plasma proteins. If protein binding is altered by disease, as is frequent in critically ill patients, drug levels may change substantially. The bound fraction of drug is generally not accessible to the central nervous system (CNS), making the free drug level a more reliable measure of active compound. This measurement becomes important when multiple drugs compete for protein binding, and in metabolic states such as renal failure, where a metabolic by-product displaces bound drug, altering free serum and consequently brain drug levels. An important example of this phenomenon is the displacement of phenytoin from albumin by urea in patients with renal failure. This displacement results in increased free phenytoin levels and greater potential drug toxicity. There are a number of conditions, such as renal and hepatic failure, and in multiple-drug therapy in which the free levels of agents, such as phenytoin and valproic acid, may be useful. These conditions are discussed in the section on specific diseases below (34).

Booker and Darcey have demonstrated that free levels correlate much better with clinical toxicity than do total drug levels (35). At present, in many centers free levels may be difficult to obtain in a timely enough fashion to be clinically useful in the acute setting. Free level monitoring may become more useful as its timely availability increases.

VOLUME OF DISTRIBUTION AND REDISTRIBUTION

The apparent volume of distribution (V_d) is the ratio of total drug in the body to the concentration of drug in plasma, or the effective volume in which the drug is distributed in the steady state. Antiepileptic drugs may go through different phases of distribution after administration. In the first phase, dependent upon cardiac output, the drug is distributed to organs receiving high blood flow, such as the brain, liver, and kidneys. In the second phase the drug is distributed to other viscera, skin, muscle, and fat. This phase is called redistribution and may trigger a decrease in brain concentration and, consequently, activity of the drug. In a third phase, fat-soluble agents build up in adipose tissue and release drug slowly into the general circulation over time. A number of AEDs used in the acute setting, particularly diazepam, have a rapid second phase of distribution. Valproic acid is an AED that is very fat-soluble and has a significant third phase of distribution.

FIRST-ORDER AND SATURATION KINETICS

Most of the AEDs used in the acute setting obey *first order kinetics* within the therapeutic range: they are metabolized at a constant rate by their degrading enzymes. Some agents, phenytoin in particular, obey *saturation kinetics*. The enzyme that degrades them becomes saturated when the drug is within the therapeutic range, causing serum, then brain levels, to increase rapidly at higher doses. For example, the serum level of phenytoin increases proportionally to the administered dose up to a serum level of approximately 10 μg/ml. Above this value the serum level increases exponentially for the same unit dose that resulted in a linear increase at levels below 10. This is an important point when estimating the amount of drug to administer to patients in different circumstances and in trying to avoid drug toxicity (30).

DRUG LEVELS AND THE CONCEPT OF THERAPEUTIC LEVELS

Therapeutic AED levels are based upon clinical studies that have determined the range of serum concentration at which the majority of seizures were prevented in a population without producing a significant incidence of side effects. What constitutes the "majority of seizures" and an "acceptable range of side effects" are statistically defined. Therapeutic levels for AEDs commonly used in the ICU are recorded in the section on antiepileptic drugs (AEDs) below. Also included are values for the ICU "target level" after an appropriate loading dose, and the usual maximum level, the level beyond which the patient is unlikely to gain any more benefit, or is likely to encounter intolerable side effects.

In practice, "therapeutic level" is defined as the level of medication at which the patient stops seizing.

Often, patients may not reach a "therapeutic level" because a particular AED is not effective for their condition, or side effects limit the amount of the medication they can receive. In the ICU, toxicity is often difficult to assess, because many critically ill patients are debilitated, confused, or unconscious. Levels should be high in the standard therapeutic range and may often exceed the maximum value for ambulatory patients (2, 36). In patients with repeated seizures, but not status epilepticus, medications are usually pushed until either the patient stops having seizures or some maximum blood level

is obtained, before another agent is added. In patients with status epilepticus, stopping seizure activity is the primary concern, and more significant side effects are tolerated, usually for a short time, than in the ambulatory population. The protocol for treatment of status epilepticus written below gives some useful guidelines for antiepileptic drug management.

AED levels are also useful to determine patient compliance, to assess for overdose and effective absorption, and to calculate a patient's rate of metabolism and further dosage requirements.

ANTIEPILEPTIC DRUGS: THE MAJOR AGENTS

Our philosophy in treating the acute seizure patient is to know a few drugs from each class well, particularly their action, administration, side effects, and interactions. While there are many useful agents that could be presented, we have chosen the ones we feel to be most useful, those with which virtually any critically ill seizure patient may be managed. The drugs we have described in depth are diazepam, lorazepam, midazolam, phenytoin, phenobarbital, valproic acid, carbamazepine, and pentobarbital. This section contains a brief discussion of each drug, with important points about its effective and safe use, followed by a series of tables that allow rapid access to useful information on pharmacologic characteristics, dosing, and interactions.

PHENYTOIN

A highly insoluble compound, phenytoin is suspended in a vehicle that contains propylene glycol, ethanol, and sodium hydroxide. With intravenous administration, even at recommended rates, this carrier may cause hypotension, bradycardia, arrhythmias and, rarely, asystole refractory to defibrillation (particularly if it is given as a rapid bolus).

Saturation kinetics:	First order up to level of 10, then 0 order above. Acute dosing depends upon blood level. If level is ~10 or greater, then small increases in dosage yield relatively large increases in blood level.
Binding:	90% protein bound, mostly albumin
V_d:	0.6 to 0.7 liters/kg
Enzyme inducer:	Yes
Metabolism:	95% conjugated in liver, 5% excreted unchanged in urine
Half life:	i.v.: 10 to 15 hr, peak blood levels 20 to 30 min after i.v. dose
	i.m.: Not advised
	p.o.: 22 hr, peak levels 4 to 8 hr after dose
	p.r.: Not advised

Excretion is increased with alkalization of the urine

Fat soluble:	Yes
Target Levels:	
Acute Load	15 to 25 μg/ml
Maintenance	10 to 20 μg/ml
Status epilepticus	20 to 25 μg/ml
Ataxia usually	≥30 μg/ml, usually there is no additional clinical benefit above this level
Lethargy	Usually, ≥40 μg/ml

Administration:

i.v.: Guarantees absorption. Give only in 0.9% saline, no faster than 50 mg/min

p.o.: GI absorption is variable, less useful acutely

i.m.: Slow absorption, crystallizes; not recommended

p.r.: Not recommended

Loading dose = 18 to 20 mg/kg, lean body weight.
Maintenance dose = average of 4 mg/kg/day divided t.i.d. This may vary widely.

Distribution

Peak levels occur 20 to 30 minutes after intravenous dose. Levels decrease rapidly as secondary binding to albumin, muscle, liver, and lung occurs. Levels increase again as these systems saturate. Level in brain is 1 to 3 times total plasma, and 6 to 10 times plasma free levels. Distribution in brain is uneven, more in temporal lobes, hippocampus, superior colliculus.

Mechanisms

Clinical. In animals, phenytoin blocks tonic phase of seizures and blocks the epileptic focus from recruiting surrounding neurons and thereby spreading activity through the cortex. Does not inhibit spread to diencephalon (37, 38).

Biochemical. Blocks sodium channels (inhibiting depolarization), increases Na-K ATPase activity (restores resting potential faster), blocks calcium uptake during depolarization (inhibiting excitation and calcium-dependent second messenger systems), inhibits cyclic AMP- and GMP-dependent processes (second messenger systems), increases Cl⁻-conductance (increases hyperpolarization).

Toxicity

Ataxia, nausea, vomiting, involuntary movements, hypersensitivity, (hepatitis, rash, fever, Stevens-Johnson syndrome, etc.), sedation, confusion may occur. At very high levels (usually ≥30): paralysis, ophthalmoplegia, hallucinations, psychosis, paradoxical excitability and agitation (rare), coma, precipitation/aggravation of systemic lupus erythematosus (SLE), seizures (rare) occur. For drug interactions, see Table 29.2.

PHENOBARBITAL: "THE OLDEST ANTIEPILEPTIC DRUG" (since 1912)

Preparation

The sodium salt is freely soluble in water and has low lipid solubility, so that dosage should be based on "lean mass" in obese patients. The i.v. preparation usually uses a vehicle composed of alcohol and propylene glycol, because phenobarbital is not stable in aqueous solution. The pH of this solution is usually high (8.5 to 10.5) (41) and may be used with any standard i.v. solution (D5, ringers, 0.45% saline, NS etc.). Intravenous preparations are usually not compatible with acidic solutions and may precipitate.

First-order kinetics: Increase in serum level per unit dose is independent of serum concentration.

Binding: 45% protein-bound, mostly to albumin. Rarely displaces or is displaced.

V_d: 0.5 liter/kg, in adults

Enzyme inducer: Yes. *Very potent* microsomal inducer

Note: Induction of microsomal enzymes usually is clinically evident within days to several weeks after starting this potent inducing agent. The amount of enzyme induction varies with the individual and is believed to be genetically determined.

Metabolism: 25% excreted unchanged in the urine, 75% parhydroxylated and conjugated in liver to glucuronic acid, then secreted in bile, reabsorbed, and actively excreted in the urine (42).

Half-life: Mean 90 to 110 hours by all routes.

i.v.:   Onset of action within 5 min, i.v. Maximum effect by 30 min.

i.m.:   Peak plasma concentration usually by 4 hr

p.o.:   Peak plasma concentration usually by 2 hr (longer with decreased GI motility or poor circulation).

p.r.:   More rapid than p.o. if i.v. solution is used. Absorbed in colon. Commercial suppositories may take longer than p.o.

Excretion

Increased with alkalization of the urine, increased urinary flow (42, 43). Activated charcoal via nasogastric tube (NGT) decreases half-life for i.v. phenobarbital from 110 hours to 45 hours (41). Also helps to clear phenobarbital given by other routes. Elimination is slowed in renal or hepatic failure, or when urine is acidified.

Target Levels:		
	Acute load	20 to 25 μg/ml
	Maintenance	10 to 25 μg/ml
	Coma	≥50 μg/ml
	Lethal	≥80 μg/ml

Note: All levels above are approximate guidelines. Levels and effects may vary greatly in tolerant individuals and those on other microsomal enzyme-inducing agents.

Administration:

i.v.:   Most rapid and guaranteed absorption. Give no faster than 100 mg/min.

p.o.:   Slower but complete absorption

i.m.:   Slower absorption than p.o.

p.r.:   May be more rapid than p.o. if i.v. preparation is used.

Loading dose = 20 mg/kg. May require more in acute setting. Beware of respiratory depression and hypotension.

Distribution

Distribution is very sensitive to pH. With alkalosis, phenobarbital is forced extracellularly, and urinary excretion is increased. With acidosis, more drug goes intracellularly, and urinary excretion is decreased. Phenobarbital is not extremely fat-soluble and requires 12 to 15 minutes after administration for maximal brain penetration. The steady-state concentration in brain is equal to the serum-free level. Distribution in brain is more in gray matter at first, then is uniform after several hours. Rate of entry into brain is inversely related to age (37).

Table 29.2. Phenytoin Interactions[a]

Action *Increased by*	*Action* *Decreased by*	*Increases* *Action of*	*Decreases* *Action of*
AEDs			
Pentobarbital	Phenobarbital	Phenobarbital	Phenobarbital
Valproic acid	Valproic acid	Valproic acid	Valproic acid
Carbamazepine	Carbamazepine		Carbamazepine
Primidone	Primidone	Primidone	
Clonazepam	Clonazepam		Clonazepam
Diazepam	Diazepam		
Ethosuxamide			
Methsuxamide			
Felbamate			
Other drugs			
Acute alcohol intake	Antacids with calcium		Antipyrine
Calcium carbimide	Chronic alcohol abuse		Corticosteroids
Cimetidine	Dioxide		Coumarin
Chloramphenical	Folate		Digitoxin
Chlordiazepoxide	Molindone HCl with calcium		Doxycycline
Chlorpheniramine	Pyridoxine		Estrogens
Clofibrate	Reserpine		Furosemide
Dicoumarol			Haloperidol
Disulfiram			Nortryptiline
Estrogens			Oral contracept
Furosemide			Phenylbutazone
Halothane			Pyridoxine
Imipramine			Quinidine
Isoniazid			Rifampin
Methylphenidate			Theophylline
Nortryptiline			Vitamin D
Pheneturide			
Phenothiazines			
Phenylbutazone			
Phenyramidol			
Propoxyphene			
Salicylates			
Sulfonamides			
Tolbutamide			
Trazodone			
Warfarin			

[a] Data taken from references 2, 39, and 40; AEDs, antiepileptic drugs.

Mechanisms

Clinical. Suppresses the discharge of epileptic foci and stops the spread of epileptiform activity to adjacent cortex **AND** the diencephalon (37, 38, 44).

Biochemical. Phenobarbital stimulates GABA-ergic responses and inhibits glutamate-related responses in animals (37, 45, 46), increases mean open time of GABA-sensitive chloride ion channels, increasing chloride conductance and hyperpolarizing the cell membrane (27), it inhibits presynaptic, voltage-dependent calcium uptake in vitro (37, 47, 48), and may decrease cerebral energy metabolism.

Administration

Loading dose is 20 mg/kg.. Give no faster than 60 to 100 mg/min i.v. (bolus may result in severe hypotension or acute respiratory depression). Many sources advocate treating with boluses of 200 mg every 10 to 15 min (each given no faster than over 5 min), and titrating to effect or side effects. Subcutaneous extravasation may cause local reactions from irritation to necrosis. Infiltration with SQ 0.5% procaine hydrochloride in affected region is recommended (41). Intraarterial injection may cause necrosis. Use extreme caution in patients with nephritis (41).

Toxicity

Toxicity primarily results from respiratory depression, coma, and hypotension. Effects are synergistic with those of benzodiazepines. Whenever one administers barbiturates in the ICU, invasive blood pressure, heart rate, and respiratory monitoring must be employed. The majority of patients loaded with this drug emergently require mechanical ventilation. Many require blood pressure support.

Other side effects include confusion and/or paradoxical excitement, insomnia, hyperkinetic activity (elderly and children), nystagmus, dysarthria, ataxia, confusion, depression, hypersensitivity (beware in patients with nephritis), sleepiness, stupor, and coma. Side effects are worse in patients previously unexposed to this drug or cross-reacting compounds (e.g., alcohol, benzodiazepines). Rarely, phenobarbital can precipitate systemic lupus erythematosus (SLE) or aggravate established SLE. Phenobarbital inhibits production of vitamin K-dependent clotting factors, can induce acute attacks of porphyria, and may be hepatotoxic to susceptible individuals. For drug interactions, see Table 29.3.

BENZODIAZEPINES

Agents in this class are usually the first choice for the treatment of ongoing seizures and status epilepticus. They are very lipophilic, efficacious, have rapid onset of action, and are virtually universally available. The three agents discussed below—diazepam, lorazepam, and midazolam—are all very useful and approximately equally effective in the acute care setting. They differ in their duration of anticonvulsant action, amount and duration of sedation, modes of administration and incidence of side effects (50–53). All potentiate the sedative, hypotensive anticonvulsant and respiratory depressant effects of other agents, particularly those that are CNS depressants. Under normal circumstances benzodiazepines are >80% protein bound, and are not dialyzable.

Benzodiazepines are antagonized by flumazenil, a benzodiazepine receptor antagonist, which competitively inhibits benzodiazepines directly at their receptors. As experience with this drug grows, flumazenil may eventually reduce the incidence of side effects, such as respiratory depression and hypotension, resulting from acute seizure therapy (54).

Clinically, benzodiazepines act primarily by inhibiting seizure spread, though there is some evidence that they suppress activity in seizure foci as well. Biochemically, benzodiazepines facilitate both pre- and postsynaptic GABAergic inhibition. They bind to the benzodiazepine receptor of GABA-sensitive chloride channels, increasing mean open time, hyperpolarizing the cell membrane, and enhancing inhibitory function (2, 50, 55, 56).

The benzodiazepines described below are poorly soluble in water, and their carriers may have cardiac depressant or hypotensive effects. Toxicity is similar in all benzodiazepines, and includes ataxia, dysarthria, sedation, fatigue, vertigo, syncope, respiratory depression, coma, cardiac arrest, and anterograde amnesia. Toxicity is worse in children and geriatric patients. Side effects are synergistic with alcohol, barbiturates, narcotics, and other CNS depressants, especially respiratory depression. Rarer side effects include agitation, aggression, paranoid ideation, auditory and visual hallucinations, increased muscle spasticity, hyperreflexia, acute rage reactions, sialorrhea, hiccups, and increased bronchial secretions.

The benzodiazepines discussed below all exhibit biexponential kinetics. In the first phase the drug penetrates rapidly into tissues that are lipid rich and receive high blood flow (e.g., brain). Later, the drug is redistributed to other tissues, resulting in a rapid drop in brain levels. This phenomenon is especially important in the case of diazepam, in which redistribution 15 to 30 after administration frequently results in rapid recurrence of seizures (50).

Target levels are not of much use in the acute administration of benzodiazepines, given the usual lack of rapidly available levels, and the wide variation of tolerance to these medications in the general population.

Table 29.4 below contains important pharmacokinetic and administration information on diazepam, lorazepam, and

Table 29.3.   Phenobarbital Drug Interactions[a]

Action Increased by	Action Decreased by	Increases Action of	Decreases Action of
AEDs			
Phenytoin	Phenytoin	Phenytoin	Phenytoin
Methsuximide		Methsuximide	
Valproate			Valproate
			Clonazepam
			Carbamazepine
Other drugs			
Amitriptyline	Ammponium chloride		Alprenolol
Antihistamines	Dicoumarol		Aminopyrine
Corticosteroids	Folate		Bishydroxycoumarin
Imipramine	Phenylbutazone		Chloramphenicol
MAO inhibitors	Pyridoxine		Chlorpromazine
Narcotics			Dexamethasone
Propoxyphene			Digitoxin
Rauwolfia alkaloids			Dipryone
(e.g., reserpine)			
Tranquilizers			Doxycycline
			Griseofulvin
			Isoniazid
			Metoprolol
			Oral contraception
			Phenylbutazone
			Propranolol
			Quinine
			Tricyclic antidepressants
			Vitamin D
			Warfarin

[a] Data taken from references 2 and 49; AEDs, antiepileptic drugs; MAO, monoamine oxidase.

Table 29.4. Benzodiazepines: Parameters and Administration

Parameter	Diazepam	Lorazepam	Midazolam
V_d (liter/kg)[2, 3a]	1.0–2.0	1.0	2.5
Lipid sol[2, 3]	Very	Yes	Very
Protein-bound[2, 3]	95%	90%	97%
Metabolism/liver[2, 3]	95%	90%	95%
Alkaline urine increases excretion	No	No	No
Half-life[3–6] clearance	36 hr	18 hr	2.8 hr
Anticonvulsant	20–30 min	4–12 hr	?
Onset effect[8, 9]	1/2–2 min	3–5 min	1–2.5 min
Time to peak level[1–3, 8, 9]			
i.v.	8 min	23 min	30 min
i.m.	30–60 min	90 min	45 min
p.o.	30–90 min	90–120 min	N/A
p.r.	65 min (mean)	Unclear	Unclear
Dilute[1, 3]	No	Yes	Optional
Bolus dose[6, 7, 10]	5 mg	2 mg	1 mg
Rate of administration[3, 6, 7, 10]	2 mg/min	1 mg/min	1/2–1 mg/min
Time between boluses[6, 7, 10]	2–5 min	2–5 min	2–5 min
Maximum dose (nontolerant)[5, 6, 10]	0.25 mg/kg	0.1 mg/kg	0.08 mg/kg
Continuous[5, 6, 11] infusion	Yes	Yes	Yes Efficacy not studied
Fluid	All i.v. fluids (may precipitate in NaCl solutions at high concentrations)	All i.v. fluids	All i.v. fluids
Suggested concentration[5, 11–13]	20 mg/250 ml i.v. fluids	?	50 mg/250 ml. (may be less concentrated)
Bolus before infusion[6, 12, 13]	0.25 mg/kg	?	0.1–0.3 mg/kg
Rate of infusion[1, 6, 12, 13]	2 mg/kg/24 hr	?	0.05–0.40 mg/kg/hr
Remix[14] preparation	q 6–8 hr at > 1.0 mg/ml q24 hr < 1.0 mg/ml	?	24 hr

[a] Table notes, by reference number: 1, 57; 2, 30; 3, 39; 4, 41; 5, 50; 6, 58; 7, 12; 8, 53; 9, 52; 10, 59; 11, 60; 12, 61; 13, 62; 14, Johns Hopkins Hospital Pharmacy Protocol.

Table 29.5. Diazepam Interactions[a]

Action Increased by	GI Absorption Decreased by	Action Decreased by	Decreases Action of
Valproic acid	Metoclopramide	Aminophylline	Levodopa
Digoxin			
Disulfiram	Ethanol		
Cimetidine	Antacids		
Ethanol	Theophylline		
Cimetidine			

[a] Data taken from references 63, 66–71.

midazolam. Following the table is a brief section on each drug containing references and important points.

Diazepam

Beware of recurrent seizures 20 to 30 minutes after administration due to rapid redistribution. When continuous infusion is used look for tolerance beginning on day 2 (50, 61, 62). Rectal use was 80% effective at 15 minutes in one study (see references 6 and 64). Information on the onset of action is available in references 50, 51, and 57. Care must be taken to avoid vascular thrombosis due to injection into small veins or extravasation into adjacent tissues (65).

For drug interactions, see Table 29.5.

Lorazepam

Lorazepam is not FDA-approved for treatment of status epilepticus, though this is the agent of choice for many epileptologists in the treatment of this condition (72). This agent

should be diluted and given in large veins to prevent thrombophlebitis (41). Next to midazolam, lorazepam is the next most rapidly and reliably intramuscularly absorbed benzodiazepine used in the acute treatment of seizures (73). Increased half-life has been noted when probenecid is given due to inhibition of glucuronidation.

Clonazepam

This drug is useful in both the chronic and acute treatment of seizures. Its application in the critically ill patient is limited in the U.S. because it is unavailable intravenously in this country. Its properties, in general, are similar to those of other benzodiazepines. It is of interest due to its rapid onset of action (within minutes), its relatively long half-life of 30 to 40 hours, and its greater effectiveness than diazepam (50, 74). It may also be given rectally for the acute treatment of status epilepticus (75).

Midazolam

Not yet FDA recommended for use in the treatment of seizures, midazolam is the only benzodiazepine that is stable when frozen. It stores this way for up to 2 years. The sedative potency of midazolam is approximately 3 to 4 times that of diazepam. An increased incidence of acute respiratory failure has been reported with midazolam as compared to other benzodiazepines. It should be administered with caution in the very young, very old, or critically ill for this reason (39). Midazolam is the most rapidly effective intramuscularly administered benzodiazepine in the acute treatment of seizures (58, 76).

The following two medications are included because of their great usefulness in treating specific seizure disorders. They are not available parenterally at present but are nonetheless useful in the ICU, at times.

CARBAMAZEPINE

Carbamazepine is chemically related to the tricyclic antidepressants and is available only in oral preparations (tablets and elixir) at present. It is a drug of choice for complex partial seizures. Important potential side effects, related to drug use, are leukopenia (dose-related), idiosyncratic pancytopenia (not dose-related), thrombocytopenia, and hyponatremia, which may be similar to the syndrome of inappropriate antidiuretic hormone secretion (30, 39, 41). Though the use of this drug in the ICU setting is limited, many patients admitted to the ICU with a history of seizures will be taking, or withdrawing from, this medication.

Linear kinetics:	Serum levels are a linear function of dosage.
Binding:	78% protein-bound, mostly to albumin
V_d:	0.8–2.0 liter/kg
Enzyme inducer:	Yes
Metabolism:	97% conjugated in liver, 3% excreted unchanged in urine, metabolites excreted in urine. Approximately 78% absorbed (38).
Half-life: p.o.:	12–17 hours, peak levels 4–5 hours after administration of tablets, 1.5 hours after oral suspension.

Excretion not increased with alkalization of the urine

Fat-soluble:	No
Target levels:	4–12 μg/ml (usual adult range). Toxicity in and above this range is highly variable.

Administration:

p.o.:   GI absorption is more rapid with elixir.

Loading dose: Not clear. Usual adult maintenance dose is 800–1200 mg/day in 3 divided doses. Rapid administration of the drug may cause acute toxicity consisting of nausea, vomiting, ataxia, malaise, confusion agitation, urinary retention, hypo or hypertension (30, 39, 41).

Distribution

Level in brain is equal to the serum-free level.

Mechanisms

Clinical.   Blocks both primary foci and seizure spread.

Biochemical.   Decreases ability of neurons to fire at high frequency by enhancing sodium channel inactivation (77–81).

Toxicity

Dizziness, vertigo, drowsiness, fatigue, ataxia, confusion, decreased coordination, headache, nystagmus, blurred vision, diplopia (transient), hallucinations, hyperacusis, abnormal involuntary movements; rarely, peripheral neuritis, paresthesia, depression with agitation, tinnitus, rare exacerbation of seizures may occur. Other important side effects may include

SIADH leading to hyponatremia, pneumonitis, hypersensitivity reactions, as well as a wide range of hematologic side effects, including dose-related leukopenia, nondose-related thrombocytopenia, and idiosyncratic aplastic anemia (30, 38, 41).

For drug interactions, see Table 29.6.

VALPROIC ACID

Valproic acid is a colorless liquid, with a "characteristic odor" that is slightly water-soluble and very soluble in organic solvents. It is currently available only in capsule or elixir form, though an intravenous preparation is about to be sent to clinical trial. Currently available preparations may be administered either enterally or by retention enema (30, 39, 41).

Saturation kinetics:	Clearance is first-order but is a function of plasma concentration, particularly the free fraction. The free fraction of drug increases at high serum levels. There is a great variety in the rate of metabolism of the drug between individuals (2, 39, 83).
Binding:	80–94% protein-bound, mostly to albumin
V_d:	0.13 liter/kg
Enzyme inducer:	Not significantly
Metabolism:	97% conjugated in liver; small amounts are excreted in feces and in expired air
Half-life: p.o.:	16 hours, peak levels 1 to 4 hours after dose

Excretion is not increased with alkalization of the urine

Fat soluble:	Yes
Target levels:	Acute load 50 to 100 μg/ml, may push to higher levels as tolerated.

Administration:

i.v.:   Under investigation. Currently available only under protocol.

p.o.:   Rapidly absorbed enterally.

p.r.:   Can administer via retention enema. Rapidly absorbed.

Loading dose = 12.5 mg/kg (18, 84, 85).

Maintenance dose = 15 to 60 mg/kg/day divided into 3 doses over each day. Levels for a given dose may vary widely.

Distribution

CSF level is approximately 10% of serum level. Drug is not concentrated in brain.

Mechanism

Clinical.   In animals blocks spread of seizure activity, but not activity at seizure focus (86, 87).

Biochemical.   Raises brain GABA concentration. Exact mechanism not known. Has been shown to inhibit GABA transferase and succinic aldehyde dehydrogenase, both important in GABA catabolism. Also postulated is alteration of presynaptic release, postsynaptic receptor binding or block of reuptake. Persistence of effect after GABA levels normalize suggest another mechanism not yet discovered (2, 41, 86, 87).

Toxicity

Gastrointestinal effects are most common: nausea and vomiting. May cause ataxia, tremor, increased appetite, diarrhea,

Table 29.6. Carbamazepine Interactions[a]

Action Increased by	Action Decreased by	Increases Action of	Decreases Action of
AEDs			
Valproic acid		Valproic acid	Valproic acid
Felbamate[b]			
	Phenytoin	Phenytoin	Phenytoin
	Primidone	Primidone	
	Clonazepam		Clonazepam
	Phenobarbital		
			Ethosuxamide
Other drugs			
Calcium channel blockers			Doxycycline
Cimetidine			Haloperidol
Erythromycin			Oral contraceptives
Isoniazid			Theophylline
Lithium			Warfarin
Propoxyphene			
Triacetyloleandomycin			

[a] Adapted from references 2, 39, 41, and 82; AEDs, antiepileptic drugs.
[b] Serum level decreased but, epoxide level increases.

acute pancreatitis, sedation, drowsiness. Rarely, paresthesia, ataxia, headache, nystagmus, dysarthria, depression, or alopecia occur. Hematologic effects include platelet dysfunction, prolonged bleeding time, thrombocytopenia, hyperammonemia (with or without clinical signs) and bone marrow suppression (39, 41). Hepatotoxicity is an important, but sometimes overestimated, side effect of valproic acid in the adult population (88). In our experience, benign mild elevation of ammonia is common in patients taking valproic acid.

For drug interactions see Table 29.7.

OTHER AGENTS

Pentobarbital

This agent is very useful for the treatment of refractory seizures in the acute setting due to its ease of administration intravenously and relatively short half-life (20 hours), as compared to phenobarbital. Pentobarbital has a more potent maximum effect on GABA-sensitive chloride channels than does phenobarbital and is a potent CNS depressant. We recommend its administration, as described below, in the protocol for treatment of refractory status epilepticus quoted from Osorio and Reed (32). Pentobarbital has potent respiratory depressant and hypotensive side effects, and great care must be taken during its administration. The drug enters the brain faster and more completely than phenobarbital or diazepam and is a very potent and effective antiepileptic drug when used properly.

General Anesthetic Agents

A number of general anesthetics are used in the treatment of refractory status epilepticus.

1. Isoflurane (89);
2. Halothane (less frequently used now);
3. Propofol (90);
4. Thiopental (91).

Agents to avoid, because they increase epileptiform activity on EEG during their administration include (2, 92);

1. Methohexital (Brevital) (32, 93);
2. Enflurane;
3. Ketamine;
4. Althesin;
5. Propanidid.

ACUTE SEIZURES AND STATUS EPILEPTICUS

Status epilepticus is a retrospective diagnosis, made after acute or intermittent seizures have persisted for ≥15 minutes. For this reason, our opinion is that all acute seizure patients should be approached as if they were developing status epilepticus. In this way, if seizures persist long enough to be called status epilepticus, treatment is already underway, according to protocol, giving the patient the best chance possible for a meaningful recovery.

EPIDEMIOLOGY

There are approximately 60,000 cases of status epilepticus in the U.S. alone every year. In one-third of these cases there is a prior history of epilepsy; in one-third status epilepticus is the presentation of the patient's first unprovoked seizure or epilepsy; and in one-third there is no history of epilepsy. One-third to one-half of all cases of status occur in the setting of an acute central nervous system or metabolic insult (94). The most common causes of status epilepticus in adults are demonstrated in Figure 29.1.

CAUSES OF STATUS EPILEPTICUS IN ADULTS

Children and adults over 60 years of age form the two highest risk groups for status epilepticus. With the widespread use of effective antiepileptic drugs and intensive care units, mortality due to status epilepticus without a precipitating cause is believed to be 1 to 2%. The major cause of morbidity and mortality from status epilepticus is from the underlying cause of the disorder (94).

A USEFUL OVERSIMPLIFICATION

As explained above, there is a homeostasis in the brain between excitatory and inhibitory inputs to cortical neurons. Excitatory pathways act primarily through the neurotransmitter glutamate and its receptor subtypes, for example, those sensitive to *N*-methyl-D-aspartate (NMDA), kainic acid or quisqualate (28). These receptors act primarily by ion channels that allow the influx of sodium and/or calcium. Inhibitory pathways act primarily through GABA, which increases mean open time of chloride ion channels. GABA-mediated chloride channels also contain receptors for benzodiazepines and barbiturates, two classes of drugs used in the treatment of status epilepticus. A number of experimental animal models have been employed to determine the pathogenesis of status epilepticus. These include use of GABA antagonists, such as bicuculline and alyglycine, and glutamate agonists, such as NMDA and Kainate. Continuous hippocampal stimulation is another model in which spontaneous seizure activity and, eventually, status epilepticus can be precipitated (5).

Experiments using NMDA and kainic acid produce pathologic changes in animals that are very similar to changes found in the brains of humans after prolonged status epilepticus (5, 13, 95). This discovery has stimulated aggressive research into the mechanisms of this "excitotoxic neuronal injury" and into a number of compounds (and potential AEDs) that may antagonize these effects, such as ketamine, PCP, and MK-801 (5, 28). Several of these animal models have identified 15 minutes as the approximate time beyond which irreversible neuronal injury takes place. Based upon this information, most epileptologists use 15 minutes as the time beyond which acute seizures are considered status epilepticus (5, 12). Clinically useful NMDA antagonists are not yet approved; however, some investigators feel that these agents may be quite useful in limiting brain injury related to stroke and seizures (96).

PHYSIOLOGIC, CLINICAL, AND ELECTROENCEPHALOGRAPHIC CHANGES DURING SE

Prolonged seizure activity, particularly generalized tonic-clonic seizures, can cause neuronal injury and, eventually, cell death as greatly increased cellular metabolic demands outstrip oxygen and nutrient supply. There is some suggestion that transient MRI lesions observed in patients with status epilepticus may reflect focal neuronal injury in these patients (97). In addition to excitotoxin-mediated neuronal injury, there are systemic changes that occur during prolonged seizures that are responsible for substantial morbidity and mortality. These changes, as they occur during prolonged seizure activity, are diagrammed in Table 29.8.

As status epilepticus progresses there is also an evolution of clinical signs, particularly in the case of generalized tonic-clonic (GTC) status epilepticus. GTC seizures begin with a brief, variable phase of increased tone, followed by sustained, synchronous, rhythmic movements of the body and extremities. As GTC status progresses without treatment, there is a gradual reduction in the amplitude of movement, until the patient is left with multifocal, asynchronous, variable length myoclonic movements. These movements may consist of brief arm, jaw, or face twitches, or poorly sustained, irregular movements of the extremities. Finally, as SE continues, all movements may cease, though the patient's brain continues to seize actively. This period of electromechanical dissociation can be deceiving, making the clinician think that seizure activity has ended (5, 99). An important principle of treating these patients is that **the seizure is not over until the EEG says its over.**

The EEG also evolves as status epilepticus progresses. Figure 29.2 illustrates that seizure activity begins with discrete bursts of irregular spiking. These discharges gradually merge until they become continuous seizure activity. As SE progresses, continuous activity becomes interrupted by periods of generalized flattening (voltage depression). In the end-stages of SE the brain puts out agonal periodic epileptiform discharges (PEDs) against a flat background (5, 100). While useful as a guideline, this progression of the EEG in untreated status epilepticus has not been agreed upon universally (101). An important conclusion here is that decreased activity on the

Table 29.7.   Valproic Acid Interactions

Action Increased by	Action Decreased by	Increases Action of	Decreases Action of
AEDs			
Phenytoin	Phenytoin	Phenytoin	Phenytoin
Carbamazepine		Carbamazepine	Carbamazepine
Felbamate			
	Phenobarbital	Clonazepam	
		Barbiturates	
		Primidone	
		Ethosuxamide	
Other drugs			
Dicumarol		CNS depressants	
Phenylbutazone		MAO inhibitors	
Salicylates		Antidepressants	

*ª*Adapted from references 2, 39 and 41; AEDs, antiepileptic drugs; MAO, monamine oxidase.

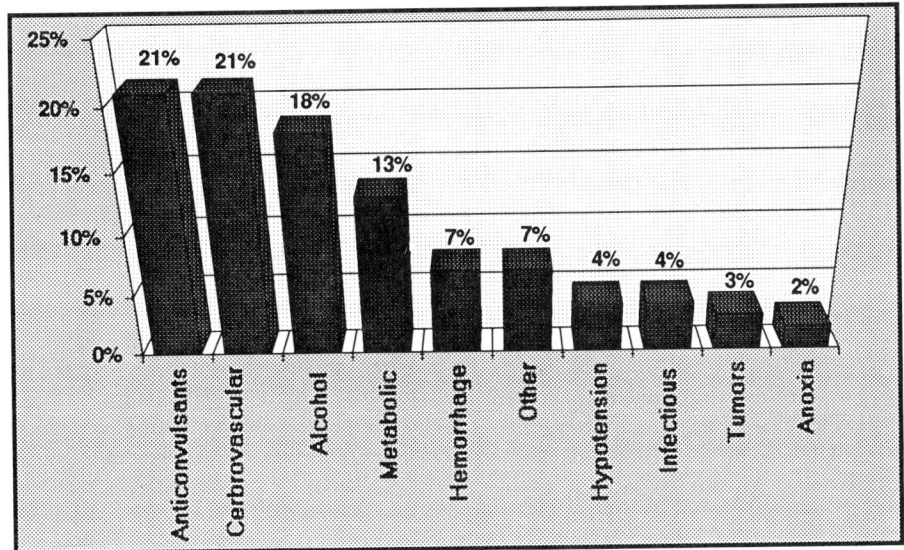

Figure 29.1.   Data collated from reference 94. "Anticonvulsants" refers to withdrawal from or noncompliance with AEDs.

Table 29.8.   Physiologic Changes during Status Epilepticus[a]

Measure	0–30 min	> 30 min	Complication
Blood pressure	Up	Down	Shock
PAO₂	Down	Down	Hypoxia
PACO₂	Up	Varies	ICP
Serum PH	Down	Varies	Acidosis
Temperature	Up	Up	Fever
Autonomic activity	Up	Up	Arrhythmias
Lung fluids	Up	Up	Atelectasis
Serum K⁺	Up	Up	Arrhythmias
Serum CPK	Nl	Up	Renal failure
Cerebral blood flow	Up (900%)	Up (200%)	Hemorrhage
Cerebral O₂ consumption	Up (300%)	Up (300%)	Neuronal death

[a] Adapted from references 97 and 98.

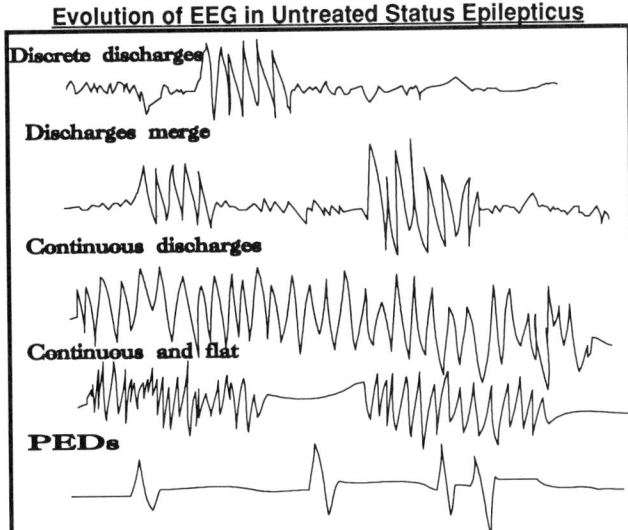

Figure 29.2.   Authors' depiction of progression of the EEG in untreated status epilepticus.

EEG does not necessarily indicate that the patient is improving, or that therapy should be withdrawn.

Finally, there are biochemical changes that have been observed as SE progresses. GABA-mediated mechanisms become less prominent, and NMDA-mediated neuronal activity grows. This may account for the diminishing utility of benzodiazepines and barbiturates, except in high concentrations, in the late stages of SE sometimes called "refractory status epilepticus" (5). At this point, beyond 30 minutes in some animal models, excitotoxic neuronal injury, mediated through NMDA channels, free radicals and other potential mechanisms, begins to have a significant effect (5, 12, 28).

Status epilepticus: Management Pearls

1. Treat the underlying cause of seizures. This has the single most important effect on outcome.
2. Have a detailed protocol for treatment.
3. Know a few drugs well, their effects, kinetics and toxicity.
4. Institute EEG monitoring early.
5. Be prepared for all complications, particularly hypoventilation and hypotension.

Table 29.9 outlines our recommended treatment protocol for status epilepticus, condensed from several sources and our personal experience (12, 59). Details of management in each time period in the protocol will be discussed below.

DISCUSSION

0 Minutes

A description of clinical presentation is important here, since seizure type affects treatment and prognosis. Make sure that proper therapeutic agents, equipment, and facilities for intubation and intensive monitoring are at hand. ***Be prepared for the worst case!!*** No matter how dire the circumstances, there is almost always a minute or two available for thought before initiating aggressive therapy. A few important points to consider are:

Brief history. Pay particular attention to:
  Known seizure disorder?
  Head trauma
  Medications, drugs, toxic exposures
  Infections, fever, rash, infected contacts (HIV)
  Anoxia, hypotension
  Known metabolic derangement (e.g., hepatic or renal failure)
  History of neoplasm, coagulation disorder
  Psychiatric history
Physical examination (to include):
  Vital signs (fever?, abnormal blood pressure?)
  Trauma survey, particularly of head/neck (battle's or raccoon's signs, hemotympanum)
  Rash, jaundice, focal general exam
  Meningismus, focal neurologic examination
  Papilledema, evidence of increased intracranial pressure
  Evidence of old neurosurgery, healed trauma
  Needle marks, pacemaker, cardiac surgery, evidence of systemic disease
  Hysterical features? (pelvic thrusting, forced eye closure, avoids hitting self when hand is dropped toward face, asynchronous or atypical movements)
If possible, establish seizure type via the following:

Clinical observation, history, It may be helpful, if available (but you should not delay treatment waiting for EEG). Treatment and prognosis may vary with seizure type.

5 Minutes

Basic Lab Information (Check or Send)

Dextrose: This is a point of some debate. Hypoglycemia is a common cause of neuronal injury and seizures. Sieber and Traystman have reviewed animal and human data, demonstrating that increased serum glucose can not only precipitate seizures but also can worsen neuronal injury in status epilepticus (102). Our recommendation is that glucose should be checked at presentation, preferably immediately, using a glucometer, and then the level should be verified by laboratory testing. Dextrose (50 mg i.v.) should be administered to hypoglycemic patients or to patients whose serum glucose is unknown or in whom measurements are felt to be unreliable.

Naloxone: An opiate antagonist, its use in SE is also controversial. Debate exists on whether or not the drug may promote seizures in rare cases. It should be given when there is a history of opiate use, or when a reliable history is not available.

Thiamine: This is given (100 mg i.v.) to prevent an acute Wernicke's encephalopathy, resulting from thiamine deficiency. Acute hyperglycemia, such as that resulting from a bolus infusion of D-50, may precipitate acute Wernicke's encephalopathy in patients who are borderline thiamine-deficient. Thiamine should always be given near the time of dextrose administration.

Send: Chemistry and electrolyte panel (especially calcium, magnesium, and sodium), arterial blood gas, blood and urine toxicology screen, liver function tests, blood urea nitrogen, creatinine, ammonia, anticonvulsant levels, and complete blood count with differential.

10 Minutes

Treat: with a first line agent to stop ongoing seizure activity and/or prevent seizure recurrence. A benzodiazepine

Table 29.9.   Protocol for Treatment of Status Epilepticus

Time (min)	Intervention
0 (min)	Recognition Airway, breathing, circulation History, trauma survey Establish intravenous access Oxygen
5 (min)	Send blood sample for lab tests Dextrose 50% 50 ml i.v. Naloxone 2 mg i.v. Thiamin 100 mg i.v.
10 (min)	Benzodiazepines[a] Phenytoin load
30 (min)	Phenobarbital; or benzodiazepine infusion (midazolam or diazepam) EEG monitoring (if not yet begun)
60 (min)	Pentobarbital coma
80 (min)	General anesthesia neuromuscular blockade

[a]Treatment with benzodiazepines should be initiated as rapidly as possible after addressing earlier items in the protocol, and always by 10 minutes, if possible.

should be administered while a phenytoin infusion is being prepared.

Benzodiazepines

Lorazepam is, in our opinion, the first choice intravenous agent for treatment of SE due to its long-lasting antiepileptic effect, short sedative half-life, and slightly lesser degree of respiratory depression (experimentally), compared to that of diazepam (50, 52, 103-106). The drug is better absorbed than diazepam when given intramuscularly, though this route is recommended only at times when i.v. access is not available (63, 107). Midazolam, a very rapidly absorbed benzodiazepine, is also effective as a first-line treatment, including intramuscularly, but its use may be limited by its relatively short effective half-life (58, 108). The specific role for midazolam in the treatment of status epilepticus, particularly as a continuous infusion, is currently being defined (58).

At the same time that benzodiazepines are being administered for acute seizure control, a full load of a longer-acting AED should be given in order to prevent seizure recurrence and establish a maintenance therapy. Drug choice will reflect physician reasoning up to that time.

Phenytoin

Usually the first choice for acute maintenance AED therapy in adults with GTC status epilepticus. Exceptions include patients with withdrawal seizures from CNS depressants, particularly barbiturates. A full load should be administered (18 to 20 mg/kg of phenytoin i.v.) at no faster than 50 mg/min, under continuous blood pressure and ECG monitoring. Physicians should be prepared to treat hypotension, and arrhythmias, usually secondary to the drug carrier. A loading dose of 20 mg/kg should give the average patient a level of around 24 to 26 μg/dl (59). Some epileptologists recommend giving another 10 mg/kg of phenytoin before proceeding to a third drug for treatment of SE. Our opinion is that the additional benefit gained by this maneuver is usually less than that gained by proceeding to the next section of the protocol, in the absence of contraindications to more aggressive therapy. *Note:* If there is a history of hypersensitivity to phenytoin, proceed directly to the next section.

30 Minutes

By this time a substantial amount of phenytoin has had time to cross the blood-brain barrier. If seizures persist, the patient should be placed in a facility equipped to provide mechanical ventilation and invasive monitoring of circulatory and cardiac function, and bedside EEG monitoring. EEG monitoring should be initiated, while treatment progresses, to determine seizure type and monitor therapeutic effect. Fixation of electrodes with standard paste several times per day or, preferably, with collodian and periodic gelling of electrodes, is suggested. The EEG guides treatment from this time on, as the clinical examination is often lost with the sedation that results from initiation of therapy with barbiturate or benzodiazepine infusions. Intubation and ventilation will be required at this point, since the agents used cause profound respiratory depression, synergistic with the benzodiazepines

given to this point. Seizure activity may itself cause apnea, independent of respiratory depressants.

Drugs of choice at this time include periodic intravenous phenobarbital or continuous infusions of diazepam or midazolam. Phenobarbital is given first as a loading dose of 20 mg/kg, administered i.v. no faster than 100 mg/min. This drug is given until seizures stop or the full load has been administered. Hypotension and respiratory depression commonly result. Dopamine should be available at the bedside for blood pressure support. Adequate fluid resuscitation with normal saline is important to maintain blood pressure in these patients, as they are often dehydrated. Phenytoin and phenobarbital maintenance therapies are continued during the acute period.

Other options include the following (see Table 29.4 in drug section above):

Benzodiazepine infusion:
1. Diazepam: Use large bore vein. Administer bolus first with 20 mg, then infuse at a rate of 2 mg/kg/day. Tolerance may develop beginning on day 2. Mix, at most, 20 mg in 250 ml i.v. fluid to help prevent precipitation (63).
2. Clonazepam: Intravenous preparation not available in the U.S.
3. Midazolam: Recent clinical protocols have been tested, although in small numbers of patients, using constant infusions of midazolam to treat status epilepticus. Kumar and Bleck suggest bolusing first with 0.05 to 0.3 mg/kg i.v., then starting an infusion at 0.05 mg/kg/hr, raising the dose as needed up to 0.4 mg/kg/hr. The higher end of this range of doses may be necessary in tolerant individuals (58).

Valproic acid therapy:
Recommended for the acute treatment of nonconvulsive status epilepticus. See special cases below.

60 Minutes

By this time irreversible neuronal injury has begun, and very aggressive measures must be employed if the patient is to make a meaningful recovery. Barbiturate coma is usually recommended at this point. It was pointed out earlier in the chapter that by this time GABA-ergic mechanisms may be having less influence on neuronal activity as status epilepticus progresses. This point in therapy would be an ideal time to employ an NMDA antagonist. Unfortunately, no clinically effective, commercially available antagonists are available at the time of this publication. Our approach is to administer large doses of barbiturates (GABA agonists), to the point of inducing coma, as well as a burst-suppression pattern on the EEG. Our drug of choice is pentobarbital, though phenobarbital and a number of anesthetic barbiturates may also be employed. Due to its long half-life (35 hours), pentobarbital does not require minute-to-minute titration, yet, it can be adjusted more rapidly than phenobarbital (half-life of 90 to 100 hours). Pentobarbital also is more potent, has a stronger maximum effect, and enters the brain more rapidly than phenobarbital (32, 101, 109, 110).

We prefer to use the protocol described by Osorio and Reed when inducing pentobarbital coma (32). This protocol is outlined in Table 29.10. Patients must be ventilated and

Table 29.10.   Pentobarbital-induced Anesthesia in Refractory Generalized Tonic-Clonic Status Epilepticus [a]

General guidelines for pentobarbital infusion
  Loading dose:[b] 5–20 mg/kg i.v. at infusion rate 25 mg/min
  Initial maintenance 2.5 mg/kg/hr
  For breakthrough seizures 59-mg bolus and increase maintenance by 0.5–1 mg/kg/hr
  Begin tapering 24 hr after last seizure
  Tapering rate (q4–6 hr) 1.0 mg/kg/hr if pentobarbital level >50 mg/liter or 0.5 mg/kg/hr if pentobarbital level <50 mg/liter
  For seizures during tapering 50-mg pentobarbital bolus; increase maintenance to closest preseizure dose
General guidelines for patient management
  Endotracheal intubation; assisted ventilation
  Continuous BP monitoring (arterial line)
  Hemodynamic monitoring (Swan-Ganz) optional
  Hypotension[c]: fluids and dopamine up to 12 μg/kg/min
  Prophylaxis of decubiti and venous thrombosis
  Daily CBC
  Maintenance of high therapeutic AED serum concentrations
  Obtain serum at least once daily
  EEG monitoring
  Baseline
  Continuous for the first 2–6 hours of anesthesia
  Ten-minute strips every 30–60 min for duration of treatment

[a] From Osorio I, Reed RC: Treatment of refractory generalized tonic-clonic status epilepticus with pentobarbital anesthesia after high-dose phenytoin. *Epilepsia* 30:464–471, 1989.
[b] Seperation of the cardiorespiratory complications of refractory generalized tonic-clonic status epilepticus from effects of pentobarbital may be difficult.
[c] In most patients 5 mg/kg was effective for induction of anesthesia.
[d] Defined as decrease in systolic blood pressure by 10 mm Hg, as compared with preanesthetic BP. Decrease or discontinue pentobarbital temporarily if dopamine requirements exceed 12 μg/kg/min.

have dopamine at the bedside for blood pressure support. Other AEDs must be kept at high concentration throughout therapy, including preadmission AEDs. Hemodynamic monitoring via Swan-Ganz catheterization may be required to ensure adequate fluid management. As with all comatose patients, it is important to prevent pressure injury (e.g., decubitus ulcers) and peripheral nerve compression (may need to pad elbows, fibular head regions, etc.). All patients should have adequate nutrition, usually by hyperalimentation, as soon as possible. Under barbiturate anesthesia, autoregulation is impaired, so that organ perfusion is directly a function of systemic blood pressure. Osorio and Reed recommend treating any drop in systemic blood pressure of ≥10 mm Hg with fluid boluses or pressor agents (32). If hypotension persists despite dopamine treatment at 12 μg/kg/min, then the pentobarbital infusion should be decreased, the patient resuscitated as appropriate, and treatment should proceed with another general anesthetic agent and neuromuscular blockade, as described below. Recurrent seizures with multiple attempts to withdraw barbiturate coma is generally felt to portend a relatively poor prognosis for meaningful recovery.

80 Minutes

By this time the chances of meaningful recovery are greatly reduced. Neuromuscular blockade should be induced and maintained, and general anesthesia should be introduced and maintained with one of the agents listed above in the section on AEDs, though the list is not meant to be exhaustive. A description of how to administer these agents is beyond the scope of this text. This treatment should be under the direction of a qualified anesthesiologist.

FOLLOW-UP TREATMENT

As treatment progresses through the above protocol and after seizures have been controlled, further evaluation to establish the cause of the seizures should be aggressively undertaken. The patient's diagnosis ultimately determines his/her prognosis for meaningful recovery. Some suggested points include:

Emergent CT scan, **after** airway has been stabilized
Culture blood, urine, sputum; check chest x-ray
Lumbar puncture (if indicated): Check cultures, opening pressure, VDRL (test for syphilis), glucose and protein, cell count, cryptococcal antigen; check cytology when appropriate.
Treat with broad spectrum CSF-penetrating antibiotic, if indicated. Do not delay antibiotic treatment while waiting to perform a lumbar puncture if CT scanning is delayed!
Try to minimize factors that increase metabolism, accelerate neuronal injury: Maintain euthermia, normoglycemia, and good oxygenation. Consider treatment with new agents designed to combat neuronal injury due to excitatory neurotoxins and free radicals as they become available for clinical use. Some experimental agents, which may be potentially useful are allopurinol, and superoxide dismutase (SOD). These agents have not yet been accepted for clinical use; however, some clinically useful agents are expected to be approved in the future.

Digital EEG Monitoring and the Critically Ill Patient

Digital EEG technology now allows the continuous monitoring of cerebral function in patients with status epilepticus and other disease states affecting the brain. Scalp or intracranial EEG can be monitored without the need for a paper recording. Data can be manipulated to display trends in the frequency (compressed spectral array, or CSA) and amplitude of cortical activity over long periods of time. Computer programs already exist that can detect interictal epileptiform activity (111–114). Altafulla et al have demonstrated that CSA display of EEG data in patients with status epilepticus promptly detected breakthrough seizures (115). Reiher et al recently have shown that on-line computer analysis of patients in status epilepticus could not detect breakthrough seizures but could detect patient patterns of high risk for developing recurrent seizures and alert physicians to treat these conditions prophylactically (116). These devices may soon become the accepted standard for monitoring patients in status epilepticus; however, the technology is expensive, still under development, and only now becoming widely available.

SPECIAL CASES

Nonconvulsive Status Epilepticus

This condition is defined by continuous or intermittent seizure activity lasting 30 minutes or more without the patient regaining consciousness and without the presence of convulsive activity. Different from generalized tonic-clonic status, nonconvulsive status is considered a "walking emergency." It may be difficult to diagnose, and the cost-benefit analysis of potentially dangerous therapies, such as barbiturate coma, have yet to be fully assessed in this condition. Nonconvulsive status epilepticus may be divided into complex partial status and absence status.

Complex-Partial Status Epilepticus

Complex-partial seizures are the most common type of seizures in adults, but complex partial status epilepticus (CPSE) is the rarest form of SE. First described by Gastaut in 1956, patients with CPSE are confused, and display automatisms, such as lip smacking, picking movements of the hands, fumbling, swallowing, and repetitive verbalizations. The EEG is necessary to distinguish CPSE from absence status and toxic-metabolic disorders and shows repetitive discharges over the temporal and, sometimes, the frontal regions. Presentation with psychiatric symptoms has been described (117, 118). Patients usually have a history of complex partial seizures and respond to treatment with benzodiazepines, phenytoin, and/or barbiturates. Left untreated there is a significant risk for long-term impairment of memory and cognition (10). Treatment should proceed according to the protocol for status epilepticus given above. As with absence status, the risk-benefit profile of barbiturate coma in CPSE has not yet been determined (26).

Absence Status Epilepticus

This condition may present in children or adults with a history of absence seizures, with a characteristic 3 to 4/second generalized spike and slow-wave pattern on EEG. However, absence status epilepticus (ASE) usually occurs in adults with no prior history of seizures (119). Clinically, this presents with "... variable degrees of impaired consciousness, disorientation, perseveration, monosyllabic speech, fluctuating amnesia, fuge-states, hallucinations, psychosis-like behavior, clumsy

motor function, or even a catatonia-like waxy flexibility" (26, 120). The physical examination and EEG are not always reliable and must be used together for diagnosis (121). The EEG often shows a characteristic 1.5 to 2.5/sec generalized slow-spike and slow-wave pattern that may or may not have some focality (19, 26, 122). Common causes are toxic and metabolic derangements; drug withdrawal, including alcohol and AEDs; and hepatic or renal failure. The condition can occur in endocrinopathies, CNS infections, carcinomas, after myelography, or without an obvious cause.

Treatment of ASE consists of the above SE protocol up to the choice of treatment after benzodiazepines. Phenytoin and carbamazepine are not thought to be effective in ASE and may actually precipitate it (26, 123). After benzodiazepines have been administered, the patient should be treated with valproic acid (12.5 mg/kg per nasogastric tube or retention enema) (26, 84, 85). Target levels are in the high therapeutic range (75 to 100 µg/ml). Even with cessation of ASE with benzodiazepine therapy, valproic acid is useful for preventing recurrence of ASE (26, 124). A new intravenous valproic acid preparation, which is currently being tested for other uses, may prove to be useful for patients with ASE. As with complex partial SE, the cost-benefit profile of barbiturate-induced coma in these patients has not yet been determined and, left untreated, this disorder may result in long-term cognitive and memory impairment. There is some recent interest in benzodiazepine infusions as treatment for this condition; however, prospective studies have not yet been published.

Myoclonic Status

This condition is characterized by persistent asynchronous, multifocal myoclonic jerking that may be generalized or affect only one or several regions of the body at once (segmental myoclonus). Typical movements are eye opening, chewing, facial twitching, asynchronous limb jerking, or brief generalized shuddering. The point at which myoclonus becomes myoclonic status epilepticus (MSE) is, at present, poorly and perhaps arbitrarily defined (26). Celesia defines MSE as "... a fixed and enduring state lasting at least 30 minutes" (125). The most common causes of MSE in the critical care setting are toxic-metabolic conditions, postanoxic encephalopathy and, rarely, patients with a history of myoclonic epilepsy. Patients with a history of myoclonic epilepsy usually respond rapidly to treatment with benzodiazepines and may recover fully. Patients with toxic or metabolic disorders may recover with treatment of the underlying disorder. Post-anoxic MSE carries a poor prognosis for recovery. Celesia reported mortality of 68% and 21% left in a persistent vegetative state (125). Krumholz et al report an incidence of MSE in 17% of cardiac arrests leading to coma, with a dismal prognosis for meaningful recovery (126). MSE is notoriously refractory to treatment and may be refractory to multiple-drug therapy or barbiturate coma. Evidence suggests that in postanoxic MSE treatment has little effect on outcome (22, 126). EEGs show variants of either a burst-suppression pattern or periodic generalized epileptiform discharges. Treatment with benzodiazepines may cause electromechanical dissociation, stopping movements but not altering EEG epileptiform activity. Krumholz et al (126) suggest that patients who present with MSE after anoxic-ischemic injury rarely survive. No survivors were reported in the anoxic-ischemic group who had MSE and loss of cranial nerve reflexes (corneal reflexes, pupillary responses, etc.), or had eye opening at the onset of myoclonic jerks along with a suppression or burst-suppression EEG pattern.

Pseudoseizures

Psychogenic seizures, described above, may result from a number of disorders, most commonly, conversion disorder, somatization disorder and, rarely, malingering. They may be continuous and present as status epilepticus. Movements may persist during treatment until consciousness is lost, giving the appearance of refractory status epilepticus. Iatrogenic injury may result from the administration of large doses of CNS depressants and the ensuing hypotension, respiratory depression, and intubation. As Leis points out, clues to psychogenic seizures include a psychiatric history, an unusual medical history, multiple normal EEGs despite frequent spells, and atypical responses to AEDs. The most common clinical presentation is a patient who is unresponsive, with minor irregular movements. Less commonly patients will present with generalized tonic clonic movements, forward pelvic thrusting, asynchronous generalized limb movements, or side-to-side head movements (25). Clinical signs may be helpful, such as forced eye closure when the examiner tries to open the patient's eyes, facial guarding to threat or the patient's arm held over his or her face, or observed visual fixation on or following people in the room. A confusing aspect of this disorder is that up to 13 to 20% of patients with psychogenic seizures may have epileptic seizures as well (24, 127, 128). The single most useful test in the diagnosis of psychogenic seizures is the EEG. The presence of normal background activity and the absence of epileptiform activity in the EEG in the presence of generalized motor "seizure" activity rules out a diagnosis of convulsive status epilepticus (25).

PHARMACOLOGIC EFFECTS OF DISEASE

An important general point is that a variety of chronic or severe systemic illnesses may increase active free fractions of anticonvulsant, especially when hypoalbuminemia is present (e.g., hepatic dysfunction, malnutrition, chronic illness). Free fractions of phenytoin, carbamazepine and valproic acid are typically about 10%, that is, a phenytoin blood level of 15 mg/liter, typically includes a free level of 1.5 mg/liter. In chronic or severe illness free fractions may increase. For example, in acute renal failure, the free fractions of both phenytoin (14 to 45%) and diazepam (2 to 10%) have an inverse correlation with serum albumin level, irrespective of the etiology of renal failure (129). Free levels are useful in evaluating unexplained medication toxicity. Occasional patients with poor seizure control with anticonvulsants may have unexpectedly low free levels. For example, a phenytoin blood level of 30 mg/liter may occasionally be necessary to obtain target free levels of 2.0 mg/liter.

RENAL DYSFUNCTION

Reduced renal clearance alters renal excretion of several anticonvulsants; however, other changes associated with renal dysfunction also may alter drug levels, and AED dosing must be individualized. For example, renal dysfunction may be associated with fluid retention, electrolyte shifts, and hypoalbuminemia—all of which may alter dosing requirements by altering the volume of distribution or free-drug fractions. Some important individual drug considerations are as follows:

1. Phenytoin: Dosage does not usually need to be altered, as decreased protein binding due to displacement of phenytoin from albumin by urea is usually balanced by decreased half-life and an increased volume of distribution. Free levels should be followed, though a reduced total serum therapeutic range of 4 to 8 µg/ml may be used as a general guideline in severe renal disease. Administration 3 times/day is recommended (130, 131).
2. Carbamazepine: Maintenance dosage should be lowered to 75% of normal when the glomerular filtration rate reaches 10 ml/min (130, 132). Carbamazepine occasionally triggers increased water and sodium retention, with hyponatremia, which could aggravate fluid-electrolyte disturbances. Reduced renal excretion rates may reduce the clearance of epoxide and transdiol metabolites; which may increase toxicity.
3. Phenobarbital: 20 to 30% of administered dose is usually excreted unchanged in the urine. In the setting of renal failure the maintenance dosage interval should be increased from 1.5 to 2 times the patient's usual dosage interval (130–132).
4. Valproic acid: This drug is highly protein bound and displaced from albumin by urea. Free levels are the most useful guide in this circumstance, with the target range of 8 to 12 µg/ml (130–132).

DIALYSIS

Most anticonvulsants have moderately large volume distribution, are highly protein-bound, and redistribution appears to occur following dialysis, with arterial serum concentrations reduced only slightly by chronic dialysis. This class of AEDs includes phenytoin, carbamazepine, and valproic acid. For example, dialysis clearance of carbamazepine following a single dose (53 ± 10 ml/min) is roughly twice endogenous clearance (133). Because carbamazepine is lipophilic and has a moderately large volume of distribution (approximately 1 to 2 liters), redistribution appears to occur following dialysis, and arterial serum concentrations are reduced only slightly (134). Somewhat similarly, serum valproate levels decrease rapidly during dialysis, but due to decreased protein binding with increased drug clearance, free drug clearance is not altered. Only 20% or less is removed; therefore, a supplemental postdialysis dose should not be necessary (135, 136). Postdialysis supplemental phenobarbital is often necessary, and reduced maintenance doses of phenobarbital are recommended for patients receiving peritoneal or hemodialysis, particularly in those receiving long-term therapy (137).

HEPATIC FAILURE

Seizures due directly to hepatic failure and hepatic encephalopathy are not common and are sometimes due to related conditions, such as hemorrhage, alcohol-related head injuries, and hypoglycemia.

As with renal failure, intrinsic drug elimination may be reduced or altered (138); however, the volume of distribution is often increased (e.g., diazepam, clonazepam, and valproic acid), and free levels may increase due to hypoalbuminemia. For example, the free levels of phenytoin may increase in hepatic failure, but this may be balanced by an increased volume of distribution. Anticonvulsant levels, with free levels obtained when unexpected toxicity occurs, are helpful to detect the need for individual dosage changes. Recognition of the effects of hepatic dysfunction is important in individual cases—for example, occasional patients with severe hepatic failure may develop prolonged obtundation when benzodiazepines are poorly metabolized and administered repeatedly. Lower doses or longer dosing intervals—as with renal failure—may be necessary. For example, the half-life of phenobarbital is significantly prolonged in patients with cirrhosis, (139) and several-day dosing intervals may be required.

Pharmacologic effects of hepatic dysfunction are variable: no significant alteration in carbamazepine pharmacokinetics is reported in cases of moderate alterations in liver function (140). In severe disease, the reduction in microsomal metabolism is more significant than changes in protein binding, and toxicity may occur in occasional patients.

Increased GABA neurotransmission has been implicated in the pathogenesis of hepatic encephalopathy, possibly due to increases in diazepam-binding inhibitor; however, this interaction may not directly influence treatment with benzodiazepines (141).

OTHER CONSIDERATIONS

AED pharmacokinetics may be altered in malnutrition (reduced absorption), fever, (increased catabolism) and pulmonary disease (reduced catabolism).

ANTICONVULSANT DRUG MANAGEMENT FOR SPECIFIC DISORDERS

POSTHYPOXIC SEIZURES

A subgroup of patients who have both coma and myoclonic seizures following hypoxic injury are often treated with anticonvulsants, although this has not been shown to improve survival. These seizures are usually treated first with phenytoin; however, valproic acid may be given rectally, usually 400 to 600 mg pr q 6h initially, for generalized seizures. Despite aggressive therapy, these seizures are usually refractory to medical treatment. This topic is covered in more depth in the section on special cases of status epilepticus above.

SURGERY

Plasma binding of antiepileptic drugs may be reduced postoperatively and increases in free levels may occur. This change is often coupled with changes in fluid volume, dosing changes, etc. Perioperative seizure prophylaxis appears worthwhile for several subgroups of injury processes that place patients at high risks for seizures. These processes include cerebral aneurysm repair, with or without hemorrhage; resection of destructive tumors located near the cerebral hemisphere surfaces or suprasellar regions (e.g., large meningiomas); and other individual cases where the risk of anticonvulsant side effects are outweighed by the consequences of seizures, such as in patients with significant cerebral edema or risk for hemorrhage. Phenytoin loading is usually necessary, and levels should be targeted to recommended ranges to avoid treatment failures.

Patients who have intracranial procedures are at a significant risk for post-operative seizures. Of previously seizure-free patients, 15% had seizures following operation for unruptured intracranial aneurysms, which is similar to the incidence for craniotomy for other indications (142).

Postoperative seizures following supratentorial procedures occurred in 17% of patients in a study by Shaw, with most of the risk in the first 6 months. Seizures were especially common following operation for arteriovenous malformations, meningiomas, and suprasellar lesions. Prophylactic anticonvulsant treatment did not reduce the incidence of postoperative seizures; however, only one-third of the patients studied had adequate anticonvulsant levels prior to surgery (143).

Mathew et al found a 13% incidence of seizures in their previously seizure-free patients in the first week following craniotomy. They recommended that anticonvulsants be considered in patients with factors predisposing to postoperative seizures, such as a history of prior seizures or lesions affecting the cerebral hemispheres. The study suggests intravenous loading with phenytoin (18 mg/kg) in 0.9% saline before or immediately after craniotomy, with careful monitoring of cardiopulmonary condition and targeting to recommended levels (10 to 20 µg/ml) (144). Contrary to this study, Kvam et al reported only a 4.3% (23 of 538 patients) incidence of seizures in postoperative neurosurgical patients who had inadequate antiepileptic drug levels prior to surgery (145).

Patients with a history of seizures who are undergoing elective surgery should have high levels of antiepileptic drugs (AEDs) maintained before, during, and after their procedures. There are many processes active during surgery which may lower the seizure threshold, such as hyperadrenergic states, pro-convulsant anesthetic agents and other medications, and lowering of AED levels due to aggressive fluid management. In patients on AEDs that are available only in oral form (e.g., carbamazepine, primidone), pre-/peri-operative loading with intravenous phenytoin or phenobarbital is recommended. These patients should be maintained on their intravenous AED therapy until therapeutic levels of their previous agents are restored.

TRAUMA

Acute anticonvulsant treatment following head injury did not appear to reduce the subsequent risk of developing epilepsy; in a study by Tempkin, however, it decreased the risk of seizures within 1 week of trauma from 14% in the placebo group to 3.6% in a phenytoin-treated group. AED treatment is recommended for patients with serious head injuries, as evidenced by post-traumatic seizures, head CT evidence of cortical contusion, hemorrhage, or hematoma, a penetrating head wound, or a Glasgow Coma Scale of 10 or less (146). In patients who develop epilepsy, seizures occur in the first week of injury approximately half the time (147).

Boucher et al found pharmacokinetic variables in the disposition of phenytoin to be similar in trauma patients and control subjects (V_d 0.76 ± 0.15 liter/kg, V_{max} 568 ± 197 mg/day and K_m 4.5 ± 1.8 mg/liter). Unbound phenytoin ranged from 7.3 to 25%. A standard loading dose of phenytoin (15 mg/kg) provided study patients with an average total serum concentration of 20 mg/liter. They recommended an initial maintenance dose of 5 mg/kg/day, which should be adjusted according to serum levels obtained over 2 to 3 days, as they found a tendency for levels to decrease after several days. Dosage once per day was associated with daily serum level fluctuations of approximately 5 µg/ml, and b.i.d. dosing was recommended (148).

STROKE

Seizures occur in approximately 3 to 6% of patients with strokes (cerebral hemorrhage, subarachnoid hemorrhage, ischemic infarcts), in most cases occurring within 48 hours of the event as solitary seizures. A small group of patients who develop partial or generalized status epilepticus need aggressive treatment and are treated similarly to other patients with these conditions. Careful hemodynamic control is vital to avoid worsening ischemic injury (149). Periodic lateralized epileptiform discharges (PLEDs) on the EEG are common following stroke and usually warrant anticonvulsant prophylaxis; however, clinical seizures—not PLEDs—should be followed in adjusting treatment. The relationship between PLEDs and status epilepticus is a source of debate among epileptologists and remains under study (150).

ALCOHOL-RELATED SEIZURES

Withdrawal seizures tend to occur within 72 hours after discontinuing alcoholic drinking and are usually tonic-clonic seizures. Alcoholic patients frequently have histories of focal brain injuries (16% in one study) and may also develop partial seizures (151). Generalized alcohol withdrawal seizures do not appear to be prevented by phenytoin (152). Delirium tremens (DTs) usually occurs later than seizures in patients who develop this withdrawal syndrome (72 hours to 2 weeks after abstaining) and is associated with autonomic instability, delirium and, occasionally, seizures. Simple withdrawal symptoms and DTs are treated with benzodiazepines (oxazepam, diazepam). Rarely, metabolism of benzodiazepines is decreased in patients with severe hepatic dysfunction, and prolonged oversedation may result if doses are not titrated carefully to sedation side effects (138). Due to poor nutrition and liver dysfunction, alcoholic patients may have hypoalbuminemia and increased free levels of protein-bound drugs, although this is usually not clinically significant.

ECLAMPSIA/PREECLAMPSIA

The optimal pharmacologic treatment of preeclampsia (toxemia) of pregnancy is controversial. Current treatment in the U.S. is usually with large (up to several grams) intravenous doses of magnesium sulfate (and, if feasible, delivery of the baby). Magnesium sulfate has been shown to have no anticonvulsant effect in animal models of epilepsy (153); however, the pathophysiology of eclampsia may include vasoconstriction and other mechanisms that could be influenced by magnesium sulfate. When seizures develop (eclampsia), conventional anticonvulsants (usually phenytoin) are recommended. Effects of magnesium sulfate may include neuromuscular blockade with associated hyporeflexia, osmotic diuresis, and hypotension.

REFERENCES

1. Bleck TP, Smith MC, Pierre-Louis SJC, Jares JJ, Murray J, Hansen CA: Neurologic complications of critical medical illness. *Crit Care Med*, accepted for publication, 1992.
2. Engel J Jr: *Seizures and Epilepsy*. F.A. Davis, Philadelphia, 1989.
3. Commission on Classification and Terminology of the International League Against Epilepsy: Proposal for Revised Clinical and Electroencephalographic Classification of Epileptic Seizures. *Epilepsia* 22:489–501, 1981.
4. Commission on Classification and Terminology of the International League Against Epilepsy: Proposal for Revised Clinical and Electroencephalographic Classification of Epilepsies and Epileptic Syndromes. *Epilepsia* 26:268–278, 1985.
5. Lothman E: The biochemical basis and pathophysiology of status epilepticus. *Neurology* 40(Suppl 2):13–22, 1990.
6. Kreisman NR, Lamanna JC, Rosenthal M, Sick TJ: Oxidative metabolic responses with recurrent seizures in rat cerebral cortex: role of systemic factors. *Brain Res* 218:175–188, 1981.
7. Todd RB: *Clinical Lectures on Paralysis, Disease of the Brain and Other Affections of the Nervous System*. Lindsay Y & Blakiston, Philadelphia, 1955.
8. Treiman DM, Delgado-Escueta AV: Complex partial status epilepticus. *Adv Neurol* 34:69–81, 1983.
9. Wieser HG, Hailemariam S, Regard M, Landis T: Unilateral limbic epileptic status activity: stereo EEG, behavioral and cognitive data. *Epilepsia* 26:19–29, 1985.
10. Krumholz A, Fisher RS, Weiss HD: Persistent neurological deficits following complex partial status epilepticus (CPSE) *Epilepsia* October: 1986.
11. Dodrill CB, Wilensky AJ: Intellectual impairment as an outcome of status epilepticus. *Neurology* 40(Suppl 2):23–27, 1990.
12. Leppik IE: Status epilepticus: the next decade. *Neurology* 40(Suppl 2):4–9, 1990.
13. Degiorgio CM, Tomiyasu U, Gott PS, Treiman DM: Hippocampal pyramidal cell loss in human status epilepticus. *Epilepsia* 33(1):23–27, 1992.
14. Niedermeyer E, Lopes da Silva F: *Electroencephalography: Basic Principles, Clinical Applications and Related Fields*, ed 2. Urban & Schwarzenberg, Munchen, Federal Republic Germany, 1987.
15. Fujiwara T, Watanabe M, Nakamura H, Kudo T, Yagi K, Seino M: A comparative study of absence status epilepticus between adults and children. *Jpn J Psychiatry Neurol* 42:497–508, 1988.
16. Schwartz MS, Scott DF: Isolated petit mal status presenting de novo in middle age. *Lancet* ii:1399–1402, 1971.
17. Van Zandycke M, Orban LC, Vander Eecken H: Acute prolonged ictal confusion (resembling petit mal status) presenting "de novo" in later life. *Acta Neurol Belg* 80:174–179, 1980.
18. Fisher RS: Non-convulsive Status Epilepticus. Neurology Grand Rounds, The Johns Hopkins Hospital, 1991.
19. Ellis JM, Lee SI: Acute prolonged confusion in later life as an ictal state. *Epilepsia* 19:119–128, 1978.
20. Yeo PT, Wodak J, Roe CJ, Gilligan BS: Absence status: a report of two cases. *Aust NZ J Med* 14:53–55, 1984.
21. Daly R, Pedly D (eds): *Clinical Electroencephalography*. Raven Press, New York, 1990.
22. Jumao-as A, Brenner RP: Myoclonic status epilepticus: a clinical and electrographic study. *Neurology* 40(8):1199–1202, 1990.
23. Gates JR, Ramani V, Whalen S, Loewenson R: Ictal characteristics of pseudoseizures. *Arch Neurol* 42:1183–1187, 1985.
24. Meierkord H, Will B, Fish D, Shorvon S: The clinical features and prognosis of pseudoseizures diagnosed using video-EEG telemetry. *Neurology* 41:1643–1646, 1991.
25. Leis AA, Ross MA, Summers AK: Psychogenic seizures: ictal characteristics and diagnostic pitfalls. *Neurology* 42:95–99, 1992.
26. Fisher RS (ed): *Neurotransmitters and Epilepsy*. Raven Press, New York, 1991.
27. Kandel ER, Schwartz JH, Jessel TM: *Principles of Neuroscience*, ed 3. Elsevier Science Publishing Company Inc, New York, 1991.

28. Clark GD: Role of excitatory amino acids in brain injury caused by hypoxia-ischemia, status epilepticus and hypoglycemia. *Clin Perinatol* 16(2):459–474, 1989.
29. Walton NY, Treiman DM: Motor and electroencephalographic response of refractory experimental status epilepticus in rats to treatment with MK-801, diazepam, or MK-801 plus diazepam. *Brain Res* 553:97–104, 1991.
30. Gillman AG, Goodman LS, Gilman A: *The Pharmacologic Basis of Therapeutics.* Macmillan, New York, 1990.
31. Scheyer RD, Cramer JA: Pharmacokinetics of antiepileptic drugs. *Semin Neurol* 10(4):414–421, 1990.
32. Osorio I, Reed RC: Treatment of refractory generalized tonic-clonic status epilepticus with pentobarbital anesthesia after high-dose phenytoin. *Epilepsia* 30:464–471, 1989.
33. Gallagher BB, Freer, LS: Barbituric acid derivatives. In Frey H-H and Janz D (eds): *Antiepileptic Drugs,* Springer-Verlag, New York, pp 421–447, 1985.
34. Lenn NJ, Robertson M: Clinical utility of unbound antiepileptic drug blood levels in the management of epilepsy. *Neurology* 42:988–990, 1992.
35. Booker HE, Darcey B: Serum concentrations of free diphenylhydantoin and their relationship to clinical intoxication. *Epilepsia* 14:177–184, 1973.
36. Treiman DM: General principles of treatment: responsive and intractable status epilepticus in adults. *Adv Neurol* 34:377–384, 1983.
37. Prichard JW, Ransom BR: Phenobarbital: mechanisms of action. In Levy RH, Dreifuss FE, Mattson RH, Meldrum BS, Penry JK (eds): *Antiepileptic Drugs,* ed 3. Raven Press, New York, 1989.
38. Morrell F, Bradley W, Ptashne M: Effects of drugs on discharge characteristics of chronic epileptogenic lesions. *Neurology* 9:492–498, 1959.
39. *Physicians Desk Reference (PDR) 1992:* Medical Economics Data, a division of Medical Economics Company, Inc, Montvale NJ, 1992.
40. Kutt H: Phenytoin: Interactions with other drugs. In Levy RH, Dreifuss FE, Mattson RH, Meldrum BS, Penry JK (eds): *Antiepileptic Drugs,* ed 3. Raven Press, New York, 1989.
41. McEvoy GK (ed): *American Hospital Formulary Service (AHFS) Drug Information 1990:* American Society of Hospital Pharmacists, Bethesda, MD, 1990.
42. Rust RS, Dodson WE: Phenobarbital: absorption, distribution, and excretion. In Levy RH, Dreifuss FE, Mattson RH, Meldrum BS and Penry JK (eds): *Antiepileptic Drugs,* ed 3. Raven Press, New York, 1989.
43. Giotti A, Maynert EW: The renal clearance of barbital and the mechanism of its reabsorption. *J Pharmacol Exp Ther* 101:296–309, 1951.
44. Oliver AP, Hoffer BJ, Wyatt RJ: The hippocampal slice: a system for studying the pharmacology of seizures and for screening anticonvulsant drugs. *Epilepsia* 18:543–548, 1977.
45. MacDonald RL, Barker JL: Different actions of anticonvulsant and anesthetic barbiturates resolved by use of cultured mammalian neurons. *Science* 200:775–777, 1978.
46. Schulz DW, MacDonald RL: Barbiturate enhancement of GABA-mediated inhibition and activation of chloride ion conductance. *Brain Res* 209:177–188, 1981.
47. Sohn RS, Ferrendelli JA: Anticonvulsant drug mechanisms. *Arch Neurol* 33:626–629, 1976.
48. Blaustein MP, Ector A: Inhibition of calcium uptake by depolarized nerve in vitro. *Mol Pharmacol* 11:369–378, 1975.
49. Kutt H: Phenobarbital: interactions with other drugs. In Levy RH, Dreifuss FE, Mattson RH, Meldrum BS, Penry JK (eds): *Antiepileptic Drugs,* ed 3. Raven Press, New York, 1989.
50. Treiman DM: Pharmacokinetics and clinical use of benzodiazepines in the management of status epilepticus. *Epilepsia* 30(Suppl 2):S4–S10, 1989.
51. Greenblatt DJ, Shader RI: Pharmacokinetics of antianxiety agents. In Meltzer HY (ed): *Psychopharmacology: the Third Generation of Progress.* Raven Press, New York, p 1377–1385, 1987.
52. Greenblatt DJ, Ehrenberg BL, Gunderman J, Locniskar A, Scavone JM, Harmatz JS, Shader RI: Pharmacokinetic and electroencephalographic study of intravenous diazepam, midazolam and placebo. *Clin Pharmacol Ther* 45:356–365, 1989.
53. Greenblatt DJ, Ehrenberg BL, Gunderman J, Scavone JM, Tai NT, Harmatz JS, Shader RI: Kinetic and dynamic study of intravenous lorazepam: comparison with intravenous diazepam. *J Pharm Exp Ther* 250(1):134–139, 1989.
54. Geller E, Thomson D (eds): Proceedings of the International Symposium on flumazenil—the first benzodiazepine antagonist. *Eur J Anaesthesiol* (Suppl 2):1–332.
55. Greenblatt DJ, Miller LG: Mechanism of the anticonvulsant action of benzodiazepines. *Cleveland Clin J Med* 57(Suppl 7):S6–S8, 1990.
56. Olsen RW: Drug interactions at the GABE receptor-ionophore complex. *Annu Rev Pharmacol Toxicol* 22:245–277, 1982.
57. Levy RH, Dreifuss FE, Mattson RH, Meldrum BS and Penry JK (eds): *Antiepileptic Drugs,* ed 3. Raven Press, New York, 1989.
58. Kuman A, Bleck TP: Intravenous midazolam for the treatment of refractory status epilepticus. *Crit Care Med* 20(4):483–488, 1992.
59. DeLorenzo RJ: Status epilepticus: concepts in diagnosis and treatment. *Semin Neurol* 10(4):396–405, 1990.
60. King J: *King's Guide to Parenteral Admixtures.* Pacemarq, Inc., St. Louis, 1992.
61. Delgado-Escueta AV, Enrile-Bacsal F: Combination therapy for status epilepticus: intravenous diazepam and phenytoin. *Adv Neurol* 34:477–485, 1983.

62. Bell DS, Bertino Jr JS: Constant diazepam infusion in the treatment of continuous seizure activity. *Drug Intell Clin Pharmacol* 18:965–970, 1984.
63. Schmidt D: Benzodiazepines. In Levy RH, Dreifuss FE, Mattson RH, Meldrum BS, Penry JK (eds): *Antiepileptic Drugs,* ed 3. Raven Press, New York, 1989.
64. Knudsen FU: Rectal administration of diazepam in solution in the acute treatment of convulsions in infants and children. *Arch Dis Child* 66:563–567, 1979.
65. Langdon DE, Harlan JR, Bailey RL: Thrombophlebitis with diazepam used intravenously. *JAMA* 223:184–185, 1973.
66. MacLeod SM, Giles HG, Patzalek G, Thiessen JJ, Sellers EM: Diazepam actions and plasma concentrations following ethanol ingestion. *Eur J Clin Pharmacol* 11:345–349, 1977.
67. Klotz U, Anttila VJ, Reimann I: Cimetidine/diazepam interaction. *Lancet* ii:699, 1979.
68. Kulkarni SK, Jog MV: Facilitation of diazepam action by anticonvulsant agents against picrotoxin induced convulsions. *Psychopharmacology* 81:332–334, 1983.
69. Czuczwar SJ, Turski WA, Ikonomidou C, Turski L: Aminophylline and CGS 8216 reverse the protective action of diazepam against electroconvulsions in mice. *Epilepsia* 26(6):693–696, 1985.
70. Dhillon S, Richens A: Valproic acid and diazepam interaction in vivo. *Br J Clin Pharmacol* 13:553–560, 1982.
71. Marrosu F, Marchi A, De Martino MR, Saba G, Gessa GL: Aminophylline antagonizes diazepam-induced anesthesia and EEG changes in humans. *Psychopharmacology* 85:69–70, 1985.
72. Levy RJ, Krall RL: Treatment of status epilepticus with lorazepam. *Arch Neurol* 41:605–611, 1984.
73. Meberg A, Langslet A, Bredesen JE, Lunde PKM: Plasma concentration of diazepam and *N*-desmethyldiazepam in children after a single rectal or intramuscular dose of diazepam. *Eur J Clin Pharmacol* 14:273–276, 1978.
74. Sato S: Clonazepam. In Levy RH, Dreifuss FE, Mattson RH, Meldrum BS, Penry JK (eds): *Antiepileptic Drugs,* ed 3. Raven Press, New York, 1989.
75. Rylance GW, Poulton J, Cherry RC, Cullen RE: Plasma concentrations of clonazepam after single rectal administration. *Arch Dis Child* 61:186–188, 1986.
76. Elgi M, Albani C: Relief of status epilepticus after IM administration of the new short-acting benzodiazepine midazolam (abstr.). In *Program and Abstracts of the 12th World Congress of Neurology.* Princeton, NJ, Excerpta Medica, p 44, 1981.
77. Schauf CL, Floyd AD, Marder J: Effects of carbamazepine in the ionic conductances of myxicola giant axons. *J Pharmacol Exp Ther* 189:538–543, 1974.
78. McLean MJ, Macdonald RL: Carbamazepine and 10,11-epoxycarbamazepine produce use- and voltage-dependent limitation of rapidly firing action potentials of mouse central neurons in cell culture. *J Pharmacol Exp Ther* 238:727–738, 1986.
79. Courtney KR, Etter EG: Modulated anticonvulsant block of sodium channels in nerve and muscle. *Eur J Pharm* 88:1–9, 1983.
80. Willow M, Gonoi T, Catterall WA: Voltage clamp analysis of the inhibitory actions of diphenylhydantoin and carbamazepine on voltage-sensitive sodium channels in neuroblastoma cells. *Mol Pharmacol* 25:228–234, 1985.
81. Macdonald RL: Carbamazepine: mechanisms of action. In Levy RH, Dreifuss FE, Mattson RH, Meldrum BS, Penry JK (eds): *Antiepileptic Drugs,* ed 3. Raven Press, New York, 1989.
82. Pitlick WH, Levy RH: Carbamazepine: interactions with other drugs. In Levy RH, Dreifuss FE, Mattson RH, Meldrum BS, Penry JK (eds): *Antiepileptic Drugs,* ed 3. Raven Press, New York, 1989.
83. Levy RL, Shen DD: Valproate: absorption, distribution, and excretion. In Levy RH, Dreifuss FE, Mattson RH, Meldrum BS, Penry JK (eds): *Antiepileptic Drugs,* ed 3. Raven Press, New York, 1989.
84. Rosenfeld WE, Leppik IE, Gates JR, Mireles RE: Valproic acid loading during intensive monitoring. *Arch Neurol* 44:709–710, 1987.
85. Snead OC III, Miles MV: Treatment of status epilepticus in children with rectal valproate loading. *J Pediatr* 106:323–325, .
86. Fariello R, Smith MC: Valproate mechanisms of action. In Levy RH, Dreifuss FE, Mattson RH, Meldrum BS, Penry JK (eds): *Antiepileptic Drugs,* ed 3. Raven Press, NY, pp 567–582, 1989.
87. Van Diujn H, Beckman MKF: Dipropylacetic acid (Depakine) in experimental epilepsy in the alert cat. *Epilepsia* 16:83–90, 1975.
88. Tennison MB, Miles MV, Pollack GM, Thorn MD, Dupuis RE: Valproate metabolites and hepatotoxicity in an epileptic population. *Epilepsia* 29:543–547, 1988.
89. Kofke WA, Young RS, Davis P, Woelfel SK, Gray L, Johnson D, Gelb A, Meeke R, Warner DS, Pearson KS, Gibson JR, Koncelik J, Wessel HB: Isoflurane for Refractory Status Epilepticus: a clinical series. *Anesthesiology* 71:653–659, 1989.
90. Mackenzie SJ, Kapadia F, Grant IS: Propofol infusion for control of status epilepticus. *Anaesthesia* 45:1043–1045, 1990.
91. Tasker RC, Boyd SG, Harden A, Matthew DJ: EEG monitoring of prolonged thiopentone administration for intractable seizures and status epilepticus in infants and young children. *Neuropediatrics* 20:147–153, 1989.
92. Messing RO, Closson RG, Simon RP: Drug-induced seizures: a 10-year experience. *Neurology* 34:1582–1586, 1984.

93. Rockoff MA, Goudsouzian NG: Seizures induced by methohexital. *Anesthesiology* 54:333–335, 1981.

94. Hauser WA: Status epilepticus: epidemiologic considerations. *Neurology* 40(Suppl 2):9–13, 1990.

95. Leifer D, Cole DG, Kowall NW: Neuropathologic asymmetries in the brain of a patient with a unilateral status epilepticus. *J Neuro Sci* 103:127–135, 1991.

96. Albers GW, Goldberg MP, Choi DW: Do NMDA Antagonists Prevent Neuronal Injury? Yes. *Arch Neurol* 49(4):418–419, 1992.

97. Riela AR, Sires BP, Penry JK: Transient magnetic resonance imaging abnormalities during partial status epilepticus. 6:143–145, 1991.

98. Fisher RS: Emergency treatment for status epilepticus. *J Crit Illness* 2(4):27–38, 1987.

99. Aminoff M, Simon RP: Status epilepticus: causes, clinical features and consequences in 98 patients. *Am J Med* 69:657–665, 1980.

100. Treiman DM, Walton NY, Kendrick A: A progressive sequence of electroencephalographic changes during generalized convulsive status epilepticus. *Epilepsy Res* 5:49–60, 1990.

101. Lowenstein DH, Aminoff MJ: Clinical and EEG features of status epilepticus in comatose patients. *Neurology* 42:100–104, 1992.

102. Sieber FE, Traystman RJ: Special issues: glucose and the brain. *Crit Care Med* 20(1):104–114, 1992.

103. Leppik IE, Derivan AT, Homan RW, et al: Double-blind study of lorazepam and diazepam in status epilepticus. *JAMA* 249:1452–1454, 1983.

104. Giang DW, McBride MC: Lorazepam versus diazepam for the treatment of status epilepticus. *Pediatr Neurol* 4:358–361, 1988.

105. Walker JE, Homan RW, Crawford IL: Lorazepam: a controlled trial in patients with intractable partial complex seizures. *Epilepsia* 25(4):464–466, 1984.

106. Walker JE, Homan RW, Vasko MR, Crawford IL, Bell RD, Tasker WG: Lorazepam in status epilepticus. *Ann Neurol* 6:207–213, 1979.

107. Homan RW, Unwin DH: In Levy RH, Dreifuss FE, Mattson RH, Meldrum BS, Penry JK (eds): *Antiepileptic Drugs*, ed 3. Raven Press, New York, 1989.

108. Richens JS, Oxley J: Pharmacodynamic and clinical evaluation of midazolam in epilepsy. *Acta Neurol Scand* 70:219, 1984.

109. Asconape JJ, Penry JK: Use of antiepileptic drugs in the presence of liver and kidney diseases: a review. *Epilepsia* 23(S1):S65–S79, 1982.

110. Van Ness PC: Pentobarbital and EEG burst suppression in treatment of status epilepticus refractory to benzodiazepines and phenytoin. *Epilepsia* 31(1):61–67, 1990.

111. Bankman I, Webber WRS, Waechter M, Fisher RS, Lesser RP: On-line detection of epileptic spikes on multi-channel recordings. *Epilepsia* 29:711, 1988.

112. Hostetler WE, Doller HJ, Homan RW: Assessment of a computer program to detect epileptiform spikes. *Electroencephalogr Clin Neurophysiol* 83:1–11, 1992.

113. Frost Jr JD: Automatic recognition and characterization of epileptiform discharges in the human EEG. *J Clin Neurophysiol* 2:231–249, 1985.

114. Gotman J, Gloor P: Automatic recognition and quantification of interictal epileptic activity in the human scalp EEG. *Electroencephalogr Clin Neurophysiol* 41:513–529, 1976.

115. Altafullah I, Asaikar S, Torres F: Status epilepticus: clinical experience with two special devices for continuous cerebral monitoring. *Acta Neurol Scand* 84:374–381, 1991.

116. Reiher J, Maison FG, Leduc CP: Partial status epilepticus: short-term prediction of seizure outcome from on-line EEG analysis. *Electroencephalogr Clin Neurophysiol* 82:17–22, 1992.

117. Engel J, Ludwig BI, Getell M: Prolonged partial complex status epilepticus: EEG and behavioral observations. *Neurology* 28:863–869, 1978.

118. Wells CE: Transient ictal psychosis. *Arch Gen Psychiatry* 32:1201–1203, 1975.

119. Thomas P, Beaumanoir A, Genton P, Dolisi C, Chatel M: "De novo" absence status of late onset: report of 11 cases. *Neurology* 42:104–110, 1992.

120. Anderman F, Robb MP: Absence status. *Epilepsia* 13:177–187, 1972.

121. Lowenstein DH, Aminoff MJ, Simon RP: Barbiturate anesthesia in the treatment of status epilepticus: clinical experience with 14 patients. *Neurology* 38:395–400, 1988.

122. Niedermeyer E, Fineyre F, Riley T, Uematsu S: Absence status (petit mal status) with focal characteristics. *Arch Neurol* 36:417–421, 1979.

123. Snead III OC, Hosey LC: Exacerbation of seizures in children by carbamazepine. *N Engl J Med* 313:916–921, 1985.

124. Berkovic SF, Andermann F, Guberman A, Hipola D, Bladin PF: Valproate prevents the recurrence of absence status. *Neurology* 39:1294–1297, 1989.

125. Celesia GG, Grigg MM, Ross E: Generalized status myoclonicus in acute anoxic and metabolic encephalopathies. *Arch Neurol* 45:781–784, 1988.

126. Krumholz A, Stern BJ, Weiss HD: Outcome from coma after cardiopulmonary resuscitation: relation to seizures and myoclonus. *Neurology* 38:401–405, 1988.

127. Krumholz A, Niedermeyer E: Psychogenic seizures: a clinical study with follow-up data. *Neurology* 33:498–502, 1983.

128. Lesser RP, Lueders H, Dinner DS: Evidence for epilepsy is rare in patients with psychogenic seizures. *Neurology* 33:502–504, 1983.

129. Tiula E, Haapanen J, Neuvonen PJ: Factors affecting serum protein binding of phenytoin, diazepam and propranolol in acute renal diseases. *Int J Clin Pharmacodyn Ther Toxicol* 25:469–475, 1987.

130. Scheuer ML: Medical patients with epilepsy. In Resor Jr SR, Kutt H (eds): *The Medical Treatment of Epilepsy*. Marcel Dekker, Inc, New York, 1992.

131. Asconape JJ, Penry JK: Use of antiepileptic drugs in the presence of liver and kidney diseases: a review. *Epilepsia* 23 (Suppl 1):65–79, 1982.

132. Bennett WM, Aronoff GR, Morrison G, et al: Drug prescribing in renal failure: dosing guidelines for adults. *Am J Kidney Dis* 3:155–193, 1983.

133. Lee CS, Marbury TC: Drug therapy in patients undergoing hemodialysis. *Clin Pharmacokinet* 42:42–66, 1984.

134. Kandrotas RJ, Oles KS, Gal P, Love JM: Carbamazepine clearance in hemodialysis and hemoperfusion. *DICP* 23:137–140, 1989.

135. Marbury TC, Lee CS, Bruni J, Wilder BJ: Hemodialysis of valproic acid in uremic patients. *Dial Transpl* 9:961–964, 1980.

136. Kandrotas RJ, Love JM, Gal P, Oles KS: The effect of hemodialysis and hemoperfusion on serum valproic acid concentration. *Neurology* 40:1456–1458, 1990.

137. Painter JP: In Levy RH, Dreifuss FE, Mattson RH, Meldrum BS, Penry JK (eds): Phenobarbital: clinical use *Antiepileptic Drugs*, ed 3. Raven Press, New York, 1989.

138. Kuhara T, Inoue Y, Matsumoto M, Shinka T, Matsumoto I, Kawahara N, Sakura N: Markedly increased omega-oxidation of valproate in fulminant hepatic failure. *Epilepsia* 31:214–217, 1990.

139. Alvin J, McHorse T, Hoyumpa A, Bush M, Schenker S: The effect of liver disease in man on the disposition of phenobarbital. *J Pharmacol Exp Ther* 192:224–235, 1974.

140. Morselli PL: Carbamazepine: absorption, distribution and excretion. In Levy RH, Dreifuss FE, Mattson RH, Meldrum BS, Penry JK (eds): *Antiepileptic Drugs*, ed 3. Raven Press, New York, 1989.

141. Basile AS, Hughes RD, Harrison PM, Murata Y, Pannell L, Jones EA, Williams R, Skolnick P: Elevated brain concentrations of 1,4-benzodiazepines in fulminant hepatic failure. *N Engl J Med* 325:473–478, 1991.

142. Rabinowicz AL, Ginsburg DL, DeGiorgio CM, Gott P, Gianotta SL: Unruptured intracranial aneurysms: seizures and antiepileptic drug treatment following surgery. *J Neurosurg* 75:371–373, 1991.

143. Shaw MDM: Post-operative epilepsy and the efficacy of anticonvulsant therapy. *Acta Neurochirur* Suppl (Wien):50:55–57, 1990.

144. Mathew E, Sherwin AL, Weiner SA, Odusote K, Stratford JG: Seizures following intracranial surgery: incidence in the first post-operative week. *J Can Sci Neurol* 7:285–288, 1980.

145. Kvam DA, Loftus CM, Copeland B, Quest DO: Seizures during the immediate postoperative period. *Neurosurgery* 12:14–17, 1983.

146. Tempkin NR, Nikmen SS, Wilensky AJ, Keihm J, et al: A randomized, double-blind study of phenytoin for the prevention of post-traumatic seizures. *N Engl J Med* 323(8):497–502, 1990.

147. Pagni CA: Posttraumatic epilepsy. Incidence and prophylaxis. *Acta Neurochirurg* Suppl (Wien):50:38–47, 1990.

148. Boucher BA, Rodman JH, Fabian TC, et al: Disposition of phenytoin in critically ill trauma patients. *Clin Pharm* 6:881–887, 1987.

149. Kilpatrick CJ, Davis SM, Tress BM, Rossiter SC, Hopper JL, Vandendriesen ML: Epileptic seizures in acute stroke. *Arch Neurol* 46:157–160, 1990.

150. Snodgrass SM, Tsuburaya K, Ajmone-Marsan C: Clinical significance of periodic lateralized epileptiform discharges: relationship with status epilepticus. *J Clin Neurophysiol* 6:159–172, 1989.

151. Krauss G, Niedermeyer E: Electroencephalogram and seizures in chronic alcoholism. *Electroencephalog Clin Neurophysiol* 78:7–104, 1991.

152. Alldredge BK, Lowenstein DH, Simon RP: Placebo-controlled trial of intravenous diphenylhydantoin for short-term treatment of alcohol withdrawal seizures. *Am J Med* 87(6):645–648, 1989.

153. Krauss GL, Fisher RS, Kaplan P: Parenteral magnesium sulfate fails to control electroshock and pentylenetetrazol seizures in mice. *Epilepsy Res* 4:201–206, 1989.

CHAPTER 30

Pharmacologic Approach to Stroke and Related Neurologic Emergencies

BARNEY J. STERN, M.D.
MICHAEL N. DIRINGER, M.D.

Optimal management of the stroke patient requires definition of the pathophysiology of the event. Once the mechanisms responsible for the neurologic condition are understood, pharmacologic and other therapeutic strategies can be tailored to the individual patient. Stroke should be considered an emergency and evaluation and treatment should be urgently pursued.

There are many causes of stroke. Broadly considered, the end result of disease leading to stroke can be either a predominantly ischemic or hemorrhagic process. This distinction is not absolute, but usually a differentiation can be made from clinical and neuroimaging information.

ISCHEMIC DISEASE

Ischemic stroke can be caused by cardiogenic emboli, large artery extracranial or intracranial disease, and small artery "penetrating branch" disease. Systemic illness, especially hematologic conditions, can lead to stroke by promoting either arterial or venous thrombosis.

Patients with cerebrovascular disease can be asymptomatic, intermittently symptomatic, relatively stable and symptomatic, or progressively deteriorating. Besides consideration of the tempo of the illness, management decisions must take into account the extent of brain injury, the nature of the underlying vascular lesion, and concurrent medical conditions, such as fever and infection and cardiopulmonary disease. Unfortunately, many treatment strategies remain of unproved

benefit, even if based on a reasonable interpretation of stroke pathophysiology and clinical observation (1, 1a, 1b).

CARDIOGENIC EMBOLUS

A cardiac embolus produces sudden neurologic dysfunction by lodging in an artery and impeding local circulation (1c). The neurologic manifestations depend on the arterial territory compromised; the middle cerebral artery and the distal basilar artery and its branches are most commonly involved.

The most important cause of cardiogenic emboli is nonvalvular atrial fibrillation (2). Other conditions include an akinetic left ventricular segment, prosthetic heart valve, cardiomyopathy, and endocarditis (3). A more complete listing of conditions associated with cardiogenic emboli is presented in Table 30.1 (3).

Evaluation of the patient with a suspected cardiogenic embolus often includes transthoracic echocardiography (4). Transesophageal echocardiography is more sensitive and therefore can provide additional information regarding left atrial anatomy, valvular structures, atrial septal abnormalities, and aortic lesions (5) for patients in whom transthoracic echocardiography is unrevealing (4, 6). Occasionally arrhythmia monitoring can detect an otherwise occult rhythm disturbance, such as paroxysmal atrial fibrillation, that predisposes to embolization (3). Lastly, a search for a hypercoagulable state is warranted in patients with sterile valvular vegetations;

Table 30.1. Selected Conditions Associated with Ischemic Stroke

Cardiogenic emboli
  Atrial fibrillation
  Recent myocardial infarction
  Cardiac thrombus
  Akinetic ventricular segment
  Dilated cardiomyopathy
  Valvular disease
  Prosthetic heart valve
  Patent foramen ovale
  Atrial septal defect
  Atrial septal aneurysm
  Infective endocarditis
  Nonbacterial thrombotic endocarditis
  Left atrial spontaneous echo contrast
  Myxoma
Large artery disease
  Atherosclerosis
  Dissection
  Fibromuscular dysplasia
  Takayasu's disease
  Moya Moya disease
  Radiation-induced damage
Small artery disease
  Microatheroma
  Lipohyalinosis
  Inflammation
    Sterile
    Infectious
Systemic and hematologic conditions
  Polycythemia
  Sickle cell disease
  Hypercoagulable states
    Malignancy
    Pregnancy
    Inflammatory bowel disease
    Nephrotic syndrome
    Antiphospholipid syndrome
    Protein S and C deficiencies
    Antithrombin III deficiency
    Dysfibrinogenemia
Miscellaneous conditions
  Migraine
  Drug use and abuse
    Cocaine (including "crack")
    Alcohol
    L-asparaginase
    Birth control pills
    Sympathomimetics

an antiphospholipid syndrome (7) or cancer-associated hypercoagulable state is occasionally found.

The presence of, for instance, atrial fibrillation, mitral valve prolapse, a patent foramen ovale, or an akinetic ventricular segment is only suggestive evidence of a cardiac embolus as the cause of the patient's stroke. The demonstration of an intracardiac thrombus is much more convincing evidence. Lastly, cardiac disease can coexist with other potential causes of stroke; for example, severe large artery occlusive disease, appropriate in location for the patient's symptoms, is present in 11% of patients with a potential source of cardiac embolism (8).

Management of patients with stroke resulting from cardiac emboli is directed toward prevention of additional embolic events by the use of anticoagulants. Critical to this approach is the concept that an ischemic infarction can convert to a hemorrhagic infarction because of lysis of the embolus and reperfusion of an already compromised vascular territory.

Hemorrhagic transformation occurs in up to 69% of cardioembolic infarctions and is usually not a cause of clinical worsening (8a). However, bleeding into infarcted brain can exacerbate mass effect, sometimes already present from the ischemic infarction, and lead to increased intracranial pressure. Large ischemic infarctions are most prone to hemorrhagic conversion (8a, 9), which typically occurs 48 to 96 hours after the ictus (3). Hypertension and advanced age may increase the risk of hemorrhagic transformation.

With the demonstration that antiplatelet or anticoagulation therapy decreases the risk of embolic events in patients with nonvalvular atrial fibrillation (10–12), an increase in the use of these agents can be expected. The impact this therapy will have on the incidence of hemorrhagic stroke remains to be seen (13).

Management (14)

Conventional wisdom dictates that patients with a suspected cardiogenic embolus should have a brain computed tomographic (CT) scan to evaluate the possibility of hemorrhage (Fig. 30.1). If no blood is apparent on brain imaging done approximately 48 hours after infarction, if the stroke is not massive (for instance, infarction of the entire middle cerebral artery territory), if the patient's blood pressure is <180/100 mm Hg, and if there is no contraindication to anticoagulation, heparin therapy should be started.

If early anticoagulation is contraindicated, the patient's status should be reviewed after 5 to 7 days. If a reasonable clinical recovery is expected and if there is no hemorrhagic infarction on CT scan, anticoagulation with heparin or warfarin therapy should be reconsidered at this time. If the patient deteriorates neurologically while on heparin treatment, a CT scan should be obtained to evaluate for bleeding. If a hemorrhagic infarction is detected at any time, anticoagulation is probably best deferred and reconsidered in another week's time. If an intracerebral hematoma is present, anticoagulation should not be attempted.

Subsequent reports have noted that patients with hemorrhagic infarction on imaging studies can remain clinically stable (15, 15a). Furthermore, anticoagulation can be safely maintained in many of these patients, though perhaps at a less intense level (15a). If a hemorrhagic infarction is large, a 6-week wait prior to anticoagulation may be prudent (16). Serial imaging studies, clinical observation, and weighing the risk of repeat embolization may help guide therapy. Patients who sustain an embolic stroke in spite of a reasonable intensity of anticoagulation with warfarin, can be treated temporarily with heparin so that anticoagulation can be quickly interrupted if the patient deteriorates.

When the underlying cause of the cardiogenic embolus cannot be eliminated, consideration should be given to chronic warfarin treatment. Potential contraindications include the patient's expected compliance, propensity to fall, and level of overall function.

Patients with recurrent cardiogenic emboli in spite of adequate anticoagulation occasionally are treated with both warfarin and antiplatelet agents; typically these are patients with prosthetic heart valves (17, 18). During the first and third trimesters of pregnancy, warfarin should not be used and subcutaneous heparin therapy is preferred to avoid the teratogenic and hemorrhagic complications associated with warfarin (19).

Septic Emboli

The risk of cerebral emboli from native valve endocarditis is greatest at the onset of illness, before antibiotic therapy has made much of an impact (20). The more virulent bacteria are most prone to embolize (21). In general, anticoagulation is not advised to prevent septic emboli in patients with native valve endocarditis (22).

Patients with prosthetic valve endocarditis are often already anticoagulated when their infection develops. Anticoagulation management in this situation is more problematic, but the consensus seems to be to continue anticoagulation unless severe intracranial bleeding develops (23, 24).

LARGE ARTERY DISEASE

Arterial disease can be classified as principally involving the large extracranial or intracranial vessels. Atherosclerosis is the most common cause of either extracranial or intracranial arterial disease, but there are other causes of arterial pathology (Table 30.1). This discussion focuses on selected aspects of the management of atherosclerotic disease, although other causes of arterial pathology are mentioned (Fig. 30.2).

Asymptomatic Extracranial Carotid Artery Disease

A cervical bruit is correlated with hemodynamically significant stenosis of the origin of the internal carotid artery in approximately 75% of patients. Atherosclerosis at the origin of the internal carotid artery is a risk factor for stroke and coronary artery disease (25). Approximately one-third of patients with internal carotid artery atherosclerosis have progressive disease, and these patients are at highest risk for stroke (26).

Management of patients with internal carotid artery disease involves modification of risk factors for atherosclerosis. Particular attention should be directed to detection and treatment of coronary artery disease, since this is a major source of morbidity and mortality (27, 28, 28a). Optimal management of asymptomatic atherosclerotic narrowing at the origin of the internal carotid artery has yet to be defined (28b–e). Until the results of the Asymptomatic Carotid Artery Study are known, disease that is not hemodynamically significant is best treated by education of the patient about warning signs of cerebral ischemia, serial assessments of the degree of stenosis, perhaps on an every-6-month basis and, perhaps, aspirin. Patients with a hemodynamically significant stenosis of the internal carotid artery origin may benefit from an elective carotid endarterectomy, if their general medical condition is good and the surgery can be performed with a morbidity and mortality of less than 3 to 5% (29). However, until the results of the Asymptomatic Carotid Artery Study are known, surgery should be considered to be of unproven value and probably should be deferred (28e). Efforts should be made to avoid hypotension in patients with a critical stenosis so as not to cause an infarction from hypoperfusion.

Management of patients undergoing coronary artery surgery who have asymptomatic disease of the internal carotid artery origin should be dictated by the aforementioned principles (30).

Intermittently Symptomatic Arterial Disease

Extracranial Carotid Artery. Transient ischemic attacks (TIAs) are commonly associated with atherosclerotic disease at the origin of the internal carotid artery. Neurologic manifestations result from emboli arising from an atheroma and lodging at a distal site or a hemodynamically significant stenosis producing distal hypoperfusion. Cardiogenic emboli, atherosclerosis at other sites, other large artery disorders, penetrating small artery disease, and neurologic disorders such as seizures, tumors, and subdural hematoma can also cause brief

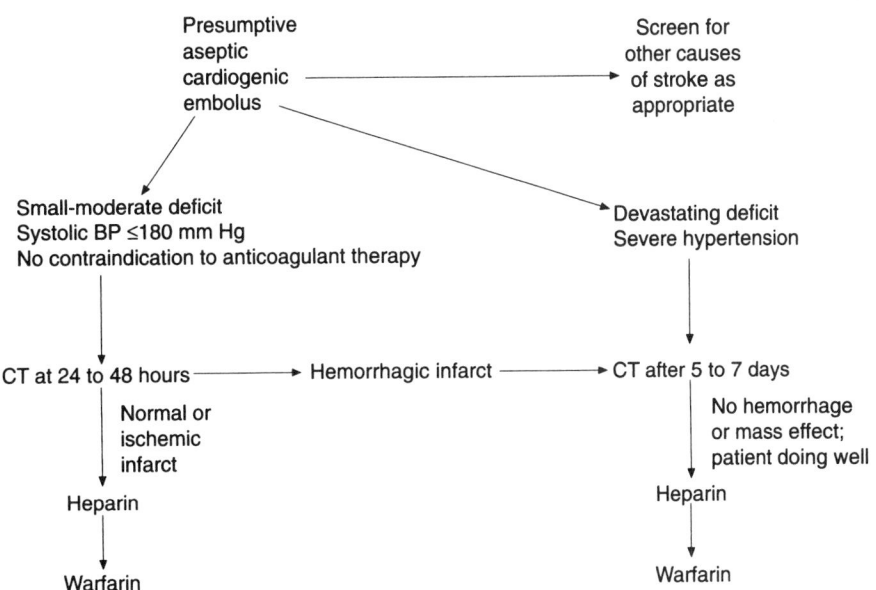

Figure 30.1. Management of cardiogenic embolic stroke.

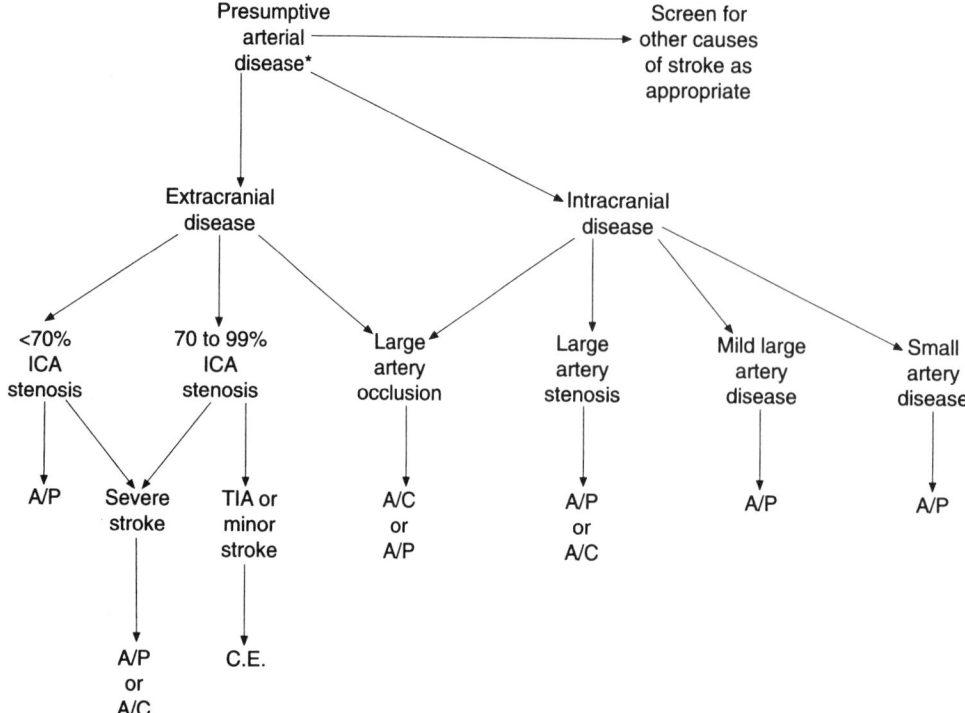

Figure 30.2. Management of arterial disease causing an acute ischemic event. (*A/P*, antiplatelet therapy; *A/C*, anticoagulant therapy; *C.E.*, carotid endarterectomy; *ICA*, internal carotid artery; *, consider A/C if patient is deteriorating).

neurologic events and should be considered. Symptoms referable to the carotid artery territory include transient monocular blindness (amaurosis fugax), aphasia, and weakness or numbness contralateral to the diseased artery that involves the face more than the arm, and, in turn, more than the leg.

General medical management of patients with atherosclerosis at the origin of the internal carotid artery includes control of risk factors, assessment for coronary artery disease, and prevention of cerebral ischemia. Carotid endarterectomy is superior to medical management, including antiplatelet therapy, in preventing stroke in symptomatic patients with a 70 to 99% stenosis at the internal carotid artery origin (31–33). Surgery provides a 17% absolute reduction in the risk of ipsilateral stroke after 2 years (31). Patients should be in good medical condition and the surgeon should have a morbidity and mortality rate of less than 5%. Optimal management of patients with TIAs and 30 to 69% stenosis at the internal carotid artery origin has yet to be defined (31–33). Surgery does not appear to be preferable to medical management to prevent stroke in patients with 0 to 29% stenosis (32).

Patients with TIAs requiring carotid endarterectomy and having either no risk factors for coronary artery disease or risk factors for coronary artery disease but no symptoms, can first undergo carotid artery surgery and then be evaluated for coronary artery disease (34). However, patients with symptomatic coronary artery disease and TIAs should have their coronary artery disease assessed and, if coronary artery disease is severe, undergo simultaneous carotid endarterectomy and coronary artery bypass surgery (30, 34). This approach carries a combined morbidity and mortality appreciably higher than that of either surgery done separately. If the patient has stable angina pectoris and relatively mild coronary artery disease,

carotid artery surgery can be performed prior to cardiac surgery (30).

Aspirin is commonly used to treat carotid territory TIAs in nonsurgical patients with atherosclerosis at the internal carotid artery origin. Many studies have examined the potential benefit of aspirin, or aspirin combined with another platelet antiaggregant drug, such as dipyridamole or sulfinpyrazone, for stroke prevention following TIA or stroke (35). The Antiplatelet Trialists Collaboration concluded that aspirin decreases the risk of stroke by 22% (35). However, another metaanalysis of seven randomized controlled trials revealed a nonsignificant 15% reduction in stroke with aspirin therapy (odds ratio 0.85, 95% confidence interval 0.60 to 1.19) (36). The dose of aspirin is an important variable (36a). Studies employing low doses of aspirin (≤300 mg/day) provide a stroke and death risk reduction of 3 to 18%, whereas a risk reduction of 25 to 42% is achieved with doses of 975 to 1300 mg/day (36a). The optimal dose of aspirin continues to be debated along with the relative efficacy of aspirin in men and women, the dose-related adverse effects of aspirin, the need to combine aspirin with other platelet antiaggregant agents, and the appropriateness of performing platelet aggregation studies to monitor aspirin effects (35–40b). Even at aspirin doses of 1300 mg/day, some patients do not have full inhibition of platelet aggregation (40b).

Low-dose (30 mg/day) aspirin, which presumably blocks thromboxane A_2 synthesis to a greater degree than prostacyclin synthesis, may be as effective as a moderate dose (283 mg) of aspirin in the prevention of stroke following TIA (39). Aspirin at a dose of 75 mg/day is also effective in reducing stroke risk (41). Other trials have employed aspirin doses as high as 1300 mg/day or more (36). It has been difficult to demonstrate any beneficial effect of aspirin therapy for women, though there is a trend toward efficacy in men (36). Although several studies have failed to demonstrate a benefit from adding dipyridamole to aspirin (35, 42), the European Stroke Prevention Study, using aspirin 330 mg three times daily and dipyridamole 75 mg three times daily, demonstrated an approximately 40% reduction in stroke risk in men *and* women with an intention-to-treat analysis (37). Aspirin-dipyridamole therapy is less effective in diabetic than in nondiabetic patients (43). The authors usually begin platelet antiaggregant therapy with aspirin, 325 mg/day (1, 35), though if severe disease is present, aspirin 325 mg three times daily is prescribed (36a).

Ticlopidine is a recently available antiplatelet agent. For the endpoint of fatal or nonfatal stroke, ticlopidine yielded a 3-year stroke rate of 10% compared with a 13% stroke rate for aspirin (650 mg twice daily) (44). Therefore, the risk reduction is 21% when ticlopidine is compared with aspirin. Both men and women benefit from ticlopidine 250 mg orally twice daily (44). Patients who are intolerant of aspirin, have neurologic symptoms in spite of aspirin therapy, have hypertension or diabetes mellitus, are of nonwhite racial origin, or are at risk for gastrointestinal bleeding may do particularly well with ticlopidine treatment (45–46a).

Future studies and experience will dictate how platelet antiaggregant agents will be used. For instance, it is not known how ticlopidine therapy compares with carotid endarterectomy for a TIA caused by a 70 to 99% stenosis at the internal carotid artery origin. Should ticlopidine be the primary platelet antiaggregant used in women (42)? Should an aspirin-ticlopidine combination be employed (46, 47)?

Other Arterial Lesions.   Stenosis of the intracranial internal carotid artery and atherosclerotic disease of the anterior, middle, or posterior cerebral arteries can cause TIAs or stroke. Lesions of the extracranial or intracranial vertebral artery or the basilar artery cause symptoms referable to their perfusion territory. Optimal medical management of patients with these arterial lesions has yet to be defined. Some clinicians will begin therapy with antiplatelet agents and reserve anticoagulation for treatment failures. The European Stroke Prevention Study demonstrated a decline in the risk of stroke in patients with vertebrobasilar TIAs from 10.8% to 5.7% with aspirin-dipyridamole treatment (48). Ticlopidine therapy seems to be particularly effective in preventing stroke in patients with vertebrobasilar TIAs (45). Other physicians will initiate anticoagulation for patients with critical arterial stenosis or occlusion and consider antiplatelet therapy if the patient remains stable for several months (49). Lesions at the vertebral artery origin can be treated with surgery or transluminal angioplasty (49a).

Acute Management.   Optimal treatment of patients immediately after a TIA, a period during which diagnostic investigations and plans for long-term therapy are often being pursued, is not well-defined. There is no significant advantage to either aspirin or intravenous heparin treatment in preventing TIA or stroke in this setting (50). Recurrent TIAs developed in 29% of patients treated with heparin and 25% of patients managed with aspirin (50). Stroke occurred in 3.7% of heparin-treated patients and 14.2% of the aspirin group (50). Nonetheless, anticoagulation is often employed in patients with "crescendo" TIAs (51). Of concern is the occasional patient, typically with large artery occlusive disease, who will deteriorate when heparin is discontinued (52, 53). Patients may benefit from having antiplatelet or warfarin therapy started prior to stopping heparin (53).

The Stable Symptomatic Patient

Because of the wide range of clinical manifestations of ischemic stroke, it is difficult to make broad statements about management. Firstly, "stable" is a relative term; many patients have a changing neurologic status over the first hours of their stroke. Fortunately, 52% of patients demonstrate changes for the better within 18 hours of ictus, though 7% deteriorate (54).

If the patient appears to be relatively stable, efforts should be made to define the cause of the patient's infarction (Table 30.1), prevent further deterioration, and optimize rehabilitation. Large artery disease causes ischemic stroke by two mechanisms: a hemodynamically significant stenosis results in cerebral hypoperfusion, and an intimal lesion can be the source of emboli that migrate and compromise circulation through a distal artery.

Blood pressure control is a critical factor, especially in the early management of ischemic stroke (55, 55a). Many stroke patients have an increased blood pressure at presentation (56). Unless the degree of elevation is severe enough to cause myocardial or renal compromise, hypertensive encephalopathy, or a blood pressure greater than 220 mm Hg systolic or 130 mm Hg diastolic, aggressive, acute lowering of the blood pressure is not indicated for fear of compromising distal perfusion, especially through collateral vessels (57, 58). If the blood pressure needs to be decreased, a modest reduction, to a mean arterial pressure of 120 to 130 mm Hg, is preferable to a more extreme adjustment that might result not only in impaired distal perfusion but also in cerebral hypoperfusion because the lower limit of cerebral autoregulation is exceeded (59). There are acute increases in circulating catecholamines following stroke that resolve over several days, and this occurrence is associated with a decrease in blood pressure. Although acute hypertension might worsen cerebral edema (59), in a stable patient without severe hypertension this effect does not usually present a problem. In general, unless hypertension is extreme, the blood pressure can be brought to desirable levels (60) over weeks to months as the neurologic status is monitored so as to avoid cerebral hemodynamic compromise. If urgent antihypertensive treatment is indicated, the authors advocate using labetalol (5 to 20 mg boluses intravenously titrated to effect), an α- and β-adrenergic antagonist that has little adverse effect on intracranial pressure.

An increased blood glucose seems to be associated with a poor outcome in large artery occlusive disease, although the validity of this concept has been challenged (61–62a). Collateral circulation may bring glucose into an ischemic area, resulting in production of lactic acid and thereby increasing local acidity so as to compromise cellular function (61). Hyperglycemia during reperfusion may also be detrimental (63). Therefore, normal saline might be used in preference to glucose solutions for intravenous hydration, and diabetic patients should have good glycemic control. There is no evidence that transient, acute increases in blood glucose need to be treated (64). Hypoglycemia should be avoided (65).

Antiplatelet therapy is often begun after an ischemic stroke to prevent recurrence (46, 66). Aspirin is commonly used, although debate continues as to its efficacy (67, 67a). The authors typically prescribe aspirin, 325 to 975 mg daily orally, depending on the severity of the underlying vascular disease. Ticlopidine, 250 mg twice daily orally, decreases the likelihood of recurrent stroke in men and women from 10.7% to 8.5% per year (68). In patients with a "minor" stroke, ticlopidine may be more effective than aspirin for the prevention of recurrent stroke (68a). If neurologic symptoms develop in spite of antiplatelet treatment, if there is large artery occlusive disease, or if carotid endarterectomy is not an option, anticoagulation therapy can be started in an attempt to prevent another stroke.

Heparin therapy has not been shown to be effective in preventing neurologic deterioration in the stable ischemic stroke patient (67a, 69, 70). However, some authorities advocate heparin administration for nondevastating strokes that are the result of critical stenosis or occlusion of a large extracranial or intracranial artery (49), especially if the event is in the vertebrobasilar territory (51). Anticoagulation is thought to decrease the likelihood of artery-to-artery embolism and maintain the patency of collateral channels. Therefore, even if the tempo of the stroke does not suggest a fluctuating process, if early interventional or magnetic resonance angiography or carotid duplex or transcranial Doppler studies suggest severe large artery occlusive disease, immediate anticoagulation is deemed desirable. This treatment may be followed by a several-months-long course of warfarin therapy and, if circumstances allow, carotid endarterectomy or eventual antiplatelet treatment (49). The likelihood of intracranial hemorrhage is approximately 1% with heparin treatment; other hemorrhagic complications occur in 2% of patients (51). Subcutaneous heparin therapy is commonly employed during the acute phase of an ischemic stroke to decrease the probability of venous thrombosis in an immobile leg (67a).

The patient's overall fluid volume and blood viscosity status should be considered, especially since one-third of stroke patients are dehydrated on admission (71). Patients with a hematocrit ≥0.45 may have a better outcome with hydration to achieve a pulmonary capillary wedge pressure of 12 mm Hg, whereas patients with a hematocrit of <0.45 may benefit from a reduction of hematocrit to 0.32 ± 0.02 and a pulmonary capillary wedge pressure of 12 mm Hg (71). Thus, the clinical outcome of patients may be improved with hemodilution (72).

Carotid endarterectomy is effective in decreasing the risk of recurrent stroke in patients who have suffered a minor stroke ipsilateral to a 70 to 99% stenosis of the internal carotid artery (31, 33). The efficacy of surgery for patients with 30 to 69% stenosis is under study.

The Deteriorating Patient

Optimal management of the deteriorating stroke patient has yet to be defined. The issue here is the characterization of the fluctuations: Is only deterioration evident, or does the patient improve at times? Are changes slow or rapid? What is the time course of changes, especially as related to systemic blood pressure and the development of cerebral edema? Do changes reflect compromise of additional neuronal structures within the arterial territory first involved or different arterial territories from the initial insult?

Assuming that the patient is deteriorating in spite of optimal blood pressure control and that increased intracranial pressure is not evident, many physicians will administer heparin intravenously (51, 73). However, anticoagulation has never been rigorously demonstrated to be effective treatment in this setting (67a, 69). Nonetheless, if anticoagulation is not contraindicated, continuous heparin treatment is advocated to increase the activated partial thromboplastin time (aPTT) to 1.5 to 2.0 times control values, although there are no critical data to define an optimal aPTT range. If the patient continues to deteriorate, the possibility of intracranial hemorrhage secondary to anticoagulation should be considered, as should the rare occurrence of heparin-induced thrombosis (51, 74).

Although normotensive or hypertensive hypervolemic therapy generally is not employed for ischemic infarction, it has been suggested for use in deteriorating ischemic stroke patients to maximize perfusion to an area of threatened infarction (75, 76). The degree of hydration should be individualized by monitoring of hemodynamic parameters (71). Although collateral circulation may be improved, cerebral edema can worsen and raise intracranial pressure, thereby endangering the patient (75). The principles of hypervolemic therapy are discussed in the section entitled, "Vasospasm" following subarachnoid hemorrhage.

Aggressive treatment of increased intracranial pressure in patients with ischemic infarction is controversial (77). Intracranial pressure monitoring in patients with mass effect from ischemic infarction may be helpful in guiding therapy, but it is also useful to indicate when intervention is *not* needed. Techniques to lower intracranial pressure in patients with large ischemic strokes may not be successful and may be at odds with other principles of ischemic stroke management. For instance, hyperventilation decreases cerebral blood flow to intact brain for a few hours, but arteries in ischemic brain regions are dilated and not responsive to hypocarbia. Therefore, edema in the infarcted area is not reduced by hyperventilation. Dehydration therapy may compromise cerebral perfusion, especially in regions of marginal blood flow (the "ischemic penumbra"), and thereby worsen the patient's status. Craniectomy and brain decompression have been used successfully in patients with nondominant hemisphere infarction with massive edema (78). Surgical resection of swollen, infarcted brain, especially cerebellum (79, 80) or anterior temporal lobe, can be effective. These aggressive measures must be tempered by the expected residual deficits, especially the language functions of the dominant hemisphere. Many ethical issues must be examined if aggressive measures are pursued.

Urgent carotid endarterectomy occasionally is recommended for the patient with a hemispheric stroke if (a) the neurologic deficits are minor, (b) the patient is deteriorating in spite of optimal medical management and there is no infarction on CT scan, and (c) a critical stenosis is present at the origin of the appropriate internal carotid artery. Patients with minor neurologic deficits and an intraluminal clot at the internal carotid artery origin may also benefit from surgery if there is no hypercoagulable state (81). Importantly, carotid endarterectomy in these situations carries considerable risk and should be done only after a careful analysis of the patient's plight.

Arterial Dissection

Extracranial arterial dissection can involve the internal carotid or vertebral arteries. Dissection is caused by penetrating or nonpenetrating local trauma, extremes of neck movement, or as a spontaneous occurrence, as in association with fibromuscular dysplasia. Patients often have ipsilateral neck or head pain, and internal carotid artery dissections can be associated with Horner's syndrome. Neurologic sequelae occur at the time of injury or may be delayed for hours or even days. Brain damage results from artery-to-artery emboli or hemodynamic compromise distal to a critical stenosis or occlusion.

Emergent anticoagulation with heparin is usually recommended for treatment of extracranial arterial dissection, if there is no contraindication (82, 83). A 6-month course of warfarin treatment is advised, with a vascular imaging procedure then being obtained to guide future treatment (83a). Rarely is acute surgery done for internal carotid artery dissection.

Rarely, an arterial dissection can involve the intracranial carotid or vertebral territories. Intracranial hemorrhage can occur and therefore anticoagulation should be considered only if there is no evidence of intracranial bleeding (83).

SMALL ARTERY DISEASE

Occlusion of an intraparenchymal small artery is often a result of chronic hypertension, and discrete neurologic syndromes such as pure motor or sensory ischemic stroke can occur. Brain magnetic resonance imaging (MRI) or CT can show an infarct, a lacune, less than 1.5 cm in diameter, deep in the cerebral hemispheres. Importantly, this clinical picture can also be caused, on occasion, by cardiogenic emboli, large artery occlusive disease, inflammatory arterial disease, and hematologic disorders (84, 85). Therefore, treatment should be based on the underlying disease process; assuming hypertension to be the cause of all "lacunar" strokes is not appropriate (86).

HEMATOLOGIC CONDITIONS

Sickle cell disease, polycythemia vera, and thrombotic thrombocytopenic purpura are well-known causes of stroke. There is a growing appreciation that conditions affecting the coagulation system are associated with arterial and venous thrombosis (Table 30.1) (87). Deficiencies of antithrombin III, protein C, and possibly, free protein S (87a) can lead to ischemic stroke, as can disorders of fibrinolysis. A family history of early thrombosis, thrombosis before age 30, a history of repeated thrombosis, thrombosis in "unusual" locations such as the arms or neck, and thrombosis in spite of "adequate" anticoagulation should raise the suspicion of a disordered coagulation system (88).

Antiphospholipid, including anticardiolipin and the lupus anticoagulant, is an important cause of ischemic stroke in patients of all ages (89). A positive anticardiolipin assay is present in 9.7% of stroke patients, yielding an odds ratio for stroke of 2.33 (89). Presentations include large and small artery occlusion, cardiac valvular lesions, venous thrombosis, retinal ischemia, and multiinfarct dementia. Optimal treatment is not defined but antiplatelet agents and anticoagulation are commonly used. Corticosteroids or other immunosuppressives and plasmapheresis are occasionally tried.

VENOUS THROMBOSIS

Superior sagittal sinus or venous thrombosis is associated with dehydration, hyperviscosity, hypercoagulable states, Behcet's syndrome, and obstruction to intracranial venous outflow. Patients often do well with supportive care, including anticonvulsant medications. In the comatose patient, aggressive treatment of increased intracranial pressure is critical (90). In spite of hemorrhagic venous infarction, heparin therapy is beneficial (91). Thrombolytic therapy has also been used for sagittal sinus thrombosis (92).

SPINAL CORD STROKE

Arterial infarction of the spinal cord is associated with hypotension, aortic aneurysm, hyperviscosity, and arterial inflammation. Therapy is directed at the underlying condition and optimization of hemodynamics. Other than supportive care, optimal treatment has yet to be defined (93, 94).

THE YOUNG STROKE PATIENT

There are numerous causes of stroke in the young (88). Hemorrhagic processes are more common in patients younger than age 45 years than in older individuals. Also, ischemic infarction in this age group is more likely a result of cardiogenic emboli and hematologic and systemic disorders than in an older patient cohort. Attention to historical clues, the physical examination, and laboratory tests, including toxicology screens, can often uncover critical information that allows accurate diagnosis. Early definition of the vascular anatomy can often provide valuable information. Therapy is based on the cause of the stroke.

FUTURE THERAPEUTIC OPTIONS

As our understanding of the pathophysiology of stroke has increased (94a), new therapeutic routes are being explored. Attention has focused on maintaining arterial patency, preventing calcium entry into ischemic cells, blocking the effects of excitatory amino acids, and ameliorating the damaging effects of free radicals.

Heparinoids are derivatives of heparin that have a comparatively greater antithrombotic than anticoagulant effect (42, 95). These glycosaminoglycans have a relatively selective antifactor X activity. ORG-10172 has been used to treat acute ischemic stroke, with relatively little risk for serious hemorrhagic complications (42, 95).

Thrombolysis with streptokinase, urokinase, and tissue plasminogen activator has been used to treat acute ischemic infarction (96). Intervention has been by both intraarterial and intravenous infusion (96). Some studies have required angiography to define an arterial occlusion prior to therapy, whereas other series allow treatment of the acute stroke patient without angiographic documentation of the occlusive lesion to reduce the time interval from onset of symptoms to treatment (96). Recanalization of obstructed arteries has been shown and patients can improve clinically, sometimes quite dramatically (97–99). Patients with basilar artery occlusion may be particularly good candidates for thrombolytic therapy. Hacke et al treated 43 patients with acute stroke and angiographically proved vertebrobasilar artery occlusion with intraarterial urokinase or streptokinase 100,000 U/hr for up to 4 hours. Of the 19 patients who had arterial recanalization, 13 survived, whereas none of the 24 patients who did not recanalize survived (100).

The most feared complication of thrombolytic therapy is that of intracranial hemorrhage (96, 100a). Bleeding can occur within the confines of the index ischemic infarction and cause transformation to a hemorrhagic infarction, which usually does not cause clinical deterioration. In other cases, a parenchymal hematoma can develop that will likely lead to clinical worsening. A parenchymal hematoma can also develop at a site distant to the index stroke and lead to an adverse outcome. Early treatment (less than 6 hours, and preferably less than 90 minutes, from ictus) seems to decrease the risk of hemorrhage (15, 96, 101), as does a dose of less than 0.85 to 0.95 mg/kg of recombinant tissue plasminogen activator infused intravenously over 60 to 90 minutes (102). Overall, hemorrhagic infarction is a relatively frequent complication of thrombolytic therapy but seems to convey an acceptable risk (99, 100a). Intraparenchymal hematoma, on the other hand, is less common but portends a poor outcome (96). Heparin can be administered with intravenous tissue plasminogen activator, though fatal hemorrhage occurred in 9% of patients (3 of 32) (103). Studies are underway to define the safety and efficacy of thrombolytic therapy for acute ischemic stroke (103a).

Because calcium entering damaged neurons through both voltage-dependent and neurotransmitter-mediated channels leads to further cell injury, considerable investigation has been directed at ways to limit this process (104). Calcium antagonists decrease neuronal injury in stroke models and improve the outcome of ischemic stroke (104). Patients with moderate to severe stroke treated with nimodipine within 24 hours of stroke onset seem to have a diminished mortality and improved outcome compared with those given placebo (105). Prognosis is best in patients older than age 65 treated within 12 hours (105). The American Nimodipine Study Group failed to demonstrate any overall benefit for nimodipine 60 to 240 mg daily administered orally within 48 hours of stroke, though a subgroup analysis showed a significantly better outcome for patients with an initially normal CT scan treated with nimodipine 120 mg daily within 18 hours of becoming ill (106). Nicardipine, which may soon be available in the U.S., has been used safely in acute stroke patients (107). Calcium antagonists promise to be beneficial in the treatment of acute ischemic stroke.

A high concentration of the excitatory neurotransmitter glutamate develops under ischemic or hypoxic conditions because of increased synaptic release and impaired neuronal reuptake (108). Neurotoxic effects follow an influx of ions into

neurons, with sodium entry causing early cellular swelling and calcium having a more delayed adverse effect (108). Antagonists of the glutamate N-methyl-D-aspartate (NMDA) and amino-3-hydroxy-5-methyl-4-isoazole proprionic acid (AMPA) receptors decrease neuronal damage in experimental stroke models and, it is hoped, will be of benefit in humans (109–111).

Ischemic insults produce free radicals, which damage membrane lipids. Inhibitors of lipid peroxidation, such as the 21-aminosteroids, decrease neuronal injury in stroke models (112). Efforts to increase superoxide dismutase activity at sites of experimental stroke can also ameliorate damage (113–115).

Research is needed to define which intervention will be most effective in a given clinical setting (116, 116a). Key issues relate to the pathogenesis of the stroke, drug safety, the timing of drug administration, and multidrug protocols directed at various components of the cell injury cascade. Given the enormous complexity of the problem, it will be necessary to consider the interrelationships among the many molecular species affected by ischemia. A single therapeutic intervention may have a widespread effect, both desirable and not (116b).

HEMORRHAGIC DISEASE

Nontraumatic intracranial hemorrhages account for approximately 20 to 25% of acute cerebrovascular disease and are classified based on the distribution of blood as either intracerebral (parenchymal or ventricular) or subarachnoid. Intracerebral hemorrhages usually present with the acute onset of focal neurologic deficits that vary with the location of the hematoma. Subarachnoid hemorrhage, on the other hand, presents with the sudden onset of headache, often associated with syncope, followed by nuchal rigidity and confusion, and occasionally a focal neurologic deficit. Since the pathophysiologic consequences of these two types of hemorrhage differ significantly, they require very different approaches to management.

NONTRAUMATIC INTRACEREBRAL HEMORRHAGE

Nontraumatic intracerebral hemorrhage accounts for approximately 10% of strokes (117). It was generally believed that active bleeding lasted less than 1 hour. However, recent ultra-early CT scans suggest that bleeding may continue for several hours, especially in patients with early clinical deterioration (118). The primary injury results from the dissection of blood along white matter fibers, which compresses and displaces tissue. Secondary injury is caused by cerebral edema and hydrocephalus, which further compress and displace brain tissue and, if unchecked, can result in brain herniation. Although the etiology of hemorrhages differs, it is the location and volume of the hemorrhage that has the major impact on outcome (119) and guides therapeutic interventions.

Etiology

Nontraumatic intracerebral hemorrhage can occur spontaneously, in association with underlying pathologic conditions (vascular abnormality, tumor, bleeding disorder), or as a result

Table 30.2. Causes of Nontraumatic Intracerebral Hemorrhage

Vascular
   Hypertension
   Vascular malformation
   Saccular aneurysm
   Arteritis
   Amyloid angiopathy
Surgical
   Carotid endarterectomy
   Postcraniotomy
Sympathomimetic drugs
   Cocaine hydrochloride
   "Crack" cocaine
   Methylphenidate
   Phenylpropanolamine
   Amphetamine
Coagulopathy
   Endogenous
   Anticoagulants
   Thrombolytic drugs
Infection
   Meningitis
   Encephalitis
Miscellaneous
   Hemorrhage into tumor
   Venous occlusion
   Severe migraine
   Exposure to cold

of drugs (Table 30.2). Spontaneous hemorrhages are often attributed to chronic hypertension and classically occur in the putamen, thalamus, cerebellum, and pons. In other patients spontaneous hemorrhage occurs without a history of hypertension, often following an acute increase in cerebral blood flow (120).

Bleeding from arteriovenous malformations (AVMs) can result in both intracerebral and subarachnoid bleeding. Hemorrhages associated with vascular malformations tend to occur in young patients (121). Therefore, young normotensive patients or hypertensive individuals with a hematoma in a location atypical for hypertensive hemorrhage should be evaluated for the presence of a vascular malformation or aneurysm (see below). Cerebral amyloid angiopathy is a cause of lobar intracerebral hemorrhage in the elderly (122) that increases in frequency with increasing age and recurs in 10% of patients (123).

Drugs appear to produce intracerebral hemorrhage principally through one of two mechanisms: coagulopathy or acute hypertension. Bleeding as a result of heparin or warfarin therapy accounts for approximately 10% of intracerebral hemorrhage (124). Intracerebral hemorrhage occurs in approximately 1% of patients treated with thrombolytic agents for acute myocardial infarction (125, 126). The use of recreational drugs, including cocaine hydrochloride (127, 128), "crack" cocaine (129, 130), amphetamines, and other sympathomimetics (127), is a major cause of intracerebral hemorrhage in young adults. Phenylpropanolamine, an over-the-counter sympathomimetic drug, also causes intracerebral hemorrhage (131). These hemorrhages can be associated with vascular abnormalities, including AVMs, aneurysms, or drug-induced vasculitis (121).

Other causes of intracerebral hemorrhage include hemorrhage into a tumor, bleeding diatheses, severe migraine, exposure to cold, surgery for trigeminal neuralgia, evacuation of subdural hematomas, and carotid endarterectomy.

Presentation

The various sites of intracranial hemorrhage are associated with typical clinical features, and the hemorrhage generally is not preceded by transient ischemic attacks. The usual sites of bleeding and their approximate proportion of cases include putamen (35%), thalamus (10%), caudate (5%), lobar (30%), cerebellum (15%), and pons (5%) (121).

Putaminal hemorrhages present with contralateral hemiparesis, hemisensory loss, and, occasionally, dysphasia or neglect. Thalamic bleeding produces a similar picture but may also have forced downgaze, upgaze palsy, and unreactive pupils. Hemorrhage into the head of the caudate produces confusion, memory loss, hemiparesis, and gaze paresis and often is accompanied by intraventricular blood and hydrocephalus. Lobar hemorrhages produce signs that depend on the region involved. Cerebellar hemorrhages classically present with the sudden onset of headache, vomiting, and gait ataxia. Large pontine hemorrhages are usually devastating and present with quadriplegia, pinpoint pupils, and coma. Seizures occur more frequently in hemorrhage than in ischemic stroke and are seen in approximately 10 to 15% of patients (132). Two-thirds of all seizures occur within 48 hours of the hemorrhage and are not necessarily predictive of a chronic seizure disorder (121). Although headaches are a nonspecific symptom in intracerebral hematoma, they are more frequent in lobar hematomas (133).

Evaluation and Initial Management

The initial steps in evaluating a patient with a suspected intracranial hemorrhage should always include assessment of level of consciousness, ability to protect the airway, blood pressure, and baseline neurologic exam (Table 30.3). However, the need for urgent intubation in comatose patients may take precedence over performing a complete neurologic exam. Patients with a Glasgow Coma Scale score of 8 or less (Table 30.4) should be intubated prior to further diagnostic evaluation (134). Since these patients have potentially elevated intracranial pressure (ICP), intubation should be smooth and rapid and should not produce an increase in ICP. This goal can be accomplished by administering ultra-short-acting barbiturates with rapid-acting neuromuscular blocking agents. Although the usual recommended dose of intravenous thiopental for induction of anesthesia is 2.5 to 4.5 mg/kg (135), often less than 50% of the recommended dose is effective in these patients. Although it poses a theoretic risk of increasing ICP (136), succinylcholine (10 mg/kg intravenously) is preferred by some practitioners because of its rapid onset of action. Others recommend use of the short-acting nondepolarizing agents atracurium besylate (3 to 4 mg/kg intravenously) or vecuronium bromide (0.1 mg/kg intravenously) (137). Muscle paralysis should not be continued, so that the patient's neurologic status can be monitored. Lidocaine (1 to 2 mg/kg intravenously) is also useful in blunting the response to intubation (137). Any

Table 30.3. Initial Management of Obtunded Patients with Suspected Intracerebral Hematoma

1. Assess level of consciousness, airway reflexes, blood pressure, and neurologic exam
2. If Glasgow Coma Score is ≤8, intubate and premedicate with thiopental 1 to 3 mg/kg i.v. and rapid-acting paralytic agent
3. Hyperventilate to $PaCO_2$ 25 to 30 mm Hg and administer mannitol 0.25 to 1.0 g/kg i.v.
4. Treat severe hypertension and reduce mean arterial blood pressure to 125 to 135 mm Hg (see Table 30.5 for agents)
5. Nonenhanced CT scan and neurosurgical evaluation

Table 30.4. Glasgow Coma Scale

Test	Finding	Score
Eye opening	No response	1
	Response to pain	2
	Response to voice	3
	Spontaneously	4
Verbal response	No response	1
	Incomprehensible sounds	2
	Inappropriate words	3
	Disoriented conversation	4
	Oriented and appropriate	5
Motor response	No response	1
	Decerebrate posturing	2
	Decorticate posturing	3
	Flexion withdrawal	4
	Localizes pain	5
	Obeys commands	6
	Maximum total score	15

patient who requires intubation should initially be hyperventilated to an arterial PCO_2 of approximately 25 to 30 mm Hg (3.3 to 4 kPa) and receive mannitol (0.25 to 1.0 g/kg intravenously) prior to CT scan (134). Extreme increases in blood pressure should be stabilized prior to transport (see below).

Coagulation status should be checked and, if necessary, correction initiated. For patients in whom the hemorrhage resulted from heparin, intravenous protamine 1 mg/100 U of heparin should be administered. In those patients who were recently administered thrombolytic agents and are deteriorating, 5 g of ε-aminocaproic acid over 15 to 30 minutes and 10 to 15 bags of cryoprecipitate are recommended (138). Patients on Coumadin should be reversed with vitamin K (3 doses of 10 mg intravenously slowly) and enough fresh frozen plasma to correct the PTT. Alternatively, factor IX concentrate (minimum dose of 50 U/kg intravenously) (139) or prothrombin complex concentrate (0.43 ml/kg intravenously) (139a) in addition to vitamin K (25 mg intravenously) has been recommended.

At present, the best diagnostic test to evaluate an intracerebral hemorrhage is a nonenhanced CT scan (140). The hemorrhage will appear as a high-density lesion (141) except in patients with very severe anemia (142). Administration of contrast may demonstrate an underlying AVM, aneurysm, or tumor. However, if only a contrast CT scan is performed, it may be impossible to differentiate hemorrhage from tumor or AVM. Although MRI is sensitive to detection of intracerebral hemorrhage, the findings depend on when the scan is performed (143). In addition, care of an acutely ill patient in an MRI scanner is difficult (144).

When the patient has no history of hypertension and the hemorrhage is lobar or otherwise atypical, angiography should be performed to search for an underlying vascular lesion (145). The timing of angiography depends on the clinical concerns.

If an aneurysm is suspected, acute angiography is indicated. Otherwise, angiography should be delayed unless urgent surgery is contemplated to remove the hematoma, since a large hematoma may compress a vascular malformation and render it invisible. In the near future, high-quality MRI and magnetic resonance angiography may substitute for conventional angiography.

Neurosurgical consultation is recommended for all patients with intracerebral hemorrhage. This consultation is critical for patients with a cerebellar hematoma, as emergent evacuation may be indicated. The role of surgery for hemorrhage in other locations remains controversial (see below).

Medical Management

General guidelines for management of patients with intracerebral hemorrhage follow. Whenever possible, the recommendations are based on experimental and clinical evidence. However, our understanding of many of these issues is incomplete, and, therefore many of the recommendations are based on theoretic considerations, extrapolation from limited data, and management protocols employed in centers that specialize in care of critically ill neurologic patients. When one is employing these therapies, it is extremely important to titrate the therapy to the patient's clinical status. The criterion used to judge the efficacy of therapies should not be a specific physiologic variable such as osmolality or ICP, but the patient's overall neurologic status.

To develop an appropriate management strategy for patients with intracerebral hemorrhage, several pathophysiologic issues must be considered. The hematoma has acutely raised the intracranial volume, resulting in reduced intracranial compliance and, possibly, increased ICP. The hematoma also stimulates the formation of edema, which increases for several days following the hemorrhage. Therefore, patients are very susceptible to the potential effects of hypercarbia, hypoxia, edema, or further bleeding on ICP (146). Whereas sustained hypertension can promote edema formation (147, 148), pressure autoregulation of cerebral blood flow (Fig. 30.3) may be disturbed and lower blood pressures may be inadequate to maintain cerebral perfusion. Intraventricular blood can produce obstructive hydrocephalus. In addition, hydrocephalus can result from tissue shifts compressing a foramen of Monro, the sylvian aqueduct, or the fourth ventricle (Fig. 30.4).

Management of intracerebral hemorrhage involves limiting the primary injury and preventing or minimizing secondary damage. Although the bulk of the primary injury has already occurred before the patient reaches medical attention, avoidance of severe hypertension may help limit the amount of bleeding, since some patients may continue bleeding for several hours (118). Rapid correction of coagulation defects also helps limit bleeding.

Secondary injury may occur as a result of seizures, hydrocephalus, edema, or increased ICP. Anticonvulsants should be administered to any patient with lobar or subcortical bleeding or any patient who has had a seizure. Phenytoin is the preferred agent, since it can be given parenterally and does not alter consciousness (see below). Use of benzodiazepines and barbiturates should be avoided, if possible, because they impair the ability to monitor the patient's neurologic condition.

Neurologic Monitoring

Monitoring of neurologic status is achieved with serial neurologic exams and/or measurement of ICP. Standardized exams should be performed by nursing staff, including at least the Glasgow Coma Scale score (Table 30.4), cranial nerve function, and motor function of each extremity.

Although ICP is a useful indicator of outcome in head trauma (149), the ability of ICP monitoring to improve outcome unequivocally in a controlled trial has not been demonstrated (150, 151). However, monitoring of ICP in intracerebral hemorrhage may be helpful in selected patients when used to guide medical therapy and to help decide when to intervene surgically. In general, if the Glasgow Coma Scale is 8 or less, many clinicians elect to monitor ICP. In addition, if a patient is agitated, unmanageable, and requires sedation, ICP should be monitored.

Blood Pressure Management

Most patients are hypertensive following an intracerebral hemorrhage, even those without a history of hypertension. Acute normalization of blood pressure is extremely dangerous because: (a) ICP may be increased and a reduction of blood pressure may reduce cerebral perfusion pressure (ICP minus mean blood pressure) to ischemic levels (Fig. 30.3); (b) the autoregulatory curve is shifted to higher pressures in chronically

hypertensive patients (152) and cerebral blood flow may decrease at "normal" blood pressures; and (c) patients with atherosclerotic disease may have focal stenoses that can critically limit flow if blood pressure is too low. Although definitive data are lacking, in general, blood pressure should not be treated unless mean arterial blood pressure exceeds 125 to 135 mm Hg or diastolic pressure exceeds 120 mm Hg. Immediately following presentation, somewhat lower pressures may be desirable to reduce the likelihood of continued bleeding, but no clear cause-and-effect relationship has been demonstrated.

Hypertension should be treated in the early stages of the illness with short-acting, easily titrated agents to allow flexibility as the patient's condition evolves (Table 30.5). The use of agents such as nitrates and sodium nitroprusside that produce venodilation are contraindicated, as they raise ICP even when cerebral compliance is normal (153). The combined α- and β-blocker labetalol is a useful agent since it can be given intravenously, is easily titrated, and does not adversely affect ICP (154). Large doses (up to 100 mg/hr intravenously) may be required. Hydralazine is a useful second agent, as it produces little venodilation and the prior use of β-blockers will prevent reflex tachycardia. The ganglionic blocker trimethaphan is useful for blood pressure control; however, since it can mask changes in pupil size, it has been replaced by the aforementioned agents.

Hydrocephalus

Hydrocephalus can produce a gradual decline in global neurologic function and, if untreated, have disastrous consequences. Therefore, drugs that may limit the caregiver's ability to monitor the patient's level of consciousness should be avoided. A decline in a patient's neurologic function should prompt a CT scan. Patients with CT evidence of enlarging ventricles and a decline in level of consciousness require ventriculostomy. This procedure will allow for both drainage of cerebrospinal fluid (CSF) and monitoring of ICP.

The optimal location for catheter placement is not clear. Some argue that in the presence of intraventricular blood the catheter should be placed, if possible, in the ventricle with the least amount of blood. However, others believe that this approach could be problematic when there is a large hematoma because of the possibility of worsening tissue shift across the midline. Obstruction of the catheter with clotted blood may be remedied temporarily by flushing the system, but breaks in the drainage system carry risk of infection (155, 156). There are reports of the use of fibrinolytic agents to dissolve intraventricular blood (157), but this technique has not yet been fully evaluated.

Ventricular catheters are prone to infection. The rate of infection rises rapidly after a catheter has been in place more than 5 days, and a climbing white blood cell count in the CSF is a good indicator of potential infection (155, 156). Therefore, routine monitoring of CSF white blood cell count, Gram stain, and culture may be useful. It is recommended that catheters be removed or replaced after 7 days or if the CSF white blood cell count rises. Although the use of prophylactic antibiotics is routine in some centers, its efficacy has not been established and it carries the risk of selecting resistant organisms.

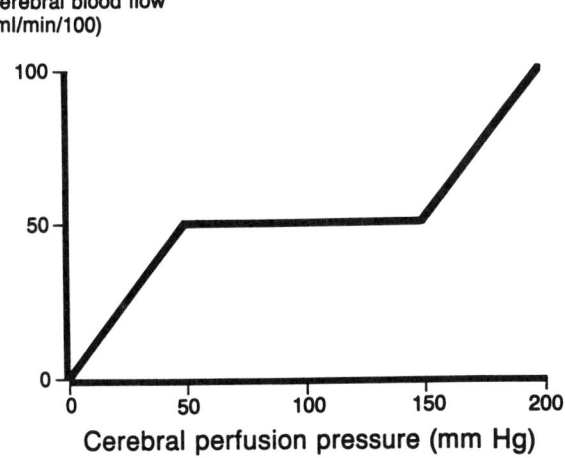

Figure 30.3. Cerebral perfusion pressure autoregulation curve. Cerebral blood flow remains stable over a wide range of cerebral perfusion pressure but becomes pressure passive as the limits of autoregulation are exceeded at both extremes. This curve is shifted to the left in newborns and to the right in chronically hypertensive adults. (Reprinted with permission of CV Mosby from Kirsch JR, Haelfer MA: Intracranial vault physiology. *Crit Care Rep* 1:12-21, 1989.)

Figure 30.4. Computed tomographic scan of a patient following an acute cerebellar hemorrhage. The upper left panel shows the hematoma in the posterior fossa obliterating the fourth ventricle and enlargement of the temporal horns of the lateral ventricles. The upper right panel shows the hematoma, subarachnoid blood in the basal cisterns, and enlargement of the temporal horns and the third ventricle. The lower panels show enlargement of the third and lateral ventricles.

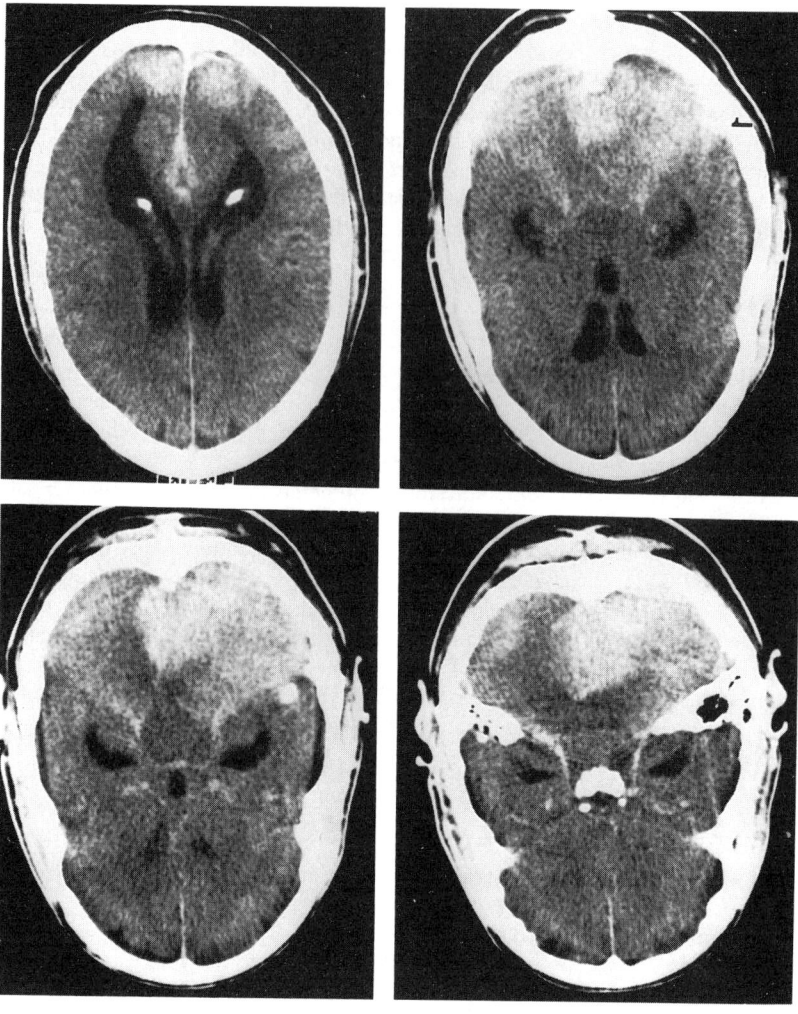

Table 30.5. Acute Blood Pressure Management in Patients with Intracerebral Hematomas

1. Avoid rapid "normalization" of mean arterial blood pressure; keep mean arterial blood pressure at 125 to 135 mm Hg
2. Avoid cerebral venodilators (nitrates and sodium nitroprusside)
3. Administer labetalol in 5 to 20 mg i.v. boluses to reach goal, then continue periodic boluses or infusion
4. If refractory, add hydralazine in 2.5 to 10 mg i.v. boluses

Treatment of Increased Intracranial Pressure and Cerebral Edema

Hyperventilation is useful in the acute control of increased ICP. Because the effectiveness of hyperventilation is short-lived (Fig. 30.5), other measures to decrease ICP, such as CSF drainage or osmotic therapy, should be instituted rapidly. The patient should be weaned as soon as ICP is controlled by other means to avoid the systemic complications of alkalemia. Furthermore, prolonged CSF alkalosis secondary to hyperventilation may worsen the neurologic outcome (158). However, there is a potential for a rebound rise in ICP if hyperventilation is discontinued quickly. Therefore, weaning should be accomplished in small steps while monitoring ICP or the neurologic examination. The rate of weaning should be guided by the clinical response, and normocarbia usually can be achieved safely in 4 to 24 hours.

The management of cerebral edema depends on the severity and location of the hemorrhage. Because of its small size and the vital structures it contains, the posterior fossa does not tolerate edema very well. Therefore, cerebellar hemorrhages larger than 2 cm in diameter may require surgical evacuation, and hematomas larger than 3 cm probably should always be evacuated (159). On the other hand, the edema around small lobar hemorrhages may not produce any significant adverse effects. In a randomized controlled trial, corticosteroids were never shown to improve neurologic recovery from intracerebral hemorrhage but did increase the rate of complications and, therefore, are not recommended (160).

The mainstay of treatment of cerebral edema and increased ICP in intracerebral hemorrhage is the use of osmotic therapy in an attempt to dehydrate the brain. In small hemorrhages the usual approach is passive dehydration by restriction of fluid intake. However, the efficacy of this therapy has never been clearly established, and studies have been unable to demonstrate a relationship between fluid balance and ICP or brain water content (161). With larger hematomas, treatment of brain edema and increased ICP is directed toward actively raising extracellular fluid osmolality.

The goal of osmotic therapy is to a achieve a state of euvolemia and hyperosmolality. Raising extracellular fluid osmolality creates an osmotic gradient between the intracellular and extracellular compartments and results in movement of water out of the brain. Hyperosmolality can be achieved by administering osmotically active agents or promoting free water clearance. Intravascular volume contraction probably adds no additional benefit and should be prevented in order to avoid systemic complications. The degree and rate of elevation of extracellular fluid osmolality is guided by the patient's clinical condition and the size and location of the hematoma.

Loop diuretics are effective in lowering ICP (162, 163). When administered in doses sufficient to produce a diuresis of 3 to 4 liters/day, osmolality will begin to rise in 24 to 48 hours. This process can be accelerated by concurrent administration of hypertonic saline. Therapy can be monitored by following urine output and serum osmolality. Measurement of serum sodium concentration, which may be available more rapidly from some clinical laboratories, will reflect serum osmolality in patients who have not recently received mannitol and who do not have elevated glucose or blood urea nitrogen.

Mannitol, in addition to acting as an osmotic diuretic, has additional effects that are of theoretic benefit. A 1 g/kg intravenous dose of mannitol reduces ICP in 10 to 20 minutes (164, 165) by means of an effect that appears to be independent of diuresis. This effect probably occurs as a result of drawing water out of brain regions with an intact blood-brain barrier into the hyperosmolal vascular space (166). This dose is usually administered every 6 hours. Lower, more frequent doses (0.25 g/kg every 3 to 4 hr) appear to be equally effective (165). As with all treatments for elevated ICP, the dosage and frequency should be guided by the clinical response. Mannitol also improves cerebral blood flow, possibly by reducing blood viscosity (167). Although mannitol has been implicated in producing a rebound increase in ICP by leaking through a damaged blood-brain barrier, experimental evidence does not support this mechanism, and the increase in ICP is probably a result of premature discontinuation of therapy (166). In patients without severe increases in ICP, osmotic agents such as mannitol may be reserved for acute deteriorations.

The usual recommendation is to increase osmolality to 310 to 320 mosm/liter. However, this choice is somewhat arbitrary. If this goal is reached, there is no clinical response, and ICP is not controlled, it would seen prudent to raise osmolality further. Once an effective osmolality is achieved, regular additional doses of loop diuretics or mannitol are needed to maintain the state. The optimal dose is determined by finding one that will maintain adequate urine output and stable osmolality.

Intramuscular volume contraction should be prevented by adequate replacement with normal saline. In addition, 50 to 100 mEq of sodium (as chloride or bicarbonate) can be added to a liter of normal saline to produce a slightly hypertonic solution (358 to 408 mosm) to be used for fluid replacement. Some advocate the use of colloids (5% or 25% albumin in

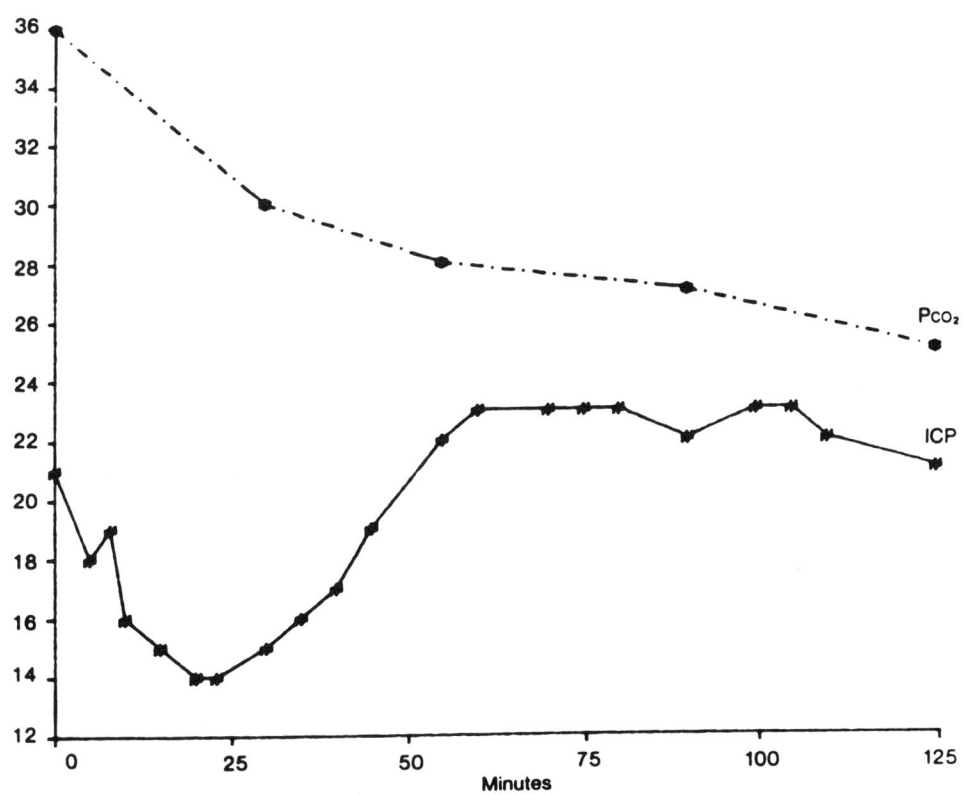

Figure 30.5. Typical temporal profile of intracranial pressure (*ICP*) change after acute and sustained hyperventilation. Hyperventilation is begun at time zero. There is an initial rapid fall in ICP with hyperventilation; however, despite a slight further lowering of arterial CO_2 tension (*PCO_2*), ICP has returned to its initial value by 1 hour. (Reprinted from Ropper AH and Kennedy SK: *Neurosurgical Intensive Care*, ed 2, p 24, with permission of Aspen Publisher, Inc. 1988.)

normal saline) to avoid volume contraction. Hypotension can usually be avoided if volume replacement is appropriate. However, if fluids are not rapidly effective in treating hypotension, appropriate vasopressors should be employed to avoid cerebral hypoperfusion.

Hyperosmolality should be maintained for several days after the patient has stabilized. When extracellular fluid osmolality is raised, water moves out of cells to reestablish osmotic equilibrium, and therefore cells shrink. The brain responds by increasing the number of intracellular osmotically active particles (potassium, proteins) and the rate of formation of idiogenic osmols (168). Therefore, caution should be exercised when reversing the hyperosmolal state to avoid massive cellular swelling and a rebound increase in ICP. Corrections of osmolality should take place over 1 to 2 weeks.

When osmotic therapy is employed, careful attention to the patient's electrolyte status is required. Use of diuretics can result in depletion of potassium, magnesium, and phosphate. These losses should be anticipated and blood levels should be monitored daily during the early phase of therapy. Oral supplementation alone may be inadequate to maintain normal levels, and frequent intravenous administration is often necessary. This therapy is important not only because of the systemic effects but also because recent evidence suggests that magnesium may be protective in brain injury (169).

Surgical Management

The role of surgical intervention in intracerebral hemorrhage has not yet been clearly defined. No randomized, controlled trial has shown an unequivocal benefit of surgery. In general, the size and location of the hemorrhage are used in predicting the utility of surgical intervention. For example, cerebellar hemorrhages, unless small and producing mild deficits, are usually evacuated emergently (159). This strategy is used because of the potential for sudden clinical deterioration from a mass in a site that is easily reached without disruption of eloquent brain regions. Deep lesions, especially in the dominant hemisphere, are usually not considered for conventional surgery. Some clinicians advocate surgery if ICP cannot be controlled by medical means (134); however, the outcome in these patients is usually poor since they probably have already suffered severe damage.

The recent advent of CT-guided stereotactic techniques has provided a new approach that may significantly affect outcome from intracerebral hemorrhage (170–172). This approach theoretically lessens the mass effect and reduces the stimulus for edema (173). CT coordinates are used to guide a cannula into the hematoma, and the blood is aspirated by one of several techniques. Thrombolytic agents may be instilled to aid removal of residual hematoma. Initial reports on this approach are promising, (174), but randomized, controlled trials have not been performed.

Prognosis

Outcome is determined primarily by the size and location of the hemorrhage and the patient's initial neurologic condition. If the total volume of the hematoma is less than 20 mm³, mortality is less than 10%, whereas if the volume is greater than 60 mm³, mortality exceeds 90% (175). Patients who are

Table 30.6.   Causes of Subarachnoid Hemorrhage

Saccular aneurysm
Vascular malformation
Moya Moya disease
Head trauma
Extension of intracerebral hematoma
Spinal vascular malformation
Ruptured superficial cortical artery
Angiopathy
Venous thrombosis
Coagulopathy (endogenous or iatrogenic)
Infection (meningitis, encephalitis)
Toxins
Idiopathic hemorrhage

unconscious on presentation have a mortality rate of 60% (176). Cerebellar and thalamic hemorrhages larger than 3 cm in diameter (159) and pontine hemorrhages larger than 1 cm in diameter (177) have a very high mortality rate. Lobar hemorrhages tend to have a lower mortality rate and better functional recovery. The presence of intraventricular blood is a poor prognostic sign, but this may be related to the overall size of the hemorrhage (178).

Multivariate analysis has identified three variables that can accurately identify 30-day survival: the Glasgow Coma Scale score, hemorrhage size, and pulse pressure (119). If hematoma volume was small (<1/2 of one lobe), Glasgow Coma Scale score was >9, and pulse pressure was <40 mm Hg, there was a 0.98 probability of 30-day survival. However, when the hematoma was large, the patient was comatose, and the pulse pressure was >65 mm Hg, the probability of 30-day survival was 0.08.

ANEURYSMAL SUBARACHNOID HEMORRHAGE

Subarachnoid hemorrhage is a devastating disease; approximately one-quarter to one-third of patients die before reaching the hospital (179). Until recently, more than one-half of those who reached medical attention either died or were left with major neurologic deficits as a result of delayed complications (180). Fortunately, over the last 10 years, innovative management strategies have been developed that appear to reduce mortality and morbidity. Widely accepted strategies now include early surgery to obliterate the aneurysm combined with the use of calcium channel antagonists and hypertensive hypervolemic therapy to reduce the impact of vasospasm. Recently, cerebral angioplasty has been introduced for the treatment of vasospasm.

Etiology

Subarachnoid hemorrhage results from rupture of an intracranial aneurysm in approximately 50 to 75% of patients (181). Other causes of subarachnoid hemorrhage include bleeding from other vascular abnormalities (AVM, Moya Moya syndrome), head trauma, extension of an intracerebral hematoma, and idiopathic subarachnoid hemorrhage (Table 30.6). Intracranial aneurysms are present in 2 to 5% of autopsy cases (182, 183) but rupture with an incidence of only 10 to 12 per 100,000 individuals per year (179, 184, 185). Aneurysms are usually located at the bifurcation of the large arteries at the base of the brain, with approximately 85% occurring in the anterior circulation (186). They are thought to result from herniation of the intima through a fragmented internal elastic membrane. Factors that may contribute to rupture include large size of the aneurysm (187–189) and a sudden increase in blood pressure (190). The hemorrhage rate of unruptured aneurysms is approximately 1 to 2% per year (191) but much more frequent if the size is larger than 1 cm in diameter (189). Therefore it is recommended that incidentally discovered aneurysms larger than 7 mm in diameter be treated surgically (187–189). A recently available alternative is to occlude unruptured aneurysms with balloons or coils via an endovascular approach (191a)

Presentation

Prodromal symptoms of intracranial aneurysms include headache and focal neurologic deficits. Third cranial nerve palsy, with or without eye pain, can result from expanding aneurysms involving the posterior communicating artery or the termination of the internal carotid artery (192). Occasionally, TIA-like symptoms are present (193, 194) and are thought to result from thrombus embolizing from the aneurysm. Sentinel bleeds, intermittent leakage of small amounts of blood, may occur in patients prior to their definitive hemorrhage (193–195). Therefore, very sudden unexplained headaches with or without neurologic signs should raise the suspicion of subarachnoid hemorrhage and be evaluated; a contrast enhanced CT scan, MRI, magnetic resonance angiogram, or conventional angiogram may reveal an aneurysm and permit diagnosis prior to a severe subarachnoid hemorrhage (Fig. 30.6).

Following acute aneurysm rupture, ICP can briefly reach mean BP (196), which may account for the transient loss of consciousness seen in approximately 45% of cases (197). The bleed is almost always associated with a sudden severe headache which the patient often describes as "the worst headache of my life." There may a report of a seizure; however, it is not clear whether these episodes represent a true epileptic phenomenon or posturing resulting from the sudden rise in ICP (196). Occasionally, focal neurologic deficits are seen. In addition to ocular palsies, they may include hemiparesis, aphasia, abulia, or hemineglect. These deficits may result from parenchymal hemorrhage, subdural hematoma, or a large localized subarachnoid clot.

Evaluation and Initial Management

The initial steps in the evaluation of the patient should include assessment of level neurologic function, ability to protect the airway, and blood pressure (Table 30.7). The Hunt and Hess Scale (198) and the more recently developed World Federation of Neurological Surgeons Scale (Table 30.8) provide standardized indicators of the patient's clinical condition. The best initial diagnostic test for any patient presenting with symptoms and signs of subarachnoid hemorrhage is a CT scan. Patients with a Glasgow Coma Score of 8 or less should be intubated, with appropriate precautions taken regarding increased ICP (see discussion under the section entitled "Nontraumatic Intracerebral Hemorrhage"), prior to performing the CT scan. Blood pressure may be increased as a

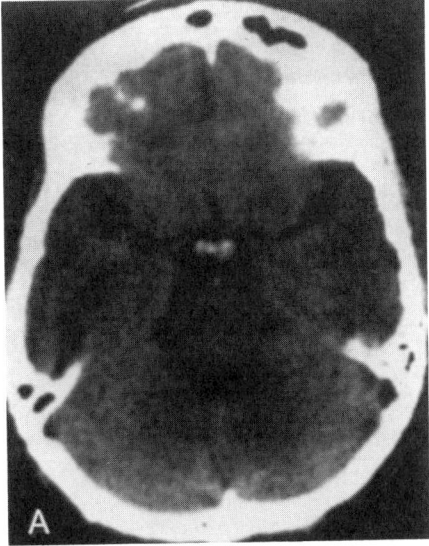

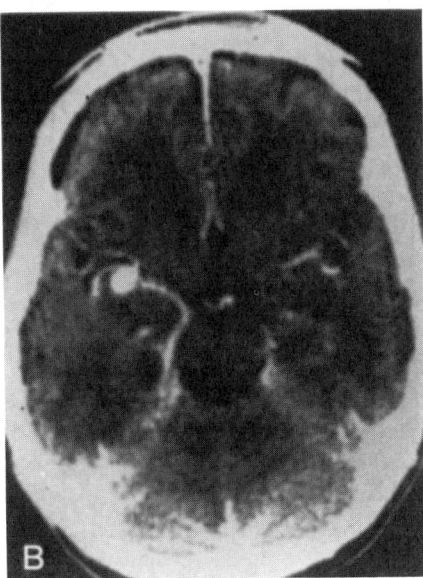

Figure 30.6. Computer tomographic scan of a patient with sudden onset of headache whose lumbar puncture revealed bloody cerebrospinal fluid. The unenhanced scan (*A*) shows a small hypodense region at the terminal portion of the middle cerebral artery that is enhanced following the administration of contrast (*B*). The presence of a saccular aneurysm in that location was confirmed with angiography. (Reprinted with permission from Weisberg L, Nice C: *Cerebral Computed Tomography,* ed 3. WB Saunders, Philadelphia, 1989, p 168.)

result of pain or anxiety, as a response to intracranial blood, or because of increased intracranial pressure. In stuporous patients, dramatic lowering of blood pressure should be avoided, as it may result in a critical decrease in cerebral perfusion pressure. On the other hand, hypertension can result in rebleeding (190). Therefore, clinical judgment must be used to weigh these two risks and arrive at a management strategy. In general, the optimal blood pressure is probably the patient's normal blood pressure. If this information is unavailable, the mean arterial blood pressure should be kept below 100 to 110 mm Hg. The principles for pharmacologic management of blood pressure are the same as those outlined previously for intracerebral hemorrhage.

Table 30.7. Early Management of Patients with Subarachnoid Hemorrhage

1. Assess level of consciousness and airway reflexes
2. Treat hypertension to patient's normal BP; if unknown, keep mean arterial blood pressure at 100 to 110 mm Hg
3. CT scan (nonenhanced)
4. Lumbar puncture only if CT is negative
5. Selective four-vessel angiography; general anesthesia for agitated uncooperative patients
6. Monitor electrocardiogram
7. Normal saline at somewhat above maintenance requirements
8. Load with phenytoin 18 to 20 mg/kg i.v.
9. Dexamethasone 4 mg every 6 hours i.v. or p.o. (optional)
10. Avoid excessive stimulation; sedate agitated patients with i.v. midazolam 1 to 3 mg, fentanyl 25 to 100 μg, or morphine 1 to 2 mg; titrate to effect; avoid long-acting agents
11. Prepare for surgery as soon as possible (most patients)

Table 30.8. Hunt and Hess Classification and World Federation of Neurological Surgeons Scale

Hunt and Hess Classification

Grade I:	Asymptomatic or with slight headache
Grade II:	Moderate to severe headache and nuchal rigidity but no focal or lateralizing neurologic signs
Grade III:	Drowsiness, confusion, and mild focal deficits
Grade IV:	Stupor, hemiparesis, early decerebrate rigidity, and vegetative disturbances
Grade V:	Deep coma and decerebrate rigidity

World Federation of Neurological Surgeons Subarachnoid Hemorrhage Scale

Grade	GCS Score	Motor Deficit
I	15	Absent
II	13–14	Absent
III	13–14	Present
IV	7–12	Present or absent
V	3–6	Present or absent

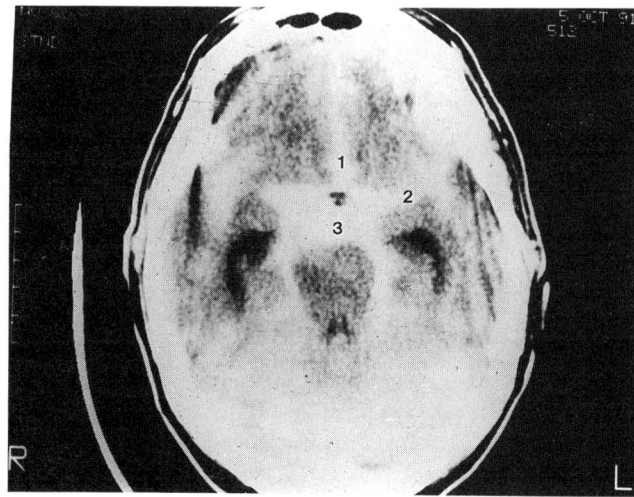

Figure 30.7. Computed tomographic scan of a patient with acute subarachnoid hemorrhage. A large amount of subarachnoid blood fills the (*1*) interhemispheric fissure, (*2*) Sylvian fissure, and (*3*) suprasellar cistern.

Almost 90% of hemorrhages are detected by a noncontrast CT scan (199). The subarachnoid blood appears as high-density (white) signal in spaces that are normally filled with CSF and thus normally appear dark (Fig. 30.7). These areas include the perimesencephalic and interpeduncular cisterns that surround the brainstem, the basal cisterns, the sylvian fissure, sulci, and the ventricles. The extent of bleeding helps predict the likelihood of developing vasospasm (200–205). Early hydrocephalus is suggested by enlargement of the third ventricle and the temporal horns of the lateral ventricles (Fig. 30.8). If clinical suspicion is strong and the CT scan is unremarkable, a lumbar puncture should be performed to search for bloody or xanthochromic CSF. However, if the diagnosis is made by CT scan, lumbar puncture is not indicated, since it may rarely induce aneurysmal rerupture (206). MRI is not very sensitive for detection of acute subarachnoid hemorrhage.

Recently, the timing of surgery has shifted toward an emphasis on early obliteration of the aneurysm in most patients (207). Angiography therefore should be performed rapidly and the patient prepared for surgery, especially in patients with subarachnoid hemorrhage complicated by intracerebral hemorrhage (208). Patients who are uncooperative and difficult to manage should have angiography performed under general anesthesia. Selective four-vessel angiography is necessary to check for multiple aneurysms, present in up to 20% of cases (209). At present, magnetic resonance angiography is not sensitive enough to replace conventional angiography.

Cardiac abnormalities are common in the first 24 hours after subarachnoid hemorrhage. Electrocardiographic changes similar to those seen with cardiac ischemia are seen and have been linked to elevated levels of circulating catecholamines (210, 211). Whether these changes represent true myocardial ischemia is unclear; however, myofibrillar degeneration has been reported (212). Significant arrhythmias, including ventricular tachycardia, have been reported (213); therefore, continuous cardiac monitoring is prudent.

Initial management (Table 30.7) focuses on prevention of rebleeding by avoiding situations that produce sudden changes in the transmural pressure across the wall of the aneurysm—sudden increases in blood pressure or decreases in ICP. Cough and Valsalva maneuvers should be avoided and hypertension treated. Patients are administered stool softeners and are treated with bed rest in a dark, quiet room, with excess stimulation avoided. Agitated patients should be sedated, but not to the point at which clinical deterioration would not be recognized. Short-acting reversible agents such as midazolam (1 to 3 mg intravenously), fentanyl (25 to 100 μg intravenously), or morphine (1 to 2 mg intravenously) can be administered in intermittent boluses and titrated to effect. The goal is to sedate the patient to the point at which he or she tends to fall asleep when left alone but can easily be aroused and examined. Opiates have the added benefit of treating head-ache. Use of longer-acting agents such as phenobarbital make this titration difficult, and the effects of the drug cannot be reversed. In addition, the loading doses of phenobarbital that would provide protection as an anticonvulsant are uniformly sedating. Thus, it becomes impossible to differentiate drug effect from deterioration resulting from hydrocephalus. When lumbar puncture is performed, a sudden decrease in ICP should be avoided by slowly removing small amounts of fluid through a small (22-gauge) needle. If a ventriculostomy is performed, the amount of CSF drained should be limited to that required to lower ICP to 15 to 20 mm Hg. Drugs with antiplatelet activity (aspirin, ibuprofen) are usually avoided.

Phenytoin is usually administered following subarachnoid hemorrhage for seizure prophylaxis but is not required long-term in the majority of patients. The loading dose should be administered intravenously. Its use is discussed in detail later in the chapter in the section entitled "Pharmacology." Dexa-methasone (4 mg every 6 hours orally or intravenously) is often used to reduce meningeal irritation and intra- and post-operative edema, although there is no specific evidence dem-onstrating efficacy. Since subarachnoid hemorrhage is associ-ated with volume contraction and hyponatremia (see below), somewhat greater than maintenance volumes of isotonic saline are appropriate in the initial management.

In approximately 15 to 20% of cases, cerebral panangiogra-phy fails to demonstrate a cause of nontraumatic subarachnoid hemorrhage (214, 215). Some of these failures may result from

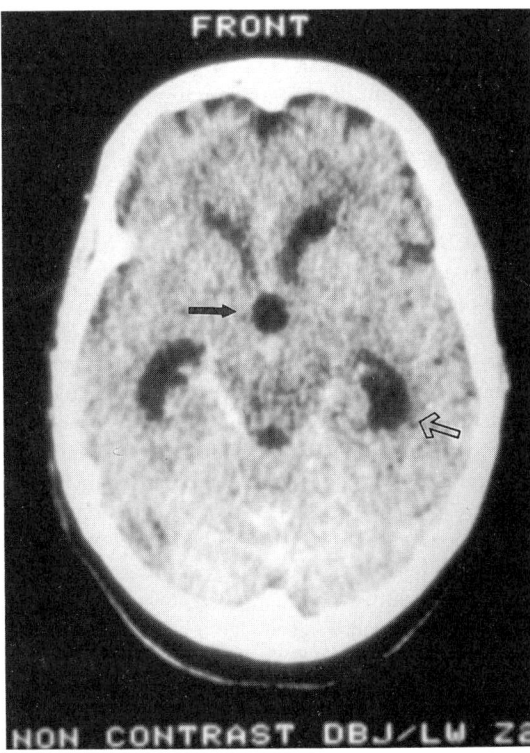

Figure 30.8. Computed tomographic scan of a patient several hours after acute subarachnoid hemorrhage. A small amount of blood is visible in the basal cisterns. Note the enlarged rounded appearance of the third ventricle (*solid arrow*) and enlarged temporal horns of the lateral ventri-cles (*open arrow*) indicating early hydrocephalus, in this case without intraventricular blood.

vasospasm or inadequate views to detect a subtle aneurysm, especially in the regions of the anterior communicating artery and posterior circulation. Therefore, repeat angiography is often recommended in 1 to 2 weeks. The natural history of "negative" high-quality angiograms is favorable, with a very low incidence of rebleeding (185, 214, 216). A subgroup of patients with blood in the perimesencephalic cisterns and normal angiograms usually has a benign clinical course (217, 218). Other rare causes of "angionegative" subarachnoid hem-orrhage include rupture of a small superficial cortical artery (219) or spinal cord AVM (220).

Management

Management of subarachnoid hemorrhage patients is ori-ented toward preventing or ameliorating major complications, which can include rebleeding, hydrocephalus, and vasospasm. Since these complications may evolve slowly over several days or longer, it is important to establish the patient's status clearly. Baseline data should include a complete neurologic exam, and a CT scan to assess amount and distribution of subarachnoid blood and ventricular size. An angiogram will indicate the aneurysm's location and whether vasospasm is present. If transcranial Doppler is used to monitor for vaso-spasm, baseline studies are needed to detect changes in blood flow velocity over time. Serum electrolytes, blood pressure, central venous pressure, and weight are needed to monitor for potential hyponatremia and intravascular volume contraction.

Routine monitoring of all patients in the intensive care unit initially should include serial neurologic exams, continu-ous EKG monitoring, and frequent determinations of blood pressure, electrolytes, body weight, fluid balance, and, in many centers, transcranial Doppler. The frequency of these measurements is determined based on the clinical condition of the patient. Initially, neurologic exams should be performed every 2 to 4 hours until the patient is stable. However, the exams should be continued several times a day for the next 1 to 2 weeks, since neurologic complications are often delayed. In neurologically unstable patients, more frequent or continu-ous blood pressure monitoring is used to determine whether there is a correlation between blood pressure and neurologic function.

Electrolytes, weight, and fluid balance should be moni-tored daily to assess for hyponatremia and intravascular vol-ume contraction. Serial measurements of central venous pres-sure or pulmonary capillary wedge pressure are also very useful. This measurement is particularly important since pa-tients tend to become volume contracted after subarachnoid hemorrhage (221), and this hypovolemia exacerbates vaso-spasm (222). Thus, weight loss, persistent negative fluid bal-ance, and decrease in central venous or pulmonary capillary wedge pressures indicate intravascular volume contraction, and intravenous fluids should be increased to correct the situation. This increase may require administration of fluids at rates of up to 200 to 400 ml/hr.

Rebleeding. The incidence of rebleeding peaks immedi-ately following hemorrhage and then declines over the first few days, but remains high for several weeks (Fig. 30.9) (223). Rates of rebleeding are highest in women, patients with poor clinical grade at presentation, patients in poor overall medical condition, and those with high systolic blood pressure (224).

DAILY RISK OF REBLEEDING

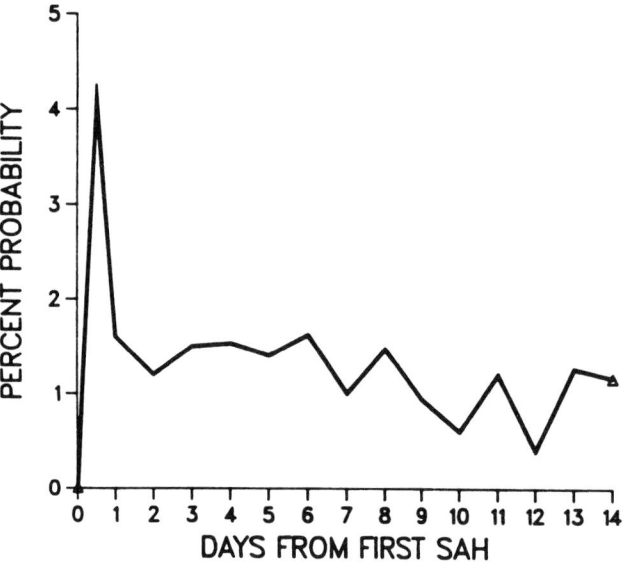

Figure 30.9. Daily risk of rebleeding following acute aneurysmal subarachnoid hemorrhage. (Reprinted with permission of The Congress of Neurological Surgeons from Kassell NF, Torner JC: Aneurysmal rebleeding: a preliminary report from the Cooperative Aneurysm Study. *Neurosurgery* 13:479-481, 1983.)

Rerupture is fatal in more than 30% of instances (225). Prior to the advent of early surgery, the antifibrinolytic agents ε-aminocaproic acid or tranexamic acid were routinely administered. Although there was a reduction in the incidence of rebleeding (226), this reduction was offset by a similar increase in ischemic infarctions from vasospasm (227) and hydrocephalus. This increase occurred even if antifibrinolytics were administered only for 2 to 3 days while the patient was awaiting surgery (228). Therefore, when early surgery is undertaken, these agents are not administered.

Definitive prevention of rebleeding is accomplished with surgical clipping of the aneurysm. The concept that surgery is more difficult and results in a worse outcome when performed early (within 3 days of subarachnoid hemorrhage) has not been supported by careful analysis (229–232). In addition, recent review of the Cooperative Aneurysm Study database found that outcome in Hunt and Hess grade II and III patients was improved with early surgery (207). Clipping of the aneurysm has the additional advantage of safely allowing elevation of blood pressure to treat vasospasm. It is expected that future analyses will demonstrate an even greater benefit as hypertensive hypervolemic therapy for vasospasm becomes more widely employed. Aneurysms can also be treated with endovascular balloon occlusion or metallic coil-induced thrombosis, but these approaches are not currently recommended for recently ruptured aneurysms (191a)

Hydrocephalus.   Hydrocephalus results from obstruction of CSF flow by intraventricular or subarachnoid blood, impedance of normal CSF flow dynamic by fibrosis, or a failure of CSF resorption. It can develop within hours of hemorrhage (233) or may not appear until weeks later (179). Acute hydrocephalus that is asymptomatic should not be treated prior to surgery, since the increase in transmural pressure across the

aneurysm wall induced by CSF drainage may precipitate rebleeding (234). Patients with hydrocephalus who are clinically deteriorating should have their ICP lowered gradually with a ventricular drain to 15 to 20 mm Hg. Postoperatively, the need for CSF drainage may be transient or protracted and should be tested by periodically stopping drainage while monitoring ICP.

Delayed hydrocephalus should be considered as an etiology for any decline in neurologic status and is easily diagnosed by CT scan. Postoperative hydrocephalus can be treated safely with ventriculostomy (235). Alternatively, if the ventricular system is patent, hydrocephalus can be treated with a lumbar drain or frequent lumbar punctures (1 to 3 per day) (236) until the need for permanent shunting is determined. Routine management of intraventricular catheters is discussed in the section entitled "Nontraumatic Intracerebral Hemorrhage."

Vasospasm.   Classically, vasospasm is defined both clinically and angiographically. Clinical symptoms of vasospasm develop in approximately one-third of patients following subarachnoid hemorrhage (225) and are more common in those with large amounts of subarachnoid blood (200–205). It usually develops in 6 to 14 days but may occur anywhere from 2 days to 3 weeks after hemorrhage (237). The clinical picture usually shows a gradual decline in consciousness or focal neurologic deficits that may fluctuate and are exacerbated by hypovolemia or hypotension. Angiographic vasospasm occurs in up to 80% of patients, follows a time course similar to that of clinical vasospasm, and appears as focal or diffuse narrowing of cerebral vessels (238). The phenomenon is incompletely understood but appears to consist of both vascular smooth muscle contraction (239) and structural changes in the vessel wall (240) that result in focal or diffuse narrowing of the vessel lumen. Although clinical symptom are more likely when there is angiographic vasospasm, symptoms can occur in the absence of angiographic changes, and vice-versa.

Recently, transcranial Doppler has been used to diagnose vasospasm (241–243). Narrowing of the blood vessels at the base of the brain is inferred from increases in linear blood flow velocities. When compared with angiography, transcranial Doppler has a sensitivity of about 80%, partly because it samples only a small segment of the vasculature (244).

Treatment of vasospasm involves both prophylaxis and intervention during deteriorations. All patients should receive prophylactic therapies. More aggressive interventions are usually reserved for patients with clinical vasospasm, but not for those patients with angiographic or transcranial Doppler-defined vasospasm. When angiographic or transcranial Doppler evidence of vasospasm is present without clinical symptoms, most clinicians will use that as an indicator to continue prophylactic measures and be on guard for clinical symptoms that would require more aggressive measures.

Prophylactic measures (Table 30.9) include mechanical removal of subarachnoid blood at the time of aneurysm surgery (245), administration of the centrally acting calcium channel antagonist nimodipine (246–250), and volume expansion (222, 230). The subarachnoid administration of tissue plasminogen activator during surgery to aid in removal of blood is currently under investigation (251, 252).

Administration of nimodipine in the recommended dose 60 mg orally every 4 hours for 3 weeks after hemorrhage reduces the incidence of ischemic infarctions and improves outcome (231, 246–248, 250). It is not yet clear whether this beneficial effect results from action on cerebral vessels or prevention of calcium influx into ischemic neurons. Although nimodipine administration can be associated with hypotension, this effect can usually be ameliorated by fluid administration prior to beginning the medication. However, in patients whose symptomatic vasospasm is being treated with hypovolemic hypertensive therapy, it is particularly important to avoid hypotension following nimodipine administration. Therefore, if such a pattern develops, adjusting the dose to 30 mg every 2 hours or 15 mg every hour is useful. In difficult cases in which there is a clear clinical response to hypertension and it is not possible to avoid hypotension with nimodipine administration, it may be necessary to increase the dose of vasopressors or discontinue the use of nimodipine.

Treatment of symptomatic vasospasm in patients with surgically clipped aneurysms is accomplished with hypervolemic hypertensive therapy (230, 253–255). Acute volume expansion is begun with isotonic crystalloid or colloid (230). The initial goal is a central venous pressure of 10 to 15 mm Hg or a pulmonary capillary wedge pressure of 15 to 18 mm Hg. It may require administration of large volumes of fluid to achieve (1 to 2 liters) and maintain (200 to 500 ml/hr) these goals. Although normal (isotonic) saline is usually effective, some patients appear to respond better to colloid-containing solutions such as 5% albumin. Packed red blood cells are very useful in volume expansion, but hematocrit should be maintained at 30 to 35% to achieve a compromise between decreasing blood viscosity while maintaining oxygen carrying capacity. If there is no clinical response in 2 to 4 hours, mean blood pressure should be increased to 10 to 20% above baseline. This increase can be achieved by means of a combination of intravenous dopamine at 5 to 15 μg/kg/min and phenylephrine 10 to 300 μg/min. If there is no improvement in the neurologic exam, further elevation of blood pressure can be effective; the decision depends on a risk-benefit analysis of neurologic improvement versus the potential for complications. The use of hypervolemic hypertensive therapy is usually not recommended in patients with unclipped aneurysms.

Patients with known or suspected cardiac disease should be monitored with a Swan-Ganz catheter to avoid precipitating fluid overload or congestive heart failure and serial electrocardiograms to monitor for cardiac ischemia. Another potential side effect is ischemia to intestinal organs, which can, in rare cases, lead to infarction. Therefore, the levels of hemodynamic augmentation should be titrated continuously based on the patient's neurologic condition. The minimal amount of vasopressors required to maintain a stable neurologic status should be administered. If a ventricular catheter is present, cerebral perfusion can be augmented by draining CSF to reduce ICP to 0 to 5 mm Hg.

Table 30.9. Prophylactic Therapies for Vasospasm

1. Volume expansion with isotonic saline ± colloids
2. Nimodipine 60 mg orally every 4 hours
3. Mechanical removal of subarachnoid blood at surgery
4. Intrathecal tissue plasminogen activator at surgery (experimental)

Weaning from hypertensive hypervolemic therapy should be performed gradually, usually over several days. Again, the neurologic exam should guide the rate of withdrawal. Vasopressors should be weaned first in steps. Later hypervolemic therapy is weaned over several days to a week.

Patients who are unable to tolerate hypervolemic hypertensive therapy or who do not respond to it may benefit from angioplasty of vasospastic arteries. Early reports are encouraging (256–259), though angioplasty carries a small risk of hemorrhage (260) and the optimal timing has not yet been established.

Altered Cerebrovascular Reactivity.   Some subarachnoid hemorrhage patients suffer from an impairment in cerebrovascular pressure autoregulation and CO_2 reactivity (261–265). This impairment is more common in patients who are more severely affected by the hemorrhage (266). Disturbed autoregulation results in pressure-passive cerebral blood flow, and neurologic function may be linked directly to blood pressure. This relationship can be assessed by determining the relationship between the neurologic exam and blood pressure. Although this phenomenon often occurs concurrently with vasospasm, it may occur independently.

Hyponatremia.   Hyponatremia occurs in up to one-third of patients after subarachnoid hemorrhage (267, 268). The hyponatremia initially was attributed to the syndrome of inappropriate secretion of antidiuretic hormone (SIADH) (269–273). However, it was noted that subarachnoid hemorrhage patients became volume contracted and had a negative sodium balance (221, 274). In addition, when hyponatremic patients were treated with fluid restriction, the standard therapy for SIADH, they had a higher incidence of cerebral infarctions (275). Thus, treating hyponatremia based on the assumption that it resulted from SIADH appeared to worsen outcome by allowing hypovolemia to exacerbate vasospasm. Although the etiology of the volume wasting and hyponatremia has not been clearly defined (268, 276, 277), it has been shown that administration of large volumes of intravenous fluids (6 to 8 liters/day of isotonic saline) can prevent volume contraction (278).

ANOXIC ISCHEMIC ENCEPHALOPATHY

There is as yet no specific therapy for the damage caused by profound cardiorespiratory compromise (279). General supportive measures are indicated, as appropriate to the clinical status of the patient. Barbiturate and calcium antagonist therapy do not benefit patient outcome (279–281).

Seizures and myoclonus can develop shortly after cardiopulmonary arrest. Seizures or myoclonus do not affect prognosis; there is no consensus as to optimal therapy with anticonvulsant medications, but phenytoin, barbiturates, and benzodiazepines are often used. However, prolonged (longer than 30 minutes) seizures, myoclonus, or a combination of seizures and myoclonus (myoclonic status epilepticus) conveys a poor prognosis for survival and functional recovery (282–285). Aggressive anticonvulsant protocols have been employed to stop convulsive or myoclonic status, but there seems to be no improvement in prognosis (282–285).

COMMENTS ON SYSTEMIC CARE

RESPIRATORY SYSTEM

In patients with an impaired level of consciousness, the ability to protect the airway must always be evaluated. This analysis should include evaluation of airway patency, gag and cough reflexes, ability to handle oral secretions, and clearance of pulmonary secretions. Compromise of the airway leads to aspiration, atelectasis, pulmonary shunting, and hypoxemia. Hypoxemia is detrimental to poorly perfused cerebral tissue and causes vasodilation, which can increase ICP. Therefore, oxygenation should be maintained within a margin of safety to avoid hypoxemia should respiratory status deteriorate. Increasing residual lung volumes with positive end-expiratory pressure is useful but increases intrathoracic pressure, which may impede cerebral venous return and theoretically increase ICP. Although some studies have found no effect of positive end-expiratory pressure on ICP in patients with normal and reduced intracranial compliance (286), it is probably best to assess the ICP response and change in PaO_2 to positive end-expiratory pressure in each individual patient. This response is easily determined if ICP is being monitored. Otherwise, the potential risk of increasing ICP should be weighed against the risk of oxygen toxicity and hypoxemia; in general, if the patient did not require ICP monitoring, then use of positive end-expiratory pressure is probably safe.

Hyperventilation, if indicated, can be achieved using intermittent mandatory ventilation or assist/control ventilation. Once hyperventilation has been weaned, pressure support ventilation is usually effective, as respiratory drive is generally intact. Some patients may hyperventilate spontaneously. Usually it is best not to attempt to correct this by increasing dead space or sedation, since it resolves as the patient improves neurologically.

Pulmonary toilette for clearance of retained secretions is essential. Unfortunately, the standard practices of deep tracheal suctioning, inducing cough, chest percussion, and postural drainage almost always increase ICP. Blocking the ICP response to these maneuvers is important. Maneuvers to accomplish this blockage include positioning the patient head up with the neck in neutral position, and hyperventilation with 100% oxygen before and after suctioning. Lidocaine 1 mg/kg intravenously or thiopental 0.5 to 1.0 mg/kg intravenously may also be effective (287).

Intubation is usually maintained until the patient is awake, has adequate cough and gag reflexes, and consistently follows commands. These criteria must be individualized; for example, a patient with receptive aphasia may be unable to follow commands. Patients who are slow to improve may require tracheostomy.

METABOLIC MANAGEMENT

Following brain injury, patients tend to be hypermetabolic and hypercatabolic. This state is exacerbated by infection, corticosteroids, seizures, and posturing. Adequate nutritional support is crucial in maintaining immunocompetence, respiratory muscle mass, and skin and mucosal surface integrity, and in minimizing exacerbation of the stress response. Therefore, early institution of nutritional support is important. Patients may require up to 35 to 45 kcal/kg/day. The diet should include an adequate supply of fat to minimize excess CO_2 production, avoid hyperglycemia, and satisfy essential fatty acid requirements. Protein requirements are high, often 1.3 to 1.8 g/kg/day. This requirement can be assessed by calculating 24-hour nitrogen balance. Careful attention to hepatic and renal function is important when administering such high protein loads.

Since most patients have intact gastrointestinal tracts, enteral feeding is the appropriate route for nutritional support. Enteral feeding offer the advantages of maintenance of the integrity and immunologic role of the gut, prophylaxis against stress ulceration, and elimination of the risks of pneumothorax and sepsis associated with parenteral nutrition. The risk of pulmonary aspiration of gastric contents is reduced by using continuous feeding and metaclopramide 10 to 20 mg every 6 hours. Patients with poor motility may benefit from placement of postpylorus tubes, which allow feeding of elemental formulas directly into the small intestine. Patients who cannot tolerate tube feedings should receive total parenteral nutrition. Care must be used in ordering the formula to avoid hypoosmolal solutions.

Prophylaxis against gastrointestinal bleeding can be achieved with continuous tube feeding or sucralfate. Use of sucralfate requires interruption of tube feeding, so rates must be adjusted accordingly. Histamine antagonists may increase the incidence of Gram-negative pneumonia (288), produce undesirable CNS side effects, and displace anticonvulsants from albumin.

Blood glucose may be elevated as a result of diabetes, corticosteroid administration, stress, or infection. Evidence is mounting that hyperglycemia has detrimental effects during ischemia; however, the effects vary depending on whether the ischemia is focal or global (65). Although it has not yet been demonstrated to alter outcome, it seems prudent to avoid hyperglycemia in patients with brain injury. This goal may be accomplished by withholding glucose-containing solutions during ischemia, or by controlling hyperglycemia with insulin. In patients with prolonged illness, it would be unwise to withhold glucose at the expense of nutrition, and judicious use of insulin is preferable. In diabetics, glucose should be controlled in the range of 150 to 200 mg/dl. Care must be taken to avoid hypoglycemia. Oral hypoglycemic agents are best avoided until the patient is on a stable, well-tolerated diet.

Disturbances in magnesium, calcium, and phosphate are common in brain-injured patients. Excretion of these electrolytes is increased as a result of a patient's catabolic state, infection, use of diuretics, or hypervolemic therapy. The patient may require daily intravenous supplement to maintain normal serum concentrations.

REHABILITATION

Traditional techniques of physical, occupational, and speech therapy are utilized to improve the patient's functioning following stroke (289, 289a). Concerns have been raised about the possible adverse effects of commonly used medications on cerebral recovery. These drugs, which include clonidine, prazosin, neuroleptics, benzodiazepines, and phenytoin, may impair neuronal long-term potentiation and neuronal rearrangements (290).

There is no generally accepted pharmacologic treatment that improves brain recovery after stroke. However, preliminary studies with amphetamine suggest a better outcome with treatment (291, 292).

Depression following stroke is quite common, especially in patients with a left frontal ischemic lesion, and can impair recovery (293). Symptoms can be relieved with pharmacologic interventions, including nortriptyline and trazodone (294, 295). Nortriptyline is started at a level of 10 to 25 mg orally at bedtime; the dose is titrated upward over several weeks. Blood levels of nortriptyline can be monitored to help ensure a therapeutic response. Trazodone can be initiated at 50 mg orally daily and the dose increased every 3 days, as tolerated, until a dose of 200 mg/day is achieved (295). Attention to adverse medication effects such as postural hypotension and urinary retention is important.

PHARMACOLOGY

HEPARIN

Heparin interacts with antithrombin III and increases its activity, thereby inhibiting the activity of thrombin and factors IX, X, XI, and XII (296). Heparin can also decrease platelet function (42). Heparin can be administered as a constant intravenous infusion, without a loading dose, to achieve an aPTT of 1.5 times that of control (16). A dosage of 6000 units of heparin can be mixed with 250 ml of normal saline, and initially 1000 units per hour (40 ml/hr) can be delivered. The aPTT is checked after 4 hours and the infusion rate adjusted to achieve the target aPTT (16). The aPTT should be checked daily and the platelet count at least every 3 days to screen for heparin-associated thrombocytopenia (74). Of note, however, is that aPTT reagents can vary, thereby leading to inaccuracies in assessing the degree of anticoagulation (296a).

WARFARIN

Warfarin adversely affects vitamin K metabolism by inhibiting vitamin K epoxide reductase and perhaps vitamin K reductase (19). There is a subsequent depletion of vitamin K-dependent proteins, including prothrombin, factors VII, IX, and X, and proteins C and S. For stroke patients, oral warfarin is often started after 3 to 7 days of heparin therapy. A 10-mg dosage of warfarin daily can be prescribed and the prothrombin time (PT) checked on the 3rd day of warfarin treatment. When the generally accepted therapeutic PT elevation to 1.3 to 1.5 times that of control (international normalized ratio = 1.83 to 2.54) is reached, heparin can be discontinued (14, 19). However, the optimal intensity of anticoagulation for most neurologic indications is not well defined; a target international normalized ratio of 2.0 to 3.0 may be more appropriate (296b). For the first few days of warfarin treatment, the PT should be monitored daily. If warfarin therapy is begun without concurrent heparin administration, as might be the case

if anticoagulation is deferred because of a hemorrhagic infarction, a paradoxic thrombogenic state can develop because of the early depletion of proteins C and S (19).

With chronic warfarin treatment, the risk of bleeding complications is greatest in the first three months of therapy; the risk of fatal bleeding is 1% at one year and 2% at three years (296c). At a prothrombin ratio of 1.3 to 1.5, there are eleven serious bleeding events per 100 patient-years (relative risk, 3.0 [95% confidence interval, 1.9 to 4.7]) (296c). The odds ratio of sustaining an intracerebral hemorrhage while on warfarin therapy is 6.7 (95% confidence interval, 4.5 to 9.9) compared to the general population (296d).

ASPIRIN

Aspirin irreversibly acetylates the active site of cyclooxygenase in platelets, thereby blocking synthesis of thromboxane A_2 and inhibiting platelet aggregation (297). Prostacyclin, an endothelial cell-derived platelet antiaggregant, also has its synthesis blocked by aspirin, albeit at a higher dose than is required to decrease thromboxane A_2 production (298, 298b). The ability of aspirin to inhibit platelet activity exhibits a dose dependency that is inversely related to the strength of the stimulus used to produce aggregation (298a). Thus, although aspirin (40 mg/day) can block platelet aggregation caused by a strong stimulus, doses up to 1280 mg/day are needed to diminish platelet aggregation induced by weaker stimuli, especially when whole blood is present in the assay system (298a).

As shown by metaanalysis, the risk of gastrointestinal hemorrhage and peptic ulcer is increased 350% (odds ratio 3.5) if aspirin is combined with another antiplatelet agent; surprisingly, in one metaanalysis use of aspirin alone did not increase the risk of serious gastrointestinal adverse effects (36). When low- and moderate-dose aspirin therapy are compared with the risk of major bleeding complications, low-dose aspirin yields a hazard ratio of 0.84 (39). When compared with placebo, aspirin 75 mg/day led to severe gastrointestinal bleeding in 1.3% of patients, compared with 0.6% of control individuals (41). Dyken et al point out that the percent of patients with gastrointestinal bleeding requiring transfusion is actually quite low at two aspirin doses: 0.73% at 1200 mg/day and 0.99% at 300 mg/day, compared to 0.12% of individuals on placebo (36a).

TICLOPIDINE

Ticlopidine inhibits platelet aggregation by irreversibly blocking the adenosine diphosphate pathway. The activity of cyclooxygenase is not affected (44). Ticlopidine also decreases erythrocyte aggregability and blood fibrinogen concentration (298b).

Diarrhea develops in about 20% of patients treated with ticlopidine (44, 299). A decrease in dose can improve diarrhea and abdominal cramps (44). Rash occurs in 3.5 to 11.9% of ticlopidine-treated patients; if the rash is serious, discontinuation of therapy leads to resolution (44, 68, 300). Severe neutropenia (absolute neutrophil count <450/mm^3) develops in up to 0.9% of patients within 1 to 3 months of beginning ticlopidine therapy (44). The neutropenia resolves within 3 weeks of discontinuing the drug (44). Therefore, a complete blood count and white blood cell differential should be obtained at baseline and every 2 weeks during the first 3 months of ticlopidine therapy. More frequent monitoring is indicated for those patients with a declining neutrophil count or a count less than 30% of baseline. If the absolute neutrophil count drops below 1200/mm³, ticlopidine should be discontinued (300).

Gastrointestinal hemorrhage occurred in 0.5% of patients treated with ticlopidine, compared with 1.4% of aspirin-treated patients (44). When any bleeding event is considered, 9% of ticlopidine- and 10% of aspirin-treated patients experienced an adverse event (44).

PHENYTOIN

A loading dose of phenytoin 18 to 20 mg/kg should be administered intravenously no faster than 50 mg/min to avoid hypotension or heart block. To avoid precipitation, the drug should be administered through an intravenous line containing saline without dextrose. Oral loading is not recommended because of slow (6 to 24 hour), unpredictable absorption. Because distribution is rapid, a blood level obtained 1 hour after an intravenous loading dose will reflect the adequacy of the dose. The therapeutic anticonvulsant range in most clinical laboratories is 10 to 20 μg/dl. Daily intravenous administration of 5 mg/kg in single or divided doses usually maintains total drug levels in the therapeutic range. However, the elixir preparation is poorly absorbed from the gastrointestinal tract, especially if the patient is receiving nasogastric feeding. The dose may need to be increased by 50 to 100% to maintain therapeutic blood levels. Blood levels should be checked every 1 to 2 days to assess the adequacy of the maintenance dose. Free (unbound) phenytoin levels may be useful in avoiding toxicity (301) in patients who are albuminemic or who are receiving drugs such as warfarin and histamine blockers, which can displace phenytoin from albumin. Free drug levels are normally 10% of total drug levels (301).

REFERENCES

1. Rothrock JR, Hart RG: Antithrombotic therapy in cerebrovascular disease. *Ann Intern Med* 115:885–895, 1991.
1a. Marshall RS, Mohr JP: Current management of ischemic stroke. *J Neurol Neurosurg Psychiat* 56:6–, 1993.
1b. National Stroke Association Consensus Statement: Stroke: the first six hours. *Stroke Clinical Updates* 4:1–12, 1993.
1c. Caplan LR: Brain embolism, revisited. *Neurology* 43:1281–1287, 1993.
2. Wolf PA, Abbott RD, Kannel WB: Atrial fibrillation as an independent risk factor for stroke: the Framingham study. *Stroke* 22:983–988, 1991.
3. Cerebral Embolism Task Force: Cardiogenic brain embolism. The second report of the Cerebral Embolism Task Force. *Arch Neurol* 46:727–743, 1989.
4. Tegeler CH, Downes TR: Cardiac imaging in stroke. *Stroke* 22:1206–1211, 1991.
5. Amarenco P, Duyckaerts C, Tzourio C, Henin D, Bousser M-G, Hauw J-J: The prevalence of ulcerated plaques in the aortic arch in patients with stroke. *N Engl J Med* 326:221–225, 1992.
6. Fisher EA, Goldman ME: Transesophageal echocardiography: a new view of the heart. *Ann Intern Med* 113:91–93, 1990.
7. Coull BM, Goodnight SH: Antiphospholipid antibodies, prethrombotic states, and stroke. *Stroke* 21:1370–1374, 1990.
8. Bogousslavsky J, Cachin C, Regli F, Despland PA, Van Melle G, Kappenberger L: Cardiac sources of embolism and cerebral infarction—clinical consequences and vascular concomitants: the Lausanne stroke registry. *Neurology* 41:855–859, 1991.
8a. Hornig CR, Bauer T, Simon C, Trittmacher S, Dorndorf W: Hemorrhagic transformation in cardioembolic cerebral infarction. *Stroke* 24:465–468, 1993.

9. Okada Y, Yamaguchi T, Minematsu K, et al: Hemorrhagic transformation in cerebral embolism. *Stroke* 20:598–603, 1989.
10. Albers GW, Sherman DG, Gress DR, Paulseth JE, Peterson P: Stroke prevention in nonvalvular atrial fibrillation: a review of prospective randomized trials. *Ann Neurol* 30:511–518, 1991.
11. Albers GW, Atwood JE, Hirsh J, Sherman DG, Hughes RA, Connolly SJ: Stroke prevention in nonvalvular atrial fibrillation. *Ann Intern Med* 115:727–736, 1991.
12. Pritchett ELC: Management of atrial fibrillation. *N Engl J Med* 326:1264–1271, 1992.
13. Clark WM, Madden KP, Lyden PD, Zivin JA: Cerebral hemorrhagic risk of aspirin or heparin therapy with thrombolytic treatment in rabbits. *Stroke* 22:872–876, 1991.
14. Cerebral Embolism Task Force: Cardiogenic brain embolism. *Arch Neurol* 43:71–84, 1986.
15. Pessin MS, Teal PA, Caplan LR: Hemorrhagic infarction: guilt by association? *AJNR* 12:1123–1126, 1991.
15a. Pessin MS, Estol CJ, LaFranchise F, Caplan LR: Safety of anticoagulation after hemorrhagic infarction. *Neurology* 43:1298–1303, 1993.
16. Yatsu FM, Hart RG, Mohr JP, Grotta JC: Anticoagulation of embolic strokes of cardiac origin: an update. *Neurology* 38:314–316, 1988.
17. Saour JN, Sieck JO, Mamo LAR, Gallus AS: Trial of different intensities of anticoagulation in patients with prosthetic heart valves. *N Engl J Med* 322:428–432, 1990.
18. Stein PD, Collins JJ, Kantrowitz A: Antithrombotic therapy in mechanical and biological prosthetic heart valves and saphenous vein bypass grafts. *Chest* 89(suppl):46S–53S, 1986.
19. Hirsh J: Oral anticoagulant drugs. *N Engl J Med* 324:1865–1875, 1991.
20. Hart RG, Foster JW, Luther MF, Kanter MC: Stroke in infective endocarditis. *Stroke* 21:695–700, 1990.
21. Salgado AV, Furlan AJ, Keys TF, Nichols TR, Beck GJ: Neurologic complications of endocarditis: a 12-year experience. *Neurology* 39:173–178, 1989.
22. Kanter MC, Hart RG: Neurologic complications of infective endocarditis. *Neurology* 41:1015–1020, 1991.
23. Keyser DL, Biller J, Coffman TT, Adams Jr HP: Neurologic complications of late prosthetic valve endocarditis. *Stroke* 21:472–475, 1990.
24. Davenport J, Hart RG: Prosthetic valve endocarditis 1976–1987. Antibiotics, anticoagulation, and stroke. *Stroke* 21:993–999, 1990.
25. Craven TE, Ryu J, Espeland MA, et al: Evaluation of the associations between carotid artery atherosclerosis and coronary artery stenosis. A case-control study. *Circulation* 82:1230–1242, 1990.
26. Bornstein NM, Norris JW: The unstable carotid plaque. *Stroke* 20:1104–1106, 1989.
27. Sirna S, Biller J, Skorton DJ, Seabold JE: Cardiac evaluation of the patient with stroke. *Stroke* 21:14–23, 1990.
28. Chimowitz MI, Mancini GB: Asymptomatic coronary artery disease in patients with stroke. Prevalence, prognosis, diagnosis, and treatment. *Stroke* 23:433–436, 1992.
28a. Love BB, Grover-McKay M, Biller J, Rezai K, McKay CR: Coronary artery disease and cardiac events with asymptomatic and symptomatic cerebrovascular disease. *Stroke* 23:939–945, 1992.
28b. Hobson II RW, Weiss DG, Fields WS, Goldstone J, Moore WS, Towne JB, Wright CB, and the Veterans Affairs Cooperative Study Group: Efficacy of carotid endarterectomy for asymptomatic carotid stenosis. *N Engl J Med* 328:221–227, 1993.
28c. The CASANOVA Study Group: Carotid surgery versus medical therapy in asymptomatic carotid stenosis. *Stroke* 22:1229–1235, 1991.
28d. Mayo Asymptomatic Carotid Endarterectomy Study Group: Results of a randomized controlled trial of carotid endarterectomy for asymptomatic carotid stenosis. *Mayo Clin Proc* 67:513–518, 1992.
28e. Barnett HJM, Haines SJ: Carotid endarterectomy for asymptomatic carotid stenosis. *N Engl J Med* 328:276–279, 1993.
29. Freischlag JA, Hanna D, Moore WS: Improved prognosis for asymptomatic carotid stenosis with prophylactic carotid endarterectomy. *Stroke* 23:479–482, 1992.
30. Graor RA, Hetzer NR: Management of coexistent carotid artery and coronary artery disease. *Stroke* 19:1441–1444, 1988.
31. North American Symptomatic Carotid Endarterectomy Trial Collaborators: Beneficial effect of carotid endarterectomy in symptomatic patients with high-grade carotid stenosis. *N Engl J Med* 325:445–453, 1991.
32. European Carotid Surgery Trialists' Collaborative Group: MRC European carotid surgery trial: interim results for symptomatic patients with severe (70–99%) or with mild (0–29%) carotid stenosis. *Lancet* 337:1235–1243, 1991.
33. Mayberg MR, Wilson SE, Yatsu F, et al: Carotid endarterectomy and prevention of cerebral ischemia in symptomatic carotid stenosis. *JAMA* 266:3289–3294, 1991.
34. Mackey WC, O'Donnell TF, Callow AD: Cardiac risk in patients undergoing carotid endarterectomy: impact on perioperative and long-term mortality. *J Vasc Surg* 11:226–234, 1990.
35. Antiplatelet Trialists' Collaboration: Secondary prevention of vascular disease by prolonged antiplatelet treatment. *Br Med J* 296:320–331, 1988.

36. Sze PC, Reitman D, Pincus MM, Sacks HS, Chalmers TC: Antiplatelet agents in the secondary prevention of stroke: meta-analysis of the randomized control trials. *Stroke* 19:436–442, 1988.

36a. Dyken ML, Barnett HJM, Easton JD, Fields WS, Fuster V, Hachinski V, Norris JW, Sherman DG: Low-dose aspirin and stroke. "It ain't necessarily so." *Stroke* 23:1395–1399, 1992.

37. Sivenius J, Laakso M, Penttila IM, Smets P, Lowenthal A, Riekkinen PJ: The European stroke prevention study: results according to sex. *Neurology* 41:1189–1192, 1991.

38. Weksler BB, Pett SB, Alonso D, et al: Differential inhibition by aspirin of vascular and platelet prostaglandin synthesis in atherosclerotic patients. *N Engl J Med* 308:800–805, 1983.

39. The Dutch TIA Trial Study Group: A comparison of two doses of aspirin (30 mg vs. 283 mg a day) in patients after a transient ischemic attack or minor ischemic stroke. *N Engl J Med* 325:1261–1266, 1991.

40. The European *Stroke* Prevention Study Group: European stroke prevention study. *Stroke* 21:1122–1130, 1990.

40a. van Grijn J, Warlow CP, Norrving B: Low-dose aspirin and stroke. *Stroke* 24:476, 1993.

40b. Helgason CM, Tortorice KL, Winkler SR, Penney DW, Schuler JJ, McClelland TJ, Brace LD: Aspirin response and failure in cerebral infarction. *Stroke* 24:345–350, 1993.

41. The SALT Collaborative Group: Swedish aspirin low-dose trial (SALT) of 75 mg aspirin as secondary prophylaxis after cerebrovascular ischaemic events. *Lancet* 338:1345–1349, 1991.

42. Biller J, Love BB, Gordon DL: Antithrombotic therapy for ischemic cerebrovascular disease. *Semin Neurol* 11:353–367, 1991.

43. Sivenius J, Laakso M, Riekkinen Sr P, et al: European stroke prevention study: effectiveness of antiplatelet therapy in diabetic patients in secondary prevention of stroke. *Stroke* 23:851–854, 1992.

44. Hass WK, Easton JD, Adams Jr HP, et al: A randomized trial comparing ticlopidine hydrochloride with aspirin for the prevention of stroke in high-risk patients. *N Engl J Med* 321:501–507, 1989.

45. Grotta JC, Norris JW, Kamm B, TASS Baseline and Angiographic Data Subgroup: Prevention of stroke with ticlopidine: who benefits most? *Neurology* 42:111–115, 1992.

46. Albers GW: Role of ticlopidine for prevention of stroke. *Stroke* 23:912–916, 1992.

46a. Weisberg LA, for the Ticlopidine Aspirin Stroke Study Group: The efficacy and safety of ticlopidine and aspirin in nonwhites: analysis of a patient subgroup from the Ticlopidine Aspirin Stroke Study. *Neurology* 43:27–31, 1993.

47. Uchiyama S, Sone R, Nagayama T, et al: Combination therapy with low-dose aspirin and ticlopidine in cerebral ischemia. *Stroke* 20:1643–1647, 1989.

48. Sivenius J, Riekkinen Sr PJ, Smets P, Laakso M, Lowenthal A: The European Stroke Prevention Study (ESPS): results by arterial distribution. *Ann Neurol* 29:596–600, 1991.

49. Estol CJ, Pessin MS: Anticoagulation: is there still a role in atherothrombotic stroke? *Stroke* 21:820–824, 1990.

49a. Higashida RT, Tsai FY, Halbach VV, Dowd CF, Smith T, Fraser K, Hieshima GB: Transluminal angioplasty for atherosclerotic disease of the vertebral and basilar arteries. *J Neurosurg* 78:192–198, 1993.

50. Biller J, Bruno A, Adams Jr HP, et al: A randomized trial of aspirin or heparin in hospitalized patients with recent transient ischemic attacks. A pilot study. *Stroke* 20:441–447, 1989.

51. Miller VT, Hart RG: Heparin anticoagulation in acute brain ischemia. *Stroke* 19:403–406, 1988.

52. Petty GW, Tatemichi TK, Sacco RL, Owen J, Mohr JP: Fatal or severely disabling cerebral infarction during hospitalization for stroke or transient ischemic attack. *J Neurol* 237;306–309, 1990.

53. Slivka A, Levy DE, Lapinski RH: Risk associated with heparin withdrawal in ischaemic cerebrovascular disease. *J Neurol* Neurosurg Psychiatry 52:1332–1336, 1989.

54. Biller J, Love BB, Marsh III EE, et al: Spontaneous improvement after acute ischemic stroke. A pilot study. *Stroke* 21:1008–1012, 1990.

55. Yatsu FM, Zivin J: Hypertension in acute ischemic strokes. Not to treat. *Arch Neurol* 42:999–1000, 1985.

55a. Powers WJ: Acute hypertension after stroke: the scientific basis for treatment decisions. *Neurology* 43:461–467, 1993.

56. Carlberg B, Asplund K, Hagg E: Factors influencing admission blood pressure levels in patients with acute stroke. *Stroke* 22:527–530, 1991.

57. Hachinski V: Hypertension in acute ischemic strokes. *Arch Neurol* 42:1002, 1985.

58. Lavin P: Management of hypertension in patients with acute stroke. *Arch Intern Med* 146:66–68, 1986.

59. Spence JD, Del Maestro RF: Hypertension in acute ischemic strokes. Treat. *Arch Neurol* 42:1000–1002, 1985.

60. Fletcher AE, Bulpitt CJ: How far should blood pressure be lowered? *N Engl J Med* 326:251–254, 1992.

61. Helgason CM: Blood glucose and stroke. *Stroke* 19:1049–1053, 1988.

62. Kushner M, Nencini P, Reivich M, et al: Relation of hyperglycemia early in ischemic brain infarction to cerebral anatomy, metabolism, and clinical outcome. *Ann Neurol* 28:129–135, 1990.

62a. Matcher DB, Divine GW, Heyman A, Feussner JR: The influence of hyperglycemia on outcome of cerebral infarction. *Ann Intern Med* 117:449–456, 1992.

63. Yip PK, He YY, Hsu CY, Garg N, Marangos P, Hogan EL: Effect of plasma glucose on infarct size in focal cerebral ischemia-reperfusion. *Neurology* 41:889–905, 1991.

64. O'Neill PA, Davies I, Fullerton KJ, Bennett D: Stress hormone and blood glucose response following acute stroke in the elderly. *Stroke* 22:842–847, 1991.

65. Sieber FE, Traystman J: Special issues: glucose and the brain. *Crit Care Med* 20:104–114, 1992.

66. Bousser MG, Eschwege E, Haguenau M, et al: "AICLA" controlled trial of aspirin and dipyridamole in the secondary prevention of athero-thrombotic cerebral ischemia. *Stroke* 14:5–14, 1983.

67. A Swedish Cooperative Study: High-dose acetylsalicylic acid after cerebral infarction. *Stroke* 18:325–334, 1987.

67a. Sandercock PAG, van den Belt AGM, Lindley RI, Slattery J: Antithrombotic therapy in acute ischaemic stroke: an overview of the completed randomized trials. *J Neurol Neurosurg Psychiatry* 56:17–25, 1993.

68. Gent M, Easton JD, Hachinski VC, et al: The Canadian American ticlopidine study (CATS) in thromboembolic stroke. *Lancet* i:1215–1220, 1989.

68a. Harbison JW, for the Ticlopidine Aspirin Stroke Study Group: Ticlopidine versus aspirin for the prevention of recurrent stroke. Analysis of patients with minor stroke from the Ticlopidine Aspirin Stroke Study. *Stroke* 23:1723–1727, 1992.

69. Jonas S: Anticoagulant therapy in cerebrovascular disease: review and meta-analysis. *Stroke* 19:1043–1048, 1988.

70. Phillips SJ: An alternative view of heparin anticoagulation in acute focal brain ischemia. *Stroke* 20:295–298, 1989.

71. Goslinga H, Eijzenbach V, Heuvelmans JHA, et al: Custom-tailored hemodilution with albumin and crystalloids in acute ischemic stroke. *Stroke* 23:181–188, 1992.

72. Strand T: Evaluation of long-term outcome and safety after hemodilution therapy in acute ischemic stroke. *Stroke* 1992:23:657–662, 1992.

73. Slivka A, Levy D: Natural history of progressive ischemic stroke in a population treated with heparin. *Stroke* 21:1657–1662, 1990.

74. Becker PS, Miller VT: Heparin-induced thrombocytopenia. *Stroke* 20:1449–1459, 1989.

75. Heros RC, Korosue K: Hemodilution for cerebral ischemia. *Stroke* 20:423–427, 1989.

76. Koller M, Haenny P, Hess K, Weniger D, Zangger P: Adjusted hypervolemic hemodilution in acute ischemic stroke. *Stroke* 21:1429–1434, 1990.

77. Ropper A, Shafran B: Brain edema after stroke. Clinical syndrome and intracranial pressure. *Arch Neurol* 41:26–29, 1984.

78. Delashaw JB, Broaddus WC, Kassell NF, et al: Treatment of right hemispheric cerebral infarction by hemicraniectomy. *Stroke* 21:874–881, 1990.

79. Chen H-J, Lee T-C, Wei C-P: Treatment of cerebellar infarction by decompressive suboccipital craniectomy. *Stroke* 23:957–961, 1992.

80. Heros RC: Surgical treatment of cerebellar infarction. *Stroke* 23:937–938, 1992.

81. Heros RC: Carotid endarterectomy in patients with intraluminal thrombus. *Stroke* 19:667–668, 1988.

82. Bogousslavsky J, Despland PA, Regli F: Spontaneous carotid dissection with acute stroke. *Arch Neurol* 44:137–140, 1987.

83. Hart RG: Vertebral artery dissection. *Neurology* 38:987–989, 1988.

83a. McCormick GF, Halbach VV: Recurrent ischemic events in two patients with painless vertebral artery dissection. *Stroke* 24:598–602, 1993.

84. Millikan C, Futrell N: The fallacy of the lacune hypothesis. *Stroke* 21:1251–1257, 1990.

85. Horowitz DR, Tuhrim S, Weinberger JM, et al: Mechanisms in lacunar infarction. *Stroke* 23:325–327, 1992.

86. Chimowitz MI, Furlan AJ, Sila CA, Paranandi L, Beck GJ: Etiology of motor or sensory stroke: a prospective study of the predictive value of clinical and radiological features. *Ann Neurol* 30:519–525, 1991.

87. Hart RG, Kanter MC: Hematologic disorders and ischemic stroke. A selective review. *Stroke* 21:1111–1121, 1990.

87a. Mayer SA, Sacco RL, Hurlet-Jensen A, Shi T, Mohr JP: Free protein S deficiency in acute ischemic stroke. A case-control study. *Stroke* 24:224–227, 1993.

88. Stern BJ, Kittner S, Sloan M, et al: Stroke in the young (parts I and II). *MMJ* 40:453–462, 565–571, 1991.

89. Antiphospholipid Antibody and Stroke Study (APASS) Group: Anticardiolipin antibodies are an independent risk factor for first ischemic stroke. *Neurology* 43:2069–2073, 1993.

90. Hanley DF, Feldman E, Borel CO, Rosenbaum AE, Goldberg AL: Treatment of sagittal sinus thrombosis associated with cerebral hemorrhage and intracranial hypertension. *Stroke* 19:903–909, 1988.

91. Einhaupl KM, Villringer A, Meister W, et al: Heparin treatment in sinus venous thrombosis. *Lancet* 338:597–600, 1991.

92. Di Rocco C, Iannelli A, Leone G, Moschini M, Valori VM: Heparin-urokinase treatment in aseptic dural sinus thrombosis. *Arch Neurol* 38:431–435, 1981.

93. Satran R: Spinal cord infarction. *Stroke* 19:529–532, 1988.

94. Sandson TA, Freidman JH: Spinal cord infarction. Report of 8 cases and review of the literature. *Medicine* 68:282–291, 1989.

94a. Siesjö BK: Pathophysiology and treatment of focal cerebral ischemia. Part I: Pathophysiology. Part II: Mechanisms of damage and treatment. *J Neurosurg* 77:169–184, 337–354, 1992.

95. Massey EW, Biller J, Davis JN, et al: Large-dose infusions of heparinoid ORG 10172 in ischemic stroke. *Stroke* 21:1289–1292, 1990.

96. del Zoppo GJ, Pessin MS, Mori E, Hacke W: Thrombolytic intervention in acute thrombotic and embolic stroke. *Semin Neurol* 11:368–384, 1991.

97. Mori E, Tabuchi M, Yoshida T, Yamadori A: Intracarotid urokinase with thromboembolic occlusion of the middle cerebral artery. *Stroke* 19:802–812, 1988.

98. del Zoppo GJ, Ferbert A, Otis S, et al: Local intra-arterial fibrinolytic therapy in acute carotid territory stroke. A pilot study. *Stroke* 19:307–313, 1988.

99. Mori E, Yoneda Y, Tabuchi M, et al: Intravenous recombinant tissue plasminogen activator in acute carotid artery territory stroke. *Neurology* 42:976–982, 1992.

100. Hacke W, Zeumer H, Ferbert A, Bruckmann H, del Zoppo GJ: Intra-arterial thrombolytic therapy improves outcome in patients with acute vertebrobasilar occlusive disease. *Stroke* 19:1216–1222, 1988.

100a. del Zoppo GJ, Poeck K, Pessin MS, et al: Recombinant tissue plasminogen activator in acute thrombotic and embolic stroke. *Ann Neurol* 32:78–86, 1992.

101. Haley Jr EC, Levy DE, Brott TG, et al: Urgent therapy for stroke. Part II. Pilot study of tissue plasminogen activator administered 91–180 minutes from onset. *Stroke* 23:641–645, 1992.

102. Brott TG, Haley Jr EC, Levy DE, et al: Urgent therapy for stroke. Part I. Pilot study of tissue plasminogen activator administered within 90 minutes. *Stroke* 23:632–640, 1992.

103. von Kummer R, Hacke W: Safety and efficacy of intravenous tissue plasminogen activator and heparin in acute middle cerebral artery stroke. *Stroke* 23:646–652, 1992.

103a. Haley EC, Brott TG, Sheppard GL, Barsan W, Broderick J, Marler JR, Kongable GL, Spilker J, Massey S, Hansen CA, Torner JC; for the TPA Bridging Study Group: Pilot randomized trial of tissue plasminogen activator in acute ischemic stroke. *Stroke* 24:1000–1004, 1993.

104. Wong MCW, Haley Jr EC: Calcium antagonists: stroke therapy coming of age. *Stroke* 21:494–501, 1990.

105. Gelmers H, Hennerici M: Effect of nimodipine on acute ischemic stroke. Pooled results from five randomized trials. *Stroke* 21(suppl IV):IV-81–IV-84, 1990.

106. The American Nimodipine Study Group: Clinical trial of nimodipine in acute ischemic stroke. *Stroke* 23:3–8, 1992.

107. Rosenbaum D, Zabramski J, Frey J, et al: Early treatment of ischemic stroke with a calcium antagonist. *Stroke* 22:437–441, 1991.

108. Rothman SM, Olney JW: Glutamate and pathophysiology of hypoxic-ischemic brain damage. *Ann Neurol* 19:105–111, 1986.

109. Albers GW, Goldberg MP, Choi DW: *N*-methyl-*D*-aspartate antagonists: ready for clinical trial in brain ischemia? *Ann Neurol* 25:398–403, 1989.

110. Albers GW, Goldberg MP, Choi DW: Do NMDA antagonists prevent neuronal injury? Yes. *Arch Neurol* 49:418–420, 1992.

111. Buchan AM: Do NMDA antagonists prevent neuronal injury? No. *Arch Neurol* 49:420–421, 1992.

112. Schmidley JW: Free radicals in central nervous system ischemia. *Stroke* 21:1086–1090, 1990.

113. Matsumiya N, Koehler RC, Kirsch JR, Traystman RJ: Conjugated superoxide dismutase reduces extent of caudate injury after transient focal ischemia in cats. *Stroke* 22:1193–1200, 1991.

114. Chan PH, Yang GY, Chen SF, Carlson E, Epstein CJ: Cold-induced brain edema and infarction are reduced in transgenic mice overexpressing CuZn-superoxide dismutase. *Ann Neurol* 29:482–486, 1991.

115. Imaizumi S, Woolworth V, Fishman RA, Chan PH: Liposome-entrapped superoxide dismutase reduces cerebral infarction in cerebral ischemia in rats. *Stroke* 21:1312–1317, 1990.

116. Scheinberg P: The biologic basis for the treatment of acute stroke. *Neurology* 41:1867–1873, 1991.

116a. Hsu CY: Criteria for valid preclinical trials using animal stroke models. *Stroke* 6:633–636, 1993.

116b. Hallenbeck JM, Frerichs KU: Stroke therapy. It may be time for an integrated approach. *Arch Neurol* 50:768–770, 1993.

117. Mohr JP, Caplan LR, Melski JW, et al: The Harvard Cooperative *Stroke* Registry: a prosective registry. *Neurology* 28:754–762, 1978.

118. Broderick JP, Brott T, Tomsick T, Barsan W, Spilker L: Ultra-early evaluation of intracerebral hemorrhage. *J Neurosurg* 72:195–199, 1990.

119. Tuhrim S, Dambrosia JM, Price TR, et al: Prediction of intracerebral hemorrhage survival. *Ann Neurol* 24:258–263, 1988.

120. Caplan LR: Intracerebral hemorrhage revisited. *Neurology* 38:624–627, 1988.

121. Feldmann E: Intracerebral hemorrhage. *Stroke* 22:684–691, 1991.

122. Kalyan-Raman UP, Kalyan-Raman K: Cerebral amyloid angiopathy causing intracranial hemorrhage. *Ann Neurol* 16:321–329, 1984.

123. Vinters HV: Cerebral amyloid angiopathy: a critical review. *Stroke* 18:311–324, 1987.

124. Kase CS: Intracerebral hemorrhage: non-hypertensive causes. *Stroke* 17:590–594, 1986.

125. Kase CS, O'Neal AM, Fisher M, Girgis GN, Ordia JI: Intracranial hemorrhage after use of tissue plasminogen activator for coronary thrombolysis. *Ann Intern Med* 112:17–21, 1990.

126. Sloan MA, Price TR, Randall AM, Solomon RE, Terrin ML, TIMI Investigators: Intracerebral hemorrhage after rTPa and heparin for acute myocardial infarction: the TIMI II pilot and randomized trial experience [Abstract]. *Stroke* 21:182, 1990.

127. Sloan MA, Kittner SJ, Rigamonti D, Price TR: Occurrence of stroke associated with use/abuse of drugs. *Neurology* 41:1358–1364, 1991.

128. Levine SR, Welch KMA: Cocaine and stroke. *Stroke* 19:779–783, 1989.

129. Peterson PL, Moore PM: Hemorrhagic cerebrovascular complications of crack cocaine abuse [Abstract]. *Neurology* 39(suppl I):302, 1989.

130. Green RM, Kelly KM, Gabrielsen T, Levine SR, Vanderzant C: Multiple intracerebral hemorrhages after smoking "crack" cocaine. *Stroke* 21:957–962, 1990.

131. Kase CS, Foster TE, Reed JE, Spatz EL, Girgis GN: Intracerebral hemorrhage and phenylpropanolamine use. *Neurology* 37:399–404, 1987.

132. Faught E, Peters D, Bartolucci A, Moore L, Miller PC: Seizures after primary intracerebral hemorrhage. *Neurology* 39:1089–1093, 1989.

133. Ropper AH, Davis KR: Lobar cerebral hemorrhages: acute clinical syndrome in 26 cases. *Ann Neurol* 82:141–147, 1980.

134. Borges LF: Management of non-traumatic brain hemorrhage. In Ropper AH, Kennedy SF (eds): *Neurological and Neurosurgical Intensive Care*, ed 2. Aspen Publications, Rockville, MD, 1988, pp 209–211.

135. Fragen RJ, Avram MJ: Barbiturates. In Miller RD (ed): *Anesthesia*, ed. 3. Churchill Livingstone, New York, 1990, pp 225–242.

136. Halldin M, Wahlin A: Effect of succinylcholine on intraspinal fluid pressure. *Acta Anaesth Scand* 3:155–161, 1959.

137. Frost EAM: Anesthesia for trauma: head trauma. In Rogers MC (ed): *Current Practice in Anesthesiology*. BC Decker, St. Louis, 1990, pp 372–378.

138. Eleff SM, Borel C, Bell WR, Long DM: Acute management of intracranial hemorrhage in patients receiving thrombolytic therapy: case reports. *Neurosurgery* 26:867–869, 1990.

139. Andrew M: Vitamin K-dependent coagulation factor deficiency. In Kassirer JP (ed): *Current Therapy in Internal Medicine*, ed 3. Philadelphia, BC Decker, Philadelphia, 1991, pp 877–880.

139a. Fredriksson K, Norrving B, Stromblad L-G: Emergency reversal of anticoagulation after intracerebral hemorrhage. *Stroke* 23:972–977, 1992.

140. Drury I, Whisnant JP, Garraway M: Primary intracerebral hemorrhage: impact of CT on incidence. *Mayo Clin Proc* 34:653–657, 1984.

141. Scott WR, New PFH, Davis KR, et al: Computerized axial tomography of intracerebral and intraventricular hemorrhage. *Radiology* 112:73–79, 1974.

142. Kasdon DL, Scott RM, Adelman LS, et al: Cerebellar hemorrhage with decreased absorption values on computed tomography. A case report. *Neuroradiology* 131:265–267, 1977.

143. Zyed A, Hayman LA, Bryan RN: MR imaging of intracerebral blood: diversity in the temporal pattern at 0.5 and 1.0 T. *AJNR* 12:469–474, 1991.

144. Barnett GH, Ropper AH, Johnson K: Physiologic support and monitoring of critical patients during MR imaging. *J Neurosurg* 68:246–250, 1988.

145. Toffol GJ, Biller J, Adams HP, Somker WRK: The predicted value of arteriography in non-traumatic intracerebral hemorrhage. *Stroke* 17:881–886, 1986.

146. Statham PF, Todd NV: Intracerebral haematoma: aetiology and haematoma volume determine the amount and progression of brain oedema. *Acta Neurochir Suppl* 51:289–291, 1990.

147. Mchedlishvili G: Pathogenetic role of circulatory factors in brain edema development. *Neurosurg Rev* 11:7–13, 1988.

148. Durward QJ, Del Maestro RF, Amacher AL, et al: The influence of systemic arterial pressure and intracranial pressure on the development of cerebral vasogenic edema. *J Neurosurg* 59:803–809, 1983.

149. Marshall LF, Smith RW, Shapiro HM: The outcome with aggressive treatment in severe head injuries. Part I: the significance of intracranial pressure monitoring. *J Neurosurg* 50:20–25, 1979.

150. Bower SA, Marshall LF: Outcome in 200 consecutive cases of severe head injury treated in San Diego county: a prospective analysis. *Neurosurgery* 6:237–242, 1980.

151. Unwin DH, Giller CA, Kopitnik TA: Central nervous system monitoring. What helps, what does not. *Surg Clin North Am* 71:733–747, 1991.

152. Strandgaard S: Autoregulation of cerebral blood flow in hypertensive patients. *Circulation* 53:720–727, 1976.

153. Rogers MC, Traystman RJ: Cerebral hemodynamic effects of nitroglycerin and nitroprusside. *Acta Neurol Scand* 60(suppl 72):600, 1980.

154. Orlowski JP, Shiesley D, Vidt DG, Barnett GH, Little JR: Labetalol to control blood pressure after cerebrovascular surgery. *Crit Care Med* 16:765–768, 1988.

155. Mayhall CG, Archer NH, Lamb VA, et al: Ventriculostomy-related infections, a prospective study. *N Engl J Med* 310:553–559, 1984.

156. Rosner MJ, Becker DP: ICP monitoring: complications and associated factors. *Clin Neurosurg* 23:494–519, 1976.

157. Braus DF, Strobel J, Myers A, Mohadjer M: Stereotactic evacuation and early rehabilitation in space-occupying cerebral hemorrhage. *Wien Med Wochenschr* 141:136, 136–138, 140, 1991.

158. Muizelaar JP, Marmarou A, Ward JD, et al: Adverse effects of prolonged hyperventilation in patients with severe head injury: a randomized clinical trial. *J Neurosurg* 75:731–739, 1991.

159. Ito Z, Nakajima K: Surgical treatment of acute cerebellar hemorrhage. In Mizukami M (ed): *Hypertensive Intracerebral Hemorrhage*. Raven Press, New York, 1983, pp 215–223.

160. Poungvarin N, Bhoopat W, Viriyavejakul A, et al: Effects of dexamethasone in primary supratentorial intracerebral hemorrhage. *N Engl J Med* 316:1229–1233, 1987.

161. Shackford SR: Fluid resuscitation in head injury. *J Intensive Care Med* 5:59–68, 1990.

162. Cottrell JE, Robustelli A, Post K, et al: Furosemide- and mannitol-induced changes in intracranial pressure and serum osmolality and electrolytes. *Anesthesia* 47:28–30, 1977.

163. Clasen RA, Pandolfi S, Casey D: Furosemide and pentobarbital in cryogenic cerebral injury and edema. *Neurology* 24:642–648, 1974.

164. Mendelow AD, Teasdale GM, Russel T, et al: Effect of mannitol on cerebral blood flow and cerebral perfusion pressure in human head injury. *J Neurosurg* 63:43–48, 1985.

165. Marshall LF, Smith RW, Rauscher A, et al: Mannitol dose requirements in brain-injured patients. *J Neurosurg* 48:169–172, 1978.

166. Go KG: The fluid environment of the central nervous system. In Go KG (ed): *Cerebral Pathophysiology*. Elsevier, New York, 1991, pp 66–171.

167. Muizelaar JP, Wei EP, Kontos HA, et al: Mannitol causes compensatory cerebral vasoconstriction and vasodilation in response to blood viscosity changes. *J Neurosurg* 59:822–828, 1983.

168. McDowell ME, Wolf AV, Steer A: Osmotic volumes of distribution. Idiogenic changes in osmotic pressure associated with administration of hypertonic solutions. *Am J Physiol* 180:545–558, 1955.

169. McIntosh TK, Vink R, Yamakami I, Faden AI: Magnesium protects against neurological deficit after brain injury. *Brain Res* 482:252–260, 1989.

170. Ito H, Muka H, Kitamura A: Stereotactic aqua stream and aspirator for removal of intracerebral hematoma. *Stereotact Funct Neurosurg* 54–55:457–460, 1990.

171. Liu ZH, Kang GQ, Chen XH, et al: Evacuation of hypertensive intracerebral hematoma by a stereotactic technique. *Stereotact Funct Neurosurg* 54–55:451–452, 1990.

172. Ito H, Mukai H, Kitamura A, Yamashita J: Stereotactic aqua stream and aspirator for hypertensive intracerebral hematoma. *Stereotact Funct Neurosurg* 53:77–84, 1989.

173. Kaufman HH, Herschberger JE, Maroon JC, Wilberger JE, Onik GM: Mechanical aspiration of hematomas in an in vitro model. *Neurosurgery* 25:347–349, 1989.

174. Niizuma H, Shimizu Y, Yonemitsu T, Nakasato N, Suzuki J: Results of stereotactic aspiration in 175 cases of putaminal hemorrhage. *Neurosurgery* 24:814–819, 1989.

175. Kase CS, Mohr JP: General features of intracerebral hemorrhage. In Barnett HJM, Mohr JP, Stein BM, Yatsu FM (eds): *Stroke: Pathophysiology, Diagnosis, and Management*. Churchill Livingstone, New York, 1968, pp 497–523.

176. Steiner L, Gomori JM, Melamed E: The prognostic value of the CT scan in conservatively treated patients with intracerebral hematoma. *Stroke* 15:279–282, 1984.

177. Sano K, Ochiai C: Brainstem hematomas: clinical aspects with reference to indications for treatment. In Pia HW, Lanjmaid C, Zierski J (eds): *Spontaneous Intracerebral Hematomas*. Springer-Verlag, New York, 1980, pp 366–371.

178. Young WB, Lee KP, Pessin MS, Kwan ES, Rand WM, Caplan LR: Prognostic significance of ventricular blood in supratentorial hemorrhage: a volumetric study. *Stroke* 40:616–619, 1990.

179. Weir B: Intracranial aneurysms and subarachnoid hemorrhage: an overview. In Wilkins RW, Rengachary SS (eds): *Neurosurgery*. New York, McGraw-Hill, 1985, pp 1308–1329.

180. Mohr JP, Kistler JP, Zabromski JM, et al: Intracranial aneurysms. In Barnett HJM, Mohr JP (eds): *Stroke: Pathophysiology, Diagnosis and Management*. Churchill Livingstone, London, 1985, pp 643–677.

181. Weir B: *Aneurysms Affecting the Nervous System*. Baltimore, Williams & Wilkins, Baltimore, 1987.

182. Chason JM, Hindman WM: Berry aneurysms of the circle of Willis. *Neurology* 8:41–44, 1958.

183. Housepian EM, Pool JL: A systemic analysis of intracranial aneurysms from the autopsy file of the Presbyterian Hospital, 1914 to 1956. *J Neuropathol Exp Neurol* 17:409–423, 1958.

184. Kassell NF, Sasaki T, Colohan ART, Nazar G: Cerebral vasospasm following aneurysmal subarachnoid hemorrhage. *Stroke* 16:562–572, 1985.

185. Phillips LH, Whisnant JP, O'Fallon WM, et al: The unchanging pattern of subarachnoid hemorrhage in a community. *Neurology* 30:1034–1046, 1980.

186. Wilkins RH: Subarchnoid hemorrhage and saccular intracranial aneurysm. An update. *Surg Neurol* 15:92–101, 1981.

187. Ojemann RG: Management of the unruptured intracranial aneurysm. *N Engl J Med* 304:725–726, 1981.

188. Wiebers DO, Whisnant JP, O'Fallon WM: The natural history of unruptured intracranial aneurysms. *N Engl J Med* 304:696–698, 1981.

189. Dell S: Asymptomatic cerebral aneurysm: assessment of its risk of rupture. *Neurosurgery* 36:34–42, 1982.

190. Tomonaga M, Fukushima T, Tanaka A, et al: Clinical and pathological study of rebleeding of intracranial aneurysm-based on 7 cases expired by rebleeding during hospital stay. *Med J Aust* 1:514–516, 1983.

191. Winn HR, Almaani WS, Berger SL, et al: The longterm outcome in patients with multiple untreated cerebral aneurysms: incidence of late hemorrhage and implications for treatment of incidental aneurysms. *J Neurosurg* 59:642–651, 1983.

191a. Guglielmi G, Vinuela F, Dion J, et al: Electrothrombosis of saccular aneurysms via endovascular approach. Part 2. Preliminary clinical experience. *J Neurosurg* 75:8–14, 1991.

192. Soni RC: Aneurysm of the posterior communicating artery and oculomotor paresis. *J Neurol Neurosurg Psychiatry* 37:475–484, 1974.

193. King RB, Saba MI: Forewarning of major subarachnoid hemorrhage due to congential berry aneurysm. *NY State J Med* 74:638–639, 1974.

194. Waga S, Ohtsubo K, Handa H: Warning signs in intracranial aneurysms. *Can Med Assoc J* 112:78–79, 1975.

195. Chan BS, Dorsch NW: Delayed diagnosis in subarachnoid haemorrhage. *Med J Aust* 154:509–511, 1991.

196. Nornes H, Magnaes B: Intracranial pressure in patients with ruptured saccular aneurysm. *J Neurosurg* 36:536–547, 1972.

197. Fisher CM: Clincial syndromes in cerebral thrombosis, hypertensive hemorrhage and ruptured saccular aneurysm. *Clin Neurosurg* 22:117–147, 1975.

198. Hunt WE, Hess RM: Surgical risk as related to time of intervention in the repair of intracranial aneurysms. *J Neurosurg* 28:14–20, 1968.

199. Adams HP, Kassell NF, Torner JC, et al: CT and clincial correlations in recent aneurysmal subarachnoid hemorrhage: preliminary report of cooperative aneurysm study. *Neurology* 33:981–985, 1983.

200. Fisher CM, Kistler JP, Davis JM: Relation of cerebral vasospasm to subarachnoid hemorrhage visualized by computerized tomographic scanning. *Neurosurgery* 6:1–9, 1980.

201. Fujita S: Computed tomographic grading with Hounsfield number related to delayed vasospasm in cases of ruptured cerebral aneurysm. *Neurosurgery* 17:609–612, 1985.

202. Gurusinghe NT, Richardson AE: The value of computerized tomography in aneurysmal subarachnoid hemorrhage. *J Neurosurg* 60:763–770, 1984.

203. Kistler JP, Crowell RM, Davis KR, et al: The relationship of cerebral vasospasm to the extent and location of subarachnoid blood visualized by CT scan: a prospective study. *Neurology* 33:424–436, 1983.

204. Mizukami M, Takemae T, Tazawa T, et al: Value of computed tomography in the prediction of cerebral vasospasm after aneurysm rupture. *Neurosurgery* 7:583–586, 1980.

205. Pasqualin A, Rosta L, DaPian R, et al: Role of computed tomography in the management of vasospasm after subarachnoid hemorrhage. *Neurosurgery* 15:344–353, 1984.

206. Nornes H: The role of intracranial-pressure in the arrest of hemorrhage in patients with ruptured intracranial aneurysm. *J Neurosurg* 39:226–234, 1973.

207. Haley EC, Kassell NF, Torner JC, Participants: The international cooperative study on the timing of aneurysm surgery. The North American experience. *Stroke* 23:205–214, 1992.

208. Heros RC: Preoperative management of the patient with a ruptured intracranial aneurysm. *Semin Neurol* 4(4):430–438, 1984.

209. Bigelow NH: Multiple intracranial arterial aneurysms: an analysis of their significance. *Arch Neurol Psychiatry* 73:76–99, 1955.

210. Benedict CR, Loach AB: Sympathetic nervous system activity in patients with subarachnoid hemorrhage. *Stroke* 9:237–244, 1978.

211. Cruickshank J, Neil-Dwyer G, Stott AW: Possible role of catecholamines, corticosteroids, and potassium in production of electrocardiographic abnormalities associated with subarachnoid hemorrhage. *Br Heart J* 36:697–706, 1974.

212. Reichenbach DD, Benditt EP: Catecholamines and cardiomyopathy: the pathogenesis and potential importance of myofibrillar degeneration. *Hum Pathol* 1:125–150, 1970.

213. Estanol BV, Dergal EB, Cesarman E, San Martin OM, Loyo M, Ortego RP: Cardiac arrhythmias associated with subarachnoid hemorrhage: prospective study. *Neurosurgery* 5:675–680, 1969.

214. Hayward RD: Subarachnoid hemorrhage of unknown etiology. A clinical and radiologic study of 51 cases. *J Neurol Neurosurg Psychiatry* 40:926–931, 1977.

215. Alexander MSM, Dias PS, Uttley D: Spontaneous subarachnoid hemorrhage and negative cerebral panangiography. Review of 140 cases. *J Neurosurg* 64:537–542, 1986.

216. Shepard RH: Prognosis of spontaneous nontraumatic subarachnoid hemorrhage of unknown cause. A personal series 1958–1980. *Lancet* i:777–779, 1984.

217. van Gijn J, van Dongen KJ, Vermeulen M, et al: Perimesencephalic hemorrhage: a nonaneurysmal and benign form of subarachnoid hemorrhage. *Neurology* 35:493–497, 1985.

218. Rinkel GE, Wijdicks EMF, Vermeulen M, et al: The clincial course of perimesencephalic nonaneurysmal subarachnoid hemorrhage. *Ann Neurol* 29:463–468, 1991.

219. Hochberg FH, Fisher CM, Robertson GH: Subarachnoid hemorrhage caused by rupture of a small superficial artery. *Neurology* 24:319–321, 1974.

220. Herdt Jr D, Chiro G, Doppman JL: Combined arterial and arteriovenous aneurysms of the spinal cord. *Radiology* 99:589–593, 1971.

221. Wijdicks EMF, Vermeulen M, ten Haaf JA, et al: Volume depletion and natriuresis in patients with a ruptured intracranial aneurysm. *Ann Neurol* 18:211–216, 1985.

222. Solomon RA, Post KD, McMurtry III JG: Depression of circulating blood volume in patients after subarachnoid hemorrhage: implications for the management of symptomatic vasospasm. *Neurosurgery* 15:354–361, 1984.

223. Kassell NF, Torner JC: Aneurysm rebleeding: a preliminary report from the cooperative aneurysm study. *Neurosurgery* 13:479–481, 1983.

224. Winn HR, Almaani WS, Berger SL, et al: The longterm outcome in patients with multiple untreated cerebral aneurysms: incidence of late hemorrhage and implications for treatment of incidental aneurysms. *J Neurosurg* 59:642–651, 1983.

225. Sundt TM, Whisnant JP: Subarachnoid hemorrhage from intracranial aneurysms. *N Engl J Med* 299:116–122, 1978.

226. Adams HP: Antifibrinolytic therapy for prevention of recurrent aneurysmal subarachnoid hemorrhage. *Semin Neurol* 3:309–315, 1986.

227. Kassell NF, Torner JC, Adams Jr HP: Antifibrinolytic therapy in the acute period following aneurysmal subarachnoid hemorrhage. *J Neurosurg* 61:224–230, 1984.

228. Wijdicks EFM, Hasan D, Lindsay KW, et al: Short-term tranexamic acid treatment in aneurysmal subarachnoid hemorrhage. *Stroke* 20:1674–1679, 1989.

229. Disney L, Weir B, Petruk K: Effect on management mortality of a deliberate policy of early operation on supratentorial aneurysms. *Neurosurgery* 5:695–701, 1987.

230. Solomon RA, Fink ME, Lennihan L: Early aneurysm surgery and prophylactic hypervolemic hypertensive therapy for the treatment of aneurysmal subarachnoid hemorrhage. *Neurosurgery* 23:699–704, 1988.

231. Seiler RW, Reulen HJ, Huber P, et al: Outcome of aneurysmal subarachnoid hemorrhage in a hospital population: a prospective study including early operation, intravenous nimodipine, and transcranial Doppler ultrasound. *Neurosurgery* 23:598–604, 1988.

232. Solomon RA, Onesti ST, Klebanoff L: Relationship between the timing of aneurysm surgery and the development of delayed cerebral ischemia. *J Neurosurg* 75:56–61, 1991.

233. van Gijn J, Hijdra A, Wijdicks EFM, et al: Acute hydrocephalus after aneurysmal subarachnoid hemorrhage. *J Neurosurg* 63:355–362, 1985.

234. Pare L, Delfino R, Leblanc R: The relationship of ventricular drainage to aneurysmal rebleeding. *J Neurosurg* 76:422–427, 1992.

235. Heros RC: Preoperative management of the patient with a ruptured intracranial aneurysm. *Semin Neurol* 4(4):430–438, 1984.

236. Hasan D, Lindsay KW, Vermeulen M: Treatment of acute hydrocephalus after subarachnoid hemorrhage with serial lumbar puncture. *Stroke* 22:190–194, 1991.

237. Fisher CM, Robertson GH, Ojemann RG: Cerebral vasospasm with ruptured saccular aneurysm: the clinical manifestations. *Neurosurgery* 1:245–248, 1977.

238. Weir B, Grace M, Hansen J, et al: Time course of vasospasm in man. *J Neurosurg* 48:173–178, 1978.

239. Nagasawa S, Handa H, Naruo Y, et al: Experimental cerebral vasospasm. Part 2. Contractility of spastic arterial wall. *Stroke* 14:579–584, 1983.

240. Vorkapic P, Bevan JA, Bevan RD: Two indices of functional damage of the artery wall parallel the time course of irreversible narrowing in experimental vasospasm in the rabbit. *Blood Vessels* 28:179–182, 1991.

241. Aaslid R, Huber P, Nornes H: A transcranial Doppler method in the evaluation of cerebrovascular spasm. *Neuroradiology* 28:11–16, 1986.

242. Seiler RW, Grolimund P, Aaslid R, et al: Cerebral vasospasm evaluated by transcranial ultrasound correlated with clinical grade and CT-visualized subarachnoid hemorrhage. *J Neurosurg* 64:594–600, 1986.

243. Lindegaard KF, Nornes H, Bakke SJ, et al: Cerebral vasospasm after subarachnoid haemorrhage investigated by means of transcranial Doppler ultrasound. *Acta Neurochir Suppl (Wien)* 42:81–84, 1988.

244. Sloan MA, Haley EC Jr, Kassell NF, et al: Sensitivity and specificity of transcranial Doppler ultrasonography in the diagnosis of vasospasm following subarachnoid hemorrhage. *Neurology* 39:1514–1518, 1989.

245. Mizukami M, Kawasi T, Usami T, et al: Prevention of vasospasm by early operation with removal of subarachnoid clot. *Neurosurgery* 10:301–307, 1982.

246. Tettenborn D, Porto L, Ryman T, et al: Survey of clinical experience with nimodipine in patients with subarachnoid hemorrhage. *Neurosurg Rev* 10:77–84, 1987.

247. Kostron H, Twerdy K, Grunert V: The calcium entry blocker nimodipine improves the quality of life of patients operated on for cerebral aneurysms. A 5-year follow-up analysis. *Neurochirurgia* 31:150–153, 1988.

248. Mee E, Dorrance D, Lowe D, et al: Controlled study of nimodipine in aneurysm patients treated early after subarachnoid hemorrhage. *Neurosurgery* 22:484–491, 1988.

249. Espinosa F, Weir B, Overton T, et al: A randomized placebo-controlled double-blind trial of nimodipine after SAH in monkeys. Part 1. Clinical and radiological findings. *J Neurosurg* 60:1167–1175, 1984.

250. Allen GS, Ahn HS, Preziiosi TJ, et al: Cerebral arterial spasm. A controlled trial of nimodipine in patients with subarachnoid hemorrhage. *N Engl J Med* 44:585–593, 1976.

251. Seifert V, Eisert WG, Stolke D, et al: Efficacy of single intracisternal bolus injection of recombinant tissue plasminogen activator to prevent delayed cerebral vasospasm after experimental subarachnoid hemorrhage. *Neurosurgery* 25:590–598, 1989.

252. Findlay JM, Weir BK, Kassell NF, et al: Intracisternal recombinant tissue plasminogen activator after aneurysmal subarachnoid hemorrhage. *J Neurosurg* 75:181–188, 1991.

253. Kassell NF, Peerless SJ, Durward QJ, et al: Treatment of ischemic deficits from vasospasm with intravascular volume expansion and induced arterial hypertension. *Neurosurgery* 11:337–343, 1982.

254. Montgomery EBJ, Grubb RLJ, Raichle ME: Cerebral hemodynamics and metabolism in postoperative cerebral vasospasm and treatment with hypertensive therapy. *Ann Neurol* 9:502–506, 1981.

255. Archer DP, Shaw DA, Leblanc RL, et al: Haemodynamic considerations in the management of patients with subarachnoid haemorrhage. *Can J Anaesth* 38:454–470, 1991.

256. Zubkov YN, Nikiforov BM, Shustin VA: Balloon catheter technique for dilatation of constricted cerebral arteries after aneurysmal SAH. *Acta Neurochir (Wien)* 70:65–79, 1984.

257. Konishi Y, Maemura E, Sato E, et al: A therapy against vasospasm after subarachnoidal haemorrhage: clinical experience of balloon angioplasty. *Neurol Res* 12:103–105, 1990.

258. Grimes CM: Cerebral balloon angioplasty for treatment of vasospasm after subarachnoid hemorrhage. *Heart Lung* 20:431–435, 1991.

259. Pistoia F, Horton JA, Sekhar L, et al: Imaging of blood flow changes following angioplasty for treatment of vasospasm. *Am J Neuroradiol* 12:446–448, 1991.

260. Linskey ME, Horton JA, Rao GR, et al: Fatal rupture of the intracranial carotid artery during transluminal angioplasty for vasospasm induced by subarachnoid hemorrhage. Case report. *J Neurosurg* 74:985–990, 1991.

261. Meyer CH, Lowe D, Meyer M, et al: Progressive change in cerebral blood flow during the first three weeks after subarachnoid hemorrhage. *Neurosurgery* 12:58–76, 1983.

262. Ritchie WL, Overton TR: Vasospasm and cerebral blood flow after subarachnoid hemorrhage. *J Can Assoc Radiol* 31:230–233, 1980.

263. Dernbach PD, Little JR, Jones SC, et al: Altered cerebral autoregulation and CO_2 reactivity after aneurysmal subarachnoid hemorrhage. *Neurosurgery* 22:822–826, 1988.

264. Seiler RW, Nirkko AC: Effect of nimodipine on cerebrovascular response to CO_2 in asymptomatic individuals and patients with subarachnoid hemorrhage: a transcranial Doppler ultrasound study. *Neurosurgery* 27:247–251, 1990.

265. Hassler W, Chioffi F: CO_2 reactivity of cerebral vasospasm after aneurysmal subarachnoid haemorrhage. *Acta Neurochir* 98:167–175, 1989.

266. Ishii R: Regional cerebral blood flow in patients with ruptured intracranial aneurysms. *J Neurosurg* 50:587–594, 1979.

267. Wijdicks EFM, Vermeulen M, van Gijn J: Hyponatraemia and volume status in aneurysmal subarachnoid haemorrhage. *Acta Neurochir Suppl* 47:111–113, 1990.

268. Diringer MN, Ladenson PW, Stern BJ, et al: Plasma atrial natriuretic factor and subarachnoid hemorrhage. *Stroke* 19:1119–1124, 1988.

269. Fox JL, Falik JL, Shalhoub RJ: Neurosurgical hyponatremia: the role of inappropriate antidiuresis. *J Neurosurg* 34:506–514, 1971.

270. Wise BL: Syndrome of inappropriate antidiuretic hormone secretion after spontaneous subarachnoid hemorrhage: a reversible cause of clinical deterioration. *Neurosurgery* 34:412–414, 1978.

271. Joynt RJ, Afifi A, Hardison J: Hyponatremia in subarachnoid hemorrhage. *Arch Neurol* 13:633–638, 1965.

272. Doczi T, Bende J, Huska E, et al: Syndrome of inappropriate secretion of antidiuretic hormone after subarachnoid hemorrhage. *Neurosurgery* 4:394–396, 1981.

273. Lester M, Nelson PB: Neurological aspects of vasopressin release and the syndrome of inappropriate release of antidiuretic hormone. *Neurosurgery* 8:735–740, 1981.

274. Nelson PB, Seif SM, Maroon JC, et al: Hyponatremia in intracranial disorders: perhaps not the syndrome of inappropriate secretion of antidiuretic hormone (SIADH). *J Neurosurg* 55:936–941, 1981.

275. Wijdicks EFM, Vermeulen M, Hijdra A, et al: Hyponatremia and cerebral infarction in patients with ruptured intracranial aneurysms: is fluid restriction harmful? *Ann Neurol* 17:137–140, 1985.

276. Diringer MN, Lim JS, Kirsch JR, et al: Suprasellar and intraventricular blood predict elevated plasma atrial natriuretic factor in subarachnoid hemorrhage. *Stroke* 22:577–581, 1991.

277. Diringer MN, Kirsch JR, Ladenson PW, et al: Cerebrospinal fluid atrial natriuretic factor in intracranial disease. *Stroke* 21:1550–1554, 1990.

278. Diringer MN, Wu KC, Verbalis JG, et al: Hypervolemic therapy prevents volume contraction but not hyponatremia following subarachnoid hemorrhage. *Ann Neurol* 31:543–550, 1992.

279. Plum F: Vulnerability of the brain and heart after cardiac arrest. *N Engl J Med* 324:1278–1280, 1991.

280. Brain Resuscitation Clinical Trial I Study Group: Randomized clinical study of thiopental loading in comatose survivors of cardiac arrest. *N Engl J Med* 314:397–403, 1986.

281. Brain Resuscitation Clinical Trial II Study Group: A randomized clinical study of a calcium-entry blocker (lidoflazine) in the treatment of comatose survivors of cardiac arrest. *N Engl J Med* 324:1225–1231, 1991.

282. Krumholz A, Stern BJ, Weiss HD: Outcome from coma after cardiopulmonary resuscitation: relation to seizures and myoclonus. *Neurology* 38:401–405, 1988.

283. Celesia GG, Grigg MM, Ross E: Generalized status myoclonicus in acute anoxic and toxic-metabolic encephalopathies. *Arch Neurol* 45:781–784, 1988.

284. Young GB, Gilbert JJ, Zochodne DW: The significance of myoclonic status epilepticus in postanoxic coma. *Neurology* 40:1843–1848, 1990.

285. Jumao-as A, Brenner RP: Myoclonic status epilepticus: a clinical and electroencephalographic study. *Neurology* 40:1199–1202, 1990.

286. Frost EAM: Effect of positive end-expiratory pressure in intracranial pressure and compliance in brain-injured patients. *J Neurosurg* 47:195–200, 1977.

287. White PF, Schlobohm RM, Pitts LH, et al: A randomized study of drugs for preventing increases in intracranial pressure during endotracheal suctioning. *Anesthesiology* 57:242–244, 1982.

288. Driks MR, Craven DE, Celli BR, et al: Nosocomial pneumonia in intubated patients given sucralfate as compared with antacids or histamine type 2 blockers. *N Engl J Med* 317:1376–1382, 1987.

289. Ernst E: A review of stroke rehabilitation and physiotherapy. *Stroke* 21:1081–1085, 1990.

289a. Ottenbacher KJ, Jannell S: The results of clinical trials in stroke rehabilitation research. *Arch Neurol* 50:37–44, 1993.

290. Goldstein LB, Davis JN: Restorative neurology. Drugs and recovery following stroke. *Stroke* 21:1636–1640, 1990.

291. Hurwitz BE, Dietrich WD, McCabe PM, et al: Amphetamine promotes recovery from sensory-motor integration deficit after thrombotic infarction of the primary somatosensory rat cortex. *Stroke* 22:648–654, 1991.

292. Crisostomo EA, Duncan PW, Propst M, Dawson DV, Davis JN: Evidence that amphetamine with physical therapy promotes recovery of motor function in stroke patients. *Ann Neurol* 23:94–97, 1988.

293. Parikh RM, Robinson RG, Lipsey JR, Starkstein SE, Fedoroff JP, Price TR: The impact of poststroke depression on recovery in activities of daily living over a 2-year follow-up. *Arch Neurol* 47:785–789, 1990.

294. Lipsey JR, Robinson RG, Pearlson GD, Rao K, Price TR: Nortriptyline treatment of post-stroke depression: a double-blind study. *Lancet*:297–300, 1984.

295. Reeding MJ, Orto LA, Winter SW, Fortuna IM, Di Ponte P, McDowell FH: Antidepressant therapy after stroke. A double-blind trial. *Arch Neurol* 43:763–765, 1986.

296. Hirsh J: Heparin. *N Engl J Med* 324:1565–1574, 1991.

296a. Brill-Edwards P, Ginsberg JS, Johnston M, Hirsh J: Establishing a therapeutic range for heparin therapy. *Ann Intern Med* 119:104–109, 1993.

296b. Albers GW: Laboratory monitoring of oral anticoagulant therapy: are we being misled? *Neurology* 43:468–470, 1993.

296c. Fihn SD, McDonell M, Martin D, Henikoff J, Vermes D, Kent D, White RH; for the Warfarin Optimized Outpatient Follow-up Study Group: Risk factors for complications of chronic anticoagulation. A multicenter study. *Ann Intern Med* 118:511–520, 1993.

296d. Fogelholm R, Eskola K, Timinkinen T, Kunnamo I: Anticoagulant treatment as a risk factor for primary intracerebral hemorrhage. *J Neurosurg Psychiatry* 55:1121–1124, 1992.

297. Tohgi H, Tamura K, Kimura B, Kimura M, Suzuki H: Individual variation in platelet aggregability and serum thromboxane B_2 concentrations after low-dose aspirin. *Stroke* 19:700–703, 1988.

298. Hirsh J: Progress review: the relationship between dose of aspirin, side-effects and antithrombotic effectiveness. *Stroke* 16:1–4, 1985.

298a. Tohgi H, Konno S, Tamura K, Kimura B, Kawano K: Effects of low-to-high doses of aspirin on platelet aggregability and metabolites of thromboxane A_2 and prostacyclin. *Stroke* 23:1400–1403, 1992.

298b. Tanahashi N, Fukuuchi Y, Tomita M, Matsuoka S, Takeda H: Ticlopidine improves the enhanced erythrocyte aggregability in patients with cerebral infarction. *Stroke* 24:1083–1086, 1993.

299. Janzon L, Bergqvist D, Boberg J, et al: Prevention of myocardial infarction and stroke in patients with intermittent claudication: effects of ticlopidine. Results from STIMS, the Swedish Ticlopidine Multicentre Study. *J Intern Med* 227:301–308, 1990.

300. Ticlid (Ticlopidine hydrochloride). Package insert. Palo Alto, CA, Syntex Laboratories, 1991.

301. Lenn NJ, Robertson M: Clinical utility of unbound antiepileptic drug blood levels in the management of epilepsy. *Neurology* 42:988–990, 1992.

CHAPTER 31

Drugs Acting at the Cholinergic Receptor

JEFFREY S. KELLY, M.D.
DREW A. MacGREGOR, M.D.

INTRODUCTION

The autonomic nervous system functions to maintain the internal environment of the body, with innervation in nearly every organ system, by way of two major divisions, sympathetic and parasympathetic (1–3). The preganglionic nerve fibers of both divisions arise in the central nervous system (CNS), with sympathetic fibers originating in the thoracolumbar segments of the spinal cord, whereas the preganglionic fibers of the parasympathetic system arise from cranial and sacral sources. Transmission of neuronal impulses across synaptic junctions is chemically mediated, and the receptors for the autonomic nervous system are classified as noradrenergic or cholinergic based upon the type of neurotransmitter, norepinephrine or acetylcholine, respectively. Acetylcholine (ACh) is the most widespread neurotransmitter in the body, present in all preganglionic autonomic nerve fibers (both sympathetic and parasympathetic), all postganglionic parasympathetic neurons, and a portion of postganglionic sympathetic neurons, including sweat glands. ACh is also the chemical mediator that transmits impulses at the neuromuscular junction and within the central nervous system. Improved understanding of the cholinergic nervous system has allowed development of a number of pharmacologic agents that can modulate the function of the parasympathetic autonomic nervous system. This chapter reviews the physiology and pharmacology of the cholinergic and anticholinergic drugs and reviews the clinical uses of these agents within critical care.

CHOLINERGIC NERVOUS SYSTEM

The sympathetic and parasympathetic nervous systems can be considered physiologic antagonists, as many of the responses seen following cholinergic (parasympathetic) stimulation are antagonized or inhibited by noradrenergic (sympathetic) stimulation (1, 3–5). Because of the widespread distribution of the parasympathetic nervous system, cholinergic stimulation results in a wide variety of end-organ responses (Table 31.1). There are two types of cholinergic receptor systems, muscarinic and nicotinic, based upon the response of these receptors to the alkaloids muscarine and nicotine. Recent research has demonstrated that there are at least five different muscarinic receptors, each with slightly different response to pharmacologic stimulation (1, 6–12). Similarly, the nicotinic receptors at the neuromuscular junction are chemically different from those at autonomic ganglia, and as newer, subtype-specific agents are developed, a more refined approach to receptor pharmacotherapy may become possible.

Muscarinic receptors mediate the actions of ACh on a number of organ systems in the human body, including the heart (bradycardia), lungs (increased secretions, bronchial smooth muscle contraction), and exocrine glands (increased secretions). The primary antagonist of these cholinergic receptors is the antimuscarinic agent atropine. Nicotinic receptors are widely distributed in tissues and modulate the effects of ACh in the neurons of autonomic ganglia (including adrenal medulla), in striated muscle, and within the CNS (Table 31.2). Activation of nicotinic receptors at the neuromuscular junction

534

results in depolarization and eventual contraction of the muscle (see below). Blockade of these nicotinic receptors results in neuromuscular paralysis and is the mechanism of action of most commonly used neuromuscular blocking agents (tubocurarine, metocurine, pancuronium, and others), as is discussed later in this chapter. Antagonism of the nicotinic receptors within autonomic ganglia results in sympathetic blockade and is the mechanism of action of trimethaphan, hexamethonium, and other sympathetic blocking agents (13).

Drugs and other agents (including toxins and other poisons) that increase the effect of the cholinergic nervous system are classified as cholinergic agonists or cholinomimetics. These agents may augment cholinergic stimulation by mimicking the presence of ACh, causing the release of ACh, or preventing destruction or reuptake of ACh at the synaptic junction (1, 3). Conversely, cholinergic antagonists may function by depleting presynaptic stores of ACh, preventing ACh release, or blocking the cholinergic receptors. Table 31.3 shows the mechanisms of actions of different classes of cholinomimetic and anticholinergic agents and a representative drug (or agent) from each class.

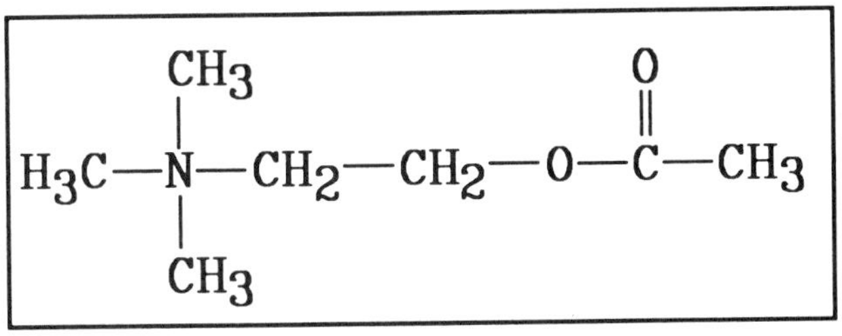

Figure 31.1. Acetylcholine.

CHOLINERGIC AGONISTS

The cholinergic agonists can be classified into (*a*) choline esters, which include ACh and a number of synthetic analogs, (*b*) cholinomimetic alkaloids, which include the naturally occurring alkaloids, muscarine, pilocarpine, and arecoline, as well as synthetic analogs, and (*c*) anticholinesterase agents. Although the mechanisms of these agents differ, the net effect is an increase in the activity of cholinergic receptors in the body.

CHOLINE ESTERS

Acetylcholine is a quaternary ammonium compound formed by the esterification of a choline base with an acetyl group (Fig. 31.1). Other choline esters (methacholine, carbechol, bethanechol) are modifications of this same quaternary ammonium compound. The major pharmacologic differences among these choline esters are their relative muscarinic activity, relative nicotinic activity, and resistance to enzymatic hydrolysis (Table 31.4). For example, although ACh has a high degree of muscarinic activity relative to carbachol and bethanechol because of the presence of the acetyl group, carbachol and bethanechol are more resistant to enzymatic degradation by the cholinesterases. Although the choline esters rarely are used in routine clinical practice today, methacholine is commonly used in bronchoprovocation tests of pulmonary function and bethanechol occasionally is administered to treat urinary retention in patients with neurogenic bladder dysfunction (1, 3, 14, 15).

CHOLINOMIMETIC ALKALOIDS

The three major naturally occurring choline alkaloids are pilocarpine, muscarine, and arecoline. Metoclopramide,

Table 31.1. End-Organ Responses to Cholinergic Stimulation

Tissue	Response
Heart	Decreased heart rate, decreased contractility, decreased conduction velocity, A-V block
Lung	Bronchoconstriction, increased secretions
Adrenal medulla	Secretion of epinephrine and norepinephrine
Exocrine glands (pancreas, salivary, and lacrimal glands)	Increased secretions
Gastrointestinal tract	Increased motility and tone, relaxation of pylorus and gastroesophageal sphincter, relaxation of cecal valve and other sphincters, increased secretions, gallbladder contraction
Bladder	Relaxation of internal sphincter (micturition)
Sweat glands	Increased secretion
Male reproductive system	Erection
Eye	Contraction of iris (miosis), contraction of ciliary muscle for accommodation-convergence

Table 31.2. Nicotinic and Muscarinic Receptors

	Nicotinic	Nicotinic	Muscarinic
Location	Autonomic ganglia	Neuromuscular junction	Autonomic effector cell
Effectors	Sympathetic ganglia	Striated muscles	Heart, exocrine glands, smooth muscle
Agonist	ACh, nicotine, succinylcholine	ACh, nicotine, succinylcholine	ACh, muscarine
Antagonist	*d*-Tubocurarine, trimethaphan, hexamethonium	*d*-Tubocurarine, metocurine, pancuronium	Atropine, hyoscine

Table 31.3. Cholinomimetic and Anticholinergic Actions and Agents

Mechanism of Action	Drug or Other Agent	Effect
Mimics effect of ACh	Methacholine, nicotine	Cholinomimetic
	Succinylcholine	Muscle paralysis
Causes release of ACh	Black widow spider venom	Initially cholinomimetic
Inhibits enzymatic destruction of ACh	Anticholinesterase drugs	Cholinomimetic
Prevents ACh synthesis	Hemicholinium	Blocks ACh reuptake with eventual depletion of ACh
Prevents ACh release	Botulinum toxin	Anticholinergic
Blocks ACh receptors	Atropine	Anticholinergic
	d-Tubocurarine	Muscle paralysis
	Hexamethonium	Sympathetic blockade

Table 31.4. Pharmacologic Properties of Choline Esters

Choline Ester	Resistance to Hydrolysis	Muscarinic Effects		Nicotinic Effects
		C-V	CNS	
Acetylcholine	−	++	++	++
Methacholine	+	+++	++	+
Carbachol	+++	+	+++	+++
Bethanechol	+++	±	+++	−

Table 31.5. Anticholinesterase Agents

Reversible	Irreversible
Physostigmine	"Nerve gases" (tabun, sarin, soman)
Neostigmine	Insecticides
Edrophonium	malathion, parathion, fenthion
Pyridostigmine	paraoxon (diazinon)
Demecarium	TEPP, others
Ambenonium	Echothiophate

cisapride, aceclidine, and oxotremorine are synthetic analogs of the choline alkaloids. The major differences among these agents include their relative activity at muscarinic and nicotinic receptors and their affinity for specific organ systems (3, 16–18). Pilocarpine and aceclidine are used clinically in the topical treatment of narrow-angle glaucoma, and rarely are used in critical care. Metoclopramide, however, is used in intensive care units, primarily for its gastrointestinal-stimulating properties, including its use to facilitate passage of enteral feeding tubes into the small bowel. Metoclopramide is also used as an antiemetic because of its antagonism of dopamine receptors in the CNS, but its use for this purpose is limited as a result of the potential for extrapyramidal symptoms occasionally seen with this drug (19). Cisapride is another prokinetic drug used in Europe and Canada that does not have the antidopaminergic properties of metoclopramide.

ANTICHOLINESTERASES

Acetylcholine is hydrolyzed rapidly at the nerve synapse by the enzyme acetylcholinesterase (AChE), which is located in the region of the cholinergic synaptic cleft and within red blood cells (1–3). No AChE exists in the plasma (2). Pseudocholinesterase (butyrocholinesterase, nonspecific cholinesterase) is found circulating in the plasma and also within the liver, kidney, and intestines. Although the exact physiologic function of pseudocholinesterase is unknown, it is responsible for the hydrolysis of depolarizing neuromuscular

blockers such as succinylcholine. Most of the available anticholinesterase agents (anti-ChE agents) inhibit or inactivate both cholinesterases, allowing acetylcholine to accumulate at cholinergic receptors throughout the body (20, 21).

Anticholinesterases are divided into reversible (competitive) active site inhibitors and "irreversible" (noncompetitive, structure-altering) inhibitors (Table 31.5). Reversible anti-ChE agents compete with ACh for the active site on the cholinesterase molecule, increasing the relative concentration of ACh. Reversible agents do not alter the function of the cholinesterase enzymes, and once the inhibitor is removed, enzymatic function returns to normal. The irreversible agents bind to the cholinesterase molecule at sites distant from the active site and cause chemical alterations in the enzyme, inhibiting its physiologic function. Chemical alterations include the transfer of carbamyl groups (neostigmine), or the phosphorylation of cholinesterase (organophosphates). Once a noncompetitive (irreversible) agent has altered the structure of AChE, regeneration of the active enzyme is required before physiologic function is restored. This regeneration can be accelerated by nucleophilic agents such as pralidoxime, which cause rapid regeneration of AChE and reversal of the anticholinesterase effects.

The main clinical uses of anti-ChE agents are in the treatment of diseases of the neuromuscular junction (such as myasthenia gravis), gastrointestinal tract, and eye (Table 31.6). They are also used to reverse the effects of nondepolarizing (competitive) neuromuscular blocking agents. Physostigmine occasionally is used in conjunction with alkalinization and detoxification measures in severely symptomatic overdoses of tricyclic antidepressants (22, 23). Because anticholinesterase agents are common components of insecticides, toxic exposure to these agents commonly is encountered in critical care medicine. Clinical signs of excessive cholinergic activity (bradycardia, profuse sweating, bronchorrhea, diarrhea, etc.) should raise suspicion of anticholinesterase toxicity. Treatment of anticholinesterase toxicity requires large doses of atropine (1 to 4 mg or more) to block the effects of ACh overload, followed

Table 31.6. Clinical Uses of Cholinesterase Inhibitors

Drug	Uses	Usual Dose	Duration
Edrophonium	Myasthenia gravis	2–8 mg i.v. test	5–10 min
	Reversal of competitive neuromuscular blockade	30–50 mg i.v.	
Physostigmine	Glaucoma	Topical drops	2–6 hr
	TCA overdose	2–12 mg i.v.	10–20 min
Pyridostigmine	Myasthenia gravis	60–120 mg p.o.	3–6 hr
		2–4 mg i.v.	2–4 hr
	Reversal of competitive neuromuscular blockade	10–20 mg i.v.	
Neostigmine	Myasthenia gravis	15 mg p.o.	2–4 hr
	Reversal of competitive neuromuscular blockade	2.5–5 mg i.v.	

Table 31.7. Dose-dependent Effects of Antimuscarinic Drugs

Low dose	Decreased salivary secretions
	Decreased bronchial secretions
	Decreased sweating
	Minimal CNS effects
Medium dose	Mydriasis, cycloplegia
	Vagolytic cardiac effects
	Increased respiratory rate
	Increased tidal volume
High dose	Inhibition of bladder tone
	Decreased gut motility
	Confusion/delirium

by the administration of the AChE-regenerating drug pralidoxime. The dose of pralidoxime is usually 1 g in 100 cc of saline, given no faster than 200 mg/min. This dose may be repeated after 1 hour, and atropine should be continued for at least 24 to 48 hours (1, 19).

CHOLINERGIC ANTAGONISTS: ANTIMUSCARINIC DRUGS

Cholinergic antagonists are classified as antimuscarinic or antinicotinic based upon the class of receptor that is antagonized. Atropine is the prototype drug used to block the effects of ACh on muscarinic receptors, with little effect on nicotinic receptors (except in very high concentrations). The effects of muscarinic blockade are dose-dependent, as outlined in Table 31.7. The major distinguishing feature among the different antimuscarinic drugs is the chemical structure of each (i.e., tertiary or quaternary amines). Tertiary amines, including atropine and scopolamine, readily cross the blood-brain barrier and can cause central antimuscarinic actions, whereas quaternary amines such as glycopyrrolate do not penetrate the CNS and produce primarily peripheral effects (Table 31.8). All of the currently available antimuscarinic drugs are competitive antagonists, and thus the effects of these drugs may be overcome by increasing the availability of ACh (or structurally

similar agonists) at the receptor sites. Table 31.9 summarizes the clinical uses and major side effects of drugs that primarily affect the muscarinic receptors.

NICOTINIC RECEPTOR AGENTS: NEUROMUSCULAR BLOCKING DRUGS

Neuromuscular blocking drugs are quarternary ammonium compounds that reversibly interfere with ACh-mediated neuromuscular transmission. They traditionally are classified as depolarizing (noncompetitive) or nondepolarizing (competitive) agents, based on their respective mechanism of action at the neuromuscular junction.

DEPOLARIZING NEUROMUSCULAR BLOCKING DRUGS

Depolarizing neuromuscular blocking drugs such as succinylcholine mimic the action of ACh at the nicotinic cholinergic receptor located on the motor end-plate of the neuromuscular junction (24, 25). The resultant opening of membrane-bound sodium and calcium channels causes intracellular influx of these two ions along their concentration gradients, with simultaneous efflux of potassium into the extracellular space. Miniature end-plate potentials develop, culminating in rapid depolarization of the adjacent muscle membrane and subsequent muscle contraction. In the native state, ACh molecules are metabolized quickly by AChE in the synaptic cleft. The muscle membrane rapidly repolarizes, and the muscle again becomes available for neurochemical stimulation and contraction. Succinylcholine, however, is metabolized much more slowly than ACh and persistently subjects the motor end-plate to ongoing depolarizing stimulation (24–27). Repolarization cannot occur, and the muscle loses its ability to contract in response to ACh-mediated neural stimulation. The flaccid

Table 31.8. Comparison of Antimuscarinic Agents

Drug	Cardiovascular Effects	CNS Effects	Primary Uses	Other Uses
Atropine	+++	+	Bradycardia	Decrease bronchial secretions
Scopolamine	++	+++	Motion sickness	Amnestic agent (anesthesia)
Propantheline	+	±	Incontinence	
Glycopyrrolate	+	0	Antisialogogue	Adjunct for neuromuscular blockade reversal

muscle paralysis that results from succinylcholine administration is thus similar to the cholinergic-induced muscle weakness caused by cholinesterase-inhibiting agents such as pyridostigmine and organophosphate insecticides.

The neuromuscular blockade described above is also known as phase I depolarizing blockade and is the typical response expected from the usual intubating dose of succinylcholine (1.0 to 1.5 mg/kg i.v.). Onset of action occurs within 60 seconds and is heralded by the presence (and subsequent extinction) of muscle fasciculations (24, 27). Areas where fasciculations may be particularly pronounced include the small muscle groups of the hands, feet, and face. Succinylcholine's duration of action after a single intubating dose is about 5 to 9 minutes due to its rapid ester hydrolysis by pseudocholinesterase in plasma (24, 26, 28). The maximum rate of this hydrolysis is thought to be approximately 100 μg/kg/min (24, 29). States in which quantitative decreases in serum pseudocholinesterase activity occur (i.e., in severe prolonged liver disease, pregnancy, cholinesterase-inhibitor exposure, malignancies, myxedema, corticosteroid therapy, newborns) can prolong succinylcholine's duration of action by 50 to 100% (24, 28, 30, 31). In addition, about 1 in every 2500 individuals is

homozygous for an atypical pseudocholinesterase that metabolizes succinylcholine poorly and leads to 1 to 3 hours of neuromuscular blockade (24, 30, 31). A serum pseudocholinesterase level will rule out the former condition, whereas genetic defects are diagnosed using the dibucaine number. Dibucaine is an amide local anesthetic that inhibits normal pseudocholinesterase activity by approximately 80% (i.e., a dibucaine number ≥80). In contrast, this same local anesthetic exhibits only 20 to 30% inhibition of atypical pseudocholinesterase (i.e., a dibucaine number ≤30). Individuals who are heterozygous for the atypical gene have dibucaine numbers between 45 and 70, with only a modest prolongation in succinylcholine's neuromuscular blocking effects (24, 30–32).

As the cumulative succinylcholine dose begins to exceed 2 mg/kg i.v., the character of its neuromuscular blockade progressively changes to that of a nondepolarizing (i.e., competitive) agent. This is referred to as phase II depolarizing blockade and may arise from the use of a single large succinylcholine bolus, multiple repetitive smaller doses, or continuous infusions (24, 27, 29, 30, 33). A small dose of a short-acting cholinesterase inhibitor (such as edrophonium 0.1 to 0.2 mg/kg i.v.) may be both diagnostic as well as therapeutic in this

Table 31.9.   Clinical Uses and Side Effects of Commonly Used Cholinergic Drugs

Drug	Clinical Uses	Side Effects	Notes
Choline esters			
Methacholine	Supraventricular tachycardia, methachol challenge	Bradycardia, heart block, hypotension, syncope	Used in pulmonary function testing
Carbachol	Stimulation of bladder and GI tract	Abdominal cramps, urinary urgency, bradycardia, hypotension	Relatively long duration
Bethanechol	Stimulation of bladder and GI tract	Less cardiovascular effects	Long duration of activity
Choline alkaloids			
Pilocarpine	Glaucoma	Diaphoresis, salivation	
Aceclidine	Topical treatment of glaucoma		Not available in U.S.
Metoclopramide	Antiemetic, treatment of gastroparesis	Dystonic reactions, extrapyramidal symptoms	
Anticholinesterases			
Physostigmine	Glaucoma, atropine intoxication, tricyclic antidepressant poisoning	Confusion, nausea, bradycardia, hypotension	Tertiary amine
Neostigmine	Reversal of nondepolarizing paralytics, treatment of gastroparesis and bladder atony	Severe bradycardia, arrhythmias, increased oral and bronchial secretions	Quaternary amine
Pyridostigmine	Reversal of nondepolarizing paralytics, myasthenia gravis	Bradycardia, oropharyngeal and bronchial secretions	Fewer arrhythmias than with neostigmine
Edrophonium	Differentiation of myasthenic crises, reversal of nondepolarizing paralytics; PSVT	Less bradycardia than with other agents	
Echothiophate	Glaucoma	May prolong neuromuscular blockade of succinylcholine	Irreversible, with long duration of action
AChE regenerators			
Pralidoxime	Organophosphate poisoning, anticholinesterase overdose	High dose may cause cholinergic blockade	Used in conjunction with atropine (see text)
Antimuscarinics			
Atropine	Symptomatic bradycardias, rarely used as mydriatic, cholinesterase-inhibitor poisoning	Tachycardia, central anti-ACh syndrome	Tertiary amine
Scopolamine	Anesthesia (amnestic), antinausea (motion sickness)	Dry mouth, sedation	Tertiary amine
Propantheline	Delays gastric emptying, augments bladder control	Urinary retention	Few CNS effects (quaternary amine)
Glycopyrrolate	Anesthesia (antisialogogue)	Dry mouth	Quaternary amine

Table 31.10. Adverse Effects of Succinylcholine

Cardiac arrhythmias
Skeletal muscle myalgias
Sustained skeletal muscle contraction
Myoglobinemia
Hyperkalemia
Increased intraocular pressure
Increased intragastric pressure
Increased intracranial pressure
Malignant hyperthermia
Allergic reactions

Table 31.11. Conditions Associated with Succinylcholine-induced Hyperkalemia

Upper motor neuron lesions
Lower motor neuron lesions
Muscle denervation
Trauma/severe tissue damage
Muscle immobilization and atrophy
Thermal burns
Muscular dystrophy
Clostridial infections
? Severe prolonged infections (>1 week)
? Anterior horn cell disease
? Diffuse CNS insult (head injury, aneurysmal rupture, encephalitis)

?, Possible.

circumstance, because these agents augment phase I blockade while antagonizing phase II blockade. This approach mimics the tensilon test used to differentiate myasthenic crisis from cholinergic excess and is most appropriate when guided by peripheral nerve stimulation monitoring. The mechanism responsible for the development of phase II depolarizing blockade is currently unknown.

Adverse effects of succinylcholine administration are listed in Table 31.10. The drug's cholinomimetic action at cardiac muscarinic receptors can lead to sinus bradycardia, junctional rhythms, or even sinus arrest. This effect occurs most often in children or following a second i.v. dose administered within 3 to 5 minutes of the first succinylcholine dose in adults (24, 34, 35). Less commonly, nicotinic stimulation at sympathetic ganglia can cause tachycardia and/or hypertension (24, 34, 35). The unsynchronized skeletal muscle fasciculations from succinylcholine are presumably the reason for the myalgias experienced by some patients as well as the myoglobinemia seen commonly in children (although rarely in adults) (24, 36, 37). Although succinylcholine does increase intragastric pressure in adults, a greater increase in lower esophageal sphincter tone causes the so-called "barrier pressure" for regurgitation (and subsequent aspiration) of stomach contents to increase as well (24, 35, 38, 39). Increases in intraocular pressure as a result of succinylcholine may be a manifestation of the sensitivity of small extraocular muscles to the agonist, resulting in tonic muscle contraction (24, 35, 40). Although this effect lasts only 5 to 6 minutes, it has led to the avoidance of succinylcholine in patients with open eye injuries, for fear of vitreous extrusion. A recent retrospective study from a leading eye center, however, suggests that succinylcholine can, indeed, be used safely in this setting (41). The increase in intracranial pressure caused by succinylcholine is of unclear clinical significance and must be weighed against the known

detrimental effects of hypercarbia and hypoxemia when airway compromise occurs in the face of intracranial hypertension (24, 35, 42, 43). Patients with certain rare muscle diseases such as myotonia congenita and myotonia dystrophica can respond to succinylcholine with sustained muscle contraction, potentially interfering with pulmonary ventilation (44). Allergic reactions to succinylcholine are uncommon, may occur with first-time exposure to the drug, and are manifested clinically as sudden hypotension and tachycardia (often in the absence of classic findings such as angioneurotic edema, bronchospasm, and urticaria) (24, 45, 46). Succinylcholine is a potent trigger of malignant hyperthermia in the operative setting and should be avoided in patients with either individual risk factors or a family history of this disorder (44, 47). Whether the masseter muscle spasm occasionally observed from succinylcholine administration in children is a harbinger for the subsequent development of malignant hyperthermia is controversial (47).

The depolarizing action of succinylcholine leads to potassium efflux into the extracellular space and typically increases the serum potassium level by approximately 0.5 to 1.0 mEq/liter (24, 48, 49). In certain disease states, this potassium shift is markedly exaggerated and can be life-threatening (Table 31.11) (24, 44, 49–51). The presumed mechanism involves the proliferation of nicotinic cholinergic receptors outside the confines of the neuromuscular junction (50, 51). Administration of an agonist such as succinylcholine to these patients results in diffuse muscle membrane depolarization, with the extrajunctional receptors providing multiple additional channels for potassium extrusion into extracellular fluid. This so-called "extrajunctional chemosensitivity" may develop within 72 to 96 hours in the case of muscle denervation, upper and lower motor neuron lesions, and burn injuries, and potentially can persist for years (50–52). Skeletal muscle myalgias, bradyarrhythmias, increased intragastric pressure, and increased intracranial pressure due to succinylcholine administration may be attenuated by preceding succinylcholine with a small nonparalytic dose of a nondepolarizing drug (approximately 10% of the typical intubating dose) (24, 38, 40, 43, 53). Such "pretreatment" also necessitates increasing the initial succinylcholine dose to 1.5 mg/kg because of the antagonism of depolarizing blockade by prior administration of the nondepolarizing agent (24, 54).

NONDEPOLARIZING (COMPETITIVE) NEUROMUSCULAR BLOCKING DRUGS

Nondepolarizing neuromuscular blocking drugs also bind to the nicotinic cholinergic receptor of the neuromuscular junction, but they elicit no ion channel activation or electrolyte fluxes. Progressive inhibition of normal ACh-mediated neuromuscular transmission occurs as a result of competitive receptor occupancy by the pharmacologically inactive nondepolarizing agent (20). Because of the wide safety margin of neuromuscular transmission, approximately 75% of the nicotinic receptors must be competitively occupied before evidence of nondepolarizing neuromuscular blockade can be identified clinically. Between 80 and 90% receptor occupancy is required for total failure of neuromuscular transmission to occur (20, 55).

Chemically, nondepolarizing agents are either benzyl isoquinolinium or steroid compounds. Because of these structural variations, a measure of equal potency is useful for comparing the pharmacokinetics and pharmacodynamics of specific agents. The drug dose required to depcrease the height of a single motor twitch from peripheral nerve stimulation by 95% (the so-called ED_{95}) conventionally has been used for this purpose (Table 31.12) (20, 56). Nondepolarizing neuromuscular blocking drugs are classified clinically as either short-, intermediate-, or long-acting, with the choice of specific agent dictated by such variables as speed of onset, duration of action, undesirable side effects, cost, and the presence of renal or hepatobiliary disease. Two times the ED_{95} dose of each drug represents the typical intubating dose, unless this larger amount leads to an unacceptable side effect profile (see below). The slow onset of intubating conditions with these drugs compared to succinylcholine can be accelerated either by giving a much larger initial dose ($\geq$three times the ED_{95}) or by using the "priming" principle (57, 58). With the latter technique, approximately 10% of an intubating dose is administered initially, followed in 3 to 4 minutes by two to three times the ED_{95} dose of the same agent (57, 59). Using either method, adequate intubating conditions can be achieved within 2 minutes and, in the case of mivacurium "priming," may approach those seen with succinylcholine. This relative advantage must be weighed against the obligatory prolongation in the drug's duration of action, the unpleasant sensation of weakness experienced by some patients, as well as an increased potential for deleterious hemodynamic side effects with certain agents (Table 31.13) (57–59). In addition, the upper airway musculature is very sensitive to small degrees of neuromuscular paralysis, and aspiration has occurred following administration of the initial priming dose (60). Long-term maintenance of neuromuscular paralysis typically is accomplished using either a continuous infusion of a short- or intermediate-acting drug or by intermittent administration of one-quarter to one-third of the intubating dose of a long-acting agent (61–64). Maintenance therapy is best guided by evaluating the patient for evidence of spontaneous recovery, using either clinical parameters or the motor response to peripheral nerve stimulation. Such monitoring possibly may aid in avoiding extended neuromuscular paralysis from excess drug accumulation, particularly in the case of vecuronium and the long-acting agents. Accumulation of atracurium and mivacurium is unlikely to occur because of these drugs' unique metabolic pathways (see below) (61–65). Critical care use of the new long-acting agents doxacurium and pipecuronium has not been reported, and the latter drug's manufacturer specifically recommends against its use in this setting (66, 67). Pertinent clinical properties of the various nondepolarizing neuromuscular blocking drugs are summarized in Table 31.12.

In general, vagal blockade is the most noteworthy side effect of the steroid-based relaxants, whereas histamine release is the main significant side effect of the benzyl isoquinolinium relaxants (Table 31.13). These adverse effects are particularly prominent when doses three times the ED_{95} or larger are rapidly administered (as in a rapid intubation technique). Thus, hypotension secondary to histamine release can be seen as a result of administering an intubating dose of *d*-tubocurarine, as well as from large doses of metocurine, atracurium, and mivacurium (58, 61, 68–70). Hypotension and tachycardia may also result from nicotinic ganglionic blockade with *d*-tubocurarine and, less commonly, metocurine (61, 71, 72). Vagal blockade from pancuronium can also elicit a tachycardiac response (68, 73). Use of these agents in critically ill patients can contribute to hypotension via loss of basal muscle tone, leading to venous pooling in the extremities and decreases in preload. Laudanosine, a Hofmann metabolite of atracurium, is known to have CNS-stimulating properties and has the potential to elicit such responses in the absence of concomitant CNS depressant administration. This theoretical concern does not appear to be a clinical problem even with prolonged use of atracurium infusions (61, 74, 75). Allergic reactions to nondepolarizing neuromuscular blocking drugs are rare and, in general, are seen most commonly with agents known to cause histamine release. The symptom complex manifested is identical to that seen with succinylcholine allergy. Cross-sensitivity as a result of their common quarternary ammonium moiety can occur, although reactions may be less likely with non-histamine-releasing monoquarternary steroid compounds such as vecuronium (45, 46, 61, 76). Certain patients may manifest resistance or increased sensitivity to the effects of nondepolarizing agents as a result of concurrent drug administration, metabolic abnormalities, or specific disease processes (Table 31.14) (44, 51, 77–83). Recent case reports suggest that extended use of steroid-based nondepolarizing neuromuscular blocking drugs in the intensive care setting may induce devastating myopathies in such patients (84, 85). It appears prudent to avoid chronic use of the steroidal agents and to monitor the motor response to peripheral nerve stimulation when long-term administration of neuromuscular blocking drugs is required in critically ill patients.

Because of their charged quarternary ammonium structure, nondepolarizing neuromuscular blocking drugs are cleared from the body primarily by glomerular filtration and cannot be passively reabsorbed by the renal tubules or cross other lipid membranes such as the placenta (61, 82, 86–88). Certain agents also undergo biliary excretion, the relative amount varying inversely to a limited extent with renal function (61, 82, 87, 89). The limited hepatic metabolism of the steroid relaxants vecuronium and pancuronium results from their more lipophilic nature and yields active metabolites with 30 to 60% the potency of their parent compounds (61, 82, 88, 90). Atracurium and mivacurium are unique in that they are rapidly metabolized in peripheral plasma by nonspecific esterases and pseudocholinesterase, respectively, with the rate of mivacurium metabolism approaching 70 to 88% that of succinylcholine (61, 63, 91–95). In addition, atracurium undergoes pH- and temperature-dependent, nonenzymatic degradation in plasma (so-called Hofmann elimination) and is not dependent on pseudocholinesterase activity for dissipation of its effects (61, 92–96). These two agents may prove useful in patients with severe liver or kidney disease when prolonged neuromuscular paralysis is undesirable (82, 97, 98). As with succinylcholine, quantitative and qualitative decreases in pseudocholinesterase activity have the potential to extend the duration of competitive neuromuscular blockade with mivacurium (91). Pertinent information concerning the metabolism and excretion of nondepolarizing relaxants is summarized in Table 31.15.

Table 31.12 Classification, Recommended Doses, and Usual Clinical Effects of Nondepolarizing Relaxants

	Short-Acting	Intermediate-Acting				Long-Acting		
	Mivacurium	*Atracurium*	*Vecuronium*	*d-Tubocurarine*	*Metocurine*	*Pancuronium*	*Pipecuronium*[a]	*Doxacurium*
Structure	BZ-ISO[b]	BZ-ISO[b]	Steroid	BZ-ISO[b]	BZ-ISO[b]	Steroid	Steroid	BZ-ISO[b]
ED_{95} (mg/kg)	0.08	0.20–0.25	0.05	0.50	0.28	0.07	0.05	0.025–0.030
Intubation dose (mg/kg)	0.15–0.20	0.40–0.50	0.10	0.50–0.60	0.40	0.10	0.10	0.05–0.075
Onset intubating conditions (min)	2–3	3–4	3–4	3–5	3–5	3–5	3–5	4–6
Intubation dose duration (min)	12–20	20–40	20–40	60–90	60–90	90–120	90–120	120–150
Onset rapid intubation (sec)[c]	60–90	90	90	NA[d]	NA[d]	90–120	90–120	120–150
Duration rapid intubation (min)[c]	20–25	50–60	50–60	NA[d]	NA[d]	150–200	150–200	>200
Infusion rate (mg/kg/min)	5–15	5–9	1–2	NA	NA	NA	NA	NA
Cost	Moderate	High	High	Low	Moderate	Very low	Very high	Very high

[a] Manufacturer specifically recommends against ICU administration.
[b] BZ-ISO, benzyl isoquinolinium.
[c] "Priming," followed by 3 times the ED_{95} (see text).
[d] NA, not applicable. Use in this fashion limited by accentuated histamine release (see text).

Table 31.13. Side Effect Profiles of Nondepolarizing Neuromuscular Blocking Drugs

Drug	*Cardiac Muscarinic Effects*	*Sympathetic Nicotinic Effects*	*Histamine Release*
Mivacurium	NS[a]	NS	Slight-modest
Atracurium	NS	NS	Slight-modest
Vecuronium	NS	NS	NS
d-Tubocurarine	Mild-modest blockade	Moderate blockade	Moderate
Metocurine	NS	Mild blockade	Modest
Pancuronium	Modest blockade	NS	NS
Pipecuronium	NS	NS	NS
Doxacurium	NS	NS	NS

[a] NS, not significant.

Table 31.14. Conditions Associated with Altered Responsiveness to Nondepolarizing Neuromuscular Blocking Agents

Increased sensitivity	
Hypothermia	Drug therapy
Hypokalemia	Inhalation anesthetics
Hypocalcemia	Local anesthetics
Hypermagnesemia	Aminoglycosides
Acidosis	Clindamycin
Myasthenia gravis	Polymyxin
Myasthenic syndrome	Calcium channel blockers
Paraplegia	Procainamide
Neurofibromatosis	Quinidine
Amyotrophic lateral sclerosis	Magnesium
Poliomyelitis	Trimethaphan
Neonates[a]	Cyclophosphamide
? Myotonia	Cyclosporine
? Muscular dystrophy	Furosemide
	Dantrolene
	? Lithium
Increased resistance	
Hemiplegia	Drug therapy
Thermal burns	Corticosteroids
Peripheral neuropathies	Carbamazepine
Peripheral nerve transection	Phenytoin
Hyperkalemia	? Aminophylline/theophylline
Hypercalcemia	? Azathioprine
Clostridial infections	? Nondepolarizing relaxants (chronic)
Cirrhosis with ascites	

[a] Sensitivity effects are offset by neonates' increased volume of distribution.

Rapid reversal of nondepolarizing neuromuscular blockade via pharmacologic antagonism of acetylcholinesterase is possible once spontaneous recovery of neuromuscular function is evident clinically or by peripheral nerve stimulation. Neostigmine, 50 to 70 µg/kg (up to a maximum of 5 mg) or edrophonium (0.5 to 1.0 mg/kg) can be used for this purpose and has maximal effect within 5 to 8 minutes. Atropine 20 µg/kg or glycopyrrolate 15 µg/kg must be administered with the cholinesterase inhibitor in order to avoid excessive muscarinic side effects such as bradyarrhythmias, increased secretions, and bronchospasm. The rate of reversal of short- and intermediate-acting relaxants is faster than that of long-acting agents, since the effect of the antagonist is additive to the rate of the drug's spontaneous recovery. Monitoring of neuromuscular function is useful in assessing the reversal process (see below) (99–101).

CLINICAL MONITORING OF NEUROMUSCULAR BLOCKADE

The degree of neuromuscular blockade caused by muscle relaxants has been traditionally monitored in the operative setting using the motor response to peripheral nerve stimulation. This technique allows for an assessment of neuromuscular function independent of confounding variables such as residual sedation and communication difficulties. Most commonly, the ulnar nerve at the wrist is stimulated while the clinician evaluates the motor response of the adductor pollicis brevis muscle at the thumb. Alternatively, the peroneal nerve at the neck of the fibula (foot dorsiflexion) or the facial nerve just anterior to the tragus of the ear (contraction of the orbicularis oculi muscle) may be used (Figure 31.2). The latter site, however, is more resistant to electrical stimulation, may elicit some direct muscle stimulation, and thus may lead to underestimation of the degree of block (102–105). Patients with hemiplegia, paraplegia, peripheral neuropathies, and transected peripheral nerves should be monitored on an unaffected extremity if possible, since their affected limbs often manifest altered responses to nondepolarizing agents (Table 31.14) (44, 51, 102). The skin over the stimulating nerve should be clean and dry, with the jelled electrocardiogram (ECG) electrodes applied so as to maximize nerve stimulation while minimizing direct stimulation of underlying muscle beds (103, 104, 106).

In a peripheral nerve containing many axons of differing sensitivities, the number of axons firing and the subsequent force of muscle contraction have a sigmoidal relationship to delivered current. The plateau of this sigmoid curve represents simultaneous stimulation of all nerve axons and contraction of all recruitable muscle fibers (102–104, 107). Delivery of such a "supramaximal" stimulus is important in monitoring for neuromuscular blockade, since it will most closely mimic normal muscle physiology (i.e., "all-or-none" contraction). Nerve stimulator characteristics required to elicit such a supramaximal stimulus are listed in Table 31.16. A stimulus pulse duration less than the peripheral nerve refractory period (0.5 to 1.0 msec) is necessary so that only a single nerve action potential is generated. Reliable delivery of a supramaximal stimulus to the ulnar nerve at the wrist typically requires 30 to 60 ma of current delivered over 0.2 msec. This requirement necessitates delivering a 200 to 400 volt impulse, depending on the resistance characteristics between the stimulating electrodes (102–104, 107, 108).

The train-of-four ratio (TOFR) is the most convenient and reliable method for monitoring neuromuscular blockade and represents a compromise between sensitivity and avoidance

Table 31.15. Metabolism and Clearance of Nondepolarizing Neuromuscular Blocking Drugs

Drug	% Renal Excretion	% Biliary Excretion	% Hepatic Metabolism	% Plasma Hydrolysis	Active Metabolites	Duration in Renal Disease	Duration Hepatic Disease
Mivacurium	5	NS[a]	NS	95[b]	No	Minimal increase	Mild to modest increase[c]
Atracurium	5–10	NS	NS	90–95[d]	Laudanosine[e]	No change	No change
Vecuronium	50	35–50	15–30	None	3-hydroxyvecuronium[f]	Minimal increase	Mild to modest increase
d-Tubocurarine	45	10–40	NS	None	No	Modest increase	? Mild to modest increase
Metocurine	46–58	<2	NS	None	No	Moderate increase	No change to mild increase
Pancuronium	85	10–15	10–15	None	3-hydroxypancuronium[g]	Modest increase	Mild to modest increase
Pipecuronium	70	20	10	None	No	Modest increase	?
Doxacurium	70	Present (significance unknown)	?	Minimal	? None	Modest increase	? No change to slight increase

[a] NS, not significant.
[b] Plasma pseudocholinesterase.
[c] Only when significant (>70%) decreases in plasma pseudocholinesterase activity occur.
[d] Nonspecific plasma esterases plus Hofmann degradation.
[e] ? CNS stimulation.
[f] 60% potency of parent compound.
[g] 33–50% potency of parent compound.

of posttetanic facilitation. This method entails delivery of four supramaximal stimuli at a frequency of 2 stimuli per second (i.e., 2 Hz) every 10 to 12 seconds and evaluating the ratio of the fourth twitch height (T_4) to that of the first twitch (T_1) (102–104, 109). Depolarizing blockade causes a similar decrement in the height of all four twitches (i.e., a TOFR > 0.7), whereas nondepolarizing blockade is characterized by a progressive decrement in successive twitch heights, or "fade" (i.e., a TOFR <0.7) (Figure 31.3). The latter phenomenon is attributable to decreased ACh release from motor nerve terminals at high rates of nerve stimulation (103). Evaluation of the TOFR more often than every 10 seconds may cause T_1 to continue to manifest fade from the preceding TOFR measurement. This effect falsely increases the TOFR, leading to underestimation of the degree of block and potential excess administration of nondepolarizing drug (103). Furthermore, excessive TOFR stimulation may overestimate the onset of blockade as a result of augmented drug delivery to the monitored muscle from physiologic increases in muscle blood flow (102, 110). Visual and/or tactile evaluation of the TOFR, although somewhat imprecise, is clinically adequate in the majority of cases (102, 111).

A 50-Hz tetanic stimulus delivered over 5 seconds closely mimics maximal voluntary muscle activity and occasionally is used to detect small amounts of residual nondepolarizing neuromuscular blockade (102–104, 112). Because tetanic stimulation may potentiate the response to nontetanic nerve stimulation for several minutes (i.e., posttetanic facilitation), the degree of nondepolarizing blockade may be underestimated due to augmentation of subsequent TOFR measurements (102–104). It is also extremely painful in conscious patients. Thus, tetanic stimulation should be applied sparingly and only when clinically necessary to detect incomplete recovery from nondepolarizing blockade. Tetanic fade may also be seen in certain diseases (such as myasthenia gravis) in which the margin of safety for neuromuscular transmission is diminished by the underlying disease process.

The main shortcoming of using peripheral nerve stimulation monitoring is that it infers global muscle function based on a single muscle group and does not take into account sensitivity differences between the peripheral musculature and the respiratory muscles. Although the diaphragm and laryngeal muscles are more resistant to neuromuscular blockade than is the adductor pollicis brevis and thus recover more quickly, their onset of action is paradoxically faster from higher blood flow and accelerated drug delivery to these sites (102, 113–115). Alternatively, the accessory muscles of respiration may be more sensitive to nondepolarizing relaxants than is the diaphragm (115, 116). As a result, respiratory embarrassment and apnea may ensue before TOFR decrements are observed at the adductor pollicis brevis with adequate doses of competitive relaxants. Furthermore, inadequate doses of nondepolarizing relaxants over time may elicit no response to peripheral train-of-four stimulation, even though the diaphragm and larynx remain incompletely blocked. Subsequently, the onset of apnea is a poor clinical indicator of acceptable conditions for endotracheal intubation (102, 113). Alternatively, monitored evidence of adequate recovery from nondepolarizing neuromuscular paralysis (adductor pollicis brevis TOFR >0.7, sustained tetanic response without "fade")

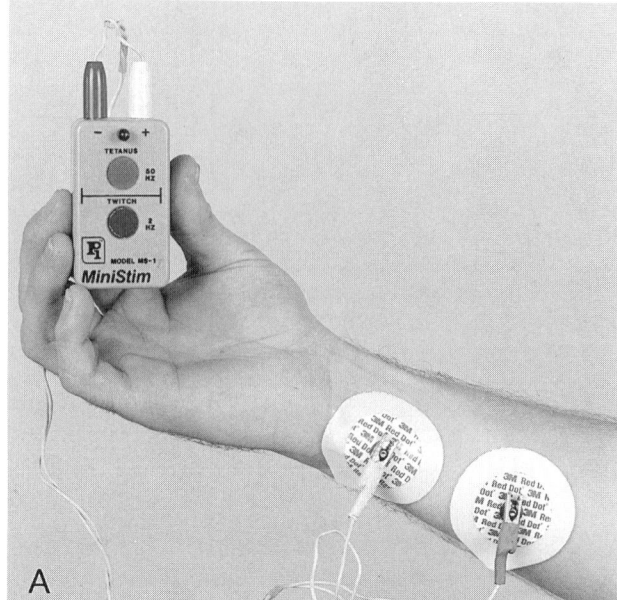

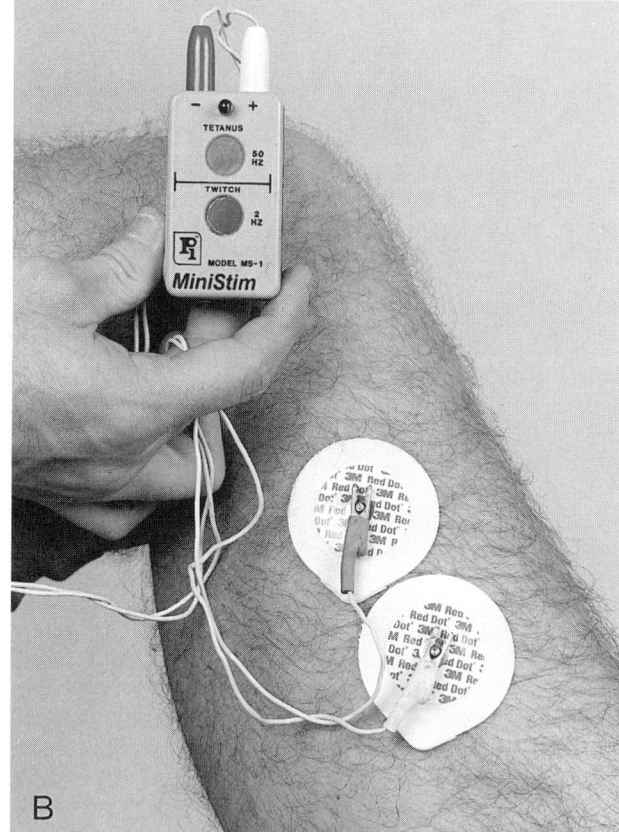

Figure 31.2.   Examples of appropriate neuromuscular blockade monitor positioning. **A,** Ulnar nerve at the wrist. **B,** Peroneal nerve at the neck of the fibula.

corresponds to clinical signs of acceptable recovery, such as sustained head lift for 5 seconds, a negative inspiratory pressure ≤-20 to 25 cm H_2O, and a forced vital capacity ≥15 to 20 ml/kg (102, 117). The supporting musculature of the upper airway, however, is very sensitive to small degrees of muscle relaxation, and the ability to maintain a patent airway in the

Table 31.16. Desirable Nerve Stimulator Traits

1. Constant current, supramaximal output[a]
2. Variable voltage delivery[b]
3. Rectangular (square wave) pulse
4. Pulse duration 0.1–0.3 msec
5. Ability to deliver train-of-four stimulation at 2 hz
6. Ability to deliver tetanic stimulus[c]
7. Stimulator polarity labelled

[a] ≥50–60 mA.
[b] Between 200 and 400 volts, ensuring that a supramaximal stimulus will be delivered over a wide range of impedances.
[c] 30–50 hz.

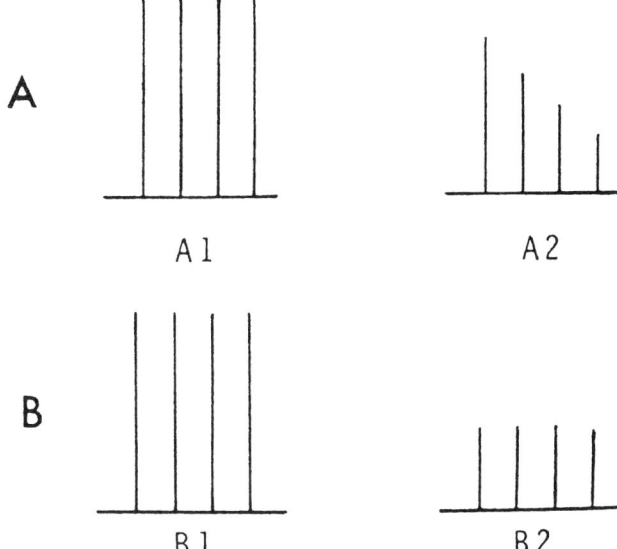

Figure 31.3. Schematic representation of train-of-four ratio changes after nondepolarizing (*A2*) and depolarizing (*B2*) drug administration. *A1* and *B1* represent respective predrug baseline measurements. (From Hudes E, Lee KC: Clinical use of peripheral nerve stimulators in anaesthesia. *Can J Anaesth* 34:525–534, 1987. Reproduced with permission.)

presence of residual sedation or the absence of an endotracheal tube is not addressed by these parameters (115, 118, 119). A study in normal volunteers suggests that sustained head lift (≥5 seconds) correlates with a negative inspiratory pressure of −55 cm H_2O and the ability to spontaneously maintain a patent protected airway (118). Thus, it is important to utilize a combination of peripheral nerve stimulation monitoring with clinical evidence of adequate neuromuscular and CNS recovery before electively extubating patients who previously have been maintained on neuromuscular blockade therapy. Furthermore, a full reassessment immediately after extubation is also mandatory.

CRITICAL CARE USE OF NEUROMUSCULAR BLOCKING DRUGS

Neuromuscular blocking agents possess no sedative or analgesic properties. Thus, administration of muscle relaxants to critically ill patients must be accompanied by appropriate doses of sedative-hypnotics and/or analgesic agents in order to avoid the profoundly unpleasant experience of awake "therapeutic" paralysis (120–123).

The primary use of succinylcholine in critical care is to facilitate rapid airway control and immediate endotracheal intubation. Loss of protective airway reflexes (CNS depressant drugs, pathologic intracranial processes, etc.), swift institution of therapeutic hyperventilation for intracranial hypertension, and severe refractory upper airway obstruction immediately post-extubation represent some examples in which succinylcholine may be indicated. Hyperkalemic cardiac arrest has been reported following administration of succinylcholine in the critically ill, and cautious assessment of succinylcholine's risks and benefits on an individual basis is warranted (124, 125).

The main indication for administering nondepolarizing relaxants to critically ill patients is to facilitate mechanical ventilation, although the establishment of adequate sedation and analgesia makes adjunctive use of neuromuscular blocking agents an infrequent necessity in most critical care units (121–123, 126). Other indications for competitive relaxant administration in this population include therapeutic hyperventilation for intracranial hypertension, diminishing total body oxygen consumption, and facilitation of bedside procedures and diagnostic studies (123). Pancuronium and vecuronium are the two agents most frequently utilized, with intermittent i.v. administration being the most common mode of delivery. A significant minority of clinicians, however, use a continuous infusion technique with or without administration of a preceding bolus (122, 123). The degree of blockade is typically monitored using clinical criteria (spontaneous movement or ventilatory effort), with only 21 to 34% using peripheral nerve stimulation monitoring. Even those physicians who use the latter monitoring modality do so infrequently (122, 123). Whether routine peripheral nerve stimulation monitoring to less dense degrees of paralysis would lower the incidence of postrelaxant myopathic weakness is not clear. The possibility exists that confounding drug therapy (antibiotics such as aminoglycosides and clindamycin, high-dose glucocorticoids) may play a role independent of the relaxant used (84, 85, 123, 127). It is likewise unknown whether these myopathic changes would result from similar durations of profound neuromuscular blockade using benzyl isoquinolinium relaxants. The effect of "drug holidays" from neuromuscular blockade therapy also requires further investigation.

REFERENCES

1. Weiner N, Taylor P: Neurohumoral transmission: the autonomic and somatic motor nervous systems. In Gilman AG, Goodman LS, Rall TW, Murad F (eds): *Goodman and Gilman's The Pharmacological Basis of Therapeutics*, ed 7. MacMillan, New York, 1985, pp 67–99.
2. Berne RM, Levy MN: The autonomic nervous system and its central control. In *Physiology*. CV Mosby, St. Louis, 1988, pp 280–296.
3. Wood M: Cholinergic and parasympathomimetic drugs. Cholinesterases and anticholinesterases. In Wood M, Wood AJJ (eds): *Drugs and Anesthesia*. Williams & Wilkins, Baltimore, 1982, pp 111–140.
4. Tabatabai M, Casper CT, Sanders CA, Price GS, Drobycki TE: Autonomic nervous system: clinical applications and anesthetic considerations. *Anesth Rev* 15:15–26, 1988.
5. Guyton AC: The autonomic nervous system: the adrenal medulla. In *Textbook of Medical Physiology*. WB Saunders, Philadelphia, 1981, pp 710–723.
6. Goyal RK: Muscarinic receptor subtypes. Physiology and clinical implications. *N Engl J Med* 321:1022–1029, 1989.
7. Goyal RK: Identification, localization and classification of muscarinic receptor subtypes in the gut. *Life Sci* 43(2):2209–2220, 1988.
8. Bonner TI, Young AC, Brann MR, Buckley NJ: Cloning and expression of the human and rat M_5 muscarinic acetylcholine receptor genes. *Neuron* 1:403–410, 1988.

9. Bonner TI, Buckley NJ, Young AC, Brann MR: Identification of a family of muscarinic acetylcholine receptor genes. *Science* 237:527–532, 1987.

10. Eglen RM, Whiting RL: Muscarinic receptor subtypes: a critique of the current classification and a proposal for a working nomenclature. *J Auton Pharmacol* 6:323–346, 1986.

11. Levine R, Birdsall NJM, North RA, Holman M, Watanabe A, Iversen LL: Subtypes of muscarinic receptors III. *Trends Pharmacol Sci* 9(suppl):1–93, 1988.

12. Liao CF, Themmen AP, Joho R, Barberis C, Birnbaumer M, Birnbaumer L: Molecular cloning and expression of a fifth muscarinic acetylcholine receptor. *J Biol Chem* 264:7328–7337, 1989.

13. Rand MJ: Neuropharmacological effects of nicotine in relation to cholinergic mechanisms. *Prog Brain Res* 79:3–11, 1989.

14. Braman SS, Corrao W, Fregault R, et al: Methacholine bronchoprovocation: adverse effects and clinical safety. *Am Rev Respir Dis* 129(part 2):A28–A37, 1984.

15. Irwin RS, Pratter MR: The clinical value of pharmacologic bronchoprovocation challenge. *Med Clin North Am* 74:767–778, 1990.

16. Davidson M, Stern RG, Bierer LM, Horvath TB, Zemishlani Z, Markofsky R, Mohs RC: Cholinergic strategies in the treatment of Alzheimer's disease. *Acta Psychiatr Scand* 366(suppl):47–51, 1991.

17. Bartlett JD: Adverse effects of antiglaucoma medications. *Optom Clin* 1:103–126, 1991.

18. Kalsner S: Cholinergic constriction in the general circulation and its role in coronary artery spasm. *Circ Res* 65:237–257, 1989.

19. AMA Division of Drugs: *AMA Drug Evaluations*, ed 5. American Medical Association, Chicago, 1983.

20. Bevan DR, Bevan JC, Donati F: The neuromuscular junction: structure and function. In *Muscle Relaxants in Clinical Anesthesia*. Yearbook Medical Publishers, Chicago, 1988, pp 13–48.

21. Pantuck EJ, Pantuck CB: Cholinesterases and anticholinesterases. In Katz RL (ed): *Muscle Relaxants: Monographs in Anesthesiology*. Elsevier North-Holland, New York, 1975, pp 143–162.

22. Newton RW: Physostigmine salicylate in the treatment of tricyclic antidepressant overdosage. *JAMA* 231:941–943, 1975.

23. Rumack BH: Anticholinergic poisoning: treatment with physostigmine. *Pediatrics* 52:449–451, 1973.

24. Bevan DR, Bevan JC, Donati F: Depolarizing agents: succinylcholine. In *Muscle Relaxants in Clinical Anesthesia*. Year Book, Chicago, 1988, pp 247–277.

25. Waud DR: The nature of "depolarization block." *Anesthesiology* 29:1014–1024, 1968.

26. Litwiller RW: Succinylcholine hydrolysis: a review. *Anesthesiology* 31:356–360, 1969.

27. Waud DR, Waud BE: Depolarization block and phase II block at the neuromuscular junction. *Anesthesiology* 43:10–20, 1975.

28. Viby-Mogensen J: Correlation of succinylcholine duration of action with plasma cholinesterase activity in subjects with genotypically normal enzyme. *Anesthesiology* 53:517–520, 1980.

29. Donati F, Bevan DR: Long-term succinylcholine infusion during isoflurane anesthesia. *Anesthesiology* 58:6–10, 1983.

30. Viby-Mogensen J: Cholinesterase and succinylcholine. *Dan Med Bull* 30:129–150, 1983.

31. Ostergaard D, Viby-Mogensen J: Prolonged apnea after succinylcholine: etiology, diagnosis, and management. *Probl Anesth* 3:455–464, 1989.

32. Viby-Mogensen J: Succinylcholine neuromuscular blockade in subjects heterozygous for abnormal plasma cholinesterase. *Anesthesiology* 55:231–235, 1981.

33. Lee C: Dose relationships of phase II, tachyphylaxis and train-of-four fade in suxamethonium-induced dual neuromuscular blockade in man. *Br J Anaesth* 47:841–845, 1975.

34. Williams CH, Deutsch S, Linde HW, Bullough JW, Dripps RD: Effects of intravenously administered succinyldicholine on cardiac rate, rhythm, and arterial blood pressure in anesthetized man. *Anesthesiology* 22:947–954, 1961.

35. Gibb DB: Suxamethonium—a review. Pharmacologic actions of suxamethonium apart from its neuromuscular blocking effect. *Anaesth Intensive Care* 2:9–26, 1974.

36. Ryan JF, Kagen LJ, Hyman AI: Myoglobinemia after a single dose of succinylcholine. *N Engl J Med* 285:824–827, 1971.

37. Stewart KG, Hopkins PM, Dean SG: Comparison of high and low doses of suxamethonium. *Anaesthesia* 46:833–836, 1991.

38. Miller RD, Way WL: Inhibition of succinylcholine-induced increased intragastric pressure by nondepolarizing muscle relaxants and lidocaine. *Anesthesiology* 34:185–188, 1971.

39. Smith G, Dalling R, Williams TIR: Gastro-oesophageal pressure gradient changes produced by induction of anaesthesia and suxamethonium. *Br J Anaesth* 50:1137–1143, 1978.

40. Cunningham AJ, Barry P: Intraocular pressure—physiology and implications for anesthetic management. *Can Anaesth Soc J* 33:195–208, 1986.

41. Libonati MM, Leahy JJ, Ellison N: The use of succinylcholine in open eye surgery. *Anesthesiology* 62:637–640, 1985.

42. Minton MD, Grosslight K, Stirt JA, Bedford RF: Increases in intracranial pressure from succinylcholine: prevention by prior nondepolarizing blockade. *Anesthesiology* 65:165–169, 1986.

43. Stirt JA, Grosslight KR, Bedford RF, Vollmer D: "Defasciculation" with metocurine prevents succinylcholine-induced increases in intracranial pressure. *Anesthesiology* 67:50–53, 1987.

44. Azar I: The response of patients with neuromuscular disorders to muscle relaxants: a review. *Anesthesiology* 61:173–187, 1984.

45. Schatz M, Fung DL: Anaphylactic and anaphylactoid reactions due to anesthetic agents. *Clin Rev Allergy* 4:215–227, 1986.

46. Fisher MM: Anaphylaxis. *Dis Mon* 33:438–479, 1987.

47. Fisher DM: Should succinylcholine continue to be used routinely in pediatric anesthesia? *Probl Anesth* 3:394–404, 1989.

48. Weintraub HD, Heisterkamp DV, Cooperman LH: Changes in plasma potassium concentration after depolarizing blockers in anaesthetized man. *Br J Anaesth* 41:1048–1052, 1969.

49. Fung DL, White DA, Jones BR, Gronert GA: The onset of disuse-related potassium efflux to succinylcholine. *Anesthesiology* 75:650–653, 1991.

50. Gronert GA, Theye RA: Pathophysiology of hyperkalemia induced by succinylcholine. *Anesthesiology* 43:89–99, 1975.

51. Martyn JAJ, White DA, Gronert GA, Jaffe RS, Ward JM: Up-and-down regulation of skeletal muscle acetylcholine receptors. Effects on neuromuscular blockers. *Anesthesiology* 76:822–843, 1992.

52. Brown TCK, Bell B: Electromyographic response to small doses of suxamethonium in children after burns. *Br J Anaesth* 59:1017–1021, 1987.

53. McLoughlin C, Elliott P, McCarthy G, Mirakhur RK: Muscle pains and biochemical changes following suxamethonium administration after six pretreatment regimens. *Anaesthesia* 47:202–206, 1992.

54. Freund FG, Rubin AP: The need for additional succinylcholine after d-tubocurarine. *Anesthesiology* 36:185–187, 1972.

55. Waud BE, Waud DR: The margin of safety of neuromuscular transmission in the muscle of the diaphragm. *Anesthesiology* 37:417–422, 1972.

56. Shanks CA: Pharmacokinetics of the nondepolarizing neuromuscular relaxants applied to calculation of bolus and infusion dosage regimens. *Anesthesiology* 64:72–86, 1986.

57. Rupp SM: The priming principle. *Probl Anesth* 3:436–446, 1989.

58. Lennon RL, Olson RA, Gronert GA: Atracurium or vecuronium for rapid sequence endotracheal intubation. *Anesthesiology* 64:510–513, 1986.

59. Glass PSA, Wilson W, Mace JA, Wagoner R: Is the priming principle both effective and safe? *Anesth Analg* 68:127–134, 1989.

60. Musich J, Walts LF: Pulmonary aspiration after a priming dose of vecuronium. *Anesthesiology* 64:517–519, 1986.

61. Bevan DR, Bevan JC, Donati F: Nondepolarizing relaxants. In *Muscle Relaxants in Clinical Anesthesia*. Year Book, Chicago, 1988, pp 133–246.

62. Diefenbach C, Mellinghoff H, Grond S, Buzello W: Atracurium and vecuronium: repeated bolus injection versus infusion. *Anesth Analg* 74:519–522, 1992.

63. Savarese JJ, Ali HH, Basta SJ, Embree PB, Scott RP, Sunder N, Weakly JN, Wastila WB, el Sayad HA: The clinical neuromuscular pharmacology of mivacurium chloride (BW B1090U). A short-acting nondepolarizing ester neuromuscular blocking drug. *Anesthesiology* 68:723–732, 1988.

64. Brandom BW: Is there a place for infusion of muscle relaxants in clinical anesthesia? *Probl Anesth* 3:421–435, 1989.

65. Ali HH, Savarese JJ, Basta SJ, Sunder N, Gionfriddo M: Evaluation of cumulative properties of three new nondepolarizing neuromuscular blocking drugs BW A444U, atracurium, and vecuronium. *Br J Anaesth* 55(suppl):107S–111S, 1983.

66. Basta SJ, Savarese JJ, Ali HH, Embree PB, Schwartz AF, Rudd GD, Wastila WB: Clinical pharmacology of doxacurium chloride. A new long-acting nondepolarizing muscle relaxant. *Anesthesiology* 69:478–486, 1988.

67. Larijani GE, Bartkowski RR, Azad SS, Seltzer JL, Weinberger MJ, Beach CA, Goldberg ME: Clinical pharmacology of pipecuronium bromide. *Anesth Analg* 68:734–739, 1989.

68. Stoelting RK: The hemodynamic effects of pancuronium and d-tubocurarine in anesthetized patients. *Anesthesiology* 36:612–615, 1972.

69. Basta SJ: Release of histamine by nondepolarizing neuromuscular blocking agents. *Anesthesiol Rev* 16:19–23, 1989.

70. Savarese JJ, Ali HH, Basta SJ, Scott RP, Embree PB, Wastila WB, Abou-Donia MM, Gelb C: The cardiovascular effects of mivacurium chloride (BW B1090U) in patients receiving nitrous oxide-opiate-barbiturate anesthesia. *Anesthesiology* 70:386–394, 1989.

71. McCullough LS, Reier CE, Delaunois AL, Gardier RW, Hamelberg W: The effects of d-tubocurarine on spontaneous postganglionic sympathetic activity and histamine release. *Anesthesiology* 33:328–334, 1970.

72. Savarese JJ: The autonomic margin of safety of metocurine and d-tubocurarine in the cat. *Anesthesiology* 50:40–46, 1979.

73. Kelman GR, Kennedy BR: Cardiovascular effects of pancuronium in man. *Br J Anaesth* 43:335–338, 1971.

74. Chapple DJ, Miller AA, Ward JB, Wheatley PL: Cardiovascular and neurological effects of laudanosine. Studies in mice and rats, and in conscious and anaesthetized dogs. *Br J Anaesth* 59:218–225, 1987.

75. Yate PM, Flynn PJ, Arnold RW, Weatherly BC, Simmonds RJ, Dopson T: Clinical experience and plasma laudanosine concentrations during the infusion of atracurium in the intensive therapy unit. *Br J Anaesth* 59:211–217, 1987.

76. Harle DG, Baldo BA, Fisher MM: Cross-reactivity of metocurine, atracurium, vecuronium, and fazidinium with IgE antibodies from patients unexposed to

these drugs but allergic to other myoneural blocking drugs. *Br J Anaesth* 57:1073–1076, 1985.

77. Hunter JM: Resistance to non-depolarizing neuromuscular blocking agents [Editorial]. *Br J Anaesth* 67:511–514, 1991.

78. Buzello W, Noeldge G, Krieg N, Brobmann GF: Vecuronium for muscle relaxation in patients with myasthenia gravis. *Anesthesiology* 64:507–509, 1986.

79. Ono K, Nagano O, Ohta Y, Kosaka F: Neuromuscular effects of respiratory and metabolic acid-base changes in vitro with and without nondepolarizing muscle relaxants. *Anesthesiology* 73:710–716, 1990.

80. Robinson BJ, Lee E, Rees D, Purdie GL, Galletley DC: Betamethasone-induced resistance to neuromuscular blockade: a comparison of atracurium and vecuronium in vitro. *Anesth Analg* 74:762–765, 1992.

81. Dwersteg JF, Pavlin EG, Heimbach DM: Patients with burns are resistant to atracurium. *Anesthesiology* 65:517–520, 1986.

82. Bevan DR, Bevan JC, Donati F: Renal and hepatic disease. In *Muscle Relaxants in Clinical Anesthesia.* Year Book, Chicago, 1988, pp 317–344.

83. Bevan DR, Bevan JC, Donati F: Drug interactions. In *Muscle Relaxants in Clinical Anesthesia.* Year Book, Chicago, 1988, pp 389–413.

84. Partridge BL, Abrams JH, Bazemore C, Rubin R: Prolonged neuromuscular blockade after long-term infusion of vecuronium bromide in the intensive care unit. *Crit Care Med* 18:1177–1179, 1990.

85. Op de Coul AAW, Lambregts PC, Koeman J, van Puyenbroek MJ, Ter Laak HJ, Gabreels-Festen AA: Neuromuscular complications in patients given Pavulon (pancuronium bromide) during artificial ventilation. *Clin Neurol Neurosurg* 87:17–22, 1985.

86. Caldwell JE: Muscle relaxants in renal failure. *Probl Anesth* 3:489–499, 1989.

87. Meijer DK, Weitering JG, Vermeer GA, Scaf AH: Comparative pharmacokinetics of d-tubocurarine and metocurine in man. *Anesthesiology* 51:402–407, 1979.

88. Agoston S, Vermeer GA, Kertsten UW, Meijer DK: The fate of pancuronium bromide in man. *Acta Anaesthesiol Scand* 17:267–275, 1973.

89. Magorian T, Lynam DP: Clinical use of muscle relaxants in patients with hepatic disease. *Probl Anesth* 3:500–509, 1989.

90. Marshall IG, Gibb AJ, Durant NN: Neuromuscular and vagal blocking actions of pancuronium bromide, its metabolites, and vecuronium bromide (ORG NC 45) and its potential metabolites in the anesthetized cat. *Br J Anaesth* 55:703–714, 1983.

91. Cook DR, Stiller RL, Weakly JN, Chakravorti S, Brandom BW, Welch RM: In vitro metabolism of mivacurium chloride (BW B1090U) and succinylcholine. *Anesth Analg* 68:452–456, 1989.

92. Merrett RA, Thompson CW, Webb FW: In vitro degradation of atracurium in human plasma. *Br J Anaesth* 55:61–66, 1983.

93. Nigrovic V, Pandya JB, Auen M, Wajskol A: Inactivation of atracurium in human and rat plasma. *Anesth Analg* 64:1047–1052, 1985.

94. Fisher DM, Canfell PC, Fahey MR, Rosen JI, Rupp SM, Sheiner LB, Miller RD: Elimination of atracurium in humans: contribution of Hofmann elimination and ester hydrolysis versus organ-based elimination. *Anesthesiology* 65:6–12, 1986.

95. Stiller RL, Cook DR, Chakravorti S: In vitro degradation of atracurium in human plasma. *Br J Anaesth* 57:1085–1088, 1985.

96. Baraka A, Wakid N, Noueihed R, Karam H, Bolotova N: Pseudocholinesterase activity and atracurium versus suxamethonium block. *Br J Anaesth* 58(suppl):91S–95S, 1986.

97. Ward S, Neill EAM: Pharmacokinetics of atracurium in acute hepatic failure (with acute renal failure). *Br J Anaesth* 55:1169–1172, 1983.

98. Fahey MR, Rupp SM, Fisher DM, Miller RD, Sharma M, Canfell C, Castagnoli K, Hennis PJ: The pharmacokinetics and pharmacodynamics of atracurium in patients with and without renal failure. *Anesthesiology* 61:699–702, 1984.

99. Bevan DR, Bevan JC, Donati F: Pharmacology: antagonists. In *Muscle Relaxants in Clinical Anesthesia.* Year Book, Chicago, 1988, pp 293–316.

100. Kopman AF: Antagonism of profound neuromuscular blockade. *Probl Anesth* 3:405–420, 1989.

101. Ferguson A, Egerszegi P, Bevan DR: Neostigmine, pyridostigmine, and edrophonium as antagonists of pancuronium. *Anesthesiology* 53:390–394, 1980.

102. Bevan DR, Bevan JC, Donati F: Clinical measurement. In *Muscle Relaxants in Clinical Anesthesia.* Year Book, Chicago, 1988, pp 49–70.

103. Lee C, Tran BK: Clinical monitoring of neuromuscular function. *Probl Anesth* 3:379–393, 1989.

104. Hudes E, Lee KC: Clinical use of peripheral nerve stimulators in anaesthesia. *Can J Anaesth* 34:525–534, 1987.

105. Caffrey RR, Warren ML, Becker KE Jr: Neuromuscular blockade monitoring comparing the orbicularis oculi and adductor pollicis muscles. *Anesthesiology* 65:95–97, 1986.

106. Kopman AF: A safe surface electrode for peripheral-nerve stimulation. *Anesthesiology* 44:343–345, 1976.

107. Kopman AF, Lawson D: Milliamperage requirements for supramaximal stimulation of the ulnar nerve with surface electrodes. *Anesthesiology* 61:83–85, 1984.

108. Epstein RA, Jackson SH: Repetitive muscle depolarization from single indirect stimulation in anesthetized man. *J Appl Physiol* 28:407–410, 1970.

109. Ali HH, Utting JE, Gray TC: Quantitative assessment of residual antidepolarizing block (part I). *Br J Anaesth* 43:473–477, 1971.

110. Curran MJ, Donati F, Bevan DR: Onset and recovery of atracurium and suxamethonium-induced neuromuscular blockade with simultaneous train-of-four and single twitch stimulation. *Br J Anaesth* 59:989–994, 1987.

111. Viby-Mogensen J, Jensen HH, Engbaek J, Ording H, Skovgaard LT, Chraemmer-Jorgensen B: Tactile and visual evaluation of the response to train-of-four nerve stimulation. *Anesthesiology* 63:440–443, 1985.

112. Merton PR: Voluntary strength and fatigue. *J Physiol* 123:553–564, 1954.

113. Donati F, Antzaka C, Bevan DR: Potency of pancuronium at the diaphragm and the adductor pollicis muscle in humans. *Anesthesiology* 65:1–5, 1986.

114. Chauvin M, Lebrault C, Duvaldestin P: The neuromuscular blocking effect of vecuronium on the human diaphragm. *Anesth Analg* 66:117–122, 1987.

115. Donati F, Bevan DR: Not all muscles are the same [Editorial]. *Br J Anaesth* 68:235–236, 1992.

116. de Troyer A, Bastenier J, Delhez L: Function of respiratory muscles during partial curarization in humans. *J Appl Physiol* 49:1049–1056, 1980.

117. Ali HH, Wilson RS, Savarese JJ, Kitz RJ: The effect of tubocurarine on indirectly elicited train-of-four muscle response and respiratory measurements in humans. *Br J Anaesth* 47:570–574, 1975.

118. Pavlin EG, Holle RH, Schoene RB: Recovery of airway protection compared with ventilation in humans after paralysis with curare. *Anesthesiology* 70:381–385, 1989.

119. Isono S, Kochi T, Ide T, Sugimori K, Mizuguchi T, Nishino T: Differential effects of vecuronium on diaphragm and geniohyoid muscle in anaesthetized dogs. *Br J Anaesth* 68:239–243, 1992.

120. Parker MM, Schubert W, Shelhamer JH, Parrillo JE: Perceptions of a critically ill patient experiencing therapeutic paralysis in an ICU. *Crit Care Med* 12:69–71, 1984.

121. Aitkenhead AR. Analgesia and sedation in intensive care. *Br J Anaesth* 63:196–206, 1989.

122. Hansen-Flaschen JH, Brazinsky S, Basile C, Lanken PN: Use of sedating drugs and neuromuscular blocking agents in patients requiring mechanical ventilation for respiratory failure: a national survey. *JAMA* 266:2870–2875, 1991.

123. Klessig HT, Geiger HJ, Murray MJ, Coursin DB: A national survey on the practice patterns of anesthesiologist intensivists in the use of muscle relaxants. *Crit Care Med* 20:1341–1345, 1992.

124. Horton WA, Ferguson NV: Hyperkalaemia and cardiac arrest after the use of suxamethonium in intensive care (letter). *Anaesthesia* 43:890–891, 1988.

125. Hemming AE, Charlton S, Kelly P: Hyperkalaemia, cardiac arrest, suxamethonium, and intensive care (Letter). *Anaesthesia* 45:990–991, 1990.

126. Sun X, Quinn T, Weissman C: Patterns of sedation and analgesia in the postoperative ICU patient. *Chest* 101:1625–1632, 1992.

127. Griffin D, Fairman N, Coursin D, Rawsthorne L, Grossman JE: Acute myopathy during treatment of status asthmaticus with corticosteroids and steroidal muscle relaxants. *Chest* 102:510–514, 1992.

CHAPTER 32

Parkinson's Disease and Other Disorders of Movement and Tone

HOWARD D. WEISS, M.D.

The cortico-striatal-pallido-thalamo-cortical system (extrapyramidal system) provides the subconscious inputs that help plan and execute the voluntary motor activity of the pyramidal tracts. Disorders that damage structures in the extrapyramidal system can "uncouple" the pyramidal tracts from this important modulation, resulting in difficulty with rapid and appropriate sequencing of tone and movement (e.g., bradykinesia, rigidity, postural instability) or hyperkinesias (e.g., tremor, chorea) (1, 2).

There has been a tremendous growth in our understanding of the physiology and neuropharmacology of the extrapyramidal pathways. The major excitatory and inhibitory neurotransmitters have been identified and localized (3) (Fig. 32.1). This explosion of knowledge has resulted in major advances in the treatment of Parkinson's disease, tremor, spasticity, and other disorders that affect movement and tone. Familiarity with the diagnosis and pharmacologic management of these commonly encountered neurologic disorders is important in treating outpatients or the critically ill hospitalized patient.

PARKINSON'S DISEASE

Parkinson's disease (PD) usually begins in middle to late adult life. Although the cause is unknown, by age 70 approximately 2% of the population is afflicted with PD, making it one of the most common neurologic disorders (4, 5). As a result of therapeutic breakthroughs during the past two decades, patients with PD who were once condemned to a shortened

life and complete invalidism can now anticipate a nearly normal life expectancy (6).

The cardinal clinical signs of PD—tremor at rest, bradykinesia, "cogwheel" rigidity, and loss of postural reflexes—were first described in the 19th century (7). These neurologic abnormalities lead to the "shuffling" gait, unsteadiness, "masked facies," drooling, micrographia, and impairment of speech that characterize PD. The clinical expression of the disease is variable. Some patients have tremor as the dominant clinical symptom, whereas others have little or no tremor but manifest marked postural instability and gait difficulty (8). The neuropathologic changes accompanying the condition—degeneration of pigmented neurons in the substantia nigra, and eosinophilic intraneuronal inclusions (Lewy bodies)—were described in the early 20th century. However, PD was viewed as a hopeless neurodegenerative disorder until the landmark neurochemistry discoveries of the 1960s (9). Studies of the regional concentration of dopamine in the brain revealed a striking deficiency (less than 10% of normal) in the caudate and putamen of patients dying with PD (10). Dopamine was identified as the neurotransmitter of the nigrostriatal tract, and PD became recognized as a disease of central dopamine depletion (11). Striatal dopamine replacement using the dopamine precursor levodopa produced dramatic amelioration of the cardinal signs and symptoms of PD (12, 13). PD became the first neurodegenerative disorder to be palliated by neurotransmitter replacement therapy, a true revolution in neurotherapeutics. Now, in addition to levodopa, newer strategies, including the use of direct-acting dopamine receptor agonists (bromocriptine, pergolide) and treatments that might possibly slow progression of the disease (selegiline), have broadened our ability to improve the quality of life for patients with PD (14).

In the early 1980s, a group of heroin addicts in California developed an acute illness closely resembling PD. These patients had injected themselves with a synthetic meperidine analog that was contaminated by 1-methyl-4-phenyl-1,2,3,6-tetrahydropyridine (MPTP) (15, 16). Injection of MPTP in humans and monkeys causes selective destruction of nigrostriatal dopamine neurons. The neurotoxicity of MPTP is caused by a metabolite, 1-methyl-4-phenylpyridine (MPP+), that selectively accumulates in dopamine terminals. MPTP is converted to MPP+ by the enzyme monoamine oxidase-B (MAO-B). Pretreatment with MAO-B inhibitors (such as selegiline, also known as deprenyl) can prevent the neurotoxic effects of MPTP in animals (17, 18).

These observations have led to an extensive search for naturally occurring MPTP-like chemicals that might lead to spontaneously occurring PD. Although at present there is little evidence to suggest that an exogenous environmental toxin causes PD (19), endogenous oxidative mechanisms in the brain may be a factor (20). There is evidence of mitochondrial oxidative phosphorylation defects in PD. An increase in substantia nigra lipid peroxidation by free radicals has been implicated as a factor in the selective death of dopamine neurons in PD (21, 21a).

The possibility that antioxidant therapy with the MAO-B inhibitor selegiline might exert a neuroprotective effect and slow the progression of PD has been explored in a large prospective trial (22). Selegiline, when administered to newly diagnosed patients with very mild PD, delayed the need for

levodopa therapy by about 1 year compared with placebo. By implication, selegiline may slow disease progression (23, 23a, 23b). Newly diagnosed patients with PD are now being treated routinely with selegiline. Research efforts are being directed at detecting PD at its very earliest stages (or even before symptoms are clinically apparent), when treatment with a neuroprotective agent would theoretically be of most benefit (24).

Selegiline is administered in a dose of 5 mg twice daily. At this dose it is a potent, selective, and irreversible inhibitor of MAO-B. After stopping the drug, MAO-B activity is >50% inhibited at 1 week and does not return to normal for 2 to 3 weeks. At the dose of 5 mg twice daily the drug does not inhibit monoamine oxidase-A (MAO-A), unlike the nonspecific MAO-A and -B inhibitors that are used to treat depression (such as phenelzine, pargyline, or isocarboxazid) (25). The inhibition of MAO-A is responsible for the severe hypertensive crises associated with sympathomimetic medications or the ingestion of foods containing tyramine ("cheese effect"). No special dietary restrictions are necessary in patients taking selegiline 5 mg twice daily (26). However, at higher doses, selegiline will lose its "selectivity" and also inhibit MAO-A, resulting in the potential for serious adverse reactions as with the other nonselective MAO inhibitors.

MAO-B is one of the catabolic enzymes of dopamine, and consequently, inhibition of this enzyme will prolong the action of levodopa. This effect may be beneficial in patients with advancing PD who have fluctuations in motor function resulting from the progressively shorter duration of action of levodopa (27, 28). However, patients who are already taking levodopa and are then started on selegiline often require a modest reduction of levodopa dosage (perhaps by 10 to 30%)

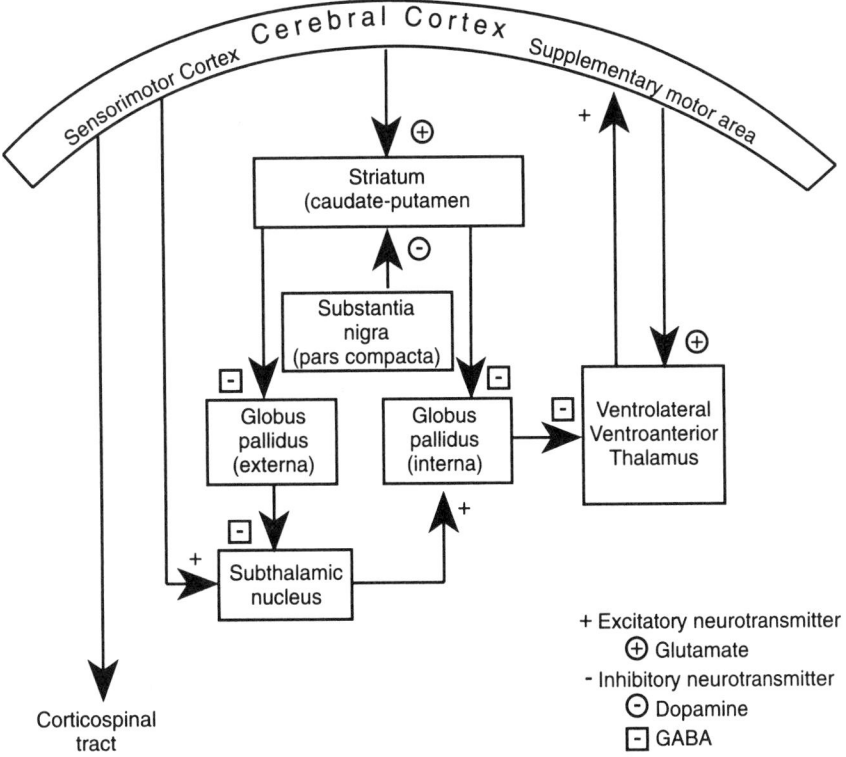

Figure 32.1. Simplified diagram of basal ganglia-thalamocortical circuitry and neurotransmitters.

Table 32.1.   Medications Currently Used in Parkinson's Disease

Type of Medication	Major Uses	Disadvantages
Dopamine precursor		
Levodopa	Most effective therapy to reverse clinical features	GI and psychiatric side effects; dyskinesia and
Carbidopa-levodopa	of Parkinson's disease (PD)	"on-off" symptoms with chronic use
Controlled release		
carbidopa-levodopa		
Dopamine agonists		
Bromocriptine	Adjunct to levodopa in patients with fluctuating	Less effective than levodopa as monotherapy;
Pergolide	motor symptoms; monotherapy in early PD	dose-related psychiatric side effects
MAO-B inhibitor		
Selegiline	"Neuroprotective therapy" to retard progression	Enhances dose-related levodopa side effects
	of PD; extends duration of levodopa effect in	
	patients with fluctuating motor symptoms	
Amantadine	Very mild PD to delay use of levodopa; drug-induced parkinsonism	Limited efficacy
Anticholinergics	Severe tremor; drug-induced parkinsonism	Limited efficacy; central and peripheral anticholinergic side effects

to avert choreiform movements, visual hallucinations, and other symptoms of dopamine excess (as outlined later in this chapter) (29).

Depression is a common accompaniment of PD. Selegiline is not an antidepressant. Some patients may experience a sense of well-being as a result of *l*-amphetamine metabolites, which are very mild stimulants (in contrast to the more potent *d*-amphetamine, which is not a metabolite of selegiline) (30, 31). For this reason, the drug can cause insomnia, and the two daily doses should be taken during the first half of the day and not at night. Clinical experience suggests that the tricyclic antidepressants may be used safely concomitantly with selegiline. There is an anecdotal report of an adverse reaction between fluoxetine and selegiline (32).

When used alone, selegiline has no particular effect in palliating the symptoms of PD. Many newly diagnosed PD patients have minimal disability and do not require immediate symptomatic treatment. However, with time, when the patient begins to experience increasing symptoms (e.g., slowing of gait, increasing rigidity, difficulty with daily activities), symptomatic treatment is indicated and usually is highly effective (Table 32.1) (33). For relatively mild symptoms, amantadine 100 mg twice a day might be considered as initial therapy (34). In patients with prominent parkinsonian tremor but little other symptomatology, anticholinergic agents (e.g., benztropine, trihexyphenidyl, or ethopropazine) would be a reasonable first consideration (35). The benefit of these drugs in PD is modest but may allow a delay in the introduction of levodopa or dopamine agonist therapy for several months to a year (36), or may serve as an adjunct for patients with advanced PD in whom levodopa therapy is losing efficacy (37).

Levodopa is unquestionably the most effective drug in palliating the cardinal symptoms of PD (38). However, there is a theoretic concern that the metabolic products of levodopa may contribute to neuronal damage in the substantia nigra as well as the development of late motor complications in PD (20). If this were the case, one could argue for delaying treatment with levodopa as long as possible (39). Clinical evidence clearly suggests that levodopa is not neurotoxic, and that the late complications of PD reflect the severity of the illness rather than the duration of levodopa treatment (40, 41). Postponing treatment with levodopa has no long-term benefit and merely deprives the patient of several years of optimal

therapeutic response (42). Current strategies involve the use of relatively low-dose levodopa, adding direct-acting dopamine receptor agonists (bromocriptine or pergolide) if necessary to achieve an optimal clinical response (43).

Levodopa is the metabolic precursor of dopamine, being decarboxylated to dopamine by the enzyme aromatic amino acid decarboxylase. Levodopa is a large neutral amino acid (LNAA) and is absorbed via the LNAA active transport system in the duodenum and proximal small intestine. Gastric emptying, changes in pH, the physical barrier of recently ingested food, and competition for active transport with other LNAA all affect the ultimate blood levels of levodopa following a dose (44, 45). There is considerable variability in the absorption of levodopa. Peak levodopa blood levels are usually reached 30 to 60 minutes after a dose, and the plasma half-life is 1 to 2 hours (46). Levodopa must then survive passage through the portal circulation to enter the systemic circulation.

Levodopa ultimately reaches the blood-brain barrier, where it competes for entry to the brain with other LNAAs via an active transport mechanism (47). Once in the brain, surviving nigrostriatal nerve terminals (and perhaps glial cells) convert the levodopa to dopamine (48). The dopamine is stored and released close to available striatal dopamine receptors to exert its clinical effects (49). Dopamine itself, when administered systemically, will not palliate PD, as it does not cross the blood-brain barrier. Aromatic amino acid decarboxylase is present in gut epithelial cells and will convert levodopa to dopamine. This action not only greatly limits the amount of levodopa available to the brain, but dramatically increases the systemic side-effects of levodopa. Nausea, vomiting, and anorexia caused by peripherally formed dopamine were major dose-limiting problems in the initial clinical trials of levodopa therapy (12, 50). Consequently, levodopa is now used exclusively in combination with drugs that inhibit peripheral aromatic amino acid decarboxylase but do not cross the blood-brain barrier to inhibit the CNS aromatic amino acid decarboxylase. Peripheral decarboxylase inhibitors increase the proportion of levodopa that enters the brain and thereby allow the dose of levodopa to be reduced 4- to 5-fold (51). At the same time, concurrent levodopa-decarboxylase inhibitor therapy reduces the amount of dopamine produced systemically, resulting in a marked reduction of gastrointestinal side-effects.

The plasma half-life of levodopa is increased to 2 to 3 hours when administered with a decarboxylase inhibitor.

The peripheral aromatic amino acid decarboxylase inhibitors used in combination with levodopa are carbidopa (in the U.S.) and benserazide (in Europe). Three fixed dose carbidopa/levodopa combinations are available: 10 mg/100 mg, 25 mg/100 mg, and 25 mg/250 mg. Most patients require at least 75 to 100 mg of carbidopa per day for optimal inhibition of the peripheral decarboxylase (52).

Carbidopa/levodopa is introduced gradually. There is considerable variation, but most patients with mild to moderate PD will have an excellent therapeutic response to a dose of 25/100 mg 1 to 1 1/2 tablets three times daily. The strategy is to administer the lowest dose possible that will provide adequate symptomatic relief, as many of the acute and late side-effects of carbidopa/levodopa therapy are dose related (53, 54). In general, the drug should be given on an empty stomach 15 to 30 minutes before meals to ensure reliable drug absorption. Nighttime doses are not necessary in most patients with mild to moderate PD and can be associated with visual hallucinations and sleep disruption (55). If the patient is already receiving amantadine or an anticholinergic, these drugs may be tapered and withdrawn once an optimal response to carbidopa/levodopa is attained.

A small proportion of patients will experience intense nausea or anorexia despite the use of carbidopa with levodopa. These patients may benefit from taking the carbidopa/levodopa with or after meals, or may require extra doses of carbidopa (25 mg) in addition to the fixed dose carbidopa/levodopa to inhibit more completely the aromatic amino acid decarboxylase. Domperidone, a peripheral dopamine antagonist without central effects, is useful in alleviating the gastrointestinal side-effects of levodopa and the direct-acting dopamine agonists (56), but it is not currently available in the U.S.

A controlled release preparation is now available, containing 50 mg of carbidopa and 200 mg of levodopa (57, 58). This preparation has the advantage of longer half-life, the ingredients being released over 4 to 6 hours, with a slower increase and decrease in blood levodopa levels compared with standard carbidopa/levodopa (59). This preparation is particularly advantageous in patients with advanced PD but theoretically may also reduce the possibility of late motor fluctuations in patients with mild to moderate disease (60). A typical dose in a patient with mild to moderate PD would be controlled release carbidopa/levodopa two or three times daily, with doses being taken 5 to 6 hours apart. The controlled release preparation should not be crushed or chewed, as it would then lose its sustained release pharmacokinetic property. The absorption of levodopa from the controlled release preparation is 10 to 30% less than that from standard carbidopa/levodopa. Therefore, patients may require 20 to 30% more controlled release carbidopa/levodopa to achieve a therapeutic response equivalent to that of standard carbidopa/levodopa (59).

Failure of a patient with early PD to respond favorably to initial treatment with levodopa may simply reflect insufficient dosage. In the absence of a drug interaction, it is appropriate to reconsider the diagnosis of PD when initial treatment is of no benefit (61).

Most patients with mild to moderate PD experience several years of "honeymoon" during which time levodopa produces sustained benefit throughout the day. The patient will not notice if a dose is late or missed entirely (61b). It is estimated that 80% of striatal dopamine is already depleted by the time the earliest signs of PD appear, with virtually total depletion in the posterior putamen (62). Nevertheless, there are enough remaining nigral neurons so that the dopamine synthesized from the exogenous levodopa can be stored in the striatum and released when necessary (48). This storage provides a "buffering" effect so that in mild PD the clinical symptoms are not dependent on moment-to-moment fluctuations in available brain levodopa.

Unfortunately, as years go by and additional nigral neurons degenerate, the striatal "buffering" capacity is lost (63), and many patients develop fluctuations in the severity of their PD symptoms (64). After 5 years of levodopa treatment, 50% of patients experience motor response fluctuations, and by 15 years 80% of patients have this problem.

The first manifestation of motor response fluctuation is that the patient may find him- or herself to be slower than usual in the early morning. This manifestation usually resolves 30 to 60 minutes after the morning dose of carbidopa/levodopa. The patient may notice that 2 to 3 1/2 hours after a dose of carbidopa/levodopa, he or she again feels more "parkinsonian" (slower, increased difficulty walking, more tremulous, loss of dexterity). This pattern of motor fluctuation is known as "end-of-dose wearing off", because the worsening symptoms seem to correlate with the decline of levodopa levels in the blood (65). The patient feels better again 30 to 60 minutes after another dose.

Appropriate strategies at this point might be to increase the frequency of carbidopa/levodopa (e.g., give 4 or 5 small doses/day each 3 to 4 hours apart, rather than 3 doses/day), switch to the controlled release preparation (66), or add a synthetic dopamine receptor agonist (Table 32.2) (67). If the patient is not already receiving selegiline, this drug might be added, as inhibition of MAO-B will delay the catabolism of dopamine to provide a longer duration of action (27, 28). When selegiline is given to patients already receiving carbidopa/levodopa, the dose of levodopa may need to be decreased by 10 to 30% to prevent symptoms of dopamine excess.

During this time patients may also begin to experience intermittent choreoathetoid movements of the head, hands, or face ("dyskinesias"). Occasionally, the involuntary muscle hyperactivity can involve the diaphragm, creating a sense of dyspnea that can be misinterpreted as resulting from a cardiopulmonary problem. These involuntary movements do not result from PD *per se* but are central side-effects of chronic dopaminergic therapy, perhaps an iatrogenic manifestation of dopamine receptor supersensitivity (64). The involuntary movements usually appear during the period of maximum benefit from levodopa, which is often 1 to 2 hours after each dose ("peak dose dyskinesia"). As the disease progresses, the dyskinesias can persist throughout the period of therapeutic benefit from levodopa. In a small number of cases, the choreoathetoid movements come and go in a diphasic pattern, beginning shortly after a dose starts to exert its clinical effect and recurring as the effects of the dose begin to wear off (68).

Table 32.2. Treatment of Motor Fluctuations in Parkinson's Disease

Problem	*Management*
Middle-of-night or early morning akinesia	Bedtime dose of CD/LD-CR[a]; middle-of-night dose of CD/LD
End-of-dose deterioration doses; ("wearing off")	Decrease interval between CD/LD
	Use controlled release CD/LD; add dopamine agonist; add selegiline
Unpredictable periods of akinesia or dyskinesia ("on-off" reactions)	Controlled release CD/LD; frequent (q 2 hr) small doses of CD/LD; add dopamine agonist; add selegiline; daytime low-protein diet
Drug-resistant prolonged "off" periods	Apomorphine injections; levodopa infusion
Peak dose dyskinesias (choreoathetosis)	Decrease each dose of CD/LD and add dopamine agonist if necessary
Diphasic dyskinesias	Decrease interval between CD/LD doses and reduce each dose

[a] Abbreviations: CD/LD, carbidopa/levodopa; CD/LD-CR, controlled release carbidopa/levodopa.

There have been no reports of irreversible induction of choreoathetosis resulting from levodopa therapy. Many patients also experience akathisia, the subjective feeling of restlessness and the need to "move around," as a complication of chronic levodopa therapy (69).

Levodopa-induced dyskinesias are dose-related and will abate with dosage reduction. However, lowering the dose to decrease the choreoathetoid movements may increase the parkinsonian symptoms. When given a choice, most patients, even those with severe drug-induced dyskinesias, would rather have the abnormal choreic movements than experience increased parkinsonian bradykinesia, rigidity, tremor, or postural instability (38). Increasing the frequency of carbidopa/levodopa administration while at the same time lowering each dose can help reduce the peaks in plasma (and brain) levodopa levels that predispose to the dyskinesias, without sacrificing antiparkinsonian efficacy. Another helpful therapeutic strategy in patients with severe dyskinesias is to combine lower doses of carbidopa/levodopa with a dopamine agonist (69b).

Eventually, many patients begin to notice that the motor fluctuations that they experience become unpredictable in relationship to doses of levodopa. These fluctuations are referred to as the "on-off" phenomenon, as patients may abruptly go from a condition of feeling relatively mobile ("on") to a state of parkinsonian immobility ("off") (64, 70). Fortunately, the "off" periods can end just as quickly as they arrive. The changes can be very dramatic, with severe hypertonus, akinesia ("freezing"), falls, or even transient catatonia. Long-term studies of PD patients treated with levodopa for more than 10 years have shown that improvement in bradykinesia, rigidity, and tremor are relatively well-maintained, whereas gait instability, sudden immobility ("freezing"), "on-off" reactions, and speech impairment are the major sources of disability late in the disease (71, 72).

The pathophysiology of these severe, seemingly random fluctuations in parkinsonian symptoms is not completely understood (73, 74). It clearly bears some relationship to striatal availability of dopamine, since "off" periods can be abolished by intravenous levodopa infusions, or acute injection of apomorphine, a direct-acting dopamine agonist (75). The pathophysiology of the motor complications and "on-off" reactions is related to complex pharmacokinetic and pharma codynamic factors (64). The pharmacokinetic problems include erratic peripheral absorption of levodopa and the central kinetics of dopamine synthesis and storage. The pharmacodynamic problems involve variables that alter striatal dopamine receptor responsiveness (76). Secondary postsynaptic dysfunction may occur, perhaps as a result of the chronic intermittent excitation of striatal dopamine receptors that normally are tonically stimulated. If this is the case, treatment of early PD with drugs that provide a relatively constant level of central dopamine stimulation (dopamine agonists or controlled release carbidopa/levodopa instead of regular carbidopa/levodopa) might delay or diminish the development of motor fluctuations (77).

The palliation of patients who are experiencing severe motor fluctuations and "on-off" reactions is difficult and often unsatisfactory. The absorption of levodopa across the intestinal tract and passage through the blood brain barrier competes with other LNAAs. High-protein meals can interfere with levodopa absorption from the gastrointestinal (GI) tract (73), and the LNAAs block delivery of levodopa from blood to brain (78). A "very low daytime protein diet" will result in a marked decrease in plasma concentration of other amino acids that compete for these active transport systems, ensuring more predictable plasma (and brain) levodopa levels after each dose. A "very low daytime protein diet" will reduce many of the motor fluctuations and increase the proportion of "on" time in patients with "on-off" reactions (79, 80, 81).

Other tactics that are employed in patients with "on-off" reactions include very frequent administration of very small doses of carbidopa/levodopa (e.g., 25/100-mg 1/2 tablet every 2 hours), use of the controlled release carbidopa/levodopa, combination therapy with a synthetic dopamine receptor agonist (bromocriptine, pergolide), and concomitant administration of selegiline. Continuous intravenous infusion of levodopa (82, 83), continuous intraduodenal infusion of levodopa, and administration of liquid suspensions of levodopacarbidopa. (84) are experimental methods of palliating some of the motor fluctuations in very advanced PD that might become clinically important techniques in the coming years.

Management of PD patients who require surgery or are unable to eat or swallow for various reasons (e.g., stroke) can be difficult, since the most effective medications (levodopa or the dopamine agonists) are not available in parenteral form. For patients with mild to moderate disease, missing several doses or even a day or two of levodopa or dopamine agonist therapy may not cause dramatic changes (61b). However, patients with more advanced disease will, after several days without treatment, become increasingly immobile, rigid, and unable to care for their bodily needs. Aspiration pneumonia, compression neuropathies, contractures, decubitus ulcers, and, in rare cases, a state resembling "neuroleptic malignant syndrome" are potential complications of drug withdrawal (85, 86). Of interest, a "drug-free holiday" had been advocated in the past for patients with advanced PD who had experienced either loss of benefit from levodopa therapy or intolerable drug-induced side-effects (87, 88). The "drug holiday" carries risks without long-term benefits (89), and there is seldom an indication for voluntary complete withdrawal of all antiparkinsonian medication in patients with moderate to severe PD.

In patients who are unable to swallow, it is important to resume the antiparkinsonian medication as soon as possible, by nasogastric or nasoduodenal tube if necessary. Unfortunately, levodopa is not absorbed through the rectal mucosa and cannot be administered by that route (90). Intravenous infusions of levodopa or levodopa methyl ester can be used to treat PD in postoperative patients who will be unable to take medication via the gastrointestinal tract for prolonged periods of time (82, 83). Unfortunately, these solutions are not commercially available. The dopamine agonists apomorphine and lisuride can be administered parenterally, but unfortunately these agents are not available in the U.S. Some of the anticholinergic medications that have modest benefit in PD are available for intramuscular administration (e.g., benztropine, biperiden) and could be helpful for the patient who is unable to take any medication via the GI tract.

Levodopa and carbidopa/levodopa do not interact adversely with other drugs. One important caveat is that nonspecific MAO inhibitors should be withdrawn at least 2 weeks before levodopa therapy to avoid serious hypertensive crises or hyperpyrexia (91). Neuroleptics (e.g., haloperidol, chlorpromazine, prochlorperazine, etc.) or other drugs with central dopamine blocking effects (e.g., metoclopramide or amoxapine) should be avoided in patients with PD. These drugs can block the efficacy of levodopa and seriously exacerbate parkinsonian symptomatology (see the section of this chapter entitled "Drug-induced Parkinsonism") (92).

The cardiovascular side-effects of levodopa therapy are seldom of clinical importance. Although cardiac arrhythmias (sinus tachycardia and atrial extrasystoles) were reported in patients receiving levodopa alone, the incidence is low when patients concomitantly receive carbidopa. Cardiac arrhythmia and acute coronary insufficiency do not contraindicate levodopa therapy (93).

Levodopa can induce modest postural hypotension via both peripheral and central mechanisms. This problem is less likely to occur with combined carbidopa/levodopa therapy and tends to decrease with time (94). PD patients may be predisposed to postprandial hypotension (95). Recent studies showed no significant change in blood pressure or heart rate in the lying and standing position in patients with mild PD being treated chronically with levodopa compared with controls (95b). When postural hypotension is a severe problem in a patient with parkinsonism, the possibility of an underlying autonomic disturbance (e.g., Shy-Drager syndrome or "multiple system atrophy") (96) and the role of other concomitantly administered medications must be considered before attributing the problem to levodopa.

Pyridoxine (vitamin B$_6$) is a cofactor for aromatic acid decarboxylase. Pyridoxine supplements diminish the therapeutic effectiveness of levodopa in PD by enhancing the peripheral production of dopamine, making less levodopa available to enter the CNS. This is not a problem in patients who are taking adequate amounts of carbidopa to inhibit peripheral aromatic acid decarboxylase (51).

Table 32.3. Management of Drug-Induced Hallucinations and Psychosis in Parkinson's Disease

"Preventive"—keep medication doses as low as possible, especially in elderly or confused patients
Taper and withdraw anticholinergic agents or amantadine
Reduce dose of dopamine agonists
Reduce dose of levodopa
Drug intervention only if absolutely necessary: thioridazine or clozapine

Anecdotal reports have suggested a possible relationship between levodopa therapy and malignant melanoma. Levodopa can be metabolized to melanin by melanoma cells. The influence of levodopa on the behavior of melanoma is probably minimal, and the drug should not necessarily be withheld in PD patients who have pigmentary skin lesions (97, 98).

An important complication of levodopa therapy is the induction of sleep disturbances and altered behavioral states. Sleep fragmentation, nightmares, somnambulism, and night terrors are common in PD and may be exacerbated by levodopa in a dose-related fashion (99). Evening and nighttime doses of carbidopa/levodopa should be avoided in mild cases of PD, or kept as low as possible in more advanced cases to reduce the likelihood of sleep disorders.

Many patients on levodopa for several years will begin to experience visual hallucinations. These are usually nonthreatening and mild, and tend to occur during the evening in the setting of an alert sensorium. Most patients are aware that they are hallucinating and will be able to discuss their visions (faces, small animals, insects) rationally with their physician. The hallucinations may be more stressful for the family than the patient. Although patients with underlying cognitive impairment have an increased susceptibility to this problem, medication-induced hallucinosis can occur in any patient with PD. This phenomenon is dose-related, and slight decreases in carbidopa/levodopa dosage (particularly in evening doses) can often palliate this problem (100, 101). In a small proportion of patients, visual hallucinosis will be accompanied by severe agitation, paranoia, progressive confusion, and frank psychosis (92 102). Although dementia and altered mental states can occur as part of PD itself, the possibility of drug-induced delirium should be a prime consideration (Table 32.3). Unfortunately, all of the drugs used to treat PD, including carbidopa/levodopa, dopamine agonists, anticholinergics, and amantadine, can cause delirium (103). In this setting, medications should be reduced or eliminated to the greatest extent possible, and other structural or metabolic causes for delirium should be investigated.

Occasionally, administration of a neuroleptic drug will be necessary to control the abnormal behavior. Thioridazine traditionally has been the neuroleptic of choice in PD, as it has less propensity to exacerbate extrapyramidal symptoms than do the higher-potency agents such as haloperidol (92, 100). The new antipsychotic drug clozapine does not block striatal dopamine receptors and therefore should not induce or exacerbate PD. Clozapine may become a useful adjunct in management of the severely agitated PD patient, but serious hematologic side-effects (agranulocytosis) that require close monitoring have limited its widespread use (104, 104b).

To be effective, the levodopa preparations require enzymatic conversion to dopamine by the presynaptic terminals in the striatum. There have been major research efforts to find direct-acting postsynaptic dopamine receptor agonists that would bypass the progressively degenerating presynaptic terminals and thereby palliate PD. Currently, two direct-acting dopamine agonists are available in the U.S. for the treatment of PD: the ergot alkaloids bromocriptine and pergolide (Table 32.4) (67, 105). Both of these medications substantially reduce the symptoms of PD, although not quite as effectively as levodopa.

There are several potential roles for the dopamine agonists in the treatment of PD. Some experts have proposed that initial therapy of PD with a dopamine agonist (rather than carbidopa/levodopa), or initial use of low-dose combinations of both, might result in fewer long-term complications such as choreoathetosis and "on-off" reactions (39). Treating new mild PD with a combination of dopamine agonist and levodopa offers no immediate symptomatic benefit compared with levodopa alone; it remains to be determined whether there are any long-term benefits to warrant the extra expense of early combination therapy (105b).

The addition of dopamine agonists is clearly beneficial in patients who are already experiencing "wearing off" of carbidopa/levodopa effect between doses. The dopamine agonists reduce disability, increase the percent of "on" time, and permit a reduction of levodopa dose when used as an adjunct to carbidopa/levodopa in patients with moderate to advanced PD (106–108). The combined use of dopamine agonist and carbidopa/levodopa may be particularly helpful in allowing reduction of the levodopa dose in patients who are experiencing psychiatric or motor side-effects of antiparkinsonian therapy.

There are neuropharmacologic differences between bromocriptine and pergolide. Bromocriptine is a D2 dopamine receptor agonist, whereas pergolide is an agonist at both D1- and D2-receptors. This finding may confer some theoretic advantage to the use of pergolide (109). As the bromocriptine dose is increased and levodopa decreased, the complete cessation of relatively small doses of levodopa may result in a marked increase in parkinsonism. This finding may relate to the need to stimulate both D1- and D2-receptors for optimum clinical benefit. Bromocriptine and pergolide have a longer half-life than levodopa, but since the doses of these drugs must be increased very slowly, it is not unusual for clinical benefits to be delayed for many weeks after initiation of therapy. Both drugs are more than 90% bound to plasma proteins, an important consideration if they are administered concurrently with other drugs known to affect protein binding (110). Pergolide is a more potent drug than bromocriptine (1 mg of pergolide is roughly equivalent to 10 mg of bromocriptine) (111).

A major side-effect of these drugs is postural hypotension, and up to 1/3 of patients receiving these drugs experience lightheadedness, giddiness, or even syncope (95b, 112). Occasionally, there is a dramatic "first-dose" hypotensive effect, so that therapy must be initiated with very small doses (1.25 mg of bromocriptine and 0.05 mg of pergolide) and increased very gradually over several weeks. Particular caution must be exercised in patients who are already receiving antihypertensive drugs. Tolerance to the hypotensive effect develops with time in most patients, so that hypotension is seldom a major persistent problem unless there is concomitant underlying autonomic dysfunction (110).

Nausea, dyspepsia, and abdominal discomfort are also common side-effects. These symptoms can be alleviated by temporarily reducing the dosage or administering the drug with food. As with levodopa, antinauseants such as prochlorperazine or metoclopramide should not be used, as these drugs are dopamine receptor blocking agents and will exacerbate extrapyramidal symptomatology.

The "optimal" dose is highly variable and depends in part on whether these drugs are being used alone (in which case typical dose ranges of bromocriptine might be from 10 to 60 mg/day, and those of pergolide, from 1 to 5 mg/day in three divided doses) (113–115) or in combination with levodopa, in which case substantially smaller doses (1/4 to 1/2 as much) are generally used (116, 117). The doses are gradually titrated upward to achieve optimal clinical benefit. The amount of carbidopa/levodopa can often be reduced cautiously as the dose of the dopamine agonist is increased, to avert side-effects of overmedication (e.g., hallucinosis, choreoathetosis).

There is no definite relationship between dopamine agonist therapy and cardiac arrhythmias. Asymptomatic atrial and ventricular arrhythmias have been associated with the use of these drugs. However, studies have not shown clinically important changes on electrocardiogram (ECG) or Holter monitoring in patients with stable heart disease and PD who are on pergolide (118, 119).

Both bromocriptine and pergolide can induce visual hallucinosis, agitation, depression, nightmares, and confusional states (similar to that seen with levodopa) (120). These are dose-related phenomena that may occur in any patient. However, drug-induced confusional states occur most commonly in patients with advanced PD and concomitant dementia who are on multiple medications. The dopamine agonists, when used alone, have less propensity than carbidopa/levodopa to induce choreoathetosis, but will exacerbate levodopa-induced involuntary movements when the drugs are used together if the carbidopa/levodopa dose is not reduced.

There are some unusual side-effects of bromocriptine and pergolide therapy that are not encountered with carbidopa/levodopa. These drugs are both ergot alkaloids, and symptoms of ergotism such as paresthesias, muscle cramps, cold extremities, vasospasm, and Raynaud's phenomenon sometimes occur. Pulmonary infiltrates, pleural fibrosis, and retroperitoneal fibrosis have also been reported after long-term use of these drugs (121). Pleuropulmonary disease associated with ergot derivatives is related to cumulative dosage and improves after drug withdrawal (122). Livedo reticularis, erythematous leg swelling, and, rarely, erythromelalgia, a painful reddish skin discoloration, may also be seen as side-effect of bromocriptine or pergolide.

Table 32.4.   Dopamine Agonists Used in Parkinson's Disease

Name	Initial Dose	Maintenance Dose Range	
		As Monotherapy	When Used with Levodopa
Bromocriptine	1.25 mg	10–80 mg/day	7.5–40 mg/day
Pergolide	0.05 mg	1–5 mg/day	0.5–4 mg/day

Table 32.5. Causes of "Secondary" Parkinsonism

Drugs and medications
    Neuroleptics
    Dopamine-depleting drugs
Toxins
    Carbon monoxide
    Manganese
    MPTP
Postencephalitic states
Postanoxic states
Multiinfarct states
Pugilistic encephalopathy
Normal pressure hydrocephalus
The "multiple system degenerations" (parkinsonism-plus"
    syndromes)

Table 32.6. Common "Parkinsonism-Plus" Syndromes

Name	Major Nonparkinsonian Features
Shy-Drager syndrome ("multiple system atrophy")	Marked orthostatic hypotension General autonomic failure Ataxia
Progressive supranuclear palsy	Supranuclear ophthalmoparesis Axial hypertonus Marked postural instability
Olivopontocerebellar atrophy	Cerebellar ataxia
Corticobasal ganglionic degeneration	Apraxia Dementia
Striatonigral degeneration	Hyperreflexia, Babinski signs Pseudobulbar dysfunction

Bromocriptine and pergolide reduce serum prolactin concentrations by stimulating dopamine receptors in the hypothalamus to release prolactin inhibitory factor. Consequently, these drugs are useful in treating disorders associated with hyperprolactinemia, such as amenorrhea, hypogonadism, and prolactin-secreting pituitary adenomas (123). These neuroendocrine effects have little clinical significance in the patient with PD, with the exception that some patients who are receiving levodopa or dopamine agonist therapy will experience renewed interest in sexual activity. In rare cases these medications have caused marked hypersexuality (124).

PARKINSONISM AND "PARKINSONISM-PLUS" SYNDROMES

There are a large number of conditions that cause akinetic-rigid clinical syndromes resembling PD (125). These disorders may account for more than 20% of all "parkinsonian" patients. Some patients with parkinsonian clinical features have "secondary" parkinsonism resulting from multiple infarcts, trauma, communicating hydrocephalus, viral infections, tumors, toxins, or medications (Table 32.5). Another group of patients have degenerative disorders that cause symptoms resembling PD but that also affect other areas of the nervous system ("multiple system degenerations" or "parkinsonism-plus syndromes") (Table 32.6).

The presence of ophthalmoplegia, cerebellar ataxia, pyramidal tract signs, dementia early in the course of the illness, or significant autonomic dysfunction is clues that a patient does not have PD but one of the "parkinsonism-plus syndromes" (126). Tremor at rest is one of the hallmarks of PD but is often an intermittent phenomenon that may be absent in up to 30% of PD patients at a given point of time. However, the persistent absence of tremor throughout the course of the illness is another important clue that the patient may have parkinsonism rather than PD (127).

The impressive initial clinical response of parkinsonian symptoms to treatment with levodopa or dopamine agonists in PD has led to the speculation that this might be a useful criterion to separate patients with PD from those with "multiple system degenerations" or other disorders that resemble PD (61). In practice, many of the disorders that resemble PD show modest clinical benefit to levodopa or dopamine agonist therapy, at least in the early stages of illness (128). Therefore these drugs are worth a trial in patients with progressive supranuclear palsy, multiple system atrophy, or other "parkinsonism-plus syndromes." However, the progressive postsynaptic cell loss in the striatum that is seen in these conditions usually means that any therapeutic benefit will be incomplete or not sustained for many years.

DRUG-INDUCED PARKINSONISM

The widespread use of neuroleptics and other drugs with central dopamine receptor blocking activity has made "drug-induced parkinsonism" a common clinical disorder (129). Although psychiatrists are usually alert to the possibility of neuroleptic-induced parkinsonism, several drugs that are not used for psychiatric indications also have a great propensity to cause drug-induced parkinsonism (Table 32.7). For example, the use of prochlorperazine for nausea, metoclopramide for GI motility disorders, and the cardiovascular medications flunarizine and cinnarizine may all cause parkinsonism. The antihypertensive drugs reserpine and α-methyldopa are dopamine-depleting agents that can also cause parkinsonian symptoms.

All of the clinical manifestations of PD may be seen in drug-induced parkinsonism, but akinesia is often the earliest and most notable feature, with slowness and expressionless facies that could be confused with psychomotor retardation of psychiatric origin (130). The signs of drug-induced parkinsonism are generally symmetric from the onset, whereas those of PD are more likely to be asymmetric. The typical PD "pill-rolling" tremor at rest generally is not a prominent sign in drug-induced parkinsonism. However, a focal perioral tremor ("rabbit syndrome"), which is very unusual in PD, is commonly seen in drug-induced parkinsonism.

Drug-induced parkinsonism usually begins within several weeks to months of starting treatment (131). The incidence of drug-induced parkinsonism is usually dose dependent for each drug: the higher the dose, the greater the incidence and the more severe the extrapyramidal symptomatology. The most potent neuroleptics (such as haloperidol or the halogenated and piperazine phenothiazines) have a greater likelihood of causing parkinsonism than do the lower-potency drugs (such as thioridazine). This observation may be related to the degree of inherent anticholinergic activity of the drug (e.g., low in haloperidol, high in thioridazine) or selectivity in the sites where dopamine is blocked (132).

It is uncertain why some patients develop drug-induced parkinsonism and others do not. Drug-induced parkinsonism is more common in women than men, unlike PD, in which

Table 32.7.   Common Causes of Drug-Induced Parkinsonism

Drugs used in psychiatry
  Neuroleptics with high incidence of DIP
    Haloperidol
    Fluphenazine
    Perphenazine
    Trifluoperazine
  Neuroleptics with moderate incidence of DIP
    Thorazine
    Mesoridazine
    Promazine
    Loxapine
    Chlorprothixene
    Thiothixene
  Neuroleptics with lower incidence of DIP
    Thioridazine
    Molindone
  Dopamine-blocking antidepressant
    Amoxapine
Drugs used for nonpsychiatric purposes
  Antinausea, antiemetic
    Prochlorperazine
    Trimethobenzamide
    Droperidol
  Gastric motility
    Metoclopramide
  Cardiovascular medications
    Flunarizine
    Cinnarizine
  Antihypertensive agents
    Reserpine
    α-methyldopa

there is no predilection for sex. There may be a hereditary susceptibility to developing drug-induced parkinsonism. The risk of developing drug-induced parkinsonism increases with advancing age, which suggests that subclinical idiopathic PD or other age-related phenomena play a role (133).

The neuroleptic drugs are extremely lipophilic and are present in the brain much longer than is reflected by their serum half-lives. Once the drug is discontinued, the duration of parkinsonism depends on the total dose, the nature of the drug (e.g., long-acting depot versus oral preparation), and the age of the patient. Drug-induced parkinsonism generally resolves over a period of several weeks to months (134), but cases lasting longer than a year have been reported (135). In a small number of cases the parkinsonism is permanent, but it is likely that these patients had underlying preclinical PD before neuroleptic treatment was initiated.

If parkinsonism develops and the dopamine-blocking drug cannot be discontinued, one should consider reducing the dose of the offending drug, switching to a drug that has a lower incidence of drug-induced parkinsonism (such as thioridazine) (92, 100), or using clozapine (104). If this approach is not possible or not beneficial, antiparkinsonian therapy with amantadine or one of the anticholinergic agents may be helpful (129). Levodopa or dopamine agonists (bromocriptine, pergolide) are not used for treating drug-induced parkinsonism because: (*a*) there is a risk of exacerbating the underlying psychiatric disorder with these drugs, and (*b*) theoretically, high doses would be required because of the neuroleptic-induced dopamine receptor blockade. The therapeutic response to levodopa in drug-induced parkinsonism is generally disappointing (136).

Amantadine was introduced as an antiviral agent for the prophylaxis of influenza A and unexpectedly was found to cause symptomatic improvement in patients with PD (35). The drug has modest benefits and occasionally is still used in the early stages of PD to allow for a delay in the introduction of levodopa or to synergize the effects of levodopa in patients with advanced disease. The most widespread neurologic use of amantadine is in treating drug-induced parkinsonism and acute dystonic reactions. The drug acts as an indirect dopamine agonist and has some mild anticholinergic effects (137). Recent studies also show that the therapeutic benefits of amantadine may be mediated in part by N-methyl-D-aspartate receptor blockade (138).

The usual dose of amantadine is 100 mg twice daily. Higher doses increase the risk of side-effects without substantial additional clinical benefits. The drug is quickly and almost totally absorbed from the GI tract, leading to a rapid onset of action. The half-life of amantadine is approximately 12 hours. The drug is not catabolized and is eliminated exclusively by the kidneys. Therefore, patients with renal impairment must be given lower doses to avoid intoxication (139). The most common manifestation of amantadine overdose is an acute paranoid psychosis (140). Amantadine in nontoxic doses does not exacerbate psychosis in schizophrenic patients.

Amantadine is equally as effective as the anticholinergic drugs used to treat drug-induced parkinsonism but has fewer side-effects (141–143). The long-term use of amantadine can often cause livedo reticularis and edema in the lower extremities (144). Visual hallucinations, confusion, agitation, insomnia, and nightmares can occur as an idiosyncratic reaction to nontoxic doses of amantadine, particularly in patients with underlying cognitive impairment. The drug is free of significant cardiovascular side-effects, although sudden death and malignant cardiac arrhythmias have been reported in amantadine overdoses (139, 145).

The anticholinergic drugs were the mainstay of treatment for PD before the introduction of levodopa and the dopamine agonists. Acetylcholine is a major neurotransmitter of striatal interneurons, and the anticholinergics are thought to exert their beneficial effects in PD by restoring a more normal balance of acetylcholine/dopamine neurotransmission (146). More recent investigations suggest that N-methyl-D-aspartate receptor blockade may also be an important central action of the anticholinergic agents (138). Their use in PD is now relatively limited, although patients with severe parkinsonian tremor may benefit greatly from the use of anticholinergics alone or in combination with dopaminergic therapy (147). Some PD patients with severe drooling benefit from decreased salivary secretions as a side-effect of anticholinergic therapy. The major current role of the anticholinergic drugs is in the treatment of drug-induced parkinsonism and acute dystonic reactions.

Many synthetic compounds with anticholinergic effects are available, the most commonly used being trihexyphenidyl, benztropine mesylate, biperiden, and ethopropazine (Table 32.8). Although theoretically the therapeutic differences among the various anticholinergics are negligible, in practice some patients find one anticholinergic to be more effective than another (148). Ethopropazine may be better tolerated by

Table 32.8. Anticholinergic Drugs Used in Parkinsonism

| Name | Typical Dose Range | | Modes of Administration |
	Initial Dose	Maintenance	
Trihexyphenidyl	1 mg/day	2–15 mg/day	Oral tablet, liquid, sustained release capsule
Benztropine	0.5 mg/day	1–6 mg/day	Tablet, injection
Biperiden	1 mg/day	2–8 mg/day	Tablet, injection

patients who are sensitive to the adverse effects of anticholinergics. Benztropine and biperiden can be administered parenterally, which is important for patients with parkinsonism who are unable to take medications by mouth. Treatment should be started with very small doses and subsequently increased gradually in increments to avert serious dose-related side-effects. The half-life of the anticholinergic antiparkinsonian drugs is between 6 and 12 hours, so twice- or thrice-daily dosing is appropriate for most patients (148).

In the peripheral nervous system, these drugs block the muscarinic receptors of the parasympathetic nervous system. Dry mouth and constipation are common symptoms, even at low dosage. Urinary retention caused by decreased detrusor muscle contraction, blurred vision resulting from impaired ocular accommodation, tachycardia resulting from vagal blockade, decreased sweating, and impaired gut motility are more serious side-effects that are commonly encountered at moderate to higher doses. The anticholinergics should not be used in patients with closed angle glaucoma, as permanent visual loss may result. Men with prostatic hypertrophy are highly susceptible to developing urinary retention and should avoid anticholinergic medications. Thermoregulation may become impaired by a combination of peripheral (impaired sweating) and central (hypothalamic) mechanisms, resulting in severe hyperpyrexia (149).

Even when the peripheral nervous system side-effects are tolerable, the central side-effects of the anticholinergic agents may be dose limiting. Sedation, memory loss, delirium, and visual hallucinations can all occur as complications of anticholinergic therapy (150). The study of the memory loss associated with anticholinergic drugs led to the "cholinergic hypothesis of memory" (151, 152): there is a linear relationship between the dose of anticholinergic agent and the degree of recent memory impairment. Even those PD patients who appear to be cognitively intact are more susceptible to the cognitive side-effects of the anticholinergics than are normal subjects.

Older patients are more susceptible to the peripheral and central side-effects of anticholinergics and should be treated with extreme caution, if at all. Patients with underlying dementia or memory loss are not suitable candidates for anticholinergic therapy. Attention must be paid to anticholinergic effects of medications that the patient is already receiving (e.g., antidepressants, antihistamines, neuroleptics, antiarrhythmics), as the adverse effects may be additive.

The side-effects of anticholinergic medications for parkinsonism are eliminated by reducing or discontinuing the drug. An important caveat is that abrupt discontinuation of anticholinergics after long-term use in patients with parkinsonism can result in a dramatic "rebound" effect, with sudden worsening of the extrapyramidal symptoms (153, 154). This problem can be avoided by tapering the dosage over several days to weeks.

Some patients with drug-induced parkinsonism may experience a spontaneous remission of parkinsonian symptoms without a change in neuroleptic dosage. The long-term pharmacologic effects of the neuroleptics on brain receptors may differ considerably from the acute and short-term effects. Therefore, it may be appropriate to taper cautiously and try to eliminate the amantadine or anticholinergic medications after 6 months in patients with drug-induced parkinsonism (155).

DRUG-INDUCED ACUTE DYSTONIC REACTIONS

Acute dyskinesias and dystonic reactions occur in 2 to 10% of patients shortly after initiating treatment with neuroleptic drugs or metoclopramide (156). Involuntary movements sometimes appear within hours of the first dose. Generally, more than 50% of patients who develop acute dystonic reactions will do so within 36 hours, and 90% will do so within 5 days of initiating treatment with neuroleptics (131). When patients on long-term neuroleptic treatment develop acute dystonic reactions, it is often related to an increase in dosage or change in neuroleptic medication.

The acute dystonic reactions have a variety of clinical features but mainly exhibit intermittent or continuous muscular spasms and abnormal postures affecting the eyes, face, neck, throat, or trunk. The classic "oculogyric crisis" of sustained upward or lateral deviation of the eyes is but one possible presentation. Trismus, forced jaw opening, grimacing, distortions of the lips or tongue, torticollis, opisthotonos, respiratory stridor, and writhing movements of the extremities are other potential manifestations. Milder forms of acute dystonic reaction may cause tightness in the jaw or tongue, with difficulty chewing, speaking, or swallowing (129).

The involuntary movements are often painful and very frightening to the patient. The ensuing emotional stress may further exacerbate the dyskinesias. Physicians without prior experience with acute dystonic reactions will find the syndrome bizarre. The signs can spontaneously wax and wane, or temporarily respond to reassurance and suggestion, leading to the mistaken diagnosis of hysterical reaction. Severe acute dystonic reactions can also be easily confused with focal seizures, status epilepticus, tetanus, tetany, or meningismus.

Unlike drug-induced parkinsonism, acute dystonic reactions occur more commonly in children and young adults than in older patients (131, 156). Males are more likely to experience dystonic reactions to neuroleptics than are females, although this gender difference has not been observed with metoclopramide (157). In a given individual, the likelihood of an acute dystonic reaction is dose-related. The incidence is higher with the most potent neuroleptics, such as haloperidol or piperazine phenothiazines (e.g., perphenazine, fluphenazine) than with the less potent neuroleptics. Dehydration and hypocalcemia increase the risk of experiencing acute dystonic reactions (158). There may be a familial susceptibility to dystonic reactions (159).

The pathophysiology of drug-induced dystonic reactions is uncertain. Increased central cholinergic activity is an important factor in dystonia (160). Neuroleptic-induced increases in dopamine turnover and postsynaptic dopamine receptor supersensitivity may play a role in precipitating the muscle spasms (161).

The acute dyskinesias and dystonia eventually resolve spontaneously if the drug that precipitated the problem is discontinued. The duration depends on the half-life of the drug, but very prolonged reactions can occur (162). Treatment generally is warranted because of the distressing and disabling nature of the involuntary movements. Diphenhydramine 50 mg intravenously usually aborts acute dystonic reactions within 2 to 5 minutes of administration. Benztropine 1 mg intravenously works equally well and is less sedating than diphenhydramine. Milder reactions can be treated with oral diphenhydramine or oral benztropine, but the therapeutic effect will be delayed. The effectiveness of these medications in terminating acute dystonic reactions is attributed to their central anticholinergic effects. Intravenous diazepam (5 to 10 mg) is also effective but must be used with caution because of the risk of respiratory depression, especially in patients being treated with other sedatives (163).

If the offending drug can be discontinued, oral therapy with diphenhydramine (e.g., 25 mg three times a day) or benztropine (e.g., 1 mg three times a day) should be given for an additional 24 to 48 hours to avert recurrence of the dystonic reaction. In patients who require continued neuroleptic treatment, it would be appropriate to reduce the dose or switch to a neuroleptic with fewer extrapyramidal side-effects, if possible. Amantadine 100 mg twice daily, or one of the antiparkinsonian anticholinergic drugs (Table 32.9), may need to be administered concurrently with neuroleptic therapy for several weeks to prevent return of the dystonia (141).

NEUROLEPTIC MALIGNANT SYNDROME

Neuroleptic malignant syndrome is an uncommon but potentially life-threatening disorder that can occur in the pharmacologic setting of: (*a*) administration of drugs that block central nervous system dopamine receptors, or (*b*) following withdrawal of levodopa or dopamine agonist therapy in patients with PD (164). Clinically, neuroleptic malignant syndrome can occur in psychiatric patients who are receiving short-term or long-term neuroleptic therapy, medical patients who are receiving neuroleptics (e.g., as antiemetics, preoperatively, or for agitation), during metoclopramide treatment for GI motility disorders (165), and in PD patients whose therapy is intentionally or inadvertently discontinued (85, 86). The syndrome has been reported as a potential complication of treatment with all of the neuroleptic drugs, including phenothiazines, butyrophenones, thioxanthenes, and the "atypical" antipsychotic agent loxapine

Table 32.9. Diagnostic Criteria for Neuroleptic Malignant Syndrome

Appropriate clinical setting
  Neuroleptic use
    Phenothiazines
    Butyrophenones
    Thioxanthenes
  Dopamine-blocking drugs
    Metoclopramide
  Discontinuation of antiparkinsonian medications
Mandatory clinical features (100% of cases)
  High fevers
  Marked rigidity
Frequent accompanying features
  Autonomic dysfunction
    Tachycardia
    Diaphoresis
    Labile blood pressure
  Extrapyramidal dysfunction
    Tremulousness
    Involuntary movements
    Catatonic akinesia
  Abnormal mental status
    Mutism
    Agitation
    Stupor/coma
  Laboratory abnormalities
    Elevated CPK
    Leukocytosis
    Dehydration

(166). More cases of neuroleptic malignant syndrome have been reported with the use of haloperidol than any other drug, but this finding may simply reflect the fact that haloperidol is the most widely prescribed neuroleptic.

The incidence of neuroleptic malignant syndrome has been difficult to assess, particularly because there is an absence of rigorous diagnostic criteria, and milder cases may go undiagnosed (167). A recent prospective surveillance for adverse drug reactions suggested a frequency of neuroleptic malignant syndrome of 0.15% among hospitalized psychiatric patients receiving neuroleptics (168).

The clinical features of neuroleptic malignant syndrome evolve over 24 to 72 hours (Table 32.9). The cardinal signs, present in virtually all cases, are marked hypertonus of the limbs ("lead pipe" or pronounced "cogwheeling") in association with high fevers (often more than 40°C) (164). The rigidity and fever are generally accompanied by a host of other signs of autonomic and extrapyramidal dysfunction. Common autonomic disturbances include labile blood pressure, tachycardia, cardiac arrhythmias, and profuse diaphoresis. The hypertonus of skeletal muscles may be accompanied by fluctuating tremors, involuntary movements, or profound immobility and akinesia resembling catatonia. The increased muscle tone may decrease chest wall compliance, producing tachypneic hypoventilation severe enough to require mechanical ventilatory support. Mental status changes are common during neuroleptic malignant syndrome, and the sensorium may fluctuate from agitation to wakeful mutism to stupor or coma (167).

Laboratory abnormalities are often, but not invariably, encountered in neuroleptic malignant syndrome. There may be marked increases in serum CPK concentrations, reflecting myonecrosis from intense sustained muscle contraction. Rhabdomyolysis and acute myoglobinuric renal failure can ensue.

Leukocytosis and mild liver enzyme abnormalities are often encountered. The rigid-akinetic-poorly responsive state predisposes the patient to dehydration, secondary infections (e.g., aspiration pneumonia), thrombophlebitis, and pulmonary embolism. Postmortem examination of brain and muscle reveals no specific pathologic abnormalities in neuroleptic malignant syndrome (169).

Neuroleptic malignant syndrome has occurred in all age groups and both sexes. The onset of this disorder is highly variable after exposure to neuroleptics. It has been reported in patients who have been on stable doses of neuroleptics for months or years, as well as in patients who were recently started on therapy or whose doses were changed. Severe agitation, dehydration, infection, and underlying organic brain dysfunction may predispose a patient to neuroleptic malignant syndrome. The degree of psychomotor agitation, use of higher doses of neuroleptics, or concomitant administration of other drugs (such as lithium) were not independent risk factors for neuroleptic malignant syndrome in a recent case-control study. Only the number of intramuscular injections of neuroleptics distinguished cases from controls (170).

The pathogenesis of neuroleptic malignant syndrome is probably related to the role of dopamine in parkinsonism and hypothalamic thermoregulatory mechanisms. Patients with PD have been found to have abnormalities of sweating and heat dissipation (171, 172). Striatal dopaminergic blockade induced by neuroleptics can trigger parkinsonian rigidity and tremor, which is thermogenic as a result of increased muscle activity. If the hypothalamus is then unable to dissipate the heat effectively through normal autonomic mechanisms, hyperthermia and the full-blown picture of neuroleptic malignant syndrome can ensue (164). "Parkinsonian hyperpyrexia syndrome" may be a more accurate appellation than "neuroleptic malignant syndrome" (164).

The possibility of neuroleptic malignant syndrome should be considered in any patient who is receiving neuroleptics or other dopamine-blocking drugs, or who has been withdrawn from antiparkinsonian therapy and develops unexplained fever and rigidity. The differential diagnosis is extensive. Underlying infection (pneumonia, sepsis, urinary tract infection, meningitis, etc.) is the most likely possibility, and antibiotic coverage is often appropriate until culture results are available. Drug withdrawal syndromes (e.g., alcohol, benzodiazepines) can produce similar fever, involuntary movements, autonomic instability, and altered mental states. Drug fever and heat stroke may also be considered but are usually not associated with the muscle rigidity that characterizes neuroleptic malignant syndrome.

The disorder "malignant hyperthermia," which occurs within hours of exposure to inhalational anesthetics in genetically susceptible individuals, shares the clinical features of fever and rigidity with neuroleptic malignant syndrome. However, these are completely distinct and unrelated disorders. There is no genetic predisposition to neuroleptic malignant syndrome, and patients who have had this disorder are not at increased risk for adverse effects to inhalational anesthetics (173). The rigidity of neuroleptic malignant syndrome is mediated centrally and can be abolished by curare or pancuronium. In malignant hyperthermia, the defect is in the muscle sarcoplasmic reticulum, and curare does not relax the muscles.

Since neuroleptic malignant syndrome is a relatively rare disorder, the literature contains case reports rather than controlled studies regarding optimal treatment. Supportive therapy should be initiated immediately, including hydration, measures to control hyperthermia, and elimination of dopamine-blocking medication. The current treatment of choice for reducing the rigidity, obtundation, tremulousness, and fever in neuroleptic malignant syndrome is bromocriptine in combination with dantrolene (174, 175). PD patients who develop neuroleptic malignant syndrome as a result of discontinuation of therapy should be restarted immediately on levodopa or dopamine agonists.

The centrally acting dopamine agonist bromocriptine is not available parenterally and is administered by mouth or by nasogastric tube. Unlike patients with PD, in whom bromocriptine is started in very low dosage and slowly titrated upward, patients with neuroleptic malignant syndrome should be started immediately on therapeutic doses of 5 to 10 mg four times daily. Improvement in fever and rigidity is often noted within 24 hours of initiating therapy, but it may take a week or more until the illness completely resolves. Bromocriptine should be continued until all of the signs and symptoms have resolved before being slowly tapered and discontinued (176).

Dantrolene was initially used in neuroleptic malignant syndrome based on its effectiveness in treating malignant hyperthermia and heat stroke (175, 177). The therapeutic effect of dantrolene occurs directly on contractile mechanisms within skeletal muscle. Dantrolene inhibits the release of calcium ions from the sarcoplasmic reticulum, thereby preventing activation of the contractile apparatus and diminishing the mechanical force of contraction (178). The reduction of tonic skeletal muscle contraction reduces thermogenesis, and the fever may diminish within hours of initiating dantrolene. The drug does not alter the underlying abnormal dopaminergic mechanisms in neuroleptic malignant syndrome. Therefore, it seems logical to use dantrolene in combination with bromocriptine rather than as monotherapy.

Dantrolene can be administered intravenously or orally. The dose requires titration according to the clinical response. A typical initial dose in neuroleptic malignant syndrome would be 2 to 3 mg per kg of body weight infused intravenously over an hour, followed by intravenous dantrolene 1 mg/kg, or oral dantrolene 1 to 2 mg/kg, four times a day for several days. The pharmacology and side-effects of dantrolene are reviewed later in this chapter in the section entitled "Spasticity."

Long-term follow-up of patients with neuroleptic malignant syndrome reveals that the syndrome usually does not recur when patients are rechallenged with neuroleptics (179, 180). Neuroleptic use within 1 month of an index episode of neuroleptic malignant syndrome is more likely to precipitate a recurrence than is rechallenge at a later date. Individual predisposition contributes only modestly to the risk for this disorder, since patients do not regularly or predictably manifest neuroleptic malignant syndrome upon reexposure to neuroleptics.

TREMOR

Tremor is an involuntary rhythmic oscillation of a body part produced by alternating or synchronous contractions of reciprocally innervated antagonistic muscles (181). Tremor is the most common movement disorder, and can occur in a variety of medical or neurologic disorders. There are many types of tremor, and appropriate diagnosis and therapy depends on the clinical analysis of the involuntary movements.

Tremors can be initially subdivided into those that appear at rest, and those that appear with movement of the affected body part. "Tremor at rest" is the typical tremor associated with PD or other parkinsonian syndromes. This tremor is seen when the patient is at repose (e.g., hand tremor when the patient is sitting or lying, or when the hands are passively held at the side while walking), but disappears with the onset of voluntary movement. Tremor at rest usually improves with the dopaminergic therapy given for PD. Severe or refractory rest tremors may benefit from the use of anticholinergic agents (147).

Tremors associated with movement of the affected body part can be divided into (*a*) those occurring with maintained posture (e.g., tremor of the outstretched hands), often referred to as "postural" or "static" tremors, and (*b*) those seen with movement from point to point to point, often referred to as "kinetic" or "intention" tremors (182). Postural tremor can be seen in normal people exposed to extreme stress or certain medications ("exaggerated physiologic tremor") and is also the typical tremor associated with the common neurologic disorder "essential tremor" (183). Kinetic tremors are usually associated with disorders affecting the cerebellar outflow (superior cerebellar peduncle) or midbrain. Many disorders may be accompanied by more than one type of tremor, and there are overlap syndromes (184). For example, some patients with PD will have a prominent postural tremor in addition to tremor at rest.

Tremor frequently is associated with metabolic brain dysfunction (e.g., uremia, hepatic encephalopathy, drug withdrawal syndromes, hyponatremia, dialysis dysequilibrium, hypoglycemia, acute intoxications, hyperosmolar nonketotic hyperglycemia, etc.). The tremor of metabolic encephalopathy is usually a coarse irregular postural tremor. Multifocal myoclonus (sudden, nonrhythmic, brief muscle jerks affecting various parts of the body) (185) and asterixis (sudden flapping movements of the extended outstretched hands or dorsiflexed feet) (186) may accompany the tremulousness in many metabolic disorders. The presence of tremor, multifocal myoclonus, and bilateral asterixis is a strong indication of metabolic or diffuse brain dysfunction and is rarely associated with focal cerebral disturbances.

"Physiologic tremor" is a postural tremor that can be measured in normal individuals using sensitive recording devices. Several mechanisms have been proposed to explain physiologic tremor, including the inherent properties of motor neuron firing, and oscillations in the stretch reflex (181, 182). Under most circumstances physiologic tremor is not noticeable. However, physiologic tremor can become very apparent when exacerbated by hyperadrenergic states (e.g., anxiety, thyrotoxicosis) or certain medications ("exaggerated physiologic tremor") (Table 32.10). A variety of medications, toxins, chemicals, and endocrine disorders may induce postural tremors: an "exaggerated physiologic tremor" in normal patients or exacerbation of an underlying essential tremor. Drug-induced tremor is usually a dose-related phenomenon, but there is a wide range of individual susceptibility. Postural tremor is

Table 32.10. Medications and Conditions that Commonly Induce Postural Tremor

Emotional factors
  Anxiety
  Stress
  Fatigue
  Fright
Psychoactive drugs
  Lithium
  Neuroleptics
β-agonists and bronchodilators
  Theophylline
  Terbutaline
  Isoproterenol
  Metaproterenol
  Isoetharine
  Epinephrine
Antiarrhythmic drugs
  Mexiletine
  Amiodarone
  Tocainide
Stimulants
  Caffeine
  Amphetamine
Anticonvulsants
  Valproic acid
Drug withdrawal syndromes
  Alcohol withdrawal
  Benzodiazepine withdrawal
  Opiate withdrawal
  Barbiturate withdrawal
Endocrine disorders
  Thyrotoxicosis
  Hypoglycemia
  Pheochromocytoma
Metabolic encephalopathy
Heavy metal intoxication
  Mercury
  Lead
  Arsenic
  Bismuth

regularly seen with toxic doses of theophylline, terbutaline, metaproterenol, isoproterenol, valproic acid, or lithium, but some individuals will experience tremor with "therapeutic" doses (187, 188). Tremulousness is also a prominent feature of withdrawal syndromes from alcohol, benzodiazepines, opiates, or barbiturates. A withdrawal phenomenon should be considered in the differential diagnosis of patients who develop tremor and altered mental status during hospitalization (189, 190, 191).

Anxiety, extreme stress, and fright will elicit a rapid postural tremor in normal individuals ("exaggerated physiologic tremor"). Tremor is an additive phenomenon. The larger-than-usual tremor experienced by a patient with PD or essential tremor when on stage or otherwise frightened results from a combination of the preexisting tremor plus enhanced physiologic tremor. All tremors disappear during sleep. The persistence of involuntary movements during sleep would suggest seizure activity or myoclonus rather than tremor.

Essential tremor (ET) is the most common movement disorder, with prevalence rates of from 0.5 to 5% in the general population (183, 192). The disorder may begin in adolescence or adulthood, increasing in incidence with advancing age. ET often occurs in families as an autosomal dominant trait with variable penetrance.

Patients with ET have a postural tremor that affects the hands or the head. Although the condition slowly worsens over the years, in many cases ET remains more embarrassing than disabling and therefore has been referred to as "benign ET." Unfortunately, some patients also develop dramatic kinetic tremors that interfere with writing, drinking, or other fine manipulations (193). The vocal cords can be affected, giving a tremorous quality to the voice. In severe cases, a rest tremor and mild cogwheeling hypertonus may be seen in ET, leading to some confusion with PD. Epidemiologic studies have not suggested that patients with ET are predisposed to PD, although this point remains somewhat controversial (194, 195).

ET is thought to be caused by rhythmic neuronal bursts (an "oscillator") in the cerebello-rubral-thalamo-cortical circuit. Morphologic studies of autopsied cases have revealed no macroscopic abnormalities in the central or peripheral nervous system of patients with ET (183). Although the postural tremor of ET resembles "exaggerated physiologic tremor" clinically, the conditions can be distinguished pharmacologically and physiologically (196). For example, deafferentation of a limb by ischemia or procaine will reduce physiologic tremor but not ET (implying a "peripheral" mechanism for the former and a "central" mechanism for the latter).

The postural tremor of ET often improves transiently after ingestion of small amounts of alcohol (197). Some patients will use alcohol to reduce their tremor in stressful circumstances (198). The action of alcohol on ET is mediated centrally, as alcohol is ineffective in palliating tremor when infused directly into the brachial artery (196).

In many patients for whom ET is not causing disability, reassurance rather than medical treatment may be all that is indicated. Many patients with ET have been misdiagnosed or self-diagnosed as having PD and are relieved to learn that they have a condition with a much more favorable long-term prognosis.

β-2 receptor antagonists are often effective for patients who require palliation of ET. Propranolol was serendipitously noted to reduce postural tremor dramatically. This initial observation was followed by double-blind cross-over studies demonstrating the efficacy of propranolol in ET (199). Subsequent studies with some of the newer cardioselective β-receptor antagonists have suggested that although β-1 antagonists are better than placebo, they are not as effective as β-2 antagonists in ET (200, 201). No drug has shown greater efficacy than propranolol in ET. There are two modes of action to account for the antitremor effects of propranolol. Doses of propranolol act rapidly at intramuscular β-receptors to reduce enhanced physiologic tremor associated with stress or anxiety. There are also less well-defined central effects to explain the reduction in amplitude of chronic ET (184).

Propranolol doses of 80 to 320 mg per day are usually required for optimal palliation of ET (202). The antitremor effect does not correlate with plasma levels (203). About 75% of patients with ET will benefit substantially from propranolol. A rapid postural tremor of the hands responds most favorably. Head tremor, voice tremor, and kinetic tremors (affecting writing, drinking) improve to a much lesser extent (193). Long-acting propranolol is beneficial for those who prefer once-daily dosing (204). Sporadic single oral doses of propranolol

(40 to 120 mg) can also be effective in ET for several hours and may be used by patients who do not wish to take medication on a regular basis (205). Metoprolol may be used instead of propranolol in patients in whom cardioselectivity is necessary (e.g., asthmatics); however, at the higher doses usually necessary to palliate tremor metoprolol may be a nonselective β-adrenoreceptor antagonist (206).

The anticonvulsant primidone has therapeutic benefit in ET comparable to that of propranolol (207). The mechanism of action of primidone in tremor is unknown. The drug is metabolized to phenobarbital and phenylethylmalonamide. Phenobarbital has some antitremor efficacy, but not to the same extent as primidone (208). In patients with asthma, chronic obstructive pulmonary disease, congestive heart failure, or insulin-dependent diabetes, primidone is a useful alternative to propranolol or other β-blockers for treating ET.

The major side-effect of primidone is sedation. Some patients experience an unusually severe first-dose reaction, with lethargy, nausea, ataxia, and vertigo. This reaction usually can be averted by initiating treatment with very low doses (e.g., 25 mg at bedtime for three or four nights). The dose should be increased very slowly to a therapeutic range (e.g., 50 mg two or three times a day) to allow time for hepatic enzyme induction and more efficient metabolism of primidone. The dose of primidone used to treat tremor (100 to 150 mg/day) is much lower than the usual anticonvulsant dose (750 mg/day or higher). Low doses of primidone (150 mg/day) are as effective against tremor as high doses, so that there is no reason to go beyond 250 mg/day for additional benefit (209). Propranolol and primidone may have additive effects and can be used together in patients with ET who have not had an optimal response to monotherapy (193, 207).

Propranolol and primidone have also been used to palliate "exaggerated physiologic tremors." These medications can reduce symptomatic postural tremors resulting from thyrotoxicosis, lithium, valproic acid, theophylline, and the like (210, 211). Actors have successfully used single doses of propranolol to suppress the tremor associated with stage fright. Sedatives and minor tranquilizers have also been used in patients with ET or "exaggerated physiologic tremor." Their effect is nonspecific and the benefit is generally modest.

The carbonic anhydrase inhibitor methazolamide, which is used to treat glaucoma, may also provide palliation for some patients with ET (211a). The relative benefits of carbonic anhydrase inhibitors as compared with those of β-blockers or primidone in ET have not been fully studied.

Unfortunately, there is no satisfactory pharmacologic palliation for most patients with the severe kinetic tremors associated with cerebellar dysfunction. Carbamazepine and isoniazid have been advocated as potential treatments for cerebellar tremors (212, 213), but there is only a limited effect and little functional improvement.

SPASTICITY

The term *spasticity* refers to the various disorders of motor control resulting from damage to the corticospinal tract (the "upper motor neuron syndrome"). The syndrome includes weakness, exaggerated muscle-stretch reflexes, "clasp-knife" hypertonus, and Babinski responses. The antigravity muscles are predominantly affected, and consequently the arm often assumes a flexed and pronated position, the leg, an extended and adducted position. Involuntary spasms of the flexor muscles can occur spontaneously, in response to cutaneous stimuli, or during attempts to move.

There are many sites where the corticospinal pathways can be injured: from the cerebral cortex, to the subcortical white matter, to the internal capsule, to the brainstem, to the spinal cord. Other tracts (e.g., vestibulospinal, reticulospinal, thalamocortical, etc.) may be impaired concomitantly with the corticospinal tract. As a result, the form and degree of spasticity can vary considerably, depending both on the level of the neuraxis and which other tracts are affected (214).

In most patients with spasticity, paresis and loss of dexterity contribute significantly to the degree of neurologic disability. In some situations spasticity can be beneficial. For example, hemiplegic contraction of antigravity muscles with extension of the leg provides an intrinsic bracing effect that allows some patients to ambulate despite weakness. Eliminating the spastic hypertonus in this situation would be detrimental. However, when painful spastic muscle spasms or severe hypertonus are adding to the patient's discomfort and disability, it is appropriate to consider pharmacologic approaches to the management of spasticity (215).

Physiologically, damage to the descending corticospinal pathways leads to excessive excitation or decreased inhibition of the segmental spinal motor neurons. The drugs used clinically to alleviate spasticity act in various ways to decrease the excitability of spinal reflexes. They work by either enhancing presynaptic inhibition (baclofen, diazepam) or diminishing muscular contraction (dantrolene) (216).

Baclofen suppresses monosynaptic and polysynaptic excitation of motor neurons and interneurons. Although baclofen initially was thought to function as a γ-aminobutyric acid (GABA) agonist, its electrophysiologic and pharmacologic profiles are quite different from those of GABA. The drug may act via presynaptic mechanisms to reduce the release of excitatory neurotransmitters (217).

Baclofen is especially effective in reducing the frequency and severity of the painful flexor or extensor spasms that commonly occur in patients with spinal lesions (218). Flexor spasms can occur spontaneously or be provoked by cutaneous stimuli or attempts to move. The spasms can awaken patients from sleep and are often very unpleasant. Baclofen palliates flexor spasms in patients with complete spinal transections as well as less complete lesions, suggesting a local site of action directly in the spinal cord (219). Baclofen reduces the prolonged tonic flexor dystonias of the legs in patients with spinal spasticity. Baclofen also has antinociceptive effects and can alleviate the pain associated with spasticity (as well as other pain syndromes such as trigeminal neuralgia). Despite these benefits, baclofen does not improve the stiff gait associated with spinal spasticity and is not particularly beneficial in spastic hemiplegia of cerebral origin.

The dose of baclofen must be individualized to produce an optimal response. Treatment is initiated with half of a 10-mg tablet two or three times daily and increased every several days to 30 to 80 mg/day in three or four divided doses. The drug is absorbed rapidly and has a half-life of 3 to 4 hours. Sedation, confusion, ataxia, or hallucinations can occur in elderly patients with cerebral lesions or when large doses are given suddenly. These side-effects are uncommon in patients with spinal lesions in whom the dose is slowly titrated upward. Abrupt withdrawal of baclofen should be avoided, as it may produce a temporary increase in the severity of flexor spasms or precipitate an acute confusional syndrome.

Although the maximum recommended dose of baclofen is 80 mg/day, there are some patients who benefit from and tolerate doses well beyond 100 mg/day to alleviate severe muscle spasms of spinal origin (220). Baclofen has also been administered safely by direct infusion into the lumbar subarachnoid space using an implanted drug pump (221). Long-term continuous intrathecal infusion of baclofen can be highly effective for patients with severe spinal spasticity who do not tolerate or respond to high-dose oral baclofen.

Benzodiazepines, such as diazepam, enhance presynaptic inhibition in the spinal cord by facilitating the effects of GABA (216). Diazepam is useful as adjunct therapy for patients with spasticity as well as other nonspastic types of involuntary muscle activity, such as tetanus, torsion dystonia, the stiff-man syndrome, or local posttraumatic muscle spasms. Treatment should be initiated in low doses (e.g., 2 mg twice a day) and increased slowly every few days up to as much as 20 mg three times a day to control spastic muscle spasms. Patients can tolerate such high doses of diazepam if the drug is introduced very gradually. However, sedation, weakness, dizziness, physical dependence, and interactions with other CNS-active medications are major drawbacks to the use of benzodiazepines in patients with spasticity (217).

Unlike baclofen and diazepam, which act centrally to alleviate spasticity, dantrolene acts directly on skeletal muscle. Dantrolene inhibits the release of calcium ions from the sarcoplasmic reticulum, thereby preventing activation of the contractile apparatus and diminishing the mechanical force of contraction (178). Dantrolene produces its muscle relaxing and antispastic effects by producing mild to moderate weakness. Therefore, this drug is useful only in treating patients with spasticity whose nursing care is made difficult by severe, prolonged muscle contraction, and who will not be further incapacitated by additional loss of strength (e.g., bedridden patients).

In treating spasticity, dantrolene is started at a dose of 25 mg/day by mouth. The dose is titrated upward by an additional 25 mg/day once or twice weekly. Benefits may not be apparent for several days after a dose change, so that frequent dose increments are inappropriate. Weakness, diarrhea, or both, will eventually occur as higher doses are reached. Maximum doses above 100 mg four times a day are seldom indicated. Concomitant use of diazepam and dantrolene might control the symptoms of spasticity better than either drug alone, with smaller doses and fewer side-effects (215). Although dantrolene has relatively little effect on cardiac or smooth muscle, patients with severe myocardial disease or borderline pulmonary function should be monitored closely if they are to receive this drug.

Dantrolene is absorbed slowly and incompletely from the gastrointestinal tract and has a half-life of 9 hours. It is metabolized by the liver and excreted in the urine. In addition to its oral use in spasticity, dantrolene is available for intravenous administration for the treatment of malignant hyperthermia, neuroleptic malignant syndrome, and heat stroke (175, 177).

A severe hepatitis can occur as an idiosyncratic reaction during dantrolene therapy, and fatalities have been reported (222). Chemical abnormalities of liver function occur in 1%, and symptomatic hepatitis (including anorexia, nausea, vomiting, and abdominal discomfort) occur in 0.5% of patients who have been receiving dantrolene for more than 2 months. Liver function should be tested periodically during dantrolene administration. In view of the potential for hepatic injury, dantrolene should be discontinued if no clear-cut benefit for spasticity is seen within several weeks of the maximum tolerated dose.

Dizziness, lightheadedness, drowsiness, and fatigue are common symptoms when dantrolene is being initiated, but are usually transient. Diarrhea is also a common side-effect and occasionally necessitates withdrawal of treatment.

REFERENCES

1. Marsden CD: The mysterious motor function of the basal ganglia. *Neurology* 32:514–539, 1982.
2. Watts RL, Mandir AS: The role of the motor cortex in the pathophysiology of voluntary movement deficits associated with parkinsonism. *Neurol Clin* 10:451–470, 1992.
3. Young AB, Penney JB: Neurochemical anatomy of movement disorders. *Neurol Clin* 2:417–433, 1984.
4. Rajput AH, Offord KP, Beard CM, et al: Epidemiology of parkinsonism: incidence, classification, and mortality. *Ann Neurol* 16:278–282, 1984.
5. Stern M, Dulaney E, Gruber SB, et al: Epidemiology of Parkinson's disease. A case control study of young onset and old onset patients. *Arch Neurol* 48:903–907, 1991.
6. Kurtzke JF, Murphy FM: The changing patterns of death rates in Parkinson's disease. *Neurol* 40:42–49, 1990.
7. Duvoisin RC: A brief history of parkinsonism. *Neurol Clin* 10:301–316, 1992.
8. Zetusky WJ, Jankovic J, Pirozzolo FJ: The heterogeneity of Parkinson's disease: clinical and prognostic implications. *Neurol* 35:522–526, 1985.
9. Hoehn MM, Yahr MD: Parkinsonism: onset, progression, and mortality. *Neurology* 17:427–442, 1967.
10. Hornykiewicz O: Dopamine and brain function. *Pharmacol Rev* 18:925–964, 1966.
11. Bernheimer H, Birkmeyer W, Hornykiewicz O, et al: Brain dopamine and the syndrome of Parkinson and Huntington. *J Neurol Sci* 20:414–445, 1973.
12. Cotzias GC, VanWoert MH, Schiffer LM: Aromatic amino acids and modification of parkinsonism. *N Engl J Med* 276:374–378, 1967.
13. Lees AJ: L-dopa treatment and Parkinson's disease. *Q J Med* 59:535–547, 1986.
14. Marsden CD: Parkinson's disease. *Lancet* 1:948–952, 1990.
15. Langston JW, Ballard P, Tetrud JW, et al: Chronic parkinsonism in humans due to a product of meperidine analog synthesis. *Science* 219:979–980, 1983.
16. Burns RS, LeWitt PA, Ebert MH, et al: The clinical syndrome of striatal dopamine deficiency. Parkinsonism induced by MPTP. *N Engl J Med* 312:1418–1421, 1985.
17. Langston JW, Irwin I, Langston EB, et al: Pargyline prevents MPTP-induced parkinsonism in primates. *Science* 225:1480–1482, 1984.
18. Cohen G, Pasik P, Cohen P, et al: Pargyline and deprenyl prevent the neurotoxicity of MPTP in monkeys. *Eur J Pharmacol* 106:209–210, 1985.
19. Tanner CM, Langston JW: Do environmental toxins cause Parkinson's disease? *Neurol* 40(suppl 3):17–30, 1990.
20. Olanow CM: Oxidative reactions in Parkinson's disease. *Neurology* 40(suppl 3):32–37, 1990.
21. Boyson SJ: Parkinson's disease and the electron transport chain. *Ann Neurol* 30:330–332, 1991.
21a. Shoffner JM, Watts RL, Juncos JL, et al: Mitochondrial oxidative phosphorylation defects in Parkinson's disease. *Ann Neurol* 30:332–339, 1991.
22. The Parkinson Study Group: Effect of deprenyl on the progression of disability in early Parkinson's disease. *N Engl J Med* 321:1364–1371, 1989.
23. Tetrud JW, Langston JW: The effect of deprenyl (selegiline) on the natural history of Parkinson's disease. *Science* 245:519–522, 1989.
23a. Langston JW: Selegiline as neuroprotective therapy in Parkinson's disease. *Neurology* 40(suppl 3):61–66, 1990.
23b. Olanow CW, Calne D: Does selegiline act by symptomatic or protective mechanisms? *Neurology* 42(suppl 4):13–26, 1992.
24. Langston JW, Koller WC: The next frontier in Parkinson's disease: presymptomatic detection. *Neurology* 41(suppl 2):5–7, 1991.
25. Knoll J: Deprenyl (selegiline): the history of its development and pharmacologic action. *Acta Neurol Scand* 95:57–80, 1983.
26. Elsworth JD, Glover V, Reynolds GP, et al: Deprenyl administration in man: a selective MAO-B inhibitor without the "cheese effect." *Psychopharmacology* 57:33–38, 1987.
27. Lieberman A: Long-term experience with selegiline and levodopa in Parkinson's disease. *Neurology* 42(suppl 4):32–36, 1992.
28. Golbe LI, Lieberman AN, Muenter MD, et al: Deprenyl in the treatment of symptom fluctuations in advanced Parkinson's disease. *Clin Neuropharmacol* 11:45–55, 1988.
29. Golbe LI: Long-term efficacy and safety of deprenyl (selegiline) in advanced Parkinson's disease. *Neurology* 39:1109–1111, 1989.
30. Karoum F, Chaung L-W, Eisler T, et al: Metabolism of deprenyl to amphetamine and methamphetamine may be responsible for deprenyl's therapeutic benefit. A biochemical assessment. *Neurology* 32:503–509, 1982.
31. Mayeux R, Stern Y, Cote L, et al: Altered serotonin metabolism in depressed patients with Parkinson's disease. *Neurology* 31:645–650, 1984.
32. Suchowersky O, de Vries JH: Interaction of fluoxetine and selegiline. *Can J Psychiatry* 35:571–572, 1990.
33. Lieberman A: An integrated approach to patient management in Parkinson's disease. *Neurol Clin* 10:553–565, 1992.
34. Schwab RS, England AC, Poskanzer DC, et al: Amantadine in the treatment of Parkinson's disease. *JAMA* 208:1168–1170, 1969.
35. Koller WC: Pharmacologic treatment of parkinsonian tremor. *Arch Neurol* 43:126–127, 1986.
36. Rajput AH, Stern W, Loverty WH: Chronic low dose levodopa therapy in Parkinson's disease: an argument for delaying levodopa therapy. *Neurology* 34:991–996, 1984.
37. Shannon KM, Goetz CG, Carroll VS, et al: Amantadine and motor fluctuations in chronic Parkinson's disease. *Clin Neuropharmacol* 6:522–526, 1987.
38. Koller WC, Hubble JP: Levodopa therapy in Parkinson's disease. *Neurology* 40(suppl 3):40–47, 1990.
39. Lesser RP, Fahn S, Snider SR, et al: Analysis of the clinical problems in parkinsonism and complications of long-term levodopa therapy. *Neurology* 29:1253–1260, 1979.
40. Markham CH, Diamond SG: Evidence to support early levodopa therapy in Parkinson's disease. *Neurology* 31:125–131, 1981.
41. Cedarbaum JM, Gandy SE, McDowell FH: "Early" initiation of levodopa treatment does not promote development of motor response fluctuations, dyskinesia, or dementia in Parkinson's disease. *Neurology* 41:622–629, 1991.
42. Diamond SG, Markham CH, Hoehn MM, et al: Multicenter study of parkinson mortality with early versus later treatment with L-dopa. *Ann Neurol* 22:8–12, 1987.
43. Rinne UK: Early combination of bromocriptine and levodopa. *Neurology* 37:826–828, 1987.
44. Bianchine JR, Shaw GM: Clinical pharmacokinetics of levodopa in Parkinson's disease. *Clin Pharmacokinet* 1:313–358, 1976.
45. Evans MA, Broe GA, Triggs EJ, et al: Gastric emptying rate and the systemic availability of levodopa in elderly parkinsonian patients. *Neurology* 31:1288–1294, 1981.
46. Nutt JG, Fellman JH: Pharmacokinetics of levodopa. *Clin Neuropharmacol* 7:35–50, 1984.
47. Wade LA, Katzman R: Synthetic amino acids and the nature of L-dopa transport at the blood-brain barrier. *J Neurochem* 25:837–842, 1975.
48. Melamed E, Hefti F, Wurtman RJ: Nonaminergic striatal neurons convert exogenous L-dopa to dopamine in parkinsonism. *Ann Neurol* 8:558–563, 1980.
49. Melamed E, Hefti F: Mechanism of short and long-term L-dopa treatment in parkinsonism: role of the surviving nigro-striatal dopaminergic neurons. *Adv Neurol* 40:149–157, 1983.
50. Muenter MD, Tyce GM: L-dopa in Parkinson's disease: plasma l-dopa concentration, therapeutic effects, and side-effects. *Mayo Clin Proc* 46:231–239, 1971.
51. Reid JL, Calne DB, Vakil SD, et al: Plasma concentration of levodopa in parkinsonism before and after inhibition of peripheral decarboxylase. *J Neurol Sci* 47:45–51, 1972.
52. Ward CD, Trombley IK, Calne DB, et al: L-dopa decarboxylation in chronically treated patients. *Neurology* 34:198–201, 1984.
53. Poewe WH, Lees AJ, Stern GM: Low dose L-dopa therapy in Parkinson's disease. *Neurology* 36:1528–1530, 1986.
54. Pfeiffer R: Optimization of levodopa therapy. *Neurology* 44(suppl 1):39–43, 1992.
55. Nausieda PA, Weiner WJ, Kaplan LR, et al: Sleep disruption in the course of chronic L-dopa therapy. *Clin Neuropharmacol* 5:183–194, 1982.
56. Parkes JD: Domperidone and Parkinson's disease. *Clin Neuropharmacol* 9:517–532, 1986.
57. Koller WC, LeWitt PA: Clinical studies and pharmacologic considerations of sustained release levodopa. *Neurology* 42(suppl 1):29–32, 1992.
58. Rodnitzky RL: Use of Sinemet CR in management of mild to moderate Parkinson's disease. *Neurology* 42(suppl 1):44–50, 1992.
59. Cedarbaum JM, Kutt H, McDowell F: A pharmacologic and pharmacodynamic comparison of Sinemet CR and standard Sinemet. *Neurology* 39(suppl 2):38–44, 1989.

60. Feldman RG, Mosbach PA, Kelly MR, et al: Double blind comparison of standard Sinemet and Sinemet CR in patients with mild to moderate Parkinson's disease. *Neurology* 39(suppl 2):96–101, 1989.

61. Duvoisin RG: Management of patients who fail to respond to levodopa therapy. *Clin Neuropharmacol* 5(suppl 2):13–18, 1982.

61b. Koller WC: Alternate day levodopa therapy in parkinsonism. *Neurology* 32:324–326, 1982.

62. Kish SJ, Shannak K, Hornykiewicz O: Uneven pattern of dopamine loss in the striatum of patients with idiopathic Parkinson's disease. *N Engl J Med* 318:876–880, 1988.

63. Fabbrini G, Mouradian MM, Juncos JL, et al: Motor fluctuations in Parkinson's disease: central pathophysiological mechanisms. *Ann Neurol* 24:366–371, 1988.

64. Cedarbaum JM: Pharmacokinetic and pharmacodynamic considerations in management of motor response fluctuations in Parkinson's disease. *Neurol Clin* 8:31–49, 1990.

65. Nutt JG, Woodward WR, Hammerstad JD, et al: Do the pharmacokinetics of L-dopa explain the on-off phenomenon? *Neurology* 33(suppl 2):91, 1983.

66. Goetz CG, Tanner CM, Gilley DW, et al: Development and progression of motor fluctuations and side-effects in Parkinson's disease: comparison of Sinemet CR versus carbidopa/levodopa. *Neurology* 39(suppl 2):63–66, 1989.

67. Goetz CG: Dopaminergic agonists in the treatment of Parkinson's disease. *Neurology* 40(suppl 3):50–54, 1990.

68. Muenter MD, Sharpless NS, Tyce GM, et al: Patterns of I-D-I and D-I-D in response to L-dopa therapy for Parkinson's disease. *Mayo Clin Proc* 52:163–174, 1977.

69. Lang AE, Johnson K: Akathisia in idiopathic Parkinson's disease. *Neurology* 37:477–481, 1987. 69b. Jankovic J: Management of motor side-effects of chronic levodopa therapy. *Clin Neuropharmacol* 5(suppl 1):19–27, 1982.

70. Obeso JA, Gvandas F, Vaamonde J, et al: Motor complications associated with chronic levodopa therapy in Parkinson's disease. *Neurology* 39(suppl 2):11–19, 1989.

71. Bonnet AM, Loria Y, Saint-Hilaire MH, et al: Does long-term aggravation of Parkinson's disease result from non-dopaminergic lesions? *Neurology* 37:1539–1542, 1987.

72. Klawans HL: Individual manifestations of Parkinson's disease after 10 or more years of treatment. *Mov Disord* 1:187–192, 1986.

73. Nutt JG, Woodward WR, Hammerstad JP, et al: The "on-off" phenomenon in Parkinson's disease. Relation to levodopa absorption and transport. *N Engl J Med* 310:483–488, 1984.

74. Nutt JG: On-off phenemenon: relation to levodopa pharmacokinetics and pharmacodynamics. *Ann Neurol* 22:535–540, 1987.

75. Granda F, Obesa JA: Motor responses following repeated apomorphine are reduced in Parkison's disease. *Clin Neuropharmacol* 12:14–22, 1989.

76. Wooten GF: Progress in understanding the pathophysiology of treatment-related fluctuations in Parkinson's disease. *Ann Neurol* 24:366–371, 1988.

77. Chase TN, Baronti T, Fabbrini G, et al: Rationale for continuous dopamimetic therapy of Parkinson's disease. *Neurology* 39(suppl 2):7–10, 1989.

78. Tsui JK, Ross S, Poulin K, et al: The effect of dietary protein on the efficacy of L-dopa. *Neurology* 39:549–552, 1989.

79. Pincus JH, Barry K: Influence of dietary protein on motor fluctuations in Parkinson's disease. *Arch Neurol* 44:270–272, 1987.

80. Pincus JH, Barry K: Protein redistribution diet restores motor function in patients with dopa-resistant "off" periods. *Neurology* 38:481–483, 1988.

81. Carter JH, Nutt JG, Woodward WR, et al: Amount and distribution of dietary protein affect clinical response to levodopa in Parkinson's disease. *Neurology* 39:552–556, 1989.

82. Juncos JL, Mouradian MM, Fabbrini G, et al: Levodopa methyl ester treatment of Parkinson's disease. *Neurology* 37:1242–1245, 1987.

83. Mouradian MM, Juncos JL, Fabbrini G, et al: Motor fluctuations in Parkinson's disease. Pathogenetic and therapeutic studies. *Ann Neurol* 22:475–479, 1987.

84. Sage JI, Trooskin S, Sonsalla PK, et al: Experience with continuous enteral levodopa infusions in the treatment of 9 patients with advanced Parkinson's disease. *Neurology* 39(suppl 2):60–63, 1989.

85. Sechi GP, Tanda F, Mutani R: Fatal hyperpyrexia after withdrawal of levodopa. *Neurology* 34:249–251, 1984.

86. Friedman JH, Feinberg SS, Feldman RG: A neuroleptic-malignant-like syndrome due to L-dopa withdrawal. *Ann Neurol* 10:126–127, 1984.

87. Weiner WJ, Koller WC, Perlik S, et al: Drug holiday and management of Parkinson's disease. *Neurology* 30:1257–1261, 1980.

88. Mayeux R, Stern Y, Mulvey K, et al: Reappraisal of temporary levodopa withdrawal (drug holiday) in Parkinson's disease. *N Engl J Med* 313:724–728, 1985.

89. Feldman RG, Kaye JA, Lannon MC: Parkinson's disease: follow-up after "drug holiday." *J Clin Pharmacol* 26:662–667, 1986.

90. Eisler T, Eng M, Plotkin C, et al: Absorption of levodopa after rectal administration. *Neurology* 31:215–217, 1981.

91. Teychenne PF, Calne DB, Lewis PJ, et al: Interactions of levodopa with inhibitors of monoamine oxidase and L-aromatic amino acid decarboxylase. *Clin Pharmacol Ther* 18:273–277, 1975.

92. Friedman JH: The management of the levodopa psychoses. *Clin Neuropharmacol* 14:283–295, 1991.

93. Jenkins RB, Mendelson SH, Lamid S, et al: Levodopa therapy of patients with parkinsonism and heart disease. *Br Med J* 3:512–514, 1972.

94. Liebowitz M, Lieberman A: Comparison of carbidopa combined with levodopa and levodopa alone on the cardiovascular system of patients with Parkinson's disease. *Neurology* 25:917–921, 1975.

95. Micieli G, Martignoni E, Cavalini A, et al: Postprandial and orthostatic hypotension in Parkinson's disease. *Neurology* 37:383–393, 1987. 95b. Durrieu G, Senard JM, Tran MA, et al: Effects of levodopa and bromocriptine on blood pressure and plasma catecholamines in Parkinson's disease. *Clin Neuropharmacol* 14:84–90, 1991.

96. McLeod JG, Tuck RR: Disorders of the autonomic nervous system. *Ann Neurol* 21:419–430, 519–529, 1987.

97. Rampen FHJ: Levodopa and melanoma: three cases and review of the literature. *J Neurol Neurosurg Psychiatry* 48:585–588, 1985.

98. Kochar AS: Development of malignant melanoma after levodopa therapy for Parkinson's disease. *Am J Med* 79:119–121, 1985.

99. Nausieda PA, Weiner WJ, Kaplan LR, et al: Sleep disruption in the course of chronic levodopa therapy. *Clin Neuropharmacol* 5:183–194, 1982.

100. Goetz CG, Tanner CM, Klawans HL: Pharmacology of hallucinations induced by long term drug therapy. *Am J Psychiatry* 139:494–498, 1982.

101. Sweet RD, McDowell FH, Ferguson JS, et al: Mental symptoms in Parkinson's disease during chronic treatment with levodopa. *Neurology* 26:305–310, 1976.

102. Moskovitz C, Moses H, Klawans HL: Levodopa-induced psychosis: a kindling phenomenon. *Am J Psychiatry* 135:669–675, 1978.

103. Klawans HL: Behavioral alterations and the therapy of parkinsonism. *Clin Neuropharmacol* 5(suppl 1):29–36, 1982.

104. Friedman JH, Lannon MC: Clozapine in the treatment of psychosis in Parkinson's disease. *Neurology* 39:1219–1221, 1989.

104b. Baldessarini RJ, Frankenburg FR: Clozapine—a novel antipsychotic agent. *N Engl J Med* 324:746–754, 1991.

105. Goetz CG, Diederich NJ: Dopaminergic agonists in the treatment of Parkinson's disease. *Neurol Clin* 10:527–540, 1992.

105b. Zimmerman T, Sage JI: Comparison of combination pergolide and levodopa to levodopa alone after 63 months of treatment. *Clin Neuropharmacol* 14:165–169, 1991.

105c. Koller WC: Initiating treatment of Parkinson's disease. *Neurology* 42(suppl 1):33–38, 1992.

106. Hoehn MM, Elton RL: Low doses of bromocriptine added to levodopa in Parkinson's disease. *Neurology* 35:199–206, 1985.

107. Goetz CG, Tanner CM, Glantz RH, et al: Chronic agonist therapy for Parkinson's disease: a five year study of bromocriptine and pergolide. *Neurology* 35:749–751, 1985.

108. Jankovic J: Long-term study of pergolide in Parkinson's disease. *Neurology* 35:296–299, 1983.

109. Walters JR, Bergstrom DA, Carlson DH, et al: D1 dopamine receptor activation required for postsynaptic expression of D2 agonist effects. *Science* 236:719–722, 1987.

110. Langtry HD, Clissold SP: Pergolide—a review of its pharmacologic properties and therapeutic potential in Parkinson's disease. *Drugs* 39:491–506, 1990.

111. Lieberman A, Neophytides A, Leibowitz M, et al: Comparative efficacy of pergolide and bromocriptine in patients with advanced Parkinson's disease. *Adv Neurol* 37:95–108, 1983.

112. Linch DC, Shaw KM, Muhlemann MF, et al: Bromocriptine induced postural hypotension in acromegaly. *Lancet* 1:320, 1978.

113. Teychenne PF, Bergsrud D, Elton R, et al: Bromocriptine: low dose therapy in Parkinson's disease. *Neurology* 32:573–583, 1982.

114. Lieberman AN, Goldstein M, Gopinathan G, et al: Further studies with pergolide in Parkinson's disease. *Neurology* 32:1181–1184, 1982.

115. Rinne UK: Dopamine agonists as primary treatment in Parkinson's disease. *Adv Neurol* 45:519–523, 1988.

116. Rinne UK: Early combination of bromocriptine and levodopa in treatment of Parkinson's disease: 5 year follow-up. *Neurology* 37:826–828, 1987.

117. Kurlan R, Miller C, Levy R, et al: Long term experience with pergolide in advanced parkinsonism. *Neurology* 35:738–742, 1985.

118. Tanner CM, Chablani R, Goetz CG, et al: Pergolide mesylate—lack of cardiac toxicity in patients with cardiac disease. *Neurology* 35:918–921, 1985.

119. Kurlan R, Miller C, Knapp R, et al: Double-blind assessment of potential pergolide-induced cardiotoxicity. *Neurology* 36:993–995, 1986.

120. Stern Y, Mayeux R, Ilson J, et al: Pergolide therapy for Parkinson's disease: neurobehavioral changes. *Neurology* 34:201–204, 1984.

121. Bhatt MH, Keenan SP, Fleetham JA, et al: Pleuropulmonary disease associated with dopamine agonist therapy. *Ann Neurol* 30:613–616, 1991.

122. McElvaney NG, Wilcox PG, Churg A, et al: Pleuropulmonary disease during bromocriptine treatment of Parkinson's disease. *Arch Intern Med* 148:2231–2236, 1988.

123. Vance ML, Evans WS, Thorner MO: Bromocriptine. *Ann Intern Med* 100:78–91, 1984.

124. Vitti RJ, Tanner CM, Rajput AH, et al: Hypersexuality with antiparkinson therapy. *Clin Neuropharmacol* 12:375–383, 1989.

125. Ropper AH, Hedley-Whyte ET: Case records of the Massachusetts General Hospital. *N Engl J Med* 308:1406–1414, 1983.

126. Jankovic J: Parkinsonism-plus syndromes. *Mov Disord* 4(suppl 1):95–119, 1989.

127. Rajput AH, Razdilsky B, Ang L: Occurrence of resting tremor in Parkinson's disease. *Neurology* 41:1298–1299, 1991.

128. Rajput AH, Rozdilsky B, Rajput A, et al: Levodopa efficacy and the pathological basis of Parkinson syndrome. *Clin Neuropharmacol* 13:553–558, 1990.

129. Tarsy D: Neuroleptic-induced extrapyramidal reactions: classification, description, and diagnosis. *Clin Neuropharmacol* 6(suppl 1):9–26, 1983.

130. Rifkin A, Quitkin F, Klein DF: Akinesia: a poorly recognised drug-induced extrapyramidal behavioral disorder. *Arch Gen Psychiatry* 32:672–674, 1975.

131. Ayd FJ Jr: A survey of drug-induced extrapyramidal reactions. *JAMA* 175:1054–1060, 1961.

132. Miller RJ, Hiley CR: Antimuscarinic properties of neuroleptic and drug-induced parkinsonism. *Nature* 248:596–597, 1974.

133. Rajput A, Rozdilsky B, Hornykiewicz O, et al: Reversible drug-induced parkinsonism. Clinicopathologic study of two cases. *Arch Neurol* 39:644–646, 1982.

134. Stephen PJ, Williamson J: Drug-induced parkinsonism in the elderly. *Lancet* 2:1082–1083, 1984.

135. Klawans HL, Bergen D, Bruyn GW: Prolonged drug-induced parkinsonism. *Confin Neurol* 35:368–377, 1973.

136. Hardie RJ, Lees AJ: Neuroleptic-induced Parkinson's syndrome. Clinical features and results of treatment with levodopa. *J Neurol Neurosurg Psychiatry* 51:850–854, 1988.

137. Allen RM: Role of amantadine in the management of neuroleptic induced extrapyramidal syndromes: overview and pharmacology. *Clin Neuropharmacol* 6(suppl 1):64–73, 1983.

138. Greenamyre TJ, O'Brien CF: N-methyl-D-aspartate antagonists in the treatment of Parkinson's disease. *Arch Neurol* 48:977–981, 1991.

139. Ing TS, Daugirdas JT, Soung LS, et al: Toxic effects of amantadine in patients with renal failure. *Can Med Assoc J* 120:695–698, 1979.

140. Fahn S, Craddock G, Kumin G: Acute toxic psychosis from suicidal overdose of amantadine. *Arch Neurol* 25:45–48, 1971.

141. Borison RL: Amantadine in the management of extrapyramidal side-effects. *Clin Neuropharmacol* 6(suppl 1):57–63, 1983.

142. Fann WE, Lake CR: Amantadine versus trihexyphenidyl in the treatment of neuroleptic-induced parkinsonism. *Am J Psychiatry* 8:940–943, 1976.

143. Gelenberg AJ: Amantadine in the treatment of benztropine refractory extrapyramidal disorders induced by antipsychotic drugs. *Curr Ther Res* 23:375–380, 1978.

144. Shealy CN, Weath JB, Mercier DA: Livedo reticularis in patients receiving amantadine. *JAMA* 212:1522–1523, 1970.

145. Sartori M, Pratt CM, Yound JB: Torsade de pointes—malignant cardiac arrhythmia induced by amantadine poisoning. *Am J Med* 77:388–391, 1984.

146. Duvoisin RC: Cholinergic-anticholinergic antagonism in parkinsonism. *Arch Neurol* 17:124–136, 1967.

147. Koller W: The pharmacologic treatment of parkinsonian tremor. *Arch Neurol* 43:126–127, 1986.

148. Duvoisin RC: A review of drug therapy in parkinsonism. *Bull NY Acad Med* 41:898–910, 1965.

149. Korczyn AD, Rubenstein AE: Autonomic nervous system complications of therapy. In Silverstein A (ed): Neurological Complications of Therapy. New York, Futura, 1982, pp 405–418.

150. Klawans HL: Behavioral alterations and the therapy of parkinsonism. *Clin Neuropharmacol* 5(suppl 1):29–37, 1982.

151. Drachman D, Leavitt J: Human memory and the cholinergic system. *Arch Neurol* 30:113–121, 1974.

152. Drachman D: Memory and cognitive function in man: does the cholinergic system have a specific role? *Neurology* 27:783–790, 1977.

153. Calne DB: The role of various forms of treatment in the management of Parkinson's disease. *Clin Neuropharmacol* 5(suppl 1):538–543, 1982.

154. Hughes RC, Polyar JG, Weightman D, et al: Levodopa in parkinsonism. The effect of withdrawal of anticholinergic drugs. *Br Med J* 2:487–491, 1971.

155. Manos N, Gziouzepar J, Logothetis J: The need for continuous use of antiparkinsonian medication in chronic schizophrenics receiving long-term neuroleptic therapy. *Am J Psychiatry* 138:184–188, 1981.

156. Swett C: Drug-induced dystonia. *Am J Psychiatry* 132:532–534, 1975.

157. Bateman DN, Rawlins MD, Simpson JM: Extrapyramidal reactions to metoclopramide. *Br Med J* 291:930–932, 1985.

158. Schaaf M, Payne CA: Dystonic reactions to perphenazine in hypoparathyroidism. *N Engl J Med* 275:991–995, 1966.

159. Gatrad AR, Gatrad AH: Familial incidence of dystonic reactions to metoclopramide. *Br J Clin Prac* 33:111–115, 1979.

160. Rupniak N, Jenner P, Marsden CD: Acute dystonia induced by neuroleptic drugs. *Psychopharmacology* 88:403–419, 1986.

161. Kolbe H, Clow A, Jenner P, et al: Neuroleptic-induced acute dystonic reactions may be due to enhanced dopamine release onto supersensitive postsynaptic receptors. *Neurology* 31:434–439, 1981.

162. Leopold NA: Prolonged metoclopramide-induced dyskinetic reaction. *Neurology* 34:238–239, 1984.

163. Gagrat D, Hamilton J, Belmaker RH: Intravenous diazepam in the treatment of neuroleptic-induced acute dystonia and akathisia. *Am J Psychiatry* 135:132–133, 1978.

164. Granner MA, Wooten GF: Neuroleptic malignant syndrome or parkinsonism hyperpyrexia syndrome. *Semin Neurol* 11:228–235, 1991.

165. Friedman LS, Weinrauch LA, D'Elia JA: Metoclopramide-induced neuroleptic malignant syndrome. *Arch Intern Med* 147:1495–1497, 1987.

166. Levenson JL: Neuroleptic malignant syndrome. *Am J Psychiatry* 142:1137–1145, 1985.

167. Guze BH, Baxter LR: Neuroleptic malignant syndrome. *N Engl J Med* 313:163–166, 1985.

168. Keck PE, Pope HG, McElroy SJ: Declining frequency of neuroleptic malignant synrome in a hospital population. *Am J Psychiatry* 148:880–882, 1991.

169. Jones EM, Dawson A: Neuroleptic malignant syndrome: a case report with post-mortem brain and muscle pathology. *J Neurol Neurosurg Psychiatry* 52:1006–1009, 1989.

170. Keck PE, Pope HG, Cohen BM, et al: Risk factors for neuroleptic malignant syndrome. *Arch Gen Psychiatry* 46:914–918, 1989.

171. Turkka JT, Myllya VV: Sweating dysfunction in Parkinson's disease. *Eur Neurol* 26:1–7, 1987.

172. Goetz CG, Lutge W, Tanner CM: Autonomic dysfunction in Parkinson's disease. *Neurology* 936:73–75, 1986.

173. Gibb WG, Lees AJ: The neuroleptic malignant syndrome—a review. *Q J Med* 56:421–429, 1985.

174. Granato JE, Stern BJ, Ringel A, et al: Neuroleptic malignant syndrome: successful treatment with dantrolene and bromocriptine. *Ann Neurol* 19:89–90, 1983.

175. Rosenberg MR, Green M: Neuroleptic malignant syndrome—review of response to therapy. *Arch Intern Med* 149:1927–1931, 1989.

176. Dhib-Jalbut S, Hesselbrock R, Mouradian MM, et al: Bromocriptine treatment in neuroleptic malignant syndrome. *J Clin Psychiatry* 48:69–73, 1987.

177. May DC, Morris SW, Stewart M, et al: Neuroleptic malignant syndrome: response to dantrolene sodium. *Ann Intern Med* 98:183–184, 1983.

178. Davidoff RA: Antispasticity drugs: mechanisms of action. *Ann Neurol* 17:107–116, 1985.

179. Rosebush PI, Stewart TD, Gelenberg AJ: Twenty neuroleptic rechallenges after neuroleptic malignant syndrome in 15 patients. *J Clin Psychiatry* 50:295–298, 1989.

180. Pope HG, Aizley HG, Keck PE, et al: Neuroleptic malignant syndrome: long-term follow up of 20 cases. *J Clin Psychiatry* 52:208–212, 1991.

181. Jankovic J, Fahn S: Physiologic and pathologic tremors: diagnosis, mechanism, and management. *Ann Intern Med* 93:460–465, 1980.

182. Hallett M: Classification and treatment of tremor. *JAMA* 266:1115–1117, 1991.

183. Findley LJ, Koller WC: Essential tremor: a review. *Neurology* 37:1194–1197, 1987.

184. Young RR: Essential-familial tremors and other action tremors. *Semin Neurol* 2:386–391, 1982.

185. Fahn S, Marsden CD, VanWoert MH: Definition and classification of myoclonus. *Adv Neurol* 43:1–5, 1986.

186. Young RR, Shahani BT: Asterixis: one type of negative myoclonus. *Adv Neurol* 43:137–156, 1986.

187. Karas BJ, Wilder BJ, Hammond EJ, et al: Valproate tremors. *Neurology* 32:428–432, 1983.

188. Schou M, Baastrup PC, Grof P, et al: Pharmacologic problems of lithium prophylaxis. *Br J Psychiatry* 116:615–619, 1970.

189. Neiman J, Lang AE, Fornazzari L, et al: Movement disorders in alcoholism: a review. *Neurology* 40:741–746, 1990.

190. Wikler A: Diagnosis and treatment of drug dependence of the barbiturate type. *Am J Psychiatry* 125:758–765, 1968.

191. Mackinnon GL, Parker WA: Benzodiazepine withdrawal syndrome: a literature review and evaluation. *Am J Drug Alcohol Abuse* 9:19–33, 1982.

192. Larsen TA, Calne DB: Essential tremor. *Clin Neuropharmacol* 6:185–206, 1983.

193. Koller W, Biary N, Cone S: Disability in essential tremor: effect of treatment. *Neurology* 36:1001–1004, 1986.

194. Findley LJ, Cleeves L: The relation of essential tremor to Parkinson's disease. *J Neurol Neurosurg Psychiatry* 48:192–196, 1985.

195. Geraghty JJ, Jankovic JJ, Zetusky WJ: Association between essential tremor and Parkinson's disease. *Ann Neurol* 17:329–333, 1985.

196. Shahani BT, Young RR: Physiological and pharmacological aids in the differential diagnosis of tremor. *J Neurol Neurosurg Psychiatry* 39:772–783, 1976.

197. Koller WC, Biary N: Effect of alcohol on tremor: comparison to propranolol. *Neurology* 34:280–282, 1984.

198. Koller WC: Alcoholism in essential tremor. *Neurology* 33:1074–1076, 1983.

199. Winkler GF, Young RR: Efficacy of chronic propranolol in action tremors of the familial, senile, or essential variety. *N Engl J Med* 290:984–988, 1974.

200. Cleeves LA, Findley LJ: Beta adrenoreceptor mechanisms in essential tremor. *J Neurol Neurosurg Psychiatry* 47:976–982, 1984.

201. Leigh PN, Jefferson D, Twomey A, et al: Beta adrenoreceptor mechanisms in essential tremor: a double-blind placebo controlled trial of metoprolol, sotalol, and atenolol. *J Neurol Neurosurg Psychiatry* 46:710–715, 1983.

202. Koller WC: Dose response relationship of propranolol in treatment of essential tremor. *Arch Neurol* 43:42–43, 1986.

203. Sorenson PS, Paulson G, Steiness E, et al: Essential tremor treated with propranolol: lack of correlation between clinical effect and plasma propranolol levels. *Ann Neurol* 9:53–57, 1981.

204. Koller WC: Long-acting propranolol in essential tremor. *Neurology* 35:108–110, 1984.

205. Koller WC, Royse VL: Time course of a single oral dose of propranolol in essential tremor. *Neurology* 35:1494–1497, 1985.

206. Newman RP, Jacobs L: Metoprolol in essential tremor. *Arch Neurol* 37:596–597, 1980.
207. Koller WC, Royse VL: Efficacy of primidone in essential tremor. *Neurology* 36:121–124, 1986.
208. Findley LJ, Cleeves L: Phenobarbitone in essential tremor. *Neurology* 35:1784–1787, 1985.
209. Sasso E, Perucca E, Fava R, et al: Primidone in the long-term treatment of essential tremor. A prospective study with computerized quantitative analysis. *Clin Neuropharmacol* 13:67–76, 1990.
210. Karas BJ, Wilder BJ, Hammond EJ, et al: Treatment of valproate tremors. *Neurology* 33:1380–1382, 1983.
211. Kirk L, Baastrup PC, Schou M: Propranolol and lithium-induced tremor. Lancet 1:839, 1972.
211a. Muenter MD, Daube JR, Caviness JN, Miller PM: Treatment of essential tremor with methazolamide. *Mayo Clin Proc* 66:991–997, 1991.
212. Hallett M, Lindsley JW, Adelstein RD, et al: Controlled trial of isoniazid therapy for severe postural tremor in multiple sclerosis. *Neurology* 35:1374–1377, 1985.
213. Sechi GP, Zuddas M, Piredda M, et al: Treatment of cerebellar tremors with carbamazepine: a controlled trial with long-term follow up. *Neurology* 39:1113–1115, 1989.
214. Landau WM: Spasticity: the fable of a neurological demon and the emperor's new therapy. *Arch Neurol* 31:217–219, 1974.
215. Young RR, Delwaide PJ: Drug therapy: spasticity (part 1). *N Engl J Med* 304:28–33, 1981.
216. Davidoff RA: Antispasticity drugs: mechanism of action. *Ann Neurol* 17:107–116, 1985.
217. Young RR, Delwaide PJ: Drug therapy: spasticity (part 2). *N Engl J Med* 304:96–99, 1981.
218. Duncan GW, Shahani BT, Young RR: An evaluation of baclofen treatment for certain symptoms of patients with spinal cord lesions: a double-blind cross-over study. *Neurology* 26:441–446, 1976.
219. Young RR: Treatment of spastic paraparesis. *N Engl J Med* 320:1553–1555, 1989.
220. Smith CR, LaRocca NG, Giesser BS, et al: High dose oral baclofen: experience in patients with multiple sclerosis. *Neurology* 41:1829–1831, 1991.
221. Penn RD, Savoy SM, Corcos D, et al: Intrathecal baclofen for severe spinal spasticity. *N Engl J Med* 320:1517–1521, 1989.
222. Wilkinson SP, Portman B, Williams R: Hepatitis from dantrolene sodium. *Gut* 20:33–36, 1979.

CHAPTER 33

Bronchodilators

MARISSA SELIGMAN, PHARM.D.

The use of drugs with potent bronchodilator action has proved to be highly effective therapy for the treatment of reversible airway obstruction. This effectiveness has been documented most extensively in patients with acute, severe asthma. In intensive care patients with bronchospasm, bronchodilator therapy may reverse hypoxia and normalize acid-base abnormalities, thereby helping to improve tissue perfusion and oxygenation. Additionally, these drugs may be used prophylactically to prevent the development of bronchospasm. In an evaluation of drug use in a trauma intensive care unit, bronchodilators accounted for 66% of all scheduled medications (7).

Effective use of bronchodilators requires a knowledge of the basic pathophysiology responsible for airway obstruction and the effect of drugs on airway caliber. Clinicians should also employ a systematic approach to the use of the various bronchodilators in patients with reversible airway obstruction.

AIRWAY OBSTRUCTION

Airway caliber and tone are regulated by the parasympathetic and sympathetic divisions of the autonomic nervous system (4, 5, 59). The vagally mediated mechanisms of the parasympathetic nervous system are the primary determinants of normal bronchomotor tone and bronchial submucosal gland secretion (4, 20, 59). On stimulation of vagal efferent nerves, the neurotransmitter acetylcholine is released from the presynaptic nerve terminal. The acetylcholine then diffuses through the synaptic cleft and binds to muscarinic cholinergic receptors found on postsynaptic tissue cell membranes throughout the respiratory tree. Stimulation of the cholinergic receptors results in an increase in intracellular levels of cyclic guanosine monophosphate (cGMP) in the cytoplasm, thereby increasing the activity of the effector mechanism (59). Acetylcholine receptors are located in or adjacent to the respiratory epithelium, submucosal glands, mast cells, and airway smooth muscle (4, 5, 20, 59). The highest number of receptors is found within the trachea and large bronchi (68). Stimulation of the acetylcholine receptors in the lung causes bronchoconstriction and decreased airway caliber (maximally in the small bronchi, but none in the small bronchioles), as well as mast cell degranulation and increased glandular secretion (8).

Direct sympathetic nervous system innervation of the respiratory tree is sparse (68). Nevertheless, bronchial smooth muscle cells, especially those located in the smaller airways (68), are well populated with noninnervated β_2-adrenergic receptors. β_1-Adrenergic receptors are also found in the lung but have only a minimal role in lung physiology (39). β_2-Adrenergic receptors are stimulated by adrenergic agonists, either endogenous (the presynaptic neurotransmitter norepinephrine, or epinephrine released by the adrenal medulla) or exogenous (drugs). This stimulation results in activation of membrane-bound adenylate cyclase to catalyze the conversion of adenosine triphosphate to cyclic adenosine monophosphate (cAMP) (38). A cascade of enzymatic reactions then progresses, resulting in bronchodilation and possibly in increased secretion of mucus (72).

α-Adrenergic receptors are also found in the lung (59). Postsynaptic α1-receptors are located predominantly in the bronchial and vascular smooth muscle and submucosal glands. Stimulation of these receptors by α-adrenergic agonists such as norepinephrine activates phosphatidylinositol turnover in the cytoplasm (63). The resulting bronchial smooth muscle and submucosal gland tissue responses are bronchoconstriction and increased mucus secretion. In the lung, α2-receptors are located on the postsynaptic nerve terminal, although they are also located presynaptically elsewhere in the body. Presynaptic α2-receptors regulate the release of norepinephrine from the presynaptic nerve terminal (63).

To summarize, the primary autonomic innervation of bronchial smooth muscle and the respiratory epithelium is via the parasympathetic (cholinergic) nervous system. This system is excitatory to the lungs; its activation causes bronchial smooth muscle contraction and bronchial gland secretion. This tonic activity is opposed, albeit minimally, by the sympathetic (adrenergic) nervous system. Bronchodilation results from activation of the β2-receptors of the sympathetic nervous system.

In addition to autonomic nervous system control of airway tone, respiratory tree caliber may be altered by a third neural innervation pathway, the so-called "purinergic" or "nonadrenergic noncholinergic (NANC)" nervous system (1, 4, 20, 68). Stimulation of this pathway produces bronchial smooth muscle contraction. The exact role of the NANC nervous system remains to be defined, but further investigation of this system eventually might lead to novel forms of treatment of airway diseases (60).

Various endogenous substances, such as histamine, prostaglandins, platelet activating factor, bradykinin, and the leukotrienes, also have documented inflammatory effects on smooth muscle tone, which have been documented to cause bronchoconstriction (1, 9).

Nonneurogenic factors may alter airway caliber by affecting either airway anatomy or physiology. The most common causes of increased airway resistance are asthma (acute or chronic), emphysema, chronic bronchitis, and cystic fibrosis. Mechanical factors, such as tumors, mucous plugging, and foreign bodies, are also frequent causes of airway obstruction (1). Less commonly, airway obstruction develops from inhalation of toxic materials and resultant airway injury, drug-induced bronchoconstriction, infectious bronchitis, or bronchiolitis (1). Acute left ventricular failure infrequently may present as airway obstruction, as can pulmonary emboli. When airway obstruction occurs as a result of immunologic disorders (e.g., collagen-vascular disorders, sensitivity to dust) or aspiration, bronchoconstriction is often not involved (1). Accordingly, drug-induced bronchodilation may not reverse the resistance to airflow associated with these conditions.

Clinically, patients with airflow obstruction usually manifest tachypnea, labored respiration with accessory muscle use, pulsus paradoxus, thoracic overinflation, and ventilation-perfusion mismatching (1). Auscultation of the airways commonly demonstrates rales and prolongation of the expiratory phase. Wheezing is a prominent sign but may be absent if airway obstruction is so severe that a wheeze cannot be generated (1). Most patients with airway obstruction demonstrate abnormalities in peak expiratory flow measurements and spirometry. For example, if presenting with an forced expiratory volume in 1 second (FEV-1) of less than 800 ml or a peak expiratory flow rate of less than 100 ml/min, the patient usually should receive aggressive pharmacotherapy (1).

Critically ill patients who are mechanically ventilated may experience airflow obstruction as a result of abnormalities in lung compliance, thoracic deflation, laryngeal spasm, laryngeal edema, epiglottitis, blunt laryngeal trauma, and tracheal avulsion (1). Thus, when assessing these patients, the clinician should take care to evaluate artificial airway position and upper airway function.

CLASSIFICATION OF BRONCHODILATOR DRUGS

The classification system used to group bronchodilator drugs is based on their mechanism of action: (*a*) direct respiratory smooth muscle relaxants—theophylline and related salts; (*b*) β-adrenergic agonists—isoetharine, isoproterenol, epinephrine, metaproterenol, albuterol, terbutaline, bitolterol, and pirbuterol; and (*c*) anticholinergics—atropine, glycopyrrolate, and ipratropium. Their sites of action are depicted in Figure 33.1 (64).

THEOPHYLLINE

Theophylline, a naturally occurring methylxanthine closely related to caffeine and found in tea, has been used to treat bronchospasm for more than 100 years (46). An enormous number of pharmacokinetic and pharmacodynamic data relative to this drug have been generated during the past 20 years. These findings have contributed to renewed interest in theophylline and the introduction of a wide variety of theophylline products into clinical use. Because of conflicting reports of efficacy and safety, however, use of theophylline in the initial treatment of acute bronchospasm remains controversial (48). Still, theophylline has become one of the most extensively prescribed drugs for the treatment of reversible airway obstruction. The development of methods to monitor serum theophylline concentrations in patients has contributed to the safe and effective clinical use of this drug.

Pharmacology

The exact mechanism by which theophylline exerts its pharmacologic effects is unclear (30). It is well-established that theophylline competitively inhibits the activity of cytoplasmic phosphodiesterase, the enzyme that catalyzes the degradation of cAMP to 5'-AMP (73). This inhibition increases intracellular levels of cAMP, resulting in smooth muscle relaxation. However, this effect is unlikely to be responsible for the bronchodilating effects of theophylline such as can be demonstrated only in vitro using very high concentrations of theophylline (6, 30). Additionally, unlike theophylline, other, more potent phosphodiesterase inhibitors do not produce bronchodilation (30). Other postulated mechanisms of action include inhibition of intracellular calcium activity (26), prostaglandin inhibition (25), indirect β-adrenergic stimulation via release of catecholamines (53), and increased binding of cAMP to cAMP-binding protein (10, 50). Adenosine receptor antagonism has also been proposed

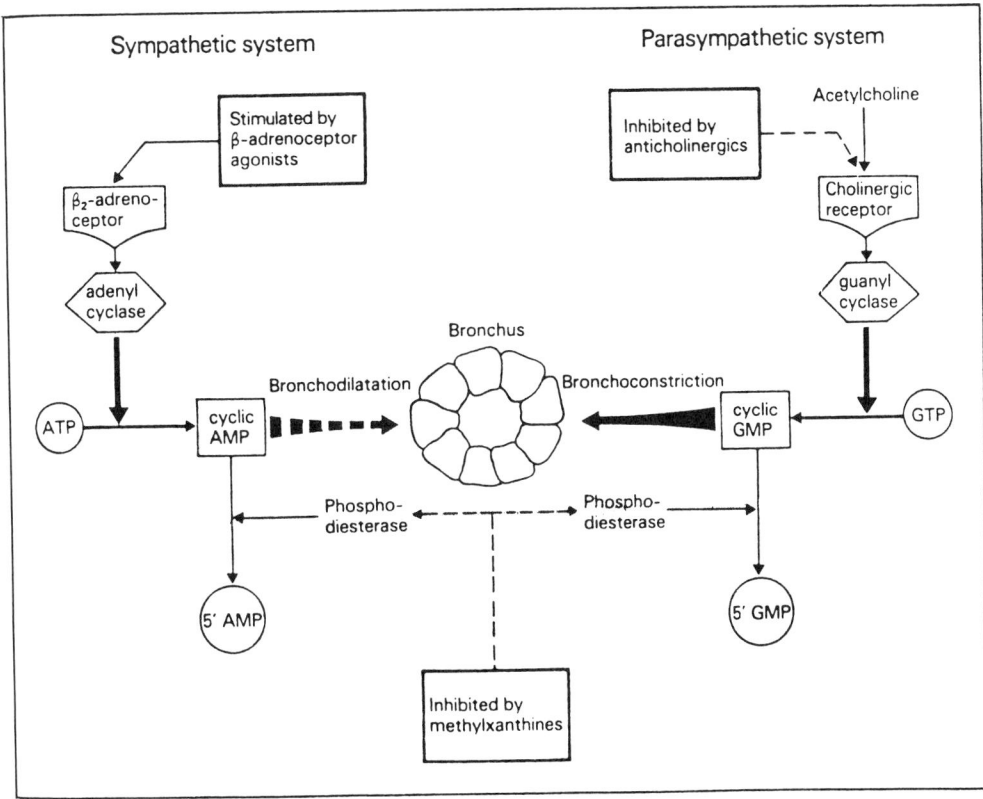

Figure 33.1. Mechanism of action of bronchodilator drugs. (Originally published in Kelly HW: Controversies in asthma therapy with theophylline and the β-2-adrenergic agents. *Clin Pharm* 3:386–395, 1984. Copyright 1984, American Society of Hospital Pharmacists, Inc. All rights reserved. Reprinted with permission.)

as the primary mediator of the pharmacologic and therapeutic actions of methylxanthines (24, 75).

Regardless of its mechanism of action, theophylline is a direct bronchial smooth muscle relaxant (21). If bronchospasm is not present, its effects on air flow and respiratory mechanics are minimal. The drug may also act by decreasing mucosal edema and reducing the production of excessive secretions (21). Other effects of theophylline include direct augmentation of myocardial inotropy and chronotropy (43, 54); stimulation of respiratory muscle contractility (3, 37, 52); dilation of the coronary, pulmonary, renal, and systemic arterioles and veins (2); diuresis (30, 44); stimulation of epinephrine and norepinephrine synthesis and release by the adrenal medulla (61); stimulation of the medullary respiratory center; relaxation of the smooth muscle of the gallbladder and gastrointestinal tract (44); stimulation of gastric acid secretion (26); and decreased cerebral blood flow (75).

Side Effects

The most common side effects of theophylline include gastrointestinal effects that are both locally and centrally mediated (44). Frequently reported side effects include nausea, vomiting, and anorexia. Central nervous system effects include headache, irritability, restlessness, nervousness, dizziness, and seizures (6, 22). The incidence and severity of all of these adverse reactions usually decrease with reduction in the daily theophylline dosage (44). Gastrointestinal adverse effects associated with oral use can be minimized by administering the drug with food (53). Unfortunately, mild side effects such as nausea and vomiting do not necessarily manifest before serious life-threatening problems such as seizures develop (22, 23, 78). Theophylline-induced seizures are often unresponsive to standard anticonvulsive therapy, and the mortality rate associated with this problem has been estimated to be as high as 50% (6, 78). Theophylline may cause a number of cardiovascular side effects that are often poorly tolerated by critically ill patients. These effects include palpitations, sinus tachycardia, extrasystoles, and multifocal atrial tachycardia (6). Flushing, hypotension, circulatory collapse, and ventricular arrhythmias have also been reported.

Prior to 1983, the only parenteral form of theophylline was aminophylline. Aminophylline is theophylline compounded with ethylenediamine, which confers water solubility to the insoluble theophylline molecule. By weight, aminophylline is 80% theophylline (e.g., 100 mg of aminophylline is equivalent to 80 mg of theophylline). Interestingly, ethylenediamine contributes to both the efficacy and toxicity of theophylline. Ethylenediamine may augment the respiratory and cardiac stimulant effects of theophylline, but the significance of these effects is questionable (44). More importantly, it is well-established that ethylenediamine can induce hypersensitivity reactions characterized by urticaria, generalized pruritus, angioedema, and bronchospasm (44). A premixed intravenous solution of theophylline in 5% dextrose in water is available for clinical use. Although adverse reactions to ethylenediamine occur rarely, theophylline therapy in critically ill patients can be simplified by use of these premixed theophylline solutions.

Because the rapid intravenous injection of aminophylline or theophylline may cause dizziness, palpitations, flushing, hypotension, and profound bradycardia, these drugs must be administered by slow intravenous injection or, preferably, by use of an infusion pump (21, 26). Cardiac arrest may also occur with the rapid administration of aminophylline. Intramuscular injections of theophylline salts are painful and the free drug is absorbed slowly and erratically from the site of administration. Therefore, this route of administration is not recommended (22, 44).

Pharmacokinetics

Theophylline is manufactured as a variety of salts for oral, rectal, and parenteral administration (in excess of 150 different products in the U.S. alone!) (22, 23, 26, 44, 78). Although rectal preparations of theophylline and its related salts are available, their absorption, especially from suppositories, into the systemic circulation is very erratic and unreliable. Use of the suppositories should be avoided in all patients (74). Fixed-dose combinations of theophylline with other drugs such as ephedrine should also be avoided (15). The intravenous forms of theophylline are limited primarily to hospitalized patients, particularly those who are critically ill and unable to take oral medications.

The pharmacokinetics of theophylline have been well described (21, 26, 44, 45). Following oral administration, gastric acidity prompts the release of free theophylline from the theophylline salt or compound preparation. The rate of this release and the subsequent absorption of theophylline into the systemic circulation depends on the theophylline product used. For example, theophylline is absorbed rapidly from any of the many available oral solutions and uncoated tablet formulations. Peak serum levels are obtained 1 to 2 hours after administration. In contrast, extended-release and slow-release tablets are designed to release theophylline over a longer period of time (thereby decreasing the number of required drug doses per day); peak serum levels usually are reached 4 hours after administration. The actual rate of theophylline absorption from slow-release or extended-release formulations varies among formulations and routes of administration (e.g., oral route with or without food).

Administration of theophylline by intravenous infusion produces the highest and most rapidly achieved peak serum concentration. In healthy, nonsmoking adults, a theophylline dose of 5 mg/kg infused over 30 minutes produces an average peak serum concentration of 10 μg/ml (44).

Theophylline achieves a volume of distribution of 0.3 to 0.7 liters/kg in children and adults (22, 24, 44). In premature infants, the volume of distribution increases almost 2-fold. The drug is 56% bound to plasma proteins in children and adults and 36% in premature infants (26, 44, 45).

Hepatic metabolism of theophylline, via the cytochrome P-450 system, is the principal method of elimination. Eighty-eight to 92% of a theophylline dose is metabolized to three inactive metabolites: 1,3-dimethyluric acid, 1-methyluric acid, and 3-methylxanthine (44). In premature infants, a high percentage of theophylline is metabolized to caffeine. Theophylline and its metabolites are excreted from the body by the kidneys. Small amounts of unchanged theophylline may be excreted in the feces.

The metabolism of theophylline varies widely owing to differing rates of metabolism in different patient populations (19, 26, 27, 44). In otherwise healthy, nonsmoking asthmatic adults, the elimination half-life averages between 7 and 9 hours; in children, between 1.5 and 9.5 hours; and in premature infants, between 15 and 58 hours (26, 44). Patients who are cigarette or marijuana smokers have a much shorter average elimination half-life of 4 to 5 hours (21). In contrast, patients with congestive heart failure, cor pulmonale, chronic obstructive pulmonary disease, or liver disease may have a markedly prolonged elimination half-life (i.e., more than 12 hours) (22, 44).

Because theophylline has a low therapeutic ratio, the drug must be administered by careful dosage titration. Dosages should be calculated by use of lean body weight and consideration of underlying disease states and smoking history (Table 33.1) (22, 26). In addition, a variety of analytic techniques have been used to assess plasma or serum levels of theophylline and assist in reducing clinical toxicity (Table 33.2).

In isolated tracheal and bronchial smooth muscle preparations, theophylline induces bronchodilation in proportion to the log of the serum or plasma concentration over the range of 5 to 25 μg/ml (30, 51). Based on this relationship, a clinical "therapeutic range" for theophylline has been generated; the most frequently cited range is 10 to 20 μg/ml (22). Within this range, serious side effects of theophylline, including seizures and cardiac arrhythmias, are reduced in incidence and severity, while efficacy is maintained. Most patients do not require levels in excess of 25 μg/ml to obtain adequate bronchodilation (47). This therapeutic range represents only the serum levels at which the majority of patients respond to theophylline; some patients respond outside this range. For example, bronchodilation can be produced at the lower end of the therapeutic range (i.e., serum concentrations of 2 to 10 μg/ml) in chronic asthmatic children (21). However, some patients may require levels in excess of 20 μg/ml (47). Marked interpatient and intrapatient variability exists for the dose-response curves for theophylline (6). Consequently, the ideal use of serum theophylline determinations is as an adjunct for titrating patient response and in determining the optimal drug level and drug dosage that are necessary to achieve maximal bronchodilation.

Drug Interactions

Theophylline clearance may be altered by a number of disease states and drugs (Table 33.3). Theophylline is reported to augment myocardial sensitivity to digitalis glycosides (44). In addition, theophylline may act synergistically with the β-adrenergic agonists to induce cardiac arrhythmias (30, 44).

Clinical Use

The primary role of theophylline is the prevention of bronchospasm in patients with either hyperactive airway disease or chronic obstructive pulmonary disorders (21, 26). For treatment of chronic bronchospasm in patients older than 1 year of age, theophylline may be given initially at 16 mg/kg/day or 400 mg/day, whichever is less (22, 23). Depending on the patient's response, the dose may be increased up to the following maximum daily doses (22, 23):

Table 33.1. Initial Intravenous Theophylline Maintenance Dosages[a]

Patient Population	Age	Theophylline Infusion Rate[b] (mg/kg/hr)
Neonates	Postnatal age up to 24 days	1 mg/kg q. 12 hours[c]
	Postnatal age above 24 days	1.5 mg/kg q. 12 hours[c]
Infants	6–52 weeks	0.008 × (age in weeks) + 0.21
Young children	1–9 yr	0.8
Older children	9–12 yr	0.7
Adolescents (smokers)	12–16 yr	0.7
Adolescents (nonsmokers)	12–16 yr	0.5[d]
Adults (healthy, smokers)	16–50 yr	0.7[d]
Adults (healthy, nonsmokers)	Above 16 years (including the elderly)	0.4[d]
Adults with cardiac decompensation, cor pulmonale, or liver dysfunction	Above 16 years	0.2[e]

[a] Originally published in Iafrate RP, Massey KL, Hendeles L: Current concepts in clinical therapeutics: asthma. *Clin Pharm* 5:206–227, 1986. Copyright 1986, American Society of Hospital Pharmacists, Inc. All rights reserved. Reprinted with permission.
[b] Assumes that an appropriate loading dose has been given. To achieve a target concentration of 10 μg/ml. Use lean body weight for obese patients. Although these doses generally are safe, many patients will require higher infusion rates as determined by serial serum measurements. These dosages differ from the current FDA recommendations, which include a higher infusion rate for the first 12 hours. Further dosage reductions may be required for patients who are receiving other drugs that decrease theophylline clearance.
[c] For a target concentration of 7.5 μg/ml (for neonatal apnea).
[d] Not to exceed 900 mg/day unless clinical symptoms and/or serum levels indicate the need for a larger dose.
[e] Not to exceed 400 mg/day unless clinical symptoms and/or serum levels indicate the need for a larger dose.

Table 33.2. Adverse Effects of Theophylline[a]

Serum Concentration	Symptoms	Frequency	Duration	Comments
5–20 μg/ml	Nausea, cramps, insomnia headache	Rare—if dose is slowly titrated over 1–2 weeks	Transient	
		Common—if therapeutic serum concentrations are attained rapidly	Transient	Avoided by dose titration
	Tremor	Rare—with concurrent administration of oral β₂-adrenergic	Unknown	Avoided if β₂-agonist is administered by inhalation
	Excessive gastric acid secretion	Rare		
15–35 μg/ml	Nausea, vomiting, diarrhea, stomach ache, headache, irritability, nervousness, insomnia, sinus tachycardia	Common—at serum concentrations >20 μg/ml	Persistent	Decrease dose
	Hyperglycemia	Rare—may occur in neonates	Persistent	
>35 μg/ml	Seizures, cerebral hypoxia, arrhythmias, cardiorespiratory arrest, death	Common	Persistent	Minor adverse effects often do not precede life-threatening toxicity

[a] Adapted from Hendeles L, Weinberger M: Theophylline: therapeutic use of serum concentration monitoring. In Taylor WJ, Finn AL (eds): *Individual Drug Therapy: Practical Applications of Drug Monitoring.* Gross, Townsend, Frank, Hoffman, New York, 1981, vol 1, pp 32–65. Used with permission of the publishers.

Age (yr)	Dosage (mg/kg/day)
1–9	24
9–12	20
12–16	18
>16	13, or 900 mg/day (whichever is less)

Note that in the prophylaxis of chronic bronchospasm, measurement of serum theophylline levels is usually necessary only (*a*) when these daily dosage recommendations are exceeded, (*b*) when drug toxicity is suspected, (*c*) when poor patient compliance to the prescribed regimen is suspected, or (*d*) to assess why a patient may not be responding to theophylline (e.g., rapid metabolism of the drug) (44, 47). In patients who are able to take medications orally, treatment should be started with an oral preparation of theophylline. The products that should be used are those with consistent 100% bioavailability: uncoated tablets, microcrystalline dosage forms, or oral solutions. Once the patient's response has been demonstrated and dosages titrated, the daily drug dosage may then be converted to an equivalent amount of an extended-release theophylline product (73). For example, if a patient is taking theophylline oral tablets, 100 mg every 4 hours, the total daily dose of 600 mg may be given as two 300-mg tablets of an extended-release product and manufacturer's recommendations followed as to the method of administration. Theophylline products should be chosen in accord with patient age and underlying disease state (51). At present a number of extended-release or slow-release theophylline products are available, each with different absorption profiles (26); not all clinicians consider these products to be interchangeable (26).

No theophylline product, oral or intravenous, should be used for the initial treatment of acute bronchospasm. Rather, only if repeated administration of inhaled β-adrenergic

Table 33.3. Factors that Affect Theophylline Clearance[a]

Increase theophylline clearance	Decrease theophylline clearance
Smoking (cigarettes or marijuana)	Hepatic cirrhosis
	Cor pulmonale
Phenobarbital	Congestive heart failure
High-protein/low-carbohydrate diet	Propranolol
	Allopurinol (>600 mg/day)
Charcoal-broiled diet	Erythromycin
Phenytoin	Cimetidine
Carbamazepine	Troleandomycin
Rifampin	Oral contraceptives

[a] Originally published in Iafrate RP, Massey KL, Hendeles L: Current concepts in clinical therapeutics: asthma. *Clin Pharm* 5:206–227, 1986. Copyright 1986, American Society of Hospital Pharmacists, Inc. All rights reserved. Reprinted with permission.

agonists (e.g., isoetharine or albuterol) produces a suboptimal effect should theophylline be administered (21, 22, 26). Of note, one well-designed randomized, double-blind, placebo-controlled trial of intravenous aminophylline in asthmatic adult patients with acute bronchospastic disease demonstrated that although there was no difference between the two treatment groups in clinical response or adverse events, there was a significant decrease in the rate of hospital admissions for patients treated with aminophylline compared with placebo (48, 76).

Theophylline therapy in an acutely bronchospastic patient (assuming normal volume of distribution) can be initiated as follows (26). Either intravenous or oral liquid theophylline can be used; the former is more commonly used in critically ill patients (21, 22, 26). If the patient has not received any theophylline during the previous 24 hours, 5 mg/kg of theophylline should be administered as a loading dose over 30 minutes. If the patient has received theophylline within the past 24 hours, the loading dose should be reduced to 2.5 mg/kg. Subsequent intravenous infusion rates should be titrated based on the patient's response, using the dosing recommendations in Table 33.1. Theophylline levels can be used to maximize therapy, in that each additional 1 mg/kg of theophylline will produce a 2 μg/ml rise in the serum concentration. For example, if a 70-kg bronchospastic patient has a serum concentration of 8 μg/ml, the administration of an additional 210 mg of theophylline will, in the majority of patients, elevate the serum drug concentration to 14 μg/ml, well within the "therapeutic range" for theophylline.

β-ADRENERGIC RECEPTOR AGONISTS

The value of β-adrenergic agonist therapy in the treatment of reversible airway obstruction was documented at the turn of the century when Solis-Cohen (67) reported the use of desiccated adrenal glands for the treatment of asthma. This discovery was followed by the isolation of ephedrine and the synthesis of isoproterenol. Subsequently, a variety of β-adrenergic agonists have been introduced into clinical use, which vary in affinity for the β₁- and β₂-adrenergic receptors and duration of action. These drugs have become well-established as effective medications in the treatment of both acute and chronic reversible airway obstruction.

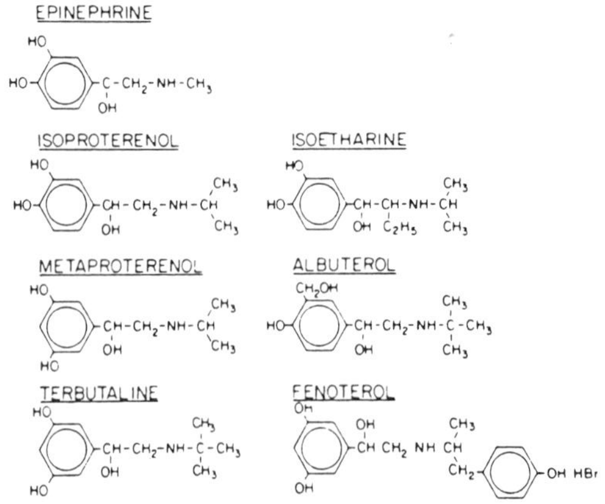

Figure 33.2. Structures of β-adrenergic agonists. (Originally published in Kelly HW: New β-2-adrenergic agonist aerosols. *Clin Pharm* 4:393–403, 1985. Copyright 1985, American Society of Hospital Pharmacists, Inc. All rights reserved. Reprinted with permission.)

Pharmacology

All β-adrenergic receptor agonists act by binding to β₁ and β₂ cell membrane receptors (Fig. 33.1), which results in activation of adenyl cyclase; accordingly, intracellular levels of cAMP are increased (63). This action induces a relaxation of bronchial and vascular smooth muscle. β-Adrenergic agonists may also induce increased mucociliary transport of respiratory secretions (72, 73). Stimulation of β₂-receptors on mast cells inhibits the release of mediators of bronchospasm (i.e., histamine and slow-reacting substances of anaphylaxis) (39).

Distinctions between the β-adrenergic agonists are based on differences in chemistry and selectivity for the β₂-receptor over the β₁-receptor. Chemically, all β-adrenergic agonists except pirbuterol are structural derivatives of phenylethylamine (Fig. 33.2). Structural modifications of the phenylethylamine nucleus result in compounds with differing durations of action and receptor activity (Table 33.4).

The catecholamine agents possess adjacent hydroxyl groups on positions 3 and 4 of the benzene ring of the catechol molecule (63). All catecholamines are capable of acting on both β₁- and β₂-adrenergic receptors. Whereas epinephrine and isoproterenol have equal β₁- and β₂-adrenergic receptor activity, isoetharine, pirbuterol, terbutaline, albuterol, salmeterol, and bitolterol are reported to have greater affinity for the β₂-receptor than for the β₁-receptor (45). All catecholamines are readily inactivated by the enzymes catechol-*O*-methyltransferase (COMT), found in high concentrations in the liver and kidney, and monoamine oxidase (MAO), located in the presynaptic neurons (63). The duration of action of the catecholamines is short because of their rapid metabolism. The exception to this rule among β-agonists is bitolterol (70). Bitolterol is actually a prodrug; hydrolysis by plasma esterases results in the generation of the active drug colterol, which is a catecholamine (26). Because colterol must be generated in the systemic circulation, the duration of action of bitolterol is longer than that of other catecholamines. Catecholamines usually are not administered orally because they are conjugated and inactivated rapidly in the mucosa of the gastrointestinal tract (45).

The substitution of the catecholamine nucleus with resorcinol or saligenin has resulted in the development of drugs with longer durations of action than the catecholamines because they are resistant to the actions of both COMT and MAO (26). In addition, they are effective after oral administration and have relatively greater affinity for the β_2-receptor than for the β_1-receptor. The resorcinols include metaproterenol, terbutaline, and the investigational agent fenoterol. The only currently available saligenin is albuterol. Salmeterol is an investigational β_2 agonist that is structurally related to albuterol but due to a long lipoploslic side chain has a 12-hour duration of action (11a). Pirbuterol (whose official international generic name is salbutamol) is not chemically related to any of the other adrenergic agonists but is similar in clinical pharmacology to albuterol.

Pharmacokinetics

As previously discussed, the catecholamines are ineffective following oral administration. Accordingly, their only route of enteral administration is oral inhalation, either as a powder in a metered-dose inhaler or as a solution for nebulization. However, the noncatecholamine β-adrenergic agonists metaproterenol, terbutaline, and albuterol are also available as oral tablets, and metaproterenol and albuterol are also manufactured as oral liquids.

Epinephrine, isoetharine, isoproterenol, metaproterenol, albuterol, and bitolterol are the only β-adrenergic agents available as solutions for administration by nebulization. The only parenteral β-adrenergic agonists are epinephrine, isoproterenol, and terbutaline; the latter is available for subcutaneous administration only. Isoetharine, metaproterenol, terbutaline, albuterol, and pirbuterol are available as a metered dose inhaler. Not all dosage forms of each drug are marketed in the U.S. For example, terbutaline is not approved for use by nebulization, despite its documented efficacy and the availability in Europe and Canada for such use.

The inhaled route of administration is the preferred method of administration for β-adrenergic agonists (26, 31, 45, 55, 64); nebulization is one of the most common methods of administration used in intensive care units. The reason for this strong interest in oral inhalation of these drugs is 3-fold (31, 55). First, inhalation delivers the drug directly to the site of activity, the airways. Second, administration by inhalation requires a smaller dose of drug to achieve a desired therapeutic response, and the drug is distributed over the large tissue surface area of the lungs, up to 70 m². Last, onset of action is very rapid following oral inhalation, within 5 minutes, and 80 to 90% of the maximal response occurs within 10 minutes (49); side effects are minimal (55). There are disadvantages to this route of administration, however. In non-mechanically ventilated patients, a great deal of patient cooperation is required to deliver the drug adequately (55). However, spacer devices may improve drug delivery in patients who may have difficulty coordinating the discharge of medication from the inhaler with inhalation (15). Additionally, a high percentage of each drug dose commonly gets trapped in the upper airways or is swallowed; only 13% of a dose from a metered-dose inhaler and 1 to 5% of a dose administered by nebulization reach the lower respiratory tract (55). Administration by inhalation can result in mouth irritation and dryness. One particular disadvantage occurs in patients with severe bronchospasm: the drug may not be administered to the lower airways, where it is needed. In this circumstance, much larger doses of drug are required to achieve a satisfactory response (55).

Few pharmacokinetic data are available on β-adrenergic agonists owing to the very low serum levels of drugs that are achieved after dosing, particularly following inhalation. However, it is well-established that most of these drugs have short plasma half-lives (26). For all inhaled catecholamine β-adrenergic agonists (except bitolterol), peak effects occur 5 to 15 minutes after administration and persist for 1 to 3 hours. Bitolterol's actions are maximal at 0.5 to 2 hours after administration and continue for up to 6 hours (31). Metaproterenol has a slow onset of action, up to 30 minutes after administration, and peak effects occur within 1 hour. The duration of action of metaproterenol is usually 3 to 5 hours. Terbutaline, albuterol, and pirbuterol have a rapid onset of action (5 to 15 minutes after administration), with peak effects in 0.5 to 2 hours and a duration of action of 4 to 6 hours.

Side Effects

The side effects of the β-adrenergic agonists are similar; the majority are transient (31, 40, 55, 58). The most common

Table 33.4. β-Adrenergic Agents[a]

Drug	Route of Administration			Duration of Action (hr)	Receptor		
	Injection	Inhaled	Oral		β_2	β_1	α
Catecholamines							
Epinephrine	Yes	Yes	No	1–2	+	+	+
Isoproterenol	Yes	Yes	No	2–3	+	+	−
Isoetharine	No	Yes	No	2–3	++	+	−
Bitolterol	No	Yes	No	4–6	++	+	−
Resorcinols							
Metaproterenol	No	Yes	Yes	3–5	++	+	−
Terbutaline	Yes	No	Yes	4–6	++	+	−
Fenoterol	No	Yes	No	4–6	++	+	−
Saligen							
Albuterol	No	Yes	Yes	4–6	++	+	−
Salmeterol	No	Yes	No	1–2	++	±	−
Miscellaneous							
Pirbuterol (Salbutamol)	No	Yes	No	4–6	++	±	−

[a] Adapted from Iafrate RP, Massey ICL, Hendeles L: Current concepts in clinical therapeutics: asthma. *Clin Pharm* 5:206-227, 1986. Copyright 1986, American Society of Hospital Pharmacists, Inc. All rights reserved. Used with permission.

adverse effects are fine skeletal muscle tremor, nervousness, insomnia, tachycardia, and palpitations (65). The cardiac effects result primarily from direct β_1-receptor stimulation. In critically ill patients, this stimulation can result in arrhythmias, most commonly supraventricular tachycardia and ventricular tachycardia (13, 69). Reflex tachycardia may also result owing to β_2-mediated peripheral vasodilation (26, 31). Hypokalemia has also been reported (14), but its clinical significance is unclear (53). Less commonly reported side effects of these drugs include paradoxic bronchoconstriction, skin flushing, headache, and dizziness (58).

Although the incidence of all side effects is very low following inhalation, the oral and parenteral routes commonly induce side effects. The side effects may be so severe that the drugs may have to be discontinued (65). For example, muscle tremor is believed to result primarily from β_2-stimulation and appears to be dose related (26, 31). In some patients, the tremor can be so serious as to be disabling. Use of oral β-adrenergics should be reserved for patients who are unable or unwilling to use the inhalation dosage forms. Some patients who achieve only suboptimal effects with the inhalant products may benefit from supplementation with an oral β-adrenergic (26).

Because intravenous epinephrine and isoproterenol are associated with myocardial ischemia, infarction, and death (36, 42), their use generally is limited to patients with drug-unresponsive bronchospasm (i.e., status asthmaticus).

Following chronic use of β-adrenergic agonists, decreased responsiveness may develop. Commonly referred to as tolerance or tachyphylaxis, this effect has been documented to occur in both animals and humans (46). Tolerance with β-agonists may result from desensitization of β_2-receptors. Desensitization is theorized to result from down-regulation and/or phosphorylation (and hence unavailability for agonist interaction) of the receptors (38, 53). Interestingly, although tolerance has been demonstrated to develop to the nonbronchial β-adrenergic responses (e.g., heart rate, tremor (56a)), conflicting information exists regarding the bronchial response. Most data indicate that repeated and prolonged use of high dose β-adrenergic agonists, either oral or inhaled, can result in a decrease in the duration of drug effect (26, 46). Thus, it has been recommended to avoid tolerance by using the lowest effective dose only on an as-needed basis (53). However, continuous albuterol therapy (i.e., one to three standard treatments per hour) has been shown to be safe and effective in acutely ill patients and may prevent acute respiratory failure (32, 69).

Recent reports from New Zealand and Canada (67a) suggest that chronic use of long-acting inhaled β-adrenergic agonists (specifically fenoterol) may negatively affect clinical outcome of asthmatics (9, 18, 62). It has been postulated that these agents may mask symptoms of the disease so that patients are unable to assess their own disease accurately. As a result, more data are needed on the safety of chronic use of the longer-acting agents, especially in asthmatics.

Drug Interactions

β-Adrenergic agonists may act synergistically when administered concurrently either with other β-adrenergic agonists or with theophylline (30, 56). The most important risk of these combinations would be in patients with underlying cardiac

disease, who have a limited capacity to tolerate high heart rate or arrhythmias (65).

Clinical Use

Despite the fact that most studies of inhaled bronchodilators have been conducted only in patients with acute asthma, bronchodilators are used extensively in intensive care unit patients (7) and have proved beneficial. Therefore, as previously discussed, inhaled β-adrenergic agonists are the drug therapy of choice for the treatment of acute bronchospasm, particularly in critically ill patients (26). Other indications for their usage include prophylaxis of chronic asthma and exercise-induced asthma (26).

Practically, all of the inhaled β-adrenergics can be considered to be equally effective in treating bronchospasm, although it has been suggested that metaproterenol and the catecholamines are less effective than albuterol, terbutaline, and isoproterenol (45). In critically ill patients, individualization of therapy is very important, as the variation in response among patients with bronchospasm is very large, owing to the heterogeneity of both the etiology of acute bronchospasm and the patients affected. Data are available that demonstrate that in acutely ill asthmatic patients, higher doses of inhaled β-adrenergics are needed compared with stable outpatient asthmatics (32). Choice of an individual agent reflects both clinician and patient preference, as well as economic factors. In hospitalized patients, isoetharine, metaproterenol, and albuterol are the most commonly used inhaled agents for administration by nebulization (26). Patients with moderate symptoms of acute bronchospasm typically benefit from nebulized β-agonist therapy every hour. Depending on their underlying cardiovascular status and the drug used, more severely ill patients may require two to three standard treatments per hour (32).

Dosing

The dosages of the various β-adrenergic agents are listed in Table 33.5.

ANTICHOLINERGIC AGENTS

In the early 1800s, the practice of inhaling burning powders of the anticholinergic alkaloids stramonium and belladonna for the treatment of asthma was introduced to Great Britain by travelers from India (77). Although effective, this practice was accompanied by a high number of adverse effects such as tachycardia, urinary retention, inspissation of secretions, and delirium. Following the development of inhaled bronchodilators, the use of anticholinergic agents for treatment of asthma was abandoned.

During the last 25 years, interest in the use of anticholinergic drugs for treatment of bronchospasm has been renewed. This interest derives from documentation of the effective use of atropine by inhalation in the treatment of asthma. Additionally, two synthetic anticholinergics have been developed that are much safer and easier to use than atropine: glycopyrrolate

Table 33.5. β₂-Adrenergic Aerosol Preparations and Dosages[a]

Drug	Preparations	Pediatric Dosages	Adult Dosages
Isoproterenol hydrochloride and sulfate			
Various manufacturers	0.25% (1:400) 2.5 mg/ml 0.50% (1:200) 5 mg/ml 1.0% (1:100) 10 mg/ml	0.05–0.1 mg/kg q. 2–4 hr	One to two inhalations of 0.25% solution by hand-bulb nebulizer; via nebulizer q. 2–4 hr
Isuprel Mistometer Norisodrine Aerotrol Medihaler-Iso Norisodrine sulfate	131 μg/spray 120 μg/spray 80 μg/spray 110 μg/spray	One to two inhalations q. 4–6 hr	One to two sprays q. 2–4 hr
Isoetharine			
Isoetharine hydrochloride for inhalation	0.1%, 0.125%, 0.2%	0.1–0.2 mg/kg q. 2–4 hr	3–5 mg undiluted via nebulizer with oxygen at 4–6 liters/min over 15–20 min q. 2–4 hr
Bronkosol	0.25%, 0.5%, 1%		0.5% and 1% solutions diluted 1:3 with 0.9% sodium chloride q. 2–4 hr
Bronkometer	340 μg/spray	One to two sprays q. 4–6 hr	One to two sprays q. 4–6 hr
Metaproterenol			
Alupent	5% (50 mg/ml) solution for nebulization	0.25–0.5 mg/kg q. 2–4 hr (15 mg maximum single dose)	0.3 ml (15 mg) diluted with 2.5 ml of 0.9% sodium chloride nebulized q. 2–4 hr
Metaprel	0.6% (15 mg/2.5 ml)		
Alupent MDI, Metaprel MDI	0.65 mg/puff, powder suspension	One to two puffs q. 4–6 hr and before exercise	Two to three puffs q. 4–6 hr and before exercise
Albuterol			
Ventolin Proventil	90 μg/puff, powder suspension	One to two puffs q. 4–6 hr and before exercise	One to two puffs q. 4–6 hr and before exercise
	0.5% (2.5 mg/ml)	0.05–0.15 mg diluted with 1–2 ml 0.9% normal saline q. 4–6 hr	2.5–5 mg diluted with 0.9% normal saline q. 4–6 hr
Terbutaline			
Brethaire	0.2 mg/puff, powder suspension	One to two puffs q. 4–6 hr and before exercise	One to two puffs q. 4–6 hr and before exercise
Brethine	0.1% (1 mg/ml) (not FDA approved for this use)	0.1–0.3 mg/kg q. 2–6 hr	5–7 mg undiluted q. 4–6 hr
Bitolterol			
Tornalate	0.37 mg/spray	One to three sprays q. 4–6 hr	One to three sprays q. 4–6 hr
Pirbuterol			
Maxair	0.2 mg/puff, powder suspension	One to two puffs q. 4–6 hr	One to two puffs q. 4–6 hr
Fenoterol hydrobromide[b]			
Berotec	0.16 mg/puff, powder suspension	One to two puffs q. 4–6 hr	One to two puffs q. 4–6 hr
Salmeterol[b]			
Serevent	0.25 mg/puff, powder suspension	One to two puffs q. 12 hr	One to two puffs q. 12 hr

[a] Originally published in Kelly HW: New beta-2-adrenergic agonist aerosols. *Clin Pharm* 4:393–403, 1985. Copyright 1985, American Society of Hospital Pharmacists, Inc. All rights reserved. Used with permission.
[b] Pending FDA approval.

and ipratropium. However, anticholinergics have been reported to reverse only bronchospasm resulting from cholinergic stimulation and thus may not be beneficial in all patients with reversible airway obstruction (33).

Pharmacology

Atropine is a naturally occurring tertiary ammonium alkaloid obtained from plants of the Solanaceae family, including *Atropa belladonna* (deadly nightshade) and *Datura stramonium* (jimsonweed) (55, 65). Also known as *dl*-hyoscyamine, atropine is the prototypic anticholinergic (antimuscarinic) agent. Other antimuscarinic drugs used in the treatment of bronchospasm—glycopyrrolate and the newly marketed compound ipratropium—are synthetic quaternary ammonium derivatives of atropine (20, 77). Atropine methylnitrate is a quaternary ammonium compound that is available only for

investigational use in the U.S., but it is available commercially in Europe as methylatropine nitrate (77).

All of the antimuscarinic drugs produce their effects by inhibiting competitively the effects of acetylcholine on muscarinic receptors. Specifically, these drugs act by inhibiting the generation of intracellular cGMP (Fig. 33.1) (64). This action results in bronchodilation, especially in the large airways, and decreased tracheobronchial secretions. Of these available antimuscarinic agents, only ipratropium is approved by the Food and Drug Administration for inhalation in the treatment of bronchospasm.

Pharmacokinetics

Atropine is a tertiary ammonium alkaloid (Fig. 33.3), most commonly used as the sulfate salt. Inasmuch as atropine readily crosses epithelial mucosa, it may be administered via the gastrointestinal tract, by inhalation, and parenterally (35, 77). In contrast, atropine methylnitrate, glycopyrrolate, and ipratropium are quaternary ammonium antimuscarinics. The quaternary structure confers an electrical charge on these drugs, resulting in their poor absorption into the systemic circulation following administration by mouth or inhalation (20, 77).

The comparative pharmacokinetics of the inhaled anticholinergic agents are shown in Table 33.6. Following an aerosol dose, onset of action of atropine sulfate occurs within 15 to 30 minutes; peak effects occur 30 to 170 minutes after administration. The duration of action of atropine sulfate is 3 to 5 hours (20, 77). Atropine is widely distributed in the body, including the central nervous system. The plasma half-life is 2 to 3 hours, and the drug is eliminated by hepatic metabolism. About 30 to 50% of a given dose is metabolized to a variety of inactive metabolites, with the remainder of the dose being eliminated unchanged in the urine. Atropine methylnitrate exhibits a pharmacokinetic profile similar to that of atropine but has a slightly longer duration of action, 4 to 6 hours. In addition, this drug does not diffuse through the pulmonary epithelium, nor does it cross the blood-brain barrier (20, 77).

Glycopyrrolate is a quaternary ammonium antimuscarinic, but it is also a complex aminoalcohol ester. Following inhalation, glycopyrrolate, like atropine, has an onset of action of 15 to 30 minutes; peak effects occur between 30 and 45 minutes after administration (20, 77). The drug has a longer duration of action than atropine, up to 8 hours (77). Like all quaternary ammonium salts, glycopyrrolate does not cross the blood-brain barrier or the pulmonary mucosa.

Ipratropium, also known as *N*-isopropylnortropine tropic acid ester, is a quaternary methyl derivative of atropine. As with other inhaled antimuscarinic drugs, the onset of action of ipratropium occurs within 15 to 30 minutes. Peak effects are noted 90 to 120 minutes after administration and last for at least 4

hours and up to 6 hours in some patients (77). Systemic absorption is minimal after inhalation, and because of the drug's quaternary structure, tissue distribution is limited. Ipratropium does not cross the blood-brain barrier (20, 77).

Side Effects

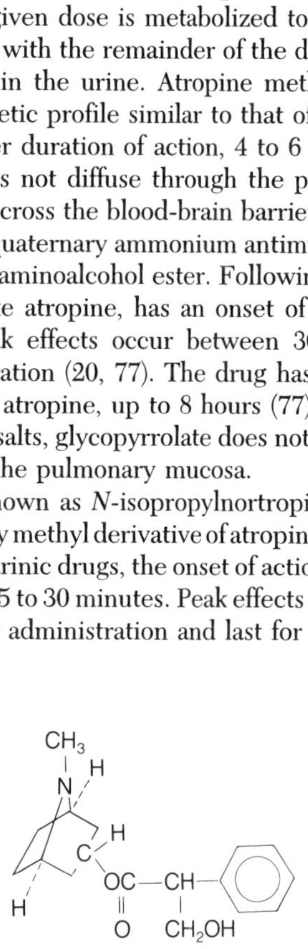

As previously discussed, the side effect profile of the antimuscarinics is determined largely by their chemical structure and route of administration. Atropine, being a tertiary ammonium compound, readily crosses the mucosal epithelium into the systemic circulation (35). Accordingly, systemic side effects are common following oral and systemic administration; these effects tend to be dose-related. Because low doses of the drug are used for inhalation, however, side effects are greatly reduced in number and severity with this route of administration (35). Following inhalation of atropine most patients develop dryness of the mouth. Other possible side effects include flushing, lightheadedness, and slight tachycardia (35, 77). Urinary retention and blurred vision are rare, as are tremors, arrhythmias, and blood pressure changes (77).

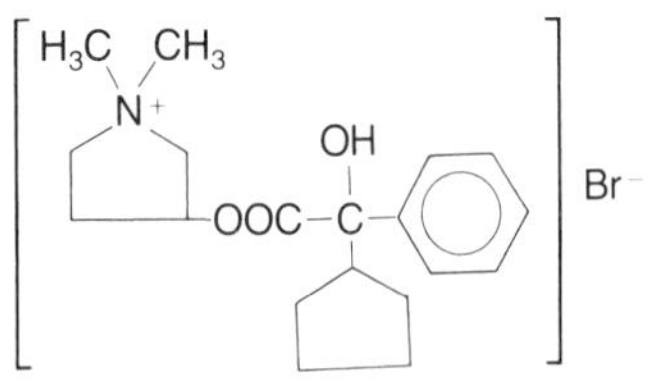

For all of the quaternary ammonium compounds, the incidence of systemic side effects is extremely low following inhalation. As previously mentioned, these compounds diffuse poorly across the pulmonary epithelium and therefore have minimal systemic absorption. They do not cross the blood-brain barrier and are therefore devoid of central nervous system effects (20, 77).

Theoretically, the inhaled anticholinergics should alter mucociliary clearance and increase the viscosity of secretions. In practice, these side effects occur most commonly with atropine and not at all with ipratropium (71).

Clinical Use

Data are available on the efficacy of atropine (11, 12, 34, 41, 50), but there is only limited information regarding the use of glycopyrrolate as bronchodilator (16, 17, 28, 35). The most information generated concerns the efficacy and safety of ipratropium in the treatment of bronchospasm (57).

Based on controlled and noncontrolled clinical trials, the use of inhaled anticholinergic drugs appears to be primarily as an alternative therapy in the treatment of bronchospastic diseases (20, 46). In contrast to inhaled β-adrenergic drugs, the anticholinergic bronchodilators have been demonstrated to be most effective in decreasing bronchial smooth muscle tone in patients with chronic bronchitis and emphysema. Their efficacy in asthma is generally considered inferior to that of β-adrenergic agonists (26). However, in one study, nebulized glycopyrrolate was as effective as nebulized metaproterenol in acutely ill asthmatic patients (17). Nebulized ipratropium was reported to improve pulmonary function similarly to nebulized metaproterenol (29). Nevertheless, because the onset of action of inhaled anticholinergics is slower than that of the inhaled β-adrenergics, the anticholinergics should not be used in the treatment of acute bronchospasm. In addition, although they have a longer duration of action than most inhaled β-adrenergics, the anticholinergics produce less bronchodilation and relief of symptoms in asthma (26, 57, 77).

Based on efficacy studies, the use of inhaled anticholinergic drugs generally should be limited to those patients who do

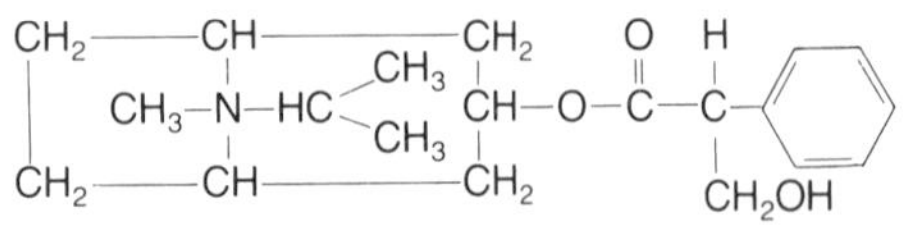

Figure 33.3.   Structure of anticholinergic agents.

Table 33.6. Bronchodilator Properties of Anticholinergic Drugs[a]

Drug	Dosages	Route of Administration	Time of Onset (min)	Peak Effect (min)	Duration (hr)
Atropine sulfate	0.025–0.075 mg/kg	Inhalation	15–30	30–170	3–5
	0.4–1 mg	Oral	NA	NA	NA
Atropine methonitrate	1–1.5 mg	Inhalation	15–30	40–60	4–6
Glycopyrrolate	0.0044 mg/kg	Inhalation	15–30	30–45	2–8
		Intramuscular Subcutaneous	15–30	30–45	2–7
	0.2 mg	Intravenous	1	NA	NA
Ipratropium	20–40 μg	Inhalation	3–30	90–120	3–8

[a] Adapted from Ziment I, Au JP: Anticholinergic agents: *Clin Chest Med* 7:355–366, 1986.

not respond adequately to maximal β-adrenergic therapy (26). These patients usually are afflicted with chronic obstructive pulmonary disease, including emphysema and chronic bronchitis. In addition, because of the longer duration of action of these agents, anticholinergics may be found to be useful in special circumstances, such as the prevention of nocturnal asthma, but such potential roles remain to be defined.

Acknowledgment: The author would like to thank Eva Wilford and Lisa Bednarik for their invaluable assistance in the preparation of this chapter.

Dosing

The dosages of anticholinergics by inhalation are listed in Table 33.5.

REFERENCES

1. Adair NE: Airflow obstruction. In *Current Therapy In Critical Care Medicine*. BC Decker, Philadelphia, 1987, pp 164–169.
2. Andersson KE, Persson CG: Extra-pulmonary effects of theophylline. *Eur J Respir Dis* 61(S109):17–28, 1980.
3. Aubier M, DeTroyer A, Sampson M, et al: Aminophylline improves diaphragmatic contractility. *N Engl J Med* 305:249–252, 1981.
4. Barnes PJ: State of the art: neural control of human airways in health and disease. *Am Rev Respir Dis* 134:1289–1314, 1986.
5. Barnes PJ: New concepts in the pathogenesis of bronchial hyperresponsiveness and asthma. *J Allergy Clin Immunol* 83:1013–1026, 1989.
6. Bergstrand H: Phosphodiesterase inhibition and theophylline. *Eur J Respir Dis* 61(S109):37–44, 1980.
7. Boucher BA, Kuhl DA, Coffey BC, Fabian TC: Drug used in a trauma intensive-care unit. *Am J Hosp Pharm* 47:805–810, 1990.
8. Boushey HA, Holtzman MJ, Sheller JR, et al: State of the art: bronchial hyperactivity. *Am Rev Respir Dis* 121:389–413, 1980.
9. Burgess C, Crane J, Pearce N, Beasley R: β₂-agonists and New Zealand asthma mortality. *Lancet* 337:982–983, 1991.
10. Brisson GR, Malaisse-Lagal F, Malaisse-Lagal WJ: The stimulus-secretion coupling of glucose-induced insulin release. 7. A proposed site of action for adenosine 3;pr-5;pr-cyclic monophosphate. *J Clin Invest* 51:232–241, 1972.
11. Cavanaugh MJ, Cooper DM: Inhaled atropine sulfate: dose-response characteristics. *Am Rev Respir Dis* 114:517–524, 1976.
11a. Cheung D. et al. Long term effects of a long-acting β₂-adrenoceptor agonist, salmeterol, on airway hyperresponsiveness in patients with mild asthma. *N Engl J Med* 327:1198–1203, 1992.
12. Chick TW, Jenne JW: Comparative bronchodilator response to atropine and terbutaline in asthma and chronic bronchitis. *Chest* 72:719–723, 1977.
13. Cochrane GM: Bronchial asthma and the role of β₂-agonists. *Lung* (suppl):66–70, 1990.
14. Crane J, Burgess C, Beasley R: Cardiovascular and hypokalemic effects of inhaled salbutamol, fenoterol and isoprenaline. *Thorax* 44:136–140, 1989.
15. Drugs used in treatment of asthma. *Med Lett Drugs Ther* 29:11–16, 1987.
16. Gal TJ, Suratt PM, Lu JY: Glycopyrrolate and atropine inhalation: comparative effects on normal airway function. *Am Rev Respir Dis* 129:871–873, 1984.
17. Gilman MJ, Meyer L, Carter J, Slovis C: Comparison of aerosolized glycopyrrolate versus metaproterenol in acute asthma. *Chest* 98:1095–1098, 1990.
18. Grainger J, Woodman K, Pearce N, Crane J, Burgess C, Keane A: Prescribing fenoterol and death from asthma in New Zealand 1981-7: a further case-controlled study. *Thorax* 41:105–111, 1991.

19. Ginchansky E, Weinberger M: Relationship of theophylline clearance to oral dosage in children with chronic asthma. *J Pediatr* 91:655–660, 1977.
20. Gross NJ, Skorodin MS: The place of anticholinergic agents in the treatment of airways obstruction. *Immunol Allergy Pract* 7:224–231, 1986.
21. Hendeles L, Weinberger M: Theophylline: a state of the art review. *Pharmacotherapy* 3:2–44, 1983.
22. Hendeles L, Weinberger M: Theophylline: therapeutic use of serum concentration monitoring. In Taylor WJ, Finn AL (eds): *Individualizing Drug Therapy: Practical Application of Drug Monitoring*, vol 1. Gross, Townsend, Frank, Hoffman, New York, 1981, pp 32–65.
23. Hendeles L, Weinberger M, Wyatt R: A guide to oral theophylline therapy for treatment of chronic asthma. *Am J Dis Child* 132:876–880, 1978.
24. Holgate ST, Mann JS, Cushey MJ: Adenosine as a bronchoconstriction mediator in asthma and its antagonism by methylxanthines. *J Allergy Clin Immunol* 74:302–306, 1984.
25. Horrobin DF, Manku MS, Franks DJ, et al: Methylxanthine phosphodiesterase inhibitors behave as prostaglandin antagonists in a perfused rat mesenteric artery preparation. *Prostaglandins* 13:33–40, 1977.
26. Iafrate RP, Massey KL, Hendeles L: Current concepts in clinical therapeutics: asthma. *Clin Pharm* 5:206–227, 1986.
27. Jenne JW, Wyze E, Rood FS, MacDonald IM: Pharmacokinetics of theophylline: application to adjustment of clinical dose of aminophylline. *Clin Pharmacol Ther* 13:349–368, 1972.
28. Johnson BE, Suratt PM, Gal TJ, Wilhort SL: Effects of inhaled glycopyrrolate and atropine in asthma precipitated by exercise and cold air inhalation. *Chest* 85:325–328, 1984.
29. Karpel JP: Bronchodilator responses to anticholinergic and β-adrenergic agents in acute and stable COPD. *Chest* 99:871M–876, 1990.
30. Kelly HW: Controversies in asthma therapy with theophylline and the beta-2-adrenergic agonists. *Clin Pharm* 3:386–395, 1984.
31. Kelly HW: New beta-2-adrenergic agonist aerosols. *Clin Pharm* 4:393–403, 1985.
32. Kelley HW, Murphy S: Beta-adrenergic agonists for acute, severe asthma. *DICP* 26:81–91, 1991.
33. Kelly HW, Murphy S: Should anticholinergics be used in acute severe asthma? *DICP* 4:409–416, 1990.
34. Klock LE, Miller TD, Morris AH, et al: A comparative study of atropine sulfate and isoproterenol hydrochloride in chronic bronchitis. *Am Rev Respir Dis* 112:371–376, 1975.
35. Kradjan WA, Lakshminarayan S, Hayden PW, et al: Serum atropine concentration after inhalation of atropine sulfate. *Am Rev Respir Dis* 123:471–472, 1981.
36. Kurland G, Williams J, Lewiston N: Fatal myocardial toxicity during continuous infusion of intravenous isoproterenol therapy for asthma. *J Allergy Clin Immunol* 63:407–411, 1979.
37. Landsberg KE, Vaughan LM, Heffner JE: The effect of theophylline on respiratory muscle contractility and fatigue. *Pharmacotherapy* 10:271–279, 1990.
38. Lefkowitz RJ: Clinical physics of adrenoreceptor regulation. *Am J Physiol* 243:E43–E47, 1982.
39. Lofdahl CG, Svedmyr N: Selectivity of beta-adrenergic stimulant and blocking agents. *Eur J Respir Dis* 65(S136):101–113, 1984.
40. Lourenco RV, Eotromanes E: Clinical aerosols II. Therapeutic aerosols. *Arch Intern Med* 142:2299–2308, 1982.
41. Marini JJ, Lakshminarayan S: Inhaled atropine improves airflow in irreversible chronic bronchitis. *Am Rev Respir Dis* 119:148, 1979.
42. Matson JF, Coughlin G, Strunk R: Myocardial ischemia complicating the use of isoproterenol in asthmatic children. *J Pediatr* 92:776–778, 1978.
43. Matthay RA, Berger JH, Loke J, et al: Effects of aminophylline on right and left ventricular performance in chronic obstructive pulmonary disease—noninvasive assessment by radionuclide angiography. *Am J Med* 65:903–910, 1978.
44. McEvoy GK: Theophylline. In McEvoy GK (ed): *AHFS Drug Information 1993*. American Society of Hospital Pharmacists, Bethesda, MD, 1993, pp 2278–2285.
45. McFadden ER Jr: Beta-2 receptor agonist: metabolism and pharmacology. *J Allergy Clin Immunol* 68:91–97, 1981.

46. McFadden ER: Clinical use of beta-adrenergic agonists. *J Allergy Clin Immunol* 76:352–356, 1985.

47. McFadden ER: Introduction: methylxanthine therapy and reversible airway obstruction. *Am J Med* 79(S6A):1–4, 1985.

48. McFadden ER Jr: Methylxanthines in the treatment of asthma: the rise, the fall, and the possible rise again [Editorial]. *Ann Intern Med* 115:323–324, 1991.

49. Meltzer DL, Kemp JP: β_2-agonists: pharmacology and recent developments. *J Asthma* 28:179–186, 1991.

50. Miech RP, Niedzwick JG, Smith TR: Effect of theophylline on the binding of c-AMP to soluble protein from tracheal smooth muscle. *Biochem Pharmacol* 28:3687–3688, 1979.

51. Mitenko PA, Ogilvie RI: Rational intravenous doses of theophylline. *N Engl J Med* 289:600–603, 1973.

52. Murciano D, Aubier M, Lecocguic Y, Pariente R: Effects of theophylline on diaphragmatic strength and fatigue in patients with chronic obstructive pulmonary disease. *N Engl J Med* 311:349–353, 1984.

53. Murphy CM, Coonce SL, Simon PA: Treatment of asthma in children. *Clin Pharm* 10:685–703, 1992.

54. Nassif EG, Weinberger M, Thompson R, et al: The value of maintenance theophylline in steroid-dependent asthma. *N Engl J Med* 304:71–75, 1981.

55. Newhouse MT, Dolovich MB: Control of asthma by aerosols. *N Engl J Med* 315:870–874, 1986.

56. Nicklas RA, Whitehurst VE, Donohue RF, et al: Concomitant use of beta-adrenergic agonists and methylxanthines. *J Allergy Clin Immunol* 73:20–24, 1984.

56a. O'Connor BJ, Aikman SL, Baines PJ. Tolerance to the non-bronchodilator effects of inhaled β_2-agonists in asthma. *N Engl I Med* 327:1204–1209, 1992.

57. Pakes GE, Brogden RN, Heel TM, et al: Ipratropium bromide: a review of its pharmacologic properties and therapy efficacy in asthma and chronic bronchitis. *Drugs* 20:237–266, 1980.

58. Paterson JW, Woolcock AJ, Shenfield GM: State of the art: bronchodilator drugs. *Am Rev Respir Dis* 120:1149–1188, 1979.

59. Richardson JB, Farguson CC: Neuromuscular structure and function in the airways. *Fed Proc* 38:202–208, 1979.

60. Sackner MA: Effect of respiratory drugs on mucociliary clearance. *Chest* 73:958–966, 1978.

61. Salter H: On some points in the treatment and clinical history of asthma. *Edinburgh Med J* 4:1109–1115, 1858.

62. Sears MR, Taylor DR, Print CG, et al: Regular inhaled β-agonist treatment in bronchial asthma. *Lancet* 336:1391–1396, 1990.

63. Seligman M, Chernow B: Use of adrenergic agents in the critically ill patient. *Hosp Formul* 223:348–360, 1987.

64. Shenfield GM: Combination bronchodilator therapy. *Drugs* 24:414–439, 1982.

65. Sly RM, Anderson JA, Bierman CW, et al: Adverse effects and complications of treatment of beta-adrenergic agonist drugs. *J Allergy Clin Immunol*: 75:443–449, 1985.

66. Snow RM, Miller WC, Blair HT, et al: Inhaled atropine in asthma. *Ann Allergy* 42:286–289, 1979.

67. Solis-Cohen S: The use of adrenal substance in the treatment of asthma. *JAMA* 34:1164–1168, 1900.

67a. Spitzer WO, Suissa S, Ernst P. et al: The use of β-agonists and the risk of death and near death from asthma. *N Engl J Med* 326:501–506, 1992.

68. Theodore AC, Beer DJ: Pharmacotherapy of chronic obstructive pulmonary disease. *Clin Chest Med* 7:657–671, 1986.

69. Truit JD: Toxic effects of bronchodilators. *Crit Care Clin* 7:639–657, 1991.

70. Walker SB, Kradgan MA, Bierman CW: Bitolterol mesylate: a beta-adrenergic agent. *Pharmacotherapy* 5:127–137, 1985.

71. Wanner A: Clinical aspects of mucociliary transport. *Am Rev Respir Dis* 116:73–125, 1977.

72. Wanner A: Effects of methylxanthines on airway mucociliary function. *Am J Med* 79(S6A):16–21, 1985.

73. Weinberger M, Hendeles L: Slow-release theophylline: rationale and basis for product selection. *N Engl J Med* 308:760–64, 1983.

74. Weinberger MM, Hendeles L: Theophylline use: an overview. *J Allergy Clin Immunol* 76:277–284, 1985.

75. Winn HR: Methylxanthines, adenosine, and the pulmonary system. *Chest* 91:800–801, 1987.

76. Wrenn K, Slovis CM, Murphy F, Greensberg RS: Aminophylline therapy for acute bronchospastic disease in the emergency room. *Ann Intern Med* 115:241–247, 1991.

77. Ziment I, Au JP: Anticholinergic agents. *Clin Chest Med* 7:355–366, 1986.

78. Zwillich CW, Sutton TD, Neft TA, et al: Theophylline-induced seizures in adults: correlations with serum concentration. *Ann Intern Med* 82:784–787, 1975.

CHAPTER 34

Oxygen Therapy and Pharmacologic Modulation of Respiratory Drive

SERGEI ERMAKOV, M.D.
JOHN W. HOYT, M.D., F.C.C.M., F.C.C.P.

This textbook on pharmacologic agents used in critical care discusses many typical "drugs" used in the intensive care unit (ICU), from antibiotics to thrombolytics. Clinicians will think of most of these agents in terms of their chemical properties and preparation, dose, uptake and distribution, elimination, and therapeutic response. Rarely is oxygen, the subject of this chapter, thought of in those terms. Even though oxygen is one of the oldest agents used for medicinal purposes discussed in this book, physicians view it differently since it is a natural part of the atmosphere that we live in and is not purchased and dispensed by the pharmacy.

The authors of this chapter have attempted to rectify the common misclassification of oxygen and place it within the full pharmacologic armamentarium of the intensivist. Oxygen is a drug with physical properties that must be prepared in a very special way and dispensed in a unique fashion. Oxygen is given in doses with a predictable response that can be monitored. Oxygen has toxicity but a clear life-saving benefit when used correctly. We begin with a review of the history of oxygen, first as a scientific phenomenon, and finally as a therapeutic agent. From there we move to a classic pharmacologic description of oxygen as a pharmacologic gas that is the most frequently used therapeutic agent in all of critical care.

HISTORY

Joseph Priestley (1733–1804) of England, a nonconformist Unitarian minister, Warrington Academy tutor, and gifted amateur chemist, was credited with the isolation of oxygen in 1774. Focusing the rays of the sun through a 1-foot-diameter "burning lens" on red mercuric oxide within a bell jar, he liberated the colorless gas, which he collected in small containers. He wrote: "But what surprised me more than I can yet well express, was that a candle burned in this air with a remarkably vigorous flame . . . and a piece of red-hot wood sparkled in it" (1). He placed a mouse in the atmosphere of this gas and noted that it could remain alive much longer than in an equal volume of common air.

Prior to Priestley's experiments, the "phlogiston theory" (G.E. Stahl, 1659–1734) dominated all theoretic conceptions about combustion and respiration. Phlogiston was believed to be a part of all combustible material and was deemed to account for the process of burning. Ever an ardent phlogistonist, Priestley himself was unable to step aside from current beliefs and convictions. He believed that his finding strengthened that theory. In 1774, in Paris at a dinner at the Arsenal organized by Antoine Lavoisier, he announced that he had just discovered a new gas that was highly combustible and respirable, and which he called "dephlogisticated air."

Without knowledge of the work of Priestley, no less of a phlogistonist, Carl Wilhelm Scheele (1742–1786) of Pomerania (Sweden), published in 1777 the description of different methods for preparing what he called "fire-air," which he apparently obtained as early as 1771. He is believed to be an absolutely independent discoverer of oxygen, and many historians describing the isolation of oxygen credit his name together with Priestley's. Before Scheele and Priestley, among

579

the scientists who had approached the issue of burning and respiration, the closest to the discovery of oxygen was John Mayow (1643–1679) of England. Almost 100 years before Priestley's experiments, Mayow was studying the survival of mice placed with a burning candle under a bell jar. He also placed a moat of water around mice inside the bell jar and observed a rising water level. The substance that disappeared during combustion and respiration, causing the water level to rise, he called "nitro aerial spirit" and believed it to be a part of room air (2).

Antoine Lavoisier, who was an extremely industrious, multitalented scientist and administrator, repeated Priestley's experiments and in 1778 showed that this gas discovered by Priestley was able to combine with carbon to form CO_2, that this new gas was necessary for the maintenance of life, and that carbon dioxide was given off in expired air. He also noted that the new gas was taken up by metals during oxidation, and was going to call it "acidifying principle," but instead chose to use the Greek roots—"oxus geinomai" (I beget acid)—or, in French, oxygen (3). In refuting the phlogiston theory, Lavoisier knocked down the wall of old dogmas and doctrines, providing an alternative theory to the "vital heat" of Hippocrates and Galen. His experiments were the first investigations on respiration in which accurate and reproducible methods were applied. By his work on respiration and metabolism, using direct and indirect calorimetry, he established not only modern chemistry but laid the foundation for biochemistry. Some historians believe that Priestley isolated a new gas but that Lavoisier discovered oxygen.

The first person to use oxygen for medical purposes was probably Francois Chaussier, who employed it in 1780 to alleviate cyanosis in newborns and relieve shortness of breath in patients with tuberculosis (4, 5). However, the first person who established the discipline of oxygen therapy was Thomas Beddoes (1760–1808) of Bristol, England. His publication "Considerations of the Medicinal Use and Production of Factitious Airs" (6) in 1798 can be considered the pioneer manuscript on inhalation and oxygen therapy. Carried away with the idea of treating all kinds of serious diseases with the administration of oxygen and nitrous oxide, Beddoes established the Pneumatic Institute in Clifton, England (1798), where he attempted to stem scrofula, dyspnea, ulcers, asthma, and even leprosy, cholera, and paralysis. His Institute was the earliest prototype of a modern medical center for treatment and research, which included a clinic, hospital, laboratory, and lecture theater (7). With his collaborator James Watt, engineer and inventor of the steam machine, they succeeded in devising a special apparatus for oxygen storage and delivery. It was an oiled silk bag with a face piece of oiled silk connected by a valve box of wood containing inspiratory and expiratory check valves. Because of an outbreak of typhus in 1800, the clinical facility of the Institute became overcrowded with patients and gradually ousted the research and laboratory divisions. The volume of patients and the absence of expected cures from oxygen therapy eventually reestablished conventional remedies and led to the demise of this prestigious institution. Indiscriminate therapeutic applications of oxygen to various diseases brought about numerous failures and disappointments in the life of Beddoes, and he died a disconsolate man.

Almost the entire subsequent 19th century appeared to be silent about and uninterested in the use of this gas for medical purposes. It was only following fractional distillation of liquid air by Carl Von Linde in 1895, who first started commercial manufacturing of oxygen, that the interest in therapeutic uses of oxygen was revived. The increasing availability of O_2 and the use of chlorine gas on the battlefields of World War I forced its utilization for the treatment of acute chlorine poisoning.

At the turn of the century, John Scott Haldane started to employ O_2 in various clinical areas, including the treatment of bronchopneumonia. He developed the first therapeutic indications for administration of O_2, dividing them into short-term use for symptomatic relief of acute respiratory problems, and long-term use for severe chlorine poisoning and chronic hypoxemia (8).

Alvan Barach placed oxygen therapy on a more sound physiologic basis. He was the first to recognize that pulmonary edema could result from left heart failure and laid the physiologic background for oxygen administration (9). He was an advocate of the prolonged use of oxygen for the treatment of chronic cardiopulmonary diseases (10), and his insights and developments led to the institution of long-term therapy for chronic obstructive pulmonary disease (COPD) patients. He and David W. Richards further expanded on the original ideas of L.A. Hill, the first to introduce the use of oxygen tents (11), to utilize oxygen chambers and tents with patients who had chronic respiratory insufficiency on a continuous basis (12). Barach introduced the concept of portable oxygen and inspired the development of oxygen-conserving devices.

The contemporary therapeutic use of oxygen, based on physiologic principles, became possible after pioneering investigations of Barcroft, Krogh, L.J. Henderson, and Y. Henderson (7). Despite two centuries of scientific history, oxygen today is rarely recognized as a drug with specific therapeutic indications, an expected dose-response curve, and predictable complications when used in excessive dosage.

PHYSICOCHEMICAL PROPERTIES

Oxygen is estimated to be the third most abundant element in outer space, following hydrogen (more than 50%) and helium (40%). Our atmospheric oxygen is most likely to have been produced as a result of photosynthetic reactions about 2 billion years ago. Photosynthesis is a very powerful tool for oxygen generation, and it can replenish the entire interior atmospheric pool in a negligible geologic time span—2500 years (13). At the top of the atmosphere, abiotic oxygen was being added to the inner pool by the photo dissociation of H_2O by ultraviolet sun, followed by escape of hydrogen.

The oxygen atom exists in three stable isotopic forms, ^{16}O, ^{17}O, and ^{18}O, which occur in nature in the ratios 1000:3.7:20, respectively (3). Oxygen atoms can combine in two allotropic molecular forms, O_2 (molecular oxygen) and O_3 (ozone). Medical oxygen is derived from air and consists mainly of $^{16}O_2$, with some ^{16}O, ^{17}O, $^{17}O_2$, and so on, which is the natural mixture of isotopes, and it is usually referred to as O_2. It is a colorless, odorless gas at ordinary room temperature and pressure, and condenses to a very pale blue liquid on cooling to -183.1°C at 1 atmosphere absolute pressure.

Three properties of oxygen allow it to be measured rapidly and reliably at the bedside: its paramagnetic property, its polarographic property, and its ionic mass. Oxygen in all its three forms is paramagnetic, or attracted to regions of high flux in a magnetic field. This property, which was first observed by Michael Faraday in 1848, results from a specific electron configuration of oxygen, in which there are two unpaired electrons with parallel spins. Oxygen greatly increases a magnetic field, whereas nonmagnetic gases such as nitrogen and carbon dioxide do not. This quality forms the basis for paramagnetic analysis, which allows measurement of inspired oxygen concentration in respiratory support equipment with an accuracy of ±0.2%. The ionic mass of oxygen and its charge are used as the basis for mass spectrometry. The polarographic property of oxygen is such that it will migrate to a cathode, resulting in a flow of current. It was this quality of oxygen that gave Leland C. Clark the idea for his oxygen electrode, which is used in blood gas machines today.

OXYGEN FORMULATIONS

In the U.S. and many other countries gases are required by law to conform to specifications of concentration and impurity. In the U.S., The Food, Drugs & Cosmetics Act requires that medical gases conform to specifications of the U.S. Pharmacopoeia and National Formulary. Substantial therapeutic benefit from acute and long-term administration of oxygen has stimulated the development of many formulations of oxygen and oxygen delivery systems for inpatient and outpatient settings. Medical oxygen can be prescribed for hospital, home, and ambulatory use and is supplied in two forms: a compressed gas in cylinders and a liquid in a stationary or portable reservoir.

The majority of hospitals utilize a piping system of oxygen delivery from a central supply area to the station outlets at each point of use. Central supplies may be located in the open air with the control panel protected from the weather or inside a specially constructed room. The central supply of O_2 ordinarily consists of several banks of cylinders, with the number determined by the usage rate. In the central area, oxygen can be stored in two sizes: bulk and smaller systems. A bulk oxygen system (liquid and/or gas) is defined as an assembly of equipment containing more than 13,000 cubic feet ready for use of oxygen, or totaling 25,000 cubic feet or more of oxygen including unconnected reserves on hand at the site. When large quantities of oxygen are required for hospital use, liquid oxygen usually is preferred.

Design, construction, testing, marking, handling, filling, and transportation of compressed gases in cylinders are regulated by the Motor Carrier Safety Division of the Department of Transportation. Oxygen is supplied in green steel or aluminum alloy cylinders, in which oxygen is stored at a pressure of 1800 to 2400 pounds per square inch (PSIG). Cylinders are opened initially by means of a key-operated valve in the neck of the cylinder from which the gas emerges at cylinder pressure. A pressure gauge shows the cylinder pressure of the gas and provides an indication of gas content in the cylinder. The gas passes through a pressure regulator that is designed to reduce the pressure to a manageable and safe level (60 PSIG) and to further control its rate of delivery. There

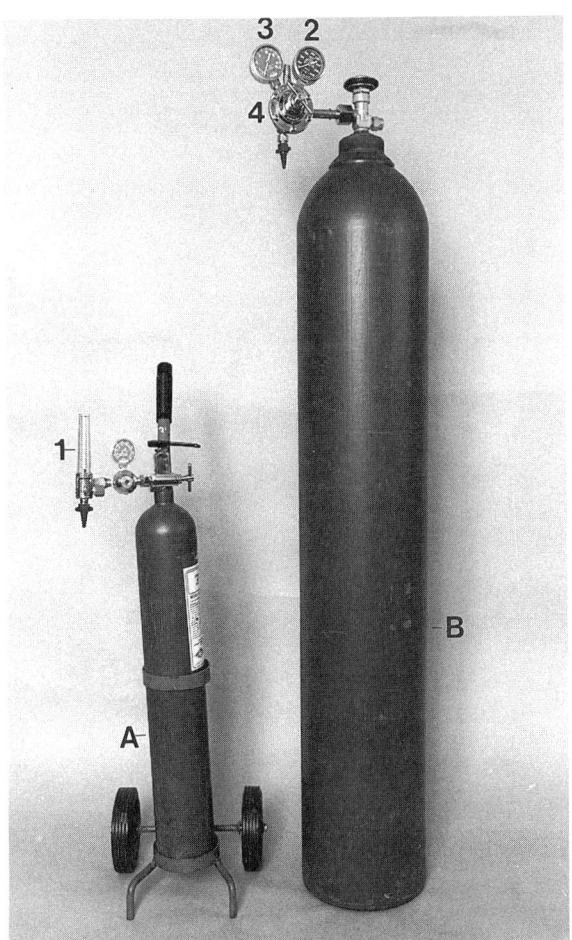

Figure 34.1. Oxygen as gas compressed in cylinders. Among nine different sizes of oxygen cylinders, E (*A*) and H (*B*) are most common for hospital use. The molybdenum steel E cylinder weighs about 25 pounds full with a two-wheel cart, regulator, and flowmeter (*1*), and can provide about 5 hours of oxygen at 2.0 liters/min. It is preferentially employed during patient transport. H cylinders currently are used as a source of gaseous oxygen for small hospitals or sections of hospitals not completely piped with oxygen, and as backup to a hospital pipeline system. One gauge (*2*) indicates the pressure in a cylinder when the valve is opened. The other (*3*) measures the pressure of oxygen after passing through a pressure reducing valve (*4*).

are nine different sizes of oxygen cylinders, containing from 76 liters to 7500 liters of gas (Fig. 34.1). A working knowledge of the volume of gas in each cylinder is helpful for planning transport of a patient (Table 34.1).

In the recent past, several hazards with cylinders were reported in the literature (14, 15). These included contamination of contents, faulty check valves, improper identification, and improper cylinder testing (16). Among others were errors in color coding and perforation of the cylinder thermal relief plug (17). As a result of these and many other (15) problems and incidents, standards and safety recommendations were developed and implemented. The cylinders must be appropriately labelled and sealed with valves that are specific for oxygen. For the small oxygen cylinders (size E or less), a Pin-Index Safety System is used on the cylinder valve to ensure that only an oxygen cylinder can be connected to an oxygen

Table 34.1.   Volumes of Various Gas Cylinders

Size of Cylinder	Liters of Gas	Duration of Use	
		At 5 liters/min	At 10 liters/min
A	76	15/min	8 min
B	196	39 min	20 min
D	396	1.3 hours	40 min
E	659	2.1 hours	1.1 hours
F	2062	6.8 hours	3.4 hours
M	3000	10.0 hours	5.0 hours
G	5331	17.7 hours	8.8 hours
H	5570	18.5 hours	9.2 hours
K	7500	25.0 hours	12.5 hours

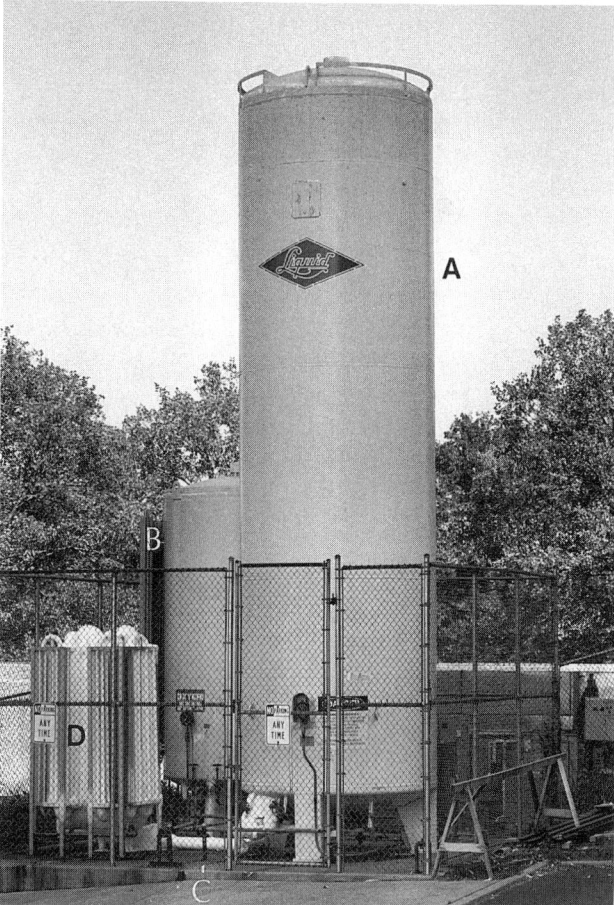

Figure 34.2.   Liquid oxygen central supply system. When large amounts of oxygen are required, it is less expensive and more convenient to store it as a liquid. Liquid oxygen containers (*A* and *B*) are constructed in a fashion similar to that of a large thermos bottle and mounted on noncombustible supports or foundations (*C*). They are refilled from trucks without interruption of service. Oxygen gas is extracted from a liquefied gas reservoir through a vaporizer (*D*), which supplies heat to convert the liquid to gaseous form.

yoke. For cylinders larger than size E, there is a similar safety protection based on a valve-threaded system.

The structure of liquefied-gas reservoirs is regulated by recommendations from the National Fire Protection Association (NFPA) and the American Society of Mechanical Engineers. The storage container for liquefied oxygen is structured in a fashion similar to that of a large thermos bottle (Fig. 34.2).

The temperature, near absolute zero, maintains the oxygen as liquid so that the high pressure that is required to store compressed gas oxygen is unnecessary. Several layers of insulation and, usually, a layer of near-vacuum are utilized to retard external heat transfer into the cold liquid. Liquid oxygen containers are constructed from materials that meet impact test requirements and are mounted on noncombustible supports or foundations. Oxygen gas is extracted from the liquefied oxygen reservoir through a vaporizer that is attached to the unit. This vaporizer acts similarly to a large radiator so that heat can be absorbed from the environment into the gas, thus allowing gas expansion with temperature stability. Because liquid oxygen is constantly being "boiled off," generating dangerous pressure, the containers are constructed to vent some of the gas to the atmosphere, a major disadvantage over compressed gas in cylinders.

After passing through a pressure-reducing valve, oxygen is distributed throughout the hospital via a central pipeline system, which delivers gas to the bedside at pressure 50 to 55 PSIG. Again, as in the case of cylinders, there are noninterchangeable connectors at the patient's bedside to ensure the safe delivery of gas. The most common of these is the Diameter Index Safety System, which ensures that only an oxygen flowmeter or oxygen high-pressure hose can be connected to an oxygen wall outlet from a hospital pipeline system. In comparison with cylinders, a bulk oxygen container with a central pipe system is safe, cost-effective, and convenient because large amounts of oxygen in liquid form can be stored in a relatively small container. Cylinders, historically a primary source of oxygen, nowadays are being used preferentially during patient transport (mostly cylinder E) to sections of the hospital that are not completely piped for oxygen and as backup to a hospital pipeline system (mainly cylinder H). All anesthesia machines manufactured in the U.S. have standard inlet connections for the oxygen pipeline, as well as a hanger yoke, which is used to connect D or E oxygen cylinders (18).

Three systems are in common use for home oxygen therapy: compressed gas oxygen in cylinders, liquid oxygen, and oxygen concentrators. Each system has advantages and disadvantages that provide compelling reasons to prescribe a particular system for specific conditions. Portable oxygen cylinders are usually of a size smaller than E cylinders. These molybdenum-steel cylinders weigh about 25 pounds with their two-wheeled cart, regulator, and flowmeter and can provide about 5 hours of oxygen at 2.0 liters/min. D cylinders weigh about 9 pounds and have a longevity of about 2 hours at 2.0 liters/min of continuous flow oxygen (5). Even smaller cylinders, constructed of thinner aluminum wound with fiberglass, lasting about 1 hour at 2.0 liters/min and weighing about 4 pounds, are practical only if coupled with oxygen-conserving devices that extend their use-time by reducing the required liter-flow. Most patients transfill their portable gas cylinders from their larger H cylinders (19).

The portable container used to store liquid oxygen is known as a Dewar flask. It is a type of thermos bottle in which liquid oxygen is constantly being converted to its gaseous state at the driving pressure of 20 PSI. Oxygen concentrators recently have become the method of choice for home and ambulatory oxygen therapy, replacing oxygen cylinders in many cases. Oxygen concentrators employ a molecular sieve method or a polymeric membrane to provide enriched oxygen from ambient air (20). The molecular sieve concentrators are capable of delivering oxygen concentrations of 85 to 95% at flow rates of 2 to 4 liters/min by removing nitrogen and water from air. The membrane oxygen enricher allows oxygen and water vapor to pass through the membrane, thus providing an oxygen concentration of 30 to 40% at a flow rate of 5 to 10 liters/min.

MODES AND TECHNIQUES OF OXYGEN DELIVERY

Oxygen is clearly a therapeutic agent, which is traditionally quantified from a dosage perspective as the fraction of inspired gas that is oxygen (FiO_2). Administration of oxygen to the critically ill patient can be divided into two separate techniques, invasive and noninvasive. Invasive oxygen therapy refers to either translaryngeal (oral or nasal) or tracheostomy tube administration of enriched oxygen mixtures. Noninvasive oxygen therapy includes nasal prongs, face tents, and a variety of face masks. Noninvasive oxygen can be delivered by either fixed or variable patient-dependent performance modes. With a low-flow-rate (<4 liters/min), low-capacitance device such as a nasal cannula, oxygen flow is insufficient for patient peak inspiratory flow and the patient must inspire some room air. This air entrainment is a function of patient inspiratory flow rate and oxygen flow rate, making tracheal FiO_2 unpredictable. With a high flow rate and an adequate capacitance device such as a face mask or tent, sufficient to provide the total inspired volume, a predictable and consistent tracheal FiO_2 can be delivered independent of fluctuations in the patient's breathing pattern.

FLOWMETERS

The flow of oxygen from either a wall or cylinder source is measured by flowmeter (Fig. 34.1). The flowmeter produces a pressure drop from 50 PSIG at the gas inlet to atmospheric pressure at the outlet. In a Thorpe tube flowmeter, a needle valve attached to a vertical tube of gradually increasing diameter controls the flow of oxygen, and the rate of gas flow is indicated by the level of a ball float suspended in the airstream within the flow tube. The needle valve can be placed upstream—between the gas inlet and the ball float—creating a non-pressure-compensated system. The most commonly employed system is a pressure-compensated flowmeter, in which the needle valve is located downstream between the ball and the gas outlet. The kinetic flowmeter is similar to the Thorpe tube but instead has a plunger.

NASAL CANNULA

Supplemental oxygen at low flow rates for critically ill patients is most often prescribed for delivery through a nasal cannula, which consists of two short plastic prongs that fit into the external nares and are connected by a length of oxygen tubing to a flowmeter (Fig. 34.3). The continuous flow of oxygen into the oral pharynx utilizes the pharyngeal anatomy as an internal reservoir, increasing oxygen concentration above ambient during inspiration. At a flow rate of 6 liters/

min, the reservoir in the oropharynx optimally is filled with oxygen and the FiO_2 is at maximum, 0.35 to 0.45. Further increase in flow does not enlarge the reservoir capacity and FiO_2 tends to remain the same. The final concentration of oxygen reaching the trachea is a function of oxygen flow rate, inspiratory flow rate, and minute ventilation. For the same oxygen flow, the final tracheal FiO_2 will be high if the minute ventilation is low, and low if the minute ventilation is high. A rule-of-thumb for a nasal cannula or catheter system is that each liter per minute of oxygen flow increases inspired oxygen concentration by approximately 3 to 4%.

FACE MASKS

The fraction of inspired oxygen can be augmented further by utilizing a face mask. The extent to which the inspired oxygen concentration can be increased by a face mask is dependent on total flow and FiO_2 delivered to the mask, the reservoir size of the mask, the presence of a reservoir bag, and the use of mask side ports with directional valves. Four types of face masks are used to supplement oxygen delivery (Fig. 34.4): simple, partial rebreather, nonrebreather, and air-entrainment (high-flow oxygen-enrichment masks).

Simple oxygen masks provide an FiO_2 of about 0.35 to 0.55 at oxygen flow rates of 6 to 10 liters/min. The addition of a reservoir bag expands the oxygen volume available for inhalation and increases FiO_2 to 0.50 to 0.80 when oxygen flow rate is 8 to 10 liters/min. Partial rebreathing masks are expected to deliver up to 60% oxygen. Oxygen from the source flowmeter is directed into the face mask reservoir bag and is inhaled with some entrained room air through the face mask exhalation ports. During exhalation the first third of exhaled gas, which is not exposed to a respiratory gas exchange area (from the anatomic dead space), goes back into the bag, mixing with fresh 100% oxygen. This system allows high FiO_2 while conserving oxygen supply. Non-rebreathing masks have directional valves to prevent the flow of room air into the face mask during inspiration and to block the passage of expired air into the reservoir bag. Since virtually all of the inspired gas comes from the reservoir bag and mask, it is critical to use high-flow oxygen, in the range of 12 to 15 liters/min. When this type of mask fits the patient's face snugly, it can deliver the highest concentration to a nonintubated patient, nearly 100%.

The most commonly prescribed high-flow oxygen device in current clinical practice is an oxygen powered air entrainment or venturi mask. The venturi mask employs Bernoulli's principle of air entrainment. A jet of gas passing through an orifice creates a lateral negative pressure as a result of viscous shearing between moving and static gas layers. By controlling the jet orifice size and the air entrainment port dimension, precise percentages of oxygen can be obtained. By employing a combination of these two variables a variety of exact oxygen concentrations between 24 and 50% can be delivered to the trachea independent of the patient's minute ventilation. Commercial air entrainment masks are supplied with a number of color-coded and appropriately labeled jets with markings for FiO_2 output and oxygen flow rate. This precision of FiO_2 is the major advantage of "ventimasks" over low-capacitance devices such as nasal cannula.

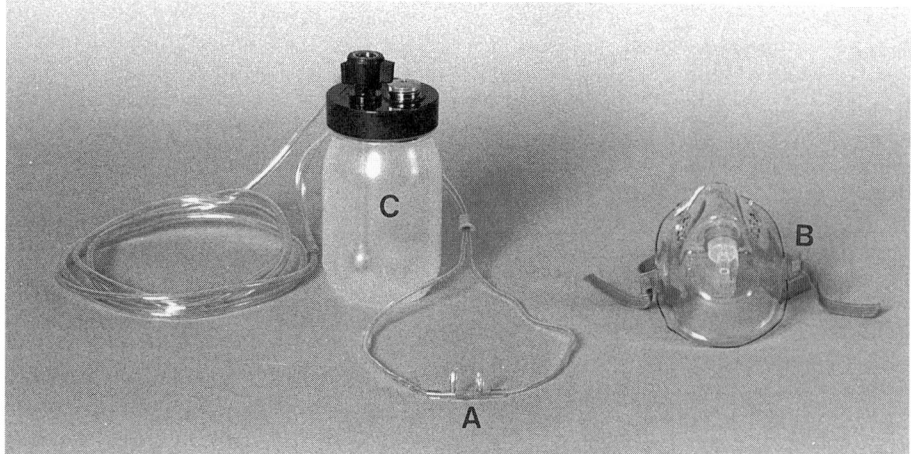

Figure 34.3.   Noninvasive oxygen can be delivered by the variable, patient-dependent mode using nasal cannula or simple mask. A nasal cannula (*A*) is a low-flow, low-capacitance device that consists of two short plastic prongs that fit into the external nares. A simple mask (*B*) can provide an FIO$_2$ of about 0.35 to 0.55 at oxygen flow rates of 6 to 10 liters/min. A cold-water bubble humidifier (*C*) has a limited efficiency because bubbling oxygen through water generates significant resistance. Therefore, it cannot be utilized to humidify high-flow oxygen and is used most commonly with supplemental oxygen administered to a spontaneously breathing patient via nasal prongs or simple mask.

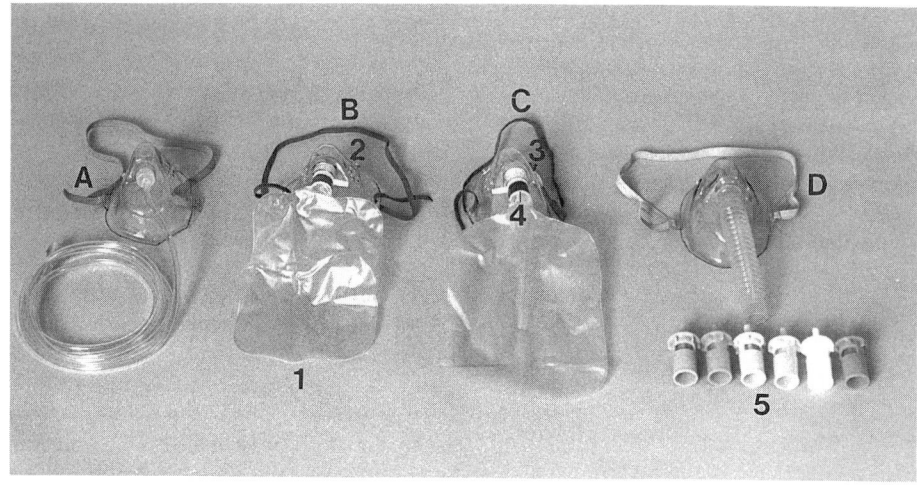

Figure 34.4.   Four types of face masks are used for oxygen delivery: simple (*A*), partial rebreather (*B*), nonrebreather (*C*), and air-entrainment (*D*) (high-flow, oxygen-enrichment). The addition of a reservoir bag (*1*) to the simple mask expands the oxygen volume available for inhalation and increases FIO$_2$ to 0.50 to 0.80. In a partial rebreathing mask, oxygen from the flowmeter is directed into a reservoir bag (*1*) and then inhaled with some entrained room air from the exhalation ports (*2*). During expiration, the first third of exhaled gas, which comes from the anatomic dead space, goes back into the bag, conserving oxygen supply. In comparison with a partial rebreathing mask, a nonrebreather has two valves. One (*3*) valve prevents air entrainment during inspiration and the other (*4*) blocks the passage of expired air into the bag. The major advantage of a venturi mask is the precision of FIO$_2$ delivery. These masks are supplied with six color-coded jets (*5*) with labeled FIO$_2$ output and required oxygen flow rate (0.24, 0.28, 0.31, 0.35, 0.40, 0.50).

Continuous transtracheal delivery of oxygen at low flow recently has gained popularity in some patients with chronic obstructive and restrictive pulmonary disease who cannot be saturated adequately on high-flow nasal cannula therapy. Transtracheal oxygen flow has been shown to decrease minute ventilation and inspiratory work in this group of patients (21). This mode of oxygen administration allows reduced oxygen requirement and decreased cost. Transtracheal oxygen is well-tolerated by most patients and provides adequate safety (22).

HUMIDIFICATION

During nasal breathing inspired gas is warmed to body temperature and saturated with water vapor so that it has 100% relative humidity by the time it reaches the trachea (23). Normally, this saturation occurs when inspired air reaches a point just below the carina, known as the isothermic saturation boundary (24). During expiration, the upper airway and nasal mucous membranes conserve heat and moisture, minimizing losses. Oxygen from both wall and cylinder sources has absolutely no water vapor. It can produce mucosal dehydration with increased mucus viscosity and reduced mucociliary clearance. When dry oxygen is delivered through an artificial airway, it can cause irritation and fissuring of mucous membranes with subsequent ciliary paralysis. Mechanical ventilation with dry gas leads to a significant loss of moisture, producing an occult dehydration of the body (25). Impairment of both structure and function may develop after as little as 10 minutes of ventilation with dry gas (26). Vaporization of water from the respiratory tract is associated with heat loss, which can have considerable impact on vulnerable groups of patients such as infants, young children (27), and critically ill patients with compromised thermoregulatory mechanisms.

In order to counteract the negative effects of breathing dry gas, humidifiers have been developed to improve the quality of O_2 delivery. Based on water output, all humidifiers can be categorized in three groups (25): those intended to reproduce environmental humidity delivering 10 g/m³ of water; those delivering at least 30 g/m³ of water when the natural airway is bypassed; and finally, devices designed to deliver moisture in excess of 44 g/m³.

A cold-water "bubble" humidifier (Fig. 34.3), representing the first group of devices, is most commonly used with supplemental oxygen administered via nasal prongs to a spontaneously breathing patient. From the flowmeter, oxygen passes down a tube and through a porous head submerged under water, forming small bubbles. The length of time of contact between oxygen and water is crucial in humidification. Therefore, this system is flow dependent and efficient only if oxygen flow rate does not exceed 6 liters/min. When gas is warmed to 37°C at a low flow rate, this device is capable of generating a relative humidity between 38 and 48% (28). However, the routine practice of employing a bubble humidifier when using gas flows of less than 4.0 liters/min through a nasal cannula recently has been called into question (29). Present data suggest that there is neither objective nor subjective benefit to humidifying oxygen at flow rates less than 4.0 liters/min (30). Humidity delivered at room temperature reduces but does not prevent water loss from the tracheobronchial tree, since relative humidity of inhaled oxygen drops as gases are warmed during inhalation.

Heated humidifiers produce fully saturated gas without particulate water and further abate water loss from the tracheobronchial tree. Based on the principle of forcing bubbles through heated water or passing gas through a low-resistance wick-type device with a large surface area, heated humidifiers are the most popular way of supplying humidity during prolonged mechanical ventilation in an intensive care unit. The wick, which can be a sponge or a paper, absorbs water by capillary action and provides an increased surface area for water evaporation. The Bennett Cascade humidifier, which has been employed in respiratory therapy since the 1960s, is an advanced, heated bubble-type humidifier in which gas travels down a tower and passes through a grid (31). High resistance to gas flow is a major disadvantage of this type of device, and it has been gradually replaced by low-resistance, servo-controlled, wick-type humidifiers that employ a "blow over" principle.

Servo-controlled, heated humidification devices that produce 100% relative humidity without aerosol have a minimal chance of causing a pulmonary infection (32) (Fig. 34.5). However, there is some risk of microbiologic contamination of the water reservoir (33).

NEBULIZERS

A nebulizer (Fig. 34.6) is a device that generates an aerosol and is designed to produce a suspension of water particles of selected diameter for the purpose of delivery and deposition in the airways of the lung. Aerosol can be used as a vehicle for administering medications and/or humidity to increase the mucus volume and mobilize dried retained secretions. Aerosol can be generated in three ways: (*a*) A mechanical nebulizer employs a rotating disc to spin water radially onto pillars designed to break droplets into the small aerosol particles (34). (*b*) An ultrasonic nebulizer utilizes a submerged diaphragm to produce water cavitation and break water on the surface into a fine aerosol (35). (*c*) Finally, an oxygen-driven nebulizer employs the Bernoulli principle to aspirate water from a reservoir into a gas jet (36). This type of nebulizer is most commonly used in critical care medicine to deliver 35 to 100% oxygen, heated and humidified, to an aerosol mask or face tent.

Humidification at a 100% level is guaranteed if gas contains 50 ml of water per liter of gas volume at 37°C (37). An even greater delivery of water to the tracheobronchial mucosal surface can be achieved by administering a heated aerosol mist that contains 100 mg/liter of particulate water.

Both underhumidification and excessive humidification are associated with detrimental effects. There have been several reports in the literature of water intoxication with intensive aerosol humidification (38, 39). Condensation of excessive water particles within the airways may lead to atelectasis and make the mucociliary elevator work less efficiently (27). This problem happens when humidity aids the production of large quantities of mucus that exceed the capacity of the mucociliary elevator to transport viscid mucus (40). Another problem with humidity was discovered via the inhalation therapy experience that aerosol equipment could harbor bacteria and that water particles could be the vehicle of bacterial translocation to the lung (41), producing pneumonitis (42). In 1970, Pierce et al demonstrated that 84% of samples from reservoir nebulizers were contaminated with Gram-negative bacteria (42).

It is important to remember that because of the inherent jet restrictions of a wall mounted nebulizer, oxygen flow should be 14 to 15 liters/min at 50 PSIG for optimum function. This nebulizer frequently is used to administer humidified oxygen to a patient with an artificial airway through a T-adaptor or tracheostomy collar. Nebulizers also can be used to humidify gas provided to large-volume tents or hoods (25), and for high-frequency jet ventilation (43).

OTHER MODES OF OXYGEN DELIVERY

A mechanical ventilator also can be regarded as an oxygen delivery system that uses the energy of the mechanical pump to perform the task usually done by respiratory muscles. A wide range of respiratory modes is offered by current ventilator technology to deliver any desired fraction of inspired oxygen, temperature, humidity, tidal volume, frequency, inspiratory-to-expiratory ratio, and end-expired pressure. Oxygen administered by a positive pressure ventilation mode is the most widely used technique in respiratory intensive care and generally is performed by means of an endotracheal or tracheostomy tube.

Percutaneous transtracheal jet ventilation is a desperate choice for oxygen delivery when the patient cannot be intubated in an emergency situation (44, 45). This method, which uses a large i.v. catheter inserted through the cricothyroid

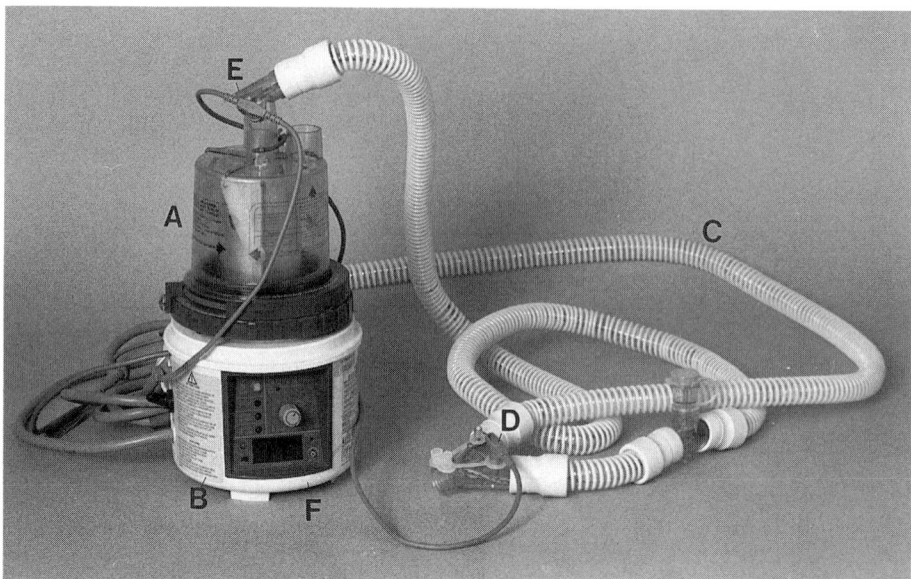

Figure 34.5.   A servo-controlled, heated humidifier is a preferred device to supply humidity to a patient during mechanical ventilation in the intensive care unit. Based on the passage of oxygen through a low-resistance, wick-type device (*A*) with a large surface area, the humidifier produces 100% relative humidity without aerosol. The humidifying unit (*A*) is attached to a heater-controller module (*B*). In order to prevent cooling of humidity and condensation of water, a heated wire is incorporated along the entire inspiratory breathing circuit (*C*) to maintain the temperature inside the tubing at a preset value. Probes mounted in the proximal (*D*) and distal (*E*) ends of the circuit allow one to display (*F*) the temperature difference as a digital readout.

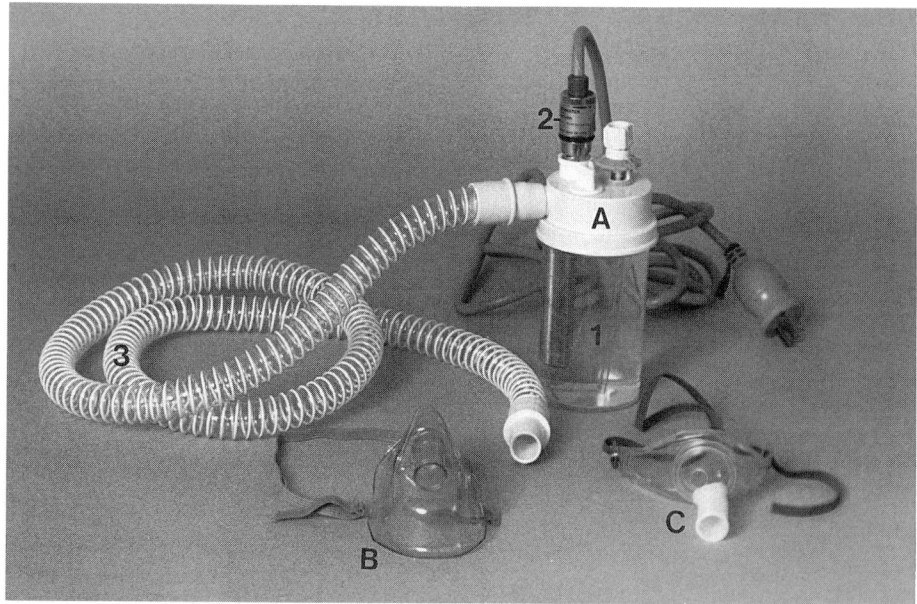

Figure 34.6.   An oxygen-driven nebulizer (*A*) is used most commonly in critical care medicine to deliver 35 to 100% humidified oxygen to an aerosol face mask (*B*) or tracheostomy mask (*C*). Oxygen passes through the narrow inlet tube at a high flow rate, aspirating water from a reservoir (*1*) into a gas jet. By incorporating a heater (*2*) into the nebulizer, the water can be heated to a temperature 10 to 15°C higher than body temperature to compensate for temperature loss as the gas passes along the tubing (*3*) to the patient.

membrane, has been recognized as advantageous to cricothyroidotomy and tracheostomy because of speed and technical simplicity (46).

The anesthesia machine, composed of a gas delivery unit, ventilator, patient breathing circuit, vaporizer, humidifier, mask, and endotracheal tube for airway management, is another type of oxygen delivery system (47). Oxygen flow through a vaporizer enables an anesthesiologist to produce variable concentrations of an anesthetic vapor to which more oxygen and nitrous oxide are added. The resultant mixture is supplied to the patient through the breathing circuit, for spontaneous breathing or mechanical ventilation. Oxygen to the anesthesia machine is provided from either a central hospital supply or small storage cylinder, located in yokes attached to the anesthesia apparatus. The latter can be utilized as either the main source, when central supply does not exist, or as a backup for central supply failure.

Hyperbaric oxygen therapy (HBO), the administration of oxygen at a pressure greater than 1 atmosphere, requires the construction of a special pressure-resistant chamber. A monoplace chamber (Fig. 34.7), which is designed for a single supine patient, can be pressurized to 3 atmospheres, a pressure sufficient for most, but not all, patients who require HBO therapy (48). Indications for hyperbaric oxygen therapy are regulated by the Undersea and Hyperbaric Medical Society. In critical care settings, the monoplace chamber is most suitable for hyperbaric oxygen treatment of carbon monoxide poisoning, compartment syndrome or crush injury, anaerobic gangrene infections, radiation necrosis, refractory osteomyelitis, acute severe anemia, and skin grafts (49). Multiplace chambers are large units that allow treatment of up to six patients at a time. Most multiplace chambers, unlike monoplace devices, are designed to achieve up to 7 ata of pressure, so that diseases requiring more than 3 ata pressure during treatment, such as diver's decompression sickness and air embolism, can be treated effectively (50).

NORMAL OXYGENATION: OXYGEN UPTAKE AND DELIVERY

OXYGEN CASCADE

Oxygen delivery refers to a physiologic journey that begins with the uptake of oxygen from the atmosphere and ends with the distribution of oxygen to the mitochondria of the cell for oxidative phosphorylation. This process starts with inhalation of atmospheric air, which is 20.093% oxygen. According to Dalton's law, total atmospheric pressure is the sum of individual gas pressures. The partial pressure of inspired oxygen at sea level and 760 mm Hg barometric pressure is 159 mm Hg. The progressive decrease of this partial pressure of oxygen

as it traverses the lungs, blood, and tissues is known as the oxygen cascade (51).

The first decrease occurs when inspired air is warmed and humidified by mucous membranes in the airway. Water vapor, exerting its partial pressure, which is equal to 47 mm Hg at 37.5°C, reduces PIO_2 from 159 to 149 mm Hg, as seen from the equation:

$$PIO_2 = (760 - 47)\,0.209 \qquad (Equation\ 1)$$

The second decrease occurs as the tracheal air passes into the terminal bronchioles and alveoli and is further diluted by carbon dioxide. Solving the alveolar air equation, alveolar oxygen tension (PaO_2) is equal to 99 mm Hg (13.2 kPa), assuming a respiratory exchange ratio of 0.8 (R = volume of carbon dioxide produced (VCO_2) divided by volume of oxygen consumed (VO_2)).

$$PaO_2 = (Pb - PH_2O)\,FIO_2$$
$$-\ _2/R = (760 - 47)\,0.209 \qquad (Equation\ 2)$$
$$-\ 40/0.8 = 99\ mm\ Hg$$

RESPIRATORY MEMBRANE AND OXYGEN DIFFUSION

Gaseous exchange between alveolar air and pulmonary capillary blood occurs by the process of diffusion across the membranes of individual acinar units, collectively known as the respiratory membrane. Diffusion refers to the net movement of molecules from one area to another by virtue of random motion of molecules imparted to them by kinetic energy. In order to reach the erythrocyte, oxygen must diffuse from alveolar air with a partial pressure of 99 mm Hg to pulmonary venous blood with a partial pressure of 40 mm Hg through layers of respiratory membrane. These layers include surfactant, alveolar epithelium (pneumocytes I and II) with basement membrane, capillary basement membrane, and

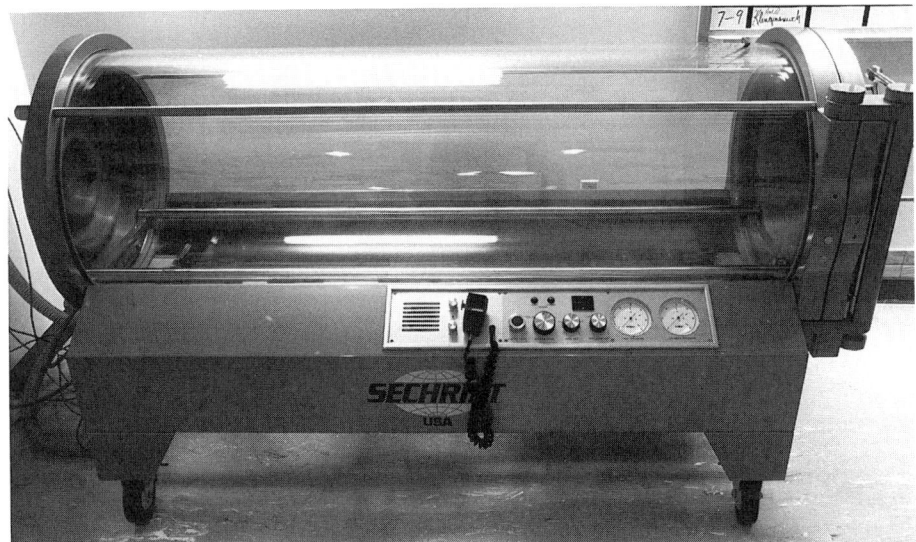

Figure 34.7. A monoplace chamber for hyperbaric oxygen (HBO) therapy is designed for a single supine patient and can be pressurized to 3 atmospheres.

endothelial membrane associated with the pulmonary capillary (52). The total surface area of the respiratory membrane is 70 to 100 m² with an average thickness of 0.6 μm.

At a gas-liquid interface, diffusion establishes an equilibrium between the number of molecules of gas entering and leaving the surface of a solution. The partial pressure of gas in the liquid equals the partial pressure of gas above the surface of the solution. According to Henry's law, the amount of gas that will dissolve in a liquid at a given temperature is directly proportional to the partial pressure of gas in the liquid. It is also dependent on the specific solubility of the gas, which is expressed as a Bunsen coefficient, milliliters of gas at 0°C dissolved in 1 ml of liquid at 1 atm partial pressure. The specific solubility of oxygen in blood is 0.0230, which accounts for 0.31 ml of physically dissolved oxygen in 100 ml of blood at partial pressure 100 mm Hg. Factors that determine diffusion of gas across the respiratory membrane include thickness and total surface area of the membrane, diffusion coefficient of gas, and partial pressure difference of the gas across the membrane. The ability of the respiratory membrane to exchange oxygen between the alveoli and the pulmonary capillary blood can be expressed in terms of diffusion capacity, which averages 21 ml/min/mm Hg. If the mean oxygen pressure difference across the respiratory membrane under normal conditions is 11 mm Hg, 230 ml of oxygen will diffuse across the membrane each minute, a volume equal to total body oxygen consumption.

Quantitatively, the rate of passive diffusion of oxygen from alveoli to red blood cells could be determined by summarizing the aforementioned factors into Fick's Law of Diffusion (53):

$$V\ oxygen = K\ A/T\ D\ (P_1 - P_2)$$
$$D = K\ Sol/Mw$$

(Equation 3)

where:

V = volume of gas diffusing per minute
K = a constant that includes temperature and diffusion coefficient of oxygen
A = surface area of diffusion
T = thickness of the diffusion barrier
D = diffusion ability
$(P_1 - P_2)$ = partial pressure difference on both sides of the membrane
Sol = solubility of oxygen
Mw = molecular weight of the oxygen

HEMOGLOBIN AND OXYHEMOGLOBIN DISSOCIATION CURVE

Low physical solubility of oxygen in water was a crucial limiting factor for the further evolution of oxygen-dependent vertebrates after the evolution of the circulatory system. A capacity for binding and carrying oxygen was absolutely necessary for the appearance of complex mammalian life. The evolution of hemoglobin, as a primary oxygen carrier, and myoglobin, as a muscle oxygen reservoir, served this function in higher vertebrates. Hemoglobin is an oligomeric conjugated protein with four peptide chains joined by noncovalent bonds

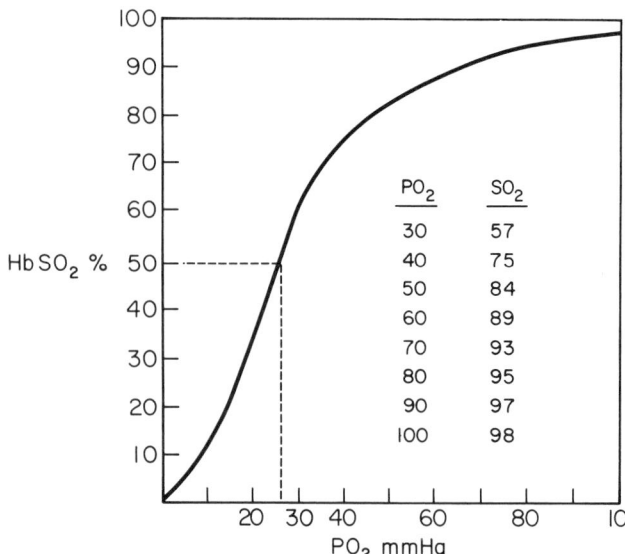

Figure 34.8. Oxyhemoglobin dissociation curve.

as a tetramer. Each hemoglobin subunit contains a pocket for heme that provides the nonpolar environment needed by the heme-iron combination to bind oxygen reversibly. As an oxygen carrier in blood, hemoglobin must have a high affinity for oxygen at the relatively high oxygen tension in the lungs and be able to release oxygen at the relatively low oxygen tension in the tissues. Therefore, the oxygen-binding curve for hemoglobin is sigmoidal in shape (Fig. 34.8), which results from conformational changes in the hemoglobin molecule that occur during uptake and release of oxygen (54). The flat portion of the curve is in the area of high PO₂, greater than 100 mm Hg, and the steep portion is in the physiologic range of PO₂, 30 to 100 mm Hg. The shape of the curve also reflects the kinetics of oxygen binding, which are cooperative in nature; that is, as the first molecule of oxygen is taken up, the hemoglobin molecule becomes structurally altered such that each subsequent oxygen molecule combines more easily.

The position of the oxyhemoglobin saturation curve is best described by examining the 50% saturation point, where there is a partial pressure of 27 mm Hg (P_{50} = 27) in normal adult Hemoglobin (Hb). The value of P_{50} can be used as an expression of affinity of Hb for oxygen. This affinity can be decreased by acidosis and hyperthermia, producing a corresponding rightward shift of the oxyhemoglobin dissociation curve and an increase in the partial pressure of oxygen in blood at 50% hemoglobin saturation. At a constant pH and temperature, the curve is also moved to the right by hypercarbia and increased 2,3-diphosphoglycerate (2,3-DPG) in the red cell. Leftward shift in the curve results from a decreased temperature, decreased 2,3-DPG, hypocarbia, and alkalosis. These physiologic changes have an opposite effect on P_{50} (55). Under normal physiologic conditions, near maximal hemoglobin saturation and content are achieved at an oxygen partial pressure of 75 to 80 mm Hg.

OXYGEN DELIVERY

After oxygen dissolves in the plasma of the pulmonary capillaries, it diffuses into the red blood cell, where it combines reversibly with the iron atom of hemoglobin and converts deoxyhemoglobin into oxyhemoglobin. The biconcave disc shape of the erythrocyte increases surface-to-volume ratio by 70% and is very advantageous for gas diffusion, as the 7.4-μm diameter erythrocyte passes through the 5- to 6-μm diameter pulmonary capillary.

Each Hb molecule binds four oxygen molecules, and each gram of hemoglobin is capable of transporting 1.36 ml of oxygen when fully saturated. Arterial oxygen content (CaO_2) represents the sum of both the oxygen physically dissolved in the plasma and the oxygen chemically bound by hemoglobin at 1 ata and 37°C. Therefore, the arterial oxygen content can be estimated by the equation (56):

$$CaO_2 = Bound\ O_2 + dissolved\ O_2$$
$$= (Hb \times 1.36 \times SaO_2) + (PaO_2 \times 0.0031)$$

(Equation 4)

where 0.0031 is Bunsen coefficient.

Under ideal circumstances arterial blood with a PaO_2 of 100 mm Hg (13.3 kPa) and complete saturation of hemoglobin at a concentration of 15 g/dl would contain approximately 200 ml of oxygen per 1 liter of blood.

$$CaO_2 = [(15 \times 1.36 \times 10) + (100 \times 0.0031)] \times 10$$
$$= 200\ ml/liter$$

(Equation 5)

One can see the insignificant contribution of oxygen physically dissolved in plasma that does not play a meaningful role in oxygen transport unless there is a substantially increased cardiac output in the presence of severe anemia or in the case of hyperbaric oxygen (56). Therefore, oxygen content is very sensitive to hemoglobin concentration and SaO_2 and is less dependent on the variability of oxygen partial pressure in blood.

Total oxygen transport or oxygen delivery (DO_2) can be expressed as a product of CaO_2 and cardiac output:

$$DO_2 = CaO_2 \times 10 \times CO$$
$$= 200\ ml/liter \times 5\ liters/min$$
$$= 1000\ ml$$

(Equation 6)

Approximately 1000 ml of oxygen leaves the left ventricle each minute and is distributed to the various regional vascular beds. When supply is adequate, oxygen consumption is a function of metabolic rate. Normally, systemic oxygen consumption is approximately 250 ml/min or 25% of oxygen transport. The remaining 750 ml of oxygen returns to the right side of the heart in the venous blood with an oxygen content of about 16 ml/dl, saturation (SvO_2) of 75%, and PvO_2 of 40 mm Hg. Four physiologic situations of oxygen supply/demand imbalance cause cells to convert from aerobic metabolism to anaerobic metabolism, with the resultant formation of lactic acid. The first of these physiologic situations is increased metabolic demand or oxygen consumption, as seen in fever, shivering, seizure activity, or strenuous exercise. If oxygen supply is unable to meet demand, acidosis will occur. Deficient oxygen transport as seen in hypoxia, pump failure, or severe anemia is a second situation of oxygen supply/demand imbalance. Third is uncoupling of oxidative phosphorylation,

as seen in cyanide poisoning, which blocks cellular metabolism and stops oxygen utilization. Finally, microcirculatory autoregulation can be lost as postulated for sepsis, leaving the tissues with inadequate oxygen supply to meet metabolic demands for oxygen.

OXYGEN METABOLISM AND CELLULAR O_2 CONSUMPTION

When systemic arterial blood reaches tissue capillaries, oxygen diffuses down a concentration gradient to the mitochondria. The tissue capillary is believed to be the main unloading location for oxygen; however, some oxygen diffusion takes place at the precapillary and arteriolar level (57). As in the case of the pulmonary capillary, the rate of oxygen diffusion follows Fick's law and is proportional to the tissue area and inversely proportional to the barrier thickness. Normally, oxygen delivery maintains an interstitial PO_2 between 20 and 40 mm Hg (2.7 and 5.3 kPa). Because the diffusion distances are broader in some tissues than others, the intracellular PO_2 usually will range from as much as 40 mm Hg (5.3 kPa) to as little as 10 mm Hg (1.3 kPa) (54). However, isolated mitochondrial enzyme systems are capable of adequate functioning at a PO_2 as low as 6.5 mm Hg (.86 kPa) (58). Within the cell, oxygen metabolism can be divided into mitochondrial and nonmitochondrial components (59). Normally, 80 to 90% of total oxygen is consumed by mitochondria and 10 to 20% by a variety of other subcellular organs.

Difficulties in energy transport and the need for energy to be converted immediately to the other forms forced the development during evolution of complete cellular energy separatism within tissue cohabitation. This energy is necessary for the maintenance of cell membrane integrity and intracellular function. Oxygen, being the only gas used for combustion of nutrients within the cell, produces that energy through the process of oxidative phosphorylation. Glucose and free fatty acids converted to acetyl-CoA are metabolized in the tricarboxylic acid cycle, yielding four electron pairs and carbon dioxide (60):

$$C_6H_{12}O_6 + 6O_2 = 6CO_2 + 6H_2O + energy$$

(Equation 7)

Reduced nicotinamide adenine dinucleotide (NAD) and flavin adenine dinucleotide (FAD) then transport these electrons to the series of respiratory enzymes located at the inner mitochondrial membrane. It is postulated that the electron pairs move down the chain of oxidation-reduction reactions to progressively lower energy levels and thus reduce molecular oxygen to water. Large quantities of energy are produced during these reactions, which are captured for synthesis of ATP from ADP and inorganic phosphate (Pi):

$$ADP + Pi + energy = ATP$$

(Equation 8)

Because the two substrate electrons pass through three coupling sites, generating three moles of ATP per electron pair, one can generalize the equation of oxidative phosphorylation in the form (61):

$$NADH + 1/2\ O_2 + H + 3ADP + 3Pi =$$
$$3ATP + NAD + H_2O$$

(Equation 9)

In the case of NADH, as much as 222.6 kJ of free energy is generated by this process of oxidative phosphorylation. There is no excess store of ATP in the cell, and it must be synthesized continuously as used. The rate of reaction is controlled at key points by the concentration of oxygen and ADP. When ATP concentration is too high, the reaction moves back to the left in order to match energy phosphate generation to metabolic need. Therefore, the ADP:ATP ratio is an accurate metabolic index of cellular oxygen consumption.

The optical properties of various members of the electron transport chain make them useful for monitoring tissue oxygen metabolism (62). The more oxygen available for oxidative phosphorylation, the greater the percentage of cytochrome aa_3 and NAD that are present in their oxidized form. Absorption of light in the near infrared region by cytochrome aa_3 forms the basis for a noninvasive method of monitoring of oxygen metabolism-niroscopy (63). It has been particularly successful in monitoring of cerebral oxygen sufficiency, brain metabolism, (64) and cerebral blood flow in anesthesia (65) and intensive care (66).

Nonmitochondrial oxygen metabolism includes a variety of biosynthetic, degradative, and detoxifying oxidation reactions that require a higher oxygen supply than does oxidative phosphorylation and are more vulnerable to oxygen deprivation (67). Synthesis of such neurotransmitters as catecholamines (68) and serotonin (69) is oxygen dependent. Both tyrosine-hydroxylase (conversion of tyrosine to dihydroxyphenylalanine) and tryptophan-hydroxylase (conversion to 5-hydroxytryptamine) are considered to be rate-limiting and oxygen-regulated enzymes in the synthesis of these monoamines. Oxygen serves as a substrate for oxygen transferases in hydroxylation reactions and is required for synthesis of collagen (70). Hypoxemia might be a cause of a decreased or defective collagen synthesis in wounds (71). Presence of oxygen is crucial for the function of mixed-oxidase systems of the microsomal fraction of hepatic and adrenal glands, where it is incorporated in the reduced form of cytochrome P-450 (72). Oxygen participates in the respiratory burst of phagocytes, resulting in production of singlet oxygen, hydrogen peroxide, and hydroxyl radicals, which are necessary for the intracellular killing of bacteria (73).

OXYGEN DEPRIVATION: INDICATIONS FOR O₂

Several central and local mechanisms exist to protect tissue oxygenation, the major ones being regulation of local blood flow and shifts in the oxyhemoglobin dissociation curve. When these mechanisms fail, hypoxia ensues. Tissue hypoxia hypothetically could be defined as an intracellular PO_2 below 10 mm Hg (1.3 kPa) or a mitochondrial PO_2 less than 6 to 7 mm Hg (0.80 to 0.93 kPa) (52, 58). Insufficient oxygen delivery may result from either hypoxemia or inadequate blood flow. As early as 1920, Barcroft (74) distinguished four types of hypoxia. He proposed anoxic hypoxia, which he defined as inadequate delivery of oxygen from the lungs to the blood (hypoxemia); anemic hypoxia,

Table 34.2. Barometric Pressure (Pb) and Partial Pressure of Inspired Oxygen (PIO₂) at Various Altitudes

Altitude (feet)	Pb	PIO₂[a]
Sea level	760	159
5,000	632	132
10,000	523	109
20,000	349	73
30,000	225	47

[a] $PIO_2 = Pb \times 20.9$.

reduced or abnormal oxygen-carrying capacity; stagnant hypoxia, low-flow phenomenon; and histotoxic hypoxia, a failure of oxygen utilization by the cells.

Hypoxemia, or reduced arterial oxygen content, results from one or a combination of five mechanisms: reduced FIO_2, alveolar hypoventilation, diffusion block, ventilation/perfusion mismatch, and right-to-left shunt. The distinction between hypoxia and hypoxemia is more than academic, since either can exist without the other (61).

A low PIO_2 is seen most commonly at high altitudes (Table 34.2) and is also associated with mining or industrial accidents. In the hospital environment, a low PIO_2 can occur in the operating room if nitrous oxide is delivered to a patient from an anesthesia machine without an appropriate blend of oxygen or in the absence of a safety system.

Other accidents can occur with hospital oxygen-nitrous oxide piping systems. These accidents have been reported in the medical literature in the recent past (15, 75–79). They include contamination of oxygen by nitrous oxide (77, 78), cross-connection of oxygen-nitrous oxide lines after system modification (79), inadvertent filling of an oxygen tank with nitrogen (76), malfunction of oxygen-air mixing valves with loss of oxygen (77), and drop of oxygen pressure and flow secondary to supply and distribution problems (15). The treatment of hypoxia caused by low PIO_2 is the administration of oxygen. In all other types of arterial hypoxemia, oxygen deficiency is secondary to a pathophysiologic mechanism that responds less favorably to supplemental oxygen.

In alveolar hypoventilation, carbon dioxide displaces oxygen in the poorly ventilated alveoli, resulting in a decrease of PaO_2. Although oxygen administration temporarily can relieve this type of hypoxia by increasing alveolar oxygen, mechanical ventilation eventually is needed for correction of respiratory acidosis and elimination of CO_2.

Diffusion defect is another entity like V_A/Q mismatch that must be considered in the critically ill. The most classic exception to the efficacy of therapeutic oxygen is hypoxemia caused by intrapulmonary right-to-left shunting. Under normal physiologic circumstances, average alveolar ventilation is about 4 liters/min and the perfusion is approximately 5 liters/min, so that the average V_A/Q for the entire lung is about 0.8. Because of the higher density of blood compared with lung tissue, the change in blood flow is much greater than the change in ventilation per unit distance. Thus, the lung base is overperfused and the apex is underperfused when compared with the ventilation. Therefore, the V_A/Q normally ranges from about 0.6 at the base to about 3 at the apex of the lung. Pulmonary shunt is defined as that portion of pulmonary blood flow that is not exposed to ventilated alveoli. One can quantify the shunt as a percentage of cardiac output that returns to the left heart unoxygenated. Anatomic shunt, venous admixture through the true venoarterial communications such as bronchial, pleural, and Thebesian veins, constitutes 3 to 5% of cardiac output. However, ventilation/perfusion mismatch in the critically ill patient may cause a physiologic shunt substantially above this 5% level.

This nonuniformity between ventilation and perfusion, which was first described by Riley and Cournand (80), can take several forms (Fig. 34.9). When ventilation predominates over perfusion, as seen in pulmonary embolism, a high V_A/Q ratio and wasted ventilation occur. The highest V_A/Q ratio occurs with ventilation in the absence of perfusion, which is known as dead space. A low V_A/Q represents an inadequate supply of oxygen to the alveolar-capillary units in the presence of normal perfusion, as might be seen in asthma or emphysema. The lowest V_A/Q ratio can be observed when perfusion occurs in the absence of ventilation, the situation known as right-to-left intrapulmonary shunting. Since shunted blood does not come in contact with alveolar air, its oxygen content cannot be augmented by an increase in alveolar air FIO_2. However, if loss of alveolar gas volume is reversed by positive end-expiratory pressure (PEEP), oxygen administration regains its therapeutic efficacy. Therapeutic oxygen may also benefit patients with low V_A/Q ratios.

Anemic hypoxia results from an inadequate quantity of hemoglobin (Hb) to transport a sufficient supply of oxygen for metabolism. Another form of anemic hypoxia occurs when Hb is present in adequate quantities but is rendered nonfunctional by some conformational changes in the Hb molecule or by blockage of access to the heme component where oxygen must temporarily and reversibly bind. An example of nonfunctional hemoglobin is methemoglobin (MetHb), in which iron normally in the ferrous state (Fe^{2+}) is oxidized to the ferric state (Fe^{3+}) and is no longer capable of binding oxygen. Methemoglobin is formed spontaneously at a slow rate within the red blood cell. It is produced by autooxidation of α-chains preferentially to β-chains and is converted back to functional hemoglobin by the presence of reducing compounds produced in the red cell by metabolic reactions.

Chemicals and drugs that are nitrates or aniline derivatives can cause acquired methemoglobinemia (81). Among them, mafenide acetate (82), ferricyanide, hydrogen peroxide, sulfonamides, phenacetin (83), primaquine, and amyl, butyl, and isobutyl nitrates (84, 85) have been reported to produce methemoglobinemia. The most common drug used in the ICU that is known to cause methemoglobinemia is nitroglycerine (86). Some local anesthetics such as benzocaine and prilocaine can cause methemoglobinemia (87). The degree of cyanosis induced by 1.5 g/dl of MetHb is equal in effect to 5 g/dl of reduced hemoglobin (83).

There are two forms of hereditary methemoglobinemia. In one form an abnormal Hb, hemoglobin M, has a crucial amino acid substitution (88). A second hereditary cause is NADH cytochrome b_5 reductase deficiency (89). This enzyme is the most important for reducing normally oxidized hemoglobin.

Methemoglobinemia up to 15 to 20% is usually well-tolerated. Levels above 30% produce a full-blown symptom complex of anemic hypoxia with gray cyanosis, dyspnea, and severe headaches. Toxic levels of methemoglobin (above 40%) are a life-threatening emergency and necessitate the urgent administration of methylene blue 1 to 2 mg/kg i.v. for activation of NADH-dehydrogenase (80, 83).

Access to the iron component of the Hb molecule can be blocked by both carbon monoxide and sulfur. Carbon monoxide has 218 times the affinity for hemoglobin that oxygen has, therefore forming a rather stable molecule of HbCO. In addition, the CO combines with the most reactive hemoglobin molecules, which are those that have the highest P_{50}. Therefore, the hemoglobin available for O_2 transport has low P_{50} or high O_2 affinity, which shifts the hemoglobin dissociation curve to the left and lowers the tissue PO_2 even further. Poisoning with carbon monoxide commonly occurs by accident or suicide attempt and is associated with smoke inhalation of organic burned material, such as vehicle exhaust, gas stove, and kerosene heaters. As in the case of methemoglobinemia, the clinical syndrome of anemic hypoxia starts to appear when the level of HbCO is above 20% (90). Severe carbon monoxide poisoning is associated with blood levels of HbCO between 30 and 40% (91). Currently, prompt administration of hyperbaric oxygen is the only efficient treatment of carbon monoxide poisoning. Time to initiation of hyperbaric oxygen therapy is crucial for prevention of hypoxic encephalopathy and myocardial injury (91, 92). Sulfur from such compounds as sulfonamides and sulfur-containing ointments can also bind to the Hb molecule and prevent oxygen from forming oxyhemoglobin (93). Sulfhemoglobin is an irreversibly blocked Hb, whereas carboxyhemoglobin can be treated by hyperbaric oxygen where the high concentration of oxygen is more competitive with carbon monoxide at the heme iron.

Stagnant hypoxia is inadequate oxygen delivery to the tissues caused by low flow, resulting from either ventricular pump failure (acute myocardial infarction, cardiogenic shock) or loss of total circulating blood volume (hemorrhage, intravascular dehydration). Stagnant hypoxia is best corrected not by oxygen administration but by intravascular volume resuscitation and improved cardiac function.

Finally, histotoxic hypoxia also does not respond to oxygen therapy but requires a metabolic correction. An example would be the use of nitroprusside in the ICU. Nitroprusside metabolism yields cyanide, which poisons the electron transport system. This poisoning makes the cell unable to use oxygen and creates metabolic acidosis. The cyanide must be

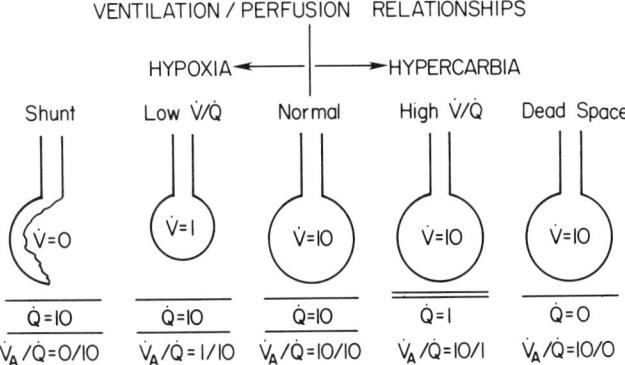

VENTILATION / PERFUSION RELATIONSHIPS

HYPOXIA ◄─────┼─────► HYPERCARBIA

Shunt	Low $\dot{V}/\dot{Q}$	Normal	High $\dot{V}/\dot{Q}$	Dead Space
$\dot{V}=0$	$\dot{V}=1$	$\dot{V}=10$	$\dot{V}=10$	$\dot{V}=10$
$\dot{Q}=10$	$\dot{Q}=10$	$\dot{Q}=10$	$\dot{Q}=1$	$\dot{Q}=0$
$V_A/\dot{Q}=0/10$	$V_A/\dot{Q}=1/10$	$V_A/\dot{Q}=10/10$	$V_A/\dot{Q}=10/1$	$V_A/\dot{Q}=10/0$

Figure 34.9. Ventilation-perfusion (V/Q) abnormalities are the etiology of hypoxia and carbon dioxide retention in most critically ill patients in the intensive care unit.

removed from the cell in order to correct this form of histotoxic hypoxia.

MONITORING OF OXYGEN THERAPY

OXYGEN ELECTRODE

The solution to the problem of measuring the partial pressure of oxygen (PO_2) in liquids is attributed to Leland C. Clark, Jr., a biochemist, physiologist, and inventor. In 1956 he developed the polarographic oxygen electrode (94). The original Clark electrode consisted of a platinum cathode and silver chloride anode mounted with a polyethylene membrane and immersed in a buffered potassium chloride solution (95). The membrane was selectively permeable to oxygen. Oxygen diffused through the membrane and reacted at the platinum cathode with water to produce hydroxyl ions. A battery induced a negative potential of 0.6 V between the anode and the cathode, ensuring that all oxygen molecules would be reduced by electrons obtained from the platinum surface:

$$O_2 + 2H_2O + 4e- \rightarrow 4\ OH^-$$

(Equation 10)

The electrons drawn from the cathode caused a current to flow, which was measured by an ammeter and proportional to the PO_2 of the sample. Clark's polarographic oxygen electrode has been used for 30 years and remains the basis of the electrochemical measurement of oxygen today. Modern arterial blood gas equipment (Fig. 34.7) combines analysis of oxygen with blood carbon dioxide and pH, providing data with an accuracy of ±2 to 3% (96).

Under ordinary conditions ($FIO_2 - 0.21$; Pb = 760 mm Hg), the normal value of PaO_2 ranges between 70 and 100 mm Hg (9.3 and 13.3 kPa), depending on age. The effect of age on oxygen partial pressure tension can be estimated approximately by the formula (97):

$$PaO_2 = 102 - 0.33 \times age\ in\ years$$

(Equation 11)

Measurement of arterial PO_2 with PCO_2 and pH has become the most commonly performed blood test to assess the adequacy of pulmonary function in the critically ill. The test ordinarily is referred to as "arterial blood gases" (ABGs). Arterial PO_2 commonly is measured on an intermittent basis to direct changes in invasive or noninvasive oxygen administration. However, in the early stages of acute respiratory failure, adequate oxygenation may be achieved at the expense of multiple compensatory mechanisms. Therefore, an observed decrease in PaO_2 may reflect not only oxygenation failure but also a failure of compensatory mechanisms. Measurement of arterial PO_2 and calculation of the alveolar-arterial oxygen partial pressure difference (A-a gradient) is a more sensitive clinical tool for early detection of oxygenation problems. Normally, while the patient is breathing room air, the gradient does not exceed 5 to 10 mm Hg but increases to 50 to 70 mm Hg on FIO_2 of 1.0. An increased gradient at a constant FIO_2 may indicate diffusion block, ventilation/perfusion mismatching, or intrapulmonary or intracardiac shunting.

INTRAARTERIAL CONTINUOUS MEASUREMENT OF PO_2

Further development of Clark's electrode has occurred in two directions (98), miniaturization (99) and continuous in vivo PO_2 measurement (100). Kreuzer and Nessler (100, 101) were the first to report an intraarterial continuous measurement of PO_2 in dogs, utilizing the Clark electrode modified by encasing it in polyethylene thrombosis-resistant tubing. The major problem encountered in the development of continuous intraarterial oxygen tension monitoring was the reduction of the size of the Clark electrode to fit into an arterial cannula. Two approaches have been attempted: one, to utilize only the platinum cathode inside the cannula and to fix the reference anode on the surface of the skin; the other, to employ the entire miniature electrode for intraarterial insertion (102, 103). However, technical problems such as catheter clotting, changes in oxygen pressure resulting from body temperature, and calibration drift have limited further development.

A new fiberoptic oxygen sensor has been developed as a substitute for the polarographic Clark electrode (104) (Fig. 34.10). Fiberoptic measurement of PO_2 is based on the principle of fluorescence quenching by oxygen. The electrons of the fluorescent dye are excited to higher energy levels by incident light. When they return to their ground state, they emit fluorescent light, which has a longer wavelength than that of the stimulating light. Oxygen interferes with the intensity of this emitted fluorescent light by consuming some of its photon energy (105). The first optical sensor for oxygen tension determination was developed by Lubers and Opitz in 1975 and is referred to as an "optode" (106). The fiberoptic fluorescence quenching optode is a new step in technology that could provide a clinician with continuous, real-time oxygen data. The experimental intraarterial optode consistently yielded the most rapid and reliable detection of inadvertent endobronchial intubation when compared with transcutaneous and pulse oximetry methods, particularly at high FIO_2 values (107). The detectable changes in PO_2 measurement could be seen within 15 seconds of every endobronchial intubation. Other in vitro and in vivo animal studies have shown excellent correlation between fiberoptic PO_2 measurements and traditional blood sampling (105, 108). The first human clinical study utilizing the intraarterial optode sensor was reported in 1987 by S.J. Barker (109). Fiberoptic oxygen measurements performed on 12 surgical patients correlated very closely (0.97) with the data obtained by traditional methods.

PULSE OXIMETRY

For more than 30 years intensive care physicians have relied on intermittent measurements of oxygen partial pressure for adjusting oxygen therapy and respiratory care. The introduction of pulse oximeters has made oxygen therapy monitoring a continuous, noninvasive, real-time evaluation process. Oximeters read oxygen saturation or percentage of oxyhemoglobin in blood based on the Lambert-Beer law: the transmission of light is a logarithmic function of the density or concentration of the absorbent, since each absorbing molecule consumes an equal fraction of a particular wavelength of the incident light (110). The arterial vascular bed is positioned

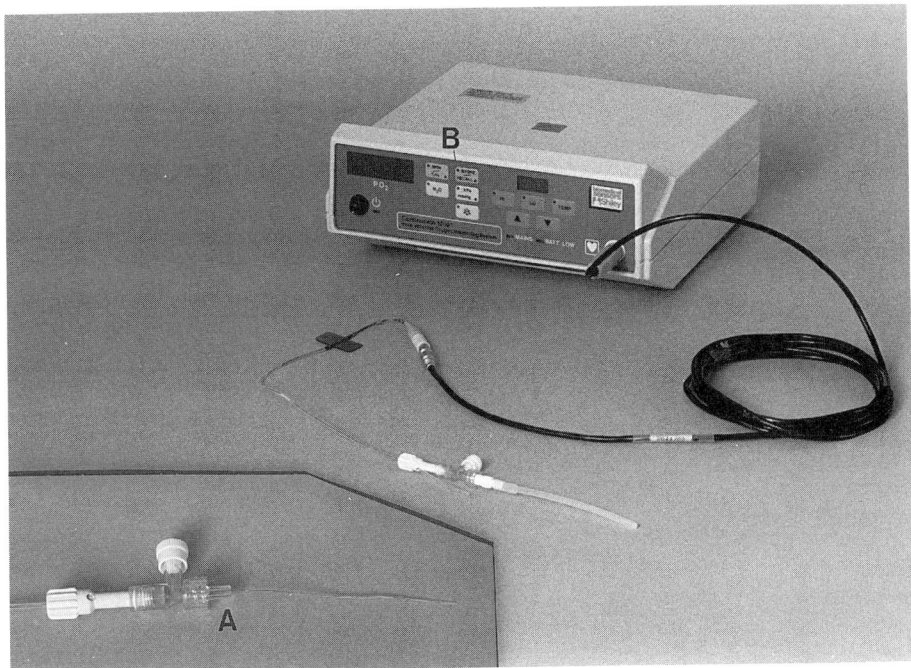

Figure 34.10. The intraarterial, fiberoptic, fluorescence-quenching optode (A) is a monitoring technology that will provide a clinician with continuous, real-time oxygen partial pressure data displayed on the bedside monitor (B) as a digital readout.

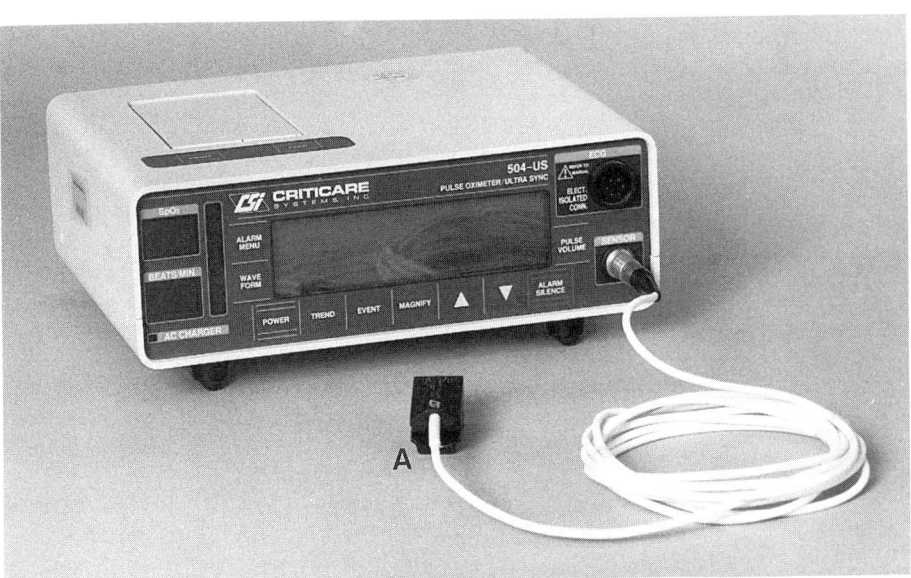

Figure 34.11. The pulse oximeter, which uses a finger probe (A) with a light-emitting diode to measure continuously pulse and arterial oxygen saturation of hemoglobin, has become a standard bedside monitor in most intensive care units for patients receiving oxygen therapy.

between a two-wavelength light source and a detector that measures the absorption of specific wavelengths of light relative to the ratio of oxyhemoglobin and deoxygenated hemoglobin. The pulsating vascular bed alters the amount of the detected light and results in a characteristic plethysmographic waveform, which is utilized by the oximeter to measure the pulse rate. The development of oximeters began in the 1930s, but not until the last 10 years, when new light-emitting diodes permitted miniaturization of ear and finger probes, did pulse oximetry find its place in the ICU (Fig. 34.11). The reader is referred to a history of the development of blood gas analysis,

the impact of the Clark electrode, and the evolution of oximetry and pulse oximetry published by Severinghaus and Astrup in 1987 (111). Pulse oximeters have become the "gold standard" for monitoring of oxygen therapy in virtually every operating room and most critical care areas (112). Several extensive reviews recently have been published updating methodologic developments, technical aspects, clinical issues, problems, accuracy, safety, and effects of pulse oximetry on other monitoring methods (113–116).

Clinical indications for pulse oximetry can be divided into oximetric and plethysmographic (114). Oximetric application has gained widespread recognition as a tool for early detection of hypoxemia in various clinical settings. Pulse oximetry is broadly used in adult, pediatric, and neonatal intensive care units (117), emergency departments (118), and recovery rooms (119) and during regional or general anesthesia (113, 116, 120). It is exceptionally helpful during transport of postoperative patients to the intensive care unit or recovery room. Substantial numbers of desaturation episodes have been shown to occur during transport of patients as a result of ventilatory failure from postanesthetic effects of analgesics, sedatives, and muscle relaxants (121–124). In the outpatient setting, pulse oximetry is irreplaceable equipment for monitoring of sedation and anesthesia during oral and dental surgery as well as radiographic and invasive procedures. During sedation for endoscopy, desaturation events have been shown to occur in as many as 45% of cases (125). The use of a pulse oximeter has been extended to titration of home-oxygen therapy in patients with severe obstructivelung disease (5).

Accuracy of pulse oximetry was established by comparison with cooximetry on arterial blood specimens, with an excellent correlation coefficient (r^2 = 0.96) (126). Numerous studies have verified the claims of most manufacturers that the oximeter errors do not exceed more than 3% at SaO_2 >70% (127, 128). However, some studies challenge the statement that the accuracy of the pulse oximeter decreases when SaO_2 is equal to 80% or less (129). Despite the ubiquitous presence of pulse oximeters in the critical care setting, limited information is available regarding clinical usefulness and cost-effectiveness in the intensive care setting (130).

It is important to point out that the pulse oximeter measures the functional saturation of hemoglobin and not the fractional saturation. Fractional SO_2 can be expressed as the proportion of oxyhemoglobin to the total hemoglobin:

$$Fractional\ SO_2 = HbO_2/\ HbO_2 + Hb + MetHb + HbCO$$
$$(Equation\ 12)$$

A four-wavelength type oximeter is required for identification of all forms of hemoglobin. However, if MetHb and HbCO are assumed to be absent, the formula can be simplified to that of functional hemoglobin, which requires an ordinary two-wavelength oximeter:

$$Functional\ SO_2 = HbO_2/HbO_2 + Hb$$
$$(Equation\ 13)$$

Thus, based on the functional equation, pulse oximeters utilize two wavelengths of light, one red (660 nm), which is absorbed more by deoxygenated hemoglobin, and the other infrared (940 nm), which is absorbed more by the oxyhemoglobin. Therefore, the presence of an abnormal hemoglobin species such as HbCO and MetHb will lead to erroneous overestimation of the arterial saturation. Another important limitation of pulse oximetry results from the shape of the oxyhemoglobin dissociation curve. Because of the flatness of the oxyhemoglobin dissociation curve at high PaO_2, it is evident that SaO_2 will not decrease until PaO_2 drops below 100 mm Hg. Therefore, a pulse oximeter is a sensitive tool for early detection of hypoxemia, and is a poor instrument for any recognition of hyperoxia. It should not be used as the only oxygen monitoring device for control of oxygen administration to neonates at risk

for retinopathy. Other limitations of pulse oximetry, as pointed out by Severinghaus (116), can be divided into two broad categories, those associated with signal-to-noise ratio and those connected with interference from the outside. Loss of a signal can occur as a result of reduction of the arteriolar pulsation (hypothermia) (131), low perfusion (132, 133), shock, infusion of vasoconstrictive drugs (134), improper probe placement on the finger (135), and motion artifacts (136). Erroneous readings can result from optical interference with ambient lights (137), especially fluorescent (138) and xenon operating room lights, magnetic resonance imaging (139), infrared heating or bilirubin lamps, and injection of intravenous dyes such as fluorescein, methylene blue, indigo carmine, and indocyanine green.

The pulsatile plethysmographic principle of pulse oximetry hypothetically can be utilized for monitoring of circulatory adequacy. No controlled, documented studies have been performed (116) to verify accuracy of this method. However, there have been a significant number of reports of the successful use of pulse oximetry for monitoring the adequacy of circulation in the hyperabducted patient arm during anesthesia and surgery (120), determining circulation in reimplanted grafts (140), assessing patency of ductus arteriosus (141), confirming patency of major arterial grafts (142), and estimating the level of ischemia in peripheral vascular disease (143).

TRANSCUTANEOUS OXYGEN TENSION

Transcutaneous measurement of oxygen tension ($PTCO_2$) utilizes a miniaturized, heated Clark polarographic electrode (Fig. 34.12), applied directly to the skin, which measures tension of oxygen that diffuses through the dermal stratum corneum to the sensor directly from the arterioles. Heating to a temperature 43 to 45°C allows faster O_2 diffusion as a result of arteriolar vasodilation and arterialization of the capillary blood. Temperature also produces alterations in lipid structure of the stratum corneum that enhance permeability of this barrier for oxygen molecules. A lag period of approximately 10 to 15 minutes is needed to achieve a steady state of reading. Repositioning of the electrode every 4 to 6 hours is necessary to avoid thermal skin damage and burns in adults and every 2 hours in neonates.

Peripheral blood flow in dermal vasculature is of crucial importance for validity and accuracy of transcutaneous PO_2 measurements. Therefore, this method has the same limitations as seen in pulse oximetry, as a result of low-flow states. Neither transcutaneous nor pulse oximetry can replace the need for an invasive arterial catheter in the critically ill patient with significant hemodynamic instability. It is interesting that the ratio of transcutaneous O_2 to arterial O_2 ($PTCO/PaCO_2$) can be used as an index of adequacy of peripheral oxygen delivery in circulatory shock states and low perfusion conditions (144). It indicates the extent to which the transcutaneous oxygen tension value is PO_2-dependent or flow-dependent (115). If a decrease in transcutaneous oxygen tension has occurred, arterial blood gas sampling is necessary to determine whether that change results from a circulatory or a respiratory problem. The transcutaneous oxygen tension value is very close to arterial oxygen tension value if peripheral circulation is adequate. However, in low-flow states, the transcutaneous

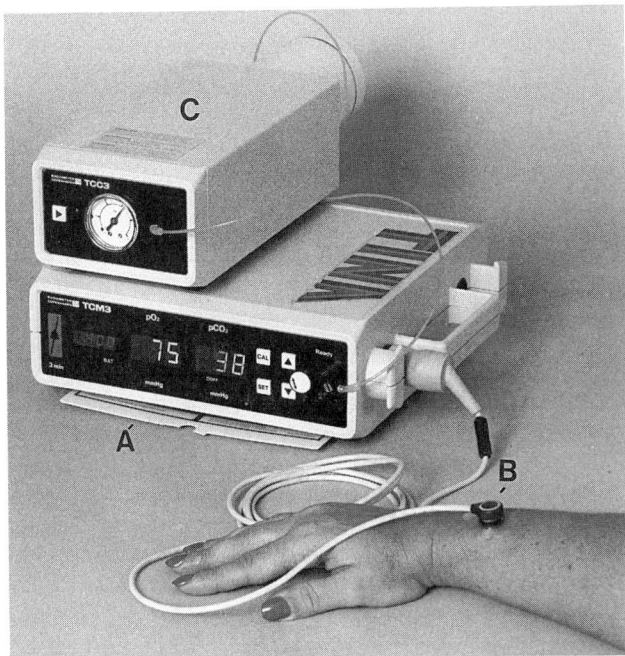

Figure 34.12. A transcutaneous oxygen tension monitor (*A*) with miniaturized heated Clark polarographic electrode (*B*) and calibration device is seen in this photograph (*C*). The electrode, which is applied directly to the skin, measures the tension of oxygen that diffuses from capillaries through cutaneous tissue. Transcutaneous PO₂ and PCO₂ are displayed continuously on the monitor.

oxygen value follows cardiac output. If both flow and oxygenation are compromised, then the transcutaneous oxygen tension reflects systemic oxygen transport.

MIXED VENOUS OXYGEN MONITORING

The introduction into critical care of the technology for continuous monitoring of mixed venous saturation has opened a new era in assessment of oxygen transport (112). It has produced a tremendous practical diagnostic, monitoring, prognostic, and therapeutic contribution to the care of patients with marginal oxygen delivery or acute oxygen supply/demand imbalance (145). Currently available systems for continuous venous oximetry are based on the principle of reflection spectrophotometry. The conventional fiberoptic, thermodilution pulmonary artery catheter has an extra channel that encloses two fiberoptic bundles for transmission of light (Fig. 34.13). A narrow-waveband light signal is emitted down one of the bundles and the reflected light is transmitted back through the second optical fiber to a photodetector in a computer optical module. Depending on the amount of reduced or oxygenated hemoglobin in the blood, different amounts of emitted light are absorbed, refracted, and reflected. This information is processed by a computer optical module, which calculates the ratio of hemoglobin saturated with oxygen and displays it continuously as a digital readout on a bedside monitor. Almost all current models are manufactured with a built-in cardiac output computer capable of calculations for a hemodynamic profile. Measured and computer-derived oxygen and hemodynamic parameters can be printed out for convenience and placed in the patient's chart.

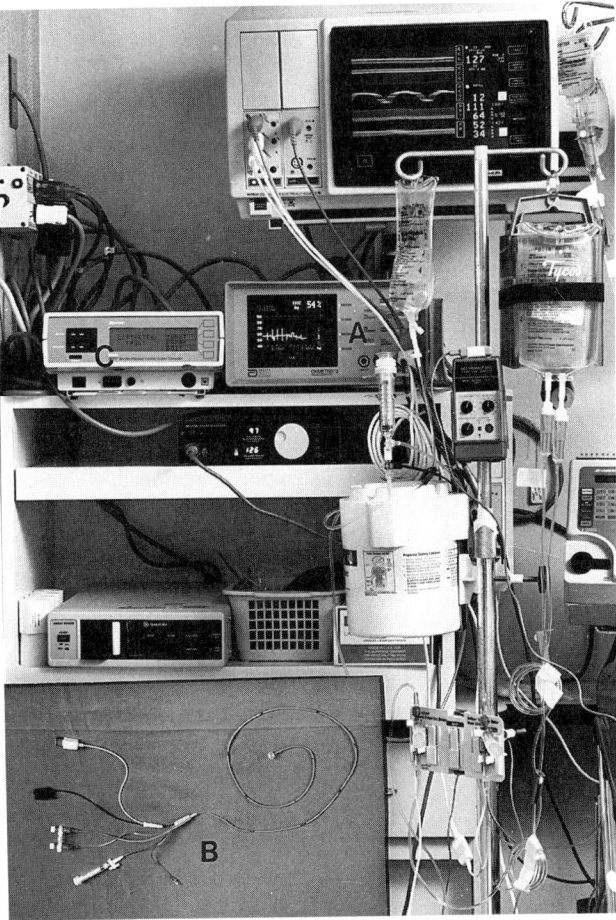

Figure 34.13. Among the variety of bedside devices for cardiorespiratory monitoring in the intensive care unit, one of the most important is the mixed venous oximeter (*A*), which is connected to a fiberoptic, thermodilution pulmonary artery catheter (*B*). The information from this device, when matched with data from a bedside pulse oximeter (*C*), provides the ICU clinician with a helpful assessment of oxygen transport. The simultaneous monitoring of arterial and mixed venous oxygen saturation is known as dual oximetry.

Since oxygen transport normally is about 1000 ml (Equation 6) and systemic oxygen consumption is usually 250 ml/min, one can calculate oxygen content of mixed venous blood ($C\bar{v}O_2$):

$$C\bar{v}O_2 = 1000 - 250/Cardiac\ output = 750/50\ dl = 15\ ml/liter/dl$$

(Equation 14)

Neglecting the amount of oxygen dissolved in plasma, the value of $S\bar{v}O_2$ can be calculated from the venous oxygen content formula:

$$C\bar{v}O_2 = (Hb \times S\bar{v}O_2 \times 1.36) + (P\bar{v}O_2 \times 0.0031)\ S\bar{v}O_2$$
$$= 15/15 \times 1.36 = 0.75 \times 100 = 75\%$$

(Equation 15)

In clinical practice the range of mixed venous oxygen saturation from 65 to 77% has been recognized as normal (146–148). As one can see from the aforementioned equations, mixed venous saturation is interrelated with three major processes of oxygen metabolism: arterial oxygenation, oxygen delivery (flow and its regulation), and oxygen consumption. Since 22 to 25% of delivered oxygen is utilized by the tissues to meet the requirements of aerobic metabolism, an abundant reserve of oxygen exists to prevent tissue hypoxia in case of low delivery. A normal exercising individual can increase oxygen delivery as much as three times by augmenting cardiac output, and can increase oxygen extraction by three times without switching to anaerobic metabolism (149). The exact value of $S\bar{v}O_2$ at which anaerobic metabolism begins varies, but an $S\bar{v}O_2$ of less than 53% most likely suggests the limits of compensation and represents impending lactic acidosis (150). Nelson (151) suggests a decrease of $S\bar{v}O_2$ of 10% as significant, regardless of its initial value, and recommends an investigation into the cause of the oxygen transport imbalance. As a rule, a decrease of venous oxygen saturation in a critically ill patient to a level below 60%, lasting longer than 5 minutes, represents a failure in at least one of the oxygen delivery determinants or indicates an uncompensated increase in oxygen consumption (152, 153).

However, some patients with chronic congestive heart failure can sustain an $S\bar{v}O_2$ level of 40% without clinical signs of decompensation (154). The adaptive mechanisms include a significant enlargement of the capillary compartment and a right shift in the oxyhemoglobin dissociation curve. Precise interpretation of $S\bar{v}O_2$ requires consideration of each individual determinant of oxygen transport in the application to a particular clinical situation.

Generally, lower values of $S\bar{v}O_2$ indicate a decrease in oxygen delivery relative to demand. Diminished oxygen supply may occur as a result of left ventricular failure, hypoxemia, significant loss of oxygen carrying capacity, or hypovolemia. Increased uncompensated oxygen consumption can be seen in patients with marked hyperthermia, violent shivering, severe agitation, and seizures. A high level of $S\bar{v}O_2$ may indicate increased levels of oxygen delivery as seen in the hyperdynamic phase of sepsis or delirium tremens, or may suggest diminished oxygen extraction as a result of neuromuscular paralysis, hypothermia, hyperoxia, peripheral arteriovenous shunting (cirrhosis, renal failure), or maldistribution of peripheral blood flow (sepsis, pancreatitis, burns).

Although the questions of clinical efficacy of mixed venous monitoring and its impact on long-term mortality have not yet been elucidated, monitoring of mixed venous saturation provides the clinician with a reliable tool for vigilant monitoring of oxygen transport and metabolism.

OXYGEN TOXICITY

Oxygen, like any other drug administered in doses that exceed biotransformation and clearance, causes toxicity. Moreover, oxygen itself is a very potent drug. The fact that oxygen serves as an efficient electron acceptor in respiration and has a powerful oxidizing effect requires that oxygen be prescribed with all pharmacokinetic dosage regimen precautions. When mitochondrial and nonmitochondrial metabolism of oxygen is saturated and its clearance becomes limited, excessive accumulation of toxic oxygen intermediates occurs. The most important toxic oxygen metabolites are superoxide

(O_2-), hydrogen peroxide (HOOH), hydroperoxide (ROOH), and hydroxyl radical (HO·). All of these species have different reactivities, but they share a common property, their very strong oxidizing power that results from the presence of the single electron in the outer orbital. A substantial body of fundamental and clinical research exits to prove that oxygen radical generation is the basis of oxygen toxicity (155–158).

Since free toxic oxygen radicals constantly are being produced at a low level during the normal process of metabolism, intrinsic protective mechanisms have evolved as an antioxidant defense system. It is well-documented that superoxide radicals and hydrogen peroxide are generated from the electron transport chain and from intact mitochondria during normal oxidative phosphorylation (159). Approximately 1% of oxygen is reduced only partially, resulting in formation of superoxide, which may be further converted into perhydroxyl radical, hydrogen peroxide, or hydroxyl radical. From an evolutionary standpoint, cellular generation of oxygen radicals emanates from stimulated phagocytic cells, primarily leukocytes and pulmonary macrophages, via the action of an NADPH-dependent, membrane-bound oxidase.

$$O_2 + e^- \rightarrow OO^- \text{ (superoxide)}$$
$$O_2 + 2e^- + 2H^+ \rightarrow HOOH \qquad \text{(Equation 16)}$$
$$OO^- + HOOH \rightarrow OH^- + OH\cdot$$

Therefore, cytosolic superoxide dismutase, which promotes the conversion of superoxide into hydrogen peroxide, may be considered the first line of defense against oxygen toxicity. Lipchik, for example, in his extensive and recent review of normobaric oxygen toxicity (160), believes that the cytochrome oxidase system itself should be regarded as a primary defense mechanism against oxygen toxicity by avoiding the mere process of generation of toxic oxygen metabolites. The second line of defense is provided by catalase and glutathione peroxidase to clear hydrogen peroxide, which is produced by the dismutases or by reoxidation of reduced flavoenzymes.

Hydroxyl radicals, generated from superoxide dismutase by redox cycling through a Fenton-catalyzed Haber-Weiss reaction (161), are the most powerful of the three partially reduced oxygen moieties. Therefore, the role of superoxide radicals and hydrogen peroxide, which are the common byproducts of cellular oxygen metabolism, appear to be significant only as precursors of OH^-.

Recent evidence suggests that singlet oxygen may be the most damaging of all the free oxygen radicals (160, 161). It may be formed in a number of ways:

$$OO^- + OO^- + 2H^+ \rightarrow HOOH + 1O_2$$
$$OO^- + HO\cdot \rightarrow OH^- + 1O_2 \qquad \text{(Equation 17)}$$
$$HOOH + HOO\cdot \rightarrow HOH + 1O_2 + OH\cdot$$

In normal oxygen metabolism the enzymes superoxide dismutase, glutathione peroxidase, and catalase and the free radical scavengers such as ascorbate, α-tocopherol, *n*-acetylcysteine and β-carotene are able to remove these reactive oxygen intermediates (162). However, when the level of metabolites is increased as a result of hyperoxia or the presence of oxygen radical generators, the protective capacity of these enzymes becomes inadequate to prevent the destructive oxidizing reactions initiated predominantly by hydroxyl radical and singlet oxygen.

Lipid peroxidation of cell membranes is the major destructive means of all oxygen free radicals, resulting in the loss of the cell membrane integrity. Oxidation of sulfhydryl groups alters enzyme function and damages protein structure. Oxygen toxicity impairs the process of transcription and replication of RNA, leading to the defects of DNA cross-linking and nucleic acid damage.

Considerable research interest is focused on the possibility of manipulating the cellular antioxidant defense system. Experimental administration of vitamin E has been shown to increase pulmonary protection against hyperoxia (155). Dexamethasone, by decreasing the activity of the antioxidant enzymes, potentiated experimental hyperoxic injury (163). However, the role of steroids has not yet been clarified. Dexamethasone in high doses has been found to have therapeutic value in the late stages of experimental pulmonary oxygen toxicity (164). The activity of catalase and superoxide dismutase correlates with increased tolerance of oxygen toxicity (165, 166). The natural approach of copying the normal cellular defense mechanism by increasing the concentration of enzymes and free radical scavengers by exogenous administration has been attempted in numerous experimental models (156, 167). The results are controversial, probably because of technical and methodologic difficulties and the complexity of the studied models. Rapid degradation of exogenous antioxidants in the recipient plasma and compartmentalization of biochemical events are the major problems of the in vivo studies. Iron-chelating agents such as deferoxamine that facilitate conversion of oxygen to the superoxide anion and catalyze the Haber-Weiss reaction may prove to have a beneficial role beyond their use in hemachromatoses and acute iron poisoning (168).

A consideration of the pulmonary system shows that the lung has the highest level of tissue PO_2 in the body. It is the most exposed and vulnerable tissue to oxygen toxicity. The morphologic changes of hyperoxic lung injury include endothelial capillary damage, destruction of alveolar lining cells, hyalinization of basement membrane, interstitial edema followed by later fibrosis, and, in advanced cases, airway mucosal infiltration with inflammatory cells. The pulmonary capillary endothelium appears to be most sensitive to high concentrations of oxygen (169), and its injury initiates the pathophysiologic mechanism of lung oxygen toxicity resulting from progressive accumulation of interstitial and alveolar fluid. Proliferation of type I epithelial cells prevails over the cytologic differentiation of type II cells, which seem to be more resistant to oxygen-induced damage (162). Type II pneumocytes are believed to produce the majority of antioxidants available in the pulmonary tissue (170).

Except for cytotoxicity, another deleterious effect of oxygen administration in high concentrations is the development of absorption atelectasis. If nitrogen in alveoli is totally or nearly totally replaced by oxygen as a result of increased FiO_2 (>60%), there is a tendency for these alveoli to collapse when the oxygen is rapidly taken up into pulmonary blood. Atelectasis tends to develop in zones of the lung with low ventilation:perfusion ratios, complicating the issue of oxygen administration in oxygenation failure as a result of ventilation/perfusion mismatch. Possible decrements in surfactant functioning may be an additional factor that predisposes toward atelectasis in high FiO_2 (171).

Of the extrapulmonary manifestations of normobaric oxygen toxicity, retrolental fibroplasia of the newborn is the most clinically important. However, direct correlation between PaO_2 and the incidence of retrolental fibroplasia has not been found (172). Other factors such as gestational age and birth weight have been reported to be associated with occurrence of this pathology without oxygen administration. Therefore, normobaric hyperoxia currently is believed to be a contributive factor that facilitates development of retrolental fibroplasia in certain predisposed newborns but not the sole cause.

Altered sensitivity to oxygen in patients with pulmonary pathology complicates the issue of practical recommendations on the duration of oxygen tolerance in high concentrations. Acutely injured pulmonary tissue, as in adult respiratory distress syndrome (ARDS), seems to be more sensitive to the high oxygen concentrations, accelerating lung fibrosis (173). Histologic changes start to appear when cultured human pulmonary artery endothelial cells are exposed to an FiO_2 of 0.6 or greater (174).

Low-flow and low-capacitance oxygen delivery devices are unable to reach a high level of FiO_2 and are safe for oxygen administration. Even with the high-flow and face mask delivery systems, it is difficult to achieve toxic oxygen concentrations for prolonged periods of time. Invasive methods of oxygen administration with mechanical ventilation are more likely to be associated with potential oxygen toxicity. Although the sensitivity of each individual patient to oxygen varies depending on underlying pulmonary pathology, most patients can be expected to sustain oxygen-induced pulmonary injury after exposure to 24 to 48 hours of FiO_2 1.0 (160, 162, 175). In the case of severe hypoxemia, which requires invasive oxygen administration in patients with high intrapulmonary shunt fractions, application of PEEP can reduce the fraction of inspired oxygen. Careful titration of oxygen therapy to an FiO_2 of 0.6 or below, optimizing oxygen delivery by cardiovascular manipulations and application of PEEP, is the best approach to avoid oxygen toxicity.

MODULATION OF RESPIRATORY DRIVE

The automatic basic rhythm of respiration is generated within the medulla by two groups of neurons, a ventral respiratory group and a dorsal respiratory group. These centers are influenced by nervous activity in other areas of the brain such as the pons, the reticular activating system (RAS), and the cerebral cortex as well as by afferent activity in the vagus, glossopharyngeal, and somatic nerves. The dorsal respiratory group is a bilateral set of cells that lies within the nuclei of the tractus solitarius and is composed primarily of inspiratory cells. Afferent input to the dorsal respiratory group comes mainly from the vagus and glossopharyngeal nerves, which carry information from the peripheral chemoreceptors and mechanical receptors in the lungs. The activity of the dorsal respiratory group is influenced through these nerves by low PO_2, high PCO_2, and low pH as well by changes in lung volume and the neural activity within the RAS.

The ventral respiratory group contains neurons that are active during both inspiration and expiration and is comprised of the upper motor neurons of the vagus and the nerves to the accessory muscles of respiration. The pontine pneumotaxic and apneustic centers modify the activity of the medullary respiratory centers. Central chemoreceptors lie just beneath the ventral surface of the medulla and respond to the H^+ concentration in the cerebrospinal fluid and the surrounding interstitial fluid. It is postulated that CO_2, but not H^+, crosses the blood-brain barrier and that an increase in CO_2 stimulates the central chemoreceptors after hydration to carbonic acid and dissociation into H^+ and HCO_3^-. About 85% of the resting ventilatory drive is attributed to the stimulatory effect of CO_2 on the central chemoreceptors (176).

Peripheral chemoreceptors are located in the carotid and aortic bodies and are believed to be the only site in the body that monitors changes in PO_2. Decreases in oxygen content of blood caused by anemia, methemoglobinemia, and carbon monoxide poisoning do not stimulate the peripheral chemoreceptors, since PO_2 or partial pressure of oxygen remains normal. These central and peripheral receptors intensify their firing rate to create a decrease of PO_2 below 100 mm Hg or an increase of PCO_2 and H^+ concentration of arterial blood. Impulses are transmitted to the brain via the vagal and glossopharyngeal nerves and result in enhanced rate and depth of respiration.

Failure of central receptors to respond to carbon dioxide and/or hydrogen ion is one of the major causes of respiratory failure in patients with metabolic alkalosis, COPD, and the obesity hypoventilation syndrome. A variety of therapeutic agents have been used to modify and enhance respiratory drive; the most common are doxapram, amitrine bismesylate, and medroxyprogesterone acetate.

The effect of doxapram infusion on peripheral chemoreceptors was studied in normal volunteers and patients with chronic bronchitis and emphysema (177). Doxapram was reported to increase chemosensitivity to hypoxia and enhance the response to hypercapnia, implying that it acts primarily through stimulation of peripheral chemoreceptors. In experimental halothane anesthesia, infusion of doxapram has been shown to decrease arterial carbon dioxide tension and increase pH and arterial blood pressure (178). It also lightened the plane of anesthesia but did not effect the recovery.

The effect of doxapram on hypercapnic response during weaning from mechanical ventilation in COPD recently has been reported in 13 patients (179). Failure of weaning from mechanical ventilation in COPD patients generally is related to a peripheral cause, diaphragmatic fatigue, or left ventricular dysfunction (180, 181). The purpose of the study was to analyze respiratory drive fatigue and reserve of excitability in COPD patients, using doxapram as a peripheral chemoreceptor stimulant. The results showed variable neuromuscular (P 0.1/$P_{ET}CO_2$) and low ventilatory ($\dot{V}E/P_{ET}CO_2$) response to hypercapnia after a short doxapram infusion. Doxapram did not change the slopes of these relations but increased the end-respiratory volume. The authors believe that doxapram is useless and may even be detrimental in COPD patients. Although doxapram has not been studied extensively in infants, it is deemed to be a viable therapy in neonatology for the treatment of refractory apnea and congenital hypoventilation syndrome (182).

A variety of drugs have been used to antagonize the respiratory depression caused by narcotic analgesics. Some of these drugs, such as nalorphine, naloxone, butorphanol, and nalbuphine, are opiates that interact directly with opiate receptors (178). Others, such as physostigmine, doxapram, and aminophylline, probably act indirectly by stimulating neuronal pathways involved in the regulation of ventilation. Cardiovascular stimulation and eradication of analgesia have been troublesome, especially with the use of naloxone. The newer mixed agonist-antagonist agents butorphanol and nalbuphine may have significant advantages compared with naloxone (183).

A double-blind, cross-over volunteer trial has been carried out to determine whether oral doxapram reduces the respiratory depression caused by morphine 0.12 mg/kg i.m. (184). Doxapram was given to subjects 90 minutes before the morphine and substantially reduced the displacement of the ventilatory response to carbon dioxide caused by morphine. However, doxapram administered alone in doses of 300 mg and 600 mg did not alter significantly respiratory variables measured in this study.

Almitrine bismesylate is a pharmacologically unique respiratory stimulant that enhances respiration by acting as an agonist of peripheral chemoreceptors located in the carotid bodies (185). It also appears to affect blood gases through mechanisms other than stimulation of ventilation, such as changing the lung ventilation/perfusion relationship or creating a metabolic effect for which there is, as yet, no firm evidence (186). In comparison with traditional centrally acting respiratory stimulants, almitrine has the advantages of oral activity, prolonged duration of effect, and an improved adverse effect profile. Almitrine generally is well-tolerated, with headache and minor gastrointestinal disturbances being the most frequently observed side effects. The data supporting the efficacy of almitrine in the treatment of different chronic pulmonary pathologies are conflicting.

The effectiveness and safety of almitrine bismesylate were assessed in patients with the hypoxemic form of chronic respiratory insufficiency caused by chronic bronchitis and emphysema (187). The multicenter trial of 12 weeks' duration was double-blinded and placebo-controlled, with individual and group comparisons. A significant decrease in $_2$ was observed in the almitrine group after 12 weeks of drug administration. No correlation was found among the plasma almitrine concentration, PaO_2, and $PaCO_2$.

The effects of oral almitrine bismesylate were studied in patients with COPD and hypoxemic cor pulmonale. Twenty-three patients admitted to the hospital with an acute exacerbation of ventilatory failure were randomized to receive either almitrine 100 mg twice a day reduced to 50 mg twice a day over 48 hours or placebo in addition to conventional treatment. The results showed no benefit from oral almitrine in this group of patients. However, plasma almitrine concentrations were often below the optimum therapeutic range, suggesting impaired drug absorption.

In the earlier studies, almitrine was shown to increase arterial oxygen tension while decreasing arterial carbon dioxide tension in patients with COPD, both at rest and during exercise (185). The drug has also been suggested to have benefit in the treatment of nocturnal oxygen desaturation because of its ability to reduce the frequency and severity of nocturnal hypoxemia without impairing the quality of sleep (185).

Naloxone has been shown to produce beneficial effects on various parameters of pulmonary function (188). These effects were evaluated after a single i.v. dose of naloxone. There has been no documentation of long-term effectiveness of naloxone in COPD. Naloxone and naltrexone recently have been reported to be useful as respiratory stimulants in two patients who failed traditional medical therapy for COPD (189). Both patients demonstrated improvement while receiving the drugs but developed respiratory failure when the drugs were discontinued abruptly.

Some recent experimental data have supported the hypothesis that serotonin enhances central ventilatory activity (190, 191) and that ventilatory stimulation preferentially may activate upper airway muscle activity relative to that of the diaphragm (192, 193). Hanzel suggested that a serotonin agonist preferentially could stimulate the activity of upper airway inspiratory muscles. A specific serotonin inhibitor, fluoxetine, was evaluated in the treatment of patients with obstructive sleep apnea (OSA) (194). It has been hypothesized that fluoxetine preserves upper airway patency during sleep by enhancing upper airway muscle activity (195). Another report shows that L-tryptophan, a serotonin precursor, was beneficial for obstructive sleep apnea (196). In a prospective, cross-over, unblinded study, fluoxetine was compared with protriptyline (a common drug used to treat OSA) in 12 patients with OSA (194). The response to fluoxetine was found to be equivalent to that of protriptyline. No significant improvement in the number of arterial desaturation events or the number of arousals was noted with either agent. Fluoxetine was reported to be better tolerated than protriptyline because of the absence of anticholinergic side effects. The authors concluded that fluoxetine is beneficial to some, but not all, patients with obstructive sleep apnea.

Thyrotropin releasing hormone (TRH) stimulates ventilation in experimental animals when applied at central nervous system sites that affect respiratory motor output (197). One part of the respiratory response, the shortening of inspiratory time, seems to be elicited from the raphe obscurus in the medulla. The other response involves an immediate tachypnea after injection of thyroid stimulating hormone (TSH) into the region of the interpeduncular nucleus of the midbrain. The location of the sites responsible for respiratory stimulation corresponded to those of the reticular activating system, where electrical stimulation induced hyperventilation in experimental animals (197). Rapid reversal of significant experimental respiratory depression caused by various general anesthetics has been reported after a 2 mg/kg i.v. injection of TRH (198). The associated hemodynamic response to TRH is consistent with a pattern of sympatho-adrenal-medullary activation. Short intravenous infusions of 200 μg/kg and 400 μg/kg of TRH administered to human volunteers initiated an increase in minute volume, ventilatory air-flow, and alveolar oxygen tension during both basal and CO_2-stimulated breathing (199). This is accompanied by general effects of central nervous system excitation such as dizziness, nausea, restlessness, palpitation, and hypervigilance. The mode of action of TRH's effects on respiration after peripheral administration is still speculative. It was concluded that an enhanced sympathetic output or a direct receptor-mediated action at central nervous system sites may be responsible, although a peripheral effect cannot be excluded.

Sex hormones currently are recognized to play an important role in maintaining normal respiratory function; in particular, progesterone has respiratory stimulant effects. Progesterone is widely known to enhance alveolar ventilation during pregnancy and the luteal phase of the menstrual cycle (200). Dysrhythmic respiratory patterns and oxygen desaturation during sleep are observed more frequently in men than in women (201). Therefore, progesterone was used for the treatment of COPD (202), alveolar hypoventilation syndrome (203), and obstructive sleep apnea (204).

Chlormadinone acetate is a potent synthetic progesterone whose luteinizing action is 10 times stronger than that of medroxyprogesterone acetate and has been used in respiratory studies (205, 206). Its effect on ventilatory stimulation in patients with COPD was studied in a randomized, double-blind, cross-over, placebo-controlled clinical trial (207). The results indicate that chlormadinone augmented not only respiratory neuromuscular response to hypercapnia and hypoxia but also flow-resistant load compensation in patients with COPD.

The effect of chlormadinone on the degree of hypoxemia during sleep recently has been used by the same group of researchers in another clinical trial on 12 patients with COPD (188). This study demonstrated that the therapeutic effectiveness of chlormadinone on sleep disorders in COPD patients depends upon the magnitude of change in $PaCO_2$ during wakefulness. Patients whose $PaCO_2$ decreased by more than 4 mm Hg (0.53 kPa) during wakefulness (correctors) suffered less desaturation during sleep. On the other hand, in patients who had no decrease of their $PaCO_2$ while awake (noncorrectors), a beneficial effect on sleep disorders was not observed. It was concluded that chlormadinone is effective in certain patients with COPD.

Chlormadinone therapy was also used in 9 patients with sleep apnea syndrome and was observed to be effective in those patients whose load response and respiratory control activity were augmented during wakefulness (208).

OXYGEN-CARRYING BLOOD SUBSTITUTES

Oxygen-carrying blood substitutes are intravenous fluids that have both oxygen-carrying capacity and volume expansion capability. Oxygen-transporting agents must load oxygen in the pulmonary circulation and unload oxygen in the peripheral tissues. They should be nontoxic, not interfere with immunity and hemostasis, and have no oncogenic properties. They should be excreted unchanged or metabolized without toxic by-products. Solutions of stroma-free hemoglobin and perfluorochemical emulsions have been investigated as possible oxygen-carrying fluids. Although the oxygen affinities of hemoglobin solutions and perfluorochemicals are totally different, they both offer advantages over natural blood components. These advantages include rapid availability since there is no need for blood typing, easy long-term storage, no disease transmission, low viscosity, and lack of microaggregates.

Perfluorochemical Emulsions

Perfluorocarbons (PFCs) are biologically inert, artificially synthesized 8- to 10-carbon-fluoronated molecules with a high solubility for gases. Oxygen solubility in the pure perfluorochemicals is about 20 times higher than in water. Unfortunately, PFCs are insoluble in water and can be manufactured only as emulsions. The commercially available perfluorochemical Fluosol-DA 20%, which was first developed by Yokoyama and co-workers in the mid-1970s (209), contains a 20% weight:volume emulsion of perfluorodecalin and tripropylomine with pluronic F-68 and egg yolk phospholipids as emulsifying detergents. A whole-body half-life of the first perfluorocarbon-perfluorodecalin is about 7 days. The half-life of the second ingredient, tripropylomine, can be unacceptably long, significantly extending the total body clearance of the entire emulsion for up to 65 days (210). It is interesting to note that the primary pathway for elimination of PFCs is via the expired air and possibly a transcutaneous route (211). The emulsion, consisting of 15.2% of perfluorodecaline and 7.6% of methylcyclopiperidine as a stabilizer emulsified with pluronic F68, has also been made in the former Soviet Union. Fluosol-DA 20% has been broadly investigated in Japan and the U.S. in both animal and human studies (212–215).

In the presence of perfluorocarbons, oxygen in blood is transported by three separate oxygen carriers: hemoglobin, plasma, and fluorochemicals. The total oxygen content is then equal to the sum of three individual oxygen vehicles where 0.0034 and 0.0057 are oxygen solubility coefficients in plasma and PFC, respectively, and FCT is fluorocrit, or the volume concentration of fluorocarbon in the emulsion (216):

$$O_2 \; Content = O_2 \; bound \; to \; Hb + O_2 \; dissolved \; in \; plasma + O_2 \; dissolved \; in \; PFC$$

$$O_2 \; Content = (1.34 \times Hb \times \%Sat) + (0.0034 \times PO_2) + (0.0057 \times PO_2 \times FCT)$$

(Equation 18)

Several striking limiting factors of perfluorocarbons as oxygen-carrying blood substitutes recently have been summarized by Gould (217) and Tremper (216). First, addition of a stabilizer and detergent to the PFC emulsion dramatically reduces the amount of perfluorocarbon available as an oxygen transport vehicle. Fluosol-DA, administered to the level of fluorocrit 5% at a PaO$_2$ of 430 mm Hg (57.3 kPa), is capable of transporting only 0.7 ml O$_2$/dl of blood, which is approximately half the oxygen carried by plasma. It appears that the maximum commercially available concentration of PFC, Fluosol-DA 20%, cannot provide an adequate fluorocrit and therefore has limited oxygen transport capability. The second limiting factor is the poor oxygen loading of Fluosol-DA (218). Therefore, a very high FIO$_2$ concentration (FIO$_2$ = 0.7 – 1.0) is necessary to maximize dissolved oxygen in PFC. Therefore, it is apparent that Fluosol-DA 20% as an oxygen carrier does not contribute significantly to the total oxygen content unless hemoglobin is reduced dramatically. A final limiting factor is the fact that Pluronic F-68, an emulsifying agent, has been associated with reactions involving complement activation (219, 220).

Clinical trials in the U.S. have been strictly limited to acutely anemic Jehovah's Witness patients who refused blood transfusions on a religious basis (212, 217, 218, 221). These studies have shown that Fluosol-DA can be administered safely in doses up to 30 ml/kg but does not improve clinical outcome. The latest randomized, controlled study performed on 46 acutely anemic patients (212) demonstrated an increase in oxygen content 12 hours after infusion that did not persist long enough to affect survival. There was a failure to maintain a steady fluorocrit as a result of a limited dose of Fluosol-DA and rapid elimination of perfluorodecalin, which has an intravascular half-life of 12 to 24 hours. In conclusion, it seems that perfluorocarbon emulsions in their present form are inadequate oxygen-carrying blood substitutes when anemia is significant and are unimportant when anemia is moderate (217). New generations of PFCs with a prolonged intravascular half-life and a substantially higher fluorochemical concentration must evolve to permit further progress in fluorocarbon blood substitutes. Perflubron, which has a single bromide atom at the end of the perfluorinated eight-carbon chain, is a new step in the evolution of PFCs (222, 223).

HEMOGLOBIN SOLUTIONS

Hemoglobin solutions can be divided into two categories, modified and unmodified. Unmodified hemoglobin is prepared from the lysis of erythrocytes and is utilized as an initial product for further modifications. Normally, hemoglobin released from ruptured red blood cells is phagocytosed by the monocyte-macrophage system and processed to liberate iron for further recirculation via binding to transferrin. The porphyrin portion of the hemoglobin molecule is converted by macrophages into bilirubin, which is first released into the blood and later secreted by the liver into the bile. Therefore, free hemoglobin ordinarily is present in plasma in very small quantities, less than 0.6 mg/100 ml (224).

Unmodified hemoglobin is produced from outdated blood by washing the red blood cells with pyrogen-free water. Subsequent filtration of the lysate separates membrane debris from stroma-free hemoglobin molecules. The hemoglobin solution does not have red blood antigens and is universally compatible. It can be stored for substantial lengths of time depending on the temperature: 10 months at 80°C and 6.5 months at 4°C (222, 225). Unmodified Hb solutions have a substantial intrinsic oncotic pressure but low viscosity. A Hb solution of 14 g/dl has a colloid oncotic pressure of 60 mm Hg, whereas a Hb solution of 7 g/dl is isooncotic and theoretically acceptable for clinical use (217). In comparison with normal human blood, unmodified hemoglobin solutions have a much greater affinity for oxygen, with a resultant decrease in P50 (to 12 to 14 mm Hg) that is attributed to the loss of the organic ligand 2,3-diphosphoglycerate (226).

Attempts to increase P$_{50}$ have led to the modification of the hemoglobin molecule by the addition of pyridoxal-phosphate, which is an organic analog of 2,3-diphosphoglycerate that decreases oxygen affinity. Pyridoxalated hemoglobin has been reported to have P$_{50}$ values of 22 to 26 mm Hg (227). This finding is of substantial physiologic importance because oxygen unloading, as shown by in vivo experiments, can occur at higher tissue PO$_2$ (217, 228).

One of the major disadvantages of stroma-free hemoglobin and pyridoxalated hemoglobin solutions is an extremely short plasma half-life, which ordinarily does not exceed 4 hours

(222, 229). Hemoglobin spontaneously breaks into two dimers in plasma and is filtered through the renal glomeruli and excreted in the urine. Incomplete removal of red cell stroma during preparation of hemoglobin solutions and associated renal abnormalities are significant obstacles to the introduction of Hb solutions into clinical practice. In addition, nephrotoxicity may also be related to the mere filtration of free Hb through the glomerular apparatus (217).

Molecular polymerization of pyridoxalated Hb using glutaraldehyde has been attempted to extend intravascular half-life and results in a preparation with a hemoglobin concentration of 7.4 g/dl, a P_{50} of 19 to 25 mm Hg, and a half-life of 25 hours (227). Another polymerized hemoglobin formulation has a concentration of 14 to 16 g/dl, a P_{50} of 16 to 20 mm Hg, and a plasma half-life of 38 hours (226). The results of the first clinical trial of polyhemoglobin solutions seem optimistic (230).

An interesting alternative approach to Hb modification includes encapsulation of hemoglobin molecules in liposomes (231) that are termed *neohemocytes*. They have been reported to have a P_{50} value of 26 to 28 mm Hg and a plasma half-life of about 6 hours (232).

SUMMARY

In addition to the topics set forth in the introduction, this chapter has included discussions about the pharmacologic modulation of respiratory drive and blood substitutes for the uptake and distribution of oxygen. Since oxygen is both a pharmacologic agent and an essential part of normal human physiology, it is essential to discuss the full range of oxygen uptake and distribution. Respiratory drive is an essential part of the uptake process, and blood substitutes may someday be part of a new technique for improving oxygen transport in critical care.

ACKNOWLEDGMENTS

The authors express their appreciation to Patrick Yorio, R.R.T., Michael Bridges, R.R.T., R.P.F.T., and Dennis DiGiacomo, C.R.T.T., Department of Respiratory Therapy, St. Francis Medical Center, for providing expert technologic assistance. They also acknowledge the help of Christine Sedlack, Administrative Assistant, Pittsburgh Critical Care Associates, and Bonnie Eichinger, R.N., C.C.R.N., Nursing and Education Development, St. Francis Medical Center, in preparing this manuscript. The authors also express their appreciation to the Department of Visual Communications at St. Francis Medical Center (Jerry Hinkes, Department Head, Dan Mohan, Photographer, and Maryanne DeJames, Photographic Technician) for their invaluable cooperation in producing the illustrations for this chapter.

REFERENCES

1. McKie D: *Antoine Lavoisier: Scientist, Economist, Social Reformer.* Schuman, New York, 1952.
2. Mayow J: Opera Omnia Medico-Physica Tractatibus Quinque Comprehensa. The Hague, 1681. In *Medico-Physical Works.* Alembic Club Reprints, Edinburgh, No. 17, 1907.
3. Stokes MA: Antoine Lavoisier and the study of respiration: 200 years old. *Aust N Z J Surg* 61(3):229–232, 1991.
4. Campbell A, Poulton EP: *Oxygen and Carbon Dioxide Therapy*, ed 2. Oxford University Press, London, 1938.
5. Tiep BL: *Portable Oxygen Therapy: Including Oxygen Conserving Methodology.* Futura Publishing Company, New York, 1991, p 21.
6. Beddoes T, Watt J: *Considerations of the Medicinal Effects of Factitious Airs. Parts I and II.* Bristol, England, 1798.
7. Sachner MA: A history of oxygen usage in chronic obstructive pulmonary diseases. *Am Rev Respir Dis* 110:25–34, 1974.
8. Haldane JS: Recent developments in the therapeutic use of oxygen. *Contributions to Medical and Biological Research Dedicated to Sir William Osler* 1:549, 1919.
9. Barach AL: The therapeutic use of oxygen. *JAMA* 79:693–698, 1922.
10. Barach AL: The therapeutic use of oxygen. *JAMA* 79:693–698, 1922.
11. Petty TL, Nett LM: The history of long-term oxygen therapy. *Respir Care* 28:859–865, 1983.
12. Richards DW, Barach AL: Prolonged residence in high oxygen atmosphere. Effects on normal individuals and on patients with chronic cardiac and pulmonary insufficency. *Q J Med* 27:437, 1934.
13. Gilbert DL: Significance of oxygen on earth. In Gilbert DL (ed): *Oxygen and Living Processes: an Interdisciplinary Approach.* Springer-Verlag, New York, 1981, pp 73–101.
14. Feeley TW, Bancroft ML, Brooks RA, et al: Potential hazards of compressed gas cylinders: a review. *Anesthesiology* 48:72–74, 1978.
15. Calkins JM: *Anesthesia equipment: help or hindrance?* Year Book, Chicago, 1985, pp 377–406.
16. Dinnick OP: More problems with piped gases. *Anaesthesia* 31:790–792, 1976.
17. Rendell-Baker L: Standards for anesthesia: the issues. Future Anesthesia Delivery. *Contemp Anesth Pract* 8:59–86, 1984.
18. Ducey JP, Culling RD: Oxygen monitoring in anesthesia. *Probl Crit Care* 5(1):99–109, 1991.
19. Petty TL: *Prescribing Home Oxygen.* Thieme-Stratton, New York, 1982, pp 83–97.
20. Gould GA, Scott W, Hayhurst MD, et al: Technical and clinical assessment of oxygen concentrators. *Thorax* 40:811–816, 1985.
21. Couser JI, Make BJ: Transtracheal oxygen decreases inspired minute ventilation. *Am Rev Respir Dis* 139:627, 1989.
22. McCarty DC, Goodman JR, Petty TL: A program for transtracheal oxygen delivery: assessment of safety and efficacy. *Ann Intern Med* 107:802, 1987.
23. Walker JEC, Wells RE, Merrill GW: Heat and water exchange in the respiratory tract. *Am J Med* 30:259–267, 1961.
24. Shelly MP, Lloyd GM, Park GR: A review of the mechanisms and methods of humidification of inspired gases. *Intensive Care Med* 14:1–9, 1988.
25. Shelly MP: Inspired gas conditioning. *Respir Care* 37(9):1070–1080, 1992.
26. Dalhamn T: Mucus flow and ciliary activity in the trachea of healthy rats and rats exposed to respiratory irritant gases. *Acta Physiol Scand* 131(suppl):60, 1956.
27. Fonkalsrud EW, Calmes S, Barcliff LT, et al: Reduction of operative heat loss and pulmonary secretions in neonates by use of heated and humidified anesthetic gases. *J Thorac Cardiovasc Surg* 80:718–723, 1980.
28. Helmholz HF, Saposnick AB: Applied humidity and aerosol therapy. In Burton GG (ed): *Respiratory Care. A Guide to Clinical Practice.* JB Lippincott, Philadelphia, 1977, p 376.
29. Fulmer JD, Snider GL: ACCP-NHLBI national conference on oxygen therapy. *Chest* 86:234–247, 1984.
30. Simmons D, Elliot CG, Greenway L, et al: Results of change to dry low-flow oxygen delivery. *Respir Care* 33:921, 1988.
31. McPherson SP: *Respiratory Therapy Equipment.* CV Mosby, St Louis, 1981, p 109.
32. Vesley D: Bacterial output from three respiratory humidifying devices. *Respir Care* 24:228, 1979.
33. Ahlgren RW, Chapel JF, Dorn GL: *Pseudomonas aeruginosa* infection potential of oxygen humidifier devices. *Respir Care* 22:383–385, 1977.
34. Heironimus TW, Eastwood DW: Humidifying the air-shields respirator. *Anesthesiology* 26:573–575, 1965.
35. Evaluation of humidifiers for medical use: ultrasonic humidifiers. Health Equipment Information, Department of Health and Social Security, 1984, p 128.
36. Humidifiers for medical use. Part 1. Heated humidifiers. International standard (ISO/IS 8185, 1985). International Organization for Standardization, Technical Committee, 1985.
37. Shapiro BA, Cane RD: Respiratory care. In RD Miller (ed): *Anesthesia*, ed 3. Churchill Livingstone, New York, pp 2169–2209, 1990.
38. Klein EF, Graves SA: "Hot pot" tracheitis. *Chest* 65:225–226, 1974.
39. Tamer MA, Modell JH, Rieffel CN: Hyponatremia secondary to ultrasonic aerosol therapy in the newborn infant. *J Pediatr* 77:1051–1054, 1970.
40. Eckerbom B: The airways during artificial respiration. In *Acta Universitatis Upsaliensis. Comprehensive Summaries of Uppsala Dissertations from the Faculty of Medicine.* Almqvist & Wiksell International, Stockholm, Sweden, 1990, p 253.
41. Moffet HL, Allan D, Williams T: Survival and dissemination of bacteria in nebulizers and incubators. *Am J Dis Child* 114:13–20, 1967.

42. Pierce AK, Sanford JP, Thomas GD, et al: Long-term evaluation of decontamination of inhalation therapy equipment and the occurrence of necrotizing pneumonia. *N Engl J Med* 282:528, 1970.

43. Carlon GC, Barker RL, Benua RS, et al: Airway humidification with high-frequency jet ventilation. *Crit Care Med* 13:114–117, 1985.

44. Holmgreen WC: Difficult intubation: suspected. In Brandy L, Smith RB (eds): *Decision Making in Anesthesiology.* BC Decker, Philadelphia, pp 16–17, 1987.

45. Gammage GW: Airway management. In Civetta JM, Taylor RW, Kirby RR (eds): *Critical Care.* JB Lippincott, Philadelphia, pp 197–199.

46. Benumof JL, Scheller MS: The importance of transtracheal jet ventilation in the management of the difficult airway. *Anesthesiology* 71:769–778, 1989.

47. Waterson CK: The anesthesia machine: current design and alternatives. *Med Instrum* 17:379–382, 1983.

48. Grim PS, Gottlieb LJ: Hyperbaric medicine in critical care. In Hall JB, Schmidt GA, Lawrence DH (eds): *Principles of Critical Care.* McGraw-Hill, 1989, pp 175–180.

49. Grim PS, Gottlieb LJ, Boddie A, et al: Hyperbaric oxygen therapy. *JAMA* 263:2216, 1990.

50. Sheffield PJ, David JC, Bell GC, et al: Hyperbaric chamber clinical support: multiplace. In Davis JC, Hunt TK (eds): *Hyperbaric Therapy.* Hyperbaric Medical Society, Bethesda, MD, 1977, p 25.

51. Nunn JF: *Applied Respiratory Physiology.* Butterworths, London, 1987, pp 242–283.

52. Guyton AC: *Textbook of Medical Physiology,* ed 8. WB Saunders, Philadelphia, 1991, pp 422–432.

53. West JB: Respiratory physiology. In *The Essentials.* Williams & Wilkins, Baltimore, 1990, p 26.

54. Perutz MF: Stereochemistry of cooperative effects in Hgb. *Nature* 228:726, 1970.

55. Babior RM, Stossel TP: *Hematology: a Pathophysiological Approach.* Churchill Livingstone, New York, 1984, pp 21–36.

56. Snyder JV: Oxygen transport: the model and reality. In Snyder JV (ed): *Oxygen Transport in the Critically Ill.* Year Book Medical Publishers, Chicago, 1987, pp 3–15.

57. Klitzman B, Popel AS, Duling BR: Oxygen transport in resting and contracting hamster muscles: experimental and theoretic microvascular studies. *Microvasc Res* 25:108, 1983.

58. Jobsis FF: Oxidative metabolism at low PO_2. *Fed Proc* 31:1404, 1972.

59. Brenner M, Ahdout JJ, Finegan RF: The transport of oxygen to tissues: lung to mitochondria. *Probl Crit Care (Oxygen Monitoring)* 5(1):21–35, 1991.

60. Harold FM: *The Vital Force: a Study of Bioenergetics.* Freeman, New York, 1986, pp 28–56.

61. Ayres SM, Schlichtig R, Sterling MJ: *Care of the Critically Ill.* Year Book, Chicago, 1988, pp 13–17.

62. Cone JB: Tissue oxygen monitoring. *Probl Crit Care (Oxygen Monitoring)* 5(1):36–43, 1991.

63. Jobsis-Vander Vliet FF: NIROS-SCOPY: non-invasive, near infrared monitoring of cellular oxygen sufficiency in vivo. *Adv Exp Med Biol* 191:833, 1985.

64. Proctor HJ, Cairns C, Fillipo D, et al: Brain metabolism during increased intracranial pressure as assessed by niroscopy. *Surgery* 96:273, 1984.

65. Fox E, Jobsis FF, Mitnick MH: Monitoring cerebral oxygen sufficiency in anesthesia and surgery. *Adv Exp Med Biol* 191:849, 1985.

66. Brazy JE, Lewis DV, Mitnik S, et al: Noninvasive monitoring of cerebral oxygenation in preterm infants: preliminary observation. *Pediatrics* 75:217, 1985.

67. Cone JB: Cellular oxygen utilzation. In Snyder JV, Pinsky MR (eds): *Oxygen Transport in the Critically Ill.* Year Book Medical Publishers, Chicago, 1987, pp 157–163.

68. Davis JN, Carlsson A: The effect of hypoxia on monoamine synthesis, levels and metabolism in rat brain. *J Neurochem* 21:783, 1973.

69. Davis JD, Carlsson A, MacMillan V, et al: Brain tryptophan hydroxylation: dependence on arterial oxygen tension. *Science* 182:72, 1973.

70. Stryer L: *Biochemistry.* Freeman, New York, 1988, pp 261–274.

71. Niinikoski J: Oxygen and wound healing. *Clin Plast Surg* 4:361, 1977.

72. Omura T, Sato R, Cooper CY, et al: Function of cytochrome P-450 of microsomes. *Fed Proc* 24:1181, 1965.

73. Bagioline M: Phagocytes use oxygen to kill bacteria. *Experientia* 40:906, 1984.

74. Barcroft J: Physiologic effects of insufficient oxygen supply. *Nature* 106:125–143, 1920.

75. Rendell-Baker L: Problems with anesthetic gas machines and their solutions. Problems with anesthetic and respiratory therapy equipment. *Int Anesthesiol Clin* 20:1–82, 1982.

76. Sprague DH, Archer GW: Intraoperative hypoxia from an erroneously filled liquid oxygen reservoir. *Anesthesiology* 42:360–362, 1975.

77. Thorp JM, Railton R: Hypoxia due to air in the oxygen pipeline: a case for oxygen monitoring in the theatre. *Anaesthesia* 37:683–687, 1982.

78. Wetzner SW: Equipment hazards: malfunction and misuse. *Semin Anesthesiol* 2:205–212, 1983.

79. Spurring PW, Shenolikar BK: Hazards in anesthetic equipment. *Br J Anaesth* 50:641, 1978.

80. Riley RL, Cournand A: Ideal alveolar air and the analysis of ventilation-perfusion relationships in the lung. *Alveolar Air Relations* 1:825, 1979.

81. Curry S: Methemoglobinemia. *Ann Emerg Med* 11:214–221, 1982.

82. Ohlgisser M, Adler M, Ben-Dor D: Methaemoglobinemia induced by mafedine acetate in children. *Br J Anaesth* 50:299, 1978.

83. Jaffe ER: Methaemoglobinemia. *Clin Lab Haematol* 10:99, 1981.

84. Wason S, Detsky AS, Platt OS, et al: Isobutyl nitrate toxicity by ingestion. *Ann Intern Med* 92:637, 1980.

85. Horne MK III, Waterman MR, Simon LM, et al: Methemoglobinemia from sniffing butyl nitrate. *Ann Intern Med* 91:417, 1979.

86. Zurick AM, Wagner RH, Starr NJ, et al: Intravenous nitroglycerine, methemoglobinemia, and respiratory distress in postoperative cardiac surgical patient. *Anesthesiology* 61:464–466, 1984.

87. Kellet PB, Copeland CS: Methemoglobinemia associated with benzocaine-containing lubricant. *Anesthesiology* 59:463–464, 1983.

88. Mansouri A: Review: methemoglobinemia. *Am J Med Sci* 289:209–220, 1985.

89. Hegesh E, Hegesh J, Kaftory A: Congenital methemoglobinemia with a deficiency of cytochrome b5. *N Engl J Med* 314:757–761, 1986.

90. Deppe SA: Co-oximetry and its applications in critical care medicine. *Probl Crit Care (Oxygen Monitoring)* 5(1):82–90, 1991.

91. Raper RF, Fisher MMcD: Poisoning and toxic exposure. In Civetta JM, Kirby RR (eds): *Critical Care.* JB Lippincott, Philadelphia, 1988, p 713.

92. Anderson RF, Allensworth DC, DeGrout WJ: Myocardial toxicity from carbon monoxide poisoning. *Ann Intern Med* 67:1172, 1967.

93. Park CM, Nagel RL: Sulfhemoglobinemia: clinical and molecular aspects. *N Engl J Med* 310:1579–1584, 1984.

94. Clark LC: Monitor and control of tissue O_2 tensions. *Trans Am Soc Artif Intern Organs* 2:41–48, 1956.

95. Severinghous JW, Astrup PB: History of blood gas analysis. *Int Anesthesiol Clin* 25(4):131, 1987.

96. Durbin CG: Monitoring arterial blood gases and acid-base balance. In Lake CL (ed): *Clinical Monitoring.* WB Saunders, Philadelphia, 1990, pp 575–614.

97. Linton RAF: Pulmonary gas exchange and acid-base status. In Churchill-Davidson HC (ed): *A Practice of Anesthesia.* Year Book Publishers, Chicago, 1984, p 122.

98. Ducey JP, Harris S: Landmarks in the development of blood oxygen monitoring. *Probl Crit Care (Oxygen Monitoring)* 5(1):1–21, 1991.

99. Staub NC: A simple small oxygen electrode. *J Appl Physiol* 16:192, 1961.

100. Kreuzer F, Nessler CG Jr: Method of polarographic in vivo continuous recording of blood oxygen tension. *Science* 128:1005, 1958.

101. Kreuzer F, Harris ED Jr, Nessler CB Jr: A method for continuous recording in vivo of blood oxygen tension. *J Appl Physiol* 15:77, 1960.

102. Tremper KK, Barker S: Oxygen monitors. *Adv Anesth* 6:97–130, 1989.

103. Bratanow N, Polk K, Bland R, et al: Continuous polarographic monitoring of intra-arterial oxygen in the perioperative period. *Crit Care Med* 13:859–860, 1985.

104. Mahutte K, Sassoon SH, Muro JR, et al: Progress in the development of a fluorescent intravascular blood gas system in man. *J Clin Monit* 6:147, 1990.

105. Barker SJ, Tremper KK, Hyatt J, et al: Continuous fiberoptic arterial oxygen tension measurements in dogs. *J Clin Monit* 3(1):48–52, 1987.

106. Lubers DW, Opitz N: Die pCO_2/pO_2-Optode: eine neue pCO_2 bzw. pO_2-Messonde zur Messung des pCO_2 oder pO_2 von Gasen and Flussigkeiten. *Z Naturforsch* 30:523–523, 1975.

107. Barker SJ, Tremper KK, Hyatt J, et al: Comparison of three oxygen monitors in detecting endobronchial intubation. *J Clin Monit* 4:240–243, 1988.

108. Shapiro BA, Koy DC, Chomka CM, et al: Evaluation of a new intraarterial blood gas system in dogs. *Crit Care Med* 15:361, 1987.

109. Barker SJ, Tremper KK, Heitzmann HA, et al: A clinical study of fiber-optic arterial oxygen tension (abstr). *Crit Care Med* 15:403, 1987.

110. Severinghaus JW, Astrup PB: History of blood gas analysis. VI. *J Clin Monit* 2:270–288, 1986.

111. Severinghaus JW, Astrup AB: History of blood gas analysis. *Intern Anesthesiol Clin* 25(4)167–214, 1987.

112. Hoyt JW: Controversies in oxygen monitoring. *Probl Crit Care (Tissue Oxygenation)* 6(3):443–450, 1992.

113. Temper KK, Barker SJ: Pulse oximetry. *Anesthesiology* 70:98–108, 1989.

114. Kelleher JF: Pulse oximetry. *J Clin Monit* 5:37–62, 1989.

115. Brown M, Vender JS: Noninvasive oxygen monitoring. *Crit Care Clin* 4:493–509, 1988.

116. Severinghaus JW, Kelleher JF: Recent developments in pulse oximetry. *Anesthesiology* 76:1018–1038, 1992.

117. Lamiell JM: Pulse oximetry. *Probl Crit Care (Oxygen Monitoring)* 5(1):44–54, 1991.

118. Galdun JP, Paris PM, Stewart RD: Pulse oximetry in the emergency department. *Am J Emerg Med* 7:422, 1989.

119. Smith DC, Canning JJ, Crul JF, et al: Pulse oximetry in the recovery room. *Anaesthesia* 44:345, 1989.

120. Hovagim AR, Backus WW, Manecke G, et al: Pulse oximetry and patient positioning: a report of eight cases. *Anesthesiology* 71:454–456, 1989.

121. Tyler IL, Tantisira B, Winter PM, et al: Continuous monitoring of arterial oxygen saturation with pulse oximetry during transfer to the recovery room. *Anesth Analg* 64:1108, 1985.

122. Canet J, Ricos M, Vidal: Early postoperative arterial desaturation: determining factors and response to oxygen therapy. *Anesth Analg* 69:207–212, 1989.

123. Brown LT, Purcell GJ, Traugott FM: Hypoxaemia during postoperative recovery using continuous pulse oximetry. *Anaesth Intensive Care* 18:509–516, 1990.

124. Thompson KD, Inoue T, Payne JP: The use of pulse oximetry in post-operative hypoxaemia in patients after propofol induction of anaesthesia. *Int J Clin Monit Comput* 6:7–10, 1989.

125. O'Connor KW, Jones S: Oxygen desaturation is common and clinically under-appreciated during elective endoscopic procedures. *Gastrointest Endosc* 36 (suppl):S2–S4, 1990.

126. Chapman KR, D'Urzo A, Rebuck AS: The accuracy and response characteristics of a simplified ear oximeter. *Chest* 83:860, 1983.

127. Raltson AC, Webb RK, Runciman WB: Potential errors in pulse oximetry. I. Pulse oximeter evaluation. *Anaesthesia* 46:202–206, 1991.

128. Taylor MB, Whitwam JG: The accuracy of pulse oximeters. A comparative clinical evaluation of five pulse oximeters. *Anaesthesia* 43:229–232, 1988.

129. Nickerson BG, Sarkisian C, Tremper KK: Bias and precision of pulse oximeters and arterial oximeters. *Chest* 93:515, 1988.

130. Jubran A, Tobin MJ: Noninvasive oxygen monitoring. *Probl Crit Care (Tissue Oxygenation)* 6(3):394–407, 1992.

131. Langton JA, Lassey D, Hanning CD: Comparison of four pulse oximeters: effects of venous occlusion and cold-induced peripheral vasoconstriction. *Br J Anaesth* 65:245–247, 1990.

132. Morris RW, Nairn M, Torda TA: A comparison of fifteen pulse oximeters: I. A clinical comparison. II. A test of performance under conditions of poor perfusion. *Anaesth Intensive Care* 17:62–73, 1989.

133. Severinghaus JW, Spellman MJ Jr: Pulse oximeter failure thresholds in hypotension and ischemia. *Anesthesiology* 73:532–537, 1990.

134. Wilkins CJ, Moores M, Hanning CD: Comparison of pulse oximeters: effects of vasoconstriction and venous engorgement. *Br J Anaesth* 62:439–444, 1989.

135. Kelleher JF, Ruff RH: The penumbra effect: vasomotion-dependent pulse oximeter artifact due to probe malposition. *Anesthesiology* 71:787–791, 1989.

136. Langton JA, Hanning CD: Effect of motion artifact on pulse oximeters: evaluation of four instruments and finger probes. *Br J Anaesth* 65:564–557, 1990.

137. Costarino AT, Davis DA, Keon TP: Falsely normal saturation reading with the pulse oximeter. *Anesthesiology* 67:830–831, 1987.

138. Amar D, Neidzwski J, Wald A: Fluorescent light interferes with pulse oximetry. *J Clin Monit* 5:135–136, 1989.

139. Tommasino C, Beretta L, Cozzi S, et al: Monitoring of pediatric patients undergoing magnetic resonance diagnosis with a superconducting magnet. *Minerva Anestesiol* 57:7–11, 1991.

140. Menick FJ: The pulse oximeter in free muscle flap surgery: "a microvascular surgeon's sleep aid." *J Reconstr Microsurg* 4:331–334, 1988.

141. Meier-Strauss P, Bucher HU, Hurlimann R, et al: Pulse oximetry used for documenting oxygen saturation and right-to-left shunting immediately after birth. *Eur J Pediatr* 149:851–855, 1990.

142. Lindsey LA, Watson JD, Quaba AA: Pulse oximetry in postoperative monitoring of free muscle flaps. *Br J Plast Surg* 44:27–29, 1991.

143. Joyce WP, Walsh K, Gough DB, et al: Pulse oximetry: a new non-invasive assessment of peripheral arterial occlusive disease. *Br J Surg* 77:1115–1117, 1990.

144. Tremper KK, Shoemaker WC: Transcutaneous oxygen monitoring of critically ill adults, with and without low flow shock. *Crit Care Med* 9:706–709, 1981.

145. Ermakov S, Hoyt JW: Pulmonary artery catheterization. *Crit Care Clin* 8(4):773–806, 1992.

146. Snyder JV: Oxygen transport: the model and reality. In Snyder JV, Pinsky MR (eds): *Oxygen Transport in the Critically Ill*. Year Book Publishers, Chicago, 1987, pp 3–21.

147. Byrne MP: Mixed venous oxygen saturation monitoring. *Probl Crit Care* 5(1):55–68, 1991.

148. Oritz CR, Lund N: Invasive oxygen monitoring. *Probl Crit Care* 6(3):408–422, 1992.

149. Aberman A: Fundamentals of oxygen transport physiology in a hemodynamic monitoring context. In Fahey PH (ed): *Continuous Measurement of Blood Oxygen Saturation in the High Risk Patient*. Beach International, San Diego, 1–14, 1985.

150. McMichan JC: Continuous monitoring of mixed venous oxygen saturation: theory applied to practice. In Schweiss JF (ed): *Continuous Measurement of Blood Oxygen Saturation in the High Risk Patient*. Beach International, San Diego, 1983, p 27.

151. Nelson LD: Mixed venous oximetry. In Snyder JV, Pinsky MR (eds): *Oxygen Transport in the Critically Ill*. Year Book Publishers, Chicago, 1987, p 235.

152. Bael PL, McMichan JC, Marsh HM, et al: Continuous monitoring of mixed venous oxygen saturation in critically ill patients. *Anesth Analg* 61:513, 1982.

153. Divertie MB, McMichan JC: Continuous monitoring of mixed venous oxygen saturation. *Chest* 85:423–428, 1984.

154. Schlichtig R, Cowden WL, Chaitman BR: Tolerance of unusually low mixed venous saturation. *Am J Med* 80:813–818, 1986.

155. Jamieson D: Oxygen toxicity and reactive oxygen metabolites in mammals. *Free Radic Biol Medicine* 7:87–108, 1989.

156. Turrens JF, Freeman BA, Crapo JD: Hyperoxia increases H_2O_2 release by lung mitochondria and microsomes. *Arch Biochem Biophys* 217:411–421, 1982.

157. Bronchopulmonary dysplasia: a longitudinal study of 23 cases. *Ir J Med Sci* 160(10):315–316, 1991.

158. Bostek CC: Oxygen toxicity: an introduction. *AANA-J* 57(3):231–237, 1989.

159. Autor AP: Oxygen toxicity in eukaryotes. In Bannister JV, Bannister WH (eds): *The Biology and Chemistry of Active Oxygen*. Elsevier, New York, 1984, pp 139–145.

160. Lipchik RJ, Presberg KW, Jacobs ER: Pulmonary normobaric toxicity. *Probl Crit Care* 6(3):375–393, 1992.

161. Buechter DD: Free radicals and oxygen toxicity. *Pharmacol Res* 5(5):253–269, 1988.

162. Nunn JF: *Applied Respiratory Physiology*. Butterworths, London, 1987, pp 482–494.

163. Yam J, Roberts RJ: Pharmacological alterations of oxygen-induced lung toxicity. *Toxicol Appl Pharmacol* 47:367–375, 1979.

164. Koizumi M, Frank L, Massaro D: Oxygen toxicity in rats: varied effect of dexamethasone treatment depending on duration of hyperoxia. *Am Rev Resp Dis* 131:907, 1985.

165. Crapo JD, Tierney DF: Superoxide dismutase and pulmonary oxygen toxicity. *Am J Physiol* 226:1401–1407, 1974.

166. Frank L: Protection from O_2 toxicity by preexposure to hypoxia: lung antioxidant role. *J Appl Physiol* 53:475–482, 1982.

167. van Asbeck S, Hoidal J, Schwartz B, et al: Insufflated red blood cells protect lungs from hyperoxic damage: role of red cell glutathione in scavenging toxic O_2 radicals. *Trans Assoc Am Physicians* 97:365–368, 1984.

168. Gutteridge JMC, Rowley DA, Griffiths E, et al: Low molecular weight iron complexes and oxygen radical reactions in idiopathic hemochromatosis. *Clin Sci* 68:463, 1985.

169. Crapo JD, Barry BE, Foscue HA, et al: Structural and biochemical changes in rat lungs occurring during exposures to lethal and adaptive doses of oxygen. *Am Rev Respir Dis* 122:123–143, 1980.

170. Fisher AB, Forman HJ: Oxygen utilization and toxicity in the lungs. In Fishman AP, Fisher AB (eds): *The Respiratory System*, vol 1. *Circulation and Nonrespiratory Functions*. American Physiological Society, Bethesda, MD, 1985, pp 231–254.

171. Holm BA, Notter RH, Siegle J, et al: Pulmonary physiological and surfactant changes during injury and recovery from hyperoxia. *J Appl Physiol* 59:1402–1409, 1985.

172. Kinsey VE, Arnold HJ, Kalina RE: PaO_2 levels and retrolental fibroplasia: a report of the cooperative study. *Pediatrics* 60:655–666, 1977.

173. Haschek WM, Reiser KM, Klein-Szanto AJ, et al: Potentiation of butylated hydroxytoluene-induced acute lung damage by oxygen. *Am Rev Respir Dis* 127:28–34, 1983.

174. Martin WJ, Kachel DL: Oxygen-mediated impairment of human pulmonary endothelial cell growth: evidence for a specific threshold toxicity. *J Lab Clin Med* 113(4):413–421, 1989.

175. Smith RA: Oxygen therapy. In Civetta JM, Taylor RW, Kirby RR (eds): *Critical Care*. JB Lippincott, Philadelphia, 1990, pp 1143–1149.

176. Mitchell RA, Berger AJ: Neural regulation of respiration. *Am Rev Respir Dis* 111:206, 1975.

177. Yoshikawa T, Yamamoto H, Nishimura M, et al: Doxapram on blunted respiratory chemosensitivity to hypoxia in hypoxemic, chronic obstructive pulmonary disease. *Jpn J Med* 26(2):194–202, 1987.

178. Flecknell PA, Liles JH, Wootton R: Reversal of fentanyl/fluanisone neurolept-analgesia in the rabbit using mixed agonist/antagonist opioids. *Lab Anim* 29(2):147–155, 1989.

179. Pourriat JL, Baud M, Lamberto C, et al: Effects of doxapram on hypercapnic response during weaning from mechanical ventilation in COPD patients. *Chest* 102(6):1639–1643, 1992.

180. Pourriat JL, Lamberto CH, Hoang PH, et al: Diaphragmatic fatigue and breathing pattern during weaning from mechanical ventilation in COPD patients. *Chest* 90:703–707, 1986.

181. Lemair F, Teboul JL, Cinotti L, et al: Acute left ventricular dysfunction during unsuccessful weaning from mechanical ventilation. *Anesthesiology* 69:157–160, 1988.

182. Locke RG, Salvia JV: Pharmacologic manipulation of the respiratory control center in the infant. *J Am Osteopath Assoc* 90(7):602–604, 1990.

183. Bowdle TA: Clinical pharmacology of antagonists of narcotic-induced respiratory depression. A brief review. *Acute Care* 12 (Suppl 1):70–76, 1988.

184. Randall NP, Pleury BJ, Fazackerley EJ, et al: Effect of oral doxapram on morphine-induced changes in the ventilatory response to carbon dioxide. *Br J Anaesth* 62(2):159–163, 1989.

185. Smith PD, Gotz VP, Ryerson GG: Almitrine bismesylate. *Drug Intell Clin Pharm* 21(5):417–421, 1987.

186. Tweney J, Howard P: Almitrine bismesylate. *Z Erkr Atmungsorgane* 168(3):197–215, 1987.

187. Barkan I, Vrhovac B, Stangl B, et al: Double-blind placebo controlled clinical trial of almitrine bismesylate in patients with chronic respiratory insufficiency. *Eur J Clin Pharmacol* 38(3):249–253, 1990.

188. Tatsumi K, Kimura H, Kunitomo F, et al: Effect of chlormadione acetate on sleep arterial oxygen desaturation in patients with chronic obstructive pulmonary disease. *Chest* 91(5):688–692, 1987.

189. Reents SB, Beck CA: Naloxone and naltrexone. Application in COPD. *Chest* 93(1):217–219, 1988.

190. Holtman JR, Dick TE, Berger AJ: Involvement of serotonin in excitation of phrenic motorneurons evoked by stimulation of the raphe obscurus. *J Neurosci* 6:1185–1193, 1986.

191. Milhorn DE, Eldridge FL, Waldrop TG: Prolonged stimulation of respiration by endogenous central serotonin. *Respir Physiol* 42:171–188, 1980.
192. Parisi RA, Nuebauer JA, Frank MM, et al: Correlation between genioglossal and diaphragmatic responses to hypercapnia during sleep. *Am Rev Respir Dis* 135:378–382, 1987.
193. Haxhiu MA, van Lunteren E, Mitra J, et al: Responses to chemical stimulation of upper airway muscles and diaphragm in awake cats. *J Appl Physiol* 56:397–403, 1984.
194. Hanzel DA, Proia NG, Hudgel DW: Response of obstructive sleep apnea to fluoxetine and protriptyline. *Chest* 100:416–421, 1991.
195. Hudgel DW, Chapman KR, Faulks C, et al: Changes in inspiratory muscle electrical activity and upper airway resistance during periodic breathing induced by hypoxia during sleep. *Am Rev Respir Dis* 135:899–906, 1987.
196. Schmidt HS: L-tryptophan in the treatment of impaired respiration during sleep. *Bull Eur Physiol Respir* 19:625–629, 1982.
197. Hedner J, McCown TJ, Mueller RA, et al: Respiratory stimulant effects by TRH into the mesencephalic region in the rat. *Acta Physiol Scand* 130 (1):69–75, 1987.
198. Schaefer CF, Brackett DJ, Biber B, et al: Respiratory and cardiovascular effects of thyrotropin-releasing hormone as modified by isoflurane, enflurane, pentobarbital and ketamine. *Regul Pept* 243:269–282, 1989.
199. Nink M, Krause U, Lehnert H, et al: Thyrotropin-releasing hormone has stimulatory effects on ventilation in humans. *Acta Physiol Scand* 141(3):309–318, 1991.
200. Takano N, Sakai A, Iida Y: Analysis of alveolar pCO_2 control during the menstrual cycle. *Pflugers Arch* 390:56–62, 1981.
201. Kunimoto F, Kimura H, Tatsumi K, et al: Sex differences in awake ventilatory drive and sleep abnormal breathing in eucapnic obesity. *Chest* 93:968–976, 1988.
202. Tyler JM: The effect of progesterone on the respiration of patients with emphysema and hypercapnea. *J Clin Invest* 39:34–41, 1960.
203. Wittels EH: Obesity and hormonal factors in sleep and sleep apnea. *Med Clin North Am* 69(6):1265–1280, 1985.
204. Hensley MJ, Saunders NA, Strohl KP: Medroxyprogesterone treatment of obstructive sleep apnea. *Sleep* 3:441–446, 1980.
205. Skatrud JB, Dempsey JA, Kaiser DG: Ventilatory response to medroxyprogesterone acetate in normal subjects: time course and mechanism. *J Appl Physiol* 44:439–444, 1978.
206. Kimura H, Hayashi F, Yoshida A, et al: Augmentation of CO_2 drives by chlormadione acetate, a synthetic progesterone. *J Appl Physiol* 56:1627–1632, 1984.
207. Tatsumi K, Kimura H, Kunitomo F, et al: Effect of chlormadione acetate on ventilatory control in patients with chronic obstructive pulmonary disease. *Am Rev Respir Dis* 133:552–557, 1986.
208. Kimura H, Tatsumi K, Kunitomo F, et al: Progesterone therapy for sleep apnea syndrome evaluated by occlusion pressure responses to exogenous loading. *Am Rev Respir Dis* 139:1198–1206, 1989.
209. Yokoyama K, Yamanouchi K, Watanabe M, et al: Preparation of perfluorodecalin emulsion, an approach to the red cell substitute. *Fed Proc* 34:1478, 1975.
210. Yokoyama K, Yamanouchi K, Ohyanagi H, et al: Fate of perfluorochemicals in animals after intravenous injection of hemodilution with their emulsions. *Chem Pharm Bull* 26(3):956, 1978.
211. Biro GP, Blais P, Rosen A: Perfluorocarbon blood substitutes. *CRC Crit Rev Oncol Hematol* 6(4): 311, 1987.
212. Spence RK, McCoy S, Costabile J, et al: Fluosol DA-20 in the treatment of severe anemia: randomized, controlled study of 46 patients. *Crit Care Med* 18(11):1227–1230, 1990.
213. Fuhrman BP, Paczan PR, DeFrancisis M, et al: Perfluorocarbon-associated gas exchange. *Crit Care Med* 19(5):712–722, 1991.
214. Elliot LA, Ledgerwood AM, Luas CE, et al: Role of Fluosol-DA 20% in prehospital resuscitation. *Crit Care Med* 17(2):166–172, 1989.
215. Mitsuno T, Ohyoanagi H, Yokoyama K, et al: Recent studies on perfluorochemical emulsion as an oxygen carrier in Japan. In Chang TMS, Geyer RP (eds): *Blood Substitutes. III. Perfluorochemicals.* Marcel Dekker, New York, 1989, pp 365–373.
216. Tremper KK, Barker SJ, Waxman KS: Oxygen transporting solutions: stroma-free hemoglobin and perfluorochemical emulsions. In Schoemaker WC, Ayres S, Grenvik A, et al (eds): *Textbook of Critical Care.* WB Saunders, Philadelphia, 1989, pp 932–935.
217. Gould SA, Moss GS, Rosen AL: Red cell substitutes. In Civetta JM, Taylor RW, et al (eds): *Critical Care 1992.* JB Lippincott, Philadelphia, 1992, pp 1719–1725.
218. Gould SA, Rosen AL, Sehgal LR, et al: Fluosol-DA as a red cell substitute in acute anemia. *N Engl J Med* 314(26):1653–1656.
219. Vercellotti G, Hammerschmidt DE, Craddock P: Activation of plasma complement by perfluorocarbon artificial blood: probable mechanism of adverse pulmonary reaction in treated patients and rationale for corticosteroid prophylaxis. *Blood* 59:129, 1982.
220. Hong F, Shastri KA, Logue GL, et al: Complement activation by artificial blood substitute Fluosol: in vitro and in vivo studies. *Transfusion* 31(7):642–647, 1991.
221. Tremper KK, Friedman AE, Levine EM, et al: The preoperative treatment of severely anemic patients with a perfluorochemical oxygen-transport fluid, Fluosol-DA. *N Engl J Med* 307:277, 1982.
222. Faithfull N: Oxygen-carrying blood substitutes. *Probl Crit Care (Tissue Oxygenation)* 6(3):423–442, 1992.
223. Long DM, Long DC, Mattrey RF, et al: An overview of perfluorocytlbromide: application as a synthetic oxygen carrier and imaging agent for x-ray, ultrasound, and nuclear magnetic resonance. *Biomater Artif Cells Artif Organs* 16(1–3):411, 1988.
224. Hanks GE, Cassel M, Ray RN, et al: Further modification of the benzine method for measurement of hemoglobin in plasma. *J Lab Clin Med* 56:486, 1960.
225. Greenberg AG, Ginsberg K, Peskin GW: Preservation of stroma-free haemoglobin. *Surg Forum* 28:5, 1977.
226. Gould SA, Sehgal LR, Rosen AL, et al: Artificial oxygen carriers. In Dutcher JP (ed): *Modern Transfusion Therapy.* CRC Press, Boca Raton, FL, 1990, pp 107–123.
227. De Venuto F, Zegna A: Preparation and evaluation of pyridoxalated-polymerized human hemoglobin. *J Surg Res* 34:205, 1983.
228. Gould SA, Rosen AL, Sehgal L, et al: The effect of altered hemoglobin-oxygen affinity on oxygen transport by hemoglobin solution. *J Surg Res* 28:246, 1980.
229. Savitsky JP, Doczi J, Black J, et al: A clinical safety trial of stroma-free hemoglobin. *Clin Pharmacol Ther* 23:73, 1978.
230. Moss GS, Gould SA, Rosen AL, et al: Results of the first clinical trial with a polymerized hemoglobin solution. Presented at the International Symposium on Red Cell Substitutes: Design and Clinical Applications, San Francisco, CA, May 1989.
231. Djordjevich L, Ivankovich AD: Half-life of synthetic erythrocytes in vivo. *Anesthesiology* 65(3A):A94, 1986.
232. Hunt CA, Burnette RR, MacGregor RD, et al: Synthesis and evaluation of a prototypical artificial red cell. *Science* 230:1165, 1985.

CHAPTER 35

Clinical Pharmacology of Mucokinetic Drugs

DANIEL J. LEBOVITZ, M.D.
MICHAEL D. REED, Pharm.D., F.C.C.P., F.C.P.

Compromised lung function exacerbated by excessive pulmonary secretions is a common clinical challenge in intensive care practice. The potential to improve airway integrity by pharmacologically influencing the rate, amount, and viscosity of respiratory secretions as well as their rate of expectoration has, for decades, represented a seductive focus for laboratory and clinical research. Properly performed pulmonary toilet with frequent suctioning to remove accumulating pulmonary secretions (1, 2) clearly benefits a number of patients cared for in the intensive care unit (ICU). Extrapolating from this experience, some clinicians and investigators have touted the many possible benefits that may be achieved from the addition of a mucokinetic drug to this tried and true procedure (3–7). Unfortunately, most of the proposed benefits and indications for mucokinetic drugs are based upon preliminary studies performed in vitro combined with descriptions obtained from uncontrolled clinical trials. This chapter reviews the physiology and pathophysiology of respiratory secretions and then provides a critical evaluation of available data addressing the clinical pharmacology of mucokinetic agents. The focus of this chapter is the possible role of these agents in the care of critically ill patients. For completeness, the use of mucokinetic drugs as adjunctive therapies in various lung diseases is also addressed.

PRODUCTION OF RESPIRATORY SECRETIONS

The primary respiratory secretion, mucus, is a complex substance that serves a number of extremely important physiologic functions, including airway lubrication and waterproofing (3, 4, 8). Respiratory mucus also serves a cleansing function by trapping cellular debris and inhaled particulate matter for subsequent removal via the mucociliary transport system. Often referred to as the "mucociliary escalator," this system provides constant upward movement of mucus for removal by swallowing or expectoration and is one of the most important host defenses of the lung (3, 4, 9). When this cleansing and removal system is compromised, local accumulation of debris and cellular wastes combined with increasingly dehydrated mucus often results in airway plugging and mechanical obstruction of the airways. A number of diseases are associated with abnormalities in mucus and/or the function of the mucociliary transport system, including asthma, bronchitis, cystic fibrosis, and emphysema (3, 4, 9, 10). In ICU practice, many treatment modalities may adversely affect these important processes, including the administration of unhumidified oxygen, which increases the viscosity of respiratory secretions (dehydration); the presence of an endotracheal/nasotracheal tube, which stimulates mucus secretion; and the use of drugs that may interfere with or ablate the cough reflex and/or mucociliary function. All of these therapies, either alone or in combination, can adversely affect production and removal of respiratory secretions. Factors that have been identified as impairing ciliary function are outlined in Table 35.1.

The human airways are lined by many different cell types that perform a wide range of physiologic functions (3, 4). The epithelial cell types lining the tracheobronchial tree and their relative distribution vary depending upon location. The cellular structure of the bronchiolar epithelium appears very similar to that of the bronchi and trachea, with the exception of fewer goblet and epithelial serous cells and increasing numbers of Clara cells (3, 4). Mucus-producing cells are absent from the more distal terminal airways. Cell types that are essential to mucus production and mucociliary transport include surface epithelial cells, pseudostratified columnar ciliated cells, surface goblet (secretory) cells, Clara cells, and the subepithelial submucosal gland.

Ultrastructurally, lung goblet cells are very similar to goblet cells located in the gastrointestinal tract. In response to irritation, the goblet cell surface membrane dehisces, secreting mucus granules onto the airway surface (3, 4). The number and secretory activity of goblet cells is increased in many respiratory diseases. Irritation resulting from allergy, infection, pollution, smoke, and the like stimulates goblet cell function and proliferation, worsening the disease process (3, 4, 9, 10). Goblet cells do not appear to be innervated or influenced by hormones and thus are poorly responsive to pharmacologic intervention. In contrast, submucosal glands are innervated by the parasympathetic nervous system (see Figure 35.1).

The submucosal glands are responsible for the majority of mucus secretion onto the airways. The cells secrete ~40 times the amount normally secreted by goblet cells. The submucosal glands are comprised of two cell types: mucus and serous cells. Granules from mucus cells contain an acid glycoprotein similar to that found in goblet cell granules, whereas serous cell granules contain a neutral glycoprotein. The granular contents of these two cells combine, mixing within the submucosal gland prior to secretion upward through a ciliated duct onto the lumenal surface of the airway. In healthy adults, the submucosal glands secrete ~100 ml mucus/24 hr onto the airway lumen. Under normal circumstances, the majority of this mucus is reabsorbed by bronchial mucosa, with <15 ml reaching the glottis. In the presence of disease, the rate and overall amount of mucus that reaches the glottis can increase

Table 35.1. Factors That Can Impair Ciliary Function[a]

Mechanical and environmental
Endotracheal tubes
Temperature extremes
High oxygen concentration
High carbon dioxide concentration
Dusts, fumes, smoke (cigarette and other)
Lack of humidity
Over-liquefaction of mucus
Inflammation
Trauma (e.g., suctioning)
Chemical and physical burns
Bacterial and viral infections
Drugs (in relatively high concentrations)
Local and general anesthetics
Codeine
Pentobarbital
Alcohol
Acetylcysteine
Nicotine
Cromolyn

[a] Adapted from Ziment I: Pathophysiology and pharmacology of sputum. In *Respiratory Pharmacology and Therapeutics.* WB Saunders, Philadelphia, 1978, pp 41–59.

dramatically; it is either swallowed, expectorated, or both (3, 4). In the critically ill, intubated, pharmacologically paralyzed, and/or heavily sedated ICU patient, these secretions can accumulate, exacerbating already compromised lung function. Although the use of mucokinetic drugs as an adjunctive therapy for these patients would appear desirable, their use is associated with numerous undesirable effects that may worsen (e.g., decrease mucociliary clearance) rather than improve the patient's already compromised lung function (see below).

PHYSICAL PROPERTIES OF MUCUS

As mentioned previously, *mucus* is a term commonly used to describe respiratory secretions. Although the terms *mucus* and *sputum* are often used interchangeably, in fact they denote different secretions (3, 4). The term *sputum* refers to an abnormally viscous product of the lower respiratory tract that is in contrast to the normal, more liquid respiratory secretions bathing the airways. The chemical composition of respiratory secretions obtained from patients with cystic fibrosis, bronchiectasis, and laryngectomy are shown in Table 35.2 (8). Despite decades of intense interest in the characteristics and composition of respiratory secretions, no complete definition that is acceptable to all parties yet exists for the terms *respiratory mucus* or *sputum* (4). For the purposes of this chapter, the term *mucus* is used to describe normal respiratory secretions found on the airway surface. In contrast, sputum will be defined as a heterogeneous viscous fluid originating from the lower respiratory tract. Furthermore, uninfected respiratory secretions are usually white in color, only slightly viscous, and composed primarily of glycoproteins with little or no DNA. Infected secretions are often yellow or green in color and viscous as a result of the added constituents of pathogens, host defense debris, and increased DNA. The presence of DNA increases viscosity by interfering with normal host proteolytic activity; it does so by decreasing local pH (slightly acidic) and by the DNA's direct interference with proteolytic enzyme activity (3, 4, 8, 11–13). This characteristic of DNA's augmenting respiratory secretion viscosity underscores the continued interest in identifying mucokinetic drugs that catabolize this DNA (e.g., proteolytic enzymes, DNase; see below).

An understanding of respiratory mucus infrastructure is essential to appreciate the various mechanisms by which drug therapy attempts to influence the physical and chemical characteristics of respiratory mucus. Respiratory mucus is comprised of multiple cross-linked mucus strands that form a macromolecular gel. These mucus strands consist of a simple amino acid foundation to which oligosaccharide side chains are attached. The mucus strands are very flexible and are cross-linked by disulfide, hydrogen, and electrophysical bonds that form this macromolecular secretion (3, 4, 13). The structure and cross-linking of mucus strands are depicted in Figure 35.2. Disulfide bonding appears to be the primary mechanism by which mucus strands are cross-linked. The importance of these disulfide cross-links was emphasized by early research efforts searching for pharmacologic agents that disrupt these cross-links as a means to reduce viscosity. The use of thiol reducing agents (e.g., *N*-acetylcysteine) to disrupt disulfide bonds and thereby reduce mucus viscosity is an example of such research strategies. However, simple destruction of the

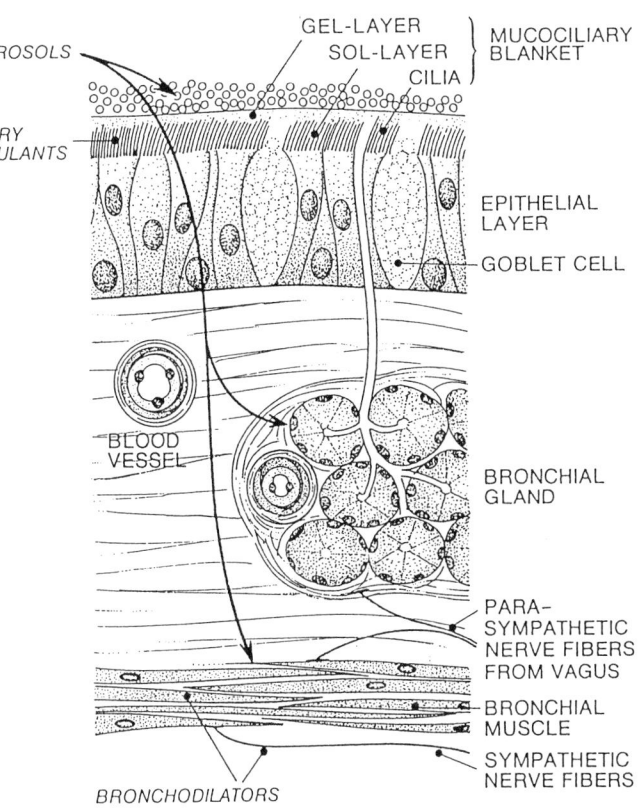

LUMEN OF AIRWAY

GEL-LAYER
SOL-LAYER } MUCOCILIARY BLANKET
CILIA

AEROSOLS

CILIARY STIMULANTS

EPITHELIAL LAYER

GOBLET CELL

BLOOD VESSEL

BRONCHIAL GLAND

PARA-SYMPATHETIC NERVE FIBERS FROM VAGUS

BRONCHIAL MUSCLE

SYMPATHETIC NERVE FIBERS

BRONCHODILATORS

Figure 35.1. Cross-sectional view of an airway revealing various types of mucus-producing cells and sites for drug action. (Adapted from Ziment I: Pathophysiology and pharmacology of sputum. In *Respiratory Pharmacology and Therapeutics*. WB Saunders, Philadelphia, 1978, p 46.)

Table 35.2. Chemical Composition of Pulmonary Secretions from Selected Patients

	"Normal"	*Cystic Fibrosis*	*Bronchiectasis*
Water	94.79	89.36	94.79
Ash	1.13	0.73	0.88
Deoxyribonucleic acid	0.028	0.408	0.084
Carbohydrate	0.951	1.137	1.050
Protein	1.000	5.570	2.040
Lipid	0.840	3.140	1.170
Total	98.739	100.345	100.014

[a] Data presented as amount per 100 g wet weight. (Adapted from Matthews LW, Spector S, Lemon J, Potter JL: Studies on pulmonary secretions. I. The over-all chemical composition of pulmonary secretions from patients with cystic fibrosis, bronchiectasis, and laryngectomy. *Am Rev Respir Dis* 88:199–204, 1963.)

mucus complex by disruption of cross-links may exacerbate, rather than ameliorate, pulmonary compromise. These important mechanistic issues and their clinical ramifications are discussed in detail in the section below entitled "The Mucokinetic Drugs."

The cross-linking of mucus produces a macromolecular gel with sponge-like properties. Water organized around the mucus strands confers this sponge-like viscoelastic characteristic to respiratory mucus. Needed water is acquired during mucus production within the submucosal and goblet cells. Despite the high water content and hydrophilic nature of respiratory mucus, topically applied water (e.g., via aerosol) is poorly, if at all, incorporated into preformed mucus. In contrast, water may evaporate from airway mucus as a result of the inhalation of unhumidified air or aerosols, supporting the clinical use of humidified oxygen and fluid-based aerosols. Other substances found in respiratory secretions influence

the physical characteristics of mucus, including serum proteins (e.g., albumin, immunoglobulins, α-1 antitrypsin) and electrolytes (e.g., sodium, potassium, chloride, calcium). As in other cells and tissues, normal electrolyte concentrations are necessary for proper water transport and hydration (Figure 35.2).

THE SOL-GEL LAYER OF RESPIRATORY MUCUS

As already discussed, the ciliated epithelium of the tracheobronchial tree is bathed continuously by mucoid fluid secreted onto the airway lumen by the bronchial glands and goblet cells (3, 4, 9). Under normal conditions, the thickness of this so-called "mucociliary blanket" fluid approximates 5 to 10 microns. The deepest layer bathing the cilia is watery (i.e., a *sol layer*) and accounts for the majority of the lumenal fluid,

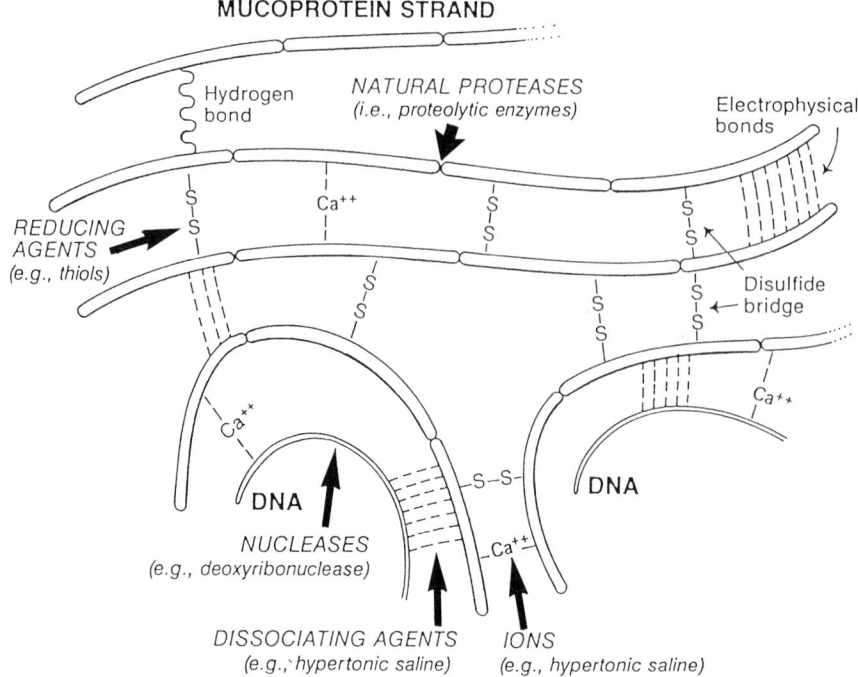

Figure 35.2. Schematic representation of the physical-chemical characteristics of the mucoprotein complex. (Adapted from Ziment I: Pathophysiology and pharmacology of sputum. In *Respiratory Pharmacology and Therapeutics.* WB Saunders, Philadelphia, 1978, p 46.)

approximating 4 to 8 microns in thickness (3, 4). Superficially "floating" atop this sol layer is the 1- to 2-micron thick, sticky gelatinous *gel layer*, which serves to trap inhaled foreign particles for removal via the mucociliary transport/escalator system. This gel layer is also extremely important in providing force for the normal upward movement of respiratory secretions.

Upward movement of the mucus bathing the airway lumen is dependent upon a competent mucociliary transport system (9). The cilia beat freely in the sol layer, stimulating a fluid-like movement. During forward movement, the cilia come into direct contact with the gel layer, causing it to stretch; because of the viscoelastic characteristics of mucus, elastic recovery causes the mucus to snap forward, providing power for upward movement. The importance of this viscoelastic property of mucus cannot be overemphasized (3, 4, 13–16), as the majority of available mucolytic drugs reduce viscosity by destroying this elasticity. Similarly, too viscous a secretion will also prevent forward movement by impeding or paralyzing ciliary activity. Without this elastic property, forward movement cannot be achieved.

THE MUCOKINETIC DRUGS

Over the years, a large number of drugs have been used, suggested, or recommended as mucolytic/mucokinetic agents (3, 5). Despite this long but often convoluted history, only limited data document any true clinical benefit from their use. Nevertheless, strong research and clinical interests persist in this area of drug therapy. To add to the confusion, drugs used to modulate respiratory secretions classically have been termed "mucolytics." The term *mucolytic* refers to the breakdown or lysis of mucus, which does not reflect accurately the different mechanisms by which many of these agents are

Table 35.3. Selected Compounds Used via Aerosol to Modulate Respiratory Secretions[a]

"Bland" agents
Water
Saline
Hypotonic (0.45% NaCl)
Normal saline (0.9% NaCl)
Hypertonic (2–20% NaCl)
Sodium bicarbonate
Mucolytics
N-acetylcysteine (20%)
Pancreatic dornase
rh DNase
Anticholinergics
Atropine
Glycopyrrolate
Ipratropium

[a] See text for specific details regarding administration techniques, dose ranges, and associated adverse effects.

believed to exert their drug effects. Thus, for the purposes of this chapter, we will refer to this class of agents as mucokinetic drugs, to reflect the diversity of agents and possible mechanism(s) of action.

Three main classes of drugs have long been considered as mucokinetic agents: the "bland" aerosols, enzymes, and mucolytics (Table 35.3). These drugs are believed to reduce the viscosity of airway mucus, hence the former term *Mucolytics.* These agents are administered as aerosols, which places another important variable in considering published descriptions of their effectiveness: Were they administered correctly? Were adequate drug concentrations achieved at the desired anatomic site in lung? A consideration of the importance of appropriate aerosol administration techniques and the various methods and equipment available to administer aerosols is beyond the scope of this chapter. The interested reader is referred to excellent reviews that critically address aerosol drug dynamics (17–21). A final group of drugs that influence respiratory secretions are those drugs that possess anticholinergic properties. These agents may reduce the rate of mucus secretion from the submucosal glands rather than alter viscosity, and they may represent the most important mucokinetic agents used in the ICU (Table 35.3).

THE BLAND AEROSOLS

This group of mucokinetic agents includes distilled water, physiologic saline, and hyper- or hypotonic saline (5, 22). These agents are most often used as diluents or carrier solvents for the aerosolization of other medications. In addition, it has long been believed that the aerosolization of these solutions will hydrate thick, tenacious airway secretions. This goal of hydrating airway secretions has, for decades, served as the foundation supporting their clinical use. However, and as discussed above, the mucus gel layer that insulates airway surfaces is very resistant to hydration, particularly from topically applied water. In contrast, the bland agents do provide humidity to aerosol particles and the ambient air, reducing or preventing further dehydration of respiratory secretions.

WATER

Historically, water has been used in the form of steam or vapor and is widely believed to "thin" respiratory secretions (3, 5, 22, 23). As already discussed, the mucus gel layer is relatively resistant to the topical incorporation of water. Nevertheless, mist tent therapy is still commonly prescribed in some centers to help "hydrate" thick, tenacious secretions in patients with certain lung diseases such as cystic fibrosis. Although an early study described come clinical benefit to the use of mist tents in children with cystic fibrosis (24), other investigators have been unable to duplicate these early findings (25). Similarly, in vitro experiments by Dulfano et al (26) with expectorated sputum from patients with chronic bronchitis exposed to 100% humidity for 3 hours failed to demonstrate any change in viscosity. When the same sputum was exposed directly to a water aerosol for 3 hours, these investigators reported a slight (29%) increase in water content and a 30 to 40% decrease in sputum viscosity. Although these data are often used to support the belief that directly applied water may enhance the hydration and/or reduce viscosity of preformed respiratory secretions, these results must be interpreted with caution. The interpretation of these data and their clinical applicability is very difficult considering the unphysiologic environment in which the studies were performed. In addition, these investigators applied the water aerosol directly to the sputum constantly for 3 hours, which is obviously not physically or anatomically possible in the clinical setting, particularly considering the dynamics of aerosol particle deposition in the airway. Wolfsdorf and colleagues (25), using radiolabeled water aerosols via both jet and ultrasonic nebulizers, found relatively small amounts of particle deposition in the small airways. These investigators reported 92% and 83% of the mass from the jet and ultrasonic nebulizers, respectively, in the upper airway with nose breathing. Changing their experimental conditions to include the use of a mouthpiece reduced the aerosol deposition in the upper airway by <40%. In a subsequent study, Wolfsdorf and Swift (27) measured transglottic airflow resistance in animals with induced upper airway inflammation and found water aerosols to be no different from humidified air. From these experiences it would appear that water aerosols would be of most benefit to patients with upper airway inflammation and in the maintenance of airway humidification. The importance of this latter indication for bland mucokinetic agents cannot be overemphasized and supports their continued use in patients receiving aerosol drug and/or oxygen therapy.

SALINE

Saline solutions used as mucokinetic aerosols range in concentrations from hypotonic (e.g., 0.45 or 0.5%) to extremely hypertonic (1.8 to 20%). A common perception is that the more abnormal the osmolality, the more irritating the substance, and that irritation reduces mucus viscosity. Irritation of mucus-secreting cells may stimulate mucus secretion, but an actual reduction in mucus viscosity (i.e., a dilutional effect) is questionable. Similar to the beliefs regarding hydration of respiratory secretions with water aerosols, no data exist that document the potential clinical benefits from airway irritation (5, 22, 28). In contrast, irritation of airways does stimulate the cough reflex, which can facilitate expectoration.

Isotonic (0.9%) saline is essentially inert in the airway. Isotonic or normal saline aerosols are well-tolerated by patients because no significant osmotic gradient exists. In contrast, hypotonic saline solutions appear to lose some of their moisture in the airways, thus reducing aerosol particle size. This characteristic may be of benefit in aerosol particle generation by enhancing particle penetration into the smaller airways. Again, specific data supporting this possible mechanical or clinical benefit are lacking.

Hypertonic saline solutions are used primarily as irritants to stimulate mucus secretion and coughing. Some investigators speculate that hypertonic saline may enhance the breakdown of sputum DNA-mucoprotein complexes, thus enhancing the penetration of more specific mucolytic drugs (29). Further speculation has suggested that the high osmotic nature of these aerosol solutions can cause fluid shifts within the airways, possibly adding water to respiratory secretions and enhancing their mobilization. However, because the salt concentration of the aerosol solution is high, substantial sodium absorption may occur, thus promoting systemic fluid retention, which may be detrimental to many of the fluid-restricted patients cared for in the ICU. Additionally, hypertonic saline aerosols can precipitate coughing, gagging, emesis, skin and mucosal irritation, bronchospasm, hypernatremia, and edema. Lastly, hypertonic saline solutions can also be very damaging to the equipment used for their administration.

pH ALTERATION

Altering the pH of the local environment within the lungs or the pH of respiratory secretions will alter mucus viscosity

(5, 30). Alkalinity weakens the intrinsic bonding of the saccharide side chains of mucus molecules (see Fig. 35.2). This influence of pH adjustment on mucus can occur following direct topical application or aerosolization of an alkaline solution. The most common solution used for this purpose is sodium bicarbonate in concentrations usually exceeding 2%. In addition to weakening mucus strand cross-linking, an alkaline environment enhances the activity of normal proteases present in the mucus, enhances ciliary activity, and augments the activity of *N*-acetylcysteine. Minimal to no systemic effects have been described from the use of sodium bicarbonate solutions as a mucokinetic or diluent aerosol (30). However, like hypertonic saline solutions, bicarbonate solutions are irritating to the airways, frequently precipitating bronchospasm limiting their clinical usefulness. To overcome this common adverse effect, concurrent administration of a β2-adrenergic agonist has been advocated if this approach is to be attempted. In particular, if the adrenergic agent is to be co-mixed and administered together with the bicarbonate solution, the aerosol solution should be used immediately to avoid drug inactivation. β-adrenergic drugs are unstable in alkaline environments and will decompose. A pinkish color to the aerosol solution may indicate the decomposition of the adrenergic drug.

DRUGS THAT DISRUPT DISULFIDE BONDS OF MUCUS

Initial attempts to identify drugs that could modulate the physicochemical characteristics of respiratory secretions focused on reducing viscosity. Proteolytic compounds were studied in the early 1950s because of their inherent ability to catabolize protein, and they are discussed in greater detail below. The findings from these early studies with proteolytic compounds stimulated research directed at reducing viscosity by disrupting mucus strand cross-linking bonds (see Fig. 35.2). Disulfide bonds are the most prominent cross-links, providing internal support for the mucus macromolecule, and thus have represented the primary target for mucokinetic (mucolytic) drug research. The first compound that demonstrated promising results was cysteine. Sheffner in the early 1960s evaluated various cysteine derivatives in vitro for their ability to reduce the viscosity of respiratory mucus and sputum (31). Cysteine and many of its derivatives were relatively toxic and unstable in solution, severely limiting their medicinal utility. Subsequent work identified the *N*-acetyl derivative of cysteine, *N*-acetylcysteine, as one of the more stable, soluble, and least irritating derivatives. Since these early studies, *N*-acetylcysteine (NAC) has emerged as one of the most popular and widely used mucokinetic drugs in the world.

N-acetylcysteine is one of a group of cysteine derivatives (e.g., S-carboxymethylcysteine) that are capable of interacting with disulfide bridges of mucoprotein (32). Two molecules reacting with one disulfide bond are necessary to disrupt a disulfide bridge in mucus (sputum). With sufficient disulfide bond disruption, the mucoprotein becomes fragmented and thus less viscous (33). In addition to a reduction in viscosity, these smaller, fragmented mucus particles exhibit decreased binding capacity to DNA from infected secretions, further reducing airway secretion viscosity (7).

The mucolytic properties of NAC are easily demonstrated in vitro, where the drug can liquefy sputum and thus decrease viscosity (34). Despite these clear in vitro relationships, demonstration of a similar effect in vivo with resultant clinical benefit is much more difficult. The majority of published studies evaluating the clinical utility of NAC therapy are uncontrolled and depend heavily upon subjective determinations as their primary outcome determinant (4, 5, 7, 30, 34–36). The results from these studies are highly variable and, because of their study design, severely restrict comparative analysis. Despite these limitations, these data have served to fuel and maintain the controversy regarding the clinical utility of NAC therapy. To add further to controversy and confusion, clinical results may differ depending upon the route of NAC administration. *N*-acetylcysteine may be administered via the more conventional topical route as an aerosol or by direct tracheal instillation, but it can also be administered orally and intravenously. The oral route for NAC is most commonly used as a component of the long-term care of ambulatory patients with chronic lung diseases such as chronic bronchitis, whereas the topical route remains the most appropriate for the ICU patient (37–39).

Administered orally, NAC has begun to enjoy a resurgence in popularity. In Europe, the most common method for NAC administration is via the oral route. Adult doses usually range from 400 to 800 mg daily (i.e., 200 to 300 mg NAC orally 2 to 3 times daily); a slow-release formulation is also available, permitting 300 mg NAC dosed twice daily. This popularity of oral NAC emanates from studies that describe a decrease in the number of pulmonary exacerbations during the winter months in patients with mild and more severe chronic bronchitis who are receiving the drug (40, 41). Although chronic oral administration of NAC may be beneficial in certain patient populations as a component of their long-term care, a role for oral NAC in the ICU is doubtful. In the U.S. the only commercially available oral NAC formulation is the solution used in the treatment of acetaminophen intoxication, with its unpleasant taste and intense sulfur odor.

In contrast to the European experience, in the U.S. NAC is most commonly administered as an aerosol when used for its mucokinetic properties. In the original studies of Sheffner, a 30% NAC solution was used. Numerous other NAC concentrations have been studied, though a consensus of most published reports finds a 10 to 20% NAC solution optimal relative to clinical effect and patient tolerance (42). As discussed previously in the section on pH alteration, optimal conditions for NAC mucolysis appear to include a pH between 7 and 9 (6), which contrasts with the more acidic environment in diseased lungs (e.g., pH 6 to 6.5+).

When administered for its mucokinetic properties, NAC is most often dosed as 2 to 5 ml of a 10 to 20% aerosol solution administered every 4 to 6 hours. The use of ultrasonic nebulizers to administer NAC aerosols should be avoided, as this method appears to increase associated drug-induced pulmonary irritation. From available experience, it would appear that an optimal method of NAC administration would deliver NAC along with a bronchodilator (e.g., albuterol aerosol) to prevent or treat NAC-induced bronchospasm. Occasionally, sodium bicarbonate may be admixed with the aerosol solution to promote a more alkaline environment. Caution should be exercised when co-mixing other drugs with the NAC aerosol, as NAC exhibits a very limited compatibility and stability profile. Many antibiotics, including ampicillin, erythromycin, tetracycline, and the antifungal agent amphotericin B, are physically incompatible with NAC. This incompatibility follows direct mixing of the compounds in the same vial and does not preclude co-administration of any of these drugs to the same patient using different, separate routes for their administration.

Obstruction of airways by mucus impaction can compromise lung function in ICU patients. If this obstruction is more localized and persists despite aggressive pulmonary toilet and suctioning, dissolution of mucus plugs may be accomplished by direct topical instillation of NAC. The drug may be instilled via a bronchoscope or an endotracheal tube to the specific location. Five to 10 ml of a 10 to 20% NAC solution are commonly used. Following administration, the NAC solution is permitted to remain in the area for 2 to 3 minutes, after which time the drug and respiratory secretions are promptly removed by suctioning.

Numerous clinically important adverse effects have been associated with the use of NAC. Their incidence and severity appear to be relative to the route of NAC administration. Nausea and vomiting are most common adverse effects following oral and aerosolized NAC, most likely because of the drug's strong offensive (thiol) odor. The most serious adverse effect of NAC is drug-induced bronchospasm, which can be severe. The incidence of NAC-induced bronchospasm is unclear, but reports in the literature suggest a common occurrence, particularly in patients with hyperactive airways. As a result, most clinicians will co-administer a bronchodilator along with NAC in an attempt to avoid this complication. Lastly, if NAC is effective in "liquefying" tenacious respiratory secretions, a ready means of rapidly removing these secretions following drug administration is necessary to prevent acute pulmonary decompensation. This adverse effect profile, along with the fact that only limited published data from critically designed investigations suggest a real clinical benefit, is the primary reason NAC finds very limited clinical use in or outside the ICU.

DEOXYRIBONUCLEASE-ASES (DNases)

The use of enzymatic agents (e.g., trypsin, chymotrypsin) to reduce the viscosity of respiratory secretions has represented a primary research focus for decades. Considering the high protein and amino acid content present in respiratory secretions from diseased lungs (Table 35.2), such a strategy to reduce mucus viscosity would appear highly effective and relatively specific. In 1958, Merck Sharp and Dohme Pharmaceuticals (43) developed a bovine pancreatic DNase formulation. Like NAC, the drug was able to "liquefy" (purulent) sputum in vitro and was described to be of moderate clinical benefit in uncontrolled trials. Aerosolized pancreatic DNase, commonly referred to as pancreatic dornase, was reported to enhance the clearance of airway secretions of patients with mucus obstructions from varying etiologies, including postoperative atelectasis, chronic bronchitis, pneumonia, and cystic fibrosis (44, 45). However, these early encouraging clinical successes were quickly tempered by the high incidence of

associated adverse effects (3, 4, 19, 30). Pharyngeal irritation, hemoptysis, and bronchospasm occurred commonly with the use of dornase. After only brief periods of use, many patients developed antibodies to the bovine proteins and some experienced serious anaphylactic reactions, particularly after 4 to 7 days of use. As a result of these frequent and potentially life-threatening side effects, the drug was removed from the U.S. market in 1977.

More recently, new attempts to reevaluate DNase mucokinetic drug therapy have emerged with the development and availability of a recombinant human deoxyribonuclease rh DNase formulation (13, 46). Like the early dornase preparation, rh DNase is without effect on mucoid specimens, affecting only purulent secretions. Because of this specificity for purulent secretions, a safe compound that is easily tolerated by patients may find some use in the ICU setting. No controlled clinical evaluations in ICU patients have been reported with the use of human recombinant rh DNase at the time of this writing. Furthermore, concern persists regarding an effective means of quickly removing large volumes of more liquid secretions and avoiding acute pulmonary decompensation. This latter concern may severely restrict the clinical utility of rh DNase to select patient populations.

ANTICHOLINERGIC AGENTS

The recognition that anticholinergic drugs have a beneficial role in the treatment of reversible airway disease has stimulated new interest in their clinical use (47, 48). In asthma, the use of cholinergic antagonists such as atropine and ipratropium has been shown to promote bronchodilation (47–50). These agents can reverse guanine monophosphate (GMP)-mediated bronchoconstriction initiated by cholinergic stimulation. In addition, these drugs can antagonize vagally mediated hypersecretion of respiratory fluids from the submucosal gland. Atropine is the drug that has been studied most extensively for this application in patients with various pulmonary diseases. In both animal and human studies, atropine has been shown to antagonize submucosal gland mucus production in response to cholinergic stimulation (48, 49, 51). Although these pharmacologic properties may appear desirable for the treatment of patients with excessive pulmonary secretions, anticholinergic drugs should be used with caution and in only a select group of patients. Anticholinergic drugs may enhance the viscosity of respiratory secretions, thus compromising mucus transport. The exact influence atropine may have on sputum viscosity remains debatable. However, and more importantly, atropine has been shown clearly to decrease mucus transport. This alteration of mucus transport most likely results from a direct depressant effect of atropine on mucociliary function (e.g., decreased cilia beating frequency) (48, 49, 51–53). In contrast to atropine, quaternary ammonium compounds (e.g., ipratropium bromide) have similar effects upon hypersecretion but do not appear to influence ciliary activity (48–51, 52).

The precise role for anticholinergic drugs as mucokinetic agents remains to be elucidated. Those patients with vagally mediated increases in airway secretions may benefit from their use. These agents should be used cautiously, and a quaternary ammonium compound should be used in preference to atropine to avoid associated adverse effects. Systemic adverse effects, including dry mouth, blurred vision, and tachycardia, occur commonly with atropine and are independent of the route of drug administration. In addition and as mentioned previously, atropine adversely effects mucociliary function. In contrast, the incidence of these effects is decreased markedly or absent with quaternary ammonium compounds (49, 54). When these drugs are used in the ICU, they are administered most often as aerosols or by intermittent intravenous injection. At present in the U.S., ipratropium bromide is available only as a metered dose inhaler (MDI), limiting its use in the ICU. However, adapters for the ventilator tubing are available, permitting the use of MDIs in ventilated patients, and this may represent the preferred route for aerosol administration to ICU patients. The dose of atropine used clinically as an aerosol is 0.1 mg per kg of body weight per dose, up to a total single maximum dose of 2.0 mg administered every 6 hours or 0.01 mg/kg administered intravenously, up to a single maximum dose of 0.5 mg. The dose of glycopyrrolate for both aerosol and intravenous administration is 0.005 to 0.01 mg per kg of body weight per dose, to a single maximal dose of 0.4 mg administered every 4 to 6 hours.

CONCLUSION

Accumulation of respiratory secretions in the critically ill, intubated, pharmacologically paralyzed ICU patient is a common occurrence. Aggressive pulmonary toilet with frequent suctioning is often all that is clinically necessary to prevent or minimize mucus impaction of airways and/or to mobilize tenacious secretions. Less frequently, respiratory secretions may be overly viscous and abundant, compromising lung function to a point at which mucokinetic therapy may appear advantageous. Although a number of agents are available to modulate the physical and chemical characteristics of respiratory secretions, very limited data describe any clinical benefit from their use. Most importantly, adverse effects that can seriously compromise a patient's lung function are often associated with their use. As a result, mucokinetic drugs are used only rarely in the care of select ICU patients. More data obtained from critically designed, well-controlled studies clearly are needed before recommendations for the use of these drugs in the ICU can be developed.

REFERENCES

1. Kiriloff LH, Owens GR, Rogers RM, Mazzocco MC: Does chest physical therapy work? *Chest* 88:436–444, 1985.
2. Pavia D: The role of chest physiotherapy in mucus hypersecretion. *Lung* 128(suppl): 614–621, 1990.
3. Richardson PS, Phipps RJ: The anatomy, physiology, pharmacology and pathology of tracheobronchial mucus secretion and the use of expectorant drugs in human disease. *Pharmacol Ther* 3:441–479, 1978.
4. Ziment I: Pathophysiology and pharmacology of sputum. In *Respiratory Pharmacology and Therapeutics*. WB Saunders, Philadelphia, pp 41–59, 1978.
5. Ziment I: Pathophysiology and pharmacology of sputum. In *Respiratory Pharmacology and Therapeutics*. WB Saunders, Philadelphia, pp 60–104, 1978.
6. Lieberman J: The appropriate use of mucolytic agents (Editorial). *Am J Med* 49:1–4, 1970.
7. Ziment I: Acetylcysteine: a drug that is much more than a mucokinetic. *Biomed Pharmacother* 513–520, 1988.
8. Matthews LW, Spector S, Lemm J, Potter JL: Studies on pulmonary secretions. I. The overall chemical composition of pulmonary secretions from patients with cystic fibrosis, bronchiectasis, and laryngectomy. *Am Rev Respir Dis* 88:199–204, 1963.
9. Satir P. The physiology of cilia and mucociliary interactions. *Annu Rev Physiol* 52:137–155, 1990.
10. Schlesinger RB: The interaction of inhaled toxicants with respiratory tract clearance mechanisms. *Crit Rev Toxicol* 20:257–286, 1990.
11. Potter JC, Spector S, Matthews LW, Lemm J: Studies on pulmonary secretions. II. The reactive acids in whole pulmonary secretions from patients with cystic fibrosis, bronchiectasis and laryngectomy. *Am Rev Respir Dis* 99:906–916, 1969.
12. Lieberman J, Kurnick NB: Influence of deoxyribonucleic acid content on the proteolysis of sputum and pus. *Nature* 196:988–990, 1962.
13. Shak S, Capon DJ, Hellmiss R, Marsters SA, Baker CL: Recombinant human DNase I reduces the viscosity of cystic fibrosis sputum. *Proc Natl Acad Sci USA* 87:9188–9192, 1990.
14. Marriott C, Davis SS: Sputum elasticity: a frog in the throat? (Editorial). *Thorax* 33:545–546, 1978.
15. Gelman RA, Meyer FA: Mucociliary transference rate and mucus viscoelasticity dependence on dynamic storage and loss modulus. *Am Rev Respir Dis* 120:553–557, 1979.
16. Hachenberg T, Wendt M, Deitmer T, Lawin P: Viscoelasticity of tracheobronchial secretions in high-frequency ventilation. *Crit Care Med* 15:95–98, 1987.
17. Brain JD, Valberg PA: State of the art: deposition of aerosol in the respiratory tract. *Am Rev Respir Dis* 120:1325–1373, 1979.
18. Clay MM, Pavia D, Newman SP, Clarke SW: Factors influencing the size distribution of aerosols from jet ventilators. *Thorax* 38:755–759, 1983.
19. Newman SP, Clarke SW: Therapeutic aerosols. I. Physical and practical considerations. *Thorax* 38:881–886, 1983.
20. Schlesinger RB: Comparative deposition of inhaled aerosols in experimental animals and humans: a review. *J Toxicol Environ Health* 15:197–214, 1985.
21. Aherns RC, Ries RA, Popendork W, Wiese JA: The delivery of therapeutic aerosols through endotracheal tubes. *Pediatr Pulmonol* 2:19–26, 1986.
22. Wanner A, Rao A: Clinical indications for and effects of bland, mucolytic, and antimicrobial aerosols. *Am Rev Respir Dis* 122(Part 2):79–87, 1980.
23. Brain J: Aerosol and humidity therapy. *Am Rev Respir Dis* 122(Part 2):17–21, 1980.
24. Matthews LW, Doershuk CF, Spector S: Mist tent therapy of the obstructive pulmonary lesion of cystic fibrosis. *Pediatrics* 39:176–185, 1967.
25. Wolfsdorf J, Swift DL, Avery ME: Mist therapy reconsidered: an evaluation of the respiratory deposition of labelled water aerosols produced by jet and ultrasonic nebulizers. *Pediatrics* 43:799–808, 1969.
26. Dulfano JJ, Adler KG, Wooten O: Physical properties of sputum. IV. Effects of 100 percent humidity and water mist. *Am Rev Respir Dis* 107:130–132, 1973.
27. Wolfsdorf J, Swift DL: An animal model simulating acute infective upper airway obstruction of childhood and its use in the investigation of croup therapy. *Pediatr Res* 12:1062–1065, 1978.
28. Sutton PP, Gemmell HG, Innes N, Davidson J, Smith FW, Legge JS, Friend JAR: Use of nebulized saline and nebulized terbutaline as an adjunct to chest physiotherapy. *Thorax* 43:57–60, 1988.
29. Zanjanian MH: Expectorants and antitussive agents—are they helpful? *Ann Allergy* 44:290–295, 1980.
30. Rau Jr JL: Mucus-controlling, surface-active, and cold and cough agents. In Respiratory Care Pharmacology, ed 3. Chicago, Year Book, pp 144–179, 1989.
31. Sheffner AL: The reduction in vitro in viscosity of mucoprotein solutions by a new mucolytic agent, N-acetylcysteine. *Ann NY Acad Sci* 106:298, 1963.
32. Livingstone CR, Andrews MA, Jenkins SM, Marriott C: Model systems for the evaluation of mucolytic drugs: acetylcysteine and S-carboxymethylcysteine. *J Pharm Pharmacol* 42:73–78, 1990.
33. Dorow P: Mucolytics: when dispensable, when necessary? *Lung* 168(suppl):622–626, 1990.
34. Aylward M, Maddock J, Dewland P: Clinical evaluation of acetylcysteine in the treatment of obstructive bronchitis: a balanced double-blind trial with placebo control. *Eur J Respir Dis* 111(suppl):81–89, 1980.
35. Millar AB, Pavia D, Agnew JE, Lopez-Vidriero MT, Lanque D, Clarke JW: Effect of oral N-acetylcysteine on mucus clearance. *Br J Dis Chest* 79:262–266, 1985.
36. Todisco T, Polidori R, Rossi F, Jannacci L, Bruni B, Fedeli L, Palumbo R: Effect of N-acetylcysteine in subject with slow pulmonary mucociliar clearance. *Eur J Respir Dis* 66:136–141, 1985.
37. Richardson P: Oral N-acetylcysteine: how does it act (editorial)? *Eur J Respir Dis* 70:71–72, 1987.
38. Cotgreave IA, Eklund A, Larsson K, Moldéus PW: No penetration of orally administered N-acetylcysteine into bronchoalveolar lavage fluid. *Eur J Respir Dis* 70:73–77, 1987.
39. Holdiness MR: Clinical pharmacokinetics of N-acetylcysteine. *Clin Pharmacokinet* 20:123–134, 1991.
40. Multicenter Study Group: Long-term oral acetylcysteine in chronic bronchitis. A double-blind controlled study. *Eur J Respir Dis* 61(suppl III):93–108, 1980.
41. Boman G, Bäcker U, Larsson S, Melander B, Wahlander L: Oral acetylcysteine reduces exacerbation rate in chronic bronchitis: report of a trial organized by the Swedish Society for Pulmonary Diseases. *Eur J Respir Dis* 64:405–415, 1983.
42. Hirsch SR, Kory RC: An evaluation of the effect of nebulized N-acetylcysteine on sputum consistency. *J Allergy* 39:265–273, 1967.

43. Chernick WS, Barbero GJ, Eichel HJ: In vitro evaluation of the effect of enzymes on tracheobronchial secretions from patients with cystic fibrosis. *Pediatrics* 27:589–596, 1961.

44. Spier R, Witebsky E, Paine JR: Aerosolized pancreatic dornase and antibiotics in pulmonary infections. Use in patients with postoperative and nonoperative infections. *JAMA* 178:878–886, 1961.

45. Liberman J: Dornase aerosol effect on sputum viscosity in cases of cystic fibrosis (letter). *JAMA* 205:114–115, 1968.

46. Hubbard RC, McElvaney NG, Birrer P, et al. A preliminary study of aerosolized recombinant human deoxyribonuclease I in the treatment of cystic fibrosis. *N Engl J Med* 326:812–815, 1992.

47. Cavanaugh MJ, Cooper DM: Inhaled atropine sulfate: dose response characteristics. *Am Rev Respir Dis* 114:517–524, 1976.

48. Gross NJ, Skorodin MS: Anticholinergic, antimuscarinic bronchodilators. *Am Rev Respir Dis* 129:856–870, 1984.

49. Wanner A: Effect of ipratropium bromide on airway mucociliary function. *Am J Med* 81(suppl 5A):23–27, 1986.

50. Cugell DW: Clinical pharmacology and toxicology of ipratropium bromide. *Am J Med* 81(suppl 5A):18–22, 1986.

51. Miyata T, Matsumoto N, Yuki H, Oda Y, Takahama K, Kai H: Effects of anticholinergic bronchodilators on mucociliary transport and airway secretions. *Jpn J Pharmacol* 51:11–15, 1989.

52. Foster WM, Bergofsky EH: Airway mucus membrane: effects of beta-adrenergic and anticholinergic stimulation. *Am J Med* 81(Suppl 5A):28–35, 1986.

53. Corssen G, Allen CF: Acetylcholine: its significance in controlling ciliary activity of human respiratory epithelium in vitro. *J Appl Physiol* 14:901–904, 1959.

54. Gal TJ, Suratt PM, Lu J-Y: Glycopyrolate and atropine inhalation: comparative effects on normal airway function. *Am Rev Respir Dis* 129:871–873, 1984.

CHAPTER 36

Clinical Pharmacology of Drugs Used in GI Disorders of Critically Ill Patients

SUDHIR K. DUTTA, M.D.
RAJAT SOOD, M.D.

In the critical care setting, a large number of drugs are used for the management of gastrointestinal (GI) disorders. An in-depth knowledge of clinical pharmacology of these drugs is crucial for the effective management of critically ill patients. A vast array of GI disorders is encountered in the acutely ill patient, ranging from stress gastritis and bleeding ulcers to impaired gastric emptying and copious diarrhea. Frequent development of multiorgan failure, sepsis, and cardiopulmonary complications make careful selection of appropriate drug, optimal dosing, and close monitoring of drug interactions an essential part of the management of critically ill patients.

The purpose of this chapter is to provide the intensive care physician with a concise, succinct description of drugs commonly used for GI disorders in critically ill patients with frequent concomitant multiorgan system problems.

DRUGS FOR STRESS ULCERS, ACID PEPTIC DISEASE, AND GASTROESOPHAGEAL REFLUX

Gastric mucosal erosions are commonly seen in intensive care unit (ICU) patients. Severe trauma, burn injury, major surgical procedures, sepsis, serious medical illnesses, CNS disease, and drug overdose frequently are associated with stress-induced gastritis (1, 2). Acute hemorrhagic gastritis generally is seen 3 to 7 days after the initial injury. Development of stress gastritis is associated with persistent low intraluminal gastric pH in the majority of critically ill patients (3). Correction of intraluminal acidic pH in the stomach has been recommended for prevention of hemorrhage from stress gastritis.

A large number of pharmacologic compounds are used to keep gastric pH higher than 5.0 to protect gastric mucosa from acid-induced injury in the critically ill patient.

ANTACIDS

Mechanism of Action. Antacids are basic salts of aluminum, magnesium, or calcium that neutralize acid in the gastric lumen and help to maintain an intraluminal gastric pH of 5.0 or higher. Antacids at this pH are also known to inhibit the proteolytic activity of pepsin. In addition, they have a local astringent effect and can increase the lower esophageal sphincter pressure to some degree. Most commonly used antacids have few systemic effects and do not cause systemic alkalosis. The various antacid preparations are compared on the basis of their acid neutralizing capacity. Acid neutralizing capacity of an antacid is defined as the quantity of 1 N HCl in mEq that can be brought to pH 3.5 in 15 minutes.

Route of Administration, Frequency, and Dosage. Antacids generally are administered orally or through a gastrostomy tube. The usual doses of an antacid in stress gastritis in critically ill patients are as follows: children, 5 to 15 ml every 1 to 2 hours; adults, 30 to 60 ml every 3 to 6 hours. In general, the aim is to provide enough antacid to neutralize a total of 1000 mEq of gastric acid every day (4). When ingested in the fasting state, antacids reduce the acidity for about 30 minutes. However, when antacids are administered about 1 hour following meal ingestion, its effect lasts for approximately 3 hours. Longer duration of action by the antacids during the

Table 36.1. Composition and Neutralizing Capacity of Commercially Available Antacids[a]

Antacids	Composition (mg/5 ml)				Acid Neutralizing Capacity (per 5 ml)
	$Al(OH)_3$	$Mg(OH)_2$	$CaCO_3$	Other	
Maalox	225	200	0	Na (1.4)	13
Mylanta	200	200	0	Simeth[b] (20) Na (0.7)	13
Gelusil	200	200	0	Simeth[b] (25) Na (0.7)	12
Amphojel	320	0	0	Na (2.0)	10
Milk of Magnesia	0	390	0	Na (0.1)	14
Gaviscon	32	0	0	$MgCO_3$ (137) Na Alginate	4
Riopan	0	0	0	Magaldrate (540) Simeth[b] (40)	15

[a] Adapted from Brunton LL: Agents for control of gastric acidity and peptic ulcer. In Gilman AG, Rall TW, Nies AS, Taylor P (eds): *The Pharmacological Basis of Therapeutics*, ed 8. McGraw-Hill, New York, 1990, pp 897–913.
[b] Simeth, simethicone.

postprandial period is related to slower gastric emptying as compared with the fasting state (5). Several studies with antacids indicate that total acid neutralization up to 180 to 400 mEq is effective in healing inflammation and ulceration of gastroduodenal mucosa in most clinical settings. In Zollinger-Ellison syndrome, a much higher dose of antacids is often needed in conjunction with H_2-antagonists or omeprazol (6).

Drug Interactions. (*a*) Antacids increase the intraluminal gastric pH and can alter the solubility, ionization, and gastric emptying of various drugs and their metabolites. As a result of antacid ingestion, absorption of acidic drugs (digitalis, phenytoin, chlorpromazine) may be reduced. (*b*) Adsorption or binding of drugs to the surface of antacids can result in decreased bioavailability of some drugs (i.e., tetracycline, ranitidine, isoniazid, ethambutol, etc.). (*c*) Antacids can affect the rate of elimination of many drugs by increasing urinary pH. Antacid ingestion potentially can increase the rate of urinary excretion of salicylates and phenobarbital and decrease the elimination of amphetamine, quinidine, and pseudo-ephedrine.

Most commercially available antacids contain sodium bicarbonate, aluminum hydroxide, magnesium hydroxide, or calcium carbonate. A comparison of contents and neutralizing capacity of the commercially available antacids is summarized in Table 36.1 (7).

Aluminum Compounds

Aluminum hydroxide gel is actually a mixture of aluminum hydroxide and other oxide hydrates. Aluminum hydroxide usually is marketed in combination with magnesium hydroxide to offset its constipating effect. Aluminum compounds are used alone or in combination with H_2-blockers for prevention of bleeding from stress gastritis.

Adverse Effects. (*a*) Administration of aluminum-containing antacids except aluminum phosphate over a period of time can cause clinically significant hypophosphatemia resulting from acid binding of aluminum to indigenous phosphates (8, 9). This binding property of aluminum hydroxide frequently is used in patients with renal failure to lower plasma phosphate levels. (*b*) Aluminum antacids can also cause an increase in calcium absorption, with resultant hypercalcemia

and bone resorption. (*c*) In addition, administration of aluminum-containing antacids can result in an increase of aluminum levels in renal failure patients (10).

Special Considerations. Aluminum-containing antacids can be used to reduce hyperphosphatemia in patients with chronic renal failure. However, this approach should be done with caution, as aluminum-containing antacids can induce disequilibrium syndrome.

Magnesium Compounds

Magnesium-containing antacids generally include magnesium hydroxides and magnesium oxide. Magnesium salts are also used for treatment of hypomagnesemia resulting from starvation, alcoholism, and malnutrition. About 5% of orally administered magnesium-containing antacids is absorbed systemically (11). Cathartic action of magnesium salts results from an increase in the osmotic load and stimulation of intestinal secretions and motility.

Adverse Effects. In renal failure, administration of magnesium-containing antacids can result in fatal hypermagnesemia. All magnesium compounds have also been implicated in causing the milk alkali syndrome. This is an acute illness characterized by headaches, nausea, irritability, weakness, and azotemia with hypercalcemia.

Calcium Compounds

Calcium carbonate was the first antacid used and still remains popular. Calcium-containing antacids are highly soluble and interact avidly with gastric acid, resulting in production of calcium chloride. In the small intestine, 90% of calcium chloride is converted by pancreatic bicarbonate to insoluble calcium salts. Approximately 9 to 16% of calcium is absorbed from normal human intestines, and up to 34% in patients with peptic ulcer disease (12). The main route of absorbed calcium excretion is through the kidney, the amount of which varies with creatinine clearance. It has been estimated that the amount of calcium absorbed from the intestine increases with a higher dose. Transient hypercalcemia has been observed with a single 4-g dose of calcium carbonate. Furthermore, of all the antacids, calcium carbonate has been shown to produce acid rebound, which is defined as sustained hypersecretion of gastric acid after calcium-containing antacid has been emptied from the stomach (13).

Adverse Effects.   Long-term use of calcium-containing antacids is associated with a positive phosphate balance, decreased magnesium absorption, and development of milk alkali syndrome (14–17).

SUCRALFATE

Sucralfate is a complex compound of aluminum hydroxide and sucrose sulfate. It is approved for treatment of acute duodenal ulcers and prevention of their recurrence (18–21). Several studies have examined the healing rates of duodenal ulcers in patients treated with sucralfate and cimetidine, an H_2-blocker antagonist. These healing rates have been reported to be 57%, 88%, and 96% at weeks 4, 8, 12, respectively, and compare favorably with those rates of cimetidine (22–24). Sucralfate is not approved for either acute or maintenance therapy of gastric ulcers.

Similar to antacids and H_2-blockers, the benefit of sucralfate therapy in patients with bleeding ulcers lies in healing the ulcers and not in stopping the bleeding (25, 26). There is no significant difference in the mortality rates of patients treated with sucralfate or H_2-antagonists or antacid-treated patients with stress-induced erosive gastritis and bleeding. However, sucralfate has been demonstrated to be just as effective in preventing stress gastritis-related bleeding in critically ill patients receiving mechanical ventilation. In treatment of patients with NSAID induced duodenal ulcers, sucralfate is just as efficacious as ranitidine (27–29). Sucralfate, however, does not prevent nonsteroidal antiinflammatory drug (NSAID)-associated gastric or duodenal ulcers. Furthermore, in patients with gastroesophageal reflux, sucralfate seems to be only modestly effective in nonerosive esophageal disease (30, 31). Controlled trials of its efficacy in healing esophageal ulcers after sclerotherapy as well as other esophageal ulcers have not shown clinically important benefit (32, 33).

Mechanism of Action

Sucralfate forms a viscous suspension that binds with high affinity to both injured and normal mucosa. At a pH less than 4.0 there is extensive polymerization and cross-linking of sucralfate. The condensed polymer is a very sticky, viscid, yellowish-white gel. Even though the pH in the duodenum is well above 4.0, the gel retains its viscid demulcent properties in the duodenal bulb. Endoscopic studies have demonstrated that the gel remains adherent to the ulcerated epithelium for more than 6 hours. The binding of sucralfate to the ulcer crater probably represents its main therapeutic action. In addition, sucralfate releases the aluminum moiety in the presence of gastric acid and binds positively charged molecules, such as peptides, proteins, glycoproteins, drugs, and metals. It seems that various physical, mechanical, absorbent, ion exchange, and buffering properties of sucralfate may all contribute to its actions to protect gastric mucosa. It has also been suggested that sucralfate stimulates formation of prostaglandins by the gastric mucosa, thus exerting a cytoprotective effect by a mechanism similar to that of misoprostol (34). This effect is particularly relevant because sucralfate has

only minimal acid neutralizing capability. It is noteworthy that in vitro studies indicate that sucralfate absorbs bile acids (35).

Pharmacokinetics

Sucralfate is poorly soluble in water, and little is absorbed from the GI tract. It is a very safe medication, and studies in animals using oral doses up to 1 g/kg have failed to establish a lethal dose (36). Aluminum absorption during sucralfate therapy is comparable to antacid therapy with aluminum hydroxide (37). Most of the aluminum (98%) is excreted in feces, and some in the urine. Sucralfate lowers the plasma phosphate level in uremic patients. However, sucralfate also results in increased plasma concentration of aluminum in these patients. Like aluminum-containing antacids, sucralfate can cause severe hypophosphatemia (38). Aluminum retention associated with sucralfate may be a problem in patients with renal insufficiency.

Drug Interactions

Sucralfate reduces the bioavailability and absorption of certain drugs when given simultaneously with them. Important drugs involved in this interaction include ciprofloxacin (39), norfloxacin (40, 41), theophylline (42), tetracycline (43), phenytoin (44), digoxin (45), and amitriptyline (46). The effect of combined therapy of sucralfate with antacids or H_2-blockers has not been evaluated in humans. However, since sucralfate is activated by acids, antacids should not be administered 30 minutes before or after sucralfate in the treatment of duodenal ulcer. Sucralfate does not seem to affect the bioavailability of acetaminophen, aspirin, diazepam, erythromycin, ethinyl estradiol, ibuprofen, imipramine, indomethacin, naprosyn, prednisone, propranolol, quinidine, and warfarin.

Dosage and Route of Administration

In the treatment of duodenal ulcer the recommended adult dosage of sucralfate is 1 g four times a day, administered orally. Interestingly, a dose of 2 g of sucralfate twice a day also appears to be equally effective in short-term treatments of duodenal ulcer (47). Sucralfate tablets can be dissolved in 15 to 30 ml of water and administered orally to patients with esophageal stricture or mucosal inflammation.

Side Effects

Because of minimal systemic absorption, side effects of sucralfate are rare (48, 49). In placebo-controlled clinical studies designed to evaluate the efficacy of sucralfate in duodenal ulcer healing, the most common side effect was constipation, which occurred in 0 to 15% of patients. Other side effects included dry mouth (0.7%), dizziness (0.4%), nausea, vomiting, headache, urticaria, and rashes. Rare side effects of sucralfate include gastric bezoar formation (50), aluminum intoxication (51), and hypophosphatemia (38). There have been no prospective safety studies of sucralfate in pregnant women, lactating women, children, and the elderly.

Special Considerations

Although sucralfate has no effect on gastric acid secretion, it is as effective as antacids or H_2-receptor antagonists in prevention of acute stress gastritis and bleeding in critically ill patients. It is interesting to note that, contrary to earlier claims, the frequency of nosocomial pneumonia is not significantly lower with sucralfate therapy than with antacid therapy in critically ill patients (52, 53).

OMEPRAZOLE

Chemically, omeprazole is a substituted benzimidazole (5-methoxy-2-(4-methoxy)-3-5-dimethyl-2-pyridinyl-sulfinyl-14-benzimidazole). It is a prototype of H^+K^+ ATPase (proton pump) inhibitor, which is being used pharmacologically as a potent inhibitor of gastric acid secretion. At present, omeprazole is the treatment of choice for patients with Zollinger-Ellison syndrome and severe gastroesophageal (GE) reflux disease.

The secretion of HCl by gastric parietal cells ultimately depends on the function of the hydrogen ion pump, which transport H^+ ions across the cell membrane in exchange for K^+ ions (54, 55). On activation of parietal cells by appropriate hormonal stimuli (i.e., histamine, gastrin, or acetylcholine), the proton pump, located in the apical portion of the parietal cell, is translocated to the plasma membrane of the acid-secreting canaliculi of the cell (56, 57). Within the acidic milieu of the parietal cells (pH $\leq$ 3) it is converted to its active form, sulfenic acid and sulfonamide (58, 59). The end products react with the sulfhydryl group in the enzyme H^+K^+ ATPase, forming an irreversible enzyme-inhibitor complex. Omeprazole is a weak base and is absorbed at an alkaline pH in the small intestine. After intestinal absorption, it is carried to the parietal cells in the stomach through the bloodstream. Thus, the resumption of acid secretion after the administration of omeprazole requires synthesis of new H^+K^+ ATPase protein (60), which takes about 72 hours. Since omeprazole is a weak base, its exposure to acid in the stomach decreases its bioavailability (61). Consequently, it is administered in a pH-sensitive enteric coated form that releases omeprazole in the small intestine. Peak plasma concentration of omeprazole occurs within 2 to 3 hours, and its duration of action exceeds 24 hours. Plasma levels tend to increase during the first few days of treatment as increasing inhibition of gastric acid results in less degradation of omeprazole and more absorption from the small intestine (62). No significant correlation is seen between the absolute plasma level of the drug and decreased acid secretion, but it correlates well with the area under the curve (63).

Dosage and Route of Administration

Omeprazole inhibits acid secretion in a dose range of 5 to 30 mg/day by the oral route. Although omeprazole may have only little effect on acid secretion on the first day of oral ingestion, it significantly inhibits gastric HCl secretion by day 5. In human studies, oral administration after 7 days of 10, 20, or 30 mg of omeprazole caused reduction in acid secretion by 27%, 90%, and 97%, respectively (64). Inhibition of gastric acid secretion with 10 mg of omeprazole ranges between 10 and 90% (64, 65). A standard 20-mg dose of omeprazole given orally causes steady-state inhibition of acid secretion between 35 and 65% within 24 hours after drug administration. Larger doses of omeprazole reduce variations in acid inhibition among patients and inhibit acid secretion more profoundly (63, 64, 66). It takes at least 3 days for acid secretion to return to pretreatment levels on cessation of omeprazole therapy. Omeprazole is metabolized extensively by the hepatic cytochrome P-450 system and is secreted in bile. About 20% of an orally administered dose of omeprazole is excreted in the feces, and 80% in urine.

Adverse Effects

The main side effect of omeprazole is related to development of hypergastrinemia and carcinoid tumors in rats. Several studies have shown that plasma gastrin levels do not increase in humans as much as in rats (67). Additional clinical trials must be performed to examine more carefully the long-term side effects of omeprazole. Oral administration of omeprazole reversibly increases the bacterial cell counts and nitrosamine levels in the stomach (68), which potentially can lead to GI infections (69) and cancers (70).

Drug Interactions

As a result of its interaction with cytochrome P-450, competitive inhibition of hepatic metabolism of certain drugs by omeprazole has been reported. Hepatic clearance of diazepam is reduced by about 50%, necessitating administration of smaller doses of the drug. Similarly, omeprazole also reduces elimination of phenytoin and Coumadin.

H_2-BLOCKERS (HISTAMINE$_2$-RECEPTOR ANTAGONISTS)

The H_2-blockers act by competitively and selectively blocking the histamine receptors on the basolateral membrane of the acid secreting parietal cells in the stomach. These histamine receptors are called H_2-type because they are not blocked by conventional H_1-type antihistamines such as diphenhydramine (71). The blockade of H_2-receptors, in turn, inhibits a cascade of reactions involving activation of adenyl cyclase, which decreases cyclic adenosine monophosphate (cAMP) concentration. In the parietal cell, cAMP is essential for optimal functioning of the hydrogen potassium ATPase pump and acid secretion. H_2-receptors are found at many other sites, including the atrium, ilium, uterus, adipocytes, T-suppressor cells, and mesenteric and percutaneous vascular beds. Structurally, all clinically approved H_2-blockers (i.e., cimetidine, ranitidine, nizatidine, and famotidine) are analogues of histamine with a bulky side chain in place of the ethylamine moiety. The relative potency of H_2-blockers varies 20- to 50-fold, with cimetidine being the least potent, and famotidine the most. A comparison of the potency of various H_2-blockers is shown in Table 36.2 (182). It is noteworthy that magnesium- and aluminum-containing antacids reduce the bioavailability of all H_2-blockers (cimetidine, ranitidine, and famotidine) by 30 to 50% and should be administered about 2 hours after the dose of the H_2-blocker (72, 73).

Table 36.2.   Comparison of H$_2$-Receptor Antagonists[a]

Variable	Cimetidine	Ranitidine	Nizatidine	Famotidine
1. Absorption				
Bioavailability (%)	30–80 (60)	30–88 (50)	75–100 (98)	37–45 (43)
Time to peak plasma concentration (hr)	1–2	1–3	1–3	1–3.5
2. Distribution				
Volume (liters/kg of body weight)	0.8–1.2	1.2–1.9	1.2–1.6	1.1–1.4
Protein binding in plasma (%)	13–26	15	25–35	16
3. Elimination				
Total systemic clearance (ml/min)	450–650	568–709	667–850	417–483
Half-life in plasma (hr)	1.5–2.3	1.6–2.4	1.1–1.6	2.5–4
Hepatic clearance (%)				
Oral	60	73	22	50–80
Intravenous	25–40	30	25	25–30
Renal clearance (%)				
Oral	40	27	57–65	25–30
Intravenous	50–80	50	75	65–80
4. Relative potency	1	4–10	4–10	20–50
Dose to heal duodenal ulcer (mg)	300 q.i.d.	150 b.i.d.	150 b.i.d.	40 h.s.
	400 b.i.d.	300 h.s.	300 h.s.	
	800 h.s.			
Dose to prevent recurrence (mg)	400 h.s.	150 h.s.	150 h.s.	20 h.s.

[a]Adapted from Feldman M, Burton ME: Comparison of H$_2$-receptor antagonists. *N Engl J Med* 323:1672–1680, 1990.

Cimetidine

Cimetidine shares the imidazole ring structure of histamine and inhibits all phases of gastric acid secretion. Both basal and nocturnal acid secretions are reduced by 60 to 70% with a 300-mg dose of cimetidine (74). Fasting serum gastrin levels are unaffected by cimetidine, but postprandial levels are raised because of the reduction in acid feedback and inhibition of gastrin release (75). Pepsin secretion by chief cells of gastric glands also decreases in parallel with the reduction in volume of gastric juice.

Pharmacokinetics.   The bioavailability of an orally ingested cimetidine dose ranges between 30 and 80% and has a plasma half-life of 2 hours. About 50% of the ingested dose is excreted unchanged by the kidneys, and the remainder is metabolized to sulfoxide prior to renal excretion. Only a very small amount of the ingested dose of cimetidine is excreted in the bile. Cimetidine easily crosses the placental barrier and blood-brain barrier and is excreted in breast milk. It is widely distributed in all organs of the body, and 70% of the total body content of cimetidine is found in the skeletal muscles. In the presence of renal failure, the dose of cimetidine is calculated by using the creatinine clearance formula. Hemodialysis decreases the level of circulating drug by at least 50%, and the dosage schedule should be adjusted to coincide with the hemodialysis (76, 77). With increasing age, a decline in volume of distribution resulting from a decrease in body mass has also been observed (78). Consequently, a one-third reduction of the cimetidine dose is justified in patients older than 65 years of age. Cimetidine can be given parenterally, and parenteral administration achieves higher peak levels than does an oral dose. After administration of a high dose of cimetidine parenterally, a clinically effective drug level is observed for approximately 4 hours (79).

Adverse Effects and Contraindications.   The reported incidence of adverse effects of cimetidine is approximately 5%. Most commonly, headaches, dizziness, skin rash, and myalgia are observed. Cimetidine crosses the blood-brain barrier and can cause mental confusion. This effect may result from blockage of the H$_2$-receptors in the brain tissue and consequent partial inhibition of the neurotransmitters. Blockage of histamine receptors in the brain has been shown to interfere with endogenous enkephalins (80). Symptomatic adverse effects of cimetidine tend to be more frequent in the elderly and in those patients with hepatic and renal failure.

Cimetidine increases the serum concentration of prolactin and causes galactorrhea in women and gynecomastia in men. In addition, cimetidine binds to androgen receptors and reduces sperm counts in young males. Cimetidine also inhibits cytochrome P-450 and catalyzes hydroxylation of estradiol. It is also shown to inhibit release of aldosterone in vivo (81, 82).

Adverse hematologic reactions of cimetidine are uncommon (0.01 to 0.07%) and include leukopenia, thrombocytopenia, anemia, and pancytopenia (83). Reversible increases of serum aminotransferase are also seen in patients taking i.v. cimetidine (84, 85). Rarely, bradycardia has been reported with cimetidine as a result of the effect on cardiac H$_2$-receptors (86, 87).

Drug Interactions.   Impairment of the hepatic metabolism of several drugs by cimetidine is caused by its inhibition of the P-450 enzyme system. Most importantly, hepatic metabolism of warfarin, theophylline, phenytoin, phenobarbital, and the benzodiazepines is prolonged. Consequently, smaller doses of these drugs may be required when they are administered with an oral dose of cimetidine. Other drugs such as digoxin, mexiletine, nifedipine, propranolol, and tricyclic antidepressants also are shown to have prolonged actions as a result of cimetidine.

Dosage.   For oral use, cimetidine is available in tablet form in 200-, 300-, 400-, or 800-mg doses. Cimetidine is also available in liquid form as 60 mg/ml. For duodenal ulcers or benign gastric ulcers, the usual dose of cimetidine is 800 mg q.h.s. or 300 mg q.i.d. to 400 mg b.i.d. to be administered for 4 to 8 weeks. A much higher dose of cimetidine is required in patients with Zollinger-Ellison syndrome. For parenteral administration, the drug is given as 300 mg i.v. every 6 hours or as a continuous i.v. infusion of 40 to 50 mg every hour.

Special Considerations. Cimetidine is shown to augment cell-mediated immunity in vitro because of H_2-receptor blockade of T-lymphocytes (88). In uncontrolled studies, cimetidine has been reported to accelerate healing of herpetic skin lesions in immunocompromised patients (89). The dose of cimetidine may need to be reduced in patients with renal function impairment. Furthermore, very small amounts of cimetidine are removed from plasma by peritoneal dialysis as a result of tight binding to plasma proteins (90).

Overdosage. Physostigmine has been reported to arouse obtunded patients, with evidence of cimetidine-induced central nervous system toxicity. Assisted renal excretion over a period of time reduces cimetidine toxicity.

Ranitidine

Structurally, ranitidine contains a furan ring instead of the imidazole ring of histamine. Ranitidine is considered effective in the treatment of both duodenal and gastric ulcers. Ranitidine is preferred over cimetidine because it binds minimally to other sites such as androgen receptors, the hepatic P-450 system, and peripheral lymphocytes (91). Furthermore, ranitidine is five to 12 times more potent than cimetidine on a molar basis in inhibiting stimulated gastric acid secretion in humans (92).

Pharmacokinetics. Ranitidine is absorbed rapidly from the small intestine and its absorption is not influenced by food ingestion. A single oral dose (150 mg) achieves a peak plasma concentration within 1 to 3 hours. In most cases, 50% inhibition of gastric acid output can be achieved with a plasma ranitidine concentration of 100 to 200 ng/ml (93). Bioavailability is influenced by hepatic function, since the drug is taken up and metabolized by the liver by first-pass kinetics. Up to 30% of ranitidine is metabolized by the liver to sulfuric oxide, nitrogen oxide, and desmethyl derivatives (94). About 50% or more of absorbed ranitidine is excreted unchanged by the kidney. In patients with liver disease, bioavailability of ranitidine is increased and serum half-life prolonged as a result of reduced hepatic metabolism. Ranitidine, however, is essentially free of dose-related adverse effects (95).

Dosage and Route of Administration. Ranitidine is available in tablet form (150 or 300 mg) and in liquid form (15 mg/ml). The usual dose for treatment of active duodenal ulcer is 150 mg b.i.d. or 300 mg q.h.s. Ranitidine can be given intravenously at a dose of 50 mg q.8 h. or as a continuous infusion (6 mg/hr). The dose of i.v. ranitidine should be adjusted to intragastric pH, which should be maintained at 5.0 or higher. With ranitidine, ulcer healing has been documented endoscopically in 70% of patients by the end of 4 weeks and in 85 to 90% by the end of 8 weeks (96, 97). In patients with Zollinger-Ellison syndrome in whom cimetidine produced ineffective control of symptoms, suppression of gastric acid secretion was achieved with high doses (600 to 1200 mg) of ranitidine daily (98).

Side Effects. Side effects of ranitidine are quite infrequent and include minor events such as rash, malaise, or constipation. Sinus bradycardia has been reported with rapid i.v. infusion of ranitidine (99–101). Ranitidine does not increase basal levels of testosterone and is devoid of antiandrogenic activity, as it does not bind to androgen receptors (102).

In patients with cimetidine-induced impotence, complete remission of impotence was observed with ranitidine after discontinuation of cimetidine (103). Furthermore, unlike cimetidine, ranitidine does not inhibit metabolism of estradiol (104). Anicteric hepatitis and mild increase of transaminase have been observed rarely with ranitidine administration. Mental confusion and other CNS symptoms have also been reported rarely with ranitidine, as it minimally crosses the blood-brain barrier and binds minimally to brain receptors. Ranitidine does not bind to the cells of the hemopoietic system, and thus anemia, thrombocytopenia, and other hematologic abnormalities are not observed with ranitidine, which is another advantage over cimetidine (105). It minimally alters hepatic metabolism of diazepam, warfarin, and propranolol. It predisposes to bezoar formation (106) and achlorhydria, which can lead to breakdown of the gastric barrier with proliferation of enteric and nitrate-producing bacteria. The proliferation of enteric bacteria is a common side effect of all H_2-blockers and is a matter of concern on a long-term basis (107–109).

Famotidine

Famotidine is a chemically distinct H_2-blocker with a thiazole ring structure. It is 50 to 80 times more potent than cimetidine and 5 to 8 times more potent than ranitidine. It is indicated for short-term treatment (4 to 8 weeks) of acute duodenal ulcer and maintenance of healed duodenal ulcer. It has also been used for hypersecretory states such as Zollinger-Ellison syndrome.

Pharmacokinetics. Famotidine is rapidly but incompletely absorbed on oral administration, with bioavailability of 35 to 45%. Seventy percent of the drug is eliminated intact in the urine (110). With renal failure (CrCl <10 ml/min), the daily dose of famotidine should be reduced from 40 mg to 20 mg. Famotidine dosage adjustment is not required with hepatic failure. Peak antisecretory activity is reached within 1 to 3 hours after oral administration and persists for 10 to 12 hours.

Dosage and Route of Administration. Famotidine can be given intravenously, with a similar time for onset of antisecretory effects but twice the potency of the oral dose. Famotidine is available in tablet (20 mg or 40 mg) or liquid form (40 mg/5 ml).

Drug Interactions and Side Effects. No drug interaction has been reported so far, but experience with this medication is limited at the present time. Famotidine does not interfere with compounds that are metabolized by hepatic microsomal enzyme processes, including diazepam, phenytoin, theophylline, and warfarin. Furthermore, no adverse effects on the central nervous, endocrine, or renal systems have been reported (111). Several minor side effects have been documented with famotidine and include headaches, dizziness, constipation, and diarrhea (112, 113). However, the frequency of these side effects is exceedingly low (1 to 4%) and the drug is very well-tolerated.

Overdosage. Doses up to 640 mg/day have been given with no reported untoward effects. Symptomatic treatment and gastric lavage within the first few hours are warranted.

Nizatidine

Nizatidine has a substituted imidazole ring compared with the other H_2-blockers. It is available in 150-mg and 300-mg capsules for oral use. Because it has little first-pass hepatic metabolism, the bioavailability of the oral dose is close to 100% (114, 115). In patients with renal failure its effect is prolonged, as renal excretion is the principal pathway for its elimination. It is the only H_2-blocker whose active metabolite (N_2 monodesmethyl nizatidine) has about 60% of the activity of the parent drug. Nizatidine does not bind notably to the cytochrome P-450 enzyme system and thus has no drug interactions with drugs that are metabolized by the hepatic route.

Adverse Reactions.   Sweating (1%), hyperuricemia unassociated with gout or nephrolithiasis, and asymptomatic ventricular tachycardia can be seen.

Overdosage.   If overdosage of nizatidine is encountered, renal dialysis should be initiated within the first 4 to 6 hours. This increases plasma clearance of the drug by 84%.

Misoprostol

Misoprostol is a synthetic prostaglandin E_1 analog which has antisecretory (gastric acid inhibition) and mucosal protection properties (116, 117).

Mechanisms of Action.   Misoprostol produces a definite decrease in gastric acid secretion and a moderate decrease in pepsin secretion. It does not seem to affect fasting or postprandial gastrin levels. Furthermore, misoprostol does not interfere with the antiinflammatory and analgesic actions of the NSAIDs. NSAIDs act by inhibiting prostaglandin synthesis, and a deficiency of prostaglandins in the gastric mucosa leads to diminished mucus and bicarbonate secretion. These diminished defense barriers are presumed to be responsible for NSAID-induced peptic ulcerations.

Indications for Use.   Prevention of NSAID- and aspirin-induced gastric ulcerations is an indication for use of misoprostol. People on high doses of NSAID have a high risk of GI bleeding (118).

Pharmacokinetics.   Misoprostol is absorbed extensively and undergoes rapid change to its free acid, misoprostic acid. Misoprostic acid is responsible for the clinical activity of misoprostol and can be measured in the plasma. Peak concentration of the drug on oral administration is achieved in 12 minutes, and it has a plasma half-life of 20 to 35 minutes. Mean plasma levels of misoprostol are linearly correlated in the dose range of 200 to 400 μg. Eighty percent of the drug is excreted in the urine. The serum protein binding of misoprostol is about 80 to 90%, and the binding is concentration independent in the therapeutic range. It is noteworthy that misoprostol and its active metabolite have no effect on the cytochrome P-450 system.

Dosage and Route of Administration.   Misoprostol is generally recommended for the full duration of the NSAID intake. The usual dose is 200 μg four times a day with food (119). It is advisable to start with a much smaller dose and increase it gradually over a period of time.

Contraindications.   (a) The most important and definite contraindication is pregnancy. Misoprostol has abortifacient properties. Misoprostol is relatively contraindicated in all women of child-bearing age unless the risk : benefit ratio truly warrants its use. All patients who are sexually active should be warned of this risk and be advised to use adequate contraception. (b) A history of severe allergic reaction to misoprostol and other synthetic prostaglandins is a contraindication.

Adverse Reactions.   (a) Development of diarrhea is seen in 13 to 40% of all patients who are started on misoprostol therapy. Diarrhea is dose-related and usually appears within the first 6 weeks after initiation of misoprostol therapy. Diarrhea usually is self-limiting and resolves in 1 to 2 weeks. Because of abdominal cramps and diarrhea, misoprostol therapy is discontinued in a small percentage of patients. Development of diarrhea can be minimized by administration of the drug after meals and at bedtime, and by starting with a small dosage of the medication. Concomitant use of magnesium-containing antacids should be avoided to minimize the problem of diarrhea (120). (b) Other adverse effects include headaches (2 to 3%), vaginal spotting (1%), abdominal cramps, and dysmenorrhea. Postmenopausal vaginal bleeding has also been reported in about 5.5% of female patients.

Overdosage.   The toxic dose of misoprostol has yet to be determined. A cumulative total oral dose of 1600 μg has been tolerated, with some GI symptoms. Higher doses may cause cardiac arrhythmias, hepatic and renal tubular necrosis, and testicular atrophy. Treatment of misoprostol overdose is mainly supportive.

ANTIDIARRHEAL AGENTS

Management of diarrhea should be directed mainly at treating the underlying cause. Most commonly, the underlying causes of diarrhea in the ICU setting include infection, malabsorption, drugs, endocrine disorders, or enterocolitis. In the critical care setting, symptomatic relief of diarrhea with prevention of fluid losses and electrolyte imbalance assumes prime importance. Apart from the nonspecific antidiarrheal drugs, oral or parenteral replacement of fluid and electrolytes is essential and life-saving. Salient pharmacologic compounds that reduce diarrhea promptly include the drugs discussed below.

OPIATES

Hydroalcoholic solutions of opium (opium tincture and paregoric) and synthetic opiates (diphenoxylates and loperamide) are the principal drugs in this class. Opioid agonists act at the μ- and possibly δ-receptors on enteric neurons and disrupt aboral peristaltic movements, which results in prolonged transit time of intestinal contents. These agents also reduce interstitial fluid secretion and enhance mucosal absorption, ameliorating abdominal cramps and diarrhea.

Loperamide

Loperamide is a piperidine opioid that is slowly and partially absorbed from the gastrointestinal tract after oral ingestion.

Mechanism of Action.   Loperamide slows intestinal motility via its direct effects on the circular and longitudinal muscles of the intestinal wall. It also slows the intestinal transit of water and electrolytes (121).

Pharmacokinetics. After oral administration, 40% of loperamide is absorbed from the GI tract. Peak plasma levels occur 5 hours after oral administration of the capsular form and 2.5 hours after intake of the liquid form. Elimination half-life of loperamide is 9 to 12 hours.

Dosage and Route of Administration. Loperamide is administered orally and is available as a 2-mg capsule or a liquid preparation (1 mg/ml). Because the drug is long-acting, it is given initially as a 4-mg dose followed by a 2-mg dose after each unformed stool, up to a maximum of 16 mg/day.

Contraindications. (*a*) Loperamide should not be used if infectious (i.e., *Salmonella, Campylobacter, Shigella,* etc.) enterocolitis is suspected (122). (*b*) Pseudomembranous colitis contraindicates its use. (*c*) Hypersensitivity to opioids is a third contraindication.

Adverse Reactions. Reactions include dry mouth, nausea, vomiting, abdominal pain, and distension. All adverse reactions are self-limiting and are seen only after months of chronic use.

Special Considerations. Loperamide is relatively devoid of central nervous system effects, as it does not cross the blood-brain barrier. It can be given to the elderly with negligible neurologic effects. Safety and efficacy of opioid analogues has not been established clearly for pregnant patients and lactating mothers.

Overdosage. Up to 60 mg of the drug has been tolerated, with minimal side effects such as constipation and CNS depression. These side effects can be reversed by naloxone. In addition, activated charcoal and gastric lavage are recommended to reduce intestinal absorption of loperamide.

Diphenoxylate HCl with Atropine Sulfate

Diphenoxylate is a piperidine opioid related to meperidine but lacking analgesic activity. To discourage abuse of this preparation, atropine is added.

Mechanism of Action and Pharmacokinetics. Diphenoxylate is metabolized rapidly and extensively to diphenoxylic acid, which is the biologically active metabolite. Fifty percent of a single orally ingested dose is excreted in the feces and 14% in the urine over a 4-day period. Elimination half-life of diphenoxylate is 12 to 14 hours.

Dosage and Route of Administration. Orally, the dose is 2.5 to 5 mg every 3 to 4 hours. In combination with atropine, the drug is called lomotil, which has 25 μg atropine for every 2.5 mg of diphenoxylate.

Adverse Reactions. Adverse reactions occur mainly because of the anticholinergic actions of atropine, which include dry skin, dry mouth, dry eyes, hyperesthesia, and urinary retention. Anorexia, nausea, vomiting, and paralytic ileus are the other common GI side effects. Allergic reactions ranging from mild pruritus to angioneurotic edema can also be seen. CNS side effects include dizziness, headaches, malaise, and lethargy (120).

Contraindications. (*a*) Pregnant and lactating mothers should not take the drug. (*b*) Neonates should not be given diphenoxylate, as it has been shown to cause cholestatic jaundice in them.

Drug Interactions. When administered with monoamine oxidase inhibitors, diphenoxylate may precipitate hypertensive crisis. Furthermore, diphenoxylate can potentiate the depressant actions of alcohol, barbiturates, and tranquilizers.

Overdosage. Anticholinergic overactivity and respiratory depression are the main toxic effects of diphenoxylate overdosage. GI lavage, naloxone, and physostigmine may be considered to reduce and reverse its toxic effect.

BISMUTH SALICYLATES

Bismuth salicylates are a mixture of trivalent bismuth and salicylates that frequently are used to treat mild to moderate diarrhea.

Mechanism of Action. Local antiinflammatory action of salicylates is thought to be the primary mode of action, as a result of inhibition of prostaglandins, which have been implicated as the cause of various forms of diarrhea (123). Bismuth has antimicrobial activity, which contributes to its antidiarrheal action in cases of infectious diarrhea.

Dosage and Route of Administration. Orally, 2 tablets (15 mg each) or 30 ml (1 mg/ml) generally are given every 30 minutes to 1 hour as needed, for a maximum of 8 doses in 24 hours.

Side Effects. Salicylism may be observed and is characterized by tinnitus. Caution should be exercised in administering this drug simultaneously with anticoagulants, oral hypoglycemic agents, and colchicine.

Drug Interactions. Bismuth salicylate may decrease GI absorption and bioavailability of tetracycline, thus reducing its antimicrobial activity. Concomitant use of aspirin can further increase the likelihood of developing salicylism.

Special Considerations. Along with ampicillin and metronidazole, bismuth subsalicylate is used as adjunctive treatment for *Helicobacter pylori*-associated gastritis and ulcer disease.

MISCELLANEOUS

In the past, a variety of starches, talcs, and chalks have been used to treat diarrhea. Kaolin or pectin, alone and in combination, have been used extensively for the treatment of diarrhea. Presumably, these compounds absorb water from the intestine and produce a more formed stool. There is little evidence that Kaopectate diminishes the number of evacuations or decreases intestinal fluid losses (124–126). In addition, α_2 central agonists such as clonidine have also been used to treat diarrhea in patients with diabetes mellitus (127). The dose of clonidine is 0.5 mg every 12 hours orally.

SOMATOSTATIN

Somatostatin is a neuropeptide that has a potent growth hormone inhibitory action. It has been demonstrated to have strong antisecretory and antimotility effects. The long-acting somatostatin analog octreotide is considered to be the new drug of choice in the treatment of secretory diarrhea, carcinoid syndrome, and vasointestinal peptide secreting tumors (128). The commercially used preparation octreotide is effective in the treatment of endocrine tumors of the gastroenteropancreatic axis. These tumors are well-known to cause accumulation of fluid in the intestinal lumen and produce voluminous diarrhea by secreting vasoactive intestinal polypeptide, serotonin, and/or prostaglandins.

Mechanism of Action. Somatostatin exerts its effects by binding to specific receptors on the surface of target cells, which then mediate a number of intracellular events. The most important intracellular event is the inhibition of adenylate cyclase activity and accumulation of cyclic AMP. Another effect is enhanced potassium conduction, causing cell membrane hyperpolarization. Either of these events could lead to reduction in the intracellular concentration of calcium necessary for cell secretion.

Pharmacokinetics. Somatostatin has a short half-life of about 2 minutes. Octreotide, the specific analog of somatostatin, has a longer half-life in plasma (90 to 115 minutes). Octreotide has a smaller ring and contains a *d*-amino acid side chain, which decreases the rate of degradation. Octreotide currently is available only for parenteral administration. Octreotide attains peak plasma concentration within 1 hour, and the height of plasma concentration is proportional to the dose administered. Injection of 50 to 100 μg results in a plasma concentration of 2 to 4 μg/liter. Clinical effects are seen within 2 hours of administering the dose (129, 130).

Dosage and Route of Administration. Octreotide is available in ampules containing 0.05, 0.10, or 0.5 mg/ml. It is administered subcutaneously two to four times a day for a total dose of 50 to 1500 μg/day. A starting dose is generally 50 μg twice a day and can be increased gradually to 600 to 1000 μg/day or as tolerated by the patient.

Side Effects. The major effect of somatostatin analog is minor pain at the injection site and abdominal cramping on initiation of therapy. Glucose intolerance, diabetes, gallstone development as a result of decreased contraction of the gallbladder, and malabsorption resulting from decreased pancreatic secretions have all been shown to be clinically significant side effects in patients on long-term (>4 to 6 months) use of this medication. None of these side effects has resulted in cessation of Sandostatin when indicated.

Special Consideration. Somatostatin has been shown to decrease basal and stimulated gastric acid secretion. In addition, somatostatin decreases plasma gastrin levels and pepsin secretion. It also stimulates mucus production in the stomach and thus may act as a cytoprotective agent (131, 132). Somatostatin has been used in clinical trials for control of variceal hemorrhage because of its effect on decreasing splanchnic circulation. Somatostatin has also been advocated as a treatment for acromegaly, thyrotropinomas, carcinoid syndrome, VIPoma, and glucagonomas (133).

DRUGS FOR GASTROPARESIS AND COLONIC INERTIA

METOCLOPRAMIDE

Metoclopramide is a procainamide analog (methoxy-2-chlor-5-procainamide) that was developed as an antiemetic

agent for the treatment of nausea and vomiting during pregnancy (134). Although structurally related to procainamide, it has no local anesthetic or antiarrhythmic effects.

Mechanism of Action. Metoclopramide is a dopamine antagonist that causes dopamine receptor blockade. Its antiemetic effect against drugs such as apomorphine and ergotamine is achieved by this mechanism. In addition to being an antiemetic agent, metoclopramide is also a prokinetic agent that promotes motility of the GI tract by stimulating the smooth muscle. Dopaminergic blockade by metoclopramide improves gastric emptying by decreasing relaxation in the upper part of the stomach and increasing antral contractions. In addition, pylorus and duodenum are relaxed while the lower esophageal sphincter tone is enhanced. It also increases peristalsis of the jejunum and accelerates intestinal transit time from duodenum to ileocecal valve (135).

These pharmacologic actions of metoclopramide accelerate gastric emptying and reduce gastroesophageal reflux. Metoclopramide has minimal effect on gastric secretion or colonic motility. Apart from its antidopaminergic effect on gut smooth muscle, metoclopramide is also intrinsically cholinergic for the intramural neurons and augments acetylcholine release from postganglionic nerve terminals.

Dosage. The oral dosage is 10 to 15 mg 30 minutes before each meal and at bedtime for 2 to 8 weeks. The parenteral dose for antiemetic effect in cancer chemotherapy patients is 1 mg/kg diluted with normal saline or 5% dextrose solution administered intravenously over 15 minutes.

Pharmacokinetics. Onset of action is within 1 to 3 minutes following an i.v. dose, 10 to 15 minutes after an i.m. dose, and 30 to 60 minutes after an oral dose. The clinical effect of metoclopramide persists for 1 to 2 hours. It is well-absorbed from the GI tract but is subject to first-pass metabolism, with a total bioavailability of 50 to 70%. After oral ingestion on an empty stomach, intestinal absorption of metoclopramide is rapid. It is weakly protein bound (13 to 22%) and rapidly distributed in all tissues.

Adverse Reactions. Mild and transient side effects of the drug are observed in 20 to 30% of cases. Principal CNS effects include fatigue, restlessness, extrapyramidal reactions, and dystonia. Common GI side effects include nausea and diarrhea. Transient hypertension may also be seen at times. Metoclopramide is known to increase serum prolactin levels, causing gynecomastia in males and amenorrhea in females.

Special Considerations. Caution should be applied when metoclopramide is given to a patient with previously detected breast cancer. Chronic administration raises prolactin levels, and one-third of breast cancers are prolactin dependent in vitro. Metoclopramide readily enters breast milk and thus should be used cautiously in nursing mothers. In infants, methemoglobinemia has been reported with the use of metoclopramide.

BETHANECHOL

Bethanechol is a cholinomimetic drug that seems to augment the prokinetic effects of metoclopramide. This observation supports the idea that enhanced responsiveness to acetylcholine (ACH) may also be a mechanism of action by which metoclopramide acts on target tissues. Bethanechol is not usually used as a single agent in the treatment of gastroparesis.

Pharmacokinetics. Bethanechol is rapidly and completely absorbed after oral administration. Sulfate conjugation during the first pass through the liver is the principal determinant of bioavailability of the oral form (136). Thirty percent of the drug is excreted unchanged in the urine, and the rest after conjugation with sulfate or glucuronic acid, also in the urine. Bethanechol is distributed rapidly into most tissues and readily crosses the blood-brain barrier. It also crosses the placental barrier and is secreted in breast milk in high concentrations.

Onset of action of bethanechol takes 1 to 15 minutes after i.v. administration, 10 to 30 minutes after i.m. injection, and 30 to 60 minutes after an oral dose. Plasma half-life of bethanechol is about 4 to 6 hours.

Dosage. Bethanechol is available in tablet (5 and 10 mg) and syrup form (5 mg/ml) and as an injectable solution (5 to 10 mg/ml). The usual dose of bethanechol is 10 mg q.i.d. orally, taken 15 to 30 minutes prior to meals and at bedtime. It has also been shown to be effective subcutaneously with sustained plasma levels.

Side Effects. The frequency of various side effects ranges between 15 and 20%. Most frequently, drowsiness, restlessness, and anxiety are observed with bethanechol therapy. Extrapyramidal reactions such as opisthotonus, torticollis, and oculogyric crisis are seen infrequently (1%). Extrapyramidal reactions secondary to bethanechol can be treated with diphenhydramine or benzotropine administration. Hyperprolactinemia with breast tenderness and menstrual irregularities has also been reported in patients treated with bethanechol.

Contraindications. Bethanechol is contraindicated in patients with suspected intestinal obstruction or perforation. In patients with pheochromocytoma, bethanechol can exacerbate a hypertensive crisis, necessitating reversal by phentolamine (137). Similarly, bethanechol should not be used in patients with Parkinson's disease. Simultaneous use of anticholinergic and dopamine agonist drugs must be monitored very closely for potentiation of action and side effects.

DOMPERIDONE

Domperidone is a benzimidazole derivative that possesses both prokinetic and antiemetic properties. It is a specific dopamine antagonist that stimulates the GI tract smooth muscle. It does not cross the blood-brain barrier and acts on the chemoreceptor trigger zone to provide antiemetic properties. Its mode of action on the chemoreceptor trigger zone may account for the absence of extrapyramidal and other CNS side effects. Domperidone's action is not blocked by atropine, suggesting that it may have no intrinsic cholinergic activity.

Pharmacokinetics. Domperidone is absorbed rapidly after oral intake, and its bioavailability is about 10 to 15% of a single oral dose. Bioavailability of domperidone increases to 90% on intravascular administration. About 70% of the drug and its metabolites are excreted in the feces, while the rest passes through the urine. Plasma half-life of domperidone is about 7 to 8 hours. This drug is shown to have a high affinity for the tissue in the GI tract, and high concentrations of the

drug have been reported in the esophagus, stomach, and small intestine of humans and animals.

Dosage. The optimal dose of domperidone is 20 to 30 mg orally four times daily. This dose has been shown to improve gastric motility in patients with idiopathic gastric stasis (138).

Side Effects. Breast enlargement, nipple tenderness, galactorrhea, and amenorrhea secondary to hyperprolactinemia are observed more commonly with domperidone than with metoclopramide. Fatal cardiac arrhythmias have been reported from Japan after intravenous administration of domperidone. In the U.S., domperidone has not been released for routine clinical use. Phase IV clinical trials are currently in progress to evaluate and establish clinical efficacy of the drug in the U.S.

CISAPRIDE

Cisapride is a benzamide derivative that is currently undergoing clinical trials in the U.S. Animal data suggest a prokinetic effect of cisapride on esophagus, stomach, and small bowel. In addition, unlike other prokinetic agents, cisapride has a stimulating effect on the colonic smooth muscle as well. It is devoid of any antidopaminergic actions but acts by facilitating acetylcholine release in the myenteric plexus. Cisapride is also demonstrated to be an effective serotonin antagonist in guinea pig intestinal mucosa (139). Because of its prokinetic action on the colon, cisapride promises to be an effective drug in patients with colonic inertia. Cisapride has also been used in patients with idiopathic gastric stasis, diabetic gastroparesis, and intestinal pseudoobstruction.

Pharmacokinetics. On oral administration, cisapride has a bioavailability of 30 to 40%. Peak plasma levels were observed after a standard oral dose at 1.5 to 2 hours. After intravenous administration, cisapride has been shown to disappear exponentially, with a half-life of approximately 19 hours.

Dosage. Clinical trials of cisapride are currently in progress. No consensus has been reached about its precise dose in various disorders. Cisapride is available in 4- and 16-mg tablets and in 2-, 4-, and 8-mg vials for intravenous administration. All of these doses have been shown to increase gastric emptying and intestinal peristalsis. The drug has no effect on plasma prolactin levels and is shown to have fewer side effects than domperidone.

ERYTHROMYCIN

Erythromycin is a macrolide antibiotic that can be both bacteriostatic or bactericidal, depending on the microorganism and the concentration of the drug. Erythromycin is most effective against Gram-positive cocci, and it is used frequently in patients who are allergic to penicillin. It is the drug of choice against *Legionella* and *Mycoplasma* infections. More recently, erythromycin in small doses has been shown to be an effective agent in promoting motility in patients with diabetic gastroparesis.

Mechanism of Action. (*a*) Erythromycin acts as an antibiotic by inhibiting protein synthesis. It does so by binding reversibly to the 50S ribosomal subunits of sensitive microorganisms (140). (*b*) Erythromycin mimics the effect of the gastrointestinal polypeptide motilin by binding to motilin receptors and acts as an agonist to enhance gastrointestinal motility.

Dosage and Route of Administration.   As an antibiotic, doses of erythromycin vary from 250 to 500 mg every 6 hours orally or intravenously. The dose of erythromycin for patients with gastroparesis has not been clearly established. In a study from Belgium that demonstrated the efficacy of erythromycin in the treatment of diabetic gastroparesis, 250-mg tablets of erythromycin were administered twice a day (141). There is a general consensus that the dose of erythromycin needed for promoting motility is much less than its dose as an antibiotic.

Pharmacokinetics.   When given orally, erythromycin base is incompletely but adequately absorbed from the upper part of the small intestine. It is inactivated by gastric juice and thus has to be taken as enteric coated tablets. A dose of 250 mg in estolate form produces peak plasma concentration after 2 hours of administration. Only 2 to 5% of orally administered erythromycin is excreted in the active form in the urine, whereas 12 to 15% is excreted in the urine after i.v. infusion. Most of the drug is concentrated in the liver and excreted in an active form in the bile.

Plasma half-life of erythromycin is approximately 1 to 6 hours. The drug diffuses rapidly into intercellular fluids but does not cross the blood-brain barrier.

Side Effects.   Allergic reactions include fever, eosinophilia, and skin eruptions, which disappear in a few days after cessation of therapy. (*b*) Cholestatic hepatitis is caused primarily by the estolate salt of erythromycin. (*c*) GI side effects are commonly seen if the drug is administered on an empty stomach. These commonly include epigastric distress, cramping, nausea, vomiting, and diarrhea.

Drug Interactions.   Erythromycin is reported to potentiate the effect of carbamazepine and cyclosporine.

DRUGS FOR TREATMENT OF VARICEAL HEMORRHAGE

In the ICU setting, variceal hemorrhage is encountered frequently and presents a potentially life-threatening condition. Variceal hemorrhage usually results from portal hypertension from chronic liver disease and frequently is associated with concomitant encephalopathy, coagulopathy, and/or renal insufficiency. Bleeding from esophageal varices usually occurs from the lower 5 cm of the esophagus as a result of disruption of a varix (142, 143). Because of accompanying coagulopathy, encephalopathy, and ascites, the management of these patients presents a special challenge. The diagnosis of variceal hemorrhage generally is established by endoscopic evaluation of the esophagus following the diagnosis. Several pharmacologic agents are used to control variceal bleeding.

VASOPRESSORS

Vasopressin

Vasopressin is a neurohypophyseal peptide that has a potent vasoconstrictor action on mesenteric circulation. Because of its effect on mesenteric blood flow, vasopressin is commonly used as an adjunctive therapy not only in control of variceal bleeding but also in hemorrhagic gastritis and in patients with portal hypertension undergoing abdominal surgery (144).

Mechanism of Action.   The principal clinical effect of vasopressin is caused by marked splanchnic vasoconstriction when the drug is administered by the intravenous or intraarterial route. A single bolus of vasopressin administered intravenously causes a marked reduction in portal blood flow and portal pressure, lasting for about 30 minutes. In patients with suspected coronary artery disease, vasopressin should be administered with caution and, if necessary, in combination with nitrates to decrease the incidence of serious myocardial ischemia (145, 146).

Dosage and Route of Administration.   Vasopressin is administered initially at a dose of 0.2 to 0.4 U/min intravenously, but higher doses up to 1 to 3 U/min have been used in cases with unmanageable bleeding. Close hemodynamic monitoring is essential during intravenous infusion of vasopressin. Although vasopressin can acutely slow down or stop bleeding, it does not prevent recurrence of bleeding from varices.

Side Effects.   The most important limiting factor for the use of vasopressin is reduced coronary blood flow in patients with coronary artery disease. Vasopressin also causes some peripheral vasoconstriction, with increased systemic afterload. In addition, cardiac arrhythmias and direct impairment of cardiac contractility have also been reported. Nausea, belching, and abdominal cramps frequently are observed as a result of increased gut motility secondary to smooth muscle stimulation. Furthermore, allergic reaction ranging from a mild rash to severe anaphylaxis have also been reported (147).

Glypressin

More recently, a synthetic analogue of vasopressin, glypressin, has become available (148). Glypressin has a much longer duration of action after administration of a single bolus (2 mg) intravenously. The pharmacologic effect of glypressin lasts for 6 hours, and consequently a continuous infusion is not necessary. Availability of glypressin may reduce the duration of ICU stay for patients with variceal hemorrhage.

SCLEROSING AGENTS

Injection sclerotherapy of esophageal varices commonly is used for control of acute variceal bleeding. Injection sclerotherapy of esophageal varices is effective in controlling variceal hemorrhage in 90 to 95% of all patients and seems to be superior to balloon tamponade or pharmacologic therapy alone (149–151). In one study, definitive control of variceal bleeding was achieved in 95% of patients with a single sclerotherapy session (152). A large number of pharmacologic compounds have been used as sclerosing agents.

Sodium Morrhuate

Sodium morrhuate is a mixture of sodium salts of the saturated and unsaturated fatty acids present in cod liver oil. On venous injection, sodium morrhuate causes inflammation of the intima layer of the blood vessels, leading to the formation of a thrombus. Intimal inflammation leads to the occlusion of the vein followed by fibrosis around it. In most cases of variceal hemorrhage, 1 to 2 ml of a solution of sodium morrhuate (5%) is injected locally, with an average total volume of 15 to 25 ml per endoscopic sclerotherapy session. The principal side effects of sodium morrhuate include hypersensitivity reaction, fever, chest pain, and mucosal ulceration. There have been concerns about sodium morrhuate's role in causing acute respiratory distress syndrome (ARDS) in patients with variceal hemorrhage. However, it has now become evident that the pulmonary endothelium is relatively safe, as only 20% of injected sodium morrhuate reaches the lungs and causes no change in diffusing capacity of the lungs (153).

Sodium Tetradecyl Sulfate

Sodium tetradecyl sulfate is a synthetic anionic surfactant that causes variceal thrombosis when injected locally. Sodium tetradecyl sulfate is available as a 1 to 5% solution containing 10 to 30 mg of drug in benzyl alcohol along with diabasic sodium phosphate. This compound has been used extensively in the management of variceal hemorrhage and is considered to be relatively safe from a clinical viewpoint. Impairment of pulmonary function has not been observed with this agent (154).

Ethanolamine Oleate

The oleic acid component of the ethanolamine oleate molecule is responsible for the inflammatory response in the intima varices and activation of coagulation cascade by release of tissue factor and activation of Hageman factor. It has been suspected that the ethanolamine component of the compound may act by inhibiting fibrin clot formation as a result of chelation of calcium ions. Generally, 1.5 to 2 ml of a solution of ethanolamine oleate is injected at one site. The pharmacologic preparation is available in 2-ml vials as a 5% solution. More than 20 ml of ethanolamine oleate should not be used at one sclerotherapy session.

Several adverse effects have been reported with the use of ethanolamine in clinical trials. These side effects include pleural effusion, pulmonary edema, and pneumonia. Case reports of anaphylactic reactions, acute renal failure, pyrexia, and retrosternal discomfort have also been recorded.

LAXATIVES

Constipation is a common clinical condition in the ICU setting. It is related primarily to lack of oral intake and impaired intestinal motility resulting from associated physical and emotional stress. Consequently, a large number of patients need laxatives to initiate defecation during their recovery from critical illness. A large variety of laxatives currently is available, ranging from stimulant laxatives to saline and bulk laxatives (Table 36.3). Stimulant or saline laxatives are used at cathartic doses prior to radiologic exam of the GI tract, kidneys, and other abdominal organs, and prior to bowel surgery. Saline laxatives are also used for emptying the large bowel prior to colonoscopy and a variety of surgical procedures.

BULK LAXATIVES

Dietary fiber is plant cell wall that escapes digestion by enzymatic secretions of the human GI tract. It can bind water in the colonic lumen, thus softening feces and increasing its bulk. In addition, some components of dietary fiber are digested by colonic bacteria to metabolites that contribute to the laxative action by increasing the osmotic activity of the luminal fluid. Dietary fiber and bulk-forming laxatives are also used for symptomatic relief of acute diarrhea in patients with ileostomy or colostomy.

Adverse Effects. Bulk laxatives generally are safe, and few side effects have been reported with their use. However, abdominal fullness, flatulence, and borborygmi are observed frequently. These agents can bind and reduce intestinal absorption of cardiac glycosides, salicylates, nitrofurantoin, and a variety of other drugs. Bulk laxatives should be taken with caution when taking other medications that affect GI motility (155).

Preparations and Dosages. (*a*) Psyllium husk is rich in mycelioid, which, on reaction with water, forms a sticky gelatinous mass. The usual dose is 2.5 to 4 g orally two to three times a day in 250 ml of fruit juice, water, or other liquid. (*b*) Methylcellulose and carbomethylcellulose sodium are also available as capsules and oral solution. The usual dose is 2 to 6 g/day in two or three divided doses. (*c*) Polycarbophil and calcium polycarbophil are polyacrylic resins with maximal water-binding capacity. As calcium polycarbophil contains calcium, its use should be avoided in patients with disorders of hypercalcemia. The dose is 1 g once a day, to four times a day. Each dose should be taken with 250 ml of water.

SALINE AND OSMOTIC LAXATIVES

The saline and osmotic laxatives include various magnesium salts, lactulose, glycerine, and sorbitol. These laxatives act via their osmotic properties in the luminal fluids, as they are poorly absorbed. In addition, the magnesium salt can stimulate cholecystokinin, which, in turn, stimulates fluid secretion and mobility (156). Lactulose is metabolized by bacteria in the colon to lactate, which is partially absorbed and augments lactulose's osmotic effects. Lactulose also causes reduction in the intestinal absorption of ammonia as a result of its decreased production and increased utilization by intestinal bacteria. Furthermore, fecal secretion of ammonia is enhanced because lactulose traps ammonia as ammonium ions and helps to lower ammonia concentration in patients with hepatic encephalopathy associated with chronic liver disease.

Adverse Effects. Administration of magnesium salts should be avoided in patients with impaired renal function because there is a greater likelihood of accumulation and toxicity. Similarly, sodium salts should be avoided in patients with congestive heart failure. Furthermore, hypertonic solutions of saline laxatives can lead to dehydration and should be administered with a sufficient quantity of water. Lactulose can cause abdominal discomfort, flatulence, cramps, and, occasionally, nausea and vomiting. Since lactulose contains glucose and fructose, it should also be used with caution in patients with diabetes mellitus.

Preparation and Dosages. (*a*) *Magnesium sulfate:* The usual dose is 10 to 15 g (5 g contains 40 mEq of magnesium).

Table 36.3.   Classification and Comparison of Representative Laxatives[a]

	Onset of Action (hr)	Site of Action	Mechanism of Action	Comments
1. Bulk producing				
Methylcellulose	12–24	Small and	Holds water in stool;	Safest and most
Psyllium	(up to 72)	large	mechanical distension	physiologic
Polycarbophil		intestine	reduces fecal pH	
2. Saline and osmotic				
Magnesium sulfate	0.5–3	Small and	Retains water in intestinal	May alter fluid and
Magnesium hydroxide		large	lumen, increasing	electrolyte balance;
Magnesium citrate		intestine	intraluminal pressure;	sulfate salts are
			cholecystokinin release	considered potent
Sodium phosphate/biphosphate enema	0.03–0.25	Colon		
Glycerin suppository	0.25–0.5	Colon	Local irritation; hyperosmotic action	
Lactulose	24–48	Colon	Delivers osmotically active molecules to colon	Also indicated in portal systemic encephalopathy
3. Irritant/stimulant				
Phenolphthalein	6–10	Colon	Direct action on intestinal	Bile must be present
Bisacodyl tablets			mucosa; stimulates	for phenolphthalein
			myenteric plexus; alters	to produce its effect
			water and electrolyte	
			secretion	
Bisacodyl suppository	0.25–1			
Senna				
Castor oil	2–6	Small intestine	Converted to ricinoleic acid (active component) in the gut	
Docusate	24–72	Small and large intestine	Detergent activity; facilitates admixture of fat and water to soften stool	Beneficial when feces is hard or dry

[a] Adapted from Olin BR: Gastrointestinal drugs. In *Drug Facts and Comparisons.* JB Lippincott, St Louis, 1990, pp 1355–1462.

This compound has a bitter taste and should be taken with citrus fruit juice. (*b*) *Milk of Magnesia* (*aqueous suspension of magnesium hydroxide*): The usual dose for adults is 15 to 40 ml and contains 40 to 110 mEq of magnesium. Magnesium hydroxide in tablet form has a dose of 1.8 to 3.6 g, which contains 62 to 124 mEq of magnesium. (*c*) *Sodium phosphate:* This is a pleasant-tasting bulk laxative. The usual dose is 1.8 g in 20 to 30 ml, to be taken with plenty of water. (*d*) *Polyethylene glycol (solution):* This laxative provides 67 g polyethylene glycol per liter and contains a mixture of sodium sulfate, sodium bicarbonate, sodium chloride, and potassium chloride in an isotonic solution. The patient drinks 4 liters of this solution over a 4-hour period to clean the bowel. Dehydration does not occur, as the fluid administered is isotonic. (*e*) *Lactulose:* This preparation is available as lactulose syrup. Each 15 ml of lactulose syrup contains 10 g of lactulose, 2.2 g of galactose, 1.2 g of lactose, and 1.2 g of other sugars. Doses vary from 7 to 10 g to 40 g/day. For chronic hepatic encephalopathy, the maintenance dose is 20 to 30 g (i.e., 30 to 45 ml) given three or four times a day and adjusted to provide a fecal pH of 5 to 5.5. (*f*) *Glycerin:* This agent acts as an osmotic to soften and lubricate the passage of inspissated feces. It may also stimulate rectal contraction. Rectal suppositories of glycerin promote colonic motility within 30 minutes and are available in strengths of 4 to 10 ml per suppository. (*g*) *Sorbitol:* This agent acts as an osmotic when administered rectally as an enema (120 ml of a 25 to 30% solution for adults and 30 to 60 ml for children). Sorbitol can also be administered as a 70% solution (60 ml every 2 hours to induce osmotic diarrhea)

and can counteract the constipating effects of sodium polystyrene sulfonate used in the treatment of hyperkalemia.

STIMULANT LAXATIVES

These compounds stimulate accumulation of water and electrolytes in the colonic lumen and enhance intestinal motility. These pharmacologic agents also increase the permeability of the intestinal mucosa by making tight junctions leaky. Stimulant laxatives also increase the synthesis of prostaglandins and cAMP and thus contribute to increased secretion of water and electrolytes. Diphenylmethane derivatives (i.e., phenolphthalein and bisacodyl) act primarily on the colon.

Phenolphthalein. The onset of laxative action takes at least 6 hours. Fifteen percent of the dose is absorbed and eliminated by the kidney, mostly in a conjugated form. The urine becomes pink if sufficiently alkaline. Phenolphthalein needs bile to produce its laxative effect. It is available in tablet form for adults in doses of 30 to 200 mg, and 15 to 60 mg for children.

Bisacodyl. Five percent of the orally administered dose of bisacodyl is absorbed and excreted in urine as glucuronidase. Bisacodyl commonly is marketed in 5-mg enteric coated tablets, 10-mg suppositories, and suspension (10 mg/30 ml). The recommended oral dose of bisacodyl is 10 to 15 mg for adults and 5 to 10 mg for children. Adverse effects of both derivatives of diphenylmethane include fluid and electrolyte deficits resulting from excessive and chronic laxative abuse. Allergic reactions include fixed drug eruption, Steven Johnson syndrome, lupus-like syndrome, osteomalacia, and protein-losing gastroenteropathy.

ANTHRAQUINONE DERIVATIVES

The anthraquinone derivatives are glycoside derivatives of 1,8-dihydroxyanthraquinone and are poorly absorbed from the small intestine. Their adverse effects include excessive laxative effect and abdominal pain. As the anthraquinone is secreted in breast milk, nursing mothers should be warned against its usage. In high doses, these pharmacologic agents can cause nephritis. Senna produces bowel evacuation within 6 hours, with considerable griping abdominal pain. The adult dose is 30 mg, which is available in both tablet and liquid form.

Castor Oil

In the intestine, pancreatic lipase hydrolyzes castor oil to glycerol and ricinoleic acid. Ricinoleic acid and its salts reduce net absorption of fluid and electrolytes in the colon and stimulate intestinal peristalsis. Castor oil stimulates uterine contractions and can cause abortions in pregnancy. The adult dose is 15 to 60 ml orally at bedtime.

Docusates

Docusates are used primarily as stool softeners. These compounds hydrate and soften the stool by emulsifying the feces and also facilitate admixture of water and fat. Occasionally, these compounds can cause nausea. Available as capsules, the daily dose is 50 to 500 mg, with a usual dose of 100 mg twice daily.

ANTIEMETICS

Symptomatic relief of nausea and vomiting is frequently a very important issue with critically ill patients. Proper control of nausea and vomiting is essential to prevent fluid and electrolytes imbalances in the presence of other illnesses. Although the underlying causes of vomiting should be treated primarily, antiemetic agents prove invaluable to tide over the acute illness. Available antiemetic agents can be divided into four classes: (*a*) phenothiazines, (*b*) benzamides, (*c*) cannabinoids, and (*d*) antihistaminics. The important role of dopamine in the function of the chemoreceptor trigger zone and as a mediator of motor reflexes in the stomach presumably is the basis for the antiemetic effect of dopamine antagonists.

PHENOTHIAZINE

Representative drugs of this group are prochlorperazine (compazine) and chlorpromazine (thorazine). These drugs constitute an important group of antiemetic agents that are commonly used to counteract vomiting secondary to radiation exposure, gastroenteritis, cancer chemotherapy, exposure to anesthetic agents, and ingestion of drugs such as estrogens and tetracycline (157). Phenothiazines also have antihistaminic and anticholinergic properties. These compounds reduce the dopamine transmission in the chemoreceptor trigger zone

(CTZ) area and decrease afferent signals to the vomiting center. Prochlorperazine has a high incidence of dystonia, especially when given intramuscularly. Administration of phenothiazine can mask diagnostic symptoms in acute surgical conditions. Sedation, dysphagia, and jaundice have been described as side effects of these drugs.

ANTIHISTAMINICS

These drugs have H_1-receptor antagonistic activity and occasionally are used in the treatment of nausea associated with pregnancy (morning sickness). Antihistaminics have also been shown to be very useful in motion sickness or vomiting resulting from other vestibular disorders. Scopolamine, another H_1-antihistamine, is widely used for motion sickness and is available as a transdermal patch.

CANNABINOLS

Tetrahydrocannabinoid is the active ingredient in marijuana and is quite effective in preventing nausea and vomiting after cancer chemotherapy. It has also been shown to be more effective than phenothiazine in such instances (158, 159). Side effects of these drugs include drowsiness, orthostatic hypotension, tachycardia, and dry mouth. Less common side effects include anxiety, depression, visual hallucinations, and manic psychosis. These symptoms have been seen more in elderly patients.

BENZAMIDE

The primary agent of the benzamide class is metoclopramide, which was discussed in detail in the section on Drugs for Gastroparesis and Clonic Inertia.

MISCELLANEOUS AGENTS

High-dose dexamethasone and adrenocorticotropic hormone (ACTH) have also been shown to be effective in counteracting emesis in chemotherapy patients (160). Furthermore, neither ACTH nor dexamethasone is particularly effective as a single agent, but each is very effective in combination with any of the agents described previously (161).

DRUGS FOR INFLAMMATORY BOWEL DISEASE

SULFASALAZINE AND AMINOSALICYLATES

Indications. Sulfasalazine is indicated for the treatment of ulcerative colitis and Crohn's colitis. In patients with ulcerative colitis, sulfasalazine is also used to maintain remission (162–164).

Pharmacokinetics and Mechanism of Action. Sulfasalazine is partially absorbed in the proximal jejunum, and a small fraction of the absorbed drug is excreted unchanged in the urine. The remaining portion of the absorbed drug is returned to the intestine unchanged in the bile, while a portion of the drug traverses the intestine intact until it encounters bacterial flora in the distal ileum and colon (165, 166). The intestinal bacteria initiate the first step in the metabolism of sulfasalazine, cleaving the azo bond that joins the sulfapyridine and the 5-amino-salicylic acid (5-ASA) moieties (167, 168). The sulfa portion is largely absorbed and, after achieving high blood levels, is metabolized by the liver and excreted in the urine. Most of the intolerance associated with sulfasalazine can be attributed to the serum sulfapyridine level. The 5-ASA portion remains largely intact and acts on the colonic mucosa until excreted in the stool. If either sulfapyridine or 5-ASA is orally ingested separately, each is absorbed in the proximal small bowel, metabolized by the liver, and excreted in the urine, thus never achieving substantial levels in the distal intestine (169). Therefore, the parent drug sulfasalazine may be merely a vehicle for the delivery of the active component, 5-ASA, to the distal ileum and colon. Both 5-ASA and sulfasalazine act as inhibitors of the initial enzyme lipoxygenase in arachidonic acid metabolism, and this results in the lowering of leukotriene levels in patients with inflammatory bowel disease (170, 171). 5-ASA may also act as a scavenger of oxygen-derived free radicals that are known to be toxic to the cell. As a possible inhibitor of antibodies, its action may be directed at colonic antigens that promote intestinal cell destruction (172).

Dosage and Route of Administration.   A comparison of 5-ASA enemas with sulfapyridine and sulfasalazine enemas has shown that significant clinical and sigmoidoscopic improvement occurred in 5-ASA and sulfasalazine groups as compared with response in the sulfapyridine group. Some additional trials have documented the efficacy of 5-ASA enemas (dose 1 to 4 g/day) in patients with distal ulcerative colitis. In addition, 5-ASA suppositories (dose 200 mg to 1 g two or three times daily) in patients with active proctitis and/or distal colitis provide high doses to the most distal bowel and are effective.

Sulfasalazine is available in 500-mg tablets and a suspension of 250 mg/5 ml. The initial therapy begins with a total dose of 1 or 2 g and then is slowly brought up to the dose of 3 to 4 g (173, 174). Oral forms of 5-ASA have been developed (i.e., olsalazine) (175) and currently are available in the U.S. (dose 500 mg twice daily, orally). 5-ASA enemas are also commercially available.

Adverse Reactions.   The sulfapyridine moiety is considered to be responsible for most of the adverse effects of sulfasalazine. Adverse effects of sulfasalazine include Heinz body anemia, acute hemolysis in patients with glucose-6-phosphatase deficiency (G_6PD) and agranulocytosis. Nausea, fever, arthralgia, and rash occur in up to 20% of patients treated with sulfasalazine. More recently, several patients have been reported to have an exacerbation of colitis with 5-ASA enemas that presumably may be related to sulfides used as preservatives in them. Furthermore, several side effects have been reported with oral 5-ASA, which include perimyocarditis and pancreatitis (176, 177). Ten to twenty percent of patients will experience a reaction to 5-ASA identical to that to sulfasalazine which clearly implicates 5-ASA, rather than sulfur, as the offending agent. Therefore, care must be taken when placing any patient who is allergic to sulfasalazine on 5-ASA.

Special Considerations.   The disappointment in drug therapy for inflammatory bowel disease has been the inability

of sulfasalazine to show efficacy in maintaining remission in patients with Crohn's disease. Although topical steroids have proved to be effective for patients with distal colitis, oral prednisone continues to be the principal medication against moderate or severely active ulcerative colitis and Crohn's disease. Neither sulfasalazine nor steroids are effective in maintaining remission in patients with Crohn's disease. Both azathioprine and 6-mercaptopurine appear to be effective agents in patients with Crohn's disease and ulcerative colitis that is in remission (175, 178, 179). However, the use of these two drugs is limited by adverse side effects such as development of lymphoma and occurrence of life-threatening neutropenia in patients with hematologic malignancy and rheumatoid arthritis (180, 181). At present, azathioprine or 6-mercaptopurine should be considered only in patients with Crohn's disease that is refractory to treatment with other agents such as sulfasalazine and corticosteroids. In recent years, metronidazole has been demonstrated to be effective in patients with Crohn's disease involving the perineal area and colon. Furthermore, metronidazole is also currently recommended for patients with Crohn's colitis or ileocolitis of mild to moderate severity who do not respond to or tolerate sulfasalazine therapy.

REFERENCES

1. Lucas CE, Sugawa C, Ridelle J, et al: Natural history and surgical dilemma of "stress" gastritis bleeding. *Arch Surg* 102:266–273, 1971.
2. Skillimann JJ, Bushnell LS, Silen W, et al: Respiratory failure, hypotension, sepsis and jaundice: a clinical syndrome associated with lethal hemorrhage from acute stress ulceration of the stomach. *Am J Surg* 117(4):523–530, 1969.
3. Fiddian-Green RG, McGough E, Pittenger G, et al: Predictive value of intramural pH and other risk factors for massive bleeding from stress ulceration. *Gastroenterology* 85:613–620, 1983.
4. Peterson WL, Sturdervant R, McCallum RW, et al: Healing of a duodenal ulcer with antacid regimen. *N Engl J Med* 227:341–347, 1977.
5. Lam SK: Antacids: the past, the present, the future. In Bayless TM (ed): *Current Therapy in Gastroenterology and Liver Disease* 2:641–654; BC Decker, Philadelphia, 1988.
6. Kumar N, Vij J, Kamal A, et al: Controlled therapeutic trial to determine the optimum dose of antacids in duodenal ulcer. *Gut* 25:1199–1202, 1984.
7. Brunton LL: Agents for control of gastric acidity and peptic ulcer. In Gilman AG, Rall TW, Nies AS, Taylor P (eds): The Pharmacological Basis of Therapeutics, ed 8. McGraw-Hill, New York, pp 897–913, 1990.
8. Ansari A: Antacid induced phosphorous depletion and repletion. *Minn Med* 53:837–838, 1970.
9. Harvey SC: Gastric antacids and digestants. In Gilman AG, Goodman LS (eds): A Pharmacologic Basis of Therapeutics, ed 6. MacMillan New York, pp 988–1001, 1980.
10. Berlyne GM, Ben Air J, Pist D, et al: Hyperaluminemia from aluminum resins in renal failure. *Lancet* 2:494–496, 1970.
11. Drake D, Hollander D: Neutralizing capacity and cost effectiveness of antacids. *Ann Intern Med* 94:215–217, 1981.
12. Ivanovich P, Fellows H, Ruth C: The absorption of calcium carbonate. *Ann Intern Med* 60:917–923, 1967.
13. Fordtran JS: Acid rebound. *N Engl J Med* 279:900–905, 1968.
14. Clarkson EM, McDonald SJ, DeWardner HW: The effect of high intake of calcium carbonate in normal subjects and patients with chronic renal failure. *Clin Sci* 30:425–438, 1966.
15. Makoff DZ, Gordon A, Franklin AS, et al: Chronic calcium carbonate therapy in uremia. *Arch Intern Med* 123:15–21, 1969.
16. McMillan DE, Freeman RB: The milk alkali syndrome: a study of the acute disorder with comments on development of the chronic condition. *Medicine (Baltimore)* 44:485–501, 1965.
17. Orwell ES: The milk alkali syndrome: current concepts. *Ann Intern Med* 97:242–248, 1982.
18. Elsborg L, Boysen K, Bruusgaard A, et al: Sucralfate versus placebo treatment in duodenal and prepyloric ulcer: a clinical endoscopic double-blind controlled investigation. *Hepatogastroenterology* 31:269–271, 1984.
19. Hollander D: Efficacy of sucralfate for duodenal ulcers: a multicenter double-blind trial. *J Clin Gastroenterol* 3(suppl 2):153–157, 1981.
20. McHardy GG: A multicenter double-blind trial of sucralfate and placebo in duodenal ulcer. *J Clin Gastroenterol* 3(suppl 2):147–152, 1981.

21. Lam SK, Hui WM, Lau WY, et al: Sucralfate overcomes adverse effect of cigarette smoking on duodenal ulcer healing and prolongs subsequent remission. *Gastroenterology* 92:1193–1201, 1987.

22. Martin F, Farley A, Gagnon M, et al: Short-term treatment with sucralfate or cimetidine in gastric ulcer: preliminary results of a controlled randomized trial. *Scand J Gastroenterol Suppl* 83:37–41, 1983.

23. Hallerback H, Anker-Hansen O, Carling I, et al: Short-term treatment of gastric ulcer: a comparison of sucralfate and cimetidine. *Gut* 27:778–783, 1986.

24. Hjortrup A, Svendsen LB, Beck H, et al: Two daily doses of sucralfate or cimetidine in the healing of gastric ulcer: a comparative randomized study. *Am J Med* 86(suppl 6A):113–115, 1989.

25. Peterson WL: Pharmacotherapy of bleeding peptic ulcer–is it time to give up the search? *Gastroenterology* 97:796–797, 1989.

26. Jensen DM, Osterhaus J, You S, et al: Health and economic impact of ranitidine in a randomized controlled study of patients with a recent severe duodenal ulcer hemorrhage [Abstract]. *Gastroenterology* 98(suppl):A5, 1990.

27. Barrier CH, Hirshowitz BI: Controversies in the detection and management of nonsteroidal and antiinflammatory drug-induced side effects of the upper gastrointestinal tract. *Arthritis Rheum* 32:926–932, 1989.

28. Caldwell JR, Roth SH, Wu WC, et al: Sucralfate treatment of nonsteroidal antiinflammatory drug-induced gastrointestinal symptoms and mucosal damage. *Am J Med* 83(suppl 3B):74–82, 1987.

29. Wu WC, Semble EL, Castell DO, et al: Sucralfate therapy of nonsteroidal antiinflammatory drug-induced gastritis [Abstract]. *Gastroenterology* 88:1636, 1985.

30. Carling L, Cronstedt J, Engqvist A, et al: Sucralfate versus placebo in reflux esophagitis: a double-blind multicenter study. *Scand J Gastroenterol* 23:1117–1124, 1988.

31. Weiss W, Brunner H, Buttner GR, et al: Treatment of reflux esophagitis with sucralfate. *Dtsch Med Wochenschr* 108:1706–1711, 1983.

32. Singal AK, Sarin SK, Misra SP, et al: Ulceration after esophageal and gastric variceal sclerotherapy—influence of sucralfate and other factors on healing. *Endoscopy* 20:238–240, 1988.

33. Tabibian N, Smith JL, Graham DY: Sclerotherapy associated esophageal ulcers: lessons from a double-blind, randomized comparison of sucralfate suspension versus placebo. *Gastrointest Endosc* 35:312–315, 1989.

34. Lingusky M, Karmski F, Ruchmilewitz D: Sucralfate stimulation of gastric PGE synthesis: possible mechanism to explain its effective cytoprotective mechanism. *Gastroenterology* 86:1164, 1984.

35. Nagishumo R: Mechanisms of action of sucralfate. *J Clin Gastroenterol* 3(suppl 2):117–127, 1981.

36. Carafate (Sucralfate): Package insert. Marion Laboratories, Kansas City, MO, 1985.

37. Leung ACT, Henderson IS, Halls DJ, et al: Aluminum hydroxide versus sucralfate as a phosphate binder in uremia. *BMJ* 286:1379–1381, 1983.

38. Sherman RA, Hwang ER, Walker JA, et al: Reduction in serum phosphorus due to sucralfate. *Am J Gastroenterol* 78:210–211, 1983.

39. The effect of sucralfate pretreatment on the pharmacokinetics of ciprofloxacin. *Pharmacotherapy* 9:377–380, 1989.

40. Nix DE, Wilton JH, Schentag JJ, et al: Inhibition of norfloxacin absorption by antacids and sucralfate [Abstract]. *Rev Infect Dis* 11(suppl 5):S1096, 1989.

41. Parpia SH, Nix DE, Hejmanowski LG, et al: Sucralfate reduces the gastrointestinal absorption of norfloxacin. *Antimicrob Agents Chemother* 33:99–102, 1989.

42. Cantral KA, Schaaf LJ, Jungnickel PW, et al: Effect of sucralfate on theophylline absorption in healthy volunteers. *Clin Pharm* 7:58–61, 1988.

43. Lacz JP, Groschang AG, Giesing DH, et al: The effect of sucralfate on drug absorption in dogs [Abstract]. *Gastroenterology* 82:1108, 1982.

44. Hall TG, Cuddy PG, Glass CJ, et al: Effect of sucralfate on phenytoin bioavailability. *Drug Intell Clin Pharm* 20:607–611, 1986.

45. Giesing DH, Lanman RC, Dimmit DC, et al: Lack of effect of sucralfate on digoxin pharmacokinetics [Abstract]. *Gastroenterology* 84:1165, 1983.

46. Ryan R, Carlson J, Farris F: Effect of sucralfate on the absorption and disposition of amitriptyline in humans [Abstract]. *Fed Proc* 45:205, 1986.

47. Brandstaetter G, Kratochvil P: Comparison of two sucralfate dose (2 gm bid vs 1 gm bid) in duodenal ulcer healing. *Am J Med* 79(suppl 2C):18–20, 1985.

48. Ishimori A: Safety experience with sucralfate in Japan. *J Clin Gastroenterol* 3(suppl 2):169–173, 1981.

49. Konturek SJ, Bizozowski T, Bielanski W, et al: Epidermal growth factor in the gastroprotective and ulcer-healing actions of sucralfate in rats. *Am J Med* 86:(suppl 6A):32–37, 1989.

50. Algozzine GJ, Hill G, Scoggins WG, et al: Sucralfate bezoar. *N Engl J Med* 309:1387, 1983.

51. Campistol JM Cases A, Botey A, et al: Acute aluminum encephalopathy in an uremic patient. *Nephron* 51:103–106, 1989.

52. Driks MR, Craven DE, Celi BR, et al: Nosocomial pneumonia in intubated patients given sucralfate as compared with antacids or histamine type 2 blockers: the role of gastric colonization. *N Engl J Med* 317:1376–1382, 1987.

53. Tryba M: Risk of acute stress bleeding and nosocomial pneumonia in ventilated intensive care unit patients: sucralfate versus antacids. *Am J Med* 83(suppl 3B):117–124, 1987.

54. Sachs G: The parietal cell as a therapeutic target. *Scand J Gastroenterol Suppl* 118:1–10, 1986.

55. Sachs G, Carllson E: H^+K^+ ATPase as therapeutic target. *Annu Rev Pharmacol* 28:269–284, 1988.

56. Helander NF, Herschowitz BI: Quantitative ultrastructural studies on inhibited and on partly stimulated gastric paretial cells. *Gastroenterology* 67:447–452, 1974.

57. Smotke A, Helander NF, Sachs G: Monoclonal antibodies against gastric H^+K^+ ATPase. *Am J Physiol* 245:6589–6596, 1983.

58. Lundberg P, Nordberg P, Almenger T, et al: The mechanism of action of the gastric acid secretion inhibitor—omeprazole. *J Med Chem* 24:1327–1329, 1986.

59. Lorentizen P, Jackson R: Inhibition of H^+K^+ ATPase by omeprazole in isolated gastric vesicles requires proton transport. *Biochem Biophys Acta* 897:41–51, 1987.

60. Im WB, Blakeman D, Davis JP: Irreversible inactivation of the rate of gastric acid secretion in vivo by omeprazole. *Biochem Biophys Res Com* 126:78–82, 1985.

61. Reganth CB: Pharmacokinetics and metabolism of omeprazole in man. *Scand J Gastroenterol Suppl* 118:99–104, 1986.

62. Pichard PJ, Yeomans NK, Mihly GW: Omeprazole: a study of its inhibition of gastric pH and oral pharmacokinetics after morning or evening doses. *Gastroenterology* 88:64–69, 1985.

63. Lind T, Cederburg C, Ebenved G, et al: Effect of omeprazole—a gastric proton pump inhibitor—on pentagastrin stimulated acid secretion in man. *Gut* 24:2470–276, 1983.

64. Sharma BK, Walt RP, Pounder RE, et al: Optimal dose of oral omeprazole for maximal 24 hr decrease of intragastric acidity. *Gut* 25:957, 1984.

65. Gowden CW, Derodra JK, Burget DW, Hunt RN: Effects of low dose omeprazole on gastric secretion and plasma gastrin in patients with healed duodenal ulcer. *Hepatogastroenterology* 33:267, 1986.

66. Festen HPM, Tuynman NA, Defizi T, et al: Effect of single and repeated doses of oral omeprazole on gastric acid and pepsin secretion and fasting serum gastrin and serum pepsinogen I levels. *Dig Dis Sci* 23:1259–1266, 1986.

67. Carlsson E, Larsson H, Mattsson N, et al: Pharmacology and toxicology of omeprazole with special reference to effects on the gastric mucosa. *Scand J Gastroenterol Suppl* 118:31–38, 1986.

68. Sharma BK, Santana IA, Wood EC: Intragastric bacterial activity and nitrosation before, during and after treatment with omeprazole. *BMJ* 289:717–719, 1984.

69. Howden CW, Hurt RH: Relationship between gastric secretion and infection. *Gut* 28:96–107, 1987.

70. Wormsley KG: Assessing the safety of drugs for long term treatment of peptic ulcers. *Gut* 25:1416–1423, 1984.

71. Wolfe MM, Soll AH: The physiology of gastric acid secretion. *N Engl J Med* 319:1707–1715, 1988.

72. Steinberg HM, Lewis JH, Katz DM: Antacids inhibit absorption of cimetidine. *N Engl J Med* 98; 307(2):400–404.

73. Gugler R, Brand M, Somogyi A: Impaired cimetidine absorption due to antacids and metoclopramide. *Eur J Clin Pharmacol* 20:225–228, 1981.

74. Binder HJ, Donaldson RM Jr: Effect of cimetidine on intrinsic factor and pepsin secretion in man. *Gastroenterology* 74:371–375, 1978.

75. Longstreth AF, Go CLW, Malagelada JR: Postprandial gastric, pancreatic and biliary response to histamine H_2 receptor antagonists in active duodenal ulcer. *Gastroenterology* 72:9–13, 1977.

76. Ma KW, Brown D, Masler DS, et al: Effects of renal failure on blood levels of cimetidine. *Gastroenterology* 74(2):473–477, 1978.

77. Vaziri ND, Ness RL, Barton CH: Peritoneal dialysis clearance of cimetidine. *Am J Gastroenterol* 71(6):572–576, 1979.

78. Somogyi A, Gugler R: Clinical pharmacokinetics of cimetidine. *Clin Pharmacokinet* 8:463–495, 1983.

79. Festen HPM, Diemel J, Lamers CBH: Is the measurement of blood cimetidine levels useful? *Br J Clin Pharmacol* 12:417–421, 1981.

80. Bulkard WP: Histamine H_2 receptor binding with ^3H-cimetidine in brain. *Eur J Pharmacol* 50:449–450, 1978.

81. Sancho JM, Garcia-Robles R, Mancheno E, et al: Interference by ranitidine with aldosterone secretion in vivo. *Eur J Clin Pharmacol* 27:495–497, 1984.

82. Fujimura A, Ohashi K, Sudo T, et al: Effects of H_2 receptor antagonists on plasma aldosterone response to angiotensin II in healthy subjects. II. Comparison of cimetidine and ranitidine. *J Clin Pharmacol* 29:230–233, 1989.

83. Aymard J-P, Aymard B, Netter P, et al: Haematological adverse effects of histamine H_2 receptor antagonists. *Med Toxicol Adverse Drug Exp* 3:430–448, 1988.

84. Brogden RN, Heel RC, Speight TM, et al: Cimetidine: a review of its pharmacological properties and therapeutic efficacy in peptic ulcer disease. *Drugs* 15:93–131, 1978.

85. Lewis JH: Hepatic effects of drugs used in the treatment of peptic ulcer disease. *Am J Gastroenterol* 82:987–1003, 1987.

86. Matthews SJ, Michelson PA, Cersosimo RJ: Cimetidine-induced sinus bradycardia. *Clin Pharm* 11:556–558, 1982.

87. Hughes DG, Dowling EA, DeMeesman RE, et al: Cardiovascular effects of H_2 receptor antagonists. *J Clin Pharmacol* 29:472–477, 1989.

88. Mavligit GM: Immunologic effects of cimetidine: potential uses. *Pharmacotherapy* 7(suppl 2):120S–124S, 1987.

89. Kurzrock R, Auber M, Mavligit GM: Cimetidine therapy of herpes simplex virus infections in immunocompromised patients. *Clin Exp Dermatol* 12:326–331, 1987.

90. Kogan FJ, Sampliner RE, Mayersohn M, et al: Cimetidine disposition in patients undergoing continuous ambulatory peritoneal dialysis. *J Clin Pharmacol* 23:252–256, 1983.

91. Binder HJ, Cocco A, Crossley RJ, et al: Cimetidine in the treatment of duodenal ulcer: a multicenter double blind study. *Gastroenterology* 74:380–388, 1978.

92. Brogden RN, Carmine AA, Heel RC, et al: Ranitidine: a review of its pharmacology and therapeutic use in peptic ulcer disease and other allied diseases. *Drugs* 24:267–303, 1982.

93. Peden NR, Saunders JHB, Wormsley KG: Inhibition of pentagastrin-stimulated and nocturnal gastric secretion by ranitidine: a new H_2 receptor antagonist. *Lancet* 1:690–692, 1979.

94. Martin LE, Oxford J, Tanner RJN: Use of high-performance liquid chromatography-mass spectrometry for the study of the metabolism of ranitidine in man. *J Chromatogr* 251:215–224, 1982.

95. Young CJ, Daneshmend TK, Roberts CJC: Effects of cirrhosis and aging on the elimination and bioavailability of ranitidine. *Gut* 23:819–823, 1982.

96. Berner BD, Conner CS, Sawyer DR, et al: Ranitidine: a new H_2 receptor antagonist. *Clin Pharm* 1:499–509, 1982.

97. Langman MJS, Henry DA, Bell GD, et al: Cimetidine and ranitidine in duodenal ulcer. *Br Med J* 281:473–474, 1980.

98. Mignon M, Vallot T, Bonfils S: Use of ranitidine in the management of Zollinger-Ellison syndrome. In: The clinical use of ranitidine. Misiewicz JT, Wormsley KG: Oxford, *Medicine Publishing Foundation.* pp 281–282, 1982.

99. Jack D, Richards DA, Granata F: Side effects of ranitidine. *Lancet* 2:264–265, 1982.

100. Jack D, Smith RN, Richards DA: Histamine H_2 antagonists and the heart. *Lancet* 2:1281, 1982.

101. Camarri E, Chirone E, Fanteria G, et al: Ranitidine induced bradycardia. *Lancet* 2:160, 1982.

102. Grant SM, Langtry ND, Brogden RN: Ranitidine: an updated review of its pharmacodynamic and pharmacokinetic properties and therapeutic use in peptic ulcer disease and other allied diseases. *Drugs* 38:551–590, 1989.

103. Jensen RT, Collen MJ, Pandol SJ, et al: Cimetidine-induced impotence and breast changes in patients with gastric hypersecretory states. *N Engl J Med* 308:883–887, 1983.

104. Galbraith RA, Michnovicz JJ: The effects of cimetidine on the oxidative metabolism of estradiol. *N Engl J Med* 321:269–274, 1989.

105. deGalocsy C, van Ypersele de Strihou C: Pancytopenia with cimetidine. *Ann Intern Med* 90:274, 1979.

106. Nichols TW Jr: Phytobezoar formation: a new complication of cimetidine therapy. *Ann Intern Med* 95:70, 1981.

107. Reed PI, Smith PLR, Haines K, et al: Effect of cimetidine on gastric juice *N*-nitrosamine concentration. *Lancet* 2:553–556, 1981.

108. Stockbrugger RW, Cotton PB, Eugenides N, et al: Intragastric nitrites, nitrosamines, and bacterial overgrowth during cimetidine treatment. *Gut* 23:1048–1054, 1982.

109. Milton-Thompson CGJ, Lightfoot NF, Ahmet Z, et al: Intragastric acidity, bacteria, nitrite, and N-nitroso compounds before, during, and after cimetidine treatment. *Lancet* 1:1091–1095, 1982.

110. Campoli S, Richards DM, Clissold SP: Famotidine: pharmacodynamic and pharmacokinetic properties and preliminary review of its therapeutic use in peptic ulcer disease and Zollinger-Ellison syndrome. *Drugs* 32:197–221, 1986.

111. Burck JD, Myka JA, Kokelman DK: Famotidine: summary of preclinical safety assessment. *Digestion* 32:7–14, 1985.

112. Drug Information File: Merck Sharp & Dohme, West Point, PA, 1988.

113. Smith J, Torey C: Clinical pharmacology of famotidine. *Digestion* 32:15–23, 1985.

114. Knadler MP, Bergstrom RF, Callaghan JT, et al: Absorption studies of the H_2 blocker nizatidine. *Clin Pharmacol Ther* 42:514–520, 1987.

115. Aronoff GR, Bergstom RF, Bopp RJ, et al: Nizatidine disposition in subjects with normal and impaired renal function. *Clin Pharmacol Ther* 43:688–695, 1988.

116. Konturek SJ: Gastric cytoprotection. *Scand J Gastroenterol* 20:543–553, 1985.

117. Robert A: Cytoprotection of the gastrointestinal mucosa. *Adv Intern Med* 28:325–337, 1983.

118. Stern WC: Summary of the 33rd meeting of the FDA's Gastrointestinal Drugs Advisory Committee, September 15–16, 1988. *Am J Gastroenterol* 84:351–354, 1989.

119. Graham DY, Agrawal NM, Roth SM: Prevention of NSAID induced gastric ulcer with misoprostol: multi-center double-blind, placebo-controlled trial. *Lancet* 2:1277–1280, 1988.

120. Olin BR: Gastrointestinal drugs. In Drug Facts and Comparisons. JB Lippincott, St Louis, MO, pp 1355–1462, 1990.

121. Binder HJ: Absorption and secretion of water and electrolytes by small and large intestine. In Sleisinger MH, Fordtran JS (eds): *Gastrointestinal Disease,* ed 4. WB Saunders, Philadelphia, pp 1022–1045, 1984.

122. DuPont NL: Nonfluid therapy and selected chemoprophylaxis of acute diarrhea. *Am J Med* 78(suppl 6B):81–90, 1985.

123. Gorbach SL (ed): Pathophysiology of gastrointestinal infections: the role of bismuth subsalicylate. *Rev Infectious Dis* 112:580–586, 1990.

124. Durrington PN, Manning AP, Bolton CH, et al: Effect of pectin on serum lipids and lipoproteins, whole gut transit time and stool weight. *Lancet* 2:394–396, 1976.

125. Cummings TN, Southgate DAT, Branch WJ, et al: The digestion of pectin in the human gut and its effect on calcium absorption and large bowel function. *Br J Nutr* 41:477–485, 1979.

126. Portnoy BL, Dupont HL, Pruitt D, et al: Antidiarrheal agents in the treatment of acute diarrhea in children. *JAMA* 236:844–846, 1976.

127. Fedorak RN, Field M, Chang EB: Treatment of diabetic diarrhea with clonidine. *Ann Intern Med* 102:197, 1985.

128. Bauer W, Briner U, Doepfrier W, et al: SMS 201-995. A very potent and selective octapeptide analogue of somatostatin with prolonged actions. *Life Sci* 31:1133–1140, 1982.

129. Davies RR, Miller M, Turner SJ, et al: Effects of somatostatin analogue SMS 201-995 in normal man. *Clin Endocrinol Oxford* 24:665–674, 1986.

130. Kutz K, Neusch E, Rosenthaler J: Pharmacokinetics of SMS 201-995 on healthy subjects. *Scand J Gastroenterol* 119(suppl 21):84–85, 1986.

131. Schrezenmier J, Plewe G, Sturmer W, et al: Treatment of APUDomas with the long acting somatostatin analogue (SMS 201–995). Investigation of therapeutic use and digestive side effects. *Scand J Gastroenterol* 21(suppl 119):223–227, 1986.

132. Buchanan KD, Johnston CV, O'Hare MM, et al: Neuroendocrine tumors. A European view. *Am J Med* 81(suppl B):14–22, 1986.

133. Ruskone A, Rene E, Chayville JA, et al: Effect of somatostatin on diarrhea and on small intestinal water and electrolyte transport in a patient with pancreatic cholera. *Dig Dis Sci* 27:459–466, 1982.

134. Justin-Besancon L, Laville L: Le metoclopramide et ses homologues. *CR Acad Sci* (Paris) 258:4384, 1964.

135. Johnson AG: Gastroduodenal motility and synchronization. *Postgrad Med J* 4:649, 1968.

136. McCallum RW, Albibi R: Metoclopramide: pharmacology and clinical application. *Ann Intern Med* 98:86, 1983.

137. Maddern GT, Chatterton BE, Collins PT, et al: Solid and liquid gastric emptying in patients with gastroesophageal reflux. *Br J Surg* 72:344, 1985.

138. McCallum RW, Ricci D, Du Boric S, et al: Effect of domperidone on gastric emptying and symptoms in patients with idiopathic gastric stasis [Abstract]. *Gastroenterology* 66:1179, 1984.

139. Cooke HT, Carey HV: The effects of cisapride on serotonin-evoked mucosal responses in guinea pig ileum. *Eur J Pharmacol* 98:148, 1984.

140. Brisson-Noel A, Trieu Chot P, Courralis P: Mechanism of action of spiramycin and stress macrolides. *J Antimicrob Chemother* 22(suppl B):13–23, 1988.

141. Janssens J, Peeters TL, Vantrappen et al: Improvement of gastric emptying in diabetic gastroparesis by erythromycin. *N Engl J Med* 322(15):1028–1031, 1990.

142. Spence RAJ, Sloan JM, Johnston GW: Esophagitis in patients undergoing esophageal transection for varices: a histological study. *Br J Surgery* 70:332–334, 1983.

143. Garcia-Tsao G, Grozman RJ, Fisher RL, et al: Portal presence of gastroesophageal varices and variceal bleeding. *Hepatology* 5:419–424, 1985.

144. Hays MR: Agents affecting the renal conservation of water. In Goodman LS, Gilman, AG, Rall TW, Nies AS, and Taylor P (eds): Goodman & Gilman's *The Pharmacologic Basis of Therapeutics,* ed 6. Macmillan, New York, pp 732–790, 1985.

145. Tsia Y-T, Lay CS, Lai K-N, et al: Controlled trial of vasopressin plus NTG versus vasopressin alone in the treatment of bleeding esophageal varices. *Hepatology* 6:406–409, 1986.

146. Gimson AES, Westaby D, Hegarty J, et al: A randomized trial of vasopressin and vasopressin and nitroglycerin in the control of cute variceal hemorrhage. *Hepatology* 6:410–413, 1986.

147. Recter WG: Drug therapy for portal hypertension. *Ann Intern Med* 105:96–107, 1986.

148. Freeman TG, Cobden I, Leshman AN, et al: Controlled trial of Terlipressin (glypressin) versus vasopressin in the early treatment of esophageal varices. *Lancet* 2:202–204, 1982.

149. Barsoum MS, Bolous FI, El Rooby AA, et al: Tamponade and injection sclerotherapy in the treatment of bleeding esophageal varies. *Br J Surg* 69:76–78, 1982.

150. Paquet K-J, Feussner H: Endoscopic sclerosis and esophageal balloon tamponade in acute hemorrhage from esophagogastric varies: a prospective controlled randomized trial. *Hepatology* 5:580–583, 1985.

151. Lasson A, Cohen H, Zweiban B, et al: Acute esophageal variceal sclerotherapy. Results of prospective randomized controlled trial. *J Am Med Assoc* 255:497–500, 1986.

152. Tarblanche J, Yakoob HJ, Bornman PC, et al: Acute bleeding varices. A 5 year prospective evaluation of tamponade and sclerotherapy. *Ann Surg* 194:521–530, 1981.

153. Connors AF, Bacon BR, Miron SD: Sodium morrhuate delivery to the lung during endoscopic variceal sclerotherapy. *Arch Intern Med* 105:539–542, 1986.

154. Korula J, Baydur A, Sasoon C, et al: Effect of esophageal variceal sclerotherapy on lung function: a prospective controlled study. *Arch Intern Med* 14:1517–1520, 1986.

155. Brunton LL: Agents effecting water flux and motility, digestants and bile acids. Goodman and Gilman's The Pharmacological Basis of Therapeutics, ed 8. Macmillan, New York, pp 918–923, 1990.

156. Harvey RF, Read AE: Mode of action of the saline purgatives. *Am Med J* 89:810–812, 1975.

157. Wapler G: The pharmacology and clinical effectiveness of phenothiazines and related drugs for managing chemotherapy induced emesis. *Drugs* 25(suppl 1):35, 1983.

158. Synthetic marijuana for nausea and vomiting due to cancer chemotherapy. *Med Lett Drug Ther* 27:97, 1985.

159. Ott LE, McKernan JF, Bloome B: Antiemetic effect of tetrahydrocannabinol. *Arch Intern Med* 140:1431, 1980.

160. Markman L, Sheidler V, Ettinger DS, et al: Antiemetic efficacy of dexamethasone in a randomised double blinded crossover study with prochlorperazine in patients receiving cancer chemotherapy. *N Engl J Med* 311:549, 1984.

161. Eyre HJ, Ward JH: Control of cancer chemotherapy induced nausea and vomiting. *Cancer* 54:2642, 1984.

162. Baron JH, Connell PM, Lennard-Jones JE, et al: Sulphasalazine and salicylazo-sulphadimidine in ulcerative colitis. *Lancet* 1:1094–1096, 1962.

163. Dissanayake AS, Truelove SC: A controlled therapeutic trial of long term maintenance treatment of ulcerative colitis with sulphasalazine (salazophyrin). *Gut* 14:923–926, 1973.

164. Goldstein F, Murdock MG: Clinical and radiologic improvement of regional enteritis and enterocolitis after treatment with salicylazosulfapyridine. *Am J Dig Dis* 16:421–431, 1981.

165. Schroder H, Campbell DE: Absorption, metabolism, and excretion of salicyla-zosulfapyridine in man. *Clin Pharmacol Ther* 13:539–551, 1972.

166. Das KM, Chowdhury JR, Zapp B, et al: Small bowel absorption of sulfasalazine and its hepatic metabolism in human beings, cats, and rats. *Gastroenterology* 77:280–284, 1979.

167. Peppercorn MA, Goldman P: The role of intestinal bacteria in the metabolism of salicylazosulfapyridine. *J Pharmacol Exp Ther* 181:555–562, 1972.

168. Das KM, Eastwood MA, McManus JP, et al: The role of the colon in the metabolism of salicylazosulfapyridine. *Scand J Gastroenterol* 9:137–141, 1974.

169. Peppercorn MA, Goldman P: Distribution studies of salicylazosulfapyridine and its metabolites. *Gastroenterology* 64:240–245, 1973.

170. Stenson WF, Lobos E: Sulfasalazine inhibits the synthesis of chemotactic lipids by neutrophilis. *J Clin Invest* 69:494–497, 1982.

171. Nielsen OH, Bukhave K, Elmgreen J, et al: Inhibition of 5-lipoxygenase pathway of arachidonic acid metabolism in human neutrophils by sulfasalazine and 5-aminosalicylic acid. *Dig Dis Sci* 6:577–582, 1987.

172. MacDermott RP, Schloemann SR, Bertovich MJ, et al: Inhibition of antibody secretion by 5-aminosalicylic acid. *Gastroenterology* 96:442–448, 1989.

173. Willoughby CP, Campieri M, Lanfranchi G, et al: 5-Aminosalicylic acid (Pentasa) in enema form for the treatment of active ulcerative colitis. *Ital J Gastroenterol* 18:15–17, 1986.

174. Danish 5-ASA Group: Topical 5-aminosalicylic acid versus prednisolone in ulcerative proctosigmoiditis. A randomized, double-blind multicenter trial. *Dig Dis Sci* 32:598–602, 1987.

175. O'Donoghue DP, Dawson AM, Powell-Tuck J, et al: Double-blind withdrawal trial of azathioprine as maintenance treatment for Crohn's disease. *Lancet* 2:955–957, 1987.

176. Bernstein LH, Frank MS, Brandt LJ, et al: Healing of perineal Crohn's disease with metronidazole. *Gastroenterology* 79:357–365, 1980.

177. Brandt LJ, Bernstein LH, Boley SJ, et al: Metronidazole therapy for perineal Crohn's disease: a follow-up study. *Gastroenterology* 83:383–387, 1982.

178. Nyman M, Hansson I, Eriksson S: Long-term immunosuppressive treatment in Crohn's disease. *Scand J Gastroenterol* 20:1197–1203, 1985.

179. Korelitz BI: The treatment of ulcerative colitis with "immunosuppressive" drugs. *Am J Gastroenterol* 76:297–298, 1981.

180. Kinlen LF: Incidence of cancer in rheumatoid arthritis and other disorders after immunosuppressive treatment. *Am J Med* 78(suppl 1A):44–49, 1985.

181. Present DH, Meltzer SJ, Wolke A, et al: Short-and long-term toxicity to 6-mercaptopurine in the treatment of inflammatory bowel disease [Abstract]. *Gastroenterology* 88:1545, 1985.

182. Feldman M, Burton ME: Comparison of H_2-receptor antagonists. *N Engl J Med* 323:1672–1680, 1990.

CHAPTER 37

Diuretics, Erythropoietin, and Other Medications Used in Renal Failure

ROBERT CHASSE, M.D.

The cogent use of diuretics in the critically ill patient requires an understanding of the sites and mechanisms of action of the various agents. This information is useful for choosing the appropriate diuretic for an individual patient. The diuretic can then be administered to achieve a desired effect.

Urine formation is the result of renal blood flow and glomerular filtration. Subsequent tubular secretion and reabsorption of solute and water alter both quantity and quality of the urine. Normally, 99% of filtered sodium is reabsorbed: 50 to 55% in the proximal tubule, 35 to 40% in the loop of Henle, 5 to 8% in the distal tubule, and 2 to 3% in the collecting tubules. The primary effect of most diuretics is to induce a natriuresis with subsequent excretion of water. The different classes of diuretics interfere with the reabsorption of sodium at different segments of the nephron. Diuretics can be divided into five groups based on site and mechanism of action: carbonic anhydrase inhibitors; loop diuretics; thiazides; potassium-sparing diuretics; and osmotic diuretics (Table 37.1).

All of the diuretics, with the exception of spironolactone, work from inside the tubular lumen. They are highly protein-bound and are actively secreted into the proximal tubule via an organic-anion exchanger (1). The magnitude of the diuretic effect is dependent on the delivery of the drug to the kidney and its concentration within the tubule. Hypoalbuminemia can decrease diuretic efficacy by decreasing drug binding and increasing the volume of distribution. This effect decreases the rate of drug delivery to the kidney. Proteinuria may likewise decrease diuretic effect by binding the drug in the tubular lumen. Increased diuretic efficacy has been reported, in patients with hypoalbuminemia, by mixing 40 mg of furosemide with 6.25 g of albumin prior to administration (2).

CARBONIC ANHYDRASE INHIBITORS

Carbonic anhydrase is an enzyme that is widely distributed throughout the body. In the kidney, it is found in tubular cells and in the luminal brush border of the proximal tubules. The enzyme is involved in the exchange of sodium (Na) for hydrogen (H) ion and the reclamation and regeneration of filtered bicarbonate. Acetazolamide is the only carbonic anhydrase inhibitor with a significant diuretic effect (3). It binds reversibly to the enzyme, 99% of which must be inhibited for a physiologic effect to occur. Administration of acetazolamide leads to a decrease in Na-H exchange and an increase in the excretion of sodium bicarbonate and sodium chloride. The diuresis attainable from acetazolamide is limited by reabsorption of sodium in distal tubule segments, particularly the loop of Henle, where reabsorption is flow-dependent. Diuresis is also limited by the development of a metabolic acidosis, which limits the amount of filtered HCO^3 available for exchange.

Acetazolamide is readily absorbed from the gastrointestinal tract. Peak serum levels occur within 2 hours of ingestion. It is excreted by the kidney but does not undergo significant metabolism. Acetazolamide is available in 125- and 250-mg tablets. A sustained release preparation is also available (500 mg). Acetazolamide is available for parenteral use (3).

Table 37.1.   Diuretic Classes

Agents	Site of Action	Usual Dose (24 hr)	$T_{1/2}$	Metabolism
Carbonic anhydrase inhibitors (acetazolamide)	Proximal tubule	250–500 mg	5 hr	Excreted unchanged in urine
Osmotic diuretics (mannitol)	Proximal tubule; loop of Henle	0.25 g/kg	Dependent on GFR; usually 30–60 mins	Excreted unchanged in urine
Loop diuretics	Loop of Henle			Both hepatic and renal metabolism
furosemide		20–80 mg	1 to 2 hr	
bumetanide		1–2 mg	1 to 2 hr	
ethacrynic acid		50–200 mg	1 to 2 hr	
Thiazides	Distal tubule	See Table 37.2		
Potassium-sparing Diuretics	Collecting duct			Hepatic and renal metabolism
spironolactone		25–200 mg	20 hr	
triamterene		50–200 mg	3–5 hr	
amiloride		5–10 mg	6–9 hr	

When used as a diuretic, acetazolamide is usually administered once per day or every 48 hours. To achieve and sustain a metabolic acidosis (i.e., in the treatment of metabolic alkalosis), it should be administered every 8 hours. The usual dose is 250 to 500 mg.

Acetazolamide is of little efficacy in renal failure because decreased serum HCO_3 and metabolic acidosis are already present. Its primary use in the ICU is in the treatment of metabolic alkalosis when further sodium chloride repletion would cause volume overload. With a concurrent infusion of $NaHCO_3$, acetazolamide can be used to alkalinize the urine to aid the excretion of weakly acidic drugs (e.g., salicylates).

Acetazolamide must be used carefully in patients with chronic obstructive pulmonary disease and CO_2 retention. A decrease in serum HCO_3 decreases the buffering capacity of the plasma. Marked pH changes can occur if $PACO_2$ suddenly rises. Carbonic anhydrase is also found in erythrocytes, where it is involved in the transport of CO_2. Carbonic anhydrase inhibitors can increase tissue CO_2 levels while decreasing CO_2 tension in expired gas. This effect may be magnified during metabolic acidosis or exercise [4]. The drug may also precipitate hepatic encephalopathy in patients with cirrhosis by decreasing renal excretion of ammonia.

Carbonic anhydrase inhibitors decrease the urinary excretion of citrate, predisposing patients to nephrocalcinosis and nephrolithiasis during prolonged use. They are teratogenic in animals and are contraindicated during pregnancy [3].

LOOP DIURETICS

Loop diuretics inhibit the sodium-potassium-chloride cotransport mechanism in the thick ascending limb of the loop of Henle. This is the primary mechanism for sodium absorption in this segment of the nephron. Loop diuretics bind reversibly to one of the Cl^- binding sites of the cotransport system, located on the luminal side of the tubule cell. The energy for this process is provided by a Na/K ATPase, that is located on the basolateral membrane. The Na-K-2Cl transport system is inhibited in a dose dependent fashion by loop diuretics, depending on the concentration of drug in the tubule [5]. This inhibition leads to a decrease in energy consumption in

these cells [6]. There may be a protective effect from these agents during renal ischemia. In most patients a plateau in the dose-response curve, measured as sodium excretion, is attainable and represents complete enzyme inhibition [5]. The magnitude of this effect is dependent on the concentration of drug in the tubules and not on serum levels. Loop diuretics are also weak inhibitors of carbonic anhydrase.

Diuresis with loop diuretics is considerable since the loop of Henle is responsible for 20 to 30% of Na reclamation. In addition, inhibition of Na transport decreases interstitial hypertonicity in the medulla, leading to reduced water reabsorption in the collecting tubule. Loop diuretics also increase the excretion of potassium, magnesium, and calcium.

The three most commonly used loop diuretics are furosemide, bumetanide, and ethacrynic acid. Ethacrynic acid is associated with an increased incidence of gastrointestinal side effects, which has led to a decrease in its utilization. Ethacrynic acid is available in 25- and 50-mg tablets. The usual oral dose in adults is 50 to 200 mg/day. For intravenous use, the dose is 50 mg or 0.5 to 1.0 mg/kg every 6 to 24 hours.

Bumetanide and furosemide are both sulfonamides. They are well absorbed orally. The bioavailability of oral furosemide is approximately 60%. The bioavailability of bumetanide is essentially 100%. Fifty percent of a dose of furosemide is excreted unchanged in the urine, while another 20% is metabolized and appears as furosemide glucuronide. On the other hand, bumetanide undergoes extensive hepatic metabolism via the cytochrome P_{450} enzyme system. This metabolism has implications for dosing since bumetanide is less likely to accumulate in renal failure. Bumetanide's metabolism may be inducible or inhibited by drugs that interact with the cytochrome P_{450} system (i.e., phenytoin and cimetidine). There is also the potential for phenotypic variation in its metabolism [7]. The half life of both diuretics is 1 to 2 hours in patients with normal renal function. The half-life of furosemide is increased up to threefold in renal failure. The half-life of bumetanide does not increase as much because of an increase in extrarenal metabolism. Ethacrynic acid, a phenoxyacetic acid derivative, is best used in patients who are allergic to sulfa compounds.

The acute administration of loop diuretics alters renal hemodynamics by increasing renal blood flow by up to 40% (8). They also result in a redistribution of renal blood flow from the inner to the outer renal cortex. This effect is thought to result from the intrarenal production of both vasodilatory prostaglandins and angiotensin II. The increase in renal blood flow can be blocked by the administration of indomethacin while the redistribution of blood flow can be blocked by the administration of angiotensin converting inhibitors (see Refs. 9, 10).

In acute left ventricular failure, furosemide has been reported to have a vasodilatory effect that precedes the onset of diuresis (11). However, studies in patients with chronic heart failure have demonstrated systemic vasoconstriction after the administration of loop diuretics. This vasoconstriction can have negative hemodynamic consequences. These vasoactive effects precede the onset of diuresis and can last as long as 2 hours (12).

Loop diuretics are used in conditions of volume overload that are refractory to more conservative measures (i.e., less potent diuretics, bed rest, and sodium restriction). Loop diuretics are also the drugs of choice for diuresis in patients whose creatinine clearance has dropped below 30 ml/min. Most diuretics can increase the fractional excretion of sodium and induce a natriuresis. However, in patients with end stage renal disease, only loop diuretics by themselves will produce a clinically significant diuresis (13). Loop diuretics are also used in the treatment of hypercalcemia to increase urinary calcium excretion and hyponatremia (from syndrome of inappropriate antidiuretic hormone secretion (SIADH)) to increase free water excretion.

Both furosemide and bumetanide are available for oral, intramuscular, and intravenous use. The potency ratio, in patients with normal renal function, is approximately 40 to 1, or 40 mg of furosemide is equivalent to 1 mg of bumetanide. In advanced renal failure, because of increased extrarenal metabolism of bumetanide, this ratio falls to 20 to 1 (14). In general, the oral dose of furosemide should be twice the intravenous dose due to incomplete enteral absorption.

The usual initial oral dose for furosemide is 20 to 80 mg every 6 to 24 hours, while that for bumetanide is 0.5 to 2.0 mg. The total dose and dosing interval should be adjusted to achieve the desired clinical effect. The maximum effective doses will vary, depending on the clinical situation and the type and severity of the renal disturbance. In chronic renal failure, little additional diuretic effect is likely to be gained at doses of intravenous furosemide greater than 200 mg. However, acute oliguric renal failure may require doses up to 500 mg (15).

The major adverse consequences of loop diuretics result from their alterations of fluid, electrolyte, and acid-base balance. Uncontrolled diuresis can result in volume depletion and hypotension. Hypokalemia, hyponatremia, hypomagnesemia, and metabolic alkalosis are common. Ototoxicity, in the form of deafness, may or may not be reversible. It is usually the result of the rapid or repeated administration of loop diuretics in patients with decreased clearance mechanisms. Rare adverse effects include interstitial nephritis, hypoglycemia, and the development of bullous skin lesions. Chronic use of furosemide in patients with congestive heart failure has resulted in

biochemical evidence of thiamine deficiency (16). Replacement of thiamine led to a 13% improvement in ejection fraction in 4 of 5 patients who were studied by echocardiography.

THIAZIDES

Thiazide diuretics act in the early distal convoluted tubule to inhibit the Na^+/Cl^- cotransport system. The diuresis promoted by these agents is usually fairly limited since this area of the nephron is only responsible for approximately 5% of sodium reabsorption. Some thiazides, in high doses, are inhibitors of carbonic anhydrase, but this effect is usually not clinically significant. The acute administration of thiazides leads to a decrease in glomerular filtration rate secondary to vasoconstriction and a subsequent decrease in renal blood flow. This effect may be of clinical importance in patients with decreased renal reserve.

There are multiple drugs in this group of diuretics that vary in regard to dose, bioavailability, and half-life (Table 37.2). Chlorothiazide is the only compound available for intravenous use. Metolazone has a slightly more pronounced diuretic effect because of concomitant inhibition of sodium reabsorption in the proximal tubule. This effect of metolazone is independent of carbonic anhydrase.

Thiazides are used for the treatment of hypertension and mild degrees of volume overload in patients with normal renal function. Their effectiveness decreases sharply as creatinine clearance decreases below 30 ml/min. Thiazides decrease renal calcium excretion and are used in the setting of recurrent calcium stones when sodium restriction is not effective. Because of their effect on calcium excretion, it has been suggested that thiazides may have a protective effect in patients at risk for osteoporosis and long bone fractures. (17–20) They are also used in the treatment of diabetes insipidus, where they paradoxically decrease urinary volume loss. This effect results from mild volume depletion, which increases proximal tubule sodium reabsorption.

The adverse effects of thiazides are primarily dose-dependent. Metabolic effects include hypokalemia, hyponatremia, and hypomagnesemia. In addition, thiazides impair glucose tolerance and increase serum lipids. Maintenance of normal serum potassium levels attenuates thiazide effects on glucose and lipid metabolism (21, 22). Rare side effects include pancreatitis, purpura, vasculitis, blood dyscrasias, and pulmonary edema.

POTASSIUM SPARING DIURETICS

The potassium sparing agents act primarily in the collecting tubule. The collecting tubule has sodium and potassium channels. Sodium is absorbed passively, creating a negative gradient across the luminal membrane. This gradient and the activity of Na-K-ATPase act together to promote potassium excretion. Potassium excretion is flow-dependent and linked to sodium reabsorption. Aldosterone increases the number of sodium and potassium channels and stimulates Na-K-ATPase activity. The potassium-sparing diuretics fall into two groups. Spironolactone competes with aldosterone for its cytosolic receptor while triamterene and amiloride block luminal sodium channels. All

Table 37.2.   Thiazide Diuretics

Thiazides	*Dose*	*Frequency*	*Route*	*Comments*
Bendroflumethizide	25–200 mg	qd–bid	po	
Benzthiazide	25–200 mg	qd	po	
Chlorothiazide	500 mg–2 g	qd–bid	po	Only IV thiazide
			IV	
Chlorthalidone	12.5–150 mg	qd	po	
Cyclothiazide	1–2 mg	qd	po	
Hydrochlorothiazide	12.5–150 mg	qd	po	
Hydroflumethiazide	25–200 mg	qd–bid	po	
Indapamide	2.5–5 mg	qd	po	? Less effect on lipids
Methyclothiazide	2.5–10 mg	qd	po	
Metolazone	0.5–10 mg	qd	po	Marked differences between formula tions
Polythiazide	1–4 mg	qd	po	
Quinethazone	25–200 mg	qd–bid	po	
Trichloromethiazide	1–4 mg	qd–bid	po	

of these agents produce a modest natriuriesis and decrease the excretion of potassium and hydrogen ion (3, 23).

Spironolactone is the only diuretic available in the U.S. that does not require tubular secretion to be effective. It is ineffective in the absence of aldosterone. Spironolactone is 70 to 90% absorbed from the gastrointestinal tract and undergoes extensive hepatic metabolism. Some of its metabolites are pharmacologically active. The normal starting dose in adults is 100 mg, given in single or divided doses every 6 to 8 hours. When used alone, onset of diuresis usually takes 1 to 2 days. This delay may be overcome by giving 2 to 3 times the normal daily dose as a loading dose. Spironolactone is most useful in situations characterized by excessive aldosterone secretion. These include cirrhosis, congestive heart failure, and hyperaldosteronism (24).

Triamterene is well absorbed from the gastrointestinal tract and undergoes hepatic metabolism. Amiloride is approximately 50% absorbed and is excreted intact in the urine. Both of these agents accumulate in renal failure and are used most often in combination with kaluretic diuretic agents.

The primary adverse effect of all agents in this class is hyperkalemia. Triamterene can serve as a nidus for nephrolithiasis and in combination with indomethacin has produced acute renal failure. The decrease in potassium excretion makes these medications unsuitable for use in renal failure. Great care must be taken when they are used in combination with angiotensin-converting enzyme inhibitors, due to potentiation of hyperkalemia.

OSMOTIC DIURETICS

There are two primary osmotic diuretics available in the U.S.: mannitol and urea. Other osmotic agents, such as isosorbide and glycerin, are used in ophthalmic surgery to reduce intraocular pressure. Urea has a higher incidence of side effects than mannitol and is not used often in clinical practice. Mannitol is the 6-carbon alcohol of mannose and is similar in structure to sorbitol and glucose. It possesses the basic qualities of all osmotic diuretics. It is freely filterable at the glomerulus, poorly reabsorbed, and metabolically inert. Mannitol's half-life is dependent on glomerular filtration. It is usually given as a hypertonic solution and is available for intravenous administration.

Mannitol has little effect on sodium reabsorption in the proximal tubule. It is a nonresorbable solute that primarily inhibits the reabsorption of water. This effect results in a low tubular concentration of sodium and decreases the gradient for sodium reabsorption. Mannitol also increases renal blood flow to the medulla, producing a partial washout of medullary hypertonicity with a resultant decrease in sodium reabsorption (23). Mannitol is administered as a hypertonic solution. It pulls water into the intravascular space, expanding the extracellular fluid compartment. This results in hemodilution, hyponatremia, hypochloremia, and a decrease in serum bicarbonate. The use of mannitol may result in volume overload, hyperkalemic metabolic acidosis, and hypernatremia. The hyperkalemia is thought to be a result of solvent drag as potassium-rich intracellular fluid is drawn from cells. Changes in mental status can result from mannitol intoxication.

Mannitol is used to reduce intracellular volume in the treatment of increased intracranial pressure. It has also been used prophylactically to prevent acute renal failure in patients during angiography (i.e., diabetics), cardiopulmonary bypass, and aortic surgery (23–27). Its role in the treatment of acute renal failure is less well-defined. Theoretically, it should be advantageous: it increases renal blood flow: redistributes blood flow to the medulla; increases tubular flow; and may prevent tubular obstruction by cellular debris and may act as a free radical scavenger (25). Combined with loop diuretics, mannitol may convert oliguric to nonoliguric renal failure. This strategy, while improving fluid management, has never been shown to impact mortality (28). Mannitol is also used to reduce intraocular pressure.

Mannitol has been reported to cause acute renal failure (29). Patients who developed acute renal failure received between 350 and 900 g mannitol over 2 to 5 days. Although the mechanism is unclear, animals with serum levels of mannitol greater than 1000 mg/dl demonstrated renal vasoconstriction (30).

For the treatment of increased intracranial pressure, mannitol should be given in doses of approximately 0.25 g/kg. This dose can be repeated every 4 hours if needed. The serum osmolality is often followed as a measure of mannitol dosage. One usually attempts to achieve a serum osmolality of 310 to 315 mosm/kg water, assuming a normal starting osmolality. It is important to realize that blood urea nitrogen increases serum osmolality but has little effect on fluid shifts between intracellular and extracellular compartments (i.e., it distributes in total body water). Thus, osmolality is elevated secondary to urea. The osmolal gap (i.e., the difference between measured and calculated osmolality) may be a more accurate monitor of mannitol action. An osmolal gap of 55 is the equivalent of a serum mannitol level of 1000 mg/dl. Mannitol may result in a paradoxical increase in intracranial pressure several hours after a dose. The mechanism of this rebound is not yet known but may result from delayed entry of mannitol into cells. This effect is greater with high mannitol doses and prolonged administration. Mannitol should be used with great care, if at all, in patients with decreased renal function. If volume overload or other complications of mannitol use occur in patients with decreased renal function, mannitol can be removed by hemodialysis.

DIURETIC RESISTANCE

Before the first dose of a diuretic has worn off, mechanisms are activated to counteract its effects. The processes activated result in avid sodium retention by the kidney. After the effect of the diuretic has worn off, sodium excretion drops below baseline levels. One frequently sees a decrease in urine output (below baseline levels) and low urine sodium values. If sodium intake is not restricted or diuretic continuously administered, there may be no net sodium excretion. The restriction of sodium intake to less than 100 mEq/day is a key determinant of diuretic efficacy (1). Even with sodium restriction, at the same daily dose of a diuretic, sodium excretion comes into balance with intake. There are several reasons for this result. Extracellular fluid volume depletion results in increased reabsorption of water and sodium proximal to the site of action of a particular diuretic. Some of this response is due to proximal tubule stimulation by angiotensin and norepinephrine. However, blockade with an angiotensin converting enzyme inhibitor and prazosin, an α-blocker, does not eliminate the effect (31). Extracellular volume depletion also results in a decrease in the amount of sodium that is filtered by the glomerulus. Finally, in the case of loop diuretics, there is evidence that increased sodium delivery to the distal tubule results in hypertrophy and increased resorptive capacity of distal tubular cells (32). These adaptive mechanisms are probably beneficial, as continued volume loss would eventually result in hypotension.

The understanding of diuretic mechanisms, sites of action, and renal compensation allow for the development of effective strategies to combat diuretic resistance. Twenty-four hour urine sodium reveals whether sodium intake is high. The excretion of more than 100 mEq/day indicates that diuresis is adequate but that sodium intake is excessive. Medications should be reviewed and agents that compete for secretion with diuretic agents in the proximal tubule stopped, if possible. One of the mechanisms responsible for diuretic resistance in end-stage renal disease and cirrhosis may be competition of uremic toxins and bile acids with diuretics for secretion into the tubule (1). Increasing the frequency of dosing or continuous infusions of diuretic may also be efficacious in overcoming diuretic resistance. It has recently been shown that a continuous infusion of bumetanide leads to the excretion of greater amounts of sodium than the equivalent amount given by bolus (33). We have had good success using continuous furosemide infusions in critically ill patients. Posture may have an effect on diuresis. Having the patient supine decreases venous pooling and may increase creatinine clearance and sodium excretion.

DOPAMINE

Dopamine infusions are often used for the treatment of oliguria in the ICU despite the lack of controlled trials demonstrating efficacy in this situation (34). Dopamine's effects are dose-dependent and subject to variability. At low doses (0.5 to 2 µg/kg/min), dopamine receptors are predominantly stimulated. Increasing the dopamine dose to between 2.0 and 4.0 µg/kg/min results in effects mediated by activation of β-receptors (i.e., increases in inotropy and chronotropy). At higher doses (>10 µg/kg/min), the predominant effects of dopamine result from activation of α-adrenergic receptors. These dose-receptor effects are only approximate and vary as a result of receptor down-regulation, renal function, disease, and age. Dopamine is used most often at low doses for "selective" stimulation of dopamine receptors.

Two receptor subtypes for dopamine have been identified: Da_1 and Da_2. Both are found in various locations in the kidney. Da_1 receptors are found in the renal microvasculature, the proximal convoluted tubule, and the cortical collecting ducts. Da_2 receptors have been localized to the presynaptic membrane of sympathetic nerve terminals in the kidney and also to the glomerulus. In addition, dopamine is produced intrarenally.

Dopamine administration to normal subjects who are volume replete results in an increase in renal blood flow of approximately 30 to 35% and an increase in glomerular filtration rate (GFR) of approximately 10 to 15% (35). Additionally, there is an increase in sodium excretion above that which would be predicted by the increase in GFR alone (36). Dopamine inhibits the reabsorption of sodium in the proximal tubule, probably by inhibiting Na-K-ATPase (37). It inhibits aldosterone secretion from the adrenal gland and may inhibit sodium resorption in the cortical collecting ducts. Both these effects appear to be mediated by Da_1 receptors. The role of Da_2 receptor stimulation has been less well-defined. The natriuretic effect of dopamine on the kidney diminishes over time and is blunted in patients who are volume or sodium-depleted (38). The decrease in efficacy over time is probably attributable to the activation of counterregulatory responses.

The renal vasodilatory response to dopamine is blunted in patients with chronic renal insufficiency, but the natriuretic response is maintained (35). Multiple trials of dopamine in both experimental and clinical acute renal failure have produced conflicting results. No clearly defined role for dopamine exists in this situation.

ERYTHROPOIETIN

Anemia is common in patients with renal failure, and approximately 25% of patients on hemodialysis are transfusion-dependent (39). The etiology of this anemia is often multifactorial. There are obligate blood loss with hemodialysis, an increased incidence of gastrointestinal blood loss, shortened red blood cell survival and, in certain patients, impaired erythropoiesis secondary to aluminum toxicity. However, the most common cause for anemia is a relative lack of erythropoietin.

Erythropoietin is a 165-amino acid glycoprotein hormone that is produced primarily in the kidneys. The molecular weight is approximately 30,400 daltons. Carbohydrate residues are necessary for its biologic activity in vivo but not in vitro (40). Erythropoietin is produced by peritubular interstitial cells of the inner renal cortex in the vicinity of the proximal tubule. It is also synthesized by the liver, the primary producer of erythropoietin in the antenatal period. Postnatally, the liver produces 10 to 15% of erythropoietin (41). Interestingly, erythropoietin messenger RNA is also expressed by macrophages (42). This finding suggests that there may be some role for local production of erythropoietin in the regulation of bone marrow production of red blood cells. The gene for erythropoietin has been cloned, and in humans it is located on chromosome 7.

Erythropoietin functions as a hematopoietic growth factor for the erythroid cell line. It stimulates the erythroid and colony-forming units (committed red blood cell progenitors). It has no effect on pluripotent stem cells or mature red blood cells. No consistent effects have been demonstrated on megakaryocyte or white blood cell progenitors (43).

The production of erythropoietin is increased in response to tissue hypoxia (i.e., anemia, chronic obstructive pulmonary disease (COPD), right-to-left shunting, high altitude). This increase in production is brought about by the recruitment of cells in the peritubular renal cortex (44). There are no preformed stores of erythropoietin (45). The tissue oxygen sensor is a heme containing protein that is subject to rapid turnover (46). Secondary increases in production can come from erythropoietin-producing tumors, including renal cell carcinomas, hepatomas, cerebellar hemangiomas, and uterine leiomyomas.

Erythropoietin levels are usually measured by radioimmunoassay. Normal levels range from 10 to 25 mU/ml. There is an inverse relationship between hematocrit and erythropoietin concentrations in otherwise normal subjects. The erythropoietin response to anemia is variable between subjects. At a hematocrit of 30%, erythropoietin levels range from 50 to 200 mU/ml (47). The production of erythropoietin in response to anemia is blunted by infection, inflammation, and malignancy. The inverse linear relationship between erythropoietin and hemoglobin is lost once renal function declines to about 30% of normal (48).

Erythropoietin is produced via recombinant DNA techniques in Chinese hamster ovary cells. It is clinically useful in the treatment of symptomatic anemia in patients with renal failure. Blood transfusions are associated with immunosuppression, transmission of infection, iron overload, transfusion reactions, and the development of cytotoxic antibodies that may limit the potential for kidney transplantation. Indications for erythropoietin therapy include symptomatic anemia or a hemoglobin less than 6 g/dl. Other indications are related primarily to the hazards of transfusion mentioned above. In clinical trials of erythropoietin, greater than 95% of patients respond with increases in the hemoglobin level (39, 41, 49, 53). Both the rate of rise and the total increase in hemoglobin are dose-dependent (39). The effective dose can vary markedly among patients. A reasonable starting dose is 50 U/kg erythropoietin 2 to 3 times/week. Erythropoietin is available in 2000, 4000, and 10,000 unit vials. It is effective when given intravenously or subcutaneously (39, 49). Intraperitoneal dosing has not been found to be effective (50). Subcutaneous dosing results in a prolonged half life of erythropoietin when compared to intravenous dosing (43). Sustained serum levels of erythropoietin make it possible for many patients to decrease the dose of erythropoietin when switching from intravenous to subcutaneous dosing.

Before beginning therapy with erythropoietin, patients require an assessment of their iron stores. Serum iron, transferrin saturation, and ferritin levels should be measured. In patients with low iron stores, the response to erythropoietin is blunted, and target hematocrits are difficult to achieve. Transferrin saturations less than 20% and ferritin levels less than 100 μg/ml are indicative of iron deficiency of a degree that results in suboptimal hematopoietic responses (51). Iron can be given orally or parenterally. In patients on hemodialysis, gastrointestinal toxicity may preclude the administration of sufficient quantities of iron. Intravenous iron may be required when oral supplementation is inadequate to replete iron stores. Iron dextran (in doses of 100 mg) may be administered at the completion of dialysis. The total dose of iron is determined by the estimated deficit and the hematopoietic response. One suggested strategy for following iron status is weekly hematocrits, monthly transferrin saturations, and quarterly ferritin levels (52). Nomograms for predicting estimated iron needs and deficits have been published (51). Approximately two thirds of patients receiving erythropoietin will require iron supplementation (53).

Patients often have an increase in reticulocyte counts within a week of beginning therapy with erythropoietin. The rate of increase in hematocrit is dose-dependent. The target hematocrit should be individualized for every patient based on symptoms. The usual goal is a hematocrit between 30 and 35%. Increases in hematocrit above this level have been associated with an increased incidence of complications. If no response is seen in 3 to 4 weeks, then the dosage of erythropoietin should be increased. Most patients will respond to dosages of 50 to 150 U/kg.

Failure to respond to erythropoietin is multifactorial. The most common reason is iron deficiency. Another cause is occult blood loss from excessive clotting of dialyzers or gastrointestinal bleeding. Aluminum toxicity interferes with the incorporation of iron into heme and is a cause of erythropoietin resistance (54). It is suggested by finding elevated serum aluminum levels. Aluminum toxicity often causes hypochromic microcytic anemia, and erythropoietin therapy can result in elevated erythrocyte protoporphorin levels (55). Aluminum toxicity is treated by withholding aluminum-containing antacids, by increasing the erythropoietin dose, or by administering chelation therapy with desferoxamine. However, the use of desferoxamine in patients with end-stage renal disease has been associated with the development of mucormycosis. Hyperparathyroidism resulting in osteitis fibrosa can also cause resistance to erythropoietin. Acute and chronic inflammation from infections, collagen vascular diseases, malignancy, and surgery will also blunt the response to erythropoietin (45). If an acute medical problem develops, erythropoietin therapy should be continued because it may lessen the decrease in hematocrit and prevent the bone marrow from becoming quiescent. Resistance to erythropoietin that develops during therapy should be investigated.

Patients who respond to erythropoietin have objective improvement in exercise tolerance, appetite, and mentation. The correction of anemia reduces heart rate, stroke volume, and cardiac output. It has also led to reductions in left ventricular mass and end-diastolic volume. Patients also report improved libido, sense of well-being, sleep patterns, and overall quality of life. 41 Low-dose erythropoietin therapy led to a decrease in histamine levels and improvement in symptoms of pruritus associated with uremia (56). The use of erythropoietin in predialysis patients with chronic renal failure does not increase the rate of decline in kidney function (57).

The most common adverse effect from erythropoietin therapy is hypertension. Approximately 25% of patients require the initiation or adjustment of antihypertensive therapy. Seizures have also been reported and appear to be related to rapid rises in hematocrit and associated increases in blood pressure. The increase in hematocrit may reduce dialyzer efficiency and increase heparin requirements. Some studies have reported an increase in vascular access thrombosis. Improved appetite can also lead to problems with hyperkalemia, and hyperphosphatemia, as well as to an increase in dialysis requirements (39, 41).

Erythropoietin has been used to treat anemia associated with rheumatoid arthritis, HIV, and malignancy. 58 It can also be used to increase the rate of blood donation for autologous transfusions for surgery and for iron overload. The commercial availability of recombinant erythropoietin represents the single greatest improvement in the care of patients with end stage renal disease in the last decade.

REFERENCES

1. Rose BD. Diuretics. *Kidney Int* 39:336–352, 1991.
2. Inoue M, Okajima K, Itoh K, et al: Mechanism of furosemide resistance in analbuminemic rats and hypoalbuminemic patients. *Kidney Int* 32:198–203, 1987.
3. Weiner IM: Drugs affecting renal function and electrolyte metabolism. In Goodman Gilman A, Rall TW, Nies AS, Taylor P (eds): *The Pharmacological Basis of Therapeutics*. Pergamon Press, Elmsford, NY, 1990, pp. 713–731.
4. Kowalchuk JM, Heigenhauser GJF, Sutton JR, Jones NL. Effect of acetazolamide on gas exchange and acid base control after maximal exercise. *J Appl Physiol* 72:278–287, 1992.
5. Brater DC, Anderson SA, Brown-Cartwright D. Response to furosemide in chronic renal insufficiency: rationale for limited doses. *Clin Pharm Ther.* 40:134–139, 1986.
6. Mohaupt M, Kramer HJ. Acute ischemic renal failure: review of experimental studies on pathophysiology and potential protective interventions. *Renal Failure* 11:177–185, 1990.
7. Brater DC: Clinical pharmacology of loop diuretics. *Drugs* 1991. 41(Suppl 3):14–22.
8. Eknoyan G, Suki WN. Renal consequences of antihypertensive therapy. *Semin Nephrol* 11:129–137, 1991.
9. Spitaleqitz S, Chou SY, Faubert PF, Porush JG: Effects of diuretics on inner medullary hemodynamics in the dog. *Circ Res* 51:703–710, 1982.
10. Gerber JG: Role of prostaglandins in the hemodynamic and tubular effects of furosemide. *Fed Proc* 42:1707–1710, 1983.
11. Kruck F: Acute and long term effects of loop diuretics in heart failure. *Drugs* 41(Suppl 3):60–68, 1991.
12. Francis GS, Siegel RM, Goldsmith SR, Olivari M, Levine TB, Cohn JN: Acute vasoconstrictor reponse to intravenous furosemide in patients with chronic congestive heart failure: activation of the neurohumoral axis. *Ann Intern Med* 103:1–6, 1985.
13. Knauf H, Mutschler E: Pharmacodynamic and kinetic considerations on diuretics as a basis for differential therapy. *Klin Wochenschr* 69:239–250, 1991.
14. Voelker JR, Cartwright–Brown D, Anderson S, et al: Comparison of loop diuretics in patients with chronic renal insufficiency. *Kidney Intl* 32:572–578, 1987.
15. Brater DC: Voelker JR. Use of diuretics in patients with chronic renal failure. In Bennett WM, McCarron DA (eds): *Contemporary Issues of Nephrology: Pharmacotherapy of Renal Disease and Hypertension*, vol 17. Churchill-Livingstone, New York, 1987, pp 115–147.
16. Seligmann H, Halkin H, Rauchfleisch S, et al: Thiamine deficiency in patients with congestive heart failure receiving long term furosemide therapy: a pilot study. *Am J Med* 91:151–155, 1991.
17. Heidrich FE, Stergachis A, Gross KM: Diuretic drug use and the risk for hip fracture. *Ann Intern Med* 115:1–6, 1991.
18. Wasnick R, Davis J, Ross P, Vogel J. The effect of thiazide on the rates of bone mineral loss: a longitudinal study. *Br Med J* 301:1303–1305, 1990.
19. Felson DT, Sloutskis D, Anderson JJ, Anthony JM, Kiel DP. Thiazide diuretics and the risk of hip fracture: results from the Framingham study. *JAMA* 265:370–373, 1991.
20. LaCroix AZ, Wienpahl J, White LR, et al: Thiazide diuretic agents and the incidence of hip fracture. *N Engl J Med* 322:286–290, 1990.
21. Andersson OK, Gudbrandsson T, Jamerson K. Metabolic adverse effects of thiazide diuretics: the importance of normokalemia. *J Intern Med* 735:89–96, 1991.
22. Langford HG, Cutter G, Oberman A, Kansal P, Russelll G. The effect of thiazide therapy on glucose, insulin, and cholesterol metabolism and of glucose on potassium: results of a cross-sectional study in patients from the hypertension detection and follow up program. *J Hum Hypertens* 4:491–500, 1990.
23. Wilcox CS: Diuretics. In Brenner BM, Rector FC (eds): *The Kidney.* WB Saunders, Philadelphia, 1991.
24. American Society of Hospital Pharmacists: Diuretics. In McEvoy GK, Litvak K (eds): *American Hospital Formulary Service Drug Information '91.* Bethesda, MD, 1991.
25. Warren SE, Blantz R. Mannitol. *Arch Int Med* 141:493–497, 1981.
26. Paganinni EP, Bosworth CR. Acute renal failure after open heart surgery: newer concepts and current therapy. *Semin Thorac Cardiovasc Surg* 3:63–70, 1991.
27. Anto H, Chou SY, Porush JG, Shapiro WB. Infusion intravenous pyelography and renal function: effects of hypertonic mannitol in patients with chronic renal insufficiency. *Arch Intern Med* 131:1652–1659, 1981.
28. Corwin JV, Bonventre JV. Acute renal failure in the intensive care unit. Part 2. *Intens Care Med* 14:86–96, 1988.
29. Dorman HR, Sondheimer JH, Cadnapaphornchai P: Mannitol-induced renal failure. *Medicine* 69:153–159, 1990.
30. Temes SP, Lilien OM, Chamberlin W: A direct vasoconstrictor effect of mannitol on the renal artery. *Surg Gynecol Obstet* 141:223–226, 1975.
31. Wilcox CS, Guzman NJ, Mitch WE et al: Na, K, and BP homeostasis in man during furosemide: effects of prazosin and captopril. *Kidney Int* 31:135–141, 1987.
32. Stanton BA, Kaissling B: Adaptation of distal tubule and collecting duct to increased sodium delivery II: Na and K transport. *Am J Physiol* 255:F1269–F1275, 1988.
33. Rudy DW, Voelker JR, Greene PK, Esparza FA, Brater DC: Loop diuretics for chronic renal insufficiency: a continuous infusion is more efficacious than bolus therapy. *Ann Intern Med* 115:360–366, 1991.
34. Szerlip HM: Renal dose dopamine: fact and fiction. *Ann Intern Med* 115:153–154, 1991.
35. Smit AJ: Dopamine in chronic renal failure. *Am J Hypertens* 3:75s–77s, 1990.
36. Hegde SS, Lokhandwala MF: Renal dopamine and sodium excretion. *Am J Hypertens* 3:78s–81s, 1990.
37. Aperia A, Bertorello A, Seri I: Dopamine causes inhibition of Na-K ATPase activity in rat proximal convoluted tubule segments. *Am J Physiol* 252:F39–F45, 1987.
38. Carey RM, Siragy HM, Felder RA. Physiological modulation of renal function by the renal dopaminergic system. *J Auton Pharmacol* 10:547–551, 1990.
39. Eschbach JW, Egrie JC, Downing MR, Browne JK, Adamson JW: Correction of the anemia of end-stage renal disease with recombinant human erythropoietin. *N Engl J Med* 316:73–78, 1987.
40. Dube S, Fisher JW, Powell JS: Glycosylation at specific sites of erythropoietin is essential for biosynthesis, secretion, and biological function. *J Biol Chem* 263:17516–17521, 1988.
41. Nissenson AR, Nimer SD, Wolcott DL: Recombinant human erythropoietin and renal anemia: molecular biology, clinical efficacy, and nervous system effects. *Ann Intern Med* 114:402–416, 1991.
42. Sytkowski AJ. Control of erythropoietin production. *Blood Rev* 5:015–018, 1991.
43. Spivak JL, Watson AJ. Hematopoiesis and the kidney. In Seldin DW and Giebisch G (eds): *The Kidney: Physiology and Pathophysiology*, ed 2. Raven Press, New York 1992, pp 1553–1593.

44. Koury ST, Bondurant MC, Caro J, Graber SE: Quantitation of erythropoietin producing cells in kidneys of mice by in situ hybridization: correlation with hematocrit, renal erythropoietin mRNA, and serum erythropoietin concentration. *Blood* 74:157–164, 1989.

45. Spivak JL: Serum immunoreactive erythropoietin in health and disease. *Int J Cell Cloning* 8 (Suppl 1):211–226, 1990.

46. Goldberg MA, Dunning SP, Bunn HF. Regulation of the erythropoietin gene: evidence that the oxygen sensor is a heme protein. *Science* 242:1412–1415, 1988.

47. Erslev AJ: Erythropoietin titers in health and disease. *Semin Hematol* 28 (Suppl 3): 2–8, 1991.

48. Radtke HW, Claussner A, Erbes PM, Scheuermann EH, Schoeppe W, Koch KM: Serum erythropoietin concentration in chronic renal failure: relationship to degree of anemia and excretory renal function. *Blood* 54:877–884, 1979.

49. Piraino B, Johnston JR. The use of subcutaneous erythropoietin in COPD Patients. *Clin Nephrol* 33:200–202, 1990.

50. Macdougall IC, Neubert P, Coles GA, et al: Pharmacokinetics of recombinant human erythropoietin in patients on continous ambulatory hemodialysis. *Lancet* i:425, 1989.

51. Van Wyck DB, Stivelman JC, Ruiz J, Kirlin LF, Katz MA, Ogden DA: Iron status in patients receiving erythropoietin for dialysis associated anemia. *Kidney Int* 35:712–716, 1989.

52. Van Wyck DB: Suboptimal response to epoetin therapy in dialysis patients with anemia. Global Medical Publications, New York. 1991.

53. Muirhead N: Recombinant human erythropoietin patient dosing algorithm. *Semin Nephrol* 10:59–65, 1990.

54. Mladenovic J. aluminum inhibits erythropoiesis in vitro. *J Clin Invest* 81:1661–1665, 1988.

55. Bia MJ, Cooper K, Schnall S, et al. Aluminum induced anemia: Pathogenesis and treatment in patients on chronic hemodialysis. *Kidney Int* 36:852–858, 1989.

56. De marchi S, Cecchin E, Villalta D, Sepiacci G, Santini G, Bartoli E. Relief of pruritus and decreases in plasma histamine concentrations during erythropoietin therapy in patients with uremia. *N Engl J Med* 326:969–974, 1992.

57. Eschbach JW, Kelly MR, Haley NR, Abels RI, Adamson JW. Treatment of the anemia of progressive renal failure with recombinant human erythropoietin. *N Engl J Med* 321:158–163, 1989.

58. Graber SE, Krantz SB. Erythropoietin: biology and clinical use. Heme/Onc *Clin North Am* 3:369–399, 1989.

CHAPTER 38

Analgesics

FRANK BALESTRIERI, D.D.S., M.D., F.C.C.P.
SHERRY FISHER, R.N.

PAIN SENSATION

Pain is defined as "an unpleasant sensory and emotional experience associated with actual or potential tissue damage, or described in terms of such damage" (1). Pain is a personal and subjective experience that each individual encounters throughout life, as actual or potential tissue-damaging experiences are encountered. Pain is also an unpleasant experience with an associated emotional response. The emotional or psychologic state of the patient may result in pain in the absence of tissue damage or other pathology. The emotional or psychologic state of the patient may modify the character of the pain.

The nociceptor activity initiated by a noxious stimulus is not pain. It consists of sensory, emotional, and cognitive elements that arise from very complex and, as yet, incompletely understood activities within the central nervous system.

Although pain is subjective and difficult to define, it is clear that critically ill and even unconscious patients experience pain. The critically ill not only are often subjected to major physical injury, but also suffer sleeplessness, extreme auditory stimulation, frequent handling, and fear. Our knowledge of patients' experiences during a critical illness is mostly anecdotal. In describing his own intensive care unit (ICU) experience following three heart operations, Ian Donald, a gynecologist-obstetrician, points out that the patient's state of mind is paramount and of more importance than the most

powerful analgesics (2, 3). Other factors that modify the experience of pain are past experience, knowledge of the postoperative routine, and fear. Donald stresses the importance of the preoperative anesthetist's visit, the need for sympathy from attendants, and the importance of preventing pain or treating it early. Fortunately, he points out, the memory of pain fades mercifully and quickly. Similar anecdotal reports are those of Henschel (4) who describes his ICU experience with Guillain-Barré syndrome, and Shovelton (5), who had a thymectomy for myasthenia gravis. Since Donald's experience in 1969, very little has changed in our critical care units.

The treatment of postoperative surgical pain has received much attention, and present-day pain regimens have been widely criticized (6). Effective pain management in the critical care setting requires effective use of narcotic analgesia (7, 8), better use of established techniques of regional anesthesia (9), and further study and use of new techniques such as continuous narcotic infusions (10) and epidural, intrathecal, and transcutaneous methods of narcotic administration (11–15).

PAIN MECHANISMS

PERIPHERAL RECEPTORS

It is known that three categories of cutaneous receptors are present: high-threshold mechanoreceptors, thermoreceptors, and nociceptors. These peripheral receptors have been classified on the basis of their morphology and the correlation

Table 38.1. Classification of Nerve Fibers and Peripheral Receptors with Conduction Velocities

Class	Function	Diameter (μm)	Conduction Velocity (m/sec)
A$_\alpha$	Motor	12–20	70–120
A$_\beta$	Pressure/touch	5–12	30–70
A$_\gamma$	Proprioception	5–12	30–70
A$_\delta$	Pain/temperature (mechanical, heat and cold sensation)	1–4	12–30
B	Preganglionic autonomic (sympathetic)	1–3	14
C			
Cutaneous nociceptors	Pain/temperature (polymodal, mechanical, and cold sensation)	0.5–1	1.2
Cutaneous mechanoreceptors	Sense skin indentation		55
Type I			
Type II			
Meissner corpuscle	Sense skin indentation		55
Pacinian corpuscle	Sense pressure changes		50
Warm	Sense increased temperature		0.5

of structure with function (e.g., pacinian corpuscles, Golgi-Mazzoni receptors, hair follicle receptors, Meissner corpuscles, Merkel "touch spots," and Ruffini endings). Nevertheless, there are no anatomic structures defined for most sensory cutaneous functions. However, one can classify nerve fibers and human peripheral receptors (18–20) (Table 38.1). The cutaneous mechanoreceptors are supplied by large myelinated fibers, whereas the cutaneous nociceptors are supplied by fine myelinated (A$_\delta$) and unmyelinated (C) fibers. Animal studies indicate that the cutaneous nociceptors have two characteristic features: a progressive augmenting response to repeated or increasing noxious stimuli (sensitization) and a high threshold to all natural stimuli relative to other receptors in the same tissue (21). Sensitization is produced by a number of chemicals (21–24) (histamine, serotonin, kinins, norepinephrine, epinephrine, and arachidonic acid metabolites) and can be reduced by the nonsteroidal antiinflammatory drugs (25–28). Substance P has also been postulated to have an influence on the peripheral afferent nociceptors. It is speculated that substance P may mediate noxious thermal and chemical stimuli, possibly at the first afferent synapse (29, 30).

CENTRAL MECHANISMS

The cell bodies of primary afferent fibers are located in the dorsal root ganglia and trigeminal sensory ganglia. Normally, activity begins in the periphery, and the action potential travels past the dorsal root ganglia cells, which may depolarize, before entering the dorsal horn layers. The dorsal roots provide the pathway by which axons from the peripheral somatic nerves enter the spinal cord. A dermatomal distribution of the dorsal roots exists, and overlapping of primary afferent fibers occurs within the dorsal horn. Axons in any given dorsal root may extend over five or more spinal cord segments. This fact implies that any point on the body is supplied by two adjoining dorsal roots. As the large and small fibers enter the dorsal horn, the large fibers separate and enter the dorsal columns, with collaterals entering the dorsal horn. The small fine fibers enter separately, forming a longitudinal tract bearing Lissauer's name. The dorsolateral fasciculus (Lissauer's

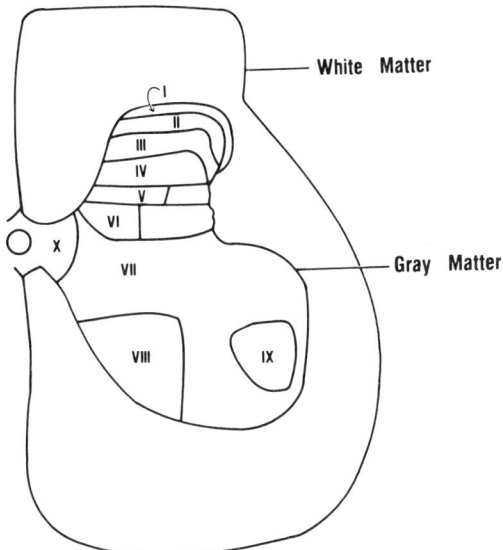

Figure 38.1. Spinal cord laminae. *I*, Marginal zone. *II* and *III*, Substantia gelatinosa. *IV*, *V*, and *VI*, Nucleus proprius. *VII*, *VIII*, *IX*, and *X*, Motor areas. (Adapted from Rexed B: Cytoarchitectonic organization of the spinal cord in the cat. Comp Neurol 96:415–495, 1952.)

tract) contains mainly fine primary afferent fibers (31) and fibers from the substantia gelatinosa (32). Afferent input into the substantia gelatinosa is by way of collaterals of large primary afferents and fine primary afferents and their collaterals. Numerous complex synaptic connections occur in the region of the substantia gelatinosa, which functions as an integrator of sensory input. The ventral roots also contain myelinated and unmyelinated sensory fibers (33). These fibers arise from the dorsal root ganglion cells and represent 15 to 30% of axons in the ventral roots (34). The presence of these sensory fibers in the ventral roots may provide a portion of the explanation for the failure of dorsal rhizotomy to result in complete relief of pain.

The spinal cord comprises a central gray zone and an outer white zone. The central gray matter can be divided into 10 groups based on cell morphology (Fig. 38.1) (35). The cell groups I and VI are involved in sensory transmission and make up the dorsal horn. The marginal zone of Waldeyer, lamina I, receives excitatory input from primary afferents, and receives inhibitory input from the substantia gelatinosa (36). The marginal zone cells respond to noxious mechanical, thermal, and polymodal stimulation, as well as innocuous thermal change (37).

ASCENDING PATHWAYS OF THE SPINAL CORD

The spinothalamic and spinoreticular tracts are the most significant ascending pathways for the transmission of nociceptive input in humans. Axons from second-order neurons in laminae I, IV, V, and VI cross the midline to ascend as the lateral and ventral spinothalamic tracts. The spinothalamic tracts travel to the posterior thalamic nuclei and the ventroposterolateral nuclei of the thalamus and then to the cerebral cortex. They relay tactile information as well as nociception. It is clear that mechanisms of pain transmission involve extremely complex connections in diverse areas of the central nervous system, many of which have yet to be defined.

MECHANISMS OF ANALGESIA

The use of nonnarcotic analgesics in the critical care setting has been hindered as a result of problems relating to route of administration and a lack of familiarity with their use in severe pain states. Nonsteroidal antiinflammatory drugs (NSAIDs) represent a group of useful analgesics, either alone or, more frequently, to enhance the effects and diminish the side effects of narcotic analgesics. These drugs possess antiinflammatory, antipyretic, antiplatelet, and analgesic properties. The mechanism of their activity is via inhibition of prostaglandin synthetase (38). This prostaglandin effect is reversible within 2 or 3 days after discontinuation of the drug. As with any prostaglandin synthetase inhibitor, some degree of interference with platelet function may be expected; therefore, patients receiving NSAIDs should be monitored carefully. The antiinflammatory action of the NSAIDs appears to occur peripherally at the site of injury. The antipyretic action appears to be centrally modulated in the hypothalamus (39). Ketorolac tromethamine is the first available parenteral form of a nonsteroidal antiinflammatory, and acetaminophen and indomethacin currently are available for rectal administration. The NSAIDs demonstrate a ceiling effect for their analgesic properties; that is, there exists a limiting dose of NSAID beyond which no further analgesic effect is obtained, but side effects continue to appear and may be increased. This ceiling dose varies from individual to individual.

Morphine and other narcotic analgesics produce their major effects on the central nervous system and the gastrointestinal tract. The major effects of opiates include analgesia, mood changes (euphoria or dysphoria), drowsiness, respiratory depression, cough suppression, decreased gastrointestinal motility, nausea, vomiting, and alterations of endocrine and autonomic nervous system function. Depending upon the route of administration, the site of action of the analgesic effect is in the brain or the spinal cord. The sites of action of the side effects are both central and peripheral. It is now clear that

opiates act as agonists, interacting with saturable, stereospecific binding sites or receptors in the central nervous system and other sites (40). These binding sites are distributed unevenly throughout the central nervous system. They are present in highest concentration in the limbic system (frontal and temporal cortex, amygdala, and hippocampus), thalamus, corpus striatum, hypothalamus, midbrain, and spinal cord (41).

Narcotic analgesic compounds demonstrate stereospecific receptor binding and reversal of effects by narcotic antagonists. Structurally, narcotics are complex, three-dimensional compounds that usually exist as optical isomers (42). Significant variation in pharmacologic activity may result from conformational changes in the molecule produced by a changing pH (43). Most narcotics have a relatively rigid T-shaped conformation, an electron-rich hydroxyl or ketone group, a positively charged basic nitrogen, a quaternary carbon that is separated from the basic nitrogen by an ethane chain, and a flat benzene or 2-thienyl ring, which is 4.58 Å from the nitrogen (42).

It is now known that there is more than one type of opiate receptor, and that different receptors may be involved in different functions (44). Opiate receptors may differ in both their affinity for various opiates and opiate antagonists and thereby in their physiologic significance. Various classifications have been proposed to distinguish among receptor types. Opiate receptors may be classified into four groups: (*a*) the μ-receptor (morphine receptor), (*b*) the κ-receptor (cyclazocine receptor), (*c*) the σ-receptor, and (*d*) the δ-receptor. The μ receptor mediates supraspinal analgesia, respiratory depression, feelings of well-being, euphoria, and a morphine-type physical dependence. The σ-receptor mediates feelings of dysphoria, hallucinations, mydriasis, hypotension, and respiratory stimulation. Finally, the δ-receptor mediates some of the in vitro pharmacologic effects of the enkephalins and endorphins. There is also a claim for a possible fifth narcotic receptor, the ϵ-receptor. The current classification of opioid-type drugs into agonists, antagonists, and agonists-antagonists has been based on this receptor concept.

NARCOTIC ANALGESICS

Narcotics are either naturally occurring, semisynthetic, or synthetic (Table 26.2). Morphine, codeine, and papaverine (the only naturally occurring clinically significant narcotics) are obtained from the poppy plant, *Papaver somniferum.* Opium is the dried powdered mixture of alkaloids obtained from the unripe seed capsules of the poppy plant, which contain more than 20 pharmacologically active natural alkaloids. These alkaloids are of two chemical classes, the phenanthrenes (morphine and codeine) and the benzylisoquinolines (papaverine).

The semisynthetic narcotics are derivatives of morphine. Codeine results from the etherification of one hydroxyl group; heroin, from the esterification of both hydroxyl groups; and hydromorphone (Dilaudid), from oxidation of the alcoholic hydroxyl group to a ketone group, or saturation of a double bond on the benzene ring (45).

The synthetic narcotics resemble morphine but usually are entirely synthesized. They include the morphinians (levorphanol), the propionanilides (methadone, *d*-propoxyphene), the

Table 38.2.   Classification and Dosage of Some Narcotic Agonists and Antagonists

Drug (Trade Name)	Dose (in 70-kg adult)		Dose Interval (hr)	Comparative Narcotic Potency
	i.v. (mg)	i.m./s.c. (mg)		
Natural Alkaloids of opium				
Morphine	2–10 (titrate)	5–10	2–4	1
Codeine	30–60	60–120	2–4	0.1
Semisynthetic derivatives				
Hydromorphone (Dilaudid)	0.5–1 (titrate)	2	3–4	5
Oxymorphone (Numorphan)	0.5 (titrate)	1	3–4	10
Synthetic derivatives				
Meperidine (Demerol, etc.)	25–100 (titrate)	50–100	2–4	0.1
Methadone (Dolophine, etc.)	2–5 (titrate)	2–10	2–4	1.2
Pentazocine (Talwin)	10–30 (titrate)	30	3–4	0.25
Fentanyl (Sublimaze)	0.05–0.1 (titrate)	0.1	½–2	150
Narcotic antagonists				
Naloxone (Narcan)	0.2–0.4	0.4	½–¾	
Nalorphine (Nalline)	5–10		p.r.n.	
Levallorphan (Lorfan)	1		p.r.n.	

benzomorphans (pentazocine, phenazocine, cyclazocine), and the phenylpiperidines (meperidine, fentanyl, sufentanil, alfentanil).

NARCOTIC AGONISTS

MORPHINE

Morphine (Fig. 38.2) is the prototypic narcotic analgesic and the most widely used. It is examined here in detail and serves as a basis for understanding the pharmacology of other narcotic analgesics.

Absorption

Morphine may be administered via the oral, subcutaneous, intramuscular, intravenous, epidural, or intrathecal routes. When given orally, as in Brompton's solution, a 10-mg dose in the average adult patient results in a plasma concentration of about 10 ng/ml within 15 minutes (46) (Fig. 38.3). Plasma concentration is maintained between 8 and 10 ng/ml for 45 to 60 minutes and then gradually decreases to about 1 ng/ml at 8 hours.

Morphine is absorbed readily from the gut, but plasma levels are considerably lower after oral administration than after parenteral administration. This finding is secondary to uptake and metabolism of the morphine by the liver and intestinal mucosa prior to reaching the central circulation (first-pass effect). There also exists an enterohepatic circulation for morphine that accounts for the observed second peak in plasma concentration in humans and animals that occurs about 30 to 40 minutes after oral ingestion (46).

Subcutaneously administered morphine results in rapid absorption, with plasma levels of unchanged morphine of about 70 ng/ml 15 minutes after injection of 10 mg in a 70-kg subject (46). The plasma levels decline progressively from the peak (Fig. 38.3).

Intramuscular injection also results in rapid absorption, with plasma concentrations of 80 ng/ml 15 minutes after administration. As with subcutaneous injection, plasma concentration decreases rapidly. Since muscle blood flow varies greatly in humans at rest (47), and even more so during activity, the rate of absorption varies. This fact explains the wide variations observed in time-to-peak plasma levels following intramuscular injection and the reports of poor pain control after intramuscular narcotic injections (48).

Intravenous injection of morphine bypasses the absorption process. Peak plasma levels are higher than by any of the other routes (46). Metabolism and distribution are more rapid, since first-order kinetics operate. Plasma levels decrease rapidly, since there is no sustained absorption phase. Plasma levels after 10 mg of intravenously administered morphine in 70-kg subjects are about 50 ng/ml 15 minutes after injection, which is lower than after intramuscular or subcutaneous administration (46). They subsequently remain lower for 3 to 4 hours (Fig. 38.3).

Morphine has been injected into the epidural and spinal subarachnoid spaces (12, 49). On the whole, the plasma levels of morphine are proportional to the dose, but there is wide variation (49). These routes of administration provide a highly useful method of pain relief, especially in the ICU, where continuous epidural and intrathecal catheters can be employed readily. The epidural route of narcotic analgesic administration has been shown to improve ventilatory function in patients with blunt chest trauma (50) and may reduce morbidity in high-risk surgical patients (51). Epidurally administered morphine has an onset of analgesic action within 60 to 90 minutes following administration.

Distribution

In addition to the central nervous system, morphine is readily taken up and concentrated by the parenchymal tissues of the lungs, kidney, liver, spleen, and muscle. The amount of morphine found in the brain is much smaller than that found in the parenchymal tissues. Morphine has a low oil/water partition coefficient and therefore penetrates cellular barriers more slowly and accumulates to a lesser degree in the lipid compartment. Morphine therefore tends to distribute more to tissues in which it is ionized, bound, or actively transported.

Excretion

Hepatic metabolism is by far the most important route for the elimination of morphine in humans and animals. Minor routes for excretion include the urine, bile, and saliva. Biotransformation of morphine occurs mainly via glucuronic acid conjugation. Morphine-3-glucuronide, the principal metabolite, essentially is not active because of its polarity and is excreted readily by both glomerular filtration and active tubular transport (46). Morphine-6-glucuronide is an active metabolite that is dependent upon renal excretion, and in patients with renal impairment possible accumulation of this metabolite must be considered (52).

Respiratory System

Morphine exerts a direct depressant effect on the medullary respiratory centers and affects the pontine centers involved in respiratory rhythmicity. Initially, respiratory rate is affected more than tidal volume, but as the dose of morphine is increased, tidal volume and minute ventilation decrease and periodic breathing and apnea occur (53, 54). A 10-mg dose of morphine (0.15 mg/kg) decreases tidal volume and respiratory rate while increasing resting $PACO_2$ by about 3 torr (0.4 kPa) in normal subjects (55). Respiratory depression is even more marked when evaluated in terms of the expected ventilatory response to hypercarbia (55, 56). At higher doses of morphine (e.g., 2 mg/kg), not only is the $PACO_2$ ventilation response curve displaced to the right, but the slope is reduced (Fig. 38.4) and can be partially reversed by naloxone (57). The administration of large doses of morphine for cardiac surgical operations may prolong the postoperative length of assisted ventilation. This effect is particularly important for patients undergoing valve replacement and is not observed in patients having myocardial revascularization procedures (58). These observed differences likely result from different rates of excretion of morphine, secondary to the overall lower cardiac indices and therefore lower hepatic and renal blood flows in patients that have valve surgery (59).

Although patients demonstrate respiratory depression after morphine administration, they usually can increase their tidal volume and respiratory rate on command if they are still

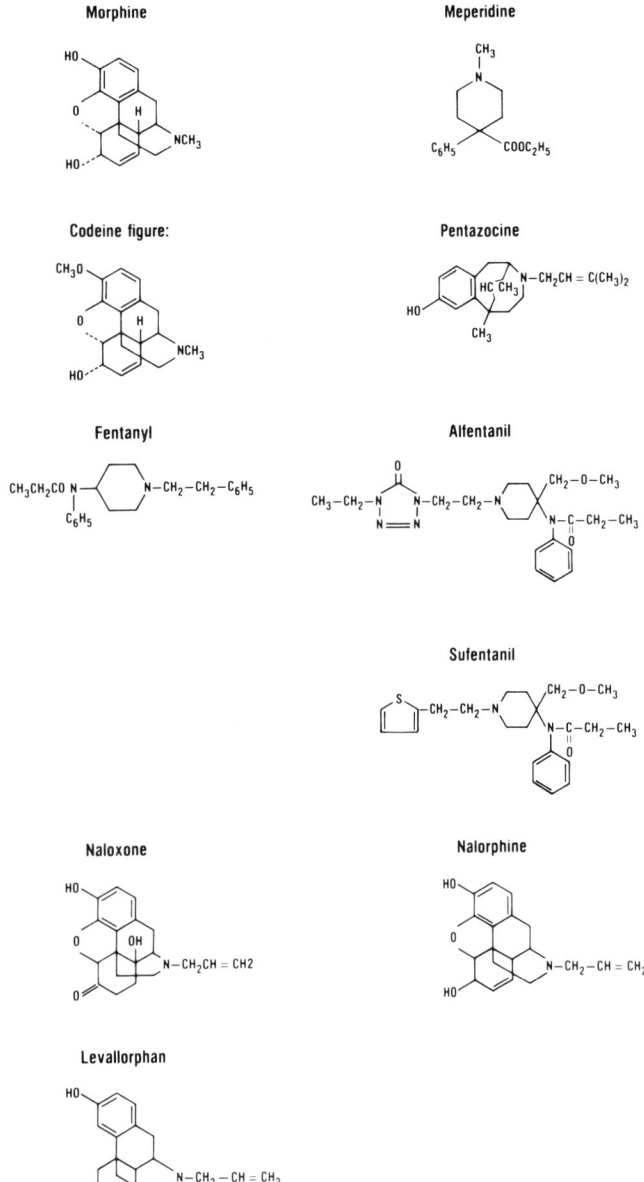

Figure 38.2.   Morphine and narcotic agonists and antagonists.

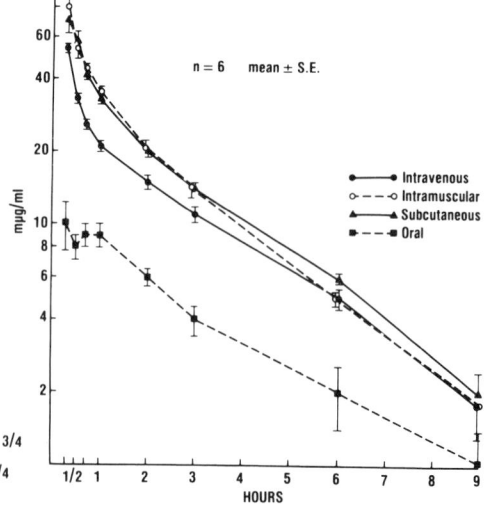

Figure 38.3.   Plasma concentrations of unchanged morphine in volunteers after a dose of approximately 10 mg (5.75 mg/m²). (Adapted from Brunk SF, Delle M: Morphine metabolism in man. Clin Pharmacol Ther 16:51–57, 1974.)

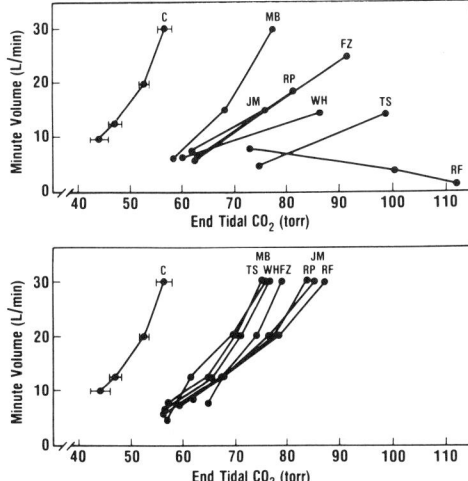

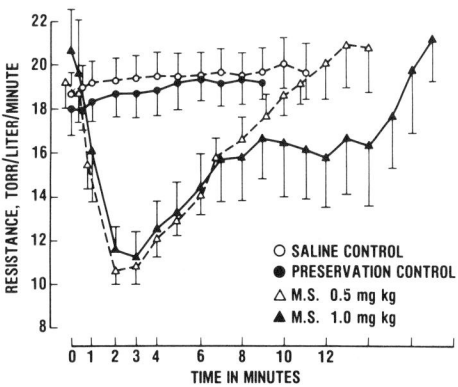

Figure 38.5. Peripheral vasculature resistance and morphine. Dosages of morphine 0.5 mg/kg and 1 mg/kg decreased peripheral vascular resistance in humans, whereas the injection of saline solution or the preservatives in morphine solution did not ($P < 0.01$). Data points are means ± SE. (Adapted from Hsu HO, et al: Morphine decreases peripheral vascular resistance and increases capacitance in man. Anesthesiology 50:98–102, 1979.)

Figure 38.4. Naloxone reversal of morphine: $PACO_2$/ventilation response curves after morphine 2mg/kg. *Curve C,* Averaged control. *Top,* Before naloxone. *Bottom,* after antagonism by naloxone. (Adapted from Johnstone RE, et al: Reversal of morphine anesthesia with naloxone. Anesthesiology 41:361–367, 1974.)

conscious, demonstrating that voluntary respiratory control remains intact. Morphine may be dangerous in those critically ill patients with respiratory compromise (e.g., asthma, chronic obstructive pulmonary disease, severe pneumonia, restrictive lung disease) and should be used cautiously. Morphine also has central antitussive properties and may interfere with pulmonary toilet in the critically ill patient.

Cardiovascular System

The effect of morphine on the circulation depends upon several factors, including the patient's illness, dose, route of administration, position, activity of the patient, and the presence of other medications. Clinical doses of morphine (0.1 to 0.2 mg/kg) in normal supine patients have little effect, but postural hypotension may occur as a result of peripheral vasodilation and venous pooling. With larger doses used in cardiovascular anesthesia (1 to 2 mg/kg) the cardiovascular system is stable so long as ventilation, oxygenation, and blood volume are maintained. Lowenstein et al (60) administered 1 mg/kg of morphine to eight healthy normal patients and to seven patients with aortic valve disease. Minimal cardiovascular effects were observed in the normal patients, whereas the patients with valve disease showed increases in cardiac index, stroke index, and pulmonary artery and central venous pressures and a decrease in systemic vascular resistance. Morphine may improve myocardial dynamics in patients with elevated left ventricular end diastolic pressures by dilating venous capacitance vessels. Intravenous injections of morphine (0.5 to 1 mg/kg) during cardiopulmonary bypass decreases peripheral vascular resistance by about 50% within 2 minutes (61) (Fig. 38.5). This decrease is followed by a return to control levels after about 10 minutes. Hypotension following morphine administration can be treated by rapid infusion of fluids to increase the intravascular volume.

The vasodilation observed with morphine is attributed to (*a*) histamine release, (*b*) direct vasodilation, and (*c*) neural

mediation. Histamine is reported to play a major role in morphine-induced vasodilation, and a dose-dependent increase in plasma histamine levels is associated with a decrease in mean arterial pressure (62). Meperidine and codeine also increase plasma histamine levels, whereas methadone and probably fentanyl do not (62). Morphine also has direct vasodilator properties (63) and may decrease central α-adrenergic activity.

The peripheral vascular and analgesic effects of morphine are beneficial in pulmonary edema, congestive heart failure, and myocardial infarction. Morphine causes a rapid decrease in pulmonary artery flow and pressure and left ventricular end diastolic pressure, and results in increased myocardial contractility (Fig. 38.6) (64). Vismara et al (65) have given intravenous injections of morphine (0.1 mg/kg) to patients with congestive heart failure and pulmonary edema. They attribute the beneficial effects of morphine to splanchnic pooling, decreased preload and afterload, and decreased work of breathing. Morphine attenuates the sympathetic efferent discharge associated with pulmonary edema and the pain of myocardial ischemia (66, 67). Morphine (4 to 8 mg every 5 to 15 minutes until pain relief or respiratory depression occurs) remains the drug of choice for the treatment of pain associated with myocardial infarction or ischemia.

Morphine and other narcotics have a negative chronotropic effect and act by central effects and by a direct effect on the sinoatrial node (68). Morphine in analgesic doses (0.1 to 0.2 mg/kg i.v.) has little effect on the sinus node and may protect against ventricular fibrillation (69). In higher doses such as those used for anesthesia, morphine and other narcotics may decrease heart rate. Fentanyl (5 to 10 μg/kg i.v.) decreases heart rate by 60 to 70% that of control (70).

Morphine should be used with caution in patients with a history of blood loss or other illness associated with a reduced intravascular volume, because of the likelihood of hypotension. Sudden postural changes should be avoided and adequate intravenous access should be present so that fluids can be administered rapidly should hypotension occur. Because of an increased risk of hypotension, morphine should be used with caution in patients with cor pulmonale and when phenothiazines are also in use.

Gastrointestinal Tract

Narcotic substances were used for the relief of dysentery and diarrhea long before they were used as analgesics. Morphine delays gastric emptying time mainly via its action on the stomach and duodenum (71). Morphine and meperidine in equianalgesic doses have the same qualitative effects on the gastrointestinal (GI) tract—that is, diminished propulsive activity and an increase in resting tone and incidence of spasm (71). Meperidine's effects peak at 1 to 1½ hours, whereas morphine's effects are prominent at 4 hours. Morphine also decreases intestinal motility in the terminal ileum (72) and diminishes activity in the colon. These effects account for the constipating effects of morphine and other narcotics. These effects are of little concern in healthy subjects, but in patients with ulcerative colitis and possibly other diseases of the GI tract, narcotics may have serious deleterious effects. Garrett et al (73) studied patients with ulcerative colitis and found marked hypermotility and increased tone. In their retrospective analysis of 18 patients with ulcerative colitis who developed toxic megacolon, they found that 17 of the 18 patients had symptoms associated with recent administration of narcotics. Morphine also decreases secretions of the salivary glands, stomach, pancreas, and biliary tract. When given alone, morphine (0.2 mg/kg, up to 15 mg) causes a 20% increase in splanchnic blood flow and a 13% decrease in splanchnic vascular resistance (74). This effect results mainly from arteriolar dilation, which may be advantageous in patients with compromised intestinal blood flow.

Morphine has been linked with biliary spasm and symptoms of biliary colic (75). Equianalgesic doses of morphine (0.125 mg/kg), meperidine (1.0 mg/kg), fentanyl (1.25 μg), and pentazocine (0.15 mg/kg) given intraoperatively increase common bile duct pressures by 52.7%, 61.3%, 99.5%, and 15% respectively, after injection. Whether or not all narcotics uniformly increase biliary pressure is not clear, but any abnormal cholangiogram or other study of the biliary tree obtained in association with administration of narcotics should be suspect.

Renal Considerations

In unstressed surgical patients, morphine (0.11 mg/kg) is associated with a decrease in glomerular filtration rate but no alteration in urine volume or composition (76). The addition of anesthesia with nitrous oxide further decreases glomerular filtration rate and urine output. Although antidiuretic hormone (ADH) may be a factor, the major effect appears to be a renal hemodynamic one, via decreased cardiac output, sympathetic stimulation, and vasoconstriction. The addition of surgical stress to nitrous oxide-narcotic anesthesia may result in very high plasma ADH levels (77). Patients with renal failure may accumulate morphine and demonstrate an enhanced narcotic effect.

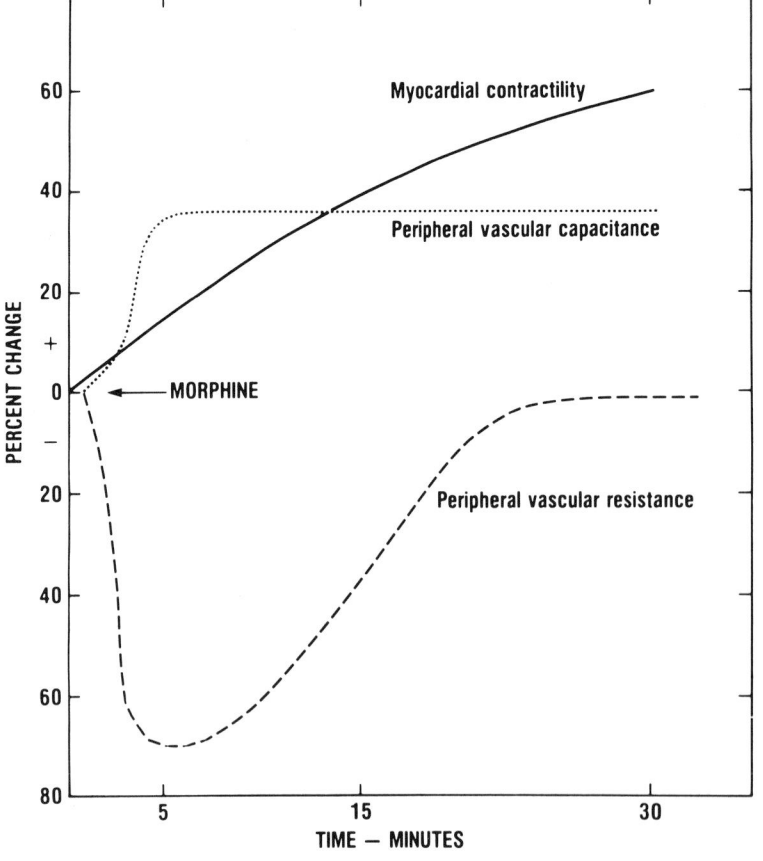

Figure 38.6. Diagrammatic representation of the interdependent effects of morphine upon the contractile state of the heart and upon the peripheral vascular bed. (Adapted form Vasko JS, et al: Mechanisms of action of morphine in the treatment of experimental pulmonary edema. Am J Cardiol 18:876–883, 1966.)

Other Considerations

It is frequently stated that elderly patients are more sensitive to the CNS effects of narcotic analgesics. Berkowitz et al (78) noted that serum levels of morphine are about 1.5 times higher in patients older than 50 years of age than in younger patients at 2 minutes after an intravenous injection of 10 mg/70 kg. The differences in plasma morphine concentrations were less at 5 minutes and absent at 10 minutes. Factors causing the higher serum morphine levels have not been identified, but a slower titration of narcotic analgesics to obtain the desired effect is advised in those older than 50 years of age.

Only free morphine is capable of penetrating biologic membranes and reaching its site of action. Approximately one-third of unchanged morphine is bound to albumin in normal humans, with a much lower amount bound to globulin (79). Protein-bound morphine is pharmacologically inactive, but the complex can dissociate readily. Alkalosis increases the percentage of morphine bound to plasma proteins. For each increase in pH of 0.2 unit, the percentage of protein-bound morphine increases by 3% (79), and likewise a decrease in pH releases more free active morphine. The percentage of morphine bound to protein is also related directly to protein concentration and to other drugs that compete for albumin binding. Therefore, in the critically ill patient who is on numerous medications and has a low albumin, normal doses of morphine may have a much greater effect. Morphine also has been reported as a cause of immune thrombocytopenia (80).

Dosage and Administration

Morphine is available as the salts morphine sulfate and morphine hydrochloride. The optimal dose is stated as being up to 10 mg/70 kg of body weight via subcutaneous or intravenous routes. The dose should be modified according to the disease and age of the patient. Subsequent doses should be titrated depending on the analgesic effect and side effects observed. Intravenous or epidural is the preferred route of administration in the ICU. Administration by continuous intravenous infusion (81) can sustain effective blood levels and pain relief, and avoid periods of depressed level of consciousness associated with peak blood levels after intramuscular or subcutaneous injections. The technique of patient-controlled analgesia in appropriate patients is highly effective and may improve patient satisfaction and decrease nursing demands (82, 83). Table 38.2 lists dosage and duration of action of narcotic agonists and antagonists used parenterally.

CODEINE

Codeine is an alkaloid of opium and is considered a mild analgesic. Codeine is two-thirds as effective orally as parenterally, both as a respiratory depressant and analgesic. Codeine is metabolized in the liver and about 10% is demethylated to form morphine, which may be responsible for codeine's major analgesic effect, since codeine itself has an exceptionally low affinity for the opioid receptor (84, 85). Codeine sulfate usually is given by mouth in a dose of 15 to 60 mg and may be given by intramuscular injection.

HYDROMORPHONE (SEMISYNTHETIC)

Hydromorphone (Dilaudid) is a semisynthetic modification of morphine. It is five times as potent as morphine and can be given orally or parenterally. It has no apparent advantages over morphine in the intensive care setting when delivered by the intravenous route. When delivered by the epidural route, hydromorphone yields similar pain relief with fewer side effects than morphine (86).

MEPERIDINE (SYNTHETIC)

Meperidine, a synthetic analgesic, is a piperidine derivative whose major actions are similar to those of morphine. Meperidine is lipophilic and exhibits a close correlation between its plasma levels and the intensity of its analgesic and ventilatory depressant actions (87, 88).

Meperidine demonstrates a dose-dependent cardiac depressant action, especially at doses above 5 mg/kg (89). Meperidine is metabolized in the liver to normeperidine, a potent CNS stimulant, and convulsions in humans have been attributed to the *N*-demethylated metabolites after large doses (90). Typical critical care patients receiving usual doses of meperidine over long periods may demonstrate accumulation and concomitant toxicity. This factor may be significant if meperidine is taken orally (first-pass effect) or administered in the presence of renal failure, or if meperidine and chlorpromazine are given together (91). Besides its toxic interaction with chlorpromazine, meperidine also should not be given with monoamine oxidase (MAO) inhibitors (92).

FENTANYL

Fentanyl is a synthetic opioid related to the phenylpiperidines. Fentanyl is approximately 7000 times more lipophilic than morphine (93). Fentanyl penetrates biologic membranes quite rapidly and has a rapid onset of action. There exists an extremely close relationship between brain and plasma concentrations and between plasma fentanyl levels and its intensity of effect (94). Fentanyl is considered 75 to 200 times more potent than morphine. This fact results in part from its ready access to the brain, and possibly also from a greater activity at opioid receptors (93). Fentanyl is highly protein bound in both the plasma (67%) and the brain (90%), and it has a high affinity for fat such that prolonged exposure may result in its accumulation in fat and a prolonged recovery. Fentanyl demonstrates a proportional, dose-related increase in its duration of action, and this factor explains why initial doses are of short duration of action, whereas repeated doses increase the concentration and duration of action (95). In equianalgesic doses fentanyl and morphine produce approximately the same degree of respiratory depression. Because of its minimal effect on the cardiovascular system (96), short duration of action, and rapid effect, fentanyl is a very useful analgesic for use during potentially painful procedures (e.g., placement of vascular catheters, balloon pumps, and endotracheal tubes). Addition of diazepam or other sedative to fentanyl may result in decreased cardiac output, blood pressure, and peripheral vascular resistance (96). Fentanyl usually is administered intravenously, with 1 to 3 μg/kg being the usual dose for analgesia. Up to 10 μg/kg may be given in the absence of other sedative, analgesic medications if ventilation is controlled. Fentanyl is supplied for injection as 50 μg/ml. Another delivery option is transdermal fentanyl. It is available in transdermal patches that release 25, 50, 75, or 100 μg/hr. Optimal blood levels require 6 to 10 hours to be attained, and blood levels remain in the analgesic range for as long as 6 to 10 hours after patch removal (97).

ALFENTANIL AND SUFENTANIL

Sufentanil was synthesized in 1974 as a result of manipulation of fentanyl structure. Sufentanil is five to 10 times more potent than fentanyl. In the tail withdrawal reflex in rats, sufentanil is 4521 times as potent as morphine, and there is minimal effect on the cardiovascular system (98). Sufentanil is highly protein bound (92.5%), predominantly to the α_1-acidic glycoprotein. It is highly lipophilic and has a faster onset of action than does fentanyl. Sufentanil has a shorter elimination half-life (148 minutes), and this, combined with its somewhat lesser volume of distribution, may explain the reported shorter duration of respiratory depression with sufentanil than with fentanyl. The clearance and hepatic extraction ratio of sufentanil are similar to those of fentanyl, and the effect of small doses is likely to be terminated by redistribution to the peripheral compartment. With larger doses, as with fentanyl, the plasma concentrations of sufentanil may not be rendered subtherapeutic by redistribution. When this redistribution occurs, hepatic biotransformation is the limiting factor for termination of the clinical effect.

Alfentanil is the result of a chemical modification of fentanyl. As compared with fentanyl, alfentanil has a methyleneoxymethyl group added at the C4 position of the piperidine ring and a tetrazolinone ring substituted for a phenyl ring. Alfentanil is approximately one-fourth as potent as fentanyl but has a faster onset and shorter duration of action than fentanyl. Alfentanil is significantly less lipophilic than fentanyl and has a significantly smaller volume of distribution at steady state. Alfentanil is highly bound to plasma proteins (92%) and is approximately 10% ionized at a pH of 7.4. Alfentanil is metabolized rapidly by the liver, but the clearance of alfentanil is less than that of fentanyl; however, the small volume of distribution of alfentanil at steady state results in an elimination half-life considerably less than that of fentanyl ($t_{1/2}\beta$ for alfentanil = 2.0 hr; $t_{1/2}\beta$ for fentanyl = 7.9 hrs) (99). In the intensive care unit, alfentanil may be a highly useful medication for performing short procedures in either spontaneously breathing patients or intubated patients. For short procedures, a bolus of 8 to 20 μg/kg may provide analgesic protection against hemodynamic responses to the stress associated with performing needed procedures. Should the procedure last longer than 20 to 30 minutes, incremental doses of 3 to 5 μg/kg given as a bolus or 0.5 to μg/kg/min by continuous infusion, titrated to patient response, may be useful in continued alleviation of the stress associated with surgical or other procedures.

NARCOTIC AGONIST-ANTAGONISTS

Pentazocine is a benzomorphan derivative with both agonist and weak opioid antagonist activity. In equianalgesic doses pentazocine produces a degree of respiratory depression similar to that of morphine (e.g., 30 mg of pentazocine and 10 mg of morphine). Increasing the dose beyond 30 mg does not result in a proportional increase in respiratory depression (100), and respiratory depression is maximal at 60 mg pentazocine. Pentazocine may cause an increase of mean arterial pressure, left ventricular end-diastolic pressure, and mean pulmonary artery pressure, resulting in an increase in myocardial work load. Pentazocine has weak opioid antagonist properties. It will not reverse the respiratory depression of other "pure" agonists but may precipitate opioid withdrawal in patients who are receiving narcotics on a regular basis. For the aforementioned reasons pentazocine has little use in the critical care setting. Butorphanol and nalbuphine are two other mixed agonist-antagonist medications with strong analgesic properties. Butorphanol may have adverse effects in patients with congestive heart failure or myocardial infarction (101). These drugs currently are undergoing study for use in epidural analgesia. Butorphanol may be useful in decreasing the side effects seen with epidural morphine (102). Dezocine is a recently introduced synthetic agonist-antagonist with a dosage and analgesic effect similar to those of morphine (103).

NARCOTIC ANTAGONISTS

The narcotic antagonists comprise nalorphine, levallorphan, and naloxone. Nalarophine and levallorphan have both antagonist and agonist actions, whereas naloxone is a pure antagonist.

In the absence of opioid drugs naloxone produces almost no clinical effect. Naloxone antagonizes the effects of both the narcotic agonists and agonist-antagonists. Narcotic reversal with naloxone has been associated with ventricular tachycardia and fibrillation in patients following cardiac surgery (104) and causes premature ventricular contractions, increased heart rate, increased cardiac output, and increased mean blood pressure and decreased stroke volume in animals anesthetized with morphine (105). It is clear that the acute withdrawal of narcotic anesthesia in the wide variety of postoperative patients presenting to ICUs (e.g., cardiac surgical patients, neurosurgical patients, general surgical patients) could result in disastrous hemodynamic effects. Furthermore, naloxone may have specific agonist effects of its own (106), and until further data are available, careful titration of naloxone in small increments for the purpose of known narcotic reversal is advised. Naloxone may be used very effectively to reverse the respiratory effects of narcotics; however, the duration of action of a single bolus of intravenously administered naloxone is short, having a half-life of about 20 minutes (107). Prolonged reversal of narcotic anesthesia has been reported with intramuscular injection of naloxone; however, because of the unreliable uptake of intramuscular medications, this route is not advised. Repeated boluses or a continuous closely monitored infusion will more reliably prevent renarcotization of postoperative patients while avoiding abrupt narcotic reversal.

Tolerance and Dependence

Tolerance to some of the effects of narcotic analgesics may develop rapidly. It develops most quickly to the depressant actions (respiratory depression, sedation, analgesia) and more slowly to the excitatory effects. Tolerance is evident 4 hours after commencement of a morphine infusion in the experimental animal (108) and is likely after six to eight consecutive administrations in humans. The mechanisms of tolerance are unclear. Cross-tolerance occurs within members of the narcotic analgesics but does not extend to other centrally acting medications. Tolerance may be considerable; a narcotic addict may tolerate up to 500 times the clinical dose of morphine.

A study by Mather and Phillips (109) has defined some common misconceptions held by health care professionals concerning analgesic use. A few of these are as follows: (*a*) doses should be as small and infrequent as possible to avoid the development of addiction; (*b*) doses larger than standard do not increase pain relief and cause heavy sedation and respiratory depression; and (*c*) nursing and/or medical staff know best when and how much pain relief each patient needs. Physical dependence on opiates is of minor importance in patients who are receiving morphine for postoperative pain, in patients in critical care units, and in those who are receiving opiates for relief of terminal cancer pain. Many physicians and nurses are unnecessarily reluctant to utilize therapeutically effective doses of opiates in acute pain, for fear of inducing severe physical dependence. Tolerance may be an early sign of physical dependence. After a 1- to 2-week course of clinical doses of opiates, mild withdrawal symptoms may be detected, but in most patients the symptoms pass unnoticed. Should a narcotic antagonist or agonist-antagonist be administered, more severe withdrawal may be precipitated. The symptoms of withdrawal generally are opposite to the effects of the narcotic analgesics (e.g., diarrhea, hyperventilation, mydriasis), except for nausea and vomiting, which may be both an effect of opiates and a withdrawal symptom. Deaths have occurred during narcotic withdrawal but probably did not result from the withdrawal symptoms *per se* (110).

REFERENCES

1. International Association for the Study of Pain Subcommittee on Taxonomy: Pain terms: a list with definitions and notes on usage. *Pain* 6:249–252, 1979.
2. Donald I: At the receiving end, a doctor's personal recollections of valve replacement. *Scott Med J* 2:1129–1131, 1969.
3. Donald I: At the receiving end, a doctor's personal recollection of second time valve replacement. *Scott Med J* 21:49–57, 1976.
4. Henschel EO: The Guillain-Barré syndrome, a personal experience. *Anesthesiology* 47:228–231, 1977.
5. Shovelton DS: Reflections on an intensive therapy unit. *Br Med J* 1:737–738, 1979.
6. Marks RM, Sachar EJ: Undertreatment of medical inpatients with narcotic analgesics. *Ann Intern Med* 78:173, 1973.
7. Mitchel RWD, Smith G: The control of acute postoperative pain. *Br J Anaesth* 63:147–158, 1989.
8. Jones NH: Postoperative pain control: solving a long standing problem. *Today's OR Nurse* 10:10–16, 1988.
9. Bonica JJ, Buckley FP: Regional analgesia with local anesthetics. In Bonica JJ (ed): *The Management of Pain*, 2nd ed. Lea & Febiger, Philadelphia, pp 1183–1966, 1990.
10. Church JJ: Continuous narcotic infusions for relief of postoperative pain. *Br Med J* 1:977–979, 1979.
11. Bromage PR, Camporessi E, Chestnut D: Epidural narcotics for postoperative analgesia. *Anesth Analg* 59:473–480, 1980.
12. Wang JK, Nauss LA, Thomas JE: Pain relief by intrathecally applied morphine in man. *Anesthesiology* 50:149–151, 1979.
13. Yaksh TL, Rudy TA: Analgesia mediated by a direct spinal action of narcotics. *Science* 192:1357–1358, 1976.
14. Yeager MP, Glass DD, Neff RK, Brinck-Johnsen T: Epidural anesthesia and analgesia in high risk surgical patients. *Anesthesiology* 66:729–736, 1987.

15. Gourlay GK, Kowalski SR, Plummer JL, Cherry DA, Gaukroger P, Cousins MJ: The transdermal administration of fentanyl in the treatment of postoperative pain: pharmacokinetics and pharmacodynamic effects. *Pain* 37:193–202, 1989.
16. Iggo A: Peripheral and spinal "pain" mechanisms and their modulation. In Bonica JJ, Albe-Fessard (eds): *Advances in Pain Research and Therapy*. Raven Press, New York, pp 381–394, 1976.
17. Iggo A: Is the physiology of cutaneous receptors determined by morphology? *Prog Brain Res* 43:15–31, 1976.
18. Perl ER, Kumazawa T, Lynn B, et al: Sensitization of high threshold receptors with unmyelinated (c) afferent fibers. *Prog Brain Res* 43:263–277, 1976.
19. Price DD, Dubner R: Neurons that observe the sensory discriminative aspects of pain. *Pain* 3:307–338, 1977.
20. Torebjork HE: Afferent C units responding to mechanical thermal and chemical stimuli in human non-glabrous skin. *Acta Physiol Scand* 92:374–390, 1974.
21. Perl ER: Sensitization of nociceptors and its relation to sensitization. In Bonica JJ, Albe-Fessard DG (eds): *Advances in Pain Research and Therapy*. Raven Press, New York, pp 17–28, 1976.
22. Hodge CJ, Woods CI, Delatizky J: Noradrenalin, serotonin, and the dorsal horn. *J Neurosurg* 52:674–685, 1980.
23. Messing RB, Lytle LD: Serotonin-containing neurons: their possible role in pain and analgesia. *Pain* 4:1–21, 1977.
24. Sagen J, Proudfit HK: Evidence for pain modulation by pre- and postsynaptic noradrenergic receptors in the medulla oblongata. *Brain Res* 331:285–291, 1985.
25. Juan H: Prostaglandins as modulators of pain. *Gen Pharmacol* 9:403–409, 1978.
26. King JS, Gallant P, Myerson V, et al: The effects of antiinflammatory agents on the responses and the sensitization of unmyelinated (c) fiber polymodal nicoceptors. In Zotterman Y (ed): *Sensory Functions of the Skin in Primates with Special Reference to Man*. Pergamon Press, Oxford, UK, pp 441–461, 1976.
27. Kenny GN, McArdle CS, Aitken HH: Parenteral ketorolac: opiate-sparing effect and lack of cardiorespiratory depression in the perioperative patient. *J Pharmacother* 10:127S–131S, 1990.
28. Stanski DR, Cherry C, Bradley R, Sarnquist FH, Yee JP: Efficacy and safety of single doses of intramuscular ketorolac tromethamine compared with meperidine for postoperative pain. *J Pharmacother* 10:40S–44S, 1990.
29. Hokfelt T, Ljungdahl A, Terenius L, et al: Immunohistochemical analysis of peptide pathways possibly related to pain and analgesia: enkephalin and substance. *P Proc Natl Acad Sci USA* 74:3081–3085, 1977.
30. Henry JL: Relation of substance P to pain transmission: neurophysiological evidence. In *Substance P and the Nervous System*, Ciba Foundation Symposium. Pitman, London, 16:206–224, 1982.
31. Chung K, Langford LA, Applebaum AE, et al: Primary afferent fibers in the tract of Lissauer in the rat. *J Comp Neurol* 184:587–598, 1979.
32. Merrill EG, Wall PD, Yaksh TL: Properties of the two unmyelinated fibre tracts of the central nervous system: lateral Lissauer tract and parallel fibres of the cerebellum. *J Physiol* (Lond) 284:127–145, 1978.
33. Coggeshall RE, Coulter JD, Willis WD: Unmyelinated fibers in the ventral root. *Brain Res* 57:229–233, 1973.
34. Maynard CW, Leonard RB, Coulter JD, et al: Central connections of ventral root afferents as demonstrated by the HRP method. *J Comp Neurol* 17:601–608, 1977.
35. Rexed B: Cytoarchitectonic organization of the spinal cord in the cat. *J Comp Neurol* 96:415–495, 1952.
36. Narotzky RA, Kerr FWL: Marginal neurons of the spinal cord: types, afferent synaptology and functional considerations. *Brain Res* 139:1–20, 1978.
37. Kumazawa T, Perl ER: Excitation of marginal and substantia gelatinosa neurons in the primate spinal cord: indications of their place in dorsal horn functional organization. *J Comp Neurol* 177:417–434, 1978.
38. Vane JR: Inhibition of prostaglandin synthesis as a mechanism of action for aspirin-like drugs. *Nature* 231:232–235, 1973.
39. Sunshine A, Olson NZ: Non-narcotic analgesics. In Wall PD, Melzack R (eds): *Textbook of Pain*. Churchill Livingstone, Edinburgh, pp 670–685, 1991.
40. Peter CB, Snyder SH: Opiate receptor: its demonstration in nervous tissue. *Science* 179:1011–1014, 1973.
41. Simon EJ, Hiller JM: The opiate receptors. *Annu Rev Pharmacol Toxicol* 18:371–384, 1978.
42. Snyder SH: Opiate receptors and internal opiates. *Sci Am* 236:44–56, 1977.
43. Beckett AH: Analgesics and their antagonists: some steric and chemical considerations. Part I. The dissociation constants of some tertiary amines and synthetic analgesics, the conformations of methadone-type compounds. *J Pharm Pharmacol* 8:848–853, 1956.
44. Lord JAH, Waterfield AA, Hughes J, et al: Endogenous spinal peptides: Multiple agonists and receptors. *Nature* 267:495–500, 1977.
45. Goodman LS, Gilman A (eds): The Pharmacological Basis of Therapeutics, 7th ed. Macmillan, New York, pp 491–531, 1985.
46. Brunk SF, Delle M: Morphine metabolism in man. *Clin Pharmacol Ther* 16:51–57, 1974.
47. Evans FF, Proctor JD, Fratkin MJ: Blood flow in muscle groups and drug absorption. *Clin Pharmacol Ther* 17:44–47, 1975.

48. Austin KL, Stapleton JV, Mather LE: Multiple intramuscular injections: a major source of variability in analgesic response to meperidine. *Pain* 8:47–62, 1980.

49. Weddell SJ, Ritter RR: Epidural morphine: serum levels and pain relief. *Anesthesiology* 53:S419, 1980.

50. Mackersie RC, Shackford SR, Hoyt DB, Karagaines TG: Continuous epidural fentanyl analgesia: ventilatory function improvement with routine use in treatment of blunt chest trauma. *J Trauma* 27:1207–1212, 1987.

51. Yeager MP, Glass DD, Neff RK, Brinck-Johnsen T: Epidural anesthesia and analgesia in high risk surgical patients. *Anesthesiology* 66:729–736, 1987.

52. Hagen NA, Foley KM, Carbone DJ, Portenoy RK, Inturrisi CE: Chronic nausea and morphine-6-glucuronide. *J Pain Symptom Manage* 6:125–128, 1991.

53. Glynn CJ, Mather LE, Cousins MJ, et al: Spinal narcotics and respiratory depression. *Lancet* 2:356–357, 1979.

54. Weil J, McCullough R, Kline J, et al: Diminished ventilatory response to hypoxia and hypercapnia after morphine in normal man. *N Engl J Med* 292:1103–1106, 1975.

55. Eckenhoff J, Helrich M: The effects of narcotics, thiopentone and nitrous oxide upon respiration and the respiratory response to hypercapnia. *Anesthesiology* 19:240–253, 1958.

56. Smith T, Stephen G, Zeigler L: Effects of premedicant drugs on respiration and gas exchange in man. *Anesthesiology* 28:883–890, 1967.

57. Johnstone RE, Jobes DR, Kennell EM: Reversal of morphine anesthesia with naloxone. *Anesthesiology* 41:361–367, 1974.

58. Bedford R, Woolman H: Postoperative respiratory effects of morphine and halothane anesthesia: a study of patients undergoing cardiac surgery. *Anesthesiology* 43:1–9, 1975.

59. Stanley T, Lathrop G: Urinary excretion of morphine during and after valvular and coronary artery surgery. *Anesthesiology* 46:166–169, 1977.

60. Lowenstein E, Hallowell P, Levine FH, et al: Cardiovascular response to large doses of intravenous morphine in man. *N Engl J Med* 281:1389–1393, 1969.

61. Hsu HO, Hickey RF, Forbes AR: Morphine decreases peripheral vascular resistance and increases capacitance in man. *Anesthesiology* 50:98–102, 1979.

62. Thompson WL, Walton RP: Elevation of plasma histamine levels in the dog following administration of muscle relaxants, opiates, and macromolecular polymers. *J Pharmacol Exp Ther* 143:131–136, 1966.

63. Lowenstein E, Whiting RB, Bittar DA, et al: Local and neurally mediated effect of morphine on skeletal muscle vascular resistance. *J Pharmacol Exp Ther* 180:359–367, 1972.

64. Vasko J, Henney R, Oldham HN: Mechanisms of action of morphine in the treatment of experimental pulmonary edema. *Am J Cardiol* 18:876–883, 1966.

65. Vismara LA, Leaman DM, Zelis R: The effects of morphine on venous tone in patients with acute pulmonary edema. *Circulation* 54:335–337, 1976.

66. Zelis R, Flaim SF, Eisele JH: Effects of morphine on reflex arteriolar constriction induced in man by hypercapnia. *Clin Pharmacol Ther* 22:172–178, 1977.

67. Zelis R, Mansour EJ, Capone RJ, et al: The cardiovascular effects of morphine: the peripheral capacitance and resistance vessels in human subjects. *J Clin Invest* 54:1247–1258, 1974.

68. Urthaler F, Isobe JH, Gilmour KE, et al: Morphine and autonomic control of the sinus node. *Chest* 64:203–212, 1973.

69. DeSilva RA, Verrier RL, Lown B: Protective effect of the vagotonic action of morphine sulfate on ventricular vulnerability. *Cardiovasc Res* 12:167–172, 1978.

70. Reitan JA, Stengert KB, Wymore ML, et al: Central vagal control of fentanyl-induced bradycardia during halothane anesthesia. *Anesth Analg* 57:31–36, 1978.

71. Chapman WP, Rowlands EN, Jones CM: Multiple-balloon kymographic recording of the comparative action of demerol, morphine and placebos in the motility of the upper small intestine in man. *N Engl J Med* 243:171–177, 1950.

72. Daniel EE, Sutherland WH, Bogoch A: Effects of morphine and other drugs on motility of the terminal ileum. *Gastroenterology* 36:510–523, 1959.

73. Garrett JM, Sauer WG, Moertel CG: Colonic motility in ulcerating colitis after opiate administration. *Gastroenterology* 53:93–100, 1967.

74. Leaman DM, Levenson L, Zelis R, et al: Effect of morphine on splanchnic blood flow. *Br Heart J* 40:569–571, 1978.

75. Butsch WL, McGowan JW: Clinical studies on the influence of certain drugs in relation to biliary pain and to the variations in intrabiliary pressure. *Surg Gynecol Obstet* 63:451–456, 1936.

76. Deutsch S, Bastron RD, Pierce EC, et al: The effects of anesthesia with thiopentone, nitrous oxide, narcotics and neuromuscular blocking drugs on renal function in normal man. *Br J Anaesth* 41:807–815, 1969.

77. Philbin DM, Coggins CH: Plasma antidiuretic hormone levels in cardiac surgical patients during morphine and halothane anesthesia. *Anesthesiology* 49:95–98, 1978.

78. Berkowitz BA, Cerreta K, Spector S: Influence of physiologic and pharmacologic factors on the disposition of morphine as determined by radioimmunoassay. *J Pharmacol Exp Ther* 191:527–534, 1974.

79. Olsen GD: Morphine binding to human plasma proteins. *Clin Pharmacol Ther* 17:31–35, 1975.

80. Cimo PL, Hammond JJ, Moake JL: Morphine-induced immune thrombocytopenia. *Arch Intern Med* 142:832–834, 1982.

81. Greenblatt DJ: Predicting steady state concentrations of drugs. *Annu Rev Pharmacol Toxicol* 19:347–356, 1979.

82. Parker RK, Holtmann B, White PF: Patient controlled analgesia. *JAMA* 266:1947–1952, 1991.

83. Urquhart ML, Klapp K, White PF: Patient controlled analgesia: a comparison of intravenous versus subcutaneous hydromorphone. *Anesthesiology* 69:428–432, 1988.

84. Jaffe JH, Martin WR: Opioid analgesics and antagonists. In Goodman LS, Gilman A: *The Pharmacological Basis of Therapeutics*, 7th ed. Macmillan, New York, p 506, 1985.

85. Lasagna L, Beecher KH: The analgesic effectiveness of codeine and meperidine. *J Pharmacol Exp Ther* 112:306–311, 1954.

86. Shulman MS, Wakerlin G, Yamaguchi L, Brodsky JB: Experience with epidural hydromorphone for post-thoracotomy pain relief. *Anesth Analg* 66:1331–1333, 1987.

87. Austin KL, Stapleton JV, Mather LE: Relationship between blood meperidine concentrations and analgesic response: a preliminary report. *Anesthesiology* 53:460–466, 1980.

88. Stapleton JV, Austin KL, Mather LE: A pharmacokinetic approach to postoperative pain: continuous infusion of pethidine. *Anaesth Intensive Care* 7:25–32, 1979.

89. Stambaugh JE, Wainer IW, Stanstead JK, et al: The clinical pharmacology of meperidine: comparison of routes of administration. *J Clin Pharmacol* 16:245–256, 1976.

90. Szeto HH, Inturrisi CE, Houde R, et al: Accumulation of normeperidine, an active metabolite of meperidine, in patients with renal failure or cancer. *Ann Intern Med* 86:738–741, 1977.

91. Stambaugh JE, Wainer IW: Drug interaction: meperidine and chlorpromazine, a toxic combination. *J Clin Pharmacol* 21:140–146, 1981.

92. Eade NR, Renton KW: Effect of monoamine oxidase inhibitors on the *N*-demethylation and hydrolysis of meperdine. *Biochem Pharmacol* 19:2243–2250, 1970.

93. Herz A, Teschenmacher HJ: Activities and sites of antinociceptive action of morphine-like analgesics and kinetics of distribution following intravenous, intracerebral and intraventricular application. *Adv Drug Res* 6:79–119, 1971.

94. McClain DA, Hug CC: Intravenous fentanyl kinetics. *Clin Pharmacol Ther* 17:21–30, 1975.

95. Hug CC, Murphy MR: Fentanyl disposition in cerebrospinal fluid and plasma and its relationship to ventilatory depression in the dog. *Anesthesiology* 50:342–349, 1979.

96. Stanley TH, Webster LR: Anesthetic requirements and cardiovascular effects of fentanyl-oxygen and fentanyl-diazepam-oxygen anesthesia in man. *Anesth Analg* 57:411–416, 1978.

97. Caplan RA, Ready LB, Oden RV, Matsen III FA, Nessly ML, Olsson GL: Transdermal fentanyl for postoperative pain management. *JAMA* 261:1036–1040, 1989.

98. Dubois-Primo J, Dewatcher B, Massaut J: Analgesic anesthesia with fentanyl and sufentanil in coronary surgery. *Acta Anaesthesiol Belg* 2:113–126, 1979.

99. Stanski DR, Hug CC: Alfentanil—a kinetically predictable narcotic analgesic. *Anesthesiology* 57:435–438, 1982.

100. Sinclair DC: Cutaneous sensation and the doctrine of specific energy. *Brain* 78:584–614, 1955.

101. Popio KA, Jackson DH, Ross AM, et al: Hemodynamic and respiratory effects of morphine and butorphanol. *Clin Pharmacol Ther* 23:281–287, 1978.

102. Lawhorn CD, McNitt JD, Fibuch EE, Joyce JT, Leadley RJ: Epidural morphine with butorphanol for post operative analgesia after Cesarean delivery. *Anesth Analg* 72:53–57, 1991.

103. Pandit UA, Kothary SP, Pandit SK: Intravenous dezocine for postoperative pain: a double-blind, placebo controlled comparison with morphine. *J Clin Pharm* 26:275–280, 1986.

104. Michaelis LL, Hickey PR, Clark TA: Ventricular irritability associated with the use of naloxone hydrochloride. *Ann Thorac Surg* 18:608–614, 1974.

105. Patschke D, Eberlein HJ, Hess W, et al: Antagonism of morphine with naloxone in dogs: cardiovascular effects with special reference to the coronary circulation. *Br J Anaesth* 49:525–533, 1977.

106. Dashwood M, Feldbert W: A pressor response to naloxone. Evidence for release of endogenous opioid peptides. *J Physiol* 281:30P–31P, 1978.

107. Anderson R, Dobloug I, Refstad S: Postanesthetic use of naloxone hydrochloride after moderate doses of fentanyl. *Acta Anaesth Scand* 20:255–258, 1976.

108. Cox BM, Ginsburg M, Osman OH: Acute tolerance to narcotic analgesic drugs in rats. *Br J Pharmacol* 33:245–256, 1968.

109. Mather LE, Phillips GD: Opioids and adjuvants: principles of use. In Cousins MJ, Phillips MJ (eds): *Acute Pain Management*. Churchhill Livingstone, New York, pp 77–103, 1986.

110. Glaser FB, Ball JC: Death due to withdrawal from narcotics. In Ball JC, Chambers CD (eds): *The Epidemiology of Opiate Addiction in the United States*. Charles C Thomas, Springfield, IL, pp 263–287, 1970.

CHAPTER 39

Psychopharmacology in the ICU

EDWIN H. CASSEM, M.D.
C. RAYMOND LAKE, M.D., Ph.D.
WILLIAM F. BOYER, M.D.

This chapter concerns the diagnosis and pharmacologic treatment of emotional disorders in the intensive care unit (ICU). Emphasis is on commonly used drugs, although some newer, alternative forms of therapy are mentioned. Problems are divided into three groups: delirium/psychosis, anxiety, and depression. In some patients two or all three of these problems may coexist. As in every other medical specialty, the treatment depends on the diagnosis.

APPROACH TO THE PATIENT

When confronted by a patient with disturbed thought, feeling, and/or behavior, the physician should decide whether the illness or its treatment has produced these symptoms or whether the patient has, in addition to a medical illness, developed a psychiatric disorder. Psychiatric symptoms frequently accompany physical illness and often resolve when the physical condition is treated effectively and is getting better. Table 39.1 lists illnesses that are associated with psychiatric symptoms.

Of all organic causes of altered mental status in intensive care settings, drugs are probably the most common contributor. Table 39.2 lists the drugs associated with psychiatric symptomatology. Some, like lidocaine, are predictable in their ability to cause an encephalopathic state, and the relationship is clearly dose related. Others, like the antibiotics, very rarely are causes of delirium and usually occur only in someone whose brain is already vulnerable, as in a patient with a low seizure threshold. The number of drugs that can be involved either in direct toxic reactions or in toxic effects because of drug interactions is large, potentially bewildering, and constantly changing. Certain sources provide regular reviews of published summaries and updates (86).

DELIRIUM AND PSYCHOSIS

The term *ICU psychosis* is a popular diagnosis often applied to patients exhibiting abnormal behavior in an ICU. In fact, the occurrence of acute functional psychosis in an ICU is rare. The term implies that the environmental features of critical care settings are themselves capable of inducing psychosis. The rationale given for this entity is usually either sensory deprivation or sensory monotony. In point of fact, use of this diagnosis usually indicates that the etiology of a delirium is simply unknown. Hence, making the diagnosis of a functional psychosis has more risks than benefits because it tends to discourage a thorough differential diagnosis.

DIAGNOSIS

Making a psychiatric diagnosis must begin by excluding organic factors that could cause symptoms in the realm of thought, emotion, and/or behavior. Throughout such an evaluation, it is helpful to have in mind a systematic schema for exclusion of organic causes of these psychiatric abnormalities.

651

Table 39.1.   Physical Illnesses Associated with Psychiatric Symptoms[a]

Illness	Anxiety	Despondency	Delirium or Psychosis
Circulatory			
Cerebral insufficiency or anoxia	+	+	+
Paroxysmal atrial tachycardia	+		
Coronary insufficiency	+		
Hypertensive encephalopathy		+	+
Electrolyte disturbance			
Hypernatremia	+ (hyperactivity, irritability)		
Hyponatremia		+	+
Hyperkalemia			
Hypokalemia	+	+	+
Hypercalcemia		+	+
Hypocalcemia	+		+
Hypomagnesemia	+	+	+
Hypophosphatemia	+		
Endocrine			
Hyperfunction or hypofunction of thyroid, parathyroid or pituitary	+	+	+
Pancreas			
Pancreatitis		+	+
Carcinoma	+	+	
Hyperinsulinism (any cause)	+	+	+
Diabetes mellitus	+	+	+
Adrenals			
Addison's or Cushing's disease	+	+	+
Pheochromocytoma	+		+
Hyperaldosteronism		+	
Gastrointestinal			
Ulcerative colitis		+	
Regional enteritis		+	
Whipple's disease		+	
Postgastrectomy		+ (fatigue, weakness)	
Hematologic			
Anemia	+	+	
Polycythemia vera	+	+	+
Thrombocytopenia (TTP)			+
Hepatic			
Cirrhosis		+	
Failure			+
Infections (other)			
Malaria	+	+	+
Lyme disease	+	+	+
Pneumonia	+	+ (especially viral)	+ (especially bacterial)
Infectious mononucleosis	+	+	+
Brucellosis	+	+	
Tuberculosis	+	+	+
Viral hepatitis	+	+ (especially in convalescence)	
Subacute bacterial endocarditis			+
Septicemia			+
Malignancies (other)			
Disseminated carcinomatosis		+	
Lymphomas		+	+
Carcinoid	+	+	+
Other (especially oat cell)		+	+
Neurologic			
Parkinson's disease		+ (may be early dementia)	
Stroke, space-occupying lesion, encephalitis, neurosyphilis, multiple sclerosis, Wilson's disease, Huntington's chorea	+	+	+
Partial complex seizures (temporal lobe epilepsy, right hemisphere focus)		(especially nondominant hemisphere focus)	(especially dominant hemisphere focus)
Postconcussive syndrome	+	+	+
Polyneuritis	+		
Combined systems disease	+		
Posterolateral sclerosis	+		
Meningitis			+
Normal pressure hydrocephalus			+

Table 39.1. *(Continued)*

Illness	*Anxiety*	*Despondency*	*Delirium or Psychosis*
Nutritional (deficiency)			
B₆, B₁₂, folic acid, niacin, thiamine, ascorbic acid		+	+
Renal			
Nephritis	+		
Uremia			+
Rheumatic or Collagen Vascular			
Systemic lupus	+	+	+
Rheumatoid arthritis, polyarteritis nodosa, temporal arteritis	+		
Other			
Acute intermittent porphyria		+ (between attacks)	+
Sarcoidosis		+	
Amyloidosis		+	

^{a} Data from references 29, 48, 52, 53, 94, 97, 98, 117, 118, and 120.

Figure 39.1 presents a decision tree, or quasi-algorithm, according to which the diagnosis and treatment of specific abnormalities in the ICU can proceed. Usually, the diagnostic and therapeutic considerations contained in the summary algorithm have already been considered by the ICU physicians and failure to reach any specific answer may be the reason that a psychiatric diagnosis has been entertained. Even at the point when that question is raised, however, it is the obligation of the physician to reconsider all organic possibilities that may have caused the psychiatric symptoms of the patient. Sometimes the psychiatric symptomatology is so bizarre or so offensive, as when a belligerent, delirious patient strikes a nurse, that the prior diagnostic efforts are disrupted and left incomplete.

The most common organic syndrome is delirium. Patients with this syndrome typically are older and have no previous psychiatric history. Delirium is often preceded by a "lucid interval" of 1 to 3 days in which no abnormality is noted in the patient, and thereafter the abrupt onset of agitation signals that delirium is present. Delirium may include disordered or incoherent speech, sensory misperceptions (hallucinations, illusions, or misidentifications), psychomotor retardation or agitation, alterations in the sleep-wake cycle, irritability, and fluctuations in arousal and somnolence, with variable disturbance in orientation, concentration, and memory. Therefore, the physician who suspects delirium should test the full range of the patient's cognitive functions (orientation, short-term memory, calculations, naming, repetition, praxis, and ability to think abstractly). Delirium usually worsens when external stimuli are reduced, characteristically at night. Prior dementia and any other CNS disturbance increase the likelihood of delirium in the ICU setting.

As Tables 39.1 and 39.2 indicate, specific diseases and drugs may be the culprit or make a contribution to the disturbances in the patient's mental state. Anticholinergic agents can be devastating, and some elderly patients who receive eye drops may absorb more because of corneal abrasions or simply absorb the drops through the tear ducts. Adrenocortical steroids, in doses of 40 mg/day or more of prednisone or its equivalent, will produce abnormalities in 5% of patients, and when the dose reaches 80 mg/day, in nearly 20% of patients. Analgesics may be culprits, none more than meperidine, whose first metabolic product, normeperidine, causes tremors, myoclonus, delirium, and, ultimately, seizures (60).

Not only are medications potentially toxic in themselves, but withdrawal states must always be considered. Patients may be heavy drinkers who have ceased to drink on their admission to hospital, or in other instances have simply stopped agents to which they were habituated, such as barbiturates, meprobamate, and alprazolam (8, 9, 15). A critical review of the literature on postcardiotomy delirium concluded that cardiac status, the severity of physical illness, the complexity of the surgical procedure, and preoperative organic brain disease are the determining factors in the prediction of this disturbance (29). It is not possible to discuss each one of the headings in the two aforementioned tables. Often several factors coincide to cause some sort of decompensation in the patient and a final encephalopathic state.

Patients with chronic functional psychoses such as schizophrenia or manic-depressive disorder may also be patients in an ICU. Schizophrenic patients are known to do well clinically under such settings. Patients with stable manic-depressive psychosis maintained on lithium may be less stable, and a psychiatric consultation should be sought if abnormalities arise while the patient is in the ICU.

NONPHARMACOLOGIC INTERVENTION

Drugs are not the only means to reduce the risk of physical harm to the patient or others. Most ICU nurses are extremely proficient in their efforts to make the ICU a nonthreatening place to the patient, orienting them to time and place, and trying to manipulate the lighting so as to help reinstate normal biologic rhythms. Physical restraints are usually necessary in agitated patients to protect vital indwelling arterial or venous catheters, Foley catheters, intraaortic balloon pumps, pacing wires, chest tubes, nasogastric and feeding tubes, and other devices that assist the patient. A night light, clock, window, radio, and belongings from home are helpful, but when agitation begins, it is usually the sign that these items have failed. Presence of the family at the bedside can be very reassuring to the patient, and in some cases a family member's presence at night may be sufficient to keep the patient out of difficulty. It is helpful to assess the patient's medication and care schedules to ensure that the longest possible period of uninterrupted sleep at night is obtained (71).

Table 39.2. Medications with Psychiatric Side Effects

Drug	Anxiety	Despondency	Delirium or Psychosis
Analgesics + antiinflammatories (nonsteroidal)			
Morphine + congeners		+	+
Meperidine, especially normeperidine		+	+
Pentazocine		+	+
Salicylates (severe abuse)			+
Acetaminophen			+
Fenoprofen	+	+	+
Indomethacin		+	+
Naproxen		+	
Phenylbutazone		+	
Propoxyphene		+	
Tolmetin sodium			+
Zomepirac sodium		+	+
Ibuprofen		+	+
Sulindac		+	+
Anticonvulsants			
Barbiturates	+	+	+
Hydantoins		+	+
Primidone		+	+
Sodium valproate		+	+
Succinimides (ethosuximide, phensuximide, methsuximide)	+	+	+
Antibiotics, antifungals, antihelminthics			
Ampicillin		+	
Sulfonamides		+	
Cephalosporins			+
Chloroquine			+
Ciprofloxacin			+
Clotrimazole		+	+
Cycloserine		+	+
Dapsone		+	+
Ethionamide		+	
Griseofulvin		+	
Isoniazid			+
Mefloquine		+	
Metronidazole		+	
Nitrofurantoin		+	
Nalidixic acid		+	
Ofloxacin			+
Para-aminosalicylic acid		+	
Quinacrine			+
Streptomycin		+	
Ketoconazole	+		
Aminoglycosides		+	+
Amodiaquine		+	+
Amphotericin-B		+	+
Chloramphenicol		+	+
Colistin sulfate		+	+
Ethambutol HCl		+	+
Rifampin		+	+
Tetracycline		+	+
Ticarcillin		+	+
Trimethoprim-sulfamethoxazole		+	+
Tobramycin		+	+
Flucytosine		+	+
Thiabendazole			+
Anticholinergics (numerous drugs)	+	+	+
Antihistamines			
Cimetidine	+	+	+
Promethazine		+	+
Ranitidine	+	+	+
Antineoplastics			
Chlorambucil			+
Cyclosporine			+

Table 39.2. (Continued)

Drug	Anxiety	Despondency	Delirium or Psychosis
Fluorouracil		+	+
Aminoglutethimide		+	+
Vinblastine		+	
Vincristine		+	+
Azathioprine		+	
Asparaginase		+	
Bleomycin		+	
Mithramycin		+	
Trimethoprim		+	
Azacitidine		+	+
Cytarabine (high dose)		+	+
Dacarbazine		+	+
Methenamine		+	+
Methotrexate (high dose)		+	+
Procarbazine		+	+
Tamoxifen		+	+
Interferon		+	+
Interleukin-2	+	+	+
Ifosfamide			+
Etopside		+	
Antivirals			
Acyclovir	+	+	+
Azidothymidine (AZT)	+	+	+
Didanosine			+
Foscarnet			+
Gancyclovir			+
Suramin		+	
Endocrine			
Adrenocorticosteroids (including ACTH)	+	+	+
Anabolic steroids	+	+	+
Clomiphene			+
Erythropoietin			+
Estrogens	+	+	+
Oral hypoglycemics			+
Thyroid	+	+	+
Sympatholytics (e.g., methysergide)	+	+	
Sympathomimetics (including theophylline preparations)			
Vitamins			
A	+		+
B complex	+	+	
D		+	
Folic acid			+
Other			
Aminocaproic acid			+
Baclofen	+		
Bupropion			+
Cyclobenzaprine			+
DEET			+
Diphenoxylate	+		
Disulfiram		+	+
Metrizamide	+		+
Orphenadrine		+	
Prarastatin		+	
Halothane		+	
Coumarin		+	
Metoclopramide	+	+	+
Antiparkinsonians			
Anticholinergic (e.g., procyclidine)	+	+	+
Amantadine	+	+	+
Bromocriptine	+	+	+
Pergolide	+	+	+
Carbidopa	+	+	+
Levodopa	+	+	+

Table 39.2. *(Continued)*

Illness	Anxiety	Despondency	Delirium or Psychosis
Cardiovascular			
Antiarrhythmics			
Amiodarone			+
Lidocaine	+	+	+
Procainamide		+	+
Disopyramide	+	+	+
Mexiletine	+	+	+
Quinidine			+
Digitalis			+
Antihypertensives			
Captopril	+		+
Carbonic anhydrase inhibitors			+
Ethacrynic acid			+
Furosemide		+	+
Hydrochlorothiazide		+	+
Spironolactone			+
β-Blockers		+	+
Ganglionic blockers (mecamylamine, pentolinium, trimethaphan)			+
Rauwolfia alkaloids	+	+	+
Guanethidine		+	+
Methyldopa		+	+
Hydralazine	+	+	+
Clonidine	+	+	+
Prazosin		+	+
Calcium blockers			
Diltiazem		+	+
Nifedipine	+	+	+
Verapamil			+
Narcotic Antagonists			

When patients have delusions, it is seldom helpful to manage it on intellectual grounds. If patients have delusional explanations for how they got to the ICU, it does not help to agree with them. If they believe that there is a plot to kill them, they must be reassured that this is not the case, but argument of the facts or attempted proofs are not helpful. The best approach is probably a calm, reassuring stance wherein the physician listens to the patient but repeatedly reassures him or her that he or she is in the ICU and that everything possible is being done to help. Talking should not delay treatment.

DRUG TREATMENT

A specific, careful etiology sometimes rewards a diagnostic search. If this is the case and one of the conditions in Figure 39.1 is realized, specific treatment can proceed. Occasionally, a history of heavy alcohol use emerges and treatment of alcohol withdrawal can proceed. In such circumstances, management with benzodiazepines is preferred.

Sometimes it is clear that a drug is causing the confusional state but stopping or reducing it is not possible. For example, in a patient with life-threatening ventricular irritability for whom a high rate of lidocaine infusion seems essential, there may be no way that one can immediately reduce the dosage even though the etiologic connection with agitation is clear. In such a case, treatment of nonspecific delirium, specifically

with intravenous haloperidol, can proceed while lidocaine is being given. However, the CNS derangement will not cease until the drug is reduced to a nontoxic level or stopped.

Occasionally, one may want to establish the diagnosis of an anticholinergic psychosis by administering physostigmine intravenously in a dose of 0.5 to 2 mg parenterally. Caution is essential for patients in critical care settings; however, because the cholinergic reaction to intravenously administered physostigmine can cause profound bradycardia and hypotension, complications may be multiplied instead of reduced. It should be noted, on the other hand, that a continuous intravenous infusion of physostigmine has been used successfully to manage a case of anticholinergic poisoning (126). If one were to use an intravenous injection of 1 mg of physostigmine, protection against excessive cholinergic reaction would be provided by preceding this injection with an intravenous injection of 0.2 mg of glycopyrrolate. This anticholinergic agent does not cross the blood-brain barrier and should protect the patient from the peripheral cholinergic actions of physostigmine.

ANTIPSYCHOTIC PHARMACOKINETICS

An intramuscular dose of an antipsychotic is about 1.5 times as potent as the equivalent oral dose. These drugs are absorbed quickly and reliably after intramuscular administration, reaching peak blood levels in as few as 10 to 20 minutes (23, 88). Maximum blood levels are obtained more rapidly after deltoid than after gluteal injection (83). There is considerable interindividual variation in antipsychotic blood levels following an equal oral dose. Antipsychotics are absorbed primarily in the jejunum (75), and peak blood levels are attained in roughly 2 to 6 hours (54). Cholestyramine, gel acids, and anticholinergic agents may inhibit absorption (9). Hence, an oral antipsychotic should precede these agents whenever possible. Liquid concentrates are the best absorbed of oral forms but also can form an insoluble precipitate with milk, fruit juice, coffee, or tea, with which they are frequently mixed. Chlorpromazine (CPZ) undergoes extensive metabolism by enzymes in the gut wall.

Antipsychotics are metabolized by the liver and excreted in both the urine and bile (8). There is significant enterohepatic circulation (88). CPZ is predicted to have more than 100 metabolites, many of which are active (83). Estimates of the half-life of CPZ in the body range from 2 to 60 days, although the longer estimate is probably more accurate (23). Haloperidol, by contrast, has no active metabolites and its half-life is between 12 and 36 hours (37). For comparison, mean half-lives of the oral preparation and the intramuscular and intravenous routes are 24, 21, and 14 hours, respectively. The long half-lives of antipsychotic drugs mean that once-a-day dosing is rational for chronic maintenance use. Acute treatment of delirium requires more frequent dosing.

CHOICE OF DRUG

There are some helpful guidelines in choosing an antipsychotic. These guidelines include side effect profile (other than sedation), available dosage forms, and history of response in

Figure 39.1. Decision tree for diagnosis and treatment of abnormalities in ICU setting. (From Cassem NH: The setting of intensive care. In Hackett TP, Cassem NH (eds): *MGH Handbook of General Hospital Psychiatry,* ed 2. PSG Publishing, Littleton, MA, 1987, p 362.)

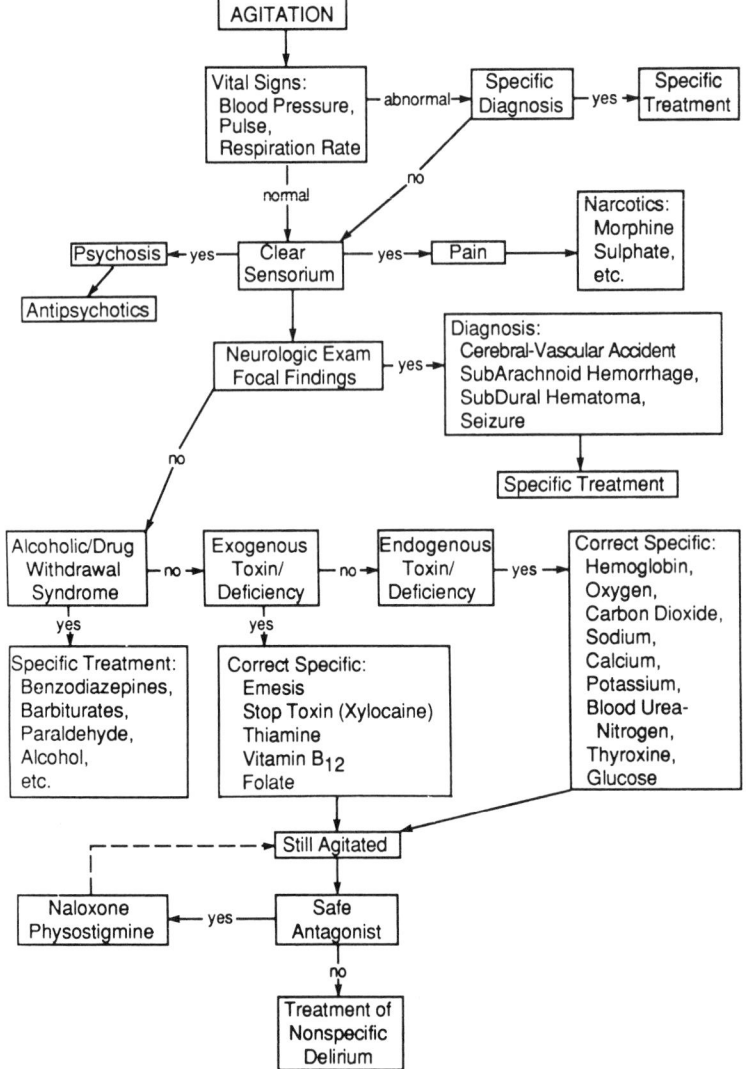

the patient or family member (4). Side effect information is summarized in Table 39.3.

There is no convincing evidence that one antipsychotic is more effective than another for particular psychotic symptoms (83), nor are there substantial data that a drug with more sedative side effects is better for agitated patients than a more "activating" drug that is assumed to be useful in treating someone who is withdrawn, although these unproved hypotheses are often adhered to in clinical practice (4, 26, 84).

Potency refers to the amount of drug needed to achieve a certain level of antipsychotic effect. The higher the potency, the less is needed for the same clinical effect. In general, the lower a drug's potency, the more likely it is to produce sedative, anticholinergic, and hypotensive effects, whereas the higher-potency drugs are more likely to produce neurologic (extrapyramidal) side effects. In most medically ill patients, undue sedation, hypotension, and anticholinergic effects are more troublesome than an extrapyramidal reaction. The latter, such as dystonia, akathisia, or parkinsonian effects, although distressing, are rarely life threatening. Rarely, the respiratory muscles may become involved (4, 50, 58, 89).

Patients with acquired immune deficiency syndrome (AIDS), like patients with Parkinson's disease, may be more susceptible to the extrapyramidal side effects of neuroleptics. Some consultants therefore prefer oral molindone or thioridazine for treating delirium in these patients. The newly approved neuroleptic clozapine should be considered for the parkinsonian patient with psychotic or delirious symptoms, despite the cumbersome but necessary precautions for initiating the drug and following the patient with weekly leukocyte counts. It is less likely to be helpful for AIDS patients because of its tendency to induce leukopenia.

Low-potency drugs are usually more anticholinergic and therefore more likely to exacerbate delirium. The effect of CPZ in blocking total peripheral resistance can be devastating, and severe hypotension can result. The intramuscular injection of CPZ is more painful than, for example, that of haloperidol. Among the low-potency antipsychotic drugs, thioridazine and mesoridazine both have quinidine-like side effects with significant potential for causing serious ventricular arrhythmias (66, 113).

Table 39.3 contains dosage recommendations for treatment of delirium with various antipsychotic drugs. The best guide

Table 39.3. Psychoactive Drugs[a]

Drugs	Dosage Forms Available[b]	Usual Dose Range for Agitation	Comments
ANTIPSYCHOTICS			
Low-potency			
		(up to q.i.d.)	
Chlorpromazine	t, c, i, s	25–100	See text
Thioridazine	t, c	25–100	Similar to chlorpromazine; drug most frequently associated with ECG changes
Mid-potency			
Perphenazine	t, c, i	4–12	Moderately sedating
High-potency			
Trifluoperazine	t, c, i	1–5	
Haloperidol	t, c, i	1–10	Often recommended for medically ill patients
Molindone	t, c	5–25	Virtually no hypotensive effects
Loxapine	t, c	2–10	Metabolized to amoxapine, an antidepressant
SEDATIVE/HYPNOTICS			
Benzodiazepines (BDZs)			
Long-acting			
		(up to q.i.d.)	
Diazepam	t, i	2–10	Only BDZ with proved muscle relaxant, anticonvulsant, and analgesic properties
Chlordiazepoxide	t, i	5–25	This drug and diazepam rarely have been associated with increased hostility and rage
Clorazepate	t	3.75–15	Like diazepam and chlordiazepam, useful for alcohol withdrawal
Flurazepam	t	15–30	Used only for sleep; cumulative effects sometimes responsible for undue sedation or disorientation
Short-acting			
Oxazepam	t	10–30	Especially well-tolerated by patients with liver disease and the elderly
Lorazepam	t, i	1–2	Strong amnesic effect; used to sedate ventilator patients, same as above
Temazepam	t	30	Marketed as a hypnotic; molecularly similar to oxazepam
Alprazolam	t	0.5–2	May have significant antidepressant effects
Midazolam	i	1–5	Use only in monitored setting
Nonbenzodiazepines			
Propranolol	t, i	30–120	Affects autonomic symptoms of anxiety; little, if any, effect on psychic symptoms
Phenobarbital	t	15–30	Barbiturates are noted for inducing respiratory failure
Secobarbital	t	30–50	
Chloral hydrate	t, c	250	
Hydroxyzine	t, c	100	Ineffective unless given in large doses

[a] Data from references 4, 8, 9, 53, 70, 82, 96, and 105.
[b] Dosage forms: t, tablets; c, oral concentrate; i, injectable; s, suppositories.

to the dose and drug required for a schizophrenic or manic-depressive patient is the patient's current drug treatment regimen. In this situation a psychiatric consultation is indicated. In general, whereas a schizophrenic may require 10 to 30 mg of haloperidol or its equivalent daily, a delirious patient may be calmed down by as little as 0.5 mg of haloperidol, especially if the patient is elderly.

Haloperidol is the recommended agent, mostly because of more extensive experience with this agent than with other high-potency neuroleptic drugs. Its effect on blood pressure, pulmonary artery pressure, heart rate, and respiration are milder than those of the benzodiazepines, making it an excellent agent for severely ill patients with impaired cardiorespiratory status (6, 122). Although haloperidol can be administered orally or parenterally, acute delirium with extreme agitation requires parenteral medication. Intravenous administration is preferable to intramuscular administration, for the following reasons:

1. Drug absorption may be poor in distal muscles if a patient's delirium is associated with circulatory compromise or borderline shock.

2. The agitated patient commonly is paranoid, and repeated, painful intramuscular injections may increase the patient's sense of being attacked by hostile forces.
3. Intramuscular injections can complicate interpretations of muscle enzyme studies if such studies are important clinically and if enzyme fractionation cannot solve the source of elevation.
4. Finally, and most importantly, intravenously administered haloperidol is less likely to produce extrapyramidal side effects.

In contrast to the immediate, observable sedation produced by intravenous diazepam, intravenous haloperidol has a mean distribution time of 11 minutes in normal volunteers, and perhaps even longer in critically ill patients. Because of this unusually long distribution time there is no reason to give an intravenous bolus of haloperidol slowly. A rapid push of the dose is safe.

The initial bolus dose of haloperidol varies from 0.5 to 20 mg: 0.5 to 2 mg for mild agitation, 2 to 5 mg for moderate agitation, and 10 mg or more for severe agitation. The only time a consultant would use a higher initial dose is when the patient has already been treated unsuccessfully with reasonable doses of haloperidol. To allow for haloperidol's delayed onset, doses usually are staggered by at least a 30-minute interval. If a 5-mg dose does not calm an agitated patient after 30 minutes, 10 mg should be administered. Partial control of agitation usually is not adequate and only prolongs the delirium. Therefore, it is recommended that haloperidol be given every 30 minutes until the patient is calm. Agitation will respond first, followed closely by hallucinations and extreme anxiety. Delusions, if present, usually take the longest to disappear.

After calm is achieved, agitation should be the sign for a repeat dose. Ideally, the total dose of haloperidol on the 2nd day should be a fraction of that on day 1. After complete lucidity has been achieved, the patient needs to be protected from delirium only at night, by small doses of haloperidol (0.5 to 3 mg), which can be given orally. This therapy is seldom necessary for more than 2 or 3 nights. As in the treatment of delirium tremens, the consultant is advised to stop the agitation completely at the outset rather than barely keeping up with it over several days. The maximum total intravenous dose of haloperidol to be used as an upper limit has not been established, although single-bolus intravenous doses of 150 mg have been administered, inasmuch as 945 mg total dose has been used in a 24-hour period (127).

Hypotensive episodes following the administration of intravenous haloperidol are rare and almost invariably caused by hypovolemia. Ordinarily this problem is easily checked in ICU patients who have indwelling pulmonary artery catheters, but since agitation is likely to return, volume replacement is necessary before administration of further doses. There are no local caustic effects on veins. Intravenous haloperidol is generally safe for epileptics and patients with head trauma. Although intravenous haloperidol may be used without mishap in patients who are receiving epinephrine drips, after very large doses of haloperidol a pressor other than epinephrine, such as norepinephrine, should be used to avoid unopposed β-adrenergic activity.

Intravenous haloperidol does not block the dopamine-mediated increase in renal blood flow. It also appears to be the safest agent for patients with chronic obstructive pulmonary disease.

Combining haloperidol with a benzodiazepine in the treatment of a nonspecific delirium may, at times, be quite helpful. When, for example, repeated doses of haloperidol fail to give a therapeutic response, another agent, preferably lorazepam or midazolam, can be tried. Adams has recommended a regular treatment regimen with alternating doses of haloperidol (10 mg) and lorazepam (1 mg) for the treatment of nonspecific delirium (1). When the agitated patient is a hospitalized psychiatric patient, lorazepam has been found to be more effective than haloperidol in decreasing acutely aggressive behavior and significantly freer of extrapyramidal symptom exacerbation (116).

Although there is now extensive experience with intravenous administration of haloperidol (15, 30, 89, 90, 114–116, 127), the Food and Drug Administration (FDA) has not given approval for the administration of the drug via that route. Protecting patients from extrapyramidal side effects makes this route extremely attractive. The less frequent appearance of these extrapyramidal effects after intravenous administration in medically ill patients may result from the fact that (a) many of these patients are receiving other medications that are protective, especially the benzodiazepines and β-blockers, (b) patients with psychiatric disorders, especially schizophrenia, are more susceptible to extrapyramidal side effects of the drugs, or (c) the patients are elderly and therefore at a lower risk for acute dystonia and akathisia. The low incidence of these effects in medical patients continues to be documented clinically (34, 89, 90, 99, 114, 115).

Alternative agents to haloperidol have been sought. Droperidol, an agent already approved for intravenous administration by the FDA, is a far more potent α-adrenergic antagonist than haloperidol, and it is more likely to lead to difficulties with hypotension, particularly when combined with other agents. One such reaction has been noted in several instances when droperidol was used as an intravenous antiemetic for cancer patients who were simultaneously receiving oral tetrahydrocannabinol. On the other hand, in a group of agitated, combative emergency room patients, droperidol resulted in more rapid control of the patient, with no increase in undesirable side effects, than did equal doses of haloperidol when the two were administered intramuscularly. The two agents were equally effective when administered intravenously (129). Perphenazine is a neuroleptic approved for intravenous use as an antiemetic. It can be also be very effective in treating acute nonspecific delirious states.

Finally, some clinicians find that very small doses of CPZ, such as 10 mg, can be administered intravenously without adverse hypotensive effects. Intravenous diazepam is used routinely to treat agitated states, particularly delirium tremens, as are intravenous chlordiazepoxide and lorazepam. Any one of these intravenous benzodiazepines may be a useful adjunct in the treatment of acute nonspecific delirium. Intravenous alcohol is also extremely effective in the treatment of alcohol withdrawal states. Its disadvantage is that it is toxic in itself to both liver and brain, although its use can be safe if these organs do not already show extensive damage (and sometimes is safe even when they do). A 5% solution of alcohol mixed with 5% dextrose and water, run at 1 ml/min, brings a calming effect amazingly quickly. Other parenteral neuroleptic drugs for treatment of agitation are thiothixene, trifluoperazine hydrochloride, and fluphenazine.

Midazolam maleate is available in the U.S. for intravenous sedation. It acts even faster than diazepam and is three to four times as potent. Its rapid onset, short elimination half-life (from 1 to 4 hours), and amnesic potency make it an ideal short-term sedative and anesthetic agent. Clinical experience with this agent is still not sufficient to evaluate its usefulness for the treatment of acute delirium. Respiratory depression and hypotension have both been reported with midazolam; the latter was particularly severe when the drug was combined with large doses of fentanyl citrate. Some have found these side effects to have been inexplicably delayed; as a result, the use of midazolam commonly is confined to a monitored setting. Midazolam is the most expensive of the benzodiazepine agents.

FEAR AND ANXIETY

DIAGNOSIS

Admission to an intensive care setting is invariably associated with a life-threatening disease. Even after the fear of death has ceased to haunt their consciousness, patients may fear that they will be maimed by the illness or by its treatments. This fear may assume many guises; verbosity, outbursts of anger, paranoia, and silent withdrawal are all behaviors typically produced by fear.

If the patient has a past history of a specific anxiety disorder, such as panic disorder, agoraphobia, a specific phobia such as claustrophobia, or obsessive-compulsive disorder, a psychiatric consultation is indicated. All of these specific disorders can, in their own way, interfere with the patient's treatment and recovery.

NONPHARMACOLOGIC INTERVENTION

Anxiety is treated both with medication and quiet reassurance. Much more is often gained by listening to the patient rather than by asking specific questions, especially open-ended questions about fears. Clarification, explanation, and reassurance are highly effective when fear stems from threatening or erroneous misconceptions about the disease or the ICU itself. After false ideas have been corrected, it is important to mention positive aspects of the treatment plan. For example, the cardiac patient might be assured that myocardial healing is complete in 5 to 6 weeks, and that normal activities will be resumed along with an exercise program. Even when the prognosis is grave, the calm statement of the treatments planned to counteract and contain the patient's suffering is of value to the anxious patient. The more ominous the prognosis, the more important it is to encourage the patient to specify the fear, so that specific and valid reassurances (e.g., that medication can control pain) can be given. False reassurance is not recommended because it robs the physician of credibility and therefore the ability to reassure the patient later in the illness.

When an anxiety persists despite explanations, further questions such as, "Have you ever known anyone with these symptoms (or this disease)?" or, "What is your idea of a heart attack (pulmonary embolus, AIDS)?" can be used to uncover misconceptions. When a family member has died of the same condition, his or her age at death may figure heavily in the patient's fear; often patients expect that fate will take them at the same age.

Equanimity has a most soothing effect on the patient. Anxious patients have a way of making people who take care of them anxious, and a vicious cycle may develop. A calm person can prevent that deleterious interaction.

DRUG TREATMENT

Unless panic has begun to encroach on rationality, the drugs of choice are the benzodiazepines (Table 39.4). If the patient's condition is one in which autonomic lability may be a hazard (e.g., myocardial infarction), routine prescription of one of these agents is recommended whether or not the patient looks anxious. Even when autonomic lability is not a hazard, the anxiety that accompanies severe acute medical illness is the most common indication for the prescription of benzodiazepines. The benzodiazepines have a wide therapeutic margin, about 10 times that of the barbiturates (21); little tendency to induce hepatic enzymes; few interactions with other drugs;

little effect on respiratory cardiovascular status in well patients; and relatively low potential for dependency or addiction, with the exception of alprazolam (37).

Of the benzodiazepines available, diazepam probably produces a high blood level most rapidly and is of particular value for the patient who needs to feel tranquilization quickly. If tranquilizers are given routinely to all patients, about 8% of them will complain of feeling sedated (18). Some of these patients may be reacting to a drug's rapid absorption and would better tolerate the slow, steady accumulation of one of the less lipid-soluble benzodiazepines, such as oxazepam or prazepam.

Clorazepate and prazepam are two long-acting benzodiazepines that are not active in their original form. They both have the same active metabolite, *n*-desmethyldiazepam, which is the only metabolite that produces psychotropic effects. However, clorazepate produces high blood levels within the first hour, whereas prazepam enters the system slowly. These differences result from the lipophilic nature of the two drugs. By 4 hours, the concentration of desmethyldiazepam is essentially the same for both of these agents (49). According to this rationale, a clinician would choose diazepam, clorazepate, lorazepam, or alprazolam if the patient wanted to experience tranquilization quickly. Oxazepam, prazepam, and temazepam are better for the patient who prefers to get the benefits slowly and imperceptibly. When using longer-acting agents such as diazepam, whose half-life varies between 20 and 60 hours, the physician can assume that saturation has been attained after 2 or 3 days and administer the drug only at bedtime or in a twice-daily dose thereafter. However, if the patient's anxiety responds best to the impacts of repeated dosing, three or four divided doses a day may remain clinically preferable. In fact, the latter is the most common way of prescribing the agent for both inpatients and outpatients. Parenteral forms of chlordiazepoxide, diazepam, lorazepam, and midazolam are available, but intramuscular absorption of the first two agents is erratic and less complete than absorption of oral doses. For this reason, oral or cautious intravenous administration is recommended. Chlordiazepoxide, diazepam, and alprazolam can, on rare occasions, produce paradoxic hostility or rage (9, 111). Hence, oxazepam, lorazepam, or temazepam may be more appropriate if the patient already seems hostile.

Among the short-acting benzodiazepines—oxazepam, lorazepam, temazepam, alprazolam, triazolam, and midazolam—only lorazepam and midazolam are currently available for parenteral use and, for this reason, have special value in critical care units. Otherwise, the major advantage of the first three (oxazepam, lorazepam, temazepam) is that they have no active metabolites and therefore do not accumulate in the blood. These shorter-acting agents are metabolized by glucuronidation, a metabolic process that is well-preserved not only in the elderly but in patients with impaired hepatic function. Since both advanced age and impaired liver function are associated with increased benzodiazepine half-lives (65, 99), these agents are very useful for these groups of patients.

A general rule is to prescribe the simplest and shortest-acting effective drug, for example, 15 mg of oxazepam three or four times a day. With the physician's permission, the nurse can withhold this drug if it seems excessive or report it if the patient seems undermedicated. One of the most sensitive

Table 39.4.   Side Effects of Psychotropic Drugs: Presentation and Management[a]

Organ System	AP[b]	TCA[b]	BDZ[b]	Presentation	Management
Central nervous system					
Dystonias	Common	Rare		Sudden, dramatic muscle contractions, especially upper trunk, head and neck; young males most susceptible; occurs early in treatment; may be precipitated by emotional stress	Benadryl 50, benztropine 2–10 mg, p.o., i.m., or i.v.; for prophylaxis same dose b.i.d.-q.i.d.
Pseudoparkinsonism	Common	Very rare		Indistinguishable from Parkinson's disease; occurs especially in elderly; mostly with high-potency APs	Benadryl 50 mg or benztropine 1–2 mg p.o. q.d.-q.i.d.
Akathisia	Common	Rare		Mostly with high-potency APs; vague sense of need to move; can be confused with psychotic agitation	Reduce dose, change or stop AP; can give propranolol 10 mg b.i.d. or t.i.d.
Seizures	Rare	Rare		Possibly more common with low-potency APs, especially in high doses, and patients with known seizure disorder	Reduce dose, stop AP, or raise dose of anticonvulsant
Tremor		Rare		More common with stimulating TCAs (e.g., imipramine, desipramine)	Usually requires no treatment
Hematologic					
Leukopenia/ agranulocytosis	Rare	Rare	Very rare	Rapid onset of sore throat and fever; periodic WBC counts of little value	Stop drug, routine management
Gastrointestinal					
Jaundice	Rare	Very rare	Very rare	Most often with low-potency APs in first month of treatment	Stop drug, routine management

[a] Data from references 29, 44, 56, 59, 75, 80, and 83.
[b] AP, antipsychotic; TCA, tricyclic antidepressant; BDZ, benzodiazepine.

measures of the dose's adequacy is the perception of the ICU nurse. The nurse, who attends the patient for an entire 8-hour shift, generally is able to see whether the patient appears to be growing more anxious or has begun to sleep all the time and is becoming harder to arouse and engage.

Slow accumulation of benzodiazepine metabolites is a problem worth worrying about. It is especially likely with flurazepam, diazepam, and all agents in which desmethyldiazepam is a metabolite. In addition, since the metabolism of these agents requires oxidative processes, patients with hepatic impairment are even more likely to accumulate excessive doses. There are those clinicians who maintain that flurazepam, despite its long half-life, is the most effective sleeping medication available to them. This claim appears to be correct in some cases, but one must still be vigilant for effects of accumulation.

DRUG INTERACTIONS

Benzodiazepines rarely interact with other compounds. All sedative/hypnotics have added effects when administered with CNS depressants. Disulfiram decreases the clearance of chlordiazepoxide, although these two drugs are unlikely to be administered concurrently in an ICU (38). Cimetidine may increase the clearance of benzodiazepines (54) but can also potentiate the sedative effects and double the plasma levels of diazepam (107). The dose of benzodiazepines, except for the three short-acting agents metabolized by glucuronidation, should be less in patients receiving cimetidine.

OTHER AGENTS

If the patient's fear is sufficiently intense to impair reason, or if the patient appears to be in a state of panic or transient psychosis, an antipsychotic drug is the agent of choice. Panicked individuals are barely in control; the benzodiazepines sometimes can further compromise an already diminished ability to cope. The preferred neuroleptic is again haloperidol, which can be administered in oral or parenteral form.

SPECIAL SITUATIONS

In some patients, anxiety may inhibit weaning from the mechanical ventilator. Multimodal treatment of this anxiety often begins with a benzodiazepine such as lorazepam, administered prior to weaning periods, or a neuroleptic such as haloperidol if the patient appears to be in a near panic state. Persons who suffer acute and chronic respiratory failure and therefore require prolonged mechanical ventilation may become so anxious when the weaning process begins that psychiatric assistance is requested. Even though the patient is physically ready for weaning, anxiety transiently can increase metabolic demands and cardiac work until further weaning becomes impossible.

Most behavioral exercises for relaxation encourage the subject to take slow, deep, easy breaths. This technique is one of the quickest and surest ways of inducing relaxation for most people, but it is precisely what patients with respiratory problems cannot do and precisely what makes them so anxious. The multimodal treatment of their anxiety usually begins with a drug, as mentioned above. Patients themselves can indicate whether the drug has been effective or which drug is most helpful. In some cases it may be possible to use a mixture of nitrous oxide if the respiratory specialist or anesthesiologist is present to administer it. Hypnosis or relaxation techniques are often helpful in distracting the patient from the weaning process. When these techniques are used, the instruction to breathe easily is best omitted from the hypnotic suggestion; the patient should be encouraged to concentrate either on a tranquil scene such as a beach or a single concept (mantra) (10). Since despondency and major depression, as well as anxiety, can impede weaning, the treatments for depression may apply here as well.

DEPRESSIVE DISORDERS

DIAGNOSIS

In any serious illness the mind sustains an injury of its own, as though the illness (for example, myocardial infarction) produced an ego infarction.

DESPONDENCY

The psychic damage known as "despondency" is distinct from depression, which is a major affective disorder. Even when recovery of the diseased organ is complete, recovery of self-esteem appears to take somewhat longer, and despondency tends to become a serious problem in ICU patients the longer they stay in a unit (19). In uncomplicated myocardial infarction patients, the myocardial scar is fully formed in 5 to 6 weeks, but recovery of psychologic well-being often requires 2 to 3 months.

Despondency is a mixture of dread, sadness, bitterness, and despair that causes patients to see themselves as broken, scarred, or even ruined. Functioning relationships seem jeopardized. Disappointment with what has and has not been accomplished haunts the individual, who now may feel old and a failure. The disease may not have killed the patient, but the patient may feel it has crippled his or her career and personal aspirations. Concerns of this kind become apparent rather early in acute illness and may prompt concern even by the 2nd or 3rd day of hospitalization.

Feeling better is the best antidote for illness-induced acute despondency. In the interim, the patient should be encouraged, but never forced, to express any concerns about the damage done by the illness. Some patients are upset merely to find such depressive concerns in their consciousness and even worry that this signals a "nervous breakdown." It is essential to let them know that such concerns are normal emotional counterparts to physical illness, which fluctuate in their intensity and usually disappear gradually as health returns. It is also reassuring for patients to hear about any rehabilitation plans while they are still in the recovery phase.

When progress is slow and intangible, minor interventions sometimes can be helpful. For example, getting a patient with severe congestive heart failure out of bed and into a reclining chair not only relieves cardiovascular strain but also provides reassurance and boosts confidence.

MAJOR DEPRESSION

There are various types of depression, but pharmacologic help is required only in those mood states that meet specific diagnostic criteria (i.e., major depression, depression with mania or manic symptoms, and depression with psychotic symptoms). The diagnostic criteria for a depressive episode are as follows:

1. Depressed mood most of the day, nearly every day;
2. Markedly diminished interest or pleasure in all, or almost all, activities;
3. Significant weight gain or weight loss when not dieting, or decrease or increase in appetite;
4. Insomnia or hypersomnia;
5. Psychomotor agitation or retardation;
6. Fatigue or loss of energy;
7. Feelings of worthlessness or excessive or inappropriate guilt;
8. Diminished ability to think or concentrate, or indecisiveness;
9. Recurrent thoughts of death (not just fear of dying), recurrent suicidal ideation without a specific plan, or a suicide attempt or a specific plan for committing suicide.

Ordinarily, the patient must possess at least five of these nine symptoms for a duration of 2 weeks to qualify for the diagnosis of major depression. Even if a patient has not been in the ICU this long, he or she may have been depressed prior to admission.

The patient actually may deny being depressed, ascribing symptoms of fatigue, anorexia, and sleep disturbance to the medical condition. When it is not clear whether an individual symptom such as anorexia or fatigue results from the primary medical illness or from a superimposed depression, the recommendation is to take an inclusive approach and count every symptom that actually is present, regardless of etiology. The true concern with every ICU patient is that, even though the treatment of the primary medical illness has been maximized, something is retarding the process of the patient toward recovery. Unless the clinician is confident that the patient does not meet the criteria for depression, a drug trial is warranted.

DRUG TREATMENT

A wide variety of agents is available to treat major depression, all of them potentially able to treat the depressed patient in an ICU. The drugs include polycyclic antidepressants, monoamine oxidase inhibitors (MAOI), lithium, carbamazepine, and psychostimulants. The approach described in the section that follows is recommended in the ICU setting.

PSYCHOSTIMULANTS

If the patient is lethargic, hard to mobilize, and listless and seems to show no investment in a caretaking regimen, an excellent, safe choice for treatment would be to start with a psychostimulant: either 5 mg of dextroamphetamine sulfate once a day or 5 mg of methylphenidate. These drugs can be extremely helpful in mobilizing a person who appears to be recovering physiologically from a long illness but lacks motivation.

For example, a patient could be given 5 mg of dexedrine once in the morning. If the patient shows considerable brightening, treatment should continue. There is no need to switch to a tricyclic or conventional antidepressant immediately. Some patients improve with psychostimulant therapy alone, become mobilized, and achieve recovery. Other patients require the addition of a traditional antidepressant. Dexedrine is administered once a day, usually first thing in the morning, to prevent the side effect of insomnia. The dose is increased daily until a beneficial effect is seen or an unwanted side effect (such as feeling tense) appears. The half-life of dexedrine varies from 7 to 30 hours, and some patients may need it twice a day (e.g., at 8 AM and noon). Methylphenidate, whose half-life varies from 2 to 4 hours, needs to be given at least twice and sometimes three times daily. Patients tolerate these drugs well. In medically ill patients, the incidence of tachycardia, increased blood pressure, or increased agitation even in demented patients has been mild (135). Nearly 90% of the patients who responded to stimulants reached their maximum response by the second day. The advantage, of course, is that one does not have to wait 2 to 3 weeks for an antidepressant treatment response to occur.

PHARMACOKINETICS OF POLYCYCLIC ANTIDEPRESSANTS

The polycyclic antidepressants (PCAs) are are well-absorbed early, generally reaching peak concentration in 2 to 6 hours. Anticholinergics and antacids may impede absorption. The PCAs are highly lipophilic and are taken up rapidly by the brain and peripheral tissues. PCAs are metabolized in the liver through oxidation and glucuronidation. They are excreted primarily in the urine, but there is significant enterohepatic circulation (102). Estimates of their half-lives generally range from 12 to 24 hours, and the most common method of dosing is once a day at bedtime.

CHOICE OF DRUG

The few clear reasons for selecting one PCA over another involve side effects more than specific depressive symptoms. A more sedating agent, such as doxepin, is often recommended for patients with severe insomnia, whereas a less sedating agent such as desipramine is used more commonly with a withdrawn, psychomotor retarded patient. It is important to remember that none of these agents appears to be superior to any other in the overall treatment of depression, but that the side effect profile of each drug provides a reasonable rationale for its selection. This side effect profile (Table 39.5) and a history of previous response by the patient or family member can provide a relative indication for a particular drug.

The PCAs have three major side effects, which, if understood, provide the ICU physician with an excellent knowledge of what to expect from each drug.

ORTHOSTATIC HYPOTENSION

The potencies of the various PCAs are listed in Table 39.5. Imipramine, clomipramine, amitriptyline, and desipramine are the tricyclics most often associated with orthostatic mishaps, such as falling and sustaining a fracture or head injury. Ordinarily in the ICU the patients are bedridden and orthostatic effects are not as worrisome. For imipramine, the orthostatic effect appears earlier than the therapeutic effect and will be objectively verifiable at roughly half the therapeutic plasma level. The clinical consensus is that nortriptyline is the tricyclic least likely to cause orthostatic hypotension clinically. However, three newer cyclic agents, fluoxetine, bupropion, and sertraline, appear to be free of this side effect.

Cardiac status is related to tricyclic-induced orthostatic hypotension. For the normal patient with normal electrocardiogram (ECG), the incidence of this side effect with imipramine will be around 7 to 10%. For the patient with bundle branch block, the incidence increases to 33%, and the patient with congestive heart failure will become orthostatic 50% of the time (101).

ANTICHOLINERGIC EFFECTS

Urinary retention, constipation, dry mouth, confusional states, and tachycardia are the most common unwanted side effects of the PCAs. The increase in heart rate is a sinus tachycardia resulting from the ability of these drugs to oppose vagal tone in the heart. Amitriptyline is the most anticholinergic of the tricyclics, with protriptyline a rather close second. These two agents regularly will cause tachycardia in medically ill patients, and the clinician should check the heart rate as the dose is increased. If significant tachycardia results, another agent may have to be used. Many hospitalized patients, particularly those with ischemic heart disease, are already being treated with β-adrenergic blockers, such as propranolol, which usually will protect the patient from developing a significant tachycardia from the antidepressant.

Among all the PCAs, trazodone, fluoxetine, bupropion, and sertraline are unique in their relative freedom from anticholinergic side effects. When urinary retention develops with a tricyclic agent, switching to one of these newer agents, alprazolam, or an MAOI is likely to treat depression without creating further concerns about the bladder.

CARDIAC CONDUCTION EFFECTS

The tricyclics, amoxapine, and maprotiline appear capable of producing cardiac arrhythmias. The mechanism is related to their ECG, a lengthening of the P-R and Q-R-S intervals, as well as the Q-T interval, corrected for heart rate (QTc). This effect makes the PCAs resemble the class IA antiarrhythmic drugs such as quinidine and procainamide hydrochloride (42). In practical terms, the depressed patient with ventricular premature contractions, when started on an antidepressant such as imipramine, is likely to experience a therapeutic reduction in ventricular irritability.

Ordinarily, this property does not pose a problem for medically ill patients who are free of disease in the conduction system. Conditions that are most worrisome, therefore, are those in patients with impaired conduction in the His Purkinje system such as bifascicular block, bundle branch block with prolonged P-R, alternating bundle branch block, and second- or third-degree atrioventricular block. First-degree heart

Table 39.5. Antidepressant Drugs

	Relative Potencies for Producing Certain Clinical Effects			Cardiac Conduction/ Arrhythmia	Target Dose (mg/day)	Dosage Range (mg/day)	Therapeutic Plasma Level (ng/ml)
	Sedative	Orthostatic	Anticholinergic				
Tricyclic agents							
Doxepin	High	Moderate	Moderate	Yes	200	25–400	
Amitriptyline	High	Moderate	Highest	Yes	150	25–300	
Imipramine	Moderate	High	Moderate	Yes	200	50–400	≥200
Trimipramine	High	? Moderate	Moderate	Yes	150	50–300	
Clomipramine	Moderate	High	High	Yes	150	75–300	
Protriptyline	Lowest	Low	High	Yes	30	5–60	
Nortriptyline	Moderate	Lowest	Moderate	Yes	100	25–150	50–150
Desipramine	Lowest	Low	Moderate	Yes	150	75–300	≥125
Other cyclic agents							
Amoxapine	Moderate	Low	Moderate	Lower	200	50–300	
Maprotiline	Moderate	Low	Moderate	Lower	150	50–200	
Trazodone	Moderate	Moderate	Very Low	Lower	200	50–600	
Fluoxetine	Low	Lowest	Low	Low	20	10–80	
Sertraline	Low	Lowest	Low	Low	50	50–200	
Paroxetine	Low	Lowest	Low	Low	20	10–20	
Bupropion	Low	Lowest	Low	Low	200	75–300	
Benzodiazepine							
Alprazolam	High	None	None	None	3	0.5–10	
MAOI							
Phenelzine	Low	High	None	Very rare	60	30–90	
Tranylcypromine	Low	High	None	Very rare	30	10–60	
Isocarboxazid	Low	Moderate	None	Very rare	30	10–60	
Psychostimulants							
Dextroamphetamine	None	None	None	Rare	10	2.5–30	
Methylphenidate	None	None	None	Rare	20	5–60	

block and right bundle branch block ordinarily present little problem with PCAs, especially if the patient is stable. The patient with unstable atrial fibrillation is always a concern. Cardiology consultation will almost always be present for these patients. Electrolyte abnormalities, particularly hypokalemia or hypomagnesemia, increase the danger of arrhythmia and require careful monitoring. There is some evidence that the hydroxymetabolites of the traditional tricyclics are related more specifically to the production of slowing in HV conduction (136). Even though trazodone appears not to prolong conduction in the His Purkinje system, aggravation of preexisting ventricular irritability has been reported with its use. Clinical caution therefore must be maintained.

Fluoxetine, bupropion, and sertraline have not been associated with significant cardiac arrhythmias. If a patient were to have a serious conduction disease, one of these agents or a psychostimulant or alprazolam might be helpful for depression and be less likely to produce cardiac conduction disturbances.

THE QUESTION OF MYOCARDIAL DEPRESSION

Some individuals have been concerned about the ability of PCAs to depress left ventricular function. Left ventricular ejection fractions have been measured before and during imipramine, doxepin, and nortriptyline treatment of cardiac patients with major depression. These tricyclics showed no adverse effects on ventricular function even in patients who demonstrated impaired ventricular function before treatment (41, 104). In fact, the use of PCAs has also been found to be safe in patients with congestive heart failure (42, 109).

CLINICAL USE

For an ICU patient who appears to be depressed, a psychostimulant trial is a reasonable beginning. If it is effective, it can be maintained. If the success is absent, the stimulant should be stopped. If it is incomplete but partially helpful, the stimulant can be maintained. In either case, an antidepressant with a low side effect profile can be started at a low dose: for example, 10 to 25 mg/day of nortriptyline, 10 mg of fluoxetine, 75 mg of bupropion, or 50 mg of sertraline, increased toward the recommended therapeutic dose. Nortriptyline, which is sedating, can be given once at night. The others, which are not, can be given once in the morning. If no improvement is noted in 7 to 10 days on the initial dose, further increases are in order. Only imipramine, desipramine, and nortriptyline have reliable plasma levels (Table 39.5), which is reassuring information if one wants to keep the patient within therapeutic range for a 3- to 4-week period of time.

SUMMARY

Psychiatric problems are a frequent occurrence in an ICU, and most often they probably come and go without anyone having taken notice of their presence. At other times, however, appearance of a psychiatric disorder may prolong and complicate the patient's ICU stay or even threaten the patient's very existence. When abnormalities of thought, feeling, and behavior arise, it is important to diagnose the cause of these problems and prescribe the proper treatment. Drug interactions and knowledge of pharmacokinetics and reasonable dosage schedules allow for effective use of psychotropic drugs

Table 39.6. Psychotropic Drugs

Chemical	Trade
Antipsychotics	
Chlorpromazine	Thorazine, Promapar, Chlor-PZ
Thioridazine	Mellaril
Perphenazine	Trilafon
Trifluoperazine	Stelazine
Haloperidol	Haldol
Molindone	Moban, Lidone
Loxapine	Loxitane, Daxolin
Clozapine	Clozaril
Benzodiazepine Sedative/Hypnotics	
Alprazolam	Xanax
Chlordiazepoxide	Librium, generics
Clonazepam	Klonopin
Clorazepate	Tranxene
Diazepam	Valium, generics
Estazolam	ProSom
Flurazepam	Dalmane
Halazepam	Paxipam
Lorazepam	Ativan, generics
Midazolam	Versed
Oxazepam	Serax
Prazepam	Centrax
Quazepam	Doral
Temazepam	Restoril
Triazolam	Halcion
Antidepressants	
Imipramine	Tofranil, Antipress, Imavate, Jamimine, Presamine, Ropramine, SK-Pramine
Desipramine	Norpramin, Pertofrane
Amitriptyline	Elavil, Endep, Amitril, Rolavil
Nortriptyline	Pamelor, Aventyl
Doxepin	Sinequan, Adapin
Trimipramine	Surmontil
Amoxapine	Asendin
Maprotiline	Ludiomil
Trazodone	Desyrel
Phenelzine	Nardil
Tranylcypromine	Parnate
Isocarboxazid	Marplan
Dextroamphetamine	Dexedrine
Methylphenidate	Ritalin
Protriptyline	Vivactil
Clomipramine	Anafranil
Fluoxetine	Prozac
Sertraline	Zoloft
Bupropion	Wellbutrin

in the critically ill patient. Trade names of drugs mentioned in this chapter are given in Table 39.6.

REFERENCES

1. Adams F, Fernandez F, Andersson BS: Emergency pharmacotherapy of delirium in the critically ill cancer patient. *Psychosomatics* 27:33–37, 1986.
2. Anderson WH: Differential diagnosis of acute psychosis. In Manschreck TC: *Psychiatric Medicine*. Elsevier/North Holland, New York, 1979.
3. Atkinson K, Biggs J, Darveniza P, et al: Cyclosporine-associated central nervous system toxicity after allogeneic bone-marrow transplantation. *N Engl J Med* 310:527, 1984.
4. Aubree JC, Lader MH: High and very high dosage antipsychotics. *J Clin Psychiatry* 41:341–350, 1980.
5. Ayd Jr FJ: Guidelines for using intramuscular haloperidol for rapid neuroleptization. In Ayd FJ (ed): *Haloperidol Update: 1959–1980*. Ayd Medical Communications, Baltimore, MD, 1980.
6. Ayd Jr, FJ: Intravenous haloperidol therapy. *Int Drug Ther Newslett* 13:20–23, 1978.
7. Ayd Jr FJ: Trazodone cardiac effects. *Int Drug Ther Newslett* 20:29–32, 1985.
8. Baldessarini RJ: Drugs effective in the treatment of psychiatric disorders. In Gilman AG, Goodman LS, Gilman A (eds): *Goodman and Gilman's The Pharmacologic Basis of Therapeutics*, ed 6. Macmillan, New York, 1980.
9. Ban T: *Psychopharmacology for the Aged*. Karger, New York, 1980.
10. Benson HA: *The Relaxation Response*. William Morrow & Co, New York, 1975.
11. Borison RL: Amantadine-induced psychosis in a geriatric patient with renal disease. *Am J Psychiatry* 136:111–112, 1979.
12. Brophy JJ: Psychiatric disorders. In Krupp MA, Chatton MJ (eds): *Current Medical Diagnosis and Therapy*. Lange, Los Altos, CA, 1980.
13. Byrd GJ: Acute organic brain syndrome associated with gentamycin therapy. *JAMA* 238:53–54, 1977.
14. Cantu TG, Korek JS: Central nervous system reactions to histamine-2 receptor blockers. *Ann Intern Med* 114:1027–1034, 1991.
15. Cassem EH, Hackett TP: Psychiatric medicine in intensive care settings. In Manschreck TC (ed): *Psychiatric Medicine*. Elsevier/North Holland, New York, 1979.
16. Cassem N: Cardiovascular effects of antidepressants. *J Clin Psychiatry* 43:22–28, 1982.
17. Cassem NH, Depression. In: TP Hackett and NH Cassem (eds): *MGH Handbook of General Hospital Psychiatry*, ed 2. PSG Publishing, Littleton, MA, 1987, pp 227–260.
18. Cassem NH, Hackett TP: Psychiatric consultation in a coronary care unit. *Ann Intern Med* 75:9–14, 1971.
19. Cassem NH: Psychiatric problems. In Parrillo JE (ed): *Current Therapy in Critical Care Medicine*. Decker, Philadelphia, 1987, pp 331–340.
20. Cassem NH, The setting of intensive care. In Hackett TP, Cassem NH (eds): *MGH Handbook of General Hospital Psychiatry*, ed 2. PSG Publishing, Littleton, MA, 1987, pp 353–379.
21. Cohen S: *The Drug Abuse Problem*. Harvorth Press, New York, 1981.
22. Cole JO: Drug treatment of anxiety. In Cole JD (ed): *Psychopharmacology Update*. Collamore Press, Lexington, MA, 1980.
23. Cressman WA, Blanchine JR, Slotnick VB, et al: Plasma level profile of haloperidol in man following intramuscular administration. *Eur J Clin Pharmacol* 7:99–103, 1974.
24. Dager SR, Heritch AJ: A case of bupropion-associated delirium. *J Clin Psychiatry* 51:307–308, 1990.
25. Davidson J, Turnbull CD: The effects of isocarboxazid on blood pressure and pulse. *J Clin Psychopharmacol* 6:139–143, 1986.
26. Davis JM: Antipsychotic drugs. In Kaplan HI, Freedman AM, Sadock BJ (eds): *Comprehensive Textbook of Psychiatry*, ed 3. Williams & Wilkins, Baltimore, 1980.
27. Devaul RA, Hall RCW: Hallucinations. In Hall RCW (ed): *Psychiatric Presentations of Medical Illness*. Spectrum Publications, New York, 1980.
28. Director KL, Muniz CE: Diazepam in the treatment of extrapyramidal symptoms: a case report. *J Clin Psychiatry* 43:160–161, 1982.
29. Dubin WR, Field HL, Gastfriend DR: Postcardiotomy delirium: a critical review. *J Thor Cardiovasc Surg* 77:586–594, 1979.
30. Dudley DL, Rowlett DB, Loebel PJ: Emergency use of intravenous haloperidol. *Gen Hosp Psychiatry* 1:240–246, 1979.
31. Dysken MW, Merry W, Davis JM: Anticholinergic psychosis. *Psychiatr Ann* 8:30–40, 1978.
32. Eisendrath SJ, Sweeney MA: Toxic neuropsychiatric effects of digoxin at therapeutic serum concentrations. *Am J Psychiatry* 144:506–507, 1987.
33. Ekholm S, Fischer H: Neurotoxicity of metrizamide. *Arch Neurol* 42:24–25, 1985.
34. Fernandez F, Holmes VF, Adams F, et al: Treatment of severe, refractory agitation with a haloperidol drip. *J Clin Psychiatry* 49:239–241, 1988.
35. Eikayam U, Frishman W: Cardiovascular effects of phenothiazines. *Am Heart J* 100:397–401, 1980.
36. Forsman A, Ohman R: Pharmacokinetic studies on haloperidol in man. *Curr Ther Res* 20:319–336, 1976.
37. Fyer HA, Liebowitz MR, Gorman JM, et al: Discontinuation of alprazolam treatment in panic patients. *Am J Psychiatry* 144:303–308, 1987.
38. Gaultieri CT, Powell SF: Psychoactive drug interactions. *J Clin Psychiatry* 39:720–729, 1978.
39. Georgotas A, McCue RE, Friedman E, et al: Electrocardiographic effects of nortriptyline, phenelzine, and placebo under optimal treatment conditions. *Am J Psychiatry* 144:798–801, 1987.
40. Giardina EG-V, Bigger JT Jr, Johnson LL: The effect of imipramine and nortriptyline on ventricular premature depolarization and left ventricular function [Abstract]. *Circulation* 64(suppl)4:316, 1981.
41. Glassman AH: Cardiovascular effects of tricyclic antidepressants. *Annu Rev Med* 35:503–511, 1984.
42. Glassman AH, Johnson LL, Giardina EG-V, et al: The use of imipramine in depressed patients with congestive heart failure. *JAMA* 250:1997–2001, 1983.
43. Goff DC, Garber HJ, Jenike MA: Partial resolution of ranitidine-associated delirium with physostigmine: case report. *J Clin Psychiatry* 46:400–401, 1985.
44. Goldman LS, Hudson JI, Weddington WW: Lupus-like illness associated with chlorpromazine. *Ann J Psychiatry* 137:1613–1614, 1980.
45. Good MI, Shader RI: Behavioral toxicity and equivocal suicide associated with chloroquine and its derivatives. *Am J Psychiatry* 134:798–801, 1977.
46. Good MI, Shader RI: Lethality and behavioral side effects of chloroquine. *J Clin Psychopharmacol* 2:40–47, 1982.
47. Goodwin JS, Regan M: Cognitive dysfunction associated with naproxen and ibuprofen in the elderly. *Arthritis Rheum* 25:1013–1015, 1982.
48. Granacher RP: Agitation in the elderly. *Postgrad Med* 72:83–96, 1982.
49. Greenblatt DJ: Pharmacokinetic comparisons. *Psychosomatics* 21(suppl):9–14, 1980.
50. Johnson AL, Hollister LE, Berger PA: The anticholinergic, syndrome: diagnosis and treatment. *J Clin Psychiatry* 42:313–317, 1981.
51. Kaiko RF, Foley KM, Grabinski PY, et al: Central nervous system excitatory effects of meperidine in cancer patients. *Ann Neurol* 13:180–185, 1983.
52. Kane JM, Smith JM: Tardive dyskinesia: prevalence and risk factors, 1959-1979. *Arch Gen Psychiatry* 39:473–481, 1982.
53. Katon W, Raskin M: Treatment of depression in the medically ill elderly with methylphenidate. *Am J Psychiatry* 137:963–965, 1980.

54. Katz IR, Greenberg WH, Barr GA, et al: Screening for cognitive toxicity of anticholinergic drugs. *J Clin Psychiatry* 46:323–326, 1985.

55. Kaufman MW, Murray GB, Cassem NH: Use of psychostimulants in medically ill elderly with methylphenidate. *Am J Psychiatry* 137:963–965, 1980.

56. Kaufman MW, Murray GB, Cassem NH: Use of psychostimulants in medically ill depressed patients. *Psychosomatics* 23:817–819, 1982.

57. Kiriike N, Maeda Y, Nishiwaki S, et al: Iatrogenic torsade de pointes induced by thioridazine. *Biol Psychiatry* 22:99–103, 1987.

58. Klotz U, Avant GR, Hoyumpa A, et al: The effects of age and liver disease on the disposition and elimination of diazepam in adult men. *J Clin Invest* 55:347–359, 1975.

59. Knox SJ: Severe psychiatric disorders in postoperative period: five-year survey of Belfast hospitals. *J Ment Sci* 107:1078, 1961.

60. Koepke HH, Lion JR, Gold RL, et al: Multicenter controlled study of oxazepam in anxious elderly outpatients. *Psychosomatics* 23:641–645, 1982.

61. Kolin IS, Linet OI: Double-blind comparison of alprazolam and diazepam for subchronic withdrawal from alcohol. *J Clin Psychiatry* 42:169–173, 1981.

62. Kornfeld DS: Psychiatric problems of an intensive care unit. *Med Clin North Am* 55:1353–1363, 1971.

63. Krupp LB, Masur D, Schwartz J, et al: Cognitive functioning in late Lyme borreliosis. *Arch Neurol* 48:1125–1129, 1991.

64. Kulig K, Rumeck BH, Sullivan JB Jr, et al: Amoxapine overdose: coma and seizures without cardiotoxic effects. *JAMA* 248:1092–1094, 1982.

65. Kuntzer T, Bogousslavsky J, Miklossy J, et al. Borrelia rhombencephalomyelopathy. *Arch Neurol* 48:832–836, 1991.

66. Lader M: *Introduction to Psychopharmacology.* Upjohn, Kalamazoo, MI, 1980.

67. Lader MH, Petursson H: Benzodiazepine derivatives—side effects and dangers. *Biol Psychiatry* 16:1195–1201, 1978.

68. Lechleitner M, Hoppichler F, Konwalinka G, et al: Depressive symptoms on hypercholesterolemic patients treated with pravastatin. *Lancet* 340:910, 1992.

69. Linn L, Kahn RL, Coles R: Patterns of behavior disturbances following cataract extraction. *Am J Psychiatry* 110:281–289, 1953.

70. Lipowski ZJ: Delirium updated. *Comp Psychiatry* 21:190–197, 1980.

71. Lowry MR, Dunner FJ: Seizures during tricyclic therapy. *Am J Psychiatry* 137:1461–1462, 1980.

72. Luft BJ, Steinman CR, Neimark HC, et al: Invasion of the central nervous system by *Borrelia burgdorferi* in acute disseminated infection. *JAMA* 267:1364–1367, 1992.

73. Lydiard RB: Temazepam (Restoril)—a new short-acting benzodiazephine hypnotic. *Biol Ther Psychiatry* 4:37–38, 1981.

74. Mason A, Granacher RP: *Clinical Handbook of Antipsychotic Drug Therapy.* Brunner/Mazel, New York, 1980.

75. May PRA, Goldberg SC: Prediction of schizophrenic patients' response to pharmacotherapy. In Lipton MA, DiMascio AD, Killam KF (eds): *Psychopharmacology: A Generation of Progress.* Raven Press, New York, 1978.

76. McGrath PJ, Blood DK, Stewart JW, et al: A comparative study of the electrocardiographic effects of phenelzine, tricyclic antidepressants, mianserin, and placebo. *J Clin Psychopharmacol* 7:335–339, 1987.

77. Medical Letter: Drugs that cause psychiatric symptoms. *Med Lett* 35:65–70, 1993.

78. Drugs for viral infections. *Med Lett* 34:31–36, 1992.

79. Menuck M, Vioneskos G: Rapid parenteral treatment of acute psychosis. *Comp Psychiatry* 22:351–361, 1981.

80. Menza MA, Murray GB, Holmes VF, Rafels WA: Decreased extrapyramidal symptoms with intravenous haloperidol. *J Clin Psychiatry* 48:278–280, 1987.

81. Menza MA, Murray GB, Holmes VF, Rafuls WA: Controlled study of extrapyramidal reactions in the management of delirious, medically ill patients: intravenous haloperidol vs. intravenous haloperidol plus benzodiazepines. *Heart Lung* 17:238–241, 1988.

82. Moeller H, Kissling W, Lang C, et al: Efficacy and side effects of haloperidol in psychotic patients: oral versus intravenous administration. *Am J Psychiatry* 139:1571–1575, 1982.

83. Moore DP: Rapid treatment of delirium in critically ill patients. *Am J Psychiatry* 134:1431–1432, 1977.

84. Murray GB: Atrial fibrillation/flutter associated with amoxapine: two case reports. *J Clin Psychopharmacol* 5:124–125, 1985.

85. Nadelson T: The psychiatrist in the surgical intensive care unit: postoperative delirium. In Guggenheim FG, Nadelson C (eds): *Major Psychiatric Disorders.* Elsevier Biomedical, New York, 1982.

86. Newman G: Intermittent recurring psychoses. In Hall RCW (ed): *Psychiatric Presentations of Medical Illness.* Spectrum Publications, New York, 1980.

87. Noyes R: Beta-blocking drugs and anxiety. *Psychosomatics* 23:155–169, 1981.

88. Paykel ES, Fleminger R, Watson JP: Psychiatric side effects of anti-hypertensive drugs other than reserpine. *J Clin Psychopharmacol* 2:14–39, 1982.

89. Peterson LG, Perk M: Psychiatric presentations of cancer. *Psychosomatics* 23:601–604, 1982.

90. Plotnick EK, Brwon GR. Intravenous haloperidol treatment of severely regressed, nonviolent psychiatric inpatients. *Gen Hosp Psychiatry* 13:358–390, 1991.

91. Pluss JL, DiBella NJ: Reversible central nervous system dysfunction due to tamoxifen in a patient with breast cancer. *Ann Intern Med* 101:652, 1984.

92. Pratt TH: Rifampin-induced organic brain syndrome. *JAMA* 241:2421–2422, 1979.

93. Preskorn SH, Irwin HA: Toxicity of tricyclic antidepressants—kinetics, mechanism, intervention: a review. *J Clin Psychiatry* 43:151–156, 1982.

94. Pumariega AJ, Muller B, Rivers-Bulkeley N: Acute renal failure secondary to amoxapine overdose. *JAMA* 248:331–341, 1982.

95. Raskin M, Veith RC, Barnes R, et al: Cardiovascular and antidepressant effects of imipramine in the treatment of secondary depression in patients with ischemic heart disease. *Am J Psychiatry* 139:1114–1117, 1982.

96. Richelson E: Biological basis of depression and Therapeutic relevavel. *J Clin Psychiatry* 52:6 (suppl):4–10, 1991.

97. Rickels K: Discussion. *Psychosomatics* 21:26–32, 1980.

98. Risch SC, Green GP, Janowsky DS: Interfaces of psychopharmacology and cardiology—part two. *J Clin Psychiatry* 42:47–59, 1981.

99. Roberts RK, Wilkinson GR, Branch RA, et al: Effect of age and parenchymal liver disease on the disposition and elimination of chlordiazepoxide. *Gastroenterology* 75:419–485, 1978.

100. Roose SP, Glassman AH, Giardina et al: Nortriptyline in depressed patients with left ventricular impairment. *JAMA* 256:3253–3257, 1986.

101. Roose SP, Glassman AH, Giardina EGV, et al: Tricyclic antidepressants in depressed patients with cardiac conduction disease. *Arch Gen Psychiatry* 44:273–275, 1987.

102. Rosenbaum JF, Woods SW, Gross JE, et al: Emergence of hostility during alprazolam treatment. *Am J Psychiatry* 141:792–793, 1984.

103. Sadeh M, Brahman J: Effects of anticholinergic drugs on memory in Parkinson's disease. *Arch Neurol* 39:666–667, 1982.

104. Salama AA: Complete heart block associated with mesoridazine in lithium combination. *J Clin Psychiatry* 48:123, 1987.

105. Sanders KM, Minnema AM, Murray GB: Low incidence of extrapyramidal symptoms in treatment of delirium with intravenous haloperidol and lorazepam in the intensive care unit. *J Intensive Care Med* 4:201–204, 1989.

106. Sanders KM, Stern TA, O'Gara PT, et al: Delirium after intra-aortic balloon pump therapy. *Psychosomatics* 33:35–41, 1992.

107. Salzman C, Solomon D, Miyawaki E, et al: Parenteral lorazepam versus parenteral haloperidol for the control of psychotic disruptive behavior. *J Clin Psychiatry* 52:177–180, 1991.

108. Scully JH: *Psychiatric Problems in Surgery.* Roche Products, Nutley, NJ, 1982.

109. Seymour-Shove R: Labile hypertension presenting as affective disorder. *Br J Clin Pract* 35:124–127, 1981.

110. Shader RI, Greenblatt DJ: Management of anxiety in the elderly: the balance between therapeutic and adverse effects. *J Clin Psychiatry* 43:8–15, 1982.

111. Sherwin I, Peron-Magnan P, Bancard J, et al: Prevalence of psychosis in epilepsy as a function of the laterality of the epileptogenic lesion. *Arch Neurol* 39:621–623, 1982.

112. Silberman EK, Reus VI, Jimerson DC, et al: Heterogeneity of amphetamine response in depressed patients. *Am J Psychiatry* 138:1302–1307, 1981.

113. Snavely SR, Hodges GR: The neurotoxicity of antibacterial agents. *Ann Intern Med* 101:92–104, 1984.

114. Sos J, Cassem NH: Managing postoperative agitation. *Drug Therapy* 10:103–106, 1980.

115. Sovner R, McGorril S: Stress as a precipitant of neuroleptic-induced dystonia. *Psychosomatics* 23:707–709, 1982.

116. Steinberg H: Erythropoietin and visual hallucinations. *N Engl J Med* 325:285, 1991.

117. Stern TA: Continuous infusion of physostigmine in anticholinergic delirium: case report. *J Clin Psychiatry* 44:462–464, 1983.

118. Tesar GE, Murray GB, Cassem NH: Use of high-dose intravenous haloperidol in the treatment of agitated cardiac patients. *J Clin Psychopharmacol* 5:344–347, 1985.

119. Tesar GE, Rosenbaum JF, Biederman J, et al: Orthostatic hypotension and antidepressant pharmacotherapy. *Psychopharmacol Bull* 23:182–186, 1987.

120. Thomas H, Jr, Schwartz E, Petrilli R: Droperidol versus haloperidol for chemical restraint of agitated and combative patients. *Ann Emerg Med* 21:407–413, 1992.

121. Thornton TL: Delirium associated with sulindac. *JAMA* 243:1630–1631, 1980.

122. Trohman RG, Castellanos D, Castellanos A, et al: Amiodarone-induced delirium. *Ann Intern Med* 108:68–69, 1988.

123. Wade JC, Meyers JD: Neurologic symptoms associated with parenteral acyclovir treatment after marrow transplantation. *Ann Intern Med* 98:921–925, 1983.

124. Walker WR: Phenothiazine therapy and latent organic brain syndrome. *Psychiatr Ann* 8:452–456, 1978.

125. Weddington WW Jr: Delirium and depression associated with amphotericin B. *Psychosomatics* 23:1076–1078, 1982.

126. Weisman AD, Hackett TP: Psychosis after eye surgery. Establishment of a specific doctor-patient relationship and treatment of "black-patch" delirium. *N Engl J Med* 258:1284–1289, 1958.

127. Woods S, Tesar G, Murray GB, et al: Psychostimulant treatment of depressive disorders secondary to medical illness. *J Clin Psychiatry* 47:12–15, 1986.

128. Young RC, Alexopoulos GS, Shamoian CA, et al: Plasma 10-hydroxy-nortriptyline and ECG changes in elderly depressed patients. *Am J Psychiatry* 142:866–868, 1985.

129. Zaret BS, Cohen RA: Reversible valproic acid-induced dementia: a case report. *Epilepsia* 27:234–240, 1986.

130. Zavodnick S: Atrial flutter with amoxapine: a case report. *Am J Psychiatry* 138:1503–1505, 1981.

CHAPTER 40

Anticoagulants in Critical Care Medicine

JOHN J. NANFRO, M.D.

Maintaining normal hemostatic integrity is a central issue in the management of the critically ill. Optimal hemostasis requires a complex interaction of the vascular endothelium, platelets, and coagulation factors. This well-balanced system may be perturbed by an underlying systemic disorder or a therapeutic intervention. It is essential that the clinician involved in the care of critically ill patients understand the normal physiology of hemostasis. This information enables one to manage a hemorrhagic or thrombotic disorder. This chapter reviews the aspects of normal hemostatic events, pathologic states, and finally, the pharmacology of anticoagulants and related substances.

NORMAL HEMOSTASIS

Vascular injury may occur in a direct or an indirect manner. Initially when the vascular endothelium is damaged, vasoconstriction occurs promptly. The exposed collagen fibrils in the subendothelial region attract circulating platelets (Fig. 40.1). The platelets adhere to the collagen fibrils closing the endothelial defect and undergo significant metabolic changes that promote continued hemostasis (87, 97, 102). Upon exposure to the collagen, the platelet begins a release reaction from the dense-core granules, generating serotonin and adenosine diphosphate (ADP). The release of these substances promotes aggregation by attracting further circulating platelets to the

damaged endothelial collagen-platelet complex. Plasma coagulation factors, in close association with the platelet membrane, as well as factors in other platelet organelles (α-granules), are also activated (85). The contact factors (XII, XI) are activated by collagen and ADP and subsequently lead to the formation of activated factor X (X_a) in the common pathway of the coagulation schema. X_a in the presence of activated factor V (V_a) and calcium convert prothrombin (II) to thrombin (IIa). The generated thrombin converts fibrinogen to fibrin monomer, and fibrin monomers subsequently bind to each other. Thrombin also activates many other factors, including factor XIII (fibrin stabilizing factor), V, VIII, and protein C. The soluble fibrin monomer is stabilized to an insoluble polymer by the action of factor XIII_a. Thrombin also promotes contraction of the platelet mass by its action on platelet actomyosin. This action further controls the hemostatic defect. If fibrin polymerization were inadequate, the initial platelet plug would disaggregate.

The coagulation schema is outlined in Figure 40.2. The initiating vascular injury may be traumatic, vasculitic, or related to endotoxin. The intrinsic pathway requires the presence of adequate concentrations of coagulation factors, calcium, and phospholipid. High-molecular-weight kininogen (HMWK) and prekallikrein (PK), released during vascular injury, augment the initial contact activation and formation of XII_a. Platelets and endothelium act as a matrix upon which the coagulation complex forms. Each coagulation factor is activated by an enzymatic reaction, which results in a functional factor in close apposition to cofactors. The extrinsic

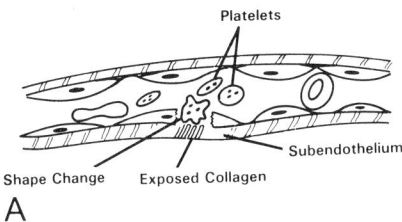

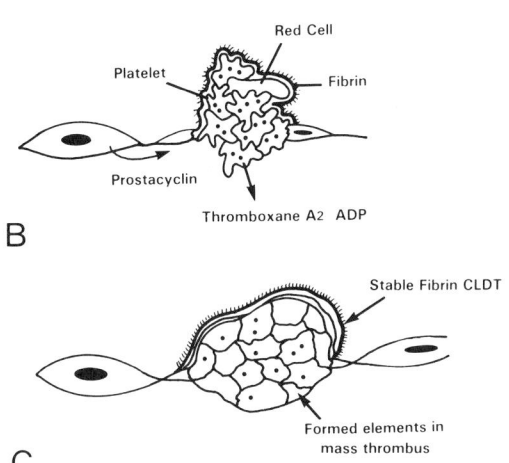

Figure 40.1. **A,** blood vessel is injured, collagen is exposed, and platelets undergo prompt shape change. **B,** platelet plug forms and coagulation schema results in fibrin formation in association with platelet plug. **C,** hemostatic plug becomes organized.

pathway predominantly involves factor VII. This factor is activated by tissue thromboplastin as well as XIIa. Kinins are generated during inflammatory states and by the activation of factor XII. These substances promote tissue contraction, hypotension, and vascular permeability.

The fibrin clot must be controlled by the fibrinolytic system (10, 66), or diffuse thrombosis develops. This system is activated by factor XIIa, the kallikreins, and tissue plasminogen activator. The resulting reaction converts plasminogen to plasmin. Plasmin may also be formed by exogenous compounds such as streptokinase. Plasmin converts fibrin to fibrin degradation products (FDPs) and dissolves clot. The FDPs inhibit further conversion of fibrinogen to fibrin by thrombin (Fig. 40.2). The procoagulant system (intrinsic and extrinsic) must be complemented by the fibrinolytic system to maintain normal hemostasis. Alterations in either limb may result in hemorrhage or thrombosis. Plasmin and factor XIIa generate the formation of complement. Complement components promote chemotaxis and the release of leukotrienes contained within leukocytes. During the inflammatory response associated with sepsis, many of these factors circulate and promote localized fibrin deposition in the form of disseminated intravascular coagulation (DIC). Circulating antiplasmins can inactivate the fibrinolytic system. An absence of the antiplasmins may result in hemorrhage. There are also circulating inhibitors of the procoagulants. The predominant inhibitor is antithrombin III. This serine protease is referred to as "heparin cofactor." Antithrombin III naturally inhibits thrombin activity, and to a

lesser degree, factors XIIA and XA. However, in the presence of heparin, this activity is markedly increased, and coagulation is prevented (Fig. 40.3).

Platelets are critical for adequate coagulation (Fig. 40.4). Platelet-released ADP activates factors XII and XI in the presence of collagen. Platelets release phospholipid and platelet factor 4 (PF4), which alters heparin function. Platelets also liberate fibrinogen, factors V, and VIII. Platelets store the phospholipid platelet factor 3 (PF3), which is necessary for modulation of the intrinsic pathway. The platelets act as a substrate for complex coagulation reactions.

Platelet metabolism is also critical to adequate hemostasis and platelet function. Platelets passively absorb glucose and produce lactic acid, with the energy thus formed stored as adenosine triphosphate (ATP). Lipid degradation provides energy as well. Glucose and lipids may be stored in granules in the platelet cytosol. When the release reaction and aggregation occurs, the platelet metabolic rate markedly escalates. ATP is converted to ADP and cyclic AMP. ADP is a critical component of the platelet release reaction. Stored ADP is localized in the dense-core granules of the platelets. The platelet metabolic machinery attempts to maintain stores of the adenosine phosphates for catabolism and the release reaction.

Prostaglandins play a critical role in platelet function (64, 74). The exposure to collagen and subsequent release of thrombin initiate metabolism of arachidonic acid. Arachidonic acid is converted enzymatically into the eicosatrienoic acids (HPETE and HETE). These components are involved in prostaglandin feedback mechanisms and the inflammatory response. The enzyme cyclooxygenase promotes the production of the prostaglandins PGI_2 (prostacyclin) and thromboxane A_2 (TXA_2). TXA_2 is a potent platelet-aggregating agent and promotes further release of ADP. TXA_2 causes profound vasoconstriction and may play a role in coronary vasospasm and other vasospastic events. PGI_2 is produced by the endothelium in contact with the platelet and is a vasodilating substance that counteracts TXA_2 activity. The relative quantities of TXA_2 and PGI_2 are currently believed to play a role in thrombotic thrombocytopenic purpura (TTP), DIC, and some antiplatelet drug activity. The by-products of arachidonic acid metabolism are actively being studied for potential use in treating thrombotic events.

Coagulation factors may critically affect platelet function. Thrombin acts on platelets by promoting aggregation, release, and clot retraction. The von Willebrand's factor VIII complex associates with the vessel wall and platelet. These complex associations point out the necessity of intact components of hemostasis: vessels, platelets, coagulation factors, and the fibrinolytic system. In the critical care setting, each of these elements may be perturbed. Vessels may be disrupted by trauma, surgery, toxic damage to the endothelium, or a vasculitic process. Platelets may be diminished in number by decreased production or increased destruction. This thrombocytopenia may be due to sepsis, surgery, endotoxins, or autoimmune phenomenon. Coagulation factors may be dysfunctional or inadequately produced as in hepatic disease. Rarely, patients in the intensive care unit may present with a previously undiagnosed congenital coagulopathy. Finally, thrombotic events may occur secondary to systemic disease or on the basis of alterations in the fibrinolytic system.

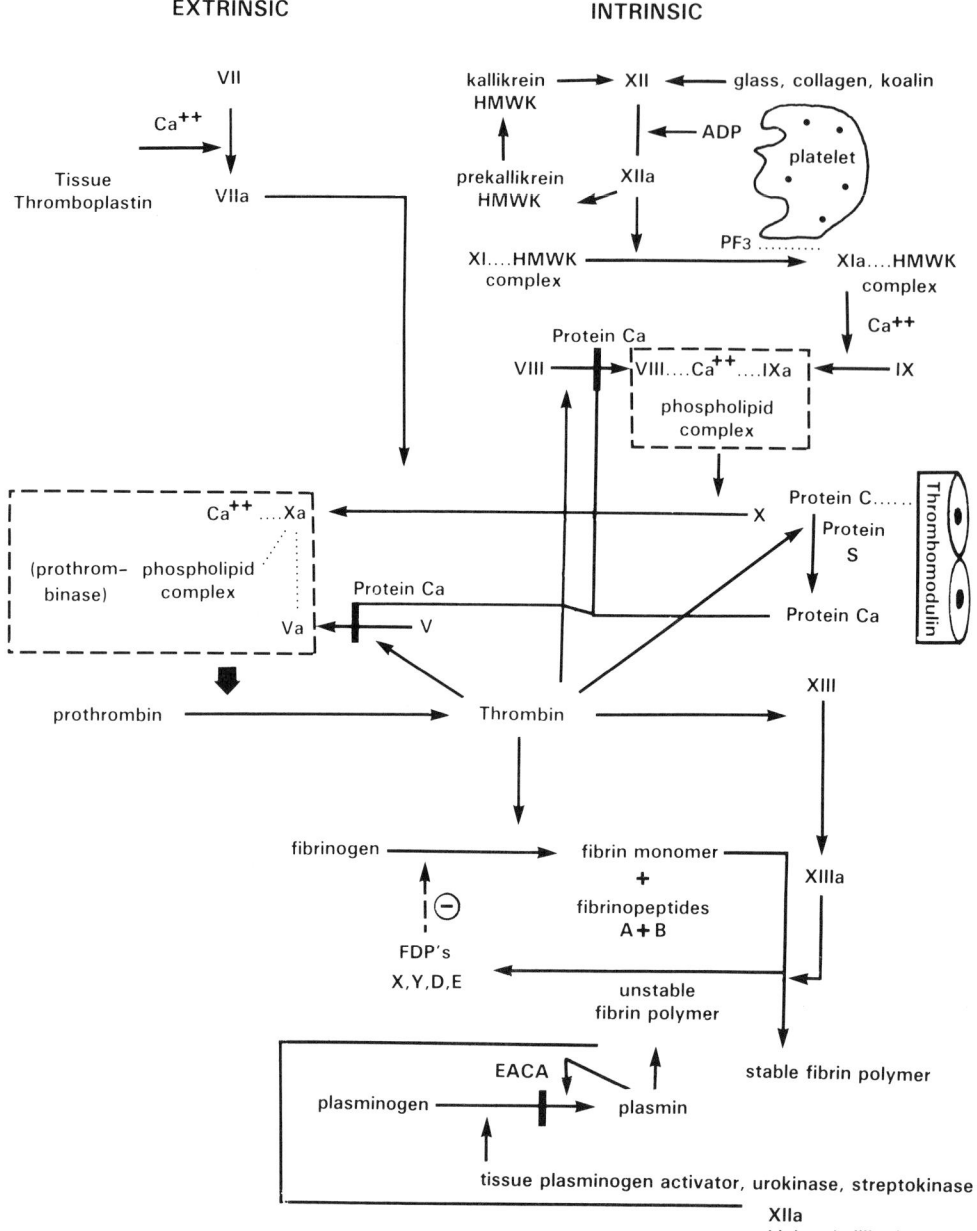

Figure 40.2.   The coagulation-fibrinolytic schema.

TESTS OF HEMOSTASIS

Tests of hemostasis are performed by drawing venous blood into commercially available test tubes containing either an anticoagulant [(EDTA, citrate, oxalate) which binds calcium and prevents clot formation] or heparin [which promptly binds to antithrombin 3 (AT^{III}) preventing coagulation via thrombin modification]. The tubes may also be siliconized to prevent activation of contact factors. Platelet function tests are performed on fresh platelet-rich plasma.

Microscopic review of the peripheral blood smear from a patient in the intensive care unit with a coagulopathy is imperative. Information obtained may be useful in clinical management and helpful in determining etiology. For example, one may note a diminished platelet count from the

hematology lab. A review of the peripheral smear will rule out artifactual platelet "satelliting" and clumping. The presence of schistocytes supports microangiopathy in patients with burns, severe organ trauma, TTP, or DIC. Microangiopathy implies fibrin deposition and may support early use of heparin as well as fresh-frozen plasma.

A normal platelet count is between 150,000 and 400,000 thrombocytes. An increase or decrease in the count may result in hemorrhage or thrombosis, depending on platelet function. A bleeding time (Simplate II) by the technique of Ivy-Mielke is the most widely used means of assessing platelet function (54, 79). The bleeding time progressively prolongs as the platelet count falls below 100,000/mm³. Performing a bleeding time on patients with platelets less than 50,000/mm³ is rarely

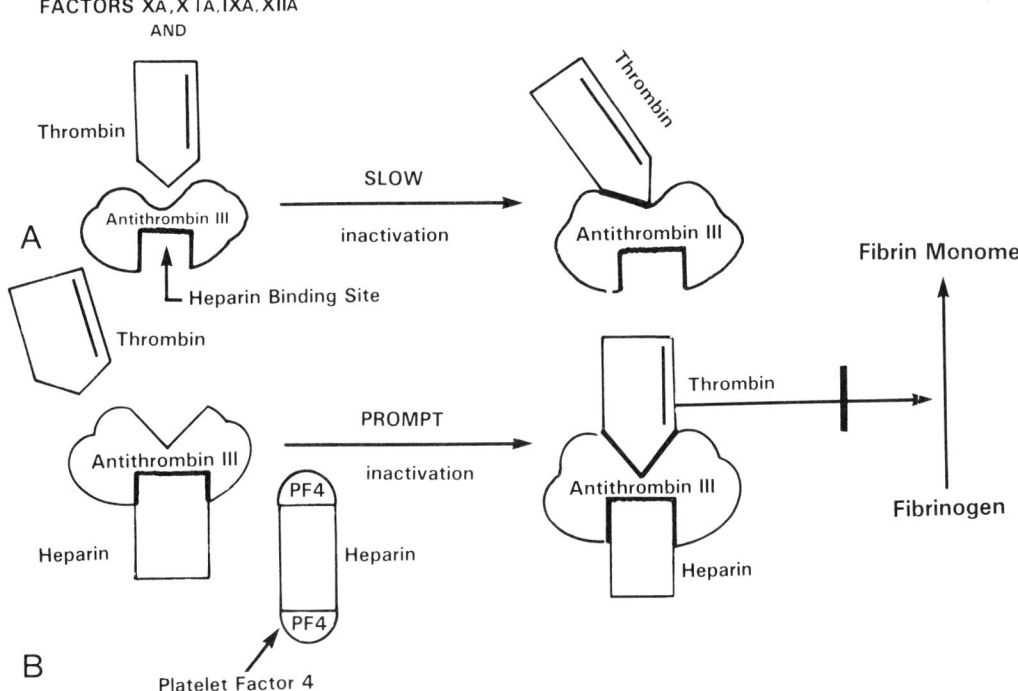

Figure 40.3. **A,** Thrombin interacts with antithrombin III and slow inactivation of thrombin occurs. **B,** In the presence of heparin, antithrombin undergoes a molecular alteration and promptly inactivates thrombin.

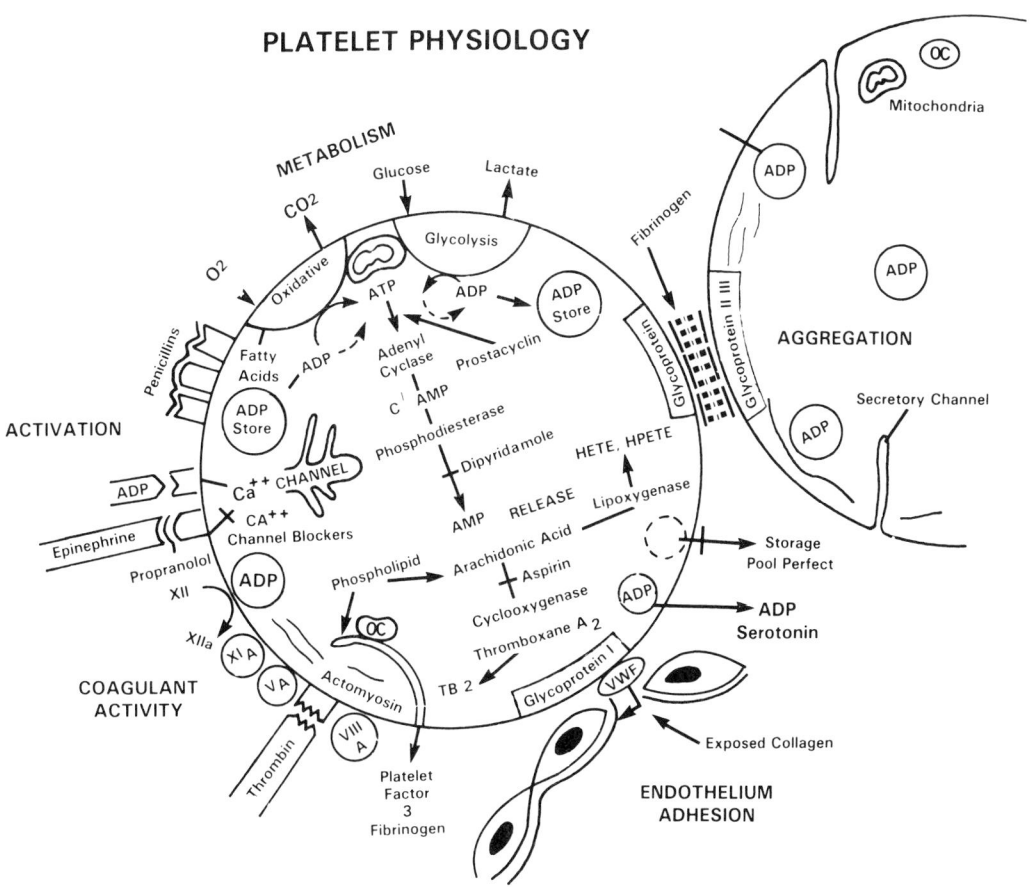

Figure 40.4. Platelet physiology and function.

of benefit unless one is using the bleeding time to assess a therapeutic manipulation to improve platelet function. The most important clinical utility of the bleeding time is in patients with normal platelet counts. Bleeding times greater than 9 minutes imply a qualitative defect, either congenital or acquired. Bleeding times are often used to evaluate platelet function following cardiopulmonary bypass or in bleeding patients with liver or renal dysfunction (3). Platelet aggregometry is reserved for the outpatient setting and is not of great utility in the ICU (16).

The more common tests in critical care are the coagulation tests. These include the prothrombin time (PT), activated partial thromboplastin time (aPTT), thrombin time (TT), whole-blood clotting time (WBT), and a measure of fibrin degradation products (FDP). The prothrombin time is performed by adding a source of tissue thromboplastin to plasma and observing the time required for a clot to form. The test screens the integrity of the extrinsic limb of coagulation (II, V, VII, X, fibrinogen) and is reported as a time compared with control values. A prolonged PT suggests a deficiency of these factors, the presence of heparin, FDPs, or low or dysfunctional fibrinogen. To perform the aPTT one adds a contact agent (kaolin, ellagic acid) to plasma and observes the time necessary for clot to form. This screens the intrinsic schema (II, V, VIII, IX, X, XI, XII, fibrinogen). A prolonged aPTT suggests the same defects as the PT (except factor VII). In addition, aPTT detects a deficiency of VIII, IX, XI, XII, prekallikrein, and HMWK. The PT and aPTT do not detect deficiency of factor XIII, low level FDPs, or fibrinolytic defects. A routine admission PT or PTT may be unnecessary if an adequate history and physical examination rule out a hemorrhage or thrombotic process. The critical care setting differs, however, in that these tests are generally monitored serially. The severity of the systemic illness and drugs used in the ICU may affect the PT and aPTT and result in altered hemostasis. The thrombin time is performed by adding measured amounts of thrombin to plasma and measuring time to clot formation. The test therefore does not rely on the presence of endogenous thrombin. Thrombin acts on fibrinogen to cleave fibrinopeptides A and B and promotes fibrin monomer polymerization. Abnormal fibrinogens (produced in liver disease), fibrin split products, or a low fibrinogen may prolong the thrombin time. Renal disease, autoimmune disorders, and hepatic dysfunction may also result in a prolonged thrombin time. Heparin is a significant cause of a prolonged thrombin time. This abnormality may be present secondary to indwelling arterial catheters, right atrial catheters, or hemodialysis. It may be difficult to distinguish systemic DIC from a heparin effect. Reptilase time (RT) (venom of *Bothrops atrox*) cleaves fibrinopeptide A from fibrinogen and is unaffected by the presence of heparin (22). Thus, a prolonged TT with a normal RT suggests heparin, whereas a prolonged RT suggests FDPs, dysfibrinogenemia, or low fibrinogen.

Other tests that may be used in an attempt to distinguish DIC from primary fibrinolysis and include the euglobulin clot lysis and the protamine paracoagulation tests. These tests must be interpreted in light of the peripheral blood smear and clinical setting. This point is important since ε-aminocaproic acid (EACA) is used in the treatment of primary fibrinolysis,

while it is contraindicated in DIC. FDPs are measured by a semiquantitative test of latex agglutination.

BLEEDING

The manifestation of inadequate hemostasis, regardless of the cause, is bleeding. In the critical care setting, the control of bleeding is imperative. Many of these patients are monitored with right atrial and pulmonary artery flotation catheters and arterial "lines." Loss of blood exacerbates volume control and promotes hypotension. Hypotension leads to end-organ dysfunction. The management of these patients must be aggressive, not only in regard to cardiopulmonary, central nervous system (CNS), hepatic, and renal support, but also in maintaining hemostasis. Disorders of hemostasis are common and may go undetected unless bleeding is apparent. Bleeding may be grossly evident from the gastrointestinal tract or a surgical wound. The possibility of occult blood loss must be considered in patients with hypotension or a decreasing hematocrit. Patients should have hemostasis parameters studied if invasive procedures (such as lumbar puncture, thoracentesis, pericardiocentesis, bronchoscopy with biopsy, and Swan-Ganz catheterization) are to be performed. Baseline studies should include PT, aTT, platelet count, hemoglobin, and hematocrit. Tamponade of the bleeding site may control acute bleeding. However, the evacuation of blood in the setting of a coagulopathy or platelet disorder may result in continued bleeding unless the abnormalities are corrected. A knowledge of the interaction of medications with the hemostatic system is critical.

QUANTITATIVE AND QUALITATIVE PLATELET DISORDERS

Platelet abnormalities occur in many intensive care patients. Surgical units tend to see thrombocytopenia due to the dilutional effects of red cell transfusion or decreased production due to sepsis and drugs. Qualitative disorders may also be seen, either as acquired or previously undetected congenital disorders (28, 75). Medical intensive care units tend to see a much broader range of platelet abnormalities both quantitative and qualitative.

Quantitative abnormalities must first be confirmed by a review of the peripheral smear. Relying on an automated counter valve may result in premature calls to the blood bank for platelet support. In the bleeding patient, an incorrect assumption of thrombocytopenia as the cause for hemorrhage may be made. Platelet transfusions will not correct a significant coagulopathy or a wound requiring surgical intervention. Having confirmed thrombocytopenia on the examination of the blood smear, one must determine etiology (Table 40.1). The presence of petechiae suggests thrombocytopenia.

Patients may have decreased platelet production caused by exposure to a toxin such as benzene (24). In these patients one should avoid platelet transfusion to prevent allosensitization. If the aplastic patient is not bleeding, platelets are not indicated on a prophylactic basis. Patients with irreversible decreased platelet production should not be transfused platelets unless actively bleeding. If patients have decreased production because they have received cytotoxic agents, or drugs such as cimetidine or heparin, platelets can be given for bleeding or counts less than 20,000. In general, it is the precipitous reduction of the platelet count as seen in cytotoxic therapy that is associated with severe life-threatening bleeding. Patients who have received intensive chemotherapy for acute leukemia may occasionally be transferred to the ICU for fluid management, or for treatment of respiratory failure, hyperuricemia or septic shock. Sepsis may induce transient bone marrow failure and decreased production of all bone marrow-generated cellular elements. Platelet replacement therapy for circulating platelet counts less than 20,000 may benefit these patients. Performing a bleeding time in thrombocytopenic patients is of minimal clinical benefit. Corticosteroids are generally not used to treat chemotherapy-induced thrombocytopenia, as they may exacerbate gastrointestinal bleeding, and promote vascular fragility without increasing the platelet count. For these patients, strict bed rest, avoidance of drugs that alter platelet function or reduce the platelet count are indicated. Invasive procedures are avoided unless clinically indicated and supported by platelet transfusion and adequate surgical technique. Intramuscular injection and vigorous dental care are also contraindicated. Thrombocytopenia due to decreased production from leukemia and induction chemotherapy is common. Platelets are given prophylactically to these patients for counts less than 20,000. If this is difficult to attain then, at least for counts less than 10,000/ml[3]. Intubation or mechanical ventilation of such patients is exceedingly difficult and excessive bleeding may occur into the respiratory tract regardless of intervention. The use of ϵ-aminocaproic acid (EACA) to decrease bleeding in this setting is not without risk.

Increased destruction of platelets may also be noted in sepsis (70). Platelet transfusions are withheld unless the platelet count gets low or bleeding occurs. Autoimmune disorders may cause thrombocytopenia by different mechanisms (8, 60, 62). An examination of the bone marrow is usually required. Increased platelet destruction on an immune basis is treated with corticosteroids (e.g., prednisone 100 mg daily or an intravenous equivalent). Corticosteroids may also be used for drug-induced thrombocytopenias. If the platelet count has not corrected within 2 weeks, other measures are indicated. Patients may be treated with intravenous immunoglobulin 0.4 g/kg/day for 5 days and subsequently by splenectomy, or splenectomy alone (41, 95). The mechanism of action of intravenous

immunoglobulin is immune thrombocytopenia is unclear but presumably involves macrophage inhibition. The clinical situation dictates which of these approaches is appropriate. Platelet transfusions are contraindicated for the treatment of immune thrombocytopenia, except for acute uncontrolled bleeding or the need for surgical intervention. Platelet sequestration may occur in hypersplenism due to chronic lymphocytic leukemia. Splenectomy may be indicated if tests with ^{51}chromium red blood cell labeling documents sequestration, and the clinical condition merits such an approach. Giant hemangioma may be another site of platelet sequestration.

During cardiopulmonary bypass, platelets are altered to a degree that depends on the type of oxygenator used (2). Platelets may be sequestered by the pump or may be reduced by heparin therapy and/or by dilutional effects. Platelet dysfunction may also develop because of platelet degranulation. A review of the peripheral blood smear and bleeding time may help to determine the etiology. Bleeding postpump usually occurs from the sternotomy drain. The cardiothoracic surgeon and hematologist monitor these parameters, as well as the rate of bleeding. Rapid bleeding suggests the need for prompt surgical reexploration. A slow stable bleed allows time for evaluation of other causes. If the PT, $_a$PTT, TT, platelets, and bleeding time are normal, then surgical reexploration is indicated for hemodynamic instability.

Thrombocytopenia is frequently caused by drugs (Table 40.2). Quinine derivatives, such as quinidine, are a common cause of drug-related thrombocytopenia. The treatment is prompt discontinuation of the offending agent. The abnormality usually corrects itself within a few days. The use of a short course of prednisone at 100 mg daily may be of benefit, as this disorder is often immunologically mediated. Patients with the acquired immune deficiency syndrome have a high rate of marrow dysfunction with thrombocytopenia (91, 100). Trimethoprim sulfamethoxazole often worsens this phenomenon. The treatment of these patients is similar to that of patients with idiopathic thrombocytopenic purpura.

Qualitative platelet defects may be caused by numerous drugs or systemic disorders (Tables 40.3 and 40.4). Collagen vascular disorders, such as systemic lupus erythematosus, may cause a prolonged bleeding time. Uremia may induce a qualitative defect. This thrombopathy may be corrected by the use of cryoprecipitate, desmopressin (dDAVP), or conjugated estrogens (42, 55, 58). Aspirin acetylates serine residues on platelet cyclooxygenase preventing the formation of TXA_2. This action of aspirin results in a prolongation of the bleeding time. The alternate products, HETE and HPETE, are produced. Aspirin blocks cyclooxygenase for the life of the platelet or approximately 7 to 10 days. With no further aspirin therapy there is a gradual improvement in the bleeding time that coincides with the generation of new platelets. At higher doses, aspirin inhibits endothelial prostacyclin synthetase and prevents generation of PGI_2. At lower doses (less than 300 mg) aspirin prevents TXA_2 generation, which results in decreased aggregation, release, and vasoconstriction (71). This observation explains the theoretic utility of aspirin in vasospastic disorders or fixed atheromatous lesions. However, with the inhibition of PGI_2 at higher doses, this effect may be negated. Nonsteroidal antiinflammatory drugs such as indomethacin and ibuprofen inhibit cyclooxygenase but not irreversibly. The

Table 40.1. Causes of Thrombocytopenia

Viral infections
   cytomegalovirus, HTLV III, rubella, adenovirus, mumps
Vaccines
   Rubella, rubeola
Nonimmune platelet destruction
   Infection, shock, surgery, DIC, malignancy, obstetrical
      complictions, cardiac prostheses, burns, vasculitis, TTP,
      hemolytic uremic syndrome
Immune thrombocytopenia
   Idiopathic, alloantibodies, collagen vascular disorders, viral
      infections, malignancy, drug mediated (Quinidine)
Radiation
Aplastic anemia
Preleukemia, leukemia, neoplastic involvement of marrow
Drug-induced myelosuppression (benzene, mycotoxin)

Table 40.2. Some Drugs That Cause Thrombocytopenia[a]

Antimicrobials
  Chloramphenicol
  Sulphonamides
  Amphotericin
  Quinacrine
  Pyrimethamine
  Streptomycin
  Tetracycline
  Penicillins
  Cephalosporins
  Isonayid
Anticonvulsants
  Diphenylhydantoin (Dilantin)
  Primidone (Mysoline)
  Trimethadione (Tridione)
  Ethosuximide (Zarontin)
  Mephenytoin (Mesantoin)
  Carbamazepine (Tegretol)
  Paramethadime
Diuretics
  Thiazides
  Furosemide
  Acetazolamide
  Ethacrynic Acid
Oral hypoglycemics
  Tolbutamide (Orinase)
  Chlorpropamide (Diabinase)
Chemicals
  Arsenicals
  Benzene
Rheumatologic medications
  Aspirin
  Phenylbutazone
  Indomethacin
  Gold salts
  Colchicine
  Phenacetin
Tranquilizers
  Meprobamate
  Chlorpromazine
  Chlordiazepoxide
  Chloral hydrate
  Alcohol
Others
  Allopurinol
  Cimetidine
  Estrogens
  Lipid infusions
  Cytotoxic agents
  Corticosteroids
  Heparin
  Inferferon
  Quinidine

[a] May be due to an immune mechanism or decreased production.

Table 40.3. Drugs That Cause a Qualitative Platelet Defect

Alteration of prostaglandin metabolism
  Aspirin
  Indomethacin, ibuprofen
  Corticosteroids
  Sulfinpyrazone
  Furosemide
  Vitamin E
Alteration of surface receptors
  Penicillins (carbenicillin, ticarcillin)
  Cephalosporins
  β-Lactams (moxalactam)
  Nitrofurantoin
  Ristocetin
Alteration of epinephrine receptors
  α-Blockers (phentolamine)
  β-Blockers (propranolol)
  Ca^{2+} channel blocker (verapamil)
Phosphodiesterase inhibitors
  Dipyridamole?
  Xanthines (theophylline, caffeine)
  Papaverine
Membrane stabilizers
  Anesthetics (Xylocaine)
  Tricyclics
  Antihistamines (diphenhydramine)
Other
  Dextran
  Heparin
  Ethanol
  Glyburide
  Clofibrate
  Reserpine
  Methylsergide
  Glyceryl Guaiacolate
  Phenothiazines
  Fish oils
  Amiodarone

Table 40.4. Acquired Qualitative Platelet Defects

Drugs[a]
Aged platelets
Antiplatelet antibodies
Cardiopulmonary bypass
Myelodysplastic syndromes
Acute leukemia
Myeloproliferative syndromes
Acquired storage pool defect
Acquired von Willebrand's disease
Hepatic dysfunction
Uremia
Paraproteinemias
Disseminated intravascular coagulation

[a] See Table 40.3.

inhibition of platelet aggregation depends on the half-life of the nonsteroidal drugs. Choline magnesium trisalicylate maintains the antiarthritic effect of aspirin and in some studies did not alter platelet aggregation. This compound may be useful in arthritics predisposed to a bleeding diathesis.

Some antibiotics may alter platelet function, predominating by altering response to aggregating agents. Classically, this platelet dysfunction occurs with carbenicillin and, to a lesser degree, with ticarcillin and other penicillins (66). Should the patient be predisposed to bleeding for other reasons, these agents are best avoided. Many drugs may affect platelet function alone or in conjunction with other drugs. A bleeding time and platelet aggregometry are useful measures of this effect.

Congenital qualitative disorders are occasionally seen in the ICU in patients without a past history of bleeding (75). Von Willebrand's disease is a complex disorder involving a protein complex (VWF-VIII). Many variants exist, and it is critical that the specific subtype of von Willebrand's disease be defined. The use of agents such as arginine vasopressin (dDAVP) may precipitate fatal thrombotic events if used in certain von Willebrand variants. In general, it is appropriate to use cryoprecipitate in suspected von Willebrand's disease unless the dDAVP-responsive subtype has been previously diagnosed. Aspirin-like thrombopathy or poorly defined qualitative platelet disorders may occasionally respond to low-dose prednisone (63). The severe qualitative disorders, such as Glanzmann's or Bernard-Soulier, are best treated with platelet transfusion for bleeding events. If surgical intervention is planned in these patients, platelets should be administered prophylactically. ∈-Aminocaproic acid can be used to diminish postoperative bleeding.

When a patient presents with either a quantitative or qualitative platelet disorder, procoagulant activity should be studied as well. Disorders such as DIC, liver disease, and renal disease may affect both hemostatic parameters. For adequate hemostasis, it is necessary to correct platelet abnormalities, as well as coagulation defects.

COAGULATION DISORDERS

In the critical care unit, bleeding due to a coagulopathy is a common event. Coagulopathy is most often due to an acquired rather than congenital defect. Patients with gastrointestinal bleeding may be heavily transfused, resulting in dilutional effects on platelets and coagulation factors. It is important to address platelet and coagulation factor replacement routinely in the massively transfused patient. One should prophylactically replace with FFP after 4 to 6 U of red cells have been administered and monitor the platelet count, PT, and $_a$PTT.

The clinician should first assess the site of bleeding. Purpura, ecchymoses, and hemarthroses suggest coagulation defects. The laboratory tests obtained should include a hematocrit, PT, $_a$PTT, platelet count, and review of the peripheral blood smear. If these tests are all normal and the bleeding is accounted for by a surgical wound, packed red cell transfusion therapy as needed is initiated. However, if the bleeding is unusual (i.e., protracted bleeding from mucous membranes, intravenous sites, urinary tract, joints, skin), a more thorough investigation is indicated. Blood oozing from multiple sites is very suggestive of DIC or primary fibrinolysis. The clinician should obtain hepatic and renal function test parameters, which may suggest an etiology of the coagulopathy (90).

If the PT and $_a$PTT are prolonged, a thrombin time and a 1 : 1 dilution of the PT and PTT (with a mix of the patient's and normal plasma) are recommended. A 1 : 1 mixture with normal plasma corrects the PT and $_a$PTT if there is an absence of a coagulation factor. If these tests do not correct, an inhibitor is implied (e.g., FDPs, heparin, lupus anticoagulant VIII, or IX inhibitors). First, one must rule out inadvertent administration of heparin. The RT should be normal in the setting of heparin effect. A normal thrombin time and a normal 1 : 1 mix of the PT, $_a$PTT implies a defect above the level of thrombin in either the common, intrinsic, or extrinsic pathway. In DIC, the platelet count would be low unless there is a chronic compensated consumptive coagulopathy secondary to liver disease, primary fibrinolysis, or underlying neoplasia.

Disseminated intravascular coagulation is a common event in the critically ill patient and is often a therapeutic dilemma. It represents an uncontrolled stimulation of the coagulation schema by various causes (Table 40.5) (21). The coagulation cascade proceeds unabated, consuming factors and platelets in the process. Often, the bone marrow of the ICU patient is suppressed and does not adequately respond to bleeding and thrombocytopenia with increased megakaryopoiesis. Liver disease may compound this process, resulting in the

Table 40.5. Precipitating Events for Disseminated Intravascular Coagulation

Pancreatitis
Prostatic surgery
Cardiopulmonary bypass
Extensive surgery
Trauma
Burns
Obstetrical complications (eclampsia, placenta previa)
Cavernous hemangioma
Heat stroke
Peritoneovenous shunts
Aneurysmal rupture
Hematotoxic snake venoms
Activated concentrates of vitamin K-dependent factors
Acute myelogenous leukemia
Mitomycin
Neoplasia
Liver disease
Viral infections
Systemic vasculitis
Rhabdomyolysis

inability to produce coagulation factors. The fibrinolytic system is activated by the kallikreins and other inflammatory byproducts. Generated plasmin degrades the fibrinogen and fibrin to the degradation products (FDPs). The FDPs subsequently inhibit coagulation at multiple points of the cascade. If fibrin deposition in the vasculature is diffuse, red cell fragmentation or microangiopathic changes may be seen in the peripheral smear. Fibrinogen levels decrease markedly. The acute inflammatory state may have induced high fibrinogen levels; hence, the relative value must be taken into account. Thrombotic events may occur because of the stimulus to coagulation. The titer of the FDP by latex agglutination may correlate with the severity of DIC. Chronic DIC as seen in liver disease and neoplasia may have low levels of FDPs without frank bleeding. However, these patients are at risk of conversion to high-grade DIC with the proper stimulus (surgery, shock, sepsis, and chemotherapy). Because of diffuse fibrin deposition, organ dysfunction may progress to hepatic, renal, and CNS dysfunction. This fibrin deposition may further release products of inflammation, compounding the fibrinolytic and procoagulant dysfunction. Tests of DIC have been described and are useful in monitoring a response to therapy.

The treatment of DIC is aimed primarily at the elimination of the precipitating cause. Rhabdomyolysis and associated shock are best treated with intense fluid and electrolyte management. Hemodialysis may be required if acute renal failure occurs. Should bleeding occur, the use of fresh-frozen plasma (FFP) and platelet transfusions is indicated. These components are given to control bleeding; one should attempt to maintain platelet counts greater than 20,000/mm^3 and normalize the PT and $_a$PTT if possible. Gestational causes of DIC are best treated by removing the thromboplastic products, fetal or placental. If bleeding persists, FFP and platelets with heparin coverage may be used. However, in a patient suffering from irreversible liver disease or a terminal neoplastic disorder, the overvigorous use of these products is expensive and may limit their use in other critically ill patients. The ICU team must assess the utility of such component therapy on an individual basis. Patients requiring surgical intervention in the setting of DIC should be supported with FFP and platelets. Sepsis is a common cause of DIC in the critically ill patient. Treatment involves aggressive cardiopulmonary support, antimicrobials, and monitoring of hemostasis. If bleeding is occurring from intravenous sites, an initial trial of FFP and platelets is indicated; however, should DIC persist, some hematologists would recommend a trial of heparin.

Heparin use remains a controversial therapy in the management of DIC (29). The use of heparin is established for specific entities, is contraindicated in some patients, and is often a final intervention to reverse DIC in others. One indication for the use of heparin includes acute promyelocytic leukemia. However, there are some hematologists who have successfully induced acute promyelocytic leukemia patients into complete remission without the use of heparin. They achieved this goal by closely monitoring clinical hemostasis, fibrinogen levels, platelets, PT, and PTT. However, since most patients with promyelocytic leukemia, and occasionally monocytic leukemia, have large amounts of thromboplastic material released into the circulation during induction, heparin is recommended. In acute leukemia, the dose of heparin generally recommended is lower than the dose used for pulmonary embolus and other cases of DIC (14, 15). In general, patients are given 100 to 200 U/kg/day by continuous infusion: a bolus is not given. Heparin may be used in cases of gestational DIC in which the excessive bleeding persists after removal of the thromboplastic material. One parameter used to determine benefit from heparin is review of the peripheral blood smear. The presence of microangiopathy and thrombocytopenia supports intravascular fibrin deposition. The use of heparin may prevent further fibrin deposition, decrease the microangiopathy, and increase the platelet count. Heparin is often augmented with the use of FFP and platelets. In a burn patient with DIC, heparin may be of benefit. Heparin is generally contraindicated in cases of surgical bleeding with DIC. These cases must be treated by surgical intervention, if feasible. Brisk bleeding from a peptic ulcer in an ICU patient with DIC is not benefited by heparin use. Finally, patients with intractable DIC, in which the underlying cause is adequately treated, can be given a trial of heparin. Occasionally, the hemostatic parameters may correct. In these situations, heparin is given as a 5000- to 10,000-U bolus followed by 1000 to 1200 U/hr; however, lower doses, as for promyelocytic leukemia, have also been used .The heparin dose is adjusted based upon the fibrinogen concentration, FDP level and platelet count, as well as the peripheral blood smear. As the fibrinogen level and platelets increase and FDPs decrease, the dose of heparin may be decreased, and the need for component replacement diminishes. The use of Amicar (ε-aminocaproic acid) in DIC is generally contraindicated, as there is a risk of EACA-induced diffuse thrombosis.

Primary fibrinolysis is a rare entity (48). A secondary fibrinolytic state may be seen in the continuum of DIC. The common causes of primary fibrinolysis are prostatic surgery, malignancy and, rarely, sepsis. The ability to distinguish primary fibrinolysis from DIC with the secondary state may be difficult. In the proper clinical setting of primary fibrinolysis, one sees bleeding, a relatively normal platelet count, elevated FDPs, fibrin monomer, minimal microangiopathy, low fibrinogen, and a positive euglobulin clot lysis. The treatment of primary fibrinolysis is with Amicar (EACA), with close hemostatic monitoring.

Coagulopathy may be due to an individual factor or to a combination of factor defects. The vitamin K-dependent factors (II, VII, IX, X) are markedly affected by alterations in vitamin K metabolism (72). If there is a deficiency of vitamin K or an interfering substance (warfarin), these factors are not produced, and a coagulopathy results. These factors are synthesized in the liver, and liver disease represents a common cause of coagulopathy (49). Vitamin K must be provided to ICU patients as part of their nutritional support. In normal individuals, the gastrointestinal tract bacterial flora provide adequate amounts of vitamin K. If an antimicrobial is used, the gut may be sterilized, inadequate vitamin K production occurs, and vitamin K replacement therapy becomes necessary. If acute bleeding has developed, patients should be given oral or intravenous vitamin K replacement, as well as FFP to replace vitamin K-dependent factors while hepatic synthesis resumes.

Calcium replacement must also be addressed in ICU patients. As the exogenous source of calcium diminishes and bone reabsorption occurs, patients may develop diminished ionized calcium stores. Calcium is critical to the function of the coagulation cascade. Lipid must also be provided for adequate platelet production of the necessary phospholipids. Although hypocalcemia and decreased phospholipid production play an insignificant clinical role in coagulopathy, they may certainly compound decreased hepatic synthesis of coagulation factors. Patients with severe liver disease may not adequately respond to vitamin K replacement and may respond only to FFP. Patients with severe viral hepatitis progressing to atrophy are monitored for the production of vitamin K-dependent factors by determination of the PT and $_a$PTT. These tests as well as factor assays are sensitive measures of hepatic synthetic abilities.

Acquired anticoagulants may be seen in collagen vascular disease, viral illness, chronic factor replacement, and idiopathic causes (13, 33). Factor VIII inhibitors usually occur in the setting of hemophilia A with prolonged factor replacement (104). However, occasionally during pregnancy, childhood, or in the elderly, inhibitors to factor VIII develop spontaneously. The anticoagulant may result in a severe bleeding event requiring intervention. The administration of greater than 75 U/kg/12 hours of factor VIII with corticosteroids (prednisone (60 to 100 mg)) plasmapheresis, or the use of activated procoagulant (IXa) may be necessary. Lupus anticoagulant represents an inhibitor to the phospholipid and is manifested by a prolonged $_a$PTT (5, 65). It occurs in children, the elderly, and in collagen vascular disease. It is associated with thrombotic events in the hospitalized patient and spontaneous abortion. Lupus anticoagulant production may decrease following the administration of corticosteroids (I recommend 30 mg prednisone daily). In healthy outpatients, lupus anticoagulant represents a laboratory phenomenon, and its clinical importance is still being defined. Endogenous inhibitors to factor IX may develop and are treated in a way similar to that of factor VIII inhibitor. In liver disease with decreased production of vitamin K-dependent factors, procoagulants induced by vitamin K absence (PIVKA) may form. PIVKA represent the K-dependent precursors that lack a second carboxyl moiety introduced on a glutamine residue. Hence, each vitamin K-dependent factor has its own PIVKA antecedent. Some of the PIVKAs inhibit the coagulation schema. Hypotension with a dysfunctional liver may result in PIVKA formation and precipitate a coagulopathy. Coumadin may also allow for the expression of PIVKA. As previously mentioned, fibrin degradation products also act as inhibitors to coagulation. Plasmin converts fibrinogen to fibrinopeptide fragments X, Y, D, and E. Fragments X and Y are extremely efficient inhibitors of fibrin polymerization. These fragments result in the prolongation of the PT, $_a$PTT, TT, and RT. The FDPs may also adversely affect platelet function.

The maintenance of hemostasis in the critically ill patient involves an extremely complex interaction between cellular components, proteins, and exogenous factors. Most cases of platelet disorders and coagulopathies in the ICU are multifactorial. They require an understanding of the physiologic aspects of hemostasis and appropriate intervention.

THROMBOSIS

In general, the endothelium is thromboresistant and normally nonreactive to platelets, coagulation factors, or the fibrinolytic system (99). However, in the ICU patient the endothelium may be damaged, resulting in decreased thromboresistance. The result may be a thrombotic event such as a superficial phlebitis or a massive pulmonary embolus. Patients in the ICU for a systemic disease may be predisposed to recurrent thrombotic events. These patients may be best managed by prophylactic measures to reduce the risk of thrombosis. Major thrombotic events are life-threatening and result in ICU admission. Arterial thrombosis can be induced by mechanical, toxic, or immune-mediated events. Small vessel thrombosis may be a platelet- and endothelium-mediated event. Disorders such as TTP, hemolytic uremic syndrome, malignant hypertension, and eclampsia are examples. Antiplatelet drugs such as aspirin, dipyridamole, or heparin have been used with some success in small vessel disease. Endotoxic shock can induce endothelial injury and subsequent microangiopathy in experimental models. Venous thrombosis was originally defined by Virchow. The etiology has not been altered since that time. Trauma and stasis remain the predominant causes of venous thrombotic events.

HYPERCOAGULABILITY

Hypercoagulability is an ill-defined state that lags behind bleeding disorders in clinical comprehension. This clinical state represents the predisposition of patients to thromboembolic phenomenon (46, 83). There are idiopathic, as well as defined, hypercoagulable disorders (Table 40.6). The best example of hypercoagulability is Antithrombin^{III} (AT^{III}) deficiency (98). This may be congenital or acquired. AT^{III} is the predominant circulating anticoagulant, inhibiting thrombin and controlling exuberant hemostasis. Patients with AT^{III} deficiency experience recurrent deep venous thrombosis and pulmonary emboli. It is inherited as an autosomal dominant disorder (86). The incidence in the general population may be as high as 1 in 2000. Thromboembolic events in AT^{III} deficiency are treated initially with heparin, followed by long-term oral anticoagulation. As expected, heparin resistance is seen in this deficiency state. To document AT^{III} deficiency, one must

Table 40.6. Hypercoagulable States

Congenital	Acquired
Antithrombin III deficiency	Malignancy
Protein C deficiency	Estrogens
Protein S deficiency	Activated procoagulant
Dysfibrinogenemia	complex
Factor XII deficiency?	Pregnancy
Dysplasminogenemia	Lupus anticoagulant
Low plasminogen	Nephrotic syndrome
Homocystinuria	Hepatic dysfibrinogenemia
Sickle cell disease	Vasculitis
	Diabetes mellitus
	Paroxysmal nocturnal
	hemoglobinuria
	Thrombotic
	thrombocytopenic
	purpura
	Venous stasis
	Myeloproliferative syndromes

measure AT^{III} levels. Patients with systemic diseases may acquire AT^{III} deficiency. Severe liver disease prevents the synthesis of AT^{III} and compounds dysfunction of platelets and deficiency of coagulation factors with low-grade DIC. Patients with the nephrotic syndrome may excrete large amounts of AT^{III} in the urine and are predisposed to renal vein occlusion and other thrombotic events (43).

Protein C deficiency is another cause of thromboembolism and dermal necrosis associated with coumadin use (12, 26). Protein C is a vitamin K-dependent factor converted to protein Ca (activated protein C) by the action of thrombin. Protein S, a protein CA cofactor, may also predispose to venous thrombosis when deficient. Protein CA is an anticoagulant that inactivates factors V$_a$ and VIII$_a$. Inactivation may not occur initially with warfarin sodium therapy. Protein C-deficient patients are treated with chronic warfarin sodium therapy. However, when initiating the warfarin sodium, serious skin necrosis involving the breast and the extremities may occur. Coumadin acutely lowers protein C levels commensurate with factor VII, prior to factors X, IX, and II. In suspected or documented cases of protein C deficiency it is recommended that lower starting doses of warfarin sodium (2.5 to 5 mg/day) be initiated.

Other causes of hypercoagulability include disorders in the fibrinolytic system. Dysfibrinogenemia in liver disease and the lupus anticoagulant may cause thromboses. Acquired hypercoagulable states are seen in malignancy (Trousseau's syndrome), pregnancy, estrogen usage, paroxysmal nocturnal hemoglobinuria, myeloproliferative syndromes, and diabetes mellitus (37). Many ICU patients may in fact have acquired hypercoagulability compounded by venous stasis and endothelial trauma. The key to proper management is to maintain vascular integrity. Other patients develop thromboembolic events without known hypercoagulability. These events include deep venous thrombosis, pulmonary emboli, and cerebrovascular and cardiovascular thromboembolic events.

PULMONARY EMBOLISM AND DEEP VENOUS THROMBOSIS

Pulmonary embolus is a serious life-threatening event in most patients (80); however, if diagnosed promptly and treated effectively, the outcome is favorable. It remains a leading undiagnosed acute illness. It is estimated that it is the third most common cause of death in the U.S. (more than 600,000 cases/year) and the incidence is increasing. The increased incidence relates to the increasing age of the population, increase in oral estrogen use, more extensive surgery, increase in malignancy, and increased awareness of the disorder. The difficulty in diagnosis correlates with the lack of pathognomonic physical findings, lab data, and noninvasive diagnostic parameters. More than 90% of pulmonary emboli arise from deep venous thrombosis (DVT) in the pelvis and thighs. Air, tumor, amniotic fluid and fat emboli are much less common.

Deep venous thrombosis (DVT) occurs in patients at prolonged bed rest. Patients with stasis due to congestive heart failure, recent myocardial infarction, immobilization, hypotension, and malignancy are at significant risk. Most patients with DVT are older than age 60. DVT in younger patients should lead one to consider AT^{III} deficiency. The incidence of DVT, as detected by ^{125}I-fibrinogen scanning, is 30% in myocardial infarction and as high as 50% in hip surgery. Surgery to the abdomen and thorax predisposes the patient to a high risk of DVT due to endothelial damage, stasis, and immobilization. Venous stasis is central to the development of DVT. If an inflammatory process ensues, the thrombosis may be clinically detected; however, in approximately 50% of cases DVT may be silent. The factors predisposing to embolization are unclear. The tests used to diagnose DVT are institution-dependent and include Doppler, plethysmography, ^{125}I-fibrinogen scanning, and venography (38, 39). Venography remains the definitive test. The clinical utility of the venogram decreases with previous episodes of DVT, and one must occasionally rely on clinical impression.

Pulmonary embolus is a serious complication of DVT. Most pulmonary emboli are multiple (85%). The embolus itself contains those materials previously discussed under "Hypercoagulability", such as platelets, fibrin, and thromboxane. Arterial blood gases are useful but not diagnostic. Patients who have pulmonary embolism may have a PAO$_2$ > 90 mm Hg (12 kPa), and patients with a PAO$_2$ < 80 mm Hg (10.7 kPa) may not have had an embolus. The alveolar-arterial O$_2$ gradient is a much more useful parameter. Ventilation-perfusion (V̇/Q̇) scans require strict interpretation to determine probability of an embolus. Pulmonary angiography remains the standard diagnostic test for pulmonary embolus (40). The patients undergoing a V̇/Q̇ scan are assigned a probability. This probability, as well as the clinical condition, dictate the need for angiography. With a normal V̇/Q̇ scan, the frequency of pulmonary embolus is extremely low. With multiple subsegmental defects and mismatch on V̇/Q̇, the odds of a pulmonary embolus are approximately 90%. The intermediate or indeterminate results require pulmonary angiograms. Angiography should be performed within 24 to 48 hours of a suspected embolus; otherwise, the activated fibrinolytic system may alter clot consistency and appearance. The angiogram should reveal luminal filling abnormalities or vessel cutoff. False-negative results are extremely rare at most centers.

The therapy of DVT or pulmonary embolus is well-established (27, 30, 31, 78). Prophylactic heparin may be given to high-risk patients. The prophylactic heparin dose is 5000 units every 8 to 12 hours. Therapeutic heparin is usually given as a 5000- to 10,000-U intravenous bolus followed by the continuous infusion of 1000 to 1200 U/hour. DVT or pulmonary embolus should be initially treated with heparin or a heparin derivative. The dose of heparin should be adjusted to maintain the $_a$PTT or the Lee-White clotting time at 1½ to 2 ½ times normal or 2 or 3 times normal, respectively. Bleeding occurs in 3 to 8% of patients receiving heparin, depending on the presence of other underlying disorders such as liver disease and malignancy. Elderly females are statistically at an increased risk for bleeding (25). Aspirin and other antiplatelet drugs are contraindicated. Platelet counts should be monitored at least ever 2 to 3 days while the patient is on heparin in order to detect heparin-associated thrombocytopenia. If the pulmonary embolus is acute and life-threatening, patients should also be given oxygen and dopamine for circulatory support, if necessary. If these measures are unsuccessful and a massive pulmonary embolus is suspected, fibrinolytic therapy or embolectomy are indicated. The pulmonary embolus should be confirmed by angiography prior to the use of streptokinase or urokinase therapy. Recent surgery, peptic ulcer, cerebrovascular accident, or history of hemorrhagic event are relative contraindictions to fibrinolytic therapy. Active bleeding is an absolute contraindication to this therapy. Arterial blood gas monitoring and other invasive techniques should be kept to a minimum. Tamponade must be maintained at all intravenous-access sites. Streptokinase is given as 250,000 IU over 30 minutes, followed by 100,000 IU/hr. This is continued for 24 to 72 hours. Most centers employ streptokinase for 24 to 48 hours, then initiate heparin. The agents are not administered simultaneously. Patients are usually discontinued from streptokinase for 3 to 4 hours prior to heparin initiation. The thrombin time (TT) and, occasionally, the FDP level are used to monitor streptokinase activity.

Thrombin time is maintained at two to three times normal, and heparin should not be instituted until the TT is less than two times normal. The use of streptokinase or urokinase requires clinical experience in thrombotic disorders. The clinical utility of streptokinase continues to increase. Coumarin derivatives are used after heparin therapy to prevent recurrent thromboembolic disease. Patients may be started on warfarin, once stable on heparin therapy. The coumarin derivatives require 2 to 7 days to adequately anticoagulate. The prothrombin time is maintained at 1½ to 2½ times normal (35). Warfarin is continued from 6 weeks to 6 months, depending on the severity of the thromboembolic process and underlying disease process. Patients with congenital or acquired hypercoagulable states may require lifelong warfarin therapy and require counseling on drug interactions. Low-dose heparin is not effective in preventing recurrent DVT.

If properly treated, DVT and pulmonary embolus have a favorable outcome (36). Patients with prior thromboembolic disease are predisposed to recurrence and should be counseled regarding prophylactic measures. These patients should avoid immobilization, avoid crossing the legs, and employ elastic compression stockings. The same measures may be carried out in patients with prolonged ICU stays, adding passive leg exercise.

RENAL VEIN THROMBOSIS

Renal vein thrombosis may be unilateral or bilateral. It may be associated with nephrotic syndrome, paroxysmal nocturnal hemoglobinuria, malignancy, or congestive heart failure. Oliguria and renal failure may result from bilateral thromboses, necessitating dialysis. The treatment may require thombectomy, if there is no improvement with conventional anticoagulants. Heparin resistance may be present because of low AT^{III} levels. Higher doses of heparin may be required to reach the therapeutic range of the $_aPTT$.

MYOCARDIAL INFARCTION

Recent studies in the field of myocardial infarction have led to the conclusion that coronary artery thrombosis is critical to the development of ischemic events. The known risk factors to coronary artery disease (e.g., smoking, hyperlipidemia, obesity, and diabetes mellitus) may alter platelet function and the fibrinolytic system (18, 23). The major physiologic activator of fibrinolysis is tissue plasminogen activator (TPA). Recent data suggest that reduced levels of TPA may be due to a circulating inhibitor. Pharmacologic manipulation of TPA may alter the outcome of myocardial infarction patients. Coronary angioscopy has documented that unstable angina may be related to thrombi in association with atheromatous plaques refractory to medical management (89). This pathophysiologic information has led to the use of anticoagulants, antiplatelet agents, and fibrinolytic therapy in patients with myocardial disease. However, studies have been slow to document significant survival advantage of such therapeutic intervention.

The use of anticoagulants to alter the course of myocardial ischemia is not recommended. An exception is crescendo angina. In this disorder, therapeutic heparin may be beneficial (92). For large infarctions the risk of pericardial bleeding with tamponade has been a concern, although this risk is not as common as might be expected. The presence of a pericardial rub is considered to be a contraindiction to the use of heparin. Heparin has been recommended on a prophylactic basis at low dose (5000 U every 8 to 12 hours) for patients felt to be at risk for DVT or pulmonary embolus. Patients with congestive heart failure, marked peripheral edema, and those confined to bed are at particular risk. Patients with chronic atrial fibrillation, ventricular aneurysms, and massive cardiomegaly may present on coumadin because of a history of recurrent thromboembolic disease. The drug is usually maintained during the early infarction period, avoiding the higher therapeutic range. It is critical to keep in mind the cardiac medications that alter coumadin action or binding. The role of coumadin and heparin in reducing infarct size or affecting overall survival remains unanswered despite a number of trials.

There is widespread use of aspirin, dipyridamole, sulfinpyrazone, and other antiplatelet drugs in clinical practice despite conflicting evidence showing benefit. Studies have revealed a trend toward benefit in reducing the incidence of reinfarction with these agents. However, the use of these antiplatelet drugs is generally not recommended in this setting. Doses of aspirin used in some trials have been those that would reduce both platelet TXA_2 and endothelial prostacyclin levels. Proper dosage and scheduling of aspirin remain to be established. Experimental data in animal models would suggest that coronary artery thrombosis and atherogenesis may be altered by the use of antiplatelet drugs or fish oils. Recent data suggest that platelet inhibition of prostaglandin synthesis

may require continued blood levels of aspirin and that a slow-release formulation may be more appropriate. The patients found most likely to benefit from low-dose (300-mg) aspirin are those with recurrent bouts of unstable angina. Postmortem studies of these patients have shown fresh thrombi in association with atheromata.

Thrombolytic therapy in myocardial infarction has become routine in critical care patients. Coronary angiography during early infarction or unstable angina reveals thrombi in the coronary arteries. In laboratory animals, fibrinolytic therapy has resulted in reperfusion and reduction in infarct size. In human trials, intracoronary perfusion with streptokinase has resulted in increased patency of obstructed coronary arteries (67). However, improvement in survival and left ventricular function as a result of thrombolytic therapy have not been demonstrated. Because of the difficulty of intracoronary streptokinase, the intravenous route has been advocated (84). Some early trials have not shown benefit from thrombolytic therapy, perhaps because of the delays in the initiation of streptokinase. If streptokinase is administered early in myocardial infarction (within hours), progressive ischemic damage may be avoided. However, bleeding of a severe nature may occur. Routine use of streptokinase in myocardial infarction awaits confirmation by larger definitive trials. Compared with intravenous streptokinase, newer formulations such as acylated streptokinase, plasminogen activator, or tissue plasminogen activator may prove to be of benefit with a lower incidence of complications.

CEREBROVASCULAR THROMBOEMBOLIC DISEASE

The mechanisms described for coronary vasospasm, ischemia, and thrombosis are similar in the cerebral circulation (69). Cerebrovascular accidents may be thrombotic or hemorrhagic. In the event of a cerebrovascular accident, an emergent computer tomography scan with contrast is generally performed. If this scan is indicative of thrombosis, lumbar puncture does not reveal frank blood or xanthochromia; the patient does not have marked meningeal findings; and neurologic examination is progressive, a trial of heparin is usually indicated. Heparin is used intravenously at conventional therapeutic doses. Subsequent cerebral angiography may detect a surgically amenable lesion. The role of the fibrinolytic system in cerebral vessels is less well-defined than in coronary vessels, and the role of thrombolytic therapy is not defined. The use of antiplatelet drugs has not been of therapeutic benefit in the management of thrombotic stroke.

Transient ischemic attacks (TIA) result from atheromatous material or small emboli dislodging from major vessels in the neck and lodging in the brain. Antiplatelet drugs are used in the management of TIAs. Their use relates to the shift in the thromboxane A2/prostacylin balance in favor of diminished thrombosis and atherogenesis. In a large trial of aspirin and sulfinpyrazone (200 mg four times/day), it was concluded that aspirin (325 mg four times/day) significantly reduced the incidence of stroke in men with a history of cerebral or retinal ischemic attacks. The same study revealed a decreased incidence of coronary death. Other trials have shown benefit to both sexes and no added benefit from dipyridamole (100 to 200 mg four times/day). Some investigators feel that women may benefit as well as men from the use of aspirin. Trials on low-dose vs. high-dose aspirin are pending. There is currently a trend to use low-dose aspirin, because conceptually bleeding and gastric irritation may be less. Low-dose aspirin may not impair prostacyclin production.

Hemorrhagic stroke implies different pathologic events than thrombotic processes. In this setting, a cerebral bleed has recurred and will progress unless adequate hemostasis occurs. The diagnosis may be confirmed by an early CT scan of the head and lumbar puncture. Altered hemostatic integrity may be detected by studying the platelet count, PT, and $_a$PTT. A drug history should be obtained to rule out drugs that may compromise hemostasis. Drugs that promote bleeding are absolutely contraindicated in the treatment of hemorrhagic stroke. Rebleeding is a frequent complication of hemorrhagic stroke and theoretically may be prevented with antifibrinolytic therapy. The antifibrinolytic agent available for stabilizing cerebral clot is ε-aminocaproic acid (EACA). This drug can reduce the incidence of rebleeding and may improve overall survival in hemorrhagic stroke. However, the routine use of EACA in stroke remains controversial. Other trials have concluded that antifibrinolytic therapy does not alter the outcome of subarachnoid hemorrhage. One of the problems in proving efficacy of antifibrinolytic therapy is the inability to monitor EACA therapy. One proposed method is cerebrospinal fluid FDP levels, but this method may be tedious (82). When EACA is used, a loading dose of 5 g is given and followed by a continuous intravenous infusion at 2 g/hr. Complications include thrombosis and cerebral rebleeding.

PHARMACOLOGY OF DRUGS AFFECTING HEMOSTASIS AND THROMBOSIS

Anticoagulants have been in clinical use for over 40 years in the management of thromboses. Numerous trials have documented their efficacy. More recent studies have attempted to reduce complications and maintain therapeutic effect. The utility of anticoagulants is established for the treatment of systemic thromboembolic disease, prosthetic cardiac valves, mitral valve disease, and atrial fibrillation (51). There are other areas in which the benefit needs to be documented. Although doses are not totally agreed upon, a table of accepted doses is included (Table 40.7).

HEPARIN AND HEPARIN-LIKE SUBSTANCES

Heparin prolongs clotting in vivo or in vitro. Knowledge of the action of heparin remains incomplete because of its heterogeneous nature (20). Heparin is a naturally occurring mucoitin polysulfuric acid consisting of equal amounts of hexuronic acid and acetylated glycosamine with sulfuric acid ester groups. The heterogeneous molecule has a significant electronegative charge. Naturally occurring heparin is stored within mast cells. The exact role of endogenous heparin is unclear, but it is thought to affect platelet function and coagulation factors. Isoelectric focusing of heparin has detected 21 components. These components differ in their affinity for AT^{III} and PF 4. The anticoagulant effect of heparin results from the cumulative effect of these components. Recently, attempts have been made to separate these components, resulting in

a more specific mode of action with decreased complications. Further description of these derivatives follows.

The commercial source of heparin is the lungs or intestinal mucosa of domestic animals. The heparins obtained in this fashion have different potency and must be standardized. The biologic effect is analyzed by comparing the activity of the preparation with a USP reference standard. The standard heparin is used to prevent clotting of citrated sheep plasma to which calcium has been added. The USP guidelines state that sodium heparin must contain no less than 120 USP units/mg but allows the manufacturer a 10% margin of error. The heparin available in the U.S. is labeled with activity in units and weight of heparin. In clinical use, 1 unit of heparin activity is equivalent to 0.01 mg of sodium heparin. The USP-standard heparin sodium injection may contain an antimicrobial agent and materials to prevent absorption. The most common preparation is 10,000 U (100 mg) in 10 ml water; more concentrated solutions are available.

Heparin is an ineffective anticoagulant via the oral or rectal route; it must be given parenterally. Intramuscular injections are painful and should be avoided. Heparin is usually given intravenously or subcutaneously. Depot injections have been given, but absorption is erratic and clinically unreliable. Following intravenous administration, 20 to 25% of the dose is recovered active in the urine. Radiolabeled heparin has revealed uptake of heparin within mast cells and subsequent storage. The heparin may bind to plasma proteins or may be degraded in the liver.

Heparin inhibits blood coagulation by a number of mechanisms (7). The predominant effect at therapeutic levels is to act in conjunction with AT^{III} as an inhibitor of activated coagulation factors. AT^{III} inhibits factors XII$_a$, XI$_a$, IX$_a$, X$_a$, and II$_a$ at a serine residue. AT^{III} in combination with the serine residue irreversibly undergoes esterification at an arginyl site. The binding site on AT^{III} for heparin is in a lysine residue. Heparin promotes a conformational change allowing for enhanced binding to activated factors, in particular XII$_a$, X$_a$, and thrombin. Factors XI$_a$ and IX$_a$ are relatively insensitive to the heparin-AT^{III} complex. A second cofactor, heparin cofactor II, may also act like an antithrombin (93). Heparinoids may act via heparin cofactor II. Heparin also inhibits the activation of prothrombin by X$_a$. Heparin affects platelet aggregation in a nonspecific manner and heparin-induced bleeding may be on the basis of altered platelet function (57). Low-molecular-weight heparin (enoxaparin) has a high affinity for AT^{III} compared with high molecular weight fractions (34).

Low molecular weight heparins are as effective as unfractionated standard heparin in preventing deep venous thrombosis in animal models. In one trial, patients were given 30 mg enoxaparin subcutaneously twice per day as compared with placebo administration. This therapy was effective in preventing DVT in patients undergoing elective hip surgery and resulted in few complications. Enoxaparin may have less antiplatelet effect and hence less bleeding complications.

Heparin can be used in either a prophylactic regimen or the therapy of DVT or pulmonary embolus (32). Low-dose subcutaneous heparin is usually given in a dose of 5000 U 2 hours preoperatively, then 5000 U every 8 to 12 hours postoperatively for the period of decreased ambulation. This method is extremely effective in preventing calf and proximal

Table 40.7. Dosage and Route of Administration of Anticoagulants, Antiplatelet Drugs, and Related Compounds

Drug	Route	Loading Dose	Maintenance Dose	Test Monitored
Heparin	i.v.	5000–10,000 USP U i.v.	1000–1200 USP U/hr by continuous infusion	$_A$PTT
	s.c.		5000 USP U every 8–12 hours	$_A$PTT
Protamine	i.v.	1 mg/100 U of heparin[a]		
Streptokinase	i.v.	250,000 U over 30 min	100,000 U/hr for 24–48 hours[b]	TT, FDP, $_A$PTT
Urokinase	i.v.	4400 U/kg	4400 U/kg/hr	TT, FDP, $_A$PTT
ε-Aminocapriotic acid (Amicar)	i.v.	4–5 g	1 g/hr i.v.	Clinical response
	p.o.	5 g	1 g/hr	
Warfarin	p.o.	5–10 mg/day	2–5 mg/day	PT
Aspirin	p.o.		15–1300 mg/day	
Dipyridamole	p.o.		200–400 mg/day	

[a] Calculated based on $t_{1/2}$ and dose of heparin given.
[b] Follow by therapeutic heparin when streptokinase or urokinase has been discontinued for 3 hr.

vein thromboses; hence, pulmonary emboli are decreased in incidence. Prophylactic low-dose heparin is the treatment of choice in most high-risk surgical and medical patients. This group of patients includes those with prolonged bed rest, congestive heart failure, and general surgery patients. In extremely high-risk patients, such as those undergoing hip surgery and amputations, a higher dose may be required. Recently, low molecular weight heparin was shown in a randomized trial to prevent DVT in hip surgery and to be more effective than placebo (with fewer complications) (94). The risk of bleeding with low molecular weight heparin is considered low. Prophylactic low-dose heparin in conjunction with dihydroergotamine (Embolex) was found to be effective as well, but a consensus has not been reached regarding its use (0.5 mg dihydroergotamine/5000 U heparin intravenous 2 hours preoperatively, then every 12 hours for 5 days). The presence of platelet dysfunction, primary coagulopathy, or a neurosurgical procedure are contraindications to low-dose heparin. Most patients on low-dose heparin are not monitored with laboratory tests. However, in patients undergoing elective hip surgery, if the $_A$PTT is maintained between 31.5 and 36 seconds with heparin therapy for 8 days postoperatively, the incidence of DVT and bleeding is statistically reduced. The final recommendations regarding high-risk patients await larger trials.

For patients with DVT or pulmonary embolus, treatment with heparin is routine. Untreated pulmonary embolus has a mortality rate approaching 25%. Thromboembolism is treated with a constant infusion of intravenous heparin. Patients are given an intravenous bolus of heparin 5000 to 10,000 USP units followed by a continuous infusion of 1000 to 1200 U/hr (20,000 U of heparin in 500 ml of ⅔ dextrose, ⅓ saline at 30 ml/hr). The dose is adjusted in an attempt to reach an endpoint of 1½ to 2½ times the $_A$PTT control. Heparin is usually administered for 7 to 10 days. Oral anticoagulants are begun on day 4 or 5 from the start of heparin. The therapy of heparin and warfarin should overlap by 4 to 5 days. This dual therapy potentially counteracts the thrombotic potential of inducing protein C deficiency.

The complications of heparin therapy are often overstated and perhaps have led to decreased usage. Heparin-induced bleeding usually occurs at large heparin doses and may be life-threatening. The risk of heparin-induced hemorrhage is from 1 to 33%. Prophylactic low-dose heparin has a very low rate of bleeding complications in most patients. Heparin-induced bleeding can be reversed with protamine sulfate. Protamines are low molecular weight proteins containing large amounts of arginine. These compounds are strongly basic and are derived from fish. Protamine functions as an anticoagulant but is not as potent as heparin. Five milliliter vials of protamine contain 50 mg/vial of the basic protein. Protamine sulfate is given intravenously and forms a stable salt with heparin, which inactivates the conformational change of AT^{III}. This effect occurs within 5 minutes of administration. Patients may develop a hypersensitivity reaction; the role of fish allergy has not been defined. The appropriate dose of protamine depends on the heparin dose administered. To reverse recent heparin administration, an intravenous dose of 1 mg of protamine for every 100 USP U of heparin is given slowly over 10 minutes to prevent hypotension. Heparin has a plasma half-life of 60 minutes, and 50 mg (maximum dose, may be repeated based on normalization of the $_A$PTT) of protamine reverses 15,000 U of heparin.

If 30 minutes have elapsed since administration of heparin, 25 mg of protamine may be given; if 60 minutes have elapsed, then 12.5 mg of protamine sulfate is given. One attempts to err on a lower dose of protamine to avoid overdosing and exacerbating bleeding. The dose of protamine may need to be repeated as heparin may dissociate from the salt complex. The $_A$PTT may be monitored to determine decreasing heparin effect. Another complication of heparin therapy is thrombocytopenia (45, 88). This adverse reaction is an idiosyncratic reaction and the frequency of this drug-induced problem is less than 6%. The likelihood of heparin-induced thrombocytopenia is independent of the route of administration; however, the source of heparin does affect the frequency of this problem. Thrombocytopenia is seen more frequently with bovine lung than porcine intestinal mucosa heparin (1). Thrombocytopenia generally occurs 6 to 12 days after initiation of heparin therapy but may occur throughout the course of therapy. Platelet-associated immunoglobulin has been implicated as the cause of heparin-related thrombocytopenia; however, the immunoglobulin is not a universal finding (57). Heparin-associated thrombocytopenia is thought to be immune-mediated. Occasionally, patients may also develop thrombotic complications (11). Patients with heparin-induced thrombocytopenia should avoid a similar heparin source if retreatment is required (44). Patients are begun on oral anticoagulants, and heparin is stopped as soon as possible. Platelet counts are carefully monitored during this period.

Heparin is rarely associated with an anaphylactic reaction (53). Patients with a history of hypersensitivity should be given a test dose. Patients with hypersensitivity or heparin-induced thrombocytopenia may be considered for low molecular weight heparin. Theoretically, the antigenic stimulus is not a component of this formulation. Osteoporosis is a rare complication of heparin therapy. This complication occurs in women who are treated with 20,000 U/day for more than 6 months. Heparin also has an antichylomicronemic action, the significance of which is unknown This action is being studied with regard to the development of atherosclerotic lesions.

Heparin has been a critical therapeutic tool for many years and will remain so. Continued research into its mode of action, clinical utility, components, and complications is imperative.

ORAL ANTICOAGULANTS

The first oral anticoagulants were synthesized approximately 40 years ago. The first compound was bishydroxycoumarin. Other derivatives have since been synthesized, including sodium warfarin (Coumadin). These compounds are similar in structure to vitamin K. Sodium warfarin is the only product currently used because of its reliable pharmacokinetics. The half-life of warfarin is about 35 hours. The metabolism and excretion rates vary among individuals. Many systemic disorders and drugs alter the absorption, metabolism, excretion, and plasma binding of warfarin (Table 40.8). Approximately 99% of warfarin is bound to plasma albumin. Only the free warfarin is biologically active. Hence, drugs that alter warfarin binding affect free warfarin and its biologic action.

These vitamin K antagonists inhibit the effect of vitamin K on posttranslational liver synthesis of factors II, VII, IX, and X; protein C; and protein S. This inhibition results in the

Table 40.8.   Drugs or Disease States That Affect Warfarin Action

Potentiation

Drugs
  Androgens, chloral hydrate, chloramphenicol, clofibrate, glucagon, indomethacin, neomycin, acetaminophen, allopurinol, diazoxide, disulfiram, ethacrynic acid, heparin, 6-mercaptopurine, α-methyldopa, monoamine oxidase inhibitors, nalifixic acid, sulfinpyrazone, thyroid drugs, tolbutamide, sulfa drugs, phenylbutazone, phenytoin, quinidine, salicylates, thyroxine, alcohol, anesthetics, metronidazole, cimetidine
Disease states
  Collagen vascular disorders, congestive heart failure, hepatitis, hyperthyroidism, vitamin K deficient diet, malignancy, malabsorption, narcotic abuse

Inhibition

Drugs
  Barbiturates, glutethimide, griseofulvin, haloperidol, corticosteroids, estrogens, meprobamate, colchicine, rifampin, tetracyclines, carbamazepine, alcohol, cholestyramine.
Disease states
  Hereditary resistance to coumadin, hypothyroidism.

formation of inactive compounds referred to previously as PIVKA. Vitamin K promotes carboxylation of factors II, VII, IX, and X; protein C; and protein S to the active procoagulant or anticoagulant. The activated factors have reactive sites for calcium and phospholipid. The vitamin K antagonists inhibit the cyclic conversion of vitamin K and its 2,3 epoxide. This action results in increased amounts of the vitamin K epoxide, as compared to vitamin K amounts. The nonepoxide is necessary for activation of vitamin K-dependent factors.

Protein C is converted to its active form by the action of thrombin. Protein C binds to thrombomodulin on the endothelium, markedly increasing its conversion by thrombin to active protein C_a. Protein C_a inhibits factors V_a and VIII_a. The thrombin bound to thrombomodulin is rendered ineffective in further activating factors V and VIII. This functions as an important anticoagulant system. This system is affected by the action of warfarin. Hence, thrombotic potential exists if the anticoagulant protein C is not synthesized. The anticoagulant effect of warfarin is first seen at 24 hours by suppression of factor VII. However, it is not until 96 hours when factors II, IX, and X are inhibited that maximal effect is seen. Protein C activity is also reduced concomitantly with factor VII. This fact has clinical importance in patients with underlying protein C deficiency (105). After warfarin has been initiated the prothrombin time begins to prolong at 24 hours because of loss of factor VII activity. Because of the risks of rapidly reducing protein C, smaller starting doses are recommended. Warfarin is begun with a 4- to 5-day overlap with heparin therapy for deep venous thrombosis or pulmonary embolus. This overlap prevents the thrombogenic risk of reducing protein C_a acutely.

Vitamin K antagonists are monitored with the prothrombin time (19). In general, the doses of vitamin K antagonists are adjusted to maintain the PT at $1\frac{1}{2}$ to $2\frac{1}{2}$ times that of the control. However, the effect of these agents on the PT is still being studied. The source of tissue thromboplastin may alter the relationship of PT to control values. The controls used to adjust the warfarin sodium dose may differ, depending on the source of tissue thromboplastin. One must inquire as to the methods of standardizing the control values.

The use of oral anticoagulants in unstable angina has not been established in well-designed studies. In patients with cerebrovascular disease there is evidence that suggests that oral anticoagulants may be of benefit in progressive thrombotic stroke. In patients with cardiac disease (congestive heart failure, cardiomyopathy) anticoagulant therapy can prevent reembolization to the cerebral circulation. Patients with mitral valve disease with resultant or chronic atrial fibrillation clearly benefit from long-term anticoagulation. Patients with prosthetic valves in the mitral position are at high risk of embolization; aspirin alone in these patients is not of benefit. Combining warfarin with antiplatelet drugs in these patients decreases embolization, compared with warfarin alone; however, when warfarin and aspirin are combined, bleeding episodes are increased. Clearly, a safer prophylactic measure is necessary. One should avoid the combination of warfarin sodium and aspirin since the plasma kinetics of warfarin sodium are altered by aspirin.

Persantine does not have a similar effect. Hence, patients who experience embolization while on Coumadin may benefit from the addition of dipyridamole.

The complications of oral anticoagulant therapy, particularly bleeding, can be life-threatening. Clinicians must be aware of the numerous drug interactions. The bleeding complications relate to the dosage of the oral anticoagulants, the underlying systemic disease, particularly hepatic dysfunction, and other factors, such as trauma, surgery, and drugs. Minor bleeding occurs in 18% of patients in large anticoagulation clinics; major bleeding occurs in less than 5% of patients. Minor bleeding is predominantly from mucous membranes and includes epistaxis and gingival bleeding. When evaluating patients with bleeding as a result of receiving sodium warfarin, one promptly orders a PT, ₐPTT, and a platelet count. If PT is in the therapeutic range, another cause of bleeding should be sought. Bleeding due to Coumadin is managed with vitamin K, as well as by the administration of FFP. Occasionally, one encounters patients who have inadvertently or purposefully ingested Coumadin. Coumadin and PIVKA levels may be used for documentation of occult usage; the activity of factors II, VII, IX, and X may also be measured.

In Coumadin overdose, if the PT and ₐPTT are markedly prolonged and bleeding is uncontrolled, prompt administration of FFP is indicated. Vitamin K can be given intravenously slowly at a dose of 10 to 25 mg (rate no faster than 1 mg/min). The response of the PT is used to determine the frequency of subsequent doses of vitamin K. The preferred route of administration of vitamin K is subcutaneous or intramuscular; however, with a markedly prolonged PT this route of administration may be contraindicated. Intravenously administered vitamin K has resulted in anaphylaxis, and anaphylaxis precautions (epinephrine, antihistamines, steroids at the bedside) are necessary, even with slow administration. The PT is affected within 1 to 2 hours of vitamin K administration.

If the PT is only marginally outside the therapeutic range (two to three times) and no bleeding is present, Coumadin is discontinued and the patient observed. If the PT is further prolonged, 2.5 to 5 mg of vitamin K may be given. If the bleeding occurs in the setting of acute DVT and further use of Coumadin is contraindicated, subcutaneous heparin for the duration of therapy (3 to 6 months) is indicated.

Numerous drugs alter the pharmacokinetics of warfarin (Table 40.8). These drug alterations result in varying levels of vitamin K-dependent factors. The production of these vitamin K-dependent factors directly relates to the plasma level of free warfarin. The plasma level of warfarin may be dependent on the rate of biotransformation or the binding of warfarin to plasma proteins. The liver microsomal enzyme system inactivates the coumarin derivative. A drug that increases activity of this system biodegrades warfarin at an increased rate. This biodegradation necessitates increasing the warfarin dose in order to maintain the anticoagulant effect. If this class of drug is stopped suddenly, warfarin levels markedly increase, and hemorrhagic complications may ensue. Drugs that induce activation of the liver microsomal enzyme system include phenobarbital, chloral hydrate, haloperidol, and griseofulvin. These drugs decrease the plasma warfarin level. Some drugs may inhibit the microsomal enzyme system and increase warfarin levels. Warfarin promptly binds to plasma proteins upon administration. Salicylates, diphenylhydantoin, and phenylbutazone displace warfarin from plasma proteins and increase free warfarin levels. Certain antibiotics, such as chloramphenicol and neomycin, interfere with the synthesis of vitamin K by inhibiting bacterial intestinal flora and may potentiate the warfarin effect. Warfarin responsiveness is increased with anabolic steroids and thyroxine.

Certain disease states may also alter warfarin action. Thyrotoxicosis enhances the mode of action of warfarin, predisposing to bleeding. Congestive heart failure prolongs the warfarin half-life. Neoplastic diseases may be associated with decreased production of vitamin K-dependent factors. Acute viral hepatitis is associated with a hypoprothrombinemic state, if hepatic dysfunction is significant. Warfarin compounds the reduced levels of factors II, VII, IX, and X in these patients. Patients on vitamin K-deficient diets may be more susceptible to a warfarin effect.

An important clinical entity seen with Coumadin therapy is dermal necrosis (59, 61). Coumadin causes other dermatological reactions as well. Bleeding into the skin with ecchymoses and purpura are commonly seen. Urticaria, macules, and papules are seen in patients allergic to Coumadin. Dermal skin necrosis is a very rare, severe complication of warfarin therapy that occurs about 1 week after therapy has begun. Dermal necrosis begins as macules and papules and progresses to hemorrhagic bulli and, finally, skin sloughing occurs. The lesions are seen in areas of adipose tissue, (e.g., breasts, buttocks and thighs). The histopathology reveals dermal vein fibrin deposition. Some of the cases have been associated with protein C deficiency. Treatment consists of warfarin withdrawal, prompt heparin therapy, and local skin care. The syndrome of Coumadin dermal necrosis has proved to be fatal in some patients.

ANTIPLATELET DRUGS

The action of platelets and endothelium in maintaining hemostasis has been described (68, 101, 102). Salicylates were first used therapeutically in 1763. Aspirin-induced prolongation of bleeding was first noted in 1954. This observation has been subsequently confirmed, and the use of aspirin to alter hemostasis has become commonplace. The predominant effect of aspirin is the acetylation of cyclooxygenase and subsequent inhibition of TXA_2 synthesis. Nonsteroidal antiinflammatory drugs act by a similar mechanism. Eicosatrienoic acid has recently been introduced to alter platelet function and reduce atherogenesis. Eicosatrienoic acid causes platelets to produce thromboxane A_2, an ineffective aggregating compound, and endothelium to produce prostaglandin I_3, a potent antiaggregating agent. Dipyridamole is a coronary vasodilator that is found to alter platelet function; the mode of action is still unclear. Dipyridamole inhibits adhesion of platelets to the subendothelium. The mechanism has been attributed to increased platelet cyclic AMP. Aspirin synergistically acts with dipyridamole to prevent platelet aggregation. Xanthines, such as theophylline, inhibit platelet phosphodiesterase and increase platelet cyclic AMP.

Antibiotics such as penicillin, carbenicillin, and ticarcillin inhibit platelet responsiveness by coating platelets and blocking binding sites on which aggregating substances act. These drugs also interfere with the release reaction. This phenomenon may have clinical importance in the critically ill patient with uncontrolled bleeding. Propranolol and other β-blockers inhibit second-wave aggregation by ADP and epinephrine. Propranolol also effects platelet clot retraction. Clofibrate, used in the treatment of hyperlipidemia, can inhibit aggregation to epinephrine and ADP. Other drugs known to inhibit platelet function include corticosteroids, furosemide, cyproheptadine, hydroxychloroquine, and heparin.

THROMBOLYTIC THERAPY

Streptokinase and urokinase activate the fibrinolytic system by complexing with plasminogen and forming plasmin (17, 81). Streptokinase is the most widely employed plasminogen activator, probably because of cost. Urokinase is isolated from human urine, is costly, and has a shorter half-life.

The action of streptokinase varies in individual patients. However, its utility in patients with pulmonary embolus, deep venous thrombosis (DVT), and early myocardial infarction is unquestioned. Patients treated for DVT with streptokinase have rapid clot resolution and increased reversal of altered hemodynamics in response to pulmonary embolus, when compared with heparin. Thrombolytic therapy can also clear microthrombi from the pulmonary circulation. Thrombolytic therapy may, in the case of DVT, preserve venous valvular function. The National Institutes of Health have strongly endorsed the use of streptokinase for treatment of thromboembolic disease. Streptokinase has been advocated for *early* treatment of pulmonary emboli, as well as for proximal deep vein thrombosis. The diagnosis of thromboembolic disease should be confirmed by venogram or pulmonary angiogram. For thrombolytic therapy to be considered, the duration of thromboembolic disease should be less than 1 week, since clot organization has begun by this time. The action of streptokinase on organized clot is limited.

Contraindications to streptokinase use include active bleeding, a cerebrovascular accident, or surgery less than 2 months prior to therapy. Other traumatic events, such as organ biopsy, pregnancy, and pericardiocentesis, are relative contraindications. Invasive techniques should be avoided while the patient is receiving streptokinase. For each patient considered for streptokinase, a risk-vs.-benefit algorithm should be established.

Streptokinase is prepared from group C streptococci; hence, allergic reactions may occur due to development of neutralizing antibodies. The molecular weight of streptokinase is 47,000 and the half-life is approximately 10 to 12 minutes. Streptokinase is prepared in sodium chloride or dextrose and should be stored at 2 to 4° C if not used immediately.

Patients are given 250,000 U of intravenous streptokinase over 30 minutes, then begun on 100,000 U/hr continuous infusion for 24 to 72 hrs. If patients have had a recent streptococcal infection, higher doses may be needed to overcome blocking antibodies. However, more than 90% of patients respond to the loading dose. Should inadequate response to streptokinase be noted, urokinase may be used. Urokinase (4400 U/kg) is given intravenously over 10 minutes followed by 4400 U/kg/hr for 24 hours. Laboratory monitoring is used to ensure that systemic fibrinolysis is occurring. If the systemic clots are less than 7 days old, prompt lysis should be seen and improvement detected by impedance plethysmography,

or pulmonary hemodynamics. It is important to document lysis because if patients are refractory to fibrinolytic therapy, reembolization may occur. Monitoring the thrombin time, euglobulin clot lysis, fibrinogen, and FDPs have all been employed. Prolongation of the PT and ₐPTT also reflect the presence of plasmin-generated FPDs. If no evidence of fibrinolysis is detected, streptokinase should be discontinued and heparin begun promptly. Heparin is not begun simultaneously with thrombolytic therapy because of the increased risk of bleeding. When the TT is less than two times the normal level, heparin is begun at conventional continuous infusion doses (1000 to 1200 U/hr). Treatment with heparin is continued for 7 to 10 days and overlapped for 4 to 5 days with warfarin.

While the patient is receiving streptokinase, it is best to avoid antiplatelet drugs, invasive techniques, intramuscular injections, or physical handling. Bleeding is the major complication of thrombolytic therapy. In one series, only 4% of patients required transfusion, and there were no fatalities from bleeding. In order to prevent bleeding complications, one gives attention to meticulously avoiding trauma. Minor bleeding can be managed with an ε-aminocaproic acid-soaked pledget and compression. If major bleeding does occur, thrombolytic therapy should be stopped. Because of the short half-lives of thrombolytics, this approach is usually successful. If transfusion is needed, packed RBCs with the use of cryoprecipitate or FFP may be in order. In episodes of severe bleeding, an oral dose of ε-aminocaproic acid has been given in 5-g courses every 4 to 6 hours, or 1 to 2 g/hr by continuous infusion after a loading dose of 5 g.

Febrile reactions occur in 20% of patients receiving streptokinase; skin allergic reactions are reported in 5% of patients. Febrile reactions are managed with acetaminophen. Allergic phenomenon can be treated with corticosteroids and antihistamines. Repeat therapy with thrombolytic therapy is usually avoided for 6 months.

Streptokinase has been administered intravenously to patients with early myocardial infarction (within 3 hours). Patients were given 750,000 U of streptokinase over 30 minutes, followed by heparin infusion and oral nitrates. Long-term anticoagulation was maintained with oral anticoagulants. Given in this manner, severe bleeding occurred in only 2 of 53 patients. Reduction in the infarct size and subsequent myocardial preservation were documented. Further randomized trials are indicated to determine effects on long-term survival.

PHARMACOLOGIC AGENTS EMPLOYED TO ENHANCE HEMOSTASIS

Antifibrinolytic therapy is currently available in the form of ε-aminocaproic acid (56), which is used clinically to counteract excessive fibrinolysis. ε-Aminocaproic acid (EACA) is a synthetic monoaminocarboxylic acid with properties similar to those of lysine, is readily absorbed from the gastrointestinal tract, and is water-soluble. EACA promptly distributes to the intravascular and extravascular spaces. Peak circulating EACA levels are seen within 2 hours of oral administration, and excretion is mainly via the kidneys. Greater than 50% is cleared in 24 hours, and 1 g of EACA inhibits the activation of plasminogen to plasmin. EACA competitively inhibits plasminogen conversion by its effect on the arginine-lysine moiety. EACA at high dose also exerts an antiplasmin effect. EACA can be employed in cases of primary fibrinolysis, altered hemostasis following cardiac surgery, amegakaryocytic thrombocytopenia, and after prostatic surgery. EACA has also been used to decrease factor requirements in hemophiliacs undergoing surgical or dental procedures. EACA should not be administered in the presence of active disseminated intravascular coagulation. Adverse reactions to EACA include myopathy (rarely rhabdomyolysis) and thrombosis, particularly in the setting of consumptive coagulopathy.

Thrombin is available only for topical use. It is used when a surgical wound continues to ooze, and ligation or pressure is unsuccessful. Allergic reactions to thrombin have been reported. Thrombin may be used in conjunction with a gelatin sponge. Sclerosing agents such as sodium tetradecyl sulfate have been employed for bleeding esophageal varices. Upon injection, this compound acts by irritating the endothelium and causing prompt thrombus formation. The risk of extensive thrombosis exists and requires use by experienced gastroenterologists.

In summary, hemorrhage and thrombosis are frequent complications in the ICU setting. These events require knowledge of the pathophysiology in order to elect proper therapeutic management. The hematologist may be of assistance to the critical care team in this regard.

REFERENCES

1. Bell WR, Royall RM: Heparin-associated thrombocytopenia: a comparison of three heparin preparations. *N Engl J Med* 303:902–907, 1980.
2. Bick RL: Hemostasis defects associated with cardiac surgery, prosthetic devices, and other extracorporeal circuits. *Semin Thromb Hemost* 11:249–279, 1985.
3. Bick RL: Alterations of hemostasis associated with cardiopulmonary bypass: pathophysiology, prevention, diagnosis, and management. *Semin Thromb Hemost* 3:59–82, 1979.
4. Bick RL: Clinical relevance of antithrombin III. *Semin Thromb Hemost* 8:276–284, 1982.
5. Branch DW, Scott JR, Kochenour N, et al: Obstetric complications associated with the lupus anticoagulant. *N Engl J Med* 313:1322–1326, 1985.
6. Brown C, Natelson E, Bradshaw M, et al: The hemostatic defect produced by carbenicillin. *N Engl J Med* 291:265–270, 1976.
7. Buchanan MR, Boneu B, Ofosu F, et al: The relative importance of thrombin inhibition and factor X_A inhibition to the antithrombotic effects of heparin. *Blood* 65:198–201, 1985.
8. Burns T, Saleem A: Idiopathic thrombocytopenic purpura. *Am J Med* 75:1001–1007, 1983.
9. Cains J, Gent M, Singer J, et al: Aspirin, sulfinpyrazone or both, unstable angina. *N Engl J Med* 313:1369–1375, 1985.
10. Castellino FJ: Biochemistry of human plasminogen. *Semin Thromb Hemost* 10:18–23, 1984.
11. Cimo PL, Moake J, Weinger R: Heparin-induced thrombocytopenia. *Am J Hematol* 6:1298–1304, 1979.
12. Clouse LH, Comp PC: The regulation of hemostasis. The protein C system. 314:1298–1304, 1986.
13. Cohen A, Philips T, Kessler C: Circulating coagulation inhibitors in the acquired immunodeficiency syndrome. *Ann Intern Med* 104:175–180, 1986.
14. Cordonnier C, Vernant JP, Brun B, et al: Acute promyelocytic leukemia in 57 previously untreated patients. 18–25, 1983.
15. Daly P, Schriffer C, Wiernik P: Acute promyelocytic leukemia—clinical management of 15 patients. *Cancer* 55:18–25, 1985.
16. Day HJ, Rao A: Evaluation of platelet function. *Semin Hematol* 23:89–101, 1986.
17. Duckert F: Thrombolytic therapy. *Semin Thromb Hemost* 10:87–102, 1984.
18. Eichner E: Platelets, carotids and coronaries. *Am J Med* 77:513–523, 1984.
19. Errichetti A, Holden A, Ansell J: Management of oral anticoagulant therapy. *Arch Intern Med* 144:1966–1968, 1984.
20. Fareed J: Heparin, its fractions, fragments and derivatives. *Semin Thromb Hemost* 11:1–8, 1985.
21. Feinstein D: Diagnosis and management of disseminated intravascular coagulation: the role of heparin therapy. *Blood* 60:284–287, 1982.
22. Fekete L, Bick R: Laboratory modalities for assessing hemostasis during cardiopulmonary bypass. *Semin Thromb Hemost* 3:83–89, 1976.
23. Fuster V, Chesebro J: Antithrombotic therapy: role of platelet-inhibitor drugs. *Mayo Clin Proc* 56:102–112, 1981.
24. Gardner F, Bessman J: Thrombocytopenia due to defective platelet production. *Clin Heme* 12:23–38, 1983.
25. Gore J, Appelbaum J, Greene H, et al: Occult cancer in patients with acute pulmonary embolism. *Ann Intern Med* 96:556–560, 1982.
26. Griffin JH: Clinical studies of protein C. *Semin Thromb Hemost* 10:162–167, 1984.
27. Halkin H, Goldberg J, Modan M, et al: Reduction of mortality in general medical in-patients by low dose heparin. *Ann Intern Med* 96:561–565, 1982.
28. Hardisty R: Hereditary disorders of platelet function. 12:153–173, 1983.
29. Harlan J: Thrombocytopenia due to non-immune platelet destruction. 12:39–68, 1983.
30. Hattersby P, Mitsuoka C, King J: Sources of error in heparin therapy of thromboembolic disease. *Arch Intern Med* 140:1173–1175, 1980.
31. Hattersby P, Mitsuoka C, King J: Heparin therapy for thromboembolic disorders. 11:1413–1416, 1983.
32. Hayes A, Baker WH: Heparin prophylaxis trials of venous thrombosis. A critical review. *Semin Thromb Hemost* 11:222–226, 1985.
33. Herbst K, Rapaport S, Kenoyer D, et al: Syndrome of an acquired inhibitor of factor VIII responsive to cyclophosphamide and prednisone. 95:575–578, 1981.
34. Hirsch J, Ofosu F, Buchanan M: Rationale behind the development of low molecular weight heparin derivatives. *Semin Thromb Hemost* 11:13–16, 1985.
35. Hirsch J: Mechanism of action and monitoring of anticoagulants. *Semin Thromb Hemost* 12:1–11, 1980.
36. Hirsch J: Effectiveness of anticoagulants. *Semin Thromb Hemost* 12:21–37, 1986.
37. Hirsch J: Hypercoagulability. *Semin Thromb Hemost* 14:409–422, 1977.
38. Huisman M, Buller M, Ten Cate J: Serial impedance plethysmography for suspected deep venous thrombosis in outpatients. *N Engl J Med* 314:823–828, 1986.
39. Hull R, Hirsch J, Sackett D, et al: Replacement of venography in suspected venous thrombosis by impedance plethysmography and ^{125}I fibrinogen leg scanning. *Ann Intern Med* 94:12–15, 1981.
40. Hull R, Hirsch J, Carter C, et al: Pulmonary angiography, ventilation lung scanning, and venography for clinically suspected pulmonary embolism with abnormal perfusion lung scan. *Ann Intern Med* 98:891–899, 1983.
41. Imbach P: A multicenter European trial of intravenous immune globulin in immune thrombocytopenic purpura in childhood. *Vox Sang* 49(suppl):25–31, 1985.
42. Janson P, Jubelner S, Weinstein M, et al: Treatment of the bleeding tendency in uremia with cryoprecipitate. *N Engl J Med* 303:1318–1322, 1980.
43. Kaufmann R, Veltkamp J, Van Tilburg N, et al: Acquired AT III deficiency and thrombosis in the nephrotic syndrome. *Am J Med* 65:607–613, 1978.
44. Kalton J, Levine M: Heparine-induced thrombocytopenia. *Am J Med* 12:59–61, 1986.
45. King D, Kelton J: Heparin-associated thrombocytopenia. *Ann Intern Med* 100:535–540, 1984.
46. Kitchens C: Concept of hypercoagulability: a review of its development, clinical application and recent progress. *Semin Thromb Hemost* 11:293–312, 1985.
47. Knapp H, Reilly I, Alessandrini P, et al: In vivo indexes of platelet and vascular function during fish-oil administration in patients with atherosclerosis. *N Engl J Med* 314:937–942, 1986.
48. Kwaan H: The role of fibrinolysis in disease processes. *Semin Thromb Hemost* 10:71–79, 1984.
49. Lechner K, Niessener H, Thaler E: Coagulation abnormalities in liver disease. *Semin Thromb Hemost* 4:40–52, 1977.
50. Lerner W, Caruso R, Faig D, et al: Drug-dependent and non drug-dependent antiplatelet antibody in drug-induced immunologic thrombocytopenic purpura. *Blood* 66:306–311, 1985.
51. Levine M: Risks and benefits of anticoagulant therapy. *Semin Thromb Hemost* 12:67–71, 1986.
52. Levine M, Hirsch J: Hemorrhagic complications of anticoagulant therapy. *Semin Thromb Hemost* 12:39–57, 1986.
53. Levine M: Nonhemorrhagic complications of anticoagulant therapy. *Semin Thromb Hemost* 12:63–66, 1986.
54. Lind S: Prolonged bleeding time. *Am J Med* 77:305–312, 1984.
55. Livio M, Manmucci P, Vigano C, et al: Conjugated estrogens for the management of bleeding associated with renal failure. *N Engl J Med* 315:731–735, 1986.
56. Lucas O, Albert T: Epsilon aminocaproic acid in hemophiliacs undergoing dental extractions, a concise review. *Oral Surg* 51:115–120, 1981.
57. Lynch D, Howe S: Heparin-associated thrombocytopenia antibody binding specificity to platelet antigens. *Blood* 66:1176–1181, 1985.
58. Mannucci P, Remuzzi G, Pusineri F, et al: DDAVP shortens the bleeding time in uremia. *N Engl J Med* 308:8–12, 1983.
59. Marcinak E, Wilson H, Marlar R: Neonate purpura fulminans: a genetic disorder related to the absence of protein C in blood. *Blood* 65:15–20, 1985.

60. Martin J, Morrison J, Files J: Autoimmune thrombocytopenic purpura: current concepts and recommended practices. *Am J Obstet Gynecol* 150:86–97, 1984.
61. McGehee W, Klotz T, Epstein D, et al: Coumarin necrosis associated with hereditary protein C deficiency. *Ann Intern Med* 101:59–60, 1984.
62. McMillan R: Immune thrombocytopenia. *Clin Heme* 12:69–88, 1983.
63. Mielke C, Levine P. Zucker S: Preoperative prednisone therapy in platelet function disorders. *Thrombosis Res* 21:655–662, 1981.
64. Moncada S, Vane T: Arachidonic acid metabolites and interactions between platelets and blood vessel walls. *N Engl J Med* 300:1142–1148, 1979.
65. Mueh T, Herbst K, Rapaport S: Thrombosis in patients with the lupus anticoagulant. *Ann Intern Med* 156–159, 1980.
66. Mulberty S: Fibrinolysis: an overview. *Semin Thromb Hemost* 10:1–5, 1984.
67. O'Neill W, Timmis G, Bourdillon P: A prospective randomized clinical trial of intracoronary streptokinase versus coronary angioplasty for acute myocardial infarction. *N Engl J Med* 314:812–818, 1986.
68. Packham M, Mustard J: The role of platelets in the development and complications of atherosclerosis. *Semin Hematol* 23:8–26, 1986.
69. Pizzo S, Petruska D, Doman K, et al: Releasable vascular plasminogen activator and thrombotic strokes. *Am J Med* 79:407–411, 1985.
70. Poskitt T, Poskitt P: Thrombocytopenia of sepsis. *Arch Intern Med* 145:891–894, 1985.
71. Preston F, Whipps S, Jackson C, et al: Inhibition of prostacyclin and thromboxane A_2 after low-dose aspirin. *N Engl J Med* 304:76–79, 1981.
72. Prydz H: Vitamin K-dependent clotting factors. *Semin Thromb Hemost* 4:1–10, 1977.
73. Ramirez-Lassepas M: Antifibrinolytic therapy in subarachnoid hemorrhage caused by ruptured intracranial aneurysm. *Neurology* 31:316–322, 1981.
74. Ramwell P: Biologic importance of arachadonic acid. *Arch Intern Med* 141:275–278, 1981.
75. Rao A, Holmsen H: Congenital disorders of platelet function. *Semin Hematol* 23:102–118, 1986.
76. Rao A, Walsh P: Acquired qualitative platelet disorders. *Clin Heme* 12:201–238, 1983.
77. Robertson RM, Robertson D, Roberts J, et al: Thromboxane A_2 in vasotonic angina pectoris. *N Engl J Med* 304:998–1003, 1981.
78. Rooke T: Heparin and the in-hospital management of deep venous thrombosis: cost considerations. *Mayo Clin Proc* 61:198–204, 1986.
79. Roper-Drewinko P, Drewinko B, Corrigan G: Standardization of platelet function tests. *Am J Hematol* 11:183–203, 1981.
80. Rosenow E, Osmandsan P, Brown M: Pulmonary embolism. *Mayo Clin Proc* 56:161–178, 1981.
81. Sasahara A, Sharma V, Trow D: Clinical use of thrombolytic agents in venous thromboembolism. *Arch Intern Med* 142:684–688, 1982.
82. Sawaya R, Sonnino V, McLaurin R, et al: Monitoring of antifibrinolytic therapy following subarachnoid hemorrhage. *J Neurosurg* 58:699–707, 1983.
83. Schafer A: The hypercoagulable states. *Ann Intern Med* 102:814–828, 1985.
84. Schroder R, Neuhaus K, Leizorovicz A, et al: A prospective trial of intravenous streptokinase in acute myocardial infarction. *N Engl J Med* 314:1465–1471, 1986.
85. Seegers WH: Basic principles of blood coagulation. *Semin Thromb Hemost* 7:180–198, 1981.
86. Shaprio ME, Rodvien R, Bauer K, et al: Acute aortic thrombosis in antithrombin III deficiency. *JAMA* 245:1759–1761, 1981.
87. Shattil S, Bennett J: Platelets and their membranes in hemostasis: physiology and pathophysiology. *Ann Intern Med* 94:108–118, 1980.
88. Sheridan D, Carter C, Kelton J: A diagnostic test for heparin induced thrombocytopenia. *Blood* 67:27–30, 1986.
89. Sherman C, Litrack F, Grundfest W, et al: Coronary angioscopy in patients with unstable angina pectoris. *N Engl J Med* 315:913–919, 1986.
90. Straub PW: Diffuse intravascular coagulation in liver disease? *Semin Thromb Hemost* 4:29–39, 1977.
91. Stricker R, Abrams D, Corash L, et al: Target platelet antigen in homosexual men with immune thrombocytopenia. *N Engl J Med* 313:1375–1380, 1985.
92. Telford A, Wilson C: Trial of heparin versus atenolol in prevention of myocardial infarction in intermediate coronary syndrome. *Lancet* 1225–1226, 1981.
93. Tollefson D, Peska C: Heparin cofactor II activity in patients with disseminated intravascular coagulation and hepatic failure. *Blood* 66:769–774, 1985.
94. Turpir A, Levine M, Hirsch J: A randomized trial of a low molecular weight heparin (enoxaprin) to prevent deep vein thrombosis in patients undergoing elective hip surgery. *N Engl J Med* 315:925–929, 1986.
95. Uchino H, Yasunaga K. Akatsuka: A cooperative clinical trial of high dose immunoglobulin therapy in 177 cases of idiopathic thrombocytopenic purpura. *Thromb Haemostas* 51:182–185, 1984.
96. VonDem Borne AK, Pegels J, VanDer Stadt R: Thrombocytopenia associated with bold therapy: a drug-induced autoimmune disease? *Br J Haematol* 63:509–516, 1986.
97. Vermylin J, Badenhorst P, Deckmyn H, et al: Normal mechanisms of platelet functions. *Clin Heme* 12:107–151, 1983.
98. Vikydal R, Korringer C, Kyrle PA, et al: The prevalence of hereditary antithrombin III deficiency in patients with a history of venous thromboembolism. *Thromb Haemostas* 1985.
99. Wall R, Harker L: The endothelium and thrombosis. *Annu Rev Med* 31:361–371, 1980.
100. Walsh C, Krigel R, Lennette E, et al: Thrombocytopenia in homosexual patients. *Ann Intern Med* 103:542–545, 1985.
101. Wautier J, Caen JP: Pharmacology of platelet suppressive agents. *Semin Thromb Hemost* 5:293–315, 1979.
102. Weiss HJ: Platelet physiology and abnormalities of platelet function. *N Engl J Med* 293:531–588, 1975.
103. Weiss HJ: Antiplatelet therapy. *N Engl J Med* 298:1344–1407, 1978.
104. White III G, McMillan C, Blatt P, et al: Factor VIII inhibitors: a clinical overview. *Am J Hematol* 13:335–342, 1982.
105. Zauber N, Stark MW: Successful warfarin anti-coagulation despite protein C deficiency and a history of warfarin necrosis. *Ann Intern Med* 104:659–660, 1986.

CHAPTER 41

Antimicrobials

HENRY MASUR, M.D.

Infection is frequently suspected or documented in critically ill patients either as the primary process that brings the patient to an intensive care unit (ICU) or as a complication of diagnostic procedures, surgical intervention, drug therapy, or nosocomial exposure in patients who originally entered the ICU for other indications. Therapy of suspected infections in critically ill patients must often be more empiric than in other hospitalized patients, because the critically ill patient may be too sick to tolerate diagnostic procedures. Treatment must also be more encompassing since the critically ill patient may not survive if a causative organism is not treated immediately, whereas a less ill patient may be able to tolerate inadequately treated infection for a few days until the specific pathogens are identified.

Another major consideration for treating critically ill patients is the route of drug administration and the dose and interval that are required. Oral and intramuscular routes usually must be avoided because of uncertainty of absorption. Hepatic and renal dysfunction must be monitored carefully and the fluid and colloid status assessed so that drug levels are maintained in therapeutic but nontoxic ranges.

The focus of this chapter is the antimicrobial agents commonly employed for critically ill patients in the U.S. In the early 1990s a plethora of antimicrobial agents has become available, and a major issue is which of these agents really represent an advance in terms of improved efficacy, lower cost, or reduced toxicity, and which agents should no longer be used (57, 69, 80). These newer drugs vary greatly in antimicrobial spectrum, toxicity, doses, distribution, half-lives, and routes of elimination. It is probably preferable for intensivists to be very familiar with a limited number of antimicrobial drugs so that these drugs are used correctly rather than to attempt the use of numerous costly agents, many of which are quite similar to each other (3, 46, 58).

SPECIFIC ANTIMICROBIAL AGENTS

ANTIBACTERIAL AGENTS

Penicillins

The penicillins are a group of natural and semisynthetic compounds that share a basic structure that consists of a thiazolidine ring connected to a β-lactam ring with an attached side chain (83). The biologic activity of the penicillins is determined by the integrity of the thiazolidine and β-lactam structures. The antibacterial and pharmacologic properties of penicillin are modified by altering the side chain, resulting in a wide variety of available penicillin compounds (Table 41.1). These penicillins are most usefully classified according to their antibacterial spectrum. They all have similar, though not necessarily identical, mechanisms of action, the details of which are currently being elucidated. Penicillins kill bacteria by interfering with synthesis of the peptidoglycan component of the bacterial cell wall. Without effective cell walls the bacteria either fail to divide or swell and rupture.

Table 41.1.   Antimicrobial Agents for Bacterial, Fungal, and Viral Infections in Critically Ill Patients

Drug	Usual Adult Daily Dose (recommended dose interval)	Route of Administration	Peak Serum Concentration (μg/ml) (i.v. dose)	Hepatic Metabolism/ Excretion	Dose Alteration with Renal Dysfunction	Serum Concentration Altered by: Hemodialysis	Serum Concentration Altered by: Peritoneal Dialysis
Penicillins							
Aqueous crystalline penicillin G	0.6–20 million units/day (continuous q. 4 hr)	i.v.	18(1×10^6 U/hr)	No	Major	No	No
Ampicillin	4–12 g/day (q. 4–6 hr)	i.v.	6 (0.5 g)	Yes	Major	Yes	No
Ampicillin-sulbactam	4–12 g/day^a (q. 4–6 hr)	i.v.	6 (0.5 g)	Yes	Major	Yes	No
Carbenicillin	0.5 g/kg/day (q. 4 hr)	i.v.	150 (2 g)	Yes	Major	Yes	Yes
Ticarcillin	0.25 g/kg/day (q. 4 hr)	i.v.	140 (3 g)	Yes	Major	Yes	Yes
Ticarcillin-clavulanate	6–18.0 g/day (q. 4–6 hr)^b	i.v.		Yes	Major	Yes	Yes
Piperacillin	0.2–0.5 g/kg/day (q. 4 hr)	i.v.	320 (4 g)	Yes	Minor	Yes	No
Oxacillin	4–8 g/day (q. 4–6 hr)	i.v.	50 (0.5 g)	No	Minor	No	No
Nafcillin	4–8 g/day (q. 4 hr)	i.v.	11 (0.5 g)	Yes	Minor	No	No
Methicillin	6–12 g/day (q. 4–6 hr)	i.v.	72 (2.0 g)	No	Minor	No	No
Cephalosporins and cephamycins							
Cephalothin	4–12 g/day (q. 4–6 hr)	i.v.	100 (2 g)	Yes	Minor	Yes	Yes
Cefazolin	2–6 g/day (q. 4–6 hr)	i.v.	188 (1 g)	Yes	Major	Yes	No
Cefoxitin	4–12 g/day (q. 4–6 hr)	i.v.	110 (1 g)	Yes	Major	Yes	
Cefamandole	4–12 g/day (q. 4–6 hr)	i.v.	80 (1 g)	Yes	Major	No	No
Cefoperazone-sulbactam	4–16 g/day (q. 6–12 hr)			Yes	Minor	No	No
Cefotaxime	4–12 g/day (q. 6–8 hr)	i.v.	214 (2 g)	Yes	Minor	No	Yes
Ceftazidime	4–6 g/day (q. 6–8 hr)	i.v.	130 (2 g)	No	Major	Yes	Yes
Ceftriaxone	2–4 g/day (q. 12 hr)	i.v.	250 (2 g)	Yes	Minor	No	No
Other β-Lactams							
Imipenem/cilastatin	3 g/day (q. 6–8 hr)	i.v.	70 (1 g)	No	Major	Yes	Yes
Aztreonam	8 g/day (q. 8–12 hr)	i.v.	125 (1 g)	Yes	Major	Yes	Yes
Aminoglycosides							
Gentamicin	3–6 mg/kg/day (q. 6–8 hr)	i.v.	3–6 (1 mg/kg)	No	Major	No	Yes
Tobramycin	3–6 mg/kg/day (q. 6–8 hr)	i.v.	4–10 (1 mg/kg)	No	Major	No	Yes
Amikacin	15 mg/kg/day (q. 12 hr)	i.v.	20 (1.0 g)	No	Major	No	Yes
Antimycobacterial agents							
Isoniazid	300 mg/day (q. 24 hr)	p.o., i.m.	1.0 (10 mg/kg)	Yes	Minor	Yes	No
Rifampin	600 mg/day (q. 24 hr)	p.o., i.v.	7 (600 mg)	Yes	Minor	No	
Ethambutol	15 mg/kg/day (q. 24)	p.o.		No	Major	Yes	
Pyrazinamide	25 mg/kg/day (q. 24)	p.o.			Minor		
Ofloxacin	400–800 mg (q. 12 hr)	i.v., p.o.			Minor	Yes	Yes

Agent	Daily dose	Route					
Other antibacterial agents							
Trimethoprim/ sulfamethoxazole	320–960 mg trimethoprim/day	i.v.	100–150 S (25 mg/kg)	Yes	Major	Yes	Yes
Vancomycin	2 g/day (q. 6 hr or q. 12 hr)	i.v.	20–40 (0.5 g)	No	Major	Yes	No
Erythromycin lactobionate	2 g/day (q. 6 hr)	i.v.	9.9 (0.50 g)	Yes	No	No	No
Clindamycin	2–4 g/day (q. 6 hr)	i.v.	14 (0.6 g)	Yes	Minor	No	No
Chloramphenicol	2–6 g/day (q. 6 hr)	i.v.	11 (1.0 g)	Yes	Minor	No	No
Metronidazole	2.25 g/day (q. 6 hr)	i.v.	26 (0.5 g)	Yes	Major	Yes	No
Tetracycline	2 g/day (q. 6 hr)	i.v.	8.5 (0.5 g)	Yes	Avoid	Yes	No
Antiprotozoal/ antipneumocystis agents							
Pentamidine	4 mg/kg/day (q. 24 hr)	i.v.	0.612 (4 mg/kg)	?	No	No	No
Trimethoprim/ sulfamethoxazole	15–20 mg/kg/day (T) and 75–100 mg/kg/day (S) (q. 6 hr)	i.v., p.o.	100–150 S (25 mg/kg)	Yes	Major	Yes	Yes
Sulfadiazine	4–8 g/day (q. 6 hr)	i.v.		Yes	Yes	Yes	Yes
Pyrimethamine	25–100 mg/day (q. 24 hr)	p.o.		No			
Antifungal agents							
Amphotericin B	0.6–1.5 mg/kg/day (q. 24 hr)	i.v.	75 (2.0 g)	No	Minor	No	
Flucytosine	150 mg/kg/day (q. 6 hr)	p.o.	1.0 (50 mg)	No	Yes	Yes	Yes
Fluconazole	100–800 mg/day	p.o., i.v.		Yes	Major	Yes	Yes
Antiviral agents							
Acyclovir	15–30 mg/kg/day (q. 8 hr)	i.v.	20 (10 mg/kg)	No	Yes	Yes	
Amantadine	100–200 mg/day (q. 24 hr)	p.o.	0.3 (100 mg)	No	Yes		
Dideoxyinosine	Variable by weight	p.o.		Yes			
Azidothymidine	600 mg/day (q. 8 hr)	p.o.					
Ribavirin	1.1 g/day	aerosol					
Ganciclovir	10 mg/kg/day (q. 12 hr)	i.v.		No	Major		
Foscarnet	180 mg/kg/day (q. 8 hr)	i.v.			Major		

[a] Ampicillin component with 2 to 6 g sulbactam.

[b] Ticarcillin component.

Table 41.2.   Antimicrobial Drugs of Choice for the Treatment of Specific Infectious Agents in Critically Ill Patients

Organism	Antimicrobial Agent of Choice	Alternative Agents
BACTERIA		
Gram-positive cocci (aerobic)		
Staphylococcus aureus		
Non-penicillinase-producing	Penicillin	Vancomycin, cephalosporin
Penicillinase producing	Nafcillin, oxacillin	Vancomycin, cephalosporin
α-Streptococci (S. viridans)	Penicillin	Erythromycin, clindamycin, cephalosporin
β-Streptococci (A, B, C, G)	Penicillin	Cephalosporin, erythromycin
Streptococcus faecalis		
Serious infection	Ampicillin + aminoglycoside	Vancomycin + aminoglycoside
Uncomplicated urinary infection	Ampicillin	Vancomycin
Streptococcus bovis	Penicillin	Cephalosporin, vancomycin
Streptococcus pneumoniae	Penicillin	Erythromycin, vancomycin cephalosporin
Gram-negative cocci (aerobic)		
Neisseria meningitidis	Penicillin	Cefotaxime
Neisseria gonorrhoeae	Penicillin	Ceftriaxone
Gram-positive bacilli (aerobic)		
Corynebacterium JK	Vancomycin	
Gram-negative bacilli (aerobic)		
Acinetobacter sp.	Aminoglycoside + carbenicillin	Trimethoprim-sulfamethoxazole
Campylobacter sp.	Erythromycin	Tetracycline
Enterobacter sp.	Aminoglycoside	Third-generation cephalosporin
Escherichia coli	Ampicillin	Cephalosporin, aminoglycoside
Haemophilus influenzae	Second- or third-generation cephalosporin	Trimethoprim-sulfamethoxazole
Klebsiella pneumoniae	Aminoglycoside	Cephalosporin, aztreonam
Legionella sp.	Erythromycin + rifampin	Quinolone
Proteus mirabilis	Ampicillin	Aminoglycoside, cephalosporin
Other *Proteus* species	Aminoglycoside	Cephalosporin, aztreonam
Providencia sp.	Aminoglycoside (amikacin)	Cephalosporin, aztreonam
Pseudomonas aeruginosa	Aminoglycoside + piperacillin	Third-generation cephalosporin, aztreonam
Salmonella sp.	Trimethoprim-sulfamethoxazole	Ampicillin, quinolone, third-generation cephalosporins
Serratia marcescens	Aminoglycoside	Third-generation cephalosporin
Shigella sp.	Ampicillin	Third-generation cephalosporin, quinolone
Anaerobes		
Anaerobic streptococci	Penicillin	Clindamycin, metronidazole
Bacteroides sp.		
Oropharyngeal strains	Penicillin	Clindamycin
Gastrointestinal strains	Clindamycin	Metronidazole, cefoxitin
Clostridium sp. (except *C. difficile*)	Penicillin	Clindamycin, metronidazole
Clostridium difficile	Vancomycin	Metronidazole
Other bacteria		
Actinomyces and *Arachnia*	Penicillin G	Tetracycline
Nocardia sp.	Trimethoprim-sulfamethoxazole	Minocycline
Mycobacterium tuberculosis	INH + rifampin + pyrizinamide + ethambutol	Streptomycin
FUNGI		
Aspergillus sp.	Amphotericin B	
Blastomyces dermatitidis	Amphotericin B	
Candida sp.	Amphotericin B	Fluconazole
Coccidioides immitis	Amphotericin B	
Cryptococcus neoformans	Amphotericin B + flucytosine	Fluconazole
Histoplasma capsulatum	Amphotericin B	
Mucor-Absidia-Rhizopus	Amphotericin B	
PROTOZOA		
Pneumocystis carinii	Trimethoprim-sulfamethoxazole	Pentamidine, trimetrexate
Toxoplasma gondii	Sulfadiazine + pyrimethamine	Clindamycin-pyrimethamine
VIRUSES		
Herpes simplex	Acyclovir	Foscarnet
Influenza A	Amantadine	
Herpes zoster	Acyclovir	Foscarnet

Table 41.2. *(Continued).*

Organism	Antimicrobial Agent of Choice	Alternative Agents
OTHER ORGANISMS		
Mycoplasma pneumoniae	Erythromycin	Tetracycline, Quinolone
Chlamydia psittaci	Tetracycline	Quinolone
Chlamydia trachomatis	Erythromycin	Tetracycline
Leptospira sp.	Penicillin G	Tetracycline
Rickettsia sp.	Tetracycline	

Penicillins do not kill or inhibit all bacteria. Bacteria may be intrinsically resistant or may acquire resistance to the penicillins. Differential permeability to penicillins and differential binding of a specific penicillin to receptor proteins account for different activity of various penicillin compounds against specific bacteria. Other bacteria contain enzymes that inactivate the drugs. In Gram-positive bacteria, for instance, the peptidoglycan polymer is near the cell surface and is thus readily acted upon. In Gram-negative bacteria, however, the cell wall is protected from the hydrophilic penicillins by a complex surface structure. Whereas some microorganisms are inherently resistant to the penicillins, other microorganisms produce enzymes that can inactivate various β-lactam drugs. Gram-positive organisms generally secrete extracellular enzymes, whereas Gram-negative organisms produce small quantities of enzymes that remain in the periplasmic space between the inner and outer cell membranes. Each bacterial species produces a somewhat different β-lactamase, and each specific penicillin, or cephalosporin, varies in its susceptibility to the particular enzyme produced. The information for penicillinase is encoded on a plasmid that can be transferred by phages to other organisms. Ability to produce the enzyme is often inducible by exposure to the appropriate substrate. Some of the β-lactamases secreted by Gram-negative bacteria are inducible, whereas others are constitutive (19). In recent years, β-lactam drugs have been combined with β-lactam inhibitors such as clavulanate acid and sulbactam to produce drug combinations that are stable in the presence of β-lactamase drugs. Ampicillin-sulbactam (Unasyn) and ticarcillin-clavulanate (Timentin) are examples that are finding increasing clinical utility.

Penicillins are most readily classified for clinical purposes on the basis of their antimicrobial spectrum. Table 41.1 lists the most commonly used penicillins and their major routes of excretion. Table 41.2 indicates organisms for which penicillin drugs are effective therapy.

Distribution and Elimination. Most penicillins are widely distributed throughout the body, though local concentrations may vary substantially. In cerebrospinal fluid (CSF), levels generally are well below serum concentrations, though the presence of fever or meningeal inflammation usually augments penetration such that subarachnoid concentrations are therapeutic for the most common community-acquired organisms that cause meningitis. Concentrations in obstructed bile and in prostatic tissue are often subtherapeutic for the most likely pathogens.

Adverse Reactions. The most common adverse reactions to the penicillins are hypersensitivity reactions. All of the penicillin compounds have potential to cause allergic phenomena (61, 77). In order of decreasing frequency, these reactions include maculopapular rash, urticaria, fever, bronchospasm,

vasculitis, serum sickness, exfoliative dermatitis, and anaphylaxis. The true incidence of such reactions is probably between 0.5 and 10%, although some hypersensitivity reactions may occur particularly frequently with one penicillin compound. A hypersensitivity response after one administration of a drug does not guarantee a similar response for each of its subsequent administrations. It is not safe clinical practice to give a patient a penicillin compound if the patient has a reliable history of immediate hypersensitivity response to any drug in the β-lactam group, with the exception of aztreonam, a monobactam that does not appear to cross-react. Whether or not desensitization of the patient to the penicillin compound decreases the likelihood of a subsequent allergic response is uncertain, but desensitization in a controlled medical setting, such as an ICU, is a standard practice for patients who have no therapeutic alternative to penicillin. Skin testing with both major and minor determinants of penicillin is useful for predicting which patients are most likely to have a hypersensitivity response. Reliable preparations of antigens should be used for skin testing. Both major and minor determinants must be employed.

Serious toxic reactions to the penicillins are unusual events. The drugs provoke an inflammatory response that appears to be concentration dependent: inflammation at injection sites and thrombophlebitis occasionally occur. Very high serum concentrations, which may occur if doses are not adjusted appropriately for severe renal dysfunction, are associated with confusion, lethargy, and seizures, especially in those patients with preexisting cerebral disorders. Intrathecal administration of penicillins can cause arachnoiditis, and such administration is almost never warranted. Other toxic reactions reported include nephritis (especially with methicillin), bone marrow depression (especially with methicillin or nafcillin), hepatitis (especially with oxacillin), and impaired platelet aggregation (especially with carbenicillin and ticarcillin).

Clinical Use. Because of their proven clinical efficacy and their safety, penicillins are commonly used in critically ill patients. Table 41.1 indicates the recommended doses for the commonly used penicillin drugs.

Numerous new penicillin compounds have appeared in recent years. The acylamino penicillins, for example (azlocillin, mezlocillin, piperacillin), are broad-spectrum penicillins with activity against many enterobacteriaceae and *Pseudomonas aeruginosa*. Piperacillin is widely used because of its excellent in vitro activity against *P. aeruginosa*, but the major determinant of the drug of choice among these acylamino penicillins is probably cost rather than efficacy or safety, because the efficacy and safety profiles of these drugs are so similar. Ticarcillin has been marketed as a combination with potassium clavulanate, a noncompetitive inhibitor of many β-lactamases. The combination is available as Timentin and has increased in vitro activity against a variety of organisms. Similarly, ampicillin has been marketed as a combination with clavulanate (Unasyn). This drug combination may be useful against certain aerobic Gram-negative bacilli, anerobes, and *Staphylococcus aureus* that produce β-lactamase.

Cephalosporins

Cephalosporins are a group of natural and semisynthetic compounds with broad antibacterial activity (20, 29). They are structurally similar to penicillins and inhibit bacterial cell wall synthesis in much the same manner as the penicillins. Cephamycins are structurally similar to cephalosporins and act in a similar manner and thus are also considered in this section.

A large and expanding number of cephalosporin and cephamycin compounds are available, which vary considerably in antibacterial spectrum, pharmacokinetics, and cost (20, 29). For most clinicians it is necessary to be knowledgeable about only a few of these many compounds but to be aware that if the cephalosporin they are accustomed to using does not have the desired antimicrobial spectrum or tissue penetration, other cephalosporin compounds should be considered. The availability of new, extended-spectrum cephalosporins may make it possible to use a relatively nontoxic cephalosporin drug as a single agent rather than a multiple-drug regimen that includes an aminoglycoside. The relative role of newer cephalosporins compared with imipenem, Timentin, aztreonam, or the quinolones and the role of monotherapy vs. combination therapy for life-threatening infection are currently matters of great debate (16, 38, 51).

Cephalothin and cefazolin are the prototype compounds against which subsequent cephalosporins should be judged. They have wide activity against almost all aerobic cocci, including *Staphylococcus aureus* (but not *Streptococcus faecalis*), and against many enteric Gram-negative bacilli (but not against *Pseudomonas aeruginosa*). Cefazolin is less phlebogenic than cephalothin and can be given either intramuscularly or intravenously, unlike cephalothin, which should not be given intramuscularly.

Cefoxitin offers the advantage, compared with cephalothin or cefazolin, of outstanding activity against almost all anaerobic organisms, including *Bacteroides fragilis*, and more activity for indole-positive *Proteus* and *Serratia*. Thus, it can be of particular use for purulent pulmonary infections such as empyemas and abscesses and for mixed abdominal infections. Cefotetan and cefmetazole are newer agents with similar spectra (28). The choice of which agent among cefoxitin, cefotetan, and cefmetazole to use often is determined by cost. The former has a longer half-life. Cefamandole has excellent activity against *Haemophilus influenzae* as well as aerobic Gram-positive cocci and an extended spectrum of enteric bacilli. Cefuroxime, however, probably has more activity than cefamandole and is preferred over cefamandole by some experts. Its usefulness is primarily for mixed upper and lower respiratory infections that are likely to involve Gram-positive cocci and *H. influenzae.*

The extended-spectrum cephalosporins (the so-called third generation) offer improved in vitro activity compared with second-generation cephalosporins for aerobic Gram-negative bacilli. As a group these drugs are active against most aerobic Gram-positive cocci (but not *S. faecalis*, methicillin-resistant *S. aureus*, or many *Staphylococcus epidermidis*), *Neisseria meningitidis*, *Neisseria gonorrhoeae*, and many anaerobic Gram-negative bacilli including, for a few cephalosporins, *P. aeruginosa*. Cefotaxime, ceftizoxime, and ceftriaxone are the most commonly used third-generation cephalosporins that have broad-spectrum activity, which includes good activity against most aerobic Gram-positive cocci (except enterococci), but which does not include *P. aeruginosa*. Ceftriaxone has the advantage of a longer half-life (10). Ceftazidime has a similar (but not identical) spectrum of activity to these latter drugs. Ceftazidime is also active against *P. aeruginosa* but has weak activity against aerobic streptococci. Cefoperazone has been combined with sulbactam to extend its spectra: it may have a role for broad-spectrum therapy that needs to include *P. aeruginosa*. All the third-generation cephalosporins mentioned above cross-inflamed meninges. The emergence of resistance during therapy has been reported for third-generation cephalosporins. The major advantage of this group of cephalosporins is their low toxicity compared with aminoglycosides, activity against certain unusual multiple-drug-resistant bacilli, and the opportunity in many situations to administer a single drug rather than multiple agents. These drugs clearly are effective clinically, but their relative efficacy compared with older antibiotic combinations has not been clearly established, particularly when these agents are used as monotherapy for immunologically abnormal patients (e.g., the efficacy of ceftazidime compared with combination regimens for therapy of sepsis and neutropenia has not been established unequivocally).

Distribution and Elimination.   Therapeutic cephalosporin levels can be found in most body sites, including bile, synovial fluid, and pericardial fluid. Cephalothin, cefazolin, cefoxitin, and cefamandole penetrate the subarachnoid space poorly, ut several of the third-generation cephalosporins appear to penetrate sufficiently to have therapeutic potential. These include cefotaxime, ceftriaxone, ceftizoxime, and ceftazidime. The elimination of cephalosporins varies with the specific agent (Table 41.1).

Adverse Effects.   Hypersensitivity reactions are the most common adverse effects for the cephalosporins and cephamycins (77). No single cephalosporin or cephamycin seems to cause dramatically more hypersensitivity responses than the others. Clinical manifestations of hypersensitivity are similar to those described with the penicillins. Clinically, about 5 to 10% of patients with a penicillin allergy demonstrate an allergic response when challenged with a cephalosporin. Skin test antigen is not available to assess cephalosporin hypersensitivity. It is imprudent to administer a cephalosporin to any patient with a history of immediate hypersensitivity reactions to a penicillin drug.

Other serious adverse effects are uncommon. They include positive Coombs test, hemolytic anemia, nephrotoxicity (especially when cephalosporins are used in combination with aminoglycosides), thrombocytopenia, and granulocytopenia (59).

Carbapenems

Imipenem is a β-lactam antibiotic that is sold in a fixed combination with cilastatin (33). Cilastatin inhibits the renal metabolism of imipenem and is included to decrease the production of potentially nephrotoxic compounds. Imipenem has the broadest activity of any β-lactam drug, including extended-spectrum cephalosporins: its spectrum includes Gram-positive cocci (except some *Enterococcus fecium*, a few *E. fecalis*, *S. epidermidis*, and methicillin-resistant staphylococci), most aerobic Gram-negative bacilli, including *P. aeruginosa* (but excluding *Pseudomonas capacia* and *Pseudomonas maltophilia*), and many anaerobic bacteria, including *B. fragilis*; it does not cover *Corynebacterium JK*. Emergence of resistance during therapy, particularly for *P. aeruginosa*, is a concern, as is superinfection and the induction of β-lactamases, which would make Gram-negative bacilli more resistant to other β-lactam drugs. The role for imipenem is similar to that for extended-spectrum cephalosporins, but imipenem should not be used as a single agent for *P. aeruginosa* infections because of the possible emergence of resistance (7). Patients who are allergic to other β-lactam drugs are likely to be allergic to imipenem. Imipenem should be avoided in patients with seizures or high seizure potential.

Monobactams

Aztreonam is a synthetic β-lactam antibiotic that is structurally different from cephalosporins and penicillins (9, 47). It is the first monobactam approved for clinical use. Aztreonam has broad activity against aerobic Gram-negative organisms, including *N. gonorrhoeae*, most enteric Gram-negative rods, and *P. aeruginosa*. It has no activity against Gram-positive organisms or anerobes. Aztreonam is clinically effective against a broad range of Gram-negative organisms (64). It crosses the blood-brain barrier adequately. Adverse effects are similar to those of other β-lactam drugs. There appears to be little cross-allergenicity with penicillins and cephalosporins (62). The major advantage of aztreonam is that it has potent activity against Gram-negative bacilli without the toxicity of aminoglycosides.

Aminoglycosides

The aminoglycosides are a group of natural and semisynthetic compounds that have broad activity against Gram-negative bacilli (21, 42). The clinically useful drugs are gentamicin, tobramycin, amikacin, and netilmicin. The group also includes streptomycin, neomycin, and kanamycin, which are used infrequently in the 1990s. Because aminoglycosides have broad activity against Gram-negative bacilli and because they are proved to be clinically efficacious, they are a major component of the antimicrobial armamentarium for the critically ill. They are widely used as part of multiple-drug empiric therapy and as specific therapy for infections caused by organisms not susceptible to less toxic drugs.

Gentamicin, tobramycin, netilmicin, and amikacin have excellent activity against aerobic Gram-negative bacilli including most *Pseudomonas* species. These drugs have no activity against anaerobic organisms and limited activity against aerobic Gram-positive cocci. *S. faecalis* are susceptible to aminoglycosides in the presence of penicillins. Aminoglycosides have excellent activity against most *P. aeruginosa*; they act synergistically against these organisms and against some Enterobacteriaceae when used in combination with ticarcillin or piperacillin. Aminoglycosides are active in vitro against most *S. aureus* and *S. epidermidis*, but clinical efficacy against staphylococci has never been proved, and staphylococci rapidly become resistant when treated with aminoglycosides alone. The aminoglycosides act at the 30S bacterial ribosomal unit, where they inhibit protein synthesis and interfere with the translation of mRNA. These mechanisms do not, however, explain the bactericidal effects of these drugs. Bacterial resistance to aminoglycosides is usually caused by elaboration of enzymes that inactivate the drugs, though failure to penetrate into the bacteria and low affinity of the drug for ribosomes are also factors. These enzymes are located in the bacterial membrane. They adenylate, acetylate, and phosphorylate the aminoglycosides at numerous sites. Aminoglycosides that are poor substrates for these enzymes are active against more organisms. Thus, amikacin, a compound that is a substrate for only one of the common enzymes, an acetylase, is active against more Gram-negative bacilli than are the other aminoglycosides. However, it is not clear whether clinicians should use this semisynthetic compound in preference to the other aminoglycosides, since resistance to amikacin could spread if this drug were used more commonly. Many consultants prefer to withhold amikacin for the treatment of microorganisms that are suspected or documented to be resistant to other aminoglycosides (66).

Distribution and Elimination. Aminoglycoside concentrations are high in the renal cortex. Levels are low in other tissues, and aminoglycosides do not reliably penetrate into the subarachnoid space. Concentrations in bile are about 30% of serum levels unless the biliary system is obstructed, in which case levels are even lower. Aminoglycosides are eliminated by glomerular filtration. Some tubular reabsorption of these agents probably occurs.

Adverse Effects. Aminoglycosides are toxic to renal, auditory, and cochlear function (44, 45, 67, 68). Toxicity is concentration dependent, and the predilection for site of toxicity varies with each specific drug. Ototoxicity occurs as a result of progressive destruction of vestibular or cochlear sensory cells when the aminoglycoside is concentrated in the perilymph of the inner ear. Ototoxicity can occur abruptly or gradually. Gentamicin and streptomycin primarily affect auditory function, and tobramycin affects both equally. All the aminoglycosides are nephrotoxic. The frequency of clinical nephrotoxicity is influenced by the frequency and severity of concurrent nephrotoxic insults and by preexisting renal pathology. Nephrotoxicity characteristically occurs after 5 to 7 days of therapy: proteinuria and tubular casts initially occur, followed by a reduction in glomerular filtration. The process is usually reversible. Tobramycin is slightly less nephrotoxic than gentamicin; the difference is probably not clinically important. In patients who are seriously ill it is important to measure serum levels of aminoglycosides in order to avoid drug accumulation and toxicity, and, conversely, to avoid inappropriately low levels and ineffectiveness. Peak serum levels of 2 to 3 μg/ml usually are needed to produce concentrations greater than the minimum inhibitory concentration of most *Pseudomonas* and many Enterobacteriaceae. Gentamicin or tobramycin levels greater than 12 mg/ml are associated with toxicity. There is controversy concerning the optimal peak and trough levels to maximize efficacy but avoid toxicity. It seems reasonable to try to maintain peak gentamicin or tobramycin levels of 6 to 12 μg/ml, and trough levels of 1 to 2 μg/ml. Peak amikacin levels should be maintained at 25 to 30 μg/ml. Serum aminoglycoside levels (peak and trough) should be measured at least two or three times weekly in seriously ill patients regardless of renal function. Many factors affect serum level, including the underlying disease and fever. Although nomograms and formulas are available, measurement of serum levels is the only accurate method of ensuring the desired range. Either the total daily dose or the interval between doses can be altered. A useful method of estimating the appropriate interval between 1 mg/kg doses of gentamicin or tobramycin while awaiting laboratory results is to estimate the interval in hours to be equal to the product of eight times the serum creatinine. Thus, if the serum creatinine is 3 mg/dl, 1 mg/kg of gentamicin should be given every 24 hours (8 × 3). Peak and trough levels should then be measured and the dose readjusted as indicated by the levels. Recent interest has focused on once daily dosing regimens; while these are promising, they cannot yet be recommended for critically ill patients.

Quinolones

Fluoroquinolones. Fluoroquinolones have become recent additions to the antibiotic armamentarium of intensivists with the introduction of intravenous preparations of ciprofloxacin and ofloxacin (34, 76). These agents inhibit the enzyme deoxyribonucleic acid (DNA) gyrase, and members of this class may have broad activity against many aerobic Gram-positive cocci, aerobic Gram-negative bacilli including *P. aeruginosa*, and some mycobacteria. These drugs have found wide application in outpatient settings, but their role in seriously ill patients is still being defined.

Ciprofloxacin has broad activity against Gram-negative bacilli, including most Enterobacteriaceae, *P. aeruginosa*, and *H. influenzae*. For Gram-negative bacilli, it is the most active of the fluoroquinolones and is generally more active than ofloxacin. Ciprofloxacin is active against many aerobic Gram-positive cocci, including *S. aureus*, and some enterococci, but has poor activity against *Streptococcus pyogenes* and some pneumococci, and no activity against anaerobes. There is increasing resistance among Gram-positive cocci against fluoroquinolones so that this class is not a first- or second-line drug for Gram-positive cocci, especially in the respiratory tract. Ofloxacin has better activity than ciprofloxacin against Gram-positive cocci. Both ciprofloxacin and ofloxacin have excellent activity against *Legionella* species.

The development of resistance to fluoroquinolones by Gram-negative bacilli as well as Gram-positive cocci is a major problem. Their major role in the intensive care unit is in the therapy of Gram-negative bacilli that are resistant to other drugs, in patients with cystic fibrosis, and perhaps in the therapy of legionellosis (48). These agents probably should not be used in prepubertal children, since evidence in some animal models indicates that they cause arthropathies. In adults, the major toxicity of fluoroquinolones is nausea.

Macrolide Antibiotics

The macrolide antibiotics are a group of compounds that contain a lactone ring to which are attached one or more deoxy

sugars. Because of their excellent gastrointestinal absorption, erythromycin and clindamycin are widely used antibiotics in ambulatory medicine. In critically ill patients, their use as intravenous preparations relates primarily to their excellent activity against agents that cause atypical pneumonia and anaerobic infections, respectively.

Erythromycin. Erythromycin is either bacteriostatic or bactericidal, depending on the microorganism and the serum concentration. The drug is effective in vitro for almost all *Streptococcus pyogenes*, *S. pneumoniae*, and *Streptococcus viridans*, though a few strains of these organisms may be resistant, particularly if the patient has been exposed recently to a macrolide antibiotic. The antibiotic is also useful against all *Mycoplasma pneumoniae*, *Legionella pneumophila*, and *N. gonorrhoeae*. Erythromycin is active against only some *S. aureus* and *H. influenzae*, and thus is not recommended as first-line therapy for infections involving these organisms. Erythromycin has little activity against most Gram-negative bacilli, with the exception of *Campylobacter* species. In critically ill patients the major role for erythromycin is to treat suspected *Legionella* or *Mycoplasma* pneumonias.

Erythromycin binds to the 50S subunit of bacterial ribosomes and thus interferes with protein synthesis.

Newer macrolides with more extended spectra (azithromycin and clarithromycin) are available as oral agents, but they are not available in parenteral form and thus are seldom used in intensive care units.

Distribution and Elimination. Erythromycin diffuses into intracellular fluids, and adequate concentration is attained in almost all tissues except the brain and CSF. It penetrates the prostate well, though its antimicrobial spectrum renders it of little utility in prostatic infections.

Erythromycin is concentrated in the liver and excreted in the bile. About 15% of the intravenous form is excreted in the urine.

Adverse Effects. Serious adverse effects caused by erythromycin are rare. The drug is irritating in its intravenous form and frequently causes phlebitis. Fever, eosinophilia, and rashes occasionally occur. Cholestatic hepatitis rarely occurs with the intravenous preparations. This complication is more often observed with the oral estolate. Erythromycin causes reversible hearing loss, a complication that intensivists using high doses must be aware of (36).

Clindamycin. Clindamycin is a macrolide antibiotic that, like erythromycin, has excellent activity against *S. pyogenes*, *S. pneumoniae*, and *S. viridans* (65). It is active against many but not all *S. aureus*. Because clindamycin is bacteriostatic only against *S. aureus*, and because resistance develops during experimental infection, clindamycin is not first-line antistaphylococcal therapy. Clindamycin differs from erythromycin in that it has excellent activity against almost all anaerobic bacteria except for a few peptococci, a few *Clostridium perfringens*, a few *B. fragilis*, and many nonperfringens clostridia. The major role for clindamycin in the treatment of critically ill patients is to provide therapy for anaerobic infections.

Clindamycin inhibits protein synthesis by binding to the 50S subunit of bacterial ribosome.

Distribution and Elimination. Clindamycin penetrates most body sites well, particularly bone. It does not reliably enter the CSF. Only about 10% of clindamycin is excreted unchanged in the urine. The rest of the drug is metabolized in the liver and excreted in the bile and urine.

Adverse Effects. The most prominently described adverse effect of clindamycin is pseudomembranous colitis, which is a serious inflammatory process caused by the toxin of *Clostridium difficile*, a normal bowel organism. The frequency of its occurrence differs sharply in various series, from 0.2 to 20% of patients. It must be recognized, however, that pseudomembranous colitis has been reported with almost every currently used antibiotic, not just clindamycin, and concern about this potential complication should not be an important factor in deciding whether or not to include clindamycin in an antibiotic regimen.

Skin rashes, transaminasemia, and bone marrow suppression occasionally have been associated with clindamycin administration. Diarrhea without pseudomembrane formations is quite common. This form of diarrhea probably results from alteration of bowel flora. It usually resolves when antimicrobial therapy is stopped.

Vancomycin and Teicoplanin

Vancomycin is a natural compound that is structurally unlike the other antimicrobial compounds (79). It is bactericidal against essentially all staphylococci (both *S. aureus* and *S. epidermidis*), all *Streptococcus pneumoniae*, *S. pyogenes*, and *S. viridans*. It is bacteriostatic against most *faecalis* and most *Corynebacterium* species. A few anaerobes are susceptible, but virtually no Gram-negative organisms are susceptible to vancomycin. Vancomycin has a prominent role in therapy of critically ill patients. To an increasing extent, critically ill patients have temporary or permanent foreign bodies implanted as pacemakers, vascular access, valves, or shunts. These devices are especially predisposed to infection by staphylococci, including *S. aureus* and *S. epidermidis*, an increasing fraction of which are methicillin resistant (1, 50). In addition, the importance of *S. epidermidis* and diphtheroid species in patients with prosthetic valves or malignant tumors and the emergence of drug-resistant *S. pneumoniae* have made vancomycin a particularly useful bactericidal antibiotic. Vancomycin is also useful for patients with Gram-positive infection and a history of serious penicillin allergy (24). Enterococci and staphylococci resistant to vancomycin are being reported in increasing numbers in Europe, and occasionally in North America (32, 35). Teicoplanin and daptomycin may have a role in treating some vancomycin-resistant strains (35, 39, 43, 63).

Distribution and Elimination. Vancomycin penetrates most body tissues well, including the brain and inflamed meninges. It is excreted almost unchanged by the kidneys.

Adverse Effects. Nephrotoxicity and ototoxicity are uncommon with the modern drug preparation if peak serum levels are maintained below 50 μg/ml (25, 82). Phlebitis is common with intravenous vancomycin. Flushing, tingling, and erythema ("red man syndrome") are usually associated with rapid infusion, especially if 1-g doses are used (18, 49). Leukopenia occasionally occurs.

Sulfonamides, Trimethoprim, and Pyrimethamine

Sulfonamides are a large group of compounds that were the first chemotherapeutic agents employed systematically for the prevention and treatment of bacterial infection in humans. They have a wide antibacterial spectrum that includes Gram-positive cocci, Gram-negative rods, *Chlamydia*, *Nocardia*, *Neisseria*, and Protozoa (*Toxoplasma*, *Pneumocystis*, malaria). More effective drugs have taken the place of sulfonamides for the treatment of most bacterial processes. They have an important role for treating uncomplicated urinary tract infections. They are also first-line therapy for *Nocardia*, *pneumocystis*, and *Toxoplasma* infections, particularly when combined with trimethoprim and pyrimethamine.

The sulfonamides are structural analogs and competitive antagonists of *para*-aminobenzoic acid and thus interfere with the production of folic acid. Sulfonamides exert a synergistic effect when they are combined with agents such as trimethoprim or pyrimethamine that act at sequential steps in folic acid synthesis. For this reason a fixed combination preparation of two of these sequential blockers, trimethoprim-sulfamethoxazole (in a ratio of 1 : 5), has proved to be an effective and widely used therapeutic product (13). It is the drug of choice for pneumocystosis. Sulfadiazine or sulfisoxazole are still preferred for nocardiosis. Pyrimethamine is the preferred choice in combination with sulfadiazine for toxoplasmosis, although both of these drugs must be given orally.

Distribution and Elimination. Sulfonamides are widely distributed throughout the body, including the CSF. They are metabolized in the liver to varying degrees depending on the compound involved. The parent drug and the metabolites are excreted in the urine.

Adverse Effects. For most patient groups, about 5% of recipients have adverse reactions to sulfonamides. Hypersensitivity reactions, especially those of the skin and mucous membranes, and vasculitic lesions can be life-threatening. Acute hemolytic anemia, often associated with glucose-6-phosphate dehydrogenase deficiency, and agranulocytosis, thrombocytopenia, aplastic anemia, crystalluria, and hepatic necrosis are also seen. For HIV-infected adults, up to 70% can have fever, leukopenia, hepatitis, nephritis, or rash when treated with trimethoprim-sulfamethoxazole; these reactions appear to be related to the sulfamethoxazole rather than the trimethoprim and may necessitate cessation of therapy. Clinicians are becoming more familiar with completing courses of therapy despite the presence of non-life-threatening reactions.

Metronidazole

Metronidazole is a synthetic nitroimidazole that has an increasingly important role in the treatment of serious anaerobic infections as well as in the treatment of certain protozoal infections (65). Metronidazole is active against almost all anaerobes; some cocci and a few non-spore-forming Gram-positive bacilli are resistant. *Amoeba*, *Giardia*, and *Trichomonas* generally are susceptible. Because metronidazole is the only bactericidal drug available for most anaerobic organisms, it has a potentially important role for critically ill patients with anaerobic infections. Its role compared with that of clindamycin or chloramphenicol is currently being defined. With regard to mechanism of action, the nitro group of metronidazole is reduced by electron transport proteins with low redox potentials. The cell is thus deprived of reducing equivalents, and the reduced form of metronidazole is able to alter the helical structure of DNA.

Although metronidazole is well-absorbed after oral administration, it should be given intravenously to seriously ill patients.

Distribution and Elimination.   Good drug levels are attained in most tissues; particularly high levels are found in the CSF. Both metabolized and unmetabolized metronidazole are excreted in the urine.

Adverse Effects.   Metronidazole causes considerable headache and gastrointestinal symptoms, including anorexia, nausea, vomiting, diarrhea, epigastric pain, and cramps. Neurotoxic effects such as dizziness, vertigo, and ataxia and peripheral neuropathy may occur. Reversible neutropenia may be noted during therapy.

ANTIMYCOBACTERIAL THERAPY

Although many antituberculosis drugs are available, the most important drugs for therapy of critically ill patients are isoniazid, rifampin, streptomycin, and ethambutol (73). The first three are available for intramuscular administration. As the tuberculosis epidemic spreads in the U.S., intensivists are likely to use these drugs with increasing frequency.

Isoniazid (INH) is the hydrazide of isonicotinic acid. It is bactericidal against dividing typical mycobacteria (*Mycobacterium tuberculosis*) and some atypical mycobacteria. It appears to work by inhibiting synthesis of the cell wall. About one in 10^5 *M. tuberculosis* are genetically impermeable to INH.

Isoniazid is readily absorbed orally. The drug penetrates all body tissues, including the CSF. The drug is acetylated and hydrolyzed and then excreted in the urine. The rate of acetylation is racially dependent. The serum INH concentration of rapid acetylators is 50 to 80% less than that of slow acetylators.

About 5% of patients develop INH-induced untoward reactions, including rash, jaundice, peripheral neuritis, fever, seizures, bone marrow depression, hypersensitivity reactions, and arthritis. The peripheral neuritis is quite common if pyridoxine is not given concurrently. The most common concern with isoniazid therapy is hepatic injury. Mild transaminasemia (SGOT and SGPT two to three times normal) is a common occurrence that does not predict more serious injury. Bridging necrosis can be caused by isoniazid. The drug should be stopped immediately in patients with symptoms of hepatitis (anorexia, nausea, malaise, and jaundice) and in those whose transaminases are more than three times normal. Older patients are more likely to have substantial hepatic damage than are younger patients.

Rifampin is a zwitterion that inhibits many Gram-positive and Gram-negative organisms by inhibiting DNA-dependent RNA polymerase, leading to suppression of the initiation of RNA chain synthesis. In vitro and in vivo resistance develops rapidly.

The drug is well-absorbed orally; the parenteral form is available only as an investigational drug. Rifampin is metabolized in the liver via an active deacetylation and ultimately excreted via bile in the gastrointestinal tract. Rifampin is widely distributed in body tissue, including the CSF.

Less than 4% of patients suffer fever, rash, jaundice, various gastrointestinal complaints, and hypersensitivity reactions.

Ethambutol is an oral compound with excellent tuberculostatic activity. The drug is widely distributed. About 50% is excreted unchanged in the urine. Optic retinitis occurs only rarely in patients who are receiving 15 mg/kg or less of the drug. Other adverse effects are rare.

Pyrizinamide is an oral agent that is bactericidal for intracellular organisms. This drug can cause hepatitis, arthralgias, and nausea.

Streptomycin is tuberculocidal. Vestibular toxicity, auditory toxicity, and nephrotoxicity are not uncommon.

A variety of other antimycobacterial drugs are available for the therapy of multiple-drug-resistant *M. tuberculosis* or atypical mycobacteria such as *M. avium intracellulare*. Clofazimine and rifabutin (investigational agents) and azithromycin, clarithromycin, and amikacin have been used in human immunodeficiency virus (HIV)-infected patients to treat *M. avium intracellulare*, but their efficacy or the efficacy of any other agents for the treatment of this organism is not entirely clear.

ANTIFUNGAL AGENTS

Amphotericin B

Amphotericin B is a polyene antibiotic that is fungistatic or fungicidal for a wide variety of fungi but has no activity against bacteria or viruses (4, 71). Amphotericin B is active against most *Candida* species, *Cryptococcus neoformans*, and *Torulopsis glabrata* as well as some *Aspergillus* and *Rhizopus* species, and most *Histoplasma capsulatum*, *Coccidioides immitis*, *Blastomyces dermatiditis*, and *Sporotrichum schenkii*. Amphotericin B binds to the sterol component of fungal membranes, creating channels that increase the permeability of the membrane. Amphotericin B does not bind to the membranes of resistant organisms. Fungi do not become resistant to amphotericin B in vivo.

Amphotericin B must be administered by slow intravenous infusion after the amphotericin B has been dissolved in 5% dextrose in water. The drug precipitates in solutions containing acids, preservatives, or electrolytes. Because of the serious adverse effects, a 1-mg test dose is usually given in 20 ml of 5% dextrose solution over 1 hour. The next dose can be given immediately if there are no adverse effects. Although some experts suggest a gradual increase in dosage by 5-mg steps, it is prudent in critically ill patients to proceed directly to 0.6 mg/kg/day administered in 500 ml of 5% dextrose solution over 2 to 8 hours (4 hours is commonly used). Few patients tolerate higher daily doses, although for life-threatening infections, especially those caused by *Aspergillus* or *Mucor*, doses as high as 1.0 to 1.5 mg/kg/day have been used. Alternate-day therapy may be useful for some critically ill patients, especially after their fungal disease is clearly controlled. Hypersensitivity effects can be diminished by premedication with meperidine (50 mg i.v.) and diphenhydramine HCl (50 mg i.v.), and heparin (1000 units) added to the infusion (11). Premedication with hydrocortisone (10 to 100 mg i.v.) may be necessary to reduce the adverse effects, but this immunosuppressive agent should not be given automatically unless the other premedications are not effective. Amphotericin B can be administered intrathecally, although there are few cases where this is warranted. Coccidioidomycosis meningitis may be one such indication.

Amphotericin B is a highly tissue-bound drug that penetrates most body compartments, though concentrations in CSF and vitreous humor are low. Its metabolic pathways are incompletely understood. Very little of the drug is excreted in the urine, though the drug can be detected in the urine for 6 to 8 weeks after the last dose is given. Altered renal function or hemodialysis do not necessitate changes in drug dosage.

Adverse Effects. Amphotericin B is associated with a substantial number of adverse reactions such as flushing, chills, fever, anorexia, and headache. When severe, these untoward effects can be associated with tachypnea, hypoxemia, and hypotension. Slowing the infusion and premedicating the patient can diminish or eliminate these untoward effects.

Renal function is impaired by long courses of amphotericin B in more than half of patients. Renal dysfunction can be reduced in severity and frequency by maintaining good hydration for the patient, and perhaps by using concomitant pentoxifylline (8). Often the patient's serum creatinine, initially normal, will plateau in the 2 to 3 mg/dl range. In most cases, the renal dysfunction is largely (but not completely) reversible. If the serum creatinine rises beyond 3.0 mg/dl, the amphotericin B should be discontinued or the dose should be reduced if the danger of uremia outweighs the acute danger of the fungal process. Renal tubular function is often impaired by amphotericin B, resulting in hypokalemia, hypomagnesemia, and renal tubular acidosis that may be permanent. Anemia is also reported as a consequence of amphotericin B therapy, but leukopenia and thrombocytopenia are rare.

Flucytosine

Flucytosine, or 5-fluorocytosine, is a fluorinated pyrimidine that has activity against *C. neoformans*, some *Candida* species, and occasional isolates of other fungal species. Because 30% of cryptococci develop resistance during therapy, and resistance has also been observed to develop during therapy of *Candida* infection, flucytosine has no role as a single agent except perhaps in the treatment of chronic blastomycosis. Its primary use is in combination with amphotericin B for cryptococcal infections and some *Candida* infections (5).

Flucytosine is converted to fluorouracil by fungal cells, but not by host cells. The fluorouracil ultimately inhibits thymidylate synthetase.

Flucytosine is well-absorbed orally and is widely distributed in body tissues, penetrating CSF and aqueous humor quite well. About 80% of the drug is excreted unchanged in the urine.

Adverse Effects. Bone marrow depression is a common occurrence in patients receiving flucytosine, especially those whose marrows have been compromised previously by malignancy, radiation, or myelosuppressive drugs. Bone marrow suppression can be minimized by maintaining peak serum levels below 100 to 125 μg/ml. Hepatomegaly, transaminasemia, nausea, rash, emesis, diarrhea, and enterocolitis are also seen occasionally.

Fluconazole

There are an expanding number of imidazoles and triazoles with excellent antifungal activity. Fluconazole is the only member of the group that is currently available as an intravenous drug (27). Fluconazole has excellent activity against *C. neoformans* and many *Candida* species, but not *Candida krusei*. Fluconazole does not have activity against molds such as *Aspergillus* or *Mucor*. Some drugs in this class are active against these fungi (e.g., itraconazole), but these agents are not approved or readily available as parenteral products. Fluconazole is very well-tolerated, although nausea, rash, and hepatotoxicity can occur. Fluconazole penetrates the cerebrospinal fluid well (72).

Fluconazole is an excellent drug for treating mucosal candidiasis, including esophageal disease. At the doses tested for treating cryptococcal meningitis, fluconazole is not as effective as optimal doses of amphotericin B (70). Fluconazole has not yet been shown to be as effective as amphotericin B for the therapy of disseminated candidiasis. Thus, its role in treating serious, life-threatening disease has not yet been established.

Itraconazole has been used to treat some cases of aspergillosis, often in conjunction with amphotericin B. The utility of this oral investigational drug for treating serious infections needs further documentation.

Ketoconazole

Ketoconazole is an oral agent that is effective against mucosal candidiasis as well as less common fungal diseases such as histoplasmosis, coccidiomycosis, and blastomycosis. For patients with life-threatening fungal disease, ketoconazole has no role as a single agent. Nausea is the major adverse effect; numerous endocrinologic effects have also been described, although their clinical importance when conventional doses are used is unclear. Ketoconazole is not absorbed unless there is gastric acidity.

Miconazole

The indications to use miconazole in an intensive care setting are extremely rare, although this imidazole does have activity against yeasts and filamentous fungi.

ANTIVIRAL AGENTS

Ribavirin

Aerosolized ribavirin is effective therapy for severe respiratory syncytial virus (RSV) infections in children (17, 31, 37, 40, 55). Precipitation of the aerosolized drug on the valves and tubing of mechanical ventilators can lead to potentially hazardous malfunctions, especially if prefilters are not used. Other adverse effects associated with its use include anemia. There is no clear role for ribavirin in adults.

Acyclovir

Acyclovir is a purine nucleoside analog that has excellent activity against herpes simplex and herpes zoster but not against cytomegalovirus or Epstein-Barr virus (2, 37, 78). The drug acts by inhibiting viral DNA synthesis. An increasing number of herpesviruses are resistant by virtue of thymidine kinase deficiency as well as other mechanisms. Resistance developing during therapy has been described. Intravenous acyclovir is the drug of choice for life-threatening herpes simplex or herpes zoster infections such as disseminated disease or herpes simplex encephalitis. Because herpes zoster is less sensitive to acyclovir than is herpes simplex, serious herpes zoster disease requires higher doses of acyclovir than does serious herpes simplex. Acyclovir is excreted largely unchanged by the kidney, so dose adjustments must be made in the presence of renal dysfunction. Acyclovir-resistant strains of herpes simplex and herpes zoster are being reported with increasing frequency.

Adverse Effects.   Intravenous acyclovir is well-tolerated; phlebitis, rash, hypotension, nausea, headache, and encephalopathic changes can occur, as can reversible renal dysfunction (60). The dosage must be adjusted in the presence of severe renal dysfunction (6, 60).

Ganciclovir

Ganciclovir (9-1,3-dihydroxy-2-propoxymethyl-guanine, or DHPG) inhibits the replication of all herpes viruses in vitro, including cytomegalovirus, herpes zoster, and herpes simplex. Ganciclovir is highly bone marrow suppressive in the doses employed clinically, so it is less desirable than acyclovir for therapy of herpes simplex and herpes zoster infections. Its major clinical role is for therapy of cytomegalovirus disease. In acquired immune deficiency syndrome (AIDS) patients it has been used successfully to treat cases of cytomegalovirus retinitis, pneumonia, esophagitis, and colitis (15). It is also being used with increasing frequency in other populations of immunosuppressed patients, often in conjunction with immune globulin (22, 23, 53). Granulocyte colony-stimulating factor (G-CSF) may be needed in some patients to reduce neutropenia. Cytomegalovirus (CMV), herpesvirus (HSV), and varicella-zoster virus (VZV) isolates resistant to ganciclovir are being reported with increasing frequency.

Foscarnet

Trisodium phosphonoformate, or foscarnet, is a pyrophosphate analog that inhibits viral DNA polymerases. It has activity against HIV, but its major current clinical use derives from its virustatic activity against the herpesviruses, especially cytomegalovirus and acyclovir-resistant herpes simplex or herpes zoster (12, 24).

Foscarnet is widely distributed and penetrates the central nervous system well. It is eliminated by the kidneys. Its major toxicities are renal failure, seizures, and chelation of ions, especially calcium. Nausea and vomiting also occur. Toxicity can probably be reduced by vigorous hydration. Foscarnet is not bone marrow toxic, although anemia can be caused by the drug.

Foscarnet is effective for treating CMV retinitis in AIDS patients and likely has good efficacy for treating CMV disease in other patient populations as well. Its role in intensive care units is to be an alternative to ganciclovir, probably with comparable efficacy but with a very different toxicity profile.

Azidothymidine/Dideoxyinosine/Dideoxycytidine

Azidothymidine (AZT, zidovudine) is a synthetic nucleoside that has activity against HIV. It was the first drug shown

clearly to prolong the lives of patients with AIDS (26,75). It is currently available commercially only in oral form. There is no evidence that therapy during life-threatening illness improves short-term survival. Major adverse effects include neutropenia, anemia, and headache. Few data are available about its interaction with other marrow suppressive drugs. Dideoxyinosine (DDI) and dideoxycytidine are newer nucleosides with antiviral efficacy. Their role in the ICU is uncertain. Both can cause life-threatening pancreatitis.

Vidarabine

Vidarabine (adenosine arabinoside) is a derivative of adenosine. It is effective for herpes simplex encephalitis and keratoconjunctivitis, but there is almost no occasion to use it since intravenous acyclovir has become available. Acyclovir is at least as effective and considerably less toxic. The vidarabine must be administered intravenously in large volumes of fluid (15 mg/kg dissolved in 25 liters) given over 12 to 24 hours. This fluid bolus presents a management problem for patients with increased intracranial pressure or renal failure.

ANTIPNEUMOCYSTIS AGENTS

PENTAMIDINE

Pentamidine is a diamidine compound that is effective for the therapy of *Pneumocystis* pneumonia (56). For protozoa the mechanism of action of pentamidine is unclear; it may inhibit replication of protozoan kinetoplast DNA.

Pentamidine isethionate should be reconstituted in sterile water and administered by slow intravenous infusion (30 to 60 minutes). Clinically important hypotension is not frequently associated with slow intravenous infusion, despite older reports to the contrary. Intramuscular administration often causes painful sterile abscesses and is no longer recommended. Aerosolized pentamidine is well-tolerated and effective as prophylaxis for *Pneumocystis* pneumonia, but the drug should rarely, if ever, be delivered by this route for the therapy of acute *Pneumocystis* pneumonia.

Distribution and Elimination

Concentrations of drug are detectable for at least 24 hours after a 4 mg/kg intravenous dose. The half-life after intravenous administration is about 6.5 hours. The routes of metabolism and elimination are not well-worked out.

Adverse Effects

Parenteral pentamidine is associated with renal failure in a high percentage of patients, as well as dysglycemia (hypoglycemia followed by hyperglycemia, both of which can be clinically severe) and pancreatitis. HIV-infected patients appear to be particularly predisposed to leukopenia, which is usually reversed quickly when drug is discontinued. Because trimetrexate is better tolerated than pentamide, there may be a role for this newer agent for treating patients who need parenteral therapy and cannot tolerate trimethoprim-sulfa methoxazole.

CLINICAL USE OF ANTIMICROBIAL AGENTS IN CRITICALLY ILL PATIENTS

GENERAL CONSIDERATIONS

The successful use of antimicrobial therapy in the critically ill depends on an understanding of the pharmacology of the agents employed (54, 57, 74, 80). For optimal therapy of an infectious process, the drug must have good activity against the suspected or documented pathogen, it must be administered in such a way that active forms of the drug reach the site of infection at concentrations greater than the minimum inhibitory concentration (MIC) of the organism, and adverse effects must be avoided. The activity of the drug against the presumed pathogens must be based on both in vitro susceptibility testing and clinical trials. Certain antibiotics have excellent in vitro activity but poor clinical efficacy. For example, polymyxins may be quite active against Gram-negative bacilli, yet clinical response is unimpressive. *Salmonella* species may be susceptible to cephalothin, and *S. aureus* may be susceptible to chloramphenicol, yet patients do not have dramatic clinical response to these drugs compared with ampicillin and methicillin, respectively. Similarly, drugs may fail because organisms quickly develop resistance, as with *S. aureus* and rifampin or *P. aeruginosa* and carbenicillin.

The mechanism of antimicrobial action is frequently considered in the choice of an antimicrobial agent. Common sense deems it preferable to use an agent that is bactericidal rather than bacteriostatic, especially if the patient's immune function is abnormal. In bacterial endocarditis, bactericidal agents are much more efficacious than bacteriostatic compounds (14, 30, 81). For the treatment of other infections, the importance of microbicidal as opposed to microbistatic drugs is unconvincing. Thus, the optimal antibiotic is probably best chosen on the basis of activity against the pathogen, distribution, and toxicity rather than mechanism of action.

Additive or synergistic drug combinations are popular approaches to the treatment of infectious processes (41, 52). For bacterial endocarditis the addition of an aminoglycoside to a penicillin enhances serum bactericidal activity and the likelihood of clinical cure. These observations have been applied to other clinical situations where in vitro testing shows synergy for the offending microbe. In fact, there are few data, except for endocarditis, that document the clinical usefulness of these drug combinations, and in many situations, toxicity of the second drug can outweigh its usefulness. In some situations, however, the addition of a second drug may provide sufficient synergy that the dose of the first drug can be reduced, thus decreasing the toxicity. This is the case when flucytosine is added to amphotericin B for the treatment of cryptococcal meningitis.

Antagonism between bactericidal and bacteriostatic drugs is another in vitro phenomenon that frequently is applied to clinical situations. With the exception of a trial of penicillin plus tetracycline for the treatment of pneumococcal meningitis, however, there is little documentation that antibiotic antagonism should be an important consideration in the choice of antibiotics. To ascertain that adequate antibiotic concentration reaches the site of infection is an essential consideration. An antibiotic must be present at a concentration equal to or greater than the MIC of the organism. Measuring antibiotic levels or measuring bacteriostatic activity in joint fluid, CSF, or bone may help determine the adequacy of drug dose. For anesthetic agents or for pressors, augmented clinical responses can be obtained by augmenting drug concentrations. With antibiotics, however, drug concentrations increased over the MIC for the pathogen do not correlate with enhanced clinical response in any predictable manner. The clinician often takes solace in attaining serum or body fluid drug levels that are much higher than the MIC of the causative organism. Attaining very high serum levels at peak and trough periods may, in fact, be useful—they assure the clinician that sufficient antibiotic will be available if renal or hepatic drug excretion suddenly increases or if the infection occurs at a site where drug diffusion is poor. Only in bacterial endocarditis, however, does a specific measurement of serum killing activity correlate with clinical efficacy.

Measuring serum levels of antibiotics is important for ensuring adequate dosing and for preventing toxicity. In critically ill patients, renal and hepatic function may be difficult to assess and may fluctuate rapidly. Formulas and nomograms may help to estimate proper drug dose. Drug levels should be measured on a regular basis, particularly if the drug is potentially toxic, such as an aminoglycoside or vancomycin. Measuring drug levels several times weekly may be expensive on an absolute basis, yet such measurements represent a small fraction of total patient cost and prevent distressing and expensive complications.

EMPIRIC THERAPY

When patients are critically ill their survival is often dependent on the prompt initiation of appropriate antimicrobial therapy. If the identity of the etiologic microorganism(s) is uncertain, empiric therapy must be initiated to cover the full range of likely pathogens pending the outcome of diagnostic procedures. For many critically ill patients, however, the optimal diagnostic procedure cannot be performed because the patient is too hypoxic for a bronchoscopy, too thrombocytopenic for a biopsy, or too hemodynamically unstable to be transported to radiology or the operating suite. This scenario is especially common when dealing with immunosuppressed patients.

Traditionally, empiric antimicrobial regimens were likely to include multiple drugs, since no one agent has broad coverage that includes aerobic and anaerobic organisms, Gram-positive and Gram-negative bacteria, rods, and cocci. The past few years have been characterized by the appearance of third-generation cephalosporins, thienamycin, quinolones, and β-lactam/β-lactamase inhibitor combinations that can provide broad coverage. Single agents have the advantage of being less time-consuming to administer. Moreover, several of these drugs are considerably less toxic than the aminoglycosides that were previously included in most multiple-drug empiric regimens, particularly those used for neutropenic patients. In the middle 1980s a major unresolved issue was whether single agents such as ceftazidime, imipenem, or Timentin would be as effective as multiple-drug regimens, thus allowing clinicians the ease of monotherapy and the diminution in direct toxicity. Whether these benefits will outweigh the high absolute cost of many of these newer drugs remains to be determined.

EPIDEMIOLOGIC AND OTHER FACTORS

The epidemiology of highly pathogenic multiple-antibiotic-resistant organisms is an important consideration in the choice of antimicrobial agents in critically ill patients. Many patients who are critically ill have been exposed to hospital flora during previous hospitalization. Many critically ill patients are hospitalized in an ICU, where they can acquire resistant organisms and become superinfected. Substantial antibiotic pressure on these patients can also select out endogenous flora that are multiply antibiotic resistant. These organisms can cause serious disease in the infected patient, and they can be transmitted to other patients. A physician caring for a critically ill patient is obligated to use the most efficacious antimicrobial therapy available. The physician must also, however, introduce antibiotics appropriately so that resistance to newer antibiotics is delayed, thus saving these drugs for unusual situations in which they are uniquely useful. For instance, amikacin has decided advantages over gentamicin and tobramycin because it is often more active against more Gram-negative bacilli. Gram-negative bacilli that are resistant to gentamicin and tobramycin will sometimes be susceptible to amikacin, yet the more frequently this latter drug is used, the more amikacin-resistant organisms will likely appear. Thus, amikacin should probably be used only if the organism is known to be resistant to other therapeutic agents, or if there is some reason to suspect strongly such resistance. Similarly, some third-generation cephalosporins appear to be useful nontoxic agents for the treatment of organisms that previously required toxic agents such as the aminoglycosides. If they are used indiscriminately to treat organisms that are susceptible to more conventional agents, however, resistance may develop rapidly, thus decreasing their usefulness and the usefulness of other β-lactam drugs.

The cost of newer antibiotics should also influence the drug selected. Newer drugs are often much more expensive than older, generically available agents, and their routine use can dramatically increase a hospital's pharmacy expenditure.

Finally, the choice of antimicrobial agent must be influenced by a physician's familiarity with the drug. The rapid explosion of penicillin, cephalosporin, and quinolone agents makes it impossible for physicians to be familiar with the doses, pharmacokinetics, and adverse effects of all agents. Errors in selection and administration are more frequent if the physician attempts to use too large an armamentarium of drugs, especially when dealing with critically ill patients with changing hepatic and renal function and when considering the interaction of the drug with other medications. It seems preferable for the physician to be very familiar with the pharmacology of a limited antibiotic armamentarium and to select other agents or newer agents only when clearly indicated, judiciously using specific information from convenient handbooks or calling consultants (3, 46, 58).

REFERENCES

1. Archer GL: Molecular epidemiology of multiresistant *Staphylococcus epidermidis. J. Antimicrob Chemother* 21(suppl):133–138, 1988.
2. Balfour Jr HH, et al: Burroughs Wellcome Collaborative Acyclovir Study Group. Acyclovir halts progression of herpes zoster in immunocompromised patients. *N Engl J Med* 308:1448–1453, 1983.
3. Bartlett JG: *1991 Pocketbook of Infectious Disease Therapy.* Baltimore, Williams & Wilkins, 1991.
4. Bennett JE, et al: Amphotericin B-flucytosine in cryptococcal meningitis. *N Engl J Med* 301:126–131, 1979.
5. Bennett JE: Antifungal agents. In: Mandell GL, Douglas Jr RG, Bennett JE (eds): *Principles and Practice of Infectious Diseases*, 3rd ed. New York, Churchill Livingstone, pp 361–370, 1990.
6. Blum RM, Liao SHT, De Miranda P: Overview of acyclovir pharmacokinetic disposition in adults and children. *Am J Med* 73(suppl):186–192, 1982.
7. Bodey GP, Alvarez ME, Jones PG et al: Imipenem/cilastatin as initial therapy for febrile cancer patients. *Antimicrob Agents Chemother* 30:211–214, 1986.
8. Branch RA: Prevention of amphotericin B-induced renal impairment. *Arch Intern Med* 148:2389–2394, 1988.
9. Brewer NS, Hellinger WC: The monobactams. *Mayo Clin Proc* 66:1152–1157, 1991.
10. Brogden RN, Ward A: Ceftriaxone: a reappraisal of its antibacterial activity and pharmacokinetic properties, and an update on its therapeutic use with particular reference to once-daily administration. *Drugs* 35:604–645, 1988.
11. Burks LC, Aisner J, Fortner CL, Wiernik PH: Meperidine for the treatment of shaking chills and fever. *Arch Intern Med* 140:483–484, 1980.
12. Chatis PA, Miller CH, Schrager LE, Crumpacker CS: Successful treatment with foscarnet of an acyclovir-resistant mucocutaneous infection with herpes simplex virus in a patient with acquired immunodeficiency syndrome. *N Engl J Med* 320:297–300, 1989.
13. Cockerill FR, Edson RS: Trimethoprim-sulfamethoxazole. *Mayo Clin Proc.* 66:1260–1269, 1991.
14. Coleman DL, Horowitz RI, Andriole VT: Association between serum inhibitory and bactericidal concentrations and therapeutic outcome in bacterial endocarditis. *Am J Med* 73:260–267, 1982.
15. Collaborative DHPG Treatment Study Group: Treatment of serious cytomegalovirus infections with 9-(1,3-dihydroxy-2-propoxymethyl) guanine in patients with AIDS and other immunodeficiencies. *N Engl J Med* 314:801–805, 1986.
16. Collins T, Gerding DN: Aminoglycosides versus betalactams in Gram-negative pneumonia. *Semin Respir Infect* 6:136–146, 1991.
17. Connor JD, Hintz M, Van Dyke R, McCormick JB, McIntosh K: Ribavirin pharmacokinetics in children and adults during therapeutic trials. In: Smith RA, Knight V, Smith JAD (eds): *Clinical Applications of Ribavirin.* Orlando, FL, Academic Press, pp 107–123, 1984.
18. Davis RL, Smith AL, Koup JR: The "redman's syndrome" and slow infusion of vancomycin. *Ann Intern Med* 104:285–286, 1986.
19. Doern GV, Jergensen JH, Thornsberry C, et al: National collaborative study of the prevalence of antimicrobial resistance among clinical isolates of *Hemophilus influenzae. Antimicrob Agents Chemother* 32:185, 1988.
20. Donowitz GR, Mandell GL: Beta-lactam antibiotics. *N Engl J Med* 318:419–426, 490–500, 1988.
21. Edson RS, Terrell CL: The aminoglycosides. *Mayo Clin Proc* 66:1158–1164, 1991.
22. Emanuel D, et al: Cytomegalovirus pneumonia after bone marrow transplantation successfully treated with the combination of ganciclovir and high-dose intravenous immune globulin. *Ann Intern Med* 109:777–782, 1988.
23. Erice A, Chou S, Biron KK, Stanat SC, Balfour HH, Jordan MC: Progressive disease due to ganciclovir-resistant cytomegalovirus in immunocompromised patients. *N Engl J Med* 320:289–293, 1989.
24. Erlich KS, Facobson MA, Koehler JE, Follansbee SE, Drennan DP, Gooze L, Safrin S, Mills J: Foscarnet therapy for severe acyclovir-resistant herpes simplex virus type-2 infections in patients with the acquired immunodeficiency syndrome (AIDS): an uncontrolled trial. *Ann Intern Med* 110:710–713, 1989.
25. Farber B, Moellering Jr RC: Retrospective study of the toxicity of preparations of vancomycin from 1974–1981. *Antimicrob Agents Chemother* 23:138–141, 1983.
26. Fischl MA, et al: The efficacy of azidothymidine (AZT) in the treatment of patients with AIDS and AIDS-related complex. *N Engl J Med* 317:185–191, 1987.
27. Grant SM, Clissold SP: Fluconazole—a review of its pharmacologic and pharmacokinetic properties, and therapeutic potential in superficial and systemic mycoses. *Drugs* 39:877–916, 1990.
28. Griffith DL, Novak E, Greenwald CA, Metzler CM, Paxton LM: Clinical experience with cefmetazole sodium in the United States—an overview. *Antimicrob Agents Chemother* 23(suppl D):21–23, 1989.
29. Gustaferro CA, Steckelberg JM: Cephalosporin antimicrobial agents and related compounds. *Mayo Clin Proc* 66:1064–1073, 1991.
30. Hackbarth CJ, Chambers HF, Sande MA: Serum bactericidal titer as a predictor of outcome in endocarditis. *Eur J Clin Microbiol* 5:93–97, 1986.
31. Hall CB, McBride JT, Walsh EE, Bell DM, Gala C, Hildreth S, TenEyck LG, Hall WJ: Aerosolized ribavirin treatment of infants with respiratory syncytial viral infection. *N Engl J Med* 308:1443, 1983.
32. Handwerger S, Perlinar DC, Aharac D, Mc Auliffe V: Concomitant high-level vancomycin and penicillin resistance in clinical isolates of enterococci. *Clin Infect Dis* 14:655–61, 1992.
33. Hellinger WC, Brewer NS; Imipenem. *Mayo Clin Proc* 66:1074–1081, 1991.
34. Hooper DC, Wolfson JS: Fluoroquinolone antimicrobial agents. *N Engl J Med* 324:384–394, 1991.
35. Johnson AP, Uttley AH, Woodford N, George RC: Resistance to vancomycin and teicoplanin: an emerging clinical problem. *Clin Microbiol Rev* 3:280–291, 1990.

36. Karmody CS, Weinstein L: Reversible sensorineural hearing loss with intravenous erythromycin lactobionate. *Ann Otol Rhinol Laryngol* 86:9–11, 1977.

37. Keating MR: Antiviral agents. *Mayo Clin Proc* 66:160–178, 1992.

38. Klastersky J, Hensgens C, Meunier-Carpentier F: Comparative effectiveness of combinations of amikacin with penicillin G and amikacin with carbenicillin in Gram-negative septicemia double blind clinical trial. *J Infect Dis* 134(suppl):433, 1976.

39. Kenny MT, Dulworth JK, Brackman MA: Comparative in vitro activity of teicoplanin and vancomycin against United States clinical trial isolates of Gram-positive cocci. *Diagn Microbiol Infect Dis* 14:29–31, 1991.

40. Knight V, Yu CP, Gilbert BE, Divine GW: Estimating the dosage of ribavirin aerosol according to age and other variables. *J Infect Dis* 158:443–448, 1988.

41. Lepper MH, Dowling HF: Treatment of pneumococcal meningitis with penicillin plus aureomycin: studies including observations on apparent antagonism between penicillin and aureomycin. *Arch Intern Med* 88:489–494, 1951.

42. Lietman PS: Aminoglycosides and spectinomycin: aminocyclitos. In: Mandell GL, Douglas Jr RG, Bennett JE (eds): *Principles and Practices of Infectious Diseases*, ed 3. New York, Churchill Livingstone, pp 269–284, 1990.

43. Livornese LL, Dias SC, et al: Hospital acquired infection with vancomycin-resistant enterococcus faecium transmitted by electronic thermometers. *Ann Intern Med* 117:112–116, 1992.

44. Moore RD, Smith CR, Lietman PS: Risk factors for the development of auditory toxicity in patients receiving aminoglycosides. *J Infect Dis* 149:23–30, 1984.

45. Moore RD, Smith Cr, Lipsky JJ, Mellits D, Leitman PS: Risk factors for nephrotoxicity in patients with aminoglycosides. *Ann Intern Med* 100:352–357, 1984.

46. Nelson JD: *1991–1992 Pocketbook of Pediatric Antimicrobial Therapy*, ed 9. Williams & Wilkins, Baltimore, 1991.

47. Neu HC: Aztreonam activity, pharmacology, and clinical uses. *Am J Med* 88:25–65, 1990.

48. Neu HC: Synergy and antagonism of combinations with quinolones. *Eur J Clin Microbiol Infect Dis* 10:255–261, 1991.

49. Newfield P, Roizen MF: Hazards of rapid administration of vancomycin. *Ann Intern Med* 91:581, 1979.

50. Peacock JE, Moorman DR, Wenzel RP, et al: Methicillin resistant *Staphylococcus aureus*: microbiologic characteristics, antimicrobial susceptibility, and assessment of virulence of an epidemic strain. *J Infect Dis* 144:575, 1981.

51. Pizzo PA, et al: A randomized trial comparing ceftazidime alone with combination antibiotic therapy in cancer patients with fever and neutropenia. *N Engl J Med* 315:552–558, 1986.

52. Rahal Jr J: Antibiotic combinations: the clinical relevance of synergy and antagonism. *Medicine (Baltimore)* 57:179–195, 1978.

53. Reed EC, Bowden RA, Dandliker PS, Lilleby KE, Meyers JD: Treatment of cytomegalovirus pneumonia with ganciclovir and intravenous cytomegalovirus immunoglobulin in patients with bone marrow transplants. *Ann Intern Med* 109:783–788, 1988.

54. Rhodes KH, Henry NK: Antibiotic therapy for severe infections in infants and children. *Mayo Clin Proc* 66:59–68, 1992.

55. Rodriguez WJ, Kim HW, Brandt CD, Fink RJ, Getson PR, Arrobio J, Murphy TM, McCarthy V, Parrott RH: Aerosolized ribavirin in the treatment of patients with respiratory syncytial virus disease. *Pediatr Infect Dis J* 6:159–163, 1987.

56. Rosenblatt JE: Antiparasitic agents. *Mayo Clin Proc* 66:276–287, 1992.

57. Rosenblatt JE: Laboratory tests used to guide antimicrobial therapy. *Mayo Clin Proc* 66:942–948, 1991.

58. Sanford JP: *Guide to Antimicrobial Therapy 1992*. Antimicrobial Therapy, Dallas, TX, 1992.

59. Sattler FR, Weitekamp MR, Ballard JO: Potential for bleeding with the new beta-lactam antibiotics. *Ann Intern Med* 105:924–931, 1986.

60. Sawyer MH, Webb DE, Balow JE, Straus SE: Acyclovir-induced renal failure: clinical course and histology. *Am J Med* 84:1067–1071, 1988.

61. Saxon A, Beall GN, Rohr AS, Adelman DC: Immediate hypersensitivity reactions to beta-lactam antibiotics. *Ann Intern Med* 107:204–215, 1987.

62. Saxon A, Hassner A, Swabb EA, Wheeler B, Adkinson Jr NF: Lack of cross-reactivity between aztreonam, a monobactam antibiotic, and penicillin in penicillin-allergic subjects. *J Infect Dis* 149:16–22, 1984.

63. Schwalbe RS, Stapleton JT, Gilligan PH: Emergence of vancomycin resistance in coagulase-negative staphylococci. *N Engl J Med* 316:927–931, 1987.

64. Scully BE, Neu HC; Use of aztreonam in the treatment of serious infections due to multiresistant Gram-negative organisms including *Pseudomonas aeruginosa*. *Am J Med* 78:251–261, 1985.

65. Smilak JD, Wilson WR, Cockerill FR: Tetracyclines, chloramphenicol, erythromycin, clindamycin, and metronidazole. *Mayo Clin Proc* 66:1270–1280, 1991.

66. Smith CR, Baughman KL, Edwards CQ, Rogers JF, Leitman PS: Controlled comparison of amikacin and gentamicin. *N Engl J Med* 296:349–353, 1977.

67. Smith CR, Lietman PS: Effect of furosemide on aminoglycoside-induced nephrotoxicity and auditory toxicity in humans. *Antimicrob Agents Chemother* 23:133–137, 1983.

68. Smith CR, Lipsky JJ, Laskin OL, Hellman DB, Mellits ED, Longstreth J, Lietman PS: Double-blind comparison of the nephrotoxicity and auditory toxicity of gentamicin and tobramycin. *N Engl J Med* 302:1106–1109, 1980.

69. Standiford HC: Tetracyclines and chloramphenicol. In: Mandell GL, Douglas Jr RG, Bennett JE (eds): *Principles and Practices of Infectious Diseases*, ed 3. John Wiley & Sons, New York, pp 284–295, 1990.

70. Stern JJ, Hartman BJ, Sharkey P, Rowland V, Squires KE, Murray HW, Graybill JR: Oral fluconazole therapy for patients with acquired immunodeficiency syndrome. *Am J Med* 297:178–179, 1988.

71. Terrell CL, Hughes CE: Antifungal agents used for deep-seated mycotic infections. *Mayo Clin Proc* 66:69–91, 1992.

72. Tucker RM, Williams PL, Arathoon RG, Levine BE, Harstein AL, Hanson LH, Steven DA: Pharmacokinetics of fluconazole in cerebrospinal fluid and serum in human coccidioidal meningitis. *Antimicrob Agents Chemother* 32:369–373, 1988.

73. Van Scoy RE, Wilkowske CJ: Antituberculous agents. *Mayo Clin Proc* 66:179–187, 1992.

74. Van Scoy RE, Wilkowske CJ: Prophylactic use of antimicrobial agents in adult patients. *Mayo Clin Proc* 66:288–292, 1992.

75. Volberding PA, Lagakos SW, Koch MA, et al: Zidovudine in asymptomatic human immunodeficiency virus infection—a controlled trial in persons with less than 500 CD4 positive cells. *N Engl J Med* 322:941, 1990.

76. Walker RC, Wright AJ: The fluoroquinolones. *Mayo Clin Proc* 66:1249–1259, 1991.

77. Weiss ME, Adkinson NF: Beta-lactam allergy. In Mandell GI, Douglas Jr RG, Bennett JE (eds): *Principles and Practice of Infectious Diseases*, ed 3. Churchill Livingstone, New York, pp 264–269, 1990.

78. Whitley RJ, Gnann JW: Drug therapy: Acyclovir: a decade later. *N Engl J Med* 327:782–789, 1992.

79. Wilhelm MP: Vancomycin. *Mayo Clin Proc* 66:1165–1170, 1991.

80. Wilkowske CJ: General principles of antimicrobial therapy. *Mayo Clin Proc* 66:931–941, 1991.

81. Wolfson JS, Swartz MN: Serum bactericidal activity as a monitor of antibiotic therapy. *N Engl J Med* 312:968–975, 1985.

82. Woods CA, Kohlhepp SJ, Houghton DC, Gilbert DN: Vancomycin enhancement of experimental tobramycin nephrotoxicity. *Antimicrob Agents Chemother* 30:20–24, 1986.

83. Wright AJ, Wilkowske CJ. The penicillins. *Mayo Clin Proc* 66:1047–1063, 1991.

CHAPTER 42

Hormones: Vasopressin, Growth Hormone, Glucagon, Somatostatin, Prolactin, G-CSF, GM-CSF

GARY P. ZALOGA, M.D., F.A.C.P.

A variety of hormones are used as therapeutic agents. Recent discovery of a large number of peptides with physiologic activity suggests that peptide "hormonal" agents may become a major part of the pharmaceutical treatment of disease in the near future. This chapter reviews the use of vasopressin, growth hormone, glucagon, somatostatin, prolactin G-CSF, and GM-CSF. Thyroid hormones and insulin are reviewed in other chapters.

VASOPRESSIN

Arginine vasopressin is a 9-amino acid peptide produced in the supraoptic and paraventricular nuclei of the hypothalamus. It is the primary hormone regulating water balance. The hormone is released from the pituitary under conditions of water deprivation (when plasma osmolality is elevated) or when extracellular volume is depleted. An increase of approximately 2% in blood osmolality is sufficient to increase vasopressin secretion. On the other hand, isotonic contraction of intravascular volume causes little change in plasma vasopressin until losses approach 10%. Other stimuli for vasopressin secretion include pain, nausea, and hypoxia.

The primary site of vasopressin action in humans is the renal collecting duct (water reabsorption). However, the hormone also is a potent vasoconstrictor. Indeed, its name was chosen on the basis of its vascular activity. Vasopressin also acts as a neurotransmitter. It plays a role in modulating adrenocorticotropic hormone (ACTH) secretion, temperature, and other visceral functions. In addition, vasopressin promotes the release of coagulation factors by the vascular endothelium.

A large number of pharmacologic agents alter vasopressin secretion. Stimulators of secretion include vinca alkaloids, cyclophosphamide, clofibrate, tricyclic antidepressants, nicotine, isoproterenol, carbamazepine, insulin, morphine, and colchicine (1). Inhibitors of vasopressin secretion include ethanol and phenytoin. Lithium and demeclocycline inhibit the effect of vasopressin on the kidney and are used to treat the syndrome of inappropriate antidiuretic hormone secretion (SIADH). Chlorpropamide, acetaminophen, and indomethacin enhance the action of vasopressin on the kidney (in part by inhibiting renal prostaglandin synthesis).

Vasopressin receptors are found throughout the body, including the kidney, liver, brain, pituitary gland, vascular smooth muscle, and platelets. There are two types of vasopressin receptors (1, 2). Receptors mediating the pressor effects (via phosphatidylinositol turnover) are designated V1. V1 receptors are found on vascular smooth muscle, hepatocytes, platelets, and some renal cells (i.e., glomerular mesangial cells, vasa recta, and medullary interstitial cells). Renal V1 receptors participate in control of the glomerular filtration rate, medullary blood flow, and renal prostaglandin synthesis. Receptors in the kidney (i.e., renal collecting duct, thick ascending limb of Henle) that mediate the antidiuretic effects of vasopressin (via production of cyclic AMP) are designated V2. V2 receptors increase the permeability of renal collecting ducts to water. They also cause vasodilation. Desmopressin, a vasopressin analog, has a relative affinity for V2 receptors 12 times that

Table 42.1. Relative Activity of Vasopressin Peptides

Receptor	Antidiuretic (V2)	Pressor (V1)
8-Arginine vasopressin	100	100
8-Lysine vasopressin	80	60
1-desamino-8-D-arginine vasopressin (dDAVP)	1200	0.40

of arginine-vasopressin. Its V2:V1 receptor binding affinity is 3000:1 (Table 42.1) (1). Synthetic peptides with selective pressor activity have also been developed (i.e., 2-phenylalanine-8-lysine vasopressin). In addition, a series of antagonists of antidiuretic action have been synthesized (1).

The pressor effect of vasopressin occurs at concentrations significantly higher than those required for maximal antidiuresis. Vasoconstriction occurs in most vascular beds (i.e., skin, gastrointestinal tract, coronary vessels, pulmonary arteries). Thus, angina, myocardial infarction, pulmonary hypertension, and bowel ischemia may be adverse effects of systemic administration.

Insufficient hypothalamic secretion of vasopressin results in central or neurogenic diabetes insipidus (3–9). This disease is caused by hypothalamic or pituitary tumors, hypothalamic or pituitary surgery, head trauma, congenital central nervous system anatomic abnormalities, infiltrative diseases of the central nervous system (i.e., malignancy), granulomatous diseases (i.e., sarcoidosis, histiocytosis), vascular disease, infection, and autoimmune disease. The most common etiologies seen in the intensive care setting are brain tumors, neurosurgery, head trauma, or pituitary/hypothalamic infarction following cardiopulmonary arrest or stroke. Nephrogenic diabetes insipidus results from diseases characterized by renal resistance to the effects of vasopressin, rather than insufficient secretion. Causes include hypercalcemia, hypokalemia, drug administration (i.e., lithium), and renal tubular disease.

Excessive production of vasopressin that does not result from hypovolemia or hyperosmolality causes SIADH. The most common causes of this syndrome are pain, nausea, and hypoxia. Other causes include CNS disorders, pulmonary disease, and drug administration. Excess vasopressin results in water retention, hyponatremia, and diminished urine output (10, 11).

Clinically, vasopressin insufficiency does not present with vascular insufficiency but rather as defective urinary concentration, polyuria, thirst, and polydipsia. If access to water is limited, dehydration and hypovolemia can result. The diagnosis of diabetes insipidus is based upon the demonstration of inappropriately dilute urine in the presence of plasma hyperosmolality (i.e., >295 to 300 mOsm/kg water) (6–8). Hyperosmolality may be induced by fluid deprivation or infusion of hypertonic saline. Neurogenic diabetes insipidus is distinguished from nephrogenic diabetes insipidus by the response to exogenous vasopressin or desmopressin (following a period of water deprivation to cause hyperosmolality). Failure to respond adequately to vasopressin (i.e., by increasing urine osmolality to levels above plasma osmolality) indicates resistance and confirms the diagnosis of nephrogenic diabetes insipidus (12).

The goals of treatment of neurogenic diabetes insipidus are water and electrolyte replacement to restore hydration status and hormonal replacement (2–4). Most awake and alert adult patients with a normal thirst sensation are able to drink

sufficient water to maintain hydration. However, if water intake is interrupted or thirst sensation is impaired, severe dehydration, hypernatremia, weakness, circulatory collapse, and death may occur. Infants are very susceptible to dehydration, hypernatremia, and circulatory collapse. Despite adequate fluid intake, polyuria may interfere with sleep and lead to hydronephrosis, megaloureters, megalobladder, and impairment of renal function.

Hormonal replacement can be accomplished with desmopressin (dDAVP), aqueous vasopressin, or lysine vasopressin (Table 42.2) (2–4). The half-lives of arginine and lysine vasopressin range from 3 to 24 minutes. The liver and kidneys are the chief sites of metabolic inactivation of vasopressin. Vasopressin is inactivated by pancreatic enzymes in the gut and should be administered by the intravenous, intramuscular, subcutaneous, or intranasal routes.

Desmopressin (1-desamino-8-D-arginine vasopressin) is the drug of choice in most situations (2, 3). It may be given intranasally, subcutaneously, or intravenously. However, recently an oral form of desmopressin has been used to control polyuria in children effectively (more than 20 times the intranasal dose is required). Desmopressin is devoid of clinically significant vasopressor activity (it is primarily a V2 receptor agonist). Deamination of cysteine at position 1 and substitution of the D-isomer of arginine for L-arginine at position 8 decrease its degradation and prolong its half-life. The half-life after intravenous injection is 50 to 158 minutes. Biologic half-life is about 4 hours and duration of action approximately 12 hours. Twice-daily administration is adequate in most patients (2.5 to 20 μg b.i.d.).

Aqueous arginine and lysine vasopressin have significant hypertensive activity (V1 and V2 receptor agonists) and can cause angina pectoris, myocardial infarction, stroke, and bowel infarction. Because of these side effects, these agents should not be employed as primary pressor agents. The author and colleagues rarely use these agents for treating neurogenic diabetes insipidus, since they prefer desmopressin.

Hormonal replacement is tapered to urine output. Patients must be monitored for dilutional hyponatremia and water intoxication (overtreatment) and hypernatremia (undertreatment). Because vasopressin administration may lead to fluid retention, intravascular volume expansion, hyponatremia, and cerebral or pulmonary edema, some clinicians prefer to treat patients with intravenous fluid replacement alone rather than hormonal replacement. However, in the absence of vasopressin, the need for large volumes of fluids and close monitoring of electrolyte levels makes management difficult. Failure to give enough fluids can result in hypernatremia, dehydration, and intravascular volume depletion. Administration of large volumes of dextrose-containing fluids can result in hyperglycemia and an osmotic diuresis. The authors and colleagues have found hormonal replacement to be technically easier and less dangerous in treating patients with diabetes insipidus; again, desmopressin is preferred. To avoid undesired fluid retention, the next dose of desmopressin should be delayed until urine output increases.

Pregnant patients may develop a transient form of diabetes insipidus. Some of these patients respond poorly to arginine vasopressin but respond well to desmopressin. Excess degradation of vasopressin by increased levels of vasopressinase

Table 42.2.   Vasopressin Analogues[a]

Agent	Dose	Duration	Formulation
Desmopressin (dDAVP)	10 μg i.n. b.i.d.	12–24 hr	2.5 and 5.0 ml for i.n. (100 μg/ml)
	or		
	1–2 μg i.v. or s.q. q. 12 hr	12–24 hr	1- and 10-ml vials for i.v. or s.q. (4 μg/ml)
Aqueous vasopressin	1.6–2 mIU/kg/hr i.v. or 5–10 U s.q. q. 4–6 hr; (children 3–5 U s.q.)	3–6 hr 4–8 hr	Pitressin 0.5- and 1.0-ml ampules; (20 U/ml)
Lysine vasopressin (lypressin)	2–4 U i.n. q. 4–6 hr	3–6 hr	5-ml bottle (50 U/ml)

[a] Abbreviations: hr = hour; i.n. = intranasal; i.v. = intravenous; s.q. = subcutaneous.

produced by the placenta is believed to be the cause. Onset of diabetes insipidus during pregnancy could also be related to hypothalamic-pituitary tumors. Neurogenic diabetes insipidus developing after delivery may result from pituitary infarction (Sheehan's syndrome). Vasopressin does not cross the placenta. However, administration of vasopressin to the mother may produce detrimental vasopressor and uterotonic effects. Thus, the author and colleagues prefer to administer desmopressin for the treatment of diabetes insipidus during pregnancy.

Approximately one-third of patients with brain death develop neurogenic diabetes insipidus. In patients who may serve as organ donors, management is facilitated by treating the diabetes insipidus with hormonal agents rather than intravenous fluids. Desmopressin is the agent of choice, since it lacks vasopressor activity and is less likely to cause organ ischemia.

A number of agents are available for nonhormonal treatment of diabetes insipidus. Chlorpropamide is an oral hypoglycemic agent (sulfonylurea) that enhances vasopressin action in patients with partial neurogenic diabetes insipidus. The usual dose is 100 mg orally daily. Its major side effect is hypoglycemia. Thiazide diuretics can decrease urine output in patients with both neurogenic and nephrogenic diabetes insipidus. They act by causing volume depletion, decreased glomerular filtration, and increased proximal tubular fluid reabsorption. Major side effects include hypotension, hypokalemia, and hypomagnesemia. Thiazide diuretics are used primarily to treat nephrogenic diabetes insipidus. Less effective agents for treating partial diabetes insipidus include carbamazepine and clofibrate. These drugs stimulate release of endogenous vasopressin. Orally administered agents (i.e., chlorpropamide, clofibrate) may also prolong the action of desmopressin (2).

Vasopressin analogs (desmopressin) have been used to treat and prevent bleeding in patients with hemophilia A, in type 1 von Willebrand's disease, following cardiac surgery, and in patients with uremia (2, 13–22). Hemophilia A and von Willebrand's disease are characterized by inadequate levels of factor VIII coagulant activity. Intravenous infusion of desmopressin, 0.3 μg/kg over 15 to 30 minutes, usually increases levels of factor VIII activity, von Willebrand antigen, and ristocetin cofactor activity and can correct elevated bleeding times. Maximal correction of bleeding time is usually achieved in 15 to 30 minutes. Desmopressin is believed to release endogenous factor VIII stores and decreased effectiveness is seen with closely spaced repeated doses. Responsiveness returns after a treatment-free interval (24 to 48 hours).

Bleeding after cardiac surgery results in reexploration of approximately 3% of patients. Abnormal platelet function contributes to the bleeding. Intraoperative desmopressin can reduce operative and early postoperative blood loss in patients undergoing complex cardiopulmonary bypass surgery (23). In many patients, desmopressin may reduce the need for blood products and the risk of acquired infection (i.e., hepatitis; acquired immune deficiency syndrome, or AIDS) or allergic reactions (13, 14, 16).

Desmopressin can also improve bleeding time (19) enough to stop bleeding following trauma or to permit minor surgery in patients with bleeding disorders. Desmopressin has been shown to elevate factor VIII:C and factor VIII:VF in patients with mild to moderate disease (hemophilia A and von Willebrand's disease), and to allow elective oral surgery, cholecystectomy, and open thoracotomy (13, 15). The effect is mediated by the V2 receptor. Desmopressin can cause platelet aggregation and thrombocytopenia in type IIB von Willebrand's disease and should not be used for that disorder. In addition, desmopressin can release plasminogen activator. Thus, some clinicians also administer ε-amino caproic acid along with desmopressin to prevent clot lysis (2).

Sickle cell crisis results from capillary plugging by sickled erythrocytes, with resulting ischemia and infarction of tissue. The sickling process (which results from polymerization of abnormal hemoglobin S) is inhibited by a hypotonic plasma environment. Desmopressin-induced hyponatremia has been shown to prevent and shorten sickle cell crises (24). However, larger studies are needed to confirm these results.

Vasopressin possesses vasopressor activity, and intraarterial (0.2 to 0.5 U/min) and intravenous (0.3 to 1.5 U/min) infusion have been used to decrease bleeding from esophageal varices (25–28). Vasopressin decreases blood flow in the splanchnic bed and decreases portal venous blood flow and pressure. Intraarterial and intravenous routes of administration produce similar therapeutic effects (27, 28). Major complications from vasopressin administration for bleeding include hypertension, decreased cardiac output, bradycardia, arrhythmias, angina pectoris, myocardial infarction, small bowel infarction, local gangrene, and abdominal cramps. Simultaneous administration of nitroglycerin has been reported to reverse the cardiotoxic effects of vasopressin while enhancing the beneficial splanchnic effects of the drug (29, 30). Vasopressin has been shown to decrease blood transfusion requirements and control hemorrhage in patients with bleeding esophageal varices but has not been shown to prolong survival. Intraarterial vasopressin infusions have also been used to treat other types of gastrointestinal bleeding (31). These include Mallory-Weiss tears, gastritis, bleeding diverticuli, and ulcers. Once bleeding is controlled, vasopressin therapy is usually continued for 12 to 24 hours and then slowly tapered (i.e., by 0.1 U/min every 6 to 12 hours).

GROWTH HORMONE

Growth hormone (a 191-amino-acid protein) is produced in the anterior pituitary gland and its secretion is stimulated by growth hormone releasing hormone, hypoglycemia, arginine, exercise, and stress. The hormone coordinates the distribution of nutrients in the body, supporting tissue growth. Growth hormone is secreted in a pulsatile pattern; each day approximately 0.5 mg is released in six to eight bursts. Measurement of plasma growth hormone at a single point in time is a poor reflection of growth hormone secretion.

Growth hormone is regulated by two hypothalamic factors: growth hormone releasing hormone (GHRH) and growth hormone release-inhibiting hormone (somatostatin). Secretion is stimulated by dopamine, 5-hydroxytryptamine (5-HT), and α-adrenergic agonists. It is inhibited by β-adrenergic agonists, free fatty acids, insulin growth factor-1 (IGF-1), and growth hormone. Provocative tests to evaluate growth hormone secretion include intravenous infusion of arginine (30 g over 30 minutes in adults), insulin-induced hypoglycemia, levodopa, apomorphine, and 5-HT antagonists.

Growth hormone is inactivated by enzymes in the gastrointestinal tract. It is well-absorbed after intramuscular or subcutaneous administration. Maximal plasma concentrations are found 2 to 6 hours after injection. Plasma half-life is 20 to 30 minutes. Peak IGF-1 plasma concentrations occur approximately 20 hours after growth hormone administration. Growth hormone is degraded primarily in the liver, kidneys, and peripheral tissues. Little is excreted intact in the urine.

Growth hormone is available as recombinant-DNA-derived preparations (i.e., Protropin, Humatrope). Both are supplied in 5-mg vials as a lyophilized powder. The usual dose for growth promotion is 0.06 to 0.1 mg/kg intramuscularly three times per week.

Growth hormone is approved for replacement therapy in growth hormone deficient children. The body responds to growth hormone by a proportional increase in size of most organs and tissues. In most tissues, growth hormone increases cell number rather than size. It is under investigation as an adjunct in the treatment of catabolic states such as burns, trauma, and fractures.

Deficiency of growth hormone may result from disease processes that impair hypothalamic or pituitary function (i.e., tumors, neurosurgery, head trauma). Lack of growth hormone early in life results in short stature. Loss of growth hormone secretion later in life (after attainment of adult height) is not associated with any significant medical problems. Excess secretion of growth hormone (usually the result of a pituitary adenoma) results in gigantism (early in life) or acromegaly (after adulthood).

Growth hormone possesses a number of metabolic actions that may be beneficial to critically ill patients (32). It decreases protein catabolism (reduces blood urea nitrogen), promotes protein synthesis (nitrogen retention), promotes fat mobilization, enhances the conversion of fatty acids to acetyl co-enzyme A, decreases glucose oxidation, and stimulates glycogen deposition. Growth hormone may be important in the adaptation to lack of food by switching fuel metabolism from carbohydrate to fat.

Injury is associated with the catabolism of body protein-carbohydrate-fat stores and negative nitrogen balance. Prolonged hypercatabolism results in the loss of organ mass and function, organ failure, and, eventually, death. Nutritional therapies alone can blunt this catabolic response but are not able to overcome it. Growth hormone, along with nutritional support, may be capable of improving nitrogen balance, inducing anabolic metabolism, improving wound healing and immune function, and improving outcome.

Many of the anabolic effects of growth hormone are mediated by somatomedins, especially somatomedin C (also known as IGF-1). This peptide has numerous anabolic actions. It decreases protein degradation, increases lipogenesis, increases amino acid uptake, and stimulates cell proliferation and growth. Serum levels result primarily from hepatic synthesis and secretion of IGF-1. IGF-1s are also synthesized in kidney, muscle, and other organs, where they act locally.

Malnutrition and fasting cause an increase in levels of circulating growth hormone. During malnutrition and fasting, growth hormone promotes the release of fatty acids from lipid stores and helps preserve protein stores. However, the anabolic actions of growth hormone are diminished during malnutrition. Growth hormone fails to stimulate growth in children with severe malnutrition and fails to improve cartilage growth in protein-restricted rats (33). Nutritional repletion restores growth hormone effects. Concomitant with increases in growth hormone concentrations during malnutrition, IGF-1 levels decrease. This inverse relationship reflects an acquired peripheral defect in tissue production of IGF-1. This peripheral defect may result from decreased levels of growth hormone receptors (34). Low levels of IGF-1 increase toward normal during protein-calorie repletion and may be useful as an indicator of nutritional recovery. Both the quantity of protein and calories are important for restoring IGF-1 levels to normal. Critical illness and metabolic stress also decrease the production of IGF-1, despite increases in growth hormone (32, 35–42).

Technology recently has made available biosynthetic human growth hormone. Adequate nutritional intake is important for the anabolic actions of growth hormone. With adequate protein intake, growth hormone can increase protein synthesis and improve nitrogen balance. However, when protein intake is reduced, growth hormone stimulates lipolysis and fails to improve nitrogen balance.

In normal subjects, growth hormone decreases nitrogen excretion, improves nitrogen balance, increases protein synthesis, decreases forearm amino acid efflux, increases free fatty acid and glycerol levels, and increases IGF-1 concentrations (43). Growth hormone improves nitrogen balance in normal subjects receiving hypocaloric total parenteral nutrition (50% calories, adequate protein) (44). Growth hormone improves nitrogen retention in elderly patients (45, 46) and obese patients during dietary restriction (47). In an uncontrolled study (48), growth hormone also improved weight gain, nitrogen balance, and maximal inspiratory pressure in malnourished patients with chronic obstructive pulmonary disease.

Ziegler et al (49) studied 11 stable malnourished surgery patients. Patients were randomized to receive growth hormone or placebo in a cross-over designed study while receiving hypocaloric total parenteral nutrition (1100 kcal/day and 1.3 g protein/kg/day). Growth hormone resulted in a significant improvement in nitrogen balance.

Growth hormone (0.1 mg/kg/day) administered with hypocaloric nutrition (average of 400 kcal/day) improved nitrogen balance in patients following gastrointestinal surgery for cancer (50). In another study of gastrointestinal surgery patients receiving hypocaloric nutrition (20 kcal/kg/day plus 1 g protein/kg/day), growth hormone (0.06 mg/kg/day) decreased protein breakdown and improved nitrogen balance (51). Body composition analysis indicated that weight loss in the growth hormone treated patients was restricted to the fat compartment, preserving lean body mass.

In early studies of burn injury, Soroff et al (52) reported greater nitrogen losses during growth hormone treatment in the catabolic phase of burn (1500 calories/m² and 9 g nitrogen/day). In a later study, Soroff et al (53) reported improved nitrogen balance during growth hormone administration to burned patients (hypocaloric feedings) during the anabolic but not the catabolic phase. Wilmore et al (54) extended these findings in burn patients receiving adequate nutritional support (4025 kcal/day and 28 g nitrogen/day). Growth hormone decreased nitrogen loss in the urine and improved nitrogen balance during the catabolic phase. Belcher et al (55) randomized 12 burn patients to placebo or growth hormone treatment. All were fed enterally and received adequate calories and protein. There was no significant difference between groups for nitrogen balance, protein oxidation, or increases in prealbumin or retinol binding protein levels. The IGF-1 response to growth hormone was variable and indicated the existence of peripheral defects in IGF-1 production. When higher doses of growth hormone were administered to burned patients receiving adequate nutrition, improved wound healing was noted (56). These data suggest that growth hormone can improve nitrogen economy in burned patients. However, response to growth hormone is dependent upon concomitant nutritional support and the dose of growth hormone administered.

Growth hormone improves weight gain and growth during uremia. Mehls et al (57) reported improved growth in uremic rats. Tönshoff et al (58) noted improved growth in children with chronic renal failure when they received growth hormone.

Growth hormone has also been shown to promote wound healing in experimental perioperative (59), fasted (60), and tumor-bearing rats (61). Belcher et al (62) evaluated the effects of growth hormone on wound healing in animals following abdominal surgery and burn. Growth hormone improved wound strength in animals following surgery alone but had no effect on wound healing in animals with combined surgery plus burn. The anabolic effect of growth hormone appeared to be abolished by the combined injury, perhaps as a result of impaired synthesis of IGF-1. Additionally, growth hormone is reported to enhance healing of stress ulcers (63) and improve postoperative immune function (64).

The anabolic actions of growth hormone may be dose-dependent, with higher doses required as severity of illness increases. Growth hormone (0.03 to 0.06 mg/kg/day) failed to improve nitrogen balance in enterally fed burn patients (55). However, higher doses of growth hormone (0.2 mg/kg/day) in burn patients receiving adequate nutrition resulted in improved wound healing (56). Decreased response to low doses of growth hormone may result from injury-induced impairment of IGF-1 production.

IGF-1 production is dependent upon nutritional intake, and adequate levels of thyroid hormone, cortisol, and insulin (33, 65, 66). Thyroid hormone levels are known to decrease during critical illness as part of the "euthyroid sick syndromes" (67, 68). It is unclear whether these alterations affect growth hormone responses and IGF-1 production. One group has found that decreased IGF-1 levels follow low thyroid hormone levels during nonthyroidal illnesses (35).

Because levels of IGF-1 are influenced by nutritional intake, some researchers have suggested that circulating levels of IGF-1 may be useful as a monitor of nutritional status. IGF-1 levels decrease during fasting and return toward normal with refeeding in normal and obese subjects (69, 70). IGF-1 levels also improve during nutritional support in malnourished patients (71, 72). However, IGF-1 levels may be diminished during critical illness (i.e., sepsis, burns, trauma, renal failure, hepatic failure), independent of nutritional support. Thus, IGF-1 levels are a poor indicator of nutritional support during critical illness.

Since many of the anabolic effects of growth hormone are mediated by IGF-1 and IGF-1 synthesis is impaired in critical illness, it would seem logical to administer IGF-1 to critically ill subjects. IGF-1 administration to malnourished rats improved weight gain (73) but decreased growth hormone levels (negative feedback). IGF-1 decreases protein breakdown and increases protein synthesis (74). Further studies are needed to evaluate the actions of IGF-1 during metabolic stress. This includes studies of IGF-1 effects on nitrogen balance, protein synthesis, wound repair, and immune function. It is also possible that improved anabolic effects in critically ill patients would be found by combining growth hormone with IGF-1 administration.

Side effects from the administration of growth hormone and IGF-1 are minimal. Transient hypoglycemia has been reported immediately following administration of these hormones. It is believed to result from stimulation of glucose uptake and utilization by tissues. The effects of IGF-1 on protein catabolism and anabolism occur at doses that are lower than those that stimulate significant glucose uptake. Repeated administration of growth hormone may result in hyperglycemia. In the nondiabetic patient with normal pancreatic reserve, growth hormone has little, if any, effect on blood glucose. On the other hand, clinically important hyperglycemia and ketosis can occur in the diabetic patient.

In conclusion, growth hormone is capable of stimulating protein synthesis, reducing protein catabolism, and augmenting lipid oxidation in normal, obese, postoperative, and burn patients. These growth hormone effects are primarily related to IGF-1 production. Growth hormone responses are blunted during malnutrition and severe hypercatabolic illness, primarily because of impaired synthesis of IGF-1. Overall, available data do not support the routine use of growth hormone in critically ill patients. Further studies of wound healing and recovery from illness are needed.

GLUCAGON

Glucagon is a 29-amino-acid polypeptide hormone produced in the α-cells of the pancreas, the gastrointestinal tract, salivary glands, and CNS (75, 76). It is a major hormone involved in glucose homeostasis. Glucagon also has a variety of effects upon the cardiovascular, gastrointestinal, and urinary systems.

ENDOGENOUS FUNCTIONS

Glucagon raises blood glucose levels by stimulating hepatic glycogenolysis (inhibits glycogen synthesis) and gluconeogenesis (inhibits glycolysis). Maintenance of blood glucose is essential for energy supply to many tissues (especially the brain, renal medulla, and white blood cells). Glucagon also stimulates lipolysis, proteolysis, and ketogenesis (75, 77). These actions are mediated through a cell surface glucagon receptor and intracellular generation of cyclic adenosine monophosphate (cAMP). Glucagon's metabolic actions are antagonized by insulin and potentiated by insulin deficiency. Regulation of hepatic glucose production and ketogenesis depends upon the insulin:glucagon ratio rather than the absolute levels of either hormone.

After protein feeding, insulin ensures cellular uptake of nutrients and utilization of amino acids, whereas glucagon limits the degree of insulin-induced hypoglycemia. The brain is dependent upon a constant supply of glucose. Glucagon maintains a constant supply of glucose, and during starvation states it stimulates hepatic ketogenesis. Ketones may substitute for glucose as a cerebral fuel.

Glucagon is important for maintaining plasma glucose concentrations and preventing hypoglycemia during fasting and stress states. Along with epinephrine, glucagon is responsible for "moment-to-moment" regulation of circulating glucose. Energy requirements during stress are met by glucose and free fatty acids. Both catecholamines and glucagon stimulate hepatic glucose output and free fatty acid release. In turn, glucagon secretion is stimulated by epinephrine, growth hormone, cortisol, and endorphins (i.e., "stress hormones"). These stress hormones are responsible for "stress hyperglycemia" by blocking hyperglycemic suppression of glucagon secretion.

Glucagon is also responsible for hyperglycemia and ketoacidosis in patients with diabetes mellitus. With loss of pancreatic β-cells and insulin secretion, there is an inappropriate increase in the glucagon/insulin ratio. This increase is perpetuated by the loss of insulin inhibition of glucagon secretion. When glucagon is suppressed with somatostatin in patients with type I diabetes mellitus, hyperglycemia and ketosis are attenuated (78, 79). Glucagon secretion and epinephrine are also important for the prevention of hypoglycemia in patients receiving exogenous insulin.

Hypoglucagonemia is a rare disorder in which hypoglycemia occurs in patients with glucagon insufficiency. Hypoglycemia can be controlled with frequent feedings or with exogenous glucagon administration. Hypoglucagonemia may contribute to hypoglycemia in patients who develop pancreatic insufficiency following pancreatitis or pancreatectomy.

Physiologic stimuli for glucagon secretion (75, 77) include hypoglycemia, protein ingestion, amino acid infusion, exercise, epinephrine (β-adrenergic agonists), growth hormone, endorphins, acetylcholine, and cortisol. Glucagon secretion is inhibited by atropine, β-adrenergic antagonists, calcitonin, free fatty acids, glucose (i.e., hyperglycemia), insulin, ketones, somatostatin, and verapamil. Glucagon is degraded in the liver, kidney, plasma, and peripheral tissues. Its plasma half-life is 3 to 6 minutes. Clearance is reduced in patients with liver or renal insufficiency.

CLINICAL USES

Glucagon is extracted from beef and pork pancreas or synthesized using recombinant DNA techniques. It is supplied as a lyophilized powder, and some forms must be reconstituted in a phenol diluent prior to use. It is insoluble in water. It may be administered subcutaneously, intramuscularly, or intravenously.

Hypoglycemia

Glucagon may be used in the treatment of hypoglycemia (80). Carbohydrate administration is the treatment of choice for hypoglycemia. However, when glucose is not available or feasible, glucagon (1 mg intramuscularly; Table 42.3) can increase blood glucose levels. Because this immediate antihypoglycemic effect of glucagon results from its potent hepatic glycogenolytic properties, glucagon is not effective in states of hepatic glycogen depletion (e.g., starvation, adrenal insufficiency, chronic hypoglycemia). Glucagon also works poorly in patients with hepatic insufficiency (e.g., hepatitis, cirrhosis, congestive heart failure). The hyperglycemic action of exogenous glucagon is poorly maintained during continuous infusion because of insulin release. The hyperglycemic effect of glucagon is greater in patients with type I diabetes mellitus than in those with type II.

Glucagon is effective in preventing hypoglycemia during insulin excess and has been used to overcome hypoglycemia following lethal injection of insulin (81). It is minimally effective in treating hypoglycemia resulting from sulfonylureas, insulinomas, nesidioblastosis, glycogen storage disease, and alcohol abuse.

Glucagon may be administered subcutaneously, intramuscularly, or intravenously in a dose of 1 to 5 mg (82). Its onset of action occurs 1 minute after intravenous injection and 8 to 10 minutes after intramuscular or subcutaneous administration. Glucagon's hyperglycemic effect usually lasts only 10 to 30 minutes. The antihypoglycemic action of glucagon is of little use in the critical care setting, where intravenous glucose is the preferred treatment for hypoglycemia. However, because it is packaged in a small volume, it is useful in field situations in which intravenous glucose is not practical. It may be administered subcutaneously or intramuscularly by nonmedical personnel (i.e., patients or relatives), and it is useful in the semiconscious or convulsing hypoglycemic patient. If glucagon fails to restore consciousness within 20 to 30 minutes, intravenous glucose must be given to avoid CNS

Table 42.3. Glucagon Therapy

Indication	Dose (mg)	Time for Response	Duration of Action	Comments[a]
Hypoglycemia	1–5 mg s.c., i.m., or i.v. bolus	<20 min	Depends on liver glycogen	Start i.v. glucose; may repeat dose
Cardiogenic shock or heart failure	1–5 mg i.v. bolus every 30–60 min or 1–10 mg/hr i.v. infusion	5–10 min	20–30 min for bolus	Use antiemetic; watch glucose and K⁺
β-Blocker overdose	1–5 mg i.v. bolus every 30–60 min or 1–10 mg/hr i.v. infusion	5–10 min	20–30 min for bolus	Repeat dose every 30 min as needed; watch glucose and K⁺
Esophageal meat impaction	1 mg i.v. bolus	5 min	30 min	Repeat every 30 min; follow with barium
Diverticular disease	1 mg i.v. bolus every 4 hr	3–12 hr	2–4 hr	Repeat as needed
Renal or biliary calculi	1 mg i.v. bolus every 4 hr	1–2 hr	2–4 hr	Repeat as needed

[a] Administer cautiously to patients with suspected pheochromocytoma or insulinoma.

damage from prolonged hypoglycemia. Recovery of consciousness produced by glucagon should be followed by ingestion of a meal or oral glucose.

The insulinemic response to glucagon can be used in the differential diagnosis of fasting hypoglycemia. Insulinoma patients have an exaggerated insulin response to glucagon characterized by initial hyperglycemia followed by rebound hypoglycemia (90 to 150 minutes later) (77). Patients with fasting hypoglycemia resulting from other causes (i.e., extrapancreatic tumors, alcohol) have a reduced glycemic and insulinemic response to glucagon. Patients with glycogen storage disease fail to show a glycemic response to glucagon. Glucagon unresponsiveness may also result from chronic carbohydrate deprivation. This entity can be ruled out by repeating the test after a period of carbohydrate repletion.

Cardiovascular Effects

Glucagon has both inotropic and chronotropic cardiac effects in animals and humans (75, 77, 83–90). It is also a peripheral vasodilator (84, 90). Glucagon's cardiotonic effects are not dependent on catecholamines or adrenergic receptors, and they are not affected by α- or β-adrenergic blockade (87, 88, 91). Glucagon produces its cardiac effects by interacting with glucagon receptors, which increase intracellular cAMP (via stimulation of adenylyl cyclase or inhibition of phosphodiesterase) and improve calcium fluxes (77, 91–96). Its chronotropic actions are antagonized by ionized hypocalcemia and hypercalcemia (97). In addition, glucagon has been reported to possess opiate antagonistic properties (98).

A variety of clinical studies have evaluated the effect of glucagon for the treatment of cardiac insufficiency. Glucagon has been shown to increase heart rate, the rate of pressure change (dP/dT), cardiac index, and oxygen delivery with little change in left ventricular diastolic pressure or systemic vascular resistance. These effects have been demonstrated in patients with coronary artery disease, heart failure, and cardiogenic shock (77, 86, 88, 99–103). In heart failure, the chronotropic effect of glucagon is blunted. Maximal cardiac output effects from glucagon are obtained with 5 to 10 mg of intravenous glucagon per hour. Overall, however, glucagon is less effective in increasing cardiac output and blood pressure than other inotropic drugs such as dobutamine, epinephrine, amrinone, or dopamine.

Glucagon improves hemodynamics in experimental endotoxin (104–107) and hypovolemic shock (104, 108–111). Glucagon increases glucose levels and improves survival in swine following endotoxin (107). Glucagon also improves survival in rat hemorrhagic shock (111). Glucagon demonstrates protective effects during the anaphylactic response in guinea-pig isolated hearts (112). In these hearts, glucagon exerts antiarrhythmic activity, reduces histamine and creatine phosphokinase (CPK) release, and improves coronary flow. The hemodynamic and metabolic effects of glucagon have not been sufficiently studied in human shock.

Glucagon decreases atrioventricular conduction time and may improve heart block (77, 84, 113). It increases the rate of discharge of atrioventricular pacemaker cells and spontaneously beating Purkinje fibers (77). Glucagon has restored sinus rhythm and effective circulation in animals following cardiac arrest (114).

Glucagon's inotropic and chronotropic actions are independent of the β-adrenergic receptor. It effectively antagonizes heart block, bradycardia, hypotension, and decreased contractility resulting from overdose of β-adrenergic blockers (77, 91, 115–121). Glucagon has also been reported to reverse the cardiotoxic effects of procainamide (122), ouabain (77, 123, 124), slow calcium channel antagonists (125–128), and quinidine (122, 129). It is important to note that calcium fails to antagonize the atrioventricular conduction abnormalities produced by slow calcium channel antagonists (126), although it may relieve hypotension. Glucagon effectively reverses these conduction disturbances. However, there have been no human controlled trials of the efficacy of glucagon in these states.

Glucagon has been administered to patients with the adult respiratory distress syndrome and pulmonary hypertension (130). Glucagon (0.5 mg/min) improved PO₂, with little change in pulmonary shunt. Cardiac output, oxygen delivery, and pulmonary artery pressures increased slightly. A larger dose of glucagon may have been more effective. On the other hand, nitroprusside decreased PO₂, pulmonary artery pressures, cardiac output, and oxygen delivery.

Glucagon's cardiac effects begin in 1 to 5 minutes, peak in 5 to 15 minutes, and last 20 to 30 minutes after a single 5-mg bolus. It may be administered in 1- to 5-mg boluses every 20 to 30 minutes or as a continuous infusion of 1 to 10 mg/hr (131).

In summary, glucagon is a moderately effective inotropic and chronotropic agent in humans. Its effects are independent of the β-adrenergic receptor and it is effective in treating β-blocker overdose. Glucagon is also effective in overcoming bradycardia and myocardial depression resulting from slow calcium channel antagonist overdose.

Vascular Effects

Glucagon is a potent vasodilator of the systemic and splanchnic vascular bed (77, 84). Relaxations induced by glucagon follow the order renal → mesenteric → femoral → cerebral = coronary (132). Hyperglucagonemia also impairs systemic vascular sensitivity to norepinephrine, angiotensin, and vasopressin (133, 134). Hyperglucagonemia, found in patients with portal hypertension, may contribute to systemic and splanchnic vasodilation, and increased portal pressure in cirrhosis (133, 135, 136).

Mesenteric ischemia results from either occlusive disease (i.e., thrombus, embolus) or nonocclusive disease (i.e., vasoconstriction). Mortality from mesenteric ischemia is high, approaching 70%. Vasodilators have been used to treat nonocclusive disease. Papaverine, prostaglandin E_1 (PGE$_1$), and phenoxybenzamine are the most frequently used agents. Glucagon is a potent vasodilator of the splanchnic circulation and may be administered intravenously (most other agents are given intraarterially) (137). Glucagon increases celiac and superior mesenteric blood flow and liver perfusion (via portal venous and hepatic arterial blood flow). The hormone significantly enhances intestinal villous tip blood flow. Glucagon also reduces intestinal motility and lowers the bowel's energy requirements. Glucagon increases mesenteric blood flow and survival in experimental models of acute mesenteric ischemia (77, 138–141). Only 21% of rats receiving saline survived 85 minutes of superior mesenteric artery occlusion (140). Neither an angiotensin-converting enzyme inhibitor, allopurinol, or a vasopressin antagonist improved survival. Intravenous glucagon (given after occlusion) improved survival to 86%, while dopamine improved it to 67% (140). Following intestinal strangulation, glucagon improved mucosal blood flow and viability of the intestine (141). Glucagon was more effective than heparin, urokinase, superoxide dismutase/catalase, or a thromboxane synthetase inhibitor (141). It is important to note that glucagon administration prior to experimental mesenteric ischemia worsened eventual reperfusion injury (142). Injury was most likely worsened as a result of glucagon-induced increases in intestinal metabolism prior to the ischemic event. Glucagon may be useful in treating human mesenteric ischemia.

Glucagon causes renal vasodilation and a resulting diuresis and natriuresis. These effects are similar to those of low-dose dopamine. Glucagon increases renal blood flow and glomerular filtration rate. It preferentially dilates the afferent arteriole (143). Glucagon may increase renal blood flow during ischemic states (144). However, the renal effects of glucagon have not been studied in human shock states.

Gastrointestinal Effects

Glucagon relaxes smooth muscle in the lower esophageal sphincter (LES), stomach, small intestine, colon, gallbladder, and biliary ducts (75, 77). Glucagon reduces LES pressure without interfering with esophageal peristalsis (145), and a 1-mg dose can relieve obstruction from esophageal impaction (i.e., meat) (146–149). Glucagon relieves elevated LES pressure and dysphagia in patients suffering from achalasia (77). Glucagon decreases LES pressure and suppresses gut motility and gastric secretion. It has been used to aid in the treatment of esophageal perforation by diminishing reflux of esophagogastric contents (150).

Glucagon is frequently administered to relax gut smooth muscle during endoscopic visualization of the intestine and bile ducts (151–153). Glucagon reduces bile duct sphincter pressure and bile duct pressure (154). It has been used to relieve pain and help the passage of gallstones (77, 155, 156). Glucagon has also been used to relieve narcotic-induced choledochoduodenal sphincter spasm and improve visualization of the bile ducts during operative cholangiography (157).

An intravenous infusion or bolus of glucagon can relieve the pain from acute diverticulitis (158). Glucagon has been used to relieve intestinal spasm and aid in surgical end-to-end anastomosis during gastrointestinal surgery (159).

Glucagon inhibits gastric and pancreatic secretions. It has not proved to be of benefit in altering the severity or outcome of pancreatitis (75). However, it may aid in the closure of pancreatic fistula (160).

Urologic Effects

Pharmacologic doses of glucagon increase urine flow and ion excretion. These effects result from an increase in glomerular filtration rate (dilation of afferent arterioles), a natriuretic effect, and decreased tubular reabsorption. Glucagon also depresses ureteral peristalsis. It has been used to relieve the pain from renal calculi and aid in their passage (161, 162).

Radiologic Effects

Glucagon-induced gut relaxation and decreased motility can aid in the visualization of gastrointestinal lesions during radiologic procedures (i.e., neoplasms, early Crohn's disease) (75, 77). Glucagon has resulted in less discomfort, faster procedures, and better radiologic images during barium enema examination. During fluoroscopy, glucagon helps separate functional spasm from organic lesions. Glucagon may also aid in the resolution of intussusception by barium enema. Glucagon relieves pain and spasm, aids in the passage of gallstones, and improves visualization of the gallbladder during cholangiography. Glucagon has been used to reverse spasm during hysterosalpingography and urography. Peristalsis-induced artifacts can be reduced by glucagon during abdominal angiography.

SIDE EFFECTS

The most common side effects from the administration of glucagon are nausea and vomiting. Antiemetic therapy can minimize these side effects. Glucagon may also cause hyperglycemia, hypokalemia, vasodilation and hypotension, and tachycardia. Severe hypertension can be precipitated in patients with an underlying pheochromocytoma (163). Hypoglycemia is common in patients with insulinoma. Glucagon is

Table 42.4.   Biologic Actions of Somatostatin

Endocrine Effects	*Nonendocrine Effects*
Inhibits secretion of:	Inhibits:
Gastrointestinal	Gastrointestinal
Gastrin	Gastric acid secretion and
Pancreoxymin	emptying
Secretin	Pancreatic secretion
Human pancreatic peptide	Gallbladder contraction
Vasoactive intestinal peptide	Splanchnic blood flow
Gastric inhibitory peptide	Intestinal transit
Motilin	Macronutrient absorption
Glucagon	Serotonin secretion
Insulin	
Pepain	
Neurotensin	
Cholecystokinin	
Lipase	
Trypsin	
Amylase	
Pituitary	
Growth hormone	
TSH	

insoluble in saline or water and should be solubilized in the accompanying diluent. Many diluents contain small amounts of phenol and glycerin. Large doses or prolonged infusion of these glucagon preparations can result in phenol toxicity (i.e., CNS and myocardial depression). To avoid these complications, glucagon should be solubilized in the smallest amount of diluent possible.

PRESCRIBING INFORMATION

Most glucagon for clinical use is extracted from beef and pork pancreas. It is insoluble in water unless the pH is less than 3 or greater than 10. Glucagon is supplied as a lyophilized powder (1 and 10 mg) mixed with lactose and is stable at room temperature. It is usually solubilized in a phenol diluent prior to administration.

Glucagon may be administered by the intravenous, subcutaneous, or intramuscular routes. Boluses of 1 to 5 mg/hr are frequently used for patients with cardiac failure (Table 42.3). Doses of 1 mg are used for gastrointestinal, urologic, or radiologic procedures. Hypoglycemia is treated with boluses of 1 to 5 mg.

Glucagon potentiates the anticoagulant effects of warfarin by depressing vitamin K-dependent clotting factors and/or increasing warfarin receptor affinity. Glucagon does not affect the actions of heparin.

SOMATOSTATIN

Somatostatin is an endogenous peptide hormone (14 amino acids) that inhibits the secretion of a variety of hormones (164–170) (Table 42.4). It inhibits the secretion of vasoactive intestinal peptide (VIP), gastrin, glucagon, growth hormone, insulin, pancreatic polypeptide, motilin, neurotensin, cholecystokinin, serotonin, secretin, gastric acid, intestinal lipase, and pepsin. Because this agent was discovered for its ability to inhibit growth hormone secretion, it was named "somatostatin." Somatostatin also increases intestinal transit time and water and electrolyte absorption. It decreases splanchnic

blood flow and nutrient absorption. Somatostatin secretion is stimulated by glucose, arginine, leucine, glucagon, VIP, and cholecystokinin.

Somatostatin is found throughout the body. It has been isolated from cells in the hypothalamus, pancreas, cerebral cortex, heart, eye, thyroid, thymus, skin, genitourinary system, gastric and intestinal epithelium, and salivary glands. Somatostatin binds to specific cell surface receptors, interacts with G proteins, and inhibits adenyl cyclase (decreases cAMP). It enhances potassium conductance and decreases function of voltage-sensitive calcium channels.

Use of somatostatin is limited by its short half-life (several minutes) and lack of selectivity. Octreotide acetate is an 8-amino-acid synthetic peptide that possesses pharmacologic actions similar to those of native somatostatin. However, it is more resistant to degradation and has a longer duration of action.

Octreotide decreases tumor secretions from growth hormone secreting pituitary adenomas, insulinomas, glucagonomas, carcinoid tumors, and VIPomas. It decreases flushing and diarrhea associated with metastatic carcinoid tumors and diarrhea associated with VIP-secreting tumors. Somatostatin has been reported to improve glucose control and diminish ketosis in diabetes mellitus. It also can improve symptoms in dumping syndrome.

Octreotide is absorbed incompletely following oral administration. Thus, it is administered intravenously or subcutaneously (171). Peak serum concentrations occur within 30 minutes of subcutaneous injection and within a few minutes after intravenous administration. It is 65% protein bound (mainly to lipoproteins). Its elimination half-life from plasma is 1.5 hours. It is metabolized by the liver, kidneys, and peripheral tissues. Approximately 33% is excreted unchanged in the urine. Some is excreted in bile. Plasma clearance is significantly reduced in patients with renal impairment, and dosage should be reduced (164, 172).

Compared with native somatostatin, octreotide has a longer duration of action and is more potent for inhibiting growth hormone release, glucagon release, and insulin secretion.

PITUITARY EFFECTS

Octreotide suppresses growth hormone secretion under both stimulated (i.e., exercise, food) and basal conditions (173). Nocturnal and pulsatile release of growth hormone is inhibited (167). Octreotide suppresses the growth hormone response to insulin-induced hypoglycemia (165). However, there is no suppression of the ACTH or cortisol response to hypoglycemia. Octreotide also suppresses arginine-stimulated growth hormone release (173). Octreotide inhibits thyroid-stimulating hormone (TSH) release in response to thyroid releasing hormone (TRH) (165, 173).

GASTROINTESTINAL EFFECTS

Octreotide increases intestinal transit time, decreases gut fluid secretion, and increases gut absorption of fluid and electrolytes. Intravenous infusion of 1 μg/kg/hr increases intestinal transit time through 30 cm of jejunum from 4 to 17 minutes in normal subjects (174).

Octreotide inhibits secretion of many gastrointestinal hormones (i.e., insulin, glucagon, pancreatic polypeptide, gastric inhibitory polypeptide, gastrin, neurotensin, secretin, motilin) (168, 170). Postprandial hyperglycemia and an increase in fasting plasma glucose may result (probably from diminished insulin secretion) (167, 170, 175). Octreotide also inhibits pancreatic secretion of lipase, trypsin, and amylase. It inhibits gallbladder contraction and bilirubin secretion. In addition, octreotide reduces hepatic, splanchnic, and gastric mucosal blood flow.

Octreotide has been effective in reducing diarrhea in patients with VIP-secreting tumors (50 μg subcutaneously). It reduces secretion and improves fluid absorption. Octreotide has also been used to treat diarrhea resulting from many other causes (i.e., short gut syndrome, AIDS, inflammatory bowel disease, dysfunctional gut following shock) (176, 177). Disorders of the gastrointestinal tract are common in patients with AIDS. These patients often develop diarrhea caused by various pathogens. Octreotide decreased stool output in patients with AIDS-associated diarrhea unresponsive to antidiarrheal medication (176). Stool output decreased from 1640 ± 183 ml/day to 1084 ± 162 ml/day. Forty-one percent of patients had >50% reduction in stool volume.

Although octreotide is effective in decreasing stool output in some patients, it is unclear whether the drug improves the disease process. Octreotide decreases stool output by decreasing the secretion of gut digestive enzymes (i.e., pepsin, trypsin, amylase, lipase) and tropic factors (i.e., glucagon, neurotensin, gastrin). Although it increases fluid and electrolyte absorption, somatostatin decreases macronutrient absorption (178). In addition, it also decreases the secretion of growth hormone, insulin, and TSH. The net result is gut atrophy and decreases in circulating anabolic hormones. The impact of these changes on nitrogen balance, protein synthesis, gut bacterial translocation, wound repair, and recovery from illness requires further evaluation.

Somatostatin and octreotide are used to treat patients with gastrointestinal fistulas (179–181). A multicenter randomized trial (179) found no differences in overall fistula closure rate in patients randomized to parenteral nutrition versus parenteral nutrition plus somatostatin. However, somatostatin shortened the time for fistula closure and reduced morbidity.

NEUROENDOCRINE TUMORS OF THE GUT

A major objective in the treatment of endocrine tumors of the gut is to reduce the amount of hormone produced and reduce symptoms. Octreotide is effective in reducing hormone secretion and controlling symptoms (flushing and diarrhea) in patients with carcinoid tumors (182, 183) and VIPomas (184, 185). Dosage requirements range from 100 to 1100 μg/day. Octreotide is currently approved for control of symptoms associated with metastatic carcinoid and VIP-secreting tumors. The drug is not effective in reducing tumor mass.

MISCELLANEOUS USES

Octreotide antagonizes endogenous insulin release and has been used to treat sulfonylurea overdose (186). Somatostatin inhibits glucagon secretion and delays glucose absorption. It may be useful as an adjunct to insulin in the treatment of diabetes mellitus. It must be given with exogenous insulin since it also inhibits insulin secretion from the pancreas. Administration of somatostatin along with insulin was more effective than insulin alone in controlling hyperglycemia and allowed for reduction in insulin requirements (187). Somatostatin attenuates the development of hyperglycemia and ketosis after acute insulin withdrawal in type I diabetes mellitus (187). The long-term effects of somatostatin in the treatment of diabetes mellitus are unknown. Somatostatin reduces splanchnic blood flow and decreases portal pressures in patients with esophageal varices (188, 189). Both gastrin and gastric acid are reduced by somatostatin. It has been used to treat hypergastrinemia in patients with Zollinger-Ellison syndrome (190) and peptic ulcer disease (191). In one study (191), somatostatin was more effective than cimetidine in controlling hemorrhage in patients with peptic ulcer disease who were not surgical candidates.

PREPARATIONS AND SIDE EFFECTS

Octreotide is supplied in 1-ml ampules containing 0.05, 0.1, or 0.5 mg. Treatment is usually initiated at 50 μg subcutaneously b.i.d. The dose is increased to 50 to 100 μg subcutaneously t.i.d. and then tapered to effect. Average dose requirements for treating carcinoid tumors and VIPomas is 200 to 300 μg/day.

Octreotide is associated with both hyperglycemia (resulting from decreased insulin secretion) and hypoglycemia. It potentiates the hypoglycemic effect of exogenous insulin. Insulin doses should be reduced in diabetic patients.

Cholelithiasis may occur as a result of altered fat absorption and decreased gallbladder motility. Fat malabsorption may result in depletion of fat-soluble vitamins (i.e., A, D, E, K). Drug and nutrient absorption are also altered. Drugs should be monitored with blood levels where appropriate.

Hypothalamic-pituitary function is poorly studied. A decrease in thyroxine is reported and patients rarely may develop hypothyroidism. The drug has the potential to decrease wound healing, diminish gut mass, and reduce nitrogen balance.

PROLACTIN

Prolactin was named based upon its stimulation of milk secretion from the breast. It is a 198-amino-acid protein secreted by the adenohypophysis. Prolactin stimulates growth and development of the breast during pregnancy (also requires cortisol, thyroxine, estrogens, progestins). It is responsible for proliferation and differentiation of mammary ductal and alveolar epithelium and synthesis of milk proteins. Suckling is a potent stimulus for prolactin secretion. Prolactin is believed to have an inhibitory effect on gonadotropin action and may be responsible for the lack of ovulation and infertility during breast feeding and in patients with pituitary prolactinomas.

Normal levels of prolactin in serum are 5 to 10 μg/liter. Plasma half-life is 15 to 20 minutes. Secretion of prolactin is normally under negative control by the hypothalamus. The major inhibitor of secretion is dopamine. Secretion is also inhibited by ergot derivatives, bromocriptine, and levodopa.

Dopamine antagonists (i.e., haloperidol, phenothiazines, metoclopramide), TRH, opioid peptides, sleep, stress, hypoglycemia, and exercise raise circulating prolactin levels.

A number of regulatory interactions among the CNS, neuroendocrine axis, and immune system have been described. Several lines of evidence suggest that prolactin may be an important immunoregulatory hormone (192). In rats, hypophysectomy and treatment with the dopamine agonist bromocriptine inhibits development of delayed cutaneous hypersensitivity, experimental allergic encephalitis, and adjuvant-induced arthritis. Prolactin reverses these immunosuppressive effects (192–194). Cyclosporin, an immunosuppressive peptide, inhibits prolactin binding to lymphocytes. Immunodeficiency in hypopituitary mice is prevented with injections of milk (a source of prolactin). Injection of bromocriptine, to suppress serum prolactin, prevents induction of tumoricidal macrophages by *Mycobacterium bovis*, *Listeria monocytogenes*, or *Propionibacterium acnes* (192). Simultaneous injection of prolactin restores induction of tumoricidal macrophages. Antiprolactin antibodies inhibit lymphocyte proliferation in response to T- and B-cell mitogens (195), IL-2, and IL-4. Bromocriptine suppresses serum prolactin and splenocyte proliferation responses to concanavalin A and lipopolysaccharide (192). Prolactin reverses these effects. Prolactin is also required for normal production of macrophage activating factors such as γ-interferon (192). Thus, hypoprolactinemia may be a cause of suppressed immune function.

Suppression of prolactin with bromocriptine resulted in a 67% mortality in mice following injection with Listeria. When prolactin was administered with bromocriptine, mortality from *Listeria* was only 33% (192). Thus, suppression of prolactin can compromise host defenses and increase the lethality of an infectious challenge. The implications of these findings for the treatment of critically ill and immunosuppressed patients requires further study.

G-CSF AND GM-CSF

Four colony-stimulating factors influence the survival, proliferation, differentiation, and functional activation of myeloid hematopoietic cells (196, 197). They are macrophage colony-stimulating factor (M-CSF), granulocyte colony-stimulating factor (G-CSF), granulocyte-macrophage colony-stimulating factor (GM-CSF), and interleukin-3. Only G-CSF and GM-CSF are commercially available for clinical use. G-CSF has been approved in the U.S. for the reduction of infection from myelotoxic chemotherapy in patients with nonmyeloid tumors. GM-CSF has been approved in the U.S. for use during reconstitution after autologous bone marrow transplantation in patients with lymphoid tumors.

The endogenous physiologic functions of colony-stimulating factors remain unclear. It would seem reasonable that these factors are part of the normal homeostatic systems that maintain and alter leukocyte counts. However, such a relationship remains unproved. Deficiency states for these factors have not been recognized. Thus, therapeutic administration of colony-stimulating factors is supplementary to endogenous factor production. The basis for the use of colony-stimulating

factors is the belief that the severity and duration of neutropenia correlates with the risk of infection. G-CSF and GM-CSF are manufactured using recombinant DNA technology.

Colony-stimulating factors should not be given immediately prior to or overlapping with chemotherapy. The cycling of hematopoietic progenitor cells stimulated by the factors may increase their susceptibility to cytotoxic drugs, increasing myelotoxicity.

G-CSF

The biologic effects of G-CSF have been studied following intravenous and subcutaneous administration in normal subjects and patients with cancer. G-CSF (3 to 10 μg/kg/day) results in an immediate transient decrease in leukocytes with a nadir at 5 to 15 minutes after intravenous administration and 30 to 60 minutes after subcutaneous administration. Leukopenia results from a decrease in circulating neutrophils and monocytes. Thus, blood samples for monitoring the hematologic effects of G-CSF should be obtained just prior to the dose. The decrease in leukocytes following G-CSF is followed by a sustained dose-dependent increase in circulating neutrophils. High doses of G-CSF may induce excessive leukocytosis and bone pain. With high doses of G-CSF (>10 μg/kg/day), there is also a slight increase in monocytes and lymphocytes. The neutrophilia is characterized by a left shift toward more immature cells. Neutrophilia results from increased input of precursor cells into the myeloblast compartment, increased neutrophil production, and shortening of the time for neutrophil precursors to mature and appear in the circulation (i.e., from 5 days to 1 day). Following discontinuation of G-CSF, neutrophils return to baseline over 4 to 7 days. G-CSF does not alter reticulocyte, erythrocyte, or platelet counts when given at recommended doses. At very high doses (i.e., 30 to 40 μg/kg/day), platelet counts may decrease slightly.

Neutrophils from patients treated with G-CSF have normal activity. Numerous studies have demonstrated beneficial effects of G-CSF on neutrophil recovery (197). The prophylactic (to prevent infections) administration of G-CSF was beneficial in a randomized, placebo-controlled, double-blind study of patients receiving chemotherapy for small cell lung cancer (198). G-CSF administration (230 μg/m²/day) for 8 to 13 days reduced the duration of neutropenia, infections, antibiotic usage, and hospitalization time. It is unknown whether chemotherapy patients who have not received G-CSF prophylactically will benefit from G-CSF once they become infected and have neutropenia.

Following autologous bone marrow transplantation, G-CSF accelerates recovery of neutrophils (197). Benefits have included reduced hospitalization time and use of parenteral nutrition. However, no definitive randomized clinical trial of G-CSF in patients undergoing bone marrow transplantation has been reported. G-CSF may also be useful in treating neutropenia and reducing infections in patients with chronic neutropenic diseases (197).

G-CSF usually is administered at doses of 1 to 20 μg/kg/day. A common regimen gives G-CSF at a dose of 5 μg/kg/day subcutaneously 1 day after the last dose of cytotoxic drug. G-CSF is stopped when the neutrophil count rises to 7000 cells/mm³ (so as to avoid rebound leukocytosis). The terminal elimination half-life of intravenous G-CSF, at doses of 3 to 60 μg/kg over 20 to 30 minutes, ranges from 1.3 to 7.2 hours (196). Side effects include bone pain and, rarely, vasculitis or anaphylaxis. Bone pain usually responds to analgesics.

GM-CSF

GM-CSF has been studied in patients with cancer. It is less potent than G-CSF on the neutrophil. However, GM-CSF also increases eosinophil and monocyte counts. Administration of GM-CSF is followed by transient leukopenia caused by a decrease in eosinophils, neutrophils, and monocytes. The effect of GM-CSF on the bone marrow is similar to that of G-CSF. In addition, GM-CSF increases eosinophil production rate. GM-CSF does not shorten the time required for neutrophils to appear in the circulation (as does G-CSF), but the circulating half-life of neutrophils is increased (8 to 48 hours).

GM-CSF has improved neutrophil counts in uncontrolled studies of cytotoxic chemotherapy (197). However, prospective controlled trials documenting clinical efficacy (i.e., fewer infections) have not been performed. GM-CSF has also been studied in patients receiving autologous bone marrow transplantation. Allogenic bone marrow transplantation is more complicated and GM-CSF may induce graft-vs.-host disease in these patients. In a randomized, placebo-controlled study of GM-CSF (250 μg/m² as a 2-hour infusion daily for 21 days) in patients undergoing autologous bone marrow transplantation after myeloablative therapy for malignant hematologic diseases, the administration of GM-CSF accelerated recovery of neutrophils (reduced from 26 days to 19 days), shortened duration of antibiotic chemotherapy, and reduced hospital stay (199). GM-CSF also reduced duration of neutropenia and infections when used as an adjunct to autologous hematopoietic stem cell transplantation for lymphoma (200). In addition, GM-CSF reduced duration of neutropenia, platelet-transfusion dependency, hospital stay, and total hospital charges when used as adjunct therapy in the treatment of relapsed Hodgkin's disease (randomized, placebo-controlled trial) (201).

At doses of 0.3 to 10 μg/kg/day, GM-CSF causes lethargy, myalgias, bone pain, anorexia, skin eruptions, and flushing. GM-CSF also causes fever and chills. The first dose of GM-CSF has been reported to induce a syndrome characterized by flushing, tachycardia, hypotension, musculoskeletal pain, dyspnea, nausea/vomiting, and arterial oxygen desaturation. This first-dose reaction occurs with doses >1 μg/kg and is more common after intravenous injection than subcutaneous administration. High doses (>20 μg/kg/day) may cause fluid retention, pleural and pericardial inflammation and effusions, and venous thrombosis. These adverse effects may be induced by cytokine production from stimulated leukocytes.

Recommended doses of GM-CSF are 1 to 6 μg/kg/day. In bone marrow transplantation, a dose of 250 μg/m² over 2 to 4 hours intravenously per day for 21 days is recommended. The terminal-phase elimination half-life for GM-CSF, after intravenous bolus doses of 0.3 to 3 μg/kg, are 0.2 to 1.2 hours (0.6 to 9.1 hours after 20- to 30-minute intravenous infusions of 3 to 30 μg/kg) (196). Many of the adverse effects of GM-CSF

adminstration can be reduced with low-dose subcutaneous administration (i.e., 125 μg/m² twice daily).

Patients should receive monitoring of blood counts, renal function, and hepatic function. GM-CSF should not be given to patients with a history of idiopathic thrombocytopenia purpura (since reactivation has been reported), and it should be given cautiously to patients with autoimmune or inflammatory diseases (i.e., thyroiditis, rheumatoid arthritis, autoimmune hemolysis).

REFERENCES

1. Hays RM: Agents affecting the renal conservation of water. In Gilman AG, Rall TW, Nies AS, Taylor P (eds): *The Pharmacological Basis of Therapeutics,* ed 8. Pergamon Press, New York, p 732, 1990.
2. Richardson DW, Robinson AG: Desmopressin. *Ann Intern Med* 103:228, 1985.
3. Chanson P, Jedynak CP, Czernichow P: Management of early postoperative diabetes insipidus with parenteral desmopressin. *Acta Endocrinol* 117:513, 1988.
4. Chanson P, Jedynak CP, Dabrowski G, et al: Ultralow doses of vasopressin in the management of diabetes insipidus. *Crit Care Med* 15:44, 1987.
5. Greger NG, Kirkland RT, Clayton GW, Kirkland JL: Central diabetes insipidus: 22 years' experience. *Am J Dis Child* 140:551, 1986.
6. Robertson GL: Diagnosis of diabetes insipidus. *Front Hormone Res* 13:176, 1985.
7. Hall J, Robertson G: Diabetes insipidus. *Probl Crit Care (Endocrine Emergencies)* 4:372, 1990.
8. Zaloga GP: Hyperosmolar states. In Civetta JM, Taylor RW, Kirby RR (eds): *Critical Care,* ed 2. JB Lippincott, Philadelphia, p 447, 1992.
9. Miller M, Dalakos T, Moses AM, Fellerman H, Streeten DH: Recognition of partial defects in antidiuretic hormone secretion. *Ann Intern Med* 73:721, 1970.
10. Sterns RH: The management of hyponatremic emergencies. *Crit Care Clin* 7:127, 1991.
11. Zaloga GP: Electrolyte disorders. In Civetta JM, Taylor RW, Kirby RR (eds): *Critical Care,* ed 2. JB Lippincott, Philadelphia, p 481, 1992.
12. Vokes TJ, Robertson GL: Disorders of antidiuretic hormone. *Endocrinol Metab Clin North Am* 17:281, 1988.
13. Mannucci PM, Ruggeri ZM, Pareti FI, Capitanio A: 1-desamino-8-D-arginine vasopressin: a new pharmacological approach to the management of haemophilia and von Willebrand's disease. *Lancet* 1:869, 1977.
14. Warrier AI, Lusher JM: DDAVP: a useful alternative to blood components in moderate hemophilia A and von Willebrand disease. *J Pediatr* 102:228, 1983.
15. Mariana G, Ciavarella N, Mazzucconi MG, et al: Evaluation of the effectiveness of DDAVP in surgery and in bleeding episodes in haemophilia and von Willebrand's disease. A study on 43 patients. *Clin Lab Haematol* 6:229, 1984.
16. de la Fuente B, Kasper CK, Rickles FE, Hoyer LW: Response of patients with mild and moderate hemophilia A and von Willebrand's disease to treatment with desmopressin. *Ann Intern Med* 103:6, 1985.
17. Kohler M, Hellstern P, Miyashita C, von Blohn G, Wenzel E: Comparative study of intranasal, subcutaneous and intravenous administration of desamino-D-arginine vasopressin (DDAVP). *Thromb Haemost* 55:108, 1986.
18. Nilsson IM, Holmberg L, Aberg M, Vilhardt H: The release of plasminogen activator and factor VIII after injection of DDAVP in healthy volunteers and in patients with von Willebrand's disease. *Scand J Haematol* 24:351, 1980.
19. Kobrinsky NL, Israels ED, Gerrard JM, et al: Shortening of bleeding time by 1-deamino-8-D-arginine vasopressin in various bleeding disorders. *Lancet* i:1145, 1984.
20. Mannucci PM, Remuzzi G, Pusineri F, et al: Deamino-8-D-arginine vasopressin shortens the bleeding time in uremia. *N Engl J Med* 308:8, 1983.
21. Watson AJ, Keogh JA: 1-deamino-8-D-arginine vasopressin (DDAVP): a potential new treatment for the bleeding diathesis of acute renal failure. *Pharmatherapeutic* 3:618, 1984.
22. Rose EH, Aledort LM: Nasal spray desmopressin (DDAVP) for mild hemophilia A and von Willebrand disease. *Ann Intern Med* 114:563, 1991.
23. Salzman EW, Weinstein MJ, Weintraub RM, et al: Treatment with desmopressin acetate to reduce blood loss after cardiac surgery. A double-blind randomized trial. *N Engl J Med* 314:1402, 1986.
24. Rosa RM, Bierer BE, Thomas R, et al: A study of induced hyponatremia in the prevention and treatment of sickle-cell crisis. *N Engl J Med* 303:1138, 1980.
25. Conn HO, Ramsby GR, Storer EH, et al: Intraarterial vasopressin in the treatment of upper gastrointestinal hemorrhage: a prospective, controlled clinical trial. *Gastroenterology* 68:211, 1975.
26. Schweitzer EJ, Kerr JC, Swan KG: Clinical use of vasopressin in the management of bleeding esophageal varices. *Am Surg* 48:558, 1982.
27. Chojkier M, Groszmann RJ, Atterbury CE, et al: A controlled comparison of continuous intraarterial and intravenous infusions of vasopressin in hemorrhage from esophageal varices. *Gastroenterology* 77:540, 1979.

28. Johnson WC, Widrich WC, Ansell JE, Robbins AH, Nabseth DC: Control of bleeding varices by vasopressin: a prospective randomized study. *Ann Surg* 186:369, 1977.

29. Bush HL Jr, Nabseth DC: Intravenous nitroglycerin to improve coronary blood flow and left ventricular performance during vasopressin therapy. *Surg Forum* 30:226, 1979.

30. Groszmann RJ, Kravetz D, Bosch J, et al: Nitroglycerin improves the hemodynamic response to vasopressin in portal hypertension. *Hepatology* 2:757, 1982.

31. Robinette C, Gerlock AJ: Intraarterial vasopressin infusion in treating acute gastrointestinal bleeding. *South Med J* 73:209, 1980.

32. Chwals WJ, Bistrian BR: Role of exogenous growth hormone and insulin-like growth factor I in malnutrition and acute metabolic stress: a hypothesis. *Crit Care Med* 19:1317, 1991.

33. Phillips LS, Unterman TG: Somatomedin activity in disorders of nutrition and metabolism. *Clin Endocrinol Metab* 13:145, 1984.

34. Bornfeldt KE, Arnqvist HJ, Enberg B, Mathews LS, Norstedt G: Regulation of insulin-like growth factor-I and growth hormone receptor gene expression by diabetes and nutritional state in rat tissues. *J Endocrinol* 122:651, 1989.

35. Valimaki M, Liewendahl L, Karonen SL, Helenius T, Suikkari AM: Concentrations of somatomedin-C and triiodothyronine in patients with thyroid dysfunction and nonthyroidal illnesses. *J Endocrinol Invest* 13:155, 1990.

36. Brandl M, Pscheidl E, Amann W, Barjasic A, Pasch T: Biochemical and hormonal parameters in patients with multiple trauma. *Prog Clin Biol Res* 308:743, 1989.

37. Coates CL, Burwell RG, Carlin SA, et al: Somatomedin activity in plasma from burned patients with observations on plasma cortisol. *Burns* 7:425, 1981.

38. Coates CL, Burwell RG, Carlin SA, et al: The somatomedin activity in plasma from patients with multiple mechanical injuries: with observations on plasma cortisol. *Injury* 13:100, 1981.

39. Frayn KN, Price DA, Maycock PF, Carroll SM: Plasma somatomedin activity after injury in man and its relationship to other hormonal and metabolic changes. *Clin Endocrinol* 20:179, 1984.

40. Hawker FH, Stewart PM, Baxter RC, et al: Relationship of somatomedin-C/insulin-like growth factor I levels to conventional nutritional indices in critically ill patients. *Crit Care Med* 15:732, 1987.

41. Anand KJ: The stress response to surgical trauma: from physiological basis to therapeutic implications. *Prog Food Nutr Sci* 10:67, 1986.

42. Dahn MS, Lange MP, Jacobs LA: Insulin-like growth factor I production is inhibited in human sepsis. *Arch Surg* 123:1409, 1988.

43. Manson JM, Smith RJ, Wilmore DW: Growth hormone stimulates protein synthesis during hypocaloric parenteral nutrition. Role of hormonal-substrate environment. *Ann Surg* 208:136, 1988.

44. Manson JM, Wilmore DW: Positive nitrogen balance with human growth hormone and hypocaloric intravenous feeding. *Surgery* 100:188, 1986.

45. Binnerts A, Wilson JH, Lamberts SW: The effects of human growth hormone administration in elderly adults with recent weight loss. *J Clin Endocrinol Metab* 67:1312, 1988.

46. Rudman D, Feller AG, Nagraj HS, et al: Effects of human growth hormone in men over 60 years old. *N Engl J Med* 323:1, 1990.

47. Clemmons DR, Snyder DK, Williams R, Underwood LE: Growth hormone administration conserves lean body mass during dietary restriction in obese subjects. *J Clin Endocrinol Metab* 64:878, 1987.

48. Pape GS, Friedman M, Underwood LE, Clemmons DR: The effect of growth hormone on weight gain and pulmonary function in patients with chronic obstructive lung disease. *Chest* 99:1495, 1991.

49. Ziegler TR, Young LS, Manson JM, Wilmore DW: Metabolic effects of recombinant human growth hormone in patients receiving parenteral nutrition. *Ann Surg* 208:6, 1988.

50. Ward HC, Halliday D, Sim AJ: Protein and energy metabolism with biosynthetic human growth hormone after gastrointestinal surgery. *Ann Surg* 206:56, 1987.

51. Jiang ZM, He GZ, Zhang SY, et al: Low-dose growth hormone and hypocaloric nutrition attenuate the protein-catabolic response after major operation. *Ann Surg* 210:513, 1989.

52. Soroff HS, Pearson E, Green NL, Artz CP: The effect of growth hormone on nitrogen balance at various levels of intake in burned patients. *Surg Gynecol Obstet* 111:259, 1960.

53. Soroff HS, Rozin RR, Mooty J, Lister J, Raben MS: Role of human growth hormone in the response to trauma. I. Metabolic effects following burns. *Ann Surg* 166:739, 1967.

54. Wilmore DW, Moylan JA Jr, Bristow BF, Mason AD Jr, Pruitt BA Jr: Anabolic effects of human growth hormone and high caloric feedings following thermal injury. *Surg Gynecol Obstet* 138:875, 1974.

55. Belcher HJ, Mercer D, Judkins KC, et al: Biosynthetic human growth hormone in burned patients: a pilot study. *Burns* 15:99, 1989.

56. Herndon DN, Barrow RE, Kunkel KR, Broemeling L, Rutan RL: Effects of recombinant human growth hormone on donor-site healing in severely burned children. *Ann Surg* 212:424, 1990.

57. Mehls O, Ritz E, Hunziker EB, Eggli P, Heinrich U, Zapf J: Improvement of growth and food utilization by human recombinant growth hormone in uremia. *Kidney Int* 33:45, 1988.

58. Tönshoff B, Mehls O, Schauer A, Heinrich U, Blum W, Ranke M: Improvement of uremic growth failure by recombinant human growth hormone. *Kidney Int* 36(Suppl 27):S201, 1989.

59. Hollander DM, Devereux DF, Marafino BJ, Hoppe H: Increased wound breaking strength in rats following treatment with synthetic human growth hormone. *Surg Forum* 35:612, 1984.

60. Zaizen Y, Ford EG, Costin G, Atkinson JB: The effect of perioperative exogenous growth hormone on wound bursting strength in normal and malnourished rats. *J Pediatr Surg* 25:70, 1990.

61. Pessa ME, Bland KI, Sitren HS, Miller GJ, Copeland EM III: Improved wound healing in tumor-bearing rats treated with perioperative synthetic human growth hormone. *Surgery* 36:6, 1985.

62. Belcher HJ, Ellis H: Somatatropin and wound healing after injury. *J Clin Endocrinol Metab* 70:939, 1990.

63. Winawer ST, Sherlock P, Sonenberg M, Vanamee P: Beneficial effect of human growth hormone on stress ulcers. *Arch Intern Med* 135:569, 1975.

64. Saito H, Taniwaka K, Hiramatu T, Morioka Y: Growth hormone treatment enhances immune function in surgically stressed rats. *J Parenter Enteral Nutr* 14(Suppl 1):10S, 1990.

65. Schalch DS, Heinrich UE, Draznin B, Johnson CJ, Miller LL: Role of the liver in regulating somatomedin activity: hormonal effects on the synthesis and release of insulin-like growth factor and its carrier protein by the isolated perfused rat liver. *Endocrinology* 104:1143, 1979.

66. Wolf M, Ingbar SH, Moses AC: Thyroid hormone and growth hormone interact to regulate insulin-like growth factor-I messenger ribonucleic acid and circulating levels in the rat. *Endocrinology* 125:2905, 1989.

67. Zaloga GP, Smallridge RD: Thyroidal alterations in acute illness. *Semin Resp Med* 7:95, 1985.

68. Zaloga GP, Chernow B, Smallridge RC, et al: A longitudinal evaluation of thyroid function in critically ill surgical patients. *Ann Surg* 201:456, 1985.

69. Isley WL, Underwood LE, Clemmons DR: Dietary components that regulate serum somatomedin-C concentrations in humans. *J Clin Invest* 71:175, 1983.

70. Clemmons DR, Klibanski A, Underwood LE, et al: Reduction of plasma immunoreactive somatomedin C during fasting in humans. *J Clin Endocrinol Metab* 53:1247, 1981.

71. Donahue SP, Phillips LS: Response of IGF-1 to nutritional support in malnourished hospital patients: a possible indicator of short-term changes in nutritional status. *Am J Clin Nutr* 50:962, 1989.

72. Unterman TG, Vazquez RM, Slas AJ, Martyn PA, Phillips LS: Nutrition and somatomedin. XIII. Usefulness of somatomedin-C in nutritional assessment. *Am J Med* 78:228, 1985.

73. Schalch DS, Yang H, Ney DM, DiMarchi RD: Infusion of human insulin-like growth factor I (IGF-I) into malnourished rats reduces hepatic IGF-I mRNA abundance. *Biochem Biophys Res Commun* 160:795, 1989.

74. Jacob R, Barrett E, Plewe G, Fagin KD, Sherwin RS: Acute effects of insulin-like growth factor I on glucose and amino acid metabolism in the awake fasted rat. Comparison with insulin. *J Clin Invest* 83:1717, 1989.

75. Zaloga GP, Malcolm DS, Holaday JW, Chernow B: Glucagon. In Chernow B (ed): *The Pharmacologic Approach to the Critically Ill Patient*, ed 2. Baltimore, Williams & Wilkins, pp 659, 1988.

76. Kahn CR, Schechter Y: Insulin, oral hypoglycemic agents, and the pharmacology of the endocrine pancreas. In Gilman AG, Rall TW, Nies AS, Taylor P (ed): *The Pharmacologic Basis of Therapeutics*, ed 8. Pergamon Press, New York, pp 1463, 1990.

77. Lefebvre PJ: *Glucagon*, vols. 1 and 2. Springer-Verlag, Berlin, 1983.

78. Gerich JE, Lorenzi M, Bier DM, et al: Prevention of human diabetic ketoacidosis by somatostatin. Evidence for an essential role of glucagon. *N Engl J Med* 292:985, 1975.

79. Lickley HL, Kemmer FW, Doi K, Vranic M: Glucagon suppression improves glucoregulation in moderate but not chronic severe diabetes. *Am J Physiol* 245:E424, 1983.

80. MacCuish AC, Munro JF, Duncan LJ: Treatment of hypoglycaemic coma with glucagon, intravenous dextrose, and mannitol infusion in a hundred diabetics. *Lancet* ii:946, 1970.

81. Elrick H, Witten TA, Arai Y: Glucagon treatment of insulin reaction. *N Engl J Med* 258:476, 1958.

82. Muhlhauser I, Koch J, Berger M: Pharmacokinetics and bioavailability of injected glucagon: differences between intramuscular, subcutaneous, and intravenous administration. *Diabetes Care* 8:39, 1985.

83. Farah A, Tuttle R: Studies on the pharmacology of glucagon. *J Pharmacol Exp Ther* 129:49, 1960.

84. Farah AE: Glucagon and the circulation. *Pharmacol Rev* 35:181, 1983.

85. Klein SW, Morch JE, Mahon WA: Cardiovascular effects of glucagon in man. *Can Med Assoc J* 98:1161, 1968.

86. Lvoff R, Wilcken DE: Glucagon in heart failure and in cardiogenic shock. Experience in 50 patients. *Circulation* 45:534, 1972.

87. Lucchesi BR: Cardiac actions of glucagon. *Circ Res* 22:777, 1968.

88. Parmley WW, Glick G, Sonnenblick EH: Cardiovascular effects of glucagon in man. *N Engl J Med* 279:12, 1968.

89. Siegel JH, Levine MJ, McConn R, del Guercio LR: The effect of glucagon infusion on cardiovascular function in the critically ill. *Surg Gynecol Obstet* 131:505, 1970.

90. Jolly SR, Jordan JC, Rose GC: Stimulation of myocardial function after brief regional ischemia by glucagon. *Drug Dev Res* 22:125, 1991.

91. Glick G, Parmley WW, Wechsler AS, Sonnenblick EH: Glucagon. Its enhancement of cardiac performance in the cat and dog and persistence of its inotropic action despite beta-receptor blockade with propranolol. *Circ Res* 22:789, 1968.

92. Sutherland EW, Robison GA, Butcher RW: Some aspects of the biological role of adenosine 3′,5′-monophosphate (cyclic AMP). *Circulation* 37:279, 1968.

93. Nayler WG, McInnes I, Chipperfield D, Carson V, Daile P: The effect of glucagon on calcium exchangeability, coronary blood flow, myocardial function and high energy phosphate stores. *J Pharmacol Exp Ther* 171:265, 1970.

94. MacLeod KM, Rodgers RL, McNeill JH: Characterization of glucagon-induced changes in rate, contractility and cyclic AMP levels in isolated cardiac preparations of the rat and guinea pig. *J Pharmacol Exp Ther* 217:798, 1981.

95. Barritt GJ, Spiel PF: Effects of glucagon on Ca outflow exchange in the isolated perfused rat heart. *Biochem Pharmacol* 30:1407, 1981.

96. Mery PF, Brechler V, Pavoine C, Pecker F, Fischmeister R: Glucagon stimulates the cardiac Ca^{2+} current by activation of adenylyl cyclase and inhibition of phosphodiesterase. *Nature* 345:158, 1990.

97. Chernow B, Zaloga GP, Malcolm D, Willey SC, Clapper M, Holaday JW: Glucagon's chronotropic action is calcium dependent. *J Pharmacol Exp Ther* 241:833, 1987.

98. Malcolm D, Zaloga G, Chernow B, Holaday J: Glucagon is an antagonist of morphine bradycardia and antinociception. *Life Sci* 39:399, 1986.

99. Deraney MF: Glucagon? One answer to cardiogenic shock. *Am J Med Sci* 261:149, 1971.

100. Drucker MR, Pindyck F, Brown RS, Elwyn DH, Shoemaker WC: The interaction of glucagon and glucose on cardiorespiratory variables in the critically ill patient. *Surgery* 75:487, 1974.

101. Eddy JD, O'Brien ET, Singh SP: Glucagon and haemodynamics of acute myocardial infarction. *Br Med J* 4:663, 1969.

102. Parmley WW, Matloff JM, Sonnenblick EH: Hemodynamic effects of glucagon in patients following prosthetic value replacement. *Circulation* 39(suppl 5):I163, 1969.

103. Parmley WW, Sonnenblick EH: A role for glucagon in cardiac therapy. *Am J Med Sci* 258:224, 1969.

104. Bower MG, Okude S, Jolley WB, Smith LL: Hemodynamic effects of glucagon following hemorrhage and endotoxic shock in the dog. *Arch Surg* 101:411, 1970.

105. Guillen J, Pappas G: Improved cardiovascular effects of glucagon in dogs with endotoxin shock. *Ann Surg* 175:535, 1972.

106. Teich S, Malcolm D, Zaloga GP, Holaday J, Chernow B: Beneficial effects of glucagon in endotoxic shock in rats (abstr.). *Circ Shock* 16:95, 1985.

107. Weingand KW, Fettman MJ, Phillips RW, Hand MS: Metabolic effects of glucagon in endotoxemic minipigs. *Circ Shock* 18:289, 1986.

108. Bowman HM, Cowan D, Kovach G Jr, Hook JB: Renal effects of glucagon in rhesus monkeys during hypovolemia. *Surg Gynecol Obstet* 134:937, 1972.

109. Schumer W, Miller B, Nichols RL, McDonald GO, Nyhus LM: Metabolic and microcirculatory effects of glucagon in hypovolemic shock. *Arch Surg* 107:176, 1973.

110. VanderWall DA, Stowe NT, Spangenberg R, Hook JB: Effect of glucagon in hemorrhagic shock. *J Surg Oncol* 2:177, 1970.

111. Jain KM, Rush BF Jr, Hastings OM, Ghosh A, Slotman G, Abousam S: Glucagon treatment of hemorrhagic shock: improved survival and metabolic parameters in a murine shock model. *Adv Shock Res* 1:149, 1978.

112. Andjelkovic I, Zlokovic B: Protective effects of glucagon during the anaphylactic response in guinea-pig isolated heart. *Br J Pharmacol* 76:483, 1982.

113. Steiner C, Wit AL, Damato AN: Effects of glucagon on atrioventricular conduction and ventricular automaticity in dogs. *Circ Res* 24:167, 1969.

114. Neimann JT, Haynes KS, Garner D, Jagels G, Rennie CJ III: Postcountershock pulseless rhythms: hemodynamic effects of glucagon in a canine model. *Crit Care Med* 15:554, 1987.

115. Whitsitt LS, Lucchesi BR: Effects of beta-receptor blockade and glucagon on the atrioventricular transmission system in the dog. *Circ Res* 23:585, 1968.

116. Agura ED, Wexler LF, Witzburg RA: Massive propranolol overdose—successful treatment with high-dose isoproterenol and glucagon. *Am J Med* 80:755, 1986.

117. Chernow B, Reed L, Geelhoed GW, et al: Glucagon: endocrine effects and calcium involvement in cardiovascular actions in dogs. *Circ Shock* 19:393, 1986.

118. Kosinski EJ, Malindzak GS Jr: Glucagon and isoproterenol in reversing propranolol toxicity. *Arch Intern Med* 132:840, 1973.

119. Peterson CD, Leeder JS, Sterner S: Glucagon therapy for β-blocker overdose. *Drug Intell Clin Pharm* 18:394, 1984.

120. Zaloga GP, DeLacey W, Holmboe E, Chernow B: Glucagon reversal of hypotension in a case of anaphylactoid shock. *Ann Intern Med* 105:65, 1986.

121. Furukawa Y, Saegusa K, Ogiwara Y, Chiba S: Different effectiveness of glucagon on the pacemaker activity and contractility in intact dog hearts and in isolated perfused right atria. *Jpn Heart J* 27:215, 1986.

122. Prasad K, Weckworth P: Glucagon in procainamide induced cardiac toxicity. *Toxicol Appl Pharmacol* 46:517, 1978.

123. Cohn KE, Agmon J, Gamble OW: The effect of glucagon on arrhythmias due to digitalis toxicity. *Am J Cardiol* 25:683, 1970.

124. Prasad K, DeSousa HH: Glucagon in the treatment of ouabain-induced cardiac arrhythmias in dogs. *Cardiovasc Res* 6:333, 1972.

125. Zaloga GP, Malcolm D, Holaday J, Chernow B: Glucagon reverses the hypotension and bradycardia of verapamil overdose in rats (abstr.). *Crit Care Med* 13:273, 1985.

126. Sabatier J, Pouyet T, Shelvey G, Cavero I: Antagonistic effects of epinephrine, glucagon and methylatropine but not calcium chloride against atrio-ventricular conduction disturbances produced by high doses of diltiazem, in conscious dogs. *Fundam Clin Pharmacol* 5:93, 1991.

127. Zaritsky AL, Horowitz M, Chernow B: Glucagon antagonism of calcium channel blocker-induced myocardial dysfunction. *Crit Care Med* 16:246, 1988.

128. Jolly SR, Kipnis JN, Lucchesi BR: Cardiovascular depression by verapamil: reversal by glucagon and interactions with propranolol. *Pharmacology* 35:249, 1987.

129. Prasad K: Use of glucagon in the treatment of quinidine toxicity in the heart. *Cardiovasc Res* 11:55, 1977.

130. Weigelt JA, Gewertz BL, Aurbakken CM, Snyder WH III: Pharmacologic alterations in pulmonary artery pressure in the adult respiratory distress syndrome. *J Surg Res* 32:243, 1982.

131. Vanderark CR, Reynolds EW Jr: Clinical evaluation of glucagon by continuous infusion in the treatment of low cardiac output states. *Am Heart J* 79:481, 1970.

132. Okamura T, Miyazaki M, Toda N: Responses of isolated dog blood vessels to glucagon. *Eur J Pharmacol* 125:395, 1986.

133. Pizcueta MP, Casamitjana R, Bosch J, Rodes J: Decreased systemic vascular sensitivity to norepinephrine in portal hypertensive rats: role of hyperglucagonism. *Am J Physiol* 258:G191, 1990.

134. Richardson PD, Withrington PG: The inhibition by glucagon of the vasoconstrictor actions of noradrenaline, angiotensin, and vasopressin on the hepatic arterial vascular bed of the dog. *Br J Pharmacol* 57:93, 1976.

135. Silva G, Navasa M, Bosch J, et al: Hemodynamic effects of glucagon in portal hypertension. *Hepatology* 11:668, 1990.

136. Romeo JM, Lopez-Farre A, Martin-Paredero V, Lopez-Novoa JM: Role of glucagon in the splanchnic and systemic hemodynamic changes induced by portal-system blood shunting. *Clin Physiol Biochem* 8:144, 1990.

137. Wright CD, Kazmers A, Whitehouse WM Jr, Stanley JC: Comparative hemodynamic effects of selective superior mesenteric arterial and peripheral intravenous glucagon infusions. *J Surg Res* 39:230, 1985.

138. Cronenwett JL, Ayad M, Kazmers A: Effect of intravenous glucagon on the survival of rats after acute occlusive mesenteric ischemia. *J Surg Res* 38:446, 1985.

139. Kazmers A, Zwolak R, Appleman HD, et al: Pharmacologic interventions in acute mesenteric ischemia: improved survival with intravenous glucagon, methylprednisolone, and prostacyclin. *J Vasc Surg* 1:472, 1984.

140. Boorstein JM, Dacey LJ, Cronenwett JL: Pharmacologic treatment of occlusive mesenteric ischemia in rats. *J Surg Res* 44:555, 1988.

141. Oshima A, Kitajima M, Sakai N, Ando N: Does glucagon improve the viability of ischemic intestine? *J Surg Res* 49:524, 1990.

142. Clark ET, Gewertz BL: Glucagon potentiates intestinal reperfusion injury. *J Vasc Surg* 11:270, 1990.

143. Aki Y, Shoji T, Hasui K, Fukui K, Tamaki T, Iwao H, Abe Y: Intrarenal vascular sites of action of adenosine and glucagon. *Jpn J Pharmacol* 54:433, 1990.

144. Levy M: The effect of glucagon on glomerular filtration rate in dogs during reduction of renal blood flow. *Can J Physiol Pharmacol* 53:660, 1975.

145. Hogan WJ, Dodds WJ, Hoke SE, Reid DP, Kalkhoff RK, Arndorfer RC: Effect of glucagon on esophageal motor function. *Gastroenterology* 69:160, 1975.

146. Ferrucci JT Jr, Long JA Jr: Radiologic treatment of esophageal food impaction using intravenous glucagon. *Radiology* 125:25, 1977.

147. Handal KA, Riordan W, Siese J: The lower esophagus and glucagon. *Ann Emerg Med* 9:577, 1980.

148. Marks HW, Lousteau RJ: Glucagon and esophageal meat impaction. *Arch Otolaryngol* 105:367, 1979.

149. Pillari G, Bank S, Katzka I, Fulco JD: Meat bolus impaction of the lower esophagus associated with paraesophageal hernia. Successful noninvasive treatment with intravenous glucagon. *Am J Gastroenterol* 71:287, 1979.

150. Pickard R: Glucagon in management of perforated oesophagus (letter). *Br Med J* 4:232, 1974.

151. Carsen GM, Finby N: Hypotonic duodenography with glucagon. A clinical comparison study. *Radiology* 118:529, 1976.

152. Qvigstad T, Larsen S, Myren J: Comparison of glucagon, atropine, and placebo as premedication for endoscopy of the upper gastrointestinal tract. *Scand J Gastroenterol* 14:231, 1979.

153. Ferrucci JT Jr, Wittenberg J, Stone LB, Dreyfuss JR: Hypotonic cholangiography with glucagon. *Radiology* 118:466, 1976.

154. Carr-Locke DL, Gregg JA, Aoki TT: Effects of exogenous glucagon on pancreatic and biliary ductal and sphincteric pressures in man demonstrated by endoscopic manometry and correlation with plasma glucagon. *Dig Dis Sci* 28:312, 1983.

155. Doman DB, Ginsberg AL: Glucagon infusion therapy for biliary tree stones (abstr.). *Gastroenterology* 80:1137, 1981.

156. Stower MJ, Foster GE, Hardcastle JD: A trial of glucagon in the treatment of painful biliary tract disease. *Br J Surg* 69:591, 1982.

157. Jones RM, Fiddian-Green R, Knight PR: Narcotic-induced choledochoduodenal sphincter spasm reversed by glucagon. *Anesth Analg* 59:946, 1980.

158. Daniel O, Basu PK, Al-Samarrae HM: Use of glucagon in the treatment of acute diverticulitis. *Br Med J* 3:720, 1974.

159. Harford FJ Jr: Use of glucagon in conjunction with the end-to-end anastomosis (EEA) stapling device for low anterior anastomoses. *Dis Colon Rectum* 22:452, 1979.

160. Fallingborg J, Andersen SP, Laustsen J, Christensen LA: Glucagon treatment of external pancreatic fistula. A case report. *Acta Chir Scand* 151:183, 1985.

161. Lowman RM, Belleza NA, Goetsch JB, Finkelstein HI, Berneike RR, Rosenfield AT: Glucagon (letter to the editor). *J Urol* 118:128, 1977.

162. Morishima MS, Ghaed N: Glucagon and diuresis in the treatment of ureteral calculi. *Radiology* 129:807, 1978.

163. Schorr RT, Rogers SN: Intraoperative cardiovascular crisis caused by glucagon. *Arch Surg* 122:833, 1987.

164. Lamberts SW: Non-pituitary actions of somatostatin. A review on the therapeutic role of SMS 201-995 (sandostatin). *Acta Endocrinol Suppl* 276:41, 1986.

165. Lightman SL, Fox P, Dunne MJ: The effect of SMS 201-995, a long acting somatostatin analogue, on anterior pituitary function in healthy male volunteers. *Scand J Gastroenterol Suppl* 119:84, 1986.

166. Vance ML, Asplin CM, Chitwood J, Frohman LA, O'Dorisio T, Thorner MO: SMS 201-995: studies in acromegaly and in normal men. *Scand J Gastroenterol* 21(suppl 119):243, 1986.

167. Johnston DG, Davies RR, Turner SJ: Effects of somatostatin and SMS 201-995 on carbohydrate metabolism in normal man. *Scand J Gastroenterol Suppl* 119:158, 1986.

168. Williams G, Fuessl H, Kraenzlin M, Bloom SR: Postprandial effects of SMS 201-995 on gut hormones and glucose tolerance. *Scand J Gastroenterol Suppl* 119:73, 1986.

169. Takemura J, Kwok YN, Brown JC: Comparison of the effect of somatostatin and an analogue, SMS 201-995, on gastrin and insulin secretion from isolated perfused rat stomach and pancreas. *Am J Med* 81:65, 1986.

170. Creutzfeldt W, Lembcke B, Folsch UR, Schleser S, Koop I: Effect of somatostatin analogue (SMS 201-995, sandostatin) on pancreatic secretion in humans. *Am J Med* 82:49, 1987.

171. Kutz K, Nuesch E, Rosenthaler J: Pharmacokinetics of SMS 201-995 in healthy subjects. *Scand J Gastroenterol Suppl* 119:65, 1986.

172. Editorial: Somatostatin: hormonal and therapeutic roles. *Lancet* ii:77, 1985.

173. Del Pozo E, Kutz K: SMS 201-995, a new somatostatin analogue: pharmacological profile. *Neuroendocrinol Lett* 7:111, 1985.

174. Dueno MI, Bai JC, Santangelo WC, Krejs GJ: Effect of somatostatin analog on water and electrolyte transport and transit time in human small bowel. *Dig Dis Sci* 32:1092, 1987.

175. Davies RR, Miller M, Turner SJ, et al: Effects of somatostatin analogue SMS 201-995 in normal man. *Clin Endocrinol* 24:665, 1986.

176. Cello JP, Grendell JH, Basuk P, et al: Effect of octreotide on refractory AIDS-associated diarrhea. A prospective, multicenter clinical trial. *Ann Intern Med* 115:705, 1991.

177. Rosen GH: Somatostatin and its analogs in the short bowel syndrome. *Nutr Clin Pract* 7:81, 1992.

178. Katz MD, Erstad BL: Octreotide, a new somatostatin analogue. *Clin Pharm* 8:255, 1989.

179. Torres AJ, Landa JI, Moreno-Azcoita M, et al: Somatostatin in the management of gastrointestinal fistulas. A multicenter trial. *Arch Surg* 127:97, 1992.

180. Nubiola-Calonge P, Badia JM, Sancho J, Gil M, Sitges-Segura M: Blind evaluation of the effect of octreotide (SMS 201-995), a somatostatin analogue, on small-bowel fistula output. *Lancet* ii:672, 1987.

181. Pederzoli P, Bassi C, Falconi M, Albrigo R, Vantini I, Micciolo R: Conservative treatment of external pancreatic fistulas with parenteral nutrition alone or in combination with continuous infusion of somatostatin, glucagon or calcitonin. *Surg Gynecol Obstet* 163:428, 1986.

182. Kvols LK, Moertel CG, O'Connell MJ, Schutt AJ, Rubin J, Hahn RG: Treatment of the malignant carcinoid syndrome. Evaluation of a long-acting somatostatin analogue. *N Engl J Med* 315:663, 1986.

183. Vinik A, Moattari AR: Use of somatostatin analog in management of carcinoid syndrome. *Dig Dis Sci* 34:14S, 1989.

184. Maton PN, O'Dorisio TM, Howe BA, et al: Effect of long-acting somatostatin analogue (SMS 201-995) in a patient with pancreatic cholera. *N Engl J Med* 312:17, 1985.

185. Vinik AI, Tsai ST, Moattari AR, Cheung P, Eckhauser FE, Cho K: Somatostatin analogue (SMS 201-995) in the management of gastroenteropancreatic tumors and diarrhea syndromes. *Am J Med* 81:23, 1986.

186. Justice KM, Boyle PJ, Krentz AJ, Nagy RJ, McKinley M, Schade DS: Intravenous octreotide reverses hypoglycemia and hyperinsulinemia caused by sulfonylurea overdose (abstr.). *Clin Res* 39:101A, 1991.

187. Rizza RA, Gerich JE: Somatostatin and diabetes. *Med Clin North Am* 62:735, 1978.

188. Bosch J, Kravetz D, Rodes J: Effects of somatostatin on hepatic and systemic hemodynamics in patients with cirrhosis of the liver: comparison with vasopressin. *Gastroenterology* 80:518, 1981.

189. Thulin L, Tyden G, Samnegard H, Muhrbeck O, Efendic S: Treatment of bleeding oesophageal varices with somatostatin. *Acta Chir Scand* 145:395, 1979.

190. Bloom SR, Mortimer CH, Thorner MO, et al: Inhibition of gastrin and gastric acid secretion by growth-hormone release-inhibiting hormone. *Lancet* ii:1106, 1974.

191. Kayasseh L, Gyr K, Keller U, Stalder GA, Wall M: Somatostatin and cimetidine in peptic ulcer hemorrhage. A randomized controlled trial. *Lancet* i:844, 1980.

192. Bernton EW, Meltzer MS, Holaday JW: Suppression of macrophage activation and T-lymphocyte function in hypoprolactinemic mice. *Science* 239:401, 1988.

193. Nagy E, Berczi I: Immunodeficiency in hypophysectomized rats. *Acta Endocrinol* 89:530, 1978.

194. Nagy E, Berczi I, Wren GE, Asa SL, Kovacs K: Immunomodulation by bromocriptine. *Immunopharmacology* 6:231, 1983.

195. Hartmann DP, Holaday JW, Bernton EW: Inhibition of lymphocyte proliferation by antibodies to prolactin. *FASEB J* 3:2194, 1989.

196. Lieschke GJ, Burgess AW: Granulocyte colony-stimulating factor and granulocyte-macrophage colony-stimulating factor—part 1. *N Engl J Med* 327:28–35, 1992.

197. Lieschke GJ, Burgess AW: Granulocyte colony-stimulating factor and granulocyte-macrophage colony stimulating factor—part 2. *N Engl J Med* 327:99–106, 1992.

198. Crawford J, Ozer H, Stoller R, et al: Reduction by granulocyte colony stimulating factor of fever and neutropenia induced by chemotherapy in patients with small-cell lung cancer. *N Engl J Med* 325:164–170, 1991.

199. Nemunaitis J, Rabinowe SN, Singer JW, et al: Recombinant granulocyte-macrophage colony stimulating factor after autologous bone marrow transplantation for lymphoid cancer. *N Engl J Med* 324:1773–1778, 1991.

200. Advani R, Chao NJ, Horning SJ, et al: Granulocyte-macrophage colony stimulating factor (GM-CSF) as an adjunct to autologous hemopoietic stem cell transplantation for lymphoma. *Ann Intern Med* 116:183–189, 1992.

201. Gulati SC, Bennett CL: Granulocyte-macrophage colony-stimulating factor (GM-CSF) as adjunct therapy in relapsed Hodgkin disease. *Ann Intern Med* 116:177–182, 1992.

CHAPTER 43

Corticosteroids

ROBERT CHIN, Jr., M.D., F.C.C.P.
DONALD CHARLES EAGERTON, M.D.
MICHAEL SALEM, M.D.

The native adrenocorticosteroids are a family of structurally related hormones secreted by the adrenal glands that are essential for normal homeostasis and the endocrine response to stress. They are classified, based on their major physiologic action, either as glucocorticoids, mineralocorticoids, or sex hormones. Cortisol is the major endogenous glucocorticoid, and aldosterone, the major mineralocorticoid. Synthetic compounds that have either glucocorticoid or mineralocorticoid activity frequently are encountered and used in the critically ill patient. Therefore, this chapter concentrates on their pharmacology and clinical use.

GLUCOCORTICOIDS (19a)

THE HYPOTHALAMUS-PITUITARY-ADRENAL AXIS

Adrenal glucocorticoid secretion is controlled centrally by the hypothalamus and pituitary glands through the release of corticotropin releasing factor (CRF) and adrenocorticotropic hormone (ACTH), respectively. CRF, a 41 amino acid peptide, after release by the hypothalamus, reaches the anterior pituitary gland through communicating vascular channels and stimulates pituitary corticotrophs to secrete ACTH. ACTH enters into the systemic circulation and stimulates the adrenal glands to produce cortisol. Both CRF and ACTH, after binding to specific target cellular surface receptors, activate the enzyme adenyl cyclase, producing cyclic adenosine monophosphate, which drives an intracellular phosphorylation-dependent activation cascade.

Normally, ACTH and cortisol secretion follow a diurnal rhythm that is linked to an individual's sleep-wake habits. Cortisol secretion increases sharply during the 3rd through 5th hours of sleep in response to an increased number of ACTH secretory bursts, reaches a maximum just after awakening, and then decreases through the day to a nadir around the hour of sleep (Fig. 43.1). The normal unstressed daily production of cortisol is estimated to be 13 to 20 mg/day (13). This rhythm may be lost in the critically ill or stressed individual (145) and in those with Cushing's disease (hypercortisolism) or blunted in chronic inflammatory disease such as rheumatoid arthritis (160a).

The activity of the hypothalamus-pituitary-adrenal axis (HPA axis) is influenced by the free unbound or active cortisol fraction to keep glucocorticoid activity within a normal range. Decreased plasma cortisol levels lead to an increase in ACTH and CRF secretion and, subsequently, cortisol secretion. Increased cortisol levels, conversely, exert negative feedback on the HPA axis and decrease ACTH release and cortisol secretion. This servomechanism maintains the plasma cortisol concentration within a normal range in the normal unstressed individual (Fig. 43.2). This regulatory system is also, however, subject to both stimulatory and inhibitory input ("positive" and "negative" feedback) outside the normal feedback system to meet the needs of the organism (Fig. 43.1).

Stresses such as surgery, trauma, hypoglycemia, and sepsis can override the normal regulatory influences and diurnal rhythm and lead to sustained increases in ACTH secretion and plasma cortisol concentrations. The stress response probably is

715

Figure 43.1. The diurnal rhythm of cortisol secretion. Cortisol levels peak in the early morning just after awakening, then fall to a minimum in the evening hours. Therefore, "normal" cortisol levels depend on the time of day when samples are drawn and the state of "stress" the patient is in.

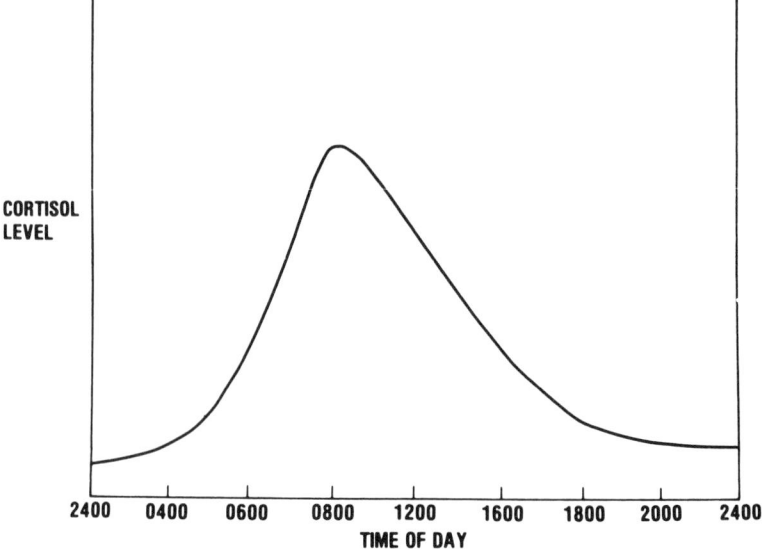

Figure 43.2. The hypothalamic-pituitary-adrenal system. The anatomic and physiologic interrelationships that are responsible for control of glucocorticoid production and their secondary effects are depicted. Cortisol production provides negative feedback at multiple levels to maintain homeostasis. This system operates to produce the optimum level of glucocorticoid activity required by the organism. (From Munck A, Mendel D, Smith L, Orti E: Glucocorticoid receptors and actions. *An Rev Respir Dis* 141:S2, 1990. Reproduced with permission.)

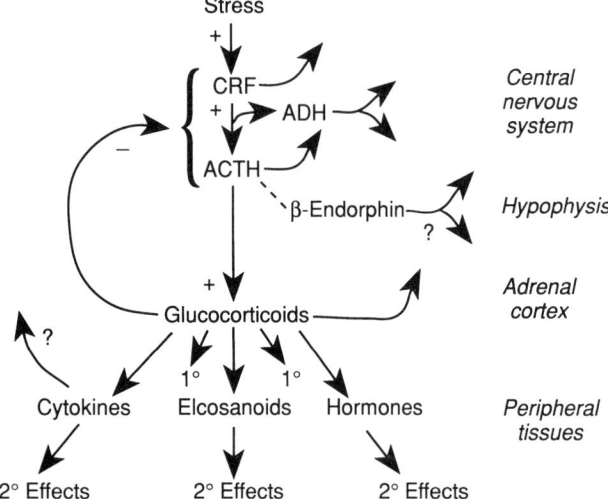

mediated primarily by the central nervous system through the release of CRF, although other hormones may also be involved (37). On the molecular level, several cytokines including platelet activating factor, gamma-interferon, interleukin-1 (IL-1), IL-2, and IL-6 and tumor necrosis factor can activate the HPA axis (160a). The maximum stress-induced output of cortisol is estimated to be 200 to 300 mg/day (36), with corresponding circulating plasma levels of more than 60 µg/dl (1650 nmol/liter) (186). Plasma cortisol levels in critically ill patients usually are increased above 20 µg/dl (552 nmol/liter) but exhibit a wide baseline range as well as a variable response to ACTH (50). Low premorbid cortisol levels may be the consequence of overwhelming stress and subsequent adrenal failure (13). Finlay and McKee found that 18 of 57 severely stressed patients had cortisol levels less than 13 µg/dl (293 nmol/liter) within 24 hours of death (67). They suggested that those patients with a morning (8 AM) cortisol level less than 13 µg/dl (350 nmol/liter) and a negative ACTH stimulation test may be relatively adrenal insufficient and may benefit from "replacement" doses of hydrocortisone, 100 mg twice daily (112). However, based on the available studies, the incidence of de novo adrenal insufficiency in the intensive care setting, based on provocative testing and excluding those with known adrenal insufficiency and those already on glucocorticoid therapy, is in the range of 3% (36, 50, 51, 97). Nevertheless, in one of these the studies, 31% of 300 patients admitted to the intensive care unit had to be excluded based on preexisting or existing conditions requiring steroid therapy (50). Therefore, the potential for catastrophic adrenal insufficiency is common in this setting. Stimulatory testing should be done with baseline levels obtained if adrenal insufficiency is suspected in critically ill patients. Empiric stress coverage may be given while awaiting the results but should discontinue if adequate function is found.

Exogenous glucocorticoid therapy suppresses the normal function of the HPA axis by inhibiting normal CRF and ACTH secretion through negative feedback on the hypothalamus and pituitary, respectively. ACTH suppression can be seen soon after glucocortocoid administration and may be progressive with continued therapy. HPA recovery may be prolonged in a manner that may be dose- and time-dependent on the glucocorticoid therapy. Unfortunately, a recent study has shown a poor correlation between tests of normal HPA function and dose or duration of glucocorticoid therapy or basal cortisol levels (147). In order for the axis to recover, a plasma cortisol nadir needs to occur to allow for endogenous ACTH release and adrenal stimulation. Therefore, when a patient has received glucocorticoids for more than 2 weeks, a tapering regimen is recommended to permit the HPA axis to recover its normal function. The tapering time should be proportional to the length of time on systemic steroid therapy and the dose. Sudden withdrawal may precipitate adrenal crisis or an exacerbation of the underlying disease. Once the need for exogenous glucocorticoids diminishes, the glucocorticoid dosage can be lowered progressively and consolidated to a single morning dose in order to simulate the normal cortisol circadian rhythm. For example, if a patient is receiving dexamethasone (a long-acting glucocorticoid preparation) 2 mg every 6 hours, the dose may be reduced to 1 mg every 6 hours and then switched to a single daily dose. Using an equivalency chart (Table 43.1), the clinician can then utilize an equivalent dose of a shorter-acting steroid, for example, hydrocortisone 75 mg each morning. This regimen, it is hoped, will allow the return of a normal nocturnal cortisol nadir and an ACTH surge. From here, the hydrocortisone dosage is then lowered progressively to 20 to 30 mg or less daily and can be discontinued when the morning fasting plasma cortisol concentration is >10 μg/dl and/or the ACTH stimulation test is normal (Fig. 43.3) (26). Alternate-day therapy with a relatively short-acting glucocorticoid also allows the HPA axis to recover and may maintain normal HPA function but it does not accelerate the recovery phase after suppression (1, 52). Although the duration and dose of glucocorticoid therapy may influence HPA recovery, the underlying disease that necessitates exogenous glucocorticoid therapy frequently dictates the rapidity of the taper.

PHARMACOLOGY OF CRH AND ACTH

CORTICOTROPIN RELEASING HORMONE

CRH is a 41 amino acid neuropeptide that, when delivered to the pituitary, stimulates the release of ACTH. Immunoreactive CRH can be found outside the central nervous system and may be involved in the integration of the neuroendocrine system and autonomic nervous system during stressful stimuli (164). Intravenously administered CRH can stimulate ventilation (132) and cause mild dyspnea in humans (164). Additionally, CRH may be responsible for the behavioral and physiologic responses of the central nervous system that are adaptive during stress (160a).

There is animal evidence that CRH can potentiate acetylcholine release at cholinergic nerve terminals (164) and that CRH mutually participates in a positive feedback loop with the locus coeruleus-norepiphrine system (the latter appears to potentiate an arousal state when stimulated) (160a). Clearance of human CRH is more rapid than that of ovine CRH and explains the longer and more potent response of ACTH and cortisol to ovine CRF (37).

Long-acting ovine CRH can be used diagnostically to differentiate hypercortisolism from a pituitary adenoma, ectopic ACTH syndrome, or ACTH-independent hypercortisolism of adrenal origin. Patients with a pituitary adenoma usually demonstrate an increase in plasma ACTH and cortisol in response to CRH, whereas patients with ectopic ACTH syndrome usually have no ACTH or cortisol response. Patients with ACTH-independent hypercortisolism will have low or undetectable levels of ACTH and fail to respond to CRH (37). Recently, Schlaghecke compared the HPA response to human CRH with the insulin tolerance test (ITT) in patients on chronic glucocorticoid therapy (147). Twenty-four hours after the last glucocorticoid dose, patients demonstrated comparable results (stimulated cortisol level) on both tests. Thus, CRH may be as accurate as an ITT in demonstrating the functional adequacy of the HPA axis (147) and a safer alternative.

ACTH

ACTH is synthesized in response to CRF as part of a larger prohormone, proopiomelanocortin (POMC), in the anterior pituitary gland. POMC includes the amino acid sequences of melanocyte stimulating hormone (MSH), lipotropin (LPH), and β-endorphin (86) and is cleaved enzymatically by tissue-specific serine proteases into smaller peptides such as ACTH (86). ACTH is a 39 amino acid polypeptide whose amino terminal (amino acids 1 through 24) is responsible for its biologic activity, whereas its carboxy terminal (amino acids 25 through 39) is considered the antigenic determinant (71). A shortened peptide (α-1-24-corticotropin) consisting of the biologically active amino acid sequence 1 through 24 is available clinically and can be used in place of ACTH, decreasing the potential antigenic complications (86). Because of this property, 1-24-corticotropin (cosyntropin) has supplanted biologic ACTH for clinical adrenal stimulation. Naturally occurring ACTH, derived from mammalian pituitaries, is still available in a lyophilized powder as well as in a repository form; 0.25 mg of 1-24-corticotropin is equivalent to 25 USP units of animal-derived ACTH. ACTH is metabolized rapidly by enzymatic hydrolysis, with a plasma half-life of roughly 15 minutes (86).

ACTH promotes cortisol secretion by the adrenal cortex through stimulation of adenyl cyclase, leading to an increase in the level of intracellular cyclic adenosine monophosphate

Table 43.1. Properties of Commonly Prescribed Corticosteroids[a]

Agent	Dose (mg)	Mineralocortical Potency[b]	Glucocorticoid Potency[c]	Duration of Action (hr)
Dexamethasone	0.75	0	25	72
Methylprednisolone	4.0	0.5	5	36
Prednisolone	5.0	0.8	4	24
Prednisone	5.0	0.8	4	24
Cortisol	20.0	1.0	1	8
Hydrocortisone	25.0	1.0	0.8	8
Cortisone	25.0	1.0	0.8	8

[a] From Chernow B: Hormonal and metabolic considerations in critical care medicine. In *Critical Care: State of the Art.* Society of Critical Care Medicine, Fullerton, CA, 1982, vol 3, pp J1.
[b] The higher the number in this column, the more likely the use of the agent will cause metabolic alkalosis.
[c] The higher the number in this column, the more likely the agent will cause suppression of hypothalamic corticotropin-releasing factor (CRF) and pituitary ACTH.

(cAMP). Intramitochondrial cAMP leads to oxidative cleavage of a cholesterol side chain, producing pregnenolone and initiating steroidogenesis (86). ACTH also stimulates steroid synthesis by promoting transfer of intracellular cholesterol from the outer mitochondria membrane to the inner membrane (86). These effects not only foster cortisol secretion and production but also lead to the synthesis of corticosterone, aldosterone, and weak androgens. In addition, ACTH causes an increase in adrenal blood flow (170), maintains adrenal weight, and induces the enzymes responsible for steroidogenesis (86). The adrenal effects of ACTH may be calcium dependent.

ACTH can cause lipolysis, insulin resistance, and skin pigmentation (86). These effects usually occur with large supraphysiologic doses. The hyperpigmentation seen in primary adrenal insufficiency (adrenal gland failure) results from increased levels of circulating ACTH whose amino acid sequence 1 through 13 is identical to that of α-melanocyte stimulating hormone (86).

Currently, ACTH is used infrequently therapeutically because of the widespread availability of its end products, the corticosteroids. Requirements for parenteral injection, an inconsistent cortisol response, the absence of benefit in HPA axis recovery, and the lack of distinct advantages over the corticosteroid preparations have led to its limited use. However, use of ACTH should not be considered equivalent to glucocorticoid therapy, since ACTH also stimulates the adrenal secretion of mineralocorticoids and androgens as well as glucocorticoids, and the combination of ACTH effects may be different from those effects produced by use of glucocorticoids alone (86). The major use of ACTH or corticotropin today is in the diagnosis of adrenal insufficiency, although some still advocate its traditional use in the treatment of multiple sclerosis and gout.

CHARACTERIZATION OF THE CORTICOSTEROIDS

The adrenal cortex is dividided histologically into three zones: outer (zona glomerulosa), middle (zona fasciculata), and inner (zona reticularis). The zona glomerulosa is responsible for the production of aldosterone, the major adrenal mineralocorticoid, whereas the zona fasciculata and zona reticularis synthesize the glucocorticoids and the sex hormones (androgens, progestins, and estrogens). The layers are characterized by the presence or absence of certain key enzyme systems in the biosynthetic pathway of the adrenocortical steroids (Fig. 43.4) that lead to a relatively segregated production of the hormones. The initial substrate in corticosteroid synthesis is cholesterol, which usually is derived from circulating sources (60 to 70%) (e.g., low-density lipoproteins), although the adrenal cortex does have a limited ability to produce it from acetate (86). The major adrenal corticosteroids include cortisol, corticosterone, 11-deoxycorticosterone, aldosterone, and the androgens. Corticosteroids are not stored in the adrenal gland in significant amounts, and secretion rates are related directly to the rate of synthesis (86).

The corticosteroids are characterized structurally by three six-carbon rings and one five-carbon ring with a side chain, for a total of 18 to 21 carbons in the skeleton (Fig. 43.4). The C4-C5 double bond and C3 ketone group are required for adrenocorticoid activity. However, modifications at the other carbon groups can alter antiinflammatory and carbohydrate (CHO)-regulating properties, sodium retention properties, bioavailability, half-life, membrane penetration, and affinity for the cell receptors.

Corticosteroids can be classified as a glucocorticoids or mineralocorticoids based on their predominant effects on either glucose metabolism or sodium retention, respectively (Table 43.1). Glucocorticoid activity promotes hepatic gluconeogenesis and glycogen deposition. Further, glucocorticoid activity causes negative nitrogen balance by stimulating protein catabolism. Amino acids are released and used as substrate by the liver for synthesis of glucose (86). Peripheral utilization of glucose is blocked, except in the liver, heart, brain, and red blood cells (86, 170). Consequently, blood glucose levels and urinary nitrogen excretion increase.

In addition to their contribution to glucose homeostasis; the glucocorticords are important endogenous modulators of the native immune-inflammatory response. The antiinflammatory actions of the corticosteroids invariably are tied to their relative effects on glucose metabolism. Both require an oxygen group at C11 in ring C (Fig. 43.4). Modifications of the sterol nucleus, which increase antiinflammatory properties, usually also cause a concomitant change in carbohydrate and protein metabolism (49, 86). Pharmacologically, the antiinflammatory activity is the desired effect and the accompanying metabolic changes are considered side effects.

Glucocorticoids also affect lipid metabolism indirectly by suppressing lipolysis and lipogenesis through the actions of counterregulatory hormones, principally insulin. Altered lipid

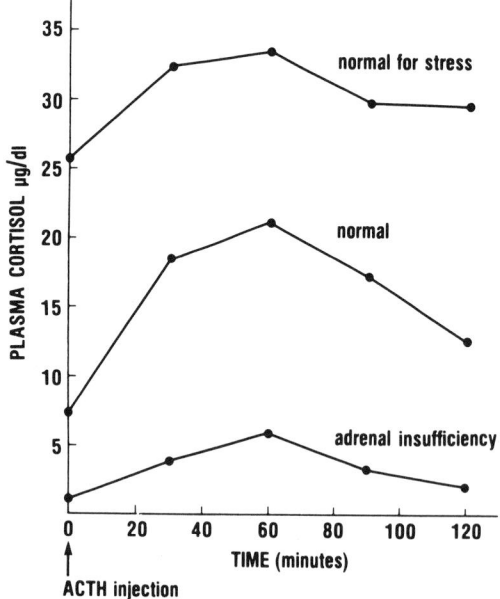

Figure 43.3. The ACTH stimulation test. If synthetic ACTH (250 μg of Cortrosyn) is given at time zero, normally a rise in plasma cortisol of at least 7 μg/dl should occur and the cortisol level should rise to ≥18 μg/dl by 60 minutes. In stress, the response is exaggerated. It is blunted in adrenal insufficiency. (From Chernow B: Hormonal and metabolic considerations in critical care medicine. In *Critical Care: State of the Art.* Fullerton, CA, Society of Critical Care Medicine, 1982.)

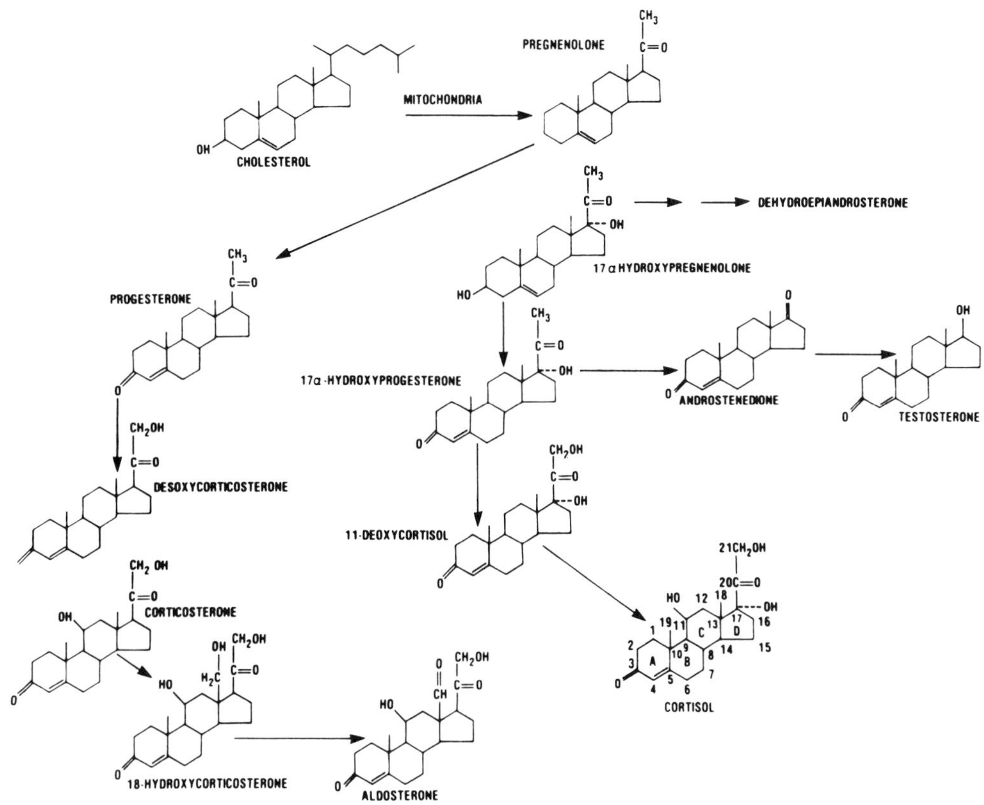

Figure 43.4. The biosynthetic pathway of the corticosteroids. Cholesterol is the precursor of the various endogenous corticosteroids. Pregnenolone is the first intermediate. The pathway pregnenolone then enters to form cortisol, aldosterone, or testosterone is determined by the presence or absence of certain key enzymes in each of the different zones of the adrenal. Cortisol is the major endogenous glucocorticoid. Modification in its structure as shown alters its properties quantitatively in terms of potency and half-life, or qualitatively (e.g., mineralocorticoid vs. glucocorticoid, vs. androgen activity).

deposition results in truncal obesity, "moon faces," and "buffalo humps" seen in Cushing's syndrome (hypercortisolism). The mechanism behind these changes is unknown but may be secondary to a differential response of adipose tissue to the effects of insulin and the glucocorticoids that leads to the central obesity (86). An increase in appetite leads to the overall obesity that is also seen in hypercortisolism (169). The lipolytic effects of epinephrine, norepinephrine, and other adipokinetic agents in fat tissue may be facilitated by glucocorticoid potentiation of the tissue's response to cAMP (86).

The primary action of the mineralocorticoids is to enhance ion transport in secretory cells. The principal target of the mineralocorticoids is the renal tubular cell. Sodium reabsorption is facilitated, whereas potassium and hydrogen ion excretion are increased. Endogenous mineralocorticoid activity is essential for the normal regulation of intravascular fluid volume. Addison's disease, or primary adrenocortical failure, is a corticosteroid deficient state that is characterized by hyponatremia resulting from renal sodium loss and decreased free water excretion (a cortisol action), hyperkalemia, and extracellular volume contraction. Although glucocorticoid activity is also missing, the disturbances in fluid and electrolyte balance because of mineralocorticoid deficiency pose the most immediately life-threatening problems and the predominant presenting feature. Other secretory cells (e.g., salivary glands, sweat glands, and exocrine, pancreatic, and gastrointestinal

cells) are also affected by mineralocorticoid activity and can contribute to fluid and electrolyte changes.

The secretion of the principal mineralocorticoid, aldosterone, is regulated primarily by potassium balance and the renin-angiotensin axis, with only limited influence from ACTH. Therefore, in secondary adrenocorticoid insufficiency (in which only ACTH input is lost) and mineralocorticoid secretion is preserved, major problems with fluid and electrolyte balance generally are not encountered and usually do not require exogenous mineralocorticoid replacement.

On a cellular level, the corticosteroids passively enter the cytoplasm of a target cell and bind to cytoplasmic receptors, forming a steroid-receptor complex (Fig. 43.5) (125). Upon binding, the glucocorticoid receptor-steroid (GR-H) dislocates from the cytoplasm and migrates to the nucleus (125). Binding also activates the steroid-receptor complex, changing it into a highly specific gene regulator that induces or suppresses the expression of cell-specific target genes (125).

The cytoplasmic glucocorticoid receptor (GR) contains at least three functional domains: an immunogenic domain, a DNA-binding domain, and a steroid-binding domain (121). The amino terminal is strongly immunogenic and contains a section that appears to increase the receptor's ability to activate transcription (121). The DNA-binding domain is a highly conserved sequence of 65 amino acids (amino acids 421 through 486) that is required for GR interaction with nuclear

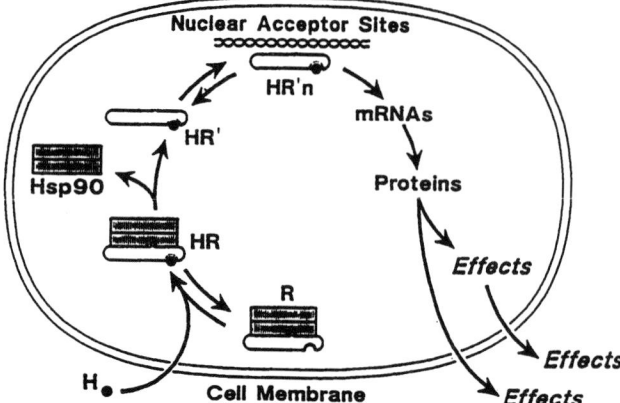

Figure 43.5. Cellular events of corticosteroid interaction. After the steroid hormone (*H*) binds to its specific cytoplasmic receptor (*R*), the complex (*HR*) is activated (*HR'*) and migrates to the nucleus. At the nuclear level, the activated complex (*HR'*) interacts with specific areas of the genetic DNA, leading to mRNA production that induces distinctive protein production. The proteins that are synthesized are the final genetic expression of steroid activity. (From Munck A, Mendel D, Smith L, Orti E: Glucocorticoid receptors and actions. *Am Rev Respir Dis* 141:S2, 1990. Reproduced with permission.)

DNA (121). The carboxy terminal contains the steroid-binding domain (121). The unbound GR exists as a heteromer of two 90-kdalton proteins complexed with the GR (121). In the native state, the GR has very little affinity for DNA (121). After binding with the steroid, the 90-kdalton proteins dissociate from the GR, uncovering the DNA domain and activating the complex (121). The activated complex migrates into the nucleus and the open DNA domain binds to glucocorticoid regulatory elements (GRE) that are responsible for the transcription of specific sequences of DNA to mRNA (121). Depending on the specific GRE that the steroid receptor complex binds to, the transcription rate of a specific protein's mRNA can be either induced (genomic upregulation) or suppressed (genomic downregulation).

Glucocorticoid expression is mediated by the synthesis and actions of specific proteins that are encoded by the GR-H receptive genes in the target cell. Initially, several similar proteins were described to be responsible for the antiinflammatory cellular response after glucocorticoid exposure (134). However, these proteins are likely to represent the active fragments of a similar precursor molecule (134). The name lipocortin has been assigned to this family of proteins (134). The lipocortins described so far share a common core structure comprised of four repeats of a 70-amino acid unit that appears to be important for calcium- and lipid-binding activity. The amino terminal may be different in all these proteins and may confer distinct biologic activites. Not all antiinflammatory actions of glucocorticoids, though, can be explained solely by the actions of the lipocortins, and production of other cellular calcium-binding proteins may be responsible (182).

Since protein synthesis is involved, a lag time may occur between administration of drug and the phenotypic expression. In addition, the duration of action may be more dependent on the breakdown of the steroid-induced mRNA and synthesized protein than on the clearance of the steroid itself. Clinically, in obstructive airway disease, the beneficial steroid effects may be delayed approximately 4 hours after initiation

of therapy (42) and may persist well beyond the half-life of the glucocorticoid. Some effects, however, have a faster response (e.g., ACTH suppression) and may be mediated by mechanisms other than protein synthesis (e.g., changes in membrane-based Ca^{2+} transport (123), activation of preformed proteins (123), and increased cellular cAMP (46)).

The corticosteroids, although defined by their effects on glucose metabolism or the maintenance of fluid and electrolyte balance, have broader systemic effects. Importantly, glucocorticoids also influence the normal function of the cardiovascular system, the central nervous system, skeletal muscle, lymphoid tissue, blood cells, the supportive tissue cells, and the immune system. These effects are discussed further in later sections of this chapter.

GLUCOCORTICOID PHARMACOLOGY

Although cortisol is the primary endogenous glucocorticoid, a number of synthetic glucocorticoid compounds are available. The relative advantages of each depend on the desired clinical effect, the glucocorticoid/mineralocorticoid activity ratio, the duration of action, and the mode of administration.

Oral glucocorticoid preparations are well-absorbed in patients with intact gastrointestinal function, but concomitant administration of antacids may decrease absorption. Intravenous administration ensures systemic delivery and results in rapid increases in concentrations of the steroid in body fluids. Intramuscular or subcutaneous injections are used primarily as depot forms and result in gradual absorption and longer duration of activity. The advantage of inhalational, topical, rectal, or intraarticular preparations is their ability to deliver high levels of the drug to local areas for the antiinflammatory effect, minimizing deleterious systemic effects. However, clinically significant absorption can occur; for example the use of plastic occlusive dressings over topically applied glucocorticoid products on the skin, the use of large topical doses, or prolonged use may lead to systemic effects. HPA axis suppression has also been reported with increased dosing of inhalational beclomethasone (174).

Circulating corticosteroids are carried both reversibly and competitively bound to plasma proteins and in a free, metabolically active state (8%) (13). Eighty percent of endogenous cortisol is bound to corticosteroid binding globulin (CBG, or transcortin) and 10% to other plasma proteins, such as albumin (10). CBG, a hepatically synthesized protein, has a high affinity for cortisol but a low capacitance and is saturated at a plasma cortisol level of 40 μg/dl (10). Above this level, more is bound to albumin (low affinity, large capacitance) and found in the free state. Because the free fraction is responsible for the biologic activity of cortisol, hypoproteinemia can lead to an increased incidence of "cushingoid" side effects with exogenous glucocorticoid therapy (10, 105). Additionally, since the clearance of corticosteroids is primarily hepatic, liver dysfunction with decreased enzyme activity and decreased hepatic protein synthesis (e.g., cirrhosis) can also contribute to the increased frequency of side effects (10). Bound cortisol acts as a reservoir for the free hormone, and equilibrium between the two states is reached quickly (13). The normal HPA axis is remarkably sensitive to changes in the free cortisol level and can maintain normal homeostasis provided there is no interference.

Cortisol is metabolized both intrahepatically and extrahepatically into biologic inactive metabolites primarily through reduction of the C4-C5 double bound and/or hydroxylation of the C3 ketone group (Fig. 43.4) (86). These products are then conjugated with either sulfate or glucuronic acid, making them water soluble, and subsequently are excreted via the kidneys (86). A small amount of unmetabolized cortisol is also excreted renally (170). Structural changes in the sterol nucleus may result in slower metabolism and extend the drug's half-life and potency. Rapid intravenous bolus administration can lead to early saturation of CBG, with an increased fraction of unbound hormone available for activity and clearance (90). Induction of hepatic microsomal enzymes by other drugs may also increase clearance. However, the chemical half-life of the corticosteroid present in the plasma or tissues may not correlate with its biologic or physiologic half-life. The biologic activity of corticosteroids depends on induction or inhibition of specific promoter genes, leading to enhanced or diminished mRNA transcription of unique DNA sequences and, subsequently, a change in rate of protein synthesis. This change leads to a delayed onset of response and prolonged activity that may not correlate directly with plasma levels of the corticosteroids. An estimate of the biologic half-lives of hydrocortisone, prednisone, and dexamethasone based on duration of adrenal suppression is 1.5 to 2 times their plasma half-life (114). The durations of physiologic action of the common commercial preparations are listed in Table 43.1.

Different glucocorticoids have different avidity for the cytoplasmic steroid receptors, and this, in part, contributes to their relative potencies. Dexamethasone and prednisolone have eight times and two times, respectively, the affinity of cortisol for these receptors (8). However, other factors such as the route and rapidity of administration, clearance, bioassays used to evaluate activity, and time after administration can also influence the overall estimated relative potencies of specific glucocorticoids (114, 169). Mineralocorticoid activity is measured by its ability to sustain life in adrenalectomized animals and its effects on sodium retention, whereas glucocorticoid activity is judged by the amount of liver glycogen deposited, which parallels its lymphoid tissue involution and antiinflammatory actions, or by adrenal gland suppression (86). Meikle and Tyler showed that the relative ability of hydrocortisone, prednisone, and dexamethasone to suppress the adrenal gland varied significantly from time of administration (114). Mean weighted estimates of relative potencies of hydrocortisone, prednisone, and dexamethasone were 1, 3, and 52, respectively, at 8 hours and 1, 5.2, and 154, respectively, at 14 hours (114). Duration of glucocorticoid exposure to tissues rather than actual dose or plasma levels may, in fact, be more important in ultimate gene expression (18). In addition, local cellular events may greatly bias the expression of steroid activity. Although cortisol and aldosterone have similar affinity for the mineralocorticoid receptor, the kidneys have an active 11-β-hydroxysteroid dehydrogenase enzyme system that rapidly oxidizes cortisol to inactive metabolite but does not affect aldosterone (74). Because of this and despite significantly higher levels of circulating cortisol than of aldosterone, the kidneys, colon, and salivary glands are much more responsive to aldosterone than to cortisol (86). Thus, the relative potencies of the various corticosteroid compounds may be only rough guides to their biologic activities and equivalencies.

Consideration of the aforementioned kinetics and the relative glucocorticoid to mineralocorticoid activity is important in the choice of a steroid. An agent with increasing mineralocorticoid activity increases the risk of steroid-mediated metabolic alkalosis and sodium and fluid retention. The former can be clinically important in the treatment of patients with chronic obstructive lung disease. Many of these patients develop a metabolic alkalosis while on glucocorticoid therapy and may compensate with alveolar hypoventilation to maintain a normal pH. This compensation can lead to a hypercapnic respiratory acidosis (31, 33) and interfere with weaning from mechanical ventilation. A preparation such as methylprednisolone, with relatively less mineralocorticoid activity, may be preferable to cortisol in these instances, although with high doses similar problems can occur. Fluid and sodium retention are major concerns in states characterized by fluid overload, such as congestive heart failure, the nephrotic syndrome, and cirrhosis, and in conditions in which further sodium and fluid retention might aggravate the process under treatment as is seen with increased intracranial pressure secondary to cerebral edema. Again, an agent with little or no mineralocorticoid activity such as dexamethasone is preferred in these situations. Conversely, hydrocortisone is preferable to methylprednisolone in acute adrenal crisis, since cortisol can provide needed mineralocorticoid activity. In active liver disease, prednisolone is preferred over prednisone because the latter requires hepatic hydroxylation of the C11 ketone group to gain agonist activity (7). Additionally, abnormal liver function may require lower doses of a glucocorticoid for the desired effect because of decreases in hepatic clearance and protein binding secondary to hypoproteinemia (7, 103).

Drug interactions between steroids and other medications can be important. Estrogens can increase CBG levels and total plasma cortisol (86). Troleandomycin, a macrolide antibiotic, reportedly extends the beneficial action of methylprednisolone by prolonging its half-life, allowing lower daily doses to be used in patients with asthma (163). The exact clinical benefit of this is unclear. Ketoconazole can decrease endogenous cortisol production through a partial block of the hydroxylation of 11-deoxycortisol to cortisol (92). Drugs such as phenytoin, barbiturates, and rifampin increase the clearance of synthetic corticosteroids by inducing hepatic microsomal enzymes (33, 55, 170). Corticosteroid therapy lessens the anticoagulation produced by ethylbiscoumacetate (29) and can augment renal clearance of salicylates (101). In addition, hydrocortisone prolongs the half-life of nortriptyline (172).

STEROID PREPARATIONS

A number of commercial steroid preparations are available for topical, aerosol, intravenous, intramuscular, subcutaneous, rectal, and oral administration. Steroids have also been applied to hardware such as pacemaker electrodes so that small amounts can be eluted over time to prevent fibrosis at the site of attachment. Because of their wide range of clinical applicability, both proved and empiric, they invariably are encountered by most physicians. A short summary of the most commonly used products in the critical care setting follows.

HYDROCORTISONE

Hydrocortisone is the synthetic equivalent to cortisol, the principal endogenous glucocorticoid. Because of this fact, it is assigned the relative glucocorticoid activity of 1.0 and is the standard with which other glucocorticoids are compared. The quality that separates it from the other major glucocorticoid agents is its mineralocorticoid activity (approximately 1% that of aldosterone) (10). It is, therefore, the preferred glucocorticoid in the physiologic replacement of corticosteroids (20 mg in the morning and 10 mg in the evening) in primary adrenocortical failure. This same property hinders its use as an antiinflammatory agent because of the fluid and electrolyte imbalances it can engender. It is available in intravenous and oral forms with different ester conjugates (sodium succinate, sodium phosphate, and cypionate; the latter is poorly soluble and used only orally) (186). It also can be used in topical (skin and ophthalmologic), rectal, depot, and intravaginal forms. Its plasma half-life is 80 to 115 minutes (7) and it has a relatively short duration of action of 8 hours.

CORTISONE

Cortisone is the 11-keto form of cortisol. It is essentially equivalent to hydrocortisone but requires hepatic hydroxylation at C11 to form cortisol, its active metabolite, and as a result is 25% less potent (186). It is unsuitable for local use because it is inactive in its native state, but it can be given systemically either orally or in an intramuscular injection.

PREDNISOLONE

A double bond in position C1-C2 increases the glucocorticoid activity of prednisolone relative to its mineralocorticoid activity. This quality allows lower doses to be given compared with cortisol, for the same antiinflammatory response, with less sodium retention. The unsaturated bond in C1-C2 also slows the metabolism of the drug (86). Its plasma half-life is 115 to 252 minutes (7) and the duration of action is 24 hours. The half-life may be prolonged significantly in renal failure (98). It has four times the glucocorticoid potency of cortisol but only 80% of cortisol's mineralocorticoid action. It is available in oral, topical, and parenteral forms (conjugated with either acetate, or sodium phosphate, esters) (86).

METHYLPREDNISOLONE

This congener of prednisolone has a methyl group added to C6 that further enhances its antiinflammatory activity. The plasma half-life is between 78 and 188 minutes (7) and its duration of action is 24 to 36 hours. Methylprednisolone has five times the glucocorticoid activity of cortisol and 50% the potency of mineralocorticoid. It may be better concentrated in the lungs than prednisolone because it has a larger volume of distribution, longer mean residence time, and greater retention in the epithelial lining fluid of the alveoli (80). It is one of the most common intravenous steroids used in the U.S. today. It is available in intravenous (acetate or sodium succinate esters), oral, and depot forms.

PREDNISONE

Hepatic hydroxylation of the C11 keto group is necessary to convert prednisone from a weak steroid antagonist to a potent agonist. It has a relative activity similar to that of prednisolone. The plasma half-life is 160 minutes and the duration of action is 24 hours. It is available only in an oral form and is well-absorbed from the gastrointestinal tract (186).

DEXAMETHASONE

Dexamethasone is a fluorinated hydrocarbon with a fluorine radical at C9, a double bond between C1 and C2, and a methyl group at C16 that distinguish it from cortisol. Each of these modifications serves to increase the antiinflammatory action and decrease the mineralocorticoid activity. Available in the parenteral (acetate or sodium phosphate ester), oral, and topical form, it has 25 times the glucocorticoid strength of cortisol and negligible mineralocorticoid activity. The plasma half-life is 110 to 120 minutes and the duration of action is 72 hours (7). However, in renal failure its clearance may be increased, whereas in hepatic dysfunction it is decreased (98). Dexamethasone is best utilized in situations in which a potent antiinflammatory agent is required but fluid or sodium retention is undesirable (e.g., cerebral edema secondary to tumor). A distinct disadvantage is its long duration of action, which extends HPA axis suppression and makes it a poor choice when recovery of the HPA axis is wanted.

DEFLAZACORT

Deflazacort or oxazacort is a relatively new synthetic heterocyclic glucocorticoid. Currently, it is not available commercially in the U.S. It has a therapeutic potency (antiinflammatory and immunosuppresive) 83% that of prednisone (1.2 mg = 1 mg, respectively) (79). Recent studies suggest that deflazacort has fewer adverse effects than prednisone or prednisolone at doses with equivalent antiinflammatory activity. It has been found to have significantly less diabetogenic effect in normal as well as diabetic patients (lower glucose levels, lower hemoglobin A_{1c} levels, and lower insulin dosage requirement) (9, 24, 79, 108). Adverse effects on calcium balance and on the hypothalamus-pituitary-adrenal axis are also decreased (79). Deflazacort has reduced short-term effects on intestinal calcium absorption and urinary excretion of calcium. It induces less bone loss as assessed by photon absorptiometry or by bone histiomorphometry than other glucocortcoids (9). Deflazacort also seems to have less detrimental impact on the growth rate of children on chronic corticosteroids as compared with other steroids (79). Cortisol secretion is not inhibited acutely by deflazacort as it is by prednisone, consistent with a decreased suppressive influence on the HPA axis.

TRIAMCINOLONE, FLUNISOLIDE, BUDESONIDE, BETAMETHASONE, AND BECLOMETHASONE

Triamcinolone, flunisolide, budesonide, and beclomethasone are halogenated glucocorticoids with greater antiinflammatory activity compared to cortisol. Triamcinolone, betamethasone, and flunisolide are fluorinated, whereas beclomethasone is chlorinated. They are long-acting agents. Triamcinolone and betamethasone are marketed in oral, parenteral, or topical forms. Triamcinolone, flunisolide, and beclomethasone are available for inhalation through metered dose inhalers. Utilization of topical antiinflammatory agents in asthma has been shown to reduce or even eliminate the need for systemic steroids to control bronchial hyperreactivity and airway inflammation (30).

Beclomethasone dipropionate is the best studied of the topical inhalational agents. Compared with the topical activity of dexamethasone, beclomethasone dipropionate has 500 times its topical activity (30). When given intravenously, bypassing absorption and first-pass degradation, beclomethasone dipropionate has a suppressive effect on the HPA axis similar to that of dexamethasone (30). Harris and his associates evaluated the HPA suppressive effects of beclomethasone and dexamethasone (30, 83). Twenty-four hour urinary secretion of 17-oxogenic steroids was greater (less adrenal suppression) after 4 mg/day of oral beclomethasone or 1000 μg/day inhaled beclomethasone dipropionate than after 2 mg/day of dexamethasone (30, 83). Reduced bioavailability after oral ingestion, rapid first-pass hepatic metabolism, and its significantly higher topical activity explain its major advantages as an inhalational agent in the control of airway inflammation in asthma and its much reduced systemic effects compared with other agents (30). The usual recommended daily dose is 400 to 600 μg/day (2 to 4 puffs two to four times a day; each puff equals approximately 40 μg). Four hundred μg/day of inhaled beclomethasone dipropionate is roughly the therapeutic equivalent of 5 to 10 mg of oral prednisone (30).

Use of spacer devices with the metered-dose steroid inhalers promotes airway deposition. This technique can lead to an increase in effectiveness and reduction of unwanted side effects such as oropharyngeal candidiasis.

Despite the advantages of inhaled steroid preparations, significant HPA repression can be seen in those patients who require high-dose therapy (>1500 μg/day) and/or prolonged therapy (23, 174). Many of the systemic effects of beclomethasone dipropionate, principally HPA axis repression, are believed to result from absorption of the agent and its active metabolites through the lung (30, 83).

In addition, beclomethasone and flunisolide are available for nasal inhalation for the control of allergic rhinitis.

PHYSIOLOGIC EFFECTS OF GLUCOCORTICOID THERAPY

Glucocorticoids have been used therapeutically in a variety of clinical disorders (Table 43.2). Much of the knowledge gained on the effects of the corticosteroids on different organ systems is derived from clinical observations of hyperadrenalism and/or hypoadrenalism and their response to treatment. The exact mechanisms by which glucocorticoids or mineralocorticoids exert many of their effects on tissue function are unknown. However, in therapies other than adrenal replacement, the antiinflammatory and/or immunosuppressive actions of the glucocorticoids are the principal desired qualities.

The discovery of lipid and peptide cellular mediators, which are responsible not only for intrinsic cell activity but also for communication among cells, has helped to explain the glucocorticoids' effects on the inflammatory process (Fig. 43.6). Many of the glucocorticoids' antiinflammatory and immune-modulating properties have been linked to a family of closely related calcium-binding cellular proteins, called the lipocortins, that are induced by the GR-H nuclear interaction. Through inhibition of the enzyme phospholipase A_2, which cleaves arachidonic acid (the precursor of the eicosanoid mediators of both the cyclooxygenase and lipooxygenase pathways) from membrane phospholipids, the lipocortins can influence the activity of this class of inflammatory mediators. Phospholipase A_2 also plays a role in signal transduction by PMNs that enables the PMNs to respond to a stimulus (70). Changes induced by steroids in membrane-bound Ca^{2+} may also affect mediator release (123). In addition, lipocortins have been shown to inhibit the ability of neutrophils to release active oxygen metabolites and impair Fc receptor function (134). However, other antiinflammatory activities have not been explained through the actions of lipocortins, implying that other peptides or other systems may be involved in the antiinflammatory actions of the glucocorticoids. An alternate theory involves the inhibition of the synthesis and effects of interleukin-1 (IL-1α and IL-1β), a proinflammatory mediator, by glucocorticoids (Fig. 43.6) (3). In addition, glucocorticoids inhibit IL-6 transcription; reduce the half-life of MRNA of IL-3 as well as IL-1; and down regulate most cytokines and growth factors. The relative contributions of these effects to the overall immunosuppresive effects of steroids are speculative, but they provide a cellular and subcellular theoretic model for this action. By interfering with the normal immune response to an antigen/stimulus and the resultant cell mediator release, glucocorticoids may interrupt the cascade that promulgates the inflammatory response.

Most, if not all, of the effector cells of inflammation can be influenced by the presence of glucocorticoids. Unlike other inflammatory cells, glucocorticoids cause an expansion of the circulating pool of neutrophils. In part, this results from the glucocorticoids' stimulation of bone marrow production and release, and the reduction of neutrophilic egress from the intravascular space (148, 149). However, the reduction in the expression of neutrophilic surface receptors seen after incubation with glucocorticoids may contribute to diminished adherence to the vascular endothelium and explain the "demargination" and leukocytosis seen clinically with the administration of glucocorticoids (148). In addition, pretreatment of endothelial cells with glucocorticoids inhibits transendothelial migration of neutrophils in vitro (148). In high concentrations, glucocorticoids may stabilize neutrophilic lysosomes, inhibit the release of lysosomal enzymes, and inhibit chemotaxis. By constraining neutrophilic priming either by direct action on the cell or by interference with the local release of priming agents and blockage of the release of cellular recruitment factors and other factors, glucocorticoids can further disrupt the normal amplification of an inflammatory response. Glucocorticoids also reduce binding of complement and

Table 43.2.   Clinical Applications of Glucocorticoid Therapy in Critical Care

Cardiovascular
  Shock states
    Anaphylactic
    Mixed[a]
  Elution from pacemaker wires to prevent fibrosis
Altered immune states
  Collagen-vascular diseases
    Systemic lupus erythematosus
    Polymyositis/dermatomyositis
    Rheumatoid arthritis
    Mixed connective tissue disease
  Disorders characterized by a predominant vasculitis
  Sarcoidosis
  Hypersensitivity reactions
    Drug and contrast dye reactions
    Serum sickness
    Urticaria
    Allergic rhinitis
    Bee stings
    Anaphylaxis
Dermatologic
  Pemphigus
  Pemphigoid
  Erythema multiforme
  Toxic epidermolysis necrosis
  Contact dermatitis
Endocrine
  Adrenal insufficiency: primary and secondary
  Hypercalcemia
Gastrointestinal
  Alcoholic hepatitis
  Inflammatory bowel disease
    Crohn's disease
    Ulcerative colitis
	Hematologic
	  Hemolytic anemias
	  Idiopathic thrombocytopenic purpura
	Infections
	  Pneumocystis carinii pneumonia in AIDS
	    Meningeal and pericardial tuberculosis
	Malignancy
	  Multiple myeloma
	  Lymphomas
	  Acute lymphocytic leukemias
	  Breast cancer
	Neonatalogy
	  Neonatal respiratory distress syndrome (antenatal)
	Neurologic
	  Multiple sclerosis[a]
	  Cord compression
	  Cerebral edema (vasogenic edema)
	  Myasthenia gravis
	  Guillain-Barre[a]
	Ophthalmologic
	  Acute uveitis
	  Choroiditis
	  Optic neuritis
	Pulmonary
	  Asthma/reversible obstructive disease
	  Fibroproliferative ARDS
	  Interstitial pneumonitis
	  Vasculitic disorders of the respiratory tract (e.g., Wegener's
	    granulomatosis, Churg-Strauss, Goodpasture's syndrome, etc.)
	  Bronchiolitis obliterans
	  Nitrous dioxide gas exposure
	Renal
	  Certain glomerulonephritis syndromes
	Transplant
	  Transplant rejection

[a] Areas of controversy in the clinical efficacy of glucocorticoid therapy.

Figure 43.6.   Glucocorticoid's effects on the immune/inflammatory response. The antiinflammatory action of the glucocorticoids results partially from their ability to regulate cytokine production after activation of the cellular and immune response to antigen challenge. (From Munck A, Mendel D, Smith L, Orti E: Glucocorticoid receptors and actions. *Am Rev Respir Dis* 141:S2, 1990. Reproduced with permission.)

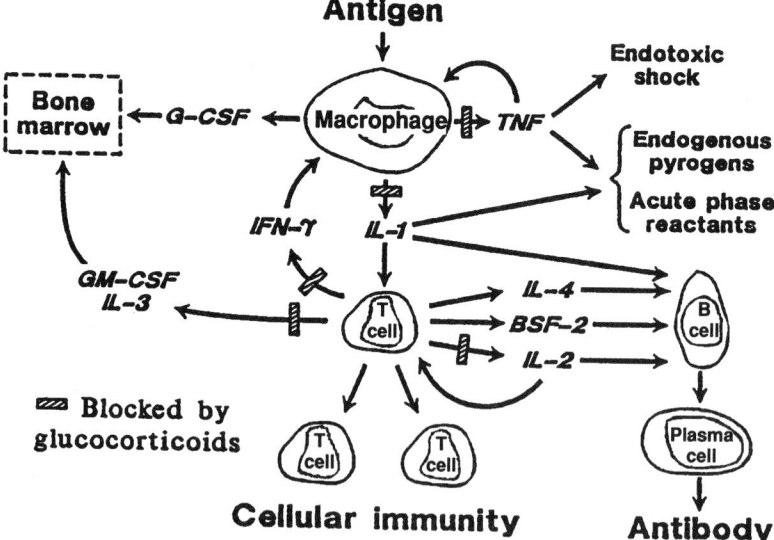

immunoglobulin E (IgE) and G (IgG) antibodies to inflammatory cell receptor sites (123). The net result is a neutrophilic granulocytosis but reduced migration and accumulation at inflammatory sites. However, isolated neutrophilic function and chemotaxis are preserved with treatment with steroids. Steroid-induced granulocytosis may be differentiated from the leukocytosis associated with infections by reviewing the peripheral blood smear. Schoenfeld and associates showed

that an increase in premature white cell forms (bands) of > 6% and the appearance of toxic granulations favored the diagnosis of infection (149). Clinically, fever is also suppressed by glucocorticoid therapy as a result of reduced leukocyte pyrogen production (demonstrated in vitro) and/or the inhibition of the release of interleukin-1, an endogenous pyrogen, from monocytes (13). The contribution of steroid-induced granulocytic lysosomal stabilization to the glucocorticoids' antiinflammatory effects is unclear. Most authors believe that steroid influence on the migratory patterns of inflammatory cells and the release of their mediators (such as prostaglandins and their derivatives) are the most significant effects.

In contrast, steroids cause the circulating mononuclear, eosinophilic, and basophilic populations to decrease with a maximum lymphocytopenia occuring 4 to 6 hours after administration of glucocorticoids and recovery within 24 hours (63). Pharmacologic doses of glucocorticoids result in a striking reduction in thymic weight and spleen and peripheral lymph node size in corticosteroid-sensitive species (e.g., mouse, rat, and rabbit) (38). Although cell cultures of chromium-tagged mouse thymus cells admixed with cortisol succinate undergo cell lysis, human (a corticosteroid-resistant species) thymus cells do not (38). Apoptosis (programmed cell death) of lymphocytes may be steroid hormone receptor mediated and contribute to the lymphocytopenia seen with glucocorticoids. Cellular redistribution of recirculating intravascular lymphocytes into the extravascular space (probably bone marrow), may be primarily responsible for the observed lymphocytopenia (46). Both B- and T-cell lymphocytes are affected, but the T-cells more so, perhaps because the subcellular rate of metabolism of cortisol is greater in the B-cell than in the T-cell (46). The changes in the migratory patterns may be mediated through steroid-induced changes on the lymphocyte surface (46, 63).

Lymphocytic function is also affected by glucocorticoid therapy. Clinically, delayed hypersensitivity is impaired and there is a subsequent development of anergy. Various theories have been proposed to explain this phenomenon. The most recent data suggest that interference with soluble mediators (e.g., cytokines, macrophage inhibition factor, eicosanoids) released from activated lymphocytes or monocytes/macrophages alters the recruitment of and collaboration between other lymphocytes and mononucleur cells (Fig. 43.6) (63). T-cell processing of antigen is normal after steroid administration, but lymphocyte migration and attraction to an inflammatory site is not (180). Proliferation of lymphocytes after a stimulus is also reduced both in vitro and in vivo, as is interleukin-1 stimulation of interleukin-2 production (46). Interleukin 1 is a macrophage-derived mediator that contributes to the activation of T-cells upon antigen presentation; interleukin-2 is a T-cell growth factor that is required for cytotoxic T-cell development (133). Expression of the IL-2 receptor on T-cells is also reduced by glucocorticoids. The corticosteroids' effects on the humoral system and B-cell function are less clear. Studies have shown that serum IgG levels (25, 63), and complement (6, 63) levels, are diminished after steroid administration. Cupps and Fauci suggest that the glucocorticoids' effects on monocytes, T-lymphocytes, and B-cells all can influence the B-lymphocyte response (46). Inhibition of immune complex movement across basement membranes in rabbits by steroids has also been reported (63). The reticuloendothelial system is impaired, with less than optimum removal of opsinized and nonopsinized substances (5,6). Circulating monocytes and tissue macrophages are reduced in number (148). Although phagocytosis is intact, the intracellular killing of microorganisms is abnormal. However, the release of eico-

sanoids, lytic enzymes, and cytokines from monocytes and macrophages is reduced markedly by glucocorticoids (148).

Eosinopenia also occurs and again is likely to be secondary to redistribution of these cells as opposed to destruction; it follows the same time course as for lymphocytopenia (148). Inhibition of release of eosinophilic chemotactic factors, decreased eosinophilic chemotaxis and diapedesis, and decreased activation of eosinophils occurs with steroid treatment (148). The inhibition by glucocorticoids of basophil and mast cell inflammatory function probably also results from alteration in cellular communication through the effects on cytokine release and response. The mechanisms of steroid influence and their importance on eosinophilic migration, and basophilic and mast cell function (particularly histamine release) in type I immediate allergic reactions (anaphylaxis), are not fully understood. The clinical efficacy of steroids in allergic responses may be based more on their effects on the late phases of the allergic response rather than their effects on the immediate phase (148).

Local factors induced by glucocorticoid treatment may also further modify the inflammatory response. Reduction in both local mediator (eicosanoids and other cytokines) generation and neutrophil accumulation and inhibition of the endothelial response to permeability-increasing mediators interfere with the increased capillary permeability brought on by acute inflammation, reducing plasma and protein exudation (185). Furthermore, the release of vasoactive kinins is blocked by steroids, and this action may lessen the local immune response to a stimulus (41). Endothelial cells contribute to the initiation and maintenance of the inflammatory response. Glucocorticoids affect the endothelial cells by interfering with local eicosanoid formation by blocking the release of arachidonic acid and by alternating the expression of histocompatibility antigens (148). Moreover, glucocorticoids inhibit the expression of the inducible enzyme nitric oxide synthase that is responsible for nitric oxide (endothelium-derived relaxing factor) production following stimulation by cytokines or lipopolysaccharide (LPS) (139). These actions, combined with the effects on the effector cells (PMNs, lymphocytes, eosinophils, basophils, and monocytes/macrophages), markedly alter the normal inflammatory response. In summary, glucocorticoids inhibit the normal immune cascade at almost all levels from macrophage processing to effector cell function (160a). Most of the inhibition results from supression of cytokines at the gene level and the inhibition of phospholipase A_2 activity responsible for eicosanoids generation at the cell level.

Glucocorticoids can be tumoricidal in certain tumor cell lines such as the lymphoproliferative malignancies, but the mechanism is unknown. Glucocorticoids may act by inhibiting mitogen-stimulated production of IL-2 by blocking the lipoxygenase pathway that helps to promote lymphocyte proliferation (72). Steroid efficacy in the treatment of other tumors (breast carcinoma, juvenile hemangiomas) is also puzzling but perhaps is related to steroid-induced inhibition of cellular growth and, at least in breast cancer, through adrenocorticoid repression of androgen production (20, 86, 169).

The cardiovascular system in Addison's disease is characterized by a hypodynamic state. Corticosteroid replacement returns the cardiac function to normal, but it is not clear whether this action results from glucocorticoid activity or mineralocorticoid activity that leads to the reestablishment of a normal volume status. The independent actions of glucocorticoids on cardiac inotropy and/or chronotropy, and smooth muscle vascular tone, are not fully elucidated. They could play a "helper" role in the interactions of other vasoactive hormones (e.g., catecholamines) with their target organs. Hypertension commonly is seen in hypercortisol states and is not necessarily related to mineralocorticoid effects. The mechanism of benefit of glucocorticoids when used in large doses in shock states is equally unclear. Reasonable postulates are interference with the propagation of the inflammatory cascade, allowing stabilization of the circulatory system, and, possibly, an increase in the sensitivity of the cardiovascular tree to sympathomimetic stimulation. These effects could lead to preservation of capillary wall integrity and tissue oxygen delivery, thus arresting tissue destruction. An alternate theory is that POMC, the parent compound of ACTH as well as the endorphins and enkephalins (both opioid-like vasodilators), is secreted by the pituitary gland in response to sepsis, hemorrhage, or other stresses and may contribute to hypotension from vasodilatation (178). POMC secretion, and thus endorphin and enkepalin release, may be inhibited by elevated levels of glucocorticoids through their negative feedback on ACTH precursor secretion (81).

The presence of steroid activity is essential for normal β-adrenergic function (22). Steroids have taken a prime role in the treatment of asthma where sufficient β-adrenergic stimulation is necessary for acute bronchodilation. Delayed improvement in airflow obstruction is seen in severe asthmatics after glucocorticoid therapy in conjuction with other direct bronchodilators. Mechanisms that may be responsible for these effects include an increased sensitivity to β-adrenergic agents caused by up-regulation of β-receptors, with an accompanying increase in their numbers and sensitivity; an antiinflammatory effect that reduces cellular infiltrates and exudates, especially in the late phase of asthma; a reduction in target tissue responsiveness to inflammatory mediators (e.g., histamine, platelet-activating factor, leukotrienes, and cyclooxygenase prostaglandin derivatives) (123); an inhibition of mucous production (110); a decrease in epithelial cell permeability (148); a decrease in IgE receptor binding (186); and altered Ca^{2+} transmembrane movement and decreasing smooth muscle reactivity (123). Glucocorticoids have not been found to have a direct effect on airway resistance or spirometry in normal subjects (140, 172).

Glucocorticoids may reduce circulating calcium levels in hypercalcemic patients. Reduced calcium absorption from the intestines, inhibition of 1,25-dihydroxycholecalciferol (vitamin D) production, increased renal excretion of calcium, and redistribution of calcium from the extracellular to the intracellular space contribute to the lowering of the serum calcium (7, 86). These effects are best observed in the hypercalcemia associated with sarcoidosis and are less effective in hypercalcemia secondary to increased parathyroid hormone levels. The use of glucocorticoids with salmon-derived calcitonin lengthens the calcium-lowering effects of the latter (12).

The most apparent and least controversial indication for corticosteroid use is in adrenocorticoid hormone replacement therapy. The corticosteroids have a variety of complex interactions with many of the other endogenous hormones and other organ systems that maintain homeostasis and a normal response to stress. The musculoskeletal system appears to be dependent on the physiologic presence of steroid activity for normal function (86). Glucocorticoids have a "permissive" function in the sympathetic nervous system and cross the blood-brain barrier to interact with the central nervous system (170). Maintenance of the plasma glucose for nutritional needs of the CNS and erythrocytes and fluid and electrolyte balance depends on corticosteroid influences. Dallman showed that in rats subjected to hemorrhagic stress, fasted adrenalectomized rats had a much higher mortality rate than fed adrenalectomized rats and fasted sham-adrenalectomized rats (47). Plasma glucose levels decreased immediately after hemorrhage in the fasted adrenalectomized rats but were well-maintained in the other groups (47). This study reinforces the importance of corticosteroids in the metabolic response to stress.

CLINICAL COMPLICATIONS OF GLUCOCORTICOID THERAPY

The side effects of therapy (Table 43.3) can be divided into those that are expected to occur with physiologic replacement doses, those that are more common with pharmacologic doses, and those that are unexpected. They can be further subdivided into those seen with acute therapy and those that are associated more with chronic therapy. Proper choice of steroid, dosage, dosing interval, and length of therapy along with an intelligent choice of endpoints of therapy can minimize the complications. Some toxicities are so intertwined with the disease process being treated that it is difficult to ascertain an independent effect from the glucocorticoids. Although the intensivist is more concerned with the side effects of acute glucocorticoid therapy, the metabolic changes induced by chronic therapy must be anticipated and recognized.

Although there is usually little danger in a short course of high-dose steroid therapy, even in the critically ill patient, there may be unforseen deleterious effects. Massive rapid bolus doses of 1 g or more have been associated with sudden death and cardiovascular collapse when given concurrently with furosemide (111, 161). Although the exact reason for this problem is not known (maybe secondary to rapid electrolyte shifts), it is prudent to give large doses slowly. In Bone's cooperative study of high-dose methylprednisolone (30 mg/kg) in septic shock, an increase in mortality related to secondary infections was noted in those patients receiving methylprednisolone compared with those in the placebo group (15). Glucose intolerance with glycosuria, metabolic alkalosis, sodium and fluid retention, the risk of peptic ulceration, psychosis, and an impairment of host immune defenses are troublesome when durations of treatment are more prolonged than 1- or 2-day high-dose therapy.

Many of the complications seen with glucocorticoid therapy are magnified with higher doses and longer duration of therapy. Steroid myopathy involves the proximal musculature, especially the pelvic girdle. It commonly develops after prolonged therapy (weeks to months) but can be seen with shorter courses. It is generally, but not always, reversible with the cessation of therapy. Muscle enzymes (creatinine phosphokinase (CPK), aldolase) (52, 86) are not increased and can be used to distinguish steroid myopathy from a primary myositis

Table 43.3. Deleterious Effects of Glucocorticoid Therapy[a]

Cardiovascular
Cardiovascular collapse and sudden death associated with rapid
  intravenous administration
Hypertension
Fluid and sodium retention with edema
Hypokalemic metabolic alkalosis
Accelerated atherosclerosis leading to coronary vascular disease
Musculoskeletal
Proximal myopathy
Osteoporosis of trabecular bones
Aseptic necrosis of bones
Gastrointestinal
Peptic ulceration, hemorrhage, and perforation
Pancreatitis
Intestinal perforation
Central nervous system
Psychiatric disturbances
  Mild euphoria
  Psychosis
  Dementia
Pseudotumor cerebri
Ophthalmologic
Ocular hypertension
Subcapsular cataracts
Infectious keratitis
Delayed healing of the cornea
Dermatologic
Hirsutism
Atrophy of the skin and subcutaneous tissue
Acne
Striae
Telangiectasias
Hematologic and Immunologic
Neutrophilic granulocytosis
Monocytopenia
Eosinopenia
Erythrocytosis and thrombocytosis
Suppression of immune and inflammatory response
  (immunosurveillance)
  Effects on circulating inflammatory cells
  Effects on the local mediators, including prostaglandins
  Effects on the reticuloendothelial system
Hypersensitivity reactions
ACTH
Glucocorticoid preparations
Metabolic and endocrinologic
Glucose intolerance (hepatic gluconeogenesis, glycogen
  deposition, and inhibition of peripheral glucose utilization)
Increased appetite and weight gain
Altered lipid metabolism and deposition
Peripheral protein catabolism
Impaired skeletal growth in children
Poor wound healing
Secondary amenorrhea
HPA suppression leading to secondary adrenal insufficiency

[a] Adapted from Melby JC: Systemic corticosteroid therapy: pharmacology and endocrinologic considerations. *Ann Intern Med* 81:505, 1974.

(e.g., polymyositis). In those patients who require chronic therapy, isokinetic exercise may partially reverse the muscle wasting and atrophy (89). In animal studies, short courses (2 weeks or less) of corticosteroids have also been shown to be associated with diaphragmatic atrophy, altered biochemistry, and a reduction in normalized diaphragmatic tetanic force (65, 175). Therefore corticosteroids could contribute to clinical respiratory muscle fatigue and/or weakness. However, in a study performed with healthy male subjects, a 2-week course on 20 mg of prednisone daily had no significant effects on measures of respiratory muscle strength or endurance (177).

Prolonged muscle paresis following the combined use of high-dose corticosteroids and nondepolarizing neuromuscular blockers in critically ill patients requiring paralysis has been reported (115). Although several reports suggesting an association anecdotally, a definite correlation has not been proved or excluded (41a).

The incidence of osteoporosis associated with corticosteroid therapy was found to be at least 50% in a recent review by Lukert (107). With prednisone doses of more than 7.5 mg/day, significant loss of trabecular bone can be seen in most patients; however, postmenopausal women and men may lose bone even with lower doses (107). After analyzing the longitudinal and cross-sectional data, Lukert believed that bone loss was accelerated during the initial weeks of glucocorticoid therapy and that the rate slowed subsequently (107). Potential mechanisms of the glucocorticoid-induced osteoporosis include reduction of sex hormone (both estrogens and testosterone) production, impairment of intestinal absorption of calcium, interference with vitamin D activity, secondary hyperparathyroidism resulting from glucocorticoid-induced negative calcium balance, inhibition of osteoblast function, and interference with prostaglandin EID_2 and insulin-like growth factor I production (both cytokines help bone formation/growth) (107). Certain populations may be at more risk of developing bone loss, such as those with rheumatoid arthritis and those who are immobilized for a protracted period. Recommended prevention and treatment strategies involve minimizing the dose and duration of glucocorticoid therapy, limiting immobility, maintaining adequate nutritional status and restricting sodium intake to 2 to 3 g/day, using thiazide diuretics if hypercalciuria is present, replacing gonadal hormones in postmenopausal or glucocorticoid-induced amenorrheic women, and replacing testosterone in men with low endogenous levels if not contraindicated (107). In addition, it is also advisable to maintain serum 25-hydroxy vitamin D concentrations within the normal range with supplements, to track bone density at 6-month intervals for the first 2 years if possible, and to consider the use of sodium fluoride 50 mg/day, calcitonin, and anabolic hormones in more severe cases or in those not responsive to conservative therapy (107).

Aseptic necrosis of the bone is also linked to chronic steroid therapy, occurring in approximately 1% of a steroid-dependent population (52, 142), with a higher incidence (14 to 50%) occurring in certain populations, such as patients with systemic lupus erythematosis (SLE) (187). Sites at risk for aseptic necrosis include the femoral heads, knees, and shoulders. Higher daily steroid doses, cushingoid changes, and Raynaud's phenomenon are associated with an increased incidence of ischemic necrosis in patients with SLE (187). Early detection may be accomplished using bone scans or magnetic resonance imaging.

The frequency of steroid-induced peptic ulceration of the gastrointestinal tract remains controversial, but 40 mg of prednisone for more than 2 weeks probably predisposes to ulcer formation. Conn and Blitzer in 1976 (43) reviewed the literature at the time and did not find a significant increase in the incidence of peptic ulceration, hemorrhage, and/or perforation in a steroid-treated group compared with controls. A divergence between the groups did appear when the total dose of steroids was considered (with >1 g of prednisone, the ulcer rate was

5.3% in contrast to 2.5% in the placebo group). Although Conn did not find a proclivity toward peptic ulceration in his retrospective study, he emphasized that "... one must not conclude that steroids are in no way associated with the development of peptic ulcer ..." (43); individual cohorts treated with steroids, such as those with cirrhotic or nephrotic disease and those receiving large total doses of steroids, may indeed have an increased tendency toward ulceration (43). Messer and associates in 1983 reexamined the literature and found an increased incidence of peptic ulceration and gastrointestinal hemorrhage in patients receiving corticosteroid treatment (120). More recently, Piper et al, using a case-control study to estimate the relative risk for peptic ulcer disease associated with the use of oral corticosteroids, found that the estimated relative risk in users of corticosteroids without concomitant nonsteroidal antiinflammatory drugs (NSAIDs) for peptic ulcer disease was 1.1 (137). The overall relative risk for corticosteroids users, including those on NSAIDs, was 2.0. The subgroup of patients receiving concurrent corticosteroids and NSAIDs had a risk of peptic ulcer disease 15 times higher than that of nonusers of either drug (137). Proposed avenues for the pathogenesis of steroid-related ulcers include increased acid production (as documented in dogs) (64), decreased mucus production by the gastric lining cells (64, 119), a defective capacity of the mucosal cells to repair and regenerate themselves (64), decreased gastric mucus production (137), gastrin and parietal cell hyperplasia (137), delayed healing and enlargement of experimental ulcers (137), and reulceration of previously healed ulcers (137). The addition of antacids (85), sucralfate, or, perhaps, enteral feedings (136) may protect the gastric cell lining. Unfortunately, raising the gastric pH in the critically ill patient with antacids, H_2-blockers, or enteral feedings may allow microbial colonization of the stomach and increase the risk of nosocomial infections.

Pancreatitis occurs with an increased frequency in those on steroid therapy but is not a common clinical problem. A direct relationship between corticosteroids and intestinal perforation remains unproved since reported cases have occurred in patients with inflammatory bowel disease (52).

Psychiatric disturbances seen with glucocorticoid therapy range from mild euphoria to frank psychosis and dementia (173). These reactions are reversible with discontinuation of the steroid and are not necessarily related to the pretreatment psyche (52). Larger doses (≥40 mg of prednisone/day) are associated with a higher frequency of psychiatric problems but not with the severity or duration of the symptoms (121a). Onset of the mental disturbances usually occurs within 10 days of starting therapy (135). Lithium prophylaxis may help prevent the development of steroid-induced psychosis if continued therapy is required (76), but decreasing the daily dose to less than 40 mg is also very effective in avoiding psychiatric side effects (121a). Dexamethasone may cause fewer problems in this regard than either cortisol or prednisone (68). Cognitive impairment may also be seen with high doses of prednisone (greater than 50 mg/day) (121a).

Uncommon cases of pseudotumor cerebri have been reported in children and adults on glucocorticoid therapy (49, 93, 176). Ocular hypertension and posterior subcapsular cataracts are ophthalmologic manifestations of chronic therapy; the former is reversible with the cessation of therapy, but the latter is not. Additionally, topical ophthalmologic preparations can lead to fungal keratitis, worsening of herpes keratitis, and delayed healing of the cornea.

Hirsutism, thinning of the skin with atrophy, poor wound repair, acne, striae, and telangiectasias are common skin complications of steroid administration. Wound healing is especially problematic in the postoperative patient. The effects of glucocorticoids on the immune-effector cells, the inflammatory response, and the cellular mediators probably all contribute to the poor wound healing seen with corticosteroid therapy. In addition, glucocorticoids alter normal collagen metabolism during wound healing, leading to a decrease in collagen deposition with a decrease in fibroblastic procollagen synthesis at the gene expression level (73). This leads to a decrease in wound integrity, as can be demonstrated by a decrease in the breaking strength and breaking energy of healing wounds (73). Moreover, glucocorticoids are associated with a reduction in several enzymes that are required for the posttranslational processing of collagen (73). However, concurrent administration of vitamin A (retinoids) may be capable of reversing the negative effects of cortisol on collagen synthesis and deposition and wound tensile strength (73). Vitamin A may reverse cortisol-induced macrophage changes but may be less effective with methylprednisolone (91). Sandberg showed that the timing of steroid administration also affects wound healing (146). Cortisone given to rats 2 days or more after wounding had no significant effect on tensile strength or hydroxyproline content (146). However, when the rats were given cortisone prior to wounding, there was a significant decrease in these parameters (146).

The effects of glucocorticoids on the hematologic and immune systems have already been discussed. Neutrophilic granulocytosis, monocytopenia, and eosinopenia are common laboratory findings. An increase in the circulating erythrocyte and platelet levels may also be seen (170). Because of the reduction in immune surveillance, especially in the cell-mediated response, infections with bacteria, viruses, fungi, and parasites (especially *Pneumocystis carinii*) complicate long-term therapy. Fauci and associates (63) reported that the incidence and frequency of infections rose with higher doses of steroids in patients with SLE. Using a meta-analysis of pooled data from 71 controlled studies, Stuck estimated that the relative risk of infectious complications in those receiving corticosteroid therapy (overall rate of infectious complications, 12.7%) was 1.6 compared with that of controls (overall rate of infectious complications, 8.0%) (162). The relative risk was especially high in patients with neurologic diseases. Potential problems from steroid therapy also result from the masking of the usual signs of inflammation (rubor, calor, dolor, and tumor) and delaying early recognition of a clinically significant infection.

The frequency of reactivation tuberculosis with steroid therapy remains unclear. However, at least in asthmatics on chronic steroid therapy there appears to be no major increase in reactivation tuberculosis (54). Additionally, only one of 25 patients with chronic active hepatitis treated with steroids in Hong Kong (where tuberculosis is likely to be more endemic than in the U.S.) developed tuberculosis (104). Still, it is suggested that isoniazid (INH) 300 mg/day for 1 year be given prophylactically to chronic steroid patients who have a known positive tuberculin skin test and have not been treated previously (61, 62). Cutaneous anergy is common while a patient is on daily doses of prednisone, developing within a few days of therapy and resolving after 10 to 14 days of steroid cessation (57).

Hypersensitivity to commercial glucocorticoid products is known (71, 171). Reactions include urticaria, angioedema, bronchospasm and anaphylactoid reactions (118). Rarely, aspirin sensitive asthmatics may demonstrate cross-sensitivity to intravenous esters of hydrocortisone. Desensitization may be required if steriod therapy is felt to be imperative (39).

Normal metabolism can be altered markedly by steroid therapy. Skeletal growth is impaired in children on chronic therapy. Switching to alternate-day administration may allow improvement. Because of the effect of the steroid on glucose metabolism and stimulation of glucagon secretion (109), hyperglycemia commonly is encountered, but the development of ketosis or acidosis associated with absolute insulin deficiency is uncommon. Treatment strategies to control blood sugar levels consist of dietary manipulation and insulin therapy and do not differ from those of nonsteroid-induced hyperglycemia. Control of the hyperglycemia is especially imperative in the critically ill patient to avoid glucosuria (with loss calories) and an osmotic diuresis, which complicates the interpetation of the hourly urine output as marker of renal perfusion. Exogenous glucocorticoid therapy may also contribute to the abnormal glucose production and utilization seen in burn patients (184). The cushingoid appearance (moon facies, buffalo hump, and centripetal obesity) is a result of altered lipid metabolism. Abnormal accumulation of fat can be seen in the mediastinum (thoracic lipomatosis), which can be distinguished from malignant mass by its fat density on computerized tomography imaging (102). Thoracic lipomatosis may also suggest a pericardial effusion (124). Weight gain and an increased appetite typically are seen with chronic therapy. In addition, it has been speculated that accelerated atherosclerosis may be a complication of long-term steroid administration leading to an increased mortality from cardiovascular disease (127).

Fluid and salt retention occur because of excessive mineralocorticoid activity and can lead to edema and hypertension. This effect is greater with the preparations that have a high mineralocorticoid:glucocorticoid ratio. Sodium retention at the expense of hydrogen ion excretion can lead to a metabolic alkalosis and consequently hypercapnia resulting from respiratory compensation (31–33). This effect may lead to difficulty in weaning patients from the ventilator. Substitution of an agent with less mineralocorticoid activity, such as prednisone or dexamethasone, may ameliorate the problem (32).

Glucocorticoid use in human pregnancy is relatively safe. Although animal data have suggested an increased prevalence of fetal wastage and cleft palates in corticosteroid-treated rats (48, 168), a recent report found no fetal malformations, neonatal deaths, or maternal death in 56 women with severe asthma requiring systemic glucocorticoids and/or inhaled steroids (69). Neonatal adrenal insufficiency is also a rarity despite maternal use of pharmacologic doses of steroids (48). Poor penetration of prednisone and/or prednisolone through the placenta may account for this observation (168). Despite this fact, careful monitoring of the newborn for signs of adrenal insufficiency is indicated because of its potential devastating effects but ease of treatment. Glucocorticoids are excreted in breast milk and nursing infants should be observed for hypercortisol effects (57).

An important consequence of exogenous glucocorticoid therapy is adrenal insufficiency caused by HPA axis suppression. Although numerous studies have been performed regarding this aspect, the data are difficult to interpret because of the heterogeneity of the patient populations, the steroid dose, the frequency of administration, the length of therapy, and the means used to assess adrenal insufficiency (7). It is clear, however, that prolonged therapy with glucocorticoids can cause suppression of the HPA axis for several months to a year after withdrawal of therapy (78) and that it is often asymptomatic. The hypothalamic-pituitary axis recovers first with the return of a normal diurnal secretion of ACTH. This ACTH secretion is followed by recovery of the adrenal gland (78, 169). The exogenous administration of ACTH does not hasten the recovery (86, 57). Streck and Lockwood (160) reported a reduced response to synthetic ACTH for up to 5 days after stopping a brief 5-day course of prednisone 25 mg orally twice a day. Larger doses over longer periods of time may suppress the normal axis for up to a year (57). However, the daily dose, cumulative dose, or duration of therapy as well as a single basal cortisol level are not accurate predictors of HPA suppression as tested by the CRF stimulation testing or insulin tolerance testing (147). Certainly, patients who currently are on glucocorticoids should be considered to have HPA suppression.

Symptoms of secondary adrenal insufficiency resulting from HPA axis suppression may be more subtle (e.g., malaise, lethargy, fatigue, hypoglycemia, and hypothermia) than those of classic Addison's disease (primary adrenal failure). There is an absence of both major fluid and electrolyte disturbances (e.g, hypotension, hyperkalemia, and dehydration) and increased skin pigmentation. Adequate physiologic replacement with an agent that has both glucocorticoid and mineralocorticoid activity (e.g., hydrocortisone 30 to 40 mg/day in two divided doses) corrects both states, although mineralocorticoid activity may not to be supplemented in secondary adrenal insufficiency because of the preservation of aldosterone secretion.

Even with normal HPA axis function, occasionally patients may experience steroid withdrawal symptoms, which consist of anorexia, malaise, nausea with emesis, headache, lethargy, orthostatic hypotension, myalgias, and weight loss (7, 48). Laboratory testing in these patients shows "normal" plasma cortisol levels and normal responses to stimulatory testing (7, 48). The reason for these symptoms is unknown, but it is important not to confuse them with documented adrenal insufficiency with low basal and stimulated cortisol levels, because education and counseling may be all that is required to deal with the problem. However, a physical dependence on higher levels of glucocorticoids may exist, requiring reinstitution of physiologic dosages and a slower and longer tapering schedule (57). Not only is HPA axis suppression a problem after stopping corticosteroid administration, but reactivation of the primary disease process for which therapy was initiated further complicates the process. Both respond to restarting the medication at least at physiologic doses or at the last dose that controlled the disease manifestations and following a more protracted tapering schedule.

Secondary adrenal insufficiency resulting from exogenous glucocorticoid therapy is often asymptomatic and may not be manifested clinically until a stress situation (e.g., surgery, general anesthesia, trauma, or critical illness) disastrously intervenes; therefore, provocative testing may be necessary to detect patients with suspected impairment in the HPA axis. The insulin tolerance test (ITT) is a standard method for testing the HPA axis, but it is hazardous in critically ill patients. A safe and practical test, though less sensitive, is the cosyntropin (ACTH) stimulation test (16). A baseline cortisol level is drawn, then 250 μg of cosyntropin (1-24 corticotropin) is injected intravenously. An increase in the plasma cortisol level of at least 7 μg/dl and an absolute level above 18 μg/dl at 60 minutes occurs with an intact axis. In adrenal insufficiency the response curve is blunted, whereas it is exaggerated in stress situations (Fig. 43.3). Although the cosyntropin test should discriminate normal from abnormal adrenocorticol function in terms of glucocorticoid activity, it does not necessarily pinpoint the locus of pathology (33). This simplified test may also miss patients with inadequate ACTH-cortisol response to physiologic stress. Thus, a subnormal test is more informative than a normal one (16, 45, 129). Recently, provocative testing with CRF has been shown to be almost as useful as an ITT (147) in the assessment of pituitary-adrenal function (147). A bolus of intravenous human CRF of 100 μg is given and serial plasma levels of corticotropin (ACTH) and cortisol are obtained before and after the administration of CRF (60 and 120 minutes). A normal response is a 1.5-fold increase in the peak plasma cortisol level and a level greater than 10 μg/dl (147). Further testing with an insulin tolerance test producing hypoglycemic stress, a metyrapone test (enzymatic blocker of the biosynthetic cascade for cortisol synthesis), a 3-day cosyntropin test, or ACTH and aldosterone levels may be required to localize the site of adrenal insufficiency (primary vs secondary). Because obtaining the results of these tests may not be readily available prednisolone or dexamethasone and other supportive measures (fluid and electrolyte replacement) should be administered coincident with testing. Plasma cortisol levels measured by the radioimmunoassay technique have little cross-reactivity with other synthetic steroids (170). If mineralocorticoid activity is also believed to be absent, hydrocortisone and/or 9-α-fludrocortisol (0.05 to 0.1 mg/day orally) should be administered after drawing blood for hormonal levels.

Surgery and general anesthesia normally increase glucocorticoid secretion. Thus, preoperative patients who are suspected of adrenal insufficiency (previous or current steroid therapy) should undergo provocative testing. If time does not permit diagnostic procedures, then patients who currently are on steroids or who have been on glucocorticoids within the preceding 6 months to 1 year for at least 1 week, and those with known adrenal insufficiency (primary or secondary) should be provided with stress coverage (Table 43.4) (181). In acute stress situations, the total steroid dose should be equivalent to 200 to 300 mg/day of hydrocortisone. Although these doses probably exceed the minimum required, they should provide a more than satisfactory safety factor to avoid adrenal insufficiency. Recent evidence supports the concept that the amount of glucocorticoid "stress coverage" can be titrated to the degree of stress (34). If mineralocorticoid activity is required, it is important to choose an agent that has both glucocorticoid and mineralocorticoid activities, such as hydrocortisone.

Since the unwanted effects of the glucocorticoids are inexorably tied to the desired effects, a healthy respect for the balance between the two is paramount. These drugs can both be life saving and life threatening in the critically ill patient.

MINERALOCORTICOIDS

Mineralocorticoids are defined by their action on ion transport (10). Aldosterone and deoxycorticosterone (DOC) are the major endogenous mineralocorticoids. About 55% of aldosterone is carried bound to protein, chiefly albumin, but only the free state is active (170). DOC is more than 95% bound to plasma proteins and, therefore, under normal physiologic conditions contributes little to the overall mineralocorticoid activity, despite its potency in the free state (170). Although cortisol has only approximately 1% of the mineralocorticoid activity of aldosterone because of local inactivation, it circulates freely in the bloodstream at concentrations 15 to 750 times higher than those of aldosterone (10) and thus may participate in normal fluid and electrolyte balance. Aldosterone is cleared hepatically and has a circulating half-life of 15 minutes (170).

The kidney is the major target organ for the mineralocorticoids, and excess or depleted states are reflected by abnormal renal fluid and electrolyte homeostasis. However, the gastrointestinal tract, salivary glands, and sweat glands are also affected. Like glucocorticoids, the mineralocorticoids bind to a cytosol receptor, inducing DNA transcription and the production of specific proteins. After a delay of up to 2 hours (10), reabsorption of sodium ions in exchange for potassium and hydrogen ions occurs in the distal renal tubules. In the absence of mineralocorticoid activity (e.g., primary adrenal insufficiency), hyperkalemia, hyponatremia, extracellular dehydration, and metabolic acidosis ensue (10). Conversely, in an excess state (Conn's syndrome or primary hyperaldosteronism), hypokalemia, fluid retention with hypertension, and metabolic alkalosis are seen.

Aldosterone secretion is regulated by the renin-angiotensin system. This axis is sensitive to changes in the effective intravascular volume, blood pressure, β-adrenergic stimulation, sodium depletion, and the extracellular potassium level. Salt depletion and/or hypotension stimulate renin release by the kidney's juxtaglomerular cells. Through a series of enzymatic cleavages, angiotensin II is produced. Angiotension II increases aldosterone biosynthesis after binding to receptors in the zona glomerulosa and altering intracellular Ca^{2+} transport and phospholipid metabolism. In addition Angiotensin II exerts a trophic effect on the zona glomerulosa. The role of ACTH in aldostersone secretion is not well-understood. Administered ACTH results in a nonsustained increase in aldosterone (167) and induces steroidogenic enzymes, but ACTH repression by dexamethasone does not impair basal aldosterone levels or their response to sodium depletion (10). Hypophysectomized animals can survive without salt therapy, and the zona glomerulosa is the zone least affected by the withdrawal of ACTH (86). Therefore, ACTH has a limited role in aldosterone secretion but other pituitary factors may

Table 43.4. Recommended Steroid Coverage for Preoperative Patients with First- or Second-Degree Adrenocortical Insufficiency[a]

Day	Hydrocortisone Sodium Succinate or Equivalent	
Preoperative day 1	25 mg at 1800 and 2400, i.v. or i.m.	
Day of operation	100 mg i.v. during surgery	
Postoperative	100 mg i.v. q. 8 hr times 24 hr	
	50 mg i.v. q. 8 hr times 24 hr }	may be switched to p.o. if the patient is able
	25 mg i.v. q. 8 hr times 24 hr	to tolerate oral medications

[a] Modified from White VA, Kumagai LF: Preoperative endocrine and metabolic considerations. Symposium on medical evaluation by the preoperative patient. *Med Clin North Am* 63:1321, 1979.

be more important. Potassium balance affects aldosterone secretion both through the renin-angiotensin pathway and independently. Hyperkalemia amplifies production of aldosterone, whereas hypokalemia diminishes it. Atrial natriuretic hormone release causes a decrease in both aldosterone synthesis and renin release (36). Dopamine is said to inhibit aldosterone secretion, especially in sodium-depleted individuals, whereas dopamine antagonists (e.g., metoclopramide) have the opposite effect (13, 170). However, under normal conditions aldosterone is usually under maximal dopamine inhibition and further increases in dopamine levels have a minor additional inhibiting effect (36). Hypoxemia can also decrease aldosterone levels (36). Thus, the overall secretion rate of aldosterone is the result of an integrated response.

Aldosterone causes an alteration in sodium permeability, increases the energy stores (ATP) for the Na^+/K^+ pump, effects the Na^+/K^+ pump itself so as to augment sodium reabsorption, and establishes an electrical gradient that promotes potassium and hydrogen ion excretion (10, 170). In this regard, kaliuresis is tied to delivery of sodium to the distal tubule (10). Clinically, the use of the urine Na^+/K^+ ratio can reflect the level of aldosterone activity. A low ratio indicates a high aldosterone state, and a high ratio indicates the reverse. In addition, aldosterone stimulates the citric acid cycle enzymes and alters cellular lipid metabolism (36).

Therapeutic uses of exogenous mineralocorticoids are limited to primary adrenal insufficiency, hyporeninemic hypoaldosteronism, and primary orthostatic hypotension. The primary commercial mineralocorticoid (excluding hydrocortisone) is 9-α-fludrocortisone (fludrocortisone acetate). It usually is administered in doses of 0.05 to 0.1 mg/day orally (up to 0.4 mg/day in hyporeninemic hypoaldosteronism). It has 125 times the mineralocorticoid activity of cortisol (86). Deoxycorticosterone and aldosterone, because of their rapid hepatic clearance, are not suitable for oral use; however, deoxycorticosterone is available in the parenteral form as an acetate or pivalate ester. In primary adrenal dysfunction, hydrocortisone may provide an adequate amount of mineralocorticoid activity, but additional fludrocortisone commonly is needed.

Antagonists of aldosterone such as spironolactone have wider clinical application. By competitive inhibition (competitive binding to the aldosterone cystol receptors without agonist activity), spironolactone promotes diuresis, sodium loss, and potassium retention. It is used in the management of hypertension, edematous states (especially those associated with excessive aldosterone activity, such as cirrhosis, nephrosis, and congestive heart failure), and certain hypokalemic states. Since only 10% of the filtered sodium load reaches the distal tubule, where aldosterone has its action, spironolactone

is not a potent diuretic and its effects are dependent on the filtered sodium load and state of aldosterone activity. It is available only in the oral form, and the usual daily dose is 100 to 200 mg/day in divided doses. Edematous states usually require the higher doses. Side effects include hyperkalemia, gynecomastia, and androgen-like effects (86).

The angiotensin-converting enzyme inhibitors such as captopril and enalapril work by preventing the conversion of angiotensin I into angiotensin II, a powerful vasoconstrictor and a stimulator of aldosterone. They are useful in the management of hypertension and cardiac failure, especially the latter, since congestive heart failure usually leads to secondary hyperaldosteronism and therefore, fluid retention. Recently, the use of enalapril has been shown to improve survival in patients with reduced left ventricular ejection fractions and congestive heart failure (157).

Isolated hypoaldosteronism can occur in conjunction with specific adrenocorticol enzyme deficiency states, with both hyporeninemia and hyperreninemia, and prolonged heparin use. Hyporeninemic hypoaldosteronism usually occurs in the setting of mild renal insufficiency and diabetes mellitus. Heparin can suppress aldosterone synthesis and secretion and usually is associated with elevated plasma renin activity. Hyperreninemic hypoaldosteronism has been reported in the critically ill population and appears to result from the dissociation of renin from aldosterone (a presumed adaptive mechanism to severe stress) (67). The relative shift away from androgen and mineralocorticoid synthesis may allow for greater production of the "stress" hormones (67).

INDICATIONS FOR CORTICOSTEROID THERAPY: SPECIFIC CRITICAL CARE IMPLICATIONS

The majority of the clinical indications for corticosteroid therapy (Table 43.2) involve their ability to alter the immune response and decrease inflammation, hopefully, leading to a decrease in tissue injury and dysfunction. Other aspects of corticosteroid activity are capitalized on in special circumstances: physiologic replacement in adrenocorticol insufficiency, decreased calcium absorption and increased renal excretion in hypercalcemia, and tumor control in certain malignant cell lines. In many instances steroid use is empiric, based on anecdotal evidence or theoretic grounds, and almost always is palliative, except in the treatment of adrenal insufficiency.

Doses to achieve clinical remission in disease processes vary from replacement doses of 30 mg/day of hydrocortisone for adrenocortical failure to supraphysiologic doses of 1 to 2 g

Table 43.5. Usual Dosages of Glucocorticoids

Treatment	Dose Equivalent
Physiologic glucocorticoid replacement	Hydrocortisone 20 mg in the AM; 10 mg in the PM p.o.
Mineralocorticoid replacement	Fludrocortisone acetate 0.1 mg p.o. every 24–48 hr
Antiinflammatory	Prednisone 0.5–2 mg p.o. every day in single or divided doses *or* Prednisolone 0.5–2 mg/kg p.o. every day in single or divided doses
Suprapharmacologic	Prednisolone ≥ 1 g i.v. bolus or in divided doses every day

Table 43.6. NHLBI Recommended Dosage Schedules for Intravenous Steroids in Acute Exacerbations of Asthma

Methylprednisolone	60–80 mg i.v. bolus	q. 6–8 hr
Hydrocortisone	2.9 mg/kg i.v. bolus	q. 4 hr
Hydrocortisone	2.0 mg/kg i.v. bolus	Then 0.5 mg/kg/ hr continuous i.v. infusion

of intravenous prednisolone for transplant rejection (Table 43.5). If steroids are to be used, a sufficient amount should be given to induce a clinical remission based on predetermined clinical signs and symptoms. The difficulty is in determining the minimum adequate dose to obtain the anticipated end result. If the literature supports the use of steroids in a disease process, then the doses and products used in the studies should be employed in the clinical arena. The usual doses implemented to control hypersensitivity or autoimmune disorders (connective tissue diseases, vasculitis, etc.) are in the range of 40 to 150 mg or 0.5 to 2 mg/kg of prednisone equivalent per day in single or divided doses. Higher doses, pulse doses, and more frequent administration (divided daily doses) may be required initially to control an acute inflammatory process before tapering back to a single daily dose. Even some rather chronic disorders (SLE or temporal arteritis) may require twice (or more) daily doses to achieve and maintain remission. High-dose pulse therapy with methylprednisolone has been advocated in some disease processes (transplant rejection, SLE, rapidly progressive glomerulonephritis) to attain rapid and longer-lasting therapeutic activity with fewer side effects. This type of drug dosing may also have the advantage of achieving the effects that are associated only with very high doses of glucocorticoids (stabilization of lysosomes, inhibition of chemotaxis and cell receptor expression, etc.). Once disease control has been obtained, dropping to the lowest single daily dose or alternate-day therapy, if possible, should provide maximum benefit with the lowest risk of side effects (especially of HPA axis suppression). It is important before embarking on steroid treatment to maximize adjunctive therapy and establish specific endpoints.

OBSTRUCTIVE LUNG DISEASES

Asthma is considered primarily an inflammatory disease of the airways. Specific allergens or irritants and nonspecific irritants lead to airway inflammation in susceptible individuals. Airway narrowing occurs as a consequence of airway inflammation from bronchial hyperreactivity, airway edema, and mucus secretion and plugging. Acute attacks of asthma are characterized by an exacerbation of bronchial smooth muscle contraction (bronchoconstriction), airway inflammation with edema, and mucus plugging. Because the glucocorticoids reduce inflammatory mediator release, mucus secretion (123), and migration of inflammatory cells, potentiate responses to β-adrenergic agonists (123), reduce bronchial epithelial cell

endothelin 1 secretion (a potent bronchial smooth muscle constrictor) (175a) and may have direct effects on smooth muscle reactivity by way of membrane bound Ca^{2+} (123), they are considered a cornerstone in the treatment of mild asthma as well as status asthmaticus. Glucocorticoids also attenuate the late asthmatic response to an antigen challenge which is ordinarily characterized by local inflammatory cell influx. Inhaled, topically administered steroid preparations are available for use in patients with stable disease to minimize exacerbations by reducing the airway inflammation that is responsible for bronchial hyperreactivity. Inhaled steroids allow freedom from systemic therapy with its attendant complications, or at least a reduction in systemic doses. Devices such as spacers for metered-dose inhalers (MDI) improve topical lung deposition by reducing droplet size and velocity. Spacers are especially helpful in those who have difficulty in coordinating the use of the MDI with their breathing pattern; they may also limit complications such as oral thrush.

A recent expert panel from the National Heart, Lung, and Blood Institute has emphasized the role of glucocorticoids in the treatment of asthma (128). The major questions remaining in the use of steroids in acute asthma deal with the dose, type, timing, frequency and length of administration, and subpopulations who require systemic therapy. Fanta et al (60) suggest a 2 mg/kg bolus of hydrocortisone followed by a continuous infusion of 0.5 mg/kg/hr for 24 hours as the initial regimen in acute asthma. However, no correlation between plasma cortisol levels and spirometric lung function was found (60). Haskell et al demonstrated that 40- and 120-mg doses of methylprednisolone intravenously every 6 hours were effective in relieving status asthmaticus, whereas 15-mg doses were not (84). They favored the use of the higher dose because of a more rapid response within the first 3 days (84). Others have noted no difference in response between low and high doses (15 mg vs 125 mg of methylprednisolone) (165). In a review of the use of glucocorticoids in acute severe asthma, Engel noted that eight of 13 placebo-controlled studies found glucocorticoid therapy superior to placebo in terms of improvement in pulmonary function, blood gas analysis, or hospital admission rate (59). In only two of 10 studies was there evidence for a dose-response relationship (59). Frequent administration of doses (four times daily) and initial doses in the range of 100 to 200 mg/day of methylprednisolone appeared to be important for success in most of the studies (Table 43.6) (59). The time course of response to steroids was usually on the order of 4 to 6 hours (123). Therefore, the decision to employ steroids should be made early during the clinical course. After control is established usually within 36–48 hours, one should convert to a single daily dose, usually in the morning, and gradually taper the dose following pulmonary function tests (peak flows or forced expiratory volume in one second (FEV_1)). Long-term systemic glucocorticoid therapy may be required in some patients (53). A minority of asthmatics appear to be steroid resistant. Resistance does not result from abnormal glucocorticoid clearance or an abnormality in the cellular glucocorticoid receptor, but from a relative insensitivity of T-lymphocytes to glucocorticoids in these patients (44).

The use of steroids in chronic obstructive pulmonary disease (COPD) is less clear than that in the asthmatic. However, since most patients with COPD have some "reversible" obstructive component during an exacerbation, a trial of glucocorticoids is indicated if there is not an adequate response to conventional bronchodilators (β-adrenergic agonists and theophylline). Albert has shown a beneficial effect from methylprednisolone 0.5 mg/kg every 6 hours intravenously during the first 72 hours of treatment in patients with chronic bronchitis and acute respiratory insufficiency (2). Murata showed that treatment with a regimen of intravenous and oral corticosteroids reduced the rate of relapse after emergency room treatment of decompensated COPD in those with a history of multiple relapses compared with matched controls (126). However, Emerman and his colleagues found that a single dose of methylprednisolone (100 mg) given one-half hour after arrival in the emergency room did not improve FEV₁ or rate of hospitalization in COPD patients (56). Long-term glucocorticoids may be of benefit in stable COPD patients (117). However, in both asthma and chronic obstructive pulmonary diseases, objective evidence of improvement (e.g., spirometric values) is important because not all patients show a significant response (e.g., primary emphysematous patients with little or no bronchitic component) and some chronic asthmatics are resistant to steroid therapy (28). Therefore, these individuals should not be subjected to the risks of corticosteroid therapy. A recent metaanalysis of studies dealing with the use of oral steroids in stable patients with COPD could document improvement of the FEV₁ (20% or greater) in only 10% of the study population (27). The efficacy of inhaled topical steroids in COPD is even less clear. Several studies have shown that inhaled topical steroids (beclomethasone and budesonide) do not alter symptomatology, pulmonary function, or response to nonspecific airway challenge compared with placebo in patients with COPD (58, 152, 179). More recently, though, the use of inhaled steroids has been shown to reduce symptoms and measure of bronchial hyperreactivity as well as visual appearance of bronchitis and bronchial lavage indices of airway inflammation (99a, 166a).

SEPSIS AND THE ADULT RESPIRATORY DISTRESS SYNDROME

Because of their antiinflammatory effects, the glucocorticoids were thought early on to improve the course and mortality of septic shock and the adult respiratory distress syndrome (ARDS). Glucocorticoids had been reported to be able to perform a number of "beneficial" functions: disaggregate clumps of granulocytes (82, 155), stabilize lysosomal enzymes and capillary membranes, minimize capillary permeability (21), improve oxygenation by altering ventilation/perfusion mismatches (123), increase cardiac contractility (87), antagonize complement (87) and reduce complement-mediated granulocytic aggregation (155), diminish coagulopathy (87), antagonize endotoxin effects (87), decrease local inflammatory responses and release of mediators, including the prostaglandin derivatives (70, 122), alter the migratory patterns of inflammatory cells, reduce toxic oxygen radical release (82), and vasoconstrict the capillary bed either directly or indirectly through the potentiation of the adrenergic system (57). Most of these effects were thought to be mediated through the effects of glucucorticoids on cellular lipocortins, which interfere with the release and metabolism of arachidonic acid.

In 1976, a prospective study of septic patients by Schumer (151) indicated that methylprednisolone (30 mg/kg) or dexamethasone (3 mg/kg) given once or twice in 24 hours reduced the mortality from 38.4% to 10.5%. Later, in 1984, Sprung et al (158) also conducted a prospective, controlled study of steroids in sepsis. Methylprednisolone- (30 mg/kg) and dexamethasone- (6 mg/kg) treated patients were more likely to have their shock reversed, but the overall survival rate was similar in both groups (steroid treated, 23%; control, 31%). The survival rates were considerably lower than those Schumer reported (151) but more in line with those from other studies and clinical practice (158). Sibbald et al (153) reported reduced accumulation of radiolabelled serum albumin in pulmonary edema fluid in patients with septic ARDS given methylprednisolone. Cheyney et al (35) reported that methylprednisolone increased the resolution of oleic acid-induced pulmonary injury in dogs. Several other experimental animal studies further suggested that early glucocorticoid therapy could blunt the effects of sepsis, improve survival, reduce pulmonary hypertension, and decrease pulmonary permeability edema associated with endotoxin infusion (77). These animal studies (though not always applicable to human trials) suggested that early administration of glucocorticoids (e.g., at the time of challenge with endotoxin or *Escherichia coli*) could improve survival. In Sprung's study an average of 17.5 ± 5.4 hours passed between the onset of shock and the first dose of glucocorticoid therapy, and perhaps the cascade of events that may have been responsive to steroid therapy had already been initiated. It was noted in Sprung's study that those who had received steroids within 4 hours of shock had a higher incidence of reversal of shock, although the overall mortality was again not changed (158). Parenthetically, there appeared to be no significant reduction in the cases of ARDS in either of the steroid-treated groups compared with the control group (27% vs 15%, respectively) (158).

The clinical efficacy of steroid therapy in sepsis was then reevaluated in two newer well-designed cooperative clinical trials by Bone and his colleagues and the Veteran's Administration Systemic Sepsis Cooperative Study Group. These two studies had a combined total of 605 patients. Both studies concluded that high-dose corticosteroids (methylprednisolone sodium succinate 30 mg/kg in four doses every 6 hours or 30 mg/kg as the initial dose followed by 5 mg/kg/hr for 9 hours) had no benefit in the treatment of severe sepsis (15, 166). Mortality secondary to infectious complications was found to be higher in the steroid cohort than in the control group in Bone's study (15). Moreover, Bone et al, after analyzing the subgroup with ARDS, reported that the group with sepsis receiving methylprednisolone had an increased tendency toward the development of ARDS (32%) compared with the placebo group (25%) (14). The 14-day mortality rate with combined sepsis and ARDS was significantly higher in the group receiving methylprednisolone (52%) than in the controls (22%) (14). Two other studies also failed to demonstrate an improved outcome with early steroid therapy in ARDS; one examined acute lung injury associated with sepsis, and the other included other predisposing factors in addition to sepsis (11, 106). Glucocorticoids also have not been effective in the treatment of acid aspiration or fresh-water drowning, both of which can lead to ARDS. Furthermore, although large doses of glucocorticoids given in a short course generally have been free of major complications, there have been reports of cardiac arrhythmias and sudden death after rapid bolus intravenous administration (111, 161). Bolus administration can also aggravate acute lung damage during the early phase of repair in experimental lung injury (99). The current consensus is that steroids are of no benefit in the management of the sepsis or acute lung injury/ARDS.

On the other hand, Schonfeld et al published a study showing that prophylactic methylprednisolone (7.5 mg/kg every 6 hours for a total of 12 doses) prevented the fat emboli syndrome (a predisposing cause of ARDS) in patients with long bone fractures (150). Glucocorticoids have also been shown to increase surfactant synthesis (144) and may prevent bronchopulmonary dysplasia when given antenatally in threatened premature birth (159). Methylprednisolone has been shown to prevent excessive collagen deposition in an experimental model of hypoxemic respiratory failure (96). Ashbaugh and Maier, Hooper and Kearl, and Meduri et al have suggested that glucocorticoids may help resolve fibrosis and improve survival in chronic ARDS patients in fibroproliferative stage (4, 88, 113).

Overall, corticosteroids are believed to be of limited clinical value in the acute treatment of sepsis/ARDS. The early enthusiasm for corticosteroids has now given way to the study of other agents such as prostaglandin agonists and antagonists, antioxidants, heavy metal chelators, oxygen radical scavengers, surfactant replacement (94), and monoclonal antibodies in the treatment of the septic syndrome and acute lung injury. The role of glucocorticoid therapy in the late fibroproliferative phase of ARDS is awaiting further documentation of efficacy in a randomized double-blinded study, but it is rather clear that steroids are not helpful in the early management of acute lung injury.

ACQUIRED IMMUNE DEFICIENCY SYNDROME

One of the more contemporary and important clinical uses of corticosteroids has been in the treatment of *P. carinii* pneumonia (PCP) in the acquired immune deficiency syndrome (AIDS) population. Current studies have demonstrated clinical benefits from glucocorticoids in reducing respiratory impairment in moderate to severe PCP in these patients (17). PCP is at present the most common life-threatening opportunistic infection in AIDS. Despite directed therapy, 5 to 30% of patients will develop acute respiratory failure, and most will die. The Pneumocystis organism and the secondary host inflammatory response can cause acute and potentially irreversible destruction of the lung architecture. The inflammatory response results in mononuclear cell invasion of the lung interstitium, subsequent arrival of other potent effector cells and their mediators, and accumulation of proteinaceous fluid

and organisms in the alveoli. Although clearance of the organism is poor, significant lung damage can occur. Initiation of glucocorticoids could blunt the inflammatory process and limit subsequent lung damage, improving oxygenation and outcome.

A recent National Institutes of Health panel reviewed the current literature on the use of corticosteroids in PCP and issued a consensus recommendation (130). The panel concluded that adjunctive corticosteroid therapy may reduce the likelihood of death, respiratory failure, and oxygen desaturation in patients with moderate to severe PCP (PaO$_2$ <70 mm Hg or an alveolar-arterial O$_2$ gradient >35 mmHg) (130). Adjunctive corticosteroid therapy should be started as soon as specific anti-Pneumocystis therapy is initiated, since most studies showed the greatest benefit when corticosteroid therapy was begun within 24 to 72 hours of anti-Pneumocystis therapy (130). No benefit was noted when corticosteroids were used late in the course of PCP or in severe respiratory failure that required assisted mechanical ventilation (130). Studies have not demonstrated an advantageous effect in patients with mild PCP (defined as PaO$_2$ >70 mm Hg or an alveolar-arterial O$_2$ gradient <35 mm Hg) (130). Recently "rescue therapy" (higher doses of corticosteroids in those who are not responding to standard doses or the institution of therapy in patients who are failing nonsteroid therapy) may also be effective in improving outcome on patients with PCP and acute respiratory failure (104a). The recommended schedule of corticosteroids as adjunctive therapy in PCP is 40 mg of oral prednisone twice a day for days 1 through 5, 40 mg daily for days 6 through 10, and 20 mg daily for days 11 through 21 (130). If intravenous therapy is required, methylprednisolone can be used (30 mg b.i.d. for days 1 through 5, 30 mg qd for days 6 through 10, and 15 mg qd for days 11 through 21) (130). This schedule is somewhat arbitrary, as there have been no definitive studies to determine the optimal dose, route, or schedule of corticosteroids in PCP.

Some concern has been raised about the use of corticosteroids in AIDS patients. Studies in which higher doses of corticosteroids were used suggested an increase in the frequency and severity of both life-threatening opportunistic infections and less common invasive fungal infections such as aspergillosis (40, 100). Other studies noted an excess of mucocutaneous herpes simplex virus and oral thrush lesions, but there were no reports of increases in the incidence of Kaposi's sarcoma or other life-threatening opportunistic infections (130). Noninfectious complications have been reported, but the serious adverse effects such as psychosis, peptic ulcer disease, and metabolic abnormalities are not common and do not seem to outweigh the overall beneficial effects (130).

Biochemical and clinical evidence of adrenal insufficiency is common in patients with AIDS. Some of the cases may result from disseminated infectious complications or neoplastic involvement, autoimmune phenomena, or changes consistent with chronic disease or malnutrition. However, more than half of 74 stable hospitalized AIDS patients who completed treatment for opportunistic infections had subnormal cortisol responses to both the short and 3-day ACTH stimulation test (116). Moreover, in an autopsy study on 41 AIDS patients, almost all patients had evidence of partial adrenal necrosis (75). These studies suggest that AIDS patients could be at risk of developing adrenal insuffiency if subjected to "stress." In addition, a small group of patients with AIDS recently has been identified to have a cortisol resistance that has been characterized by abnormal lymphocytic glucocorticoid receptors (131).

CEREBRAL EDEMA

In the treatment of cerebral edema (vasogenic edema) secondary to tumor, an initial 10-mg dose of dexamethasone followed by 4 mg every 6 hours generally is recommended (68). Dexamethasone is particularly well-suited to treatment of this condition because of its minimal fluid-retaining properties. The use of dexamethasone in other forms of cerebral edema, such as that seen after intracerebral hemorrhage (mixed vasogenic and cytotoxic edema), may not be warranted and could be harmful (138). A retrospective study from the database of the Brain Resuscitation Clinical Trial 1 Study Group found no benefit from steroids (either low dose, 1 to 20 mg of dexamethasone; medium dose, 21 to 76 mg of dexamethasone; or high dose, >70 mg of dexamethasone) in mean group survival rate or neurologic recovery rate in comatose cardiac arrest survivors with global brain ischemia after restoration of spontaneous circulation (95).

SPINAL CORD INJURY

In a recent controlled study, an immediate dose of 30 mg/kg methylprednisolone followed by an infusion of 5.4 mg/kg/hr for the ensuing 23 hours reduced the degree of subsequent neurologic dysfunction in acute traumatic paraplegia (19). If treatment was delayed for more than 8 hours, there was no demonstrable benefit (19).

TRANSPLANTATION

Large doses of steroids (0.5 to 1 g of methyprednisolone i.v.) are given to treat acute organ rejection in allogenic transplants. In addition to steroids, other immunomodulating agents are utilized to reduce chronic rejection or graft-versus-host disease in bone marrow transplants. In some cases, such as lung transplantation, preoperative steroids may be weaned and withheld perioperatively to avoid the adverse effects on wound healing. Steroids are then restarted to avoid rejection a few weeks after transplantation. Just as the beneficial effects of steroids arise from the their ability to alter the host's response to foreign antigen, so also do the most serious complications in these patients stem from this ability. Infectious problems haunt organ transplant patients because of the necessity for immunosuppression. Because of steroids' effects on lymphocytic function, cell-mediated immunity is reduced and infections caused by *P. carinii*, fungal organisms, mycobacterial species, and other protozoal agents are common.

Despite the discovery of newer and more specific immunosuppressive agents, glucocorticoids are still used in most chronic antirejection regimens.

OTHER INFLAMMATORY STATES

A number of inflammatory and autoimmune diseases can be palliated by the use of corticosteroids (see Table 43.2).

Common to these disorders is an undesirable inflammatory or immune response. The usual dose of glucocorticoids ranges from 0.5 to 2 mg/kg/day in single or divided doses. The dose is tapered to the lowest dose that controls the process. The duration of therapy depends on the response to therapy and the underlying disease. Although the recommended dose and length of therapy may be somewhat empiric, successful regimens described in the literature for the specific process should be followed to ensure similar results.

Following control of the underlying disease process, the lowest corticosteroid dose required to maintain a remission should be used and adjunctive therapy maximized. If the requirement for steroid therapy is short lived, a rapidly tapering schedule can be instituted (Table 43.7). If chronic therapy is required and the disease is amenable to alternate-day therapy, such a regimen should be considered. Alternate-day therapy usually is initiated by doubling the daily maintenance dose and giving it as a single dose in the morning every other day. The dose is reduced in daily decrements of 5 to 10 mg over a gradual period until a 20-mg every-other-day dose is reached. The dose is then reduced by 2.5 mg every other day until the requirement for therapy has resolved or the disease flares (57). Once the disease has flared, doubling the last dose given usually suppresses the disease activity, although full doses occasionally are again required. After reinduction of remission, weaning back to alternate-day therapy can be attempted and a slower tapering schedule begun. This type of regimen allows recovery of the HPA axis and reduction of some of the undesirable effects (1, 52).

HYPERCALCEMIA

Hypercalcemia secondary to hematologic malignancies such as lymphoma and myeloma generally responds to the administration of glucocorticoids in doses equivalent to 200 to 300 mg of hydrocortisone (183). Calcium reduction may result from steroid-induced growth inhibition of neoplastic lymphoid tissue (183). Because glucocorticoids interfere with the effects of vitamin D on serum calcium, the hypercalcemia that results from sarcoidosis is very sensitive to glucocorticoids and can be controlled with relatively low oral doses. Conversely, hypercalcemia that results from primary hypoparathyroidism and nonhematologic cancers does not respond well to glucocorticoids (143). Biphosphonates, calcitonin, gallium nitrate, and mithramycin are more effective in controlling malignant hypercalcemia, as are hydration, furosemide, and treatment of the underlying disorder.

ADRENAL INSUFFICIENCY

New cases of adrenal insufficiency presenting to the intensivist are uncommon. Nonetheless, specific groups may be at risk for developing clinically significant adrenal insuffiency, such as those patients who have received exogenous glucocorticoid therapy within the preceding year and patients with AIDS. Although adrenal hemorrhage with resulting adrenocortical failure classically has been described in severe meningococcal or pseudomonal septicemia, sepsis-induced adrenal

Table 43.7. Schedule for Glucocorticoid Withdrawal[a]

Step	Interval	Observation	Result	Glucocorticoid Dose
I	Variable	Underlying disease	Clinical improvement	Variable
II	Variable	Underlying disease	Stable	Switch from divided doses to single daily doses. Gradual decrements to the equivalent of 20 mg/day of hydrocortisone
			Decline in status or signs and symptoms of steroid withdrawal	Raise dosage for flare-ups of disease; supplement for stress; recontinue tapering when disease is quiescent
III	4 wk	8 AM plasma cortisol	Plasma cortisol: <10 μg/dl	When tapered to the equivalent of 20 mg of hydrocortisone per day, start hydrocortisone at 20 mg/day and then taper by 2.5 mg/day once a week to 10 mg each morning and continue this dosage; supplement for stress
			Plasma cortisol: >10 μg/dl	Stop maintenance hydrocortisone Supplement for stress
IV	4 wk to indefinite	8 AM Cortrosyn 250 μg test[b]	when plasma cortisol increment is <6 μg/dl or maximum <18 μg/dl at 60 min (or both)	Supplement for stress
V	4 wk to indefinite	8 AM Cortrosyn 250 μ g test[b]	When plasma cortisol increment is >6 μg/dl and maximum >18 μg/dl at 60 min	Stop supplementation for stress
VI	Indefinite	Routine		As indicated

[a] Adapted from Byyny RL: Withdrawal from glucocorticoid therapy. *N Engl J Med* 295:30, 1976.
[b] See Fig. 43.3 for explanation of the ACTH (Cortrosyn: synthetic ACTH) stimulation test.

insufficiency in adults is relatively uncommon. However, bilateral adrenal hemmorhage from other potential causes has become increasingly recognized. Rao et al identified risk factors associated with the development of adrenal insufficiency from adrenal hemorrhage. Indicators of possible adrenal hemorrhage were a history of thromboembolic disease or recent surgery, the use of anticoagulants, or the presence of a coagulopathy along with the development of abdominal or back pain, a precipitous drop in the hemoglobin level, and fever (141). Siu et al also reported the presence of a lupus anticoagulant as a risk factor for this syndrome (154). Recognition is particularly difficult in the severely ill patient because of coexistent disease and masking of characteristic laboratory abnormalities or clinical features.

In adrenal crisis, prompt therapy is life saving. Corticosteroid replacement is essential; dexamethasone (10 mg), methylprednisolone (50 mg), or hydrocortisone (200 to 300 mg) is given intravenously over 10 to 20 minutes (33). Fluid replacement with isotonic saline should be instituted simultaneously. Hypertonic saline should be avoided, since this fluid worsens intracellular dehydration and may precipitate coma (33). Hypoglycemia is prevented via the administration of 5% dextrose in normal saline (30). Sodium bicarbonate rarely is needed to correct metabolic acidosis, and hyperkalemia usually resolves with mineralocorticoid and fluid replacement. For maintenance therapy, hydrocortisone may be given in 100-mg doses every 6 to 8 hours or as a continuous drip of 200 mg over 16 hours. At this dose further mineralocorticoid activity generally is not needed; however, with smaller hydrocortisone doses or with other glucocorticoids, fludrocortisone (0.1 to 0.2 mg/day orally) may be required (156). If hypothyroidism coexists with hypoadrenalism (e.g., Schmidt's syndrome), corticosteroid replacement should occur first so as to avoid aggravation of the adrenal insufficiency by thyroid hormone replacement.

PERIOPERATIVE GLUCOCORTICOID ADMINISTRATION (19a)

In 1952, Fraser and his colleagues reported the first case of surgery-associated adrenal insufficiency as a consequence of preoperative withdrawal from glucocorticoid therapy (72a). The following year Lewis and co-workers (105a) described a similar glucocorticoid-dependent patient (in whom the cortisone was discontinued the day before surgery) who died several hours after a minor orthopaedic surgical procedure had been performed. A postmortem examination in both cases revealed atrophy and hemorrhage of the adrenal glands, and the diagnosis of secondary adrenal insufficiency was made. The Lewis case report concluded with a list of recommendations for perioperative glucocorticoid treatment that has become the standard of therapy for perioperative glucocorticoid coverage for the past 40 years (105a). They recommended that any glucocorticoid-dependent patient requiring anesthesia or surgery should receive 350 to 450 mg of cortisol daily in the perioperative period. It is worth noting (for the sake of perspective) that the average cortisol production rate in patients with Cushing's syndrome is 36 mg/day (56b). Knowledge of adrenal cortical responses to physical stressors such as surgery has been refined during the past 20 years (2a, 11a, 22a, 34a, 34b, 49a, 56a, 98a, 99a, 100a, 101a, 103a, 104, 110a, 137a, 140a, 170a, 170b) and, therefore, perioperative glucocorticoid management can be prescribed in a more rational fashion.

Though perioperative adrenal insufficiency is an uncommon complication of surgery, a review (98a) of all the reported putative instances of death and hypotension attributed to perioperative adrenal insufficiency (in glucocorticoid treated patients) suggests that the problem is real and does occur. Many glucocorticoid-dependent patients will undergo major surgery, however, without having perioperative glucocorticoid coverage provided, or while just receiving their baseline glucocorticoid dose (for their primary disease process). One explanation for this paradox is that these patients had normal preoperative biochemical indices of hypothalamic-pituitary-adrenal (HPA) axis function. Glucocorticoid-dependent patients whose preoperative biochemical indices of HPA axis function are normal (i.e., an intact stress system response) will not require perioperative glucocorticoid coverage beyond that determined by their baseline disease process.

The assessment of the functional states of the HPA axis is based upon laboratory determinations. In most cases a random cortisol value of >500 nmol/liter suggests adequate adrenal function; however, to ensure that the plasma cortisol value reflects adrenal competence, a maximally stimulated value is important. The 30-minute ACTH test (see Adrenal Insufficiency) is the most convenient and accurate diagnostic tool for preoperative evaluation of HPA axis function. The authors believe that the ACTH stimulation test is very useful as an initial screening test for preoperative evaluation of HPA integrity.

Perioperative glucocorticoid therapy should be based on the magnitude of the surgical stress and the glucocorticoid production rate associated with it. For *minor* surgery (i.e., inguinal heriorraphy, excisional biopsy) the daily cortisol secretion rate and static plasma cortisol measurements (170a, 170b) suggest that the glucocorticoid target is about 25 mg of hydrocortisone equivalent. For example, most patients should simply take their baseline glucocorticoid dosing regimen 2 hours prior to their surgery. In most cases the patient can return (unless complications arise) to his or her normal dosing regimen the next day.

For *moderate* surgery (i.e., cholecystectomy, lower extremity revascularization, segmental colon resection, total joint replacement), cortisol production rates suggest that the glucocorticoid target is about 50 to 75 mg of hydrocortisone equivalent daily for 2 days. The authors suggest that 75 mg of hydrocortisone (25 mg every 8 hours) shoud be administered intravenously (with the first dose of 25 mg of intravenous hydrocortisone administered preoperatively within 2 hours) on the operative and first postoperative days. The patient may return to his or her preoperative glucocorticoid dose (enterally or parenterally) on postoperative day 2.

Finally, for *major* surgery (esophagogastrectomy, cardiac surgery involving cardiopulmonary bypass) the glucocorticoid target should be 100 to 150 mg of hydrocortisone equivalent per day for 2 to 3 days. For example, a patient who has been receiving 10 mg of prednisone every other day for asthma who is undergoing *major* surgery would require 10 mg of oral prednisone (or 50 mg of intravenous hydrocortisone) preoperatively within 2 hours of surgery, with 50 mg of hydrocortisone to be administered intravenously every 8 hours for the next 48 to 72 hours.

To the authors' knowledge, there is no experimental or clinical evidence that these recommended equivalent doses need be exceeded; therefore, a patient who is receiving a maintenance dose of glucocorticoid therapy that exceeds the estimated stress requirement will not need more glucocorticoid coverage during the perioperative period. After uncomplicated surgery (in most patients), circulating cortisol concentrations decrease rapidly to normal values by 24 to 48 hours

(34a, 94a, 110b). There is little evidence in support of a "steroid taper," with the exception of those patients who have been on high-dose glucocorticoids for an extended period of time. In the case of postoperative complications, continued glucocorticoid administation consistent with the postoperative stress response is appropriate.

SUMMARY

Corticosteroid activity is required for normal day-to-day living. Stress situations increase the demand for corticosteroids, and the HPA axis responds accordingly. Corticosteroid therapy in patients with a normal HPA axis provides therapeutic benefit in many circumstances. Oftentimes, it does not cure the underlying disease but instead ameliorates the pathophysiology until more definitive therapy can be given or the inciting insult can be removed. However, corticosteroids have revolutionized the care of patients in many instances.

In the critically ill patient, one encounters advantages and disadvantages from both acute and chronic steroid therapy. The intensivist must be aware of the benefits, shortcomings, and controversies of steroid therapy. Steroids have wide application but should not be given without an appreciation of their adverse effects. Refinement in our knowledge of the pharmacology and physiology of steroids may introduce broader application with more specific effects and finer definition of their benefits and toxicities.

REFERENCES

1. Ackerman GL, Nolan CM: Adrenocortical responsiveness after alternate day corticosteroids. *N Engl J Med* 278:405, 1968.
2. Albert RK, Martin TR, Lewis SW: Controlled clinical trial of methylprednisolone in patients with chronic bronchitis and acute respiratory insufficiency. *Ann Intern Med* 92:753, 1980.
2a. Alford WCJr, Meador CK, Mihalevich J, et al: Acute adrenal insufficiency following cardiac surgical procedures. *J Thorac Cardiovasc Surg* 78:489–493, 1979.
3. Allison AC, Lee SC: The mode of action of anti-rheumatic drugs. 1. Anti-inflammatory and immunosuppressive effects of glucocorticoids. *Prog Drug Res* 33:63, 1989.
4. Ashbaugh DG, Maier RV: Idiopathic pulmonary fibrosis in adult respiratory distress syndrome. *Arch Surg* 120:539, 1985.
5. Atkinson, JP, Schreiber AD, Frank MM: Effects of corticosteroids and splenectomy on immune clearance and destruction of erythrocytes. *J Clin Invest* 52:1509, 1973.
6. Atkinson JP, Frank MM: Effect of cortisone therapy on serum complement components. *J Immunol* 111:1061, 1973.
7. Axelrod L: Glucocorticoid therapy. *Medicine* 55:39, 1976.
8. Ballard PL, Carter JP, Graham BS, et al: A radioreceptor assay for the evaluation of the plasma glucocorticoid activity of natural and synthetic steroids in man. *J Clin Endocrinol Metab* 41:290, 1975.
9. Balson S, Steru D, Bourdeau A, Grimberg E, Lenoir G: effects of lung term therapy with a new glucocorticoid, deflazacort, on mineral metabolism and statural growth. *Calcif Tissue Int* 40:303, 1987.
10. Baxter JD, Tyrell JB: The adrenal cortex. In Felig P, et al (eds): Endocrinology and Metabolism. McGraw-Hill, New York, 1981, pp 385–510.
11. Bernard GR, Luce JM, Sprung CL, et al: High dose corticosteroids in patients with the adult respiratory distress syndrome. *N Engl J Med* 317:1565, 1987.
11a. Beyer HS, Parker L, Li CH, Stuart D, Sharp BM: β-endorphin attenuates the serum cortisol response to exogenous adrenocorticotropin. *J Clin Endocrinol Metab* 62:808–811, 1986.
12. Binstock ML, Mundy GR: Effect of calcitonin and glucocorticoids in combination on the hypercalcemia of malignancy. *Ann Intern Med* 93:269, 1980.
13. Bondy PK: Disorder of the adrenal cortex. In Wilson JD, Foser DW (eds): Williams Textbook of Endocrinology, ed 7. WB Saunders, Philadelphia, 1985, pp 816–880.
14. Bone RC, Fisher CJ, Clemmer TP, et al: Early methylprednisolone treatment for septic syndrome and the adult respiratory distress disease syndrome. *Chest* 92:1032, 1987.
15. Bone RC, Fisher CJ, Clemmer TP, et al: A controlled clinical trial of high-dose methylprednisolone in the treatment of severe sepsis and septic shock. *N Engl J Med* 317:653, 1987.

16. Borst G, Michenfleder JHJ, O'Brian JT: Discordant cortisol response to exogenous ACTH and insulin-induced hypoglycemia in patients with pituitary disease. *N Engl J Med* 306:1462, 1982.

17. Borzette SA, Sattler, Chiu J, et al: A controlled trial of early adjunctive treatment with corticosteroids for *Pneumocystis carinii* in the acquired immunodeficiency syndrome. *N Engl J Med* 323:1451, 1990.

18. Boudmot JH, D'Ambrosio R, Jusko WJ: Receptor-mediated pharmacodynamics of prednisolone in the rat. *J Pharmacokinet Biopharm* 14:469, 1986.

19. Bracken MB, Shepard MJ, Hellenbrand KG, et al: A randomized, controlled trial of methylprednisolone or naloxone in the treatment of spinal cord injury. *N Engl J Med* 322:1405, 1990.

19a. Brattsand R: Glucocorticoids. *Am Rev Respir Dis* 149:1360, 1993.

20. Brennan MJ: Corticosteroids in the treatment of solid tumors: symposium on steroid therapy. *Med Clin North Am* 57:1225, 1973.

21. Brigham KL, Bowers RE, McKeen CR: Methylprednisolone prevention of increased lung vascular permeability following endotoxemia in sheep. *J Clin Invest* 67:1103, 1981.

22. Brodie BB, Davies JI, Hynie S, Krishna G, Weiss B: Interrelationships of catecholamine with other endocrine systems. *Pharmacol Rev* 18:273, 1966.

22a. Bromberg JS, Alfrey EJ, Barker CF, Chavin KD, Dafoe DC, Holland T, Naji A, Perloff LJ, Zellers LA, Grossman RA: Adrenal suppression and steriod supplementation in renal transplant recipients. *J Transplant* 51:385–390, 1991.

23. Brown PH, Blundell G, Greening AP, Crompton GK: Hypothalamo-pituitary-adrenal axis suppression in asthmatics inhaling high dose corticosteroids. *Respir Med* 85:501, 1991.

24. Bruno A, Cavallo-Perin P, Cassader M, Pagnano G: Deflazacort vs. prednisone. Effect on blood glucose control in insulin-treated diabetics. *Arch Intern Med* 147:679, 1987.

25. Butler WT, Rossen RD: Effect of corticosteroids on immunity in man. I. Decreased serum IgG concentration caused by 3 or 5 days of high dose methylprednisolone. *J Clin Invest* 52:2629, 1973.

26. Byyny RL: Withdrawal from glucocorticoid therapy. *N Engl J Med* 295:30, 1976.

27. Callahan CM, Dittus RS, Katz BP: Oral corticosteroid therapy for patients with stable chronic obstructive pulmonary disease. *Ann Intern Med* 114:216, 1991.

28. Carmichael J, Paterson IC, Diaz P, Crompton GK, Kay AB, Grant IWB: Corticosteroid resistance in chronic asthma. *Br Med J* 282:1419, 1981.

29. Chatterjea JB, Salmon L: Antagonistic effect of ACTH and cortisone on the anticoagulant activity of ethyl biscoumacetate. *Br Med J* 2:790, 1954.

30. Check WA, Kaliner MA: Pharmacology and pharmokinetics of topical corticosteroid derivatives used for asthma therapy. *Am Rev Respir Dis* 141:544, 1990.

31. Chernow B, Zwillich CW: Is hypercapnia complicating metabolic alkalosis, a rare clinical entity? *Chest* 70:421, 1976.

32. Chernow B, Vernoski BK, Zaloga GP, et al: Dexamethasone causes less steroid-induced alkalemia than methylprednisolone or hydrocortisone. *Crit Care Med* 12:384, 1984.

33. Chernow B: Hormonal and metabolic considerations in critical care medicine. In Critical Care: State of the Art, vol 3. Society of Critical Care Medicine, Fullerton, CA, 1982, p J1.

34. Chernow B, Alexander HR, Smallridge RC, et al: Hormonal responses to graded surgical stress. *Arch Intern Med* 147:1273–1278, 1987.

34a. Chernow B, Alexander HR, Thompson WR, Cook D, Beardsley D, Fink MP, Smallridge RC, Fletcher JR: The hormonal responses to surgical stress. *Arch Intern Med* 147:1273–1278, 1978.

34b. Chernow B, Anderson DM: Endocrine responses to critical illness. *Semin Respir Med* 7:1–10, 1985.

35. Cheyney FW, Huang TH, Gronka R: Effects of methylprednisolone on experimental pulmonary injury. *Ann Surg* 190:236, 1979.

36. Chin R: Adrenal crisis. *Crit Care Clin* 7:23, 1991.

37. Chrousos GP, Schuermeyer TH, Doppman J, et al: Clinical applications of corticotropin releasing factor. *Ann Intern Med* 102:344, 1985.

38. Claman HN: Corticosteroids and lymphoid cells. *N Engl J Med* 287:388, 1972.

39. Clee MD, Ferguson J, Browning MCK, Jung RT, Clark RA: Glucocorticoid hypersensitivity in an asthmatic patient: presentation and treatment. *Thorax* 40:477, 1985.

40. Clement M, Edison R, Turner J, et al: Corticosteroids as adjunctive therapy in severe *Pneumocystis* pneumonia: a prospective placebo controlled trial. *Am Rev Respir Dis* 139:A250, 1989.

41. Cline MJ, Melmon KL: Plasma kinins and cortisol: a possible explanation of the anti-inflammatory action of cortisol. *Science* 153:1135, 1966.

41a. Coakley JH, Nagemdran K, Ormerod IEC, Ferguson CN, Hinds CJ: Prolonged neurogenic weakness in patients requiring mechanical ventilation for airflow limitation. *Chest* 101:1413, 1992.

42. Collins JV, Clark TJH, Brown D, et al: The use of corticosteroids in the treatment of acute asthma. *Q J Med* 44:259, 1975.

43. Conn HO, Blitzer BL: Nonassociation of adrenalcorticosteroid therapy and peptic ulcer. *N Engl J Med* 294:473, 1976.

44. Corrigan CJ, Brown PH, Barnes NC, et al: Glucocorticoid resistance in chronic asthma: glucocorticoid pharmacokinetics, glucocorticoid receptor characteristics, and inhibition of peripheral blood T cell proliferation by glucocorticoids in vitro. *Am Rev Respir Dis* 144:1016, 1991.

45. Cunningham SK, Moore A, McKenna J: Normal cortisol response to corticotropin in patients with secondary adrenal failure. *Arch Intern Med* 143:2276, 1983.

46. Cupps TR, Fauci AS: Corticosteroid-mediated immunoregulation in man. *Immunol Rev* 65:133, 1982.

47. Dallman MF, Darlington DN, Suemaru S, et al: Corticosteroids in homeostasis. *Acta Physiol Scand* 136:583:S27, 1989.

48. David DS, Grieco MH, Cushman P: Adrenal glucocorticoids after twenty years: a review of their clinically relevant consequences. *J Chronic Dis* 22:637, 1970.

49. Dhuly RG, Lauler DP, Thorn GW: Pharmacology and chemistry of adrenal glucocorticoids: symposium of steroid therapy. *Med Clin North Am* 57:1155, 1973.

49a. Downing R, Davis I, Black J, Windson CWO: Effect of intrathecal morphine on the adrenocorticoid and hyperglycemic responses to upper abdominal surgery. *Br J Anaesth* 58:858–861, 1986.

50. Drucker D, Shandling M: Variable adrenocortical function in acute medical illness. *Crit Care Med* 13:477, 1985.

51. Drucker D, Shanding M: Variable adrenocortical function in acute medical illness. *Crit Care Med* 14:789, 1986.

52. Dujovne CA, Azarnoff DL: Clinical complication of corticosteroid therapy: symposium on steroid therapy. *Med Clin North Am* 57:1331, 1973.

53. Dykewicz M, Greenberger PA, Patterson R, Halwig M: Natural history of asthma in patients requiring long-term systemic corticosteroids. *Arch Intern Med* 146:2369, 1986.

54. Tuberculosis in corticosteroid treated asthmatics [Editorial]. *Br Med J* 2:266, 1976.

55. Elias AN, Gwinup G: Effects of some clinically encountered drugs on steroid synthesis and degradation. *Metabolism* 29:583, 1980.

56. Emerman CL, Connors AF, Lukens TW, May ME, Effron D: A randomized controlled trial of methylprednisolone in the emergency treatment of acute exacerbations of COPD. *Chest* 95:563, 1989.

56a. Engquist S, Brandt MR, Fernandes A, Kehlet H: The blocking effect of epidural analgesia on the adrenocortical and hyperglycemic response to surgery. *Acta Anaesth Scand* 21:330–335, 1977.

56b. Esteban N, Loughlin T, Yergey A, Zawadski J, Booth J, Winterer J, Loriaux L: Daily cortisol production rate in man determined by stable isotope dilution, mass spectrometry. *J Clin Endocrinol Metab* 71:39–45, 1991.

57. Fauci AS: Glucocorticoid therapy. In Wyngaarden JB, Smith LH (eds): Cecil's Textbook of Medicine, ed 17. WB Saunders, Philadelphia, 1985, pp 111–116.

58. Engel T, Heinig JM, Madsen O, Hansen M, Weeke ER: A trial of inhaled budesonide on airway responsiveness in smokers with chronic bronchitis. *Eur Respir J* 2:935, 1989.

59. Engel T, Henig JH: Glucocorticosteroid therapy in acute severe asthma. Critical review. *Eur Respir J* 4:881, 1991.

60. Fanta CH, Rossing TH, McFadden ER: Glucocorticoids in acute asthma. A critical controlled trial. *Am J Med* 74:845, 1983.

61. Farer LS: Chemoprophylaxis: Kock centennial supplement. *Am Rev Resp Dis* 125:102, 1982.

62. Farer LS: Chemoprophylaxis against tuberculosis. *Clin Chest Med* 1:203, 1980.

63. Fauci AS, Dale DC, Lalow JE: Glucocorticoid therapy: mechanisms of action and clinical considerations. *Ann Intern Med* 84:304, 1976.

64. Fenster KF: The ulcerogenic potential of glucocorticoids and possible prophylactic measures: symposium on steroid therapy. *Med Clin North Am* 57:1289, 1972.

65. Ferguson GT, Irwin CG, Cherniak RM: Effect of corticosteroids on diaphragm function and biochemistry in the rabbit. *Am Rev Respir Dis* 144:156, 1990.

66. Findling JW, Waters VO, Raff H: The dissociation of renin and aldosterone during critical illness. *J Clin Endocrinol Metab* 64:592, 1987.

67. Finlay WE, McKee J: Serum cortisol levels in severely stressed patients. *Lancet* 1:414, 1982.

68. Fishman RA: Brain edema. *N Engl J Med* 293:706, 1975.

69. Fitzsimmons R, Greenberger PA, Patterson R: Outcome of pregnancy in women requiring corticosteroids for severe asthma. *J Allergy Clin Immunol* 78:349, 1986.

70. Flower RJ: The mediators of steroid action. *Nature* 320:20, 1986.

71. Foresman O, Mulder J: Hypersensitivity to different ACTH peptides. *Acta Med Scand* 193:557, 1973.

72. Goodwin JS, Atluru D, Sierakowski S, Lianos EA: Mechanism of action of glucocorticoids: inhibition of T cell proliferation and interleukin 2 production by hydrocortisone is reversed by leukotriene B4. *J Clin Invest* 77:1244, 1986.

72a. Fraser CG, Preuss FS, Bigford WD: Adrenal atrophy and irreversible shock associated with cortisone therapy. *JAMA* 149:1542–1543, 1952.

73. Fuller GC, Cutroneo KR: Pharmacological interventions. In Cohen IK, Diefelmann RF, Lindblad WJ (eds): Wound Healing: Biochemical and Clinical Aspects. WB Saunders, Philadelphia, 1992.

74. Funder JW, Pearce PT, Smith R, Smith AI: Mineralocorticoid action: Target tissue specificity vs. enzyme, not receptor mediated. *Science* 242:583, 1988.

75. Glaslow BJ, Steinsaper AD, Anders K: Adrenal pathology in AIDS. *Am J Clin Pathol* 84:594, 1985.

76. Goggans FC, Weisberg LJ, Koran LM: Lithium prophylaxis of prednisone psychosis: a case report. *J Clin Psychiatry* 44:3, 1983.

77. Goldstein G, Luce JM: Pharmacologic treatment of the adult respiratory distress syndrome. *Clin Chest Med* 11:773, 1990.

78. Graber AL, Ney RL, Nicholson WE, et al: Natural history of pituitary-adrenal recovery following long-term suppression with corticosteroids. *J Clin Endocrinol Metab* 25:11, 1965.

79. Gray RES, Doherty SM, Galloway J, Coulton L, deBroe M, Kanis JA: A double-blind study of deflazacort and prednisone in patients with chronic inflammatory disorders. *Arthritis Rheum* 34:287, 1991.

80. Greos LS, Vichyanond P, Bloedow DC, et al: Methylprednisolone achieves greater concentrations in the lung than prednisolone: a pharmacokinetic analysis. *Am Rev Respir Dis* 144:586, 1991.

81. Guillemin R, Bargo T, Rossier J, et al: Beta-endorphin and adrenocortico-tropin are secreted concomitantly by the pituitary gland. *Science* 197:1367, 1977.

82. Hammerschmidt DE, White JG, Craddok PR, et al: Corticosteroids inhibit complement-induced granulocyte aggregation: four possible mechanisms for their efficacy in shock states. *J Clin Invest* 63:798, 1979.

83. Harris DM, Martin LE, Harrison C, Jack D: The effect of oral and inhaled beclomethasone dipropionate on adrenal function. *Clin Allergy* 3:243, 1973.

84. Haskell RJ, Wong BM, Hansen JE: A double-blind, randomized clinical trial of methylprednisolone in status asthmaticus. *Arch Intern Med* 143:1324, 1983.

85. Hastings PR, Skillman JJ, Bushnell LS, et al: Antacid titration in the prevention of acute gastrointestinal bleeding. A controlled, randomized trial in 100 critically ill patients. *N Engl J Med* 298:1041, 1978.

86. Haynes RC: Adrenocorticotropic hormone: adrenocortical steroids and their synthetic analogs; inhibitors of the synthesis and actions of adrenocortical steroid hormones. In Gilman AG, Goodman LS, Rall TW, Neis AS, Taylor P (eds): The Pharmacological Basis of Therapeutics, ed 8. Macmillan, New York, 1990, p 1431.

87. Hess ML, Hastillo A, Greenfield LJ: Spectrum of cardiovascular function during Gram-negative sepsis. *Prog Cardiovasc Dis* 23:279, 1981.

88. Hooper RG, Kearl RA: Established ARDS treated with a sustained course of adrenocortical steroids. *Chest* 97:138, 1990.

89. Horber FF, Scheidegger JR, Grunig BE, Frey FJ: Evidence that prednisone-induced myopathy is reversed by physical training. *J Clin Endocrinol Metab* 61:83, 1985.

90. Hsueh WA, Pas-Guevara A, Bledsoe T: Studies comparing the metabolic clearance rate of 11-beta-17,21-trihydroxypregn 1,4-diene-3,20-dione (prednisolone) after oral 17,21-dihydrooxypregn-1,4-diene-3,11,20-trione and intravenous prednisolone. *J Clin Endocrinol Metab* 48:748, 1979.

91. Hunt TK: Vitamin A and wound healing. *J Am Acad Dermatol* 15:817, 1986.

92. Iranmanesh A, Ovetsky RM, Lizzarralde G, Schleuper CJ: Effect of ketoconazole on the 11-hydroxylation step of adrenal steroidogenesis. *South Med J* 80:735, 1987.

93. Ivey KJ, Den Besten L: Pseudotumor cerebri associated with corticosteroid therapy in an adult. *JAMA* 208:1698, 1969.

94. Jacobs ER, Bone RC: Therapeutic implications of acute lung injury. *Crit Care Clin* 2:615, 1986.

94a. Jasani M, Freeman P, Boyle J, Reid A, Diver M, Buchanan W: Studies of the rise in plasma 11-hydroxycorticosteroids (11-HOCS) in corticosteroid-treated patients with rheumatoid arthritis during surgery: correlations with the functional integrity of the hypothalamo-pituitary-adrenal axis. *Q J Med* 37:407–421, 1968.

95. Jastremski M, Sutton-Tyrrell K, Vaagenes P, et al: Glucocorticoid treatment does not improve neurological recovery following cardiac arrest. *JAMA* 262:3427, 1989.

96. Jones RL, King EG, et al: The effects of methylprednisolone on oxygenation in experimental hypoxemic respiratory failure. *J Trauma* 15:297, 1975.

97. Jurney TH, Cockrell JL, Lindberg JS, Lamiell JM, Wade CE: Spectrum of serum cortisol response to ACTH in ICU patients. *Chest* 92:292, 1987.

98. Kawai S, Ichikawa Y, Homma M: Differences of metabolic properties among cortisol, prednisolone, and dexamethasone in liver and renal diseases: accelerated metabolism of dexamethasone in renal failure. *J Clin Endocrinol Metab* 60:848, 1985.

98a. Kehlet H: Clinical Course and Hypothalamic-Pituitary-Adrenocortical Function in Glucocorticoid-Treated Surgical Patients. FADL's Forlag, Copenhagen, 1976.

98b. Kehlet K, Binder C: Value of an ACTH test in assessing hypothalamic-pituitary-adrenocortical function in glucocorticoid-treated patients. *Br Med J* 2:147–149, 1973.

98c. Kehlet H, Binder C: Adrenocortical function and clinical course during and after surgery in unsupplemented glucocorticoid-treated patients. *Br J Anaesth* 45:1043–1048, 1973.

98d. Kehlet H, Binder C, Engbaek C: Imitation of the adrenocorticoid response to surgery by intravenous infusion of synthetic human ACTH. *Acta Endocrnol (Copenh)* 72:75–80, 1973.

99. Kehrer JP, Klein-Szanto AJP, Sorensen EMB, Pearlman R, Rosner MH: Enhanced acute lung damage following corticosteroid treatment. *Am Rev Respir Dis* 130:256, 1984.

99a. Kerstjens HAB, Brand PLP, Hughes MD, et al: A comparison of bronchodilator therapy with or without inhaled corticosteriod therapy for obstructive airways disease. *N Engl J Med* 327:1413, 1992.

99b. Khilnani P, Munoz R, Salem M, Gelb C, Todres ID, Chernow B: Prolactin and response to surgical stress in children. *J Pediatr Surg* 28:1–4, 1993.

100. Klapholz A, Saloman N, Perlman DC, Talavera W: Aspergillosis in the acquired immunodeficiency syndrome. *Chest* 100:1614, 1991.

100a. Kleg HK, Peerenboom H, Strohmeyer G, Druskemper HL: Cortisol excretion into gastric juice—studies in health, in digestive ulcer disease and in surgery stress. *Dig Dis Sci* 28:494–501, 1983.

101. Klinenberg JR, Miller R: Effect of corticosteroids on blood salicylate concentrations. *JAMA* 194:601, 1965.

101a. Knudsen L, Christiansen LA, Lorentzed JE: Hypotension during and after operation in glucocorticoid-treated patients. *Br J Anaesth* 53:295–301, 1981.

102. Koener JH, Sun DC: Mediastinal lipomatosis secondary to steroid therapy. *AJR* 98:461, 1966.

103. Kozower N, Veatch L, Kaplan MM: Decreased clearance of prednisolone, a factor in the development of corticosteroid side effects. *J Clin Endocrinol Metab* 38:407, 1974.

103a. Lacoumenta S, Paterson JL, Burrin J, Cavson RC, Brown MJ, Hall GM: Effects of two differing halothane concentrations on the metabolic and endocrine responses to surgery. *Br J Anaesth* 58:844–850, 1986.

104. Lam KC, Lai CL, Trepo C, et al: Deleterious effect of prednisolone in HBsAg-positive chronic active hepatitis. *N Engl J Med* 304:380, 1981.

104a. LaRocco A, Amundson DE, Wallace MR, Malone J, Oldfield EC. Corticosteroids for *Pneumocystis carinii* pneumonia with acute respiratory failure. *Chest* 102:892, 1992.

104b. Lehtinen AM, Fyhrquist F, Kivalo I: The effect of fentanyl on arginine vasopressin and cortisol secretion during anesthesia. *Anesth Analg* 63:25–30, 1984.

105. Lewis GP, Jusko WJ, Burke CW, et al: Prednisone side effects and serum protein levels. *Lancet* 2:778, 1971.

105a. Lewis L, Robinson RF, Yee J, Hacker LA, Eisen G: Fatal adrenal cortical insufficiency precipitated by surgery during prolonged continuous cortisone infusion. *Ann Intern Med* 39:116–125, 1953.

106. Luce JM, Montgomery AB, Marks JD, Turner J, Metz CA, Murray JF: Ineffectiveness of high-dose methylprednisolone in preventing parenchymal lung injury and improving mortality in patients with septic shock. *Am Rev Respir Dis* 138:62, 1988.

107. Lukert BP, Raisz LG: Glucocorticoid-induced osteoporosis: pathogenesis and management. *Ann Intern Med* 112:352, 1990.

108. Lund B, Egsmose C, Jorgensen S, Krogsgaard MR: Establishment of the relative anti-inflammatory potency of deflazacort and prednisone in polymyalgia rheumatica. *Calcif Tissue Int* 41:316, 1987.

109. Marco J, Colle C, Roman D, et al: Hyperglucagonism induced by glucocorticoid treatment in man. *N Engl J Med* 288:128, 1973.

110. Marom Z, Shelhamer, Alling D, Lainer M: The effects of corticosteroids on mucous glycoprotein secretion from human airways in vitro. *Am Rev Respir Dis* 129:62, 1984.

110a. Masala A, Satta G, Alagna S, Anania V, Frassetto GA, Rovasio PP, Semiani A: Effect of clonidine on stress-induced cortisol release in man during surgery. *Pharmacol Res Commun* 17:293–298, 1985.

110b. Mattingly D, Tyler C: Plasma 11-hydroxycorticoid levels in surgical stress. *Proc R Soc Med* 58:24–26, 1965.

111. McDougal BA, Whittier FC, Cross DE: Sudden death after bolus steroid therapy for acute rejection. *Transplant Proc* 8:493, 1976.

112. McKee JI, Finlay WE: Cortisol replacement in severely stressed patients [Letter]. *Lancet* 1:484, 1986.

113. Meduri G, Belenchia JM, Estes RJ, et al: Fibroproliferative phase of ARDS. *Chest* 100:943, 1991.

114. Meikle AW, Tyler F: Potency and duration of action of glucocorticoids: effects of hydrocortisone, prednisone, and dexamethasone on human pituitary-adrenal function. *Am J Med* 63:200, 1977.

115. Danon MJ, Carpenter S: Myopathy with thick filament (myosin) loss following prolonged paralysis with vecuronium during steroid treatment. *Muscle Nerve* 14:1131, 1991.

116. Membreno L, Irony I, Dere W, et al: Adrenocortical function in AIDS. *J Clin Endocrinol Metab* 65:482, 1987.

117. Mendella LA, Manfreda J, Warren CP, Anthonisen NR: Steroid response in stable chronic pulmonary disease. *Ann Intern Med* 96:17, 1982.

118. Mendelson LM, Meltxer EO, Hamburger RN: Anaphylaxis-like reactions to corticosteroid therapy. *J Allergy Clin Immunol* 54:125, 1974.

119. Menguy R, Masters YF: Effect of cortisone on mucoprotein secretion by gastric antrum of dogs: pathogenesis for steroid ulcer. *Surgery* 54:19, 1963.

120. Messer J, Reitman D, Sacks HS, Smith H, Chalmers TC: Association of adrenocorticosteroid therapy and peptic ulcer disease. *N Engl J Med* 309:21, 1983.

121. Miesfeld R: Molecular genetics of corticosteroid action. *Am Rev Respir Dis* 141:S11, 1990.

121a. Milgrom H, Bender BG: Psychologic side effects of therapy with corticosteriods. *Am Rev Respir Dis* 147:471, 1993.

122. Moore PK, Hoult JRS: Anti-inflammatory steroids reduce tissue prostaglandin synthetase activity and enhance prostaglandin breakdown. *Nature* 288:269, 1980.

123. Morris HG: Mechanisms of glucocorticoid action in pulmonary disease. *Chest* 88(suppl):133S, 1985.

124. Mulrow CD, Corey GR: Pericardial pseudoeffusion due to steroid-induced lipomatosis. *N C Med J* 46:179, 1985.

125. Munck A, Mendel D Smith L, Orti E: Glucocorticoid receptors and actions. *Am Rev Respir Dis* 141:S2, 1990.

126. Murata GH, Gorby MS, Chick MW, Haperin AK: Intravenous and oral corticosteroids for the prevention of relapse after treatment of decompensated COPD. *Chest* 98:845, 1990.

127. Nashel DJ: Is atherosclerosis a complication of long-term corticosteroid treatment? *Am J Med* 80:925, 1986.

128. National Asthma Education Program, Expert Panel, NHBLI, NIH: Publication Number 91-3042. Executive Summary: Guidelines for the diagnosis and management of Asthma. US Department of Health and Human Services, Bethesda, MD, 1991.

129. Newmark SR: Can the pituitary release adrenocorticotropic hormone during stress? *Arch Intern Med* 143:2248, 1983.

130. NIH Panel: Consensus statement on the use of corticosteroids as adjunctive therapy for *Pneumocystis pneumonia* in the acquired immunodeficiency syndrome? *N Engl J Med* 323:1500, 1190.

131. Norbiato G, Bevilacqua M, Vago T, et al: Cortisol resistance in acquired immunodeficiency syndrome. *J Clin Endocrinol Metab* 74:608, 1992.

132. Opperman D, Huber I, Nink M, Schultz V: Human corticotropin-releasing hormone in man. Dose response of minute ventilation and end tidal partial pressures of carbon dioxide and oxygen. *J Clin Endocrinol Metab* 64:292, 1987.

133. Paul WE: Introduction: the immune system. In Wyngaarden JB, Smith LH (eds): Cecil Textbook of Medicine, ed 17. WB Saunders, Philadelphia, 1984, pp 1846-1852.

134. Peers SH, Flowers RJ: The role of lipocortin in corticosteroid actions. *Am Rev Respir Dis* 141:S18, 1990.

135. Perry PJ, Tsuang MT, Hwang MH: Prednisolone psychosis: clinical observations. *Drug Intell Clin Pharm* 18:603, 1984.

136. Pingleton SK: Gastrointestinal hemorrhage. In Bone RC (ed): Critical Care: A comprehensive approach. American College of Chest Physicians, Park Ridge, Ill 1984, pp 82–97.

137. Piper JM, Ray WA, Daugherty JR, Griffin MR: Corticosteroid use and peptic ulcer disease: role of nonsteroidal anti-inflammatory drugs. *Ann Intern Med* 114:735, 1991.

137a. Rittmaster RS, Cutler GBJr, Sobel DO, Goldstein DS, Koppelman MCS, Loriaux DL, Chrousos GP: Morphine inhibits the pituitary-adrenal response to ovine corticotropin-releasing hormone in normal subjects. *J Clin Endocrinol Metab* 60:891–895, 1985.

138. Poungvarin N, Bhoopat W, Viriyavejakul A, et al: Effects of dexamethasone in primary supratentorial intracerebral hemorrhage. *N Engl J Med* 316:1229, 1987.

139. Radomski MW, Palmer MJ, Moncada S: Glucocorticoids inhibit the expression of an inducible, but not the constitutive, nitric oxide synthase in vascular endothelial cells. *Proc Natl Acad Sci USA* 87:10043, 1990.

140. Ramsdell JW, Berry CC, Clausen JL: The immediate effects of cortisol on pulmonary function in normals and asthmatics. *J Allergy Clin Immunol* 71:69, 1983.

141. Rao RH, Vagnucci AH, Amico JA: Bilateral massive adrenal hemorrhage. Early recognition and treatment. *Ann Intern Med* 110:227, 1989.

142. Richards JM, Santiago SM, Klaustermyer WB: Aseptic necrosis of the femoral head in corticosteroid-treated pulmonary disease. *Arch Intern Med* 140:1473, 1980.

142a. Rittmaster RS, Cutler GB Jr, Sobel DO, Goldstein DS, Koppelman MCS, Loriaux DL, Chrousos GP: Morphine inhibits the pituitary-adrenal response to ovine corticotropin-releasing hormone in normal subjects. *J Clin Endocrinol Metab* 60:891–895, 1985.

143. Percival RC, Yates AJP, Gray RES, Neal FE, Forrst ARW, Kanis JA: Role of glucocorticoids in the management of malignant hypercalcaemia. *British Medical Journal* 289:287, 1984.

144. Rooney SA: The surfactant system and lung phospholipid biochemistry. *Am Rev Respir Dis* 131:439, 1985.

145. Sainsberg JRC, Stoddard JC, Watson MJ: Plasma cortisol levels: a comparison between sick patients and volunteers given intravenous cortisol. *Anaesthesia* 36:16, 1981.

146. Sandberg N: Time relationship between administration of cortisone and wound healing in rats. *Acta Chir Scand* 127:446, 1964.

147. Schlaghecke R, Kornely E, Santen RT, Ridderskamp P: The effect of long-term glucocorticoid therapy on pituitary-adrenal responses to exogenous corticotropin-releasing hormone. *N Engl J Med* 326:226, 1992.

148. Schleimer RP: Effects of glucocorticosteroids on inflammatory cells relevant to their therapeutic applications in asthma. *Am Rev Respir Dis* 141:559, 1990.

149. Schoenfeld Y, Gurewich Y, Gallant LA, et al: Prednisone-induced leukocytosis: influence of dosage, method and duration of administration on the degree of leukocytosis. *Am J Med* 71:773, 1981.

150. Schonfeld SA, Polysongsang Y, DiLisio R, et al: Fat embolism prophylaxis with corticosteroids. A prospective study in high-risk patients. *Ann Intern Med* 99:438, 1983.

151. Schumer W: Steroids in the treatment of clinical septic shock. *Ann Surg* 184:333, 1976.

152. Shin CS, Williams MH: Aerosol beclomethasone in patients with steroid responsive chronic obstructive pulmonary disease. *Am J Med* 78:655, 1985.

153. Sibbald WJ, Anderson RR, Reid B, et al: Alveoli-capillary permeability in human septic ARDS: effect of high-dose corticosteroid therapy. *Chest* 79:133, 1981.

154. Siu SCB, Kitzman DW, Sheedy PF, et al: Adrenal insufficiency from bilateral adrenal hemorrhage. *Mayo Clin Proc* 65:664, 1990.

155. Skubitz KM, Craddock PR, Hammershmidt DE, et al: Corticosteroids block binding of chemotactic peptide to its receptor in granulocytes and cause disaggregation of granulocyte aggregates in vitro. *J Clin Invest* 67:1103, 1981.

156. Smith SJH, MacGregor GA, Markandu ND, et al: Evidence that patients with Addison's disease are undertreated with fludrocortisone. *Lancet* 1:11, 1984.

157. SOLVD Investigators: Effect of enalapril on survival in patients with reduced left ventricular ejection fractions and congestive heart failure. *N Engl J Med* 325:293, 1991.

158. Sprung CL, Caralis PV, Marcial EH, et al: The effects of high-dose corticosteroids in patients with septic shock. A prospective, controlled study. *N Engl J Med* 311:1137, 1984.

159. Vanmarter LJ, Lenton A, Kuun KCK, Pagano M, Allred EN: Maternal glucocorticoid therapy and reduced bronchopulmonary dysplasia. *Pediatrics* 86:331, 1990.

160. Streck WK, Lockwood DH: Pituitary adrenal recovery following short-term suppression with corticosteroids. *Am J Med* 66:910, 1979.

160a. Sternberg EM, Chrousos GP, Wilder RL, Gold PW: The stress response and the regulation of inflammatory disease. *Ann Intern Med* 117:854, 1992.

161. Stubs SS, et al: Intravenous methylprednisolone sodium succinate: adverse reactions reported in association with immunosuppressive therapy. *Transplant Proc* 5:1145, 1976.

162. Stuck AE, Minder CE, Frey FJ: Risk of infectious complications in patients taking glucocorticoids. *Rev Infect Dis* 11:954, 1989.

163. Szefler SJ, Rose JQ, Ellis EF, et al: The effect of troleandomycin on methylprednisolone elimination. *J Allergy Clin* 66:447, 1980.

164. Tamoki J, Sakai N, Kobayashi T, et al: Corticotropin-releasing factor potentiates the contractile response of rabbit airway smooth muscle to electrical field stimulation but not to acetylcholine. *Am Rev Respir Dis* 140:1331, 1989.

165. Tanaka RM, Santiago SM, Kuhn GJ, et al: Intravenous methylprednisolone in adults and in status asthmaticus: comparison of two dosages. *Chest* 82:438, 1982.

166. The Veterans Administration Systemic Sepsis Cooperative Study Group: Effect of high-dose glucocorticoid therapy on mortality in patients with clinical signs of systemic sepsis. *N Engl J Med* 317:659, 1987.

166a. Thompson AB, Mueller MB, Heires AJ, et al: Aerosolized beclomethasone in chronic bronchitis. *Am Rev Respir Dis* 146:389, 1992.

167. Tucci JR, Espiner EA, Jagger PL, et al: ACTH stimulation of aldosterone secretion in normal subjects and in patients with chronic adrenocortical insufficiency. *J Clin Endocrinol Metab* 27:568, 1967.

168. Turner ES, Greenberger PA, Patterson RP: Management of the pregnant asthmatic patient. *Ann Intern Med* 6:905, 1980.

169. Tyrell JB, Baxter JD: Glucocorticoid therapy. In Felig P, et al (eds): Endocrinology and Metabolism. McGraw-Hill, New York, 1981, p 559.

170. Tyrell JB, Baxter JD: Disorders of the adrenal cortex. In Wyngaarden JB, Smith LH (eds): Cecil Textbook of Medicine, ed 17. WB Saunders, Philadelphia, 1985, pp 1300–1320.

170a. Udelsman R, Goldstein DS, Loriaux DL, Chrousos GP: Catecholamine-glucocorticoid interactions during surgical stress. *J Surg Res* 539–545, 1987.

170b. Udelsman R, Ramp J, Gallucci WT, Gordon A, Lipford E, Norton JA, Loriaux DL, Chrousos GP: Adaptation during surgical stress—a re-evaluation of the role of glucocorticoids. *J Clin Invest* 44:1377–1381, 1986.

171. VanArsdel PP: Drug allergy, an update. Symposium on clinical allergy. *Med Clin North* Am 65:1089, 1981.

172. VanBahr C, Sjoquist F, Orrenius S: The inhibitory effect of hydrocortisone and testosterone in plasma disappearance of nortriptyline in the dog and perfused rat liver. *Eur J Pharmacol* 9:106, 1970.

173. Varney NR, Alexander B, MacIndoe JH: Reversible steroid dementia in patients without steroid psychosis. *Am J Psychiatry* 143:3, 1984.

174. Vaz R, Sencor B, Morris M, et al: Adrenal effects on beclomethasone inhalation therapy in asthmatic children. *J Pediatr* 100:660, 1982.

175. Viires N, Pavlovic D, Pariente R, Aubier M: Effects of steroids on diaphragmatic function in rats. *Am Rev Respir Dis* 132:34, 1990.

175a. Vittori E, Marini M, Fasoli A, DeFranchis R, Mattoli S: Increased expression of endothelin in bronchial epithelial cells of asthmatic patients and effect of corticosteriods. *Am Rev Respir Dis* 146:1320, 1992.

176. Walker AE, Adamkiewicz JJ: Pseudotumor cerebri associated with prolonged corticosteroid therapy: report of four cases. *JAMA* 188:779, 1964.

177. Wang Y, Zintel T, Vasquez A, Gallagher CG: Corticosteroid therapy and respiratory muscle function in humans. *Am Rev Respir Dis* 144:108, 1991.

178. Weissglas IS: The role of endogenous opiates in shock: experimental and clinical studies in vitro and in vivo. *Adv Shock Res* 10:87, 1983.

179. Wesseling GJ, Quadvlieg M, Wouters EFM: Inhaled budesonide in chronic bronchitis. Effects on respiratory impedance. *Eur Respir J* 4:1101, 1991.

180. Weston WI, Mandel MJ, Yeckley JA, et al: Mechanism of cortisol inhibition of adoptive transfer of tuberculin sensitivity. *J Lab Clin Med* 82:366, 1973.

181. White VA, Kumagai LF: Preoperative endocrine and metabolic considerations. Symposium on medical evaluation of the preoperative patient. *Med Clin North Am* 63:132, 1979.

182. Whitehouse BJ: Lipocortins, mediators of the anti-inflammatory actions of corticosteroids. *J Endocrinol* 123:363, 1989.

183. Bilezikian JP: Management of acute hypercalcemia. *N Engl J Med* 326:1196, 1992.

184. Wolfe R: Carbohydrate metabolism in the critically ill patient. Implications for nutritional support. *Crit Care Clin* 3:11, 1987.

185. Williams TJ, Yarwood H: Effects of glucocorticoids on microvascular permeability. *Am Rev Respir Dis* 141:S39, 1990.

186. Ziment I: Steroids. *Clin Chest Med* 7:341,1986.

187. Zizic TM, Maroux C, Hungerford DS, Dansereau J-V, Stefens MB: Corticosteroid therapy associated with ischemic necrosis of bone in systemic lupus erythematosus. *Am J Med* 79:596, 1985.

CHAPTER 44

Thyroid Hormones[a]

KENNETH D. BURMAN, M.D., Col., M.C.

In the last several years, our understanding of thyroid physiology and the mechanism of thyroid hormone action has progressed at an unheralded rate. As a result, we can now apply these newly acquired principles to clinical settings and, thus, appropriately alter our approach to patients with thyroid disease. We have accrued an understanding of the pathophysiologic alterations in thyroid metabolism that occur in ambulatory patients. This chapter reviews basic thyroid hormone physiology, the laboratory tests available to assess thyroid hormone function, and the therapeutic agents employed to treat patients with altered thyroid hormone function. Unfortunately, however, our knowledge of the critically ill individual is still clouded by a lack of understanding of the mechanism for the perturbations in thyroid function tests and the lack of a definitive tissue marker denoting thyroid hormone action at the cellular level. This chapter also reviews the findings relative to thyroid function in the critically ill subject and gives the author's opinion concerning the interpretation of these tests and how to apply them to systemically ill patients. These opinions, of course, are subject to modification as further research and experience evolve.[b]

[a] The opinions or assertions contained herein are the private views of the author and are not to be construed as official or as reflecting the views of the Department of the Army or the Department of Defense.

[b] A useful aid in understanding the action, kinetics, and adverse effects of the drugs mentioned in this chapter is the Rocky Mountain Drug Consultation Center, West 8th and Cherokee, Denver, CO 80204. Many of the data in this chapter were checked with that source.

THYROID HORMONE PHYSIOLOGY

Although thyroid function tests and clinical examination are extremely useful in ascertaining whether an individual is euthyroid, these parameters are less useful and perhaps even misleading when applied to a patient in the intensive care unit (23, 30, 33, 59, 148). The interpretation of the appropriateness of these tests is dependent upon an understanding of the basic physiology of the hypothalamic-pituitary-thyroid axis. Hypothalamic thyrotropin releasing hormone (thyrotropin, or TRH) stimulates pituitary synthesis and release of thyroid stimulating hormone (TSH), a hormone that then stimulates thyroidal synthesis and release of 3,5,3′,5′-L-tetraiodothyronine (T_4) and 3,5,3′-L-triiodothyronine (T_3) (Figs. 44.1 and 44.2) Circulating T_4 is derived entirely from direct thyroidal secretion, whereas only approximately 25% of circulating T_3 is derived from glandular release, the remainder being derived from peripheral conversion of T_4 to T_3 (19, 21, 83, 136). Another metabolite, reverse T_3 (rT_3), is also principally derived from T_4. These conversions of T_4 to T_3 and rT_3 are dependent upon an enzyme(s) that resides in many tissues, including brain, liver, and kidney. In normal subjects about 40% of the T_4 secreted eventually is monodeiodinated, resulting in about 80% of all serum T_3 being derived from this extrathyroidal source. Pituitary conversion of T_4 to T_3 probably accounts for approximately 50% of the local pituitary T_3, the remainder being derived from circulating T_3 that is transported to the pituitary (83). The deiodination enzymes recently have been cloned and characterized (11, 12). In either case, it is probably

741

the local pituitary T_3 content that regulates TSH synthesis and release. Of course, other factors are capable of stimulating TSH release, such as TRH (Fig. 44.3) and hypothermia, whereas inhibitory factors include dopamine, somatostatin, hyperthermia, glucocorticoids, and, of course, T_4/T_3 (55, 78, 97).

In the serum, T_4 and T_3 circulate tightly bound to serum proteins (thyroxine-binding globulin, or TBG; thyroxine-binding prealbumin, or TBPA) and albumin, and only about 0.3% of T_3 and 0.03% of T_4 are unbound. This unbound fraction is believed to be the major portion of the hormone that is capable of traversing membranes and exerting its influence upon nuclear receptors (e.g., to increase protein synthesis) (76, 109, 116, 123). Since nuclear receptors have affinities for T_3 about 10 times greater than for T_4, and since T_3 is also less tightly bound to serum proteins than T_4, one can account for most, if not all, of thyroid hormone action by T_3 alone. In selected circumstances T_4 may be active, albeit less so than T_3, but in most situations T_4 can be thought of as a prohormone. It recently has been shown that the T_3 receptor is similar to an oncogene protein, C-erb A. These receptors may be slightly different in various tissues and have been found to have mutations that can result in altered T_3 binding and relative resistance to thyroid hormone action. These rare resistance syndromes are familial, and it is not yet known whether similar abnormalities occur in more common clinical circumstances (43, 48, 106b, 127, 153). Understanding these considerations helps us conceptualize why the serum T_4 concentration may

not always be an accurate reflection of the tissue effects by thyroid hormones.

Peripheral deiodination proceeds enzymatically (Fig. 44.1), and in some circumstances this conversion is altered in such a way that less T_3 (active hormone) and more rT_3 (inactive metabolite) is formed (5, 19, 26, 65, 112, 120). This decrease in conversion to T_3 may be homeostatic, as it would reduce catabolism, thus theoretically being beneficial during critical illness. Several of the conditions or agents that decrease conversion of T_4 to T_3 are listed in Table 44.1.

Although a great deal is understood about the physiology of thyroid hormone and its mechanism of action, no accurate, reproducible parameters are available for assessing the metabolic state of any patient, especially one in the intensive care unit. A physician must depend to a large degree on his or her clinical skills to assess the thyroid status of a systemically ill patient. A complete medical history, including family history of thyroid disease, medications ingested, and a physical examination of the neck revealing a surgical scar or enlarged gland, are extremely helpful and crucial to the correct interpretation of the thyroid function test results. Of course, specific findings such as exophthalmos or pretibial myxedema are also important, reflecting the likelihood of hyperthyroidism (present or past). However, commonly used parameters such as hand tremor, reflex return phase, and skin condition are nonspecific and difficult to assess in the ambulatory patient, much less in the critically ill subject. No laboratory tests are available that can assess accurately the action of T_3/T_4 at the

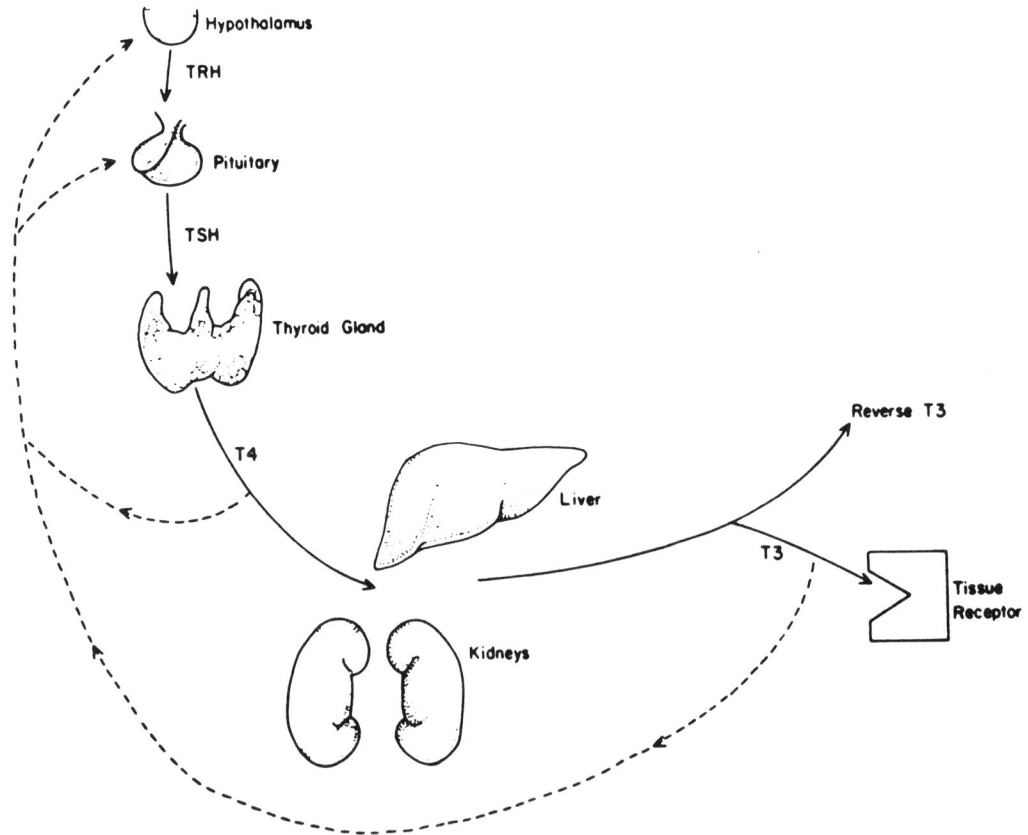

Figure 44.1.   Hypothalamic-pituitary-thyroid axis in a euthyroid individual. (From Burman KD: *Thyroid: University Case Reports,* vol 3. Parke-Davis, Morris Plains, NJ, 1981.)

DEIODINATIVE PATHWAYS
OF IODOTHYRONINES

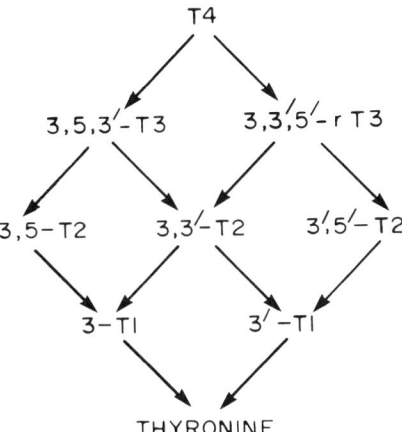

THYROXINE (T4)

T4

3,5,3′-T3   3,3′,5′-r T3

3,5-T2   3,3′-T2   3′,5′-T2

3-TI   3′-TI

THYRONINE

Figure 44.2. The deiodinative cascade of T_4/T_3 to lesser iodinated iodo-thyronines. (Adapted from Smallridge RC: *Heart and Heart-like Organs.* Academic Press, New York, 1980.)

Table 44.1. Conditions or Agents Associated with Decreased T_4-to-T_3 Conversion

Systemic illnesses
   Chronic renal failure, malignancy, thermal injury, diabetes melli-tus, acute infections, and chronic hepatic disease
Fasting or caloric deprivation
Surgery and the postoperative period
β-Adrenergic blockers
Propylthiouracil
Glucocorticoids
Lithium[a]
Amiodarone
Radiopaque dyes (e.g., ipodate, iopanoic acid)
Neonatal period

[a] Studies indicate that lithium may decrease T_4 disappearance and theo-retically may decrease T_4-to-T_3 conversion.

cellular level. Indeed, development of such tests is crucial to our understanding, interpretation, and treatment of thyroid function tests in the critically ill patient.

LABORATORY TESTS THAT REFLECT THYROID FUNCTION

T_4 ASSAY

Most clinical T_4 laboratory tests analyze the serum T_4 con-centration by a specific radioimmunoassay (RIA), in which

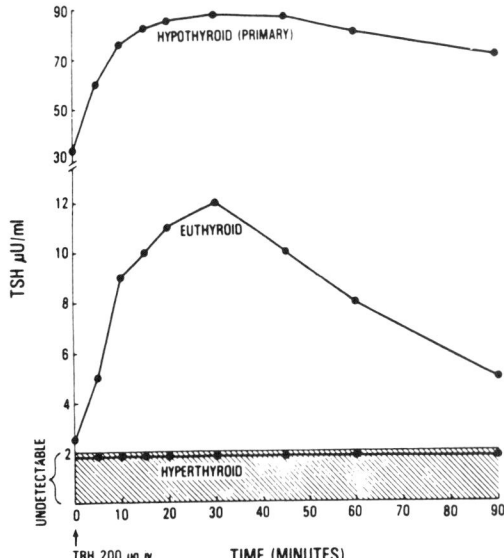

Figure 44.3. Idealized representation of the serum TSH response to the intravenous administration of TRH in a euthyroid, hypothyroid (primary), and hyperthyroid patient.

there are few known factors that may artifactually influence the results (152). The normal range for serum T_4 is approximately 4 to 12 μg/dl. Although this range is useful as a guideline in the majority of cases, not every patient who has a serum T_4 outside the normal range has a metabolic derangement in thyroid hormone function and action. In addition, some pa-tients with "normal" T_4 values may actually be hyperthyroid or hypothyroid at the tissue level. Alterations in the serum T_4 level can be caused by disturbed thyroid function resulting from increases or decreases in serum iodothyronine levels; in addition, changes in serum binding proteins may result in values outside the normal range, despite normal free thyroxine (FT_4) levels and euthyroidism. Situations that are associated with an acquired increase in TBG, with an increased serum T_4 and lowered resin T_3 uptake (RT_3U) yet clinical euthyroid-ism, are summarized in Table 44.2 (15). Euthyroidism with an increased serum total T_4 also can occur in conditions other than those that have increased TBG (Table 44.3). During the acute phase of any systemic illness serum T_4 may be increased transiently (15, 40, 77, 94). This increase is seen infrequently, and the great majority of patients with systemic illnesses have decreased serum T_4 levels and an increased RT_3U. Psychiatric illness of any type may also be associated with increases in serum T_4; these alterations seem to normalize after several days to weeks.

T_3 ASSAY

The serum T_3 assay is also performed by RIA and is specific; it measures total serum T_3 and not simply the small unbound fraction. The normal serum T_3 range is about 80 to 220 ng/dl. Serum T_3 levels frequently are increased in thyrotoxic subjects but commonly are in the normal range in hypothyroid individuals. As a result, a serum T_3 by RIA would not be expected to aid in the differentiation of hypothyroid and euthyroid patients but is useful in diagnosing hyperthy-roidism.

Table 44.2.   Conditions That Increase or Decrease Serum Thyroxine-binding Globulin Levels[a]

Increase serum thyroxine-binding globulin (TBG) concentrations[b]
  Physiologic
    Inherited
    Pregnancy
    Newborn
  Nonthyroidal illness
    Infectious hepatitis
    Chronic active hepatitis
    Primary biliary cirrhosis
    Acute intermittent porphyria
    Estrogen-producing tumors
    Hydatidiform mole
    Lymphosarcoma
  Drug-induced
    Exogenous estrogens
    Oral contraceptives
    Heroin and methadone
    Perphenazine
    Clofibrate
    Carbamazepine[c]
Decrease serum thyroxine-binding globulin levels or decrease
  binding of T_4 or T_3 to TBG
  Systemic illness (e.g., nephrotic syndrome)
  Glucocorticoids
  Androgens
  Danazol
  L-asparaginase
  Salicylates
  Phenylbutazone
  Halofenate
  Mitotane

[a] Adapted with permission from Borst GC, et al: Euthyroid hyperthyroxinemia. *Ann Intern Med* 98:366–378, 1983.
[b] Patients with an increased TBG concentration would be expected to have an increased serum T_4, a lowered RT_3U, a normal free T_4, and clinical and biochemical euthyroidism. Similarly, patients with decreased TBG would have a decreased T_4, increased RT_3U, and also a normal free T_4.
[c] Carbamazepine may increase TBG but also most commonly decreases serum T_4 and T_3 (1), possibly because it also enhances extrathyroidal iodothyronine metabolism (1).

Table 44.3.   Situations Associated with Elevated Serum Thyroxine Concentrations yet with Clinical and Biochemical Euthyroidism[a]

Acquired or inherited increase in serum thyroxine-binding globulin
Peripheral resistance to thyroid hormones
Transient hyperthyroxinemia of acute medical illness (e.g., hepatitis)
Transient hyperthyroxinemia of acute psychiatric illness
Drug-related hyperthyroxinemia
  Iopanoic acid
  Ipodate
  Amiodarone
  Propranolol

[a] Adapted from Borst GC, et al: Euthyroid hyperthyroxinemia. *Ann Intern Med* 98:366–378, 1983.

RESIN T_3 UPTAKE

This test is performed most appropriately as an accompaniment to the T_4 assay. It is not an immunoassay, and the test consists of incubating serum with ^{125}I-T_3. The isotope binds to the available hormone binding sites, and then a resin is added, which nonspecifically binds the ^{125}I-T_3 that had not been bound in the serum; the number of resin-bound counts is then determined. The resin T_3 uptake test does not measure hormone levels directly but simply assesses indirectly the number of serum thyroid binding sites available. The results of this test show increased numbers in hyperthyroid and decreased numbers in hypothyroid subjects, but in the author's view, it is an insensitive indicator of thyroid hormone levels and action. Indeed, its major utility lies in the simple fact that it reflects the number of unavailable binding sites. Generally, if the RT_3U values are discordant with serum T_4 levels (e.g., serum T_4 increased and RT_3U decreased), then a binding abnormality probably is present rather than a true metabolic derangement in thyroxine action. For example, if a patient does have increased TBG levels secondary to estrogen administration, the T_4 level would be increased and the RT_3U would be decreased. Of course, a patient with an altered TBG level and a normal free T_4 index is believed to be metabolically euthyroid (1, 148). On the other hand, if the T_4 level and the RT_3U level are altered concordantly (i.e., in the same direction), then one preliminarily can assume that altered thyroid function may be present.

REVERSE T_3 (rT_3)

The serum reverse T_3 level is measured by RIA and has a normal range of about 20 to 40 ng/dl. Reverse T_3, levels frequently are increased in thyrotoxic and decreased in hypothyroid individuals. In addition, rT_3 concentrations are increased in euthyroid critically ill subjects, either as a result of enhanced conversion from T_4 or decreased rT_3 clearance (76).

SERUM-FREE T_4

Free T_4(FT_4) concentrations may be performed by estimating the total T_4 concentration by RIA and then multiplying this value by the dialyzable percentage of T_4. This dialyzable percentage figure is obtained by placing serum in dialysis tubing along with ^{125}I-T_4. The amount of ^{125}I-T_4 that crosses the membrane then is determined and used to derive the serum-free T_4 value, normally about 1.5 to 5.0 ng/dl (123, 146). This method of analysis yields excellent discrimination among hypothyroidism, euthyroidism, and hyperthyroidism in the ambulatory patient. Most euthyroid critically ill subjects have a normal or even elevated FT_4 by dialysis, despite low total T_4 levels. The problem is that this method of analysis is relatively expensive and time-consuming, and generally is performed only in research or specific reference laboratories, causing it to have a turnaround time of about 2 to 5 days. Because of these limitations, several newer tests that measure free T_4 directly have been manufactured commercially. There is a controversy as to the validity of each of the marketed kits; the debate centers on their ability to obtain "normal values" in most critically ill subjects (34, 77, 93, 118). Although the argument is somewhat circular, it is reasonable to assume that most critically ill subjects are euthyroid and, thus, that the FT_4 should be normal. However, many commercial FT_4 kits obtain low values in this setting, a fact that allows investigators to conclude that such a kit would be inappropriate when applied to critically ill patients. In one or two separate studies (34, 77, 93) the Clinical Assays (Cambridge, MA), Corning (Medfield, MA), or Damon kits (Needham Heights, MA) were relatively consistent in obtaining normal FT$_4$ values in most critically ill subjects. It is expected that these controversies will subside as FT$_4$ kits are analyzed in more detail and as further studies are performed. Of course, the availability of accurate FT$_4$ kits with a rapid turnaround time would be extremely useful in the interpretation of thyroid function tests in critically ill subjects. A free T$_4$ kit that actually employs equilibrium dialysis in small, specially designed tubes has been developed (100, 101). This kit is clinically applicable; as the assay time is approximately 24 hours, the values seem reflective of the "classic" dialysis method, and the cost is reasonable (higher than that for total T$_4$ but less than that for "classic" dialysis method). Further investigation of this kit and analysis in the critical care setting would be important. Unfortunately, it is in the critically ill subjects in whom indirect estimates of FT$_4$, such as the "FT$_4$ index," are thought to be misleadingly low (33). Since most conditions associated with altered thyroid hormone binding to their serum binding proteins also have discordantly altered serum T$_4$ and RT$_3$U, it seems reasonable that multiplying these two measurements might lead to an accurate estimate of the FT$_4$. This derived number has been called an "FT$_4$ index." This index correlates well with the serum FT$_4$ level by dialysis in most conditions, except in systemically ill patients, in whom it appears to be inappropriately low, erroneously suggesting hypothyroidism in a presumed euthyroid patient.

SERUM-FREE T$_3$

At present, the most accurate method of assessing FT$_3$ is by equilibrium dialysis (114, 146). Several new kit methods that measure FT$_3$ (and FT$_4$) recently have been used to detect low FT$_3$ levels in the "euthyroid sick syndrome" (146). Further studies with these methods should help determine whether they will be useful clinically.

THYROID-STIMULATING HORMONE

Within the last several years, highly sensitive commercial TSH assay kits have been developed and their use has become routine (86, 111, 122, 133). The most highly sensitive methods employ chemiluminescence techniques and have a minimal sensitivity of about 0.05 μU/ml. In these assays, normal subjects virtually always have detectable TSH levels, and all patients with thyrotoxicosis are expected to have undetectable levels (61, 160). The normal range varies by each assay but is usually about 0.5 to 4.0 μU/ml. Primary hypothyroid subjects are expected to have increased TSH concentrations and euthyroid patients with "nonthyroid" illnesses are expected to have detectable levels that are usually within the normal range. Serum TSH may decrease to undetectable levels in patients with systemic illness, although a summary of reports indicates that TSH levels usually are normal or only slightly low in these patients. TSH can increase during recovery from systemic illness, generally resulting in TSH levels as high as about 15 μU/ml that may persist for several days (60). The serum T$_4$ also increases slightly, suggesting the biologic relevance of this TSH increase, and when such patients are followed, their TSH and T$_4$ concentrations usually remain normal.

TRH responsiveness, as determined by these highly sensitive TSH assays, is interpreted in a manner similarly to that of the older assays; thyrotoxic patients do not respond, euthyroid patients have a normal response, and patients with primary hypothyroidism hyperrespond (121). Although further studies are required, it seems that normal subjects have a TSH level between 5 and 30 μU/ml at 15 or 30 minutes after TRH administration (usually 500 μg administered intravenously). Each laboratory should assess its own assay, but a hyperresponsive patient usually has a level greater than 30 or 40 μU/ml.

RADIOIODINE UPTAKE

The radioiodine uptake (RAIU) test is performed by administering radioactive iodine orally and determining how much is accumulated by the thyroid gland. The normal range is about 8 to 30%. The major drawback of this test, as applied to the critically ill subject, is the lack of practicality of measuring thyroidal uptake in the intensive care unit because of the immobility of the equipment required to detect accurately the amount of isotope residing in the thyroid gland. Furthermore, there is a large amount of overlap in RAIU values in hypothyroid and euthyroid subjects, although this test is useful in discriminating hyperthyroid from euthyroid individuals. The RAIU can be artifactually lowered by recent administration of radioopaque dyes, which contain large amounts of iodine, a factor that especially must be considered after enhanced computed tomographic (CT) scans. This effect upon the RAIU may last for 6 weeks to 6 months after a scan, depending upon the type of scan and contrast agent used.

HYPERTHYROIDISM

THERAPEUTIC AGENTS COMMONLY USED IN HYPERTHYROIDISM

The prescribing physician should be familiar with the mechanisms of action and patient warnings or adverse effects of therapeutic agents for treatment of hyperthyroidism prior to their use. Table 44.4 lists several of these agents. The physician should also be familiar with the varying treatments of Graves' disease in various countries (91, 149).

Propylthiouracil

Propylthiouracil (PTU) is an effective inhibitor of thyroidal synthesis of T$_4$ and/or T$_3$ (36, 137). This agent frequently is employed either in the short-term situation to decrease thyroidal secretion, or over the long term to maintain euthyroidism in a patient with Graves' disease (or other causes of hyperthyroidism) or to induce a remission. PTU also has a peripheral effect in that it decreases extrathyroidal deiodination of T$_4$, such that serum T$_3$ levels decrease. PTU (and methimazole) may also have a direct immunologic effect in decreasing the synthesis of TSH receptor antibodies (25, 144, 145). This agent usually is administered orally, although the tablets may be crushed and the pills placed down a nasogastric tube. Alternatively, the drug theoretically can be given rectally (as may methimazole) (99), although the author is unaware of

Table 44.4.   Pharmacology of Agents Used to Treat Hyperthyroidism[a]

Agent	Maintenance Dose	Mechanism of Action	Common or Serious Adverse Effects
Commonly used			
Propylthiouracil (6-propyl-2-thiouracil)	50–300 mg t.i.d., p.o.	Inhibits thyroid hormone synthesis; inhibits T_4 extrathyroidal conversion to T_3	Skin rash, nausea, epigastric distress, agranulocytosis, granulocytopenia, hepatitis, lupus-like syndrome
Methimazole (1-methyl-2-mercapto imidazole)	5–30 mg t.i.d., p.o.	Inhibits thyroid hormone synthesis	As above
DL-propranolol or Atenolol[b]	10–80 mg q.i.d., p.o. 50–100 mg, once daily, p.o.	Decreases β-adrenergic mediated activity and helps ameliorate signs and symptoms of thyrotoxicosis	Cardiovascular, bronchospasm, central nervous system; must be used with care in patients with congestive heart failure or asthma
Nonroutine agents[c]			
Lithium carbonate	600 mg t.i.d., p.o., to produce blood levels between 0.5 and 1.3 mEq/liter	Probably decreases thyroidal secretion and possibly inhibits extrathyroidal T_4 to T_3 conversion	Hand tremor, polyuria, drowsiness, lack of coordination, ataxia, blurred vision; may cause increased thyroid size and in certain subjects may cause either hypothyroidism or, rarely, hyperthyroidism
Iodides[d]	5 drops SSKI t.i.d., p.o., or 5 drops Lugol's solution t.i.d., p.o.	Decreases thyroidal secretion	Parotitis or skin rash or serum sickness-like reaction; prolonged use may lead to unabated hypersecretion of thyroid hormone
Ipodate sodium[d]	3 g p.o. every 2–3 days or 1 g daily	Decreases thyroidal secretion and extrathyroidal T_4 to T_3 conversion	Skin rash, agranulocytosis, liver disease; should not be used in patients with history of iodide allergy

[a] The prescribing physician should be very knowledgeable with regard to the mechanism of action and potential warnings and side effects of these agents, and appropriately detailed textbooks or articles should be consulted prior to their use.

[b] Any β-adrenergic blocking agent can be used. DL-propranolol has been utilized for the longest time and thus is preferred in some unusual circumstances (e.g., pregnancy). On the other hand, a cardioselective, long-acting blocker (e.g., atenolol) may have advantages in the routine thyrotoxic patient.

[c] None of these agents has been studied adequately in the prolonged treatment of hyperthyroidism. As a general rule these agents should not be utilized for longer than 1 month, since the potential complications have not been investigated and the likelihood of causing unabated thyrotoxicosis exists, especially with iodide-containing substances.

[d] SSKI (1 g/ml) contains 76.4% iodine. Five drops t.i.d. (assuming 20 drops/ml) gives about 573 mg iodine. Lugol's solution (125 mg/ml) of total iodine contains 5 g iodine and 10 g potassium iodide in each 100 ml. Five drops t.i.d. gives about 94 mg iodine daily. It is assumed at present that the antithyroid action of ipodate is related partly to the release of iodides and partly to the ipodate molecule itself. Contains 61.4% iodine, so one 3-g dose of ipodate has 1842 mg iodine. For purposes of this chapter, iodide and iodine are used interchangeably.

such usage of PTU being reported in the literature. Cooper and his colleagues (39, 41) have developed a specific, sensitive RIA for PTU. A single 150-mg oral dose of PTU is absorbed rapidly, appearing in serum of both normal and thyrotoxic subjects within 5 minutes and peaking at 65 ± 10 minutes (level 3.3 ± 0.3 μg/ml) in the former group and at 54 ± 6 minutes (level 4.5 ± 0.6 μg/ml) in the latter (39). In both groups, detectable PTU was observed to be present in the serum for as long as 6 to 8 hours after a single dose. In further studies using various doses of PTU, Cooper et al (41) noted that comparable serum PTU serum levels were obtained in thyrotoxic and normal subjects after 50- and 200-mg doses of PTU, but after 300 mg of oral PTU the serum PTU concentrations were significantly higher in the thyrotoxic subjects. The explanation for this difference possibly relates to enhanced intestinal absorption of PTU in thyrotoxic subjects; this theoretic explanation, however, requires scientific validation. Ingestion of food did not appear to influence the amount of PTU absorbed, although further studies in this area seem warranted because of the variable and inconsistent results obtained.

PTU is concentrated within the thyroid gland, and the serum PTU level may correlate with its ability to block thyroidal organification (41). However, the actual duration of effect of PTU within the thyroidal gland is unknown. In contrast, even a single PTU dose can inhibit T_4 conversion such that serum T_3 decreases as early as 1 hour following the dose, reaching its nadir at about 6 to 10 hours and gradually returning toward basal levels (41). After doses of 50, 200, and 300 mg of PTU in euthyroid subjects, the serum T_3 levels after 24 hours were quite close to basal, pretreatment levels (38). In the hyperthyroid subjects, 50- and 300-mg doses resulted in a return to or near baseline by 20 to 24 hours, whereas 200 mg of PTU still resulted in significantly decreased T_3 levels after 24 hours (41). Thus, even though the serum PTU concentration and its effect on thyroidal organification are correlated with the oral dose given, apparently the influence on extrathyroidal conversion is not dose-related, since T_3 levels decreased further after a single dose of 200 mg of PTU than after 300 mg of PTU. These data obtained by RIA are similar to those obtained by other types of assays. Earlier studies also indicated that PTU absorption was delayed significantly in euthyroid elderly subjects compared with euthyroid younger individuals. Vesell et al (142) used a spectrophotometric assay to estimate that the plasma half-life of PTU was 6.7 ± 1.0 hours in normal subjects, 4.3 ± 0.7 hours in thyrotoxics, and 24.7 ± 34.5 hours in hypothyroid subjects. Schuppan et al (117) and Sitar and Hunninghake (120) used gas-liquid chromotography techniques to estimate that the plasma half-life of PTU is about 1 hour, an estimate similar to that obtained from observations of other investigators (72–75, 92). Conceivably, spectrophotometric assays might result in a longer estimated half-life by measuring metabolites; gas-liquid chromotography and specific RIA techniques should be able to measure directly the parent compound alone. Cooper et al (39) specifically tested the major metabolites of PTU (propyluracil, S-methyl PTU, and PTU-S-glucuronide) and concluded that there was no significant cross-reaction in their PTU assay.

A mildly hyperthyroid subject generally is started on 100 to 300 mg of PTU daily in three or four divided doses; a moderately thyrotoxic patient, on 300 to 600 mg daily; and a severely hyperthyroid subject, on 600 to 900 mg PTU daily. Serum T_4 is monitored frequently (about every 1 to 3 weeks) and PTU doses are adjusted to keep the T_4 value in the normal range. Adverse effects of PTU are thought to increase with increasing PTU doses, the most common side effects being skin rash and a metallic taste in the mouth. More severe, and fortunately less common, adverse effects include hepatotoxicity, granulocytopenia, and agranulocytosis (2, 4, 108, 123, 140). PTU and methimazole should be used with caution in nursing women. Tegler and Lindstrom (129) proposed that the estimated dose to the child would be less with PTU; however, recent studies find no evidence of hypothyroidism in nursing infants exposed to low-dose carbimazole. Cooper et al (36–39) concluded that the mean methimazole serum and breast milk levels were both about equal, with an approximate total of 70 μg excreted in 8 hours after a single 40-mg dose, representing about 0.75% of the ingested amount. Further, they calculated that a 70-μg dose was the equivalent of about 17.5 μg/kg in a 4-kg infant and could possibly have antithyroid effects. Since methimazole is 10 times more active than PTU on a milligram-for-milligram basis, and because the researchers believed that breast milk concentrations of PTU were only about 10% of PTU serum levels (73), PTU may be preferred in breastfeeding women (82). The frequency of serious untoward effects from PTU is less than 1%, whereas skin rashes may occur in 5 to 10% of patients (37, 154). Some clinicians monitor the hematocrit and white blood count in patients who are taking PTU; the author generally obtains a hemogram and "SMAC-20" prior to and during therapy, although the time of onset of adverse effects (e.g., agranulocytosis or hepatotoxicity) is unpredictable (61). Clinical findings or complaints such as sore throat or infection could indicate agranulocytosis. In those circumstances a hemogram, including total white blood cell and differential counts as well as a peripheral blood smear, is indicated, in conjunction with an appropriate history and physical examination. Interestingly, there is one report of a 12-year-old girl who was taking PTU for thyrotoxicosis. She acutely ingested at least 5000 mg of PTU prior to admission, and she excreted more than 90 mg/dl of PTU within the first 12 hours after admission (69). Her T_4 level dropped only from 6.5 μg/dl to 4.8 μg/dl, and she had no symptoms referable to this dose of PTU.

Methimazole

Methimazole is an effective inhibitor of thyroidal hormone synthesis, and this drug may also be used either short term to induce the euthyroid state or long term to attempt to induce a remission in patients with hyperthyroidism. Despite similar effects on the thyroid gland, this drug differs from PTU in that it does not inhibit peripheral T_4 conversion to T_3. Its serum half-life is probably longer than that of PTU, although it is also concentrated within the thyroid gland, and the duration of its influence upon secretion generally is unknown. A mildly thyrotoxic patient may require a total of 10 to 30 mg daily, and a severely thyrotoxic patient may require a total of 60 to 90 mg daily, each in divided doses. Methimazole also can be administered via nasogastric tube or rectally (99).

Methimazole's pharmacokinetics have been investigated less thoroughly than those of PTU. In 1969, Alexander and associates (3) administered 35-S-labeled methimazole to one patient with thyrotoxicosis and to another with inoperable carcinoma of the cervix, renal failure, and a goiter. The distribution space, plasma half-life, and renal clearance were 34.2 liters, 13.8 hours, and 20 ml/min in the hyperthyroid patient and 35.7 liters, 20.7 hours, and 11.9 ml/min in the euthyroid patient. Cooper et al (38), using an RIA to document that peak methimazole levels were comparable in normal and thyrotoxic subjects, found the serum half-life to be about 6 to 7 hours. Cirrhotic patients had a prolonged serum half-life (about 21 hours). In other reports (6, 106, 142), the half-life ranged from 6.4 to 13.6 hours in normal subjects. Obviously, further studies investigating methimazole's kinetics with more sensitive and specific techniques (e.g., RIA) are warranted. Absorption of methimazole occurs within 30 to 60 minutes of either oral or rectal administration. Nabil and associates (99) also observed that a 60-mg dose of methimazole resulted in comparable plasma levels in six healthy volunteers whether given orally or rectally.

Although controversial, it is the author's opinion that PTU and methimazole are essentially interchangeable with regard to their clinical use, as they have basically the same mechanism of action and the same types and frequency of adverse reactions. Despite this general clinical statement, methimazole may be more effective in inducing euthyroidism rapidly and in causing long-term remissions (9). The initial use of PTU or methimazole is arbitrary except if a patient has a known hypersensitivity to one agent, if a woman is pregnant, or if a woman is breastfeeding, in which case PTU may be preferred.

Administration of methimazole has been associated with the following adverse reactions: skin rash, hepatic toxicity, fever, leukopenia, agranulocytosis, adenopathy, lupus-like syndrome, circulating immune complexes, nausea, vomiting, and hypothyroidism (108).

In a retrospective study, Cooper and associates (42) gave new insight into the likelihood of a patient's developing agranulocytosis with PTU or methimazole. They compared the clinical characteristics of hyperthyroid patients who had untoward hematologic reactions and those who did not. The mean age of 14 subjects who had an untoward hematologic reaction was 50.6 ± 16 years, a value significantly higher than that of 35.7 ± 13.7 years in patients who had no reaction. Also, the mean dose of methimazole was higher in the patients who had a reaction (43.8 ± 9.9 mg/day vs. 29.5 ± 10.5 mg/day). They concluded that there was an 8.6-fold increased risk of agranulocytosis with methimazole doses >40 mg/day. The mean doses of PTU, however, were not different in patients who did or did not have a reaction. Low-dose methimazole (<30 mg/day) may be safer with regard to the development of agranulocytosis than conventional dose PTU. However, agranulocytosis is rare and probably occurs in 0.3 to 0.6% of hyperthyroid patients who ingest either PTU or methimazole. When agranulocytosis does occur, it usually becomes manifest within 2 months of the initiation of therapy (42). If a patient has a mild adverse reaction (e.g., skin rash) to either PTU or methimazole, the author recommends that the patient be switched immediately to the other agent. The frequency of cross-allergies to these agents is unknown, but it is estimated to be about 20 to 30%. A recent collaborative study of a total of 309 patients with Graves' disease showed that there were 39 patients (of 251) (15.5%) that had an adverse drug reaction when they received 10 mg/day for a year and 67 (of 258) (26%) who had an adverse reaction in the 40 mg/day group. One patient in each group had agranulocytosis; 15 people had a skin rash in the 10 mg/day group and 18 in the 40 mg/day group (106b).

In a pregnant thyrotoxic subject it is preferable to use PTU, since only methimazole has been associated with a rare scalp condition in the infant called "aplasia cutis" (96, 98). A retrospective review, however, questions this effect of methimazole (139). In addition, Momotani et al (95) studied 643 neonates from mothers with Graves' disease and concluded that the risk of malformation in the infants was 1.7% or less if the mother had received methimazole during pregnancy. Further, it appeared that thyrotoxicosis itself seemed to be more related to the development of malformation than did euthyroidism, even with administration of antithyroid drugs.

Hashizume et al (64) recently have reported on the combined use of methimazole and thyroxine in the treatment of Graves' disease. These studies suggested that such therapy resulted in decreased recurrence of hyperthyroidism when compared with methimazole therapy alone. This article has received much attention, but, in the author's view, further confirmatory studies are required before such therapy can be recommended on a routine clinical basis.

β-Adrenergic Receptor Blockers. β-Adrenergic receptor antagonists (β-blockers) are very helpful in ameliorating the signs or symptoms of thyroidal hyperthyroidism, but they do not alter thyroid hormone synthesis or action (119, 132). The β-blockers, however, result in prompt improvement in tachycardia, fever, sweating, anxiety, and muscle weakness. Propranolol, but probably not other β-blockers, has a slight ability to decrease conversion of T_4 to T_3, so that serum T_3 levels may drop by about 10 to 20% (49, 50, 62, 71, 141, 156). Although β-blockers are very useful in the treatment of hyperthyroidism, there are reports of individuals developing thyroid storm when only β-blockers and no other agents, such as PTU or methimazole, were used (46). The author believes that, in an ordinary case of thyrotoxicosis, patients should not be treated solely with β-blockers.

Propranolol is the most studied and most commonly employed of the β-blockers, and the usual oral dose for a mildly thyrotoxic patient is 20 to 80 mg daily. A severely thyrotoxic subject may require as much as a total of 160 to 320 mg daily (in three or four divided doses) (47, 57). Feely and associates (49) noted that propranolol doses of 160 mg/day or more were required to achieve adequate β-adrenergic blockade. Moreover, they emphasize that resting heart rate alone does not always provide as accurate an estimate of the full effect of β-adrenergic blockade in hyperthyroidism as does the effect of β-adrenergic blockade upon exercise-induced tachycardia. Plasma propranolol levels appear to depend upon the age of a patient: they were lower in younger subjects. Levels also tend to be lower in smokers than nonsmokers. Rubenfeld et al (112) noted that after a single oral 80-mg dose there were variable plasma propranolol levels in both normal and thyrotoxic subjects; the former group achieved peak levels between 59 and 226 ng/ml and the latter group had peak levels between 54 and 211 ng/ml. The peak was achieved at 125 ± 16 minutes, with a plasma half-life of 4.5 ± 0.5 hours in the normal subjects; the thyrotoxic patients had peak levels achieved at 108 ± 11 minutes, with a plasma half-life of 3.7 ± 0.4 hours. These values were not significantly different in the two groups. Plasma propranolol concentrations after the 22nd dose of 40 mg of propranolol given every 6 hours orally were also studied in thyrotoxic subjects (112). Peak levels varied from 48 to 169 ng/ml, and levels at the end of the interval varied from 16 to 118 ng/ml. Plasma propranolol levels between 50 and 100 ng/ml probably result in adequate β-adrenergic blockade and seem to be associated with a 25 to 50% reduction in the exercise-induced increase in heart rate. Intravenous doses have a shorter half-life (2.4 hours) than do oral doses (3.3 hours). Chronic renal insufficiency was reported in one study to have no effect on half-life, but in another the half-life increased with decreasing creatinine clearance (15, 77). Hemodialysis does not significantly remove propranolol and thus essentially leaves the half-life unaltered, whereas plasmapheresis in one reported case appeared to remove significant amounts of propranolol, so that the half-life was about 25% of the initial value (128).

In special circumstances, propranolol can be administered intravenously to severely thyrotoxic patients. The dose by this route is 1 mg given slowly, with careful monitoring of cardiovascular function (e.g., electrocardiogram and central venous pressure). The major side effects of all β-blockers include precipitation or aggravation of congestive heart failure or asthma. Propranolol is contraindicated for use in patients with bronchial asthma, sinus bradycardia, preexisting heart block greater than first degree, cardiogenic shock, congestive heart failure, right ventricular failure secondary to pulmonary hypertension, or Raynaud's disease. In addition, propranolol should not be given to patients who are receiving myocardial depressant anesthetics, psychotropic drugs with adrenergic augmenting properties, or MAO inhibitors (and during the 2-week withdrawal period of such agents). Propranolol should be used cautiously in patients with renal or hepatic dysfunction, cardiac failure, angina pectoris, and Wolff-Parkinson-White syndrome, and during anesthesia or surgery. In general, β-blockers should not be discontinued abruptly but decreased gradually, since rapid tapering might exacerbate catechola-mine-mediated actions (110). The author now prefers to use a cardioselective, long-acting agent in the treatment of thyro-toxicosis. β-Blockers other than propranolol have not been studied as extensively in the treatment of hyperthyroidism, but they appear to be equally effective in the treatment of thyrotoxicosis (for comparable effect of β-blockade).

Other Agents.   In an unusual or particularly resistant case of hyperthyroidism, one can employ lithium or iodine (14, 29, 81, 130). Both of these agents decrease thyroidal secretion. Lithium may also inhibit adenyl cyclase generation in the thyroid and decrease extrathyroidal conversion of T_4 to T_3. Serum lithium concentrations of 0.5 to 1.3 mEq/liter appear optimal; if higher levels are achieved, adverse reactions such as renal and CNS effects (e.g., tremor, drowsiness, blurred vision, and tinnitus) may occur (4).

Iodides decrease thyroid hormone synthesis by inhibiting directly the organization of iodide in the thyroid gland (14). This effect occurs rapidly, so that a 30 to 50% decrease in serum T_4 may be observed after only 5 to 10 days of treatment in a thyrotoxic subject. In a study by Wartofsky et al (150), after a control period, hyperthyroid patients were administered Lugol's solution five drops three times a day for 6 to 7 days; the mean serum T_4 concentration decreased by about 20 to 50%. Boehm and associates (14) performed a similar study using the same dose of Lugol's solution; the mean serum T_4 decreased in four thyrotoxic subjects from 26 μg/dl during the control period to 14 μg/dl after about 5 days of Lugol's solution. Unfortunately, in some patients this effect of iodides upon inhibition of T_4 secretion may be overcome gradually by the thyroid gland, resulting in subsequent increased thyroidal synthesis and release (135). This untoward effect may be ex-tremely difficult to control and represents the rationale for most clinicians' recommendation that iodides should not be utilized alone or in the routine management of thyrotoxic subjects. Iodides should not be administered to individuals with a known allergy; other adverse effects may include paroti-tis and skin rash. Some physicians prefer to administer iodides in the 7- to 10-day period prior to surgery; this short-term use should not worsen the course of thyrotoxicosis and would likely lower the serum T_4 level. The author does not generally prefer this approach, especially in an unreliable subject, be-cause of the possibility that the patient might not return in 10 days but would still continue taking iodide, a circumstance that might lead to unabated thyroidal secretion. It would be much more desirable to produce euthyroidism by agents that block thyroid gland synthesis (e.g., PTU or methimazole). Iodides have also been used for 1 to 2 weeks after radioactive iodine administration, usually starting on days 3 to 5. This regimen may allow the radioactive iodine to be trapped within the thyroid gland but not released, resulting in more effective thyroidal destruction. Further, the unlabelled iodine will in-duce rapid euthyroidism, and it is expected, but not proved, that iodine-induced hyperthyroidism would be infrequent be-cause of the concomitant effect of cellular destruction induced by the radioactive iodine. In the author's opinion, this treat-ment plan is rational but largely empiric and should be re-served for special circumstances. Radiocontrast agents (e.g., ipodate) have not been studied extensively in the treatment

of thyrotoxicosis but may be useful antithyroid agents as well (20, 52, 79, 124, 125, 141, 142).

Lithium carbonate is an effective second-line agent for the treatment of thyrotoxicosis. Although lithium has not been studied extensively in this role, its major use appears to be limited to the short-term treatment of thyrotoxic subjects who may be allergic to PTU and/or methimazole. However, in one study, Boehm et al (14) administered lithium carbonate in a total daily dose of 300 to 3000 mg (average 2100 mg daily) to maintain a total therapeutic serum lithium level in the therapeutic range of 1.0 to 1.5 mEq/liter (blood samples for lithium determination were drawn 1 hour after the early morn-ing dose). After only about 5 days of lithium carbonate therapy, the mean serum T_4 in four thyrotoxic patients decreased from 22 μg/dl to 13 μg/dl. In this study lithium carbonate appeared to act by decreasing thyroidal secretion and also may have decreased T_4 disappearance. Kristensen et al (81) observed comparable results, as the mean percentage fall in T_4 was 24% after 10 days of lithium carbonate administration to thyrotoxic subjects. All workers also observed a high frequency of adverse reactions to lithium carbonate and strongly urge that the serum lithium level be maintained between 0.5 and 1.3 mEq/liter. Further studies investigating the use of lithium carbonate in the treatment of thyrotoxicosis are warranted, but at present its use is limited to certain specific short-term settings; careful attention to serum levels and potential adverse effects is neces-sary. On rare occasions long-term lithium use may be associ-ated with the development of thyrotoxicosis (90).

Hyperthyroidism in a Critically Ill Subject.   Hyperthy-roidism, of course, can occur in critically ill subjects, and some of the usual history and physical findings are similar to those noted in an ambulatory patient (7, 27, 44, 45, 89). How-ever, because of the age of the patient as well as the accompa-nying systemic illness, hyperthyroidism can be extremely diffi-cult to recognize in an intensive care unit setting. So-called apathetic hyperthyroidism may occur, a situation in which the customary findings of heightened anxiety and nervousness and stare may be subtle or lacking (131). In addition, tachycar-dia as a discriminating parameter is less helpful than in an ambulatory patient, since there are so many other reasons for the presence of an elevated heart rate in a systemically ill patient. The condition of hepatic coma may be difficult to differentiate from thyrotoxicosis or thyroid storm because many of the physical findings (e.g., hand tremor or disorienta-tion) may be similar. In the intensive care setting greater reliance must be placed upon interpretation of the thyroid function tests and the examination of the thyroid gland.

A radioactive iodide uptake test, assessing thyroid gland activity, is a useful test in discriminating hyperthyroidism from euthyroidism in a critically ill patient. Also, administration of 200 to 500 μg of TRH (Fig. 44.3) is an excellent indicator of thyrotoxicosis, since a metabolically hyperthyroid subject essentially always demonstrates no rise (compared with base-line) in the serum TSH level when measured at 0, 15, and 30 minutes after TRH injection, whereas a euthyroid individ-ual has an increase in serum TSH from less than 5 μU/ml basally to about 10 to 25 μU/ml after TRH. The finding of an undetectable TSH concentration basally that remains undetectable after TRH injection is highly suggestive of thyro-toxicosis, especially in the presence of physical findings (e.g., enlarged thyroid gland) and historic findings compatible with overproduction of thyroid hormones. In the author's view, a "blunted" TSH response to TRH injection (e.g., TSH increases from less than 2.5 to 6 μU/ml) does not necessarily indicate the presence of thyrotoxicosis, assuming that sensitive TSH assay is used. Also, occasionally, a patient who has had hyperthyroidism in the recent past (1 to 3 months) but who is clinically and metabolically euthyroid when studied may demonstrate no TSH response to TRH. Recently, third-generation TSH assays have been developed that can discriminate even subnormal TSH values from undetectable ones. These assays generally have a normal range of approximately 0.5 to 4.0 μU/ml, with a lower limit of detectability of about 0.05 μU/ml. These assays have been found to be reliable and useful and largely have supplanted the use of less sensitive methods. With these third-generation assays a TRH stimulation test rarely needs to be performed, as an undetectable TSH level implies the presence of biochemical hyperthyroidism (or rarely, pituitary or hypothalamic deficiency).

It appears that several alterations in thyroid function tests can occur in thyrotoxic systemically ill patients, but these perturbations *per se* should not obscure the diagnosis of thyrotoxicosis. The serum FT_4 level by dialysis or kit method and the serum T_4 usually are increased in a thyrotoxic critically ill patient, although the total T_4 may be less increased (as a result of altered binding proteins) than if the patient were healthier. On occasion, the total T_4 may be in the upper part of the normal range in a thyrotoxic critically ill patient. The resin T_3 uptake is expected to be high in most critically ill patients whether or not they are hyperthyroid; the serum T_3 may not be increased, since critical illness may decrease extrathyroidal conversion of T_4 to T_3. In sum, a hyperthyroid critically ill patient should have appropriate physical findings (e.g., enlarged thyroid gland), elevated RAIU and/or an undetectable TSH level in a third-generation assay, and an elevated or high normal T_4 and free T_4. The treatment of a thyrotoxic critically ill patient who is not in impending thyroid storm should probably proceed as described above. The pharmacologic parameters for essentially all drugs or agents mentioned in this chapter have not been studied in critically ill subjects. At present, we can only assume that the doses, half-lives, and mechanisms of action are comparable in ambulatory and critically ill patients. Furthermore, the issue of definitive (surgery or radioactive iodine) therapy may be addressed after the patient has become euthyroid with antithyroid medications (58).

THYROID STORM

A patient with thyroid storm displays an exaggeration of the customary findings of thyrotoxicosis and, in addition, exhibits temperature increase, diarrhea, and central nervous system symptoms (e.g., disorientation) (56). Because of the potentially lethal nature of this disorder, thyroid storm should be anticipated, since it generally can be avoided by the early and appropriate diagnosis and treatment of thyrotoxicosis. Frequently, thyroid storm is precipitated by a major stressful event such as surgery or anesthesia. The treatment of thyroid storm depends primarily upon its early diagnosis and is directed at the systemic signs or symptoms (e.g., a cooling

Table 44.5. Pharmacology of Agents Used to Treat Hypothyroidism[a]

Medication	Maintenance Dose	Common or Serious Adverse Effects
L-thyroxine	0.075–0.200 mg daily (75–200 μg)	Precipitation or aggravation of cardiac disease, arrhythmias, angina pectoris; may aggravate diabetes mellitus and adrenal insufficiency
T-triiodothyronine	25 μg t.i.d. or q.i.d.	As above

[a]These guidelines apply to the routine ambulatory patient with hypothyroidism; the text should be consulted for the treatment of myxedema coma.

blanket and acetaminophen for hyperthermia) and at the thyroid hormone excess. PTU (800 to 1200 mg daily in four to six divided doses) or methimazole (80 to 100 mg daily in four to six divided doses) is the mainstay of therapy, even though their maximal effects may not be achieved for 7 to 14 days. Propranolol is given orally (120 to 400 mg daily in four to six divided doses) but alternatively might be administered intravenously (1 to 2 mg given slowly with careful monitoring of cardiovascular function). The author also administers sodium iodide intravenously (1 g in 1 liter); 2 to 3 liters may be given over a 24-hour period, although oral iodide (8 drops every 6 hours of potassium iodide (SSKI) daily) may be given instead. It seems increasingly difficult to obtain sodium iodide as a sterile preparation. Adequate fluids (3 to 4 liters daily) are administered and there should be careful monitoring for cardiac or renal decompensation. Most clinicians also give glucocorticoids (hydrocortisone 200 mg every 8 hours), partly because they decrease conversion of T_4 to T_3 and partly because of the theoretic possibility of the precipitation of adrenal insufficiency by the hypermetabolic state. Indeed, the coexistence of Graves' disease and other autoimmune endocrine disease (e.g., Type I diabetes mellitus, Addison's disease) is thought to occur relatively frequently. On rare occasions, thyroid storm has been treated effectively with charcoal plasma perfusion (28), although in the author's opinion further studies of such techniques must be performed before this technique should be considered in this condition. The best treatment of thyroid storm, however, lies in realizing the circumstances that predispose to it and adequately treating thyrotoxic subjects prior to their having medical or surgical interventions.

HYPOTHYROIDISM

As previously mentioned, the prescribing physician should, once again, be familiar with mechanisms and adverse effects of agents used in treating hypothyroidism (Table 44.5).

PATHOPHYSIOLOGY

Hypothyroidism is a disease of inadequate levels of T_4 and/or T_3 characterized by malaise, intolerance to cold, dyspnea, bradycardia, constipation, weakness, dry skin, central nervous system findings, and, occasionally, pleural, pericardial, or peritoneal effusions (26, 147, 154). Hypothyroidism can be either primary (that is, as a consequence of thyroid gland failure) or secondary (as a result of hypothalamic-pituitary gland failure). In all patients with hypothyroidism, pituitary disease must be excluded. Generally, the finding of an increased serum TSH concentration is adequate for this purpose, but if the patients have either other significant signs or symptoms related to the cranial area (e.g., headache or impairment of the visual field) or lack of normal secretion of other pituitary hormones, further appropriate laboratory and radiologic studies should be performed to rule out a pituitary or cranial tumor. The most common causes of primary hypothyroidism are either chronic thyroiditis or idiopathic disease. About 10 to 15% of patients with primary hypothyroidism have disease caused by antibodies against the TSH receptor (80). Recent studies indicate that hypothyroidism occasionally may result from TSH receptor blocking antibodies and that these antibodies may change their character over time, even resulting in remission of the previous hypothyroidism (126). Until further investigation is performed to analyze this phenomenon, the author prefers to continue L-thyroxine therapy indefinitely for all patients diagnosed with primary hypothyroidism. The routine ambulatory patient with primary hypothyroidism should have a complete evaluation, including a thorough physical examination and measurement of serum T_4, RT_3U, and TSH levels; RAIU; or thyroid scan and thyroid antibodies. A hemogram and screening chemical profile are also of value. The overall prevalence of overt hypothyroidism is about 1% in females and somewhat less in males. Nevertheless, among elderly patients perhaps 5% of females and 2% of males have serum TSH values between 5 and 10 μU/ml and 2.5% of females and 1.9% of men have TSH values > 10 μU/ml (7, 84). In the elderly, many of the symptoms of hypothyroidism may be absent and the clinician must rely increasingly on thyroid function tests. One should initiate therapy gradually using L-thyroxine, starting with oral daily doses of 0.0125 to 0.050 mg and gradually increasing to maintenance doses of about 0.10 to 0.15 mg daily (Table 44.5) (26, 65, 147). The average L-thyroxine replacement dose is about 1.7 μg/kg body weight. Clinical findings and serum T_4 and TSH levels are monitored to assess adequacy of treatment. The serum TSH may require as long as several months to normalize but may start to decrease within several days of initiation of therapy. Although TSH and T_4 values probably are the most sensitive laboratory indicators of adequacy of therapy, clinical findings such as heart rate and nervousness and personal history relative to such factors as anxiety or palpitations also represent important parameters to assess whether the therapeutic dose is optimal. The doses recommended are adequate for adults; however, specific texts should be consulted for the treatment of hypothyroid children.

MYXEDEMA COMA

Myxedema coma is a condition that represents an exaggeration of the usual symptoms and signs of hypothyroidism. A patient with myxedema coma may also have the following characteristics: coma or stupor, hypothermia, hypoventilation, hypotension, hypothermia, hyponatremia, or hypoglycemia (8, 26, 154, 161, 162). This condition should be suspected especially in patients with a known history of thyroid abnormalities (regardless of type), a family history of thyroid problems, a surgical scar in the lower anterior neck, or proptosis (suggesting a history of Graves' disease, which frequently evolves into hypothyroidism), or in a patient who appears to be unusually sensitive to medications or narcotics.

The treatment of myxedema coma involves thyroid replacement, alleviation of any possible precipitating cause, and amelioration of hypotension, hypothermia, hypercapnia, or hypoxia (25, 147). The possibility of a pericardial effusion must be borne in mind and excluded appropriately. Because definitive laboratory diagnosis may require several days, and because these patients are extremely ill, in an appropriate setting, therapy should be instituted immediately based upon clinical, historic, and available laboratory data, even though definitive thyroid tests may have been drawn but have not yet returned from the laboratory.

Alleviation of the hypotension should be performed with any conventional regimen, and adrenal steroids probably should be given because of the potential coexistence of adrenal insufficiency and because, theoretically, initiation of thyroid hormone treatment may increase the clearance of endogenous steroids. Definitive testing for the presence of adrenal insufficiency can be performed at a later date. In many patients, hyponatremia is observed and may be secondary to inappropriate secretion of antidiuretic hormone; this hyponatremia is treated optimally by water restriction. Hypoxia frequently is noted and is treated by conventional means. The treatment of hypothermia is more controversial; some have suggested that warming the patient is unnecessary and potentially dangerous, since it may shunt blood to the smaller vessels in the skin.

Thyroid hormone replacement regimens in a patient with myxedema coma are different from those in a routine ambulatory hypothyroid patient. Although some thyroidologists may approach such a patient differently, the author usually begins therapy with 50 to 75 μg L-thyroxine daily orally or intravenously (26). This medicine can be given orally or crushed and placed into a nasogastric tube. The serum half-life of L-thyroxine in a euthyroid subject is 7 days, and preliminary studies suggest an absorption rate of about 50 to 75% in systemically ill individuals, although this rate may be decreased with specific gastrointestinal diseases. Parenteral L-thyroxine preparation can be administered intravenously in a critically ill patient (50 to 75 μg L-thyroxine daily). Clinical findings and serum T_4 and TSH levels should be followed to assess the adequacy of treatment. As noted earlier, however, a systemically ill patient may have decreased binding of thyroid hormones to serum proteins and the serum T_4 may even be below the usual normal range, yet the dose employed still may represent adequate therapy. Therefore, it becomes a complicated matter to assess the adequacy of therapy in systemically ill subjects. Since serum T_4 level may be misleading, and because serum TSH values may be a better indicator but may require several days or weeks to return to normal, the only practical solution is to pick a dose of L-thyroxine that is reasonable and to continue this dose (which is enough to treat myxedema coma but not sufficient to cause hypermetabolism) until definitive testing can be achieved. This time, of course, may occur only when the patient has improved significantly and is out of the intensive care unit.

Some clinicians prefer to treat myxedema coma with T_3 (12.5 to 25 μg every 6 to 8 hours), which has a serum half-life of 24 to 30 hours in a euthyroid subject. It should also be noted that some clinicians give 300 to 500 μg L-thyroxine intravenously initially followed by 50 to 100 μg intravenously daily (67). The author does not prefer these approaches and believes that they may be dangerous in some patients, theoretically helping to induce cardiac arrhythmias. Hylander and Rosenquist (68) recently conducted a retrospective study of patients with myxedema coma. Patients who died were older (78.9 yrs vs 66.8 yrs) and had initial heart rates that were lower (43 vs 50 beats/min). Although only 11 patients were studied (7 died, 4 survived), it seemed that the surviving patients had a lower serum T_3 level during treatment compared with those in the nonsurviving patients (1.7 ± 0.6 nmol/liter vs 3.3 ± 0.4 nmol/liter). Many contributing factors led to death, but circulatory failure was frequent. Although larger studies need to be performed, this preliminary study supports using low-dose T_4 treatment for myxedema coma.

Regardless of the treatment plan employed, the physician should be familiar with the usage and possible complications of thyroid medications and should be current in his or her understanding of the interpretation of thyroid function tests in systemically ill patients. Further, as a general rule, administration of thyroid medications to a patient with cardiac disease (either ambulatory or in myxedema coma) should be instituted gradually and with careful attention to monitoring for the possibility of arrhythmias and increasing angina. Only in life-threatening emergencies should initial vigorous thyroid hormone replacement be given to a hypothyroid patient with cardiac disease. Lastly, clearances and, thus, half-lives of other medications may change as the hypothyroid patient becomes euthyroid.

INTERPRETATION OF THYROID FUNCTION TESTS IN EUTHYROID CRITICALLY ILL SUBJECTS: "EUTHYROID SICK SYNDROME"

Interpretation of thyroid function tests in a critically ill patient is complex (Tables 44.6–44.9) (4, 8, 10, 13, 53–55, 148, 159). The important question the clinician wants answered is, Which patients are hypothyroid and require treatment, and which patients are euthyroid? However, these decisions are extremely difficult, largely because normal ranges for thyroid function tests obtained in ambulatory patients generally are not applicable to the critically ill patient, and because at present there are no sensitive tissue markers to help determine whether there is adequate thyroid hormone at a tissue level. A full discussion of the "euthyroid sick syndrome" is beyond the scope of this chapter, and the interested reader is referred to several reviews (148, 154). However, summarized in Tables 44.6 through 44.9 are the commonly observed changes in thyroid function tests associated with various systemic illnesses or with several drugs known to affect thyroid function tests (148). In addition to those noted, hyperemesis gravidarum may elevate free T_4 and decrease TSH response to TRH (13), and carbamazepine has also been associated with lowered total and free T_4 and T_3 (1). Although the cause(s) of the "euthyroid sick syndrome" is unknown, it has been suggested that tumor necrosis factor-α plays an important role in the pathophysiology of this condition (30, 138).

Special emphasis should be given in the intensive care unit patient to the relationship of dopamine to thyroid hormone levels. Endogenous dopamine decreases TSH secretion physiologically. In the intensive care setting, the constant intravenous administration of dopamine (6.5 ± 0.4 μg/kg/min) for 48 hours decreased serum TSH to 0.9 ± 0.04 μU/ml, compared with 2.3 ± 0.4 μU/ml in non-dopamine-treated subjects (78, 115). Total and free T_4 indexes were not altered significantly, although both parameters were decreased markedly compared with those of normal subjects. It also appears

Table 44.6. Effect of Miscellaneous Conditions on Thyroid Hormone Parameters[a]

	TOTAL T_4	FREE T_4	TOTAL T_3	FREE T_3	REVERSE T_3	BASAL TSH	TSH RESPONSE to TRH
PRIMARY DEPRESSION	↑, N.C.	↑, N.C.	N.C.	N.C.	↑	N.C.	↓
INFECTION	↓	↑	↓	N.C.	↑	N.C., ↓	N.C.
MALIGNANCY	N.C.	↑, N.C.	↓	N.S.	↑	N.C.	N.S.
THERMAL INJURY	↓	↓	⬇	↓, N.C.	⬆	N.C.	N.C., ↑
CRITICAL ILLNESS	⬇	N.C. *	⬇	⬇*	⬆	N.C.	N.S.

[a] Adapted with permission from Wartofsky L, Burman KD: Alterations in thyroid function in patients with systemic illness: "The euthyroid sick syndrome." *Endscrinol Rev* 3:164–217, 1982. N.C., no change; N.S., not adequately studied. Arrows indicate direction of alterations compared with values observed in euthyroid individuals. A broad arrow indicates a marked change, and a narrow arrow, a change. Symbols for a given parameter are listed in decreasing frequency of likelihod of occurrence. Free T_4 and free T_3 indicate dialysis measurements or calculated indices. Notations indicated were derived by extrapolation of data from what the authors believe to be the majority of reports.

Table 44.7. Conditions Associated with Commonly Observed Changes in Thyroid Function Tests[a]

	TOTAL T$_4$	FREE T$_4$	TOTAL T$_3$	FREE T$_3$	REVERSE T$_3$	BASAL TSH	TSH RESPONSE to TRH
FASTING	N.C.	N.C., ↑	⇓	⇓	⇑	↓	↓
ANOREXIA NERVOSA	↓	Probably N.C.	⇓	N.S.	↑	N.C.	Late Peak
PROTEIN-CALORIE MALNUTRITION	↓	N.C.	⇓	↓	⇑	N.C., ↑	Exaggerated Delayed
OBESITY	N.C.	N.C.	N.C., ↑	N.C.	N.C.	N.C.	N.C.
DIABETES MELLITUS, CONTROLLED	N.C.	N.C.	N.C., ↑	N.S.	N.C., ↑	N.C.	N.C.
DIABETES MELLITUS, KETOACIDOSIS	↓	N.C., ↑	⇓	N.S.	⇑	N.C.	Blunted

[a] Adapted with permission from Wartofsky L, Burman KD: Alterations in thyroid function in patients with systemic illness: "The euthyroid sick syndrome." *Endscrinol Rev* 3:164–217, 1982. N.C., no change; N.S., not adequately studied. Arrows indicate direction of alterations compared with values observed in euthyroid individuals. A broad arrow indicates a marked change, and a narrow arrow, a change. Symbols for a given parameter are listed in decreasing frequency of likelihod of occurrence. Free T$_4$ and free T$_3$ indicate dialysis measurements or calculated indices. Notations indicated were derived by extrapolation of data from what the authors believe to be the majority of reports.

Table 44.8. Drugs Known to Affect Thyroid Function Tests[a]

	TOTAL T$_4$	FREE T$_4$	TOTAL T$_3$	FREE T$_3$	REVERSE T$_3$	BASAL TSH	TSH RESPONSE to TRH
DOPAMINE	↓	↓	↓	↓	N.C.	↓	↓
GLUCOCORTICOIDS	↓	N.C.	⇓	N.S.	⇑	↓	↓
RADIO-OPAQUE DYES	N.C., ↑	N.C.	⇓	↓	⇑	N.C., ↑	↑ , N.C.
PROPRANOLOL	N.C.	N.C.	↓	N.S.	↑	N.C.	N.C.
AMIODARONE	↑	↑	⇓	↓	⇑	↑	↑

[a] Adapted with permission from Wartofsky L, Burman KD: Alterations in thyroid function in patients with systemic illness: "The euthyroid sick syndrome." *Endscrinol Rev* 3:164–217, 1982. N.C., no change; N.S., not adequately studied. Arrows indicate direction of alterations compared with values observed in euthyroid individuals. A broad arrow indicates a marked change, and a narrow arrow, a change. Symbols for a given parameter are listed in decreasing frequency of likelihod of occurrence. Free T$_4$ and free T$_3$ indicate dialysis measurements or calculated indices. Notations indicated were derived by extrapolation of data from what the authors believe to be the majority of reports.

that dopamine infusion could even suppress basal serum TSH levels and the TSH response to TRH to within the normal ranges in hypothyroid subjects, thus obscuring the diagnosis of primary hypothyroidism.

In addition to the effect of dopamine in a "typical euthyroid" critically ill subject, there are profound alterations in serum thyroid function tests. Serum T$_4$ levels are decreased, probably secondary to alterations in binding to serum proteins, and serum T$_3$ by RIA is low because of decreased extrathyroidal conversion of T$_4$ to T$_3$ (35). The alteration in binding of iodothyronine to binding proteins may be related to increased levels of free fatty acids. Serum levels determined by equilibrium dialysis are either normal or even increased, whereas free T$_4$ calculation estimates generally are decreased. Commercial kits are now available that are capable of measuring free T$_4$ directly; investigations have demonstrated that some of these kits may be capable of differentiating hypothyroid from euthyroid critically ill subjects (34, 78, 94). However, more studies in this area must be performed, and it appears that some commercial kits are more effective discriminators than others. The question also remains as to the extent to which free T$_4$ and T$_3$ in the serum of critically ill subjects is available for uptake into tissues (113). Although there may be alterations in the regulation of TSH secretion even in

Table 44.9. Factors or Conditions That Affect Thyroid-stimulating Hormone Levels[a]

Decrease
Dopamine agonists
Corticosteroids
Diphenylhydantoin
Low caloric intake (<500 cal/day)
Somatostatin
Opioids
Serotonin antagonists
Increase
Hypothermic cardiovascular surgery
Recovery from systemic illness
Dopamine antagonists
Iodide
Lithium
Cimetidine
Theophylline
Amphetamines

[a] Artifactual elevation resulting from the presence of heterophilic antibodies to rabbit or mouse immunoglobulins may also have an effect on TSH levels.

Table 44.10. Symptoms That Distinguish Patients with Primary Hypothyroidism from Those Who Are Euthyroid or Hypothyroid[a]

Symptom	Primary Hypothyroidism	Euthyroid Critically Ill	Hypothyroid Critically Ill
Intolerance to cold	+	+	+
Dry skin	+	+	+
Edema	+	+	+
Malaise	+	+	+
Pallor	+	+	+
Anemia	+	+	+
Constipation	+	+	+
Mental slowing	+	+	+
Enlarged thyroid gland	+	−	+/−
Serum T$_4$	Low	Normal/Low	Low
Serum TSH	Elevated	Normal	Elevated
Serum reverse T$_3$	Low	Normal/Elevated	Low
Free T$_4$ (dialysis)	Low	Normal/High	Low
Free T$_3$ (dialysis)	Low	Normal/Low	Low

[a] From Burman KD: *Thyroid: University Case Reports,* vol 3. Parke-Davis, Morris Plains, NJ, 1981.

euthyroid critically ill subjects, the basal serum TSH concentration still appears to be the best laboratory aid in discriminating hypothyroidism from euthyroidism. In the author's view, serum TSH values >10 μU/ml are evidence of biochemical hypothyroidism, whereas basal TSH concentrations <5 μU/ml indicate that the patient is euthyroid. In the author's opinion, values between 5 and 10 μU/ml are in a borderline zone and in a critically ill transient subject may reflect only mild tissue hypothyroidism or simply physiologic alterations. Caloric deprivation, dopamine, and systemic illness itself can lower TSH in hypothyroid subjects (5, 15, 23, 151) (Table 44.10). Recovery from systemic illness transiently could increase TSH to as high as about 15 to 20 μU/ml even in euthyroid subjects (60). The use of third-generation TSH assays largely have supplanted the necessity of performing a TRH stimulation test. However, if such a test still needs to be performed, it may be helpful (Fig. 44.3) (121) in that a patient with an increased basal TSH level would probably hyperrespond (i.e., have TSH levels greater than about 30 μU/ml). Practically,

if a basal serum TSH is >10 μU/ml, a TRH test probably need not be performed in a routine case; if the TSH is between 5 and 10 μU/ml, a TRH test may be useful. A serum free T$_4$ by dialysis that is low may also be helpful in indicating hypothyroidism, since in most euthyroid critically ill patients the FT$_4$ level is either normal or high; lastly, a serum rT$_3$ that is low suggests hypothyroidism, since most euthyroid critically ill patients have a normal or increaed rT$_3$. Thus, in the author's view, only three thyroid function tests are primarily capable of helping to discriminate the hypothyroid from the euthyroid critically ill subject: the serum TSH, free T$_4$ by dialysis (or specific kit method), and the rT$_3$ level. If the serum TSH level is >10 μU/ml, the serum FT$_4$ is low, the rT$_3$ level is low, and there is a compatible clinical picture, then the author would start treatment with exogenous L-thyroxine in a dosage plan detailed herein, which depends on the clinical severity of the patient's illness. If only one or two of these tests are consistent with hypothyroidism, in a proper clinical setting, judicious and gradual therapy with L-thyroxine might be instituted if, in the physician's view, the likelihood of hypothyroidism is great and the circumstances urgent. In the great majority of cases, a serum TSH value can be obtained within 1 or 2 days, and if the TSH is less than 5 μU/ml replacement therapy usually is not indicated (assuming that secondary hypothyroidism is not a consideration). If, however, this value is >10 μU/ml, most clinicians would institute L-thyroxine therapy as detailed herein, even if the FT$_4$ and rT$_3$ values had not returned. TSH regulation may be altered in critically ill subjects (88). The author's comments regarding TSH depend on the use of a newer, highly sensitive TSH assay that has a normal range of about 0.5 to 4.0 μU/ml.

It does appear that mortality is higher in "euthyroid" critically ill subjects with a decreased serum T$_4$. Indeed, mortality rates of about 70 to 80% have been found in those patients with a serum T$_4$ less than 3 μg/dl. The question of whether T$_3$ or T$_4$ treatment might benefit these patients remains largely unanswered. However, oral T$_3$ given to extensively burned patients did not reduce mortality (8). Further, Brent and Hershman (18) published a randomized prospective study in which critically ill patients with serum T$_4$ levels less than 5 μg/dl were assigned either to a control group or to a treatment group that received 1.5 μg/kg of L-thyroxine intravenously daily for 2 weeks. Even though the free T$_4$ index increased in the treatment group, the free T$_3$ index was comparable in the control and treatment group, as was mortality.

Thyroid function test "abnormalities" that have been observed to occur in euthyroid critically ill patients may also occur in all hospitalized patients as well as in most ambulatory patients who have systemic illnesses. Further, although the generally observed alterations in thyroid function tests in systemically ill subjects have just been outlined, there are exceptions based upon the specific illness a patient may have or agents he or she may be receiving (Tables 44.6–44.9). The reader is referred to appropriate reviews for specific details of specific diseases (148, 154). Thyroid function tests in patients with HIV infection, however, deserve special attention, since the associated alterations seem unique. Serum total T$_4$ levels remained normal or even increased in patients with various stages of HIV infection managed as outpatients, but when those patients were admitted to the ICU, both survivors and nonsurvivors had lower serum total T_4 levels than normal (51, 85). Serum total T_3 usually was normal until hospitalization, when concentrations decreased significantly in nonsurvivors. Survivors had decreased values compared with normal, but these concentrations were higher than those of nonsurvivors. Reverse T_3 concentrations generally decreased and TBG increased with increasing stage of disease. Thus, in sum, it seems that HIV patients in the ICU have minimal changes compared with those of other patients. LoPresti et al speculate that the relatively minimal decrease in total T_3 (except in very ill patients) may contribute to the weight loss seen in these patients (85). Feldt-Rasmussen et al (51) generally confirmed these findings, although the total T_4 levels were not increased despite the increases in TBG. Further studies are needed to identify these changes in a large number of patients with different stages of HIV disease.

There are also interesting studies using cardiopulmonary bypass patients as a model for the "euthyroid sick syndrome" (66). In this circumstance, T_3 may be useful in increasing cardiac output, although further clinical trials and confirmation are required prior to such usage on a clinical basis (102–104).

Finally, the author emphasizes that the question of whether a systemically ill patient is hypothyroid and therefore requires therapy arises quite frequently. However, the majority of these patients, when fully evaluated, are deemed euthyroid and do not require therapy. Indeed, the observed changes in thyroid function tests (e.g., decreased serum T_3) are thought even to be beneficial because they probably represent homeostatic alterations for conserving energy by reducing catabolic expenditure. Despite these cautions, a patient who may be truly hypothyroid should be diagnosed and treated as rapidly as possible, since undue delays may be detrimental, and treatment in these subjects should be instituted without hesitation. There are no ideal methods to help select patients who have a high likelihood of being hypothyroid, but the following findings may be helpful: a history of thyroid surgery or radioiodine therapy, enlarged thyroid gland, hypothermia, macroglossia, unexplained pleural or peritoneal effusions, and/or presence of other autoimmune endocrine hypofunction (Table 44.10).

ACKNOWLEDGMENTS

The author is grateful to Dr. Robert C. Smallridge and Dr. Leonard Wartofsky for their assistance in the preparation of this chapter. Alice Jacobson provided editorial assistance.

REFERENCES

1. Aanderud S, Myking OL, Strandjord RE: The influence of carbamazepine on thyroid hormones and thyroxine binding globulin in hypothyroid patients substituted with thyroxine. *Clin Endocrinol* 15:247–252, 1981.
2. Aksoy M, Erdem S: Aplastic anemia after propylthiouracil. *Lancet* i:1379, 1968.
3. Alexander WO, Evans V, MacAulay A, et al: Metabolism of 5S-labeled antithyroid drugs in man. *Br Med J* 2:290–291, 1969.
4. American Medical Association Council on Drugs: *Drug Evaluations*. American Medical Association, Chicago, 1980.
5. Azizi F: Effect of dietary composition of fasting-induced changes in serum thyroid hormones and thyrotropin. *Metabolism* 27: 935–942, 1978.
6. Balzer J, Lahrtz HG, van Zwieten PA: Serum level and urinary excretion of ^{14}Cthiamol in patients with hyperthyroidism. *Dtsch Med Wochenschr* 100: 548–552, 1975.
7. Bastenie PA, Bonnyns M, VanHaelst L: Natural history of primary myxedema. *Am J Med* 79:91–100, 1985.
8. Becker RA, Vaughan GM, Ziegler MG, et al: Hypermetabolic low triiodothyronine syndrome of burn injury. *Crit Care Med* 10:870–875, 1982.
9. Berglund J, Christensen SB, Dymling JF, Hallengren B: The incidence of recurrence and hypothyroidism following treatment with antithyroid drugs, surgery or radioiodine in all patients with thyrotoxicosis in Malmö during the period 1970–1974. *J Intern Med* 229:435–442, 1991.
10. Bermudez F, Surks MI, Oppenheimer JH: High incidence of decreased serum triiodothyronine concentration in patients with nonthyroidal disease. *J Clin Endocrinol Metab* 41:27–40, 1975.
11. Berry MJ, Banue L, Larsen PR: Type I iodothyronine deiodinase is a selenocysteine-containing enzyme. *Nature* 349:438–440, 1991.
12. Berry MJ, Kieffer JD, Harney JW, Larsen PR: Selenocysteine confers the biochemical properties characteristic of the type I iodothyronine deiodinase. *J Biol Chem* 266:14155–14158, 1991.
13. Bober SA, McGill AC, Tunbridge WMG: Thyroid function in hyperemesis gravidarum. *Acta Endocrinol* 111:404–410, 1986.
14. Boehm TM, Burman KD, Barnes S: Synergism of lithium and iodide in the treatment of thyrotoxicosis. *Acta Endocrinol* 94:174–183, 1980.
15. Borst GC, Eil C, Burman KD: Euthyroid hyperthyroxinemia. *Ann Intern Med* 98: 366–378, 1983.
16. Borst GC, Osburne RC, O'Brian JT, George LP, Burman KD: Fasting decreases thyrotropin responsiveness to thyrotropin-releasing hormone: a potential cause of misinterpretation of thyroid function tests in the critically ill. *J Clin Endocrinol Metab* 57:380–383, 1983.
17. Branch RA, Jaes J, Read AE: A study of factors influencing drug disposition in chronic liver disease, using the model drug propranolol. *Br J Clin Pharmacol* 2:243–249, 1976.
18. Brent GA, Hershman JM: Thyroxine therapy in patients with severe nonthyroidal illnesses and low serum thyroxine concentration. *J Clin Endocrinol Metab* 63:1–8, 1986.
19. Brown J, Chopra IJ, Cornell JS, et al: Thyroid physiology in health and disease. *Ann Intern Med* 81:68–81, 1974.
20. Burgi H, Wimpfheimer C, Burger A, et al: Changes of circulating thyroxine, triiodothyronine and reverse triiodothyronine after radiographic contrast agent. *J Clin Endocrinol Metab* 43:1203–1210, 1976.
21. Burman KD: Recent developments in thyroid hormone metabolism: interpretation and significance of measurements of reverse 3,3',5'-triiodothyronine, 3,3'-diiodothyronine, and thyroglobulin. *Metabolism* 27:615–630, 1978.
22. Burman KD, Dimond RC, Harvey GS, et al: Glucose modulation of alterations in serum iodothyronine concentrations induced by fasting. *Metabolism* 28:291–299, 1979.
23. Burman KD, Smallridge RC, Osburne R, et al: Nature of suppressed TSH secretion during undernutrition: effect of fasting and refeeding on TSH responses to prolonged TRH infusion. *Metabolism* 29:46–52, 1980.
24. Burman KD: Interpretation of thyroid function tests in critically ill patients. In Wilber JF (ed): *Thyroid: University Case Reports*, vol 3. Parke-Davis, Morris Plains, NJ, 1981.
25. Burman KD, Baker JR Jr: Immune mechanisms in Graves' disease. *Endocrinol Rev* 6:183, 1985.
26. Burman KD: Hypothyroidism. In Conn HF (ed): *Current Therapy*. WB Saunders, Philadelphia, 1986, p 521.
27. Burrow GN: The management of thyrotoxicosis in pregnancy. *N Engl J Med* 313:562–565, 1985.
28. Candrina R, Di Stefano O, Spandrio S, Giustina G: Treatment of thyrotoxic storm by charcoal plasmaperfusion [Letter to the Editor]. *J Endocrinol Invest* 12:133–134, 1989.
29. Carlson HE, Temple R, Robbins J: Effect of lithium on thyroxine disappearance in man. *J Clin Endocrinol Metab* 36:1251–1254, 1973.
30. Chopra IJ, Sakane S, Choateco GN: Study of the serum concentration of tumor necrosis factor-α in thyroidal and nonthyroidal illnesses. *J Clin Endocrinol Metab* 72:1113–1116, 1991.
31. Chopra IJ, Solomon DH, Chopra U, et al: Pathways of metabolism of thyroid hormones. *Recent Prog Horm Res* 34:521–567, 1978.
32. Chopra IJ, Solomon DH, Chua-Teco GN, et al: An inhibitor of the binding of thyroid hormones to serum proteins is present in extrathyroidal tissues. *Science* 215:407–409, 1982.
33. Chopra IJ, Solomon DH, Hepner GS, et al: Misleadingly low free thyroxine index and usefulness of reverse triiodothyronine measurement in nonthyroidal illnesses. *Ann Intern Med* 90:905–912, 1979.
34. Chopra IJ, Van Herle AJ, Chua-Teco GN, et al: Serum free thyroxine in thyroidal and nonthyroidal illnesses: comparison of measurements by radioimmunoassay, equilibrium dialysis, and free thyroxine index. *J Clin Endocrinol Metab* 51:135–143, 1980.
35. Chopra IJ, Huang T-S, Solomon DH, Chaudhuri G, Chua-Teco GN: The role of thyroxine (T_4)-binding serum proteins in oleic acid-induced increase in free T_4 in nonthyroidal illness. *J Clin Endocrinol Metab* 63:776–779, 1986.
36. Cooper DS: Antithyroid drugs. *N Engl J Med* 311:1353–1362, 1984.
37. Cooper DS, Halpen R, Wood L, Levin AA, Ridgway EC: L-thyroxine therapy in subclinical hypothyroidism: a double-blind placebo-controlled trial. *Ann Intern Med* 101:18–24, 1984.
38. Cooper DS, Bode HH, Nath B, Saxe V, Maloof F, Ridgway EC: Methimazole pharmacology in man: studies using a newly developed radioimmunoassay for methimazole. *J Clin Endocrinol Metab* 58:473, 1984.
39. Cooper DS, Saxe VC, Maloff F, et al: Studies of propylthiouracil using a newly developed radioimmunoassay. *J Clin Endocrinol Metab* 52:204–213, 1981.
40. Cooper DS, Daniels GH, Landenson PW, et al: Hyperthyroxinemia in patients treated with high-dose propranolol. *Am J Med* 73:867–871, 1982.

41. Cooper DS, Saxe VC, Meskell M, et al: Acute effects of propylthiouracil (PTU) on thyroidal iodide organification and peripheral iodothyronine deiodination: correlation with serum PTU levels measured by radioimmunoassay. *J Clin Endocrinol Metab* 54:101–107, 1982.

42. Cooper DS, Goldminz D, Levin AA, et al: Agranulocytosis associated with antithyroid drugs: effects of patient age and drug dose. *Ann Intern Med* 98:26–29, 1983.

43. Cugini CD Jr, Leidy JW Jr, Chertow BS, Berard J, Bradley WEC, Menke JB, Hao E-H, Usala SJ: An arginine to histidine mutation in codon 315 of the c-erb A beta thyroid hormone receptor in a kindred with generalized resistance to thyroid hormones results in a receptor with significant 3,5,3'-triiodothyronine binding activity. *J Clin Endocrinol Metab* 74:1164–1170, 1992.

44. Davis PJ, Davis FB: Hyperthyroidism in patients over the age of 60 years: clinical features in 85 patients. *Medicine* 53:161–181, 1974.

45. Engler D, Donaldson EB, Stockigt JR, et al: Hyperthyroidism without triiodothyronine excess: an effect of severe non-thyroidal illness. *J Clin Endocrinol Metab* 46:77–82, 1978.

46. Eriksson M, Rubenfeld S, Garber AJ, et al: Propranolol does not prevent thyroid storm. *N Engl J Med* 296:263–264, 1977.

47. Evans GH, Shand DG: Disposition of propranolol. VI. Independent variations in steady-state circulating drug concentrations and half-life. *Clin Pharmacol Ther* 14:494–500, 1973.

48. Evans RM: The steroid and thyroid hormone receptor superfamily. *Science* 240:889–895, 1988.

49. Feely J, Forrest A, Gunn A, et al: Propranolol dosage in thyrotoxicosis. *J Clin Endocrinol Metab* 51:658–661, 1980.

50. Feely J, Isles TE, Ratcliffe WA, et al: Propranolol, triiodothyronine, reverse triiodothyronine and thyroid disease. *Clin Endocrinol* 10:531–538, 1979.

51. Feldt-Rasmussen U, Sestoft L, Berg H: Thyroid function tests in patients with acquired immune deficiency syndrome and healthy HIV$_1$-positive outpatients. *Eur J Clin Invest* 21:59–63, 1991.

52. Felicetta JV, Green WL, Nelp WB: Inhibition of hepatic binding of thyroxine by cholecystographic agents. *J Clin Invest* 65:1032–1040, 1980.

53. Finucane JF, Griffiths TS: Thyroid function in non-thyroidal illness. *Int J Med Sci* 146:103–107, 1977.

54. Gardner DF, Carithers RL, Galen EA, et al: Thyroid function tests in patients with acute and resolved hepatitis B infection. *Ann Intern Med* 96:450–452, 1982.

55. Gavin LA, McMahon FA, Castle JN, et al: Alterations in serum thyroid hormones and thyroxine-binding globulin in patients with nephrosis. *J Clin Endocrinol Metab* 46:125–130, 1978.

56. Gavin LA: Thyroid crises. *MCNA* 75:179–193, 1991.

57. George CF, et al: Pharmacokinetics of dextro, laevo, and racemic propranolol in man. *Eur J Clin Pharmacol* 4:74–76, 1972.

58. Graham G, Burman KD: Radioiodine treatment of Graves' disease: an assessment of its potential risks. *Ann Intern Med* 105:901–905, 1986.

59. Gregerman RI, Davis PJ: Effects of intrinsic and extrinsic variables on thyroid hormone economy. In: Werner SC, Ingbar SH (eds): *The Thyroid: a Fundamental and Clinical Text.* Harper & Row, New York, 1978, p 223.

60. Hamblin PS, Dyer SA, Mohr VS, LeGrand BA, Lim C-F, Tuxen DV, Topliss DJ, Stockigt JR: Relationship between thyrotropin and thyroxine changes during recovery from severe hypothyroxinemia of critical illness. *J Clin Endocrinol Metab* 62:717–722, 1986.

61. Hanson JS: Propylthiouracil and hepatitis. *Arch Intern Med* 144:994–996, 1984.

62. Harrower ADB, Fyffe JA, Horn DB, et al: Thyroxine and triiodothyronine levels in hyperthyroid patients during treatment with propranolol. *Clin Endocrinol* 7:41–44, 1977.

63. Hashimoto T, Matsubara F, Nishibu M, Kawai K: Evaluation of a new chemiluminescence technique for human thyrotropin (BeriLux hTSH): diagnostic value of five immunometric assay methods. *Eur J Clin Chem Clin Biochem* 29:753–757, 1991.

64. Hashizume K, Ichikawa K, Sakurai A, Suzuki S, Takeda T, Kobayashi M, Miyamoto T, Arai M, Nagasawa T: Administration of thyroxine in treated Graves' disease: effects on the level of antibodies to thyroid-stimulating hormone receptors and on the risk of recurrence of hyperthyroidism. *N Engl J Med* 324:947–990, 1991.

65. Hennessey JV, Evaul JE, Tseng Y-C, Burman KD, Wartofsky L: L-thyroxine dosage: a reevaluation of therapy with contemporary preparations. *Ann Intern Med* 105:11–15, 1986.

66. Holland FW, Brown PS Jr, Weintraub BD, Clark RE: Cardiopulmonary bypass and thyroid function: a "euthyroid sick syndrome." *Ann Thorac Surg* 52:46–50, 1991.

67. Holvey DN, Goodner CJ, Nicoloff JT, et al: Treatment of myxedema coma with intravenous thyroxine. *Arch Intern Med* 113:89–96, 1964.

68. Hylander B, Rosenquist U: Treatment of myxoedema coma factors associated with fatal outcome. *Acta Endocrinol* 108:65, 1985.

69. Jackson GL, Flickinger FW, Wells LW: Massive overdosage of propylthiouracil. *Ann Intern Med* 91:418–419, 1979.

70. Jonckheer MH: Amiodarone and the thyroid gland: a review. *Acta Cardiol* 36:199–205, 1981.

71. Jones MK, John R, Jones GR: The effect of oxprenolol, acebutolol, and propranolol on thyroid hormones in hyperthyroid subjects. *Clin Endocrinol* 13:343–347, 1980.

72. Kampmann JP: Pharmacokinetics of propylthiouracil in man after intravenous infusion. *J Pharmacokinet Biopharm* 5:435–443, 1977.

73. Kampmann JP, Johansen K, Hansen JM, Helweg J: Propylthiouracil in human milk. Revision of a dogma. *Lancet* ii:736, 1980.

74. Kampmann JP, Skovsted L: The kinetics of propylthiouracil in hyperthyroid subjects. *Acta Pharmacol* 37:201–210, 1975.

75. Kampmann JP, Skovsted L: The pharmacokinetics of propylthiouracil. *Acta Pharmacol Toxicol* 35:361–369, 1974.

76. Kaptein EM, Grieb DA, Spencer C, et al: Thyroxine metabolism in the low thyroxine state of critical nonthyroidal illnesses. *J Clin Endocrinol Metab* 53:764–771, 1981.

77. Kaptein EM, MacIntyre SS, Weiner JM, et al: Free thyroxine estimates in nonthyroidal illness: comparison of eight methods. *J Clin Endocrinol Metab* 52:1073–1077, 1981.

78. Kaptein EM, Spencer CA, Kamiel MB, et al: Prolonged dopamine administration and thyroid hormone economy in normal and critically ill subjects. *J Clin Endocrinol Metab* 51:387–393, 1980.

79. Kleinmann RE, Vagenakis AG, Braverman LE: The effect of iopanoic acid on the regulation of thyrotropin secretion in euthyroid subjects. *J Clin Endocrinol Metab* 51:399–403, 1980.

80. Konishi J, Iida Y, Kasagi K, Misaki T, Nakashima T, Endo K, Mori T, Shinpo S, Nohara Y, Matsuura N, Torizuka K: Primary myxedema with thyrotropin-binding inhibitor immunoglobulins: clinical and laboratory findings in 15 patients. *Ann Intern Med* 103:26–31, 1985.

81. Kristensen O, Anderson HH, Pallisgaard G: Lithium carbonate in the treatment of thyrotoxicosis: a controlled study. *Lancet* i:603–605, 1976.

82. Lamberg B-A, Ikonen E, Osterlund K, et al: Antithyroid treatment of maternal hyperthyroidism during lactation. *Clin Endocrinol* 21:81–87, 1984.

83. Larsen PR: Thyroid pituitary interaction: feedback regulation of thyrotropin secretion by thyroid hormones. *N Engl J Med* 30:623–632, 1982.

84. Levy EG: Thyroid disease in the elderly. *Med Clin North Am* 75:151–167, 1991.

85. LoPresti JS, Fried JC, Spencer CA, Nicoloff JT: Unique alterations of thyroid hormone indices in the acquired immunodeficiency syndrome (AIDS). *Ann Intern Med* 110:970–975, 1989.

86. Lowenthal DT, et al: Pharmacokinetics of oral propranolol in chronic renal disease. *Clin Pharmacol Ther* 16:761–769, 1974.

87. Martino E, Bambini G, Bartalena L, Mammoli C, Aghini-Lombardi F, Baschieri L, Pinchera A: Human serum thyrotropin measurement by ultrasensitive immunoradiometric assay as a first-line test in the evaluation of thyroid function. *Clin Endocrinol* 24:141–148, 1986.

88. Maturlo SJ, Rosenbaum RL, Pan C, et al: Variable thyrotropin response to thyrotropin-releasing hormone after small decreases in plasma free thyroid hormone concentrations in patients with nonthyroidal disease. *J Clin Invest* 66:451–456, 1980.

89. Mayfield RK, Sagel J, Colwell JA: Thyrotoxicosis without elevated serum triiodothyronine levels during diabetic ketoacidosis. *Arch Intern Med* 140:409–410, 1980.

90. McDermott MD, Burman KD, Hofeldt FD, Kidd GS: Lithium-associated thyrotoxicosis. *Am J Med* 80:1245–1248, 1986.

91. McDougall IR: Graves' disease: current concepts. *Med Clin North Am* 75:79–95, 1991.

92. McMurry JF, Gilliland PF, Ratliff CR, Bourland PD: Pharmacodynamics of propylthiouracil in normal and hyperthyroid subjects after a single dose. *J Clin Endocrinol Metab* 41:362–364, 1975.

93. Melmed S, Geola FL, Reed AW, et al: A comparison of methods for assessing thyroid function in nonthyroidal illness. *J Clin Endocrinol Metab* 54:300–306, 1982.

94. Melmed S, Nademanee K, Reed AW, et al: Hyperthyroxinemia with bradycardia and normal thyrotropin secretion after chronic amiodarone administration. *J Clin Endocrinol Metab* 53:997–1001, 1981.

95. Momotani N, Ito K, Hamada N, Ban Y, Nishikawa Y, Mimura T: Maternal hyperthyroidism and congenital malformation in the offspring. *Clin Endocrinol* 20:695–700, 1984.

96. Momotani N, Noh J, Oyanagi H, Ishikawa N, Ito K: Antithyroid drug therapy for Graves' disease during pregnancy: optimal regimen for fetal thyroid status. *N Engl J Med* 315:24–28, 1986.

97. Morley JE: Neuroendocrine control of thyrotropin secretion. *Endocrinol Rev* 2:396–436, 1981.

98. Mujtaba Q, Burrow GN: Treatment of hyperthyroidism in pregnancy with propylthiouracil and methimazole. *Obstet Gynecol* 46:282–286, 1975.

99. Nabil N, Miner DJ, Amatruda JM, et al: Methimazole: an alternative route of administration. *J Clin Endocrinol Metab* 54:180–181, 1982.

100. Nelson JC, Tomei RT: Direct determination of free thyroxin in undiluted serum by equilibrium dialysis radioimmunoassay. *Clin Chem* 34:1737–1744, 1988.

101. Nelson JC, Wilcox RB: Further studies on thyroxin-binding globulin-dependence in equilibrium dialysis assays of free thyroxin [Letter to the Editor]. *Clin Chem* 37:128–130, 1991.

102. Novitzky D, Cooper DKC, Barton CI, et al: Triiodothyronine as an inotropic agent after open heart surgery. *J Thorac Cardiovasc Surg* 98:972–977, 1989.

103. Novitzky D, Human PA, Cooper DKC: Effect of triiodothyronine (T$_3$) on myocardial high energy phosphates and lactate after ischemia and cardiopulmonary bypass. An experimental study in baboons. *J Thorac Cardiovasc Surg* 96:600–607, 1988.

104. Novitzky D, Human PA, Cooper DKC: Inotropic effect of triiodothyronine following myocardial ischemia and cardiopulmonary bypass. *J Thorac Cardiovasc Surg* 45:50–55, 1988.

105. Pilo A, Zucchelli GC, Masini S, Calvo S: A new luminescence immunoassay for thyrotropin using coated tubes: evaluation and comparison with immunoradiometric assay. *J Biolumin Chemilumin* 4:185–190, 1989.

106. Pittman JA, Beschi RJ, Smitherman TC: Methimazole: its absorption and excretion in man and tissue distribution in rats. *Endocrinology* 33:182–185, 1971.

106a. Refetoff S, Weiss RE, Usala SJ: The syndromes of resistance to thyroid hormone. *Endocrinol Rev* 14:348–399, 1993.

106b. Reinwein D, Benker G, Lazarus JH, Alexander WO, and the European Multicenter Study Group on Antithyroid Drug Treatment. A prospective randomized trial of antithyroid drug dose in Graves' disease therapy. *J Clin Endocrinol Metab* 76:1516–1521, 1993.

107. Reus VI, Gold P, Post R: Lithium-induced thyrotoxicosis. *Am J. Psychiatry* 136:191–194, 1974.

108. Reveno WS, Rosenbaum H: Observations on the use of antithyroid drugs. *Ann Intern Med* 60:982–989, 1964.

109. Robbins J, Rall JE: The interaction of thyroid hormones and proteins in biological fluids. *Recent Prog Horm Res* 13:161–208, 1957.

110. Ross TJ, Jones MK, John R: The effect of propranolol withdrawal on thyroid hormones in normal and hyperthyroid subjects. *Clin Endocrinol* 13:27–31, 1980.

111. Ross DS: New sensitive immunoradiometric assays for thyrotropin. *Ann Intern Med* 104:718–720, 1986.

112. Rubenfeld S, Silverman VE, Welch KMA, et al: Variable plasma propranolol levels in thyrotoxicosis. *N Engl J Med* 300:353–354, 1979.

113. Sarne DH, Refetoff S: Measurement of thyroxine uptake from serum by cultured human hepatocytes as an index of thyroid status: reduced thyroxine uptake from serum of patients with nonthyroidal illness. *J Clin Endocrinol Metab* 61:1046–1052, 1985.

114. Sawin CT, Chopra D, Albano J, et al: The free triiodothyronine (T_3) index. *Ann Intern Med* 88:474–477, 1978.

115. Scanlon MF, Weightman DR, Shale DJ, et al: Dopamine is a physiological regulator of thyrotropin (TSH) secretion in normal man. *Clin Endocrinol* 10:7–15, 1979.

116. Schimmel M, Utiger RD: Thyroidal and peripheral production of thyroid hormones. Review of recent findings and their clinical implications. *Ann Intern Med* 87:760–768, 1977.

117. Schuppan D, et al: Preliminary pharmacokinetic studies of propylthiouracil in humans. *J Pharmacokinet Biopharm* 1:307–318, 1973.

118. Schussler GC: Thyroid function tests in patients with non-thyroidal disease. In *Thyroid Today*, vol 3, no 3. Flint Laboratories, Morton Grove, IL, 1980.

119. Shand DG: Propranolol. *N Engl J Med* 293:280–285, 1976.

120. Sitar DS, Hunninghake DB: Pharmacokinetics of propylthiouracil in man after a single oral dose. *J Clin Endocrinol Metab* 40:26–29, 1975.

121. Snyder PJ, Utiger RD: Response to thyrotropin-releasing hormone (TRH) in normal man. *J Clin Endocrinol Metab* 34:380–385, 1972.

122. Spencer CA, Lai-Rosenfeld AO, Guttler RB, Lopresti J, Marcus A, Nimala-suriya A, Eigen A, Doss RG, Green BJ, Nicoloff JT: Thyrotropin secretion in thyrotoxic and thyroxine-treated patients: assessment by a sensitive immunoenzymometric assay. *J Clin Endocrinol Metab* 63:349–355, 1986.

123. Sterling K, Brenner MA: Free thyroxine in human serum: simplified measurement with the aid of magnesium precipitation. *J Clin Invest* 45:155–163, 1966.

124. Suzuki H, Kadena N, Taekuchi K, et al: Effects of three-day oral cholecystography on serum iodothyronines and TSH concentrations: comparison of the effects among some cholecystographic agents and the effects of iopanoic acid on the pituitary-thyroid axis. *Acta Endocrinol* 92:477–488, 1979.

125. Suzuki H, Noguchi K, Nakahata M, et al: Effect of iopanoic acid on the pituitary-thyroid axis: time sequence of changes in serum iodothyronines, thyrotropin, and prolactin concentrations and responses to thyroid hormones. *J Clin Endocrinol Metab* 53:779–788, 1981.

126. Takasu N, Yamada T, Takasu M, Komiya I, Nagasawa Y, Asawa T, Shinoda T, Aizawa T, Koizumi Y: Disappearance of thyrotropin-blocking antibodies and spontaneous recovery from hypothyroidism in autoimmune thyroiditis. *N Engl J Med* 326:513–518, 1992.

127. Takeda K, Balzano S, Sakurai A, De Groot LJ, Refetoff S: Screening of nineteen unrelated families with generalized resistance to thyroid hormone for known point mutations in the thyroid hormone receptor beta gene and the detection of a new mutation. *J Clin Invest* 87:496–502, 1991.

128. Talbert RL, Wong YY, Duncan RB: Propranolol plasma concentrations and plasmapheresis. *Drug Intell Clin Pharm* 15:993–995, 1981.

129. Tegler L, Lindstrom B: Antithyroid drugs in milk [Letter]. *Lancet* 2:591, 1980.

130. Temple R, Berman M, Robbins J, et al: The use of lithium in the treatment of thyrotoxicosis. *J Clin Invest* 51:2746–2756, 1972.

131. Thomas FB, Mazzaferri IL, Skillman G: Apathetic thyrotoxicosis: a distinctive clinical and laboratory entity. *Ann Intern Med* 72:679–685, 1970.

132. Toft AO, Irvine WJ, Sinclair I, et al: Thyroid function after surgical treatment of thyrotoxicosis: a report of 100 cases treated with propranolol before operation. *N Engl J Med* 298:643–647, 1978.

133. Tseng Y-C, Burman KD, Baker JR Jr, Wartofsky L: A rapid, sensitive enzyme-linked immunoassay for human thyrotropin. *Clin Chem* 31:1131–1134, 1985.

134. Utiger RD: Decreased extrathyroidal triiodothyronine production in non-thyroidal illness: benefit or harm. *Am J Med* 69:807–810, 1980.

135. Vagenakis AF, Braverman LE: Adverse effects of iodine on thyroid function. *Med Clin North Am* 59:1075–1088, 1975.

136. Vagenakis AG, Portnay GI, O'Brian JT, et al: Effect of starvation on the production and metabolism of thyroxine and triiodothyronine in euthyroid obese patients. *J Clin Endocrinol Metab* 45:1205–1309, 1977.

137. Vanderlaan WP: Antithyroid drugs in practice. *Mayo Clin Proc* 47:962–965, 1972.

138. Van der Poll M, Romijn JA, Wiersinga WM, Werwein HP: Tumor necrosis factor: a putative mediator of the sick euthyroid syndrome in man. *J Clin Endocrinol Metab* 71:1567–1572, 1990.

139. Van Dijke CP, Heydendael RJ, DeKleine MJ: Methimazole, carbimazole and congenital skin defects. *Ann Intern Med* 106:60–61, 1987.

140. Vasily BD, Tyler WB: Propylthiouracil-induced cutaneous vasculitis: case presentation and review of the literature. *JAMA* 243:458–461, 1980.

141. Verhoeen RP, Visser TJ, Docter R, et al: Plasma thyroxine, 3,3',5'-triiodothyronine during beta-adrenergic blockade in hyperthyroidism. *J Clin Endocrinol Metab* 44:1002–1005, 1977.

142. Vesell ES, Shapiro JR, Passananti GT, et al: Altered plasma half-lives of antipyrine, propylthiouracil and methimazole in thyroid dysfunction. *Clin Pharmacol Ther* 17:48–52, 1975.

143. Visser TJ: A tentative review of recent in vitro observations of the enzymatic deiodination of iodothyronines and its possible physiological implications. *Mol Cell Endocrinol* 35:241, 1978.

144. Volpe R, Karlsson A, Jansson R, Dahlberg P: Evidence that antithyroid drugs induced remissions in Graves' disease by modulating thyroid cellular activity. *Clin Endocrinol* 25:453–462, 1986.

145. Wall JR, Fang SL, Kuroki T, Ingbar SH, Braverman LE: In vitro immunoreactivity to propylthiouracil methimazole, and carbimazole in patients with Graves' disease: a possible cause of antithyroid drug-induced agranulocytosis. *J Clin Endocrinol Metab* 58:868–872, 1984.

146. Wang Y-S, Pekary AE, England MS, Hersaman JM: Comparison of a new ultrafiltration method for serum-free T_4 and free T_3 with two RIA kits in eight groups of patients. *J Endocrinol Invest* 8:495–500, 1985.

147. Wartofsky L, Burman KD: Hypothyroidism. In Conn HF (ed): *Current Therapy*. WB Saunders, Philadelphia, 1979.

148. Wartofsky L, Burman KD: Alterations in thyroid function in patients with systemic illness: "The euthyroid sick syndrome." *Endocrinol Rev* 3:164–217, 1982.

149. Wartofsky L, Glinoer D, Solomon B, Lagasse R: Differences and similarities in the treatment of diffuse goiter in Europe and the United States. *Exp Clin Endocrinol* 97:243–251, 1991.

150. Wartofsky L, Ransil BJ, Ingbar SH: Inhibition by iodine of the release of thyroxine from the thyroid glands of patients with thyrotoxicosis. *J Clin Invest* 49:78–86, 1970.

151. Weetman RE, Gregerman RI, Burns WH, Saral R, Santos GW: Suppression of thyrotropin in the low-thyroxine state of severe nonthyroidal illness. *N Engl J Med* 312:546–552, 1985.

152. Weinberger C, Thompson CC, Ong ES, Lebo R, Gruol DJ, Evans RM: The c-erb A beta gene encodes a thyroid hormone receptor. *Nature* 324:641–646, 1986.

153. Wenzel KE: Pharmacological interference with in vitro tests of thyroid function. *Metabolism* 30:7171–7232, 1981.

154. Werner SC: Thyroid function tests in non-thyroidal illness are diagnostically and prognostically important. *Ariz Med* 38:356–358, 1981.

155. Werner SC, Ingbar SH (eds): In The Thyroid: A Fundamental and Clinical Text. Harper & Row, Hagerstown, MD, 1978.

156. Wiersinga WM, Touber JL: The influence of β-adrenoceptor blocking agents on plasma thyroxine and triiodothyronine. *J Clin Endocrinol Metab* 45:293–298, 1977.

157. Wu SY, Chopra IJ, Solomon DH, et al: Changes in circulating iodothyronines in euthyroid and hyperthyroid subjects given ipodate (Oragrafin), an agent for oral cholecystography. *J Clin Endocrinol Metab* 46:691–697, 1978.

158. Wu SY, Shyh TP, Chopra IJ, et al: Comparison of sodium podate (Oragrafin) and propylthiouracil in early treatment of hyperthyroidism. *J Clin Endocrinol Metab* 54:630–634, 1982.

159. Zaloga GP, Chernow B, Smallridge RC, Zajtchuk R, Hall-Boyer K, Hargraves R, Lake CR, Burman KD: A longitudinal evaluation of thyroid function in critically ill surgical patients. *Ann Surg* 201:456–464, 1985.

160. Zucchelli GC, Pilo A, Masini S, Chiesa MR, Masi A: Methodological evaluation of a new chemiluminescence immunoassay for thyrotropin using acridinium ester-labelled antibody. *J Biolumin Chemilumin* 4:185–190, 1989.

161. Zwillich CW, Pierson DK, Hofeldt FD, et al: Ventilatory control in myxedema in hypothyroidism. *N Engl J Med* 292:662–665, 1975.

162. Zwillich CW, Sahn SA, Weil JV: Effects of hypermetabolism on ventilation and chemosensitivity. *J Clin Invest* 60:900–906, 1977.

CHAPTER 45

Insulin and Oral Hypoglycemics

GARY P. ZALOGA, M.D., F.A.C.P.
BART CHERNOW, M.D., F.A.C.P.

Insulin is a polypeptide hormone that is essential for normal metabolic activity. Deficiency of the hormone results in diabetes mellitus. This chapter details the pharmacology of insulin and the application of insulin therapy in the treatment of diabetic ketoacidosis, hyperglycemic nonketotic syndromes, alcoholic ketoacidosis, parenteral nutrition, and the diabetic surgical patient.

Insulin, which consists of two polypeptide chains connected by disulfide bridges, is synthesized by the β-cells of the islets of Langerhans. The pancreas secretes insulin into the portal vein and the liver removes 50 to 60% before it reaches the peripheral circulation. The normal fasting venous immunoreactive insulin concentration in healthy individuals is 10 to 20 μU/ml and represents a basal secretory rate of 0.25 to 1.5 U/hour.

Insulin secretion is regulated by the coordinated interplay of various nutrients, gastrointestinal hormones, pancreatic hormones, and autonomic neurotransmitters (1). Glucose, amino acids, fatty acids, and ketones all stimulate the secretion of insulin. However, glucose is the primary regulator of the β-cell and stimulates insulin secretion by a process that involves an increase in intracellular calcium availability (enhanced by adenosine 3′:5′-cyclic monophosphate, or cAMP) (1, 2). Glucose-induced insulin release is biphasic. The first phase of insulin secretion is brief (0 to 5 minutes) and involves release of stored insulin, whereas the second phase of insulin release (which is more gradual, lasting 5 to 60 minutes) involves the secretion of newly synthesized insulin. The plasma insulin response to an oral glucose load is greater than that after an intravenous glucose load. The oral administration of glucose also reduces hepatic extraction of insulin compared with intravenous glucose (1). Part of the reason for the enhanced insulin secretion and decreased metabolism following oral glucose loads involves the release of gastrointestinal hormones (3). Gastric inhibitory polypeptide (GIP), pancreozymin-cholecystokinin, gastrin, secretin, gut glucagon, and vasoactive intestinal polypeptide have been shown to stimulate insulin secretion (4). Protein, amino acids, and fatty acids also stimulate insulin secretion, an effect enhanced by gastrointestinal hormones. Adrenergic agents affect insulin release via α- and β-adrenergic receptors involving cAMP (5). α-Adrenergic action is inhibitory and predominates over the β-stimulatory effect. As a result, epinephrine and norepinephrine inhibit, whereas isoproterenol stimulates, insulin secretion. Propranolol blocks the isoproterenol effect. Catecholamine effects are responsible for the hypoinsulinemia that accompanies "stress" hyperglycemia (e.g., in severe burns). Such states may occur when the autonomic nervous system is activated during hypoxia, hypothermia, surgery, and burns. Parasympathetic stimulation increases insulin secretion, an effect that is partially antagonized by atropine. Dopamine diminishes insulin release in vitro (6). Prostaglandins are inhibitory to insulin release and may play a role in insulin-dependent diabetes (7). Prostaglandin inhibitors (e.g., acetylsalicylic acid) augment (8--10), whereas prostaglandin stimulators (e.g., furosemide) reduce, insulin secretion (9). A variety of other hormones affect insulin action. Glucagon, growth hormone, glucocorticoids, estrogens, progestins, and parathyroid hormone

Table 45.1. Insulin Action

	Liver	Adipose	Muscle	Periphery
Glucose uptake		+[a]	+	+
Glycogen synthesis	+		+	
Fatty acid synthesis	+	+		
Protein synthesis			+	
Glycerol synthesis		+		
Amino acid uptake			+	
Glycogenolysis	−			
Gluconeogenesis	−			
Ketogenesis	−			
Lipolysis		−		
Protein catabolism			−	

[a] Abbreviations: Increases (+); decreases (−).

(PTH) each increase insulin levels. Somatostatin inhibits both insulin and glucagon secretion. Agents that destroy the β-cells induce hypoinsulinemic diabetes mellitus (e.g., alloxan and streptozotocin). Some of these agents have been used to treat insulin-secreting tumors.

Insulin elicits a vast array of biologic responses and is the primary hormone controlling the storage and utilization of cellular nutrients (i.e., glucose, amino acids, fatty acids). Insulin also inhibits catabolic processes. The immediate effects of insulin (seconds to minutes) include activation of glucose and ion transport systems and phosphorylation/dephosphorylation of enzymes (1). The intermediate effects (3 to 6 hours) involve new protein synthesis (i.e., enzymes). The long-term effects of insulin (hours to days) include stimulation of cell proliferation and differentiation. The actions of insulin are initiated by binding to a cell surface receptor (present on virtually all cells). The number of receptors varies depending upon cell type (i.e., approximately 40 per cell on erythrocytes and 300,000 per cell on adipocytes and hepatocytes) (1). The insulin receptor is a ligand-activated tyrosine protein kinase (1, 11). Following activation, the receptor catalyzes phosphorylation of cellular proteins. Hormonal stimulation also activates phospholipase C. Insulin stimulates glucose transport into muscle and adipose tissue (requires ATP). Insulin does not stimulate glucose uptake into liver (1).

Insulin controls the storage and metabolism of a variety of metabolic fuels including glucose, fat, and amino acids (Table 45.1). Insulin lowers the concentration of glucose in the blood by inhibiting hepatic glucose production (i.e., glycogenolysis and gluconeogenesis) and by stimulating the uptake and metabolism of glucose in muscle and adipose tissue. Glucose production is inhibited half-maximally by an insulin concentration of 20 to 30 μU/ml, whereas glucose utilization is stimulated half-maximally by a concentration of 100 μU/ml (1). Thus, hepatic glucose output is suppressed when glucose utilization is only minimally stimulated. This fact explains why type II diabetics can have normal fasting glucose concentrations despite postprandial hyperglycemia. Glucagon opposes the effect of insulin on the liver by stimulating glycogenolysis and gluconeogenesis but has little effect upon peripheral glucose uptake. Diabetics with insulin deficiency/resistance and hyperglucagonemia demonstrate an increase in gluconeogenesis and glycogenolysis, a decrease in peripheral glucose uptake, and a decrease in the conversion of glucose to glycogen in the liver. The net result is hyperglycemia.

Insulin suppresses ketogenesis by inhibiting fatty acid release from adipose tissue and hepatic oxidation of fatty acids to ketones. It accelerates muscle uptake and oxidation of ketone bodies. Insulin also stimulates fatty acid synthesis and increases the concentration of malonyl CoA. Malonyl CoA inhibits the enzyme, acylcarnitine transferase, that is responsible for transport of fatty acids into mitochondria (the site of ketone body production). All of these insulin effects decrease ketone body production and occur at insulin concentrations below those required to stimulate glucose uptake. Conversely, glucagon stimulates ketone body production by stimulating lipolysis and fatty acid oxidation, and by decreasing malonyl CoA (1).

Insulin activates lipoprotein lipase on capillary endothelium (1). This enzyme hydrolyzes the triglycerides present in very-low-density lipoproteins (VLDL) and chylomicrons. During insulin insufficiency, hypertriglyceridemia may result from decreased metabolism of VLDL.

Insulin stimulates amino acid uptake and protein synthesis and inhibits protein breakdown in muscle and other tissues. Insulin effects also cause hypokalemia, hypophosphatemia, and antinatriuresis (2). The antinatriuretic action may account for edema occasionally seen during insulin treatment of patients with diabetic ketoacidosis.

Most long-term complications (i.e., premature atherosclerosis, glomerulosclerosis, retinopathy, neuropathy) of diabetes are believed to result from prolonged exposure of tissues to elevated concentrations of glucose. The toxic effects of hyperglycemia may result from the accumulation of nonenzymatically glycosylated products and osmotically active sugar alcohols (i.e., sorbitol) (1, 12).

Insulin circulates in plasma predominantly as the free unbound hormone and distributes in the extracellular fluid (13). Under fasting conditions, the pancreas secretes 40 μg (1 unit) of insulin per hour into the portal vein; the concentration in portal blood is 2 to 4 ng/ml (50 to 100 μU/ml) and that in the peripheral circulation is 500 pg/ml (12 μU/ml) (1, 13). The plasma half-life of insulin is 5 to 9 minutes. The major sites of degradation are the liver (40 to 60%), kidney (15 to 20%) and muscle (14). Fifty percent of insulin that reaches the liver via the portal vein is destroyed in a single passage. The decrease in insulin requirements in patients with renal failure results from decreased renal degradation of insulin.

INSULIN PREPARATIONS

Insulin is available as pure beef, pork, beef-pork, fish, or human insulin. Porcine insulin is most similar to that of humans and differs only in the substitution of alanine for threonine at the carboxy-terminus of the β-chain. Human insulin is obtained either by synthesis from pork insulin or by recombinant DNA techniques using *Escherichia coli*. All newly diagnosed patients with insulin-dependent diabetes and patients requiring insulin for control of hyperglycemia should be treated with human insulin. Other indications include lipoatrophy and insulin resistance resulting from insulin antibodies. It is not necessary to change stable patients receiving animal insulins to human insulin.

Insulin is available in a variety of forms that differ in onset of action and duration of effects (Table 45.2) (1, 15–17). Insulin preparations are classified as rapid-, intermediate-, and long-acting based upon their duration of action. Insulin is mixed with solutions containing protamine and zinc to slow absorption and prolong duration of action. The Lente insulins employ different concentrations of zinc, whereas neutral protamine Hagedorn (NPH) and protamine zinc insulin (PZI) employ both zinc and protamine. NPH insulin is formulated by mixing together regular and PZI in proportions to maintain action throughout the day. PZI should not be given with regular insulin, since excess zinc slows the absorption of the regular insulin. Premixed combinations of rapid- and intermediate-acting insulins are also available. However, these preparations do not provide flexibility in altering the dose of one insulin component independent of the other. Most insulin today is marketed as U-100 (100 units/ml) insulin. Insulin is supplied at neutral pH, which improves its stability. Refrigeration is no longer required, but extremes of temperature and exposure to sunlight should be avoided. Regular insulin is the only form approved for intravenous use (Table 45.2). It may also be given intramuscularly (18, 19), where it has faster and more predictable absorption than subcutaneous injection. Insulin should not be mixed with sodium bicarbonate, since insulin is unstable in the presence of alkali (20).

Doses and concentrations of insulin are expressed in units. One unit of insulin is equal to the amount required to reduce the blood glucose level in a fasting rabbit to 45 mg/dl (1). Most commercial preparations of insulin are supplied at a concentration of 100 U/ml (about 3.6 mg of insulin per ml).

Insulin production by the normal healthy pancreas is between 0.2 and 0.5 U/kg/day (21). Usually, half is secreted in the basal state and about half in response to meals. Thus, basal secretion is about 0.5 to 1 U/hr. The average type I diabetic patient requires 0.6 to 0.7 U/kg/day (range 0.2 to 1.0 U/kg per day). Obese and stressed patients require more insulin because of tissue insulin resistance.

The principal goal of insulin therapy in the critically ill patient is to relieve clinical signs and symptoms of diabetes, prevent severe hyperglycemia, and avoid hypoglycemia. The attainment of euglycemia, in an attempt to prevent chronic complications, is not a primary goal in these patients. One frequently utilizes the intravenous, intramuscular, and subcutaneous routes for administration of insulin in the critically ill patient. When using the subcutaneous route, the author and colleagues find that glucose control is improved by combining a short- and intermediate-acting insulin. Use of a short-acting insulin alone (i.e., regular insulin every 4 to 6 hours by

sliding scale) usually results in large fluctuations of circulating blood glucose levels.

FACTORS THAT INFLUENCE RESPONSE TO INSULIN

There is a marked individual variability in insulin absorption and half-life. Duration of effect and magnitude of hypoglycemic response (at peak action) vary with the dose (22); the larger the dose, the longer the duration of action and the greater the hypoglycemic effect. Rate of absorption varies with the site and depth of injection (23). Absorption is more rapid from the deltoid area and abdomen than from thighs and buttocks. Deep intramuscular injections are absorbed more rapidly than superficial intramuscular injections, and both are absorbed more rapidly than subcutaneous injections.

Increased subcutaneous blood flow (i.e., from massage, exercise, heating of the skin) increases the rate of insulin absorption. Cooling decreases subcutaneous absorption. Mixing different insulin preparations can alter absorption. When regular insulin is mixed with Lente insulin, some of the regular insulin becomes modified, causing a partial loss of the rapidly acting component (1). Alterations in action also occur when regular insulin is mixed with ultralente insulin. Thus, injections of mixtures of insulin should be made without delay. The authors prefer to mix regular with NPH insulin, since there is less reaction between these two preparations. Some patients are insensitive to subcutaneous or intramuscular insulin but sensitive to intravenous insulin (24, 25). This sensitivity may be related to excessive protease activity in the subcutaneous tissue, resulting in excessive insulin degradation at the injection site (26, 27). The effectiveness of subcutaneously administered insulin in these patients can be increased by mixing the insulin with aprotinin, a protease inhibitor (26, 27).

Changes in insulin receptors are important in insulin-resistant states (28) and states of increased insulin sensitivity. In circumstances of hyperinsulinemia (such as obesity) the insulin receptor concentration (sites/cell) is reduced (downregulated), whereas the reverse occurs in hypoinsulinemia.

The most common cause of insulin resistance is obesity (29). In obesity, the defect is at the target cell (decreased number of insulin receptors) and is proportional to the degree of basal hyperinsulinemia (30, 31). Several weeks of a low-carbohydrate diet corrects this abnormality. Insulin resistance may be seen in association with acanthosis nigricans because of a decrease in the number of insulin receptors, or with antireceptor antibodies

Table 45.2. Insulin Preparations

Type of Insulin	Action	Protein	Peak s.q. Action (hr)	Duration s.q. (hr)	Route	Concentration (U/ml)
Regular (crystalline)[a]	Rapid	None	1–3	5–7	i.v., s.c., i.m.[b]	100
Semilente	Rapid	None	2–4	10–16	s.c.	100
NPH[a]	Intermediate	Protamine	6–14	18–28	s.c.	100
Lente[a]	Intermediate	None	6–14	18–28	s.c.	100
Ultralente[a]	Prolonged	None	18–24	30–40	s.c.	100
PZI	Prolonged	Protamine	18–24	30–40	s.c.	100

[a] Available as human insulin.
[b] Abbreviations: i.v., intravenous; s.c., subcutaneous; i.m., intramuscular.

that decrease insulin binding (31). Additional causes of decreased insulin binding include glucocorticoid excess (e.g., Cushing's disease), growth hormone excess (e.g., acromegaly), and lipoatrophic diabetes mellitus. Increased insulin binding (augmented sensitivity) is seen in trained athletes and in cases of starvation and glucocorticoid or growth hormone deficiency. Insulin resistance may also result from postreceptor deficits (e.g., type II diabetes mellitus).

Patients who take insulin develop antibodies to the insulin molecule (29). These antibodies may cause a slower onset and longer duration of insulin action, insulin resistance, or insulin allergy (28). Initial treatment consists of switching to a less antigenic insulin. Pork is less immunogenic than beef insulin, and single component is less immunogenic than single peak. Lente and protamine (NPH) insulins produce higher antibody titers than does regular insulin (NPH > Lente > regular). Human insulins are least immunogenic. The authors use only human insulin in their intravenous insulin infusions and in patients in whom short-term insulin therapy is contemplated (e.g., after surgery) so as to avoid antigenicity. If this treatment fails, systemic steroids (prednisone 60 to 80 mg/day for 10 days) usually results in a marked reduction in insulin requirements (2, 29). Additional therapeutic approaches include the use of sulfated insulins (32), fish insulin (33), immunosuppressants (34), and U-500 regular insulin (35). Other factors to consider with insulin resistance include stress, infection, ketosis, and drug interactions.

COMPLICATIONS

The most common complication of insulin therapy is hypoglycemia. Symptoms include neuroglucopenic (e.g., confusion, blurred vision, weakness, hunger, bizarre behavior, depression, seizures, coma) and hyperadrenergic manifestations (e.g., tachycardia, palpitations, diaphoresis, vasoconstriction, piloerection, anxiety). Localizing neurologic symptoms (e.g., hemiplegia or visual disturbances) may occur secondary to underlying vascular disease. Hypothermia may be an important clue to hypoglycemia in a comatose patient (36). In normal volunteers given insulin, hypoglycemic symptoms occur when blood glucose decreases to 40 to 45 mg/dl. This threshold may be lower in patients with diabetes mellitus. Symptoms may also occur with rapid decreases in blood glucose, even though the plasma glucose value may be normal (60 to 120 mg/dl) (37). Hypoglycemic symptoms may be difficult to detect in comatose patients or those who are receiving sedative medications, or during sleep. Bedside glucose monitoring is useful in these patients. The most common causes of hypoglycemia are excessive insulin dosage, omission of or delay in meals, heavy exercise, and poor injection technique (e.g., failure to mix insulin properly or accidental injection into muscle). When recurrent hypoglycemic episodes develop, one should consider progressive renal insufficiency, failure to reduce dosage after resolution of a stress, onset of adrenal insufficiency, pregnancy, and drug interactions (e.g., with propranolol). Glucagon and epinephrine are the major hormones preventing hypoglycemia in the normal state. Secretion of these hormones frequently is impaired in patients with diabetes mellitus. In addition, the glycemic threshold for symptoms commonly is diminished in diabetics. These factors increase the risk of severe hypoglycemia.

The "Somogyi effect" is the occurrence of posthypoglycemic hyperglycemia and ketonuria after excessive insulin administration. Rebound hyperglycemia results from the release of counterregulatory hormones (e.g., cortisol, catecholamines, glucagon, growth hormone). Widely varying urine glucose values suggest the Somogyi effect. Detection is accomplished by frequent blood glucose monitoring. Treatment consists of decreasing the insulin dose.

Occasionally, a patient will develop edema during insulin therapy. The edema partially results from reduced urinary sodium excretion induced by insulin. Insulin allergy results from production of immunoglobulin E (IgE) antiinsulin antibodies (28, 38–40), antigen-antibody complexes, or cell-mediated hypersensitivity responses. These reactions usually result from small amounts of aggregated or denatured insulin in the preparations, minor contaminants, or sensitivity to one of the components added to insulin during its formulation (i.e., protamine, zinc, phenol). Local symptoms manifest as induration, pruritus, erythema, or pain at the injection site. Systemic symptoms of insulin allergy include generalized pruritus and urticaria, angioneurotic edema, anaphylaxis, and bronchospasm. Symptoms appear 30 minutes to several hours after injection and usually disappear spontaneously within a few weeks. Many patients exhibit allergic responses following an interval during which insulin therapy had been discontinued and reinstituted (41, 42).

The allergy may at times be attributed to exogenous contaminants (from the extraction process) rather than to the insulin (42). Protamine found in many insulins can be antigenic. If allergic symptoms persist, treatment may be required (Table 45.3) (28, 38, 41). One must first rule out contamination of the insulin. Sources include a dirty bottle, poor injection technique, or reaction to material used in the commercial process of preparing the insulin (e.g., acid, alcohol). Before treating with other agents one should review the requirements for insulin therapy. If insulin is required, the patient should be switched to a less antigenic form. The authors recommend using *E. coli* recombinant human insulin. A trial of antihistamines (43) or systemic steroids (44–46) may decrease adverse reactions. Corticosteroids have been given as oral prednisone (30 mg daily) (45) or as injectable hydrocortisone (10 mg) mixed with the insulin (44). Slow desensitization occurs under corticosteroid coverage, which can be discontinued at a future time. At times desensitization is required (38, 40, 42, 47). Patients should be skin tested against different insulin preparations and the least antigenic form used. Insulin injection should be begun intradermally, and if a local reaction occurs, the dose should be repeated or lowered before proceeding (Table 45.3). Once desensitization is completed, insulin should be given at frequent intervals (e.g., two to four times a day).

Other adverse effects of insulin include lipoatrophy and lipohypertrophy at injection sites (28). Lipoatrophy is more frequent with animal insulins. It can be treated by injection of human insulin into the border of the atrophied area. Lipohypertrophy is caused by repeated injections into the same subcutaneous site and results from the lipogenic effects of insulin.

Table 45.3.   Treatment of Insulin Allergy

1. Rule out foreign material being injected; switch to new bottle of insulin, review injection technique, and check for sensitivity to solvent.
2. Consider diet and oral hypoglycemics.
3. Switch to a less antigenic insulin:
   Escherichia coli (human) < fish < pork < beef
   Regular < Lente < NPH
   Single component < single peak
4. Antihistamines
5. Corticosteroids
6. Desensitization
   a. Use insulin preparation with least skin test reactivity
   b. Slow desensitization:

Day	Time	Units of Insulin	Route[a]
1	0730 AM	0.00001	i.d.
	1200	0.0001	
	0430 PM	0.001	
2	0730 AM	0.01	i.d.
	1200	0.1	
	0430 PM	1	
3	0730 AM	2	s.c.
	1200	4	
	0430 PM	8	
4	0730 AM	12	s.c.
	1200	16	
	0430 PM	20	
5	0730 AM	25	s.c.
6	0730 AM	30	s.c.

   c. Fast desensitization: double dose every 30–60 minutes and cover with steroids

[a] Abbreviations: i.d., intradermal; s.c., subcutaneous.

DIABETES MELLITUS

Insulin insufficiency results in the production of diabetes mellitus and can be classified, based upon the cause, into various groups: insulin-dependent diabetes mellitus (type I), non-insulin-dependent diabetes mellitus (type II), secondary diabetes mellitus (e.g., drug induced, pancreatic disease, hormonal), carbohydrate intolerance, and gestational diabetes mellitus. Insulin insufficiency may result from inadequate secretion (i.e., deficiency) or decreased response (i.e., resistance). Long-term management of these patients with insulin is discussed elsewhere (48). Major surgery and critical illness are stressful events that stimulate the secretion of "antiinsulin" hormones. Normally, these changes in metabolism are balanced by an increase in insulin secretion. Patients with a diminished ability to secrete insulin may be unable to counterbalance the antiinsulin hormonal effects, and hyperglycemia and ketosis may result. Acute metabolic decompensation in these patients may result in diabetic ketoacidosis or diabetic hyperglycemic nonketotic states.

Stress increases the need for insulin. It is important that the usual dose of insulin not be withheld during illness or surgery, although it may be reduced. Withholding insulin may precipitate severe hyperglycemia or ketoacidosis.

DIABETIC KETOACIDOSIS

The most severe manifestation of insulin lack is diabetic ketoacidosis (DKA). Mortality from DKA has declined since the advent of insulin therapy; however, it may still be as high as 5 to 15% (2, 49). Major causes of death include irreversible circulatory shock, myocardial infarction, sepsis, cardiac arrest, stroke, renal failure, pulmonary aspiration, cerebral edema, adult respiratory distress syndrome, thrombosis, pulmonary embolism, gastrointestinal hemorrhage, and electrolyte abnormalities (50).

Hyperglycemia and ketoacidosis result from an imbalance between the actions of anabolic (insulin) and catabolic (glucagon, cortisone, growth hormone, catecholamines) hormones (51, 52). The importance of glucagon in the pathogenesis of DKA forms the basis of the bihormonal theory of diabetes mellitus (48, 53–55). In this theory glucagon is thought of as the major agent responsible for the massive production of ketones and glucose.

Glucagon, when unopposed by insulin in the liver, increases glycogenolysis, gluconeogenesis, and ketogenesis (Table 45.4). In humans about 75% of hepatic glucose production is mediated by glucagon, whereas only about 40% of glucose utilization occurs in insulin-sensitive tissues. If both glucagon and insulin were lacking, glucose production would decline by 75%, utilization would decline by 40%, and serum glucose levels would most likely decline (48). The major direct effect of insulin on the liver is to oppose the effects of glucagon, and insulin has minimal influence on hepatic glucose and ketone metabolism unless glucagon is present (48). Diabetic patients fail to suppress glucagon normally during hyperglycemia. The loss of glucose-induced glucagon suppression can be improved by infusion of insulin (48). A decrease in the insulin/glucagon ratio (i.e., during DKA) causes increased glucose production by the liver, whereas the absolute decline in insulin levels or action reduces glucose utilization in peripheral tissues. Insulin deficiency is the mechanism by which substrates for hepatic glucose and ketone production (e.g., amino acids and free fatty acids) are delivered to the liver in increased quantities; glucagon is the switch that activates the production machinery for glucose and ketones (48).

In DKA, hyperglycemia results from decreased utilization of glucose (reduced rate of entrance of glucose into cells) and glucose overproduction by the liver (Table 45.4). Insulin does not influence the rate of glucose transfer across the cell membrane in hepatocytes, brain cells, erythrocytes, leukocytes, and cells of the renal medulla (13). It does affect transfer in muscle and fat cells. Insulin deficiency also impairs the activity of glycogen synthetase, activates lipolysis, accelerates protein catabolism, causes hyperglucagonemia, intensifies glucagon's effects in the liver, and stimulates hepatic gluconeogenesis. Protein is degraded to amino acids and converted to glucose in the liver. Insulin reverses these effects. Ketones accumulate as a result of increased lipolysis, decreased fatty acid synthesis in adipose tissue, increased hepatic ketogenesis, and decreased ketone utilization in the periphery. In the absence of insulin, lipolysis, facilitated by various counterregulatory hormones, proceeds unchecked. The liver picks up liberated free fatty acids and converts them to ketones (since insulin deficiency impairs their conversion to triglycerides) (Fig. 45.1) (51, 52). In the absence of glucagon, insulin deficiency leads to only a modest increase in glucose and ketones (53–55). Suppression of glucagon by somatostatin (48, 56–59) results in attenuation of hyperglycemia and hyperketonemia in diabetes. Hyperglycemia and ketonemia appear readily when glucagon

Table 45.4. Effect of Insulin and Glucagon on Glucose and Ketone Metabolism in Diabetes

	Insulin Deficiency	*Relative Glucagon Excess*
Hyperglycemia		
Decreased glucose utilization	++++	0
Hepatic glucose production	+	++++
Ketonemia		
Lipolysis	++++	+
Hepatic ketogenesis	+	++++

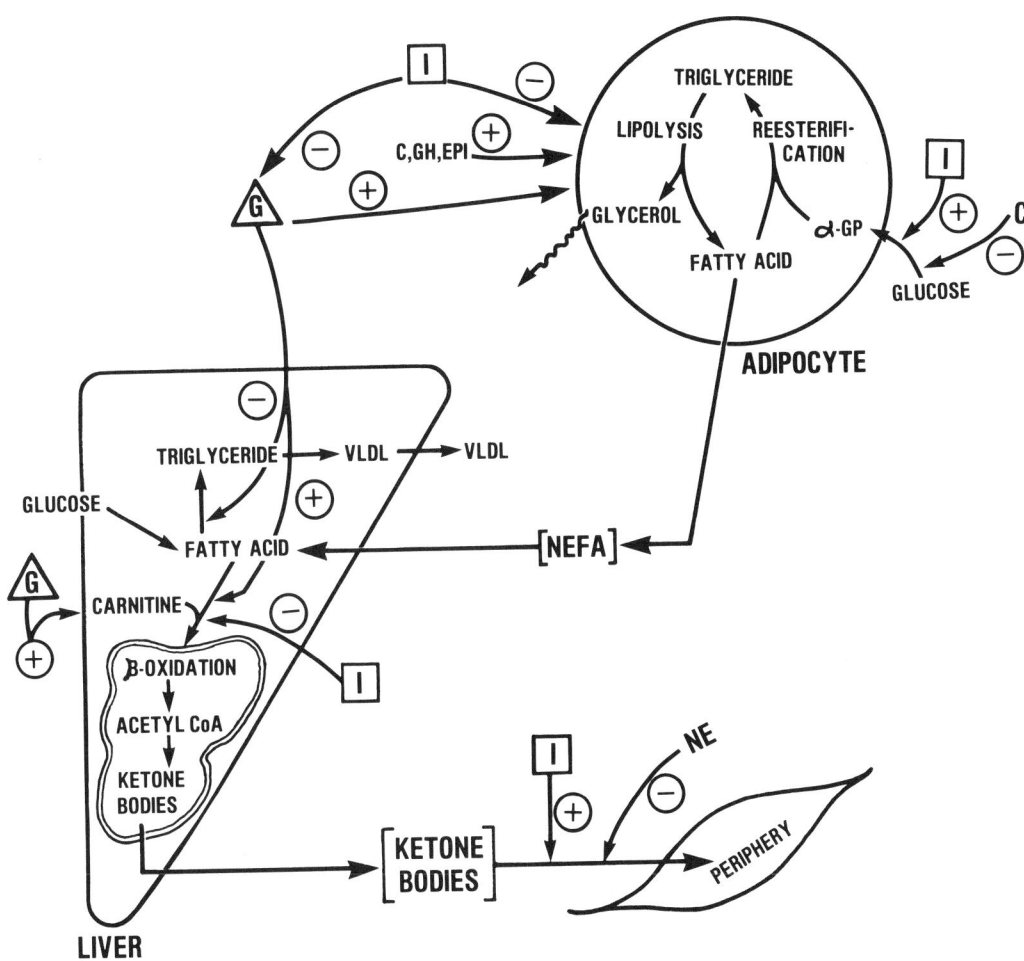

Figure 45.1. Hormonal control of ketogenesis.

is infused (48). However, somatostatin offers no advantage over insulin alone in the treatment of established DKA (60). Hyperglycemia in diabetic rats may be decreased by blocking glucagon action with a glucagon receptor antagonist (61). Glucagon-suppressing agents someday may provide an additional therapeutic agent in the treatment of diabetes mellitus.

Most cases of DKA are not a result of simple insulin deficiency but result from identifiable precipitating factors that alter antiinsulin hormonal levels (e.g., epinephrine, cortisol, norepinephrine, and growth hormone). These counterregulatory hormones oppose insulin action and stimulate glucagon release and action. Hypovolemia resulting from glucose-induced diuresis also increases glucagon secretion and release of catecholamines and other stress hormones. The most common

precipitating factor for DKA is infection followed by myocardial infarction, cerebrovascular accidents, and trauma (49). Many patients will present with DKA as the initial clinical manifestation of diabetes mellitus.

Signs and symptoms of DKA relate to the presence of hyperglycemia (e.g., osmotic diuresis, dehydration, hyperosmolality, or electrolyte depletion) or ketoacidosis (e.g., acidosis or osmotic diuresis) (52). The major presenting symptoms and signs of DKA include nausea, vomiting, labored (Kussmaul) breathing, polyuria, polydipsia, depressed mental function, dehydration, tachycardia, fruity odor of breath, abdominal pain, and hypotension (Table 45.5). Laboratory examination characteristically shows hyperglycemia, metabolic acidosis with an increased anion gap, ketonemia, glucosuria, ketonuria, hemoconcentration with hyperosmolality, and leukocytosis. Other causes of an anion gap acidosis include alcoholic ketoacidosis, lactic acidosis, renal failure, and certain poisons (e.g., ethylene glycol, or methyl alcohol). Ketoacidosis can be distinguished by the presence of ketonemia. Diabetic ketoacidosis is suggested by the concomitant presence of hyperglycemia.

The cause of the altered consciousness in DKA is uncertain and correlates poorly with blood glucose, ketone bodies, hydrogen ions, or electrolyte levels. Plasma hyperosmolality provides the best correlation to date. The explanation for nausea, vomiting, gastric stasis, and ileus is also unknown. They may be secondary to intracellular potassium and/or magnesium deficiency. Acute abdominal pain occurs in 20 to 25% of decompensated diabetics (62) and may be the result of intestinal distension. Differentiation from an acute intraabdominal problem may be difficult. Leukocytosis is common and correlates with the degree of ketosis but not with infection (63). In addition, many DKA patients with infection fail to mount a fever.

An understanding of the nitroprusside reaction (NTPR) (e.g., Acetest) for measuring ketones is essential in the therapy of DKA to avoid inappropriate use of insulin (64). Nitroprusside reacts with acetoacetate (AcAc) and weakly with acetone but not with β-hydroxybutyrate (βOHB). Normally, ketones are present in low concentration with a βOHB/AcAc ratio of 3:1. During DKA, total ketones increase and the βOHB/AcAc ratio may approach 30:1. Hence, a negative or trace NTPR may mislead the clinician to underestimate the severity of ketoacidosis when most of the ketones are in the βOHB form.

Table 45.5. Clinical Features of Diabetic Ketoacidosis

General
    Malaise, weakness
    Dehydration (dry mucous membranes, decreased skin turgor)
    Polyuria, polydipsia
    Muscle aches
Neurologic
    Depressed mental function
    Drowsiness, stupor, coma
    Headache
Cardiac
    Tachycardia
    Hypotension
    Heart failure
Gastrointestinal
    Anorexia
    Nausea, vomiting
    Gastric stasis, distention
    Ileus
    Abdominal pain
Respiratory
    Hyperpnea
    Kussmaul breathing
    Fruity odor on breath
Laboratory
    Metabolic acidosis
    Ketonemia, ketonuria
    Hyperglycemia, glucosuria
    Hyperosmolality
    Hypokalemia
    Hypomagnesemia
    Hyponatremia
    Hypophosphatemia
    Leukocytosis
    Elevated serum amylase, creatine phosphokinase, transaminases

When the NTPR is used to assess response to insulin therapy one can be misled in the opposite direction. With insulin therapy βOHB decreases more rapidly than AcAc. In addition, βOHB is reoxidized to AcAc and the absolute levels of AcAc may rise while total ketones are falling and metabolic status is improving. Nitroprusside results may erroneously indicate a worsening of ketosis, and the insulin dosage may be increased unnecessarily. Indirect measures of ketonemia (e.g., anion gap and blood pH) may be useful in these situations.

DKA must be distinguished from other causes of metabolic acidosis and altered mental function (Table 45.6). Hypoglycemia should be ruled out quickly with bedside blood glucose test strips (65). Cerebrovascular accidents may lead to glycosuria and ketonuria but usually can be distinguished on clinical grounds and by obtaining blood glucose and ketone levels. Nonketotic hyperosmolar syndrome and alcoholic ketoacidosis are discussed in later sections.

Therapy in DKA (Table 45.7) is aimed at correction of fluid and electrolyte abnormalities, correction of the metabolic consequences of insulin lack, and identification of precipitating factors (66, 67). The airway must be protected, and if the patient is obtunded with vomiting, nasogastric suctioning should be undertaken. A comprehensive flow sheet of vital signs, laboratory data, and treatment given aids in proper assessment of therapy. Routine bladder catheterization should not be performed, unless the patient does not void in 3 to 4 hours or has cardiovascular depression. DKA develops over a number of days and should not be corrected all at once, since rapid changes may be harmful by creating harmful osmotic and biochemical gradients (e.g., resulting in cerebral edema and pulmonary edema).

Fluid replacement (Table 45.7) is the first step in the therapy (66) of DKA. Dehydration and intravascular volume depletion (average 6 to 10 liters) result from glucosuria (osmotic diuresis) and vomiting. The circulating volume should be restored with normal saline to promote proper organ function and to ensure insulin action. Volume repletion alone can lower plasma glucose levels and decrease counterregulatory hormone concentrations but does not reverse the acidosis. Thus, insulin is also required. Arguments abound regarding the type of fluid replacement. The body is deficient in hypotonic (0.7 N) saline, and many centers replace fluid losses with 0.5 N saline or an equivalent hypotonic fluid. The authors favor the use of isotonic saline. Despite losses of water, plasma sodium concentration is usually normal (25%) or low (67%) (68) and the hypernatremic effect of an isotonic saline infusion is small. Isotonic saline dampens the fall in extracellular osmolality that occurs during fluid and insulin treatment and may lessen the chance of cerebral and pulmonary edema (caused by unfavorable osmotic gradients). However, if the plasma sodium rises above 150 to 155 mEq/liter, hypotonic fluid should be substituted. Large amounts of sodium chloride may contribute to hyperchloremic acidosis during treatment (69). The authors usually give 1 liter of isotonic saline when the patient is admitted, followed by 1 liter over 1 hour, 1 liter over 2 hours, and finally 150 to 300 ml/hr depending on the clinical response. A positive fluid balance should be achieved. Excessive urinary losses resulting from an osmotic diuresis will continue until plasma glucose levels decrease below the

Table 45.6. Serum Changes in the Differential Diagnosis of Diabetic Ketoacidosis

Diagnosis	Glucose	Ketones	pH	Anion Gap	Sodium	Blood Urea Nitrogen
Diabetic ketoacidosis	3 +^a (400–800 mg/dl)	3+	3−	2+	N to −	3 + (30–60 mg/dl)
Hyperglycemic hyperosmolar nonketotic syndrome	4 + (>600 mg/dl)	0 to +	−	N	N to 3+	4 + (70–90 mg/dl)
Alcoholic ketoacidosis	− to + (50–250 mg/dl)	+	+−	+	+	N
Lactic acidosis	N	0 to +	3−	+	N to −	N to 3+
Hypoglycemia	2−	0 to +	N	N	N	N

^a Abbreviations: Increased (+, 2+, 3+, 4+); decreased (−, 2−, 3−); normal (N).

Table 45.7. Treatment of Diabetic Ketoacidosis

Fluids
  Give 1 liter isotonic saline on admission followed by 1 liter in 1 hour, 1 liter in 2 hours, then 150–300 ml/hr. If serum sodium rises above 150–155 mEq/liter, switch to 0.5 N saline. When plasma glucose falls below 250 mg/dl, switch to D_5W. Central hemodynamic monitoring may be required in elderly or in patients with cardiac or renal disease.
Insulin
  Begin with continuous i.v. infusion of 0.5–1.0 U/hr regular insulin for each 100 mg/dl increase in blood glucose above 100 mg/dl (in isotonic saline). Increase infusion rate if glucose does not fall by 10%/hr. When plasma glucose drops to 250 mg/dl, decrease i.v. infusion to 1–3 U regular insulin per hour and continue until acidosis is corrected (glucose "clamp").
    Alternative
      Use 0.3 U regular insulin per kg i.m. or s.c. initially, then 5–10 U regular insulin i.m. or s.c. per hour; when glucose drops to 250 mg/dl, continue i.m. or s.c. injections at 2 to 4 hour intervals using glucose clamp until acidosis clears. Give injections into deltoids.
Potassium
  Give 20 mEq/hr; if the patient is oliguric, give 5–10 mEq/hour; if K^+ above 6 mEq/liter, stop infusion; if K^+ below 4 mEq/liter, increase infusion. Use continuous ECG monitoring.
Phosphorus
  Oral: Neutra-Phos 250 mg every 6 hr.
  i.v.: potassium phosphate 0.08–0.16 mmol/kg/6 hr. Measure serum phosphorous levels.
Bicarbonate
  If arterial pH <7.1 or bicarbonate <5–7 mEq/liter, give 1/2 ampule bicarbonate (22 mEq); if pH <7.0, give one ampule bicarbonate (44 mEq); monitor arterial or venous pH hourly.
Magnesium
  If less than 1.2 mg/dl, give:
  Oral: Mg oxide 35 mEq every 6–24 hr
  i.v.: $MgSO_4$ or $MgCl_2$ 20–80 mEq/day
  Monitor serum glucose, electrolytes, arterial blood gas, anion gap, and hemodynamic and mental status.

renal threshold. Young children are more vulnerable to cerebral edema than adults. Fluid deficits usually are replaced at a slower rate in children. Average rates of replacement are around 5 ml/kg/hr.

When the blood glucose falls below 250 mg/dl, the intravenous infusion is switched to 5% dextrose in water (D_5W), 5% dextrose in 0.5 normal saline (D_5NS), or 5% dextrose in normal saline (D_5NS), depending on the serum sodium concentration. For example, if the patient is hypernatremic (>150 mEq/liter), the authors use D_5W, whereas if the patient is hyponatremic (<135 mEq/liter), D_5NS is used. When the serum sodium is between 135 and 150 mEq/liter, D_5NS is the best choice. The importance of administering glucose is not only to avoid hypoglycemia but to protect against the development of cerebral edema (discussed later in this section). Hemodynamic monitoring may be required in the elderly and in patients with cardiac or renal disease.

Total body potassium (K^+) and phosphorus (PO_4^{2-}) are depleted in DKA, despite normal or elevated plasma levels on admission (68, 70, 71). Assessment and monitoring of circulating potassium is essential to the management of patients treated with insulin. Life-threatening complications frequently result from hypokalemia or hyperkalemia. Life-threatening hypokalemia may develop within 1 to 2 hours of initiating insulin therapy, even in patients with initial hyperkalemia.

K^+ deficits average 3 to 10 mEq/kg of body weight. In 4 to 10% of patients with DKA serum K^+ may be decreased on presentation, implying severe K^+ deficiency. The serum K^+ falls with therapy, reaching a nadir at 1 to 4 hours. The decrease is a result of (a) dilution from rehydration, (b) continued urinary K^+ loss because of volume expansion and hyperaldosteronism, (c) correction of acidosis with reentry of K^+ into the cell, and (d) increased cellular K^+ uptake as a result of insulin therapy (less with low-dose insulin). During treatment of DKA 20 to 50% of administered K^+ is lost in the urine (68). If bicarbonate is used, K^+ will reenter cells at an accelerated rate in exchange for hydrogen ions. Extra potassium may be required. The authors recommend adding K^+ to bicarbonate therapy (13 to 20 mEq K^+/100 mEq bicarbonate). K^+ requirements are reduced with renal insufficiency. However, these patients still require K^+ because other factors responsible for hypokalemia (discussed earlier in this section) are still operative. The authors withhold K^+ only when the serum K^+ is increased. Otherwise, 20 mEq K^+/hour is used to begin treatment as the chloride and/or PO_4^{2-} salt (Table 45.7). If the patient is oliguric, the K^+ dose is reduced by 20 to 50%. Potassium should be given along with insulin, since without insulin potassium cannot enter cells effectively and hyperkalemia may result. Decreases in serum potassium levels may not parallel changes in blood glucose. Both levels must be monitored during treatment. Adjustments in potassium are made based on serum K$^+$ measurements at intervals of 2 to 4 hours. Occasionally, patients may require 60 to 80 mEq/hour. Electrocardiogram (ECG) monitoring is also used as an index of hypokalemia or hyperkalemia (72). Hypokalemia is suggested by prominent U waves with apparent Q-T prolongation, T wave inversion, and sagging ST segments. Hyperkalemia produces peaked T waves, P-R prolongation, ST depression, QRS widening, P wave disappearance, and, finally, a sine wave configuration.

PO$_4^{2-}$ deficiency (deficits range from 0.5 to 1.5 mmol/kg) results from increased urinary losses, increased tissue catabolism, and impaired tissue uptake caused by insulin deficiency. Despite PO$_4^{2-}$ deficiency, only 11% of patients with DKA show hypophosphatemia when admitted to the hospital (73). PO$_4^{2-}$ decreases in the first 4 to 5 hours of DKA therapy as a result of insulin-induced shifts into cells and may reach levels less than 1 mg/dl (68, 74). PO$_4^{2-}$ deficiency is associated with insulin resistance (75, 76), decreased 2,3-diphosphoglycerate (2,3-DPG) (68, 75, 77), and decreased intracellular ATP. Depletion of 2,3-DPG alters the oxygen-hemoglobin dissociation curve and may contribute to tissue ischemia. This effect is important since patients with DKA have elevated hemoglobin A$_{1c}$ levels, a hemoglobin with very high affinity for oxygen. PO$_4^{2-}$ supplementation can restore 2,3-DPG levels to normal within 12 to 24 hours (78), whereas without supplementation it takes 72 to 96 hours (77). PO$_4$ deficiency is also associated with cardiac insufficiency, hemolysis, respiratory failure, and rhabdomyolysis. Although studies have not clearly demonstrated a benefit of PO$_4^{2-}$ therapy in DKA, some researchers (79, 80) have suggested more prompt recovery. In addition, if one evaluates all patients with severe hypophosphatemia who develop symptoms, insulin treatment of DKA is a common cause of the hypophosphatemia. K$^+$ deficits (3 to 10 mEq/kg) exceed PO$_4^{2-}$ deficits (1 mmol/kg); thus, to avoid hyperphosphatemia one should replace K$^+$ with a combination of KCl and K$_2$PO$_4$. The authors recommend giving PO$_4^{2-}$ orally (Neutra-Phos 250-mg capsule every 6 hours) if possible, and if parenteral therapy is required the dosage should be 0.08 to 0.16 mmol/kg/6 hr as potassium phosphate. Serum PO$_4^{2-}$ and calcium levels should be monitored every 6 hours and the PO$_4^{2-}$ dosage adjusted accordingly. Complications of PO$_4^{2-}$ therapy include hyperphosphatemia, hypocalcemia, hypotension, and metastatic calcification (81, 82).

Insulin treatment alone will gradually reverse the metabolic acidosis of diabetic ketoacidosis by inhibiting lipolysis and ketogenesis. Thus, routine administration of bicarbonate is usually unnecessary. Bicarbonate therapy should be withheld unless the arterial pH is less than 7.1, since acidosis is well-tolerated in patients with DKA (83). Acidosis shifts the oxygen-hemoglobin dissociation curve to the right (increases tissue oxygenation) and counteracts the effect of lowered 2,3-DPG levels; therefore, rapid correction of the pH may augment tissue hypoxia. In addition, rapid correction of pH with bicarbonate exaggerates hypokalemia and can lead to a paradoxic fall in CNS pH (84). Upon initiation of insulin, AcAc and βOHB are metabolized to bicarbonate and thus the pH will correct on its own. If alkali is given, there may be an overshoot and late alkalosis. On the other hand, severe acidosis

(pH <7.1) should also be prevented, since it produces cardiovascular, CNS, and respiratory depression. The authors suggest treating a pH less than 7.1 or a serum bicarbonate level less than 5 to 7 mEq/liter. One-half ampule of bicarbonate (22 mEq) should be given for a pH less than 7.1, and one ampule of bicarbonate (44 mEq) for a pH less than 7.0. It is also recommended that serum magnesium levels be checked since hypomagnesemia is common in DKA (as a result of renal losses and intracellular shift with insulin) and treated if they are low.

Low-dose intravenous insulin infusion regimens (3 to 10 U regular insulin/hr) are as effective as high-dose insulin in reducing blood sugar and correcting acidosis in DKA and are associated with a decreased incidence of hypoglycemia, hypokalemia, hypophosphatemia, and hypomagnesium (19, 68, 85–90). Lipolysis begins to be inhibited by an insulin concentration of 5 μU/ml, proteolysis by 10 μU/ml, and hepatic glucose production by 20 μU/ml (67). Peripheral glucose utilization is not maximally stimulated until an insulin concentration of 100 μU/ml is achieved. To allow for insulin resistance, a circulating insulin concentration of 200 μU/ml is desired. These levels are achieved with intravenous insulin infusion rates of 3 to 10 U/hr (0.1 U/kg/hr). Insulin suppresses glucagon levels, reestablishing hepatic glycogenesis and preventing glycogenolysis. Insulin causes an increase in fructose 2,6-bisphosphate, which blocks hepatic gluconeogenesis and activates hepatic glycolysis. An increase in malonyl CoA inhibits ketogenesis. In adipocytes insulin inhibits lipolysis, and in the periphery insulin increases glucose uptake (Fig. 45.1). The blood glucose decreases at a rate of 70 to 75 mg/dl/hr in most patients with DKA, reaching a level of 250 mg/dl in 4 to 8 hours. Correction of acidosis usually takes 8 to 12 hours because of the slower metabolism of ketone bodies.

In the critical care setting regular insulin should be given intravenously in the initial phases of therapy. Intramuscular or subcutaneous insulin injections may be poorly and erratically absorbed in the dehydrated patient and may produce undesirable tissue depots. In addition, in the event of complications (i.e., hypokalemia or hypoglycemia) the intravenous infusion can be stopped, allowing for quick reversal of the insulin effect (plasma half-life of 3 to 5 minutes). Intravenous insulin should be given as a continuous infusion rather than by bolus injection, since bolus administration results in stimulation of counterregulatory hormones (49, 91). A loading dose of insulin is also unnecessary in view of the rapid rate at which insulin values reach a plateau with an infusion (91). Despite this fact, there may be a theoretic advantage of a small intravenous bolus (1 U regular insulin for each 100 mg/dl increase in blood glucose above 100 mg/dl) to saturate insulin receptors. The authors recommend starting with a continuous infusion of 0.5 to 1.0 U/hr regular insulin for each 100 mg/dl increase in blood glucose above 100 mg/dl (in isotonic saline). In children, a dose of 0.1 U/kg/hr may be used. If serum glucose does not decrease by at least 10% each hour, the infusion rate should be increased by 3 to 5 U/hr and the process repeated. In evaluating the effectiveness of the insulin dose, the clinician should remember that blood glucose falls 35 to 70 mg/dl in the first hour from hydration alone. On rare occasions patients with DKA may have insulin resistance and require larger doses of insulin. Failure to respond to 5 to 7 U/hr, however, should suggest infection. The dosages just discussed apply to DKA; however, insulin infusions are also used to treat non-DKA hyperglycemia in critically ill patients. In this latter group, who may be receiving 50% dextrose (in total parenteral nutrition), corticosteroids, or catecholamines, large insulin infusion dosages (>20 U/hr) may be required (92).

There is usually no need to give less than 3 to 4 U regular insulin per hour during the initial few hours of DKA therapy. Use of too little insulin may be dangerous in that it may delay correction of metabolic abnormalities. Doses below 2.4 U regular insulin per hour have not been found to correct metabolic derangements with acceptable rapidity (93, 94), and if insulin resistance is present such doses are insufficient (95). Maximal biologic effect of insulin requires serum insulin concentrations in the 100 to 200 μU/ml range (91, 96). This level is usually obtained with an insulin infusion rate of approximately 0.1 U/kg/hr.

A small amount of insulin added to infusions is absorbed to glassware and plastic tubing (97, 98). Absorption during the initial period of infusion can be minimized by running 20 to 30 ml of insulin solution through the intravenous tubing before connecting it to the patient (99). This infusion will saturate all "insulin-binding" sites on the tubing. However, the quantity of insulin absorbed to tubing is small and not clinically significant. The practice of adding a small amount of albumin to infusion bottles is not cost-effective and has been abandoned at most hospitals. Once the plasma glucose level reaches 250 mg/dl, the insulin infusion is decreased to 1 to 3 U/hr and 5% dextrose is administered to maintain a serum glucose concentration of 200 to 250 mg/dl. The intravenous insulin infusion should be continued until acidosis is corrected, an effect that usually takes twice as long as normalization of the blood glucose. It is important to maintain blood glucose in the 150 to 200 mg/dl range for 24 to 48 hours in order to avoid potential complications of cerebral and pulmonary edema and hypoglycemia.

Cerebral edema (50, 100, 101) is a rare complication of DKA. It becomes clinically apparent 6 to 10 hours after therapy has begun, at a time when severe acidosis has been partially corrected, the blood glucose level is falling, adequate circulation has been restored, and all indications suggest that the patient is recovering satisfactorily. Cerebral edema is believed to result largely from the development of unfavorable osmotic gradients that favor intracellular movement of water (68). During sustained hyperglycemia the brain makes "idiogenic osmoles" that protect it from continued dehydration (102, 103). Cerebral edema develops when the osmotic gradient between brain and plasma exceeds 35 mosm/kg of water. If blood glucose concentration remains above 200 to 250 mg/dl (with initial values of 800 mg/dl) and the serum osmolality is not reduced faster than 2 to 3 mosm/kg/hr, the osmolar gradient usually remains below 30 mosm/kg water (103). Thus, it is recommended that blood glucose not be reduced faster than 100 mg/dl/hr or below 200 to 250 mg/dl during early therapy.

The clinical picture of cerebral edema is characterized by deteriorating mental status, abnormal neurologic signs, coma, papilledema, headache, dilated or unequal pupils, hyperpyrexia, nausea/vomiting, and, occasionally, diabetes insipidus. Respiratory arrest may occur in association with brainstem herniation. Cerebral edema complicating DKA has a mortality rate of about 90%. Treatment with glucocorticoids or mannitol is recommended, although there is little experience with this approach. Subclinical brain swelling is believed to be common during treatment of DKA (17), even though most patients fail to develop symptoms of cerebral edema.

Pulmonary edema (104) also results from unfavorable osmotic gradients and may cause hypoxia in more than 50% of those treated for DKA (105). Supplemental use of oxygen should be administered to these patients. Volume loading with crystalloid produces an acute hypooncotic state and may contribute to the development of pulmonary and cerebral edema (49). Most instances appear to be subclinical.

Stupor and coma in DKA correlate best with osmolality and not acidosis (106, 107). If the plasma osmolality does not exceed 340 to 350 mosm/liter, other causes of coma should be sought. Plasma osmolality (mosm/liter) may be measured directly or calculated according to the following equation:

$$P_{osm} = (2 \times [Na^+ + K^+ \ mEq/liter]) + \text{glucose (mg/dl)}/18 + \text{BUN (mg/dl)}/2.8$$

where normal = 285 to 300 mosm/liter.

To minimize wide swings in the blood glucose concentrations during intravenous insulin therapy, the carbohydrate substrate should be fixed at a given rate. To avoid intermittent boluses of dextrose, all intravenous additives should be in saline. By fixing carbohydrate substrate while infusing insulin, one can achieve a glucose "clamp" and avoid hypoglycemia and hyperglycemia.

The endpoint in the therapy of DKA is attainment of a desirable blood glucose level (usually, 150 to 250 mg/dl) and correction of acidosis. A blood glucose in this range offers protection from sudden drops in glucose, which may cause hypoglycemia. Based on the volume of the glucose space (approximately that of extracellular fluid) and rate of glucose decline, it is possible to approximate the rate of glucose administration. For example, in a 70-kg individual (glucose space = 21 liters) with a glucose disappearance rate of 100 mg/dl/hr the rate of glucose administration is 21 g/hr.

If staffing is short or close monitoring of the rate of intravenous insulin infusion cannot be achieved, it can be administered intramuscularly (half-life of 2 hours) or subcutaneously (half-life of 4 hours) (19, 85, 88). However, the initial decline in glucose and ketones will be slower in the first 2 hours when compared with intravenous insulin (88). Both of these routes carry the risk of erratic absorption (especially if the patient is dehydrated) and tissue depot accumulation (which can lead to late hypoglycemia). Another potential problem is the injection site. Injections into the buttocks can give variable absorption as a result of underperfusion (especially in supine patients). If intravenous administration is impossible or impractical, the authors suggest giving injections into the deltoid (19). The authors recommend giving 0.3 U regular insulin per kilogram initially, then 5 to 10 U regular insulin intramuscularly or subcutaneously hourly until the blood glucose level is less than 250 mg/dl. At that point, fluids should be switched to D_5NS, $D_5\frac{1}{2}NS$, or D_5W (glucose clamp) and intramuscular or subcutaneous insulin should be continued at 2- to 4-hour intervals until acidosis resolves.

Table 45.8. Adjustment of NPH Insulin[a]

Day	NPH Insulin	Regular Insulin	Sliding Scale
1	24 U NPH s.c. at 0600 AM; continue insulin infusion for 4–6 hours following NPH	0600 AM 1200 1800 PM 2400	4 U 0 U 6 U 4 U 14 U/2 = 7 U
2	24 U + 7 U = 31 U NPH s.c. at 0600 AM	0600 AM 1200 1800 PM 2400	4 U 0 U 4 U 0 U 8 U/2 = 4 U
3	31 U + 4 U = 35 U NPH s.c. at 0600 AM	0600 AM 1200 1800 PM 2400	0 U 0 U 0 U 0 U 0 U
4	35 U NPH at 0600 AM		

[a] Patient receiving continuous insulin infusion at 2 U/hr (48 U/day).

The response to treatment (e.g., normalization of plasma glucose, electrolytes, arterial blood gases, hemodynamic and mental status) must be monitored carefully (at least hourly) and therapy adjusted accordingly. The authors follow blood glucose at the bedside using dry chemistry blood glucose test strips (64, 65) and find them to reflect accurately the measured serum glucose levels. Urine glucose is inaccurate in estimating the serum glucose concentration in many patients because of variations in renal glucose threshold. Urine glucose also reflects plasma glucose at the time the urine is produced, not when it is excreted. Urine glucose does not provide a measure of hypoglycemia (108).

As soon as the DKA is under control, NPH insulin is begun and is supplemented with regular insulin given subcutaneously according to a sliding scale (Table 45.8). The insulin infusion is continued for 4 to 6 hours after the NPH insulin is given to keep the insulin receptors saturated, thereby preventing rebound hyperglycemia. The authors begin the subcutaneous NPH insulin by giving half of the patient's previous daily maintenance dose. Supplemental regular insulin is given at 6-hour intervals depending on plasma glucose. The next day's NPH insulin is increased by half the amount of supplemental regular insulin used in the preceding 24 hours (Table 45.8). There is tremendous variability in the total dose of insulin required by any patient, depending on whether one is dealing with a type I or type II diabetic; the presence of insulin-binding antibodies; the patient's diet, activity level, and stress state; and other factors (15). Most newly diagnosed type I diabetics require approximately 0.5 U/kg/day of insulin, whereas established type I diabetics usually require 0.6 to 0.7 U/kg/day. Some patients may be controlled on a single dose of intermediate-acting insulin per day (with or without concomitant short-acting insulin); others require twice-daily injections of intermediate/short-acting insulin. Dosage decisions are based upon fasting and postprandial serum or blood glucose concentrations. Patients who eat three meals during the day and who require multiple insulin injections usually require two-thirds of their total insulin dose before breakfast and one-third of their insulin dose before dinner (15).

Treatment of DKA must not be confined to correction of biochemical abnormalities alone. Precipitating factors and complications must be sought and treated. Common precipitating factors include infection (109), myocardial infarction, pancreatitis, and discontinuation of insulin therapy. Common sites of infection (109) include the urinary tract, respiratory tract, sinuses, middle ear, skin, soft tissues, and gallbladder. Shock may develop as a consequence of hypovolemia and reduced myocardial contractility. Cerebral and pulmonary edema were discussed previously. Disseminated intravascular coagulation is also being recognized increasingly (49).

HYPERGLYCEMIC HYPEROSMOLAR NONKETOTIC SYNDROME

The hyperglycemic hyperosmolar nonketotic syndrome (HHNS) typically develops in middle-aged and elderly patients in the setting of previously mild, non-insulin-dependent (type II) diabetes mellitus or as the first manifestation of diabetes (110–114). The syndrome can also occur in nondiabetic patients as a complication of extensive burns, heat stroke, myocardial or cerebral infarction, acute pancreatitis, infections, surgery, thyrotoxicosis, trauma, and acromegaly (112). In addition, it may occur in association with dialysis or intravenous hyperalimentation. Mortality is between 5 and 40%. Most patients experience polydipsia and polyuria during a prodromal phase of several days to a few weeks, culminating in severe dehydration and altered consciousness. The syndrome occurs most frequently in older patients in whom an intercurrent illness increases glucose production (from stress hormones) and impairs the capacity to ingest fluids. Drugs most frequently associated with the syndrome include thiazide diuretics, phenytoin, corticosteroids, cimetidine, furosemide, propranolol, chlorpromazine, and L-asparaginase (see "Drug Interactions"). The pathophysiology involves an imbalance between glucose production and its excretion in the urine. Maximal hepatic production of glucose results in a plateau of plasma glucose in the 400 to 500 mg/dl range provided urine output is maintained. Severe hyperglycemia results when there is renal impairment (progressive glucose accumulation resulting from impaired renal glucose excretion) and dehydration (110, 111, 114, 115). The exact mechanism by which ketoacidosis is suppressed despite extreme hyperglycemia is unknown but appears to result from impaired lipolysis and liver ketogenesis. Joffe and associates (116) suggest that the syndrome occurs because the liver is insulinized while the periphery is diabetic. Others have postulated a defect in ketone synthesis within the liver.

Symptoms (Table 45.9) last longer (12 days) than in DKA (3 days) (111, 112). Transient, focal neurologic signs may occur (117), and occasionally the patient is misdiagnosed as having had a stroke. Some patients present with seizures, since hyperosmolality may activate epileptogenic foci (112). It is important to recognize the hyperosmolar nature of the etiology, since treatment with phenytoin may be hazardous because it impairs insulin release. The depressed sensorium parallels the hyperosmolarity and requires prompt treatment (113). Therapeutic delay is a primary cause of mortality (110). Osmolarity may be measured by the freezing point depression technique or calculated, and values above 350 mosm/liter typically are seen. Hyperglycemia is usually severe (>600 mg/dl), with levels as high as 4800 mg/dl recorded. Total absence of ketonuria is not essential, but when present it is mild and may result from starvation. Patients are severely dehydrated on presentation despite adequate (>0.5 ml/kg/hr) urine output, because of the glucosuria-induced osmotic diuresis. The serum sodium concentration may be low, normal, or increased when the patient is admitted. However, one must remember that serum sodium is lowered by about 1.5 mEq/liter for each 100 mg/dl of glucose above normal. The hematocrit usually is increased as a result of hemoconcentration. Nearly all HHNS patients present with azotemia, which may be of both renal and prerenal origin. A metabolic acidosis is often present with a large anion gap. Unmeasured anions are thought to result from lactate, renal insufficiency, and other unidentified organic acids.

Therapy of HHNS (Table 45.10) is aimed at correction of the volume depletion and metabolic abnormalities (e.g., hyperosmolarity) and detection of precipitating factors (67). The first priority is immediate restoration of intravascular volume, which is accomplished with 0.9% saline. Once hypotension is abolished, hypotonic saline should be given to replace free water losses. The glucose-induced osmotic diuresis results in large urinary losses of both water and electrolytes.

Contraction of intravascular volume is partially compensated for by movement of intracellular and interstitial fluid and electrolytes into the intravascular space. The result is a contraction of the intracellular compartment and depletion of sodium, potassium, phosphorus, and magnesium. Balance studies suggest that the fluid lost in HHNS contains about 60 mEq/liter of sodium plus potassium (110), which closely approximates half-normal saline. Use of isotonic saline and isotonic glucose are associated with higher mortality rates (113).

The authors assume that the patient with HHNS is depleted of about 25% of his or her total body water on presentation (110). Using the patient's usual weight, the body water deficit is estimated (mean total body water in elderly patients is about 50% of body weight in kilograms). Half of the estimated water deficit is administered as 0.45% saline (including urinary losses) in the first 12 hours and the remainder in the next 24 hours. The authors usually give 2 to 3 liters of 0.45% saline over the first 2 hours followed by one-half the body water deficit over the next 12 hours. Usual deficits range from 6 to 18 liters of fluid (110, 111, 113). Water can shift abruptly into cells as the plasma glucose concentration decreases. Patients must be observed closely, and adjustments in the rate of fluid administration must be made as indicated. Dangers inherent in aggressive fluid therapy (especially in the elderly) can be reduced with central hemodynamic monitoring.

Patients with HHNS are depleted of potassium, phosphorous, and magnesium (see the section entitled "Diabetic Ketoacidosis"). Hypokalemia in patients who have just been admitted indicates severe depletion and occasionally is associated with acute quadriplegia (118). The potassium requirements in the first 36 hours usually average 200 to 300 mEq (110, 113). Precipitous decreases in serum potassium occur as a result of hemodilution, insulin therapy, correction of acidosis, and continued urinary losses. If the patient is hyperkalemic, potassium therapy is withheld until the serum potassium concentration normalizes. Otherwise, 10 to 20 mEq of potassium are given per hour, mostly as the chloride, and to a lesser degree as the phosphate salt. The potassium replacement dose is reduced by 50% if the patient is oliguric. Further therapy with phosphorus, magnesium, and bicarbonate are the same as for DKA.

Intravenous regular insulin should be administered by continuous infusion. Patients with HHNS usually are more sensitive to insulin than those with DKA and therefore less total insulin is required. The authors begin the insulin infusion at 0.5 to 1.0 U regular insulin for each 100 mg/dl increase in blood glucose above 100 mg/dl (mixed in hypotonic saline) and taper accordingly (see the section entitled "Diabetic Ketoacidosis"). When the blood glucose concentration reaches 250 to 300 mg/dl, the intravenous fluid is switched to D$_5$W and the insulin infusion rate decreased to 1 to 3 U/hr. A glucose clamp is established and maintained for 24 to 36 hours to avoid the possibility of cerebral edema. The endpoint of the initial therapy is correction of hyperglycemia, normalization of serum osmolality (to less than 310 mosm/liter), and stabilization of the hemodynamic status (e.g., urine output and blood pressure). The change from

Table 45.9. Clinical Features of Hyperglycemic Hyperosmolar Nonketotic Syndrome

General
  Polydipsia, polyuria
  Dehydration
  Gastric distension
  Hyperthermia
  Ileus
Neurologic
  Seizures
  Mental obtundation (lethargy to coma)
  Focal neurologic signs (hemiparesis, unilateral hyperreflexia, aphasia, hemianopsia)
Cardiovascular
  Hypotension, shock
  Thromboses
Respiratory
  Tachypnea (no Kussmaul breathing)
Laboratory findings
  Hyperglycemia (>600 mg/dl)
  Hyperosmolality (>350 mosm/liter)
  Azotemia (blood urea nitrogen 70–90 mg/dl)
  Absent or mild ketonemia
  Glycosuria (4+)
  Acidosis (lactate)
  Hemoconcentration

Table 45.10.   Treatment of Hyperglycemic Hyperosmolar Nonketotic Syndrome

Fluids
    Restore intravascular volume with isotonic saline, then:
    Give 2–3 liters hypotonic saline (0.45%) in first 2 hours followed by one-half of the body water deficit (0.25 × total body water (kg) +
    urinary losses) over the next 12 hours; give the remainder of the body water deficit over the next 24 hours; central hemodynamic
    monitoring may be required in elderly or in those with cardiac or renal disease.
Insulin
    Begin with i.v. infusion of 0.5–1.0 U regular insulin for each 100 mg/dl increase in blood glucose above 100 mg/dl (in hypotonic saline).
    When serum glucose drops to 250 mg/dl, switch fluid to D_5W and decrease infusion rate of regular insulin to 1–3 U/hour (glucose
    clamp technique). Maintain infusion for 24–36 hours. Increase infusion rate if glucose does not fall by 10%/hr.
        Alternative
            5–7 U regular insulin i.m. or s.c. per hour; when glucose drops to 250 mg/dl, continue i.m. or s.c. injections at 2–4 hour intervals
            using glucose clamp.
Potassium
    Give 15–20 mEq/hr; if the patient is oliguric, give 5–10 mEq/hour; if K^+ above 6 mEq/liter, stop infusion of K^+; if K^+ below 4 mEq/
    liter, increase infusion rate. Use continuous ECG monitoring.
Phosphorus
    Oral: Neutra-Phos 250 mg every 6 hours.
    i.v.: potassium phosphate 0.08–0.16 mmol/kg/6 hr.
Bicarbonate
    If arterial pH <7.1 or bicarbonate <5–7 mEq/liter, give ½ ampule bicarbonate (22 mEq); if pH <7.0, give one ampule bicarbonate (44
    mEq); monitor arterial or venous pH hourly.
Magnesium
    If less than 1.2 mg/dl, give:
    p.o.: Mg oxide 35 mEq every 6–24 hr.
    i.v.: $MgSO_4$ or $MgCl_2$ 20–80 mEq/day.
    Monitor serum glucose, electrolytes, arterial blood gas, anion gap, and hemodynamic and mental status.

intravenous to subcutaneous insulin is similar to that for DKA. Complications of therapy include hypokalemia, hypophosphatemia, hypomagnesemia, hypoglycemia, cerebral edema, pulmonary edema (from aggressive fluid resuscitation and unfavorable osmotic gradients), and, rarely, intravascular hemolysis. As in DKA, careful monitoring of the plasma glucose and electrolytes, ECG, and hemodynamic status are essential.

NON-INSULIN-DEPENDENT DIABETES MELLITUS

Non-insulin-dependent diabetes mellitus (NIDDM) is a heterogeneous disorder of glucose metabolism with a strong genetic component. This disorder frequently is precipitated by obesity, stress, and aging (119). These patients manifest hyperglycemia as a result of insulin resistance and insufficient insulin secretion.

Acute complications in these patients are caused by hyperglycemia and infections. Chronic complications result from macrovascular disease, microvascular disease (i.e., kidneys, retina), and neuropathies. Fifty to sixty percent of deaths result from coronary heart disease. Cerebrovascular complications are also common.

Treatment consists of diet therapy, exercise, and use of pharmacologic agents to control blood sugar. Goals of diet therapy are weight reduction (if the patient is obese), lowering of blood glucose levels, and improvement in serum lipid profile. The recommended nutritional content of the diet for patients with NIDDM is 50 to 60% of total calories as complex carbohydrate, less than 30% of total calories as fat, and 12 to 20% as protein. Pharmacologic therapy is adjusted to match dietary intake.

Pharmacologic treatment of patients with NIDDM consists of oral hypoglycemic agents (see section in this chapter), insulin, or, rarely, combinations of insulin and oral hypoglycemics (119).

ALCOHOLIC KETOACIDOSIS

Alcoholic ketoacidosis is seen in the setting of recently discontinued heavy alcohol use (68, 120–123). Differentiation from DKA with a low blood glucose may be difficult (especially if it occurs in a known diabetic). Typically, these patients are chronic alcoholics with diminished food intake. There is usually little or no ethanol in the blood at the time of presentation. The mechanism responsible for alcoholic ketoacidosis is only partially understood. Ethanol is metabolized by alcohol dehydrogenase to acetaldehyde, which is metabolized to acetyl-CoA. The process generates reduced nicotinamide adenine dinucleotide (NADH) from NAD^+. Gluconeogenesis is impaired because this process requires NAD^+. When glycogen is exhausted, hypoglycemia results. The resultant low insulin state promotes lipolysis and ketogenesis. A "reduced" environment also inhibits the tricarboxylic acid cycle and favors the formation of lactate instead of pyruvate and βOHB instead of AcAc, contributing to acidosis. A variety of lipolytic hormones are released, possibly because of the hypoglycemia that results from inhibited gluconeogenesis and depleted glycogen stores. Released growth hormone, cortisol, glucagon, and catecholamines increase the availability of free fatty acids, which results in the formation of ketones. Low blood insulin levels, as well as alcohol itself, augment the ketotic state. The final result is augmented hepatic ketogenesis and decreased peripheral ketone utilization.

When metabolic acidosis occurs in an alcoholic with high blood alcohol concentrations, it is likely to be lactic acidosis. However, when it occurs in the presence of falling, low, or absent blood ethanol concentrations, the acidosis is usually the result of alcoholic ketoacidosis (68).

Patients with alcoholic ketoacidosis present with normal or altered mental status, tachycardia, tachypnea, dehydration, and signs of alcohol abuse (e.g., hepatomegaly, jaundice, and portal hypertension). Laboratory studies show a metabolic acidosis (mean anion gap 25 mEq/liter) with ketosis. The arterial pH is usually less than 7.20. The predominant ketone in this condition is βOHB, and thus the nitroprusside reaction underestimates the degree of ketosis. Blood glucose concentrations vary from those of hypoglycemia (≤50 mg/dl) to mild hyperglycemia (300 mg/dl). Blood ethanol is usually absent, and most patients have azotemia and hemoconcentration as a result of dehydration. Patients may also have increased serum transaminases, alkaline phosphatase, bilirubin, and amylase. Management (121–124) consists of replacement of intravascular volume, in addition to the administration of glucose, electrolytes, and thiamine (100 mg administered intravenously). In diabetics or in patients with hyperglycemia, insulin may also be required (121–124). Sodium bicarbonate is given only if the pH is less than 7.10. Glucose stimulates phosphorylation of ADP to ATP and reduces lactate production. The intracellular availability of glucose and thiamine produces NADPH via the pentose phosphate shunt. NADPH, in turn, decreases fatty acid metabolism to ketones. During correction of alcoholic ketoacidosis there is a decrease in the serum potassium, phosphate, and magnesium concentrations. Hypophosphatemia (123) results from phosphaturia and phosphate utilization in metabolic processes.

CARE OF THE DIABETIC SURGICAL PATIENT

Preoperative evaluation of the diabetic includes identification of other underlying diseases (125, 126). Such patients frequently have coronary artery disease, a major cause of perioperative mortality, and peripheral vascular disease. Those patients with renal disease require careful fluid and electrolyte management and adjustment of drug dosages. Some diabetics have autonomic neuropathy that may predispose them to respiratory depression, cardiac arrest, urinary retention, and postural hypotension (127). Diabetics often have an increased risk of infection and poor wound healing.

Cardiac bypass surgery may present special problems for the diabetic (128). The bypass pump may have glucose-containing fluids, and as a result patients may receive up to 500 g of extra glucose during surgery. In addition, hypothermia and use of sympathomimetic drugs cause insulin resistance.

The objective of the management of diabetes before, during, and after operations is to prevent excessive hyperglycemia and glycosuria, to prevent ketosis, and to prevent hypoglycemia. Prior to surgery the diabetic's blood glucose level should be well-controlled (150 to 200 mg/dl range) and the patient should be free of acidemia (125). The patient should not have symptoms of polydipsia, polyuria, or hypoglycemia. Slight hyperglycemia is desirable to protect against hypoglycemia during surgery. Electrolyte concentrations and volume status should also be normalized.

For minor surgery, in the diet-controlled diabetic in good glycemic control, no insulin therapy is required. Glucose-containing solutions should be avoided and if control deteriorates, insulin may be given. In patients taking oral hypoglycemic agents, the medication should be stopped 3 days prior to surgery. If glycemic control is good on diet alone, no insulin is required for minor surgery. If glucose control becomes poor or major surgery is required, insulin may be needed.

In the diabetic undergoing major surgery or in insulin-dependent diabetics, the combined administration of glucose-insulin-potassium is often effective (117) (Table 45.11). Intravenous glucose is needed to avoid starvation ketosis. Patients are stabilized preoperatively on twice-daily subcutaneous injections of insulin, with only regular insulin (every 6 hours) being given on the day prior to surgery. No subcutaneous insulin is given on the day of surgery. On the morning of surgery, an insulin infusion at 2 to 3 U regular insulin per hour with 100 ml/hr of 10% dextrose and 2 mEq potassium chloride per hour is begun and continued until the patient resumes oral feeding and subcutaneous insulin. Glucose, electrolytes, and ketones are monitored at 2- to 3-hour intervals and intravenous insulin adjusted accordingly. Insulin requirements are increased with infection and decreased in patients undergoing adrenalectomy or hypophysectomy and in postdelivery patients.

An alternative form of perioperative therapy includes the use of subcutaneous insulin and intravenous glucose. Patients are stabilized on subcutaneous injections of regular insulin (128, 129). On the operative day, oral carbohydrate is replaced with an equivalent amount of 5% or 10% dextrose by intravenous infusion. Insulin therapy (regular) is given by subcutaneous injection every 6 hours. Additional perioperative insulin is given intramuscularly or intravenously as needed, and electrolytes are replaced as required.

Another method for managing the diabetic in the perioperative period is to give one-half of the usual dose of insulin (NPH + Reg) as NPH on the morning of surgery and to cover the patient with a short-acting insulin at frequent intervals. The authors give regular insulin by the subcutaneous route (every 4 to 6 hours). However, one must remember that subcutaneous insulin may be poorly absorbed in the perioperative period. Hypoglycemia is prevented by intravenous administration of dextrose.

Close monitoring of blood/serum potassium levels is important during perioperative support of diabetic patients. Hypokalemia may result from insulin-induced translocation of potassium into cells and ongoing urinary/gut losses. Intracellular shift of potassium may also result from use of sympathomimetic drugs (e.g., epinephrine, dobutamine) and rewarming following intraoperative hypothermia. On the other hand, these patients may develop hyperkalemia as these drugs are tapered in the postoperative period. Other factors that predispose to hyperkalemia include sympathetic neuropathies, renal insufficiency, and hypoaldosteronism. Thus, the authors frequently see hypokalemia in diabetic patients early following

Table 45.11. Glucose-Insulin-Potassium During Surgery

Preoperative
  Switch to twice-daily s.c. insulin; give short-acting insulin only on day prior to surgery (every 6 hours).
Operation
  Begin i.v. infusion of 100 ml D_{10} plus 2–3 U regular insulin plus 2–3 mEq K per hour on morning of surgery. Monitor glucose and K^+ at 2–3 hour intervals and readjust as required. Use dry chemistry reagent strips for quick evaluation of bedside blood glucose.
Postoperative
  Continue glucose-insulin-potassium until oral feeding is resumed. Check glucose and electrolytes at 4–6 hour intervals. When feeding resumes, return to preoperative s.c. insulin.

surgery (i.e., after cardiac or major vascular surgery). These patients are stabilized using a combination of insulin, glucose, and potassium infusions. Many patients are managed with inotropic and vasoactive drugs. Hyperkalemia is not uncommon 24 to 48 hours after surgery when the infusion rates of the cardiovascular drugs and insulin are being decreased.

The most important factor in managing the diabetic in the perioperative period is careful and frequent monitoring. Blood glucose must be monitored (every 2 to 3 hours) so as to avoid marked hyperglycemia or hypoglycemia. This step is particularly important in the early perioperative period when counter-regulatory hormones are elevated. The authors use dry chemistry blood glucose test strips (64, 65) for rapid evaluation of blood glucose and find them to be more reliable than urine glucose measurements. The renal threshold for glucose may be elevated (as a result of renal insufficiency) and lead to an underestimation of blood glucose (64). In addition, a number of drugs interfere with urine measurements. For Clinitest, Clinstix, or Diastix these include cephalosporins, chloramphenicol, tetracycline, sulfonamides, and salicylates. Ketones should also be monitored (every 4 to 6 hours) so as to avoid ketoacidosis. Hypoglycemia during surgery is uncommon with these regimens, since the stress of surgery leads to hyperglycemia because of the action of counterregulatory hormones.

INSULIN-INFUSION PUMP THERAPY

Two types of insulin-infusion pumps exist for improvement of diabetic control (130–133): closed loop systems (artificial pancreas), in which the rate of insulin administration is controlled by changes in plasma glucose; and open loop systems, in which predetermined amounts of insulin are administered on the basis of previous estimates of insulin requirement. In the critically ill patient with fluctuating metabolic status, a closed loop system would be required. At present, these units are large, bulky, and expensive, and they have not been shown to be superior to continuous intravenous insulin infusion therapy for short-term diabetic control.

TOTAL PARENTERAL NUTRITION

Serum glucose should not exceed 150 to 200 mg/dl during total parenteral nutrition (TPN) to allow for maximal cellular glucose utilization. Glucosuria should be prevented, since it produces an osmotic diuresis (with loss of fluid and electrolytes) and calorie loss. Glucosuria also prevents the clinician from using urine output as an index of tissue perfusion. As TPN is started, the pancreas responds by increasing insulin secretion. Exogenous insulin is required when the rate of glucose administration exceeds the ability of the pancreas to respond. In some patients, insulin administration may be reduced after 3 to 6 days as endogenous insulin secretion becomes adequate and insulin resistance (e.g., malnutrition, stress, or infection) decreases (18). Sudden discontinuation of TPN may cause hypoglycemia because of high rates of endogenous insulin secretion, and thus TPN should be tapered as oral intake increases or intravenous dextrose should be administered. To avoid large fluctuations in blood glucose,

exogenous insulin should be administered by continuous infusion in the parenteral nutrition fluid. The authors recommend following the schedule of Grant (18) by adding regular insulin to parenteral nutrition fluid based upon the blood glucose level (Table 45.12). Blood glucose is monitored and additional insulin added as required. Insulin requirements may vary from 5 to 40 U/hr, and at very high rates of dextrose administration normoglycemia may be unobtainable (as a result of downregulation of insulin receptors). Decreasing the infusion rate may allow for return of insulin sensitivity. Insulin, as an anabolic hormone, may also help the severely catabolic patient convert from negative to positive nitrogen balance.

Table 45.12.   Initial Insulin Requirements for Parenteral Nutrition

Blood Glucose (mg/dl)	Regular Insulin (U/250 g dextrose)
<120	0
120–150	6–10
150–200	10–20
>200	21 (or more)

Table 45.13.   Insulin-Drug Interactions

Inhibit insulin secretion
  Prostaglandin E (furosemide)
  Thiazides
  Phenytoin
  Diazoxide
  α-Adrenergic agonists
  β-Adrenergic antagonists
  Pentamidine
  Verapamil
  Somatostatin
  Dopamine
Suppress insulin action or increase insulin requirements
  Glucocorticoids
  Oral contraceptives
  L-Asparaginase
  Growth hormone
  Obesity
  Pregnancy
  Infection
  Hyperthyroidism
  Hyperadrenocorticalism
Stimulate insulin secretion
  Sulfonylureas
  Salicylates
  Phentolamine
  Prostaglandin inhibitors
  Glucagon
  β-Adrenergic agonists
Potentiate insulin action or decrease insulin requirements
  Sulfonylureas
  Clonidine
  Dicumarol
  Terramycin
  Monoamine oxidase inhibitors
  Endotoxin
  Weight loss
  Exercise
  Renal insufficiency
  Pentamidine
  Hypothyroidism
  Hypoadrenocorticalism

Table 45.14. Sulfonylurea Oral Hypoglycemic Agents

	Tolbutamide	*Acetohexamide*	*Tolazamide*	*Chlorpromide*	*Glipizide*	*Glyburide*
Relative potency	1	2.5	5	5	100	150
Duration (hr)	6–8	8–12	12–18	24–72	12–18	16–24
Daily dose	0.5–3 g	0.25–1.5 g	0.1–1 g	0.1–0.5 g	2.5–30 mg	1.25–20 mg
Doses per day	2–3	1–2	1–2	1	1–2	1–2
Inactivation	Hepatic	Renal	Hepatic	Hepatic/renal	Hepatic	Hepatic
Diuretic	Yes	Yes	Yes	No	No	Yes
Antidiuretic	Yes?	No	No	Yes	No	No
Antabuse effect	No	No	No	Yes	No	No
Frequency of hypoglycemia	Rare	<1%	<1%	2–3%	3–5%	4–6%

DRUG INTERACTIONS

A number of drugs affect insulin secretion or action (Table 45.13). Prostaglandin E (PgE) inhibits insulin secretion (9, 134, 135). Furosemide, by stimulating PgE, inhibits insulin secretion, whereas tolbutamide, phentolamine, and salicylates stimulate insulin secretion by inhibiting PgE synthesis (8–10, 134, 135). Thiazides, phenytoin, α-adrenergic receptor agonists (e.g., norepinephrine), verapamil, somatostatin, dopamine, diazoxide, and β-adrenergic antagonists decrease insulin secretion (5, 62, 80, 136–141). Epinephrine and other β-adrenergic agonists stimulate insulin secretion. However, these agents usually cause hyperglycemia by impairing peripheral insulin action, stimulating gluconeogenesis, and increasing glycogenolysis. β-Adrenergic antagonists have the opposite effects and predispose to hypoglycemia. Pentamidine (an antiprotozoal agent) can cause both hypoglycemia (destruction of β-cells with release of insulin) and hyperglycemia (continued β-cell destruction with resultant hypoinsulinemia).

A variety of agents interfere with peripheral insulin action (Table 45.13). Corticosteroids decrease hepatic and extrahepatic insulin sensitivity (142), enhancing gluconeogenesis while they decrease peripheral glucose utilization by decreasing the insulin receptor concentration (143). In addition, estrogens, growth hormone, and L-asparaginase (144) also decrease insulin binding to insulin receptors. Sulfonylureas increase insulin secretion and receptor binding (145). Sulfonylureas cross the placenta and stimulate hypersecretion of insulin in neonates. Neonates of mothers who receive these agents may require intravenous glucose for 3 to 4 days after delivery to prevent hypoglycemia.

In hyperthyroidism there is decreased insulin sensitivity (146), whereas in endotoxemia there is increased sensitivity as well as decreased gluconeogenesis (124). These effects of endotoxemia are responsible for the hypoglycemia occasionally seen with sepsis. In sepsis, antagonism of insulin by dexamethasone and ATP improves survival (124). Ethanol enhances insulin action (147) by impairing gluconeogenesis and secretion of counterregulatory hormones. In renal insufficiency and malnutrition, decreased gluconeogenesis and slowed insulin degradation contribute to enhanced insulin effect (148).

ORAL HYPOGLYCEMIC AGENTS

A variety of oral agents (Table 45.14) are available for the treatment of diabetes mellitus that stimulate insulin secretion

Table 45.15. Drugs that Alter the Effect of Oral Hypoglycemic Agents

Potentiate	*Antagonize*
Alcohol	Chronic ethanolism
Anabolic steroids	Corticosteroids
β-Adrenergic blockers	Diazoxide
Bishydroxycoumarin	Estrogens
Chloramphenicol	Furosemide
Clofibrate[a]	Nicotinic acid
Cyclophosphamide	Phenytoin (decreased insulin)
Diphenylhydantoin[a]	Rifampin
Guanethidine	Thiazides
Halofenate	Thyroid hormone
Methysergide	
Monoamine oxidase inhibitors	
Oral anticoagulants	
Oxyphenbutazone[a]	
Phenylbutazone[a]	
Salicylates[a]	
Sulfonamides	
Tetracyclines	

[a] Decrease binding to plasma proteins.

and improve insulin action. Sulfonylurea drugs are the only oral agents available in the U.S. These agents are well-absorbed from the gastrointestinal tract (1, 149), and peak levels occur 1 to 4 hours after ingestion. Sulfonylureas are divided into two generations. The first-generation drugs include tolbutamide, acetohexamide, tolazamide, and chlorpropamide. Second-generation drugs are more potent than first-generation drugs and include glipizide, glyburide, and gliclazide (available in Europe).

Sulfonylurea compounds (Table 45.14) acutely stimulate the islet tissue to secrete insulin and are primarily effective in patients who retain the capacity to secrete insulin (e.g., those patients with type II diabetes mellitus). However, during chronic therapy a significant portion of their hypoglycemic action results from increases in the number of insulin receptors and postreceptor effects (149, 150). Sulfonylureas act synergistically with insulin to enhance glucose disposal, with little effect on glucose production. Sulfonylureas are ineffective in type I insulin-dependent diabetes mellitus and in pancreatectomized animals, suggesting that their major mechanism of action is dependent upon β-cell function. Sulfonylureas also stimulate release of somatostatin and may suppress the secretion of glucagon (1). These drugs bind to cell surface receptors on the pancreatic β-cell and decrease potassium conductance, similar to glucose (151). Reduced potassium conductance causes an influx of calcium and subsequent insulin secretion. The most important differences among the sulfonylureas, for clinical purposes, are their different potencies, duration of action (13, 15, 48, 149, 150), and metabolism.

These drugs are relatively contraindicated in patients with type I diabetes mellitus; in patients during pregnancy or lactation; in patients with hepatic or renal disease, because of the importance of the liver in metabolizing these drugs and the kidney in excreting them; in patients with known allergy to sulfa drugs; and during stressful conditions in diabetics (such as during infection, myocardial infarction, or surgery, when the ability to increase insulin secretion is diminished).

The major complication from sulfonylurea drugs is hypoglycemia (149, 150). Hypoglycemia is more likely in the elderly and in patients with diminished hepatic/renal function. Hypoglycemic episodes may last for several days because of the long duration of action of these drugs, and prolonged or repeated glucose administration may be required. Chlorpropamide and tolbutamide potentiate antidiuretic hormone action in the kidney and may cause water retention and hyponatremia. They may also cause an antabuse-like reaction. Sulfonylurea drugs have also been associated with a small incidence of hematologic (leukopenia, pancytopenia, and bone marrow depression), cutaneous, endocrine (e.g., hypothyroidism), and gastrointestinal (e.g., cholestatic jaundice and nausea) side effects. Drugs that may potentiate the action of sulfonylurea drugs (Table 45.15) are alcohol, β-adrenergic blockers, monoamine oxidase inhibitors, phenylbutazone, oxyphenbutazone, clofibrate, bishydroxycoumarin, sulfonamides, salicylates, and diphenylhydantoin (13, 15, 149). Drugs that may antagonize the action of sulfonylureas are thiazide and loop diuretics, estrogens, and corticosteroids (15).

Most authorities believe that there is little indication for use of sulfonylureas together with insulin (152–154). However, some patients may not respond well to insulin because of severe resistance. Such patients may show better glucose regulation using a combination of insulin and sulfonylureas (119, 155, 156). Allen et al. (155) treated six patients with non-insulin-dependent diabetes mellitus and insulin resistance with combination insulin-glipizide therapy. Four patients had considerable improvement in glycemic control when the sulfonylurea was added to their insulin treatment program. The authors have used combined sulfonylurea-insulin therapy on occasion to treat severely stressed (e.g., sepsis or trauma) non-insulin-dependent diabetics in the intensive care unit who demonstrated resistance to infusions of insulin and have also noted improvement in their glycemic control.

REFERENCES

1. Kahn CR, Schechter Y: Insulin, oral hypoglycemic agents, and the pharmacology of the endocrine pancreas. In Gilman AG, et al (eds): *The Pharmacological Basis of Therapeutics*, 8th ed. New York, Pergamon Press, 1990, pp 1463–1495.
2. Felig P: The endocrine pancreas: diabetes mellitus. In Felig P, et al (eds): *Endocrinology and Metabolism*. New York, McGraw-Hill, 1981, pp 761–868.
3. Creutzfeldt W: The incretin concept today. *Diabetologia* 16:75–85, 1979.
4. Brown JC, Otte SC: Gastrointestinal hormones and the control of insulin secretion. *Diabetes* 27:782–787, 1977.
5. Porte D Jr, Smith PH, Ensinck JW: Neurohumoral regulation of the pancreatic islet A and B cells. *Metabolism* 25 (suppl 1):1453–1456, 1976.
6. Lebovitz HE, Feldman JM: Pancreatic biogenic amines and insulin secretion in health and disease. *Fed Proc* 32:1797–1802, 1973.
7. Robertson RP, Chem M: A role for prostaglandin E in defective insulin secretion and carbohydrate intolerance in diabetes mellitus. *J Clin Invest* 60:747–753, 1977.
8. Chen M, Robertson RP: Restoration of the acute insulin response by sodium salicylate. A glucose dose-related phenomenon. *Diabetes* 27:750–756, 1978.
9. Giugliano D, Torella R, Sgambato S, Donofrio F: Acetylsalicylic acid restores acute insulin response reduced by furosemide in man. *Diabetes* 28:841–845, 1979.
10. Giugliano D, Torella R, Siniscalchi N, Improta L, Donofrio F: The effect of acetylsalicylic acid on insulin response to glucose and arginine in normal man. *Diabetologia* 14:359–362, 1978.
11. Kahn CR, White MF: The insulin receptor and the molecular mechanism of insulin action. *J Clin Invest* 82:1151–1156, 1988.
12. Brownlee M, Cerami A, Vlassara H: Advanced products of nonenzymatic glycosylation and the pathogenesis of diabetic vascular disease. *Diabetes Metab Rev* 4:437–451, 1988.
13. Larner J: Insulin and oral hypoglycemic drugs: glucagon. In Gilman AG, Goodman LS, Rall TW, Murad F (eds): *The Pharmacological Basis of Therapeutics*. New York, Macmillan, 1985, pp 1490–1516.
14. Duckworth WC, Kitabchi AE: Insulin metabolism and degradation. *Endocr Rev* 2:210–233, 1981.
15. Fajans SS: The adult diabetic patient. In Krieger DT, Bardin CW (eds): *Current Therapy in Endocrinology and Metabolism*. Toronto, BC Decker, 1985, pp 245–254.
16. Grossman LD, Zinman B: Insulin-dependent diabetes mellitus in adults. In Bardin CW (ed): *Current Therapy in Endocrinology and Metabolism*, 4th ed. Philadelphia, BC Decker, 1991, pp 338–342.
17. Krane EJ, Rockoff MA, Wallman JK, Wolfsdorf JI: Subclinical brain swelling in children during treatment of diabetic ketoacidosis. *N Engl J Med* 312:1147–1151, 1985.
18. Grant JP: Administration of parenteral nutrition solutions. In Grant JP (ed): *Handbook of Total Parenteral Nutrition*. Philadelphia, WB Saunders, 1980, pp 92–117.
19. Kitabchi AE, Ayyagari V, Guerra SM: The efficacy of low-dose versus conventional therapy of insulin for treatment of diabetic ketoacidosis. *Ann Intern Med* 84:633–638, 1976.
20. Grant JP: Preparation of parenteral nutrition solutions. In Grant JP (ed): *Handbook of Total Parenteral Nutrition*. Philadelphia, WB Saunders, 1980, pp 118–124.
21. Polonsky KS, Rubenstein AH: Current approaches to measurement of insulin secretion. *Diabetes Metab Rev* 2:315–329, 1986.
22. Brownlee M: Insulin treatment in diabetes. *Hosp Pract* 14:85–94, 1979.
23. Galloway JA, Spradlin CT, Nelson RL, Wentworth SM, Davidson JA, Swarner JL: Factors influencing the absorption, serum insulin concentration, and blood glucose responses after injections of regular insulin and various insulin mixtures. *Diabetes Care* 4:366–376, 1981.
24. Kitabchi AE, Stentz FB, Cole C, Duckworth WC: Accelerated insulin degradation: an alternate mechanism for insulin resistance. *Diabetes Care* 2:414–417, 1979.
25. Paulsen EP, Courtney JW III, Duckworth WC: Insulin resistance caused by massive degradation of subcutaneous insulin. *Diabetes* 28:640–645, 1979.
26. Berger M, Cuppers HJ, Halban PA, Offord RE: The effect of aprotinin on the absorption of subcutaneously injected regular insulin in normal subjects. *Diabetes* 29:81–83, 1980.
27. Freidenberg GR, White N, Cataland S, O'Dorisio TM, Sotos JF, Santiago JV: Diabetes responsive to intravenous but not subcutaneous insulin: effectiveness of aprotinin. *N Engl J Med* 305:363–368, 1981.
28. Shuldiner AR, Roth J: Insulin allergy and insulin resistance. In Bardin CW (ed): *Current Therapy in Endocrinology and Metabolism*, 4th ed. Philadelphia, BC Decker, 1991, pp 400–407.
29. Galloway JA, Bressler R: Insulin treatment in diabetes. *Med Clin North Am* 62:663-680, 1978.
30. Bar RS, Roth J: Insulin receptor status in disease states in man. *Arch Intern Med* 137:474–481, 1977.
31. Flier JS, Kahn CR, Roth J: Receptors, antireceptor antibodies and mechanisms of insulin resistance. *N Engl J Med* 300:413–419, 1979.
32. Davidson JK, DeBra DW: Immunologic insulin resistance. *Diabetes* 27:307–318, 1978.
33. Yalow RS, Berson SA: Reaction of fish insulins with human insulin antiserums. Potential value in the treatment of insulin resistance. *N Engl J Med* 270:1171–1178, 1964.
34. Merimee TJ: Insulin resistance: study of effect of 6-mercaptopurine. *Lancet* 1:69–71, 1965.
35. Nathan DM, Axelrod L, Flier JS, Carr DB: U-500 insulin in the treatment of antibody-mediated insulin resistance. *Ann Intern Med* 94:653–656, 1981.
36. Carter WP Jr: Hypothermia—a sign of hypoglycemia. *J Am Coll Emerg Phys* 5:594–595, 1976.
37. DeFronzo RA, Hendler R, Christensen N: Stimulation of counterregulatory hormonal responses in diabetic man by a fall in glucose concentration. *Diabetes* 29:125–131, 1980.
38. Mattson JR, Patterson R, Roberts M: Insulin therapy in patients with systemic insulin allergy. *Arch Intern Med* 135:818–821, 1975.

39. Patterson R, Mellies CJ, Roberts M: Immunologic reactions against insulin. II. IgE anti-insulin, insulin allergy and combined IgE and IgG immunologic insulin resistance. *J Immunol* 110:1135–1145, 1973.

40. Witters LA, Ohman JL, Weir GC, Raymond LW, Lowell FC: Insulin antibodies in the pathogenesis of insulin allergy and resistance. *Am J Med* 63:703–709, 1977.

41. Bucholtz HK: Insulin allergy: an approach to therapy. *South Med J* 69:1118–1120, 1976.

42. Lieberman P, Patterson R, Metz R, Ucena G: Allergic reactions to insulin. *JAMA* 215:1106–1112, 1971.

43. Klein SP: Insulin allergy: treatment with the histamine antagonists. *Arch Intern Med* 81:316, 1948.

44. Cockel R, Mann S: Insulin allergy treated by low-dosage hydrocortisone. *Br Med J* 3:722, 1967.

45. Oakley WG, Jones VE, Cunliffe AC: Insulin resistance. *Br Med J* 2:134–138, 1967.

46. Shipp JC, Cunningham RW, Russell RO, Marble A: Insulin resistance. Clinical features, natural course and effects of adrenal steroid treatment. *Medicine* 44:165–186, 1965.

47. Davidson JA, Galloway JA, Petersen BH, Wentworth SM, Crabtree RE: The use of purified insulins in insulin allergy [Abstract]. *Diabetes* 23(suppl 1):352, 1974.

48. Unger RH, Foster DW: Diabetes mellitus. In Wilson JD, Foster DW (eds): *Williams Textbook of Endocrinology*, 7th ed. Philadelphia, WB Saunders, 1985, pp 1018–1080.

49. Alberti KGMM, Nattrass M: Severe diabetic ketoacidosis. *Med Clin North Am* 62:799–814, 1978.

50. Fein IA, Rachow EC, Sprung CL, Grodman R: Relation of colloid osmotic pressure to arterial hypoxemia and cerebral edema during crystalloid volume loading of patients with diabetic ketoacidosis. *Ann Intern Med* 96:570–575, 1982.

51. McGarry JD, Foster DW: Regulation of hepatic fatty acid oxidation and ketone body production. *Annu Rev Biochem* 49:395–420, 1980.

52. Zaloga GP, Chernow B: The use of hormones as therapeutic agents. *Semin Respir Med* 7:39–51, 1985.

53. Raskin P, Unger RH: Effects of exogenous hyperglucagonemia in insulin-treated diabetes. *Diabetes* 26:1034–1039, 1977.

54. Raskin P, Unger RH: Glucagon and diabetes. *Med Clin North Am* 62:713–722, 1978.

55. Unger RH: Role of glucagon in the pathogenesis of diabetes: the status of controversy. *Metabolism* 27:1691–1709, 1978.

56. Gerich JE: Metabolic effects of long-term somatostatin infusion in man. *Metabolism* 25(suppl 1):1505–1507, 1976.

57. Gerich JE, Lorenzi M, Bier DM, et al: Prevention of human diabetic ketoacidosis by somatostatin. Evidence for an essential role of glucagon. *N Engl J Med* 292:985–989, 1975.

58. Gerich JE, Raptis S, Rosenthal J: Somatostatin symposium. *Metabolism* 27(suppl 1):1, 1978.

59. Raskin P, Unger RH: Hyperglucagonemia and its suppression. Importance in the metabolic control of diabetes. *N Engl J Med* 299:433–436, 1978.

60. Lundbaek K, Hansen AP, Orskov H, et al: Failure of somatostatin to correct manifest diabetic ketoacidosis. *Lancet* 1:215–218, 1976.

61. Johnson DG, Goebel CU, Hruby VJ, Bregman MD, Trivedi D: Hyperglycemia of diabetic rat decreased by a glucagon receptor antagonist. *Science* 215:1115–1116, 1982.

62. Campbell IW, Duncan LJP, Innes JA, MacCuish AC, Munro JF: Abdominal pain in diabetic metabolic decompensation. Clinical significance. *JAMA* 233:166–168, 1975.

63. Alberti KGMM, Hockaday TDR: Diabetic coma: a reappraisal after five years. *Clin Endocrinol Metab* 6:421–455, 1977.

64. Zaloga GP: Bedside reagent testing: blood, CSF, and bacterial cultures. *J Crit Illness* 3:85–94, 1988.

65. Chernow B, Diaz M, Cruess D, et al: Bedside blood glucose determinations in critical care medicine: a comparative analysis of two techniques. *Crit Care Med* 10:463–465, 1982.

66. Zaloga GP, Chernow B: Diabetes and diabetic coma. In Parrillo JE (ed): *Current Therapy in Critical Care Medicine*. Toronto, BC Decker, 1987, pp 297–299.

67. Genuth SM: Diabetic ketoacidosis and hyperglycemic hyperosmolar coma. In Bardin CW (ed): *Current Therapy in Endocrinology and Metabolism*, 4th ed. Philadelphia, BC Decker, 1991, pp 348–353.

68. Kreisberg RA: Diabetic ketoacidosis: new concepts and trends in pathogenesis and treatment. *Ann Intern Med* 88:681–695, 1978.

69. Oh MS, Carroll HJ, Goldstein DA, Fein IA: Hyperchloremic acidosis during the recovery phase of diabetic ketosis. *Ann Intern Med* 89:925–927, 1978.

70. Beigelman PM: Potassium in severe diabetic ketoacidosis. *Am J Med* 54:419–420, 1973.

71. Podolsky S, Emerson K Jr: Potassium depletion in diabetic ketoacidosis (KA) and in hyperosmolar nonketotic coma (HNC) [Abstract]. *Diabetes* 22:299, 1973.

72. Marriott HJL: Miscellaneous conditions. In *Practical Electrocardiology*, 6th ed. Baltimore, Williams & Wilkins, 1977, pp 290–318.

73. Munro JF, Campbell IW, McCuish AC, Duncan LJ: Euglycaemic diabetic ketoacidosis. *Br Med J* 2:578–580, 1973.

74. Keller U, Berger W: Prevention of hypophosphatemia by phosphate infusion during treatment of diabetic ketoacidosis and hyperosmolar coma. *Diabetes* 29:87–95, 1980.

75. DeFronzo RA, Lang R: Hypophosphatemia and glucose intolerance: evidence for tissue insensitivity to insulin. *N Engl J Med* 303:1259–1263, 1980.

76. Harter HR, Santiago JV, Rutherford WE, Slatopolsky E, Klahr S: The relative roles of calcium, phosphorus, and parathyroid hormone in glucose- and tolbuta-mide-mediated insulin release. *J Clin Invest* 58:359–367, 1976.

77. Alberti KGMM, Emerson PM, Darley JH, Hockaday TD: 2,3-Diphosphoglyc-erate and tissue oxygenation in uncontrolled diabetes mellitus. *Lancet* 2:391–395, 1972.

78. Guest GM, Rapoport S: Electrolytes of blood plasma and cells in diabetic acidosis and during recovery. *Proc Am Diabetes Assoc* 7:97, 1947.

79. Ditzel J: Importance of plasma inorganic phosphate on tissue oxygenation during recovery from diabetic ketoacidosis. *Horm Metab Res* 5:471–472, 1973.

80. Franks M, Berris RF, Kaplan NO, et al: Metabolic studies in diabetic acidosis. II. The effect of the administration of sodium phosphate. *Arch Intern Med* 81:42, 1948.

81. Chernow B, Rainey TG, Georges LP, O'Brian JT: Iatrogenic hyperphospha-temia: a metabolic consideration in critical care medicine. *Crit Care Med* 9:772–774, 1981.

82. Winter RJ, Harris CJ, Phillips LS, Green OC: Diabetic ketoacidosis. Induction of hypocalcemia and hypomagnesemia by phosphate therapy. *Am J Med* 67:897–900, 1979.

83. Morris LR, Murphy MB, Kitabchi AE: Bicarbonate therapy in severe diabetic ketoacidosis. *Ann Intern Med* 105:836–840, 1986.

84. Ohman JL Jr, Marliss EB, Aoki TT, Munichoodappa CS, Khanna VV, Kozak GP: The cerebrospinal fluid in diabetic ketoacidosis. *N Engl J Med* 284:283–290, 1971.

85. Alberti KGMM: Low-dose insulin in the treatment of diabetic ketoacidosis. *Arch Intern Med* 137:1367–1376, 1977.

86. Alberti KGMM, Hockaday TDR, Turner RC: Small doses of intramuscular insulin in the treatment of diabetic "coma." *Lancet* 2:515–522, 1973.

87. Bendezu R, Wieland RG, Furst BH, Mandel M, Genuth SM, Schumacher OP: Experience with low-dose insulin infusion in diabetic ketoacidosis and diabetic hyperosmolarity. *Arch Intern Med* 138:60–62, 1978.

88. Fisher JN, Shahshahani MN, Kitabchi AE: Diabetic ketoacidosis: low-dose insulin therapy by various routes. *N Engl J Med* 297:238–241, 1977.

89. Heber D, Molitch ME, Spirling MA: Low-dose continuous insulin therapy for diabetic ketoacidosis. Prospective comparison with "conventional" insulin therapy. *Arch Intern Med* 137:1377–1380, 1977.

90. Kitabchi AE: Low-dose insulin therapy in diabetic ketoacidosis: fact or fiction? *Diabetes Metab Rev* 5:337–363, 1989.

91. Sonksen PH, Srivastava MC, Tompkins CV, Nabarro JD: Growth-hormone and cortisol responses to insulin infusion in patients with diabetes mellitus. *Lancet* 2:155–159, 1972.

92. Byrne WJ, Lippe BM, Strobel CT, Levin SR, Ament ME, Kaplan SA: Adapta-tion to increasing loads of total parenteral nutrition: metabolic, endocrine, and insulin receptor responses. *Gastroenterology* 80:947–956, 1981.

93. Piters K, Goodman J, Bessman A: Treatment of diabetic ketoacidosis with continuous low-dose intravenous insulin [Abstract]. *Diabetes* 24(suppl 2):396, 1975.

94. Semple PF, White C, Manderson WG: Continuous intravenous infusion of small doses of insulin in treatment of diabetic ketoacidosis. *Br Med J* 2:694–698, 1974.

95. Field JB, Johnson P, Herring B: Insulin-resistant diabetes associated with increased endogenous plasma insulin followed by complete remission. *J Clin Invest* 40:1672–1683, 1961.

96. Schade DS, Eaton RP: Dose response to insulin in man: differential effects on glucose and ketone body regulation. *J Clin Endocrinol Metab* 44:1038–1053, 1977.

97. Kraegen EW, Lazarus L, Meler H, Campbell L, Chia YO: Carrier solutions for low-level intravenous insulin infusion. *Br Med J* 3:464–466, 1975.

98. Weisenfeld S, Podolsky S, Goldsmith L, Ziff L: Adsorption of insulin to infusion bottles and tubing. *Diabetes* 17:766–771, 1968.

99. Peterson L, Caldwell J, Hoffman J: Insulin absorbance to polyvinylchloride surfaces with implications for constant-infusion therapy. *Diabetes* 25:72–74, 1976.

100. Metzger AL, Rubenstein AH: Reversible cerebral oedema complicating dia-betic ketoacidosis. *Br Med J* 3:746–747, 1970.

101. Young E, Bradley RF: Cerebral edema with irreversible coma in severe dia-betic ketoacidosis. *N Engl J Med* 276:665–669, 1967.

102. Arieff AI, Kleeman CR: Studies on mechanisms of cerebral edema in diabetic comas. Effects of hyperglycemia and rapid lowering of plasma glucose in normal rabbits. *J Clin Invest* 52:571–583, 1973.

103. Guisado R, Arieff AI: Neurologic manifestations of diabetic comas: correlation with biochemical alterations in the brain. *Metabolism* 24:665–679, 1975.

104. Sprung CL, Rackow EC, Fein IA: Pulmonary edema: a complication of diabetic ketoacidosis. *Chest* 77:687–688, 1980.

105. Goldstein DA, Oh MS, Fein A, Carroll HJ: Transient hypoxemia in diabetic ketoacidosis [Abstract]. *Kidney Int* 10:499, 1976.

106. Fulop M, Rosenblatt A, Kreitzer SM, Gerstenhaber B: Hyperosmolar nature of diabetic coma. *Diabetes* 24:594–599, 1975.

107. Fulop M, Tannenbaum H, Dryer N: Ketotic hyperosmolar coma. *Lancet* 2:635–639, 1973.
108. Zaloga GP, Chernow B, McFadden E, Soldano S, Lyons P, O'Brian JT: Urine glucose testing in the critically ill: a comparison of two enzymatic test strips. *Crit Care Med* 12:188–190, 1984.
109. File TM Jr, Tan JS: Infection in the diabetic. In Bardin CW (ed): *Current Therapy in Endocrinology and Metabolism*, 4th ed. Philadelphia, BC Decker, 1991, pp 394–398.
110. Arieff AI, Carroll HJ: Nonketotic hyperosmolar coma with hyperglycemia: clinical features, pathophysiology, renal function, acid-base balance, plasma-cerebrospinal fluid equilibria and the effects of therapy in 37 cases. *Medicine* 51:73–94, 1972.
111. Gerich JE, Martin MM, Recant L: Clinical and metabolic characteristics of hyperosmolar nonketotic coma. *Diabetes* 20:228–238, 1971.
112. Khardori R, Soler NG: Hyperosmolar hyperglycemic nonketotic syndrome. Report of 22 cases and brief review. *Am J Med* 77:899–904, 1984.
113. Podolsky S: Hyperosmolar nonketotic coma in the elderly diabetic. *Med Clin North Am* 62:815–828, 1978.
114. Turpin BP, Duckworth WC, Solomon SS: Simulated hyperglycemic hyperosmolar syndrome. Impaired insulin and epinephrine effects upon lipolysis in the isolated rat fat cell. *J Clin Invest* 63:403–409, 1979.
115. Joffe BI, Seftel HC, Goldberg R, Van As M, Krut L, Bersohn I: Factors in the pathogenesis of experimental nonketotic and ketoacidotic diabetic stupor. *Diabetes* 22:653–657, 1973.
116. Joffe BI, Goldberg RB, Krut LH, Seftel HC: Pathogenesis of nonketotic hyperosmolar diabetic coma. *Lancet* 1:1069–1071, 1975.
117. Maccario M: Neurological dysfunction associated with nonketotic hyperglycemia. *Arch Neurol* 19:525–534, 1968.
118. Manzano F, Kozak GP: Acute quadriplegia in diabetic hyperosmotic coma with hypokalemia. *JAMA* 207:2278–2281, 1969.
119. Lebovitz HE: Noninsulin-dependent diabetes mellitus. In Bardin CW (ed): *Current Therapy in Endocrinology and Metabolism*, 4th ed. Philadelphia, BC Decker, 1991, pp 343–348.
120. Fulop M, Hoberman HD: Alcoholic ketosis. *Diabetes* 24:785–790, 1975.
121. Goldfrank L, Starke CL: Metabolic acidosis in the alcoholic. *Hosp Physician* 4:34, 1979.
122. Levy LJ, Duga J, Girgis M, Gordon EE: Ketoacidosis associated with alcoholism in nondiabetic subjects. *Ann Intern Med* 78:213–219, 1973.
123. Miller PD, Heinig RE, Waterhouse C: Treatment of alcoholic acidosis: the role of dextrose and phosphorus. *Arch Intern Med* 138:67–72, 1978.
124. Filkins JP, Figlewicz DP: Increased insulin responsiveness in endotoxicosis. *Circ Shock* 6:1–6, 1979.
125. Goldmann DR: Surgery in patients with endocrine dysfunction. *Med Clin N Am* 71:499–509, 1987.
126. White VA, Kumagai LF: Preoperative endocrine and metabolic considerations. *Med Clin North Am* 63:1321–1334, 1979.
127. Page MM, Watkins PJ: Cardiorespiratory arrest and diabetic autonomic neuropathy. *Lancet* 1:14–16, 1978.
128. Johnston DG, Alberti KGMM: Diabetic emergencies: practical aspects of the management of diabetic ketoacidosis and diabetes during surgery. *Clin Endocrinol Metab* 4:437–460, 1980.
129. Alberti KGMM, Thomas DJB: The management of diabetes during surgery. *Br J Anaesth* 51:663–710, 1979.
130. Gamblin GT, Clapper M, Chernow B, O'Brian JT: Insulin infusion pump therapy: a review. *Military Med* 147:747–749, 1982.
131. Nathan DM, Lou P, Avruch J: Intensive conventional and insulin pump therapies in adult type I diabetes. A crossover study. *Ann Intern Med* 97:31–36, 1982.
132. Rizza RA: Treatment options for insulin-dependent diabetes mellitus: a comparison of the artificial endocrine pancreas, continuous subcutaneous insulin infusion, and multiple daily insulin injections. *Mayo Clin Proc* 61:796–805, 1986.
133. Rizza RA, Gerich JE, Haymond MW, et al: Control of blood sugar in insulin-dependent diabetes: comparison of an artificial endocrine pancreas, continuous subcutaneous infusion, and intensified conventional therapy. *N Engl J Med* 303:1313–1318, 1980.
134. McRae JR, Metz SA, Robertson RP: A role for endogenous prostaglandins in defective glucose potentiation of nonglucose insulin secretagogues in diabetes. *Metabolism* 30:1065–1075, 1981.
135. Robertson RP, Metz SA: Sounding board. Prostaglandins, the glucoreceptor, and diabetes. *N Engl J Med* 301:1446–1447, 1979.
136. Gerich JE: Somatostatin and diabetes. *Am J Med* 70:619–626, 1981.
137. Podolsky S, Pattavina CG: Hyperosmolar nonketotic diabetic coma: a complication of propranolol therapy. *Metabolism* 22:685–693, 1973.
138. Porte D Jr: A receptor mechanism for the inhibition of insulin release by epinephrine in man. *J Clin Invest* 46:86–94, 1967.
139. Porte D Jr: Inhibition of insulin release by diazoxide and its relation to catecholamine effects in man. *Ann NY Acad Sci* 150:281–291, 1968.
140. Porte D Jr, Williams RH: Inhibition of insulin release by norepinephrine in man. *Science* 152:1248–1250, 1966.
141. Seltzer HS, Allen EW: Hyperglycemia and inhibition of insulin secretion during administration of diazoxide and trichlormethiazide in man. *Diabetes* 18:19–28, 1969.
142. Rizza RA, Mandarino LJ, Gerich JE: Cortisol-induced insulin resistance in man: impaired suppression of glucose production and stimulation of glucose utilization due to a postreceptor defect of insulin action. *J Clin Endocrinol Metab* 54:131–138, 1982.
143. dePirro R, Bertoli A, Fusco A, Testa I, Greco AV, Lauro R: Effect of dexamethasone and cortisone on insulin receptors in normal human male. *J Clin Endocrinol Metab* 51:503–507, 1980.
144. Carpentieri U, Balch MT: Hyperglycemia associated with the therapeutic use of *l*-asparaginase: possible role of insulin receptors. *J Pediatr* 93:775–778, 1978.
145. Olefsky JM, Reaven GM: Effects of sulfonylurea therapy on insulin binding to mononuclear leukocytes of diabetic patients. *Am J Med* 60:89–95, 1976.
146. Wennlund A, Arner P, Ostman J: Changes in the effects of insulin on human adipose tissue metabolism in hyperthyroidism. *J Clin Endocrinol Metab* 53:631–635, 1981.
147. Wright J, Marks V: Alcohol-induced hypoglycaemia. *Adv Exp Med Biol* 126:479–483, 1980.
148. Peitzman SJ, Agarwal BN: Spontaneous hypoglycemia in end-stage renal failure. *Nephron* 19:131–139, 1977.
149. Shen SW, Bressler R: Clinical pharmacology of oral antidiabetic agents. *N Engl J Med* 296:493–497, 787–793, 1977.
150. Gerich JE: Sulfonylureas in the treatment of diabetes mellitus–1985. *Mayo Clin Proc* 60:439–443, 1985.
151. Boyd AE III: Sulfonylurea receptors, ion channels, and fruit flies. *Diabetes* 37:847–850, 1988.
152. Peters AL, Davidson MB: Insulin plus a sulfonylurea agent for treating type 2 diabetes. *Ann Intern Med* 115:45–53, 1991.
153. Lewitt MS, Yu VK, Rennie GC, et al: Effects of combined insulin-sulfonylurea therapy in Type II patients. *Diabetes Care* 12:379–383, 1989.
154. Simonson DC, Delprato S, Castellino P, Groop L, DeFronzo RA: Effect of glyburide on glycemic control, insulin requirement, and glucose metabolism in insulin-treated diabetic patients. *Diabetes* 36:136–146, 1987.
155. Allen BT, Feinglos MN, Lebovitz HE: Treatment of poorly regulated non-insulin-dependent diabetes mellitus with combination insulin-sulfonylurea. *Arch Intern Med* 145:1900–1903, 1985.
156. Longnecker MP, Elsenhans VD, Leiman SM, Owen OE, Boden G: Insulin and a sulfonylurea agent in non-insulin-dependent diabetes mellitus. *Arch Intern Med* 146:673–676, 1986.

Divalent Ions: Calcium, Magnesium, and Phosphorus

GARY P. ZALOGA, M.D., F.A.C.P.
BART CHERNOW, M.D., F.A.C.P.

Calcium (Ca^{2+}), magnesium (Mg^{2+}), and phosphorus (PO_4) are divalent ions that are essential for normal body function. Disorders involving these ions are common in critically ill patients because of their underlying illnesses and the effects of administered drugs. This chapter discusses the pharmacology, homeostasis, causes, clinical features, and treatment of disorders involving these ions. The emphasis is placed upon those disorders most commonly seen in the critical care setting.

CALCIUM

Ca^{2+} is important in humans for both structural and biochemical integrity. The normal adult body contains approximately 1000 to 1400 g of Ca^{2+}, of which 99% is in the skeleton and 1% is in the soft tissues and extracellular spaces. Ca^{2+} is the most abundant electrolyte in the human body. Skeletal Ca^{2+} supports and protects body tissues and serves as a storehouse, providing Ca^{2+} for physiologic requirements when dietary Ca^{2+} is unavailable.

Ca^{2+} movement into the cell and release from intracellular sites is vital for the coupling of receptor-stimulated cell surface events to cellular responses (i.e., stimulus-response coupling). Thus, calcium is an important second and third messenger. Ca^{2+} is required for muscle contraction (e.g., excitation-contraction coupling), hormonal and neurotransmitter secretion (e.g., stimulus-secretion coupling), cell division, cell motility, axonal flow, enzyme activity, cell membrane structure, and blood coagulation. In general, calcium is required for cellular activities that involve movement. It also plays a vital role in the cardiac action potential and is essential for cardiac pacemaker automaticity.

MEASUREMENT OF BLOOD CALCIUM

Ca^{2+} circulates in the blood in three forms: an ionized fraction (50%), a protein-bound (mostly to albumin) fraction (40%), and a diffusible but nonionized fraction in chelates with other circulating ions (10%). It is the ionized fraction that is thought to be physiologically active and homeostatically regulated. A determination of the total serum calcium concentration is the measurement that is performed in most hospital laboratories. However, alterations in the amount of protein present, the percentage of Ca^{2+} bound to protein, and the amount of Ca^{2+} bound in chelates may affect the total Ca^{2+} value independent of the ionized Ca^{2+} concentration (1–6).

A variety of factors can alter the serum total and ionized Ca^{2+} levels (5–7). Protein-bound Ca^{2+} (primarily albumin) represents a large proportion (40%) of the total serum Ca^{2+} concentration. Thus, alterations in a patient's serum albumin concentration can change that person's total serum Ca^{2+} measurement. Critically ill patients with low serum albumin levels characteristically have a low total serum Ca^{2+} value, while serum ionized Ca^{2+} measurements may be normal (6). On the other hand, a normal total serum Ca^{2+} level in the face of hypoalbuminemia may indicate ionized hypercalcemia. Increases in serum protein levels (e.g., from albumin infusions, venostasis as a consequence of prolonged tourniquet use during phlebotomy, and, rarely, myeloma) may also raise the total serum Ca^{2+} value and mask ionized hypocalcemia.

Blood pH alters Ca^{2+} binding to serum proteins: acute acidosis decreases protein binding (increases the serum ionized Ca^{2+} concentration), whereas alkalosis increases protein binding (decreases ionized Ca^{2+}). Measurement of the total serum Ca^{2+} concentration in critically ill patients with acid-base changes may therefore give deceptive results. For example, a patient being therapeutically hyperventilated (e.g., in an attempt to reduce intracranial pressure following head injury) may develop ionized hypocalcemia, without abnormalities in the total serum Ca^{2+} concentration, as a result of an alkalosis-induced increase in Ca^{2+} binding to proteins. Patients given bicarbonate for control of metabolic acidosis can also develop acute ionized hypocalcemia. Shifts in ionized Ca^{2+} induced by changes in arterial pH are usually small; however, occasionally, they may be associated with clinically important ionized hypocalcemia. Patients who are most susceptible to ionized hypocalcemia are those with an underlying abnormality in parathyroid hormone (PTH) and vitamin D metabolism.

Fatty acids (FFA) constitute a major metabolic fuel for the body and are carried in the circulation bound to the albumin molecule. The authors (7) and others (8) have found that FFAs increase Ca^{2+} binding to albumin. Serum FFA levels increase during critical illness as a result of illness-induced elevations in plasma concentrations of epinephrine, glucagon, growth hormone, and corticotropin, as well as decreases in serum insulin concentrations. Elevations in FFA levels, sufficient to alter calcium binding, may also occur after the administration of heparin sodium, intravenous lipids, epinephrine, norepinephrine, and isoproterenol, as well as with alcohol ingestion. These pharmacologic agents are commonly used in critically ill patients. Normal individuals have serum FFA concentrations of approximately 250 μmol/liter. Values of FFAs increase to 400 to 600 μmol/liter after an overnight fast and may increase further to 1000 μmol/liter after prolonged fasting (72 hours). Severely stressed patients (e.g., those with acute pancreatitis, diabetic ketoacidosis, sepsis, or acute myocardial infarction) may have serum levels of 3000 μmol/liter. Increases in serum FFA levels in acutely ill and stressed patients may alter the distribution of Ca^{2+} between bound and unbound states (4, 7). FFAs may act as modulators of free Ca^{2+} levels in various pathologic states.

The timing and technique of venipuncture are important in the interpretation of serum Ca^{2+} values. Postprandial increases in serum Ca^{2+} levels of 0.5 to 1 mg/dl may occur. Postprandial increases in serum Ca^{2+} are higher and more prolonged in hyperabsorptive states such as hyperparathyroidism, vitamin D excess, and hypothyroidism. To avoid these changes, one should measure serum Ca^{2+} in the fasting state.

Changes in the concentration of chelating ions (e.g., phosphate, bicarbonate, albumin, and citrate) may also lower the circulating ionized Ca^{2+} level. Citrate is used as a blood preservative and anticoagulant. Citrate-induced decreases in ionized Ca^{2+} are usually transient, and without hemodynamic effect in most blood transfusion situations. Howland et al (9) studied 100 patients who received blood during a variety of surgical procedures. Mean ionized Ca^{2+} levels decreased from 4.06

to 3.22 mg/dl (1.01 to 0.80 mmol/liter) while patients were receiving an average of 18.6 ml of blood per minute. Twenty of the 100 (20%) patients who received blood at this rate had ionized Ca^{2+} levels that fell below 2.5 mg/dl (0.62 mmol/liter), and 10 of the 100 patients (10%) had levels below 2 mg/dl (0.50 mmol/liter). Only one patient (1%) developed hypocalcemia-induced cardiovascular problems (e.g., hypotension). Kahn et al (10) studied 53 patients undergoing a variety of surgical procedures. Serum-ionized Ca^{2+} levels decreased from a mean of 4.14 to 3.04 mg/dl (1.03 to 0.76 mmol/liter) during transfusion of blood at an average rate of 0.5 ml/kg/min. However, hemodynamic variables remained stable throughout the period of observation, and ionized Ca^{2+} values returned to normal after discontinuation of the transfusion.

Decreases in ionized Ca^{2+} values during blood transfusion correlate with elevations in circulating citrate levels and speed of transfusion. Denlinger et al (11) administered citrated blood to anesthetized patients at rates of 50, 100, and 150 ml/70 kg/min and found decreases in serum-ionized Ca^{2+} levels of 14%, 31%, and 41%, respectively. After a 5-minute blood transfusion period, ionized Ca^{2+} values returned to normal within 15 minutes, and this normalization correlated with metabolism of the citrate.

The metabolism of citrate is affected by tissue perfusion, acid-base status, and the activity of the rate-limiting enzyme aconitase, which is present in muscle, kidney, and liver. When transfusion rate exceeds citrate metabolism, citrate levels rise and ionized Ca^{2+} levels fall. Citrate may also chelate Mg^{2+}, causing hypomagnesemia, which in turn may accentuate hypocalcemia. Thus, when citrate clearance is impaired (e.g., in hypothermia or with renal or hepatic disease) or blood transfusion is rapid, plasma citrate levels may rise and cause clinically important hypocalcemia and cardiovascular insufficiency. The effect of citrate and other chelators on Ca^{2+} is accentuated in patients with underlying defects of the parathyroid-vitamin D axis. Decreases in ionized Ca^{2+} levels may also occur after volume resuscitation with albumin, after intravenous injection of radiocontrast media, and after the intravenous administration of phosphates (4).

Heparin is capable of chelating with Ca^{2+}; however, heparin dosages capable of causing Ca^{2+} chelation are not usually obtained in vivo except during cardiopulmonary bypass. On the other hand, adding heparin to syringes used to collect blood samples for measurement of ionized Ca^{2+} can lower the ionized Ca^{2+} concentration significantly. Thus, samples used for measurement of plasma or blood Ca^{2+} should use the smallest amount of heparin that will adequately anticoagulate blood. The amount of heparin added should be standardized and each laboratory performing ionized Ca^{2+} measurements should use its own normal values.

The serum-ionized Ca^{2+} value may be altered during hemodialysis, depending on the calcium concentration of the dialysate (4, 12, 13). Patients with renal failure are vulnerable to the hypocalcemic effects of dialysis because they have an impaired ability to hydroxylate vitamin D within the kidney and mobilize calcium. Maynard et al (13) showed that the drop in blood pressure induced by hemodialysis was reduced when a high-Ca^{2+} dialysate was used. Henrich et al (12) demonstrated that ionized Ca^{2+} values during dialysis were key factors affecting left ventricular contractility, an increase in ionized Ca²⁺ being associated with improved contractility. These studies indicate that the Ca²⁺ composition of the dialysate baths can affect hemodynamics during dialysis. In fact, hypotensive episodes are common in critically ill patients dialyzed against low Ca²⁺ baths. Currently, the authors recommend use of a high-Ca²⁺ bath (7.5 mg/dl) in unstable critically ill patients, unless the patient is hypercalcemic.

Many attempts have been made to correct mathematically the total serum Ca²⁺ concentration for alterations in circulating albumin levels and pH. Despite these attempts, total serum Ca²⁺ and calculated ionized Ca²⁺ levels have been poor predictors of the physiologically active ionized Ca²⁺ fraction (6, 14). The authors have found abnormally low total and calculated ionized Ca²⁺ values in 50 to 60% of critically ill patients (6). However, when ionized Ca²⁺ levels were measured directly, only about 10% of critically ill patients had hypocalcemia. Despite high sensitivity, total serum and calculated ionized Ca²⁺ values lack specificity in predicting ionized hypocalcemia. On the other hand, an increased total serum Ca²⁺ level in a critically ill patient usually indicates ionized hypercalcemia, whereas a normal total serum Ca²⁺ measurement is strong evidence against ionized hypocalcemia (6). The authors have found that the amount of Ca²⁺ bound to albumin varies widely between patients (e.g., 40 to 60%) and that alterations in binding that result from blood pH and FFA changes differ significantly between normal and ill patients (implying differences in the physicochemical properties of their binding proteins) (6, 7). At present, the authors believe that the serum-ionized Ca²⁺ level remains the best measure of Ca²⁺ delivery in critically ill patients, and it is recommended that all centers caring for critically ill patients measure ionized Ca²⁺ concentrations. Ionized calcium analysis is available on most state-of-the-art blood gas analyzers (15). When ionized Ca²⁺ measurements are not available, an ultrafilterable Ca²⁺ level may be substituted (16). Ultrafilterable Ca²⁺ levels can be measured easily by passing a plasma or serum sample through a small filter, which prevents the passage of protein through it. The Ca²⁺ in the ultrafiltrate can be measured in the hospital laboratory.

Different laboratories have different ways of measuring serum-ionized Ca²⁺ levels. Many laboratories correct the serum pH to 7.4 to correct for losses in carbon dioxide that may have occurred between the time of blood drawing and Ca²⁺ measurement. Since many critically ill patients have alterations in blood pH, the authors do not correct the pH to 7.4; they have also found that present methods for correcting the pH to 7.4 work poorly in critically ill patients. The authors are extremely careful to collect blood samples anaerobically and measure the ionized Ca²⁺ level immediately after drawing.

CALCIUM HOMEOSTASIS

The daily recommended oral dietary intake of Ca²⁺ is 1000 to 1500 mg. Of this intake, 30 to 35% is absorbed, primarily in the small intestine, by both active (vitamin D-dependent) and passive (concentration-dependent) absorption. Loss of Ca²⁺ via the gastrointestinal tract (150 to 200 mg/day) and urine (150 mg/day) is balanced by gastrointestinal absorption.

The serum Ca²⁺ concentration is maintained within normal limits by the combined effects of PTH and vitamin D (Fig.

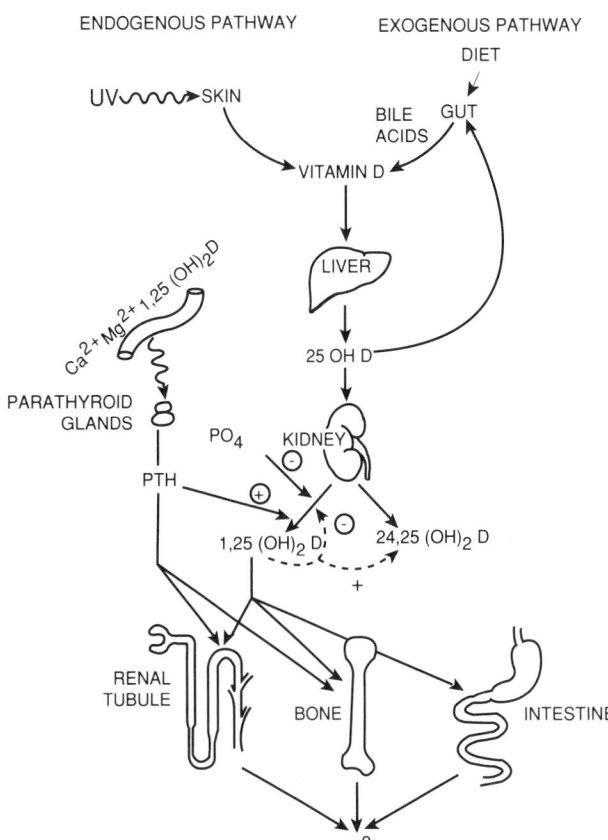

Figure 46.1. Regulation of the serum calcium level.

46.1). Dietary Ca²⁺ is usually not required, since these hormones can maintain a normal serum Ca²⁺ level via their skeletal effects. However, with chronic Ca²⁺ deficiency the skeletal Ca²⁺ mobilizing response to PTH or 1,25-dihydroxyvitamin D is diminished and predisposes the patient to hypocalcemia. This decrease in PTH and vitamin D responsiveness results from receptor desensitization caused by high levels of the hormones and depletion of the mobilizable pool of Ca²⁺ in bone (17). A deficiency in either hormone, however, may lead to hypocalcemia. Deficiency in PTH may result from parathyroid gland damage (as may occur after neck surgery) or from parathyroid gland suppression. The parathyroid glands may be suppressed by hypercalcemia, hypomagnesemia, hypermagnesemia, or 1,25-dihydroxyvitamin D. PTH increases bone resorption and renal tubular Ca²⁺ absorption by stimulating the renal conversion of 25-hydroxyvitamin D to 1,25-dihydroxyvitamin D (17). The action of PTH on bone osteoclasts may be mediated through an intermediary monocyte rather than by direct action (17).

Vitamin D can enter the body through the gastrointestinal tract (dietary vitamin D) or can be synthesized in the skin under the influence of ultraviolet light. Either source is sufficient to maintain normal vitamin D levels. However, when exposure to sunlight is minimal and dietary intake is poor, vitamin D deficiency may develop. These circumstances are commonly found in elderly, debilitated, and chronically ill patients. Many of these patients are admitted to intensive care units (ICUs) and, under the increased metabolic demands of severe illness, may be unable to maintain normal serum Ca²⁺

levels. Vitamin D is a fat-soluble vitamin, and its absorption is dependent on intact lipolytic activity, biliary secretion, and functional intestinal mucosa. Thus, diseases of the pancreas, liver, biliary system, or intestine may cause vitamin D malabsorption and deficiency (18).

Vitamin D is 25-hydroxylated in the liver and then 1-hydroxylated in the kidneys to 1,25-dihydroxyvitamin D, the active form of the vitamin. The renal hydroxylation of vitamin D is stimulated by both PTH and hypophosphatemia and is suppressed by hyperphosphatemia, acidosis, and 1,25-dihydroxyvitamin D (negative feedback). Synthesis of 25-hydroxyvitamin D within the liver is poorly regulated, and its measurement serves as a good indicator of dietary/skin vitamin D supply. Disease of the kidneys or liver can disrupt Ca^{2+} homeostasis by impairing vitamin D activation. Intestinal and renal tubular Ca^{2+} absorption and bone resorption are stimulated by 1,25-dihydroxyvitamin D. The osteoclast action of 1,25-dihydroxyvitamin D may result from the recruitment and differentiation of precursor cells (17) rather than from action on mature cells.

Thyroid hormone also has effects on the skeleton that affect Ca^{2+} homeostasis. Hyperthyroidism increases bone resorption and may cause hypercalcemia. Hypothyroidism causes a decrease in bone resorption and may cause hypocalcemia.

HYPOCALCEMIA

Causes

Hypocalcemia (ionized calcium <1 mmol/liter or 4 mg/dl) develops when Ca^{2+} leaves the vascular space or is chelated faster than it can be replaced. A frequent underlying problem in critically ill patients who become hypocalcemic is their impaired ability to mobilize skeletal Ca^{2+} because of PTH or vitamin D deficiency. In general, the etiologies of ionized hypocalcemia can be grouped into four major categories: impaired PTH secretion or action, impaired vitamin D synthesis or action, calcium chelation/precipitation, and decreased bone turnover (Table 46.1). Ionized hypocalcemia has been reported to occur in 15 to 50% of critically ill patients. The exact incidence reflects the type of patients studied.

HYPOPARATHYROIDISM

Primary (usually autoimmune) hypoparathyroidism is seen rarely, whereas secondary hypoparathyroidism after neck surgery is a common cause of hypocalcemia (19). Hypocalcemia is usually seen when surgery involves removal of a parathyroid adenoma, total or near-total thyroidectomy, or bilateral neck surgery for cancer. Hypocalcemia may occur immediately or 1 to 2 days after surgery and is transient (lasting less than 5 days) unless permanent parathyroid damage has occurred. Parathyroid insufficiency may result from gland suppression after removal of an adenoma, interference with parathyroid blood supply, or intraoperative release of calcitonin (20). Watson et al (21) found a close correlation between decrements in serum Ca^{2+} and increases in calcitonin after thyroidectomy.

Table 46.1. Causes of Hypocalcemia

I.   Impaired PTH secretion or action
A.   Primary hypoparathyroidism
B.   Secondary (acquired) hypoparathyroidism
1.   After neck surgery or trauma
2.   Radioiodine
3.   Infiltrative disease (i.e., hemochromatosis, malignancy)
4.   Neonatal
5.   Hypomagnesemia, hypermagnesemia
6.   Sepsis, burns
7.   Pancreatitis
8.   Rhabdomyolysis
9.   Post-hypercalcemia
II. Impaired vitamin D synthesis or action
A.   Poor dietary vitamin D intake
B.   Malabsorption
C.   Liver disease
D.   Renal disease
E.   Hypomagnesemia
F.   Sepsis, rhabdomyolysis
G.   Pseudohypoparathyroidism
III. Calcium chelation/precipitation
A.   Phosphate
B.   Citrate (i.e., blood)
C.   EDTA, EGTA[a]
D.   Albumin
E.   Hungry bone syndromes
F.   Fat embolism
G.   Pancreatitis
H.   Sepsis
I.   Rhabdomyolysis
J.   Ethylene glycol
K.   Protamine
L.   Sodium sulfate, sodium fluoride
IV. Decreased bone turnover
A.   Calcitonin
B.   *Cis*-platinum
C.   Diphosphonates
D.   Mithramycin
E.   Gallium nitrate
F.   WR-2721

[a] EGTA, ethylenebisoxyethylenenitrilo tetraacetic acid.

No significant changes in PTH levels were observed, which suggests that calcitonin release accounted for the decrease in serum Ca^{2+}. Serum Ca^{2+} returned to normal as calcitonin levels decreased. With convalescence, there is resolution of edema or revascularization, which results in the reestablishment of parathyroid gland integrity.

Most patients who develop hypocalcemia after neck surgery remain asymptomatic; however, occasionally patients may develop paresthesias, laryngeal spasm, or tetany. The authors recommend that the serum-ionized Ca^{2+} level be monitored every 12 hours in patients after neck surgery—more frequently if hypocalcemic symptoms develop—until the serum-ionized Ca^{2+} level begins to rise (indicating recovery of the parathyroid glands). Symptomatic or severely hypocalcemic (ionized Ca^{2+} <3 mg/dl) patients should receive supplemental Ca^{2+}. When Ca^{2+} is replaced in these patients, it is important that the Ca^{2+} level be maintained in the low normal ranges so as not to suppress the recovering parathyroid glands. Postoperative hypoparathyroidism may manifest late after neck surgery (months to years), and patients at risk should have their serum ionized Ca^{2+} levels serially monitored. Other patients may have latent hypoparathyroidism after neck surgery, which manifests only with stress. Thus, critically ill patients with a previous history of neck surgery should have a serum Ca^{2+} determination performed.

Overt hypoparathyroidism rarely occurs after radioiodine treatment for thyroid disease (19); however, a significant number of these patients may have latent hypoparathyroidism, as measured by a diminished PTH response to ethylenediamine-tetraacetic acid (EDTA)-induced hypocalcemia. The serum Ca^{2+} should be monitored in these patients during stress in order to avoid hypocalcemia. Infrequent causes of hypoparathyroidism are metastasis to the parathyroid glands and iron deposition resulting from hemochromatosis.

Neonates have lower serum Ca^{2+} concentrations than do older infants; the limits for pathologic hypocalcemia have been set at 8 mg/dl in full-term infants and 7 mg/dl in premature infants (19). Two types of hypocalcemia have been described in newborn infants. The first occurs early after birth (1 to 3 days) and is called "early neonatal hypocalcemia." It is attributed to parathyroid immaturity and/or physiologic maternal hyperparathyroidism (causing neonatal parathyroid gland suppression) and usually resolves within the first week of life. Predisposing factors for neonatal hypocalcemia include prematurity, maternal diabetes mellitus, perinatal complications, and birth asphyxia. Late-onset neonatal hypocalcemia occurs 6 to 8 days after birth and is associated with hyperphosphatemia and hypomagnesemia. These infants frequently present with metabolic convulsions, and the hypocalcemia likely results from high PO_4 intake (from milk). High-serum PO_4 levels decrease the serum Ca^{2+} concentration by increasing Ca^{2+} deposition in bone. Hypomagnesemia results from decreased intestinal Mg^{2+} absorption. The hypomagnesemia augments the hypocalcemia via inhibition of PTH secretion and skeletal resistance. Other causes of hypoparathyroidism and hypocalcemia in infants include maternal hyperparathyroidism and excessive Ca^{2+} or vitamin D intake in the mother (both agents cross the placenta).

Parathyroid gland immaturity is believed to occur in some infants, especially premature infants, immediately following birth. Maturation of the parathyroid glands following birth is poorly studied. The authors recently evaluated PTH secretion in infants and young children following cardiopulmonary bypass-induced hypocalcemia (22). PTH secretion was reduced slightly in infants less than 1 month of age, but in older infants and young children it was similar to that in adults. Thus, it appears that most infants have adequate parathyroid gland function to maintain normal ionized calcium homeostasis.

Postoperative hypocalcemia may also occur in patients after parathyroid or thyroid surgery, unrelated to hypoparathyroidism. After removal of the stimulus for elevated bone turnover (such as PTH or thyroid hormone), high rates of bone formation may develop and result in a lowering of the serum Ca^{2+} concentration ("recalcification hypocalcemia"). The incidence and severity of symptoms depends on the degree of postoperative bone involvement. These patients also frequently develop hypomagnesemia and hypophosphatemia.

Ionized hypocalcemia is common in patients undergoing cardiopulmonary bypass surgery (23). Hypocalcemia results from dilution and chelation of circulating calcium. Parathyroid gland secretion is normal in these patients, and ionized calcium levels usually return to normal following bypass.

MAGNESIUM

Mg^{2+} abnormalities are common in critically ill patients and may cause hypocalcemia (16, 24–29). The serum Mg^{2+} level influences both PTH secretion and action. Mild hypomagnesemia stimulates PTH secretion, whereas severe hypomagnesemia ($Mg^{2+} < 1.0$ mg/dl) and hypermagnesemia inhibit PTH secretion. Hypomagnesemia also impairs PTH action at its receptor (i.e., skeletal resistance) and causes vitamin D resistance (20, 28, 30, 31). Since Mg^{2+} is an important cofactor for the activation of adenylate cyclase, it is possible that severe Mg^{2+} deficiency leads to an impairment of adenylate cyclase resulting in deranged PTH release and skeletal resistance. A variety of diseases and medications can cause hypomagnesemia and hypermagnesemia (see the section entitled "Magnesium"). Hypomagnesemic hypocalcemia responds poorly to calcium therapy alone but does respond to Mg^{2+} repletion.

PHOSPHATE

Hyperphosphatemia (see the section entitled "Phosphorus") may cause hypocalcemia as a result of calcium precipitation, inhibition of bone resorption, and suppression of renal 1-hydroxylation of vitamin D (32, 33). The most common causes of this syndrome in the ICU include PO_4 administration (e.g., during the treatment of diabetic ketoacidosis), tumor lysis syndromes following chemotherapy, renal failure, and rhabdomyolysis. Hypocalcemia during rhabdomyolysis is complex and appears to result from a combination of factors that include tissue Ca^{2+} deposition, hyperphosphatemia, impaired 1,25-dihydroxyvitamin D synthesis, and skeletal resistance to PTH (34). The serum PO_4 level should be measured in all hypocalcemic patients, since administration of Ca^{2+} to hyperphosphatemic patients may increase Ca^{2+} precipitation and cause further harm. The hypocalcemia in hyperphosphatemic patients is treated by lowering the serum PO_4 level.

CHELATORS

Chelators are anions that are capable of forming complexes with Ca^{2+}. The most common chelators that cause hypocalcemia in critically ill patients are citrated blood, albumin, and radiocontrast dyes.

VITAMIN D DEFICIENCY

Vitamin D deficiency is being recognized increasingly as an important cause of hypocalcemia in patients in the ICU. Approximately 20% of the hypocalcemic patients seen by the authors in the ICU have a defect in the vitamin D axis. Many of these patients are chronically ill, malnourished, and have minimal exposure to sunlight. They have low serum 25-hydroxyvitamin D levels, suggestive of dietary vitamin D deficiency. Vitamin D deficiency may also occur in patients with a normal dietary intake as a result of gut malabsorption, defects in fat digestion, impaired biliary secretion or disrupted intestinal integrity (e.g., gastrectomy, gastrojejunostomy, celiac disease, Crohn's disease, intestinal bypass surgery, pancreatic insufficiency, hepatobiliary disease) (18). Excessive amounts of vitamin D bound to its transport protein may be lost in the urine of patients with the nephrotic syndrome.

Acquired defects in the hepatic 25-hydroxylase enzyme have not been shown to cause pathologic vitamin D deficiency (e.g., hypocalcemia). Although hypocalcemia is found in patients with advanced liver disease, the primary cause for low vitamin D levels appears to be malabsorption (failure of biliary secretion) rather than failure of hydroxylation.

Other patients have renal insufficiency with deficiency of the renal 1-hydroxylase system, which is responsible for the production of 1,25-dihydroxyvitamin D. These vitamin D-deficient patients frequently have normal serum Ca^{2+} levels as outpatients; however, they may be unable to mobilize sufficient Ca^{2+} to maintain normal circulating levels during critical illness (35). Pseudohypoparathyroidism (20) is a rare disorder that results from resistance to PTH. Resultant suppression of the 1-hydroxylase system leads to deficiency of 1,25-dihydroxyvitamin D and hypocalcemia.

PANCREATITIS

Hypocalcemia is commonly seen in patients with acute pancreatitis and is associated with a poor prognosis (5, 36). The exact etiology of the hypocalcemia in pancreatitis is uncertain. Saponification of Ca^{2+} is inadequate to explain the degree and length of hypocalcemia. PTH has been reported to be elevated (37), normal (38, 39), or decreased (38, 40). Bone and kidney can respond to exogenous PTH when it is given to patients with pancreatitis (39). Although this observation rules out complete end-organ resistance to PTH, it does not rule out partial PTH resistance. Analysis of the data on hypocalcemia in pancreatitis suggests that there are at least two groups of patients who develop hypocalcemia in this disorder. The majority of these patients have relative hypoparathyroidism (20) with normal or low PTH during hypocalcemia, whereas the remainder have appropriately increased levels of PTH. The group with elevated PTH levels may suffer from a defect in the vitamin D axis or from tissue resistance to PTH or vitamin D. In one study (37), serum 1,25-dihydroxyvitamin D levels were measured in six pancreatitis patients with hypocalcemia. In these patients serum vitamin D levels were low when the patients were admitted (during hypocalcemia) but increased in parallel with increases in PTH during recovery. Pancreatitis-associated hypomagnesemia and renal failure may also contribute to hypocalcemia.

SEPSIS

The hypocalcemia occurring in patients with sepsis appears to have multiple causes (41). Some patients have dietary vitamin D deficiency, whereas others have acquired parathyroid gland insufficiency, renal 1-hydroxylase insufficiency, or peripheral resistance to 1,25-dihydroxyvitamin D (41). Renal 1-hydroxylase deficiency usually occurs when renal insufficiency accompanies sepsis.

HUNGRY BONE SYNDROMES

Hypocalcemia may occur after parathyroidectomy or thyroidectomy in patients with "overactive glands." These patients have accelerated bone resorption and formation. When the stimulus for resorption is removed at surgery, bone formation may exceed mineral supply and hypocalcemia results. The hypocalcemia is usually accompanied by hypophosphatemia and hypomagnesemia. Increased bone formation and hypocalcemia may also occur during osteoblastic metastasis from prostate, breast, and lung malignancies (20).

FAT EMBOLISM SYNDROME

Hypocalcemia is seen occasionally in trauma patients with fat embolism. The hypocalcemia probably results from a combination of Ca^{2+} chelation and increases in protein binding of Ca^{2+} induced by release of fatty acids. Transient episodes of ionized hypocalcemia associated with respiratory distress, in a patient after trauma, suggest the presence of this syndrome.

MISCELLANEOUS

Hypocalcemia is associated with the toxic shock syndrome. Although circulating calcitonin levels are elevated in this syndrome, the exact pathogenesis of the hypocalcemia remains undefined (4). Ionized hypocalcemia occurs in patients with burns; however, the etiology remains to be defined. Hypothyroidism affects Ca^{2+} homeostasis by decreasing bone turnover and may also cause hypocalcemia. Hypothyroid patients usually have elevated levels of PTH and 1,25-dihydroxyvitamin D (5). A large number of drugs have been reported to cause hypocalcemia, although clear documentation of ionized hypocalcemia is lacking with many. Listed in Table 46.1 are those drugs in which a clear association with hypocalcemia has been documented. Phosphates, citrate, magnesium, radiocontrast dye, albumin, and heparin have already been discussed. Aminoglycosides, *cis*-platinum, and loop diuretics may cause hypocalcemia by producing hypomagnesemia. *Cis*-platinum also can inhibit bone resorption (42–44). EDTA and sodium sulfate (45) are potent Ca^{2+} chelators and have been used clinically to treat hypercalcemia. Mithramycin (46), calcitonin (47), estrogens, protamine (48), gallium nitrate (49), and diphosphonates (50–52) decrease bone resorption and are also used to treat hypercalcemia. WR-2721 is a radioprotective agent that inhibits PTH secretion (53, 54). Anticonvulsants such as phenytoin and phenobarbital have been associated with hypocalcemia and reduced bone mass. Although they increase the hepatic metabolism of vitamin D, this effect does not appear to be adequate to explain the hypocalcemia. These anticonvulsant drugs may also decrease intestinal Ca^{2+} absorption and reduce PTH-induced bone resorption (20). Ethylene glycol intoxication causes hypocalcemia, presumably by means of the complexation of oxalate (a metabolic product of ethylene glycol metabolism) with Ca^{2+} (55). Sodium fluoride forms an insoluble salt with Ca^{2+} (56) and may induce hypocalcemia when taken in large doses (as may be used in the treatment of osteoporosis).

Clinical Manifestations

Hypocalcemia may present with a variety of clinical signs and symptoms (Table 46.2) that relate to increased neuronal irritability (5). Cardiovascular manifestations are the most

Table 46.2. Clinical Manifestations of Hypocalcemia

Cardiovascular
   Hypotension
   Cardiac insufficiency
   Bradycardia
   Arrhythmias
   Insensitivity to catecholamines and digitalis
   Cardiac arrest
ECG
   Q-T and S-T interval prolongation
   T-wave inversion
Respiratory
   Laryngeal spasm
   Apnea
   Bronchospasm
   Weakness
Neuromuscular
   Tetany
   Chvostek's and Trousseau's signs
   Muscle spasm
   Paresthesias
   Seizures
   Weakness
   Extrapyramidal manifestations
Psychiatric
   Anxiety
   Dementia
   Depression
   Irritability
   Psychosis
   Confusion
Miscellaneous
   Coarse, dry, scaly skin
   Brittle nails
   Thin, brittle hair
   Cataracts

commonly encountered features of hypocalcemia seen in critically ill patients. Patients may develop hypotension, cardiac insufficiency, bradycardia, arrhythmias (e.g., ventricular fibrillation), and failure to respond to drugs that act through calcium-related mechanisms (e.g., digoxin, catecholamines, glucagon) (57–62). Hypocalcemia should always be considered in patients with hypotension that responds poorly to fluids and/or to pressor agents. Restoration of a normal circulating Ca^{2+} level may restore vascular tone and improve cardiac contractility. It is important to note that mild degrees of ionized hypocalcemia (e.g., ionized calcium >0.8 mmol/liter) rarely cause cardiovascular insufficiency. Most patients with cardiovascular insufficiency have levels of ionized calcium below 0.7 mmol/liter. Ca^{2+} may also be an effective inotropic agent in patients with advanced cardiac disease (62, 63) who have β-adrenergic receptor down-regulation as a result of chronic sympathetic stimulation. In some patients, digitalis may be ineffective, at normal levels, in controlling supraventricular arrhythmias (59), and catecholamines and glucagon (58) may be ineffective in raising blood pressure or heart rate caused by hypocalcemia. Agents that decrease cellular Ca^{2+} availability (e.g., β-adrenergic blockers and slow calcium channel antagonists) may exacerbate hypocalcemia-induced cardiac insufficiency. Hypocalcemia may inconsistently cause Q-T and S-T interval prolongation; however, these electrocardiogram (ECG) changes cannot be relied upon to exclude a diagnosis of hypocalcemia.

Hypocalcemia may also present as laryngospasm or bronchospasm in critically ill patients. Tetany and muscle spasms

are the classical signs of hypocalcemia, but these signs may be absent in hypocalcemic ICU patients. Chvostek's and Trousseau's signs are nonspecific indicators of hypocalcemia. Chvostek's sign is present in 25% of normal adults, whereas Trousseau's sign is present in 4% of the normal population (20). In addition, Trousseau's sign may be negative in 30% of subjects with hypocalcemia. Anticonvulsant drugs, sedation, and paralysis may eliminate signs of neuronal irritability. The intubated, sedated, or paralyzed patient may be unable to express symptoms such as anxiety and paresthesias. Psychiatric manifestations of hypocalcemia (Table 46.2) are nonspecific and are frequently seen in critically ill patients as a result of their illness.

The authors routinely monitor serum-ionized Ca^{2+} levels in all critically ill patients and treat all patients with hypocalcemic symptoms or severe hypocalcemia. Life-threatening arrhythmias develop when the ionized Ca^{2+} level approaches 2.0 to 2.5 mg/dl (0.5 to 0.65 mmol/liter); thus, the authors recommend that all patients with an ionized Ca^{2+} concentration below 3.2 mg/dl (0.8 mmol/liter) receive treatment.

Treatment

Patients with suspected hypocalcemia should have an ionized Ca^{2+} level measured to confirm the diagnosis (Fig. 46.2). Once this diagnosis is confirmed, these patients should have a blood sample sent for measurement of serum magnesium and phosphorus levels. Levels of these ions should be corrected. Blood samples should be saved for plasma PTH and vitamin D levels, should these tests later become necessary (Fig. 46.2).

Acute symptomatic hypocalcemia is a medical emergency that necessitates intravenous Ca^{2+} therapy (Table 46.3). Initial therapy in adults consists of the administration of a Ca^{2+} bolus (100 to 200 mg of elemental Ca^{2+} over 10 minutes) followed by a maintenance infusion of 1 to 2 mg/kg/hr of elemental Ca^{2+}. A 100 to 200 mg bolus of elemental Ca^{2+} will usually raise the serum total Ca^{2+} by 1 mg/dl, with levels returning to baseline by 30 minutes after injection. To maintain levels above baseline a continuous infusion or intermittent boluses of Ca^{2+} are necessary. The amount of calcium required to maintain normal circulating levels varies among patients and must be individualized. The serum Ca^{2+} usually normalizes in 6 to 12 hours with this regimen, and the maintenance rate may need to be decreased to 0.3 to 0.5 mg/kg/hr. Serum Mg^{2+} and PO_4 levels should be measured and restored to normal values. Administration of Ca^{2+} to hyperphosphatemic patients may cause Ca^{2+} precipitation. Hypomagnesemic and hypermagnesemic hypocalcemia responds poorly to Ca^{2+} therapy but does respond to normalization of the serum Mg^{2+} level. Potassium deficiency protects the patient from hypocalcemic tetany and arrhythmias, and correction of the hypokalemia without correction of the hypocalcemia may provoke these disorders (56). Administration of drugs that may be aggravating hypocalcemia (e.g., furosemide) should be discontinued or another drug substituted if possible. Intravenous Ca^{2+} preparations are irritating to veins, and Ca^{2+} should be diluted in 50 to 100 ml of 5% dextrose in water. Ca^{2+} chloride should never be injected into tissues; however, Ca^{2+} gluceptate may be given intramuscularly when intravenous access is not possible (56). Ca^{2+} salts should not be administered with bicarbonate, since the two precipitate. Ca^{2+} must be administered cautiously to patients receiving digitalis, since hypercalcemia predisposes to digitalis toxicity. Adequacy of treatment can be monitored at the bedside by following Chvostek's and Trousseau's signs, the ECG, and hemodynamic parameters. Optimal therapy requires frequent monitoring of the serum Ca^{2+}, Mg^{2+}, PO_4, potassium, and creatinine levels. Once serum Ca^{2+} is stable in the low normal range, the patient may be started on enteral Ca^{2+} (Table 46.3). Most patients require 2 to 4 g of calcium per day in divided doses. Ca^{2+} carbonate is converted in the stomach to a soluble calcium salt by hydrochloric acid. It is ineffective in patients with achlorhydria (20).

A large body of evidence suggests that cellular calcium overload contributes to cellular dysfunction and death after ischemia and shock (64–67). Patients with a large number of diseases may have increased intracellular free calcium concentrations, even when circulating ionized calcium is low (68).

Administration of calcium to these patients may be detrimental by activating proteases, lipases, nucleases, or free radical production. Thus, calcium should be given after confirmation of ionized hypocalcemia so as to avoid unnecessary and potentially injurious therapy in patients with low total calcium levels but normal ionized calcium concentrations.

Mild degrees of hypocalcemia (i.e., ionized calcium >0.8 mmol/liter) are usually well-tolerated in critically ill patients. Animal studies suggest that mild hypocalcemia may be protective during ischemic and shock states. Thus, the authors do not usually treat patients with mild hypocalcemia but rather observe the ionized calcium level closely and treat only if it falls below 0.8 mmol/liter.

When Ca^{2+} alone is insufficient in normalizing the serum Ca^{2+} concentration, vitamin D metabolites (Table 46.4) may be added (56). Vitamin D is rarely required during the period

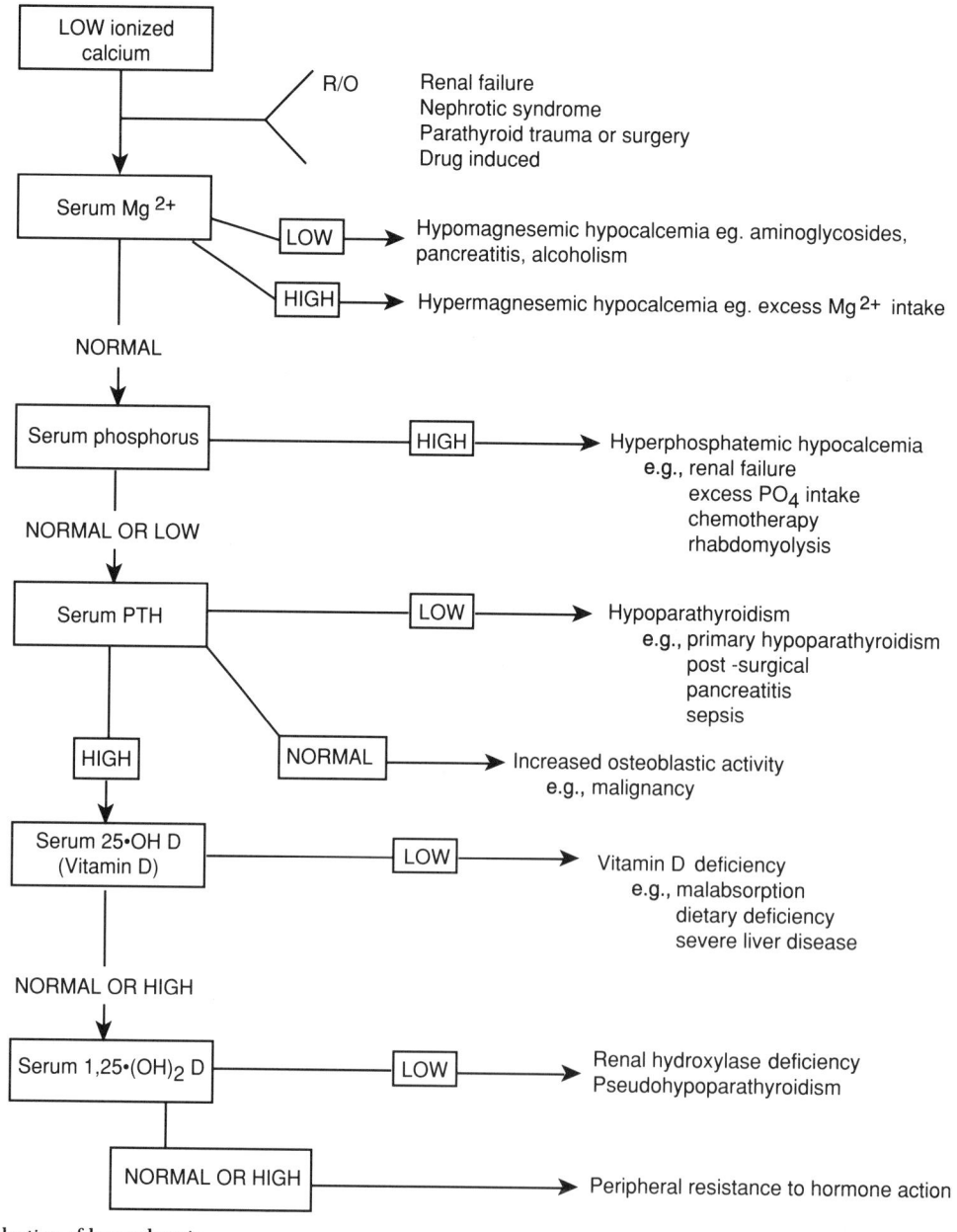

Figure 46.2.   Evaluation of hypocalcemia.

Table 46.3.   Calcium Preparations

	Dosage/Form	Contents[a]
Parenteral		
Ca^{2+} gluconate (10%)	10 ml	93 mg Ca^{2+} (4.6 mEq)
Ca^{2+} gluceptate	5 ml	90 mg Ca^{2+} (4.5 mEq)
Ca^{2+} chloride (10%)	10 ml	272 mg Ca^{2+} (13.6 mEq)
Oral		
Ca^{2+} carbonate (e.g., Os-cal 500)	Tablets	500 mg Ca^{2+}
Ca^{2+} gluconate	Tablets	500 mg Ca^{2+}
Ca^{2+} lactate	Tablets	650 mg Ca^{2+}
Ca^{2+} glubionate (e.g., Neo-calglucon)	Syrup	115 mg Ca^{2+}/5 ml

[a] Elemental Ca^{2+}.

Table 46.4.   Vitamin D Preparations

	Ergocalciferol (Vit D_2)	Calcifediol (250HD)	Dihydrotachysterol (1-OHD)	Calcitriol (1,25(OH)2D)
Concentration in serum	10 ng/ml	30 ng/ml		0.03 ng/ml
Physiologic dose (µg/day)	10	5	20	0.5
Pharmacologic dose (µg/day)	1200	50	200–800	0.25–1
Onset of maximal effect (days)	30	15	15	3
Dosage forms	Tablets	Capsules	Tablets	Capsules
	625 µg	20 µg	125 µg	0.25 µg
	1250 µg	50 µg	200 µg	0.50 µg
			400 µg	
	Solution		Solution	
	8000 U/ml		200 µg/ml	
	Oil for injection			
	500,000 U/ml			
Commercial products	Calciferol	Calderol	Hytakerol	Rocaltrol
Serum half-life (days)	30	15		0.2
Time for reversal of effect (days)	17–60	7–30	3–14	2–10
Advantages	Low cost, prolonged action, parent compound	Liver disease	Renal disease, hypoparathyroidism	Renal disease, liver disease, hypoparathyroidism, rapid onset, rapid offset
Disadvantages	Instability, long toxicity	Expense	Expense	Expense

of critical illness while the patient is in the ICU. It is usually reserved for chronic treatment of hypocalcemia. The principal effect of vitamin D is to increase gut Ca^{2+} absorption, although it also has effects on bone resorption. The earliest calciferol metabolite that is deficient should be administered first. This approach allows the body to regulate activation of the vitamin and replenishes other vitamin D metabolites, which may have some as yet unknown physiologic function. When the 1-hydroxylase enzyme is deficient (as in renal failure) or when patients are resistant to ergocalciferol, they may respond to 1,25-dihydroxyvitamin D. This analogue is more potent than other vitamin D metabolites (Table 46.4), has a quicker onset of action, and has a greater tendency to induce hypercalcemia and hypercalciuria but a shorter duration of toxicity. Vitamin D requirements vary and must be adjusted based on disease activity, interacting drugs, and dietary Ca^{2+} intake.

Hypercalciuria with its attendant problems (e.g., nephrocalcinosis and renal stones) may occur before eucalcemia is reached. In these situations, a thiazide diuretic may be helpful in reducing Ca^{2+} excretion. Serum Ca^{2+} and PO_4 levels and urinary Ca^{2+} excretion should be measured at regular intervals. The therapeutic goal is to restore the serum Ca^{2+} to nearly normal levels (which alleviate symptoms) and avoid complications (e.g., hypercalcemia and hypercalciuria).

Definitive treatment of hypocalcemia involves recognition and correction of the underlying disorder. Frequently, however, acute measures are required to stabilize the serum Ca^{2+} level within safe ranges before addressing the primary problem.

HYPERCALCEMIA

Causes

Hypercalcemia (ionized calcium >1.3 mmol/liter or 5.2 mg/dl) occurs when Ca^{2+} enters the vascular space faster than it can be excreted or sequestered. The most common causes (Table 46.5) of hypercalcemia seen in the critical care setting are malignancy, hyperparathyroidism, immobilization, exogenous Ca^{2+} administration, hypercalcemia of renal failure, and posthypocalcemic hypercalcemia. Except in the case of exogenous calcium administration, the hypercalcemia results primarily from increased bone resorption.

MALIGNANCY

Hypercalcemia (69) occurs in approximately 10 to 20% of patients with malignancy because of direct tumor osteolysis

Table 46.5.   Causes of Hypercalcemia

Malignancy
Hyperparathyroidism
Immobilization
Calcium administration
Renal causes
   Chronic renal failure
   Recovery from acute renal failure
   After renal transplantation
Posthypocalcemic hypercalcemia
Hypocalciuric hypercalcemia
   Familial
   Hypothyroidism
   Lithium
   Thiazides
   Adrenal insufficiency
   Bartter's syndrome
Granulomatous disease
   Sarcoidosis
   Histoplasmosis
   Coccidiomycosis
   Tuberculosis
Hyperthyroidism
AIDS
Phosphorus depletion syndrome
Multiple endocrine neoplasia syndromes
Pheochromocytoma
Acromegaly
Drug-induced
   Calcium
   Estrogens or progestins for malignancy
   Lithium
   Milk-alkali syndrome
   Theophylline
   Thiazides
   Vitamin D or A

of bone and because of the secretion of humoral substances that stimulate bone resorption (20). Humoral bone resorbing substances include PTH-like substances (69–73), 1,25-dihydroxyvitamin D (74, 75), osteoclast activating factor (76), and prostaglandins (77). PTH-like substances cross-react in the radioimmunoassay for PTH but are not identical to PTH. They are at present thought to be responsible for most instances of humoral hypercalcemia of malignancy and most likely represent a heterogeneous group of molecules. These molecules stimulate bone resorption and frequently are capable of stimulating the renal adenylate cyclase system and inhibiting phosphate resorption, similar to PTH. They have little activity on the renal 1-hydroxylase enzyme that is responsible for the renal synthesis of 1,25-dihydroxyvitamin D. Tumor synthesis of 1,25-dihydroxyvitamin D is a less common cause of hypercalcemia but has been described in patients with lymphoma (74) and Hodgkin's disease (75). Osteoclast activating factor, a lymphokine released by stimulated peripheral blood leukocytes, may be released into the circulation in neoplasia of lymphoid origin (e.g., multiple myeloma, lymphoma, and leukemia) and, like 1,25-dihydroxyvitamin D, is antagonized by glucocorticoids. Hypercalcemia resulting from prostaglandins is a rare cause of hypercalcemia, usually occurs with solid tumors, and may respond to cyclooxygenase inhibitors. Tumor-related hypercalcemia occurs most commonly with breast, lung, kidney, prostate, and hematologic malignancies. Primary hyperparathyroidism also occurs with a higher frequency in hypercalcemic patients with malignancy (20).

HYPERPARATHYROIDISM

Primary hyperparathyroidism is found in the general population with a prevalence that ranges from 0.03 to 0.1% (5, 69, 78–81). The most common causes of primary hyperparathyroidism are single adenomas (75 to 87%), hyperplasia of multiple glands (12 to 22%), and carcinoma of the parathyroid glands (3%). Hypercalcemia in hyperparathyroidism results from the combined effects of increased PTH and 1,25-dihydroxyvitamin D on bone, intestine, and kidneys. Many hyperparathyroid patients are asymptomatic, and the hypercalcemia is noted only when a serum Ca^{2+} level is measured for other reasons. Most of these patients do not require emergency treatment for their hypercalcemia, but some type of treatment is frequently required to prevent accelerated bone loss. Surgery remains the only definitive treatment for patients with hyperparathyroidism (81), although some patients may have slight decreases in plasma Ca^{2+} and decreased bone turnover with estrogen or progestogen therapy (82, 83). Estrogens and progestins appear to work by antagonizing PTH action upon the skeleton. When one encounters a patient with hyperparathyroidism caused by glandular hyperplasia, a search for other endocrine tumors should be sought as part of the multiple endocrine neoplasia syndromes (e.g., tumors of the pituitary, pancreas, adrenal, and thyroid).

IMMOBILIZATION

Immobilization hypercalcemia (69) occurs following immobilization in patients with rapid bone turnover. The patients most at risk are children, adolescents, postfracture patients, patients with Paget's disease of bone, and patients with underlying malignancy or hyperparathyroidism. Patients with renal failure are also at risk because of their inability to excrete an increased Ca^{2+} load. Most immobilized patients have increased urinary Ca^{2+} and PO_4 levels, but only a few develop hypercalcemia (5). Serum PTH and 1,25-dihydroxyvitamin D levels are usually suppressed, and hypercalcemia probably results from a relative increase in osteoclastic activity. Symptoms relate to the degree of hypercalciuria and hypercalcemia. The primary therapeutic modality in these patients is mobilization. Quiet standing for a few hours a day is superior to supine bed exercise. Serum Ca^{2+} levels may also be reduced by saline diuresis, calcitonin, oral phosphates, and diphosphonates. Dietary Ca^{2+} restriction has little effect, since most circulating Ca^{2+} is derived from bone.

RENAL-RELATED CAUSES

Hypercalcemia is seen occasionally in patients with uremia and may be iatrogenic, resulting from excess Ca^{2+} or vitamin D supplementation, the use of high Ca^{2+} dialysate, or immobilization. These patients are prone to hypercalcemia because they lack the ability to excrete Ca^{2+} through the kidneys, and many have a defect in bone mineralization. Patients with secondary hyperparathyroidism may become hypercalcemic after the institution of dialysis. Dialysis may render the bone more responsive to PTH or may lead to hypercalcemia by lowering PO_4 levels. Other causes of hypercalcemia in these patients include the use of Ca^{2+}-containing cation exchange resins, PO$_4$ depletion with aluminum hydroxide compounds, or the use of thiazide diuretics. Hypercalcemia may also occur during the recovery phase of acute renal failure or following renal transplantation (20). The cause of hypercalcemia in these patients relates to the presence of secondary hyperparathyroidism, reduction in circulating PO$_4$ concentrations, tapering of steroids, and, perhaps, increased sensitivity of bone to PTH during resolution of uremia (20). Hyperplastic parathyroid glands usually involute within 6 months of renal transplantation. At times, hyperplastic glands may persist and parathyroidectomy may be necessary to avoid renal graft dysfunction (20) and persistent bone loss.

POSTHYPOCALCEMIC HYPERCALCEMIA

Transient hypercalcemia is not uncommon in patients after a period of hypocalcemia (84). The hypercalcemia most likely results from increased PTH and 1,25-dihydroxyvitamin D levels that were stimulated by the hypocalcemia. Hypocalcemia resolves faster than the Ca^{2+}-mobilizing hormones can readjust, resulting in a transient period of rebound hypercalcemia. A review of cases of transient hypercalcemia of unknown etiology in the authors' ICU revealed a period of hypocalcemia preceding the hypercalcemia in each case. The hypercalcemia resolved without treatment in all cases.

HYPOCALCIURIC HYPERCALCEMIA

Hypercalcemia may occur in patients associated with decreased urinary Ca^{2+} excretion (85, 86). The hypercalcemia appears to result from the combination of altered parathyroid gland function and altered ion transport in the kidneys. Marx and associates (85) described the inherited syndrome of familial hypocalciuric hypercalcemia (FHH). This disease rarely causes symptoms and is usually discovered when a serum Ca^{2+} level is obtained for other reasons. Serum Ca^{2+}, PTH, 1,25-dihydroxyvitamin D, and urinary cyclic adenosine monophosphate (cAMP) levels (an index of PTH activity) overlap with normal and hyperparathyroid patients; however, urinary Ca^{2+} excretion is less than 150 mg/day and the Ca^{2+}/creatinine clearance ratio is less than 0.01. These patients generally do well without treatment and do not develop bone disease. Hypocalciuric hypercalcemia may also occur in patients with hypothyroidism (87), with lithium therapy, after thiazide administration, with adrenal insufficiency, and with Bartter's syndrome.

GRANULOMATOUS DISEASE

Hypercalcemia (10 to 20%) and hypercalciuria (30 to 50%) are commonly seen in patients with sarcoidosis (20, 69, 78, 88). Most hypercalcemic sarcoid patients have an abnormal chest radiograph, abnormal pulmonary function tests, increased bone turnover, and increased gut absorption of Ca^{2+}. Parathyroid function is suppressed; however, these patients produce excess amounts of 1,25-dihydroxyvitamin D within their granuloma (89–91). Lymphocytes in granulomata (69, 88) associated with histoplasmosis, coccidiomycosis, tuberculosis (92), silicone injections, and berylliosis are also capable of producing excessive amounts of active vitamin D metabolites and hypercalcemia. The hypercalcemia in these patients improves with glucocorticoids.

MISCELLANEOUS

Thyroid hormone has direct effects on the skeleton, increasing bone turnover and Ca^{2+} release. Although severe hypercalcemia is rare in patients with hyperthyroidism, mild asymptomatic hypercalcemia is encountered frequently (20). PTH and 1,25-dihydroxyvitamin D levels are suppressed in these patients. Hypercalcemia in patients with hyperthyroidism may respond to calcitonin, glucocorticoids, propranolol, and lowering of thyroid hormone levels. Hypercalcemia associated with suppressed PTH and 1,25-dihydroxyvitamin D levels also may occur in patients with the acquired immune deficiency syndrome (AIDS) and probably results from increased bone turnover (93). Phosphorus depletion may occur in patients given phosphate-binding antacids. Stimulation of 1,25-dihydroxyvitamin D synthesis may lead to increased gut Ca^{2+} absorption and bone resorption and thereby cause hypercalcemia. Catecholamines may increase PTH secretion and stimulate bone turnover. In fact, hypercalcemia is seen occasionally in patients with pheochromocytoma (20). These patients may respond to therapy with β-adrenergic blockers. Growth hormone can enhance the formation of 1,25-dihydroxyvitamin D, and hypercalcemia has been reported in patients with acromegaly (20). Patients with breast cancer may rarely develop progressive hypercalcemia after receiving treatment with estrogens or progestins, as a result of tumor necrosis with release of bone-resorbing substances. A variety of drugs may cause hypercalcemia (Table 46.5). Administration of vitamin D or A increases bone turnover and causes hypercalcemia (69, 88). Vitamin D also increases intestinal Ca^{2+} absorption. Hypervitaminosis D or vitamin A-induced hypercalcemia responds to glucocorticoid administration. The milk-alkali syndrome (94) consists of hypercalcemia, alkalosis, and renal impairment and is seen in patients who ingest excessive amounts of Ca^{2+} and alkali (e.g., Ca^{2+} carbonate or milk plus sodium bicarbonate for treatment of peptic ulcers). The alkali lowers the urine solubility for Ca^{2+}, decreases Ca^{2+} excretion, and may cause progressive hypercalcemia and renal insufficiency. Ca^{2+} depresses PTH secretion and increases renal bicarbonate resorption, further worsening alkalosis. Thiazides and lithium enhance renal Ca^{2+} resorption and decrease renal Ca^{2+} excretion (20). Lithium may also stimulate parathyroid gland activity. Theophylline causes an elevation of the serum Ca^{2+} level that is mediated through adrenergic mechanisms and is compatible with enhancement of PTH action (95). Serum Ca^{2+} levels fall after the administration of β-adrenergic blockers.

Clinical Manifestations

Hypercalcemia causes a variety of effects on multiple organ systems (Table 46.6). In addition, many of the clinical features of hypercalcemia reflect features of the underlying disease (i.e., malignancy) and not the hypercalcemia itself. Ca^{2+} may form stones within the kidneys or disrupt tubular or glomerular function. Reduction in glomerular filtration results from

Table 46.6. Clinical Features of Hypercalcemia

Cardiovascular
    Hypertension
    Arrhythmias
    Digitalis sensitivity
    Catecholamine resistance
    Q-T shortening
Urinary system
    Nephrocalcinosis
    Nephrolithiasis
    Tubular dysfunction
        Renal tubular acidosis
        Impaired Na resorption
        Free water loss
    Glomerular disorders
    Interstitial nephritis
Gastrointestinal
    Peptic ulcers
    Pancreatitis
    Constipation
    Anorexia
    Nausea/vomiting
Neuromuscular
    Weakness, atrophy
    Hyporeflexia
Neuropsychiatric
    Depression
    Personality change
    Psychomotor retardation
    Memory impairment
    Psychosis
    Disorientation
    Obtundation
    Coma
    Seizures
    EEG abnormalities
Skeletal
    Osteopenia
    Osteitis fibrosa cystica
Miscellaneous
    Skin necrosis
    Corneal calcification
    Conjunctivitis
    Pruritus
    Decreased bronchial clearance of secretions
    Hypomagnesemia

volume depletion and a reduction in the ultrafiltration coefficient (20). Impairment of sodium resorption results from inhibition of sodium-potassium ATPase in the ascending limb of Henle and distal tubules. Ca^{2+} antagonism of antidiuretic hormone activity within the kidney can lead to a state of nephrogenic diabetes insipidus (impaired renal concentration), progressive dehydration, and further hypercalcemia. Neuromyopathic manifestations are common and may contribute to the failure to wean a hypercalcemic patient from the ventilator. Neuropsychiatric changes are frequent but are not specific for hypercalcemia.

The cardiovascular effects of hypercalcemia include hypertension and arrhythmias. These effects may respond to Ca^{2+} channel antagonists (96). Electrocardiographic changes are not reliable indicators of the degree of hypercalcemia, and Q-T shortening is seen in only a minority of cases (97). Hypercalcemia increases cardiac sensitivity to digitalis and may lead to digitalis-related toxicity. Calcium administration decreases the response to β-adrenergic agonists in both animal (98) and

human studies (64, 99–101). Ca^{2+} may work in these situations by inhibiting adenyl cyclase activity (102).

Anorexia is common in hypercalcemic patients. These patients are also prone to develop pancreatitis and peptic ulcer disease. Skeletal disease may occur secondary to direct tumor invasion or secretion of bone-resorbing substances. Hypomagnesemia may result from Ca^{2+}-induced inhibition of Mg^{2+} resorption in the renal tubules (20). The threshold for the development of hypercalcemic symptoms varies; however, most asymptomatic patients have a total serum Ca^{2+} level below 12 mg/dl (3 mmol/liter) with a normal albumin concentration. Ionized calcium levels are usually below 1.5 mmol/liter (6 mg/dl) in asymptomatic patients. Factors such as the rapidity with which the serum Ca^{2+} rises, accompanying renal failure, electrolyte disturbances, cardiovascular status, and the general state of debilitation of the patient can alter the threshold for symptoms. The most common causes of death as a result of hypercalcemia relate to renal failure, arrhythmias, and central nervous system impairment.

Evaluation

Hypercalcemia should be documented by measuring a fasting serum calcium level (Fig. 46.3) to exclude exogenous causes of hypercalcemia (e.g., orally or intravenously administered Ca^{2+}). Once this has been established, a careful history, physical examination, and review of the patient's chart, including drugs, may uncover the cause of the hypercalcemia in most cases. Renal function and phosphate levels should be measured to rule out renal causes. Measurement of thyroid hormone and TSH concentrations can detect hypothyroidism or hyperthyroidism. A 24-hour urine collection for Ca^{2+} and creatinine determinations helps to separate hypocalciuric from hypercalciuric syndromes.

Frequently, one must differentiate between primary hyperparathyroidism and malignancy (Table 46.7). The best tests that distinguish between these two entities are PTH and 1,25-dihydroxyvitamin D measurements. PTH is elevated in primary hyperparathyroidism and normal or low in patients with hypercalcemia of malignancy. The 1-hydroxylase enzyme is stimulated by PTH and 1,25-dihydroxyvitamin D levels are usually high in patients with hyperparathyroidism. On the other hand, 1,25-dihydroxyvitamin D values are low in malignancy unless they are caused by rare tumors that contain a 1-hydroxylase enzyme. The development of assays for circulating PTH-related peptide may also prove to be useful for distinguishing hyperparathyroidism from malignancy (71). PTH and factors released from certain tumors are both capable of raising nephrogenous cAMP levels (17). An elevated nephrogenous cAMP level cannot distinguish between hypercalcemia resulting from hyperparathyroidism or malignancy; however, low levels can help to exclude hyperparathyroidism. A careful search for malignancy using chest roentgenograms, bone and liver scans, and computed tomography scanning may also help to establish a definitive diagnosis. If no malignancy can be found after a careful search and laboratory data are compatible with primary hyperparathyroidism, then neck exploration should be performed. In high-risk patients, selective venous catheterization with analysis of serum for PTH or nuclear medicine scanning may help to localize the site of overactive parathyroid tissue.

Treatment

Definitive treatment of hypercalcemia lies in the correction of the cause (e.g., surgery for hyperparathyroidism; chemotherapy, surgery, or radiotherapy for malignancy) (69, 81); however, while evaluation is taking place it may be necessary to treat the patient to avoid complications and symptoms of hypercalcemia (3, 69, 103, 104). Ca^{2+} enters and exits the circulation from the gastrointestinal, skeletal, or renal routes. The goal of therapy is to minimize Ca^{2+} entry and maximize Ca^{2+} exit. General measures of treatment (Table 46.8) include hydration, correction of electrolyte abnormalities, removal of offending drugs, dietary Ca^{2+} restriction, and mobilization of the patient. Concomitant electrolyte disturbances (e.g., potassium, Mg^{2+}, PO_4) are common in patients with hypercalcemia. Aldinger and Samaan (105) found a 16.9% incidence of hypokalemia in patients with primary hyperparathyroidism and a 52.3% incidence in patients with hypercalcemia of malignancy. Serum potassium levels were lowest in patients with the highest serum Ca^{2+} concentrations. Hypokalemia or hypomagnesemia increase the arrhythmogenic potential of hypercalcemia. Diuresis for treatment of hypercalcemia may further lower the serum Mg^{2+} and potassium concentrations.

Renal Ca^{2+} excretion can be enhanced with the use of saline (which inhibits proximal tubule resorption) and furosemide (which inhibits distal Ca^{2+} resorption) (Table 46.8). Sodium competes with Ca^{2+} in the kidney and inhibits its resorption. In addition, expansion of intravascular volume dilutes the Ca^{2+} concentration in the blood and promotes renal flow. Furosemide and saline are adjusted to maintain a urine output of 200 to 300 ml/hr. Sodium, Mg^{2+}, PO_4, and potassium should be monitored and replaced as necessary. Central hemodynamic monitoring may be necessary in patients with heart or renal disease. Ca^{2+} may also be removed from the plasma with dialysis (106) in patients with oliguric renal disease. Hemodialysis can clear up to 682 mg Ca^{2+}/hr as compared with 124 mg/hr for peritoneal dialysis and 82 mg/hr for forced diuresis (106).

Ca^{2+} may be lowered by agents that decrease bone resorption (Table 46.8). These agents work best in patients with hyperresorptive disease such as hyperparathyroidism, Paget's disease, and malignancy. Calcitonin (47) inhibits osteoclastic bone resorption and can be given to patients with hyperphosphatemia and before hydration is complete. It is particularly useful in treating patients with congestive heart failure or renal failure in whom large quantities of saline or PO_4 cannot be used. A hypocalcemic effect (average decrease of 2 to 3 mg/dl) may be seen in 6 to 10 hours. Calcitonin has low toxicity but occasionally may cause nausea, vomiting, abdominal cramps, skin rash, flushing, and diarrhea. The major disadvantages of calcitonin are its unpredictability (25% do not respond) and drug resistance. Calcitonin resistance frequently develops in patients after 48 to 72 hours of use as a result of receptor down-regulation and uncoupling of adenyl cyclase (20); resistance may be delayed by the co-administration of glucocorticoids (20 to 40 mg prednisone every 6 hours) or oral phosphates. Discontinuation of the drug for 24 to 48 hours can also restore effect.

Osteoclastic bone resorption may be decreased by mithramycin (46) (Table 46.8). This drug is almost always effective but takes 12 to 24 hours to produce a hypocalcemic effect, and its maximal hypocalcemic effect occurs at 5 to 7 days. If a response is not seen within 24 to 48 hours the dose may be repeated until a response is seen. Hypocalcemia may be seen following its use, and it has renal, hepatic, and hematologic toxicities (especially thrombocytopenia).

Cis-platinum is able to lower serum Ca^{2+} levels in cancer-associated hypercalcemia in animals (43) and humans (44). Lad et al (44) treated 13 patients with severe cancer-induced hypercalcemia refractory to rehydration with a 24-hour infusion of *cis*-platinum (100 mg/m² of body surface area). Nine patients achieved normocalcemia. The maximal lowering occurred 10 days after treatment and persisted for a mean duration of 38 days. *Cis*-platinum inhibits PTH and tumor extract-induced osteolysis in vitro in the mouse calvarium bone resorption assay (42), suggesting that it controls hypercalcemia by inhibiting bone resorption. Gallium nitrate (49) is an antitumor compound that decreases Ca^{2+} resorption from bone and causes hypocalcemia. Warrell et al (49) treated 10 patients with cancer-related hypercalcemia with gallium nitrate (200 mg/m²/day by continuous infusion for 5 to 7 days). Total serum Ca^{2+} concentrations decreased from 13.8 mg/dl to 8.0 mg/dl. Gallium nitrate produced few side effects, although nephrotoxicity has been reported. Nausea and myelosuppression do not occur.

Glucocorticoids decrease osteoclastic bone resorption, inhibit osteoclast activating factor, block prostaglandin synthesis, and antagonize vitamin D action. They are the agents of choice in vitamin D excess states and in treating hypercalcemia resulting from granulomatous disease (e.g., sarcoidosis).

Table 46.7. Primary Hyperparathyroidism vs. Hypercalcemia of Malignancy

	Hyperparathyroidism	*Malignancy*
Clinical course	Chronic	Acute
Serum Ca^{2+}	<12.5 mg/dl	>12.5 mg/dl
Serum Cl	>102 mEq/liter	<102 mEq/liter
Serum PO_4	Normal or low	Normal or high
Cl/PO_4	>33	<33
Acid-base	Hyperchloremic acidosis	Metabolic alkalosis
Renal calculi	Frequent	Rare
Osteitis fibrosa	Present	Absent
Urinary Ca^{2+}	High	Very high
PTH	Elevated	Low or normal
1,25(OH)2D	High	Low
TmP/glomerular filtration rate	Low	Variable
Nephrogenous cAMP	High	Variable
PTH-related peptide	Normal	Elevated

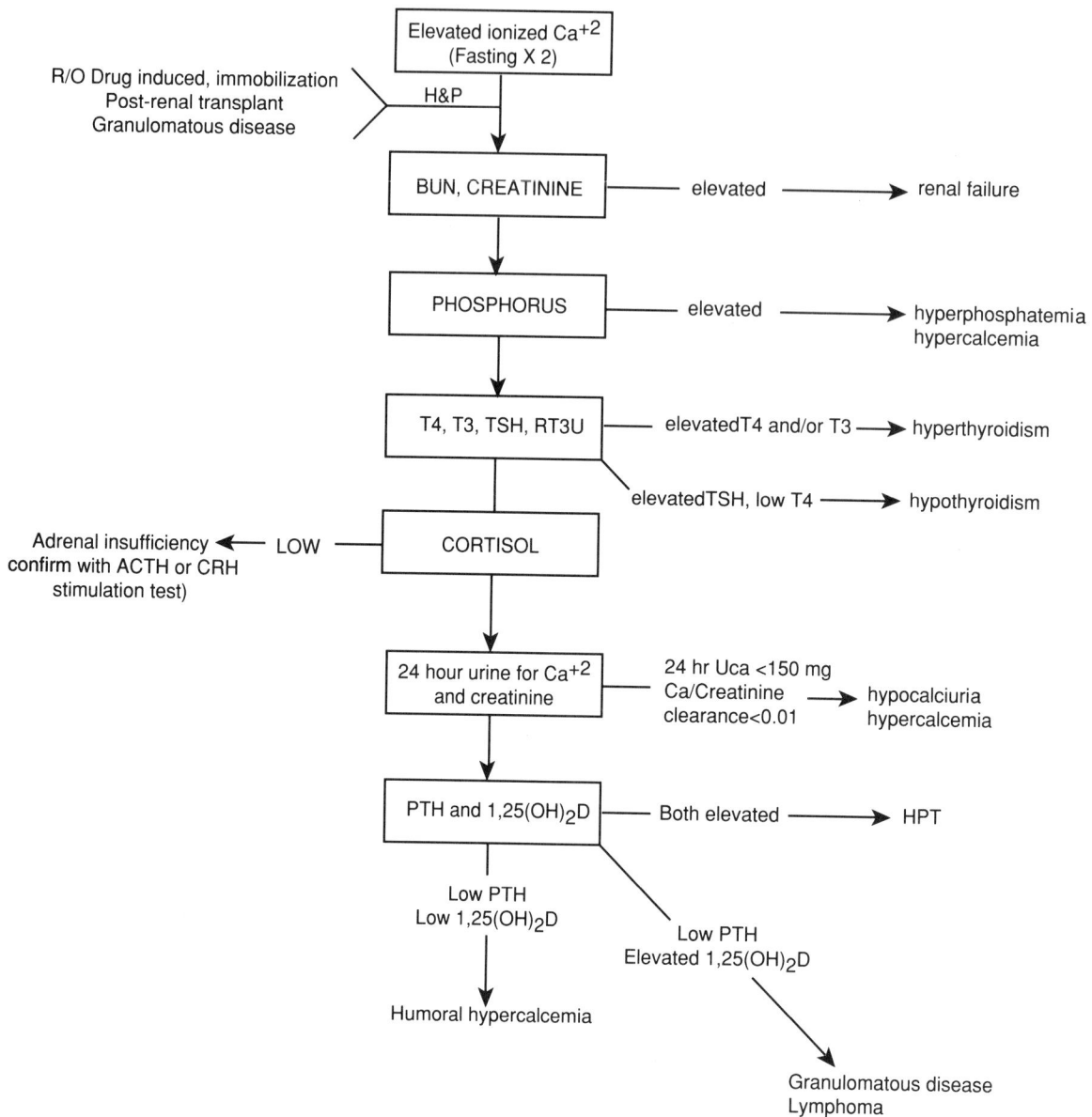

Figure 46.3. Evaluation of hypercalcemia.

Glucocorticoids are also effective in control of hypercalcemia in patients with multiple myeloma and lymphoid malignancies. They are ineffective in patients with hyperparathyroidism.

Indomethacin has been used to treat hypercalcemia in patients with some tumors that produce prostaglandins (e.g., hypernephroma and lung cancer). Propranolol has been used to treat hypercalcemia in patients with pheochromocytoma. Hypercalcemia in patients with hyperthyroidism responds to treatment of the thyroid disease. Diphosphonates decrease bone resorption by binding to hydroxyapatite and by inhibiting osteoclast function (50–52). Etidronate disodium (52), 7.5 mg/kg/day administered intravenously, reduced Ca^{2+} to normal in 3 days in 19 of 26 patients with hypercalcemia of malignancy (mean decrease in Ca^{2+} of 2.2 mg/dl). It is minimally effective when administered orally. Side effects occasionally may occur and include nausea, vomiting, diarrhea, hyperphosphatemia, renal dysfunction, and defective bone

mineralization. Oral and intravenous dichloromethylene diphosphonate is also effective in lowering serum Ca^{2+} levels in patients with malignancy and hyperparathyroidism (20, 50, 51). Large doses of protamine cause acute hypocalcemia in animals by blocking efflux of Ca^{2+} from bone (48). Further studies are needed to examine its potential clinical utility in control of hypercalcemia resulting from diseases associated with increased bone turnover.

Chelators (e.g., phosphates and EDTA) are indicated for the management of life-threatening hypercalcemic emergencies when an immediate lowering of the ionized Ca^{2+} level is required (Table 46.8). Phosphates (oral, rectal, or intravenous) are extremely effective agents for lowering circulating Ca^{2+}. They work by binding and precipitating Ca^{2+}, inhibiting bone resorption, and decreasing renal activation of vitamin D. Their major disadvantage is the potential for extraskeletal calcification in vital structures (e.g., heart, retina, and kidney).

Orally and rectally administered phosphates are safer than intravenously administered phosphates but require several days for maximal effect. Intravenous phosphates work rapidly (maximal effect 6 to 24 hours) but should not be given in doses exceeding 50 mM over 6 to 8 hours. Serum Ca^{2+} may fall from 1 to 6 mg/dl depending upon the dose of PO_4 administered. Patients should be well-hydrated and blood pressure and electrolytes should be monitored closely. Phosphates are contraindicated in the hyperphosphatemic hypercalcemic patient and should be withheld if the total serum $Ca^{2+} \times PO_4$ product exceeds 60 to 70. EDTA forms complexes with Ca^{2+} as well as Mg^{2+} and is excreted in the urine. It is very effective in lowering circulating Ca^{2+} levels. Hydration is important so as to minimize renal toxicity. EDTA is best given centrally and should be diluted in saline. A dose of EDTA of 50 mg/kg usually lowers the serum Ca^{2+} concentration by 2 to 3 mg/dl. Infusion of albumin, sodium citrate, or sodium sulfate (45) can also be used to lower acutely the ionized Ca^{2+} level. However, these agents have not been tested in clinical trials for the treatment of hypercalcemia and should not be used as primary therapy.

The chemoprotective and radioprotective agent WR-2721 lowers serum Ca^{2+} when administered to patients with malignancy (53, 54). Reduction of PTH secretion plays a role in the hypocalcemic action of WR-2721, and this agent has been used to treat refractory hypercalcemia in a patient with parathyroid cancer (54). Further studies are needed before widespread use of this agent is recommended. Conjugated estrogens (1.25 mg daily) and norethindrone (5 mg daily) may lower serum Ca^{2+} and inhibit bone resorption by antagonizing PTH in patients with mild hyperparathyroidism (83, 107).

Ca^{2+} may have toxic life-threatening effects upon the cardiovascular system (e.g., arrhythmias, heart block, and cardiac arrest). These effects may be antagonized by calcium channel blockers such as verapamil (96) while the patient is awaiting definitive therapy.

Saline, furosemide, phosphates, EDTA, sodium citrate, sodium sulfate, and dialysis have a rapid hypocalcemic effect (within hours) and should be used for life-threatening hypercalcemic emergencies. WR-2721 and protamine are experimental agents that also work within hours of administration. Calcitonin and mithramycin work within 1 to 3 days of administration, whereas glucocorticoids, prostaglandin inhibitors, gallium nitrate, diphosphonates, and *cis*-platinum take 4 to 7 days to elicit a maximal hypocalcemic effect.

CARDIOVASCULAR ACTIONS OF CALCIUM

Calcium has a variety of effects on the cardiovascular system (64, 101, 108). Although calcium possesses inotropic activity, most studies indicate that in humans calcium acts primarily as a vasopressor. Cardiac output and oxygen delivery do not increase significantly in most patients following calcium administration (64, 99, 100). Patients most likely to demonstrate an improvement in cardiac output following calcium are those with severe ionized hypocalcemia (ionized calcium <0.7 mmol/liter). Recent studies also indicate that calcium impairs β-adrenergic actions in the heart (64, 99, 100). This negative interaction between calcium and β-adrenergic receptor agonists appears to result from calcium's inhibition of agonist-induced cAMP generation (102).

MAGNESIUM

Magnesium is the second most common intracellular cation, next to potassium. It is essential for the activity of many metabolic pathways and is vital to a number of enzyme systems. It is required for the activity of phosphatases, which are essential for splitting high-energy ATP bonds and providing energy for the sodium-potassium ATPase pump, proton pump, calcium ATPase pump, neurochemical transmission, muscle contraction, glucose-fat-protein metabolism, oxidative phosphorylation, and DNA synthesis (27, 109, 110). Mg^{2+} is also required for the activity of adenylate cyclase.

The total body content of Mg^{2+} in the average adult is 2000 mEq, about 50 to 60% of which is in the skeleton and 20% in muscle (110). Less than 1% of total body Mg^{2+} is found in the serum; thus, serum levels may not reflect intracellular stores accurately (27). The total serum Mg^{2+} concentration ranges from 1.7 to 2.4 mg/dl (1.4 to 2.0 mEq/liter) in normal adults and is composed of three fractions: a protein-bound fraction (30%), a chelated fraction (15%), and an ionized fraction (55%). It is the ionized fraction that is physiologically active and homeostatically regulated. Recently, an ionized magnesium electrode has been developed. Patient studies are needed to confirm its clinical usefulness. A simple filter method is available for measuring ultrafilterable (ionized plus chelated) levels (16). Ultrafilterable levels adjust the Mg^{2+} concentration for variations in serum protein levels.

The normal dietary intake of Mg^{2+} is approximately 25 to 30 mEq/day (0.3 - 0.4 mEq/kg/day), which is close to the amount required to maintain Mg^{2+} balance (111). Mg^{2+} is ubiquitous in foods, and dietary Mg^{2+} deficiency is rare unless food intake is severely limited. Mg^{2+} is absorbed in the small intestine and excreted in the urine and stool (110). Normally, 30 to 40% of dietary Mg^{2+} is absorbed; however, this amount may increase during deficiency states. Gut Mg^{2+} absorption occurs by both a vitamin D-dependent and -independent mechanism. Gastrointestinal absorption is inhibited by phosphates, calcium, and fats. Mg^{2+} homeostasis is regulated primarily in the kidney by tubular resorption (110, 112–115). The kidneys possess a remarkable ability to conserve Mg^{2+} and can decrease excreted Mg^{2+} to less than 1 to 2 mEq/day in deficiency states. Failure of the kidneys to conserve Mg^{2+} during hypomagnesemia suggests that the cause is renal Mg^{2+} wasting. Mg^{2+} resorption in the renal tubule is enhanced by PTH, vitamin D, extracellular fluid depletion, Mg^{2+} depletion, hypothyroidism, and hypocalcemia (110). Renal Mg^{2+} excretion is increased by extracellular fluid expansion, hypermagnesemia, hypercalcemia, loop and osmotic diuretics, PO_4 depletion, metabolic acidosis, and protein and alcohol intake (110). However, the majority of resorption is independent of hormonal influences. Urinary Mg^{2+} resorption is linked to resorption of Ca^{2+} and sodium, and renal loss of either of these electrolytes causes Mg^{2+} loss. A tubular maximum (Tm) for Mg^{2+} resorption occurs at serum concentrations of 1.5 to 2.0 mg/dl. This Tm is close to the normal serum Mg^{2+}

Table 46.8. Treatments of Hypercalcemia: Alternatives

General measures
    Hydration
    Remove offending drugs
    Dietary Ca^{2+} restriction
    Treat underlying disorder
    Mobilization
    Correct electrolyte abnormalities
Increase renal Ca^{2+} excretion
    Saline: 2–3 liters over 3–6 hr, maintain urine output >200–300 ml/hr
    Furosemide: 10–40 mg i.v. every 2–4 hr
    Dialysis
Decrease bone resorption
    Calcitonin: 1–2 MRC[a] U/kg i.v. or i.m. every 6 hr
    Mithramycin: 25 μg/kg i.v. over 4 hr every 2–7 days
    Glucocorticoids: Hydrocortisone 3 mg/kg/day in divided doses every 6 hr or prednisone 40–60 mg/day
    Indomethacin: 25 mg p.o. every 6 hr
    Etidronate disodium: 7.5 mg/kg/day i.v. in 250-ml saline over 2 hr for 1–4 days or 5–10 mg/kg/day p.o.
    Cis-platinum: 100 mg/m² over 24 hr
    Gallium nitrate: 200 mg/m²/day by continuous infusion for 5–7 days
Ca^{2+} chelators
    Phosphates
        p.o.: 500–1000 mg every 6 hr
        i.v.: 50 mM PO_4 over 8–12 hr
        Rectal: Phosphosoda 5 ml every 6 hours; Fleets enema 100 ml twice daily
    EDTA: 10–50 mg/kg over 4 hr
    Sodium citrate
    Sodium sulfate
Ca^{2+} antagonists
    Verapamil 5–10 mg i.v.
    Nifedipine 10–20 mg sublingually
PTH antagonists
    WR-2721 430-910 mg/m² over 20–60 min

[a] MRC, Medical Research Council.

concentration, and small changes in the serum level rapidly alter renal Mg^{2+} excretion. Thus, in Mg^{2+} overload, the kidneys can rapidly excrete excess Mg^{2+}. During correction of Mg^{2+} deficiency, despite cellular Mg^{2+} depletion, much of the administered Mg^{2+} is lost in the urine and repletion usually takes 5 to 7 days (e.g., to replete intracellular stores). With a normal functioning kidney, obligate loses of Mg^{2+} in stool, sweat, urine, and secretions amount to about 0.3 mEq/kg/day.

Although PTH and vitamin D can increase renal and gastrointestinal absorption of Mg^{2+}, this ion also has potent effects upon the parathyroid glands (24, 26–29, 116). Hypermagnesemia and severe hypomagnesemia decrease PTH secretion, whereas mild hypomagnesemia stimulates secretion. Hypomagnesemia may also impair end-organ response to PTH and vitamin D (27, 28, 30, 117).

Magnesium is important for the maintenance of normal potassium metabolism (27, 118–121). It is a cofactor for sodium-potassium transport. Magnesium deficiency results in cellular potassium deficiency and renal potassium wasting. Repletion of cellular potassium requires magnesium. Thus, it is important to correct magnesium deficiency in patients with concomitant potassium deficiency.

HYPOMAGNESEMIA

Causes

Hypomagnesemia usually occurs when Mg^{2+} losses exceed dietary intake and usually results from a defect in renal Mg^{2+} conservation or excessive stool losses (Table 46.9). Prevalence rates for hypomagnesemia range from 10 to 65% depending upon the type of patients studied (16, 25, 27, 29, 109, 122, 123). Since there is an obligate daily Mg^{2+} loss, severe malnutrition or inadequate supplementation in parenteral nutrition or intravenously administered fluids may also cause hypomagnesemia. Hypomagnesemia may develop when Mg^{2+} requirements are increased but intake remains constant (e.g., in pregnancy). Decreased gut absorption of Mg^{2+} and/or excessive stool losses may occur in a variety of diseases (e.g., inflammatory bowel disease, gastroenteritis, pancreatic insufficiency, fistulas, short-bowel syndromes, ileal bypass, intestinal resection, and cholestatic liver disease). Hypomagnesemia results from a combination of reduced mucosal surface area, increased intestinal secretions, and formation of insoluble Mg^{2+} soaps in the stool caused by complexation with unabsorbed fat. Secretions from the lower gastrointestinal tract are richer in Mg^{2+} (10 to 14 mEq/liter) than are secretions from the upper tract (1 to 2 mEq/liter).

Acute hypomagnesemia can result from internal redistribution of Mg^{2+}. Mg^{2+} shifts into cells following the administration of glucose or amino acids (111, 124). This shift is more pronounced when intracellular Mg^{2+} depletion is coupled to an anabolic state, as may occur with refeeding after starvation or protein-calorie malnutrition; with administration of parenteral nutrition to depleted patients; and with insulin treatment of hyperglycemic disorders. Increased catecholamines from endogenous or exogenous sources, correction of acidosis, and hungry bone syndromes may also lower the serum Mg^{2+} levels by shifting Mg^{2+} into cells.

Table 46.9. Causes of Hypomagnesemia

Gastrointestinal losses
  Reduced absorption
    Malabsorption
    Laxative abuse
    Fistulas
    Prolonged nasogastric suction
  Reduced intake
    Malnutrition
    Hyperalimentation
    Prolonged i.v. therapy
Drug-induced losses
  Diuretics
    Furosemide
    Thiazides
    Mannitol
    Glucose
    Urea
  Aminoglycosides
  Amphotericin B
  Cis-platinum
  Carbenicillin
  Cyclosporine
  Thyroid hormone
  Digoxin
  Calcium
  Ethanol
  Insulin[a]
  Saline
  Citrate (blood)
  Catecholamines[a]
Renal losses
  Renal disease
    Glomerulonephritis
    Tubular disorders
    Interstitial nephritis
    Diuretic phase of acute tubular necrosis
  Hypercalcemia
  Hyperaldosteronism
  Hyperthyroidism
  PO_4 deficiency
  Diabetic ketoacidosis
  Syndrome of inappropriate antidiuretic hormone secretion (SIADH)
Miscellaneous losses
  Lactation
  Pregnancy
  Severe sweating
  Hungry bone syndrome[a]
  Burns
  Sepsis
  Hypothermia
  Cardiopulmonary bypass
  Administration of glucose, amino acids, and insulin[a]
  Mg^{2+} free dialysis
  Refeeding after starvation[a]

[a] Redistribution of Mg^{2+}.

A large number of diseases may disrupt renal conservation of Mg^{2+} and result in hypomagnesemia. However, when advanced renal disease develops, hypermagnesemia usually occurs. Medications that alter renal Mg^{2+} conservation (Table 46.9) include the diuretics, aminoglycoside antibiotics, amphotericin B, *cis*-platinum, cardiac glycosides, calcium, and saline (27). Aminoglycosides cause hypomagnesemia in 38% of patients receiving a standard intravenous course (29). Cardiac glycosides may cause hypomagnesemia by blocking the action of the sodium-potassium ATPase pump in the renal tubule.

This effect is important in view of the fact that hypomagnesemia may also potentiate digitalis toxicity. Thyroid hormone excess causes loss of Mg^{2+} in the urine as a result of increases in glomerular filtration and may also shift Mg^{2+} intracellularly. Citrate (found in blood products) can lower the serum ionized Mg^{2+} concentration by chelation.

Hypomagnesemia is encountered frequently in patients admitted to the hospital for ethanol withdrawal. Although acute ethanol intake results in increased renal Mg^{2+} excretion, chronic ethanol exposure has no lasting effect. Hypomagnesemia in alcoholic patients results primarily from poor dietary intake, ketosis, emesis, diarrhea, and hyperaldosteronism. Many alcoholic patients have a normal serum Mg^{2+} level on admission, which decreases during hospitalization because of metabolic changes induced during hospitalization (e.g., insulin secretion induced by dextrose infusion and anabolism). These patients may benefit from careful monitoring of the serum Mg^{2+} concentration. Despite the occurrence of hypomagnesemia in many patients with delirium tremens, there are no convincing data to suggest a cause-and-effect relationship. Mg^{2+} supplementation has not been shown to prevent delirium tremens.

Hypomagnesemia is common in patients undergoing cardiac bypass surgery (23). The etiology is multifactorial and results from dilution/chelation, redistribution, and renal losses. Magnesium repletion can decrease the incidence of arrhythmias in these patients.

Clinical Manifestations

Signs and symptoms of Mg^{2+} deficiency (Table 46.10), like those of hypocalcemia, relate to increased neuronal irritability and tetany. Symptoms are rare when the total serum Mg^{2+} concentration is above 1.5 mg/dl, and most symptomatic patients have levels below 1.0 mg/dl. Most symptomatic patients with hypomagnesemia have concomitant hypocalcemia or hypokalemia, and it is unclear whether hypomagnesemia alone causes symptoms (125, 126). Hypomagnesemic patients may complain of muscle spasms, paresthesias, and weakness. Correction of hypomagnesemia can improve respiratory muscle strength (127). Central nervous system effects range from coma, disorientation, apathy, and depression to irritability and seizures.

Cardiovascular consequences of Mg^{2+} depletion may include heart failure, coronary artery spasm, arrhythmias, and hypotension (124, 128–137). Hypomagnesemia increases cardiac sensitivity to the effects of digitalis and pressor agents (111) and can lead to toxicity at lower serum digitalis levels (138). This effect may result from the synergistic effects of magnesium and digitalis on the cardiac sodium-potassium pump. Mg^{2+} deficiency is thought to lead to increased vascular tone and reactivity by modulating uptake, content, and distribution of Ca^{2+} in the smooth muscle cell (124). Hypomagnesemia may contribute to vasospasm and hypertension. Standard antiarrhythmic therapy and defibrillation may be ineffective in controlling ventricular arrhythmias associated with Mg^{2+} deficiency (129).

Hypomagnesemia may cause hypokalemia and intracellular potassium depletion. Repletion of intracellular and extracellular potassium may be impaired unless concurrent Mg^{2+} deficits

Table 46.10. Clinical Manifestations of Hypomagnesemia

Cardiovascular
 Heart failure
 Arrhythmias
 Coronary artery spasm
 Vasospasm
 Hypertension
 Digitalis sensitivity
 Decreased pressor response
 ECG: Prolonged P-R and Q-T interval, S-T depression, tall
  peaked T-waves (early), broadening and decreased amplitude of
  T-waves (late), wide QRS (late)
Gastrointestinal
 Dysphagia
 Anorexia
 Nausea
 Abdominal cramps
Neuromuscular
 Tetany
 Muscle spasm, tremor
 Seizures
 Confusion, disorientation
 Obtundation, coma
 Ataxia, nystagmus
 Apathy
 Depression
 Paresthesias
 Irritability
 Weakness
 Psychosis
Miscellaneous
 Hypokalemia
 Hypocalcemia
 Hypophosphatemia

are treated simultaneously (111, 118–121, 124). Hypomagnesemic hypokalemia results from impaired renal potassium conservation caused by diminished activation of the sodium-potassium adenosine triphosphatase pump and altered cell membrane permeability to potassium (29, 139).

Hypomagnesemia-induced hypocalcemia results from impaired PTH secretion, end-organ resistance to PTH, and vitamin D resistance (24, 28, 30, 31, 116, 117). Impaired Mg^{2+}-dependent adenyl cyclase generation of cAMP may be responsible for some of these effects (124). These patients present with clinical features of hypocalcemia (Table 46.2). Hypocalcemia may be difficult to correct until Mg^{2+} is replaced.

Evaluation

Hypomagnesemia is usually diagnosed when the serum Mg^{2+} level is below normal limits. However, since Mg^{2+} is 30% protein bound, low total serum levels may occur in patients with hypoalbuminemia despite the occurrence of normal ionized concentrations (16). Mg^{2+} is primarily an intracellular ion, and circulating levels may not always reflect the status of the intracellular environment. However, most patients with chronic hypomagnesemia have cellular Mg^{2+} depletion (111). At present, clinicians remain dependent upon the serum level, until new methods become available for assessing intracellular Mg^{2+} activity.

Measurement of urine Mg^{2+} excretion (24-hour urine measurement) is helpful in separating renal from nonrenal causes of hypomagnesemia. Normal kidneys are capable of decreasing Mg^{2+} excretion to 1 to 2 mEq/day in deficiency states.

High urinary Mg^{2+} excretion (>3 mEq/day) in the presence of a low serum Mg^{2+} level suggests increased renal loss of Mg^{2+} as the mechanism for Mg^{2+} depletion. Low urinary Mg^{2+} excretion (<1 to 2 mEq/day) in the presence of hypomagnesemia suggests renal conservation of Mg^{2+} and a Mg^{2+} deficient state resulting from decreased intake, redistribution, or nonrenal losses. If Mg^{2+} depletion is suspected in patients with a normal serum Mg^{2+} concentration and low renal Mg^{2+} excretion (e.g., intact renal Mg^{2+} conservation), a Mg^{2+} load test may be helpful. After a baseline 24-hour urine collection, 30 mmol of Mg^{2+} sulfate are administered in 500 ml of 5% dextrose in water over 12 hours; urine is collected for 24 hours from the beginning of the infusion. Individuals with normal Mg^{2+} stores excrete more than 60 to 80% of the administered load within 24 hours, whereas Mg^{2+}-deficient patients excrete less than 50% (111, 124, 140). Decreased fractional Mg^{2+} excretion occurs in Mg^{2+} deficiency because of enhanced resorption of Mg^{2+} in the renal tubules as a result of resetting of Mg^{2+} transport (110). This test should be used with caution in patients with renal insufficiency, disturbances in cardiac conduction, or advanced respiratory insufficiency.

Treatment

Mg^{2+} deficiency is treated by correcting the cause (if possible) and replacing body Mg^{2+} deficits with exogenous Mg^{2+} (Table 46.11). Maintenance doses of Mg^{2+} for adults are 0.4 mEq/kg/day orally or 0.1 to 0.2 mEq/kg/day parenterally. These requirements assume no unusual losses and must be augmented accordingly. For maintenance intravenous therapy or parenteral nutrition, the authors give the sulfate salt so as to provide needed sulfate ions as well (141).

Mild Mg^{2+} deficiency may be treated with diet alone. Patients with symptomatic or severe hypomagnesemia (Mg^{2+} <1 mg/dl) are best treated with intravenous magnesium (27, 109, 112, 114, 142, 143). In the treatment of acute life-threatening arrhythmias, the authors recommend giving 1 to 2 g (8 to 16 mEq) of intravenous magnesium sulfate over 5 minutes (using ECG monitoring). This bolus should be followed with an infusion of 1 to 2 g magnesium sulfate per hour for the next few hours and then reduced to 0.5 to 1.0 g magnesium sulfate per hour as a maintenance infusion (in patients with normal renal function). Potassium should also be monitored and replaced if necessary. Serum magnesium levels should be monitored during therapy to avoid severe hypermagnesemia. In the treatment of severe but non-life-threatening hypomagnesemia, the authors recommend beginning an infusion of 1 to 2 g/hr magnesium sulfate for 3 to 6 hours and then decreasing the rate to 0.5 to 1.0 g/hr as a maintenance infusion.

In less urgent situations and in patients with prolonged magnesium depletion, the authors recommend administering 50 to 100 mEq magnesium sulfate per day (600 to 1200 mg elemental magnesium). These dosages should be reduced in patients with renal insufficiency. Treatment is usually carried out over 3 to 5 days so as to replace intracellular stores, and then the patient is placed on maintenance doses of magnesium (which depend on magnesium losses from the body). Bolus doses of intravenous magnesium, which raise serum magnesium concentration above physiologic levels, are excreted quickly by the kidneys. Thus, it is better to administer magnesium by continuous intravenous infusion, intramuscularly

Table 46.11. Magnesium Supplements[a]

Parenteral
  Mg^{2+} chloride
    1 g = 118 mg Mg^{2+} = 9 mEq   Loading: 1–2 gms i.v. over 5–10 min
  Mg^{2+} sulfate   Maintenance: 0.5–2 gm/hr by infusion
    1 g = 98 mg Mg^{2+} = 8 mEq
Enteral
  Mg^{2+} oxide tablets   20–80 mEq/day in divided doses
    Tablet = 241 mg Mg^{2+} = 20 mEq
  Mg^{2+} gluconate tablets   20–80 mEq/day in divided doses
    500-mg tablet = 27 mg Mg^{2+} = 2.3 mEq

[a] 1 mEq = 0.5 mmol = 12.3 mg Mg^{2+}

(magnesium sulfate only), or via the enteral route (so as to maintain an elevated blood magnesium concentration). If magnesium is given enterally, one usually gives two to three times the intravenous dose to compensate for incomplete absorption (usually 30 to 50% absorbed). It is also important to replace deficits plus ongoing losses.

Magnesium is excreted by the kidneys, and its dose should be reduced in patients with renal insufficiency. During magnesium repletion, the authors frequently monitor the serum magnesium and calcium level, potassium concentration, serum creatinine, blood pressure, ECG, respiratory status, and neurologic status (mental alertness, deep tendon reflexes).

Once the patient is stable, Mg^{2+} can be replaced by the oral route (Table 46.11). Mg^{2+} oxide is the preferred Mg^{2+} preparation. Mg^{2+}-containing antacids are poorly absorbed and should not be used to replace Mg^{2+} unless other preparations are not available.

MAGNESIUM AND THE HEART

Intractable ventricular arrhythmias associated with hypomagnesemia may respond to Mg^{2+} therapy (111, 121, 129–134, 136, 137, 144). Magnesium administration has been shown to decrease cardiac arrhythmias during states of myocardial ischemia and improve survival in patients with myocardial infarctions (130–137). Mg^{2+} therapy has also been useful in suppressing ventricular tachycardia and fibrillation in patients with ischemic heart disease who have normal serum Mg^{2+} levels (134, 145). Abraham et al (134) treated a group of patients with acute myocardial infarction with Mg^{2+} sulfate (2.4 g administered intravenously over 20 minutes daily for 3 days). Potentially lethal arrhythmias were reduced from 34.8% to 14.6% when compared with placebo. The authors have used Mg^{2+} sulfate (1 g administered intravenously over 20 minutes every 6 hours) effectively in the ICU to treat ventricular arrhythmias. Mg^{2+} depletion interferes with sodium-potassium ATPase and causes ionic imbalance and electrical instability. Mg^{2+} administration prolongs the effective refractory period, depresses conduction, increases the membrane potential (makes it more negative), and can control ventricular tachyarrhythmias. Thus, when ventricular fibrillation or malignant ventricular arrhythmias cannot be controlled with conventional antiarrhythmic drugs, the authors recommend infusing Mg^{2+}. Iseri et al (145) give 16 mEq slowly over 1 minute followed by 80 mEq over the next 5 hours. Potassium chloride at 10 mEq/hr is also infused, since there is evidence that Mg^{2+} and potassium depletion frequently occur together. It may be necessary to continue a maintenance infusion of Mg^{2+} to

prevent recurrence of arrhythmias. The authors usually aim for a serum Mg^{2+} concentration of 3 to 4 mg/dl in patients with refractory arrhythmias.

Intravenous administration of Mg^{2+} (50 mmol MgCl$_2$ in 1000 ml isotonic dextrose at 100 ml/hr for 6 hours followed by 22 ml/hr for 18 hours) has been reported to reduce both mortality and arrhythmias (137) when given to patients with acute myocardial infarction. Placebo- (n=74) and Mg^{2+}-treated (n=56) patients had similar admission serum Mg^{2+} levels. However, 4 weeks after myocardial infarction the patients given Mg^{2+} had a lower mortality (7% versus 19%). The proportion of patients requiring treatment for arrhythmias was also lower (21% versus 47%). In another study, Rasmussen et al (136) found that the serum Mg^{2+} concentrations of patients with acute myocardial infarctions dropped over the first 32 hours after infarction. The drop appeared to result from an extracellular to intracellular shift in Mg^{2+}. Kafka et al (146) noted a 6% incidence of hypomagnesemia in patients with acute myocardial infarction, whereas Dyckner (135) reported a 46% incidence. Hypomagnesemia was associated with a higher frequency of major ventricular arrhythmias. Kafka et al (146) also found a 17% incidence of hypokalemia in their patients with myocardial infarction. Ventricular arrhythmias occurred in all patients with both hypokalemia and hypomagnesemia.

Whang and colleagues (147) found a 19% incidence of hypomagnesemia and a 9% incidence of hypokalemia in patients receiving digitalis. Hypomagnesemia and hypokalemia are important since both predispose to digitalis toxicity (124, 129, 148). Mg^{2+} deficiency may also enhance digoxin uptake by myocardial cells (149). Iseri et al (129) reported the efficacy of intravenously administered Mg^{2+} in treating hypomagnesemic patients with toxic reactions to digitalis and recurrent ventricular tachycardia. Mg^{2+}-responsive ventricular arrhythmias may also occur in normomagnesemic patients receiving digitalis (145, 150). A decrease in serum Mg^{2+} after cardiopulmonary bypass surgery has been reported (23, 128). Suppression of cardiac arrhythmias after heart surgery may be assisted by Mg^{2+} therapy.

Magnesium has a variety of effects upon hemodynamic status (101, 151). Magnesium antagonizes calcium entry into cells through the slow calcium channels. Large doses of magnesium can impair myocardial and smooth muscle function. However, magnesium administration at clinically relevant (i.e., antiarrhythmic) doses has little detrimental hemodynamic actions (101, 151–153). Cardiac output is usually well-maintained. Systemic vascular resistance and arterial pressure are maintained or slightly decreased. When combined with epinephrine, magnesium was found to blunt epinephrine's hypertensive actions but not its cardiotonic effects (i.e., cardiac output) (151).

MAGNESIUM AND BRONCHOSPASM

Relief of dyspnea and stridor after Mg^{2+} infusion has been observed on occasion. The Mg^{2+} ion has an inhibitory action on smooth muscle contraction, histamine release from mast cells, and acetylcholine release from cholinergic nerve terminals (154, 155). Okayama et al (155) studied the bronchodilating effect of Mg^{2+} sulfate infusion (0.5 mmol/min for 20 minutes) in 10 patients with mild asthma. Serum Mg^{2+} concentrations rose from 2.1 mg/dl (0.86 mmol/liter) to 5.1 mg/dl (2.08 mmol/liter) with this dose. Mg^{2+} infusion decreased respiratory resistance by 30%, improved forced vital capacity by 17%, and improved forced expiratory volume at 1 second by 18%. There were no adverse effects on blood pressure or heart rate. The magnitude of these effects was similar to that of those found with albuterol inhalation. The same authors also administered Mg^{2+} to three patients with severe asthma who were treated with dexamethasone, aminophylline, and inhaled albuterol. They noted an improvement in wheezing, dyspnea, and sputum expectoration. Other investigators (156) have reported bronchodilation using inhaled magnesium. In preliminary studies, the authors have been unable to confirm these findings. More studies (prospective, blinded, and randomized) are needed before this therapy can be recommended. Extreme caution must be used, since hypermagnesemia can depress neuromuscular and cardiovascular function.

HYPERMAGNESEMIA

Spontaneous hypermagnesemia (serum magnesium >3 mg/dl or 2.4 mEq/liter or 1.2 mmol/liter) is rare in clinical practice, and most cases result from iatrogenic causes (26, 27, 73, 114, 141, 157). The most common etiology of hypermagnesemia is the administration of Mg^{2+}-containing antacids, enemas, or parenteral nutrition to patients with renal insufficiency. Hypermagnesemia is rare in patients with normal renal function. Other causes of hypermagnesemia include hypothyroidism, Addison's disease, lithium intoxication, familial hypocalciuric hypercalcemia, and the administration of Mg^{2+} to patients with premature labor or preeclampsia/eclampsia. Hypermagnesemia may also occur in infants born to mothers who received Mg^{2+} for these problems.

Hypermagnesemia diminishes neuromuscular transmission and can depress skeletal muscle function and cause neuromuscular blockade (Table 46.12). Mg^{2+} excess inhibits prejunctional release of acetylcholine and decreases motor end plate sensitivity to acetylcholine (110). Excess Mg^{2+} may also cause vasodilation and hypotension. Hypermagnesemia increases neuromuscular sensitivity to the effects of skeletal muscle relaxants and can result in more prolonged and potent effects of these drugs. Hypocalcemia may result from hypermagnesemia-induced parathyroid gland suppression (26).

The neuromuscular and cardiac toxicity of hypermagnesemia can be antagonized transiently by the administration of intravenous Ca^{2+} (5 to 10 mEq). Definitive therapy to lower

Table 46.12.   Clinical Manifestations of Hypermagnesemia

	Serum Mg^{2+} Level (mg/dl)
Normal level	1.7–2.4
Decrease in DTR	4–5
ECG changes (e.g., prolonged P-R, QRS, S-T)	4–6
Bradycardia	4–7
Hypotension	5–7
Somnolence	6–8
Respiratory insufficiency	10–12
Heart block	15
Respiratory paralysis	18
Cardiac arrest	15–24

the serum Mg^{2+} level consists of stopping all drugs and supplements containing Mg^{2+} and administering saline and furosemide to enhance renal excretion. In patients with renal failure, Mg^{2+} may be removed by dialysis.

PHOSPHORUS

The adult body contains about 700 to 800 g of PO_4. PO_4 is the major intracellular anion (concentration 100 mEq/liter) and is essential for a large variety of biochemical processes (33, 158–162). It is required in protein, fat, and carbohydrate metabolism and is the source of high-energy bonds in adenosine triphosphate and phosphocreatine. PO_4 high-energy bonds provide the energy for maintenance of cellular integrity, muscle contraction, neurologic function, hormonal secretion, and cell division. PO_4 is also a component of 2,3-diphosphoglycerate, which functions as a regulator of oxygen release from hemoglobin. PO_4 is a component of cyclic nucleotides, nicotinamide diphosphate, phospholipids, and nucleic acids, and it participates in the urinary buffering of acids.

Phosphorus circulates in the blood in three major forms: a protein-bound form (12%), a complexed form (33%), and an ionized form (55%). It is the ionized form that is physiologically active and regulated. However, most clinical laboratories measure total phosphorus. Since phosphorus is an intracellular ion, circulating levels may not always reflect the status of intracellular stores.

The normal serum PO_4 level is 4.0 to 7.1 mg/dl in children and 2.7 to 4.5 mg/dl in adults (33). The average dietary intake of PO_4 ranges from 800 to 1200 mg/day, with most being absorbed in the small intestine by both passive (50%) and active (vitamin D-dependent) transport. Thus, even in vitamin D-deficient states the gut is able to absorb enough PO_4 to maintain normal serum levels. PO_4 is excreted in the urine and stool. PO_4 is regulated primarily by the kidneys (162), with most PO_4 resorption occurring in the proximal tubules. Tubular resorption increases to a maximum (TmP), with further increases in PO_4 being excreted in the urine. This system is analogous to that seen with glucose. The set point for the TmP determines one's fasting serum PO_4 level and is affected by a large number of drugs. It is reduced by aminohippurate sodium, amino acids, dextrose, acetoacetate, sodium bicarbonate, saline, acute hypercapnia, thyroid hormone, estrogen, digoxin, long-term corticosteroids, and renal vasodilation (33, 163). Infusion of dextrose in amounts sufficient to cause glycosuria decreases tubular resorption of PO_4 by 20%, and both may share a common resorptive pathway (163). Extracellular volume expansion is associated with decreases in the proximal tubular resorption of both PO_4 and sodium (163), resulting in phosphaturia. Growth hormone increases the TmP and thus decreases the amount of PO_4 excreted in the urine. Higher growth hormone levels in children may explain their higher serum PO_4 concentrations.

The amount of PO_4 excreted in urine also depends upon PTH and its effects upon tubular PO_4 resorption. PTH produces phosphaturia by decreasing TmP via the adenyl cyclase system. This phosphaturic effect is important in Ca^{2+} homeostasis. PTH increases bone resorption and releases Ca^{2+} and PO_4. Hyperphosphatemia is avoided via the renal action of PTH. Acute hypercalcemia and hypermagnesemia decrease the renal excretion of PO_4 by inhibiting PTH secretion, whereas hypocalcemia and hypomagnesemia do the reverse. PO_4 has no direct effect upon the parathyroid glands, but rather affects PTH secretion through its effects upon the ionized Ca^{2+} level.

PO_4 affects the 1-hydroxylation of 25-hydroxyvitamin D within the kidney, and this effect is independent of PTH. Hypophosphatemia stimulates the 1-hydroxylase, whereas hyperphosphatemia inhibits it. 1,25-Dihydroxyvitamin D can stimulate PO_4 mobilization from bone and enhance absorption from the intestine. It plays a minor role in regulating renal PO_4 resorption.

Insulin causes glucose and PO_4 to move into cells and is responsible for the hypophosphatemia seen during insulin administration or high-carbohydrate feedings. PO_4 is trapped in the cell when glucose is converted to glucose-6-phosphate.

HYPOPHOSPHATEMIA

Causes

Hypophosphatemia (33, 158–161, 164) results from three primary mechanisms (Table 46.13): intracellular shift of PO_4, increased loss of PO_4 through the kidneys, and decreased gastrointestinal absorption of PO_4.

Carbohydrate loading (e.g., intravenous dextrose solutions and parenteral nutrition) causes hypophosphatemia by shifting PO_4 into the cell and accounts for about half of the cases of hypophosphatemia seen in hospitalized patients. PO_4 is trapped in the cell when glucose is converted to glucose-6-phosphate (33, 165). Inadequate PO_4 in parenteral nutrition or rapid refeeding of severely starved patients elicits a similar response. Acute respiratory and metabolic alkalosis stimulates intracellular glycolysis, consuming PO_4 in the process (159). Sepsis, central nervous system disorders, and salicylate poisoning cause hyperventilation and respiratory alkalosis. Salicylate poisoning may also stimulate glycolysis directly. Reversal of hypothermia causes a shift of PO_4 into the cell and may cause hypophosphatemia (166). Hypophosphatemia is common after severe burns and results from a combination of increased metabolism, anabolism, respiratory alkalosis, sepsis, inappropriate phosphaturia, excess catecholamine and cortisol secretion, and nutritional repletion.

Epinephrine and glucagon, like insulin, can also cause a reduction in the circulating PO_4 level, presumably by stimulating the cellular utilization of glucose and accelerating the formation of intracellular PO_4 esters. The intravenous infusion

Table 46.13. Causes of Hypophosphatemia

Transcellular shift
  Recovery from malnutrition[a]
  Carbohydrate loading[a]
  Recovery from hypothermia[a]
  Recovery from burns[a]
  Acute alkalosis[a]
  Alcoholism[a]
  Diabetic ketoacidosis[a]
  Sepsis
  Salicylate poisoning
  Hungry bone syndrome
  Anabolic steroids
Gastrointestinal losses
  Malabsorption
  Emesis
  Diarrhea
  Prolonged nasogastric suction
  PO_4-binding resins
  Vitamin D deficiency
Drug-induced
  Anabolic steroids
  Antacids[a]
  Calcitonin
  Corticosteroids
  Diuretics
  Epinephrine
  Glucagon
  Insulin[a]
  Sodium bicarbonate
  Saline diuresis
  Salicylates
Renal losses
  Renal tubular defects (e.g., myeloma, heavy metals, renal tubular acidosis, Fanconi syndrome)
  Hyperparathyroidism
  Hypomagnesemia
  Hypokalemia
  Acidosis
  Pregnancy
  Vitamin D deficiency or resistance
  Reye's syndrome
  Recovery from acute tubular necrosis
  After renal transplant
  Diuresis
  Oncogenic hypophosphatemia
Miscellaneous
  Hemodialysis
  Inadequate PO_4 in i.v. fluids

[a] Most common causes of severe hypophosphatemia (PO_4 <1 mg/dl).

of epinephrine at a rate of 10 μg/min for 10 minutes results in a 25% fall in the serum PO_4 concentration (167).

Hypomagnesemia augments renal PO_4 excretion; however, hypomagnesemia alone rarely causes hypophosphatemia, since it also suppresses parathyroid hormone secretion, causing hypocalcemia and a reduction in PO_4 excretion. The two effects balance out. However, hypophosphatemia may occur in these patients when magnesium is replaced without PO_4, resulting in a surge in parathyroid hormone release and augmented phosphaturia. Diuretic therapy, renal tubular defects (e.g., from myeloma or heavy metals), primary and secondary hyperparathyroidism, vitamin D deficiency, and acidemia are other causes of renal PO_4 wasting and hypophosphatemia. Vitamin D deficiency causes hypophosphatemia via its effects on increasing PTH secretion (induced by hypocalcemia) and reduced intestinal PO_4 absorption. Posttransplantation hypophosphatemia develops in more than 50% of patients with a transplanted kidney and results from a combination of renal phosphaturia, persistent hyperparathyroidism, glucocorticoid therapy, 1,25-dihydroxyvitamin D deficiency, and use of antacids (159). Hypophosphatemia has also been associated with a variety of tumors (159). These tumors appear to elaborate substances that interfere with renal PO_4 resorption, bone mineralization, and renal 1,25-dihydroxyvitamin D synthesis.

Inadequate PO_4 intake alone rarely causes hypophosphatemia. However, hypophosphatemia may occur in patients on a marginally adequate PO_4 intake when another cause for hypophosphatemia occurs (Table 46.13). A frequently seen clinical situation is that of a chronically ill patient admitted to the hospital and placed on intravenous dextrose solutions (containing little PO_4) or given nonabsorbable PO_4-binding antacids. PO_4-binding antacids, such as aluminum or magnesium hydroxide, are common causes of hypophosphatemia. These antacids bind PO_4 that is found in enteral nutrition as well as PO_4 that is secreted into the gut. Thus, they produce hypophosphatemia even in patients who are not fed enterally. Malabsorption states, such as those seen with pancreatic disease or diarrhea, may also cause hypophosphatemia by impairing PO_4 absorption and increasing gut losses.

Hypophosphatemia is commonly seen during the treatment of diabetic ketoacidosis and hyperglycemic hyperosmolar nonketotic syndromes. Serum PO_4 levels are usually normal at the time the patient is admitted, despite total body depletion of PO_4 (158, 168). After the initiation of insulin therapy, PO_4 shifts into the cells along with glucose and potassium. Plasma

levels may decrease to less than 1 mg/dl within 24 hours of initiation of therapy (158, 169). PO_4 deficiency is associated with insulin resistance, decreased levels of 2,3-diphosphoglycerate, and decreased intracellular ATP. Low 2,3-diphosphoglycerate shifts the hemoglobin dissociation curve to the left, decreasing oxygen off-loading to the tissues. This alteration in the oxyhemoglobin dissociation curve may be important clinically in some patients, since elevated levels of glycosylated hemoglobin (found in diabetics) also impair oxygen off-loading. As acidosis is corrected during the treatment of ketoacidosis, the ability of hemoglobin to release oxygen is decreased even further. PO_4 supplementation can more quickly restore 2,3-diphosphoglycerate levels and intracellular ATP concentrations to normal. Although deleterious effects of hypophosphatemia on the clinical course of diabetic ketoacidosis have not been shown conclusively (170, 171), the authors have seen a number of diabetic patients develop complications believed to be secondary to hypophosphatemia (e.g., seizures and respiratory failure). In addition, if one looks at all patients with hypophosphatemia, diabetic ketoacidosis is a common cause. For the aforementioned reasons, the authors recommend administering PO_4 for the treatment of hyperglycemic states, provided that hyperphosphatemia can be avoided.

Hypophosphatemia is common in alcoholics admitted to the hospital (159, 172). These patients frequently are malnourished and suffer from malabsorption processes. When admitted to the hospital, they are given intravenous or oral carbohydrate loads that shift PO_4 into the cells. Respiratory alkalosis may develop,

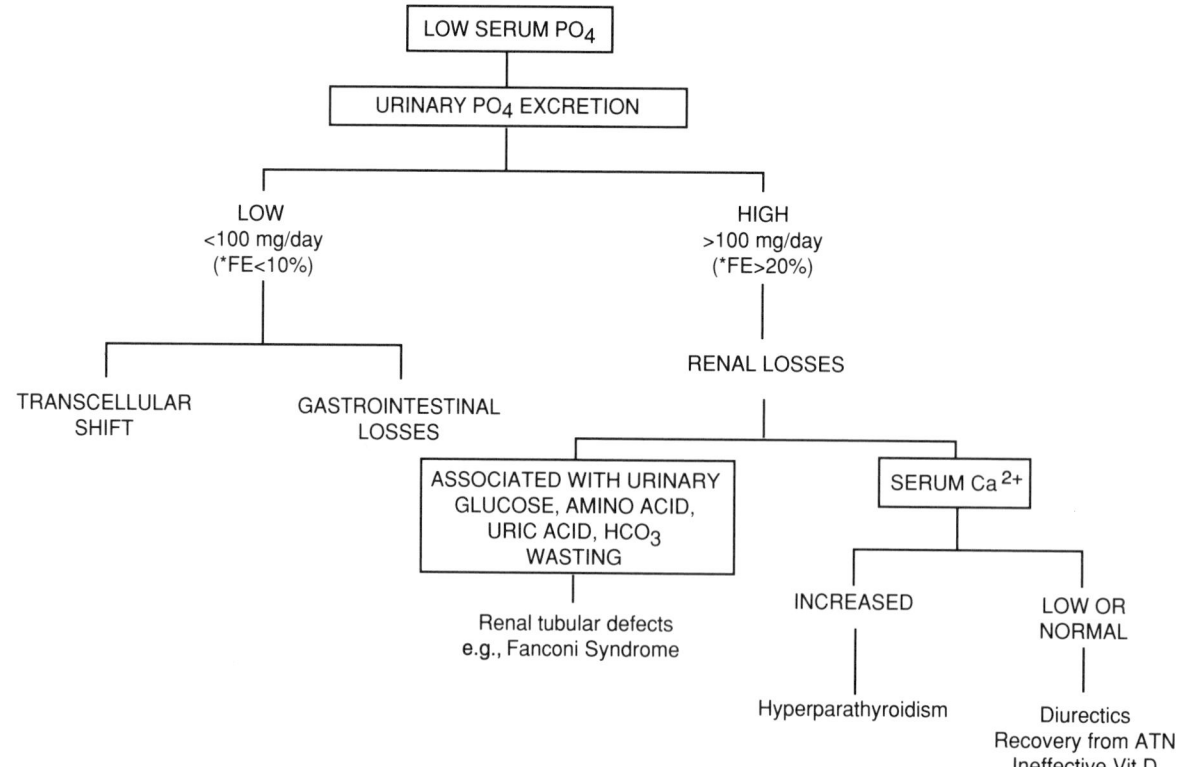

* FE = Excreted PO_4 (mg/day)/Filtered PO_4
Filtered PO_4 = GFR X 0.95 (Serum PO_4)

Figure 46.4. Evaluation of hypophosphatemia.

especially during withdrawal, and further exacerbate hypophosphatemia. Hypomagnesemia, hypokalemia, alcohol, and acidosis may lead to impaired renal conservation of PO_4.

Hypophosphatemia (PO_4 <2.4 mg/dl) occurs in approximately 29% of surgical patients (173). Hypophosphatemia develops 24 hours after surgery and results from glucose infusions, increased tissue metabolism, increased catecholamine secretion, and renal PO_4 losses (159, 174, 173). It is not known whether routine PO_4 supplementation in these patients would improve outcome.

Table 46.14. Clinical Features of Hypophosphatemia

General
  Weakness
  Malaise
Myocardial insufficiency
Impaired pressor reponses
Respiratory insufficiency
Rhabdomyolysis
Hepatocellular damage
Hematologic
  Hemolysis
  Platelet dysfunction
  Leukocyte dysfunction
Skeletal
  Osteomalacia
  Fractures
  Increased bone resorption
Metabolic
  Impaired glucose tolerance
  Impaired gluconeogenesis
  Impaired phospholipid synthesis
  Hypercalciuria
  Hypermagnesemia
Neurologic
  Ataxia
  Confusion
  Obtundation
  Coma
  Delirium
  Dysarthria
  Encephalopathy
  Muscle weakness
  Irritability
  Myopathy
  Paresthesias
  Seizures
  Tremor
Gastrointestinal
  Anorexia
  Nausea
  Vomiting

The cause of hypophosphatemia can usually be determined from the medical history and clinical setting. When in doubt, measurement of urinary PO_4 excretion may be helpful (Fig. 46.4). Transcellular shifts of PO_4 and gastrointestinal loss of PO_4 evoke avid renal PO_4 resorption, decreasing the fractional excretion of PO_4 in the urine to less than 10%. Renal causes of hypophosphatemia result in PO_4 wasting in the urine and a fractional excretion of PO_4 greater than 20%.

Clinical Manifestations

Severe hypophosphatemia is associated with decreased levels of PO_4-containing metabolites (e.g., ATP, 2,3-diphosphoglycerate) and membrane phospholipids and may cause a variety of clinical problems (Table 46.14). Patients rarely may develop cardiac insufficiency (159, 175–177). The cause for cardiac insufficiency is uncertain but may relate to depleted intracellular PO_4 stores (e.g., ATP, creatine phosphate), impaired action of the sodium-potassium ATPase pump, decreased calcium flux, or impaired catecholamine action (159, 178).

Patients with serum PO_4 levels of less than 2 mg/dl may complain of muscle weakness, anorexia, or tremor. As PO_4 levels approach 1 mg/dl, respiratory weakness or insufficiency may occur (179–184). Respiratory failure is more likely to occur in patients with underlying lung disease. In addition, hypophosphatemia may decrease muscle strength and impair weaning from ventilators. PO_4 supplementation in these patients may improve muscle strength (179, 181). The authors have treated a few patients with advanced pulmonary disease who could not be weaned off the ventilator because of respiratory muscle fatigue. After PO_4 supplementation, these patients were weaned from the ventilator. Hypophosphatemia has been reported to produce a large number of neurologic symptoms that include ataxia, tremor, paresthesias, myopathy, seizures, coma, and death.

Muscle cell integrity depends upon PO_4, and severe hypophosphatemia (<1 mg/dl) may injure the cell and cause rhabdomyolysis. Severe hypophosphatemia may also affect blood cells and cause hemolysis, platelet dysfunction, and leukocyte dysfunction (185). Hemolytic anemia rarely is seen unless the plasma PO_4 falls below 0.5 mg/dl. Depressed erythrocyte levels of 2,3-diphosphoglycerate shift the oxyhemoglobin dissociation curve to the left (reduces P_{50}), decreasing oxygen delivery to the tissues. Depressed leukocyte chemotaxis, phagocytosis, and bactericidal activity may impair recovery from infection. Metabolic consequences of hypophosphatemia

Table 46.15. Phosphate Preparations

Preparation	PO_4 Content[a]	Daily Dose
Enteral		
Whole milk	1 mg/ml	1200 ml
Skim milk	0.9 mg/ml	1330 ml
Neutra-Phos[b]	250-mg/capsule	1–2 t.i.d.
Potassium-PO_4 (K-Phos)	125-mg tablet	3–4 t.i.d.
	250-mg tablet	1–2 t.i.d.
Parenteral		
Potassium-PO_4	93 mg/ml (4 mEq/ml K^+)	1000 mg/day
Sodium-PO_4	93 mg/ml (4 mEq/ml Na^+)	1000 mg/day

[a] 31 mg PO_4 = 1 mmol PO_4.
[b] Also available as a solution.

include insulin resistance (186), impaired gluconeogenesis, impaired bone mineralization, and liver dysfunction. Hypercalciuria results from release of Ca^{2+} from bone in an attempt to maintain normal serum PO_4 concentrations (159) and decreased renal absorption of Ca^{2+}. Hypermagnesuria also results from increased mobilization of Mg^{2+} from bone and reduced Mg^{2+} resorption in the kidney (159).

PO_4 depletion is associated with three major alterations in renal acid-base regulation: proximal tubular bicarbonate wasting, impaired distal acidification, and decreased buffer excretion (diminished renal ammoniagenesis and hypophosphaturia) (159). Acid-base stability is usually well-preserved because of the balance of acidifying and alkalinizing forces (e.g., alkali released from bone). However, prolonged and severe PO_4 depletion may exhaust bone stores of alkali and result in a metabolic acidosis.

Therapy

The potential consequences of severe hypophosphatemia necessitate prompt recognition and treatment so as to avoid potentially devastating consequences. Serious life-threatening consequences usually do not occur until the serum PO_4 concentration falls below 1 mg/dl. Primary therapy should be oriented toward preventing hypophosphatemia. Serum PO_4 levels, like those of other primarily intracellular ions, may not reflect body stores adequately. Thus, initial therapy is usually empiric, and one must monitor the serum level to avoid hyperphosphatemia.

Initially, all drugs that are contributing to hypophosphatemia should be stopped (if possible). The list of drugs must include PO_4-binding antacids, intravenous glucose, and diuretics.

For immediate correction of profound hypophosphatemia (<1 mg/dl) or symptomatic hypophosphatemia, intravenous therapy (187–189) is necessary (Table 46.15), since oral PO_4 preparations, when given in large amounts, usually cause diarrhea. The rate of administration of PO_4 varies in the literature from 0.3 mg/kg/hr to 4 mg/kg/hr (187–189).

Based upon experience, the authors recommend the following: If depletion is recent and uncomplicated, the clinician should give 0.6 mg (0.02 mmol)/kg/hr; if it is prolonged and multifactorial, he or she should give 0.9 mg (0.03 mmol)/kg/hr. The serum PO_4 level should be checked every 6 to 12 hours until the level has stabilized, so as to avoid hyperphosphatemia. Hyperkalemia may result from excessive administration of potassium phosphate, especially in patients with impaired renal function. If the patient is also hypocalcemic or hypercalcemic, PO_4 should be administered at a slower rate and both PO_4 and Ca^{2+} should be monitored. Risks of treatment include hyperphosphatemia, hypocalcemia, hypotension, hyperkalemia (with potassium PO_4), hypomagnesemia, hyperosmolality, metastatic calcification, and renal failure. Extreme caution must be used when administering PO_4 to patients with renal insufficiency or failure, since these patients have a diminished ability to excrete PO_4. Parenteral solutions of PO_4 are hypertonic and should be diluted before use or given by central line. The addition of calcium to PO_4-containing solutions or administration of both through the same intravenous line may cause precipitation. Parenteral PO_4 may be discontinued and enteral therapy (Table 46.15) started

when the serum PO_4 level exceeds 2 mg/dl. Repletion should be carried out over 5 to 7 days to replace intracellular stores, after which the patient should be placed on a maintenance dose (e.g., 1200 mg/day orally or 1000 mg/day intravenously in the adult). Additional PO_4 may be required if excess losses are present. A major side effect of enteral phosphate is diarrhea. Hypomagnesemia is common in patients with PO_4 deficiency and should always be measured and replaced as needed (189).

HYPERPHOSPHATEMIA

Causes

Hyperphosphatemia (33, 159, 160) results from three basic mechanisms (Table 46.16): reduced renal excretion, increased entrance of PO_4 into the extracellular space from the intracellular space, and increased PO_4 or vitamin D intake.

Levels of PO_4 remain within normal ranges until the glomerular filtration rate falls below 20 to 25 ml/minute. Hyperphosphatemia, as well as renal failure, impairs the renal conversion of 25-hydroxyvitamin D to 1,25-dihydroxyvitamin D. Impaired synthesis of 1,25-dihydroxyvitamin D contributes to hypocalcemia and secondary hyperparathyroidism. PO_4 levels rise in patients with acute renal failure and frequently does so before the increase in blood urea nitrogen or creatinine. Elevated PO_4 levels are also seen in patients with hypoparathyroidism resulting from the loss of the phosphaturic action of parathyroid hormone. Hyperphosphatemia and hypercalcemia occur in hyperthyroidism as a result of increased bone resorption, parathyroid gland suppression, and increased tubular resorption of PO_4. Diphosphonates are used to treat patients with Paget's disease of bone and hypercalcemia. These agents cause hyperphosphatemia by reducing PO_4 excretion and altering its distribution among cellular compartments.

Hyperphosphatemia may occur when PO_4 enters the extracellular space after cellular damage induced by chemotherapy

Table 46.16. Causes of Hyperphosphatemia

Reduced renal excretion
Renal insufficiency
Hypoparathyroidism
PTH resistance
Hyperthyroidism
Acromegaly
Diphosphonates
Tumoral calcinosis
Increased PO_4 or vitamin D intake
Ingestion of PO_4 (e.g., laxatives)
Intravenous PO_4
PO_4 enemas
Vitamin D
Increased PO_4 entrance into extracellular fluid
Acidosis
Tumor lysis
Rhabdomyolysis
Sepsis
Malignant hyperpyrexia
Fulminant hepatitis
Severe hypothermia
Hemolysis

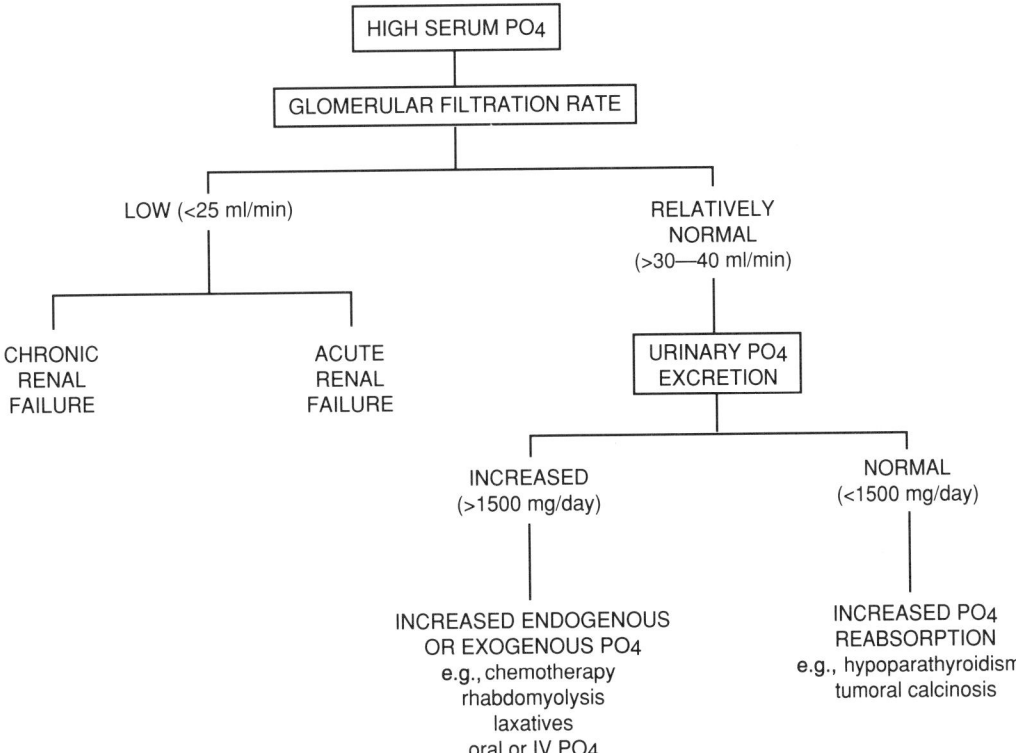

Figure 46.5. Evaluation of hyperphosphatemia.

(tumor lysis syndrome), rhabdomyolysis, malignant hyperthermia, hypothermia, sepsis, or hepatic necrosis. The hyperphosphatemia is exaggerated when there is concomitant renal insufficiency. Hyperphosphatemia may also occur from overzealous administration of PO_4-containing compounds (32) or from laxative abuse. Serum PO_4 levels may be increased artificially as a result of hemolysis during blood drawing.

Measurement of glomerular filtration and urinary PO_4 excretion are helpful in evaluating the etiology of hyperphosphatemia (Fig. 46.5). A glomerular filtration rate less than 20 to 25 ml/min suggests renal failure as the cause. Relatively normal glomerular filtration with a PO_4 excretion >1500 mg/day suggests increased PO_4 loading from either endogenous or exogenous sources. Normal renal filtration with a PO_4 excretion less than 1500 mg/day indicates increased renal PO_4 resorption as the cause.

Symptoms of hyperphosphatemia relate primarily to the hypocalcemia that it induces and ectopic calcification. Soft tissue calcification usually occurs when the calcium-phosphate product exceeds 75. In addition, alkalosis favors calcification.

Therapy

The therapy of hyperphosphatemia is aimed at eliminating the PO_4 source, removing PO_4 from the circulation, and correcting any associated hypocalcemia. Dietary PO_4 intake should be restricted. PO_4 excretion in the urine can be increased by hydration with saline (250 to 500 ml/hr) and diuresis with acetazolamide (500 mg every 6 hours) (190). Intestinal PO_4 absorption can be minimized and PO_4 removed from the body via the gastrointestinal tract with oral PO_4 binders (e.g., aluminum hydroxide), which are beneficial even if no oral

PO_4 is given. If renal insufficiency is not a problem, alternating aluminum hydroxide with magnesium salts can decrease aluminum-induced constipation. If symptomatic hypocalcemia is present, the patient should be given calcium. Hemodialysis or peritoneal dialysis are effective in removing PO_4 in renal failure.

REFERENCES

1. Moore EW: Ionized calcium in normal serum, ultrafiltrates and whole blood determined by ion exchange electrodes. *J Clin Invest* 49:318–334, 1970.
2. Robertson WG: Measurement of ionized calcium in body fluids—a review. *Ann Clin Biochem* 13:540–548, 1976.
3. Zaloga GP: Calcium disorders. In Zaloga GP (ed): Endocrine Emergencies. *Probl Crit Care* 4:382–401, 1990.
4. Zaloga GP, Chernow B: Hypocalcemia in critical illness. *JAMA* 256:1924–1929, 1986.
5. Zaloga GP, Chernow B: Stress-induced changes in calcium metabolism. *Semin Respir Med* 7:52–68, 1985.
6. Zaloga GP, Chernow B, Cook D, Snyder R, Clapper M, O'Brian JT: Assessment of calcium homeostasis in the critically ill surgical patient. The diagnostic pitfalls of the McLean-Hastings nomogram. *Ann Surg* 202:587–594, 1985.
7. Zaloga GP, Willey SC, Tomasic P, Chernow B: Free fatty acids alter calcium binding: a cause for misinterpretation of serum calcium values and hypocalcemia in critical illness. *J Clin Endocrinol Metab* 64:1010–1014, 1987.
8. Aguanno JJ, Ladenson JH: Influence of fatty acids on the binding of calcium to albumin. Correlation of binding and conformation studies and evidence for distinct differences between unsaturated fatty acids and saturated fatty acids. *J Biol Chem* 257:8745–8748, 1982.
9. Howland WS, Schweizer O, Jascott D, Ragasa J: Factors influencing the ionization of calcium during major surgical procedures. *Surg Gynecol Obstet* 143:895–900, 1976.
10. Kahn RC, Jascott D, Carlon GC, Schweizer O, Howland WS, Goldiner PL: Massive blood replacement: correlation of ionized calcium, citrate, and hydrogen ion concentration. *Anesth Analg* 58:274–278, 1979.
11. Denlinger JK, Nahrwold ML, Gibbs PS, Lecky JH: Hypocalcaemia during rapid blood transfusion in anaesthetized man. *Br J Anaesth* 48:995–1000, 1976.
12. Henrich WL, Hunt JM, Nixon JV: Increased ionized calcium and left ventricular contractility during hemodialysis. *N Engl J Med* 310:19–23, 1984.

13. Maynard JC, Cruz C, Kleerekoper M, Levin NW: Blood pressure response to changes in serum ionized calcium during hemodialysis. *Ann Intern Med* 104:358–361, 1986.

14. Ladenson JH, Lewis JW, Boyd JC: Failure of total serum calcium corrected for protein, albumin, and pH to correctly assess free calcium status. *J Clin Endocrinol Metab* 46:986–993, 1978.

15. Zaloga GP: Evaluation of bedside testing options for the critical care unit. *Chest* 97:185S–190S, 1990.

16. Zaloga GP, Wilkens R, Tourville J, Wood D, Klymer DM: A simple method for determining physiologically active calcium and magnesium concentrations in critically ill patients. *Crit Care Med* 15:813–816, 1987.

17. Marx SJ, Bourdeau JE: Calcium metabolism. In Maxwell MH, Kleeman CR, Narins RG (eds): *Clinical Disorders of Fluid and Electrolyte Metabolism*, 4th ed. New York, McGraw Hill, 1987, pp 207–244.

18. Zaloga GP, Chernow B, Hodge J, Eil C: Hypocalcemia and altered vitamin D metabolism in patients with small intestinal disease. *Military Med* 153:34–37, 1988.

19. Nagant De Deuxchaisnes C, Krane SM: Hypoparathyroidism. In Avioli LV, Krane SM (eds): *Metabolic Bone Disease*, vol 2. Orlando, FL, Academic Press, 1978, pp 217–445.

20. Benabe JE, Martinez-Maldonado: Disorders of calcium metabolism. In Maxwell MH, Kleeman CR, Narins RG (eds): *Clinical Disorders of Fluid and Electrolyte Metabolism*, 4th ed. New York, McGraw Hill, 1987, pp 758–788.

21. Watson CG, Steed DL, Robinson AG, Deftos LJ: The role of calcitonin and parathyroid hormone in the pathogenesis of post-thyroidectomy hypocalcemia. *Metabolism* 30:588–589, 1981.

22. Robertie PG, Butterworth JF, Prielipp RC, Tucker WY, Zaloga GP: Parathyroid hormone responses to marked hypocalcemia in infants and young children undergoing repair of congenital heart disease. *J Am Coll Cardiol* 20:672–677, 1992.

23. Robertie PG, Butterworth JF IV, Royster RL, et al: Normal parathyroid hormone responses to hypocalcemia during cardiopulmonary bypass. *Anesthesiology* 75:43–48, 1991.

24. Anast CS, Winnacker JL, Forte LR, Burns TW: Impaired release of parathyroid hormone in magnesium deficiency. *J Clin Endocrinol Metab* 42:707–717, 1976.

25. Chernow B, Barmberger S, Stoiko M, et al: Hypomagnesemia in patients in postoperative intensive care. *Chest* 95:391–397, 1989.

26. Cholst IN, Steinberg SF, Tropper PJ, Fox HE, Segre GV, Bilezikian JP: The influence of hypermagnesemia on serum calcium and parathyroid hormone levels in human subjects. *N Engl J Med* 310:1221–1225, 1984.

27. Zaloga GP, Roberts JE: Magnesium disorders. In Zaloga GP (ed): Endocrine emergencies. *Probl Crit Care* 4:425–436, 1990.

28. Rude RK, Oldham SB, Singer FR: Functional hypoparathyroidism and parathyroid hormone end-organ resistance in human magnesium deficiency. *Clin Endocrinol* 5:209–224, 1976.

29. Zaloga GP, Chernow B, Pock A, Wood B, Zaritsky A, Zucker A: Hypomagnesemia is a common complication of aminoglycoside therapy. *Surg Gynecol Obstet* 158:561–565, 1984.

30. Medalle R, Waterhouse C, Hahn TJ: Vitamin D resistance in magnesium deficiency. *Am J Clin Nutr* 29:854–858, 1976.

31. Miravet L, Ayigbede O, Carre M, Rayssiguier Y, Larvor P: Lack of vitamin D action on serum calcium in magnesium deficient rats. In Catin M, Seelig MS (eds): *Magnesium in Health and Disease*. New York, SP Medical and Scientific Books, 1980, pp 281–289.

32. Chernow B, Rainey TG, Georges LP, O'Brian JT: Iatrogenic hyperphosphatemia: a metabolic consideration in critical care medicine. *Crit Care Med* 9:772–774, 1981.

33. Zaloga GP: Phosphate disorders. In Zaloga GP (ed): Endocrine emergencies. *Probl Crit Care* 4:416–424, 1990.

34. Zaloga GP, Chernow B: Hypocalcemia and rhabdomyolysis. *J Am Med Assoc* 257:626, 1987.

35. Prielipp RC, Zaloga GP: Life-threatening hypocalcemia after abdominal aortic aneurysm repair in patients with renal insufficiency. *Anesth Analg* 73:638–641, 1991.

36. Jacobs ML, Daggett WM, Civetta JM, et al: Acute pancreatitis: analysis of factors influencing survival. *Ann Surg* 185:43–51, 1977.

37. Hauser CJ, Kamrath RO, Sparks J, Shoemaker WC: Calcium homeostasis in patients with acute pancreatitis. *Surgery* 94:830–835, 1983.

38. Haldimann B, Goldstein DA, Akmal M, Massry SG: Renal function and blood levels of divalent ions in acute pancreatitis. A prospective study in 99 patients. *Miner Electrolyte Metab* 3:190–199, 1980.

39. Robertson GM Jr, Moore EW, Switz DM, Sizemore GW, Estep HL: Inadequate parathyroid response to acute pancreatitis. *N Engl J Med* 294:512–516, 1976.

40. Condon JR, Ives D, Knight MJ, Day J: The aetiology of hypocalcemia in acute pancreatitis. *Br J Surg* 62:115–118, 1975.

41. Zaloga GP, Chernow B: The multifactorial basis for hypocalcemia during sepsis. Studies of the parathyroid hormone-vitamin D axis. *Ann Intern Med* 107:36–41, 1987.

42. Chang J, Abramson EC, Mayer M, et al: Mechanism of *cis*-platinum effectiveness in hypercalcemia of malignancy. *Clin Res* 33:888A, 1985.

43. Kukla LJ, Abramsom EC, McGuire WP, Shevrin DH, Lad T, Kukreja SC: *Cis*-platinum treatment for malignancy-associated humoral hypercalcemia in an athymic mouse model. *Calcif Tissue Int* 36:559–562, 1984.

44. Lad TE, Mishoulam HM, Shevrin DH, Kukla LJ, Abramson EC, Kukreja SC: Treatment of cancer-associated hypercalcemia with cisplatin. *Arch Intern Med* 147:329–332, 1987.

45. Heckman BA, Walsh JH: Hypernatremia complicating sodium sulfate therapy for hypercalcemic crisis. *N Engl J Med* 276:1082–1083, 1967.

46. Singer FR, Neer RM, Murray TM, Keutmann HT, Deftos LJ, Potts JT Jr: Mithramycin treatment of intractable hypercalcemia due to parathyroid carcinoma. *N Engl J Med* 283:634–636, 1970.

47. Silva OL, Becker KL: Salmon calcitonin in the treatment of hypercalcemia. *Arch Intern Med* 132:337–339, 1973.

48. Potts M, Doppelt S, Taylor S, Folkman J, Neer R, Potts JT Jr: Protamine: a powerful in vivo inhibitor of bone resorption. *Calcif Tissue Int* 36:189–193, 1984.

49. Warrell RP Jr, Bockman RS, Coonley CJ, Isaacs M, Staszewski H: Gallium nitrate inhibits calcium resorption from bone and is effective treatment for cancer-related hypercalcemia. *J Clin Invest* 73:1487–1490, 1984.

50. Jacobs TP, Siris ES, Bilezikian JP, Baquiran DC, Shane E, Canfield RE: Hypercalcemia of malignancy: treatment with intravenous dichloromethylene diphosphonate. *Ann Intern Med* 94:312–316, 1981.

51. Jung A: Comparison of two parenteral diphosphonates in hypercalcemia of malignancy. *Am J Med* 72:221–226, 1982.

52. Ryzen E, Martodam RR, Troxell M, Benson A, Paterson A, Shepard K, Hicks R: Intravenous etidronate in the management of malignant hypercalcemia. *Arch Intern Med* 145:449–452, 1985.

53. Glover DJ, Shaw L, Glick JH, et al: Treatment of hypercalcemia in parathyroid cancer with WR-2721, S-2-(3-aminopropylamino) ethyl-phosphorothioic acid. *Ann Intern Med* 103:55–57, 1985.

54. Glover D, Riley L, Carmichael K, et al: Hypocalcemia and inhibition of parathyroid hormone secretion after administration of WR-2721 (a radioprotective and chemoprotective agent). *N Engl J Med* 309:1137–1141, 1983.

55. Turk J, Morell L: Ethylene glycol intoxication. *Arch Intern Med* 146:1601–1603, 1986.

56. Haynes RC, Murad F: Agents affecting calcification: calcium, parathyroid hormone, calcitonin, vitamin D, and other compounds. In Gilman AG, Goodman LS, Rall TW, Murad F (eds): *The Pharmacological Basis of Therapeutics*. New York, Macmillan, 1985, pp 1517–1543.

57. Chaimovitz C, Abinader E, Benderly A, Better OS: Hypocalcemic hypotension. *J Am Med Assoc* 222:86–87, 1972.

58. Chernow B, Zaloga GP, Malcolm D, Willey SC, Clapper M, Holaday JW: Glucagon's chronotropic action is calcium dependent. *J Pharmacol Exp Ther* 241:833–837, 1987.

59. Chopra D, Janson P, Sawin CT: Insensitivity to digoxin associated with hypocalcemia. *N Engl J Med* 296:917–918, 1977.

60. Connor TB, Rosen BL, Blaustein MP, Applefeld MM, Doyle LA: Hypocalcemia precipitating congestive heart failure. *N Engl J Med* 307:869–872, 1982.

61. Drop LJ: Ionized calcium, the heart and hemodynamic function. *Anesth Analg* 64:432–451, 1985.

62. Ginsburg R, Esserman LJ, Bristow MR: Myocardial performance and extracellular ionized calcium in a severely failing human heart. *Ann Intern Med* 98:603–606, 1983.

63. Bristow MR, Schwartz HD, Binetti G, Harrison DC, Daniels JR: Ionized calcium and the heart. Elucidation of in vivo concentration-response relationships in the open-chest dog. *Circ Res* 41:565–574, 1977.

64. Prielipp R, Zaloga GP: Calcium action and general anesthesia. *Adv Anesth* 8:241–278, 1991.

65. Zaloga GP, Malcolm D: Calcium as a mediator in septic shock. In Neugebauer E, Holaday J (eds): *Handbook of Mediators in Septic Shock*. CRC Press, Boca Raton, FL, 1993, 475–485.

66. Malcolm DS, Zaloga GP, Holaday JW: Calcium administration increases the mortality of endotoxic shock in rats. *Crit Care Med* 17:900–903, 1989.

67. Zaloga GP, Soger A, Prielipp R, Ward K: Low dose calcium administration increases mortality during septic peritonitis. *Circ Shock* 37:226–229, 1992.

68. Zaloga GP, Washburn D: Multiorgan failure is associated with elevated free intracellular calcium in human sepsis. *Chest* 94(suppl):6S, 1988.

69. Mundy GR: *Calcium Homeostasis: Hypercalcemia and Hypocalcemia*. London, Martin Dunitz, 1989, pp 1–240.

70. Benson RC Jr, Riggs BL, Pickard BM, Arnaud CD: Radioimmunoassay of parathyroid hormone in hypercalcemic patients with malignant disease. *Am J Med* 56:821–826, 1974.

71. Insogna KL: Humoral hypercalcemia of malignancy. The role of parathyroid hormone-related protein. *Endocrinol Metab Clin North Am* 18:779–794, 1989.

72. Buckle R: Ectopic PTH syndrome, pseudohyperparathyroidism, hypercalcaemia of malignancy. *Clin Endocrinol* 3:237–251, 1974.

73. Stewart AF, Horst R, Deftos LJ, Cadman EC, Lang R, Broadus PE: Biochemical evaluation of patients with cancer-associated hypercalcemia: evidence for humoral and nonhumoral groups. *N Engl J Med* 303:1377–1383, 1980.

74. Breslau NA, McGuire JL, Zerwekh JE, Frenkel EP, Pak CY: Hypercalcemia associated with increased serum calcitriol levels in three patients with lymphoma. *Ann Intern Med* 100:1–6, 1984.

75. Zaloga GP, Eil C, Medbery CA: Humoral hypercalcemia in Hodgkin's disease. Association with elevated 1,25-dihydroxycholecalciferol levels and subperiosteal bone resorption. *Arch Intern Med* 145:155–157, 1985.

76. Mundy GR, Raisz LG, Cooper RA, Schechter GP, Salmon SE: Evidence for the secretion of an osteoclast stimulating factor in myeloma. *N Engl J Med* 291:1041–1046, 1974.

77. Seyberth HW, Segre GV, Morgan JL, Sweetman BJ, Potts JT Jr, Oates JA: Prostaglandins as mediators of hypercalcemia associated with certain types of cancer. *N Engl J Med* 293:1278–1283, 1975.

78. Habener JF, Potts JT: Parathyroid physiology and primary hyperparathyroidism. In Avioli LV, Krane M (eds): *Metabolic Bone Disease*, vol. 2. New York, Academic Press, 1978, pp 1–147.

79. Heath DA: Primary hyperparathyroidism. Clinical presentation and factors influencing clinical management. *Endocrinol Metab Clin North Am* 18:631–646, 1989.

80. Marcus R: Laboratory diagnosis of primary hyperparathyroidism. *Endocrinol Metab Clin North Am* 18:647–658, 1989.

81. Clark OH, Duh QY: Primary hyperparathyroidism. A surgical perspective. *Endocrinol Metab Clin North Am* 18:701–714, 1989.

82. Gallagher JC, Wilkinson R: The effect of ethinyloestradiol on calcium and phosphorus metabolism of post-menopausal women with primary hyperparathyroidism. *Clin Sci Mol Med* 45:785–802, 1973.

83. Horowitz M, Wishart J, Need AG, Morris H, Philcox J, Nordin BE: Treatment of postmenopausal hyperparathyroidism with norethindrone. *Arch Intern Med* 147:681–685, 1987.

84. Forster J, Querusio L, Burchard KW, Gann DS: Hypercalcemia in critically ill surgical patients. *Ann Surg* 202:512–518, 1985.

85. Marx SJ, Attie MF, Levine MA, Spiegel AM, Downs RW Jr, Lasker RD: The hypocalciuric or benign variant of familial hypercalcemia: clinical and biochemical features in fifteen kindreds. *Medicine* 60:397–412, 1981.

86. Heath H III: Familial benign (hypocalciuric) hypercalcemia. A troublesome mimic of mild primary hyperparathyroidism. *Endocrinol Metab Clin North Am* 18:723–740, 1989.

87. Zaloga GP, Eil C, O'Brian JT: Reversible hypocalciuric hypercalcemia associated with hypothyroidism. *Am J Med* 77:1101–1104, 1984.

88. Adams JS: Vitamin D metabolite-mediated hypercalcemia. *Endocrinol Metab Clin North Am* 18:765–778, 1989.

89. Bell NH, Stern PH, Pantzer E, Sinha TK, DuLuca HF: Evidence that increased circulatory 1α,25-dihydroxyvitamin D is the probable cause for abnormal calcium metabolism in sarcoidosis. *J Clin Invest* 64:218–225, 1979.

90. Cushard WG Jr, Simon AB, Canterbury JM, Reiss E: Parathyroid function in sarcoidosis. *N Engl J Med* 286:395–398, 1972.

91. Mason RS, Frankel T, Chan YL, Lissner D, Posen S: Vitamin D conversion by sarcoid lymph node homogenate. *Ann Intern Med* 100:59–61, 1984.

92. Abbasi AA, Chemplavil JK, Farah S, Muller BF, Arnstein AR: Hypercalcemia in active pulmonary tuberculosis. *Ann Intern Med* 90:324–328, 1979.

93. Zaloga GP, Chernow B, Eil C: Hypercalcemia and disseminated cytomegalovirus infection in the acquired immune deficiency syndrome. *Ann Intern Med* 102:331–333, 1985.

94. Orwoll ES: The milk-alkali syndrome: current concepts. *Ann Intern Med* 97:242–248, 1982.

95. McPherson ML, Prince SR, Atamer ER, Maxwell DB, Ross-Clunis H, Estep HL: Theophylline-induced hypercalcemia. *Ann Intern Med* 105:52–54, 1986.

96. Zaloga GP, Malcolm DS, Holaday J, Chernow B: Verapamil reverses calcium cardiotoxicity. *Ann Emerg Med* 16:637–639, 1987.

97. Ellman H, Dembin H, Seriff N: The rarity of shortening of the QT interval in patients with hypercalcemia. *Crit Care Med* 10:320–322, 1982.

98. Zaloga GP, Willey S, Malcolm D, Chernow B, Holaday JW: Hypercalcemia attenuates blood pressure response to epinephrine. *J Pharmacol Exp Ther* 247:949–952, 1988.

99. Zaloga GP, Strickland RA, Butterworth JF IV, Mark LJ, Mills SA, Lake CR: Calcium attenuates epinephrine's β-adrenergic effects in postoperative heart surgery patients. *Circulation* 81:196–200, 1990.

100. Butterworth JF IV, Zaloga GP, Prielipp RC, Tucker WY Jr, Royster RL: Calcium inhibits the cardiac stimulating properties of dobutamine but not amrinone. *Chest* 101:174–180, 1992.

101. Butterworth JF, Strickland RA, Zaloga GP: Hemodynamic actions and drug interactions of calcium and magnesium. In Zaloga GP (ed): Endocrine emergencies. *Probl Crit Care* 4:402–415, 1990.

102. Prielipp RC, Hill T, Washburn D, Zaloga GP: Circulating calcium modulates adrenaline induced cyclic adenosine monophosphate production. *Cardiovasc Res* 23:838–841, 1989.

103. Davis KD, Attie MF: Management of severe hypercalcemia. *Crit Care Clin* 7:175–190, 1991.

104. Attie MF: Treatment of hypercalcemia. *Endocrinol Metab Clin North Am* 18:807–828, 1989.

105. Aldinger KA, Samaan NA: Hypokalemia with hypercalcemia. Prevalence and significance in treatment. *Ann Intern Med* 85:571–573, 1977.

106. Cardella CJ, Birkin BL, Rapoport A: Role of dialysis in the treatment of severe hypercalcemia: report of two cases successfully treated with hemodialysis and review of the literature. *Clin Nephrol* 12:285–290, 1979.

107. Marcus R, Madvig P, Crim M, Pont A, Kosek J: Conjugated estrogens in the treatment of postmenopausal women with hyperparathyroidism. *Ann Intern Med* 100:633–640, 1984.

108. Zaloga GP: Hypocalcemia in critically ill patients. *Crit Care Med* 20:251–262, 1992.

109. Salem M, Munoz R, Chernow B: Hypomagnesemia in critical illness. A common and clinically important problem. *Crit Care Clin* 7:225–252, 1991.

110. Quamme GA, Dirks KJ: Magnesium metabolism. In Maxwell MH, Kleeman CR, Narins RG (eds): *Clinical Disorders of Fluid and Electrolyte Metabolism*, 4th ed. New York, McGraw Hill, 1987, pp 297–316.

111. Brauthbar N, Massry SG: Hypomagnesemia and hypermagnesemia. In Maxwell MH, Kleeman CR, Narins RG (eds): *Clinical Disorders of Fluid and Electrolyte Metabolism*, 4th ed. New York, McGraw Hill, 1987, pp 831–849.

112. Cronin RE, Knochel JP: Magnesium deficiency. *Adv Intern Med* 28:509–533, 1983.

113. Massry SG, Seelig MS: Hypomagnesemia and hypermagnesemia. *Clin Nephrol* 7:147–153, 1977.

114. Rude RK, Singer FR: Magnesium deficiency and excess. *Annu Rev Med* 32:245–259, 1981.

115. Wacker WEC, Parisi AF: Magnesium metabolism. *N Engl J Med* 278:658–663, 712–717, 772–776, 1968.

116. Brown EM, Chen CJ: Calcium, magnesium and the control of PTH secretion. *Bone Miner* 5:249–257, 1989.

117. Freitag JJ, Martin KJ, Conrades MB, et al: Evidence for skeletal resistance to parathyroid hormone in magnesium deficiency. Studies in isolated perfused bone. *J Clin Invest* 64:1238–1244, 1979.

118. Whang R, Flink EB, Dyckner T, Wester PO, Aikawa JK, Ryan MP: Magnesium depletion as a cause of refractory potassium repletion. *Arch Intern Med* 145:1686–1689, 1985.

119. Whang R, Morosi HJ, Rodgers D, Reyes R: The influence of sustained magnesium deficiency on muscle potassium repletion. *J Lab Clin Med* 70:895–902, 1967.

120. Ryan MP, Whang R, Yamalis W, Aikawa JK: Effect of magnesium deficiency on cardiac and skeletal muscle potassium during dietary potassium restriction. *Proc Soc Exp Biol Med* 143:1045–1047, 1973.

121. Dyckner T, Wester PO: Relation between potassium, magnesium and cardiac arrhythmias. *Acta Med Scand* Suppl 647:163–169, 1981.

122. Ryzen E, Wagers PW, Singer FR, Rude RK: Magnesium deficiency in a medical ICU population. *Crit Care Med* 13:19–21, 1985.

123. Fiaccadori E, Del Canale S, Coffrini E, et al: Muscle and serum magnesium in pulmonary intensive care unit patients. *Crit Care Med* 16:751–760, 1988.

124. Berkelhammer C, Bear RA: A clinical approach to common electrolyte problems: hypomagnesemia. *Can Med Assoc J* 132:360–368, 1985.

125. Kingston ME, Al-Siba'i MB, Skooge WC: Clinical manifestations of hypomagnesemia. *Crit Care Med* 14:950–954, 1986.

126. Zaloga GP: Interpretation of the serum magnesium level. *Chest* 95:257–258, 1989.

127. Molloy DW, Dhingra S, Solven FR, Wilson A, McCarthy DS: Hypomagnesemia and respiratory muscle power. *Am Rev Respir Dis* 129:497–498, 1984.

128. Burch GE, Giles TD: The importance of magnesium deficiency in cardiovascular disease. *Am Heart J* 94:649–657, 1977.

129. Iseri LT, Freed J, Bures AR: Magnesium deficiency and cardiac disorders. *Am J Med* 58:837–846, 1975.

130. Rasmussen HS, Suenson M, McNair P, Norregard P, Balslev S: Magnesium infusion reduces the incidence of arrhythmias in acute myocardial infarction. A double-blind placebo-controlled study. *Clin Cardiol* 10:351–356, 1987.

131. Smith LF, Heagerty AM, Bing RF, Barnett DB: Intravenous infusion of magnesium sulfate after acute myocardial infarction: effects on arrhythmias and mortality. *Int J Cardiol* 12:175–183, 1986.

132. Morton BC, Nair RC, Smith FM, McKibbon TG, Poznanski WJ: Magnesium therapy in acute myocardial infarction—a double blind study. *Magnesium* 3:346–352, 1984.

133. Bigg RPC, Chia R: Magnesium deficiency. Role in arrhythmias complicating acute myocardial infarction. *Med J Aust* 1:346–348, 1981.

134. Abraham AS, Rosenmann D, Kramer M, et al: Magnesium in the prevention of lethal arrhythmias in acute myocardial infarction. *Arch Intern Med* 147:753–755, 1987.

135. Dyckner T: Serum magnesium in acute myocardial infarction. Relation to arrhythmias. *Acta Med Scand* 207:59–66, 1980.

136. Rasmussen HS, Aurup P, Hojberg S, Jensen EK, McNair P: Magnesium and acute myocardial infarction. Transient hypomagnesemia not induced by renal magnesium loss in patients with acute myocardial infarction. *Arch Intern Med* 146:872–874, 1986.

137. Rasmussen HS, McNair P, Norregard P, Backer V, Lindeneg O, Balslev S: Intravenous magnesium in acute myocardial infarction. *Lancet* 1:234–236, 1986.

138. Beller GA, Hood WB Jr, Smith TW, Abelmann WH, Wacker WEC: Correlation of serum magnesium levels and digitalis intoxication. *Am J Cardiol* 33:225–229, 1974.

139. Webb S, Schade DS: Hypomagnesemia as a cause of persistent hypokalemia. *JAMA* 233:23–24, 1975.

140. Bohmer T, Mathiesen B: Magnesium deficiency in chronic alcoholic patients uncovered by an intravenous load test. *Scand J Clin Lab Invest* 42:633–636, 1982.

141. Chernow B, Zaloga GP: SCCM—ions for society members (sulfate, chloride calcium, magnesium). In *Critical Care—State of the Art*, vol. 4. Fullerton, CA, Society of Critical Care Medicine, 1984, pp K1–K43.

142. Flink EB: Therapy of magnesium deficiency. *Ann NY Acad Sci* 162:901–905, 1969.

143. Heath DA: The emergency management of disorders of calcium and magnesium. *Clin Endocrinol Metab* 9:487–502, 1980.

144. Loeb HS, Pietras RM, Gunnar RM, Tobin JR Jr: Paroxysmal ventricular fibrillation in two patients with hypomagnesemia. Treatment by transvenous pacing. *Circulation* 37:210–215, 1967.

145. Iseri LT, Chung P, Tobis J: Magnesium therapy for intractable ventricular tachyarrhythmias in normomagnesemic patients. *West J Med* 138:823–828, 1983.

146. Kafka H, Langevin L, Armstrong PW: Serum magnesium and potassium in acute myocardial infarction. Influence on ventricular arrhythmias. *Arch Intern Med* 147:465–469, 1987.

147. Whang R, Oei TO, Watanabe A: Frequency of hypomagnesemia in hospitalized patients receiving digitalis. *Arch Intern Med* 145:655–656, 1985.

148. Seller RH, Cangiano J, Kim KE, Mendelssohn S, Brest AN, Swartz C: Digitalis toxicity and hypomagnesemia. *Am Heart J* 79:57–68, 1970.

149. Goldman RH, Kleiger RE, Schweizer E, Harrison DC: The effect on myocardial ³H-digoxin in magnesium deficiency. *Proc Soc Exp Biol Med* 136:747–749, 1971.

150. Cohen L, Kitzes R: Magnesium sulfate and digitalis-toxic arrhythmias. *JAMA* 249:2808–2810, 1983.

151. Prielipp RC, Zaloga GP, Butterworth JF IV, et al: Magnesium inhibits the hypertensive but not the cardiotonic actions of low-dose epinephrine. *Anesthesiology* 74:973–979, 1991.

152. Mroczek WJ, Lee WR, Davidov ME: Effect of magnesium sulfate on cardiovascular hemodynamics. *Angiology* 28:720–724, 1977.

153. James MFM, Cork RC, Dennett JE: Cardiovascular effects of magnesium sulfate in the baboon. *Magnesium* 6:314–324, 1987.

154. Altura BM, Altura BT, Carella A: Magnesium deficiency induced spasms of umbilical vessels: relation to preeclampsia, hypertension, growth retardation. *Science* 221:376–378, 1983.

155. Okayama H, Aikawa T, Okayama M, Sasaki H, Mue S, Takishima T: Bronchodilating effect of intravenous magnesium sulfate in bronchial asthma. *JAMA* 257:1076–1078, 1987.

156. Rolla G, Bucca C, Arossa W, Bugiani M: Magnesium attenuates methacholine-induced bronchoconstriction in asthmatics. *Magnesium* 6:201–204, 1987.

157. Mordes JP, Wacker WE: Excess magnesium. *Pharmacol Rev* 29:273–300, 1977.

158. Knochel JP: The pathophysiology and clinical characteristics of severe hypophosphatemia. *Arch Intern Med* 137:203–220, 1977.

159. Brauthbar N, Kleeman CR: Hypophosphatemia and hyperphosphatemia: clinical and pathophysiologic aspects. In Maxwell MH, Kleeman CR, Narins RG (eds): *Clinical Disorders of Fluid and Electrolyte Metabolism*, 4th ed. New York, McGraw Hill, 1987, pp 789–830.

160. Peppers MP, Geheb M, Desai T: Endocrine crises. Hypophosphatemia and hyperphosphatemia. *Crit Care Clin* 7:201–214, 1991.

161. Stoff JS: Phosphate homeostasis and hypophosphatemia. *Am J Med* 72:489–495, 1982.

162. Lee DBN, Kurakowa K: Physiology of phosphorus metabolism. In Maxwell MH, Kleeman CR, Narins RG (eds): *Clinical Disorders of Fluid and Electrolyte Metabolism*, 4th ed. New York, McGraw-Hill, 1987, pp 245–295.

163. Massry SG, Friedler RM, Coburn JW: Excretion of phosphate and calcium. Physiology of their renal handling and relation to clinical medicine. *Arch Intern Med* 131:828–259, 1973.

164. Knochel JP: The clinical status of hypophosphatemia: an update. *N Engl J Med* 313:447–449, 1985.

165. Fitzgerald FT: Hypophosphatemia. *Adv Intern Med* 23:137–157, 1978.

166. Levy LA: Severe hypophosphatemia as a complication of the treatment of hypothermia. *Arch Intern Med* 140:128–129, 1980.

167. Massara F, Camanni F: Propranolol block of adrenaline-induced hypophosphataemia in man. *Clin Sci* 38:245–250, 1970.

168. Kreisberg RA: Diabetic ketoacidosis: new concepts and trends in pathogenesis and treatment. *Ann Intern Med* 88:681–695, 1978.

169. Riley MS, Schade DS, Eaton RP: Effects of insulin infusion on plasma phosphate in diabetic patients. *Metabolism* 28:191–194, 1979.

170. Keller U, Berger W: Prevention of hypophosphatemia by phosphate infusion during treatment of diabetic ketoacidosis and hyperosmolar coma. *Diabetes* 29:87–95, 1980.

171. Wilson HK, Keuer SP, Lea AS, Boyd AE III, Eknoyan G: Phosphate therapy in diabetic ketoacidosis. *Arch Intern Med* 142:517–520, 1982.

172. Ryback RS, Eckardt MJ, Paulter CP: Clinical relationship between serum phosphorus and other blood chemistry values in alcoholics. *Arch Intern Med* 140:673–677, 1980.

173. Swaminathan R, Bradley P, Morgan DB, Hill GL: Hypophosphatemia in surgical patients. *Surg Gynecol Obstet* 148:448–454, 1979.

174. Hessov I, Jensen NG, Rasmussen A: Prevention of hypophosphatemia during postoperative routine glucose administration. *Acta Chir Scand* 146:109–114, 1980.

175. Darsee JR, Nutter DO: Reversible severe congestive cardiomyopathy in three cases of hypophosphatemia. *Ann Intern Med* 89:867–870, 1978.

176. Fuller TJ, Nichols WW, Brenner BJ, Peterson JC: Reversible depression in myocardial performance in dogs with experimental phosphorus deficiency. *J Clin Invest* 62:1194–1200, 1978.

177. O'Connor LR, Wheeler WS, Bethune JE: Effect of hypophosphatemia on myocardial performance in man. *N Engl J Med* 297:901–903, 1977.

178. Kreusser W, Vetter HO, Mittmann U, Horl WH, Ritz E: Haemodynamics and myocardial metabolism of phosphorus depleted dogs: effects of catecholamines and angiotensin II. *Eur J Clin Invest* 12:219–228, 1982.

179. Aubier M, Murciano D, Lecocguic Y, et al: Effect of hypophosphatemia on diaphragmatic contractility in patients with acute respiratory failure. *N Engl J Med* 313:420–424, 1985.

180. Newman JH, Neff TA, Ziporin P: Acute respiratory failure associated with hypophosphatemia. *N Engl J Med* 296:1101–1103, 1977.

181. Varsano S, Shapiro M, Taragan R, Bruderman I: Hypophosphatemia as a reversible cause of refractory ventilatory failure. *Crit Care Med* 11:908–909, 1983.

182. Zaloga GP: Hypophosphatemia in patients with chronic obstructive pulmonary disease. *J Crit Illness* 7:364–375, 1992.

183. Agusti AG, Torres A, Estopa R, Agustividal A: Hypophosphatemia as a cause of failed weaning: the importance of metabolic factors. *Crit Care Med* 12:142–143, 1984.

184. Gravelyn TR, Brophy N, Siegert C, Peters-Golden M: Hypophosphatemia associated respiratory muscle weakness in a general inpatient population. *Am J Med* 84:870–876, 1988.

185. Craddock PR, Yawata Y, VanSanten L, Gilberstadt S, Silvis S, Jacob HS: Acquired phagocyte dysfunction: a complication of the hypophosphatemia of parenteral hyperalimentation. *N Engl J Med* 290:1403–1407, 1974.

186. DeFronzo RA, Lang R: Hypophosphatemia and glucose intolerance: evidence for tissue insensitivity to insulin. *N Engl J Med* 303:1259–1263, 1980.

187. Kingston M, Al-Siba'i MB: Treatment of severe hypophosphatemia. *Crit Care Med* 13:16–18, 1985.

188. Lentz RD, Brown DM, Kjellstrand CM: Treatment of severe hypophosphatemia. *Ann Intern Med* 89:941–944, 1978.

189. Vannatta JB, Whang R, Papper S: Efficacy of intravenous phosphorus therapy in the severely hypophosphatemic patient. *Arch Intern Med* 141:885–887, 1981.

190. Agus ZS, Goldfarb S, Wasserstein A: Disorders of calcium and phosphate balance. In Brenner BM, Rector FC (eds): *The Kidney*, 2nd ed. Philadelphia, WB Saunders, 1981, pp 940–1022.

CHAPTER 47

Vitamins

LAWRENCE BORTENSCHLAGER, M.D.
GARY P. ZALOGA, M.D., F.A.C.P.

Vitamins are substances that are essential for the maintenance of normal metabolic functions. Most are not synthesized in the body. Therefore, the body is dependent upon an exogenous supply. Healthy individuals who consume normal diets receive adequate quantities of vitamins. However, during states of abnormal body metabolism (i.e., critical illness) and malnutrition, multiple vitamin deficiencies may develop. Vitamin deficiencies impair cellular and organ function and recovery from illness. A knowledge of their properties is important when these agents are administered to patients. This chapter presents a brief review of both the fat-soluble (A, D, E, K) and water-soluble vitamins (Table 47.1), discussing their basic chemistry, metabolism, sources, requirements, manifestations of deficiency, and therapeutic administration.

VITAMIN C (ASCORBIC ACID) (1–13)

CHEMISTRY

Ascorbic acid is a simple carbohydrate (L-ascorbic acid) that is soluble in water, stable in acid, and destroyed by alkali and oxygen. In the body, L-ascorbic acid is reversibly oxidized to dehydroascorbic acid, a form possessing full biologic activity. Further metabolism of dehydroascorbic acid yields derivatives that are void of vitamin C activity.

METABOLISM

Ascorbic acid is readily absorbed in the small intestine by facilitated diffusion and active transport. Absorption of ascorbic acid occurs in both intestinal cells and renal tubular cells. In the intestine, dehydroascorbic acid can be reduced to ascorbic acid and subsequently absorbed. Ascorbic acid is excreted in the urine as ascorbic acid, dehydroascorbic acid, or one of several metabolites. Small amounts appear in feces and sweat. The efficiency of intestinal absorption decreases with large daily intakes (i.e., >180 mg). Renal tubular reabsorption also varies with intake. Complete tubular reabsorption occurs when the plasma concentration is <15 mg/liter. Consequently, large quantities of ascorbic acid in the intestine and kidney tubule result in poor absorption and tubular reabsorption respectively, and in significant fecal and renal losses. Following absorption, all organs and tissues take up ascorbic acid. Concentrations are highest in glandular tissues (i.e., adrenals, liver), averaging up to 50 times higher than the plasma concentration. The body pool of ascorbic acid averages 1500 mg in normal individuals (i.e., receiving about 80 mg of the vitamin per day). Approximately 3% is catabolized daily. Plasma concentrations reflect dietary intake and are variable. White blood cell ascorbic acid levels are used as an indicator of cellular and tissue levels.

Ascorbic acid is a reducing agent involved in numerous oxidation-reduction reactions and the transfer of protons. It is important in the synthesis of collagen, catecholamines, and corticosterone, and in the metabolism of tyrosine. It helps maintain the integrity of connective tissue, osteoid tissue of bone, and dentin of teeth. Vitamin C enhances iron absorption and is needed for the conversion of folic acid to folinic acid (it protects folic acid reductase). Wound healing, vascular

Table 47.1. Fat-Soluble and Water-Soluble Vitamins

Vitamin	Functions	Deficiency	Usual Therapeutic Dosage
A	Epithelial integrity Photoreceptors	Night blindness Perifollicular hyperkeratosis Xerophthalmia Keratomalacia Panophthalmitis Blindness	10,000–20,000 µg or 30,000–60,000 IU per day
D	Maintenance of calcium homeostasis, bone mineralization	Rickets Osteomalacia Hypocalcemia	Ergocalciferol 20–125 µg per day
E	Antioxidant, integrity of membranes	Hemolysis Neural abnormalities	30–100 mg/day or 45–150 IU per day
K	Blood coagulation	Hemorrhage Bruising	Phytonadione 2.5–20 mg p.o., s.q., or i.m. per day
C (ascorbic acid)	Reducing agent, collagen and catecholamine synthesis, iron absorption, wound healing, immune function, vascular integrity	Scurvy (loose teeth, gingivitis, hemorrhages, anemia, poor healing)	50–1000 mg/day
B_{12} (cyanocobalamin)	DNA synthesis, maturation of RBCs, neural function, folate metabolism	Pernicious anemia, glossitis, diarrhea, peripheral neuropathy, posterior column disease (CNS), dementia	50 µg/day i.m. first 2 weeks, 100 µg twice weekly for next 2 months, then 100 µg/month
Folic acid	Synthesis of DNA, RBC maturation, growth	Pancytopenia, stomatitis, diarrhea	1 mg/day
Riboflavin (B_2)	Energy and protein metabolism, integrity of mucous membranes	Cheilitis, stomatitis, corneal vascularization, dermatitis	5–25 mg/day
Thiamine (B_1)	Carbohydrate metabolism Myocardial function Central and peripheral nerve function	Beriberi, peripheral neuropathy, cardiac failure, Wernicke-Korsakoff	30–90 mg/day
Pyridoxine (B_6)	Nitrogen metabolism, transamination, porphyrin and heme synthesis, tryptophan conversion to niacin, linoleic acid metabolism	Seizures in infancy, anemia, neuropathy, skin lesions	25–100 mg/day
Niacin	Oxidation-reduction reactions Carbohydrate metabolism	Pellagra (dermatosis, glossitis, GI and CNS dysfunction)	50–500 mg nicotinic acid daily
Biotin	Carboxylation, amino acid and fatty acid metabolism	Dermatitis Glossitis	100–300 µg/day
Pantothenic acid	Component of CoA, carbohydrate and fatty acid metabolism	"Burning foot syndrome"	10 mg/day

integrity, and immune function are also under the influence of ascorbic acid. With the exception of collagen synthesis, the mechanism of action for most of these activities is poorly understood.

SOURCES

Vitamin C is widely distributed in foods. The best dietary sources are citrus fruits and green vegetables, especially broccoli, green peppers, tomatoes, cabbage, oranges, grapefruits, and lemons. Variation in content depends upon the degree of ripeness, storage conditions, and food preparation.

REQUIREMENTS

The recommended dietary allowance (RDA) for ascorbic acid is 60 mg/day for adults. Patients who smoke as well as those who are febrile, undergoing surgery, subjected to trauma or burns, on total parenteral nutrition, pregnant or lactating, or have thyrotoxicosis may require increased amounts of daily vitamin C intake. Vitamin C requirements are increased in patients with malabsorption, inflammatory diseases, and achlorhydria. The RDA for pregnant females is increased to 70 mg/day, while lactating females should receive 95 mg/day of ascorbic acid.

DEFICIENCY STATES

Clinical vitamin C deficiency (scurvy) is uncommon in the western world, but when seen it usually results from dietary inadequacy in the chronically ill, the poor, or the elderly, or in chronic alcoholics. The manifestations of scurvy are initially nonspecific and include malaise and weakness. Progression of the deficiency state is evidenced by perifollicular hemorrhages, petechiae, bruising, follicular hyperkeratosis and purpura, bleeding and swollen gums, loosened teeth, joint hemorrhage, subperiosteal hemorrhage, and bone fractures. Pallor and anemia are common and wound healing is markedly impaired. As the disease advances, edema, oliguria, and neuropathy are common. Intracerebral hemorrhage is usually followed by death.

Assessment of vitamin C status may be accomplished by measuring plasma ascorbic acid levels (normal >1.30 mg/dl) and leukocyte ascorbic acid concentrations (normal >15 mg/dl). Vitamin C deficiency usually occurs when plasma ascorbic acid levels are <0.20 mg/dl and leukocyte ascorbic acid levels are <7 mg/dl. The diagnosis of scurvy is usually made on the basis of clinical manifestations in conjunction with low plasma and leukocyte ascorbic acid levels.

THERAPY

For prophylaxis against scurvy or correction of deficiency, 40 to 60 mg of vitamin C are administered daily. The oral route is preferred. However, vitamin C may also be given parenterally (i.v. or i.m.). For treatment of scurvy, 300 mg to 1.0 g should be administered daily parenterally for 1 week followed by 100 mg daily for several weeks until tissue stores are replenished. For disease states requiring increased intake (i.e., surgery, trauma, febrile state), 150 mg of vitamin C should be administered daily. For severe burns, 500 mg to 2.0 g should be administered parenterally daily until healing has occurred.

PREPARATIONS AND ADVERSE EFFECTS

Vitamin C is available in tablet, capsule, and parenteral forms. It is also a component of most multivitamin preparations. Large doses of vitamin C may cause diarrhea or renal stones (i.e., cystine, oxalate, or urate). Renal stones are more likely when the urine is acidic. Lightheadedness and dizziness may occur following rapid i.v. administration.

VITAMIN B₁₂ (COBALAMIN, CYANOCOBALAMIN) (1–13)

CHEMISTRY

Vitamin B$_{12}$ is composed of a central cobalt ion within a porphyrin-like ring (corrin ring), linked to a nucleotide base, ribose, and phosphoric acid. In its natural form the vitamin usually occurs in combination with protein. Vitamin B$_{12}$ exists in several forms. Cyanocobalamin, hydroxocobalamin, 5′-deoxyadenosylcobalamin, and methyl cobalamin serve as coenzymes and are essential for cell growth and replication. Cyanocobalamin and hydroxocobalamin are both available commercially for therapeutic use, in part because of their stable structure. Vitamin B$_{12}$ is produced commercially as a by-product of the cultivation of *Streptomyces griseus* used in the preparation of the antibiotic streptomycin. Vitamin B$_{12}$ is freely soluble in water and somewhat resistant to boiling in neutral solution but is unstable in alkali.

METABOLISM

After ingestion, vitamin B$_{12}$ is bound to intrinsic factor, a protein secreted by gastric parietal cells. This intrinsic factor-cobalamin complex transits the intestine and attaches to a specific receptor in the ileal mucosa, where it is absorbed. Following absorption, the vitamin is bound by a plasma protein, transcobalamin II, for transport to the tissues. The liver is the major storage site for vitamin B$_{12}$, containing approximately 2 mg. Normal individuals on a standard American diet excrete about 1.3 μg/day of vitamin B$_{12}$. Small quantities of the vitamin are secreted in bile. However, most of this vitamin B$_{12}$ is reabsorbed with intrinsic factor via an enterohepatic cycle. Since daily losses of vitamin B$_{12}$ are 1 to 2 μg/day, the body has sufficient stores to last more than 3 years after vitamin B$_{12}$ absorption ceases. Thus, vitamin B$_{12}$ deficiency states are unusual unless gut absorption is diminished for long periods of time.

Vitamin B$_{12}$ is required for normal hematopoiesis and for maintenance of the integrity of the nervous system (especially myelin formation). It is an important cofactor for the metabolism of folate. Both folate and B$_{12}$ are required for DNA synthesis.

SOURCES

The average U.S. diet supplies 5 to 15 μg/day of vitamin B$_{12}$. Vitamin B$_{12}$ content of vegetables is low. The usual dietary sources are meat and meat products, fish, eggs, and, to a lesser extent, milk and milk products. Vitamin B$_{12}$ is present in several forms in food. The main forms are deoxyadenosyl- and hydroxocobalamin, of which one-third to one-half is absorbed. Methylcobalamin is found in egg yolk and cheese, while little or no cyanocobalamin occurs in foods.

REQUIREMENTS

The RDA of vitamin B$_{12}$ for adults is 3 μg/day. The minimum daily requirement is 2 μg/day. Pregnant females have a slightly higher RDA of 4 μg/day. Vitamin B$_{12}$ requirements are higher in patients with diminished intrinsic factor production and altered ileal absorption.

DEFICIENCY STATES

Dietary vitamin B_{12} deficiency is rare and seen only in strict vegetarians who avoid all dairy products as well as meat and fish. Secondary causes of vitamin B_{12} deficiency are more common, with pernicious anemia (i.e., lack of intrinsic factor) accounting for the majority of such cases. Other causes include malabsorption syndromes (i.e., celiac disease, sprue, drugs, malignancy), gastrectomy, blind loop syndrome, tapeworms, surgical resection of the ileum, Chron's disease, transcobalamin II deficiency (rare), and liver and kidney disease.

The manifestations of vitamin B_{12} deficiency are usually insidious. The hallmark of the deficiency is megaloblastic anemia. Weakness, fatigue, and dyspnea are usually related to anemia. Other signs and symptoms include glossitis, anorexia, diarrhea, and loss of taste. Vitamin B_{12} deficiency also leads to the development of a complex neurologic syndrome. Peripheral nerves are affected first in the lower extremities and manifest as numbness and tingling. The posterior columns are affected next, with patients complaining of difficulty in balance during walking along with loss of vibratory and positional sense. Dementia and psychoses may also become evident with progressive deficiency.

Assessment of vitamin B_{12} status is usually accomplished by measuring serum levels of the vitamin (normal 150 to 900 pg/ml) by radioimmunoassay and clinical assessment of red blood cell indices (especially mean corpuscular volume (MCV)), peripheral blood smear, and bone marrow aspirate. Findings of a macrocytic anemia, hypersegmented leukocytes, megaloblastic bone marrow, and a serum B_{12} level <100 pg/ml are indicative of B_{12} deficiency. Vitamin B_{12} absorption may be assessed with the Schilling test ($>30\%$ normal).

THERAPY

Vitamin B_{12} deficiency secondary to pernicious anemia is treated with 50 to 100 μg of vitamin B_{12} i.m. daily for 14 days or 1000 μg every 7 days for 3 weeks. This regimen is followed by 100 μg i.m. twice a week for 2 months, then monthly maintenance injections of 100 μg for life.

Patients with vitamin B_{12} deficiency who present with neurologic symptoms are treated with 100 μg of vitamin B_{12} i.m. daily for 14 days followed by 100 μg of B_{12} i.m. every 2 weeks for 6 months. This is followed by 100 μg i.m. vitamin B_{12} per month for life in patients with impaired absorption. Neurologic signs and symptoms may be reversible if they are of relatively short duration (i.e., <6 months). For megaloblastic anemia, both vitamin B_{12} and folate should be administered until results of folate/B_{12} levels have returned. Vitamin B_{12} may be administered orally (25 to 100 μg/day), intramuscularly, or subcutaneously. Intramuscular or subcutaneous routes are preferred during initial therapy. Doses are 30 μg/day for 5 to 10 days followed by a monthly maintenance dose of 100 to 200 μg. Normal vitamin B_{12} absorption must be documented before relying on oral administration. Higher doses may be required in critically ill patients or in those with hyperthyroidism or disease states of increased metabolic activity.

PREPARATIONS AND ADVERSE EFFECTS

Vitamin B_{12}, as cyanocobalamin crystalline, is available in oral (25 to 1000 μg tablets) and injectable forms (for i.m. injection 30, 100, and 1000 μg/ml). Vitamin B_{12}, as hydroxocobalamin crystalline, is available in an injectable form (for i.m. injection 1000 μg/ml). Vitamin B_{12} liver preparations are available in oral (0.5 unit vitamin B_{12} with intrinsic factor concentrate and 25 μg cobalamin) and parenteral forms (i.m. only—2, 10, and 20 μg B_{12}/ml). The i.v. route of administration should be avoided because of the occurrence of hypersensitivity reactions. However, if i.v. vitamin B_{12} is required, multivitamin preparations containing B_{12} are available. Adverse effects from vitamin B_{12} administration include hypersensitivity reactions (i.e., anaphylaxis, urticaria, pruritus), pulmonary edema, congestive heart failure, vascular thrombosis, diarrhea, hypokalemia, polycythemia vera, and local pain at the injection site.

FOLIC ACID (PTEROYLGLUTAMIC ACID, FOLATE; FOLACIN) (1–13)

CHEMISTRY

Folic acid (i.e., folate) is composed of a pteridine ring attached to *p*-aminobenzoic acid and conjugated to one molecule of glutamic acid. Pteroylglutamic acid is the pharmaceutical form of folic acid but not the active co-enzyme or the primary form found in food. Replacement of the glutamic acid residue renders the vitamin inactive. This water-soluble vitamin is unstable when heated in a neutral or alkaline medium.

METABOLISM

Three-quarters of the folate in foods is in the reduced polyglutamyl form, which is normally hydrolyzed to free folate in small intestinal epithelium. Free folate is actively absorbed from the upper small intestine, during which time it is reduced and methylated to dihydro- and tetrahydrofolates, the active forms of folate that are delivered to all tissues. Some vitamin remains unreduced and is metabolized by the liver. After conversion in the liver to 5-methyl-tetrahydrofolate, the vitamin enters the plasma, is stored in tissue, or is excreted in bile. Folate stores are maintained by the diet. Folate excreted in bile is reabsorbed via an enterohepatic circulation. Total body folate stores are approximately 70 mg, with 20 to 25 mg found in the liver. About one-fifth of ingested folate is excreted in the urine. An additional 60 to 90 μg/day is excreted in bile and lost into the stool (i.e., not reabsorbed).

Folic acid is essential for growth. It is required for carbon transfer, purine and pyrimidine biosynthesis, amino acid conversions, and maturation of blood cells.

SOURCES

Dietary folic acid exists largely as reduced polyglutamates. The average U.S. diet contains 30 to 1000 μg of folic acid per day. Foods rich in folate are green leafy vegetables, organ meats, yeast, and some fruits. Boiling, steaming, or frying of foods can destroy 80 to 95% of the folate content.

REQUIREMENTS

The RDA for folic acid in adults is 400 μg per day. The RDA for pregnant and lactating females is 600 to 800 μg per day. Daily requirements are based on the amount of oral pteroylglutamic acid needed to preserve body stores. In adults this requirement is 50 to 100 μg per day of folic acid, and in pregnant or lactating females the requirement is increased to 200 to 600 μg per day.

DEFICIENCY STATES

Causes of folate deficiency include chronic alcoholism, total parenteral nutrition, poor dietary intake, malabsorption syndromes (i.e., celiac sprue, sprue), drugs that cause inadequate absorption (i.e., phenytoin, barbiturates, cycloserine), increased utilization of folate (i.e., hemolytic anemia, leukemia, chronic exfoliative dermatitis, chronic myelofibrosis, hyperthyroidism), folic acid antagonists (i.e., methotrexate, triamterene, trimethoprim, pyrimethamine), and pregnancy.

Symptoms of deficiency develop 2 to 4 months after stores have been depleted. Deficiency of folate manifests as anorexia, nausea, diarrhea, stomatitis, alopecia, glossitis, megaloblastic anemia, thrombocytopenia, leukopenia, and fatigue.

Assessment of folate status and diagnosis of deficiency may be accomplished by measuring folate levels in plasma and in red blood cells. Plasma folate is a poor predictor of tissue folate levels but reflects dietary intake. Red blood cell folate levels correlate better with tissue levels. Normal plasma levels of folate are 6 to 20 ng/ml, and normal red blood cell levels of folate are 160 to 600 ng/ml. Folate deficiency is usually present when plasma folate levels are <3 to 4 ng/ml. A more definitive diagnosis is made when both plasma and red blood cell levels of folate are decreased (i.e., plasma folate <3 to 4 ng/ml and red blood cell folate <140 ng/ml).

THERAPY

Unreduced pteroylglutamic acid is the form of folic acid used therapeutically. Deficiency states are treated by giving 1 to 2 mg folic acid orally per day. Once symptoms have subsided, a maintenance dose of 0.4 mg/day in adults and 0.8 mg/day in pregnant and lactating females is advised. Parenteral administration is advisable for the treatment of patients with malabsorption.

For treating overdosage of folic acid antagonists (i.e., methotrexate), leucovorin calcium 10 mg/m² should be given orally or parenterally every 6 hours for 72 hours (i.e., leucovorin "rescue"). If the 24-hour postmethotrexate serum creatinine is 50% greater than premethotrexate creatinine levels, the dose of leucovorin should be increased to 100 mg/m² every 3 hours until serum methotrexate levels are below 5×10^{-8} M. For hematologic toxicity from folic acid antagonists, leucovorin calcium 5 to 15 mg orally should be given daily. Doses > 25 mg/day should be administered via the parenteral route.

Adequate hydration and urinary alkalization with sodium bicarbonates should be employed to increase urinary elimination of the antagonists.

PREPARATIONS AND ADVERSE EFFECTS

Folic acid is available in oral (0.1, 0.4, 0.8, and 1 mg tablets) and injectable forms (1, 5, and 10 mg/ml). Leucovorin calcium (folinic acid) is available in oral (5, 10, 15, and 25 mg) and injectable forms (1, 3, and 10 mg/ml). Adverse effects for both folic acid and leucovorin calcium preparations are infrequent, but hypersensitivity reactions have been reported.

VITAMIN D (1–13)

CHEMISTRY

Vitamin D is a fat-soluble vitamin whose name is used as a generic term for a number of distinct but closely related sterols possessing antirachitic properties. The two sterol forms important in nutrition and therapeutics are vitamin D_2 (ergocalciferol) and D_3 (cholecalciferol).

Vitamin D_3 is the natural form of vitamin D, which is synthesized in skin under the influence of ultraviolet irradiation in sunlight. Vitamin D_2, a synthetic vitamin D compound, is manufactured by exposing the provitamin ergosterol, found in fungi and yeasts, to ultraviolet irradiation. This active ingredient is used in a number of commercial vitamin preparations. Ergocalciferol (D_2) differs from cholecalciferol (D_3) by the presence of a methyl group at C-24 and a double bond between C-22 and C-23. D_2 and D_3 possess similar physiologic actions in humans.

METABOLISM/FUNCTION

Dietary vitamin D is absorbed in the small intestine. Normal absorption requires intact fat digestion and presence of bile salts. Once absorbed, it is carried by chylomicrons to the liver. Vitamin D (of skin or dietary origin) is converted to 25-hydroxy-vitamin D (calcifediol), the major circulating form of the vitamin, in the liver. In the kidney, calcifediol is 1-hydroxylated by a mitochondrial 1-hydroxylase enzyme to 1,25-dihydroxy-vitamin D (calcitriol). Calcitriol is the primary active form of vitamin D.

Calcitriol functions as a hormone and, along with parathyroid hormone and calcitonin, regulates calcium and phosphate metabolism. In the upper small intestine and kidney it promotes calcium absorption. In bone, calcitriol (along with parathyroid hormone) stimulates reabsorption of calcium and phosphorus. These processes are important for maintenance of normal calcium and phosphorus concentrations in plasma. Normal ion concentrations are essential for normal cardiovascular function, neuromuscular activity, mineralization of bone, and other calcium-dependent processes. Vitamin D deficiency results in hypocalcemia, osteomalacia, or rickets. Vitamin D excess causes hypercalcemia, bone loss, renal stones, and tissue calcinosis. Recent evidence also suggests a role for vitamin D metabolites in cell differentiation and immune function.

The primary route of excretion of vitamin D is the bile, with small amounts found in the urine.

SOURCES

Endogenous production of vitamin D is the most important source of the vitamin. More than 90% of circulating 25-hydroxycholecalciferol is derived from skin synthesis in normal healthy individuals. The rate of synthesis in the skin is determined by the degree of exposure to ultraviolet light and by the amount of skin pigment.

The major dietary sources supplying vitamin D_3 (cholecalciferol) are liver, oils, egg yolk, and butter. Milk and other foods fortified with vitamin D_2 (ergocalciferol) are another major dietary source.

REQUIREMENTS

The recommended daily allowance of vitamin D in adults is 200 to 400 IU (510 μg). Intakes above the recommended levels are potentially dangerous and should be avoided. Many chronically ill patients lack sunlight exposure and may require higher dietary amounts of the vitamin (i.e., especially patients with fat malabsorption, liver disease, and renal disease).

DEFICIENCY STATES

Primary nutritional deficiency of vitamin D in the U.S. is rare. However, ill patients with inadequate exposure to sunlight and inadequate dietary intake may develop vitamin D deficiency. An absolute or relative deficiency may occur secondary to malabsorption syndromes, liver and/or cholestatic diseases, prolonged anticonvulsant usage (phenytoin, phenobarbital), rare metabolic disorders (i.e., vitamin D-dependent rickets), hypoparathyroidism, renal diseases (i.e., chronic renal disease, Fanconi syndrome, renal tubular acidosis), and chronic corticosteroid use. Vitamin D status may be assessed by measuring calcifediol (nl 25 to 50 ng/ml) and calcitriol (nl 20 to 45 pg/ml) serum levels. Calcifediol levels primarily reflect dietary intake and skin synthesis of vitamin D. Calcitriol levels reflect renal 1-hydroxylase activity. The vitamin D status can also be assessed indirectly by measuring serum calcium (ionized form) and phosphorus, 24-hour urine calcium, alkaline phosphatase levels, and radiographic bone density.

Vitamin D deficiency may manifest clinically as poor bone mineralization in children (rickets) or adults (osteomalacia). In severe deficiency states, hypocalcemia may occur. Muscle cramps, tetany, and seizures may result from hypocalcemia, while muscle weakness may result from decreased muscle phosphate levels (see Chapter 46, "Divalent Ions: Calcium, Magnesium, and Phosphorus").

THERAPY

Adequate calcium and phosphorus intake must accompany vitamin D replacement therapy. Vitamin D is available in various forms (Table 47.2) that differ in their metabolism, dose, half-lives, and cost. Ergocalciferol is the vitamin D form most commonly used to treat dietary deficiency, malabsorption syndromes, and hypoparathyroidism. Dietary vitamin D deficiency states are treated with 25 to 125 μg/day orally; malabsorption syndromes with 2.5 to 7.5 mg/day orally or 250 μg/day i.m.; hypoparathyroidism with 0.625 to 2.5 mg/day orally. Calcifediol may be useful in patients whose vitamin D deficiency results from severe liver disease or in a patient with chronic renal failure. Calcifediol is usually started at a dose of 50 μg/day or 100 μg on alternate days orally. The dose is increased every 4 weeks until the desired effect is achieved.

Calcitriol is used primarily in patients with chronic renal failure or other renal disease states. It is also useful in the treatment of hypoparathyroidism and is the preferred treatment for vitamin D-dependent rickets. Calcitriol is initiated at a dose of 0.25 μg/day orally. The dose is increased by 0.25 μg/day every 2 to 4 weeks until the desired effect is achieved. An injectable form of calcitriol is also available.

PREPARATIONS AND ADVERSE EFFECTS

Ergocalciferol (calciferol, vitamin D capsules, Deltalin Gelseals, Drisdol) is available in capsule (0.625 mg, or 25000 IU; 1.25 mg, or 50,000 IU), liquid (8000 IU/ml), and injectable forms (12.5 mg, or 500,000 IU, per ml). Calcifediol (25 hydroxyvitamin D, Calderol) is available as capsules (20 and 50 μg). Calcitriol (1,25-dihydroxyvitamin D, Rocaltrol, Calcijex) is available in capsule (0.25 and 0.5 μg) and injectable forms (1 and 2 μg/ml). The major toxicities from vitamin D administration are hypercalcemia, hypercalciuria, renal stones, bone loss, and tissue calcium deposition. Clinical features of hypercalcemia include headache, ataxia, irritability, somnolence, convulsions, hypertension, dysrhythmias, bradycardia, dry mouth, conjunctivitis, pruritus, anorexia, nausea, vomiting, constipation, polyuria, renal insufficiency, and weakness.

VITAMIN K (1–13)

CHEMISTRY

Vitamin K is a fat-soluble naphthaquinone. It occurs naturally in two forms, differing from one another only in their side chains. The most active form, vitamin K_1, (phytonadione), is the only form found in plants and is the only natural vitamin K available for therapeutic use. Vitamin K_2 (menaquinone) is synthesized by the normal intestinal flora and also found in some animal tissues. Vitamin K_3 (menadione) is the water-soluble parent compound of the vitamin K series. It is not found naturally but rather represents an artificial provitamin that can be alkylated in vivo to menaquinone.

METABOLISM

The naturally occurring vitamin K derivatives are absorbed only in the presence of bile salts, like other lipids, and are distributed in the bloodstream via the lymphatics (i.e., in chylomicrons). Menadione is absorbed in the absence of bile

Table 47.2. Vitamin D Preparations

	Ergocalciferol (Vit D₂)	*Calcifediol (250HD)*	*Dihydrotachysterol (1-OHD)*	*Calcitriol (1,25(OH)₂D)*
Concentration in serum	10 ng/ml	30 ng/ml		0.03 ng/ml
Physiological dose (μg/day)	10	5	20	0.5
Pharmacological dose (μg/day)	1200	50	200–800	0.25–1
Onset of maximal effect (days)	30	15	15	3
Dosage forms	Tablets 625 μg 1250 μg Solution 8000 U/ml Oil for injection 500,000 U/ml	Capsules 20 μg 50 μg	Tablets 125 μg 200 μg 400 μg Solution 200 μg/ml	Capsules 0.25 μg 0.50 μg
Commercial products	Calciferol	Calderol	Hytakerol	Rocaltrol
Serum half-life (days)	30	15		0.2
Time for reversal of effect (days)	17–60	7–30	3–14	2–10
Advantages	Low cost, prolonged action, parent compound	Liver disease	Renal disease, hypoparathyroidism	Renal disease, liver disease, hypoparathyroidism, rapid onset, rapid offset
Disadvantages	Instability, long toxicity	Expense	Expense	Expense

salts and enters directly into the bloodstream. The absorption of phytonadione occurs in an energy-dependent, saturable process in the proximal small bowel, whereas menaquinone and menadione are absorbed via a diffusional process in the distal small bowel and colon. Once absorbed, vitamin K is stored in the liver and other tissues; however, its storage is limited. Vitamin K is metabolized in the liver and excreted in the urine and bile after conjugation with glucuronate and sulfate.

Vitamin K is required for normal blood clotting. It acts as a cofactor for a liver carboxylase that activates factors II (prothrombin), VII (proconvertin), IX (plasma thromboplastin component), and X (Stuart factor). The carboxylase converts glutamate residues to α-carboxyglutamate. Carboxyglutamate is also found in other proteins such as bone osteocalcin, protein S, and protein C.

SOURCES

The best dietary sources of vitamin K are green leafy vegetables (i.e., broccoli, lettuce, cabbage, and spinach). Beef liver is a good source, but most other animal foods, cereals, and fruits are poor sources unless they have undergone extensive bacterial putrefaction. The average diet in the U.S. contains approximately 300 to 500 μg/day of vitamin K. It should be noted that approximately half of the vitamin K in the body is derived from gut bacteria, while the other half comes from the diet.

REQUIREMENTS

The RDA for vitamin K in normal adult males is 70 to 80 μg/day and in normal adult females 60 to 65 μg/day, assuming that half of the vitamin made by bacteria is absorbed and the rest supplied by the diet. The RDA would double (i.e., 140 μg/day) in cases in which bacterial vitamin is not synthesized or absorbed (i.e., patients on broad-spectrum antibiotics).

DEFICIENCY STATES

Primary deficiency states occur in newborn babies as a result of poor placental transport of lipids, sterile intestines, and breast feeding (a poor source of vitamin K). Deficiency states also result from fat malabsorption (i.e., biliary obstruction, malabsorption syndromes), from the use of broad-spectrum antibiotics with little enteral nutrition, as a result of severe liver disease, from the use of oral anticoagulants such as warfarin, and from long-term total parenteral nutritional support.

Clinically, vitamin K deficiency results in delayed blood clotting and is manifested by easy bruising and/or an increased tendency to bleeding. A diagnosis of vitamin K deficiency is suggested by finding a prolonged prothrombin time. A specific diagnosis is made by radioimmunoassay measurement of one or more of the four vitamin K-dependent clotting factors.

THERAPY

Phytonadione (vitamin K_1) is the preparation of choice for treating vitamin K deficiency, remembering that vitamin K deficiency will respond rapidly to administration of vitamin K only if liver function is normal. For prophylaxis against hemorrhagic disease of the newborn, a single i.m. dose of phytonadione 0.5 to 1 mg should be administered immediately after birth. A dose of 1 to 2 mg/day i.m. or s.q. is administered to treat hemorrhagic disease of the newborn.

Anticoagulant-induced hypoprothrombinemic states should be treated with phytonadione 2.5 to 20 mg p.o., s.q. or i.m. (titrated to effect). Menadiol is ineffective in reversing anticoagulant-induced hypoprothrombinemic states. In more severe hemorrhagic states secondary to anticoagulant overdose, 10 to 50 mg of phytonadione dissolved in 5% dextrose or 0.9% sodium chloride may be given i.v. at a rate not to exceed 1 mg/min. Additional doses may be given at 6- to 8-hour intervals and therapy may be monitored by following prothrombin times. In such situations, the transfusion of plasma may also be indicated. Vitamin K deficiency secondary to other causes may be treated adequately with menadiol or phytonadione preparations. Oral, s.q., or i.m. doses of 5 to 10 mg/day or twice daily are usually sufficient. Whenever possible, phytonadione should be given s.q. or i.m. If oral phytonadione is used in patients with biliary insufficiency, a bile salt preparation must be administered concomitantly. Lastly, for patients on long-term total parenteral nutrition, phytonadione 5 to 10 mg/wk s.q. or i.m. is sufficient to prevent deficiency.

PREPARATIONS AND ADVERSE EFFECTS

Phytonadione (K_1) (AquaMEPHYTON, Konakion, Mephyton) is a lipid-soluble synthetic preparation. It is available in 5-mg tablets (Mephyton) and 2 and 10 mg/ml injection (AquaMEPHYTON for i.v. use, Konakion for i.m. use). Menadiol sodium diphosphate (K_4) is a water-soluble derivative. It is available as an oral preparation (Synkayvite—5 mg tablets), and injectable (Synkayvite solution—5, 10, and 37.5 mg/ml). Menadiol may be administered i.v. (slow push) in doses of 5 to 20 mg. Adverse effects following oral administration are rare. Hypersensitivity reactions may occur following i.v. administration. Hemolysis has been reported in individuals with G6PD deficiency. Anemia, hyperbilirubinemia, and kernicterus may occur with large doses in the newborn.

VITAMIN A (1–13)

CHEMISTRY

Vitamin A is a fat-soluble vitamin, found in animal tissues as retinol. It exists in several isomeric forms. Naturally occurring vitamin A is found only in animal tissues and not in vegetables. However, many vegetables contain carotenoid pigments that have a similar chemical structure to that of vitamin A and hence act as provitamins for conversion to vitamin A in the liver. The most important of these carotenoids with provitamin A activity is β-carotene. In nature, the esterified form of vitamin A is often found as the acetate or the palmitate ester.

METABOLISM

Foods containing retinol or carotenoids are digested by gastric and intestinal enzymes, and both forms are absorbed by the intestinal mucosa. Eighty to ninety percent of dietary vitamin A is actively absorbed as retinol esters, while 40 to 60% of β-carotene is absorbed. Following absorption, β-carotene is cleaved to two molecules of retinal (retinaldehyde), which is then reduced to retinol. Most of the retinol is esterified with saturated fatty acids and incorporated into lymph chylomicrons, which enter the bloodstream. Chylomicrons are metabolized and taken up by the liver together with their content of retinol. Retinol is stored as retinol esters in the parenchymal cells of the liver (which contains about 90% of total body reserves). These esters subsequently are hydrolyzed and release free alcohol (i.e., retinol). Retinol is transported to peripheral tissues by a specific transport protein, retinol-binding protein. Vitamin A is important for epithelia integrity and is a component of photoreceptors in the retina.

SOURCES

Animal tissues and products (i.e., liver, fish, dairy products, margarine) are responsible for the daily intake of preformed vitamin A. Vegetable sources supply carotenoid provitamins. Carotenoid compounds, mainly β-carotenes, form part of the yellow and orange pigments of most fruits and vegetables (i.e., carrots, leafy green vegetables, cantaloupes, and papaya).

REQUIREMENTS

Daily intake of vitamin A is expressed as μg retinol equivalents (RE), where one RE is defined as 1 μg of retinol or 6 μg of β-carotene (making the overall utilization of β-carotene one-sixth that of retinol, attributed to the relative inefficiency by which it is absorbed and converted to vitamin A). The RDA for vitamin A is 1000 μg (1.0 mg) of retinol equivalents (RE) for adult males and 800 μg (0.8 mg) for adult females (pregnancy 1000 μg, lactation 1200 μg). Vitamin A allowances may also be expressed as the international unit (IU). One RE is equivalent to 3.33 IU retinol and 10 IU μ-carotene. Thus, the RDA expressed in IUs for vitamin A is 5000 for adult males and 4000 for adult females.

DEFICIENCY STATES

Vitamin A deficiency, a common problem worldwide (especially in developing countries), may account for the majority of cases of blindness in the young. In the U.S., vitamin A deficiency usually results from fat malabsorption syndromes (i.e., sprue or intestinal bypass surgery), alcoholism, long-term parenteral nutrition, laxative abuse (mineral oil based), and prolonged use of drugs such as cholestyramine, colestipol, neomycin, or colchicine. The clinical manifestations of these deficiency states include night blindness, dryness of the conjunctivae (xerosis) and of the cornea (xerophthalmia), development of small white patches on the sclera (Bitots' spots), ulceration and necrosis of the cornea (keratomalacia), prolapse of the iris, and panophthalmitis leading to blindness. In such patients, keratinization of epithelial tissues of the eyes, lungs, gastrointestinal, and genitourinary tracts may occur and increase the propensity to infection. Except for keratomalacia, most of the manifestations of vitamin A deficiency are reversible with adequate replacement therapy.

THERAPY

When vitamin A is used for therapy, it is provided entirely in the form of retinol, and its biologic potency is given in IUs. Night blindness and other signs of early deficiency can be treated effectively with 30,000 IU of vitamin A daily for 1 week. Clinical features of advanced disease (i.e., corneal damage) are best treated by the administration of 20,000 IU/kg body weight for at least 5 days followed by a maintenance dose of 10,000 to 20,000 IU (3000 to 6000 µg)/day p.o. in three divided doses. Vitamin A is available in a liquid form that contains an emulsifier that solubilizes the vitamin. However, these forms require bile acids for absorption. When bile acids are deficient, the water-soluble forms may be of greater benefit (i.e., better absorbed).

PREPARATIONS AND ADVERSE EFFECTS

Vitamin A capsules (oil preparation) are available in 10,000, 25,000, and 50,000 IU doses. Aquasol A (water-miscible form; may be used parenterally) is supplied in 25,000 IU (7.5 mg retinol/ml) and 50,000 IU (15 mg retinol/ml) doses; Del-Vi-A is supplied in 50,000 IU doses. Adverse effects include anaphylaxis (after i.v. administration), increased intracranial pressure, cutaneous desquamation, liver damage, hypercalcemia, bone pain, arthralgias, nausea, vomiting, anorexia, malaise, headache, irritability, alopecia, leukopenia, polyuria, and polydipsia.

VITAMIN E (1–13)

CHEMISTRY

Vitamin E is an alcohol derived from phytol and trimethyl hydroquinone, soluble in fat solvents, readily oxidized, and most stable in the acetate form. Eight tocopherols and tocotrienols with vitamin E activity have been identified, differing from each other in the number and position of methyl groups around the phenol ring of the molecule. α-Tocopherol is the most widely distributed and most active of the tocopherols. Although its exact function and mechanisms of action are somewhat unclear, the most widely accepted function of vitamin E is as an antioxidant that protects membranes and other cellular structures from attack by free radicals.

METABOLISM

The absorption of vitamin E, like that of all fat-soluble vitamins, is linked to fat absorption and requires biliary (bile salt micelles) and pancreatic (esterase) secretions. Normally, 20 to 50% of dietary tocopherols are absorbed. This amount is decreased by excess fat in the intestinal lumen. Most ingested vitamin E is d-α-tocopherol acetate. It is hydrolyzed in the intestine, enters the blood via the lymph, and is bound to lipoproteins. There is no specific carrier protein for vitamin E. Plasma levels correlate with plasma lipid levels. Vitamin E is stored in all tissues. However, adipose tissue, liver, and muscle are the most important sites of storage. The major excretory route is through the feces (about 75% is excreted in bile), with the remainder excreted as glucuronides in the urine. Vitamin E functions as an antioxidant in the body.

SOURCES

The richest sources of vitamin E are vegetable oils (i.e., wheat germ, sunflower seed, cotton seed, safflower, palm, and other oils). Shortening and margarine are major sources in the diet. Eggs, butter, whole-grain cereals, and broccoli are moderately good sources, while meats, fruits, and vegetables provide small amounts of vitamin E. Breast milk contains four times as much vitamin E as cow's milk. Total daily ingestion varies from 2.6 to 15.4 mg of tocopherol.

REQUIREMENTS

Vitamin E requirements must take into account the intake of natural oxidants such as polyunsaturated fatty acids (which increase the requirement) and of dietary antioxidants (which decrease the requirement). In general, approximately 1 mg of vitamin E is needed for each 600 mg of polyunsaturated fatty acid. It should be remembered, however, that the food sources highest in vitamin E content are also high in polyunsaturated fatty acids.

The RDA for vitamin E is expressed in terms of milligrams of α-tocopherol equivalents and is 10 mg/day (15 IU) for adult males and 8 mg/day (12 IU) for adult females. Pregnant females require between 10 and 12 mg/day of vitamin E.

DEFICIENCY STATES

In view of the wide distribution of vitamin E in foods, primary dietary deficiency of the vitamin is unlikely. However, in the setting of severe malabsorption (i.e., celiac sprue, Crohn's disease, etc.), clinical deficiency may appear. Severe deficiency occurs in patients with abetalipoproteinemia in whom both intestinal absorption and serum transport of the vitamin are defective. Vitamin E deficiency may also accompany chronic cholestatic liver disease, biliary atresia, cystic fibrosis, and use of infant formulas that contain large amounts of polyunsaturated fats and iron. Diagnosis of vitamin E deficiency is made by measuring plasma levels of the vitamin (normal >0.5 to 0.7 mg/dl). The concentration of vitamin E correlates with plasma lipid levels. Approximately 1 µg α-tocopherol is present per milligram of total lipid.

Clinical features of vitamin E deficiency include areflexia, reduced proprioception and vibratory sense, gait disturbance, and ophthalmoplegia. In premature infants, deficiency of the vitamin has been associated with retrolental fibroplasia, hemolytic anemia, intraventricular hemorrhage, edema, and thrombocytosis.

THERAPY

Vitamin E supplementation is indicated in patients with serum vitamin E levels <0.5 mg/dl or when a clinical deficiency state has been diagnosed. In those individuals in whom severe malabsorption is the cause of the deficiency, vitamin E 30 to 100 mg/day should be given i.m. as *dl*-α-tocopherol acetate (1 mg = 1 IU). Deficiency presenting as neuropathy may be corrected with oral administration of high doses of vitamin E (50 to 200 IU/kg/day). If oral therapy fails, i.m. administration of *dl*-α-tocopherol acetate (1 to 2 mg/kg/day) should be tried. Retrolental fibroplasia in premature infants may be prevented with the prophylactic use of oral vitamin E (100 mg/kg/day).

PREPARATIONS AND ADVERSE EFFECTS

Vitamin E may be obtained in the *d* or the *dl* isomers of α-tocopherol, α-tocopherol acetate, or α-tocopherol succinate. Oral preparations of the fat-soluble form of tablets or capsules range from 50 to 1000 IU. The water-miscible preparation, Aquasol E, comes in 100- and 400-IU capsules. Parenteral forms of vitamin E are also available (200 IU/ml). Adverse effects include fatigue, nausea, vomiting, weakness, headache, blurred vision, and diarrhea.

RIBOFLAVIN (VITAMIN B₂) (1–13)

CHEMISTRY

Riboflavin consists of a heterocyclic isoalloxazine ring attached to a sugar alcohol side chain, ribitol. It is water soluble and heat stable but unstable in alkali solution.

METABOLISM

Riboflavin is rapidly absorbed from the upper gastrointestinal tract by a site-specific and saturable transport process. During absorption it is phosphorylated in the intestinal mucosa to the co-enzyme flavin mononucleotide (FMN). Phosphorylation also takes place in the liver and other tissues. The vitamin is stored in small concentrations in all tissues, with varying amounts being bound to serum proteins. Riboflavin is excreted in the urine. As ingestion increases, a larger proportion is excreted unchanged. Small quantities of the vitamin are found in sweat. Riboflavin is important for normal energy metabolism. It is a component of two tissue co-enzymes, FMN and flavin adenine dinucleotide (FAD). FMN and FAD also serve as the prosthetic groups for several enzyme systems concerned with hydrogen transport (oxidation) and metabolism of amino acids.

SOURCES

Riboflavin is widely distributed in leafy vegetables, milk, cheese, meat, fish, egg whites, kidney, liver, and whole grain and enriched cereals. In the U.S., milk and dairy products account for nearly half of the daily intake. Its biologic activity can be lost by exposing it to light during cooking. Small quantities of riboflavin are also synthesized by colonic bacteria.

REQUIREMENTS

The recommended daily allowance for riboflavin is 1.4 to 1.7 mg/day in adult males and 1.2 mg/day in adult females. The RDA is increased to 1.6 to 1.8 mg/day during pregnancy and lactation. Riboflavin requirements vary with caloric intake (0.6 mg/1000 kcals) and increase during strenuous exercise (i.e., energy expenditure). Needs may be increased during hypermetabolic illness.

DEFICIENCY STATES

Riboflavin deficiency usually results from chronic malnutrition or use of parenteral nutrition solutions containing inadequate vitamin. Other factors such as drugs (i.e., phenothiazines, tricyclic antidepressants) and disease states such as hypothyroidism, chronic alcoholism, trauma, burns, dialysis, and malignancy may also lead to deficiency.

Early symptoms of riboflavin deficiency manifest as soreness of the mouth, burning and itching of the eyes, photophobia, and personality alteration. With progression of the deficiency, cheilosis, angular stomatitis, seborrheic dermatitis, glossitis, corneal vascularization, anemia, and retarded intellectual development can occur. In addition to these disorders, metabolism of a number of drugs can be altered by deficiency of this vitamin.

Laboratory evaluation of riboflavin status may be assessed by measuring urinary excretion of riboflavin or erythrocyte activity of glutathione reductase (a riboflavin-dependent enzyme). Excretion of <50 μg of riboflavin per day is indicative of deficiency. Glutathione reductase activity is expressed as an activity coefficient (i.e., the ratio of enzyme activity after incubation with FAD in vitro to that before incubation). A value >1.3 is considered to indicate deficiency.

THERAPY

For treatment of deficiency states, 5 to 25 mg/day of oral riboflavin should be given until clinical findings resolve. A prophylactic dose of 3 mg/day is useful when malabsorption is present. Since riboflavin deficiency usually co-exists with other vitamin B deficiencies, many clinicians recommend replacement therapy in the form of B complex vitamins.

PREPARATIONS AND ADVERSE EFFECTS

Riboflavin is available in oral tablet (5, 10, 25, 50, and 100 mg) and injectable forms (35 mg/ml). The taking of riboflavin can result in bright yellow urine. Clinical toxicity has not been reported.

THIAMINE (VITAMIN B₁) (1–13)

CHEMISTRY

Thiamine is a water-soluble organic molecule consisting of a pyrimidine ring joined to a sulfur-containing thiazole ring by a methylene bridge.

METABOLISM

Thiamine is absorbed rapidly from the upper small intestine by a Na^+-dependent active transport system (low concentrations) and by passive diffusion (high concentrations). Oral absorption ranges from 8 to 15 mg/day. During absorption, the vitamin is phosphorylated to thiamine pyrophosphate (TPP) within the mucosal cells of the intestine. This phosphorylated form is found in all cells and comprises the majority (80%) of stored vitamin. Other forms, stored in lesser amounts, are thiamine triphosphate, thiamine monophosphate, and free vitamin. The major site of thiamine storage is skeletal muscle, with heart, liver, kidneys, and brain serving as secondary storage sites. Tissue stores are saturated by approximately 1 mg of thiamine per day. As the intake exceeds this minimal requirement, excess appears in the urine (either as metabolite or unchanged vitamin). Thiamine is an important precursor for TPP, the co-enzyme responsible for the decarboxylation of α-keto acids and carbohydrate metabolism (i.e., pyruvate to acetyl CoA). Additionally, thiamine modulates neuromuscular transmission.

SOURCES

Humans are almost entirely dependent on dietary sources for thiamine. The best dietary sources are beef, pork, whole grains, enriched cereal grains, peas, potatoes, beans, and nuts. The refining of sugar and many cereal products may lead to the removal of this vitamin. Some foods such as raw fish, coffee, and tea contain thiaminases, which can destroy the dietary supply of thiamine. Thiamine is destroyed rapidly at alkaline pH and is heat sensitive. Because of its water-soluble properties, much of the vitamin is extracted from dry foods when cooked in liquids.

REQUIREMENTS

The RDA for thiamine in adult males is 1.4 mg/day and in adult females 1.1 mg/day. Given that thiamine is essential for energy metabolism, especially that of carbohydrates, the RDA is related to caloric intake (0.5 mg/1000 kcal). This requirement increases when carbohydrates form the major dietary component; in the elderly, who utilize thiamine less efficiently; in states of increased metabolism (i.e., hyperthyroidism, fever, increased activity); and during pregnancy and lactation. Needs frequently increase by 50% in these situations.

DEFICIENCY STATES

Deficiency of the vitamin results from decreased intake, increased tissue utilization, or both. In the U.S., chronic alcoholism is the most common cause of thiamine deficiency. Other important causes include malabsorption syndromes, diuretic therapy, dialysis, increased metabolic rate, diarrhea, chronic malnutrition, folate deficiency, diets in which refined grains make up the major caloric source (mainly in developed countries), the placement of patients on i.v. dextrose solutions, and chronic ingestion of food high in thiaminases.

Early manifestations of thiamine deficiency include weight loss, muscle cramps, anorexia, irritability, and paresthesias. Advanced deficiency affects the cardiovascular system (wet beriberi) and/or the nervous system (dry beriberi). Wet beriberi is characterized by a reduced systemic vascular resistance and augmented venous return, resulting in high-output cardiac failure characterized by dyspnea, tachycardia, biventricular failure, QT prolongation, pulmonary and peripheral edema, wide pulse pressure, sweating, and warm extremities. A rare low-output state (Shoshin disease) may occur and is characterized by hypotension, tachycardia, absence of edema, and lactic acidosis.

Nervous system involvement includes both the peripheral and central nervous systems. Typically, peripheral nerve involvement is manifested by symmetrical motor and sensory neuropathy with pain, paresthesias, and loss of reflexes. Lower extremity distal segments are commonly involved. However, arm involvement may occur after leg signs are well-established. Involvement of the central nervous system results in Wernicke-Korsakoff's syndrome. Wernicke's encephalopathy consists of horizontal nystagmus, unilateral or bilateral ophthalmoplegia, fever, ataxia, and confusion. Korsakoff's syndrome is characterized by retrograde amnesia, confabulation, and an impaired ability to learn. Thiamine deficiency is best diagnosed by assessing erythrocyte transketolase activity (normal <15%; mild deficiency 15 to 25%; severe deficiency > 25%). Other indicators of deficiency include increased blood pyruvate levels and diminished urinary thiamine excretion (< 50 μg/day). In most instances, however, the clinical response to empirical thiamine therapy is used to support a diagnosis.

THERAPY

Thiamine deficiency may be treated with thiamine 10 to 20 mg i.m. q. 8 hours for 1 to 2 weeks followed by an oral daily maintenance dose (usually in the form of a multivitamin containing 5 to 10 mg thiamine). Severe deficiency, in the form of beriberi heart disease ("wet beriberi"), is a medical emergency. Thiamine 10 to 30 mg i.v. q. 8 hours for 1 to 2 weeks followed by 25 mg orally per day may lead to dramatic improvement. Wernicke's encephalopathy may require up to 1 g thiamine i.v. for acute control, followed by 25 to 100 mg every 12 hours orally for maintenance. Thiamine deficiency may be prevented by administration of 1 to 2 mg thiamine per day.

PREPARATIONS AND ADVERSE EFFECTS

Thiamine hydrochloride is available in tablets (5, 10, 25, 50, 100, 250, and 500 mg), elixir (2.25 mg/5 ml), and injectable forms (100 and 200 mg/ml). Adverse effects include restlessness, allergic reactions (especially following rapid i.v. administration), nausea, vomiting, hemorrhage, and diarrhea.

PYRIDOXINE (VITAMIN B₆) (1–13)

CHEMISTRY

The term *vitamin B₆* or *pyridoxine* is used to refer to three closely interrelated compounds: pyridoxine (alcohol), pyridoxal (aldehyde), and pyridoxamine (amine) and their corresponding phosphates. Pyridoxal-5′-phosphate is the major coenzyme and active form of the vitamin. All are soluble in water and alcohol. They are resistant to normal heat but degradable by alkali and ultraviolet light.

METABOLISM

Vitamin B₆ is absorbed rapidly in the small intestine by passive transport following hydrolysis of their phosphorylated derivatives. It is distributed throughout the tissues as the coenzyme pyridoxal phosphate. In addition, this form makes up about 60% of the circulating vitamin. The various forms of pyridoxine are readily interconverted in the liver and by erythrocytes. Excretion of pyridoxine occurs in the urine mainly as the metabolite 4-pyridoxic acid. Vitamin B₆, as the coenzyme pyridoxal phosphate, functions in many chemical reactions related to amino acid and protein metabolism. Its most important role is as a co-enzyme for transamination in the synthesis of amino acids. Pyridoxal phosphate is also involved in the metabolism of several vitamins and in the biosynthesis of heme and sphingosine.

SOURCES

Low concentrations of vitamin B₆ are widespread in the food supply (both plants and animals). Liver, meat, wholegrain cereals, legumes, fruits, and vegetables are good sources. Substantial losses of the vitamin occur during prolonged cooking.

REQUIREMENTS

Vitamin B₆ requirements are estimated by using a ratio of 0.02 mg of the vitamin per gram of protein ingested. The RDA is 2.0 mg/day for adult males and 1.6 mg/day for adult females, providing a reasonable margin of safety and allowing for daily intakes of more than 100 g of protein per day. During pregnancy and lactation, a 0.5 mg/day increase is recommended. The use of estrogens and diets high in protein may also necessitate an increased allowance of vitamin B₆.

DEFICIENCY STATES

Deficiency of pyridoxine rarely results from dietary restrictions, since it is found in many foods. The major causes of vitamin B₆ deficiency are related to malabsorption syndromes,

alcoholism, pregnancy, and use of medications such as isoniazid, l-Dopa, estrogens, cycloserine, and penicillamine.

Deficiency may manifest as seborrhea-like lesions about the eyes, nose, and mouth, stomatitis, glossitis, nausea, vomiting, seizures, peripheral neuritis, and hypochromic anemia. Laboratory diagnosis of pyridoxine deficiency may be accomplished by measuring urinary levels of metabolites or by direct assay of pyridoxal phosphate in the blood (normal >50 ng/ml). Urinary excretion of <1.0 mg/day of 4-pyridoxic acid suggests deficiency. One may also measure the activity of erythrocyte transaminases. An activity coefficient >1.5 for aspartate aminotransferase and >1.25 for alanine aminotransferase indicates pyridoxine deficiency.

THERAPY

Pyridoxine deficiency is treated with 25 to 100 mg of pyridoxine daily for 3 weeks followed by a maintenance dose of 2.0 to 2.5 mg daily in a multivitamin preparation. Prophylaxis in patients receiving isoniazid consists of 25 to 50 mg pyridoxine daily. Pyridoxine deficiency in patients receiving isoniazid (i.e., peripheral neuritis) is best treated with 50 to 200 mg pyridoxine daily. Isoniazid poisoning (i.e., >10 g) is treated with an equal quantity of pyridoxine (i.e., 4 g i.v. followed by 1 g i.m. every 30 minutes × 6).

PREPARATIONS AND ADVERSE EFFECTS

Pyridoxine hydrochloride is available in oral (10, 25, 50, 100, 200, 250, and 500 mg) and injectable forms (100 mg/ml). Adverse effects include paresthesias, somnolence, headache, decreased sensation (to touch, temperature, and vibration), unstable gait, seizures, nausea, burning or stinging at injection sites, allergic reactions, and decreased serum folate levels.

NICOTINIC ACID (NIACIN) (1–13)

CHEMISTRY

Niacin is the generic name for nicotinic acid and nicotinamide, either of which may act as a source of the vitamin in the diet. Nicotinic acid is a monocarboxylic acid derivative of pyridine, and nicotinamide is the corresponding amide. Both are water soluble and heat stable but labile in air, alkali, or light.

METABOLISM

Both forms of niacin are nearly completely absorbed from the intestinal tract by facilitated and passive diffusion. After absorption, co-enzymes are formed and distributed in all tissues. Little vitamin is stored. A small quantity of niacin is also formed from dietary tryptophan. The major metabolites are *N*-methylnicotinamide and 2-pyridine. Metabolites and unchanged vitamin are excreted in the urine. Nicotinic acid functions as a precursor for the co-enzymes nicotinamide adenine dinucleotide (NAD) and nicotinamide adenine dinucleotide phosphate (NADP). These co-enzymes are essential for a variety of oxidation-reduction reactions (i.e., carbohydrate, protein, fat metabolism). In addition, nicotinic acid has therapeutic functions as a result of its ability to lower serum cholesterol and triglyceride levels.

SOURCES

Niacin is present in whole-grain cereals, meats, liver, fish, legumes, and many vegetables. Tryptophan from protein sources is also an important precursor for endogenous niacin production.

REQUIREMENTS

The RDA for niacin in adult males is 15 to 19 mg and in adult females 13 to 15 mg daily. Allowances are dependent upon the protein intake (i.e., 60 mg of dietary tryptophan are required to form 1 mg of niacin). Niacin requirements depend upon caloric intake (6.6 mg of niacin/1000 kcal). An additional 5 mg niacin per day may be required in pregnant and lactating females.

DEFICIENCY STATES

Niacin deficiency occurs when the diet is poor in both niacin and tryptophan. Historically, niacin deficiency occurred when corn, a poor source of both niacin and tryptophan, was the major source of calories. Today, niacin deficiency results more commonly from secondary causes such as alcoholism, drugs (i.e., isoniazid and 6-mercaptopurine), rare inborn errors of metabolism (Hartnup's disease), and malnourishment in patients with malignant carcinoid syndrome.

The manifestations of nicotinic acid deficiency are collectively known as "pellagra." Early manifestations are vague and nondescript. However, with advanced deficiency, the classic triad of pellagra (dermatitis, diarrhea, and dementia) may present. The characteristic dermatitis is symmetrical and involves areas exposed to sun. Skin lesions are dark, dry, and scaling. The diarrhea can be severe, recurrent, and bloody. It may result in malabsorption caused by atrophy of the intestinal villi. Dementia may begin as headache, dizziness, irritability, and insomnia that progresses to confusion, memory loss, hallucinations, seizures, and psychosis. Death ultimately follows in an untreated patient.

Diagnosis of pellagra, especially in early cases, requires a high index of suspicion. Measurement of the niacin metabolite *N*-methylnicotinamide in the urine may be helpful. Low levels suggest deficiency. Blood concentrations of NAD and NADP are reduced. However, these are variable and nonspecific indicators of deficiency.

THERAPY

Niacin deficiency may be prevented by administering 5 to 20 mg nicotinic acid daily as a dietary supplement. Niacin deficiency is treated with 50 to 100 mg oral nicotinic acid daily. Pellagra is treated with 300 to 500 mg oral nicotinic acid daily in divided doses, or 25 to 100 mg nicotinic acid i.v. every 2 to 3 hours (maximum 1 g/day). It should be given very slowly and diluted in 0.9% sodium chloride to run at a rate of 2 mg/min. Nicotinic acid may also be given i.m. (50 to 100 mg) in divided doses. For treatment of hyperlipidemia, 1 to 2 g nicotinic acid should be administered in three divided oral doses daily.

PREPARATIONS AND ADVERSE EFFECTS

Nicotinic acid is available in oral prolonged-release capsules (125 to 500 mg), tablets (25 to 50 mg) and injectable forms (100 mg/ml). Nicotinamide is manufactured as oral tablets (50 to 500 mg), timed-release capsules (1000 mg), or as an injectable (100 mg/ml). Adverse effects include headache, dizziness, syncope, flushing, burning, tingling, tachycardia, hypotension, nausea, vomiting, diarrhea, flatulence, peptic ulcers, hepatotoxicity, hyperglycemia, hyperuricemia, and blurred vision.

BIOTIN (1–13)

CHEMISTRY

Biotin is an imidazole derivative consisting of eight isomers, of which only *d*-biotin is found naturally and has vitamin activity. This vitamin is soluble in water and alcohol, stable to heat, and unaffected by acid or alkali.

METABOLISM

Ingested biotin is absorbed rapidly from the small intestine and distributed widely in all tissues. It is also synthesized by intestinal bacteria and absorbed from the colon. The intact vitamin is the major form excreted in the urine, with the metabolites biotin sulfoxide and bis-norbiotin appearing in smaller amounts. Biotin acts as a cofactor for carboxylating enzymes essential to the metabolism of both fat and carbohydrates.

SOURCES

Biotin is found in low concentrations in most animal and vegetable foodstuffs. Good sources are organ meats, yeast extracts, egg yolks, dairy products, meat, grains, fruits, and vegetables.

REQUIREMENTS

The recommended daily requirement for biotin is 100 to 200 μg in adults. A specific RDA has not been established. The average U.S. diet provides 100 to 300 μg of biotin per day. Bacterial synthesis in the large intestine provides additional quantities of the vitamin.

DEFICIENCY STATES

Causes of biotin deficiency include severe malnutrition, consumption of large quantities of raw egg whites (egg white contains avidin, a biotin antagonist), disruption of normal intestinal flora by broad-spectrum antibiotics, and long-term total parenteral nutrition. Biotin deficiency manifests as maculopapular dermatitis, glossitis, lingual atrophy, muscle pain, lassitude, alopecia, paresthesias, nausea, and anorexia. Biotin status is assessed by measuring the vitamin in plasma (normal 1.47 mg/ml, range 0.82 to 2.7) or urine (24-hour urinary excretion; normal 42.4 mg, range 24 to 81).

THERAPY

Most of the symptoms of deficiency are reversible with large doses of biotin (100 to 300 μg/day). Deficiency may be prevented by administering a multivitamin preparation containing biotin.

PREPARATIONS AND ADVERSE EFFECTS

Biotin is available as oral tablets (1, 5, and 10 mg). It is also available in various multivitamin preparations. No significant adverse effects are reported.

CHOLINE (1–13)

CHEMISTRY

Choline (trimethylethanolamine or trimethyl-β-hydroxyethylammonium hydroxide), is a lipotropic quaternary amine that is water soluble, strongly alkaline, and hygroscopic. It is classified as being "vitamin-like," since this substance is synthesized within the body. The endogenous synthesis of choline, however, requires adequate amounts of the amino acids serine and methionine, along with adequate amounts of folic acid and vitamins B_{12} and B_6.

METABOLISM

Choline is absorbed from the intestinal tract. Most of the free choline is metabolized by intestinal bacteria to trimethylamine, whereas dietary choline derived from lecithin is absorbed and extracted by the liver and peripheral tissues. Choline is excreted in urine and feces. The functions of choline are many. It is an important component of membrane phospholipids (i.e., lecithin and sphingomyelin), essential for the synthesis of the neurotransmitter acetylcholine, and an integral component of normal lung development (i.e., as a component of surfactant); it also functions as a methyl donor for synthesis of compounds such as methionine.

SOURCES

Choline is found in most foods, with egg yolk, liver, soybean, and fish providing a rich source. Foods high in fat contain more choline than those low in fat (i.e., vegetables and fruits).

REQUIREMENTS

No deficiency state attributable to choline has been identified in humans. Given that the average U.S. diet contains 300 to 900 mg/day of choline and that it is readily available endogenously, no RDA has been established.

PANTOTHENIC ACID (1–13)

CHEMISTRY

Pantothenic acid is a dimethyl derivative of butyric acid (pontic acid) joined by a peptide linkage to the amino acid β-alanine. It is a water-soluble vitamin that is unstable in acid, alkali, and heat.

METABOLISM

Pantothenic acid is readily absorbed from the intestinal tract and subsequently transformed to 4′-phosphopantetheine. In the tissues, this derivative forms the prosthetic group for both co-enzyme A and acyl carrier protein. The vitamin does not appear to be degraded in the body, with 70% of absorbed vitamin being excreted in the urine unchanged. Pantothenic acid is an essential component of co-enzyme A, which participates in enzymatic reactions important in metabolism of carbohydrates, gluconeogenesis, fatty acid oxidation, and synthesis of sterols, steroid hormones, and porphyrins. Its contribution to acyl carrier protein is important for fatty acid synthesis.

SOURCES

Pantothenic acid is widely distributed in foods. Good sources include organ meats, beef, yeast, egg yolk, whole-grain cereals, and legumes.

REQUIREMENTS

A recommended daily intake of 4 to 7 mg is considered an adequate intake for adults. There is no established RDA for pantothenic acid. A well-balanced 2500 kcal diet contains about 10 mg of the vitamin. During pregnancy and lactation, daily intake of the vitamin should be increased.

DEFICIENCY STATES

The occurrence of pantothenic acid deficiency is rare because of its wide distribution in foods. Spontaneous clinical deficiency has not been described but may occur as a constellation of symptoms in association with other B-vitamin deficiencies. Experimental deficiency has produced the following symptoms and signs: heel and foot pain, fatigue, paresthesias, weakness, leg cramps, and the so-called "burning foot syndrome." In clinical practice, these symptoms rarely respond to vitamin supplementation. Assessment of pantothenic acid status is accomplished by measuring blood levels (normal 100 to 180 μg/dl).

THERAPY

For deficiency presenting as the "burning foot syndrome," 10 mg pantothenic acid per day should be given orally.

PREPARATIONS AND ADVERSE EFFECTS

Pantothenic acid is available as a calcium salt preparation (oral, 10 to 500 mg). It is also present in many of the multivitamin and B complex preparations. Adverse effects have not been reported.

REFERENCES

1. Marks J: The individual vitamins. In Marks J (ed): *The Vitamins: Their Role in Medical Practice*, part 3. MTP Press Limited, Boston, pp 111–193, 1985.
2. Feldman EB: *Essentials of Clinical Nutrition*. Philadelphia, FA Davis, Philadelphia, pp 24–42, 333–361, 1988.
3. Suter PM, Russel RM: Vitamin nutriture and requirements of the elderly. In Munro HN, Danford DE (eds): *Human Nutrition. A Comprehensive Treatise: Nutrition, Aging, and the Elderly*, vol 6. Plenum Press, New York, pp 245–291, 1989.
4. Gibson RS: *Principles of Nutritional Assessment*. Oxford University Press, New York, pp 377–486, 1990.
5. Herbert V: Vitamins and minerals. In Herbert V, Subak-Sharpe GJ (eds): *The Mount Sinai School of Medicine Complete Book of Nutrition*. St. Martin's Press, New York, pp 89–105, 1990.
6. Suter PM: Vitamin requirements. In Chernoff R (ed): *Geriatric Nutrition. The Health Professional's Handbook*. Aspen Publications, Gaithersburg, MD, pp 25–51, 1991.
7. Chaney SG: Principles of nutrition. II. Micronutrients. In Devlin TM (ed): *Textbook of Biochemistry with Clinical Correlations*, ed 2. John Wiley & Sons, New York, pp 962–983, 1986.
8. Kissane JM: *Anderson's Pathology*, ed 9. CV Mosby, St. Louis, pp 550–561, 1377–1378, 1990.
9. Gilman AG, Rall TW, Nies AS, Taylor P: *Goodman and Gilman's The Pharmacological Basis of Therapeutics*, ed 8. Pergamon Press, New York, pp 1510–1522, 1530–1571, 1990.
10. Wyngaarden JB, Smith LH Jr, Bennett JC: *Cecil Textbook of Medicine*, ed 19. Saunders, Philadelphia, pp 1170–1183, 1404–1406, 1992.
11. Bennett DR: Choline [chapter 16]; Vitamins and minerals [chapter 92]. In *Annual Drug Evaluations*. American Medical Association, Chicago, pp 368, 2017–2032, 1992.
12. Olin BR, Hebel SK, Dombek CE, Kastrup EK: *Drug Facts and Comparisons*, ed 46. Facts and Comparisons, St. Louis, pp 4–28, 169, 223–233, 1992.
13. Viteri FE: Vitamin deficiencies. In Paige DM (ed): *Clinical Nutrition*, ed 2. CV Mosby, St. Louis, pp 547–578, 1988.

CHAPTER 48

Topical Therapy I: Dermatology

STANFORD I. LAMBERG, M.D.

This chapter focuses on topical therapy for acute dermatologic conditions commonly encountered in the hospital or in the acute care unit. Comprehensive descriptions of these skin disorders should be sought in standard dermatology texts. To assist the reader in reaching a differential diagnosis, tables for patients who present with a rash in the acute care unit (Table 48.1) and for patients who develop a rash while in the hospital (Table 48.2) are provided. A list of cutaneous disorders associated with AIDS also is included (Table 48.3). Drug eruptions are described in detail because of their frequency in hospitalized patients. To assist the nondermatologist, both the algorithms and the section on drug eruptions are arranged by clinical sign.

Supportive dermatologic therapy, such as compresses and soothing pastes, may be initiated in the acute care unit without a specific diagnosis. However, if a major dermatologic component, such as blisters or shedding of skin, overshadows the rest of the clinical problem, or if longer-term therapy is being planned, clarification of the underlying disorder, which usually requires dermatologic consultation, should be initiated promptly. Because many skin disorders resemble each other, an experienced diagnostic eye and perhaps a skin biopsy or another diagnostic procedure may yield earlier recognition of a primary cutaneous disorder, an evolving complication of therapy, or an important underlying systemic disorder.

DRUG-INDUCED ERUPTIONS

Drug-induced eruptions are the most common acute skin disorder encountered in the hospital, particularly in patients who develop a new eruption after entering the hospital.

Although almost any dermatologic pattern may be induced by drugs, some patterns are more relevant in critical care practice. Vasculitis, erythema multiforme, urticaria, and serum sickness often appear suddenly and require prompt attention, as they may be life-threatening. By contrast, diffuse hair thinning from β-blockers, psoriasis worsened by lithium administration, or sun sensitivity induced by tetracycline are neither life-threatening nor likely to develop in the hospital.

Drug eruptions may appear shortly after reexposure or may develop 1 to 2 weeks after a period of sensitization. Occasionally, the eruption appears many days or even weeks after the drug is stopped.

Although it is possible to classify some drug eruptions as allergic or toxic in origin, the mechanism of most drug eruptions is too poorly understood to group them. Far more practical is recognizing that a drug-induced reaction probably is present and then trying to identify and discontinue the offending agent (1, 2). It is unwise to attempt to suppress a drug reaction with systemic corticosteroids or antihistamines without discontinuing the offending drug. Persistent exposure to the offending drug may have life-threatening consequences, even if the cutaneous manifestations appear controlled (3).

PENICILLIN SKIN TEST

The association of a drug with a reaction must be presumptive since there is little justification to reexpose the patient to the drug deliberately to confirm the association. However, a penicillin skin test (Pre-Pen) is available which, if negative,

Table 48.1. Patient Admitted with a Cutaneous Eruption

1. Redness, with or without scaling	a) Exfoliative erythroderma
	   (1) psoriasis
	   (2) atopic dermatitis
	   (3) seborrheic dermatitis
	   (4) contact dermatitis
	   (5) cutaneous T-cell lymphoma
	b) Viral exanthems
	c) Toxic shock syndrome
	d) Kawasaki's disease
	e) Rocky Mountain spotted fever
	f) Erythema multiforme
	g) Collagen vascular disease
	h) Drug eruption

2. Blisters (clear fluid)	a) Infections
	   (1) bacterial
	   (2) rickettsial
	   (3) viral
	      (a) Herpes simplex
	      (b) Herpes zoster
	b) Pemphigus/bullous pemphigoid
	c) Erythema multiforme/
	   Stevens-Johnson syndrome
	d) Toxic epidermal necrolysis

3. Pustules (purulent fluid)	a) Infection
	   (1) bacterial
	      (a) impetigo
	      (b) septic emboli
	      (c) gonococcemia
	      (d) meningococcemia
	      (e) Gram-negative
	   (2) viral
	   (3) fungal
	b) Acneform
	   (1) acne/rosacea
	   (2) halide ingestion
	c) Pustular psoriasis

4. Pruritus	a) with a rash
	b) without a rash
	   (1) psychogenic
	   (2) xerosis
	   (3) liver disease
	   (4) renal disease
	   (5) hyperthyroidism
	   (6) diabetes mellitus
	   (7) lymphoma/leukemia
	   (8) pediculosis corporis
	   (9) polycythemia vera
	   (10) drugs
	   (a) opiates
	   (b) opioides
	   (c) phenothiazines

5. Purpura or petechia	a) Infections
	   (1) bacterial
	      (a) septic emboli
	      (b) gonococcemia
	      (c) meningococcemia
	      (d) Gram-negative
	         (erythemagangrenosum)
	   (2) rickettsial
	      (a) RMSF
	   (3) viral
	      (a) hepatitis
	b) Disseminated intravascular coagulation
	c) Palpable purpura (vasculitis)
	   (1) collagen vascular disease
	   (2) hypersensitivity angiitis
	   (3) Henoch-Schoenlein purpura
	   (4) hepatitis
	   (5) paraproteinemia/leukemia

Table 48.1. *Continued*

	d) Hematologic (platelet/coagulation) disorder
	   (1) platelet disorder
	   (2) coagulation defect
	   (3) cryoglobulin/paraprotein
	   (4) leukemia
	e) Drug reaction
	f) Amyloidosis
	g) Vitamin C (scurvy) or vitamin K deficiency

6. Nodules and/or plaques	a) Urticaria/angioedema/anaphylaxis
	b) Sweet's syndrome
	c) Cellulitis/erysipelas
	   (1) bacterial
	   (2) fungal
	d) Malignant infiltrate
	   (1) lymphoma
	   (2) metastatic tumor
	   (3) Kaposi's sarcoma

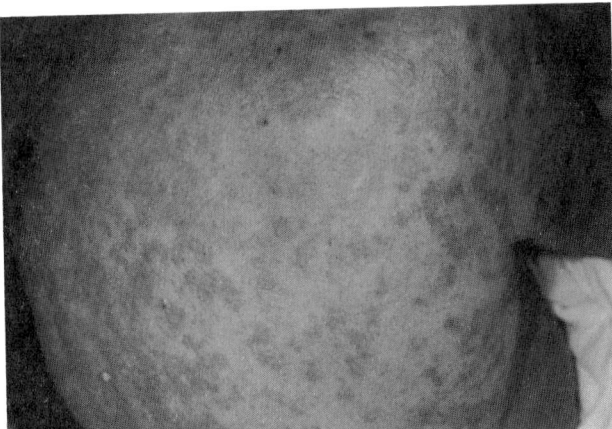

Figure 48.1. Drug eruption: morbilliform rash (Pronestyl).

substantially reduces the likelihood of an urticarial- or anaphylactic-type allergic reaction to penicillin (4). Penicillin testing should only be performed if the patient has a strong history of penicillin allergy; if penicillin is the only suitable agent; and if the decision has been made to give the drug if the test is negative. Results of a penicillin skin test are not predictive of a reaction to a course of penicillin given much later, nor is it useful for nonurticarial, nonanaphylactic types of penicillin reactions. The test may be falsely negative for weeks after a penicillin reaction due to the formation of blocking antibodies. Furthermore, the clinical value of Pre-Pen with semisynthetic penicillins, in pediatric patients and in adult patients with no history of penicillin hypersensitivity, has not been determined. The packaging material provides full directions for conducting the test.

TYPES OF DRUG-INDUCED ERUPTIONS

Maculopapular, morbilliform, or exanthematous dermatitis are the most common drug-induced eruptions in hospitalized patients. These eruptions typically start on the trunk and spread peripherally (Fig. 48.1). They are less pruritic than urticarial eruptions. A low-grade fever also may develop, sometimes obscuring the diagnosis when fever accompanies the underlying disease. A viral exanthem, for example, closely resembles a drug eruption, and both may be accompanied by fever. The most common causes of such eruptions are antibiotics, allopurinol, barbiturates, carbamazepine, gold salts, hydantoin derivatives, phenothiazines, phenylbutazones, and thiazides.

URTICARIA

Urticarial eruptions (hives) are IgE-mediated; therefore, they also may be associated with anaphylactic and serum sickness reactions. Urticarial lesions are intensely itchy geographic wheals or plaques, and they are transient, with each wheal lasting only minutes to a few hours (Fig. 48.2). The most common causes of acute hives are antibiotics, barbiturates, phenothiazines, radiographic contrast media, and agents that cause direct histamine release, such as aspirin and opiates.

SERUM SICKNESS

Serum sickness is caused by immune complex reactions that develop during administration of the offending drug. Common clinical manifestations are palpable purpuric lesions, malaise, fever, arthralgia, and lymphadenopathy. Neurologic, renal, and even myocardial involvement may develop as well.

ACNE-LIKE DRUG ERUPTIONS

Acne from medication, more accurately termed drug-induced folliculitis, can be distinguished from typical teenage acne by its lack of comedones and the uniformity of the lesions, usually either papules or pustules. The lesions are found scattered about the face and upper trunk, rather than being confined to the central parts of the face, back, and chest, as seen in typical teenage acne. Unexpectedly, acne associated with drugs often improves with standard acne topical therapy without discontinuation of the offending medication. Frequently associated drugs are prednisone, androgenic hormones, isoniazide, lithium, and phenytoins.

PURPURA

Patients with drug-associated purpura may have either low (less than 20,000/mm^3) or normal platelet counts. The differential diagnosis of purpura in a patient with low platelet counts is extensive and includes sepsis, amyloid, hemophilia, disseminated intravascular coagulation, collagen vascular disease, and some heritable disorders. Thrombocytopenia from drugs may result directly from the effect of a chemocytotoxic agent or indirectly from an allergic mechanism that induced platelet aggregation and platelet clearing. Several in vitro tests are available to examine platelet function in the presence of the suspected offending drug if platelet counts are seriously depressed (5). The most common drugs associated with purpura and low platelet counts are allopurinol, antibiotics, cimetidine, furosemide, phenytoin, quinidine, gold, and nonsteroidal antiinflammatory agents.

If platelet counts are normal, the most likely cause of the purpura is **vasculitis**, leakage through an inflamed vessel wall. Purpuric lesions with underlying vasculitis often are elevated and palpable, but the clinical suspicion of vasculitis must be confirmed with a skin biopsy (Fig. 48.3). Although most instances of cutaneous vasculitis are not associated with systemic disorders, scrutiny of the patient for systemic disease,

Table 48.2.   Patient Developed an Eruption in the Hospital

1. Redness, with or without scaling	a) Toxic shock syndrome b) Erythema multiforme c) Drug eruption

2. Blisters (clear fluid)	a) Miliaria crystallina
	b) Infections
	  (1) bacterial
	    (a) bullous impetigo
	    (b) *Staphylococcus* scalded skin syndrome
	  (2) rickettsial
	  (3) viral
	    (a) Herpes simplex
	    (b) Herpes zoster
	c) Diabetes mellitus
	d) Bullous drug eruption
	e) Erythema multiforme/Stevens-Johnson syndrome
	f) Toxic epidermal necrolysis

3. Pustules (purulent fluid)	a) Infection
	  (1) bacterial
	    (a) impetigo
	    (b) septic emboli
	    (c) gonococcemia
	    (d) meningococcemia
	    (e) Gram-negative
	  (2) viral
	  (3) fungal
	b) Miliaria
	c) Acneform
	  (1) acne/rosacea
	  (2) halide ingestion

4. Pruritus	a) with a rash b) without a rash

5. Purpura or petechia	a) Infections
	  (1) bacterial
	    (a) septic emboli
	    (b) gonococcemia
	    (c) meningococcemia
	    (d) Gram-negative
	  (2) viral
	    (a) hepatitis
	b) Disseminated intravascular coagulation
	c) Palpable purpura (vasculitis)
	  (1) drug-associated
	  (2) collagen vascular disease
	  (3) hypersensitivity angiitis
	  (4) hepatitis
	  (5) paraproteinemia/leukemia
	d) Hematologic (platelet/coagulation) disorder
	  (1) platelet disorder
	  (2) coagulation defect
	  (3) cryoglobulin/paraprotein
	  (4) leukemia
	e) Drug reaction

6. Nodules and/or Plaques	a) Urticaria/angioedema/anaphylaxis
	b) Cellulitis/erysipelas
	  (1) bacterial
	  (2) fungal

Table 48.3.   AIDS-associated Skin Eruptions

1. Acute exanthem: 1–4 wk after infection

2. Infections that develop with the onset of clinical AIDS
   - a) Viral infections
     - (1) Herpes simplex
     - (2) Herpes zoster
     - (3) Oral "hairy" leukoplakia
     - (4) Warts and condyloma accuminata
     - (5) Molluscum contagiosum
     - (6) Cytomegalovirus
   - b) Fungal infections
     - (1) *Candida*
     - (2) *Der*matophytes
     - (3) cryptococcosis
     - (4) histoplasmosis
     - (5) coccidioidomycosis
     - (6) sporotrichosis
   - c) Bacterial infections
     - (1) Gram-positive infections
     - (2) Bacillary (epithelioid) angiomatosis
   - d) Mycobacterial infections
   - e) Treponemal infections (syphilis)
   - f) Arthropod infections (scabies, lice)

3. Eruptions that may appear with clinical AIDS
   - a) seborrheic dermatitis
   - b) folliculitis
   - c) xerosis and ichthyosis
   - d) psoriasis
   - e) Reiter's disease
   - f) hair thinning and alopecia areata
   - g) hyperpigmentation
   - h) folliculitis
   - i) pityriasis rosea
   - j) rosacea
   - k) drug eruptions
   - l) papular urticaria
   - m) atopic dermatitis
   - n) granuloma annulare
   - o) papular lesions, undefined
   - p) vascular lesions
     - (1) cutaneous vasculitis
     - (2) idiopathic thrombocytopenic purpura
     - (3) telangiectasias
     - (4) macular purpura, undefined
   - q) Neoplasms
     - (1) Kaposi's sarcoma
     - (2) squamous/basal cell cancer
     - (3) melanoma
     - (4) lymphoma (usually B cell)

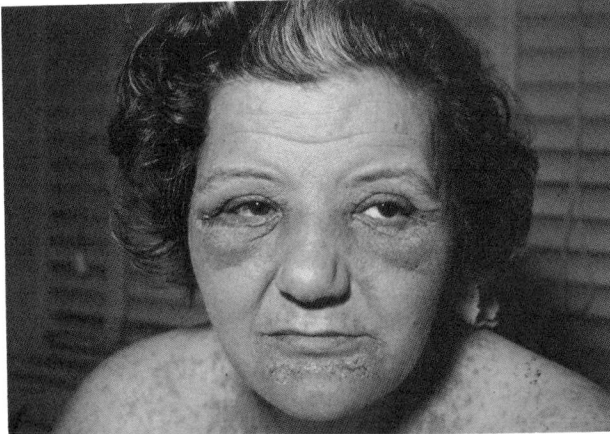

Figure 48.2.   Drug eruption: urticaria and angioneurotic edema (penicillin).

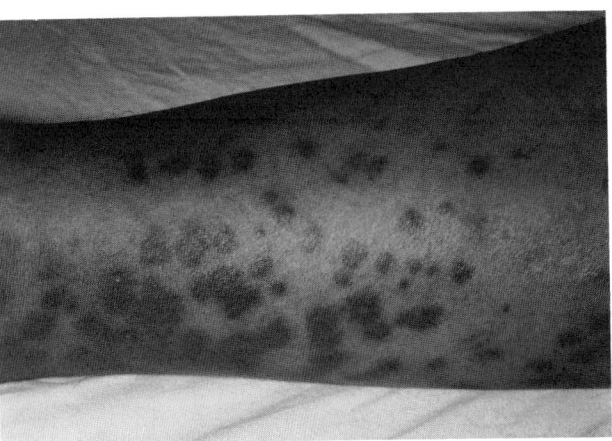

Figure 48.3.   Vasculitis: leukocytoclastic.

especially infectious disease, rheumatoid arthritis, inflammatory bowel disease, and lymphoproliferative disorders, should be made (6). Drugs most commonly associated with vasculitis are hydantoins, indomethasone, phenylbutazones, sulfonamides, and thiouracils, but the list of drugs that have been implicated is long. A nonthrombocytopenic macular purpura has been associated with AIDS, but the cause is unclear.

ERYTHEMA NODOSUM

Erythema nodosum is an inflammation of the vessels and septa of the subcutaneous tissue. It has a distinctive clinical pattern with tender, erythematous, deep nodules usually restricted to the anterior tibial area of adult women (Fig. 48.4). A skin biopsy is needed to confirm the diagnosis. Although some cases are associated with drugs, other causes are more likely, including infections such as *Streptococcus*, TB, and deep fungal infections, as well as sarcoidosis, ulcerative colitis, and lymphoma. Erythema nodosum induced by a drug is less likely to be accompanied by fever, malaise, and joint pains than when it is associated with a systemic disease. Episodes resolve spontaneously in a few weeks but may recur, especially if there is an underlying condition. The most common drug causes are gold salts, halides, oral contraceptives, and sulfonamides. Treatment, necessary only in persistent cases, is less important than seeking the underlying cause. Analgesics and bed rest generally give symptomatic relief.

BULLOUS ERUPTIONS

Blisters associated with drugs may appear as scattered blisters without a distinctive pattern or may assume the more distinctive patterns of erythema multiforme or toxic epidermal necrolysis described below (Fig. 48.5). Sometimes, they appear at pressure points, particularly in a comatose patient or after a narcotic overdose. Blisters also may arise from a reaction between light and a medication; nonsteroidal antiinflammatory agents and nalidixic acid are examples, but such reactions are only likely to be encountered in outpatients.

Evaluation of a blistering disorder should include a search for viral and bacterial causes and include culture, Gram-stained smears, and cytologic examination for multinucleated cells. A biopsy and serologic tests for circulating antiepidermal antibodies distinctive for pemphigus and pemphigoid also may be indicated.

ERYTHEMA MULTIFORME

Erythema multiforme is characterized by a variety of lesions, as the name implies, but the most distinctive are erythematous plaques, more frequent on the extensor surfaces of the extremities than the trunk, with a tendency to bull's eye or display target centers, as well as urticarial and, if severe, bullous lesions (Fig. 48.6). Those lesions on the palms and soles often are tender. Mucosal erosions may be severe and interfere with eating. Prodromal symptoms of a viral respiratory syndrome precede the eruption in about half the cases.

Most cases of erythema multiforme are idiopathic, but up to 20% of cases, particularly if recurrent, are preceded by a flare of herpes simplex virus, and about 10% are drug-related (7). The relationship between a specific drug and the appearance of erythema multiforme often is confused because patients may have been given the suspected offending medication for the flu-like prodromal symptoms of erythema multiforme. Nevertheless, it is not wise to attempt to prove the relationship between erythema multiforme and a drug by rechallenge, as a severe flare may develop (8). Typical cases of erythema multiforme run their course, with or without treatment, in 2 or 3 weeks, although some patients have recurring episodes. The most common drugs implicated in erythema multiforme are antibiotics, especially sulfonamides, as

well as allopurinol, barbiturates, carbamazepine, hydantoins, nonsteroidal antiinflammatory agents, phenothiazines, and phenylbutazones.

Severe skin lesions, especially bullae, and mucosal involvement in an acutely ill, febrile patient comprises the **Stevens-Johnson syndrome,** generally considered an extreme variant of erythema multiforme. The syndrome may be life-threatening because of electrolyte loss and organ failure.

TOXIC EPIDERMAL NECROLYSIS

The eruption is dramatic, frequently preceded by a febrile prodrome with pharyngitis and malaise, resembling that prodrome preceding erythema multiforme. Extensive areas of exquisitely tender erythematous patches develop and evolve into large flaccid blisters, or they simply peel, like a burn, without blistering (Fig. 48.7). Patients appear acutely ill. Toxic epidermal necrolysis may be a variant of erythema multiforme, but it usually can be separated from erythema multiforme because there are no target lesions, the mucosal surfaces are uninvolved, and a causal drug or toxin usually can be directly implicated. The histology of the skin also has a distinctive pattern. The fatality rate is high, perhaps as high as 30% of adult cases, as compared to about 10% in those with the Stevens-Johnson syndrome. Drugs implicated in toxic epidermal necrolysis are the same as those that lead to erythema multiforme.

Patients with Stevens-Johnson syndrome or toxic epidermal necrolysis should be treated similarly to patients with severe burns, even in a burn unit if one is available. The role of systemic corticosteroids is controversial, but these drugs are now generally avoided (9). A recent report showed dramatic benefit using cyclophosphamide in patients with toxic epidermal necrolysis (10).

Another acute blistering disorder in the differential diagnosis is the **staphylococcal scalded skin syndrome,** which is restricted to young children with immature kidneys and adults with renal insufficiency or major immunosuppression. The cause is accumulation of a phage type 2 staphylococcal toxin ordinarily eliminated in the urine (11). Increased levels of the toxin induce a split within the epidermis, leading to peeling of the skin which, like a burn, is noticeably tender (Fig. 48.8).

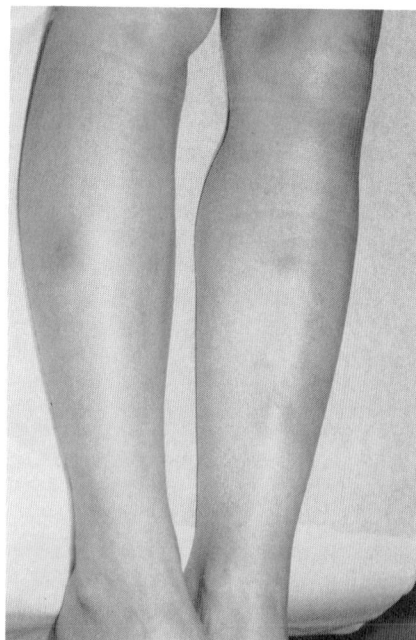

Figure 48.4.   Erythema nodosum.

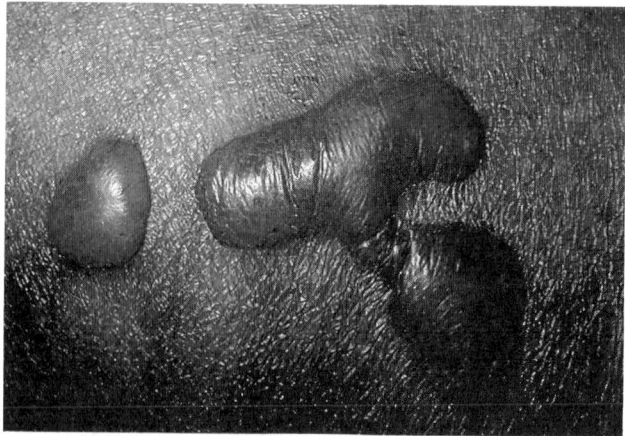

Figure 48.5.   Drug eruption: bullous (sulfa).

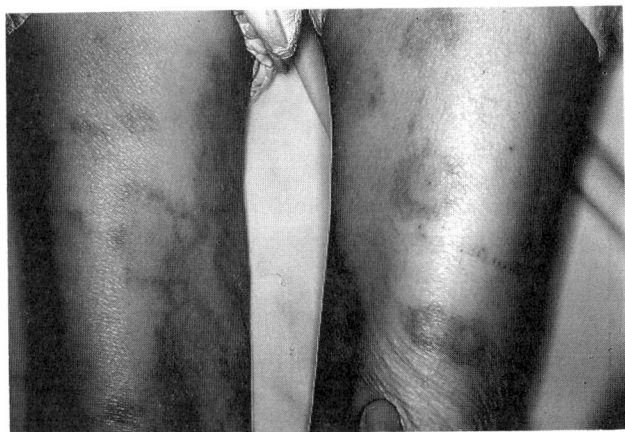

Figure 48.6. Erythema multiforme: "target" lesions.

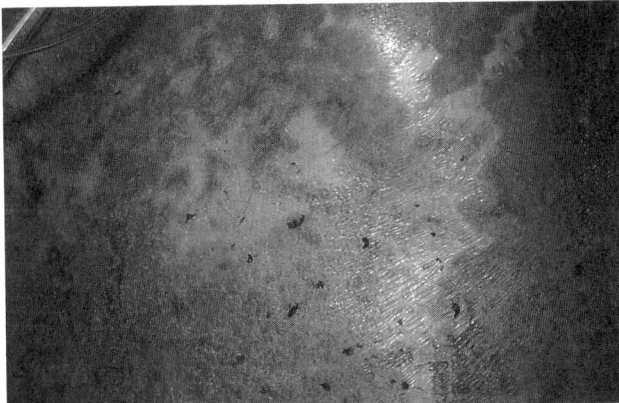

Figure 48.7. Toxic epidermal necrolysis: sheets of denuded skin.

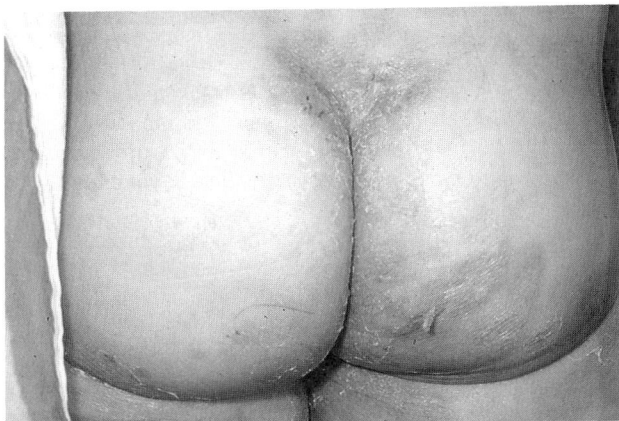

Figure 48.8. Staphylococcal scalded skin syndrome.

It is important to identify the syndrome since therapy of the infection provides rapid resolution.

TOPICAL THERAPY

COMPRESSES (WET DRESSINGS)

Compresses, the repeated application of moist dressings, are safe and effective as initial therapy for *any* acute skin condition, especially those that are crusty, oozy, red, and painful. A compress is distinguished from a soak (i.e., simple immersion of the area). Compressing removes crusts and debris, cools, and reduces skin inflammation, while soaking is more effective to reduce inflammation in muscles or joints.

The most readily available compressing solution is physiologic saline, available in the hospital as a sterile solution or made easily with 1 teaspoon of table salt in a pint of water. Lukewarm or room temperature water usually is satisfactory, but cold compresses, even with added ice cubes, provide additional relief in patients with particularly painful or itchy dermatitis. Acetic acid (0.25 to 1%) compresses may be useful for the treatment of *Pseudomonas* skin infections (12, 13).

To perform a compress, one wets a soft cloth in the solution, squeezes it so it is not dripping wet, and applies it to the affected area. The compress is left in place for 2 to 3 minutes, removed, wet again, and squeezed out again. The process is repeated for about 20 minutes. As the debris softens, it can be wiped gently away. Compressing may be repeated as often as every 2 hours during the day for acute dermatitis or as infrequently as twice a day for a crusty, chronic leg ulcer. A "wet-to-dry" dressing is a compromise that eases nursing: dry gauze is applied over wet gauze that sticks to skin debris, and both are removed when the dressing is changed. This technique is not as effective as sustained compressing.

Once the area is clean and inflammation has been reduced, which usually takes a day or two; compressing should be stopped, as continuation may lead to excessive dryness and uncomfortable cracking. If large areas are compressed, the cooling effect may even reduce body temperature and lead to electrolyte imbalance. These complications are more likely in patients with extensive burns or with extensive denuding dermatitis, such as pemphigus.

PASTES

Pastes are useful for any acute or subacute oozing dermatitis, such as diaper dermatitis, intertrigo, or pruritus ani. Pastes provide protection while absorbing serous drainage. The most commonly available paste is zinc oxide paste, also called Lassar's paste. It is most effective when applied thickly with a tongue blade, like icing a cake, following compressing to first remove debris.

TOPICAL CORTICOSTEROIDS

Corticosteroids are the most widely prescribed topical medication. Because they are potent inhibitors of inflammation, the effect of topical corticosteroids is most dramatic for acute dermatitis but they are also beneficial in a variety of nonmalignant proliferative disorders, such as psoriasis, cutaneous sarcoid, and granuloma annulare.

Topical corticosteroids interfere with fibroblastic proliferation and connective tissue synthesis, however, and chronic use may lead to vascular wall weakness and cutaneous atrophy. Local side effects are most likely when these agents are used for many weeks or months on the face and when occluded in intertriginous areas. There is little danger of overuse of topical corticosteroids in the acute hospital setting, as it is unlikely that short-term use will seriously mask allergic contact or

Table 48.4. Topical Corticosteroid Potency

Very high potency	Diproline cr, lotion, oint[a]
	Psorcon cr, oint
	Temovate cr, oint
	Ultravate cr, oint
High potency	Cyclocort cr, lotion, oint
	Diprosone cr, lotion, oint
	Florone cr, oint
	Halog cr, oint, sol[a]
	Lidex cr, gel, oint, sol
	Maxiflor cr, oint
	Maxivate cr, lotion, oint
	Topicort cr, gel, oint
	Valisone oint
Intermediate potency	Cordran cr, lotion, oint
	Elocon cr, lotion, oint[b]
	Locoid cr, oint[b]
	Synalar cr, oint, sol
	Triamcinolone cr, lotion, oint
	Valisone cr, lotion
Low potency	Westcort cr, oint[b]
	Aclovate cr, oint[b]
	Desonide cr, oint[b]
	Hydrocortisone cr, lotion, oint[b]
	Hytone (non-generic HC)[b]
	Tridesilon cr, oint[b]

[a] cr, cream; oint, ointment; sol, solution.
[b] Nonfluorinated preparations. The more potent fluorinated steroids may cause telangiectasias when used on the face and atropy with permanent striae, when used in the groin or axilla.

drug eruptions or encourage the spread of cutaneous viral or bacterial infections.

Systemic absorption occurs after skin application, but systemic effects are unusual even with long-term, widespread use. However, growth retardation and hypertension have been reported in small children using potent topical corticosteroids (14).

Dozens of brands of topical corticosteroids are marketed, most in various bases and strengths. All are expensive. A large volume is needed to treat the skin; for example, 10 g of cream applied sparingly are needed to cover the thighs and legs one time (30 g are needed for the entire body). If the prescription is written for TID application, simple calculation shows that ½ lb is needed per week, far more than most physicians prescribe.

Table 48.4 shows the relative potency of many of the topical corticosteroids. Topical corticosteroids in cream bases are the preparations of choice for acute or subacute dermatitis, as they are miscible with exudate. Ointments are better for chronic, dry conditions. Solutions or lotions are preferred in hairy areas.

SYSTEMIC CORTICOSTEROIDS

The use of systemic corticosteroids in critical care settings should be restrained to avoid suppressing or hiding an underlying immune or infectious cause. As is well-known, systemic corticosteroids are particularly hazardous in patients with diabetes mellitus, hypertension, infection, peptic ulcer disease, osteoporosis, renal stones, or glaucoma. Glucocorticoids often are required for conditions that are the consequence of undesirable immune reactions such as acute lupus or pemphigus, but a definitive diagnosis should be sought before steroid

therapy is initiated. While teratogenicity from systemic corticosteroids has not been shown in humans, their use during pregnancy generally is avoided, particularly during the first trimester.

Oral forms are well-absorbed by the intestines. Glucocorticoids have differing biologic half lives: they are grouped as short (less than a day, cortisol, cortisone); intermediate (a day, prednisone, prednisolone); or long (about 2 days), betamethasone, dexamethasone). In addition, preparations differ in their antiinflammatory, sodium retention, and nitrogen-wasting properties (15). Prednisone, the most frequently prescribed systemic corticosteroid, has a high ratio of antiinflammatory-to-sodium retention properties, as do the long-acting forms. Prednisolone, rather than prednisone, is used intravenously, as prednisone must be converted to prednisolone in the liver. While dosages of oral and parenteral preparations are comparable, intravenous administration gives high levels faster.

Dividing the dose during the day gives the greatest antiinflammatory effect but also the highest frequency of side effects. A single daily dose early in the morning is less likely to suppress the normal nighttime surge of ACTH. Larger doses on alternate days further reduce side effects, except cataracts and osteopenia, while providing satisfactory antiinflammatory effects in most clinical situations, but this schedule works best in long-term, noncritical conditions (16). Obviously, alternate-day therapy is not suitable if long-acting steroids are used.

Clearance of systemic corticosteroids occurs faster, and their therapeutic effect is reduced by coadministration of drugs that induce hepatic microsomal enzymes, such as phenytoin and phenobarbital.

ANTIHISTAMINES

Antihistamines compete for H_1 or H_2 histamine receptor sites. H_1 antihistamines are used widely for their antipruritic effect but, except for urticaria, a therapeutic role beyond sedation has not been proven. There are six chemically distinct groups of H_1 blockers: alkylamines; ethanolamines; ethylenediamines; phenothiazines; piperidines; and piperazines. The H_2 blockers, most commonly used to inhibit gastric acid secretion, appear to have an antipruritic effect if combined with H_1 blockers (17).

Generally, antihistamines are rapidly absorbed after oral administration and are metabolized in the liver for excretion by the kidneys within 24 hours. The most common side effect is sedation, particularly in elderly individuals, while children may become hyperexcitable. Anticholinergic side effects are also common. These side effects include dry mouth, tachycardia, blurred vision, and urinary retention. Alcohol and barbiturates exaggerate CNS effects while monamine oxidase inhibitors intensify the anticholinergic effects. H_2 blockers interfere with hepatic microsomal enzyme function and potentiate the effects of warfarin, phenobarbital, diazepam, and phenytoin. Tetracycline absorption is decreased by H_2 blockers. None of the antihistamines are proven safe for use in pregnancy. Antihistamines should not be used in topical preparations, as they can induce contact allergy.

Generally, antihistamines should be started at a low dose and increased slowly every day or two until improvement occurs or troublesome side effects develop. If a satisfactory response is not achieved in 1 or 2 weeks, an antihistamine from another chemical group should be tried.

TOPICAL ANTIBACTERIAL AGENTS

Topical antibiotics are effective only with superficial infections, having no value if tissue invasion has occurred. Even with impetigo, it is difficult to demonstrate that topical antibiotics are more effective than simple soap and water. However, when applied to nasal passages, they are useful in reducing the carriage rate of pathogenic staphylococci and may be useful to reduce bacterial contamination around intravenous catheters. The topical antibiotics most useful in the treatment of mild inflammatory acne vulgaris include clindamycin and erythromycin. Topical antibiotics are sold widely in combinations of bacitracin, polymyxin B, and neomycin. Topical preparations of gentamicin also are available.

As a result of widespread exposure, topical allergy to neomycin is common. When applied topically, gentamycin reduces the number of Gram-negative organisms in infected burns and stasis ulcers, and allergic reactions are unusual. However, topical gentamycin is not frequently used, as it is absorbed systemically, particularly from large denuded areas, and may increase the risk of developing gentamicin-resistant organisms.

Mupirocin is a newer topical antibiotic effective against staphylococci, including methicillin-resistant strains, and streptococci but not against Gram-negative organisms or fungi. Topical mupirocin has been shown to be as effective as oral erythromycin in the treatment of impetigo (18) and is useful in reducing nasal carriage of *Staphylococcus aureus*. However, when used for extensive open wounds, such as burns, absorption has been associated with renal damage.

TOPICAL AGENTS USED FOR BURN TREATMENT

Silver nitrate inhibits growth of a wide spectrum of pathogenic bacteria and fungi and until recently was used on burn units as compresses of a 0.5% aqueous solution to help prevent burn wound infections. The major danger of its use is its binding to chloride ions, complicating the electrolyte imbalance of burn patients. Its major inconvenience is the blackening of the skin of the patient, hospital personnel, and hospital floor and bed area from reduction of the solution to silver metal by light.

More often used now, except in patients allergic to sulfa, is **silver sulfadiazine.** Sulfadiazine, as well as silver, is released, and serum levels of sulfa can be substantial, leading to depressed white blood cell counts in some cases. The preparation is applied once or twice daily after compressing and is used thickly, like frosting a cake. Application often is followed by discomfort that usually subsides within an hour.

Mafenide is another topical sulfonamide also useful in the treatment of burns to prevent bacterial colonization. However, it is less effective than silver sulfadiazine in controlling yeasts. Mafenide also is applied after compressing. It is rapidly absorbed and more often induces local discomfort or allergic reactions than does silver sulfadiazine. Therefore, it usually is reserved for deep eschars and small areas. Bacitracin also

is widely used in burn units, but topical gentamicin is avoided for the reasons previously stated.

TOPICAL ANTIVIRAL AGENTS

Topical acyclovir is useful for primary herpes simplex infections, although the oral form is more effective. Double-blind studies did not confirm the value of topical acyclovir in recurrent eruptions (19).

TOPICAL ANTIFUNGAL AGENTS

Cutaneous infection with *Candida albicans* is common in critical care units because of superinfection during antibiotic therapy and the hot, moist conditions of bedridden febrile patients. Cutaneous dermatophyte infections, such as tinea cruris or capitis, generally do not require prompt treatment in this setting.

Nystatin

Nystatin is a specific and effective treatment of *Candida* infections of the skin, vagina, and GI tract. It is inexpensive and rarely causes allergic or irritant reactions; as it is not absorbed, side effects are rare. Successful treatment of superficial candidal infection requires correction of underlying causes, including excess moisture and hyperglycemia, and discontinuance of antibiotics. Nystatin does not work well in immunocompromised patients.

Broad-Spectrum Antifungal Agents

Newer agents that demonstrate broad activity against both dermatophytes and *Candida* are available. These agents include the imidazoles and triazoles (such as butoconazole, clotrimazole, econazole, ketoconazole, miconazole, oxiconazole, sulconazole, and terconazole), as well as ciclopirox olamine, haloprogin, and naftifine.

Application to the skin once or twice a day usually clears the infection within a week; applications once or twice weekly afterward reduces the frequency of recurrence in susceptible persons. Side effects are uncommon, although contact allergies have been reported.

SYSTEMIC ANTIFUNGAL AGENTS (20, 21)

Griseofulvin

Oral griseofulvin is a useful systemic agent for cutaneous dermatophyte infections that are resistant or too widespread to be treated topically. It is not effective for systemic *Candida,* tinea versicolor, or deep fungal infections.

Griseofulvin is absorbed variably from the GI tract, with improved absorption after a fatty meal. It reaches the epidermis by reabsorption following excretion in the sweat, as well as directly from the blood. Griseofulvin is fungistatic, deposited only in newly keratinized structures, so failure to respond to the drug occurs frequently, especially in chronic tinea infections of thick areas such as the palms, soles, and nails. Therefore, therapy for infections of the hair may take months and for infections of the nails, a year or more. The usual adult dose is 250 to 500 mg of the ultrafine form and is best absorbed if taken with a fatty food, such as milk.

Serious reactions are uncommon although high doses may cause headache and nausea, usually corrected by lowering the dose. Patients who are on griseofulvin for more than 3 months should be monitored for hepatic and bone marrow toxicity, although the incidence of such side effects is quite low (22). Rare instances of a lupus erythematosus-like syndrome or porphyria have been reported. Griseofulvin stimulates hepatic enzyme activity and decreases the activity of warfarin-type anticoagulants. Griseofulvin should not be given to pregnant women, particularly in the first trimester.

Ketoconazole has a broader spectrum than griseofulvin and is effective against dermatophytes, *Candida*, tinea versicolor, and some deep fungal infections, including blastomycosis, histoplasmosis, coccidioidomycosis, pseudoallescheriasis, and paracoccidioidomycosis. It is the drug of choice for chronic mucocutaneous candidiasis. Ketoconazole is not effective when there is meningeal involvement or in the immunosuppressed patient (23), nor in treating sporotrichosis, cryptococcosis, chromomycosis, eumycetoma, or mucormycosis (23).

Ketoconazole is best absorbed if taken on an empty stomach or with an acidic citrus juice. Gastric acidity facilitates absorption, while antacids and H_2 blockers reduce it (24). Ketoconazole reduces the serum level of rifampin, increases the anticoagulant effect of warfarin-like drugs, increases the blood levels of cyclosporin, and affects the serum levels of phenytoin, increasing the need to monitor serum levels.

Mild reversible elevations in serum hepatic enzyme levels are seen in up to 5% of patients, and a potentially fatal hepatitis develops in up to 1 of every 10,000 to 20,000 persons. The most common side effects are dose-dependent mild GI symptoms and headache. These side effects usually do not occur at doses below 400 mg/day. The usual dose for superficial infections is 200 mg/day for 3 weeks. Ketoconazole inhibits steroid synthesis both in fungi and in humans; long-term use can lead to menstrual irregularities, gynecomastia, and impotence. It should not be used during pregnancy or in nursing mothers.

Amphotericin B is the treatment of choice for aspergillosis, blastomycosis, coccidiodomycosis, crytococcosis, histoplasmosis, mucormycosis, paracoccidiodomycosis, and sporotrichosis, especially if it is invasive, rapidly progressive, or in an immunosuppressed person (23). It must be given intravenously in dextrose, rather than in saline, which aggregates the commercial preparation. The drug is toxic to most organ systems, especially the kidneys, which limits its use. Careful guidelines must be followed (21).

Flucytosine is rapidly absorbed after oral administration and is excreted by the kidneys. It generally is used in combination with amphotericin B because of rapid emergence of resistant strains when used alone. However, it is effective when used alone for chromoblastomycosis. The combination (amphotericin B [0.3 mg/kg/day] and flucytosine [100 to 150 mg/kg/day]) is active against candidiasis and cryptococcosis, including meningitis, and *Torulopis* (*Candida*) *glabrata*, agents that cause chromomycosis (25). The most serious side effect of flucytosine is bone marrow depression, particularly white blood cells and platelets. Reversibly elevated liver enzymes

occur in 5% of patients. AIDS and renal insufficiency, including that caused by amphotericin B, increase toxicity (26).

ANTIPARASITICS

Persons with cutaneous infestations are seen frequently in hospital emergency rooms, usually with itching as their chief complaint. Infestations often accompany alcoholism, drug abuse, or homelessness, and quickly spread between persons who live together, share clothing, or have sexual relations. Lice (pediculosis) and scabies are the usual culprits. Lice are wingless insects that are species specific to humans. Head lice and body lice are similar in appearance: elongated, 2 to 4 mm gray bodies with three pairs of legs. Head lice, or their egg cases (called nits) can be found on the scalp and hair shafts, while body lice live in clothing and are most easily found in seams, rather than on the skin surface. Pubic lice are shorter and wider than head and body lice, resemble a crab, and often are so firmly attached to the skin they look like freckles.

Scabies are mites about a millimeter in size with four pairs of legs. Most infestations are passed between humans via close personal contact or shared clothing, but animal scabies (mange) can be acquired from pets. Animal scabies is not passed between humans. Scabies mites are difficult to find because generally only 5 to 15 are present, hidden deep within the horny layer. A mite may be sought by scraping the edge of a suspected burrow with a scalpel blade, just deep enough to get a little blood. A small drop of mineral oil over the area to be scraped helps keep the debris together for transfer to a microscope slide. Burrows are most likely in the genital area, buttocks, elbows, and fingerwebs. Scabies is contagious to hospital personnel who have direct physical contact with the infested patient; even lifting a patient with scabies may spread the infestation. Such exposure of staff justifies prophylactic treatment. However, hospital personnel are unlikely to get scabies if treatment of the infested patient was completed the previous day. Clothing can be cleansed of parasites by washing, dry cleaning, ironing, or tumble drying on the hot cycle. Changing bed linens and towels and normal cleaning constitute sufficient decontamination of the hospital room.

Pyrethrins and permethrines have replaced lindane as the treatments of choice for pediculosis (27). Permethrine works as well or better than lindane for scabies (28). Lindane is now used less often because up to 10% is absorbed, occasionally leading to CNS toxicity, particularly in infants. Pyrethrins and permethrines are safe in children older than 2 months of age, but safety in pregnant and nursing mothers has not been proven. Response to treatment of pediculosis usually is prompt, but patients with scabies may continue to itch for weeks after the mites are killed, because the pruritus, an irritant and allergic response to the mites, subsides slowly.

Method of Treatment

Pediculosis capitis.   Advise patients to shampoo with pyrethrin or permethrin (10 minutes), or with lindane (4 minutes). Treat eyebrows, eye lashes, or nipples, if involved.

Pediculosis pubis.   Advise patients to apply pyrethrin, permethrin, or lindane cream or lotion to the pubic area and leave on for 8 to 12 hours before showering. Pediculi in the pubic area often spreads to the thighs, trunk, and axillae. If symptomatic, treat from the neck to the toes. A shower immediately before treatment should be avoided, as it may increase irritation from the medication.

Scabies. Permethrin and lindane are effective against scabies and ticks, as well as against lice. Advise patients to apply 1 ounce of the cream or lotion from neck to toes and between all crevices between, then leave on for 8 to 12 hours. Although both drugs are ovicidal, they are not 100% effective, and a second application a week later often must be made.

Ticks. Ticks are large mites. The common dog tick, when engorged with blood, may be the size of a flattened pea. It is best removed by grabbing it with forceps near its attachment to the skin and lifting it upward and out. Applying glycerin or solvent to the tick or heating it with a match are ineffective. Dog ticks may carry rickettsia (Rocky Mountain spotted fever) and virus (encephalitis) and should be saved in case later laboratory examination would prove useful. The deer tick associated with Lyme disease is about the size of a small pinhead and is not easily seen.

REFERENCES

1. Bigby M, Jick S, Jick H: Drug induced cutaneous reactions: a report from the Boston Drug Collaborative Drug Surveillance Program on 15,438 consecutive inpatients, 1975–1982. *JAMA* 256:3358–3363, 1986.
2. Bruinsma WA: *A Guide to Drug Eruptions: the European File of Side Effects in Dermatology*, ed 5. The File of Medicines, Oosthuizen, The Netherlands, 1990.
3. Mullick FG, McAllister Jr HA, Wagner BM, et al. Drug related vasculitis. *Hum Pathol* 10:313–325, 1979.
4. Adkinson Jr NF: Tests for immunoglobulin drug reactions. In Rose NF, Friedman H (eds): *Manual of Clinical Immunology*. American Society for Microbiology, Washington, DC, pp 692–697, 1986.
5. Rao AK, Walsh PN: Acquired qualitative platelet disorders. *Clin Haematol* 12:201–205, 1983.
6. Gibson LE: Cutaneous vasculitis: approach to diagnosis and systemic associations. *Mayo Clin Proc* 65:226–229, 1990.
7. Huff JC, Weston WL, Tonnesen MC: Erythema multiforme: a critical review of characteristics, diagnostic criteria, and causes. *J Am Acad Dermatol* 8:763–775, 1983.
8. Girard M: Oral provocation: limitations. *Semin Dermatol* 8:192–195, 1989.
9. Avakian R, Flowers FP, Araujo OE, Ramos-Caro FA: Toxic epidermal necrolysis: a review. *J Am Acad Dermatol* 25:69–79, 1991.
10. Heng MCY, Allen SG: Efficacy of cyclophosphamide in toxic epidermal necrolysis. *J Am Acad Dermatol* 25:778–786, 1991.
11. Melish ME, Glasgow LA, Turner MD: The staphylococcal scalded skin syndrome. *J Infect Dis* 125:129–140, 1972.
12. Phillips I, Lobo AZ, Fernandes R, et al: Acetic acid in the treatment of superficial wounds infected by *Pseudomonas aeruginosa. Lancet* ii:11–13, 1968.
13. Leyden JJ, Kligman AM: The role of microorganisms in diaper dermatitis. *Arch Dermatol* 114:56–59, 1978.
14. Gallant C, Kenny P: Oral glucocorticoids and their complications. *J Am Acad Dermatol* 14:161–177, 1986.
15. Haynes Jr RC: Adrenocorticosteroids. In Gilman AG, Rall TW, Nies AS, Taylor P (eds): *Goodman and Gilman's, The Pharmacological Basis of Therapeutics*. Pergamon Press, New York, pp 1447–1451, 1990.
16. Harter JG, Reddy WJ, Thorn GW: Studies on an intermittent corticosteroid dosage regimen. *N Engl J Med* 269:591–596, 1963.
17. Matthews CNA, Boss JM, Warin RP, Storari F: The effect of H1 and H2 histamine antagonists on symptomatic dermographism. *Br J Dermatol* 101:57–61, 1979.
18. Leyden JS: Review of mupirocin ointment in the treatment of impetigo. *Clin Pediatr* 31:549–553, 1992.
19. Nilsen AE, Aasen T, Halsos AM, Kinge OR, Tiotta EA, Wikstrom K, Fiddian AP: Efficacy of oral acyclovir in the treatment of initial and recurrent genital herpes. *Lancet* ii:571–573, 1982.
20. Utz JP: Chemotherapy of the systemic mycoses. *Med Clin North Am* 66:221–230, 1986.
21. Bodey GP: Topical and systemic antifungal agents. *Med Clin North Am* 72:637–659, 1988.
22. Lesher JL, Smith Jr JG: Antifungal agents in dermatology. *J Am Acad Dermatol* 17:383–394, 1987.
23. Bennett JE: Antimicrobial agents. In Gilman AG, Rall TW, Nies AS, Taylor P (eds): *Goodman and Gilman's, The Pharmacological Basis of Therapeutics*. Pergamon Press, New York, pp 1168, 1171, 1990.
24. Blum RA, D'Andrea DT, Florentino BM, et al: Increased gastric pH and the bioavailability of fluconazole and ketoconazole. *Ann Intern Med* 114:755–775, 1991.
25. Bennett JE, Dismukes WE, Duma RJ, et al: A collaborative study: amphotericin B-flucytosine in cryptococcal meningitis. *N Engl J Med* 301:126–131, 1979.
26. Stamm AM, Diasio RB, Dismukes WE, Shadomy S, Cloud GC, Bowles CA, Karam GH, Espinel-Ingroff A: Toxicity of Amphotericin B plus flucytosine in 194 patients with cryptococcal meningitis. *Am J Med* 83:236–242, 1987.
27. Taplin D, Meinking DL: Pyrethins and pyrethroids in dermatology. *Arch Dermatol* 126:213–221, 1990.
28. Schultz MW, Gomez M, Hansen RC: Comparative study of 5% pyrmethrin cream and 1% lindane lotion for the treatment of scabies. *Arch Dermatol* 126:167–170, 1990.

CHAPTER 49

Topical Therapy II: Burns

COLLEEN M. RYAN, M.D.
RONALD G. TOMPKINS, M.D., Sc.D.

The cutaneous nature of burn injury makes the topical application of pharmaceutical agents an obvious treatment that has been used for centuries (1). Topical application enables drugs to be delivered directly to the affected areas in high concentrations independent of plasma protein binding or biodistribution inequalities. Topical application has advantages because potential systemic toxicity can be limited by selecting drugs that are poorly absorbed through the burn eschar but maintain their active concentrations at the wound site. In general, drugs with high molecular weight, poor water solubility, or the ability to be precipitated by wound products are less likely to be absorbed systemically.

Successful topical therapy for the burn wound includes not only the application of pharmaceutical agents (antiseptics, antibiotics, enzymes, and recombinant protein products) but also the topical management of the wound. This topical management includes the surgical preparation of the wound bed and the immediate closure of the open wound with autologous skin or wound closure materials when autologous skin is insufficient. Great improvement in survival rates has occurred since the 1940s and 1950s, because effective topical agents were developed to suppress the colonization of the burn wounds with bacteria or fungi. This successful control of wound flora has allowed surgical treatments to advance and skin replacement technologies to be developed.

There are multiple goals for topical agents for burn injuries, including (*a*) the prevention of invasive infections; (*b*) the relief of pain; (*c*) the optimization of long-term functional and cosmetic results; and (*d*) the normalization of the patient's

metabolic and immunologic responses to the injury. The ideal topical agent should accomplish these goals with limited or minimal risk and toxicity to the patient. Unfortunately, there is no ideal agent, and most agents usually achieve only a single goal. In modern burn care, the most important of these goals is the prevention of invasive burn wound infections. Topical agents are intended to restore and support the body's natural defense against infection; however, an established burn wound infection and its devastating consequences cannot be eradicated by the simple application of a topical pharmaceutical agent alone. The complete treatment usually requires debridement of the burn wound eschar in combination with topical and systemic antibiotics.

For superficial burn injuries in which only the epidermal and very superficial dermal elements have been destroyed, most any effective antibacterial topical agent will suffice, because the major goals are limited to the prevention of wound infection and the relief of pain. As long as infection does not supervene, these wounds will heal satisfactorily regardless of the particular topical treatment selected.

On the other hand, when substantial portions of the dermis have been destroyed by the burn injury, topical antimicrobial agents alone will not solve the problems presented by the burn wound. Since dermis does not regenerate, the most effective and successful treatment for these injuries includes surgical excision of the destroyed and nonviable tissue and immediate closure of the open wound with autologous skin. In these deep partial-thickness or full-thickness burns, definitive surgical closure of the wound with skin grafting prevents

Table 49.1.   Commonly Used Topical Antimicrobial Agents[a]

	Povidone-Iodine	*Silver Nitrate*	*Silver Sulfadiazine*	*Mafenide Acetate*
Class	Halogen	Heavy metal	Heavy metal/antibiotic	Antibiotic
Microbial spectrum	Gram-negative Gram-positive Fungal Viral Protozoan	Gram-negative Gram-positive Fungal	Gram-negative Gram-positive Fungal (weak)	Gram-negative Gram-positive
Forms	Ointment	0.5% liquid	1% cream	11.1% cream
Advantages	Broad-spectrum Rare resistant organisms	Decreased free water and heat loss No allergic reactions Least toxic	Minimal nursing effort Least pain Minimal eschar penetration	Excellent eschar penetration Excellent Gram-negative activity
Disadvantages	Environmental staining	Environmental staining Substantial nursing effort	Expensive Delays epithelialization	Painful application Expensive Delays epithelialization
Potential complications	Cutaneous hypersensitivity Hyperthyroidism	Argyria Hyponatremia Hypochloremia Methemoglobinemia	Argyria Cutaneous hypersensitivity Methemoglobinemia Granulocytopenia Hyperosmolality Hemolysis in G6PD deficiencies	Cutaneous hypersensitivity Carbonic anhydrase inhibition Methemoglobinemia Erythema multiforme Hemolysis in G6PD deficiencies

[a] None of these agents alone will eradicate established burn wound infections.

infection, relieves pain, and improves long-term cosmetic and functional results when compared with healing by regeneration of epidermal elements overlying a limited residual or absent dermis. Unfortunately, the surgical excision and grafting approach is limited by the availability of donor sites and the concomitant morbidity of pain and scarring associated with donor sites. Newer developing therapies, including biologic, bioartificial, and artificial wound devices, begin to address these limitations with partial success and are discussed in this chapter.

Grease, oil, tar, loose skin, burned clothing, and other wound contaminants should be removed before any topical agent other than cool water is applied. Of the antimicrobial agents available, the most commonly used agents in burn centers in the U.S., along with their advantages, disadvantages, and potential complications, are shown in Table 49.1. Among these agents, two are antiseptic and two are antibiotic agents. The agents differ in their spectrum of antimicrobial activity and method of application, and each has a fundamentally different mode of action. One of these agents, silver nitrate, decreases bacterial and fungal growth on the burn wound, minimizes evaporative free water loss through the burn wound, and can be applied with equal facility to eschar, debrided wounds, donor sites, and freshly grafted wounds. Although silver nitrate stains most everything it contacts, its potential complications occur rarely and are the least toxic and most easily managed of the four commonly used agents. Most importantly, there has been no reported association of silver nitrate with any allergic reactions. Methemoglobinemia is a potentially serious complication, but it has also been reported with silver sulfadiazine and mafenide acetate, and it has been rare with any of these drugs. Argyria, which is a brown discoloration of the oral mucosa and the skin resulting from the ingestion of silver, has been reported with silver nitrate; it can be decreased significantly by avoiding application to the face. Argyria is primarily a cosmetic issue, is not known to be otherwise harmful, and has been reported to occur with silver sulfadiazine as well as silver nitrate.

The three additional topical agents frequently used are mafenide acetate (Sulfamylon), silver sulfadiazine (Silvadene, SSD), and povidone-iodine (Betadine). Although povidone-iodine has a broad spectrum of activity, it is the least frequently used of the four agents because severe hypersensitivity reactions can occur. In addition, hyperthyroidism can result when povidone-iodine is used in extensive wounds. Mafenide acetate is the most effective agent against Gram-negative bacteria and penetrates the wound eschar with the greatest efficiency; however, its application in the cream base is extremely painful when applied to wounds that are sensate. The cream base also contains sodium metabisulfite, which can precipitate asthmatic attacks. Its use can promote overgrowth by fungi and antibiotic-resistant Gram-negative and staphylococcal organisms. Since mafenide acetate and its major metabolite are carbonic anhydrase inhibitors, it also causes a metabolic acidosis, particularly when used on extensive wounds. Silver sulfadiazine is probably the most commonly used agent because it is the least painful of these agents and requires the least effort. Unfortunately, its application can result in granulocytopenia or allergic reactions. Both mafenide acetate and silver sulfadiazine may cause hemolysis in patients deficient in glucose-6-phosphate dehydrogenase (G6PD).

TOPICAL ANTIMICROBIAL THERAPY

The development of effective topical antimicrobial agents for use in burn care parallels the development of surgical antiseptics and antibiotics. These agents are categorized by chemical groups to facilitate an understanding of their general mechanisms of action (Table 49.2), with the realization that agents such as silver sulfadiazine may be appropriate for more than one category. The first three categories, astringents and resins, acids and alkalis, and phenols, are mainly of historical interest; however, features of these agents demonstrate important pitfalls to be avoided by an ideal topical agent for a large burn wound. The five remaining categories feature agents that have important roles in the management of burn wounds in the future.

ASTRINGENTS AND RESINS

Astringents and resins are among the oldest forms of topical burn care. Their use began as early as 500 BC, when tea was used as an ancient Chinese remedy (1). Other examples of astringents and resins include myrrh, zinc oxides, and tannic acid. These agents are not directly antimicrobial; however, they do decrease fluid loss from the wound, shrink edematous tissues, close off dilated blood vessels, and create a protective coagulated protein film that provides an external physical barrier and allows the wound to heal undisturbed. Astringents and resins are the active ingredients in many folk remedies; however, it is difficult to evaluate most home remedies because the composition and active components are not well-known and the impurities have not been well-controlled.

Tannic acid is an example of an astringent. Tannic acid occurs widely in nature, chiefly in the bark and woody parts of plants, and is a major component of tea leaves. It is an internal polyester, made up of 10 molecules of gallic acid (3,4,5-trihydroxybenzoic acid) and one molecule of glucose. When used on burns, as in the 1920s and 1930s, it produced a thick, hard eschar that decreased fluid losses and was intended to precipitate the proteins of the degrading wound, preventing systemic absorption of these toxins and protecting the wound from bacterial invasions while it healed (2). Unfortunately, however, absorption of the drug occurred over large areas of open wound and caused massive centrilobular necrosis of the liver (3). Furthermore, the development of a thick, tanned eschar over an infected wound bed enclosed the infection within the wound, promoted the bacterial invasion, and guaranteed the development of invasive systemic sepsis. Mortality from burn wound infections was particularly common when tannic acid was used; therefore, tannic acid is no longer recommended for burned patients.

ACIDS AND ALKALIS

Organic and inorganic acids can each have antiseptic properties. Boric acid is an example of a simple inorganic acid that has weak germicidal potency and yet does not irritate or devitalize tissues. However, boric acid has important disadvantages in that it inhibits phagocytosis in concentrations greater than 2% and can be absorbed systemically through burned skin, resulting in severe systemic toxicities and death (4).

Organic acids also have antiseptic properties, but the effect of increasing hydrogen ion concentration is probably not critical to the germicidal activities above the pH of 2.6. In this pH region, the undissociated molecule contributes to the germicidal action; this effect increases with molecular weight and by the introduction of a hydroxyl group (4).

Sour wines, vinegar (acetic acid), nalidixic acid, and salicylic acid are examples of organic acids used in burn care.

Table 49.2. Chemical Classes and Examples of Antimicrobial Agents

Astringents/Resins	*Acids/Alkalis*	*Phenols*
Tannic acid	Boric acid	Picric acid
Myrrh	Nalidixic acid	
Zinc oxide	Wood ash leaching	
Halogens	Heavy metals	Rare earth elements
Iodine	Silver	Cerium
Povidone-iodine	Silver nitrate	Cerium nitrate
	Silver sulfadiazine	Cerium sulfadiazine
Chlorine	Mercury	
Dakin's solution	Merbromin	
Chlorhexidine	Merthiolate	
Bromine		
Merbromin		
Dyes	Antibiotics	
Scarlet red	Mafenide acetate	
Triple dye therapy	Silver sulfadiazine	
	Gentamicin	
	Mupirocin	
	Nalidixic acid	
	Neosporin	
	Bacitracin	

Nalidixic acid analogues (pefloxacin) have been used in combination with other topical therapies and may be effective therapy in the case of colonization with resistant *Pseudomonas* (5). Alkalis have only weak antiseptic properties and are rarely used. Wood ash leachings provide the sole example.

PHENOLS

Picric acid (2,4,6-trinitrophenol), a phenol analog, has been used in burn therapy because as a 1% solution, it exerts antibacterial and local anesthetic actions; however, systemic absorption can occur. Absorption occurs particularly when it is used on large surface areas and can result in hemolytic anemia, liver failure, central nervous system depression, and glomerular nephritis (6).

HALOGENS

Halogens have a high affinity for protoplasm and are highly effective antibacterial agents.

Iodine

Povidone-iodine, one of the most important antiseptics in this class, is an example of a halogen agent (Table 49.1). It is composed of iodine combined with the polymer polyvinylpyrrolidone. The most important advantage of povidone-iodine is its highly effective toxicity against bacteria, fungi, amebae, and viruses. Povidone-iodine has the broadest spectrum of activity of any antiseptic agent, and its potency kills bacteria in vitro within 15 to 30 seconds. Even so, it is ineffective in eradicating an established infection in a burn wound because it penetrates thick eschar very poorly. Serious allergic and idiosyncratic reactions can occur, including fever and generalized skin eruptions (7). Induction of hyperthyroidism has been associated with the use of povidone-iodine on large burn wounds, despite the slow release of iodine from the polyvinyl-pyrrolidone complex into the large open wounds (8). Other disadvantages include: (*a*) it stains everything it contacts; (*b*) pain is elicited during its application; and (*c*) in higher concentrations, it tends toward cytotoxicity to the regenerating tissue elements (9). The use of povidone-iodine to treat burn wounds has been largely abandoned in most burn centers except in limited and very specific instances.

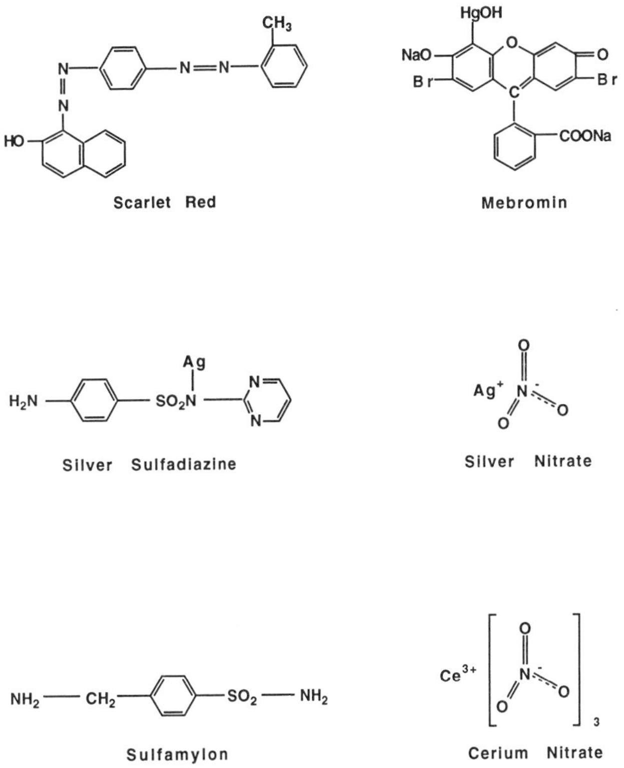

Chlorine

Chlorine is also a highly effective antimicrobial agent that comes in two main forms, Dakin's solution and chlorhexidine. It kills bacteria at 0.0002% concentration by inhibiting enzymes, including those enzymes involved in glucose oxidation and enzymes containing sulfhydryl groups (4).

Dakin's solution, freshly prepared at a full strength of 0.5% sodium hypochlorite in water, has germicidal and cytotoxic activities dependent on concentration (10). At 0.0125% (1/40 strength), Dakin's solution is bactericidal to Gram-positive but not Gram-negative organisms. Between 0.25% and 0.025% NaOCl (1/2 and 1/20 strengths), it is bactericidal to Gram-positive and Gram-negative bacteria as tested in vitro to *Escherichia coli, Pseudomonas aeruginosa, Enterobacter cloacae, Staphylococcus aureus, S. epidermidis,* and *Enterococcus faecalis.* Unfortunately, it is cytotoxic in vitro to fibroblasts at 0.25% or higher concentrations. Therefore, the clinically useful treatment concentration range is between 0.025% and 0.125% solution (1/20 to 1/4 strengths). The disadvantages of Dakin's solution are important and include (*a*) instability in solution, (*b*) skin irritation, (*c*) cytotoxicity to fibroblasts at increased concentrations, and, interestingly, (*d*) interference with thrombin formation and possible dissolution of clots. This latter feature may play a possible role in the decreased "take" of skin grafts secondary to an inhibition of the fibrin glue that is considered critical to stabilize grafts during the first 72 hours after operation (11).

Chlorhexidine (0.2% chlorhexidine digluconate) is commonly used in Canadian burn centers in combination with silver sulfadiazine (12). The addition of chlorhexidine may improve the overall activity of silver sulfadiazine against *S. aureus.* More concentrated chlorhexidine (4%, Hibiclens) can be applied directly to the wound by scrubbing the wound with a sponge saturated with 4% chlorhexidine.

Bromine

Mebromin (Fig. 49.1) contains both the halogen bromine and the heavy metal mercury. It is discussed in the next section of this chapter.

HEAVY METALS

Heavy metals such as mercury and silver have been useful in the treatment of burns because the salts of heavy metals are highly toxic to bacteria and fungi. The metallic ion combines with certain ionogenic groups ($-SH$) on protein surfaces and destroys the normal proteins' activities (4). The ability of extremely minute quantities of metals to kill bacteria is known as their oligodynamic action and may represent quantities as little as 10^{-3} to 10^{-6} mg per liter of silver. Arsenic and mercury

Figure 49.1. Chemical structures of some commonly used topical antimicrobial agents.

are also effective to a similar extent; however, their toxicity to humans is well-known. To a far lesser extent, copper, nickel, and cobalt are also germicidal.

Silver

The antiseptic activity of atomic silver and its soluble salts is very dramatic and prolonged; therefore, silver therapy, in its many forms, is currently widely used in modern burn care. Atomic silver and silver complexes, including silver proteinates and silver oxide, are formed on the wound surface and are bacteriostatic in low concentrations and bactericidal in higher ones. The atomic form of silver that is required for in vivo bacteriostasis remains unknown. Moyer, in his original description of silver nitrate in burn patients, reported in vitro bacteriostatic activity against both *S. aureus* and *P. aeruginosa* by $AgNO_3$, $AgCl$, Ag_2O, $Ag_3C_6H_5O_7$, $AgC_2H_3O_2$, silver proteinates, and colloidal silver (13). Moyer anticipated that $AgNO_3$, $AgCl$, Ag^+, $(AgCl)Ag^+$, and $NaAgCl$ might also be involved in the in vivo bacteriostasis of silver nitrate on burn wounds. One mechanism for bacterial toxicity proposed by recent investigators working with silver sulfadiazine is that the silver ion replaces the hydrogen ion involved in the cross-linking of the DNA double helix (14).

Silver has a broad spectrum of antimicrobial activity; however, determinations of in vivo sensitivities of bacteria to various topical agents containing silver have been hampered by the ability to predict reliably the outcome of in vivo action by an in vitro assay. Minimal inhibitory concentration (MIC) predicts the clinical outcome in only 72% of cases, whereas Nathan's agar well diffusion test (NAWD) is more accurate

(15). Studies of both silver nitrate and silver sulfadiazine sensitivities in vitro have also been complicated by the precipitation of the silver complex with saline and other ingredients in the gels. Fortunately, however, bacterial resistance to the activities of silver has been rare. There are a few reports of organisms resistant to silver; these species include particular strains of *Pseudomonas, Klebsiella, Enterobacter,* and *Providencia* (16–18). Interpreting these reports is difficult because the investigators must satisfactorily eliminate the possibility of cross-contamination and reinfection by the same organism. In studies of silver sulfadiazine, the resistance to the sulfadiazine component can be transmitted via a plasmid, and resistance to the silver component has been shown to be unstable on passage in culture (19).

Silver is relatively nontoxic and generally is not absorbed in substantial quantities through the burn wound; however, the exact amount of silver that is actually absorbed systematically remains controversial. Radiolabeled silver applied as liquid nitrate remains mostly in the eschar, and in at least one study, the radiolabeled silver was not detectable in other organs such as liver or spleen (20). On the other hand, silver levels were mildly increased in the urine of burn patients treated with silver sulfadiazine (21), and organ deposition of silver has been noted on autopsy examinations (22) and in body fluids (13) of burn patients treated with silver nitrate. Argyria, or a bronze discoloration of the skin and mucous membranes, can occur, usually with the chronic ingestion of liquid silver nitrate applied around the mouth. Although possible, ingestion is less likely to occur with silver sulfadiazine in the cream base, although one study using silver sulfadiazine in a 10% cream reported a significant frequency of argyria (23). A toxicity concern, on a theoretic basis, is that chronically increased silver levels may interfere with the function of selenium; however, the clinical relevance of this concern is unknown (24). Selenium is necessary for glutathione peroxidase, an enzyme that takes part in the cellular antioxidant enzyme defense system.

Multiple attempts have been made to deliver the silver molecule to the wound. Silver lactate (25) and silver kaolin (26) administration have been attempted, with no great improvement over current practices. Synthetic and biologic substances have been complexed with silver with the intent of producing a slow delivery of silver to the wound (27). It has been hypothesized that complexing silver with the sulfadiazine molecule does, in fact, simply create a better vehicle for the delivery of silver to the wound via an organic base (19). Silver nitrate and silver sulfadiazine remain the most commonly used topical silver agents in burn care. Silver sulfadiazine is discussed in the section of this chapter entitled "Antibiotics."

Silver Nitrate

Silver nitrate (Fig. 49.1) (0.5% in aqueous solution, 29.4 mEq Ag⁺/liter) is useful for the prophylaxis of burn wound infection (Table 49.1). Because it precipitates on the surface of the wound and does not penetrate the eschar, it has no efficacy in the treatment of an established invasive burn wound infection. It is, however, highly effective in suppressing wound colonization. It has a broad spectrum of activity against Gram-negative bacteria, Gram-positive bacteria, and yeast.

Resistance, as discussed above, is rare. The clear, colorless solution is applied to thick gauze (six to eight layers of four-ply gauze) covering the wound as a wet dressing. The solution is applied in excess every 2 hours to maintain a concentration of silver nitrate of 0.5% at the level of the wound. The dressings may be changed two or three times daily. It is relatively inexpensive, readily available, and easy to use, although it does require substantial nursing effort. It stains everything that it contacts black; however, this staining can be removed by washing with polyethoxy-polypropoxy-ethanol-iodine (Wescodyne) and hot soapy water prior to prolonged exposure to light. It can be removed from skin with lanolin.

The application of silver nitrate is associated with no discomfort to the patient; however, patients with reepithelializing wounds may experience brief periods of discomfort after application of the solution. The application of this thick, wet dressing to the burn patient, followed by a warm, dry blanket, decreases fluid loss through the wound, reduces evaporative heat and water loss, and potentially decreases the metabolic demands on the patient (13, 28).

Silver nitrate solution is hypotonic. Failure to recognize this feature and to replace sodium losses adequately can result in hyponatremia. Burke et al (29) measured sodium transit across burn wounds treated with silver nitrate solution in patients with burns covering more than 15% of the total burn surface area and reported that sodium effluxes ranged from 190 to 920 mEq/m²/day; infections of the wound may result in even higher sodium losses. Administration of 350 mEq/m² open area/day of sodium chloride above normal maintenance prevents sudden derangements in serum sodium. In addition, with ion exchange between Ag^+ cation and Cl^-, HCO_3^-, CO_3^-, and protein anions at the wound surface, relatively insoluble silver salts are formed, which tend to deplete the body of anions relatively more than cations (30). Jelenko and Anderson studied ion selection by the burn eschar and suggested that the eschar acts as a passive dialysis membrane in the presence of hypotonic silver nitrate solutions (31). Therefore, electrolytes should be monitored closely when silver nitrate is used on large burn surfaces to ensure adequate replacement. More specifically, resuscitation formulas that involve the administration of free water during the second 24 hours should be modified to account for the electrolyte changes caused by silver nitrate as well as for the decreased free water loss.

Methemoglobinemia, which is hemoglobin oxidized from the ferrous to ferric state, results from the conversion of nitrates to nitrites in the burned surfaces and can be associated with the use of silver nitrate (32, 33). In small amounts, methemoglobin causes cyanosis, and if the concentration of methemoglobin exceeds 60% of the available hemoglobin, cardiovascular collapse and circulatory arrest can result. Administration of 1% methylene blue dye solution (1 mg/kg up to 7 mg/kg) can reverse these effects. Methemoglobinemia has also been reported with both silver sulfadiazine and mafenide acetate, as sulfonamides can also cause the oxidation of hemoglobin (34).

Allowing the dressing to dry out or allowing the fluid to collect and evaporate (such as in the heel of a posterior ankle splint or underneath a stitch under tension) may cause the concentration of the solution locally to increase substantially above 0.5%, which places the patient at risk for localized necrobiosis. Moyer et al, in their original description of 0.5%

silver nitrate therapy, noted that use of 1% silver nitrate solutions interfered with epithelialization and healing of grafts. Silver nitrate, however, is not toxic to regenerating epithelial cells in vivo at 0.5% solution concentration (13). Scapicchio et al (35) reported on epidermal regeneration under application of silver nitrate and mafenide acetate. Full-thickness defects on the inner surfaces of the ears of white male rabbits were created and treated with saline, silver nitrate, or mafenide acetate. The defects treated with silver nitrate epithelialized comparable to the controls, whereas wounds treated with mafenide acetate showed significant delays in the rate of epithelialization. Similar effects were seen on donor site healing (36).

Mercury

Mercury is another example of a heavy metal used for its antiseptic activity. Merbromin (Mercurochrome; see Fig. 49.1) was introduced in 1919 and was the first organic mercurial to be used. It has weak antiseptic properties and penetrates eschars poorly, and its activity is greatly influenced by pH and the presence of organic matter. When it is used on large wounds, sufficient absorption of mercury causes systemic toxicity. Thimerosal (Merthiolate) is a white crystalline solid that contains about 49% mercury in an organic combination. It is used in an aqueous or an alcohol-acetone-water solution colored with eosin and is an effective, safe antiseptic for small open wounds. It is incompatible with acids, heavy metal salts, and iodine and should not be used at the same time as other common topical agents (4).

RARE EARTH ELEMENTS: LANTHANIDE SERIES

Elements of the lanthanide series have long been known to have antimicrobial activity in vitro to both bacteria and fungi, and their utility in clinical situations is currently under investigation (37–45). Cerium nitrate (Fig. 49.1) and cerium sulfadiazine as well as cerium nitrate-silver sulfadiazine combinations are currently under investigation.

Cerium

Cerium nitrate-silver sulfadiazine provides excellent coverage for most Gram-positive and Gram-negative organisms and good antifungal activity, and may be superior to silver sulfadiazine alone. It is provided as a cream, and complications are similar to those of silver sulfadiazine. Munster et al reported a prospective, randomized trial that demonstrated no difference in mortality rates between burn patients treated with cerium nitrate-silver sulfadiazine cream and those treated only with silver sulfadiazine (41). However, in their study, the density of the colonizing bacteria was reduced. Another study (42) has also shown improved control of bacterial levels with this combination. However, Bowser et al (44) reported the opposite result in a study of children that showed a significantly greater percentage of Gram-negative pathogens in patients treated with the cerium mixture. Peterson and co-workers showed that the treatment of burned mice with cerium nitrate alone or in combination with silver sulfadiazine prevented postburn alterations in cell-mediated immunity (37). Fox et al reported a predominance of Gram-positive

bacteria in patients treated with cerium nitrate (45). Trivalent cerium is oxidized to yellow ceric ions on a wound eschar, changing the color of the eschar to yellow-green. This color change potentially might be mistaken as a wound infection by inexperienced personnel.

DYES

Gentian violet, an aniline dye, was found by Aldrich in 1933 to be effective in the in vitro killing of streptococci. He subsequently reported a reduction in burn wound mortality and ushered in the era of modern topical therapy of burn wounds (46). Unfortunately, promptly thereafter, bacterial resistance was reported (47). Brilliant green, acriviolet, and acriflavine were the three components of triple dye therapy that he introduced later to circumvent drug resistance. Triple dye therapy was the contemporary topical agent undergoing trials at the time of the Coconut Grove fire in 1942 in Boston (48). The dye therapy-induced improvement in outcome over treatment with tannic acids made the use of tannic acids obsolete. Unfortunately, the antibacterial action of the dyes is, in general, feeble and insufficient for the prevention of infection in burn wounds. Of the dyes, only scarlet red (*o*-tolylazo-*o*-tolylazo-β-naphthol) (Fig. 49.1) is currently in use, because it stimulates tissue proliferation and improves wound healing in donor sites and not because it has weak antibacterial activity.

In 1935, the red dye Prontosil (sulfachrysoidine) was found by Dogmagk to be highly active against bacteria in vivo although ineffective in the test tube. This drug was the first synthetic antibacterial agent reported. The active component, sulfanilamide, was finally isolated from the red urine of patients treated with Prontosil. This was the result of the in vivo cleavage of the complex red dye's azo ($-N=N-$) linkage between two aromatic compounds. Thereafter, chemists synthesized many sulfanilamide derivatives, including sulfadiazine, all of which are active both in vitro and in vivo. Dogmagk later synthesized sulfamylon (49).

ANTIBIOTICS

The use of antibiotics topically has the certain advantage that the antibiotic can be applied directly to the wound and therefore does not rely upon biodistribution to deliver the drug to the site in concentrations high enough for antibacterial activity. Therefore, local factors are less important, including blockade of the microcirculation by coagulation after thermal trauma, inflammatory edema, or tissue ischemia that would otherwise prevent transfer of the drug from the blood to the wound and decrease the effective concentration at the wound site. In addition, high molecular weight antimicrobial agents that are poorly soluble are more effective when applied topically and are less readily absorbed. Drugs are more readily absorbed from partial-thickness burns than from unexcised full-thickness burns because of the physical barrier of the dead tissue. The major disadvantage of topical antibiotics, as described by Aldrich, is the development of resistant organisms (46, 47).

Sulfamylon

Sulfamylon (mafenide) is 4-amino-methyl-benzene-sulfon-amide (Fig. 49.1). It is available in the chloride or acetate form. Mafenide acetate (Table 49.1) is sulfamylon 11.1% in a water-soluble suspension (cream). The actual mechanism of its antimicrobial action is not known. Initially, it was expected to have a mechanism similar to that of sulfonamides, but apparently that is not the case. Sulphonamides are structural analogues of *para*-aminobenzoic acid (PABA) and compete with PABA for the same binding site on dihydropteroate synthase. It was expected that mafenide, similar to sulfonamides in structure, would interfere directly with the synthesis of dihydropteroic acid, a precursor of tetrahydrofolic acid, which is the co-enzyme form of folic acid. However, the inhibitory action of mafenide is not antagonized by PABA, serum, pus, or tissue exudates. Furthermore, there is no correlation of bacterial sensitivities between mafenide and sulfon-amides (50).

Mafenide penetrates the wound eschar and is absorbed systematically and readily metabolized to an inactive acid salt that is excreted through the kidneys. The active component of the drug is deaminated shortly after systemic absorption and rendered inactive against bacteria (51). The absorption through the burn wound is rapid and results in depletion of the compound in the wound below effective antibacterial levels within 8 to 10 hours (52). Therefore, application of mafenide is recommended twice daily; more frequent applications can result in systemic toxicity. It is applied in a thin layer and covered with a single layer of gauze dressing or treated openly. Some centers also use a 5% slurry that is applied as a solution over thick dressings (53).

Mafenide acetate provides excellent coverage for Gram-negative and Gram-positive bacteria. It is bacteriostatic at the concentrations available clinically, yet much higher concentrations are bactericidal. It is especially effective against *P. aeruginosa* and *Clostridia* and has only limited activity against some *S. aureus*, particularly the methicillin-resistant strains. It has minimal activity against fungi. Resistance of Gram-negative organisms is rare. The combination of topical antibiotics with topical nystatin has led to important progress in the prevention of fungal wound overgrowth (54).

There are certain disadvantages to the use of mafenide acetate. It is supplied in a carrier cream containing sodium metabisulfite, which can cause allergic reactions, including anaphylaxis, and life-threatening or less severe episodes of asthmatic reactions, particularly in asthmatic patients (55). It has been associated with erythema multiforme and cutaneous reactions. The frequency of maculopapular rash associated with the use of mafenide has been reported to range from 10 to 50%, but treatment with antihistamines and continuation of the drug are usually recommended (56–59). Mafenide is painful on application, and the pain is considered to be related to its hypertonicity. The cream (11.2% mafenide acetate, os-molality 2,180 mOsm/kg) is composed of a base agent (1080 mOsm/kg) and the mafenide acetate (1065 mOsm/kg). The 5% solution, which is less hypertonic, is considered less painful (60). Pain relief occurs 20 to 30 minutes after application and correlates with the depletion of mafenide in the cream layer closest to the skin.

Methemoglobinemia (34) and carbonic anhydrase inhibition (61) have been associated with mafenide acetate. The carbonic anhydrase inhibition is particularly common in patients with renal failure. Both mafenide acetate and its primary metabolite, *para*-carboxybenzene sulfonamide, are potent carbonic anhydrase inhibitors. Application results in increased $PACO_2$, tissue and plasma CO_2, and acidosis, despite relatively high minute alveolar ventilation. Fortunately, treatment can be specific because both drug and metabolite are removed easily by dialysis. Because of its carbonic anhydrase effects and the osmotic effects of the breakdown products, an osmotic diuresis occurs that may result in hypernatremia in addition to the hyperchloremic metabolic acidosis (61). G6PD-deficiency-associated hemolysis has been reported with mafenide as has previously been reported with sulfonamides (62).

In addition to the excellent Gram-negative coverage and penetration of the eschar, mafenide acetate has other theoretic and practical advantages. The initial adherence of a skin graft to its prepared bed may be a result of fibrin deposition secondary to local coagulation. It is the fibrin bonding of the graft to the wound bed that may be important early after graft placement (14). Sulfamylon demonstrates a potent antifibrinolytic property by competitively inhibiting plasmin through interaction with its lysine site (63). Therefore, mafenide acetate may have at least a theoretic advantage in the prevention of early graft failure. The ability to penetrate the burn eschar is particularly important and is a major advantage in the management of ear burns in which cartilage is at risk for infection (64). It may also, however, cause an allergic reaction simulating chondritis (65).

Jelenko et al (66) and Zawacki et al (67) studied the effects of sulfamylon on water loss through the burn eschar. Sulfamylon reduced water loss over the eschar when compared with un-treated eschar, although not to the levels achieved with silver nitrate wet dressings. The effectiveness of mafenide acetate therapy on the eradication of an established burn wound infection is debatable; however, because of its ability to penetrate the burn wound eschar, the chances of success are considered to be better with this agent than with other agents. Despite the eschar-penetrating property of mafenide acetate, debridement of the wound of devitalized tissue and bacteria-packed granulations remains the standard of care for an established burn wound infection.

Silver Sulfadiazine

Silver sulfadiazine (Table 49.1), introduced by Fox et al (14) in 1969, is currently the most widely used topical agent for the treatment of burn injury. It is available as a 1% suspension in a water-soluble base. It is easily applied as a thin film over the wound and covered with a thin layer of gauze. It is recommended that this agent be applied every 24 to 48 hours and every 24 hours in larger burns. Its application is painless and allows for unrestricted joint motion. The drug reacts with proteinaceous exudates in the wound, and if the silver sulfadiazine is not removed adequately between dressings, a yellow-gray build-up appears that can be confused with a deeper tissue injury. The silver sulfadiazine exudate separates within a few days.

The empiric formula of silver sulfadiazine is shown in Figure 49.1. X-ray diffraction studies suggest, however, an intermolecular association resulting in a polymeric structure composed of six silver atoms bonded to six sulfadiazine molecules by linkage of the silver atoms to the nitrogens of the pyrimidine ring (68). In contrast to silver nitrate, silver sulfadiazine does not react rapidly with chloride, sulfhydryl groups, or protein and therefore allows for the greater availability of the silver ion. Silver sulfadiazine reacts rapidly with DNA and releases sulfadiazine. The silver replaces the hydrogen bonding between strands of DNA and prevents replication (18). In addition, silver sulfadiazine can modify the cell membranes (69). It has moderate penetration into the burn wound eschar, and it is contraindicated in pregnancy.

The low solubility and large molecular size of silver sulfadiazine impair its absorption and facilitate relatively high concentrations in wound exudates. In wound exudates in patients, measurements of sulfadiazine levels 24 hours after topical application were 90 to 100 mg% (more than 1000 times the MIC). Simultaneous blood levels were less than 0.2 to 1.0 mg%, and urine levels were 40 to 60 mg% (14). Harrison, using radiolabeled silver sulfadiazine, demonstrated that 81 to 98.7% of the labeled silver was in the most superficial layers of the rat eschar at 24 hours (70). In patients, the 24-hour urinary excretion of silver appears to be a very sensitive indicator of cutaneous absorption of the drug in burn patients (21).

The drug has an excellent spectrum of antimicrobial action in vitro, including *S. aureus, E. coli, Klebsiella, P. aeruginosa, Proteus, Enterobacteriaceae,* and *Candida albicans.* Resistance to silver sulfadiazine has been demonstrated and may be transmitted within a plasmid that confers resistance to other important antibiotics as well (71). Resistance occurs mainly in Gram-negative organisms such as *P. aeruginosa* and *E. cloacae* (71–73). Combination of the silver sulfadiazine with other agents such as sodium piperacillin may be effective in resistant *Pseudomonas* cases (74). Addition of trimethoprim to silver sulfadiazine has resulted in more resistant organisms, with no prophylactic benefit (75).

Hypersensitivity reactions to silver sulfadiazine are considered infrequent at 1.5%. A maculopapular rash occurs in less than 5% of patients, and withdrawal of the drug is rarely required (76). Neutropenia may occur, presenting as granulocytopenia within the first 5 days after injury; this problem may be accompanied by thrombocytopenia. These abnormalities usually improve (77–81). Others have indicated, however, that this transient decrease in the white blood cell count may be a response to the burn wound itself and unrelated to the use of the drug (82). The incidence of methemoglobinemia is rare (76). Hyperosmolality induced by the propylene glycol carrier of the silver sulfadiazine cream has been reported in an 8-month-old infant (83). Nephrotic syndrome has also been reported to be attributed to silver sulfadiazine therapy (84).

Silver sulfadiazine is toxic to human fibroblasts in culture (85). However, in an animal study, Geronemus et al (86) reported an increase in the rate of reepithelialization of clean wounds with silver sulfadiazine when compared with neosporin and povidone-iodine.

Other Antibiotics

Zinc sulfadiazine is less potent than silver sulfadiazine in vitro but may be better than silver sulfadiazine in burned animals infected with *Pseudomonas* (87). Clinical trials have been limited; however, they suggest that it is very effective in controlling these infections (88). A more recent study (89) suggests that zinc sulfadiazine has a greater activity against *S. aureus* than does silver sulfadiazine.

Gentamicin (0.1% gentamicin sulfate in a cream base) enjoyed a brief period of popularity in the topical treatment of burns in the mid-1960s. Although this agent initially was highly effective, resistant organisms soon developed; therefore, antibiotic resistance became an important problem in its continued use (90). Absorption of the drug through the burn wound did not lead to toxicity in the absence of renal failure.

Other poorly absorbed topical antibiotics have also been used on burn wounds. Neomycin is effective against staphylococci, and bacitracin has been useful for streptococci. Polymyxin B is useful for most Gram-negative organisms except *Proteus* and *Serratia* (4). Nitrofurazone is bactericidal for many Gram-negative and Gram-positive organisms, but *Pseudomonas* and *Proteus* are often resistant (4). The main disadvantage of the topical antibiotics is that after the elimination of one bacterium, a second organism, which is often worse than the first one, overgrows and dominates the wound flora.

One notable exception, mupirocin, is a new antistaphylococcal drug. Often, with long-term treatment of seriously burned patients with silver nitrate, silver sulfadiazine, or mafenide acetate, small remaining open areas become colonized and infected with *S. aureus,* which may be resistant to methicillin and many other Gram-positive antibiotics. This problem usually presents as a gradually expanding wound within previously grafted skin. These patients may have positive blood cultures and intermittent fevers and often have greatly increased lengths of hospital stay. Mupirocin, derived from *P. fluorescens,* inhibits protein synthesis by binding irreversibly to bacterial isoleucyl transfer RNA synthetase (91). It has been highly effective in eradicating burn wound infections from multiply resistant *S. aureus* (92). Its major problem, poor activity toward *Pseudomonas,* could lead to overgrowth of the wound by this organism with continued use; therefore, mupirocin is not recommended early in the treatment of large burns. Also, when mupirocin is applied to large surface areas, the carrier substance, polyethylene glycol, can be absorbed and lead to osmolality problems (93).

TOPICAL WOUND MANAGEMENT

WOUND DEBRIDEMENT

Surgical Excision

The advent of effective topical antibacterial agents revolutionized burn care; however, their control of burn wound sepsis is not complete. The technique of primary excision and grafting was carefully evaluated by Cope et al prior to 1950 (94) and was rejected as routine therapy because of the physiologic and bacterial problems that were associated with the primary excision. Development of effective topical agents allowed for the successes of later studies with this therapy (95–97), and primary excision and grafting is now accepted as the treatment of choice in most burn centers. Surgical excision of the burn wound, either tangentially (removal of the eschar in sequential thin layers until viable tissue is identified) or fascially (removal of eschar and fat in toto down to the fascial layer) removes the persistent stimulus of dead tissue and, in an infected wound, drains the abscess. Excisional treatment in combination with intravenous antibiotics is the only effective therapy available for management of infected burn wounds.

Early (primary) excision and closure of the wound with autologous split-thickness skin grafts accomplishes all the goals mentioned earlier in this chapter more completely than does any topical agent (95). Primary excision and closure of the wound reduces mortality, restores the natural barriers to infection, relieves pain, allows for an improved cosmetic result, and decreases hospital stay (95–97). Disadvantages include the necessity of donor sites, physiologic stresses, and blood loss associated with a major surgical procedure and the risks of graft failure. Fascial excision minimizes length of anesthesia, blood loss, and the risk of graft failure secondary to inadequately excised dead tissue, or graft failure secondary to problems associated with securing a graft onto poorly vascularized, poorly stabilized fat. Despite the cosmetic defect, accentuated in obesity, fascial excision remains the operation of choice in a severely burned critically ill patient where graft failure or invasive infection compromises survival. A properly performed tangential or sequential excision with autografting improves the cosmetic and often the functional outcome of the resulting scar, and this approach is the procedure of choice when the patient's mortality is not at issue (98).

Dressing Debridement

Debridement of the wound with gauze dressings remains a mainstay in the topical therapy of burn wounds. Gauze allows for debriding action by trapping proteinaceous debris and bacteria and removing them from the wound. Changing the dressing more frequently can be helpful in the treatment of invasive infections when all other measures, including surgical excision, have failed to relieve the infection. This debridement facilitates the effects of intravenous antibiotics. Dressing changes are painful and should be accompanied by adequate pain medication.

Hydrotherapy

Hubbard tanks and whirlpool immersion should be considered obsolete in modern burn care. Popular as a debridement measure in the 1970s, particularly for partial-thickness burns, the tubs were responsible for serious outbreaks of *Pseudomonas* and other resistant organisms from cross-infections, which would spread insidiously through entire wards of patients (99). The use of disposable sterile liners in the tubs has decreased the frequency of outbreaks in some centers but does not protect the patient against bacteria and fungi borne by the local water supply or from rapid colonization of all wound surfaces with organisms from the patient's own perineal or other area. Immersion in the tub is extremely painful, and similar debriding activity can be accomplished more safely and humanely in an operating room environment under general anesthesia.

Enzymatic Debriding Agents

Enzymatic debriding agents were popular in the 1970s; however, an ideal agent is not yet available. This therapy involves the application of pharmaceutical enzymes that digest the dead tissue of the eschar. Often, this therapy involves cross-hatching or scoring of the eschar to allow penetration of the agent into the eschar to the vital tissue-eschar interface. It has often been used in combination with tubing or frequent dressing debridements. The use of enzymatic agents on the face can cause conjunctivitis; its use near major nerves, tendons, or communications with body cavities is contraindicated. Enzymatic agents have been reported to increase fluid losses, especially if applied to more than 20% of the body surface area at one time (100), and their use is not recommended in pregnancy. Travase, the most popular agent, is usually applied on the day of admission at the time of the initial dressing and is applied daily for 4 to 6 days. Many agents, including iodine and hexachlorophene, may interfere with its enzymatic action. Side effects including transient burning pain, paresthesias, and dermatitis; bleeding from previously thrombosed capillaries can occur. Zawacki showed in animals that enzyme therapy destroys skin epithelium that otherwise might have survived (101). Although some have reported success with the use of this therapy when it is used in combination with a topical antimicrobial agent such as silver sulfadiazine (100), the incorporation of sulfamylon or silver sulfadiazine did not protect against burn wound sepsis and death in an experimental burn wound infection model (102).

WOUND CLOSURE

Autografts

Once the wound bed is prepared either by surgical excision or other proper debridement methods, immediate and definitive closure of the burn wound with split-thickness skin grafts is most appropriate and highly desirable. Immediate wound closure reduces the level of physiologic stress, relieves pain in sensate wounds, and reduces the risk of infection. In patients with burns that cover more than 30% of the body surface area, these grafts should be thin to allow healing of the donor sites for repeated harvesting as necessary. The autograft may be meshed 2 : 1 or 3 : 1 to allow for egress of tissue fluid and to cover a larger area of the burn wound. In the seriously injured patient (>90% total body surface area burned (TBSA)), in whom total donor sites may include only the posterior scalp, axillary patches, and groin area, harvested skin may be expanded as much as 6 : 1 or 9 : 1. In patients with less severe injuries, wounds can and should be grafted with an unmeshed sheet of skin to provide superior functional and cosmetic results.

Graft failures usually occur for four reasons, which include wound infections, inadequate excision of the burn eschar, early mechanical sheer forces that have disrupted the placement of the graft during the first few days of attachment, or poor vascularity of the wound bed. Poor nutritional status or systemic illnesses such as cancer or diabetes mellitus, as well as technical problems with the handling of the autograft, may also account for the occasional graft failure.

Biologic Dressings

Allografts, or skin from living donors and cadavers, are ideal biologic dressings. They reduce heat as well as evaporative water and protein loss through the open wound; prevent desiccation of wounds, thus preserving valuable functional structures such as nerves, vessels, and tendons; and promote granulation tissue angiogenesis (103). When used on partial-thickness wounds, they can limit edema and produce a more organized deposition of collagen in the wound as it heals. They are remarkable in their ability to relieve pain. They promote mobility of the injured area and decrease blood loss associated with debriding dressing changes. Viable allografts, when left on an excised or granulating wound bed, will derive a blood supply from the wound bed (103). Immunologic rejection of the graft may take weeks or months to occur in a patient with a serious injury because of the natural immuno-suppression from the burn itself. Rejection of the vascularized allograft generally occurs piecemeal and is detected clinically by wrinkling of the epidermal layers of the graft followed by blistering and eventual sloughing. It can be treated easily by excision of the allograft and replacement with a split-thickness autograft. There is some evidence that the dermis part of the allograft may be nonimmunogenic (104).

The antibacterial effects of allografts that are replaced frequently in combination with intravenous antibiotics and topical antimicrobials may be the final resort to control a life-threatening invasive infection once the burn eschar is removed (98). Allografts are often useful in testing the readiness of a wound bed for staging a major excision and grafting operations, and they are particularly useful for temporary wound closure in the very young or elderly patient or patients with a severe medical illness such as a new myocardial infarction. Transmission of viruses from the allograft to the patient, such as hepatitis or human immunodeficiency virus (HIV), has not been documented but remains a serious theoretic concern (105). Meticulous skin banking techniques and protocols are essential to avoid this potential catastrophe.

Xenografts, usually from pigs or dogs, and amnion are less effective but remain important biologic dressings. These grafts attach to the wound by ingrowth of granulation tissue and do not derive a blood supply from the patient (106). Porcine xenograft is readily available in meshed or sheet forms. These grafts are nonviable and are provided sterile commercially, after the collagen has been cross-linked with an aldehyde (E·Z DERM). They are extremely useful in decreasing edema, promoting healing, and reducing pain in partial-thickness injuries. They are also invaluable in the management of patients with extensive toxic epidermal necrolysis (TENS) or Stevens-Johnson's syndrome (107). Xenografts should be removed when they no longer attach, which generally occurs anywhere between 6 hours and 1 week after grafting depending on the patient's previous exposure to the pigskin and the condition of the wound bed.

Particular care must be exercised in the use of biologic dressings. One should avoid the placement of a nonviable biologic dressing over an infected wound bed or the failure to remove these dressings when infection develops. This circumstance creates the equivalent of an undrained abscess and may result in death from invasive sepsis. Health care professionals who are unfamiliar with this technique should be cautious in its use.

Skin Substitutes

Three different approaches to skin replacement have been taken: first, the development of a totally artificial device to mimic the three-dimensional structure and character of dermis; second, the development of culture methods to replace the keratinocytes of epidermis; and third, emergence of a strategy that combines these techniques to create a composite graft material (Fig. 49.2). The totally artificial matrix approach successfully solves the problem of dermal replacement with a permanent solution, whereas the cultured epidermal cell approach addresses the epidermal problem alone. The composite materials hold promise and are currently in the stages of early clinical testing.

Yannas et al reported the first and most successful dermal matrix device (108). This device was constructed out of a bilayer, polymeric membrane that consisted of an upper layer of medical-grade silastic (epidermal layer) and a lower layer (dermal layer) of highly porous cross-linked bovine collagen co-precipitated with shark-derived chondroitin 6-sulfate (a glycosaminoglycan, or GAG). The upper layer of silastic is important in that its porosity is sufficient to control water loss and to prevent invasion of microbes. The lower layer has been designed with pore sizes (20 to 125 μm) that have been optimized to allow the migration of the patient's own endothelial cells and fibroblasts into the matrix. The artificial dermis in effect provides a lattice for the invasion of host cells, which provide vascularization of this "neodermis." This dermal component is required for the success of this product, because it is the dermis that provides mechanical integrity and stability to the skin and that eliminates the host's inflammatory response. Dermis does not generate its normal anatomy during usual wound healing without a template (a collagen-GAG matrix with a three-dimensional structure resembling that of normal dermis). If the fibroblasts that synthesize new connective tissue in a healing open wound could be induced to produce the three-dimensional structure of dermis and not the three-dimensional structure of scar, a tissue could be produced that performed like dermis. The scaffolding is slowly degraded. After 2 weeks and up to 12 weeks, the upper silicone layer is peeled away and a very thin (0.003-inch thickness) epidermal autograft is placed on this neodermis. This stage I product, Integra, is now in the final stages of FDA approval. It may be used in the sheet or meshed form and is placed on the freshly excised wound bed in a manner similar to that used for autografts.

Clinical experience with Integra in burn injuries in an 11-center prospectively randomized trial has been reported (109). The "take" of the Integra was a very acceptable 80%, as compared with 95% for meshed autograft. In these patients, donor sites healed an average of 4 days sooner because they were harvested more superficially at an average of 0.006 inches (0.15 mm), as compared with the usual depth of 0.013 inches (0.33 mm) for standard split-thickness donor skin. At the completion of the study, there was less hypertrophic scarring, and more patients preferred the areas covered with Integra to the control areas with meshed autograft. The conclusion of this multicenter trial was that Integra provided a permanent cover that was at least as satisfactory as that produced by currently available skin grafting techniques, and that it allowed donor grafts that were thinner and donor sites that healed more rapidly.

The use of cultured keratinocytes to close wounds has gained recent attention and involves either the culture of the patient's own epidermal cells using methods described by Green et al (110) or the transplantation of cultured allogenic keratinocytes for wound closure (111). Although these methods generate considerable enthusiasm in the lay and business communities, opinion as to their success is more reserved in the medical and scientific arenas. In 1981, the first reported experience in patients using cultured autologous epidermal cells described two thermally injured patients who received autologous epidermal cell transplantations to very limited body surface areas (112). Two years later, two extensively burned patients, who were also receiving multiple other therapeutic modalities, received transplants of cultured epidermal autografts to an extent that reportedly covered 50% of the body surface area (113). Other reports soon appeared (114). Additional experience with this technology has been reported from Europe (115, 116), Japan (117), and the U.S. (118–124). These studies are summarized in Table 49.3 (125).

Several controversies surround this cultured cell approach. First, the degree of "take" of the cultured epidermal autografts (the efficiency with which the cultured cells adhere and persist in vivo); second, the long-term morphology of the dermal-epidermal junction in the development of normal histologic features of this junction; and third, the long-term cosmetic and functional results. The efficiency of "take" has been reported to vary widely between 0 and 85% in burned patients (Table 49.3) and to be 68% when used in a purely elective circumstance in the excision of congenital hairy nevi (122). Conflicting reports exist concerning the presence and temporal development of normal dermal-epidermal structures, including hemidesmosomes and anchoring fibrils, which are considered necessary for long-term adherence of the cultured cell grafts. In a report by Compton et al (121) in follow-up of 21 pediatric patients with burn injuries, hemidesmosomes and anchoring fibrils were completely reconstituted within 3

to 4 weeks after transplantation. In contrast, Woodley et al reported that in four patients the formation of these same structures remained abnormal (120) and was associated with abnormal keratinocyte differentiation (124). Investigators have recognized that formation of a proper dermal-epidermal junction is not only highly desirable but likely is necessary to develop a pliable and durable long-term result. Further analysis of studies using this skin replacement strategy will be necessary to resolve these issues.

In addition to the application of cultured autologous epidermal cells, in a parallel effort investigators have transplanted cultured allogenic keratinocytes using methods described by Eisinger and co-workers (126) to accelerate wound healing by repopulating the wound with epidermal cells. In initial studies (127), acceleration of healing of partial-thickness wounds was seen; however, in later studies (128), essentially no "take" of these transplanted epidermal cells was found in full-thickness wounds. In later studies in patients with partial-thickness excisions of tattoos (129) and full-thickness wounds in burned patients (130), the transplanted allogenic cells were found not to persist in the wound beyond the first few weeks posttransplantation by using gender chromosomal analysis of the cells remaining in the wound (Table 49.3). Therefore, the beneficial effects of allogenic epidermal cells on the acceleration of partial-thickness wound healing must be dependent upon effects unrelated to the persistence of the transplanted cells within the wound.

The best example of a composite device is a system described by Boyce and Hansbrough (131) that is a modification of the collagen-chondroitin 6-sulfate matrix of Burke and Yannas. This composite is a nonporous surface of collagen and GAG that is laminated to the upper layer of the dermal membrane to provide a nonporous, planar surface. The nonporous

BIOARTIFICIAL MATERIALS

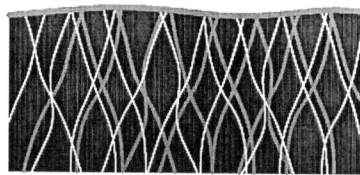

COMPOSITE MATERIALS

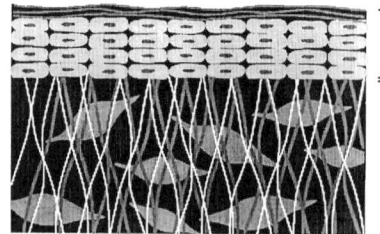

CULTURED EPITHELIAL AUTOGRAFTS

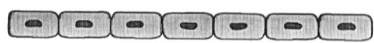

Figure 49.2. Approaches to skin replacement.

Table 49.3.   Cultured Epidermal Cells

Author (Ref. No.)	*Year*	*No. of Patients*	*Comments from Text of Articles*[a]
Autologous epidermal cells			
O'Conner (112)	1981	1	Initial clinical report
Gallico (113)	1984	2	Early clinical studies with extensive coverage
Gallico (114)	1985	5	Additional follow-up study
Pittelkow (118)	1986	1	Use of two-phase culture method
Eldad (115)	1987	25	Combination of allografts and autografts yielding "disappointing results"
Latarjet (116)	1987	2	"Disappointing take"
Herzog (119)	1988	8	No anchoring fibrils; 0–85% "take"
Kamagai (117)	1988	7	Lack of rete ridge and elastin
Woodley (120)	1988	4	"Defective anchoring fibrils"
Compton (121)	1989	21	Normal dermal-epidermal junction
Gallico (122)	1989	8	Fascial excision of giant hairy nevi; 68% "take"
Munster (123)	1990	7	75% "take"
Peterson (124)	1990	3	"Abnormal keratinocyte differentiation"
Allogenic epidermal cells			
Hefton (127)	1983	3	Partial-thickness wounds; accelerated healing
Madden (128)	1986	26	Accelerated healing on partial-thickness; no "take" on full-thickness
Brain (129)	1989	19	Partial-thickness excision of tattoos; last grafts ≤3 weeks
Burt (130)	1989	20	Last grafts ≤1 week

[a] Adapted with permission from Tompkins RG, Burke JF: Burn wound closure using permanent skin replacement materials. *World J Surg* 16:47–52, 1992.

surface is seeded with cultured, proliferating autologous epidermal cells, and the porous dermal collagen-chondroitin 6-sulfate matrix is seeded with proliferating autologous (or potentially allogenic) fibroblasts.

Another composite graft has been described by Bell et al (132) that is a "living skin equivalent" consisting of a gelled collagen matrix that is seeded with cultured fibroblasts and keratinocytes. Although many in vitro and animal studies have investigated the living skin equivalent properties, clinical results of this composite material have not been reported. The composite material is currently available from Organogenesis, Inc. (Cambridge, MA) exclusively for in vitro testing purposes.

Biobrane is a bilaminate temporary wound coverage material that has been used clinically. It consists of collagen and a silastic membrane. The membrane does not become incorporated into the patient's skin via cellular invasion of the collagen layer. Because of the bacteriologically unprotected surface location of skin, the constant exposure to the environment can result in bacterial colonization within the implant and at the interface of the implant and the host tissue. Since host antibacterial defenses usually are defective at the prosthesis-tissue interface, eventual failure from sepsis can be inevitable. Biobrane therefore should be used like xenograft for pain control in superficial second-degree burns (98).

Growth Factors

Once injured, the body responds to repair this injury with a defined order of events. Immediate response to the injury involves formation of thrombi and an increase in the presence of granulocytes and mononuclear cells in the area of the wound. A secondary phase is then entered, which is characterized by the formation of granulation tissue with angiogenesis, collagen production, and fibroblast proliferation. Once the wound is closed, the process of remodeling persists for a prolonged period. Growth hormones have been identified in the wound early in the healing process and are assumed to have a significant role in the mediation of this process. These

peptides are produced by platelets, macrophages, and epidermal and dermal cells. Newly synthesized recombinant growth factors and highly purified natural substances are now available for study. The direct topical application of these substances to burn wounds and donor sites is currently under study in many centers and holds some promise for future therapy.

Preliminary studies using epidermal growth factor, transforming growth factors α and β, insulin-like growth factor I, platelet derived growth factors 1 and 2, and fibroblast growth factors have been reported (133–142). The topical therapy of burn wounds with growth hormones holds modest promise in the future therapy of burns. The long-term benefits and risks of this therapy, including the possibility of metaplasia or neoplasia, must be investigated before these methods are incorporated into the clinician's routine armamentarium.

REFERENCES

1. Pinnegar MD, Pinnegar FC: History of burn care: a survey of important changes in the topical treatment of thermal injuries. *Burns* 12:508–517, 1986.
2. Davidson EC: Tannic acid in the treatment of burns. *Surg Gynecol Obstet* 41:202–221, 1925.
3. Wells DB, Humphrey HD, Coll JJ: The relation of tannic acid to the liver necrosis occurring in burns. *N Engl J Med* 226:626–636, 1942.
4. Oster KA: Chemotherapy of bacterial infections I: antiseptics and germicides. In Drill VA, Dipalma JR (eds): *Pharmacology in Medicine*, ed 4. McGraw-Hill, New York, pp 1631–1656, 1971.
5. Modak S, Stanford J, Friedlaender J, Fox P, Fox CS: Control of burn wound infections by pefloxacin and its silver derivative. *Burns* 10:170–178, 1983.
6. Moncrief JA: The development of topical therapy. *J Trauma* 11:906–910, 1971.
7. Rath T, Meissi G: Induction of hyperthyroidism in burn patients treated topically with povidone-iodine. *Burns* 14:320–322, 1988.
8. Robson MC, Schaerf RHM, Krizek TJ: Evaluation of topical povidone-iodine ointment in experimental burn wound sepsis. *Plast Reconstr Surg* 54:328–334, 1974.
9. Cooper ML, Laxer JA, Hansbrough JF: The cytotoxic effects of commonly used topical antimicrobial agents on human fibroblasts and keratinocytes. *J Trauma* 31:775–784, 1991.
10. Heggers JP, Sazy JA, Stenberg BD, et al. Bactericidal and wound-healing properties of sodium hypochlorite solutions: the 1991 Lindberg award. *J Burn Care Rehabil* 12:420–424, 1991.
11. Teh BT: Why do skin grafts fail? *Plast Reconstr Surg* 63:323–332, 1979.

12. Gray JH, Henry DA, Forbes M, et al: Comparison of silver sulfadiazine 1 per cent, silver sulfadiazine 1 per cent plus chlorhexidine digluconate 0.2 per cent and mafenide acetate 8.5 per cent for topical antibacterial effect in infected full skin thickness rat burn wounds. *Burns* 17:37–40, 1991.

13. Moyer CA, Brentano L, Gravens DL, Margraf HW, Monafo WW Jr: Treatment of large human burns with 0.5% silver nitrate solution. *Arch Surg* 90:812–867, 1965.

14. Fox CL, Rappole BW, Stanford W: Control of *Pseudomonas* infection in burns by silver sulfadiazine. *Surg Gynecol Obstet* 128:1021–1026, 1969.

15. Heggers JP, Velanovich V, Robson MC, et al: Control of burn wound sepsis: a comparison of in vitro topical antimicrobial assays. *J Trauma* 27:176–179, 1987.

16. McHugh GL, Moellering RC, Hopkins CC, Swartz MN: *Salmonella typhimurium* resistant to silver nitrate, chloramphenicol and ampicillin. *Lancet* 1:235–240, 1975.

17. Bridges K, Kidson A, Lowbury EJL, Wilkins MD: Gentamicin- and silver-resistant *Pseudomonas* in a burns unit. *BMJ* 1:446–449, 1979.

18. Monafo WW: Bacteriological studies of burn wounds treated with silver nitrate solution. *J Trauma* 7:99–105, 1967.

19. McManus AT, Denton CL, Mason AD: Mechanisms of in vitro sensitivity to sulfadiazine silver. *Arch Surg* 118:161–166, 1983.

20. Constable JD, Morris PJ, Burke JF: Absorption pattern of silver nitrate from open wounds. *Plast Reconstr Surg* 39:342–348, 1967.

21. Boosalis MG, McCall JT, Ahrenholz DH, Solem LD, McClain CJ: Serum and urinary silver levels in thermal injury patients. *Surgery* 101:40–43, 1987.

22. Bader KF: Organ deposition of silver following silver nitrate therapy of burns. *Plast Reconstr Surg* 37:550–551, 1966.

23. Wang XW, Wang NZ, Zhang OZ, Sapata-Sirvent RL, Davies JWL: Tissue deposition of silver following topical use of silver sulfadiazine in extensive burns. *Burns* 11:197–201, 1985.

24. Boosalis MG, Solem LD, Ahrenholz DH, McCall JT, McClain CJ: Serum and urinary selenium levels in thermal injury. *Burns* 12:236–240, 1986.

25. Hoopes JE, Butcher HR, Margraf HW, Gravens DL: Silver lactate burn cream. *Surgery* 70:29–37, 1971.

26. Linares HA, Fadert RC: Evaluation of topical therapy with silver-kaolin (argostop) in an experimental model of burn wound sepsis. *Burns* 13:281–285, 1987.

27. Deitch EA, Sittig K, Heimbach D, et al: Results of a multicenter outpatient burn study on the safety and efficacy of Dimac-SSD, a new delivery system for silver sulfadiazine. *J Trauma* 29:430–434, 1989.

28. Jelenko C, Buxton RW: The caloric significance of postburn surface water loss. *Surgery* 62:994–999, 1967.

29. Burke JF, Bondoc CC, Morris PJ: Metabolic effects of topical silver nitrate therapy in burns covering more than fifteen percent of the body surface. *Ann NY Acad Sci* 150:674–682, 1968.

30. Polk HC, Tessler RH: Sodium transit across burn wounds treated with silver solution (0.5%). *Ann NY Acad Sci* 150:682–684, 1968.

31. Jelenko C, Anderson AP: Ion selection by burn eschar. *South Med J* 63:1393–1399, 1970.

32. Cushing AH, Smith S: Methemoglobinemia with silver nitrate therapy of a burn: report of a case. *J Pediatr* 74:613–615, 1969.

33. Strauch B, Buch W, Grey W, Laub D: Successful treatment of methemoglobinemia secondary to silver nitrate therapy. *N Engl J Med* 281:257–258, 1969.

34. Ohlgisser M, Adler M, Ben-Dov D, et al: Methaemoglobinaemia induced by mafenide acetate in children. *Br J Anaesth* 50:299–301, 1978.

35. Scapicchio AP, Constable JD, Opitz B: Comparative effects of silver nitrate and sulfamylon acetate on epidermal regeneration. *Plast Reconstr Surg* 41:319–322, 1968.

36. Bellinger CG, Conway H: Effects of silver nitrate and sulfamylon on epithelial regeneration. *Plast Reconstr Surg* 45:582–585, 1979.

37. Peterson VM, Hansbrough JF, Wang XW, Zapata-Sirvent R, Boswick JA: Topical cerium nitrate prevents postburn immunosuppression. *J Trauma* 25:1039–1044, 1985.

38. Wassermann D, Schlotterer M, Lebreton F, Levy J, Guelfi MC: Use of topically applied silver sulfadiazine plus cerium nitrate in major burns. *Burns* 15:257–260, 1989.

39. Boeckx W, Focquet M, Cornelissen M, Nuttin B: Bacteriological effect of cerium-flamazine cream in major burns. *Burns* 11:337–342, 1985.

40. Helvig EI, Munster AM, Su Ct, Oppel W: Cerium nitrate-silver sulfadiazine cream in the treatment of burns: a prospective, randomized study. *Am Surg* 45:270–272, 1979.

41. Munster AM, Helvig E, Rowland S: Cerium nitrate-silver sulfadiazine cream in the treatment of burns: a prospective evaluation. *Surgery* 88:658–660, 1980.

42. Herman RP: Topical treatment of serious infections with special reference to the use of a mixture of silver sulphadiazine and cerium nitrate: two clinical studies. *Burns* 11:59–62, 1984.

43. Monafo WW, Tandon SN, Ayvazian VH, et al: Cerium nitrate: a new topical antiseptic for extensive burns. *Surgery* 80:465–473, 1976.

44. Bowser BH, Caldwell FT, Cone JB, Eisenach KD, Thompson CH: A prospective analysis of silver sulfadiazine with and without cerium nitrate as a topical agent in the treatment of severely burned children. *J Trauma* 21:558–563, 1981.

45. Fox CL, Monafo WW, Ayvazian VH, et al: Topical chemotherapy for burns using cerium salts and silver sulfadiazine. *Surg Gynecol Obstet* 144:668–672, 1977.

46. Aldrich RH: The role of infection in burns: the theory and treatment with special reference to gentian violet. *N Engl J Med* 208:299–309, 1933.

47. Aldrich RH: Treatment of burns with a compound of aniline dyes. *N Engl J Med* 217:911–914, 1937.

48. Clowes GHA, Lund CC, Levenson SM: The surface treatment of burns: a comparison of results of tannic acid, silver nitrate, triple dye, and Vaseline or boric ointment as surface treatments in 150 cases. *Ann Surg* 118:761–779, 1943.

49. Fox CL: Topical therapy and the development of silver sulfadiazine. *Surg Gynecol Obstet* 157:82–88, 1983.

50. Eagon RG, McManus AT: The effect of mafenide on dihydropteroate synthase. *J Antimicrob Chemother* 25:25–29, 1990.

51. White MG, Asch MJ: Acid-base effects of topical mafenide acetate in the burned patient. *N Engl J Med* 284:1281–1286, 1971.

52. Harrison H, Blackmore W, Bales H, et al: The absorption of ^{14}C labelled sulfamylon acetate through burned skin. *J Trauma* 12:986–993, 1972.

53. Shuck JM, Thorne LW, Cooper G: Mafenide acetate solution dressings: an adjunct in burn wound care. *J Trauma* 15:595–599, 1975.

54. Heggers JP, Robson MC, Herndon DN, Desai MH: The efficacy of nystatin combined with topical microbial agents in the treatment of burn wound sepsis. *J Burn Care Rehabil* 10:508–511, 1989.

55. Mathison DA, Stevenson DD, Simon RA: Precipitating factors in asthma: aspirin, sulfites, and other drugs and chemicals. *Chest* 871(suppl):505–545, 1985.

56. Yaffee HS, Dressler DP: Topical application of mafenide acetate: its association with erythema multiforme and cutaneous reactions. *Arch Dermatol* 100:277–281, 1969.

57. Bandmann HJ, Breit R: Contact dermatitis XXIII: the mafenide story. *Br J Dermatol* 89:219–221, 1973.

58. Velasco JE, Africk JA: Contact dermatitis to mafenide acetate. *Arch Dermatol* 103:61–63, 1971.

59. Shuck JM, Moncrief JA: Safeguards in the use of topical mafenide (sulfamylon) in burned patients. *Am J Surg* 118:864–870, 1969.

60. Harrison HN, Shuck JM, Caldwell E: Studies of the pain produced by mafenide acetate preparation in burns. *Arch Surg* 110:1446, 1975.

61. Asch MJ, White MG, Pruitt BA: Acid-base changes associated with topical sulfamylon therapy. *Ann Surg* 172:946–950, 1970.

62. Marsicano AR, Hutton JJ, Bryant WM: Fatal hemolysis from mafenide treatment of burns in a patient with glucose-6-phosphate dehydrogenase deficiency. *Plast Reconstr Surg* 52:197–199, 1973.

63. Weisdorf DJ, Aldridge JH: Mafenide (sulfamylon) inhibits plasmin fibrinolytic activity. *Thromb Haemost* 59:440–444, 1988.

64. Purdue GF, Hunt JL: Chondritis of the burned ear: a preventable complication. *Am J Surg* 152:257–259, 1986.

65. Kroll SS, Gerow FJ: Sulfamylon allergy simulating chondritis. *Plast Reconstr Surg* 80:298–299, 1987.

66. Jelenko C, Wheeler ML, Anderson AP: The effect of topical sulfamylon on water loss through burn eschar: a re-evaluation. *J Trauma* 10:1123–1131, 1970.

67. Zawacki BE, DiVincentri FC, Moncrief JA: The effect of topical sulfamylon on the insensible weight loss of burned patients. *Ann Surg* 169:249–252, 1969.

68. Baenziger NC, Struss AW: Crystal structure of 2-sulfanilamidopyrimidine-silver(1). *Inorg Chem* 15:1807–1809, 1976.

69. Coward JE, Carr HS, Rosenkranz HS: Silver sulfadiazine: effect on the growth and ultrastructure of staphylococci. *Chemotherapy* 19:348–353, 1973.

70. Harrison HN: Pharmacology of sulfadiazine silver. *Arch Surg* 114:281–285, 1979.

71. McManus AT, Denton CL, Mason AD: Mechanisms of in vitro sensitivity to sulfadiazine silver. *Arch Surg* 118:161–166, 1983.

72. Gayle WE, Mayhall CG, Lamb VA, Apollo E, Haynes BW: Resistant *Enterobacter cloacae* in a burn center: the ineffectiveness of silver sulfadiazine. *J Trauma* 18:317–323, 1978.

73. Bridges K, Lowbury EJL: Drug resistance in relation to use of silver sulfadiazine cream in a burns unit. *J Clin Pathol* 30:160–164, 1977.

74. Modak S, Fox CL: Synergistic action of silver sulfadiazine and sodium piperacillin on resistant *Pseudomonas aeruginosa* in vitro and in experimental burn wound infections. *J Trauma* 25:27–31, 1985.

75. Lowbury EJL, Jackson DM, Ricketts CR, Davis B: Topical chemoprophylaxis for burns: trials of creams containing silver sulfadiazine and trimethoprim. *Injury* 3:18–24, 1971.

76. Monafo WW, West MA: Current treatment recommendations for topical burn therapy. *Drugs* 40:364–373, 1990.

77. Smith-Choban P, Marshall WJ: Leukopenia secondary to silver sulfadiazine: frequency, characteristics and clinical consequences. *Am Surg* 53:515–517, 1987.

78. Fraser GL, Beaulieu JT: Leukopenia secondary to sulfadiazine silver. *JAMA* 241:1928–1929, 1979.

79. Wilson P, George R, Raine P: Topical silver sulphadiazine and profound neutropenia in a burned child. *Burns* 12:295–296, 1986.

80. Chan CK, Jarrett F, Moylan JA: Acute leukopenia as an allergic reaction to silver sulfadiazine in burn patients. *J Trauma* 16:395–396, 1976.

81. Kiker RG, Carvajal HF, Mlcak RP, Larson DL: A controlled study of the effects of silver sulfadiazine on white blood cell counts in burned children. *J Trauma* 17:835–836, 1977.

82. Fuller FW, Engler PE: Leukopenia in non-septic burn patients receiving topical 1% silver sulfadiazine cream therapy: a survey. *J Burn Care Rehabil* 9:606–609, 1989.

83. Fligner CL, Jack R, Twiggs GA, Raisys VA: Hyperosmolality induced by propylene glycol. *JAMA* 253:1606–1609, 1985.

84. Owens CJ, Yarbrough DR, Brackett NC: Nephrotic syndrome following topically applied sulfadiazine silver therapy. *Arch Intern Med* 134:332–335, 1974.

85. McCauley RL, Linares HA, Pelligrini V, et al: In vitro toxicity of topical antimicrobial agents to human fibroblasts. *J Surg Res* 46:267–274, 1989.

86. Geronemus RG, Mertz PM, Eaglstein WH: Wound healing: the effects of topical antimicrobial agents. *Arch Dermatol* 115:1311–1314, 1979.

87. Fox CL, Modak SM, Stanford JW: Zinc sulfadiazine for topical therapy of *Pseudomonas* infection in burns. *Surg Gynecol Obstet* 142:553–558, 1976.

88. Fox CL, Parsa MH: Treatment of infected burns and wounds with zinc sulfadiazine. *Iran J Surg* 2:113–121, 1979.

89. Fox CL, Rao TNV, Azmeth R, Gandhi SS, Modak S: Comparative evaluation of zinc sulfadiazine and silver sulfadiazine in burn wound infection. *J Burn Care Rehabil* 11:112–117, 1990.

90. Snelling CFT, Ronald AR, Waters WR, et al: Comparison of silver sulfadiazine and gentamicin for topical prophylaxis against burn wound sepsis. *Can Med Assoc J* 119:466–470, 1978.

91. Parenti MA, Hatfield SM, Leyden JJ: Mupirocin: a topical antibiotic with a unique structure and mechanism of action. *Clin Pharm* 6:761–769, 1987.

92. Strock LL, Lee MM, Rutan RL, et al: Topical Bactroban (mupirocin): efficacy in treating burn wounds infected with methicillin-resistant staphylococci. *J Burn Care Rehabil* 11:454–459, 1990.

93. Rode H, deWet PM, Cywes S, Millar AJ: Mupirocin in a polyethylene glycol carrier base. *J Antimicrob Chemother* 24:78–79, 1989.

94. Cope O, Langhor JL, Moore FD, Webster RC: Expeditious care of full-thickness burn wounds by surgical excision and grafting. *Ann Surg* 125:1–122, 1947.

95. Tompkins RG, Remensnyder JP, Burke JF, et al: Significant reductions in mortality for children with burn injuries through the use of prompt eschar excision. *Ann Surg* 208:577–585, 1988.

96. Burke JF, Quinby WC, Bondoc CC: Primary burn excision and immediate grafting as routine therapy for the treatment of thermal burns in children. *Surg Clin North Am* 56:477–494, 1976.

97. Burke JF, Bondoc CC, Quinby WC: Primary burn excision and immediate grafting: a method shortening illness. *J Trauma* 14:389–395, 1974.

98. Pruitt BA, Goodwin CW: Thermal injuries. In Davis JH (ed): *Clinical Surgery.* St. Louis, CV Mosby, pp 2823–2904, 1987.

99. McGuckin MB, Thorpe RJ, Abrutyn E: Hydrotherapy: an outbreak of *Pseudomonas aeruginosa* wound infections related to Hubbard Tank treatments. *Arch Phys Med Rehabil* 62:283–285, 1981.

100. Dimick AR: Experience with the use of proteolytic enzyme (Travase) in burn patients. *J Trauma* 17:948–955, 1977.

101. Zawacki BE: The effect of Travase on heat-injured skin. *Surgery* 77:132–136, 1975.

102. Krizek TJ, Robson MC, Groskin MG: Experimental burn wound sepsis: evaluation of enzymatic debridement. *J Surg Res* 17:219–227, 1974.

103. Pruitt BA, Silverstein P: Methods of resurfacing denuded skin areas. *Transplant Proc* 3:1537–1545, 1971.

104. Heck EL, Bergstresser PR, Baxter CR: Composite skin graft: frozen dermal allografts support the engraftment and expansion of autologous epidermis. *J Trauma* 25:106–112, 1985.

105. Gottesdiener KM: Transplanted infections: donor to host transmission with allograft. *Ann Intern Med* 110:1001–1016, 1989.

106. Silverstein P: Evaluation of formalin fixed skin as a temporary dressing for granulation wounds. *Surg Forum* 22:60–62, 1971.

107. Taylor JA, Grube B, Heimbach DM, Bergman AB: Toxic epidermal necrolysis. A comprehensive approach. Multidisciplinary management in a burn center. *Clin Pediatr* 28:404–407, 1989.

108. Yannas IV, Burke JF, Orgill DP, Skrabut EM: Wound tissue can utilize a polymeric template to synthesize a functional extension of skin. *Science* 215:174–176, 1982.

109. Heimbach D, Luterman A, Burke J, et al: Artificial dermis for major burns: a multicenter randomized clinical trial. *Ann Surg* 208:313–320, 1988.

110. Green H, Kehinde O, Thomas J: Growth of cultured human epidermal cells into multiple epithelia suitable for grafting. *Proc Natl Acad Sci USA* 76:5665–5668, 1979.

111. Madden MR, Finkelstein JL, Staiano-Coico L, et al: Grafting of cultured allogeneic epidermis on second- and third-degree burn wounds on 26 patients. *J Trauma* 26:955–962, 1986.

112. O'Conner NE, Mulliken JB, Banks-Schlegel S, Kehinde O, Green H: Grafting of burns with cultured epithelium prepared from autologous epidermal cells. *Lancet* i:75–78, 1981.

113. Gallico GG, O'Conner NE, Compton CC, Kehinde O, Green H: Permanent coverage of large burn wounds with autologous cultured human epithelium. *N Engl J Med* 311:448–451, 1984.

114. Gallico GG, O'Conner NE: Cultured epithelium as a skin substitute. *Clin Plast Surg* 12:149–157, 1985.

115. Eldad E, Burt A, Clarke JA: Cultured epithelium as a skin substitute. *Burns* 13:173–180, 1987.

116. Latarjet J, Gangolphe M, Hezez G, et al: The grafting of burns with cultured epidermis as autografts in man. *Scand J Plast Reconstr Surg* 21:241–244, 1987.

117. Kamagai N, Nishina H, Tanabe H, et al: Clinical application of autologous cultured epithelia for the treatment of burn wounds and burn scars. *Plast Reconstr Surg* 82:99–108, 1988.

118. Pittelkow MR, Scott RE: New techniques for the in vitro culture of human skin keratinocytes and perspectives on their use for grafting of patients with extensive burns. *Mayo Clin Proc* 61:771–777, 1986.

119. Herzog SR, Meyer A, Woodley D, Peterson HD: Wound coverage with cultured autologous keratinocytes: use after burn wound excision, including biopsy followup. *J Trauma* 28:195–198, 1991.

120. Woodley DT, Peterson DT, Herzog SR, et al: Burn wounds resurfaced by cultured epidermal autografts show abnormal reconstitution of anchoring fibrils. *JAMA* 259:2566–2571, 1988.

121. Compton CC, Gill JM, Bradford DA, et al: Skin regenerated from cultured epithelial autografts on full-thickness burn wounds from 6 days to 5 years after grafting. *Lab Invest* 60:600–612, 1989.

122. Gallico GG, O'Conner NE, Compton CC, et al: Cultured epithelial autografts for giant congenital nevi. *Plast Reconstr Surg* 84:1–9, 1989.

123. Munster AM, Weiner SH, Spence RJ: Cultured epidermis for the coverage of massive burn wounds. *Ann Surg* 211:676–680, 1990.

124. Peterson MJ, Lessane B, Woodley DT: Characterization of cellular elements in healed cultured keratinocyte autografts used to cover burn wounds. *Arch Dermatol* 126:175–180, 1990.

125. Tompkins RG, Burke JF: Burn wound closure using permanent skin replacement materials. *World J Surg* 16:47–52, 1992.

126. Eisinger M, Lee JS, Hefton JM, et al: Human epidermal cell cultures: growth and differentiation in the absence of dermal components and medium supplements. *Proc Natl Acad Sci USA* 76:5340–5344, 1979.

127. Hefton JM, Finkelstein JL, Madden MR, Shires GT: Grafting of burn patients with allografts of cultured epidermal cells. *Lancet* 2:428–430, 1983.

128. Madden MR, Finkelstein JL, Staiano-Coico L, et al: Grafting of cultured allogeneic epidermis on second- and third-degree burn wounds on 26 patients. *J Trauma* 26:955–962, 1986.

129. Brain A, Purkis P, Coates P, et al: Survival of cultured allogeneic keratinocytes transplanted to deep dermal bed assessed with probe specific for Y chromosome. *BMJ* 298:917–919, 1989.

130. Burt AM, Pallett CD, Sloane JP, et al: Survival of cultured allografts in patients with burns assessed with probe specific for Y chromosome. *BMJ* 298:915–917, 1989.

131. Boyce ST, Hansbrough JF: Biologic attachment, growth, and differentiation of cultured human epidermal keratinocytes on a graftable collagen and chondroitin-6-sulfate substrate. *Surgery* 103:421–431, 1988.

132. Bell E, Ehrlich HP, Buttle DJ, Nahatsuji T: Living tissue formed in vitro and accepted as skin-equivalent tissue of full thickness. *Science* 211:1052–1054, 1981.

133. Lynch SE, Colvin RB, Antoniades HN: Growth factors in wound healing: single and synergistic effects on partial thickness porcine skin wounds. *J Clin Invest* 84:640–646, 1989.

134. Brown GL, Curtsinger L, Brightwell JR, et al: Enhancement of epidermal regeneration by biosynthetic epidermal growth factor. *J Exp Med* 163:1319–1324, 1986.

135. Brown GL, Nanney LB, Griffen J, et al: Enhancement of wound healing by topical treatment with epidermal growth factor. *N Engl J Med* 321:76–79, 1989.

136. Boyce ST, Foreman TJ, English KB, et al: Skin wound closure in athymic mice with cultured human cells, biopolymers, and growth factors. *Surgery* 110:866–876, 1991.

137. Jones SC, Curtsinger LJ, Whalen JD, et al: Effect of topical recombinant TGF-β on healing of partial thickness injuries. *J Surg Res* 51:344–352, 1991.

138. Schultz G, Rotatori DS, Clark W: EGF and TGF-α in wound healing and repair. *J Cell Biochem* 45:346–352, 1991.

139. Varani J, Mitra RS, Gibbs D, et al: All-trans retinoic acid stimulates growth and extracellular matrix production in growth-inhibited cultured human skin fibroblasts. *J Invest Dermatol* 94:717–723, 1990.

140. Schultz GS, White M, Mitchell R, et al: Epithelial wound healing enhanced by transforming growth factor-α and vaccinia growth factor. *Science* 235:350–352, 1987.

141. Jijon AJ, Gallup DG, Behzadian MA, Metheny WP: Assessment of epidermal growth factor in the healing process of clean full-thickness skin wounds. *Am J Obstet Gynecol* 161:1658–1662, 1991.

142. Hennessey PJ, Nigiotis JG, Shinn MN, Andrassy RJ: Continuous EGF application impairs long-term collagen accumulation during wound healing in rats. *J Pediatr Surg* 26:362–366, 1991.

SECTION FOUR

Special Considerations in Critical Care Pharmacology

CHAPTER 50

Pharmacologic Approach to the Critically Ill Obstetric Patient[a]

MICHAEL W. GALLAGHER, M.D.

JOHN T. REPKE, M.D.

PHILLIP J. GOLDSTEIN, M.D.

The past 20 years have seen significant advances in the field of obstetrics. With the development of the subspecialty of Maternal-Fetal Medicine came a new concentration on the understanding of the medical and surgical problems affecting the pregnant patient. This understanding, accompanied by advances in ultrasound, genetics, and the rapidly growing discipline of fetal diagnosis and therapy, has done much to reduce the morbidity and mortality once associated with childbearing. Yet, care of the pregnant patient continues to pose a difficult challenge, especially when she is critically ill. Physiologic changes induced by pregnancy and the very presence of a fetus can seriously affect critical care decisions. Potentially life-saving interventions can fail to yield expected results or can have adverse affects on an embryo or fetus. The welfare of the mother and the developing fetus must be constantly balanced as care is planned.

It is the purpose of this chapter to examine the pharmacologic approach to the critically ill pregnant patient. Consideration will be given to how pregnancy affects serious illness and to how therapeutic interventions might affect the pregnancy. Important physiologic changes brought about by pregnancy will be discussed as they pertain to each area of discussion. The reader is referred elsewhere for a complete discussion of these changes (1). Because of space limitations, discussion will be limited to maternal disease. In utero treatment of the

critically ill fetus is just beginning to emerge as a science, and its principles are treated elsewhere (2).

Although several institutions have developed dedicated obstetrical critical care areas (3), critical care of the obstetric patient will be delivered, in the vast majority of cases, not in an obstetric unit but in a hospital's central critical care area, where resources for monitoring and special interventions are readily available. Care in these areas may still be managed by an obstetrician with varying amounts of involvement from the critical care unit team. It is essential, therefore, that all who are involved in critical care have some understanding of the special requirements of the pregnant patient so that optimum cooperation can be achieved.

Before examining specific areas it is necessary to make explicit certain general principles involved in the care of an obstetric patient. Primary among these principles is that the pregnant patient deserves the same considerations for critical care as does her nonpregnant counterpart. The presence of a developing embryo or fetus must be kept in mind but should not result in delay or denial of life-saving interventions. The well-being of the fetus is totally dependent on the life of the mother. Thus, the evaluation and treatment of the mother should be a primary concern in an emergency and a prominent part of any critical care scenario. Ongoing evaluation and consideration of fetal well-being must be undertaken but only after immediate threats to maternal life have been addressed.

Indications for intervention in critical care situations are not necessarily changed by pregnancy. Invasive monitoring

[a]The views expressed in this chapter are those of the authors and do not reflect the official policy or position of the Department of the Navy, the Department of Defense, or the United States Government.

847

Table 50.1.   U.S. Food and Drug Administration Ratings for Drug Use in Pregnancy

Category	Explanation
A	Controlled studies that show no risk to the fetus are available.
B	Either animal findings show risk and human studies do not or, if no human studies are available, animal studies show no risk.
C	There are no human studies available, and animal studies either show fetal risk or are not available. Potential benefits may justify fetal risk.
D	There is investigational evidence of some risk of harm to the fetus, but potential benefits may outweigh risks.
X	Animal or human studies or postmarketing investigation show fetal risk that outweighs possible benefits.

can and should be used to gain the valuable physiologic information required for care. Diagnostic radiology should be employed if indicated. Surgical procedures should not be automatically ruled out. How these interventions should be used must be determined in close conjunction with obstetricians who themselves must be knowledgeable of critical care requirements.

An important concern present among all who treat pregnant patients is the potential effects on the fetus of pharmacologic agents administered to the mother. Because of the difficulty involved in conducting well-designed, randomized clinical trials of drugs in pregnant patients, there is often little concrete information provided about effects of agents when used during pregnancy. The Food and Drug Administration has attempted to class drugs according to the information available (Table 50.1) to aid practitioners who are faced with decisions concerning prescribing for the pregnant patient. These classifications are assigned by the manufacturer, and they are not provided for all drugs. There are other sources which collect and update data about drug effects in pregnancy (4). The practitioner is often faced with weighing potential risks against required therapeutic results. The severity of the situation and availability of alternative agents will affect clinical decisions.

With these principles in mind we shall now consider specific situations of critical illness in pregnancy and concentrate on the pharmacologic interventions used in their treatment.

CARDIAC DISEASE

While significant cardiac disease is rare in the reproductive age group, it can be an important source of morbidity for the pregnant patient and could require intensive care admission. The physiologic changes of pregnancy can alter relationships among hemodynamic factors, which can cause a compensated state to shift to decompensation. Likewise, pregnancy can unmask previously undetected cardiac disease as new demands are made on the maternal cardiovascular system. In either case it is necessary for the critical care team to understand the nature of the underlying disease and how pregnancy affects maternal cardiovascular physiology.

The New York Heart Association classification of cardiac disease symptoms is useful in predicting how women with cardiac disease will function during pregnancy. In general those patients who begin pregnancy as Class I or II will be at lower risk for morbidity and mortality than those who are III or IV. It is important to note, however, that 40% of patients who develop congestive heart failure during pregnancy were Class I prior to the onset of pregnancy (5).

A number of investigators have characterized mortality risk for specific disorders. Pregnant patients at low risk (<1%) are those patients with simple atrial or ventricular septal defects, pulmonic or tricuspid valvular heart disease, tetralogy of Fallot (corrected), mitral stenosis functional Class I or II, and patients with porcine valves. Those patients at moderate risk (5 to 15%) include patients with mitral stenosis (Class III and IV), aortic stenosis, tetralogy of Fallot (uncorrected), coarctation of the aorta, and recent myocardial infarction. Finally, the highest-risk patients (25 to 50%) are those with Marfan syndrome and pulmonary hypertension (5).

CONGENITAL HEART DISEASE

Through much of this century the incidence of congenital heart disease has been almost 4% (6). In recent decades this statistic has declined somewhat as the incidence of rheumatic heart disease has decreased. Because of early detection and improved methods of support and repair, more women with congenital heart disease are reaching reproductive age. Most of these patients have had some treatment and are compensated to various degrees. Their health during pregnancy will depend largely on their specific disease, on their functional class, and on how the changes of pregnancy affect them hemodynamically. Those patients who experience sudden decompensation and whose underlying congenital heart disease may be unmasked by pregnancy will frequently require a critical care approach.

Pharmacologic intervention in these patients will depend upon the nature of their decompensation. The drug classes most widely used in these settings are antiarrhythmics, anticoagulants, and antibiotics. The first two classes will be treated later in this chapter. Antibiotics are important in these patients since they are at significant risk for bacterial endocarditis. The American Heart Association recommendations for prophylaxis should be followed carefully when any invasive procedure is undertaken (Table 50.2) (7). Antibiotic allergies should be noted and appropriate substitutions made. If possible, interventions should be anticipated and dosage timed so that there are adequate circulating levels of antibiotics at the time of the planned procedure.

There is one class of congenital heart lesion that bears special consideration. This is Eisenmenger's complex, which results from any situation that produces left-to-right shunting causing pulmonary hypertension. Compensation is achieved when the pulmonary pressure exceeds the systemic pressure, and shunt reversal or bidirectional flow results. Pregnancy causes a decrease in systemic vascular resistance, especially in the second trimester. This change is due in part to the effects of increased estrogen, progesterone, prostaglandins, and prolactin. This effect is augmented by the large, low-resistance A-V shunt effect, which increases as the placenta

Table 50.2. American Heart Association Recommendations for Prophylaxis against Bacterial Endocarditis

Agents	Dose
Ampicillin, gentamicin, amoxicillin	Ampicillin (2.0 g i.m. or i.v. plus gentamicin (1.5 mg/kg) (not exceeding 80 mg), given 30 min prior to procedure. Amoxicillin (15 g 6 hrs after initial dose). (Alternatively, ampicillin-gentamicin administration can be repeated 8 hr after initial dose.)
Penicillin-allergic patients:	
Vancomycin, gentamicin	Vancomycin (1.0 g i.v. over 1 hr plus i.m. or i.v. gentamicin 1.5 mg/kg as above. Repeat 8 hr after initial dose.
Low-risk patient:	
Amoxicillin	3.0 g given orally 1 hr before procedure; 1.5 g given 6 hr after initial dose.

grows. This decrease in systemic pressure can cause right-to-left shunting to increase and dramatically decrease oxygenation. Pregnancy mortality associated with this lesion is 30 to 70%.

The avoidance of hypotension is one of the primary concerns in the treatment of these patients. Diuretics should be used with great caution, even in the face of fluid overload. When conduction anesthesia is employed, care must be taken to avoid hypotension.

Termination of pregnancy will often be recommended to the decompensating Eisenmenger's patient, given the high risk of pregnancy-associated mortality. The use of prostaglandins should be avoided in these patients since there is evidence that prostaglandin E (an agent with both uterotonic and smooth muscle-relaxing properties often used to induce an abortion (8)) can cause a significant increase in maternal cardiac output and place more stress on an already compromised cardiovascular system (9). Prostaglandin F (used as 15-methyl prostaglandin $F_{2\alpha}$, a potent uterotonic agent that is injected into the uterine cavity (10)) has been seen to cause acute maternal arterial oxygen desaturation and should also be avoided (11). Use of oxytocin for pregnancy termination may avoid these complications in the Eisenmenger's patient.

MITRAL STENOSIS

This lesion, often rheumatic in origin, is the leading cause of cardiac death during pregnancy (12). The stenotic mitral valve causes a relatively fixed cardiac output that can be reasonable but is not readily adaptable to increases in oxygen demand. Maternal blood volume increases 50% in pregnancy with increases in heart rate and stroke volume. A concomitant increase in cardiac output is usually seen. In the pregnant patient with mitral stenosis there is a shorter amount of time to transport an increased amount of blood across a noncompliant valve. The result is increased left atrial pressure, which translates into increased right heart pressure and right-sided failure. Pulmonary edema can be seen, especially postpartum, when an autotransfusion of blood resulting from a suddenly smaller uterus causes a dramatic increase in blood volume over a short period of time.

One of the important underlying problems in this disease is decreased diastolic filling times. This problem can be treated by slowing the heart rate with β-blockers, especially the more cardioselective classes. The goal of therapy should be a rate less than 90 beats/min.

β-blockers are safe and effective agents for use in pregnancy. Propranolol and atenolol have been used effectively. Pregnancy has little effect on the pharmacokinetics of propranolol. It readily crosses the placenta, resulting in fetal serum concentrations equal or slightly less than maternal concentrations (13). Since the fetus has a relatively less efficient hepatic metabolism and altered protein binding, the half-life of propranolol will be increased. This increase could result in some blunting of fetal catecholamine response, as evidenced in decreased heart rate variability. Animal studies have demonstrated decreased tolerance for hypoxia in fetuses affected by propranolol (14). There has also been some suggestion that mothers taking propranolol are at higher risk for growth-retarded fetuses (15). Many of these studies are retrospective, however, and there is not wide agreement as to their conclusions. Nonetheless, close monitoring of fetal growth is indicated.

Another theoretical risk of β-blockers is the possibility of preterm labor. Since stimulation of β-receptors leads to smooth muscle relaxation, β-adrenergic agents are sometimes employed to effect uterine relaxation in the face of premature contractions. Theoretically, blockade of this β-effect could cause contractions in those patients at risk for preterm labor (16). While this seems to make empiric sense, in fact, the pregnant uterus is fairly refractory to the effects of β-blocking drugs.

Atenolol is 50 to 60% absorbed when given orally. The drug is eliminated principally in the urine, so adjustments must be made for renal function. Like propranolol, atenolol freely crosses the placenta. Similar concerns about fetal growth have been raised (17). While caution should be employed in the use of these and any drug in pregnancy, it is necessary to weigh the benefits against the theoretical risks.

Preload reduction can be achieved by the judicious use of furosemide and fluid restriction. Hypotension should be avoided. Because of the nature of the lesion, pulmonary artery occlusion pressure measured by a Swan-Ganz catheter will not necessarily reflect left ventricular filling pressure. Too low a filling pressure will also result in decompensation. Experience has shown that these patients do best with wedge pressures of 12 to 14 mm Hg (5).

Digoxin therapy is indicated for the prevention and treatment of atrial fibrillation (which can worsen an already precarious situation) and for its effect on slowing ventricular response, should this dysrhythmia occur. Digoxin is only 60 to 80% absorbed when given orally. This rate is further slowed by the delayed gastric emptying time seen in pregnancy. In the circulation digoxin is only 20 to 25% protein-bound, so the hypoalbuminemic state accompanying pregnancy will not affect its concentration. Oral administration results in peak levels in 2 to 3 hours, with the maximum effect at 4 to 6 hours. Intravenous infusion leads to a rapid peak serum concentration at 5 to 20 minutes, with maximum effect at 1.5 to 2 hours. Digoxin half-life is 36 to 40 hours.

Maternal volume of distribution increases during pregnancy. Although the recommended digitalizing dose is still 0.75 to 1.5 mg given intravenously, it will be necessary to adjust subsequent dosing to account for changes as pregnancy progresses. Since digoxin is excreted by the kidneys, dosage should be adjusted in those with renal compromise.

Serum digoxin levels can be misleading in some pregnant patients. There have been reports of the presence of an endogenous digoxin-like substance in pregnancy that interferes with radioimmune assays for digoxin, resulting in erroneous values (18). Concentrations of this digoxin-like substance have been seen to increase in maternal serum with gestational age (19). To ensure accuracy in determination of digoxin levels, a serum sample should be obtained before treatment and analyzed for the presence of this endogenous substance. Fortunately, newer assay methods have largely eliminated this problem.

HYPERTROPHIC, OBSTRUCTIVE CARDIOMYOPATHY (IDIOPATHIC HYPERTROPHIC SUBAORTIC STENOSIS)

This autosomal dominant disorder may be recognized for the first time when a woman becomes pregnant. The hypertrophied cardiac muscle causes a pressure gradient between the left ventricle and its outflow tract. This is a dynamic gradient that may vary in the same patient over time or with increased physical exertion. Mitral regurgitation may result from left ventricular back pressure.

The increased blood volume associated with pregnancy tends to enhance left ventricular filling. Most patients tolerate pregnancy well. The major cause of morbidity and mortality is dysrhythmia. Angina can be a serious problem that can result in an intensive care admission to rule out myocardial infarction.

Symptomatic angina and dysrhythmias are indications for pharmacologic intervention. Digoxin should be avoided since it can worsen the situation by increasing the outflow gradient. Propranolol can be useful for its antiarrhythmic effect and for increasing myocardial compliance. The calcium channel blocker verapamil has been successfully employed in the nonpregnant patient with this disease. This agent is very well absorbed orally with 90% protein binding. More free drug may, therefore, be seen in pregnancy when albumin is decreased. Peak serum levels are seen in 1 to 2 hours. Bioavailability is only 10 to 35%, however, because of extensive first-pass elimination in the liver. The half-life of verapamil is 2 to 5 hours, and that of norverapamil, the most active hepatic metabolite, is 8 to 10 hours. This condition can be altered by liver disease. Intravenous administration yields onset of action in 5 to 15 minutes with duration of about 6 hours. Intravenous dosage is 0.15 mg/kg infused at 1 mg/min (20).

Some adverse side effects have been described in connection with the use of verapamil in the treatment of hypertrophic cardiomyopathy (21). Conduction disturbances and hypotension can result. There is little information about the chronic use of verapamil in pregnancy. It has been employed to treat maternal and fetal dysrhythmias. Some concern has been raised over a report on fetal death after maternal administration of verapamil to treat fetal tachycardia (22).

The use of prostaglandins should be avoided in the patient with hypertrophic cardiomyopathy since these tend to have a vasodilating effect that can compromise venous return and left ventricular pressure. Conduction anesthesia should be used with caution to avoid hypotension and maintain sufficient cardiac output. β-mimetic tocolytic agents (terbutaline, ritodrine) should be avoided because of the possibility of augmenting the pressure gradient across the lesion.

PERIPARTUM CARDIOMYOPATHY

This condition is defined as the relatively sudden onset of fatigue, dyspnea, and pulmonary edema in the last month of pregnancy or the first 6 weeks post partum in a woman with no prior cardiac disease and without evidence of another cause of symptoms (valvular, infectious, metabolic, embolic). The incidence is 1/1500 to 1/4000 live births, and the cause remains unknown. A typical clinical picture is a woman in the final weeks of her pregnancy or the first weeks after birth who suddenly develops congestive heart failure with a dilated cardiomyopathy. Mortality can be 20 to 50%. Intensive and aggressive care can result in successful recovery, but there is significant risk of recurrence in the next pregnancy. If the myocardium has returned to normal size in the interim, the mortality risk in a recurrence is 11 to 14%. If the heart remains dilated the risk is 40 to 80%. Therefore, avoidance of future pregnancy is usually advised (23).

Treatment consists of supportive care and symptomatic relief. Digoxin can play an important role as a positive cardiac inotrope, but there seems to be an increased tendency to toxicity in these patients (24). Diuretics such as furosemide can be used to control volume. Hydralazine can be used for arterial dilatation and improvement of cardiac output. There is considerable experience with use of this agent in pregnancy (see Hypertensive Crisis), and its safety is recognized.

Nitrates can be employed for venodilatation to ease preload, but consideration must be made in the undelivered patient of the association of organic nitrate use with hypotension and fetal heart rate decelerations and fetal bradycardia (24).

Angiotensin-converting enzyme inhibitors can have a benefit in afterload reduction. They are contraindicated in pregnancy, however, because of reports of fetal renal toxicity and fetal death, the latter presumably due to reduced uteroplacental perfusion (25).

As the patient recovers from the acute event, maintenance therapy with digoxin, diuretics, and vasodilators is recommended. Some form of anticoagulant therapy is recommended since the risk of intracardiac thrombus formation is increased. If the patient is still pregnant, heparin would be the agent of choice. It could be administered intravenously while the patient is being stabilized and then given by subcutaneous injection later. The usual dose is 8000 units q.i.d., to be adjusted as necessary according to the values of the patient's partial thromboplastin time. If the patient is postpartum, warfarin can be used in the usual dosage (see discussion under Thromboembolic Disease). The postoperative patient should be watched closely for the development of pelvic hematoma.

Some recent studies have suggested that myocarditis may be an underlying cause for many cases of peripartum cardiomyopathy. These studies report successful resolution of symptoms with good overall outcomes after use of a treatment regimen of prednisone (1 mg/kg/day) combined with azathioprine (1.5 mg/kg/day) for 6 to 8 weeks (26). This evidence is not accepted by all, however, and it is not clear that there is any successful treatment for this disease.

As was noted, future pregnancy is not advisable, given the mortality with recurrences. The patient should not be started on oral contraceptives, however, because of the increased risk of thrombotic disease.

MYOCARDIAL INFARCTION

This is not a common event in the reproductive-age woman (less than 1/10,000 pregnancies), but its occurrence during pregnancy can result in serious problems for the critical care team. One study places the mortality rate at 37% (43% in women over age 35) (27).

Emergency treatment should proceed in the usual manner. Attention should be given to maternal stabilization. Fetal monitoring can be instituted after stabilization has been achieved. Ventricular dysrhythmias are controlled by using lidocaine, with atropine used to control bradycardia. When given intravenously, lidocaine has an immediate onset of action with a 100-minute half-life. The loading dose is 1 to 1.5 mg/kg. A continuous infusion at 1 to 4 mg/min will then provide a therapeutic level of 1 to 5 μg/ml in 7 to 10 hours. Lidocaine is well-tolerated in pregnancy. It crosses the placenta and can induce central nervous system toxicity in the fetus at high doses. This action has usually been associated with its use for regional or local analgesia, however, and not with antiarrhythmic doses.

Recent recommendations by the American Heart Association caution against the *routine* use of lidocaine for prophylaxis against dysrhythmias in the acute myocardial infarction patient (27a). These recommendations are based on studies that have shown no improvement in mortality when lidocaine is administered routinely (27b, 27c). Lidocaine therapy may be of benefit to young patients without left ventricular dysfunction who are within 6 hours of onset of symptoms (27a, 27d). Although many pregnant patients will fall into this group, the use of lidocaine should be tailored to the individual situation.

Caution must also be used in the application of thrombolytic therapy in the pregnant myocardial infarction patient. While early administration of streptokinase or tissue plasminogen activators has shown benefits in patients with acute transmural infarctions, these drugs are not without potentially serious side effects (27a). Experience with the use of these agents during pregnancy is extremely limited, and extreme caution is warranted.

Morphine sulfate can be used for pain relief and control of catecholamine release. Doses of up to 10 mg can be administered intravenously over a 30-minute period in 2- to 4-mg increments over 5 minutes. The drug can cross the placenta and result in loss of fetal heart rate variability and occassional sinusoidal patterns in the fetal heart rate tracing. These effects are transient, however, and are without sequelae (28).

DISTURBANCES IN RHYTHM

Mild rhythm disturbances are not uncommon in pregnancy. They can range from occasional "skipped beats" (premature atrial contractions) to supraventricular tachycardia. In most cases they are benign and self-limiting. There are cases, however, in which a pregnant patient will present with an unstable or life-threatening dysrhythmia. She will then require treatment and diagnostic studies to rule out underlying cardiac disease.

The treatment of dysrhythmias in the pregnant patient is the same as in the nonpregnant patient. Digoxin, as was noted above, is well-tolerated and can be used as indicated. Again, it should be noted that pretreatment levels should be drawn to allow for the presence of endogenous digoxin-like substance in maternal serum (see above).

Quinidine is also useful in treating dysrhythmias in pregnancy. After oral dosing 70 to 80% absorption is noted with maximum serum levels within 60 to 90 minutes. Since quinidine is highly protein-bound (80%), the free fraction increases during the hypoalbuminemic state of pregnancy. The therapeutic level is 3 to 6 μg/ml with toxicity seen at 7 to 8 μg/ml.

Quinidine's side effects of nausea, vomiting, diarrhea, and possible skin rash may make its use undesirable. It has also been associated with syncope accompanied by ventricular tachycardia with "torsade de pointes" seen on electrocardiography.

Both quinidine and digoxin cross the placenta, and both have been used to treat fetal tachydysrhythmias. In these cases the drug is usually given to the mother in doses as high as she can tolerate. Fetal effects are monitored closely, and the mother is maintained on the lowest dose that effects fetal cardiac conversion (29).

Procainamide is also an effective antiarrhythmic, especially in the face of reciprocating tachydysrhythmias associated with Wolff-Parkinson-White syndrome (17). It can be given orally and intravenously. Absorption is 75 to 95% orally but can be slowed by decreased gastric emptying and intestinal motility, as is seen in pregnancy. Protein binding is only 10 to 20%, so the lower albumin in pregnancy does not exert as much of an effect in this case. Therapeutic levels are attained in 45 to 70 minutes, and elimination is through the kidney. Dosage should be altered in patients with impaired renal function (e.g., preeclamptics). The major active metabolite is *N*-acetylprocainamide (NAPA), which is formed in the liver. This, too, is eliminated by the kidneys. The therapeutic level of procainamide is 4 to 10 μg/ml and of NAPA 9.4 to 19.5 μg/ml. Levels of both entities should be followed to avoid toxic symptoms of QT interval prolongation, hypotension, dysrhythmias, and central nervous system disturbances. Side effects can include nausea, vomiting, and diarrhea. Procainamide administration has also been associated with a lupus-like syndrome.

Procainamide crosses the placenta freely and has also been used to treat fetal dysrhythmias (30).

Disopyramide was approved as a class IA antiarrhythmic in 1977 after a long history of European use as an alternative drug to quinidine. There is little information as to its use in pregnancy. There have been isolated case reports of successful use without adverse fetal effects (31). One case report cites the onset of preterm labor after administration of disopyramide. Labor resolved after discontinuation of the drug (32). Because of the paucity of information on this agent in pregnancy it is recommended that its use be limited to those cases in which potentially life-threatening dysrhythmias (i.e., ventricular tachydysrhythmias) have proven refractory to other agents.

Mexiletine is a lidocaine-like agent used as a class Ib antiarrhythmic. Oral doses are almost completely absorbed in the proximal small bowel, and the delayed gastric emptying seen in pregnancy can delay its uptake. Peak level is usually reached in 1.5 hours. It is 75% protein-bound, so hypoalbuminemia may be a factor in the concentration of free drug seen. Mexiletine is metabolized in the liver. Clearance of the nonmetabolized drug through the kidney is increased by acidifying the urine. The loading dose is 400 mg orally with daily doses of 400 to 1200 mg to achieve therapeutic levels of 0.72 to 2.0 μg/ml. Adverse effects of nausea, vomiting, tremulousness, dizziness, and paresthesias can be seen in 30 to 40% of patients. "Torsades de pointes" rhythm has also been reported.

Reports of successful use of mexiletine in pregnancy do exist, but concerns about reported fetal bradycardia, growth disturbances, and neonatal hypoglycemia make this agent unsuitable for primary use (17).

Amiodarone is a class III antiarrhythmic approved for oral treatment of life-threatening dysrhythmias. Its absorption is variable, and bioavailability is reported to be 22 to 86%. Peak plasma levels are seen in 10 hours, but therapeutic effects can take as long as 21 days to become evident. Metabolism is not fully understood, but there is an hepatic metabolite, desethylamiodarone, which is seen in the plasma after long-term use. Amiodarone is 96% protein-bound with a half-life of from 13 to 100 days. Loading dose of 800 to 1600 mg/day is given for 1 to 3 weeks. Doses are then decreased to 800 mg/day for 2 to 4 weeks, 600 mg/day for 4 to 8 weeks, and then maintenance of 400 mg/day. Therapeutic level is 1 to 2.5 μg/ml.

Cases of AV block, QT alterations, and "torsades de pointes" have been reported to accompany amiodarone administration. Pulmonary fibrosis with an associated mortality of 10% has also been seen. Since there can be up to 75 mg of elemental iodine in a 200-mg dose of this drug, thyroid effects are also noted. Amiodarone can potentiate digoxin, quinidine, procainamide, and phenytoin. Adverse effects can persist for long periods after discontinuation of the drug.

Amiodarone crosses the placenta, and its levels in fetal serum and amniotic fluid have been studied (33). Fetal levels reach 10 to 25% of maternal levels. Of concern for the fetus is an increase in the concentrations of iodine found in umbilical cord blood of fetuses of mothers taking amiodarone. This finding has been associated with neonatal hypothyroidism and is a theoretical risk for fetal goiter. This and the other adverse effects mentioned above make amiodarone an agent that should be reserved for life-threatening situations. If used, there should be close monitoring of fetal thyroid size antenatally and observation of neonatal thyroid function.

The calcium channel blocker verapamil has been discussed above. It should be noted again that there is insufficient data to guarantee the safety of chronic usage in pregnancy.

β-blockers can be safely used in pregnancy as has been stated, but concerns for fetal growth disturbances, blunted fetal catecholamine responses, and neonatal hypoglycemia should prompt close monitoring of the patient using these agents.

Esmolol is a selective β_1 antagonist with an extremely short duration of action. This agent has been very useful in many intensive care settings in which rapid reversal of its effects is desirable. Esmolol is given only intravenously. Loading dose is 500 μg/kg over 1 minute. This dosage is followed by 50 μg/kg/min for 4 minutes. If an adequate result is not seen within 5 minutes, another loading dose is given, and maintenance is increased to 100 μg/kg/min. To date, there is little data on use of this agent in pregnancy, but it appears to be a safe and effective means of heart rate control.

Recently, the American Heart Association, in its new guidelines for emergency cardiac care, recommended adenosine as a first-line agent in the treatment of symptomatic paroxysmal supraventricular tachycardia (33a). Adenosine is an endogenous nucleoside that inhibits the automaticity of the sinus node, depresses AV node conduction, and prolongs AV node refractoriness. One of its major advantages is its extremely short half-life (approximately 10 seconds). After intravenous injection it is taken up by erythrocytes and endothelial cells and is immediately converted to the inactive metabolites inosine and adenosine monophosphate. Because adenosine can be used without regard to hepatic or renal function, and because it does not produce hypotension as can verapamil, it is a useful agent in the treatment of paroxysmal supraventricular tachycardia (PSVT) in critically ill patients. It is contraindicated in patients with sick sinus syndrome or second- or third-degree AV block. Methylxanthines antagonize adenosine, and larger doses may be required in their presence. Dipyridamole and carbamazepine potentiate the effects of adenosine.

Recommended initial dose of adenosine is 6 mg given intravenously as a rapid bolus. If no effect is seen in 1 to 2 minutes, a second rapid bolus of 12 mg may be given. This latter dose can be repeated if necessary. Sixty-two percent of patients will respond to the initial dose and 91% by the second. Initial dose should be reduced to 1 to 2 mg if given through a central line.

Although there are few studies specifically addressing adenosine's safety in pregnancy, its extremely short half-life ensures that virtually no active drug reaches the fetus (33b). Adenosine has been used successfully in the treatment of fetal tachycardia in utero. Administration must be directly intravenous requiring access to the fetal circulation, usually by percutaneous entry into the umbilical vein (33c).

In the case of severe rhythm disturbances, as in any other cardiac problem requiring critical care of the pregnant patient, therapy should be carefully planned, with full cooperation between the critical care and the obstetric specialist. Plans must be made for fetal monitoring in critical care settings when it is deemed appropriate.

ASTHMA

Asthma is defined by the American College of Chest Physicians as "a disease characterized by an increased responsiveness of the airways to various stimuli and manifested by prolongation of forced expiration, which changes in severity either spontaneously or with treatment" (34). Asthma is responsible for approximately 1 million emergency room visits each year and more than 130,000 hospitalizations. Mortality is quoted as 1 to 3%, with 4000 deaths each year. The prevalence among pregnant patients is estimated at 0.4 to 1.5% (35).

During pregnancy there is a 50% increase in minute ventilation that is probably hormonally mediated. Oxygen consumption also increases. Because of slight hypoventilation the PCO_2 is decreased, causing a mild respiratory alkalosis with normal pH 7.40 to 7.45. One must remember this when the arterial blood gas of an acute asthmatic is evaluated, since asthmatic changes will be superimposed. Total lung capacity is increased 4 to 6%, and residual volume and functional residual capacity are reduced 15 to 25% (36).

With careful management and good cooperation between physician and patient, it is possible for the pregnant asthmatic to have a normal pregnancy with a good outcome. Good control of asthma must be maintained, and exacerbations must be detected and treated as soon as possible. Acute onset of symptoms can lead to a cycle of declining function and to status asthmaticus, resulting in the necessity for hospitalization and, in some cases, intubation and ventilatory support. The patient with a history of frequent exacerbations or who has been identified as having potentially fatal asthma (37) must be watched closely. Early intervention can sometimes avoid the downward spiral leading to critical illness.

The patient who requires critical care will probably have been treated in an emergency room setting prior to admission. First-line therapy for acute exacerbation consists of oxygen administration, then inhalation therapy with nebulized β-mimetic agents, such as albuterol (0.5 ml in 3 ml saline nebulized and given every 20 to 30 minutes, up to three doses), or subcutaneous administration of terbutaline (0.25 mg every 15 minutes, for three doses). Some centers use epinephrine (1:1000 aqueous solution, 0.3 to 0.5 ml s.c.) in the acute setting. This treatment can be repeated every 20 to 30 minutes, up to three doses.

The endpoint for treatment should be relief of symptoms and signs of respiratory compromise. In the pregnant patient evaluation of arterial blood gas values is essential. The patient with a PO_2 less than 75 mm Hg (10 kPa) should be given supplemental oxygen. If pH falls below 7.35 with PCO_2 greater than 35 mm Hg (4.7 kPa) in the face of decreasing PO_2, admission for further treatment is necessary. Continuing acidosis and hypoxia may necessitate mechanical ventilation.

If the patient fails to improve after the first-line therapy has reached its maximum, other agents can be employed. There is growing recognition of the importance of the inflammatory component of asthma. Some practitioners describe the acute manifestation of the disease as a "desquamative eosiniphilic bronchiolitis" (38). The early use of steroids is becoming more popular as an adjunct to use of the more traditional first-line agents. Prednisone (75 to 150 mg) or methylprednisolone (60 to 150 mg) can be given intravenously. These agents can be given every 6 hours as needed. They can be helpful in the acute period and should be a part of ongoing therapy for the patient who has required admission, especially to a critical care area.

Attitudes toward the use of theophylline are changing. This agent was once considered indispensable in asthma therapy. Now, many believe that this drug may potentiate the side effects of β-mimetics without offering any distinct advantage

in the acute setting (35). Theophylline functions as a bronchodilator by relaxing smooth muscle. It also stimulates the central nervous system and cardiac muscle, as well as effecting diuresis in the kidneys. It is readily absorbed on administration by any route. It is 60% protein-bound. Theophylline is metabolized in the liver, and only about 20% is excreted in the urine. Half-life is 8 to 9 hours. The drug crosses the placenta but is tolerated well by the fetus.

Theophylline can be administered parenterally as aminophylline. Loading dose is 5.8 mg/kg (equal to 5.0 mg/kg theophylline) administered at a rate of no more than 25 mg/min. It is necessary to reduce the loading dose by 50% in the patient who has had theophylline in the past 24 hours (39). Maintenance dosage is 0.7 mg/kg/hr for the next 12 hours, then 0.5 mg/kg/hr thereafter. Serum levels should be obtained 12 hours after initial treatment. Therapeutic level is 10 to 12 μg/ml.

Maintenance and ongoing treatment of the pregnant asthmatic in the intensive care setting will often employ a combination of aminophylline and steroid therapy with use of β-mimetics as needed. As improvement is seen, dosages can be adjusted. Ongoing drug therapy will depend on the individual's response and underlying condition.

One other agent is now often employed in the asthmatic patient, but more as a prophylactic measure than as acute treatment—cromolyn sodium. This agent has been in use in the U.S. since 1973. It works as an inhibitor of pulmonary mast cell degranulation, thus lessening the concentration of the substances that contribute to the reactive asthmatic response. Cromolyn is only 1% absorbed when given orally but has excellent effects when applied topically to the lung surface. The usual route of administration is, therefore, inhalation. A nebulized preparation of 10 mg/ml can be given as two puffs (800 μg) 4 times/day. It can also be given as a nasal spray, which delivers 5.2 mg/compression. The nasal spray is given as one compression in each nostril 6 times/day.

All of the agents mentioned here for use in treating asthma are well-tolerated in pregnancy. While it is desirable to avoid any unnecessary drugs in pregnancy, these agents have proven to be without adverse effects on mother or fetus and can be of great benefit to the patient experiencing a severe exacerbation of asthma.

HYPERTENSIVE CRISIS

Hypertension in pregnancy has an incidence of 10 to 15% but is the second most common cause of maternal mortality. The American College of Obstetricians and Gynecologists defines four types of hypertensive disease in pregnancy (40). The first is called *chronic hypertension* and is defined as blood pressure of 140/90 or greater that predates pregnancy or is diagnosed before 20 weeks' gestation. Also included here is hypertension persisting more than 42 days after pregnancy.

Preeclampsia/eclampsia describes a spectrum of disease characterized by increased blood pressure, proteinuria, and edema. Definition criteria for preeclampsia call for an increase in systolic pressure of 30 mm Hg or in diastolic of 15 mm Hg over the baseline measured at the first obstetrical visit early in pregnancy. If an early pressure is not available, a reading of 140/90 after 20 weeks' gestation will meet the

Table 50.3.   Criteria for Severe Preeclampsia[a]

1. Blood pressure $\geq$ 160 mm Hg systolic or $\geq$ 110 mm Hg diastolic when recorded on at least 2 occasions 6 hr apart with patient at bed rest.
2. Proteinuria $\geq$ 5 g in 24 hr (3+ to 4+ on qualitative measure).
3. Oliguria $\leq$ 400 ml in 24 hr.
4. Visual or other CNS changes.
5. Epigastric pain.
6. Pulmonary edema or cyanosis.
7. Liver function abnormalities or uncertain etiology.
8. Thrombocytopenia.

[a] One or more required for diagnosis.

criteria. Alternatively, the diagnosis can be made on the basis of an increase in mean arterial pressure (MAP) of 20 mm Hg, or a reading of 105 mm Hg MAP. All of these readings must be present on two measurements taken at least 6 hours apart.

Proteinuria is defined as a concentration in a spot urine collection of 0.1 g/l or greater on two separate occasions 6 hours apart or 300 mg in a 24-hour collection (usually 1+ on the dipstick). Edema must be clinically measurable and not merely dependent edema or ankle edema, both of which are common in pregnancy. The best objective measure of edema is rapid weight gain.

Preeclampsia is graded from mild to severe. The criteria for severe preeclampsia are shown in Table 50.3. Eclampsia is the occurrence of seizure in the pregnant patient that cannot be attributed to other causes. The eclamptic patient may or may not exhibit the classic signs of preeclampsia prior to seizing.

The final two categories of hypertension in pregnancy are *preeclampsia superimposed on chronic hypertension* and *transient hypertension.* The latter is the onset of hypertension during pregnancy or in the first 24 hours after delivery without signs of preeclampsia or preexisting hypertension. Pressures must then return to normal within 10 days after delivery.

Although all forms of hypertension in pregnancy pose a serious problem for the obstetrician, the practitioner in the critical care setting will usually be faced only with hypertensive crises in chronic hypertensives or with the severe preeclamptic/eclamptic.

HYPERTENSIVE CRISIS IN THE CHRONIC HYPERTENSIVE

The management of hypertensive crisis in the pregnant patient is very similar to management of her nonpregnant counterpart. A useful distinction can be made between hypertensive emergencies and urgencies (41). Emergencies are those situations in which blood pressure must be lowered within the next hour to avoid serious or irreversible damage. They are usually characterized by acute, precipitous increases in pressure. Some of the more critical instances involve hypertensive encephalopathy, intracranial hemorrhage, acute left ventricular failure with pulmonary edema, and dissecting aortic aneurysm. Rapid and definitive therapy is required in these instances. The setting for this treatment is usually an intensive care unit.

Hypertensive urgencies are those instances in which blood pressure must be lowered within the next 24 hours. Sudden increases in pressure without evidence of end-organ damage and perioperative hypertension are in this category. More

gradual therapies can be applied in these situations, but the patient must be observed closely in a critical care setting for any evidence of new or worsening end-organ damage.

The most powerful agent for acute treatment of hypertensive crisis is sodium nitroprusside (42). This drug acts rapidly as an equal arterial and venous dilator. The nitroprusside molecule probably decomposes in the circulation on contact with red blood cells to form nitric oxide, which acts as a vasodilator and a platelet aggregation inhibitor. Onset of action is about 30 seconds after administration, with peak effect at 2 minutes. Duration of effect is about 3 minutes. Effective therapy requires continuous intravenous infusion beginning at 0.25 μg/kg/min. This dosage is titrated to effect in increments of 0.25 μg/kg/min every 5 minutes.

Because of the profound response to this agent, the patient must be monitored continuously in a critical care setting during therapy. The drug itself is very unstable. It is photosensitive and must be protected from light.

Adverse effects include severe hypotension, hyperdynamic cardiac response, undesired vasodilatation resulting in intrapulmonary shunting and coronary artery steal, and potential thiocyanate and cyanide toxicity of the fetus (43). Severe hypotension can cause fetal distress, and the patient undergoing treatment who has a fetus in a viable gestational age range should be monitored closely with continuous fetal monitoring. As in any critical situation, however, a threat to maternal life must be treated in the most appropriate manner.

Another valuable agent in the face of emergency hypertension is diazoxide. This agent hyperpolarizes arterial smooth muscle through activation of ATP-sensitive K^+ channels. This results in relaxation and arterial dilatation. Diazoxide is absorbed orally but is usually given intravenously for more rapid effect. Treatment was formerly initiated by a 300-mg bolus infusion, but this dosage has been found to cause maternal hypotension and fetal distress in many patients. Dosage should be 30 to 75 mg every 10 to 15 minutes. Half-life is 20 to 60 minutes. Duration of response is widely variable at 4 to 20 hours.

Adverse responses to diazoxide are maternal and fetal hyperglycemia and burning at the infusion site. Sodium and water retention may also occur.

Hydralazine is a potent arterial dilator that works on the smooth muscle of the artery, probably through release of nitric oxide in the circulation. This drug is well-absorbed through the GI tract, but systemic availability varies with the individual. Fast acetylators inactivate the compound before it reaches the circulation and have availability of only 16%. Slow acetylators show 35% availability. Systemic clearance is about 50 mg/kg/min. Metabolism is largely in the liver, but some extrahepatic metabolism must occur. Half-life is 1 hour. Peak effect is seen from 30 to 120 minutes. Duration can be up to 12 hours. Dosage is usually 5 mg given intravenously in the critical situation, followed by 5- to 10-mg doses every 20 minutes until the desired effect is reached. The total acute dose should not exceed 40 mg.

A baroreceptor-mediated sympathetic response to arterial dilatation can cause a reflex tachycardia and increase in cardiac output after administration. This response is usually not a factor in an otherwise healthy pregnant patient but can cause problems in a compromised individual. Hypotension (with

Table 50.4. Indications for Invasive Hemodynamic Monitoring in the Preeclamptic Patient

1. Persistent, profound oliguria not responsive to fluid bolus.
2. Pulmonary edema.
3. Hypertension resistant to hydralazine.
4. Induction of conduction anesthesia in a hemodynamically unstable patient.

accompanying fetal distress), chest pain, and, after chronic treatment, a lupus-like syndrome, have also been described.

Extensive clinical experience has shown the safety of administration of hydralazine during pregnancy. Animal studies show no changes in intervillous blood flow and an increase in uterine blood flow (which may slightly offset some of the hypotensive effects (44). Hydralazine crosses the placenta but seems to have no adverse effects on the fetus (45).

In the setting of dissecting aortic aneurysm during a hypertensive crisis, use of trimethaphan may be indicated. This is a ganglionic blocking agent with arterial and venous effects. It has rapid action, and effects can be achieved by minute-to-minute titration. A 0.1% solution (1 mg/ml) in 5% dextrose is administered intravenously. Infusion starts at 0.5 to 1 mg/min and is titrated until the blood pressure decreases 20 mm Hg or more. Another agent should be used after acute control has been attained.

Indiscriminate ganglionic blockade is the adverse effect seen with this agent. Paralytic ileus (both maternal and fetal), urinary retention, and hypotension are seen. Trimethaphan may also interact with succinylcholine at surgery, resulting in a prolonged muscular blockade.

Nitroglycerin is a vasodilator that can be administered sublingually or intravenously in the acute situation. An initial dose of 10 mg/min i.v. can be titrated to effect by doubling every 5 minutes. Half-life is 1 to 3 minutes. Methhemoglobinemia (methhemoglobin > 3%) is seen as doses exceed 7 mg/kg/min.

Nifedipine may be given orally as a 10-mg dose that can be repeated in 30 minutes. This dosage usually results in acute blood pressure reduction. Regular dosing can then continue at 10 to 20 mg every 3 to 6 hours. It should be noted that administration of this agent to a patient receiving magnesium sulfate (see below) can cause an exaggerated hypotension (46).

Nifedipine may become a more important agent in the control of acute hypertension in the pregnant patient since the manufacturer of hydralazine has announced its intention to discontinue manufacture of hydralazine for parenteral administration.

SEVERE PREECLAMPSIA/ECLAMPSIA

The patient meeting the criteria for severe preeclampsia or who has progressed to eclamptic seizures should be treated in an intensive care setting. Close monitoring is required. Occasionally, invasive hemodynamic monitoring will provide the only method of gaining information vital to management (Table 50.4) (47).

The only treatment for severe preeclampsia is delivery of the fetus and the placenta. The route and timing of the delivery must be determined by the condition of the patient and the fetus (who should be monitored continuously throughout evaluation and stabilization of the mother). The goals of therapy

before, during, and after delivery are stabilization of the mother, prevention of seizures, cessation of existing seizures, and control of malignant hypertension.

The agent customarily used for seizure prophylaxis in preeclampsia and eclampsia is magnesium sulfate ($MgSO_4 \cdot 7H_2O$). The exact mechanism of action of this drug is controversial. Many practitioners believe it acts as a neuromuscular blocker; others believe that it has central action. Its effectiveness as a seizure prophylaxis agent in this setting has been supported by numerous descriptive studies and long clinical experience (48).

The "classic" dosing was described by Pritchard (49): 4 g I.V., followed by 10 g i.m. Doses of 5 g i.m. are then given every 4 hours. Magnesium levels of 4 to 7 mEq/liter have been suggested for seizure suppression. Toxicity is seen at levels above this and is manifested by loss of patellar reflexes at 8 mEq and above, with respiratory arrest in patients with levels exceeding 13 mEq. Calcium gluconate (10 ml of 10% solution given intravenously) is an effective antidote.

An alternative dosing that has become more popular and results in equal efficacy is 4 to 6 g i.v. loading, followed by 2 to 3 g/hr continuous i.v. infusion (50).

Magnesium administration can cause loss of variability in the fetal heart rate tracing. Prolonged administration can also cause postnatal respiratory depression and hypotonia in the newborn.

An alternative to magnesium sulfate for seizure prophylaxis is administration of phenytoin. This agent is used widely as an anticonvulsant. Because of its erratic oral absorption, it is best given intravenously in the setting of preeclampsia. Concentrations of this drug in the serum are not linearly related to dosage. Small increases can result in large changes in serum levels. Serum half-life is approximately 24 hours, but this, too, varies. Therapeutic levels are 10 to 20 μg/ml. At concentrations above this nystagmus, ataxia, and lethargy can be seen.

The dosing for prophylaxis in preeclampsia varies with patient body habitus. Those patients weighing less than 50 kg are given a 1-g loading dose. The patient between 50 and 70 kg is given 1.2 g, while the patient over 70 kg is given 1.5 g. The first 750 mg of the loading dose is given at 25 mg/min. The remainder is given at 12.5 mg/min. A serum phenytoin level is then obtained 30 to 60 minutes after the loading dose. If a therapeutic level has been attained, no further drug is given. Another level is drawn in 12 hours. If the initial level is <10 μg/ml, an additional 500 mg of phenytoin is given. If the initial value lies between 10 and 12 μg/ml, 250 mg is given. Levels are then rechecked. The usual duration of administration is 24 hours after delivery, unless signs and symptoms of preeclampsia persist (51).

Hypotension is sometimes seen as a complication of phenytoin therapy and is thought to be related to free phenytoin levels in the serum. This situation can be encountered in the pregnant, preeclamptic patient who is relatively hypoalbuminemic. Slowing of the infusion rate is usually effective in reversing hypotension.

If the hypertension accompanying preeclampsia or eclampsia is at the urgent or emergent levels, the antihypertensive agents described above can and should be used to control blood pressure. This approach should not be viewed as

Table 50.5. Changes in Coagulation Factors Attributable to Pregnancy

Increased
    Factors V, VII, VIII, IX, X, XII
    Fibrinogen
    Placental inhibitors of fibrinolysis
Decreased
    Factors XI, XIII
    Antithrombin III
    PAPP-A (protein specific to pregnancy that neutralizes AT III)

Table 50.6. Some Features Associated with Warfarin Embryopathy

1. Nasal hypoplasia with depressed nasal bridge
2. Stippling of uncalcified epiphyses (resolves after 1st year of life)
3. Mild nail hypoplasia with shortened fingers
4. Low birth weight
5. Varying degrees of mental retardation

treatment of the underlying disease process, however, and plans for delivery should proceed.

THROMBOEMBOLIC DISEASE

DEEP VEIN THROMBOSIS AND PULMONARY EMBOLISM

During pregnancy there is an increase in factors promoting thrombosis and a decrease in thrombolytic factors (see Table 50.5). For this reason pregnancy has been called a "hypercoagulable state." The risk of thrombotic episodes increases at time of delivery and post partum. Deep vein thrombosis (DVT) is a complicating factor in only 0.018 to 0.29% of deliveries but can have dire consequences. Untreated, DVT will progress to thromboembolism in 15 to 24% of cases. Twelve to fifteen percent of these will result in maternal mortality. Early recognition and treatment can reduce these figures to 4.5 and 0.7%, respectively. Pulmonary embolism (PE) accounted for 14.3% of all maternal deaths in the U.S. from 1980 to 1985 (52).

The obstetric caregiver always maintains a high degree of suspicion of DVT in a pregnant or post partum patient but, occasionally, a thrombosis will progress quickly to embolism. Pulmonary embolism can be immediately fatal. In most patients there are some symptoms that point to the diagnosis. Dyspnea is seen in 80% of patients with PE, and pleuritic chest pain. Apprehension (60%), cough (50%), and tachypnea (90%) are also commonly seen. Once the diagnosis is established (usually by ventilation-perfusion scan or pulmonary arteriogram, which is the "gold standard"), the patient must be observed closely and treated immediately to avoid further, possibly fatal, embolization.

The drug of choice for acute and some long-term treatment is heparin. This drug is a heterogeneous acid mucopolysaccharide with a very high molecular weight (4000 to 40,000 daltons) that does not cross the placenta. It acts by binding to antithrombin III (AT III) and changes the configuration of AT III, causing it to bind more readily to thrombin and factors XIIa, IXa, Xa, and XIa and neutralize them. Small amounts of heparin can inhibit clotting, but larger amounts are required to keep an already established clot from growing.

Heparin can be given by intravenous or subcutaneous routes, but continuous intravenous infusion is more reliable in the acute situation. A bolus dose of 5000 to 10,000 units is given to load, followed by 700 to 2000 units/hr infusion. Half-life varies with dose and amount of thrombosis, and values of <1 hour to 2.5 hours are seen. Peak levels are also dose-related.

Heparin levels can be obtained, and these should be kept in the 0.2 to 0.4 IU/ml range (53). In clinical settings it is much easier and more practical to follow activated partial thromboplastin times (aPTT), which can be readily obtained in almost every hospital unit (54). The goal of therapy is a 1.5- to 2-fold increase in aPTT over that of controls. Dosage can be titrated to this endpoint. A minimum of 15 days of intravenous therapy is recommended.

The principal risk involved with heparin therapy is bleeding, which is especially dangerous in the postoperative patient who requires heparin after diagnosis of pulmonary embolism. Constant vigilance is necessary to rule out pelvic hematoma or ongoing blood loss.

The patient who survives the acute stage will require ongoing anticoagulation. The usual choice for this therapy is warfarin. This agent inhibits regeneration of vitamin K in the liver. Vitamin K is required to carboxylate glutamic acid residues on factors II, VII, IX, X, and protein C to render them active. Peak effect is achieved 36 to 72 hours after oral dosing. Action lasts 2 to 5 days. The rate of degradation is constant for each individual but varies among patients.

Therapy is monitored by following prothrombin time (PT) with a goal of a 2- to 2.5-fold rise. Dosing is 15 mg on the first day, 10 mg on the second, and 10 mg on the third. Depending on the PT at the end of this time, loading is continued or the maintenance dose of 5 to 7.5 mg/day is begun. PT is then followed at regular intervals.

Unlike heparin, warfarin's molecular weight is relatively small, allowing it to cross the placenta readily. There is a recognized embryopathy associated with administration of warfarin between the 6th and 9th weeks of gestation (Table 50.6) (52). There have also been reports of associations between warfarin therapy during the second and third trimesters of pregnancy and various central nervous system and ophthalmologic defects in the fetus (55). It is believed that up to 13% of pregnancies in which warfarin was used resulted in abnormal infants, 4% of these with the classic embryopathy. Of the latter, 30% may be developmentally retarded (56). For these reasons it is advisable to avoid the use of warfarin in pregnancy whenever possible.

Long-term treatment in the pregnant patient can be attained using heparin administered subcutaneously. Doses of 5000 to 8000 units given 3 times/day can keep the aPTT in the therapeutic range. The patient can be instructed in self-injection, and aPTT can be monitored in an outpatient setting.

Risks of long-term heparin therapy include thrombocytopenia and osteoporosis (52). The latter is reported more often in patients receiving 20,000 units/day or greater for >20 weeks (57). The mechanism is unknown but is thought to involve inhibition of hydroxylation of vitamin D, and patients on chronic heparin therapy should receive adequate amounts of vitamin D and calcium in their diets. Thrombocytopenia affects about 1% of those patients treated with heparin and is seen 5 to 10 days after the initiation of therapy. It may be caused by heparin-dependent platelet antibodies (52, 58). Platelet count should be followed closely in patients on this regime.

DISSEMINATED INTRAVASCULAR COAGULATION

Disseminated intravascular coagulation (DIC) is not itself a disease entity but rather the consequence of many disease entities. In obstetric patients the causes can be numerous (Table 50.7). The primary task of the treatment team is to make an accurate diagnosis and rectify the underlying disorder while minimizing the damage caused by this abnormal coagulation.

The initiator of DIC usually causes stimulation of platelet-activating factors, causing degranulation and activation of the intrinsic coagulation cascade. Fibrin is formed, which is in turn degraded by plasminogen. The normal controls for this process are lost in DIC, and the continued activation and degradation of clotting factors proceed throughout the body, causing acute shortage of these factors, resulting in clinical bleeding. Unless reversed, the process is fatal.

Most patients respond to support with blood products until the precipitating causes are rectified. There are some instances in which treatment of the pregnant patient may be required. In this case intravenous heparin may be employed. This treatment should be done with caution, however, as indiscriminate use of heparin in the face of low AT III levels can be ineffective and quite dangerous. AT III activity should be assessed before instituting therapy. If this activity is greater than 70%, low-dose heparin (2500 to 5000 units subcutaneously every 8 to 12 hours) can be administered (59). This therapy can often stabilize the patient until the original insult is corrected and its effects have been reversed. An intact vasculature must be ensured prior to the initiation of heparin therapy in the pregnant patient with DIC.

DIABETIC KETOACIDOSIS

Diabetic ketosis can be a very morbid state for the pregnant diabetic and can result in fetal losses of up to 50%. Although modern management of pregnant diabetics has reduced the number of patients presenting with diabetic ketoacidosis (DKA), this condition is still encountered in approximately 5% of pregnant diabetic patients (60).

DKA results from a relative or absolute lack of insulin that results in hyperglycemia and release of hormones that counterregulate metabolism opposite insulin: glucagon, cate-cholamines, growth hormone, and cortisol. In pregnancy, human placental lactogen (HPL) and prolactin also function in this latter capacity. Free fatty acids are liberated and metabolized. Ketones accumulate, and β-hydroxybutyrate and acet-oacetate levels increase. As a result, serum pH drops. The

Table 50.7. Factors Predisposing to DIC in the Obstetric Patient

Placental abruption	Amniotic fluid embolus
Pre-eclampsia/eclampsia	Saline abortion
Intrauterine fetal demise	Sepsis
Acute fatty liver of pregnancy	Mulitple transfusions

presence of increased amounts of glucose causes osmotic diuresis. Potassium and sodium ions are lost in the process.

The fetus is affected by the fluid and electrolyte shifts in the maternal system and can experience hypoxia due to decreased placental blood flow. Fetal serum levels of β-hydroxybutyrate and glucose parallel maternal levels, causing acidosis and hyperglycemia in the fetus. This change can result in fetal damage or loss unless quickly corrected (61).

Therapy is directed at correction of fluid and metabolic derangements. While blood is being obtained from the acute patient for hemogram and chemistry profiles, a challenge bolus of 25 mL D50 should be administered intravenously. This regimen will distinguish the patient in hyperinsulinemic coma from the DKA patient. Fluid replacement should then begin immediately, using isotonic solution. One liter should be given in the first hour. The infusion should then run at 250 to 500 ml/hr until 75% of the estimated volume deficit is corrected. Rates can then be reduced, but a goal of 6 to 8 liters in the first 24 hours should be met. When the blood glucose is below 250 mg/dl, 5% dextrose can be added to the fluid solution.

Potassium chloride should be administered from the start of treatment. Because intracellular K^+ exits the cell during the DKA process, false-normal levels can be obtained. As the situation is corrected, these K^+ ions will return to the cell, leaving an extracellular deficit that must be corrected. If the initial K^+ level is normal, 20 to 30 mEq should be added to each liter of fluid. If initial levels are low, 40 to 60 mEq should be given with the infusion.

Regular insulin should be infused intravenously for glucose control. A dose of 0.1 units/kg i.v. push is given immediately, as a loading dose. A continuous infusion of 8 to 10 units/hr should then be started. If no response is seen in 2 hours (at least a 25% decrease in blood glucose), the dose should be doubled, because insulin resistance can be a factor. When the glucose level reaches 250 mg/dl, 5% dextrose is added to the solution, and the insulin dose is cut in half. When the level of 150 mg/dl is reached, a constant infusion of 1 to 2 units/hr is maintained.

While this therapy is proceeding, efforts must be made to identify and correct the precipitating cause of DKA. In the pregnant patient this cause is most often infection, tocolysis with β-mimetic agents, missed insulin doses, or insulin pump failure (61, 62). Since the use of β-mimetic agents can greatly exacerbate DKA, tocolysis in the patient that is believed to be in preterm labor should be initiated with other agents.

THYROTOXICOSIS

Thyroid disease complicates about 0.2% of pregnancies (61). Graves' disease is responsible for approximately 80% of these cases. Occasionally, this disease will manifest severely, causing heart failure or the potentially fatal thyroid storm.

Thyroid hormone is known to have effects on cardiac inotropy and chronotropy. Excess thyroid hormone can cause dysrhythmias. Tachycardia at rest, increased cardiac output, and widening pulse pressures are also seen. If there is preexisting cardiac compromise, if thyroid disease is in poor control, or if unusual stress factors exist, these symptoms may progress to frank cardiac failure (63).

The thyrotoxic patient with heart failure requires rapid treatment. One of the primary goals is diagnosis of the underlying cause of thyroid excess and prompt return of thyroid hormone to normal levels. Propranolol, one of the agents often used to control dysrhythmias in the hyperthyroid state, should be discontinued if failure becomes evident. Digoxin may be helpful but may need to be administered in higher doses to be effective. Support of cardiac function should be maintained until the levels of thyroid hormone can be returned to normal levels and the precipitating factors controlled.

Thyrotoxicosis can also be manifest as thyroid storm. This is an acute and severe exacerbation of hyperthyroidism manifested by fever, agitation, tremor, alteration in mental status, tachycardia, atrial fibrillation, signs of heart failure, nausea, vomiting, and diarrhea. Rarely, it is the first manifestation of thyroid disease in an undiagnosed patient. More commonly, it is an acute worsening of preexisting disease precipitated by some stress such as emergency surgery, induction of anesthesia, infection, myocardial infarction, diabetic ketoacidosis, or pulmonary embolus.

Because of the physiologic changes imposed by pregnancy, the symptoms of hyperthyroidism may be difficult to detect. Increase in heart rate and cardiac output, nausea, and heat intolerance are commonly seen in early pregnancy. Consistent heart rate >100, accompanied by tremors, lid lag, and thyromegaly, suggests increased thyroid effects. Low serum thyroid-stimulating hormone (TSH) and increased free thyroxine are reliable indicators of hyperthyroidism not affected by pregnancy (61).

The patient in thyroid storm should be admitted to an intensive care unit. Intravenous access should be obtained and isotonic fluids administered. A thorough history and examination should be undertaken in an effort to diagnose the precipitating cause. Hemodynamic monitoring may be required. Cooling blankets can be used to control temperature. Oxygen should be administered.

Until a full picture of the patient's situation can be obtained, broad spectrum antibiotics should be administered. Fever should be controlled with acetaminophen (325 to 500 mg every 3 to 4 hours) instead of salicylates, which cause increased free thyroid hormone by inhibiting binding (64).

The goal of antithyroid therapy is to reduce the action of thyroid hormone at tissue levels as quickly as possible. Propylthiouracil (PTU) is the usual agent of choice in this situation. It inhibits the formation of new thyroid hormone and blocks conversion of T_4 to T_3 peripherally. Dosage is 300 to 600 mg orally (or by nasogastric tube) initially, then 150 to 300 mg every 6 hours. Effective levels are reached approximately 30 to 40 minutes after dosing. Half-life is 3 to 6 hours. The drug is concentrated in the thyroid gland. Sensitivity is manifested by a rash.

An alternative medication is methimazole, which has the same actions and indications as PTU but is 10 times more potent. Plasma half-life is 3 to 9 hours. Methimazole is given in a dose of 30 to 60 mg every 6 hours until the patient is euthyroid. Then it is given as 10 to 30 mg/day in divided doses.

It is recommended that administration of iodine follow treatment with PTU or methimazole in this setting. Iodides inhibit the secretion of thyroid hormone (61). Sodium iodide (Lugol's solution) or potassium iodide can be given orally or by NG tube. The former is given as 2 to 6 drops 3 times daily,

the latter as 5 drops 3 times/day. Sodium iodide can also be administered intravenously as 250 to 500 mg daily.

PTU, methimazole, and iodides cross the placenta freely (65). Ultrasound of the fetus may be able to detect a fetal goiter in more severe cases when the mother has been treated with iodides or with more than 300 mg PTU or more than 30 mg methimazole per day. This condition may hinder delivery and cause hypothyroidism in the neonate (66). Close ultrasound observation of the fetus is recommended, however, and this therapy should proceed in cooperation with an obstetrician. Since thyroid storm is potentially fatal for the pregnant patient and since the duration of acute therapy is short, the critical care practitioner should not hesitate to use iodides in this setting.

Propranolol can inhibit tachycardia and block T_4 to T_3 conversion peripherally. It is administered intravenously at a rate of 1 mg/min not to exceed 10 mg. The effects usually last 3 to 4 hours. The oral dose is 40 to 80 mg every 4 to 6 hours. This regimen can be a crucial element of initial therapy. Acute thyroid storm has also been managed using esmolol (67).

Steroids are also helpful as adjunctive therapy (61). Hydrocortisone (300 mg/day), prednisone (60 mg/day), and dexamethasone (8 mg/day) can be used. The effect is to aid inhibition of peripheral T_4 to T_3 conversion.

After the acute phase has been controlled, the iodides and the steroids can be discontinued. The antithyroid drugs should continue until the patient is euthyroid. In the nonpregnant patient, ablation of the thyroid or thyroidectomy would then be performed. It is advisable to postpone ablation of the thyroid until after pregnancy. Surgery has been accomplished successfully on pregnant patients, but this, too, should be deferred if at all possible (66).

SEPTIC SHOCK

Shock is a state of reduced tissue perfusion that results in cellular hypoxia and, eventually, hemodynamic instability and organ damage. Sepsis is the third most common cause of shock after hypovolemia and myocardial infarction (68). Until relatively recently, septic shock was an important cause of maternal death in postpartum patients. Since the development of antibiotics, the incidence of sepsis in the obstetric population has drastically declined. Today, bacteremia is seen in only 8 to 10% of obstetric infections, and progresses to shock in only about 4% of these cases (69).

Death from septic shock is much less common in the obstetric population (0 to 3%) than in other hospitalized patients (10 to 81%) (70). This is so because obstetric patients tend to be younger and have fewer concurrent diseases than other patients in a hospital population. The cause of sepsis is often more easily diagnosed and, therefore, treated more rapidly in the obstetric patient as well. The most common predisposing conditions in the pregnant and postpartum patient are given in Table 50.8.

The major cause of morbidity in septic shock is vascular collapse caused by infection by a variety of microorganisms. The most common cause is endotoxin release by Gram-negative bacteria, usually coliforms. Anaerobes such as *Bacteroides fragilis* and Gram-positive organisms that release exotoxins can also be seen. There is at least one study in animal models

Table 50.8. Conditions Predisposing to Sepsis in the Obstetric Patient

Chorioamnionitis	Postpartum endometritis
Pyelonephritis	Septic abortion
Postoperative fasciitis	Immune deficiency
Concurrent conditions requiring immunosuppressive drugs	

that suggests that pregnancy may confer an increased susceptibility to endotoxins, placing the pregnant patient at greater risk for shock (71, 72).

Treatment involves aggressive efforts to support and improve circulation by restoring volume. Isotonic crystalloid solutions are usually employed, although some practitioners advocate colloid. A reliable airway must be established and maintained. A thorough history and examination should be undertaken to determine the cause. Empiric, broad-spectrum antibiotics should be administered to cover aerobic and anaerobic infections. If *Staphylococcus* is suspected, appropriate agents should be added to cover this organism. During evaluation and treatment, fetal monitoring should be undertaken since the fetus will often show signs of intolerance of maternal hypoperfusion. Priority treatment should be given to the mother since fetal well-being will depend on her stability in the immediate situation. Delivery is not automatically indicated unless the source of the sepsis is determined to be intrauterine. In this case the uterus should be emptied only after the mother has been stabilized and antibiotic therapy has begun.

Besides volume expansion, vasoactive agents may be necessary to ensure adequate circulation. The drug most commonly employed is dopamine. The hemodynamic effects of this agent vary with dosage. Small doses (<5 μg/kg/min) act on dopaminergic receptors in the mesenteric and renal vascular beds, producing selective vasodilatation. At doses from 5 to 10 μg/kg/min, β-receptors are also activated, causing improved myocardial contractility and increased heart rate and cardiac output without increase in myocardial oxygen consumption. Doses of 10 to 20 μg/kg/min cause β-effects to predominate. Large doses (>20 μg/kg/min) bring α-receptors into play, causing vasoconstriction.

In the setting of septic shock, dopamine should be started at 2 to 5 μg/kg/min and titrated to best effect. Adverse effects include nausea, vomiting, headache, tachydysrhythmias, and angina. Dopamine has been found to cause decreased uterine blood flow in one study (73), and fetal monitoring is indicated during use.

If heart failure is noted, digoxin should be administered. Dosing begins with 0.75 mg in three doses 4 to 6 hours apart. Levels of 0.5 to 2.5 ng/ml should be the therapeutic goal.

Broad spectrum antibiotics should be given intravenously, with coverage tailored to suspected causes. The regimen most often used in obstetric populations is ampicillin (2 g every 6 hours), gentamicin (1.5 mg/kg every 8 hours), and clindamycin (600 mg every 6 hours) (68). Antibiotics that should be avoided in pregnancy include tetracyclines that cross the placenta and deposit in fetal decidual teeth and ossification centers, resulting in dental discoloration and inhibition of bone growth, and quinolones that inhibit DNA synthesis and have been

shown to deposit in fetal cartilage in animal studies, resulting in irreversible arthropathies (68).

Extensive cultures should be obtained, but should not delay therapy. The patient should be observed closely for signs of adult respiratory distress syndrome (ARDS). Supportive measures should be readily available. Surgical intervention, including evacuation of the uterus, should be undertaken as indicated but only after antibiotics have been started.

There have been indications that administrations of corticosteroids (methylprednisolone) early in the course of sepsis may improve outcome (74). The proposed mechanisms were stabilization of cell membranes, inhibition of complement-induced inflammation, improvement of myocardial performance, and improvement of the oxygen dissociation curve. Two recent randomized controlled studies have failed to prove the efficacy of steroids in this setting, however (75, 76). Many authorities currently recommend avoiding steroid use in the septic patient (68).

Other suggested methods of treatment include naloxone administration to counter endorphins, which have been seen to increase in the septic shock patient (77), and specific monoclonal antibodies aimed at cachectin, a substance implicated in many of the physiologic changes leading to vascular collapse (70). These methods may have some promise but as yet are unproven as first-line therapy.

MISCELLANEOUS SITUATIONS

HUMAN IMMUNODEFICIENCY VIRUS INFECTION

The World Health Organization estimates that in early 1990 more than 3 million females were infected by the human immunodeficiency virus (HIV). Most of them were of childbearing age (78). Many were unaware of their HIV status until during or after their pregnancy. Since transmission of the virus to the fetus is an important form of infection and since the incidence of this transmission is estimated to be from 30 to 50%, this situation is most serious.

HIV infection is also an important source of morbidity for the pregnant patient. The mean time from infection with HIV until progression to AIDS is 6 years (79). It is at present unclear whether pregnancy may accelerate this process (68).

The most common AIDS-related opportunistic infection that will place the pregnant patient in a critical care setting is *Pneumocystis carinii* pneumonia (PCP) (78). This infection is especially likely in those patients whose CD_4 (helper T-cell) counts are below 200 cells/mm³.

PCP can cause acute respiratory distress requiring assisted ventilation in an intensive care setting. Recommended treatment is oral or intravenous sulfamethoxazole/trimethoprim (68). In the pregnant patient who may have impaired gastrointestinal absorption the intravenous route is favored (80). These drugs are inhibitors of the synthesis of tetrahydrofolic acid and act at separate sites in this process. Sulfamethoxazole inhibits incorporation of para-aminobenzoic acid into folic acid. Trimethoprim inhibits reduction of dihydrofolate to tetrahydrofolate. These agents are often administered together in one preparation (Septra, Bactrim) and act in such a way that they remain in a constant ratio of 20 : 1 (sulfamethoxazole/trimethoprim). Trimethoprim attains peak levels at 2 hours

Table 50.9. American Rheumatism Association Criteria for Diagnosis of Systemic Lupus Erythematosus[a]

1. Malar rash
2. Discoid rash
3. Photosensitivity
4. Oral ulcers
5. Arthritis
6. Serositis
7. Renal disorder
8. Neurologic disorder
9. Hematologic disorder
10. Immunologic disorder
11. Antinuclear antibody

[a] Four of the symptoms must be present.

after dosing, while sulfamethoxazole requires 4 hours. Half-life of trimethoprim is 11 hours, and that of sulfamethoxazole 10 hours. Dosage for sulfamethoxazole is 100 mg/kg/day and for trimethoprim 20 mg/kg/day.

Since these agents are folate antagonists there is a theoretical possibility of teratogenic action if given in early pregnancy. While this possibility has not been conclusively proven, alternative antibiotics are usually preferred (68).

In later pregnancy these drugs can cross to the fetus and impair liver function causing postnatal icterus. While this is rarely a serious problem in term infants it can be a consideration for extremely preterm children. Given the seriousness of PCP infection in an AIDS patient, however, potential life-saving medication should not be withheld for these considerations.

For those patients who are intolerant of sulfamethoxazole-trimethoprim or who have failed therapy with these agents, treatment with pentamidine isethionate is recommended (68). This drug is an antiprotozoal medication of the diamidine class that is well-absorbed parenterally. Half-life is 6 hours. Usual dosage is 4 mg/kg/day.

There is no definitive data on the safety of pentamidine during pregnancy. The manufacturer counsels against its use in this setting. However, since this agent is potentially life-saving in severe PCP, the unknown risk of fetal effects should not delay its use.

Adverse effects of pentamidine include breathlessness, tachycardia, dizziness, fainting, headache, and vomiting. These effects may be caused by histamine release.

CONNECTIVE TISSUE DISEASES

Connective tissue diseases are a group of overlapping disease entities with the common features of inflammation of skin, joints, and other connective tissue structures, altered patterns of immune regulation, production of autoantibodies, and abnormalities of cell-mediated immunity. Systemic lupus erythematosus (SLE) is a specific disease within this group. The American Rheumatism Association has defined strict criteria for diagnosis of SLE (Table 50.9) (81). This disease can present with renal, neurologic, hematologic, and immunologic abnormalities that can cause serious illness during times of acute exacerbation (flare). Since this disease affects women more often than men, and since most of the affected women become symptomatic during the reproductive years, SLE can pose critical problems during pregnancy.

Lupus flare in the pregnant patient can be as mild as increased joint pain or rash or as serious as renal failure, psychosis, seizures, or thrombotic stroke (82). Often, SLE flare in pregnancy presents a diagnostic dilemma since its manifestations are difficult to distinguish from acute, severe preeclampsia. Since the treatment of these two entities is different and both are potentially very morbid when not treated promptly, accurate diagnosis is essential (83).

Laboratory studies are sometimes helpful in proper diagnosis of the patient presenting with proteinuria, hypertension, seizures, and mental status changes. Acute decrease in complement levels coinciding with symptom onset would indicate lupus flare (83). Decreased urinary calcium excretion in a 24-hour collection implies preeclampsia (84). Most often, however, these results cannot be obtained in time to be useful in an acute situation, and the practitioner must weigh the clinical evidence and act accordingly.

The treatment for preeclampsia has been described above. Lupus flare is usually treated with steroids (usually, prednisone, with dosage depending on the usual daily dose on which the patient had been maintained prior to flare). If seizures are present, antiseizure medication can be employed. If preeclampsia is thought to be superimposed, magnesium sulfate or phenytoin may be used (see Severe Preeclampsia/Eclampsia). If thrombotic stroke is diagnosed, heparin should be administered and continued at anticoagulation doses (see Thromboembolic Disease) (85). Heparin therapy should be delayed until after operative delivery if it is deemed necessary for treatment of severe superimposed preeclampsia.

Current evidence suggests that pregnant lupus patients are more likely than nonpregnant lupus patients to experience some flare (86). With this in mind it is recommended that the pregnant lupus patient be followed closely by an obstetrician and a rheumatologist throughout pregnancy. Early treatment at the first sign of exacerbation may avoid further severe complications.

THE ORGAN TRANSPLANT RECIPIENT

As transplantation technology advances, more women of childbearing age will be organ recipients, and some of these women will become pregnant. At the present time most of the experience with pregnant transplant recipients has been with renal patients. It is estimated that 2% of women in the reproductive age group with renal transplants become pregnant (87). Many of these pregnancies result in spontaneous or elective abortions. Of those proceeding past the first trimester, 90% result in successful delivery (88).

Renal transplant recipients are prone to pregnancy-induced hypertension, which may progress to preeclampsia/eclampsia in 30% of cases (88). Acute transplant rejection occurs in approximately 9% of pregnancies (87). Increased incidence of septicemia is also seen in these patients.

All transplant recipients require some immunosuppressive agents to protect against rejection of the organ. Most patients will be receiving prednisone and either azathioprine or cyclosporine. Azathioprine is a prodrug that is cleaved to mercaptopurine by nucleophiles such as glutathione. The purine analog mercaptopurine is incorporated into RNA and

DNA, causing dysfunctional protein products that usually result in varying degrees of bone marrow suppression and blunting of the immune-rejection system. Oral availability is 60%. Half-life is approximately 0.16 hour but can vary. The usual dose is 3 to 10 mg/kg/day before transplant and maintenance doses of 1 to 3 mg/kg/day. Adverse effects include leukopenia, thrombocytopenia, nausea, vomiting, and hepatic toxicity.

Azathioprine has been used successfully in many pregnant renal transplant patients without any apparent adverse effects on the fetus. This may be due to the fact that in the early period of development, the fetus lacks the enzyme inosinate pyrophosphorylase, which converts azathioprine to thioinosinic acid, an active metabolite (87).

Cyclosporine is a relatively new agent that is part of a family of cyclic peptides produced by the fungus *Tolypocladium inflatum Gams*. Cyclosporine is lipophilic and readily binds to circulating lipoproteins. It acts by inhibiting activation of T-cells without myelosuppression. The exact site of this action is not well-defined. Bioavailability is 20 to 50%. Peak concentrations are reached 3 to 4 hours after dosing. Half-life is thought to be 6 hours. The drug is metabolized in the liver. Agents such as phenytoin, phenobarbital, sulfamethoxazole-trimethoprim, and rifampin can effect the liver metabolism of cyclosporine, causing increased clearance and decreased circulating levels. This phenomenon has been responsible for transplant rejection in some patients.

Dosage of cyclosporine is 15 mg/kg/day for 1 to 2 weeks preceding transplant and then 3 to 10 mg/kg/day thereafter. Levels are measured for dose adjustment. In whole blood 250 to 800 ng/ml is considered adequate. Therapeutic levels in plasma are 50 to 100 ng/ml. If newer monoclonal antibody detection systems are used, levels of 100 to 150 ng/ml are sought.

Adverse effects include renal toxicity (seen in up to 25 to 75% of patients), hepatic toxicity (50% of patients will have elevated liver enzymes), and increased infections.

There is insufficient evidence to state unequivocally that cyclosporine is safe for the fetus during pregnancy. As more information is gained, its clinical safety is being clarified. Since the drug is lipophilic, it crosses the placenta. Levels are seen in the fetus, but no fetal nephrotoxicity or hepatotoxicity has been reported. Fetal levels decline to undetectable levels in about 1 week (89).

Some studies have noted that levels of cyclosporine in the pregnant patient can fluctuate. With constant dosing, levels have been seen to decrease in the second and third trimesters. Increase in dose restores therapeutic levels, but it has been noted that immediately after delivery the patient may exhibit toxic symptoms, and rapid dose reductions are necessary (90). This phenomenon may be related to the fact that cyclosporine is highly bound to erythrocytes and lipoproteins in the circulation. During pregnancy blood volume and red cell volume change drastically. This change may alter the proportion of bound and free cyclosporine, resulting in an apparent change in levels in the patient. After delivery, these volume relationships change rapidly, which could explain the sudden rebound seen in drug effect. Levels of cyclosporine should be monitored carefully during pregnancy and shortly after delivery.

There has been limited experience with pregnancy in liver transplant recipients (91, 92). The same principles of drug therapy used in renal transplant patients apply.

Heart transplantation is now practiced in many centers throughout the world. The expected 5-year survival exceeds 70% for the 2500 cases performed each year. There are now reports of experience with pregnancies in recipients of cardiac allografts (92a). Complications are similar to those seen in other transplant patients, and immunosuppressant therapy is a mainstay of successful outcome.

CONCLUSION

This discussion has presented some of the more serious situations in which the critical care practitioner might encounter the pregnant patient. It is by no means exhaustive. The critical care team is urged to solicit the advice of an obstetrician early in the care of an obstetric patient. Those clinicians who desire further information concerning the physiologic changes seen in pregnancy and their implications for the medical and surgical care of the pregnant patient are referred to more specialized texts (93).

REFERENCES

1. Hytten F, Chamberlain G (eds): *Clinical Physiology in Obstetrics*, ed 2. Blackwell Scientific Publications, Oxford, 1991.
2. Harrison MR, Golbus MS, Filly RA: *The Unborn Patient*, ed 2. WB Saunders, Philadelphia, 1990.
3. Mabie WC, Sibai BM: Treatment in an obstetric intensive care unit. *Am J Obstet Gynecol* 162:1–4, 1990.
4. Briggs GG, Freeman RK, Yaffe SJ: *Drugs in Pregnancy and Lactation*, ed 3. Williams & Wilkins, Baltimore, 1990.
5. Clark SL: Structural cardiac disease in pregnancy. In Clark SL, Cotton DB, Hankins GDV, Phelan JP (eds): *Critical Care Obstetrics*, ed 2. Blackwell Scientific Publications, Boston, pp 114–131, 1991.
6. Perloff JK: Congenital heart disease. In Gleicher N (ed): *Principles and Practice of Medical Therapy in Pregnancy*, ed 2. Appleton & Lange, Norwalk, CT, pp 788–794, 1991.
7. Dajani AS, Bisno AL, Chung KJ, et al: Prevention of bacterial endocarditis: Recommendations by the American Heart Association. *JAMA* 264:2919–2922, 1990.
8. Wigvist N, Bygdeman M, Kwon Su, et al: Effect of prostaglandin E₁ on the midpregnant human uterus: intravenous, intramuscular, intra-amniotic, and vaginal administration. *Am J Obstet Gynecol* 102:327–332, 1968.
9. Willis DC, Caton D, Levelle P, et al: Cardiac output response to prostaglandin E₂—induced abortion in the second trimester. *Am J Obstet Gynecol* 156:170–173, 1987.
10. American College of Obstetricians and Gynecologists: Methods of midtrimester abortion. *Tech Bull* #109, October 1987.
11. Hankins GDV, Berryman GK, Scott RT: Maternal arterial desaturation with 15-methyl prostaglandin F₂ alpha for uterine atony. *Obstet Gynecol* 72:367–370, 1988.
12. McAnulty JH: Rheumatic heart disease. In Gleicher N (ed): *Principles and Practice of Medical Therapy in Pregnancy*, ed 2. Appleton & Lange, Norwalk, CT, pp 783–788, 1991.
13. Pruyn SC, Phelan JP, Buchanan GC: Long-term propranolol therapy in pregnancy: maternal and fetal outcome. *Am J Obstet Gynecol* 135:485–489, 1979.
14. Hokegard KH, Karlsson K, Kjellmer I, et al: ECG changes in the fetal lamb during asphyxia in relation to beta-adrenoreceptor stimulation and blockade. *Acta Physiol Scand* 105:195–203, 1979.
15. Redmond GP: Propranolol and fetal growth retardation. *Semin Perinatol* 6:142–147, 1982.
16. Barden TP, Stauder RW: Effects of adrenergic blocking agents and catecholamines in human pregnancy. *Am J Obstet Gynceol* 102:226–235, 1968.
17. Widerhorn J, Widerhorn ALM, Elkayam U: Cardiovascular pharmacotherapy in pregnancy and lactation. In Gleicher N (ed): *Principles and Practice of Medical Therapy in Pregnancy*, ed 2. Appleton & Lange, Norwalk, CT, pp 767–783, 1991.
18. Valdes Jr R: Endogenous digoxin-like immunoreactive factors: impact on digoxin measurements and potential physiologic implications. *Clin Chem* 31:1525–1531, 1985.
19. Phelps SJ, Cochran EB, Gonzalez-Ruiz A, et al: The influence of gestational age and preeclampsia on the presence and magnitude of serum endogenous digoxin-like immunoreactive substance(s). *Am J Obstet Gynecol* 158:34–39, 1988.
20. Widerhorn J, Rubin JN, Frishman WH, et al: Cardiovascular drugs in pregnancy. *Cardiol Clin* 5:651–674, 1987.
21. Epstein SE, Rosing DR: Verapamil: its potential for causing serious complications in patients with hypertrophic cardiomyopathy. *Circulation* 64:437–441, 1981.
22. Owen J, Colvin EV, Davis RO: Fetal death after successful conversion of fetal supraventricular tachycardia with digoxin and verapamil. *Am J Obstet Gynecol* 158:1169–1170, 1988.

23. Lee W, Cotton DB: Peripartum cardiomyopathy: current concepts and clinical management. *Clin Obstet Gynecol* 32:54–67, 1989.
24. Elkayam U, Ostrzega EL, Shotan A: Peripartum cardiomyopathy. In Gleicher N (ed): *Principles and Practice of Medical Therapy in Pregnancy*, ed 2. Appleton & Lange, Norwalk, CT, pp 812–814, 1991.
25. Broughton-Pipkin F, Baker PN, Symonds EM: ACE inhibitors in pregnancy. *Lancet* ii:96–97, 1989.
26. Midei MG, DeMent SH, Feldman AM, et al: Peripartum myocarditis and cardiomyopathy. *Circulation* 81:922–928, 1990.
27. Hankins GDV, Wendel GD, Leveno KJ, Stoneham J: Myocardial infarction during pregnancy: a review. *Obstet Gynecol* 65:139–146, 1985.
27a. Emergency Cardiac Care Committee. American Heart Association: Guidelines for cardiopulmonary resuscitation and emergency cardiac care. *JAMA* 268:2231, 1992.
27b. MacMahon S, Collins R, Peto R, Koster RW, Yusuf S: Effects of prophylactic lidocaine in suspected acute myocardial infarction: an overview of results from the randomized controlled trials. *JAMA* 260:1910–1916, 1988.
27c. Berntsen RF, Rasmussen K: Lidocaine to prevent ventricular fibrillation in the prehospital phase of suspected acute myocardial infarction: the North-Norwegian lidocaine intervention trial. *Am Heart J* 124:1478–1483, 1992.
27d. Nattel S, Arenal A: Antiarrhythmic prophylaxis after acute myocardial infarction: Is lidocaine still useful? *Drugs* 45:9–14, 1993.
28. Nolan TE, Hankins GDV: Myocardial infarction in pregnancy. *Clin Obstet Gynecol* 32:68–75, 1989.
29. Hansmann M, Gembruch U, Bald R, et al: Fetal tachyarrhythmias: transplacental and direct treatment of the fetus—a report of 60 cases. *Ultrasound Obstet Gynecol* 1:162–170, 1991.
30. Dumesic DA, Silverman NH, Tobias S, et al: Transplacental cardioversion of fetal supraventricular tachycardia with procainamide. *N Engl J Med* 307:1128–1131, 1982.
31. Shaxted EJ, Milton PJ: Disopyramide in pregnancy: a case report. *Curr Med Res Opin* 6:70–72, 1979.
32. Leonard RF, Braun TE, Levy AM: Initiation of uterine contractions by disopyramide during pregnancy. *N Engl J Med* 299:84–85, 1978.
33. Foster CJ, Love HG: Amiodarone in pregnancy: a case report and review of literature. *Int J Cardiol* 20:307–316, 1988.
33a. Emergency Cardiac Care Committee, American Heart Association: Guidelines for cardiopulmonary resuscitation and emergency cardiac care. *JAMA* 268:2224–2225, 1992.
33b. Leffler S, Johnson DR: Adenosine use in pregnancy: lack of effect on fetal heart rate. *Am J Emerg Med* 10:548–549, 1992.
33c. Kleinman CS, Copel JA: Electrophysiological principles and fetal antiarrhythmic therapy. *Ultrasound Obstet Gynecol* 1:286–297, 1991.
34. ACCP-AIS: Joint committee on pulmonary nomenclature: pulmonary terms and symbols. *Chest* 67:583, 1975.
35. Barth WH, Hankins GDV: Severe acute asthma in pregnancy. In Clark SL, Cotton DB, Hankins GDV, Phelan JP (eds): *Critical Care Obstetrics*, ed 2. Blackwell Scientific Publications, Boston, pp 371–392, 1991.
36. Schatz M: Asthma during pregnancy: interrelationships and management. *Ann Allergy* 68:123–133, 1992.
37. Greenberger PA: Asthma during pregnancy. *J Asthma* 27:341–347, 1990.
38. Schreier L: Asthma. In Gleicher N (ed): *Principles and Practice of Medical Therapy in Pregnancy*, ed 2. Appleton & Lange, Norwalk, CT, pp 748–757, 1991.
39. Huff RW: Asthma in pregnancy. *Med Clin North Am* 73:653–660, 1989.
40. Davye DA, MacGillivray I: The classification and definition of the hypertensive disorders of pregnancy. *Am J Obstet Gynecol* 158:892–898, 1988.
41. Ferguson RK, Vlasses PH: Hypertensive emergencies and urgencies. *JAMA* 255:1607–1613, 1986.
42. Baker AB: Management of severe pregnancy-induced hypertension, or gestosis, with sodium nitroprusside. *Anesth Intens Care* 18:361–365, 1990.
43. Shoemaker CT, Meyers M: Sodium nitroprusside for control of severe hypertensive disease of pregnancy: a case report and discussion of potential toxicity. *Am J Obstet Gynecol* 149:171–173, 1984.
44. Jouppila P, Kirkinen P, Koivula A, et al: Effects of dihydralazine infusion on the fetoplacental blood flow and maternal prostanoids. *Obstet Gynecol* 65:115–118, 1985.
45. Liedholm H, Wahlin-Boll E, Hanson A, et al: Transplacental passage and breast milk concentrations of hydralazine. *Eur J Clin Pharmacol* 21:417–419, 1982.
46. Waisman GD, Mayorga LM, Camera MI, et al: Magnesium plus nifedipine: potentiation of hypotensive effect in preeclampsia. *Am J Obstet Gynecol* 159:308–309, 1988.
47. Dildy GA, Phelan JP, Cotton DB: Complications of pregnancy-induced hypertension. In Clark SL, Cotton DB, Hankins GDV, Phelan JP (eds): *Critical Care Obstetrics*, ed 2. Blackwell Scientific Publications, Boston, pp 251–288, 1991.
48. Pritchard JA: The use of magnesium sulfate in preeclampsia-eclampsia. *J Reprod Med* 23:107–113, 1979.
49. Pritchard JA: The use of magnesium ion in the management of eclamptogenic toxemias. *Surg Gynecol Obstet* 100:131–140, 1955.
50. Sibai BM, Graham JM, McCubbin JH: A comparison of intravenous and intramuscular magnesium sulfate regimens in preeclampsia. *Am J Obstet Gynecol* 150:728–733, 1984.
51. Repke JT, Friedman SA, Kaplan PW: Prophylaxis of eclamptic seizures: current controversies. *Clin Obstet Gynecol* 33:365–374, 1991.
52. Rutherford SE, Phelan JP: Deep venous thrombosis and pulmonary embolism in pregnancy. *Obstet Gynecol Clin North Am* 18:345–370, 1991.
53. Hyers TM, Hull RD, Weg JG: Antithrombotic therapy for venous thromboembolic disease. *Chest* 89:265–355, 1986.
54. Basu D, Gallus A, Hirsh J, et al: A prospective study of the value of monitoring heparin treatment with the activated partial thromboplastin time. *N Engl J Med* 287:324–327, 1972.
55. Ginsburg JS, Hirsh J, Turner C, et al: Risks to the fetus of anticoagulant therapy during pregnancy. *Thromb Haemost* 61:197–203, 1989.
56. Hall JG, Pauli RM, Wilson KM: Maternal and fetal sequelae of anticoagulation during pregnancy. *Am J Med* 68:122–140, 1978.
57. deSwiet M, Ward PD, Fidler I, et al: Prolonged heparin therapy in pregnancy causes bone demineralization. *Br J Obstet Gynaecol* 90:1129–1134, 1983.
58. Chang BH, Pitney WR, Castaldi PA: Heparin-induced thrombocytopenia: association of thrombotic complications with heparin-dependent IgG antibody that induces thromboxane synthesis and platelet aggregation. *Lancet* ii:1246–1249, 1982.
59. Weiner CP: Disseminated intravascular coagulopathy associated with pregnancy. In Clark SL, Cotton DB, Hankins GDV, Phelan JP (eds): *Critical Care Obstetrics*, ed 2. Blackwell Scientific Publications, Boston, pp 180–198, 1991.
60. Rodgers BD, Rodgers DE: Clinical variables associated with diabetic ketoacidosis during pregnancy. *J Reprod Med* 36:797–800, 1991.
61. Prihoda JS, Davis LF: Metabolic emergencies in obstetrics. *Obstet Gynecol Clin North Am* 18:301–318, 1991.
62. Tibaldi JM, Lorber DL, Nerenberg A: Diabetic ketoacidosis and insulin resistance with subcutaneous terbutaline infusion: a case report. *Am J Obstet Gynecol* 163:509–510, 1990.
63. Clark SL, Phelan JP, Montoro M, et al: Transient ventricular dysfunction associated with cesarean section in a patient with hyperthyroidism. *Am J Obstet Gynecol* 151:384–386, 1985.
64. Larsen PR: Salicylate-induced increases in free triiodothyroinine in human serum. *J Clin Invest* 51:1125–1134, 1972.
65. Roti E, Gnudi A, Braverman LE: The placental transport, synthesis and metabolism of hormones and drugs which affect thyroid function. *Endocr Rev* 4:131–149, 1983.
66. Kaplan MM: Thyroid diseases. In Gleicher N (ed): *Principles and Practice of Medical Therapy in Pregnancy*, ed 2. Appleton & Lange, Norwalk, CT, pp 321–338, 1991.
67. Isley WL, Dahl S, Gibbs H: Use of esmolol in managing a thyrotoxic patient needing emergency surgery. *Am J Med* 89:122–123, 1990.
68. Sweet RL, Gibbs RS: *Infectious Diseases of the Female Genital Tract*, ed 2. Williams & Wilkins, Baltimore, 1990.
69. Ledger WJ, Norman M, Gee C, et al: Bacteremia on an obstetric-gynecologic service. *Am J Obstet Gynecol* 121:205–212, 1975.
70. Gonik B: Septic shock in obstetrics. In Clark SL, Cotton DB, Hankins GDV, Phelan JP (eds): *Critical Care Obstetrics*, ed 2. Blackwell Scientific Publications, Boston, pp 289–306, 1991.
71. Beller FK, Schmidt EH, Holzgreve W, et al: Septicemia during pregnancy: a study in different species of experimental animals. *Am J Obstet Gynecol* 151:967–975, 1985.
72. Morishima HO, Niemann WH, James LS: Effects of endotoxin on the pregnant baboon and fetus. *Am J Obstet Gynecol* 131:899–902, 1978.
73. Rolbin SH, Levinson G, Shnider DM, et al: Dopamine treatment of spinal hypotension decreases uterine blood flow in the pregnant ewe. *Anesthesiology* 51:36–40, 1979.
74. Sprung CL, Caralis PV, Marcial EH, et al: The effects of high-dose corticosteroids in patients with septic shock. *N Engl J Med* 311:1137–1143, 1984.
75. Bone RC, Fisher CJ, Clemmer TP, et al: A controlled clinical trial of high-dose methylprednisolone in the treatment of severe sepsis and septic shock. *N Engl J Med* 317:653–658, 1987.
76. The Veterans Administration Systemic Sepsis Cooperative Study Group: Effect of high-dose glucocorticoid therapy on mortality in patients with clinical signs of systemic sepsis. *N Engl J Med* 317:659–665, 1987.
77. Holaday JW, Faden AI: Naloxone reversal of endotoxin hypotension suggests role of endorphins in shock. *Nature* 275:450–451, 1978.
78. Sperling RS: Human immunodeficiency virus and the acquired immunodeficiency syndrome in obstetrics. *Curr Opin Obstet Gynecol* 3:692–697, 1991.
79. Newman CL, Quinn TC: Acquired immunodeficiency syndrome. In Harvey AM, Johns RJ, McKusick VA, et al (eds): *The Principles and Practice of Medicine*, ed 32. Appleton & Lange, Norwalk, CT, pp 668–677, 1988.
80. Feinkind L, Minkoff HL: HIV in pregnancy. *Clin Perinatol* 15:189–202, 1988.
81. Tan EM, Cohen AS, Fries JF, et al: The 1982 revised criteria for the classification of systemic lupus erythematosus. *Arthritis Rheum* 25:1271–1277, 1982.
82. Out HJ, Derksen RHWM, Christiaens GCML: Systemic lupus erythematosus and pregnancy. *Obstet Gynecol Surv* 44:585–591, 1989.
83. Ramsey-Goldman R: Pregnancy in systemic lupus erythematosus. *Rheum Dis Clin North Am* 14:169–185, 1988.
84. Sanchez-Ramos L, Jones DC, Cullen MT: Urinary calcium as an early marker for preeclampsia. *Obstet Gynecol* 77:685–695, 1991.
85. Lockshin M: Pregnancy associated with systemic lupus erythematosus. *Semin Perinatol* 14:130–138, 1990.
86. Petri M, Howard D, Repke J: Frequency of lupus flare in pregnancy. *Arthritis Rheum* 34:1538–1545, 1991.
87. Davison JM, Lindheimer MD: Pregnancy in women with renal allografts. *Semin Nephrol* 4:240–251, 1984.
88. Davison JM: Renal transplantation and pregnancy. *Am J Kidney Dis* 9:374–380, 1987.
89. Flechner SM, Katz AR, Rogers AJ, et al: The presence of cyclosporine in body tissues and fluids during pregnancy. *Am J Kidney Dis* 5:60–63, 1985.
90. Ross WB, Rischards T, Williams GI: Cyclosporine and pregnancy. *Transplantation* 45:1142, 1988.
91. Laifer SA, Darby MJ, Scantlebury VP, et al: Pregnancy and liver transplantation. *Obstet Gynecol* 76:1083–1088, 1990.
92. Scantlebury V, Gordon R, Tzakis A, et al: Childbearing after liver transplanation. *Transplantation* 49:317–321, 1990.
92a. Scott JR, Wagoner LE, Olsen SL, Taylor DO, Renlund DG: Pregnancy in heart transplant recipients: management and outcome. *Obstet Gynecol* 82:324–327, 1993.
93. Gabbe SG, Niebyl JR, Simpson JL (eds): *Obstetrics: Normal and Problem Pregnancies*, ed 2. Churchill Livingstone, New York, 1991.

CHAPTER 51

Neuroprotective Therapy for Brain and Spinal Cord Injury

WISE YOUNG, PH.D., M.D.

Critical care medicine enables many patients to survive brain and spinal cord injury but traditionally has done little to improve neurologic recovery. This situation changed when the second National Acute Spinal Cord Injury Study (NASCIS 2) demonstrated that high-dose methylprednisolone (MP) given shortly after spinal cord injury can significantly improve neurologic recovery. This chapter summarizes the laboratory and clinical studies leading to the demonstration that MP is neuroprotective in spinal cord injury, discusses the research and clinical implications of this demonstration, and then presents a brief overview of neuroprotective treatments for brain and spinal cord injury.

THE NATIONAL ACUTE SPINAL CORD INJURY STUDIES

THE FIRST NATIONAL ACUTE SPINAL CORD INJURY STUDY (NASCIS 1)

In 1980, only two treatments were recognized to have potential for protecting neurons against ischemic and traumatic injury: hypothermia (1–6) and glucocorticoids (3, 6–13). Demopoulos et al (14–16) proposed that oxygen and other free radicals contribute to progressive damage in injured brain and spinal cord tissues, hypothesizing that high doses of MP prevented secondary injury by scavenging free radicals rather than acting as a glucocorticoid. The first National Acute Spinal Cord Injury Study (NASCIS 1) began in 1979 to test the free

radical hypothesis in spinal cord injury. This multicenter study randomized 330 patients to low-dose (100 mg/day for 10 days) or high-dose (1000 mg/day for 10 days) MP started within 48 hours after spinal cord injury.

NASCIS 1 (17) found no significant differences in motor or sensory recovery between high- and low-dose MP-treated patients. In retrospect, the study was seriously flawed in two respects. First, the dose of MP may have been too small. Laboratory studies suggested that higher doses of MP were required to inhibit spinal cord lipid peroxidation (18–28), to improve the histologic appearance (29) and blood flow (30), and to maximize locomotory recovery in spinal-injured cats (31, 32). Second, MP may have been given too late. Some patients were randomized as late as 24 to 48 hours after injury. By 1985, it became clear that MP should be reevaluated at a higher dose and earlier timing. In addition, naloxone (NX) was reported to improve evoked potentials, locomotory recovery, and spinal cord blood flow in animal spinal cord injury models (33–37).

NASCIS 2—CLINICAL TRIAL DESIGN

The Second National Acute Spinal Cord Injury Study (NASCIS 2) began in 1985 to compare MP, NX, and placebo treatments of spinal cord injury. Table 51.1 summarizes NASCIS 2 treatment protocols. The MP protocol was based on laboratory data showing that 30 mg/kg optimally inhibited spinal cord lipid peroxidation (18, 20–27, 38, 39) and improved blood flow (30). The dose of 5.4 mg/kg/hr maintains plasma

Table 51.1. NASCIS Treatment Protocols[a]

Treatment	n	Initial Dose	Maintenance Dose
NASCIS 1			
High-dose MP	165	MP 1000 mg (<48 hr)	MP 1000 mg/day • 10 days
Low-dose MP	165	100 mg (<48 hr)	100 mg/day • 10 days
NASCIS 2			
24h MP	162	MP 30 mg/kg (<12 hr)	MP 5.4 mg/kg/hr • 23 hr
Naloxone	154	MP 5.4 mg/kg (<12 hr)	MP 3.0 mg/kg/hr • 23 hr
NASCIS 3			
24h MP	—	MP 30 mg/kg (<8 hr)	MP 5.4 mg/kg/hr • 23 hr
48h MP	—	MP 30 mg/kg (<8 hr)	MP 5.4 mg/kg/hr • 47 hr
MP + 48h TM	—	MP 30 mg/kg (<8 hr)	TM 2.5 mg/kg/6hr • 47 hr

[a] Acronyms and abbreviations in this table denote the following: NASCIS, National Acute Spinal Cord Injury Study; MP, methylprednisolone sodium succinate, Upjohn Company; NX, naloxone hydrochloride, Dupont; TM, tirilazad mesylate, Upjohn Company; mg/day, milligrams given per day as a continuous infusion; mg/kg, mg per kilogram body weight as a single bolus; mg/kg/hr, mg per kg per hour as a continuous infusion; mg/kg/6hr, mg per kg every 6 hours as a bolus injection.

levels. The NX protocol was based on laboratory studies showing that 2 mg/kg/hr or 10 mg/kg bolus NX given shortly after injury improved recovery (33, 34, 36, 37, 40–42). In a phase I accelerated dose trial (43), spinal-injured patients tolerated 5.4 mg/kg of NX well without significant hyperalgesia or other side effects. The maintenance dose of 3.0 mg/kg/hr was based on the plasma NX clearance rate in humans.

NASCIS 2 tested two preplanned hypotheses: (*a*) that earlier treatment would be more effective than late treatment, and (*b*) that treatment would have less effect on severe spinal cord injuries. To test these two hypotheses, the patient population was stratified by treatment time and injury severity. The patient population was segregated into two roughly equal groups based on the median treatment time. The patients were categorized into three groups on admission: those with no motor or sensory function below the injury level (plegic), those with no motor and some sensory preservation, and those with some motor and variable sensory function (paretic). These categories correspond respectively to the Frankel Classifications A, B, and C-D, respectively (44).

The patients were assessed neurologically on admission and at 6 weeks, 6 months, and a year after spinal cord injury. Table 51.2 summarizes the motor scoring system. Fourteen muscles were graded on each side of the body on the standard clinical scale of 0 to 5 (Table 51.2). The right-side muscle grades were summed to obtain an "expanded" motor score of 70. Pinprick and touch sensations were assessed in 29 dermatomes on each side of the body, using a clinical scale of 0 to 2 where 0 indicates absent, 1 is abnormal, and 2 is normal sensation. Right-sided sensory grades were summed for maximum normal sensory scores of 58 for pinprick and touch. In addition, the odds that patients would convert from paraplegic or quadriplegic to paraparesis or quadriparesis, from anesthesia to hypesthesia, and analgesia to hypalgesia were calculated. Lumbosacral motor and sensory scores were analyzed separately to determine whether treatment improved distal function. Finally, the group collected detailed data on morbidity and mortality in each treatment group.

NASCIS 2—POSITIVE FINDINGS

A total of 487 patients were randomly allocated to MP (*n* = 162), NX (*n* = 154), and placebo (*n* = 171). Eligibility required

a confirmed diagnosis of spinal cord injury, absence of comorbidity, fulfillment of several entry criteria, including no high-dose MP or NX treatment before randomization, and treatment within 12 hours after injury. Half the patients were treated within and the remainder were treated ≥8 hours after spinal cord injury. Treatment timing, injury severity, or neurologic scores did not differ significantly among the three treatment groups. The MP, NX, and placebo groups respectively had 45, 37, and 43 plegic subjects; 12, 11, and 16 paretic subjects; and only 5, 11, and 6 plegic subjects with some sensation who were treated within 8 hours.

MP treatment improved motor and sensory score recovery. At 1 year after injury, irrespective of treatment times, the MP group had better pinprick sensation ($p < 0.012$) and touch ($p < 0.042$) than did the placebo group. Motor scores were also better in the MP group compared with the placebo group, but the difference was not statistically significant. Patients who received MP within 8 hours after injury had significantly better motor and sensory recovery scores than did those in the placebo group or those given MP more than 8 hours after injury. In plegic patients, early MP treatment restored 20% of motor score, compared with 8% in the placebo group ($p = 0.019$). In paretic patients, early MP treatment restored 75% motor return, compared with 59% in the placebo group ($p = 0.024$).

Analysis of lumbosacral motor scores revealed that patients receiving early MP recovered more distal motor and sensory function than did placebo-treated patients. For example, 11.8% (95% confidence limits: −2.9% to 25.5%) more early MP-treated patients had better motor scores than did placebo-treated patients. Likewise, 16.2% (95% confidence limits: 1.9% to 30.5%) and 17.9% (95% confidence limits: 3.6% to 32.2%) more early MP-treated patients recovered pinprick and touch sensation than did placebo-treated patients. MP-treated patients showed a greater propensity to convert from quadriplegia to quadriparesis, analgesia to hypalgesia, and anesthesia to hypesthesia ($p < 0.05$) than did placebo-treated patients.

The preceding analyses utilized a conservative intention-to-treat approach, including all randomized patients. About 8% of the randomized patients were not eligible and did not receive any treatments, or received the wrong treatment or dose. Exclusion of these patients from the analysis increased the significance of differences between MP and placebo groups. For example, at 6 months after injury, MP-treated had significantly better motor scores ($p = 0.011$), pinprick sensation ($p = 0.001$), and touch ($p = 0.02$) than did placebo-treated patients. The increase in outcome differences after removal of protocol violators strongly supports the hypothesis that MP treatment improved recovery.

NASCIS 2—NEGATIVE FINDINGS

Neurologic scores and distribution of injury severity did not differ significantly among the stratified treatment groups. Treatment had no effect on mortality in the patients at 6 months (log-rank test, $p = 0.465$) or 1 year ($p = 0.525$) after injury. The mortality rates in each of the treatment groups were 6 to 10% at 1 year. A vast majority (>95%) of surviving patients were examined at the 1-year follow-up period. The incidence of infection, gastrointestinal hemorrhage, decubiti, thrombophlebitis, and other potential complications of spinal cord injury or drug treatment did not differ significantly among the treatment groups.

Motor and sensory scores of NX-treated patients tended to fall between those of the MP and placebo-treated patients, but most of the differences were not significant. NX-treated patients also had greater odds of converting from quadriplegia or paraplegia to quadriparesis or paraparesis ($p < 0.05$) at 1 year after injury. However, NX-treated patients did not show improved odds of converting from analgesia to hypalgesia or from anesthesia to hypesthesia. Patients who received MP late had less neurologic recovery than did placebo-treated patients, although the difference was not significant ($p = 0.08$).

NASCIS 2 did not measure the behavioral consequences of the neurologic changes. In 1985, when the study began, no validated measure of behavioral function was available. Although motor score differences of 8 to 10 points appear modest, the changes are functionally meaningful. An 8-point improvement indicates conversion of four muscle groups on each side of the body from paralysis (muscle grade 0) to some movement (muscle grade 2), four muscle groups from trace motor activity (muscle grade 1) to antigravity strength (muscle grade 3), or four muscle groups from useless movement (muscle grade 3) to useful strength (muscle grade 4). Any of these changes would seem to be worthwhile.

Finally, NASCIS 2 did not rule out two possibilities. First, patients admitted late may have received different care in the immediate postinjury period. Second, most of the patients receiving "early" MP were treated between 4 and 8 hours after injury. Earlier therapy may yield better and more significant results. The latter hypothesis is being addressed in the third NASCIS trial, which is randomizing patients within 8 hours after injury and will be directly comparing earlier treatment times within 8 hours.

CRITICAL CARE IMPLICATIONS

NASCIS 2 has had and will continue to have an important impact on critical care treatment of central nervous system (CNS) injury for several reasons. First, it demonstrated that a drug given after the CNS injury can improve recovery, vindicating decades of animal studies showing progressive tissue damage in injured spinal cords. Second, the study emphasized the importance of treatment timing. Third, the observation that MP improves recovery in severe spinal cord injury challenged the widely accepted clinical dogma that severe spinal cord injuries cannot recover. Fourth, the NASCIS results have complicated preclinical studies of CNS injury treatments. Each of these reasons is described below.

SECONDARY INJURY

Before 1990, many clinicians and scientists were deeply skeptical about secondary injury in central nervous tissues.

Table 51.2. Key Muscles in the NASCIS and ASIA Motor Scores[a]

Level	Action	NASCIS Muscles	R	ASIA Muscles	R+L
C5	Shoulder shrug	• Deltoid	5		
	Elbow flexion	• Biceps	5	• Biceps, brachialis	5+5
C6	Wrist extension	• Extensor carpi radialis	5	• Extensor carpi radialis	5+5
C7	Elbow extension	• Triceps	5	• Triceps	5+5
C8	Finger flexion			• Flexor digitorum profundus middle	5+5
	Finger extension	• Extensor digitorum	5		
T1	Finger adduction	• 1st dorsal	5		
	Finger abduction	Interosseus		• Abductor digiti minimi	5+5
	Thumb opposition	• Opponens pollicis	5		
L2	Hip flexion	• Iliopsoas	5	• Iliopsoas	5+5
L3	Knee extension	• Quadriceps femoris	5	• Quadriceps	5+5
L4	Ankle dorsiflexion	• Tibialis anterior	5	• Tibialis anterior	5+5
L5	Long toe extension	• Extensor hallucis longus	5	• Extensor hallucis longus	5+5
	Knee flexion	• Hamstring	5		
S1-S2	Ankle plantar flexion	• Gastrocnemius	5	• Gastrocnemius, soleus	5+5
	Toe flexion	• Peroneus long and brevis	5		
		Total NASCIS Score	70	Total ASIA Score	100

[a] Key muscles in the National Acute Spinal Cord Injury (NASCIS) and American Spinal Injury Association (ASIA) motor scores are compared. Each muscle is graded on a scale of 0 to 5 where 0 is total paralysis, 1 is palpable or visible contraction, 2 is active full range of motion (ROM) under no gravity, 3 is active full ROM against gravity, 4 is active full ROM against moderate resistance, and 5 is normal. The ASIA motor index sums 10 muscle grades on both sides of the body, for a total of 100. The NASCIS motor score sums 14 muscle grades on the right side, for a total of 70. ASIA recommends grading of deltoid and lateral hamstrings, whereas NASCIS collects data on the flexor digitorum profundus and abductor digiti minimi.

Although progressive tissue damage has been observed often in animal brain and spinal cord injury models, the relevance of the models for human condition was not well-accepted. The demonstration that MP can improve recovery even when given after spinal cord injury vindicates decades of animal studies indicating that trauma initiates autodestructive mechanisms in the spinal cord.

The NASCIS 2 results provide some insights into the nature of these autodestructive mechanisms. First, the mechanisms appear to be robust and occur in all types of spinal cord injuries. MP improved neurologic recovery in both plegic and paretic patients. Second, the mechanisms must occur relatively early after injury, since MP was ineffective when started more than 8 hours after injury. Third, as much as 20% of function can be salvaged even in patients admitted with no function below the lesion level.

The finding that MP must be given within 8 hours after injury suggests that secondary injury becomes irreversible over this period. In NASCIS 2, the average patient treated with MP received about 10 g of drug over a 24-hour period. This dose transcends previous definitions of "megadose," vastly exceeding that dose necessary to activate glucocorticoid receptors. At such high concentrations the drug is an antioxidant and scavenges free radicals (45–47). However, MP may inhibit lipid peroxidation by other mechanisms (48). For example, glucocorticoids are potent inhibitors of phospholipase activity (49–57).

TREATMENT TIME WINDOWS

The hypothesis that early treatment is better than delayed treatment seems obvious. However, few investigators suspected a sharply delimited effective treatment time window. NASCIS 2 showed that patients receiving MP more than 8 hours after injury not only did not recover but may have had less recovery than placebo controls. A short time window also may explain why NASCIS 1 showed no significant difference between high- and low-dose MP treatment. The patients were randomized within 48 hours after injury. Clearly, not only was too little MP given, but the drug was given too late.

Eight hours was the median treatment time of patients in NASCIS 2. Although the study clearly showed that patients given MP more than 8 hours after injury did not have better recovery, perhaps patients treated even earlier would recover more completely. NASCIS 3 is addressing this question by randomizing patients within 8 hours after injury. Until more information is available, the 8-hour window should be considered an upper limit for beneficial effects and treatment should be delivered as soon as possible.

Before 1990, spinal cord injury was often not treated with urgency. Because no treatment was perceived to be effective, spinal-injured patients were often transported to the nearest emergency room where they might have been delayed for hours before diagnosis and treatment. Surgeons often delayed surgery for severely injured patients. NASCIS 2 has changed this situation not only for pharmacologic but other forms of therapy. If MP can improve neurologic recovery, perhaps surgical procedures should be carried out within the same time frame to have beneficial effects of recovery.

A tightly restricted treatment time window may apply to brain injury. For example, most brain injury and stroke clinical trials carried out in the past decade randomized patients with a 48-hour time window. If most secondary injury occurs shortly after injury, delaying treatment is tantamount to closing the barn doors after the horses have left. The best treatment dose may also differ depending on treatment timing. Traditionally, investigators have focused on dose-response assessments and have not systematically investigated treatment timing and duration. Such studies are now required.

CLINICAL DOGMAS

Surprisingly, MP improved recovery even in spinal-injured patients admitted with no neurologic function below the lesion level. This observation challenges a long-held clinical dogma that such patients cannot recover. The dogma has been utilized for centuries to justify conservative or no treatment of these patients. An anonymous Egyptian physician wrote more than two millennia ago in the Edwin-Smith Papyrus (58) that water should be withheld from spinal-injured warriors. Unfortunately, such dogmas can become self-fulfilling prophesies.

Patients with complete loss of function below the lesion level have the most to gain and the least to lose from treatment. Because they recover little function when left untreated, these patients have little to gain from conservative management. Since even slight gains of function can result in marked differences in lifestyle and independence of patients, the risk of MP treatment seems worthwhile. These patients should be treated aggressively.

Clinical loss of function does not necessarily imply transection of the spinal cord. Dimitrijevic et al (59–62) have shown that a majority of "complete" spinal-injured patients have residual descending control of lumbosacral reflexes. The finding that MP improves motor and sensory recovery in patients with no function below the lesion site strongly supports the concept that these patients have residual axons that can be salvaged by treatment.

RESEARCH IMPLICATIONS OF NASCIS 2

The discovery of an effective treatment has greatly complicated spinal cord injury research. Before NASCIS 2, it was sufficient to show that a drug works. Because of NASCIS 2, placebo-controlled clinical trials are difficult to justify. Treatment must be as good as or better than MP to be considered for clinical trials. Combination therapy also has become an important option. Most spinal-injury victims in the U.S. now receive an initial MP bolus shortly after injury. Patients and physicians may be reluctant to eschew a drug with known efficacy for an untried drug. Differences between any treatment and MP may be small; more subjects must be studied. Thus, preclinical studies must now be compared with both vehicle and MP controls, alone and in combination with MP.

A drug would be considered superior to MP if it had a broader dose-response curve, had fewer side effects, was less expensive, and was more effective over a wider range of injury severity. To assess these possibilities, preclinical trials must study the optimum treatment dose, timing, and duration over a range of injury severity.

Table 51.3. Preclinical Experimental Protocols[a]

Treatment	Treatment Dose	Treatment Time	Treatment Duration	Injury Severity	Groups Injured	Sham
Vehicle	• Standard	• Early • 6 hr • 24 hr	• Bolus • 24 hr • 48 hr	• Mild • Moderate • Severe • Sham	9 9 9	 9
MP	• Standard	• Early • 6 hr • 24 hr	• Bolus • 24 hr • 48 hr	• Mild • Moderate • Severe • Sham	9 9 9	 9
X	• High • Medium • Low	• Early • 6 hr • 24 hr	• Bolus • 24 hr • 48 hr	• Mild • Moderate • Severe • Sham	27 27 27	 27
MP+X	• High • Medium • Low	• Early • 6 hr • 24 hr	• Bolus • 24 hr • 48 hr	• Mild • Moderate • Severe • Sham	27 27 27	 27
Totals					216	72

[a]This table illustrates a study of two controls (vehicle and MP), a drug alone (X), and the drug combined with MP (MP+X). To test three treatment doses (high, medium, low), three times (early, 6 hr, 24 hr), and durations (bolus, 24 hr, 48 hr) at three injury severities (mild, moderate, and severe), 216 injured groups are required. Sham injury controls increase the number to 286 groups.

These requirements have placed an onerous burden on preclinical spinal cord injury studies, as illustrated in Table 51.3. To evaluate three treatment doses, three initiation times, and three durations across three injury severities, alone and in combination with MP and with appropriate sham and vehicle controls, would require more than 200 experimental groups. Systematic investigation of a drug may require several thousand experiments. Few laboratories today can assume the burden of studies involving thousand of animals. Multicenter preclinical trials will become necessary. However, multicenter preclinical trials require well-standardized outcome measures, efficient and reproducible models of neuronal injury, and cooperation among laboratories.

Progress in developing better neuroprotective treatments depends strongly on the availability of reproducible and efficient in vivo and in vitro injury models, as well as better and well-standardized outcome measures. A better understanding of secondary injury mechanisms would help alleviate the empiric testing. Unfortunately, we do not understand secondary injury or drug mechanisms well enough to predict the effects of many drugs or drug combinations on spinal cord injury. Until this capability occurs, we must test each variable empirically.

"INDUSTRIAL STRENGTH" MEDICINE

The dose of MP given in NASCIS 2 far exceeds those required for glucocorticoid actions. For example, 100 mg/day of MP is sufficient to saturate glucocorticoid receptors in humans. A decade ago, 1000 mg/day of MP was considered "megadose" treatment. NASCIS 2 gave the typical patient as much as 10,000 mg/day! Likewise, 0.5 mg of NX will reverse heroin overdoses in patients. NASCIS 2 gave more than 5000 mg/day. "Industrial-strength" medicine is a better descriptor of treatments used in this study.

The high dose of MP required for neuroprotection prompted the hypothesis that MP may be acting as a free radical scavenger (47, 63) rather than as a glucocorticoid. The

Upjohn Company developed the 21-aminosteroids, a family of antioxidant steroid compounds with no glucocorticoid activity (64–66). One 21-aminosteroid, tirilazad mesylate (TM), has significant neuroprotective effects in many traumatic and ischemic CNS injury models (67–90). Clinical trials of TM have begun in spinal cord injury, stroke, subarachnoid hemorrhage, and traumatic brain injury.

The high doses of naloxone likewise led investigators to propose that the neuroprotective effects of naloxone are the result of κ-opiate receptor blockade. Faden et al (91–94) showed that thyrotropin releasing hormone (TRH) improves recovery in spinal cord injury, suggesting that κ-opiate receptors are involved in secondary tissue damage, possibly through calcium-mediated mechanisms (95). TRH analogs (96–102) and κ-opiate receptor antagonists (103–108) appear more effective than naloxone. Finally, excitotoxic neurotransmitter receptors (103, 109–113) and serotonin receptor blockers (102, 114) have been implicated in the secondary injury process.

COMBINATION THERAPY

Many drugs have been reported to have neuroprotective effects. Table 51.4 illustrates the diversity of drugs claimed to be useful for spinal cord injury alone. Many investigators have postulated complex schemes involving a cascade of secondary injury mechanisms, starting with one or two initiating causes, such as free radicals or calcium entry into cells, leading to a broadening cascade of toxic substances, including vasoactive lipid inflammatory mediators, neurotransmitters that open membrane ionic channels, and enzymes that catalyze protein and lipid breakdown.

The cascade theory has led to the popular view that neural injuries are best treated with a "cocktail" of drugs since no single drug can block all the mechanisms participating in secondary injury. Mixtures and doses of drugs can be tailored for different injuries. Unfortunately, the knowledge base of pharmacokinetics or drug mechanisms does not yet allow

Table 51.4. Acute Spinal Cord Injury Treatments[a]

Drug	Action	Type	References
Methylprednisolone	• Glucocorticoid • Antioxidant	+RCT +Cat +Rat	16, 21, 30, 31, 45, 122, 171–175
GM1 (monosialic ganglioside)	• Stimulates protein kinase C and other protein kinases	+RCT	115, 116
Tirilazad mesylate	• 21-Aminosteroid • Antioxidant • Nonglucocorticoid	•RCT +Cat +Rat	65, 67, 75, 80, 89, 176
Thyrotropin releasing hormone	• A κ-opiate receptor blocker • Small peptide	+Cat +Rat	41, 96, 97
Vitamin E (α-tocopherol) with selenium	• Antioxidant	+Cat +Rat	120–122, 127
Naloxone	• μ-Opiate receptor blocker	−RCT +Cat +Rat	32–34, 37, 40, 42, 43
Nalmefene	• Blocks κ-opiate receptor	+Rat	107, 108
YM-14673	• TRH analog • κ-Opiate receptor blocker	+Rat	98, 102, 177
MK801	• Blocks NMDA receptor	+Rat	109–113
Mianserin	• Blocks serotonin receptor	+Rat	102, 114
BW755C	• Inhibits cyclooxygenase and lipoxygenase	+Rat	178
Ibuprofen	• Inhibits cyclooxygenase	+Cat	179
Protease inhibitors	• Prevents damage to neurofilaments	+Rat	180, 181
Nimodipine	• Blocks L-type calcium channels • Increases blood flow	±Rat	182, 183

[a] Some treatments reported to be useful in spinal cord injury are listed. Their putative actions, preparations in which the neuroprotective effects were found, and relevant literature are cited.

rational design of combination therapies. Treatment effects and side effects cannot yet be predicted reliably. For example, high doses of MP and NX given together were found to be toxic (32). Combination therapy, however, is already widely practiced. Critically ill patients already receive many drugs.

Finally, another kind of combination therapy must be considered: sequential therapy. Geisler et al (115, 116) recently reported improved motor recovery in spinal-injured patients given low-dose MP (i.e., 250 mg bolus with 125 mg every 6 hours) for 48 hours and the monosialic ganglioside GM1 (100 mg/day) for 4 to 6 weeks after injury. Likewise, one of the treatment protocols being tested by NASCIS 3 is an initial bolus of MP followed by tirilazad mesylate. Both of these are sequential therapies.

NASCIS 3 AND OTHER ONGOING CLINICAL TRIALS

The third National Acute Spinal Cord Injury Study (NASCIS 3) is underway, assessing three treatment protocols: (a) the standard 24-hour course of MP, 30 mg/kg given as a bolus followed by 23 hours of 5.4 mg/kg/hr; (b) a similar course of MP but given for 48 hours; and (c) an initial bolus dose of 30 mg/kg MP followed by tirilazad mesylate (TM) at 2.5 mg/kg every 6 hours for 48 hours. The trial will determine whether 48-hour MP treatment is as safe as or safer than 24-hour, whether TM is an effective substitute for MP, and whether the therapeutic window is shorter than 8 hours.

A trial to reexamine the effects of GM1 on neurologic recovery in human spinal cord injury is underway. Like NASCIS 2, the GM1 trial will compare three treatment protocols: (a) the standard 24-hour course of MP; (b) 24 hours of MP followed by 100 mg/day of GM1 given for 6 weeks; and

(c) 24 hours of MP followed by 200 mg/day of GM1 given daily for 6 weeks. This trial should definitively answer the question whether addition of GM1 to MP improves neurologic recovery compared with MP alone.

The main challenge for the field is to develop a rational basis for designing neuroprotective treatments. A better and detailed theoretic understanding of secondary injury mechanisms is essential. Without a better understanding of mechanisms, the field will progress slowly beyond the current situation in which many drugs are believed to influence secondary injury mechanisms but each treatment protocol must still be tested individually and empirically in preclinical and clinical trials. Better laboratory models for preclinical studies and more efficient clinical trials with better outcome measures are required.

NEUROPROTECTIVE TREATMENTS

MP is the first drug that has been shown in a large randomized clinical trial to improve recovery in human spinal cord injury. Although GM1 has also been reported to improve motor recovery, the study involved a smaller population of patients and requires further confirmation. Without doubt, other drugs will soon be shown to be neuroprotective, not only in spinal cord injury but in traumatic and ischemic brain injury. Even a brief review of the treatments that have been reported to be neuroprotective is well beyond the scope of this chapter. The tables are meant to illustrate the diversity of treatments and mechanisms that may soon be available clinically for treating spinal cord injury, traumatic brain injury, and cerebral ischemia.

SPINAL CORD INJURY

A 24-hour course of high-dose MP is currently the only pharmacologic therapy that has been shown to be effective for acute spinal cord injury. Although GM1 has been reported to be beneficial, the first study involved relatively few patients and the results need to be confirmed on a larger scale. MP is widely available, inexpensive, and has no significant side effects in large series of patients. It is neuroprotective even in patients with complete loss of function below the lesion level. The benefit-to-risk ratio is sufficiently high that its use is recommended, except for the following: First, no data support starting high-dose MP more than 8 hours after spinal cord injury. Second, the efficacy or safety of giving MP for more than 24 hours has not yet been established. Until such data are available, MP treatment of spinal cord injury must be initiated within 8 hours and should be limited to a 24-hour course.

Some physicians have extrapolated the NASCIS 2 results to prophylactic therapy. If MP is neuroprotective after injury, it should be as effective or more so when given before injury. One caveat is that NASCIS 2 excluded patients with severe comorbidity, brain injury, gunshot wounds, and pregnancy and thus did not directly demonstrate the safety of MP use before surgery. However, high-dose MP treatment does not increase morbidity or mortality of patients with severe blunt chest trauma (117–119), suggesting that it can be given safely to patients before an operation. Another caveat is that treatment duration is limited to 24 hours. Thus, the treatment is applicable only when injury is imminent. Finally, rapid drug penetration into the central nervous system is not necessary for prophylactic therapy. Other antioxidants, such as vitamin E (120–125) and tirilazad mesylate (65, 126, 127) may be as efficacious and safer.

BRAIN INJURY

An often-asked question is whether high-dose MP should be given in head injury. Many investigators have observed beneficial effects of glucocorticoids on brain injury (8, 9, 28, 128–133), and some negative laboratory studies have been reported as well (134–136). Although some experience suggests beneficial effects of high-dose (1 mg/kg) dexamethasone after head injury (137–139), others found no significant difference between low-dose (5 to 16 mg/day) versus high-dose (100 mg/day) dexamethasone (140), placebo versus high-dose dexamethasone (100 mg) (141), and placebo versus low-dose (5 mg/kg/day) MP (142). Gudeman et al (143) found that a large MP dose (2 g bolus followed by 500 mg every 6 hours for 24 hours) started after 12 hours of low-dose protocol (40 mg every 6 hours) had no effect on intracranial pressures.

Only one clinical head injury trial to date has examined MP treatments in the dose range of the NASCIS 2 protocol. Giannotta et al (144) randomized 88 patients with Glasgow coma score (GCS) of ≤8 at 6 hours after injury to either high-dose MP (30 mg/kg q 6hr × 2, then 250 mg q 6hr × 6, and then tapered over 6 days) or low-dose MP (1.5 mg/kg q 6hr × 2, 25 mg q 6hr × 6, and then tapered over 6 days). At 6 months, no significant difference in neurologic outcome was observed. However, the high-dose group had a mortality of 39%, compared with 52% in the low-dose group (P < 0.05). The mortality difference was most marked in patients younger than 40 years old (i.e., young high-dose MP-treated patients had 6% mortality compared with 43% in the young low-dose MP-treated patients). Thus, MP improved survival, but the outcome of the survivors skewed the overall neurologic scores.

The question whether high-dose steroid therapy would be beneficial in brain injury has not yet been answered adequately. The situation is similar to that faced by those in the spinal cord injury field in 1985 before NASCIS 2. Although most animal studies suggest beneficial effects when high doses are given, all but one of the clinical trials may have given too little drug too late. For example, the so-called high-dose dexamethasone (1 to 2 mg/kg) may have been insufficient. In vitro studies suggest that very high doses of dexamethasone (30 mg/kg) are necessary to inhibit lipid peroxidation (46). The accumulated data provided little or no rationale for low-dose dexamethasone (<1 mg/kg or MP <30 mg/kg) delayed more than 8 hours. Likewise, prolonged (more than 24 hours) steroid therapy of head injury may be contraindicated because chronic glucocorticoids have been reported to inhibit neurite sprouting (145–148).

STROKE

High-dose glucocorticoids should be beneficial in stroke. However, few data support or refute high-dose MP treatment of cerebral ischemia. Several investigators have reported beneficial effects of steroid therapy on cerebral ischemia (149–151) and hypoxia (152) models. However, elevations of endogenous glucocorticoid levels have been reported to be deleterious to some ischemic neurons (153). Glucocorticoids also may increase plasma glucose, which can aggravate cerebral ischemic injury (154). To date, no randomized clinical trial of any steroid therapy has been carried out in stroke.

Tirilazad mesylate has been shown to be neuroprotective in several models of cerebral ischemia (46, 47, 70, 75, 78). TM possesses several potential advantages over high-dose steroid therapy. First, it lacks glucocorticoid activity (68) and therefore should be free of the deleterious side effects of steroid therapy. Second, it is approximately 10 to 100 times more potent an antioxidant than MP (64, 66). Third, tirilazad has a much broader dose-response curve than does MP (67, 75, 89). A clinical trial of tirilazad mesylate treatment of stroke is underway.

Many other drug therapies have been reported to be neuroprotective in ischemia. A discussion of these therapies would be beyond the scope of this review. Table 51.5 lists some of these treatments that have been reported to be effective for traumatic brain injury (TBI), focal cerebral ischemia (FCI), and global cerebral ischemia (GCI). Of the drugs listed, nimodipine has undergone the most extensive clinical testing and is approved for subarachnoid hemorrhage (155, 156). The recent British trial of nimodipine in 176 head-injured patients did not show a significant outcome difference (157).

Many brain injury treatments are also effective in spinal cord injury. The overlap in treatments suggests strongly that similar mechanisms operate in spinal cord injury, brain injury, and stroke. In particular, one treatment not listed, hypothermia, appears to be effective in ischemic (158–160, 161) and

Table 51.5. Acute Ischemic and Traumatic Brain Injury Treatments[a]

Drug	Action	Type	References
Methylprednisolone	• Glucocorticoid	+FCI	45, 152
	• Antioxidant	+TBI	
Dexamethasone	• Glucocorticoid	+FCI	149–151
		+TBI	
Tirilazad mesylate	• 21-Aminosteroid	+TBI	47, 70, 78, 184, 185
	• Antioxidant	+FCI	
	• Nonglucocorticoid	+GCI	
Barbiturates	• Anesthetic	+GCI	186–191
	• Metabolic depressant	+FCI	
Naloxone	• μ-opiate receptor blocker	+GCI	35, 40, 42, 192, 193
		+TBI	
		+SCI	
Nalmefene	• Blocks κ-opiate receptor	+GCI	113, 194
		+SCI	
Monosialic ganglioside (GM1)	• Stimulates protein kinase C	+FCI	195–198
		+GCI	
Allopurinol	• Inhibits xanthine oxidase	+FCI	199, 200
Other antioxidants (dimethylthiourea, MCI-186, U-78517F)	• Scavenges free radicals	+FCI	46, 47, 200–205
		+GCI	
		+TBI	
MK801	• Blocks NMDA receptor	+FCI	113, 159, 203, 206–218
		±GCI	
		+SCI	
		+TBI	
Dextromethorphan	• Blocks NMDA receptor	+GCI	219–221
Emopamil	• Ca channel blocker	+FCI	222–224
	• Serotonin receptor antagonist	+GCI	
Indomethacin	• Blocks cyclooxygenase	+FCI	135, 225–229
		+GCI	
		+BFL	
Adenosine	• Increases cAMP	+FCI	230
Superoxide dismutase (SOD)	• Breaks down superoxide radical	+GCI	204, 231
		+FCI	
Nicardipine	• Blocks L-type calcium channels	+FCI	232, 233
Nimodipine	• Blocks L-type calcium channels	+FCI	218, 234–244
		+GCI	

[a]Treatments reported to be beneficial to focal cerebral ischemia (FCI), global cerebral ischemia (GCI), spinal cord ischemia (SCI), traumatic brain injury (TBI), and brain freeze lesion (BFL) models.

traumatic (161–163) brain injury, as well as spinal cord injury (3, 6, 164–166). The work by Busto et al (158, 167) drew attention to the neuroprotective effects of even small decreases in brain temperature. The temperature effects may be related to release of excitotoxic neurotransmitters (168–170). One interesting possibility is that moderate hypothermia is effective because it prevents hyperthermia, which is well-known to aggravate ischemic injury.

SUMMARY

Care of central nervous system injuries has come a long way. Compared with the paucity of hope and treatments for spinal cord and brain injuries only a decade ago, we have a glut of promising drugs awaiting systematic preclinical investigation and clinical trial. The day will soon come when a choice of treatments will be available to the critical care specialist caring for patients who have suffered or are in imminent danger of neural damage. The question is not if, but when, such treatments will become available. The discovery of an effective treatment for acute spinal cord injury, however, has made the task of identifying better therapy much more difficult. Converting promising drugs into practical treatments

will require a much better understanding of secondary injury mechanisms, more reproducible models and outcome measures, and well-designed clinical trials.

ACKNOWLEDGMENTS

This work was supported in part by NIH grants P01 NS10164 and R01 NS15590.

REFERENCES

1. Rosomoff HL: Effects of hypothermia on physiology of nervous system. *Surgery* 40:328, 1956.
2. Little DM: Hypothermia. *Anesthesiology* 20:842–877, 1959.
3. Black P, Markowitz RS: Experimental spinal cord injury in monkeys: comparison of steroids and local hypothermia. *Surg Forum* 22:409–411, 1971.
4. Bering EA: Effects of profound hypothermia and circulatory arrest on cerebral oxygen metabolism and cerebrospinal fluid electrolyte composition in dogs. *J Neurosurg* 39:199–205, 1974.
5. Holland CE, Olsen RE: Prevention by hypothermia of paradoxical calcium necrosis in cardiac muscle. *J Mol Cell Cardiol* 7:917–928, 1975.
6. Kuchner EF, Hansebout RR: Combined steroid and hypothermia treatment of experimental spinal cord injury. *Surg Neurol* 6:371–376, 1976.
7. Ducker TB, Hamit HF: Experimental treatments of acute spinal cord injury. *J Neurosurg* 30:693–697, 1969.
8. Lewin MG, Pappius HM, Hansebout RR: Effects of steroids on edema associated with injury of the spinal cord. In Reulen HJ, Schürmann K (eds): *Steroids and Brain Edema.* Berlin, Springer-Verlag, pp 101–112, 1972.

9. Tutt HP, Pappius HM: Studies on the mechanisms of action of steroids in traumatized brain. In Reulen HJ, Schürmann K (eds): *Steroids and Brain Edema.* Berlin, Springer-Verlag, pp 147–151, 1972.
10. Campbell JB, DeCrescito V, Tomasula JJ, Demopoulos HB, Flamm ES, Ortega BD: Effects of antifibrinolytic and steroid therapy on the contused spinal cord of cats. *J Neurosurg* 40:726–733, 1974.
11. Hedeman LS, Sil R: Studies in experimental spinal cord trauma. Part 2. Comparison of treatment with steroids, low-molecular weight dextran and catecholamine blockage. *J Neurosurg* 40:44–51, 1974.
12. Lewin MG, Hansebout RR, Pappius HM: Chemical characteristics of traumatic spinal cord edema in cats. Effects of steroids on potassium depletion. *J Neurosurg* 56:106–113, 1974.
13. Parker AJ, Smith CW: Functional recovery from spinal cord trauma following dexamethasone and chlorpromazine therapy in dogs. *Res Vet Sci* 21:246–247, 1976.
14. Demopoulos HB, Flamm ES, Seligman ML, Mitamura JA, Ransohoff J: Membrane perturbations in central nervous system injury: theoretical basis for free radical damage and a review of the experimental data. In Popp AJ, Bourke RS, Nelson LR, Kimelberg HK (eds): *Neural Trauma.* Raven Press, New York, pp 63–78, 1979.
15. Demopoulos HB, Flamm ES, Pietronigro DD, Seligman MC, Tomasula J, DeCrescito V: The free radical pathology and the microcirculation in the major central nervous system disorders. *Acta Physiol Scand* 492:91–119, 1980.
16. Demopoulos HB, Flamm ES, Seligman MC, Pietronigro DD, Tomasula J, DeCrescito V: Further studies on free radical pathology in the major central nervous system disorders: effect of very high doses of methylprednisolone on the functional outcome, morphology and chemistry of experimental spinal cord impact injury. *Can J Physiol Pharmacol* 60:1415–1424, 1981.
17. Bracken MB, Shepard MJ, Hellenbrand KG et al: Methylprednisolone and neurological function 1 year after spinal cord injury. *J Neurosurg* 63:704–713, 1985.
18. Braughler JM, Hall ED: Correlation of methylprednisolone pharmacokinetics in cat spinal cord with its effect on (Na^+-K^+)-ATPase, lipid peroxidation and motor neuron function. *J Neurosurg* 56:838–844, 1981.
19. Hall ED, Braughler JM: Acute effects of intravenous glucocorticoid pretreatment on the in vitro peroxidation of cat spinal cord tissue. *Exp Neurol* 73:321–324, 1981.
20. Braughler JM, Hall ED: Acute enhancement of spinal cord synaptosomal (Na^+-K^+)-ATPase activity in cats following intravenous methylprednisolone. *Brain Res* 219:464–469, 1981.
21. Hall ED, Braughler JM: Glucocorticoid mechanisms in acute spinal cord injury: a review and therapeutic rationale. *Surg Neurol* 18:320–327, 1982.
22. Braughler JM, Hall ED: Pharmacokinetics of methylprednisolone in cat plasma and spinal cord following a single intravenous dose of the sodium succinate ester. *Drug Metab Dispos* 10:551–552, 1982.
23. Hall ED, Braughler JM: Effects of methylprednisolone on spinal cord lipid peroxidation and (Na^+-K^+)-ATPase activity: dose response analysis during the first hour after contusion injury in the cat. *J Neurosurg* 57:247–253, 1982.
24. Braughler JM, Hall ED: Lactate and pyruvate metabolism in injured cat spinal cord before and after a single large intravenous dose of methylprednisolone. *J Neurosurg* 59:256–261, 1983.
25. Braughler JM, Hall ED: Uptake and elimination of methylprednisolone from contused cat spinal cord following intravenous injection of sodium succinate ester. *J Neurosurg* 58:538–542, 1983.
26. Hall ED, Wolf DL, Braughler JM: Dose response and time action analysis of the effects of a single large dose of methylprednisolone sodium succinate on posttraumatic spinal cord ischemia. *J Neurosurg* 58:1–22, 1983.
27. Hall ED, Wolf DL, Braughler JM: Effects of a single large dose of methylprednisolone sodium succinate on experimental posttraumatic spinal cord ischemia. Dose-response and time-action analysis. *J Neurosurg* 61:124–130, 1984.
28. Hall ED: High-dose glucocorticoid treatment improves neurological recovery in head-injured mice. *J Neurosurg* 62:882–887, 1985.
29. Anderson DK, Means ED, Waters TR, Green BS: Microvascular perfusion and metabolism in injured spinal cord after methylprednisolone treatment. *J Neurosurg* 56:106–113, 1982.
30. Young W, Flamm ES: Effect of high dose corticosteroid therapy on blood flow, evoked potentials, and extracellular calcium in experimental spinal injury. *J Neurosurg* 57:667–673, 1982.
31. Anderson DK, Saunders RD, Demediuk P, Dugan LL, Braughler JM, Hall ED, Means ED, Horrocks LA: Lipid hydrolysis and peroxidation in injured spinal cord: partial protection with methylprednisolone or vitamin E and selenium. *Cent Nerv Syst Trauma* 2:257–267, 1985.
32. Young W, DeCrescito V, Flamm ES, Blight AR, Gruner JA: Pharmacological therapy of acute spinal cord injury: studies of high dose methylprednisolone and naloxone. *Clin Neurosurg* 34:675–697, 1988.
33. Faden AI, Jacobs TP, Mougey E, Holaday JW: Endorphins in experimental spinal injury: therapeutic effect of naloxone. *Ann Neurol* 10:326–332, 1981.
34. Young W, Flamm ES, Demopoulos HB, DeCrescito V, Tomasula JJ: Effect of naloxone on posttraumatic ischemia in experimental spinal contusion. *J Neurosurg* 55:209–219, 1981.
35. Faden AI, Hallenbeck JM, Brown CQ: Treatment of experimental stroke: comparison of naloxone and thyrotropin releasing hormone. *Neurology (NY)* 32:1083–1087, 1982.
36. Faden AI, Jacobs TP, Holaday JW: Comparison of early and late naloxone treatment in experimental spinal injury. *Neurology (NY)* 32:677–681, 1982.
37. Flamm ES, Young W, Demopoulos HB, DeCrescito V, Tomasula JJ: Experimental spinal cord injury: treatment with naloxone. *Neurosurgery* 10:227–231, 1982.
38. Hall ED, Plaster M, Braughler JM: Acute cardiovascular response to a single large intravenous dose of methylprednisolone and its effects on the responses to norepinephrine and isoproterenol. *Proc Soc Exp Biol Med* 173:338–343, 1983.
39. Braughler JM, Hall ED: Effects of multi-dose methylprednisolone sodium succinate administration on injured cat spinal cord neurofilament degradation and energy metabolism. *J Neurosurg* 61:290–295, 1984.
40. Faden AI, Jacobs TP, Zivin JA: Comparison of naloxone and a delta-selective antagonist in experimental spinal "stroke." *Life Sci* 33(suppl 1):707–710, 1983.
41. Faden AI, Jacobs TP, Smith MT: Comparison of thyrotropin-releasing hormone (TRH), naloxone, and dexamethasone treatments in experimental spinal injury. *Neurology* 33:673–678, 1983.
42. Faden AI, Jacobs TP, Zivin JA: Naloxone but not TRH improves neurological recovery following spinal cord ischemia in the rabbit. *Stroke* 14:1–15, 1983.
43. Flamm ES, Young W, Collins WF, Piepmeier J, Clifton GL, Fischer B: A phase I trial of naloxone treatment in acute spinal cord injury. *J Neurosurg* 63:390–397, 1985.
44. Frankel HL, Hancock DO, Hyslop G, Melzak J, Michaelis LS, Ungar GH, Vernon JD, Walsh JJ: The value of postural reduction in the initial management of closed injuries of the spine with paraplegia and tetraplegia. I. *Paraplegia* 7:179–192, 1969.
45. Hall ED: The neuroprotective pharmacology of methylprednisolone. *J Neurosurg* 76:13–22, 1992.
46. Hall ED, Yonkers PA, Andrus PK, Cox JW, Anderson DK: Biochemistry and pharmacology of lipid antioxidants in acute brain and spinal cord injury. *J Neurotrauma* 9:S425–S442, 1992.
47. Hall ED, Braughler JM, McCall JM: Antioxidant effects in brain and spinal cord injury. *J Neurotrauma* 9:S165–S172, 1992.
48. Hsu CY, Dimitrijevic MR: Methylprednisolone in spinal cord injury: the possible mechanism of action. *J Neurotrauma* 7:115–119, 1990.
49. Flower RJ, Blackwell GJ: Anti-inflammatory steroids induce biosynthesis of a phospholipase A2 inhibitor which prevents prostaglandin generation. *Nature* 278:456–458, 1979.
50. Hirata F, Corcoran BA, Venkatasubramanian K, Schiffman E, Axelrod J: Chemoattractants simulate degradation of methylated phospholipids and release of arachidonic acid in rabbit leukocytes. *Proc Natl Acad Sci USA* 76:2640–2643, 1979.
51. Metz R, Giebler C, Forster W: Evidence for a direct inhibitory effect of glucocorticoids on the activity of phospholipase A2 as a further possible mechanism of some actions of steroid anti-inflammatory drugs. *Pharmacol Res Commun* 12:817–827, 1980.
52. Hirata F, Schiffman E, Venkatasubramanian K, Saloman D, Axelrod J: A phospholipase A2 inhibitory protein in rabbit neutrophils induced by glucocorticoids. *Proc Natl Acad Sci USA* 77:2533–2536, 1980.
53. Blackwell GJ, Carnuccio R, Di Rosa M, Flower RJ, Parente L, Persico P: Macrocortin: a polypeptide causing the anti-phospholipase effect of glucocorticoids. *Nature* 287:147–149, 1980.
54. Hirata F, Notsu Y, Iwata M, Parente L, Di Rosa M, Flower RJ: Identification of several species of phospholipase proteins by radioimmunoassay for lipomodulin. *Biochem Res Commun* 109:223–230, 1982.
55. Russo-Marie F, Duval D: Dexamethasone-induced inhibition of prostaglandin production does not result from a direct action on phospholipase activities but is mediated through a steroid-inducible factor. *Biochem Biophys Acta* 712:177–185, 1982.
56. Cirino G, Flower RJ, Browning JL, Sinclair LK, Pepinsky RB: Recombinant human lipocortin 1 inhibits thromboxane release from guinea-pig isolated perfused lung. *Nature* 328:270–272, 1987.
57. Cirino G, Flower RJ: Human recombinant lipocortin 1 inhibits prostacyclin production by human umbilical artery in vitro. *Prostaglandins* 34:59–62, 1987.
58. Breasted JH: *The Edwin Smith Papyrus.* University of Chicago Press, Chicago, IL, 1930.
59. Dimitrijevic MR, Faganel J, Lehmkuhl D, Sherwood AM: Motor control in man after partial or complete spinal cord injury. In Desmedt JE (ed): *Motor Control Mechanisms in Health and Disease.* Raven Press, pp 915–926, 1983.
60. Dimitrijevic MR, Dimitrijevic M, Faganel J, Sherwood AM: Suprasegmentally induced motor unit activity in paralyzed muscles of patients with established spinal cord injury. *Ann Neurol* 16:216–221, 1984.
61. Cioni B, Dimitrijevic MR, McKay WB, Sherwood AM: Voluntary supraspinal suppression of spinal reflex activity in paralyzed muscles of spinal cord injury patients. *Exp Neurol* 93:574–583, 1986.
62. Dimitrijevic MR: Residual motor functions in spinal cord injury. In Waxman SG (ed): *Functional Recovery in Neurological Disease.* Raven Press, New York, pp 139–155, 1988.
63. Braughler JM, Hall ED: Involvement of lipid peroxidation in CNS injury. *J Neurotrauma* 9:S1–S7, 1992.
64. McCall JM, Braughler JM, Hall ED: A new class of compounds for stroke and trauma: effects of 21-aminosteroids on lipid peroxidation. *Acta Anaesthesiol Belg* 38:417–420, 1987.
65. Braughler JM, Pregenzer JF, Chase RL, Duncan LA, Jacobsen EJ, McCall JM: Novel 21-amino steroids as potent inhibitors of iron-dependent lipid peroxidation. *J Biol Chem* 262:10438–10440, 1987.
66. Hall ED, McCall JM, Chase RL, Yonkers PA, Braughler JM: A non-glucocorticoid steroid analog of methylprednisolone duplicates its high-dose pharmacology in models of central nervous system trauma and neuronal membrane damage. *J Pharmacol Exp Ther* 242:137–142, 1987.
67. Anderson DK, Braughler JM, Hall ED, Waters TR, McCall JM, Means ED: Effects of treatment with U74006F on neurological outcome following experimental spinal cord injury. *J Neurosurg* 69:562–567, 1988.
68. Braughler JM, Chase RL, Neff GL, Yonkers PA, Day JS, Hall ED, Sethy VH, Lahti RA: A new 21-aminosteroid antioxidant lacking glucocorticoid activity blocks arachidonic acid release and stimulates adrenocorticotropin secretion from mouse pituitary tumor (AtT-20) cells. *J Pharmacol Exp Ther* 244:423–427, 1988.
69. Hall ED, Braughler JM: New pharmacological treatment of acute spinal cord trauma. *J Neurotrauma* 5:81–89, 1988.
70. Hall ED, Pazara KE, Braughler JM: 21-Aminosteroid lipid peroxidation inhibitor U74006F protects against cerebral ischemia in gerbils. *Stroke* 19:997–1002, 1988.
71. Hall ED, Travis MA: Effects of the non-glucocorticoid 21-aminosteroid U74006F on acute cerebral hypoperfusion following experimental subarachnoid hemorrhage. *Exp Neurol* 102:244–248, 1988.

72. Hall ED, Travis MA: Inhibition of arachidonic acid-induced vasogenic brain edema by the non-glucocorticoid 21-aminosteroid U74006F. *Brain Res* 451:350–352, 1988.
73. Hall ED, Yonkers PA: Attenuation of postischemic cerebral hypoperfusion by the 21-aminosteroid U74006F. *Stroke* 19:340–344, 1988.
74. Hall ED, Yonkers PA, McCall JM: Attenuation of hemorrhagic shock by the non-glucocorticoid 21-aminosteroid U74006F. *Eur J Pharmacol* 147:299–303, 1988.
75. Hall ED: Effects of the 21-aminosteroid U74006F on posttraumatic spinal cord ischemia in cats. *J Neurosurg* 68:462–465, 1988.
76. Hall ED, Yonkers PA, McCall JM, Braughler JM: Effects of the 21-aminosteroid U74006F on experimental head injury in mice. *J Neurosurg* 68:456–461, 1988.
77. Natale JE, Schott RJ, Hall ED, Braughler JM, D'Alecy LG: Effect of the aminosteroid U74006F after cardiopulmonary arrest in dogs. *Stroke* 19:1371–1378, 1988.
78. Young W, Wojak JC, DeCrescito V: 21-Aminosteroid reduces ion shifts and edema in the rat middle cerebral artery occlusion model of regional ischemia. *Stroke* 1013–1019, 1988.
79. Hall ED, Pazara KE: Effects of novel 21-aminosteroid antioxidants on postischemic neuronal degeneration. In Ginsberg MD, Dietrich WD (eds): *Cerebrovascular Diseases.* Raven Press, New York, pp 387–391, 1989.
80. Hall ED, Yonkers PA, Horan KL, Braughler JM: Correlation between attenuation of posttraumatic spinal cord ischemia and preservation of tissue vitamin E by the 21-aminosteroid U74006F: evidence for an in vivo antioxidant mechanism. *J Neurotrauma* 6:169–176, 1989.
81. Steinke DE, Weir BKA, Findlay JM, Tanabe T, Grace M, Krushelnycky BW: A trial of the 21-aminosteroid U74006F in a primate model of chronic cerebral vasospasm. *Neurosurgery* 24:179–186, 1989.
82. Vollmer DG, Kassell NF, Hongo K, Ogawa H, Tsukahara T: Effect of the nonglucocorticoid 21-aminosteroid U74006F on experimental cerebral vasospasm. *Surg Neurol* 31:190–194, 1989.
83. Zuccarello M, Anderson DK: Protective effect of a 21-aminosteroid on the blood brain barrier following subarachnoid hemorrhage in rats. *Stroke* 20:367–371, 1989.
84. Zuccarello M, Marsch JT, Schmidt G, Woodward J, Anderson DK: Effect of the 21-aminosteroid U74006F on cerebral vasospasm following subarachnoid hemorrhage. *J Neurosurg* 71:98–104, 1989.
85. Fowl RJ, Patterson RB, Gewirtz RJ, Anderson DK: Protection against postischemic spinal cord injury using a new 21-aminosteroid. *J Surg Res* 48:597–600, 1990.
86. Hall ED, Braughler JM, McCall JM: Role of oxygen radicals in stroke: effects of the 21-aminosteroid—a novel class of antioxidants. In Meldrum BS, Williams M (eds): *Current and Future Trends in Anticonvulsant, Anxiety and Stroke Therapy.* Wiley, New York, p 351, 1990.
87. Hall ED, Yonkers PA: Attenuation of the postischemic cerebral hypoperfusion by the 21-aminosteroid antioxidant U74006F. *Brain Res* 513:244–247, 1990.
88. Monyer H, Hartley DM, Choi DW: 21-Aminosteroids attenuate excitotoxic neuronal injury in cortical cell cultures. *Neuron* 5:121–126, 1990.
89. Anderson DK, Hall ED, Braughler JM, McCall JM, Means ED: Effect of delayed administration of U74006F (tirilazad mesylate) on recovery of locomotor function after experimental spinal cord injury. *J Neurotrauma* 8:187–192, 1991.
90. Holtz A, Gerdin B: Blocking weight-induced spinal cord injury in rats: therapeutic effect of the 21-aminosteroid U74006F. *J Neurotrauma* 8:239–245, 1991.
91. Faden AI, Jacobs TP, Holaday JW: Thyrotropin releasing hormone improves neurologic recovery after spinal trauma in cats. *N Engl J Med* 305:1063–1067, 1981.
92. Faden AI: Opiate antagonists and thyrotropin releasing hormone. I. Potential role in the treatment of shock. *J Am Med Assoc* 252:1177–1180, 1984.
93. Faden AI: Opiate antagonists and thyrotropin-releasing hormone. II. Potential role in the treatment of central nervous system injury. *J Am Med Assoc* 252:1452–1454, 1984.
94. Faden AI, Jacobs TP, Smith MT: Thyrotropin-releasing hormone in experimental spinal injury: dose response and late treatment. *Neurology* 34:1280–1284, 1984.
95. Krusal BA, Keith CH, Maxfield FR: Thyrotropin releasing hormone induced changes in intracellular [Ca^{2+}] measured by microspectrofluorometry on individual quin2-loaded cells. *J Cell Biol* 99:1167–1172, 1984.
96. Faden AI, Jacobs TP: Effect of TRH analogs on neurologic recovery after experimental spinal trauma. *Neurology* 35:1331–1334, 1985.
97. Arias MJ: Treatment of experimental spinal cord injury with TRH, naloxone, and dexamethasone. *Surg Neurol* 28:335–338, 1987.
98. Faden AI, Sacksen I, Noble LJ: Structure-activity relationships of TRH analogs in rat spinal cord injury. *Brain Res* 448:287–293, 1988.
99. McIntosh TK, Vink R, Faden AI: Centrally active analogs of thyrotropin-releasing hormone (TRH) improve outcome and survival following traumatic brain injury in rats: laboratory and magnetic resonance studies. *Am J Physiol* 254:R785–R792, 1988.
100. Faden AI, Vink R, McIntosh TK: Thyrotropin-releasing hormone and central nervous system trauma. *Ann NY Acad Sci* 553:380–384, 1989.
101. Faden AI, Yum SW, Lemke M, Vink R: Effects of TRH-analog treatment on tissue cations, phospholipids and energy metabolism after spinal cord injury. *J Pharmacol Exp Ther* 255:608–614, 1990.
102. Puniak MA, Freeman GM, Agresta CA, Van NL, Barone CA, Salzman SK: Comparison of a serotonin antagonist, opioid antagonist, and TRH analog for the acute treatment of experimental spinal trauma. *J Neurotrauma* 8:193–203, 1991.
103. Bakshi R, Newman AH, Faden AI: Dynorphin A-(1-17) induces alterations in free fatty acids, excitatory amino acids, and motor function through an opiate-receptor-mediated mechanism. *J Neurosci* 10:3793–3800, 1990.
104. Faden AI: Opioid and nonopioid mechanisms may contribute to dynorphin's pathophysiological actions in spinal cord injury. *Ann Neurol* 27:67–74, 1990.
105. Faden AI, Jacobs TP: Opiate antagonist WN 44,441-3 stereospecifically improves neurologic recovery after ischemic spinal injury. *Neurology* 35:1311–1315, 1985.
106. Faden AI, Takemori AE, Portghese PS: K-selective opiate antagonist nor-binaltorphimine improves outcome after traumatic spinal cord injury in rats. *Cent Nerv Syst Trauma* 4:227–234, 1987.
107. Faden AI, Sacksen I, Noble LJ: Opiate-receptor antagonist nalmefene improves neurologic recovery after traumatic spinal cord injury in rats through a central mechanism. *J Pharmacol Exp Ther* 245:742–748, 1988.
108. Vink R, McIntosh TK, Rhomhanyi R, Faden AI: Opiate antagonist nalmefene improves intracellular free Mg^{2+}, bioenergetic state, and neurologic outcome following traumatic brain injury in rats. *J Neurosci* 10:3524–3530, 1990.
109. Faden AI, Lemke M, Simon RP, Noble LJ: *N*-methyl-*D*-aspartate antagonist MK801 improves outcome following traumatic spinal cord injury in rats: Behavioral, anatomic, and neurochemical studies. *J Neurotrauma* 5:33–45, 1988.
110. Faden AI, Simon RP: A potential role for excitotoxins in the pathophysiology of spinal cord injury. *Ann Neurol* 23:623–626, 1988.
111. Bakshi R, Faden AI: Competitive and non-competitive NMDA antagonists limit dynorphin A-induced rat hindlimb paralysis. *Brain Res* 507:1–5, 1990.
112. Faden AI, Ellison JA, Noble LJ: Effects of competitive and noncompetitive NMDA receptor antagonists in spinal cord injury. *Eur J Pharmacol* 175:165–174, 1990.
113. Yum SW, Faden AI: Comparison of the neuroprotective effects of the *N*-methyl-*D*-aspartate antagonist MK-801 and the opiate-receptor antagonist nalmefene in experimental spinal cord ischemia. *Arch Neurol* 47:277–281, 1990.
114. Salzman SK, Puniak MA, Liu Z-J, Maitland-Heriot RP, Freeman GM, Agresta CA: The serotonin antagonist mianserin improves functional recovery following experimental spinal trauma. *Ann Neurol* 30:533–541, 1991.
115. Geisler FH, Dorsey FC, Coleman WP: Recovery of motor function after spinal cord injury—a randomized, placebo-controlled trial with GM-1 ganglioside. *N Engl J Med* 324:1829–1838, 1991.
116. Geisler FH, Dorsey FC, Coleman WP: GM-1 ganglioside in human spinal cord injury. *J Neurotrauma* 9:S517–S530, 1992.
117. Svennevig JL, Bugge-Asperheim B, Vaage J, Geiran O, Birkeland S: Corticosteroids in the treatment of blunt injury of the chest. *Injury* 16:80–84, 1984.
118. Svennevig JL, Pillgram-Larsen J, Fjeld NB, Birkeland S, Semb G: Early use of corticosteroids in severe closed chest injuries: a 10-year experience. *Injury* 18:309–312, 1987.
119. Svennevig JL: Blunt chest trauma. *Acta Anaesth Belg* 38:301–305, 1987.
120. Anderson DK, Waters TR, Means ED: Pretreatment with alpha tocopherol enhances neurologic recovery after experimental spinal cord compression injury. *J Neurotrauma* 5:61–67, 1988.
121. Saunders RD, Dugan LL, Demediuk P, Means ED, Horrocks LA, Anderson DK: Effects of methylprednisolone and the combination of alpha-tocopherol and selenium on arachidonic acid metabolism and lipid peroxidation in traumatized spinal cord tissue. *J Neurochem* 49:24–31, 1987.
122. Anderson DK, Means ED: Alpha-tocopherol, mannitol, and methylprednisolone prevention of $FeCl_2$ initiated free radical induced lipid peroxidation in spinal cord. In Novelli U (ed): *Oxygen Free Radicals in Shock.* Karger, Basel, pp 224–230, 1986.
123. Travis MA, Hall ED: The effects of chronic two-fold dietary vitamin E supplementation on subarachnoid hemorrhage-induced brain hypoperfusion. *Brain Res* 418:366–370, 1987.
124. Clifton GL, Lyeth BG, Jenkins LW, Taft WC, DeLorenzo RJ, Hayes RL: Effect of *d*-alpha-tocopheryl succinate and polyethylene glycol on performance tests after fluid percussion brain injury. *J Neurotrauma* 6:71–81, 1989.
125. Lemke M, Frei B, Ames BN, Faden AI: Decreases in tissue levels of ubiquinol-9 and -10, ascorbate and alpha-tocopherol following spinal cord impact trauma in rats. *Neurosci Lett* 108:201–206, 1990.
126. Hall ED: Intensive anti-oxidant pretreatment retards motor nerve degeneration. *Brain Res* 413:175–178, 1987.
127. Hall ED, Braughler JM: Role of lipid peroxidation in posttraumatic spinal cord degeneration: a review. *Cent Nerv Syst Trauma* 3:281–294, 1986.
128. Klatzo I: Experimental aspects of brain edema and therapeutic approach. In Reulen HJ, Schürmann K (eds): *Steroids and Brain Edema.* Springer-Verlag, Berlin, pp 1–8, 1972.
129. Rovit RL, Hagan R: Steroids and cerebral edema: the effects of glucocorticoids on abnormal capillary permeability following cerebral injury in cats. *J Neuropathol Exp Neurol* 27:277–299, 1968.
130. Fishman RA: Steroids in the treatment of brain edema. *N Engl J Med* 306:359–360, 1982.
131. Sztriha L, Joo F, Szerdahelyi P, Eck E, Koltai M: Effects of dexamethasone on brain edema induced by kainic acid seizures. *Neuroscience* 17:107–114, 1986.
132. Meinig G, Deisenroth K: Dose- and time-dependent effects of dexamethasone on rat brain following cold-injury oedema. *Acta Neurochir Suppl (Wien)* 51:100–103, 1990.
133. Meinig G, Deisenroth K: Dose-response relation for dexamethasone in cold lesion-induced brain edema in rats. *Adv Neurol* 52:295–300, 1990.
134. Clasen RA, Pandolfi S, Clasen JR: Massive doses of steroids in cryogenic cerebral injury and edema. *Stroke* 10:670–673, 1979.
135. Shapira Y, Davidson E, Weidenfeld Y, Cotev S, Shohami E: Dexamethasone and indomethacin do not affect brain edema following head injury in rats. *J Cereb Blood Flow Metab* 8:395–402, 1988.
136. Spillert CR, Glicini RL, Tortella BJ, Lazaro EJ: Effect of steroid therapy in experimental head trauma. *Brain Inj* 4:199–201, 1990.
137. Goblet W: Monitoring of intracranial pressure in patients with severe head injury. *Neurochirurgia (Stuttg)* 20:35–47, 1977.
138. James HE, Madauss WC, Tibbs PA, McCloskey JJ, Bean JR: The effect of high dose dexamethasone in children with severe closed head injury. A preliminary report. *Acta Neurochir (Wien)* 45:225–236, 1979.
139. Du Plessis JJ: High-dose dexamethasone therapy in head injury: a patient group that may benefit from therapy. *Br J Neurosurg* 6:145–147, 1992.
140. Cooper PR, Moody S, Clark WK, Kirkpatrick J, Maravilla K, Gould AL, Drane W: Dexamethasone and severe head injury. A prospective double-blind study. *J Neurosurg* 51:307–316, 1979.

141. Braakman R, Schouten HJ, Blaauw vDM, Minderhoud JM: Megadose steroids in severe head injury. Results of a prospective double-blind clinical trial. *J Neurosurg* 58:326–330, 1983.
142. Saul TG, Ducker TB, Salcman M, Carro E: Steroids in severe head injury: a prospective randomized clinical trial. *J Neurosurg* 54:596–600, 1981.
143. Gudeman SK, Miller JD, Becker DP: Failure of high-dose steroid therapy to influence intracranial pressure in patients with severe head injury. *J Neurosurg* 51:301–306, 1979.
144. Giannotta SL, Weiss MH, Apuzzo ML, Martin E: High dose glucocorticoids in the management of severe head injury. *Neurosurgery* 15:497–501, 1984.
145. Scheff SW, Benardo LS, Cotman CW: Hydrocortisone administration retards axon sprouting in the rat dentate gyrus. *Exp Neurol* 68:195–201, 1980.
146. Scheff SW, Cotman CW: Chronic glucocorticoid therapy alters axon sprouting in the hippocampal dentate gyrus. *Exp Neurol* 76:644–654, 1982.
147. Scheff SW, Dekosky ST: Steroid suppression of axon sprouting in the hippocampal dentate gyrus of the adult rat: dose-response relationship. *Exp Neurol* 82:183–191, 1983.
148. Scheff SW, Hoff S, Anderson KJ: Altered regulation of lesion-induced synaptogenesis by adrenalectomy and corticosterone in young adult rats. *Exp Neurol* 93:456–470, 1986.
149. Betz AL, Coester HC: Effect of steroid therapy on ischemic brain oedema and blood to brain sodium transport. *Acta Neurochir Suppl (Wien)* 51:256–258, 1990.
150. Betz AL, Coester HC: Effect of steroids on edema and sodium uptake of the brain during focal ischemia in rats. *Stroke* 21:1199–1204, 1990.
151. Dux E, Ismail M, Szerdahelyi P, Joo F, Dux L, Koltai M, Draskoczy M: Dexamethasone treatment attenuates the development of ischaemic brain oedema in gerbils. *Neuroscience* 34:203–207, 1990.
152. Kalayci O, Cataltepe S, Cataltepe O: The effect of bolus methylprednisolone in prevention of brain edema in hypoxic ischemic brain injury: an experimental study in 7-day-old rat pups. *Brain Res* 569:112–116, 1992.
153. Sapolsky RM, Pulsinelli WA: Glucocorticoids potentiate ischemic injury to neurons: therapeutic implications. *Science* 229:1397–1400, 1985.
154. Levy DE, Pulsinelli WA, Scherer PB, Plum F: Effect of admission glucose and hematocrit on recovery from acute ischemic stroke. In Battistini N, Fiorani P, Courbier R, Plum F, Fieschi C (eds): *Acute Brain Ischemia: Medical and Surgical Therapy*. Raven Press, New York, pp 151–157, 1986.
155. Pickard JD, Murray GD, Illingworth R, Shaw MD, Teasdale GM, Foy PM, Humphrey PR, Lang DA, Nelson R, Richards P: Effect of oral nimodipine on cerebral infarction and outcome after subarachnoid haemorrhage: British aneurysm nimodipine trial. *Br Med J* 298:636–642, 1989.
156. Allen GS, Ahn HS, Preziosi TJ et al: Cerebral arterial spasm-A controlled trial of nimodipine in patients with subarachnoid hemorrhage. *N Engl J Med* 308:619–624, 1983.
157. Teasdale G, Bailey I, Bell A, Gray J, Gullan R, Heiskanan O, Marks PV, Marsh H, Mendelow DA, Murray G: A randomized trial of nimodipine in severe head injury: HIT I. British/Finnish Co-operative Head Injury Trial Group. *J Neurotrauma* 2:S545–S550, 1992.
158. Busto R, Dietrich WD, Globus MY, Valdes I, Scheinberg P, Ginsberg MD: Small differences in intraischemic brain temperature critically determine the extent of ischemic neuronal injury. *J Cereb Blood Flow Metab* 7:729–738, 1987.
159. Ikonomidou C, Price MT, Mosinger JL, Olney JW: Hypothermia enhances protective effect of MK801 against hypoxic/ischemic brain damage in infant rats. *Brain Res* 487:184–187, 1989.
160. Onesti ST, Baker CJ, Sun PP, Solomon RA: Transient hypothermia reduces focal ischemic brain injury in the rat. *Neurosurgery* 29:369–373, 1991.
161. Morikawa E, Ginsberg MD, Dietrich WD et al: The significance of brain temperature in focal cerebral ischemia: histopathological consequences of middle cerebral artery occlusion in the rat. *J Cereb Blood Flow Metab* 12:380–389, 1992.
162. Clifton GL, Jiang JY, Lyeth BG, Jenkins LW, Hamm RJ, Hayes RL: Marked protection by moderate hypothermia after experimental traumatic brain injury. *J Cereb Blood Flow Metab* 11:114–121, 1991.
163. Lee MR, Sakatani K, Young W: Interaction of hypoxia and hypothermia on dorsal column conduction in adult rat spinal cord in vitro. *Exp Neurol* 119:140–145, 1993.
164. Albin MS, White RJ, Acosta RG, Yashon D: Study of functional recovery produced by delayed localized cooling after spinal cord injury in primates. *J Neurosurg* 29:113–120, 1968.
165. Albin MS, White RJ, Yashon D, Harris LS: Effects of localized cooling on spinal cord trauma. *J Trauma* 9:1000–1008, 1969.
166. Kuchney EF, Hansebout RR: Combined steroid and hypothermia treatment of experimental spinal cord injury. *Surg Neurol* 6:371–376, 1967.
167. Busto R, Dietrich WD, Globus MYT, Ginsberg MD: The importance of brain temperature in cerebral ischemic injury. *Stroke* 20:1113–1114, 1989.
168. Globus MY, Ginsberg MD, Busto R: Excitotoxic index—a biochemical marker of selective vulnerability. *Neurosci Lett* 127:39–42, 1991.
169. Globus MY, Busto R, Martinez E, Valdes I, Dietrich WD, Ginsberg MD: Comparative effect of transient global ischemia on extracellular levels of glutamate, glycine, and gamma-aminobutyric acid in vulnerable and nonvulnerable brain regions in the rat. *J Neurochem* 57:470–478, 1991.
170. Globus MY, Ginsberg MD, Busto R: Excitotoxic index—a biochemical marker of selective vulnerability. *Neurosci Lett* 127:39–42, 1991.
171. Means ED, Anderson DK, Waters TR, Kalaf L: Effect of methylprednisolone in compression trauma to the feline spinal cord. *J Neurosurg* 55:200–208, 1981.
172. Bracken MB, Collins WF, Freeman DF et al: Efficacy of methylprednisolone in acute spinal cord injury. *J Am Med Assoc* 251:45–52, 1984.
173. Braughler JM, Hall ED, Means ED, Waters TR, Anderson DK: Evaluation of an intensive methylprednisolone sodium succinate dosing regimen in experimental spinal cord injury. *J Neurosurg* 67:102–105, 1987.
174. Bracken MB, Shepard MJ, Collins WF et al: Methylprednisolone or naloxone in the treatment of acute spinal cord injury: 1 year follow-up data. Results of the second National Acute Spinal Cord Injury Study. *J Neurosurg* 76:23–31, 1992.
175. Bracken MB, Shepard MJ, Collins WF et al: A randomized controlled trial of methylprednisolone or naloxone in the treatment of acute spinal-cord injury: Results of the Second National Acute Spinal Cord Injury Study. *N Engl J Med* 322:1405–1411, 1990.
176. Hall ED: Beneficial effects of the 21-aminosteroid U74006F in acute CNS trauma and hypovolemic shock. *Acta Anaesth Belg* 38:421–425, 1987.
177. Faden AI: TRH analog YM-14673 improves outcome following traumatic brain and spinal cord injury in rats: dose-response studies. *Brain Res* 486:228–235, 1989.
178. Faden AI, Lemke M, Demediuk P: Effects of BW755C, a mixed cyclo-oxygenase-lipoxygenase inhibitor, following traumatic spinal cord injury in rats. *Brain Res* 463:63–68, 1988.
179. Hall ED, Wolf DL: A pharmacological analysis of the pathophysiological mechanisms of posttraumatic spinal cord ischemia. *J Neurosurg* 64:951–961, 1986.
180. Iizuka H, Iwasaki Y, Yamamoto T, Kadoya S: Morphometric assessment of drug effects in experimental spinal cord injury. *J Neurosurg* 65:92–98, 1986.
181. Iwasaki Y, Yamamoto H, Iizuka H, Yamamoto T, Konno H: Suppression of neurofilament degradation by protease inhibitors in experimental spinal cord injury. *Brain Res* 406:99–104, 1987.
182. Guha A, Tator CH, Piper I: Increase in rat spinal cord blood flow with the calcium channel blocker, nimodipine. *J Neurosurg* 63:250–259, 1985.
183. Tator CH, Fehlings MG: Review of the secondary injury theory of acute spinal cord trauma with emphasis on vascular mechanisms. *J Neurosurg* 75:15–26, 1991.
184. Braughler JM, Hall ED: Involvement of lipid peroxidation in CNS injury. *J Neurotrauma* 9:S1–S7, 1992.
185. Braughler JM, Hall ED, Jacobsen EJ, McCall JM, Means ED: Correlates in pharmacostructures. The 21-aminosteroids: potent inhibitors of lipid peroxidation for the treatment of central nervous system trauma and ischemia. *Drugs of the Future* 14:143–152, 1989.
186. Yatsu FM, Diamond I, Graziano C, Lindquist PC: Experimental brain ischemia: protection from irreversible damage with a rapid-acting barbiturate (methohexital). *Stroke* 3:726–732, 1972.
187. Smith AL, Hoff JT, Nielsen SL, Larson CP: Barbiturate protection in acute focal cerebral ischemia. *Stroke* 5:1–7, 1974.
188. Flamm ES, Demopoulos HB, Seligman ML, Ransohoff J: Possible molecular mechanisms of barbiturate mediated protection in regional cerebral ischemia. *Acta Neurol Scand* 64:150–152, 1977.
189. Molinari GF, Lightfotte WEI, Fein JM: Evidence for barbiturate protection in focal cerebral ischemia: a hypothesis of mechanism and clinical utility. In Fein JM, Reichman OH (eds): *Microvascular Anastomoses for Cerebral Ischemia*. Springer-Verlag, Berlin, pp 86–93, 1978.
190. Oldfield EH, Plunkett RJ, Nylander WA, Meachan WF: Barbiturate protection in acute experimental spinal cord ischemia. *J Neurosurg* 56:511–516, 1982.
191. Astrup J, Rehncrona S, Siesjo BK: The increase in extracellular potassium concentration in the ischemic brain in relation to the pre-ischemic functional activity and cerebral metabolic rate. *Brain Res* 199:161–174, 1980.
192. Holaday JW, D'Amato RJ: Naloxone or TRH fails to improve neurological deficits in gerbil models of "stroke." *Life Sci* 31:385–392, 1982.
193. Zabramski JM, Spetzler RF, Selman WF, Roessmann UR, Hershey LA, Crumrine RC, Macko R: Naloxone therapy during focal cerebral ischemia evaluation in a primate model. *Stroke* 15:621–627, 1984.
194. Faden AI, Shirane R, Chang LH, James TL, Lemke M, Weinstein PR: Opiate-receptor antagonist improves metabolic recovery and limits neurochemical alterations associated with reperfusion after global brain ischemia in rats. *J Pharmacol Exp Ther* 255:451–458, 1990.
195. Karpiak SE, Li YS, Mahadik SP: Gangliosides (GM1 and AGF2) reduce mortality due to ischemia: protection of membrane function. *Stroke* 18:184–187, 1987.
196. Borzeix MG, Cahn R, Cahn J: Effect of brain gangliosides on early and late consequences of a transient incomplete forebrain ischemia in the rat. *Pharmacology* 38:167–176, 1989.
197. Manev H, Favaron M, Vicini S, Guidotti A: Ganglioside-mediated protection from glutamate-induced neuronal death. *Acta Neurobiol Exp (Warsz)* 50: 475–488, 1990.
198. Magal E, Louis JC, Aguilera J, Yavin E: Gangliosides prevent ischemia-induced down-regulation of protein kinase C in fetal rat brain. *J Neurochem* 55:2126–2131, 1990.
199. Kanemitsu H, Tamura A, Kirino T, Oka H, Sano K, Iwamoto T, Yoshiura M, Iriyama K: Allopurinol inhibits uric acid accumulation in the rat brain following fecal cerebral ischemia. *Brain Res* 499:367–370, 1989.
200. Martz D, Rayos G, Schielke GP, Betz AL: Allopurinol and dimethylthiourea reduce brain infarction following middle cerebral artery occlusion in rats. *Stroke* 20:488–494, 1989.
201. Nishi H, Watanabe T, Sakurai H, Yuki S, Ishibashi A: Effect of MCI-186 on brain edema in rats. *Stroke* 20:1236–1240, 1989.
202. Martz D, Beer M, Betz AL: Dimethylthiourea reduces ischemic brain edema without affecting cerebral blood flow. *J Cereb Blood Flow Metab* 10:352–357, 1990.
203. Oh SM, Betz AL: Interaction between free radicals and excitatory amino acids in the formation of ischemic brain edema in rats. *Stroke* 22:915–921, 1991.
204. Kirsch JR, Helfaer MA, Lange DG, Traystman RJ: Evidence for free radical mechanisms of brain injury resulting from ischemia/reperfusion-induced events. *J Neurotrauma* 9:S157–S163, 1992.
205. Hall ED, Braughler JM, Yonkers PA et al: U-78517F: a potent inhibitor of lipid peroxidation with activity in experimental brain injury and ischemia. *J Pharmacol Exp Ther* 258:688–694, 1991.
206. Gill R, Foster AC, Woodruff GN: Systemic administration of MK-801 protects against ischemia-induced hippocampal neurodegeneration in the gerbil. *J Neurosci* 7:3343–3349, 1987.

207. McDonald JW, Silverstein FS, Johnston MV: MK-801 protects the neonatal brain from hypoxic-ischemic damage. *Eur J Pharmacol* 140:359–361, 1987.
208. Ozyurt KA, Shigeno T, Balarsky A-M, Ford I, McCulloch J, Teasdale GM, Graham DI: Protective effect of glutamate antagonist, MK801, in focal cerebral ischemia in the cat. *J Cereb Blood Flow Metab* 8:138–143, 1988.
209. Park CK, Nehls DG, Graham DI, Teasdale GM, McCullogh J: Focal cerebral isch-aemia in the cat: treatment with the glutamate antagonist MK-801 after induction of ischaemia. *J Cereb Blood Flow Metab* 8:757–762, 1988.
210. Park CK, Nehls DG, Graham DI, Teasdale GM, McCullogh J: The glutamate antago-nist MK-801 reduces focal ischemic damage in the rat. *Ann Neurol* 24:543–551, 1988.
211. Park CK, Nehls DG, Teasdale GM, McCullogh J: Effect of the NMDA antagonist MK-801 on local cerebral blood flow in focal cerebral ischemia in the rat. *J Cereb Blood Flow Metab* 9:617–622, 1989.
212. Ford LM, Sanberg PR, Norman AB, Fogelson MH: MK-801 prevents hippocampal neurodegeneration in neonatal hypoxic-ischemic rats. *Arch Neurol* 46:1090–1096, 1989.
213. McIntosh TK, Vink R, Soares H, Hayes R, Simon R: Effects of the *N*-methyl-*D*-aspartate receptor blocker MK-801 on neurologic function after experimental brain injury. *J Neurotrauma* 6:247–259, 1989.
214. Olney JW, Ikonomidou C, Mosinger JL, Frierdich G: MK-801 prevents hypobaric-ischemic neuronal degeneration in infant rat brain. *J Neurosci* 9:1701–1704, 1989.
215. Shapira Y, Yadid G, Cotev S, Niska A, Shohami E: Protective effect of MK801 in experimental brain injury. *J Neurotrauma* 7:131–139, 1990.
216. Zhang ET, Hansen AJ, Wieloch T, Lauritzen M: Influence of MK-801 on brain extracellular calcium and potassium activities in severe hypoglycemia. *J Cereb Blood Flow Metab* 10:136–139, 1990.
217. Kochhar A, Zivin JA, Mazzarella V: Pharmacologic studies of the neuroprotective actions of a glutamate antagonist in ischemia. *J Neurotrauma* 8:175–186, 1991.
218. Uematsu D, Araki N, Greenberg JH, Sladky J, Reivich M: Combined therapy with MK-801 and nimodipine for protection of ischemic brain damage. *Neurology* 41:88–94, 1991.
219. Steinberg GK, Saleh J, Kunis D: Delayed treatment with dextromethorphan and dextrorphan reduces cerebral damage after transient focal ischemia. *Neurosci Lett* 89:193–197, 1988.
220. George CP, Goldberg MP, Choi DW, Steinberg GK: Dextromethorphan reduces neocortical ischemic neuronal damage in vivo. *Brain Res* 440:375–379, 1988.
221. Prince DA, Feeser HR: Dextromethorphan protects against cerebral infarction in a rat model of hypoxia-ischemia. *Neurosci Lett* 85:291–296, 1988.
222. Nakayama H, Ginsberg MD, Dietrich WD: S-emopamil, a novel calcium channel blocker and serotonin S2 antagonist, markedly reduces infarct size following middle cerebral artery occlusion in the rat. *Neurology* 38:1667–1673, 1988.
223. Lin BW, Dietrich WD, Busto R, Ginsberg MD: (S)-emopamil protects against global ischemic brain injury in rats. *Stroke* 21:1734–1739, 1990.
224. Ginsberg MD, Lin B, Morikawa E, Dietrich WD, Busto R, Globus MY: Calcium antagonists in the treatment of experimental cerebral ischemia. *Arzneimittelforschung* 41:334–337, 1991.
225. Deluga KS, Plotz FB, Betz AL: Effect of indomethacin on edema following single and repetitive cerebral ischemia in the gerbil. *Stroke* 22:1259–1264, 1991.
226. Dempsey RJ, Roy MW, Meyer KL, Donaldson DL: Indomethacin-mediated im-provement following middle cerebral artery occlusion in cats. Effects of anesthesia. *J Neurosurg* 62:874–881, 1985.
227. Dougherty JHJ, Levy DE, Rawlinson DG, Ruff R, Weksler B, Plum F: Experimental cerebral ischemia produced by extracranial vascular injury: protection with indometh-acin and prostaglandin. *Neurology* 32:970–974, 1982.
228. Papadopoulos SM, Black KL, Hoff JT: Cerebral edema induced by arachidonic acid: role of leukocytes and 5-lipoxygenase products. *Neurosurgery* 25:369–372, 1989.
229. Yen MH, Lee SH: Effects of cyclooxygenase and lipoxygenase inhibitors on cerebral edema induced by freezing lesions in rats. *Eur J Pharmacol* 144:369–373, 1987.
230. Miller LP, Hsu C: Therapeutic potential for adenosine receptor activation in ischemic brain injury: *J Neurotrauma* 2:S563–S577, 1992.
231. Chan PH: Antioxidant-dependent amelioration of brain injury: role of CuZn-superox-ide dismutase. *J Neurotrauma* 2:S417–S423, 1992.
232. Grotta J, Spydell J, Pettigrew C, Ostrow P, Hunter D: The effect of nicardipine on neuronal function following ischemia. *Stroke* 17:213–219, 1986.
233. Hadani M, Young W, Flamm ES: Nicardipine reduces calcium accumulation and electrolyte derangements in regional cerebral ischemia in rats. *Stroke* 19:1125–1132, 1988.
234. Steen PA, Newberg LA, Milde JH, Michenfelder JD: Nimodipine improves cerebral blood flow and neurological recovery after complete ischemia in the dog. *J Cereb Blood Flow Metab* 3:38–43, 1983.
235. Steen PA, Newberg LA, Milde JH, Michenfelder JD: Cerebral blood flow and neurologic outcome when nimodipine is given after complete cerebral ischemia in the dog. *J Cereb Blood Flow Metab* 4:82–87, 1984.
236. Steen PA, Gisvold SE, Milde JH, Newberg LA, Scheithauer BW, Lanier WL, Michenfelder JD: Nimodipine improves outcome when given after complete cerebral ischemia in primates. *Anesthesiology* 62:406–414, 1985.
237. Meyer FB, Anderson RE, Yaksh TL, Sundt TM: Effect of nimodipine on intracellular brain pH, cortical blood flow, and EEG in experimental focal cerebral ischemia. *J Neurosurg* 64:617–626, 1986.
238. Fujisawa A, Matsumoto M, Matsuyama T, Ueda H, Wanaka A, Yoneda S, Kimura K, Kamada T: The effect of the calcium antagonist nimodipine on the gerbil model of experimental cerebral ischemia. *Stroke* 17:748–752, 1986.
239. Germano IM, Bartkowski HM, Cassel ME, Pitts LH: The therapeutic value of nimodipine in experimental focal cerebral ischemia: Neurological outcome and histo-pathological findings. *J Neurosurg* 67:81–87, 1987.
240. Kobayashi S, Obana W, Andrews BT, Nishimura MC, Pitts LH: Lack of effect of nimodipine in experimental regional cerebral ischemia. *Stroke* 19:147, 1988.
241. Tally PW, Sundt TMJ, Anderson RE: Improvement of cortical perfusion, intracellular pH, and electrocorticography by nimodipine during transient focal cerebral ischemia. *Neurosurgery* 24:80–87, 1989.
242. Lazarewicz JW, Pluta R, Salinska E, Puka M: Beneficial effect of nimodipine on metabolic and functional disturbances in rabbit hippocampus following complete cerebral ischemia. *Stroke* 20:70–77, 1989.
243. Mossakowski MJ, Gadamski R: Nimodipine prevents delayed neuronal death of sector CA1 pyramidal cells in short-term forebrain ischemia in Mongolian gerbils. *Stroke* 21:120–122, 1990.
244. Scriabine A, Teasdale GM, Tettenborn D, Young W (eds): *Nimodipine: Pharmacologi-cal and Clinical Results in Cerebral Ischemia*. Springer Verlag, Berlin, 1991.

CHAPTER 52

Lipid Mediators in Critical Care Medicine

MITCHELL P. FINK, M.D.

INTRODUCTION

A variety of lipid autocoids, including the prostaglandins, platelet activating factor, and other related compounds, are of considerable importance in critical care medicine. These mediators participate in the normal physiology of virtually every organ system and have been implicated as playing important roles in the pathophysiology of many life-threatening acute illnesses. In addition, several of these naturally occurring compounds (or synthetic derivatives of them) show considerable promise as therapeutic agents for treating or preventing problems encountered in critical care medicine, such as pulmonary hypertension, erosive gastritis, and the adult respiratory distress syndrome (ARDS).

Pharmacologic manipulation of the prostaglandin system is already a standard component of neonatal intensive care medicine, in which, depending upon the clinical situation, indomethacin is used to achieve pharmacologic closure of the ductus arteriosus or PGE_1 is used to maintain patency of this structure. Pediatric issues are not addressed in detail here, and the interested reader is referred to Chapters 7 and 64. Prostaglandin synthesis inhibitors also are used to control fever and pain. The reader is referred to Chapter 38 for a discussion of the use of prostaglandin synthesis inhibitors to provide analgesia. Pharmacotherapy directed at lipid autocoids may prove to be useful in the management of central nervous system disorders or asthma, but the clinical application of this approach is in its infancy and is not discussed here. This chapter provides an introduction to the biochemistry

and pharmacology of the lipid mediators and focuses on the manipulation of the lipid mediator system in the management of syndromes characterized by uncontrolled systemic inflammation, such as sepsis and ARDS.

BIOCHEMISTRY AND NOMENCLATURE

EICOSANOIDS

The term **eicosanoids** refers to a group of biologically active compounds that result from the partial oxygenation of arachidonic acid, a 20-carbon (hence, the root *eicosa*) polyunsaturated fatty acid (PUFA). By convention, the closely related oxygenation products of other fatty acids, notably eicosapentaenoic acid (EPA) and docosahexaenoic acid (DHA), also are considered "eicosanoids." Members of the eicosanoid family include the prostaglandins (PGs), thromboxanes (TXs), leukotrienes (LTs), lipoxins, hydroxy-eicosatetraenoic acids (HETEs), and epoxides.

Mammals are unable to synthesize fatty acids with double bonds distal to the ninth carbon atom (i.e., more than nine carbons away from the carboxylic acid terminus of the molecule's backbone). Therefore, long-chain PUFAs, such as linoleic acid, which is found in corn and safflower oil, are essential components of the diet. According to the standard nomenclature used by lipid biochemists, linoleic acid is a C18:2ω-6 PUFA, meaning that the molecule has an 18-carbon backbone with two double bonds, the more distal of which is located six carbons from the ω (noncarboxylated) end of the chain. In the body, linoleic acid is elongated and further unsaturated to form arachidonic acid (C20:4ω-6).

In contrast to ω-6 PUFAs like linoleic and arachidonic acids, linolenic acid (C18:3ω-3), which is another essential PUFA, is of the ω-3 type. Although linolenic acid is found in some plant oils (e.g., soybean oil), the main dietary sources of ω-3 PUFAs are the oils of marine animals, such as the mackerel, tuna, and menhaden. Both EPA and DHA are ω-3 PUFAs.

Arachidonic acid is a normal constituent of the phospholipids in cell membranes. The rate-limiting step in the synthesis of the eicosanoids is the liberation (by hydrolysis of an ester linkage) of arachidonate from phospholipids, a reaction that is catalyzed by either phospholipase A_2 or phospholipase C. Once free arachidonic acid is generated, it can be acted upon by other enzymes, leading to the formation of biologically active products.

There are two main pathways of arachidonate metabolism (Fig. 52.1). In the first, cyclooxygenase catalyzes the addition of oxygen to arachidonic acid to form an unstable cyclic endoperoxide (PGG_2). This compound is then acted upon by a hydroperoxidase to form PGH_2, which, in turn, can be metabolized into several different products, notably PGD_2, PGE_2, PGF_{2a}, PGI_2 (i.e., prostacyclin), and TXA_2. Different cell types tend to be highly selective in their metabolism of PGH_2. For example, endothelial cells preferentially metabolize the cyclic endoperoxide to prostacyclin, whereas platelets preferentially convert PGH_2 into TXA_2.

The first step in the other main pathway for the metabolism of arachidonic acid is catalyzed by the enzyme 5-lipoxygenase. This enzyme converts arachidonate to 5S-hydroperoxy-6,8-*trans*-11,14-*cis*-eicosatetraenoic acid (5-HPETE). The same enzyme also catalyzes the metabolism of 5-HPETE to LTA_4, which then can be further converted to LTB_4 by an epoxide hydrolase or, in a reaction catalyzed by glutathione-S-transferase, conjugated with reduced glutathione to form LTC_4. Sequential reactions catalyzed by γ-glutamyl transpeptidases and dipeptidases convert LTC_4 into LTD_4 and LTE_4. These latter three compounds have been identified as the "slow-reacting substance of anaphylaxis" (1) and, because of their chemical structures, are referred to as cysteinyl LTs or sulfidopeptide LTs.

In addition to the cyclooxygenase and 5-lipoxygenase pathways, other pathways of arachidonate metabolism have been identified. Among these are the reactions initiated by the enzymes 12-lipoxygenase and 15-lipoxygenase. The 5- and 15-lipoxygenase pathways are predominant in neutrophils and mononuclear cells, whereas the 12-lipoxygenase pathway is more important in platelets (2). The lipoxins (A and B) are products of the 5- and 15-lipoxygenase pathways, via the intermediate 5(S)hydroperoxy-15(S)-hydroxytetraenoic acid (2).

The cyclooxygenase-derived metabolites of arachidonic acid are referred to as bisenoic prostanoids, which means that their chemical structure is characterized by the presence of two double bonds. This structure is denoted by the subscript 2 in their names (e.g., PGE_2). Related compounds derived

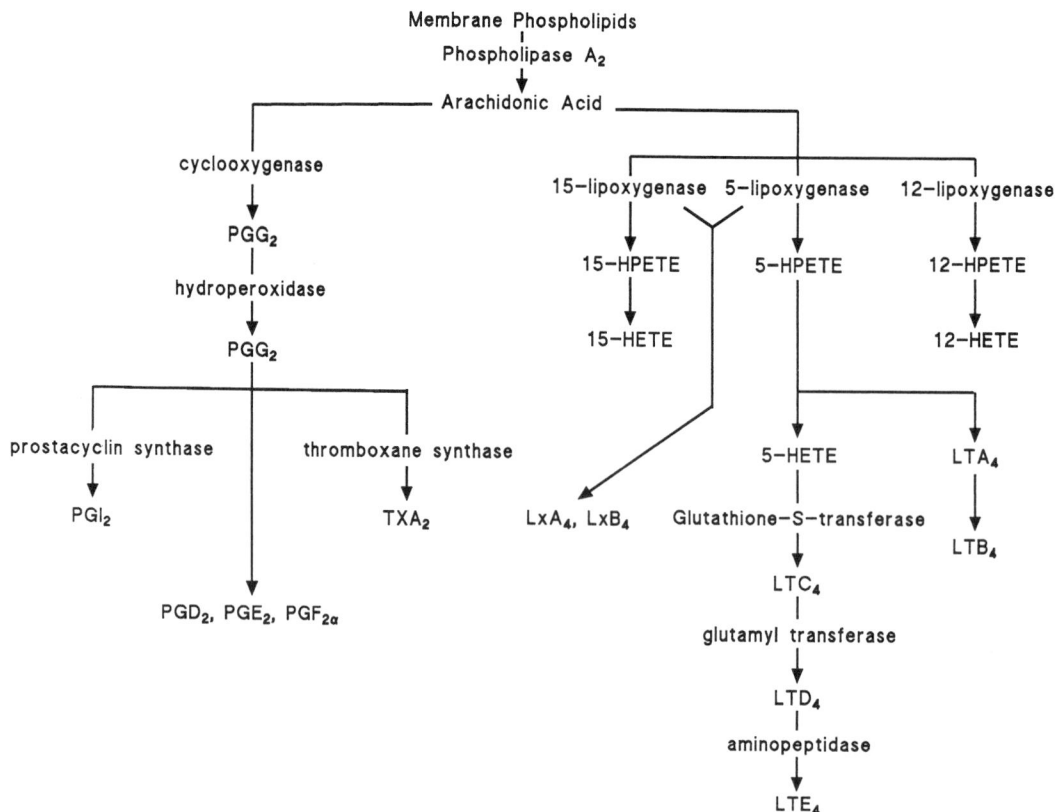

Figure 52.1. Pathways of arachidonate metabolism. Abbreviations: PG=prostaglandin; TX=thromboxane; HPETE=hydroperoxyeicosatetraenoic acid; HETE=hydroxyeicosatetraenoic acid; LT=leukotriene; Lx=lipoxin.

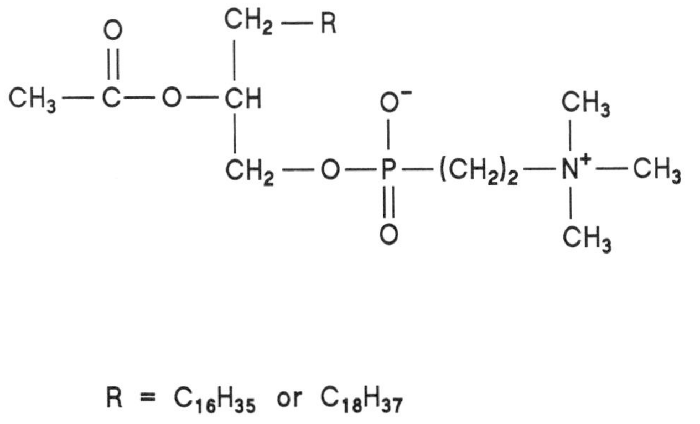

$$R = C_{16}H_{35} \text{ or } C_{18}H_{37}$$

Figure 52.2. Strucure of platelet activating factor.

Table 52.1. Key Biologic Effects of Lipid Mediators

Mediator(s)	Actions
PGE_1, PGE_2	Vasodilation, inhibition of neutrophil function, inhibition of T-cell activation, gastric mucosal cytoprotection
PGI_2	Vasodilation, inhibition of platelet aggregation
TXA_2	Vasoconstriction, platelet aggregation
LTB_4	Neutrophil activation and chemotaxis, enhanced activation and differentiation of B lymphocytes, stimulation of IL-2 and γ-interferon production
LTC_4, LTD_4, LTE_4	Bronchoconstriction, increased microvascular permeability, vasoconstriction
PAF	Increased microvascular permeability, activation of neutrophils, bronchoconstriction, coronary vasoconstriction

from dihomo-γ-linolenic acid are referred to as monoenoic prostanoids and are denoted by the subscript 1 (e.g., PGE_1). The trienoic prostanoids (e.g., TXA_3) are cyclooxygenase-derived products of EPA. Metabolites of EPA derived via the 5-lipoxygenase pathway are denoted by a subscript 5 (e.g., LTB_5). The 1-series and 3-series prostanoids and the 5-series LTs are assuming increasing importance in clinical medicine. A monoenoic prostanoid, PGE_1, is being used as a therapeutic agent. The cyclooxygenation and 5-lipoxygenation products of ω-3 fatty acids are much less active as biological mediators than are the corresponding derivatives of arachidonic acid. Therefore, maneuvers that increase the ratio of ω-3 to ω-6 PUFAs in the diet are being investigated as a means for modifying disease processes in which eicosanoids are believed to be important mediators.

PLATELET ACTIVATING FACTOR

In addition to the eicosanoids, there is another biologically active lipid that assumes great importance as an inflammatory mediator. This compound is called platelet activating factor (PAF). Chemically, PAF is 1-O-alkyl-2(R)-acetyl-glycero-3-phosphorylcholine (Figure 52.2). The ether-linked alkyl group in the 1 position is either a C16 or C18 straight-chain aliphatic residue.

Like the eicosanoids, PAF is not stored by cells in its active form, but rather as a precursor molecule, namely 1-O-alkyl-2-acyl-glycero-3-phosphorylcholine (alkyl-acyl-GPC). The acyl group in this molecule is often arachidonate. In a reaction catalyzed by phospholipase A_2, the acyl group in the 2 position of alkyl-acyl-GPC is cleaved, yielding the precursor of PAF, which is called lyso-PAF. The rate-limiting step in the formation of PAF is the acetylation of lyso-PAF, a reaction catalyzed by an acetyltransferase. Lyso-PAF, which is biologically inactive, is also the principal metabolite of PAF.

BIOLOGIC ACTIVITIES OF LIPID MEDIATORS

The main biologic effects of the most important lipid mediators are summarized in Table 52.1. This tabulation is necessarily an oversimplification, and more detailed information is presented below.

THE PROSTANOIDS

TXA_2, the principal cyclooxygenase product synthesized by platelets, is a potent inducer of platelet aggregation. TXA_2 also stimulates contraction of bronchial and vascular smooth muscle (3, 4). In addition to platelets, both endothelial cells (5) and neutrophils (6) reportedly are capable of releasing TXA_2. By way of an incompletely defined mechanism that also involves LTB_4, the release of TXA_2 appears to play an important role in the attachment of neutrophils to the endothelium and their subsequent diapedesis in response to inflammatory stimuli (7). After being released, TXA_2 is rapidly hydrolyzed to an inactive metabolite (TXB_2). Because of its short in vivo half-life (~30 sec), TXA_2 functions as a locally acting mediator, rather than as a circulating hormone.

Prostacyclin (PGI_2), which is the main prostanoid produced by vascular endothelium, causes biologic effects that generally are the opposite of those produced by TXA_2. By activating adenylate cyclase and increasing intracellular concentrations of cyclic adenosine monophosphate, PGI_2 functions as a potent inhibitor of platelet aggregation (8). Prostacyclin also is a potent relaxant of vascular smooth muscle, inducing large- and small-vessel arteriolar vasodilation in the cerebral, mesenteric, renal, and pulmonary circulations (9). The vasodilation induced by prostacyclin is an endothelium-independent phenomenon (10).

Prostacyclin and PGs of the E series manifest both proinflammatory and antiinflammatory properties. The idea that E series PGs are proinflammatory mediators was first proposed by Vane, who discovered that aspirin and other nonsteroidal antiinflammatory drugs (NSAIDs) inhibit PG biosynthesis and proposed that this was their mechanism of action (11). Subsequent studies confirmed the presence of E series PGs (and other eicosanoids) in inflammatory exudates (12).

When present at the local site of inflammation, the vasodilating PGs (i.e., PGE_1, PGE_2, and prostacyclin) tend to act as proinflammatory "modulators" rather than as true inflammatory mediators, since, by themselves, these compounds are not capable of causing extravasation of plasma (13, 14). PGEs (or prostacyclin), however, can potentiate the pain- and edema-promoting effects of other inflammatory mediators, such as histamine and bradykinin (15–18). The proinflammatory effects of the PGEs or prostacyclin result from their vasodilating properties. Arteriolar dilation increases blood flow, which promotes edema formation by augmenting the delivery of inflammatory cells, elevating venular hydrostatic pressure and increasing microvascular surface area (18).

Although PGs of the E series and prostacyclin can potentiate local inflammation caused by other mediators, it is increasingly apparent that the predominant effect of these compounds is to down-regulate a variety of inflammatory and immunologic responses. Thus, in vitro, PGE_2 decreases T-cell activation by inhibiting the production of the regulatory cytokine IL-2 (19). PGE_2 also inhibits the generation and proliferation of immunoglobulin-secreting cells by B cells (20, 21). Both the E series PGs and prostacyclin are potent inhibitors of a variety of neutrophil functions, including enzyme release, chemotaxis, membrane depolarization, and oxygen radical production (22–24). In the murine system, PGE_2 down-regulates Ia antigens on antigen-presenting cells (25).

Proinflammatory cytokines, including interleukin-1 and tumor necrosis factor α, trigger the release of PGs, leukotrienes, and PAF from various cell types, both in vivo and in vitro (26–34). Indeed, release of PGs, particularly PGE_2, in the anterior hypothalamus is responsible for the pyrogenic effect of interleukin-1 (35, 36), and inhibition of this phenomenon accounts for the antipyretic action of aspirin and related drugs. Recent findings, however, indicate the existence of an important negative feedback loop, whereby PGEs inhibit the release of proinflammatory cytokines from mononuclear cells (37–41). Interruption of this negative feedback loop with NSAIDs has been shown to increase cytokine release (39, 42–44). Since high circulating cytokine levels have been associated with adverse outcomes in sepsis (45–47), the tendency of NSAIDs to increase plasma concentrations of tumor necrosis factor α and interleukin-6 suggests that inhibitors of PG biosynthesis may have deleterious effects in septic patients. The role of NSAIDs in sepsis is discussed in greater detail below.

Most of the inhibitory effects of PGEs and prostacyclin on immune and inflammatory functions appear to result from activation of adenylate cyclase, leading to increased intracellular concentrations of adenosine 3′:5′-cyclic phosphate (cAMP) (48, 49). Another important mechanism, however, may be PGE-mediated inhibition of the release of another eicosanoid, LTB_4, since the latter lipid mediator tends to up-regulate many inflammatory and immunologic responses (50).

THE LEUKOTRIENES

Mononuclear cells and neutrophils are the main sources of LTB_4, although certain other cell types, such as tracheal mucosal cells (51), are capable of synthesizing this eicosanoid. LTB_4 is a potent chemokinetic and chemotactic agent for polymorphonuclear leukocytes (PMNLs) (52). Exposure of PMNLs to LTB_4 leads to aggregation, release of lysosomal enzymes, and production of reactive oxygen metabolites (52–55). LTB_4 also promotes the attachment of PMNLs to vascular endothelium, an action that apparently results from an effect of the eicosanoid on endothelial cells rather than neutrophils (56–60). Numerous other aspects of the immune response tend to be up-regulated by LTB_4. For example, LTB_4 has been shown to enhance the activation, proliferation, and differentiation of B-cells (61), the production of IL-2 by T-cells

(62), and the synthesis of interleukin-1 by mononuclear cells (63). In addition to its immunologic and proinflammatory actions, LTB_4 also increases pulmonary arterial pressure, an effect that apparently occurs independent of any action on neutrophils (64, 65).

Eosinophils and monocytes are major sources of the cysteinyl leukotrienes (LTC_4, LTD_4, and LTE_4) (66–68). Although endothelial cells do not contain 5-lipoxygenase, they are able to synthesize LTC_4 by means of a process known as transcellular metabolism (1). In this process, LTA_4 is generated and exported by neutrophils and subsequently converted into LTC_4 in adjacent endothelial cells. This represents a potential mechanism for the amplification of the inflammatory response. LTC_4, LTD_4, and LTE_4 increase microvascular permeability (69–70) and cause arteriolar constriction in a variety of vascular beds (71–75). The cysteinyl LTs also affect myocardial contractility. At very low doses, a positive inotropic effect can be demonstrated (76). At higher doses, the cysteinyl LTs decrease contractility, a phenomenon that is caused by both coronary vasoconstriction and a direct negative ionotropic effect of the eicosanoids on the myocardium (74, 76, 77). LT-mediated decrements in myocardial contractility may play a role in some forms of shock (e.g., systemic anaphylaxis). Perhaps the most important biologic action of the cysteinyl LTs is contraction of bronchial smooth muscle. When administered to human volunteers by nebulization, LTC_4 and LTD_4 are more than 1000 times as potent as histamine in inducing bronchoconstriction (1).

PLATELET ACTIVATING FACTOR

PAF is released by numerous cell types, including platelets, monocytes, macrophages, PMNLs, and endothelial cells (78). PAF is a classic proinflammatory mediator and has been shown to induce enhanced PMNL-endothelial adhesion, increased microvascular permeability, and arteriolar constriction (79–82). When injected into experimental animals, PAF causes hypotension, diminished cardiac output, increased microvascular permeability, and bronchoconstriction (78). PAF is capable of exerting direct effects on certain cell types, such as platelets (83), endothelial cells (84), and myocardial cells (85). Nevertheless, many PAF-induced phenomena (e.g., bronchoconstriction or coronary vasoconstriction) seem to be caused by the release of secondary mediators, including TXA_2, LTB_4, and the cysteinyl LTs (86–92).

NONSTEROIDAL ANTIINFLAMMATORY DRUGS (NSAIDS)

The actions of lipid mediators can be pharmacologically down-regulated in four main ways. First, drugs can be used to inhibit key synthetic enzymes, such as phospholipase A_2, cyclooxygenase, thromboxane synthase, or 5-lipoxygenase. Second, drugs can be used to block the specific membrane receptors responsible for the actions of the lipid mediators. Third, dietary maneuvers, such as substituting ω-3 for ω-6 PUFAs in the diet, can be used to deplete cells of the substrate (arachidonic acid) necessary for the generation of biologically active eicosanoids. Fourth, drugs can be used to stimulate the production of naturally occurring inhibitors of a key enzyme in the

Table 52.2. Nonsteroidal Antiinflammatory Drugs

Class	Examples
Acetylated carboxylic acid	Aspirin
Nonacetylated carboxylic acids	Choline salicylate, sodium salicylate
Acetic acid derivatives	Indomethacin, tolmetin, sulindac
Propionic acids	Ibuprofen, naproxen, fenoprofen
Feramic acids	Meclofenamate
Enolic acids	Phenylbutazone, piroxicam
Nonacid compounds	Nabumetone

biosynthetic pathway for the eicosanoids. This action appears to be a mechanism of action responsible for the down-regulation of eicosanoid biosynthesis caused by the administration of pharmacologic doses of glucocorticoids. Antiinflammatory steroids have been shown to induce the production of proteins, which inhibit the activity of phospholipase A_2 (93, 94).

Glucocorticoids are discussed separately in Chapter 43. Dietary maneuvers are discussed in Chapters 60 and 61. A variety of drugs that interfere with the biosynthesis or action of lipid mediators, although undergoing extensive preclinical (in some cases, clinical) evaluation, remain experimental. Drugs in this category include TX synthase inhibitors, phospholipase A_2 inhibitors, 5-lipoxygenase inhibitors, so-called dual (i.e., lipoxygenase plus cyclooxygenase) inhibitors, TX receptor antagonists, and PAF receptor antagonists. Some of the data obtained with these studies are discussed in later sections of this chapter. At present, the agents that are being used clinically and hence warrant special attention here are the aspirin-like drugs, or NSAIDs.

As noted previously, the predominant mechanism of action of the NSAIDs appears to be inhibition of the cyclooxygenase enzyme complex and the production of PGs and TXA_2. This notion is supported by studies showing that the rank order of potency of NSAIDs as antiinflammatory agents in vivo correlates with their potency as inhibitors of PG synthesis (95). Numerous classes of drugs (Table 52.2), with differing biochemical mechanisms of action, have clinically useful activity as inhibitors of the cyclooxygenase enzyme complex.

Aspirin, or acetylsalicylic acid, is the prototypical NSAID. In platelets, this agent inhibits cyclooxygenase by acetylating the enzyme (96). Since platelets are incapable of synthesizing new protein, aspirin-induced blockade of TXA_2 biosynthesis persists for the lifetime of the cell. In other tissues, notably vascular endothelium, the recovery of prostanoid biosynthesis after exposure to aspirin is more rapid (97). When aspirin is administed in low doses (<100 mg), the production of TXA_2 is inhibited much more than is the synthesis of prostacyclin (98). Therefore, in low doses aspirin provides a measure of selectivity that fosters its antithrombotic actions. Although the mechanism underlying this selectivity has not been established with certainty, it may result from the fact that after oral administration, aspirin undergoes substantial hydrolysis to salicylic acid. This latter compound is much less potent than the parent compound as an inhibitor of cyclooxygenase. Low doses of aspirin may lead to "presystemic" irreversible blockade of cyclooxygenase in platelets traversing capillaries in the stomach and gut prior to the hydrolysis of the drug to its much less active metabolite (99). Recently, the use of a "controlled-release" preparation of aspirin that releases 10

mg/hr of the drug was shown to inhibit TX synthesis markedly without affecting production of prostacyclin (100).

In addition to aspirin, indomethacin and ibuprofen are among the NSAIDs receiving the most attention as agents with applications or potential applications in critical care medicine. Indomethacin is a substituted acetic acid derivative. The intravenous form of the drug has been approved by the Food and Drug Administration for use as an agent for pharmacologically closing a persistently patent ductus arteriosis (PDA) in premature infants (see Chapter 64). Intravenous indomethacin also has been used experimentally to inhibit PGE-mediated immunosuppression in elective surgical and trauma patients (101, 102). Ibuprofen is currently undergoing evaluation in humans for the adjuvant therapy of septic shock and ARDS. Although indomethacin and ibuprofen are inhibitors of cyclooxygenase, these agents also have other pharmacologic actions that may be important under some circumstances. Indomethacin inhibits phospholipase A_2, various lipoxygenases, and superoxide production by neutrophils (93, 103–105). Ibuprofen has been shown to scavenge hydroxyl radicals and chelate iron (106, 107), effects that would tend to limit oxidant-mediated damage to tissues and might help to explain the beneficial effects of this drug observed in many models of septic shock and acute lung injury (see below).

The NSAIDs are among the most widely used drugs. Although these agents are relatively safe, side effects are common (108). The most common serious reactions are peptic ulceration and renal dysfunction. Other serious, but rare, side effects include blood dyscrasias, hepatic dysfunction, and allergic skin reactions.

It is not surprising that peptic ulceration is a potentially serious side effect of pharmacologically inhibiting cyclooxygenase, since PGs are known to play a key role in protecting the gastrointestinal (GI) mucosa against damage caused by a number of noxious agents (109). Although serious GI complications are clearly a concern when NSAIDs are used to manage outpatients with rheumatic diseases (110), an increased incidence of erosive gastritis or peptic ulceration has not been noted in the few reported studies using parenteral NSAIDs in critically ill adults (111, 112).

Perhaps the greatest concern regarding the use of NSAIDs in critically ill patients is the potential for adverse effects on renal function. PGs play an important role in maintaining renal perfusion and glomerular filtration, particularly when arterial perfusion pressure and/or cardiac output are diminished (113). Renal production of PGs also affects tubular functions (114). Although NSAIDs have little or no effect on glomerular filtration rate or urine flow in normal volunteers, numerous clinical studies and case reports amply document that inhibition of PG biosynthesis can lead to marked decrements in renal function in patients with conditions associated with low "effective arterial volume" (e.g., ascites, congestive heart failure, or intravascular volume depletion secondary to diuretic therapy) (113, 115). In animal models of syndromes in which NSAIDs might be used in critically ill patients, such as hyperdynamic sepsis and endotoxic shock (116–119), inhibition of PG synthesis has been shown to diminish renal perfusion and glomerular filtration rate (GFR). Some studies have suggested that one NSAID, sulindac, has "renal-sparing" properties (120–122), but subsequent reports have discounted this notion (115, 123, 124).

Experience regarding the renal effects of parenteral NSAIDs in the critical care setting is limited. Although reversible decrements in GFR have been reported in neonates treated with indomethacin to achieve closure of PDAs (125), this problem has not been noted in the trials of ibuprofen or indomethacin for the treatment of sepsis in adults (111, 112). In addition to causing reversible decrements in GFR on a hemodynamic basis, NSAIDs also have been associated with other renal complications, including papillary necrosis, nephrotic syndrome, and interstitial nephritis (113, 115). These complications typically occur after prolonged administration and would not be expected to present a major problem when NSAIDs are used for short durations in patients with acute, critical illnesses.

ROLE OF LIPID MEDIATORS IN SEPSIS, SEPTIC SHOCK, AND THE ADULT RESPIRATORY DISTRESS SYNDROME (ARDS)

In 1962, Northover and Subramanian reported that aspirin prevents hypotension in dogs challenged with lipopolysaccharide (LPS; endotoxin) (126). Since that initial report, overwhelming evidence has accumulated indicating that the eicosanoids and PAF play key roles in the pathophysiology of shock states induced by injecting experimental animals with LPS or live bacteria. Lipid mediators also have been shown to be important mediators in many experimental models of acute lung injury. At present, it is less clear that lipid mediators play an important role in human sepsis and septic shock, although the best available data are certainly consistent with this notion.

Consistent with Koch's postulates, the evidence implicating the eicosanoids and PAF in sepsis and/or ARDS belongs to three general categories: (*a*) data showing that the mediator is released in animals or humans with the condition; (*b*) data showing that infusing animals with the mediator leads to pathophysiologic changes (e.g., pulmonary edema) similar to those observed in sepsis or ARDS; and (*c*) data showing that blocking the release or action of the mediator ameliorates one or more features of sepsis or ARDS.

PROSTANOIDS

Elevated levels of PGE_2, 6-keto-$PGF_1\alpha$ (stable hydrolysis product of prostacyclin), $PGF_2\alpha$, and TXB_2 (stable hydrolysis product of TXA_2) have been detected in plasma, pulmonary lymph, and bronchoalveolar lavage fluid in a wide range of animal models of sepsis or endotoxicosis (127). Cyclo-oxygenase-derived metabolites of arachidonic acid are also released in many models of ARDS caused by agents other than endotoxin or live bacteria (128–130). Elevated circulating levels of some of these prostanoids also have been detected in septic patients, particularly those with shock or a lethal outcome (131–135). Data reported by Bernard et al (111) are particularly compelling in this regard, since these authors used gas chromatography and mass spectrometry to measure urinary concentrations of 2,3-dinor-TXB_2 (TXA_2 metabolite) and 2,3-dinor-6-keto-PGF_1 (prostacyclin metabolite) in septic

patients. The use of urinary levels of 2,3-dinor-TXB_2 and 2,3-dinor-6-keto-PGF_1 as markers of systemic production of TXA_2 and prostacyclin, respectively, avoids artifacts introduced by the ex vivo synthesis of these prostanoids. In this study, using previously reported values from healthy subjects as historical controls, urinary concentrations of 2,3-dinor-TXB_2 and 2,3-dinor-6-keto-PGF_1 were elevated approximately 15-fold and 20-fold above normal, respectively, in septic patients. Moreover, urinary levels of 2,3-dinor-TXB_2 correlated with peak airway pressure ($r = 0.43$, P <0.05), a finding that is consistent with data obtained in animal models of sepsis-induced ARDS indicating that TXA_2 is an important mediator of diminished pulmonary compliance in this syndrome (136, 137). In addition, elevated plasma levels of TXB_2 also have been observed in patients with ARDS secondary to multiple trauma or acute pancreatitis (138), suggesting that TXA_2 may be an important mediator of acute lung injury associated with a variety of predisposing conditions. The mechanisms responsible for prostanoid release in sepsis have not been completely elucidated, but complement-dependent (139) and cytokine-dependent (140, 141) mechanisms have been implicated. Endotoxin also can directly stimulate the release of eicosanoids from numerous cell types (127).

Pharmacologic inhibition of PG biosynthesis is beneficial in experimental sepsis or ARDS (including ARDS resulting from noxious stimuli other than LPS or bacteria). In animal models of these conditions, treatment with cyclooxygenase inhibitors has been shown to improve survival, arterial blood pressure, and visceral perfusion and to ameliorate pulmonary hypertension, pulmonary edema, pulmonary transvascular protein sieving, arterial hypoxemia, tissue lipid peroxidation, and bronchoconstriction (128–130, 136, 137, 142–150). Some studies suggest that certain cyclooxygenase inhibitors, particularly ibuprofen, may be more active in protecting against acute lung injury than are other chemically dissimilar NSAIDs (e.g., indomethacin or meclofenamate) (149–151). This observation suggests that some of the protection afforded by ibuprofen may be related to antiinflammatory properties, such as iron chelation or radical scavenging that are unrelated to cyclooxygenase inhibition (see above). Salutary effects on hemodynamics or survival are also observed in some animal models of sepsis when synthesis of biologically active eicosanoids is diminished by dietary maneuvers, such as inducing a state of essential PUFA deficiency or substituting ω-3 for ω-6 PUFAs (152–154).

In experimental models of endotoxicosis or ARDS, TXA_2 seems to be a particularly important mediator. Important beneficial effects, including improved survival, can be demonstrated when the generation or action of TXA_2 is blocked using specific inhibitors of TX synthase or antagonists of the TXA_2 receptor (147, 155, 156). In experimental models of ARDS, the early phase of pulmonary hypertension is mediated primarily by TXA_2, although other mediators seem to be responsible for the more delayed and persistent phase of increased pulmonary vascular resistance (136, 157–159). The role of TXA_2 as a mediator of increased pulmonary microvascular permeability remains controversial (136, 160–162).

At present, data are quite limited regarding the effects of inhibiting PG or TXA_2 biosynthesis in humans with sepsis or ARDS. Disappointing results were obtained in two separate small-scale trials of adjuvant therapy with a TX synthase inhibitor (163, 164). Based upon the results of two limited randomized prospective trials, the administration of ibuprofen to patients with sepsis appears to be safe. Ibuprofen clearly reduces fever and tachycardia and may have beneficial effects on pulmonary compliance and the reversal of shock (111, 112). A large-scale clinical study of ibuprofen for the adjuvant therapy of sepsis is currently in progress.

LEUKOTRIENES

In 1984, Matthay et al reported that LTD_4 concentrations were significantly higher in bronchoalveolar lavage fluid from patients with ARDS than in fluid from those with cardiogenic pulmonary edema (165). Subsequently, other investigators have confirmed that sulfidopeptide LT concentrations are elevated in bronchoalveolar lavage fluid or urine samples from patients with ARDS or those at high risk for developing ARDS (166–169). Recent data suggest that increased levels of sulfidopeptide LTs in bronchoalveolar lavage samples may reflect damage to the tracheobronchial epithelium rather than ARDS per se, since $LTC_4/D_4/E_4$ concentrations are also elevated in tracheal aspirates from patients with inhalation or aspiration injuries but without ARDS (170). LTB_4 production by neutrophils is increased in ARDS patients, and the increase in production of this eicosanoid seems to precede the development of acute lung injury (171, 172). LTB_4 or its ω-oxidized metabolites have been detected in elevated quantities in bronchoalveolar lavage samples from patients with ARDS (167, 168, 173). Increased production of LTs has been documented in numerous experimental models of endotoxicosis and/or ARDS (174–180).

In experimental animals or isolated perfused lung preparations, infusions of authentic sulfidopeptide LTs cause pulmonary hypertension and an increase in lymph flow or extravascular lung water accumulation (181–183). Some results suggest that this phenomenon may be due more to an increase in pulmonary microvascular pressure than to a change in microvascular permeability (184), although other results indicate that sulfidopeptide LTs are capable of increasing the leakiness of pulmonary capillaries (185, 186). Infusions of LTB_4 also induce pulmonary hypertension and microvascular sieving in experimental animals, apparently via a PMNL-independent mechanism (64, 65, 186).

Many studies have documented beneficial effects following inhibition of LT biosynthesis or selective blockade of LT receptors in animal models of septic shock or ARDS. In endotoxic rats, pretreatment with 5-lipoxygenase inhibitors or sulfidopeptide LT receptor antagonists has been shown to improve survival, ameliorate hypotension, improve regional blood flow, and prevent hemoconcentration and extravasation of plasma proteins (187–191). In one study using an ovine model of LPS-induced acute lung injury, pre- and posttreatment with LY171883, a selective LTD_4 receptor antagonist, attenuated the pulmonary hypertensive response to endotoxin and prevented increased airway resistance (192). In this model, neither LPS-induced hypoxemia nor increased pulmonary capillary permeability was affected by treatment with LY171883. In another study using the ovine endotoxicosis paradigm, a selective 5-lipoxygenase inhibitor, L-651,392, was shown to ameliorate

LPS-induced pulmonary hypertension, hypoxemia, diminished dynamic compliance, and capillary hyperpermeability (193). In a canine endotoxicosis model, pre- and posttreatment with LY171883 (LTD_4 receptor antagonist) were shown to improve systemic and renal hemodynamics (194). Olson and colleagues have reported that, in pigs, pharmacologic inhibition of LTD_4 receptors has little effect on physiologic responses to endotoxin (195), whereas the present author has found that LTD_4 receptor blockade prevents pulmonary edema and transiently ameliorates pulmonary hypertension and mesenteric hypoperfusion (196). The author's results are supported by recent findings obtained in a rat model of ARDS induced by aerosolized endotoxin, which indicate that blockade of LTD_4 receptors improves survival and ameliorates pulmonary edema (197).

Because specific LTB_4 receptor antagonists have not been available until quite recently, relatively little is known regarding the importance of this particular 5-lipoxygenase product in experimental models of sepsis or ARDS. Nevertheless, Li and colleagues now have reported that treatment with LY255283, an LTB_4 receptor antagonist, prevents some of the hematologic sequelae of endotoxin administration in rats (198). Furthermore, Hechtman and colleagues have accumulated a large body of circumstantial evidence that implicates LTB_4 as a pivotal mediator of pulmonary hyperpermeability induced by the infusion of cytokines or caused by lower extremity ischemia-reperfusion (199-203). Observations from the author's laboratory similarly indicate that LTB_4 is a key mediator of endotoxin-induced lung injury in pigs (204).

PLATELET ACTIVATING FACTOR

For several reasons, PAF is difficult to assay in complex biological fluids, such as plasma, blood, or urine. First, PAF is metabolized in a time-dependent fashion by acetylhydrolases, present in plasma and tissues, to a biologically inactive metabolite, lyso-PAF (205, 206). Second, bioassays for the detection of PAF can be confounded by the presence of naturally occuring lipids, which co-extract with and inhibit the biologic actions of PAF (207, 208). Third, PAF binds to circulating lipoproteins, and detectable levels of this bound PAF are found even in normal individuals (209). Despite these methodologic problems, convincing evidence has been obtained that pathologic quantities of PAF are released in sepsis and other shock states. Thus, Diez and colleagues showed that the number of unoccupied receptors for PAF was diminished on platelets obtained from septic patients as compared with nonseptic patients or normal volunteers (210). Moreover, these investigators were able to extract significant quantities of PAF from platelets obtained from septic donors, whereas this mediator could not be isolated from platelets of patients without sepsis or platelets from normal volunteers. Recently, Pittman and colleagues have obtained indirect evidence that pathologic levels of PAF are present in the circulation of burn patients (211). Rather than assaying PAF directly, these authors showed that serum samples from burn victims (but not controls) primed neutrophils to undergo an exaggerated oxidative burst when stimulated by another agonist, and further showed that this priming effect was largely blocked by a specific PAF receptor antagonist.

In addition to these data from human studies, elevated PAF levels have been detected in animal models of shock, ischemia, or trauma. In these studies, various bioassays, such as PAF-induced platelet aggregation or serotonin release, have been utilized to document increased circulating and/or tissue concentrations of PAF in rats subjected to endotoxin infusion (212-214), hypoxia (206), Noble-Collip drum trauma (215), and tumor necrosis factor infusion (216). Recently, circulating PAF also has been detected in a large-animal model of acute endotoxicosis (217).

Infusing animals or isolated organ preparations with PAF elicits a variety of pathologic effects, which are similar to those observed in septic shock or endotoxin-induced organ injury. In intact animals, the biologic effects of PAF infusions include: systemic arterial hypotension, pulmonary arterial hypertension, increased pulmonary and gastrointestinal microvascular permeability, diminished pulmonary dynamic compliance, arterial hypoxemia, hyperglycemia, hyperlactatemia, and increased glucose turnover (90, 218-221).

In an isolated, blood-perfused small intestine preparation, infusion of PAF leads to increased microvascular permeability, an effect that depends upon PAF-induced adherence of neutrophils to the endothelium and production of reactive oxygen metabolites (222). In isolated lung preparations perfused with a cell-free buffer, infusion of PAF leads to pulmonary hypertension, but the effects of the mediator on capillary permeability are minimal (184, 223). However, in this preparation, if the lung is primed by prior exposure to bacterial LPS, subsequent infusion of PAF leads to a marked increase in alveolar capillary permeability (223).

This synergy between PAF and other mediators, such as endotoxin and tumor necrosis factor, has been observed in other model systems as well. For example, in rats, small doses of LPS or PAF, when given alone, fail to alter blood pressure or lung function and histology (224). However, the combined administration of low doses of PAF and LPS leads to hypotension, hemoconcentration, and pulmonary leukocyte sequestration and edema. Similarly, neither LPS nor PAF causes gut mucosal necrosis when given alone in low doses to rats, but co-administration of these substances leads to development of necrotizing lesions in the gastrointestinal tract (225).

Pretreatment with various PAF antagonists has been shown to ameliorate hypotension and improve survival in rats, rabbits, and dogs challenged with intravenous LPS (213, 226-232). Pharmacologic antagonism of PAF receptors also has been shown to diminish pulmonary hypertension, brochoconstriction, and pulmonary microvascular hyperpermeability in animal models of acute lung injury induced by infusion of endotoxin or live bacteria (213, 226, 227, 233-236). In contrast to the effect of NSAIDs in many of these models, most studies have documented that PAF receptor blockade produces only a modest (or sometimes no) beneficial effect on arterial hypoxemia. Interestingly, PAF does not appear to be a major mediator of acute lung injury induced by infusion of activated complement (221) or tumor necrosis factor (237). Pharmacologic blockade of PAF receptors attenuates gut mucosal lesions induced by LPS (214) tumor necrosis factor (216) or mucosal hypoxia (206). Pretreatment with a PAF receptor antagonist also has been shown to ameliorate LPS-induced myocardial depression (238).

EXOGENOUS PROSTAGLANDINS AS THERAPEUTIC AGENTS

PGI_2 AND PGE_1 AS PHARMACOLOGIC AGENTS

When infused into animals or humans, both PGI_2 and PGE_1 are potent vasodilators and platelet antiaggregants. Both agents have short half-lives (estimated to be 30 seconds to about 5 minutes) (239, 240). For PGI_2, the threshold dose for vasodilation and inhibition of platelet aggregation in humans is about 2 ng/kg/min, and the dose-response curve is steep. Infusion of 8 ng/kg/min is about the maximal dose that can be tolerated by conscious humans, because larger doses cause excessive hypotension and tachycardia. The principal side effects of PGI_2 infusion are headache, abdominal cramps, nausea, and restlessness. Ventricular ectopy can occur at higher infusion rates. PGE_1 is less potent than PGI_2, particularly with respect to effects on platelet function. Threshold effects with PGE_1 are detectable at an infusion rate of 10 μg/kg*min and doses as high as 60 ng/kg*min have been employed in clinical trials (241). The principal side effect of PGE_1 is diarrhea. Discontinuation of therapy with PGI_2 and PGE_1 can cause rebound platelet activation, a side effect that tends to be more pronounced with the latter drug (242).

INFUSIONS OF PGI_2 OR PGE_1 IN SEPTIC SHOCK OR ARDS

In various experimental models of sepsis, endotoxicosis, or acute lung injury, infusions of PGI_2 or PGE_1 have been shown to improve survival (243, 244), ameliorate pulmonary hypertension (245–249), and attenuate pulmonary microvascular hyperpermeability (245, 247, 249, 250). Salutary effects also have been observed in experimental sepsis or endotoxicosis models following treatment with long-acting analogues of PGE or PGI_2 (251–253). Despite these beneficial actions, infusion of vasodilating prostaglandins in experimental models of acute lung injury typically has been associated with exacerbation of pulmonary venous admixture (i.e., shunting); thus, arterial hypoxemia generally has been observed to remain unchanged or even to worsen (245, 249, 253-255). In some studies, infusion of PGE has potentiated inflammatory injury to the lung, presumably on the basis of pulmonary microvascular dilation (257, 258). In a primate model of *Escherichia coli*-induced ARDS, therapy with PGE_1 did not affect the development of pulmonary edema, arterial hypoxemia, or mortality (259). In a rabbit model of acute lung injury induced by hyperoxia, treatment with PGE_1 attenuated alveolar infiltration by neutrophils but failed to improve survival (260). Findings from one recent study suggest that the salutary effects of PGE on pulmonary hypertension in models of acute lung injury result from diminished right ventricular preload, rather than pulmonary vasodilation (261).

Several studies have investigated the effects of PGI_2 or PGE_1 on outcome in patients with ARDS. In a single-center prospective trial, Holcroft et al randomized 41 patients with acute respiratory failure to receive either placebo or an infusion of PGE_1 (30 ng/kg/min) for 7 days (262). Thirty-day survival, the predetermined endpoint of the study, was significantly improved in the group treated with PGE_1. In a subsequent multicenter trial (263), 100 patients with ARDS were randomized to placebo or PGE$_1$, using a study design similar to that employed by Holcroft et al. In this study, treatment with PGE$_1$ did not enhance survival. Recently, Holcroft's group has completed another prospective, randomized trial of adjuvant therapy with PGE$_1$ (264). In this study, therapy with PGE$_1$ or placebo was administered to high-risk trauma patients prior to the development of frank ARDS, and although a statistically significant difference between groups was not detected, there was a trend toward a lower incidence of severe respiratory failure in the treated group (13%) as compared with the control group (28%). Survival was similar in both groups.

In addition to these large-scale studies investigating the effect of PGE$_1$ on survival, numerous smaller studies have assessed the effect on hemodynamics and oxygen transport of infusing PGI$_2$ or PGE$_1$ into patients with sepsis and/or ARDS. In general, infusion of either of these potent vasodilators increases cardiac output and decreases mean arterial blood pressure, systemic vascular resistance, and mean pulmonary artery pressure (265–269). Some (269, 270), but not all (271), studies suggest that systemic oxygen delivery (DO$_2$) is increased with PGI$_2$ or PGE$_1$ infusion in patients with ARDS or sepsis. The effect of these prostanoids on systemic consumption (VO$_2$) also is variable, but both Silverman et al and Bihari et al have reported that an increase in VO$_2$ after vasodilator prostanoid infusion identifies a group of patients with higher mortality (272, 273). This finding has been interpreted as indicating that these agents improve microvascular perfusion, which "uncovers" a previously inapparent oxygen debt. Most studies indicate that infusions of PGE$_1$ or PGI$_2$ decrease arterial oxygenation and/or increase intrapulmonary shunt flow in postoperative patients or patients with ARDS (265, 266, 268). Findings from one study suggest that PGE$_1$ infusion decreases superoxide production by neutrophils in patients with ARDS (264), but discrepant findings have been obtained in another similar trial (274).

INFUSIONS OF PGE$_1$ OR PGI$_2$ TO TREAT PULMONARY HYPERTENSION

In addition to their use in pulmonary hypertension associated with ARDS and sepsis, PGE$_1$ and PGI$_2$ have been used to treat primary pulmonary hypertension, as well as pulmonary hypertension related to mitral stenosis, chronic lung disease, and protamine reactions. Since PGE$_1$ and PGI$_2$ are short-lived agents and are not active orally, these drugs are not useful for the long-term outpatient management of primary pulmonary hypertension. Nevertheless, a large number of studies suggest that acute infusions of PGI$_2$ (and, to a lesser extent, PGE$_1$) predict the responsiveness of patients to subsequent therapy with orally active vasodilators, such as nifedipine, hydralazine, or diltiazem (275, 276). Prolonged infusions of PGI$_2$ have been shown to be safe, and this agent may provide clinically significant palliation to patients awaiting heart-lung transplantation (275, 277). In patients with decompensated chronic lung disease, infusions of PGE$_1$ have been shown to improve cardiac output and systemic DO$_2$ (277, 278). Afterload reduction (of both the right and left ventricles) with PGE$_1$ or PGI$_2$ has been shown to improve cardiac output dramatically in patients with refractory congestive heart failure (275). As in

the case of primary pulmonary hypertension, prolonged infusions of these vasodilating PGs may provide valuable palliation in patients awaiting transplantation.

Refractory right heart failure associated with severe pulmonary hypertension can occur after mitral valve replacement. In particularly severe cases, this problem can prevent weaning from cardiopulmonary bypass. D'Ambra et al have shown that this life-threatening problem often can be successfully managed by infusing large doses of PGE$_1$ (30 to 150 μg/kg/min) into the pulmonary artery to dilate the pulmonary vascular bed, while using norepinephrine, infused via a left atrial catheter, to control PGE$_1$-induced systemic arterial hypotension (280). In a similar fashion, Esmore and colleagues have reported the use of PGI$_2$ plus a mechanical right ventricular assist device to manage right heart failure successfully after cardiac transplantation (281). PGE$_1$ also has been used to manage severe pulmonary hypertension resulting from an allergic reaction following protamine reversal of heparin anticoagulation after cardiopulmonary bypass (282).

In the pediatric age group, the responsiveness of the pulmonary vasculature to an infusion of PGI$_2$ has been used to help assess operability in patients with pulmonary hypertension secondary to congenital heart diseases (283). PGI$_2$ and PGE$_1$ also have been used to manage severe pulmonary hypertension in the perioperative period after cardiac surgery in pediatric patients (283, 284).

INHIBITION OF PLATELET ACTIVATION DURING CARDIOPULMONARY BYPASS

Blood flow through extracorporeal tubing and oxygenators during cardiopulmonary bypass leads to platelet activation and consumption. This phenomenon is thought to contribute to excessive bleeding after cardiac operations. Since PGI$_2$ inhibits platelet aggregation and activation, several investigators have tested the hypothesis that infusion of this agent (285, 286) or a stable analog (287) might improve platelet counts and diminish postoperative hemorrhage. These studies all have shown beneficial effects in patients receiving heparin plus PGI$_2$ (or a PGI$_2$ analogue) as compared with those receiving heparin alone, but the benefits have been mild, and, as a result, PGI$_2$ is not used routinely during cardiopulmonary bypass.

PREVENTION OR TREATMENT OF EROSIVE GASTRITIS IN CRITICALLY ILL PATIENTS

In a variety of animal models, therapy with exogenous PGs has been shown to confer protection against gastric mucosal damage induced by a number of different noxious agents or conditions (288). Multiple mechanisms have been postulated as being responsible for this protection, including inhibition of acid secretion, stimulation of mucus secretion, augmentation of mucosal blood flow, stimulation of alkaline secretion by nonparietal cells, stabilization of tissue lysosomes, inhibition of cytokine release, and prevention of depletion of sulfhydryl compounds with antioxidant activity (288–290).

In general, PGs (and their stable analogues) have been disappointing as agents for the treatment of chronic gastric or duodenal ulcers (291). Relatively high (i.e., antisecretory) doses of PG derivatives are required to achieve healing rates similar to those achieved with H_2-receptor antagonists, and these doses are often complicated by side effects, such as diarrhea (292). Nevertheless, stable prostaglandin E analogues, particularly misoprostol have been shown to overcome the adverse effect of smoking on ulcer healing (293), to heal duodenal ulcers that are resistant to H_2-blockers (294), and to prevent gastroduodenal mucosal injury in patients being treated with NSAIDs (295, 296).

Given these considerations, several studies have sought to determine whether prophylactic therapy with PGE (or a stable analogue) is useful for preventing stress ulcers in critically ill patients. In an early prospective randomized trial, Skillman and colleagues compared treatment with 15(R)-15-methyl PGE_2 to gastric alkalinization to a pH >3.5 with antacids (297). Using gastric bleeding (determined by assessing the nasogastric aspirate for frank or occult blood) as the endpoint, these authors concluded that antacids provide significantly better prophylaxis than does 15(R)-15-methyl PGE_2. In another early trial, intragastric administration of PGE_2 was no more effective than placebo in preventing upper gastrointestinal bleeding in critically ill patients (298). Two more recent multicenter, prospective trials used both bleeding and endoscopic grading of the gastric mucosa as study endpoints and concluded that prophylactic administration of misoprostol (200 μg per nasogastric tube every 4 hours) is as effective as either antacid (299) or H_2 blocker (300) administration.

TREATMENT OF THE HEPATORENAL SYNDROME

The hepatorenal syndrome (HRS) occurs in patients with cirrhosis and refractory ascites. It is characterized by intense vasoconstriction in the renal vascular bed, leading to azotemia and impaired sodium and water excretion. It has been hypothesized that HRS is caused by insufficient production of vasodilating PGs in the kidneys (301, 302). In view of this hypothesis, investigators have tried to treat HRS by infusing exogenous vasodilator PGs. In general, results have not been encouraging (303–305), although in one recent report of four cases of HRS treated with oral misoprostol plus volume loading, marked improvements were observed in glomerular filtration rate, urine flow, and sodium excretion (306).

SUMMARY

The lipid autocoid system can be manipulated pharmacologically by inhibiting the synthesis of these mediators, blocking their receptors, or administering these compounds as therapeutic agents. New classes of compounds, such as phospholipase A_2 inhibitors, are undergoing development. Manipulation of lipid mediators in adult critical care medicine is done routinely for controlling fever or pain, but, at present, this strategy is used only rarely to improve hemodynamics or blunt systemic inflammation. Nevertheless, lipid mediators remain a prime focus of investigation by many researchers interested in critical care medicine, and it seems quite likely that the use of agents such as ibuprofen or the PAF antagonists will be common in the intensive care unit in the near future.

REFERENCES

1. Lewis RA, Austen KF, Soberman RJ: Leukotrienes and other products of the 5-lipoxygenase pathway. Biochemistry and relation to pathobiology in human diseases. *N Engl J Med* 323:645–55, 1990.
2. Lefer AM: Significance of lipid mediators in shock states. *Circ Shock* 27:3–12, 1989.
3. Oates JA, FitzGerald GA, Branch RA, Jackson EK, Knapp HR, Roberts LJ: Clinical implications of prostaglandin and thromboxane A_2 formation [first of two parts]. *N Engl J Med* 319:689–698, 1988.
4. Hamberg M, Svensson J, Samuelsson B: Thromboxanes—a new group of biologically active compounds derived from prostaglandin endoperoxides. *Proc Natl Acad Sci USA* 72:2994–2998, 1975.
5. Dunham B, Shepro D, Hechtman HB: Leukotriene induction in TxB_2 in cultured bovine endothelial cells. *Inflammation* 8:13–321, 1984.
6. Spagnulo PJ, Ellinger JJ, Hassid A, Dunn MJ: Thromboxane A_2 mediates augmented polymorphonuclear leukocyte adhesiveness. *J Clin Invest* 66:406–414, 1982.
7. Palder SB, Huval W, Lelcuk S, Alexander F, Shepro D, Mannick JA, Hechtman HB: Reduction of polymorphonuclear leukocyte accumulations by inhibition of cyclooxygenase and thromboxane synthase in the rabbit. *Surgery* 99:72–81, 1986.
8. Vane JR, Anggard EE, Botting RM: Regulatory functions of the endothelium. *N Engl J Med* 323:27–36, 1990.
9. Wittle BJR, Moncada S: Pharmacological interactions between prostacyclin and thromboxanes. *Br Med J* 39:232–238, 1983.
10. Furchgott RF, Vanhoutte PM: Endothelium-derived relaxing and contracting factors. *FASEB J* 3:2007–2018, 1989.
11. Vane JR: Inhibition of prostaglandin synthesis as a mechanism of action for aspirin-like drugs. *Nature* 231:232–235, 1971.
12. Vane J, Botting R: Inflammation and the mechanism of action of anti-inflammatory drugs. *FASEB J* 1:89–96, 1987.
13. Komoriya K, Ohmori H, Azuma A, Kurozumi S, Hashimoto Y, Nicolaou KC, Barnette WE, Magolda RL: Prostaglandin I_2 as a potentiator of acute inflammation in rats. *Prostaglandins* 15:557–564, 1978.
14. Williams TJ: Prostaglandin E_2, prostaglandin I_2 and the vascular changes of inflammation. *Br J Pharmacol* 65:517–524, 1979.
15. Williams TJ, Morley J: Prostaglandins as potentiators of increased vascular permeability in inflammation. *Nature* 246:215–217, 1973.
16. Ferreira SH, Nakamura M, Abreau–Castro MS: The hyperalgesic effects of prostacyclin and PGE_2. *Prostaglandins* 16:31–37, 1978.
17. Ferreira SH: Prostaglandins, aspirin–like drugs and analgesia. *Nature New Biol* 240:200–203, 1973.
18. Williams TJ: Interactions between prostaglandins, leukotrienes, and other mediators of inflammation. *Br Med Bull* 39:239–242, 1983.
19. Chouaib S, Fradelizi D: The mechanism of inhibition of interleukin 2 production. *J Immunol* 129:2463–2468, 1982.
20. Jelinek DF, Thompson PA, Lipsky PE: Regulation of human B cell activation by prostaglandin E_2. Suppression of the generation of immunoglobulin secreting cells. *J Clin Invest* 75:1339–1349, 1985.
21. Thompson PA, Jelinek DF, Lipsky PE: Regulation of human B cell proliferation by prostaglandin E_2. *J Immunol* 133:2446–2450, 1984.
22. Fantone JC, Kinnes DA: Prostaglandin E_1 and prostaglandin I_2 modulation of superoxide production of human neutrophils. *Biochem Biophys Res Commun* 113:506–512, 1983.
23. Fantone JC, Marasco WA, Elgas LJ, Ward PA: Stimulus specificity of prostaglandin inhibition of rabbit polymorphonuclear leukocyte lysozomal enzyme release and superoxide production. *Am J Physiol* 115:9–16, 1984.
24. Fletcher MP: Prostaglandin E_1 inhibits N-formyl-methionyl-leucyl-phenylalanine-mediated depolarization responses by decreasing the proportion of responsive cells without affecting chemotaxin-induced forward light scatter changes. *J Immunol* 139:4167–4173, 1987.
25. Snyder SD, Beller DI, Unanue ER: Prostaglandins modulate macrophage Ia expression. *Nature* 299:163–165, 1982.
26. Raz A, Wyche A, Siegel N, Needleman P: Regulation of fibroblast cyclooxygenase synthesis by interleukin-1. *J Biol Chem* 263:3022–3028, 1988.
27. Chang J, Gilman SC, Lewis AJ: Interleukin-1 activates phospholipase A_2 in rabbit chondrocytes: a possible signal for interleukin-1 action. *J Immunol* 136:1283–1287, 1986.
28. Zucali JR, Dinarello CA, Oblon DJ, Gross MA, Anderson L, Wiener RS: Interleukin-1 stimulates fibroblasts to produce granulocyte-macrophage colony-stimulating activity and prostaglandin E_2. *J Clin Invest* 77:1857–1863, 1986.
29. Albrightson CR, Baenziger NL, Needleman P: Exaggerated human vascular prostaglandin biosynthesis mediated by monocytes. Role of monokines and interleukin-1. *J Immunol* 135:1872–1877, 1985.
30. Libby P, Warner SJC, Friedman GB: Interleukin-1, a mitogen for human vascular smooth muscle cells that induces the release of inhibitory prostanoids. *J Clin Invest* 81:487–498, 1988.
31. Cominelli F, Nast CC, Lierena R, Dinarello CA, Zipser RD: Interleukin-1 suppresses inflammation in rabbit colitis: mediation by endogenous prostaglandins. *J Clin Invest* 85:582–586, 1990.
32. Huber M, Beutler B, Keppler D: Tumor necrosis factor a stimulates leukotriene production in vivo. *Eur J Immunol* 18:2085–2088, 1988.
33. Camussi G, Bussolino F, Salvidio G, Baglioni C: Tumor necrosis factor cachectin stimulates peritoneal macrophages, polymorphonuclear neutrophils, and vascular endothelial cells to synthesize and release platelet activating factor. *J Exp Med* 166:1390–1396, 1987.
34. Bachwich PR, Chensue SW, Larrick JW, Kunkel SL: Tumor necrosis factor stimulates interleukin-1 production and prostaglandin E_2 production in resting macrophages. *Biochem Biophys Res Commun* 136:94–101, 1986.

35. Sirko S, Bishai, Coceani F: Prostaglandin formation in the hypothalamus in vivo: effect of pyrogens. *Am J Physiol* 246:R616–R624, 1989.
36. Coceani F, Lees J, Bisnai I: Further evidence complicating prostaglandin E_2 in the genesis of pyrogen fever. *Am J Physiol* 254:R463–R469, 1988.
37. Scales WE, Chensue SW, Otterness I, Kunkel SL: Regulation of monokine gene expression: prostaglandin E_2 suppresses tumor necrosis factor but not interleukin-1a or β-mRNA and cell-associated bioactivity. *J Leukoc Biol* 45:416–421, 1989.
38. Kunkel SL, Spengler M, May MA, et al: Prostaglandin E_2 regulates macrophage-derived tumor necrosis factor gene expression. *J Biol Chem* 263:5380–5384, 1988.
39. Ertel W, Morrison MH, Wang P, Ba ZF, Ayala A, Chaudry IH: The complex pattern of cytokines in sepsis: association between prostaglandins, cachectin, and interleukins. *Ann Surg* 214:141–148, 1991.
40. Bahl AK, Foreman JC, Dale MM: The effect of prostaglandin E_2 and nonsteroidal anti-inflammatory drugs on cell-associated interleukin one. *Adv Prostaglandin Thrombox Leukot Res* 21:513–515, 1990.
41. Chouaib S, Bertoglio JH: Prostaglandins E as modulators of the immune response. *Lymphokine Res* 7:237–245, 1988.
42. Ertel W, Morrison MH, Ayala A, Perrin MM, Chaudry IH: Blockade of prostaglandin production increases cachectin synthesis and prevents depression of macrophage functions after hemorrhagic shock. *Ann Surg* 213:265–271, 1991.
43. Spengler RN, Spengler ML, Strieter RM, Remick DG, Larrick JW, Kunkel SL: Modulation of tumor necrosis factor alpha gene expression. *J Immunol* 263:5380–5384, 1989.
44. Spinas GA, Bloesch D, Keller U, Zimmerli W, Cammisuli S: Pretreatment with ibuprofen augments circulating tumor necrosis factor-α, interleukin-6 and elastase during acute endotoxemia. *J Infect Dis* 163:89–95, 1991.
45. Offner F, Phillipe J, Vogelaers D, Colardyn F, Baele G, Baudrihaye M, Vermeulen A, Leroux-Roels G: Serum tumor necrosis factor levels in patients with infectious disease and septic shock. *J Lab Clin Med* 116:100–105, 1990.
46. Marks JD, Marks CB, Luce JM, Montgomery AB, Turner J, Metz CA, Murray JF: Plasma tumor necrosis factor in patients with septic shock: mortality rate, incidence of adult respiratory distress syndrome, and effects of methylprednisolone administration. *Am Rev Respir Dis* 141:94–97, 1990.
47. Hack CE, DeGroot ER, Felt-Bersma JF, Nuijens JH, Strack van Schijndel RJM, Eerenberg-Belmer AJM, Thijs LG, Aarden LA: Increased plasma levels of interleukin-6 in sepsis. *Blood* 74:1704–1710, 1989.
48. Marone G, Thomas LL, Lichtenstein LM: The role of agonists that activate adenylate cyclase in the control of cAMP metabolism and enzyme release by human polymorphonuclear leukocytes. *J Immunol* 125:2277–2283, 1980.
49. Goodwin JS, Kaszubowski PA, Williams RC: Cyclic adenosine monophosphate response to prostaglandin E_2 on subpopulations of human lymphocytes. *J Exp Med* 150:1260–1264, 1979.
50. Ham EA, Soderman DD, Zanetti ME, Dougherty HW, McCauley E, Kuehl FA: Inhibition by prostaglandins of leukotriene B_4 release from activated neutrophils. *Proc Natl Acad Sci USA* 80:4349–4353, 1983.
51. Holtzman MJ, Aizawa H, Nadel JA, Goetzl EJ: Selective generation of leukotriene B_4 by tracheal epithelial cells from dogs. *Biochem Biophys Res Commun* 114:1071–1076, 1983.
52. Ford-Hutchinson AW, Bray MA, Doig MV, Shipley ME, Smith MJH: Leukotriene B_4, a potent chemokinetic and aggregating substance released from polymorphonuclear leukocytes. *Nature* 286:264–265, 1980.
53. Serhan CN, Radin A, Smolen JE, Korchak H, Samuelsson B, Weissmann G: Leukotriene B_4 is a complete secretagogue in human neutrophils: a kinetic analysis. *Biochem Biophys Res Commun* 107:1006–1010, 1982.
54. Palmblad J, Gyllenhammer H, Lindgren JA, Malmsten CL: Effects of leukotrienes and fMet-Leu-Phe on oxidative metabolism of neutrophils and eosinophils. *J Immunol* 132:3041–3045, 1984.
55. Rae SA, Smith MJH: The stimulation of lysozomal enzyme secretion from human polymorphonuclear leukocytes by leukotriene B_4. *J Pharm Pharmacol* 33:616–617, 1981.
56. Gimbrone MA Jr, Brock AF, Schafer AI: Leukotriene B_4 stimulates polymorphonuclear leukocyte adhesion to cultured vascular endothelial cells. *J Clin Invest* 74:1552–1555, 1984.
57. Hoover R, Karnovsky MJ, Austen KF, Corey EJ, Lewis RA: Leukotriene B action on endothelium mediates augmented neutrophil/endothelial adhesion. *Proc Natl Acad Sci USA* 81:2191–2193, 1984.
58. Palmblad J, Lindstrom P, Lerner R: Leukotriene B_4 induced hyperadhesiveness of endothelial cells for neutrophils. *Biochem Biophys Res Commun* 166:848–851, 1990.
59. Lewis RE, Granger HJ: Diapedesis and the permeability of venous microvessels to protein macromolecules: the impact of leukotriene B_4. *Microvasc Res* 35:27–47, 1988.
60. Dahlen S-E, Bjork J, Hedqvist P, Arfors K-E, Hammarstrom S, Lindgren J-A, Samuelsson B: Leukotrienes promote plasma leakage and leukocyte adhesion in postcapillary venules: in vivo effects with relevance to the acute inflammatory response. *Proc Natl Acad Sci USA* 78:3887–3891, 1991.
61. Dugas B, Paul-Eugene N, Cairns J, Gordon J, Calenda A, Mencia-Huerta JM, Braquet P: Leukotriene B_4 potentiates the expression and release of FCeRII/CD23, and proliferation and differentiation of human B lymphocytes induced by IL-4. *J Immunol* 145:3406–3411, 1990.
62. Rola-Pleszczynski M, Chavaillaz PA, Lemaire I: Stimulation of interleukin 2 and interferon gamma production by leukotriene B_4 in human lymphocyte cultures. *Prostaglandins Leukot Med* 23:207–210, 1986.
63. Rola-Pleszczynski M, Lemaire I: Leukotrienes augment interleukin 1 production by human monocytes. *J Immunol* 135:3958–3961, 1985.
64. Burgess CA, McCandless BK, Cooper JA, Malik AB: Leukotriene B_4 increases pulmonary transvascular filtration by a neutrophil-independent mechanism. *J Appl Physiol* 68:1260–1264, 1990.
65. Noonan TC, Selig WM, Burhop KE, Burgess CA, Malik AB: Pulmonary microvascular responses to LTB_4: effects of perfusate composition. *J Appl Physiol* 64:1989–1996, 1988.
66. Weller PF, Lee CW, Foster DW, Corey EJ, Austen KF, Lewis RA: Generation and metabolism of 5-lipoxygenase pathway leukotrienes by human eosinophils: predominant production of leukotriene C_4. *Proc Natl Acad Sci USA* 80:7626–7630, 1983.
67. Owen WF Jr, Soberman RJ, Yoshimoto T, Sheffer AL, Lewis RA, Austen KF: Synthesis and release of leukotriene C_4 by human eosinophils. *J Immunol* 138:532–538, 1987.
68. Williams JD, Czop JK, Austen KF: Release of leukotrienes by human monocytes on stimulation of their phagocytic receptor for particulate activators. *J Immunol* 132:3034–3040, 1984.
69. Drazen JM, Austen KF, Lewis RA, et al: Comparative airway and vascular activities of leukotrienes C and D in vivo and in vitro. *Proc Natl Acad Sci USA* 77:4354–4358, 1980.
70. Joris I, Majno G, Corey EJ, Lewis RA: The mechanism of vascular leakage induced by leukotriene E_4. *Am J Pathol* 126:19–24, 1987.
71. Cohn SM, Kruithoff KL, Rothschild HR, Wang H, Antonsson JB, Heard SO, Fink MP: Leukotriene C_4 induces mesenteric hypoperfusion and intestinal intramural acidosis in pigs. *J Surg Res* 50:303–307, 1991.
72. Piper PJ, Stanton AWB, McLeod LJ: The actions of leukotrienes C_4 and D_4 in the porcine renal vascular bed. *Prostaglandins* 29:61–73, 1985.
73. Schumacher WA, Heran CL, Allen GT, Ogletree ML: Leukotrienes cause mesenteric vasoconstriction and hemoconcentration in rats without activating thromboxane receptors. *Prostaglandins* 38:335–345, 1989.
74. Bittl JA, Pfeffer MA, Lewis RA, Mehrotra MM, Corey EJ, Austen KF: Mechanisms of the negative inotropic action of leukotrienes C_4 and D_4 on isolated rat heart. *Cardiovasc Res* 19:426–432, 1985.
75. Roth DM, Lefer AM: Studies on the mechanism of leukotriene induced coronary artery constriction. *Prostaglandins* 26:573–581, 1983.
76. Karmazyn M, Moffat MP: Positive inotropic effects of low concentrations of leukotrienes C_4 and D_4 in rat heart. *Am J Physiol* 259:H1239–H1246, 1990.
77. Hattori Y, Levi R: Negative inotropic effects of leukotrienes: leukotrienes C_4 and D_4 inhibit calcium-dependent contractile response in potassium-depolarized guinea pig myocardium. *J Pharmacol Exp Ther* 230:646–651, 1984.
78. Braquet P, Touquil L, Shen TY, Vargaftig BB: Perspectives in platelet-activating factor research. *Pharmacol Rev* 39:97–145, 1987.
79. Tomeo AC, Duran WN: Resistance and exchange microvessels are modulated by different PAF receptors. *Am J Physiol* 261:H1648–H1652, 1991.
80. Garcia JGN, Azghani A, Callahan KS, Johnson AR: Effect of platelet activating factor on leukocyte-endothelial interactions. *Thromb Res* 51:83–96, 1988.
81. Tomeo AC, Egan RW, Duran WN: Priming interactions between platelet activating factor and histamine in vivo microcirculation. *FASEB J* 5:2850–2855, 1991.
82. Dillon PK, FitzPatrick MF, Ritter AB, Duran WN: The effect of platelet activating factor on leukocyte adhesion to microvascular endothelium: time course and dose-response relationships. *Inflammation* 12:563–573, 1988.
83. Braquet P, Bourgain R, Mencia-Huerta JM: Effect of platelet-activating factor on platelets and vascular endothelium. *Semin Thromb Hemost* 15:184–196, 1989.
84. Bussolino F, Camussi G, Aglietta M, Braquet P, Bosia A, Pescarmona G, Sanavio F, D'Urso N, Marchisio PC: Human endothelial cells are target for platelet activating factor. I. Platelet activating factor induces changes in cytoskeleton structures. *J Immunol* 139:2439–2446, 1987.
85. Pugsley MK, Salari H, Walker MJA: Actions of platelet-activating factor on isolated rat hearts. *Circ Shock* 35:207–214, 1991.
86. Chilton FH, O'Flaherty JT, Walsh CE, Thomas MJ, Wykle RL, DeChatelet LR, Waite BM: Platelet activating factor. Stimulation of the lipoxygenase pathway in polymorphonuclear leukocytes by 1-*O*-alkyl-sn-glycero-3-phosphocholine. *J Biol Chem* 257:5402–5407, 1982.
87. Lin AH, Morton DR, Gorman RR: Acetyl glyceryl ether phosphocholine stimulates leukotriene B_4 synthesis in human polymorphonuclear leukocytes. *J Clin Invest* 70:1058–1065, 1982.
88. Chung KF, Aizawa H, Leikauf GD, Ueki IF, Evans TW, Nadel JA: Airway hyperresponsiveness induced by platelet-activating factor: role of thromboxane generation. *J Pharmacol Exp Ther* 236:580–584, 1986.
89. Hsueh W, Gonzales-Crussi F, Arroave JL: Platelet-activating factor-induced bowel necrosis. An investigation of secondary mediators in its pathogenesis. *Am J Pathol* 122:231–239, 1986.
90. Burhop KE, Garcia JGN, Selig WM, Lo SK, van der Zee H, Kaplan JE, Malik AB: Platelet-activating factor increases lung vascular permeability to protein. *J Appl Physiol* 61:2210–2217, 1986.
91. Bruijnzeel PLB, Kok PTM, Hamelink ML, Kijne AM, Verhagen J: Plateletactivating factor induces leukotriene C_4 synthesis by purified human eosinophils. *Prostaglandins* 34:205–214, 1987.
92. Voelkel NF, Worthen S, Reeves JT, Henson PM, Murphy RC: Nonimmunological production of leukotrienes induced by platelet-activating factor. *Science* 218:286–288, 1982.
93. Blackwell GJ, Flower RJ: Inhibition of phospholipase. *Br Med J* 39:260–264, 1983.
94. Hirata F, Hirata A: Biology of phospholipase inhibitory proteins. In Mukherjee AB (ed): *Biochemistry, Molecular Biology, and Physiology of Phospholipase A_2 and its Regulatory Factors*. New York, Plenum Press, pp 211–218, 1990.
95. Brooks PM, Day RO: Nonsteroidal antiinflammatory drugs—differences and similarities. *N Engl J Med* 324:1716–1725, 1991.
96. Roth GJ, Majerus PW: The mechanism of the effect of aspirin on human platelets. I. Acetylation of a particulate fraction protein. *J Clin Invest* 56:624–632, 1975.
97. Jaffe EA, Weksler BB: Recovery of endothelial cell prostacyclin production after inhibition by low doses of aspirin. *J Clin Invest* 63:532–535, 1979.
98. FitzGerald GA, Oates JA, Hawiger J, et al: Endogenous synthesis of prostacyclin and thromboxane and platelet function during chronic administration of aspirin in man. *J Clin Invest* 71:676–678, 1983.
99. Pederson AK, FitzGerald GA: Dose-related kinetics of aspirin. Presystemic acetylation of platelet cyclooxygenase. *N Engl J Med* 311:1206–1211, 1984.

100. Clarke RJ, Mayo G, Price P, FitzGerald GA: Suppression of thromboxane A_2 but not of systemic prostacyclin by controlled-release aspirin. *N Engl J Med* 325:1137–1141, 1991.
101. Faist E, Markewitz A, Fuchs D, Lang S, Zarius S, Schildberg F-W, Wachter H, Reichart B: Immunomodulatory therapy with thymopentin and indomethacin. Successful restoration of interleukin-2 synthesis in patients undergoing major surgery. *Ann Surg* 214:264–275, 1991.
102. Faist E, Ertel W, Salmen B, et al: The immunoprotective effects of cyclooxygenase inhibition in patients with major surgical trauma. *J Trauma* 30:8–18, 1990.
103. Abramson S, Korchak HM, Ludewig R, et al: Modes of action of aspirin-like drugs. *Proc Natl Acad Sci USA* 82:7227–7231, 1985.
104. Minta JO, Williams MD: Some nonsteroidal antiinflammatory drugs inhibit the generation of superoxide anions by activated polymorphs by blocking ligand-receptor interactions. *J Rheumatol* 12:751–757, 1985.
105. Kitchen EA, Dawson W, Rainsford KD, Cawston T: Inflammation and possible modes of action of anti-inflammatory drugs. In Rainsford KD (ed): *Antiinflammatory and Antirheumatic Drugs*. Vol. 1. *Inflammation Mechanisms and Actions of Traditional Drugs*. Boca Raton, Fla., CRC Press, 1985, pp 21–87.
106. Kennedy TP, Rao NV, Noah W, Michael JR, Jafri MH Jr, Gurtner GH, Hoidal JR: Ibuprofen prevents oxidant lung injury and in vitro lipid peroxidation by chelating iron. *J Clin Invest* 86:1565–1573, 1990.
107. Aruoma OI, Halliwell B: The iron-binding and hydroxyl radical scavenging action of antiinflammatory drugs. *Xenobiotica* 18:459–470, 1988.
108. Committee on Safety of Medicines: Nonsteroidal antiinflammatory drugs and serious gastrointestinal adverse reactions. *Br Med J* 292:614, 1986.
109. Euler AR: Gastroenterology: eicosanoids and the gastrointestinal tract. In Watkins WD, Peterson MB, Fletcher JR (eds): *Prostaglandins in Clinical Practice* New York, Raven Press, 1989, pp 97–129.
110. Fries JF, Miller SR, Spitz PW, Williams CA, Hubert HB, Block DA: Towards an epidemiology of gastropathy associated with nonsteroidal antiinflammatory drug use. *Gastroenterology* 96(suppl 2):647–655, 1989.
111. Bernard GR, Reines HD, Halushka PV, Higgins SB, Metz CA, Swindell BB, Wright PE, Watts FL, Vrbanac JJ: Prostacyclin and thromboxane A_2 formation is increased in human sepsis syndrome: effects of cyclo-oxygenase inhibition. *Am Rev Respir Dis* 144:1095–1101, 1991.
112. Haupt MT, Jastremski MS, Clemmer TP, Metz CA, Goris GG: The Ibuprofen Study Group: Effect of ibuprofen in patients with severe sepsis: a randomized, double-blind, multicenter study. *Crit Care Med* 19:1339–1347, 1991.
113. Clive DM, Stoff JS: Renal syndromes associated with nonsteroidal antiinflammatory drugs. *N Engl J Med* 310:563–572, 1984.
114. Kokko JP: Effects of prostaglandins on renal epithelial electrolyte transport. *Kidney Int* 19:791–796, 1981.
115. Murray MD, Brater DC: Adverse effects of nonsteroidal antiinflammatory drugs on renal function. *Ann Intern Med* 112:559–560, 1990.
116. Fink MP, MacVittie TJ, Casey LC: Effects of nonsteroidal antiinflammatory drugs on renal function in septic dogs. *J Surg Res* 36:516–525, 1984.
117. Cryer HM, Unger LS, Garrison RN, Harris PD: Prostaglandins maintain renal microvascular blood flow during hyperdynamic bacteremia. *Circ Shock* 26:71–88, 1988.
118. Henrich WL, Hamasaki Y, Said SI, Campbell WB, Cronin RE: Dissociation of systemic and renal effects in endotoxemia: prostaglandin inhibition uncovers an important role of renal nerves. *J Clin Invest* 69:691–697, 1982.
119. Fink MP, Nelson R, Roethel R: Low-dose dopamine preserves renal blood flow in endotoxin shocked dogs treated with ibuprofen. *J Surg Res* 38:582–591, 1985.
120. Ciabattoni G, Cinotti GA, Pierucci A, Simonetti GM, Manzi M, Pugliese F, Barsotti P, Pecci G, Taggi F, Patrono C: Effects of sulindac and ibuprofen in patients with chronic glomerular disease. Evidence for the dependence of renal function on prostacyclin. *N Engl J Med* 310:279–283, 1984.
121. Ciabattoni G, Pugliese F, Cinotti GA, Patrono C: Renal effects of antiinflammatory drugs. *Eur J Rheumatol Inflamm* 3:210–221, 1980.
122. Bunning DG, Barth WF: Sulindac. A potentially renal-sparing nonsteroidal antiinflammatory drug. *JAMA* 248:1864–1867, 1984.
123. Brater DC, Anderson S, Baird B, Campbell WB: Effects of ibuprofen, naproxen, and sulindac on prostaglandins in men. *Kidney Int* 27:66–73, 1985.
124. Zambraski EJ, Chremos AN, Dunn MJ: Comparison of the effects of sulindac with other cyclooxygenase inhibitors on prostaglandin excretion and renal function in normal and chronic bile duct-ligated dogs and swine. *J Pharmacol Exp Ther* 228:560–566, 1984.
125. Gersony W, Peckham G, Ellison R, Miettenen O, Nadas A: Effects of indomethacin in premature infants with patent ductus arteriosus: results of a national collaborative study. *J Pediatr* 102:895–906, 1983.
126. Northover BJ, Subramanian G: Analgesic–antipyretic drugs as antagonists of endotoxin shock in dogs. *J Pathol Bacteriol* 83:463–468, 1962.
127. Ball HA, Cook JA, Wise WC, Halushka PV: Role of thromboxane, prostaglandins and leukotrienes in endotoxic and septic shock. *Intensive Care Med* 12:116–126, 1985.
128. Zanaboni PB, Bradley JD, Baudendistel LJ, Webster RO, Dahms TE: Cyclooxygenase inhibition prevents PMA-induced increases in lung vascular permeability. *J Appl Physiol* 69:1494–1501, 1990.
129. Zanaboni PB, Bradley JD, Webster RO, Dahms TE: Cyclooxygenase inhibitors prevent ethchlorvynol-induced injury in rat and rabbit lungs. *J Appl Physiol* 71:43–49, 1991.
130. Wang D, Chou C-L, Hsu K, Chen HI: Cyclooxygenase pathway mediates lung injury induced by phorbol and platelets. *J Appl Physiol* 70:2417–2421, 1991.
131. Fletcher JR: The role of prostaglandins in sepsis. *Scand J Infect Dis* (suppl 31):55–60, 1982.
132. Halushka PV, Reines HD, Barrow SE, Blair IA, Dollery CT, Rambo W, Cook JA, Wise WC: Elevated plasma 6-keto-prostaglandin F_1 in patients in septic shock. *Crit Care Med* 13:451–453, 1985.
133. Reines HD, Cook JA, Halushka PV, Wise WC, Rambo W: Plasma thromboxane concentrations are raised in patients dying with septic shock. *Lancet* 2:174–175, 1982.
134. Oettinger WKE, Walter GO, Jensen UM, Beyer A, Peskar A: Endogenous prostaglandin F_2 in the hyperdynamic state of severe sepsis in man. *Br J Surg* 70:237–239, 1983.
135. Oettinger W, Berger D, Beger HG: The clinical significance of prostaglandins and thromboxane as mediators of septic shock. *Klin Wochenschr* 65:61–68, 1987.
136. Kuhl PG, Bolds JM, Loyd JE, Snapper JR, FitzGerald GA: Thromboxane receptor-mediated bronchial and hemodynamic responses in ovine endotoxemia. *Am J Physiol* R310–R319, 1988.
137. Byrne K, Carey PD, Sielaff TD, Jenkins JK, Blocher CR, Cooper KR, Fowler AA, Sugerman HJ: Ibuprofen prevents deterioration in static transpulmonary compliance and transalveolar protein flux in septic porcine acute lung injury. *J Trauma* 31:155–166, 1991.
138. Deby-Dupont G, Braun M, Lamy M, Deby C, Pincemail J, Faymonville ME, Damas P, Bodson L, Lecart MP, Goutier R: Thromboxane and prostacyclin release in adult respiratory distress syndrome. *Intensive Care Med* 13:167–174, 1987.
139. Fink MP, Rothschild HR, Deniz YF, Cohn SM: Complement depletion with Naje haje cobra venom factor limits prostaglandin release and improves visceral perfusion in porcine endotoxic shock. *J Trauma* 29:1076-1085, 1989.
140. Johnson J, Meyrick B, Jesmok G, Brighmam KL: Human recombinant tumor necrosis factor alpha infusion mimics endotoxemia in awake sheep. *J Appl Physiol* 66:1448–1454, 1989.
141. Kreil EA, Greene E, Fitzgibbon C, Robinson DR, Zapol WM: Effects of recombinant human tumor necrosis factor alpha, lymphotoxin, *Escherichia coli* lipopolysaccharide on hemodynamics, lung microvascular permeability, and eicosanoid synthesis in anesthetized sheep. *Circ Res* 65:502–514, 1989.
142. Schulman LL, Lennon PF, Ratner SJ, Enson Y: Meclofenamate enhances blood oxygenation in acute oleic acid lung injury. *J Appl Physiol* 64:710–718, 1988.
143. Gnidec AG, Sibbald WJ, Cheung H, Metz CA: Ibuprofen reduces the progression of permeability edema in an animal model of hyperdynamic sepsis. *J Appl Physiol* 65:1024–1032, 1988.
144. Snapper JR, Hutchinson AA, Ogletree ML, Brigham KL: Effects of cyclooxygenase inhibitors on the alterations in lung mechanics caused by endotoxemia in the unanesthetized sheep. *J Clin Invest* 72:63–76, 1983.
145. LaLonde C, Knox J, Daryani R, Zhu D, Demling RH, Nuemann M: Topical flurbiprofen decreases burn wound-induced hypermetabolism and systemic lipid peroxidation. *Surgery* 109:645–651, 1991.
146. Fink MP, Rothschild HR, Deniz YF, Wang H, Lee PC, Cohn SM: Systemic and mesenteric O_2 metabolism in endotoxic pigs: effect of ibuprofen and meclofenamate. *J Appl Physiol* 67:1950–1957, 1989.
147. Turner CR, Lackey MN, Quinlan MF, Schwartz LW, Wheeldon EB: Therapeutic intervention in a rat model of adult respiratory distress syndrome. III. Cyclooxygenase pathway inhibition. *Circ Shock* 34:270–277, 1991.
148. Carey PD, Leeper-Woodford SK, Walsh CJ, Byrne K, Fowler AA, Sugerman HJ: Delayed cyclo-oxygenase blockade reduces the neutrophil respiratory burst and plasma tumor necrosis factor levels in sepsis-induced acute lung injury. *J Trauma* 31:733–741, 1991.
149. Perlman MB, Johnson A, Malik AB: Ibuprofen prevents thrombin-induced lung vascular injury: mechanism of effect. *Am J Physiol* 252:H605–H614, 1987.
150. Shinozawa Y, Hales C, Jung W, Burke J: Ibuprofen prevents synthetic smoke-induced pulmonary edema. *Am Rev Respir Dis* 134:1145–1148, 1986.
151. Perkowski SZ, Havill AM, Flynn JT, Gee MH: Role of intrapulmonary release of eicosanoids and superoxide anion as mediators of pulmonary dysfunction and endothelial injury in sheep with intermittent complement activation. *Circ Res* 53:574–583, 1983.
152. Heard SO, McGuire K, Haw MP, Forse RA, Blackburn GL, Fink MP: Dietary enrichment with omega-3 fatty acids partially protects against lipopolysaccharide-induced atrial depression in rats. *Circ Shock* 36:140–146, 1992.
153. Murray MJ, Svingen BA, Holman RT, Yaksh TL: Effects of a fish oil diet on pigs' cardiopulmonary response to bacteremia. *J Parenter Enter Nutr* 15:152–158, 1991.
154. Mascioli EA, Iwasa Y, Trimbo S, Leader L, Bistrian BR, Blackburn GL: Endotoxin challenge after menhaden oil diet: effects on survival of guinea pigs. *Am J Clin Nutr* 49:277–282, 1989.
155. Cook JA, Wise WC, Halushka PV: Elevated thromboxane levels in the rat during endotoxic shock: protective effects of imidazole, 13-azaprostanoic acid, or essential fatty acid deficiency. *J Clin Invest* 65:227–230, 1980.
156. Taneyama C, Sasao J, Senna S, Kimura M, Kiyono S, Goto H, Arakawa K: Protective effects of ONO 3708, a new thromboxane A_2 receptor antagonist, during experimental endotoxin shock. *Circ Shock* 28:69–77, 1989.
157. Redl G, Abdi S, Traber LD, Nichols RJ, Flynn JT, Herndon DN, Traber DL: Inhibition of thromboxane synthesis reduces endotoxin-induced right ventricular failure in sheep. *Crit Care Med* 19:1294–1302, 1991.
158. Svartholm E, Bergqvist D, Hedner U, Ljungberg J, Haglund U: Thromboxane A_2-receptor blockade and prostacyclin in porcine *Escherichia coli* shock. *Arch Surg* 124:669–672, 1989.
159. Henry CL, Ogletree ML, Brigham KL, Hammon JW Jr: Attenuation of the pulmonary vascular response to endotoxin by a thromboxane synthesis inhibitor (UK-38485) in unanesthetized sheep. *J Surg Res* 50:77–81, 1991.
160. Wakerlin GE, Benson GV, Pearl RG: A thromboxane analog increases pulmonary capillary pressure but not permeability in the perfused rabbit lung. *Anesthesiology* 75:475–480, 1991.
161. Price S, Harlan J, Carrico CJ, Hildebrandt J, Winn R: Indomethacin, dazoxiben and extravascular lung water after *Escherichia coli* infusion. *J Surg Res* 41:189–197, 1986.
162. Wisner D, Sturm J, Sutter G, Ellendorf B, Nerlich M: Thromboxane receptor blockade in an animal model of ARDS. *Surgery* 104:91–97, 1988.
163. Reines HD, Halushka PV, Olanoff LS, Hunt PS: Dazoxiben in human sepsis and adult respiratory distress syndrome. *Clin Pharmacol Ther* 37:391–395, 1985.

164. Leeman M, Boeynaems J-M, Degaute J-P, Vincent J-L, Kahn RJ: Administration of dazoxiben, a selective thromboxane synthetase inhibitor, in the adult respiratory distress syndrome. *Chest* 87:726–730, 1985.
165. Matthay MA, Eschenbacher WL, Goetzl EJ: Elevated concentrations of leukotriene D_4 in pulmonary edema fluid of patients with the adult respiratory distress syndrome. *J Clin Immunol* 4:479–483, 1984.
166. Stephenson AH, Lonigro AJ, Hyers TM, Webster RO, Fowler AA: Increased concentrations of leukotrienes in bronchoalveolar lavage fluid of patients with ARDS or at high risk for ARDS. *Am Rev Respir Dis* 138:714–719, 1988.
167. Antonelli M, Lenti L, Bufi M, et al: Differential evaluation of bronchoalveolar lavage cells and leukotrienes in unilateral acute lung injury and ARDS patients. *Intensive Care Med* 15:439–445, 1989.
168. Antonelli M, Bufi M, De Blasi RA, et al: Detection of leukotrienes B_4, C_4 and of their isomers in arterial, mixed venous blood and bronchoalveolar lavage fluid from ARDS patients. *Intensive Care Med* 15:296–301, 1989.
169. Bernard GR, Korley V, Chee P, Swindell B, Ford-Hutchinson AW, Tagari P: Persistent generation of peptido leukotrienes in patients with the adult respiratory distress syndrome. *Am Rev Respir Dis* 144:263–267, 1991.
170. Sala A, Murphy RC, Voelkel NF: Direct airway injury results in elevated levels of sulfidopeptide leukotrienes, detectable in airway secretions. *Prostaglandins* 42:1–7, 1991.
171. Davis JM, Yurt RW, Barie PS, Hudgins LC, Verma M, Dineen P, Shires GT: Leukotriene B_4 generation in patients with established pulmonary failure. *Arch Surg* 124:1451–1455, 1989.
172. Davis JM, Meyer JD, Barie PS, Yurt RW, Duhaney R, Dineen P, Shires GT: Elevated production of neutrophil leukotriene B_4 precedes pulmonary failure in critically ill surgical patients. *Surg Gynecol Obstet* 170:495–500, 1990.
173. Seeger W, Grimminger F, Barden M, Becker G, Lohmeyer J, Heinrich D, Lasch H-G: Omega-oxidized leukotriene B_4 detected in the broncho-alveolar lavage fluid of patients with noncardiogenic pulmonary edema, but not in those with cardiogenic edema. *Intensive Care Med* 17:1–6, 1991.
174. Morel DR, Skoskiewicz M, Robinson DR, Bloch KJ, Hoaglin DC, Zapol WM: Leukotrienes, thromboxane A_2, and prostaglandins during systemic anaphylaxis in sheep. *Am J Physiol* 261:H782–H792, 1991.
175. Perlman MB, Johnson A, Jubiz W, Malik AB: Lipoxygenase products induce neutrophil activation and increase endothelial permeability after thrombin-induced pulmonary microembolism. *Circ Res* 64:62–73, 1989.
176. Olson NC, Dobrowsky RT, Fleisher LN: Dexamethasone blocks increased leukotriene B_4 production during endotoxin-induced lung injury. *J Appl Physiol* 64:2100–2107, 1988.
177. Ball HA, Cook JA, Spicer KM, Hsu CY, Halushka PV: Oleic acid-induced pulmonary injury in rats: potential role of sulfidopeptide leukotrienes. *Circ Shock* 26:59–70, 1988.
178. Sprague RS, Stephenson AH, Dahms TE, Lonigro AJ: Production of leukotrienes in phorbol ester-induced acute lung injury. *Prostaglandins* 39:439–450, 1990.
179. Hagmann W, Denzlinger C, Keppler D: Production of peptide leukotrienes in endotoxin shock. *FEBS Lett* 180:309–313, 1985.
180. Stephenson AH, Sprague RS, Dahms TE, Lonigro AJ: Increased leukotriene C4 in ethchlorvynol-induced acute lung injury in dogs. *J Appl Physiol* 62:732–738, 1987.
181. Voelkel NF, Stenmark KR, Reeves JT, Mathias MM, Murphy RC: Actions of lipoxygenase in isolated rat lungs. *J Appl Physiol* 47:860–867, 1984.
182. Shapiro JM, Mihm FG, Trudell JR, Stevens JH, Feeley TW: Leukotriene D_4 increases extravascular lung water in the dog. *Circ Shock* 21:121–128, 1987.
183. Noonan TC, Kern DF, Malik AB: Pulmonary microcirculatory responses to leukotrienes B_4, C_4 and D_4 in sheep. *Prostaglandins* 30:419–435, 1985.
184. Sakai A, Chang S-W, Voelkel NF: Importance of vasoconstriction in lipid mediator-induced pulmonary edema. *J Appl Physiol* 66:2667–2674, 1989.
185. Farrukh IS, Sciuto AM, Spannhake EW, Gurtner GH, Michael JR: Leukotriene D_4 increases pulmonary vascular permeability and pressure by different mechanisms in the rabbit. *Am Rev Respir Dis* 134:229–232, 1986.
186. Noonan TC, Selig WM, Kern DF, Malik AB: Mechanism of peptidoleukotriene-induced increases in pulmonary transvascular fluid filtration. *J Appl Physiol* 61:1928–1934, 1986.
187. Smith EF III, Kinter LB, Jugus M, Wasserman MA, Eckardt RD, Newton JF: Beneficial effects of the peptidoleukotriene receptor antagonist, SK&F 104353, on the responses to experimental endotoxemia in the conscious rat. *Circ Shock* 25:21–31, 1988.
188. Cook JA, Li EJ, Spicer KM, Wise WC, Halushka PV: Effect of leukotriene receptor antagonists on vascular permeability during endotoxic shock. *Circ Shock* 32:209–218, 1990.
189. Rogers F, Dunn R, Nolan P, Phunangsab A, Barrett J: Diethylcarbamazine, a leukotriene inhibitor, improves survival of endotoxemia in the rat. *Circ Shock* 16:52–57, 1985.
190. Cook JA, Wise WC, Halushka PV: Protective effect of a leukotriene antagonist in endotoxic shock. *J Pharmacol Exp Ther* 235:470–474, 1985.
191. Etemadi AR, Temple GE, Farah BA, Wise WC, Halushka PV, Cook JA: Beneficial effects of a leukotriene antagonist on endotoxin-induced acute hemodynamic alterations. *Circ Shock* 22:55–63, 1987.
192. Gross D, Dahan JB, Landau EH, Krausz MM: Effect of leukotriene inhibitor LY-171883 on the pulmonary response to *Escherichia coli* endotoxemia. *Crit Care Med* 18:190–197, 1990.
193. Coggeshall JW, Christman BW, Lefferts PL, Serafin WE, Blair IA, Buttersfield MJ, Snapper JR: Effect of inhibition of 5-lipoxygenase metabolism of arachidonic acid on response to endotoxemia in sheep. *J Appl Physiol* 65:1351–1359, 1988.
194. Young JS, Passmore JC: Hemodynamic and renal advantages of dual cyclooxygenase and leukotriene blockade during canine endotoxic shock. *Circ Shock* 32:243–255, 1990.
195. Olson NC, Kruse-Elliott KT, Johnson L: Effect of LY171883 on endotoxin-induced lung injury in pigs. *J Appl Physiol* 69:1315–1322, 1990.
196. Fink MP, Kruithoff KL, Antonsson JB, Wang H, Rothschild HR: Delayed treatment with an LTD_4/LTE_4 antagonist limits pulmonary edema in endotoxic pigs. *Am J Physiol* 260:R1007–R1013, 1991.
197. Turner CR, Lackey MN, Quinlan MF, Griswold DE, Schwartz LW, Wheeldon EB: Therapeutic intervention in a rat model of adult respiratory distress syndrome. II. Lipoxygenase pathway inhibition. *Circ Shock* 34:263–269, 1991.
198. Li EJ, Cook JA, Wise WC, Jackson WT, Halushka PV: Effect of LTB_4 receptor antagonists in endotoxin shock in the rat. *Circ Shock* 34:385–392, 1991.
199. Klausner JM, Paterson IS, Valeri CR, Shepro D, Hechtman HB: Limb ischemia-induced increase in permeability is mediated by leukocytes and leukotrienes. *Ann Surg* 208:755–760, 1988.
200. Anner H, Kaufman RP, Kobzik L, Valeri CR, Shepro D, Hechtman HB: Pulmonary leukosequestration induced by hind limb ischemia. *Ann Surg* 206:162–167, 1987.
201. Klausner JM, Paterson IS, Kobzik L, Valeri CR, Shepro D, Hechtman HB: Leukotrienes but not complement mediate limb ischemia-induced lung injury. *Ann Surg* 209:462–470, 1989.
202. Goldman G, Welbourn R, Paterson IS, Klausner JM, Kobzik L, Valeri CR, Shepro D, Hechtman HB: Ischemia-induced neutrophil activation and diapedesis is lipoxygenase dependent. *Surgery* 107:428–433, 1990.
203. Klausner JM, Goldman G, Skornick Y, Valeri R, Inbar M, Shepro D, Hechtman HB: Interleukin-2-induced lung permeability is mediated by leukotriene B_4. *Cancer* 66:2357–2364, 1990.
204. Wollert PS, Menconi MJ, O'Sullivan BP, Wang H, Larkin V, Fink MP: LY255283, a novel leukotriene B_4 receptor antagonist, limits activation of neutrophils and prevents acute lung injury induced by endotoxin in pigs. *Surgery* 114:191–198, 1993.
205. Hanahan DJ: Platelet activating factor: abiologically active phosphoglyceride. *Ann Rev Biochem* 55:483–509, 1986.
206. Caplan MS, Sun X-A, Hsueh W: Hypoxia causes ischemic bowel necrosis in rats: the role of platelet-activating factor (PAF-acether). *Gastroenterology* 99:979–986, 1990.
207. Miwa M, Hill C, Kumar R, Sugatani J, Olson ML, Hanahan DJ: Occurrence of an endogenous inhibitor of platelet activating factor in rat liver. *J Biol Chem* 262:527–530, 1987.
208. Nakayama R, Yasuda K, Saito K: Existence of endogenous inhibitors of platelet-activating factor (PAF) with PAF in rat uterus. *J Biol Chem* 262:13174–13179, 1987.
209. Benveniste J, Nunez D, Duriez P, Korth R, Bidault J, Frutchard JC: Preformed PAF-acether and lyso-PAF acether are bound to blood lipoproteins. *FEBS Lett* 226:371–376, 1988.
210. Diez FL, Nieto ML, Fernandez-Gallardo S, Gijon MA, Crespo MS: Occupancy of platelet receptors for platelet-activating factor in patients with septicemia. *J Clin Invest* 83:1733–1740, 1989.
211. Pittman JM III, Thurman GW, Anderson BO, Ketch LL, Hartford CE, Harken AH, Ambruso DR: WEB2170, a specific platelet-activating factor antagonist, attenuates neutrophil priming by human serum after clinical burn injury. *J Burn Care Rehabil* 12:411–419, 1991.
212. Doebber TW, Wu MS, Robbins JC, Choy BM, Chang MN, Shen TY: Platelet activating factor (PAF) involvement in endotoxin-induced hypotension in rats. Studies with PAF-receptor antagonist kadsurenone. *Biochem Biophys Res Commun* 127:799–808, 1985.
213. Chang S-W, Feddersen CO, Henson PM, Voelkel NF: Platelet-activating factor mediates hemodynamic changes and lung injury in endotoxin-treated rats. *J Clin Invest* 79:1498–1509, 1987.
214. Hsueh W, Gonzalez-Crussi F, Arroyave JL: Platelet-activating factor: an endogenous mediator for bowel necrosis in endotoxemia. *FASEB J* 1:403–405, 1987.
215. Stahl GL, Craft DV, Lento PH, Lefer AM: Detection of platelet-activating factor during traumatic shock. *Circ Shock* 26:237–244, 1988.
216. Sun X-M, Hsueh W: Bowel necrosis induced by tumor necrosis factor in rats is mediated by platelet-activating factor. *J Clin Invest* 81:1328–1331, 1988.
217. Dobrowsky RT, Voyksner RD, Olson NC: Effect of SRI 63-675 on hemodynamics and blood PAF levels during porcine endotoxemia. *Am J Physiol* 260:H1455–H1465, 1991.
218. Christman BW, Lefferts PL, King GA, Snapper JR: Role of circulating platelets and granulocytes in PAF-induced pulmonary dysfunction in awake sheep. *J Appl Physiol* 64:2033–2041, 1988.
219. Lang CH, Dobrescu C, Hargrove DM, Bagby GJ, Spitzer JJ: Platelet-activating factor-induced increases in glucose kinetics. *Am J Physiol* 254:E193–E200, 1988.
220. Sirois MG, Jancar S, Braquet P, Plante GE, Sirois P: PAF increases vascular permeability in selected tissues: effect of BN-52021 and L-655,240. *Prostaglandins* 36:631–644, 1988.
221. Smallbone BW, Taylor NE, McDonald JWD: Effects of L-655,731, a platelet-activating factor (PAF) receptor antagonist, on PAF- and complement-induced pulmonary hypertension in sheep. *J Pharmacol Exp Ther* 242:1035–1040, 1987.
222. Kubes P, Suzuki M, Granger DN: Modulation of PAF-induced leukocyte adherence and increased microvascular permeability. *Am J Physiol* 259:G859–G864, 1990.
223. Salzer WL, McCall CE: Primed stimulation of isolated perfused rabbit lung by endotoxin and platelet activating factor induces enhanced production of thromboxane and lung injury. *J Clin Invest* 85:1135–1143, 1990.
224. Rabinovici R, Esser KM, Lysko PG, Yue T-L, Griswold DE, Hillegass LM, Bugelski PJ, Hallenbeck JM, Feuerstein G: Priming by platelet-activating factor of endotoxin-induced lung injury and cardiovascular shock. *Circ Res* 69:12–25, 1991.
225. Gonzalez-Crussi F, Hsueh W: Experimental model of ischemia bowel necrosis. The role of platelet-activating factor and endotoxin. *Am J Pathol* 112:127–135, 1983.
226. Chang S-W, Fernyak S, Voelkel NF: Beneficial effect of a platelet-activating factor antagonist, WEB 2086, on endotoxin-induced lung injury. *Am J Physiol* 258:H153–H158, 1990.
227. Olson NC, Joyce PB, Fleisher LN: Role of platelet-activating factor and eicosanoids during endotoxin-induced lung injury in pigs. *Am J Physiol* H1674–H1686, 1990.
228. Casals-Stenzel J: Protective effect of WEB 2086, a novel antagonist of platelet activating factor, in endotoxic shock. *Eur J Pharmacol* 135:117–122, 1987.

229. Terashita Z-I, Kawamura M, Takatani M, Tshushima S, Imura Y, Nishikawa K: Beneficial effects of TCV-309, a novel potent and selective platelet activating factor antagonist in endotoxin and anaphylactic shock in rodents. *J Pharmacol Exp Ther* 260:748–755, 1992.
230. Fletcher JR, DiSimone AG, Earnest MA: Platelet activating factor receptor antagonist improves survival and attenuates eicosanoid release in severe endotoxemia. *Ann Surg* 211:312–316, 1990.
231. Moore JM, Earnest MA, DiSimone AG, Abumrad NN, Fletcher JR: A PAF receptor antagonist, BN 52021, attenuates thromboxane release and improves survival in lethal canine endotoxemia. *Circ Shock* 31:53–59, 1991.
232. Yue T-L, Farhat M, Rabinovici R, Perera PY, Vogel SN, Feuerstein G: Protective effect of BN 50739, a new platelet-activating factor antagonist, in endotoxin-treated rabbits. *J Pharmacol Exp Ther* 254:976–981, 1990.
233. Siebeck M, Weipert J, Keser C, Kohl J, Spannagl M, Machleidt W, Schweiberer L: A triazolodiazepine platelet activating factor receptor antagonist (WEB 2086) reduces pulmonary dysfunction during endotoxin shock in swine. *J Trauma* 31:942–950, 1991.
234. Christman BW, Lefferts PL, Blair IA, Snapper JR: Effect of platelet-activating factor receptor antagonism on endotoxin-induced lung dysfunction in awake sheep. *Am Rev Respir Dis* 142:1272–1278, 1990.
235. Byrne K, Sessler CN, Carey PD, Sielaff TD, Vasquez A, Tatum JL, Hirsch JI, Sugerman HJ: Platelet-activating factor in porcine *Pseudomonas* acute lung injury. *J Surg Res* 50:111–118, 1991.
236. Sessler CN, Glauser FL, Davis D, Fowler AA III: Effects of platelet-activating factor antagonist SRI 63-441 on endotoxemia in sheep. *J Appl Physiol* 65:2624–2631, 1988.
237. Chang S-W, Ohara N, Kuo G, Voelkel NF: Tumor necrosis factor-induced lung injury is not mediated by platelet-activating factor. *Am J Physiol* 257:L232–L239, 1989.
238. Baum TD, Heard SO, Feldman HS, Latka CA, Fink MP: Endotoxin-induced myocardial depression in rats: effect of ibuprofen and SDZ 64-688, a platelet activating factor receptor antagonist. *J Surg Res* 48:629–634, 1990.
239. Hamberg M, Samuelsson B: On the metabolism of prostaglandins E_1 and E_2 in man. *J Biol Chem* 246:6713–6721, 1971.
240. Lewis PJ, Dollery CT: Clinical pharmacology and potential of prostacyclin. *Br Med Bull* 39:281–284, 1983.
241. Appel PL, Shoemaker WC, Kram HB: Effects of prostaglandin E_1 in postoperative surgical patients with circulatory deficiency. *Chest* 99:945–950, 1991.
242. Sinzinger H, Reiter R: The intrafusion platelet rebound during and following PGE_1-infusion is faster and more intensive than that with PGI_2. *Prostaglandins Leukot Med* 13:281–288, 1984.
243. Fletcher JR, Ramwell PW: The effects of prostacyclin (PGI_2) on endotoxin shock and endotoxin-induced platelet aggregation in dogs. *Circ Shock* 7:299–308, 1980.
244. Krausz MM, Utsunomiya T, Feuerstein G, Wolfe JHN, Shepro D, Hechtman HB: Prostacyclin reversal of lethal endotoxemia in dogs. *J Clin Invest* 67:1118–1125, 1981.
245. Demling RH, Smith M, Gunther R, Gee M, Flynn J: The effect of prostacyclin infusion on endotoxin-induced lung injury. *Surgery* 89:257–263, 1981.
246. Modig J, Samuelsson T, Sandin R: Treatment with prostaglandin E_1 in a porcine model of early adult respiratory distress syndrome. *Acta Chir Scand* 152:569–575, 1986.
247. Brigham KL, Serafin W, Zadoff A, Blair I, Meyrick B, Oates JA: Prostaglandin E_1 attenuation of sheep lung responses to endotoxin. *J Appl Physiol* 64:2568–2574, 1988.
248. Marini CP, Woloszyn T, Coons M, Tachmes L, Nathan I, Cunningham JN, Jacobowitz IJ: Efficacy of right atrial infusion of PGE_1 in sepsis-induced pulmonary hypertension. *J Surg Res* 49:476–482, 1990.
249. Smith ME, Gunther R, Zaiss C, Demling RH: Prostaglandin infusion and endotoxin-induced lung injury. *Arch Surg* 117:175–180, 1982.
250. Gee MH, Tahamont MV, Flynn JT, Cox JW, Pullen RH, Andreadis NA: Prostaglandin E_1 prevents increased lung microvascular permeability during intravascular complement activation in sheep. *Circ Res* 61:420–428, 1987.
251. Smith EF III, Temple GE, Wise WC, Halushka PV, Cook JA: Experimental endotoxemia in the rat: efficacy of prostacyclin or the prostacyclin analog Iloprost. *Circ Shock* 16:1–7, 1985.
252. Waymack JP, Moldawer LL, Lowry SF, Guzman RF, Okerberg CV, Mason AD Jr, Pruitt BA Jr: Effect of prostaglandin E in multiple experimental models. IV. Effect on resistance to endotoxin and tumor necrosis factor shock. *J Surg Res* 49:328–332, 1990.
253. Schneider J, Matthiesen T: The prostacyclin analogue taprostene and recombinant human superoxide dismutase increase the permanent survival rate of endotoxemic rats. *Life Sci* 46:1421–1426, 1990.
254. Bolliger C, Fourie P, Coetzee A: The effect of prostaglandin E_1 on acute pulmonary artery hypertension during oleic acid-induced respiratory dysfunction. *Chest* 99:1501–1506, 1991.
255. Devitt HH, Burka JF, Jones R, Amy RWM, King EG: Hemodynamic and pathologic effects of prostacyclin on oleic acid-induced pulmonary injury. *Surgery* 103:213–220, 1988.
256. Steinberg SM, Dehring DJ, Gower WR, Vento JM, Lowery BD, Cloutier CT: Prostacyclin in experimental septic acute respiratory failure. *J Surg Res* 34:298–302, 1983.
257. Downey GP, Gumbay RS, Doherty DE, LaBrecque JF, Henson JE, Henson PM, Worthen GS: Enhancement of pulmonary inflammation by PGE_2: evidence for a vasodilator effect. *J Appl Physiol* 64:728–741, 1988.
258. Henson PM, Larson GL, Webster RO, Mitchell BC, Goins AJ, Henson JE: Pulmonary microvascular alterations and injury induced by complement fragments: synergistic effect of complement activation, neutrophil activation, neutrophil sequestration, and prostaglandins. *Ann NY Acad Sci* 384:287–300, 1982.
259. Brockmann DC, Stevens JH, O'Hanley P, Shapiro J, Walker C, Mihm FG, Collins JA, Raffin TA: The effects of prostaglandin E_1 on the adult respiratory distress syndrome in septic primates. *Am Rev Respir Dis* 134:885–890, 1986.
260. Hageman JR, Lee SE, Zemaitis J, Smith LJ, Hunt CE: Prostaglandin E infusion fails to prevent hyperoxic lung injury in adult rabbits. *Crit Care Med* 17:339–344, 1989.
261. Dervin G, Calvin JE: Role of prostaglandin E_1 in reducing pulmonary vascular resistance in an experimental model of acute lung injury. *Crit Care Med* 18:1129–1133, 1990.
262. Holcroft JW, Vassar MJ, Weber CJ: Prostaglandin E_1 and survival in patients with the adult respiratory distress syndrome. A prospective trial. *Ann Surg* 203:371–378, 1986.
263. Bone RC, Slotman G, Maunder R, Silverman H, Hyers TM, Kerstein MD, Ursprung JJ, and the Prostaglandin E_1 Study Group: Randomized double-blind, multicenter study of prostaglandin E_1 in patients with the adult respiratory distress syndrome. *Chest* 96:114–119, 1989.
264. Vassar MJ, Fletcher MP, Perry CA, Holcroft JW: Evaluation of prostaglandin E_1 for prevention of respiratory failure in high risk trauma patients: a prospective clinical trial and correlation with plasma suppressive factors for neutrophil activation. *Prostaglandins Leukot Essent Fatty Acids* 44:223–231, 1991.
265. Radermacher P, Santak B, Becker H, Falke KJ: Prostaglandin E_1 and nitroglycerin reduce pulmonary capillary pressure but worsen ventilation-perfusion distributions in patients with adult respiratory distress syndrome. *Anesthesiology* 70:601–606, 1989.
266. Radermacher P, Santak B, Wust HJ, Tarnow J, Falke KJ: Prostacyclin for the treatment of pulmonary hypertension in the adult respiratory distress syndrome: effects on pulmonary capillary pressure and ventilation-perfusion distributions. *Anesthesiology* 72:238–244, 1990.
267. Radermacher P, Santak B, Wust HJ, Falke KJ: Prostacyclin and right ventricular function in patients with pulmonary hypertension associated with ARDS. *Intensive Care Med* 16:227–232, 1990.
268. Melot C, Lejeune P, Leeman M, Moraine J-J, Naeije R: Prostaglandin E_1 in the adult respiratory distress syndrome: benefit for pulmonary hypertension and cost for pulmonary gas exchange. *Am Rev Respir Dis* 139:106–110, 1989.
269. Shoemaker WC, Appel PL: Effects of prostaglandin E_1 in adult respiratory distress syndrome. *Surgery* 99:275–283, 1986.
270. Tokioka H, Kobayashi O, Ohta Y, Wakabayashi T, Kosaka F: The acute effects of prostaglandin E_1 on the pulmonary circulation and oxygen delivery in patients with the adult respiratory distress syndrome. *Intensive Care Med* 11:61–64, 1985.
271. Russell JA, Ronco JJ, Dodek PM: Physiologic effects and side effects of prostaglandin E_1 in the adult respiratory distress syndrome. *Chest* 97:984–992, 1990.
272. Silverman HJ, Slotman G, Bone RC, Maunder R, Hyers TM, Kerstein MD, Ursprung JJ, and the Prostaglandin E_1 Study Group: Effects of prostaglandin E_1 on oxygen delivery and consumption in patients with the adult respiratory distress syndrome. Results from the prostaglandin E_1 multicenter trial. *Chest* 98:405–410, 1990.
273. Bihari D, Smithies M, Gimson A, Tinker J: The effects of vasodilation with prostacyclin on oxygen delivery and uptake in critically ill patients. *N Engl J Med* 317:397–403, 1987.
274. Rossignon M-D, Khayat D, Royer C, Rouby J-J, Jacquillat C, Viars P: Functional and metabolic activity of polymorphonuclear leukocytes from patients with adult respiratory distress syndrome: results of a randomized double-blind placebo-controlled study on the activity of prostaglandin E_1. *Anesthesiology* 72:276–281, 1990.
275. Long WA, Rubin LJ: Prostacyclin and PGE_1 treatment of pulmonary hypertension. *Am Rev Respir Dis* 136:773–776, 1987.
276. Palevsky HI, Long W, Crow J, Fishman AP: Prostacyclin and acetylcholine as screening agents for acute pulmonary vasodilator responsiveness in primary pulmonary hypertension. *Circulation* 82:2018–2026, 1990.
277. Higenbottam T: The place of prostacyclin in the clinical management of primary pulmonary hypertension. *Am Rev Respir Dis* 136:782–785, 1987.
278. Sakaguchi K, Tanaka N, Sawada N, Araki Y, Fujita K: Vasodilator therapy for right ventricular failure. *Jpn Circ J* 48:357–364, 1984.
279. Naeije R, Melot C, Mols P, Hallemans R: Reduction in pulmonary hypertension by prostaglandin E_1 in decompensated chronic obstructive pulmonary disease. *Am Rev Respir Dis* 125:1–5, 1982.
280. D'Ambra MN, LaRaia PJ, Philbin DM, Watkins WD, Hilgenber AD, Buckley MJ: Prostaglandin E_1. A new therapy for refractory right heart failure and pulmonary hypertension after mitral valve replacement. *J Thorac Cardiovasc Surg* 89:567–572, 1985.
281. Esmore DS, Spratt PM, Branch JM, Keogh AM, Lee RP, Farnsworth AE, Shanahan MX, Chang VP: Right ventricular assist and prostacyclin infusion for allograft failure in the presence of high pulmonary vascular resistance. *J Heart Transplant* 9:136–141, 1990.
282. Whitman GJR, Martel D, Weiss M, Pochanapring A, See WM, Hopeman A, Harken AH, Dauber IM: Reversal of protamine-induced catastrophic pulmonary vasoconstriction by prostaglandin E_1. *Ann Thoracic Surg* 50:303–305, 1990.
283. Bush A, Busst C, Knight WB, Shinebourne EA: Modification of pulmonary hypertension secondary to congenital heart disease by prostacyclin therapy. *Am Rev Respir Dis* 136:767–769, 1987.
284. Kermode J, Butt W, Shann F: Comparison between prostaglandin E_1 and epoprostenol (prostacyclin) in infants after heart surgery. *Br Heart J* 66:175–178, 1991.
285. Aren C, Feddersen K, Radegran K: Effects of prostacyclin infusion on platelet activation and postoperative blood loss in coronary bypass. *Ann Thoracic Surg* 36:49–54, 1983.
286. Fish KJ, Sarnquist FH, van Steennis C, Mitchell RS, Hilberman M, Jamieson SW, Linet OI, Miller DC: A prospective, randomized study of the effects of prostacyclin on platelets and blood loss during coronary bypass operations. *J Thoracic Cardiovasc Surg* 91:436–442, 1986.
287. Addonizio VP, Fisher CA, Kappa JR, Ellison N: Prevention of heparin-induced thrombocytopenia during open heart surgery with iloprost (ZK36374). *Surgery* 102:796–807, 1987.
288. Miller TA: Protective effects of prostaglandins against gastric mucosal damage: current knowledge and proposed mechanisms. *Am J Physiol* 245:G601–G623, 1983.

289. Victor BE, Schmidt KL, Smith GS, Reed RL, Thompson DA, Miller TA: Prostaglandin-induced gastric mucosal protection against stress injury. Absence of a relationship to tissue glutathione levels. *Ann Surg* 209:289–296, 1989.

290. Mahatma M, Agrawal N, Dajani EZ, Nelson S, Nakamura C, Sitton J: Misoprostol but not antacid prevents endotoxin-induced gastric mucosal injury: role of tumor necrosis factor alpha. *Dig Dis Sci* 36:1562–1568, 1991.

291. Penston JG, Wormsley KB: Histamine H$_2$-receptor antagonists versus prostaglandins in the treatment of peptic ulcer disease. *Drugs* 37:391–401, 1989.

292. Bianchi Porro G, Parente F: Side effects of anti-ulcer prostaglandins: an overview of the worldwide clinical experience. *Scand J Gastroenterol* 1989; 24(suppl 164):224–231, 1989.

293. Lam SK, Lau Wy, Choi TK, Lai CL, Lok ASF, et al: Prostaglandin E$_1$ (misoprostol) overcomes the adverse effect of chronic cigarette smoking on duodenal ulcer healing. *Dig Dis Sci* 31(suppl 2):68S–74S, 1986.

294. Newman RD, Gitlin N, Lacayo EJ, Safdi AV, Ramsey EJ, et al: Misoprostol in the treatment of duodenal ulcer refractory to H$_2$-blocker therapy: a placebo-controlled, multicenter, double-blind, randomized trial. *Am J Med* 83(suppl 1A):27–31, 1987.

295. Graham DY, Agrawal NM, Roth S: Prevention of NSAID-induced gastric ulcer with misoprotol: multicentre, double-blind placebo-controlled trial. *Lancet* 2:1277–1280, 1988.

296. Lanza FL: A double-blind placebo-controlled endoscopic comparison of the mucosal protective effects of misoprostol versus cimetidine on tolmetin-induced mucosal injury to the stomach and duodenum. *Gastroenterology* 95:289–294, 1988.

297. Skillman JJ, Lisbon A, Long PC, Silen W: 15(R)-15-methyl prostaglandin E$_2$ does not prevent gastrointestinal bleeding in seriously ill patients. *Am J Surg* 147:451–455, 1984.

298. van Essen HA, van Blankenstein M, Wilson P, van den Berg B, Bruining HA: Intragastric prostaglandin E2 and the prevention of gastrointestinal hemorrhage in ICU patients. *Crit Care Med* 13:957–960, 1985.

299. Zinner MJ, Rypins EB, Martin LR, Jonasson O, Hoover EL, Swab EA, Fakouhi TD: Misoprostol versus antacid for preventing stress ulcers in postoperative surgical ICU patients. *Ann Surg* 210:590–595, 1989.

300. Martin LF, Booth FVM, Reines HD, Deysach LG, Kochman RL, Erhardt LJ, Geis GS: Stress ulcers and organ failure in intubated patients in surgical intensive care units. *Ann Surg* 215:332–337, 1992.

301. Arroyo V, Bosch J, Mauri F, Rivera F, Navarro-Lopez F, Rodes J: Effect of angiotensin-II blockade on systemic and hepatic hemodynamics and on the renin-angiotensin system in cirrhosis. *Eur J Clin Invest* ll:221–229, 1981.

302. Rimola A, Gines P, Arroyo V, et al: Urinary excretion of 6-keto-prostaglandin-F$_l$, thromboxane A$_2$ and prostaglandin E$_2$ in cirrhosis with ascites: relationship with functional renal failure (the hepatorenal syndrome). *J Hepatol* 3:111–117, 1986.

303. Arief AI, Chidsey CA: Renal function in cirrhosis and the effects of prostaglandin A. *Am J Med* 56:695–703, 1974.

304. Zussman RM, Axelrod L, Tolkoff-Rubin N: The treatment of hepatorenal syndrome with intrarenal administration of prostaglandin E$_1$. *Prostaglandins* 13:8l9–830, 1977.

305. Arroyo V, Gines P: Prostaglandins and the treatment of hepatorenal syndrome in cirrhosis. *J Hepatol* 11:142–144, 1990.

306. Fevery J, Van Cutsem E, Nevens F, Van Steenbergen W, Verberckmoes R, De Groote J: Reversal of hepatorenal syndrome in 4 patients by peroral misoprostol (prostaglandin E$_1$-analogue) and albumin administration. *J Hepatol* 11:153–158, 1990.

CHAPTER 53

Anterior Pituitary Hormones and Critical Illnesses

JOHN W. HOLADAY, Ph.D., F.C.C.M.

INTRODUCTION

Many of the body's own powerful and selective "drugs" derive from the anterior pituitary gland and its primary regulatory structure in the brain, the hypothalamus. In response to neural, humoral, and inflammatory influences, this endogenous "medicine chest" releases a number of peptide hormones, including adrenocorticotropic hormone (ACTH), β-endorphin (BEP), thyroid stimulating hormone (TSH), prolactin, growth hormone (GH), follicle stimulating hormone (FSH) and luteinizing hormone (LH). Each of these neuroendocrine hormones plays an important role in orchestrating growth, reproduction, and metabolism, essential bodily functions that are affected by stress and disease. Adaptation to the chronic stress of critical illnesses involves significant changes in the regulation of neuroendocrine function within the brain, pituitary, and target glands. For example, chronic stress results in the sustained elevation of circulating ACTH, BEP, and glucocorticoids, whereas the secretion of gonadotropins (FSH and LH), TSH, prolactin, and GH in the plasma is often reduced (1). During shock and trauma, changes in circulating levels of these hormones may profoundly affect function at the cellular, tissue, or organismal level.

In addition to the peptide hormones of the neuroendocrine system, it is becoming increasingly evident that within the immunological network, peptide cytokines such as the interleukins (IL-1, IL-2, and IL-6), tumor necrosis factor (TNF), interferon-α and -γ (IF-α and IF-γ) and other mediators of the immune system play important roles in modulating assaults on

homeostasis brought about by trauma, infection, shock, and systemic inflammatory response syndromes. Although cytokines frequently are thought of as predominantly "local" messengers that transmit information among nearby cells, at varying times after the initiation of infection, shock, or trauma, circulating levels of these cytokines in the bloodstream may be increased or decreased in a manner that is correlated with the severity of critical illnesses (2, 3).

During the past decade, it has become apparent that many of these hormones and cytokines communicate within the brain, endocrine, and immune system network, collectively termed the "neuroendocrine-immune axis." As biological messengers, these peptide hormones and cytokines share many common targets throughout the body; furthermore, many of the hormones classically attributed to an endocrine origin may also be found in lymphocytes, and many cytokines are found in neuroendocrine networks (see below). Regardless of their origin, the body's own endocrine/immune "drugs" have both therapeutic and toxic effects. As with any drug, their actions may be beneficial (homeostatic) or detrimental (dyshomeostatic), depending on the timing and circumstances of their release.

This chapter initially focuses on specific examples of neuroendocrine-immune interactions as they affect the body's physiologic and pharmacologic responses, with emphasis on the relevance of this network to the pathophysiology and treatment of critical illnesses. In addition, the potential role of endogenous opioids (endorphins) in the pathogenesis of circulatory shock and central nervous system trauma is reviewed,

890

along with a current perspective on the therapeutic effects of naloxone (Narcan) in treating these disorders. The author asks the reader's indulgence, since the primary examples cited in this chapter evolved from the work of his many colleagues and collaborators and may not represent a thorough cross-section of this emerging field of biomedical research.

ANTERIOR PITUITARY HORMONE EFFECTS UPON IMMUNE FUNCTION

It is well-established that other anterior pituitary hormones may affect immunity by both direct and indirect actions. Although the immunosuppressant effects of endogenous or pharmacologically administered glucocorticoids have been known for almost half a century (4), the immunological effects of other steroid and peptide hormones are less well-established. For example, current research indicates that pituitary or lymphocyte-derived prolactin directly functions as an immuno-permissive hormone that may play a role in the rejection of transplanted organs (5) or in the exacerbation of autoimmune diseases (6, 7). Examples of these interactions are presented below.

As examples of indirect hormone actions on immune function, LH and FSH, the pituitary regulators of gonadal steroid hormones, can influence the growth of cancers of the prostate gland, testes, ovaries, and breast by their actions on the release of estrogen, progesterone, and testosterone. Dyhydroepiandrosterone (DHEA), a steroid hormone also under the regulation of LH and FSH, has also received attention as an immunoregulatory substance (8). Although these hormones are of significant immunologic importance, the effects of LH, FSH, and their target steroid hormones on critical illnesses are beyond the scope of this review.

GLUCOCORTICOIDS

The neuroendocrine regulation of glucocorticoid (e.g., cortisol) release involves an orchestration of events in the brain, anterior pituitary gland, and adrenal gland, collectively referred to as the hypothalamic-pituitary-adrenal (HPA) axis. Activation of this HPA system by stress initiates a sequence of events, including the hypothalamic release of corticotropin-releasing hormone (CRH) that then activates the anterior pituitary gland to result in the release of ACTH and its sister hormone, BEP. Subsequently, ACTH stimulates the adrenal cortex to release adrenal glucocorticoids such as cortisol (or corticosterone, depending upon the species). To turn off this system, the physiologic secretion (or pharmacologic administration) of glucocorticoids into the circulation feeds back upon the brain and pituitary glands to inhibit the further release of CRH, ACTH, and cortisol. In homeostatic conditions, circulating cortisol levels are maintained within physiologic limits by this feedback network. Rhythmic, circadian fluctuations of the HPA hormones result in increased cortisol concentrations in the morning, with cortisol levels subsequently declining throughout the day and night (9).

In the practice of critical care medicine, patients experience sustained increases of glucocorticoid levels due to (*a*) the effects of chronic stress on the HPA axis, as well as (*b*) the pharmacologic use of "steroids" for the treatment of disorders such as sepsis, stroke, inflammation, organ transplantation, or chronic autoimmune diseases. In these circumstances, high concentrations of glucocorticoids profoundly alter immunologic and inflammatory responses. At the leukocyte level, glucocorticoids block macrophage IL-1 and TNF release, block the inflammatory actions of IL-1, and decrease γ-interferon and IL-2 release by T-lymphocytes (10). These effects result in an impairment of both cellular and humoral immunity (Fig. 53.1).

In addition to these effects, glucocorticoids may have other, less well-recognized consequences. For example, disruption of the normal pattern of circadian cortisol rhythms brought about by the "around-the-clock" management of critical illnesses, or by the pharmacologic use of glucocorticoids, may well contribute to a disruption of the circadian pattern of lymphocyte counts and other measures of immune function influenced by this hormone and therefore compromise our interpretation of "normal" laboratory values. Thus, the cascade of immunologic responses affected by glucocorticoids provides one example of the strong influence exerted by the neuroendocrine system on host defenses (4, 11, 12).

PROLACTIN

Prolactin and growth hormone are members of a superfamily of related hormones, including proliferin, placental lactogen, and others, that share some structural similarities and biologic actions (11). As with the HPA axis and the regulation of adrenal glucocorticoids, the physiologic release of prolactin and growth hormone from the anterior pituitary fluctuates in a pulsatile, circadian fashion and is further modulated by behavioral and environmental stimuli, the reproductive cycle, steroid hormones, neurotransmitters, immunoregulatory cytokines, and various drugs (11).

The mechanisms mediating the neuroendocrine regulation of prolactin release are well-known. Prolactin secretion is tonically inhibited by the release of dopamine from the hypothalamus (or by the pharmacologic use of dopamine or dopaminergic drugs). Dopamine then acts upon dopamine-2 (DA-2) receptors located on lactotroph cells of the anterior pituitary to shut down prolactin secretion. The opposite effect occurs when dopamine antagonists, such as metoclopramide (Reglan) or haloperidol (Haldol), are used; the tonic inhibition of prolactin release is removed, resulting in prompt prolactin secretion. Prolactin, like all neuroendocrine hormones, is also altered by stress; sustained stress greatly inhibits prolactin secretion and blunts prolactin release in response to subsequent stimuli acting at a suprapituitary level (e.g., the superimposition of an acute stress or the pharmacological use of opiates) (1, 11, 12).

Although prolactin classically has been associated exclusively with lactation, prolactin subserves several additional physiologic functions, including profound effects upon the immune system. The potential importance of prolactin in immune function was first reported by Nagy et al (13), who demonstrated that either hypophysectomy or the drug bromocriptine (Parlodel), a DA-2 agonist that inhibits prolactin secretion, was shown to suppress antibody formation in a prolactin-reversible manner. The author's laboratories have extended these early findings through studies demonstrating that bromocriptine-induced hypoprolactinemia in mice results in a

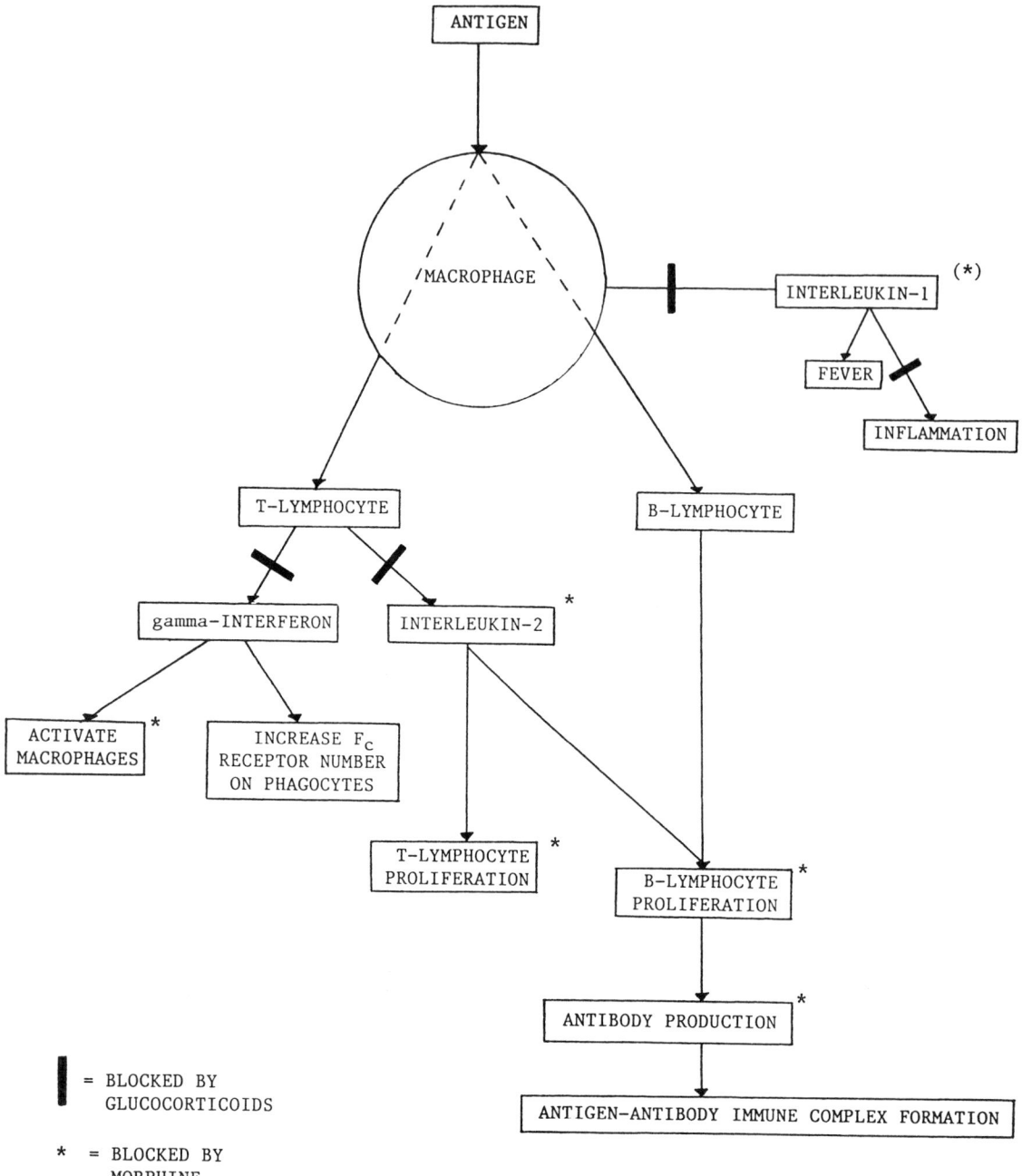

Figure 53.1.   Schematic representation of the sites of action of glucocorticoids on various aspects of immune function. The immunologic pathways that are blocked by glucocorticoids are represented by a bar. (For additional information, see reference 75.) (Reprinted with permission from Bryant HU, Bernton EW, Holaday JW: Immunomodulatory effects of chronic morphine treatment: pharmacologic and mechanistic studies. *Natl Inst Drug Abuse Monogr* 96:131–149, 1990.)

variety of immunologic effects that include (*a*) abrogation of T-lymphocyte-dependent activation of macrophages, as well as the production of lymphocyte-derived macrophage activating factor (IF-γ) following inoculation with *Listeria monocytogenes* or *Mycobacterium bovis* (strain BCG), (*b*) suppression of T-lymphocyte proliferation without affecting the production of interleukin-2, and (*c*) increased lethality of an infectious challenge with *L. monocytogenes* (14). All of the immunologic changes produced by bromocriptine were prevented by coincident administration of ovine prolactin, indicating that hypoprolactinemia played a causal role (14).

Unlike hypoprolactinemia, the stimulation of prolactin release (hyperprolactinemia) resulting from the administration of dopamine antagonists such as metoclopramide (Reglan) reverses many measures of immunosuppression brought about by cyclosporine, glucocorticoids, or chronic morphine treatment in mice (11, 12). Early work from the author's laboratories has been reinforced by more recent work by Mukherjee et al (15), who have shown that prolactin induces IL-2 receptors on rat splenic lymphocytes, and Clevenger et al (16), who have demonstrated a requirement of nuclear prolactin for IL-2 stimulation of T-lymphocyte proliferation. Taken together,

Dopamine Patients

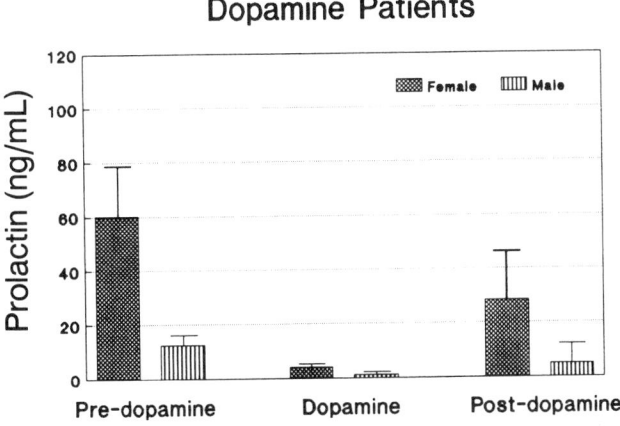

Control Patients

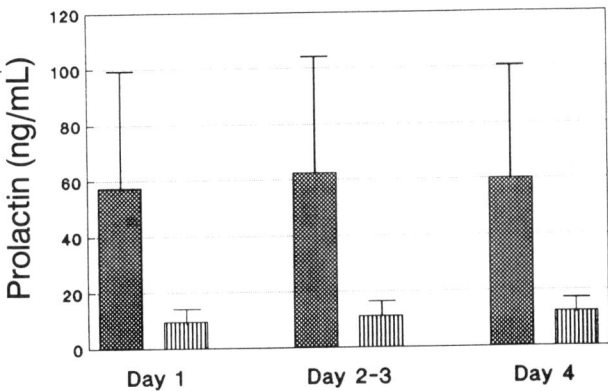

Figure 53.2. Serum prolactin levels in patients who received dopamine (*top*) (>5 μg/kg/min) (19) or control patients (*bottom*). As observed in mice (14), dopamine agonists significantly depressed circulating prolactin levels. Data are presented separately for males and females; vertical bars represent ±1 SD (19). (Reprinted with permission from Devins SS, Miller A, Herndon BL, et al: The effects of dopamine on T-cell proliferative response and serum prolactin in critically ill patients. *Crit Care Med* 20:1644–1649, 1992.

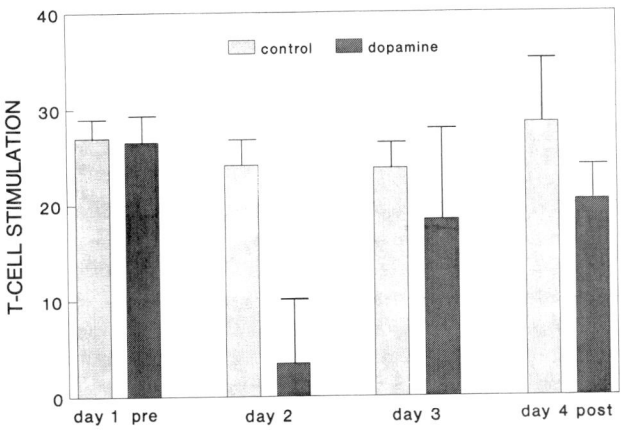

Figure 53.3. T-cell stimulation by the mitogen Concanavalin A in peripheral polymorphonuclear leukocytes obtained from patients receiving dopamine ($N = 6$) or in a similar patient population who did not receive dopamine (control; $N = 6$). As in animal studies using mice (14), dopamine or a dopamine agonist significantly depressed prolactin levels (Fig. 53.2) as well as lymphocyte proliferation, indicating a potential role for prolactin in modulating immune function. Data are presented as percent increase over unstimulated cells (19). (Reprinted with permission from Devins SS, Miller A, Herndon BL, et al: The effects of dopamine on T-cell proliferative response and serum prolactin in critically ill patients. *Crit Care Med* 20:1644–1649, 1992.)

extensive data have accumulated at the preclinical level to indicate that prolactin plays a physiologic role in modulating T-cell immunity.

Although the preclinical studies reviewed above indicate that prolactin can enhance immune function, prolactin cannot be considered to serve as an immunostimulant *per se* since pharmacologic doses of prolactin do not further enhance immune function if it is already functioning adequately (11, 17). Instead, prolactin may be an important counter-regulatory immunotropic hormone that can oppose the immunosuppression brought about by chronic stress, diseases, or medical intervention with immunosuppressive drugs such as glucocorticoids, cyclosporine, or morphine (12, 17). These observations have further importance since Russell and colleagues (18) have indicated that prolactin and cyclosporine may compete for the same binding sites on lymphocytes. Thus, the immunosuppressive actions of cyclosporine may, in part, be a consequence of its actions to inhibit prolactin's immunostimulatory effects by blocking the prolactin receptor.

Devins and colleagues recently provided evidence that the use of dopamine to improve hemodynamics in critically ill

patients results in profound hypoprolactinemia that is temporally associated with a suppression of T-cell proliferative responses (19) (Figs. 53.2 and 53.3). This very interesting clinical finding is a direct extrapolation of the aforementioned preclinical findings. From data obtained with animal experimentation, it can also be predicted that the inhibition of prolactin secretion by dopamine administration or as a result of the chronic stress of critical illnesses may, along with stress-induced increases in immunosuppressive adrenal corticosteroids, be an important co-determinant of the compromised immune function (anergy) associated with these patients.

GROWTH HORMONE

Like prolactin, GH is also affected by dopamine. Unlike prolactin, however, the effects of dopamine on GH release are stimulatory and are mediated within the hypothalamus (20). Furthermore, the hypothalamic hormone somatostatin serves to decrease GH release, whereas the release of prolactin is apparently not counter-regulated by a separate inhibitory substance. Despite these neuroendocrine differences, prolactin and GH also share some common regulatory mechanisms. The secretion of both hormones is stimulated by estrogens and inhibited by glucocorticoids (12), and in humans, both hormones are increased acutely by stress. Like prolactin, growth hormone may also play an important role in the regulation of host defenses (21, 22).

Kelley et al (23) have attempted to restore the hormonal balance in aged rats by implanting them with the prolactin and growth hormone secreting GH3 tumor line; their results indicate that the age-reduced thymic cellularity and T-cell mitogenic responses were partially reversed by this treatment. In addition to the possible positive role of prolactin in maintaining an immunohomeostatic balance, these findings may give credence to the generalized role of GH in immune function.

ENDORPHINS (ENDOGENOUS OPIATES) IN SHOCK AND TRAUMA

Three years after their discovery in 1975, the author and colleagues first proposed that endogenous opiate peptides may play a critical role in endotoxic shock (24) and other forms of critical illnesses. Since it became known that endogenous opioid peptides, including β-endorphin, were part of the HPA axis and were activated by stress, it was postulated that these "morphine-like" substances within the body could be released in excessive amounts by the severe physiologic stress of shock and trauma, resulting in a functional opiate "overdose." If this were the case, as with high doses of morphine or heroin, excess activity of the endogenous opioid system would contribute to the decreased cardiovascular function and impaired organ perfusion that characterize shock and trauma (25).

The availability of naloxone (Narcan), a competitive antagonist that selectively blocks or reverses the actions of morphine or endogenous opiates, provided an opportunity to test this hypothesis. The first several preclinical and clinical publications clearly demonstrated that naloxone, administered after the onset of shock, improved arterial pressure and other hemodynamic endpoints and, in some studies, survival (25–27). Naloxone therefore provided an inferential tool by which to suggest that the body's own endogenous opiate "painkillers" were indeed involved in the pathogenesis of endotoxic or septic shock.

Hundreds of articles and reviews have addressed the potential function of endogenous opiates and their receptors in circulatory shock resulting from endotoxemia, sepsis, hemorrhage, anaphylaxis, and neurogenic causes (25–27). Over the last few years, the scientific enthusiasm for defining the relevance of endorphins and peptides to critical illnesses has been replaced by an infatuation with studies defining the potential role of inflammatory cytokines and other potential mediators of shock and trauma. Now, we are learning that the distinctions among endocrine-derived hormones and immune-derived hormones are becoming blurred (17). Thus, it is perhaps opportune at this time to reevaluate the evidence indicating a functional role of endogenous opioids and their receptors in the pathogenesis of circulatory shock and central nervous system (CNS) trauma, emphasizing the contributions of the author and colleagues in this area, and providing an update of relevant work from other laboratories.

ENDOGENOUS OPIOID SYSTEMS

The term *"endogenous opiates"* (perhaps more correctly called *"endogenous opioids"*) serves to describe a family of different molecules, including hormonal and neurotransmitter opioid peptides as well as the recently described morphine-like molecules that are synthesized biochemically within the body. Generally speaking, there are three categories of endogenous opioid peptides—enkephalins, β-endorphin, and dynorphins—each of which derives from a distinctly different precursor molecule and each of which is characterized by distinctive patterns of distribution throughout the brain, spinal cord, the autonomic network, the endocrine system, various organs of the body, and the immune system (28).

Structurally, the first four amino acids at the "amine" end of these peptide molecules, common to all three families of endogenous opioids, are "Tyr-Gly-Gly-Phe," a sequence that is essential to their opioid-like actions. The fifth amino acid is either "Met" or "Leu," and serves to distinguish between the pentapeptide "Met-" and "Leu-" enkephalins. The remaining amino acid sequences of β-endorphin (Tyr-Gly-Gly-Phe-Met, followed by an additional 26 amino acids) and dynorphins (Try-Gly-Gly-Phe-Leu, followed by eight amino acids for dynorphin B or 12 amino acids for dynorphin A) dictate the unique pattern of pharmacological and physiological profiles that distinguishes among these endogenous opioid peptides. The "enkephalin" end of the molecule therefore provides for the "opioid" action, and the remaining amino acids on the carboxy terminus affect the differing specificities of enkephalins, endorphins, and dynorphins for the three opioid receptor types upon which they primarily act (28).

Endogenous opioid systems are compromised not only of the three different categories of opioid peptides as described above, but also of the cellular receptors to which they bind and through which they implement their biologic actions. At least five categories of opioid receptors have been characterized, among which three receptor types are most critical to endogenous opioids. None of these opioid peptides is absolutely selective for individual receptors; however, Met-enkephalin predominantly acts upon μ-receptors, Leu-enkephalin predominantly acts upon δ-receptors, β-endorphin acts upon both β- and δ-receptors, and dynorphin A or B acts predominantly upon κ-receptors. Because of the lack of absolute receptor selectivity, given adequate concentrations, these opioid peptide ligands will cross-talk with other opioid receptor types. As a further complication, evidence is also accumulating to indicate that even these three "opioid receptor" types are not biologically or biochemically distinct, but may instead be different binding surfaces that share a common macromolecular opioid receptor complex (29).

ENDOGENOUS OPIOIDS IN ENDOTOXIC AND SEPTIC SHOCK

Extensive information about the role of endogenous opioid peptides in endotoxic or septic shock has been obtained by the use of naloxone, a "universal" competitive opioid receptor antagonist that blocks or reverses opioid responses at all receptor types when adequate concentrations are used. The successful reversal of the signs of circulatory shock by naloxone has served as important inferential evidence to indicate a role of endogenous opioid systems in the pathogenesis of shock (24–28).

Endotoxic shock, resulting from the injection of lipopolysaccharide endotoxins from the cell wall of Gram-negative bacteria, is often used as an experimental model of human septic shock. Early studies involved the administration of lipopolysaccharide endotoxin, and subsequent experimentation relied upon more sophisticated animal models of sepsis, including the administration of live *Escherichia coli* or the intraperitoneal implantation of fecal pellets. In a typical experiment, once a hypodynamic response was obtained from either endotoxin or live infectious models, naloxone was administered. In the initial studies using a rat model of endotoxic hypotension (24), it was shown that naloxone injection resulted in a prompt restoration of arterial pressure to control levels. Subsequent studies using endotoxin administration to well-instrumented dogs (30) and cynomolgus monkeys (31) clearly demonstrated that naloxone at a dose of 2 mg/kg significantly improved hemodynamic variables as well as survival.

A review of the potential mechanisms by which endogenous opioids mediate their pathophysiological actions in endotoxic and septic shock requires analysis of pharmacologic data obtained from the biochemical to the organ-system level. It was first necessary to determine whether naloxone and other general opioid antagonists were exerting therapeutic actions via opioid receptors, via nonopioid receptors, or via nonspecific (i.e., membrane) effects.

Opioid receptors are stereospecific, requiring the (−) isomer to achieve opioid responses; (+) isomers are not biologically active as opioid agonists or antagonists. Through the use of (−) and (+) stereoisomers of naloxone, it was shown that only the (−) isomer successfully antagonized endotoxic shock hypotension in rats (32), providing strong pharmacologic evidence for an opioid-specific involvement in this model of circulatory shock.

One impediment to progress in this area of research has been a lack of understanding about the dose-response actions of naloxone. As little as 0.01 mg/kg naloxone successfully reverses morphine and heroin overdoses in animals and humans (25–27). However, endogenous opioids bind with greater avidity to their receptors than does morphine, and the laws of mass action require that high doses of naloxone are required to displace opioid peptide ligands from their receptors. For example, the doses of naloxone required to reverse endotoxic or hemorrhagic shock hypotension exceed by one or two orders of magnitude (1.0 mg/kg or more) the naloxone doses required to reverse the pharmacologic actions of administered opioid alkaloids such as morphine or heroin (28). Additionally, naloxone is somewhat selective for μ-receptors, as characterized by the actions of the alkaloid morphine. Since high doses of naloxone were required to elicit therapeutic effects, it was suspected that endogenous opioids were acting upon non-μ-receptors. This finding is also consonant with the knowledge that far higher concentrations of naloxone are required to reverse opioid actions at δ- and κ-receptors (28).

Following these initial studies with naloxone, the availability of more specific antagonists for the δ- and κ-receptors provided an opportunity to test directly the hypothesis that non-μ-receptors were involved. Indeed, the selective μ-antagonists naloxanazine and β-funaltrexamine (B-FNA) were without effect on endotoxic hypotension, whereas the δ-antagonists ICI-154,129 and ICI-174,864 improved arterial pressure whether administered intracerebroventricularly into the brain in microgram doses or intravenously at mg/kg doses (33). From these studies, it was concluded that δ-, not μ-, receptors are involved in endogenous opioid actions in endotoxic shock, and that these actions are at least in part mediated within the brain, since very low antagonist doses, ineffective when administered systemically, reversed endotoxic shock hypotension when injected into the ventricles of the brain in both rats and dogs (32–34). Other studies have shown that endogenous

opioids and morphine may act directly on the myocardium to depress contractility (35–37), and that the direct intracoronary arterial administration of systemically ineffective doses of naloxone can improve myocardial contractility in dogs subjected to hemorrhagic shock (see below) (35).

Attempts to define the type of endogenous opioid(s), their biologic sources, and mechanisms of action in endotoxic and septic shock have been difficult to interpret. Although circulating endorphins and enkephalins both increase dramatically during circulatory shock, and both can act upon δ-receptors, it is still unclear (a) which of these opioid molecules is predominantly responsible for the pathophysiologic effects, (b) where they are released, and (c) their precise mechanism of action in decreasing perfusion. Analysis of the extensive experimental data addressing a potential pituitary, adrenal, or autonomic origin of endogenous opioids involved in endotoxemia or sepsis has indicated that it is unlikely that pituitary-derived endorphins or adrenal-derived enkephalins are primarily involved (see references 26 and 28 for review). Yet, experimental data in a number of shock models are consistent with actions of endogenous opioids to inhibit sympathoadrenal function. Further evidence (35, 36) directly links opioids receptors with catecholamine systems. Lechner et al (35) have speculated that this interaction is at a second-messenger level within the cells of the myocardium where opioids inhibit adenosine 3':5'-cyclic phosphate (cAMP) and catecholamines stimulate cAMP. This finding is consistent with data indicating that naloxone potentiates epinephrine's hypertensive effects in endotoxemic rats (37). A direct cardiac action of naloxone in endotoxic shock is further reinforced by data obtained by Parker et al (38).

Recent work from Blalock's group (39) has indicated that circulating lymphocytes contain β-endorphin-derived peptides that are released during endotoxemia and act upon δ-receptors. This work (see below) may provide the elusive answer to the potential source of endogenous opioids that mediate the pathogenesis of circulatory shock.

ENDOGENOUS OPIOIDS IN HEMORRHAGIC SHOCK

Acute hemorrhage has long been known to produce profound neuroendocrine changes (40). As with experimental models of septic shock, the author and colleagues theorized that endogenous opioid systems would be activated by hemorrhage and could contribute to the pathophysiology of hemorrhagic shock (41). Early work in the author's laboratories demonstrated that naloxone successfully reversed the hypotension and improved survival in conscious rats subjected to a 50% lethal model of hemorrhagic shock (41). In further studies with dogs, naloxone was shown to improve inotropic function, resulting in elevations of cardiac output and mean arterial pressure (42). As with studies of canine endotoxemia, naloxone did not affect heart rate, total peripheral resistance, or portal venous pressure. Importantly, in this severe model of canine hemorrhagic shock, all saline-treated control dogs died, whereas all naloxone-treated (2 mg/kg) dogs survived (42).

Subsequent studies in a number of species, including cynomolgus monkeys, rabbits, cats, pigs, and others, have demonstrated that naloxone improves hemodynamic and metabolic variables following acute hemorrhage. Since the publication

Figure 53.4. Mean arterial pressure (*MAP*) following naloxone injection at varying doses in a canine model of hemorrhagic shock without volume resuscitation. Anesthetized dogs were bled to 45 mm Hg for 1 hour; shed blood was not reinfused. Survival time is represented on the abscissa as mean ± SEM. (For details, see Gurll NJ, Reynolds DG, Vargish T, et al: Naloxone without transfusion prolongs survival and enhances cardiovascular function in hypovolemic shock. *J Pharmacol Exp Ther* 220:621–624, 1982; reprinted with permission.)

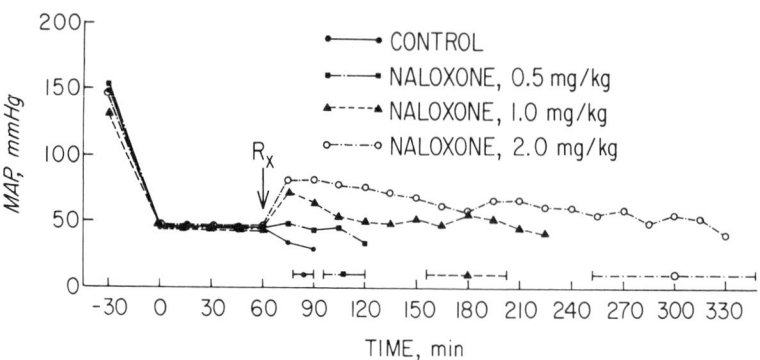

of the second edition of the present book (25), relatively few advances in understanding the mechanisms of action of naloxone and/or the site of endogenous opioid release have been made. In summary, it appears from the work of Lechner et al (35) and from the work of Parker et al (38) that endogenous opioids are released into the coronary circulation, where they locally exert a negative inotropic action. This action is stereospecific for naloxone, indicating a receptor involvement, and involves a decreased responsiveness to the vasoactive effects of catecholamines.

Although volume repletion is the primary treatment for hypovolemia resulting from acute hemorrhage, under emergency circumstances where blood, plasma, or isotonic solutions are unavailable, a drug such as naloxone may be a useful treatment until standard therapies can be administered (Fig. 53.4). Furthermore, the extensive literature (25, 35–37) indicating that naloxone restores the pressor actions of catecholamines may suggest the need for therapeutic trials to assess the value of naloxone in treating patients who have become refractory to catecholamines or in weaning patients from catecholamine drips. Nonetheless, there is extensive evidence for the value of naloxone in treating experimental hemorrhagic shock, and prospective, randomized clinical trials to assess the efficacy of naloxone in treating hypovolemic patients are needed.

ENDOGENOUS OPIOIDS IN CNS INJURY

Based upon the work just described, including a demonstration that naloxone improved spinal shock (43, 44), the author and colleagues suggested that endogenous opioids are released following traumatic spinal injury and contribute to secondary injury, in part, by reducing blood flow within the microcirculation (45, 46). This hypothesis provided the rationale for the use of opiate antagonists in experimental spinal cord injury (SCI). Subsequent investigations reviewed below also provided evidence for a pathogenic role of endogenous opioids in other forms of CNS injury, including head injury, stroke, and neurologic deficits resulting from prolonged aortic cross-clamping during aortic aneurysm repair (see below).

The earliest experiments testing the importance of endogenous opioids in CNS injury utilized a model in which the cervical spinal cord was damaged by dropping a fixed weight a fixed distance onto the exposed spinal cord of anesthetized cats (45).

The impact energy was chosen to yield a severe but incomplete degree of injury that might be amenable to pharmacologic manipulation. The injury was associated with a 10-fold increase in β-endorphin-like immunoreactivity in plasma within the first hour after trauma; during this period there was a significant reduction in both gray and white matter blood flow, particularly at the injury level (46). Treatment with naloxone 1 hour after injury resulted in significant recovery of spinal cord blood flow. Moreover, such treatment significantly improved neurologic outcome 6 weeks following injury when data were compared with those for saline-treated controls (46). In later studies, it was found that naloxone treatment significantly improved neurologic outcome, even when treatment was delayed for 4 hours following trauma (47). The neuroprotective effects of high-dose naloxone treatment in rats were subsequently confirmed by Arias (48) and others. Using a somewhat different but related feline SCI model, researchers also demonstrated naloxone's therapeutic actions, including an improvement in somatosensory evoked potentials (49, 50).

These models of spinal cord ischemia have also been useful in predicting therapeutic responses to naloxone in experimental models of stroke (51) and head injury (52, 53) and in neurologic deficits produced by protracted cross-clamping of the infrarenal aorta such as occurs during surgical procedures to correct aortic aneurysms (51, 54, 55).

The surgical repair of aneurysms, particularly aneurysms of the infrarenal aorta, may result in significant motor deficits in as many as 20–50% of patients because of protracted aortic cross-clamping. Studies were conducted to evaluate the effects of naloxone treatment in ischemic SCI produced in the lumbar region in rabbits through occlusion of the infrarenal portion of the abdominal aorta (51, 54, 55). In this model, naloxone-treated rabbits showed significantly improved motor recovery and diminished histopathological changes when compared with saline-treated controls (51, 54). The beneficial effects of naloxone in these rabbit models were dose-related, with significant effects observed at or above doses of 0.2 mg/kg and optimal effects at the highest doses tested (2 mg/kg/hr) (51, 54).

As with endotoxic and septic shock studies, the high doses of naloxone required to produce a beneficial effect in SCI suggested that the effects might result from actions at non-μ- or naloxone-resistant receptors. To investigate this possibility, the effects of more receptor-selective opiate antagonists were examined. The δ-antagonist (e.g., ICI-154,129) failed to affect neurologic outcome, whereas κ-antagonist (WIN44,441-3, nalmefene, and nor-binaltorphimine) demonstrated significant therapeutic responses. These collective data provide further support for the concept that κ-receptors mediate the pathophysiologic actions of endogenous opioids in SCI (55–58).

This concept is consistent with other experimental evidence regarding the proposed role of the κ-selective opioid peptide dynorphin in SCI. Dynorphin, but not enkephalins or β-endorphin, accumulates at the injury site following traumatic SCI in rats in concentrations that are correlated significantly with the severity of injury (59). After intrathecal administration, dynorphin causes hind-limb paralysis that clinically simulates posttraumatic paraparesis (60–62); the intact dynorphin molecule is almost equipotent with other opioids or dynorphin fragments in producing this effect (61, 62).

After condensing years of extensive experimental data, it appears that dynorphin-induced paralysis includes both opiate receptor-mediated and nonopioid components, and that the ability of opiate-receptor antagonists to inhibit motor dysfunction caused by dynorphin may therefore be critically dependent on the dynorphin dose (61, 62). In fact, the nonopioid component of dynorphin's paralytic actions likely involves the secondary pathogenic actions of excitatory amino acids (63). In more recent studies by Faden and colleagues, it has been shown that the administration of dynorphin antiserum significantly limited the neurologic deficits produced by traumatic SCI, and that the intrathecal injection of exogenous dynorphin exacerbated posttraumatic SCI (60). These studies are consistent with the hypothesis that dynorphin contributes to secondary SCI after trauma and that such effects are, at least in part, mediated by κ-opiate receptors.

"ANTERIOR PITUITARY" HORMONES LOCALIZED WITHIN LYMPHOCYTES

Conventional thinking about endocrinology and immunology has been challenged by recent evidence indicating that the origin of "hormones" may not always be restricted to classic endocrine tissues. One of the most interesting developments in the newly evolving discipline of neuroendocrine immunology has been the discovery that leukocytes are capable of producing many of the hormones usually associated with an anterior pituitary origin, including GH, TSH, ACTH, and endorphins (21).

As discussed earlier, the origin of endogenous opioids that contribute to endotoxic shock may well be the immune system. A recent series of experiments has demonstrated that the endorphins can derive directly from circulating lymphocytes. From the work of Harbour et al, it appears that endotoxin serves to release these lymphocyte-derived endogenous opioids in concentrations that cause hypotension by actions upon δ opioid receptors (39). These studies indicate the likelihood that a primary source of endogenous opioids in sepsis may be lymphocytes, and that the release of opioid peptides from these cellular mediators of immune function may be part of their orchestrated physiological or pathophysiologic actions in circulatory shock, trauma, or inflammation.

Prolactin has been added to this list of "pituitary hormones" found in lymphocytes; in a series of immunocytochemical and biochemical studies, Kenner et al (64) demonstrated that lymphocytes also produce a prolactin-like protein whose concentration is increased by exposure to mitogens. Immunocytochemical techniques using antibodies specific to pituitary prolactin revealed that 48 hours after mitogenic stimulation with the T-cell mitogen Con-A, phytohemagglutinin, or antibody to the T3 receptor, a large subpopulation of human or murine T- and B-lymphocytes contain prolactin immunoreactivity (64). Con-A increased the expression of lymphocytic prolactin more than 2.5-fold. In a manner uncharacteristic of most secreted proteins, electron microscopic studies indicated that lymphocyte prolactin was localized in discrete cytoplasmic avesicular foci. Control studies demonstrated the specificity of these antiprolactin antibodies for prolactin and confirmed that the prolactin within the lymphocytes did not derive from the media or from the pituitary (64, 65).

From these immunocytochemical results, it remains unclear whether lymphocyte prolactin is secreted by lymphocytes or acts within the lymphocyte to perform a biologic function. Evidence as to the potential biologic function of lymphocyte-derived prolactin was obtained in collaborative studies with Hartmann et al (66), where lymphocyte-derived prolactin-like-protein was indirectly shown to play a role in cell proliferation. Specifically, the addition of antiprolactin antibodies to mitogen-stimulated lymphocytes inhibited their proliferation in a prolactin-reversible manner (66). Based upon these studies and others, the author and colleagues have proposed that this lymphocyte-derived prolactin-like protein may function as an autocrine cytokine that facilitates lymphocyte proliferation (65).

Estimates of molecular weight for lymphocyte prolactin-like protein using western blot analysis indicated that this polypeptide had a molecular weight of 48 kilodaltons, approximately twice as large as pituitary prolactin (64). Similar results have been obtained more recently by Montgomery et al (67), who have reported a 46-kilodalton prolactin-like molecule in stimulated murine splenocytes.

SUMMARY AND CLINICAL PERSPECTIVES

ENDOCRINE-IMMUNE INTERACTIONS

The identification of bidirectional interactions among the brain, endocrine, and immune systems touched upon in this review may significantly alter the way we look at the body's responses to critical illnesses. The neuroendocrine axis regulates the production of hormones that modify immune function, including adrenal glucocorticoids and prolactin. Although not reviewed in this chapter, it is also becoming clear that the flow of biologic information in the neuroendocrine-immune axis is not unidirectional. Increasing emphasis is being placed on the role of inflammatory lymphokines as mediators of neuroendocrine responses. For example, the release of monokines (such as IL-1, IL-6, or TNF) from macrophages as part of immunologic responses to infection or inflammation have been shown to affect brain and neuroendocrine function by stimulating or inhibiting the release of many pituitary hormones (68–71). It has been speculated that the

Table 53.1.   Potential Immunologic Effects of Commonly Used Drugs[a]

Drug	Drug Type	Endocrine Effect	Immunologic Effect	Site of Action
Hydrocortisone Methylprednisolone Dexamethasone	Glucocorticoid	↓ Cortisol ↓ Prolactin, ↓ ACTH	Immunosuppression	Macrophage, T-cell
Dopamine Bromocryptine	DA-agonist	↓ Prolactin ↓ Growth hormone	Immunosuppression	T-cell
Haloperidol Metoclopramide	DA-antagonist	↑ Prolactin ↓ Growth hormone	Immunostimulation	T-cell
Morphine (chronic)	Opioid agonist	↑ Corticosterone, ↓ Prolactin	Immunosuppression	Macrophage, T-cell
Cysteamine	Mucolytic	↓ Prolactin	Immunosuppression	T-cell

[a] Many drugs frequently used in the critical care setting have pronounced effects on neuroendocrine function that, in turn, affect immune function as shown above. (For details, see reference 17; reprinted with permission from Holaday JW, Bryant HU, Kenner JR, Bernton EW: Brain, endocrine and immune interactions: implications in intensive care. In Holaday JW, Bihari D (eds): *Brain Failure: Series Update in Intensive Care and Emergency Medicine*, vol 9. Springer-Verlag, New York, 1989, pp 1–13.)

sick euthyroid syndrome may be a consequence of cytokine influences upon the neuroendocrine network (17, 72). A more detailed review of the effects of cytokines on the release of neuroendocrine hormones is available elsewhere (17).

Many of the drugs commonly found in the intensive care setting may have beneficial or detrimental actions well beyond their intended purpose. For example, dopamine drips used to maintain renal perfusion in septic shock patients may contribute to the anergy of critical illnesses by depriving the organism of the immunopermissive actions of prolactin. The recent work of Devins and colleagues (19) has reinforced this possibility; they indicate that the use of dopamine to improve hemodynamics in critically ill patients results in profound hypoprolactinemia that is temporally associated with a suppression of T-cell proliferative responses. Prolactin levels are also profoundly affected by many other drugs commonly used in the intensive care setting. The immunosuppressive effects of hypoprolactinemia, cyclosporin, and glucocorticoids have been shown to be reversed by prolactin or by dopamine antagonists that stimulate endogenous prolactin release (11, 12, 14). Chronically administered morphine and other opioids also affect immune responses via their actions on the endocrine system (73–75). Several examples of pharmacologic interventions that act through the anterior pituitary hormones to modulate immune responses are presented in Table 53.1.

Although much of the research reviewed in this chapter is preclinical, several clinical correlates indicates that dopamine agonists do indeed play a role in suppressing human immune responses via suppression of prolactin release. It was noted that the use of bromocriptine for the treatment of Parkinson's disease also improved autoimmune uveitis in a small population of patients with this coincident condition (76). The response was attributed to the decrease in circulating prolactin. The hypoprolactinemic effects of bromocriptine have been shown to suppress the postpartum exacerbation of collagen-induced arthritis (6), prolactin serves as a marker for rejection of transplanted hearts (5), and prolactin exacerbates systemic lupus erythematosus (7).

Future clinical research based upon animal and in vitro studies may reveal that therapy with prolactin, growth hormone, or drugs that affect their release could play a role in improving immune host defenses in a variety of chronic diseases. Without doubt, our increasing knowledge of the functional interactions within the neuroendocrine-immune

axis will also improve our knowledge of how to care for the critically ill patient. Perhaps even more fundamentally, the rapidly emerging biomedical research in this discipline forces us to rethink our definitions of classic hormones, cytokines, and other biologic mediators as their orchestrated effects upon homeostasis and dyshomeostasis become better characterized.

ENDOGENOUS OPIOIDS AND SHOCK

After more than a decade of research addressing a potential role of endogenous opioid systems in the pathophysiology of endotoxic-septic shock, an enormous amount of data using a broad range of species has amassed to indicate that opioid antagonists may be useful in treating human septic shock (25, 27, 77). Although precise mechanisms require additional clarification, the fundamental observation that naloxone and related opioid antagonists improve the shock state has been reported in more than 80% of the published investigations using a variety of animal species. According to the rigid criteria dictated by a classic meta-analysis, the vast majority of published reports provide only inferential data and do not conclusively demonstrate a cause-effect relationship between endogenous opioids and endotoxic-septic shock (27). Nonetheless, among all the mediators subjected to meta-analysis in a recent book evaluating mediator involvement in septic shock (78), endogenous opioids were among the very few mediators for which data supported a pathogenic role in this critical illness.

As reviewed above, the use of opiate-receptor antagonists such as naloxone for the treatment of CNS injury and ischemia was based upon the hypothesis that endogenous opioids are released following trauma and contribute to secondary injury by reducing blood flow within the microcirculation. Subsequent experimental studies confirmed this hypothesis by demonstrating that opiate-receptor antagonists reverse posttraumatic ischemia, improve electrophysiologic responses, limit histopathologic changes, reverse metabolic derangements, and enhance neurologic recovery in traumatic brain injury, spinal cord injury, and CNS ischemia resulting from experimental stroke or aortic cross-clamping.

Although opioid systems may play only a partial role in the dyshomeostasis that characterizes clinical shock and trauma, there is a critical need for more thorough dose-response studies to support or refute conclusively the role of endogenous opioids in these pathophysiologic circumstances. Despite many published clinical reports in which naloxone was administered to shock-trauma patients, no clinical trials have yet been reported in which adequate doses of naloxone were given. In studies in which a therapeutic action of naloxone has not been claimed, too low a dose of naloxone (77) or too high a dose was used (79). Unfortunately, little attention is paid to the extensive animal literature indicating that a dose of 2 mg/kg naloxone is optimal, and that too much or too little is without therapeutic effects.

It is perhaps unfortunate that the process of scientific research emphasizes new discoveries, often prematurely dismissing the old. Before dismissing endogenous opioids as relevant mediators of these critical illnesses, it would be timely for new research to address interactions between opioid antagonists, for instance, and other more recently described mediators, such as cytokines, eicosanoids, and growth factors. At the clinical level, it is critical that prospective, randomized studies be conducted using opioid antagonists such as naloxone in 1 to 2 mg/kg doses before firm conclusions can be drawn about the relevance of endogenous opioid systems to shock and CNS trauma.

ACKNOWLEDGMENTS

The author is grateful to his many colleagues, including Drs. Bernton, Kenner, Bryant, Malcolm, Chernow, Zaloga, Hartmann, Faden, Smith, and many others whose work is reviewed in this chapter.

REFERENCES

1. Tache Y, Du Ruisseau P, Ducharme JR, Collu R: Pattern of adenohypophyseal hormone changes in male rats following chronic stress. *Neuroendocrinology* 26:208–219, 1978.
2. Calandra T, Gerain J, Heumann D, et al: Circulating levels of IL-6 in patients with septic shock: evolution during sepsis, prognostic value, and interplay with other cytokines. *Am J Med* 91:23–29, 1991.
3. Fong Y, Tracey KJ, Moldawer LL, et al: Antibodies to cachectin/tumor necrosis factor reverse interleukin 1B and interleukin 6 appearance during lethal bacteremia. *J Exp Med* 170:1627–1633, 1989.
4. Parrillo JE, Fauci AS: Mechanisms of glucocorticoid action on immune processes. *Ann Rev Pharmacol Toxicol* 19:129–201, 1979.
5. Carrier M, Emrey RW, Wild-Moblay J, et al: Prolactin as a marker of rejection in human heart transplantation. *Transplant Proc* 19:3442–3443, 1987.
6. Whyte A, Williams R: Bromocriptine suppresses postpartum exacerbation of collagen-induced arthritis. *Arthritis Rheum* 31:927–928, 1988.
7. Jara-Quezada L, Graef A, Lavalle C: Prolactin and gonadal hormones during pregnancy in systemic lupus erythematosus. *J Rheumatol* 18:349–353, 1991.
8. Blauer KL, Poth M, Rogers WM, Bernton EW: Dehydroepiandrosterone antagonizes the suppressive effects of dexamethasone on lymphocyte proliferation. *Endocrinology* 129(6):3174–3179, 1991.
9. Holaday JW, Meyerhoff JL, Natelson BH: Cortisol secretion and clearance in the rhesus monkey. *Endocrinology* 100:1178–1185, 1977.
10. Meltzer MS, Nacy CA: Cell-cell interactions during inflammation: the role of the macrophage. In Cerra FB, Shoemaker WC (eds): *Critical Care State-of-the-Art*, vol 8. Fullerton, CA, Society of Critical Care Medicine, pp 119–132, 1987.
11. Bernton EW, Bryant HU, Holaday JW: Prolactin and immune function. In Ader R, Felten DL, Cohen N (eds): *Psychoneuroimmunology*, 2nd ed. San Diego, Academic Press, pp 403–428, 1991.
12. Bernton EW, Bryant H, Holaday J, Dave J: Prolactin and prolactin secretagogues reverse immunosuppression in mice treated with cysteamine, glucocorticoids or cyclosporin-A. *Brain Behav Immun* 6:394–408, 1992.
13. Nagy E, Berczi I, Wren GE, Asa SL, Kovacs K: Immunomodulation by bromocriptine. *Immunopharmacology* 6:231–243, 1983.
14. Bernton EW, Meltzer MS, Holaday JW: Suppression of macrophage activation and T-lymphocyte function in hypoprolactinemic mice. *Science* 239:401–403, 1988.
15. Mukherjee P, Mastro AM, Hymer WC: Prolactin induction of interleukin-2 receptors on rat splenic lymphocytes. *Endocrinology* 126:88–94, 1991.
16. Clevenger CV, Altmann SW, Prystowsky MB: Requirement of nuclear prolactin for interleukin-2 stimulated proliferation of T-lymphocytes. *Science* 253:77–79, 1991.
17. Holaday JW, Bryant HU, Kenner JR, Bernton EW: Brain, endocrine and immune interactions: implications in intensive care. In Holaday JW, Bihari D (eds): *Brain Failure: Series Update in Intensive Care and Emergency Medicine*, vol 9. New York, Springer-Verlag, pp 1–13, 1989.
18. Russell DH, Matrisian L, Kibler R, Larson DF, Poulos B, Magun BE: Prolactin receptors on human lymphocytes and their modulation by cyclosporin. *Biochem Biophys Res Commun* 121:899–906, 1984.
19. Devins SS, Miller A, Herndon BL, et al: The effects of dopamine on T-cell proliferative response and serum prolactin in critically ill patients. *Crit Care Med* 20:1644–1649, 1992.
20. Bernton EW: Prolactin and immune host defenses. *Prog Neuroendoimmunol* 2:21–29, 1989.
21. Weigent DA, Blalock JE: Interactions between the neuroendocrine and immune systems: common hormones and receptors. *Immunol Rev* 100:79–96, 1987.
22. Snow ED, Feldbush TL, Oakes JA: The effect of growth hormone and insulin upon MLC responses and the generation of cytotoxic leukocytes. *J Immunol* 126:161–164, 1981.
23. Kelley K, Brief S, Westly H, Novakofski J, Bechtel P, Simon J, Walter E: GH3 pituitary adenoma cells can reverse thymic aging in rats. *Proc Natl Acad Sci USA* 83:5663–5667, 1986.
24. Holaday JW, Faden AI: Naloxone reversal of endotoxin hypotension suggests role of endorphins in shock. *Nature* 275:450–451, 1978.
25. Holaday JW, Malcolm DS: Endogenous opioids and other peptides: evidence for their clinical relevance in shock and CNS injury. In Chernow B, Holaday JW, Zaloga G, Zaritsky A (eds): *The Pharmacologic Approach to the Critically Ill Patient*, ed 2. William & Wilkins, Baltimore, pp 718–732, 1988.
26. Bernton EW, Long JB, Holaday JW: Opioids and neuropeptides: mechanisms in circulatory shock. *Fed Proc* 44:290–299, 1985.
27. Gurll NJ: Endogenous opiates in septic-endotoxic shock. In Neugebauer E, Holaday JW (eds): *Handbook on Mediators in Septic Shock*, Boca Raton, FL, CRC Press, 1992.
28. Holaday JW: *Endogenous Opioids and Their Receptors: Current Concepts*. Kalamazoo, MI, Scope (Upjohn) Publications, pp 1–64, 1985.
29. Holaday JW, Porreca F, Rothman RB: Functional coupling among opioid receptor types. In Estefanos F (ed): *Opioids in Anesthesia II*. Butterworth-Heineman, New York, pp 50–60, 1991.
30. Reynolds DG, Gurll NJ, Vargish T, Lechner R, Faden AI, Holaday JW: Blockade of opiate receptors with naloxone improves survival and cardiac performance in canine endotoxic shock. *Circ Shock* 7:39–48, 1980.
31. Gurll NJ, Reynolds DG, Holaday JW: Evidence for a role of endorphins in the cardiovascular pathophysiology of primate shock. *Crit Care Med* 16:521–524, 1988.
32. Faden AI, Holaday JW: Naloxone treatment of endotoxin shock: stereospecificity of physiologic and pharmacologic effects in the rat. *J Pharmacol Exp Ther* 212:411–447, 1980.
33. D'Amato RJ, Holaday JW: Multiple opiate receptors in endotoxic shock: Evidence for *d* involvement and *m-d* interactions in vivo. *Proc Natl Acad Sci USA* 81:2898–2901, 1984.
34. Holaday JW: Neuropeptides in shock and traumatic injury: sites and mechanisms of action. *Neuroendocrinol Perspect* 3:161–199, 1984.
35. Lechner RB, Gurll NJ, Reynolds DG: Naloxone potentiates the cardiovascular effects of catecholamines in canine hemorrhagic shock. *Circ Shock* 16:347–361, 1985.
36. Holaday JW: Cardiovascular effects of the endogenous opiate system. *Annu Rev Pharmacol Toxicol* 23:541–594, 1983.
37. Malcolm DS, Zaloga GP, Willey SC, Holaday JW: Naloxone potentiates epinephrine's hypertensive effects in endotoxemic rats. *Circ Shock* 25:259–265, 1988.
38. Parker JL, Keller RS, Behm LL, Adams HR: Left ventricular dysfunction in early *E. coli* endotoxemia: effects of naloxone. *Am J Physiol* 259(2):H504–H511, 1990.
39. Harbour DV, Galin FS, Hughes TK, Smith EM, Blalock JE: Role of leukocyte-derived pro-opiomelanocortin peptides in endotoxic shock. *Circ Shock* 35:181–191, 1991.
40. Ganong WF: Neuroendocrine responses to injury and shock. In Biro ZA, Kovach AGB, Spitzer JJ, Stoner BH (eds): *Advances in Physiological Sciences*, vol 26. Pergamon Press, Budapest, Akademiai Kiado, 1981, pp 35–44.
41. Faden AI, Joladay JW: Opiate antagonists: a role in the treatment of hypovolemic shock. *Science* 205:317–318, 1979.
42. Vargish T, Reynolds DG, Gurll NJ, Lechner RJ, Holaday JW, Faden AI: Naloxone reversal of hypovolemic shock in dogs. *Circ Shock* 7:31–38, 1980.
43. Holaday JW, Faden AI: Naloxone acts at central opiate receptors to reverse hypotension, hypothermia and hypoventilation in spinal shock. *Brain Res* 189:295–299, 1980.
44. Faden AI, Jacobs TP, Holaday JW: Endorphin-parasympathetic interaction in spinal shock. *J Auton Nerv Syst* 2:295–304, 1980.
45. Faden AI, Jacobs TP, Holaday JW: Opiate antagonists improve neurologic recovery after spinal injury. *Science* 211:493–494, 1981.
46. Faden AI, Jacobs TP, Holaday JW: Endorphins in experimental spinal injury: therapeutic effect of naloxone. *Ann Neurol* 10:326–332, 1981.

47. Faden AI, Jacobs TP, Holaday JW: Comparison of early and late naloxone treatment in experimental spinal injury. *Neurology* 32:677–681, 1982.

48. Arias MJ: Treatment of experimental spinal cord injury with TRH, naloxone and dexamethasone. *Surg Neurol* 28:335–338, 1987.

49. Flamm ES, Young W, Demopoulos HB, DeCrescito V, Tomasula JJ: Experimental spinal cord injury: treatment with naloxone. *Neurosurgery* 10:227–231, 1982.

50. Young W, Flamm ES, Demopoulos HB, Tomasula JJ, DeCrescito V: Naloxone ameliorates posttraumatic ischemia in experimental spinal contusion. *J Neurosurg* 55:209–219, 1981.

51. Faden AI, Jacobs TP, Smith MT, Zivin JA: Naloxone in experimental spinal cord ischemia: dose-response studies. *Eur J Pharmacol* 103:115–120, 1984.

52. Hayes RL, Galinet BJ, Kulkarne P, Becker DP: Effects of naloxone on systemic and cerebral responses to experimental concussive brain injury in cats. *J Neurosurg* 58:720–728, 1983.

53. McIntosh TK, Agura VM, Hellgeth M, Rittner H, Faden AI, Hayes RL: Stereospecific efficacy of the opiate antagonist WIN44,441-3 in the treatment of head injury in the cat. *Neurosci Abstr* 1(2):1200, 1985.

54. Kinney RC, Holaday JW, Harmon JW: Naloxone decreases neurologic deficits in experimental aortic cross-clamping ischemia. *Surg Forum* 36:460–461, 1985.

55. Faden AI, Jacobs TP: Opiate antagonist WIN44,441-3 stereospecifically improves neurologic recovery after ischemic spinal injury. *Neurology* 35:1311–1315, 1985.

56. Faden AI, Jacobs TP, Zivin JA: Comparison of naloxone and a delta-selective antagonist in experimental spinal "stroke." *Life Sci* 33(suppl 1):707–710, 1983.

57. Vink R, McIntosh TK, Rhomhanyi R, Faden AI: Opiate antagonist nalmefene improves intracellular free Mg++, bioenergetic state and neurologic outcome following traumatic brain surgery in rats. *J Neurosci* 10:3524–3530, 1990.

58. Faden AI, Takemori AE, Portoghese TS: δ-Selective opiate antagonist norbinaltorphimine improves outcome after traumatic spinal cord injury in rats. *CNS Trauma* 4:227–237, 1987.

59. Faden AI, Molineaux CJ, Rosenberger JC, et al: Endogenous opioid immunoreactivity in rat spinal cord following traumatic injury. *Ann Neurol* 17:386–390, 1985.

60. Faden AI, Jacobs TP: Dynorphin induces partially reversible paraplegia in the rat. *Eur J Pharmacol* 91(2/3):321–324, 1983.

61. Long JB, Kinney RC, Malcolm DS, Graeber GM, Holaday JW: Intrathecal dynorphin A (1-13) and dynorphin (3-13) reduce spinal cord blood flow by non-opioid mechanisms. *Brain Res* 436:374–379, 1986.

62. Long JB, Martinez-Arizala A, Petras JM, Holaday JW: Endogenous opioids in spinal cord injury: a critical evaluation. *Central Nerv Sys Trauma* 3:295–306, 1986.

63. Long JB, Petras JM, Mobley WC, Holaday JW: Neurological dysfunction following intrathecal injection of dynorphin A (1-13) in the rat. II. Non-opioid mechanisms mediate loss of motor, sensory, and autonomic function. *J Pharmacol Exp Ther* 246:1167–1171, 1988.

64. Kenner JR, Holaday JW, Bernton EW, Smith PF: Prolactin in murine lymphocytes: morphologic and biochemical evidence. *Prog Neuroendoimmunol* 3:188–195, 1990.

65. Holaday JW, Kenner JR, Smith PF, et al: Is prolactin an autocrine cytokine? In Frederickson RCA, McGaugh JL, Felten DL (eds): *Peripheral Signaling of the Brain: Role in Neural-Immune Interactions, Learning and Memory.* Hogrefe & Huber, Toronto, 1990, pp 243–255.

66. Hartmann DP, Holaday JW, Bernton EW: Inhibition of lymphocyte proliferation by antibodies to prolactin. *FASEB J* 3:2194–2202, 1989.

67. Montgomery DG, Zukoski CT, Shah GN, et al: Concanavalin A-stimulated murine splenocytes produce a factor with prolactin-like bioactivity and immunoactivity. *Biochem Biophys Res Commun* 145:692–698, 1987.

68. Bernton E, Beach J, Holaday JW, Smallridge R, Fein H: Release of multiple hormones by a direct action of interleukin-1 on pituitary cells. *Science* 238:519–521, 1987.

69. Beach JE, Smallridge RC, Kinzer CA, Bernton EW, Holaday JW, Fein HG: Interleukin-1 releases multiple hormones from perfused rat pituitaries. *Life Sci* 44:1–8, 1989.

70. Berkenbosch F, van Oert J, Del Ray A, Tilders F, Besedovsky H: CRF-producing neurons in the rat are activated by interleukin-1. *Science* 238:524–526, 1987.

71. Breder C, Dinarello C, Saper C: Interleukin-1 immunoreactive innervation of the human hypothalamus. *Science* 240:321–323, 1988.

72. Dubuis JM, Dayer JM, Siegrist-Kaiser CA, Burger AG: Human recombinant interleukin-1 beta decreases plasma thyroid hormone and thyroid-stimulating hormone levels in rats. *Endocrinology* 123:2175–2181, 1988.

73. Bryant HU, Bernton EW, Holaday JW: Morphine pellet-induced immunomodulation in mice: temporal relationships. *J Pharmacol Exp Ther* 245:913–920, 1988.

74. Bryant HU, Bernton EW, Kenner JR, Holaday JW: Role of adrenal cortical activation in the immunosuppressive effects of chronic morphine treatment. *Endocrinology* 128:3253–3258, 1991.

75. Bryant HU, Bernton EW, Holaday JW: Immunomodulatory effects of chronic morphine treatment: pharmacologic and mechanistic studies. *Natl Inst Drug Abuse Monogr* 96:131–149, 1990.

76. Palestine AG, Nussenblatt RB: The effect of bromocriptine on anterior uveitis. *Am J Ophthalmol* 104(4):488–489, 1988.

77. DeMaria A, Heffeman JJ, Grindlinger GA, et al: Naloxone versus placebo in treatment of septic shock. *Lancet* June 15:1363–1365, 1985.

78. Neugebauer E, Holaday JW (eds): *Handbook of Mediators in Septic Shock.* CRC Press, Boca Raton, FL, 1993.

79. Bracken MB, Shepherd MJ, Collins WF, et al: A randomized controlled trial of methylprednisolone or naloxone in the treatment of acute spinal cord injury: results of the second national acute spinal cord injury study. *N Engl J Med* 322:1405–1411, 1990.

CHAPTER 54

Oxygen Free Radicals

JERRY J. ZIMMERMAN, Ph.D., M.D.

It has been noted that the price paid for aerobic metabolism is oxygen radical (·OR) injury. Thus, although the oxygen environment allows efficient production of ATP via the mitochondrial electron transport chain, incomplete reduction of molecular oxygen adds to the entropy of life on earth in terms of "rancid, rusty, and rotten" insults. High levels of endogenous ·OR scavengers emphasize the importance of ·OR as an injury mechanism. During the past decade, there has been a virtual explosion of interest in ·OR involvement in human disease, as documented by the exponential increase in the number of publications related to this investigative area. Physicians stand on the threshold of ·OR scavenger therapeutic realization.

This chapter presents an overview of the area of ·OR injury, particularly as it relates to the critically ill patient, and sequentially considers the types of ·OR species, ·OR sources, ·OR injury detection, ·OR molecular, cellular, and organ injury, and finally, the numerous avenues of investigation involving ·OR therapeutics. A compendium of references for this subject could fill a textbook—accordingly, the reference list frequently reflects examples of a particular point, with emphasis on more recent investigations. Certainly, the reference list does not claim to be inclusive but is meant to reflect the scope of scientific input that has been generated in this fascinating and exciting field.

OXYRADICAL SPECIES

A free radical may be defined as any species that has one or more unpaired electrons (1–3). Ground-state diatomic oxygen (O_2) is itself a diradical, with one unpaired electron in each of its outer two orbitals exhibiting parallel spin. Accordingly, if O_2 is to oxidize another species (by accepting a pair of electrons), electron spin inversion must occur. As a consequence of this spin restriction kinetic barrier, spontaneous reaction of O_2 is impeded, and as a result, biomolecules, although thermodynamically unstable in air, do not ordinarily oxidize spontaneously. All toxic oxygen species are not radicals (e.g., H_2O_2, N-chloroamines). However, for ease of discussion, all such species will be referred to as oxyradicals (·OR).

Active sites of certain enzymes (e.g., oxidases) have evolved to lower the activation energy of O_2-mediated oxidations and, hence, catalyze the controlled reduction of O_2. Complete reduction of O_2 to water requires the addition of a total of four electrons (Fig. 54.1). Single electron reductions of oxygen, shown in Figure 54.2, do not require spin inversions and occur through a variety of mechanisms. Addition of a single electron to molecular oxygen produces superoxide anion (O_2^-), which is formed by all aerobic cells. Protonation of O_2^- yields the hydroperoxyl radical (HO_2^-) characterized by a pK_a of 4.8. At physiologic pH of 7.4, the hydroperoxyl radical species would be mostly dissociated—only about 0.25% would exist as HO_2^-. In other environments such as ischemic tissue, phagosomes, or an endothelial cell/phagocyte interface, the pH may be considerably lower and, hence, the concentration of HO_2^- higher. The significance of increased concentrations of HO_2^- relates to HO_2^- increased membrane solubility and enhanced reactivity compared with O_2^-.

901

$$O_2 + 4H^+ + 4e^- \longrightarrow 2H_2O$$

Figure 54.1. Complete reduction of O_2 to H_2O.

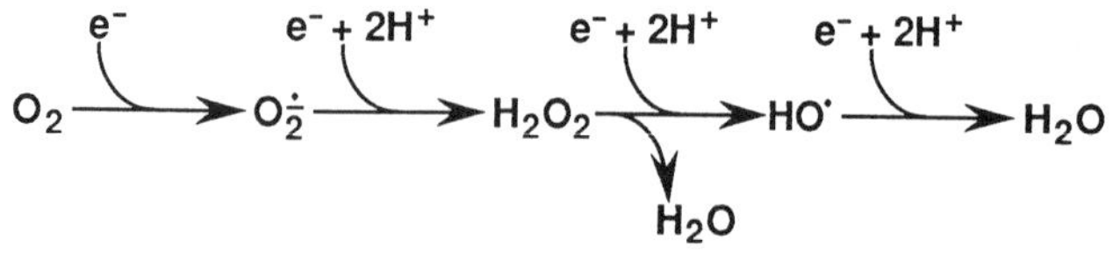

$$O_2 \xrightarrow{e^-} O_2^{\cdot-} \xrightarrow{e^- + 2H^+} H_2O_2 \xrightarrow{e^- + 2H^+} HO^{\cdot} \xrightarrow{e^- + 2H^+} H_2O$$
$$\searrow H_2O$$

Figure 54.2. Sequential one-electron reductions of O_2.

$$O_2^{\cdot-} + {}^{\cdot}NO \longrightarrow ONOO^- \xrightarrow[\overset{H^+}{\rightleftarrows}]{} ONOOH \longrightarrow "HO^{\cdot}" + NO_2$$

Figure 54.3. Formation and decomposition of peroxylnitrite radical.

$$H_2O_2 + Na\,Cl \longrightarrow NaOCl + H_2O$$

Figure 54.4. Formation of sodium hypochlorite by myeloperoxidase.

Superoxide has recently been shown to combine with endothelial derived relaxant factor (nitric oxide, NO·) to yield the peroxyl nitrite radical (ONOO·) (4). Endothelial cells, macrophages, and neutrophils have all been demonstrated to produce both $O_2^{\cdot-}$ and NO·. As shown in Figure 54.3, peroxylnitrite anion is in equilibrium with its corresponding acid—the relevant pK_a at 37°C is 6.8. The half-life of the protonated species, peroxynitrous acid, appears to be about 1 second preceding its decomposition to nitrogen dioxide (NO_2) and a hydroxyl radical-like species. Importance of this reaction is twofold: (*a*) $O_2^{\cdot-}$ may inactivate endothelial derived reactive factor; and (*b*) peroxynitrite/peroxynitrous acid has been shown to react with free sulfhydryl groups at 37°C, pH 7.4, with a rate constant of 26,000 to 28,000 $M^{-1}\cdot sec^{-1}$, which is approximately 1000 times faster than the reaction of sulfhydryls with hydrogen peroxide.

Superoxide anion is metabolized to hydrogen peroxide (H_2O_2) at a spontaneous reaction rate of $2 \cdot 10^5$ $M^{-1}\cdot sec^{-1}$. Superoxide dismutase enhances this dismutation by a factor of 10,000. It should be noted that H_2O_2 can also be generated directly, as, for example, by glucose oxidase. Hydrogen peroxide itself is not classified as a radical because it has no unpaired electrons. Its biological reactivity is limited but its half-life is relatively long, and it can cross biological membranes in the absence of anion channels, which apparently are required for $O_2^{\cdot-}$. Hydrogen peroxide represents an important substrate relative to the production of a variety of other ·OR species. Myeloperoxidase, as well as other peroxidases, can catalyze the formation of hypohalous acids in the presence of H_2O_2 (5) (Fig. 54.4). When chlorine is utilized as the halide substrate, sodium hypochlorite (NaOCl) is generated. This species (equivalent to chlorine bleach) obviously has high oxidative capacity, both in terms of killing microbes as well as mediating tissue injury. Reaction of amines with hypohalous acids yields *N*-chloroamines, which are characterized by high reactivity as well as a long half-life (6) (Fig. 54.5).

Interaction of $O_2^{\cdot-}$ and H_2O_2 may result in the formation of the highly reactive species hydroxyl radical (HO·) and hydroxyl anion via the Haber-Weiss or Fenton reactions. This

$$HClO + R-NH_2 \longrightarrow R-NH-Cl + H_2O$$

Figure 54.5. Generation of *N*-chloroamines.

$$O_2^{\cdot-} + Fe^{3+} \longrightarrow Fe^{3+} + O_2$$
$$H_2O_2 + Fe^{3+} \longrightarrow Fe^{3+} + HO^{\cdot} + HO^-$$
$$\overline{\text{Net:} \quad O_2^{\cdot-} + H_2O_2 \longrightarrow O_2 + HO^{\cdot} + HO^-}$$

Figure 54.6. Haber-Weiss/Fenton reaction catalyzed by redox cycling of transition metals.

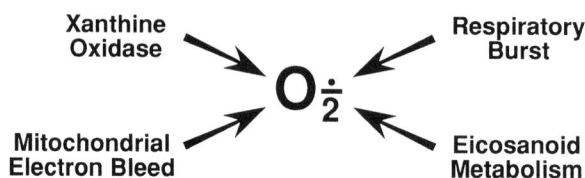

Figure 54.7. Schematic depiction of the major sources of superoxide anion.

reaction is catalyzed by redox cycling of a transition metal ion, as noted in Figure 54.6 (7, 8). Hydroxyl radical is highly unstable—reaction occurs within 1 to 5 molecular diameters and is characterized as diffusion-limited. The half-life for this species is approximately $10^{-9}sec$ (8). It has been suggested that the in vivo free iron required for the catalytic formation of hydroxyl radical comes from the $O_2^{\cdot-}$-dependent reduction and release of ferrous iron from ferritin (9, 10).

Utilizing terminal components of the mitochondrial electron transport chain, namely cytochrome aa_3 and cytochrome oxidase, O_2 can be reduced to H_2O in an organized fashion. Cytochrome oxidase, obviously in concert with the other mitochondrial electron transport chain components, allows not only an approximate 20-fold increase in energy substrate metabolism efficiency compared with anaerobic metabolism, but also under normal conditions provides an avenue for complete reduction of oxygen without massive production of the highly toxic intermediate reduced species depicted in Figure 54.2.

OXYRADICAL SOURCES

Although there are innumerable sources for the generation of ·OR species, four mechanisms have been most actively investigated, particularly because of their likely roles in the pathogenesis of human disease. Accordingly, extensive literature exists on the role of mitochrondrial electron transport chain electron bleed, eicosanoid metabolism, xanthine oxidase, and the respiratory burst of activated phagocytes in the generation of pathophysiologically relevant ·OR (Fig. 54.7).

MITOCHONDRIAL ELECTRON BLEED

As noted previously, complete reduction of oxygen can occur via the mitochondrial electron transport chain and is closely linked with ATP synthesis in aerobic organisms. However, under normal circumstances and certainly in a variety of pathologic conditions, single-electron reduction of oxygen can occur, with the result being production of $O_2^{\cdot-}$. Some estimates indicate that as much as 1% of electron flow along the mitochondrial electron transport chain may "leak" off to produce $O_2^{\cdot-}$. Most of this univalent oxygen reduction occurs at the nicotinamide adenine dinucleotide (NADH) flavoprotein dehydrogenase and ubiquinone-cytochrome b segments. Undoubtedly, the presence of a mitochondrial-specific manganese superoxide dismutase (MnSOD) in rather high concentrations represents a protective strategy for this potential ongoing insult. Synthesis of partially reduced O_2 metabolites occurs when the mitochondrial electron transport chain components are mostly in the reduced state. This state would occur under conditions of poor O_2 delivery to the mitochondria. For example, it has been shown in a Langendorf isolated rat heart model, utilizing low-temperature electron spin resonance (ESR), that the rate of $\cdot OR$ generation within mitochondria isolated from hearts was significantly higher under ischemic as compared with normal conditions (11). Similarly, septic shock is also known to impair the normal flow of electrons along the mitochondrial electron transport chain. Impaired oxygen consumption in this state may also be associated with increased production of $\cdot OR$ (12).

EICOSANOID METABOLISM

A variety of stimuli can activate the arachidonic acid pathway, leading to production of eicosanoids and generation of $O_2^{\cdot-}$ as a byproduct. For example, in the conversion of prostaglandin G_2 to prostaglandin H_2 by endoperoxidase, $O_2^{\cdot-}$ is formed (13). Similarly, other reactions involving peroxidases within the eicosanoid metabolic scheme can lead to production of $O_2^{\cdot-}$ (14).

XANTHINE OXIDASE

An important source of $\cdot OR$, particularly in the setting of ischemia/reperfusion (I/R), is xanthine oxidase (XO) (Fig. 54.8). During ischemia two important series of events unfold. Because of diminished supply of O_2 to tissues, adenosine triphosphate (ATP) synthesis is impaired. In an effort to extract all available energy from existing stores, ATP is completely hydrolyzed sequentially to adenosine diphosphate (ADP), adenosine monophosphate (AMP), adenosine, and, finally, xanthine and hypoxanthine. Simultaneously, as a result of the lack of ATP for the plasma membrane ATPases, pathologic ion fluxes occur. The cytosolic concentration of calcium increases, which is thought to activate an intracellular protease, which in turn leads to the conversion of xanthine dehydrogenase (XD) to XO. Xanthine dehydrogenase catalyzes the conversion of xanthine and hypoxanthine to uric acid, utilizing NAD^+ as an electron acceptor. Following conversion to an oxidase, the enzyme is capable of catalyzing the same reaction utilizing oxygen as the electron acceptor, with the resultant generation of either $O_2^{\cdot-}$ or H_2O_2 as reaction products, along with uric acid. With prolonged ischemia there is an accumulation of xanthine, as well as increased conversion of XD to XO. With reintroduction of oxygen, XO catalyzes a burst of $\cdot OR$ production (Fig. 54.9) (15). This sequence of events has been examined in numerous models of I/R injury in both humans and animals. As one example, in the isolated perfused rat liver, XO activity has been demonstrated to increase as a function of both the duration and the degree of hypoxia, a process that is accelerated by fasting and ischemia (16).

In addition to the "usual" series of events that can lead to activation of XO, it is also known that other events may promote this process. For instance, serum treated with cobra venom factor to activate the complement cascade has been shown to facilitate the conversion of XD to XO (17). This process requires the presence of $C5_a$ but not other complement components, and it does not require the synthesis of new protein. Similarly, activated neutrophils can activate XO (18). In this instance the conversion does not seem to depend on neutrophil $\cdot OR$ products, since oxygen radical scavengers and deferoxamine do not inhibit this process. Rather, neutrophil elastase appears to be the essential constituent in alteration of xanthine dehydrogenase in this setting. It should be noted that XO may be inactivated by H_2O_2 (20). This process appears to involve formation of hydroxyl radical and alteration of the XO active site. At least one cytokine, interferon-γ (IFN-γ), has been shown to increase the activity of XO (19). In this case the cytokine appears to mediate transcriptional activation of the XD/XO gene. Most other cytokines are inactive in this regard.

PHAGOCYTIC RESPIRATORY BURST

Activated phagocytes are also capable of generating a variety of $\cdot OR$ metabolites as products of their respiratory burst. Polymorphonuclear leukocytes are normally quiescent and utilize anaerobic metabolism. However, a variety of agents are capable of stimulating an increased oxygen consumption concomitant with production of $O_2^{\cdot-}$ and H_2O_2 and degranulation of various lysosomal constituents. Whereas baseline $O_2^{\cdot-}$ production by these cells may be essentially zero, following appropriate activation these cells may typically produce 100 million molecules of $O_2^{\cdot-}$/sec/cell. Associated with the activation

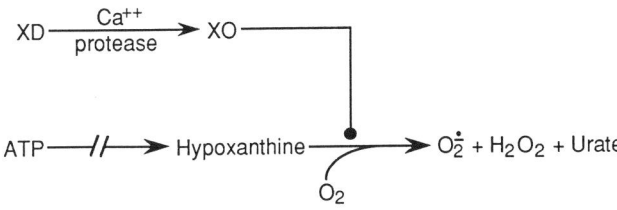

Figure 54.8. Ischemia/reperfusion events leading to conversion of xanthine dehydrogenase (*XD*) to xanthine oxidase (*XO*) and resultant production of $O_2^{\cdot-}$.

$$X + NAD^+ + H_2O \xrightarrow{XD} UA + NADH + H^+$$

$$X + 2O_2 + H_2O \xrightarrow{XO} UA + 2O_2^{\cdot-} + 2H^+$$

$$X + O_2 + H_2O \xrightarrow{XO} UA + H_2O_2$$

Figure 54.9. Various reactions of xanthine dehydrogenase (*XD*) and xanthine oxidase (*XO*) utilizing NAD^+ or O_2 as electron acceptors. *UA*, uric acid; *X*, xanthine.

$$\text{NADPH} \xrightarrow{\text{2e}^-} \text{Flavoprotein} \xrightarrow{\text{e}^-} \text{Cytochrome b-245} \xrightarrow[\substack{\text{O}_2 \\ \searrow \text{e}^-}]{} \text{O}_2^{\cdot}$$

Figure 54.10. Phagocyte respiratory burst electron transport chain.

is the occurrence of a change in transmembrane potential, which is followed by secondary signaling systems that lead to assembly of a nicotinamide adenine dinucleotide phosphate (NADPH)-dependent oxidoreductase complex (21). Absence or dysfunction of various components of this complex results in chronic granulomatous disease.

This respiratory burst electron transfer system consists of a flavin adenine dinucleotide (FAD)-containing flavoprotein, as well as a unique cytochrome, cytochrome b-245, which exhibits the lowest potential of any mammalian cytochrome and consists of a 91 kDa glycosylated protein and a 22 kDa nonglycosylated protein with two heme prosthetic groups. Cytosolic proteins with molecular weights of 47 kDa and 67 kDa translocate to the plasma membrane as part of the activation of the respiratory burst. NADPH, which provides the reducing equivalents for the production of $O_2^{\cdot}$, is generated from the hexose monophosphate shunt. A cytosolic NADPH-binding subunit with a molecular weight of 24 to 28 kDa also appears to translocate from the cytosol to the membrane active enzyme complex site (22–24) (Fig. 54.10).

As noted earlier, a variety of other ·OR metabolites can be generated from the parent ·OR species $O_2^{\cdot}$. Moreover, neutrophils are known to contain a variety of proteases, as well as lipases that may act synergistically with ·OR. All of these mediators are designed to clear foreign antigens as part of a normal inflammatory response. When any of these constituents, including ·OR, are leaked from the neutrophil through an incomplete phagosome, the potential for host autoinjury exists. Although neutrophils generally are not thought to initiate primary injury, their leukoagglutination and activation can orchestrate significant secondary inflammatory injury. Certainly a major mediator in this process is the variety of ·OR species generated by activated neutrophils.

Polymorphonuclear leukocytes and XO appear to interact (25). Mention has already been made of the capacity for neutrophils to convert XD to XO. In addition, whereas XO may be responsible for an initial injury in the I/R setting, typically neutrophils subsequently intervene to augment the ·OR injury. As an example, it has been shown in a model of hemorrhagic shock that XO, at least in part, mediates neutrophil recruitment (26). Following a 30% hemorrhage, which results in a 50% decrease in mean arterial pressure, control animals exhibit an increase in lung neutrophils as assayed by tissue myeloperoxidase. Alternately, if rats are prefed tungsten (which depletes lung and plasma XO) and then phlebotomized, a significant decrease in lung-associated myeloperoxidase is seen. It has been hypothesized that XO-derived oxidants may be involved in the generation of chemotaxins for neutrophils and, in addition, may be responsible for alteration of neutrophil receptors, which might enhance neutrophil binding.

Table 54.1.   Detection of "Oxyradicals"

1. Direct detection by electron spin resonance and spin trapping
2. Measurement of thiobarbituric acid reactive species
3. Direct detection of malondialdehyde
4. Quantification of other polyunsaturated fatty acid (PUFA) oxidative degradation products such as 4-hydroxynonenal
5. Measurement of PUFA hydroperoxides and H_2O_2 or corresponding alcohols
6. Detection of PUFA β-scission-derived volatile hydrocarbons such as ethane and pentane
7. Quantification of PUFA conjugated dienes
8. Assessment of oxidation products of methione and cysteine
9. Detection of protein-derived carbonyl-containing products
10. Determination of decreases in antioxidant compounds such as glutathione and α-tocopherol
11. Assessment of oxidized DNA bases such as thymine glycol and 8-hydroxydeoxyguanosine

OXYRADICAL/OXYRADICAL INJURY DETECTION

Parallel to the explosive interest in the pathogenic aspects of ·OR species has emerged an interest in detection and quantification of ·OR and/or corresponding macromolecular injury. Many of the numerous methodologies that have been proposed lack either sensitivity, specificity, or both. Detection of these species is not a trivial matter, since rational design of ·OR therapeutic trials should include not only demonstration of a physiologic effect, but alterations in reliable biochemical markers of the purportedly involved ·OR. Most ·OR species are fleeting in existence, and methods for their direct assessment are few and largely cumbersome. Accordingly, various investigators have proposed assays to detect "footprints" of previous ·OR presence (27, 28) (Table 54.1).

ELECTRON SPIN RESONANCE

Electron spin resonance (ESR) utilizing direct detection or the spin trapping technique has been used in a few studies to demonstrate pathologic involvement of ·OR species. Isolated perfused hearts have been examined in models of I/R (29). Tissue from this same type of model has been examined utilizing the freeze clamp technique (30). Signals indicative of semiquinones, lipid peroxyl radicals, and carbon-centered radicals have all been detected utilizing ESR technology in the I/R setting.

MALONDIALDEHYDE

It is perhaps not surprising to note that most of the techniques utilized to detect ·OR involve quantification of some lipid peroxidation product. Certainly, other macromolecules are targets for ·OR injury (see below). However, by-products of free radical attack on polyunsaturated fatty acids (PUFA) have received the most analytical interest. Probably the best known and most controversial assay for lipid peroxidation involves the detection of a 3-carbon breakdown product that occurs during lipid peroxidation, namely malondialdehyde (MDA). It may be quantified in its native state or as some derivative. It should be appreciated that MDA is extremely reactive and may bind to a variety of macromolecules such that the true quantification of MDA, generated as a result of lipid peroxidation, may be significantly underestimated. The most popular assay for detection of MDA involves its condensation with two molecules of thiobarbituric acid, which results in the production of a red chromophore termed *thiobarbituric acid reactive species* (TBARS), which exhibits a high extinction coefficient at 532 nm. This particular assay has been utilized in hundreds of investigations in an attempt to quantify lipid peroxidation (Fig. 54.11).

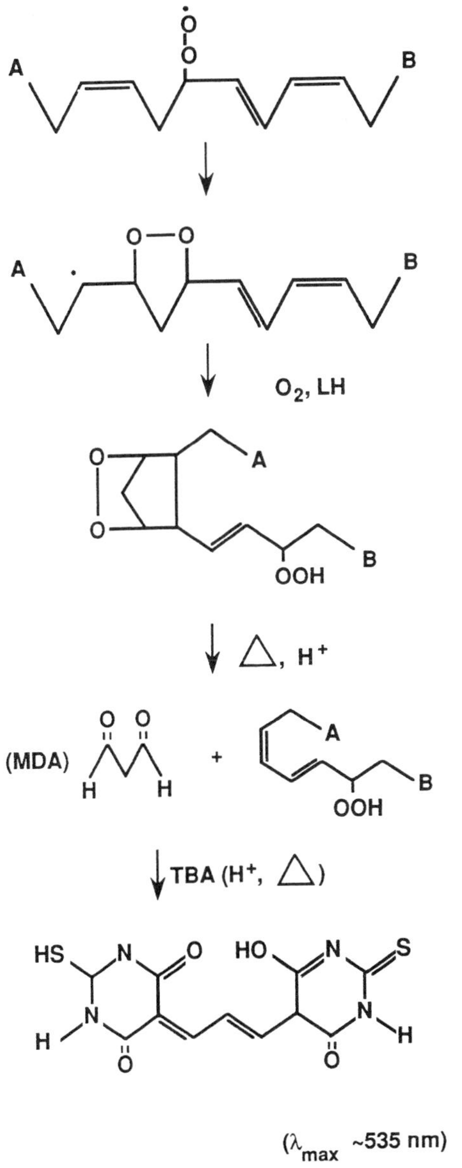

Figure 54.11. Formation of malondialdehyde from peroxidized lipids and its detection with thiobarbituric acid.

However, the TBARS assay is hardly specific for MDA. In addition to reacting with MDA, the TBARS reagent can also interact with proteins, amino sugars, 2-deoxyribose, sucrose, hemoglobin, bilirubin, pyrimidines, and hydroxyalkenals to yield colored products (31). Numerous other derivatives of MDA, (e.g., 2,4-dinitrophenylhydrazine) have also been examined (32). An attractive adjunct for any MDA assay involves separation of the reaction products utilizing high-performance liquid chromatography (33). This allows fractionation of the nonspecific reactions of the derivatization reagents and the breakdown products of the derivatization reaction, which can occur even in the absence of nonspecific adducts.

Despite their sensitivity and utility, the MDA assays have been criticized on several accounts (34): (*a*) yield of MDA depends on the nature of the PUFA and peroxidation stimulus—only certain lipid peroxidation products yield MDA; (*b*) MDA represents only one of several aldehydic end products of PUFA peroxidation and decomposition; (*c*) the peroxidation environment influences both the formation and the decomposition of various MDA precursors; (*d*) MDA itself is extremely reactive and may not be available for analytic detection; and (*e*) oxidative injury to various nonlipid macromolecules may also result in the formation of MDA, as well as MDA-like products. In well-defined in vitro systems with minimal contamination by the confounding variables outlined above, the assay of MDA, as an index of lipid peroxidation, may be both sensitive and specific. However, in complex biological systems one must at least suspect that multiple variables could be contributing to the MDA signal. As has been pointed out, "MDA may represent nothing more than an empirical indicator of potential occurrence of peroxidative lipid injury . . ." (34).

HYDROXYLALDEHYDES

Other aldehydic lipid peroxidation decomposition products also may be quantified in addition to MDA. A particularly attractive candidate in this regard is 4-hydroxynonenal, which may be assessed utilizing high-pressure liquid chromatography and gas chromatography techniques (35, 36). Quantifying this lipid peroxidation product improves the specificity of the assay considerably over MDA, since the longer-chain aldehyde quite specifically reflects a decomposition product of lipid peroxidation.

CONJUGATED DIENES

Probably the other most widely employed assay that attempts to reflect lipid peroxidation is the conjugated diene assay. In their native state, mammalian PUFAs contain double bonds that are interspersed between fully saturated methylene bridges. With lipid peroxidation, rearrangement of the double bond structure occurs in order to transiently resonance-stabilize an unpaired electron. Depending upon where the eventual peroxyl functional group locates, the fatty acid may contain a conjugated double bond system that absorbs ultraviolet light at 234 nm. With the conjugated diene assay, a lipid extraction is performed and the extract is analyzed spectrophotometrically at 234 nm (37). In performing scanning spectrophotometry of such samples, one immediately becomes aware of the imprecision of the methodology, as a steep rise in absorption of the sample typically occurs at lower and lower wavelengths. Characteristically a small shoulder around 234 nm reflects the presence of conjugated dienes. Some authors have advocated the use of the second-derivative spectrophotometry to improve detection utilizing this methodology (38). Obviously, the other important drawback with the conjugated diene assay is that numerous molecules will absorb nonspecifically at 234 nm.

HYDROPEROXYL FATTY ACIDS

Hydroperoxyl fatty acids may be quantified directly in lipid extracts of samples utilizing high-performance liquid chromatography fractionation and column effluent detection employing either chemiluminescence or electrodetection. In the chemiluminescence method, lipid peroxides are reacted with microperoxidase in the presence of isoluminal to generate light quanta that may subsequently be quantified (39, 40). The amperometric approach utilizes a channel electrochemical detector with a reducing potential generated between solid-disk electrodes (41). Since the hydroperoxyl functional groups generally display a short half-life, this approach is limited by the speed with which samples may be extracted and prepared for chromatography.

Lipid hydroperoxides are known to activate cyclooxygenase activity; this property may be utilized as an assay with a sensitivity of 10 to 150 pmol, which is approximately 50 times more sensitive than either TBARS or related fluorescence assays (42). Still another assay for hydroperoxides involves their reduction to corresponding alcohols with glutathione peroxidase GSH Px, utilizing glutathione (GSH) as the reducing agent (Fig. 54.12). Glutathione disulfide is subsequently cycled back to GSH with glutathione reductase and NADPH. This coupled enzyme assay is monitored at 340 nm as the oxidation of NADPH cofactor (43). If catalase (CAT) is added to the reaction mixture, one can differentiate H_2O_2 from lipid peroxides, since CAT will convert any H_2O_2 to H_2O and O_2 but will not act on long-chain fatty acid hydroperoxides.

GAS CHROMATOGRAPHY OF FATTY ACID ALCOHOLS

Lipid peroxides have also been quantified utilizing gas chromatography with mass spectroscopy detection. Extracted lipid peroxides are first reduced with sodium borohydride to the corresponding alcohols, which are considerably more stable (Fig. 54.13). Subsequently, the fatty acids are transesterified and any hydroxyl groups (alcohols) derivatized with trimethylsilane to increase the volatility of the samples. Fatty acid methyl ester (FAME) derivatives are fractionated utilizing gas chromatography. Individual species are identified by

their unique retention times. Confirmation of positive identification can be made by examining the mass spectroscopy molecular fragmentation pattern for a particular peak. Utilizing chemical ionization detection, specific molecular ions can be quantified with high yield and sensitivity to the pg level (44).

HEAD SPACE GAS CHROMATOGRAPHY OF ALKANES

In addition to long- and short-chain aldehydes, various volatile alkanes are also formed during decomposition of lipid peroxidation products. This observation has led to the development of other gas chromatography technology that allows quantification of these volatile lipid breakdown products. By collecting expired breath from patients and employing head space gas chromatography, a real-time indicator of lipid peroxidation may be generated (45, 46).

ANTIOXIDANT CONSUMPTION

Macromolecular oxidant stress may also be assayed as depletion of protective ·OR scavenging systems—for example, the consumption of cellular sulfhydryls, particularly GSH. Loss of GSH reflects its oxidation to glutathione disulfide for the purpose of protecting critical cysteine sulfhydryls (47–50). Depletion of other cellular constituents such as α-tocopherol, uric acid, and ascorbic acid have also been used as indicators of oxidant stress.

An extensive literature exists relative to the determination of the sulfhydryl redox state. Although a number of methods have been developed, variations of the original Ellman's assay, which monitor the interaction of 2-nitro-5-thiobenzoate anion with free sulfhydryls (with or without the use of glutathione reductase), continue to be the most frequently utilized assays (51, 52) (Fig. 54.14). This methodology may be used specifically for glutathione or, alternatively, for total acid soluble sulfhydryls or protein sulfhydryls. All reflect protein oxidant stress as quantified by the ratio of reduced to oxidized sulfhydryls.

NITROBLUE TETRAZOLIUM REDUCTION

In situ generation of O_2^- has been followed in animal models utilizing the tissue closed window technique and nitroblue tetrazolium. For example, in a model of brain I/R in newborn pigs, a closed cranial window technique with continual flush of nitroblue tetrazolium solution beneath the window revealed an enhanced production of O_2^- as detected by a change in color of the nitroblue tetrazolium from yellow to blue (53). This color change could be eliminated by including SOD in the flush solution, thus ascertaining the role of O_2^- in the dye reduction. In this case the increase in blue color attributable

$$2\ GSH + LOOH \xrightarrow{\text{GSH Px}} GSSG + ROH$$

$$GSSG + 2NADPH \xrightarrow{\text{GSH R}} 2\ GSH + NADP+$$

Figure 54.12. Assay of lipid peroxides utilizing glutathione peroxidase (*GSH Px*) and glutathione reductase (*GSH R*).

$$R\text{-}OOH \xrightarrow{\text{NaBH}_4} R\text{-}OH$$

Figure 54.13. Reduction of lipid peroxides to the corresponding alcohols by sodium borohydride.

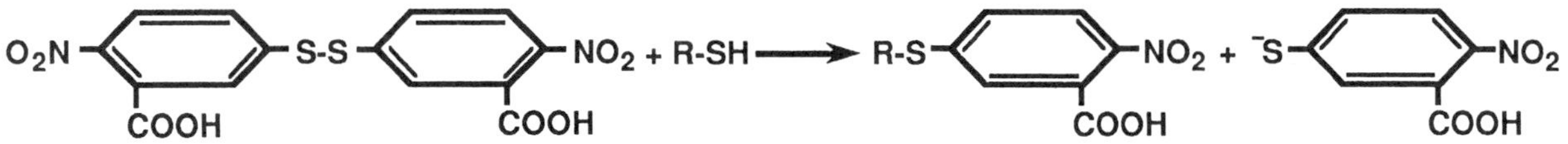

Figure 54.14. Schematic depiction of the Ellman's assay for reduced sulfhydryls.

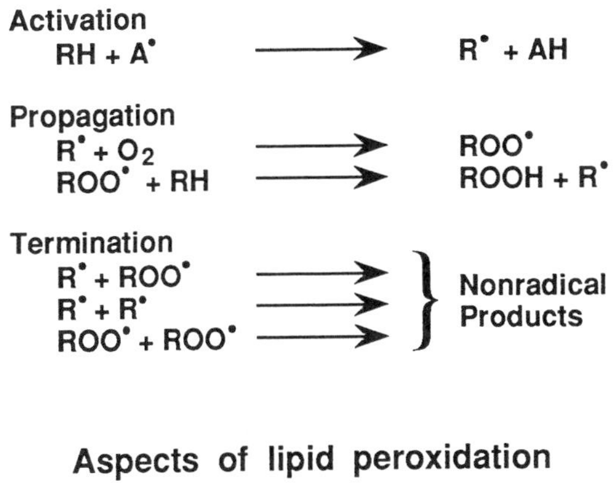

Aspects of lipid peroxidation

Figure 54.15. Lipid peroxidation reactions, including initiation, propagation, and termination.

to generation of O_2^- could also be prevented by prior administration of indomethacin to the animals. These results suggested that the O_2^- produced during reperfusion was a byproduct of the prostaglandin endoperoxide synthetase pathway.

PROTEIN CARBONYL CONTENT

Another assay that quantifies protein oxidative stress involves determination of carbonyl content. γ-Glutamyl-semialdehyde, a glutamic acid oxidation product, is thought to provide most of the substrate for this assay (54). Following tissue extraction, trititated borohydride or 2,4-dinitrophenylhydrazine is utilized to reduce or derivatize the aldehyde for detection. Considerably more sample is required with the 2,4-dinitrophenylhydrazine method than with the borohydride reduction method, since, in the former case, the hydrazone is quantified spectrophotometrically, while in the latter assay the determination is made radiometrically.

ASSAYS REFLECTING DNA ·OR INJURY

Oxidant stress upon nucleic acid, typically DNA, has also been analyzed utilizing a variety of techniques. The classic assay involves fluorometric analysis of DNA unwinding (55). Typical double-stranded mammalian DNA will intercollate the fluorescence dye, ethidium bromide, with little interference from single-stranded DNA and RNA. When DNA is subjected to oxidant stress, strand breaks occur, and under proper assay conditions these segments begin to unwind and hence intercollate less ethidium bromide. Accordingly, a decrease in fluorescence indicates oxidant stress. More direct analysis of DNA damage can also be performed by examining oxidant products of various nucleotides directly. For example, 8-hydroxy-2′-deoxyguanosine has been measured in urine samples by high-performance liquid chromatography and

electrochemical detection (56). It appears to be a marker of in vivo oxidative DNA damage reflecting oxidant stress upon guanine. Similarly, gas chromatography with mass spectrometry detection has been utilized to identify specific DNA base alterations (57). By using specific ion monitoring in this setting, a variety of specific nucleotide oxidant products can be quantified precisely (58).

Numerous other examples of assays for ·OR and corresponding tissue damage have been advocated. Some of these are mentioned below in discussing the spectrum of oxyradical injury as well as the therapeutic potential of various ·OR scavengers.

OXYRADICAL MEDIATED MOLECULAR ALTERATIONS

Oxyradical stress can mediate profound alterations in proteins, lipids, and nucleic acids. Oxidant-mediated molecular alterations can result in both structural and functional changes that may adversely affect cellular and organ physiology.

PROTEINS

Proteins are the most abundant macromolecules in living cells and constitute about one-half of the dry weight of cells. Biological functions of proteins include catalysis, transport, storage, contractility, structure, regulation, and defense. All proteins are subject to oxidative injury, which may, in turn, result in denaturation and/or fragmentation (59, 60). Primary structure of proteins involves a chain of amino acids. Although all amino acids are susceptible to ·OR modification, tryptophan, tyrosine, histidine, and cysteine are particularly sensitive (61). Alterations in amino acid primary structure are associated with alterations in protein secondary, tertiary, and quarternary structure, with potential resultant effects in all of the areas of protein function as noted previously.

Some of the most important effects of ·OR protein stress include specific alterations in amino acids. Oxidation of cysteine has been noted previously. Thiols (RSH) may be oxidized to the corresponding disulfide (RSSR) or, alternately, to sulfenic acid (RSOH), sulfinic acid (RSO_2H), or sulfonic acid (RSO_3H) by sequential losses of two electrons per step. It should be noted that the thiyl radical (RS·) may also be formed and represents a possible alternate route to lipid peroxidation (62). Other common ·OR-mediated amino acid alterations include carbonyl formation as well as the production of bityrosine. Changes in protein structure may result in alterations in isoelectric point, folding, hydrophobicity, aggregation, and active site orientation (63). Denaturation by ·OR has been shown to increase the susceptibility of proteins to proteolysis (64).

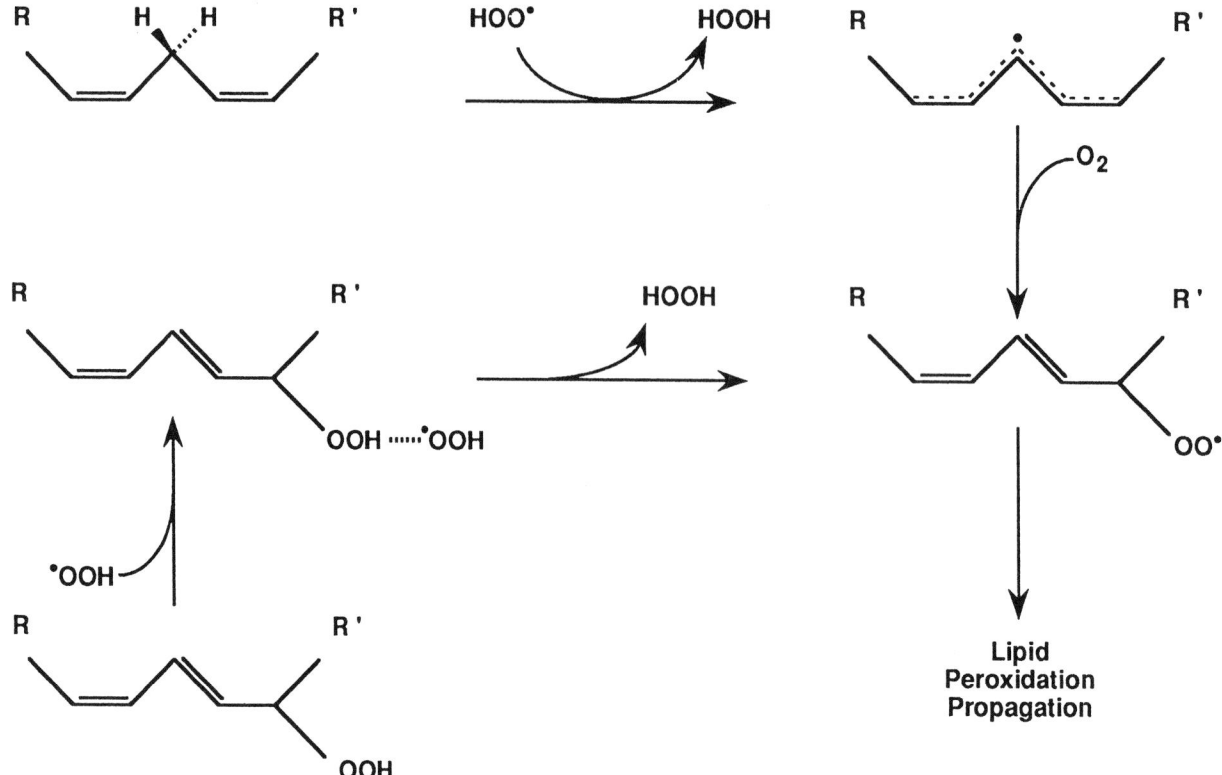

Figure 54.16. Two routes for initiation of lipid peroxidation.

LIPIDS

PUFAs are readily susceptible to ·OR stress. Like proteins, lipids, particularly those that are polyunsaturated, represent an important target of ·OR stress, since these macromolecules are prevalent throughout all tissues. Specifically, all cells are bounded by a phospholipid-rich plasmalemma and, in addition, contain numerous phospholipid-rich intracellular organelles, including endoplasmic reticulum, nuclear membrane, and mitochondria. Hydrogen abstraction from allylic or bis-allylic positions on the fatty acid side chain leads to formation of peroxyl radicals. Oxidation of PUFA has traditionally been viewed as consisting of three steps: initiation or activation, propagation, and termination (65) (Fig. 54.15).

Autocatalytic chain reactions involving PUFAs may become self-sustaining. A single initiating event may be magnified substantially through such autocatalytic events. Following introduction of the peroxyl functional group, intramolecular rearrangements and scission reactions lead to a variety of decomposition products, including aldehydes and alkanes, as discussed previously. It has been demonstrated that the peroxyl radical (HOO·), which represents the conjugate acid of O_2^-, may initiate fatty acid lipid peroxidation via two possible pathways, one that depends upon the presence of low levels of existing fatty acid hydroperoxide, and one that is hydroperoxide independent (the traditional view) (66) (Fig. 54.16).

The fatty acid hydroperoxide-dependent mechanism involving perhydroxyl radical defines a greater role for O_2^- than has been recognized previously. This fact, coupled with the observation that low levels of hydroperoxides are common in PUFA, supports this alternate reaction. Details of neutrophil

·OR-mediated PUFA peroxidation have been described (67). Peroxidized phospholipids are more susceptible to hydrolysis by phospholipase A_2 (68).

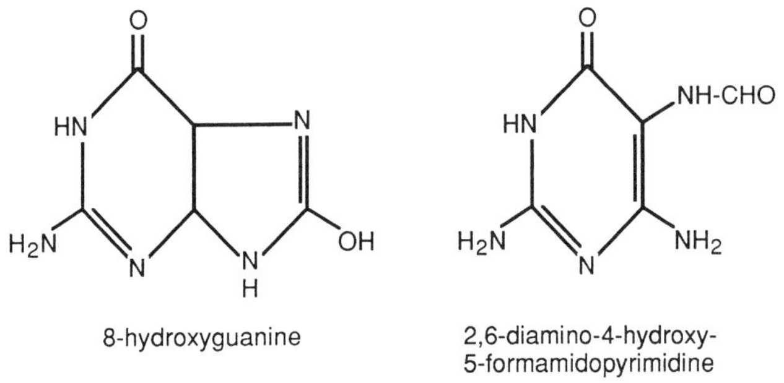

Figure 54.17. Common nucleic acid oxidation products.

8-hydroxyguanine   2,6-diamino-4-hydroxy-5-formamidopyrimidine

NUCLEIC ACID

Potentially the most ominous ·OR-mediated injury involves nucleic acid. Oxidant stress upon DNA interferes not only with the overall synthetic activity of the cell but also with its ability to replicate and repair itself. Oxyradical damage to nucleic acid has been associated with carcinogenesis and mutagenesis (69). A variety of ·OR-mediated nucleic acid products have been identified by gas chromatography/mass spectrometry. Among the most common are 2,6-diamino-4-hydroxy-5-formamidopyrimidine and 8-hydroxyguanine (70) (Fig. 54.17).

These nucleic acid base alterations may be conveniently analyzed in urine specimens (56). In a cell culture model employing Chinese hamster ovary cells, ·OR species, generated by activated phagocytes, have been shown to enhance DNA sister chromatid exchange formation (71). Such alterations were reduced by utilizing various antioxidant enzymes as well as by ensuring adequate cellular GSH concentration. In other cell culture models employing vascular endothelium, it has been demonstrated that cells exposed to either H_2O_2 or $O_2^{\cdot-}$ exhibit DNA strand breakage much earlier than overt cellular cytotoxicity (72). In cultured endothelial cells as well as murine macrophages exposed to oxidants, DNA single-strand breaks have been demonstrated concomitant with a decrease in DNA double-strandedness (73, 74). This type of injury can occur within seconds of a cell's exposure to oxidant stress. Significant DNA damage not only alters the cell's genetic repertoire but also may be associated with acute cytotoxicity. Depletion of cellular NAD^+ and ATP levels and activation of the enzyme ADP-ribose polymerase occur concomitant with ·OR-mediated DNA damage (75). The latter enzyme system utilizes NAD^+ for the production of poly(ADP)-ribose, which is used to facilitate the DNA repair process. ADP-ribose moieties are successively linked to form homopolymers that may vary in length from a few residues to long-chain polymers in excess of 100 residues. Enzyme activity has been demonstrated to depend on the number of DNA strand breaks as well as the duration of the existence of these breaks. Depletion of cellular NAD^+ may be sufficient to completely disrupt cellular metabolism, including synthesis of ATP (76). Following ·OR-mediated DNA base damage, nonspecific endonucleases may cleave a short chain of DNA or specific glycosylases may remove specific altered bases. Eventually these oxidized nucleic acids are excreted into the urine. Even in the absence of overt lipid and protein oxidant damage, depletion of cellular NAD^+ and ATP would obviously threaten cell viability.

OXYRADICAL MEDIATED CELLULAR INJURY

CELL CULTURE EXPERIMENTS

Oxidant-mediated macromolecule injury would be expected to affect various aspects of cellular biochemistry, physiology, and structure. Utilizing dihydroxyfumarate and $FeCl_3$/ADP to continuously generate $O_2^{\cdot-}$, investigators have demonstrated that C6 glioma cells manifest progressive morphologic changes, including a loss of villi, cellular blebbing, rupture, and necrosis, all of which are associated with the accumulation of TBARS and are indicative of lipid peroxidation (77). As key components of the inflammatory response, ·OR species may play roles in both cellular protection and cellular injury. On the one hand, monocyte and granulocytes are known to utilize ·OR in mediating bacterial and tumor cell destruction (78). However, on the other, this same phagocytic ·OR generating system is known to mediate cytotoxicity of nonforeign cells (79). Much of the detailed information regarding oxidant stress has been gleaned from cell culture experiments. Toxic oxygen species were first demonstrated to mediate damage to cultured endothelial cells. These same early experiments were the first to show the possible utility of various ·OR scavenging systems in ameliorating such injury (80). These types of investigations have also demonstrated the possible synergistic action of ·OR damage and proteolytic insult (81).

Alveolar type II cells represent another relevant and popular cell culture system utilized to study the subtleties of ·OR-mediated cell injury. Type II cells grown in 95% O_2 demonstrate increased release of cytosolic lactic dehydrogenase while simultaneously exhibiting decreases in both DNA synthesis and its key exocrine product, dipalmitoyl phosphatidylcholine (82). Exposure of cultured type II cells to H_2O_2 has been shown to decrease intracellular ATP concentrations by 77% within 5 minutes following exposure (83). In this setting the mitochondria appeared to be a key target of ·OR stress, particularly at the ATPase synthetase enzyme complex—mitochondrial electron transport was unaltered. Hydrogen peroxide has also been shown to cause a dose-dependent decrease in phosphatidylcholine synthesis in cultured type II cells; a 70% inhibition of synthesis of phosphatidylcholine was noted with exposure of type II cells to 300 mM H_2O_2 (84). This severe alteration in cell function was seen at a point in time when little change in cell viability could be demonstrated. This type of injury may be significantly attenuated by loading the cells with exogenous polyethylene glycol (PEG)-conjugated CAT, which increases the concentration of this apparent key antioxidant enzyme approximately 8-fold. Utilizing a somewhat more physiologic approach, it has also been demonstrated that activated neutrophils can similarly inhibit de novo synthesis of phosphatidylcholine by type II alveolar cells (85). Again, because this effect can be largely reversed with antioxidant enzymes, a significant portion of this neutrophil-mediated injury is postulated to occur via ·OR. Cultured type II cells appear to be more sensitive to ·OR stress as compared with alveolar macrophages or fibroblasts, as demonstrated by their increased lactic dehydrogenase leak, decreased DNA thymidine incorporation, and decreased synthesis of dipalmitoyl phosphatidylcholine following identical ·OR insults (86).

Specific components of type II cells have been demonstrated to be targets of ·OR. For example, exposure of surfactant protein A (SP-A) to ozone appears to impair its interaction with alveolar type II cells and to enhance its susceptibility to proteolysis (87). Alterations of SP-A could have a variety of cellular physiologic effects, including an impaired ability to inhibit phosphatidylcholine secretion, to enhance phagocytosis, and to stimulate the macrophage respiratory burst. Similarly, various characteristics of surfactant itself, including its isopycnic density, minimal surface tension, time course of absorption, compressibility, and stability index, may be adversely affected by exposure to ·OR generated by activated neutrophils or $FeCl_3$/ascorbate (88). Polyacrylamide gel electrophoresis of the surfactant proteins following these types of ·OR stress have demonstrated a decrease in the band density of SP-A that is associated with the appearance of several bands with both lower and higher molecular weights.

MEMBRANE ALTERATIONS

In vitro investigations have established that ·OR species decrease deformability of rabbit and human erythrocytes (89). Similar changes have been noted in rats in a septic shock model involving cecal ligation and puncture, in which erythrocyte deformability changes concomitant with sepsis were shown to be preventable by prior administration of α-tocopherol (90). Impaired deformability, secondary to oxidant stress,

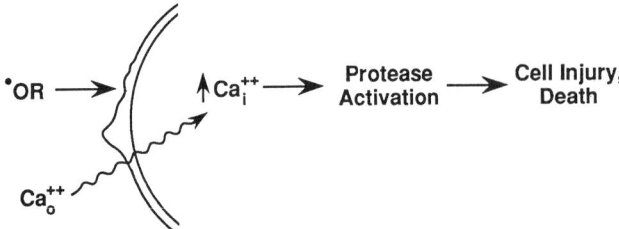

Figure 54.18. Schematic depiction of the relationship between plasma membrane ·OR injury, Ca^{2+} influx, and protease activation.

could represent an important pathophysiologic mechanism in sepsis, as such changes might be associated with impaired oxygen delivery and/or peripheral shunting, which seems to occur in the setting of sepsis. Alterations in membrane perturbation by ·OR have also been studied in cultured endothelial cells utilizing ESR and spin-trapping agents. In this model ·OR stress was associated with increased membrane fluidity (91). In the discussion of their results, the investigators point out that ·OR species have been shown both to increase and to decrease membrane order and that these changes may reflect increased disulfide interprotein linkage, increased aldehyde formation (that subsequently forms Schiff base cross-links with protein amino groups), and decreased fatty acid chain length. Liver I/R oxidant stress has been shown to increase the molecular order of microsomal membranes and is associated with an increased cholesterol-to-phospholipid ratio (92). Oxyradical stress appears to accelerate phospholipid degradation, which is associated with an increased molecular order as quantitated by ESR analysis of the anisotropic motion of 12-deoxylsteric acid within the phospholipid milieu of membrane (92). As a result of alterations in plasma membrane following ·OR stress, alterations of cell membrane potential have been demonstrated in cardiac and skeletal cells (93). Oxidant damage has also been shown to alter the steady-state background current in isolated ventricular myocytes (94). Depolarization of the cell membrane of these cultured myocytes has been postulated to occur secondary to a reduction of the inward rectifying potassium current, associated with activation of calcium-activated membrane conductants.

CELLULAR CALCIUM INFLUX

Alteration of the plasma membrane by ·OR has been shown to increase intracellular free calcium ion concentration in several cell types (e.g., see reference 95). This may occur secondary to alteration of plasma membrane components, which results in creation of calcium ionophores (96). Cultured human umbilical endothelial cells have been examined utilizing multiparameter digitalized video microscopy with fluorescent probes. Following XO stress, intracellular calcium concentration was shown to increase approximately 5-fold and was preceded by plasma membrane blebs (97). Subsequent cellular death in this system could be delayed by the protease inhibitors leupeptin or pepstatin, which implicate protease activation by the elevated intracellular calcium. Other investigators have similarly demonstrated that increased cellular protein degradation occurs as a consequence of cellular oxidant stress (98) (Fig. 54.18).

Numerous cellular enzymes have been shown to be specific targets of ·OR injury. Oxyradical-sensitive enzymes include catalase (99), aconitase (100), glycerol-3-phosphate acyltransferase (101), glyceraldehyde-3-phosphate-dehydrogenase (102), glutamine synthetase (103), Na^+/K^+ ATPase (104), xanthine oxidase (20), and various components of the mitochondrial electron transport chain, including NADH dehydrogenase, NADH oxidase, succinate dehydrogenase, succinate oxidase, and the ATP synthetase enzyme complex (105). Obviously, alteration of any of these enzyme systems would have profound implications for numerous aspects of cellular metabolism. Lipid peroxidation of cell membranes is known to decrease the number and activity of β-adrenergic receptors (106).

Another protein that has been studied in detail with respect to its ·OR inactivation is α-1-antiprotease. A critical methionine residue on the active site of α-1-antiprotease may be oxidized to the corresponding sulfoxide by lipid peroxides or the neutrophil myeloperoxidase system (see Figure 54.4), which results in a molecule that will not bind to elastase (107–109). Such a scenario has been demonstrated in human subjects exposed to nitrous oxide (110). Subsequent analysis of their bronchoalveolar lavage fluid demonstrated increased levels of conjugated dienes as well as decreased elastase inhibitory capacity. Nutritional supplementation with vitamins E and C prior to nitrous oxide exposure significantly decreased these alterations. Oxidative inactivation of α-1-protease is another example of the synergistic activity between ·OR species and proteases.

Oxyradicals have been shown to mediate damage of extracellular constituents (111). In the case of extracellular matrix proteoglycan, once again a synergistic action between the neutrophil myeloperoxidase system and proteases has been ascertained (112).

VASCULAR AND AIRWAY REACTIVITY

Oxyradicals may mediate complex roles relative to vascular reactivity (113). On the one hand they may initiate eicosanoid metabolism, which could lead to increased production of both vasodilators as well as vasoconstrictors. Hydrogen peroxide activation of guanylate cyclase is known to affect signal transduction and smooth muscle contraction directly. Similarly, ·OR species have been implicated in inducing airway hyper-responsiveness (114). It is known that H_2O_2, for example, can induce specifically the production of thromboxane A_2 without altering the synthesis of prostaglandin E_2. In related studies it has been shown in dog I/R models that ·OR species are apparently responsible, in part, for release of histamine, and this effect may be significantly attenuated with either catalase (CAT) or deferoxamine (115).

OXYRADICAL-MEDIATED CRITICAL CARE ILLNESS

It can be argued that most critical care illnesses involve the participation of ·OR pathophysiology. Accordingly, when one considers the various forms of acute lung injury, the sepsis syndrome, the numerous I/R states, including shock, myocardial infarction, stroke, acute renal failure, necrotizing enterocolitis, gastric and duodenal ulcers, and transplantation, as well as the multiple organ failure syndrome, most of what encompasses intensive care medicine is included (116). Involvement of ·OR species in the pathophysiology of all of these diseases has been implicated in either human investigations or appropriate animal models. Many of these syndromes involve activation of the host inflammatory response (117). Oxygen radicals represent a key constituent of this system that may both benefit the host and mediate autoinjury. A study examining patients with a variety of critical illnesses, including sepsis, pneumonia, cardiac disease, and central nervous system disorders, demonstrated that levels of plasma TBARS, an indicator of lipid peroxidation, are significantly increased and levels of a plasma antioxidant, α-tocopherol (αTH), are significantly decreased as compared with those in non-critically ill patients (118). These differences were most profound in those patients demonstrating disseminated intravascular coagulation.

ACUTE LUNG INJURY

Since the various pulmonary epithelial cells may be exposed to very high FiO$_2$, which is utilized therapeutically to support a variety of critical illnesses, it is not surprising that ·OR injury was first investigated in the lungs (119). In addition to mediating parenchymal lung injury, ·OR species have also been implicated in bronchoconstriction, increased mucus secretion, microvascular leak, cilia changes, and pulmonary macrophage inhibition (120). In acute lung injury associated with sepsis, histologic lung injury and associated tissue lipid peroxidation products appear to be more abundant in the lung than in the liver. Investigators have proposed that the lung may be protecting systemic tissue by clearing endotoxin (or even perhaps long-lived oxygen radical species) (121). It should be noted that hyperoxia may injure both alveolar epithelium and the pulmonary surfactant system (122). Actual evidence for the involvement of ·OR in (acute) lung injury has been demonstrated by examining markers of ·OR stress in bronchoalveolar lavage (BAL) specimens from patients with idiopathic pulmonary fibrosis. The ratio of oxidized methionine to native methionine residues was increased 5-fold in the idiopathic pulmonary fibrosis patients as compared with controls and was correlated with increased numbers of neutrophils in the BAL fluid (123). Other studies examining patients with adult respiratory distress syndrome (ARDS) have revealed increased levels of expired breath H$_2$O$_2$ (124, 125).

Increased levels of the diene-conjugated 9,11 isomer of linoleic acid have been demonstrated in BAL fluid obtained from patients with acute asthma (126). Moreover, neutrophils isolated from patients with asthma appear to produce more O$_2^{\cdot}$, an observation that has been directly correlated with the duration of chronic disease and the acute attack and inversely correlated with FEV$_1$ and V$_{25}$ (127).

Oxyradicals have also been scrutinized with regard to pathogenesis in neonatal lung disease, particularly RDS of the newborn and acute bronchopulmonary dysplasia (BPD). In a neonatal rat model resulting in 85% mortality after exposure to 100% oxygen for 72 hours, it was shown that the microsomal fraction of lung parenchyma exhibited increased

Table 54.2. Maximal Exhaled Ethane and Pentane in Critically Ill VLBW Neonates (131)

	Ethane^a	Pentane^a
Good outcome	2–32	2–19
Poor outcome	22–217	7–71

^{a} pmol/min/kg

levels of lipid peroxides. In addition, the activity of endogenous phospholipase was increased in the lungs of these animals, as was the concentration of leukotriene B4 and the density of polymorphonuclear leukocytes (128). Obviously any or all of these mediators could play a role in oxygen-mediated lung injury. Investigators and clinicians continue to argue about the relative contributions of O$_2$ toxicity and barotrauma to the development of BPD. A recent study employing a neonatal piglet model concluded that hyperoxia caused more physiologic, inflammatory, and histologic changes than did barotrauma alone (129).

In addition to the increased ·OR stress placed upon premature newborns with RDS, another problem may be inadequate ·OR defense mechanisms. At least in some models of neonatal lung injury, not only are baseline levels of various antioxidants low compared with those of adults but, in addition, preterm animals may not demonstrate the expected induction of these various antioxidant systems following exposure to hyperoxia (130). Real-time quantification of lipid peroxidation in infants with RDS and acute BPD has been performed in the neonatal intensive care setting by measuring exhaled ethane and pentane by mass spectrometry. In 19 very low birth weight infants elevated levels of these exhaled alkane lipid peroxidation decomposition products have been correlated with poor outcome, either death or bronchopulmonary dysplasia (131) (Table 54.2).

SEPSIS SYNDROME

Evidence for the involvement of ·OR injury in sepsis has been examined utilizing a variety of models, including αTH consumption (132), tissue GSH depletion (133), exhaled ethane (134), and levels of TBARS in plasma (135), BAL (136), and tissue (137). Sepsis again exemplifies the dual role of ·OR in disease. For example, although ·OR-dependent mechanisms appeared to be essential for bacterial killing in a piglet group B streptococcus sepsis model, they were also associated with pulmonary hypertension (138). Utilizing the sensitive hydroperoxide assay that involves stimulation of the cyclooxygenase system, investigators have demonstrated differential detection of plasma hydroperoxides in human sepsis. The study established the value of obtaining both mixed venous and arterial blood to improve the yield of plasma hydroperoxides generated from pulmonary versus intraabdominal infection sites (139).

ISCHEMIA-REPERFUSION STATES

The role of activation of XO in I/R syndromes has been considered in detail (140, 141). As has been discussed previously, following initial ·OR production by XO, typical I/R models demonstrate the subsequent appearance of neutrophils, which hours later leukoagglutinate into the previously ischemic area and appear to extend and/or amplify the injury initiated by ischemia and enhanced by XO-derived ·OR. All forms of shock represent aspects of I/R. Involvement of ·OR with shock has been reviewed recently (142).

Central Nervous System Disease

Oxyradicals have been implicated in all forms of central nervous system injury, including trauma, subarachnoid hemorrhage/vasospasm, peritumoral brain edema, and I/R (143). An important aspect of brain ischemia involves the progressive liberation of free fatty acids after activation of a calcium-dependent phospholipase. These free fatty acids may be cycled into eicosanoid metabolism and generate O_2^- via endoperoxidases and hydroperoxidases (144–146). This provides an additional mechanism of ·OR generation in addition to injury by O_2^- from XO.

Classic studies have outlined the morphologic changes seen with I/R injury to the brain, which include increased brain water, neurophil and neuronal cytoplasmic vacuoles, alterations of the blood-brain barrier, and neutrophil infiltration at approximately 24 hours (147). Evidence of ·OR involvement in this type of injury has been made directly utilizing ESR as well as indirectly utilizing nitroblue tetrazolium reduction, chemiluminescence, salicylate hydroxyl radical trapping, and TBARS (148–151). Some investigators have noted the enhanced vulnerability of certain areas of the brain, such as the hippocampus, striatum, and neocortex, with respect to I/R injury (e.g., reference 150). The importance of reperfusion in CNS injury was demonstrated in an elegant model using two methods of cerebral I/R. When microspheres were utilized to cause CNS infarction, little increase in tissue lipid peroxidation was noted. However, when this infarction involved carotid artery occlusion followed by reperfusion, a significant increase in TBARS was seen, particularly in the vulnerable regions outlined above (150).

Cardiac Arrest and Myocardial Infarction

Another exceedingly common event in the intensive care unit involves myocardial I/R. Tissue markers of oxidant injury, as well as amelioration of the I/R injury by various antioxidants, have been utilized to demonstrate ·OR involvement. Again, the probable importance of leukoaggregation at the infarction site has been emphasized (152, 153). Neutrophil accumulation appears to be dependent on specific neutrophil plasmalemma adherence proteins (154). Neutrophil injury may involve not only production and release of ·OR and hydrolases but also capillary plugging, which would result in a no-reflow phenomenon with possible additional ischemic injury (155).

In addition to the acute I/R event (i.e., myocardial infarction), the precursors to this phenomenon likely also involved ·OR-mediated pathogenesis. Oxidative alteration of low-density lipoprotein appears to increase its atherogenicity (156). Lipid peroxidation products modify critical cell membranes, including those of platelets and circulating lipoproteins (157–159). It should be noted that intact lipid peroxidation products as well as aldehyde breakdown products are capable of modifying lipoproteins.

Lung Ischemia Reperfusion

An added subtlety in pulmonary I/R disease involves the concentration of alveolar oxygen. A correlation has been noted between elevated alveolar PO_2 and enhanced lung fluid accumulation and lipid peroxidation (160).

Digestive Tract Diseases

Extensive research implicates the role of ·OR in I/R of intestine and liver (161, 162). Necrotizing enterocolitis of the newborn likely involves similar pathogenesis. Even gastric ulcers, which represent a common problem for patients in adult critical care units, probably involve ·OR pathogenesis (163). In a human study examining more than 300 patients, various agents were analyzed for their ability to prevent relapse of duodenal ulcer. As compared with control patients, who demonstrated a relapse rate of 65%, those treated with cimetidine showed a relapse rate of 30%. However, in the groups of patients treated with either allopurinol or dimethyl sulfoxide, the relapse rate was only 12 to 13%. Neither of the two latter antioxidants exhibited any adverse affects (164).

Acute Renal Failure

In a rat model of acute renal failure that involved reperfusion after 60 minutes of vascular occlusion, increases in plasma creatinine, decreases in renal blood flow, and increases in histologic indices of injury were noted. Renal tissue levels of MDA in control, ischemic, and I/R kidneys were 130 ± 18, 166 ± 17, and 215 ± 22 nmol/g, respectively. Protection in this animal model, both in terms of renal physiology and biochemical markers of lipid peroxidation, was noted with SOD, dimethythiourea, and allopurinol (165). It should be noted that ·OR may also be involved in progression of renal disease (166).

Skeletal Muscle Injury

Both I/R and crush injury represent components of skeletal muscle insult in patients with multiple trauma. Both have been associated with ·OR-mediated tissue injury (167). In a dog model involving 4 hours of limb ischemia and 1 hour of reperfusion, a 50% decrease in tissue GSH, reflective of protein ·OR stress, was reported (168). Much as in myocardial and brain tissue, neutrophils increased in the previously ischemic skeletal muscle tissue. In a rat model of limb I/R, dimethythiourea (a hydroxyl radical scavenger), but not urea, improved limb function following ischemia. Rats prefed tungsten or allopurinol had neglectable XO activity and, again, improved function after reperfusion. In contradistinction to control animals, no H_2O_2 accumulation was noted in rats treated with antioxidants (169).

Multiple Organ Failure Syndrome

Prolongation of low flow states and prolonged tissue oxygen debt are associated with the development of multiple organ failure syndrome. Intestinal bacteria translocation under conditions of relative gut ischemia can lead to low-grade endotoxemia and/or bacteremia. Both oxygen radicals, derived from

$$2\,O_2^{\cdot -} + 2\,H^+ \longrightarrow H_2O_2 + O_2$$

Figure 54.19. Dismutation of $O_2^{\cdot -}$ by superoxide dismutase.

activation of XO, and polymorphonuclear leukocytes are probably involved in the multifactorial pathogenesis of multiple organ failure syndrome (170).

Transplantation and Cardiopulmonary Bypass

Organ transplantation represents one example of controlled tissue I/R. Similar situations exist in which total circulatory arrest and cardiopulmonary bypass are used for surgery of congenital and acquired heart disease. The importance of ·OR in the pathogenesis of these situations has been reviewed in detail (171, 172).

ANTIOXIDANT THERAPEUTICS

Numerous studies employing cell culture technique, animal models, and clinical protocols have explored the potential use of antioxidants in a variety of disease settings. In the discussion that follows, the basic classes of antioxidants are reviewed with respect to their potential as therapeutic agents. Obviously, not all investigations have been referenced but rather representative examples are cited.

SUPPORTIVE INTERVENTION

It has been pointed out that several existing resuscitative measures, commonly used in the setting of critical care, may involve antioxidant strategy (173). For example, in any shock state, it is imperative that adequate tissue oxygenation be reestablished as soon as possible in order to eliminate tissue oxygen debt. Ongoing splanchnic ischemia may not be readily recognized. Accordingly, it may be prudent to sequentially monitor mixed venous lactate concentrations as an indicator of oxygen delivery adequacy. Moreover, it has been suggested that supranormal hemodynamic endpoints be chosen to optimize resuscitative efforts (174). Infusion of erythrocytes may be beneficial, not only in terms of improving oxygen delivery, but also because these cells contain high concentrations of endogenous enzyme antioxidants, particularly catalase and glutathione. Also, many of the commonly used inotropic agents have potent β-adrenergic agonist activity, which again will not only tend to improve oxygen delivery but also exert significant antiinflammatory effects. For example, β-agonists are known to inhibit the respiratory burst of neutrophils and β-antagonists may also suppress lipid peroxidation (175). The clinical implications of these in vitro findings have not been pursued. In summary, the initial approach to resuscitating ·OR injury should revolve around the ABCs of cardiopulmonary-cerebral resuscitation. Namely, provision of an adequate airway and oxygen and hemodynamic support as needed to deliver oxygen and energy substrate to all tissues so that aerobic metabolism may be quickly reestablished. Additional therapy aimed specifically at ·OR is discussed below.

ENZYME ANTIOXIDANTS

Superoxide Dismutase

The discovery and characterization of superoxide dismutase (SOD) probably represent the premier events that spurred initial interest in ·OR species and their possible involvement in human disease (176). This enzyme is present in all aerobic organisms and exists in several different forms. Copper-zinc SOD is a dimer with a molecular weight of 32 kDa. The Cu appears to undergo redox cycling, while the Zn is important for protein structure. Cu-Zn SOD is located in the cytosol and is particularly rich in hepatic and brain tissue and lower in concentration in erythrocytes and lung parenchyma. Manganese SOD is a tetrameric enzyme, with a molecular weight of 85 kDa, located in the mitochondria. Another copper-containing SOD, which has been isolated from both interstitial fluid and plasma, is a tetramer and has a molecular weight of 134 kDa (177). Superoxide dismutase catalyzes the dismutation of 2 moles of $O_2^{\cdot -}$ to H_2O_2 and O_2 with a rate constant on the order of 10^9 M^{-1}·sec^{-1} (Fig. 54.19).

Many animal models have demonstrated the utility of various forms of SOD in inhibiting ·OR injury. SOD with or without CAT has been shown to increase rat survival and inhibit hepatic lipid peroxide accumulation in a model of endotoxemia in rats (178). Although allopurinol, αTH, and GSH could similarly inhibit lipid peroxidation, they did not improve survival. Similarly, in a model of endotoxin-challenged mice, SOD but not N-acetylcysteine was shown to increase survival (179). Dose-response data have been generated for human recombinant SOD (rh SOD) relative to lung vascular permeability in an endotoxemic rat model. High doses of rh SOD were shown to normalize the lung vascular permeability index (180).

Human recombinant SOD has also been examined in a model of transient ischemic injury in gerbils (181). Very high doses of rh SOD or the apoenzyme devoid of metal cofactors were given to rats 1 minute before a 5-minute bilateral carotid artery occlusion. High doses of rh SOD were required to minimize vasogenic edema and permit survival. Animals were sacrificed at 7 days. In the controls, almost complete destruction of CA1 pyramidal neurons in the hippocampus was noted. However, in the group treated with rh SOD, such lesions were minimal. Interestingly, in these animals, a stress induction of endogenous SOD mRNA in the hippocampus, analyzed by in situ hybridization or Northern blot analysis, was essentially abolished by the administration of exogenous rh SOD. Liposome-entrapped SOD has also been shown to reduce cerebral infarction following cerebral ischemia in rats (181a).

Similarly, extracellular rh SOD has been shown to reduce the concentration of ·OR in I/R rat heart (182). In a related cardiac model employing microvascular immobilization, rh SOD, 2-O-octadecyl ascorbic acid, and allopurinol were all shown to attenuate the I/R-induced impairment of contractility and metabolic dysfunction and to enhance coronary artery blood flow (183).

In a rat model of superior mesenteric artery occlusion, SOD improved survival, but CAT, dimethylsulfoxide, and selenium did not (184). In another study, SOD not only increased survival time but also protected against the rise in lipid peroxidation products and suppressed the release of lysosomal enzymes (indicative of cellular injury) (185).

Table 54.3. Prevention of BPD by Administration of Bovine SOD (187)

BPD indicators	Experimental Groups	
	SOD ($n = 14$)	Control ($n = 17$)
Radiologic criteria	3/14	12/17
Clinical criteria	3/14	12/17

$$LOO^{\bullet} + HO_{\overline{2}} \longrightarrow LOOH + O_2$$

Figure 54.20. Termination of lipid peroxidation by $O_{\overline{2}}$.

Superoxide dismutase has also been utilized in human critical illness. When bovine SOD was administered at reperfusion to transplanted kidneys, it did not appear to attenuate acute renal failure, except perhaps for late implanted kidneys with long ischemic times (186). However, the drug was noted to be safe and well-tolerated. Probably the best known application of SOD in human disease relates to its use in preventing BPD in premature infants with RDS. Forty-five neonates were studied prospectively in a randomized, controlled fashion (187). The experimental group received bovine SOD at a dosage of 0.25 mg/kg subcutaneously every 12 hours until the infants were breathing room air or had been placed on continuous positive airway pressure (CPAP). The average gestational age of these infants was 28.7 weeks, and their mean weight was 1154 g. All required $FiO_2 \geq 0.70$ at 24 hours of age. As shown in Table 54.3, there were 31 survivors in this study. Both radiologic findings and clinical findings diagnostic of BPD were significantly fewer in the group that had received SOD. This group also required fewer days of CPAP following discontinuation of mechanical ventilation.

When utilized at the time of coronary thrombolysis in patients with acute myocardial infarction, SOD reduced the number of subsequent ventricular arrhythmias, although it did not appear to have any effect on left ventricular function (188). Pharmacokinetics of rh SOD in healthy volunteers have been studied in detail at doses of 1 to 45 mg/kg (189). The average half-life for this preparation was approximately 4 hours. No adverse effects were noted in any of the study participants.

A note of caution should be raised regarding the use of SOD in ·OR-mediated disease, namely that a bell-shaped dose-response curve may exist for this agent. In I/R models employing isolated rabbit hearts, the cardiac protective effect of either Cu/Zn SOD or Mn SOD appeared to be lost at high doses in the reperfused heart as assessed by physiologic as well as biochemical parameters (190, 191). It is known that the Cu/Zn SOD has weak peroxidase activity, which might contribute to injury, but this is not the case for Mn SOD. High levels of SOD could alter "baseline steady-state" levels of $O_{\overline{2}}$. Superoxide is required for inactivation of endothelial-derived relaxant factor. In addition, $O_{\overline{2}}$ or $HO_{\overline{2}}$ may be important in termination of lipid peroxidation reactions, as shown in Figure 54.20. Certain steady state levels of at least $O_{\overline{2}}$ appear to be homeostatic. Decreasing these levels with excess therapeutic radical scavenger may have undesirable consequences.

$$2\,H_2O_2 \longrightarrow O_2 + 2\,H_2O$$

Figure 54.21. Decomposition of H_2O_2 by catalase.

Catalase

Some investigations do not conclude a protective effect of SOD. Another reason for this failure, other than those noted above, may be that exogenous SOD would increase the steady-state level of H_2O_2, a membrane permeable oxidant with a "long" half-life potential. CAT augments the metabolism of H_2O_2 to O_2 and H_2O, as shown in Figure 54.21. Catalase is a tetrameric hemoprotein with a molecular weight of 240 kDa containing an iron-heme active site (192). It displays activity toward small molecules only and hence does not participate in the breakdown of high molecular weight lipid peroxides. The second-order rate constant for the decomposition of H_2O_2 by CAT is approximately 10^7 M^{-1} sec^{-1}. Catalase is characterized by a high reaction capacity but relatively low substrate affinity. It is highly compartmentalized in peroxisomes and is found in high concentration in both hepatocytes and erythrocytes, with much lower concentrations in the brain and lung.

Catalase has been studied in various cell culture models. For example, in cultured rat gastric mucosal cells, XO-mediated cytotoxicity was inhibited by exogenous CAT but not SOD (193). Depletion of intracellular GSH enhanced cytotoxicity as measured by ^{51}Cr release. In the classic sheep chronic lung lymph fistula model, CAT given intraperitoneally 30 minutes before intravenous endotoxin has been shown to attenuate the increase in protein-rich lung lymph flow (194). In addition, systemic leukopenia also was decreased with CAT. In the same model, exogenous CAT has been shown to prevent prostanoid release as well as to suppress lung lipid peroxidation when administered prior to endotoxin infusion (195). In addition to decreasing actual evidence of cell oxidant injury as ascertained by lung MDA content, exogenous CAT also decreased the release of thromboxane A_2. Recently, it was demonstrated again in a sheep endotoxemia model that inactivation of endogenous lung but not liver CAT occurred and that lipid peroxidation products in the lung increased as CAT content decreased (196). These results confirm that CAT itself may be a target of ·OR inactivation (99), and that the lung may be providing a defense mechanism for other systemic organs such as the liver.

Combined Superoxide Dismutase/Catalase

Since SOD alone may actually enhance the potential for oxygen radical injury (197), the logical combination of SOD and CAT has been examined. Numerous studies employing I/R models have demonstrated the beneficial effect of combining these two enzyme antioxidants for therapeutic intervention. Much of this work has been performed using myocardial infarction models, in which the combination of enzymes has been shown to maintain cardiac output and mean arterial pressure, attenuate the rise in products of lipid peroxidation, and reduce infarct size (e.g., references 198–200). Combined SOD/CAT has also been utilized as a retrograde bolus into the great cardiac vein prior to coronary reperfusion in dogs that had been subjected to a 90-minute occlusion of the left anterior descending coronary artery (201). In this model, which is certainly applicable to human cardiac surgery, infarct size as a percent of the area at risk was reduced approximately 4-fold in the SOD/CAT group as compared with controls. In addition, the treatment group demonstrated fewer arrhythmias and enhanced echocardiographic cardiac function. It should be noted that the combination of SOD and CAT has also been successfully utilized to decrease I/R injury following long-term hypothermic lung preservation in dogs (202). The combination of SOD/CAT presented to the lungs at reperfusion decreased extravascular lung water and modulated the rise in lung lipid peroxidation products.

Glutathione Peroxidase

Glutathione peroxidase (GSH Px) is a tetrameric protein with a molecular weight of 85 kDa that contains four selenium atoms as selenocystines at the active site (203). Glutathione represents an essential cofactor for the enzyme, which catalyzes the reduction of peroxides to the corresponding alcohols with the simultaneous conversion of reduced GSH to glutathione disulfide (Fig. 54.22). Subsequently, the glutathione disulfide is reduced by GSH reductase, a dimeric protein with a molecular weight of 105 kDa (see Fig. 54.12). Reducing equivalents for the reductase assay are provided by NADPH generated by glucose-6-phosphate dehydrogenase and 6-phospogluconate dehydrogenase. High levels of GSH Px are found in hepatocytes and red blood cells, while intermediate levels are found in the heart and lung. This peroxidase is differentiated from CAT in that it catalyzes the decomposition of high molecular weight peroxides as well as H_2O_2. The K_m for hydroperoxides is low, whereas the K_m for H_2O_2 is somewhat higher. Under normal conditions of low background levels of peroxides, GSH Px probably represents the key antioxidant. Also unlike CAT, which is largely confined to peroxisomes, GSH Px may be found in cytosol and mitochondria, as well as extracellularly in plasma.

Glutathione peroxidase has been investigated much less rigorously than either SOD or CAT. It has, however, demonstrated efficacy in decreasing myocardial I/R injury as assessed by improved contractile indices in animals treated with the exogenous peroxidase as compared with controls (204, 205).

Pharmacologic Manipulation of Enzyme Antioxidants

Significant advances have been made in innovative techniques for enzyme delivery as well as pharmacologic manipulation of endogenous antioxidant enzyme levels (206). In experiments utilizing cell culture systems, it has been determined that the level of endogenous antioxidant enzymes can be significantly enhanced by exposing the cells to exogenous enzymes encapsulated within liposomes. Liposomes fuse and/or penetrate the cell plasmalemma to deliver the exogenous protein. Such liposome-entrapped SOD or CAT has been delivered to animals intravenously (207) or endotracheally (208, 209) and has been shown to protect against pulmonary oxygen toxicity.

In a similar manner, CAT and SOD may be conjugated to PEG, which, as previously mentioned, has been used to enhance endothelial antioxidant enzyme activity and ·OR resistance in cell culture models. Polyethylene glycol moieties (see Fig. 54.23) of an average molecule weight of 5 kDa are typically condensed, with approximately 10 to 15 of the 20 ε-amino groups of exposed lysine residues of SOD. Conjugation to PEG increases the molecular weight of SOD from the native enzyme of 32 kDa to approximate 100 kDa. This alteration in the native conformation of the enzyme increases long-term stability, increases the circulating half-life from less than 10 minutes to more than 40 hours, reduces its immunogenicity, decreases its sensitivity to proteolysis, and increases endothelial cell uptake/association (210). Cultured cells augmented with exogenous enzyme antioxidants demonstrate an increased resistance to oxidant stress as assessed by cytotoxicity and ESR membrane fluidity. Animal models employing conjugated enzyme antioxidants have confirmed the utility of these modified enzymes in the in vivo setting (211, 212).

In some fetal animal models, cortisol has been shown to increase the activity of SOD, CAT, and GSH Px (213). However, thyrotropin releasing hormone may actually delay maturation of antioxidant systems (214). Such observations are important, as prematures have low levels of antioxidant enzymes that are not readily inducible by hyperoxia (130). Utilizing a low molecular weight compound to enhance the expression of endogenous antioxidant enzymes would be a simpler and less costly approach than, for example, relying on infusions of recombinant-engineered exogenous proteins. It has been shown that the induction of rat lung antioxidant enzymes during hyperoxia is actually mediated by cytokines. Lipopolysaccharide (endotoxin) appears to induce the same increase in antioxidant enzymes through a similar mechanism. Interleukin 1, tumor necrosis factor-α, and interferon-γ all appear to be effective in inducing endogenous levels of antioxidant enzymes and may, in fact, demonstrate synergy among agents (215–218). Future clinicians may be able to therapeutically titrate the genome's antioxidant responsive element(s) directly (219).

HYDROPHILIC LOW MOLECULAR WEIGHT ANTIOXIDANTS

Allopurinol

Because of the demonstration of involvement of XO in I/R injury, a logical therapeutic extension would hypothesize that allopurinol might be utilized as an XO inhibitor to ameliorate I/R injury. It is not surprising, considering the chemical structures involved in the conversion of xanthine to uric acid (see Figs. 54.24 and 54.25), that allopurinol, a pyrazolopyrimidine mimic of xanthine, would bind to the active site of XO. Allopurinol itself is oxidized to oxypurinol, which displays even tighter enzyme binding than does allopurinol.

Allopurinol/oxypurinol have been demonstrated to be effective in inhibiting ·OR injury in several model systems. In

$$LOO^{\cdot} + 2\ GSH \longrightarrow LOH + H_2O + GSSG$$

Figure 54.22. Reduction of lipid hydroperoxides by glutathione peroxidase.

$$HO\text{-}(CH_2\text{-}CH_2\text{-}O)_n\text{-}CH_3$$

Figure 54.23. Structure of polyethylene glycol (PEG).

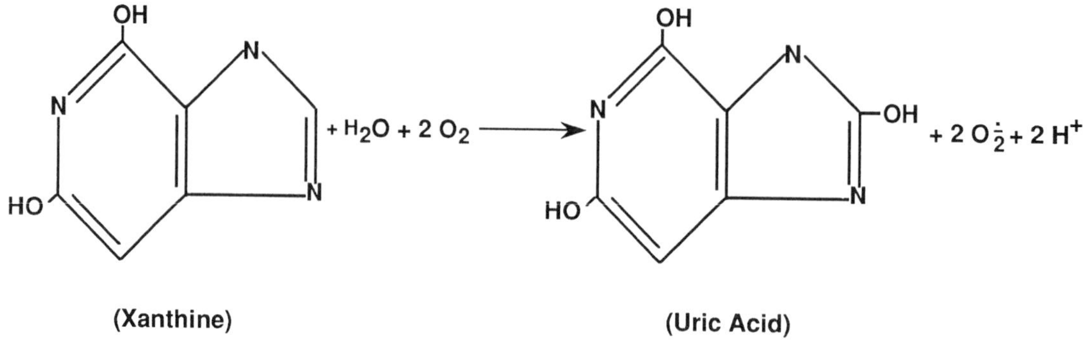

(Xanthine)   **(Uric Acid)**

Figure 54.24. Catalysis of xanthine to uric acid by xanthine oxidase.

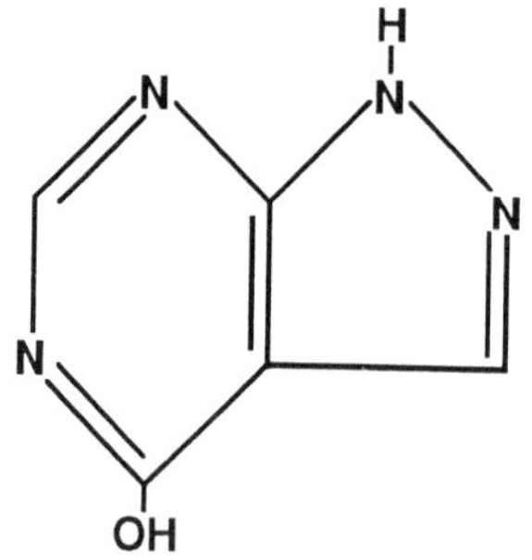

Figure 54.25. Structure of allopurinol.

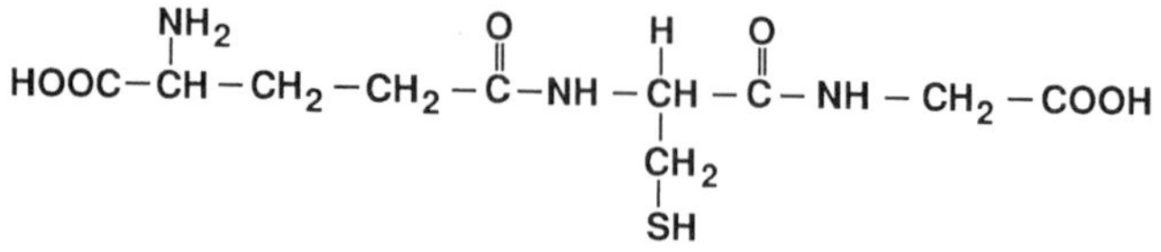

Figure 54.26. Structure of glutathione.

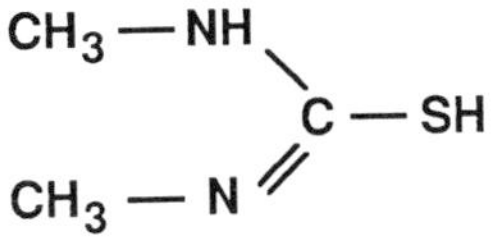

Figure 54.27. Structure of dimethylthiourea.

cultured bovine lung endothelial cells insulted with endotoxin, allopurinol (as well as dimethyl sulfoxide) decreased cytosolic lactate dehydrogenase release, alterations in cellular morphology, and various indicators of oxidant stress (220). Allopurinol has also been demonstrated to attenuate endotoxin-induced microvascular leakage in an in vivo system employing the Syrian hamster cheek pouch model (221). Many investigations have verified the effectiveness of allopurinol in traditional models of I/R, as exemplified by studies examining perinatal brain (222), liver (223), and, of course, cardiac muscle (224).

Allopurinol has also been studied in several human clinical investigations. Thirty-four paired kidneys (from brain-dead donors) preserved with hypothermic pulsatile perfusion with and without allopurinol reflected no changes in either short- or long-term function with allopurinol (225). However, two clinical trials have employed allopurinol in the setting of coronary bypass surgery, with very encouraging results (226, 227). In patients treated with allopurinol at reperfusion, mortality appeared to be decreased, cardiac performance improved, and enzyme levels indicative of myocardial injury decreased. Some hospitals now use allopurinol routinely in this setting. In organs such as the intestine and liver, where cellular concentrations of XO are very high, inhibition of XO with allopurinol is rational. The debate about the concentration of XO in cardiac muscle continues. Recent evidence suggests that the protective effect of allopurinol or its derivative oxypurinol may not be related to inhibition of XO (228), but rather to its effect as a hydroxyl radical (HO·) scavenger (229, 230).

Sulfhydryl Compounds

Glutathione is a tripeptide γ-glutamyl-cysteinyl-glycine, whose structure is shown in Figure 54.26. Concentration of

this sulfhydryl agent in the cytosol ranges between 0.10 and 1.0 mM, confirming its important role as an immediate source of cellular reducing equivalents (231). Previous mention has been made of its essential cofactor role with GSH Px. Various low molecular weight sulfhydryl agents, which may be thought of as congeners of glutathione, have been used in animal models and clinically to inhibit ·OR injury. N-2-mercaptopropionyl glycine has been shown to be protective in a model of dog myocardial I/R (232). N-acetyl-cysteine has been shown to reduce lung lymph clearance following endotoxin administration in sheep (233). These agents may be acting directly through their sulfhydryl moiety or perhaps may be involved in regenerating GSH. It should be noted that N-acetyl-cysteine has been utilized for a number of years in treatment of acetaminophen toxicity and hence has demonstrated both efficacy and safety in human disease. Glutathione appears to offer myocardial protection in patients undergoing cardiopulmonary bypass when incorporated as a constituent of the cardioplegia solution (234). Dimethylthiourea (DMTU), whose structure is shown above, has a resonance form that also includes a sulfhydryl group (Fig. 54.27). Dimethylthiourea is thought to exert its primary affect through scavenging of HO·, which arises through the transition metal-catalyzed Haber-Weiss/Fenton reactions (see Fig. 54.6). In vitro studies have shown that DMTU can prevent H_2O_2 and neutrophil damage to cultured endothelial cells (235). In various animal models, DMTU has been demonstrated to reduce activated neutrophil, I/R, and endotoxin-induced injury (236–239). Unfortunately, it is likely that the high concentrations (mM) that are required for effective HO· scavenging by DMTU are likely to be toxic and, hence, preclude its clinical usefulness.

Taurine

Taurine is an amino-sulfonic acid with the structure shown in Figure 54.28. Unlike other amino acids, taurine is abundant in its free form and is not incorporated into proteins. The intracellular concentration for taurine is higher than that for all other amino acids except glutamate (240). The antioxidant effect of taurine stems from its amino group, which reacts with hypochlorous acids to form nontoxic monochlorotaurine. When utilized as a preoperative rapid intravenous infusion prior to human myocardial revascularization, taurine decreased ·OR species as assessed by chemiluminescence and also significantly decreased the percentage of damaged mitochondria as assessed by electron microscopy of tissue samples (241). Taurine is thought to be nontoxic. Additional investigations of this promising agent are warranted.

HYDROPHOBIC LOW MOLECULAR WEIGHT ANTIOXIDANTS

Deferoxamine

Since transition metals are intimately involved in the generation of ·OR (Fig. 54.6), it is not surprising that metal-chelating agents such as deferoxamine (Fig. 54.29) might be effective in modulating ·OR injury (242). In a model of myocardial I/R performed in isolated perfused rabbit hearts and employing ESR and ^{31}P nuclear magnetic resonance (NMR), hearts treated with deferoxamine during ischemia prior to reperfusion demonstrated improved recovery of developed pressure and improved recovery of phosphocreatine as compared with control animals not treated with deferoxamine (243). In addition, there was a reduction in ·OR generation at the time of reperfusion in the animals treated with deferoxamine. Deferoxamine has been examined in the setting of cardiopulmonary bypass surgery in humans (244). The study speculated that deferoxamine might limit ·OR-mediated amplification of the inflammatory response and, hence, the harmful effects of bypass. When incorporated as part of fluid resuscitation in a sheep burn model, hetastarch-complexed deferoxamine reduced the amount of fluid resuscitation and prevented the increase in lung and liver lipid peroxidation products as compared with resuscitation with lactated Ringer's or hetastarch alone (245). Deferoxamine is not the ideal chelating agent, since its cellular membrane permeability is limited (246). By complexing the molecule to hetastarch, adverse hemodynamic affects have largely been eliminated. Other congeners of deferoxamine are currently being synthesized and investigated. It should be noted that ibuprofen, traditionally viewed as an antiinflammatory agent affecting eicosanoid metabolism, can prevent oxidant lung injury and lipid peroxidation, probably through a mechanism involving iron chelation (247). In vitro experiments have indicated that, in addition to inhibiting cyclooxygenase, ibuprofen has a number of neutrophil-relevant antiinflammatory effects and, in addition, can attenuate in vitro lipid peroxidation of arachidonic acid. Thus, ibuprofen may have a number of beneficial effects in the setting of ·OR injury.

Carotenoids

β-carotene, whose structure is shown in Figure 54.30, has an extensive conjugated double-bond system capable of stabilizing an odd electron that defines its chemical potential as a free radical scavenger. In addition, β-carotene serves as a precursor to retinol, which, when used therapeutically, may have a number of antiinflammatory effects. β-carotene is known to quench singlet oxygen (248, 249). Although β-carotene and its derivatives have been investigated much less thoroughly than many of the other lipid-soluble, low molecular weight antioxidants, β-carotene has been shown to inhibit peroxidation of linoleic acid by XO, to reduce neutrophil-mediated cell injury, and to decrease evidence of lipid peroxidation in guinea pigs exposed to carbon tetrachloride (248). Human investigations examining its potential role in the setting of critical care ·OR injury are lacking to date.

α-Tocopherol

α-Tocopherol (vitamin E, αTH) represents the primary antioxidant in hydrophobic settings, particularly membranes (250–253). The structure of αTH, shown in Figure 54.31, consists of two primary components. The chroman ring represents the radical-trapping portion of the molecule. It quenches lipid chain reactions by stabilizing an odd electron in chroman resonance structure. The long hydrophobic, aliphatic tail allows partition into lipid bilayers where lipid peroxidation is most prevalent. Native αTH may be regenerated through a tocopheroxyl radical reductase enzyme system employing ascorbate and GSH (254, 255).

In vitro investigations have ascertained the effectiveness of αTH in inhibiting membrane lipid peroxidation (256). The level of membrane αTH appears to represent an important determinant of its susceptibility to ·OR stress.

Rats administered intraperitoneal αTH demonstrated a marked improvement in survival from 0 to 45% following hepatic ischemia. Biochemical markers in this model indicated that the augmentation of levels of αTH preserved the rate of ATP generation following reperfusion while suppressing a rise in lipid peroxidation products (257). Combined administration of αTH and ascorbate has also been shown to reduce the percentage of potential myocardial necrosis from 73% to 47%

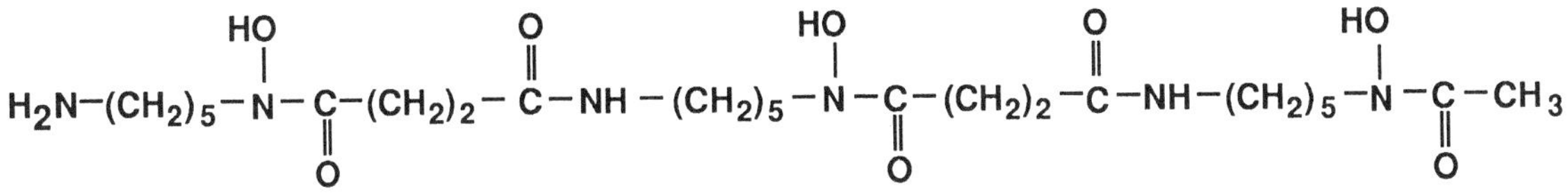

$$\overset{+}{H_3N} - CH_2CH_2 - SO_3^-$$

Figure 54.28. Structure of taurine.

$$H_2N-(CH_2)_5-N-C-(CH_2)_2-C-NH-(CH_2)_5-N-C-(CH_2)_2-C-NH-(CH_2)_5-N-C-CH_3$$

Figure 54.29. Structure of deferoxamine.

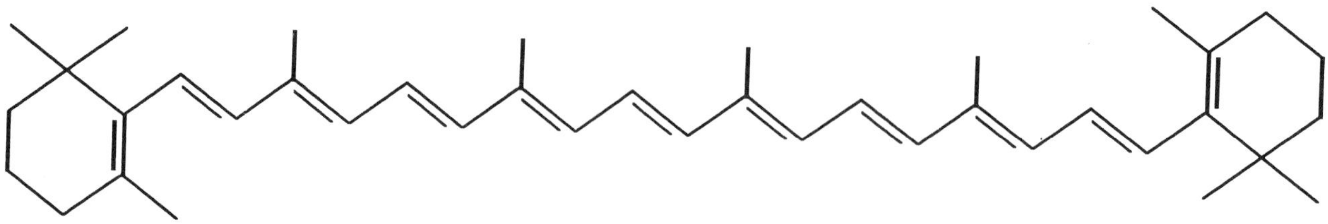

Figure 54.30.   Structure of β-carotene.

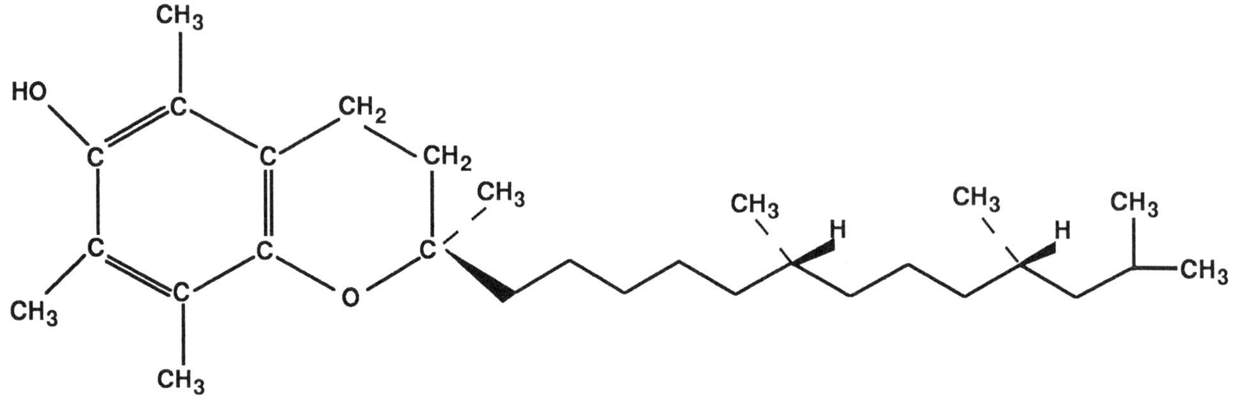

Figure 54.31.   Structure of α-tocopherol.

in a porcine model of myocardial infarction (258). It has also been reported recently that survival in guinea pigs following an *Escherichia coli*/staphylococcus peritonitis septic challenge, appeared to be significantly influenced by the level of αTH in their preceding diets (259).

Unfortunately, human trials utilizing αTH therapeutically have been less encouraging. Vitamin E, like other antioxidants, is known to increase in concentration during development. Accordingly, premature infants are typically αTH deficient and, unless supplemented with exogenous αTH, may demonstrate evidence of increased lipid peroxidation as assessed by in vitro enhanced peroxide-induced hemolysis, increased malondialdehyde production, and increased concentrations of exhaled pentane and ethane (260, 261). In the setting of a diet rich in PUFA but deficient in αTH, evidence of lipid peroxidation is further magnified.

Infants with RDS at risk for developing BPD are usually premature, with underdeveloped antioxidant systems, who typically receive high FiO$_2$ and whose endotracheal tube aspirates typically reflect a pulmonary influx of activated neutrophils. Hence, αTH supplementation as an exogenous antioxidant represented a logical intervention to investigate in this population. An initial report appeared to indicate that pharmacologic administration of αTH decreased the incidence of BPD (262). Unfortunately, three follow-up studies have failed to demonstrate any protective effect of αTH in the setting of acute BPD (263–265). However, αTH may be helpful in another common disease in premature infants, retinopathy of prematurity. Large doses of αTH (100 mg/kg/day) appear to decrease the severity but not the incidence of this serious neonatal iatrogenic eye injury thought to be mediated by ·OR (266). One investigation has also examined αTH in the setting of ARDS, where it appeared to demonstrate a beneficial effect (267). However, this particular investigation involved a small number of subjects and was uncontrolled, and the results have not been confirmed by other studies.

In a related area of ·OR injury and nutritional supplementation, it has been shown that PUFA supplementation may protect newborn rats from oxygen toxicity (268, 269). Traditionally, PUFAs have been viewed as promoting lipid peroxidation because of their susceptibility to autocatalytic chain reactions. However, an "alternate hypothesis" has been advanced that suggests that excess PUFAs may serve as free radical sinks in times of oxidant stress that protect more critical membrane lipids and proteins from oxidant damage (Fig. 54.32). In fact, this hypothesis is currently being investigated in human infants.

Coenzyme Q

Coenzyme Q (CoQ) contains both a quinone ring and a long-chain isoprenoid tail, as shown in Figure 54.33. The long isoprenoid tail provides the molecule with its hydrophobic character, which enables it to function in lipid environments. Normally, this coenzyme functions as an electron shuttle as part of the mitochondrial electron transport chain, where it is situated between the flavoproteins and cytochromes (270). A one-electron addition to the ring structure results in the formation of a relatively stable semiquinone that defines the molecule's antioxidant capacity. CoQ has been shown to be effective in improving left ventricular function during myocardial I/R (271) and has also been examined in the setting of murine endotoxemia, where pharmacologic doses increased survival from 30 to 70% (272). When used in conjunction with αTH, the combination preserved hepatic ATP levels and reduced the accumulation of MDA. In a canine endotoxin shock model, CoQ appeared to attenuate the accumulation of lactate through a mechanism hypothesized to involve the promotion of oxygen utilization under hypoxic conditions (273). Physiologic measures of pulmonary function but not circulatory function were improved with CoQ. It is difficult to ascertain whether CoQ in these model systems is functioning as an antioxidant or whether it is improving oxygen consumption by enhancing electron flow along the mitochondrial electron transport chain. CoQ has not been investigated as therapy for human ·OR-mediated illnesses, although it has been examined in a number of clinical settings, including congestive heart failure (270).

Nitrones

Nitrones or nitroxides are examples of compounds that were originally used as spin-trapping agents to detect the presence of ·OR by ESR (e.g., Figure 54.34). More recently, these and related agents have been examined for their possible therapeutic utility in various animal models of ·OR injury. In

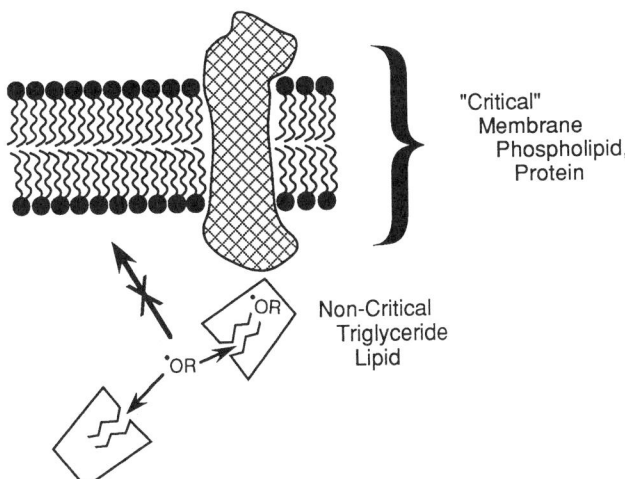

Figure 54.32. Schematic depiction of the "alternate hypothesis," in which exogenous polyunsaturated fatty acids act as free radical sinks, thus protecting critical cellular proteins and lipid.

a neonatal cardiomyocyte cell culture model in which H_2O_2 was utilized as the ·OR stress, nitrones conferred full protection as assessed by the quality and quantity of spontaneous cell beating, as well as cytotoxicity assessed as lactate dehydrogenase leak (274). The therapeutic benefit of nitrones compared very favorably with that of CAT or deferoxamine. These same types of agents are beginning to be investigated in animal models. In studies to date, nitrones have been shown to be very effective in minimizing ·OR injury in the settings of I/R (275), endotoxemia (276), and traumatic shock (277).

21-Amino Steroids

21-Amino steroids represent a novel group of low molecular weight hydrophobic antioxidants colloquially referred to as "lazaroids" (278). Structure of the prototypic compound U74006F is shown in Figure 54.35. The precise mechanism by which this class of compounds inhibits lipid peroxidation is incompletely understood, but these compounds are known to chelate iron (279). Inclusion of the steroid moiety confers considerable hydrophobicity to the overall molecular structure and probably allows it to locate within membranes where the greatest potential for lipid peroxidation occurs. When examined as direct inhibitors of lipid peroxidation, members of this class of compounds are considerably less effective than αTH in preventing peroxidative damage (280). 21-Amino steroids have been examined and shown to be effective in models of cardiopulmonary arrest (281), isolated myocardial ischemia (282), head injury (283), spinal cord trauma (284), cerebral vasospasm following subarachnoid hemorrhage (285), splenic artery occlusion (286), and hemorrhagic shock (287). In many of these studies the administration of the 21-amino steroid was timed to occur after the insult, which certainly argues favorably for the potential of these agents in human therapeutics.

FUTURE DIRECTIONS

Analysis of the preceding discussion by experts interested in the field of ·OR injury would establish that this presentation

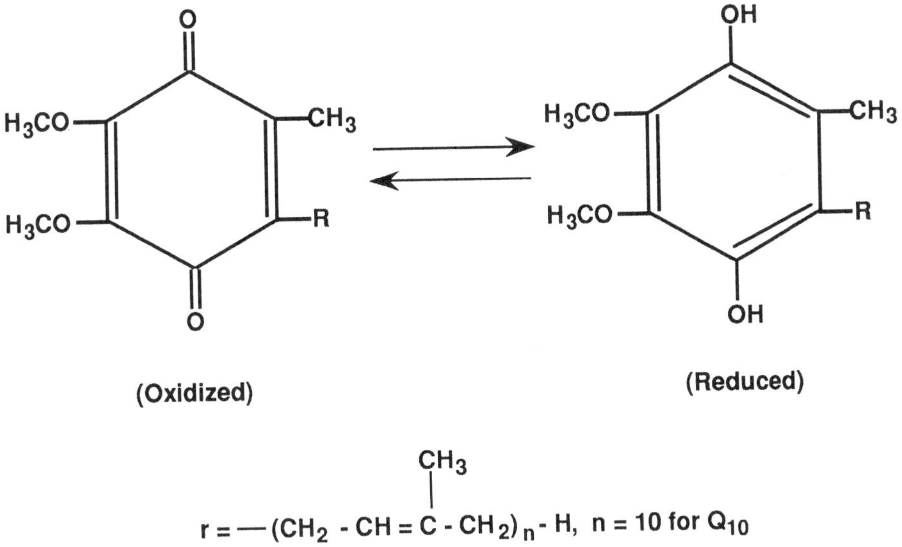

(Oxidized)

(Reduced)

$$r = —(CH_2 - CH = C - CH_2)_n - H, \quad n = 10 \text{ for } Q_{10}$$

with CH_3 substituent

Figure 54.33. Structure of coenzyme Q.

has been somewhat biased, in that many negative studies have not been cited. However, it is fair to state that the majority of studies examining the potential use of antioxidants as therapeutic agents have demonstrated at least a potential positive therapeutic benefit. An example of this presumption relates to the use of antioxidants in the setting of organ preservation and transplantation (288). Twenty-seven studies employing a variety of different animal models have been summarized, including data concerning liver, heart, and kidney transplantation. Clearly, a majority of these studies demonstrated a positive effect for the particular antioxidant under investigation. The actual number of human trials examining antioxidants is admittedly small, and most of them have been reviewed in this chapter.

It is important to point out that many studies examining antioxidants have been flawed in design and methodology (289). Drug dosing frequently has been unrealistic, with both long- and short-term toxicity often disregarded; potential differences among animal species have been largely ignored; control populations frequently have been inadequate in number and definition; and long-term benefit of a given antioxidant intervention rarely has been determined because of the short duration of most experiments. Despite this flawed history, the medical and pharmaceutical communities are beginning to consider large-scale human trials for many of the agents

discussed. This is a reasonable goal because, as previously stressed, virtually every problem associated with critical care involves ·OR pathophysiology, at least in part. The logical arenas for initial investigation of many of these agents would be in the surgical suite, where transplantation and cardiac surgery take place. In these settings, surgeons and anesthesiologists can dictate control over the parameters of both ischemia and reperfusion (290). Because ·OR injury is probably such an exceedingly common event in critical illness, exploring the therapeutic utility of various antioxidants will ultimately define the clinical basis for intensivists to intervene in ·OR-mediated pathogenic processes.

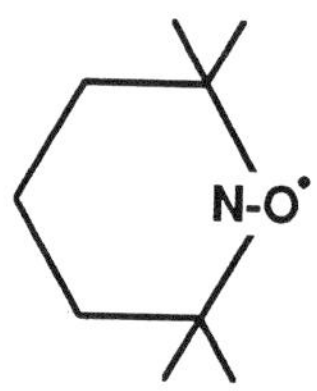

REFERENCES

1. Freeman BA, Crapo JD: Free radicals and tissue injury. *Lab Invest* 47:412–426, 1982.
2. Halliwell B, Gutteridge JMC: Role of free radicals and catalytic metal ions in human disease. *Methods Enzymol* 186:1–85, 1990.
3. Southorn P: Free radicals in medicine. I. Chemical nature and biologic reactions. II. Involvement in human disease. *Mayo Clin Proc* 63:381–389, 390–408, 1988.
4. Radi R, Beckman JS, Bush KM, Freeman BA: Peroxynitrite oxidation of sulfhydryls. *J Biol Chem* 266:4244–4250, 1991.
5. Andrews PC, Krinsky NI: A kinetic analysis of the interaction of human myeloperoxidase with hydrogen peroxide, chloride ions, and protons. *J Biol Chem* 257:13240–13245, 1982.
6. Weiss SJ, Lampert MB, Test ST: Long-lived oxidants generated by human neutrophils: characterization and bioactivity. *Science* 222:625–627, 1983.
7. Halliwell B, Gutteridge JMC: Role of iron in oxygen radical reactions. *Methods Enzymol* 105:47–56, 1984.
8. Pryor WA: Oxy-radicals and related species: their formation, lifetimes, and reactions. *Ann Rev Physiol* 48:657–667, 1986.
9. Babbs CF: Role of iron ions in the genesis of reperfusion injury following successful cardiopulmonary resuscitation. *Ann Emerg Med* 14:777–783, 1985.
10. Thomas CE, Morehouse LA, Aust SD: Ferritin and superoxide-dependent lipid peroxidation. *J Biol Chem* 260:3275–3280, 1985.
11. Houtchens BA, Westenskow DR: Oxygen consumption in septic shock: collective review. *Circ Shock* 13:361–384, 1984.
12. Ruuge EK, Ledenev AN, Lakomkin VL, Konstantinov AA, Ksenzenko MY: Free radical metabolites in myocardium during ischemia and reperfusion. *Am J Physiol* 261(suppl):81–86, 1991.

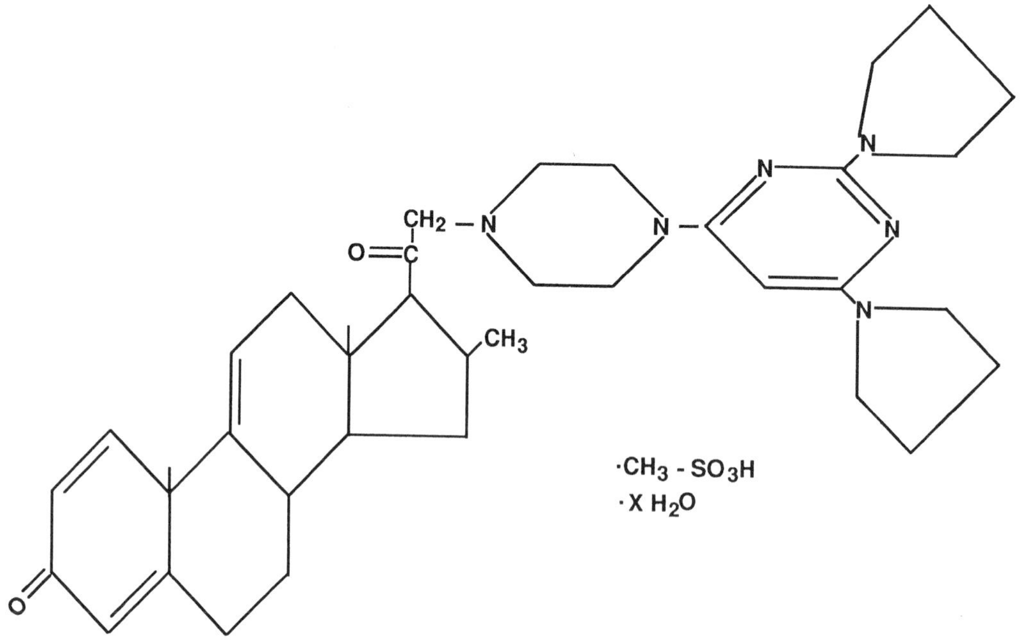

Figure 54.34.   Structure of a typical spin-trapping nitroxide, 2,2,6,6-tetramethyl-piperidinoxyl (Tempo).

Figure 54.35.   Structure of U74006F, a 21-amino steroid.

13. Oates JA, Fitzgerald GA, Branch RA, Jackson EK, Knapp HR, Roberts LJ: Clinical implications of prostaglandin and thromboxane A₂ formation. *N Engl J Med* 319:689–698, 671–767, 1988.

14. Kukreja RC, Kontos HA, Hess ML, Ellis EF: PGH synthase and lipoxygenase generate superoxide in the presence of NADH or NADPH. *Circ Res* 59:612–619, 1986.

15. McCord JM: Oxygen-derived free radicals in postischemic tissue injury. *N Engl J Med* 312:159–164, 1985.

16. Brass CA, Narciso J, Gollan JL: Enhanced activity of the free radical producing enzyme xanthine oxidase in hypoxic rat liver. *J Clin Invest* 87:424–431. 1991.

17. Friedl HP, Till GO, Ryan US, Ward PA: Mediator-induced activation of xanthine oxidase in endothelial cells. *FASEB J* 3:2512–2518, 1989.

18. Phan SH, Gannon DE, Varani J, Ryan US, Ward PA: Xanthine oxidase activity in rat pulmonary artery endothelial cells and its alteration by activated neutrophils. *Am J Pathol* 134:1201–1211, 1989.

19. Dupont GP, Huecksteadt TP, Marshall BC, Ryan US, Michael JR, Hoidal JR: Regulation of xanthine dehydrogenase and xanthine oxidase activity and gene expression in cultured rat pulmonary endothelial cells. *J Clin Invest* 89:197–202, 1992.

20. Terada LS, Leff JA, Guidot DM, Willingham IR, Repine JE: Inactivation of xanthine oxidase by hydrogen peroxide involves site-directed hydroxyl radical formation. *Free Radic Biol Med* 10:61–68, 1991.

21. Babior BM: Oxidants from phagocytes: agents of defense and destruction. *Blood* 64:959–966, 1984.

22. Cross AR, Jones OTG: Enzymatic mechanisms of superoxide production. *Biochim Biophys Acta* 1057:281–298, 1991.

23. Morel F, Doussiere J, Vignais PV: The superoxide-generating oxidase of phagocytic cells. *Eur J Biochem* 201:523–546, 1991.

24. Jesaitis A, Quinn MT, Mukherjee G, Ward PA, Dratz EA: Death by oxygen: radical views. *New Biol* 3:651–655, 1991.

25. Repine JE, Cheronis JC, Rodell TC, Linas SL, Patt A: Pulmonary oxygen toxicity and ischemia-reperfusion injury. A mechanism in common involving xanthine oxidase and neutrophils. *Am Rev Respir Dis* 136:483–485, 1987.

26. Anderson BO, Moore EE, Moore FA, et al: Hypovolemic shock promotes neutrophil sequestration in lung by a xanthine oxidase-related mechanism. *J Appl Physiol* 75:1862–1865, 1991.

27. Pryor WA: On the detection of lipid hydroperoxides in biological samples. *Free Radic Biol Med* 7:177–178, 1989.

28. Pryor WA, Godber SS: Noninvasive measures of oxidative stress status in humans. *Free Radic Biol Med* 10:177–184, 1991.

29. Arroyo CM, Kramer JH, Leiboff RH, Mergner GW, Dickens BF, Weglicki WB: Spin trapping of oxygen and carbon-centered free radicals in ischemic canine myocardium. *Free Radic Biol Med* 3:313–316, 1987.

30. Baker JE, Felix CC, Olinger GN, Kalyanaraman B: Myocardial ischemia and reperfusion: direct evidence for free radical generation by electron spin resonance spectroscopy. *Proc Natl Acad Sci USA* 85:2786–2789, 1988.

31. Valenzuela A: The biological significance of malondialdehyde determination in the assessment of tissue oxidative stress. *Life Sci* 48:301–309, 1991.

32. Tomita M, Okuyoma T: Determination of malonaldehyde in oxidized biological materials by high-performance liquid chromatography. *J Chromatogr* 515:391–397, 1990.

33. Lepage G, Munoz G, Champagne J, Roy CC: Preparative steps necessary for the accurate measurement of malondialdehyde by high-performance liquid chromatography. *Anal Biochem* 197:277–283, 1991.

34. Janero DR: Malondialdehyde and thiobarbituric acid-reactivity as diagnostic indices of lipid peroxidation and peroxidative tissue injury. *Free Radic Biol Med* 9:515–540, 1990.

35. Esterbauer H, Cheeseman KH: Determination of aldehydic lipid peroxidation products: malonaldehyde and 4-hydroxynonenal. *Methods Enzymol* 186:407–421, 1990.

36. Esterbauer H, Schaur RJ, Zollner H: Chemistry and biochemistry of 4-hydroxynonenal, malonaldehyde and related aldehydes. *Free Radic Biol Med* 11:81–128, 1991.

37. Recknagel RO, Glende EA: Spectrophotometric detection of lipid conjugated dienes. *Methods Enzymol* 105:331–337, 1984.

38. Corongiu FP, Banni S, Dessi MA: Conjugated dienes detected in tissue lipid extracts by second derivative spectrophotometry. *Free Radic Biol Med* 7:183–186, 1989.

39. Yamamoto Y, Brodsky MH, Baker JC, Ames BN: Detection and characterization of lipid hydroperoxides at picomole levels by high-performance liquid chromatography. *Anal Biochem* 160:7–13, 1987.

40. Miyazawa T, Yasuda K, Fujimoto K, Kaneda T: Presence of phosphatidylcholine hydroperoxide in human plasma. *J Biol Chem* 103:744–746, 1988.

41. Funk MO: The electroanalytical approach to lipid peroxide determinations. *Free Radic Biol Med* 3:319–321, 1987.

42. Pendleton RB, Lands WEM: Assay of lipid hydroperoxides by activation of cyclooxygenase activity. *Free Radic Biol Med* 3:337–339, 1987.

43. Heath RL, Tappel AL: A new sensitive assay for the measurement of hydroperoxides. *Anal Biochem* 76:184–191, 1976.

44. Van Kuijk FJGM, Thomas DW, Stephens RJ, Dratz EA: Gas chromatography-mass spectrometry method for determination of phospholipid peroxides. I.

Transesterification to form methyl esters. II. Transesterification to form pentafluorobenzyl esters and detection with picogram sensitivity. *Free Radic Biol Med* 1:215–225, 387–393, 1985.

45. Frankel EN, Tappel AL: Headspace gas chromatography of volatile lipid peroxidation products from human red blood cell membranes. *Lipids* 26:479–484, 1991.

46. Jeejeebhoy KN: In vivo breath alkane as an index of lipid peroxidation. *Free Radic Biol Med* 10:191–193, 1991.

47. Barsacchi R, Pelosi G, Camici P, Bonaldo L, Maiorino M, Ursini F: Glutathione depletion increases chemiluminescence emission and lipid peroxidation in the heart. *Biochim Biophys Acta* 804:356–360, 1984.

48. Andreoli S, Mallett C, Bergstein J: Role of glutathione in protecting endothelial cells against hydrogen peroxide oxidant injury. *J Lab Clin Med* 108:190–198, 1986.

49. White C, Mimmack R, Repine J: Accumulation of lung tissue oxidized glutathione GSSG as a marker of oxidant induced lung injury. *Chest* 8:3–4, 1986.

50. Beehler CJ, Simchuk ML, Toth KM, et al: Blood sulfhydryl level increases during hyperoxia: a marker of oxidant lung injury. *J Appl Physiol* 67:1070–1075, 1989.

51. Ellman G, Lysko H: A precise method for the determination of whole blood and plasma sulfhydryl groups. *Anal Biochem* 93:98–102, 1979.

52. Jaeschke H: Glutathione disulfide as index of oxidant stress in rat liver during hypoxia. *Am J Physiol* 258:499–505, 1990.

53. Pourcyrous M, Leffler CW, Mirror R, Busija DW: Brain superoxide anion generation during asphyxia and reventilation in newborn pigs. *Pediatr Res* 28:618–621, 1990.

54. Levine RL, Garland D, Oliver CN, et al: Determination of carbonyl/content in oxidatively modified proteins. *Methods Enzymol* 186:464–480, 1990.

55. Birnboim HC: Fluorometric analysis of DNA unwinding to study strand breaks and repair in mammalian cells. *Methods Enzymol* 186:550–555, 1990.

56. Shigenaga MK, Ames BN: Assays for 8-hydroxy-2'-deoxyguanosine: a biomarker of in vivo oxidative DNA damage. *Free Radic Biol Med* 10:211–216, 1991.

57. Dizdaroglu M, Galjewski E: Selected-ion mass spectrometry: assays of oxidative DNA damage. *Methods Enzymol* 186:530–545, 1990.

58. Dizdaroglu M: Chemical determination of free radical-induced damage to DNA. *Free Radic Biol Med* 10:225–242, 1991.

59. Davies KJA: Protein damage and degradation by oxygen radicals. I. General aspects. *J Biol Chem* 262:9895–9901, 1987.

60. Dean RT, Hunt JV, Grant AJ, Yamamoto Y, Niki E: Free radical damage to proteins: the influence of the relative localization of radical generation, antioxidants, and target proteins. *Free Radic Biol Med* 11:161–168, 1991.

61. Davies KJA, Delsignore ME, Lin SW: Protein damage and degradation by oxygen radicals. II. Modification of amino acids. *J Biol Chem* 262:9902–9907, 1987.

62. Schoneich C, Asmus K-D, Dillinger U, Bruchhausen FV: Thiyl radical attack on polyunsaturated fatty acids: a possible route to lipid peroxidation. *Biochem Biophys Res Commun* 161:113–120, 1989.

63. Pacifici RE, Davies KJA: Protein degradation as an index of oxidative stress. *Methods Enzymol* 186:485–502, 1990.

64. Davies KJA, Goldberg AL: Proteins damaged by oxygen radicals are rapidly degraded in extracts of red blood cells. *J Biol Chem* 262:8227–8234, 1987.

65. Gardner HW: Oxygen radical chemistry of polyunsaturated fatty acids. *Free Radic Biol Med* 7:65–86, 1989.

66. Aikens J, Dix TA: Perhydroxyl radical (HOO·) initiated lipid peroxidation. The role of fatty acid hydroperoxides. *J Biol Chem* 266:15091–15098, 1991.

67. Zimmerman JJ, Lewandoski JR: In vitro phosphatidylcholine peroxidation mediated by activated human neutrophils. *Circ Shock* 34:231–239, 1991.

68. Sevanian A, Kim E: Phospholipase A₂ dependent release of fatty acids from peroxidized membranes. *J Free Radic Biol Med* 1:263–271, 1985.

69. Imlay JA, Linn S: DNA damage and oxygen radical toxicity. *Science* 240:1302–1309, 1988.

70. Aruoma OI, Halliwell B, Dizdaroglu M: Iron-dependent modifications of bases in DNA by the superoxide radical-generating system hypoxanthine/xanthine oxidase. *J Biol Chem* 264:13024–13028, 1989.

71. Weitberg AB, Weitzman SA, Clark EP, Stossel TP: Effects of antioxidants on oxidant-induced sister chromatid exchange formation. *J Clin Invest* 75:1835–1841, 1985.

72. Spragg RG: DNA strand break formation following exposure of bovine pulmonary artery and aortic endothelial cells to reactive oxygen products. *Am J Respir Cell Mol Biol* 4:4–10, 1991.

73. Kirkland JB: Lipid peroxidation, protein thiol oxidation and DNA damage in hydrogen peroxide-induced injury to endothelial cells: role of activation of poly (ADP-ribose) polymerase. *Biochim Biophys Acta* 1092:319–325, 1991.

74. Schraufstatter IU, Hinshaw DB, Hyslop PA, Spragg RG, Cochrane CG: Oxidant injury of cells. DNA strand breaks activate polyadenosine diphosphate-ribose polymerase and lead to depletion of nicotinamide adenine dinucleotide. *J Clin Invest* 77:1312–1320, 1986.

75. Andreoli SP: Mechanisms of endothelial cell ATP depletion after oxidant injury. *Pediatr Res* 25:97–101, 1989.

76. Berger NA: Oxidant-induced cytotoxicity: a challenge for metabolic modulation. *Am J Respir Cell Mol Biol* 4:1–3, 1991.

77. Goldberg WJ, Dickens BF, Tadvalker G, Bernstein JJ, Laws ER, Weglicki WB: Free radical-induced injury to C6 glioma cells. *Neurosurgery* 29:532–537, 1991.

78. Weiss SJ, Slivka A: Monocyte and granulocyte-mediated tumor cell destruction. *J Clin Invest* 69:255–262, 1982.

79. Weiss SJ, Young J, LoBuglio AF, Slivka A: Role of hydrogen peroxide in neutrophil-mediated destruction of cultured endothelial cells. *J Clin Invest* 68:714–721, 1981.

80. Sacks TCF, Molder CF, Craddock PR, Bowers TK, Jacob HS: Oxygen radicals mediate endothelial cell damage by complement-stimulated granulocytes. *J Clin Invest* 61:1161–1167, 1978.

81. Varani J, Ginsburg I, Schuger L, et al: Endothelial cell killing by neutrophils. Synergistic interactions of oxygen products and proteases. *Am J Pathol* 135:435–438, 1989.

82. Housset B, Hurbain I, Masliah J, et al: Toxic effects of oxygen on cultured alveolar epithelial cells, lung fibroblasts and alveolar macrophages. *Eur Respir J* 4:1066–1075, 1991.

83. LaCagnin LB, Bowman L, Ma JYC, Miles PR: Metabolic changes in alveolar type II cells after exposure to hydrogen peroxide. *Am J Physiol* 259:L57–L65, 1990.

84. Holm BA, Hudak BB, Keicher L, et al: Mechanisms of H_2O_2-mediated injury to type II cell surfactant metabolism and protection with PEG-catalase. *Am J Physiol* 261:C751–C757, 1991.

85. Zimmerman JJ, Lewandoski JR: Activated polymorphonuclear leukocytes inhibit phosphatidylcholine synthesis in cultured type II alveolar cells. *Pediatr Pulmonol* 10:164–171, 1991.

86. Housset B, Hurbain I, Masliah J, Laghsal A, Chaumette-Demaugre MT, Karam H, Derenne JP: Toxic effects of oxygen on cultured alveolar epithelial cells, lung fibroblasts, and alveolar macrophages. *Eur Respir J* 4:1066–1075, 1991.

87. Oosting RS, Van Iwaarden JF, van Bree L, Verhoef J, van Golde LMG, Haagsman HP: Exposure of surfactant protein A to ozone in vitro and in vivo impairs its interactions with alveolar cells. *Am J Physiol* 262:L63–L68, 1992.

88. Ryan SF, Ghassibi Y, Liau DF: Effects of activated polymorphonuclear leukocytes upon pulmonary surfactant in vitro. *Am J Respir Cell Mol Biol* 4:33–41, 1991.

89. Hirayama T, Folmerz P, Hansson R, et al: Effect of oxygen free radicals on rabbit and human erythrocytes. *Scand J Thorac Cardiovasc Surg* 20:247–252, 1986.

90. Powell RJ, Machiedo GW, Rush BF, Dikdan G: Oxygen free radicals: effect on red cell deformity in sepsis. *Crit Care Med* 19:732–735, 1991.

91. Freeman BA, Rosen GM, Barber MJ: Superoxide perturbation of the organization of vascular endothelial cell membranes. *J Biol Chem* 261:6590–6593, 1986.

92. Petrovich DR, Finkelstein S, Waring AJ, Farber JL: Liver ischemia increases the molecular order of microsomal membranes by increasing the cholesterol-to-phospholipid ratio. *J Biol Chem* 259:13217–13223, 1984.

93. Yokota J, Chiao JJC, Shires GT: Oxygen free radicals affect cardiac and skeletal cell membrane potential during hemorrhagic shock in rats. *Am J Physiol* 262:H84–H90, 1992.

94. Matsuura H, Shattock MJ: Effects of oxidant stress on steady-state background currents in isolated ventricular myocytes. *Am J Physiol* H1358–H1365, 1991.

95. Masumoto N, Tasaka K, Miyake A, Tanizawa O: Superoxide anion increases intracellular free calcium in myometrial cells. *J Biol Chem* 265:22533–22536, 1990.

96. Franceschi D, Graham D, Sarasua M, Zollinger RM: Mechanisms of oxygen free radical-induced calcium overload in endothelial cells. *Surgery* 108:292–297, 1990.

97. Geeraerts MD, Ronveaux-Dupal M-F, Lemasters JJ, Herman B: Cytosolic free Ca++ and proteolysis in lethal oxidative injury in endothelial cells. *Am J Physiol* 261:C889–C896, 1991.

98. Davies KJA, Goldberg AL: Oxygen radicals stimulate intracellular proteolysis and lipid peroxidation by independent mechanisms. *J Biol Chem* 262:8220–8226, 1987.

99. Kono Y, Fridovich I: Superoxide radical inhibits catalase. *J Biol Chem* 257:5751–5754, 1982.

100. Gardner PR, Fridovich I: Superoxide sensitivity of the *Escherichia coli* aconitase. *J Biol Chem* 266:19328–19333, 1991.

101. Thomas PD, Poznansky MJ: Lipid peroxidation inactivates rat liver microsomal glycerol-3-phosphate acyl transferase. *J Biol Chem* 265:2684–2691, 1990.

102. Hyslop PA, Hinshaw DB, Halsey WA, et al: Mechanisms of oxidant-mediated cell injury. *J Biol Chem* 263:1665–1675, 1988.

103. Oliver CN, Starke-Reed PE, Stadtman ER, Liu GJ, Carney JM, Floyd RA: Oxidative damage to brain proteins, loss of glutamine synthetase activity, and production of free radicals during ischemia/reperfusion-induced injury to gerbil brain. *Proc Natl Acad Sci USA* 87:5144–5147, 1990.

104. Mishra OP, Delivoria-Papadopoulos M, Cahillane G, Wagerle LC: Lipid peroxidation as the mechanism of modification of the affinity of the Na+, K+-ATPase active sites for ATP, K+, Na+, and strophanthidin in vitro. *Neurochem Res* 14:845–851, 1989.

105. Zhang Y, Marcillat O, Giulivi C, Ernster L, Davies KJA: The oxidative inactivation of mitochondrial electron transport chain components and ATPase. *J Biol Chem* 265:16330–16336, 1990.

106. Kramer K, Rademaker B, Rozendal W, et al: Influence of lipid peroxidation of β-adrenoreceptors. *FEBS Lett* 198:80–84, 1986.

107. Mohsenin V, Gee JBL: Oxidation of alpha-1-protease inhibitor: role of lipid peroxidation products. *J Appl Physiol* 66:2211–2215, 1989.

108. Carp H, Janoff A: Potential mediator of inflammation. Phagocyte-derived oxidants suppress the elastase-inhibitory capacity of alpha₁-proteinase inhibitor in vitro. *J Clin Invest* 66:987–995, 1980.

109. Zaslow MC, Clark RA, Stone PJ, Calore JD, Snider GL, Franzblau C: Human neutrophil elastase does not bind to alpha₁-protease inhibitor that has been exposed to activated human neutrophils. *Am Rev Respir Dis* 128:434–439, 1983.

110. Mohsenin V: Lipid peroxidation and antielastase activity in the lung under oxidant stress: role of antioxidant defenses. *J Appl Physiol* 70:1456–1462, 1991.

111. Thomas EL, Learn DB, Jefferson M, Weatherred W: Superoxide-dependent oxidation of extracellular reducing agents by isolated neutrophils. *J Biol Chem* 263:2178–2186, 1988.

112. McGowan SE: Mechanism of extracellular matrix proteoglycan degradation by human neutrophils. *Am J Respir Cell Mol Biol* 2:271–279, 1990.

113. Gurtner GH, Burke-Wolin T: Interactions of oxidant stress and vascular reactivity. *Am J Physiol* 260:L207–L211, 1991.

114. Lansing MW, Mansour E, Ahmed A, et al: Lipid mediators contribute to oxygen-radical-induced airway responses in sheep. *Am Rev Respir Dis* 144:1291–1296, 1991.

115. Boros M, Kaszaki J, Nagy S: Histamine release during intestinal ischemia-reperfusion: role of iron ions and hydrogen peroxide. *Circ Shock* 35:174–180, 1991.

116. Cross CE, Halliwell B, Borish ET, et al: Oxygen radicals and human disease. *Ann Intern Med* 107:526–545, 1987.

117. Fantone JC, Ward PA: Role of oxygen-derived free radicals and metabolites in leukocyte-dependent inflammatory reactions. *Am J Physiol* 107:397–418, 1982.

118. Takeda K, Shimada Y, Amano M, Sakai T, Okada Y, Yoshiya I: Plasma lipid peroxides and alpha-tocoperol in critically ill patients. *Crit Care Med* 12:957–959, 1984.

119. Heffner JE, Repine JE: Pulmonary strategies of antioxidant defenses. *Am Rev Respir Dis* 140:531–554, 1989.

120. Doleman CJA, Bast A: Oxygen radicals in lung pathology. *Free Radic Biol Med* 9:381–400, 1990.

121. Demling RH, LaLonde C, Daryani R, Zhu D, Knox J, Youn Y-K: Relationship between the lung and systemic response to endotoxin. Comparison of physiologic change and the degree of lipid peroxidation. *Circ Shock* 34:364–370, 1991.

122. Matalon S, Holm BA, Loewen GM, Baker RR, Notter RH: Sublethal hyperoxic injury to the alveolar epithelium and the pulmonary surfactant system. *Exp Lung Res* 14:1021–1033, 1988.

123. Maier K, Leuschel L, Costabel U: Increased levels of oxidized methionine residues in bronchoalveolar lavage fluid proteins from patients with idiopathic pulmonary fibrosis. *Am Rev Respir Dis* 143:271–274, 1991.

124. Baldwin SR, Grum CM, Boxer LA, Simon RH, Ketai LH, Devall LJ: Oxidant activity in expired breath of patients with adult respiratory distress syndrome. *Lancet* 1:11–14, 1986.

125. Sznajder JI, Fraiman A, Hall JB, et al: Increased hydrogen peroxide in the expired breath of patients with acute hypoxic respiratory failure. *Chest* 96:606–612, 1989.

126. Galloe AM, Graudal N: Evidence of free-radical activity in asthma. *N Engl J Med* 325:586–587, 1991.

127. Kanazawa H, Kurihara N, Hirata K, Takeda T: The role of free radicals in airway obstruction in asthmatic patients. *Chest* 160:1319–1322, 1991.

128. Iwata M, Takagi K, Satake T, Sugiyama S, Ozawa T: Mechanism of oxygen toxicity in rat lungs. *Lung* 164:93–106, 1986.

129. Davis JM, Dickerson B, Metlay L, Penney DP: Differential effects of oxygen and barotrauma on lung injury in the neonatal piglet. *Pediatr Pulmonol* 10:157–163, 1991.

130. Frank L, Sosenko IRS: Failure of premature rabbits to increase antioxidant enzymes during hyperoxic exposure: increased susceptibility to pulmonary oxygen toxicity compared with term rabbits. *Pediatr Res* 29:292–296, 1991.

131. Pitkanen OM, Hallman M, Andersson SM: Correlation of free oxygen radical-induced lipid peroxidation with outcome in very low birth weight infants. *J Pediatr* 116:760–764, 1990.

132. Sugino K, Dohi K, Yamada K, et al: The role of lipid peroxidation in endotoxin induced hepatic damage and the protective effect of antioxidants. *Surgery* 101:746–752, 1987.

133. Keller GA, Barke R, Harty JT, Humphrey E, Simmons RL: Decreased levels of hepatic glutathione in septic shock. *Arch Surg* 120:941–945, 1985.

134. Peavy DL, Fairchild EJ: Evidence for lipid peroxidation in endotoxin-poisoned mice. *Infect Immun* 52:613–616, 1986.

135. Takeda K, Shimada Y, Okada T, Amano M, Saki T, Yoshiya I: Lipid peroxidation in experimental septic rats. *Crit Care Med* 14:719–724, 1986.

136. Ishizaka A, Stephens KE, Tazelar HD, Hall EW, O'Hanley P, Raffin TA: Pulmonary edema after *Escherichia coli* peritonitis correlates with thiobarbituric-acid-reactive materials in bronchoalveolar lavage fluid. *Am Rev Respir Dis* 137:783–789, 1988.

137. Demling RH, LaLonde C, Lin L-J, Ryan P, Fox R: Endotoxemia causes increased lung tissue lipid peroxidation in unanesthetized sheep. *J Appl Physiol* 60:2094–2100, 1986.

138. Bowdy BD, Marple SL, Pauly TH, Coonrod JD, Gillespie MN: Oxygen radical-dependent bacterial killing and pulmonary hypertension in piglets infected with group B streptococcus. *Am Rev Respir Dis* 141:648–653, 1990.

139. Keen RR, Stella L, Flanigan DP, Lands WE: Differential detection of plasma hydroperoxides in sepsis. *Crit Care Med* 19:1114–1119, 1991.

140. Granger DN: Role of xanthine oxidase and granulocytes in ischemia-reperfusion injury. *Am J Physiol* 255:H1269–H1275, 1988.

141. Punch J, Rees R, Cashmer B, Wilkins E, Smith DJ, Till GO: Xanthine oxidase: its role in the no-re-flow phenomena. *Surgery* 111:169–176, 1992.

142. Haglund U, Gerdin B: Oxygen-free radicals and circulatory shock. *Circ Shock* 34:405–411, 1991.

143. Ikeda Y, Long DM: The molecular basis of brain injury and brain edema: the role of oxygen free radicals. *Neurosurgery* 27:1–11, 1990.

144. Braughler JM, Hall ED: Central nervous system trauma and stroke. I. Biochemical considerations for oxygen radical formation and lipid peroxidation. II. Physiological and pharmacological evidence for involvement of oxygen radicals and lipid peroxidation. *Free Radic Biol Med* 6:289–301, 303–313, 1989.

145. Schmidley JW: Free radical in central nervous system ischemia. *Stroke* 21:1086–1089, 1990.

146. Vannucci RC: Experimental biology of cerebral hypoxia-ischemia: relation to perinatal brain damage. *Pediatr Res* 27:317–326, 1990.

147. Chan PH, Schmidley JW, Fishman RA, Longar SM: Brain injury, edema, and vascular permeability changes induced by oxygen-derived free radicals. *Neurology* 34:315–320, 1984.

148. Kirsch JR, Phelan DG, Lange DG, Traystman RJ: Evidence for free oxygen radical production during reperfusion from global cerebral ischemia. *Anesth Rev* 14:19–20, 1987.

149. Gardner TJ, Stewart JR, Casale AS, Downey JM, Chambers DE: Reduction of myocardial ischemic injury with oxygen-derived free radical scavengers. *Surgery* 94:423–427, 1983.

150. Bromont C, Marie C, Bralet J: Increased lipid peroxidation in vulnerable brain regions after transient forebrain ischemia in rats. *Stroke* 20:918–924, 1989.

151. Traystman RJ, Kirsch JR, Koehler RC: Oxygen radical mechanisms of brain injury following ischemia and reperfusion. *J Appl Physiol* 71:1185–1195, 1991.

152. Chatelain P, Latour JG, Tran D, de Lorgeril M, Dupras G, Bourassa M: Neutrophil accumulation in experimental myocardial infarcts: relation with extent of injury and effect of reperfusion. *Circulation* 75:1083–1090, 1987.

153. Ko W, Hawes AS, Lazenby WD, et al: Myocardial reperfusion injury. Platelet-activating factor stimulates polymorphonuclear leukocyte hydrogen peroxide production during myocardial reperfusion. *J Thorac Cardiovasc Surg* 102:297–308, 1991.

154. Dreyer WJ, Michael LH, West S, et al: Neutrophil accumulation in ischemic canine myocardium: insights into time course, distribution and mechanism of localization during early reperfusion. *Circulation* 84:400–411, 1991.

155. Engler RL, Dahlgren MD, Morris DD, Peterson MA, Schmid-Schonbein GW: Role of leukocytes in response to acute myocardial ischemia and reflow in dogs. *Am J Physiol* 251:H314–H322, 1986.

156. Steinberg D, Parthasarathy S, Carew TE, Khoo JC, Witztum JL: Beyond cholesterol. Modifications of low-density lipoprotein that increase its atherogenicity. *N Engl J Med* 320:915–924, 1989.

157. Yagi K: A biochemical approach to atherogenesis. *Trends in Biochemical Sciences* 11:18–19, 1986.

158. Stringer MD, Gorog PG, Freeman A, Kakkar VV: Lipid peroxides and atherosclerosis. *Br Med J* 298:281–284, 1989.

159. Liu K, Cuddy TE, Pierce GN: Oxidative status of lipoproteins in coronary disease patients. *Am Heart J* 123:285–290, 1992.

160. Fisher AB, Dodia C, Tan Z, Ayene I, Eckenhoff RG: Oxygen-dependent lipid peroxidation during lung ischemia. *J Clin Invest* 88:674–679, 1991.

161. Parks DA, Bulkey GB, Granger DN: Role of oxygen-derived free radicals in digestive tract diseases. *Surgery* 94:415–422, 1983.

162. Jaesche H, Smith C, Mitchell J: Reactive oxygen species during ischemia-reflow injury in isolated perfused rat liver. *J Clin Invest* 81:1240–1246, 1988.

163. Smith SM, Kvietys PR: Gastric ulcers: role of oxygen radicals. *Crit Care Med* 16:892–898, 1988.

164. Salim AS: Oxygen-derived free radicals and the prevention of duodenal ulcer relapse: a new approach. *Am J Med Sci* 300:1–6, 1990.

165. Paller MS, Hoidal JR, Ferris TF: Oxygen free radicals in ischemic acute renal failure in the rat. *J Clin Invest* 74:1156–1164, 1984.

166. Stratta P, Canavese C, Dogliani M, Mazzucco G, Monga G, Vercellone A: The role of free radicals in the progression of renal disease. *Am J Kidney Dis* 17(suppl 1):33–37, 1991.

167. Odeh M: The role of reperfusion-induced injury in the pathogenesis of the crush syndrome. *N Engl J Med* 324:1417–1423, 1991.

168. Smith JK, Grisham MB, Granger DN, Korthus RJ: Free radical defense mechanisms and neutrophil infiltration in postischemic skeletal muscle. *Am J Physiol* 256:H789–H793, 1989.

169. McCutchan HJ, Schwappach JR, Enquist EG, et al: Xanthine oxidase-derived H_2O_2 contributes to reperfusion injury of ischemic skeletal muscle. *Am J Physiol* 258:H1415–H1419, 1990.

170. Van Bebber T, Boekholz W, Goris D, et al: Neutrophil function and lipid peroxidation in a rat model of multiple organ failure. *J Surg Res* 47:471–475, 1989.

171. Hernandez LA, Granger N: Role of antioxidants in organ preservation and transplantation. *Crit Care Med* 16:543–549, 1988.

172. Royston D, Fleming JS, Desai JB, Westaby S, Taylor KM: Increased production of peroxidation products associated with cardiac operations. *J Thorac Cardiovasc Surg* 91:759–766, 1986.

173. Youn Y-K, LaLonde C, Demling R: Use of antioxidant therapy in shock and trauma. *Circ Shock* 35:245–249, 1991.

174. Shoemaker W, Appel P, Kram H: Hemodynamic and oxygen transport effects of dobutamine in critically ill general surgical patients. *Crit Care Med* 14:1032–1038, 1986.

175. Mak IT, Weglicki WB: Protection by β-blocking agents against free radical-mediated sarcolemmal lipid peroxidation. *Circ Res* 63:262–266, 1988.

176. McCord JM, Fridovich I: Superoxide dismutase: an enzymatic function for erythrocuprein (hemocuprein). *J Biol Chem* 244:6049–6055, 1969.

177. Hjalmarsson LK, Edlund T, Engstrom A, Marklund SL: Expression of human extracellular-superoxide dismutase in Chinese hamster ovary cells and characterization of the product. *Proc Natl Acad Sci USA* 84:6634–6638, 1987.

178. Kunimoto F, Morita T, Ogawa R, Fujita T: Inhibition of lipid peroxidation improves survival rate of endotoxemic rats. *Circ Shock* 21:15–22, 1987.

179. Broner CW, Shenep JL, Stidham GL, Stokes DC, Hildner WK: Effect of scavengers of oxygen-derived free radicals on mortality in endotoxin-challenged mice. *Crit Care Med* 16:848–858, 1988.

180. Schneider J, Friderichs E, Heintze K, Flohe L: Effects of recombinant human superoxide dismutase on increased lung vascular permeability and respiratory disorder in endotoxemic rats. *Circ Shock* 30:97–106, 1990.

181. Uyama O, Matsuyama T, Michishita H, Nakamura H, Sugita M: Protective effects of human recombinant superoxide dismutase on transient ischemic injury of CA1 neurons in gerbils. *Stroke* 23:75–81, 1992.

181a. Imaizumi S, Woolworth V, Fishman RA, Chan PH: Liposome-entrapped superoxide dismutase reduces cerebral infarction in cerebral ischemia in rats. *Stroke* 21:1312–1317, 1990.

182. Johansson MH, Deinum J, Marklund SL, Sjoquist PO: Recombinant human extracellular superoxide dismutase reduces concentration of oxygen free radicals in the reperfused rat heart. *Cardiovasc Res* 24:500–503, 1990.

183. Hori M, Gotoh K, Kitakaze M, et al: Role of oxygen-derived free radicals in myocardial edema and ischemia in coronary microvascular embolization. *Circulation* 84:828–840, 1991.

184. Dunn SP, Gross KR, Dalsing M, Hon R, Grosfeld JL: Superoxide: a critical oxygen-free radical in ischemic bowel injury. *J Pediatr Surg* 19:740–744, 1984.

185. Wang J, Chen H, Wang T, Diao Y, Tian K: Oxygen-derived free radicals induced cellular injury in superior mesenteric artery occlusion shock: protective effect of superoxide dismutase. *Circ Shock* 32:31–41, 1990.

186. Schneeberger H, Illner WD, Abendroth D, et al: First clinical experiences with superoxide dismutase in kidney transplantation—results of a double-blind randomized study. *Transplant Proc* 21:1245–1246, 1989.

187. Rosenfeld W, Evans H, Concepcion L, Jhaveri R, Schaeffer H, Friedman A: Prevention of bronchopulmonary dysplasia by administration of bovine superoxide dismutase in preterm infants with respiratory distress syndrome. *J Pediatr* 105:781–785, 1984.

188. Murohara Y, Yui Y, Hattori R, Kawai C: Effects of superoxide dismutase on reperfusion arrhythmias and left ventricular function in patients undergoing thrombolysis for anterior wall acute myocardial infarction. *Am J Cardiol* 67:765–767, 1991.

189. Tsao C, Greene P, Odlind B, Brater DC: Pharmacokinetics of recombinant human superoxide dismutase in healthy volunteers. *Clin Pharmacol Ther* 50:713–720, 1991.

190. Omar BA, Gad NM, Jordan MC, et al: Cardioprotection by Cu, Zn-superoxide dismutase is lost at high doses in the reoxygenated heart. *Free Radic Biol Med* 9:465–471, 1990.

191. Omar BA, McCord JM: The cardioprotective effect of Mn-superoxide dismutase is lost at high doses in the postischemic isolated rabbit heart. *Free Radic Biol Med* 9:473–478, 1991.

192. Deisseroth A, Dounce AL: Catalase: physical and chemical properties, mechanisms of catalysis, and physiologic role. *Physiol Rev* 50:319–375, 1970.

193. Hiraishi H, Terano A, Ota S-I, Ivey KJ, Sugimoto T: Oxygen metabolite-induced cytotoxicity to cultured rat gastric mucosal cells. *Am J Physiol* 253:G40–G48, 1987.

194. Milligan SA, Hoeffel JM, Goldstein IM, Flick MR: Effect of catalase on endotoxin-induced acute lung injury in unanesthetized sheep. *Am Rev Respir Dis* 137:420–428, 1988.

195. Seekamp A, LaLonde C, Zhu D, Demling R: Catalase prevents prostanoid release and lung lipid peroxidation after endotoxemia in sheep. *J Appl Physiol* 65:1210–1216, 1988.

196. Daryani R, LaLonde C, Zhu D, Demling RH: Changes in catalase activity in lung and liver after endotoxin in sheep. *Circ Shock* 32:273–280, 1990.

197. Scott MD, Meshnick SR, Eaton JW: Superoxide dismutase amplifies organismal sensitivity to ionizing radiation. *J Biol Chem* 264:2498–2501, 1989.

198. Jolly SR, Kane WJ, Bailie MB, Abrams GD, Lucchesi BR: Canine myocardial reperfusion injury. Its reduction by the combined administration of superoxide dismutase and catalase. *Circ Res* 54:277–285, 1984.

199. Morgan RA, Manning PB, Coran AG, et al: Oxygen free radical activity during live *E. coli* septic shock in the dog. *Circ Shock* 25:319–323, 1988.

200. Johnson DL, Horneffer PJ, Dinatale JM, Gott VL, Gardner TJ: Free radical scavengers improve functional recovery of stunned myocardium in a model of surgical coronary revascularization. *Surgery* 102:334–340, 1987.

201. Hatori N, Miyazaki A, Tadokoro H, et al: Beneficial effects of coronary venous retroinfusion of superoxide dismutase and catalase on reperfusion arrhythmias, myocardial function, and infarct size in dogs. *J Cardiovasc Pharmacol* 14:396–404, 1989.

202. Paull DE, Keagy BA, Kron EJ, Wilcox BR: Reperfusion injury in the lung preserved for 24 hours. *Ann Thorac Surg* 47:187–192, 1989.

203. Chaudiere J, Tappel AL: Purification and characterization of selenium-glutathione peroxidase from hamster liver. *Arch Biochem Biophys* 226:448–457, 1983.

204. Menasche P, Grousset C, Gauduel Y, Mouas C, Piwnica A: Enhancement of cardioplegic protection with free-radical scavengers. *Circulation* 74:138–144, 1986.

205. Menasche P, Grousset C, Gauduel Y, Piwnica A: A comparative study of free radical scavengers in cardioplegic solutions. Improved protection with peroxidase. *J Thorac Cardiovasc Surg* 92:264–271, 1986.

206. Greenwald RA: Superoxide dismutase and catalase as therapeutic agents for human diseases. *Free Radic Biol Med* 8:201–209, 1990.

207. Turrens JF, Crapo JD, Freeman BA: Protection against oxygen toxicity by intravenous injection of liposome-entrapped catalase and superoxide dismutase. *J Clin Invest* 73:87–95, 1984.

208. Padmanabhan RV, Gudapaty R, Liener IE, Schwartz BA, Hoidal JR: Protection against pulmonary oxygen toxicity in rats by the intratracheal administration of liposome-encapsulated superoxide dismutase or catalase. *Am Rev Respir Dis* 132:164–167, 1985.

209. Thibeault DW, Rezaiekhaligh M, Mabry S, Beringer T: Prevention of chronic pulmonary oxygen toxicity in young rats with liposome-encapsulated catalase administered intra-tracheally. *Pediatr Pulmonol* 11:318–327, 1991.

210. Beckman JS, Minor RL, White CW, Repine JE, Rosen GM, Freeman BA: Superoxide dismutase and catalase conjugated to polyethylene glycol increases endothelial enzyme activity and oxidant resistance. *J Biol Chem* 263:6884–6892, 1988.

211. White CW, Jackson JH, Abuchowski A, et al: Polyethylene glycol-attached antioxidant enzymes decreases pulmonary oxygen toxicity in rats. *J Appl Physiol* 66:584–590, 1989.

212. Jackson RM, Veal CF, Beckman JS, Brannen AL: Polyethylene glycol-conjugated superoxide dismutase in unilateral lung injury due to re-expansion (re-oxygenation). *Am J Med Sci* 300:22–28, 1990.

213. Walther FJ, Ikegami M, Warburton D, Polk DH: Corticosteroids, thyrotropin-releasing hormone and antioxidant enzymes in preterm lamb lungs. *Pediatr Res* 30:518–521, 1991.

214. Rodriquez MP, Sosenko IRS, Antigua MC, Frank LF: Prenatal hormone treatment with thyrotropin releasing hormone and with thyrotropin releasing hormone plus dexamethasone delays antioxidant enzyme maturation but does not inhibit a protective antioxidant enzyme response to hyperoxia in newborn rat lung. *Pediatr Res* 30:522–527, 1991.

215. White CW, Ghezzi P, McMahon S, Dinarello CA, Repine JE: Cytokines increase rat lung antioxidant enzymes during exposure to hyperoxia. *J Appl Physiol* 66:1003–1007, 1989.

216. Warner BB, Burhans MS, Clark JC, Wispe JR: Tumor necrosis factor-α increases Mn-SOD expression: protection against oxidant injury. *Am J Physiol* 260:L296–L301, 1991.

217. Tsan M-F, Lee CY, White JE: Interleukin 1 protects rats against oxygen toxicity. *J Appl Physiol* 71:688–697, 1991.

218. Harris CA, Derbin KS, Hunte-McDonough B, et al: Manganese superoxide dismutase is induced by IFN-γ in multiple cell types. *J Immunol* 147:149–154, 1991.

219. Rushmore TH, Morton MR, Pickett CB: The antioxidant responsive element. *J Biol Chem* 266:11632–11639, 1991.

220. Brigham KL, Meyrick B, Berry LC, Repine JE: Antioxidants protect cultured bovine lung endothelial cells from injury by endotoxin. *J Appl Physiol* 63:840–850, 1987.

221. Matsuda T, Eccleston CA, Rubinstein I, Rennard SI, Joyner WL: Antioxidants attenuate endotoxin-induced microvascular leakage of macromolecules in vivo. *J Appl Physiol* 70: 1483–1489, 1991.

222. Palmer C, Vannucci RC, Towfighi J: Reduction of perinatal hypoxic-ischemic brain damage with allopurinol. *Pediatr Res* 27:332–336, 1990.

223. Nordstrom G, Seeman T, Hasselgren P-O: Beneficial effect of allopurinol in liver ischemia. *Surgery* 97:679–683, 1985.

224. Stewart JR, Crute SL, Loughlin V, Hess ML, Greenfield LJ: Prevention of free radical-induced myocardial reperfusion injury with allopurinol. *J Thorac Cardiovasc Surg* 90:68–72, 1985.

225. Toledo-Pereyra LH, Simmons RL, Olson LC, Najarian JS: Clinical effect of allopurinol on preserved kidneys: a randomized double-blind study. *Ann Surg* 185:128–131, 1977.

226. Tabayashi K, Suzuki Y, Nagamine S, Ito Y, Sekino Y, Mohri H: A clinical trial of allopurinol (zyloric) for myocardial protection. *J Thorac Cardiovasc Surg* 101:713–718, 1991.

227. Johnson WD, Kayser KL, Brenowitz JB, Saedi SF: A randomized controlled trial of allopurinol in coronary bypass surgery. *Am Heart J* 121:20–24, 1991.

228. Werns SW, Grum CM, Ventura A, et al: Xanthine oxidase inhibition does not limit canine infarct size. *Circulation* 83:995–1005, 1991.

229. Moorhouse PC, Grootveld M, Halliwell B, Quinlan JG, Gutteridge JMC: Allopurinol and oxypurinol are hydroxyl radical scavengers. *FEBS Lett* 2113:23–28, 1987.

230. Das DK, Engelman RM, Clement R, Otani H, Prasad MR, Rao PS: Role of xanthine oxidase inhibitor as free radical scavenger: a novel mechanism of action of allopurinol and oxypurinol in myocardial salvage. *Biochem Biophys Res Commun* 148:314–318, 1987.

231. Meister A: Glutathione metabolism and its selective modification. *J Biol Chem* 263:17205–17208, 1988.

232. Mitsos SE, Askew TE, Fantone JC, et al: Protective effects of N-2-mercaptopropionyl glycine against myocardial reperfusion injury after neutrophil depletion in the dog: evidence for the role of intracellular-derived free radicals. *Circulation* 73:1077–1086, 1986.

233. Bernard GR, Lucht WD, Niedermeyer ME, Snapper JR, Ogletree ML, Brigham KL: Effect of *N*-acetylcysteine on the pulmonary response to endotoxin in the awake sheep and upon in vitro granulocyte function. *J Clin Invest* 73:1772–1784, 1984.

234. Amano J, Sunamori M, Okamura T, Suzuki A: Effect of glutathione pretreatment on hypothermic ischemic cardioplegia. *Jpn J Surg* 12:87–92, 1982.

235. Toth KM, Harlan JM, Beehler CJ, et al: Dimethylthiourea prevents hydrogen peroxide and neutrophil mediated damage to lung endothelial cells in vitro and disappears in the process. *Free Radic Biol Med* 6:457–466, 1989.

236. Fox RB: Prevention of granulocyte-mediated oxidant lung injury in rats by a hydroxyl radical scavenger, dimethylthiourea. *J Clin Invest* 74:1456–1464, 1984.

237. Vander Heide RS, Sobotka PA, Ganote CE: Effect of the free radical scavenger DMTU and mannitol on the oxygen paradox in perfused rat hearts. *J Mol Cell Cardiol* 19:615–625, 1987.

238. Olson NC, Anderson DL, Grizzle MK: Dimethylthiourea attenuates endotoxin-induced acute respiratory failure in pigs. *J Appl Physiol* 63:2426–2432, 1987.

239. Kennedy TP, Ras NV, Hopkins C, Pennington L, Tolley E, Hoidal JR: Role of reactive oxygen species in reperfusion injury of the rabbit lung. *J Clin Invest* 83:1326–1335, 1989.

240. Gaull GE: Taurine in pediatric nutrition: review and update. *Pediatrics* 83:433–442, 1989.

241. Milei J, Ferreira R, Llesuy S, Forcada P, Covarrubias J, Boveris A: Reduction of reperfusion injury with preoperative rapid intravenous infusion of taurine during myocardial revascularization. *Am Heart J* 123:339–345, 1992.

242. Aust SD, Morehouse LA, Thomas CE: Role of metals in oxygen radical reactions. *J Free Radic Biol Med* 1:3–25, 1985.

243. Williams RE, Zweier JL, Flaherty JT: Treatment with deferoxamine during ischemia improves functional and metabolic recovery and reduces reperfusion-induced oxygen radical generation in rabbit hearts. *Circulation* 83:1006–1014, 1991.

244. Menasche P, Pasquier C, Jaillon P, Piwnica A: Deferoxamine reduces neutrophil-mediated free radical production during cardiopulmonary bypass in man. *J Thorac Cardiovasc Surg* 96:582–589, 1988.

245. Demling R, LaLonde C, Knox J, Youn Y-K, Zhu D, Daryani R: Fluid resuscitation with deferoxamine prevents systemic burn-induced oxidant injury. *J Trauma* 31:538–544, 1991.

246. Cross CE, Halliwell B, Borish ET, et al: Oxygen radicals and human disease. *Ann Intern Med* 107:526–545, 1987.

247. Kennedy TP, Rao NV, Noah W, et al: Ibuprofen prevents oxidant lung injury and in vitro lipid peroxidation by chelating iron. *J Clin Invest* 86:1565–1573, 1990.

248. Krinsky NI: Antioxidant functions of carotenoids. *Free Radic Biol Med* 7:617–635, 1989.

249. Terao J: Antioxidant activity of β-carotene-related carotenoids in solution. *Lipids* 24:659–661, 1989.

250. Packer L: Protective role of vitamin E in biological systems. *Am J Clin Nutr* 53:1050S–1055S, 1991.

251. Chow CK: Vitamin E and oxidative stress. *Free Radic Biol Med* 11:215–232, 1991.

252. Bieri JG, Corash L, Hubbard VS: Medical uses of vitamin E. *N Engl J Med* 308:1063–1070, 1983.

253. Burton GW, Joyce A, Ingold KU: Is vitamin E the only lipid-soluble, chain breaking antioxidant in human blood plasma and erythrocyte membranes? *Arch Biochem Biophys* 221:281–290, 1983.

254. McCay PB: Vitamin E interactions with free radicals and ascorbate. *Ann Rev Nutr*, 5:323–340, 1985.

255. Packer JE, Slater TF, Wilson RL: Direct observation of a free radical interaction between vitamin E and vitamin C. *Nature* 278:737–738, 1986.

256. Fukuzawa K, Takase S, Tsukatini H: The effect of concentration on the antioxidant effectiveness of α-tocopherol induced by superoxide free radicals. *Arch Biochem Biophys* 240:117–120, 1985.

257. Marubayashi S, Kiyohiko D, Ochi K, Kawasaki T: Role of free radicals in ischemic rat liver cell injury: prevention of damage by α-tocopherol administration. *Surgery* 99:184–191, 1986.

258. Klein HH, Pich S, Lindert S, Nebendahl K, Niedmann P, Kreuzer H: Combined treatment with vitamin E and C in experimental myocardial infarction in pigs. *Am Heart J* 118:667–673, 1989.

259. Peck MD, Alexander W: Survival in septic guinea pigs is influenced by vitamin E, but not by vitamin C in enteral diets. *J Parenter Enter Nutr* 15:433–436, 1991.

260. Gutcher GR, Farrell PM: Early intravenous correction of vitamin E deficiency in premature infants. *J Pediatr Gastroenterol Nutr* 4:604–609, 1985.

261. Karp WB, Robertson AF: Vitamin E in neonatology. *Adv Pediatr* 33:127–148, 1986.

262. Ehrenkranz RA, Ablow RC, Warshaw JB: Prevention of bronchopulmonary dysplasia with vitamin E administration during the acute stages of respiratory distress syndrome. *J Pediatr* 95:873–878, 1979.

263. Ehrenkranz RA, Bonta BW, Ablow RC, Warshaw JB: Amelioration of broncho-pulmonary dysplasia after vitamin E administration: a preliminary report. *N Engl J Med* 299:564–568, 1978.

264. Saldanha R, Cepeda E, Poland R: The effect of vitamin E prophylaxis on the incidence and severity of bronchopulmonary dysplasia. *J Pediatr* 101:89–93, 1982.

265. Watts JL, Milner R, Zipursky A, et al: Failure of supplementation with vitamin E to prevent bronchopulmonary dysplasia in infants <1,500 g birth weight. *Eur Resp J* 4:188–190, 1991.

266. Hittner HM, Godio LB, Rudolph AJ, et al: Retrolental fibroplasia: efficacy of vitamin E in a double-blind clinical study of preterm infants. *N Engl J Med* 305:1365–1371, 1981.

267. Wolf HRD, Seeger HW: Experimental and clinical results in shock lung treatment with vitamin E. *Ann NY Acad Sci* 393:392–409, 1982.

268. Sosenko IRS, Innis SM, Frank L: Polyunsaturated fatty acids and protection of newborn rats from oxygen toxicity. *J Pediatr* 112:630–637, 1988.

269. Sosenko IRS, Innis SM, Frank L: Intralipid increases lung polyunsaturated fatty acids and protects newborn rats from oxygen toxicity. *Pediatr Res* 30:413–417, 1991.

270. Beyer RE: The participation of coenzyme Q in free radical production and antioxidation. *Free Radic Biol Med* 8:545–565, 1990.

271. Konishi T, Nakamura Y, Konishi T, Kawai C: Improvement in recovery of left ventricular function during reperfusion with coenzyme Q10 in isolated working rat heart. *Cardiovasc Res* 19:38–43, 1984.

272. Sugino K, Dohi K, Yamada K, Kawasaki T: The role of lipid peroxidation in endotoxin-induced hepatic damage and the protective role of antioxidants. *Surgery* 101:746–752, 1987.

273. Yasumoto K, Inada Y: Effect of coenzyme Q10 on endotoxin shock in dogs. *Crit Care Med* 14:570–574, 1986.

274. Samuni A, Winkelsberg D, Pinson A, Hahn SM, Mitchell JB, Russo A: Nitroxide stable radicals protect beating cardiomyocytes against oxidative damage. *J Clin Invest* 87:1526–1530, 1991.

275. Hearse DJ, Tosaki A: Free radicals and reperfusion-induced arrhythmias: protection by spin trap agent PBN in the rat heart. *Circ Res* 60:375–380, 1987.

276. Novelli GP, Angiolini P, Tani R, et al: Phenyl-t-butyl nitrone is active against traumatic shock in rats. *Free Radic Res Commun* 1:321–323, 1986.

277. Hamburger SA, McCay PB: Endotoxin-induced mortality in rats is reduced by nitrones. *Circ Shock* 29:329–334, 1989.

278. Braughler JM, Pregenzer JF, Chase RL, Duncan LA, Jacobsen EJ, McCall JM: Novel 21-amino steroids as potent inhibitors of iron dependent lipid peroxidation. *J Biol Chem* 262:10438–10440, 1987.

279. Braughler JM, Burton PS, Chase RL, et al: Novel membrane localized iron chelators as inhibitors of iron-dependent lipid peroxidation. *Biochem Pharmacol* 37:3853–3860, 1988.

280. Braughler JM, Pregenzer JF: The 21-amino-steroid inhibitors of lipid peroxidation: reactions with lipid peroxyl and phenoxy radicals. *Free Radic Biol Med* 7:125–130, 1989.

281. Natale JE, Schott RJ, Hall ED, Braughler JM, D'Alecy LG: Effect of the aminosteroid U74006F after cardiopulmonary arrest in dogs. *Stroke* 19:1371–1378, 1988.

282. Holzgrefe HH, Buchanan LV, Gibson JK: Effects of U74006F, a novel inhibitor of lipid peroxidation, in stunned reperfused canine myocardium. *J Cardiovasc Pharmacol* 15:239–248, 1990.

283. Hall ED, Yonkers PA, McCall JM, Braughler JM: Effects of the 21-amino steroid U74006F on experimental head injury in mice. *J Neurosurg* 68:456–461, 1988.

284. Anderson DK, Braughler JM, Hall ED, Waters TR, McCall JM, Means ED: Effects of treatment with U-74006F on neurological outcome following experimental spinal cord injury. *J Neurosurg* 69:562–567, 1988.

285. Zuccarello M, Marsch JT, Schmitt G, Woodward J, Anderson DK: Effect of the 21-aminosteroid U-74006F on cerebral vasospasm following subarachnoid hemorrhage. *J Neurosurg* 71:98–104, 1989.

286. Lefer AM, Johnson G: Protective effects of a novel 21-amino steroid during splanchnic artery occlusion shock. *Circ Shock* 30:155–164, 1990.

287. Fleckenstein AE, Smith SL, Linseman KL, Beuving LJ, Hall ED: Comparison of the efficacy of mechanistically different antioxidants in the rat hemorrhagic shock model. *Circ Shock* 35:223–230, 1991.

288. Hernandez LA, Granger DN: Role of antioxidants in organ preservation and transplantation. *Crit Care Med* 16:543–549, 1988.

289. Cohen MV: Free radicals in ischemic and reperfusion myocardial injury: is this the time for clinical trials? *Ann Intern Med* 111:918–931, 1989.

290. Menasche P, Piwnica A: Free radicals and myocardial protection: a surgical viewpoint. *Ann Thorac Surg* 47:939–945, 1989.

Radiation Injury

SHIRLEY A. FRY, M.B., B.Cн., M.P.H.
FUN H. FONG, Jr., M.D., F.A.C.E.P.

INTRODUCTION

Historically, accidental civilian overexposures to ionizing radiation (hereafter referred to as radiation) resulting in serious medical consequences have been rare. With a few notable exceptions (1–5) most of these events have involved small numbers of people and have not impacted on the health of the general public. Only a small percentage of persons exposed in these accidents have incurred acute radiation-induced injuries that were life-threatening or fatal (6, 7). The occurrence of these events and the threat of similar events in the future, however, continue to arouse public interest and concern. Although recent political changes within and between nations appear to have reduced the risk of global nuclear conflict, there is concern that the risks of serious radiation exposures have increased, occurring on a more limited scale due to the inadvertent or intentional misuse of atomic devices or nuclear materials. At the same time, industrial and medical applications of radiation and radioactive materials continue to proliferate, along with activities involving the handling and disposition of radioactive wastes from past and current nuclear industry and medical operations. During the past decade, fatal radiation accidents in industrial settings in El Salvador (8), Israel (9), and Belarus (Baranov AE, Selidovkin GD, Kontchalovckij MV, et al, 1992 personal communication), and others involving radiation therapy units in Brazil (5), the U.S. (10), and Spain (11) have further heightened public concern. Generally and in specific instances, public officials and private citizens, as well as patients, tend to seek guidance and reassurance

about radiation and its potential health effects from physicians because they are perceived as reliable and trustworthy sources of information. Thus, there is a continuing need for physicians to be knowledgeable about radiation-induced health effects, both acute and long-term, so that they can respond accurately to questions. They also need to be capable of participating in the assessment and management of individuals suspected of being overexposed to radiation or contaminated with radioactive materials. The biologic, histopathologic, and acute and long-term health effects of radiation are described in detail elsewhere (12–14), and the body of current knowledge on these topics has been extensively reviewed by several national and international scientific organizations (15-17). In this chapter we present an overview of the nature of radiation-induced injuries, the principles for their medical management, and the pathophysiologic basis for pharmacologic therapy, together with a review of recent advances in critical-care modalities for seriously irradiated patients.

OVERVIEW

IONIZING RADIATION

Ionizing radiation is a naturally occurring form of energy that exists in electromagnetic or particulate forms. All living organisms are continually exposed to low levels (low doses delivered at low-dose rates) of radiation from sources normally present in the environment; this exposure usually is referred to as natural background radiation. Approximately 82% of the dose to the population is from naturally occurring sources—primarily, radon (55%), which is a product of the radiologic decay of radioactive forms of uranium normally present in the earth's crust. Other natural sources of radiation are cosmic radiation and radioisotopes, such as potassium-40, which are normal constituents in tissue. Man-made radiation sources and radioactive materials used in medical diagnosis and therapy contribute almost all of the remaining 18% of the background dose, with less than 1% coming from all other environmental sources, including occupational, nuclear industry, and atomic testing activities (17). An individual receives an average annual dose to the whole-body of about 3.6 millisieverts (mSv) of radiation from all natural and man-made sources combined [mSv = International System (SI) unit of radiation dose equivalent. 1 mSv = 100 millirem (conventional units)]. This dose is roughly equal to that received from a total of 36 chest roentgenographies and is several orders of magnitude less than the threshold dose required to cause acute clinical symptoms of radiation exposure. Accidental radiation exposures having serious medical consequences typically have been associated with uncontrolled exposures to man-made radiation sources or radioactive materials used in industry, scientific research and development, and medical procedures (6, 7).

THE BIOLOGIC BASIS OF RADIATION INJURIES

The clinical effects of exposure to radiation are expressions of underlying biologic damage induced by radiation at cellular and molecular levels. The resulting clinical manifestations of this biologic damage may be categorized as deterministic or stochastic in nature. With few exceptions they are nonspecific and indistinguishable by existing clinical or biologic technologies from clinically similar lesions caused by other agents.

Deterministic effects, also known as threshold effects, are due to biologic damage that results in immediate or early cell death or sterilization and, thereby, to cell depletion. DNA in cell nuclei is considered to be the primary site of radiation-induced chemical reactions that can result in clinical effects, but these reactions also may involve molecules in the membrane and other cellular structures. There are threshold ranges for the doses of radiation that are required to cause lethal damage to cells sufficient to produce clinical evidence of cell depletion. If the affected cell system is essential for survival, (e.g., the hematopoietic system), then doses significantly greater than the threshold level for the system can result in a critically ill patient. The severity and the incidence of deterministic effects are related directly to the radiation dose received. Effects of this type may be clinically evident, as acute signs and symptoms during the early (1 - < 60 days) postexposure period in individuals exposed to radiation above threshold dose levels; they include acute radiation syndrome (ARS), acute local lesions (including radiation burns), and decreased fertility. Expression of other effects of acute radiation injury may be delayed for periods ranging from about 60 days to years after exposure, depending on the cell system affected and the degree of damage. These effects include fibroatrophy, cataracts, temporary infertility or sterility, and hypothyroidism. Deterministic effects in the irradiated embryo or fetus are described below.

Stochastic or nonthreshold radiation-induced effects are associated with incomplete or misrepair of sublethal radiation-induced biologic damage that can result in gene mutations. Such mutations can increase an exposed population's risk of heritable genetic effects when the affected genes are in the reproductive cells or of neoplastic effects in the case of somatic cell genes. In the absence of definitive epidemiological data for stochastic effects in the low dose range (<20 cGy), it is assumed for radiation protection purposes that there is no dose below which no biologic damage occurs [cGy = International System (SI) unit of radiation absorbed dose. 1 cGy = 1 rad (conventional unit)]. This type of injury may be clinically expressed at random among a population exposed to radiation (somatic effects) or their progeny (herited genetic effects) with the probability of clinical expression increasing above that of the nonexposed population with increasing dose above zero. However, unlike the deterministic effects, the severity of stochastic effects is independent of dose. As it takes years, even decades, for stochastic effects to present clinically, they do not account for critical illnesses in the early postexposure period. Experimental and epidemiologic studies have contributed to the extensive body of knowledge on radiogenic stochastic effects. These studies have identified the increased risk of malignant disease among populations exposed to radiation as the most notable of these effects. The reader is referred to the literature for specific details (15–17) as stochastic effects are considered further in this chapter only with respect to the use of medications in the early postexposure period aimed at minimizing the uptake and incorporation of radioactive contaminants.

Exposure of the pregnant female to radiation can induce nonspecific deterministic effects in the embryo or fetus that are related to dose, dose rate, and the period of gestation. Experimental and epidemiological studies support a threshold of 50 mSv received anytime during pregnancy, below which there is no measurable increased risk to the exposed vs. the nonexposed embryo or fetus. It is assumed, although the epidemiological data remain equivocal, that in utero exposure to radiation increases the risk of cancer in childhood.

FACTORS INFLUENCING THE CLINICAL EXPRESSION OF RADIATION INJURY

Clinical expression of radiation-induced biologic damage is influenced by several physical and biologic factors. In the context of the seriously irradiated patient, factors influencing the expression of the deterministic effects of radiation are of major interest. These factors include radiation type, radiation dose and dose rate, the radiosensitivity of the irradiated tissues, the area of the body irradiated, and variations in individuals' biologic response to radiation.

The type of radiation determines its penetrating power, a key factor in considering the medical consequences of exposure. For present purposes, distinction is made between penetrating radiations (i.e., X- and γ-rays, and neutrons), and those radiations having less penetrating power (i.e., α- and β-particles). X- and γ-rays are sparsely ionizing electromagnetic waves emitted, respectively, when a metal target is bombarded by electrons in a vacuum from the nuclear fission process or during radioactive decay of fission products. Neutrons are uncharged particles that typically are released in the fission process but that also can be produced in cyclotrons and linear accelerators. They also occur naturally in cosmic radiation. Being uncharged, neutrons do not interact directly with biologic targets. In traveling through tissue they are absorbed by interaction with the nuclei of atoms in the tissue, thereby releasing high-energy particles that cause ionization of molecular materials. α-Particles are densely ionizing; they have a penetrating power of only a few micrometers, equivalent to one or two layers of cells, and thus they are not a health hazard when external to the body. β-particles are sparsely ionizing; they may penetrate up to a few centimeters of tissue, depending on their energy. When near or in contact with skin, β-radiation can induce acute radiation burns locally but has a limited whole-body effect. Internally deposited β-particles can induce local and whole-body effects, depending on their energy and distribution.

The type, incidence, and severity of radiation-induced deterministic effects are directly related to the magnitude of the radiation dose and the rate at which it is delivered. A single dose of radiation delivered in a short period of time (i.e., acutely) will have greater biologic and clinical effects than the same dose delivered in increments at intervals over an extended period of time (i.e., fractionation, protraction). In the latter situation, the interval between exposures allows biologic repair of radiation-induced damage to occur so that the total damage will be less than if the dose had been delivered acutely, and the clinical effects will be correspondingly less severe.

The sensitivity of cell systems to radiation is directly related to their mitotic index and inversely to their level of differentiation. Thus in general, the stem cells of rapidly proliferating cell systems are highly radiosensitive (e.g., the stem cells of the hematopoietic systems and spermatocytes). Conversely, muscle and nervous tissue cells are highly radioresistant. Cells having intermediate mitotic rates and differentiation, such as those of the gastric mucosa, fall between these extremes. An important exception to this generalization is the small lymphocyte which, despite its low mitotic index and high degree of differentiation, is highly radiosensitive and is an early indicator of whole-body irradiation at acute doses higher than 200 to 250 cGy. Casarett developed a five-class system that categorizes cell systems according to their relative radiosensitivity (13).

As stem cells are highly radiosensitive, the extent to which they lie in the radiation field influences the magnitude of the whole-body effect of the exposure. Uniform exposure to penetrating radiation of the whole body, or a significant portion of it with respect to sensitive cell systems, can result in a whole-body response that is directly related to dose. If, however, the exposure is nonuniform or limited to a small area of the body, thereby exposing only a limited variety and number of stem cells, the whole body response will be less than if the same dose had been delivered to the whole-body. The ability of internally deposited sources of α- or β-radiation to induce serious whole-body effects (e.g., clinically significant bone marrow depression) is dependent on their distribution within the body and their penetrating power.

Variations in the clinical response of healthy individuals to similar doses of radiation are largely unexplained. Such

Table 55.1. Clinical Effects of External Whole-Body Irradiation at Various Dose Levels

Dose (cGy)[a]	Effect
10	Detectable increase in chromosome aberrations; no clinical effects/symptoms
≥12	Sperm count declines to minimum about day 45
20–50	Detectable bone marrow depression; mild lymphocytopenia
50–100	Fatigue, anorexia
>~120	Mild radiation sickness: anorexia, nausea, 50% within 48 hr
240	Vomiting in 50% within 48 hours, moderate lymphocytopenia
~325	Bone marrow depression; pancytopenia at 28–30 days, likelihood of death of 50% untreated exposed persons in 60 days
≥500	Radiation pneumonitis
≥600	$LD_{50/60}$ with treatment, possibly higher with improved therapies
~2000	Up to 100% death in 30–60 days
~2000–4000	Severe bone marrow depression; death in 9–11 days from electrolyte imbalance, malabsorption septicemia
>~4000	Generalized vascular damage → CNS edema, shock; death in ≤ 48 hours

[a] cGy = centigray, the international system (SI) unit of absorbed radiation dose. 1 cGy (SI unit) = 1 rad (conventional unit).

variations are taken into account by expressing threshold doses in terms of the dose that elicits a certain clinical response among 50% of those patients who receive that dose within a specified period (e.g., $ED_{50/48}$ represents the dose that is effective in causing vomiting among 50% of persons receiving that dose within 48 hours). Similarly, the $LD_{50/60}$ represents the radiation dose that would result in the deaths of 50% of those receiving it within 60 days. These values may be modified by age or the presence of preexisting disease.

CLINICAL FEATURES OF RADIATION INJURY

Depending on the disposition of the previously described factors known to influence the clinical expression of radiation injury, exposure to radiation above the threshold dose levels may elicit a whole-body or a local response that can be life-threatening or even fatal. The various types of radiation injury can occur alone, in combination with each other, or with physical trauma or other medical conditions or complications of the injury. The clinical effect of such combined injuries has been shown to be synergistic, so that the response to a given whole- or partial-body dose of radiation is apparently greater in the presence, rather than in the absence, of other radiogenic or nonradiogenic injuries or complications, such as infection.

Whole-Body Irradiation

Whole- or significant partial-body irradiation causes irreversible biologic damage that, if in excess of clinical thresholds, is expressed in a set of dose-related signs and symptoms (Table 55.1) that comprise the ARS or, more commonly, "acute radiation sickness." The ARS is characterized by an acute illness that follows a four-phase clinical course. The duration

Table 55.2. ARS: Clinical Course[a]

1. Prodromal stage: 0–48 hr
2. Latent period: hr—2/3 wk
3. Manifest illness: hr-days-wk
4. Recovery: wk-mos
Death: hr, days, wk

[a] ARS = acute radiation sundrome.

Table 55.3. Acute Whole-Body Irradiation: Predominant Clinical Response/Acute Dose

Prodromal signs and symptoms: >90 cGy
Hematopoietic syndrome: 150–1000 cGy
Respiratory syndrome: >500 cGy
Gastrointestinal syndrome: >1000–4000 cGy
Cerebrovascular (CNS) syndrome: >4000 cGy

of each phase is inversely related to radiation dose (Table 55.2). The prodromal phase is characterized by symptoms that are induced by the products of acute cell death and by direct parasympathetically mediated neurogenic effects on the gastrointestinal and central nervous systems. These symptoms include fatigue, anorexia, nausea, and apathy. At higher doses, vomiting, diarrhea, hyperexcitability, ataxia, erythema, perspiration, and fever can occur. Conjunctivitis is induced by doses to the eyes of about 200 cGy. During this phase the earliest detectable clinical signs are of bone marrow depression, beginning at doses greater than 20 to 25 cGy, with the absolute lymphocyte and granulocyte counts the parameters of interest. The development of signs and symptoms during the prodromal phase serves as a basis for radiologic triage and assessment of medically stable patients for therapeutic and prognostic purposes. Persons involved in radiation accidents should be observed and hematologically monitored for the development of such prodromata. Those who develop prodromal symptoms and have an absolute lymphocyte count of <1,000/mm^3 within 24 hours of exposure will require treatment. Medical management during the prodromal phase comprises primarily supportive care and clinical evaluations in preparation for subsequent therapy. The latent period is characterized by the disappearance or decreased severity of the prodromal symptoms and an apparent improvement in the patient's well-being. At lower doses, the patient can proceed to recovery. At higher doses, cell systems become increasingly depleted during the latent period, until they fall below levels of clinical competence. Continued observation and clinical laboratory monitoring of the patients is recommended for patients who exhibit prodromal signs and symptoms, until the direction of the injury (recovery or progression) has been determined. Supportive care and the implementation of hematopoietic stem cell replacement and stimulating therapies to be discussed later are the focus of treatment during the latent phase. The appearance of signs and symptoms of systems' incompetence mark the onset of the manifest (critical) illness. These dose-related syndromes are (a) the hematopoietic, with signs and symptoms of increasing leukopenia reaching a nadir 28 to 30 days after an acute sublethal dose; (b) gastrointestinal (GI), with radiogenic GI injury resulting in vomiting, bloody diarrhea, fluid and electrolyte shifts, malabsorption; and (c) cerebro- or cardiovascular syndrome (formerly known as the central nervous system syndrome) with early and increasingly severe signs and symptoms of increasing intracranial pressure due to cerebral edema associated with a generalized vasculitis. Supportive care and sustaining therapies play a vital role during the manifest illness period. In the absence of treatment, death can occur 48 hours to 60 days after acute exposure to doses in the lethal range (LD$_{50/60}$ 325 cGy to bone marrow). The exposure to death interval decreases with increasing dose.

Recent experience suggests that with modern therapeutic regimens the LD$_{50/60}$ can be increased up to 600 to 800 cGy (8). Table 55.3 shows the relationship between the clinical response and radiation dose in terms of the syndromes comprising the ARS. The clinical characteristics of the hematopoietic, gastrointestinal, and cerebrovascular syndromes and their management have been described and discussed in detail in several recent publications (18–20). Prior to the mid 1980s, patients irradiated in excess of about 800 cGy (whole-body) did not survive long enough to enable full expression of radiation pneumonitis, the respiratory component of ARS that is induced by whole-body doses greater than about 500 cGy. Recent advances in supportive and stem cell-stimulating therapies have prolonged survival sufficient for the clinical effects of the respiratory system injury to be expressed and to be identified as a critical component of the ARS (20). Despite recent therapeutic advances, eventual recovery of patients with whole-body doses in excess of 800 to 1000 cGy remains improbable because of the currently irreversible clinical problems associated with the respiratory, gastrointestinal, and cerebrovascular syndromes that become superimposed on those of the hematopoietic syndrome at higher doses.

Exposure of the pregnant female to radiation can give rise to radiogenic effects in the embryo or fetus that are related to dose, dose rate, and the period of gestation. Radiation doses high enough to induce ARS in the pregnant female will have a similar and possibly greater acute effect per unit dose on the fetus and can result in acute fetal death, although the mother may survive. In these situations, critical care is necessarily directed to the mother. The effect of exposure to lower doses during the embryonic or preimplantation period is described as "all or nothing," indicating that if the embryo survives—and is in the absence of other risk factors—it will continue to grow and develop normally. Threshold effects of fetal exposure include nonspecific congenital malformations, growth retardation (including microcephaly), and mental impairment or retardation (21).

Acute Local Radiation Injury

Except for doses in the range of several hundreds of grays, acute local irradiation alone is unlikely to cause a significant whole-body effect or critical illness in the immediate postexposure period. However, a patient with local radiation injuries can become critically ill several weeks or months postexposure if healing is compromised, and complications such as infection occur. Radiation accident experience has shown the frequency of local radiation injury to be greater than that for acute whole-body injury (22). It can result from external exposure to a source of penetrating radiation, close proximity to or contact with a β-radiation source, or contamination with β-emitting radionuclides.

The clinical manifestations of local radiation-induced damage at increasing doses are summarized in Table 55.4. The earliest observable effect of local exposure above threshold levels is a transient erythema that appears 2 to 3 hours later. This effect is believed to be due to an inflammatory response to the products of cell necrosis. Except for this reaction, the effects of doses of less than several hundreds of grays do not become apparent for several days or longer, depending on the dose. This characteristic of local radiogenic lesions distinguishes them from those caused by heat or corrosive chemicals and can account for the absence of a history of radiation exposure. One or more waves of erythema will follow approximately 5 or more days after moderate local doses (2000 cGy). These waves initially reflect capillary incompetence that is associated with radiation damage to the endothelial cells. With increasing dose, subsequent waves of erythema and increasing edema reflect expression of radiation damage affecting larger and deeper vessels. The deeper damage can affect other structures in the dermis and subcutaneous tissue, such as sweat glands, hair follicles, and nerve endings, as well as the vasculature. Resulting progressive endarteritis obliterans leads to ischemic pain and irreversible tissue necrosis. Management of this type of radiation injury is initially symptomatic and conservative. Frequent observations, including serial color photographs and protection of the exposed area from additional trauma, are recommended. Doses of 5000 cGy and higher can progressively effect deeper structures such as muscle and bone and require surgical intervention ranging from excision of necrotic tissue to amputation at some time in the future as the injury evolves. Extensive skin burns induced by heavy and continued contamination with β-emitters were a prominent feature among the on-site victims of the Chernobyl reactor accident and contributed significantly to the deaths of several these individuals (4).

Contamination

Contamination with radioactive materials alone is unlikely to cause symptoms of ARS, although clinical signs of bone marrow depression and oligospermia are possible, depending on the amount and radiologic characteristics of the contaminant and its disposition on or in the body. Management of any ARS-related effects resulting from contamination is the same as that for patients with ARS due to whole- or partial-body irradiation. Although there is minimal risk of critical illness related to radiation in the contaminated patient, there is a need for prompt action to minimize the risk of local radiogenic lesions on areas of skin contaminated with β- or γ-emitters and to minimize or reduce internal deposition of

radionuclides, thereby minimizing the risk of stochastic effects in the future. Internally contaminated patients or those at risk of internal contamination should be managed by principles of prompt blocking, displacement, dilution, or chelation, depending on the radionuclides involved. Details of these management approaches are beyond the scope of this chapter but are available with respect to specific radionuclides in Publication No. 65 of the National Council for Radiation Protection and Measurements (NCRP) (23).

CRITICAL CARE IMPLICATIONS

GENERAL CONSIDERATIONS

In all cases, management of patients for whom critical care is indicated because of exposure to radiation or radioactive materials presupposes their medical stability. Treatment of life-threatening trauma or medical conditions takes precedence over treatment of conditions associated with radiologic exposures. Irradiated patients who are medically stable may require specialized care because of (*a*) acute whole- or partial-body irradiation alone; (*b*) complications of acute radiation-induced injury; (*c*) any combination of radiation injuries alone or with nonradiologic injuries. Pharmaceuticals are used in these situations to (*a*) minimize acute symptoms; (*b*) support and supplement the patient's own vital systems during the period of manifest (critical) illness; and (*c*) stimulate reconstitution of the patient's stem cell pool. Management of the patient who is contaminated with radioactive materials presents a special case in that early pharmaceutical intervention must be considered, even in the absence of acute clinical effects, so as to prevent or minimize the potential for incorporation and retention of internalized contaminants, thereby minimizing the risk of inducing radiogenic stochastic effects that may be expressed years later.

In the past decade, advances in therapeutic modalities for the nonspecific syndromes of interest provide opportunities for physicians to be more proactive than previously in the treatment of patients with serious radiation-induced injuries. Many of the newer pharmaceuticals and protocols are used in the treatment of syndromes (e.g., immunosuppression) that are common to several clinical conditions, and there are no specific indications from the FDA for use in the management of radiation-induced injury. However, this has not prevented their innovative use by physicians in such cases. Actions to be considered in the medical management of patients with or at risk of acute radiation-induced illness include the following:

Supportive Care

Supportive care has been—and continues to be—a major component of the medical response to significant overexposures to radiation. Although the need for supportive care in the management of seriously irradiated patients has not changed, the development of improved and more specific therapeutic modalities in recent years has increased its effectiveness in some areas. Supportive care may be symptomatic, as well as based on the estimated dose received, and directed toward effects anticipated on specific organ systems.

Table 55.4. Acute Local Irradiation: Dose Response Relationships

>300 cGy	Epilation beginning around day 17
~600 cGy	Erythema, distinguish from thermal burn, min–wk postexposure, depending on dose.
>600 cGy	Edema
1000–2000 cGy	Blistering, 2–3 wk postexposure, depending upon dose
~3000 cGy	Ulceration, 1–2 mos postexposure, depending on dose
5000–6000 cGy	Gangrene, necrosis, deep ulceration

Prodromal symptoms of ARS (e.g., nausea, emesis, pyrexia, and attendant anxiety) are generally responsive to pharmaceuticals in general use for treatment of similar symptoms associated with nonradiogenic conditions and may be prescribed according to current protocols.

Thrombocytopenic hemorrhages and anemia associated with radiation-induced hematopoietic depression may require transfusions of platelets and red cells. If indicated, blood product replacement should be irradiated by exposure to 10 to 20 Gy before administration to minimize the risk of graft-vs.-host reaction in the radiogenically immunosuppressed patient. Empiric antibiotic therapy and fluid electrolyte resuscitation may be prescribed as needed to support the patient with evidence of immunosuppression and fluid electrolyte imbalance during the manifest illness period. The choice of antibiotics should be based on the assumption that Gram-negative bacilli are most likely to present the initial risk of infection. Toxicity and the development of resistant strains of bacteria associated with long-term antibiotic use are unlikely to be a major problem in the sublethally irradiated patient because the period of immunosuppression lasts for only 3 to 4 weeks before the patient's hematopoietic system recovers and immune competency is restored. These problems are moot if the patient does not recover (24). Reverse isolation will minimize the potential for nosocomial infection as in any immunocompromised patient. Appropriate use of these approaches has been shown to extend the human $LD_{50/60}$ from approximately 3 to 6 Gy (25, 26). Other approaches to basic supportive care are related to prevention of infection with endogenous organisms in an immunocompromised patient. Techniques that appear promising are (*a*) early enteral feeding to prevent or reduce the loss of jejunal mucosal thickness (27, 28) and (*b*) use of pirenzepine (29, 30) and sucralfate (29, 31–33), instead of H_2 blockers, to prevent stress bleeding and to reduce the incidence of aspiration pneumonia.

Pain and delayed healing experienced by patients with acute radiation burns are related to radiation-related ischemia in the exposed area. Recognition of this relationship is the basis for effective management of these injuries. In the past, narcotics have been the drugs of necessity rather than choice, but more specific pharmaceuticals, such as hemorrheologic agents, show promise for the more effective management of radiogenic pain. One such agent is pentoxifylline (Trental). It acts by decreasing red blood cell deformability, thereby reducing blood viscosity, and by stimulating release of prostacylin, a vasodilator and thrombolytic stimulant. A pilot study by Dion et al showed significantly reduced healing time in pentoxifylline-treated vs. nontreated patients with late radiation soft tissue necrosis; all of the treated patients also experienced pain relief (34). Pentoxifylline also was effective in relieving ischemic pain that developed in the fingers bilaterally following their accidental exposure to radiation emitted by a linear accelerator (Redfern, 1992, personal communication).

Dose Estimation

In the past, dose estimation in the immediate postexposure period had a low clinical priority, because treatment options during this period were limited, primarily to the management of symptoms. However, modalities for treating radiation injury that requires early clinical decisions based on the dose to the patient have increased considerably in recent years. While early treatment includes emphasis on symptomatic treatment, recent radiation accident experiences indicate that therapy using biologic response modifiers is most effective if it begins early in the postexposure period (7). This need for early dose estimation also may reflect the fact that a 1989 consensus summary conference on acute radiation injury held in Washington, D.C., accepted a treatment algorithm based on radiologic triage into four dose categories (35). In addition to physical approaches to dose estimation during the early postexposure period, collection of blood samples for dose estimation by cytogenetic analysis may be considered. This analysis takes several days to conduct but maximizes the precision of the estimate of the dose received (36).

Selective Gut Decontamination

The concept of selective gut decontamination (SGD), which has been present in some form for the past 20 or more years, is to selectively limit numbers of certain pathogenic flora while minimally affecting other benign flora in the gut. A number of antibiotics, both systemic and nonsystemic, have been used to achieve this goal. There may be an advantage to the use of nonsystemic antibiotics in that they may be less likely to result in development of antibiotic-resistant bacterial strains. Fluoroquinolones, such as ciprofloxacin, ofloxacin, and norfloxacin, provide relatively new alternatives for prophylaxis because as a general rule they are active against *Enterobacteriaceae*, *Pseudomonas*, and *Staphylococcus* but are not as effective against anaerobes (37). Norfloxacin, in particular, has the additional advantage of nonsystemic absorption. Quinolone resistance can develop, however (38).

A study of neutropenic patients showed that prophylactic norfloxacin was more effective than cotrimoxazole in reducing the incidence of Gram-negative infection but less effective in reducing the incidence of Gram-positive infection (39). In an experimental study comparing the effectiveness of oral ofloxacin in SGD with that of gentamicin prophylaxis in mice irradiated with 7.5 Gy, mortality was found to be 0% in the ofloxacin-treated group while wide variations in mortality were found after 30 days among the gentamicin-treated group, irrespective of the protocol used (37). Most reported studies of SGD have been performed on patient populations who are immunocompromised for a variety of reasons, making results difficult to extrapolate to previously healthy victims of accidental irradiation (40). Many of these studies also are performed in intensive care or burn units, which are well-known environments for the development of antibiotic-resistant strains. Consequently, the development of antibiotic resistance is a concern in the use of selective gut decontamination (41). The irradiated patient, who is immunocompromised and also has thermal burns or desquamation of the gastrointestinal epithelium, may pose a special circumstance in which SGD may be used to advantage. Experience is limited, and there is still considerable debate as to whether SGD should be used routinely in immunocompromised radiation accident patients (Brook I, 1991, personal communication). SGD with ciprofloxacin was used briefly in the treatment of the victim of the 1990 Sor-Van accident in Israel, who received a whole-body dose estimated to be between 12 and 15 Gy. Its role in prolonging the victim's survival to 36 days, from the 28 days anticipated based on what previous experience would have predicted, is unclear owing to its use in combination with other new modalities (9).

Hematopoietic Stem Cell Replacement

Bone marrow transplants (BMT) have been utilized for bone marrow reconstitution for radiation accident patients since the early 1950s. The procedure is an attempt to reconstitute the bone marrow by introduction of a healthy and compatible sample of bone marrow stem cells and cell precursors. The potential for complications is similar to that in any tissue transplantation procedure, with the additional risk of causing graft vs. host disease (GVHD). Genetically identical cells, such as the patient's own marrow or the marrow of an identical twin, are ideal and would have no possibility of tissue rejection.

A total of 13 allogeneic BMT and six fetal liver transplantations was performed in acutely injured victims of the Chernobyl disaster. In the absence of well-matched donors, deliberately mismatched bone-marrow transplants were administered to provide temporary coverage, with the intention of causing a "bridge effect" during the usual period of granulocytopenia. The concept of this approach was that, as the patient's own stem cells recovered, the transplant would be rejected, and it was hypothesized that during this time the donor's cells would provide some measure of immunocompetence until reconstitution of the patient's bone marrow. The use of deliberately mismatched BMT and fetal liver transplants is controversial, and there is no consensus among experts in the U.S. as to their role in the management of radiation accident victims. Only two of the seriously irradiated Chernobyl patients survived after BMT (42). This experience has resulted in discussions of the role of BMT in heavily irradiated accident victims. Unlike leukemia patients irradiated prior to transplantation, accidental doses can only be estimated. Underestimation of the accidental dose can lead to underestimation of the proportion of viable bone marrow remaining in the patient, thereby increasing the risk of reaction to the transplant. Fetal liver transplants have been used with success in China following therapeutic or accidental whole-body irradiation (43).

With the advent of improved immunosuppressive agents such as cyclosporin A, less than perfect matches are more successful. A 3-loci haploidentical bone marrow transplant was performed on the victim of the 1990 Israel accident on day 4 postexposure, with survival to day 36—then the longest known survival for the magnitude of dose received (9).

There appears to be a correlation between human leukocyte antigen disparity in BMT (suboptimally matched BMT) and poor post-BMT reconstitution and the development of interstitial pneumonitis (44). The possibility of this significant complication must be weighed against benefits that BMT might offer.

The use of umbilical cord blood as a source of stem cells is a therapy currently under investigation. The majority of transplants in which this modality has been used to date have used umbilical cord blood from HLA-identical siblings. Engraftment of cord blood stem cells remains untested in other children and adults (45). In a study of in vitro growth potential of human umbilical cord blood cells Hows et al (1992) found that hematopoietic progenitor cells obtained were more numerous and of better quality than those in normal bone marrow, raising hopes that umbilical cord blood may be an important source of hematopoietic stem cells for patients of all ages (46). Alternate sources of stem cell progenitors for transplant include peripheral blood, fetal liver, and cadavers (47).

Biologic Response Modifiers

Immunomodulators that cause nonspecific stimulation of the immune system are thought to have a potential role in therapy for irradiated individuals. L-Glucan, trehalose dimycolate, and acemannan (Carrington Laboratories, 1992) are examples of immune stimulators that may have therapeutic potential, but to date there are no definite clinical recommendations.

Cytokine therapy was first used in the treatment of accidentally irradiated persons in the Chernobyl disaster. Cytokines are hormone-like peptides that form the basis of communication between many different cell types. They also exert a definite influence on modulating inflammatory and repair responses. Cytokines are subclassified into interleukins and colony-stimulating factors. Selected colony-stimulating factors and interleukins are used in cases of bone marrow depression to more specifically induce stem cells or specific bone marrow cell line precursors to proliferate but not necessarily to cause general stimulation of the immune system. Their use in treating seriously irradiated victims of recent accidents has contributed to the victims' prolonged survival.

The success of cytokine therapy depends in large part on the presence of remaining cell precursors that are capable of response. It has been conservatively estimated that the bone marrow of humans in whom as few as 0.1% of the original stem-cell population survives might be reconstituted utilizing cytokine combinations without the need to resort to bone marrow transplantation (MacVittie TJ, 1992, personal communication).

One of the cytokine combinations in current usage is recombinant human granulocyte-macrophage colony-stimulating factor (GM-CSF) and interleukin-3 (IL-3). Its use in the 1990 Israel accident (in combination with BMT) and in the 1991 Belarus accident prolonged the survival of the two victims by several weeks beyond that anticipated based on experience of the management of radiation accident victims before this therapy was available (9, Baranov AE, Selidovkin GD, Kontchalovckij MR, 1992, personal communication). Both of these patients received the cytokine combination early during the postexposure period, a factor that experimental studies suggest is also important in the effectiveness of these agents.

Complications of Acute High-Dose Radiation Exposure

Interstitial pneumonitis (IP) and the more subacute process of pulmonary fibrosis are serious sequelae of acute high-dose (> 5 Gy) whole- or partial-body irradiation for which there is no truly effective treatment at this time. High doses of steroids have been used to treat IP but with only limited success. There appears to be an increased incidence of IP in certain subgroups of patients, such as cases of suboptimally matched bone marrow transplants (48, 49). Cytomegalovirus

(CMV) is often activated in seriously irradiated, immunosuppressed patients and is the organism most commonly associated with IP (50). IP appears to have an earlier onset after BMT in patients infected with CMV (90 days) than in non-CMV leukemic patients (186 days) (51). There is evidence that seropositive CMV patients are at high risk for developing IP (48). Incidence of IP is also associated with increased dose-rate (52). It has been hypothesized that certain doses of cytokine or cytokine combinations may be associated with an increased incidence of IP, although this has not been proven clinically.

Gancyclovir has now been approved by the FDA for use in cases of CMV retinitis (usually seen in AIDS patients) and eventually may have specific indications for systemic illness. A second drug, Foscarnet, also exerts action against CMV and may have application in cases of acute radiation syndrome, although it has never been used in this context, and significant toxicity has been reported.

Venoocclusive disease (VOD) of the liver may occur after high-dose irradiation. It has been a long-recognized complication of total body irradiation (53, 54) for which there is no definitive therapy at this time.

Herpes simplex virus (HSV) reactivation occurs as often as 70 to 80% of the time in cases of high-dose exposure. In the Chernobyl disaster, more than 30% of third and fourth degree combined-injury patients (modified U.S.S.R. classification) were affected by HSV, but treatment was generally successful (55). Oral acyclovir is recommended prophylactically against the herpes simplex reactivation associated with exposure to high doses of radiation.

Fungal infections are frequent complications in immunosuppressed patients. Early implementation of antifungal prophylaxis is indicated in immunosuppressed victims of accidental irradiation to prevent fungal growth and the systemic spread of any subclinical infection. Although their effectiveness in immunosuppressed patients has been proven, the use of amphotericin B and some imidazole derivatives is limited by toxicity and by absorbability in a nonacid medium, respectively (19, 49).

Combined injury is defined as concurrent conventional trauma and radiation injury occurring during a period of time before recovery from any one of the injuries (35). Combined injury is significant in that mortality is synergistically increased over that mortality expected for each type of injury alone. The synergism of combined injuries should be anticipated early, particularly if aggressive therapeutic maneuvers are being considered.

Acute radiation-induced skin lesions may be complicated by delayed or absent healing associated with the impairment of the local blood supply by progressive endarteritis obliterans. Grafts of skin or covering the affected area with natural or synthetic membranes may promote healing and minimize the risk of infection. The development of infection in radiation-induced skin lesions involving >30% of the body can lead to potentially life-threatening systemic toxicity. As was recognized among survivors of the Chernobyl accident, this development is of particular concern if the patient also is immunosuppressed as the result of concurrent significant whole-body irradiation. Early surgical intervention may be considered in order to control local infection in such patients.

Life-saving surgery and other major surgeries should be performed within the first 48 hours (before hematopoietic depression), and elective surgery should be postponed for 45 to 60 days (after hematologic recovery has occurred). Efforts to preserve and maintain barriers to infection, including skin grafting, should be considered and applied early and aggressively in the course of local radiation injury in anticipation of immunocompromise (56).

Risks to Health Care Personnel

Personnel involved in the treatment and care of persons who are or who are expected to become critically ill as the result of exposure to radiation or radioactive materials should follow universal precautions and other standard protocols for self-protection, just as they would in the case of the nonexposed patient. In addition, consideration should be given to the patient's potential to present a radiologic hazard to others or the environment in some form. In the absence of contamination, the externally irradiated patient does not present any such hazard. The risk to individual personnel of exposure to nonpenetrating radiation from contaminated patients can be minimized by wearing protective clothing such as surgical suits to which headcoverings, surgical gloves (double), and shoe covers are taped. A surgical mask will provide substantial protection against airborne contaminants. Additional protection will be provided against both penetrating and nonpenetrating radiation by (a) working as rapidly as possible; (b) remaining as far from the contaminated patient as practicable; (c) rotating personnel as frequently as necessary to minimize individual exposures; and (d) adhering to nuclear medicine department standards for disposal of contaminated wastes. Occupational and emergency radiation protection standards are federally mandated based on the recommendations of the NCRP (57).

CONCLUSIONS

The medical management of patients who have been accidentally exposed to radiation at high levels is directed toward the support and reconstitution of critical systems during the period of manifest illness when the patient is at risk from hematologic and immune suppression and fluid electrolyte imbalance. In the past decade, there have been significant advances in the treatment of these syndromes in association with the management of nonradiogenic conditions. These modalities have been implemented in the treatment of recent radiation accident victims with some success. Complications associated with high-dose radiation exposure are being identified and are becoming better understood. The advances in treatment methods and increased patient survival times have brought with them the challenge of successfully treating complications seen at higher dose ranges, such as interstitial pneumonitis and prolonged loss of integrity of the gastrointestinal lining. The preferred modalities for treatment of hematologically and immunosuppressed patients are rapidly developing and changing. The critical care specialist is advised to consult with specialists in these areas when planning treatment for accidentally irradiated victims.

ACKNOWLEDGMENT

This report is based upon work performed under Contract No. DE-ACO5-76OR00033 between the Department of Energy, Office of Health and Environmental Research and Oak Ridge Associated Universities. The submitted manuscript has been authored by a contractor of the U.S. Government under contract number DE-ACO5-76OR00033. Accordingly, the U.S. Government retains a nonexclusive, royalty-free license to publish or reproduce the published form of this contribution, or allow others to do so, for U.S. Government purposes.

REFERENCES

1. Windscale: The Committee's Report. *Nuclear Engineering* 2:510–512, 1957.
2. Medvedev ZA: *Nuclear Disaster in the Urals*. Vintage Books, New York, 1980.
3. U.S. Nuclear Regulatory Commission Contaminated Mexican Steel Accident: *Importation of Steel into the U.S. That Had Been Inadvertently Contaminated with ^{60}Co as a Result of Scrapping a Teletherapy Unit*. U.S. Nuclear Regulatory Commission, Washington 1985, NUREG 1103.
4. Linneman RE: Soviet medical response to the Chernobyl nuclear accident. *JAMA* 258:5:637–643, 1987.
5. Maletskos CJ, Lipstein JL: The Goiania Radiation Accident. *Health Physics* 60(Special Issue):1–113, 1991.
6. Lushbaugh CC, Fry SA, Hübner KF, Ricks RC: Total body irradiation: a historical review and follow-up. In Hübner KF, Fry SA (eds): *The Medical Basis for Radiation Accident Preparedness. Proceedings of the REAC/TS International Conference*, Oak Ridge, TN. Elsevier/North Holland, New York, 1980, pp 59–79.
7. Ricks RC, Fry SA, Sipe AH, Berger ME, Fong Jr FH, Lushbaugh CC: History of radiation accidents. In Mossman KL, Mills WA (eds): *The Biological Basis for Radiation Protection Practice*. Williams & Wilkins, Baltimore, 1992, pp 218–225.
8. International Atomic Energy Agency: The radiological accident in El Salvador. IAEA, Vienna, 1990.
9. International Atomic Energy Agency: The radiological accident in Soreq. IAEA, Vienna, 1993.
10. Newman HF: The malfunction "54" accelerator accidents 1985, 1986, 1987. In Ricks RC, Fry SA (eds): *The Medical Basis for Radiation Accident Preparedness II. Clinical Experience and Follow-Up Since 1979. Proceedings of an International Conference*. Oak Ridge, TN, 1988. Elsevier Science Publishing, New York, 1990, pp 165–171.
11. Craven-Bartle J: Information regarding the accident in the linear accelerator in Hospital Clinico de Zaragoza. Asociacion Espanola de Radioterapiay Oncologia, Spain, March 1991.
12. Pizzarello DJ, Colombetti LG (eds): *Radiation Biology*. CRC Press, Boca Raton, FL, 1982.
13. Casarett GW: *Radiation Hispathology*. vol. 1 and 2. Boca Raton, FL, CRC Press, 1980.
14. Mettler Jr FA, Moseley RD: *The Medical Effects of Ionizing Radiation*. Grune & Stratton, Orlando, FL, 1985.
15. Committee on the Biological Effects of Ionizing Radiation: Health risks of radon and other internally deposited alpha-emitters. National Academy of Sciences, Washington, 1988.
16. United Nations Committee on Effects of Atomic Radiation: *Sources, Effects and Risks of Ionizing Radiation. Report to the General Assembly and Annexes*. United Nations, New York, 1988.
17. Committee on the Biological Effects of Ionizing Radiation: *Health Effects of Exposure to Low Levels of Ionizing Radiation*. National Academy of Sciences, Washington, 1990.
18. Mettler Jr FA: Effects of whole-body irradiation. In Mettler Jr FA, Kelsey CA, Ricks RC, (eds): *Medical Management of Radiation Accidents*. Williams & Wilkins, Baltimore, 1990, pp 79–88.
19. Browne D, Weiss JF, MacVittie TH, Pillai MV (eds): *Treatment of Radiation Injuries*. Plenum Press, New York, 1990.
20. Wald N: The acute radiation syndromes and their management. In Mossman KL, Mills WA (eds): *The Biological Basis of Radiation Protection Practice*. Williams & Wilkins, Baltimore, 1992.
21. Brent RL: Ionizing radiation. *Contemporary Obstet/Gynecol* 8:20–29, 1987.
22. Fry SA: The United States radiation accident and other registries of the REAC/TS registry system: their functions and current status. In Hübner KF, Fry SA (eds): *The Medical Basis for Radiation Accident Preparedness*. Elsevier/North Holland, New York, 1980, pp 451–468.
23. Management of Persons Accidentally Contaminated with Radionuclides: *National Council on Radiation Protection and Measurements. Report No. 65*. Washington, 1980.
24. Hübner KF: Radiation injury. In Chernow B, Lake CR (eds): *The Pharmacologic Approach to the Critically Ill Patient*. Williams & Wilkins, Baltimore, 1983, pp 707–714.
25. Health Effects Models for Nuclear Power Plant Accidents Consequence Analysis: *Low LET Radiation. Part II. Scientific Bases for Health Effects Models*. US Nuclear Regulatory Commission, Washington. NUREG/CR-4214, Rev. 1, 1989, pp 2–38.
26. Browne D, Weiss JF, MacVittie TH, Pillai MV (eds): *Treatment of Radiation Injuries*. Plenum Press, New York, 1990, p 225.
27. Alexander JW: Influence of feeding route on metabolic response to injury. In *The Gastrointestinal Response to Injury, Starvation, and Enteral Nutrition. 8th Ross Conference on Medical Research*. Ross Laboratories, Columbus, OH, 1988, pp 41–42.
28. Moore EE, Jones TN: Benefits of immediate jejunostomy feeding after major abdominal trauma: a prospective, randomized study. *J Trauma* 25:874–880, 1986.
29. Tryba M: Pulmonary complications during the prevention of stress bleeding with drugs. In Tryba M (ed): *Prevention of Stress Bleeding in Critically Ill Patients: A New Concept*. Thieme, New York, 1988, pp 128–135.
30. Tryba M: Prevention of stress bleeding with ranitidine or pirenzepine and the risk of pneumonia. *J Clin Anesth* 1:12–20, 1988.
31. Driks MR, Craven DE, Celli BR: Nosocomial pneumonia in intubated patients randomized to sucralfate versus antacids and/or histamine type 2 blockers: the role of gastric colonization. *N Engl J Med* 17:1376–1382, 1987.
32. Tryba M, Rether J: Sucralfate versus antacids for the prevention of acute stress bleeding in risk patients receiving respiratory assistance. In Tryba M (ed): *Prevention of Stress Bleeding in Critically Ill Patients: a New Concept*. Thieme, New York, 1988.
33. Tryba M: The risk of acute stress bleeding and nosocomial pneumonia in ventilated ICU-patients: Sucralfate versus antacids. *Am J Med* 83(3B):117–124, 1987.
34. Dion MW, Hussey DH, Doornbos JF, Bigliotti AP, Wen BC, Anderson B: Preliminary results of a pilot study of pentoxifylline in the treatment of late radiation soft tissue necrosis. *Int J Radiation Oncol Biol Phys* 19:401–407, 1990.
35. Browne D, Weiss JF, MacVittie TH, Pillai MV (eds): *Treatment of Radiation Injuries*. Plenum Press, New York, 1990, p 221.
36. Littlefield LG, Joiner EE, Hübner KF: Cytogenetic techniques in biological dosimetry: overview and example of dose estimates in ten persons exposed to gamma radiation in the 1984 Mexican ^{60}Co accident. In Mettler FA, Kelsey CA, Ricks RC (eds): *Medical Management of Radiation Accidents*. CRC Press, Boca Raton, FL, 1990, pp 109–126.
37. Brook I, Ledney GD: Oral aminoglycoside and ofloxacin therapy in the prevention of gram-negative sepsis after irradiation. *J Infect Dis* 164:917–921, 1991.
38. Browne D, Weiss JF, MacVittie TH, Pillai MV (eds): *Treatment of Radiation Injuries*. Plenum Press, New York, 1990, p 137.
39. Bow EJ: Comparison of norfloxacin with cotrimoxazole for infection prophylaxis in acute leukemia. The trade-off for reduced gram-negative sepsis. *Am J Med* 84:847–854, 1988.
40. Daschner F: Emergence of resistance during selective decontamination of the digestive tract. *Eur J Clin Microbiol Infect Dis* 11:1:1–3, 1992.
41. Emmerson AM: Selective decontamination of the digestive tract: an issue open to discussion. *Hosp Originated Sepsis Ther* 4:1994.
42. Sources, effects and risks of ionizing radiation. United Nations Scientific Committee on the Effects of Atomic Radiation 1988 Report to the General Assembly. UNSCEAR, New York, 1988, p 622.
43. Ye GY, Wang GL, Huang SM, et al: The People's Republic of China Radiation Accidents, 1980, 1985, 1986, and 1987. In Hübner KF, Fry SA (eds): *The Medical Basis for Radiation Accident Preparedness. Proceedings of the REAC/TS International Conference*, Oak Ridge, TN, Elsevier/North Holland, New York, 1980, pp 81–89.
44. Latini P, Aristei C, Aversa F, et al: Lung damage following bone marrow transplantation after hyperfractionated total body irradiation. *Radiother Oncol* 22:127–132, 1991.
45. Flomenberg N, Keever CA: Cord blood transplants: potential utility and potential limitations. *Bone Marrow Transplant* 10:1:115–120, 1992.
46. Hows JM, Bradley BA, Marsh JCW, et al: Growth of human umbilical-cord in long term haemopoietic cultures. *Lancet* 340:73–76, 1992.
47. Lasky LC: The role of the laboratory in marrow manipulation. *Arch Pathol Lab Med* 115:293–298, 1991.
48. Latini P, Aristei C, Aversa F, et al: Interstitial pneumonitis after hyperfractionated total body irradiation in HLA-matched T-depleted bone marrow transplantation. *Int J Radiation Oncol Biol Phys* 23:401–405, 1992.
49. Oliveira AB: Treatment of infectious complications of the hematopoietic syndrome. In Brown D, Weiss JF, MacVittie TJ Pillai MV (eds): *Treatment of Radiation Injuries*. Plenum Press, New York 1990, pp 95–100.
50. Ljungman P, Engelhard D, Link H, et al: Treatment of interstitial pneumonitis due to cytomegalovirus and ganciclovir and intravenous immune globulin: Experience of European Bone Marrow Transplant Group. *Clin Infect Dis* 14:831–835, 1992.
51. Inoue T, Masaoka T, Shibata H: Difference in onset between cytomegalovirus and idiopathic interstitial pneumonitis following allogenic bone marrow transplantation for leukemia. *Strahlenther Onkol* 166:5:322–325, 1990.
52. Health Effects Models for Nuclear Power Plant Accidents Consequence Analysis: *Low LET Radiation. Part II. Scientific Bases for Health Effects Models*. Washington, US Nuclear Regulatory Commission, NUREG/CR-4214, Rev. 1, 1989, pp 2–38.
53. Morio S, Oh H, Hirasawa A, et al: Hepatic veno-occlusive disease in a patient with lupus anticoagulant after allogenic bone marrow transplantation. *Bone Marrow Transplant* 8:147–149, 1991.
54. Shulman HM, McDonald GB, Matthews D, et al: An analysis of hepatic veno-occlusive disease and centrilobular hepatic degeneration following bone marrow transplantation. *Gastroenterology* 79:1178–1191, 1980.
55. Sources, effects and risks of ionizing radiation. United Nations Scientific Committee on the Effects of Atomic Radiation 1988 Report to the General Assembly. UNSCEAR, New York, 1988, p 620.
56. Browne D, Weiss JF, MacVittie TH, Pillai MV (eds): *Treatment of Radiation Injuries*. Plenum Press, New York, 1990, p 229.
57. Recommendations on limits for exposure to ionizing radiation. National Council for Radiation Protection and Measurements, Washington, 1987, Report No. 91.

CHAPTER 56

Nerve Agents and Anticholinesterase Insecticides[a]

RICHARD J. GALLOWAY, M.D.
ROBERT C. SMALLRIDGE, M.D.

The military confrontation in the Middle East during Operation Desert Storm in 1991 presented the very real possibility that chemical weapons, including nerve agents, might be used against American and coalition forces. Although there is a general appreciation of nerve agents' extreme toxicity, most physicians are not experienced in either recognizing or treating patients who have been exposed to them. This chapter reviews the history, physical properties, and toxicity of known nerve agents and some of their less potent relatives, the organophosphate and carbamate insecticides. It also provides a practical approach to the recognition and treatment of insecticide and nerve gas toxicity, emphasizing some of the developments in the last decade, as well as a preview of newer developments to improve survivability.

CRITICAL CARE IMPLICATIONS

Exposure to, and death from, organophosphorus compounds are not rare. Over the last 20 years, worldwide exposure to organophosphate insecticides has been estimated at 500,000 to 2 million cases a year, with a fatality rate of 1 to 2% (1–3). In children, the fatality rate may be as high as 50% (4). In the United States there were about 200 fatalities per year in the early 1980s (5, 6). The incidence of exposure, largely restricted to California, Florida, and other agricultural

states, seems to be declining (5). This decline is due in part to regulation of concentrated insecticide solutions and careful surveillance of agricultural workers (5, 7).

Although accidental nerve agent exposure is rare, the extreme toxicity of these compounds makes the potential for mass casualties frightening. If a significant human exposure does occur, either through leakage of stored nerve agent or intentional use as an act of terrorism or war, there is the potential for hundreds to thousands of casualties to occur in a short period of time. Many of these patients would require management in an intensive care unit (ICU).

Moderate to severe exposure to organophosphorus compounds in the form of insecticides or nerve agents results in an acute, life-threatening intoxication. Aggressive supportive care, rapid and sequential use of several medications, careful dose monitoring, and close observation of cardiac and respiratory parameters are all required for a successful outcome. Appropriate diagnosis and therapy usually result in complete recovery. Delayed or incorrect diagnosis may lead to needless patient death and possible contamination of the health care provider.

ORGANOPHOSPHORUS COMPOUNDS

HISTORY

Two early investigators of organophosphorus (OP) compounds personally experienced their toxicity and yet survived.

---

[a]The opinions or assertions contained herein are the private views of the authors and are not to be construed as official or reflecting the views of the Department of the Army or Department of Defense.

In 1854, De Clermont described the synthesis of tetraethylpyrophosphate (8), the first organophosphate, but not until the 1920s was a systematic study of these compounds undertaken. Gerhard Schrader, at Farbenfabriken Bayer AG, while searching for compounds with insecticidal activity, synthesized several thousand compounds (9). Through his studies, he was able to define the relationship between structure and chemical activity. Parathion, one of his early compounds, proved to have excellent insecticidal activity. Several of his most toxic compounds (tabun, sarin, soman) were believed to have potential as weapons and were developed for use by the German military (10).

From this point the history begins to diverge. For insecticidal use, it was essential to decrease human toxicity and increase the environmental persistence of the drug, whereas for military use, extreme toxicity and low persistence were desirable.

Tabun, the first of these deadly agents, was discovered in 1936. It was put into production so rapidly that 20,000 to 30,000 tons were stockpiled by the start of World War II (11). The more toxic agents, soman and sarin, were developed after the large-scale commitment to tabun and hence were never produced in large quantities. After the war, the Soviets apparently dismantled the nerve gas plants (12), including the one at Dúhernfurt, and collected technical information that facilitated their own chemical weapons program (10).

The family of German agents was called *G agents*, and each was given a second letter to distinguish it, such as GA, GB, and GD. The abbreviation *GC* reportedly was never used to name these agents because of its association with sexually transmitted disease. Strangely enough, further pesticide research, this time in England, by Ghosh of Imperial Chemical Industries (13), led to the discovery of a new family of toxic OP compounds. Patented in 1955, these compounds were too toxic to be useful as insecticides. They were then further developed in England, the U.S., and Canada as chemical weapons and called *V*, or venom, agents. Only one of the many compounds produced, VX, is currently of military significance (14). The Soviet agent V_{55}, or VR-55, is probably not a V agent at all but a modified form of soman that has been "thickened" by the addition of petroleum or synthetic polymers (15–17). Figure 56.1 shows the structures of nerve agents and several insecticides.

The low cost, ease of production, tremendous destructive capacity, and ability to use relatively inaccurate delivery systems have made nerve agents tempting weapons. At least 22 countries, including Iran, Iraq, Syria, and Libya, are believed to possess them (18–20). The dubious distinction of being the first to use nerve agents in war belongs not to Germany but to Iraq. According to a United Nations investigating team, and supported by chemical analysis of samples collected on site, tabun was used on several occasions between 1984 and 1987 during the Iran-Iraq war (21–24).

The former Soviet Union and the United States possess the largest stockpiles of nerve agents. These agents can be used in the form of artillery shells, mines, bombs, missiles, or spray tanks (14, 25). When the United States halted production of chemical weapons in 1969, it had an estimated 18,000 tons in storage (26). Currently, nerve agents are stored in eight different states and two foreign sites (16, 27). They are being disposed of in accordance with Public Law 99-145 and

its amendments. Incineration, the favored method of disposal, is both effective and safe (18, 27). The size of the Soviet arsenal is more difficult to assess, as it was not until 1987 that the Soviet Union even admitted that they had chemical weapons (19). They estimated their supply at 45,000 tons, but estimates by outside sources were much higher (15, 18, 19). They are also destroying these weapons. Even if all these "unitary" weapons were destroyed, the threat of nerve agent use would remain, as two-component, or binary, weapons are not covered under the existing treaty. In these weapons, nerve agent precursors are placed in separate containers inside a projectile and mixed after firing. The active nerve agent is rapidly formed on the way to the target and is released upon impact (17, 18, 28).

NERVE AGENTS

Although many nerve agents have been developed (29), only four (tabun, sarin, soman, and VX) have been produced in militarily significant quantities. The physical and toxicologic properties of these agents have been reviewed in unclassified military (29, 30) and civilian (31, 32) sources. Selected characteristics are summarized in Table 56.1. Commonly called nerve gases because they stimulate cholinergic nerves and are delivered as an aerosol or fog, these compounds are actually liquids at room temperature. Their volatilities vary tremendously, with sarin being the most volatile and VX the least. In fact, VX is so nonvolatile that some authors even doubt the ability to achieve lethal inhalational concentrations of VX under combat conditions (31). Volatility has a significant impact on toxicity, as is discussed in a later section. Vapors from these agents are considerably more dense than air, causing them to settle in low-lying areas. This settling, of course, makes fortifications and settling tunnels especially vulnerable to their effects.

None of these agents is particularly well-suited to contamination of water supplies. Although sarin is completely soluble in water, it decomposes fairly quickly, especially in chlorinated water. VX, on the other hand, is relatively resistant to hydrolysis even in alkaline pH, but it is not very soluble at normal temperatures. VX has the unusual property of increasing water solubility with decreasing temperature, being poorly soluble at 25°C but completely soluble at water temperatures below 10°C (30).

Although all of the major agents can be lethal regardless of the route of exposure (inhalation, ingestion, or dermal), considerable variation in toxicity exists. The more volatile ones (tabun, sarin, and soman) are most toxic when inhaled, while VX, the least volatile, is most toxic as a skin penetrant. The effectiveness of inhalation exposure is quite variable, depending on a multitude of factors, including dose, characteristics of the agent itself, climatic conditions (temperature, wind) (14, 31), and characteristics of the soldier (respiratory rate, degree of protection). The values given are largely estimates based on animal studies and are for pure compounds (29, 30). Toxicity and persistence can be modified significantly by several methods, including microencapsulation (32), "thickening" (17), combined agents (14), and even the presence of impurities (30). Combination of VX with the skin penetrant dimethylsulfoxide, for example, increases the toxicity 6-fold (15). Significant species differences in toxicity occur, with the nonhuman primate and guinea pig being the most similar to

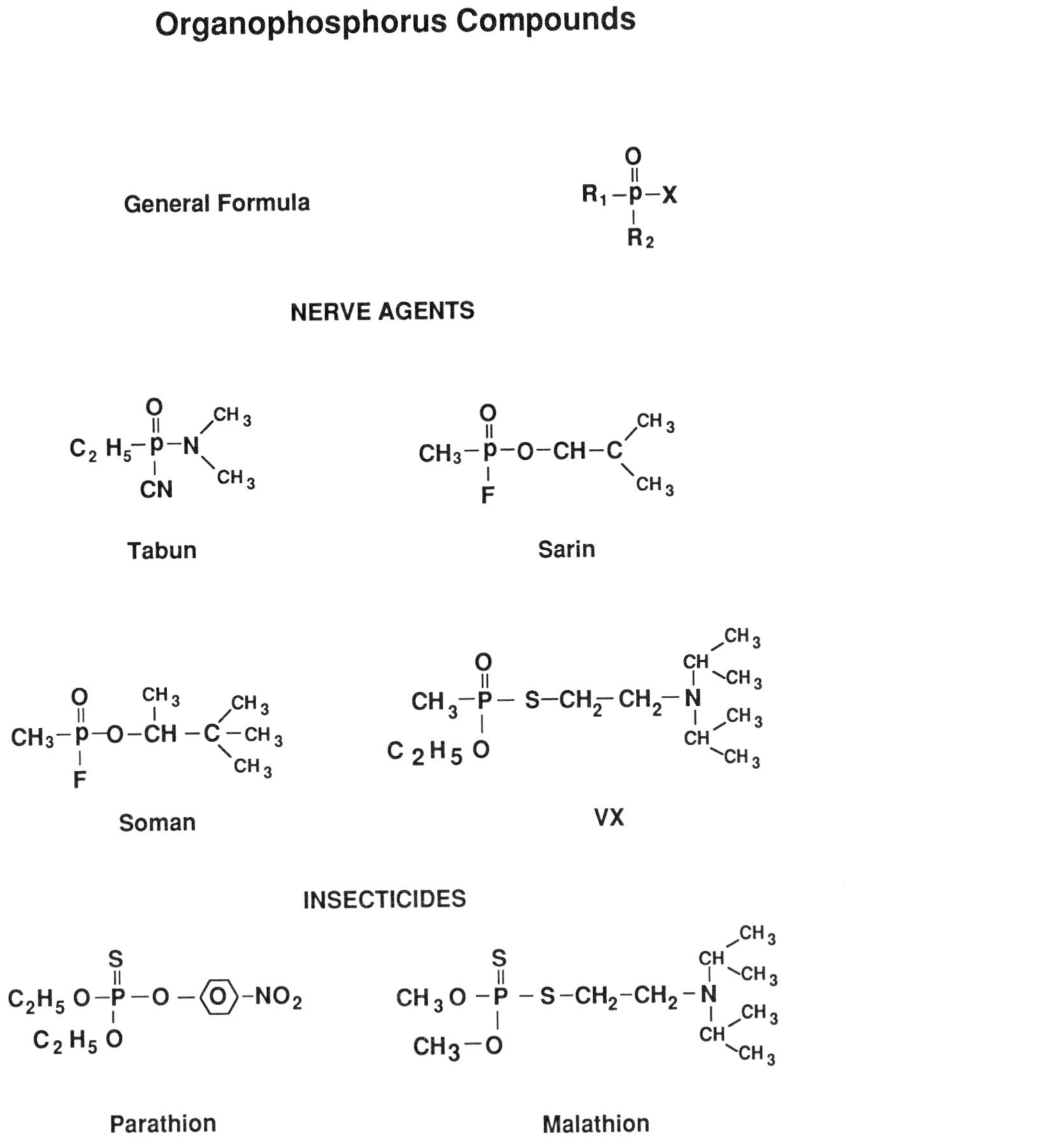

Organophosphorus Compounds

General Formula

$$R_1 - \overset{\overset{\displaystyle O}{\|}}{\underset{\underset{\displaystyle R_2}{|}}{P}} - X$$

NERVE AGENTS

$$C_2H_5 - \overset{\overset{\displaystyle O}{\|}}{\underset{\underset{\displaystyle CN}{|}}{P}} - N\begin{smallmatrix} CH_3 \\ \\ CH_3 \end{smallmatrix}$$

Tabun

$$CH_3 - \overset{\overset{\displaystyle O}{\|}}{\underset{\underset{\displaystyle F}{|}}{P}} - O - CH - C\begin{smallmatrix} CH_3 \\ \\ CH_3 \end{smallmatrix}$$

Sarin

$$CH_3 - \overset{\overset{\displaystyle O}{\|}}{\underset{\underset{\displaystyle F}{|}}{P}} - O - \overset{\overset{\displaystyle CH_3}{|}}{CH} - \overset{\overset{\displaystyle CH_3}{|}}{\underset{\underset{\displaystyle CH_3}{|}}{C}} - CH_3$$

Soman

$$\underset{\underset{\displaystyle C_2H_5O}{|}}{\overset{\overset{\displaystyle O}{\|}}{CH_3 - P}} - S - CH_2 - CH_2 - N\begin{smallmatrix} CH\begin{smallmatrix} CH_3 \\ CH_3 \end{smallmatrix} \\ \\ CH\begin{smallmatrix} CH_3 \\ CH_3 \end{smallmatrix} \end{smallmatrix}$$

VX

INSECTICIDES

$$\underset{\underset{\displaystyle C_2H_5O}{|}}{\overset{\overset{\displaystyle S}{\|}}{C_2H_5O - P}} - O - \langle O \rangle - NO_2$$

Parathion

$$\underset{\underset{\displaystyle CH_3 - O}{|}}{\overset{\overset{\displaystyle S}{\|}}{CH_3O - P}} - S - CH_2 - CH_2 - N\begin{smallmatrix} CH\begin{smallmatrix} CH_3 \\ CH_3 \end{smallmatrix} \\ \\ CH\begin{smallmatrix} CH_3 \\ CH_3 \end{smallmatrix} \end{smallmatrix}$$

Malathion

Figure 56.1.   Shown here is the general formula for organophosphorus compounds, which include the nerve agents and organophosphate insecticides. The structures of the major nerve agents and two common insecticides are depicted. In some insecticides, as illustrated by parathion and malathion, a sulfur atom is substituted for an oxygen atom.

humans (33). Leeches and birds are so sensitive to these nerve agents that they were considered as possible early warning devices by the Chinese (31). The lethal dose (LD_{50}) for skin penetration given in Table 56.1 represents values for exposure to bare skin. The ease of skin penetration depends not only on the agent but also on the affected skin site; that is, skin penetration is not uniform. The permeability of skin from the head and neck area is especially high (14). Because the stratum corneum is the major impediment to penetration, any damage to the skin such as abrasions or wounds will increase the toxicity markedly (30). Penetration, and thus toxicity, seems to be increased in individuals with little subcutaneous fat (30). VX is extremely potent as a dermal toxin because it persists on the skin (high viscosity, low vapor pressure), has a high lipid solubility, and is insensitive to dermal hydrolases. The higher vapor pressure (decreased skin contact time) of the G agents and their sensitivity to dermal hydrolases make them

less effective by this route. Because of the permeability of the conjunctiva, exposure of the eyes to liquid droplets results in rapid absorption of both G and V agents (31, 34).

Oral toxicity has been estimated in part by giving sublethal doses to human volunteers (35, 36). Except for the possibility of intentional poisoning, this toxicity is relevant primarily to VX, the most persistent agent. VX may persist in vegetation for more than a month under optimal weather conditions. In one study, four of 10 guinea pigs, fed grass cut 46 days after VX exposure, died (30).

Figure 56.2 compares the reaction of acetylcholinesterase (AchE), with its natural substrate, acetylcholine (Ach), to its reaction with carbamate (C) and OP compounds. As the figure illustrates, all involve binding via an ester linkage to a serine (S) residue at the active site. Adjacent anionic sites (-) serve to orient the substrate properly. Acetylcholine, shown in reaction sequence 1, is cleaved in a two-step process, with loss of

Table 56.1.   Physical and Toxicologic Properties of Nerve Agents

Property	Tabun (GA)	Sarin (GB)	Soman (GD)	VX
		Common Name		
Chemical name	Ethyl N, N-dimethyl-phosphoramidocyanidate	Isopropyl methyl-phosphonofluoridate	Pinacolyl methyl-phosphonofluoridate	O-ethyl S-2-diisopropylaminoethyl methylphosphonothiolate
Physical appearance	Colorless to brown liquid	Colorless liquid	Colorless liquid	Colorless to straw-colored liquid
Boiling point (°C)	245°	158°	198°	298°
Volatility (mg/m^3 at 25°C)	610	22,000	300	14
Solubility				
Water	9.8	100%	2.1	3[a]
g/100 g solvent, 25°C)				
Organic solvents	100%	100%	~100%	100%
LD$_{50}$				
Route				
Inhalation (mg min/m^3)[b]	135[c]	70	70	30
Oral (mg)	40	10	10	5
Skin (mg)[c]	1000–1500	1700	350	10
Persistence				
Soil	1–1½ days	2.5–24 hrs	Up to 2 days	2–6 days
Water (25°C)	14–28 hrs	7½ hrs–several weeks	5 min–60 hrs[d]	Up to several weeks
t½ aging	46 hrs	12 hrs	<2.4 min	>48 hrs

[a] 100% soluble in water <10°C.
[b] LCt$_{50}$ (lethal concentration for 50%).
[c] When exposure is via liquid droplets.
[d] pH dependent.

choline, and then loss of acetic acid, with the resultant regeneration of reactive AchE. This reaction is one of the most rapid ones known, as a single molecule of AchE can hydrolyze 300,000 Ach molecules per minute (5). Carbamates, shown in reaction series 2, react with AchE in a similar fashion but at a much slower rate. They are considered reversible inhibitors of AchE. OP compounds, which include both nerve agents and organophosphate insecticides, react with AchE as shown in reaction series 3. The phosphorylated or phosphonylated intermediate formed is quite stable, and as a result, the rate of spontaneous regeneration of AchE is negligible. Enzyme reactivators (oximes) usually can accelerate this regeneration to a clinically useful rate unless "aging" has occurred.

Reaction series 4 illustrates the critical concept of "aging." If the phosphorylated or phosphonylated enzyme is dealkylated, as shown in the figure by the loss of R_1, the resulting enzyme complex is essentially permanent. Once the complex is aged, even chemical reactivation is ineffective. New synthesis is required to return AchE levels to normal. The rapid aging produced by soman (see Table 56.1) and the resulting resistance to reactivation by oximes have been a major concern. A portion of this resistance may be due to steric factors rather than dealkylation (37, 38).

If these compounds had not been so strikingly toxic, their story might have ended much sooner. By the late 1940s, DuBois et al realized the possible connection between the clinical symptoms of OP toxicity and stimulation of cholinergic nerves (39). They subsequently were able to show not only that atropine antagonized these effects but also that AchE levels were decreased in tissues of poisoned animals. AchE has now been shown to be present in red blood cells (RBCs) and many other tissues. Its major role is to terminate the effects of the neurotransmitter acetylcholine (Ach) in the synaptic cleft by catalyzing its hydrolysis into acetic acid and choline. This rapid destruction of Ach allows the postsynaptic fiber to repolarize in preparation for the next nerve transmission. When AchE is inhibited, acetylcholine levels in the synaptic cleft rise, repolarization is prevented, and repetitive stimulation of the postsynaptic fiber occurs. The clinical consequence of this overstimulation depends on both the severity of the AchE inhibition and the nature of the postsynaptic fibers.

Receptors on cholinergic nerves are divided into those stimulated by muscarine (muscarinic) and those stimulated by nicotine (nicotinic). Although both types of receptors can be stimulated by Ach, the clinical consequences are different (see Table 56.2) (34, 36, 40–42). As the table shows, the effects of muscarinic and nicotinic stimulation are antagonistic on the pupil and heart. A third category of effects, those in the central nervous system (CNS), is also listed in the table. CNS effects seem to be a mixture of muscarinic and nicotinic effects.

Although cholinergic stimulation is the most striking effect of nerve agents, abnormalities in other systems, including ion channels (43, 44), cyclic peptides, and cyclic nucleotides (45), have been suggested. The neuroendocrine axis seems to be especially sensitive to these agents (46). Initial studies in rodents (47) showed a stimulation of the adrenal axis, with increased adrenocorticotropic hormone (ACTH) and corticosterone. More detailed analysis confirmed the increase in the adrenal axis and also showed a decrease in basal serum thyrotropin and a reduction in both basal and hypothalamic releasing hormone-stimulated luteinizing hormone and prolactin (48). Only the effects on the adrenal axis could be normalized by atropine.

The clinical characteristics of the 19 cases of human nerve agent exposure in the open literature have been reviewed (49). Since these were all accidental, the actual dose received was unknown. There were 12 cases of sarin exposure (five severe, four moderate, three mild) and seven cases of soman

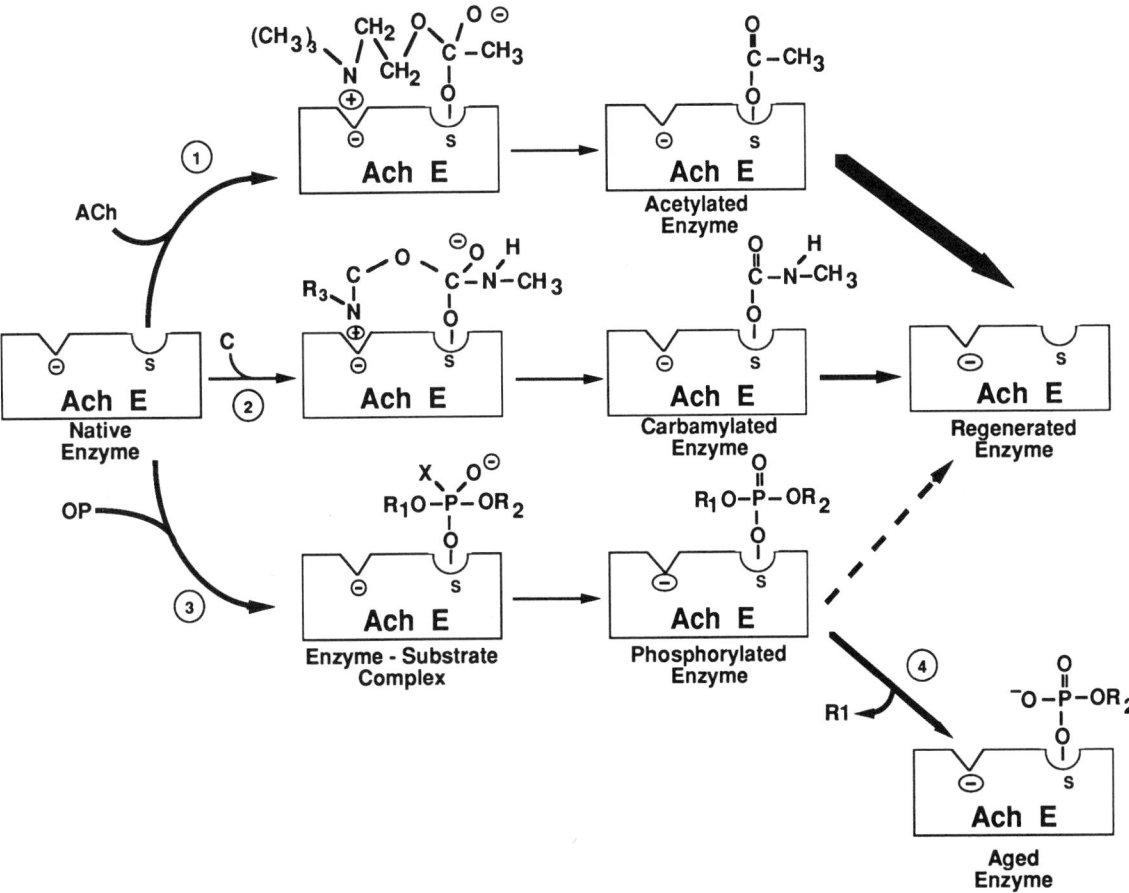

Figure 56.2.   This is a summary of the reactions of acetylcholine (*Ach*), carbamates (*C*), and organophosphorus (*OP*) compounds with acetylcholinesterase (*AchE*). In reaction series *1*, acetylcholine binds to a serine residue (*S*) at the active site and is oriented by electrostatic attraction between its quaternary nitrogen on a nearby anionic site (–). Ach is cleaved, leaving an acetylated intermediate, which is in turn hydrolyzed to regenerate the native AchE molecule. Reaction series *2* shows a similar reaction sequence with a carbamate compound. Notice that a carbamylated intermediate is formed, which again is hydrolyzed to regenerate the native AchE. The *thinner arrow* indicates that this process occurs at a much slower rate than with Ach. Reaction series *3* illustrates the interaction between AchE and organophosphorus compounds. The phosphorylated (shown here) or phosphonylated intermediate formed is very stable, and its rate of dissociation is negligible, as indicated by the *dashed arrow*. Finally, reaction *4* illustrates the dealkylation of the phosphorylated enzyme to form an even more stable, or "aged," enzyme. Once aging occurs, enzyme reactivators are of no value.

Table 56.2.   Effects of Excess Acetylcholine by Receptor Type and Location

RECEPTOR TYPE	MUSCARINIC			NICOTINIC		MUSCARINIC AND NICOTINIC
SITE OF ACTION	Smooth Muscle	Exocrine Glands	Cardiac	Ganglia	Skeletal Muscle	CNS
EFFECTS	*Wheezing* *Chest* *tightness* *Increased* *peristalsis* Vomiting Diarrhea Abdominal cramps Incontinence Urinary Fecal Miosis Blurred vision	*Wheezing* *Salivation* *Lacrimation* *Diaphoresis*	*Bradycardia* *Decreased* *blood* *pressure* Heart block	*Tachycardia* *Increased* *blood* *pressure* Hyperglycemia Mydriasis	*Weakness* *Cramps* *Fasciculations* *Local* *Generalized* Paralysis	*Tension* *Anxiety* *Insomnia* *Nightmares* Memory loss Weakness Tremor Ataxia Slurred speech Seizures Coma Depression of respiratory and circulatory centers

exposure (one severe, six mild). No cases of tabun or VX exposure are reported. The clinical symptoms reported were well-predicted (Table 56.2). Of the six cases of severe poisoning, the time of onset of symptoms was listed in only three. All three of these had symptoms within 30 minutes of exposure. The one patient with inhaled (rather than oral) exposure had symptoms within 10 seconds. Three of these four patients had seizures within 2 to 60 minutes of exposure, and four had respiratory arrest. All patients were treated with atropine (mean dose, 19.5 mg) and one-half were treated with pralidoxime chloride (2–PAM). All patients survived. Vomiting and neuromuscular weakness lasted for up to several days, blurred vision and miosis for up to a week, and neuropsychiatric symptoms from a day to more than 4 months.

INSECTICIDES

A comprehensive review of organophosphate and carbamate insecticides, although beyond the scope of this chapter, is available from other sources (5, 11, 50–51). OP agents have become the insecticide of choice because of their lack of persistence in the environment (51). Currently, more than 1 million tons of these compounds are produced worldwide each year (52). These OP insecticides represent more than 900 different compounds and a wide range of toxicities (4). They are historically, structurally, and toxicologically similar to the nerve agents.

Although all of the OP insecticides are less toxic than nerve agents, their widespread use has resulted in more cases of intoxication and death than has exposure to nerve agents. The treatment methods discussed in this chapter have proved effective in treating poisoning caused by insecticides as well as nerve agents. Where appropriate, differences in their clinical evaluation and treatment are pointed out.

MEDICATIONS

CHOLINOLYTIC AGENTS

Extracts from the belladonna plant have been used by physicians and practitioners for centuries, both as an agent of healing and as an occult poison. Atropine, the first alkaloid from this plant to be purified, has been widely studied.

Atropine

Indications.   Atropine is the mainstay of treatment for organophosphate or carbamate poisoning. It should be given as soon as the diagnosis is made. In fact, resistance to atropine may help make the diagnosis of OP toxicity when other signs are confusing.

Mechanism of Action.   Atropine is a competitive inhibitor of acetylcholine, primarily at muscarinic receptor sites. At least five subtypes of these receptors have been described and their complementary DNAs (cDNAs) cloned (53). It appears that these different receptor subtypes may be linked to different signal transduction systems, including ion channels, phosphoinositide hydrolysis, adenyl cyclase, and cytoplasmic calcium (54). Atropine is not selective among these receptor subtypes.

Pharmacokinetics.   After a single 2 mg intramuscular (i.m.) dose, the mean peak serum level is 9.1 ng/ml (range, 6.7

to 11.7), and the mean elimination half-life is 3.0 hours. A summary of the pharmacokinetic data for parenteral and oral atropine is shown in Table 56.3 (55–64). Single case reports and reports with incomplete data were excluded. Small doses (0.02 mg/kg) of atropine have also been given rectally (65).

The pharmacokinetics of atropine can be altered by a number of physiologic, pathologic, and pharmacologic conditions (Table 56.4) (56, 60, 61, 63, 66–68). Of these factors, exercise, hemorrhage, hypotension, and 2-PAM and diazepam co-administration are particularly relevant when managing military casualties. Atropine elimination is equally divided between hepatic metabolism and urinary excretion (54). Atropine penetrates the CNS poorly (54).

Dosage and Routes of Administration.   In OP poisoning the resistance to atropine is significant. Whereas the usual daily atropine dose in severely poisoned patients is about 40 mg, doses of more than 1000 mg have been given (69, 70). Carbamate exposure usually requires lower total doses of atropine (51). If the diagnosis is clear, the initial dose should be 2 to 5 mg given i.m. or intravenously (i.v.) for adults, or 0.02 to 0.05 mg/kg for children, depending on the severity of the symptoms (50, 51, 70). This dose is repeated every 15 to 30 minutes until muscarinic symptoms have resolved and there are signs of mild atropine excess (atropinization). Because of unpredictable effects on heart rate (as well as possible confounding factors such as hypovolemia, shock, etc.), the initial presence or absence of tachycardia is not helpful. In patients presenting with bradycardia, however, the development of tachycardia upon treatment is a reliable sign of atropinization (50, 51). Similarly, pupillary size is not a dependable predictor of the adequacy of the atropine dose (6, 41, 42, 71–73) if there has been any local absorption of OP. For difficult cases, some have suggested the use of atropine as a continuous infusion at 0.02 to 0.08 mg/kg/hr (69, 70, 74). It should be emphasized that patients with OP poisoning rarely receive too much atropine and frequently are given too little. This underuse of atropine has led to patients' deaths (71, 75).

A state of mild atropinization should be maintained for at least 24 to 48 hours. Therapy for as long as several weeks may be required depending on the agent involved and the severity of the exposure (71). The longer treatment periods are needed for those insecticides having a high fat solubility. In these cases, fat can act as a depot for the drug, allowing slow, continuous release (5, 76).

Adverse Effects and Contraindications.   Some authors believe that atropine is contraindicated in anoxic or hypoxic patients because of the risk of ventricular fibrillation (4, 50, 71, 77), and they suggest that oxygenation should be improved prior to atropinization. Unfortunately, these may also be the very patients with the most severe intoxication and the highest risk of death. Although the cause of death in OP poisoning is usually central respiratory failure, an effect that atropine would not be expected to improve (because of its poor penetration of the blood-brain barrier), atropine can improve ventilation by decreasing both bronchoconstriction and bronchial secretions. Delay in initiating atropine therapy can be fatal, especially when dealing with a nerve agent that ages rapidly (such as soman).

Overdose Considerations.   Atropine overdose in the setting of OP poisoning is very uncommon. Symptoms of excess

Table 56.3. Studies of Atropine Pharmacokinetic in Humans

First Author (Reference)	n[a]	Dose (mg)	Route of Administration	$t_{1/2}\beta$[b] (hrs)	C_{max}[c] (ng/ml)	Time to C_{max} (hrs)	Cl[d] (ml/min/70 kg)	V_D[e] (liters/kg)	AUC[f] (ng/hr/ml)
Metcalfe (55)	10			3.8	16.4				
Virtanen et al (56)	31	0.02/kg	i.m.[g]	3.0 ± 0.9			476.0 ± 203.0	1.6 ± 0.4	
Kanto et al (57)	10	0.01/kg	i.v.[h]	2.6 ± 0.5	29.9 ± 3.8	1.6 ± 0.2	445.2 ± 128.8	1.0 ± 0.1	
Kanto et al (57)	8	0.01/kg	i.m.	2.1 ± 0.6					
Adams et al (58)	6	1	i.v.	4.1			533.4 ± 309.6	230.8 ± 145.4	
Harrison et al (59)	8	2	i.m.	4.1	11.7 ± 2.5	0.9 ± 0.8			47.6 ± 9.2
		2	neb.[i]		11.5 ± 3.4	1.9 ± 2.1			51.8 ± 19.6
		4	neb.		16.4 ± 6.2	0.9 ± 0.8			63.1 ± 19.5
		6	neb.		18.0 ± 3.1	0.8 ± 0.3			82.0 ± 1.3
Pihlajamäki et al (60)	9	0.01/kg	i.m.		5.1 ± 1.3	0.7 ± 0.5			20.4 ± 11.3
Friedl et al (61)	20	2 mg[j]	i.m.	3.5 ± 0.3	13.2 ± 0.8	0.3 ± 0.1			50.6 ± 4
Smallridge et al (62)	6	0.5	i.v.	2.5 ± 1.1			769 ± 277	1.2 ± 0.7	10.9 ± 3.2
		1.0	i.v.	2.8 ± 0.6			616 ± 158	1.8 ± 0.4	26.1 ± 7.5
		2.0	i.v.	3.0 ± 0.8			673 ± 135	2.0 ± 0.4	46.8 ± 9.9
		2.0	i.m.	3.4 ± 1.0	10.8 ± 1.5		589 ± 196	2.3 ± 0.3	56.8 ± 18.4
Kamimori et al (63)	7	2.0	i.m.	4.2 ± 0.8	6.7 ± 0.9		738 ± 142	3.9 ± 0.4	44.1 ± 4.5
Ellinwood et al (64)	8	0.5	i.m.	3.3 ± 0.1	2.4 ± 0.3				
		1.0	i.m.	3.0 ± 0.1	4.6 ± 0.5				
		2.0	i.m.	2.3 ± 0.1	7.2 ± 0.6				
		4.0	i.m.	1.6 ± 0.1	13.5 ± 0.8				

[a] n = number of subjects studied.
[b] $t_{1/2}\beta$ = elimination half-life.
[c] C_{max} = maximum concentration reached.
[d] Cl = clearance.
[e] V_D = volume of distribution.
[f] AUC = area under the curve.
[g] i.m. = intramuscular.
[h] i.v. = intravenous.
[i] neb. = nebulized.
[j] = dose administered by Mark I autoinjector. Mean dose delivered was 2.13 mg.

Table 56.4. Factors Affecting Atropine Pharmacokinetics[a]

Condition (Reference)	Absorption Rate	$t_{1/2}\beta$[b]	C_{max}	Time to C_{max}	V_D	Cl	AUC
Physiologic							
Age (56)	-		-	-	↑	NC	-
<2 years	-	↑					
>65 years	-	↓	↑	↓	↓	NC/↓	NC
Exercise (63, 66)	↑	-					
Pathologic	-						
Hemorrhage (67) (moderate)	-	NC	NC	-	↓	NC	NC
Hypothyroidism (67)	-	NC	-	-	NC	↓	↑
Pharmacologic							
2-PAM (61)[c]	-	NC	↓	NC	NC	-	NC
Diazepam (68)[c]	-	NC	NC	↑	-	-	NC
Hypotension (60) (nitroprusside/ trimetaphan)	-	NC	NC	-	-	-	NC

[a] For explanation of column headings see Table 56.3.
[b] Species studies include human, sheep, and canine.
[c] 2-PAM and diazepam studies compared injections of both drug in separate sites (control) with co-administration of both drugs into the same tissue site by a multichambered autoinjector. NC = no change; - = not studied.

atropinization include severe tachycardia, muscle twitching, fever, restlessness, and delirium (56). Overdose can be treated with physostigmine (54).

Drug Monitoring. Atropine levels are not routinely measured, although radioimmunoassays exist (Table 56.3). Instead, the dose of atropine is determined by the clinical response. Inadequate atropine levels are suggested by continuing symptoms of acetylcholine excess, whereas excessive atropine levels are suggested by excess parasympathetic activity as described in the preceding paragraphs.

Other Cholinolytics

Many atropine-like compounds have been studied in an effort to develop a more effective nerve agent antidote. In animals, centrally acting analogs such as perpanit and benzactazine have been shown to be superior to atropine in improving survival (78). In fact, benzactazine was initially used in combination with atropine as a nerve agent antidote by both the Soviets and the U.S. (16, 17) and appears to decrease the frequency of seizures (31). The major problem with these compounds is the high incidence of CNS side effects (78). Scopolamine, which is much more potent centrally and slightly more potent peripherally than atropine, decreases both central respiratory depression and seizure activity (31). Scopolamine, when used in a human case of soman exposure, caused an improvement in concentration and computational ability rather than the decrement that was expected (42). Studies of new synthetic cholinolytic agents such as aprophen and azaprophen suggest the possibility of potent antimuscarinic activity without behavioral side effects (79).

Glycopyrrolate has been used successfully in combination with atropine to treat several cases of OP intoxication. It appeared to reduce secretions better than atropine alone and resulted in fewer ocular, cardiac, and CNS side effects. However, glycopyrrolate should not be used alone, as it is unable to control bradycardia (80).

ENZYME REACTIVATORS (OXIMES)

The oximes, a group of compounds having the general structure R=NOH, were described by Wilson and Ginsburg (81). This oxime group has a high affinity for phosphorus and is capable of removing the organophosphate moiety from acetylcholinesterase, thus reactivating the enzyme. PAM (pyridine-2-aldoxime methiodide), one of the first of these compounds to be used clinically, was effective in treating five cases of parathion poisoning (82). 2-PAM, a closely related oxime, was also found to be effective (35). A number of these compounds have now been tested and shown to have slightly different properties. Differences in effectiveness depending on agent and anatomic site have all been noted.

A critical issue is the process known as aging (see Fig. 56.2). Once an OP has "aged," oximes are no longer effective. The time required for aging is hours to days for most OP insecticides and nerve agents except soman, which ages in minutes.

Pralidoxime Chloride (2-PAM)
Indications.   2-PAM, in the form of its chloride salt, is the only oxime approved for use in the U.S. It is indicated as an antidote for OP compounds having anti-AchE activity and for the control of symptoms of overdose of drugs used in the treatment of myasthenia gravis. Its use may decrease the incidence of Wadia's late-onset paralysis (51).

Mechanism of Action.   2-PAM binds to the anionic site of AchE, thereby orienting its oxime group toward the OP bound in the adjacent active site. A preferential bond between the oxime and the OP is then formed, releasing the phosphate from the active site, and hence reactivating the enzyme. The reactivation rate varies with the source of the cholinesterase and the substituents on the phosphoryl group and is inversely related to the rate of aging. Additional benefits of 2-PAM include its ability to bind free OP and exert a direct anticholinergic effect (4, 84).

Although 2-PAM has some muscarinic effects, its most important site of action is at the nicotinic receptor of muscle, a site where atropine itself has little effect (50, 76). This action results in rapid reversal of paralysis, including paralysis of the muscles of respiration (35, 85). The ability to reverse neuromuscular blockade occurs only if atropine is also present, as 2-PAM has little effect when used alone. Although 2-PAM spinal fluid levels are measurable, CNS effects are minimal except at high doses (85). Greater CNS levels occur in OP poisoned patients, probably as a result of an increased permeability of the blood-brain barrier (86).

Pharmacokinetics.   Table 56.5 presents a summary of human and nonhuman primate data (61, 87, 88). As the table shows, in poisoned patients the maximal concentration of 2-PAM is not only higher but persists longer. This is believed to be due to decreased clearance resulting from a decrease in renal blood flow (71). The minimum effective plasma level is believed to be 4 mg/liter (71). The pharmacokinetic properties of 2-PAM are modified by exercise, heat exposure, and dehydration (Table 56.6). The drug is distributed in the extracellular water, unbound to plasma protein and actively secreted by the renal tubules, with a clearance similar to that of para-amino-hippuric acid (89).

Dosage and Routes of Administration.   For adults, an initial dose of 1 to 2 g in 100 ml of saline given by a slow infusion over 15 to 30 minutes is recommended (82). If the patient's condition requires more rapid action, a similar dose may be given i.m. or by slow i.v. push at a rate of less than 500 mg/min (6, 51). If 2-PAM is injected too rapidly (greater than 500 mg/min), there is a risk of tachycardia, headache, blurred vision, weakness, and laryngospasm (6, 76, 84). This dose should be repeated within an hour if muscular weakness persists. Additional doses, if needed, should be given cautiously at 8 to 12 hour intervals as either i.m. injections or as a repeated i.v. infusion at no more than 0.5 g/hr. The maximum daily adult dose is 12 g (50). For children, a dose of 20 to 40 mg/kg is recommended and may be given as above (50, 84). Although the timing of 2-PAM administration is somewhat controversial (4), it must be given before aging has occurred. Although 2-PAM is unlikely to be effective if given more than 48 hours after exposure, a few patients have responded to this therapy (82). If continuing absorption is occurring from a skin or bowel site, longer treatment may be needed.

Special Considerations.   Special care should be taken in treating a patient with OP poisoning who also has myasthenia gravis, as myasthenic crisis could result.

Adverse Effects and Contraindications.   2-PAM has few side effects except when given too rapidly (76, 85). Dizziness, blurred vision, sedation, weakness, tachycardia, and manic behavior have all been reported, but these often occurred in the setting of OP poisoning and concomitant atropine use (84). Occasionally, cramping of the extremities, believed to result from calcium binding, has been reported. The cramping responds well to calcium infusion (5). Several small studies using 2-PAM alone in healthy volunteers have found minimal side effects (90, 91). Transient dizziness, blurring vision, and mild increase in diastolic blood pressure have been reported, but not problems with memory or cognitive function (90, 92). With large oral doses of 2-PAM (8 to 9 g) diarrhea is a frequent side effect (93).

Table 56.5.   Studies of 2-PAM Pharmacokinetics

First Author (Reference)	n^a	Dose	Route	$t^{1/2}\,\beta$ (min)	C_{max} (μg/ml)	T_{max} (min)	Cl (ml/kg/min)	V_D (liters/kg)	AUC (μg/ml/min)
Chinn et al (87)	12	8.57 mg/kg	i.m.	~120	17	10.4	17.1	2.75	677
	12	17.4	i.m.		70.2	8.67	10.3	1.98	2299
	12	25.14	i.m.		97.5	5.55	11.1	2.18	2950
Jovanovic (88)	9	~12.5 mg/kg (1 g)	i.m.	148.9	7.5±1.7	34	9.8	2.7	1701
	6^b	~13.2 mg/kg (1 g)	i.m.	174.4	9.9±2.4	33	5.5	2.8	2594
Friedl et al (61)	20		MI^c	244.5	3.7±0.2	22.8±2.8			1864±51.8
	20		MCP^d	276.3	4.3±0.3	21.0±4.7			1792±66.0

^{a} For an explanation of column headings see Table 56.3.
^{b} These patients were being treated for OP poisoning.
^{c} i.m. injection using the Mark II injector (see text).
^{d} i.m. injection using the multichambered injector (see text).

Table 56.6.   Factors Affecting 2-PAM Pharmacokinetics^a

	$t^{1/2\,b}$	C_{max}	Renal Elimination
Exercise	↑	NC	↓
Heat	NC	Slight ↓	Slight ↑
Heat and exercise	↑	↑	↓
Dehydration	NC	↑	↓

^{a} Modified from Swartz RD, Sidell FR: Effects of heat and exercise on the elimination of pralidoxime in man. *Clin Pharmacol Ther* 14:83–89, 1973.
^{b} For an explanation of column headings see Table 56.3.

There have been some reports of liver damage, but these are probably a result of the OP rather than 2-PAM (94).

Combined use of atropine and 2-PAM has been shown to cause an additional worsening of visual accommodation and orthostatic blood pressure over that caused by atropine alone (92). Although some believe that oximes are contraindicated in all cases of carbamate poisoning (6), 2-PAM is clearly contraindicated in cases of known carbaryl poisoning because of the formation of AchE inhibitory complexes (6, 95). 2-PAM also worsened AchE inhibition in cases of soman poisoning, presumably via the same mechanism (96).

Overdose Considerations.   Few data are available on 2-PAM overdose. As 2-PAM has been shown to inhibit AchE (97) and to produce neuromuscular block when given at high doses (35), respiratory failure may occur.

Drug Monitoring.   Monitoring is again by observation of clinical effect, especially on neuromuscular blockade. Drug levels are not widely available.

Other Oximes

The protective effect of oximes depends on a number of factors, including the chemical structure of the OP itself. No oxime is equally effective against all OPs (98). Since the exact nature of the former Soviet nerve agent threat was uncertain, most of the Western European countries and the U.S. chose 2-PAM. It has a wider spectrum of activity than other oximes and fewer side effects (99). Eastern European countries, knowing that the West stockpiles only sarin and VX (15, 17, 99), have chosen obidoxime (toxogonin) or trimedoxime (TMB-4) (16) as their standard agents. These oximes, while more potent than 2-PAM, have a higher incidence of side effects (100).

A major problem with oxime therapy has been the inability to treat soman poisoning effectively, even when given prophylactically (38). The known stockpiling of soman by the former Soviet Union (16) and the inadequacy of current treatment regimens have led to the production and testing of many new oximes. Of these, one of the Hagedorn compounds, HI-6, seems most promising. It appears to have low toxicity in humans (101) and is effective against soman poisoning in primates (102, 103). The pharmacokinetics of HI-6 have been studied in primates (104) and humans (101) and appear to be unaltered by the administration of atropine or diazepam (104). Because HI-6 is unstable in solution and poorly absorbed orally, a special wet/dry autoinjector has been developed for its use (105). Although HI-6 has been shown to reactivate soman-inhibited AchE both in vitro (106) and in vivo (37), it is also believed to enhance receptor desensitization to excessive Ach by decreasing receptor affinity (44).

REVERSIBLE ACETYLCHOLINESTERASE INHIBITORS

Pyridostigmine

Indications.   In clinical medicine pyridostigmine is used to treat myasthenia gravis or to reverse the effects of curare-like muscle relaxants. Pyridostigmine appears to have value as prophylactic treatment for OP exposure, including nerve agents. It was given for the first time in large scale to humans during Operation Desert Storm in anticipation of possible nerve agent attack (107).

Mechanism of Action.   Pyridostigmine, a carbamate, is a reversible inhibitor of AchE. By reducing AchE levels, pyridostigmine might be expected to worsen the acute toxicity of nerve agents, but it does not (108). Pyridostigmine given prior to exposure protects a portion of the AchE from irreversible binding by nerve agent. The reversibly bound enzyme can then be reactivated when the concentration of nerve agent is low, resulting in just enough functional AchE to avoid

Table 56.7. Studies of Pyridostigmine Pharmacokinetics

First Author (Reference)	n^a	Dose	Route	$t\frac{1}{2}$ β (hrs)	C_{max} (mg/ml)	T_{max} (hrs)	Cl (ml/min/kg)	V_D (liters/kg)	AUC^b
Chinn et al (87)	12	0.286 mg/kg	oral	2	14.1	0.9	158	2.2	2150 mg/min/ml
	12	0.571 mg/kg	oral		26.6	1.1	149	1.98	5255
	12	1.14 mg/kg	oral		44.8	1.1	175	2.18	7665
Breyer-Pfaff et al (109)	11								13.9 μg (micrograms)/ ml/min
		60 mg	oral	3.3		1.5–5^c			6.7
	11	4 mg	i.v.	1.5		^{d}	9.7	1.03	
Cronnelly et al (110)	5^e	0.35 mg/kg	i.v.	1.9			8.6	1.1	
	5^f			1.4			10.8	1.0	
	4^g			6.3			2.1	1.0	
Technical Memo	Summary		oral	3.7		8.5	1.1		
90-4 (108)			i.v.	1.9					

^{a} For explanation of column headings see Table 56.3.
^{b} Average of lower and upper limits.
^{c} Variable kinetics suggest that GI absorption may be rate limiting.
^{d} Maximum at end of infusion (30 min).
^{e} Treated with atropine and neuromuscular block.
^{f} Post-renal transplant.
^{g} Anephric patients.

symptoms. In addition, pyridostigmine decreases receptor affinity for Ach and has some cholinergic agonist effects on both nicotinic and muscarinic receptors (43).

Pharmacokinetics. Pyridostigmine pharmacokinetics have been studied in a small number of humans who were either healthy volunteers or patients with myasthenia gravis. The effect of renal function on its metabolism has also been studied. Table 56.7 (87, 108–110) summarizes the results. Pyridostigmine, a quaternary amine, crosses the blood-brain barrier poorly (44) and as a result does not protect brain AchE (111). There is some evidence that its penetration may improve with high doses or with concomitant OP exposure (85). Single-dose oral pharmacokinetics have been quite variable, with differences in bioavailability, time to achieve peak drug level, and plateau drug concentration described (108, 109, 112, 113). There is some evidence that these variations diminish with repeated doses. Pyridostigmine is minimally bound to plasma proteins and is renally cleared, largely in an unaltered form. There are no data on the effects of heat, dehydration, concomitant illness, or injury on the pharmacokinetics of pyridostigmine. At the oral dose used by the military, AchE levels return to normal within 12 hours after the last dose (114).

Dosage and Routes of Administration. The U.S. military uses 30 mg orally every 8 hours as its standard dose. This dose was chosen because it inhibits about 30% of AchE (an amount sufficient to improve survival) and has a relatively low incidence of side effects (115). The time to start and stop prophylaxis is determined by the local commander and is guided by his assessment of the risk of nerve agent attack. Since the value of pyridostigmine is its prophylactic use, it is rarely used in nonmilitary situations.

Special Considerations. A primary consideration for a drug used prophylactically in wartime is that it should have minimal effects on performance. Physostigmine, the first known reversible cholinesterase inhibitor, has much greater CNS penetration than does pyridostigmine, and would therefore offer the possibility of better central protection (116). Unfortunately, this improved CNS penetration also results in significant performance decrements that make it unsuitable

for prophylactic use (117). On the other hand, in many studies over the last 20 years, pyridostigmine has been shown to cause no significant changes in cognitive function, memory, alertness, vision, or ability to perform complex skills, including driving, tracking moving targets, and flying an airplane (108, 118, 119). A mild decrease in heart rate has been noted (108, 120).

Although pyridostigmine does decrease sweating, it has minimal effects on the ability to tolerate heat-induced stress, even in conditions of mild dehydration (114). Thermoregulation is significantly impaired, however, during moderate or severe exercise (115).

Adverse Effects and Contraindications. When used at a dose of 30 mg every 8 hours for as long as 2 weeks, the incidence of side effects was less than 1% (108). Most of these were gastrointestinal (GI) in nature, with increased flatus and loose stools heading the list. Retrospective questioning of medical personnel stationed in Saudi Arabia during Operation Desert Storm, where more than 40,000 soldiers took the drug, suggested a much higher incidence of adverse affects: GI symptoms in more than 50%, urinary urgency in 5 to 30%, and headaches in less than 5% (107). Most of these side effects were considered to be minimal and were not believed to cause decreased performance. About 1% of those receiving the drug required a medical visit for one of the aforementioned symptoms. Other side effects were seen, including isolated cases of rash, nightmares, worsening of acute bronchitis, asthma, and unexpected hypertension. Two women (each weighing ≤50 kg) developed signs of overdose with severe abdominal cramps, excess salivation, diaphoresis, and muscle twitching. In all, <0.1% of the soldiers given pyridostigmine had to discontinue the drug as a result of side effects. It should be noted that the major problems, GI and urinary, would be expected to increase in frequency with stress alone, and hence these data, obtained without a control population, represent a worst-case situation. Possible drug interactions include bradycardia (when combined with a β-blocker), orthostasis (when combined with vasodilators or with volume-depleted patients), and bronchoconstriction with asthmatics.

Pyridostigmine might also be expected to worsen the atrioventricular (AV) block that can be produced by antimalarial drugs, gastroesophageal reflux, and peptic ulcer disease, and to increase the risk of atrial fibrillation in a hyperthyroid patient. The possible interactions of pyridostigmine with anesthetic drugs, especially neuromuscular blocking agents, is of particular concern, as these drugs are inactivated by acetylcholinesterases. A complete discussion of anesthesia, although beyond the scope of this chapter, has been reviewed recently (114). The drug is contraindicated in patients with mechanical obstructions of the GI or urinary tracts (84).

Overdose Considerations. Symptoms of overdose are largely a result of pyridostigmine's direct cholinergic activity, much like the effects of OP poisoning itself. Both muscarinic and nicotinic symptoms are seen. Pyridostigmine overdose could be confused with exposure to a nerve agent or, in peacetime, to an OP or carbamate insecticide. The lack of central nervous system effects from pyridostigmine should help differentiate these possibilities. The overdose may be treated with atropine, as long as one recalls that much smaller doses are needed (34, 84). In a patient with myasthenia gravis, it may be difficult to differentiate pyridostigmine overdose (cholinergic crisis) from myasthenic crisis. This is a critical distinction, as the treatments are opposite. Osserman and Genkins (121) have suggested the use of edrophonium to distinguish them. Myasthenic crisis can be precipitated by an overzealous use of atropine, making the treatment of OP intoxication in such patients especially difficult.

ANTICONVULSANTS

Regardless of the route of entry, all nerve agents can cross the blood-brain barrier and enter the CNS. Soman has a special affinity for the CNS, perhaps because of its high lipid solubility (37, 38). It rapidly causes central respiratory failure (38, 122) and, frequently, generalized seizure activity (123). Neuronal necrosis, especially in the limbic, corticofugal, and central motor areas of the brain, has been found in affected animals (124). Although the etiology of this neuronal damage is unknown, it is not believed to result from hypoxia (124) or a direct neurotoxic effect of the nerve agent (125). It has been suggested that an increase in the activity of the excitatory neurons or a decrease in the activity of the inhibitory neurons could result in the release of an endogenous neurotoxic substance (126). The elucidation of this mechanism has significant implications on the choice of anticonvulsant medications.

Diazepam

Indications. Diazepam (Valium) is indicated in moderate to severe OP exposure for the treatment of anxiety and seizures induced by OP poisoning (34, 71). Early observations in animals and humans exposed to nerve agents showed that even with the aggressive use of atropine and 2-PAM, many convulsed. Histologic examination showed evidence of brain lesions in nearly all of those animals (49). In the presence of atropine, diazepam (and other benzodiazepines) was able to suppress seizure activity completely in most animals. Those that did convulse, did so for a shorter time than did controls

(49, 125, 127–129). Histologic evaluation of the diazepam-treated animals showed a marked decrease in brain pathology (49, 128, 130–133).

Mechanism of Action. The mechanism of action of diazepam is unknown. In vitro, it has been shown to augment the actions of the inhibitory neurotransmitter γ-aminobutyric acid (GABA) at a number of sites (134). In brain membrane preparations, diazepam appears to increase the binding affinity of GABA, presumably making it a better inhibitor. Recently, Shih et al (135) have shown that diazepam may have a direct effect on Ach in soman-treated animals. Brain Ach levels were decreased following treatment with diazepam.

Pharmacokinetics. Diazepam is highly protein bound (> 98%) in serum and is metabolized prior to excretion. Less than 1% is excreted unchanged in the urine (136). Its major metabolite, a product of *N*-demethylation, is biologically active. The elimination half-life ($t\frac{1}{2}$) is 1.5 days and increases with liver disease or at extremes of age (137). Its volume of distribution is 1.1 liters/kg.

Dosage and Routes of Administration. In clinical medicine, diazepam is usually given either orally or intravenously. For use in the military, an i.m. delivery system is needed so that soldiers can administer the drug quickly. An autoinjector similar to that for 2-PAM was developed and filled with 10 mg of diazepam (2 ml volume). Current military doctrine specifies its use for convulsions or after three injections of atropine and 2-PAM have been given (total of 6 mg atropine and 1800 mg 2-PAM). Combat lifesavers and medics carry additional autoinjectors so that a total of as much as 30 mg of i.m. diazepam can be given prior to evacuation from the battlefield (34).

The minimum effective i.m. dose, estimated from nonhuman primate studies, is about 12 mg for a 70-kg man (138). If i.v. access is available, that route of administration is preferred. The recommended i.v. starting dose is 5 to 10 mg, which may be repeated every 15 minutes to a maximum of 30 mg if needed to control recurrent seizures (84). Nonhuman primate data suggest that concomitant use of atropine in the early phases of treatment is important for effectiveness. Diazepam has also been shown to prevent seizures if given prophylactically (127, 129).

Special Considerations. Use of diazepam in pregnant or potentially pregnant females poses additional risks in that (*a*) there is a controversial small increased incidence of cleft lip or palate and (*b*) fetal exposure may be high, as fetal ability to metabolize the drug is low and cord blood levels are high (84).

Adverse Effects and Contraindications. Diazepam used chronically is physically addictive. The CNS depressant effects (sedation, respiratory depression) of diazepam are usually of greatest concern, especially when the drug is given parenterally. This effect could augment the CNS depressive effect intrinsic to OPs themselves. However, when subjected to nerve agents, animals treated with diazepam regained alertness more quickly than did controls (128, 139, 140). A cardiodepressant effect has been described, and occasional development of bradycardia, hypotension, and cardiovascular collapse has been noted. Venous thrombosis and phlebitis have been seen with i.v. administration, especially with drug extravasation (84). For a list of the less common side effects, the reader is referred to the *Physicians' Desk Reference* (84). Drug interactions are unusual except for the additive effect on CNS depression when diazepam is given with other CNS depressants such as alcohol, barbiturates, or narcotics.

Overdose Considerations. Most overdose deaths occur when diazepam is combined with other CNS depressant drugs. Overdose of diazepam alone is an uncommon cause of death. Treatment is supportive.

Other Anticonvulsants

In animal models (rodents, nonhuman primates), other benzodiazepines have also been found to be effective in preventing or treating OP-induced convulsions. These include midazolam (128, 131, 141), clonazepam (127), and nitrazepam (127). Additionally, midazolam appears to decrease brain pathology following OP exposure (128, 141).

In the search for more effective anticonvulsants, inhibitors of excitatory amino acids (EAA) have been studied (135, 142). A possible association of EAA with the CNS effects of OP poisoning was suggested by the occurrence of both neurotoxicity and seizure activity. MK-801, an experimental noncompetitive antagonist of *n*-methyl-d-aspartate (an EAA), has been shown to prevent neuronal necrosis and to decrease the likelihood of death from soman exposure (143).

Recently, nonopioid antitussive drugs have been shown to possess anticonvulsant activity. The parent compound, dextromethorphan (DM), has specific, high-affinity binding sites in rat and guinea pig brain that do not correspond to known neurotransmitter sites. DM binding in these sites not only has inherent antiseizure properties but enhances the binding of other anticonvulsants such as diphenylhydantoin (144). Of the many compounds in this new family, carbetapentane and caramiphen (CM) have been most thoroughly studied. CM, the most potent of these compounds, is more than twice as potent as diphenylhydantoin in preventing seizures in rodents (145). It has now been shown to be effective in the treatment of soman poisoning. Seizure intensity and duration are decreased, neuronal damage is reduced, and with high CM doses the death rate is reduced. Behavioral side effects are minimal. The mechanism by which this protective effect occurs is unclear but is not a result of its cholinolytic effects (146).

DIAGNOSIS

Successful treatment of nerve agent or OP exposure first requires an accurate diagnosis. The diagnosis rests on (*a*) a history of exposure, (*b*) a constellation of characteristic signs and symptoms, (*c*) a reduced cholinesterase level in blood or plasma, and (*d*) a clear clinical response to appropriate therapy. OP intoxication is often misdiagnosed as any of a wide variety of illnesses, including gastroenteritis, pancreatitis, pulmonary edema, ataxia, arrhythmia, psychosis, or seizure disorder (51). In children, this diagnosis is missed more than half the time, as the classic symptoms are less prominent or even absent. Children usually present with severe CNS symptoms such as flaccidity, stupor, respiratory depression, and coma (147, 148).

A history of exposure will be available in a majority of cases. In others, the presence of an open chemical container, involvement in an at-risk occupation, or a garlic-like smell

could suggest exposure. Methods for identifying pesticide or nerve agent residues on skin, clothing, or bodily fluids are available but will not be helpful in the initial diagnosis or treatment, as symptoms usually occur within minutes to a few hours after exposure, depending on the agent's lipid solubility, dose, method of entry, and need for activation. For a given agent, the time of onset of symptoms decreases with increasing dose. For a given dose, respiratory exposure results in the earliest symptoms, and dermal exposure, the latest. Most agents cause symptoms within 24 hours of exposure (51). Agents such as parathion, which require metabolic activation to become toxic, have a slower onset of symptoms. Dichlofenthion, leptophos, and other fat-deposited OP agents may result in a markedly delayed onset (up to 48 hours) and a prolonged recovery (more than 30 days) (149, 150).

The characteristic signs and symptoms are predictable from the known effects of Ach excess (see Table 56.2) and are similar for both nerve agents (34, 41) and OP insecticides (4, 50). In mild poisonings, the signs and symptoms depend on the method of exposure (34, 35). If the exposure was oral, then nausea, vomiting, and diarrhea are often prominent; if inhalational, then wheezing, shortness of breath, and excessive bronchial secretions are common; and if dermal, local fasciculations and sweating are common. With larger exposures, sufficient systemic absorption occurs to cause similar symptoms regardless of the route of entry. According to Namba et al (85), the most helpful signs are miosis, fasciculations, and excessive secretions (diaphoresis, lacrimation, salivation, bronchial). Ellenhorn and Barceloux (6) cite similar signs and suggest the mnemonic DUMBELS (*d*iarrhea, *u*rination, *m*iosis, *b*ronchospasm, *e*mesis, *l*acrimation, *s*alivation) to aid in the diagnosis. Miosis is one of the most consistent signs and may affect the eyes unequally (85). Its presence does not always imply severe exposure, however, as significant miosis can occur with local exposure to the eye alone (5, 6, 73). Additionally, its absence does not rule out OP poisoning, as mydriasis has been noted in some cases (151). Carbamate poisoning produces similar signs and symptoms but they are less intense, of shorter duration, and, except in children, rarely involve the CNS (51). Other drug-related etiologies for miosis such as parasympathomimetics, phenothiazines, opiates, clonidine, phencyclidine, and the like should be considered. In cases of diagnostic uncertainty, resistance to the effects of atropine can be helpful (4).

The most useful laboratory test is the measurement of AchE activity of blood or pseudocholinesterase activity of plasma (4, 36, 35). Both of these are lowered acutely by OP or carbamate poisoning and recover slowly toward normal thereafter (40). RBC AchE is the most specific of these and is believed to mimic the enzyme from neural tissue most closely (35, 36, 40, 51, 152). Pseudocholinesterase (butyrylcholinesterase), on the other hand, is more sensitive and recovers faster (6, 36). Many authors have suggested that both should be measured (4, 6, 85). Table 56.8 presents a comparison of these two enzymes. Namba et al. (85), in reviewing cases of parathion and methyl parathion poisoning, have suggested that the degree of serum cholinesterase depression can be correlated with the severity of acute exposure, but only in the initial stages. They combined cholinesterase values with the severity of signs and symptoms to get four groups: latent,

Table 56.8.   Cholinesterase Types

	Acetylcholinesterase	*Pseudocholinesterase*
Source	RBC Neuronal tissue	Plasma
Production	Possible local synthesis	Liver synthesis
Kinetics of Change		
Decrease	Slower	Faster
Recovery	0.5–1%/day new synthesis	1–3 wks

Causes of falsely
low values
	Pernicious anemia
	Paroxysmal nocturnal
	   hemoglobinuria
	Use of antimalarial drugs
	Use of oxalated tube for
	   blood collection
		Liver disease
		   Viral hepatitis
		   Cirrhosis
		   Congestion
		   Metastasis
		Malnutrition
		Anemia
		Acute infection
		Chronic inflammation
		Pregnancy (trimesters 1 and 2)
		Post-myocardial infarction
		Genetic–3%

Table 56.9.   Grading the Severity of Exposure

	Latent	*Mild*	*Moderate*	*Severe*
Symptoms[a]	None	Yes	Yes	Yes
Ambulation	Yes	Yes	No	No
Consciousness	Yes	Yes	Yes	No
Serum Cholinesterase[b]	50–90%	20–50%	10–20%	<10%

[a] See Table 56.2. Both the number and severity of these symptoms increase as the severity of exposure increases.

[b] Percent of normal.

mild, moderate, and severe (see Table 56.9). Others believe that cholinesterase levels are useful only for diagnosis and not for judging the severity of exposure (153). With chronic exposure, AchE levels, although still valuable for diagnosis, are clearly of no value as a measure of severity.

There are several caveats in interpreting AchE levels. First, normal AchE levels do not always rule out OP or carbamate exposure. The most common reason for this effect is the wide variation of AchE found in normals (154–156). A patient whose initial value is near the top of the normal range could have a 50% reduction in cholinesterase and still be in the normal range. This variation is such a problem that California requires that individual preexposure levels be measured for each agricultural worker (7). The percent reduction can then be determined by using each worker as his or her own control. A variation in RBC AchE >23% in a single measure or >16.5% in two measures is a marker of exposure (156). Unfortunately, such preexposure cholinesterase levels would not be available for most acutely poisoned patients. A clear increase in RBC AchE after 2-PAM administration can also be used to confirm OP poisoning in those with mild AchE inhibition (6). The normal variation in AchE should not present a diagnostic problem for cases of severe poisoning, as these patients will have very low AchE levels. One possible exception is with carbamate exposure. These compounds produce a much more reversible AchE inhibition than do OP insecticides or nerve agents. As a result, using blood drawn too long after exposure or waiting too long before analysis might make it appear that AchE levels are normal (6). Second, low AchE levels do not

always imply OP or carbamate exposure. This diagnostic problem is restricted to the asymptomatic patient. Low AchE levels could, of course, imply mild chronic exposure but could also be the result of other conditions or even a genetic variation (see Table 56.8). The third problem is the poor correlation of cholinesterase levels with recovery. Although RBC cholinesterase is similar to neuronal AchE in vitro, it may not be a very good predictor in vivo. Symptomatic recovery precedes recovery of RBC or plasma cholinesterase levels (36, 40).

OTHER LABORATORY FINDINGS

The routine laboratory workup is not helpful in making the diagnosis and is usually unremarkable (4). Hyperglycemia and glycosuria (4, 85, 157) are common and may reflect increased catechols produced by direct cholinergic stimulation of the adrenal medulla. Occasional hypokalemia may be explained by this same mechanism (4). Mild proteinuria, increased hematocrit (158), leukocytosis with or without a left shift (4, 6, 85, 87), and increased prothrombin time (85, 158) have been described. Elevations of serum amylase as well as clinical pancreatitis have been reported in a number of patients (4, 159–161).

OTHER TESTS

Electrocardiogram (ECG).   Cardiac abnormalities are quite common (4). Nonspecific ST–T wave changes and atrioventricular block are seen frequently (162), while QT prolongation is less common. The most common rhythm disturbance is premature ventricular contractions, but a variety of atrial (including fibrillation) and ventricular tachycardias (especially torsade de pointes) have been reported (4, 163, 164).

Electroencephalogram (EEG). EEG abnormalities are common, even in those without clinical signs of seizure activity (43). Initially, desynchronization of the cortical EEG is seen with waves of high frequency but low amplitude. Ultimately, this pattern changes to low-frequency, high-amplitude waves and subsequent seizure activity (41, 43, 165). The most characteristic EEG abnormality resembles that of temporal lobe seizures. Generalized seizures are common. EEG abnormalities may persist for as long as a year or more after the initial exposure (166).

Chest X-ray. This is usually normal, but several cases of pulmonary edema without cardiomegaly have been reported (51, 167). This resolves rapidly with therapy of the primary intoxication and is probably neurogenic in origin (167). Aspiration pneumonia and chemical pneumonitis have also been described (51).

TREATMENT

For purposes of clarity, treatment is discussed as a series of discrete steps: decontamination, supportive care, and pharmacologic intervention. When one is actually caring for an OP- or carbamate-poisoned patient, however, the treatment sequence is determined by the severity of the patient's condition, and often many interventions are made simultaneously. Routine laboratory studies as well as both plasma and RBC cholinesterase levels should be drawn early in the hospital course, but treatment should not be delayed until the results return. The first step of treatment is to prevent exposure of the health care team. Although this step is of lesser concern in exposures to dilute OP insecticides or carbamates, it may be a matter of survival in exposure to nerve agents. The caregiver should remember that as little as one drop of VX the size of the head of a pin on unprotected skin is a lethal dose! As these agents are rapidly bound once in the body, blood and body secretions do not present an exposure hazard (168).

Ideally, the first step in treatment is to decontaminate the patient. This decreases the risk to the health care team and may decrease the total exposure dose to the patient. If the exposure was to a volatile nerve agent, the decontamination process should occur before a health care provider in full protective equipment, including a gas mask, places the patient in a closed space (such as an ambulance) (77). If the clinical presentation is severe, supportive care and early pharmacologic intervention may need to precede complete patient decontamination. In this case, decontamination should be completed as soon as the patient is stabilized. The patient's clothing should be completely removed and placed in a sealed plastic bag. Special care should be taken while handling shoes and other leather articles, as they are readily penetrated by OP agents and may act as a reservoir of contamination (34). Bleach may be added to speed detoxification (40). Burning of the clothes can release toxic smoke, and decontamination of

tabun releases cyanide, itself a toxin (31). Liquid nerve agent should be removed by gentle blotting with an absorbent material. Wiping or rubbing should be avoided, as such actions may increase agent penetration (34). The contaminated skin should be cleaned by washing with simple soap and water, followed by an alcohol wash to remove OP from the upper layers of the skin (71). The eyes should be flushed with large amounts of water if direct contact with an OP is suspected. If there is any possibility of oral ingestion, efforts to decrease GI absorption should be initiated. Although some have suggested the use of either forced emesis or gastric lavage (51), the frequent use of hydrocarbon solvents with OP compounds and the rapid loss of consciousness that can occur would make induced vomiting less desirable. Aggressive gastric lavage, usually with large volumes of water or 5% sodium bicarbonate (73, 168), should be started almost regardless of the time since exposure, since gastric retention of OP compounds may be prolonged. If the patient's consciousness is impaired, airway protection should be provided prior to gastric lavage. Administration of activated charcoal as well as cathartics such as sorbitol or sodium sulfate is recommended (51).

Supportive care is a vital part of the successful treatment of OP intoxication. Life-threatening complications are largely restricted to the respiratory, cardiovascular, and central nervous systems. Respiratory symptoms are often severe and rapidly progressive. Respiratory care is complicated by the multifactorial nature of the defect. In addition to the loss of respiratory effort that results both from depression of the respiratory center and paralysis of the respiratory muscles, obstruction of airflow is caused by severe bronchoconstriction and the accumulation of copious bronchial secretions. Respiratory care should be aggressive, with careful maintenance of the airway, frequent suctioning, close monitoring of oxygen saturation, and oxygen supplementation if necessary. Most cases of severe exposure will require assisted ventilation or intubation and ventilator support. Initially, bronchospasm may make ventilation very difficult (168). Pharmacologic intervention, discussed in a later section, is also required.

Continuous cardiac monitoring is required in all cases of severe poisoning, as a wide variety of both atrial and ventricular dysrhythmias is common (4, 6, 51, 163). Cardiac dysrhythmias are treated with the usual antiarrhythmic drugs. Those patients who present with or develop prolongation of the QT interval on surface ECG are especially susceptible to polymorphous ventricular tachycardia (torsade de pointes) (164). Although this rhythm is often resistant to therapy and has a mortality rate of more than 50% (163, 169), it may respond to ventricular overdrive pacing or isoproterenol (164). Sudden death as late as 5 days after exposure has been reported (51, 164). Hypotension, when found, usually responds to i.v. fluids and dopamine (51). Hypotension from central depression may be very difficult to treat. If hypotension is absent, fluids should be given to replace losses (51).

Supportive care required for CNS complications includes serial evaluation of mental status and appropriate seizure precautions to minimize patient injury and risk of aspiration. Administration of oxygen is, of course, important to minimize hypoxia.

Figure 56.3 summarizes the mechanisms and sites of action of the drugs used in treatment of OP poisoning. Atropine

SYNAPSE

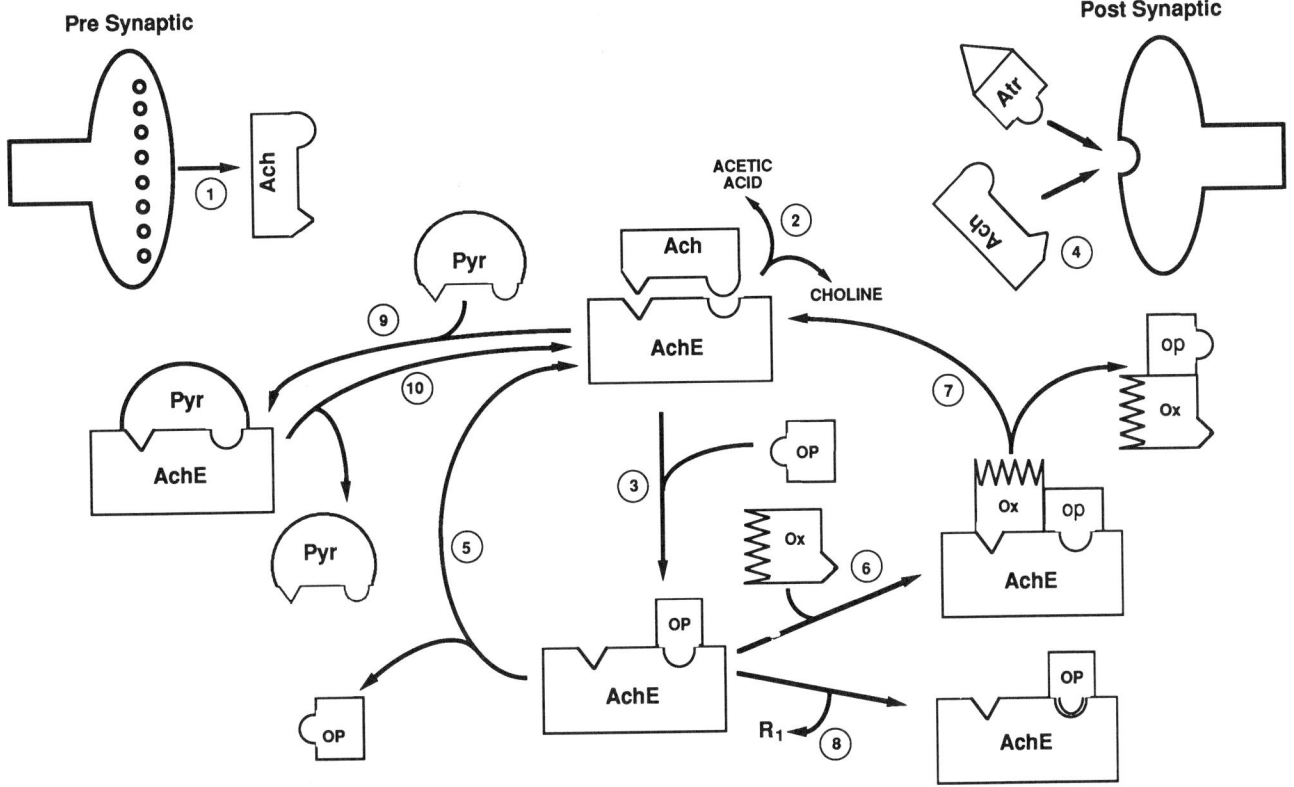

Figure 56.3. Acetylcholine (*Ach*) is released from the presynaptic nerve terminal in response to a depolarizing signal (*1*). Site *2* shows the normal binding of Ach to acetylcholinesterase (*AchE*) and its subsequent hydrolysis to acetic acid and choline. When an organophosphate (*OP*) binds to the active site of AchE (*3*), further inactivation of Ach is prevented. As Ach levels rise, the postsynaptic fiber is overstimulated, and symptoms (nicotinic, muscarinic, CNS) are produced. Atropine (*Atr*) antagonizes the effects of Ach by competing for binding (*4*) at the postsynaptic receptor. Spontaneous hydrolysis of the phosphorylated enzyme (*5*) does not occur at a perceptible rate. Hydrolysis can be facilitated, however, by the addition of an oxime (*Ox*), which binds to OP on the enzyme surface (*6*). This weakens the OP–AchE bond, resulting in regeneration of the native enzyme (*7*). If the OP–bound enzyme is dealkylated, or "aged" (*8*), the OP–AchE bond becomes so strong that 2-PAM is ineffective. Pyridostigmine (*Pyr*), given prior to OP exposure, reversibly blocks the active site on AchE (*9*), preventing subsequent OP binding. When OP levels decline, Pyr is discontinued, allowing the "protected" enzyme to return to its native state (*10*).

should be given parenterally as early as possible. If the diagnosis of OP intoxication is clear, the initial dose should be 2 to 4 mg. This dose should be repeated every 10 to 20 minutes until an appropriate clinical response has been achieved. The desired end point, mild atropinization, is evidenced by a normalization of respiration, decreased bronchial secretions, dry skin, and heart rate between 90 and 100 beats per minute. As discussed previously, pupillary response (development of mydriasis) is a poor indicator of atropinization and should not be used. If the diagnosis is unclear, an i.v. test dose (1 mg) of atropine may be given. If no signs of atropinization develop within 10 minutes, a presumptive diagnosis of OP poisoning may be made and higher doses of atropine may be given (4, 50). Severe eye involvement may present with eye pain and headache caused by spasm of the ciliary muscle. This symptom, although resistant to systemic atropine, responds to topical atropine (1% eyedrops or ointment) (34, 72) or homatropine (2% drops) (40). This treatment will, of course, disrupt vision for nearly 24 hours.

In contrast to its effectiveness against muscarinic symptoms, atropine has little effect on skeletal muscle. Since muscle weakness and paralysis are important clinical problems in

most cases of moderate to severe exposure, this is a serious drawback. Fortunately, 2-PAM, combined with atropine, has its greatest effect at this site and results in reversal of neuromuscular block within 10 to 40 minutes of administration (50, 71). In the ICU setting, adults should receive 1 to 2 g of 2-PAM i.v. given as a slow push at a rate not to exceed 500 mg/min (20 to 50 mg/kg for children) (50, 71). Alternately, 2-PAM (2.5% in saline) may be given as a continuous infusion at a rate of no more than 0.5 g/hr (51, 85). The timing of 2-PAM administration is important. It should be given after atropine, as it has little clinical effect when given alone. In addition, because of the problem of aging, it should be given as early in the course of treatment as possible. In most OP insecticide or nerve agent poisonings, it will be effective if given within 24 hours and occasionally as long as 48 hours after exposure. 2-PAM is of questionable value in treating agents that age rapidly (soman), agents whose AchE inhibition is easily reversible (carbamates), and some insecticides that are resistant to its effects (including ciodrin, dimefox, dimethoate, methyl diazinon, methyl phencapton, phorate, schradan, and wepsyn) (84). In treatment of the acute intoxication, however,

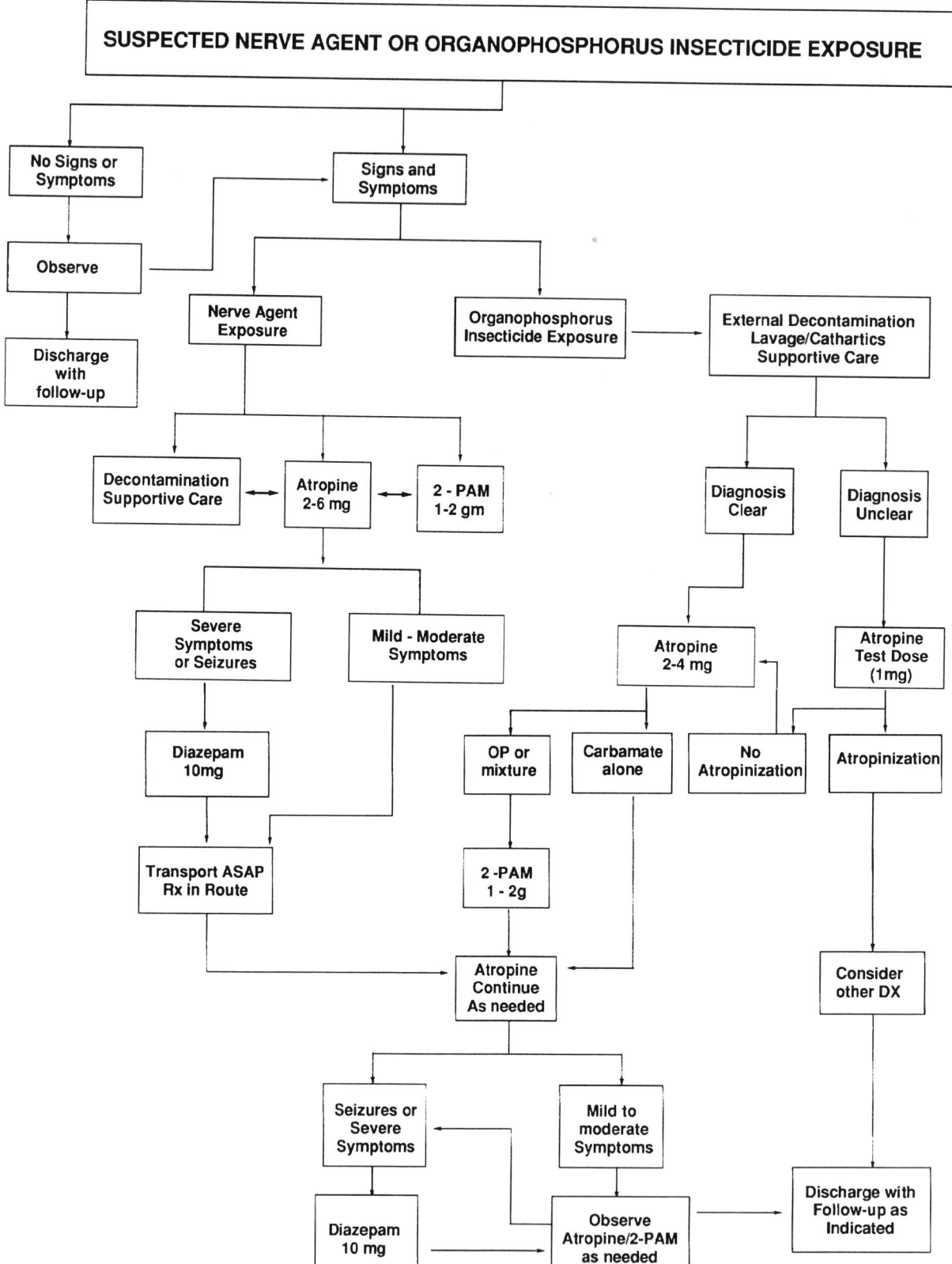

Figure 56.4. This is a flow diagram illustrating the steps in the initial diagnosis and treatment of suspected exposure to organophosphorus compounds. Carbamates, although not organophosphorus compounds themselves, are included in this diagram, since they can produce similar signs and symptoms in exposed individuals. Twenty–four hours of observation is appropriate in a patient with suspected exposure but no symptoms. If symptoms of AchE inhibition occur during that time, specific treatment should be initiated. In the absence of symptoms, the patient may be discharged, with follow–up as needed. Although aggressive decontamination and supportive care are vital to the treatment of exposed patients, the use of atropine is still the cornerstone of therapy. If the diagnosis is still uncertain, the response to a 1 mg test dose of atropine may be helpful. Resistance to atropine confirms

2-PAM is normally used, as the offending agent may be unknown or a mixture of agents may have been used. If symptoms return, repeat boluses of 0.5 to 1 g 2-PAM may be given every 8 to 12 hours for 48 hours (4, 51) or a continuous infusion of 0.5 g/hour started (85). Overzealous use or overly rapid injection of 2-PAM can cause tachycardia and brief neuromuscular block (84). This result could lead to the erroneous conclusion that the patient is atropinized and that 2-PAM is ineffective. A return of muscular strength and a rise in RBC cholinesterase activity will confirm the efficacy of 2-PAM. CNS depressant drugs, including phenothiazines, barbiturates, opiates, and alcohol, should be avoided (6, 73).

Pyridostigmine offers additional benefit by reversibly inhibiting AchE, thus protecting it from nerve agent binding. This protected AchE can then be converted back to an active enzyme and decrease Ach levels toward normal. Unfortunately, pyridostigmine must be taken prophylactically in order to be effective. Since most civilian exposures cannot be anticipated, pyridostigmine has little use in this population. Pyridostigmine pretreatment could be of benefit if a terrorist threat existed in a specific area or if a storage site for nerve agent was leaking or on fire. Physicians caring for patients who have been treated with pyridostigmine or have low AchE levels must be especially cautious in the use of anesthetics such as succinylcholine, which require AchE for metabolism (see the section entitled "Pyridostigmine"). If the use of such drugs is necessary, a small dose should be used initially and increased to the minimum effective dose. This dose is best determined by following the response to peripheral nerve stimulators (114).

Atropine is only partially effective in treating the CNS effects of OP toxicity, probably because of its poor penetration of the blood–brain barrier. Acute CNS effects are limited primarily to mental status changes and seizures. Mental status changes ranging from agitation to coma are seen, with more severe symptoms suggesting a more severe exposure. Although only limited data are available, cholinolytics with greater CNS penetration, such as scopolamine, may offer additional benefit. Seizures, a major problem in OP poisoning, are associated with a worse prognosis and, in animals, brain damage. Other than the benzodiazepines, most anticonvulsants are of limited value in treating OP–induced seizures. Of the benzodiazepines, diazepam is the most thoroughly studied. Diazepam should be given i.v. or i.m. in 5 to 10 mg increments until seizure activity stops. Special care should be taken when evaluating a paralyzed patient, as seizure activity and brain hypoxia can occur in such a patient in the absence of convulsions. Drugs that lower the seizure threshold, including theophylline, should be avoided (73).

Early deaths are largely the result of respiratory failure, and later deaths, of dysrhythmias. Recurrence of symptoms has been reported to occur after smoking, discontinuation of therapy, or exercise (34). If symptoms recur, retreatment

should be initiated immediately. Hemoperfusion, but not hemodialysis, may be of value (6, 73). Figure 56.4 summarizes the management of OP poisoning.

TREATMENT METHODS UNDER DEVELOPMENT

The current medications atropine, 2-PAM, pyridostigmine, and diazepam treat nerve agent poisoning at the muscarinic, nicotinic, and CNS sites after AchE inhibition has already occurred. Another strategy is to use drugs known as scavengers to bind or trap OP agents in the blood before tissue AchE sites are reached. Scavengers currently being studied are classified as hydrolases, β–cyclodextrans, antibodies, or exogenous cholinesterase (44, 170).

Since nerve agents are metabolized slowly in humans, an obvious approach was to isolate and study these drug-metabolizing enzymes, called hydrolases, as obtained from different sources. Mammalian hydrolase activity was first described in 1946, but progress in this research area has been slow because of the difficulty of isolating and purifying the enzymes. Recently, soman–hydrolyzing activity has been demonstrated in a clonal neuronal cell line (171). A squid hydrolase, active against organophosphorus compounds, has been isolated and purified and is now being studied in vitro (172). Paraoxon hydrolase obtained from bacteria has recently been shown to protect mice from multiple lethal doses of paraoxon (173).

Cyclodextrans are cyclic polymers of dextrose that trap soman inside a cavity in their structure. This trapping then becomes permanent as a result of the formation of a covalent bond (174). Cyclodextrans have now been shown to provide a small protective effect in vivo (guinea pigs) (174). Further studies to increase the effectiveness of these compounds are ongoing.

Monoclonal antibodies have had increasing use in clinical medicine. A monoclonal antibody specific for soman was described in 1984 (175), but its affinity was too low to be clinically useful. More recently, monoclonal antibodies with stereospecificity and catalytic properties have been produced (175a–177). Antibodies that block OP binding to AchE are also under study (178). This area of investigation is still far from being ready for use in humans, but it is very exciting. If antibodies with catalytic properties can be perfected, only a relatively low blood level would be needed for clinical efficacy. Of these new methods, the use of exogenous cholinesterase to bind and inactivate nerve agents before they reach tissue sites is the most promising. Wolfe et al (179) showed that AchE, purified from fetal bovine serum, protected mice from multiple lethal doses of soman and VX. Subsequently, purified butyrylcholinesterase (BuChE) and AchE have been shown not only to protect monkeys against death from three to five lethal doses of soman, but also to prevent a performance decrement (180–182). As a result of the recent cloning of the

exposure to AchE inhibitors, while the development of dry mouth, warm skin, and tachycardia suggests the need for an alternate diagnosis. The initial dose of atropine given increases with the severity of agent exposure. Atropine should be given parenterally every 15 to 30 minutes until the muscarinic symptoms have resolved and the patient has mild symptoms of atropine excess (atropinization). Atropine should then be repeated as needed to maintain a state of mild atropinization for at least 48 hours. 2-PAM should be given to all patients unless their exposure has been to carbamates alone. In patients with severe exposure, as indicated by significant atropine resistance or seizure activity, diazepam should be given in a dose sufficient to suppress seizure activity. (See text for a more detailed discussion.)

human genes for BuChE and AchE (183), and the expression of genes by *Escherichia coli* (184), studies of human cholinesterase are now possible. Maxwell et al (185) have shown that human BuChE protects mice from the lethal and behavioral effects of four lethal doses of soman.

MILITARY TREATMENT

The military faces a unique situation in the treatment of nerve agent exposure. Not only is the risk of exposure higher than that of a civilian population, but soldiers are also more likely to be exposed in a location without fixed hospitals and ventilatory support. To respond to these problems and the anticipated exposure of two to five LD_{50} of nerve agents on the battlefield, the U.S. military has developed an effective treatment plan (34).

The centerpiece of this plan is, of course, to avoid or minimize exposure. Protective clothing is provided to each soldier, including an effective gas mask with hood and cloth, an activated charcoal-laminated shirt and pants, and rubber gloves and boot covers. Once the protective barrier is breached and significant exposure has occurred, medical treatment is necessary. To be effective in a battlefield environment, this therapy must utilize drugs that can be administered rapidly by nonmedical personnel without removal of protective clothing, reach protective blood levels rapidly, have a prolonged therapeutic effect, and have few side effects. Atropine and 2-PAM meet many of these requirements but needed a new delivery system.

To respond to this need, autoinjectors were developed. These devices consist of a preloaded syringe with a retracted, spring-loaded needle. Upon impact against the lateral thigh, the needle extends, penetrates the clothing, and injects the contents into the muscle. At least three different types of autoinjectors have been used to date: the Mark I, which has two independently activated syringes (one of atropine and one of 2-PAM); the Mark II, with two syringes activated simultaneously with injection of atropine and 2-PAM through separate needles; and a multichambered pen injector (MCP) that allows injection of atropine and 2-PAM through the same needle. Pharmacokinetic parameters are similar or superior to those found for atropine and 2-PAM given by conventional i.m. injection. Each soldier carries an equivalent of three atropine (2 mg each) and three 2-PAM (600 mg each) doses. Medical aide personnel carry additional injectors. Current guidelines recommend the use of these autoinjectors in doses depending on the site of exposure as well as the rapidity of onset and the severity of symptoms. Diazepam injectors (10 mg in 2 cc) are also carried and should be given after the third Mark I injector (or equivalent) has been given. Because of the possibility of abuse, and because soldiers requiring diazepam are sick, diazepam autoinjectors are intended for "buddy" administration rather than self-use.

Pyridostigmine, intended for prophylactic use, is given orally in a dose of 30 mg t.i.d. It is supplied to the soldier in blister packs of 21 tablets (7-day supply).

CHRONIC EFFECTS

Although most of the effects of OP poisoning are seen acutely, some chronic effects have been described. The majority of these effects are on the nervous system, involving either the CNS or peripheral nerves. Persistent behavioral changes, including depression, increased irritability, confusion, and decreased ability to concentrate, have been described in survivors of OP poisoning (107, 186). Many of these survivors also complain of headache, weakness, numbness, and visual disturbances (6, 35, 158, 186) that may persist for 6 to 12 months or, occasionally, longer (35, 187). EEG abnormalities may also persist for more than a year (187, 188). The mechanism by which these persistent changes occur and the long-term consequences on human health are unknown.

The most well-known chronic neurotoxic effect is called *organophosphate-induced delayed neurotoxicity* (OPIDN) (189). Clinical interest in this neuropathy began with the description of a curious spastic paralysis associated with the use of Jamaican rum (190). This so-called Ginger Jake paralysis reached epidemic proportions, involving more than 20,000 cases in the U.S. Its cause was found to be a contaminant (triorthocresylphosphate, or TOCP) of Jamaican ginger used in the production of rum. A typical case presented initially as a mixed sensorimotor peripheral neuropathy of the lower extremities with muscle cramps, paresthesias, ataxia, and weakness. The weakness progressed first to a flaccid paralysis and then to a spastic paralysis with hyperreflexia, clonus, and a characteristic gait. In some exposures the involvement may appear to "ascend" to involve the upper extremities as well.

Although these early cases occurred as a result of chronic exposure, similar toxicity can be seen 2 to 4 weeks after a single exposure to certain OP insecticides and nerve agents (189, 191). Symptoms usually improve in months to years (191), but recovery is often incomplete (6). Although the etiology remains unknown, toxicity correlates with the inhibition of a nonspecific neuronal enzyme called neuropathic target esterase (6, 189, 191, 192). Histologically, there appears to be focal injury with Wallerian degeneration of the axon followed by demyelination. The injury tends to be worse distally and greater in large fibers. There is no known effective treatment. All of the nerve agents except VX have been shown to cause delayed neurotoxicity in susceptible animals when given in high doses (193). No cases have been reported in humans (27). Currently, OP insecticides are tested for delayed neurotoxicity using a hen model prior to release (191).

In addition, a so-called intermediate syndrome has been described (194–196). This syndrome presents as weakness of the proximal limbs and respiratory muscles that occurs 24 to 96 hours after the initial OP intoxication, usually at a time when the cholinergic symptoms have resolved. Cranial nerve involvement may be prominent and precedes respiratory paralysis (196). There is a significant risk of death if prompt respiratory support is not provided. Symptoms resolve spontaneously in 4 to 18 days.

The possible relationship between OP or nerve agent exposure and the subsequent risk of cancer or birth defects has not been thoroughly studied. Whereas an increased mutagenesis rate in response to some organophosporuses has been seen in vitro, no conclusive carcinogenic or teratogenic effect has been demonstrated in humans (5, 50). Initial studies of teratogenicity and carcinogenicity following nerve agent exposure have been negative (27).

SUMMARY

Four nerve agents have been developed for military use. Although their physical properties differ, they all act by a common mechanism, namely, the irreversible inhibition of AchE. The resulting inability to metabolize Ach leads to its accumulation at cholinergic nerve sites, with an overstimulation of the postsynaptic fiber (nerve or muscle) and the glands or organs that these fibers innervate. This stimulation is expressed in patients as a combination of copious secretion, intense contraction of smooth muscle (miosis, bronchospasm, abdominal pain, urinary and fecal incontinence), weakness or paralysis, mental status changes, seizures, and often death. Larger doses usually cause more severe symptoms that begin sooner and progress more rapidly.

Fortunately, experience with human exposure to nerve agents is quite limited. OP insecticides, although less toxic than nerve agents, are structurally similar to them and act by the same mechanism. Their worldwide use has led to many severe intoxications and death. Effective treatment regimens using patient decontamination, aggressive supportive care, and a combination of medications (cholinolytics, enzyme reactivators, and anticonvulsants) have been developed and successfully applied to cases of accidental nerve agent exposure.

ACKNOWLEDGMENTS

We would like to offer special thanks to Ms. Sylvia Hennighan for her tireless dedication in the preparation of this manuscript. Without her help it would not have been possible.

REFERENCES

1. World Health Organization: *Safe Use of Pesticides: Twentieth Report of the World Health Organization Expert Committee on Pesticides.* World Health Organization, Geneva, WHO Technical Report Series 513, 1973.
2. Copplestone JF: A global view of pesticide safety. In Watson DL and Brown AWA (eds): *Pesticide Management and Pesticide Resistance.* New York, Academic Press, 1977.
3. Economic and Social Commission of Asia and the Pacific (ESCAP): *Development/Environmental Trends in Asia and the Pacific: A Regional Overview.* Bangkok, ESCAP, 1983.
4. Tafuri J, Roberts J: Organophosphate poisoning. *Ann Emerg Med* 16:193–202, 1987.
5. Murphy SD: Toxic effects of pesticides. In Klaassen CD, Amdus MO, Doull J (eds): *Casarett and Doull's Toxicology,* ed 3. New York, Macmillan, 1986, pp 519–581.
6. Ellenhorn MJ, Barceloux DG: Pesticides. In *Medical Toxicology: Diagnosis and Treatment of Human Poisoning.* New York, Elsevier, 1988, pp 1069–1105.
7. Ames RG, Brown SK, Mengle DC, Kahn E, Stratton JW, Jackson RJ: Protecting agricultural applicators from over–exposure to cholinesterase–inhibiting pesticides: perspectives from the California Programme. *J Soc Occup Med* 39:85–92, 1989.
8. De Clermont P: Chimic organique–note sur la preparation de quelques ethers. *C R Acad Sci* 39:338–341, 1854.
9. Schrader G: Die Entwicklung Neuer Insektizide auf Grundlage Organischer Fluor– und Phosphoverbindungen. Monographic no 62. Weinheim, Verlag Chemic, 1952.
10. Holmstedt B: Structure–activity relationships of the organophosphorus anticholinesterase agents. In Koelle GB (ed): *Cholinesterases and Anticholinesterase Agents.* Berlin, Springer–Verlag, pp 428–485, 1963.
11. SIPRI: *The Problem of Chemical and Biological Warfare. Vol i: The Rise of CB Weapons.* New York, Humanities Press, 1976.
12. Anonymous: *Soviet Chemical Weapons Threat.* Publication DST-1620F–051–85. Washington, DC, US Defense Intelligence Agency, 1985.
13. Holmstedt B: Pharmacology of organophosphorus cholinesterase inhibitors. *Pharmacol Rev* 11:567–688, 1959.
14. SIPRI: *The Problem of Chemical and Biological Warfare. Vol II: CB Weapons Today.* New York, Humanities Press, 1973.
15. Koelle GB: Organophosphate poisoning–an overview. *Fundam Appl Toxicol* 1:129–134, 1981.
16. Robinson JP: Chemical warfare capabilities of the Warsaw and North Atlantic Treaty Organizations: an overview from sources. In SIPRI, *Chemical Weapons, Destruction and Conversion.* Crane, Russak, & Co., New York, pp 9–56, 1980.
17. Meselson M, Robinson JP: Chemical warfare and chemical disarmament. *Sci Am* 242:38–47, 1980.
18. Orient JM: Chemical and biological warfare: should defenses be researched and deployed? *JAMA* 262:644–648, 1989.
19. Apt KE: Chemical Warfare Arms Control: Issues and Challenges. Los Alamos, NM, Center for National Security Studies, Los Alamos National Laboratory, report no. 6, LA11451, 1988.
20. Norman C: CIA details chemical weapons spread. *Science* 243:888, 1989.
21. United Nations Security Council: *Report of the Specialists Appointed by the Secretary–General to Investigate Allegations by the Islamic Republic of Iran Concerning the Use of Chemical Weapons.* New York, document S16433, 1984.
22. United Nations Security Council: *Report of the Mission Dispatched by the Secretary–General to Investigate Allegations of the Use of Chemical Weapons in the Conflict Between the Islamic Republic of Iran and Iraq.* New York, document S17911, 1986.
23. United Nations Security Council: *Report of the Mission Dispatched by the Secretary–General to Investigate Allegations of the Use of Chemical Weapons in the Conflict Between the Islamic Republic of Iran and Iraq.* New York, document S18852, 1987.
24. Anderson G: Analysis of two chemical weapons samples from the Iran–Iraq War. *Nuc Biol Chem Defense Tech Inter* 62–65, 1986.
25. Robinson JP: A summary of western sources on Soviet and Warsaw Pact chemical weapons. In Meselson M (ed): *Chemical Weapons and Chemical Arms Control.* New York, Carnegie Endowment for International Peace, 1977.
26. Anonymous: Chemical and bacteriological weapons in the 1980's. *Lancet* 2:141–143, 1984.
27. Carnes SA, Watson AP: Disposing of the US chemical weapons stockpile: an approaching reality. *JAMA* 262:653–659, 1989.
28. Budiansky S: Qualified approval for binary chemical weapons. *Science* 234:930–932, 1986.
29. Anonymous: *Chemical Agent Data Sheets.* Vols I and II. Aberdeen Proving Ground, MD, Department of the Army, Headquarters, Edgewood Arsenal, Edgewood Arsenal Special Report EO–SR–74001, 1974.
30. Fielding GH: *V Agent Information Summary.* Washington, DC, US Naval Research Laboratory, NRL report 5421, 1960.
31. Zhou J: *Chinese Medical Encyclopedia: Protective Medicine Against Chemical Weapons.* Shanghai, Shaghai Science and Technology, 1985.
32. Compton JAF: Nerve agents. In *Military Chemical and Biological Agents: Chemical and Toxicological Properties.* Telford Press, Caldwell, NJ, pp 135-188, 1988.
33. Inns RH, Leadbeater L: The efficacy of bispyridinium derivatives in the treatment of organophosphate poisoning in the guinea–pig. *J Pharm Pharmacol* 35:427–433, 1983.
34. Anonymous: Nerve agents. In *Treatment of Chemical Casualties and Conventional Military Chemical Injuries.* Washington, DC, US Army Field Manual FM–8–285, pp 2–1–2–19, 1990.
35. Grob D, Johns RJ: Use of oximes in the treatment of intoxication by anticholinesterase compounds in normal subjects. *Am J Med* 24:497–511, 1958.
36. Grob D, Harvey JC: Effects in man of the anticholinesterase compound sarin (isopropyl methyl phosphonofluoridate). *J Clin Invest* 37:350–368, 1958.
37. Bŏsković B: The treatment of soman poisoning and its perspectives. *Fundam Appl Toxicol* 1:203–213, 1981.
38. Wolthuis OL, Berends F, Meeter E: Problems in the therapy of soman poisoning. *Fundam Appl Toxicol* 1:183–192, 1981.
39. DuBois KP, Doull J, Salerro PR, Coon JM: Studies on the toxicity and mechanism of action of p–nitrophenyldiethyl thionophosphate (parathion). *J Pharmacol* 95:79–91, 1949.
40. Grob D, Harvey AM: Effects and treatment of nerve gas poisoning. *Am J Med* 14:52–63, 1953.
41. Grob D: The manifestations and treatment of poisoning due to nerve gas and other organic phosphate anticholinesterase compounds. *Arch Intern Med* 98:221–239, 1956.
42. Sidell FR: Soman and sarin: clinical manifestations and treatment of accidental poisoning by organophosphates. *Clin Toxicol* 7:1–17, 1974.
43. Rickett DJ, Glenn JF, Houston WE: Medical defense against nerve agents: new directions. *Milit Med* 152:35–41, 1987.
44. Dunn MA, Sidell FR: Progress in medical defense against nerve agents. *JAMA* 262:649–652, 1989.
45. Lundy PM, Magor GR: Cyclic GMP concentrations in cerebellum following organophosphate administration. *J Pharm Pharmacol* 30:251–252, 1978.

46. Clement JG: Hormonal consequences of organophosphate poisoning. *Fundam Appl Toxicol* 5:S61–S77, 1985.

47. Sevaljević C, Marinković S, Bogojević S, Boković B: Soman intoxication–induced changes in serum acute phase protein levels, corticosterone concentration and immunosuppressive potency of the serum. *Arch Toxicol* 63:406–411, 1989.

48. Smallridge RC, Carr FE, Fein HG: Diisopropylfluorophosphate (DFP) reduces serum prolactin, thyrotropin, luteinizing hormone, and growth hormone and increases adrenocorticotropin and corticosterone in rats: involvement of dopaminergic and somatostatinergic as well as cholinergic pathways. *Toxicol Appl Pharmacol* 108:284–295, 1991.

49. Anonymous: Diazepam: anticonvulsive therapy for nerve agent intoxication. Aberdeen Proving Ground, MD, US Army Medical Research Institute of Chemical Defense, USAMRICD Tech. Memo 90–3, 1990.

50. Milton NA, Murray VSG: A review of organophosphate poisoning. *Med Toxicol* 3:350–375, 1988.

51. Haddad LM: Organophosphates and other insecticides. In Haddad LM, Winchester JF (eds): *Clinical Management of Poisoning and Drug Overdose*, ed 2. Philadelphia, W.B. Saunders, pp 1076–1087, 1990.

52. World Health Organization: *Organophosphorus Insecticides: A General Introduction*. Geneva, Switzerland, 1986.

53. Bonner TI, Buckley NJ, Young AC, Brann MR: Identification of a family of muscarinic acetylcholine receptor genes. *Science* 237:527–532, 1987.

54. Brown JH: Atropine, scopolamine, and related antimuscarinic drugs. In Gilman AG, Rall TW, Niew AS, Taylor P (eds): *Goodman and Gilman's the Pharmacological Basis of Therapeutics*, ed 8. New York, Macmillan, pp 150–165, 1991.

55. Metcalfe RF: A sensitive radioreceptor assay for atropine in plasma. *Biochem Pharmacol* 30:209–212, 1981.

56. Virtanen R, Kanto J, Iisalo E, Iisalo EUM, Salo M, Sjövall S: Pharmacokinetic studies on atropine with special reference to age. *Acta Anaesthesiol Scand* 26:297–300, 1982.

57. Kanto J, Virtanen R, Iisalo E, Mäenpää K, Liukko P: Placental transfer and pharmacokinetics of atropine after a single maternal intravenous and intramuscular administration. *Acta Anesthesiol Scand* 25:85–88, 1981.

58. Adams RG, Verma P, Jackson AJ, Miller RL: Plasma pharmacokinetics of intravenously administered atropine in normal human subjects. *J Clin Pharmacol* 22:477–481, 1982.

59. Harrison LI, Smallridge RC, Lasseter KC, et al: Comparative absorption of inhaled and intramuscularly administered atropine. *Am Rev Respir Dis* 134:254–257, 1986.

60. Pihlajamäki K, Hovi–Viander M, Kanto J: Effect of induced hypotension on serum concentrations of atropine after intramuscular administration. *Acta Anesthesiol Scand* 30:64–65, 1986.

61. Friedl KE, Hannan CJ, Schadler PW, et al: Atropine absorption after administration with 2–pralidoxime chloride by automatic injector. Fort Detrick, MD, US Army Research and Development Command, report no. 87–1, 1987.

62. Smallridge RC, Fein HG, Umstott CE, et al: Pharmacokinetics of atropine in resting normal volunteers: equivalent bioavailability by intramuscular and intravenous routes. In *Proceedings of the Sixth Medical Chemical Defense Bioscience Review*. Aberdeen Proving Ground, MD, US Army Medical Research Institute of Chemical Defense:719–722, 1987.

63. Kamimori GH, Smallridge RC, Redmond DP, Belenky GL, Fein HG: The effect of exercise on atropine pharmacokinetics. *Eur J Clin Pharmacol* 39:395–397, 1990.

64. Ellinwood Jr EH, Nikaido AM, Gupta SK, Heatherly DG, Nishita JK: Comparison of central nervous system and peripheral pharmacodynamics to atropine pharmacokinetics. *J Pharmacol Exp Ther* 255:1133–1139, 1990.

65. Bejersten A, Olsson GL, Palmér L: The influence of body weight on plasma concentration of atropine after rectal administration in children. *Acta Anaesthesiol Scand* 29:782–784, 1985.

66. Mundie TG, Pamplin CL III, Phillips YY, Smallridge RC: Effect of exercise in sheep on the absorption of intramuscular atropine sulfate. *Pharmacology* 37:132–136, 1988.

67. Smallridge RC, Chernow B, Teich S, et al: Atropine pharmacokinetics are affected by moderate hemorrhage and hypothyroidism. *Crit Care Med* 17:1254–1257, 1989.

68. Moore DH, Smallridge RC, Von Bredow JD, Lukey BJ: The pharmacokinetics of atropine and diazepam in sheep: intramuscular co-administration. *Biopharm Drug Dispos* 12:525–536, 1991.

69. Du Toit P, Muller F, Van Tonder W, et al: Experience with the intensive care management of organophosphate insecticide poisoning. *S Afr Med J* 60:227–229, 1981.

70. Golsousidis H, Kokkas V: Use of 19,590 mg of atropine during 24 days of treatment, after a case of unusually severe parathion poisoning. *Hum Toxicol* 4:339–340, 1985.

71. Lotti M: Treatment of acute organophosphate poisoning. *Med J Aust* 154:51–55, 1991.

72. Anonymous: Nerve agents. In *Medical Manual of Defense Against Chemical Agents*. London, Great Britain Ministry of Defense, Her Majesty's Stationery Office, 1972.

73. Anonymous: Parathion. In Gosselin RE, Smith RP, Hodge HC, (eds): *Clinical Toxicology of Commercial Products*, ed 5. Baltimore, Williams & Wilkins, pp III–336–III–343, 1984.

74. Le Blanc FW, Benson BE, Gilg AD: A severe organophosphate poisoning requiring the use of an atropine drug. *Clin Toxicol* 24:69–76, 1986.

75. Ferrando R: Preventable acute organophosphate poisoning deaths. *Cey Med J* 34:139–142, 1989.

76. Taylor P: Anticholinesterase agents. In Gilman AG, Rall TW, Nies AS, Taylor P (eds): *Goodman and Gilman's the Pharmacological Basis of Therapeutics*, ed 8. New York, Pergamon Press, pp 131–149, 1991.

77. Woods JR: Medical problems in chemical warfare. *JAMA* 144:606–609, 1950.

78. Rump S, Faff J: Limitations of pharmacotherapy in organophosphate intoxications. In SPIRI, *Medical Protection Against Chemical Warfare Agents*. Stockholm, Almquist & Wiksell, pp 109–116, 1976.

79. Witkin JM, Gordon RK, Chiang PK: Comparison of in vitro actions with behavioral effects of antimuscarinic agents. *J Pharmacol Exp Ther* 242:796–803, 1987.

80. Tracey JA, Gallagher H: Use of glycopyrrolate and atropine in acute organophosphorus poisoning. *Hum Exp Toxicol* 9:99–100, 1990.

81. Wilson H, Ginsburg S: Powerful reactivator of alkylphosphate–inhibited acetylcholinesterase. *Biochem Biophys Acta* 18:168–170, 1955.

82. Namba T, Hiraki K: PAM (pyridine–2–aldoxime methiodide) therapy for alkylphosphate poisoning. *JAMA* 166:1834–1839, 1958.

83. Swartz RD, Sidell FR: Effects of heat and exercise on the elimination of pralidoxime in man. *Clin Pharmacol Ther* 14:83–89, 1973.

84. Schumacher MM, Dowd AL (eds): *Physicians' Desk Reference*, ed 45. Oradell, NJ, Medical Economics Data, 1991.

85. Namba T, Nolte CT, Jackrel J, Grob D: Poisoning due to organophosphate insecticides. *Am J Med* 50:475–492, 1971.

86. Briggs CJ, Simons KJ: Recent advances in the mechanism and treatment of organophosphate poisoning. *Pharm Int* 7:155–159, 1986.

87. Chinn J, Kluwe W, Stabus A, Hayes T, Joiner R: Pharmacokinetic evaluations of atropine, pralidoxime chloride, and pyridostigmine in rhesus monkeys. In *Proceedings of the Sixth Medical Chemical Defense Bioscience Review*. Aberdeen Proving Ground, MD, US Army Medical Research Institute of Chemical Defense, pp 217–225, 1987.

88. Jovanović D: Pharmacokinetics of pralidoxime chloride: a comparative study in healthy volunteers and in organophosphate poisoning. *Arch Toxicol* 63:416–418, 1989.

89. Sidell FR: Clinical aspects of intoxication by cholinesterase inhibitors. In *Medical Protection Against Chemical Warfare Agents*. Stockholm, Almquist & Wiksell, pp 22–35, 1976.

90. Headley DB: Effects of atropine sulfate and pralidoxime chloride on visual, physiological, performance, subjective, and cognitive variables in man: a review. *Milit Med* 147:122–132, 1982.

91. Haegerstrom–Portnoy G, Jones R, Adams AJ, Jampolsky A: Effects of atropine and 2-PAM chloride on vision and performance. In *Proceedings of the Fifth Annual Chemical Defense Bioscience Review*. Aberdeen Proving Ground, MD, US Army Medical Research Institute of Chemical Defense, pp 209–228 1985.

92. Penetar DA, Haegerstrom–Portnoy G: Combined effects of atropine and 2-PAM Cl on tracking performance, physiological, psychological, and visual functions. In *Proceedings of the Sixth Medical Chemical Defense Bioscience Review*. Aberdeen Proving Ground, MD, US Army Medical Research Institute of Chemical Defense, pp 613–616, 1987.

93. Sidell FR, Groff WA, Ellin RI: Blood levels of oxime and symptoms in humans after single and multiple oral doses of 2–pyridine aldoxime methochloride. *J Pharm Sci* 58:1093–1098, 1969.

94. Erdmann WD: Success and failure of oximes therapy in acute poisoning by organophosphorus compounds. In SIPRI, *Medical Protection Against Chemical Warfare Agents*. Stockholm, Almquist & Wiksell, pp 46–52, 1976.

95. Natoff IL, Reiff B: Effect of oximes on the acute toxicity of anticholinesterase carbamates. *Toxicol Appl Pharmacol* 25:569–575, 1973.

96. Schoene K: Kinetic studies on chemical reactions between acetylcholinesterase, toxic organophosphates and pyridinium oximes. In SIPRI, *Medical Protection Against Chemical Warfare Agents*. Stockholm: Almquist & Wiksell, pp 88–100, 1976.

97. Gutmann L, Besser R: Organophosphate intoxication: pharmacologic, neurophysiologic, clinical, and therapeutic considerations. *Semin Neurol* 10:46–51, 1990.

98. Oldiges H: Comparative studies of the protective effects of pyridinium compounds against organophosphate poisoning. In SIPRI. *Medical Protection Against Chemical Warfare Agents*. Stockholm, Almquist & Wiksell, pp 101–108, 1976.

99. Stares JES: Medical protection against chemical warfare agents. In SIPRI, *Medical Protection Against Chemical Warfare Agents*. Stockholm, Almquist & Wiksell, pp 157–166, 1976.

100. Vojuodić V, Bŏsković B: A comparative study of pralidoxime, obidoxime, and trimedoxime in healthy men volunteers and in rats. In *Medical Protection Against Chemical Warfare Agents*. Stockholm, Almquist & Wiksell, pp 65–73, 1976.

101. Kusic R, Bŏskovíc B, Vojvodíc V, Jovanovíc D: HI-6 in man: blood levels, urinary excretion, and tolerance after intramuscular administration of the oxime to healthy volunteers. *Fundam Appl Toxicol* 5:S89–S97, 1985.

102. Hamilton MG, Lundy PM: HI-6 therapy of soman and tabun poisoning in primates and rodents. *Arch Toxicol* 63:144–149, 1989.

103. Lipp J, Dola T: Comparison of the efficacy of HS–6 versus HI–6 when combined with atropine, pyridostigmine, and clonazepam for soman poisoning in the monkey. *Arch Int Pharmacodyn* 246:138–148, 1980.

104. Clement JG, Lee MJ, Simons KJ, Briggs CJ: Pharmacokinetics of the acetylcholinesterase oxime reactivator, HI-6, in rhesus monkeys (Macaca mulatta): effect of atropine diazepam, and methoxyflurane anesthesia. *Biopharm Drug Dispos* 11:227–232, 1990.

105. Olson CT, Menton RG, Kiser RC, Matthews MC, Dill GS: Bioequivalence of atropine and HI-6 when delivered by wet/dry autoinjector or by syringe. In *Proceedings of the 1991 Medical Chemical Defense Bioscience Review*. Aberdeen Proving Ground, MD, US Army Medical Research Institute of Chemical Defense, pp 607–610, 1991.

106. de Jong LP, Wolring GZ: Reactivation of acetylcholinesterase inhibited by 1,2,2′–trimethyl–propyl methylphosphonofluoridate (soman) with HI-6 and related oximes. *Biochem Pharmacol* 29:2379–2387, 1980.

107. Keeler JR, Hurst CG, Dunn MA: Pyridostigmine used as a nerve agent pretreatment under wartime conditions. *JAMA* 266:693–695, 1991.

108. Anonymous: Pyridostigmine. Aberdeen Proving Ground, MD, USAMRICD technical memo 90–4, pp 2–11, 1990.

109. Breyer–Pfaff U, Maier U, Brinkmann AM, Schumm F: Pyridostigmine kinetics in healthy subjects and patients with myasthenia gravis. *Clin Pharmacol Ther* 37:495–501, 1985.

110. Cronnelly R, Stanski D, Miller RD, Sheiner LB: Pyridostigmine kinetics with and without renal function. *Clin Pharmacol Ther* 28:78–81, 1980.

111. Xia D, Wang L, Pei S: The inhibition and protection of cholinesterase by physostigmine and pyridostigmine against soman poisoning in vivo. *Fundam Appl Toxicol* 1:217–221, 1981.

112. Parker FR, Barbar JA, Forster EM, Whinnery JE: Chemical warfare prophylaxis: pyridostigmine bromide levels and acetylcholinesterase activity in single and multiple dose protocols. In *Proceedings of the Sixth Medical Chemical Defense Bioscience Review*. Aberdeen Proving Ground, MD, US Army Medical Research Institute of Chemical Defense, pp 661–664, 1987.

113. Calvey TN, Chan K: Plasma pyridostigmine levels in patients with myasthenia gravis. *Clin Pharmacol Ther* 21:187–193, 1977.

114. Keeler JR: Interactions between nerve agent pretreatment and drugs commonly used in combat anesthesia. *Mil Med* 155:527–533, 1990.

115. Kolka MA, Burgoon PW, Quigley MD, Stephenson LA: Red blood cell cholinesterase activity and plasma pyridostigmine concentration during single and multiple dose studies. Natick, MA, US Army Research Institute of Environmental Medicine, technical report T3–91, 1991.

116. Somani SM, Dube SN: Physostigmine–an overview as pretreatment drug for organophosphate intoxication. *Int J Clin Pharm Ther Toxicol* 27:367–387, 1989.

117. Herning RI, Glover BJ, Reddish R: Information processing effects of physostigmine. In *Proceedings of the 1991 Medical Chemical Defense Bioscience Review*. Aberdeen Proving Ground, MD, US Army Medical Research Institute of Chemical Defense, pp 873–876, 1991.

118. Schiflett SG, Miller JC, Gawron VJ: Pyridostigmine bromide effects on performance of tactical transport aircrews. In *Proceedings of the Sixth Medical Chemical Defense Bioscience Review*. Aberdeen Proving Ground, MD, US Army Medical Research Institute of Chemical Defense, pp 609–611, 1987.

119. Boll PA, Whinnery JE, Forster EM, Parker FR, Barber JA: Performance effects of pyridostigmine bromide during and after acceleration stress. In *Proceedings of the 1991 Medical Chemical Defense Bioscience Review*. Aberdeen Proving Ground, MD, US Army Medical Research Institute of Chemical Defense, pp 827–830, 1991.

120. Wenger CB, Latzka WA: Effects of pyridostigmine bromide on physiological responses to heat, exercise and hypohydration. In *Proceedings of the 1991 Medical Chemical Defense Bioscience Review*. Aberdeen Proving Ground, MD, US Army Medical Research Institute of Chemical Defense, pp 841–844, 1991.

121. Osserman KE, Genkins G: Studies in myasthenia gravis: reduction in mortality rate after crisis. *JAMA* 183:97–102, 1963.

122. Johanson WG, Anzweto A, Moore GT, White CD, Berdine CG: Etiology of respiratory failure in organophosphate intoxication in non–human primates. In *Proceedings of the Fifth Annual Chemical Defense Bioscience Review*. Aberdeen Proving Ground, MD, US Army Medical Research Institute of Chemical Defense, pp 32–40, 1985.

123. McLeod Jr CG: Pathology of nerve agents: perspectives on medical management. *Fundam Appl Toxicol* 5:S10–S16, 1985.

124. Petras JM: Soman neurotoxicity. *Fundam Appl Toxicol* 1:242, 1981.

125. McDonough Jr JH, McLeod Jr CG, Nipwoda MT: Direct microinjection of soman or VX into the amygdala produces repetitive limbic convulsions and neuropathology. *Brain Res* 435:123–137, 1987.

126. Shih TM, Capasio BR, Koviak TA, Cook L, Adams NC: Pharmacological mechanism of action of soman–induced convulsions. In *Proceedings of the 1991 Medical Chemical Defense Bioscience Review*. Aberdeen Proving

Ground, MD, US Army Medical Research Institute of Chemical Defense, pp 479–482, 1991.

127. Lipp JA: Effect of benzodiazepine derivatives on soman-induced seizure activity and convulsions in the monkey. *Arch Int Pharmacodyn* 202:244–251, 1973.

128. Hayward IJ, Wall HG, Jaax NK, et al: Decreased brain pathology in organophosphate–exposed rhesus monkeys following benzodiazepine therapy. *J Neurol Sci* 98:99–106, 1990.

129. Karlsson B, Lindgren B, Millquist E, Sandberg M, Sellstr§m A: On the use of diazepam and pro–diazepam (2-benzoyl-4-chloro-N-methyl-N-lysyl glycin anilide) as adjunct antidotes in the treatment of organophosphorus intoxication in the guinea–pig. *J Pharm Pharmacol* 42:247–251, 1990.

130. McDonough JH, Jaax NK, Crowley RA, Mays MZ, Modrow HE: Atropine and/or diazepam therapy protects against soman-induced neural and cardiac pathology. *Fundam Appl Toxicol* 13:256–276, 1989.

131. Harris LW, Anderson DR, Bowersox SL, Chang FCT, Baze WB: Antagonism of soman–induced convulsions by midazolam, diazepam and scopolamine. In *Proceedings of the 1991 Medical Chemical Defense Bioscience Review*. Aberdeen Proving Ground, MD, US Army Medical Research Institute of Chemical Defense, pp 461–464, 1991.

132. Martin LJ, Doebler JA, Shih T, Anthony AA: Protective effect of diazepam pretreatment on soman–induced brain lesion formation. *Brain Res* 325:287–289, 1985.

133. Baze WB, Anderson DR, Harris LW, Lennox WJ, Bowersox SL, Solana RP: Soman–induced brain and heart lesions in the rat: effects of antidotal and anticonvulsant therapy. In *Proceedings of the 1991 Medical Chemical Defense Bioscience Review*. Aberdeen Proving Ground, MD, US Army Medical Research Institute of Chemical Defense, pp 449–452, 1991.

134. Rall TW, Schleifer LS: Drugs effective in the therapy of the epilepsies. In *Goodman and Gilman's the Pharmacological Basis of Therapeutics*, ed 8. New York, Macmillan, pp 436–462, 1991.

135. Shih TM, Koviak TA, Capacio BR: Anticonvulsants for poisoning by the organophosphorus compound soman: pharmacological mechanisms. *Neurosci Biobehav Rev* 15:349–362, 1991.

136. Kaplan SA, Jack ML, Alexander K, Weinfield RE: Pharmacokinetic profile of diazepam in man following single intravenous and oral and chronic oral administrations. *J Pharm Sci* 62:1789–1796, 1973.

137. Klotz U, Avant GR, Hoyumpa A, Schenker S, Wilkinson GR: The effects of age and liver disease on the disposition and elimination of diazepam in adult man. *J Clin Invest* 55:347––359, 1975.

138. Solana RP, Corcoran KD, Von Bredow JD, Lukey BJ: Diazepam efficacy for inhibition of soman-induced convulsions: Interspecies scaling from monkey to man. In *Proceedings of the 1989 Medical Defense Bioscience Review*. Aberdeen Proving Ground, MD, US Army Medical Research and Development Command, pp 459–462, 1989.

139. Blick DW, Murphy MR, Fanton JW, et al: Incapacitation and performance recovery after high–dose soman: effects of diazepam. In *Proceedings of the 1989 Bioscience Review*. Aberdeen Proving Ground, MD, US Army Medical Research and Development Command, pp 219–222, 1989.

140. Castro CA, Finger A, Larsen T, Solana RP, McMaster SB: Behavioral efficacy of diazepam against nerve agent exposure in rhesus monkeys. In *Proceedings of the 1991 Medical Chemical Defense Bioscience Review*. Aberdeen Proving Ground, MD, US Army Medical Research Institute of Chemical Defense, pp 385–392, 1991.

141. von Bredow J, Maitland G, Adams N, et al: Control of soman induced convulsions in carbamate pretreated primates with a water soluble benzodiazepine as an adjunct to therapy. In *Proceedings of the 1991 Medical Chemical Defense Bioscience Review*. Aberdeen Proving Ground, MD, US Army Medical Research Institute of Chemical Defense, pp 519–522, 1991.

142. Olney JW, Collins RC, Sloviter RS: Excitotoxic mechanisms of epileptic brain damage. In Delgado–Escueta AV, Ward AA Jr, Woodbury DM, Porter RJ (eds): *Advances in Neurology*. New York, Raven Press, pp 857–877, 1986.

143. Braitman DJ, Sparenborg SP: MK–801 protects against seizures induced by the cholinesterase inhibitor soman. *Brain Res Bull* 23:145–148, 1989.

144. Tortella FC, Musacchio JM: Dextromethorphan and carbetapentane: centrally acting non–opioid antitussive agents with novel anticonvulsant properties. *Brain Res* 383:314–318, 1986.

145. Tortella FC, Witkin JM, Musaccio JM: Caramiphen: a non-opioid antitussive with potent anticonvulsant properties in rats. *Eur J Pharmacol* 155:69–75, 1988.

146. Sparenborg S, Brennecke LH, Braitman DJ: Prevention of soman neurotoxicity by non–opioid antitussives. *Neurol Toxicol* 11:509–520, 1990.

147. Zweiner RJ, Ginsburg CM: Organophosphate and carbamate poisoning in infants and children. *Pediatrics* 81:121–126, 1988.

148. Sofer S, Tal A, Shahak E: Carbamate and organophosphate poisoning in early childhood. *Pediatr Emerg Care* 5:222–224, 1989.

149. Davies JE, Barquet A, Freed VH, et al: Human pesticide poisoning by a fat soluble organophosphate insecticide. *Arch Environ Health* 30:608–613, 1975.

150. Merrill D, Mihm F: Prolonged toxicity of organophosphate poisoning. *Crit Care Med* 10:550–551, 1982.

151. Dixon E: Dilation of pupils in parathion poisoning. *JAMA* 163:444–445, 1957.

152. Durham W, Hayes W: Organic phosphorus poisoning and its therapy. *Arch Environ Health* 5:21–43, 1962.

153. De Wilde V, Vogelaers D, Colardyn F: Prompt recovery from severe cholinesterase–inhibitor poisoning–remarks on classification and therapy of organophosphate poisoning. *Klin Wochenschr* 68:615–618, 1990.

154. Brock A, Brock V: Plasma cholinesterase activity in a healthy population group with no occupational exposure to known cholinesterase inhibitors: relative influence of some factors related to normal inter- and intra-individual variations. *Scand J Clin Lab Invest* 50:401–408, 1990.

155. Coye MJ, Lowe JH, Maddy KT: Biological monitoring of agricultural workers exposed to pesticides. I. Cholinesterase activity determinations. *J Occup Med* 28:619–627, 1986.

156. Gage JC: The significance of blood cholinesterase activity measurements. *Residue Rev* 18:159–173, 1967.

157. Meller D, Fraser I, Kruger M: Hyperglycemia in anticholinesterase poisoning. *Can Med Assoc J* 124:745–747, 1981.

158. Holmes JH, Gaon MD: Observations on acute and multiple exposure to the anticholinesterase agents. *Trans Am Clin Climatol Assoc* 68:86–103, 1957.

159. Moore PG, James OF: Acute pancreatitis induced by acute organophosphate poisoning. *Postgrad Med J* 57:660–662, 1981.

160. Dressell TO, Goodale RL, Arneson MA, et al: Pancreatitis as a complication of anticholinesterase insecticide intoxication. *Ann Surg* 189:199–204, 1979.

161. Haubenstock A, Hruby K, Jager U: More on the triad of pancreatitis, hyperamylasemia, and hyperglycemia. *JAMA* 249:1563, 1983.

162. Wren C, Carson P, Sanderson J: Organophosphate poisoning and complete heart block. *J Royal Soc Med* 74:688–689, 1981.

163. Kiss Z, Fazekas T: Arrhythmias in organophosphate poisoning. *Acta Cardiol* 34:323–330, 1979.

164. Ludomirsky A, Klein HO, Sorelli P, et al: QT prolongation and polymorphous ("Torsade de Pointes") ventricular arrhythmias associated with organophosphorus insecticide poisoning. *Am J Cardiol* 49:1654–1658, 1982.

165. Lipp JA: Cerebral electrical activity following soman administration. *Arch Int Pharmacodyn Ther* 175:161–169, 1968.

166. Duffy FH, Burchfiel JL, Bartels PH, et al: Long–term effects of an organophosphate upon the human electroencephalogram. *Toxicol Appl Pharmacol* 47:161–176, 1979.

167. Bledsoe F, Seymour E: Acute pulmonary edema associated with parathion poisoning. *Radiology* 103:53–56, 1972.

168. Anonymous: Nerve agents: a brief reference. Aberdeen Proving Ground, MD, US Army Medical Research Institute of Chemical Defense, USAMRICD tech memo 90–1, pp 2–11, 1990.

169. Luzhikov E, Savina A, Shepelev V: On the pathogenesis of cardiac rhythm and conductivity disorders in cases of acute insecticide poisoning. *Kardiologiya* 15:126–129, 1975.

170. Anonymous: Nerve agent scavenger. In: *Medical Chemical Defense.* Aberdeen Proving Ground, MD, US Army Medical Research Institute of Chemical Defense, 3:2–12, 1989.

171. Radharaman R, Boucher LJ, Broomfield CA, Lenz DE: Specific soman–hydrolyzing enzyme activity in a clonal neuronal cell culture. *Biochim Biophys Acta* 967:373–381, 1988.

172. Rajan KS, Mainer S, Hosken FC: Systemic use–potential of DFPase in medical defense. In *Proceedings of the 1991 Medical Chemical Defense Bioscience Review.* Aberdeen Proving Ground, MD, US Army Medical Research Institute of Chemical Defense, pp 505–510, 1991.

173. Ashani Y, Bromberg A, Saxena A, et al: Monoclonal antibodies: probes of acetylcholinesterase function. In *Proceedings of the 1991 Medical Chemical Defense Bioscience Review.* Aberdeen Proving Ground, MD, US Army Medical Research Institute of Chemical Defense, pp 519–523, 1991.

174. Seltzman HH, Narula AS, Lonikar MS: Catalytic cyclodextran enzyme mimics as soman scavengers. In *Proceedings of the 1991 Medical Chemical Defense Bioscience Review.* Aberdeen Proving Ground, MD, US Army Medical Research Institute of Chemical Defense, pp 533–536, 1991.

175. Lenz DE, Brimfield A, Hunter K, Benschop R: Studies using a monoclonal antibody against soman. *Fundam Appl Toxicol* 4:S156–164, 1984.

175a. Lenz DE, Yourick J, Dawson JS, Scott J: Monoclonal antibodies against soman: characterization and stereospecificity. In *Proceedings of the 1991 Medical Chemical Defense Bioscience Review.* Aberdeen Proving Ground,

176. MD, US Army Medical Research Institute of Chemical Defense, pp 551–554, 1991.

176. Shokat KM, Schultz PG: Catalytic antibodies. *Ann Rev Immunol* 8:335–363, 1990.

177. Brimfield AA, Hunter Jr KW, Lenz DE, Benschop HP, Van Dijk C, deJong LPA: Structural and stereochemical specificity of mouse monoclonal antibodies to the organophosphorus nerve agent soman. *Mol Pharmacol* 28:32–39, 1985.

178. Gentry MK, Hur R, Brady DR, Ashani Y, Doctor BP: Isolation and characterization of monoclonal antibodies which inhibit acetylcholinesterases from various species and sources. In *Proceedings of the 1991 Medical Chemical Defense Bioscience Review.* Aberdeen Proving Ground, MD, US Army Medical Research Institute of Chemical Defense, pp 503–506, 1991.

179. Wolfe AD, Rush RS, Doctor BP, et al: Acetylcholinesterase prophylaxis against organophosphate toxicity. *Fundam Appl Toxicol* 9:266–270, 1987.

180. Blick DW, Murphy MR, Miller SA, et al: Protection of primate performance against soman by pretreatment with exogenous cholinesterases. In *Proceedings of the 1991 Medical Chemical Defense Bioscience Review.* Aberdeen Proving Ground, MD, US Army Medical Research Institute of Chemical Defense, pp 355–358, 1991.

181. Broomfield CA, Maxwell DM, Solana RP, Castro CA, Finger AV, Lenz DE: Protection by butyrylcholinesterase against organophosphorus poisoning in nonhuman primates. *J Pharmacol Exp Ther* 259:633–638, 1991.

182. Doctor BP, Brecht K, Castro C, et al: Protection against soman toxicity and prevention of performance decrement in rhesus monkeys by pretreatment with acetylcholinesterase. In *Proceedings of the 1991 Medical Chemical Defense Bioscience Review.* Aberdeen Proving Ground, MD, US Army Medical Research Institute of Chemical Defense, pp 407–413, 1991.

183. Soreq H, Ben–Aziz R, Prody CA, et al: Molecular cloning and construction of the coding region for human acetylcholinesterase reveals a G+C–rich attenuating structure. *Proc Natl Acad Sci USA* 87:9688–9692, 1990.

184. Fischer M, Gorecki M: Expression and isolation of biologically active human acetylcholinesterase from *E. coli.* In *Proceedings of the 1991 Medical Chemical Defense Bioscience Review.* Aberdeen Proving Ground, MD, US Army Medical Research Institute of Chemical Defense, pp 513–518, 1991.

185. Maxwell DM, Wolfe AD, Ashani Y, Doctor BP: Cholinesterase and carboxylesterase as scavengers for organophosphorus agents. In *Proceedings of the 3rd International Meeting on Cholinesterases.* La Grande–Motte, France, May 12–16, pp 206–209, 1990.

186. Gershorn S, Shaw FH: Psychiatric sequelae of chronic exposure to organophosphate insecticides. *Lancet* 1:1371–1374, 1961.

187. Duffy HF, Burchfiel JL, Bartels HP, Goan M, Sim VM: Long-term effects of an organophosphate upon the human electroencephalogram. *Toxicol Appl Pharmacol* 47:161–176, 1979.

188. Burchfiel JL, Duffy HF, Sim VM: Persistent effects of sarin and dieldrin upon the primate electroencephalogram. *Toxicol Appl Pharmacol* 35:365–379, 1976.

189. Abou–Donia MB: Organophosphorus ester–induced delayed neurotoxicity. *Ann Rev Pharmacol Toxicol* 21:511–548, 1981.

190. Morgan JP: The Jamaica ginger paralysis. *JAMA* 248:1864–1867, 1982.

191. Davis CS, Johnson MK, Richardson RJ: Organophosphorus compounds. In O'Donoghue JL (ed): *Neurotoxicity of Industrial and Commercial Chemicals VII.* Boca Raton, FL, CRC Press, pp 1–23, 1985.

192. Johnson MK: The target for initiation of delayed neurotoxicity by organophosphorus esters: biochemical studies and toxicological applications. *Rev Biochem Toxicol* 4:141–212, 1982.

193. Willems JL, Nicaise M, De Bisschop HC: Delayed neuropathy by the organophosphorus nerve agents soman and tabun. *Arch Toxicol* 55:76–77, 1984.

194. Wadia RS, Sadagopan C, Amin RB, Sardesai HV: Neurological manifestations of organophosphorus insecticide poisoning. *J Neurol Neurosurg Psychiatr* 37:841–847, 1974.

195. Senanayake N, Karalliedde L: Neurotoxic effects of organophosphorus insecticides: an intermediate syndrome. *N Engl J Med* 316:761–763, 1987.

196. Wadia RS: The neurology of organophosphorus insecticide poisoning: newer findings, a viewpoint. *J Assoc Phys India* 38:129–131, 1990.

CHAPTER 57

Electrolyte and Acid-Base Disorders

MAN S. OH, M.D.
HUGH J. CARROLL, M.D.

This chapter reviews electrolyte and acid-base disorders with particular reference to those problems that occur frequently in critically ill patients. Discussions stress pathophysiology, diagnosis, and pharmacologic aspects of management.

HYPONATREMIA

Hyponatremia is defined as a reduced plasma sodium concentration (less than 135 mEq/liter) and is the most common electrolyte disorder. Generally, clinical concern arises when concentration is less than 130 mEq/liter (16).

The term pseudohyponatremia is applied to a spurious reduction in serum sodium concentration due to a measurement error. The common causes include hyperlipidemia, hyperproteinemia, or increased viscosity of the plasma. The error in measurement in pseudohyponatremia results from the dilution of the sample (38). Measurements of serum sodium with a flame photometer can result in this type of error because the sample is always diluted for flame-photometric measurement. The error also occurs when an ion-specific electrode is used, if the sample is diluted (indirect method), but can be avoided with a direct method without dilution of the sample (18, 26). In pseudohyponatremia, plasma osmolality, which is customarily measured without dilution, is normal (38). However, a low plasma sodium concentration with a normal plasma osmolality need not indicate the presence of pseudohyponatremia; true hyponatremia may be accompanied by a normal plasma osmolality because of hyperglycemia, azotemia, or the presence of mannitol or alcohol

(34). In hypergammaglobulinemia, such as in multiple myeloma, on the one hand serum sodium is falsely low because of displacement of serum water by γ-globulins, but on the other hand the sodium concentration is also truly low because of the accumulation of cationic γ-globulins, which displace sodium to maintain electrical neutrality (25).

A mechanism of pseudohyponatremia not widely appreciated is in vitro hemolysis, which is also a well-known cause of pseudohyperkalemia. Since cell lysis does not change osmolality of the plasma, any rise in serum potassium must be met by a reciprocal decrease in serum sodium.

Hyponatremia usually signifies a proportionate reduction in plasma osmolality, which causes cellular overhydration by the shift of water into the cells. Cell overhydration, especially when it occurs abruptly, can cause neuromuscular dysfunction, convulsions, and death. Cellular overhydration in hyponatremia is independent of extracellular volume, since the shift of water across the cell membrane depends solely on the osmotic gradient. Accumulation of a substance such as mannitol or glucose which is restricted to the extracellular fluid can cause hyponatremia by increasing extracellular (effective) osmolality and, hence, causing the shift of water from the intracellular space to the extracellular space. In such situations, despite hyponatremia, cells are dehydrated rather than swollen. Some authors extend the definition of pseudohyponatremia to those hyponatremic states accompanied by increased effective osmolality. However, since the sodium concentration in mannitol- or hyperglycemia-induced hyponatremia is truly

957

Table 57.1. Hyponatremia according to Effective Osmolality

1. Normal effective osmolality: pseudohyponatremia (due to hyperlipidemia, hyperproteinemia, etc.), accumulation of abnormal cations (e.g., lithium, γ-globulins).
2. Increased effective osmolality: hyperglycemia, mannitol infusion
3. Low effective osmolality: usual hyponatremia

Table 57.2. Causes of Hyponatremia according to Mechanisms of Its Maintenance

A. Increased water intake, e.g., primary polydipsia
B. Reduced renal water excretion
   1. Reduced delivery of fluid to the distal nephron because of low effective arterial volume (ADH release is usually stimulated as well)
     a. Edema forming states: heart failure, nephrotic syndrome, cirrhosis of the liver
     b. Nonrenal sodium loss: gastrointestinal sodium loss, sweating
     c. Renal sodium loss: diuretic therapy, aldosterone deficiency
     d. Low solute excretion
   2. Advanced renal failure
   3. Inappropriate secretion of ADH (SIADH)
     a. Tumors
     b. Pulmonary diseases
     c. Central nervous system disorders
     d. Drugs, e.g., chlorpropamide, barbiturates, morphine, indomethacin
     e. Physical and emotional stress
     f. Glucocorticoid deficiency
     g. Myxedema
     h. Idiopathic
     i. Reset osmostat
     j. Nausea

low, such definition of pseudohyponatremia is inappropriate and also confusing.

Glucose, sodium, and mannitol are effective osmols, whereas urea and alcohol are ineffective osmols because the former can effectively cause the shift of water across the cell membrane, whereas the latter diffuse freely into the cell and therefore do not cause the water shift (14). Thus, the clinical importance of hyponatremia must be judged in the context of the effective plasma osmolality, which may be determined in two ways. It can be measured by summation of all effective osmols in plasma:

$$\text{Effective osmolality} =$$
$$\text{Plasma Na (mEq/liter)} \times 2 + \frac{\text{glucose (mg/dl)}}{18}$$
$$+ \frac{\text{mannitol (mg/dl)}}{18} + \text{any effective osmols}$$

Alternately the total osmolality can be measured and the osmolality due to ineffective osmols, usually urea (mg/dl/2.8) and ethanol (mg/dl/4.6), can be subtracted. Table 57.1 lists the categories of hyponatremia associated with increased, normal, and low effective plasma osmolality.

CAUSES AND PATHOGENESIS

The immediate mechanisms responsible for a reduction in extracellular sodium concentration are (*a*) shift of water from the cell, caused by accumulation of extracellular solutes other than sodium salts; (*b*) retention of excess water in the body; (*c*) loss of sodium; and (*d*) shift of sodium into the cells.

The appropriate physiologic response to hypotonicity is suppression of antidiuretic hormone (ADH) release, which leads to rapid excretion of excess water and correction of hyponatremia. Thus, persistence of hyponatremia indicates the failure of this compensatory mechanism. In most instances hyponatremia is maintained because the kidney fails to produce water diuresis, but sometimes ingestion of water in excess of the limits of normal renal compensation is responsible.

The reasons for inability of the kidney to excrete water include (*a*) renal failure; (*b*) reduced delivery of glomerular filtrate to the distal nephron; and (*c*) the presence of ADH. The mechanism for impaired water excretion in renal failure is obvious and needs no further explanation. Reduced distal delivery of filtrate results from the low glomerular filtration rate and enhanced proximal tubular reabsorption, and these states are most commonly caused by volume depletion.

The normal dilution of urine requires delivery of adequate amounts of fluid to the diluting segment and the reabsorption of solute without water at that segment. An increased body fluid tonicity causes release of ADH, which allows reabsorption of water in the collecting duct, helping to restore the

body fluid tonicity. Thus, the response is considered appropriate when ADH is released in response to hypertonicity of the body fluid. However, release of ADH in the presence of hyponatremia is not considered inappropriate if the effective arterial volume is reduced. The term syndrome of inappropriate ADH secretion (SIADH) is therefore reserved for ADH secretion in hyponatremia with a normal or increased effective arterial volume. The causes of SIADH include tumors; pulmonary diseases, including tuberculosis and pneumonia; central nervous system diseases; drugs, etc. (Table 57.2).

Hyponatremia in clinical states associated with reduced effective arterial volume, such as congestive heart failure and cirrhosis of the liver, is caused by a combination of reduced delivery of fluid to the distal nephron and elaboration of ADH (80). Salt restriction and diuretics increase severity of hyponatremia. ADH secretion may be present despite hyponatremia in myxedema and glucocorticoid deficiency states (27, 39, 73). It is not clear, however, whether ADH secretion in these states is truly inappropriate or is in response to reduced effective arterial volume.

Finally, mild hyponatremia may be caused by "resetting the osmostat" at an osmolality lower than the usual level. In such cases urine dilution occurs normally when the plasma osmolality is brought down below the reset level. Resetting of the osmostat is a form of SIADH, since ADH secretion occurs inappropriately at hyponatremic levels without evidence of reduced effective arterial volume. Patients with chronic debilitating disease such as pulmonary tuberculosis often manifest this phenomenon (35).

DIAGNOSIS

The presence of a low plasma sodium and normal osmolality suggests pseudohyponatremia, but does not confirm it. By coincidence true hyponatremia may be accompanied by a high concentration of urea or alcohol, resulting in a normal osmolality. A more direct proof is the demonstration of a normal sodium concentration, using a sodium specific electrode or demonstration of reduced water content of plasma. Pseudohyponatremia due to hyperlipidemia is caused by accumulation of chylomicrons, which consist mostly of triglyceride (38), and is obvious from the milky appearance of serum or plasma. Substantial hyponatremia due to hyperlipidemia requires accumulation of more than 5 to 6 g/dl of lipids, and that degree of hyperlipidemia does not occur with hypercholesterolemia alone. Each gram per deciliter of lipid causes a false reduction in serum sodium by 1.7 mEq/liter and each g/dl of protein by 1.0 mEq/liter. Pseudohyponatremia due to hyperproteinemia can be confirmed by measurement of plasma proteins. Hyponatremia caused by mannitol or glucose is easily detected from the history or by simultaneous measurements of plasma sodium, osmolality, and glucose.

In evaluating hyponatremia associated with hypoosmolality, the main concern is to distinguish between SIADH and hyponatremia due to other causes, for the most part volume depletion states and edematous states. The major distinction between SIADH and other causes of hyponatremia lies in the status of effective arterial volume (EAV). EAV is normal or increased in the former and reduced in the latter. However, there is no single diagnostic test that measures effective arterial volume with certainty. Physical examination is notoriously inaccurate in determining mild-to-moderate volume depletion. A much more reliable technique for estimating effective arterial volume is based on the renal responses to the effective arterial volume. This technique involves measurement of urinary Na, serum urea nitrogen (SUN), creatinine, and uric acid. Urinary Na excretion greater than 20 mEq/liter, SUN less than 10 mg/dl (19), serum creatinine less than 1 mg/dl, and serum urate less than 4.0 mg/dl (5) are all suggestive of normal or increased effective arterial volume. In contrast, the measurement of urine osmolality has virtually no diagnostic value and often misleads physicians. Contrary to common belief, urine osmolality in SIADH need not be greater than plasma osmolality (4). Furthermore, a high urine osmolality does not necessarily support the diagnosis of SIADH, because most other causes of hyponatremia are also accompanied by urine osmolality higher than plasma osmolality.

The only situations in which urine osmolality may be appropriately low in the presence of hyponatremia are the hyponatremia caused by primary polydipsia and low solute excretion, and these are usually apparent when a careful history reveals polyuria or low protein intake (60). In all other disorders that cause hyponatremia urine osmolality is inappropriately increased, i.e., greater than 100 mOsm/liter.

MANAGEMENT AND PHARMACOLOGY

Hyponatremia is treated either by the addition of sodium or by removal of water. Salt is given to patients with hyponatremia due to salt depletion. Water is removed in hyponatremic states with normal or increased body sodium content. The speed of correction of hyponatremia should depend on the speed of development and on the patient's symptoms.

Clearly, severe symptomatic hyponatremia is a life-threatening condition (2), but there are considerable dangers associated with treatment of hyponatremia. In the past, volume overload was thought to be the main danger associated with administration of a large quantity of salt-containing solution. Now, central pontine myelinolysis is considered the major danger associated with rapid correction of hyponatremia (46). This demyelinating disease of the central pons and the other areas of the brain is characterized by motor nerve dysfunction, including quadriplegia. The complication tends to occur more often with chronic hyponatremia than with acute hyponatremia and is more frequently observed in malnourished and debilitated patients. In order to minimize this complication, chronic hyponatremia should be corrected at a speed less than 0.5 mEq/liter/hr (79). Since the danger of central pontine myelinolysis is limited mainly to those patients with asymptomatic chronic hyponatremia, rapid correction (at a rate of 1 to 2 mEq/liter/hr) should be restricted to those patients with acute symptomatic hyponatremia. Even then, there is no advantage in a rapid increase of serum sodium to a level above 125 to 130 mEq/liter.

For patients admitted with hypotonic dehydration and chronic asymptomatic hyponatremia, the traditional recommendation has been administration of isotonic saline. As the ADH release induced by low effective arterial volume is suppressed with the volume expansion, excess water is excreted in the urine, resulting in correction of hyponatremia. This approach is feasible of course, only in patients with sufficient renal function for water excretion. Sometimes, rapid excretion of water following isotonic saline administration in these patients may leave them particularly vulnerable to the development of central pontine myelinolysis. For those patients, use of 0.45% alternating with 0.9% sodium chloride solution may be safer (49). If the salt-depleted patients require potassium replenishment, the appropriate treatment is 0.45% NaCl containing 40 mEq of potassium in each liter.

RAPID TREATMENT

For hyponatremia with sodium depletion and symptomatic hypoosmolality, i.v. administration of sodium as hypertonic saline will correct hypoosmolality effectively. The amount of sodium necessary to increase the serum sodium to a desired level is calculated as follows:

$$Sodium\ requirement\ (in\ mEq) = TBW\ (l) \times \Delta\ Na$$

where Δ Na is the desired serum sodium-actual serum sodium, and TBW is the total body water.

Sodium may be administered as a 3% or 5% NaCl solution.

When accumulation of excess water is primarily responsible for hyponatremia, as in SIADH, water may be rapidly removed by administration of i.v. osmotic diuretics, such as mannitol or urea. An easier technique to use is to administer a loop diuretic, e.g., furosemide, simultaneously with hypertonic saline. Furosemide causes loss of water and sodium, but the latter is given back as hypertonic saline; the net result is removal of water (30). The usual adult starting dose of furosemide for this purpose is 40 mg. The same dose can be repeated at 2 to 4-hour intervals while hypertonic saline is being given.

The response to this regimen cannot be predicted with precision, and frequent follow-up measurements of serum sodium level must be made. There is no theoretical advantage of replacing exactly the amount of sodium lost in urine with hypertonic saline. Administration of hypertonic saline alone usually causes a salt and water diuresis, but addition of a loop diuretic makes the correction of hyponatremia easier by preventing excretion of concentrated urine. Another advantage of addition of a diuretic is prevention of fluid overload that may result from the administration of hypertonic saline. Potassium supplements are usually needed with this therapy.

CHRONIC THERAPY

Chronic hyponatremia may be treated by a reduction in water intake or by an increase in renal water excretion. Reduction of water intake is preferable but is not always feasible. If water restriction is difficult or unsuccessful, the latter approach may be used. Increased renal water excretion can be achieved by the use of pharmacologic agents that interfere with urine concentration. Lithium and demeclocycline increase urine output by reducing the production of cyclic AMP and also by interfering with its action (21, 71, 72). Demeclocycline is more effective and has fewer side effects (22), but it may cause nephrotoxicity in patients with liver disease (13). The usual dose of demeclocycline is 300 mg b.i.d. to q.i.d., and the usual dose of lithium for this purpose is 300 mg b.i.d. or t.i.d.

Administration of a loop diuretic such as furosemide, in conjunction with increased salt and potassium intake, is safer for treating chronic hyponatremia than the above methods (30). The diuretic prevents high medullary interstitial osmolality by limiting the reabsorption of salt in Henle's loop and, hence, prevents urine concentration. Increased salt and potassium intake increases water output by increasing delivery of solutes (67). There is evidence that ethacrynic acid may impair ADH-stimulated water movement across the collecting duct, and furosemide may have the same effect. The usual dose of furosemide is 40 mg b.i.d. to q.i.d.

Finally, vasopressin antagonists, not yet commercially available, may become an important addition to the chronic, as well as acute, treatment of hyponatremia in the future. The vascular effect, as well as the antidiuretic effect of vasopressin, is antagonized by vasopressin antagonists (37). A mode of therapy that has found more favor in Europe than in the U.S. is the daily ingestion of urea (20).

HYPERNATREMIA

Hypernatremia is defined as an increased sodium concentration in plasma water. Whereas hyponatremia may not be accompanied by hypoosmolality, hypernatremia is always associated with an increased effective plasma osmolality and, hence, with a reduced cell volume. However, the extracellular volume in hypernatremia may be normal, decreased, or increased (51).

CAUSES AND PATHOGENESIS

Hypernatremia is caused by loss of water, gain of sodium, or both (Table 57.3). Loss of water could be due to increased loss or reduced intake, and gain of sodium is due either to increased intake or to reduced renal excretion. Increased loss of water can occur through the kidney (e.g., in diabetes insipidus or osmotic diuresis), the gastrointestinal tract (e.g., gastric suction or osmotic diarrhea), or the skin. Reduced water intake occurs most commonly in comatose patients or in those with a defective thirst mechanism. Less frequent causes of reduced water intake include continuous vomiting, lack of access to water, and mechanical obstruction such as esophageal tumor. The excess gain of sodium leading to hypernatremia is usually iatrogenic, e.g., from hypertonic saline infusion, accidental entry into maternal circulation during abortion with hypertonic saline, or administration of hypertonic sodium bicarbonate during cardiopulmonary resuscitation or treatment of lactic acidosis (40). Reduced renal sodium excretion leading to sodium gain and hyponatremia is most commonly observed in patients who are water-depleted.

Water depletion resulting from diabetes insipidus, osmotic diuresis, or insufficient water intake commonly leads to secondary renal sodium retention in those who continue to ingest or are given sodium. Often, hypernatremia observed in such cases is due more to sodium retention than to water loss (Table 57.3). Whether hypernatremia is the result of sodium retention or water loss can be determined by examination of the patient's volume status. For example, if a patient with a serum sodium of 170 mEq/liter is normotensive and does not have obvious evidence of dehydration, hypernatremia cannot be caused entirely by water loss. In order to increase a serum sodium to 170 mEq/liter by water deficit alone, one would have to lose more than 20% of total body water.

Whereas the most effective defense against hyponatremia is increased renal water excretion, the most effective defense against hypernatremia is increased water drinking in response to thirst. Because thirst is such an effective and sensitive defense mechanism against hypernatremia, it is virtually impossible to increase serum sodium by more than a few mEq/liter if the water-drinking mechanism is intact. Therefore, in a patient with hypernatremia, there will always be a reason for reduced water intake (Table 57.3).

MANAGEMENT

Acute Management

Hypernatremia is treated either by addition of water or removal of sodium. The choice depends on the status of the body sodium and water content. If water depletion is the cause of hypernatremia, water is added. If sodium excess is the cause, sodium needs to be removed. When the water deficit is substantial, circulatory disturbances may result from extracellular volume depletion. In this situation, isotonic (0.9%) NaCl or 0.45% NaCl may be given initially to stabilize circulatory dynamics, with subsequent administration of more hypotonic solutions to normalize the tonicity. Administration of 5% dextrose solution would also correct the extracellular volume depletion, but a larger volume than that of isotonic saline is needed to expand the extracellular volume to the same extent, and too-rapid reduction of the plasma osmolality may result in cerebral edema. In acute symptomatic hypernatremia, serum sodium may be reduced by 6 to 8 mEq/liter

Table 57.3. Pathogenetic Mechanism of Hypernatremia

A. Reduced water content of the body
    a. Reduced water intake
        1. Defective thirst
        2. Unconsciousness
        3. Inability to drink water
        4. Lack of access to water
    b. Increased water loss
        1. Gastrointestinal loss: vomiting, osmotic diarrhea
        2. Cutaneous loss: sweating and fever
        3. Respiratory loss: hyperventilation and fever
        4. Renal loss: diabetes insipidus, osmotic diuresis
B. Increased sodium content of the body
    a. Increased intake
        1. Hypertonic saline or sodium bicarbonate infusion
        2. Ingestion of sea water
    b. Renal salt retention; usually in response to primary water deficit

in the first 3 to 4 hours, but thereafter the rate of decline should not exceed 1 mEq/liter/hr. As with hyponatremia, chronic hypernatremia usually does not cause CNS symptoms and therefore does not require rapid correction. A safe rate of correction is 0.7 mEq/liter/hr, or about 10% of the serum sodium concentration each 24 hours. The amount of water needed to correct hypernatremia can be estimated with the following equation:

$$Water\ deficit\ (in\ liters) = TBW\ (Na_2/Na_1 - 1) = TBW \times \Delta Na/Na_1$$

where Na_1 is the desired serum sodium level, Na_2 the observed serum sodium, TBW the total body water, and ΔNa the difference between the desired and observed serum sodium. Total body water (in liters) can be estimated using the following formula:

$$TBW = body\ weight\ in\ lb/4 = body\ weight\ in\ kg \times 0.55$$

In hyponatremia with excess sodium, the restoration of normal volume usually initiates natriuresis, but if natriuresis does not occur promptly, sodium may be removed with diuretics. Furosemide plus 5% dextrose solution might be an appropriate regimen to treat hypernatremia associated with excess sodium, but care must be taken not to allow serum sodium concentration to decline too rapidly. Furosemide can be given at 40 to 60 mg i.v. at 2- to 4-hour intervals while 5% dextrose solution is being infused. If the patient is in renal failure, salt can be removed by dialysis.

Chronic Management

Hypernatremic disorders that require chronic preventive therapy include diabetes insipidus and primary hypodipsia. If diabetes insipidus is the primary cause of hypernatremia, the distinction should first be made between nephrogenic and neurogenic (pituitary) diabetes insipidus. Administration of pitressin or stimulation of endogenous ADH secretion is helpful only for pituitary diabetes insipidus. Exogenous pitressin is available in three forms. Pitressin tannate in oil is administered i.m. Desmopressin (dDAVP), a synthetic analog of ADH, is administered intranasally, subcutaneously, or intravenously (63). A synthetic lysine vasopressin (lypressin, Diapid) is administered as a nasal spray. The usual dose of intranasal

dDAVP is 0.2 ml b.i.d. by tube or by nasal spray, and the usual dose for Diapid is 1 to 2 sprays in each nostril 4 times a day.

A common indication for injectable antidiuretic hormone is acute central diabetes insipidus due to head trauma or neurologic procedure. Aqueous pitressin may be infused intravenously at a rate of 1 ml/min of a solution containing 4 mU/ml. Desmopressin can be injected subcutaneously or intravenously at a rate of 2 to 4 μg daily in 2 to 3 divided doses. When ADH is administered in these acute situations, free water intake must be markedly curtailed in order to avoid hyponatremia.

Some patients may prefer oral agents, and the two that have been used extensively with relatively few side effects are chlorpropamide and thiazide diuretics. Chlorpropamide (100 to 250 mg/day) stimulates the secretion of endogenous ADH and may also enhance the effect of ADH. Its use has been markedly curtailed since the advent of dDAVP. Thiazide diuretics produce vascular volume depletion and enhanced reabsorption of fluid in the proximal tubule. Thus, they increase urine concentration by reducing the delivery of fluid to the distal diluting segment of the nephron. Addition of a thiazide diuretic to chlorpropamide may prevent the hypoglycemia that may occur if the latter is used alone. Two other drugs that have been used for the treatment of neurogenic diabetes insipidus are clofibrate (the usual dose, 2 g/day) (44) and carbamazepine (600 mg/day) (59). Since both drugs are less effective than chlorpropamide and have serious side effects, they should be the last resources in the treatment of diabetes insipidus. Nephrogenic diabetes insipidus cannot be treated with ADH preparations or an agent that stimulates ADH release, but measures to reduce the distal delivery of salt and water, i.e., low-salt diet and thiazide diuretics, have been used successfully. Subjects with primary hypodipsia should be educated to drink on schedule. In some instances, stimulation of the thirst center with chlorpropamide has met with success (8).

POTASSIUM METABOLISM

Although most of the body potassium is intracellular, the plasma potassium concentrations usually reflect the total body store of potassium. However, in conditions such as periodic paralysis or acid-base disorders where abnormal shifts in potassium take place across the cell membrane, the plasma potassium concentration may not accurately reflect body stores. In both hyperkalemic and hypokalemic types of periodic paralysis, abnormal plasma potassium concentrations are explained by transmembrane potassium shifts. Similarly, in acute acidosis hyperkalemia may occur because of the shift of potassium from the cell, while acute alkalosis leads to hypokalemia because of potassium shift into the cells. Catecholamines and respiratory alkalosis are common causes of hypokalemia by transcellular shift in critical care units.

HYPOKALEMIA

Hypokalemia refers to a reduction in the plasma potassium concentration. Except for the situations where hypokalemia

Table 57.4.   Causes and Mechanisms of Hypokalemia

1. Shift into the cell
   a. Acute correction of acidosis or acute alkalosis
   b. Administration of insulin and glucose
   c. Hypokalemic periodic paralysis
   d. Barium poisoning
   e. β_2 agonists
2. Reduced intake
3. Increased Loss
   a. Renal loss
      1. Primary hyperaldosteronism
      2. Secondary hyperaldosteronism, e.g., diuretic therapy, malignant hypertension, Bartter's syndrome, renal artery stenosis
      3. Mineralocorticoids other than aldosterone, e.g., licorice, fluoroprednisolone ointment, carbenoxolone
      4. Miscellaneous: hypercalcemia, Liddle's syndrome, magnesium deficiency, L-dopa, renal tubular acidosis, acute myelocytic and monocytic leukemia, poorly reabsorbable anions, metabolic alkalosis, metabolic acidosis
   b. Gastrointestinal loss
      1. Vomiting or nasogastric suction
      2. Diarrhea or fistula drainage

is caused by intracellular shift, it usually represents depletion of cellular potassium.

CAUSES AND PATHOGENESIS

There are three basic mechanisms for hypokalemia: (*a*) intracellular shift; (*b*) reduced intake; and (*c*) increased loss (Table 57.4). An intracellular shift of potassium occurs with an increase in blood pH (68). This shift may occur when a patient develops alkalosis or when acidosis is being corrected. Administration of glucose and insulin also causes an intracellular shift of potassium, in part by stimulation of glucose metabolism but also by a direct effect of insulin on the cellular uptake of potassium (36, 65). The mechanism of intracellular shift of potassium in familial periodic paralysis is not clearly known.

The ingestion of absorbable barium salts, e.g., carbonate or chloride, causes a reduction in plasma potassium concentration by intracellular shift (64). The intracellular shift is due to decreased conductance of potassium, resulting in a decrease in passive outward diffusion of potassium (75).

The major routes of potassium loss are the kidneys and the GI tract. There are numerous causes for renal potassium loss, but the two most constant factors are increased sodium delivery to the distal nephron and increased mineralocorticoid activity. Increased sodium delivery with reduced mineralocorticoid activity (e.g., high-salt diet) or increased mineralocorticoid activity with reduced sodium delivery (e.g., low-salt diet) does not lead to increased renal potassium excretion. Conditions such as primary hyperaldosteronism or chronic diuretic therapy are associated with increased sodium delivery to the distal nephron, even though sodium intake and urinary excretion may be normal. In primary hyperaldosteronism, the proximal tubular sodium reabsorption is reduced because of volume expansion, resulting in increased delivery of sodium to the distal nephron. Enhanced sodium reabsorption at the Na-K exchange site at the collecting duct allows normal amounts of sodium to be excreted despite increased delivery of sodium to the distal nephron.

A similar mechanism is responsible for the maintenance of increased sodium delivery to the Na-K exchange site during chronic diuretic therapy. Increased urinary sodium excretion, which occurs with calcium infusion, is suggested as a possible mechanism of increased renal potassium loss in hypercalcemia (3). Hypokalemia caused by magnesium deficiency is due to increased renal loss of potassium, perhaps caused by increased production of aldosterone (24). Plasma renin activity (PRA) in magnesium deficiency is normal, and the mechanism of increased aldosterone is not known. Although the causal relationship is not entirely clear, the prevalence of hypokalemia in familial hypomagnesemia suggests that they are related (74). L-Dopa also occasionally causes hypokalemia, possibly through increased aldosterone secretion (28). Kaliuresis and hypokalemia in renal tubular acidosis are commonly attributed to secondary hyperaldosteronism caused by renal salt wasting. However, although renal salt wasting occurs in chronic metabolic acidosis, there is little convincing evidence for secondary hyperaldosteronism. There may be a specific tubular defect, causing increased potassium loss in renal tubular acidosis (69). The mechanism of hypokalemia in acute myelocytic and acute monocytic leukemias is increased renal loss of potassium, but the mechanism of this loss is not well-understood (41). Delivery to the distal nephron of poorly reabsorbable anions, such as penicillin and carbenicillin, leads to increased urinary loss of potassium because increased luminal negativity enhances potassium secretion (32). Vomiting and nasogastric suction cause hypokalemia, in part because of direct loss of potassium from the stomach but to a larger extent because of renal loss attributable to the renal bicarbonate wasting that occurs with metabolic alkalosis. Excretion of bicarbonate causes renal potassium loss in part because bicarbonate acts as a poorly reabsorbable anion, but an additional mechanism might be that alkaline pH of the urine reduces permeability to chloride, thereby enhancing luminal negativity (11). Secondary hyperaldosteronism due to volume depletion is an additional factor involved in the pathogenesis of hypokalemia in this setting.

MANAGEMENT

Hypokalemia is usually treated either by potassium administration or by prevention of the renal loss of potassium. Renal loss of potassium is prevented either by treating its cause (e.g., removal of aldosterone-producing adenoma or discontinuation of diuretics) or by the administration of potassium-sparing diuretics. The potassium-sparing diuretics in current use are aldosterone antagonists (e.g., spironolactone), triamterene, and amiloride. Aldosterone antagonists are effective in preventing renal potassium loss only if an increased mineralocorticoid concentration is responsible for hypokalemia. In Liddle's syndrome, spironolactone is ineffective because plasma aldosterone is reduced; triamterene and amiloride are effective, regardless of the plasma aldosterone concentration. The daily dose of spironolactone ranges from 25 to 400 mg. The usual doses of triamterene range from 50 to 150 mg b.i.d. Amiloride is administered at 5 mg/day and can be slowly increased up to 20 mg/day. Amiloride should be administered with food to avoid gastric irritation. Because reduced delivery of sodium to the distal nephron always reduces potassium secretion, a low-salt diet helps to reduce renal potassium loss of any cause, independent of the plasma aldosterone concentration.

In the nonemergency setting, potassium is most likely to be given orally in the form of potassium chloride or potassium phosphate or in the form of the salt of organic acids. In the critical care setting, potassium is usually given intravenously, primarily as potassium chloride. The first goal in treating severe hypokalemia is elimination of the greatest hazard—cardiac arrest or lethal cardiac arrhythmia. A decline in serum K of 1 mEq/liter generally indicates a loss of 150 to 200 mEq of potassium, and a decline of 2 mEq/liter a loss in excess of 500 mEq, but the relationship is not rigidly fixed. For example in acidotic states, serum potassium may be high in the face of potassium depletion.

To initiate rapid i.v. administration of potassium it may be useful to estimate the number of liters of extracellular fluid as body weight in kg $\times$ 0.2. This figure multiplied by desired increment in serum potassium per liter represents the amount of potassium that can safely be given in 20 to 30 minutes without danger of hyperkalemia. Although it is usually unnecessary to give potassium at a rate greater than 10 to 20 mEq/hr, a rate in excess of 100 mEq/hr may be needed in certain life-threatening situations, e.g., a patient with ketoacidosis, severe hypokalemia, and an EKG showing a dangerous arrhythmia. Glucose-containing solution should not be used as a vehicle for KCl when serum K is to be increased rapidly; glucose will stimulate release of insulin which will, in turn, drive K into the cells.

Potassium at concentrations exceeding 40 mEq/liter may produce pain at the infusion site and may lead to sclerosis of smaller vessels. When a concentration in excess of 100 mEq/liter is used, a femoral line is preferable. It is advisable to avoid central venous infusion of potassium at high concentrations lest depolarization of the conduction tissues lead to cardiac arrest.

HYPERKALEMIA

CAUSES AND PATHOGENESIS

Hyperkalemia may be caused by one of three mechanisms: (*a*) shift of potassium from the cells to the extracellular space; (*b*) increased potassium intake; and (*c*) reduced renal potassium excretion (Table 57.5). Hyperkalemic familial periodic paralysis; use of succinylcholine in paralyzed patients (17); use of cationic amino acids such as ϵ-aminocaproic acid, arginine, or lysine (15, 31); rhabdomyolysis or hemolysis; and acute acidosis all cause hyperkalemia by extracellular potassium shift. Rhabdomyolysis and hemolysis cause hyperkalemia only when they cause renal failure. Acute acidosis has long been regarded as a cause of extracellular potassium shift, irrespective of the type of acidosis, but evidence now suggests that hyperkalemia is not as predictable with organic acidosis as with inorganic acidosis (53). Furthermore, there is little change in serum potassium concentration with either respiratory acidosis or alkalosis. However, hyperkalemia is common in diabetic ketoacidosis and phenformin-induced lactic acidosis (1). The more frequent occurrence of hyperkalemia in clinical organic acidosis than in experimental organic acidosis

Table 57.5. Causes of Hyperkalemia

A. Pseudohyperkalemia
  a. Thrombocytosis, massive leukocytosis, use of tourniquet with fist exercise, in vitro hemolysis
B. True hyperkalemia
  a. Due to extracellular shift: acute acidosis (especially inorganic acidosis), catabolic states, periodic paralysis, succinylcholine, cationic amino acids
  b. Due to excessive ingestion; rare, if renal excretion is normal
  c. Decreased renal excretion:
    1. Hypoaldosteronism: Addison's disease; selective hypoaldosteronism (hyporeninemic hypoaldosteronism, heparin, congenital adrenal enzyme deficiencies, angiotensin-converting enzyme inhibitors)
    2. Tubular unresponsiveness to aldosterone (pseudohypoaldosteronism): congenital, salt-losing nephropathy, pseudohypoaldosteronism type II
    3. Potassium-sparing diuretics
    4. Severe dehydration

may be explained by the longer duration of acidosis and the presence of other factors, such as dehydration and renal failure in clinical organic acidosis. Hyperkalemia can also occur in severe digitalis intoxication by extracellular shift of potassium as digitalis inhibits the Na-K pump (6).

The kidney's ability to excrete potassium is so great that hyperkalemia rarely occurs solely on the basis of increased intake of potassium. Thus, hyperkalemia is almost always due to impaired renal excretion. There are three major mechanisms of diminished renal potassium excretion: reduced aldosterone or aldosterone responsiveness; renal failure; and reduced distal delivery of sodium.

Aldosterone deficiency may be part of a generalized deficiency of adrenal hormones (e.g., Addison's disease), or it may represent a selective process (e.g., hyporeninemic hypoaldosteronism). Hyporeninemic hypoaldosteronism is the most common cause of all aldosterone deficiency states and by far the commonest cause of chronic hyperkalemia (55). Selective hypoaldosteronism can also occur with heparin therapy (56). In patients with reduced aldosterone secretion, any agent that limits the supply of renin or angiotensin II may provoke hyperkalemia, for example, angiotensin-converting enzyme (ACE) inhibitors, nonsteroidal antiinflammatory agents, and β-blockers. The latter may compound the tendency to hyperkalemia by interfering with potassium transport into cells. Renal tubular unresponsiveness to aldosterone (pseudohypoaldosteronism) may be congenital, but it is more often an acquired defect. This defect may involve only potassium secretion (pseudohypoaldosteronism type II) (66) or sodium reabsorption, as well as potassium secretion. Most cases of socalled "salt-losing nephritis" appear to represent the latter defect (82). Severe dehydration may cause hyperkalemia despite secondary hyperaldosteronism when delivery of sodium to the distal nephron is markedly reduced (47).

Pseudohyperkalemia is defined as an increase in potassium concentration only in the local blood vessel or in vitro and has no physiologic consequences. Prolonged use of a tourniquet with fist exercises can increase the serum potassium level by as much as 1 mEq/liter (10). Thrombocytosis and severe leukocytosis cause pseudohyperkalemia through potassium release from the platelets and white blood cells, respectively, during blood clotting (9, 29).

MANAGEMENT

Hyperkalemia may be treated by removal of potassium from the body, by relocation of extracellular potassium in the cells, and by antagonism of potassium action on the membrane of the cardiac conduction system. Removal of potassium may be accomplished by several routes: through the gastrointestinal tract with a potassium exchange resin given orally or by enema; through the kidney by diuretics, mineralocorticoids, and increased salt intake; or by hemodialysis or peritoneal dialysis. A potassium exchange resin, sodium polystyrene sulfonate (Kayexalate), is more effective when it is given with agents that cause osmotic diarrhea, such as sorbitol or mannitol. One tablespoon of Kayexalate mixed with 100 ml of 10% sorbitol or mannitol can be given by mouth 2 to 4 times a day. When it is given as an enema, a larger quantity is given more frequently. Shift of potassium into cells can be accomplished with glucose and insulin or by increasing the blood pH with sodium bicarbonate. Specific β_2 agonists such as salbutamol have shown striking efficacy in driving K into cells by stimulating the Na-K-dependent ATPase. At this time no i.v. preparation is available in the U.S., but European experience is promising (43). Antagonism of the action of potassium on the heart with i.v. calcium salts or hypertonic sodium solution provides the fastest effect against hyperkalemia and is used in cases of life-threatening hyperkalemia.

Prolonged administration of diuretics and a high-salt diet is an effective treatment for hyporeninemic hypoaldosteronism. This regimen ensures the delivery of an adequate amount of sodium to the distal nephron without causing further volume expansion. Mineralocorticoid may be required as an adjunct therapy for hyporeninemic hypoaldosteronism, and the agent most commonly used is a synthetic mineralocorticoid, fludrocortisone (Florinef, 0.1 mg once or twice daily). However, since renal salt retention may be an important mechanism in the pathogenesis of hyporeninemic hypoaldosteronism (55), mineralocorticoid replacement may lead to salt retention and worsening hypertension. Reduced intake of potassium is an additional measure to be added to any of the methods recommended above in the long-term management of hyperkalemia.

METABOLIC ACIDOSIS

CAUSES AND PATHOGENESIS

Metabolic acidosis is defined as a reduction in extracellular pH resulting from a decrease in the bicarbonate concentration that is not secondary to reduction in PCO_2. The kidney plays a major role in maintaining the extracellular bicarbonate concentration, and metabolic acidosis due to the failure of the kidney in this function is referred to as renal acidosis (Table 57.6). The term extrarenal acidosis is used when factors other than defective renal acid-excretory function are responsible. Renal acidosis may occur because of specific defects of tubular function in acid excretion or bicarbonate reabsorption (renal tubular acidosis) (70) or because of reduced nephron mass due to renal parenchymal disease (uremic acidosis). Three types of metabolic acidosis that deserve special attention in critically ill patients are lactic acidosis, ketoacidosis, and uremic acidosis.

Table 57.6. Causes of Metabolic Acidosis

A. Renal acidosis
  a. Uremic acidosis
  b. Renal tubular acidosis
    1. Distal renal tubular acidosis (type I)
    2. Proximal renal tubular acidosis (type II)
    3. Aldosterone deficiency or unresponsiveness (type IV)
B. Extrarenal acidosis
  a. Gastrointestinal loss of bicarbonate
  b. Ingestion of acids or acid precursors: ammonium chloride, sulfur, toluene, salicylate, ethylene glycol, methanol, paraldehyde
C. Organic acidosis
  1. D- and L-lactic acidosis
  2. Ketoacidosis

Table 57.7. Causes of Lactic Acidosis

1. Tissue hypoxia, e.g., circulatory shock, severe hypoxemia, severe heart failure, severe anemia
2. Acute alcoholism
3. Drugs and toxins, e.g., phenformin, isoniazid
4. Diabetes mellitus
5. Leukemia
6. Idiopathic
7. Short bowel syndrome (D-lactic acidosis)

Lactic acidosis resulting from tissue hypoxia is called type A lactic acidosis (the common type). Tissue hypoxia leading to lactic acidosis is usually caused by circulatory shock, which may be due to sepsis, hypovolemia, or cardiac failure. Generalized convulsion is also a fairly common cause, but the resulting acidosis is transient. Less commonly, tissue hypoxia may result from severe hypoxemia due to respiratory failure, carbon monoxide poisoning, or severe anemia. In type B lactic acidosis, the less common variety, there is no apparent tissue hypoxia, but the possibility of subtle tissue hypoxia must be considered. The causes of type B lactic acidosis include alcoholic intoxication, various drugs (phenformin, isoniazid), cancer, and possibly diabetes (54, 61) (Table 57.7). The prognosis of both types of lactic acidosis is dismal.

Ketoacidosis occurs most frequently in diabetes mellitus, but it occasionally occurs in vomiting, binge-drinking chronic alcoholics. When ketoacidosis occurs in the presence of poor mitochondrial oxidation (e.g., ethanol intoxication, septic shock in the diabetic, use of phenformin), the ratio of the reduced form of ketoacid β-hydroxybutyrate to the oxidized form acetoacetate is increased. The usual ratio of β-hydroxybutyrate to acetoacetate in typical diabetic ketoacidosis is about 2.5 to 3, and the ratio is increased to 8 or higher in β-hydroxybutyric acidosis. Since acetoacetate is the only form measured by the nitroprusside reagent (Acetest), the patient with β-hydroxybutyric acidosis may present with a large unexplained anion gap. Lactic acidosis often coexists with β-hydroxybutyric acidosis, because the abnormal redox state of mitochondria is a sufficient condition for increased production of lactic acid. Uremic acidosis is most often a result of chronic end-stage renal failure, but in critically ill patients acute renal failure is a common cause. Lactic acidosis also commonly coexists in this setting.

Uremic acidosis is a common occurrence in patients with acute renal failure. The rate of development of uremic acidosis depends on the rate of production of endogenous acids. Because critically ill patients are often severely catabolic, the rate of reduction in serum bicarbonate in these patients is often greater than that in other patients, but the rate is still considerably slower than that in organic acidosis.

MANAGEMENT

Restoration of normal blood pH and bicarbonate concentration is the ultimate aim of therapy for metabolic acidosis. Rapid restoration of normal pH is usually unnecessary and may be undesirable for several reasons. When the pH is increased acutely, restoration of a normal concentration of the red blood cell 2,3-DPG lags behind (42). In addition, a sudden increase in extracellular pH can cause a paradoxical CSF acidosis (58). Rapid restoration of a normal serum bicarbonate level in metabolic acidosis would be undesirable, because persistent hyperventilation produces a very high blood pH (57).

The initial aim in the treatment of severe metabolic acidosis should be to increase the blood pH to a level at which adverse cardiovascular effects of severe acidemia can be avoided. Although the risk of acidosis varies with the age and the cardiovascular status of patients, it is considered prudent, at least in older subjects, to keep blood pH above 7.1 to 7.2. The blood pH may be increased by the administration of alkali or by allowing alkali to be produced endogenously by metabolism of retained organic anions (OA$^-$):

$$OA^- + H_2CO_3 \rightarrow OAH + HCO_3^-$$
$$\updownarrow$$
$$CO_2 + H_2O$$

Successful treatment of the cause of organic acidosis increases the serum bicarbonate concentration by the latter mechanisms. When ketoacidosis is treated with insulin and fluid, the outcome is usually predictable: a substantial increase in the plasma bicarbonate concentration with a concomitant increase in arterial pH. Exogenous alkali is seldom necessary in ketoacidosis.

In contrast to the favorable outcome in ketoacidosis, response to treatment in lactic acidosis is usually poor. In lactic acidosis induced by hypoxia (type A), the prognosis depends on the cause of tissue hypoxia. In most cases of circulatory shock the prognosis is extremely poor. The prognosis of lactic acidosis due to acute alcohol intoxication is fairly good. With seizure-induced lactic acidosis, recovery is usually complete within hours after the control of the seizure (52). Improvement in the microcirculation with the infusion of sodium nitroprusside may be effective in a patient with idiopathic lactic acidosis (81).

Treatment for type B lactic acidosis has consisted of the administration of alkali in the hope of spontaneous recovery, but administration of bicarbonate tends to be self-defeating because it may also lead to increased production of lactic acid (23). Increasing cell pH increases glycolysis and, therefore, increases production of lactic acid. Glucose needed for the glycolysis may come from tissue protein via gluconeogenesis in patients with insufficient caloric intake, such as those patients with cancer, and this occurrence could further aggravate cachexia.

Discouraged by the poor results of bicarbonate therapy and offering theoretical arguments against alkali therapy as discussed above, some authors have recommended not using bicarbonate in the treatment of any type of lactic acidosis (76). In contrast, others feel that the judicious use of bicarbonate is still beneficial to patients with severe metabolic acidosis (45).

Dichloroacetate, an experimental drug, offers some hope in the treatment of type B lactic acidosis (62, 77). Its main action is stimulation of pyruvate dehydrogenase, the enzyme responsible for conversion of pyruvate to acetyl-CoA. Increased conversion of pyruvate to acetyl-CoA results in a decrease in pyruvate concentration, which in turn increases utilization of lactate as well as alanine. Despite the theoretical prediction that lactic acidosis due to hypoxia should respond only to the supply of sufficient oxygen, dichloroacetate causes a striking increase in serum bicarbonate concentration in patients with type A lactic acidosis. A major drawback of the drug appears to be the frequent occurrence of central nervous system side effects with chronic use (78).

D-lactic acidosis is a disorder that occurs in patients with the short bowel syndrome. The acidosis is caused by production of *d*- and *l*-lactic acids by the colonic bacteria; *l*-lactic acid that is absorbed is rapidly metabolized, and there is no accumulation, but *d*-lactate accumulates in the body fluids. Accumulation of *d*-lactate has been attributed to its slow metabolism, but our studies showed that the rate of *d*-lactate metabolism in man is fairly fast, suggesting that there may be an additional defect in the metabolism of *d*-lactate in those patients who develop *d*-lactic acidosis (50). A neurologic syndrome characterized by mental confusion, disorientation, and staggering gait commonly accompanies the disease. Treatment consists of sterilization of the gut with antibiotics (48).

The response to the administration of alkali depends on the type of metabolic acidosis. In nonorganic acidosis, the alkali requirement can be estimated with reasonable accuracy. In contrast, in organic acidosis, the alkali requirement is usually much more than predicted in lactic acidosis and much less than predicted in ketoacidosis. In lactic acidosis, almost continuous administration of bicarbonate may be needed to maintain serum bicarbonate at a reasonable level, whereas in ketoacidosis administration of insulin and fluid usually suffices.

There are three types of alkali that can be used for the treatment of metabolic acidosis: bicarbonate; salts of organic acids; and THAM (tromethamine). Organic salts used as a bicarbonate substitute include lactate, acetate, and citrate. Each milliequivalent of the organic salts produces 1 mEq of bicarbonate. Thus, the milliequivalent doses of organic salts are the same as those of bicarbonate. However, because these salts require metabolism, an increase in bicarbonate concentration is delayed. Furthermore when metabolism is impaired (e.g., in lactic acidosis) administration of an organic salt may have no effect on the serum bicarbonate concentration. The amount and speed of administration of bicarbonate and organic salts vary widely, depending on the severity of acidosis. Shohl's solution (citric acid and sodium citrate) contains 1 mEq of alkali (as citrate) per ml.

In contrast to the delayed and sometimes uncertain responses to organic salts, THAM increases serum bicarbonate concentration promptly and predictably in the following reaction:

$$THAM + H_2CO_3 \dashrightarrow THAM\text{-}H^+ + HCO_3.$$
$$\updownarrow$$
$$CO_2 + H_2O$$

Because formation of bicarbonate by THAM occurs at the expense of carbonic acid, rapid infusion of THAM results in a marked reduction in PCO_2; the rate should not exceed 2 mmol/min.

For a given quantity of administered bicarbonate, the increase in serum bicarbonate is less in severe than in mild metabolic acidosis (i.e., the apparent volume of distribution of bicarbonate is greater in severe than mild metabolic acidosis). However, the absolute increase in pH for a given dose of bicarbonate administered is greater in more severe metabolic acidosis than in mild acidosis, because the proportionate increase in serum bicarbonate is greater with severe acidosis. In practice, however, there is no need to estimate the bicarbonate requirements to achieve a certain specific level. Since pH is determined by the ratio of bicarbonate to PCO_2 and a change in ventilation and PCO_2 following acute increase in serum bicarbonate cannot be accurately predicted, it is difficult to predict what the pH will be, even if the increase in bicarbonate concentration were accurately predicted. The best approach is to administer 2 to 3 ampules of sodium bicarbonate (44.5 or 50 mEq/ampule) by direct i.v. injection, then repeat the blood gas measurement 20 to 30 min after bicarbonate injection to determine the need for further bicarbonate administration.

For treatment of chronic acidosis, citrate is more palatable than bicarbonate, and citrate is available as Shohl's solution. For treatment of uremic acidosis, sodium acetate is the most commonly used alkali in hemodialysis fluids, sodium lactate in peritoneal dialysis fluids. Administration of THAM probably has no advantage in treatment of metabolic acidosis in most situations (7) but might be more advantageous than bicarbonate in treating metabolic acidosis complicated by respiratory acidosis. THAM is available as a 0.3 M solution, and the rate of infusion of THAM in this setting should not exceed 30 ml/min.

METABOLIC ALKALOSIS

Metabolic alkalosis is defined as an increase in extracellular pH caused by an increase in the serum bicarbonate concentration. Normally, the kidney's ability to excrete the excess bicarbonate when the serum bicarbonate is high is so great that it is virtually impossible to maintain metabolic alkalosis by a mechanism that simply causes increased generation of bicarbonate; another mechanism must coexist that prevents the rapid renal excretion of bicarbonate. Hence, there are always two abnormalities for sustained metabolic alkalosis: an abnormality that increases the extracellular bicarbonate concentration and an abnormality that increases renal bicarbonate threshold.

MECHANISMS FOR INCREASE IN SERUM BICARBONATE

There are several mechanisms for increasing the extracellular bicarbonate concentration. These mechanisms include loss of HCl (from the stomach or, rarely, in the stool), administration of bicarbonate or bicarbonate precursors, metabolism of

Table 57.8. Mechanisms and Causes of Increasing Extracellular Bicarbonate Concentration

1. Loss of HCl from the stomach, e.g. gastric suction, vomiting
2. Administration of bicarbonate or bicarbonate precursors, e.g., sodium lactate, sodium acetate, sodium citrate
3. Shift of H^+ into the cell, e.g., K^+ depletion
4. Rapid contraction of extracellular volume by loop diuretics: contraction alkalosis
5. Increased renal excretion of acid, e.g., diuretic therapy, hypermineralocorticoid state, potassium depletion, high PCO_2, secondary hypoparathyroidism

Table 57.9. Mechanisms and Causes of Maintaining High Serum Bicarbonate Concentration

1. Reduced effective arterial volume, e.g., diuretic therapy, vomiting, edema-forming states
2. Potassium deficiency
3. Chloride deficiency accompanied by low effective arterial volume, e.g., vomiting
4. High PCO_2
5. Secondary hypoparathyroidism, e.g., milk-alkali syndrome, certain malignancy-induced hypercalcemia
6. Severe renal failure

bicarbonate precursors, shift of $H+$ into the cell, contraction of extracellular volume by rapid loss of sodium chloride and water, and increased renal excretion of acid (Table 57.8). Of these, the two most frequent causes of metabolic alkalosis are increased renal generation of bicarbonate and loss of HCl from the stomach.

Gastric suction is a particularly frequent cause of metabolic alkalosis in critically ill patients, because acid secretion is often markedly stimulated in these patients because of the stress of severe illness. Considerable loss of acid may still occur in these patients, even when gastric acid secretion is inhibited by a H_2-blocker such as cimetidine or ranitidine. Diuretic therapy with complicating hypokalemia is also a common cause of metabolic alkalosis in critically ill patients. Sometimes, metabolic alkalosis is a complication of the treatment of metabolic acidosis; administration of bicarbonate to a patient with lactic acidosis increases the production of lactic acid, which is retained as lactate following titration by bicarbonate. The subsequent metabolism of the lactate can lead to a rapid increase in the serum bicarbonate concentration.

MECHANISMS FOR MAINTAINING HIGH SERUM BICARBONATE

Since the kidney is the organ responsible for excreting the excess bicarbonate when the concentration is abnormally high (83), renal failure would be the most effective mechanism for maintaining excess bicarbonate. However, in mild-to-moderate renal failure, the ability to excrete bicarbonate is still well-preserved (33). Other mechanisms of maintaining a high serum bicarbonate concentration include contraction of effective arterial volume, potassium deficiency, high PCO_2, and secondary hypoparathyroidism. Chloride deficiency is usually listed among the causes of increased renal bicarbonate threshold, but chloride deficiency without reduced effective arterial volume does not increase the bicarbonate threshold (Table 57.9). For example, in severe hyponatremia due to SIADH, total body chloride content is often reduced, but renal bicarbonate threshold is not increased because effective arterial volume is not reduced.

The commonest causes of increased renal bicarbonate threshold encountered clinically are low effective arterial volume and potassium deficiency. These two and severe renal failure are probably the mechanisms responsible for maintenance of most cases of metabolic alkalosis. In patients who develop metabolic alkalosis due to gastric suction or vomiting, the high renal bicarbonate threshold is caused by low effective arterial volume and hypokalemia. Thus, large losses of gastric fluid will not lead to metabolic alkalosis, as long as the normal renal threshold of bicarbonate is maintained by prevention of volume depletion and potassium depletion.

MANAGEMENT

Since the increased renal bicarbonate threshold in metabolic alkalosis is most often caused by reduced effective arterial volume and hypokalemia, correction of these abnormalities leads to rapid restoration of bicarbonate concentration in most patients. Correction of low effective arterial volume is accomplished by administration of normal saline or half-normal saline. Sometimes discontinuation of an offending agent (e.g., a diuretic) and restoration of normal salt intake is sufficient. If volume depletion is to be corrected, chloride must be given to replace the excreted bicarbonate; it can be given as either sodium chloride or potassium chloride. In certain clinical situations such as edema-forming states, treatment of reduced effective arterial volume with salt solution may not be feasible. A logical and effective choice in such situations is acetazolamide (Diamox), a carbonic anhydrase inhibitor, which will treat metabolic alkalosis as well as edema. Diamox can be given either i.v. or p.o. The starting dose is 250 or 500 mg and can be repeated at 6-hour intervals until a desired serum bicarbonate concentration has been achieved. Acetazolamide administration usually reduces the renal bicarbonate threshold to a subnormal level, but it may not be able to reduce bicarbonate threshold to even a normal level in the presence of severe volume depletion.

Correction of metabolic alkalosis by renal excretion of bicarbonate requires adequate renal function. In renal failure, metabolic alkalosis can be treated by administration of dilute HCl or acidifying salts or by dialysis; the latter has an advantage in that it treats uremia as well as alkalosis. HCl can be administered in 0.1 or 0.05 N solution into a central vein (84). Acidifying salts include ammonium chloride, arginine chloride and lysine chloride. Metabolism of these salts results in release of HCl, which then titrates bicarbonate. The amount of acidifying salts to be administered depends on the severity of metabolic acidosis. The optimal rate with i.v. infusion is about 1 mEq/min. If continuous acid loss from the stomach is the cause of metabolic alkalosis, an inhibitor of acid secretion, such as cimetidine or ranitidine, is useful. Considerable acid secretion, however, may still occur, even with the maximal dose of these drugs.

REFERENCES

1. Adrogue HJ, Wilson H, Boyd AE, et al: Plasma acid-base patterns in diabetic ketoacidosis. *N Engl J Med* 307:1603, 1982.
2. Arieff AI: Hyponatremia, convulsions, respiratory arrest, and permanent brain damage after elective surgery in healthy women. *N Engl J Med* 314:1529, 1986.
3. Adlinger KA, Samaan NA: Hypokalemia with hypercalcemia. Prevalence and significance in treatment. *Ann Intern Med* 87:571, 1977.
4. Bartter FC, Schwartz WB: The syndrome of inappropriate secretion of antidiuretic hormone. *Am J Med* 42:651, 1967.
5. Beck LH: Hypouricemia in the syndrome of inappropriate secretion of antidiuretic hormone. *N Engl J Med* 301:528, 1979.
6. Bismuth C, Gaultier M, Conso F, et al: Hyperkalemia in acute digitalis poisoning: prognostic significance and therapeutic implications. *Clin Toxicol* 6:153, 1973.
7. Bleich HL, Schwartz WB: Tris buffer (THAM). An appraisal of its physiological effects and clinical usefulness. *N Engl J Med* 274:782, 1966.
8. Bode HH, Harley BM, Crawford JD: Restoration of normal drinking behavior by chlorpropamide in patients with hypodipsia and diabetes insipidus. *Am J Med* 51:304, 1971.
9. Bronson WR: Pseudohyperkalemia due to release of potassium from white blood cells during clotting. *N Engl J Med* 274:369, 1966.
10. Brown JJ, Chin RH, David DL, et al: Falsely high serum potassium levels in patients with hyperaldosteronism. *Br Med J* 2:18, 1970.
11. Carlisle EJF, Donnelly SM, Ethier JH, Kamel KS, Halperin ML: Modulation of the secretion of potassium by accompanying anions in humans. *Kidney Int* 39:1206–1212, 1991.
12. Carlisle EJF, Donnelly SM, Ethier JH, Vasuvattakul S, Kamel KS, Tobe S, Halperin ML: Glue-sniffing and distal renal tubular acidosis: sticking to the facts. *J Am Soc Nephrol* 1:1019–1027, 1991.
13. Carrilho F, Bosch J, Arroyo V, et al: Renal failure associated with demeclocycline in cirrhosis. *Ann Intern Med* 87:195–197, 1977.
14. Carroll HJ, Oh MS: Electrolyte physiology and body composition. In *Water, Electrolyte and Acid-Base Metabolism.* J.B. Lippincott, Philadelphia, 1989, p 1.
15. Carroll HJ, Tice DA: The effects of epsilon aminocaproic acid upon potassium metabolism in the dog. *Metabolism* 14:499, 1966.
16. Carroll HJ, Oh MS: Hyponatremia. In Hurst JW (ed): *Medicine for the Practicing Physicians,* ed 3. Butterworth-Heinemann, London, 1992, p 1296.
17. Cooperman LH: Succinylcholine-induced hyperkalemia in neuromuscular disease. *JAMA* 213:1867, 1970.
18. Cowell DC, McGrady PM: Direct-measurement ion-selective electrodes: analytical error in hyponatremia. *Clin Chem* 31:2009, 1985.
19. Decaux G, Genette F, Mockel J: Hypouremia in the syndrome of inappropriate secretion of antidiuretic hormone. *Ann Intern Med* 93:716, 1980.
20. Decaux G, Genette F: Urea for long-term treatment of syndrome of inappropriate secretion of antidiuretic hormone. *Br Med J* 283:1081, 1981.
21. Forrest JN, Cohen AD, Torretti J, et al: On the mechanism of lithium-induced diabetes insipidus in man and rat. *J Clin Invest* 53:1115–1123, 1974.
22. Forrest JN, Cox M, Hong C, et al: Superiority of demeclocycline over lithium in the treatment of chronic syndrome of inappropriate secretion of antidiuretic hormone. *N Engl J Med* 298:173–177, 1978.
23. Fraley DS, Adler S, Bruns FJ, et al: Stimulation of lactate production by administration of bicarbonate in a patient with a solid neoplasma and lactic acidosis. *N Engl J Med* 303:1100–1102, 1980.
24. Francisco LL, Sawin LL, DiBona GF: Mechanism of negative potassium balance in the magnesium deficient rat. *Proc Soc Exp Biol Med* 168:382, 1981.
25. Frick PG, Schmid JR, Kistler HJ, et al: Hyponatremia associated with hyperproteinemia in multiple myeloma. *Helv Med Acta* 33:317–329, 1967.
26. Furhman SA, Eckfeldt JH: Hyponatremia and ion-selective electrodes. *Ann Intern Med* 102:872, 1985.
27. Graettinge JS, Muenster JJ, Checchia CS, et al: A correlation of clinical and hemodynamic studies in patients with hypothyroidism. *J Clin Invest* 37:502, 1958.
28. Granerus AK, Jagenburg R, Svanborg A: Kaliuretic effect of L-dopa treatment in Parkinsonian patients. *Acta Med Scand* 201:291–297, 1977.
29. Hartman RC, Auditore JC, Jackson DP: Studies in thrombocytosis. I. Hyperkalemia due to release of potassium from platelets during coagulation. *J Clin Invest* 37:699, 1958.
30. Hartman D, Rossier B, Zohlman R, et al: Rapid correction of hyponatremia in the syndrome of inappropriate secretion of antidiuretic hormone. *Ann Intern Med* 78:870, 1973.
31. Hertz P, Richardson JA: Arginine-induced hyperkalemia in renal failure patients. *Arch Intern Med* 130:778, 1972.
32. Hoffbrand BI, Steward JD: Carbenicillin and hypokalemia. *Br Med J* 4:746, 1970.
33. Husted FC, Nolph KD, Maher JF: NaHCO$_3$ and NaCl tolerance in chronic renal failure. *J Clin Invest* 56:414, 1975.
34. Gennari FJ: Current concepts: uses and limitations. *N Engl J Med* 310:102, 1984.
35. Hill AR, Uribarri J, Mann J, Berl T: Altered water metabolism in tuberculosis. *Am J Med* 88:357, 1990.
36. Kestens PJ, et al: The effect of insulin on the uptake of potassium and phosphate by the isolated perfused canine liver. *Metabolism* 12:941, 1963.
37. Kinter LB, Huffman WF, Stasser FL: Antagonists of the antidiuretic activity of vasopressin. *Am J Physiol* 254:F165, 1988.

38. Ladenson JK, Apple FS, Koch DD: Misleading hyponatremia due to hyperlipemia: a method-dependent error. *Ann Intern Med* 95:707, 1981.

39. Linas SL, Berl T, Robertson GL, et al: Role of vasopressin in the impaired water excretion of glucocorticoid deficiency. *Kidney Int* 18:58–67, 1980.

40. Mattar JA, Weil MH, Shubin H, Stein L: Cardiac arrest in the critically ill. Hyperosmolar states following cardiac arrest. *Am J Med* 56:162, 1974.

41. Mir MA, Brabin B, Tnag OT, et al: Hypokalemia in acute myeloid leukemia. *Ann Intern Med* 82:54–57, 1972.

42. Mitchell JH, Sildenthal K, Johnson RL: The effects of acid-base disturbances on cardiovascular and pulmonary function. *Kidney Int* 1:375, 1972.

43. Montoliu J, Lens XM, Revert L: Potassium lowering effect of albuterol for hyperkalemia in renal failure. *Arch Intern Med* 147:713, 1987.

44. Moses AM, Howanitz J, van Gemert M, et al: Clofibrate-induced antidiuresis. *J Clin Invest* 52:535, 1973.

45. Narins RG, Cohen JJ: Bicarbonate therapy for organic acidosis: the case for its continued use. *Ann Intern Med* 106:615, 1987.

46. Norenberg MD, Leslie KO, Robertson AS: Association between rise in serum sodium and central pontine myelinolysis. *Ann Neurol* 11:128, 1982.

47. Oh MS: Selective hypoaldosteronism. *Resident Staff Phys* 28:46S–62S, 1982.

48. Oh MS, Phelps K, Traube M, et al: D-Lactic acidosis in a man with the short bowel syndrome. *N Engl J Med* 301:249, 1979.

49. Oh MS, Uribarri J, Barrido D, Landsman S, Choi K-C, Carroll HJ: Danger of central pontine myelinolysis in hypotonic dehydration and recommendation for treatment. *Am J Med Sci* 296:41–43, 1989.

50. Oh MS, Uribarri J, Alveranga D, et al: Metabolic utilization and renal handling of D-lactate in man. *Metabolism* 34:621, 1985.

51. Oh MS, Carroll HJ: Hypernatremia, ed 3. In Hurst JW (ed): *Medicine for the Practicing Physicians*. Butterworth-Heinemann, London, p 1293, 1992.

52. Orlinger CE, Estace JC, Wunsch CD, et al: Natural history of lactic acidosis after grand mal seizures. *N Engl J Med* 297:796–799, 1977.

53. Oster JR, Perez GO, Vaamonde CA: Relationship between blood pH and phosphorus during acute metabolic acidosis. *Am J Physiol* 235:F345–F351, 1978.

54. Park R, Arieff AI: Lactic acidosis. *Adv Intern Med* 24:33, 1980.

55. Phelps KR, Lieberman RL, Oh MS, et al: The syndrome of hyporeninemic hypoaldosteronism. *Metabolism* 29:185, 1980.

56. Phelps KR, Oh MS, Carroll HJ: Heparin-induced hyperkalemia: report of a case. *Nephron* 25:254–258, 1980.

57. Pierce NF, Fedson DS, Brigham KL, et al: The ventilatory response to acute base deficit in humans. Time course during development and correction of metabolic acidosis. *Ann Intern Med* 172:633, 1970.

58. Posner JB, Plum E: Spinal fluid pH and neurological symptoms in acidosis. *N Engl J Med* 277:605, 1967.

59. Rado JP: Combination of carbamazepine and chloropropamide in the treatment of "hyporesponder" pituitary diabetes insipidus. *J Clin Endocrinol Metab* 38:1, 1974.

60. Raskind M, Burns RF: Water metabolism in psychiatric disorders. *Semin Nephrol* 4:316, 1984.

61. Relman AS: Lactic acidosis. In Brenner BM, Stein JH (eds): *Contemporary Issues in Nephrology: Acid-Base and Potassium Homeostasis*, vol 2. Churchill Livingstone, New York, 1978, p 65.

62. Relman ASD: Lactic acidosis and a possible new treatment. *N Engl J Med* 298:564–565, 1978.

63. Robinson AG: DDAVP in the treatment of central diabetes insipidus. *N Engl J Med* 294–507, 1976.

64. Roza O, Berman LB: The pathophysiology of barium: hypokalemic and cardiovascular effects. *J Pharmacol Exp Ther* 177:433–439, 1971.

65. Santensanio F, et al: Evidence for a role of endogenous insulin and glucagon in the regulation of potassium homeostasis. *J Lab Clin Med* 81:809, 1973.

66. Schambelan M, Sebastian A, Rector Jr FC: Mineralocorticoid-resistant renal hyperkalemia without salt wasting (type II pseudohypoaldosteronism): role of increased renal chloride reabsorption. *Kidney Int* 19:716, 1981.

67. Schrier RW, Lehman D, Zacherle B, et al: Effect of furosemide on free water excretion in edematous patients with hyponatremia. *Kidney Int* 3:30, 1973.

68. Scribner BH, Burnell JM: Interpretation of serum potassium concentration. *Metabolism* 5:468, 1956.

69. Sebastian A, McSherry E, Morris RC: Renal potassium wasting in renal tubular acidosis (RTA). Its occurrence in types I and II RTA despite sustained correction of systemic acidosis. *J Clin Invest* 50:667, 1971.

70. Sebastian A, McSherry Z, Morris RC: Metabolic acidosis with special reference to the renal acidosis. In Brenner BM, Rector FC (eds): *The Kidney*. W.B. Saunders, Philadelphia, p 615, 1976.

71. Singer I, Rotenberg D, Puschett JB: Lithium-induced nephrogenic diabetes insipidus. *J Clin Invest* 51:1081, 1972.

72. Singer I, Rotenberg D: Demeclocycline-induced nephrogenic diabetes insipidus. In vivo and in vitro studies. *Ann Intern Med* 79:679, 1973.

73. Skowsky WR, Kikuchi TA: The role of vasopressin in the impaired water excretion of myxedema. *Am J Med* 64:613, 1978.

74. Spencer PW, Voyce MA: Familial hypomagnesemia and hypokalemia. *Acta Paediatr Scand* 65:505, 1976.

75. Sperlakis N, Schneider MF, Harris EJ: Decreased K^+ conductance produced by Ba^{++} in frog sartorius fibers. *J Gen Physiol* 50:1565–1583, 1967.

76. Stacpoole PW: The lactic acidosis: the case against bicarbonate therapy (editorial). *Ann Intern Med* 105:276, 1986.

77. Stacpoole PW, Moore GW, Korhauser DM: Metabolic effects of dichloroacetate in patients with diabetes mellitus and hyperlipoproteinemia. *N Engl J Med* 298:526–530, 1978.

78. Stacpoole PW, Harman EM, Curry SH, et al: Treatment of lactic acidosis with dichloroacetate. *N Engl J Med* 309:390, 1983.

79. Sterns RH, Riggs JE, Schochet Jr, SS: Osmotic demyelinating syndrome following correction of hyponatremia. *N Engl J Med* 314:1535, 1986.

80. Szatalowicz VL, Arnold PE, Chaimovitz L, et al: Radioimmunoassay of plasma arginine vasopressin in hyponatremic patients with congestive heart failure. *N Engl J Med* 305:203, 1981.

81. Taradash MR, Jacobson LB: Vasodilatory therapy of idiopathic lactic acidosis. *N Engl J Med* 293:468, 1975.

82. Uribarri J, Oh MS, Carroll HJ: Salt-losing nephritis. *Am J Nephrol* 3:193, 1983.

83. Van Goidsenhoven GMT, et al: The effect of prolonged administration of large doses of sodium bicarbonate in man. *Clin Sci* 13:383, 1954.

84. Wilson RF, Gibson D, Percivel AK: Severe alkalosis in critically ill surgical patients. *Arch Surg* 105:197, 1972.

CHAPTER 58

Bicarbonate Therapy in the Treatment of Metabolic Acidosis

ALLEN I. ARIEFF, M.D., F.A.C.P.

The appropriate indications for use of bicarbonate in patients with metabolic acidosis have become an important topic that has spilled into the fields of critical care, internal medicine, surgery, and anesthesia. Editorials during the past 5 years have often expressed disparate opinions (1–4). The fundamental disagreements involve both the qualitative and quantitative indications, or lack of them, for the use of bicarbonate in several clinical situations. This chapter reviews the rationale for use of sodium bicarbonate in the management of patients with metabolic acidosis.

CLASSIFICATION OF METABOLIC ACIDOSIS

Metabolic acidosis has generally been broadly defined as a condition characterized by an arterial pH below 7.35 and bicarbonate below 20 mM/liter in the absence of arterial hypercapnia. However, recent evidence demonstrates that there is a separate entity, which can best be defined as "hypercapneic metabolic acidosis," in which the acidosis is secondary to "metabolic carbon dioxide" (CO_2) accumulation. This entity is not "respiratory acidosis," as the lungs are functioning well (5–8). The CO_2 accumulation is secondary to some combination of decreased cardiac output (with decreased delivery of mixed venous blood to the lungs) and increased formation of metabolic CO_2 (5, 8).

With metabolic acidosis and a decreased blood bicarbonate, the biochemical findings result from addition to the extracellular fluid of an acid load, which may be either exogenous or endogenous. The response of the body to an acid load includes its titration by various fixed buffers, both intracellular and extracellular. The intracellular buffers consist primarily of proteins and polypeptides, while extracellular buffers include hemoglobin, plasma proteins, and creatinine. In general, because of the body's buffering capacity, there will be no change in the plasma bicarbonate until almost all fixed buffers have been exhausted. Thus, when a patient with metabolic acidosis has a measurable decline in plasma bicarbonate, the interpretation is that essentially all available intra- and extracellular buffers except bicarbonate have been exhausted.

One method of classification of metabolic acidosis is based on the anion gap (9). The "anion gap" (AG) is defined as the difference between the blood concentration of sodium (Na) minus that of chloride (Cl) plus bicarbonate (HCO_3) (10, 11). Metabolic acidosis thus can be classified according to whether the anion gap is normal, low, or elevated. Increased anion gap metabolic acidosis includes those disorders in which there is acidosis because of the presence of increased quantities of organic acid(s). Such organic acids may be either endogenous (keto-acids, lactic acid) or exogenous (salicylate, paraldehyde). Those forms of metabolic acidosis with normal to low anion are primarily the renal tubular acidoses. The normal range for the anion gap is 9–14 mM/liter. It must be pointed out that with the introduction of ion-specific electrodes, the clinical use of the anion gap may be superseded in the near future (12).

Metabolic acidosis with increased anion gap can also be conveniently divided further into those clinical conditions in which there is either (*a*) the presence of tissue hypoxia, or (*b*) the absence of tissue hypoxia (13). Tissue hypoxia theoretically is present in all forms of lactic acidosis in general, the acidosis of cardiac arrest in particular, and in a substantial number of patients who are critically ill, even if blood lactate is not elevated (14). There is a critical level at which a modestly depressed total body oxygen utilization will not result in increased lactate production. When a critically low level of oxygen utilization is reached, arterial lactate may increase quite rapidly. There is often the impression of an acute disturbance of tissue oxygenation, whereas, in fact, oxygen use has been depressed for some time (14–16).

In most other forms of metabolic acidosis, in particular, diabetic ketoacidosis, uremic acidosis, acidosis resulting from most exogenous intoxicants, renal tubular acidosis, and the acidosis of diarrheal disease, tissue hypoxia is generally absent (4). A major reason for identifying those metabolic acidoses that are associated with tissue hypoxia relates to therapy. The therapy of such disorders often has included administration of sodium bicarbonate ($NaHCO_3$), which frequently makes the acidosis worse (17–19). To the contrary, administration of sodium bicarbonate to patients who have metabolic acidosis that is not associated with tissue hypoxia is often of benefit (4).

OXYGEN USE AND HYPOXIC METABOLIC ACIDOSIS

HYPOXIA AND THE CARDIOVASCULAR SYSTEM

In the development of lactic acidosis associated with tissue hypoxia, the critical factors are the performance of the heart and lungs, and the subsequent delivery of oxygen to the tissues. The critical role of the heart in the development of lactic acidosis is often not appreciated (13, 20). Total body oxygen utilization can be impaired substantially without a measurable increase in arterial lactate (14, 15). Also, measurements of arterial blood gases and lactate are often of no use in determining the acid-base and oxygenation status of either the "whole body" or the heart (7, 8, 14). A critical factor is the "oxygen extraction reserve" (Fig. 58.1). This is the difference between the arterial oxygen content (in volume %) and the mixed venous oxygen from either the "whole body" or any organ system. It is clear that the limiting factor is the oxygen supply to the heart, or the coronary venous oxygen content.

METABOLIC ACIDOSIS: HYPOXIC AND NORMOXIC

If one attempts to determine the response to therapy in patients with metabolic acidosis, it appears that a more useful classification of metabolic acidosis would be based on whether the condition is or is not associated with tissue hypoxia. In general, when there is metabolic acidosis in the presence of tissue hypoxia, available tissue oxygen is not adequate for the individual's metabolic needs (Table 58.1). Therapy of the metabolic acidosis with $NaHCO_3$ tends to limit further the available oxygen and thus lead to increased lactate production, actually worsening the metabolic acidosis. However, if the metabolic acidosis is not associated with tissue hypoxia (Table

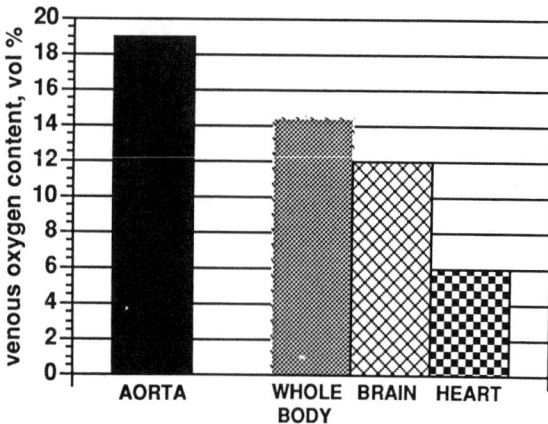

OXYGEN EXTRACTION RESERVE

Figure 58.1. The oxygen content in aorta and venous blood in normal humans. The oxygen extraction reserve can be calculated as the venous oxygen content, since in severe hypoxia, all available oxygen theoretically can be extracted. The oxygen reserve of either "whole body" or brain is at least twice that of the heart. Thus, in hypoxic states, the heart has less reserve oxygen than any other organ or tissue in the body.

Table 58.1. Therapy with $NaHCO_3$: Metabolic Acidosis Without Hypoxia

No change in oxygen utilization
No change in lactate production
Increase in arterial pH

58.1), bicarbonate may raise the arterial pH and prove beneficial (4, 21, 22).

BLOOD GASES: ARTERIAL VERSUS MIXED VENOUS

It is now clear from studies in both laboratory animals (23–25) and human subjects (7, 8, 14) that although arterial blood gases are a good indicator of pulmonary oxygenation, they are a poor indicator of the oxygenation and acid-base status of the rest of the body. Arterial blood gases evaluate the performance of the lungs, and the lungs can affect only the blood that has just passed through them. In low-flow states with impaired venous return and/or cardiac output, arterial blood may be relatively normal while mixed venous blood demonstrates severe acidosis and/or hypoxia (7, 8). In critically ill patients, measurements must be made of the arterial and mixed venous (pulmonary artery) gases, including oxygen content (which can be determined from the oxygen saturation and hemoglobin). As a practical matter, central venous gases are similar enough to mixed venous (pulmonary artery) gases that they can be used when a pulmonary artery catheter cannot be placed in the patient (8). When these measurements are available, the oxygen transport (or delivery) can be calculated using the product of the arterial oxygen content and blood flow (usually expressed as ml O_2/min) (26). It represents the quantity of oxygen available or delivered to the whole body or to individual organs or tissues, and is maintained preferentially to the "vital organs" during hypoxia by a number of adaptive mechanisms (27, 28). The ability of tissues to increase oxygen extraction when oxygen delivery is inadequate is the oxygen extraction reserve, or the oxygen utilization coefficient (29–31). Since the hypoxic states tissues theoretically are capable of extracting virtually all of the oxygen delivered, the oxygen extraction reserve represents the amount of oxygen not extracted by the tissues, which theoretically is available (32). Under normal aerobic conditions, this oxygen extraction reserve is quite large. However, because resting oxygen requirements are higher per gram of tissue in the heart than in any other organ, resting oxygen will be much higher, about 60–65%. Consequently, the heart has the smallest extraction reserve, and can increase resting oxygen extraction only by a maximum of about 50%. This reserve is in marked contrast to the body as a whole, which has an oxygen reserve three times the normal resting oxygen extraction. With increasing hypoxia, circulatory adjustments become increasingly important to maintain adequate oxygen delivery to the heart and brain. There is a generalized reduction of oxygen utilization in most of the "nonvital organs," such as skeletal muscle, liver, and gastrointestinal tract, with preferential utilization by heart and brain. The failure of such adjustments will lead to intracellular acidosis and eventual organ failure.

SODIUM BICARBONATE AND METABOLIC ACIDOSIS

GENERAL CONSIDERATIONS

Sodium bicarbonate has been used in the therapy of metabolic acidosis for more than 50 years and has almost become a matter of routine. This practice was continued without any serious question of its metabolic and systemic actions until about 1980. The rationale has been the implied logic of administering a base to correct an acidotic state. Theoretically, sodium bicarbonate should react with the hydrogen ion from an organic acid as shown below in Equation 1, where Ac− represents the anion of an organic acid.

$$HAc + NaHCO_3 \rightarrow NaAc + H_2O + CO_2 \qquad (1)$$

The preceding reaction should remove the H^+ ion by its chemical conversion to H_2O, with removal of the CO_2 via the lungs. In fact, in patients with renal tubular acidosis, diarrhea, and uremic acidosis, the arterial pH generally improves with the administration of sodium bicarbonate. Such patients generally do not have problems of tissue oxygenation. However, there are several potential negative effects of sodium bicarbonate administration, some of which are shown in Table 58.2. These include (*a*) venous hypercapnea with an increase of mixed venous CO_2 (33, 34), leading to a decrease in tissue pHi (23, 24, 35); (*b*) a decrease in the pH of cerebrospinal fluid (22, 36); (*c*) tissue hypoxia (37–39); (*d*) circulatory congestion (40); (*e*) hypernatremia (40, 41); and (*f*) hyperosmolality

Table 58.2. Therapy with NaHCO₃: Metabolic Acidosis with Hypoxia

Increase in Blood PCO₂
Decrease in blood pH
Decreased tissue O₂ delivery
Decreased coronary blood flow

with brain damage (40, 42). Whereas sodium bicarbonate is often beneficial in most patients who have metabolic acidosis without tissue hypoxia, some patients with diabetic ketoacidosis or hepatic failure will have impaired tissue oxygen delivery, and the aforementioned complications of sodium bicarbonate will be manifest. Additionally, in most patients with either cardiac arrest, shock, or sepsis, tissue oxygen delivery is impaired substantially and is the primary cause of lactate accumulation. The administration of sodium bicarbonate does not appear to affect the underlying tissue hypoxia and generally is not successful in improving either the acidotic state or clinical status. Thus, the underlying cause of lactate accumulation appears to determine whether sodium bicarbonate will be of benefit.

In an early study of patients with lactic acidosis (18) given large amounts of intravenous bicarbonate, there was essentially no change in either arterial pH or the clinical condition of these patients. None survived. In patients with cardiac arrest, sodium bicarbonate increases the mixed-venous and arterial PCO₂ (7, 34, 41) without either decreasing the blood lactate or increasing the bicarbonate. The result is either no change or a net decrease in the blood pH when compared with observations if sodium bicarbonate is not used. Moreover, the administration of large amounts of bicarbonate (mean of 180 mmol) during cardiac arrest (41) resulted in severe hypernatremia, hyperosmolality, increasing lactic acidosis, and no survival. These observations and others have apparently led to continuing recommendations of the American Heart Association to reduce the amount of bicarbonate given in cardiac arrest. Current guidelines for therapy of cardiopulmonary arrest no longer recommend the routine use of NaHCO₃ (43).

DIABETIC KETOACIDOSIS

Indications for the use of bicarbonate in diabetic ketoacidosis are currently less controversial than previously had been the case. There are at least two important studies in which the effects of bicarbonate on blood pH, glucose, bicarbonate, and ketone levels were examined in patients with diabetic ketoacidosis (44, 45). In general, it was found that administration of bicarbonate did not result in either a greater decrease in blood ketone levels or a greater increase in blood pH than was observed in patients who did not receive bicarbonate. Sodium bicarbonate administered to patients with diabetic ketoacidosis thus had no apparent effect on the rate of change of pH, the levels of blood ketones, or the change in blood bicarbonate or arterial CO₂. In addition, the ultimate survival was similar in patients who did or did not receive bicarbonate. In the cerebrospinal fluid, sodium bicarbonate administration was associated with an increase in spinal fluid PCO₂ that was not observed when bicarbonate was not given (46, 47). This resulted in a small but significant decrease in the pH of cerebrospinal fluid. Earlier studies had suggested that such a decrease in spinal fluid pH secondary to administration of bicarbonate might lead to depression of sensorium (36). However, subsequent studies have failed to confirm these earlier impressions (22). Although the decrease in spinal fluid pH may not be harmful, it is almost certainly of no benefit. Evidence that bicarbonate potentially may be detrimental in

Table 58.3. Types of Lactic Acidosis

Type A—Definite cause of tissue hypoxia
   Shock
   Hemorrhage
   Pulmonary edema
Type B—No definite cause of tissue hypoxia
   Idiopathic
   Malignancy
   Diabetes

patients with ketoacidosis is found in other studies. In animals with metabolic acidosis, administration of bicarbonate decreased delivery of oxygen to the brain, increased cerebrospinal fluid lactate levels, and decreased brain intracellular pH (35, 38). Another reason why the use of bicarbonate in patients with diabetic ketoacidosis may not be useful relates to the stoichiometry of the disorder. In ketoacidosis, there are at least 400–500 mM of available endogenous bicarbonate precursor in the form of lactate and ketoacid anions. The liver is able to metabolize these anions, and for each mM metabolized, 1 mM of H+ ion is consumed, which generates a bicarbonate ion (48, 49). Thus, in patients with diabetic ketoacidosis, the body has more than 400 mM of available bicarbonate precursor, and with insulin administration, ketogenesis (a H+ ion generating reaction) ceases. Thus, administration of the 50–100 mM of bicarbonate commonly given to patients with diabetic ketoacidosis would not be expected to affect arterial pH, and in effect, it generally does not (44). Overall, it appears that few beneficial effects are attributed to the use of bicarbonate in patients with ketoacidosis. There are several potentially harmful sequelae, but the clinical importance of these mechanisms is unclear.

LACTIC ACIDOSIS

Lactic acidosis is probably the most common form of metabolic acidosis and generally is defined as metabolic acidosis resulting from the accumulation of lactic acid, with blood lactate in excess of 5 mM and blood pH less than 7.25. Hyperlactatemia is far more than an isolated laboratory finding. It has been observed that when the blood lactate exceeds 9 mM, mortality is in excess of 75% (50). Disorders of lactate metabolism are usually divided into either anaerobic (type A) or aerobic (type B) (51) (Table 58.3). In patients with type A lactic acidosis, there is tissue hypoxia resulting in anaerobic lactic acid production. Such disorders include cardiopulmonary arrest and other states characterized by impaired cardiac performance, reduced tissue perfusion, and arterial hypoxemia. In type B lactic acidosis, on the other hand, tissue hypoxia appears not to be present, and there is increased lactic acid production for other metabolic reasons. Such disorders include diabetes mellitus, certain malignancies, and selected congenital diseases of the liver; the same is true in certain patients with AIDS and lactic acidosis (52). Of the two forms of lactic acidosis, type A is more common clinically and generally is associated with a higher morbidity and mortality.

LACTIC ACIDOSIS AND THE CARDIOVASCULAR SYSTEM

Lactic acidosis appears to have negative effects on myocardial function that are both direct and indirect, and are present when the acidosis results from either hypercapnia with hypoxia or metabolic acidosis *per se* (53–55). However, recent data strongly suggest that following myocardial ischemia (cardiac arrest, coronary occlusion), myocardial intracellular pH may fall below 6.0 (56). The H+ ion comes from a combination of the hydrolysis of ATP (57, 58) and "metabolic" hypercapnia (6, 59). Furthermore, the acid-base status of the heart and coronary circulation is not reflected accurately by the chemistries in arterial blood (8). Since effects on myocardium are determined largely by myocardial intracellular pH and not the extracellular pH, it is not appropriate to make a decision to administer $NaHCO_3$ based on arterial gases (7). The goal of cardiopulmonary resuscitation has been to correct rapidly both hypoxia and metabolic acidosis in order to help restore myocardial function. However, sodium bicarbonate has not been consistently shown to neither improve hemodynamics, increase arterial pH, or increase the blood bicarbonate concentration, and it appears to have adverse effects on both tissue oxygenation and myocardial function (17, 26, 60–62).

ALTERNATIVES TO SODIUM BICARBONATE

Because of the varied detrimental effects of sodium bicarbonate on organ function, particularly the heart, during hypoxic states, several other agents have been developed for the treatment of type A lactic acidosis. The goal has been to improve the blood pH during hypoxic states without reducing oxygen delivery, stimulating CO_2 or lactate production, or adversely affecting end-organ function. The most promising of these agents are: dichloroacetate, Carbicarb, and Tham. All have been tested in human subjects with metabolic acidosis, but currently, only Tham is approved for human use.

DICHLOROACETATE

Sodium dichloroacetate (DCA) may be an effective and safe form of therapy for reducing lactate levels and increasing pH in lactic acidosis. The effects of this drug on intermediary metabolism have been studied extensively in normal animals and in several animal models of lactic acidosis (63, 64). In animals with elevated lactate levels that have been induced by either exercise, diabetes, endotoxin, sepsis, phenformin, hepatic insufficiency, epinephrine, or hypoxia, DCA administration results in a reduction. In dogs with lactic acidosis resulting from either hypoxia, or from diabetes and phenformin, intravenous administration of DCA improved both intracellular and systemic pH (65, 66).

To date, the effects of DCA in the treatment of lactic acidosis have been described in several clinical studies (3, 61, 67, 68). More than 80% of the patients in these studies responded to treatment, with "response" defined as at least a 20% reduction in blood lactate occurring within 6 hours of the first DCA dose. DCA administration did not change the arterial or mixed venous PCO_2 levels, and thus presumably does not result in intracellular CO_2 accumulation (61, 69). There have been no reported adverse effects of oral or parenteral DCA administration in adults with lactic acidosis. Based on these preliminary data, a multicentered, controlled clinical trial to evaluate the effect of DCA therapy on mortality in adult patients with lactic acidosis recently has been completed (67). Initial results from this study should become available soon.

The mechanisms by which DCA improves cardiovascular function in hypoxic lactic acidosis are complex. However, in both patients with lactic acidosis and animal models with hypoxic lactic acidosis, administration of DCA improves cardiac output, while bicarbonate decreases both arterial pressure and cardiac output (17, 61, 65, 66). It is clear that in patients with lactic acidosis, DCA improves arterial blood gases and decreases blood lactate. Improvement in survival has not yet been demonstrated (67).

CARBICARB

Carbicarb was described in 1984 (70) as a potential replacement for $NaHCO_3$ in the therapy of metabolic acidosis (71). Carbicarb is an equimolar solution of $NaHCO_3$ and Na_2CO_3 (72). It buffers in a similar way as does $NaHCO_3$, but without increasing the blood CO_2 levels. This effect permits an evaluation of the hypothesis that generation of CO_2 after $NaHCO_3$ administration results in many of the detrimental effects on lactate metabolism and cardiovascular function (71). In normal volunteers, administration of $NaHCO_3$ resulted in a marked increase in CO_2 excretion, whereas Carbicarb actually resulted in a decrease in PCO_2 (73). These results suggested that Carbicarb actually decreased generation of CO_2 when administered systemically.

Carbicarb has been compared with $NaHCO_3$ in rats with metabolic acidosis induced by asphyxia (74). In rats with arterial pH of 7.17, $NaHCO_3$ did not increase arterial pH but resulted in significant increases in both PCO_2 and lactate. With Carbicarb, there was a significant increase in arterial pH, with no change in lactate or PCO_2. In another study in acidotic rats, Carbicarb normalized arterial pH without an increase in arterial PCO_2, and the intracellular pH (pHi) of brain was alkalinized (35). In a model of cerebral ischemia, $NaHCO_3$ administration resulted in an increase in brain PCO_2 and a decline in brain pHi (33).

In a recent large-scale study from the author's laboratory (72), 28 dogs with hypoxic lactic acidosis were treated with 2.5 mEq/kg of either $NaHCO_3$ or Carbicarb over 1 hour. After therapy, the arterial pH increased with Carbicarb and decreased with $NaHCO_3$. Mixed venous PCO_2 did not change with Carbicarb but increased with $NaHCO_3$. Arterial pressure decreased less with Carbicarb, and the cardiac output was stable with Carbicarb but decreased by 31% with $NaHCO_3$. Thus, administration of Carbicarb to dogs with hypoxic lactic acidosis results in improvement in the arterial blood gases, tissue pHi, lactate production, and cardiac hemodynamics. The response to Carbicarb contrasts to the effects of $NaHCO_3$ and may be related to less systemic CO_2 generation by Carbicarb. The author and colleagues began clinical testing in humans in 1990.

THAM

Tham (Tris buffer; 2-amino-2-hydroxymethyl-1,3-propanediol) is a synthetic buffer that has been proposed for the therapy of metabolic and respiratory acidosis. It theoretically counteracts the effects of CO_2 accumulation in respiratory acidosis (75) and has also been shown to be effective in the therapy of some forms of metabolic acidosis (76). At physiological pH (7.38), Tham has about the same buffer capacity as does normal blood (76). Unlike other buffers, such as bicarbonate, Tham penetrates cells and is an effective intracellular buffer. In dogs with metabolic acidosis, $NaHCO_3$ administration resulted in an increase in extracellular pH (pHe) from 7.30 to 7.58, but no change in pHi. However, with Tham, when pHe increased from 7.34 to 7.47, the pHi increased from 7.08 to 7.27, with an increase in intracellular bicarbonate from 11.6 to 21.4 mM/liter. Thus, Tham readily penetrates certain cells and appears to be an effective intracellular buffer (77).

In preliminary studies on patients, Tham was used in the therapy of six patients with severe diabetic ketoacidosis (mean arterial pH = 7.12, bicarbonate = 8.8 mM/liter). In all cases, Tham corrected the metabolic acidosis within 4–12 hours, without obvious toxicity (78). In additional preliminary studies in five patients with acidosis of renal failure, Tham was successful in elevating the arterial pH in all five patients, again without obvious toxicity. Thus, based on the effects of Tham on ischemic myocardium in vitro (79) and in vivo effects on metabolic acidosis of several different etiologies, Tham may be a valuable agent for the overall management of patients with lactic acidosis or cardiac arrest. Studies have not yet been carried out in either human subjects or animal models of lactic acidosis or cardiac arrest.

Thus, Tham, DCA, and Carbicarb all appear to be promising agents for the management of metabolic acidosis. All have been used in human subjects without apparent toxicity, although, as stated previously, only Tham is approved for human use. Based on data in both laboratory animals and patients with various forms of metabolic acidosis, all appear to be superior to sodium bicarbonate in the management of metabolic acidosis, and it is hoped that these agents will be available for human use in the near future.

ACKNOWLEDGMENT

This study was supported by the research service of the Veterans Affairs Medical Center, San Francisco, California.

REFERENCES

1. Ayus JC, Krothapalli RK: Effect of bicarbonate administration on cardiac function. *Am J Med* 87:5–6, 1989.
2. Narins RG, Cohen JJ: Bicarbonate therapy for organic acidosis: the case for its continued use. *Ann Intern Med* 106:615–618, 1987.
3. Stacpoole PW, Lorenz AC, Thomas RG, Harman EM: Dichloroacetate in the treatment of lactic acidosis. *Ann Intern Med* 108(1):58–63, 1988.
4. Gabow PA: Sodium bicarbonate: a cure or curse for metabolic acidosis? Acidosis type determines whether administration is appropriate. *J Crit Illness* 4(5):13–28, 1989.
5. Relman S: "Blood gases": arterial or venous? *N Eng J Med* 315:188–189, 1986.
6. von Planta M, Weil MH, Gazmuri RJ, Bisera J, Rackow EC: Myocardial acidosis associated with CO_2 production. *Circulation* 80:684–692, 1989.
7. Weil MH, Rackow EC, Trevino R, Grundler W, Falk JL, Griffel MI: Difference in acid-base state between venous and arterial blood during cardiopulmonary resuscitation. *N Engl J Med* 315(3):153–156, 1986.
8. Adrogue HJ, Rashad MN, Gorin AB, Yacoub J, Madias NE: Assessing acid-base status in circulatory failure. Differences between arterial and central venous blood. *N Engl J Med* 320:1312–1316, 1989.
9. Narins RG, Emmett M: Simple and mixed acid-base disorders: A practical approach. *Medicine (Baltimore)* 56:161–187, 1980.
10. Gabow PA, Keahny WD, Fennessey PV, Goodman SI, Gross PA, Schrier RW: Diagnostic importance of an increased anion gap. *N Engl J Med* 303:854–858, 1980.
11. Oh MS, Carroll HJ: The anion gap. *N Engl J Med* 297:814–817, 1977.

12. Winter SD, Pearson R, Gabow PA, Schultz AL, Lepoff RB: The fall of the serum anion gap. *Arch Intern Med* 150:311–313, 1990.

13. Arieff AI: Pathogenesis of metabolic acidosis with hypoxia. In Arieff AI (ed): *Hypoxia and the Circulation.* New York, Oxford University Press, pp 116–138, 1992.

14. Bihari D, Smithies M, Gimson A, Tinker J: The effects of vasodilation with prostacyclin on oxygen delivery and uptake in critically ill patients. *N Engl J Med* 317:397–403, 1987.

15. Eldridge F: Blood lactate and pyruvate in pulmonary insufficiency. *N Engl J Med* 274:878–883, 1966.

16. Arieff AI, Graf H: Pathophysiology of type A hypoxic lactic acidosis in dogs. *Am J Physiol* 253(16):E271–E276, 1987.

17. Graf H, Leach W, Arieff AI: Evidence for a detrimental effect of bicarbonate therapy in hypoxic lactic acidosis. *Science* 227(4688):754–756, 1985.

18. Waters WC, Hall JD, Schwartz WB: Spontaneous lactic acidosis. *Am J Med* 35:781–793, 1963.

19. Cooper DJ, Worthley LIG: Adverse haemodynamic effects of sodium bicarbonate in metabolic acidosis. *Intensive Care Med* 13:425–427, 1987.

20. Arieff AI: Pathogenesis of lactic acidosis. *Diabetes Metab Rev* 5(8):637–649, 1989.

21. Rosenbaum BJ, Coburn JW, Shinaberger JH, Massry SG: Acid-base status during the interdialytic period in patients maintained with chronic hemodialysis. *Ann Intern Med* 65:265, 1969.

22. Pierce NF, Fedson DS, Brigham KL, Mitra RC, Sack RB, Mondal A: The ventilatory response to acute base deficit in humans. *Ann Intern Med* 72:633–640, 1970.

23. Arieff AI, Leach W, Park R, Lazarowitz VC: Systemic effects of NaHCO$_3$ in experimental lactic acidosis in dogs. *Am J Physiol* 242(11):F586–F591, 1982.

24. Graf H, Leach W, Arieff AI: Metabolic effects of sodium bicarbonate in hypoxic lactic acidosis in dogs. *Am J Physiol* 249(18):F630–F635, 1985.

25. Mathias DW, Clifford PS, Klopfenstein HS: Mixed venous blood gases are superior to arterial blood gases in assessing acid-base status and oxygenation during acute cardiac tamponade in dogs. *J Clin Invest* 82:833–838, 1988.

26. Cooper JD, Walley KR, Wiggs BR, Russell JA: Bicarbonate does not improve hemodynamics in critically ill patients who have lactic acidosis. *Ann Intern Med* 112:492–498, 1990.

27. Cain SM: Oxygen delivery and uptake in dogs during anemic and hypoxic hypoxia. *J Appl Physiol* 42:228–234, 1977.

28. Hoffman JIE, Buckberg GD: The myocardial supply:demand ratio—a critical review. *Am J Cardiol* 41:327–332, 1977.

29. Guyton C: Transport of oxygen in the blood. In *Textbook of Medical Physiology.* WB Saunders, Philadelphia, pp 496–503, 1986.

30. Shoemaker WC: Relation of oxygen transport patterns to the pathogenesis and therapy of shock states. *Intensive Care Med* 13:230–243, 1987.

31. Chappell TR, Rubin LJ, Markham RV, Firth BG: Independence of oxygen consumption and systemic oxygen transport in patients with either stable pulmonary hypertension or refractory left ventricular failure. *Am Rev Respir Dis* 128:30–33, 1983.

32. Miller MJ: Tissue oxygenation in clinical medicine: an historical review. *Anesth Analg* 61:527–535, 1982.

33. Hope PL, Cady EB, Delpy DT, Ives NK, Gardiner RM, Reynolds EO: Brain metabolism and intracellular pH during ischaemia: effects of systemic glucose and bicarbonate administration by ^{31}P and ^{1}H nuclear magnetic resonance spectroscopy in vivo in the lamb. *J Neurochem* 50(5):1394–1402, 1988.

34. Bishop RL, Weisfeldt ML: Sodium bicarbonate administration during cardiac arrest. Effect on arterial pH, PCO$_2$, and osmolality. *J Am Med Assoc* 235:506–509, 1976.

35. Shapiro JI, Whalen M, Kucera R, Kindig N, Filley G, Chan L: Brain pH responses to sodium bicarbonate and Carbicarb during systemic acidosis. *Am J Physiol* 256:H1316–H1321, 1989.

36. Posner JB, Plum F: Spinal-fluid pH and neurologic symptoms in systemic acidosis. *N Engl J Med* 277:605–613, 1967.

37. Makisalo HK, Soini HO, Nordin AJ, Hockerstedt KAV: Effects of bicarbonate therapy on tissue oxygenation during resuscitation of hemorrhagic shock. *Crit Care Med* 17:1170–1174, 1989.

38. Bureau MA, Begin R, Berthiaume Y, Shappcott D, Khoury K, Gagnonn N: Cerebral hypoxia from bicarbonate infusion in diabetic acidosis. *J Pediatr* 96:968–973, 1980.

39. Bersin RM, Chatterjee K, Arieff AI: Metabolic and hemodynamic consequences of sodium bicarbonate administration in patients with heart disease. *Am J Med* 87(1):7–14, 1989.

40. Simmons MA, Adcock EW, Bard H, Battaglia FC: Hypernatremia and intracranial hemorrhage in neonates. *N Engl J Med* 291:6–10, 1974.

41. Mattar JA, Weil MH, Shubin H, Stein L: Cardiac arrest in the critically ill. II. Hyperosmolar states following cardiac arrest. *Am J Med* 56:162–168, 1974.

42. Snyder NA, Feigal DW, Arieff AI: Hypernatremia in elderly patients. A heterogeneous, morbid, and iatrogenic entity. *Ann Intern Med* 107(3):309–319, 1987.

43. National Conference on Cardiopulmonary Resuscitation: Standards and guidelines for cardiopulmonary resuscitation (CPR) and emergency cardiac care (ECC). Part III: Adult advanced cardiac life support. *J Am Med Assoc* 255:2933–2954, 1986.

44. Morris LR, Murphy MB, Kitabchi AE: Bicarbonate therapy in severe diabetic ketoacidosis. *Ann Intern Med* 105:836–840, 1986.

45. Lever E, Jaspan JB: Sodium bicarbonate therapy in severe diabetic ketoacidosis. *Am J Med* 75:263–268, 1983.

46. Ohman JL, et al: The cerebrospinal fluid in diabetic ketoacidosis. *N Engl J Med* 284:283, 1971.

47. Assal JP, Aoki TT, Manzano FM, Kozak GP: Metabolic effects of sodium bicarbonate in management of diabetic ketoacidosis. *Diabetes* 23:405–411, 1974.

48. Cohen RD, Iles RA, Barnett D, Howell MEO, Strunin J: The effect of changes in lactate uptake on the intracellular pH of the perfused rat liver. *Clin Sci* 41:159–170, 1971.

49. Beech JS, Williams SR, Cohen RD, Iles RA: Gluconeogenesis and the protection of hepatic intracellular pH during diabetic ketoacidosis in rats. *Biochem J* 263:737–744, 1989.

50. Peretz DL, Scott HM, Duff J: The significance of lactic acidemia in the shock syndrome. *Ann NY Acad Sci* 119:1133–1141, 1965.

51. Cohen RD, Woods F: Lactic acidosis revisited. *Diabetes* 32:181–191, 1983.

52. Chattha G, Arieff AI, Cummings C, Tierney LT: Lactic acidosis complicating the acquired immune deficiency syndrome. *Ann Intern Med* 118:37–39, 1993.

53. Walters F, Wilson GJ, Steward DJ, Domenech RJ, MacGregor DC: Intramyocardial pH as an index of myocardial metabolism during cardiac surgery. *J Thorac Cardiovasc Surg* 78:319–330, 1979.

54. Jeffrey FMH, Malloy CR, Radda GK: Influence of extracellular acidosis on contractile function in the working rat heart. *Am J Physiol* 253(22):H1499–H1505, 1987.

55. Ng ML, Levy MN, Zieske HA: Effects of changes of pH and of carbon dioxide tension on left ventricular performance. *Am J Physiol* 213:115–120, 1967.

56. Khuri SF, Marston W, Josa M, et al: Observations on 100 patients with continuous intraoperative monitoring of intramyocardial pH. *J Thorac Cardiovasc Surg* 89:170–182, 1985.

57. Zilva JF: The origin of the acidosis in hyperlactataemia. *Ann Clin Biochem* 15:40–43, 1978.

58. Johnston DG, Alberti KGMM: Acid-base balance in metabolic acidosis. *Clin Endocrinol Metabol* 12:267–285, 1983.

59. Khuri SF, Kloner RA, Karaffa SA, et al: The significance of the late fall in myocardial PCO$_2$ and its relationship to myocardial pH after regional occlusion in the dog. *Circ Res* 56:537–547, 1985.

60. Graf H, Arieff AI: The use of sodium bicarbonate in the therapy of organic acidosis. *Intensive Care Med* 12(4):285–288, 1986.

61. Stacpoole PW, Harman EM, Curry SH, Baumgartner TG, Misbin RI: Treatment of lactic acidosis with dichloroacetate. *N Engl J Med* 309:390–396, 1983.

62. Stacpoole PW: Lactic acidosis: the case against bicarbonate therapy. *Ann Intern Med* 105(2)276–279, 1986.

63. Crabb DW, Yount EA, Harris RA: The metabolic effects of dichloroacetate. *Metabolism* 30(10):1024–1039, 1981.

64. Stacpoole P: The pharmacology of dichloroacetate. *Metabolism* 38:1124–1144, 1989.

65. Park R, Arieff AI, Leach W, Lazarowitz VC: Treatment of lactic acidosis with dichloroacetate in dogs. *J Clin Invest* 70(4):853–862, 1982.

66. Graf H, Leach W, Arieff AI: Effects of dichoroacetate in the treatment of hypoxic lactic acidosis in dogs. *J Clin Invest* 76(3):919–923, 1985.

67. Stacpoole PW, Wright EC, Baumgartner TG: Dichloroacetate-Lactic Acidosis Study Group. A controlled trial of dichloroacetate for treatment of lactic acidosis in adults. *N Engl J Med* 327:1564–1569, 1992.

68. Stacpoole PW, Lactic Acidosis Study Group D-M: Causes, natural history and course of lactic acidosis in adults. *Clin Res* 39:165A, 1991.

69. Park R, Radosevich, PR, Leach WJ, Seto P, Arieff AI: Metabolic effects of dichloroacetate in diabetic dogs. *Am J Physiol* 245(8):E94–E101, 1983.

70. Filley GF, Kindig NB: Carbicarb, an alkalinizing ion generating agent of possible clinical usefulness. *Trans Am Clin Climatol Assoc* 96:141–153, 1984.

71. Kindig NB, Owens LV, Filley GF: Carbicarb as a replacement for NaHCO$_3$: Theory and in vitro experiments. *Appl Cardiopulmonary Pathophysiol* 2:231–240, 1987.

72. Bersin RM, Arieff AI: Improved hemodynamic function during hypoxia with Carbicarb, a new agent for the management of acidosis. *Circulation* 77(1):227–233, 1988.

73. Shapiro JI, Mathew A, Whalen M, et al: Different effects of sodium bicarbonate and an alternate buffer (Carbicarb) in normal volunteers. *J Crit Care* 5:157–160, 1990.

74. Sun J, Filley G, Hord K, Kindig N, Bartle E: Carbicarb: an effective substitute for NaHCO$_3$ for the treatment of acidosis. *Surgery* 102:835–839, 1987.

75. Conant JS, Hughs RE: The usefulness of THAM in metabolic acidosis. *Ann NY Acad Sci* 92:751–754, 1961.

76. Luchsinger PC: The use of 2-amino-2-hydroxymethyl-1,3-propanediol in the management of respiratory acidosis. *Ann NY Acad Sci* 92(2):743–750, 1961.

77. Robin ED, Wilson RJ, Bromberg PA: Intracellular acid-base relations and intracellular buffers. *Ann NY Acad Sci* 92:539–546, 1961.

78. Rees SB, Younger MD, Freedlender AE: Some in vivo and in vitro observations on the effects of Tris in diabetic acidosis. *Ann NY Acad Sci* 92:755–764, 1961.

79. Effron MB, Guarnieri T, Frederiksen JW, Greene HL, Weisfeldt ML: Effect of Tris (hyroxymethyl)aminomethane on ischemic myocardium. *Am J Physiol* 235:H167–H174, 1978.

CHAPTER 59

Poisoning

JAMES B. MOWRY, Pharm.D., A.B.A.T.
R. BRENT FURBEE, M.D., F.A.C.E.P., A.B.M.T.
PETER A. CHYKA, Pharm.D., A.B.A.T.

INTRODUCTION

A majority of patients with acute poisoning will be assessed, treated, and discharged from the emergency department. Twenty five percent of the 1.7 million poison exposures reported to the American Association of Poison Control Centers in 1990 were treated in a health care facility, of which only 18% required hospital admission for medical care (1). It is unknown what percentage of these 79,000 patients were admitted to an intensive care unit, but 5% of adult admissions and 3.1% of pediatric admissions to intensive care units are for poisonings or overdoses (2, 3).

The poisoned patient in the intensive care unit presents some unique aspects to clinical management (Table 59.1) (4). Antidotes and specific treatments do not take the place of routine supportive care measures that intensive care units are most skilled at providing. Good outcomes are common with only the provision of supportive care in critically ill, overdosed patients (3, 5). Close bedside and invasive monitoring in the ICU promotes the early detection and prevention of complications in overdoses. Therefore, a large number of poisoned patients are admitted to the ICU for observation, not for active intervention. Indeed, of all ICU admissions, including poisonings, only 10 to 15% require aggressive management and invasive monitoring (6).

Patients with acute reversible conditions that require intervention such as mechanical ventilation, vasopressor support, arrhythmia management, or hemodialysis clearly benefit from intensive care (7). Some criteria developed to identify poisoned patients at risk for complications include: need for intubation; unresponsiveness to verbal stimuli; seizures; $PACO_2 > 45$ mm Hg (6 kPa); systolic blood pressure < 80 mm Hg; any cardiac rhythm, except normal sinus, sinus tachycardia, or sinus bradycardia; second- or third-degree AV block; and QRS duration > 120 ms (8). Seventy-two percent of patients meeting these criteria develop one or more complications or require ICU interventions, while patients not meeting these criteria do not require ICU care. Kirk suggests ICU admission based upon end-organ toxicity and other defined criteria (Table 59.2) (4). Overdoses of substances that do not meet the above criteria, such as accidental chronic overdose on phenytoin or acetaminophen overdose requiring N-acetylcysteine administration, could well be managed on a general hospital ward. However, until further clinical studies are available to define these patients more precisely, most overdose patients will continue to be admitted to the intensive care unit.

The remainder of this chapter will be devoted to discussing the management strategies for the overdose or poisoned patient in general and for 15 of the most common serious poisonings likely to be treated in the intensive care setting, as identified by the American Association of Poison Control Center's statistics (1).

GASTRIC DECONTAMINATION

As the time between ingestion and emesis, gastric lavage, or activated charcoal administration increases, efficacy decreases.

Table 59.1. Unique Characteristics of Poisoning Cases*a*

Unreliable historical information
Multiple ingestions and interactions
Unpredictable clinical course
Continued or prolonged absorption
Delayed onset of action
Delayed complications
Survival after prolonged hypotension/hypoxia
Unfamiliar antidotes/treatments
High doses of conventional medications required

a Adapted from Kirk MA: Rational utilization of the intensive care unit in managing the poisoned patient. *Contemp Management Crit Care* 1(3):3–19, 1991.

Table 59.2. Considerations for ICU Admission

Intervention to maintain normal physiologic parameters
Signs of severe poisoning
Worsening signs of toxicity
Laboratory evidence of potential severe toxicity
Predisposing underlying medical conditions
Insufficient literature on human exposure
Potential for prolonged absorption
Potential for delayed onset of toxicity
Invasive procedures or monitoring needed
Antidotes with potential for serious side effects
Antidote with short duration of action
Evidence for drug withdrawal
Suicidal patients requiring observation

a Adapted from Kirk MA: Rational utilization of the intensive care unit in managing the poisoned patient. *Contemp Management Crit Care* 1(3):3–19, 1991.

However, prolonged absorption or formation of gastrointestinal bezoars may allow gastric decontamination to be useful late in an intoxication. Evidence to recommend one method over another remains controversial.

Ipecac syrup may be used prior to hospital presentation or, rarely, in the Emergency Department. Ipecac induces emesis in 81% to 91% of subjects in an average of 11.6 to 19.0 minutes (9–11). An additional 9% to 15% will vomit after a second dose in a total time of about 35 minutes. Recovery of ingested material in emesis averages only 19 to 62% and is inversely related to the time of administration (12–14). Ipecac produces from one to eight productive episodes of emesis lasting from 24 to 28 minutes, although emesis for more than 1 hour has been reported in up to 17% of patients (10, 11, 15–17). Side effects include drowsiness in up to 16% of children, and mild diarrhea in up to 13% (10, 15, 17, 18). Cardiomyopathy occurs only with chronic dosing, due to accumulation of emetine (19).

Gastric lavage requires 10 to 15 ml/kg water or normal saline (up to 300 ml per wash), using a large-bore orogastric tube (adult: 36 to 40 French; child: 26 to 30 French) for a minimum of 2 liters. Frequent repositioning of the tube and placing the patient in the left lateral decubitus position aids in the recovery of stomach contents (20). Using this technique, recoveries of 88%, compared to 56% for ipecac, have been reported when both procedures are started immediately after ingestion (21). Waiting even 10 minutes to initiate treatment may reduce returns by 50% (22). The 60- to 90-minute delays common in reaching emergency departments and delays in large-bore tube insertion may further limit lavage's efficacy (23, 24).

Activated charcoal adsorbs chemicals onto the internal surface of a network of pores. Desorption from charcoal can occur in the gastrointestinal tract, necessitating a high charcoal-drug ratio (10:1). In practice, dosing is empiric, with infants and children generally receiving 30 to 50 g (about 1 to 2 g/kg) and adults 50 to 100 g/dose. Commercial preparations of charcoal in water or sorbitol circumvent some administration problems, but too-rapid administration commonly results in vomiting. Potentially life-threatening pulmonary aspiration is becoming more common with increased usage (25–28). Saline cathartics or sorbitol may decrease GI transit time, although evidence of their efficacy in preventing further absorption is lacking, and evidence of adverse effects is accumulating (29, 30). Fluid and electrolyte depletion from sorbitol and excessive magnesium absorption from magnesium-containing cathartics has occurred (31, 32). Contraindications to charcoal's use include ingestions of mineral acids, alkalis, most metals (iron, lithium, lead, etc.), organic solvents, and drugs that may have a specific oral antidote.

With the value of gastric emptying procedures being questioned, activated charcoal as a single agent for gastrointestinal decontamination has been suggested. Activated charcoal is considered equal to, or more effective, than gastric lavage or ipecac-induced emesis when given at equal times after drug administration (33–39). However, inadequate time postingestion has been allowed in research trials for administration of activated charcoal, considering the common time delays expected in clinical practice. Relatively small reductions in drug absorption with both charcoal and ipecac if delayed 1 hour after ingestion cast doubt about the efficacy of either treatment, although significant lowering of acetaminophen concentrations in pediatric ingestions, compared to that in untreated controls, has been demonstrated (33, 36). Another concern with the use of ipecac and charcoal together centers on the potential for significant delays in charcoal administration when given after ipecac-induced emesis (38).

Three large prospective clinical trials, totaling 1600 patients, have evaluated activated charcoal vs. gastric emptying in the emergency department (40–42). Gastric emptying procedures plus activated charcoal did not significantly alter the clinical outcome, admission rate, mean intubation time, or length of hospital or ICU admission, compared to those of activated charcoal administration alone. Ipecac administration and lavage were associated with higher complication rates for aspiration pneumonitis (41, 42). Asymptomatic patients, as determined by strictly defined parameters, receiving no gastric decontamination did not show clinical deterioration (42). Gastric emptying was deemed unwarranted in most cases, but lack of nontreatment control groups, prolonged patient presentation times, no quantitative measurements of outcome, and small numbers of severely ill patients limit the conclusions of these studies (43). These trials also primarily deal with the adult overdose patient, limiting their application to the pediatric population (3, 23, 40).

Whole bowel irrigation may reduce absorption in selected clinical situations by mechanically flushing the gastrointestinal tract of its contents. A standard solution of polyethylene glycol electrolyte solution (Go-Lytley, OCL Solution, Co-Lyte) is administered by nasogastric tube at a rate of 0.5 liters/hour in children and 2 liters/hour in adults (44). The endpoint of therapy is clear rectal effluent, which usually occurs in 4 to 6 hours. Limited work has been done in evaluating the efficacy of this procedure. One controlled trial with ampicillin and a number of anecdotal reports have surfaced about its use in overdoses of iron, lithium, zinc sulfate, and cocaine body packers (45–49).

Any gastric emptying procedure is questionable if begun more than 1 to 2 hours after ingestion (43). Ipecac's value in the hospital is limited to compounds not absorbed by activated charcoal (e.g., iron, lithium), for sustained release or enteric-coated tablets too large to remove by lavage, or drugs inhibiting gastric emptying. Gastric decontamination for most asymptomatic patients with a history of trivial overdose seems rarely indicated for a satisfactory outcome. However, failure to empty the gut may have medicolegal implications, especially in self-poisoning cases, given their notoriously poor histories. Gastric lavage is useful for removal of liquids and small tablet particles if used within 1 to 2 hours of ingestion and possibly for severely symptomatic patients to help limit further absorption (40). Activated charcoal seems to be more effective than ipecac in the hospital setting and can be used as a single agent for gastrointestinal decontamination in symptomatic, mild-to-moderate overdose patients, assuming the substance is adsorbed by charcoal. Whole bowel irrigation should be reserved for situations in which the above techniques would not be expected to be effective: late presentations with substances not adsorbed by activated charcoal or with the potential for delayed or prolonged periods of absorption due to chemical, physical, or pharmaceutical properties or constraints.

LABORATORY STUDIES: USE AND MISUSE

The vast majority of toxins are best managed with supportive care. Contrary to popular belief, there are few antidotes or specific treatments for ingestion, inhalation, or dermal exposures. For that reason, identification and quantitation of the specific toxin are only important if management involves more than supportive care. Quantitation of serum concentrations that are of use in the management of poisoned patients includes acetaminophen, alcohols, digitalis, heavy metals, iron, lithium, salicylate, theophylline, and warfarin (prothrombin time). Toxins treated with antidotes for which concentrations are not necessary include benzodiazepines, β-blockers, calcium channel blockers, cyanide, isoniazid, opiates, organophosphates, and venoms. Occasionally, medicolegal considerations may make quantitative measurement desirable, such as in the case of attempted homicide or child abuse.

The ordering of toxicologic screens is frequently a reflex action on the part of the clinician but offers little benefit to patient management (50, 51). Many of the major groups of toxins have characteristic presentations, or toxidromes. Salicylates, antidepressants, sedative hypnotics, opiates, cholinergic, and anticholinergic agents are only a few of the poisonings that may be diagnosed by physical examination. Screening examinations, on the other hand, may identify drugs that are present in small amounts and are of little consequence. The clinician may incorrectly assume that a negative drug screen rules out certain toxins when, in fact, they are not detected

by the test even when present in large amounts (52). Antidepressant screens, for example, may only detect five or six compounds but completely miss several others in the same class. It is imperative that the physician become familiar with the sensitivity and range of the studies available in their institution (53). Some drugs, such as cocaine, are rapidly cleared from the plasma, but they or their metabolites may be detected in the urine for days. Therefore, if screens are desired, urine usually offers a wider range of detection.

FORMULAS HELPFUL IN PATIENT MANAGEMENT

Common causes of anion gap ($Na^+-(Cl^- + HCO_3^-)$) metabolic acidosis include ethanol-induced ketoacidosis, salicylates, uremia, diabetic ketoacidosis, methanol, ethylene glycol, paraldehyde, isoniazid, toluene, iron, lactic acidosis secondary to seizure, hypoxia, or shock, cyanide, and carbon monoxide. Causes of a decreased or negative anion gap include lithium or bromate intoxication. The anion gap in conjunction with the osmolal gap can be frequently used to determine the etiology of an acidotic state (54, 55).

An osmolal gap occurs due to the presence of osmotically active substances not accounted for in the common formulas utilized to calculate serum osmolality ($2 \times Na^+ + glucose/18 + BUN/2.8 + other osmotic compound/(MW/10)$), where the sodium is in millimoles/liter; glucose, BUN, and other osmotic compound are in milligrams per deciliter; and MW is the molecular weight of the osmotic compound (55). Common causes of increased serum osmolality with approximate molecular weights include methanol (MW = 32), ethylene glycol (MW = 62), ethanol (MW = 46), isopropanol (MW = 60), acetone (MW = 58), mannitol (MW = 182), and propylene glycol (MW = 76). An approximation of the concentration of a toxin in the plasma can be obtained from the formula (osmolar gap − 10) × MW/10 = serum concentration (mg/dl), where the osmolar gap equals the measured osmolality less the calculated osmolality and MW is the molecular weight of the substance sought after (55). When the plasma concentration of another osmotically active drug is present and known, it must be added into the calculated gap in order to get an accurate estimate of the specific toxin desired. For example, a patient poisoned with methanol who is being treated with an ethanol infusion may have a blood ethanol of 100 mg/dl, which can raise the serum osmolality by 22 mOsm/kg H_2O. This factor must be added into any calculation of serum osmolality to determine the methanol concentration correctly. Serum osmolality must be measured by freezing point depression osmometry, as the vapor pressure method produces false-negative results (56).

A crude estimate of the plasma level of a drug may be made if the amount of drug ingested is known by using the formula $Cp = amount/(V_d \times Wt)$, where Cp equals the plasma concentration, V_d the volume of distribution, and Wt the patient's weight in kilograms. Potential changes in absorption and volume of distribution for most drugs involved in overdoses limit the accuracy of pharmacokinetic formulas to estimate potential plasma concentrations, and knowledge of the drug's volume of distribution and therapeutic and toxic concentrations is necessary (57).

DRUG REMOVAL

Approaches to enhance the systemic elimination of a toxin include diuresis, diuresis with pH adjustment, hemodialysis, hemoperfusion, hemofiltration, and repeat-dose activated charcoal. The decision to utilize these options should be based on an assessment of its effectiveness for the specific toxin, availability and experience with the technique at the facility, condition of the patient, the patient's response to conventional therapy, the risks of the procedure, and the function of the patient's normal elimination processes. Generally, these techniques, particularly extracorporeal techniques, are reserved for poisonings that are potentially life-threatening.

Diuresis after administration of large volumes of intravenous fluid and diuretics to provide urine flow near 1 liter/hr or 2 to 4 ml/kg/hr may increase the urinary secretion of some drugs by decreasing the amount subject to tubular reabsorption. This technique is applicable only for drugs or active metabolites excreted unchanged primarily in the urine, of which there are very few of toxicologic significance. Complications such as pulmonary and cerebral edema and fluid electrolyte imbalance make this unproven therapy not generally useful (58).

Diuresis with manipulation of urinary pH theoretically can increase the clearance of weak acids and bases, but its application in current management is limited. Urinary acidification was advocated for amphetamine and strychnine, both epileptogenic agents, but acidification may promote deposition of myoglobin in the renal tubules in a patient already prone to rhabdomyolysis (59, 60). Urinary alkalinization to a urinary pH of 7 to 8 can be achieved with intravenous sodium bicarbonate 1 to 2 mEq/kg/hr over 1 to 2 hours every 3 to 4 hours; however, serum potassium deficits must be replaced to successfully achieve an alkaline pH. Alkaline diuresis may be useful for moderate salicylate or phenobarbital overdose, but severe poisonings require more efficient means of removal (61, 62). The complications of alkaline diuresis include hypernatremia, alkalosis, and fluid overload.

Dialysis should be considered when the duration of symptoms is expected to be prolonged, other pathways of excretion are unavailable, clinical deterioration is present, the drug is dialyzable, and appropriate personnel and equipment are available. In general it is more effective for drugs that possess small molecular weight (under 500 daltons), are not highly protein-bound, and are not highly distributed to tissues (63, 64). Certain drug characteristics (Table 59.3) suggest the type of dialysis that would be effective (65, 66). Hemodialysis, hemoperfusion, and hemofiltration are difficult to perform in patients who are hypotensive or perfusing poorly. Complications of hemodialysis include hypotension, nosocomial infection, and anticoagulation; complications for hemoperfusion include those and thrombocytopenia, hypocalcemia, and leukopenia. Peritoneal dialysis is a simple but slow procedure that does not require anticoagulation and may be useful when other methods are unavailable or vascular access cannot be established (67). Extracorporeal dialysis is used less frequently due to improvement in critical care approaches and monitoring, but it still has a routine place for serious poisonings with ethylene glycol, methyl alcohol, lithium, and theophylline. In situations where the dialyzability of a drug is unknown, application of the principles in Table 59.3 may provide some

Table 59.3. Kinetic Characteristics of Drugs That Make Them Amenable to Removal by Extracorporeal Procedures[a]

Hemodialysis
  Relative molecular mass <500 daltons
  Walter-soluble
  Small volume of distribution (<1 liter/kg)
  Poorly bound to plasma proteins
  Single-compartment kinetics
  Low endogenous clearance (<4 ml/min/kg)
Hemoperfusion
  Adsorbed by activated charcoal
  Small volume of distribution (<1 liter/kg)
  Poorly bound to plasma proteins
  Single-compartment kinetics
  Low endogenous clearance (<4 ml/min/kg)
Hemofiltration
  Relative molecular mass less than the cutoff of the filter fibers, usually <40,000 daltons
  Small volume of distribution (<1 liter/kg)
  Single-compartment kinetics
  Low endogenous clearance (<4 ml/min/kg)

[a] Source: Pond SM: Extracorporeal techniques in the treatment of poisoned patients. *Med J Aust* 154:618, 1991. © Copyright *The Medical Journal of Australia 1991*. Reproduced with permission.

insight. Further, if the percentage of free drug in plasma divided by the apparent volume of distribution (liters per kilogram) exceeds 80, 6 hours of hemodialysis should generally remove a significant amount (20 to 50%) of the drug (68). The pharmacokinetic data for this relationship may be obtained from several standard references (69, 70).

Therapy with repeated doses of activated charcoal has been shown to increase the systemic clearance of several compounds through a process likened to intestinal dialysis (71, 72). The mechanism of action of repeat-dose activated charcoal is unknown, but several options exist (Fig. 59.1) and may work in concert (73). It is generally indicated for moderate-to-severe poisonings, except where activated charcoal does not bind, e.g., with iron or lithium, or when bowel sounds are not present. Generally, 20 to 40 g of activated charcoal (0.5 to 1 g/kg/hr in neonates) are administered every 2 to 4 hours with a saline cathartic given once every 24 hours if needed. Several aspects of this therapy are unclear. Chief among them are which drugs are amenable to this treatment, the adverse effects during therapy, and the impact on patient outcome (74–76). Clinical studies (Fig. 59.2) to date indicate that repeat-dose activated charcoal can reduce the plasma elimination half-life in human volunteers by up to 62% and that certain drugs (Table 59.4) demonstrate no significant response to therapy (74, 77, 78). The risk of emesis in 12.5% to 56% of patients receiving charcoal and that of developing aspiration pneumonitis have prompted an outcry against its empiric universal use (25–28, 78–81). Although properties of drugs amenable to hemodialysis would seem reasonable predictors of the effectiveness of repeat-dose activated charcoal, a relationship has yet to be demonstrated (74).

ACETAMINOPHEN

Acetaminophen has been available in the U.S. as a nonprescription drug since 1955. The first case of hepatic toxicity was reported in Great Britain in 1966 (82). Today, it is found in over 200 nonprescription preparations and many prescription formulations.

Acetaminophen has strong analgesic and antipyretic effects. Though not devoid of antiinflammatory activity, animal studies have shown that doses required to reduce inflammation far exceed those required for analgesia. The exact mechanism by which acetaminophen produces analgesia and antipyretic effects is not completely clear; however, it appears to be related to a central inhibition of prostaglandin synthetase (83).

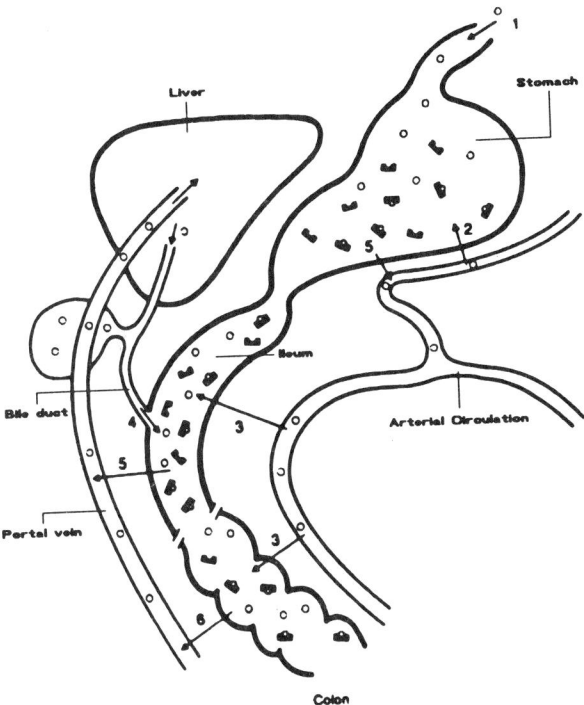

Figure 59.1. Schematic representation of the gastrointestinal tract and liver, showing points at which drug molecules (*o*) may enter or leave the gut and/or interact with activated charcoal (◼). *1*, oral absorption; *2*, gastric secretion; *3*, intestinal secretion/passive diffusion; *4*, biliary excretion; *5*, passive absorption of nonabsorbed drug; *6*, passive reabsorption of hydrolyzed drug conjugates. (From McLuckie A, Forbes AM, Ilett KF: Role of repeated doses of oral activated charcoal in the treatment of acute intoxications. *Anaesth Intens Care* 18:375–384, 1990. Used with permission.)

Table 59.4. Effect of Repeated Doses of Activated Charcoal on the Elimination of Drugs Based on Overdose Reports, Clinical Studies in Human Volunteers, and Studies in Animal Models[a]

Amitriptyline[b,c]	Disopyramide[d]	Piroxicam[c]
Atrazine[d]	*Doxepin[c]*	Porphyrine[c]
Carbamazepine[b,c]	*Imipramine[c]*	Quinine[b,c]
Chlorpropamide[c]	Meprobamate[b]	*Salicylates[b–d]*
Cyclosporine[b]	Methotrexate[c]	Satolol[c]
Dapsone[b,c]	Nadolol[c]	Tobramycin[c]
Diazepam[b]	Nortriptyline[c]	Theophylline[b–d]
Digitoxin[b,c]	Phenobarbital[b,c]	Theophylline SR[b,c]
Digoxin[b,c]	Phenylbutazone[c]	
Diltiazem[b]	Phenytoin[b,c]	*Vancomycin[b]*

[a] Drugs in italics showed no change in elimination.
[b] Overdose.
[c] Volunteers.
[d] Animals.

The toxic effects of acetaminophen are due to the metabolite, *N*-acetyl-*p*-benzoquinoneimine (NAPQI), a strong electrophile that covalently bonds within the hepatocyte, creating a pattern of central lobular necrosis. A similar mechanism in the kidney leads less frequently to renal necrosis. Infrequent reports of toxicity include subendocardial hemorrhage, focal myocardial necrosis, and pancreatitis, which has occurred with ingestions as low as 9.75 to 13 g in a chronic alcohol abuser (84, 85). The exact mechanism of these injuries is not known. Unlike phenacetin and acetanilide, acetaminophen does not produce clinically significant methemoglobinemia in humans.

The therapeutic dose of acetaminophen is 10 to 20 mg/kg in children and 0.5 to 1 g in adults given every 4 hours. Toxicity is dependent upon the dose and nutritional state of the patient. Among healthy patients there have been no reports of hepatotoxicity at doses less than 125 mg/kg. When the dose exceeds 250 mg/kg, 50% of untreated patients exhibit severe hepatic damage, while 100% of untreated patients will suffer severe injury at concentrations exceeding 350 mg/kg. Fatalities have occurred with therapeutic doses given to patients with hepatic failure (86, 87).

Absorption of acetaminophen is rapid and complete, with peak therapeutic concentrations occurring within 1 hour. In large or mixed ingestions, peak concentrations may not be seen until 4 hours postingestion. Acetaminophen is metabolized and eliminated via four different pathways (Fig. 59.3). Less than 5% is eliminated unchanged in the urine. Approximately 90% is eliminated following conjugation with sulfate or glucuronide. Although the sulfate pathway is less important in adults, it has been proposed as a more active pathway in children, which could account for their greater tolerance to higher doses. Between 5 and 10% of a dose of acetaminophen may be metabolized by a cytochrome P-450 mixed-function oxidase pathway. The intermediate metabolite of this pathway, NAPQI, is responsible for the hepatic injury associated with acetaminophen toxicity and can be detoxified by the addition of sulfhydryl groups. Ordinarily, glutathione acts as the sulfhydryl group donor but, in nutritionally depleted patients or in the presence of massive doses, it may not be present in sufficient quantity to protect the liver. Renal injury is also thought to occur via the same mechanism. The volume of distribution of acetaminophen is 0.75 to 1.0 liters/kg, with protein binding of 35 to 50%.

The classic presentation of acetaminophen toxicity includes the onset of gastrointestinal upset with nausea, vomiting, and abdominal pain. This presentation is most often seen in children but can be absent following significant ingestions in adults. For that reason, an acetaminophen concentration should be obtained in *any* intentional ingestion in patients over the age of 5 years. A quiescent or latent period occurs at 24 to 48 hours. If the ingestion of acetaminophen has been missed at that point, there is little benefit from administration of an antidote. The hepatic stage appears 3 to 4 days postingestion and includes the increase of hepatic transaminases, right upper quadrant abdominal pain, and liver dysfunction with hypoglycemia, coagulopathy, encephalopathy, and jaundice. The final stage is resolution, representing either recovery or death. Pancreatitis and myocardial damage have also been reported, as well as renal failure. Contrary to the multistep presentation above, massive overdoses have resulted in coma

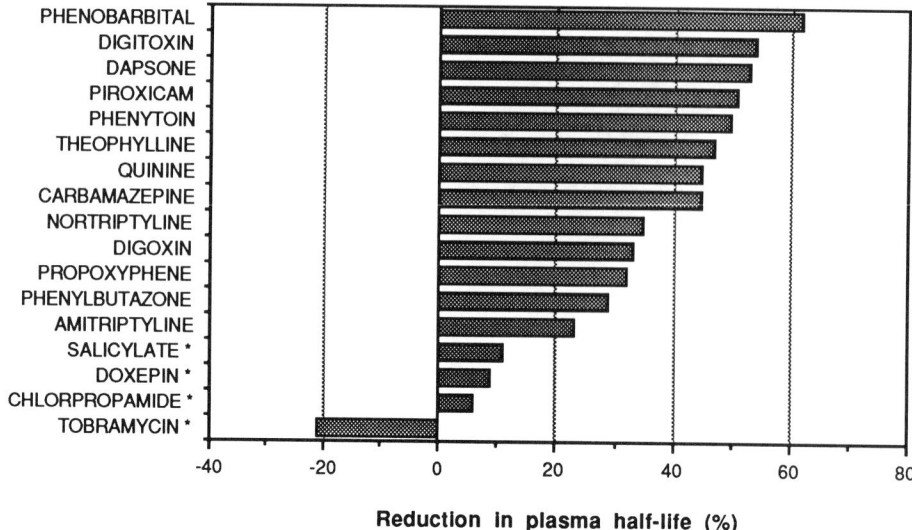

Figure 59.2.   Reduction in plasma half-life after repeated doses of activated charcoal in human volunteers. Drugs with asterisks show no significant change, others *p* < 0.05.

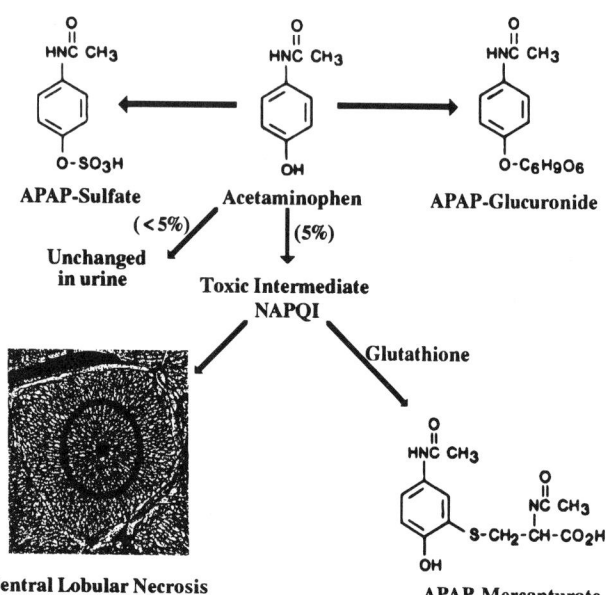

Figure 59.3.   Metabolism and elimination of acetaminophen (APAP).

and profound acidosis in the absence of the usual presenting signs (88).

Acetaminophen may be measured by colorimetric methods, immunoassays, gas chromatography, and high-performance liquid chromatography. The therapeutic level is considered to be 5 to 20 μg/ml. Acetaminophen concentrations may peak as late as 4 hours; therefore, concentrations obtained earlier than that may not be predictive. A 4-hour level of 150 μg/ml is considered "possibly toxic" while a level of 200 μg/ml at that time is designated "probably toxic." Other laboratory studies include electrolytes, blood glucose, liver function studies, BUN, creatinine, and complete blood count.

The mainstays of treatment are good supportive care and the early institution of antidotal therapy. *N*-acetylcysteine (Mucomyst, *N*-acetylcysteine (NAC)) acts as a sulfhydryl group

donor to detoxify NAPQI when glutathione is depleted. It is most effective when started within 10 hours of ingestion. Some recent studies suggest NAC may be of benefit even beyond 24 hours, especially in the presence of hepatic encephalopathy (89, 90). The institution of NAC therapy in acute ingestions is indicated by where the serum acetaminophen level falls on the Rumack-Matthews nomogram (Fig. 59.4) (91). Treatment of those patients whose serum concentrations fall upon or above the "possible toxicity" line on the nomogram has become conventional. As this nomogram has not been verified in children, children whose serum acetaminophen concentrations fall between the "possible" and "probable" toxicity lines may fare well even if they are not treated.

The Rumack-Matthews nomogram is intended for one-time, acute overdoses and cannot be applied to repeated overmedication during an extended period of time. Furthermore, serum concentrations obtained prior to 4 hours postingestion cannot be evaluated by the nomogram. A frequent area of confusion is when to stop NAC treatment. Serum acetaminophen concentrations do not reflect the concentration of the NAPQI metabolite; therefore, the full course of treatment should be carried out, regardless of any decrease in the serum concentration of acetaminophen. Secondly, glutathione is an important mechanism by which many varieties of oxidant stress are managed in vivo. The absence of acetaminophen in the serum at some time after a toxic concentration does not indicate the need to stop treatment with NAC.

Another source of confusion for clinicians is the management of poisoning when the time of ingestion is unknown. Because NAC is a relatively nontoxic antidote, some physicians choose to treat empirically for the full course. Elevations of liver function tests will also support the institution of therapy. Regional poison centers can assist in deciding which patients require acetylcysteine therapy.

Acetaminophen is also known to freely cross the placenta. While therapeutic doses are generally considered safe in pregnancy, fetal death has occurred as a result of overdose (92). *N*-acetylcysteine, however, does not appear to cross the placenta in significant amounts (93). However, the approach to acetaminophen toxicity should be the same in the pregnant patient and nonpregnant patient.

The dosage for NAC is 140 mg/kg orally as a loading dose, followed by 17 doses of 70 mg/kg given every 4 hours. NAC is commercially available as 10 and 20% solutions (10 or 20 g/100 ml). Because of the strong sulfur odor and the frequent gastrointestinal distress associated with acetaminophen ingestion, vomiting often makes oral administration difficult. Doses should be diluted to a 5% solution (1:1 or 1:3) in a cold acidic vehicle (cola, grapefruit juice, etc.) and administered in a covered container through a straw. Nasogastric or feeding tube placement may decrease vomiting, or metoclopramide

(0.1 to 1.0 mg/kg i.v.) or droperidol (2.5 to 5.0 mg i.v.) in adults may be used.

While intravenous administration of NAC is commonplace in Canada and Great Britain, it remains investigational in the U.S. A 48-hour treatment protocol begins with a loading dose of 140 mg/kg of pyrogen-free *N*-acetylcysteine (94). The initial dose is infused over an hour and, because of the risk of anaphylactoid reaction, should be administered under the direct supervision of a physician. Subsequent doses of 70 mg/kg are infused over 1 hour every 4 hours for a total of 12 additional doses. While study protocols have employed pyrogen-free *N*-acetylcysteine, that preparation is not yet commercially available. Some authors have suggested that when

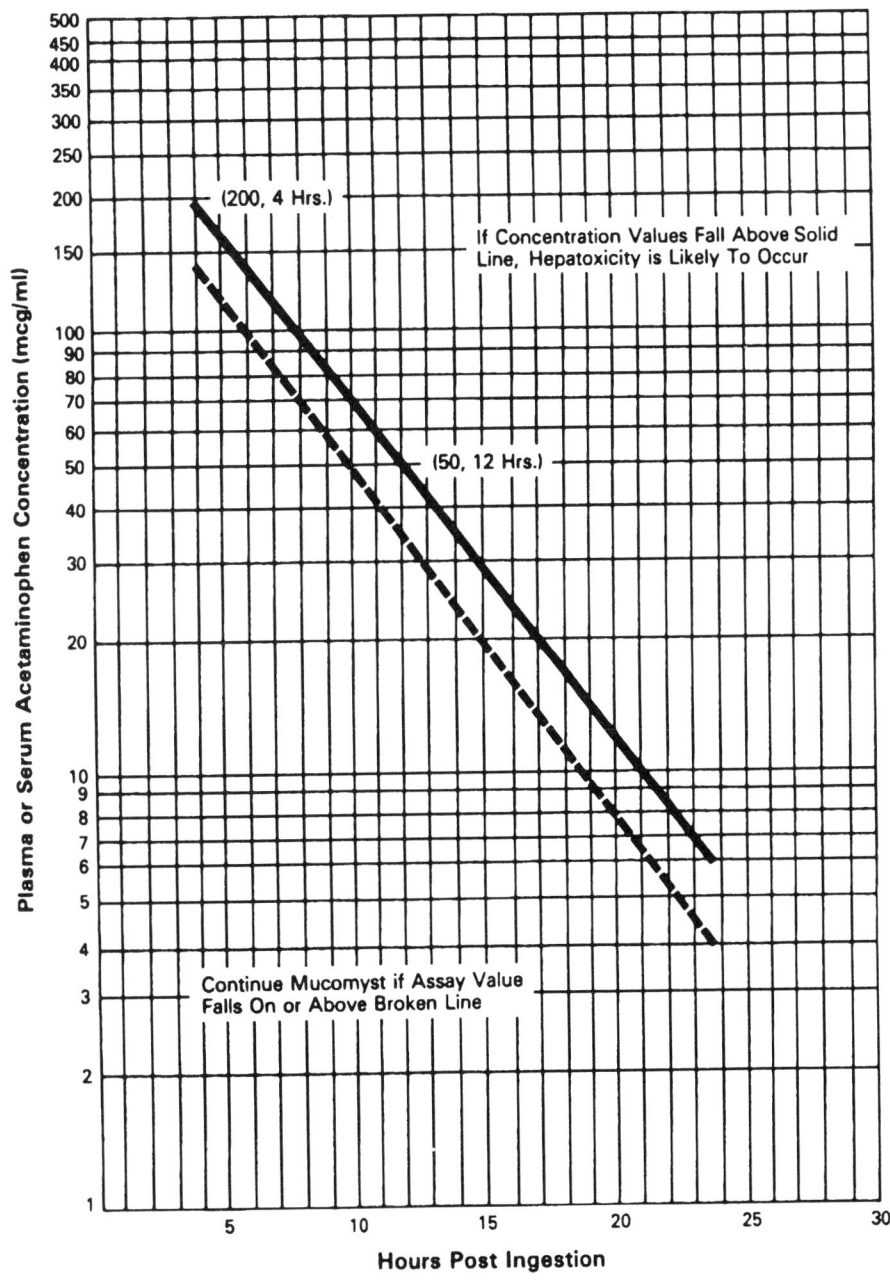

Figure 59.4. Rumack-Matthew nomogram. (Adapted from Rumack BH, Matthew H: Acetaminophen poisoning and toxicity. *Pediatrics* 55:871–876, 1975.)

patients cannot tolerate oral NAC, a study center be contacted to arrange for intravenous NAC administration. Study centers, however, cannot distribute the investigational drug and, in many cases, transfer of the patient to a study center is not practical because of the time required and the decrease in NAC efficacy when given more than 10 hours after ingestion. Because of these considerations, some clinicians extemporaneously prepare a 5% solution in 5% dextrose or normal saline from the preservative-free 20% NAC used for oral administration. The solution is then infused through a 0.22-μm filter according to the above intravenous protocol. This regimen is not FDA-approved, and to date there are no published reports of its use. Because anaphylactoid reactions and death have been reported following intravenous administration, its potential benefit should clearly outweigh the risks of its use (95–97). Information concerning intravenous administration should be obtained from a regional poison center.

Because metabolism of acetaminophen by cytochrome P-450 is responsible for its toxicity, cytochrome P-450 inhibitors have also been studied as possible antidotes (98). Cimetidine has shown promise in animal studies, but this has not been supported by the few human studies available (99–103). Ranitidine and famotidine appear to be of little use (98).

ALCOHOLS

Of the alcohol intoxications seen in the intensive care unit, ethanol and isopropyl alcohol are undoubtedly the most common. However, two other alcohols, methanol and ethylene glycol, present a greater challenge to the intensivist. In 1990, the American Association of Poison Control Centers reported 3306 exposures to ethylene glycol, of which 44% required medical treatment and 68 cases resulted in serious morbidity or death (1). Methanol accounted for 1047 exposures, of which over half were treated in a health care facility, with 32 resulting in serious morbidity or death.

ETHYLENE GLYCOL

Ethylene glycol is a straight chain-saturated polyalcohol commonly used in antifreeze and hydraulic fluids, as an industrial solvent; in pharmaceutical, food, and cosmetic manufacturing; and as an ink and lacquer solvent. It is a colorless, odorless, water-soluble liquid with a bittersweet taste that depresses the freezing point of water. The estimated lethal dose of ethylene glycol is 1.4 to 1.6 g/kg or 105 to 110 ml of most commercial antifreezes, although death has been reported with as little as 60 ml and survival with as much as 2 liters. Oral absorption is rapid, with peak concentrations occurring after 1 to 4 hours. Volume of distribution approximates total body water at 0.65 to 0.83 liters/kg with an elimination half-life ranging from 3.0 to 8.4 hours, depending on renal function (104–108). Ethanol treatment prolongs ethylene glycol's half-life to between 17 and 18 hours in patients with normal renal function and up to 102 hours in patients with renal insufficiency (106, 108, 109).

Table 59.5.   Stages of Ethylene Glycol Intoxication

Stage	Onset (hr)	Symptomatology
Central nervous system	0.5–12	Intoxication (no breath odor), nausea, vomiting, hematemesis, coma, convulsions, nystagmus, ophthalmoplegias, papilledema, optic nerve atrophy, depressed reflexes, myoclonic jerks, tetanic contractions
Cardiovascular	12–24	Rapidly progressive onset of tachypnea, tachycardia, cyanosis, pulmonary edema, congestive heart failure
Renal	24–72	Oxaluria, CVA tenderness, flank pain, acute tubular necrosis
Cranial nerve	144–432	Facial paralysis, hearing loss, dysarthria, dysphagia

Ethylene glycol is rapidly metabolized by NAD-dependent alcohol dehydrogenase to glycoaldehyde, which is then converted to glycolate via aldehyde oxidase (105). Glycolate metabolism to glyoxylate is the rate-limiting step before glyoxylate is then metabolized to oxalate (1 to 3%), glycine, glycolate, and formate and CO_2 (110). Oxalate depends upon renal excretion for its elimination, while formate requires further metabolism involving a folate-dependent system (111). Cofactors important in glyoxylate metabolism include pyridoxal phosphate and thiamine pyrophosphate.

The toxic effects of ethylene glycol are due to its metabolites and can be divided into four stages, although considerable overlap exists (Table 59.5) (112, 113). Metabolic effects include an increased anion gap metabolic acidosis due to glycolic and lactic acid accumulation, as well as hypocalcemia (108, 110, 114). Calcium oxalate crystals can be found in all major organs, and crystalluria may be detected 4 to 6 hours after ingestion, along with hematuria, proteinuria, and glycosuria. Envelope-shaped dihydrate crystals presenting early in the intoxication are replaced by the thermodynamically stable, needle-shaped monohydrate form when calcium oxalate concentrations decrease in the urine (108). While calcium oxalate crystal deposition has been implicated as a cause of renal damage, a direct effect from soluble oxalate and aldehydes is more likely (112). If large amounts of ethylene glycol are ingested, death may occur within 24 hours, although this result is uncommon. The outcome of the cranial nerve deficits appears to be variable, with significant neuropathies persisting as long as 6 months (113).

The diagnosis of ethylene glycol intoxication should be strongly considered in patients who present intoxicated or comatose with an anion gap metabolic acidosis, osmolar gap, and/or calcium oxalate crystalluria.

METHANOL

Methanol (methyl alcohol, wood alcohol) is a straight-chain, single-carbon alcohol commonly found in gasoline and windshield antifreeze. Additional uses include as a denaturant for other alcohols, a solvent, and a component of some paint removers. It is colorless, volatile, and flammable. Poisoning with methanol frequently occurs by ingestion as a substitute for ethyl alcohol (115, 116). The lethal dose of methanol has been estimated to be 60 to 70 ml or approximately 1 g/kg, with one-half that dose expected to cause visual defects. As little as 15 ml of methanol has been implicated in causing blindness.

Absorption of methanol is complete within 1 to 2 hours after oral administration and can occur from inhalation or topical application. It is distributed to total body water with a volume of distribution of approximately 0.7 liters/kg (117). Hepatic oxidation by alcohol dehydrogenase to formaldehyde has a zero-order elimination rate of about 8.5 mg/dl/hr (118). Aldehyde dehydrogenase metabolizes formaldehyde to formic acid with a half-life of 1 to 2 minutes (119). Formic acid is then eliminated by a folate-dependent one-carbon pathway to carbon dioxide. When oxidation of methanol is blocked during alcohol therapy, methanol is eliminated in the urine and by pulmonary excretion with a half-life as long as 52 hours (120, 121).

Accumulation of formic acid due to insufficient hepatic tetrahydrofolate is responsible for the toxic manifestations of methanol in humans (111, 119). Formic acid accounts for 60 to 100% of the anion gap and bicarbonate deficit in methanol poisoning, although lactic acidosis may be present late in intoxications due to formic acid inhibition of cytochrome oxidase activity (118, 122–126). The degree of acidosis but not the methanol concentration is a predictor of central nervous system damage and mortality (115, 116, 127).

A latent period of 6 to 36 hours occurs before significant symptoms are seen. Optic nerve damage secondary to central demyelination of the retrolaminar segment is due to formate inhibition of cytochrome oxidase activity and decreased perfusion of the optic nerve head (128, 129). Blurred vision, photophobia, and eye tenderness with slowly reactive, dilated pupils results. Axonal swelling and optic disc edema inhibit axoplasmic flow and may result in permanent vision loss. Other early symptoms include headache and dizziness in one-third of patients and nausea, vomiting, and abdominal pain. Abdominal pain may be secondary to pancreatitis. Physical findings include tachypnea, Kussmaul respirations, optic disc hyperemia, retinal edema, and nuchal rigidity. Bilateral hemorrhagic putaminal necrosis in association with extensive white matter necrosis can be seen in severe cases, resulting in a parkinsonian-like extrapyramidal syndrome and severe neurologic deficits (128, 130).

MANAGEMENT

Electrolytes, arterial blood gases, serum calcium, CBC with differential, urinalysis, creatinine, and indices of liver function should be monitored. The combination of increased anion gap and an increased osmolar gap are good indications of ethylene glycol or methanol intoxication (54, 55). Urine fluorescence may be noted by Wood's lamp up to 4 hours after ingestion of some ethylene glycol-containing antifreezes.

Ethylene glycol, methanol, and ethanol concentrations should be performed to aid in assessing the severity of an ingestion. Request ethylene glycol concentrations specifically as they are commonly not included in the standard "volatile" screens that report ethanol, methanol, isopropanol, and acetone. Ethylene glycol concentrations greater than 50 mg/dl

and methanol concentrations greater than 20 mg/dl are thought to be associated with toxicity, although an absolute relation is not well-documented (127). If concentrations are not readily available, an approximation of the ethylene glycol or methanol concentration in the plasma can be obtained, using the osmolar gap as described previously; however, osmolar gaps late in an intoxication may be absent due to metabolism of ethylene glycol or methanol (55, 131). Formic or glycolic acid concentrations have been suggested as reliable indicators of toxicity and the need for aggressive treatment, but these assays are not routinely available (132, 133).

Therapy is directed toward the rapid reversal of metabolic abnormalities, prevention of metabolism, and elimination of ethylene glycol or methanol and their metabolites from the body. Gastric evacuation is effective only if used soon after ingestion. Activated charcoal may be used if other substances have also been ingested; otherwise, it has not been shown to be effective.

Correction of metabolic acidosis substantially enhances survival and corrects visual defects in methanol poisoning by increasing formic acid dissociation and limiting its penetration into the CNS (122). Metabolic acidosis may be difficult to correct and large amounts of sodium bicarbonate may be needed. A bicarbonate deficit should be calculated [(0.4 × wt in kg) × (desired HCO_3 − measured HCO_3)], with half the deficit given immediately and the remainder based on arterial blood gas values. Caution must be exercised with the potentially large sodium load in the face of impending renal or cardiac failure in ethylene glycol intoxication.

Oxidation of ethylene glycol and methanol by hepatic alcohol dehydrogenase can be blocked by ethanol administration (134, 135). Indications for ethanol therapy include: (a) ingestion of greater than 0.15 ml/kg methanol or 0.25 ml/kg ethylene glycol, regardless of symptoms; (b) serum methanol concentration greater than 20 mg/dl or any amount of ethylene glycol in the serum; or (c) unexplained metabolic acidosis with anion and osmolar gaps. Blood ethanol concentrations should be maintained at least 100 mg/dl (22 mmol/liter) in patients in whom ethylene glycol or methanol concentrations are unknown. If concentrations are known, ethanol concentrations should be kept at least one-quarter the concentration of methanol or ethylene glycol (122). For initial intravenous loading, infuse the total loading dose plus a 1-hour maintenance dose over 1 hour (Table 59.6) (106, 136, 137). Intravenous solutions should be limited to 5 to 10% ethanol unless administered by central vein. Oral loading doses are best tolerated by nasogastric tube in concentrations of 30 to 50%; maintenance doses should be 20 to 30% ethanol (136). If these concentrations

Table 59.6. Initial Ethanol Dosing Guidelines

Alcohol (% v/v)	Loading Dose[a] (ml/kg)	Maintenance Dose[b] (ml/kg/hr)	Maintenance Dose + Hemodialysis[c] (ml/kg/hr)
95	0.8–1.1	0.1–0.2	0.3–0.5
40	1.9–2.5	0.3–0.4	0.8–1.1
20	3.8–5.1	0.7–0.8	1.6–2.2
10	7.6–10.1	1.4–1.6	3.2–4.4
5	15.2–20.3	2.8–3.3	6.3–8.9

[a] Loading dose: 0.6–0.8 g/kg p.o. or i.v.
[b] Maintenance dose: 110–130 mg/kg/hr p.o. or i.v.
[c] Maintenance dose with hemodialysis: 250–350 mg/kg/hr p.o. or i.v.

are not tolerated, further dilution to 10 to 15% may be needed to prevent vomiting. Adequate ethanol concentrations should be maintained for at least 24 hours, or until no ethylene glycol or methanol can be detected. Hourly adjustments may be required initially to maintain adequate concentrations.

Because of the difficulties with ethanol administration, 4-methylpyrazole (4-MP), a potent alcohol dehydrogenase inhibitor is being investigated (137, 138). Based on a volume of distribution of 1 liter/kg and a minimum inhibitory concentration of 10 μmol/liter, doses of 5 mg/kg every 12 hours are required, although current dosing regimens employ 10 mg/kg every 12 hours. Methylpyrazole's advantages include both oral and intravenous administration, rapid onset of action, a prolonged dosing interval, and lack of sedation (137).

Due to the long elimination half-life of methanol or ethylene glycol during ethanol or 4-MP therapy, extracorporeal elimination is recommended for: (*a*) visual symptoms with methanol or ingestion of potentially lethal amounts of ethylene glycol, when confirmation is lacking; (*b*) serum concentrations of greater than 50 mg/dl methanol or 100 mg/dl ethylene glycol; (*c*) presence of an arterial bicarbonate of less than 10 mmol/liter, a pH < 7.1, or acidosis refractory to treatment; or (*d*) serum formate greater than 20 mg/dl or high glycolate concentrations (132, 133, 139). Dialysis enhances the elimination of ethylene glycol and methanol and their small molecular weight metabolites. Both peritoneal dialysis and hemodialysis have been successfully used, although hemodialysis is more effective (140, 141). Elimination half-lives for methanol and ethylene glycol on hemodialysis are reported to be between 2.5 to 4.5 hours and 2.9 to 3.65 hours, respectively (106–109, 114, 117, 142, 143). Metabolite half-lives are between 2.4 to 3.55 hours for glycolate and 1.1 to 2.75 hours for formic acid on hemodialysis (108, 114, 132, 144). Hemodialysis should be continued until no ethylene glycol or methanol is detectable. Based on the above pharmacokinetic values, hemodialysis should be required for 12.5 to 22.5 hours, as compared to ethanol therapy alone, which could require 90 to 260 hours of therapy. During hemodialysis, maintenance doses of ethanol must be increased to compensate for the elimination of ethanol by dialysis (Table 59.6).

Osmotic diuresis has been advocated to increase ethylene glycol's elimination during ethanol therapy, as well as to reduce cortical and interstitial renal edema, but its efficacy is unproven (105). If used, mannitol diuresis (1.0 to 1.5 g/kg of a 20% solution over 15 to 30 minutes) should be maintained until ethylene glycol blood concentrations are nondetectable and/or crystalluria disappears (105). Other adjunctive therapy includes thiamine (100 mg i.m.) and pyridoxine (100 to 600 mg/day i.m. or i.v. daily) to ensure adequate cofactors for glyoxylate metabolism to metabolites other than oxalate in ethylene glycol poisoning. Leucovorin (50 mg i.v. every 4 hours for 24 hours) should be administered for methanol poisoning to ensure adequate formic acid metabolism (111, 145). Hypocalcemia should be managed with administration of intravenous calcium gluconate, while seizures respond well to standard anticonvulsant therapy.

CARBON MONOXIDE

Annually, at least 10,000 people seek medical attention for carbon monoxide poisoning. Add to this figure 1500 accidental

Table 59.7. Symptoms of Carbon Monoxide Poisoning

COHB (%)[a]	Symptoms
1–5	Usual range (smokers); no symptoms
5–10	Increased visual light threshold; increased chest pain in anginal patients; no symptoms in normals
10–20	Tightness across forehead; shortness of breath on severe exertion; headache; dilation of cutaneous blood vessels
20–30	Throbbing headache; shortness of breath on moderate exertion; nausea
30–40	Severe headache; nausea and vomiting; dizziness; dim vision; weakness; disturbed judgement; collapse
40–50	Deterioration of above; collapse more prominent; syncope; increased respirations and pulse
50–60	Syncope; coma with intermittent convulsions; Cheyne-Stokes respirations
60–70	Coma with intermittent convulsions; decreased cardiac and respiratory function; death
>70	Cardiac and respiratory failure; death

[a] COHB, carboxyhemoglobin.

and 2300 suicidal deaths, and one can see that carbon monoxide is one of the most common poison exposures in the U.S. (146).

Carbon monoxide is rapidly absorbed by inhalation and combines with hemoglobin to form carboxyhemoglobin (COHB). Hypoxia occurs by at least three mechanisms: (*a*) a decrease in oxygen saturation due to displacement of oxygen from hemoglobin; (*b*) a left shift in the oxyhemoglobin dissociation curve; and (*c*) interference with intracellular enzyme functions, including cytochrome oxidase, cytochrome P-450, and others (147). Carbon monoxide is excreted only through active respiration with a half-life ($t_{1/2}$) in room air of 240 to 320 minutes. Increased blood oxygen tension and atmospheric pressure enhance carbon monoxide excretion: 100% oxygen at one atmosphere results in a $t_{1/2}$ of about 80 minutes while 2.5 atmospheres decreases the $t_{1/2}$ to 24 minutes (147–149).

Symptoms of carbon monoxide intoxication depend upon the exposure time and atmospheric carbon monoxide concentration. Extremely high atmospheric concentrations will result in death before significant elevations in COHB occur. Table 59.7 summarizes the expected acute toxic effects of carbon monoxide correlated with COHB concentrations in healthy adults (147, 149). Cardiovascular disease, respiratory disease, pregnancy, and infancy result in increased susceptibility to carbon monoxide with severe toxicity possible at COHB concentrations less than 20%. Carbon monoxide readily crosses the placenta, exhibits a higher affinity for fetal hemoglobin than adult hemoglobin, and may result in fetal brain damage and subsequent developmental delays.

Delayed CNS toxicity, resulting from perivascular infarction and demyelination in the basal ganglia, and residual neuropsychiatric damage are common in patients who are comatose or acidotic upon presentation (150, 151). Sinus tachycardia, ST wave depression, atrial fibrillation, increased PR and QT_c intervals, and AV and bundle branch block are reported cardiovascular events (152). Myocardial ischemia and/or infarction can occur, especially in patients with existing coronary artery disease. The classic "cherry-red" appearance of cheeks and mucous membranes is an infrequent occurrence, as are rhabdomyolysis, renal failure, pulmonary edema, blindness, and hearing loss.

Treatment decisions should be based on history and symptomatology and secondarily on COHB concentrations. Carboxyhemoglobin concentrations at the hospital do not reliably predict toxicity, while the severity of symptoms such as headache, dizziness, muscle weakness, and visual difficulty have been found useful in the triage of victims and correlate well with the duration of exposure and recovery time (153). Laboratory investigations such as complete blood count, transaminases, electrolytes, serum creatinine, urinalysis, and arterial blood gases may be indicated. The PAO_2 may be normal in the face of significantly decreased measured oxygen saturation.

After immediate removal of the patient from the contaminated environment, complete rest should be enforced to limit tissue oxygen demands. Hospital admission is recommended for all patients with COHB > 25%, cardiovascular disease (COHB > 15%), pregnancy (COHB > 10%), impaired mentation, or metabolic acidosis (152).

Administration of 100% oxygen by means of a "tight-fitting" face mask with nonrebreathing valves should be instituted as soon as possible for any suspected carbon monoxide intoxication. Oxygen not only decreases the $t_{1/2}$ of COHB but also is dissolved directly into the blood to provide tissue oxygenation in the presence of COHB. Up to one-third of the normal arteriovenous oxygen difference can be provided with 100% oxygen at 1 atm; 100% of the arteriovenous oxygen difference can be provided with 100% oxygen at three atmospheres (147, 149). Hyperbaric oxygen (HBO) should be administered to every patient with signs and symptoms of severe intoxication, regardless of the COHB concentration (147, 154). Ideally, any patient with a COHB > 40% should receive HBO therapy. Patients with ischemic heart disease, acute ECG changes, anemia, seizure history, or pregnancy should receive HBO if the COHB is greater than 20% or any acute symptoms are present. A recent prospective evaluation of hyperbaric oxygen use found no benefit for HBO, compared to normobaric oxygen, in patients without loss of consciousness, regardless of the initial COHB level (155). In patients who had brief losses of consciousness, two HBO sessions were no more efficacious than one. The clinical applications of this study await further evaluation due to questions of study design. Oxygen therapy should be continued until the COHB is less than 5% and symptoms have resolved. In pregnancy, if HBO is not available, oxygen should be continued for five times as long as needed to reduce the maternal COHB to normal (156).

CARDIOVASCULAR DRUGS

Cardiovascular drugs contribute largely to the overdose population requiring intensive care observation and treatment. In 1990, the American Association of Poison Control Centers reported 22,378 cases of cardiovascular drug exposures, of which 55% were treated in a health care facility (1). While exposures to β-adrenergic blocking agents, calcium antagonists, and digitalis glycosides accounted for 50% of the cardiovascular drug exposures, they were also responsible for 61% of the major toxicity seen and 89% of the deaths reported. While β-blocker exposures continue to be the most prevalent, the incidence of calcium antagonist poisoning is steadily increasing as their therapeutic popularity increases. Among cardiovascular drug poisoning, calcium antagonists now account

for over 40% of fatalities (157). Ten to twenty percent of all patients treated with digitalis glycosides are expected to develop some clinical manifestation of toxicity, while ingestion of massive amounts of digitalis glycosides was formerly associated with a mortality rate of 20 to 55% (158, 159).

Before discussing the toxicity of these three classes of drugs, some basic concepts of cellular contraction must be understood. Calcium is required for contraction of smooth muscle and the generation of action potentials in myocardial contractile and pacemaker cells (157, 160). In myocardial pacemaker cells, phase 0 depolarization is primarily controlled by calcium influx into the cells. Depolarization of myocardial contractile cells by sodium during phase 0 of the action potential results in opening of voltage-dependent "slow channels," allowing calcium to enter the cells. The increased intracellular calcium results in additional calcium release from the sarcoplasmic reticulum, as well as increased calcium influx through the show channels and a decrease in a sodium/calcium exchange mechanism that is necessary for contraction. Inhibition of cardiac cell membrane bound Na^+-K^+-ATPase also results in increased intracellular sodium concentrations (161, 162). The increased intracellular sodium promotes increased calcium entry through slow channels and decreased calcium extrusion by the sodium-calcium exchange mechanism, allowing more calcium to be available for contraction (161). β-adrenergic agonists activate membrane-bound adenyl cyclase, catalyzing the production of cyclic AMP from ATP (160). Cyclic AMP, in turn, activates protein kinases in the myocardial cell, augmenting calcium influx by increasing the number of open receptor-activated calcium channels and enhancing calcium accumulation in the sarcoplasmic reticulum. The net effect is enhanced inotropic effect, relaxation, and speed of relaxation in the myocardial cell. In vascular smooth muscle, calcium enters through voltage-dependent slow channels and binds to calmodulin to activate myosin kinase and produce contraction (160). α-adrenergic agonists open receptor-operated calcium channels, resulting in increased contraction of vascular smooth muscle by increasing calcium influx. β-adrenergic stimulation, however, increases cyclic AMP concentrations, which activates protein kinases to reduce intracellular calcium and inactivate myosin kinase to result in vasodilation (160).

β-ADRENERGIC BLOCKERS

β-adrenergic blockers compete with β-adrenergic agonists for their receptor sites on all cell membranes, although the principal manifestations of toxicity are seen in the cardiovascular system. By reducing cyclic AMP concentrations in myocardial and vascular smooth muscle cells, a decrease in the chronotropic, inotropic, and vasodilator responses to β-receptor stimulation is seen (160, 163). β-blocking agents are categorized according to their receptor selectivity, intrinsic sympathomimetic activity, membrane-depressant action, and lipid solubility. In toxic doses, these properties may be important in predicting toxicity, such as membrane-stabilizing activity on QRS prolongation or seizure activity, or as in the case of $β_1$-receptor selectivity, they may be lost.

β-blocker poisoning may represent a low hazard to subjects with normal hearts, but circulatory collapse may occur in patients with preexisting cardiac failure when sympathetic drive is inhibited by even a small dose (164–167). The usual clinical course following overdose is the sudden appearance of bradycardia, followed by severe hypotension, low-output cardiac failure, cardiogenic shock, coma, seizures, respiratory depression, and peripheral cyanosis (168, 169). Typical ECG findings include sinus or nodal bradycardia, first-degree AV block, and intraventricular conduction defects. Bradycardia is not commonly seen with agents other than propranolol, oxprenolol, and alprenolol (170). Tachyarrhythmias have been reported with practolol and torsades des pointes, responsive to isoproterenol, with sotalol (167). Intraventricular conduction defects with a prolonged QRS interval are rarely seen, even with massive overdoses of agents devoid of membrane-depressant activity (164). Fatal intoxications produce gradual deterioration of left ventricular function until asystole or electromechanical dissociation occurs (171).

Bronchospasm rarely complicates β-blocker overdose unless bronchospastic disease is already present. Direct depression of CNS ventilatory response to carbon dioxide has been associated with respiratory arrest and increased cardiovascular toxicity from propranolol, with artificial ventilation significantly increasing the dose of β-blocker needed for cardiovascular collapse (164, 170). Intermittent clonic seizures are common in high-dose propranolol and oxprenolol intoxications due to their membrane-stabilizing properties. However, seizures have also been observed with sotalol, a β-blocker devoid of membrane-stabilizing effects. Decreased cerebral perfusion, hypoxia, or hypoglycemia may be indirect effects of other β-blockers, contributing to seizures and coma (164, 165, 167). β-blockers also interfere with the glycogenolysis effect of catecholamines, but hypoglycemia has not been a prominent feature of β-blocker overdose in nondiabetic patients (164, 172).

Absorption of β-blockers is rapid, with peak plasma concentrations seen within 1 to 2 hours (170). In normal doses, elimination half-lives range from 2 to 4 hours, with peak effects occurring from 1 to 4 hours (164, 168). In overdoses, critical signs of toxicity can appear within 20 minutes of ingestion but are more commonly seen within 1 to 2 hours. Lipid solubility determines a β-blocker's ability to cross the blood-brain barrier and result in CNS toxicity. Alprenolol and propranolol have the strongest degree of lipid solubility. Acebutolol, metoprolol, oxprenolol, pindolol, and practolol possess weak lipid solubility characteristics, and the other agents have no lipid solubility (164, 168). Plasma half-life may be significantly increased in overdoses due to decreased cardiac output, reducing hepatic and renal perfusion (164). Prolonged effects have been seen in patients with massive β-blocker overdose and compromised cardiac function (173).

Plasma concentrations may not reflect the degree of β-blockade due to differences in sympathetic tone, and the presence of active metabolites from agents such as alprenolol and propranolol, which are not detected in plasma assays. Therefore, plasma concentrations are of limited value in the immediate management of patients (164). Specific clinical parameters to monitor include ECG, heart rate, blood pressure, respiratory rate and rhythm, and blood glucose (172). Hemodynamic monitoring may be crucial in assessing appropriate treatment modalities.

Most patients admitted to the hospital for β-blocker poisoning will require only observation. A patient who remains asymptomatic for 12 to 24 hours after an overdose can be safely discharged, unless a sustained release preparation has been ingested (170). Since β-blocker effects may last longer than the elimination half-life, intensive care may be necessary for several days (164). Gastric decontamination, performed early to be of any value, is preferred to emesis due to the potential sudden onset of hemodynamic compromise and seizures. Multiple-dose activated charcoal may aid in the excretion of those β-blockers with small volumes of distribution (e.g., atenolol, nadolol, and sotalol). Although it has not been evaluated in overdoses, hemodialysis is unlikely to remove β-blockers due to their high percentage of protein binding (164, 168). Charcoal hemoperfusion has been reported successful in combined diltiazem and metoprolol overdose (174).

Atropine and isoproterenol inconsistently reverse the bradycardia and hypotension of β-blocker overdose (163, 168). Atropine should be given in doses of 0.5 to 3.0 mg i.v. in adults and 50 µg/kg in children to reduce unopposed vagal activity. If one dose of atropine is ineffective, an isoproterenol infusion at 4 µg/min should be started. With massive β-blockade, concentrations of isoproterenol at the receptor site must be equal to or greater than the β-blocker concentration. This requirement may dictate more than a 10,000-fold increase in dose to overcome the receptor blockade (170). Extremely high doses of isoproterenol may produce arrhythmias and excessive vasodilation, so dobutamine, a cardioselective β-agonist, can be given, although reports of its effectiveness are mixed. α-receptor agonists such as norepinephrine may be necessary for severe hypotension, as they can increase intracellular calcium by non-β-receptor activity but may worsen peripheral vasoconstriction. Wei et al have demonstrated that a combination of dopamine and isoproterenol can provide effective hemodynamic support in chronic β-blockade (175). If heart block or severe bradycardia persists despite pharmacologic means, a temporary transvenous pacemaker should be inserted (164, 168, 176).

Glucagon may be useful in patients unresponsive to isoproterenol (170, 176). Glucagon increases heart rate and improves AV node conduction through an increase in intracellular cyclic AMP. Since glucagon bypasses the β-receptor in the adenyl cyclase system, its beneficial action in β-blocker-induced myocardial failure may be superior to that of β-adrenergic receptor agonists. Glucagon is supplied as a lyophilized powder in 1- or 10-mg vials and should be reconstituted with preservative-free saline or 5% dextrose, as the diluent supplied contains phenol. An intravenous bolus of 50 to 150 µg/kg (approximately 3 to 10 mg in adults) over 1 minute is followed by a continuous infusion of 70 µg/kg/hr (3 to 5 mg/hr). Continuous administration is necessary due to a half-life of 3 to 6 minutes. Peak effects are seen within 5 minutes after an intravenous bolus and persist for about 15 to 20 minutes. Patients treated with glucagon should be monitored for hypokalemia, hyperglycemia, nausea, and profuse vomiting (164, 167, 176).

Amrinone may increase cyclic AMP concentration by inhibiting phosphodiesterase-mediated metabolism of cyclic AMP. It has been shown experimentally to reverse β-blocker-induced cardiac depression by increasing cardiac output and decreasing preload in a propranolol cardiac failure model (177). Due to the vasodilator properties of amrinone, increased total peripheral resistance in propranolol toxicity was also reduced. Higher concentrations of extracellular calcium have been shown to partially ameliorate the myocardial depression of propranolol, timolol, and sotalol (178). Calcium chloride administration in one case of propranolol overdose exhibiting seizures and electromechanical dissociation with wide QRS complexes repeatedly resulted in dramatic improvement in blood pressure and narrowing of the QRS interval (179). Further study is needed to define the role of phosphodiesterase inhibitors and calcium. If all pharmacologic attempts at management fail, use of an intraaortic balloon pump or cardiopulmonary bypass may be considered for hemodynamic support while allowing time for the β-blocker to be eliminated from the body (180).

CALCIUM ANTAGONISTS

Calcium channel blockers or calcium antagonists are a heterogenous group of compounds, of which verapamil, diltiazem, and nifedipine are the prototypes. The effects of calcium antagonist overdose differ among the three classes of drugs, but by blocking the entry of calcium into myocardial and smooth muscle cells, varying degrees of negative dromotropic, chronotropic, and inotropic effects on the heart and arterial vasodilation are seen (181). Verapamil commonly results in sinus bradycardia and combinations of AV nodal rhythms, second- and third-degree AV block, sinus arrest, and asystole (157, 181–183). Hypotension is a result of peripheral vasodilation, bradycardia, and depressed myocardial contractility. Diltiazem overdoses commonly show AV conduction defects with junctional escape rhythms and hypotension due to peripheral vasodilation (157, 181, 183, 184). Profound hypotension is seen in nifedipine overdoses due to peripheral vasodilation and decreased contractility. Tachycardia is common, and conduction defects are not seen unless very large doses are taken (157, 181, 183, 185). As most newer calcium channel blockers are dihydropyridines similar to nifedipine, their cardiac actions should closely resemble nifedipine's.

Other common symptoms in calcium antagonist overdoses include dizziness, lethargy, and slurred speech. Coma and seizures are seen rarely. Hyperglycemia secondary to calcium antagonist inhibition of insulin release from the pancreas is usually reversible within 24 hours and rarely requires treatment. Mild metabolic acidosis is probably due to hypoperfusion and clears upon correction of the hemodynamic status. Pulmonary edema has been reported frequently in severe nifedipine overdoses (185).

Calcium antagonists are well-absorbed but exhibit significant first-pass metabolism that limits their bioavailability. Absorption is usually complete within 2 to 4 hours in normal doses, but sustained-release verapamil has resulted in symptoms developing as long as 24 hours after ingestion. Sustained release forms of nifedipine and diltiazem also exist. All are greater than 80% protein-bound and, except for nifedipine, have volumes of distribution greater than 2 liters/kg. Elimination is primarily by hepatic metabolism, with verapamil and diltiazem forming the active metabolites norverapamil and desacetyldiltiazem, respectively. Elimination half-lives in normal doses range from 2 to 5 hours but may be increased with reduced hepatic blood flow, such as in overdoses. Six cases of diltiazem overdose showed linear elimination with half-lives

ranging from 4.6 to 10.2 hours (184). Two cases of verapamil overdose reported half-lives of 7.9 and 13.2 hours, and one case of nifedipine intoxication reported a half-life of 7.5 hours. No saturation of metabolism has been reported to date.

Initial management of calcium antagonist poisoning consists of gastric decontamination with gastric lavage and administration of activated charcoal. Induction of emesis with syrup of ipecac is not advised, as it may worsen or precipitate bradycardia and hypotension (157). Management of central nervous system effects should follow standard treatment, including benzodiazepines, phenytoin, and/or phenobarbital for control of seizure activity. Calcium antagonist serum concentrations are not generally available and show poor correlation with clinical outcome. They are not necessary for the management of calcium antagonist poisonings.

Management of cardiovascular effects should be based on the electrophysiologic effects of each individual calcium antagonist. Shock in nifedipine overdose is due to greater negative inotropy and hypovolemia secondary to an increase in venous capacitance, suggesting that treatment should consist of aggressive crystalloid therapy combined with calcium administration and inotropic agents (183). In verapamil and diltiazem poisoning, shock seems to correlate best with decreased heart rate and less so with negative inotropy. Treatment may require ventricular pacing, as well as calcium and inotropic agents. Calcium chloride, isoproterenol, norepinephrine, epinephrine, dopamine, phenylephrine, and 4-aminopyridine have all been shown to increase myocardial contractility. Only dopamine, isoproterenol, 4-aminopyridine, and ventricular pacing were effective in increasing the heart rate with verapamil (186, 187). Decreased peripheral vascular resistance is usually refractory to all pharmacologic therapy, with calcium, dopamine, and isoproterenol actually decreasing peripheral resistance further (186, 188).

The optimal dose of calcium is unknown, but animal studies suggest that relatively high doses are needed (186). Calcium chloride (1 g or 10 ml of a 10% solution) is administered intravenously over 5 minutes and can be repeated every 10 to 20 minutes for 2 to 3 additional doses until response is seen or until a maximum dose of 4g has been administered (182). Mild-to-moderate poisonings tend to respond well to calcium. Calcium may be repeated when the beneficial effects abate, but serum calcium concentrations should be monitored. Use of calcium gluconate will require larger doses, as it provides only one-third the calcium of the chloride salt.

Calcium will probably not be effective in correcting symptomatic bradyarrhythmias. Atropine and isoproterenol administration may be attempted temporarily until ventricular pacing can be established. Hypotension, if due to decreased myocardial contraction, should be corrected by the administration of calcium. If calcium is ineffective, β-adrenergic agonists such as isoproterenol and dobutamine may be effective by enhancing calcium influx into the cell through β-adrenergic receptor-operated channels. Hypotension primarily due to decreased peripheral vascular resistance should be managed initially with fluid replacement, but in most cases this therapy will not be effective alone. Administration of vasopressor agents with strong α-adrenergic properties, such as norepinephrine or phenylephrine, may be effective by taking advantage of the α-adrenergic-stimulated, receptor-operated calcium channels in smooth muscle, although animal studies have shown inconsistent effects (189). Combination therapy will be needed in many severe cases.

Alternative methods to increase myocardial contractility may include the use of amrinone or glucagon. One successful report of combined amrinone and isoproterenol use has been reported (190). Glucagon has been shown experimentally to increase myocardial contractility, with variable effects on heart rate in doses equivalent to 5 mg in a 70-kg individual for all three classes of calcium antagonist toxicity (191). Improved AV nodal conduction has also been reported (192). Unfortunately, little clinical benefit from glucagon administration has been reported in the literature (182). A potassium channel blocker available in Europe, 4-aminopyridine, has been shown to increase heart rate, blood pressure, cardiac output, and myocardial contractility in verapamil intoxication and has been used successfully in one patient (187). Cardiopulmonary bypass has shown some benefit in cardiac arrest from verapamil overdose, although toxicity reappeared after removal from bypass (193). A more prolonged period of bypass to allow further metabolism of the drug might have resulted in a better outcome.

Enhancement of elimination by hemodialysis or multiple-dose-activated charcoal has not been found to be an effective means of managing calcium antagonist overdoses, due to the relatively short half-lives, large volumes of distribution, and hemodynamic instability of the patients (157, 194). Charcoal hemoperfusion has been reported successful in one combined diltiazem and metoprolol overdose (174).

DIGITALIS GLYCOSIDES

While digoxin will be discussed in detail, many aspects can be extended to other digitalis glycosides. Digoxin produces its toxicologic effects by means of at least two mechanisms. Inhibition of cardiac cell membrane-bound Na^+-K^+-ATPase results in excessive intracellular calcium accumulation, producing delayed afterdepolarizations that lead to triggered arrhythmias (161, 162). Neurally mediated increased sympathetic activity facilitates the initiation of and increases the rate of ectopic impulse formation. Increased vagal tone produces bradycardia due to slow conduction and an increased refractory period in the atrioventricular (AV) node (162). In toxic doses, digoxin produces atrial arrhythmias through inhibition of sinoatrial (SA) node conduction and increased atrial automaticity with decreased conduction (161, 162, 195, 196). Intracellular potassium depletion and sodium accumulation in Purkinje fibers and the ventricles decreases the resting membrane potential, prolongs phase 0 depolarization, and increases spontaneous phase 4 depolarizations (162, 195). The net result is slowing of conduction in the specialized cardiac-conducting tissue while increasing conduction velocity and shortening the refractory period in working heart muscle (161).

Toxic doses of digoxin can produce nearly any type of arrhythmia, including atrial and ventricular premature depolarizations, ventricular fibrillation, and ventricular tachycardia (162, 195, 196). Enhancement of automaticity may be seen as tachycardia arising from atrial, ventricular, or junctional tissue. Impulse conduction disorders include AV block of any degree and sinus exit block. In general, patients without previous cardiac disease show sinus bradycardia with varying degrees

of AV block and supraventricular arrhythmias (196). Death is usually from asystole associated with a high-degree heart block, hyperkalemia, and resistance to electrical pacing. Patients with existing heart disease show exacerbation of existing arrhythmias, AV block, and ventricular arrhythmias. Death is commonly from ventricular fibrillation. Hypokalemia in chronic intoxication predisposes patients to SA and AV node block, AV junctional rhythms, and ventricular fibrillation or tachycardia. Pediatric patients most commonly exhibit sinus bradycardia or first- to second-degree AV block, although life-threatening cardiac events have also been reported (197).

Common noncardiac symptoms include nausea and vomiting due to medullary chemotrigger receptor zone stimulation and vagal stimulation, anorexia, and diarrhea (196). Neuropsychiatric manifestations, such as psychosis, lassitude, and agitation, may also be seen. Visual disturbances, including abnormal yellow-green color perception and halos, are frequent warnings of toxicity (196). Hypokalemia is common in chronic intoxication while massive digoxin ingestions result in inhibition of skeletal muscle Na^+-K^+-ATPase and marked hyperkalemia (158, 159, 195, 198). Serum potassium concentrations above 5 mEq/liter are common in acute overdose and may be easier to monitor than serum digoxin concentrations, although concentrations above 5 mEq/liter are rarely seen in children (197).

In normal doses, 60 to 80% of digoxin administered is absorbed. Absorption is usually complete within 6 hours but may be delayed for as long as 12 to 34 hours after large ingestions. Digoxin in the blood is approximately 20 to 30% protein-bound and represents less than 2% of total body stores. With a volume of distribution of approximately 7.0 ± 2 liters/kg lean body weight, highest tissue concentrations are found in the myocardium and kidney, although skeletal muscle represents the largest single store in the body (195). Approximately 60 to 70% of a dose is excreted renally, with hepatic hydroxylation accounting for the remainder and 30% of a normal dose undergoing enterohepatic recycling. Elimination is biphasic with a distribution half-life of 0.5 to 1.0 hours and a terminal elimination half-life that averages 39 ± 13 hours in patients with normal renal function (195). The effect of overdose on the elimination of digoxin is controversial, being reported as shortened, prolonged, or unchanged. Most cases report a prolongation of the initial distribution half-life with variable effects on the terminal elimination half-life. The prolonged distribution half-life may represent continued absorption.

Management of digoxin toxicity includes the prevention of further exposure, as well as symptomatic treatment with correction of electrolyte disturbances, antiarrhythmic therapy, and electrical pacemaker support (159). Factors associated with a poor prognosis are prior cardiac disease, advanced age, and disturbances in serum potassium concentrations.

In chronic intoxication, maintenance doses are withheld until all signs of toxicity clear and therapy is then restarted at a lower dose (196). In acute intoxication, gastric decontamination is important due to the possibility of delayed absorption. Multiple-dose-activated charcoal in digoxin intoxication has resulted in an elimination half-life of 1.4 days, as compared to 7.3 days before and 6.3 days after charcoal therapy (199). For this therapy to be most effective, it should be started early in intoxication while digoxin is still within the central compartment. In mild cases, these measures may be all that is necessary to alleviate signs of toxicity, in addition to careful monitoring of the patient's ECG and serum digoxin concentrations, which should ideally remain in the 0.5 to 2.0 ng/ml range. Care should be taken in the interpretation of serum digoxin concentrations in acute overdose because of the drug's slow distribution into the tissues, resulting in high initial concentrations that after 6 to 8 hours better reflect total body stores. Hemodialysis and hemoperfusion are not effective measures of decreasing the total body burden, due to digoxin's large volume of distribution (200).

Hypokalemia is associated with increased binding of digitalis to Na⁺-K⁺-ATPase, resulting in increased toxicity (196). Potassium replacement is recommended in chronic overdose with documented hypokalemia and ventricular premature depolarizations, ventricular tachycardia, and atrial tachycardia with AV block (196). Potassium should not be administered if the serum concentration is normal, as this may exacerbate AV conduction abnormalities. In acute intoxication, hyperkalemia may predominate. Sodium bicarbonate or a glucose-insulin infusion will shift potassium intracellularly, while potassium excretion can be promoted by the use of sodium polystyrene sulfonate or dialysis in life-threatening situations, although this technique is rarely indicated. Calcium salts should not be used to correct hyperkalemia, as they may worsen cardiac abnormalities due to increasing intracellular calcium concentrations.

Treatment of hemodynamically significant bradycardia and AV block may be successful with intravenous atropine (0.5 to 2.0 mg), if the patient is normokalemic (196). Phenytoin has also been shown to increase AV conduction in digoxin intoxication in this setting in doses of 25 mg. High-degree AV block with hyperkalemia, however, will require ventricular pacing. If ventricular arrhythmias persist in chronic digoxin intoxication despite potassium replacement, phenytoin or lidocaine could be tried. Both drugs have minimal effect on SA node, atrial, and AV node, as well as His-Purkinjie conduction. Phenytoin in doses of 200 to 400 mg i.v. is effective in treating premature ventricular depolarizations, ventricular tachycardia, and atrial tachycardia with AV block, but AV junctional tachycardia does not seem to respond as well to either phenytoin or lidocaine (196). Refractory digitalis-induced arrhythmias may be responsive to intravenous magnesium sulfate in doses of 1 to 2 g intravenously (201). β-blockers, while effective in controlling atrial tachycardia with block and ventricular arrhythmias from digitalis, are not recommended due to their deleterious effects on SA and AV conduction and myocardial contractility.

In severe digitalis intoxication, the use of digoxin-specific antibodies (Digoxin Immune Fab (ovine), Digibind) has proven to be successful in reversing cardiac and noncardiac toxicity. Of 125 adult and 25 pediatric patients, 80% showed full resolution of toxicity, while an additional 10% improved, and the remainder showed no response (198). Of patients who experienced cardiac arrest, 54% survived hospitalization. Poor response was due to underlying heart disease as the true cause of toxicity, insufficient antibody dose, or treatment of moribund patients.

Digoxin immune Fab rapidly binds circulating digoxin, making it unavailable for binding at membrane receptors. A rapid release of digoxin from receptor sites in the heart then results, which is immediately bound and inactivated by circulating digoxin immune Fab. Release of digoxin from Na⁺-K⁺-ATPase normalizes sodium, potassium, and calcium concentrations in the heart, resulting in restoration of normal conduction and rhythm. Seventy-five percent of patients show evidence of clinical response within 1 hour, with complete resolution of cardiac toxicity and hyperkalemia within 4 hours (198).

The volume of distribution of digoxin immune Fab in primates is approximately 0.46 liters/kg. After administration of Fab, free digoxin serum concentrations drop to 0 within 1 to 2 minutes, while total serum digoxin concentrations reach concentrations 8 to 20 times and up to 33 times the initial digoxin serum concentration in patients with normal or impaired renal function, respectively (202). Peak total serum digoxin concentrations occur in less than 12 hours but may be prolonged for up to 30 hours in patients with renal insufficiency. Elimination half-life of Fab in normal renal function is 16 to 30 hours, lengthening to an average of 98 hours in renal insufficiency (203). Rebound of free digoxin peaks between 3.5 to 24 hours, although 41 to 129 hours (average: 88 hours) may be needed in renal insufficiency (202, 203). This rebound has resulted in additional toxicity in only one patient to date but may require prolonged observation. Unless free digoxin concentrations are measured by incorporating equilibrium dialysis or ultrafiltration in the assay, once digoxin-immune Fab have been administered, serum digoxin concentrations are no longer useful, as they represent both free and inactive Fab-bound digoxin.

Indications for digoxin immune Fab include potentially life-threatening intoxications with ventricular tachycardia, ventricular fibrillation or other refractory arrhythmias, high-grade AV-block, and/or a progressive elevation of serum potassium exceeding 5 mEq/liter (197, 204, 205). Patients in cardiac arrest suspected of digitalis toxicity and those ingesting large amounts of digoxin (more than 10 mg in adults or 0.1 mg/kg in children) exhibiting cardiac symptoms or hyperkalemia are also candidates for treatment (197, 204). Patients requiring prolonged temporary pacing for bradyarrhythmias due to decreased elimination of digoxin may also benefit from antibody administration (205).

Digoxin immune Fab is available as a sterile lyophilized powder, with each vial containing 40 mg Fab, which will bind 0.6 mg of digoxin. A dose of digoxin immune Fab equimolar to the digoxin total body load is most effective in reversing the symptoms of digoxin toxicity. The dosage of digoxin immune Fab required can be calculated by estimating the total body load of digoxin in the patient (Table 59.8). Calculation of the dose of Fab fragments needed (in number of vials) can be obtained by dividing the total body load by 0.6 mg/vial. The average dose used during clinical trials was 10 to 20 vials in acute overdoses and four to six vials in chronic intoxication.

Table 59.8. Calculation of Digitalis Total Body Load

Acute ingestion
   Digoxin (mg) = dose ingested (mg) × 0.80
   Digitoxin (mg) = dose ingested (mg)
Chronic ingestion: From steady-state serum concentrations
   Digoxin (mg) = (concentration) × 5.6 × weight (in kg)/1000
   Digitoxin (mg) = (concentration) × 0.56 × weight (in kg)/1000

Contents of each vial should be dissolved in 4 ml sterile water for injection and infused intravenously over a period of 30 minutes through a 0.22-μm filter to remove any undissolved aggregates.

Adverse reactions attributed to Fab fragments include rapid hypokalemia in six patients, presumably due to reactivation of Na⁺-K⁺-ATPase and congestive heart failure from loss of digoxin's inotropic effect in an additional four (198). Allergic reactions in a postmarketing survey of 717 patients receiving digoxin immune Fab revealed only six cases (0.8%) of suspected allergic reactions consisting of rash, chills, or mild urticaria responsive to antihistamines (206). Four of the reactions however, came in the 82 patients with an atopic history (5%).

CYCLIC ANTIDEPRESSANTS

Imipramine was first developed as a phenothiazine derivative, which showed little neuroleptic effect but was found to have utility as an antidepressant. The monoamine oxidase inhibitors that were popular at the time were responsible for numerous drug and food interactions while the tricyclic antidepressants (TCAs) were effective without those adverse effects. It is understandable that these drugs would be frequent agents of suicide, as they are prescribed for the population of patients at greatest risk. By the 1970s they were one of the leading causes of drug-related deaths. Many of today's newer agents are structurally unrelated to the tricyclics. Initially, they were all thought to share similar effects; however, some of the newer agents appear to have fewer CNS and cardiovascular side effects.

The toxic effects can, for the most part, be ascribed to four mechanisms. Anticholinergic effects are responsible for tachycardia, mydriasis, dry skin, hypoactive GI tract, and urinary retention. CNS effects are noted with disorientation and rapid loss of consciousness. Blockade of the reuptake of neurotransmitters (norepinephrine, dopamine, serotonin) has been cited as the mechanism for the mood-elevating effects of the tricyclic antidepressants, but proof of that activity is still lacking. Sodium channel blockade is probably the most lethal effect of the TCAs. Manifestations of membrane stabilization include a widened QRS complex, QT prolongation, ventricular dysrhythmias, and negative inotropic effects. Although seizure activity is associated with many sodium channel-blocking agents, it is unknown if that is the cause of convulsions in tricyclic antidepressant overdose patients. α-Adrenergic blockade may cause hypotension and, in contrast to the anticholinergic effects, miosis.

Imipramine, first synthesized in 1948, was the prototype for the tricyclic antidepressants. Imipramine, amitriptyline, doxepin, trimipramine, and a newer compound, chlorimipramine, are classified on the basis of their structure as tertiary amines. Their metabolites, nortriptyline, desipramine, and protriptyline, are classified as secondary amines. Amoxapine, a metabolite of loxapine, and maprotiline, a tetracyclic compound, have greater CNS toxicity and, while amoxapine is thought to be less cardiotoxic, overdoses have resulted in intractable seizures and a higher mortality.

Two recently synthesized cyclic antidepressants are trazadone and fluoxetine. Both appear to be safer than other drugs in this class. In a recent study of fluoxetine overdoses 87 patients ingested only fluoxetine. Of those, thirty remained asymptomatic, while others reported tachycardia, drowsiness, tremor, vomiting, and nausea in that order (207).

In therapeutic doses, cyclic antidepressants are rapidly and completely absorbed. However, in toxic doses, anticholinergic effects may slow absorption, and gastric secretion and enterohepatic recirculation may also occur. Large volumes of distribution, ranging from 9 to 59 liters/kg, high-protein binding, and high lipophilicity are characteristic of these compounds. The parent compound usually undergoes hydroxylation or demethylation by microsomal enzymes before conjugation with glucuronide. Many of the metabolites are active, including desipramine (from imipramine), nortriptyline (from amitriptyline), and nordoxepin (from doxepin). Desmethylation reduces the muscarinic and antihistaminic properties of the metabolites.

Patients frequently present to the emergency department without overt evidence of toxicity. Significant ingestions are often accompanied by tachycardia and dry axilla. Rapid loss of consciousness, seizure activity, and cardiac dysrhythmias may present without warning. Pupillary response is variable and unreliable. Bowel sounds may be decreased or absent. Urinary retention may become apparent within a few hours of ingestion. Tachycardia may be absent in ingestions of secondary tricyclic compounds. Widening of the QRS to greater than 100 msec and the onset of ventricular tachycardia will usually be seen early in the clinical course; however, recurrence of symptoms may occur in patients who have suffered toxicity. Seizure activity is short-lived in most ingestions, although amoxapine, maprotiline, and desipramine have been associated with intractable seizures. Convulsions have heralded ventricular tachycardia in some cases, perhaps owing to acidosis that accompanies seizure activity (208). Structurally similar compounds, such as the muscle relaxant cyclobenzaprine, although structurally similar to amitriptyline, do not exhibit the cardiovascular toxicity of the latter. The few reported overdoses have experienced agitation, disorientation, and hallucinations. Antimuscarinic effects seem to be the major cause of toxicity. Carbamazepine structurally resembles imipramine. Anticholinergic toxicity is frequently observed, although cardiovascular effects are rare. Phenothiazines share many of the effects of the tricyclic antidepressants, including anticholinergic effects, cardiovascular toxicity (especially thioridazine), and α-blocking activity. Fortunately, phenothiazines have a much wider therapeutic index than do tricyclics.

Urine drug screens detect only a few of the available compounds. The clinical picture is usually more helpful in determining the presence of TCAs. Quantitative tests are of even less clinical value. Concentrations greater than 1000 ng/ml have been associated with severe toxicity; however, by the time of their return the clinical course has usually been recorded in the patient's chart.

Anticholinergic effects include tachycardia, which seldom requires treatment. Urinary retention is easily treated by Foley catheter, but it is important to carefully monitor patients, particularly children for this complication. Gastrointestinal hypomotility does not require treatment, but its presence should preclude more than a single dose of activated charcoal. Physostigmine has been used to reverse CNS depression but because of the incidence of physostigmine-induced seizures and asystole, it is no longer recommended, with one exception.

Patients will frequently experience disorientation, anxiety, and combativeness following coma. This condition is frequently associated with staccato perseveration of speech, in the presence of other signs of antimuscarinic activity. Diazepam is often sufficient if treatment is required. Physostigmine is a second-line drug, given in 0.5-mg doses intravenously over 1 minute, which may be repeated at 10-minute intervals to the desired effect. The total dose should not exceed 2.0 mg.

Sodium channel blockade is probably the most frequent cause of death. It results in prolongation of the QT interval, widened QRS, and ventricular dysrhythmias, including torsades des pointes. The mainstay of treatment is the administration of sodium bicarbonate. Sodium bicarbonate appears to increase available sodium in the presence of sodium channel blockade and increases the slope of phase 0 depolarization. Increasing pH also has a beneficial effect, although the exact mechanism is not understood. While hyperventilation is of benefit, it is not as effective as sodium bicarbonate (209). Indications for alkalinization include a QRS duration greater than 100 msec, ventricular dysrhythmias, and hypotension. The arterial pH should be adjusted to 7.5 by bolus injection. The pH should be maintained by adding 100 mEq of sodium bicarbonate to one liter of D5W and titrating the infusion to maintain the desired pH. Sodium chloride should be avoided to diminish the occurrence of hypernatremia. Electrolytes must be monitored, and potassium supplementation is frequently required due to intracellular shifts of potassium. Sodium bicarbonate therapy should be discontinued in the absence of all of the original indications for its use.

Lidocaine is considered as second-line therapy for ventricular tachycardia. Quinidine, procainamide, and disopyramide must be avoided because of their sodium channel-blocking properties.

Seizure activity is often of short duration and easily controlled by benzodiazepines. If longer duration of seizure control is necessary, phenobarbital (15 to 20 mg/kg i.v.) may be required. Phenytoin (15 mg/kg) administered at 20 to 40 mg/min may also be used, although there is conflicting data as to its effectiveness (210). Amoxapine, maprotiline, and desipramine may cause intractable seizures, requiring neuromuscular blockers to avoid rhabdomyolysis, and aggressive seizure management.

α-Blockade results in hypotension that should be best treated with norepinephrine, although norepinephrine has not yet been shown to be superior (211). Dopamine and various other agents have been used with some success; however, β-agonist effects of some vasopressors may lead to vasodilation and worsening of hypotension. Fluid depletion should be corrected prior to the institution of vasoactive drugs.

An asymptomatic patient with a history of cyclic antidepressant ingestion should be observed on a cardiac monitor for 6 hours. If no symptoms occur, the patient may be released for psychiatric evaluation. Symptomatic patients should be admitted to a critical care unit for cardiac monitoring. The patient should remain in that area until all symptoms resolve. The presence of anticholinergic symptoms alone is not usually of major significance by itself but represents a persistent threat of recurrence of CNS or cardiovascular toxicity.

Dialysis is of no benefit due the high volume of distribution, lipophilicity, and protein binding of these drugs.

NEWER CYCLIC ANTIDEPRESSANTS

Trazadone has been reported to cause nausea, vomiting, and CNS depression. It appears to lack the sodium channel-blocking properties and anticholinergic symptoms of the tricyclics. Fluoxetine, a serotonin reuptake blocker, also appears to have a benign course in overdose. Although death following massive overdose has been reported, it appears to be extremely rare (212). Bupropion has been associated with seizure activity in overdose but seems to lack the cardiotoxic effects of the tricyclics (213). Further evaluation of these agents is required before treatment protocols can be developed.

CYANIDE

Cyanide poisoning may result from the inhalation of, ingestion of, or skin contact with a variety of cyanide-containing or cyanide-liberating compounds. It may be found in various occupational settings, such as metal extraction, electroplating, chemical synthesis, and firefighting (214). At home it may be produced by the metabolism of acetonitrile found in some sculpted fingernail removers; in seeds of pitted fruits such as apricots, apples, or peaches; and in laetrile (215, 216). In the hospital, prolonged nitroprusside infusions or rates of 30 to 120 μg/kg/min may lead to cyanide or thiocyanate accumulation and toxicity (217, 218).

Upon skin contact, inhalation, or ingestion, cyanide is quickly detoxified by two primary enzymes that convert it to thiocyanate, which is excreted in the urine. When the exposure overwhelms this metabolism, cyanide acts to inhibit several enzymes. Cyanide's affinity for ferric iron leads to binding with cytochrome oxidase, which prevents electron transport in the cytochrome system, halts oxidative phosphorylation, and curtails the cell's ATP production (214, 219, 220). Cyanide may also inhibit glutamate decarboxylase, leading to lower γ-aminobutyric acid (GABA) concentrations in the CNS and seizures. As ATP production via oxidative phosphorylation is impaired, metabolic acidosis and decreased oxygen consumption occur. Decreased oxygen consumption can be indicated by arteriolization of venous blood (221). Severe metabolic acidosis is caused by anaerobic glycolysis, an increased NADH-NAD ratio, and a decreased hydrogen ion buffering capacity from impaired oxidative phosphorylation, that leads to lactate and ketone accumulation (214). Metabolic acidosis may not be present in some cases of nitroprusside-induced cyanide toxicity (222).

The organs most sensitive to energy deprivation, the heart and brain, are affected first. With overwhelming doses of cyanide, death occurs within minutes. Initial symptoms include nausea, vomiting, diaphoresis, agitation, lethargy, and tachycardia. In serious poisonings, coma, convulsions, apnea, hypotension, ventricular arrhythmias, and asystole develop quickly. The ECG may indicate various arrhythmias, including progressive shortening of the ST segment and the T wave originating in the R wave (223). Other complications include metabolic acidosis, rhabdomyolysis, hepatic necrosis, adult respiratory distress syndrome, and mucosal burns due to cyanide's alkaline nature. Cyanide poisoning should be suspected with sudden unexpected collapse into coma or seizures accompanied by metabolic acidosis and decreased oxygen utilization

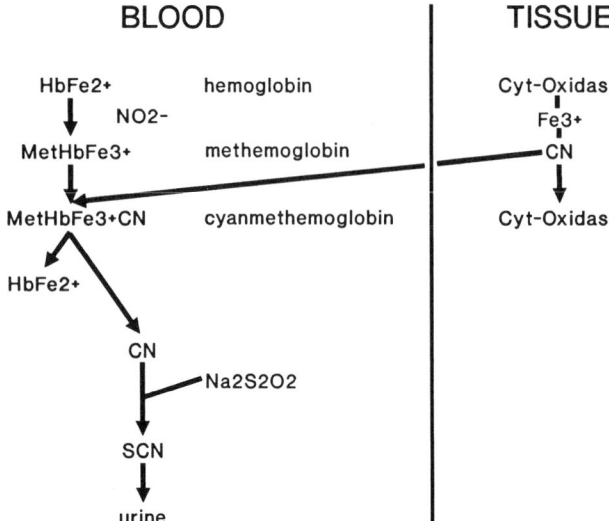

BLOOD   **TISSUE**

Figure 59.5. Antidotal strategy for cyanide poisoning. (From Curry SC: Hydrogen cyanide and inorganic cyanide salts. In Sullivan JB, Kreiger GR (eds): *Hazardous Materials Toxicology*. Williams & Wilkins, Baltimore, pp 698–710, 1992. Used with permission.)

during adequate oxygen administration (214, 219). The scent of bitter almonds may be present (224).

The treatment of cyanide poisoning exploits cyanide's high affinity for ferric ions by inducing methemoglobinemia and converting the cyanide to a renally excreted compound (Fig. 59.5 (214, 225). This conversion is accomplished by administering sodium nitrite and sodium thiosulfate, also known as the Lilly Cyanide Antidote Kit. Administration of sodium nitrite and sodium thiosulfate should be initiated in patients who have a history of exposure to cyanide and exhibit systemic symptoms. Not all cyanide exposures become symptomatic; massive exposures promptly lead to death at the scene; and supportive therapy may be sufficient for many exposures or for those patients whose poisonings are recognized several hours after the exposure (220, 226).

The mechanism of action of sodium nitrite for cyanide poisoning involves introducing an oxidant stress that causes erythrocytes to form methemoglobin. The ferric ion of methemoglobin competes with cytochrome oxidase for cyanide, dissociates cyanide from tissues, and forms cyanmethemoglobin (214, 219). Sodium thiosulfate enhances the conversion of the cyanide found in the bloodstream and contained in cyanmethemoglobin to thiocyanate (Fig. 59.5). The thiocyanate is excreted in the urine but can lead to toxicity if renal function is impaired. Sodium thiosulfate increases the conversion of cyanide to thiocyanate by more than 30-fold in dogs (227). The combination also has demonstrated a synergistic action in animals, and oxygen administration further enhances the antidotal effect (228).

Sodium nitrite's production of methemoglobin peaks within 30 to 60 minutes of intravenous administration (Fig. 59-6) (229). The pharmacokinetics of sodium nitrite and sodium thiosulfate in cyanide poisoning have not been well-characterized (230). Approximately 60% of sodium nitrite is metabolized to ammonia in volunteers, and the remainder is excreted in the urine (231). The half-life of sodium thiosulfate is approximately 15

minutes, whereas the half-life of thiocyanate is 3 days in volunteers and prolonged to 9 days or more in patients with renal dysfunction (218, 232).

The Lilly Cyanide Antidote Kit contains amyl nitrite pearls for inhalation as an immediate source of nitrite while intravenous access is established. If given a choice, it would be more important to adequately ventilate and oxygenate the patient rather than administer amyl nitrite, owning to its limited effectiveness. The pearls are crushed and the fumes inhaled for 30 seconds every minute.

Sodium nitrite is administered intravenously over 2 to 3 minutes, and the entire 10-ml ampule of 3% solution is the adult dose. The pediatric dose is 0.33 ml/kg up to 10 ml in a child without anemia. If the child's hemoglobin is known the dose can be further adjusted (Table 59.9) (233). Sodium thiosulfate (50 ml of 25% solution or 1.65 ml/kg in children) is administered intravenously over several minutes. If the systemic symptoms of cyanide poisoning persist, sodium nitrite and sodium thiosulfate may be repeated. If readily available, the extent of methemoglobinemia may guide further therapy. Generally, methemoglobinemia of 20 to 30% is tolerated in otherwise healthy individuals (225). Although a methemoglobinemia of 25 to 40% has been advocated for maximal effectiveness, current doses of sodium nitrite rarely achieve this extent and typically produce 7 to 17.5% methemoglobin (229, 234). The intramuscular administration of these agents is not effective for acute exposures (235).

Adverse reactions from the nitrites involve vasodilation and hypotension. If too much sodium nitrite is administered, fatal methemoglobinemia may result particularly in children (233). The true incidence and nature of the adverse reactions from sodium nitrite and sodium thiosulfate are hard to determine due to the serious condition of most recipients and the isolated experiences with their use.

The pharmacologic approach to the successful treatment of cyanide poisoning involves prompt resuscitation and aggressive supportive care, administration of oxygen and mechanically assisted ventilation, if needed, intravenous administration of sodium nitrite and sodium sulfate, and decontamination to prevent further absorption or exposure to others. The inhalation of 100% oxygen is relatively safe with short-term administration and is readily administered. It may increase the delivery of oxygen to tissues and may reverse the binding of cyanide with cytochrome oxidase (236, 237). Hyperbaric oxygen offers little advantage to 100% oxygen at 1 atm, but it has been advocated as a treatment (238, 239). Cyanide may bind to activated charcoal, but its benefits in cyanide-poisoned patients have not been determined (240). Generally, dialysis and forced diuresis have no role in therapy; dialysis may remove thiocyanate if renal failure is present (241, 242).

Other therapies for cyanide poisoning are used in other countries. Dicobalt EDTA is an intravenous chelating agent that works rapidly to bind and form an excretable compound, but toxicity from cobalt may limit its usefulness (243). The intravenous administration of hydroxycobalamin and sodium thiosulfate relies on the formation of water-soluble and nontoxic cyanocobalamin, vitamin B_{12} (244, 245). The low concentration of the dosage forms of hydroxycobalamin available in the U.S. make its administration impractical at this time.

IRON POISONING

Iron poisoning results from the ingestion and absorption of excessive amounts of iron from iron tablets, multiple vitamins with iron, and prenatal vitamins. It is often not recognized as a potentially serious problem by parents or victims until symptoms develop and valuable time to institute treatment is lost. Acute iron poisoning can produce death in children and adults.

The toxicity of iron is related to local effects on the gastrointestinal mucosa and systemic effects induced by excessive iron in the circulation (246–248). Iron causes variable necrosis of gastric and duodenal mucosa with associated hemorrhage and occasional perforations. Once absorbed iron is taken up by Kupffer cells, it acts as a mitochondrial poison, and occasionally causes hepatic necrosis. Iron may significantly inhibit aerobic glycolysis and perturb the electron transport system. Further, iron may shunt electrons away from the electron transport system, thereby reducing the efficiency of oxidative phosphorylation. These biochemical factors, along with the cardiovascular effects of iron, lead to metabolic acidosis. Shock ensues by means of mechanisms not well-understood but may include hypovolemia, release of endogenous vasodilators, and direct vasodepressant effects of iron and ferritin on the circulation (Fig. 59.7).

In the first few hours of ingestion of toxic amounts of iron, symptoms of gastrointestinal irritation, e.g., nausea, vomiting, and diarrhea, are common. In certain severe cases, acidosis and shock can become manifest within 6 hours of ingestion.

Some propose a quiescent phase between 6 and 48 hours after ingestion, where symptoms improve or abate, but this phenomenon is poorly characterized (249). Continued gastrointestinal symptoms, poor perfusion, mild hyperventilation, and oliguria should portend the presence of severe toxicity with other effects still to become manifest. Generally, within 24 to 36 hours after the ingestion, CNS involvement (coma and seizures), hepatic injury (jaundice, increased prothrombin time, increased bilirubin and hypoglycemia), worsening cardiovascular shock, and acidosis, ensue (250). Coagulopathy due to reduced thrombin formation has been described and appears to be biphasic, with early effects related to the serum concentration of iron and later disturbances, i.e., after 24 hours of ingestion, associated with hepatotoxicity (251).

Following the gastric mucosal injury by iron, pyloric and duodenal stenosis may occur 2 to 6 weeks after the exposure. Mucosal injury and an iron-rich circulation may promote septicemia with *Yersinia enterocolitica* during iron overdose (252).

Deferoxamine chelates iron and lessens morbidity and mortality of severe iron poisoning. It is indicated for iron-poisoned patients in shock, coma, or exhibiting gross gastrointestinal bleeding or metabolic acidosis. Further, if the serum iron concentration exceeds 500 μg/dl, serious systemic toxicity is likely, and deferoxamine is indicated (253). Its use is less clear in patients with serum iron concentrations in the range of 350 to 500 μg/dl since many of these patients do not develop systemic symptoms, but it seems prudent to remove excess iron from the circulation. The parenteral administration of deferoxamine produces an orange-red-colored urine within 3 to 6 hours that is indicative of the iron-deferoxamine complex, ferrioxamine (254–256). For mild-to-moderate cases of iron poisoning where its use is unclear, the presence of discolored urine would indicate the presence of chelatable iron and the need to continue deferoxamine. The reliability of discolored urine has been challenged because it is not sensitive and is difficult to detect (257).

Deferoxamine is a highly selective chelator of iron that theoretically binds ferric (Fe^{3+}) iron in a one-to-one molar ratio (100 mg of deferoxamine to 8.5 mg ferric iron) that is more stable than iron's binding to transferrin. Its affinity for calcium, magnesium, and copper is poor, as is its binding of iron in hemoglobin and hemosiderin. Deferoxamine removes some iron from transferrin by chelating ferric complexes in

Table 59.9. Pediatric Doses of Sodium Nitrite and Sodium Thiosulfate

Hemoglobin (g/dl)	*3% Sodium Nitrite* (ml/kg)	*25% Sodium Thiosulfate* (ml/kg)
7.0	0.19	0.95
8.0	0.22	1.10
9.0	0.25	1.25
10.0	0.27	1.35
11.0	0.30	1.50
12.0	0.33	1.65
13.0	0.36	1.80
14.0	0.39	1.95

a Adapted from Berlin CM: The treatment of cyanide poisoning in children. *Pediatrics* 46:793–796, 1970.

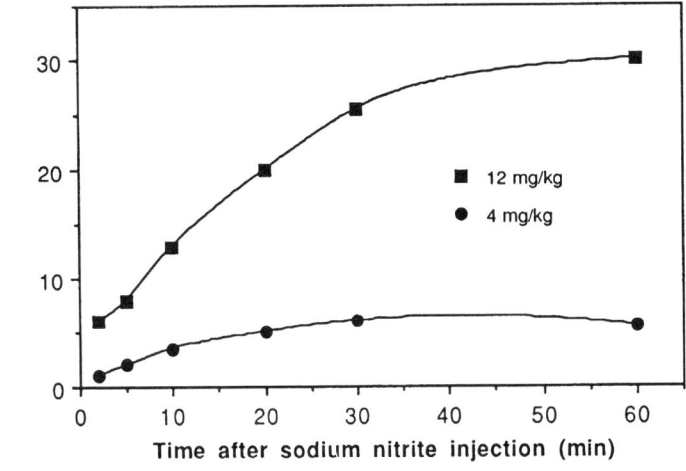

Figure 59.6. Time course of methemoglobin production after sodium nitrite administration. (Adapted from Kiese M, Weger N: Formation of ferrihemoglobin with aminophenols in the human for the treatment of cyanide poisoning. *Eur J Pharmacol* 7:97–105, 1969.)

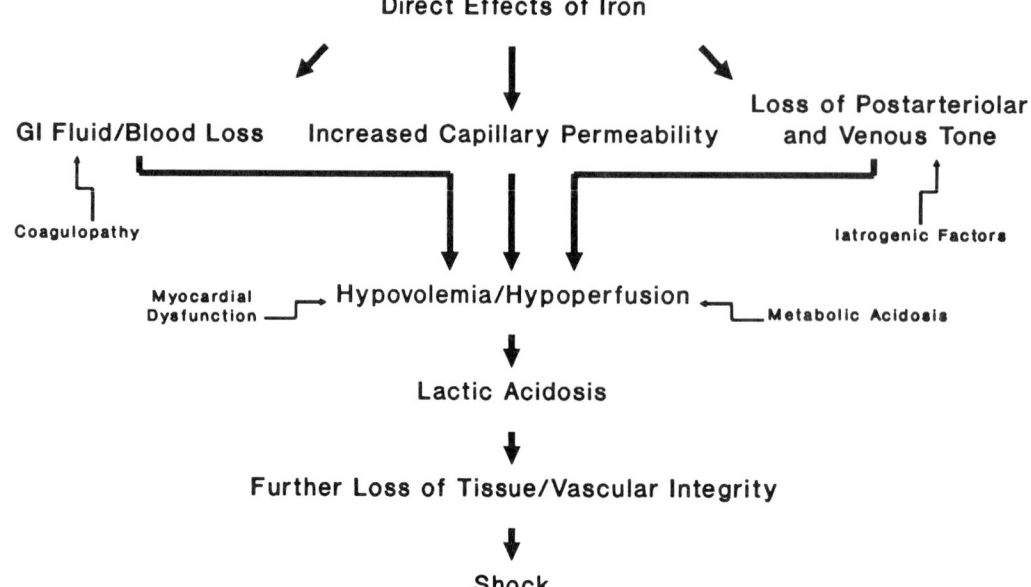

Figure 59.7.   Factors responsible for the development of shock in iron intoxication. (From Banner W, Tong TG: Iron poisoning. *Pediatr Clin North Am* 33:393–409, 1986. Used with permission.)

equilibrium with transferrin. The straight-chain deferoxamine coordinates itself around a ferric ion that becomes attached to form ferrioxamine, which is excreted in the urine. Its rate of elimination in the urine is not sufficient to account for its action, and deferoxamine may also have a protective effect cellularly or may chelate extramitochondrial iron (247, 258).

Deferoxamine has a volume of distribution of about 60% body weight and a plasma half-life of 10 to 60 minutes in dogs due to rapid metabolism (259). Ferrioxamine has a volume of distribution of 20% and is excreted in the urine. Pharmacokinetics in humans have not been characterized.

For serious poisonings, a controlled intravenous infusion of 15 mg/kg/hr is indicated. Although the manufacturer states that the total dose in 24 hours should not exceed 6 g, the basis for this recommendation is unclear, and daily doses as high as 16 to 37.1 g have been administered without incident (260, 261). Intramuscular administration of deferoxamine (90 mg/kg up to 1 g every 4 to 8 hours) may be indicated for patients with mild poisonings, asymptomatic patients with serum iron concentrations between 350 and 500 μg/dl or patients undergoing transport. Since ferrioxamine is more stable at a pH above 6, a slightly alkaline urine may be desirable (255).

The oral administration of deferoxamine has been advocated by some to reduce iron absorption, but the ferrioxamine complex is absorbable, increases the total iron body burden, is toxic in high concentrations, and may outstrip the hospital's supply that should be used for intravenous administration (262). There are teratogenic concerns based on animal studies on the use of deferoxamine during pregnancy, but the risk has not been demonstrated clearly in humans, if at all (263). The risk of fatal iron poisoning generally overshadows the potential risk of fetal malformations in a pregnant patient. In the patient who develops renal failure, hemodialysis does not remove excess iron but does remove ferrioxamine (255). Hemofiltration or exchange transfusions may prove to be also

useful in serious cases that have been treated with deferoxamine (264–266).

The rapid intravenous infusion of deferoxamine (>15 mg/kg/hr) has been associated with tachycardia, hypotension, shock, generalized erythema, and urticaria (255, 256). Anaphylaxis has also been reported (267).

The endpoint of deferoxamine therapy is not clear. Some have suggested that deferoxamine therapy should cease when the serum iron concentration decreases below the iron-binding capacity. The pitfalls of applying the total iron binding capacity as a diagnostic or monitoring tool are manifold, and its use is generally unreliable (268–271). The cessation of orange-red urine production that is indicative of ferrioxamine excretion is also not fully reliable because many can not distinguish the color (257). The decrease of serum iron concentrations to some acceptable value, e.g., 150 μg/dl, may not account for the potential cellular action of deferoxamine, irrespective of its effect on iron elimination. Given all these shortcomings, it may be prudent to continue deferoxamine therapy for 12 to 24 hours after the urine returns to normal color and the patient has been asymptomatic. Monitoring acid-base, fluid, and electrolyte balance, and perfusion are good indicators of iron toxicity.

Gastric evacuation by lavage or emesis is indicated to remove iron tablets, but activated charcoal administration is not warranted since it does not bind iron. Lavage with 1 to 2% sodium bicarbonate may increase intragastric pH and precipitate iron, but the precipitate is reversibly soluble in the acidic pH of the stomach (272). Symptomatic patients should receive deferoxamine early in the course of the poisoning. Good hydration and urine output mitigate some of the toxic effects of iron and allow good urine output of ferrioxamine. If radiographs of the abdomen reveal a large number of iron tablets remaining after gastric evacuation, removal by gastrostomy or whole bowel irrigation may be indicated (46, 273).

OPIOIDS

Acute overdosage with opioids typically produces symmetrical miosis, depressed respirations, and coma. Miosis may not be observed when anticholinergic drugs have been congested or when meperidine, hypoxia, or head trauma are involved. Other symptoms on acute overdose include nausea, vomiting, pulmonary edema, and constipation (274–276).

The toxic effects of opioids are in large part an extension of their effects on the various opioid receptors thus far identified in man. Differences among the opioid drugs depend upon their agonist and antagonist action on opioid receptors and their other pharmacologic properties (274–277).

Morphine is the prototype of a pure opioid agonist by virtue of its actions on the μ-receptor to produce supraspinal analgesia. Codeine is 20% as potent as morphine and is used as a mild analgesic and antitussive. There are few fatalities from its abuse alone due to cramping, constipation, nausea, and vomiting that limit abuse. Codeine is more stimulating to the spinal cord and may lead to delirium and seizures during coma. Heroin is rapidly taken up by the CNS and produces an intense euphoria. Illicit heroin is usually contaminated and adulterated with various agents that can lead to other complications. Methadone produces symptoms typical of opioid poisoning, but its longer duration produces prolonged intoxication. Meperidine possesses weak anticholinergic effects and its metabolite, normeperidine, possesses neurotoxic actions that can lead to seizures, myoclonus, jitteriness, and tremors in patients with renal insufficiency or those receiving high doses. Propoxyphene and its metabolite, norpropoxyphene, exhibits local anesthetic and sodium channel blocking properties that lead to a high potential for seizures and cardiac arrhythmias such as bundle-branch block (278). Pentazocine is often abused with an antihistamine such as tripelennamine that produces alternating states of sedation, wakefulness, and seizures. Diphenoxylate, marketed in combination with atropine as Lomotil, produces serious opioid poisoning, particularly in children, who may not exhibit significant symptoms for up to 12 to 24 hours (279). Fentanyl, typically used as a preoperative analgesic, has been chemically manipulated to produce illicit analogs ("designer drugs") that are typically highly lipid-soluble and lead to pulmonary edema and respiratory arrest. Since the final breakdown products of a designer drug are unknown, the effects produced may be bizarre and unexpected. Dextromethorphan may also produce coma and respiratory depression with massive doses, but the effects are reversible with naloxone (280).

Treatment of opioid overdose involves basic life support and gastric decontamination procedures, if indicated. Dialysis and diuresis are ineffective in enhancing opioid elimination. Symptoms of withdrawal may be acutely mitigated with haloperidol or diazepam with detoxification initiated after the acute stages in a noncritical care setting (281). Additional complications due to infections (e.g., skin, sepsis, hepatitis, acquired immunodeficiency disease) and adulterants such as lidocaine, quinine, stimulants, baking soda, and talc may result from the method of abuse and chronic drug abuse practices (274, 275, 282). Management of patients who have swallowed condoms or balloons filled with an opioid ("body packers") may be treated with activated charcoal and cathartics or whole bowel irrigation if asymptomatic. Surgical intervention may be warranted if serious CNS depression is present (49, 283).

Naloxone is a direct opioid receptor antagonist effective in reversing the symptoms of opioid toxicity such as respiratory depression, coma, miosis, analgesia, delayed gastric emptying, and cardiovascular depression (284–288). It may not produce a satisfactory response during a postictal period, with mixed overdoses, with concurrent head trauma, during hypoglycemic episodes, with hypoxic states, or when an insufficient dose has been given. Certain agents, such as meperidine, propoxyphene, diphenoxylate, and fentanyl analogs, may require higher doses for an acceptable response from naloxone (274, 275).

For respiratory depression caused by opioid overdosage, give naloxone 2 mg as an intravenous bolus to an adult or child (276). If there is no response in 2 to 3 minutes, the dose may be repeated up to a total dose of 10 mg before one concludes that it is ineffective (275, 289). In patients with suspected opioid dependence, 0.1- to 0.2-mg increments may avoid an abrupt withdrawal syndrome. For infants and neonates, an initial naloxone dose of 0.01 mg/kg intravenously should be given, followed by 0.1 mg/kg within 2 minutes, if the initial response is poor. Naloxone may need to be repeated several times owing to its short duration of action (20 to 60 minutes), compared to that of many opioids (290, 291). For patients requiring repeated doses of naloxone, a continuous infusion can be titrated to maintain an acceptable response (292). A continuous hourly infusion of two-thirds of the bolus dose that resulted in reversal of symptoms is a reasonable starting point (Table 59.10). Individualization of the dose should be guided by the patient's response. Patients who have had their microsomal enzymes induced, for example, by prior ethanol or barbiturate abuse, may require a faster rate, while neonates may be adequately treated with a slower rate (276).

It is desirable to give naloxone intravenously to achieve a rapid and predictable response, but intramuscular, intralingual, endotracheal, or intraosseous administration may be useful when venous access is delayed (276, 293–294). Naloxone is rapidly distributed throughout the body with an apparent volume of distribution of 3 liters/kg. The plasma half-life is 40 to 60 minutes in normal adults and approximately 25% shorter when hepatic microsomal enzymes have been induced

Table 59.10. Continuous Infusion of Naloxone for Reversal of Opioid Poisoning[a]

Initial Bolus Dose[b] (mg)	Initial Continuous Infusion (mg/hr)	Initial Infusion Rate (ml/hr)
0.4	0.25	25[c]
2	1.25	125[c]
3	1.9	190[c]
4	2.5	25[d]
5	3.2	32[d]
6	6.25	63[d]

[a] Adapted from Goldfrank L, Weisman R, Errick J, Lo M-W: A dosing nomogram for continuous infusion of intravenous naloxone. *Ann Emerg Med* 15:566–570, 1986.
[b] Total initial dose for reversal guides the initial continuous infusion.
[c] Intravenous dilution: 5 mg naloxone to 500 ml 5% dextrose in water (0.01 mg/ml).
[d] Intravenous dilution: 10 mg naloxone to 100 ml 5% dextrose in water (0.1 mg/ml).

(275, 276). In neonates, the half-life may be twice as long (295, 296).

Adverse effects of naloxone have been notably few. Several isolated cases of pulmonary edema, hypertension, dysarrhythmias, and cardiac arrest have been attributed to naloxone use (297–303). After administration of large doses (2 to 4 mg/kg) in healthy subjects, benign reversible complaints such as dizziness and numbness of extremities were followed by diaphoresis, nausea, and stomach-ache (304). In adults dependent upon opioids, a short-lived withdrawal syndrome (nausea, vomiting, diaphoresis, tachycardia) or agitation and combativeness may be induced by naloxone administration (274–276, 305). Opioid withdrawal in neonates may precipitate seizures. In the context of opioid poisoning, naloxone's use can be lifesaving and should not be withheld due to concerns about potential adverse effects, of which there are few. Naloxone has also been used in attempts to reverse coma due to ethanol, clonidine, and benzodiazepines, but results have been equivocal (306–308). The empiric use for naloxone for patients with altered mental status has also been challenged (309).

ORGANOPHOSPHATE INSECTICIDES

Organic phosphorus compounds were first developed in the mid-1800s. In 1932, the toxic effects on rats were discovered during development of organophosphate insecticides. Tetraethylpyrophosphate (TEPP) was developed when nicotine insecticides came into short supply prior to World War II. Though TEPP was toxic, it was rather unstable, leading to the search for other compounds not so rapidly hydrolyzed. At the same time organophosphates began to be developed as nerve gases (Sarin and Tabun) for use in WW II. In 1944, Parathion was developed and proved to be a very toxic but widely used organophosphate insecticide. The most common use of organophosphate compounds is for insect control. Available as fogging agents, pest strips, granules, and sprays, organophosphate compounds are available worldwide in a multitude of formulations. Use in humans include treatment of myasthenia gravis and glaucoma.

Acetylcholine (ACH) acts as a neurotransmitter at the parasympathetic neuroeffector junction, the parasympathetic and sympathetic synapses, the central nervous system, and the neuroeffector junction of sweat glands in the sympathetic system (Fig. 59.8) (310). Ordinarily, acetylcholine (ACH) that has been released into the synapse or neuroeffector junction is rapidly hydrolyzed following stimulation of the receptor site. This rapid breakdown prevents prolonged stimulation of the receptors and allows the receptor to function normally. Acetylcholinesterase provides two binding sites for ACH, an anionic site to which the acetylcholine (ACH) molecule "anchors" and an esteric site that forms a short-lived bond with the acetate moiety of the ACH molecule. The organophosphates inhibit the action of acetylcholinesterase (ACHE) by attaching to the esteric site of ACHE (Fig. 59.9A), blocking ACH attachment to the anionic site and hydrolysis (Fig. 59.9B).

Because organophosphates inhibit the action of acetylcholinesterase at several different sites, the clinical picture can be confusing. At the neuroeffector junction of the parasympathetic system, stimulation from excess ACH results in muscarinic symptoms. Bronchospasm, miosis, increased gut motility,

diaphoresis, decreased A-V conduction, and ventricular dysrhythmias result. Nicotinic stimulation from increased ACH stimulation at somatic nerve endings is responsible for fasciculations in the early excitatory stage followed by flaccid paralysis when receptor sites become refractory due to fatigue by overstimulation. Stimulation of nicotinic presynaptic ganglia of the sympathetic nervous system may produce sympathetic symptoms, including mydriasis, tachycardia, and hypertension, while stimulation of the adrenal medulla leads to increased circulating catecholamines, causing hyperglycemia and hypokalemia. Central nervous system dysfunction is manifest in lethargy and coma. Neurotoxic esterase inhibition is responsible for the delayed neurologic effects that have been described as a "dying back" of axons (311, 312). Hydrocarbon toxicity may be seen in organophosphate exposures because of the use of these compounds as a vehicle. Effects include CNS depression and pneumonitis, as discussed below.

Organophosphates are rapidly absorbed via the skin, conjunctiva, gut, and lungs. Skin absorption is normally slow, although dermatitis may greatly increase absorption. Many organophosphates undergo metabolism via cytochrome P-450 mixed-function oxidases. Some insecticides, such as chlorpyrifos, are converted to compounds that are hundreds of times more active than the parent compound (313). Storage in fat, the intestine, or other organs may be responsible for delayed mobilization and toxicity. Metabolites are excreted in the urine with wide variability in half-lives reported.

Acutely, many patients will have little or no symptoms. Although the classic presentation is a combination of muscarinic and nicotinic effects, one or the other may predominate. Therefore, some patients may present with muscle weakness and tachycardia in the absence of the traditional "SLUDGE" acronym (salivation, lacrimation, urination, defecation, gastrointestinal upset, emesis). Symptoms of the muscarinic presentation include bronchoconstriction, bronchorrhea, hypersalivation, nausea, vomiting, diarrhea, urinary incontinence, and bradycardia. Nicotinic presentations include weakness, muscle fasciculations, cramping, tachycardia, and hypertension. Hydrocarbon toxicity consists of aspiration pneumonitis, CNS depression, cardiac dysrhythmias, and dermatitis.

Delayed peripheral neurotoxicity, which later came to be known as "Ginger Jake paralysis," was noted in workers chronically exposed to tri-o-cresyl phosphate (TOCP) in the early 1930s (314, 315). More recently, a delayed neurotoxic syndrome has been described that develops 1 to 2 weeks after an acute exposure or may also be associated with multiple dermal exposures. Paresthesias with a stocking-glove distribution over lower extremities are associated with ataxia and may appear up to 3 weeks following acute exposure. Later, there is progression to the upper extremities. Improvement occurs after months to years with residual disability. Only a few of the organophosphates (mipafox, trichlorphon, phytosol, and tamaron) are associated with this syndrome, which is felt to result from the inhibition of neurotoxic esterase (NTE) and to be distinct from cholinesterase inhibition (316–318). Electromyography may be of benefit in diagnosis.

An intermediate syndrome has been described that occurs 24 to 96 hours postexposure following the resolution of cholinergic symptoms. Symptoms include muscle weakness of the proximal limbs, muscles supplied by the cranial nerves, and

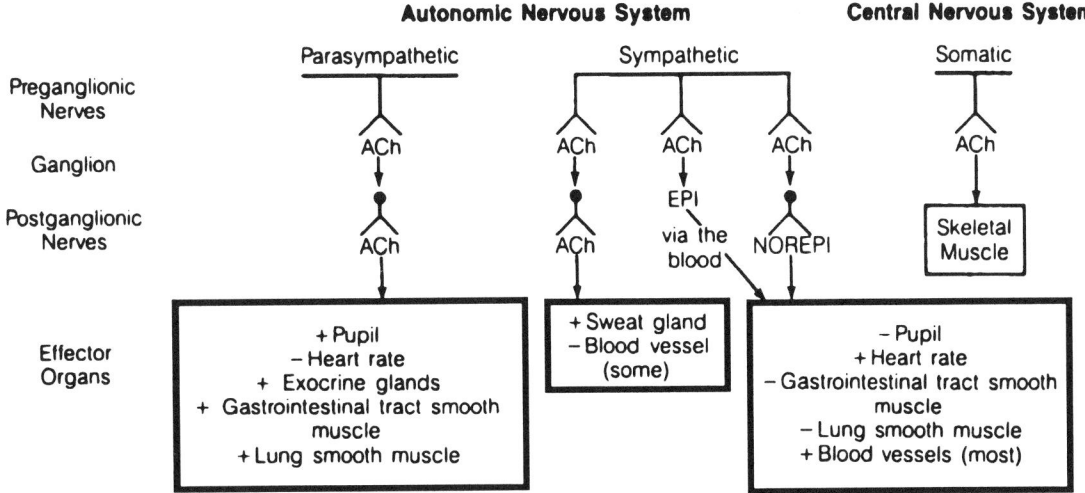

Figure 59.8. Schematic representation of the human peripheral nervous system. *ACh,* acetylcholine; *EPI,* epinephrine; *NOREPI,* norepinephrine. (From Tafuri J, Roberts J: Organophosphate poisoning. *Ann Emerg Med* 16:193–202, 1987. Used with permission.)

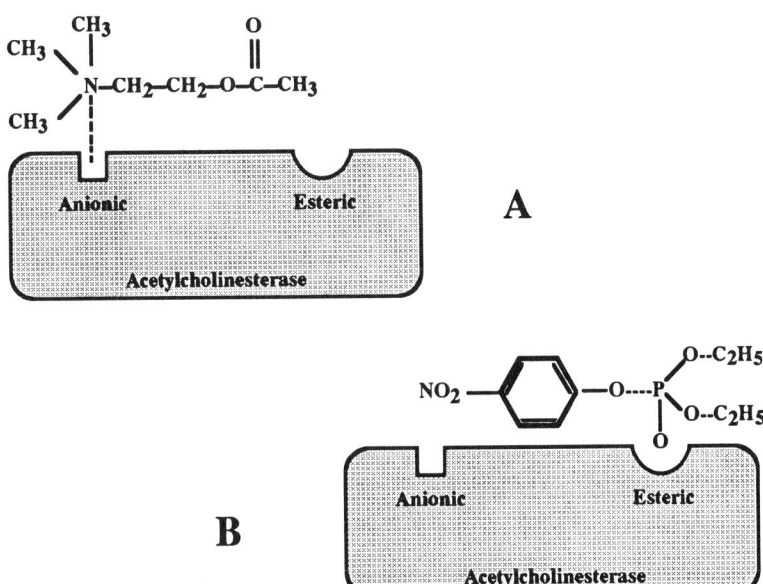

Figure 59.9. A, Attachment of acetylcholine to acetylcholinesterase. **B,** Blocking of anionic attachment site on acetylcholinesterase by attachment of organophosphate to acetycholinesterase.

muscles of respiration. This clinical picture has been observed following exposure to a few compounds including dimethoate, fenthion, methamidophos, and monocrotophos (319). As with the other neuropathies, atropine and pralidoxime have no effect. Symptoms may resolve or improve within a few weeks, but deaths have also occurred. Neuropsychologic effects mimicking cerebellar dysfunction, including mood shifts, deterioration of intellectual function, and memory loss, may be seen as late as 7 years following the last episode of a chronic exposure (320). EEG changes have been noted.

Erythrocyte cholinesterase is found in nervous tissue, red blood cells, spleen, lung, and gray matter. Because it measures the enzyme active in nervous tissue, it has been described as the preferred test over plasma (pseudo) cholinesterase. It remains depressed from a few weeks to 3 months postexposure. Erythrocyte cholinesterase activity may not be affected by some of the organophosphates, such as chlorpyrifos or chlorfenvinphos; therefore, plasma cholinesterase activity

should be obtained (321, 322). Plasma cholinesterase is frequently more easily acquired but fluctuates daily and may be depressed by liver disease, chronic inflammation, malnutrition, morphine, codeine, succinylcholine, and hypersensitivity reactions. Its activity recovers more rapidly than erythrocyte cholinesterase following exposure. Cholinesterase activity must be depressed by 50% or more of the lower end of the normal range in order to see clinical signs. Because of the wide variation of normal activity, a patient's activity may drop by 50% or more and still be within the normal range. Frequently, these activities are of little clinical assistance. Chest radiograph may show pulmonary edema or hydrocarbon-induced pneumonitis. EEG may be helpful for behavioral disorders. CBC, electrolytes, arterial blood gases, blood glucose, and ECG are also indicated.

Organophosphates saturate leather and clothing, becoming virtually impossible to remove by cleaning. A number of patients have suffered recurrent exposures by repeatedly

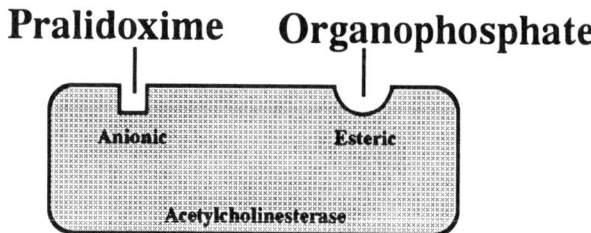

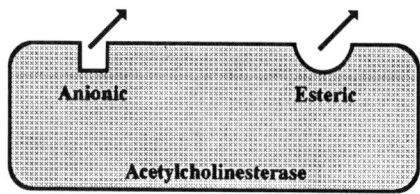

Figure 59.10. **A** and **B,** Action of pralidoxime on organophosphate binding to acetylcholinesterase.

wearing contaminated clothing. Therefore, decontamination should include removal of clothing and thoroughly washing contaminated skin. Due to the rapid absorption of organophosphates, gastric lavage and activated charcoal may be of limited benefit to decrease absorption; however, their use is encouraged. Seizures may be controlled with diazepam or phenobarbital.

Atropine is indicated for the control of muscarinic symptoms. While undertreatment should be avoided, the patient should be monitored for persistent muscarinic symptoms during administration. Atropine should be discontinued when miosis and tachycardia appear or when hypersecretion is controlled. The dose of atropine for adults is 2 to 5 mg i.v. every 15 minutes until muscarinic symptoms abate. As much as 30 g over 35 days has been needed for treatment of resistant cases (323). Pediatric doses are 0.05 mg/kg every 15 minutes until muscarinic symptoms disappear. Effects should be seen within 1 to 4 minutes, with maximal effects occurring within 8 minutes. Side effects of excessive atropine treatment include tachycardia, hypertension, marked mydriasis, restlessness, excitement, hallucinations, and delirium.

The action of oximes such as pralidoxime is to anchor to the anionic site on the acetylcholinesterase molecule and bind to the organophosphate that occupies the esteric site (Fig. 59.10). The two molecules then complex and detach from ACHE, leaving it reactivated. If the organophosphate is allowed to remain attached to the esteric site too long, the bond will age and cannot be broken by the action of oximes.

The initial dose of pralidoxime for children is 20 to 50 mg/kg and for adults 1 to 2 g over 15 to 30 minutes, which may be repeated at 1 to 2 hours. Thereafter, the dose may be administered every 8 to 12 hours as needed. This method of dosing has the potential for the concentration of pralidoxime to decrease below the putative therapeutic range of 4 to 12 µg/ml after approximately 1.5 hours. A continuous infusion of 10 to 20 mg/kg/hr for children or 0.5 g/hr for adults has been recommended to maintain serum concentrations within the therapeutic range based upon an average volume of distribution of 0.25 liter/kg for the central compartment and 0.73

liter/kg at steady state, and an elimination half-life of 1.2 hours (324). A relatively benign antidote, pralidoxime may produce hypertension, headache, ECG changes, dizziness, and GI upset at very high doses (321). Recent evidence has brought into question the utility of pralidoxime in organophosphate poisoning, as its use provided no additional benefit, compared to treatment with atropine alone, in one series of moderate-to-severe organophosphate overdoses (325).

SALICYLATES

Salicylate poisoning can become a complicated life-threatening condition in both children and adults, with the involvement of multiple-organ systems. The major pathophysiologic effects of salicylate toxicity involve: (*a*) the stimulation of the CNS respiratory center; (*b*) the stimulation of the metabolic rate; (*c*) disturbances of carbohydrate lipid metabolism; and (*d*) consequences of the patient's compensatory response to these actions (326–328). Early in the intoxication, salicylates produce gastrointestinal irritation, with resultant nausea, vomiting, and hematemesis; moreover, tachypnea and hyperpnea lead to a lowering of the PCO_2 and resultant respiratory alkalosis. This alkalosis may decrease the ionized serum calcium pool and lead to tetany. Salicylate's ability to uncouple oxidative phosphorylation leads to hyperthermia (up to 42°C) and increased tissue glycolysis, particularly in the brain. Through inhibition of dehydrogenases and aminotransferases in carbohydrate and lipid metabolic pathways, organic acids and ketones accumulate that lead to metabolic acidosis 6 to 24 hours after the acute ingestion. The effects on serum glucose concentrations are variable, but a cerebral glucopenia results.

In response to the respiratory alkalosis, there is a compensatory renal elimination of bicarbonate that reduces the buffering capacity of the blood to subsequent acid accumulation. The accumulation of organic acids and ketones promotes their excretion in the urine, thereby increasing the solute load and resulting in losses of water, sodium, and potassium. Significant dehydration can develop from increased insensible water loss through tachypnea, hyperthermia, and increased renal excretion of water. Salicylates also can produce increased prothrombin times and decreased platelet adhesion, but spontaneous hemorrhage is rare. Reversible tinnitus and deafness, noncardiogenic pulmonary edema, and facial petechial hemorrhages can occur (329). Severe poisonings exhibit coma and seizures.

Salicylate intoxication in adults, particularly in the elderly, can lead to high mortality and morbidity with late presentation or recognition. The diagnosis should be considered in older patients with nonfocal neurologic abnormalities; in patients with dyspnea or tachypnea; in patients having unexplained acid-base disturbances, particularly acidosis; or in patients with apparent sepsis syndrome without readily identifiable source of infection fever, hypotension, or multiple organ failure (330, 331). A contrast of acute and chronic salicylate poisoning in children indicates that chronic salicylism is more likely to exhibit hyperventilation, dehydration, acidemia, coma, and seizures (332).

As more salicylate enters the CNS, morbidity and mortality increase as a consequence of a cerebral glucopenia, leading to coma and seizures (333, 334). Acidosis promotes the nonionization of salicylate, allowing easier penetration through the blood-brain barrier and increased toxicity. This phenomenon parallels the increase in volume of distribution of salicylate as protein-binding decreases with increasing plasma concentrations of salicylate and increasing tissue distribution from the plasma. Both are related to worsening acidosis (335). The mixed-function biotransformation of salicylate prolongs and worsens toxicity with increasing plasma concentrations of salicylate (336). Since two major pathways of the five common metabolic routes are capacity-limited, the elimination half-life of the salicylate can increase by fivefold or more.

The management of salicylate poisoning is primarily directed toward correcting acid-base fluid and electrolyte disturbances and enhancing the elimination of salicylate in the blood. Initial intravenous fluids should be given to correct shock and establish adequate urine flow. After urine flow is established, 0.45% sodium chloride with potassium 3 to 4 mEq/kg/day should be given at a rate of 3 to 5 liters/m²/24 hr. Adequate replacement of potassium losses is necessary to correct the acidosis. Since aspirin can form concentrations in the stomach, gastric evacuation may be successful up to 8 to 12 hours after ingestion (337). Activated charcoal can adsorb aspirin in the gastrointestinal tract and should be routinely administered for acute ingestions.

Several approaches have been used to enhance the elimination of salicylate, but none is more efficient than hemodialysis (338, 339). In addition to hemodialysis, other dialysis techniques have been shown to be effective in this decreasing order: hemoperfusion; peritoneal dialysis with 5% albumin; and peritoneal dialysis with urinary alkalinization (338, 340, 341). Obvious limits of the use of dialysis involve availability and sophistication of personnel and extracorporeal techniques, but hemodialysis is generally reserved for the patient who exhibits life-threatening symptoms unresponsive to current therapy or is oliguric and has a plasma salicylate in excess of 100 to 130 mg/dl (328). Other dialytic procedures are slower (peritoneal dialysis) or not generally effective (exchange transfusion). Repeat-dose activated charcoal therapy has not been shown to be useful in enhancing salicylate elimination (77).

Alkalinization of the urine to a urinary pH of 7.5 has been promoted as a means of enhancing salicylate elimination. Its proponents posit that salicylate clearance increases at least twofold when the urine pH is raised from 7 to 7.5 (61, 342–345). The general goal of forced alkaline diuresis has been to achieve a urinary pH of 7.5 or greater and a minimum urine flow of 2 to 4 ml/kg/hr. Opponents to forced alkaline diuresis cite the difficulty in achieving an alkaline urinary pH with severely poisoned patients and the risks of the potential adverse effects (hypernatremia, hypokalemia, metabolic alkalosis, and fluid overload) and lack of effectiveness in improving patient outcome (346). For moderate poisonings, forced alkaline diuresis may safely enhance elimination, but the need for such intervention is questionable. Establishment of acceptable acid-base, fluid, and electrolyte balance is paramount.

Improvement in symptoms and acid-base, fluid, and electrolyte balance provides a good guide to successful therapy. The Done monogram, a semilogarithmic plot of plasma salicylate concentration vs. hours after ingestion, provides a rough guide to interpreting plasma concentrations, but it is based on some erroneous assumptions (zero-order kinetics with back extrapolation), a small number of patients, has not been confirmed to be well-predictive in adults, has not been evaluated in elderly adults, and is not useful for chronic exposures (347, 348).

SEDATIVE HYPNOTICS

Sedative/hypnotics are a group of pharmaceuticals originally intended to induce sleep during the medical control of anxious or disturbed patients. Within this group are barbiturates, benzodiazepines, chloral hydrate, ethchlorvinyl, glutethimide, methyprylon, meprobamate, methaqualone, and paraldehyde. In general the drugs in this class have similar presentations in overdose, and the mainstay of therapy is good supportive care. Because of some notable differences, barbiturates and benzodiazepines will be discussed here.

BARBITURATES

Since their introduction in 1903, barbiturates have been employed in the treatment of sleep disorders, convulsions, gastrointestinal disorders, and anxiety. They have also, in years past, headed the list of drugs responsible for overdose deaths. The advent of the benzodiazepines in the 1970s has been accompanied by a decrease in barbiturate-induced deaths. Recent popular publications on suicide, however, still list barbiturates as being among the "drugs of choice."

In the central nervous system, γ-aminobutyric acid (GABA) attaches to a postsynaptic receptor that controls the opening of the chloride ionophore, allowing negatively charged ions to enter the resting cell. This hyperpolarizing lowers the resting membrane potential, stabilizes the neuron, and thus exerts an inhibitory effect on firing. The GABA receptor may also be influenced to open the chloride ionophore by the attachment of benzodiazepines or barbiturates to receptors nearby. GABAergic activity is seen in many anticonvulsants and is the primary mechanism by which barbiturates and benzodiazepines act to prevent seizures.

Barbiturates are rapidly absorbed from the gastrointestinal tract. Short-acting barbiturates are more lipid-soluble than the intermediate- and long-acting preparations and enter the gray matter more quickly. Therefore, an ultrashort-acting barbiturate such as methohexital has a volume of distribution of 2.2 liters/kg while that of phenobarbital is 0.54 liters/kg. Elimination half-lives vary widely and are only roughly correlated to duration of action, with ultrashort-acting agents exhibiting half-lives of 1.8 to 10.6 hours, short-acting agents 20 to 30 hours, intermediate-acting agents 15 to 42 hours, and long-acting agents 48 to 144 hours. Lethal doses of short-acting barbiturates are 2 to 3 g, with those of the long-acting barbiturates beginning at 6 to 10 g, though again, lethal amounts vary widely (349). Serum barbiturate concentrations may be helpful in management but are not as important as the clinical picture. The nature of the ingestant and the patient's tolerance give wide variance to the clinical course. Other studies include CBC, electrolytes, CPK, urine myoglobin, glucose, BUN, creatinine, arterial blood gases, and chest radiograph.

CNS depression is the primary presentation in barbiturate overdose. Short-acting barbiturates have an onset of 15 to 20 minutes, with peak activity in 2 to 4 hours. Long-acting barbiturates, such as phenobarbital, may begin to exert toxic effects in 1 to 2 hours, which may peak as late as 18 hours postingestion. Hypotension and hypothermia may be seen late in the course. Bullae are reported in a small percentage of patients, but their cause remains a point of controversy, as they are also seen with many other CNS depressants. Another potential complication of CNS depression is rhabdomyolysis, which can result from long periods of immobilization. Patients should be monitored for increase of CPK and the presence of myoglobinuria. While early deaths are usually due to cardiorespiratory arrest, in-hospital deaths are usually the result of complications of sustained coma.

Good supportive care is the most effective treatment for barbiturate overdose. Because of CNS depression, ipecac is contraindicated. Gastric lavage is a safer procedure, once protection of the airway is ensured. Activated charcoal (25 to 50 g every 4 hours) reduces the elimination half-life of phenobarbital. If activated charcoal has been administered, the patient's gastrointestinal motility should be monitored, and the charcoal should be discontinued if bowel sounds are diminished. The clinical course may, however, be unaffected by serial-activated charcoal (76).

Alkaline diuresis may also increase the excretion of barbital, metharbital, and phenobarbital but is of no use for short- or intermediate-acting barbiturates. Fluid status should be closely monitored to avoid overload. Sodium bicarbonate may be administered in 1 to 2 mEq/kg boluses to increase the arterial pH to 7.45. An infusion of 100 mEq of sodium bicarbonate in 1 liter of 5% dextrose may be titrated to obtain a urine pH of 7.5 to 8.0. Adequate fluid maintenance and alkalinization of the urine are also helpful if rhabdomyolysis is suspected.

Hemodialysis is more effective for long-acting barbiturates with their smaller volume of distribution and lower lipid solubility. Extracorporeal extraction is, however, rarely necessary with ventilatory support, fluid balance, and maintenance of adequate blood pressure.

BENZODIAZEPINES

Much like barbiturates, benzodiazepines attach to a postsynaptic receptor site, where they influence the GABA receptor's action on the chloride ionophore. Benzodiazepines have been identified in three varieties: *agonists*, which stimulate GABA to open the chloride ionophore and "stabilize" the postsynaptic neuron. These compounds are used as sedatives and anticonvulsants. *Reverse agonists* impose a negative effect on the GABA receptor, causing it to decrease the passage of chloride ions. They are used experimentally to induce seizure activity. They are also being studied as memory-enhancing agents. *Antagonists*, such as flumazenil, can attach to the benzodiazepine receptor in the CNS. Unlike the agonists and reverse agonists, they exert no effect on the GABA receptor but block the attachment of molecules that do.

Oral absorption of benzodiazepines is rapid and complete, though intramuscular absorption is erratic. Metabolism consists of hydroxylation or demethylation to form metabolites, which may account for some or all of the activity of the drug and hepatic conjugation of amino and hydroxyl groups leading to inactivation. Some benzodiazepines (lorazepam, oxazepam, and temazepam) undergo only phase II metabolism (350). Typical elimination half-lives of short-acting benzodiazepines range from 1 to 6 hours, intermediate-acting agents from 5 to 20 hours, long-acting agents from 20 to 70 hours, and ultralong-acting agents from 30 to 300 hours. However, duration of action, especially in overdose, correlates poorly with the elimination half-life.

A lethal dose has not been established for benzodiazepines. Though deaths have been reported with single-drug ingestions of many of the benzodiazepines, they are rare and usually involve patients in the sixth decade of life or later (1, 351). Quantitative laboratory studies are of no value in the management of benzodiazepine overdose.

Slurred speech, ataxia, somnolence and, on rare occasions, respiratory depression may be seen. Even with large overdoses, patients are usually responsive to pain. There is some evidence that temazepam and shorter-acting benzodiazepines may be more toxic than their longer-acting counterparts (352, 353).

When compared to other sedative hypnotics, benzodiazepines are relatively benign. For that reason, supportive care will suffice in the vast majority of cases. In 1992, flumazenil, a benzodiazepine antagonist, became commercially available. Structurally similar to midazolam, this drug attaches to the benzodiazepine receptor but exerts no effect upon the GABA receptor. It blocks the action of benzodiazepine agonists without affecting their pharmacokinetics. Because of its short half-life, resedation occurs in approximately 65% of overdose cases, making close monitoring imperative for at least 2 hours following administration (354). Dosage in overdose patients differs from that for reversal of conscious sedation. For benzodiazepine overdose patients, 0.2 mg i.v. is given over 30 seconds, with the physician waiting 45 seconds for a response. If no response is seen, 0.3 mg i.v. is given over 30 seconds, with the physician waiting another 45 seconds. If response is inadequate, 0.5 mg may be given intravenously every minute to a total dose of 5 mg. For resedation in overdose patients, doses should not exceed 1 mg/dose or 3 mg/hr.

Flumazenil is contraindicated in the following situations, where seizure activity may be precipitated: (*a*) with patients receiving benzodiazepines for seizure control; (*b*) with patients who have been taking benzodiazepines chronically; and (*c*) with patients in whom mixed-drug overdose is suspected, and tricyclic antidepressants are known or suspected to be present. Although flumazenil appears to be a safe and effective agent when used properly, it should not be used indiscriminately for a toxin that usually has a benign clinical course.

STIMULANTS

Generally, CNS stimulants lead to increases of norepinephrine that produce varying degrees of central nervous system and cardiovascular stimulation. Acute toxicity produces a hyperactive syndrome that is characterized by restlessness, agitation, tremor, tonic-clonic seizures, hypertension, and tachycardia (355, 356). Potential complications include behavioral changes (psychosis, paranoia, formication), cardiovascular collapse, pulmonary edema, dysrhythmias, status epilepticus, hyperthermia, rhabdomyolysis, lactic acidemia, acute renal failure, coma, emboli, stroke, and hypertensive encephalopathy.

Cocaine will be discussed as the prototype, and others will be compared to it.

Cocaine is primarily available as the hydrochloride salt and the alkaloid ("free base"). Cocaine hydrochloride is typically inhaled intranasally ("snorted") or injected intravenously. It may also be taken orally, vaginally, sublingually, rectally, or injected intramuscularly or subcutaneously. "Crack" is the alkaloid form prepared by adding an alkalinizing agent such as ammonia or baking soda to an aqueous solution of the hydrochloride, forming a precipitate that is nearly pure cocaine. A purer alkaloid product, "free base," can be formed by a dangerous extraction process that typically uses ether. Both alkaloid forms are more heat-stable and exhibit a lower vaporization temperature than the hydrochloride, which allows the alkaloid to be smoked. The effects of the various forms are similar, except for a slower onset and longer duration of action after nasal insufflation of the hydrochloride (onset: 1 to 3 minutes; duration: 45 to 75 minutes), compared to smoking an alkaloid (onset: 4 to 6 seconds; duration: 5 to 7 minutes) (356–358). Cerebral infarction may be more common among alkaloidal cocaine users, whereas hemorrhagic stroke may be more common with intravenous cocaine hydrochloride use (359).

Cocaine produces local anesthesia upon contact by stabilizing neuronal membranes through sodium channel blockade. Centrally, several neurotransmitters are affected. Norepinephrine reuptake is inhibited; dopamine reuptake is decreased; and serotonin concentrations are decreased. Peripherally, cocaine blocks norepinephrine reuptake, which results in tachycardia, hypertension, vasoconstriction, pulmonary edema, and diaphoresis. Hyperthermia may result from a direct effect on the hypothalamus or indirectly from cocaine's vasoconstrictive effects (356–358).

In serious toxicity after cocaine use, one must also consider the contribution of other drugs, preexisting disease, and adulterants (360). Myocardial infarction and ischemia that become manifest within minutes or up to several hours after use have been associated with cocaine (361–363). Sudden death and cardiac arrhythmia with idioventricular rhythms and ventricular fibrillation have been reported. Seizures are common and, if solitary, are usually self-limiting.

If multiple seizures are present, the risks of hyperthermia, acidosis, and death are much greater. Intracranial hemorrhage and stroke have also been reported within minutes of cocaine use, and up to 24 hours later (364, 365). Cocaine may induce hepatotoxicity through free radical production and depletion of glutathione stores, leading to lipid peroxidation of cellular membranes (358). Rhabdomyolysis and pulmonary complications, such as pulmonary edema and respiratory arrest, in addition to pneumomediastinum and pneumothorax from a forced Valsalva maneuver from smoking crack, may also occur after cocaine use (366, 367). During the prenatal period, complications from cocaine abuse include abruptio placentae, spontaneous abortion, premature labor, and intrauterine growth retardation. Chronic intranasal cocaine use can lead to atrophy of the nasal mucosa, perforation of the nasal septum epistaxis, and persistent rhinorrhea (356–358).

Cocaine undergoes biotransformation in man by three major routes: (*a*) hydrolysis by cholinesterase to form ecgonine methylester; (*b*) *N*-demethylation for form norcocaine; and (*c*) nonenzymatic hydrolysis to form benzoylecgonine (358, 368).

Since 50% of a cocaine dose is hydrolyzed by cholinesterases, patients with decreased plasma cholinesterase activity may have a greater risk of life-threatening cocaine toxicity (369). Generally, cocaine is undetectable in the blood within 24 hours of a single dose, but metabolites may be detected in the urine for several days (358).

The treatment of a stimulant overdose involves standard life-support and gastric decontamination procedures, if indicated (356, 358). Agitation generally responds to diazepam, other benzodiazepines, or haloperidol. Status epilepticus warrants aggressive treatment with diazepam, followed by administration of phenytoin or phenobarbital. Resistant seizures may require endotracheal intubation, neuromuscular blockade, and general anesthesia. Hyperthermia should be treated aggressively with cool-water washes and blowing air or cooling blankets. Hypertension may respond to sedation and oxygen administration, but nitroprusside or phentolamine may be needed for resistant cases. Propranolol has been previously recommended for hypertensive crisis, but paradoxical hypertension may result from unopposed α-adrenergic stimulation (370). Labetolol or calcium channel blockers such as verapamil or nifedipine may be useful alternatives (371). Tachyarrhythmias usually respond to propranolol, if hypertension is not present, or to esmolol. If cardiac ischemia is suspected, intravenous administration of verapamil or nitroglycerin should be considered. Rhabdomyolysis can be managed by maintaining an alkaline urine flow with intravenous fluids and sodium bicarbonate administration (60).

The treatment of asymptomatic individuals who swallow condoms or balloons filled with cocaine ("body packers") as a smuggling or concealment technique involves administration of activated charcoal and a cathartic or employment of whole bowel irrigation. Surgical removal should be considered for patients exhibiting serious toxicity (49, 372, 373).

Other stimulants produce a similar toxic effect upon overdose with a few distinctions. Amphetamines cause adrenergic stimulation by releasing norepinephrine from neuronal storage granules and by directly stimulating α- and β-receptors (374, 375). Typically, amphetamines produce longer-lasting effects, compared to those of cocaine (355, 356). Other sympathomimetic agents, such as ephedrine or phenypropanololamine, are found in many nasal decongestants, weight loss pills, and "look-a-like" stimulants and may produce serious toxicity, such as hypertensive crisis and stroke on overdose (376).

In the past decade, illicit amphetamine derivatives such as 3,4-methylene dioxymethamphetamine ("Ecstasy," or "MDMA") and a smokable form of methamphetamine ("Ice") have been used for their stimulatory and hallucinogenic properties (377–379). At higher doses, hallucinations and adrenergic crisis are possible and can last for 12 hours.

Abstinence after chronic use of cocaine and amphetamines can be associated with neuropsychiatric symptoms such as exhaustion, anxiety, and depression. Suicidal ideation and intensive craving for the drug are common during withdrawal from stimulants (355).

THEOPHYLLINE

Theophylline, a methylxanthine structurally related to caffeine, has been used for centuries for its stimulatory properties. Derived from plant alkaloids, it was commonly extracted by brewing leaves as tea. Theophylline has been used since the 1930s in the treatment of asthma and utilized in the management of chronic obstructive pulmonary disease (COPD), apnea of the newborn, and congestive heart failure in animals. Statistics from the American Association of Poison Control Centers indicate that approximately 6000 people each year are reported to have toxic effects from theophylline. Approximately 30 fatal exposures were reported for 1989 and 1990 (1, 351).

Because theophylline metabolism follows saturable kinetics, chronic toxicity is seen at lower serum concentrations than acute toxicity. Toxicity is known to increase with age, perhaps owing to decreased hepatic function or protein binding. Possible explanations for chronic toxicity include CNS saturation or accumulation of 3-methylxanthine, an active metabolite of theophylline. Though seizures and serious dysrhythmias have been reported at concentrations of 15 to 20 $\mu g/ml$, they are more frequently seen with chronic serum theophylline concentrations of 35 to 70 $\mu g/ml$.

In patients not previously exposed to theophylline, ingestions greater than 10 mg/kg are potentially toxic. Acute serum concentrations generally correlate with toxicity, with concentrations of 20 to 40 $\mu g/ml$ producing minimal toxicity, 40 to 100 $\mu g/ml$ moderate-to-severe toxicity, and greater than 100 $\mu g/ml$ severe toxicity.

Absorption of theophylline is rapid and nearly complete. Peak effects from therapeutic doses may be seen in 1 to 2 hours but are prolonged with sustained release tablets. In overdose, peak concentrations may occur from 2 to 8 hours. Sustained-release preparations may peak between 1 and 24 hours with a mean of 11 hours. Bezoar formation has been reported with sustained-release tablets (380). The mean volume of distribution is 0.5 liters/kg with 40 to 60% protein binding. Theophylline is metabolized via cytochrome P-450 mixed-function oxidase by demethylation or hydroxylation. The only active metabolite is 3-methylxanthine. Five to 10% of a therapeutic dose is excreted unchanged. Metabolism of theophylline initially follows first-order kinetics but in overdose may become saturable. This characteristic makes dose adjustment difficult, and serum concentrations must be monitored closely when doses are changed or drugs affecting metabolism are used concomitantly.

Theophylline clearance varies with age. Newborns and adults have similar rates of clearance while children eliminate the drug much more rapidly. A number of drug interactions influence theophylline concentrations. Decreased concentrations are seen with phenytoin, rifampin, β-agonists, phenobarbital, carbamazepine, and smoking. Increased concentrations can be seen with erythromycin, oral contraceptives, allopurinol, cimetidine, and ciprofloxacin.

The exact mechanism of action is not known for theophylline at therapeutic doses. Inhibition of phosphodiesterase leading to increased cyclic AMP has been proposed but has not been substantiated. It may, however, be a mechanism of toxicity. Other theories include translocation of intracellular calcium by increased permeability to Ca^{+2} of the sarcoplasmic reticulum, inhibition of leukotriene production, blockade of adenosine receptors, reduction in the uptake or metabolism of catecholamines, stimulation of catecholamine release with

high doses, inhibition of benzodiazepine receptors at toxic doses, and prostaglandin inhibition.

Gastrointestinal, cardiovascular, and CNS symptoms predominate, particularly in acute exposures. Metabolic manifestations, though important, may be more subtle. Gastrointestinal symptoms include nausea and vomiting in 60 to 100% of cases, abdominal pain, diarrhea, and acute gastritis with GI bleeding. Cardiovascular effects include supraventricular and ventricular dysrhythmias. Ventricular tachycardia is associated with acute concentrations greater than 100 $\mu g/ml$ and chronic concentrations of 40 $\mu g/ml$ or greater (381). Atrial fibrillation is more frequently seen with chronic exposure. Hypotension is most commonly due to decreased vascular resistance. Central nervous system symptoms are seen as tremors and/or ataxia in 50% of poisonings. Headache, hallucinations, disorientation, and coma are also observed. Convulsions are seen in 50% of patients with acute exposures with serum concentrations over 120 $\mu g/ml$ or chronic concentrations of 40 $\mu g/ml$ (381). Seizure activity is associated with markedly increased mortality, and its prevention is a primary objective of therapy.

Hypokalemia, one of the metabolic effects of theophylline toxicity, may result from cyclic AMP-mediated stimulation of the Na^+-K^+-ATPase pump, resulting in decreased extracellular potassium. Hypophosphatemia, hypomagnesemia, and hypercalcemia have also been reported (382). Metabolic acidosis is a common finding in moderate-to-severe toxicity and may be related to catecholamine activity. Theophylline may also have a mild diuretic effect.

Theophylline may be detected by enzyme-mediated immunoassay (EMIT) or high-performance liquid chromatography (HPLC). Several substances may interfere with spectrophotometric measurements, including theobromine, probenecid, furosemide, barbiturates, phenytoin, and acetaminophen. Other parameters that should be monitored include electrolytes, calcium, magnesium, phosphorus, CPK, arterial blood gases, and urine pH.

Because of the associated increase in mortality and resistance to anticonvulsant therapy, prevention of seizures is essential in the management of theophylline poisoning. Though serum concentrations cannot serve as a definitive guideline, patients with chronic concentrations greater than 40 $\mu g/ml$ or acute concentrations greater than 100 $\mu g/ml$ merit consideration of anticonvulsant prophylaxis (381). Patients with lower concentrations who are symptomatic with tremor, hallucinations, or agitation should also be considered for prophylactic treatment. Though effective, the duration of benzodiazepines is generally too short to be of greatest benefit in this situation. Animal data suggest that phenytoin is of little efficacy for seizure prophylaxis in theophylline overdose and may actually lower the seizure threshold (383). Phenobarbital has proved effective in doses of 10 to 20 mg/kg intravenously.

Cardiac dysrhythmias such as supraventricular tachycardia (SVT) may require no treatment. Hemodynamically significant SVT may be treated with β-blocking drugs such as propranolol or esmolol (384). Other ventricular dysrhythmias may also respond to β-blockers or lidocaine or other antiarrhythmics. Hypotension, with an increased pulse pressure and diastolic hypotension, is often due to decreased vascular resistance and may respond to β-blockade. α-Agonists such as levarterenol may also correct hypotension.

Hypokalemia, hyperglycemia, hypophosphatemia, hypercalcemia, and metabolic acidosis have been corrected by intravenous propranolol and by specific replacement where indicated.

Multiple-dose-activated charcoal has proven effective at enhancing elimination of theophylline from the bloodstream even after intravenous overdose. Doses (20 to 50 g) repeated at 3- to 6-hour intervals have been shown to reduce theophylline half-life by 50% (385). Repeat-dose activated charcoal should be considered if serum concentrations in acute overdose are over 40 μg/ml, symptomatic patients (acute or chronic exposures), or chronic intoxication with serum concentrations over 20 μg/ml (381).

Charcoal hemoperfusion is also very effective in removal of theophylline, though frequently unnecessary when repeat-dose charcoal can be employed. It should be considered in acute overdose with serum concentrations greater than 100 μg/ml, for seizure activity or hemodynamically significant dysrhythmias not responding to conventional therapy or chronic intoxication with serum concentrations over 40 μg/ml (386). Hemodialysis will also remove theophylline but is somewhat less efficient than charcoal hemoperfusion.

Seizure activity should prompt the monitoring of creatine phosphokinase (CPK). When marked increase occurs, prophylactic treatment for rhabdomyolysis should be instituted, including alkaline diuresis, maintaining a urine pH of 8.

REFERENCES

1. Litovitz TL, Bailey KM, Schmitz BF, et al: 1990 Annual Report of the American Association of Poison Control Centers National Data Collection Program. *Am J Emerg Med* 9:461–509, 1991.
2. Stern TS, Mulley AG, Thibault GE: Life-threatening drug overdose: precipitants and prognosis. *JAMA* 251:1983–1985, 1984.
3. Lacroix J, Gaudreault P, Gauthier M: Admission to a pediatric intensive care unit for poisoning: a review of 105 cases. *Crit Care Med* 17:748–750, 1989.
4. Kirk MA: Rational utilization of the intensive care unit in managing the poisoned patient. *Contemp Management Crit Care* 1(3):3–19, 1991.
5. Elk JR, Linton DM, Potgieter PD: Treatment of acute self-poisoning in a respiratory intensive care unit. *S Afr J Med* 72:532–534, 1987.
6. Henning RJ, McClish D, Daly B, et al: Clinical characteristics and resource utilization of ICU patients: implications for organization of intensive care. *Crit Care Med* 15:264–269, 1987.
7. Ron A, Aronne LJ, Kalb PE, et al: The therapeutic efficacy of critical care units. *Arch Intern Med* 149:338–341, 1989.
8. Brett AS, Rothschild N, Gray R, Perry M: Predicting the clinical course in intentional drug overdose. *Arch Intern Med* 147:133–137, 1987.
9. Mannoguerra AS, Krenzelok EP: Rapid emesis from high-dose ipecac syrup in adults and children intoxicated with antiemetics and other drugs. *Am J Hosp Pharm* 35:1360–1362, 1978.
10. MacLean WC: A comparison of ipecac syrup and apomorphine in the immediate treatment of ingestion of poisons. *J Pediatr* 82:121–124, 1973.
11. Mowry JB, Sketris IS, Czajka PA, Sweat DL: Ipecac syrup for poisonings at home: availability, compliance, and response monitored by telephone. *Am J Hosp Pharm* 38:1028–1030, 1981.
12. Corby DG, Decker WJ, Moran MJ, Payne CE: Clinical comparison of pharmacologic emetics in children. *Pediatrics* 42:361–364, 1968.
13. Corby DG, Lisciandro RG, Lehman RH, Decker WJ: The efficacy of methods used to evacuate the stomach after acute ingestions. *Pediatrics* 40:871–874, 1967.
14. Abdullah AH, Tye A: A comparison of the efficacy of emetic drugs and stomach lavage. *Am J Dis Child* 113:571–575, 1967.
15. Veltri JC, Temple AR: Telephone management of poisonings using syrup of ipecac. *Clin Toxicol* 9:407–417, 1976.
16. Thompson WL: Poisoning: the twentieth-century black death. In *Critical Care Medicine—State of the Art, Vol 1.* Society of Critical Care Medicine, pp 1–94, 1980.
17. Czajka PA, Russell SL: Nonemetic effects of syrup of ipecac. *Pediatrics* 75:1101–1104, 1985.
18. Schofferman JA: A clinical comparison of syrup of ipecac and apomorphine in adults. *JACEP* 5:22–25, 1976.
19. Adler AG, Walinsky P, Krall RA, Cho SY: Death resulting from ipecac syrup poisoning. *JAMA* 243:1927–1928, 1980.
20. Vance MW, Selden BS, Clark RF: Optimal patient position for transport and initial management of toxic ingestions. *Ann Emerg Med* 21:243–246, 1992.
21. Auerbach PS, Osterloh J, Braun O, et al: Efficacy of gastric emptying: gastric lavage versus emesis induced with ipecac. *Ann Emerg Med* 15:692–698, 1986.
22. Tandberg D, Diven BG, McLeod JW: Ipecac-induced emesis vs. gastric lavage: a controlled study. *Am J Emerg Med* 4:205–209, 1986.
23. Robertson WO: Syrup of ipecac—a slow or fast emetic? *Am J Dis Child* 103:58–61, 1962.
24. Reid DHS: Treatment of the poisoned child. *Arch Dis Child* 45:428–433, 1970.
25. Menzies DG, Busuttil A, Prescott LF: Fatal pulmonary aspiration of oral activated charcoal. *Br Med J* 287:459–460, 1988.
26. Silberman H, Davis SM, Lee A: Activated charcoal aspiration. *NC Med J* 51:79–80, 1990.
27. Elliott CG, Colby TV, Kelly TM, et al: Charcoal lung-bronchiolitis obliterans after aspiration of activated charcoal. *Chest* 96:672–674, 1989.
28. Pollack MM, Dunbar BS, Holbrook PR, et al: Aspiration of activated charcoal and gastric contents. *Ann Emerg Med* 10:528–529, 1981.
29. Sketris IS, Mowry JB, Czajka PA: Saline catharsis: effect on aspirin bioavailability in combination with activated charcoal. *J Clin Pharmacol* 22:59–64, 1982.
30. McNamara R, Aaron CK, Gemborys M, Davidhiser S: Sorbitol catharsis does not enhance efficacy of charcoal in simulated acetaminophen overdose (abstr). *Ann Emerg Med* 16:520, 1987.
31. Farely TA: Severe hypernatremic dehydration after use of an activated charcoal-sorbitol suspension. *J Pediatr* 109:719–722, 1986.
32. Jones J, Heiselman D, Dougherty J, Eddy A: Cathartic-induced magnesium toxicity during overdose management. *Ann Emerg Med* 15:1214–1218, 1986.
33. Kirk MA, Petersen J, Kulig K, Lowenstein S, Rumack BH: Acetaminophen overdose in children: a comparison of ipecac versus activated charcoal versus no gastrointestinal decontamination (abstr). *Ann Emerg Med* 20:472–473, 1991.
34. Burton BT, Bayer MJ, Barron L, Aitchison JP: Comparison of activated charcoal and gastric lavage in the prevention of aspirin absorption. *J Emerg Med* 1:411–416, 1984.
35. Comstock EC, Boisaubin V, Comstock, et al: Assessment of the efficacy of activated charcoal following gastric lavage in acute drug emergencies. *Clin Toxicol* 19:149–165, 1982.
36. McNamara RM, Aaron CK, Gemborys M, Davidheiser S: Efficacy of charcoal cathartic versus ipecac in reducing serum acetaminophen in a simulated overdose. *Ann Emerg Med* 18:934–938, 1989.
37. Neuvonen PJ, Vartianen M, Tokola O: Comparison of activated charcoal and ipecac syrup in prevention of drug absorption. *Eur J Clin Pharmacol* 24:557–562, 1983.
38. Curtis RA, Bartone J, Giacona N: Efficacy of ipecac and activated charcoal/cathartic: prevention of salicylate absorption in a simulated overdose. *Arch Intern Med* 144:48–52, 1984.
39. Tenenbein M, Cohen S, Sitar DS: Efficacy of ipecac-induced emesis, orogastric lavage, and activated charcoal for acute drug overdose. *Ann Emerg Med* 16:838–841, 1987.
40. Kulig K, Bar-OR D, Cantrill SV, Rosen R, Rumack BH: Management of acutely poisoned patients without gastric emptying. *Ann Emerg Med* 14:562–567, 1985.
41. Albertson TE, Derlet RW, Foulke GE, Minguillon MC, Tharratt SR: Superiority of activated charcoal alone compared with ipecac and activated charcoal in the treatment of acute toxic ingestions. *Ann Emerg Med* 18:56–59, 1989.
42. Merigian KS, Woodard M, Hedges JR, Roberts JR, Stuebing R, Rashkin MC: Prospective evaluation of gastric emptying in the self-poisoned patient. *Am J Emerg Med* 8:479–483, 1990.
43. Olson KR: Is gut emptying all washed up (editorial)? *Am J Emerg Med* 8:560–561, 1990.
44. Tenenbein M: Whole bowel irrigation as a gastrointestinal decontamination procedure after acute poisoning. *Med Toxicol* 3:77–84, 1988.
45. Tenenbein M, Cohen S, Sitar DS: Whole bowel irrigation as decontamination procedure after acute drug overdose. *Arch Intern Med* 147:905–907, 1987.
46. Everson GW, Bertaccini EJ, O'Leary J: Use of whole bowel irrigation in an infant following iron overdose. *Am J Emerg Med* 9:366–369, 1991.
47. Smith SW, Ling LJ, Halstenson CE: Whole-bowel irrigation as a treatment for acute lithium overdose. *Ann Emerg Med* 20:536–539, 1991.
48. Burkhart KK, Kulig KW, Rumack B: Whole-bowel irrigation as treatment for zinc sulfate overdose. *Ann Emerg Med* 19:1167–1170, 1990.
49. Hoffman RS, Smilkstein MJ, Goldfrank LR: Whole bowel irrigation and the cocaine body-packer: a new approach to a common problem. *Am J Emerg Med* 8:523–527, 1990.
50. Sporer KA, Ernst AA: The effect of toxicologic screening on management of minimally symptomatic overdoses. *Am J Emerg Med* 10:173–175, 1992.
51. Clark RF, Harchelroad F: Toxicology screening of the trauma patient: a changing profile. *Ann Emerg Med* 20:151–153, 1991.
52. Kellerman AL, Fihn SD, LoGerfo JP: Impact of drug screening in suspected overdose. *Ann Emerg Med* 16:1206–1216, 1987.
53. Hepler BR, Sutheimer CA, Sunshine I: Role of the toxicology laboratory in the treatment of acute poisoning. *Med Toxicol* 1:61–75, 1986.

54. Jacobsen D: Anion and osmolar gaps in the diagnosis of methanol and ethylene glycol poisoning. *Acta Med Scand* 212:17–20, 1982.
55. Gabow PA: Ethylene glycol intoxication. *Am J Kidney Dis* 11:277–279, 1988.
56. Walker JA, Schwartzbard A, Krauss EA, Sherman RA, Eisinger RP: The missing gap. A pitfall in the diagnosis of alcohol intoxication by osmometry. *Arch Intern Med* 146:1843–1844, 1986.
57. Rosenberg J, Benowitz NL, Pond S: Pharmacokinetics of drug overdose. *Clin Pharmacokinet* 6:161–192, 1981.
58. Pond SM: Principles of techniques used to enhance elimination of toxic compounds. In Haddad LM, Winchester JF (eds): *Clinical Management of Poisoning and Drug Overdose*, ed 2. WB Saunders, Philadelphia, pp 21–28, 1990.
59. Eneas JF, Schoenfield PY, Humphreys MH: The effect of infusion of mannitol-sodium bicarbonate on the clinical course of myoglobinuria. *Arch Intern Med* 139:801–805, 1979.
60. Scandling J, Spital A: Amphetamine-associated myoglobinuric renal failure. *South Med J* 75:237–240, 1982.
61. Morgan AG, Polak A: The excretion of salicylate in salicylate poisoning. *Clin Sci* 41:475–484, 1971.
62. Linton AL, Luke RG, Briggs JD: Methods of forced diuresis and its application in barbiturate poisoning. *Lancet* ii:377–379, 1967.
63. Takki S, Gambertoglio JG, Honda DH, Tozer TN: Pharmacokinetic evaluation of hemodialysis in acute drug overdose. *J Pharmacokinet Biopharm* 6:427–442, 1978.
64. Pond S, Rosenberg J, Benowitz NL, Takki S: Pharmacokinetics of haemoperfusion for drug overdose. *Clin Pharmacokinet* 4:329–354, 1979.
65. Pond SM: Extracorporeal techniques in the treatment of poisoned patients. *Med J Aust* 154:617–622, 1991.
66. Golper TA, Bennett WM: Drug removal by continuous arteriovenous haemofiltration: a review of the evidence in poisoned patients. *Med Toxicol* 3:341–349, 1988.
67. Garella S: Extracorporeal techniques in the treatment of exogenous intoxications. *Kidney Int* 33:735–754, 1988.
68. Gwilt PR, Perrier D: Plasma protein binding and distribution characteristics of drugs as indices of their hemodialyzability. *Clin Pharmacol Ther* 24:154–161, 1978.
69. Benet LZ, Williams RL: Design and optimization of dosage regimens: pharmacokinetic data. In Gilman AG, Rall TW, Nies AS, Taylor P (eds): *The Pharmacological Basis of Therapeutics*, ed 8. Pergamon Press, Elmsford, NY, pp 1650–1735, 1990.
70. Bennett DR (ed): *Drug Evaluations Annual 1991.* American Medical Association, Milwaukee, 1990.
71. Levy G: Gastrointestinal clearance of drugs with activated charcoal. *N Engl J Med* 307:676–678, 1982.
72. Neuvonen PJ, Olkkola KT: Oral activated charcoal in the treatment of intoxications. *Med Toxicol* 3:33–58, 1988.
73. McLuckie A, Forbes AM, Ilett KF: Role of repeated doses of oral activated charcoal in the treatment of acute intoxications. *Anaesth Intens Care* 18:375–384, 1990.
74. Campbell JW, Chyka PA: Physicochemical characteristics of drugs and response to repeat-dose activated charcoal. *Am J Emerg Med* 10:208–210, 1992.
75. Tenenbein M: Multiple doses of activated charcoal: time for reappraisal. *Ann Emerg Med* 20:529–531, 1991.
76. Pond SM, Olson KR, Osterloh JD, Tong TG: Randomized study of the treatment of phenobarbital overdose with repeated doses of activated charcoal. *JAMA* 251:3104–3108, 1984.
77. Mayer AL, Sitar DS, Tenenbein M: Multiple-dose charcoal and whole-bowel irrigation do not increase clearance of absorbed salicylate. *Arch Intern Med* 152:393–396, 1992.
78. Smolinske SC: Activated charcoal/treatment protocol. In Rumack BH (ed): *Poisindex ® Information System*. Micromedex, Inc., Denver, (Edition expires 5/31/92.)
79. Kornberg AE, Dolgin J: Pediatric ingestions: charcoal alone versus ipecac and charcoal. *Ann Emerg Med* 20:648–651, 1991.
80. Harchelroad F, Cottingham E, Krenzelok EP: Gastrointestinal transit times of a charcoal/sorbitol slurry in overdose patients. *Clin Toxicol* 27:91–99, 1989.
81. Palatnik W, Tenenbein M: Activated charcoal in the treatment of drug overdose. *Drug Safety* 7:3–7, 1992.
82. Davidson DGD, Eastham WN: Acute liver necrosis following overdose of paracetamol. *Br Med J* 2:497–499, 1966.
83. Ameer B, Greenblatt DJ: Acetaminophen. *Ann Intern Med* 87:202–209, 1977.
84. Sanerkin NG: Acute myocardial necrosis in paracetamol poisoning. *Br Med J* 3:478, 1971.
85. Mofenson HC, Caraccio TR: Acetaminophen induced pancreatitis. *Clin Toxicol* 29:3–30, 1991.
86. Maddrey WC: Hepatic effects of acetaminophen: enhanced toxicity in alcoholics. *J Clin Gastroenterol* 9:180–185, 1987.
87. Seeff LB, Cuccherini BA, Zimmerman HJ: Acetaminophen hepatotoxicity in alcoholics. *Ann Intern Med* 104:399–404, 1986.
88. Flanagan RJ, Mant TGK: Coma and metabolic acidosis early in severe acute paracetamol poisoning. *Hum Toxicol* 5:179–182, 1986.
89. Keays R, Harrison PM, Wendon JA, et al: Intravenous acetylcysteine in paracetamol induced fulminant hepatic failure: a prospective controlled trial. *Br Med J* 303:1026–1029, 1991.
90. Harrison PM, Keays R, Bray GP, et al: Improved outcome of paracetamol-induced fulminant hepatic failure by late administration of acetylcysteine. *Lancet* 335:1572–1573, 1990.
91. Rumack BH, Peterson RG, Koch GG, et al: Acetaminophen overdose: 662 cases with evaluation of acetylcysteine treatment. *Arch Intern Med* 141:380–385, 1981.
92. Haibach H, Akhter JE, Muscato MS, et al: Acetaminophen overdose with fetal demise. *Am J Clin Pathol* 40:240–242, 1984.
93. Selden BS, Curry SC, Clark RF, Johnson BC, Meinhart RM, Pizziconi VB: Transplacental transport of N-acetylcysteine in an ovine model. *Ann Emerg Med* 20:1069–1072, 1991.
94. Smilkstein MJ, Bronstein AC, Linden CH, Augenstein WL, Kulig KW, Rumack BH: Acetaminophen overdose: a 48 hour intravenous N-acetylcysteine treatment protocol. *Ann Emerg Med* 20:1058–1063, 1991.
95. Vale JA, Wheeler DC: Anaphylactoid reactions to IV acetylcysteine. *Lancet* ii:988, 1982.
96. Ho SW, Beilin LJ: Asthma associated with N-acetylcysteine infusion and paracetamol poisoning: report of two cases. *Br Med J* 287:876–877, 1983.
97. Anonymous Death after N-acetylcysteine. *Lancet* i:1421, 1984.
98. Murase T, Hazama H, Okuno H, Shiozaki Y, Sameshima Y: Effect of H_2 receptor antagonists on acetaminophen-induced hepatic injury. *Jpn J Pharmacol* 41:467–473, 1986.
99. Davis M: Protective agents for acetaminophen overdose. *Semin Liver Dis* 6:2 138–147, 1986.
100. Jackson JE. Cimetidine protects against acetaminophen toxicity. *Life Sci* 31:31–35, 1982.
101. Ruffalo R, Thompson J: Cimetidine and acetylcysteine as antidote for acetaminophen overdose. *South Med J* 75:954–962, 1982.
102. Speeg KV: Potential use cimetidine for treatment of acetaminophen overdose. *Pharmacotherapy* 7(Part 2):125s–133s, 1987.
103. Burkhart K, Janco N, Kulig K, Rumack BH: Cimetidine as adjunctive treatment for acetaminophen overdose (abstr.). *Vet Hum Toxicol* 31:337, 1989.
104. Stokes JB, Aueron P: Prevention of organ damage in massive ethylene glycol poisoning ingestion. *JAMA* 243:2065–2066, 1980.
105. Parry MF, Wallach R: Ethylene glycol poisoning. *Am J Med* 57:143–150, 1974.
106. Peterson CD, Collins AJ, et al: Ethylene glycol poisoning. Pharmacokinetics drug therapy with ethanol and hemodialysis. *N Engl J Med* 304:21–23, 1981.
107. Jacobsen D, Ostby N, Bredesen JE: Studies on ethylene glycol poisoning. *Acta Med Scand* 212:11–15, 1982.
108. Jacobsen D, Hewlett TP, Webb R, Brown ST, Ordinario AT, McMartin KE: Ethylene glycol intoxication: evaluation of kinetics and crystalluria. *Am J Med* 84:145–152, 1988.
109. Cheng JT, Beysolow TD, Kaul P, Weisman R, Feinfeld DA: Clearance of ethylene glycol by kidneys and hemodialysis. *Clin Toxicol* 25:95–108, 1987.
110. Clay KL, Murphy RC: On the metabolic acidosis of ethylene glycol intoxication. *Toxicol Appl Pharmacol* 39:39–49, 1977.
111. McMartin KE, Martin-Amat G, Makar AB, Tephly TR: Methanol poisoning. V. Role of formate metabolism in the monkey. *J Pharmacol Exp Ther* 201:564–572, 1977.
112. Berman LB, Schreiner GE, Feys G: The nephrotoxic lesion of ethylene glycol. *Ann Intern Med* 46:611–619, 1957.
113. Spillane L, Roberts JR, Meyer AE: Multiple cranial nerve deficits after ethylene glycol poisoning. *Ann Emerg Med* 20:208–210, 1991.
114. Jacobsen D, Ovrebo S, Ostborg J, Sejersted OM: Glycolate causes the acidosis in ethylene glycol poisoning and is effectively removed by hemodialysis. *Acta Med Scand* 216:409–416, 1984.
115. Bennett IL, Freeman HC, Mitchell GL, Cooper MN: Acute methyl alcohol poisoning: a review based on experiences in an outbreak of 323 cases. *Medicine* 32:431–463, 1953.
116. Swartz RD, Millman RP, Billi JE, et al: Epidemic methanol poisoning: clinical and biochemical analysis of a recent episode. *Medicine* 60:373–392, 1981.
117. Jacobsen D, Jansen H, Wiik-Larsen E, Bredesen JE, Halvorsen S: Studies on methanol poisoning. *Acta Med Scand* 212:5–10, 1982.
118. Jacobsen D, Webb, Collins TD, McMartin KE: Methanol and formate kinetics in late diagnosed methanol intoxication. *Med Toxicol* 3:418–423, 1988.
119. McMartin KE, Martin-Amat G, Nokar PE, Tephly TR: Lack of a role of formaldehyde in methanol poisoning in the monkey. *Biochem Pharmacol* 28:645–649, 1979.
120. Jacobsen D, Ovrebo S, Arneson E, Paus PN: Pulmonary excretion of methanol in man. *Scand J Clin Lab Invest* 43:377–379, 1983.
121. Tenenbein M: Methanol half-life during ethanol administration (abstr). *Vet Hum Toxicol* 33:369, 1991.
122. Jacobsen D, McMartin KE: Methanol and ethylene glycol poisoning: mechanism of toxicity, clinical course, diagnosis and treatment. *Med Toxicol* 1:309–334, 1988.
123. McMartin KE, Ambre JJ, Tephly TR: Methanol poisoning in human subjects. Role for formic acid accumulation in the metabolic acidosis. *Am J Med* 68:414–418, 1980.
124. Smith SR, Smith SJM, Buckley BM: Combined formate and lactate acidosis in methanol poisoning. *Lancet* 2:1295–1296, 1981.
125. Sejersted OM, Jacobsen D, Ovrebo S, Jansen H: Formate concentrations in plasma from patients poisoned with methanol. *Acta Med Scand* 213:105–110, 1983.

126. Nicholls P: The effect of formate on cytochrome aa₃ and on electron transport in the intact respiratory chain. *Biochim Biophys Acta* 430:13–29, 1976.

127. Anderson TJ, Shuaib A, Becker WJ: Methanol poisoning: factors associated with neurologic complications. *Can J Neurol Sci* 16:432–435, 1989.

128. Suit PF, Estes M: Methanol intoxication: clinical features and differential diagnosis. *Cleve Clin J Med* 57:464–471, 1990.

129. Sharpe JA, Hostovsky M, Bilbao JM, Rewcastle NB: Methanol optic neuropathy: a histopathological study. *Neurology* 32:1093–1100, 1982.

130. Phang PT, Passerini L, Mielke B, Berendt R, King EG: Brain hemorrhage associated with methanol poisoning. *Crit Care Med* 16:137–140, 1988.

131. Steinhart B: Case report: severe ethylene glycol intoxication with normal osmolal gap—"a chilling thought." *J Emerg Med* 8:583–585, 1990.

132. Osterloh JD, Pond SM, Grady S, Becker CE: Serum formate concentrations in methanol intoxication as a criterion for hemodialysis. *Ann Intern Med* 104:200–203, 1986.

133. Hewlett TP, McMartin KE: Ethylene glycol poisoning. The value of glycolic acid determinations for diagnosis and treatment. *Clin Toxicol* 24:389–402, 1986.

134. Underwood F, Bennett WM: Ethylene glycol intoxication: prevention of renal failure by aggressive management. *JAMA* 226:1453–1454, 1973.

135. Peterson DI, Peterson JE, Hardings MG, Wacker WEC: Experimental treatment of ethylene glycol poisoning. *JAMA* 186:955–957, 1963.

136. Peterson CD: Oral ethanol doses in patients with methanol poisoning. *Am J Hosp Pharm* 38:1024–1027, 1981.

137. Baud FJ, Galliot M, Astier A, Vu Bein D, Garnier R, Likorman J, Bismuth C: Treatment of ethylene glycol poisoning with 4-methylpyrazole. *N Engl J Med* 319:97–100, 1988.

138. Baud FJ, Bismuth C, Garnier R, Galloit M, Astier A, Maistre G, Soffner M: 4-methylpyrazole may be an alternative to ethanol therapy for ethylene glycol intoxication in man. *Clin Toxicol* 24:463–483, 1986–1987.

139. Becker CE: Methanol poisoning. *J Emerg Med* 1:51–58, 1983.

140. Vale JA, Prior JG, O'Hare JP, Flanagan RJ, Feehally J: Treatment of ethylene glycol poisoning with peritoneal dialysis. *Br Med J* 284:557, 1982.

141. Keyvan-Larijarni H, Tannenberg AM: Methanol intoxication. Comparison of peritoneal dialysis and hemodialysis treatment. *Arch Intern Med* 134:293–296, 1974.

142. Malmlund HO, Berg A, Karlman G, Magnusson A, Ullman B: Considerations for the treatment of ethylene glycol poisoning based on analysis of two cases. *Clin Toxicol* 29:231–240, 1991.

143. LeGatt DF: Frequent determinations of methanol in serum not needed for monitoring hemodialysis therapy of methanol ingestion. *Clin Chem* 34:1371–1372, 1988.

144. Jacobsen D, Ovrebo S, Sejersted OM: Toxicokinetics of formate during hemodialysis. *Acta Med Scand* 214:409–412, 1983.

145. Noker PE, Eellis JT, Tephly TR: Methanol toxicity: treatment with folic acid and 5-formyl tetrahydrofolic acid. Alcoholism: *Clin Exp Res* 4:378–383, 1980.

146. Anonymous: Carbon monoxide intoxication—a preventable environmental health hazard. *Morbid Mortal Weekly Rep* 31:529–531, 1982.

147. Koumbourlis AC, Skoutakis VA: Carbon monoxide poisoning: diagnosis and treatment. *Clin Toxicol Consult* 4:51–69, 1982.

148. Klassen CD: Nonmetallic environmental toxicants: air pollutants, solvents and vapors, and pesticides. In Gilman AG, Rall TW, Nies AS, Taylor P (eds): *The Pharmacological Basis of Therapeutics*, ed 8. MacMillan, New York, pp 1615–1639, 1990.

149. Winter PM, Miller JN: Carbon monoxide poisoning. *JAMA* 236:1502–1504, 1976.

150. Choi IS: Delayed neurologic sequelae in carbon monoxide intoxication. *Arch Neurol* 40:433–435, 1983.

151. Smith JS, Brandon S: Morbidity from acute carbon monoxide poisoning at three-year follow-up. *Br Med J* 1:318–321, 1973.

152. Myers RA, Linberg SE, Cowley RA: Carbon monoxide poisoning: the injury and its treatment. *JACEP* 8:479–484, 1979.

153. Burney RE, Wu SC, Nemiroff MJ: Mass carbon monoxide poisoning: clinical effects and results of treatment in 184 victims. *Ann Emerg Med* 11:394–399, 1982.

154. Myers RA, Snyder SK, Linberg S, Cowley RA: Value of hyperbaric oxygen in suspected carbon monoxide poisoning. *JAMA* 246:2478–2480, 1981.

155. Raphael JC, Elkharrat D, Jars-Guincestre MC, et al: Trial of normobaric and hyperbaric oxygen for acute carbon monoxide intoxication. *Lancet* ii:414–419, 1989.

156. Van Hoesen KB, Camporesi EM, Moon RE, et al: Should hyperbaric oxygen be used to treat the pregnant patient for acute carbon monoxide poisoning? *JAMA* 261:1039–1043, 1989.

157. Pearigen PD, Benowitz NL: Poisoning due to calcium antagonists. Experience with verapamil, diltiazem and nifedipine. *Drug Safety* 6:408–430, 1991.

158. Beller GA, Smith TW, Abelman WH, Haber E, Hood WB: Digitalis intoxication: a prospective clinical study with serum level concentrations. *N Engl J Med* 284:989–997, 1971.

159. Ekins BR, Watanabe AS: Acute digoxin poisoning: review of therapy. *Am J Hosp Pharm* 34:268–277, 1978.

160. Braunwald E: Mechanism of action of calcium-channel-blocking agents. *N Engl J Med* 307:1618–1627, 1982.

161. Smith TW: Digitalis: mechanisms of action and clinical use. *N Engl J Med* 318:358–365, 1988.

162. Smith TW, Antman EM, Friedman PL, Blatt CM, March JD: Digitalis glycosides: mechanisms and manifestations of toxicity. Part II. *Prog Cardiovasc Dis* 26:495–540, 1984.

163. Agura ED: Massive propranolol overdose: successful treatment with high dose isoproterenol and glucagon. *Am J Med* 80:755–757, 1986.

164. Frishman W, Jacob H: Clinical pharmacology of the new beta-adrenergic blocking drugs. Part 8. Self poisoning with beta-adrenoreceptor blocking agents: recognition and management. *Am Heart J* 98:798–811, 1979.

165. Lewis M, Kallenbach J: Survival following massive overdose of adrenergic blocking agents (acebutolol and labetolol). *Eur Heart J* 4:328–332, 1983.

166. Nicholas F, Villers D: Severe self-poisoning with acebutolol in association with alcohol. *Crit Care Med* 15:173–174, 1987.

167. Khan MI, Miller MT: Beta-blocker toxicity—the role of glucagon. *S Afr Med J* 67:1062–1063, 1985.

168. Weinstein RS: Recognition and management of poisoning with beta-adrenergic blocking agents. *Ann Emerg Med* 13:1123–1131, 1984.

169. Gwinup GR: Propranolol toxicity presenting with early repolarization, ST segment elevation, and peaked T waves on the ECG. *Ann Emerg Med* 17:171–173, 1988.

170. Critchley JAJH, Ungar A: The management of acute poisoning due to beta-adrenoreceptor antagonists. *Med Toxicol* 4:32–45, 1989.

171. Lindvall K, Personne M: High dose prenalterol in beta-blockade intoxication. *Acta Med Scand* 218:525–528, 1985.

172. Artman M, Grayson M: Propranolol in children: safety-toxicity. *Pediatrics* 70:30–31, 1982.

173. Wallen CJ, Hulting J: Massive metoprolol poisoning treated with prenalterol. *Acta Med Scand* 214:254–255, 1983.

174. Anthony T, Jastremski M, Elliott W, Morris G, Prasad H: Charcoal hemoperfusion for the treatment of combined diltiazem and metoprolol overdose. *Ann Emerg Med* 15:1344–1348, 1986.

175. Wei J, Spotnitz HM, Spotnitz WD, et al: Pharmacologic antagonism of propranolol in dogs. *J Thorac Cardiovasc Surg* 87:732–742, 1984.

176. Peterson CD, Leeder JS: Glucagon therapy for beta-blocker overdose. *DICP* 18:394–397, 1984.

177. Alousi AA, Canter JM, Fort DJ: The beneficial effect of amrinone on acute drug-induced heart failure in the anaesthetised dog. *Cardiovasc Res* 19:483–494, 1985.

178. Langemijer J, de Wildt D, de Groot G, Sangster B: Calcium interferes with the cardiodepressive effects of beta-blocker overdose in isolated rat hearts. *Clin Toxicol* 24:111–133, 1986.

179. Brinacoumbe JR, Scully M, Swainston R: Propranolol overdose—a dramatic response to calcium chloride. *Med J Aust* 155:267–268, 1991.

180. Lane AS, Woodward AC, Goldman MR: Massive propranolol overdose poorly responsive to pharmacologic therapy: use of intra-aortic balloon pump. *Ann Emerg Med* 16:1381, 1987.

181. Ramoska EA, Spiller HA, Myers A: Calcium channel blocker toxicity. *Ann Emerg Med* 19:649–653, 1990.

182. Horowitz BZ, Rhee KJ: Massive verapamil ingestion: a report of two cases and a review of the literature. *Am J Emerg Med* 7:624–631, 1989.

183. Schoffstall JM, Spivey WH, Gambone L, Shaw RP, Sit SP: Effects of calcium channel blocker overdose-induced toxicity in the conscious dog. *Ann Emerg Med* 20:1104–1108, 1991.

184. Erickson FC, Ling LJ, Grande GA, Anderson DL: Diltiazem overdose: case report and review of literature. *J Emerg Med* 9:357–366, 1991.

185. Wells TG, Graham CJ, Moss MM, Kearns GL: Nifedipine poisoning in a child. *Pediatrics* 86:91–94, 1990.

186. Hariman RJ, Mangiardi LM, McAllister RG, Surawicz B, Shabetai R, Kishida H: Reversal of the cardiovascular effects of verapamil by calcium and sodium: differences between electrophysiologic and hemodynamic responses. *Circulation* 59:797–804, 1979.

187. Gay R, Alego S, Lee R, Olajos M, Morkin E, Goldman S: Treatment of verapamil toxicity in intact dogs. *J Clin Invest* 77:1805–1811, 1986.

188. Strubelt O: Antidotal treatment of the acute cardiovascular toxicity of verapamil. *Acta Pharmacol Toxicol* 55:231–237, 1984.

189. Strubelt O, Diedrich KW: Experimental investigations on the antidotal treatment of nifedipine overdosage. *Clin Toxicol* 24:135–149, 1986.

190. Goenen M, Col J, Compere A, Bonte J: Treatment of severe verapamil poisoning with combined amrinone-isoproterenol therapy. *Am J Cardiol* 58:1142–1143, 1986.

191. Zaritsky AL, Horowitz M, Chernow B: Glucagon antagonism of calcium channel blocker-induced myocardial dysfunction. *Crit Care Med* 16:246–251, 1988.

192. Jolly SR, Kipnis JN, Lucchesi BR: Cardiovascular depression by verapamil: reversal by glucagon and interactions with propranolol. *Pharmacology* 35:249–255, 1987.

193. Hendren WG, Schieber RS, Garrettson LK: Extracorporeal bypass for the treatment of verapamil poisoning. *Ann Emerg Med* 18:984–987, 1989.

194. Roberts D, Honcharik N, Sitar DS, Tenenbein M: Diltiazem overdose: pharmacokinetics of diltiazem and its metabolites and effect of multiple dose activated charcoal. *Clin Toxicol* 29:45–52, 1991.

195. Hoffman BF, Bigger JT: Digitalis glycosides and allied cardiac glycosides. In Gilman AG, Rall TW, Nies AS, Taylor P (eds): *The Pharmacological Basis of Therapeutics*, ed 8. MacMillan, New York, pp 814–839, 1990.

196. Smith TW, Antman EM, Friedman PL, Blatt CM, March JD: Digitalis glycosides: mechanisms and manifestations of toxicity. Part III. *Prog Cardiovasc Dis* 27:21–56, 1984.

197. Woolfe AD, Wenger TL, Smith TW, Lovejoy FH: Results of multicenter studies of digoxin-specific antibody fragments in managing digitalis intoxication in the pediatric population. *Am J Emerg Med* 9(Suppl 1):16–20, 1991.

198. Antman EM, Wenger TL, Butler VP, et al: Treatment of 150 cases of life-threatening digitalis intoxication with digoxin-specific Fab antibody fragments. *Circulation* 81:1744–1752, 1990.

199. Lake KD, Brown DC, Peterson CD: Digoxin toxicity: enhanced systemic elimination during oral activated charcoal therapy. *Pharmacotherapy* 4:161–163, 1984.

200. Slattery JT, Koup JP: Haemoperfusion in the management of digoxin toxicity: Is it warranted? *Clin Pharmacokinet* 4:395–399, 1979.

201. Reisdorf EJ, Clark MR, Walters BL: Acute digitalis poisoning: the role of intravenous magnesium sulfate. *J Emerg Med* 4:463–469, 1986.

202. Allen NM, Dunham GD, Sailstad JM, Findlay JWA: Clinical and pharmacokinetic profiles of digoxin immune Fab in four patients with renal insufficiency. *DICP* 25:1315–1319, 1991.

203. Ujhelyi MR, Robert S, Cummings M, et al: Disposition of free and total digoxin post digoxin Fab therapy in hemodialysis and acute renal failure patients (abstr). *Crit Care Med* 20(suppl):S108, 1992.

204. Bayer MJ: Recognition and management of digitalis intoxication: implications for emergency medicine. *Am J Emerg Med* 9(Suppl 1):29–32, 1991.

205. Marchlincki FE, Hook BG, Callans DJ: Which cardiac disturbances should be treated with digoxin immune Fab (ovine) antibody? *Am J Emerg Med* 9(Suppl 1):24–28, 1991.

206. Hickey AR, Wenger TL, Carpenter VP, et al: Digoxin immune Fab therapy in the management of digitalis intoxication; safety and efficacy results of an observational surveillance study. *J Am Coll Cardiol* 17:590–598, 1991.

207. Borys D, Setzer S, Ling LJ, Reisdorf JJ, Day LC, Krenzelok EP: Acute fluoxetine overdose: a report of 234 cases. *Am J Emerg Med* 10:115–123, 1991.

208. Ellison DW, Pentel PR: Clinical features and consequences of seizures due to cyclic antidepressant overdose. *Am J Emerg Med* 7:5–10, 1989.

209. Pentel PR, Benowitz NL: Tricylic antidepressant poisoning: management of arrhythmias. *Med Toxicol* 1:101–121, 1986.

210. Frommer DA, Fulig KW, Marx JA, Rumack BH: Tricyclic antidepressant overdose: a review. *JAMA* 257:521–526, 1987.

211. Vernon DD, Banner W, Garrett JS, Dean JM: Efficacy of dopamine and norepinephrine for treatment of hemodynamic compromise in amitriptyline intoxication. *Crit Care Med* 19:544–549, 1991.

212. Kincaid RL, McMullin MM, Crookham SB, et al: Report of a fluoxetine fatality. *J Anal Toxicol* 14:327–329, 1990.

213. Hayes PE, Dristoff CA: Adverse reactions to five new antidepressants. *Clin Pharm* 5:471–480, 1986.

214. Curry SC: Hydrogen cyanide and inorganic cyanide salts. In Sullivan JB, Keiger GR (eds): *Hazardous Materials Toxicology: Clinical Principles of Environmental Health*. Baltimore, Williams & Wilkins, pp 698–710, 1992.

215. Geller RJ, Ekins BR, Iknoian RC: Cyanide toxicity from acetonitrile-containing false nail remover. *Am J Emerg Med* 9:268–270, 1991.

216. Schmidt ES, Newton GW, Sanders SM, Lewis JP, Conn EE: Laetrile toxicity studies in dogs. *JAMA* 239:943–947, 1978.

217. Bennett DR (ed): AMA Drug Evaluations Annual 1992. American Medical Association, Chicago, pp 553, 1991.

218. Rindone JP, Sloane EP: Cyanide toxicity from sodium nitroprusside: risks and management. *Ann Pharmacother* 26:515–519, 1992.

219. Hall AH, Rumack B: Clinical toxicology of cyanide. *Ann Emerg Med* 15:1067–1074, 1986.

220. Graham DL, Laman D, Theodore J, et al: Acute cyanide poisoning complicated by lactic acidosis and pulmonary edema. *Arch Intern Med* 137:1051–1055, 1977.

221. Johnson RP, Mellors JW: Arteriolarization of venous blood gases: a clue to the diagnosis of cyanide poisoning. *J Emerg Med* 6:401–404, 1988.

222. Patel CB, Laboy V, Venus B, et al: Use of sodium nitroprusside in post-coronary bypass surgery. A plea for conservatism. *Chest* 89:663–667, 1986.

223. DeBush RF, Seidi LG: Attempted suicide by cyanide. *Calif Med* 110:394–396, 1969.

224. Gonzales ER: Cyanide evades some noses, overpowers others. *JAMA* 248:2211, 1982.

225. Chen KK, Rose CL: Nitrate and thiosulfate therapy in cyanide poisoning. *JAMA* 149:113–119, 1952.

226. Brivet F, Delfraissy JF, Duche M, et al: Acute cyanide poisoning: recovery with non-specific supportive therapy. *Intensive Care Med* 9:33–35, 1983.

227. Sylvester DM, Hayton WI, Morgan RL, Way JL: Effects of thiosulfate on cyanide pharmacokinetics in dogs. *Toxicol Appl Pharmacol* 69:265–271, 1983.

228. Chen KK, Rose RL, Clowes GHA: Methylene blue (methylthionine chloride), nitrites and sodium nitrosulphate against cyanide poisoning. *Proc Soc Exp Biol Med* 31:250–251, 1933.

229. Kiese M, Weger N: Formation of ferrihaemoglobin with aminophenols in the human for the treatment of cyanide poisoning. *European J Pharmacol* 7:97–105, 1969.

230. Hall AH, Doutre WH, Ludden T, Kulig KW, Rumack BH: Nitrate/thiosulfate treated acute cyanide poisoning: estimated kinetics after antidote. *J Toxicol Clin Toxicol* 25:121–133, 1987.

231. Reynolds JEF (ed): Sodium nitrite treatment. In *Martindale: The Extra Pharmacopoeia*, ed 28. The Pharmaceutical Press, London, p 392, 1982.

232. Schulz V, Bonn R, Kindler J: Kinetics of elimination of thiocyanate in 7 healthy subjects and in 8 subjects with renal failure. *Klin Wochenschr* 57:243–247, 1979.

233. Berlin CM: The treatment of cyanide poisoning in children. *Pediatrics* 46:793–796, 1970.

234. Vogel SN, Sultan TR, Ten Eyck RP: Cyanide poisoning. *Clin Toxicol* 18:367–383, 1981.

235. Vick JA, Froehlich H: Treatment of cyanide poisoning. *Milit Med* 156:330–339, 1991.

236. Isom GE, Way JL: Effect of O_2 on cyanide intoxication: reactivation of cyanide-inhibited glucose metabolism. *J Pharmacol Exp Ther* 189:235, 1974.

237. Way JL, Sylvester D, Morgan RL, et al: Recent perspectives on toxicodynamic basis of cyanide antagonism. *Fund Appl Toxicol* 4:S231–S239, 1984.

238. Way JL, End E, Sheehy MH, et al: Effect of oxygen on cyanide intoxication. IV. Hyperbaric oxygen. *Toxicol Appl Pharmacol* 22:415–421, 1972.

239. Litovitz TL, Larkin RF, Myers RAM: Cyanide poisoning treated with hyperbaric oxygen. *Am J Emerg Med* 1:94, 1983.

240. Lambert RJ, Kindler BL, Schaeffer DJ: The efficacy of superactivated charcoal in treating rats exposed to a lethal oral dose of potassium cyanide. *Ann Emerg Med* 17:595–598, 1988.

241. Wesson DE, Foley R, Sabatini S, Wharton J, Kapusnik J, Kurtzman NA: Treatment of acute cyanide intoxication with hemodialysis. *Am J Nephrol* 5:121–126, 1985.

242. Marbury TC, Sheppard JE, Gibbons K, et al: Combined antidotal and hemodialysis treatment for nitroprusside-induced cyanide toxicity. *Clin Toxicol* 19:475–482, 1982.

243. Hillman B, Bardhan KD, Bain JTB: The use of dicobalt edetate (Kelocyanor) in cyanide poisoning. *Postgrad Med J* 50:171–174, 1974.

244. Cottrell JE, Casthely P, Brodie JD, Patel K, Klein A, Turndorf H: Prevention of nitroprusside-induced cyanide toxicity with hydroxocobalamin. *N Engl J Med* 298:809, 1978.

245. Hall AH, Rumack BH: Hydroxocobalamin/sodium thiosulfate as a cyanide antidote. *J Emerg Med* 5:115–121, 1987.

246. Whitten CF, Brough AJ: The pathophysiology of acute iron poisoning. *Clin Toxicol* 4:585–595, 1971.

247. Robotham JL, Lietnams PS: Acute iron poisoning in children. *Am J Dis Child* 134:875–879, 1980.

248. Jacobs J, Greene H, Gendel BR: Acute iron intoxication. *N Engl J Med* 273:1124–1127, 1965.

249. Banner W, Tong TG: Iron poisoning. *Pediatr Clin North Am* 33:393–409, 1986.

250. Gleason WA Jr, deMello DE, deCastro FJ, et al: Acute hepatic failure in severe iron poisoning. *J Pediatr* 95:138–140, 1979.

251. Tenenbein M, Israels SJ: Early coagulopathy in severe iron poisoning. *J Pediatr* 113:695–697, 1988.

252. Melby K, Slordahl S, Gutteberg TJ, Nordbo SA: Septicaemia due to *Yersinia enterocolitica* after oral overdose of iron. *Br Med J* 285:467–468, 1982.

253. Greengard J: Iron poisoning in children. *Clin Toxicol* 8:575–577, 1975.

254. Whitten CF, Gibson GW, Good MH, et al: Studies in acute iron poisoning. I. Desferrioxamine in the treatment of acute iron poisoning: clinical observations, experimental studies, and theoretical considerations. *Pediatrics* 36:322–335, 1965.

255. Whitten CF, Chen YC, Gibson GW: Studies in acute iron poisoning. II. Further observations of desferrioxamine in the treatment of acute experimental iron poisoning. *Pediatrics* 38:102–110, 1966.

256. Westlin WF: Desferrioxamine in the treatment of acute iron poisoning: clinical experience with 172 children. *Clin Pediatr* 5:531–535, 1966.

257. Eisen TF, Lacouture PG, Woolf A: Visual detection of ferrioxamine color changes in urine. *Vet Hum Toxicol* 30:369–370, 1988.

258. Proudfoot AT, Simpson D, Dyson EH: Management of acute iron poisoning. *Med Toxicol* 1:83–100, 1986.

259. Proper R, Nathan D: Clinical removal of iron. *Annu Rev Med* 33:509–519, 1982.

260. Peck M, Rogers J, Riverbach J: Use of high doses of deferoxamine (Desferal) in an adult patient with acute iron overdosage. *J Toxicol Clin Toxicol* 19:865–869, 1982.

261. Proper R, Shurn S, Nathan D: Reassessment of the use of desferrioxamine B in iron overload. *N Engl J Med* 294:1421–1423, 1976.

262. Banner W, Czajka PA: Iron poisoning (letter). *Am J Dis Child* 135:484–485, 1981.

263. McElhatton PR, Roberts JC, Sullivan FM: The consequences of iron overdose and its treatment with desferrioxamine in pregnancy. *Hum Exp Toxicol* 4:251–259, 1991.

264. Movassaghi N, Purugganan GG, Leikin S: Comparison of exchange transfusion and deferoxamine in the treatment of acute iron poisoning. *J Pediatr* 604–608, 1969.

265. Weiss LG, Danielson BG, Fellstroem B, Wikstroem B: Aluminum removal of hemodialysis, hemofiltration and charcoal hemoperfusion in uremic patients after desferrioxamine infusion. A comparison of efficiency. *Nephron* 3:325–329, 1989.

266. Banner W, Vernon DD, Ward RM, et al: Continuous arteriovenous hemofiltration in experimental iron intoxication. *Crit Care Med* 17:1187–1190, 1989.

267. Miller KB, Rosenwasser LJ, Bessett JM, et al: Rapid desensitization for deferoxamine anaphylactic reaction. *Lancet* 1:1059, 1981.

268. Bentur Y, St. Louis P, Klein J, Koren G: Misinterpretation of iron-binding capacity in the presence of deferoxamine. *J Pediatr* 118:139–142, 1991.

269. Burkhart KK, Kulig KW, Hammond B, Pearson JR, Ambruso D, Rumack B: The rise in the total iron-binding capacity after iron overload. *Ann Emerg Med* 20:532–535, 1991.

270. Tenenbein M, Yatsoff RW: The total iron-binding capacity in iron poisoning: Is it useful? *Am J Dis Child* 145:437–439, 1991.

271. Heffer RE, Rodgerson DO: The effect of deferoxamine on the determination of serum iron and iron-binding capacity. *J Pediatr* 68:804–806, 1966.

272. Czajka PA, Konrad JD, Duffy JP: Iron poisoning: an in vitro comparison of bicarbonate and phosphate lavage solutions. *J Pediatr* 98:491–494, 1981.

273. Venturelli J, Kwee Y, Cameron G: Gastrotomy in the management of acute iron poisoning. *J Pediatr* 100:787–789, 1982.

274. Bryson P: Narcotics. In *Comprehensive Review in Toxicology*, ed 2. Rockville, MD, ASPEN, pp 323–338, 1989.

275. Ellenhorn MJ, Barceloux DG: Opiates, opioids, and designer drugs. In *Medical Toxicology*. Elsevier, New York, pp 687–762, 1988.

276. Anonymous: Drugs used in the management of poisoning. In Bennett DR (ed): *Drug Evaluations Annual 1992*. American Medical Association, Chicago, pp 62–63, 1991.

277. Synder D: Opiate receptors in the brain. *N Engl J Med* 296:266–271, 1977.

278. Krantz T, Thised B, Strom J, et al: Severe acute propoxyphene overdose treated with dopamine. *Clin Toxicol* 23:347–352, 1985.

279. McCarron MM, Challoner KR, Thompson GA: Diphenoxylate-atropine (Lomotil) overdose in children: an update. *Pediatrics* 87:694–700, 1991.

280. Schneider SA, Michelson EA, Boucek CD, Ilkanipour K: Dextromethorphan poisoning reversed by naloxone. *Am J Emerg Med* 9:237–238, 1991.

281. Freitas PM: Narcotic withdrawal in the emergency department. *Am J Emerg Med* 3:456–460, 1985.

282. Silverman SH, Turner WW Jr: Intraarterial drug abuse: new treatment options. *J Vasc Surg* 14:111–116, 1991.

283. Stewart A, Heaton ND, Hogbin B: Body packing—a case report and review of the literature. *Postgraduate Med J* 66:659–661, 1990.

284. Handal K, Schauben J, Salamone F: Naloxone. *Ann Emerg Med* 12:438–445, 1983.

285. Martin W: Clinical evidence for different narcotic receptors and relevance for the clinician. *Ann Emerg Med* 15:1026–1029, 1986.

286. Martin W: Naloxone. *Ann Intern Med* 85:765–768, 1976.

287. Goldfrank L, Weisman R, Errick J, Lo M-W: A dosing nomogram for continuous infusion of intravenous naloxone. *Ann Emerg Med* 15:566–570, 1986.

288. Nimmo WS, Heading RC, Prescott LF: Reversal of narcotic-induced delay in gastric emptying and paracetamol absorption by naloxone. *Br Med J* 10:1189, 1979.

289. Moore RA, Rumack B, Conner S, Peterson RG: Underdosage after narcotic poisoning. *Am J Dis Child* 134:156–158, 1980.

290. Barsan WG, Seger D, Danzl D, et al: Duration of antagonistic effects of nalmefene and naloxone in opiate-induced sedation for emergency department procedures. *Am J Emerg Med* 7:155, 1989.

291. Berkowitz B: The relationship of pharmacokinetics to pharmacological activity: morphine, methadone and naloxone. *Clin Pharmacol* 219–230, 1976.

292. Goldfrank L, Weisman R, Errick J, Lo M-W: A dosing nomogram for continuous infusion of intravenous naloxone. *Ann Emerg Med* 15:566–570, 1986.

293. Maio R, Gaukel B, Freeman B: Intralingual naloxone injection for narcotic-induced respiratory depression. *Ann Emerg Med* 16:572–573, 1987.

294. Tandberg D, Abercrombie D: Treatment of heroin overdose with endotracheal naloxone. *Ann Emerg Med* 11:443–445, 1982.

295. Moreland TA, Brice JEH, Walker CHM, et al: Naloxone pharmacokinetics in the newborn. *Br J Clin Pharmacol* 9:609–612, 1980.

296. Stile IL, Fort M, Wurzburger RJ, et al: Pharmacokinetics of naloxone in the premature newborn. *Dev Pharmacol Ther* 10:454–459, 1987.

297. Schwartz J, Koenigberrg M: Naloxone-induced pulmonary edema. *Ann Emerg Med* 16:1294–1296, 1987.

298. Flacke JW, Flacke WE, Williams GD: Acute pulmonary edema following naloxone reversal of high-dose morphine anesthesia. *Anesthesiology* 47:376–378, 1977.

299. Prough DS, Roy R, Bumgarner J: Acute pulmonary edema in healthy teenagers following conservative doses of intravenous naloxone. *Anesthesiology* 485–486, 1984.

300. Tanaka G: Hypertensive reaction to naloxone. *JAMA* 228:25–26, 1974.

301. Michaelis L, Hickey P, Clark T, et al: Ventricular irritability associated with the use of naloxone hydrochloride. *Ann Thorac Surg* 18:608–614, 1974.

302. Andree R: Sudden death following naloxone administration. *Anaesth Analg* 59:782–784, 1980.

303. Cuss FM, Colaco CB, Baron JH: Cardiac arrest after reversal of effects of opiates with naloxone. *Br Med J* 288:363–364, 1984.

304. Cohen MR, Cohen RM, Pickar D, et al: Behavioral effects after high dose naloxone administration to normal volunteers. *Lancet* ii:1110, 1981.

305. Gaddis GM, Watson WA: Naloxone-associated patient violence: an overlooked toxicity? *Ann Pharmacother* 26:196–198, 1992.

306. Mattila M, Neotto E, Seppala T: Naloxone is not an effective antagonist of ethanol. *Lancet* i:1775–1776, 1981.

307. Banner W, Lund ME, Clawson L: Failure of naloxone to reverse clonidine toxic effect. *Am J Dis Child* 137:1170–1171, 1983.

308. Bell E: The use of naloxone in the treatment of diazepam poisoning. *J Pediatr* 87:803–804, 1975.

309. Hoffman JR, Schriger DL, Luo JS: The empiric use of naloxone in patients with altered mental status: a reappraisal. *Ann Emerg Med* 20:246–252, 1991.

310. Tafuri J, Roberts J: Organophosphate poisoning. *Ann Emerg Med* 16:193–202, 1987.

311. Barret DS, Oehme F: A review of organophosphorus ester induced delayed neurotoxicity. *Vet Hum Toxicol* 27:22–37, 1985.

312. Johnson MK: Organophosphate neuropathy: progress in understanding. In Manzo L, Levy N, Lacasse Y, Roche L (eds): *Advances in Neurotoxicology*. Pergamon Press, New York, pp 223–235, 1980.

313. Sultatos LG, Murphy SD: Kinetic analyses of the microsomal biotransformation of the phosphorothioate insecticides chlorpyrifos and parathion. *Fund Appl Toxicol* 3:16–21, 1983.

314. Morgan JP: Jamaica ginger paralysis. *JAMA* 248:1864–1867, 1982.

315. Morgan JP, Penovich P: Jamaica ginger paralysis: a forty-seven year follow-up. *Arch Neurol* 35:530–532, 1978.

316. Bidstrup PL, Bonnell JA, Beckett AG: Paralysis following poisoning by a new organic phosphorus insecticide (mipafox): report on two cases. *Br Med J* 1:1068–1072, 1953.

317. Hierons R, Johnson MK: Clinical and toxicological investigations of a case of delayed neuropathy in man after acute poisoning by an organophosphorus insecticide. *Arch Toxicol* 40:279–284, 1978.

318. Jedrzejowska H, Rowinska-Marcinska K, Hoppe B: Neuropathy due to phytosol (Agritox). *Acta Neuropathol* 49:163–168, 1980.

319. Senanayake N, Karalliedde L: Neurotoxic effects of organophosphorous insecticides. *N Engl J Med* 316:761–763, 1987.

320. Savage EP, Keefe TJ, Mounce LM, Heaton RK, Lewis JA, Burcar PJ: Chronic neurological sequelae of acute organophosphate pesticide poisoning. *Arch Environ Health* 43:38–45, 1988.

321. Gallo MA, Lawryk NJ: Organic phosphorus pesticides. In Hayes WJ, Laws ER (eds): *Handbook of Pesticide Toxicology*, vol 2. *Classes of Pesticides*. Academic Press, San Diego, pp 917–1123, 1991.

322. Eliason DA, Cranmer MF, von Windeguth DL, et al: Dursban premises applications and their effect on the cholinesterase levels in spraymen. *Mosquito News* 9:591–595, 1969.

323. LeBlanc FN, Benson BE, Gilg AD: A severe organophosphate poisoning requiring the use of an atropine drip. *Clin Toxicol* 24:69–76, 1986.

324. Thompson DF, Thompson GD, Greenwood RB, Trammel HL: Therapeutic dosing of pralidoxime chloride. *Drug Intell Clin Pharm* 21:590–593, 1987.

325. De Silva HJ, Wijewickrema R, Senanayake N: Does pralidoxime affect outcome of management in acute organophosphorus poisoning? *Lancet* 339:1136–1138, 1992.

326. Smith M: The metabolic basis of the major symptoms in acute salicylate intoxication. *Clin Toxicol* 1:387–392, 1968.

327. Temple A: Pathophysiology of aspirin overdosage toxicity, with implications for management. *Pediatrics* 62(suppl):873–876, 1978.

328. Temple A: Acute and chronic effects of aspirin toxicity and their treatment. *Arch Intern Med* 141:364–369, 1981.

329. Hefner J, Sahn S: Salicylate-induced pulmonary edema: clinical features and prognosis. *Ann Intern Med* 95:405–409, 1981.

330. Chapman BJ, Proudfoot AT: Adult salicylate poisoning: deaths and outcome in patients with high plasma salicylate concentrations. *Q J Med* 72:699–707, 1989.

331. Leatherman JW, Schmitz PG: Fever, hyperdynamic shock, and multiple-system organ failure. A pseudo-sepsis syndrome associated with chronic salicylate intoxication. *Chest* 100:1391–1396, 1991.

332. Gaudreault P, Temple AR, Lovejoy FH: The relative severity of acute versus chronic salicylate poisoning in children: a clinical comparison. *Pediatrics* 70(4):566–569, 1982.

333. Thurston J, Pollack P, Warren S, et al: Reduced brain glucose with normal plasma glucose in salicylate poisoning. *J Clin Invest* 49:2139–2142, 1970.

334. Reed J, Palmisano P: Central nervous system salicylate. *Clin Toxicol* 8:623–631, 1975.

335. Levy G, Sumner JY: Relationship between dose and apparent volume of distribution of salicylate in children. *Pediatrics* 54:713, 1974.

336. Levy G, Tsuchiya T: Salicylate accumulation kinetics in man. *N Engl J Med* 287:430–432, 1972.

337. Matthew H, Mackintosh TF, Tompsett SL, Cameron JS: Gastric aspiration and lavage in acute poisoning. *Br Med J* 5499:1333–1337, 1966.

338. Jacobsen D, Wiik-Larsen E, Bredesen JE: Haemodialysis or haemoperfusion in severe salicylate poisoning. *Hum Toxicol* 7:161–163, 1988.

339. Kallen RJ, Zaltman S, Coe FL, et al: Hemodialysis in children: technique, kinetic aspects related to varying body size, and application to salicylate intoxication, acute renal failure and some other disorders. *Medicine* 45:2–37, 1966.

340. Etteldorf JN, Dobbins WT, Summitt RL, et al: Intermittent peritoneal dialysis using 5 per cent albumin in the treatment of salicylate intoxication in children. *J Pediatr* 58:226–236, 1961.

341. Summitt RL, Etteldorf JN: Salicylate intoxication in children—experience with peritoneal dialysis and alkalinization of the urine. *J Pediatr* 64:803–814, 1964.

342. Cumming G, Dukes D, Widdowson G: Alkaline diuresis in treatment of aspirin poisoning. *Br Med J* 4:1033–1036, 1964.

343. Lawson A, Proudfoot A, Brown S, et al: Forced diuresis in the treatment of acute salicylate poisoning in adults. *Q J Med* 38:31–48, 1969.

344. Prescott L, Balali-Moody M, Critchley J, et al: Diuresis or urinary alkalinization for salicylate poisoning? *Br Med J* 285:1383–1386, 1982.

345. Prowse K, Pain M, Marston A, et al: The treatment of salicylate poisoning using mannitol and forced alkaline diuresis. *Clin Sci* 38:327–337, 1970.

346. Done AK: Salicylate intoxication: significance of measurement of salicylate in blood in cases of acute ingestion. *Pediatrics* 26:800–807, 1960.

347. Elenbaas R: Critical review of forced alkaline diuresis in acute salicylism. *Crit Care Q* 4:89–95, 1982.

348. Dugandzic RM, Tierney MG, Dickinson GE, et al: Evaluation of the validity of the Done Nomogram in the management of acute salicylate intoxication. *Ann Emerg Med* 18:1186–1190, 1989.

349. Berman LB, Jeghers HJ, Schreiner GE, Pallotta AJ: Hemodialysis: an effective therapy for acute barbiturate poisoning. *JAMA* 161:820, 1956.

350. Gaudreault P, Guay J, Thivierge RL, Verdy I: Benzodiazepine poisoning: clinical and pharmacological considerations and treatment. *Drug Safety* 6:247–265, 1991.

351. Litovitz TL, Schmitz BF, Bailey KM: 1989 Annual Report of the American Association of Poison Control Centers National Data Collection Program. *Am J Emerg Med* 8:394–442, 1990.

352. Forrest ARW, Marsh I, Bradshaw C, et al: Fatal temazepam overdoses. *Lancet* ii:226, 1986.

353. Olson DR, Yin L, Osterloh J, et al: Coma caused by trivial triazolam overdose. *Am J Emerg Med* 3:210–211, 1985.

354. Mazicon (flumazenil): Product Information. Roche Laboratories, Nutley, NJ, 1991.

355. Gawin FH, Ellinwood Jr EH: Cocaine and other stimulants: actions, abuse, and treatment. *N Engl J Med* 318:1173–1182, 1988.

356. Bryson PD: Stimulants. In *Comprehensive Review in Toxicology*, ed 2. Aspen, Rockville, MD, pp 361–379, 1989.

357. Cregler LL, Mark H: Medical complications of cocaine abuse. *N Engl J Med* 315:1495–1500, 1986.

358. VanDette JM, Cornish LA: Medical consequences of illicit cocaine use. *Clin Pharm* 8:401–411, 1989.

359. Levine SR, Brust JC, Futrell N, Brass LM, Blake D, Fayad P, et al: A comparative study of the cerebrovascular complications of cocaine: alkaloid versus hydrochloride—a review. *Neurology* 41:1173–1177, 1991.

360. Shannon M: Clinical toxicity of cocaine adulterants. *Ann Emerg Med* 17:1243–1247, 1988.

361. Isner JM, Estes III NA, Thompson PD, et al: Acute cardiac events temporally related to cocaine abuse. *N Engl J Med* 315:1438–1443, 1986.

362. Goldfrank LR, Hoffman RS: The cardiovascular effects of cocaine. *Ann Emerg Med* 20:165–175, 1991.

363. Gitter MJ, Goldsmith SR, Dunbar DN, Sharkey SW: Cocaine and chest pain: clinical features and outcome of patients hospitalized to rule out myocardial infarction. *Ann Intern Med* 115:277–282, 1991.

364. Levine SR, Brust JC, Futrell N, et al: Cerebrovascular complications of the use of the "crack" form of alkaloidal cocaine. *N Engl J Med* 323:699–704, 1990.

365. Barth III CW, Bray M, Roberts WC: Rupture of the ascending aorta during cocaine intoxication. *Am J Cardiol* 57:496, 1986.

366. Shesser R, David C, Edelstein S: Pneumomediastinum and pneumothorax after inhaling alkaloidal cocaine. *Ann Emerg Med* 10:213–215, 1981.

367. Forrester JM, Steele AW, Waldron JA, Parsons SE: Crack lung: an acute pulmonary syndrome with a spectrum of clinical and histopathological findings. *Am Res Respir Dis* 142:462–467, 1990.

368. Hall WC, Talbert RL, Ereshefsky L: Cocaine abuse and its treatment. *Pharmacotherapy* 10:47–65, 1990.

369. Hoffman RS, Henry GC, Howland MA, Weisman RS, Weil L, Goldfrank LR: Association between life-threatening cocaine toxicity and plasma cholinesterase activity. *Ann Emerg Med* 21:247–253, 1992.

370. Ramoska E, Sacchetti AD: Propranolol-induced hypertension in the treatment of cocaine intoxication. *Ann Emerg Med* 14:1112–1113, 1985.

371. Gay GR, Loper KA: The use of labetalol in the management of cocaine crisis. *Ann Emerg Med* 17:282–283, 1988.

372. Caruna DS, Weinbach B, Goerg D, et al: Cocaine-packet ingestion: diagnosis, management, and natural history. *Ann Intern Med* 100:73–74, 1984.

373. McCarron M, Wood J: The cocaine "body packer" syndrome: diagnosis and treatment. *JAMA* 250:1417–1420, 1983.

374. Goodman S, Becker D: Intracranial hemorrhage associated with amphetamine abuse. *JAMA* 212:480–482, 1970.

375. Ginsberg M, Hartzman M, Schmidt-Nowara W: Amphetamine intoxication with coagulopathy, hyperthermia and reversible renal failure. *Ann Intern Med* 73:81–85, 1970.

376. Pentel P: Toxicity of over-the-counter stimulants. *JAMA* 252:1898–1903, 1984.

377. Dowling GP, McDonough ET, Bost RO: "Eve" and "Ecstasy": a report of five deaths associated with the use of MDEA and MDMA. *JAMA* 257:1615–1617, 1987.

378. Hong R, Matsuyama E, Nur K: Cardiomyopathy associated with the smoking of crystal methamphetamine. *JAMA* 265:1152–1154, 1991.

379. Nestor TA, Tamamoto WI, Kan TH, Schultz T: Acute pulmonary oedema caused by crystalline methamphetamine (letter). *Lancet* ii:1277–1278, 1989.

380. Coupe M: Self poisoning with sustained-release aminophylline: a mechanism for observed secondary rise in serum theophylline. *Hum Toxicol* 5:341–342, 1986.

381. Olson KR, Benowitz NL, Woo OF, Pond SM: Theophylline overdose: acute single ingestion versus chronic repeated overmedication. *Am J Emerg Med* 3:386–394, 1985.

382. Kearney TE, Manoguerra AS, Curtis GP, Ziegler MG: Theophylline toxicity and the beta adrenergic system. *Ann Intern Med* 102:766–769, 1985.

383. Blake KV, Massey KL: Relative efficacy of phenytoin and phenobarbital for the prevention of theophylline-induced seizures in mice. *Ann Emerg Med* 17:1024–1028, 1988.

384. Gaar GG, Banner W: The effects of esmolol on the hemodynamics of acute theophylline toxicity. *Ann Emerg Med* 16:1334–1339, 1987.

385. Gal P, Miller A: Oral activated charcoal to enhance theophylline elimination in an acute overdose. *JAMA* 251:3130–3131, 1984.

386. Woo OF, Pond SM, Benowitz NL, Olson KR: Benefit of hemoperfusion in acute theophylline intoxication. *Clin Toxicol* 22:411–424, 1984.

CHAPTER 60

Parenteral Nutrition

JOHN P. GRANT, M.D.
LAURENCE H. ROSS, M.D.

In normal health the adult human being is in a state of nitrogen equilibrium where daily dietary nitrogen intake equals nitrogen loss. When dietary intake is limited or interrupted, the human adapts by reducing physical activity and lowering core body temperature, with a reduction in metabolic rate. The term "basal metabolic rate" (BMR) describes the minimal energy expenditure of a trained subject at rest after an overnight fast. In chronic uncomplicated starvation, the body can reduce energy expenditure by up to 5 to 10% below the BMR. If starvation is complicated by stress or sepsis, however, energy expenditure markedly increases and may approach 200% BMR. When dietary intake does not meet energy requirements, the human resorts to catabolism of body mass to generate energy. Proteins are broken down for gluconeogenesis, and lipids are mobilized for lipid oxidation. This catabolic state is not without consequences and cannot be sustained indefinitely. The fat mass is relatively expendable. However, there are no known protein reserves; each protein molecule serves some biologic function. During acute and chronic starvation, protein used for gluconeogenesis is derived from all parts of the body, with preservation only, perhaps, of the brain. Seven-day fasting in rats produces a 30% body weight loss with 30 to 40% decrease in the protein content of the liver, kidney, lung, intestine, and heart (3, 100). Similar data have been reported in humans (123). Associated with the loss of organ mass and protein content is an impairment of organ function (77). Skeletal muscle function is decreased in chronic starvation, as demonstrated by the Minnesota Experiment in 1950 (114). Acute starvation in hospitalized patients

also decreases muscle function, independent of measured muscle mass (135). Respiratory muscle function is also impaired in chronic malnutrition, as measured by pulmonary function tests (115). Acute starvation decreases maximal inspiratory vacuum and maximal expiratory pressures in hospitalized patients (11, 151). Doekel et al (55) demonstrated that short periods of semistarvation in normal volunteers impaired the ventilatory response to hypoxia. Likewise, Weissman et al (222) demonstrated loss of chemoreceptor sensitivity to hypercarbic gas mixtures following short periods of protein-free diets in normal volunteers. Catabolism of the gastrointestinal tract leads to loss of villous height and absorptive surface with depletion of brush border enzymes and subsequent malabsorption (141). Decreased gastric acid secretion with starvation can lead to bacterial overgrowth of the upper gastrointestinal tract, contributing to diarrhea (75). Finally, delayed gastric emptying and small bowel hypermotility also occurs further aggravating diarrhea. Hepatic function is markedly altered with undernutrition. The microsomal enzyme system is severely depressed, as are protein synthetic pathways (124, 183). On the other hand, some enzyme systems, including the gluconeogenic series, increase in activity with progressive starvation. Changes in renal function during starvation include loss of concentrating ability, with progressive diuresis in the face of dehydration, and impaired ability to excrete titrable acid, leading to metabolic acidosis (119, 120). In children, impaired clearance of aminoglycosides may occur due to altered glomerular and tubular function with severe protein depletion (25). Myocardial atrophy results in decreased cardiac reserves and function (1, 93). Immune system function becomes impaired as starvation progresses with loss of chemotactic and phagocytic activity, anergy to common skin test antigens, and impairment of the humoral response (68, 72).

Because of these alterations in organ function, as well as other complex interactions, undernourished patients have an increased incidence of morbidity and mortality. Prognostic relationships exist between morbidity and mortality and serum albumin and transferrin concentrations, delayed-type hypersensitivity skin test reactions, percent weight loss from usual weight, and various combinations of these parameters (47, 89, 127, 154, 177, 218). Surveys of infectious complications in patients undergoing clean surgical procedures demonstrate malnutrition (defined as weight loss and a low serum albumin concentration) to be as important a factor as old age, obesity, diabetes, and infections in other parts of the body (47). It therefore behooves the physician in the critical care unit to consider the patient's nutritional status in the initial patient evaluation. The need for specialized nutritional support must be considered whenever a patient's nutritional status is threatened by disease or when significant preillness malnutrition is present. Whenever possible, the enteral route should be utilized to reduce costs and risks. If the enteral route cannot or should not be utilized for nutritional support, there should be no hesitancy to provide intravenous nutrition. At no time should nutritional support be withheld until some clinical parameter indicates the presence of malnutrition. Instead, emphasis should be placed on prophylactic nutritional support to avoid malnutrition. As a general rule, patients admitted to a critical care unit for evaluation and treatment should be receiving adequate nutritional support within the first 48 hours of admission.

ENDOCRINE RESPONSE TO STRESS

The endocrine response to stress is a complex feedback system that is intimately related to the metabolic response to stress. In this section only a brief discussion of the endocrine response is presented. For simplification, a division is made between the hormones of catabolism, anabolism, and fluid and electrolyte balance.

CATABOLIC HORMONES

A large number of secretory products from mononuclear phagocytes have been identified that mediate the metabolic response to injury. Some of the more well-recognized of these products include interleukins 1 and 2, tumor necrosis factor, colony-stimulating factor, platelet-derived growth factor, and γ-interferon (30, 51–53, 158, 162, 169). The extensive impact of just interleukin-1 and tumor necrosis factor is suggested by Figure 60.1. Initial investigations suggested that the intravenous infusion of a combination of the three counterregulatory "stress" hormones (cortisol, glucagon, and epinephrine) into normal healthy volunteers closely reproduced the metabolic responses observed following mild-to-moderate injury including negative nitrogen balance, hyperglycemia, and insulin resistance (16). However, fever, acute-phase protein responses,

and leukocytosis did not occur. It is now believed that the response to stress is mediated by two main cytokines, interleukin-2 and tumor necrosis factor, with tumor necrosis factor the primary cytokine (144, 145). These cytokines, in turn, cause secretion of the counterregulatory "stress" hormones with their subsequent clinical effects, as summarized below.

Glucocorticoids

Immediately after injury there is a rapid increase in cortisol secretion lasting for 34 to 48 hours (61). However, even with minor injuries, up to two to five times normal excretion of urinary hydroxycorticoids is found for 7 to 10 days (148, 149). With severe or prolonged stress, urinary hydroxycorticoids are increased for weeks to months and may be associated with hypertrophy of the adrenal cortex. Cortisol acts in concert with the catecholamines to stimulate lipolysis, inhibit protein synthesis, facilitate amino acid mobilization from muscle, induce the enzymes of gluconeogenesis, enhance secretion of glucagon while inhibiting insulin secretion, and stimulate conversion of lactic acid to glycogen.

Catecholamines

Epinephrine and norepinephrine are secreted within seconds of injury. Although their biologic half-lives are short, their continued secretion for several days and, in severe stress, for several weeks, results in a prolonged metabolic effect (80). Epinephrine induces the enzymes of hepatic glycogenolysis and gluconeogenesis, stimulates glucagon secretion, inhibits insulin secretion, stimulates lipolysis, enhances amino acid release from skeletal muscle, and inhibits the uptake of glucose by peripheral tissues. In addition, epinephrine leads to the secretion of pituitary ACTH, which stimulates glucocorticoid secretion (61).

Glucagon

Glucagon is a potent catabolic hormone secreted by pancreatic α-islet cells in response to trauma. It acts predominantly on hepatocytes to prevent hypoglycemia by stimulating gluconeogenesis and glycogenolysis. In the periphery it may also enhance lipolysis and proteolysis (212).

ANABOLIC HORMONES

Insulin

Insulin is a potent anabolic hormone secreted by pancreatic β-islet cells. It plays a central role in the regulation of glucose metabolism by inhibiting gluconeogenesis and glycogenolysis in the hepatic cells through the stimulation of glucokinase and UPDG-glycosyl transferase, and the inhibition of pyruvate carboxylase and phosphorylase. Insulin also promotes glucose and potassium uptake by peripheral tissues, inhibits lipolysis, and favors protein synthesis (149). The stress reaction (largely catecholamine-mediated) leads to a marked depression in insulin production and secretion that results in a disproportionately and persistently low serum insulin level (143). With the increase in serum glucagon, the molar insulin-glucagon ratio

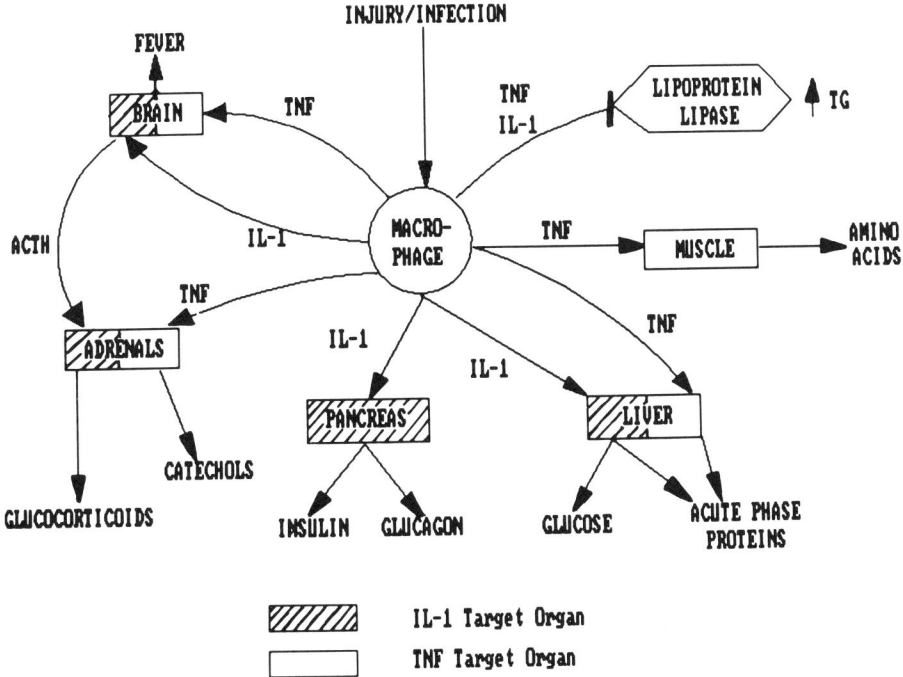

Figure 60.1. Effects of interleukin-1 (*IL-1*) and tumor necrosis factor (*TNF*) on host endocrine response and substrate metabolism during stress. (From Pomposelli JJ, Flores EA, Bistrian BR: Role of biochemical mediators in clinical nutrition and surgical metabolism. *TG,* triglyceride; *ACTH,* adrenocorticotropic hormone. *J Parenter Enteral Nutr* 12:212–218, 1988. With permission.)

is depressed, resulting in an increase in gluconeogenesis and glycogenolysis.

Growth Hormone

Stress is a strong stimulant of growth hormone secretion (228). Growth hormone supports nitrogen, phosphorus, and potassium retention, fatty acid oxidation, and ketogenesis. It also inhibits insulin and promotes amino acid uptake with protein synthesis (129).

Androgens

Testosterone, in addition to its other roles, is a potent anabolic hormone. It stimulates protein synthesis and decreases amino acid catabolism. Retention of nitrogen, potassium, phosphorus, and calcium is a manifestation of its anabolic effect. Stress and catecholamines result in a slight depression of testosterone secretion (149).

FLUID AND ELECTROLYTE HORMONES

Antidiuretic Hormone

Antidiuretic hormone (ADH) acts to maintain a proper solute-solvent ratio in the serum. Hypovolemia and hypertonicity during stress strongly stimulate ADH release from the posterior pituitary gland (149). The primary site of action of ADH is the kidney, where it promotes water reabsorption.

Aldosterone

Aldosterone promotes reabsorption of sodium bicarbonate while increasing potassium and hydrogen ion losses. Aldosterone secretion in stress is augmented by increased catecholamines and hyponatremia. In addition, isotonic hypovolemia,

by increasing renin production, leads to angiotensin release that stimulates aldosterone secretion. The endocrine response to stress can be graphically displayed, as in Figure 60.2.

METABOLIC RESPONSE TO STRESS

The metabolic response to stress and injury, as first described by Cuthbertson (49) in 1930, can be divided into three phases that have gradual transitions. The acute phase begins immediately following injury and lasts for 12 to 36 hours. It is characterized by a rapid secretion of cytokines and the stress hormones (catecholamines, glucocorticoids, glucagon, growth hormones, etc.), marked fluid shifts, acid-base imbalances, and a decrease in energy expenditure, oxygen consumption, and core temperature (61, 117). Therapeutic priorities are to provide hemostasis, cardiovascular stability, and electrolyte balance. If the injury is severe, there is an accompanying metabolic acidosis from anaerobic metabolism, development of an oxygen deficit, an increase in the acute-phase proteins, hyperglycemia due to insulin resistance, and an increase in free fatty acids in serum. Nutritional support during this initial phase is not indicated due to other priorities.

After the first 12 to 16 hours, the acutely stressed patient enters a catabolic phase. During this phase there is an increase in urea production and urinary urea nitrogen excretion due to protein catabolism. While uncomplicated starvation is associated with a loss of 3 to 7 g/day of urea nitrogen, with stress urinary urea nitrogen excretion may increase to 7 to 40 g/day, depending upon the degree of stress (20 g nitrogen/day = 171 g protein/day = 0.5 kg lean tissue/day). Other potential sources of nitrogen loss during stress include blood, transudates, exudates, and wound drainage. Protein catabolism supplies the carbon skeletons for gluconeogenesis, not obtainable

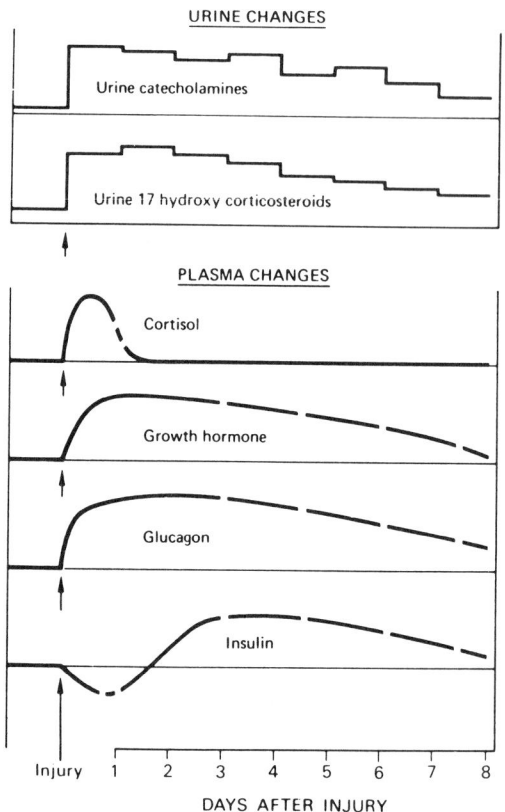

Figure 60.2. Hormone changes after injury. (Reprinted with permission from Fleck A: Metabolic response to injury. In Ledingham IM, Mackay G (eds): *Jamieson and Kay's Textbook of Surgical Physiology.* Churchill Livingstone, New York, p 45, 1978.)

from fat oxidation, and also provides substrates acutely needed for the synthesis of blood proteins, structural proteins, and enzymes. Prior to the development of intravenous feeding, it was believed that net nitrogen loss was mandatory and irreversible during this phase. However, the advent of nonvolitional tube feeding and parenteral nutrition has shown that, although the catabolic response cannot be suppressed, the negative nitrogen balance and subsequent body wasting can be reduced and, at times, overcome by infusion of specially formulated intravenous solutions (31, 113, 138).

The catabolic phase is associated with marked increases in daily caloric expenditure and nitrogen excretion. The two tend to parallel each other with increasing degrees of stress, except in the case of severe stress, where the caloric expenditure increases more than nitrogen excretion (132). An equation for estimation of BMR in healthy individuals was first developed by Harris and Benedict in 1919 (88). This equation is still valid but must be adjusted by a factor of approximately 10% to obtain the clinically more useful value of resting metabolic expenditure (RME). In stress, the energy expenditure is significantly increased above the predicted RME (Fig. 60.3). After extensive metabolic studies, Long et al (132) modified the original Harris-Benedict equation to better estimate daily caloric expenditure by adding a stress and activity factor (see Table 60.1).

In times of stress, when an individual is usually unable or unwilling to eat, the body adapts by converting from exogenous to endogenous sources of carbohydrate, fat, and protein.

Carbohydrates are stored mainly as glycogen (500 g). Mobilization by glycogenolysis can provide only about 1700 kcal, which is exhausted after 8 hours. Certain organs require glucose as their caloric source early in starvation (brain, heart, renal medulla, leukocytes, fibroblasts). To provide glucose, the body converts protein into glucose in the liver and kidney by gluconeogenesis. The conversion of body protein is an inefficient and expensive process, as it yields few calories (20 kcal gained for each gram of nitrogen excreted = 6.25 g of protein = 30 g of wet muscle tissue). Other tissues can use fatty acids for energy, which are plentiful and expendable. Up to 300 to 500 g/day of fat may be oxidized, providing 2700 to 4500 kcal/day. Even by providing large amounts of exogenous glucose through parenteral nutrition, the stressed body prefers to convert excess glucose to glycogen while the endogenous fat stores continue to be oxidized (12). In the unstressed depleted patient, extra glucose is converted into fat, and fat oxidation is suppressed. When excess glucose is given to the hypermetabolic stressed patient, gluconeogenesis is not suppressed, and protein catabolism continues (133).

The electrolyte and acid-base derangements that occur during the catabolic phase are largely due to losses from, or shifts between, various body compartments and reflect cellular destruction, proteolysis, and the body's effort to maintain an effective circulating blood volume. In the urine, excretion of potassium, phosphorus, sulfate, magnesium, creatinine, creatine, and uric acid is increased (150). Bicarbonate and sodium are retained by the kidney through the effects of aldosterone, resulting in kaluresis and a mild metabolic alkalosis with an acidic urine. The metabolic alkalosis can be further aggravated by blood transfusions (citrate metabolized to bicarbonate) and nasogastric suction (hydrogen ion loss).

If the clinical course progresses without complications, the catabolic phase gradually gives way to an anabolic phase. Urinary nitrogen excretion decreases, reflecting decreased protein catabolism. There is a diuresis of salt and water, a normalization of serum potassium and sodium, and a change in the endocrine pattern from the stress hormones (catecholamines, glucocorticoids, and glucagon) to the growth hormones (insulin, androgens, and growth hormone). The state of convalescence may continue for weeks or months, depending on the amount of body protein and fat lost during the catabolic phase. In the anabolic phase, requirements for amino acids and calories are greater than normal, but less than during the stressed period. Appropriate adjustments in the level of nutritional support must be made. An oral diet is usually well-tolerated at this point, and intensive intravenous or enteral nutritional support is usually not necessary.

SUBSTRATE REQUIREMENTS FOR NUTRITIONAL SUPPORT

FLUID REQUIREMENTS

Fluid requirements for patients on parenteral nutrition are somewhat greater than for patients on 5% dextrose solutions. The standard formulas used to calculate fluid requirements, based either on body weight or body surface area, assume a catabolic state to be present with an expected release of 300 to 500 ml of water per day from oxidation of fat and release

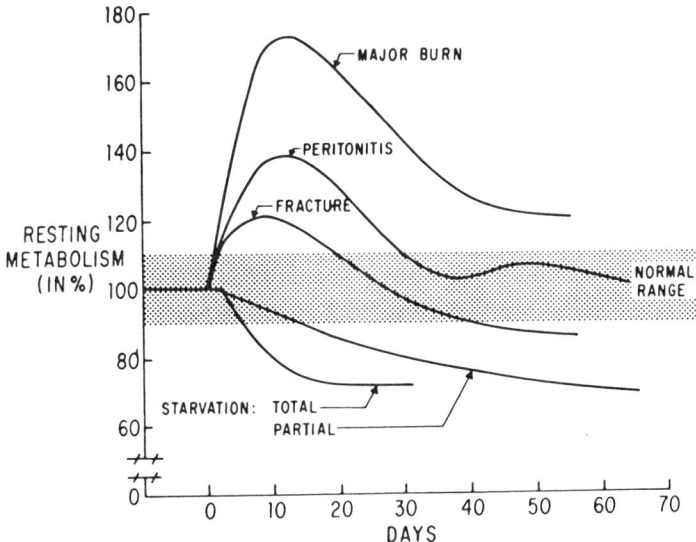

Figure 60.3. Changes in resting metabolic expenditure in six patient groups with time. (Reprinted with permission from Long CL, Schaffel N, Geiger JW et al: Metabolic response to injury and illness: estimation of energy and protein needs from indirect calorimetry and nitrogen balance. *J Parenter Enteral Nutr* 3:452–456, 1979.)

Table 60.1. Calculation of Actual Energy Expenditure (AEE)[a]

AEE (men)   = (66.47 + 13.75W + 5.011 − 6.76A) × (activity factor) × (injury factor)
AEE (women) = (6.55.10 × 9.56W + 4.8511 − 4.68A) × (activity factor) × (injury factor)
Where AEE = actual energy expenditure, W = weight in kg, 11 = height in cm, A = age in years

Activity factor	Use	Injury factor	Use
Confined to bed	1.2	Minor operation	1.20
Out of bed	1.3	Skeletal trauma	1.35
		Major sepsis	1.60
		Severe thermal burn	2.10

[a] Modified from Long CL, Schaffel N, Geiger JW: Metabolic response to injury and illness: estimation of energy and protein needs from indirect calorimetry and nitrogen balance. *J Parenter Enteral Nutr* 3:452–456, 1979.

of intracellular water. When a patient is converted to an anabolic state with parenteral nutrition, the intracellular water is no longer released and, indeed, in an anabolic state; new cells are being formed and new intracellular water must be provided. The standard fluid formulas underestimate fluid requirements during nutritional support by 500 to 800 ml/day. In addition to basic fluid requirements and requirements of an anabolic state, one must replace all measured losses, estimated insensible losses, and estimated third-space fluid losses (insensible fluid loss estimates must be increased by 360 ml/day/°C in febrile patients). Finally, fluid administration must be appropriately reduced in patients with congestive heart failure, renal failure, pulmonary edema and in those patients receiving humidified air from a ventilator.

CALORIC REQUIREMENTS

An interaction exists between caloric and nitrogen substrates (156, 224). If one increases either caloric or nitrogen supplementation, less of the other substrate is required to achieve nitrogen balance. The optimal ratio of calories-to-nitrogen for patients in the intensive care unit is likely quite variable. Usually, an estimate of optimal nitrogen supplementation is made, then caloric supplementation is given to establish positive nitrogen balance. This approach usually results in a calorie-to-nitrogen ratio between 100:1 and 200:1. Several substrates are now, or soon will be, available to meet the caloric needs of stressed patients.

Glucose

Glucose is utilized by nearly all body tissues. There are some tissues, however, which are obligate glucose users, including the brain, renal medulla, red blood cells, and fibroblasts. The sensitivity of these tissues to the availability of glucose is illustrated by the rapid alterations in mental function when excessive insulin is administered. Within minutes, confusion develops and, if glucose is not given, coma can develop, and permanent brain injury can occur. The daily consumption of glucose by these tissues alone is approximately 200 g. At least this much glucose should always be given during parenteral nutrition. As most other tissues in the body readily utilize glucose as an energy source, it is common practice to increase glucose infusion to tolerance. Determination of that endpoint is not very difficult, because it is marked by the onset of hyperglycemia and an increased respiratory quotient above 1.1, as measured by a metabolic cart.

Providing glucose in excess of maximal glucose utilization is of no clinical value and may be of some harm. In 1979, Burke et al (27) demonstrated that the conversion to carbon dioxide of labeled glucose given intravenously to burn patients was maximal at a rate of 6 mg/kg/min. They further demonstrated that a maximal benefit of glucose loading during stress with respect to whole-body protein synthesis occurred with 4.7 to 6.8 mg/kg/min glucose infusion. Infusions at lower rates resulted in a reduced protein synthesis, and infusions at a higher rate were associated with no further increase in protein synthesis.

Black et al (18) studied maximal glucose uptake and utilization in intensive care patients, as compared to that in non-stressed patients, and found a marked decrease in average maximal glucose disposal from 9.46 mg/kg/min in normal subjects to only 6.23 mg/kg/min in stressed patients. It is therefore recommended that stressed patients receive a maximum of 5 to 6 mg/kg/min glucose as a caloric substrate (500 to 600 g/day, or 1700 to 2000 kcal/day in a 70-kg patient). Attempts to improve glucose tolerance with insulin infusion during stress have met with limited success. When used, only mono-component, and preferably recombinant insulin, should be given to avoid sensitization. Although insulin can increase uptake of glucose by peripheral tissues and, therefore, lower blood glucose concentrations in stress, studies have failed to demonstrate an increase in glucose oxidation or nitrogen sparing. Potential adverse effects of insulin must be considered. Insulin (like free fatty acids associated with the neuroendocrine response to stress) inhibits the activity of pyruvate dehydrogenase, thereby limiting the entry of glucose into the Krebs cycle for oxidative metabolism (215). The increase in pyruvate favors fat synthesis, which requires energy and produces carbon dioxide. In general, use of insulin beyond 50 to 75 U/day is not recommended. If glucose intolerance persists, an alternate fuel source should be sought and carbohydrate infusion reduced to 6 mg/kg/day or less.

Long-Chain Fatty Acids

The long-chain fatty acids are satisfactory fuels for many organs in the body and provide a high amount of energy per gram of substrate. Three long-chain fatty acids are essential in the diet, because they cannot be synthesized by humans: arachidonic acid, linoleic acid, and linolenic acid. These fatty acids are necessary for cell membrane structure and stability and for synthesis and action of the prostaglandin system. A minimum of 1 to 2% of total caloric intake should be in the form of essential fatty acids to meet minimal nutritional requirements. This amounts to a minimum of 1 liter of a 10% fat emulsion per week. Whether supplementation with more than the minimum required fat is of any benefit during stress is debatable. Free fatty acids are already in relatively high concentrations in the interstitial fluids during stress, and additional intravenous fat may be of little value. Although there is increased clearance of intravenous fat from the bloodstream during stress (83), Goodenough and Wolfe (73) demonstrated that clearance of lipid did not necessarily mean utilization of the fatty acids as a fuel source. In their study of eight burned patients, only 13% of the infused lipid was oxidized within the first 7.5 hours after administration. The remaining fat was thought mainly to replace mobilized endogenous fat. Chen (38, 39) demonstrated deposition of infused lipid in the liver of experimental septic rats. Hamawy et al (84) infused lipid emulsions in an experimental animal mode at rates equivalent to a human dose of 2 kcal/min and found deposition of lipid in the reticuloendothelial system. When challenged with intravenous bacteria, phagocytosis and bacterial killing were found to be suppressed. Others have found similar deleterious effects in humans (186, 190). On the other hand, Ota et al (163) infused lipids in only moderate amounts and found no adverse effects on levels of immunoglobulins, C_3 and C_4 complement, circulating B and T lymphocytes, suppressor T lymphocytes, natural killer cell activity, monocytes, lymphocyte blastogenic response and neutrophil chemotaxis, and bactericidal activity.

As the level of stress increases, the rate of clearance of lipid from the blood decreases, suggesting poorer utilization (32, 38, 131). Coran et al (44) reported decreased oxidation of exogenous fatty acids in puppies during septic shock. Long et al (134) progressively substituted fat for glucose in an animal burn model and demonstrated a linear decrease in nitrogen balance as glucose was replaced. They found the formula for nitrogen loss to be:

$$N\ loss = 17.44 - 1.997\ ln\ (glucose\ intake \\ kcal/m^2/day) + 0.0752\ (RME\ kcal/m^2/day)$$

A possible explanation for any ineffectiveness of fat as an energy source in stressed patients is the necessity of carnitine for fatty acids to pass into mitochondria, where it undergoes β-oxidation. As stress increases, carnitine disappears from the mitochondrial membrane surface. Without adequate carnitine on the cell surface, transport of long-chain fatty acids into mitochondria is decreased. Although one clinical report during sepsis demonstrated increased losses of carnitine in the urine with low serum concentrations (157), infusion of carnitine in stressed patients has demonstrated no conclusive benefit with respect to increasing the efficiency of fat utilization as an energy source (167).

In clinical practice, a mixture of glucose and long-chain fatty acids is given in a ratio of 50 to 80% glucose to 20 to 50% fat. This ratio is adjusted based on tolerance as determined by serum concentrations. Work by Giovannini et al (71) has added further support to use of a mixed-fuel nutrient solution during stress. They found that respiratory work was significantly reduced in septic patients due to reduced carbon dioxide production. In contrast, Shaw and Holdaway (192) demonstrated a similar reduction in net protein catabolism when caloric support was given solely as glucose or as a glucose-lipid mixture, with actual results being dependent on the clinical status of the patient.

Medium-Chain Fatty Acids

Medium-chain fatty acids contain 8 to 10 carbon atoms. They can be used by most organs as a fuel. They require neither carnitine nor insulin for oxidation. Consequently, they could theoretically serve as an energy source during stress when glucose and long-chain fatty acids are poorly tolerated. Development of so-called structured lipid emulsions for intravenous use, in which the glycerol molecule contains both long-chain fatty acids (approximately 40%) and medium-chain fatty acids (approximately 60%), is in progress. Studies in the experimental animal have shown excellent tolerance and improved nitrogen balance when structured lipids are substituted for long-chain fat emulsions (138), and less interference with the reticuloendothelial system (84, 106). When administered to humans, there have been no adverse effects reported; the structured lipids are rapidly cleared from the blood (109, 223); and nitrogen balance appears to be somewhat better (14, 50).

Branched-Chain Amino Acids

There are three branched-chain amino acids: leucine, isoleucine, and valine. None of the three can be synthesized within the body. Although amino acids are not usually considered an energy source, branched-chain amino acids serve as a major energy source for skeletal muscle, especially during stress. They promote protein synthesis, reduce protein degradation, and serve as a substrate for gluconeogenesis. The liver does not have enzymes for oxidation of the branched-chain amino acids, and all metabolism is in the skeletal muscle. This fact increases their usefulness in the presence of liver dysfunction.

Provision of increased amounts of branched-chain amino acids during acute stress has been shown to improve nitrogen balance, although not all reports agree (21, 35, 102, 188). It would appear that a 45% branched-chain enrichment is the most optimal for nitrogen sparing and protein synthesis (70). If there is a benefit, it occurs during the time of maximal stress (107).

Glutamine

It has long been known that glutamine is an essential nutrient for establishment of cells in tissue culture. Yet, it has only recently been recognized that glutamine is an important nutrient in the experimental animal and, likely, in the human. It is a necessary component for protein and nucleotide synthesis and is an important respiratory substrate for most rapidly dividing cells, including the gastrointestinal tract, pancreas, alveolar cells, and white blood cells (9, 63, 160, 200, 204, 227). Particular interest has been directed to its role in maintenance of normal gut histology. With the increased metabolic demands of inflammation or injury, the consumption of glutamine as a fuel exceeds the increased release from skeletal muscle, and serum glutamine concentrations decrease dramatically (10, 67, 225). The resulting glutamine deficiency is associated with progressive intestinal atrophy resulting in decreased villous height and weight, loss of brush border enzymes, villous disruption, and bacterial invasion (7, 78, 201, 202, 225). These changes in intestinal morphology, with possible translocation of organisms or toxins across the disrupted mucosal barrier, have been implicated as an initiating step in the development of the septic syndrome and multiple organ failure (29, 225). The provision of supplemental glutamine prevents small bowel atrophy (78, 161) and reduces the incidence and severity of bacterial translocation (4, 201). Supplementation of enteral diets with glutamine has improved animal survival in several reported experiments (64, 147).

Glutamine is similarly metabolized, whether it enters the enterocyte across the brush border from the intestinal lumen or across the basolateral cell membrane from the arterial blood. Its metabolic effect appears to be the same, therefore, whether given enterally or parenterally (200). Current intravenous solutions do not contain glutamine. Ziegler et al (231) have demonstrated compatibility and stability of glutamine additives to the intravenous nutrition solution, and several manufacturers are working on adding glutamine to their formulas. Until commercial amino acid solutions become available, clinical use of glutamine is restricted to enteral administration. As an alternative, or as a supplement to the enteral formula, L-glutamine powder can be given directly, either via a feeding tube or as an oral capsule. Glutamine can be obtained commercially and packaged into 500-mg capsules by a pharmacist. Although no minimum effective dose has been established, most authors recommend that at least 6 to 8 g/day of L-glutamine be given in divided doses.

ω-3 Fatty Acids (Fish Oils)

ω-3 fatty acids have been shown to have competitive and inhibitory effects on the metabolism of linoleic acids, including the conversion of arachidonic acid to prostaglandins (24). Provision of the ω-3 fatty acids in the diet, by reducing production of the two series prostaglandins, reduce the suppression of proliferative immune responses, antibody and lymphokine production, and cell-mediated cytolysis (74). With prolonged administration of ω-3 fatty acids, cell membrane fatty acid composition changes as well, which may alter release of prostaglandins associated with cellular damage. Because these fatty acids are just as effective as an energy source as other long-chain fatty acids, they may find extensive use in parenteral nutrition when they become commercially available for intravenous infusion, especially in the stressed patient.

Short-Chain Fatty Acids

A final alternate fuel receiving increasing attention is the group of short-chain fatty acids. These fatty acids (acetate, propionate, and butyrate) are the end-products of soluble fiber metabolism in the colon and are readily absorbed. Studies by several investigators have shown them to be a major fuel of the colon and an important substrate for the small intestine as well (121, 203). Infusion of the simple fatty acids or of pectin results in an improved colonic mucosal histological pattern, with increased DNA content, increased mucosal height, increased nitrogen content and, perhaps, maintenance of the mucosal barrier. These nutrients are not available for intravenous use in humans yet, but enteral feeding products containing soluble fiber and pectin are available.

Summary of Caloric Support

Current practice is to provide stressed patients with their estimated or, preferably, measured caloric needs. When estimated, a modification of the Harris-Benedict equation is used (Table 60.1) (132). As a rule of thumb, mild stress is associated with a 30 kcal/kg/day caloric requirement, moderate stress with 35 kcal/kg/day, and severe stress with 40 kcal/kg/day. Actual measurement of caloric expenditure can be accomplished with one of several metabolic carts available that measure oxygen consumption and carbon dioxide production. An onboard computer calculates energy expenditure and respiratory quotient and estimates substrate utilization. To meet the caloric requirement, up to 1500 to 1800 kcal/day are given as carbohydrates with the rest given as long-chain fatty acids as the clinician watches carefully to ensure clearance of both from the blood. If the stress is moderate-to-severe, branched-chain enriched amino acid solutions can be used as an additional protein and caloric source. It is hoped that structured lipid emulsions and glutamine supplements will soon be available.

NITROGEN REQUIREMENTS

Minimal nitrogen supplementation to maintain nitrogen balance with adequate caloric support is estimated to be between 0.5 and 0.75 g/kg/day. However, to achieve optimal nitrogen utilization and preserve lean body mass, it is recommended that 1.0 g/kg/day be administered to the unstressed patient, 1.5 g/kg/day to the moderately stressed patient, and 2.0 g/kg/day to the severely stressed patient. Patients with protein-losing enteropathies or nephropathies, those with exudative wound losses, and those patients undergoing hemodialysis or peritoneal dialysis may have significantly increased requirements due to excessive loss of nitrogen. In practice, if there is a question concerning the adequacy of caloric and nitrogen support, a nitrogen balance study is performed by comparing total nitrogen input to total losses. The following formula is used:

$$Nitrogen\ balance = (protein\ intake \div 6.25) - TUN^a$$
$$- 5\ mg\ N/kg^b - 12\ mg\ N/kg^c$$

where: a = total urinary nitrogen excreted over 24 hours, b = estimated insensible nitrogen losses, and c = estimated nitrogen losses from the gastrointestinal tract.

For maintenance of lean body mass the nitrogen balance should be neutral. For body cell mass repletion, nitrogen balance should be between 0.04 and 0.07 g/kg/day.

ELECTROLYTE REQUIREMENTS

Electrolyte requirements during nutritional support occur in three phases. During the first 24 to 48 hours, electrolyte deficits must be replaced. Patients who are severely malnourished often have normal serum electrolyte concentrations. True whole-body deficits are not apparent until feeding is initiated, when an intravascular-to-intracellular shift occurs. Phase II occurs between 24 and 48 hours and follows conversion to an anabolic state. In this phase there are increased requirements for the intracellular electrolytes (potassium, phosphorus, and magnesium) due to formation of new intracellular water. Phase III of electrolyte requirements occurs when patients become stable after repletion of deficits and establishment of the anabolic state. In this phase, electrolyte shifts are uncommon, and requirements are fairly constant.

Requirements for sodium, chloride, and calcium are not changed from requirements during administration of 5% dextrose.

OTHER ADDITIVES

Many additives are often included in the intravenous nutrition solution, including 1000 or more units of heparin per liter, up to 25 g of albumin per liter, hydrochloric acid, cimetidine, and even occasionally antibiotics and steroids. As intravenous nutritional solutions can be extremely complex, the risk of precipitate formation or adverse interaction is high. Expertise in formulation and meticulous monitoring is critical. To be safe, additives other than those required for nutritional support should be minimized.

VASCULAR ACCESS

Solutions formulated to provide optimal calories, nitrogen, electrolytes, trace elements, and vitamins are quite hypertonic and cannot be administered through peripheral veins. Central venous access is therefore necessary for parenteral nutrition. In clinical practice, catheters are typically placed percutaneously into the superior vena cava via the subclavian vein or, less commonly, via the external or internal jugular veins. If there is no access in the neck or shoulder area due to skin lesions or draining infections, catheters can be placed via an antecubital vein and advanced into the superior vena cava (PICC lines). If the superior vena cava is not available due to thrombosis, access can be achieved via the femoral vein advancing the catheter into the inferior vena cava to the level of the renal veins. As femoral catheters carry the risk of venous thrombosis, systemic anticoagulation is recommended. On rare occasions, a port of a Swan-Ganz catheter or the central port of a dual lumen percutaneous subclavian vein dialysis catheter can be employed for feeding. Due to potential infectious complications, use of these catheters should be avoided unless no other alternative is available.

Recently, there has been increasing interest in using triple-lumen central catheters for administration of parenteral nutrition in the intensive care unit, a practice that should be discouraged. Table 60.2 summarizes the current published experience with triple-lumen catheters, as compared with single-lumen catheters. Although some studies suggest no increased risk, all studies have been poorly controlled, often using too small a sample, and frequently using an obscure definition of what constitutes a true catheter-related septic episode. The average incidence of catheter-related sepsis with the triple-lumen catheters was 8.8% in these studies, as compared with the usual catheter-related sepsis incidence of 3.8% with single-lumen catheters ($p < 0.0001$), suggesting that caution be taken in their routine use.

On the chance that the higher sepsis rate was due to treating sicker patients with triple-lumen catheters, we performed a prospective randomized, comparative study of single-lumen vs. triple-lumen catheters in which single-lumen catheters were isolated for use only in parenteral nutrition, and the triple-lumen catheters had one lumen isolated for nutrition and the other two lumina available for administration of routine fluids, as well as for blood sampling [41]. A group of 177 patients were entered into the study between June 1989 and November 1991. All required multiple intravenous access and would therefore benefit from use of a triple-lumen catheter, if it were proven to be safe. At the same time, all patients were at increased risk of developing catheter-related sepsis, owing to the presence of one or more of the following: age over 60 years; diagnosis of acute pancreatitis; altered immunocompetence, as indicated by loss of skin integrity, a white blood cell count less than 4000, or immunosuppression with steroids; severity of illness great enough to require management in an intensive care environment; presence of an infectious process, such as a wound infection, urinary tract infection, or pulmonary infection; and the presence of a tracheostomy or recent head and neck surgery. Catheter dressings were maintained by the Nutritional Support Service. In this study, there were two catheter-related episodes of sepsis in 78 patients with a single-lumen catheter (2.6%), compared

Table 60.2. Incidence of Catherer-related Sepsis during Intravenous Nutrition, Using Triple-Lumen vs. Single-Lumen Catheters

Study	*Yr*	*Single-Lumen Catheter*	*Triple-Lumen Catheter*	*p*
Crocker et al (46)[a]	1986		7.0% (42)	
Pemberton et al (166)	1986	3.0% (68)	19.0% (59)	<0.05
Kaufman et al (110)	1986		3.8% (104)	
Kelly et al (112)	1986		3.1% (96)	
Apelgren (8)	1987		14.3% (119)	
McCarthy et al (136)	1987	0% (36)	12.8% (39)	<0.05
Mantese et al (139)	1987		35.0% (69)	
Pomp et al (168)	1988	1.9% (274)	7.7% (52)	<0.05
Kovacevich et al (122)	1988	5.2% (756)	5.7% (523)	>0.70
Rose et al (180)	1988	1.6% (248)	4.9% (232)	<0.07
Powell et al (172)	1988		14.3% (126)	
Powell et al (171)[b]	1988	22.7% (22)	22.7% (22)	
Gill et al (69)	1989		6.1% (114)	
Horowitz et al (98)	1990		6.5% (214)	
Duke University (unpublished data)	1992	2.6% (78)	13.1% (99)	<0.02
Total		3.8% (1482)	8.8% (1910)	<0.0001

[a] Numbers in parentheses indicate total catheters.
[b] Used dual-lumen rather than triple-lumen catheter.

with 13 septic episodes in 99 patients with triple-lumen catheters (13.1%) ($p < 0.01$). From this study it would appear that triple-lumen catheters expose the patient to a fivefold increased risk of catheter-related sepsis when used simultaneously for intravenous nutrition and for other vascular access. Use of multilumen catheters for parenteral nutrition, especially in the patient at higher risk of catheter-related sepsis, should therefore be reserved only for the patient in whom such access is absolutely mandatory and should never be used just for convenience.

CATHETER-RELATED COMPLICATIONS OF PARENTERAL NUTRITION

Subclavian catheter insertion has the potential for numerous complications and should be performed by, or directly supervised by, experienced physicians. Full knowledge of subclavian vein anatomy and attention to minute details minimizes the occurrence of pneumothorax, arterial puncture, hemomediastinum, hemothorax, hydrothorax, and hydromediastinum and virtually eliminates injury to the brachial plexus or thoracic duct, air embolism, and catheter embolism. In large series, catheter insertion complications occur between 1% and 5% of the time, with 1% or less being major complications (76).

The majority of pneumothoraces are small and nonprogressive and usually resolve over several days without treatment. However, some are large and progressive, requiring chest tube placement. If an air leak persists for several days after chest tube placement, it may be necessary to remove the catheter, as it may be passing through lung and pleura, causing a bronchopleural fistula. An unrecognized pneumothorax is an especially serious problem in the patient receiving mechanical ventilation as the positive pressure can rapidly lead to a tension pneumothorax.

Arterial puncture is a risk associated with most approaches to the great veins. Usually, puncture of an artery does not pose a serious problem, if the needle is carefully removed, as normal muscular contraction of the artery prevents significant leakage of blood. If the direction of the needle is altered during insertion or withdrawal, however, the artery or vein may be lacerated, resulting in development of hemothorax or hemomediastinum with possible cardiac tamponade requiring emergent surgical decompression.

Air embolism is a completely avoidable and potentially lethal complication. Aspiration of air may occur during insertion of the catheter, during changing of the intravenous tubing, upon accidental separation of the intravenous tubing, or through the subcutaneous tract, which may fail to close after removal of the catheter. Treatment consists of placing the patient in a head-down, left lateral decubitus position to allow trapped air to migrate from the pulmonary outflow tract to the right ventricle. Needle aspiration of the right ventricle and even emergency thoracotomy may be necessary to remove the air in the pulmonary outflow tract.

Very rarely, catheter shearing and embolization have occurred with embolization to the subclavian or innominate vein, right atrium, right ventricle, or pulmonary artery. In all cases, the catheter must be removed promptly, usually by vascular radiology, to avoid thrombus formation, infection, cardiac arrhythmias, and possible perforation of the vessels or heart. With the development of newer and more pliable catheter materials, great vein perforation by the catheter, leading to hemothorax and hemomediastinum, or perforation of the right atrium, is very infrequent.

Another difficulty related to placement of the central venous catheter is improper catheter tip location. The catheter should be a few centimeters superior to the right atrium in the superior vena cava. Improper location can lead to thrombophlebitis, atrial or ventricular perforation, and cardiac arrhythmias. Subclavian vein phlebitis and thrombosis can result in edema of the arm, face, and neck and can be a cryptic source of infection or pulmonary emboli.

Standard treatment of subclavian vein thrombosis due to a central catheter consists of removal of the catheter. The catheter tip and blood drawn through the catheter should be cultured and appropriate antibiotics begun if the culture results are positive. Immediately upon confirmation of thrombosis by venogram, either urokinase or streptokinase can be infused through the venogram catheter or a peripheral vein on the affected side (57, 184, 185, 197, 226). The infusion should be continued for 24 hours and a repeat venogram done. If complete clearing of the clot has not occurred, the infusion can be continued for another 24 hours, and the venogram repeated. Once the clot has resolved, anticoagulation with heparin should be begun, with conversion to long-term warfarin therapy. Obstructive symptoms usually resolve in 24 to 48 hours, at which time a new catheter may be placed in the opposite subclavian vein and parenteral nutrition resumed. Alternately, if the nutritional status of the patient permits, parenteral nutrition may be delayed until heparin therapy is discontinued, rendering placement of a new catheter safer. Even if clot lysis is not attempted or if the clot does not resolve entirely, it is probably beneficial to give 7 to 10 days of heparin and then convert to warfarin, with anticoagulation continued for 6 to 8 weeks, during which time the irregular vessel wall may reepithelialize or the clot may completely reabsorb. Eventual recannulation of the subclavian vein is thought to be possible but is not documented. Atkinson et al (13) have suggested use of tissue plasminogen activator (t-PA) as a thrombolytic agent when urokinase or streptokinase fails. In six patients who failed to respond to urokinase, five were cleared with t-PA injections.

If no other access is available, including the femoral vein, and central venous access is essential for further care of the patient, the subclavian catheter can be left in place in the thrombosed vein, in spite of the thrombosis. Streptokinase or urokinase can still be given, as well as heparin and warfarin, as outlined previously.

Sepsis is a serious complication of intravenous feeding. Patients who require parenteral nutrition are already at high risk due to malnutrition, use of broad-spectrum antimicrobial therapy and corticosteroids, and concomitant infection in the lungs, urine, and wounds. Most septic problems related to parenteral nutrition can be eliminated by scrupulous attention to aseptic catheter placement, solution preparation, and administration. Primary catheter sepsis is defined as a septic episode in which no other source is found and the septic episode resolves upon catheter removal with culture-positive identification of the same microorganism on the catheter or in blood drawn through the catheter as is present in the peripheral blood. Management of patients who become febrile while receiving parenteral nutrition begins with a detailed investigation for a possible etiology of the fever. If there is a clear cause of fever unrelated to the catheter, the catheter should be left in place and appropriate care given to the unrelated cause. If the etiology of the fever is not obvious, if the fever is ≥38.5°C, often with shaking chills every 4 to 8 hours, and if leukocytosis is present with increased polymorphonuclear and immature cells, the catheter should be removed, with cultures taken from a peripheral vein and from the catheter just prior to removal. If the clinical condition is not urgent and the diagnosis of catheter-related sepsis is not obvious, cultures can be obtained through the catheter and parenteral nutrition continued until the culture results are available. If the patient's condition deteriorates while waiting for the culture results, peripheral infusion of 5% dextrose should be initiated and the central catheter removed and cultured as above.

SOLUTION PREPARATION AND ADMINISTRATION

Multiple protein sources are available for intravenous infusion. Initially, these sources were casein or fibrin hydrolysates. More recently, crystalline amino acid solutions have replaced the hydrolysate solutions and are available as 3.5 to 15% solutions. Although the various solutions have slightly different amino acid compositions, there are no apparent clinical differences between products. Specialized amino acid solutions for renal failure and liver failure, as well as branched-chain amino acid enriched solutions, are available.

Dextrose is available as a 10% to 70% solution and is mixed in various proportions with the protein solutions. Patients with volume intolerance may have special formulas mixed with 70% dextrose and 10% amino acids to reduce free water.

Since 1973 fat emulsions have been available for intravenous use. They are useful as a caloric source, as well as for meeting essential fatty acid requirements of patients during intravenous nutrition. They are available in 10% and 20% concentrations.

Multiple additives are available in combination or singly so that electrolytes, trace elements, and minerals can be added in a wide range of concentrations. Solutions of multivitamins that contain both fat-soluble and water-soluble vitamins are also available. Vitamin K is usually given orally or by intramuscular injection.

The exact order of additive injection does not appear to be important, except that phosphate should always be added before calcium. Exposure to light may result in vitamin and amino acid deterioration. Interactions between vitamin C and heparin and the various trace elements, although rarely clinically important, are theoretically possible. The following mixing sequence is satisfactory:

1. Sodium chloride (2.5 or 4 mEq/ml);
2. Sodium acetate (2 or 4 mEq/ml);
3. Potassium chloride (2 mEq/ml);
4. Potassium acetate (2 mEq/ml);
5. Sodium phosphate (4 mEq Na$^+$ and 3 mM P/ml);
6. Potassium phosphate (4.4 mEq K+ and 3 mM P/ml);
7. Magnesium sulfate (0.8, 1, and 4 mEq/ml);
8. Calcium gluconate (0.47 mEq/ml);
9. Copper, zinc, chromium, and other trace elements as indicated;
10. Heparin (1000 U/ml);
11. Recombinant human regular insulin (100 U/ml);
12. Salt-poor albumin (12.5 g/50 ml);
13. Medications;
14. Ascorbic acid;
15. Folic acid;
16. Thiamine;
17. Phytonadione;
18. Multivitamins (MVI-12).

Following each addition, the container should be agitated gently to ensure thorough mixing and to prevent electrolyte precipitation. Before distribution to the patient, the solution should be carefully inspected for precipitation or separation.

WRITING ORDERS FOR PARENTERAL NUTRITION

Patients requiring intravenous feeding should begin on approximately 2000 ml/day of a 25% dextrose solution with approximately 4% amino acids. This regimen will provide approximately 500 g of carbohydrate, (which is generally well-tolerated during initiation of intravenous support), and 80 g of protein. In patients with volume restrictions, either the solutions can be concentrated, or the starting volume of the standard solution can be reduced. If glucose intolerance has been observed on 5% dextrose solutions, or if diabetes is present, insulin should be added to the initial order. If the blood glucose concentration is above 150 mg/dl, 10 U of insulin should be added per 250 g of carbohydrate. If the blood glucose concentration is greater than 200 mg/dl, 20 to 25 units of insulin should be added and, if greater than 250 mg/dl, 30 to 40 units of insulin per 250 g carbohydrate are called for. If the patient is stable on the 2-liter infusion after the first 24 hours, the infusion rate should be advanced to the required caloric support. If glucose intolerance is observed, even with the addition of insulin, lipid calories should be substituted for carbohydrate.

When the feeding solution is to be discontinued, the amount infused should be reduced by 1000 kcal/day until the patient is receiving 1500 to 2000 kcal in 24 hours. At this point the solution should be replaced with 5% dextrose overnight and then discontinued the following morning. Whenever the solution must be suddenly interrupted, it is recommended that a 5% dextrose solution with appropriate electrolytes be substituted via a peripheral vein and administered at the same rate as the previous parenteral nutrition solution. At no time is 10% dextrose necessary. When converting to 5% dextrose by a peripheral vein, one must be careful to ensure adequate insulin coverage in those patients who are glucose intolerant.

PATIENT MONITORING

Patients in the critical care unit should have serum electrolytes, blood urea nitrogen, and glucose concentrations evaluated daily until stability is achieved. Serum calcium, phosphorus, and magnesium concentrations should be initially monitored every other day, the prothrombin time and white blood count two to three times a week. After stability has been reached, electrolytes and minerals should be monitored twice a week for the next week and then, depending on the degree of stability, reduced to once/week by monitoring. Patients are observed carefully for evidence of sepsis, which may be heralded by glucose intolerance 12 to 24 hours before obvious clinical sepsis. In addition, body weight is monitored carefully to avoid fluid overload with the expectation of no more than 0.5 kg/day weight gain in malnourished patients. Finally, careful observation of the access catheter with routine dressing changes is necessary to avoid septic complications.

OTHER TECHNIQUES OF ADMINISTRATION

New innovations in nutritional support are being evaluated in the critical care setting. The first of these is cyclic intravenous feeding, whereby for 12 to 16 hours/day patients receive parenteral nutrition, and during the remaining 8 to 12 hours they are either on protein solutions alone or converted to a heparin lock (137). Whether cyclic feeding is more advantageous from a metabolic viewpoint remains to be determined. Another valuable method in the critical care unit is modular feeding, in which some nutrition substrates are given enterally, and the rest are given parenterally. An example might be the administration of amino acids and fats through a peripheral vein with glucose via an enteric feeding tube. This technique is especially useful when the gastrointestinal tract is only partially usable, yet one wishes to avoid the risks of central venous cannulation.

METABOLIC COMPLICATIONS OF PARENTERAL NUTRITION

HYPERGLYCEMIA

Special attention must be paid to patients with stress, extremes of age, malnutrition, diabetes, and sepsis. Although these patients need nutrition the most, they are the least tolerant to glucose loading. If spillage of 2 or more g glucose per 100 ml urine occurs, a vigorous osmotic diuresis will ensue, leading to a syndrome of hyperglycemic, hyperosmolar, nonketotic acidosis with an associated mortality approaching 40 to 50% (54). Optimal therapy is prevention, but survival is improved by early intervention, replacing lost fluid with half normal saline plus 20 mEq/liter potassium chloride at 250 ml/hour. Insulin should be added to the intravenous solution at 15 to 20 units/hr while carefully monitoring blood glucose and potassium concentrations. Correction of the acidosis with sodium bicarbonate should be gradual. The goal is to achieve a slow return to normal serum glucose, permitting equilibration between the blood and the cerebral spinal fluid, preventing cerebral edema.

Normal serum glucose concentrations during parenteral nutrition should be less than 200 mg/dl with no more than 1% glucosuria. Values greater than 200 mg/dl should be treated. Normal insulin supplementation was discussed earlier, but if a patient is glucose tolerant and suddenly develops glucose intolerance, the following should be evaluated as potential causes:

1. *Medication change.* Many medications interfere with the urinary sugar determination by standard Clinitest or Tes-Tape techniques (Table 60.3). There are some medications that affect glucose metabolism directly (corticosteriods, certain diuretics, phenytoin, and phenothiazines).
2. *Error in rate of fluid administration.* A sudden increase in the infusion rate can lead to glucose overload.
3. *Impending sepsis.* Glucosuria, hyperglycemia, and hyperkalemia may occur up to 12 hours before a temperature increase or any other signs of sepsis.
4. *Insulin need.* A change in insulin requirements with persistently elevated serum glucose may indicate the formation of antibodies to insulin or resistance of peripheral tissues to the effects of insulin, possibly due to chromium deficiency (see Trace Element Deficiency). Some patients who tolerate low doses of glucose will, as doses are increased, exhibit evidence of a diabetic state and require insulin during parenteral nutrition.

Table 60.3.   Drug Interference with Urine Glucose Determinations[a]

Drug	Effect on Copper Reduction (Clinitest)	Effect on Glucose Oxidase (Tes-Tape)	Dealing with Potential Interferences
Cephalosporins Keflin Keflex Kefzol, Ancef Kafocin Loridine	False-positive (black-brown color)	No effect	Use glucose oxidase test
Vitamin C (in large doses)	False-positive	False-negative	Also may monitor blood glucose[a]
Aspirin and other salicylates (in very large doses)	False-positive	False-negative	Also may monitor blood glucose[a]
Aldomet (methyldopa) (in very large doses)	False-positive	No effect	Use glucose oxidase test
Benemid (probenecid)	False-positive	No effect	Use glucose oxidase test
Achromycin (tetracycline, injection only)	False-positive	False-negative	Also may monitor blood glucose[a]
Pyridium (phenazopyridine)	No effect	False-positive and false-negative	Use copper reduction method
Chloromycetin (chloramphenicol)	False-positive (potentially)	No effect	If in doubt, use glucose oxidase test
Levodopa (in large doses)	False-positive	False-negative	Also may monitor blood glucose[a]

[a]*Note:* Potential interferences with glucose oxidase tests (Tes-Tape) can be eliminated by careful testing. While interfering substances will prevent color development in the part of the paper actually dipped into the urine sample, they will not prevent accurate development in a band across the very highest portion of the wetted tape. A true-negative test occurs when the band remains the same color as the rest of the tape, and a true-positive test occurs when the band changes to one of the colors shown on the color chart. (Reprinted with permission from Grant JP: *Handbook of Total Parenteral Nutrition.* WB Saunders, Philadelphia, 1980.)

HYPOGLYCEMIA

Administration of hypertonic dextrose solutions to nondiabetic patients is associated with an increase in serum insulin to four to six times basal levels within 6 hours (187). As the infusion continues, serum insulin concentrations gradually decrease but are always above normal as long as the dextrose infusion continues. With sudden interruption of the infusion, serum insulin concentrations usually decrease to basal levels within 60 minutes, and blood glucose concentrations decrease to below previous basal levels but seldom to less than 60 mg/dl. In spite of a rapid decline in serum insulin, reactive hypoglycemia is occasionally observed with abrupt discontinuance of parenteral nutrition. It may occur if the infusion is interrupted for as little as 15 to 30 minutes. Therefore, in patients receiving more than 2000 kcal/day of parenteral nutrition, the solution should be tapered by 1000 kcal/day to 2000 kcal, then changed to 5% dextrose at 100 to 125 ml/hour for 12 to 24 hours, at which time the intravenous solution can be safely discontinued. If abrupt cessation of parenteral nutrition is necessary, a peripheral infusion of 5% dextrose with appropriate electrolytes at the same rate as the parenteral nutrition should be given for 12 to 24 hours.

ANABOLIC ELECTROLYTES

Potassium

Potassium is the most abundant intracellular cation. Ninety-eight percent of total body potassium is within the intracellular fluid pool, with an average intracellular concentration of 150 mEq/liter. Intravascular potassium is only 2% of total body potassium (3.5 to 5.0 mEq/liter). Serum concentration is, therefore, a poor indicator of total body potassium. The kidneys are the major route of potassium excretion, eliminating approximately 100 mEq/day in the normal healthy

Table 60.4.   Clinical Symptoms of Potassium Alterations

System	Hyperkalemia	Hypokalemia
Neuromuscular	Diarrhea, weakness, intestinal colic	Paralytic ileus, muscular weakness, possible paralysis
Cardiac	Ventricular arrhythmias, ECG changes: peaked T waves, prolonged PR interval, possible cardiac arrest	Atrial and ventricular premature contractions, myocardial fibrosis, ECG changes: flat T waves, U waves
Metabolic		Abnormal carbohydrate metabolism, negative nitrogen balance

person. In certain situations, the kidneys can preserve potassium, but not as efficiently as they can preserve sodium.

Potassium is essential to the function and operation of the cell and to the maintenance of the resting potential of the cell membrane by maintaining an extracellular/intracellular ion gradient, to various enzyme systems, to carbohydrate metabolism, and to protein metabolism. Hypokalemia (Table 60.4) reflects a decrease in extracellular potassium and is usually the result of insufficient administration or increased gastrointestinal or urinary losses. The lost potassium should be replaced with either the chloride, acetate, or phosphate salts at 10 mEq/hr to a maximum of 40 mEq/hr.

Hyperkalemia is usually the result of excessive exogenous administration or decreased urinary output. On rare occasions, hyperkalemia is factitious, resulting from red cell lysis or forearm acidosis caused by improper blood-drawing techniques. Hyperkalemia is especially prominent in renal failure when the glomerular filtration rate is below 5 ml/min but may also result from transfusion of aged blood, Addison's disease, tissue trauma, or potassium-sparing diuretics (triamterene or spironolactone). Treatment should be rapid and aggressive, as hyperkalemia can lead to cardiac arrest. Specific treatment consists of glucose and insulin administration to increase intracellular transport of potassium; correction of metabolic acidosis with sodium bicarbonate, transporting potassium intracellularly; kaluretic diuretics; ion-exchange resins; dialysis; and intravenous calcium, which lowers the threshold away from the resting potential of the cell membrane.

Phosphorus

The phosphate ion is an integral modulator of human metabolism. It participates in energy transfer through high-energy phosphates (ATP), oxygen transport and release, leukocyte phagocytosis, and microbial resistance (45, 87). Approximately 80% of the adult body's phosphorus is located in bones and teeth, while 9% is within skeletal muscle. Serum phosphorus is a small fraction of total body phosphorus (2.5 to 4.3 mg/100 ml). Serum phosphate concentrations are regulated by the kidneys and parathormone.

During parenteral nutrition, hypophosphatemia may result from insufficient administration, alkalosis with subsequent increased phosphorylation of carbohydrate (respiratory alkalosis has a greater effect than metabolic alkalosis), Gram-negative bacteremia, salicylate intoxication, impaired absorption as with the phosphate binding antacids (Mg^{2+} and Al^{2+}), increased renal clearance (hyperparathyroidism, vitamin D deficiency, Fanconi syndrome, hypomagnesemia, hypokalemia), metabolic acidosis, and alcoholism. Phosphate deficiency may develop within the first 24 hours of intravenous feeding if adequate phosphate supplementation is not provided (196, 211). Glucose administration stimulates insulin secretion, which facilitates transport of glucose and phosphate into the liver and skeletal muscle, acutely lowering blood concentrations. In general, renal losses and amino acid binding of phosphate are minimal.

Clinically, phosphate depletion rarely becomes apparent until serum concentrations decrease below 1.0 mg/100 ml. Symptoms and signs include weakness of the muscles of the extremities, neck, mastication, and respiration. There may be paresthesias, absent deep tendon reflexes, anisocoria, hyperventilation, mental obtundation, and an abnormal electromyogram (196, 211). Bone pain may mimic ankylosing spondylitis. There is a depletion of ATP that conformationally affects RBC membranes, leading to rigid spherocytes. Also seen are abnormal red blood cell and platelet survival times, a shift of the oxyhemoglobin curve to the left, and impaired white blood cell chemotaxis and phagocytosis (45, 101, 211). Phosphate replacement can be accomplished by adding sodium or potassium phosphate to the nutrition solution in excess of maintenance until normal serum inorganic phosphate concentrations are reestablished. To avoid a rapid decrease in calcium and associated tetany, phosphate supplements should be accompanied by 0.2 to 0.3 mEq/kg/day calcium infusion.

Hyperphosphatemia during parenteral nutrition is usually the result of acute and chronic renal failure. When the glomerular filtration rate is ≤20 to 25 ml/min, a large portion of the phosphate becomes nonfilterable and forms colloidal complexes with calcium. These complexes may be responsible for the development of metastatic calcifications in soft tissues and organs. Other etiologies of hyperphosphatemia include neoplastic diseases treated with cytotoxic agents, excessive

oral phosphate ingestion, and administration of phosphate-containing enemas. Hyperphosphatemia may lead to hypocalcemia with possible tetany. Effective treatment consists of the administration of phosphate-binding antacids, which decreases the gastrointestinal absorption of phosphate.

Magnesium

The adult human body contains approximately 2000 mEq of magnesium. Sixty percent is firmly bound to bone. The remaining 800 mEq is distributed in the soft tissues, with only 1.4 to 2.2 mEq/liter circulating in the blood. Of soft tissues, liver and striated muscle have the highest concentrations. Balance studies have indicated that 0.30 to 0.35 mEq/kg/day magnesium is required orally to maintain positive balance in normal persons (65). It is absorbed by the entire small intestine and by at least part of the colon. Excess dietary intake is excreted by the kidneys, with only small amounts lost in the feces. During magnesium deprivation, renal losses decrease markedly to less than 1 mEq/day (194).

Magnesium ion is important metabolically in the activation of many enzyme systems critical to cellular metabolism. It is a cofactor for oxidative phosphorylation; stabilizes macromolecular structures such as DNA, RNA, and ribosomes; assists in the binding of messenger RNA to the 70S ribosome in protein synthesis; and is active in the transfer of high-energy phosphate radicals to and from adenosine triphosphate.

Hypomagnesemia during parenteral nutrition may result from inadequate supplementation of the feeding solution. It may be preexisting due to various malabsorption syndromes, extensive small bowel resections, intestinal or biliary tract fistulas, prolonged vomiting or nasogastric suction, chronic alcoholism, pancreatitis, parathyroid disease, and diabetes, especially if large insulin doses are required. Excessive renal losses of magnesium can occur due to diuretic abuse with mercurials, ammonium chloride, and thiazides; during the diuretic phase of acute renal failure when losses can be very high; or to various intrinsic renal diseases such as glomerulonephritis, pyelonephritis, and nephrosclerosis (6). Clinical manifestations of magnesium deficiency are usually present when the serum concentrations are less than 1.0 mEq/liter. Many signs and symptoms resemble those of calcium depletion. Differentiation from calcium deficiency is essential, as tetany from hypocalcemia is only temporarily corrected by magnesium administration and vice versa. Most clinical signs of hypomagnesemia are related to increased neuromuscular irritability, such as confusion, hyperactive deep tendon reflexes, convulsions, tetany, positive Chvostek's sign, tremor, clonus, nystagmus, muscle fasciculation, paresthesias, and weakness (195). It is important for the patient in the intensive care unit that magnesium decreases cardiac irritability in ischemic disease and improves coronary artery blood flow. A deficiency of magnesium has been associated with early mitochondrial and sarcosomal damage and frank myocardial necrosis and calcification (189). There may be depression of ST segments, inverted T waves in precordial leads, tachycardia, and an accentuation of digitalis toxicity, much as in the presence of hypokalemia (191). Finally, magnesium deficiency can result in severe potassium wasting in the urine. Treatment of magnesium deficiency is by administration of up to 40

Table 60.5. Recommended Daily Intravenous Allowances for Essential Trace Elements

Element	Site of Excretion	RDA (i.v.)[a]
Chromium	7–10 μg/day urine	10–15 μg/day
Copper	25 ± 13 μg/kg/day in bile	0.5–1.5 mg/day
Iodine		1–2 μg/kg/day
Iron	0.1 mg urine 0.3–0.5 mg feces ± sweat/skin Total = 0.5–2.5 mg/day	0.5–1.0 mg/day
Manganese	Bile and pancreatic secretions	0.15–0.8 mg/day
Selenium	?	40–120 μg/day
Zinc	0.3–0.7 mg/day urine (up to 8 mg/day in stress) 17.1 mg/kg stool 12.2 mg/kg UGI drainage	2.5–4 mg/day

[a] RDA from Expert Panel for Nutrition Advisory Group, AMA Department of Food and Nutrition: guidelines for essential trace element preparations for parenteral use. *JAMA* 241:2052–2054, 1979.

mEq/day of magnesium sulfate, with the rate of administration depending on the clinical situation.

Hypermagnesemia is rare during parenteral nutrition, except in patients with renal failure, diabetic acidosis, aldosterone deficiency, hyperparathyroidism, and those who use magnesium-containing laxatives and enemas excessively (6). The clinical spectrum of hypermagnesemia usually involves impairment of neuromuscular transmission, as reflected by hypotension, nausea, vomiting, lethargy, drowsiness, hyporeflexia, weakness, respiratory depression, coma, and cardiac arrest. ECG changes reveal prolongation of the QT and PR intervals and various degrees of atrioventricular block. Intravenous calcium can temporarily reverse the depressant effects of excess magnesium, and in severe cases, hemodialysis can be used to lower serum magnesium concentrations rapidly.

TRACE ELEMENT DEFICIENCY

As the application of intravenous nutrition has increased, various deficiency syndromes of the trace elements have been observed. These deficiencies develop for several possible reasons: inadequate supplementation in the intravenous solution; increased utilization; decreased plasma binding secondary to either decrease in synthesis or loss of the plasma binding proteins; or increased excretion. Clinical symptoms may take months to become evidence because of body stores of the trace elements.

Chromium, cobalt, copper, iodine, iron, manganese, selenium, and zinc are essential to human nutrition. Cadmium, fluorine, molybdenum, nickel, silicon, tin, and vanadium are believed to be possibly needed during intravenous nutrition. In patients with renal and hepatic dysfunction, appropriate adjustments in dosage must be made. Table 60.5 details the route of excretion, recommended daily supplementation, body stores, and measured levels of the nine essential trace elements (81).

ESSENTIAL TRACE ELEMENTS

Chromium

Chromium is found in high concentrations in many proteins and nucleic acids, where it is thought to stabilize their tertiary structures. It also apparently stimulates hepatic synthesis of fatty acids and cholesterol from acetate. Of importance in parenteral nutrition, chromium plays a critical role in the metabolism of glucose through its close association with the glucose tolerance factor (GTF). In combination with GTF, chromium potentiates the effect of insulin upon muscle and fat cells, driving glucose intracellularly. Jeejeebhoy et al (104) described a case of chromium deficiency in a patient receiving home parenteral nutrition for 3 years. Symptoms included weight loss, hyperglycemia, abnormal glucose tolerance, and a diabetes-like peripheral neuropathy.

Cobalt

The only human requirement for cobalt is the amount necessary for the structure of vitamin B_{12}. Human beings are unable to incorporate cobalt into the corrinoid ring of this vitamin; therefore, the active cobalt that is absorbed is in the form of intact vitamin B_{12}.

Copper

The adult body contains 75 to 150 mg of copper, which is located mainly in brain, liver, heart, spleen, kidneys, and blood. Serum copper concentrations range from 75 to 150 μg/100 ml, of which approximately 95% is bound to a circulating α_2-globulin, ceruloplasmin. The major excretory route of copper is the biliary system, with 25 ± 13 μg/kg/day lost (15, 59).

Copper has many biologic functions similar to those of iron, including a role in the formation of hemoglobin and red blood cells. It also is involved in the activity of cytochrome oxidase, the terminal oxidase in the electron transport mechanism from which high-energy phosphate bonds are derived (130). Copper plays an essential role in connective tissue integrity. It is necessary for the maintenance of normal amine oxidase activity, which converts lysine to desmosine and isodesmosine, the amino acids required for cross-linkage of elastin. Lysyl oxidase, another enzyme required for collagen cross-linkage, is also copper-dependent. Copper is a functional part of the enzyme tyrosinase, which is essential for conversion of tyrosine to melanin. Finally, copper-containing proteins from the brain (cerebrocuprein) and from the liver (hepatocuprein and mitochondrocuprein) have been isolated. The function of these proteins, however, is unknown.

Copper deficiency during parenteral nutrition commonly presents as a hematologic abnormality consisting of anemia and neutropenia, often with marked decrease in polymorphonuclear cells (216). The precise mechanism for these changes is unclear, but it is known that in copper deficiency, iron stores are not effectively utilized for heme formation. Zidar et al (230) showed an inappropriately low level of erythropoietin for the degree of anemia during zinc deficiency and demonstrated ineffective granulopoiesis. In children, copper deficiency may lead to osteoporosis (91).

Acute copper toxicity follows ingestion of more than 15 mg of elemental copper and is associated with nausea, vomiting, intestinal cramps, diarrhea, intravascular hemolysis, and renal impairment.

Iodine

Much has been written about iodine and its deficiency syndrome of thyroid goiter. Iodine is an integral part of the thyroid hormones thyroxine and triiodothyronine, and as such plays an important role in the regulation of body metabolism.

Iron

Iron is necessary for the production of hemoglobin and myoglobin, as well as for the functioning of some essential metabolic enzymes. Deficiency is characterized by a hypochromic, microcytic anemia, by low serum iron, and by high total iron binding capacity. Its deficiency leads to increased susceptibility to helminth infections, depression of cellular immunity, and a decrease in bactericidal activity of leukocytes (37, 108, 221). If anemia is present due to iron deficiency, the following formula is useful to determine the amount of iron needed to correct iron deficiency:

$$Iron\ (mg)\ needed = 0.3\ (wt\ in\ lb) \times \frac{100 - Hgb \times 100}{14.8}$$

Manganese

Manganese participates as a cofactor in many enzyme systems, including those involved with protein synthesis via stimulation of RNA and DNA polymerase activity and chondroitin sulfate synthesis. Doisy (56) reported a case of human manganese deficiency manifested by weight loss, dermatitis, slow growth, change in hair color, poor protein synthesis, and hypocholesterolemia. Toxicity of manganese is rare, but it may damage the extrapyramidal system, causing symptoms resembling Parkinson's disease.

Selenium

Selenium is involved as a catalyst for the important enzyme glutathione peroxidase (208). This enzyme protects against oxidative stress and cellular damage by peroxides. Selenium can, therefore, function as an antioxidant and is probably important in metabolic processing of many drugs. In experimental animals, selenium deficiency can cause liver necrosis, pancreatic atrophy, and a form of muscular dystrophy. In the human, several case reports have been published describing severe muscle pain, thigh tenderness, and cardiomyopathy (22, 62, 175, 214, 219).

Zinc

Zinc was first shown to be essential in 1934 (210). It is required for both RNA and DNA synthesis, as well as for the proper functioning of a number of zinc-dependent metabolic enzymes, including aldolases, dehydrogenases, peptidases, and thymidine kinases. A deficiency of zinc in the diet has been associated with growth retardation (85), impaired wound healing (170), alopecia (111), depressed cellular immunity (165), acrodermatitis enteropathica-like skin lesions (86), anorexia with impairment of taste and smell, hypogonadism,

diarrhea, and glucose intolerance (173). Patients prone to develop zinc deficiency include those on long-term corticosteroid therapy; those patients with bilateral adrenalectomies; patients undergoing major surgical procedures; those who have experienced extensive trauma or have sepsis; patients with various malabsorption syndromes, including enterocutaneous fistulas; and patients with low dietary intake of zinc. Zinc toxicity has been associated with fever, nausea, vomiting, and diarrhea.

POSSIBLY ESSENTIAL TRACE ELEMENTS

Cadmium

Much of the importance of cadmium appears to lie in its interactions with other trace elements, competing directly with intracellular ligands. Deficiency states in the human have yet to be described, and daily requirements are unknown. Due to its long metabolic half-life, cadmium supplementation during parenteral nutrition is considered unnecessary at this time.

Fluorine

Fluorine may play an important role in fertility, growth, and maintenance of a normal hematocrit. It also is beneficial for maintenance of teeth and the bony skeleton.

Molybdenum

This metal is essential for the activity of xanthine oxidase. There are no documented deficiency syndromes in humans.

Nickel

Deficiency of nickel in animals has led to impairment of reproduction, hair loss, and hepatocyte dysfunction. There has been no documented deficiency in humans.

Silicon

Silicon appears to be involved in bone calcification, structure of cartilage matrix, and possible mucopolysaccharide metabolism. No human deficiency syndrome is known.

Tin

Tin may contribute to the tertiary structure of proteins. No deficiency syndrome is documented.

Vanadium

Deficiency of this element in animals retards growth, increases packed red blood cell values, increases plasma triglycerides, impairs reproduction, and impairs bony development. No human deficiency is documented.

VITAMIN DEFICIENCIES

Vitamins are essential components in the metabolism of carbohydrates, protein, and fat. It is only over the past 40 to 50 years that the symptoms of various vitamin deficiencies have been well-delineated. Recommended daily allowances for each vitamin are established by the National Research Council (207). Unfortunately, these values are based on oral, rather than intravenous, nutrition and changes in requirements that might occur with various disease and injury states are unknown. For convenience the various vitamins are divided into two groups: those that are fat-soluble and those that are water-soluble.

FAT-SOLUBLE VITAMINS (A, D, E, K)

Vitamin A

The activity of vitamin A is measured in international units (IU), where one IU is equal to 0.3 μg of crystalline vitamin A alcohol or 0.6 μg of β-carotene. The decreased biologic activity of carotene is due to the less efficient absorption from the intestine and to an inefficiency in converting carotene to vitamin A. In the normal healthy person there are about 600,000 IU of vitamin A, which is stored mainly in the liver. Serum vitamin A concentrations are very small, compared to the liver and serum measurements; therefore, they do not serve as a very good indicator of total body stores. The hepatic reserve could theoretically support the body's metabolic needs for 3 months to 1 year under normal health conditions. If a patient suffers an infectious process, develops hypothermia, or is exposed to other stresses, however, the liver stores of vitamin A rapidly diminish and, if adequate supplementation is not provided, deficiency symptoms may occur within much shorter periods.

Deficiencies of vitamin A usually occur when there is interference with absorption or storage, inadequate dietary intake, interference with conversion from carotene to vitamin A, and when there is rapid loss from the body. Deficiencies of vitamin A are associated with nyctalopia, xerophthalmia, phrynoderma, decreased resistance to infection, retardation of growth, decreased production of corticosteroids, and mild leukopenia with a decrease in polymorphonuclear leukocytes and an increase in juvenile forms. Vitamin A deficiency can easily be prevented by providing adequate supplementation either orally or intravenously. The recommended oral intake of vitamin A is 2667 IU/day for females and 3333 IU/day for males (207). Suggested intravenous supplementation of vitamin A is 3330 IU/day (155).

Vitamin D

The activity of vitamin D is also measured in international units, where 1 mg vitamin D equals 40,000 IU. Normally, vitamin D stores are maintained through both dietary intake and internal synthesis from the action of ultraviolet light on the skin. It is transported to the liver, where it is hydroxylated to 25-(OH)D3 and then converted by the renal mitochondria to the highly active form 1,25-(OH)2D3. In the 1,25-(OH)2D3 form, vitamin D regulates calcium and phosphorus homeostasis in conjunction with the two hormones parathormone and thyrocalcitonin. Vitamin D increases absorption of calcium and phosphate from the intestine and regulates the rate of reabsorption of phosphates by the renal tubules. Deficiency of vitamin D leads to osteomalacia (rickets), decreased serum calcium and phosphorus, and elevated alkaline phosphatase

levels. Tetany due to hypocalcemia may occur. Proposed maintenance therapy for vitamin D is 200 IU/day orally or intravenously (155, 207).

Vitamin K

Vitamin K can be either synthesized by gut flora or extracted from ingested food. Absorption requires the presence of bile salts and pancreatic juices. Vitamin K plays an essential role in synthesis of clotting factors (II, VII, IX, X). Deficiency of vitamin K leads to a prolongation of the prothrombin time. The recommended daily oral intake for vitamin K is 65 μg for females and 80 μg for males (207). During intravenous nutrition, if there is some intestinal function, vitamin K has been given orally as 5 mg twice a week with apparent adequate supplementation. Jeejeebhoy et al have suggested that 5 mg/week be administered intramuscularly (105).

Vitamin E

There is much speculation about the function of vitamin E in human nutrition. It may serve primarily as an antioxidant, thereby inhibiting the oxidation of unsaturated free fatty acids. Deficiency states of vitamin E are well-described and include anemia secondary to hemolysis, excessive creatinuria, deposition of a ceroid material in smooth muscle, lesions in skeletal muscles similar to those found in muscular dystrophy, and increased platelet aggregation (17, 125). The recommended daily oral allowance for vitamin E is 11 IU for females and 14 IU for males (207). Suggested intravenous support is 10 IU/day (155). Requirements for vitamin E are increased by the administration of polyunsaturated fatty acids, and additional vitamin E is recommended if fat emulsions are utilized to any great extent as a caloric source.

WATER-SOLUBLE VITAMINS

Tissue stores of water-soluble vitamins are small, and deficiencies can develop rapidly with any interruption of dietary intake. For that reason, patients receiving parenteral nutrition must be given ample supplementation early in their treatment. The clinical syndromes seen due to deficiency of the various water-soluble vitamins are similar. For that reason, both maintenance and replacement therapy are accomplished with a mixture of the various vitamins. Any excesses in administration of the water-soluble vitamins are excreted in the urine, making toxic complications very rare. Due to the wide therapeutic index, usually 2 to 3 times the normal RDA for water-soluble vitamins are given during parenteral nutrition.

Thiamine-Vitamin B₁

Thiamine functions as a coenzyme for the enzyme transketolase, which is important in the phosphogluconate pathway and, therefore, in the generation of reduced nicotinamide-adenine dinucleotide phosphate. Thiamine is also believed to be a structural component of nervous system membranes. Nutritional deficiencies are common, owing to its limited distribution in foods. Mild deficiency leads to peripheral neuropathy characterized by paresthesias, hyperesthesia, anesthesia, and weakness. Muscles become tender and atrophic, and there may be foot or wrist drop.

Severe deficiency of thiamine results in beriberi. Clinically, patients may develop cardiomegaly (especially right-sided), along with tachycardia, palpitations, dependent edema, and arteriovenous shunting. Acute pernicious beriberi may occur if a patient becomes acutely thiamine-deficient during parenteral nutrition. This complication is associated with a mortality rate of up to 50%. High-output cardiac failure may be severe.

In protracted thiamine deficiency, the clinical syndrome of Wernicke's encephalopathy is more commonly observed (20). Early recognition of thiamine deficiency with institution of adequate replacement usually results in a rapid and complete recovery from all symptoms. Failure to treat can result in permanent neurologic damage.

Recommended daily supplementation of thiamine in the oral diet is 1.1 mg for females and 1.5 mg for males (207). Although the intravenous requirements are really unknown, general recommendations are for administration of 3 mg/day during parenteral nutrition (155).

Riboflavin-Vitamin B$_2$

Riboflavin is a constituent of two coenzymes, riboflavin-5′-phosphate and flavin adenine dinucleotide. These coenzymes are important components of several oxidative enzyme systems involved in electron transport, including xanthine oxidase, glutathione reductase, amino acid oxidases, and succinic dehydrogenase.

There are essentially no stores of riboflavin, and deficiency symptoms develop rapidly with dietary restriction. Symptoms include inflammation of the lips, fissures at the corners of the mouth, scaliness of the skin, seborrheic dermatitis about nose and scrotum, and vascularization of the cornea—a clinical spectrum called cheilosis. The recommended daily oral requirements for riboflavin are 1.3 mg for females and 1.7 mg for males (207). Intravenous requirements are not well-established, but it is recommended that 3.6 to 7.5 mg/day be given (155).

Pantothenic Acid-Vitamin B$_3$

Coenzyme A is the only known functional form of pantothenic acid. Coenzyme A takes part in all acylation reactions. There is no documented deficiency syndrome of pantothenic acid. There is no specified daily allowance established, but recommended oral intake is 5 to 10 mg/day (207). The suggested intravenous supplementation is 10 to 29 mg/day (155).

Niacin-Vitamin B$_5$

Niacin plays an important role in body metabolism due to its incorporation into nicotinamide-adenine dinucleotide and nicotinamide-adenine dinucleotide phosphate (NAD and NADH). These coenzymes participate in the intracellular respiratory mechanism of all cells by assisting in the stepwise transfer of hydrogen from glycolysis to the flavin mononucleotide. The reduced forms of the coenzymes also participate in many biosynthetic pathways, including the synthesis of fatty acids.

Deficiency of niacin results in the disease known as pellagra. Clinical symptoms include weakness, lassitude, anorexia, dermatitis, and inflammation of the mouth. Prevention of niacin deficiency is accomplished by providing oral niacin at 15

mg/day for females and 19 mg/day for males. Intravenous supplementation has been recommended at 40 mg/day (155).

Pyridoxine-Vitamin B$_6$

Pyridoxine functions as a coenzyme for transaminases, decarboxylases, for the two enzyme systems involved in the metabolism of sulfur-containing amino acids, and for phosphorylase. Pyridoxine also function as a cofactor for hydroxylases, synthetases, and many other enzymes. Deficiency of vitamin B$_6$ is well-described. Personality changes, irritability, depression, filiform hypertrophy of the lingua papilla, and stomatitis characterize the deficiency syndrome. There is also a strong tendency to develop genitourinary infections. Prolonged vitamin B$_6$ deficiency leads to sideroblastic anemia. Vitamin B$_6$ deficiency is accentuated by certain antagonists such as isoniazid, penicillamine, and cycloserine (116). The recommended oral intake of pyridoxine is 1.6 mg/day for females and 2.0 mg/day for men (207). Suggested intravenous supplementation is 4.0 mg/day (155).

Biotin-Vitamin B$_7$

The main metabolic activity of biotin is in carboxylation reactions. As biotin can be synthesized by the intestinal flora, deficiency syndromes are rare. To date, six instances of biotin deficiency have been reported during long-term parenteral nutrition (140). Biotin deficiency can result in cutaneous, ophthalmic, and neurologic manifestations. The cutaneous symptoms include erythematous impetigo-like eruptions in cutaneomucosal transitional areas, such as the corners of the eyelid and mouth and the perineal region, and total loss of body hair. The skin may demonstrate a fine, scaly desquamation without pruritus. Ophthalmologic manifestations include blurred vision caused by diffuse keratoconjunctivitis, loss of eyebrows and eyelashes, skin eruptions around the eyes, and photophobia caused by keratitis. Neurologic symptoms have included an occasional depressive reaction, along with paresthesias, tremors, and ataxia. Other symptoms may include anemia, anorexia, nausea, lassitude, and muscle pain. Adult requirements for biotin are not determined.

Folic Acid-Vitamin B$_9$

Folate participates in the uptake and transfer of 1-carbon fragments. It is involved in a multitude of metabolic processes such as purine synthesis, pyrimidine nucleotide biosynthesis, and various 3-carbon amino acid conversions. Stores of folate can usually last 3 to 6 months upon complete dietary restriction (92); in stressed patients, depletion may be more rapid. As serum folate concentrations are normally only 5 to 16 ng/ml and body folate stores range from 5 to 10 mg, serum measurements do not accurately reflect tissue stores.

Deficiencies of folic acid can result from inadequate absorption secondary to a host of diseases or competing drugs (220); from deficiency of vitamin B$_{12}$, which participates in removal of a methyl group to form the active tetrahydrofolic acid; and from increased requirements associated with pregnancy, malignancy, sepsis, and anemia. Symptoms include megaloblastic anemia and diarrhea. Recommended oral intake for folate is 180 μg/day for females and 200 μg/day for males (207). Suggested intravenous supplementation is 400 μg/day (155).

Cyanocobalamin-Vitamin B₁₂

Vitamin B₁₂ has many metabolic functions, but primarily it acts as a transmethylating agent. Therefore, it is important in the biosynthesis of thiamine, methionine and, possibly, choline. By an unknown mechanism, vitamin B₁₂ assists in the movement of folate into cells. It is also involved in many different enzyme reactions and therefore is important in the normal metabolism of fat, carbohydrate, and protein.

Absorption of vitamin B₁₂ from the diet is dependent upon two mechanisms: separation of the vitamin from food under the action of gastric acid and intestinal enzymes and an interaction with gastric intrinsic factor. Normal stores of vitamin B₁₂ are from 1 to 2 mg, with the liver containing 50 to 90% of the total. The normal serum concentration is 200 to 900 g/ml. A deficiency of vitamin B₁₂ during short-term dietary restriction is rare because of large stores and an efficient enterohepatic circulation. When deficiencies do occur, it may take 3 to 6 years to become clinically evident. Deficiencies are characterized by a megaloblastic anemia (pernicious anemia), glossitis, impairment of myelinization of peripheral nerves, and platelet aggregation defects, resulting in a prolonged bleeding time (128). Neurologic symptoms develop insidiously with peripheral paresthesias, decreased vibratory sense, ataxia, central scotomata, confusion, and possible psychosis.

The recommended daily maintenance for vitamin B₁₂ is 2.0 μg (207). Intravenous supplementation has been estimated to be 5.0 μ/day (155). Deficiency symptoms can usually be treated with a single injection of 100 to 1000 μg of vitamin B₁₂. (Note: Begin with no more than 100 μg, as larger doses may cause severe hypokalemia.)

Ascorbic Acid-Vitamin C

Vitamin C is active in forming collagen, transporting mitochondrial electrons, metabolizing tyrosine, converting folate to tetrahydrofolic acid, and metabolizing cholesterol. Body stores of vitamin C are minimal. The small stores, coupled with the increased urinary losses associated with stress, can result in clinical symptoms of vitamin C deficiency rapidly during parenteral nutrition if adequate supplements are not given. The deficiency syndrome is termed scurvy. Scurvy is characterized by anemia, joint pain, mucous membrane hemorrhages, weakness, and emaciation. Less severe vitamin C deficiencies impair wound healing, diminish host immunity, and slow tyrosine metabolism.

The recommended daily oral intake is 60 mg (207). Suggested intravenous supplementation is 100 mg/day (155). It should be noted that ascorbic acid interferes with the anticoagulant effects of heparin: 2 mg of ascorbic acid neutralize 1 unit of heparin (164).

OTHER COMPLICATIONS OF PARENTERAL NUTRITION

ELEVATED LIVER FUNCTION TEST

A high percentage of patients receiving parenteral nutrition developed increases of serum bilirubin and hepatic enzymes in early reports. Liver biopsies obtained at these times revealed periportal fatty changes with little evidence of inflammation or other abnormalities. With utilization of mixed-fuel formulas and reduction in the infusion of glucose, the frequency of enzyme abnormalities has significantly decreased, but abnormal values are still observed (40, 79, 142, 193, 213). There is much speculation as to the etiology of these liver changes, but attempted correlation with various parameters has been unsuccessful. The liver enzyme elevations do not correlate with the initiation of feeding preoperatively vs. postoperatively, with the mean serum glucose level, or with the amount of exogenous insulin administered. Possible etiologies have included toxic conversion products of the amino acid tryptophan in the presence of sodium bisulfite, progressive intrahepatic cholestases with bile duct proliferation and bile plugging, an imbalance in the calorie-to-nitrogen ratio, a lack of essential fatty acids, excessive infusion of lipid emulsions, deficiency of lipotropic factors with a decreased ability to transport lipid away from the liver due to a deficiency of lipotropic factors, and a possible amino acid allergy. Hall et al documented abnormalities in fat synthesis, fat oxidation, fat uptake, and fat mobilization by the liver (82). The precise etiology of hepatic injury remains to be determined. Most investigators feel it is due to glucose overloading and emphasize the use of mixed fuels for caloric support (fat and glucose) and avoidance of overfeeding (181).

ELEVATION OF BLOOD UREA NITROGEN (BUN)

Most patients given parenteral nutrition demonstrate some increase of BUN, even if their renal function is normal. The elevations are due to increased protein loading and, at times, dehydration. Rarely does the BUN exceed accepted normal values if renal function is satisfactory. In patients with depressed renal function, the BUN may progressively increase and limit the amount of nitrogen that can be infused. Usually, increased BUN causes few clinical problems until it exceeds 100 mg/dl, at which time mental status and platelet function can be compromised. If the creatinine clearance is >20 ml/min, at least 9 g of nitrogen per day will be well-tolerated. With more severe renal failure, special formulas may be required to reduce nitrogen support to under 9 g/day (see later discussion of Renal Failure).

ESSENTIAL FATTY ACID DEFICIENCY

There are three polyunsaturated fatty acids that cannot be synthesized by humans (linoleic, arachidonic, and linolenic). Only linoleic acid is essential in the adult diet. Arachidonic acid can be synthesized when linoleic acid is present, and the precise role and need for linolenic acid in the adult is undetermined. The essential fatty acids (EFA) play a primary role in the structure and maintenance of cell membranes, prostaglandin synthesis, and various transport mechanisms. EFA deficiency leads to a decrease in the efficiency of calorie utilization and, possibly, the dissociation of oxidative phosphorylation and impairment of production of high-energy phosphate bonds. The clinical symptoms of EFA deficiency include diarrhea, dryness of skin, hair loss, impaired wound healing, and brittle and osteoporotic bones (97). Biochemical changes include decreased cholesterol levels, thrombocytopenia, increased platelet aggregation, increased capillary permeability, anemia, increased red blood cell fragility, elevations of serum hepatic enzymes, and fatty infiltration of the liver (198). Biochemical signs of EFA deficiency may develop early over the first few days of fat-free parenteral nutrition, whereas clinical symptoms usually require several weeks to become obvious.

EFA deficiency can be documented by an increased serum 5,8,11-eicosatrienoic:arachidonic acid ratio that is normally less than 0.4 (96, 97). All symptoms can be reversed with the administration of linoleic acid. If the oral route is available, oils high in linoleic acid, such as corn oil or safflower oil, may be administered (5 ml 2 or 3 times/day). Before intravenous lipid emulsions were available, some clinicians found the topical application of corn oil or safflower oil to the skin to be effective (15 ml three times/day) (174). With the development of safe intravenous lipid emulsions, however, intravenous infusion is preferable and appears to be fully satisfactory in preventing and correcting any deficiency. The RDA for EFA is not established, but suggested intravenous supplementation ranges from a minimum of 1% to 4% of the total caloric intake (25 to 100 mg/kg/day of linoleic acid) (96, 209).

HYPOALBUMINEMIA

Albumin is a major synthetic product of the liver. On the average, about 130 to 200 mg/kg/day is synthesized, but it may be as high as 860 mg/kg/day during maximum synthesis. Depressed serum albumin concentrations may result from decreased synthesis, increased degradation, or altered fluid status. Decreased synthesis is seen in patients with marked malnutrition, cancer, acute stress, cirrhosis, hypothyroidism, and following exposure to hepatic toxins. Increased degradation is most commonly due to the presence of a catabolic state (58). The state of hydration, in particular dehydration, can dramatically alter serum albumin concentrations. A normal value may be less than 2.5 g/dl after a rehydration is accomplished. Finally, following any stressful event, albumin is sequestered into third space fluid with serum values falling in spite of normal total body albumin. Most of the body albumin is in the extravascular space maintained in sluggish equilibrium with serum albumin. This fact, coupled with large body stores (4.5 to 5.0 g/kg), makes serum concentrations an unreliable indicator of total body albumin, except in a perfectly steady state.

Hypoalbuminemia has been associated with impairment of soft and bony tissue healing, decreased immune defenses (126), depressed gastrointestinal motility (152), and impaired intestinal absorption of water and electrolytes (153). A major function of albumin is binding and transporting various products of metabolism, serving both as a detoxifying agent and as a transport agent. Because of these later functions, an attempt should be made during intravenous nutrition to reestablish normal total body albumin content. The approximate amount of total albumin necessary to replete any deficit can be determined by the formula (23):

$$y = 0.33 + 0.003x$$

Where y = change in serum albumin concentration desired (g/100 ml) and x = amount of exogenous albumin to be given in grams.

When albumin is given alone without adequate nutritional support, a significant portion is used as a caloric substrate. When given with adequate caloric support, however, its half-life approaches normal. In patients who have acute respiratory distress or possible damage to pulmonary capillary integrity, it may not be wise to administer albumin because it may leak into the perivascular pulmonary tissues (95). Use of good clinical judgment is necessary in deciding whether or not to administer albumin during parenteral nutrition.

ACID-BASE DERANGEMENTS

Enzymatic and metabolic processes in the human body are quite pH-sensitive. It is important to monitor and maintain normal acid-base homeostasis when administering parenteral nutrition. Metabolic acidosis can usually be attributed to either abnormal acid production or to excessive loss of base. Some of the diseases or processes leading to excessive production of acid are diabetes mellitus, hyperthyroidism, high-fat diets, hepatitis, general anesthesia, sepsis, and low cardiac output syndromes leading to lactic acidosis. Disease states that may lead to excessive loss of bicarbonate include diarrhea; loss of pancreatic, biliary, or small intestinal fluid from drainage tubes or via fistulas; renal insufficiency; and the administration of acidifying salts.

Parenteral nutrition also has the potential for causing or magnifying acid-base disturbances. Although synthetic L-amino acids contain one-third to one-fifth the titratable acidity of the older protein hydrolysates, the increased amount of cationic amino acids, compared to anionic amino acids, is enough to induce metabolic acidosis in selected patients (90). In addition, metabolic acidosis may result from excessive chloride administration. In this setting, an increased quantity of chloride ions are filtered at the renal glomerulus, providing more chloride for reabsorption in the distal renal tubules, along with sodium. The increased sodium chloride reabsorption inversely effects hydrogen ion secretion into the tubules, leading to an alkaline urine, hyperchloremia, and metabolic acidosis.

Metabolic alkalosis during parenteral nutrition may result from gastric suctioning, vomiting, diarrhea, diuretic intake, excessive administration of potassium-free solution, ingestion of antacids, and hyperadrenocorticism. The main problem associated with long-term intravenous nutrition is the common need to aspirate the stomach due to gastrointestinal ileus. In addition to the loss of hydrogen ions in the aspirate, there is a loss of chloride ions, leaving less chloride for filtration by the renal glomerulus and, therefore, greater amounts of hydrogen ion secreted in the distal tubule in exchange for sodium.

To avoid complicating the clinical course of patients in the intensive care unit, it is important to take steps to avoid disturbances of acid-base balance. To avoid any difficulties of excess chloride infusion, the sodium-to-chloride ratio in the infused solution should be adjusted to 1:1 with additional anions given as acetate, lactate, or phosphate. Nasogastric losses should be replaced carefully with appropriate electrolyte solutions. Administration of an H_2 blocker may be of help, and in severe acid depletion dilute hydrochloric acid may be infused intravenously (up to 0.2 N hydrochloric acid is compatible with crystalline amino acid solutions or standard dextrose solutions and can be administered via the central venous line). Trace elements, vitamins, and other low-priority additives should be removed when hydrochloric acid is added to prevent untoward reactions.

If a metabolic acidosis is present, the nutrition solution formula can be modified to reduce the amount of chloride ion to below the sodium content, forcing the kidneys to conserve hydrogen ion. On the other hand, if a metabolic alkalosis is present, excessive chloride ion, compared to sodium ion, can force the kidneys to excrete hydrochloric acid. Normal renal function is necessary to accomplish the above metabolic manipulations (an adequate renal response can be confirmed by simply measuring the pH of the excreted urine).

LETHARGY

Patients will occasionally become weak, tired, lethargic, and even semicomatose upon initiation of intravenous nutrition. The cause of this lethargy is unknown. One suggestion is that the change from starvation to full nutritional support results in metabolic or hormonal changes that lead to sedation. Any increase in serum tryptophan resulting from infusion of the amino acid solution could enhance its passage into the brain. Increased tryptophan in the brain leads to increased serotonin production and subsequent mental depression. There is no specific therapy for any observed lethargy, and symptoms usually diminish after 6 to 10 days.

ALOPECIA

Partial and even complete loss of hair is common during parenteral nutrition but is usually not due to the nutrition solution. The most common cause is an interruption of the normal hair cycle in response to a stressful event. Hair undergoes three phases of growth. The anagen phase is the period of intense mitotic activity, formation of the hair root, and growth of the hair shaft. The catagen phase is a short period of transition when the hair follicle stops growing and regresses to a state similar to that of the embryologic follicle germ. The final resting state, the telogen phase, is when the keratinized hair shaft and hair bulb are lying within the resting follicle. At some point the follicles are reactivated, and the old hair is shed. Normally, 85% of hairs in the scalp are in the anagen phase while 15% are in the telogen phase. With stress, many hair follicles simultaneously enter the telogen phase. Shortly thereafter, the hair is shed, and the follicles start over in the anagen phase. Hair loss is therefore a temporary event. This process has been termed telogen effluvium (118). Other causes of hair loss include severe protein depletion and zinc deficiency.

REFEEDING SYNDROME

With initiation of parenteral nutrition, particularly in severely malnourished patients, acute fluxes in fluids, electrolytes (phosphorus, potassium, and magnesium), vitamins, and glucose tolerance occur, which have been termed the refeeding syndrome (199). Typically, fluid is retained in excessive amounts with edema of the dependent portions of the body.

The excessive fluid, coupled with increased basal metabolic rate, can lead to acute congestive heart failure or pulmonary edema. In addition to fluid shifts, serum potassium, phosphorus, and magnesium concentrations may decrease as the result of intracellular transport. If inadequately supplemented, severe deficiencies may develop, and clinical symptoms occur within the first 24 to 48 hours of refeeding. The syndrome is often associated with glucose intolerance, lethargy, confusion, weakness, and even coma. Careful initiation and slow advancement of nutritional support in the severely malnourished patient, with careful adjustment of electrolytes, minerals, vitamins, and occasional use of diuretics, can usually minimize the severity of this syndrome.

NUTRITIONAL SUPPORT IN SPECIAL CLINICAL SETTINGS

RENAL FAILURE

Renal failure is a frequent complication in the critically ill patient. Metabolic requirements of these patients are no different than requirements of patients without renal failure (205). Any reduction of metabolic support to avoid volume or protein intolerance should be avoided. Instead, effective dialysis should be established early to permit full nutritional support. Note should be made, however, that there is a significant loss of nitrogen during dialysis that requires additional protein loading during intravenous nutrition. Hemodialysis results in loss of up to 9 g of amino acids and 3 to 4 g of peptides over 4 hours while peritoneal dialysis is associated with loss of up to 15 g of amino acids and 40 g of protein per dialysis.

If dialysis is contraindicated or not available, intravenous feeding should not be withheld but rather the formula should be modified, reducing both volume and protein content. If intravenous protein support must be reduced to below 30 to 40 g/day to avoid problems with BUN (the minimum protein support providing adequate essential amino acids in currently available solutions), administration of supplemental essential amino acids should be considered. Renal failure solutions containing only essential amino acids can be of some use for a limited time in anuric patients who cannot tolerate dialysis. These solutions are packaged in 200- to 250-ml volume and provide approximately 6 g of protein as essential amino acids plus histidine. When mixed with 70% dextrose, caloric and essential amino acid needs can usually be met in 500 to 600 ml of solution. As soon as renal function recovers or dialysis becomes available, the more balanced routine parenteral nutrition solutions are preferable. Routine supplementation of vitamins, essential fatty acids, trace elements, and minerals must be provided, whether specialized renal failure formulas or standard products are used. As the morbidity and mortality of renal failure is due in part to the associated metabolic alterations and nutritional depletion when nutritional support is inadequate, intravenous nutritional support should be considered as an important part of the overall treatment plan whenever possible.

HEPATIC FAILURE

Providing adequate nutritional support to patients with hepatic failure poses a major metabolic problem. These patients often manifest protein intolerance, which is characterized by increased serum ammonia concentrations and hepatic encephalopathy. Studies by Fischer et al (60) suggest that the onset of hepatic encephalopathy may be due to abnormal amino acid profiles due to the altered hepatic function. In particular, straight-chain and aromatic amino acids are increased in the blood and brain, whereas branched-chain amino acids are decreased. The resulting abnormal ratio between aromatic and branched-chain amino acids contributes to altered amino acid transport through the blood-brain barrier and an abnormal neurotransmitter profile (103). Experimentation in the animal, as well as clinical trials in humans, have demonstrated that products containing high concentrations of branched-chain amino acids and low concentrations of aromatic amino acids improve or prevent hepatic encephalopathy while permitting aggressive protein supplementation of up to 100 to 150 g/day (99). Coupled with adequate caloric, vitamin, electrolyte, mineral, and trace element supplementation, anabolism can often be achieved even in the patient with significant hepatic failure (19, 34, 36, 66, 206). Some studies, however, have not confirmed these findings (2, 28, 33, 43, 146, 159, 182, 217). Current recommendations are to provide routine protein loading until or unless encephalopathy is present, at which time use of branched-chain enriched products may be considered. It appears that nutritional support plays little role in altering the course of the hepatic disease but can maintain better nutritional status allowing time for recovery.

RESPIRATORY FAILURE

Depending on the type of respiratory failure, patients require different approaches to nutritional support. If the respiratory failure is due to respiratory muscle depletion, nutritional support is necessary for recovery and should be begun early and continued until resumption of an adequate oral diet. If the patient is initially dependent on a respirator, the level of respiratory support should be adjusted to slowly wean, allowing for exercise of the respiratory muscles. Nutritional support may require an increase in the level of mechanical ventilation due to an associated slight increase in carbon dioxide production. As there is little evidence to support use of lipids to accomplish recovery of respiratory muscle mass or function, the temptation to substitute fat for glucose to reduce carbon dioxide production should be resisted.

If, on the other hand, respiratory failure is due to acute respiratory distress syndrome or pulmonary infection, nutritional support should be given with no consideration for nutrient modification, simply adjusting the respirator to clear any excess carbon dioxide production until the acute illness resolves.

If severe chronic obstructive pulmonary disease is present, a different clinical situation arises. In this setting, although respiratory muscle function is important, any excess glucose infusion, with the associated mild increase in carbon dioxide production, may so aggravate pulmonary function that respiratory support becomes mandatory, and the patient will not be able to be weaned from it (12). In this case, the nutrient solution can be modified, substituting lipid for glucose (up to 50% of the calories can be delivered as fat). Use of structured lipids in this patient population has not yet been evaluated.

CARDIAC FAILURE

Cardiac dysfunction in the malnourished, critically ill patient can occur by means of two mechanisms (94). In the first, patients have intrinsic cardiac disease, such as valvular disease or coronary artery disease, which leads to progressive cardiac failure and subsequent decreased nutritional intake, a clinical state termed cardiac cachexia. Attempts at nutritional rehabilitation without correction of the intrinsic cardiac disease, and sometimes even after correction of their cardiac disease, can be catastrophic. The additional burden on the myocardium of regenerated body cell mass can lead to an excessive demand on the damaged heart and irreversible cardiac failure. Maintenance of body cell mass should be the priority, rather than repletion. Only as myocardial function recovers should attention be turned to repeating body cell mass.

In the second mechanism, patients present with malnutrition as a primary diagnosis with subsequent nutritional injury to the myocardium and cardiac failure. Contrary to patients with cardiac cachexia, these patients require nutritional support as specific therapy. Nutritional support must be initiated slowly and advanced gradually, allowing time for recovery of myocardial function. Patients should be observed carefully for the refeeding syndrome or tachycardia and congestion, as they are quite prone to develop congestive heart failure.

SPINAL CORD INJURY

Most patients with spinal cord injury can be adequately nourished using enteral nutrition. However, some patients have associated injuries, resulting in prolonged ileus. Energy expenditure and nutrient needs, except for nitrogen, are similar to those of other patients with traumatic injuries. Studies by Rodriguez et al (179) have documented that negative nitrogen balance is unavoidable, owing to extensive muscle denervation and subsequent inactivity. Attempts at forcing positive nitrogen balance by increasing nitrogen and caloric infusion can result in overfeeding and hepatic injury. They suggested adjusting caloric loading to 1.6 times basal, preferably using indirect calorimetry to determine needs more accurately. Protein support should be about 2.0 g/Kd/day based on ideal body weight.

SEVERE HEAD INJURY

Intensive nutritional support can reduce complications and improve survival in patients with head injuries (5, 176, 229). The weight loss and severe protein wasting associated with the hypermetabolic response can be minimized if necessary carbohydrate, fat, and protein are provided. Often, it is possible to provide these metabolic substrates via the gastrointestinal tract, either with an oral diet or with nasogastric feeding tubes. When enteral feedings are contraindicated or inadequate, however, supplementary calories and nitrogen should be administered intravenously.

Robertson et al (178) determined the metabolic expenditure of the head-injured patient during the first 2 weeks following injury, using a metabolic cart, and suggested the following predictive formula:

$$\%RME = 152 - 14(GCS) + 0.4(HR) + 7(DSI)$$
$$(r = 0.7, p < 0.0001)$$

Where %RME = resting metabolic expenditure as a percentage of normal; GCS = Glasgow Coma Score; HR = heart rate; DSI = day since injury.

A major contributor to the hypermetabolic state is the associated increased muscle tone. Use of chemical paralysis may be helpful in reducing metabolic expenditure (42). Nitrogen requirements likewise are greater than expected, and nitrogen balance is often not possible until 2 to 3 weeks following injury. Generally, 10 to 15 g of nitrogen are provided during nutritional support.

MULTIPLE ORGAN FAILURE

When malfunction of more than one organ requires nutrient modifications, the ability to support metabolic processes may be severely limited. Whenever possible, dialysis, respiratory support, and cardiotonic drugs should be utilized to allow full nutritional support. The completeness of the nutrient formula should be compromised only when all other support methods fail. The value of restricted support must be questioned. At some yet to be determined point, the cost-benefit-risk ratio favors withholding of intravenous nutrition.

BURNS

There is a dramatic increase in metabolic rate in patients with body surface burns. Failure to meet the increased nutrient needs results in a rapid loss of body mass and associated organ function. It is now standard practice of burn units to initiate nutritional support early in the hospital course (48). Usually, these patients will tolerate oral or enteral nutrition, but at times supplementation via the intravenous route is required. As with volume supplementation in burn patients, formulas have been developed to calculate nitrogen and caloric requirements based on the degree and percent of body burn.

REFERENCES

1. Abel RM, Fischer JE, Buckley ML et al: Malnutrition in cardiac surgical patients. *Arch Surg* 111:45–50, 1976.
2. Achord JL: A prospective randomized trial of peripheral amino acid-glucose supplementation in acute alcoholic hepatitis. *Am J Gastroenterol* 82:871–875, 1987.
3. Addis P, Poo LJ, Lew W: The quantities of proteins lost by the various organs and tissues of the body during a fast. *J Biol Chem* 115:111–116, 1936.
4. Alexander JW, Boyce ST, Babcock GF et al: The process of microbial translocation. *Ann Surg* 212:496–512, 1990.
5. Alexander JW, MacMillan BG, Stinnett JD et al: Beneficial effects of aggressive protein feeding in severely burned children. *Ann Surg* 192:505–517, 1980.
6. Alfrey AC: Disorders of magnesium metabolism. In Shriers RW (ed): *Renal and Electrolyte Disorders.* Boston, Little, Brown, pp 223–243, 1976.
7. Alverdy JA, Aoys E, Weiss-Carrington P et al: The effect of glutamine-enriched TPN on gut immune cellularity. *J Surg Res* 52:34–38, 1992.
8. Apelgren KN: Triple lumen catheters: technological advance or setback? *Am Surg* 53:113–116, 1987.
9. Ardawi MSM: Glutamine and glucose metabolism in human peripheral lymphocytes. *Metabolism* 37:99–103, 1988.
10. Ardawi MSM: Effect of glutamine-enriched total parenteral nutrition on septic rats. *Clin Sci* 81:215–222, 1991.
11. Arora NS, Rochester DF: Respiratory muscle strength and maximal voluntary ventilation in undernourished patients. *Am Rev Respir Dis* 126:5–8, 1982.
12. Askanazi J, Carpentier YA, Elwyn DH et al: Influence of total parenteral nutrition on fuel utilization in injury and sepsis. *Ann Surg* 191:40–46, 1980.
13. Atkinson JB, Bagnall HA, Gomperts E: Investigational use of tissue plasminogen activator (t-PA) for occluded central venous catheters. *J Parenter Enteral Nutr* 14:310–311, 1990.
14. Bach AC, Storck D, Meraihi Z: Medium-chain triglyceride-based fat emulsions: an alternative energy supply in stress and sepsis. *J Parenter Enteral Nutr* 12(suppl):82S–88S, 1988.
15. van Berge Henegouwen GP, Tangedahl TN, Hofmann AF et al: Biliary secretion of copper in healthy man. *Gastroenterology* 72:1228–1231, 1977.
16. Bessey PQ, Watters JM, Aoki TT et al: Combined hormonal infusion simulates the metabolic response to injury. *Ann Surg* 200:264–281, 1984.
17. Binder HJ, Hertin DC, Hurst V et al: Tocopherol deficiency in man. *N Engl J Med* 273:1287–1297, 1965.
18. Black PR, Brooks DC, Bessey PQ et al: Mechanisms of insulin resistance following injury. *Ann Surg* 196:420–435, 1982.
19. Blackburn GL, O'Keefe SJD: Nutrition in liver failure. *Gastroenterology* 97:1049–1051, 1989.
20. Blennow G: Wernicke's encephalopathy following prolonged artificial nutrition. *Am J Dis Child* 129:1456, 1975.
21. Bower RH, Muggia-Sullam M, Vallgren S et al: Branched chain amino acid-enriched solutions in the septic patient. A randomized, prospective trial. *Am Surg* 203:13–20, 1986.
22. Brown MR, Cohen HJ, Lyons JM et al: Proximal muscle weakness and selenium deficiency associated with long term parenteral nutrition. *Am J Clin Nutr* 43:549–554, 1986.
23. Brown RO, Bradley JE, Luther RW: Response of serum albumin concentrations to albumin supplementation during central total parenteral nutrition. *Clin Pharm* 6:222–225, 1987.
24. Bruckner GG, Lokesh B, German B et al: Biosynthesis of prostanoids, tissue fatty acid composition and thrombotic parameters in rats fed diets enriched with docosahexaenoic or eicosapentaenoic acids. *Thromb Res* 34:479–497, 1984.
25. Buchanan N, Davis MD, Eyberg C: Gentamycin pharmacokinetics in kwashiorkor. *Br J Clin Pharmacol* 8:451–453, 1979.
26. Deleted in text.
27. Burke JF, Wolfe RR, Mullany CJ et al: Glucose requirements following burn injury. *Ann Surg* 190:274–285, 1979.
28. Calvey H, Davis M, Williams R: Control trial of nutritional supplementation, with or without branched-chain amino acid enrichment, in treatment of acute alcoholic hepatitis. *J Hepatol* 1:141–151, 1985.
29. Carrico CJ, Meakins JL, Marshall JC et al: Multiple-organ failure syndrome. *Arch Surg* 121:196–208, 1986.
30. Cerami A: Materials which promote and inhibit the biosynthesis of cachectin. A macrophage protein which induces catabolic state: a review. In *Mechanism of Drug Action.* Academic Press, New York, pp 175–186, 1983.
31. Cerra FB, Mazuski JE, Chute E et al: Branched chain metabolic support. A prospective randomized, double-blind trial in surgical stress. *Ann Surg* 199:286–291, 1964.
32. Cerra FB, Siegel JH, Border JR et al: The hepatic failure of sepsis: cellular versus substrate. *Surgery* 86:409–422, 1979.
33. Cerra FB: A multi-center trial of branched chain enriched amino acid infusion (FO80) in hepatic encephalopathy. *Hepatology* 2:699, 1982.
34. Cerra FB, McMillen M, Angelico R et al: Cirrhosis, encephalopathy, and improved results with metabolic support. *Surgery* 94:612–619, 1983.
35. Cerra FB, Mazuski JE, Chute E et al: Branched chain metabolic support. A prospective, randomized, double-blind trial in surgical stress. *Ann Surg* 199:286–291, 1984.
36. Cerra FB, Cheung NK, Fischer JE et al: Disease-specific amino acid infusion (F080) in hepatic encephalopathy: a prospective, randomized, double-blind, controlled trial. *J Parenter Enteral Nutr* 9:288–295, 1985.
37. Chandra RK: Reduced bactericidal capacity of polymorphs in iron deficiency. *Arch Dis Child* 48:864–866, 1973.
38. Chen WJ: Utilization of exogenous fat emulsion (Intralipid) in septic rats. *J Parenter Enteral Nutr* 8:14–17, 1984.
39. Chen WJ: Utilization of Intralipid in septic rats: effects of sepsis on the clearance of exogenous fat emulsion from various organs. *J Parenter Enteral Nutr* 10:482–486, 1986.
40. Clarke PH, Ball MJ, Kettlewell MGW: Liver function tests in patients receiving parenteral nutrition. *J Parenter Enteral Nutr* 15:54–59, 1991.
41. Clark-Christoff N, Watters VA, Sparks W et al: Use of triple-lumen subclavian catheters for administration of total parenteral nutrition. *J Parenter Enteral Nutr* 16:403–407, 1992.
42. Clifton GL, Robertson CS, Choi SC: Assessment of nutritional requirements of head injured patients. *J Neurosurg* 64:895–901, 1986.
43. Conn HO: Branched chain amino acids in hepatic encephalopathy. *Hepatology* 6:148–150, 1986.

44. Coran AG, Drongowski RA, Lee GS et al: The metabolism of an exogenous lipid source during septic shock in the puppy. *J Parenter Enteral Nutr* 8:652–656, 1984.

45. Craddock PR, Yawata Y, Van Santen L et al: Acquired phagocyte dysfunction. A complication of the hypophosphatemia of parenteral hyperalimentation. *N Engl J Med* 290:1403–1407, 1974.

46. Crocker KS, Pine RW, Steffe WP: The triple lumen central venous catheter. *Nutr Clin Pract* 1:90–96, 1986.

47. Cruse PJE, Foord R: A five-year prospective study of 23,649 surgical wounds. *Arch Surg* 107:206–210, 1973.

48. Curreri PW: Nutritional support of burn patients. *World J Surg* 2:215–221, 1978.

49. Cuthbertson DP: The disturbances of metabolism produced by bony and non-bony injury, with notes on certain abnormal conditions of bone. *Biochem J* 24:1224–1263, 1930.

50. Dennison AR, Hands LJ, Crowe PJ et al: Total parenteral nutrition using conventional and medium chain triglycerides: effect on liver function tests, complement, and nitrogen balance. *J Parenter Enteral Nutr* 12:15–19, 1988.

51. Dinarello CA: Interleukin-1 and the pathogenesis of the acute phase response. *N Engl J Med* 311:1413–1418, 1984.

52. Dinarello CA: Interleukin-1. *Rev Infect Dis* 6:51–95, 1984.

53. Dinarello CA: An update on human interleukin-1: from molecular biology to clinical relevance. *J Clin Immunol* 5:287–297, 1985.

54. Docomal M, Cantos JW: Hyperosmolar nonketotic coma complicating intravenous hyperalimentation. *Surg Gynecol Obstet* 136:729–732, 1973.

55. Doekel RC, Zwillich CW, Scoggins CH et al: Clinical semistarvation: depression of the hypoxic ventilatory response. *N Engl J Med* 295:358–361, 1976.

56. Doisy Jr EA: Micronutrient control of biosynthesis of clotting proteins and cholesterol. In Hemphill DD (ed): *Proceedings of the University of Missouri's 6th Annual Conference on Trace Substances in Environmental Health*. Columbia, MO, University of Missouri Press, p 193, 1973.

57. Druy EM, Trout HH, Giordano JM et al: Lytic therapy in the treatment of axillary and subclavian vein thrombosis. *J Vasc Surg* 2:821–827, 1985.

58. Eckart J, Tempel G, Schreiber V et al: The turnover of I-125-labeled serum albumin after surgery and injury. In Wilkinson AW (ed): *Parenteral Nutrition*. Churchill Livingstone, Edinburgh, pp 288–298, 1972.

59. Evans GW: Copper homeostasis in the mammalian system. *Physiol Rev* 53:535–570, 1973.

60. Fischer JE, Rosen HM, Ebeid AM et al: The effect of normalization of plasma amino acids on hepatic encephalopathy in man. *Surgery* 80:77–91, 1976.

61. Fleck A: Metabolic response to injury. In Ledingham IM, Mackay G (ed): *Jamieson and Kay's Textbook of Surgery Physiology*. Churchill Livingstone, New York, 1978.

62. Fleming CR, Lie JT, McCall JT et al: Selenium deficiency and fatal cardiomyopathy in a patient on home parenteral nutrition. *Gastroenterology* 83:689–693, 1982.

63. Fong Y, Minei J, Marano MA et al: Cellular injury and decreased mRNA for myofibrillar proteins: potential role of intracellular glutamine as mediator. *Surg Forum* 42:21–23, 1991.

64. Fox AD, Kripke SA, de Paula J et al: Effect of a glutamine-supplemented enteral diet on methotrexate-induced enterocolitis. *J Parenter Enteral Nutr* 12:325–331, 1988.

65. Freeman JB, Wittine MF, Stegink LD et al: Effects of magnesium infusions on magnesium and nitrogen balance during parenteral nutrition. *Can J Surg* 25:570–574, 1982.

66. Freund H, Dienstag J, Lehrich J et al: Infusion of branched-chain enriched amino acid solution in patients with hepatic encephalopathy. *Ann Surg* 196:209–219, 1981.

67. Furst P, Albers S, Stehle P: Evidence for a nutritional need for glutamine in catabolic patients. *Kidney Intern* 36(Suppl 27) 36:S287–S292, 1989.

68. Garre MA, Boles JM, Youinou PY: Current concepts in immune derangement due to malnutrition. *J Parenter Enteral Nutr* 11:309–313, 1987.

69. Gill RT, Kruse JA, Thill-Baharozian MC et al: Triple- vs single-lumen central venous catheters. *Arch Intern Med* 149:1139–1143, 1989.

70. Gimmon Z, Freund HR, Fischer JF: The optimal branched-chain to total amino acid ratio in the injury-adapted amino acid formulation. *J Parenter Enteral Nutr* 9:133–138, 1985.

71. Giovannini I, Chiarla C, Boldrini G et al: Impact of fat and glucose administration on metabolic and respiratory interactions in sepsis. *J Parenter Enteral Nutr* 13:141–146, 1989.

72. Good RA, Fernandes G, West A: Nutrition and immunity. In: *Nutrition Reviews' Present Knowledge in Nutrition*, ed 5. The Nutrition Foundation, Inc, Washington DC, pp 693–710, 1984.

73. Goodenough RD, Wolfe RR: Effect of total parenteral nutrition on free fatty acid metabolism in burned patients. *J Parenter Enteral Nutr* 8:357–360, 1984.

74. Goodwin JS, Webb DR: Regulation of the immune response by prostaglandins. *Clin Immunol Immunopathol* 15:106–122, 1980.

75. Gracey M, Suharjono S, Stone DE: Microbial contamination of the gut: another feature of malnutrition. *Am J Clin Nutr* 26:1170–1174, 1973.

76. Grant JP: *Handbook of Total Parenteral Nutrition*, ed 2. WB Saunders, Philadelphia, p 123, 1992.

77. Grant JP: Clinical impact of protein malnutrition on organ mass and function. In Blackburn GL, Grant JP, Young VR (eds): *Amino Acids Metabolism and Medical Applications*. John Wright PSG Inc, Boston, pp 347–358, 1983.

78. Grant JP, Snyder PJ: Use of l-glutamine in total parenteral nutrition. *J Surg Res* 44:506–513, 1988.

79. Greenlaw C: Liver enzyme elevations associated with total parenteral nutrition. *Drug Intell Clin Pharm* 14:702–709, 1980.

80. Groves AC, Griffiths J, Leung F et al: Plasma catecholamines in patients with serious postoperative infection. *Ann Surg* 178:102–107, 1973.

81. Guidelines for Essential Trace Element Preparations for Parenteral Use: a statement by the Nutrition Advisory Group. *J Parenter Enteral Nutr* 3:263–267, 1979.

82. Hall RI, Grant JP, Ross LH et al: Pathogenesis of hepatic steatosis in the parenterally fed rat. *J Clin Invest* 74:1658–1668, 1984.

83. Hallberg D: Studies on the elimination of exogenous lipid from the bloodstream. The effect of fasting and surgical trauma in man on the elimination rate of a fat emulsion injected intravenously. *Acta Physiol Scand* 65:151–163, 1965.

84. Hamawy KJ, Moldawer LL, Georgieff M et al: The effect of lipid emulsions on reticuloendothelial system function in the injured animal. *J Parenter Enteral Nutr* 9:559–565, 1985.

85. Hambridge RM, Hambridge C, Jacobs M et al: Low levels of zinc in hair, anorexia, poor growth, and hypogeusia in children. *Pediatr Res* 6:668–874, 1972.

86. Hambridge KM, Neldnes KH, Walravens PA: Zinc and acrodermatitis enteropathica. In Hambridge KM, Nichols BL (eds): *Zinc and Copper in Clinical Medicine*. Spectrum Publications, New York, pp 81–89, 1978.

87. Harken AH, Woods M: The influence of oxyhemoglobin affinity on tissue oxygen consumption. *Ann Surg* 183:130–135, 1976.

88. Harris JA, Benedict FG: Biometric studies of basal metabolism in man. Carnegie Institution of Washington, Publication No. 279, 1919.

89. Harvey KB, Moldawer LL, Bistrian BR et al: Biological measures for the formation of a hospital prognostic index. *Am J Clin Nutr* 34:2013–2022, 1981.

90. Heird WC, Dell RB, Driscol Jr JM et al: Metabolic acidosis resulting from intravenous alimentation mixtures containing synthetic amino acids. *N Engl J Med* 286:943–948, 1972.

91. Heller RM, Kirchner SG, O'Neill Jr JA et al: Skeletal changes of copper deficiency in infants receiving prolonged total parenteral nutrition. *J Pediatr* 92:947–948, 1978.

92. Herbert V: Experimental nutritional folate deficiency in men. *Trans Assoc Am Physicians* 75:307–320, 1962.

93. Heymsfield SB, Bethel RA, Ansley JD et al: Cardiac abnormalities in cachectic patients before and during nutritional repletion. *Am Heart J* 95:584–594, 1978.

94. Heymsfield SB, Smith J, Redd S et al: Nutritional support in cardiac failure. *Surg Clin North Am* 61:635–652, 1981.

95. Holcoft JW, Trunkey DD: Pulmonary extravasation of albumin during and after hemorrhagic shock in baboons. *J Surg Res* 18:91–97, 1975.

96. Holman RT: The ratio of trienoic-tetraenoic acids in tissue lipids as a measure of essential fatty acid requirement. *J Nutr* 70:405–410, 1960.

97. Holman RT: Essential fatty acid deficiency. *Prog Chem Fats Other Lipids* 9:329–331, 1971.

98. Horowitz HW, Dworkin BM, Savino JA et al: Central catheter-related infections: comparison of pulmonary artery catheters and triple lumen catheters for the delivery of hyperalimentation in a critical care setting. *J Parenter Enteral Nutr* 14:588–592, 1990.

99. Horst D, Graze N, Conn HO: A double-blind randomized comparison of dietary protein and an oral branched chain amino acid (BCAA) solution in cirrhotic patients with chronic protal-systemic encephalopathy. *Hepatology* 2:184, 1982.

100. Jackson CM: Effect of acute and chronic inanition upon the relative weights of the various organs and systems of adult albino rats. *Am J Anat* 18:75–116, 1915.

101. Jacob HS, Amsden T: Acute hemolytic anemia with rigid red cells in hypophosphatemia. *N Engl J Med* 285:1446–1450, 1971.

102. Jaing Z, Zhang F, Zhu Y et al: Evaluation of parenteral nutrition in the postoperative patient. *Surg Gynecol Obstet* 166:115–120, 1988.

103. James JH, Jeppsson B, Ziparo V et al: Hyperammonemia, plasma amino acid imbalance, and blood-brain amino acid transport: a unified theory of portal-systemic encephalopathy. *Lancet* ii:772–775, 1979.

104. Jeejeebhoy KN, Chu RC, Marliss EB et al: Chromium deficiency, glucose intolerance, and neuropathy reverse by chromium supplementation in a patient receiving long-term total parenteral nutrition. *Am J Clin Nutr* 30:532–538, 1977.

105. Jeejeebhoy KN, Langer B, Tsallas G et al: Total parenteral nutrition at home: studies in patients surviving 4 months to 5 years. *Gastroenterology* 71:943–953, 1976.

106. Jensen GL, Mascioli EA, Seidner DL et al: Parenteral infusion of long- and medium-chain triglycerides and reticuloendothelial system function in man. *J Parenter Enteral Nutr* 14:467–471, 1990.

107. Jimenez FJJ, Leyba CO, Mendez SM et al: Prospective study on the efficacy of branched-chain amino acids in septic patients. *J Parenter Enteral Nutr* 15:252–261, 1991.

108. Joynson DHM, Walker DM, Jacobs A et al: Defect of cell-mediated immunity in patients with iron-deficiency amaemia. *Lancet* ii:1058–1059, 1972.

109. Julius U, Leonhardt W: Elimination and metabolism of a fat emulsion containing medium chain triglycerides (Lipofundin MCT 10%). *J Parenter Enteral Nutr* 12:116–119, 1988.

110. Kaufman JL, Rodriguez JL, McFadden JA et al: Clinical experience with the multiple lumen central venous catheter. *J Parenter Enteral Nutr* 10:487–489, 1986.

111. Kay RG, Tasman-Jones C, Pybur J et al: A syndrome of acute zinc deficiency during total parenteral alimentation in man. *Ann Surg* 183:331–340, 1976.

112. Kelly CS, Ligas JR, Smith CA et al: Sepsis due to triple lumen central venous catheters. *Surg Gynecol Obstet* 163:14–16, 1986.

113. Kern KA, Bower RJ, Atamian S et al: The effect of a new branched chain-enriched amino acid solution on postoperative catabolism. *Surgery* 92:780–785, 1982.

114. Keys A, Brozek J, Hernchel A et al: *The Biology of Human Starvation.* University of Minnesota Press, Minneapolis, pp 714–718, 1950.

115. Keys A, Brozek J, Henschel A et al: *The Biology of Human Starvation.* University of Minnesota Press, Minneapolis, pp 601–606, 1950.

116. Kilsell ME: Vitamin B_6 in metabolism of the nervous system. *Ann NY Acad Sci* 166:1–364, 1969.

117. Kinney JM: The metabolic response to injury. In Richard JR, Kinney JM (eds): *Nutritional Aspects of Care in the Critically Ill.* Churchill Livingstone, New York, 1977.

118. Klingman AM: Pathologic dynamics in human hair loss. *Arch Dermatol* 83:175–198, 1961.

119. Klahr S, Tipathy K, Garcia FT et al: On the nature of the renal concentrating defects in malnutrition. *Am J Med* 43:84–95, 1967.

120. Klahr S, Tipathy K, Lotero H: Renal regulation of acid-base in malnourished man. *Am J Med* 48:325–331, 1970.

121. Koruda MJ, Rolandelli RH, Settle RG et al: The effect of a pectin-supplemented elemental diet on intestinal adaptation to massive small bowel resection. *J Parenter Enteral Nutr* 10:343–350, 1986.

122. Kovacevich DS, Faubion WC, Braunschweig CL et al: Prevalence of catheter sepsis in parenteral nutrition patients with triple lumen vs single lumen catheters. *J Parenter Enteral Nutr* 12(Suppl):23S, 1988.

123. Krieger M: Ueber die Atrophie der menschilchen Organe bei Inanition. *Z Angew Anat Konstitutional* 7:87–134, 1921.

124. Krishnaswamy K, Naidu AN: Microsomal enzymes in malnutrition as determined by plasma half life of antipyrine. *Br Med J* 1:538–540, 1977.

125. Lake AM, Stuart MJ, Iski FA: Vitamin E deficiency and enhanced platelet function. Reversal following E supplementation. *J Pediatr* 90:722–725, 1977.

126. Law DK, Dudrick SJ, Abdou HI: Immunocompetence of patients with protein-calorie malnutrition: the side effects of nutritional repletion. *Ann Intern Med* 79:545–550, 1973.

127. Lawson LJ: Parenteral nutrition in surgery. *Br J Surg* 52:795–800, 1965.

128. Levin PH: A qualitative platelet defect in severe vitamin B_{12} deficiency. Response, hyperresponse, and thrombosis after vitamin B_{12} therapy. *Ann Intern Med* 78:533–539, 1973.

129. Levin R: Analysis of the actions of the hormonal antagonists of insulin. *Diabetes* 13:362–365, 1964.

130. Linder MC, Munro HN: Iron and copper metabolism during development. *Enzyme* 15:111–138, 1973.

131. Lindholm M, Rössner S: Rate of elimination of the Intralipid fat emulsion from the circulation in ICU patients. *Crit Care Med* 10:740–746, 1982.

132. Long CL, Schaffel N, Geiger JW et al: Metabolic response to injury and illness: estimation of energy and protein needs from indirect calorimetry and nitrogen balance. *J Parenter Enteral Nutr* 3:452–456, 1979.

133. Long CL, Kinney JM, Gerger JW: Nonsuppressability of gluconeogenesis by glucose in septic patients. *Metabolism* 25:193–201, 1976.

134. Long JM III, Wilmore DW, Mason Jr AD et al: Effect of carbohydrate and fat intake on nitrogen excretion during total parenteral feeding. *Ann Surg* 185:417–422, 1977.

135. Lopes J, Russell D, Whitwell J et al: Skeletal muscle function in malnutrition. *Am J Clin Nutr* 36:602–610, 1982.

136. McCarthy MC, Shives JK, Robison RJ et al: Prospective evaluation of single and triple lumen catheters in total parenteral nutrition. *J Parenter Enteral Nutr* 11:259–262, 1987.

137. Maini B, Blackburn GL, Bistrian BR: Cyclic hyperalimentation: an optimal technique for preservation of visceral protein. *J Surg Res* 20:515–525, 1976.

138. Maiz A, Yamazaki K, Sobrado J et al: Protein metabolism during total parenteral nutrition in injured rats using medium-chain triglycerides. *Metabolism* 33:901–909, 1984.

139. Mantese VA, German DS, Kaminski DL et al: Colonization and sepsis from triple-lumen catheters in critically ill patients. *Am J Surg* 154:597–601, 1987.

140. Matsusue S, Kashihara S, Takeda H et al: Biotin deficiency during total parenteral nutrition: its clinical manifestations and plasma nonesterified fatty acid level. *J Parenter Enteral Nutr* 9:760–763, 1985.

141. Mayoral LG, Tripathy K, Bolanos O et al: Intestinal, functional, and morphologic abnormalities in severely protein-malnourished adults. *Am J Clin Nutr* 25:1084–1091, 1972.

142. Meguid MM, Akahoshi MP, Jeffers S et al: Amelioration of metabolic complications of conventional total parenteral nutrition. A prospective randomized study. *Arch Surg* 119:1294–1298, 1984.

143. Meguid MM, Brennan MF, Aoki TT et al: Hormone-substrate interrelationships following trauma. *Arch Surg* 109:776–783, 1974.

144. Michie HR, Eberlein TJ, Spriggs DR et al: Interleukin-2 initiates metabolic responses associated with critical illness in humans. *Ann Surg* 208:493–503, 1988.

145. Michie HR, Spriggs DR, Manogue KR et al: Tumor necrosis factor and endotoxin induce similar metabolic responses in humans. *Surgery* 104:280–286, 1988.

146. Millikan WJ, Henderson JM, Warren WD et al: Total parenteral nutrition with FO80 in cirrhotics with subclinical encephalopathy. *Ann Surg* 52:294–304, 1983.

147. Mochizuki H, Trocki O, Dominioni L et al: Mechanism of prevention of postburn hypermetabolism and catabolism by early enteral feeding. *Ann Surg* 200:297–310, 1984.

148. Moore FD, Steenburg RW, Ball MR et al: Studies in surgical endocrinology. I. The urinary secretion of 17-hydroxycorticoids, and associated metabolic changes in cases of soft tissue trauma of varying severity and in bone trauma. *Ann Surg* 141:145–174, 1955.

149. Moore FD, Meguid MM: Homeostasis and nutrition in the surgical patient: the metabolic and endocrine response to injury. In Byrne JJ, Goldsmith HS: *General Surgery I.* Harper & Row, Philadelphia, 1982.

150. Moore FD: Homeostasis: Bodily changes in trauma and surgery. In Sabiston DC (ed): *Davis-Christopher Textbook of Surgery,* ed 11. WB Saunders, Philadelphia, pp 27–64, 1977.

151. Moran LR, Thurlow J, Custer P et al: Nutritional assessment as a predictor of physical performance (abstr). *J Parenter Enteral Nutr* 3:514, 1980.

152. Moss G: Plasma albumin and postoperative ileus. *Surg Forum* 18:333–334, 1967.

153. Moss G: Postoperative metabolism. The role of plasma albumin in the absorption of water and electrolytes. *Pacific Med Surg* 75:355–358, 1967.

154. Mullen JL: Consequences of malnutrition in the surgical patient. *Surg Clin North Am* 61:465–487, 1981.

155. Multivitamin Preparations for Parenteral Use: A statement by the Nutrition Advisory Group. *J Parenter Enteral Nutr* 3:258–262, 1979.

156. Munro HN: General aspects of the regulation of protein metabolism by diet and hormones. In Munro HN, Allison JB (eds): *Mammalian Protein Metabolism.* Academic Press, New York, vol 1, pp 381–481, 1964.

157. Nanni G, Pittiruti M, Giovannini I et al: Plasma carnitine levels and urinary carnitine excretion during sepsis. *J Parenter Enteral Nutr* 9:483–490, 1985.

158. Nathan CF: Secretory products of macrophages. *J Clin Invest* 79:319–326, 1987.

159. Naveau S, Pelletier G, Poynard T et al: A randomized clinical trial of supplementary parenteral nutrition in jaundiced alcoholic cirrhotic patients. *Hepatology* 6:270–274, 1986.

160. Newsholm EA, Crabtree B, Ardawi MSM: Glutamine metabolism in lymphocytes: its biochemical, physiological and clinical importance. *Q J Exp Physiol* 70:473–489, 1985.

161. O'Dwyer ST, Smith RJ, Hwang TL, Wilmore DW: Maintenance of small bowel mucosa with glutamine-enriched parenteral nutrition. *J Parenter Enteral Nutr* 13:579–585, 1989.

162. Old LJ: Polypeptide mediator network. *Nature* 326:330–331, 1987.

163. Ota DM, Jessup JM, Babcock GT et al: Immune function during intravenous administration of a soybean oil emulsion. *J Parenter Enteral Nutr* 9:23–27, 1985.

164. Owen Jr CA, Tyc GM, Glock EV et al: Heparin-ascorbic acid antagonism. *Mayo Clin Proc* 45:140–145, 1970.

165. Pekarek RS, Sanstead HH, Jacob RA et al: Abnormal cellular responses during acquired zinc deficiency. *Ann J Clin Nutr* 32:1466–1472, 1979.

166. Pemberton LB, Lyman B, Lander V et al: Sepsis from triple-vs. single-lumen catheters during total parenteral nutrition in surgical or critically ill patients. *Arch Surg* 121:591–594, 1986.

167. Pichard C, Roulet M, Rössle C et al: Effects of L-carnitine supplemented total parenteral nutrition on lipid and energy metabolism in postoperative stress. *J Parenter Enteral Nutr* 12:555–562, 1988.

168. Pomp A, Varella MSN, Caldwell MD et al: Catheter-related sepsis: single lumen catheters (SLC) vs. triple lumen catheters (TLC). *J Parenter Enteral Nutr* 12(suppl):23S, 1988.

169. Pomposelli JJ, Flores EA, Bistrian BR: Role of biochemical mediators in clinical nutrition and surgical metabolism. *J Parenter Enteral Nutr* 12:212–218, 1988.

170. Pories WJ, Strain WH: Zinc and wound healing. In Prasad AS (ed): *Zinc Metabolism.* Charles C Thomas, Springfield, IL, p 378, 1966.

171. Powell C, Fabri PJ, Kudsk KA: Risk of infection accompanying the use of single-lumen vs double-lumen subclavian catheters: a prospective randomized study. *J Parenter Enteral Nutr* 12:127–129, 1988.

172. Powell C, Kudsk KA, Kulich PA et al: Effect of frequent guidewire changes on triple-lumen catheter sepsis. *J Parenter Enteral Nutr* 12:462–464, 1988.

173. Prasad AS, Miale Jr A, Farid Z et al: Zinc metabolism in patients with the syndrome of iron deficiency anemia, hepatosplenomegaly, dwarfism, and hypogonadism. *J Lab Clin Med* 61:537–549, 1963.

174. Press M, Hartop PJ, Prottey C: Correlation of essential fatty acid deficiency in man by the cutaneous application of sunflower seed oil. *Lancet* i:597–599, 1974.

175. Quercia RA, Korn S, O'Neill D et al: Selenium deficiency and fatal cardiomyopathy in a patient receiving long-term home parenteral nutrition. *Clin Pharmacol* 3:531–535, 1984.

176. Rapp RP, Young B, Twyman D et al: The favorable effect of early parenteral feedings on survival in head-injured patients. *J Neurosurg* 58:906–912, 1983.

177. Reinhardt GJ, Myscofski JW, Wilkens DB et al: Incidence and mortality of hypoalbuminemic patients in hospitalized veterans. *J Parenter Enteral Nutr* 4:357–359, 1980.

178. Robertson CS, Clifton GL, Goodman JC: Steroid administration and nitrogen excretion in the head injured patient. *J Neurosurg* 63:714–718, 1985.

179. Rodriguez DJ, Clevenger FW, Osler RM et al: Obligatory negative nitrogen balance following spinal cord injury. *J Parenter Enteral Nutr* 15:319–322, 1991.

180. Rose SG, Pitsch RJ, Karrer FW et al: Subclavian catheter infections. *J Parenter Enteral Nutr* 12:511–512, 1988.

181. Ross LH, Griffeth L, Hall RI et al: Elimination of hepatotoxicity of total parenteral nutrition using fat-carbohydrate mixture. *Surg Forum* 35:97–99, 1984.

182. Rossi-Fanelli F, Riggo O, Cangiano C et al: Branched-chain amino acids vs lactulose in the treatment of hepatic coma: a controlled study. *Dig Dis Sci* 27:929–935, 1982.

183. Rothschild MA, Oratz M, Schreiber SS: Albumin synthesis. *N Engl J Med* 286:748–757, 816–821, 1972.

184. Rubenstein M, Creger WP: Successful streptokinase therapy for catheter-induced subclavian vein thrombosis. *Arch Intern Med* 140:1370–1371, 1980.

185. Ruggiero RP, Aisenstein TJ: Central catheter fibrin sleeve—heparin effect. *J Parenter Enteral Nutr* 7:270–273, 1983.

186. Salo M: Inhibition of immunoglobulin synthesis *in vitro* by intravenous lipid emulsion (Intralipid). *J Parenter Enteral Nutr* 14:459–462, 1990.

187. Sanderson I, Deitel M: Insulin response in patients receiving concentrated infusions of glucose and casein hydrolysate for complete parenteral nutrition. *Ann Surg* 179:387–394, 1974.

188. Sax HC, Talamini MA, Fischer JE: Clinical use of branched-chain amino acids in liver disease, sepsis, trauma, and burns. *Arch Surg* 121:358–366, 1986.

189. Seelig MS, Heggtveit HA: Magnesium interrelationships in ischemic heart disease: a review. *Am J Clin Nutr* 27:59–79, 1974.

190. Seidner DL, Mascioli EA, Istfan NW et al: Effects of long-chain triglyceride emulsions on reticuloendothelial system function in humans. *J Parenter Enteral Nutr* 13:614–619, 1989.

191. Seller RH, Cangiano J, Kim KE et al: Digitalis toxicity and hypomagnesemia. *Am Heart J* 79:57–68, 1970.

192. Shaw JHF, Holdaway CM: Protein-sparing effect of substrate infusion in surgical patients is governed by the clinical state, and not by the individual substrate infused. *J Parenter Enteral Nutr* 12:433–440, 1988.

193. Sheldon GJ, Peterson SR, Sanders R: Hepatic dysfunction during hyperalimentation. *Arch Surg* 113:504–508, 1978.

194. Shils ME: Experimental human magnesium depletion. I. Clinical observations and blood chemistry alterations. *Am J Clin Nutr* 15:133–143, 1964.

195. Shils ME: Experimental human magnesium depletion. *Medicine* 48:61–81, 1969.

196. Silvis SE, Paragas Jr PD: Paresthesias, weakness, seizures, and hypophosphatemia in patients receiving hyperalimentation. *Gastroenterology* 62:513–520, 1972.

197. Smith NL, Ravo B, Soroff HS, Kahn SA: Successful fibrinolytic therapy for superior vena cava thrombosis secondary to long-term total parenteral nutrition. *J Parenter Enteral Nutr* 9:55–57, 1985.

198. Soderhjelm L, Wiese HF, Holman RT: The role of polyunsaturated acids in human nutrition and metabolism. *Prog Chem Fats Other Lipids* 9:555–585, 2970.

199. Solomon SM, Kirby DF: The refeeding syndrome: a review. *J Parenter Enteral Nutr* 14:90–97, 1990.

200. Souba WW, Herskowitz K, Salloum RM et al: Gut glutamine metabolism. *J Parenter Enteral Nutr* 14:45S–50S, 1990.

201. Souba WW, Klimberg VS, Hautamaki RD et al: Oral glutamine reduces bacterial translocation following abdominal radiation. *J Surg Res* 48:1–5, 1990.

202. Souba WW, Klimberg VS, Plumley DA et al: The role of glutamine in maintaining a healthy gut and supporting the metabolic response to injury and infection. *J Surg Res* 48:383–391, 1990.

203. Souba WW, Scott TE, Wilmore DW: Intestinal consumption of intravenously administered fuels. *J Parenter Enteral Nutr* 9:18–22, 1985.

204. Souba WW, Herskowitz K, Salloum RM et al: Gut glutamine metabolism. *J Parenter Enteral Nutr* 14(suppl):45S–50S, 1990.

205. Steffee WP: Nutritional support in renal failure. *Surg Clin North Am* 61:661–670, 1981.

206. Strauss E: Treatment of hepatic encephalopathy: a randomized clinical trial comparing a branched-chain enriched amino acid solution to oral neomycin. *Nutr Support Serv* 6:18–23, 1986.

207. Subcommittee on the Tenth Edition of the RDAs, Food and Nutrition Board, Commission of Life Sciences, National Research Council: Recommended Dietary Allowances. National Academy Press, Washington, DC, 1989.

208. Sunde RA, Hoekstra WG: Structure, synthesis and function of glutathione peroxidase. *Nutr Rev* 38:265–273, 1980.

209. Tashiro T, Ogata H, Yokoyama H et al: The effects of fat emulsion on essential fatty acid deficiency during intravenous hyperalimentation in pediatric patients. *J Pediatr Surg* 10:203–213, 1975.

210. Todd WR, Elvehjem CA, Hart EB: Zinc in the nutrition of the rat. *Am J Physiol* 107:146–156, 1934.

211. Travis SF, Sugerman JH, Ruberg RL et al: Alterations of red cell glycolytic intermediates and oxygen transport as a consequence of hypophosphatemia in patients receiving intravenous hyperalimentation. *N Engl J Med* 285:763–768, 1971.

212. Unger RH, Orci L: Physiology and pathophysiology of glucagon. *Physiol Rev* 56:778–826, 1976.

213. Valuzzi M, Meguid MM: A prospective randomized study of the optimal source of nonprotein calories in total parenteral nutrition. *Surgery* 102:711–717, 1987.

214. Van Rij AM, Thomson CD, McKenzie JM et al: Selenium deficiency in total parenteral nutrition. *Am J Clin Nutr* 32:2076–2085, 1979.

215. Vary TC, Siegel JH, Nakatani T et al: Regulation of glucose metabolism by altered pyruvate dehydrogenase activity. I. Potential site of insulin resistance in sepsis. *J Parenter Enteral Nutr* 10:351–355, 1986.

216. Vilter RW, Bozian RC, Hess EV et al: Manifestations of copper deficiency in a patient with systemic sclerosis on intravenous hyperalimentation. *N Engl J Med* 291:188–191, 1974.

217. Wahren J, Jacques D, Desurmont P et al: Is intravenous administration of branched chain amino acids effective in the treatment of hepatic encephalopathy? *Hepatology* 3:475–480, 1983.

218. Warnold I, Lundholm K: Clinical significance of preoperative nutritional status in 215 noncancer patients. *Ann Surg* 199:299–305, 1984.

219. Watson RD, Cannon RA, Kurland GS et al: Selenium responsive myositis during prolonged home total parenteral nutrition in cystic fibrosis. *J Parenter Enteral Nutr* 9:58–60, 1985.

220. Waxman S, Corcino JJ, Herbert V: Drugs, toxins and dietary amino acids affecting vitamin B_{12} or folic acid absorption or utilization. *Am J Med* 48:599–608, 1970.

221. Weinberg ED: Iron and susceptibility to infectious disease. *Science* 184:952–956, 1974.

222. Weissman C, Askanazi J, Rosenbaum S et al: Amino acids and respiration. *Ann Intern Med* 98:41–44, 1983.

223. Wicklmayr M, Rett K, Dietze G et al: Comparison of metabolic clearance rates of MCT/LCT and LCT emulsions in diabetics. *J Parenter Enteral Nutr* 12:68–71, 1988.

224. Wilmore DW: *The Metabolic Management of the Critically Ill*. Plenum Press, New York, p 197, 1977.

225. Wilmore DW, Smith RJ, O'Dwyer ST et al: The gut: a central organ after surgical stress. *Surgery* 104:917–923, 1988.

226. Wilson CM, Merritt RJ, Thomas DW: Successful treatment of superior vena cava syndrome with urokinase in an infant. *J Parenter Enteral Nutr* 12:81–83, 1988.

227. Windmueller HG, Spaeth AE: Uptake and metabolism of plasma glutamine by the small intestine. *J Biol Chem* 249:5070–5079, 1974.

228. Wright PD, Johnson IDA: The effect of surgical operation on growth hormone levels in a plasma. *Surgery* 77:479–486, 1975.

229. Young B, Ott L, Twyman D et al: The effect of nutritional support on outcome from severe head injury. *J Neurosurg* 67:668–676, 1987.

230. Zidar BL, Shaddus RK, Zeigler Z et al: Observations on the anemia and neutropenia of human copper deficiency. *Am J Hematol* 3:177–185, 1977.

231. Ziegler TR, Benfell K, Smith RJ et al: Safety and metabolic effects of l-glutamine administration in humans. *J Parenter Enteral Nutr* 14(suppl):137S–146S, 1990.

CHAPTER 61

Enteral Nutrition in the Critically Ill

GARY P. ZALOGA, M.D., F.A.C.P.

Cellular integrity is dependent upon a constant supply of nutrients. Nutrients are required for cell growth and division, enzyme activity, protein-carbohydrate-fat synthesis, muscle contraction, neurohumoral secretion, wound repair, immune competence, gut integrity, and numerous other essential cellular functions. In the absence of adequate nutritional support, protein catabolism and malnutrition can decrease organ mass and impair function of organ systems (i.e. cardiac, respiratory, gastrointestinal, hepatic, renal, immune) (1–5). Malnutrition is associated with higher morbidity and mortality following critical illness (1–6). The author and colleagues believe that optimal recovery from illness encompasses adequate metabolic as well as hemodynamic resuscitation of the patient. This chapter discusses the optimal timing of nutritional support, the optimal delivery of nutrients, effects of illness on gut function, techniques for early enteral feeding, complications of enteral feeding, and the use of specific nutrients for nutritional support.

TIMING OF NUTRITIONAL SUPPORT

It is clear that many patients can "tolerate" a short period of starvation following critical illness (i.e., coronary artery surgery). It is also clear that prolonged starvation (i.e., a few weeks) impairs organ function, predisposes to infection, increases morbidity, and can result in significant mortality. Thus, the optimal timing of nutritional support has not yet been

well-defined. The optimal timing of nutritional support is most likely disease dependent. In other words, it may be important to begin nutritional support within hours of injury in some patients (i.e., those with burns or multiple trauma), whereas in others (i.e., those having elective hernia repair) the delay of a few days may have little consequence. The preinjury nutritional status of patients (i.e., their nutritional reserve) may also be an important variable affecting the timing of nutritional support.

Our concept of nutritional support has evolved over the past decade from the mere delivery of calories and protein to metabolic resuscitation of organs. Current research is indicating that delivery of specific "nutrients" can support gut integrity, improve gut and liver blood flow, minimize liver injury, improve liver function, speed wound healing, improve immune status, decrease infection rates, and improve outcome. Although some patients "tolerate" short periods of starvation, their recovery may be improved with nutrient support.

Experimental studies of gut integrity in guinea pigs following thermal injury indicate that the bowel becomes edematous, loses mucosal integrity, and allows for bacterial translocation within 24 to 72 hours of burn injury. Initiation of enteral nutrition immediately following the burn protects the gut from such injury (7). Chiarelli et al (8) randomized 20 patients to early (average time 4 hours) or delayed (average time 57 hours) enteral feeding following burn injury (average 38% total body burn). The early-fed group was found to have a decrease in hospital stay, decrease in bacteremia, and improved nitrogen balance. Animal and human studies indicate that early enteral feeding diminishes the hypermetabolic/hypercatabolic response to burn injury (9–13). Jenkins et al reported lower infections with early versus delayed (72-hour) feeding in burned children. Recently, Jenkins et al (14) extended these results to intraoperative feeding. Burn-injured patients (40 per group) were randomized to two early feeding regimens. One group was fed following burn and throughout hospitalization, including surgery. The second group was fed following burn injury but had feedings stopped for operative procedures. The group receiving the continuous feedings demonstrated significant decreases in hospital stay and wound infection rates.

A recent study by the author and colleagues (15) found that enteral feeding protected the liver from damage following hemorrhage in rats. The enteral nutrients are believed to have improved blood flow to the gut and liver following hemorrhage. Moore and colleagues (16) randomized trauma patients to early or delayed (day 5) enteral feeding. The group fed early after injury developed fewer infections (10% vs. 28%) during their hospital course. Ryan et al (17) also reported a reduction in septic complications with early postoperative feeding. A randomized study of postoperative patients reported decreased hospital stay, decreased infections, and less weight loss with early versus delayed (day 3) feedings (18). In addition, Rapp et al (19) reported a higher mortality in neurosurgical patients (nonrandomized) when nutritional support was delayed.

Wound healing rate is increased with early enteral nutritional support. A doubling of wound strength was found in animals following abdominal surgery with early versus delayed (day 3) enteral feeding (20). Moss et al (21) reported a doubling of colorectal anastomosis strength and improved collagen synthesis in dogs receiving immediate postoperative enteral feeding. Windsor et al (22) reported improved wound healing in surgical patients with adequate food intake prior to surgery compared with patients with impaired food intake. Wound healing is also improved by early feeding with parenteral nutrition (23–26). In addition, early institution of parenteral nutrition improved total body protein stores, increased wound healing, and decreased hospital stay following surgery for ulcerative colitis (1, 26).

There is a need for additional studies evaluating the timing of nutritional support in critically ill patients. At the present time, the author and colleagues conclude that the available data support the use of early nutritional support. No studies can be found that indicate an advantage to delaying nutrient delivery.

ROUTE OF NUTRITIONAL SUPPORT

Nutrients may be administered via the enteral or parenteral routes. The body has evolved a complex processing station (i.e., gastrointestinal tract) to handle nutrient intake. Accumulating evidence from animal and human studies indicates that enteral administration of nutrients is superior to parenteral administration (27, 28).

Kudsk et al (29, 30) evaluated the effect of enteral versus parenteral delivery of nutrients in an animal model of abdominal infection. Animal survival was improved with enteral nutri-

tion in both well-nourished (60% vs. 20%) and malnourished animals (70% vs. 30%). Peterson et al (31) evaluated the route of nutrient delivery in protein-depleted animals with peritonitis. Enterally fed animals had significantly better survival. The author (32) and others (33) extended these studies to endogenous infection utilizing high-dose methotrexate. In all these studies survival was better in animals receiving enteral nutrition compared with parenteral nutrition. The author and colleagues (34) have also reported improved survival with enteral versus parenteral nutrition in animals following hemorrhagic hypotension.

Randomized prospective studies have compared enteral and parenteral nutrition in patients following trauma, surgery, and chemotherapy. Adams et al (35) randomized trauma patients to total parenteral nutrition (TPN) or enteral nutrition (EN). They found no significant differences in intensive care unit (ICU) stay, hospital stay, ventilator time, infection rate, or nutritional response between groups. However, the cost of nutritional support was 3-fold greater in patients receiving TPN. Moore et al (36) randomized abdominal trauma patients to EN or TPN. There was a significantly lower rate of infection (3% vs. 20%) and greater improvements in visceral proteins in the EN group. A recent metaanalysis (37) of results from a multicenter study of EN versus TPN in patients following trauma also reported a significant decrease in infections in the EN group (18% vs. 35%). Kudsk et al (38) studied 98 patients following traumatic injury randomized to EN or TPN. Infection rate was significantly lower in the EN group (15.7% vs. 40%). There was also a significantly lower rate of intraabdominal abscess formation (1.9% vs. 13.3%) and pneumonia (11.8% vs. 31%) in the EN group.

Young and colleagues (39) compared EN with TPN in neurosurgical patients. Despite significantly lower calories (666 vs. 1466 calories/day) and protein intake (23 vs. 54 g/day) over the first 10 days of feeding, there was no difference in outcome. Similarly, Hadley et al (40) found no differences in outcome in head trauma patients randomized to EN versus TPN.

Routine use of perioperative TPN for major surgery was evaluated in 18 controlled studies and analyzed by metaanalysis (41, 42). Routine use of perioperative TPN was found to be of no benefit over oral feeding. EN and TPN were also evaluated in malnourished patients undergoing elective surgery (43). The TPN group received a week of preoperative intravenous nutrition in an attempt to improve nutritional status prior to surgery. This study reported a significantly higher rate of sepsis (14% vs. 6%) in the TPN group. There were no significant differences in overall complications or mortality.

Route of nutritional support has also been studied in patients receiving chemotherapy for cancer. Koretz (44) analyzed 17 trials and reported no significant benefit from TPN over EN in terms of outcome, tumor response, complication rate, or cost. Klein and colleagues (45) reviewed 28 prospective randomized trials and concluded that TPN may be useful in reducing complications when used preoperatively in patients with gastrointestinal (GI) cancer. However, no significant benefit from TPN could be demonstrated in terms of survival, treatment tolerance, toxicity, tumor response, or outcome in other cancer patients receiving chemotherapy or radiotherapy.

Chemotherapy patients receiving TPN had a significantly higher incidence of infections. The American College of Physicians (46) recently published a position paper based upon a metaanalysis of 12 prospective, randomized, controlled trials of EN versus TPN in cancer chemotherapy. The use of TPN was associated with a significantly lower survival, lower tumor response, and higher infection rate.

Experimental studies have examined the effect of enteral and parenteral nutrition on organ function. TPN is poor for maintaining gut integrity. The major trophic stimulus for the gut is the presence of luminal nutrients. These nutrients directly stimulate gut growth, indirectly stimulate the gut via the production of gut trophic hormones (i.e., neurotensin, enteroglucagon), and increase gut nutrient blood flow (47–52). In the absence of luminal nutrients, gut atrophy occurs (47–56). This atrophy involves loss of mucosal mass, increased mucosal permeability, loss of the gut-associated lymphoid tissue (GALT), and loss of secretory immunoglobulin A (IgA) (57–59). These changes result in greater viability of translocating bacteria (57). TPN has also been associated with a reduced response of T-cells to mitogens (60, 61). In addition, TPN is associated with atrophy of the pancreas and liver. When compared with EN, TPN results in loss of liver function (62–65). Diminished liver function probably results from decreased secretion of intestinal trophic factors.

Compared with TPN, EN has been reported to support better body weight gain/maintenance (50–53, 66, 67), higher organ mass (i.e., gut, kidney, spleen) (50–55), and greater protein synthesis in the postoperative period (68).

Fong et al (69) evaluated the systemic response to endotoxin in individuals who were pretreated for 1 week with TPN or EN. In the TPN subjects, endotoxin injection resulted in higher body temperature (i.e., fever), lower blood pressure, higher circulating lactate levels, greater tumor necrosis factor (TNF) release, and higher hepatic amino acid release. The authors concluded that TPN "primed" the host to a more exaggerated response to endotoxin. The relevance of this observation to human sepsis awaits further study.

In summary, the available data indicate that enteral nutrition is a superior mode of nutritional support when compared with TPN. The vast majority of patients possess a functioning small intestine and should receive their nutrition via the enteral route.

GUT FUNCTION

The gastrointestinal tract may be divided into three major sections: esophagus and stomach, small intestine, and large intestine. Numerous studies have shown that gastric emptying and colonic motility are impaired in critically ill patients. On the other hand, small-bowel function (digestion, absorption, motility) remains adequate for use of enteral nutrition. True "ileus," defined as a dilated nonfunctioning small intestine, is rare. Studies demonstrating adequate small-bowel function have employed movement of radiolabeled compounds and barium, absorption of xylose and vitamin B_{12}, and measurement of small-bowel myoelectric activity. Many clinicians routinely feed patients via the small bowel following multiple trauma, burn injury, abdominal surgery, abdominal aneurysm

repair, head injury, craniotomy, cardiopulmonary arrest, and many other severe illnesses.

Bowel sounds represent the sound of air moving through the small intestine. Many critically ill patients have gastroparesis and are receiving nasogastric suctioning. Little air moves from the stomach to the small intestine in these patients. Bowel sounds are a poor monitor of small-intestinal function, and the presence of active bowel sounds better indicates active gastric emptying. Injection of air into the small bowel through small-bowel feeding tubes almost always produces bowel sounds.

True "ileus" is best diagnosed by finding a distended abdomen on clinical examination and dilated air-filled loops of small intestine on radiologic exam. These patients require evaluation for specific etiologies of the ileus. Passage of flatus or stool represents return of colonic motility. This positive result may require a week or longer following injury. Patients with decreased colonic motility tolerate enteral feeding with nonfiber formulas.

TECHNIQUES FOR ENTERAL FEEDING

Enteral feeding can be accomplished via the oral, gastric, or small-intestinal routes (70–75). Anabolic responses to enteral feeding are best using the oral route, followed by the gastric and small-intestinal routes (70); thus, the author and colleagues believe that the oral route is the preferred route of nutritional support. However, the oral route may not be feasible in many patients because of altered mentation, inability to consume adequate nutrients, and problems with swallowing (i.e., aspiration). These patients usually require gastric or small-intestinal feeding. The preferred method is to feed via the stomach in patients with intact gastric emptying and in whom aspiration is not a significant concern. When gastric emptying is delayed or aspiration is of particular concern, feeding is usually via the small intestine.

Gastric feeding is accomplished using nasogastric tubes, small-bore feeding tubes, or gastrostomy tubes. The author and colleagues prefer the larger-bore nasogastric tubes or gastrostomy tubes in patients in whom gastric residual monitoring is important. Nasogastric tubes are easily passed into the stomach through the nasal or oral cavities. Proper confirmation of gastric position (i.e., by pH, aspiration of gastric contents or bile) is essential prior to feeding. Gastrostomy tubes may be inserted using the percutaneous endoscopic gastrostomy (PEG) technique (72) or by surgery.

Small-intestinal feeding is accomplished using small-bore feeding tubes passed through the nasal or oral cavities. These tubes are passed into the stomach, through the pylorus, and into the small intestine. The author and colleagues prefer to position the tubes in the distal duodenum or proximal jejunum. They have been successful in passing small-bore feeding tubes into the small intestine in 92% of critically ill patients at the bedside using a "corkscrew" technique (71). These tubes can also be effectively placed into the small intestine using fluoroscopic or endoscopic guidance. The overall failure rate using the combination of these techniques in critically ill patients is less than 1%. Small-bowel feeding tubes may also be inserted using percutaneous endoscopic jejunostomy (PEJ) or combined PEG/PEJ techniques (73, 74).

Many clinicians place small-bore feeding tubes into the stomach and wait for them to migrate into the small intestine. Although this technique is moderately effective (30 to 70%) in ward patients, it has little efficacy (<5%) in critically ill patients. In one study, it was found that only 5 of 100 gastric feeding tubes spontaneously migrated into the small intestine in critically ill patients. Metoclopramide has not proved reliable as an agent to speed migration of feeding tubes from the stomach into the small intestine in critically ill patients. However, this agent may be useful for minimizing gastric reflux. Active placement of small-bowel feeding tubes is essential for early nutritional support.

Enteral feeding may also be accomplished using jejunal feeding tubes. These are usually placed at the time of abdominal surgery and are available in a variety of sizes. A disadvantage of the small-diameter needle catheter jejunostomy tubes is their tendency to clog with many nutritional formulas. The author and co-workers prefer larger-sized jejunal catheters.

SPECIFIC NUTRIENTS

A large number of enteral formulas are available for nutritional support. The number and variety of these formulas is increasing rapidly, and discussion of specific formulas is beyond the scope of this chapter. However, a basic understanding of the major nutrient classes should help in choosing an appropriate enteral formula.

PROTEIN

Intact Protein, Peptides, and Amino Acids

Enteral feeding formulas vary in both quantity and quality of protein. Protein content varies from 19 to 83.5 grams per liter of formula. Protein is available as free amino acids, peptides, or intact protein.

Protein normally is consumed in the diet as intact protein, and a complex process for digestion and absorption of protein has evolved over thousands of years. Protein digestion begins in the stomach under the influence of hydrochloric acid (HCl) and pepsin. However, pepsin and HCl are not essential for the digestive process. After leaving the stomach, dietary protein is further hydrolyzed by pancreatic enzymes (i.e., trypsin, chymotrypsin) and mucosal peptidases. The net result is the production of a combination of small peptides (70%) and amino acids (30%). Free amino acids, dipeptides, and tripeptides may enter the small intestine through discrete transport carriers. However, it is also clear that small quantities of larger peptides (more than three amino acids) enter the circulation through the intestine via an undefined process that may involve pinocytosis. Although this transport system is not capable of maintaining nitrogen balance, it can allow the entry of small amounts of physiologically active peptides (76–78). The author and colleagues believe that absorbed biogenic amines may have important physiologic functions that involve the stimulation of growth factors, blood flow regulation, and other activities. It appears that approximately 30 to 70% of nitrogen absorbed and appearing in the portal circulation may be in the form of peptides (79, 80).

When digestive functions are intact, dietary proteins are degraded to peptides and amino acids. These patients are best fed using intact protein diets. However, when digestion is impaired (i.e., pancreatic insufficiency, multiple trauma, shock, sepsis, severe malnutrition), there are advantages to feeding formulas containing high quantities of smaller peptides (i.e., less than seven to 10 amino acids).

The author and colleagues believe that few data support the use of amino acid based formulas over intact protein or peptide formulas (27, 81, 82). Amino acid based formulas are associated with gut atrophy (83–88), bacterial translocation (84, 89), decreased liver function (34, 90–92), poorer growth and wound repair (83, 93, 94), decreased visceral protein levels (85), greater diarrhea (85, 95), poorer nitrogen balance (82, 93), and higher mortality (32, 34, 84, 85, 90, 96–100) compared with intact protein or peptide formulas.

When compared with intact protein formulas, peptide-based formulas are associated with improved nitrogen absorption (81, 82, 101–103), decreased stool output and diarrhea (95, 104, 105), improved protein synthesis (106), better body growth (83, 93, 94) and wound healing, higher insulin growth factor 1 (somatomedin C) levels (83), better gut maintenance (107–109) and improved hepatic protein synthesis (34, 92, 103, 105, 110).

The liver is an important organ for immunologic competence, synthesis of vital proteins, and processing of cellular waste products. Gut venous blood drains into the liver. Thus, translocating bacteria/toxins as well as absorbed nutrients drain to the liver for processing. Gut failure frequently leads to hepatic dysfunction, and loss of hepatic function initiates multiple organ failure. As a result, therapy frequently is oriented toward protecting liver and gut integrity.

Hepatic function can be assessed clinically by measuring changes in circulating hepatic proteins (i.e., prealbumin, transferrin, retinol binding protein) or clearance of bilirubin. Brinson et al (111) reported better absorption and increased albumin and transferrin levels in patients receiving a peptide versus an intact protein diet. Meredith et al (105) compared a peptide with an intact protein diet in ICU patients with multiple trauma. Patients receiving the peptide diet had less diarrhea, greater increases in visceral protein levels (i.e., prealbumin, transferrin, albumin), and decreased hospital stay. Ziegler et al (103) reported better nitrogen absorption and hepatic protein levels in ICU patients receiving a peptide versus an intact protein diet. Zaloga and colleagues (110) compared a peptide diet with an intact protein diet in multitrauma patients. Patients receiving the peptide diet maintained higher levels of prealbumin, transferrin, and retinol binding protein. Hepatic protein levels were also higher with peptide than with amino acid and regular (food) diets in geriatric patients (112) and patients with inflammatory bowel disease (113). On the other hand, Mowatt-Larsen et al (114) found no difference in hepatic protein levels in trauma patients receiving a peptide versus an intact protein diet. The majority of studies suggest that peptide diets may better support liver function during critical illness.

Net nutrient absorption is higher (101, 102) and diarrhea less (95) as the concentration of peptides in the formula increases. The specific protein source may also be important.

Bounous et al (115) demonstrated improved immune responsiveness when animals were fed lactoalbumin protein hydrolysates versus casein hydrolysates.

A large number of peptides have been identified that possess biologic activities. Cyclo-histidine-proline (c-his-pro) and β-casomorphin are two examples of peptides found in current peptide formulations. C-his-pro is the active component of thyrotropin releasing hormone (TRH). This peptide is absorbed through the intestinal tract. It is capable of stimulating the release of thyroid stimulating hormone (TSH), regulating blood flow and hormone secretion, affecting neurosynaptic transmission, and improving blood pressure during shock states; it is also a physiologic opiate antagonist. β-Casomorphin is a peptide produced by trypsin/chymotrypsin hydrolysis of casein. This peptide has opiate activity and is believed to modulate gut motility, permeability (116), secretion, and absorption.

Glutamine

Glutamine is the most abundant free amino acid in plasma and body tissues. It is synthesized in most tissues of the body and has been considered a "nonessential" amino acid. However, recent data suggest that tissue demands for glutamine can outstrip endogenous synthesis during critical illness. Exogenous administration of glutamine may be beneficial in these states. Thus, glutamine is now considered to be "semiessential". The highest rate of glutamine synthesis occurs in muscle. The greatest rate of glutamine metabolism occurs in the intestine. Glutamine functions as a nitrogen transporter, carrier of ammonia, constituent of proteins, regulator of protein synthesis, precursor for gluconeogenesis, and source of cellular energy (metabolism through the Krebs cycle yields 30 ATPs per molecule). Glutamine is a precursor for the neurotransmitters glutamate and γ-aminobutyric acid.

Glutamine is consumed by replicating cells and is a major fuel for maintenance and repair of the gastrointestinal tract (117–121). Maintaining the integrity of the gastrointestinal tract is a major goal in the treatment of critically ill patients, since bacterial/toxin entry via the gastrointestinal tract is believed to be a major precursor of multiple organ failure.

Glutamine is absent from current parenteral nutritional formulas, and this absence contributes to gut atrophy. Free glutamine is unstable in solution; however, glutamine peptides are stable in solution and are undergoing clinical trials. Glutamine-supplemented TPN has been shown to improve gut mass in a number of animal studies (122–125). However, glutamine-supplemented TPN is less effective for stimulating the gastrointestinal tract than is enteral nutrition (123). Glutamine-supplemented TPN also improves nitrogen balance in patients following surgery (126, 127).

Most enteral studies of glutamine supplementation have compared a glutamine-supplemented amino acid diet with a glutamine-deficient amino acid diet (125, 128–131). These studies have demonstrated that glutamine supplementation benefits gut mass, barrier function, and survival. However, these studies have little clinical relevance since none of the available enteral diets is glutamine deficient and most diets utilize intact proteins rather than amino acids.

McAnena et al (132) evaluated the effect of polypeptide feeding versus amino acid feeding on survival following methotrexate in rats. The study design was the same as that used

by Fox et al (129, 130), who demonstrated a 100% mortality in animals fed an amino acid glutamine-deficient diet and an 80% mortality for animals fed a glutamine-supplemented amino acid diet. McAnena et al (132) found a 100% mortality in animals receiving an amino acid diet and a 30% mortality in animals receiving a polypeptide diet. Mortality increased as the quantity of amino acids in the diet increased. Shou et al (84, 97) also studied the effect of diet on gut mass, bacterial translocation, and survival in rats following methotrexate. A glutamine-supplemented amino acid diet improved gut mass when compared with a glutamine-deficient amino acid diet. However, gut mass was significantly larger in animals receiving intact protein formulas. Bacterial translocation was 100% on the amino acid glutamine-deficient diet, 70% on the glutamine-supplemented amino acid diet, and 0% on the intact protein diet. Mortality was 100% on the amino acid glutamine-deficient diet, 75% on the amino acid glutamine-supplemented diet, and 0% on the intact protein diet.

Vanderhoff et al (133) studied the effect of glutamine on gut adaptation following massive small-bowel resection in rats. A chow diet was supplemented with glutamine, glycine, or glucose. There were no differences in gut mass among groups. Wells et al (134) evaluated a chow diet, an intact protein diet, and a glutamine-supplemented intact protein diet in rats given endotoxin and metronidazole. There were no differences in gut histology or bacterial translocation among groups. Barber et al (135) studied the effect of glutamine supplemented to a peptide diet. There was no significant effect of the glutamine on gut mass, bacterial translocation, or survival after endotoxin.

Oral diets supplemented with glutamine accelerated recovery of small-bowel mucosa after injury with radiation (131, 136, 137). However, glutamine-supplemented parenteral nutrition failed to accelerate recovery of small bowel following radiation injury (138).

All marketed enteral nutritional formulas contain glutamine in the free form or as a component of peptides or intact protein. The optimal quantity and form of glutamine (i.e., free amino acids, peptides, intact protein) for gut maintenance in humans remains to be determined.

In conclusion, glutamine is an important amino acid for gut maintenance, and glutamine requirements exceed synthetic rates during severe stress. Glutamine-deficient diets result in gut atrophy and bacterial translocation during critical illness. However, there is little evidence to indicate that glutamine supplementation improves the physiologic effects of complex diets (i.e., intact protein and peptide diets).

Arginine

Arginine is an important amino acid for protein synthesis (i.e., connective tissue), creatine synthesis, and the urea cycle (139). Arginine is synthesized in the body. Although arginine was once considered a nonessential amino acid, its demand may exceed synthetic rates during growth and critical illness (139, 140). Arginine deficiency can impair the urea cycle and cause hyperammonemia and increased orotate excretion. Thus, it is now considered a "semiessential" amino acid. Arginine is also a secretagogue and in pharmacologic doses can stimulate the secretion of growth hormone, prolactin, glucagon, somatostatin, and adrenal catecholamines. Recent interest in arginine is based upon its effects on wound healing and immune function.

Traumatized animals grow and heal poorly on arginine-deficient diets (139, 141). Arginine supplementation (1% to 3%) improves nitrogen balance and decreases weight loss in animals following injury (139, 141–144). Arginine also improves wound healing when supplemented to chow (1%) (141, 144) and intravenous nutrition (7.5 g/L) (145). However, arginine failed to improve wound healing in hypophysectomized rats, suggesting that its effect was dependent upon the hypothalamic-pituitary axis (144). Arginine's effects on wound healing are not associated with increases in growth hormone (139, 146).

Liver protein synthesis was evaluated in control and septic rats (*Escherichia coli* injection) during total parenteral nutrition with arginine or glycine supplementation (147). Supplemental arginine led to increased liver protein synthesis (i.e., histone, fibrinogen, albumin, total liver protein).

Arginine supplementation (15 g/day i.v. and 25 g/day enterally) has been evaluated in humans and found to improve nitrogen balance minimally (148, 149). The effect of arginine supplementation (30 g/day for 2 weeks) on wound healing was evaluated in healthy human volunteers using subcutaneously implanted polytetrafluoroethylene tubing (150). Arginine supplementation increased the amount of collagen deposited in the wound site.

Arginine supplementation improves lymphocyte blastogenic response to mitogens in animals (139, 145, 151–153) and humans (140, 149, 154). Barbul et al (151) found that 1% arginine-supplemented chow improved thymic weight and cellularity in both healthy and injured (femoral fracture) rats. Arginine supplementation also improved mitogen stimulation of thymic lymphocytes in healthy and injured animals. In addition, arginine prevented the decrease in mitogen stimulation associated with injury. Arginine also enhanced skin allograft rejection, diminished tumor induction, and produced antitumor effects in animals (139, 141). Barbul et al (150, 154) reported improved lymphocyte mitogenic activity in healthy humans following arginine supplementation (30 g/day). Daly et al (149) found that arginine supplementation enhanced T-lymphocyte responses to concanavalin A (Con-A) and phytohemagglutinin (PHA) in postoperative cancer patients. However, there were no differences in infections or outcome between control and arginine-supplemented groups. On the other hand, parenteral arginine alone (without nutritional support) failed to enhance mitogen-stimulated lymphocyte proliferation in postoperative patients (155).

Saito et al (156) fed burned guinea pigs (30% total body burn) different amounts of arginine (1 to 4% of total calories supplemented to an intact protein diet). There were no differences between control and arginine groups for weight loss, urinary vanillylmandelic acid (VMA) concentrations, plasma cortisol levels, glucagon levels, nitrogen balance, transferrin levels, C3, carcass weights, or gastrocnemius muscle weights. Resting metabolic expenditure was higher in the arginine groups. Dinitrofluorobenzene (DNFB) dependent delayed cutaneous hypersensitivity responses were greater in the 1 to 2% arginine-supplemented group. Skin lesion size after injection of *Staphylococcus aureus* was smaller in the arginine-supplemented

groups. Mortality was 56% in the control group, 56% in the 4% arginine-supplemented group, 29% in the 1% arginine-supplemented group, and 22% in the 2% arginine-supplemented group. The mortality data demonstrated a dose effect, with the 4% arginine causing a higher mortality than the 1% and 2% arginine. Since dose responses vary between guinea pigs and humans, similar experiments should be performed in humans prior to clinical use of arginine supplementation.

Madden et al (157) examined the effect of arginine on the survival of rats with peritonitis induced by cecal ligation and puncture (CLP). Arginine had no effect on survival when given enterally starting immediately after CLP. Arginine improved survival when given enterally 3 days prior to CLP and continued after CLP. Arginine also improved survival when given intravenously after CLP. Impaired intestinal absorption or markedly increased arginine utilization may explain why the post-CLP enteral group failed to demonstrate improved survival.

Gonce et al (158) evaluated the efficacy of supplemental arginine in guinea pig peritonitis (infused *E. coli* and *S. aureus*). Survival was 54% in the 0% arginine group, 41% in the 2% and 4% groups, and 9% in the 6% arginine group. There were no differences among groups for albumin, C3, or transferrin levels. Nitrogen balance was lower in the arginine-supplemented groups. This study suggests that dietary arginine supplementation does not enhance survival in guinea pig peritonitis.

Synthesis of nitric oxide (also known as endothelium-derived relaxant factor) is arginine dependent (159). Rat aortic rings incubated with endotoxin demonstrate depressed reactivity to norepinephrine (160, 161). L-arginine potentiates this effect. An L-arginine antagonist, N^Gmonomethyl-L-arginine (NMMA), restores the contractile response to norepinephrine. L-arginine administration reverses this effect (i.e., results in a depressed contractile response). In vivo, endotoxin infusion depresses the pressor response to norepinephrine (161). This effect is abolished by NMMA. L-arginine reverses the in vivo effect of NMMA (i.e., causes norepinephrine resistance). These data indicate that endotoxin, in vivo and in vitro, acts on vascular tissue to induce norepinephrine resistance that is secondary to the activation of an L-arginine pathway (160).

Tumor necrosis factor (TNF) causes hypotension when injected intravenously and is believed to play a significant role in the hypotension and decreased organ perfusion during sepsis and other forms of shock. TNF decreases blood pressure in dogs (162). This hypotensive response is reversed with NMMA. The effect of NMMA is antagonized and hypotension restored by L-arginine. These data suggest that nitric oxide production from arginine mediates the hypotensive effect of TNF.

It is unclear whether arginine supplementation predisposes to hypotension during human sepsis. Despite predisposing to systemic hypotension, nitric oxide may also play important roles in maintaining organ perfusion (as a vasodilator) and improving blood flow for wound healing. Clearly, further studies on the effects of arginine supplementation, as well as arginine antagonism, are needed before widespread clinical use of arginine can be recommended.

FAT

Lipids are an important source of energy for the body and provide 9.3 kcal/g. In addition, lipids form structural components of cell membranes (i.e., phospholipids), participate in the regulation of cardiovascular tone (i.e., prostaglandins), and act as cell messengers (i.e., phosphoinositides). The diet contains many lipids that differ in the number of carbon atoms, the number of double bonds, and the position of the double bonds. These structural differences impart unique physiologic properties to the lipid molecules. The w-terminus is the carbon atom farthest from the carboxy end. Linoleic acid (18:2w-6) has 18 carbon atoms and two double bonds. The first double bond is at the sixth carbon atom from the w-terminus. Short-chain fatty acids have two to four carbons, medium-chain fatty acids have six to 10 carbons, and long-chain fatty acids have 12 to 26 carbons.

Linoleic acid is essential for normal growth and development and must be provided in the diet (i.e., it is an "essential" fatty acid). It is the precursor of arachidonic acid (20:4w-6), which upon metabolism produces the prostaglandins and leukotrienes. Although only approximately 3% of calories are required as linoleic acid, most nutritional formulas provide 10 to 20% of calories as linoleic acid.

The lipid composition of the diet affects the fatty acid composition of cell membranes (163–166). Dietary manipulation of fatty acid content alters lymphocyte function (163, 164), enzyme activity (167), and receptor responsiveness (168). These effects may result from dietary fatty acid induced changes in membrane structure and function.

Dietary lipids exert potent effects upon the immune system (163–165). Dietary lipids may alter immune function by affecting energy supply, essential fatty acid availability, fat-soluble vitamin supply, cell membrane fluidity, membrane receptor coupling, cytokine release, and eicosanoid synthesis.

Exogenous administration of linoleic acid or diets rich in linoleic acid (i.e., corn oil, safflower oil, soybean oil, sunflower oil, parenteral lipids) suppresses mitogen-induced (i.e., PHA, Con-A) lymphocyte proliferation (163, 166, 169–171). For example, diets containing 30% corn oil suppressed mitogenic responses of isolated monkey lymphocytes to PHA, Con-A, and pokeweed mitogen (171).

Saturated fats, monounsaturated fats, and medium-chain triglycerides have negligible effects on mitogen-induced lymphocyte stimulation. On the other hand, diets rich in saturated fats are reported to inhibit chemotaxis, phagocytosis, and bactericidal activity of isolated neutrophils (163). High-saturated-fat diets also reduce adherence and phagocytosis in macrophages.

Low quantities of linoleic acid are important for normal immune function. However, high levels suppress certain components of the immune system (163, 164). This suppressive effect may be useful for treating inflammatory states and preventing organ rejection. For example, administration of linoleic acid prolongs allograft survival in animals, whereas diets low in linoleic acid accelerate graft rejection (163, 164, 169). Animals with essential fatty acid deficiency also have a lower incidence of methylcholanthrene-induced tumors (172). On the other hand, essential fatty acid deficiency impairs antibody production and reduces delayed cutaneous hypersensitivity responses (163).

In general, diets high in long-chain polyunsaturated fatty acids (PUFA) suppress mitogenic responses of splenocytes and T-lymphocytes, promote tumorigenesis, and reduce B-lymphocyte generation of antibodies. These suppressive effects appear to be mediated through the release of cellular factors such as prostaglandins. Immune suppressive effects may be good in certain situations. They may be important for minimizing tissue damage early after injury. However, they may also predispose to infection during long-term recovery.

Eicosanoids derived from PUFA are major factors affecting the immune response. When immune cells are stimulated by antigen, arachidonic acid is released from the cells by the action of phospholipase. The quantity of arachidonic acid released is proportional to the amount in cell membranes, which is affected by dietary lipid intake (especially linoleic acid). Arachidonic acid is subsequently metabolized to a variety of eicosanoids by the cyclooxygenase and lipoxygenase pathways. Linoleic acid is the precursor of monoenoic and dienoic prostaglandins. These prostaglandins can be immunosuppressive. On the other hand, ω-3 PUFA are precursors of trienoic prostaglandins and have less potent effects on certain cells (i.e., less platelet aggregation from thromboxane A_3, less immunosuppression from prostaglandin E_3, or PGE_3).

Low concentrations of PGE_2 are permissive to portions of the immune system (i.e., promote lymphocyte differentiation). On the other hand, high levels of PGE_2 ($>10^{-8}M$) are suppressive to lymphocytes and macrophages. High levels are produced in patients with sepsis, trauma, burns, adult respiratory distress syndrome (ARDS); after major surgery; and following blood transfusion (163).

High dietary levels of ω-6 PUFA favor the production of PGE_2. Johnston and Marshall (173) fed animals with corn oil (high linoleic acid), linseed oil (rich in the ω-3 fat linolenic acid) or coconut oil (rich in medium-chain triglycerides). Mononuclear cell production of PGE_2 induced by PHA stimulation was 28.5 ng/million cells in corn oil fed animals, 9.3 ng/million cells in coconut oil fed animals, and 3.5 ng/million cells in linseed oil fed animals.

The exact physiologic role of high levels of PGE_2 is unclear. However, it may be part of a negative feedback system designed to minimize the immune response and decrease cytokine production following tissue injury. High levels of PGE_2 have antiinflammatory actions and suppress mitogen response, clonal proliferation, antigenic stimulation, lymphokine production, generation of cytotoxic cells, lymphocyte migration, and antibody production (163). Other effects of PGE_2 include inhibition of lysosomal release from neutrophils, suppression of mast cell degranulation, and vasodilation. However, chronic overproduction of PGE_2 may predispose to infection.

Leukotrienes (LT) are generated by macrophages, lymphocytes, neutrophils, mast cells, and other cells. These compounds have a variety of physiologic effects. LTC_4, LTD_4, and LTE_4 are bronchial constrictors. LTC_4 and LTD_4 also increase vascular permeability. LTB_4 is a chemoattractant for neutrophils, activator of neutrophils (i.e., aggregation, enzyme release), and stimulator of killer cell activity (163). It is also chemotactic for lymphocytes and monocytes, enhances adherence of lymphocytes to endothelium, inhibits antibody production, and can induce interleukin-2 (IL-2) production. Physiologic levels of leukotrienes tend to be immune stimulators.

Eicosapentaenoic acid (EPA) and docosahexaenoic acid (DHA) are ω-3 long-chain fatty acids present in high concentrations in fish oils. These fatty acids compete with arachidonic acid for cyclooxygenase. ω-3-derived endoperoxides and thromboxanes have attenuated activity. Animals fed diets rich in EPA and DHA (ω-3 PUFA) produce lower concentrations of PGE_2, LTB_4, LTC_4, and 6-keto-$PGF1_a$ (163, 164, 174). Dietary linolenic acid (ω-3 fat) has been reported to decrease endotoxin-induced production of thromboxane A_2 (TxA2), prostacyclin, and TNF in equine peritoneal macrophages (175, 176). The exact clinical significance of these effects is unclear.

The total fat content of the diet also alters leukotriene synthesis. LTE_4 synthesis was greater on a 5% ω-6 PUFA diet compared with a 20% diet (164). ω-3 PUFA were more effective in decreasing synthesis of eicosanoids and leukotrienes in low-fat (5%) than in high-fat (20%) diets (164).

It is important to realize that the immune system is an extremely complex system. The first line of defense involves nonspecific immunity. Important mechanisms of nonspecific immunity include macrophages, neutrophils, complement, and the acute phase response. Specific immunity recognizes invading organisms, "remembers" the invader, and destroys the invader. Important mechanisms of specific immunity include cell-mediated immunity (i.e., helper T-cells, cytotoxic T-cells, antigen-presenting cells such as the macrophage, T-cell growth factors) and humoral immunity (i.e., antibodies, helper T-cells, B-cells, macrophages). The effect of different lipids and combinations of lipids on all aspects of the immune system has not been evaluated. Thus, it is possible that a lipid that enhances one component of the immune system may suppress another component. The overall effect is difficult to predict from isolated studies, and clinical trials are needed.

Animal and Human Studies

Cytokines released from the reticuloendothelial system are believed to contribute to organ failure during shock states. Kupffer cells from rats fed ω-3 PUFA for 6 weeks had reduced secretion of tumor necrosis factor (164). Feeding of ω-3 PUFA also decreased tumor necrosis factor and interleukin-1 secretion from monocytes stimulated with endotoxin. Cerra et al (177) studied rat Kupffer cell secretion of PGE_2 and TxB_2 in response to endotoxin. Animals fed menhaden oil (ω-3 PUFA) produced less PGE_2 and TxB_2 compared with animals fed corn oil or safflower oil.

The optimal fat content (safflower oil) in burned guinea pigs for promoting protein synthesis and preserving muscle mass is 5 to 15% (178). Higher concentrations (30 to 50%) are associated with adverse effects on muscle mass, nitrogen balance, and serum transferrin levels.

Oral and intravenous administration of fish oils (ω-3 PUFA) improved survival in guinea pigs following endotoxin (163). This effect was similar to that obtained with prostaglandin synthesis inhibitors such as ibuprofen and indomethacin. In addition, mortality was higher in rats after cecal ligation and puncture as the dietary ω-6/ω-3 PUFA ratio increased (177).

Following burn injury in guinea pigs, mortality is higher in animals fed linoleic acid diets (10% lipid diet) than in those fed with safflower oil or fish oil diets (179). The fish oil group also demonstrates lower resting metabolic expenditure, less weight loss, better spleen and carcass weights, higher transferrin levels, better DNFB response, and better opsonic indexes. Trocki et al (180) also administered fish oil to burned guinea pigs. Animals receiving 5%, 15%, 30%, or 50% of nonprotein calories as fish oil had similar mortalities, resting metabolic expenditures, albumin concentrations, transferrin levels, DNFB responses, macrophage bactericidal indexes, and opsonic indexes. The 5% and 15% fat groups had slightly higher liver weights and liver nitrogen levels, and the 50% fat group had more diarrhea. In addition, thermally injured rats fed a structured lipid-containing medium-chain triglycerides (60%) and fish oil (40%) diet had better nitrogen balances, decreased energy expenditures, and reduced net protein catabolism compared with animals fed safflower oil diets (181).

Peck and colleagues (182) fed mice diets containing different fats for 2 to 3 weeks. The animals subsequently underwent a 20% burn and infection with *Pseudomonas aeruginosa*. Animals receiving a fish oil supplemented diet had a higher mortality than animals receiving a safflower oil supplemented diet (78% vs 27%). Mortality was intermediate in animals receiving oleic acid (44%) or coconut oil diets (58%). PGE_2 production was lower in the fish oil group. There were no differences in T- and B-lymphocyte function assessed by Con-A and PHA stimulation, mixed lymphocyte cultures, and Jerne plaque-forming assay (for B-cells). These results are opposite those obtained in burned but noninfected animals. It is possible that nonlymphocyte functions of the immune system (i.e., macrophages, neutrophils) were responsible for the better survival in the safflower oil group compared with the fish oil animals. It is also possible that different lipids have different effects at different times after burn injury. Immunosuppression (i.e., from PGE_2) may be beneficial early after tissue injury to minimize the inflammatory response and diminish organ injury. On the other hand, prolonged immunosuppression may predispose to infection and worsen outcome.

Clouva-Molyvdas et al (183) investigated the role of different lipid sources (coconut oil, oleic acid, safflower oil, fish oil) on survival in two models of peritonitis in mice (*P. aeruginosa* and *Salmonella typhimurium*). Animals received 5% and 40% of total calories as fat for 2 to 3 weeks. No significant differences in survival were found among groups, and the authors concluded that 2 to 3 weeks of dietary fat manipulation does not affect outcome from infection in this model. Peck and colleagues (183a) randomized guinea pigs to diets varying in fat content (3.5 to 56% of calories) and fat composition (safflower oil, fish oil, 50/50 mixture). The level of fat intake did not affect survival following experimental peritonitis. However, fat composition significantly influenced survival. The 50/50 mixture group had a 39% survival; the safflower oil group, a 20% survival; and the fish oil group, a 9% survival. The ear swelling response to DNFB was greatest in the fish oil group, intermediate in the 50/50 group, and lowest in the safflower group. PGE_2 production by splenic macrophages was highest in the safflower group, intermediate in the 50/50 group, and lowest in the fish oil group. Thus, response to DNFB and PGE_2 production did not predict survival in this model of infection. This study suggests that outcome from infection is best with fat mixtures. However, the optimal fat mixture remains to be determined.

At the present time, we have a poor understanding of the metabolic and immune response to injury and infection. It is not clear what responses are associated with optimal outcomes. Thus, one must be extremely careful when manipulating normal responses, since such manipulations may benefit one response but harm others. Clearly, more research in these areas is needed.

There has been concern over the use of intravenous lipids in parenteral nutrition because these preparations contain large quantities of linoleic acid. Hamawy et al (184) administered TPN with 50% and 0% lipid to animals following leg fracture and infection. Lipid was administered as long-chain triglycerides (LCT) or 75% medium-chain triglycerides (MCT) plus 25% LCT. Reticuloendothelial function was better in the animals receiving the MCT/LCT preparation. Reticuloendothelial dysfunction was also reported in normal and burned guinea pigs when LCT emulsions were administered (185). Intraperitoneal "Intralipid" delayed the clearance of *S. aureus* from the peritoneal cavity and increased its dissemination to other organs in mice (186). It also increased mortality in animals infected with *Streptococcus* (187). In vitro exposure of human leukocytes to lipid emulsions (high in linoleic acid) impaired leukocyte chemotaxis and decreased bactericidal capacity (187–189). Mitogen-stimulated and IL-2 activated human lymphocyte proliferation are both inhibited by lipid emulsions (190). These lipids also inhibit the generation of cytotoxic lymphokine-activated killer cells.

Intravenous lipid-supplemented nutrition has no effect on Kupffer cell phagocytosis in septic rats (191). However, supplementation with linoleic acid potentiates blood-transfusion-induced immunosuppression and prolongs graft survival (192). Linoleic acid administration also prolongs graft survival and produces additive immunosuppressive effects when combined with cyclosporin (193).

Cheney et al (194) reported an association between the amount of intravenous lipid administered to immunocompromised patients (bone marrow transplants) and the rate of infection. Freeman et al (195) found a significant association between the use of intravenous lipid and staphylococcal bacteremia in neonates. Although others have not been able to detect adverse effects from the use of high linoleic acid containing intravenous lipids, these data indicating that linoleic acid possesses immunosuppressive effects are worrisome.

Dietary supplementation with EPA and DHA alters cytokine and prostaglandin secretion by leukocytes in healthy subjects. Following 6 weeks (but not 3 weeks) of supplementation, leukotriene B4 (LTB_4) generation is lower (196). LTB_4-induced neutrophil chemotaxis is also diminished. Endres et al (197) fed ω-3 PUFA to normal subjects for 6 weeks and measured cytokine release from mononuclear cells following in vitro stimulation with endotoxin, PHA, and *Staphylococcus epidermidis*. TNF, IL-1, and PGE_2 secretion are diminished on the diet. LTB_4-induced chemotaxis of neutrophils is also reduced. These data indicate that ω-3 PUFA attenuates the release of inflammatory mediators in healthy subjects. The effect in critically ill patients requires further study. To date, there have been no human studies evaluating the effect of ω-3 PUFA alone on the course of infection.

Structured lipids are prepared by mixing triglycerides in specific proportions, allowing hydrolysis to fatty acids and random esterification into composite triglyceride molecules. These lipids contain combinations of fatty acids. Preliminary studies indicate that feeding structured lipids produces metabolic effects that differ from those produced by a physical mixture of the lipids. Further studies are required to evaluate the use of these lipids during critical illness.

Overall, the available data indicate that the lipid content of the diet alters cellular and metabolic activity. Lipids alter cell membrane composition and function, alter the generation of cytokines and prostaglandins, alter immune cell function, and may alter the body's response to infection. High linoleic acid content of the diet appears to have immunosuppressive effects. Decreasing the linoleic acid content of the diet improves immune cell function. The best method for lowering linoleic acid content while maintaining the benefits of lipids as energy sources is unclear. The optimal fat content of the diet remains unknown. The author and co-workers favor the use of balanced fat formulas that contain required amounts of linoleic acid (i.e., 5 to 10% of nonprotein calories) mixed with a variety of other lipids (i.e., MCTs, saturated fats, ω-3 fats).

CARBOHYDRATE

Carbohydrate may be provided as simple sugars or complex polysaccharides (i.e., starch and fiber). Some fibers (i.e., pectin) are not digested in the upper gastrointestinal tract and reach the colon, where they are metabolized by bacteria to short-chain fatty acids (SCFAs; acetate, propionate, butyrate) (198). SCFAs are preferential fuels for the colon, stimulate water and electrolyte absorption, increase colonic blood flow, and stimulate colonic proliferation. They are also metabolized to glutamine and ketones, providing fuel for the small intestine. SCFAs are well-absorbed and metabolized by both the small and large bowels. They are cleared principally by the liver. Acetate and butyrate are converted to acetylcoenzyme A, while propionate is converted to succinylcoenzyme A (and is gluconeogenic). In humans, SCFAs are produced principally in the large bowel by fermentation of fiber and contribute to energy needs of the host. Other fibers (i.e., cellulose, lignin) are not digested or metabolized in the gastrointestinal tract. These fibers add bulk to the stool. They act as stool softeners and help stimulate stool movement through the bowel.

Dietary fibers have a variety of effects on gut integrity (199). Pectin and guar (metabolizable fibers) stimulate proliferation and maturation of intestinal cells (199–204). Metabolizable fibers also increase gut mucosal enzyme activity and improve gut absorption (199–205). Infusion of SCFAs into the colon of animals enhances healing of colonic anastomoses (206) and increases mucosal DNA content (207). Supplementation of parenteral nutrition with SCFAs reduces the gut atrophy associated with TPN (208). Instillation of SCFAs into the colon of patients with diversion colitis reduces bowel inflammation (209). Pectin-supplementation of elemental diets improves intestinal adaptation following experimental small-bowel resection (210). Pectin-supplementation also decreases colonic inflammation following experimental colitis and improves the healing of colonic anastomoses in the rat (211). Pectin supplementation reduces the incidence of liquid stools (199, 212) and may help control diarrhea.

Bulk fiber has minimal effect on these parameters. Bulk fibers accelerate colonic transit and produce larger, softer stool (205). These fibers are useful in the treatment of constipation. They may also increase stool viscosity in patients with diarrhea. However, bulk fibers have not been shown to decrease the incidence of diarrhea (213).

Metabolizable fibers are important substrates for colonic and small-bowel structure and function. Maintenance of the gut barrier is important for minimizing bacterial/toxin translocation through the intestinal tract. Pectin-supplemented enteral and parenteral nutrition decreases the incidence of bacterial translocation compared with TPN alone and oral enteral nonfiber diets. Most liquid-formula diets do not contain these fibers and may benefit from their addition. Fermentation of carbohydrate by anaerobes occurs principally in the colon. Use of antimicrobial agents that destroy gut anaerobes reduces this fermentation and may lead to gut atrophy and bacterial translocation.

Basal glucose production is elevated in critically ill patients and is not fully suppressed by exogenously administered glucose. Hyperglycemia results from accelerated gluconeogenesis and glycogenolysis and insulin resistance (impaired glucose clearance). Substrates for glucose synthesis include lactate, glycerol, alanine, and other amino acids. Glucose and fat metabolism are usually enhanced in most critically ill patients, indicating that the body can use both fuel sources efficiently. Lipid cannot totally suppress glucose oxidation, and glucose cannot totally suppress lipid oxidation. There is no absolute preference for one fuel source over the other and no metabolic advantage for using only one fuel source (i.e., either lipid or glucose).

Both glucose and lipid administration produce nitrogen-sparing effects (214–219), in which there are plateaus (220). Once the plateau is reached, increasing the infusions further will not result in greater suppression of protein breakdown. However, addition of supplemental insulin (to prevent hyperglycemia) may aid in suppressing protein catabolism (221, 222).

An undesirable effect of carbohydrate feeding is excessive carbon dioxide production (VCO_2). Increased VCO_2 increases minute ventilation and work of breathing. Patients with impaired respiratory function may develop hypercarbia and respiratory failure. Septic patients (223) overfed with dextrose (1.5 to 2 times resting energy expenditure) demonstrated increased oxygen consumption, VCO_2, and minute ventilation.

In order to avoid hypercapnia, respiratory acidosis, and respiratory failure, lipid has been substituted for carbohydrate as a caloric source. Lipid/glucose combinations cause less CO_2 production and stimulate lower minute ventilation than does glucose alone (224–226). However, studies reporting clinically significant increases in VCO_2 administered calories in excess of needs. When carbohydrate or carbohydrate/lipid were administered at rates that matched energy expenditure, there were few significant differences in VCO_2 between diet groups. There were also no significant differences in VCO_2 when glucose-lipid diets containing 30 to 50% lipid (at rates that matched energy needs) were compared (227).

NUCLEIC ACIDS

The importance of nucleic acids as nutrients for nutritional support remains unclear. Nucleic acids are not present in parenteral nutritional formulas or most enteral formulas. They are not considered to be essential nutrients since the body can synthesize them.

A variety of studies suggest that nucleic acids may play a role in the immune response. Dietary supplementation of animals with nucleotides enhances immune responses when compared with diets lacking these substances (228, 229). Nucleotide-free diets suppress cardiac allograft rejection, graft versus host disease, delayed cutaneous hypersensitivity, mixed-lymphocyte responses, and mitogen-stimulated lymphocyte proliferation (228–232). These effects are reversed with nucleotide supplementation. Nucleotide-free diets enhance cyclosporin immunosuppression (232, 233), are associated with decreased production of IL-2, and decreased activity of natural killer cells in animals (231). However, these diets are associated with higher macrophage activation. Dietary nucleotide effects are time- and dose-dependent. Uracil is a key ingredient of nucleotide preparations (228, 232).

Nucleotide-free diets are associated with increased mortality in animals administered *Candida albicans* (229, 234) and *S. aureus* (235, 236). The role of nucleotide supplementation in human disease has not been evaluated adequately, and support for its use is lacking.

NUTRIENT COMBINATIONS

There are no randomized controlled human trials in the literature evaluating the efects of individual nutrients such as arginine, glutamine, ω-3 polyunsaturated fatty acids (PUFA), peptides, or nucleotides on infection rates and outcome in critically ill patients. However, there have been several recent controlled trials of nutrient combinations aimed at improving immune function and decreasing infection rates.

A modular tube feeding (MTF), which utilizes supplemental arginine and ω-3 long-chain fatty acids, was developed at the Shriner's Burn Institute (236a). Fifty patients with burns were allocated to the MTF or two intact protein enteral formulas. Patients with the MTF had a significant reduction in wound infections and ICU stay. There was a trend toward less pneumonia and mortality. Impact (Sandoz Nutrition) is an enteral formula containing supplemental arginine, ω-3 PUFA, and RNA. Cerra et al (236b) randomized 20 trauma patients to Impact vs. an intact protein formula. There were no differences in infections or mortality between these small groups. However, mononuclear cell mitogenic responses were greater in the Impact group. The clinical significance of these findings remains unclear. Daly et al (236c) evaluated Impact vs. an intact protein formula in patients undergoing gastrointestinal surgery for malignancy. The intact protein group received significantly less nitrogen and was in greater negative nitrogen balance. There were no significant reductions in infections or length of stay (20 vs. 19 days for all patients) between groups. However, the incidence of infections plus wound healing complications was reduced in the Impact group. Bower et al (236d) reported the preliminary results of a large multicenter double-blind randomized trial, comparing Impact with an intact protein formula in critically ill patients. Nitrogen and calorie intake were not reported. There were fewer urinary tract infections in the Impact group. However, overall infections and mortality were similar between groups.

The length of stay was shorter in the Impact group (22 vs. 26 days). Variables that influence hospital stay were not reported (i.e., Acute Physiology Score, Age, comorbid conditions, primary reason for ICU admission, surgery status, physician, mortality.

The results of these studies evaluating "immune-enhancing" formulas in critically ill patients are difficult to interpret at the current time. Many of the groups failed to receive comparable nutritional support. Variables affecting length of stay were not controlled for. However, the current data suggest that these formulas have potential for reducing infections and hospital stay, and further studies of their efficacy are warranted.

INDICATIONS FOR ENTERAL NUTRITION

An adequate supply of nutrients to cells is important for recovery from illness and injury. Results from experimental and clinical studies indicate that enteral nutrition is the preferred method for delivering nutrients (75). Compared with parenteral feeding, enteral nutrition supplies a wider variety of nutrients, delivers the nutrients in a more physiologic way, and is cheaper in cost.

Enteral nutrition is indicated in patients requiring nutritional support when there is a functioning small intestine. Patients with intact swallowing and gastric emptying may be fed orally. Patients with adequate gastric emptying may be fed via the stomach (i.e., gastric tube). Patients with gastroparesis (i.e., delayed gastric emptying) or significant gastric reflux are best fed via the small intestine so as to avoid high gastric residuals, reflux, and pulmonary aspiration. Some critically ill patients develop poor colonic motility. These patients are best fed nonfiber formulas until colonic motility returns (i.e., patients develop flatus, bowel movements). It is important to note that most critically ill patients have adequate small-intestinal function, despite gastroparesis and poor colonic motility (see the section of this chapter entitled "Gut Function").

Enteral feeding is the preferred route for nutrient administration in most patients, including those who are undergoing surgery, have cancer, are receiving chemotherapy, and have respiratory, cardiac, hepatic, or renal failure. Enteral feeding may be used safely and is well-tolerated in most patients following abdominal surgery, gastrointestinal surgery, vascular surgery, neurosurgery, cardiothoracic surgery, trauma, and burns (1, 8, 16, 36, 38, 105). These patients usually have adequate small-bowel motility and absorption, although absorption may be decreased from normal levels. Experimental data suggest that enteral feedings improve healing of injured bowel when administered immediately following intestinal surgery (21).

Most patients with pancreatitis can be fed enterally. Feeding via the proximal jejunum produces less pancreatic stimulation than does intragastric feeding. Administration of pancreatic enzymes also reduces pancreatic stimulation (237). Clinical experience indicates that small-bowel feedings are tolerated by patients with pancreatitis (238–240). It is unclear whether "bowel rest" and nasogastric suctioning improve the course of pancreatitis. Patients with pancreatitis should be monitored closely for signs of dietary intolerance (i.e., abdominal pain, abdominal distention, reflux, vomiting). Malabsorption diarrhea can be treated effectively with enzyme replacement and low fat intake. Only when patients fail enteral feeding should they be started on parenteral nutrition.

Most patients with inflammatory bowel disease (IBD) (Crohn's disease, ulcerative colitis) can tolerate enteral feeding (241–244). There are few data indicating that "bowel rest" improves the course of inflammatory bowel disease (244). Some studies suggest that defined-formula diets improve the course of IBD when compared with normal diets. It is thought that these defined-formula diets reduce antigenic stimulation and resultant bowel inflammation. Patients with Crohn's disease are characterized by small-bowel inflammation. These patients frequently have malabsorption and may benefit from hydrolyzed protein and low-fat diets. Patients with ulcerative colitis usually have an intact small bowel and usually tolerate enteral feedings.

Tolerance of enteral feeding is related to the length of the small bowel. Patients with very short guts may be unable to absorb adequate nutrients to maintain body integrity. Although these patients require parenteral nutrients to maintain adequate intake, they should also receive enteral nutrients to maintain, stimulate, and protect the integrity of the gut.

Enteral nutrients stimulate blood flow to the gastrointestinal tract and may be useful in improving gut blood flow during shock states. It is important that intravascular volume be replaced. Dilation of gut blood vessels with enteral nutrients may further decrease intravascular volume in the underresuscitated patient.

Diarrhea is not a contraindication to enteral feeding in most patients. Diarrhea may result from medications (i.e., sorbitol, magnesium), bacterial overgrowth (i.e., use of broad-spectrum antibiotics), infection of the bowel (i.e., viral, bacterial), bacterial toxins (i.e., *Clostridium* toxin, cholera toxin), gut atrophy and loss of absorptive area, gut diseases, or loss of digestive processes (245, 246). These processes do not contraindicate enteral feeding and may improve more quickly when the gut is stimulated with nutrients. However, it may be necessary to alter the diet to help control diarrhea (i.e., hydrolyzed protein diets, pancreatic enzyme supplementation, low-fat diets, reduced fiber intake). Clinical experience indicates that enteral nutrition can be used effectively in most patients with diarrhea. Most diarrhea is self-limited and will resolve over time. Fluid and electrolytes should be monitored and replaced as necessary. Antidiarrheal drugs may be used as adjuvants to control the diarrhea while the etiology is investigated. The author and colleagues have used paregoric effectively. Enteral formulas are mixed with 15 to 30 ml of paregoric administered over 4 to 6 hours. The dose is tapered to control the number of bowel movements. Antiemetic drugs are used to control nausea and vomiting. In the author's experience, diarrhea usually resolves in critically ill patients as their disease processes are controlled. Failure of diarrhea to improve or resolve frequently indicates gut failure and high mortality.

Enteral nutrition has been used effectively in patients receiving chemotherapy or radiotherapy and following transplantation. Oral nutrition is the preferred route of support. However, enteric feeding tubes have been used effectively in patients who are unable to consume adequate oral nutrients. Enteral nutrition is believed to protect the gut from the harmful effects of chemotherapy and radiotherapy. Many clinicians worry about the possibility of infections resulting from feeding tubes (especially nasal tubes). This worry is not supported by clinical data. In fact, enteral nutrition (compared with parenteral nutrition) has been shown to reduce infections in patients following chemotherapy (44–46).

In summary, enteral nutrition is the preferred mode of feeding in most critically ill patients with a functioning small intestine. Enteral access is rarely impossible but does require skill. Access is facilitated by the use of fluoroscopy, endoscopy, or surgery.

NUTRITIONAL GOALS AND MONITORING

Optimal nutritional support requires the administration of adequate nutrients. Calorie consumption in critically ill patients is reduced by bed rest, sedation, paralysis, and β-adrenergic blockade. It is increased during hypermetabolic states (i.e., sepsis, burns, trauma) and exercise (i.e., respiratory distress). Clinical studies indicate that most critically ill patients require 25 to 30 kcal/kg/day and 1.5 to 2.5 g protein/kg/day. Calories are usually administered as a combination of carbohydrate (60 to 70%) and fat (30 to 40%). The author and colleagues usually begin nutritional support with these quantities and adjust as indicated by the clinical course and nutritional monitoring. An attempt is made to avoid overfeeding. Overfeeding increases the respiratory quotient and carbon dioxide production, increases lipogenesis and fatty liver, and can impair recovery.

Enteral feeding is begun using full-strength formulas at a rate of 50 to 75 ml/hr in adults (50 to 100% of nutritional requirements). Most enteral formulas have osmolalities below 500 mosm/kg water and are well-tolerated. Diluting the formulas does not improve tolerance and slows the rate of nutrient repletion. The rate is advanced by 25 ml/hr every 4 to 6 hours until full rates are achieved. These rates of nutrient delivery are extremely slow (i.e., less than 1 ml/min) and approximate the normal rate of saliva production.

It is important to monitor the adequacy of nutritional support. The best monitor of nutritional support is the patient's clinical response. However, it is frequently difficult to determine the adequacy of nutritional support based on clinical response alone. Disease processes are complex, variable, and may progress for reasons unrelated to nutrition. For these reasons, objective criteria are often used to monitor nutritional support. Caloric needs can be determined by measuring oxygen consumption and carbon dioxide production. Oxygen consumption can be measured using a pulmonary artery catheter or indirect calorimetry (i.e., metabolic cart).

Serial changes in visceral protein levels (i.e., prealbumin, transferrin, retinol binding protein) are good measures for assessing the adequacy of nutritional support. Single measurements are less valuable. Visceral proteins reflect hepatic protein synthesis. Synthesis and secretion are depressed as a result of hypercatabolism, uncontrolled sepsis, malnutrition, and other states that impair liver function. Maintenance or improvement in visceral protein levels suggests that nutritional support is adequate. Decreasing levels indicate continued hepatic dysfunction and should prompt a search for underlying infection, continued tissue damage, or inadequate nutritional support. In the author's experience, most surviving patients demonstrate an improvement in visceral protein levels over the first 7 to 10 days of nutritional support, whereas decreasing levels usually predict progressive organ failure and death. In addition, infections are more common in patients whose visceral proteins fail to increase in response to nutritional support.

Nitrogen balance may also be used to assess the adequacy of nutritional support. However, nitrogen balance alone has many problems. Urea nitrogen fails to detect a significant amount of nitrogen lost in the urine and underestimates nitrogen losses. Thus, total nitrogen (not available in many hospitals) is a better test than urea nitrogen. In addition, most hospitals fail to measure stool or wound nitrogen losses when assessing nitrogen balance. Nitrogen is lost from muscle (i.e., atrophy) when patients are placed on bed rest or when they are paralyzed (by drug or disease). This negative nitrogen balance is appropriate. Nitrogen balance integrates all nitrogen losses into one value. However, nitrogen loss is not uniform. Thus, one tissue may lose more nitrogen than another. It is even possible for some tissues to be in negative nitrogen balance while other tissues and overall balance are positive.

The author and others have attempted to assess the effect of nutritional support on immune function by measuring delayed cutaneous hypersensitivity responses (DCH). DCH has proved valuable in assessing prognosis and risk of complications in outpatients prior to surgery. However, critical illness produces skin anergy in most patients, and the test has not been useful for assessing nutrient adequacy.

COMPLICATIONS OF ENTERAL NUTRITION

Enteral feeding may be associated with complications such as misplaced feeding tubes, diarrhea, and pulmonary aspiration (i.e., gastric contents). With the exception of pulmonary aspiration, life-threatening complications are few. Severe complications are unusual when enteral nutrition is administered by skilled clinicians.

MECHANICAL COMPLICATIONS

Tracheal placement of feeding tubes can occur. Tracheal placement is more common in patients with altered gag reflexes, dysphagia, and diminished mental status (i.e., from drugs or disease). Although the presence of an endotracheal tube reduces the chance for tracheal insertion of feeding tubes, it does not prevent this complication. Gastrointestinal placement of feeding tubes should be confirmed before the tube is fully inserted (i.e., by aspiration of gastric contents or bile, pH, myoelectric activity, or visual inspection), to avoid pulmonary damage and pneumothorax. It is important to note that pneumothorax is more common with central line placement than with feeding tube placement (1.7% vs 0.3%) (75, 247). Feeding tube position must be checked before infusion of nutrients to prevent infusion into the lung. X-ray of the chest/abdomen frequently is used for this purpose but requires time and is not cost-effective. The author and co-workers prefer aspiration of gastric/intestinal contents, measurement of gastric pH, measurement of myoelectric activity, or direct visualization of the tube passing into the esophagus with a laryngoscope. Auscultation following air injection may produce deceptive results. Feeding tubes placed into the base of the lung can produce sounds similar to those from tubes placed into the stomach.

Enteral feeding tubes may become clogged during use. Clogging can be minimized by flushing the tubes with warm water every 4 to 6 hours and avoiding the administration of medications through the tubes. Pill fragments can clog the tube, and some medications may precipitate with feeding formula. In addition, the author and co-workers have found that clogging of small-bore feeding tubes is more frequent with high-fat and high-fiber formulas.

PULMONARY ASPIRATION

Pulmonary aspiration (248–252) is one of the most serious complications of enteral feeding. It is believed that high gastric residuals predispose to gastric reflux and aspiration. The amount of gastric residual that predisposes to aspiration is unclear and depends on the competence of the lower esophageal sphincter, stomach size, and patient position (248–250). Salivary and gastric secretions contribute to gastric residuals. Most normal fasting adults have gastric residuals that range from 0 to 100 ml (253). High gastric residuals may occur as a result of gastroparesis (i.e., delayed gastric emptying) in patients not receiving enteral nutrition.

Small-bowel feeding of nutrients minimizes the risk of pulmonary aspiration (251, 252). A nasogastric feeding tube is frequently required in these patients to decompress the stomach and prevent high gastric residuals. Placement of a nasogastric tube also allows for administration of drugs for stress ulcer prophylaxis and for monitoring of duodenal reflux. Addition of dye to the feeding formula is a convenient method for detecting reflux of formula into the stomach from the small bowel. Gastric reflux and aspiration can also be minimized by keeping the head of the bed elevated (248, 249).

DIARRHEA

Diarrhea (245, 246) may occur in patients receiving enteral feeding. Diarrhea may result from the administration of drugs, gut infection (i.e., *Clostridium difficile*, cholera, *Salmonella*), gut atrophy, impaired digestion and absorption, hypersecretory states, hypoalbuminemia, and impaction. Drugs associated with diarrhea include magnesium (i.e., antacids), sorbitol (frequently used as the vehicle for many drugs), and antibiotics (which induce bacterial overgrowth). Digestion and absorption are impaired in patients with malnutrition, following injury (i.e., burn, trauma), and from diseases that decrease bile formation or enzyme secretion (i.e., pancreatitis, cystic fibrosis). Diarrhea may also be a manifestation of gut failure as part of multiple organ failure.

Diarrhea represents the production of excess stool (i.e., >250 g/day). Many critically ill patients have rectal incontinence (i.e., resulting from loss of rectal tone), which results in numerous bowel movements but not true diarrhea. In addition, stool is frequently liquid or pasty in texture because of lack of fiber intake.

Most diarrhea can be managed with enteral nutrition. Drugs that may be causing the diarrhea should be discontinued, if possible. The exact cause of the diarrhea should be determined and treated (especially with infectious diarrhea). Diarrhea frequently can be diminished by manipulating dietary intake (i.e., reducing long-chain fats, using peptide feedings) and using opiates. Stool consistency can be made more solid by the use of fiber supplementation. Stool output can be managed with diapers, fecal-incontinence bags, or rectal Foley catheters. It is important to monitor and replace lost fluids and electrolytes. Most diarrhea resolves as the patient improves. Persistence of diarrhea frequently indicates gut failure and high mortality.

OTHER COMPLICATIONS

Otitis media and sinus complications are possible from the use of nasal feeding tubes. Erosions at sites of insertion (i.e., nose and mouth) may also occur. Dislodgement of gastrostomy or jejunostomy tubes are rare complications.

CONCLUSION

Enteral feeding of nutrients is the preferred method of nutritional support in critically ill patients. Nutrient administration should be started as early as possible following hospital admission. Patients who are unable to ingest adequate nutrients safely should be fed using gastric or small-bowel feeding tubes. Enteral feeding requires careful monitoring of feeding tube position, possible complications, and nutritional response.

REFERENCES

1. Hill GL: Body composition research: implications for the practice of clinical nutrition. *J Parenter Enter Nutr* 16:197–218, 1992.
2. Windsor JA, Hill GL: Weight loss with physiologic impairment. A basic indicator of surgical risk. *Ann Surg* 207:290–296, 1988.
3. Windsor JA, Hill GL: Risk factors for postoperative pneumonia. The importance of protein depletion. *Ann Surg* 208:209–214, 1988.
4. Arora NS, Rochester DF: Respiratory muscle strength and maximal voluntary ventilation in undernourished patients. *Am Rev Respir Dis* 126:5–8, 1982.
5. Haydock DA, Hill GL: Impaired wound healing in surgical patients with varying degrees of malnutrition. *J Parenter Enter Nutr* 10:550–554, 1986.
6. Windsor JA, Hill GL: Protein depletion and surgical risk. *Aust NZ J Surg* 58:711–715, 1988.
7. Saito H, Trocki O, Alexander JW, Kopcha R, Heyd T, Joffe SN: The effect of route of nutrient administration on the nutritional state, catabolic hormone secretion, and gut mucosal integrity after burn injury. *J Parenter Enter Nutr* 11:1–7, 1987.
8. Chiarelli A, Enzi G, Casadei A, Baggio B, Valerio A, Mazzoleni F: Very early nutrition supplementation in burned patients. *Am J Clin Nutr* 51:1035–1039, 1990.
9. Dominioni L, Trocki O, Mochizuki H, Fang CH, Alexander JW: Prevention of severe postburn hypermetabolism and catabolism by immediate intragastric feeding. *J Burn Care Rehabil* 5:106–112, 1984.
10. Mochizuki H, Trocki O, Dominioni L, Brackett KA, Joffe SN, Alexander JW: Mechanism of prevention of postburn hypermetabolism and catabolism by early enteral feeding. *Ann Surg* 200:297–310, 1984.
11. McArdle AH, Palmason C, Brown RA, Brown HC, Williams HB: Early enteral feeding of patients with major burns: prevention of catabolism. *Ann Plast Surg* 13:396–401, 1984.
12. Jenkins M, Gottschlich M, Alexander JW, Warden GD: Effect of immediate enteral feeding on the hypermetabolic response following severe burn injury (abstr.). *J Parenter Enter Nutr* 13:12, 1989.
13. Mochizuki H, Trocki O, Dominioni L, Alexander JW: Reduction of postburn hypermetabolism by early enteral feeding. *Current Surgery* 42:121–125, 1985.
14. Jenkins M, Gottschlich M, Baumer T, et al: Enteral feeding during operative procedures. *J Parenter Enter Nutr* 15:225, 1991.
15. Zaloga GP, Black KW, Prielipp R: Enteral feeding minimizes liver damage following hemorrhage. *Chest* 100:135S, 1991.
16. Moore EE, Jones TN: Benefits of immediate jejunostomy feeding after major abdominal trauma—a prospective, randomized study. *J Trauma* 26:874–881, 1986.
17. Ryan JA Jr, Page CP, Babcock L: Early postoperative jejunal feeding of an elemental diet in gastrointestinal surgery. *Am Surg* 47:393–403, 1981.
18. Sager S, Harland P, Shields R: Early postoperative feeding with elemental diet. *Br Med J* 1:293–295, 1979.

19. Rapp RP, Young B, Twyman D, Bivins BA, Haack D, Tibbs PA, Bean JR: The favorable effect of early parenteral feeding on survival in head-injured patients. *J Neurosurg* 58:906–912, 1983.
20. Zaloga GP, Bortenschlager L, Black KW, Prielipp R: Immediate postoperative enteral feeding decreases weight loss and improves wound healing after abdominal surgery in rats. *Crit Care Med* 20:115–118, 1992.
21. Moss G, Greenstein A, Levy S, Bierenbaum A: Maintenance of GI function after bowel surgery and immediate enteral full nutrition. I. Doubling of canine colorectal anastomotic bursting pressure and intestinal wound mature collagen content. *J Parenter Enter Nutr* 4:535–538, 1980.
22. Windsor JA, Knight GS, Hill GL: Wound healing response in surgical patients: recent food intake is more important than nutritional status. *Br J Surg* 75:135–137, 1988.
23. Schroeder D, Gillanders L, Mahr K, Hill GL: Effects of immediate postoperative enteral nutrition on body composition, muscle function, and wound healing. *J Parenter Enter Nutr* 15:376–383, 1991.
24. Haydock DA, Hill GL: Improved wound healing response in surgical patients receiving intravenous nutrition. *Br J Surg* 74:320–323, 1987.
25. Law NW, Ellis H: The effect of parenteral nutrition on the healing of abdominal wall wounds and colonic anastomoses in protein-malnourished rats. *Surgery* 107:449–454, 1990.
26. Collins JP, Oxby CB, Hill GL: Intravenous amino acids and intravenous hyperalimentation as protein-sparing therapy after major surgery. A controlled trial. *Lancet* 1:788–791, 1978.
27. Zaloga GP: Nutrition and prevention of systemic infection. In Society of Critical Care Medicine (eds): *Critical Care State of the Art*, vol 12. Fullerton, CA, Society of Critical Care Medicine, 1991, pp 31–79.
28. Zaloga GP, Macgregor DA: What to consider when choosing enteral or parenteral nutrition. *J Crit Ill* 5:1180–1200, 1990.
29. Kudsk KA, Carpenter G, Petersen S, Sheldon GF: Effect of enteral and parenteral feeding in malnourished rats with *E. coli*-hemoglobin adjuvant peritonitis. *J Surg Res* 31:105–110, 1981.
30. Kudsk KA, Stone JM, Carpenter G, Sheldon GF: Enteral and parenteral feeding influences mortality after hemoglobin-*E. coli* peritonitis in normal rats. *J Trauma* 23:605–609, 1983.
31. Petersen SR, Kudsk KA, Carpenter G, Sheldon GF: Malnutrition and immunocompetence: increased mortality following an infectious challenge during hyperalimentation. *J Trauma* 21:528–533, 1981.
32. Zaloga GP, Prielipp RC, Ward KA: Total parenteral nutrition (TPN) increases mortality following methotrexate-induced endogenous sepsis. *Anesthesiology* 73:A1232, 1990.
33. Alverdy JC, Aoys E, Moss BS: Parenteral nutrition results in bacterial translocation from the gut and death following chemotherapy. *J Parenter Enter Nutr* 14:8S, 1990.
34. Zaloga GP, Knowles R, Black KW, Prielipp R: Total parenteral nutrition increases mortality after hemorrhage. *Crit Care Med* 19:54–59, 1991.
35. Adams S, Dellinger EP, Wertz MJ, Oreskovich MR, Simonowitz D, Johansen K: Enteral versus parenteral nutritional support following laparotomy for trauma: a randomized prospective trial. *J Trauma* 26:882–891, 1986.
36. Moore FA, Moore EE, Jones TN, McCroskey BL, Peterson VM: TEN versus TPN following major abdominal trauma—reduced septic morbidity. *J Trauma* 29:916–923, 1989.
37. Moore FA, Feliciano DV, Andrassy RJ, McArdle AH, Booth FV, Morgenstein-Wagner TB, Kellum JM Jr, Welling RE, Moore EE: Early enteral feeding, compared with parenteral, reduces postoperative septic complications. The results of a meta-analysis. *Ann Surg* 216:172–183, 1992.
38. Kudsk KA, Croce MA, Fabian TC, Minard G, Tolley EA, Poret HA, Kuhl MR, Brown RO: Enteral versus parenteral feeding. Effects on septic morbidity after blunt and penetrating abdominal trauma. *Ann Surg* 215:503–513, 1992.
39. Young B, Ott L, Twyman D, Norton J, Rapp R, Tibbs P, Haack D, Brivins B, Dempsey R: The effect of nutritional support on outcome from severe head injury. *J Neurosurg* 67:668–676, 1987.
40. Hadley MN, Grahm TW, Harrington T, Schiller WR, McDermott MK, Posillico DB: Nutritional support and neurotrauma: a critical review of early nutrition in forty-five acute head injury patients. *Neurosurgery* 19:367–373, 1986.
41. Detsky AS, Baker JP, O'Rourke K, Goel V: Perioperative parenteral nutrition: a meta-analysis. *Ann Intern Med* 107:195–203, 1987.
42. American College of Physicians: Perioperative parenteral nutrition. *Ann Intern Med* 107:252–253, 1987.
43. Veterans Affairs Total Parenteral Nutrition Cooperative Study Group: Perioperative total parenteral nutrition in surgical patients. *N Engl J Med* 325:525–532, 1991.
44. Koretz RL: Parenteral nutrition: is it oncologically logical? *J Clin Oncol* 2:534–538, 1984.
45. Klein S, Simes J, Blackburn GL: Total parenteral nutrition and cancer clinical trials. *Cancer* 58:1378–1386, 1986.
46. American College of Physicians: Parenteral nutrition in patients receiving cancer chemotherapy. *Ann Intern Med* 110:734–736, 1989.
47. Ryan GP, Dudrick SJ, Copeland EM, Johnson LR: Effects of various diets on colonic growth in rats. *Gastroenterology* 77:658–663, 1979.
48. Johnson LR, Copeland EM, Dudrick SJ, Lichtenberger LM, Castro GA: Structural and hormonal alterations in the gastrointestinal tract of parenterally fed rats. *Gastroenterology* 68:1177–1183, 1975.
49. Levine GM, Deren JJ, Steiger E, Zinno R: Role of oral intake in maintenance of gut mass and disaccharide activity. *Gastroenterology* 67:975–982, 1974.
50. Johnson LR, Copeland EM, Dudrick SJ, Lichtenberger LM, Castro GA: Structural and hormonal alterations in the gastrointestinal tract of parenterally fed rats. *Gastroenterology* 68:1177–1183, 1975.
51. Thompson JS, Vaughan WP, Forst CF, Jacobs DL, Weekly JS, Rikkers LF: The effect of the route of nutrient delivery on gut structure and diamine oxidase levels. *J Parenter Enter Nutr* 11:28–32, 1987.
52. Lickley HL, Track NS, Vranic M, Bury KD: Metabolic responses to enteral and parenteral nutrition. *Am J Surg* 135:172–176, 1978.
53. Helton WS, Jacobs DO, Bonner-Weir S, Bueno R, Smith RJ, Wilmore DW: Effects of glutamine-enriched parenteral nutrition on the exocrine pancreas. *J Parenter Enter Nutr* 14:344–352, 1990.
54. Levine GM, Deren JJ, Steiger E, Zinno R: Role of oral intake in maintenance of gut mass and disaccharide activity. *Gastroenterology* 67:975–982, 1974.
55. Kudsk KA, Stone JM, Carpenter G, Sheldon GF: Effects of enteral and parenteral feeding of malnourished rats on body composition. *J Trauma* 22:904–906, 1982.
56. Czernichow B, Galluser M, Hasselmann M, Doffoel M, Raul F: Effects of amino acids in mixtures given by enteral or parenteral route on intestinal morphology and hydrolases in rats. *J Parenter Enter Nutr* 16:259–263, 1991.
57. Alverdy JC, Aoys E, Moss GS: Total parenteral nutrition promotes bacterial translocation from the gut. *Surgery* 104:185–190, 1988.
58. Alverdy J, Chi HS, Sheldon GF: The effect of parenteral nutrition on gastrointestinal immunity. The importance of enteral stimulation. *Ann Surg* 202:681–684, 1985.
59. Alverdy JC, Weisz-Carrington P, Bushmann RJ, Kelemen PR, Aoys E, Moss GS: Effect of parenteral nutrition on gut IgA plasma. *J Parenter Enter Nutr* 14:10S, 1990.
60. Renk CM, Owens DR, Birkhahn RH, Long CL, Blakemore WS: Effect of intravenous or oral feeding on immunocompetence in traumatized rats. *J Parenter Enter Nutr* 4:587, 1980.
61. Birkhahn RH, Renk CM: Immune response and leucine oxidation in oral and intravenous fed rats. *Am J Clin Nutr* 39:45–53, 1984.
62. Lindor KD, Fleming CR, Abrams A, Hirschkorn MA: Liver function values in adults receiving total parenteral nutrition. *JAMA* 241:2398–2400, 1979.
63. Riely CA, Fine PL, Boyer JL: Progressively rising serum bile acids—a common effect of parenteral nutrition. *Gastroenterology* 77:A34, 1979.
64. Knodell RG, Spector MH, Brooks DA, Keller FX, Kyner WT: Alterations in pentobarbital pharmacokinetics in response to parenteral and enteral alimentation in the rat. *Gastroenterology* 79:1211–1216, 1980.
65. Knodell RG, Steele NM, Cerra FB, Gross JB, Solomon TE: Effects of parenteral and enteral hyperalimentation on hepatic drug metabolism in the rat. *J Pharmacol Exp Ther* 229:589–597, 1984.
66. Saito H, Trocki O, Alexander JW, Kopcha R, Heyd T, Joffe SN: The effect of route of nutrient administration on the nutritional state, catabolic hormone secretion, and gut mucosal integrity after burn injury. *J Parenter Enter Nutr* 11:1–7, 1987.
67. Rivera A Jr, Bhatia J, Rassin DK, Gourley WK, Catarau E: In vivo biliary function in the adult rat: the effect of parenteral glucose and amino acids. *J Parenter Enter Nutr* 13:240–245, 1989.
68. Hiramatu T, Saito S, Taniwaka K, Fukushima R, Moriaka Y: The beneficial effects of postoperative enteral nutrition on protein metabolism and immunocompetence in rats with gastrectomy. *J Parenter Enter Nutr* 14:10S, 1990.
69. Fong Y, Marano MA, Barber A, He W, Moldawer LL, Bushman ED, Coyle SM, Shires GT, Lowry SF: Total parenteral nutrition and bowel rest modify the metabolic response to endotoxin in humans. *Ann Surg* 210:449–457, 1989.
70. Young EA, Cioletti LA, Traylor JB, Balderas V: Gastrointestinal response to oral versus gastric feeding of defined formula diets. *Am J Clin Nutr* 35:715–726, 1982.
71. Zaloga GP: Bedside method for placing small bowel feeding tubes in critically ill patients. A prospective study. *Chest* 100:1643–1646, 1991.
72. Ponsky JL, Gauderer MW: Percutaneous endoscopic gastrostomy: a nonoperative technique for feeding gastrostomy. *Gastrointest Endosc* 27:9–11, 1981.
73. Ponsky JL, Gauderer MW, Stellato TA, Aszodi A: Percutaneous approaches to enteral alimentation. *Am J Surg* 149:102–105, 1985.
74. Baskin W: PEJ placement: a new steerable catheter technique. *Am J Gastroenterol* 84:1155, 1989.
75. Roundtable Conference: *Enteral nutritional support for the 1990s: innovations in nutrition, technology, and techniques.* Columbus, OH, Ross Laboratories, 1992, pp 1–51.
76. Amoss M, Rivier J, Guillemin R: Release of gonadotropins by oral administration of synthetic LRF or a tripeptide fragment of LRF. *J Clin Endocrinol Metab* 35:175–177, 1972.
77. Gardner MG: Intestinal assimilation of intact peptides and proteins from the diet—a neglected field? *Biol Rev* 59:289, 1984.
78. Danforth E, Moore RO: Intestinal absorption of insulin in the rat. *Endocrinology* 65:118–123, 1959.
79. Gardner ML: Absorption of intact peptides: studies on transport of protein digests and dipeptides across rat small intestine in vitro. *Q J Exp Physiol* 67:629–637, 1982.
80. Webb KE Jr: Amino acid and peptide absorption from the gastrointestinal tract. *Fed Proc* 45:2268–2271, 1986.
81. Zaloga GP: Studies comparing intact protein, peptide, and amino acid formulas. In Bounos G (ed): *Uses of Elemental Diets in Clinical Situations.* Boca Raton, FL, CRC Press, 1993, pp 201–217.
82. Zaloga GP: Physiologic effects of peptide-based enteral formulas. *Nutr Clin Pract* 5:231–237, 1990.
83. Zaloga GP, Ward KA, Prielipp RC: Effect of enteral diets on whole body and gut growth in unstressed rats. *J Parenter Enter Nutr* 15:42–47, 1991.
84. Shou J, Lieberman MD, Hofmann K, Leon P, Redmond HP, Davies H, Daly JM: Dietary manipulation of methotrexate-induced enterocolitis. *J Parenter Enter Nutr* 15:307–312, 1991.
85. Trocki O, Mochizuki H, Dominioni L, Alexander JW: Intact protein versus free amino acids in the nutritional support of thermally injured animals. *J Parenter Enter Nutr* 10:139–145, 1986.

86. Janne P, Carpenter Y, Willems G: Colonic mucosal atrophy induced by a liquid elemental diet in rats. *Am J Dig Dis* 22:808–812, 1977.

87. Morin CL, Ling V, Bourassa D: Small intestinal and colonic changes induced by a chemically defined diet. *Dig Dis Sci* 25:123–128, 1980.

88. Birke H, Thorlacius-Ussing O, Hessov I: Trophic effect of dietary peptides on mucosa in the rat small bowel. *J Parenter Enter Nutr* 14:26S, 1990.

89. Alverdy JC, Aoys E, Moss GS: Total parenteral nutrition promotes bacterial translocation from the gut. *Surgery* 104:185–190, 1988.

90. McAnena OJ, Harvey LP, Bonau RA, Daly JM: Alteration of methotrexate toxicity in rats by manipulation of dietary components. *Gastroenterology* 92:354–360, 1987.

91. Knodell RG: Effects of formula composition on hepatic and intestinal drug metabolism during enteral nutrition. *J Parenter Enter Nutr* 14:34–38, 1990.

92. Feller A, Rudman D, Caindec N: Comparison of nutritional efficacy of peptamin and vivonex TEN elemental diets in elderly tube fed subjects. *J Parenter Enter Nutr* 13:12S, 1989.

93. Poullain MG, Cezard JP, Roger L, Mendy F: Effect of whey proteins, their oligopeptide hydrolysates and free amino acid mixtures on growth and nitrogen retention in fed and starved rats. *J Parenter Enter Nutr* 13:382–386, 1989.

94. Imondi AR, Stradley RP: Utilization of enzymatically hydrolyzed soybean protein and crystalline amino acid diets by rats with exocrine pancreatic insufficiency. *J Nutr* 104:793–801, 1974.

95. Plumb JA, Gardner ML: Can elemental diets reduce the intestinal toxicity of 5-fluorouracil? *J Parenter Enter Nutr* 7:351–357, 1983.

96. Jones BJ, Lees R, Andrews J, Frost P, Silk DB: Comparison of an elemental and polymeric enteral diet in patients with normal gastrointestinal function. *Gut* 24:78–84, 1983.

97. Shou J, Lieberman M, Hofmann K, Redmond H, Leon P, Davies H, Daly JM: Dietary manipulation of methotrexate (MTX)-induced enterocolitis. *J Parenter Enter Nutr* 14:12S, 1990.

98. Fox AD, Kripke SA, DePaula J, Berman JM, Settle RG, Rombeau JL: Effect of a glutamine-supplemented enteral diet on methotrexate-induced enterocolitis. *J Parenter Enter Nutr* 12:325–331, 1988.

99. Harvey LP, McAnena OJ, Mehta BM, Daly JM: Reversibility of elemental liquid diet-induced methotrexate toxicity by refeeding with chow. *J Parenter Enter Nutr* 11:119–123, 1987.

100. Stanford JR, King D, Carey L, Anderson G: The adverse effects of elemental diets on tolerance for 5-FU toxicity in the rat. *J Surg Oncol* 9:493–501, 1977.

101. Granger DN, Brinson RR: Intestinal absorption of elemental and standard enteral formulas in hypoproteinemic (volume expanded) rats. *J Parenter Enter Nutr* 12:278–281, 1988.

102. Brinson RR, Pitts VL, Taylor AE: Intestinal absorption of peptide enteral formulas in hypoproteinemic (volume expanded) rats: a paired analysis. *Crit Care Med* 17:657–660, 1989.

103. Ziegler F, Ollivier JM, Cynober L, Masini JP, Coudray-Lucas C, Levy E, Giboudeau J: Efficacy of enteral nitrogen support in surgical patients: small peptides vs non-degraded proteins. *Gut* 31:1277–1283, 1990.

104. Brinson RR, Kolts BE: Diarrhea associated with severe hypoalbuminemia: a comparison of a peptide-based chemically defined diet and standard enteral alimentation. *Crit Care Med* 16:130–136, 1988.

105. Meredith JW, Ditesheim JA, Zaloga GP: Visceral protein levels in trauma patients are greater with peptide diet than intact protein diet. *J Trauma* 30:825–829, 1990.

106. Monchi M, Vaugelade P, Vaissade P, Rerat A: Net protein utilization after duodenal infusion of small peptides or free amino acids in growing rats. *J Parenter Enter Nutr* 15:29S, 1991.

107. Bounous G, Hugon J, Gentile JM: Elemental diet in the management of the intestinal lesion produced by 5-fluorouracil in the rat. *Can J Surg* 14:298–311, 1971.

108. Bounous G, Maestracci D: Use of an elemental diet in animals during treatment with 5-fluorouracil (NSC-19893). *Cancer Treat Rev* 60:17–22, 1976.

109. Anderson WMD, Brinson RR, Conrad SA, Robinson RH: Intestinal protein loss during enteral alimentation in critically ill patients. *J Parenter Enter Nutr* 14:24S, 1990.

110. Zaloga G, Meredith JW, Roberts P, Bortenschlager L, Black K, Henningfield M: Improved hepatic protein responses with hydrolyzed protein versus intact protein diets after trauma. *Crit Care Med* 20:S94, 1992.

111. Brinson RR, Kolts BE: Diarrhea associated with severe hypoalbuminemia: a comparison of a peptide-based chemically defined diet and standard enteral alimentation. *Crit Care Med* 16:130–136, 1988.

112. Feller A, Rudman D, Caindec N: Comparison of nutritional efficacy of peptamin and vivonex TEN elemental diets in elderly tube fed subjects. *J Parenter Enter Nutr* 13:12S, 1989.

113. Smith JL, Arteaga C, Heymsfield SB: Increased ureagenesis and impaired nitrogen use during infusion of a synthetic amino acid formula: a controlled trial. *N Engl J Med* 306:1013–1018, 1982.

114. Mowatt-Larssen CA, Brown RO, Wojtysiak SL, Kudsk KA: Enteral nutrition efficacy and tolerance: comparison of peptide with standard formulas. *J Parenter Enter Nutr* 15:32S, 1991.

115. Bounous G, Kongshavn PA: Influence of dietary proteins on the immune system of mice. *J Nutr* 112:1747–1755, 1982.

116. Brinson RR, Pitts WM, Benoit J: Effect of β-casomorphin, a casein hydrolysate derivative, on intestinal permeability in volume expanded hypoproteinemic rats. *J Parenter Enter Nutr* 14:10S, 1990.

117. Souba WW, Smith RJ, Wilmore DW: Glutamine metabolism by the intestinal tract. *J Parenter Enter Nutr* 9:608–617, 1985.

118. Wilmore DW, Smith RJ, O'Dwyer ST, Jacobs DO, Ziegler TR, Wang XD: The gut: a central organ after surgical stress. *Surgery* 104:917–923, 1988.

119. Windmueller HG, Spaeth AE: Uptake and metabolism of plasma glutamine by the small intestine. *J Biol Chem* 249:5070–5079, 1974.

120. Windmueller HG, Spaeth AE: Identification of ketone bodies and glutamine as the major respiratory fuels in vivo for postabsorptive rat small intestine. *J Biol Chem* 253:69–76, 1978.

121. Windmueller HG, Spaeth AE: Intestinal metabolism of glutamine and glutamate from the lumen as compared to glutamine from blood. *Arch Biochem Biophys* 171:662–672, 1975.

122. Klimberg VS, Souba WW, Sitren H, Plumley DA, Salloum RM, Hautamaki RD, Bland KI, Copeland EM III: Glutamine-enriched total parenteral nutrition supports gut metabolism. *Surg Forum* 15:175–177, 1989.

123. Hwang TL, O'Dwyer ST, Smith RJ, et al: Preservation of small bowel mucosa using glutamine-enriched parenteral nutrition. *Surg Forum* 38:56, 1987.

124. O'Dwyer ST, Scott T, Smith RJ, Wilmore DW: 5-Fluorouracil toxicity on small intestinal mucosa but not white blood cells is decreased by glutamine. *Clin Res* 35:369A, 1987.

125. O'Dwyer ST, Smith RJ, Kripke SA, et al: New fuels for the gut. In Rombeau JL, Caldwell MD (eds): *Clinical Nutrition: Enteral and Tube Feeding*, 2nd ed. Philadelphia, WB Saunders, 1990, pp 540–555.

126. Stehle P, Zander J, Mertes N, Albers S, Puchstein C, Lawin P, Furst P: Effect of parenteral glutamine peptide supplements on muscle glutamine loss and nitrogen balance after major surgery. *Lancet* 1:231–233, 1989.

127. Hammarqvist F, Wernerman J, Ali R, von der Decken A, Vinnars E: Addition of glutamine to total parenteral nutrition after elective abdominal surgery spares free glutamine in muscle, counteracts the fall in muscle protein synthesis, and improves nitrogen balance. *Ann Surg* 209:455–461, 1989.

128. Jacobs DO, Evans A, O'Dwyer ST, Smith RJ, Wilmore DW: Disparate effects of 5-fluorouracil on the ileum and colon of enterally fed rats with protection by dietary glutamine. *Surg Forum* 38:45–47, 1987.

129. Fox AD, Kripke SA, Berman JR, Settle RG, Rombeau JL: Reduction of the severity of enterocolitis by glutamine-supplemented enteral diets. *Surg Forum* 38:43–44, 1987.

130. Fox AD, Kripke SA, DePaula J, Berman JM, Settle RG, Rombeau JL: Effect of a glutamine-supplemented enteral diet on methotrexate-induced enterocolitis. *J Parenter Enter Nutr* 12:325–331, 1988.

131. Klimberg VS, Dolson DJ, Salloum RM, Bland KI, Copeland EM III, Souba WW: Radioprotection with a glutamine-enriched elemental diet. *J Parenter Enter Nutr* 14:9S, 1990.

132. McAnena OJ, Harvey LP, Bonau RA, Daly JM: Alteration of methotrexate toxicity in rats by manipulation of dietary components. *Gastroenterology* 92:354–360, 1987.

133. Vanderhoff JA, Park JHY, Mohammadpour H, Blackwood D: Absence of trophic effect of glutamine on intestinal adaptation following massive bowel resection. *J Parenter Enter Nutr* 14:8S, 1990.

134. Wells CL, Jechorek RP, Erlandsen SL, Lavin PT, Cerra FB: The effect of dietary glutamine and dietary RNA on ileal flora, ileal histology, and bacterial translocation in mice. *Nutrition* 6:70-83, 1990.

135. Barber AE, Jones WG III, Minei JP, Fahey TJ III, Moldawer LL, Rayburn JL, Fischer E, Keogh CV, Shires GT, Lowry SF: Glutamine or fiber supplementation of a defined formula diet: impact on bacterial translocation, tissue composition, and response to endotoxin. *J Parenter Enter Nutr* 14:335–343, 1990.

136. Souba WW, Klinberg VS, Hautamaki RD, Mendenhall WH, Bova FC, Howard RJ, Bland KI, Copeland EM: Oral glutamine reduces bacterial translocation following abdominal radiation. *J Surg Res* 48:1–5, 1990.

137. Klimberg VS, Souba WW, Dolson DJ, Salloum RM, Hautamaki RD, Plumley DA, Mendenhall WM, Bova FJ, Khan SR, Hackett RL, et al: Prophylactic glutamine protects the intestinal mucosa from radiation injury. *Cancer* 66:62–68, 1990.

138. Scott TE, Moellman JR: Intravenous glutamine fails to improve gut morphology after radiation injury. *J Parenter Enter Nutr* 16:440–444, 1992.

139. Barbul A: Arginine: biochemistry, physiology, and therapeutic implications. *J Parenter Enter Nutr* 10:227–238, 1986.

140. Barbul A: Arginine and immune function. *Nutrition* 6:53–62, 1990.

141. Seifter E, Rettura G, Barbul A, Levenson SM: Arginine: an essential amino acid for injured rats. *Surgery* 84:224–230, 1978.

142. Chyun JH, Griminger P: Improvement of nitrogen retention by arginine and glycine supplementation and its relation to collagen synthesis in traumatized mature and aged rats. *J Nutr* 114:1697–1704, 1984.

143. Sitren HS, Fisher H: Nitrogen retention in rats fed on diets enriched with arginine and glycine. I. Improved N retention after trauma. *Br J Nutr* 37:195–208, 1977.

144. Barbul A, Rettura G, Levenson SM, Seifter E: Wound healing and thymotropic effects of arginine: a pituitary mechanism of action. *Am J Clin Nutr* 37:786–794, 1983.

145. Barbul A, Fishel RS, Shimazu S, Wasserkrug HL, Yoshimura NN, Tao RC, Efron G: Intravenous hyperalimentation with high arginine levels improves wound healing and immune function. *J Surg Res* 31:328–334, 1985.

146. Barbul A, Wasserkrug HL, Yoshimura NN, Tao R, Efron G: High arginine levels in intravenous hyperalimentation abrogate post-traumatic immune suppression. *J Surg Res* 36:620–624, 1984.

147. Leon P, Redmond HP, Stein TP, Shou J, Schluter MD, Kelly C, Lanza-Jacoby S, Daly JM: Arginine supplementation improves histone and acute-phase protein synthesis during Gram-negative sepsis in the rat. *J Parenter Enter Nutr* 15:503–508, 1991.

148. Elsair J, Poey J, Issad H, Reggabi M, Bekri T, Hattab F, Spinner C: Effect of arginine chlorhydrate on nitrogen balance during the three days following routine surgery in man. *Biomedicine* 29:312–317, 1978.

149. Daly JM, Reynolds J, Thom A, Kinsley L, Dietrick-Gallagher M, Shou J, Ruggieri B: Immune and metabolic effects of arginine in the surgical patient. *Ann Surg* 208:512–523, 1988.

150. Barbul A, Lazarou SA, Efron DT, Wasserkrug DL, Efron G: Arginine enhances wound healing and lymphocyte immune responses in humans. *Surgery* 108:331–337, 1990.

151. Barbul A, Wasserkrug HL, Seifter E, Rettura G, Levenson SM, Efron G: Immunostimulatory effects of arginine in normal and injured rats. *J Surg Res* 29:228–235, 1980.

152. Barbul A, Wasserkrug HL, Sisto DA, Seifter E, Rettura G, Levenson SM, Efron G: Thymic stimulatory actions of arginine. *J Parenter Enter Nutr* 4:446–449, 1980.

153. Kirk SJ, Regan MC, Wasserkrug HL, Sodeyama M, Barbul A: Arginine enhances T-cell responses in athymic nude mice. *J Parenter Enter Nutr* 16:429–432, 1992.

154. Barbul A, Sisto DA, Wasserkrug HL, Efron G: Arginine stimulates lymphocyte immune response in healthy human beings. *Surgery* 90:244–251, 1981.

155. Sigal RK, Shou J, Daly JM: Parenteral arginine infusion in humans: nutrient substrate or pharmacologic agent? *J Parenter Enter Nutr* 16:423–428, 1992.

156. Saito H, Trocki O, Wang SL, Gonce SJ, Joffe SN, Alexander JW: Metabolic and immune effects of dietary arginine supplementation after burn. *Arch Surg* 122:784–789, 1987.

157. Madden HP, Breslin RJ, Wasserkrug HL, Efron G, Barbul A: Stimulation of T-cell immunity by arginine enhances survival in peritonitis. *J Surg Res* 44:658–663, 1988.

158. Gonce SJ, Peck MD, Alexander JW, Miskell PW: Arginine supplementation and its effect on established peritonitis in guinea pigs. *J Parenter Enter Nutr* 14:237–244, 1990.

159. Palmer RM, Rees DD, Ashton DS, Moncada S: L-arginine is the physiological precursor for the formation of nitric oxide in endothelium-dependent relaxation. *Biochem Biophys Res Commun* 153:1251–1256, 1988.

160. Fleming I, Gray GA, Julou-Schaeffer G, Parratt JR, Stoclet JC: Incubation with endotoxin activates the L-arginine pathway in vascular tissue. *Biochem Biophys Res Commun* 171:562–568, 1990.

161. Julou-Schaeffer G, Gray GA, Fleming I, Schott C, Parratt JR, Stoclet JC: Loss of vascular responsiveness induced by endotoxin involves L-arginine pathway. *Am J Physiol* 259:H1038–H1043, 1990.

162. Kilbourn RG, Gross SS, Jubran A, Adams J, Griffith OW, Levi R, Lodato RF: NG-methyl-L-arginine inhibits tumor necrosis factor-induced hypotension: implications for the involvement of nitric oxide. *Proc Natl Acad Sci USA* 87:3629–3632, 1990.

163. Kinsella JE, Lokesh B: Dietary lipids, eicosanoids, and the immune system. *Crit Care Med* 18:S94–S113, 1990.

164. Johnston PV: Dietary fat, eicosanoids and immunity. *Adv Lipid Res* 21:103–141, 1985.

165. Kinsella JE, Lokesh B, Broughton S, Whelan J: Dietary polyunsaturated fatty acids and eicosanoids: potential effects on the modulation of inflammatory and immune cells: an overview. *Nutrition* 6:24–62, 1990.

166. Wan JM, Teo TC, Babayan VK, Blackburn GL: Lipids and the development of immune dysfunction and infection. *J Parenter Enter Nutr* 12:43S-52S, 1988.

167. Swanson O, Lokesh BR, Kinsella JE: Ca²⁺-MG²⁺ ATPase of mouse cardiac sarcoplasmic reticulum is affected by membrane n-6 and n-3 polyunsaturated fatty acid content. *J Nutr* 119:364–372, 1989.

168. Alam SQ, Ren YF, Alam BS: [³H]Forskolin- and [³H] dihydroalprenolol-binding sites and adenylate cyclase activity in hearts of rats fed diets containing different oils. *Lipids* 23:207–213, 1988.

169. Meade CJ, Mertin J: Fatty acids and immunity. *Adv Lipid Res* 16:127–165, 1978.

170. Locniskar M, Nauss KM, Newberne PM: The effect of quality and quantity of dietary fat on the immune system. *J Nutr* 113:951–961, 1983.

171. Meydani SN, Nicolosi RJ, Hayes KC: Effect of long-term feeding of corn oil or coconut oil diets on immune response and prostaglandin E₂ synthesis on squirrel and cebus monkeys. *Nutr Res* 5:993–1002, 1985.

172. Mertin J, Hunt R: Influence of polyunsaturated fatty acids on survival of skin allografts and tumor incidence in mice. *Proc Natl Acad Sci USA* 73:928–931, 1976.

173. Johnston DV, Marshall LA: Dietary fat, prostaglandins and the immune response. *Prog Food Nutr Sci* 8:3–25, 1984.

174. Yoshino S, Ellis EF: Effects of a fish-oil-supplemented diet on inflammation and immunological processes in rats. *Int Arch Allergy Appl Immunol* 84:233–240, 1987.

175. Morris DD, Henry MM, Moore JN, Fischer K: Effect of dietary linolenic acid on endotoxin-induced thromboxane and prostacyclin production by equine peritoneal macrophages. *Circ Shock* 29:311–318, 1989.

176. Morris DD, Henry MM, Moore JN: Dietary alpha linolenic acid reduces endotoxin-induced tumor necrosis factor activity production by equine macrophages. *Circ Shock* 31:82, 1990.

177. Cerra FB, Alden PA, Negro F, Billiar T, Svingen BA, Licari J, Johnson SB, Holman RT: Sepsis and exogenous lipid modulation. *J Parenter Enter Nutr* 12:63S-68S, 1988.

178. Mochizuki H, Trocki O, Dominioni L, Ray MB, Alexander JW: Optimal lipid content for enteral diets following thermal injury. *J Parenter Enter Nutr* 8:638–646, 1984.

179. Alexander JW, Saito H, Trocki O, Ogle CK: The importance of lipid type in the diet after burn injury. *Ann Surg* 204:1–8, 1986.

180. Trocki O, Heyd TJ, Waymack JP, Alexander JW: Effects of fish oil on postburn metabolism and immunity. *J Parenter Enter Nutr* 11:521–528, 1987.

181. Teo TC, DeMichele SJ, Selleck KM, Babayan VK, Blackburn GL, Bistrian BR: Administration of structured lipid composed of MCT and fish oil reduces net protein catabolism in enterally fed burned rats. *Ann Surg* 210:100–107, 1989.

182. Peck MD, Alexander JW, Ogle CK, Babcock GF: The effect of dietary fatty acids on response to *Pseudomonas* infection in burned mice. *J Trauma* 30:445–452, 1990.

183. Clouva-Molyvdas P, Peck MD, Alexander JW: Short-term dietary lipid manipulation does not affect survival in two models of murine sepsis. *J Parenter Enter Nutr* 16:343–347, 1992.

183a. Peck MD, Ogle CK, Alexander JW: Composition of fat in enteral diets can influence outcome in experimental peritonitis. *Ann Surg* 214:74–82, 1991.

184. Hamawy KJ, Moldawer LL, Georgieff M, Valicenti AJ, Babayan VK, Bistrian BR, Blackburn GL: The effect of lipid emulsions on the reticuloendothelial system function in the injured animal. *J Parenter Enter Nutr* 9:559–565, 1985.

185. Sobrado J, Moldawer LL, Pomposelli JJ, Mascioli EA, Babayan VK, Bistrian BR, Blackburn GL: Lipid emulsions and reticuloendothelial system function in healthy and burned guinea pigs. *Am J Clin Nutr* 42:855–863, 1985.

186. Nugent KM: Intralipid effects on reticuloendothelial function. *J Leukoc Biol* 36:123–132, 1984.

187. Fischer GW, Hunter KW, Wilson SR, Mease AD: Diminished bacterial defenses with intralipid. *Lancet* 2:819–820, 1980.

188. Nordenstrom J, Jarstrand C, Wiernik A: Decreased chemotactic and random migration of leukocytes during Intralipid infusion. *Am J Clin Nutr* 32:2416–2422, 1979.

189. Jarstrand C, Berghem L, Lahnborg G: Human granulocyte and reticuloendothelial system function during intralipid infusion. *J Parenter Enter Nutr* 2:663–670, 1978.

190. Sedman PC, Ramsden CW, Brennan TG, Guillou PJ: Pharmacological concentrations of lipid emulsions inhibit interleukin-2-dependent lymphocyte responses in vitro. *J Parenter Enter Nutr* 14:12–17, 1990.

191. Nishiwaki H, Iriyama K, Asami H, Kihata M, Hioki T, Asakawa T, Suzuki H: Influences of an infusion of lipid emulsion on phagocytotic activity of cultured Kupffer's cells in septic rats. *J Parenter Enter Nutr* 10:614–616, 1986.

192. Perez RV, Munda R, Alexander JW: Dietary immunoregulation of transfusion-induced immunosuppression. *Transplantation* 45:614–617, 1988.

193. Perez RV, Munda R, Alexander JW: Augmentation of donor-specific transfusion and cyclosporin effects with dietary linoleic acid. *Transplantation* 47:937–940, 1989.

194. Cheney CL, Lenssen P, Aker SN: Association of intravenous lipid emulsion with risk of infection. *J Am Coll Nutr* 9:532, 1990.

195. Freeman J, Goldmann DA, Smith NE, Sidebottom DG, Epstein MF, Platt R: Association of intravenous lipid emulsion and coagulase-negative staphylococcal bacteremia in neonatal intensive care units. *N Engl J Med* 323:301–308, 1990.

196. Lee TH, Hoover RL, Williams JD, Sperling RI, Ravalese J III, Spur BW, Robinson DR, Corey EJ, Lewis RA, Austen KF: Effect of dietary enrichment with eicosapentaenoic and docosahexaenoic acids on in vitro neutrophil and monocyte leukotriene generation and neutrophil function. *N Engl J Med* 312:1217–1224, 1985.

197. Endres S, Ghorbani R, Kelley VE, Georgilis K, Lonnemann G, van der Meer JW, Cannon JG, Rogers TS, Klempner MS, Weber PC, et al: The effect of dietary supplementation with n-3 polyunsaturated fatty acids on the synthesis of interleukin-1 and tumor necrosis factor by mononuclear cells. *N Engl J Med* 320:265–271, 1989.

198. Mortensen PB, Clausen MR, Bonnen H, Hove H, Holtug K: Colonic fermentation of ispaghula, wheat bran, glucose, and albumin to short-chain fatty acids and ammonia evaluated in vitro in 50 subjects. *J Parenter Enter Nutr* 16:433–439, 1992.

199. Palaccio JC, Rolandelli RH, Settle RG, et al: Dietary fibers' physiologic effects and potential applications to enteral nutrition. In Rombeau JL, Caldwell MD (eds): *Clinical Nutrition: Enteral and Tube Feeding*, 2nd ed. Philadelphia, WB Saunders, 1990, pp 556–574.

200. Tasman-Jones C, Jones AL, Owen RL: Jejunal morphological consequences of dietary fiber in rats. *Gastroenterology* 74:1102, 1978.

201. Jacobs LR: Effect of dietary fiber on mucosal growth and cell proliferation in the small intestine of the rat: a comparison of oat bran, pectin, and guar with total fiber deprivation. *Am J Clin Nutr* 37:954–960, 1983.

202. Koruda MJ, Rolandelli RH, Settle RG, Saul SH, Rombeau JL: The effect of a pectin-supplemented elemental diet on intestinal adaptation to massive small bowel resection. *J Parenter Enter Nutr* 10:343–350, 1986.

203. Brown RC, Kelleher J, Losowsky MS: The effect of pectin on the structure and function of the rat small intestine. *Br J Nutr* 42:357–365, 1979.

204. Jacobs LR, Lupton JR: Effect of dietary fibers on rat large bowel mucosal growth and cell proliferation. *Am J Physiol* 246:G378–G385, 1984.

205. Spiller GA, Chernoff MC, Hill RA, Gates JE, Nassar JJ, Shipley EA: Effect of purified cellulose, pectin, and a low-residue diet on fecal volatile fatty acids, transit time, and fecal weights in humans. *Am J Clin Nutr* 33:754–759, 1980.

206. Rolandelli RH, Koruda MJ, Settle RG, Rombeau JL: Effects of intraluminal infusion of short-chain fatty acids on the healing of colonic anastomosis in the rat. *Surgery* 100:198–204, 1986.

207. Kripke SA, Fox AD, Berman JM, Settle RG, Rombeau JL: Stimulation of intestinal mucosal growth with intracolonic infusion of short-chain fatty acids. *J Parenter Enter Nutr* 13:109–116, 1989.

208. Koruda MJ, Rolandelli RH, Settle RG, Zimmaro DM, Rombeau JL: Effect of parenteral nutrition supplemented with short-chain fatty acids on adaptation to massive small bowel resection. *Gastroenterology* 95:715–720, 1988.

209. Harig JM, Soergel KH, Komorowski RA, Wood CM: Treatment of diversion colitis with short-chain fatty acid irrigation. *N Engl J Med* 320:23–28, 1989.

210. Rolandelli RH, Koruda MJ, Settle RG, Rombeau JL: The effect of enteral feedings supplemented with pectin on the healing of colonic anastomoses in the rat. *Surgery* 99:703–707, 1986.

211. Rolandelli RH, Saul SH, Settle RG, Jacobs DO, Trerotola SO, Rombeau JL: Comparison of parenteral nutrition and enteral feeding with pectin in experimental colitis in the rat. *Am J Clin Nutr* 47:715–721, 1988.

212. Zimmaro DM, Rolandelli RH, Koruda MJ, Settle RG, Stein TP, Rombeau JL: Isotonic tube feeding formula induces liquid stool in normal subjects: reversal by pectin. *J Parenter Enter Nutr* 13:117–123, 1989.
213. Hart GK, Dobb GJ: Effect of a fecal bulking agent on diarrhea during enteral feeding in the critically ill. *J Parenter Enter Nutr* 12:465–468, 1988.
214. Shaw JH, Wolfe RR: An integrated analysis of glucose, fat, and protein metabolism in severely traumatized patients. Studies in the basal state and the response to total parenteral nutrition. *Ann Surg* 209:63–72, 1989.
215. Bark S, Holm I, Hakansson I, Wretlind A: Nitrogen-sparing effect of fat emulsion compared with glucose in the postoperative period. *Acta Chir Scand* 142:423–427, 1976.
216. Nordenstrom J, Askanazi J, Elwyn DH, Martin P, Carpentier YA, Robin AP, Kinney JM: Nitrogen balance during total parenteral nutrition-glucose vs. fat. *Ann Surg* 197:27–33, 1983.
217. Baker JP, Detsky AS, Stewart S, Whitwell J, Marliss EB, Jeejeebhoy KN: Randomized trial of total parenteral nutrition in critically ill patients: metabolic effects of varying glucose-lipid ratios as the energy source. *Gastroenterology* 87:53–59, 1984.
218. Shaw JH, Holdaway CM: Protein-sparing effect of substrate infusion in surgical patients is governed by the clinical state, and not by the individual substrate infused. *J Parenter Enter Nutr* 12:433–440, 1988.
219. deChalain TM, Michell WL, O'Keefe SJ, Ogden JM: The effect of fuel source on amino acid metabolism in critically ill patients. *J Surg Res* 52:167–176, 1992.
220. Iapichino G, Gattinoni L, Solca M, Radrizzani D, Zucchetti M, Langer M, Vesconi S: Protein sparing and protein replacement in acutely injured patients during TPN with and without amino acid supply. *Intensive Care Med* 8:25–31, 1982.
221. Brooks DC, Bessey PQ, Black PR, Aoki TT, Wilmore DW: Insulin stimulates branched chain amino acid uptake and diminishes nitrogen flux from skeletal muscle of injured patients. *J Surg Res* 40:395–405, 1986.
222. Jahoor F, Shangraw RE, Miyoshi H, Wallfish H, Herndon DN, Wolfe RR: Role of insulin and glucose oxidation in mediating the protein catabolism of burns and sepsis. *Am J Physiol* 257:E323–E331, 1989.
223. Askanazi J, Rosenbaum SH, Hyman AI, Silverberg PA, Milic-Emili J, Kinney JM: Respiratory changes induced by the large glucose loads of total parenteral nutrition. *JAMA* 243:1444–1447, 1980.
224. Askanazi J, Nordenstrom J, Rosenbaum SH, Elwyn DH, Hyman AI, Carpentier YA, Kinney JM: Nutrition for the patient with respiratory failure: glucose vs. fat. *Anesthesiology* 54:373–377, 1981.
225. Herve P, Simmonneau G, Girard P, Cerrina J, Mathieu M, Duroux P: Hypercapnic acidosis induced by nutrition in mechanically ventilated patients: glucose vs. fat. *Crit Care Med* 13:537–540, 1985.
226. Heymsfield SB, Head CA, McManus CB III, Seitz S, Staton GW, Grossman GD: Respiratory, cardiovascular, and metabolic effects of enteral hyperalimentation: influence of formula dose and composition. *Am J Clin Nutr* 40:116–130, 1984.
227. Talpers SS, Romberger DJ, Bunce SB, Pingleton SK: Nutritionally associated increased carbon dioxide production. Excess total calories vs. high proportion of carbohydrate calories. *Chest* 102:551–555, 1992.
228. VanBuren CT, Rudolph FB, Kulkarni A, Pizzini R, Fanslow WC, Kumar S: Reversal of immunosuppression induced by a protein-free diet: comparison of nucleotides, fish oil, and arginine. *Crit Care Med* 18:S114–S117, 1990.
229. VanBuren CT, Kulkarni AD, Fanslow WC, Rudolph FB: Dietary nucleotides, a requirement for helper/inducer T-lymphocytes. *Transplantation* 40:694–697, 1985.
230. VanBuren CT, Kulkarni AD, Schandle VB, Rudolph FB: The influence of dietary nucleotides on cell-mediated immunity. *Transplantation* 36:350–352, 164, 1983.
231. Carver JD, Cox WI, Barness LA: Dietary nucleotide effects upon murine natural killer cell activity and macrophage activation. *J Parenter Enter Nutr* 14:18–22, 1990.
232. Rudolph FB, Kulkarni AD, Fanslow WC, Pizzini RP, Kumar S, VanBuren CT: Role of RNA as a dietary source of pyrimidines and purines in immune function. *Nutrition* 6:45–62, 1990.
233. VanBuren CT, Kim E, Kulkarni AD, Fanslow WC, Rudolph FB: Nucleotide-free diet and suppression of the immune response. *Transplant Proc* 19:57–59, 1987.
234. Fanslow WC, Kulkarni AD, VanBuren CT, Rudolph FB: Effect of nucleotide restriction and supplementation on resistance to experimental murine candidiasis. *J Parenter Enter Nutr* 12:49–52, 1988.
235. Kulkarni AD, Fanslow WC, Drath DB, Rudolph FB, VanBuren CT: Influence of dietary nucleotide restriction on bacterial sepsis and phagocytic cell function in mice. *Arch Surg* 121:169–172, 1986.
236. Kulkarni AD, Fanslow WC, Rudolph FB, VanBuren CT: Effect of dietary nucleotides on response to bacterial infections. *J Parenter Enter Nutr* 10:169–171, 1986.
236a. Gottschlich MM, Jenkins M, Warden GD, et al: Differential effects of three dietary regimens on selected outcome variables in burn patients. *J Parenter Ent Nutr* 14:225–236, 1990.
236b. Cerra FB, Lehmann S, Konstantinides N, et al: Improvement in immune function in ICU patients by enteral nutrition supplemented with arginine, RNA, and menhaden oil is independent of nitrogen balance. *Nutrition* 7:193–199, 1991.
236c. Daly JM, Lieberman MD, Goldfine J, et al: Enteral nutrition with supplemental arginine, RNA, and ω-3 fatty acids in patients after operation: immunologic, metabolic and clinical outcome. *Surgery* 112:56–67, 1992.
236d. Bower RH, Lavin PT, LiCari JJ, et al: A modified enteral formula reduces hospital length of stay (LOS) in patients in intensive care units (ICU) (abstr.). *Crit Care Med* 21 (suppl):S275, 1993.
237. Slaff J, Jacobson D, Tillman CR, Curington C, Toskes P: Protease-specific suppression of pancreatic exocrine secretion. *Gastroenterology* 87:44–52, 1984.
238. Sax HC, Warner BW, Talamini MA, Hamilton FN, Bell RH Jr, Fischer JE, Bower RH: Early total parenteral nutrition in acute pancreatitis: lack of beneficial effects. *Am J Surg* 153:117–124, 1987.
239. Kudsk KA, Campbell SM, O'Brien T, Fuller R: Postoperative jejunal feedings following complicated pancreatitis. *Nutr Clin Pract* 5:14–17, 1990.
240. Voitk A, Brown RA, Echave V, McArdle AH, Gurd FN, Thompson AG: Use of an elemental diet in the treatment of complicated pancreatitis. *Am J Surg* 125:223–227, 1973.
241. Culpepper-Morgan JA, Floch MH: Bowel rest or bowel starvation: defining the role of nutritional support in the treatment of inflammatory bowel diseases. *Am J Gastroenterol* 86:269–271, 1991.
242. Greenberg GR, Fleming CR, Jeejeebhoy KN, Rosenberg IH, Sales D, Tremaine WJ: Controlled trial of bowel rest and nutritional support in the management of Crohn's disease. *Gut* 29:1309–1315, 1988.
243. Cravo M, Camilo ME, Correia JP: Nutritional support in Crohn's disease: which route? *Am J Gastroenterol* 86:317–321, 1991.
244. Greenberg GR: Inflammatory bowel disease. In Kinney JM, et al (eds): *Nutrition and Metabolism in Patient Care*. Philadelphia, WB Saunders, 1988, pp. 266–280, 1988.
245. Edes TE, Walk BE, Austin JL: Diarrhea in tube-fed patients: feeding formula not necessarily the cause. *Am J Med* 88:91–93, 1990.
246. Guenter PA, Settle RG, Perlmutter S, Marino PL, DeSimone GA, Rolandelli RH: Tube feeding-related diarrhea in acutely ill patients. *J Parenter Enter Nutr* 15:277–280, 1991.
247. Roubenoff R, Ravich WJ: Pneumothorax due to nasogastric feeding tubes. Report of four cases, review of the literature, and recommendations for prevention. *Arch Intern Med* 149:184–188, 1989.
248. Torres A, Serra-Batlles J, Ros E, Piera C, Puig de la Bellacasa J, Cobos A, Lomena F, Rodriguez-Roisin R: Pulmonary aspiration of gastric contents in patients receiving mechanical ventilation: the effect of body position. *Ann Intern Med* 116:540–543, 1992.
249. Ibanez J, Penafiel A, Raurich JM, Marse P, Jorda R, Mata F: Gastroesophageal reflux in intubated patients receiving enteral nutrition: effect of supine and semirecumbent positions. *J Parenter Enter Nutr* 16:419–422, 1992.
250. Mullan H, Roubenoff RA, Roubenoff R: Risk of pulmonary aspiration among patients receiving enteral nutrition support. *J Parenter Enter Nutr* 16:160–164, 1992.
251. Lazarus BA, Murphy JB, Culpepper L: Aspiration associated with long-term gastric versus jejunal feeding: a critical analysis of the literature. *Arch Phys Med Rehabil* 71:46–53, 1990.
252. Burtch GD, Shatney CH: Feeding jejunostomy (versus gastrostomy) passes the test of time. *Am Surg* 53:54–57, 1987.
253. McClave SA, Snider HL, Lowen CC, McLaughlin AJ, Greene LM, McCombs RJ, Rodgers L, Wright RA, Roy TM, Schumer MP, et al: Use of residual volume as a marker for enteral feeding intolerance: prospective blinded comparison with physical examination and radiographic findings. *J Parenter Enter Nutr* 16:99–105, 1992.

Immunosuppressive Therapy of Transplant Patients

ALAN J. ROSENBLOOM, M.D.
DAVID J. KRAMER, M.D.
KEITH L. STEIN, M.D.
AKE N.A. GRENVIK, M.D., PH.D., F.C.C.M.

The number of transplant patients who will present to intensive care units is growing rapidly. In addition, there is an expanding list of indications for immunosuppressive therapy, making expertise in the management of these drugs increasingly necessary for the intensivist. The critically ill transplant patient presents several unique challenges and is the focus of this chapter.

The newly transplanted patient is prone to the same postoperative complications as other patients after comparable surgery. Additionally, problems with graft failure, infection, drug side effects, and the complications of immunosuppression are common. Changes in immunosuppressive therapy bear considerable risk. Decreasing or stopping immunosuppression may cause graft destruction. The loss of a grafted kidney to rejection is catastrophic to the patient, while loss of a heart, liver, or lung allograft is often fatal. On the other hand, the infectious consequences of overimmunosuppression, which may not be manifest for weeks, are also frequently very serious. Every immunosuppression regimen balances these risks. The line between them is particularly fine in liver and lung transplantation patients.

For optimizing the outcome of patients on immunosuppressive therapy, the importance of accurate diagnosis cannot be overemphasized. The multiple causes of graft failure such as technical problems, local or systemic infection, drug side effects, and rejection must be distinguished as clearly as possible before making major changes in therapy. It is particularly important to attempt to differentiate infection from rejection. These complications can mimic one another and may be very difficult to distinguish. In some cases, however, diagnostic accuracy must be sacrificed for expediency. The immunosuppressed hemodynamically unstable patient with the sepsis syndrome prompts the immediate use of empiric broad-spectrum antibiotics, including an aminoglycoside. Subsequent identification of the infectious agent with culture data and appropriate tailoring of therapy, where possible, remain important for prevention of drug side effects, selection of resistant organisms, and avoidance of diagnostic confusion.

CLINICAL PATTERNS OF REJECTION

Clinically, three distinct patterns of allograft rejection in solid organs are recognized: hyperacute, acute, and chronic (1).

Hyperacute rejection (HAR), the least common, typically occurs within hours of transplantation, is severe, and usually destroys the graft. It is believed to be mediated by antibodies formed by presensitization of the recipient to donor antigens, as a result of transfusion, pregnancy, ABO mismatching (now rare), or other unknown mechanisms. Antibody appears to play a major role, recruiting other mechanisms, especially activation of the clotting system. The pathology of HAR is remarkable for its extensive platelet aggregation and antibody deposition. Currently available immunosuppressive regimens are usually not effective against HAR.

Acute cellular rejection (ACR) occurs over days to months. Antibody appears to play a much lesser role in ACR. Biopsies of acutely rejecting grafts reveal infiltration of lymphocytes and multiple other cell types. A delayed-type hypersensitivity (DTH) mechanism is hypothesized (see below).

The mechanisms of chronic rejection (CR) are least well-defined. Long-term graft loss is often characterized by insidious damage or loss of vital structures within the graft. For example, cardiac allografts develop coronary atherosclerosis at a rate greater than that expected by normal aging. Hepatic grafts undergo the "vanishing bile duct syndrome" and transplanted lungs develop obliterative bronchiolitis. These phenomena are presumably at least partly immunologic in nature, and a variety of mechanisms have been proposed. Whatever the cause, at present there is no effective way to prevent these phenomena. Thus, current regimens of immunosuppression are actually clearly effective only in suppressing ACR. In this capacity, they are highly effective, with 1-year graft survival rates in the 80 to 90% range possible under the best of conditions. In many transplants, however, a gradual, inexorable loss of graft function, probably because of ongoing, low-grade immunologic injury, occurs over the ensuing 5 to 10 years.

IMMUNOSUPPRESSION: GENERAL CONSIDERATIONS

BASIC PRINCIPLES

Most immunosuppressive regimens combine two to four drugs, often with different modes of action and toxicities, allowing lower doses of each drug. The goal is to achieve additive or perhaps synergistic effects while reducing the severity of any one individual toxicity. The use of cyclosporine A (CyA) with steroids and azathioprine (AZA) is very common. Regimens of as many as four agents are not uncommon, combining CyA, steroids, a cytotoxic agent such as azathioprine, and an antilymphocyte antibody such as antilymphocyte globulin (ALG) or OKT3 (monoclonal antibody to CD3, the T-cell antigen receptor; "CD" denotes "Cluster Designation," the internationally agreed-upon system for designating white cell surface molecules). The exact combination of agents often depends on the philosophy and experience present at the institution.

There is significant controversy concerning the treatment of acute rejection. Some clinicians prefer to increase baseline immunosuppression simultaneously during acute antirejection therapy. Others decrease baseline drug dosages during the most intense part of treatment to decrease the probability of overimmunosuppression. The second approach may be more logical, particularly with hepatic rejection, which may cause accumulation of immunosuppressant drugs to toxic levels, even at previously acceptable doses.

INCREASED INCIDENCE OF INFECTION

Infection remains a life-long major cause of death in immunosuppressed transplant patients. The first 6 months are particularly risky because of the juxtaposition of hospitalization, surgery, and the most intense immunosuppression. As pointed out by Rubin and Cosimi (2), infections result from the cumulative effect of immunosuppression over time and follow a predictable timetable starting at the day of surgery (Fig. 62.1). In the first month, the cumulative level of immunosuppression is low and 90% of infections are of the usual type seen in postoperative patients. In the period from 1 to 6 months after transplantation, viral and opportunistic infections make their appearance. Failure of antibacterial therapy should always prompt a search for overgrowth with resistant bacteria or infection with fungal or viral organisms. Cytomegalovirus (CMV) infection is very prevalent, occurring with clinically important illness in 20 to 50% of patients in most series. Clinical manifestations include fever, interstitial pneumonia, enteritis with ulcerations, hepatitis, leukopenia and thrombocytopenia, and, possibly, central nervous system involvement. Treatment includes ganciclovir, adjusted for creatinine clearance. The major toxicities of ganciclovir are neutropenia, thrombocytopenia, and a variety of central nervous system side effects. There may be an association with renal failure as well. The combination of gancyclovir and intravenous immune globulin appears to be warranted in the setting of interstitial pneumonia after bone marrow transplantation (3). CMV can also cause a progressive chorioretinitis, generally not seen until 4 months or more after the start of immunosuppression.

Epstein-Barr virus (EBV) can cause clinical signs similar to those of CMV. An additional important aspect of EBV is its association with lymphoproliferative disorders. Because of exposure to blood products, hepatitis B and non-A, non-B (hepatitis C, etc.), and human immunodeficiency virus (HIV) occur at an increased frequency following transplantation. Herpes simplex and herpes zoster viral infections are also increased in incidence, probably because of the general embarrassment of cell-mediated immunity. These infections may be primary or result from reactivation of latent virus.

Reactivation of tuberculosis becomes 100 times more likely on immunosuppression. Isoniazid prophylaxis is recommended if any risk of latent tuberculosis is present. Dissemination of previously contained *Strongyloides* from the gastrointestinal tract can be catastrophic. Patients with a travel or residence history in tropical or subtropical regions should be screened prior to transplantation. The incidence of fungal infection is also increased. Previously localized fungal infections such as the endemic mycoses can disseminate on immunosuppression. Invasive fungal disease, often from inhaled spores of *Cryptococcus*, Mucoraceae, or *Aspergillus*, can invade the lung or sinuses, with subsequent spread to the brain. *Nocardia* disease occurs in a similar pattern, except that sinus disease is rare. *Candida*, *Torulopsis glabrata*, and *Aspergillus* can also gain entry via wound infection or intravenous lines to cause local or disseminated disease. *Toxoplasmosis* can be transmitted by cardiac transplantation from a seropositive donor, with the result of myocarditis or central nervous system invasion in the recipient. *Pneumocystis carinii* usually produces an interstitial pneumonia, which can be life-threatening.

Commonly used prophylactic antibiotic regimens prevent or decrease the incidence of some of these infections. Trimethoprim-sulfamethoxazole is very effective against *Pneumocystis*, *Nocardia*, *Legionella*, *Toxoplasmosis*, and *Listeria monocytogenes* (meningitis). The drug is continued indefinitely. In renal transplantation, acyclovir has been shown to reduce the occurrence of CMV by about 50%. Conservative dosing is often necessary because of neurologic side effects

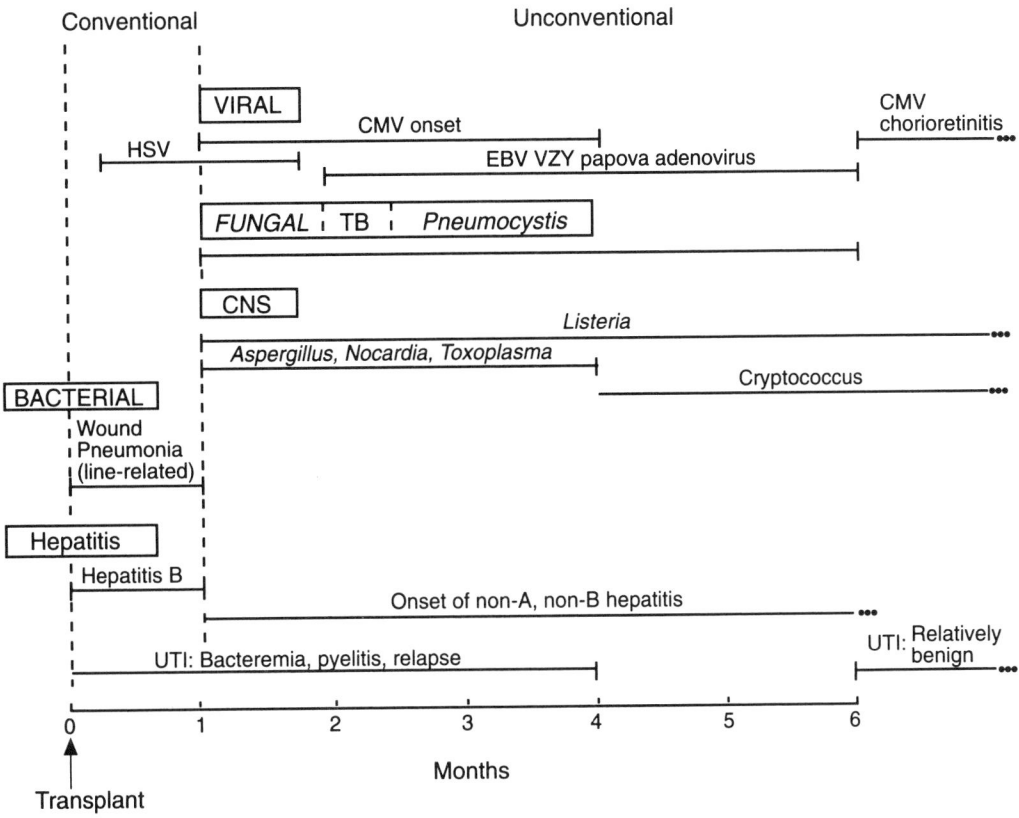

Figure 62.1. The types of infection in immunosuppressed solid organ recipients follow a predictable time course, starting at the time of transplantation. (From Rubin R, Cosimi A: Therapy, Both Immunosuppression and Antimicrobial, for the Transplant Patient in the 1990s, London, Bailliere, Tindall, 1989, pp 71–88. In Brent L, Sells R (eds): *Organ Transplantation.*

and exacerbation of renal failure. The drug is continued for 6 months after transplantation. Although the procedure is controversial, some centers use decontamination of the gastrointestinal tract as a prophylactic measure in selected patients, especially those who are critically ill. For example, a mixture of colistin 100 mg, gentamicin 80 mg, and Mycostatin 2 million units administered via the nasogastric tube four times per day is used at the University of Pittsburgh.

Beyond 6 months after transplantation, the incidence and type of infection is most dependent on the state of the host. Patients who are doing well and have good graft function generally get the infections of normal hosts (i.e., with community-acquired organisms). Those recipients who are doing poorly or require continued heavy immunosuppression continue to be at high risk for opportunistic infections.

INCREASED INCIDENCE OF MALIGNANCY (4, 5)

With any immunosuppressive agent, the occurrence of malignant tumors is increased. In a study of more than 2500 renal transplant patients in the Cincinnati Transplant Tumor Registry, mostly on azathioprine and prednisone, the findings were as follows: Skin cancer is the most common malignancy, at nearly 40% of all neoplasms and at a rate 28 times higher than that in the general population. Also, squamous cell carcinoma is more common than basal cell, which is the reverse of the trend in the general population. Non-Hodgkin's

lymphoma accounted for 12%, at 30 to 50 times the risk of the general population. Kaposi's sarcoma, otherwise rare (excluding those with acquired immune deficiency syndrome, or AIDS), accounted for 3.2% at 400 to 800 times the normal risk. Carcinoma of the cervix accounted for 18% of cancer in female recipients, at 14 times the general risk; and carcinomas of the perineum and vulva, for 6%, at 30 times the normal risk.

The introduction of potent antilymphocyte therapies such as CyA and antilymphocyte antibodies appear to have added an even higher risk of lymphocytic malignancies. For comparison, lymphoma occurs at a mean interval of 11 months on cyclosporine-based immunosuppression versus 42 months on noncyclosporine (e.g., steroid-azathioprine) immunosuppression. The term *posttransplant lymphoproliferative disorder* (PTLD) refers to a general tendency of these agents to cause abnormal lymphoid growth. These abnormalties range from benign lymphoid hyperplasia to frank invasive lymphoma. The development of PTLD is suspected to be associated with EBV infection, perhaps by blockade of lymphocyte immunity against EBV, which is known to cause proliferation of infected lymphocytes. At the University of Pittsburgh, in a review of 7 years of transplant data, PTLD was found to occur in 1.7% of patients on cyclosporine (6). Current management includes discontinuation of immunosuppression and surgical resection where appropriate. The value of acyclovir in this situation is unproved.

BASIC SCIENCE REVIEW

Early experiments showed that tissue transplanted from the individual to him- or herself (i.e., autografts) will be accepted; conversely, tissue from a genetically nonidentical donor will be rejected and repeated attempts to use tissue from the same donor will result in stronger and quicker rejection. Later experiments gave insights into the differences among individuals that trigger these phenomena. It was shown that certain protein molecules present on the surface of mammalian cells act as the identifiers of self and determine the compatibility of allografted tissue. These have been named the major histocompatibility complex (MHC) molecules, also called the human leukocyte antigens (HLA). Two classes of MHC, class I and class II, are important in allograft rejection. The more mismatching that exists between the MHC molecules of donor and recipient, the more vigorous will be the rejection response to transplanted tissue. The molecular basis of these behaviors is being defined (7).

An allograft presents foreign material to the recipient's immune system, both as a result of entry of recipient cells into the graft and exit of donor cells from the graft. Recipient lymphocytes quickly "find" the newly transplanted organ. These cells recirculate repeatedly and patrol nearly all tissues of the body. Naive (unstimulated) lymphocytes circulate randomly. After encountering antigen on their rounds they are permanently rerouted to that pathway on subsequent passes. This process utilizes cell surface "homing" molecules on lymphocytes and location identifier molecules called "addressins" on endothelium (8). The result is that lymphocytes accumulate at sites of inflammation, foreign protein, or tissue, such as allografts. At the same time, most solid tissues carry dendritic cells and "passenger" white cells. After transplantation, these cells leave the graft and enter local lymph nodes and the recipient's spleen. Hence, donor leukocytes and dendritic cells interact with recipient lymphocytes and macrophages inside recipient lymphoid tissue.

Although many cell types participate, it is the thymus-derived lymphocyte, or T-cell, that initiates and drives allograft rejection. There are different subsets of T-cells, which can be identified by distinct proteins on their surfaces. The CD4 molecule identifies "helper" T-cells, which augment the immune response through several mechanisms. For example, by the secretion of various cytokines, CD4 cells stimulate B-cell antibody production. The CD8 protein identifies T-cells with two different behaviors: so-called "suppressor" cells and "cytotoxic" cells. The suppressor CD8 T-cells antagonize CD4 help, decrease B-cell stimulation, inhibit antibody production, and generally down-regulate the immune response. The balance between T-cell "help" and T-cell "suppression" is believed to be a major regulatory mechanism of the immune response. Cytotoxic CD8 T-cells attach directly to, and kill, foreign cells. These cells are important effectors in intracellular infection and also in the destruction of rejecting allografts.

T-cells are extremely potent in the immune response by virtue of two properties, of which some of the molecular mechanisms are now understood. Firstly, they have the ability to secrete multiple hormone-like substances called cytokines. Secondly, they produce a number of cell surface molecules, allowing them to attach specifically to other cells and structures.

T-cells produce interleukins (IL) 1 through 6, 9, and 10, as well as interferons, tumor necrosis factor (TNF)-α and -β,

monocyte colony stimulating factor (M-CSF), and granulocyte monocyte colony stimulating factor (GM-CSF) (9). These substances have at least three important functions: (*a*) Cytokines can attract and activate other leukocytes. The CD4 "helper" T-cells are probably responsible for attracting CD8 cells and macrophages into rejecting allografts (10). This mechanism has been compared with DTH, to which it bears great similarity. CD4 helper T-cells are certainly responsible for the activation of B-cells and thus, indirectly, for the great majority of antibody production. (*b*) Cytokines up-regulate both MHC molecules on tissues and adhesion molecules on endothelium. This effect aids the entry and accumulation of leukocytes in the tissue and an accelerated recognition of "foreign" MHC-bearing cells. (*c*) Cytokines activate distant tissues such as the hepatic acute phase response, bone marrow phagocyte synthesis, and the hypothalamic-pituitary axis, producing the systemic signs of rejection.

T-cells have adhesion molecules on their surfaces (11). These molecules allow tissue-seeking T-cells to attach to receptors on endothelium. Next, these cells migrate to a junction between endothelial cells and move into the tissue, using different adhesion targets (e.g., fibronectin, collagen, and others) to move along the intracellular matrix inside the tissue. CD8 cytotoxic T-cells use adhesion molecules to attach to foreign cells. They can attach, deliver a fatal blow to target cells, and detach in seconds. Hence, T-cells are highly mobile and effective against their targets.

T-cells recognize foreign molecules (antigen) by a complex process (Fig. 62.2). The antigen must be presented to the T-cell by an antigen-presenting cell (APC), such as a macrophage. The cells touch, with molecules on their surfaces matching precisely, similar to a key entering a lock. The T-cell "lock" is composed of the T-cell antigen receptor (TCR) and a tightly associated accessory molecule, either CD4 or CD8. The "key" on the APC consists of a fragment of foreign protein (the processed antigen) of about 10 amino acids in length, embedded in an MHC molecule. When the cells come together, the TCR attaches to the antigen fragment and, simultaneously, the accessory molecule (CD4 or CD8) attaches to the MHC molecule. CD8 T-cells nearly always match with MHC class I-bearing cells, which are widely distributed. In fact, MHC I is present on most cell types except red blood cells. This matching of CD8 T-cells and MHC I-bearing targets is believed to grant widespread access of CD8 cytotoxic cells to viral infection or cancerous alteration, which may occur in any type of cell. Thus, the MHC I-CD8 complementarity is a global defense mechanism. In contrast, CD4 T-cells attach to cells bearing MHC class II molecules, which are limited in distribution to cells believed to be important in stimulating the immune system. These include monocytes, tissue macrophages, and dendritic cells. Other cells, such as endothelial and epithelial cells, can be induced to display class II MHC by cytokines. Access of these cells to CD4 helper lymphocytes allows them to up-regulate the immune response. Thus, the MHC II-CD4 complementarity is primarily immunoregulatory.

Although T-cells are very potent mediators of the immune response, only a small number of T-cells will recognize any one antigen. For this reason, T-cell proliferation is linked with antigen recognition. When a T-cell is stimulated by any antigen, it begins cell division. The result is a larger number

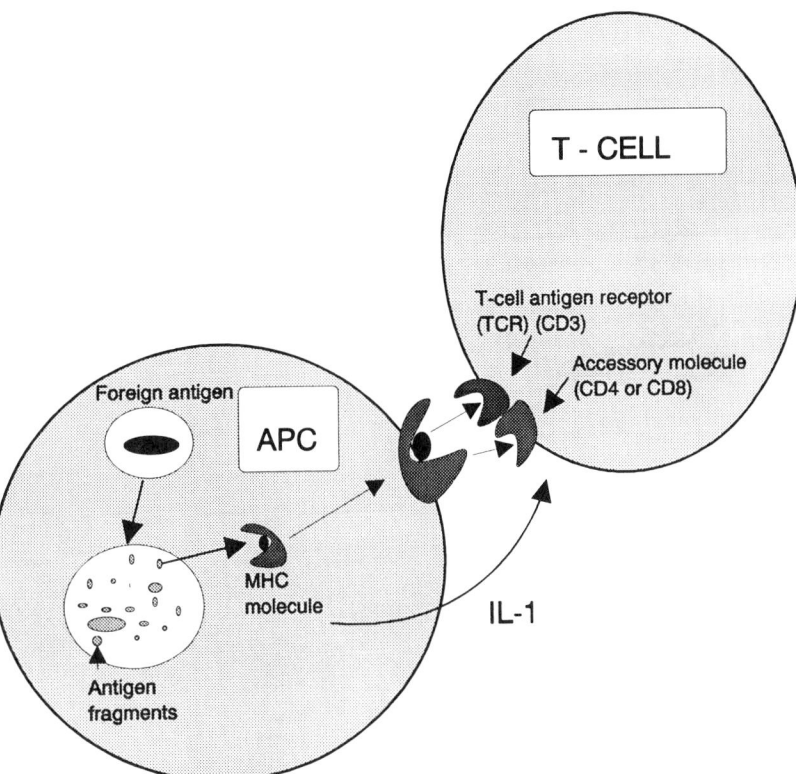

Figure 62.2. Antigen presentation. Fragments of antigen are created by intracellular processing in an antigen presenting cell (*APC*). Foreign proteins are cleaved into fragments of about 10 amino acids in length. These fragments are joined with a major histocompatibility complex (*MHC*) molecule, which moves to the cell surface, carrying the antigen fragment. The T-cell receptor (*TCR*) recognizes the antigen fragment, while an accessory molecule (*CD4* or *CD8*) recognizes the MDC molecule. MHC class I molecules are involved in the processing of foreign intracellular antigens, such as viruses, and are selectively recognized by CD8 T-cells. MHC class II molecules are involved with antigens brought into cells from the outside and are recognized by CD4. Along with IL-1, these binding interactions trigger T-cell activation.

of identical T-cells all recognizing the same antigen. This process is critical for effective immune response and is highly dependent on IL-2 (Fig. 62.3). Blockade of this proliferation is the mode of action of many of the presently useful immunosuppressant drugs. When T-cells proliferate, some of the cells produced become long-lived "memory" cells, which remain in the body for long periods and account for the stronger response on repeat exposure to antigen known as the "second set" response.

The balance between CD4 "helper" and CD8 "suppressor" activity provides one mechanism for regulation and control of the immune response. Attempts to measure help or suppression to determine the direction that an immune response is taking have been unsuccessful. One problem is that it has been impossible to find unique markers identifying suppressor cells, leading some to believe that suppression is a composite property of many different lymphocyte types, rather than belonging to a unique cell subset (12). A recent paper identifying stable markers for CD4 helpers that give help selectively to suppressor cells appears to offer the possibility of monitoring the status of T-cell overall control of help versus suppression (13).

The response to allografted tissue is a special case immunologically. Not only are antigens within the graft potentially foreign, but the MHC molecules presenting them are themselves foreign. It is unclear whether the allografted foreign

MHC itself is stimulating the donor's lymphocyte response or, alternatively, whether foreign antigen within the graft is more strongly reacted to when presented by a foreign MHC molecule. Matching of MHC molecules is the goal of tissue typing for renal transplantation. Disparities of MHC class II molecules have the greatest impact. Other molecular differences, unrelated to the MHC molecules, also exist and can cause rejection. For example, the ABO molecules must be matched to avoid severe and rapid graft rejection caused by preformed ABO antibodies. Still other, presently undefined, molecular differences exist. These defferences are demonstrated by rejection between ABO-matched, MHC-identical twins. Apparently, each individual has a unique molecular signature based in differences in other, still unknown, molecules.

CORTICOSTEROIDS

MECHANISM

Corticosteroids (CST) have broad effects on many cell types. They interfere with the production of both IL-1 and IL-2, blocking the early steps of T-cell activation. Multiple

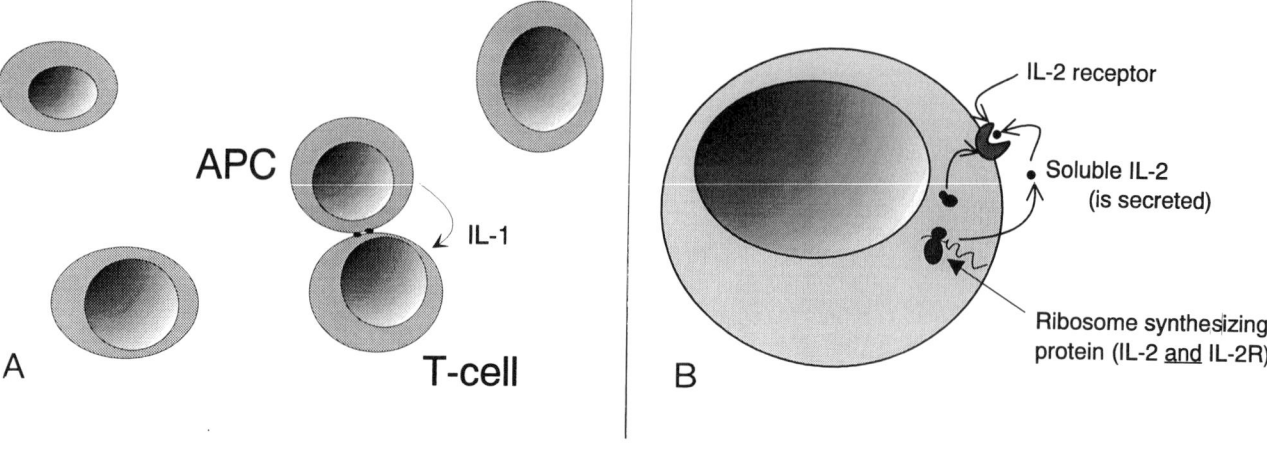

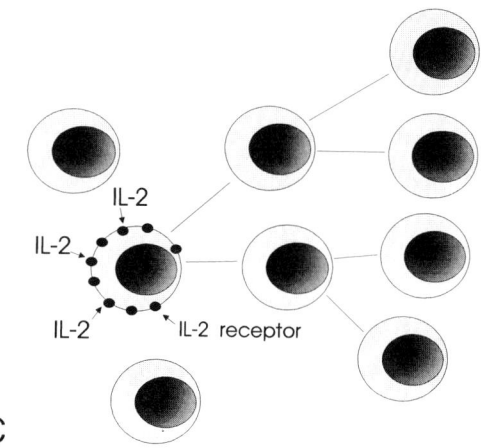

Figure 62.3.   T-cell clonal proliferation. **A,** A T-cell bearing an antigen receptor specific for a presented antigen is activated by the APC. **B,** Activation triggers synthesis of soluble IL-2 and IL-2 receptor, simultaneously. **C,** Under the influence of IL-2, the cell proliferates, creating a clone of antigen-specific cells. Nearby, unactivated T-cells do not have IL-2 receptor and thus do not respond to the IL-2 around them.

other immune effects occur, including (*a*) antagonism of inflammatory mechanisms by stabilization of leukocyte lysosomal membranes, decreased capillary permeability, and inhibition of histamine release and the kinin and complement systems; (*b*) alteration of circulating cell populations, including drastic reduction of lymphocyte traffic and circulating immunoglobulin levels, and reduction in numbers of neutrophils and eosinophils; and (*c*) inhibition of leukocyte adhesion to endothelium. The relative importance of these effects, as well as the precise mechanism responsible for the potent immunosuppression produced by steroids, is unknown.

USE (14)

Corticosteroids are used extensively in brief but high doses for the reversal of acute rejection episodes. They are also almost invariably a part of multidrug maintenance regimens. Prednisone, methylprednisolone, and prednisolone are the agents of choice for immunosuppression.

PHARMACOKINETICS

Bioavailability.   Prednisone has a somewhat variable oral bioavailability of about 80%. Peak concentrations are achieved 2 to 3 hours after oral administration.

Elimination.   CST are metabolized in all tissues but most importantly in the liver. The serum half-life of both prednisone and methylprednisolone is 3 hours. However, suppression of lymphokine production, likely to be a key effect, persists for 24 hours or more.

DOSAGE AND ADMINISTRATION

There is no fixed dosing regimen. Rather, doses are titrated by effect and local custom. A preoperative dose of 250 to 1000 mg may be given, followed by 20 to 200 mg/day during the first week. Acute rejection may be treated with one to three high doses, 250 mg to 1 g methylprednisolone i.v., or by a tapering regimen starting at 200 mg/day and reducing to baseline maintenance doses over 3 to 6 days. Evidence suggests that lower doses than those traditionally used can be equally effective but with a lower risk of subsequent infection. Because of multiple side effects and unacceptably broad suppression of immunity and inflammation, every attempt is made to minimize long-term dosages. By combination regimens, steroids can often be reduced to 10 or 20 mg/day, or less, including every-other-day therapy. In some patients, steroids can be stopped altogether without incurring rejection.

SPECIAL CONSIDERATIONS

Roughly equivalent dosages are: cortisone 25 mg, hydrocortisone 20 mg, prednisone 5 mg, prednisolone 5 mg, and methylprednisolone 4 mg. The naturally occurring glucocorticoids cortisone and hydrocortisone have significant mineralocorticoid activity. Prednisone and prednisolone have about half as much. Hence, sodium retention, edema, hypertension, potassium loss, and hypokalemic alkalosis are seen with prolonged use of these steroids. In contrast, methylprednisolone has very little mineralocorticoid effect. Adrenal suppression can be seen with all steroids but is very variable. It can develop unexpectedly if the patient is stressed, even up to 12 months after stopping steroids.

ADVERSE EFFECTS

Unfortunately, the ill effects of CST are numerous and cause considerable morbidity. An increased incidence of serious infections is well-documented. Impaired fibroblast growth and collagen synthesis contribute to poor wound healing. Hence, surgical wounds and anastomoses are at increased risk, and gastrointestinal (GI) ulcerations tend to heal slowly, with perforation and rebleeding reported. Spontaneous GI ulceration occurs in approximately 2% of patients on steroids. Because of suppression of the signs of inflammation, the diagnosis of intraabdominal infection and peritonitis can be significantly delayed, with disastrous consequences. Decompensation of glucose tolerance is often dramatic. Patients with this side effect are at risk for the long-term effects of glucose intolerance, such as cardiovascular disease. Generalized protein catabolism and bone demineralization can produce a debilitated state. Atherosclerosis is probably accelerated. The risk of cataract and increased intraocular pressure (glaucoma) is increased. Central nervous system effects such as euphoria and mood swings are well-known. Soft tissue and dermatologic changes such as fat redistribution, skin atrophy, and striae produce the characteristic "cushingoid" appearance.

CYTOTOXIC DRUGS

GENERAL MECHANISM (1, 15)

Agents commonly used for immunosuppression in transplantation include antimetabolites such as AZA and alkylating agents such as cyclophosphamide (CPM). AZA, a sulfur analog of the purine adenine, inhibits purine synthesis. Purines are required for DNA and RNA synthesis. Also, AZA can be incorporated into DNA in place of natural purines. The altered molecule does not function properly, allowing strand breaks in the chromosomes. Thus, not surprisingly, AZA is most toxic to proliferating cells that are making new DNA. In contrast, CPM nonspecifically damages cellular macromolecules by alkylating them, particularly DNA. Thus, CPM is toxic to both resting and dividing cells, but more so to the latter.

The precise mechanism of immunosuppression mediated by cytotoxic drugs is unknown. However, the antiproliferative effects on lymphocytes are believed to inhibit the generation of antigen-specific T-cell clones.

CYCLOPHOSPHAMIDE (15–18)

Mechanism

For reasons that are unclear, CPM has its greatest effect on B-cells. The order of cytotoxicity in immune cells is: B-cells > T suppressor cells > T helper cells. CPM significantly inhibits antibody production in humans, in contrast to AZA. CPM potently suppresses delayed-type hypersensitivity and cellular immunity and, also in contrast to AZA, can inhibit an ongoing immune response.

Use

CPM is the most widely used preparatory treatment for bone marrow transplantation. It is useful at high doses both to incapacitate the recipient's immune system, preventing rejection of the grafted marrow, and, in neoplastic diseases leading to marrow transplantation, as effective chemotherapy.

Pharmacokinetics

Bioavailability. Oral CPM is well-absorbed (87 to 96%), with peak concentrations being reached in 1 hour.

Elimination. The volume of distribution ranges from 0.5 to 1.1 liter/kg body weight. CPM is activated by metabolism in the liver. Several metabolites are formed. The ultimately active metabolite, phosphoramide mustard, is eliminated by spontaneous hydrolysis and has an intracellular half-life of 40 to 50 minutes.

Blood half-life is about 5 to 7 hours, and elimination proceeds similarly with the use of regular or high doses. Neither impaired renal function nor liver failure requires dosage adjustment. CPM is removed by hemodialysis: about 72% is cleared after a 6-hour treatment.

Dosage and Administration

High-dose CPM used in bone marrow conditioning regimens is administered at about 60 mg/kg/day for 2 to 4 days i.v. Doses exceeding this amount may cause severe cardiac toxicity.

Drug Interactions. Levels of CPM or its effects may be increased by concurrent administration of allopurinol and cimetidine, but not ranitidine. The neuromuscular blocking effect of succinylcholine can be prolonged significantly by a decrease in plasma pseudocholinesterase activity.

Adverse Effects

Virtually all patients develop nausea, vomiting, and hair loss with the doses used for bone marrow transplantation. Cardiac toxicity occurs commonly. At least 90% of patients have measurably reduced QRS voltage and as many as 15% develop clinically significant cardiac dysfunction. This effect appears to correlate with doses exceeding 1.55 g/m² body surface area/day for 4 days. The critical dose is lower with simultaneous irradiation or treatment with adriamycin. Hemorrhagic cystitis is a well-known side effect of CPM, but the reported incidence is very variable (0.5 to 40%). It can be limited by giving thiosulfate (e.g., mesna, or 2-mercaptoethane sulfonate) or, apparently equally successfully, with aggressive hydration. Infertility is associated with CPM therapy, especially at high doses. The syndrome of inappropriate antidiuretic hormone (SIADH) has been reported.

AZATHIOPRINE (4, 14, 19, 20)

Mechanism

AZA has a greater effect on T-cells than on B-cells. Thus, formation of antibody to new antigens, which usually requires T-cell help, is depressed. Humoral response to recall (previously sensitized) antigens is relatively spared. The T-cell suppression effects can be demonstrated by inhibition of the mixed lymphocyte reaction in vitro, and DTH in vivo. AZA has some antiinflammatory effect.

Pharmacokinetics

Bioavailability. The oral bioavailability of AZA is about 40%. Peak concentration after an oral dose is reached in 1 to 2 hours.

Elimination. The metabolism of AZA is complex. The parent drug is inactive but is rapidly converted to several metabolites. Thioinosinic acid is an inhibitor of purine synthesis. The 6-thioguanine nucleotides (TGN) are known to incorporate into DNA and probably are toxic to dividing cells. TGN has a very long tissue half-life, perhaps on the order of 13 days. A delayed and prolonged effect of the drug is therefore probable. On this basis, once-daily dosage is logical. At an incidence of one patient in 300, a genetic enzyme deficiency of thiopurine methyltransferase exists. This enzyme normally shunts drug away from the formation of TGN. Hence, its reduced action is believed to contribute to increased tissue TGN levels and toxicity. Also, in patients with renal failure, TGN accumulates, presumably accounting for the greater toxicity of AZA in these patients. The final end metabolite of all pathways is 6-thiouric acid, which is inactive. It is excreted by the kidneys.

Use

AZA is used in maintenance immunosuppressive regimens. It has no usefulness in the treatment of acute rejection episodes. Historically, the drug has been combined with corticosteroids. This two-drug regimen has been very effective in renal transplantation for many years. With the introduction of cyclosporine, the drug has remained useful in both three- and four-drug regimens, the latter including antilymphocyte antibodies.

Dosage and Administration

The drug is usually given orally. It can be started 1 to 3 days prior to transplantation. The dose is 3 to 5 mg/kg as a single daily oral dose. While the patient is unable to take oral medication, AZA can be give intravenously at half of the oral dose, for brief periods. Typical maintenance oral dosage after transplantation is 2 to 3 mg/kg daily. Tapering to 1 to 2 mg/kg/day is often possible as time goes on. In combination regimens, AZA can be reduced to as little as 0.25 to 0.5 mg/kg/day. All dosing is tempered by the white blood cell count.

Drug Interactions (21). Allopurinol interacts with AZA, probably by inhibiting xanthene oxidase, one of the enzymes involved in degradation of AZA metabolites. This interaction can cause significantly increased myelotoxicity, which appears after 1 month of therapy on both drugs.

Adverse Effects

Dose-limiting myelosuppression usually occurs 1 to 2 weeks into therapy. Pancytopenia and thrombocytopenia with megaloblastic anemia is the pattern usually seen. White counts below 3000 cells/mm³ mandate discontinuation of the drug. As with other cytotoxic drugs, nausea, vomiting, and hair loss may occur. Hepatic injury can occur in two patterns: a reversible hepatitis, and a rare, but serious, hepatic venoocclusive disease that can cause irreparable damage. AZA therapy has also been associated with an increased risk of pancreatitis, believed to result from a hypersensitivity reaction. The causality of AZA, however, has been questioned in both venoocclusive disease and pancreatitis (22, 23). Hypersensitivity to AZA has been reported to cause a variety of manifestations (24). Diagnosis of these disorders has been largely on clinical grounds.

Drug Monitoring

Levels of AZA and several of its metabolites are measurable in the blood. However, there is no correlation between these levels and the activity of the drug. The level of TGN in the tissue may turn out to be the clinically relevant level to measure. At present, however, this measurement is a research tool only.

ISOMERASE-BINDING DRUGS: CYCLOSPORINE A, FK-506, RAPAMYCIN

GENERAL MECHANISMS

When a T-lymphocyte is activated by antigen, a coordinated program of multiple gene activations is set in motion; this program eventuates in the proliferation of the activated cell. CyA blocks the transcription of 10 genes of at least 60 that are activated (25). Some of these are: IL-2, -3, and -4, GM-CSF, and γ-interferon (26). The inhibition of the production of IL-2, which acts as a potent T-cell growth factor, is a key effect and has been studied extensively. The drug is known to block the activation of the IL-2 gene, ultimately preventing the synthesis of IL-2. Both CyA and FK-506 (FK) act similarly, interfering with the binding of specific transcription factors

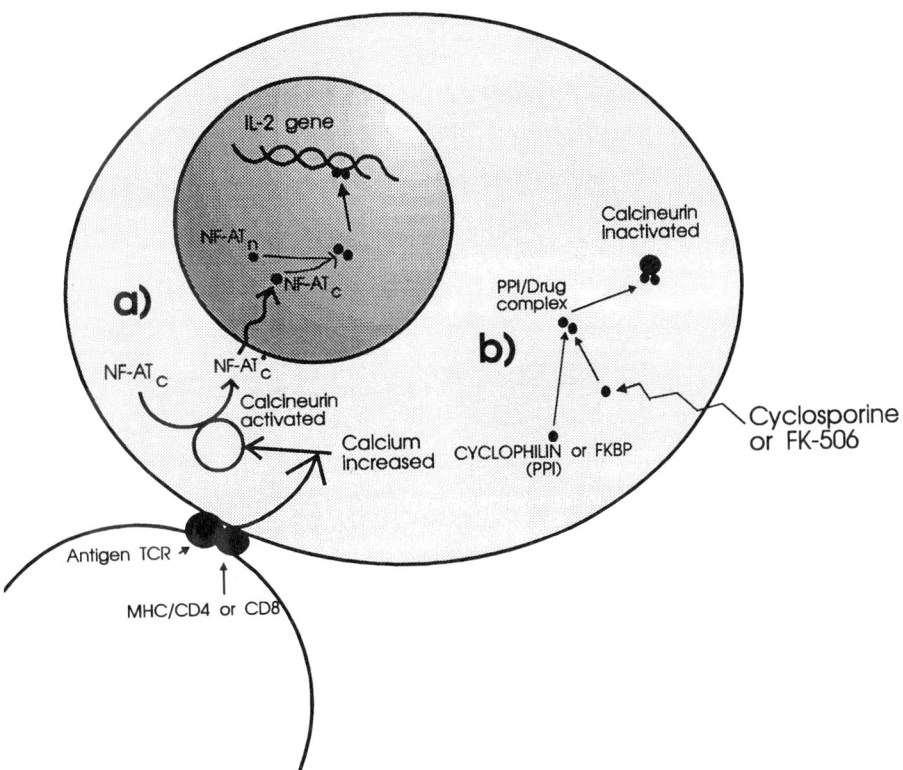

Figure 62.4. Model proposed for the blocking action of FK-506 and CyA on activation of the T-cell IL-2 gene. **A,** When a T-cell becomes activated by antigen, a signal is sent into the cell. Intracellular calcium rises. This activates calcineurin, a calcium-dependent phosphatase. Active calcineurin dephosphorylates NF-ATc, a cytoplasmic component of a DNA-binding protein. The dephosphorylated form, NF-ATc*, can enter the nucleus and join with NF-ATn, the nuclear component. Together these bind to and activate the IL-2 gene. **B,** FK-506 and cyclosporine A interfere with IL-2 gene activation. They each bind a peptidyl-prolyl *cis/trans* isomerase (*PPI*). The PPI/drug complex, in turn, binds to and inactivates calcineurin, preventing the migration of NF-ATc into the nucleus and ultimately blocking production of IL-2.

to the promoter (control region) of the IL-2 gene, preventing RNA synthesis (27–29).

When CyA and FK enter the cell, they bind to distinct proteins, cyclophilin and FK binding protein (FKBP), respectively (26, 30, 31). Both cyclophilin and FKBP were discovered to be enzymes sharing the same function. Each is a peptidyl-prolyl *cis/trans* isomerase (PPI), thought to be important in the folding of intracellular proteins. At first it was hypothesized that the drugs acted by inhibiting the activity of the PPI. Recently, it has been shown that the PPI/drug complex (32, 33) specifically binds, and inactivates, a Ca²⁺ dependent phosphatase, calcineurin. Calcineurin blockade ultimately results in the blockage of gene activation (Fig. 62.4) and not interference with PPI.

Considerable redundancy is built into the T-cell activation system. Proliferation can be initiated through different cell surface receptors (such as CD28), not just through the binding of antigen. The exact role of these alternate pathways is unknown. Some appear to be dependent on an increase in intracellular calcium, and some do not. As described above, CyA and FK block the calcium-dependent process. Although rapamycin (RPM) specifically binds the same cytoplasmic protein (FKBP) as does FK, the drugs have remarkably different effects (29, 34, 35). The RPM-FKBP complex does not bind calcineurin. Neither does it inhibit the translocation of NF-ATc (a cytoplasmic component of a DNA-binding protein) into the nucleus. RPM blocks T-cell activation at a later step

in the activation cascade, effectively inhibiting both calcium-dependent and non-calcium-dependent signals (36). In fact, RPM blocks every activation pathway so far discovered (37). The early activation events blocked by FK and CyA are left intact by RPM.

As isomerase-binding drugs are studied in greater detail, it becomes clear that they have multiple effects on many processes in lymphocytes and other cell types as well. CyA and FK-506, and rapamycin to a lesser extent, have antiinflammatory properties. FK and CyA both inhibit the release of histamine and leukotriene from basophils caused by some stimuli (38); rapamycin inhibits selectively histamine release. FK and CyA, but not rapamycin, inhibit degranulation from polymorphonuclear granulocytes as well (39). B-cell activation is inhibited, especially by FK and RPM, although less so than by T-cells.

CYCLOSPORINE A

Use

Prior to the introduction of CyA, immunosuppression protocols relied heavily on steroids and cytotoxic drugs. These regimens had the disadvantage of producing broad suppression of the immune and inflammatory cascades using relatively toxic drugs. CyA introduced a new era of immunosuppression,

Table 62.1.   Drug Interactions with Cyclosportine (CSA)[a]

Increased CSA Levels		Decreased CSA Levels	Enhance CSA Nephrotoxicity
Ketoconazole	Fluconazole	Phenytoin	Aminoglycosides
Norfloxacin	Metoclopramide	Phenobarbital	Amphotericin B
Erythromycin	Verapamil	Carbamazepine	Trimethoprim
Diltiazem	Nicardipine	Valproic acid	Melphalan
Methylprednisolone	Prednisolone	Nafcillin	Acyclovir
Methyltestosterone	Levonorgestrel	Rifampin	Ganciclovir
Warfarin	Ethanol		Doxorubicin
Imipenem/cilastatin			Digoxin
			Furosemide
			Metolazone
			Indomethacin

[a] Adapted from Kahan BD: Cyclosporine. N Engl J Med 321:1725–1738, 1989; Ptachcinski RJ, Venkataramanan R, Burckart GJ: Clinical pharmacokinetics of cyclosporine. Clin Pharmacokinet 11:107–132, 1986; and Rodighiero V: Therapeutic drug monitoring of cyclosporine. Practical applications and limitations. Clin Pharmacokinet 16:23–37, 1989; with permission.

with potent, relatively specific, noncytotoxic suppression of T-cell activation.

Pharmacokinetics (40)

Bioavailability.   The drug is insoluble in water and thus must be dissolved in an organic solvent. The carrier probably causes some of the flushing and paresthesias seen with intravenous use. The drug dose must be increased by a factor of three when going from i.v. to p.o. because of an approximate 30% oral bioavailability that is highly variable (range 10 to 60%). Small-intestinal absorption decreases with bowel dysfunction or reduced bile flow (41). The peak blood level after an oral dose is achieved at about 3.5 hours.

Elimination.   The volume of distribution of CyA is large and variable. Hepatic metabolism is the only significant elimination mechanism. Drug alteration is via the cytochrome P-450 IIIA enzymes. The mean terminal half-life with normal liver function is 19 hours. At least 17 metabolites are identifiable, and at least a few are immunosuppressive, although of considerably less potency than the parent compound. Half-life increases with hepatic failure and is changed significantly by co-administration of a large number of other drugs that can cause unexpected increased or decreased serum levels, by induction or competitive inhibition of P-450, respectively (42). Many other drugs are also additive to CyA renal toxicity (Table 62.1). For all these reasons, it is essential that levels be monitored regularly and dosage adjusted accordingly.

Dosage and Administration

CyA administration is typically begun 12 to 24 hours prior to heart or kidney transplantation, and just after graft reperfusion in liver allograft recipients. A typical dose is 4 to 5 mg/kg/day i.v. This amount can be given in two divided doses each over 2 to 6 hours. Alternatively, some centers prefer to use slow continuous infusion over 24 hours. The changeover to p.o. dosing usually requires a dose three times higher (i.e., about 12 to 15 mg/kg). After 1 to 2 weeks, the dosage can be tapered slowly, by about 5% per week (40). Many patients are tapered to doses as low as 3 mg/kg by 6 months posttransplant. Liver transplant patients with a T-tube, which diverts some of the bile flow, require higher oral doses as a result of decreased absorption.

In renal transplantation, CyA, which is nephrotoxic, may be withheld initially, to avoid injury to the fresh graft. An example of sequential, combination therapy would be to start ALG, AZA, and prednisone for the first week, adding CyA at 8 to 10 mg/kg/day p.o. in one daily dose, tapering to 2 to 4 mg/kg/day p.o. over 3 to 6 months.

Adverse Effects

Several adverse effects are seen early on with the administration of CyA. Significant nephrotoxicity, probably because of vasoconstrictive effects on the afferent arterioles of the kidney (43), is a major problem. The mechanism of this effect is under debate (43–45). The nephrotoxicity is transient and reversible with decrease of dosage or discontinuation of drug (46). The incidence of nephrotoxicity varies from 25 to 32%, 37 or 38% in kidney, heart, or liver transplant patients, respectively (40). A promising diagnostic approach to distinguishing CyA toxicity from rejection in renal allograft recipients is by the measurement of CyA levels combined with serum and urine cytokine assay, particularly of soluble IL-2 receptor (sIL-2R) (47). As T-cells are stimulated to make IL-2 receptor, a soluble form, sIL-2R, is shed into the bloodstream. Thus, levels of sIL-2R are elevated in rejection but not with CyA-induced nephrotoxicity. Hypertension occurs frequently, within weeks of commencing therapy. The incidence varies widely in different patient populations, between 10 and 80% (48, 49). It is hypothesized that this hypotension results from a vasoconstrictive effect of CyA both in the renal and systemic circulations (50), perhaps caused by antagonism of endothelium-derived relaxation factors (51) or increased synthesis of endothelin, a vasoconstrictor (52). Physiologically, the hypertension is responsive to sodium restriction; therapies incorporating diuretics or calcium channel blockers have been advocated (48, 53). Minor neurotoxicity (tremor) is common (10 to 55%) and may improve over time without a change in therapy. More severe symptoms such as seizures and encephalopathy have also been associated with CyA, but it is frequently unclear whether the association is causal (54). Several reports detail a rare syndrome of confusion and cortical blindness in both liver and bone marrow transplant patients (45). Hypomagnesemia and hypocholesterolemia are believed to be risk factors for CyA neurotoxicity (45). CyA is probably diabetogenic, although analysis of this effect is confounded by the frequent concomitant use of steroids with CyA (45). Other metabolic effects include hypochloremic alkalosis and changes in serum potassium, magnesium, prolactin, and testosterone (55). Hepatotoxicity, manifested by an increased cholestatic tendency, may be quite common (45), but a reduction in dosage often improves this effect and it does not appear to be a major problem. Connective tissue side effects of CyA are common and can be distressing to the patient. These include hirsutism, seen over 2 to 4 weeks in 20 to 45%; gingival hyperplasia in 4 to 16%; and coarsening of facial features (56). Both FK and CyA appear to cause alterations of thymic structure of unknown significance (57).

Chronic administration of CyA has been associated with a nonreversible, probably progressive, nephrotoxicity. The incidence is estimated at 15% (58). The pathologic lesion resembles that of nephrosclerosis (43, 59, 60). Rarely, a syndrome resembling thrombotic hemolytic uremic syndrome (HUS)/thrombocytic purpura (TTP) has been reported (43).

Monitoring

The dosing of CyA is complicated by variable oral bioavailability and hepatic metabolism, the presence of at least 17 metabolites, several of which are active, and differing results from measuring CyA in blood or plasma with radioimmunoassay or high-pressure liquid chromatography (HPLC). Advantages and disadvantages inherent in each method have kept many variations of assaying CyA in use and, hence, there is no universally accepted blood level; "therapeutic" levels vary widely from center to center. Roughly, desired levels, by mode of testing, are (61): (a) radioimmunoassay (RIA) in serum or plasma—150 to 250 ng/ml at the time of transplantation, tapered to 50 to 100 ng/ml at 3 to 6 months; and (b) HPLC in whole blood, 100 to 300 ng/ml initially, tapered to 80 to 200 ng/ml.

FK-506

Use

The largest experience with FK is at Pittsburgh. About 1600 patients were on FK as of March, 1992 (62). In terms of the treatment of ACR, FK appears to have at least the same immunosuppressive efficacy as CyA, and possibly more; the drug is two to three orders of magnitude more potent in vitro than in vivo. Experiences in patients after liver (63, 64), kidney (65), and heart (66) transplantation have been reported. In general, the results suggest that the drug is associated with fewer episodes of rejection and less serious rejection, allowing a lower dose of steroids than traditionally used with CyA. However, the majority of these studies were neither randomized nor blinded comparisons of FK and CyA; thus, the actual comparability of the two drugs is uncertain.

In the treatment of acute resistant or chronic rejection, experience with FK rescue has been variable, although generally favorable. Patients selected have been resistant to CyA, steroids, and usually also to antilymphocyte antibodies and AZA. Response rates of 70 to 85% have been reported for resistant ACR (67–70). Resistant chronic rejection responded less well (70). In one study (71), the response of chronic rejection depended on the degree of injury present when rescue therapy was started. The finding on biopsy of "early" chronic rejection predicted a high degree of success (four of five) with FK. More advanced changes predicted frequent failure (seven of nine).

As has been reported for CyA in some studies, FK may also decrease ischemic injury to hepatocytes (72) and may augment liver regeneration (73) through unknown mechanisms.

Pharmacokinetics

FK has extremely variable pharmacokinetics with large interindividual variations. Significant toxicity can be encountered with FK. Therefore, it is essential to follow FK levels compulsively. With decreases in liver function or inhibitors of P450, FK levels rise and a decrease of dosage will be needed. The converse may be true with inducers of P450 (74). FK inhibits the hepatic cytochrome P450 reductase, which metabolizes it, potentially decreasing its own metabolism (75, 76). The significance of this effect in humans on chronic FK therapy is unknown.

Bioavailability. Absorption of an oral dose is very variable, with some individuals reaching a peak level in 30 minutes, while others only slowly absorb the drug over many hours. Bioavailability ranged from 5 to 67% after an oral dose. FK absorption was less dependent on bile flow than was CyA; therefore, there is no need to decrease the dose when the T-tube is clamped after liver transplantation (74).

Elimination. FK is metabolized by the liver, and elimination is markedly slowed with liver dysfunction. In one study of liver transplant patients (74), the half-life ranged from 3.5 to 40.5 hours. The volume of distribution also varied widely, from 5.6 to 65 liters/kg body weight.

Dosage and Administration

FK initially is started intravenously. It appears that a slow continuous infusion over 24 hours is less toxic than infusion over 4 hours (77). The initial dose is 0.05 mg/kg/day for liver transplants, 0.10 mg/kg/day for kidney transplants, and 0.15 mg/kg/day for small bowel transplants. When the patient can take oral FK, the i.v. drug is discontinued and the oral dose is started at 0.15 mg/kg/day, in two divided doses (78). Careful following of levels is absolutely essential.

Adverse Effects

Precise quantification of FK-506 toxicity and analysis of its comparability to CyA is confounded by multiple factors. Early studies with FK used doses that were too high. The complex and variable pharmacokinetics of FK make estimation of appropriate dosing difficult. The technical difficulties in obtaining and interpreting FK levels add another uncertainty. Finally, most of the comparisons between FK and CyA have used historical controls. As the drug enters wider usage and undergoes more studies, and laboratory monitoring methodology improves, a clearer picture will inevitably emerge.

FK-506 is nephrotoxic. The mechanism is not yet clear. Increased endothelin synthesis may play a role (79). Early studies suggest that this effect reverses with lowering the dose and/or changing to the oral route (80). The incidence of long-term renal injury, as seen with CyA, is unknown.

Hypertension appears less common, perhaps only 50% of that seen with CyA (78).

Neurotoxicity appears comparable to that of CyA, with both minor and major toxicity being seen (81). Minor toxicity, such as tremor, sleep disturbance, dysesthesias, and the like, is common and, as with CyA, is seen in about 20% of cases. Major toxicities, such as encephalopathy, which can progress to coma or a peculiar state resembling akinetic mutism, seizures, psychosis, and focal neurologic deficit, are less common, being estimated at 3 to 5%. Patients after liver transplantation are particularly prone to major neurotoxicity.

Gastrointestinal side effects, including diarrhea, anorexia, bloating and flatulence, are common, as with CyA. FK is also similarly diabetogenic (15 to 20%). Both drugs inhibited insulin release in a rat model (82). Hyperkalemia requiring Florinef has been noted with FK (70). Studies in rats (83) reveal some hepatotoxicity, but the clinical significance is not known.

FK does not seem to cause the connective tissue side effects seen with CyA. If early experience with FK allowing the use of lower doses of steroids is confirmed, less steroid-induced toxicity may be associated with FK usage.

Monitoring

As with CyA, there are many ways to measure FK levels. At Pittsburgh, the current method of choice is by ELISA, using solid-phase extraction, in plasma (62). Turn-around time for FK levels is 48 hours. The drug is trapped at high concentration inside red blood cells in a temperature-dependent fashion. Thus, whole-blood levels can be 8 to 10 times higher than plasma levels, with much variability (3.6 to 39) (74). Somewhat higher, more consistent plasma levels can be obtained by equilibration of the sample at 37°C before analysis.

A 12-hour trough level of 1.0 ng/ml with a range of 0.5 to 2.0 ng/ml is desired in the early posttransplant period. Higher or lower levels are sometimes accepted depending on the clinical situation. High-pressure liquid chromatography and mass spectroscopy are being investigated, as is the use of whole blood (84). One study of whole blood versus plasma (85) showed that whole-blood levels were more stable and more reliably elevated with nephrotoxicity than were plasma levels.

RAPAMYCIN (29, 86–90)

Use

The ultimate use of RPM has yet to be determined. The drug is clearly a very potent immunosuppressant, more so than FK, and much more than CyA. It inhibits delayed-type hypersensitivity, and both B- and T-cell responses to alloantigen (37). In animal models up to nonhuman primates, it prolongs the survival of MHC-incompatible grafts and can halt ongoing rejection. There is evidence that the drug may be synergistic with CyA and perhaps additive with FK, although under some conditions RPM and FK are mutually antagonistic (91).

Pharmacokinetics

RPM has a poor bioavailability after oral administration. Very low plasma levels (currently below detection) are therapeutic. The pharmacokinetics have thus been difficult to determine. The elimination appears to be very slow, with once-weekly doses being effective. The drug is unstable in plasma, low, and neutral pH buffers.

Special Considerations

The issues of drug delivery, stability, and monitoring remain problematic and require resolution before RPM can be introduced for human use. Current detection methods cannot accurately measure blood levels in the therapeutic range.

Adverse Effects

Rodents are very resistant to any toxic effects of RPM. The drug has been tested in cynomolgus monkeys. It caused atrophy of central lymphoid tissue, lethargy, anorexia, microscopic enterocolitis, and testicular atrophy. It did not appear to cause much nephrotoxicity or to be diabetogenic. It was not bone marrow toxic in preliminary studies.

ANTILYMPHOCYTE ANTIBODIES (40, 92)

Antilymphocyte antibodies, such as ALG, were first produced by immunizing animals against purified lymphocyte preparations, producing multispecificity polyclonal antibodies. Antibodies cross-reacting with other cellular molecules in blood were removed by extensive adsorption to blood components. Because of variability among immunized animals, many ALG are pooled to produce a more homogeneous preparation. Hybridoma technology later allowed the development of single-specificity monoclonal antibodies (e.g., OKT3 directed against one particular epitope of a single cell surface molecule). These drugs are much more standardized and potent than polyclonal antibodies.

MECHANISM

Antibodies to surface molecules on lymphocytes interfere with lymphocyte function in the immune response by several possible mechanisms. Lymphocytes are known to be both removed from the circulation rapidly after treatment with antilymphocyte antibodies and also to be phenotypically and functionally altered. Antibody-directed opsonization of cells with entrapment in the reticuloendothelial system and direct cell lysis by complement fixation may each partially explain the cell removal phenomenon. Studies with monoclonal antibodies have provided other insights. Treatment with OKT3 (anti-CD3, part of the T-cell receptor complex) has been shown to alter the cell surface. After the initial disappearance of cells bearing the target molecule (the T-cell receptor complex), those lymphocytes that reappear do not display the molecule on the surface despite the fact that they are capable of producing it, unless OKT3 therapy is halted for at least 48 hours. Obviously, lymphocytes without the antigen receptor cannot react to antigen and hence are effectively immunosuppressed. Additionally, OKT3 causes a massive initial activation of T-cells, producing an uncontrolled release of cytokines. Such dysregulation appears to alter the ability of affected cells to mount a subsequent immune response in poorly understood ways.

PREPARATIONS

Polyclonal ALG and equine antithymocyte globulin (ATG) potency is variable from lot to lot. Antibodies to "innocent bystander" molecules and structures can damage other blood and tissue components. The larger amount of animal protein also bears a risk of causing serum sickness. Monoclonal antibodies, currently produced by mouse cells, are specifically targeted to one molecule and contain no extraneous antibody or protein. They are much less apt to cause serum sickness or attack nonlymphocyte structures. Potency is uniform but, unfortunately, individuals vary in the amount of endogenous antibody they form directed against the mouse antibody. Intermediate and high responders form a significant titer of blocking antibody. This antibody production can be decreased by continuing other immunosuppressive therapy during monoclonal antibody administration. Retreatment can often succeed if higher doses of antibody are used for subsequent administration. The very highest antibody responders, probably about 5 to 20% of patients, form high-titer antibodies and will fail even increased dose therapy. This problem should be greatly improved with the development of humanized, as opposed to murine, monoclonal antibodies.

USE

The place of immunoglobulin therapy in immunosuppressive regimens is in a state of flux. These agents initially were shown to be effective in the reversal of acute rejection. For this use, OKT3 has been shown to be more effective than high doses of steroids. More recently, protocols wherein antibody replaces CyA in the early phase after renal transplantation have been shown to produce less early renal toxicity. CyA is added later. Some maintenance regimens also use antibody in some combination with CyA, and/or AZA, and/or steroids.

PHARMACOKINETICS

The approximate plasma half-life of ATG polyclonal antibody is 6 days. The duration of effects on circulating cell populations is quite variable. The effects of OKT3, as measured by the absence of circulating T-cells bearing CD3, last for 48 hours after the discontinuation of therapy. However, in a successful course of therapy, immunosuppressive effects last for a much longer period.

DOSAGE AND ADMINISTRATION

Immunoglobulin therapy is given intravenously. Equine ATG is given in the dosage range of 10 to 15 mg/kg in a single daily dose. Therapy of acute rejection is usually continued for 14 days. With OKT3, the dose of 5 mg/day for 7 to 10 days is typical. Prophylactic OKT3 regimens use the same dose but for up to 30 days of therapy. Higher doses can be used to overcome the effect of antimurine antibodies.

ADVERSE EFFECTS

Polyclonal preparations cause a high incidence of febrile reactions with the first few doses. Antihistamines, antipyretics, and sometimes steroids are given in preparation. Because of antibodies reacting with other blood cells, leukopenia (about 14%) and thrombocytopenia (about 30%) are seen. Anaphylaxis occurs in less than 1%. Nonetheless, a skin test prior to use is recommended. Skin rash is a fairly frequent occurrence, seen in 10 to 30%

Monoclonal antibody treatment with OKT3 is by far the most extensively studied. On the first one or two doses a syndrome of fever, chills, tachycardia, gastrointestinal disturbance, and increased or decreased blood pressure is noted. These symptoms are probably a consequence of uncontrolled cytokine release (93) from lymphocytes and can be blocked to a large extent by pretreatment with a 1-g i.v. bolus of Solu-Medrol 15 to 60 minutes prior to OKT3 infusion.

The potent suppression of T-lymphocyte populations is known to be associated with an increased incidence of viral infection and lymphoproliferative disorders.

MONITORING

Some researchers (92) advocate following thrice-weekly CD3+ cell counts via flow cytometry in patients on OKT3. If CD3+ cells reach 10%, it is recommended that OKT3 either be increased in dosage (to as much as 15 mg/day) or discontinued.

MYCOPHENOLIC ACID AND RS-61443 (94)

MECHANISM

Interference with purine metabolism is known to cause immunosuppression. Lymphocytes are particularly sensitive to defects in the de novo synthesis pathways of purines. Adenosine deaminase allows the interconversion of adenine and guanosine nucleotide bases. Children born with a deficiency of this enzyme are severely lymphopenic, with poor function of both B- and T-lymphocytes. They have a reduced number of guanosine nucleotides. This defect can be mimicked by inhibiting inosine monophosphate dehydrogenase, which is involved in the de novo synthesis of guanosine monophosphate, with the antibiotic mycophenolic acid (MPA). A modified form of MPA designated RS-61443 (RS6) was synthesized in an attempt to provide more stability and better bioavailability. This agent inhibits B-cell humoral response and blocks the generation of cytotoxic T-cells in vivo. In comparison with FK and CyA, prevention of antibody response is much stronger. The drug has been tested in animal models and in one human trial (95). It was shown to suppress graft rejection and to be effective in treating ongoing rejection.

USE

The use of RS6 remains to be determined. It would be logical to use the drug in a fashion similar to that of AZA. The drug effect appears to be at least additive with CyA. The ability to block humoral responses effectively (96) may make the drug useful in prevention of chronic rejection.

PHARMACOKINETICS

Bioavailability. MPA, the parent compound, has been found to be slowly and variably absorbed after oral administration in cynomolgus monkeys. The derivative RS6 was prepared by Lee et al (97) to improve stability and bioavailability. Currently there are no published human data on bioavailability, but in a rat model the two drugs showed little difference (98).

DOSAGE AND ADMINISTRATION

In a human trial, RS6 was given as part of quadruple induction (antilymphocyte globulin, steroid, CyA, and RS6) with triple maintenance (steroid, CyA, and RS6). The dose range of 100 to 3500 mg/day p.o. was studied. Six patients were entered into each of eight dosage groups of RS6. At 1.5 g/day, 50% rejection was seen; at 2 g/day, 16%; and at 2.5 g/day, no episodes of rejection were seen. In a rescue study, wherein steroid and antilymphocyte antibody-resistant rejection was treated in nine patients, doses of 2 to 3 g/day were associated with improvement in six of nine patients.

ADVERSE EFFECTS

Since lymphocyte sensitivity to this antimetabolite is greater than that experienced by other cell types, the antiproliferative effect is more specific than with drugs such as AZA, with less toxicity in the bone marrow and gastrointestinal tract.

The following adverse effects were encountered in the aforementioned studies: gastritis in one of 48, ileus in three of 48, nausea and vomiting in two of 48. These findings were in contrast to previous dog studies wherein major gastrointestinal toxicity was noted. No significant nephrotoxicity, hepatotoxicity, or bone marrow suppression was noted in this small study.

MIZORIBINE (99–101)

MECHANISM

Mizoribine (MZB), also known as Bredinin, is an adenosine analog. Like RS6 and MPA, MZB is an inhibitor of the enzyme inosine monophosphate dehydrogenase. Not surprisingly, the drug has antiproliferative effects on lymphocytes and antagonizes the formation of cytotoxic cells but does not affect the function of previously formed cytotoxic cells. There is no effect on IL-2 production after lymphocyte stimulation, but the ensuing cell proliferation is potently antagonized.

USE (102–104)

MZB has been used as a maintenance agent in combination with CyA and steroids, primarily in renal transplant patients. The drug appears to have advantages over AZA (105).

PHARMACOKINETICS

Bioavailability. With a normal GI tract, peak blood levels are achieved 2 to 3 hours after an oral dose. Absorption of MZB is delayed in the presence of gastrointestinal disease.
Elimination. The major elimination pathway of MZB is renal. There is little hepatic metabolism, and 85% of a dose is excreted unchanged in the urine. Clearance of the drug is thus affected markedly by renal failure. In 26 renal transplant patients with an average creatinine clearance of 50 ml/min (range 22 to 93), the half-life was 4 hours (range 1.6 to 8.2).

DOSAGE AND ADMINISTRATION

The drug is administered once daily, at an oral dose of 50 to 300 mg/day.

ADVERSE EFFECTS

MZB has considerably less myelotoxicity and hepatic toxicity than AZA.

15-DEOXYSPERGUALIN (106–110)

MECHANISM

15-Deoxyspergualin (DSG) was discovered by a drug development program investigating antitumor agents in Japan. The drug was shown to be very active against lymphoid tumors only, and later to be immunosuppressive by antilymphocyte action. The molecular basis for the action of DSG is unknown but appears to be different from that of all previously known immunosuppressant drugs. Delayed-type hypersensitivity is suppressed and allograft survival is prolonged. The display of MHC type 2 molecules on macrophages is inhibited. IL-1 production is not affected. The formation of cytotoxic T-lymphocytes after antigen presentation is suppressed, whereas the activity of previously formed cytotoxic cells is spared. This effect can be reversed completely by exogenous interferon-γ, and partly by IL-2. There is no effect on IL-2 production by lymphocytes.The proliferative response of T-lymphocytes to IL-2 is inhibited. In multiple animal models, DSG has suppressed rejection and has been effective against ongoing rejection and graft vs. host disease. Both primary and secondary antibody responses are inhibited.

USE

DSG performed well in animal models of xenograft transplantation and was better than FK or CyA. In a human trial (110) with one haplotype matched renal transplants, the incidence of accelerated rejection was significantly decreased when DSG was combined with CyA.

PHARMACOKINETICS

Bioavailability. The drug must be given intravenously.

Elimination. In a human trial, the half-life varied between 39 and 55 hours in renal transplant patients, which was about twice that in prior studies in cancer patients.

DOSAGE AND ADMINISTRATION

In a human trial in which DSG was used for reversal of rejection, doses ranging from 80 to 220 mg/m²/day were used. The optimal dose appeared to be 180 mg/m²/day. The drug is given i.v. In other studies, in which DSG was used in combination with AZA, CyA, and steroids, doses of 2 to 5 mg/kg/day were used for maintenance of immunosuppression.

ADVERSE EFFECTS

Toxicity is decreased by slow infusion, usually over 4 to 5 hours. The toxic effects seen in transplant patients have been central nervous system (facial dysesthesias), gastrointestinal (anorexia, nausea), reversible bone marrow suppression (lymphocytes and thrombocytes), and reversible hypotension. The bone marrow suppression appears to be the most significant side effect.

BREQUINAR (111, 112)

MECHANISM

Brequinar (BQR) is an antimetabolite with broad antineoplastic activity that has been tested in humans with cancer. It is an inhibitor of dihydroorotate dehydrogenase, a mitochondrial enzyme in the de novo synthesis pathway of pyrimidines. The antiproliferative effects of the drug appear to be mediated by the depletion of pyrimidine precursors needed for DNA and RNA synthesis. BQR is a potent immunosuppressant in a rat model (113).

ADVERSE EFFECTS

Dose-limiting toxicities resulted from thrombocytopenia and a severe desquamative dermatitis.

NEW AND NOVEL APPROACHES TO IMMUNOSUPPRESSION

IMMUNE TOLERANCE

The development of specific tolerance of the host for donor tissue without the need for ongoing immunosuppression has been sought for a long time. Recently, the molecular basis for several mechanisms of immune tolerance has been elucidated. Early in life, "self"-reactive T-cells are destroyed in the thymus, preventing autoimmunity. This process, known as "thymic education," kills T-cells with antigen specificities that would damage the host. There are also nonfatal mechanisms for turning off T-cells, making them permanently nonreactive

to antigen. It was shown that stimulation of T-cells with antigen, but without the complete set of signals needed to cause full activation, actually turns them off permanently (114). Strong evidence has been provided for the natural occurrence of these "anergic" cells in vivo by other workers (115). Specific tolerance can also be achieved by certain conditions that favor the development of T-cell suppressor activity (116). This finding is particularly interesting in light of recent work that may have described the T-cell subset responsible for "help" to suppressor activity (13).

Several experimental strategies have produced effective immune tolerance in animal models. In a rat model (117) investigators injected pancreatic islet cells into the thymus, accompanied by a single dose of antilymphocyte serum (ALS). This procedure unexpectedly produced a state of donor tolerance to islet transplant in extrathymic sites. The mechanism is uncertain. It was proposed that the ALS depleted the peripheral T-cell pool and that, as fresh lymphocytes matured in the thymus, they underwent "thymic education" with the injected antigens, as T-cells do early in life. In another study (118), investigators injected anti-MHC class I antibodies into a graft of human tissue, which was transplanted into a mouse. The idea was to "mask" the MHC molecules to prevent rejection. Also surprisingly, this technique created permanent tolerance toward the graft. Another strategy (119, 120) involves the irradiation of the recipient, with subsequent bone marrow reconstitution using a mixture of both donor and recipient marrow. This irradiation produces a chimeric animal with circulating donor and recipient leukocytes, having specific immune tolerance to donor tissue transplants. A variation of this method is approaching clinical trials in humans.

BIOLOGICAL RESPONSE MODIFIERS AND MONOCLONAL ANTIBODIES

The widespread application of recombinant DNA and monoclonal antibody technology to immunology has produced a large number of cytokine agonists, antagonists, and antibodies that target dozens of soluble and cell surface molecules. These reagents are being tested and are poised to move into the clinical arena. Only a cursory review of some putative targeting strategies can be presented here.

Antibodies and receptor antagonists to the mediators of inflammation, IL-1 and TNF, have caused remarkable reductions in mortality caused by fatal bacteremia in endotoxin shock models. Because of the involvement of inflammation and multiple cytokines in ACR, many studies have been published on these mediators and ACR. Multiple cytokines (IL-1, IL-2, TNF, IL-6, and IFN-γ) have been shown to be involved in ACR and have been studied as diagnostic markers. In general, they are increased early (prior to clinical signs) and are very sensitive markers but, unfortunately, nonspecific, since they also increase in infection and other conditions. So far, a soluble form of IL-2 receptor (sIL-2R) seems to be the best single molecule to follow for the diagnosis of ACR. In the therapeutic area, IL-1 antagonists are immunosuppressive and have prolonged graft survival in a murine model (121). IL-10 appears to suppress production of IL-2 and IFN-γ. Thus, this cytokine may be a "natural" immunosuppressant.

Many studies have now demonstrated the immunosuppressive efficacy of antibodies to cell surface molecules. Antibodies can merely block a receptor, or, in more sophisticated systems, carry toxins to kill the target cell. Antibodies to IL-2 receptor have prolonged graft survival in many animal models, but have so far not been impressive in early human trials. The advantage of targeting this receptor is that it selectively appears on activated cells. The disadvantage is that it may block both helper and suppressor cell activations. Both anti-CD4 (helper cell marker) and anti-CD7 (another T-cell activation antigen) have been effective immunosuppressants in animal models and are under development for possible human trials. Antibodies to cell surface adhesion molecules will affect lymphocyte target attachment and tissue emigration. Anti-CD54 (intracellular adhesion molecule-1, or ICAM-1) has prolonged graft survival in a monkey model (122). Since ICAM-1 attaches to CD11a/CD18, known as lymphocyte function-associated antigen-1 or LFA-1, this is also a logical target. Antibodies to CD11a appeared to improve bone marrow transplant results in humans (123). Combination therapy with both anti-LFA-1 and anti-CD54 proved to be very potent immunosuppressives in a murine heart transplant model (124).

CONCLUSION

For almost 30 years, immunosuppression for transplantation has been accomplished with only four drugs. As a result of the recent explosion of molecular knowledge in immunology, many more options are now available. Drugs that interfere with lymphocyte biochemical pathways are becoming more specific. New drugs similar in action to cyclosporine are many times more potent. Biologic response modifiers and monoclonal antibodies can accurately target molecular processes. Finally, advances in the understanding of immune tolerance offer the promise of permanent graft acceptance without immunosuppression. Intensivists can expect to see more patients treated with these agents and more therapies as the number of transplants continues to increase and the usefulness of immune manipulation of other disease processes becomes increasingly apparent.

REFERENCES

1. Goust JM, Stevenson HC, Galbraith RM, Virella G: Immunosuppression and immunomodulation. *Immunol Series* 50:481–498, 1990.
2. Rubin RH, Cosimi AB: Therapy, both immunosuppressive and antimicrobial, for the transplant patient in the 1990s. In Brent L, Sells RA (eds): Organ Transplantation: Current Clinical and Immunological Concepts. London, Bailliere Tindall, 1989, pp 71–88.
3. Emanuel D, Cunningham I, Jules-Elysee K, et al: Cytomegalovirus pneumonia after bone marrow transplantation successfully treated with the combination of ganciclovir and high dose intravenous immune globulin. *Ann Intern Med* 109:777–782.
4. Boitard C, Bach JF: Long-term complications of conventional immunosuppressive treatment. Advances In Nephrology From the Necker Hospital 18:335–354, 1989.
5. Sheil AGR: Complications of immunosuppression in renal allograft recipients: malignancy. *Clin Transplantation* 5:573–579, 1991.
6. Nalesnik MA, Jaffe R, Starzl TE, et al: The pathology of posttransplant lymphoproliferative disorders occurring in the setting of cyclosporine A-prednisone immunosuppression. *Am J Pathol* 133:173–192, 1988.
7. Roitt IM, Brostoff J, Male DK: Immunology, 2nd ed. London, Gower, 1989.
8. Picker LJ, Terstappen LWMM, Rott LS, Streeter PR, Stein H, Butcher EC: Differential expression of homing-associated adhesion molecules by T cell subsets in man. *J Immunol* 145:3247–3255, 1990.
9. Male D, Champion B, Cooke A, Owen M: Advanced Immunology, 2nd ed. London, Gower, 1991.
10. Hall BM: Cells mediating allograft rejection. *Transplantation* 51:1141–1151, 1991.
11. Springer TA: Adhesion receptors of the immune system. *Nature* 346:425–434, 1990.
12. Mitchison NA: Suppressor activity as a composite property. *Scand J Immunol* 28:271–276, 1988.
13. Torimoto Y, Tothstein DM, Dang NH, Schlossman SF, Morimoto C: CD31, a novel cell surface marker for CD4 cells of suppressor lineage, unaltered by state of activation. *J Immunol* 148(2):388–396, 1992.
14. Chan GL, Gruber SA, Skjei KL, Canafax DM: Principles of immunosuppression. *Crit Care Clin* 6:841–892, 1990.
15. Ahmed AR, Hombal SM: Cyclophosphamide (Cytoxan). A review on relevant pharmacology and clinical uses. *J Am Acad Dermatol* 11:1115–1126, 1984.
16. Moore MJ: Clinical pharmacokinetics of cyclophosphamide. *Clin Pharmacokinet* 20:194–208, 1991.
17. Cunningham D, Cummings J, Blackie RB, et al: The pharmacokinetics of high dose cyclophosphamide and high dose etoposide. *Med Oncol Tumor Pharmacother* 5:117–123, 1988.
18. Goldberg MA, Antin JH, Guinan EC, Rappeport JM: Cyclophosphamide cardiotoxicity: an analysis of dosage as a risk factor. *Blood* 68:1114–1118, 1986.
19. Chan GL, Erdmann GR, Gruber SA, Matas AJ, Canafax DM: Azathioprine metabolism: pharmacokinetics of 6-mercaptopurine, 6-thiouric acid and 6-thioguanine nucleotides in renal transplant patients. *J Clin Pharmacol* 30:358–363, 1990.
20. Chan GL, Erdmann GR, Gruber SA, et al: Pharmacokinetics of 6-thiouric acid and 6-mercaptopurine in renal allograft recipients after oral administration of azathioprine. *Eur J Clin Pharmacol* 36:265–271, 1989.
18. J Intern Med 228:69–71, 1990.
19. Nephron 51:509–516, 1989.
20. Lancet 337:251–252, 1991.
21. Venkat Raman G, Sharman VL, Lee HA: Azathioprine and allopurinol: a potentially dangerous combination, *J Intern Med* 228:69–71, 1990.
22. Liano F, Moreno A, Matesanz R, et al: Veno-occlusive hepatic disease of the liver in renal transplantation: is azathioprine the cause, *Nephron*, 51:509–516, 1989.
23. Frick TW, Fryd DS, Goodale RL, Simmons RL, Sutherland DE, Najarian JS: Lack of association between azathioprine and acute pancreatitis in renal transplant patients. *Lancet* 337:251–292, 1991.
24. Saway PA, Heck LW, Bonner JR, Kirklin JK: Azathioprine hypersensitivity: case report and review of the literature. *Am J Med* 84:960–964, 1988.
25. Zipfel PF, Irving SG, Kelly K, Siebenlist U: Complexity of the primary genetic response to mitogenic activation of human T cells. *Mol Cell Biol* 9(3):1041–1048, 1989.
26. Siekierka JJ, Hung SH, Poe M, Lin CS, Sigal NH: A cytosolic binding protein for the immunosuppressant FK-506 has peptidyl-prolyl isomerase activity but is distinct from cyclophilin. *Nature* 341:755–757, 1989.
27. Brabletz T, Pietrowski I, Serfling E: The immunosuppressives FK-506 and cyclosporin A inhibit the generation of protein factors binding to the two purine boxes of the interleukin 2 enhancer. *Nucleic Acids Res* 19:61–67, 1991.
28. Banerji SS, Parsons JN, Tocci MJ: The immunosuppressant FK-506 specifically inhibits mitogen-induced activation of the interleukin-2 promoter and the isolated enhancer elements NFIL-2A and NF-AT1. *Mol Cell Biol* 11:4074–4087, 1991.
29. Henderson DJ, Naya I, Bundick RV, Smith GM, Schmidt JA: Comparison of the effects of FK-506, cyclosporin A and rapamycin on IL-2 production. *Immunology* 73:316–321, 1991.
30. Hohman RJ, Hultsch T: Cyclosporin A: new insights for cell biologists and biochemists. *New Biologist* 2:663–672, 1990.
31. Harding MW, Handschumacher RE: Cyclophilin, a primary molecular target for cyclosporine. Structural and functional implications. *Transplantation* 46:29S–35S, 1988.
32. Schreiber SL, Liu J, Albers MW, et al: Immunophilin-ligand complexes as probes of intracellular signaling pathways. *Transplant Proc* 23(6):2839–2844, 1992.
33. Ullman KS, Flanagan WM, Cothesy B, et al: Site of action of cyclosporine and FK-506 in the pathways of communication between the T lymphocyte antigen receptor and the early activation genes. *Transplant Proc* 23(6):2845, 1992.
34. Dumont FJ, Staruch MJ, Koprak SL, Melino MR, Sigal NH: Distinct mechanisms of suppression of murine T cell activation by the related macrolides FK-506 and rapamycin. *J Immunol* 144:251–258, 1990.
35. Kay JE, Doe SE, Benzie CR: The mechanism of action of the immunosuppressive drug FK-506. *Cell Immunol* 124:175–181, 1989.
36. Kay JE, Benzie CR: T lymphocyte activation through the C28 pathway is insensitive to inhibition by the immunosuppressive drug FK-506. *Immunol Lett* 23:155–159, 1989.
37. Kay JE, Kromwel L, Doe SE, Denyer M: Inhibition of T and B lymphocyte proliferation by rapamycin. *Immunology* 72:544–549, 1991.
38. de Paulis A, Cirillo R, Ciccarelli A, Condorelli M, Marone G: FK-506, a potent novel inhibitor of the release of proinflammatory mediators from human Fc epsilon RI+ cells. *J Immunol* 146:2374–2381, 1991.

39. Forrest MJ, Jewell ME, Koo GC, Sigal NH: FK-506 and cyclosporin A: selective inhibition of calcium ionophore-induced polymorphonuclear leukocyte degranulation. *Biochem Pharmacol* 42:1221–1228, 1991.

40. American Hospital Formulary Service: AHFS Drug Information 91, 33rd ed. Bethesda, American Society of Hospital Pharmacists, 1991.

41. Freeman DJ: Pharmacology and pharmacokinetics of cyclosporine. *Clin Biochem* 24:9–14, 1991.

42. Watkins PB: The role of cytochrome P-450 in cyclosporine metabolism. *J Am Acad Dermatol* 23:1301–1309, 1990.

43. Remuzzi G, Bertani T: Renal vascular and thrombotic effects of cyclosporine. *Am J Kidney Dis* 13:261–272, 1989.

44. Abraham JS, Bentley FR, Garrison RN: The role of intrarenal prostaglandins and angiotensin II in acute cyclosporine-induced vasoconstriction. *Surgery* 110:343–349, 1991.

45. Rush DN: Cyclosporine toxicity to organs other than the kidney. *Clin Biochem* 24:101–105, 1991.

46. Keown PA, Stiller CR, Wallace AC: Effect of cyclosporine on the kidney. *J Pediatr* 111:1029–1033, 1987.

47. Smith AY, Citterio F, Welsh M, Kerman RH, Kahan BD: Interleukin-2 receptor as an immunodiagnostic tool to differentiate rejection from nephrotoxicity. *Transplant Proc* 21(1):1462–1464, 1989.

48. Luke RG: Mechanism of cyclosporine-induced hypertension. *Am J Hypertens* 4:468–471, 1991.

49. Weidle PJ, Vlasses PH: Systemic hypertension associated with cyclosporine: a review. *Drug Intell Clin Pharm* 22:443–451, 1988.

50. Mason J: The pathophysiology of Sandimmune (cyclosporine) in man and animals. *Pediatr Nephrol* 4:554–574, 1990.

51. Luscher TF, Yang Z, Diederich D, Buhler FR: Endothelium-dependent vascular responses: effect of hypertension and cyclosporin A. *Z Kardiol* 78(suppl 6):132–136, 1989.

52. Bunchman TE, Brookshire CA: Cyclosporine-induced synthesis of endothelin by cultured human endothelial cells. *J Clin Invest* 88:310–314, 1991.

53. Weir MR: Therapeutic benefits of calcium channel blockers in cyclosporine-treated organ transplant recipients: blood pressure control and immunosuppression. *Am J Med* 90:32S–36S, 1991.

54. Mason J: The pathophysiology of Sandimmune (cyclosporine) in man and animals. *Pediatr Nephrol* 4:686–704, 1990.

55. Scott JP, Higenbottam TW: Adverse reactions and interactions of cyclosporin. *Med Toxicol Adv Drug Exper* 3:107–127, 1988.

56. Reznick VM, Lyons Jones K, Durham BL, Mendoza SA: Changes in facial appearance during cyclosporine treatment. *Lancet* 1:1405–1407, 1987.

57. Pugh-Humphreys RG, Ross CS, Thomson AW: The influence of FK-506 on the thymus: an immunophenotypic and structural analysis. *Immunology* 70:398–404, 1990.

58. Lorber MI: Cyclosporine: lessons learned—future strategies. *Clin Transplant* 5:505–516, 1991.

59. Kopp JB, Klotman PE: Cellular and molecular mechanisms of cyclosporin nephrotoxicity. *J Am Soc Nephrol* 1:162–179, 1990.

60. Mihatsch MJ, Thiel G, Ryffel B: Histopathology of cyclosporine nephrotoxicity. *Transplant Proc* 20:759–771, 1988.

61. Keown PA: Optimizing cyclosporine therapy: dose, levels, and monitoring. *Transplant Proc* 20:382–389, 1988.

62. Warty VS, Venkataramanan R, Zendehrouh P, et al: Practical aspects of FK-506 analysis (Pittsburgh experience). *Transplant Proc* 23(6):2730–2731, 1992.

63. Todo S, Fung JJ, Tzakis A, et al: One hundred ten consecutive primary orthotopic liver transplants under FK-506 in adults. *Transplant Proc* 23:1397–1402, 1991.

64. Fung J, Abu-Elmagd K, Jain A, et al: A randomized trial of primary liver transplantation under immunosuppression with FK-506 vs cyclosporine. *Transplant Proc* 23(6):2977–2983, 1992.

65. Shapiro R, Jordan M, Scantlebury V, et al: FK-506 in clinical kidney transplantation. *Transplant Proc* 23(6):3065–3067, 1992.

66. Armitage JM, Kormos RL, Fung J, Starzl TE: The clinical trial of FK-506 as primary and rescue immunosuppression in adult cardiac transplantation. *Transplant Proc* 23(6):3054–3057, 1992.

67. Jensen CWB, Scantlebury V, Fung J, et al: FK-506 conversion of renal allografts failing cyclosporine immunosuppression. *Transplant Proc* 23(6):3078–3081, 1992.

68. Winkler M, Ringe B, Gerstenkorn C, et al: Use of FK-506 for treatment of chronic rejection after liver transplantation. *Transplant Proc* 23(6):2984–2986, 1992.

69. D'Alessandro AM, Kalayoglu M, Pirsch JD, et al: FK-506 rescue therapy for resistant rejection episodes in liver transplant recipients. *Transplant Proc* 23(6):2987–2988, 1992.

70. Lewis WD, Jenkins RL, Burke PA, et al: FK-506 rescue therapy in liver transplant patients with drug resistant rejection. *Transplant Proc* 23(6):2989–2991, 1992.

71. Shaw BW, Markin R, Stratta R, et al: FK-506 rescue treatment of acute and chronic rejection in liver allograft recipients. *Transplant Proc* 23(6):2994–2995, 1992.

72. Sakr MF, Zetti GM, Hassanein TI, et al: FK-506 ameliorates the hepatic injury associated with ischemia and reperfusion in rats. *Hepatology* 13:947–951, 1991.

73. Francavilla A, Starzl TE, Barone M, et al: Studies on mechanisms of augmentation of liver regeneration by cyclosporine and FK-506. *Hepatology* 14:140–143, 1991.

74. Venkataramanan R, Jain A, Warty VS, et al: Pharmacokinetics of FK-506 in transplant patients. *Transplant Proc* 23(6):2736–2740, 1992.

75. Vincent SH, Wang RW, Karanam BV, Klimko M, Alvaro R, Chiu SH: Effects of the immunosuppressant FK-506 and its analog FK-520 on hepatic and renal cytochrome P450 mixed-function oxidase. *Biochem Pharmacol* 41:1325–1330, 1991.

76. Venkataramanan R, Warty VS, Zemaitis MA, et al: Biopharmaceutical aspects of FK-506. *Transplant Proc* 19:30–35, 1987.

77. Abu-Elmagd K, Fung J, Draviam R, et al: Four hour versus 24 hour intravenous infusion of FK-506 in liver transplantation. *Transplant Proc* 23(6):2767–2770, 1992.

78. Fung JJ, Abu-Elmagd K, Todo S, et al: FK-506 in clinical organ transplantation. *Clin Transplantation* 5:517–522, 1991.

79. Moutabarrik A, Ishibashi M, Kameoka H, et al: FK-506 mechanism of nephrotoxicity: stimulatory effect on endothelin secretion by cultured kidney cells. *Transplant Proc* 23(6):3133–3136, 1992.

80. McCauley J, Takaya S, Fung J, et al: The question of FK-506 nephrotoxicity after liver transplantation. *Transplant Proc* 23:1444–1447, 1991.

81. Eidelman BH, Abu-Elmagd K, Wilson J, et al: Neurologic complications of FK-506. *Transplant Proc* 23(6):3175–3178, 1991.

82. Muller MK, Wojcik M, Coone H, et al: Inhibition of insulin release by FK-506 and its prevention by rioprostil, a stable prostaglandin E1 analogue. *Transplant Proc* 23(6):2812–2816, 1992.

83. Farghali H, Sakr M, Gasbarrini A, et al: Effect of FK-506 chronic administration on bromosulphthalein hepatic excretion in rats. *Transplant Proc* 23(6):2802–2804, 1992.

84. Beysens AJ, Wijnen RMH, Beuman GH, et al: FK-506: monitoring in plasma or whole blood? *Transplant Proc* 23(6):2745–2747, 1992.

85. Japanese FK-506 Study Group: Japanese study of FK-506 on kidney tranplantation: the benefit of monitoring the whole blood FK-506 concentration. *Transplant Proc* 23(6):3085–3088, 1992.

86. Morris RE: Rapamycins: antifungal, antitumor, antiproliferative and immunosuppressive macrolides. *Trans Rev* 6(1):39–87, 1992.

87. Chang JY, Sehgal SN: Pharmacology of rapamycin: a new immunosuppressive agent. *Br J Rheumatol* 30(suppl 2):62–65, 1991.

88. Kahan BD, Chang JY, Sehgal SN: Preclinical evaluation of a new potent immunosuppressive agent, rapamycin. *Transplantation* 52:185–191, 1991.

89. Morris RE, Meiser BM, Wu J, Shorthouse R, Wang J: Use of rapamycin for the suppression of alloimmune reactions in vivo: schedule dependence, tolerance induction, synergy with cyclosporine and FK-506, and effect on host-versus-graft and graft-versus-host reactions. *Transplant Proc* 23:521–524, 1991.

90. Wu J, Palladino MA, Figari IS, Morris RE: Comparative immunoregulatory effects of rapamycin, FK-506 and cyclosporine on mitogen-induced cytokine production and lymphoproliferation. *Transplant Proc* 23:238–240, 1991.

91. Dumont FJ, Melino MR, Staruch MJ, Koprak SL, Fischer PA, Sigal NH: The immunosuppressive macrolides FK-506 and rapamycin act as reciprocal antagonists in murine T cells. *J Immunol* 144:1418–1424, 1990.

92. Kreis H, Legendre C, Chatenoud L: OKT3 in organ transplantation. *Trans Rev* 5:181–199, 1991.

93. Chatenoud L, Gerran C, Legendre C, et al: In vivo cell activation following OKT3 administration. *Transplantation* 49:697–702, 1990.

94. Sollinger HW, Eugui EM, Allison AC: RS-61443: Mechanism of action, experimental and early clinical results. *Clin Trans* 5(6):523–526, 1991.

95. Sollinger HW, Deierhoi MH, Belzer FO, Diethelm AG, Kauffman RS: RS-61443—a phase I clinical trial and pilot rescue study. *Transplantation* 53(2):428–432, 1992.

96. Burlingham WJ, Grailer APAU, Sollinger HW: Inhibition of both MLC and in vitro IgG memory response to tetanus toxoid by RS-61443. *Transplantation* 51:545–547, 1991.

97. Lee WA, Gu L, Miksztal AR, Chu N, Leung K, Nelson PH: Bioavailability improvement of mycophenolic acid through amino ester derivatization. *Pharm Res* 7:161–166, 1990.

98. Morris RE, Wang J: Comparison of the immunosuppressive effects of mycophenolic acid and the morpholinoethyl ester of mycophenolic acid (RS-61443) in recipients of heart allografts. *Transplant Proc* 23:493–496, 1991.

99. Ichikawa Y, Ihara H, Takahara S, et al: The immunosuppressive mode of action of mizoribine. *Transplantation* 38:262–267, 1984.

100. Takada K, Asada S, Ichikawa Y, et al: Pharmacokinetics of bredinin in renal transplant patients. *Eur J Clin Pharmacol* 24:457–461, 1983.

101. Turka LA, Dayton J, Sinclair G, Thompson CB, Mitchell BS: Guanine ribonucleotide depletion inhibits T cell activation. Mechanism of action of the immunosuppressive drug mizoribine. *J Clin Invest* 87:940–948, 1991.

102. Amemiya H, Suzuki S, Watanabe H, Hayashi R, Niiya S: Synergistically enhanced immunosuppressive effect by combined use of cyclosporine and mizoribine. *Transplant Proc* 21:956–958, 1989.

103. Kokado Y, Ishibashi M, Jiang H, Takahara S, Sonoda T: A new triple-drug induction therapy with low dose cyclosporine, mizoribine and prednisolone in renal transplantation. *Transplant Proc* 21:1575–1578, 1989.

104. Marumo F, Okubo M, Yokota K, et al: A clinical study of renal transplant patients receiving triple-drug therapy—cyclosporine A, mizoribine, and prednisolone. *Transplant Proc* 20:406–409, 1988.

105. Mita K, Akiyama N, Nagao T, et al: Advantages of mizoribine over azathioprine in combination therapy with cyclosporine for renal transplantation. *Transplant Proc* 22:1679–1681, 1990.

106. Takahashi K, Ota K, Tanabe K, et al: Effect of a novel immunosuppressive agent, deoxyspergualin, on rejection in kidney transplant recipients. *Transplant Proc* 22:1606–1612, 1990.

107. Nishimura K, Tokunaga T: Mechanism of action of 15-deoxyspergualin. I. Suppressive effect on the induction of alloreactive secondary cytotoxic T lymphocytes in vivo and in vitro. *Immunology* 68:66–71, 1989.

108. Ochiai T, Nakajima K, Sakamoto K, et al: Comparative studies on the immunosuppressive activity of FK-506, 15-deoxyspergualin, and cyclosporine. *Transplant Proc* 21:829–832, 1989.

109. Okazaki H, Sato T, Jimbo M, Senga S, Amada N, Oguma S: Prophylactic use of deoxyspergualin in living related renal transplantation. *Transplant Proc* 23:1094–1095, 1991.

110. Koyama I, Amemiya H, Taguchi Y, et al: Prophylactic use of deoxyspergualin in a quadruple immunosuppressive protocol in renal transplantation. *Transplant Proc* 23:1096–1098, 1991.

111. Anderson LW, Strong JM, Cysyk RL: Cellular pharmacology of DUP-785, a new anticancer agent. *Cancer Commun* 1:381–387, 1989.

112. Arteaga CL, Brown TD, Kuhn JG, et al: Phase I clinical and pharmacokinetic trial of brequinar sodium (DuP 785; NSC 368390). *Cancer Res* 49:4648–4653, 1989.

113. Cramer DV, Chapman FA, Jaffee BD, et al: The effect of a new immunosuppressive drug, brequinar sodium, on heart, liver and kidney allograft rejection in the rat. *Transplantation* 53(2):303–308, 1992.

114. Schwartz RH: A cell culture model for T lymphocyte clonal anergy. *Science* 248:1349–1356, 1990.

115. Blackman MA, Gerhard-Burgert H, Woodland DL, Palmer E, Kappler JW, Marrack P: A role for clonal inactivation in T cell tolerance to Mls-1a. *Nature* 345:540–542, 1990.

116. Sachs DH: Antigen-specific transplantation tolerance. *Clin Transplant* 4:78, 1990.

117. Posselt AM, Barker CF, Tomaszewski JE, Markmann JF, Choti MA, Naji A: Induction of donor specific unresponsiveness by intrathymic islet transplantation. *Science* 249:1293–1295, 1990.

118. Faustman D, Coe C: Prevention of xenograft rejection by masking donor HLA class I antigens. *Science* 252:1700–1702, 1991.

119. Ildstad ST, Sachs DH: Reconstitution with syngeneic plus allogeneic or xenogeneic bone marrow leads to specific acceptance of allografts or xenografts. *Nature* 307:168–170, 1984.

120. Ildstad ST, Wren SM, Oh E, Hronakes ML: Mixed allogeneic reconstitution (A+B----A) to induce donor-specific transplantation tolerance. Permanent acceptance of a simultaneous donor skin graft. *Transplantation* 51:1262–1267, 1991.

121. Fanslow WC, Sims JE, Sassenfeld H, et al: Regulation of alloreactivity in vivo by a soluble form of the interleukin-1 receptor. *Science* 248:739–742, 1990.

122. Cosimi AB, Conti D, Delmonico FL, et al: In vivo effects of monoclonal antibody to ICAM-1 (CD54) in nonhuman primates with renal allografts. *J Immunol* 144:4604–4612, 1990.

123. Fischer A, Friedrich W, Fasth A, et al: Reduction of graft failure by a monoclonal antibody (anti-LFA-1 CD11a) after HLA nonidentical bone marrow transplantation in children with immunodeficiencies, osteopetrosis, and Fanconi's anemia: a European Group for Immunodeficiency/European Group for Bone Marrow Transplantation report. *Blood* 77:249–256, 1991.

124. Isobe M, Yagita H, Okumura K, Ihara A: Specific acceptance of cardiac allograft after treatment with antibodies to ICAM-1 and LFA-1. *Science* 255:1025–1027, 1992.

CHAPTER 63

Computer Control of Vasoactive Drug Therapy

LOUIS C. SHEPPARD, PH.D.

THOMAS C. JANNETT, PH.D.

Hypertension following intracardiac operations may be the result of pain, hypothermia, reflex vasoconstriction following cardipulmonary bypass, activation of the renin-angiotensin system, ventilatory difficulties, and recovery from anesthesia. Complications of postoperative hypertension include myocardial ischemia, myocardial infarction, rupture of suture lines, increased bleeding, cerebrovascular accident, and arrhythmia. The fast-acting vasodilator sodium nitroprusside (SNP) is the most frequently used hypotensive agent in postoperative patients. With SNP infusion, the reduction of peripheral vascular resistance, and the resulting reduction in the arterial pressure, has a rapid onset and quickly subsides when the infusion is stopped. Control of arterial pressure with this drug requires frequent adjustment of the infusion rate based on measurement of systolic or mean arterial pressure (MAP). An intraarterial cannula, pressure transducer, and preamplifier system is necessary for reliable pressure measurement. The MAP signal is obtained by low-pass filtering of the arterial pressure signal, thus attenuating the signal variation during the cardiac cycle and recovering the mean, or average, arterial pressure value.

Manual regulation of MAP with hypotensive agents is difficult and time consuming. The drug infusion rate must be adjusted frequently because of spontaneous pressure variations and the changing condition of the patient. Difficulties in control are also encountered because the response of blood pressure to infusion rate changes is delayed, may change with time, and varies among patients. Inadequate adjustments of the SNP infusion rate by clinical personnel often cause poor pressure regulation. In patients in whom pressure regulation is difficult, the nurse must monitor the MAP constantly and make frequent changes in the infusion rate to avoid pressure fluctuations that could be catastrophic. In such situations, the nurse is not free to undertake other tasks, and the quality of blood pressure control may suffer because of the distraction of the nurse in an emergency, or because of the nurse's inexperience.

An automated system for infusing vasodilating agents in postoperative patients is used in the Cardiac Surgical Intensive Care Unit (CICU) of University Hospital at The University of Alabama at Birmingham (1). Automated control of MAP has the following advantages:

1. The benefits of feedback control are provided. These benefits include the control of the blood pressure response to changes in the setpoint, reduction of the effect of spontaneous pressure variations, and reduction of the sensitivity of the system to variations in the patient's response to the drug.
2. Infusion rate adjustments are based on pressure measurements made at a higher frequency than is possible with manual control.
3. A rigid set of rules is applied to calculate the infusion rate adjustments.

AUTOMATED BLOOD PRESSURE CONTROL SYSTEM

Development of the automated blood pressure control system was based on investigation of the dynamics of physiologic

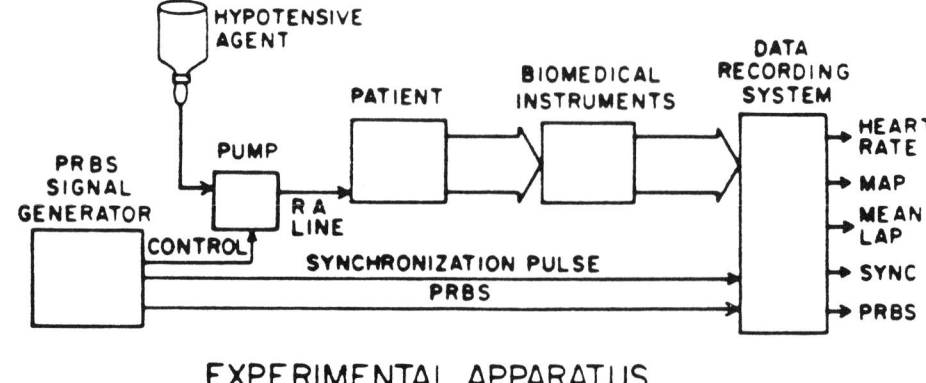

EXPERIMENTAL APPARATUS

Figure 63.1. Equipment arrangement for programming the infusion of the agent and recording the physiologic response. (Reprinted with permission from Sheppard LC: Computer control of the infusion of vasoactive drugs. *Ann Biomed Eng* 8:431, 1980. Copyright 1980, Pergamon Press, Ltd.)

responses of hypertensive patients to SNP. In computer simulations, representative patient responses were used for evaluation of the control algorithm, which determines the change in SNP infusion rate. The control algorithm was tuned further in clinical trials.

DYNAMIC RESPONSE INVESTIGATIONS

Control of a physiologic variable with a pharmacologic agent in the clinical environment requires knowledge of the dynamics of the response produced by drug infusion. The dynamic response characteristics of a linear system are described by its impulse response. The impulse response can be identified by observing the system output response to the application of an appropriate excitation signal, such as pure white noise. The impulse response is similar to the response of a biologic system to the bolus injection of a pharmacologic agent. Overdriving the system with a large input may produce an output that contains undesirable nonlinear components. It is theoretically feasible to obtain an impulse response with a cross-correlation technique, since the cross-correlation function of a white random input signal with the output signal is directly proportional to the impulse response. The advantage of the cross-correlation method is that the system response can be evaluated in the linear range near the operating state without introducing an unacceptably large disturbance.

The cross-correlation method was used to determine the dynamic response of cardiovascular system variables to vasodilating agents. Pseudo-random-binary sequences (PRBS) were used to vary the SNP infusion rate to provide an appropriate input signal for system excitation. This class of periodic signals meets the randomness criteria over the sequence length and is easy to generate by computer programming. Also, conversion of the PRBS to the appropriate system input variable is easily achieved, since there are only two states (off and on).

The dynamic responses of heart rate, MAP, and mean left atrial pressure (LAP) to the infusion of SNP through the right atrium (Fig. 63.1) were investigated. Signals were each digitized at one sample per second and recorded. For analysis, the system was considered to have a single input (SNP infusion rate) and multiple outputs. The input signal was cross-correlated with each output to determine the impulse response of each output variable to the drug infusion

rate. Subjects were selected from postoperative patients who exhibited MAP above 100 mm Hg following an open intracardiac operation. MAP was recorded from a radial artery cannula; LAP was recorded from an intracardiac cannula. Heart rate was determined from recording of the electrocardiogram (ECG).

Impulse responses were serially reproducible for a given patient and exhibited common features among patients. The duration of the impulse responses ranged from 2.0 to 3.5 minutes. The MAP response to drug infusion is delayed by a period that corresponds to one circulation time (20 to 45 seconds), reaches a minimum at 1.2 to 1.9 minutes, and rises as the drug effect dissipates.

CONTROLLER DESIGN AND SIMULATION

For controller evaluation, representative impulse responses were selected to model the patient MAP response to SNP infusion in computer simulations. The impulse response was considered to be a simple exponential for simulation of patient responses. A computer programmed version of a proportional-integral-derivative (PID) controller was selected because the impulse responses were not complicated. The control algorithm was adjusted initially in simulations to provide a simulated patient response with minimal overshoot and acceptable settling time in the reduction of MAP from 120 to a set point of 100 mm Hg. In the control algorithm an error signal (e) was calculated as the difference between the simulated MAP (P) and the setpoint (desired pressure, $P_D = 100$ mm Hg). The error signal was used to calculate the infusion rate required to reduce the error by increasing, holding constant, or decreasing the drug infusion rate in the simulations.

Further tuning of the algorithm was required in the CICU to achieve good controller performance. The following equations and coefficients gave the best clinical performance for the computerized controller:

$$e = P_D - P$$
$$A = (0.4512)e + (0.4512)(e - e')$$
$$\Delta I = KA$$
$$I = I' + \Delta I$$

where P_D is the desired pressure; P is the mean arterial pressure; e is the current error, $P_D - P$; e' is the previous error,

1 minute earlier; *A* is the calculated pressure change required; *I* is new infusion rate; *I'* is the present rate, initiated 1 minute earlier; ΔI is the incremental infusion rate; and *K* is the controller gain. P_D, *P*, *e*, *e'*, and *A* are measured in millimeters of mercury; *I*, *I'* and ΔI are measured in milliliters per hour; and *K* is measured in milliliters per hour per millimeter of mercury.

The measured MAP is filtered digitally by taking a six-point average of samples acquired at 1-second intervals to reduce disturbances produced by respiration. In the control algorithm, an incremental infusion rate change is calculated from proportional and derivative error terms where the first difference of the error signal approximates its derivative. The proportional component in the control algorithm is needed to increase the infusion rate in proportion to the degree of MAP elevation above the set point. Derivative control assists in reducing overshoot by taking into account the rate at which MAP is approaching the target value. This incremental action is multiplied by the overall controller gain and is then integrated to determine the infusion rate.

To minimize pharmacologic intervention, rules have been applied that bias the algorithm to minimize the infusion rate and the total amount of drug infused. Intentional nonlinearities are introduced into the calculation of the incremental infusion rate change using a decision table (Table 63.1). These rules were developed to improve the transient response of the PID controller and for patient safety.

The incremental infusion rate per unit of pressure correction (*K*, in milliliters per hour per millimeter of mercury) depends on the measured MAP (*P*). This gain scheduling (rules 1–4) reduces overshoot, improves the speed of response, and biases the controller to turn off the infusion if pressure is persistently below the set point. Infusion rate increases are limited to +7 ml/hr (rule 5), but infusion rate decreases are not constrained. To reduce overshoot, the increment is reduced (−2 ml/hr) if the MAP is above the set point by 5 mm Hg more than (rule 6) during the transient control phase. If MAP is more than 5 mm Hg below the set point, infusion is not allowed to increase (rule 7). Also, the infusion rate is limited to prevent negative infusion rates and to avoid exceeding the maximum recommended dose rate (10 μg/kg/min). All rules are evaluated each minute.

IMED Corporation, San Diego, California, developed a pump (IMED 929) that is digitally controlled by the authors' computer system (Hewlett-Packard 21MX). The eight infusion pumps in the unit accept numerically coded information (RS-232, serial, asynchronous, ASCII) that specifies infusion rates from 0 to 399 ml/hr in 1 ml/hr increments. The infusion rates for each patient are calculated at 1-minute intervals using the control algorithm. The incremental infusion rate adjustment is summed with the previous rate to calculate a new infusion rate that is transmitted to each pump in turn. A schematic diagram of the control loop is shown in Figure 63.2.

DISCUSSION

The automated blood pressure control system is used in the CICU to treat patients with high arterial blood pressure or high afterload (which impairs the pumping ability of the heart). Automated control may be started when the patient is moved to the intensive care unit if SNP infusion is begun in the operating room. MAP above 100 to 110 mm Hg is usually treated, and the pressure is usually maintained at a level between 75 and 110 mm Hg. Automated control of MAP exhibits approximately half the variation observed during manual control; MAP measurements are more tightly distributed about the mean (Fig. 63.3).

The incidence of transient MAP variations caused by patient care procedures is minimized by affixing a label to the pressure transducer mount at the bedside inform clinical personnel that the patient is on "computer nipride." Also, a label is placed on the patient's arm adjacent to the stopcock attached to the radial artery cannula. Clinical personnel temporarily interrupt automatic control when arterial blood samples are withdrawn for cardiac output measurements and blood gases. The computer system is directed to maintain a constant rate of SNP infusion during any event likely to disturb the MAP measurement. Since short-lived transients induced by patient care procedures or by patient movement may sometimes bring about higher or lower infusion rates than are necessary, the stability of blood pressure regulation must be observed by the bedside nurse or physician to ensure the selection of an appropriate constant infusion rate.

The use of computer-controlled drug infusion requires implementation of highly structured, complete, and explicit operating procedures that are rigidly enforced. Strict adherence to these rules is necessary to avoid operator error and to prevent negligent use of devices and systems. Training and experience are required to avoid erratic performance and to prevent system malfunctions. Clinical personnel must monitor system performance to detect malfunctions and to take corrective actions. Safeguards are employed to minimize the severity of operator errors.

The infusion pumps are equipped with air embolism detectors and empty reservoir alarms that signal malfunctions to personnel and to the computer. Two steps are required for the nurse to modify the desired pressure (P_D). First, the new value is entered by means of a bedside computer terminal. The newly entered value must then be verified by the entry

Table 63.1. Decision Table for Controller Gain and Infusion Rate Increment

Criteria	Rules						
	1	*2*	*3*	*4*	*5*	*6*	*7*
$P>P_D+5$	+					+	
$P\leq P_D+5$		+					
$P>P_D$		+			+		
$P\leq P_D$			+				
$P\geq P_D-5$			+				
$P<P_D-5$				+			+
$\Delta I>7$					+		
$\Delta I>0$							+
Action							
1 $K=-1$	1						
2 $K=-0.5$		2					
3 $K=-1$			3				
4 $K=-2$				4			
5 $\Delta I=7$					5		
6 $\Delta I=\Delta I-2$						6	
7 $\Delta I=0$							7

Figure 63.2. Schematic diagram of the control loop. (Reprinted with permission from Sheppard LC: Computer control of the infusion of vasoactive drugs. *Ann Biomed Eng* 8:431, 1980. Copyright 1980, Pergamon Press, Ltd.)

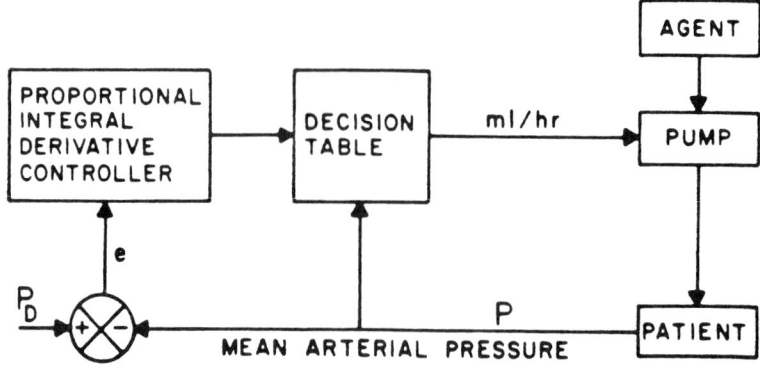

Figure 63.3. Regulation of MAP with automatic control of SNP infusion. (Reprinted with permission from Sheppard LC: Computer control of the infusion of vasoactive drugs. *Ann Biomed Eng* 8:431, 1980. Copyright 1980, Pergamon Press, Ltd.)

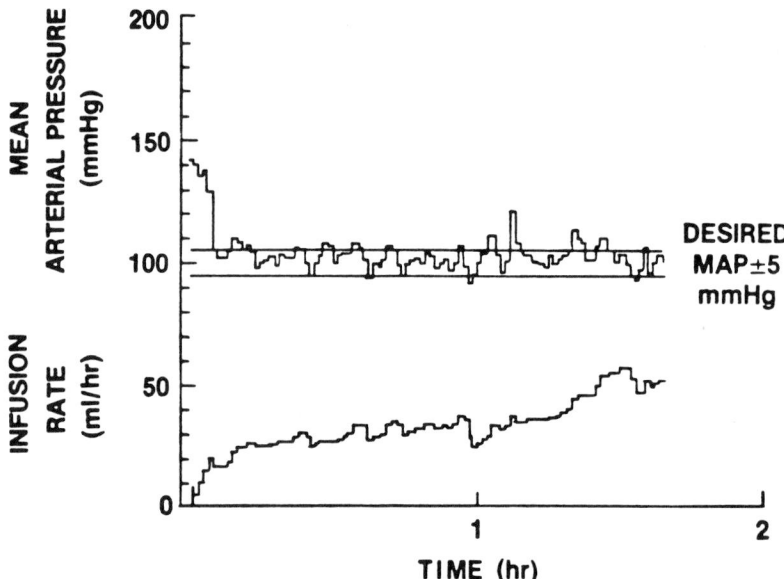

of a code before the current set point is replaced. Extremely high or low pressure measurements are identified as invalid; the infusion rate is not adjusted during that minute. The computer stops the infusion of SNP if two very low pressure measurements occur in succession.

The system can be used to control the MAP of six patients simultaneously, but the requirement seldom exceeds three patients during a 24-hour period. Typically, two or three patients are hypertensive upon arrival in the CICU or become so during the early hours following operation. The infusion of a hypotensive agent is discontinued after 12 to 24 hours of treatment in most patients.

FACTORS THAT MAY AFFECT CONTROLLER PERFORMANCE

Controller performance is influenced by several factors (Table 63.2). Time is required for the circulation to carry the agent from the infusion site to the vascular receptors, which may be located an appreciable distance away. The authors use a right atrial cannula for SNP infusion; if infusion is more

Table 63.2. Factors That May Affect Controller Performance

Infusion site
Background variation
Variable sensitivity to SNP
Reflex responses
Blood volume
Arrhythmias

peripheral, controller performance may be degraded by the additional transport delay.

Fluctuations in MAP measurements that are not attributable to drug infusion have been observed. Variations in the background pressure may be the result of spontaneous fluctuations in sympathetic nervous system activity. During routine patient care, a number of maneuvers introduce short-lived variations in the MAP. Many of these variations are directly attributable to activities such as suctioning of the endotracheal tube, bathing, chest film plate placement and withdrawal, flushing of the arterial line, administration of pain medication, extubation, and the ventilatory cycle. Nausea, restlessness, shivering, pain, and anxiety are other factors that may introduce more prolonged pressure changes. The conservative rules and limits applied to the control action tend to reduce the impact of MAP variations.

Sensitivity to SNP may vary over a 30-to-1 range among patients; the sensitivity of an individual patient may also change with time. Since SNP is photosensitive, it may appear that the patient is becoming less responsive to SNP as the drug deteriorates over a few hours.

Lowering the blood pressure may trigger reflex responses that cause changes in the background pressure; slow drifts and pressure oscillations exhibiting periods from 1 to 8 minutes have been observed (2). The reflex response model has assisted in interpreting certain clinically observed responses. Lowering the blood pressure may trigger reflex responses with relatively long time constants such as increased renal secretion of renin. For example, the requirement for a gradually increasing infusion rate for maintenance of a desired arterial pressure, which previously was not understood, is now attributed to this reflex response. Also, the patient's endogenous neurohumoral control system, which may be severely disturbed following open-heart surgery, causes pressure fluctuations and oscillations. Other reflex responses appear to be of neurohumoral origin (endogenous epinephrine and norepinephrine).

The main effect of SNP is the reduction of arteriolar resistance through the relaxation of vascular smooth muscle. However, venous capacitance is also increased. If this results in a sufficient pooling of blood, venous return and cardiac output may be reduced as ventricular filling pressure is lowered (Frank-Starling mechanism).

Cardiac arrhythmias, particularly atrial flutter and tachycardia, may cause disturbances in the MAP that degrade the performance of both manual and automatic control.

RESEARCH

Clinical experiences with the controller indicate that system performance needs improvement for patients who are relatively sensitive or insensitive to SNP and for patients whose blood pressure exhibits large fluctuations. To facilitate the design of an improved control algorithm, Slate formulated a mathematical model to represent the essential aspects of the MAP and its response to the infusion of SNP (3). The design of an adaptive controller that provides robust performance has been the topic of significant research. With adaptive control, the control algorithm adapts to individual patients to provide improved performance.

MODELING

Slate used physiologic and pharmacologic concepts in structuring model input-output relationships from patient data (3). The MAP is considered to be the sum of a background pressure (P_{ba}) and a change in the pressure resulting from drug infusion (ΔP_d), which is related to the drug infusion rate (*I*) by a linear transfer function ($G_d(s)$) (Fig. 63.4). The transfer function was derived from impulse response data obtained

using cross-correlation analysis in Sheppard's dynamic response investigations (1). A first-order transfer function provides an adequate and parsimonious representation of the human MAP response to SNP infusion:

$$G_d(s) = \frac{\Delta P_d(s)}{I(s)} = \frac{Ke^{-T_i s}(1 + \alpha e^{-T_c s})}{(1 + \tau s)}$$

The gain *K* represents the patient's sensitivity to the drug (in millimeters of mercury per milliliter per hour), while α is the recirculating fraction ($\alpha = 0.4$). The lag with time constant $\tau = 50$ s represents the uptake, distribution, and metabolism of the drug. The time delays represent the delay in response caused by transport of the drug from the infusion site ($T_i = 30$ seconds) and the recirculation time ($T_c = 45$ seconds).

The background pressure consists of a constant term, a low-amplitude sinusoid that represents activity caused by respiration or ventilation, stochastic activity, and a component representing the neurohumoral reflex response to a reduction in pressure. Other disturbances, including those associated with changes in the condition of the patient or procedures related to patient care, can be modeled approximately as step, ramp, or pulse changes in the background activity. The stochastic activity is modeled as the output of a second-order filter with a corner frequency corresponding to a period of 30 seconds and a broadband random noise input. The renin-angiotensin reflex response is modeled as a one-sided dead zone with saturation followed by a first-order lag. The effect of this model of renin-angiotensin reflex response is to increase the background pressure level when the MAP drops below a threshold value.

ADAPTIVE BLOOD PRESSURE CONTROL

Adaptation of the control algorithm allows variations in the patient's sensitivity to SNP to be accommodated. Slate used the model (Fig. 63.4) to design a controller in which an adaptive mechanism adjusts controller parameters based on the estimated sensitivity of a patient to the drug. Adaptation is performed during an initial 15-minute control period. Controller parameters are fixed after the adaptation period, which may be repeated if necessary. Improved performance of this adaptive controller was demonstrated in simulations, dog experiments, and clinical trials.

Other adaptive control methods have been investigated (4–7). If parameter values in an appropriate model of the patient are known, the control algorithm can be designed to optimize a performance index in which factors such as the control performance (pressure variance) and the cost of control (variance of the drug infusion rate) are weighed (8, 9). Such controllers usually are used in conjunction with on-line parameter estimation to form adaptive control algorithms, because the performance index is optimized only if accurate model parameter values are used to calculate the optimal control.

Although many adaptive blood pressure control systems have been tested in the laboratory, there have been few clinical applications. For the design of a clinically useful system, patient care practices and other aspects of the clinical environment must be considered. Stable operation of the adaptive

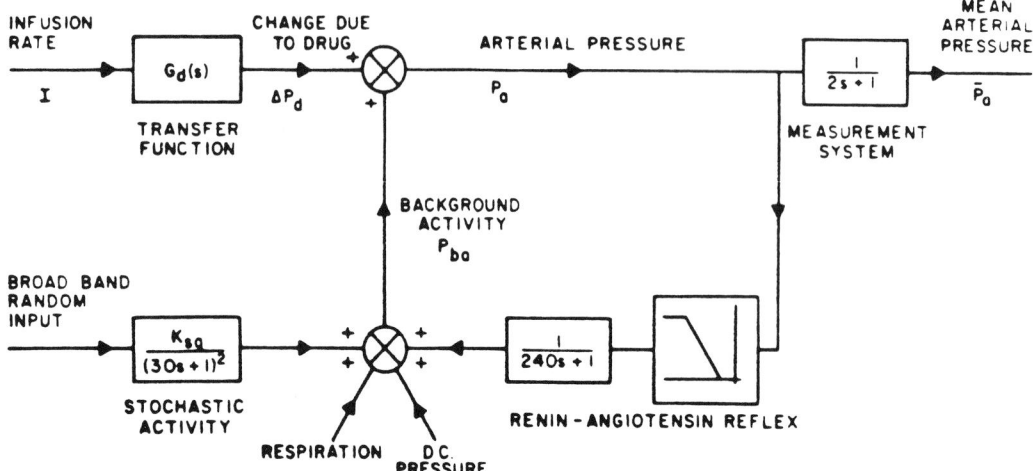

Figure 63.4.   Model of MAP and its response to SNP infusion. (Reprinted with permission from Sheppard LC: Computer control of the infusion of vasoactive drugs. *Ann Biomed Eng* 8:431, 1980. Copyright 1980, Pergamon Press, Ltd.)

controller must be ensured by the use of supervisory algorithms (3, 7).

OTHER CLINICAL EXPERIENCE

A computerized bedside system for automated delivery of SNP has been developed and clinically tested at the Mount Sinai Medical Center in New York City (4). The control algorithm is based on the work of Sheppard (1) and Slate (3). The system was used to investigate the hypothesis that automated control of SNP infusion is superior to manual control. In a group of 37 patients managed with manual control, the measured MAP was within 5 mm Hg of the desired MAP only 52% of the time; in a group of 49 patients managed by computer control, the measured MAP was within the prescribed range 94% of the time.

The use of automated SNP infusion for blood pressure control in medical emergencies has also been investigated (10). The algorithm for blood pressure control reflects a series of decision pathways that is based on clinical experience. Potentially dangerous blood pressure levels are reduced in a stepwise and predictable fashion, and long-term regulation is achieved.

CONCLUSION

The rapid and powerful action of SNP makes frequent monitoring of MAP followed by appropriate adjustment of the infusion rate necessary for MAP regulation. Because of many other nursing duties, there may not be sufficient time

available for achieving good control manually (11). Automated blood pressure control has been used at The University of Alabama at Birmingham to provide minute-by-minute monitoring and control of MAP in several thousand patients for more than 10 years. The automated controller performs satisfactorily over a wide range of conditions and is operated by personnel without knowledge of control theory. The success of the system is attributed to the fact that it was designed to reduce the workload in the clinical environment.

REFERENCES

1. Sheppard LC: Computer control of the infusion of vasoactive drugs. *Ann Biomed Eng* 8:431, 1980.
2. Slate JB, Sheppard LC: Automatic control of blood pressure by drug infusion. *IEE Proc* 129:639, 1982.
3. Slate JB: Model-based design of a controller for infusing sodium nitroprusside during postsurgical hypertension. Ph.D. thesis, University of Wisconsin, Madison, 1980.
4. de Asla RA, Benis AM, Jurado RA, et al: Management of postcardiotomy hypertension by microcomputer-controlled administration of sodium nitroprusside. *Thorac Cardiovasc Surg* 89:115, 1985.
5. He WG, Kaufman H, Roy R: Multiple model adaptive control procedure for blood pressure control. *IEEE Trans Biomed Eng* 33:10, 1986.
6. Kaufman H, Roy R, Xu X: Model reference adaptive control of drug infusion rate. *Automatica* 20:205, 1984.
7. Stern KS, Chizeck HJ, Walker BK et al: The self-tuning controller: comparison with human performance in the control of arterial pressure. *Ann Biomed Eng* 813:341, 1985.
8. Arnsparger JM, McInnis BC, Glover JR, et al: Adaptive control of blood pressure. *IEEE Trans Biomed Eng* 30:168, 1983.
9. Meline LJ, Westenskow DR, Pace NL, et al: Computer-controlled regulation of sodium nitroprusside infusion. *Anesth Analog* 64:38, 1985.
10. Hammond JJ, Kirkendall WM, Calfee RV: Hypertensive crisis management by computer controlled infusion of sodium nitroprusside: a model for the closed loop administration of short acting vasoactive agents. *Comput Biomed Res* 12:97, 1979.
11. Mitchell RM: The need for closed-loop therapy. *Crit Care Med* 10:831, 1982.

CHAPTER 64

Special Pediatric Problems

CURT M. STEINHART, M.D.

Developments in the care of critically ill infants and children have proceeded apace with those in adults. Unique clinical situations that present in the pediatric intensive care unit (PICU) are often handled differently in the young patient than in the adult. Examples covered in this chapter include status asthmaticus, status epilepticus, supraventricular tachycardia, sedation, and neuromuscular blockade. Respiratory conditions commonly seen in PICUs, including respiratory syncytial virus infections and croup syndromes, are virtually unknown in adult ICUs. Special considerations for their management are included. Three of the most common toxicologic causes for PICU admission (clonidine overdose, iron intoxication, and organophosphate poisoning) are presented because of their unique pharmacotherapy. In addition, the special role of maintaining patency of the ductus arteriosus using prostaglandin E_1 is discussed. These issues provide special challenges to caregivers in the PICU.

TREATMENT OF STATUS ASTHMATICUS

Although most children with status asthmaticus respond adequately to some combination of inhaled β-adrenergic receptor agonists, intravenous aminophylline, parenteral epinephrine, and corticosteroid administration, a small percentage develop respiratory failure and require admission to a pediatric ICU. Unlike most other lower airway causes of respiratory failure, status asthmaticus in children often is treated successfully without the need for endotracheal intubation and mechanical ventilation (1–3). Several methods, including isoproterenol by continuous intravenous infusion (4, 5), terbutaline by continuous infusion (6), and continuous inhalation of β-agonists (7, 8) have been utilized in children in an effort to avoid intubation.

Because of concerns about isoproterenol-induced tachycardia (2, 3, 9), myocardial oxygen supply and demand (10), and a previous report of myonecrosis (11), isoproterenol infusion therapy is employed more frequently for children and adolescents (1–5) than for adults (9). In pediatric patients with severe hypercarbia (arterial PCO_2 ≥55 torr (≥7.3 kPa) and/or hypoxemia, defined as arterial PO_2 ≤60 torr (≤8.0 kPa) on 60% FIO_2), continuously infused isoproterenol reverses respiratory failure without the need for mechanical ventilation in up to 85% of cases (1, 3, 5).

For administration, isoproterenol hydrochloride is diluted in 5% dextrose or dextrose 5% in 0.2 normal saline ($D_5.2NS$). The number of milligrams of isoproterenol to be diluted to 100 ml is equal to the child's weight in kilograms multiplied by 0.15. When a microdrip infusion pump is used, an initial rate of 2.0 ml/hr gives 0.05 μg/kg/min. Incremental increases in the rate of infusion of 1.0 ml/hr increase the amount infused by 0.025 μg/kg/min. The dilution and adjustment of infusion rate allow for very careful titration to the desired effect. The use of infused isoproterenol requires monitoring of the electrocardiogram (ECG), heart rate, and respiratory rate. An indwelling arterial catheter is required for continuous blood pressure measurement and also allows for frequent arterial blood gas determinations. Fluid intake and output also should be monitored carefully. The isoproterenol infusion rate is increased every 15 to 30 minutes until (*a*) the PaCO$_2$ is ≤45 torr (≤6.0 kPa), (*b*) the heart rate becomes excessive (≥200 beats/min for infants and small children; ≥180 for older children and adolescents), or (*c*) other evidence of toxicity (usually a dysrhythmia) is noted. Dose requirements usually range from 0.20 to 0.50 μg/kg/min (1, 3), but infusion rates greater than 1.0 μg/kg/min have been administered successfully without untoward occurrences (5).

Because isoproterenol has a very short plasma half-life (12), a continuous infusion is necessary to maintain effective plasma drug levels. On the other hand, dose-related toxic effects are readily controlled. Tachycardia is the most common side effect. Concomitant use of aminophylline and the presence of relative dehydration, respiratory distress, and anxiety may compound the increased chronotropy inherent with isoproterenol. Isoproterenol-induced increases in heart rate of 10 to 20 beats/min should be anticipated; however, in some cases relief of respiratory distress and anxiety after initiating isoproterenol infusion causes the heart rate to decrease. Aminophylline administration, usually as a continuous infusion, should be continued during isoproterenol therapy. Theophylline clearance increases when the drug is administered with isoproterenol (13). Therefore, in isoproterenol-treated patients, adjustments in aminophylline infusion rates should be based on frequent serum theophylline determinations. Caution is required when using β-agonists with aminophylline, based upon evidence for increased myocardial toxicity with this combination (14). It is prudent to achieve low therapeutic serum theophylline levels (10 to 15 μg/ml) when using isoproterenol.

Reports of both myocardial ischemia (15) and myonecrosis (11) indicate potentially dangerous cardiovascular consequences from isoproterenol infusion. As a nonselective β-adrenergic receptor agonist with marked inotropic and chronotropic activity, isoproterenol increases myocardial oxygen consumption that, in the presence of hypoxemia, may potentiate myocardial cell injury. Continuous ECG recording and frequent careful bedside evaluation should provide detection of overt toxicity in most instances. A daily 12-lead ECG and determination of myocardial creatine kinase (CPK-MB) concentrations are advocated by some authors to assist in this assessment (2, 5).

Because isoproterenol-induced pulmonary arteriolar dilation may occur before bronchial dilation, intrapulmonary shunting may increase. The resultant worsening of hypoxemia can be extremely troublesome but is usually transient. Frequent assessment of the arterial PO$_2$ in the first several hours after initiating isoproterenol therapy, aided by continuous pulse oximetry and coupled with additional supplemental oxygen via face mask, provides ample monitoring and therapy for this circumstance.

When an effective isoproterenol infusion rate is achieved, that rate should be continued for 24 hours unless complications occur. Subsequently, the infusion rate is reduced slowly over 24 to 48 hours with careful, repeated evaluation of clinical status and arterial blood gases.

Should respiratory failure persist or worsen despite the isoproterenol infusion, the infusion is continued during mechanical ventilation in a persistent effort to control bronchospasm.

This approach may allow for a shorter ventilator time and improve chances for successful endotracheal extubation.

In an effort to avoid some of the complications inherent in isoproterenol administration, the use of terbutaline by continuous infusion has been advocated (6). The relative β-2-selectivity of this agent theoretically makes it less toxic than isoproterenol and may minimize many of the undesirable cardiac effects of isoproterenol.

For administration, 2.0 μg/kg terbutaline should be given over 5 minutes followed by a continuous infusion of 4.5 μg/kg/hr. This regimen appears to allow maximum bronchodilation with the fewest side effects. Larger doses do not appear to offer any additional benefit. Even at this dosing level, tremors and mild tachycardia are often noted. Systolic blood pressure tends to increase, while the diastolic blood pressure decreases. Headache has also been noted. In patients receiving both aminophylline and terbutaline, a lower constant infusion rate of 2.25 μg/kg/hr is recommended.

Recently, the author and colleagues have used β-agonists by continuous inhalation. The rationale for this approach is somewhat empirical, but frequent observations that asthmatic children fare better during periods of β-agonist inhalation than between hourly doses suggest that continuous therapy might prove beneficial (unpublished observations). The author's findings have been substantiated by others (7, 8). Hence, it is recommended that continuous inhalation therapy using albuterol precede endotracheal intubation and mechanical ventilation if patient acceptance will allow.

Delivery of continuous inhalation β-agonists should be via jet nebulization. Doses of 0.15 to 0.30 mg/kg (0.03 to 0.06 ml/kg of the 5 mg/ml albuterol solution) are diluted in 4 to 8 ml normal saline such that the resulting volume is fully nebulized every hour. Albuterol by continuous jet nebulization is continued for several hours after clinical improvement is noted. Once a satisfactory response is sustained for 4 to 6 hours, conventional intermittent therapy can then be used.

STATUS EPILEPTICUS IN CHILDREN

Status epilepticus may be defined as seizures that last more than 30 minutes or recur so frequently during a given period as to be nearly continuous. Prolonged seizures in children may result from infection, drug ingestions, trauma, tumors, hypoxia, cerebral ischemia, metabolic derangements, fever, and uncertain (idiopathic) causes. A variety of effective anticonvulsant medications are currently available; however, no single method of treatment for status epilepticus has emerged. Moreover, dosage and drug-interactions warrant careful attention.

Seizures from metabolic causes (e.g., from hypoglycemia, hypocalcemia, or hyponatremia) are usually resistant to anticonvulsants and require correction of the metabolic abnormality. Proper diagnosis by blood chemistry analysis is essential in order to manage such seizures suitably.

For status epilepticus resulting from causes other than metabolic derangements, diazepam (0.1 to 0.2 mg/kg, via slow intravenous push) has become the mainstay for acute convulsive states in both children and adults (16–21). Its ready availability in nearly all emergency rooms and intensive care units, and its rapid onset of action (often less than 1 minute) makes it a nearly ideal and effective agent. Diazepam, however, has several properties that necessitate cautious use in pediatric patients. It has a relatively short anticonvulsant duration of action (20 to 30 minutes), but it may have a more prolonged effect on respiratory activity (22). For those reasons, repeated administration is often necessary to maintain seizure control but may result in cumulative respiratory depressant effects. Rectal administration of the intravenous preparation in doses of 0.5 mg/kg has also been shown to be effective (23).

A common approach is to stop the acute convulsions with diazepam and then initiate treatment with a longer-acting preparation. Phenobarbital administration following diazepam therapy results in such potent respiratory depression that their concomitant use is not advised. Providing initial anticonvulsant therapy with phenobarbital alone is safer than using it after diazepam (19, 21, 24). Children who are not receiving chronic therapy should receive an initial intravenous dose of phenobarbital of 10 mg/kg over 1 to 2 minutes. Seizures may take 5 minutes or longer to abate; therefore, careful observation of the airway and the cardiovascular system are needed while convulsions persist. Subsequently, phenobarbital doses of 5 mg/kg (maximum 20 to 30 mg/kg) are given every 5 to 15 minutes until the seizures cease. The decision to administer further therapy should be governed by serum phenobarbital levels.

The use of phenobarbital therapy after diazepam should be undertaken only when facilities and personnel can rapidly provide endotracheal intubation and subsequent ventilatory support. Numerous cases of respiratory arrest following combination therapy with diazepam and phenobarbital have been observed. Conversely, if the airway has been secured via endotracheal intubation, early use of diazepam to halt the convulsions and subsequent use of phenobarbital for maintenance therapy are appropriate.

Phenytoin is an excellent agent for use in status epilepticus (19, 20, 25). In combination with diazepam, it provides long-acting anticonvulsant activity without the respiratory depressant synergism seen with phenobarbital. It may also be used as the initial agent. A first phenytoin dose of 10 mg/kg (maximum 500 mg) is given slowly (over 10 minutes) intravenously. Subsequent doses of 5 mg/kg to a total of 20 to 25 mg/kg result in therapeutic serum levels of 10 to 25 μg/ml. If the initial dose of phenytoin stops the seizures, the remainder of the total dose should be given over 12 to 18 hours in order to reach therapeutic levels needed for chronic therapy.

To avoid potential phenytoin toxicity and to avert respiratory depression created when using phenobarbital (with or without diazepam), some clinicians use lorazepam for status epilepticus in children (26). Lorazepam has a relatively rapid onset (usually less than 3 minutes), a longer duration of action (2 to 4 hours) than that of diazepam, and less respiratory depressant activity than diazepam (27). An initial lorazepam dose of 0.05 to 0.10 mg/kg via slow intravenous push is usually effective, but subsequent similar doses every 15 minutes may be necessary in more refractory states. A maximum of three doses of lorazepam has been recommended. Anticonvulsant activity lasted more than 3 hours in 83% and more than 24 hours in 50% of the children in one study (26), with no adverse systemic or local effects. Maintenance therapy with phenobarbital or phenytoin following lorazepam administration appears

to be safe (26). Flunitrazepam has been used effectively for acute status epilepticus in Japan, but this agent is not yet available for routine use in the U.S. (28, 29).

For cases that are refractory to a combination of agents, diazepam by continuous infusion is usually effective but is used only after endotracheal intubation. Diazepam should be diluted in normal saline and administered through a large peripheral or central vein at a rate of 0.2 mg/kg/hr and titrated to achieve total seizure control. Cardiovascular depression may be noted with diazepam infusion, and inotropic support may be required.

RIBAVIRIN FOR RESPIRATORY SYNCYTIAL VIRUS

Respiratory syncytial virus (RSV) is a common respiratory pathogen in infants and young children and may be particularly troublesome in infants with underlying pulmonary or cardiovascular disease. This RNA virus causes epidemic bronchiolitis and pneumonia during yearly outbreaks (30–32). Following infection, immunity is only short-term, and no effective immunization is currently available (33, 34).

Ribavirin (1-α-D-ribofuranosyl-1,2,4-triazole-3-carboxamide), a synthetic nucleoside analog, possesses activity against several different viruses, apparently through RNA synthesis inhibition (35). It may also act by interfering with the expression of viral messenger RNA without becoming incorporated into host cell RNA or DNA. The drug was approved in 1985 by the Food and Drug Administration (FDA) in aerosol form only for respiratory infections caused by RSV. It has been administered safely to both previously well infants (31, 36) and to those patients with underlying cardiopulmonary disorders (37, 38), such as bronchopulmonary dysplasia and congenital heart diseases. Rapid diagnostic testing for RSV antigen utilizing fluorescent antibodies or enzyme immunoassay makes it possible to select patients for treatment.

Ribavirin is administered using a Collison generator to create an aerosol with a mass median diameter of 1.3 to 1.4 μm. The contents of the 6-g vial are diluted in 300 ml of sterile water and placed in a reservoir so that the solution then has a concentration of 20 mg/ml. The generator flow is adjusted to 12 to 14 liters/min and is delivered into an oxygen hood. No exact administered dosage has been determined, as this dose depends upon the patient's minute ventilation, although delivery over 18 to 21 hr/day has been recommended (31, 33). Concerns about exposure of health care workers and family members to potential teratogenic effects of ribavirin have led many centers to design and utilize special scavenging equipment and isolation techniques (39). In addition, high-dose, short-duration therapy appears to be safe (40) and can minimize nonpatient exposure.

Respiratory failure, endotracheal intubation, and mechanical ventilation do not preclude the use of ribavirin despite FDA-required product labeling, which states that therapy during mechanical ventilation is contraindicated. That warning is related to the hygroscopic nature of the drug that, when aerosolized, may deposit onto ventilator circuit tubing and the endotracheal tube. With careful monitoring and strong technical support from respiratory therapists, complications from ribavirin during mechanical ventilation can be reduced and even eliminated (41). It is crucial that aerosol flow from the Collison generator be connected to the inspiratory limb of the ventilator circuit as close to the endotracheal tube as is feasible. One-way valves between the generator and the inspiratory limb and between the humidifier and the patient aid in delivery of ribavirin without causing drug deposition into the ventilator or the circuitry. Ventilator gas flow should be well-humidified and warmed to at least 34°C. Filters should be placed on the expiratory limb of the ventilator circuit and all filters and valves must be changed frequently (every 2 to 4 hours) to avoid residue accumulation that can result in increased peak inspiratory pressure and inadvertent positive end-expiratory pressure (PEEP). Both the aerosol generator flow rate and the ventilator gas flow rate must be adjusted at frequent intervals so that most of the 300 ml of ribavirin solution is delivered from the reservoir during an 18 to 24 hour period. Close monitoring of peak inspiratory pressure and PEEP is essential, and continuous pulse oximetry or frequent measurement of arterial blood gases is important when ribavirin is given to patients requiring mechanical ventilation to ensure adequate ventilation and oxygenation.

Toxicity studies of ribavirin have shown no consistent patterns (31, 36). Minor variations in hematologic values and serum chemistries have been transient and trivial. No long-term untoward effects have yet been found. Treatment usually lasts for 3 to 5 days, but long-term therapy has been undertaken in an infant with an immunodeficiency (42).

Recommendations regarding indications for treatment are still evolving; however, recent recommendations (43) regarding candidates for ribavirin therapy include infants at high risk for severe or complicated RSV infection and infants who are already severely ill because of RSV lower respiratory tract disease. RSV often causes only mild upper respiratory tract symptoms, but lower respiratory tract disease may require hospital admission. During epidemics, it has been recommended that all hospitalized infants with a clinical presentation strongly suggesting RSV infection should receive ribavirin prior to laboratory confirmation (33, 44). Where diagnostic studies for RSV can be done without delays, it may be prudent to withhold treatment pending laboratory diagnosis. In those patients with underlying cardiac or pulmonary disease, therapy has been advocated even without diagnostic certainty. Numerous questions still remain regarding the actual efficacy and safety of ribavirin (45, 46).

SUPRAVENTRICULAR TACHYCARDIA IN CHILDREN

Supraventricular tachycardia (SVT) in infants and children can occur as a single episode or as a chronic condition (47–49). It may result from drug ingestion (50) or infection (51), as well as from an abnormal cardiac conduction pathway, both in the presence and absence of congenital heart disease (47–49, 52). Although often presenting with nonspecific symptoms (poor weight gain, poor appetite), SVT may also present as an acute, life-threatening emergency requiring admission to the PICU (53, 54). Whereas verapamil has become the treatment of choice for SVT in adults (55), controversy continues as to the proper management of SVT in pediatric patients (47, 52–54, 56–59). Careful consideration of the patient's age,

hemodynamic status, and underlying cardiac disorder is required for optimal results.

The primary consideration at the time of initial evaluation should be the hemodynamic and respiratory status of the patient. If respiratory distress is present, endotracheal intubation should be considered as the initial step. In the presence of hypotension, poor perfusion, or other evidence of a decreased cardiac output, continuous ECG and blood pressure monitoring are required. Immediate direct current (DC) cardioversion, at 0.2 to 0.5 watt-sec/kg, should be tried and repeated if necessary. Cardioversion does not preclude early attempts at vagal stimulation (carotid massage, gag reflex, Valsalva maneuver), but repeated efforts to induce vagal slowing in the hemodynamically compromised patient are discouraged.

In many pediatric centers, intravenous adenosine has become the agent of choice for SVT (59–61). This short-acting purine nucleoside is extremely effective in SVT involving the AV node whether due to overt preexcitation or due to dual pathway reentry tachycardia. Dosing should be initiated at 0.05 mg/kg (50 μg/kg) as a rapid intravenous bolus. Flushing the intravenous catheter with saline solution should be performed immediately after adenosine administration to ensure rapid delivery of the agent. Success may be noted in as few as 6 seconds. Should SVT be reinitiated, the dose may be repeated as often as necessary. If no results are obtained at 0.05 mg/kg, the dose may be increased in increments of 0.05 mg/kg until a maximum dose of 0.25 mg/kg is reached.

Side effects with adenosine are minimal and transient (flushing, dyspnea, bradydysrhythmias) because of its very short half-life of less than 10 seconds. Once SVT has been ablated, specific antidysrhythmic therapy can be started as indicated. Adenosine has been very helpful in elucidating the nature of certain tachydysrhythmias, making long-term therapy easier to gauge (61).

The role of rapid digitalization in children with SVT has become even more controversial. In the presence of ventricular tachycardia (which is often difficult to distinguish from SVT), digoxin may produce ventricular fibrillation. In addition, extreme caution must be exercised when using DC cardioversion once digoxin has been administered. With the availability of adenosine, digoxin should be reserved for selected situations wherein adenosine has aborted the SVT and long-term therapy is required. A total digitalizing dose of 20 to 40 μg/kg is used, with one-fourth to one-half given as the first dose over 1 to 2 minutes; the remainder is prescribed as two or three equal doses given 6 to 8 hours apart.

When the patient is hemodynamically stable, verapamil hydrochloride in small doses successfully converts up to 93% of pediatric patients with acute SVT to sinus rhythm or sinus tachycardia (54). Continuous ECG and blood pressure monitoring are required during verapamil administration (0.1 mg/kg), which should be infused intravenously over 30 to 60 seconds. When this method is successful, the rhythm often reverts to normal sinus rhythm or sinus tachycardia within 1 to 3 minutes. If needed, verapamil may be repeated at 15-minute intervals for a total of three doses (0.3 mg/kg total dose). Calcium chloride (10%) at 10 mg/kg must be available and administered if sudden hypotension or asystole occurs as a result of the verapamil infusion. Atropine sulfate (0.01 mg/kg, minimum 0.1 mg) may be useful if problematic bradycardia develops. However, should SVT return, the rate may be more rapid than previously noted. Since verapamil may cause peripheral vasodilation, volume expansion with normal saline or lactated Ringer's solution (10 ml/kg) may be required. Decreased inotropic activity caused by verapamil can be counteracted by dopamine or epinephrine infusion, but recurrence of SVT with these catecholamines is common. For these reasons, verapamil should be avoided in pediatric patients with hypotension, low cardiac output, or unstable second-degree atrioventricular block and third-degree atrioventricular block, as well as in those patients in the tachycardic phase of the sick-sinus syndrome (53, 62). Its use in patients who have received β-blockers (62) and in newborn infants (53) may be particularly dangerous. Numerous reports of ventricular fibrillation, asystole, and/or sudden death with verapamil make its safety margin much less than that of adenosine.

In certain instances, the electrophysiology of the child's SVT may be known from a previous electrophysiologic study. In SVT resulting from reentry (atrioventricular reentry or accessory pathway), verapamil is likely to be very effective. It is generally ineffective in SVT because of ectopic tachycardias (atrial or junctional) and may lead to further deterioration (58, 62).

Diving reflex stimulation via ice water immersion (less than 5 seconds) or application for 15 to 30 seconds to the face (e.g., an ice-water-filled bag over the patient's face) are both rapid and safe but only occasionally successful. An α-adrenergic agonist such as phenylephrine hydrochloride via intravenous infusion (0.5 to 5.0 μg/kg/min) may be utilized to induce reflex slowing of heart rate and to correct hypotension through vasoconstriction, but often does so at the expense of worsened tissue perfusion.

Should hemodynamic decompensation from SVT persist, "overdrive" pacing through the transvenous approach may be performed. The pacemaker rate is gradually increased until capture of the rate occurs. Once captured, the rate can then be reduced to achieve ventricular slowing; if SVT resumes upon a reduction of pacemaker rate, the pacemaker rate can be increased in an effort to obtain a 2:1 block with a reduced ventricular rate.

Other pacing techniques continue to gain wider acceptance for the emergency treatment of SVT. Both transesophageal (63) and transcutaneous (external) pacing (64) have been utilized successfully. These methods (not described further here) allow rapid termination of SVT and certain other tachydysrhythmias so as to avoid other more invasive and potentially more dangerous interventions.

In conclusion, the relative safety of adenosine and its rapid onset of action make it the drug of choice for the treatment of SVT. DC cardioversion should be used immediately for those patients with hemodynamic instability. Digoxin remains a useful agent for long-term management with certain forms of SVT, but its role in therapy of acute SVT has been supplanted by faster-acting and safer agents in all pediatric age groups. Concerns about DC cardioversion in patients receiving digoxin are warranted. Verapamil should be used only in the older child or adolescent in whom hypotension is not present and when other agents have not been utilized.

RACEMIC EPINEPHRINE

Acute upper airway problems are a frequent cause of admissions to PICUs. Croup syndromes (viral laryngotracheobronchitis, spasmodic croup) and postextubation subglottic edema present as stridor, which may portend respiratory distress and eventual respiratory failure. These maladies affect pediatric patients far more frequently than adults because of anatomic airway differences, particularly in the subglottic area where the narrowest portion is at the level of the cricoid cartilage.

As treatment for respiratory distress, racemic epinephrine, a mixture of the optically active epinephrine isomers L-epinephrine and D-epinephrine, can be diluted in 0.9% normal saline and then delivered as a nebulized aerosol (65–68). In this form, it is a rapidly acting, effective means of controlling acute subglottic swelling and perhaps of avoiding the need for endotracheal intubation or tracheostomy (69–71). Supplied as a 2.5% solution, 0.25 to 0.50 ml of the drug should be diluted in 3.0 to 4.0 ml of normal saline, aerosolized by jet nebulizer, and given by either face mask or simply by holding the nebulizer that delivers the mist close to the patient's face. The localized delivery to the upper airway avoids many of the side effects from parenterally administered epinephrine, such as systemic vasoconstriction. Tachycardia is not uncommon, but excessively high rates and ectopy are infrequent (65, 70–72).

Racemic epinephrine has a duration of action of 30 to 120 minutes. Therefore, discharging the patient from the emergency room after treatment with this medication without a long observation period (at least 6 hours) is contraindicated. Whether rebound swelling in excess of that already present occurs after therapy is uncertain (68, 71, 72), but there is little disagreement that despite racemic epinephrine's palliative, temporizing effect, the natural history of viral croup is not altered (71, 72). The author and colleagues believe that any child whose airway abnormality is severe enough to require racemic epinephrine should be hospitalized. A false sense of security following a single treatment and an early discharge home can lead to catastrophic results.

Treatment with racemic epinephrine should be construed as a palliative effort to avoid endotracheal intubation or tracheostomy. The croup score (73) is extremely useful for initial and repeated evaluations for those patients with subglottic swelling. A score of 5 or more should necessitate admission to a unit where direct observation is possible. Scores of 7 or 8 imply respiratory difficulty that often responds to racemic epinephrine treatment and continued use of other therapies such as cool mist and mild sedation. When the croup score is 9 or 10, impending or actual respiratory failure exists. Rapid improvement with racemic epinephrine may still be possible, but preparation for emergency intubation and/or tracheostomy in the operating room should be made, with an anesthesiologist and otolaryngologist in attendance. If a patient requires racemic epinephrine nearly continuously (more than every 30 minutes), it is prudent to establish an airway via intubation or tracheostomy and to avoid the risk of respiratory fatigue, sudden obstruction, hypoxemia, or hypercarbia.

PROSTAGLANDIN E₁

Although an understanding of prostaglandin biosynthesis and pharmacology have provided potential therapeutic modalities for sepsis and cerebral ischemia (74–77), nowhere has the ability to manipulate prostaglandin-mediated events been more profound than with therapies aimed at constricting or dilating the ductus arteriosus early in life. The premature infant may sustain prolonged cardiorespiratory failure secondary to a patent ductus arteriosus (78–80) that may respond to nonsurgical closure using the prostaglandin synthetase inhibitor indomethacin (81, 82). To the contrary, maintaining ductal patency in certain forms of cyanotic and acyanotic congenital heart disease may provide preoperative stabilization (83–86).

Since Coceani and Olley (87) showed that prostaglandins E₁ and E₂ relaxed the isolated ductus arteriosus of fetal lambs, many large clinical trials have provided ample support for the use of prostaglandin E₁ in the presence of cyanotic or acyanotic lesions in which ductal patency is required for adequate pulmonary or systemic flow (84, 85, 88, 89). Infants with pulmonary atresia, hypoplastic right ventricle, and severe pulmonic stenosis may sustain a large increase in arterial PO₂ following prostaglandin E₁ initiation. Other forms of cyanotic congenital heart disease, including transposition of the great vessels, tricuspid atresia, truncus arteriosus, and total anomalous pulmonary venous return, may also benefit from prostaglandin E₁ infusion to improve arteriovenous mixing. Since severe cyanosis with resultant acidemia and cardiovascular collapse may occur prior to diagnosis, most pediatric heart centers advocate prostaglandin E₁ therapy for all critically ill neonates in whom cyanotic congenital heart disease is strongly suspected.

Infants with systemic cardiovascular collapse resulting from aortic arch anomalies (interrupted aortic arch, juxtaductal aortic coarctation) or with hypoplastic left heart syndrome may develop severe acidemia and renal failure during spontaneous ductal closure. Many such infants show marked improvement in lower body perfusion, urine output, and arterial pH when prostaglandin E₁ is used to obtain ductal patency (83, 85). As with cyanotic lesions, prostaglandin E₁ should be instituted in all critically ill infants suspected to have aortic arch anomalies even before an exact diagnosis is established.

Prostaglandin E₁ therapy may be administered via a peripheral venous, central venous, or umbilical arterial site. The intravenous route is preferred, since cutaneous vasodilation is more pronounced with intraarterial infusion (89). The amount of prostaglandin E₁ in milligrams to be diluted in 100 mg 5% dextrose water is the product of the body weight in kilograms multiplied by 0.3. An initial dose of 0.05 μg/kg/min is achieved with an infusion rate of 1.0 ml/hr. Clinical efficacy is usually achieved at doses ranging from 0.05 to 0.20 μg/kg/min; however, both lower and higher doses have been utilized. The infusion should be continued until surgical palliation or correction is performed, or until further assessment shows no need to maintain ductal patency.

Side effects from prostaglandin E₁ infusion merit considerable attention. Apnea and/or hypoventilation, presumably attributed to central nervous system (CNS) effects, are extremely common. Provisions should be made for immediate airway management, including endotracheal intubation for all infants receiving prostaglandin E₁. Endotracheal intubation should be performed prior to transport of an infant to another center. Because there is concern about susceptibility to infection, concurrent antibiotic therapy is usually warranted. Cardiovascular effects secondary to vasodilation should be anticipated, and volume replacement and inotropic agents (usually dopamine) are often necessary to avoid systemic hypotension. Fever, even in the absence of sepsis, is not unusual, and seizures, jitteriness, hypoglycemia, hypocalcemia, diarrhea, renal failure, and clotting abnormalities have also been reported (88, 89). Despite these associated risks, prostaglandin E₁ is often life-sustaining in critically ill infants with congenital heart disease prior to surgical correction or palliation.

SEDATION AND NEUROMUSCULAR BLOCKADE

Numerous pharmacologic agents are used routinely in the PICU to relieve pain, prevent anxiety, facilitate endotracheal intubation, and provide muscle relaxation for those patients who require mechanical ventilation. The following commentary is a review of these drugs as utilized in the PICU.

Morphine sulfate is one of the more commonly used analgesics in the PICU. Its uses include (*a*) relief of postoperative pain, (*b*) sedation for infants and children who require neuromuscular blockade, (*c*) afterload reduction in patients with congestive cardiac states or low cardiac output, and (*d*) sleep in anxious patients. Morphine's popularity is based upon its easy dosing, fairly predictable responses, duration of action, and the ability to reverse its action with the opiate antagonist, naloxone.

To provide sedation for those patients who require neuromuscular blockade, an intravenous morphine dose of 0.1 mg/kg given over 1 to 5 minutes appears to be effective. Common practice is to repeat the dose every 2 to 6 hours based on evidence that desired effects have dissipated (return of tachycardia, hypertension, decreased perfusion, movement). Precautions should be taken in patients with altered cardiovascular performance, since a slight, transient reduction in blood pressure, presumably resulting from decreased peripheral vascular resistance, is quite common (unpublished observation). Relaxation of venous tone resulting in decreased preload may also result in a decreased blood pressure. Dosing for postoperative analgesia, afterload reduction, and sleep induction more commonly requires individual titration, but intravenous doses of 0.05 to 0.10 mg/kg are commonly employed. The author and colleagues prefer to avoid intramuscular administration, as this approach is painful and offers no advantage to the ICU patient, who must always have an intravenous catheter in place.

Infants and children rarely develop dependency and/or addiction when morphine is used for less than 7 days in the PICU setting. Other than cardiovascular changes, the primary concern with prolonged use is reduced gastrointestinal motility. Morphine may impair the ability to feed these patients enterally. Metoclopramide may alleviate gastric atony but seems ineffective in improving lower gastrointestinal immotility (unpublished observation). Despite its potential problems, morphine remains in frequent use in most PICUs. Morphine has been given by continuous intravenous infusion in both infants (90) and children (91). Dosages of 10 to 30 μg/kg/hr seem to provide effective analgesia and may reduce the hemodynamic variations seen with intermittent bolus infusion. Neonates develop higher serum morphine levels than do older children, and doses not exceeding 15 µg/kg/hr have been recommended for infants (90).

Some pediatric intensivists prefer the potent synthetic opioid fentanyl over morphine because of fentanyl's lack of histamine release and minimal cardiovascular effects (92). Fentanyl is approximately 100 times more potent than morphine because of its greater lipid solubility (93). Although its duration of action may be only 30 to 90 minutes following a single dose, far longer activity may be seen after higher doses or following repeated usage. Intravenous bolus doses of 1.0 to 2.0 µg/kg can be given every 1 to 2 hours or a continuous intravenous infusion at rates of 1.0 to 3.0 µg/kg/hr provide excellent analgesia in most circumstances.

Chloral hydrate provides mild sedation without analgesia. Its advantages are a lack of cardiovascular effects and minimal, or no, respiratory depression. Given as an oral or rectal dose of 20 to 50 mg/kg, chloral hydrate generally induces sleep in 20 to 30 minutes. It is not available in parenteral form and provides no pain relief, which are its two major disadvantages. Despite these shortcomings, it remains a valuable adjunct for sedation.

The benzodiazepines diazepam and lorazepam both provide effective sedation and amnesia. Diazepam in doses of 0.1 to 0.2 mg/kg given slowly via the intravenous route provides amnesia for up to 3 hours with a rapid onset of action. These properties make it an ideal agent for use during endotracheal intubation in children and adolescents and for other uncomfortable procedures such as DC cardioversion and fiberoptic bronchoscopy. Diazepam provided alternately with morphine in patients who require neuromuscular paralysis is quite satisfactory. In this setting, diazepam adds amnesia and anxiolysis to the analgesic and muscle relaxation provided by morphine and vecuronium (or pancuronium) respectively. Diazepam cannot be administered with dextrose-containing solutions and may cause hypotension if infused too rapidly. For the latter reason, lorazepam at an intravenous dose of 0.05 to 0.10 mg/kg may be preferred to diazepam for inducing amnesia with less potent cardiovascular effects (27, 94).

More recently, most PICUs have begun using midazolam instead of diazepam. Midazolam, when given in intravenous doses of 0.05 to 0.10 mg/kg, has a very short onset of action, is very reliable in providing anxiolysis and amnesia, and may have fewer cardiovascular effects than diazepam. In addition, elimination half-lifes of the parent compound and its active metabolites are far shorter than the half-lifes of diazepam and its metabolites, which allows for more rapid resolution of effects when awakening patients for neurologic examination or when weaning from ventilation is required.

A variety of neuromuscular blocking agents is available to assist with endotracheal intubation or for more prolonged use during mechanical ventilation. Succinylcholine chloride, a depolarizing neuromuscular blocker, is usually the drug of choice for endotracheal intubation, particularly in young children and infants. Adequate muscle relaxation, to facilitate intubation, occurs within 10 to 20 seconds after a dose of 1.0 to 2.0 mg/kg given as an intravenous bolus, and usually lasts 3 to 5 minutes. The higher dose (2 mg/kg) is primarily recommended for infants and young children who have a relatively greater blood volume and extracellular fluid volume than older children on a weight basis, as succinylcholine is distributed rapidly to the extracellular spaces (95–97). Elimination of succinylcholine chloride is rapid because of hydrolysis by plasma (pseudo-) cholinesterase. Succinylcholine activity is potentiated by decreased or abnormal plasma cholinesterase, alkalosis, increased extracellular potassium (hyperkalemia), decreased temperature, quinidine, concomitant magnesium sulfate administration, liver disease, and certain antibiotics (aminoglycosides, polymixins, tetracyclines). Antagonism and/or a shortened duration of action may occur with hypokalemia, acidosis, decreased cardiac output, or increased skeletal muscle blood flow (97).

Succinylcholine frequently induces vagal stimulation, which may be further augmented during laryngoscopy, resulting in clinically significant bradycardia. It should usually be administered with, or preferably after, intravenous atropine (0.01 mg/kg, minimum 0.10 mg) or glycopyrrolate (0.005 mg/kg). Older children and adolescents should be given an "obtundation dose" of thiopental (2.0 to 4.0 mg/kg), ketamine (1.0 to 2.0 mg/kg), diazepam (0.2 to 0.4 mg/kg), or as the author and colleagues prefer, midazolam (0.1 mg/kg) prior to succinylcholine administration.

The major drawbacks of succinylcholine are a very short duration of action; induction of muscle fasciculations, particularly in older children; and its contraindication in patients with burns, massive muscle trauma, and certain motor neurologic deficits (97), as well as in those patients at risk for the malignant hyperthermia syndrome (determined by history, familial predisposition, or provocative muscle testing). Succinylcholine also causes increased intracranial, intragastric, and intraocular pressures. "Crash induction" techniques, using thiopental coupled with cricoid pressure and then atropine-succinylcholine, block increases in intracranial pressure and also lessen the hazards of aspiration.

The nondepolarizing neuromuscular blockers most commonly used are *d*-tubocurarine chloride, pancuronium bromide, and vecuronium bromide, but metocurine iodide and atracurium besylate are also available. Equipotent doses for these agents have been established for both infants and children (Table 64.1). Advantages and disadvantages for each of these agents are also noted in the table, with a few requiring specific commentary.

Histamine release by *d*-tubocurarine can potentially aggravate bronchospasm in those patients with asthma or other allergic disorders. However, in newborn infants histamine appears to be a bronchodilator and vasodilator (98). This fact makes histamine release potentially helpful in early postnatal circulatory derangements caused by high pulmonary vascular resistance (persistent pulmonary hypertension syndrome), wherein pulmonary vasodilation via histamine release would be advantageous.

Pancuronium has great appeal because of its longer duration of action. This characteristic makes dosing less frequent, a major advantage to nursing personnel who must administer these agents frequently around the clock for several days or weeks. This advantage is somewhat offset by the drug's often profound cardiovascular effects, particularly tachycardia and hypertension. These responses may be particularly troublesome in patients with cardiovascular compromise or in those

Table 64.1.   Equipotent Doses of Nondepolarizing Neuromuscular Blockers

	Usual Dose (mg/kg)	*Onset of Action* (min)	*Duration of Action* (min)	*Metabolic Clearance*	*Comments*
Pancuronium	0.08–0.012	2–4	65	40% unchanged (urine) 87% bound	Somewhat longer action; tachycardia frequent
Vecuronium	0.06–0.10	2–3	35–55	35% unchanged (urine) 25–50% bile 60–80% bound	Few cardiovascular changes; shorter duration of action
Atracurium	0.4–0.5	2–2½	40–60	Hofmann elimination and ester hydrolysis	Predictable duration of renal and hepatic failure
d-Tubocurarine	0.3–0.6	2–4	50	45% unchanged (urine)	Released histamine may be beneficial in neonates
Metocurine	0.2–0.4	1½–2	40–60	50% unchanged (urine)	Somewhat shorter onset of action

in whom other pharmacologic agents may already have created or may further enhance tachydysrhythmias (methylxanthines, β-agonists, catecholamines).

For the reasons just mentioned, the author and colleagues prefer to use vecuronium as the agent of choice whenever pancuronium has elicited or may potentially elicit an untoward response. Vecuronium has almost no cardiovascular side effects, and although it is not as "long acting" as pancuronium, its duration of action is acceptable in most circumstances.

Atracurium is cleared by rapid, nonenzymatic degradation (Hoffmann elimination) (99), a potential advantage over other agents that may require renal or hepatic removal. Since many PICU patients have altered renal and hepatic function, atracurium may be more predictable in certain patients. The author's group has recently begun using atracurium via continuous infusion in rates ranging from 0.30 to 0.60 mg/kg/hr following an initial intravenous dose of 0.4 to 0.5 mg/kg. The infusion is titrated to achieve partial neuromuscular blockade in intubated patients who may benefit from less than total blockade, but in whom minimal movement is desired (i.e., epiglottitis, croup). Although other nondepolarizing neuromuscular blocking agents could be used in a similar fashion, atracurium has been keynoted for this purpose.

Ketamine hydrochloride, a so-called dissociative anesthetic, has been used for pediatric patients during dental (100) and other minor surgical procedures (101). As such, its use for minor surgical procedures in the PICU seems reasonable. Intravenous doses of 0.5 to 2.0 mg/kg have been utilized (102). Intramuscular doses of 4.0 mg/kg also appear effective but seem unnecessary when an intravenous line is already in place. Ketamine creates cardiovascular stimulation, primarily through CNS mechanisms, a fact that offers a potential advantage over morphine and other depressant agents. Paradoxically, ketamine is a direct myocardial depressant (103), which may explain the sudden, unexpected hypotension reported in critically ill patients (104). Well-described, unpleasant psychic disturbances during emergence from ketamine may make its use less preferable than that of other agents, and unpleasant dreams have been reported even weeks after its use have been reported (105). These "emergence phenomena" are less common in children than in adults. In the unfamiliar PICU environment, psychiatric stresses should be eliminated as much as possible, a drawback for ketamine usage. In nonintubated patients who require painful procedures such as central venous catheter placement, ketamine is an excellent agent when appropriate dosing (0.5 to 2.0 mg/kg i.v.) is utilized as

protective reflexes are maintained. Ketamine increases upper airway secretions, and an antisialagogue may be needed. Titration via repeat dosing every 20 to 40 minutes will often allow for a smooth procedure with minimal or no patient discomfort or recall. Ketamine probably should be avoided in those patients less than 3 months of age and in those older than 10 years. Infants appear to lose protective reflexes more readily than older pediatric patients, and adolescents are more prone to psychiatric disturbances. Recently, ketamine has been given by continuous intravenous infusion in critically ill pediatric patients via an initial bolus of 0.5 to 1.0 mg/kg followed by 10 to 15 μg/kg/min. With this regimen, effective sedation and analgesia can be achieved without cardiopulmonary compromise.

Propofol (2,6-diisopropylphenol) has been used extensively as an anesthetic agent in patients of all ages (106–109). Prepared as a soybean emulsion, it is comparatively short-acting and rapidly metabolized. These characteristics make it highly desirable for short surgical procedures. When utilized in ICUs following surgery, it provides effective sedation and analgesia with rapid recovery upon discontinuation of the agent (106, 107). The author and colleagues have employed continuous propofol infusion in postoperative patients, including open heart cardiac cases. Doses of 50 to 125 μg/kg/min are titrated to effect the degree of sedation and analgesia desired. Upon discontinuing propofol, extubation is often possible within 30 to 60 minutes, depending upon factors related to use of other anesthetic agents during operation. Few contraindications to propofol exist but include allergic hypersensitivity. Lipid emulsions alter blood coagulation, but no reports of this problem with propofol have been published. Little information is available on propofol use for more than 8 hours, but several small series reported no undesirable effects with prolonged use (107, 108). Concomitant use of a neuromuscular blocking agent may be required for successful ventilator management. It is likely that propofol will gain further utility in the PICU in the near future.

CLONIDINE INGESTION

Clonidine hydrochloride is frequently prescribed orally as an antihypertensive agent. It has been investigated for use in treating migraine headaches, for narcotic withdrawal, and for smoking cessation. More recently, a transdermal patch preparation has been made available (110). Because of its widespread popularity, it is a relatively frequent cause of drug overdose in children admitted to intensive care units (111, 112). The drug achieves its antihypertensive effect through central sympathetic mechanisms that reduce peripheral vascular tone and heart rate. Conversely, the drug may act on peripheral receptors to transiently increase vascular tone. These dual, somewhat competitive, actions can create a variety of clinical manifestations when the drug is ingested by small children or when overdose occurs in adolescents. Symptoms of overdose include drowsiness, impaired sensorium, respiratory depression, apnea, bradycardia, miosis, hypertension, and hypothermia as probable consequences of its central actions. Hypertension, resulting from peripheral α-adrenergic agonist effects, has also been reported (113–115). The balance between central sympathetic inhibition and peripheral α-adrenergic stimulation determines which effects predominate.

In infants and young children who ingest clonidine by accident, central sympathetic depression often predominates. Drowsiness often ensues within 1 hour of ingestion of even very small amounts (as little as 0.1 mg) and may progress to obtundation, coma, respiratory depression, and apnea. Cardiovascular effects range from mild bradycardia with a normal or minimally decreased blood pressure to overt hypotension (116, 117). Some who ingest an overdose of clonidine may manifest hypertension along with respiratory depression and a depressed level of consciousness.

Initial treatment must include attention to the airway and adequacy of ventilation. Endotracheal intubation may be required, especially in young children, if marked slowing of respiration occurs. Cardiovascular support may be necessary to correct either hypotension or bradycardia, and less often for hypertension. Atropine sulfate (0.01 mg/kg, minimum 0.1 mg) is generally effective for bradycardia and may improve blood pressure in the heart rate-dependent cardiovascular system of the infant. Although the α-adrenergic blocker tolazoline has been recommended in both hypotensive and hypertensive states, patients respond unpredictably to this drug (118, 119). Volume expansion with 10 mg/kg of 0.9% normal saline or lactated Ringer's solution, often accompanied by dopamine (5 to 10 μg/kg/min) or epinephrine (0.1 to 0.3 μg/kg/min) by continuous infusion, reverses both the bradycardia and hypotension. The short half-lifes of dopamine and epinephrine permit rapid discontinuation as the clonidine effects subside. The infrequent hypertensive state induced by clonidine may be better treated with tolazoline (118, 119). An initial dose of 1.0 mg/kg (followed by a continuous infusion of 1.0 to 2.0 mg/kg/hr when necessary) may be effective, but alternative therapy with a more predictable peripheral vasodilator such as sodium nitroprusside (0.5 to 5.0 μg/kg/min) should also be considered.

Such supportive and specific treatment is given in addition to routine measures for acute ingestions, which include emetics, activated charcoal, and cathartics. Clonidine is cleared mostly in the urine (114), while poorly defined extrarenal clearance mechanisms also exist, with an overall plasma half-life of approximately 12 hours. Although forced diuresis with loop and/or osmotic diuretics has been advocated, most authors believe that such treatment is not necessary and may even worsen hypotension (120). As expected from the drug's half-life, most symptoms of clonidine ingestion resolve within 12 to 24 hours.

The opiate antagonist naloxone has been debated as a specific agent for management of clonidine intoxication. Such use has some pharmacologic justification in that naloxone reverses clonidine's hypotensive effects in spontaneously hypertensive rats (121) and is efficacious in models of respiratory and cardiovascular depression (122–124). Nevertheless, Banner et al. (116) reported that five children, ages 17 months to 2 years, had no detectable response to intravenous naloxone (0.03 to 0.05 mg/kg). Although improvement with naloxone appears to be unpredictable, no adverse reactions have been reported when the drug is used to antagonize clonidine. Its efficacy remains anecdotal and unsubstantiated.

IRON INTOXICATION

The ingestion of iron-containing compounds, particularly by young children, remains a frequent cause for PICU admission (125–128). These products are widely available, and their use during pregnancy, when mothers may be less able to adequately supervise the younger children in the household, creates a scenario for accidental iron intoxication, as does an underappreciation by the general public regarding the danger associated with iron ingestion.

The clinical effects from acute iron ingestion are well-described (129, 130). The characteristic stages are (*a*) initial gastrointestinal, (*b*) relative stability, (*c*) shock, (*d*) hepatic necrosis, and (*e*) gastrointestinal scarring. Clearly, not all patients manifest each stage, but the more severe cases are likely to do so. The initial gastrointestinal stage begins shortly after the iron-containing product has been ingested. Symptoms usually include vomiting and abdominal pain, but may also include diarrhea and/or gastrointestinal hemorrhage. A quiescent stage of relative stability may ensue between 4 and 48 hours after ingestion, but in severe cases this "eye of the hurricane" period may only be a failure to recognize the subtle signs of impending cardiovascular collapse. The third stage is characterized by circulatory derangements attributed to both the direct and indirect effects of iron. A reduction in the circulating plasma volume may result from vomiting, diarrhea, hemorrhage, or "third-spacing" of fluid into the irritated gastrointestinal tract. Metabolic acidosis results from conversion of ferrous to ferric ions (131), from inhibitory effects of iron on cellular oxidative metabolism (132), and from a hypoperfusion-low cardiac output state. Coagulation defects, occasionally noted in the initial phase (133), may lead to further bleeding and continued cardiovascular deterioration. Hepatic necrosis may develop even if circulatory impairment is corrected. The liver appears to be a target organ for the direct toxic effects of iron. Fortunately, the hepatic toxicity stage occurs only rarely. The acute, corrosive injury to bowel usually heals within several weeks; however, such healing may leave stenotic areas in both the gastric outlet and the proximal small bowel that later may present as acute gastrointestinal obstruction (134, 135).

Despite the availability of deferoxamine mesylate as an effective chelating agent, some controversy persists as to the actual procedures for treating acute iron intoxication. Certain recommendations can be reasonably made. Emesis should be induced unless the sensorium precludes it. Mechanical lavage to remove iron in the neurologically depressed patient is always indicated. Some have proposed using sodium bicarbonate (136) or sodium phosphate (137) as the lavage fluid, based on the relatively water-insoluble complexes these agents form with iron (138). Because of the risk of excessive phosphate absorption (139), a 5% sodium bicarbonate solution in water is preferable, and an appropriate volume should be left in the stomach after lavage to produce poorly soluble ferrous carbonate (140). Activated charcoal is of little value in inhibiting absorption, but a cathartic should be used to assist in intestinal emptying. Although deferoxamine has been administered via the enteral route, absorption of the iron-deferoxamine complex may occur from the gastrointestinal tract (129). Thus, the author and colleagues believe that its safety has not been adequately demonstrated.

The serum iron concentration should be determined. Patients with serum values greater than 300 μg/dl usually require parenteral deferoxamine therapy. Unless there is evidence of poor tissue perfusion, deferoxamine (40 mg/kg) should be given intramuscularly. In the presence of hypotension, a secure intravenous line is required for blood volume expansion, and intravenous deferoxamine administration is indicated. A continuous infusion at 15 mg/kg/hr is generally safe, but continuous ECG and frequent blood pressure measurements are necessary. Hypotension is generally reversible with further volume expansion, although catecholamine (dopamine or epinephrine) infusion occasionally may be required. Acute renal dysfunction has also been described (141).

The iron-deferoxamine complex may produce a pink color in the urine. When present, the color serves as a simple method to assess excretion of the complex. A simple qualitative test has been proposed as a screen for iron ingestion (142) when the intoxicant is unknown. Monitoring of urine color as well as serial serum iron determinations indicates when chelation therapy may be discontinued.

Intranasal deferoxamine has been utilized experimentally for chronic iron overload (143), but irregular absorption precludes its use in acute intoxications. Deferoxamine complexed to high molecular weight carbohydrates such as hydroxyethyl starch and dextran has been utilized experimentally (144, 145). These preparations appear to avoid deferoxamine-induced hypotension, which may allow higher doses of deferoxamine to be used. The same effects were not seen when deferoxamine and the high molecular weight substances were given separately (144).

More invasive treatments aimed at removing iron have been advocated, including surgical gastrotomy (146), hemodialysis (130), and total body exchange transfusion (131). Although each of these therapies has been helpful in specific, unusual cases, their routine use generally is not advised. Continuous arteriovenous hemofiltration (CAVH) with deferoxamine infusion into the arterial limb has been utilized experimentally, but iron clearance with this method was no better than with urinary clearance (147). Further supportive care requirements should be based on the severity of the ingestion and the clinical response to initial therapy.

ORGANOPHOSPHATE POISONING

Children exposed to organophosphate insecticides through inhalation, ingestion, or skin absorption may face a serious medical emergency. Other insecticides may also cause severe toxic reactions and may occasionally prove fatal, but the relative availability of organophosphates in both household and agricultural pesticides warrants their specific mention here. Carbamate insecticides have effects that are similar to those of organophosphate compounds but milder. Their toxicologic effects and therapeutic rationales are often included together.

Organophosphate compounds bind irreversibly to the two cholinesterases found in humans. Acetylcholinesterase (true cholinesterase) is found primarily in neurons, at the neuromuscular junction, and in red blood cells, whereas pseudocholinesterase (serum cholinesterase) is found in serum, liver, and other organs. These enzymes are responsible for terminating the effects of acetylcholine, a central and peripheral neurotransmitter responsible for central respiratory and cardiovascular control and peripheral nicotinic and muscarinic receptor activity. Failure to deactivate acetylcholine at the neuroeffector junction occurs when organophosphates bind to the cholinesterase enzymes and create symptoms that can be classified as nicotinic (muscle fasciculations, cramps, incoordination, weakness, paralysis), muscarinic (miosis, sweating, salivation, lacrimation, bronchospasm, bronchorrhea, bradycardia, hypertension, nausea, vomiting, diarrhea), and central (apathy, obtundation, coma, convulsions). Several large clinical series seem to indicate that in children, central nervous system symptoms may predominate (148, 149). Other important clinical complications have been reported, including ARDS (150), chorea, depression (151), and delayed-onset respiratory failure (the intermediate syndrome) (152, 153).

Highly toxic organophosphates include tetraethyl pyrophosphate (TEPP), methyl parathion, ethyl parathion, and bomyl. Moderately toxic agents such as fenthion, diazinon, dichlorvos, and malathion are more commonly used in household products than for agricultural use (154, 155). In addition, most household products are provided in diluted formulations. Petroleum distillates may be used as the organic solvent for certain organophosphates and further complicate therapy.

Initial therapy should be administered promptly. For preparations not containing petroleum distillates, emesis should be induced. Gastric lavage, if indicated, should be performed in the usual manner. Skin cleansing with copious amounts of soap and water is required to remove the compounds from the skin. Health professionals must be careful to wear rubber gloves and other protective garments to prevent contamination by the toxin and subsequent absorption. Atropine antagonizes the central and muscarinic effects but does not reverse the nicotinic receptor-mediated muscle weakness. Dosing should be directed toward atropinization, which may require large and frequent intravenous infusions. Younger children are treated with an initial dose of 0.05 mg/kg followed by a maintenance dose of 0.02 to 0.05 mg/kg every 10 to 30 minutes until cholinergic signs are reversed. Older children (12 years of age and older) may be given 1.0 to 2.0 mg initially and then every 15 to 30 minutes until complete reversal of cholinergic signs occurs. Careful, repeated assessment of airway adequacy and respiratory muscle strength is required even in the fully atropinized patient. The presence of a dry mouth, warm, flushed skin, dilated pupils, and increased heart rate indicate adequate atropinization. Atropine therapy should be continued for at least 24 hours in moderate and severe cases to allow time for the organophosphate compound to be eliminated. Atropine toxicity manifested by fever, muscle fasciculations, and delirium requires that further atropine administration be halted. If cholinergic signs return during withdrawal of atropine therapy, it should be reinstituted.

The cholinesterase reactivating oxime pralidoxime chloride (Protopam, 2-PAM chloride) counteracts the nicotinic and muscarinic effects but not the central effects incurred with organophosphate intoxication. Atropine therapy must continue concurrently with the use of pralidoxime chloride or any other oxime. In Europe and the Middle East, obidoxime chloride appears to be preferred. An intravenous infusion of pralidoxime in a dose of 25 to 50 mg/kg prepared in 5% dextrose and 0.45% normal saline (D5.45NS) should be administered over 10 to 30 minutes. A dose of 0.5 to 1.0 g may be given to larger children or adolescents. Nausea, headache, dizziness, diplopia, respiratory depression, and hypertension are side effects of pralidoxime. The initial infusion should be followed by a second infusion using the same dose 1 to 2 hours later and then again after approximately 12 hours if cholinergic signs recur.

Alternatively, recent use of pralidoxime by continuous infusion may avoid both low circulating levels and toxic side effects created with intermittent infusions (156). When given by continuous infusion, a loading dose of 25 mg/kg over 10 to 30 minutes should be followed by a continuous infusion at a rate of 10 to 20 mg/kg/hr. Treatment for more than 24 hours generally is not required except with severe intoxication or with fenthion exposure, which undergoes very slow elimination (155). Although measurements of acetylcholinesterase and pseudocholinesterase are helpful in determining the response to therapy and in assessing the severity of organophosphate exposure, these tests often are not readily available. Delays in providing pralidoxime therapy must be avoided. This recommendation is made because the enzyme-organophosphate complexes become more resistant to the reactivating effects of pralidoxime as time passes (157). Oximes generally are not recommended for carbamate poisonings.

Morphine, methylxanthines, and loop diuretics are specifically contraindicated in organophosphate poisoning (155). Supportive care, including endotracheal intubation and mechanical ventilation, is based upon the severity of exposure, physical findings, arterial blood gases, and other laboratory assessments. When clinical improvement is noted within the first 24 hours, respiratory function must be assessed carefully for at least 96 hours to avoid the acute respiratory failure inherent with the intermediate syndrome. Prophylaxis with agents that are also capable of interacting with acetylcholinesterase in the neuroeffector junction, such as physostigmine (158), curare, and pancuronium (159), has been investigated experimentally but these agents are not, at present, part of the therapeutic regimen.

ACKNOWLEDGMENTS

The author thanks Dr. Al Pruitt for his contributions to the previous edition of this chapter and Ms. Lucinda Smith for her valuable secretarial assistance.

REFERENCES

1. Herman JJ, Noah ZL, Moody RR: Use of intravenous isoproterenol for status asthmaticus in children. *Crit Care Med* 11:716–720, 1983.
2. Kurland G, Leong AB: The management of status asthmaticus in infants and children. *Clin Rev Allergy* 3:37–67, 1985.
3. Parry WH, Martorano F, Cotton EK: Management of life-threatening asthma with intravenous isoproterenol infusions. *Am J Dis Child* 130:39–42, 1976.
4. Wood DW, Downes J: Intravenous isoproterenol in the treatment of respiratory failure in childhood status asthmaticus. *Ann Allergy* 31:607–610, 1973.
5. Wood DW, Downes JJ, Scheinkopf H, et al: Intravenous isoproterenol in the management of respiratory failure in childhood status asthmaticus. *J Allergy Clin Immunol* 50:75–81, 1972.
6. Fuglsang G, Pedersen S, Borgstrom L: Dose-response relationships of intravenously administered terbutaline in children with asthma. *J Pediatr* 114:315–320, 1985.
7. Al-Jundi S, Horowitz I, Deakers TW, Newth CJL: Continuous inhalation of full-strength albuterol in the management of severe acute asthma in a pediatric intensive care unit [Abstract]. Presented at the Fifth Annual Pediatric Critical Care Colloquium, Waterville Valley, NH, October 1990.
8. Papo MC, Frank JA, Thompson AE: A prospective randomized study of continuous versus intermittent nebulized albuterol for severe status asthmaticus in children [Abstract]. *Crit Care Med* 19 (suppl):577, 1991.
9. Klaustermeyer WB, DiBernardo RL, Hale FC: Intravenous isoproterenol: rationale for bronchial asthma. *J Allergy Immunol* 55:325–333, 1975.
10. Krasnon N, Rolett EL, Yurchak D, et al: Isoproterenol and cardiovascular performance. *Am J Med* 37:514–525, 1964.
11. Kurland G, Williams J, Lewiston NJ: Fatal myocardial toxicity during continuous infusion intravenous isoproterenol therapy of asthma. *J Allergy Clin Immunol* 64:407–411, 1979.
12. Kadar D, Tanf HY, Conn AW: Isoproterenol metabolism in children after intravenous administration. *Clin Pharmacol Ther* 16:789–795, 1974.
13. Hemstreet MP, Miles MV, Rutland RO: Effect of intravenous isoproterenol on theophylline kinetics. *J Allergy Clin Immunol* 69:360–364, 1982.
14. Lehr D, Guideri G: More on combined beta-agonists and methylxanthines in asthma. *N Engl J Med* 30:1581–1582, 1983.
15. Aelony Y, Laks MM, Beall G: An electrocardiographic pattern of acute myocardial infarction associated with excessive use of aerosolized isoproterenol. *Chest* 68:107–110, 1975.
16. Camfield PR: Treatment of status epilepticus in children. *Can Med Assoc J* 128:671–672, 1983.
17. Delgado-Escueta AV, Wasterlain C, Treiman DM, et al: Management of status epilepticus. *N Engl J Med* 306:1337–1348, 1982.
18. Gastaut H, Naquet R, Poire R, et al: Treatment of status epilepticus with diazepam (Valium). *Epilepsia* 6:167, 1965.
19. Rothner AD, Erenberg G: Status epilepticus. *Pediatr Clin North Am* 27:593–602, 1980.
20. Shaywitz BA: Management of acute neurologic syndromes in infants and children. *Yale J Biol Med* 57:83–95, 1984.
21. Trauner DA: Acute management of seizures. In James HE, Anas NG, Perkin RM (eds): *Brain Insults in Infants and Children*. Orlando, FL, Grune & Stratton, 1985, pp 213–218.
22. Schmidt D: Benzodiazepines-diazepam. In Woodburg DM, Penry JK, Pippenger CE (eds): *Antiepileptic Drugs*. New York, Raven Press, 1982, pp 771–735.
23. Albano A, Reisdorff EJ, Wiegenstein JG: Rectal diazepam in pediatric status epilepticus. *Am J Emerg Med* 70:168–172, 1989.
24. Zimmerman SS, Fish I: Status epilepticus. In Zimmerman SS, Gildea JH (eds): *Critical Care Pediatrics*. Philadelphia, WB Saunders, 1985, pp 397–400.
25. Wilder BJ, Ramsay RE, Willmore LJ, et al: Efficacy of intravenous phenytoin in the treatment of status epilepticus: kinetics of central nervous system penetration. *Ann Neurol* 6:511–518, 1977.
26. Lacey DJ, Singer WC, Horwitz SJ, et al: Lorazepam therapy of status epilepticus in children and adolescents. *J Pediatr* 108:771–774, 1986.
27. Dundee JW, McGowan WAW, Lilburn JK, et al: Comparison of the actions of diazepam and lorazepam. *Br J Anaesth* 51:439–436, 1979.
28. Ono J, Minaki T, Tagawa T, Tanaka J: Intravenous injection of flunitrazepam for status epilepticus in children—two case reports. *Brain Dev* 10:329–332, 1988.
29. Sumi K, Nagaura T, SaKata N, Nishigaki T, Akagi M: Intravenous flunitrazepam for status epilepticus. *Acta Pediatr Jpn* 31:563–566, 1989.
30. Glezen WP, Denny FW: Epidemiology of acute lower respiratory disease in children. *N Engl J Med* 288:498–505, 1989.
31. Hall CB, McBride JT, Walsh EE, et al: Aerosolized ribavirin treatment of infants with respiratory syncytial viral infection—a randomized double-blind study. *N Engl J Med* 308:1443–1447, 1983.
32. Parrott RH, Kim HW, Brandt CD, et al: Respiratory syncytial virus in infants and children. *Prev Med* 3:473, 1974.
33. Hall CB, McBride JT: Vapors viruses and views—ribavirin and respiratory syncytial virus [Editorial]. *Am J Dis Child* 140:331–332, 1986.
34. Henderson FW, Collier AM, Clyde WA, et al: Respiratory syncytial virus infections, reinfection, and immunity: a prospective, longitudinal study in young children. *N Engl J Med* 300:530–534, 1979.

35. Smith RA: Background and mechanisms of action of ribavirin. In Smith RA, Knight V, Smith JAD (eds): *Clinical Application of Ribavirin*. Orlando, FL, Academic Press, 1984, p 1.

36. Taber LH, Knight V, Gilbert BE, et al: Ribavirin aerosol treatment of bronchiolitis associated with respiratory syncytial virus infection in infants. *Pediatrics* 72:613–618, 1983.

37. Hall CB, McBride JT, Gala CL: Ribavirin therapy of respiratory syncytial virus in infants with cardiopulmonary disease. *Pediatr Res* 19:295A, 1985.

38. Spinelli, M, Ciardullo-Geraci K, Palumbo PE, et al: Efficacy of ribavirin for treating respiratory syncytial virus (RSV) pneumonia in high-risk infants. *Pediatr Res* 19:304A, 1985.

39. Fackler JC, Flannery K, Zipkin M, McIntosh K: Precautions in the use of ribavirin at the Childrens Hospital [Letter]. *N Engl J Med* 322:634, 1990.

40. Englund JA, Piedra PA, Jefferson LS, et al: High-dose, short-duration ribavirin aerosol therapy in children with suspected respiratory syncytial virus infection. *J Pediatr* 117:313–320, 1990.

41. Outwater KM, Meissner HC, Peterson MB: Ribavirin administration to infants receiving mechanical ventilation. *Am J Dis Child* 142:512–515, 1988.

42. McIntosh K, Kurachek SC, Cairns LM, et al: Treatment of respiratory viral infection in an immunodeficient infant with ribavirin aerosol. *Am J Dis Child* 138:305–308, 1984.

43. American Academy of Pediatrics Committee on Infectious Disease: Ribavirin therapy of respiratory syncytial virus. *Pediatrics* 79:475–478, 1987.

44. Hall CB: Ribavirin: beginning the blitz on respiratory viruses? *Pediatr Infect Dis J* 4:668–671, 1985.

45. Ray CG: Ribavirin—ambivalence about an antiviral agent [Editorial]. *Am J Dis Child* 142:488–489, 1988.

46. Wald ER, Dashefsky B, Green M. In re ribavirin: a case of premature adjudication. *J Pediatr* 112:154–158, 1988.

47. Benson DW Jr, Dunnigan A, Benditt DG, et al: Transesophageal study of infant supraventricular tachycardia: electrophysiologic characteristics. *Am J Cardiol* 53:1002–1006, 1983.

48. Garson A, Gillette PC: Electrophysiologic studies of supraventricular tachycardia in children. I. Clinical-electrophysiologic correlations. *Am Heart J* 102:233–350, 1981.

49. Gillette PC, Garson A, Kugler JD: Wolff-Parkinson-White syndrome in children: electrophysiologic and pharmacologic characteristics. *Circulation* 60:1487–1495, 1979.

50. Dobmeyer DJ, Stine RA, Leier CV, et al: The arrhythmogenic effects of caffeine in human beings. *N Engl J Med* 308:814–816, 1983.

51. Garson A, Gillette PC, McNamara DG: Supraventricular tachycardia in children: clinical features, response to treatment and long-term follow-up in 217 patients. *J Pediatr* 98:875–882, 1981.

52. Whitman V, Friedman Z, Berman W Jr, et al: Supraventricular tachycardia in newborn infants: an approach to therapy. *J Pediatr* 91:304–305, 1977.

53. Epstein ML, Kiel EA, Victorica BE: Cardiac decompensation following verapamil therapy in infants with supraventricular tachycardia. *Pediatrics* 75:737–740, 1985.

54. Shahar E, Barzilay Z, Frand M: Verapamil in the treatment of paroxysmal supraventricular tachycardia in infants and children. *J Pediatr* 98:323–326, 1981.

55. Heng MK, Singh BN, Roch AHG, et al: Effects of intravenous verapamil on cardiac arrhythmias and on the electrocardiogram. *Am Heart J* 90:487–498, 1975.

56. Garson A: Medicolegal problems in the management of cardiac arrhythmias in children. *Pediatrics* 79:84–88, 1987.

57. Pickoff AS, Zies L, Ferrer PL, et al: High-dose propranolol therapy in the management of supraventricular tachycardia. *J Pediatr* 94:144–146, 1979.

58. Porter CJ, Gillette PC, Garson A, et al: Effects of verapamil on supraventricular tachycardia in children. *Am J Cardiol* 48:497–491, 1981.

59. Kaminer SJ, Gelband H: Pediatric cardiac electrophysiology. *Curr Opin Cardiol* 5:101–106, 1991.

60. Till J, Shinebourne EA, Rigby ML, et al: Efficacy and safety of adenosine in the treatment of supraventricular tachycardia in infants and children. *Br Heart J* 62:204–211, 1989.

61. Overholt ED, Rheuban KS, Gutgeshell HP, et al: Usefulness of adenosine for arrhythmias in infants and children. *Am J Cardiol* 61:336–340, 1988.

62. Porter CJ, Garson A, Gillettee PC: Verapamil: an effective calcium blocking agent for pediatric patients. *Pediatrics* 71:748–755, 1983.

63. Dick M, Scott WA, Serwer GS, Bromberg BI, Beckman RH, Rocchini AP, et al: Acute termination of supraventricular tachyarrhythmias in children by transesophageal atrial pacing. *Am J Cardiol* 61:925–927, 1988.

64. Grubb BP, Temesy-Armos P, Hahn H, Elliott L: External pacing for the termination of sustained supraventricular tachycardia in children. *Int J Cardiol* 28:159–162, 1990.

65. Fogel JM, Berg IJ, Gerber MA, et al: Racemic epinephrine in the treatment of croup: nebulization alone versus nebulization with intermittent positive pressure breathing. *J Pediatr* 101:1028–1031, 1982.

66. Gardner HG, Powell KR, Roden VJ, et al: The evaluation of racemic epinephrine in the treatment of infectious croup. *Pediatrics* 52:52–55, 1973.

67. Kepes ER, Martinez LR, Andrews IC, et al: Racemic epinephrine in postintubation laryngeal edema. *NY State J Med* 7:583–584, 1972.

68. McBride JT: Stridor in childhood. *J Fam Pract* 19:782–790, 1984.

69. Postma DS, Jones RO, Pillsbury HC: Severe hospitalized croup: treatment trends and prognosis. *Laryngoscope* 94:1170–1175, 1984.

70. Singer OP, Wilson WJ: Laryngotracheobronchitis: 2 years' experience with racemic epinephrine. *Can Med Assoc J* 115:132–134, 1976.

71. Westley CR, Cotton EK, Brooks JG: Nebulized racemic epinephrine by IPPB for the treatment of croup. *Am J Dis Child* 132:484–487, 1979.

72. Taussig LM, Castro O, Beaudry PH, et al: Treatment of laryngotracheobronchitis (croup). *Am J Dis Child* 129:790–793, 1975.

73. Downes JJ, Raphaely R: Pediatric intensive care. *Anesthesiology* 43:238–250, 1975.

74. Butler RR, Wise WC, Haluska PV, et al: Thromboxane and prostacyclin production during septic shock. *Adv Shock Res* 7:133–145, 1982.

75. Fukumori T, Tani E, Maeda Y, et al: Effects of selective inhibitor of thromboxane A_2 synthetase on experimental cerebral vasospasm. *Stroke* 15:306–311, 1984.

76. Short BL, Gardiner WM, Walker R, et al: Indomethacin improves survival in gram-negative sepsis. *Adv Shock Res* 6:27–36, 1981.

77. White BC, Wiegenstein JB, Winegar CD: Brain ischemic anoxia—mechanisms of injury. *JAMA* 251:1586–1590, 1984.

78. Danilowicz D, Rudolph AM, Hoffman JIE: Delayed closure of the ductus arteriosus in premature infants. *Pediatrics* 37:74–78, 1966.

79. Kitterman JA, Edmunds LH, Gregory GA: Patent ductus arteriosus in premature infants: incidence, relation of pulmonary disease and management. *N Engl J Med* 287:473–477, 1972.

80. Levin DL, Stanger P, Kitterman JA, et al: Congenital heart disease in low-birth-weight infants. *Circulation* 52:500–503, 1975.

81. Heymann MA, Rudolph AM, Silverman, NH: Closure of the ductus arteriosus in premature infants by inhibition of prostaglandin synthesis. *N Engl J Med* 295:530–533, 1976.

82. McCarthy JS, Zies LG, Gelband H: Age-dependent closure of the patent ductus arteriosus by indomethacin. *Pediatrics* 62:706–712, 1978.

83. Freed MD, Heymann MA, Lewis AB, et al: Prostaglandin E_1 in infants with ductus arteriosus-dependent congenital heart disease. *Circulation* 64:898–905, 1981.

84. Graham TP, Atwood GF, Boucek RJ: Pharmacologic dilatation of the ductus arteriosus with prostaglandin E_1 in infants with congenital heart disease. *South Med J* 72:1238–1241, 1978.

85. Heymann MA, Berman W, Rudolph AM, et al: Dilatation of the ductus arteriosus by prostaglandin E_1 in aortic arch abnormalities. *Circulation* 59:169–173, 1979.

86. Hiraishi S, Fujino N, Saito K, Oguchi K, Kadoi N, Agata Y, et al: Responsiveness of the ductus arteriosus to prostaglandin E_1 assessed by combined cross sectional and pulsed Doppler echocardiography. *Br Heart J* 62:140–147, 1988.

87. Coceani F, Olley PM: The response of the ductus arteriosus to prostaglandins. *Can J Physiol Pharmacol* 51:220–225, 1973.

88. Cole RB, Alman S, Aziz KU, et al: Prolonged prostaglandin E_1 infusion: histologic effects on the patent ductus arteriosus. *Pediatrics* 67:815–819, 1981.

89. Lewis AB, Freed MD, Heymann MA, et al: Side effects of therapy with prostaglandin E_1 in infants with critical congenital heart disease. *Circulation* 64:893–898, 1981.

90. Koren G, Butt W, Chinyanga H, et al: Post-operative morphine infusion in newborn infants: assessment of disposition characteristics and safety. *J Pediatr* 107:963–967, 1985.

91. Lynn AM, Opheim KE, Tyler DC: Morphine infusion after pediatric cardiac surgery. *Crit Care Med* 12:863–866, 1984.

92. Sonntag H, Larsen R, Hilfiker D, et al: Myocardial blood flow and oxygen consumption during high dose fentanyl anesthesia in patients with coronary artery disease. *Anesthesiology* 56:417–422, 1982.

93. Mather LE, Phillips GD: Opioids and adjuvants: principles of use. In Cousins MJ, Phillips GD (eds): *Acute Pain Management*. New York, Churchill Livingstone, 1986, pp 77–103.

94. Fragen RJ, Caldwell N: Lorazepam premedication—lack of recall and relief of anxiety. *Anesth Analg* 55:792–796, 1976.

95. Cook DR: Muscle relaxants in infants and children. *Anesth Analg* 60:335–343, 1981.

96. Cook DR, Fischer CG: Neuromuscular blocking effects of succinylcholine in infants and children. *Anaesthesia* 42:662–665, 1975.

97. Nugent SK, Laravuso R, Rogers MC: Pharmacology and use of muscle relaxants in infants and children. *J Pediatr* 94:481–487, 1979.

98. Levin DL, Heymann MA, Kitterman JA, et al: Persistent pulmonary hypertension of the newborn infant. *J Pediatr* 89:626–630, 1976.

99. Basta SJ, Ali HH, Savarese JJ, et al: Clinical pharmacology of atracurium besylate (BW 33A). *Anesth Analg* 61:723–729, 1982.

100. Cohenhour K, Gamble JW, Metzgar MT, et al: A composite general anesthesia for pediatric outpatients. *J Oral Surg* 36:594–598, 1978.

101. Carrel R: Ketamine: a general anesthetic for unmanageable ambulatory patients. *ASDC J Dent Child* 40:288–292, 1973.

102. White PF, Way WL, Trevor AJ: Ketamine—its pharmacology and therapeutic uses. *Anesthesiology* 56:119–136, 1982.

103. Schwartz DA, Horwitz LD: Effects of ketamine on left ventricular performance. *J Pharmacol Exp Ther* 194:410–414, 1975.

104. Waxman K, Shoemaker WC, Lippmann M: Cardiovascular effects of anesthetic induction with ketamine. *Anesth Analg* 59:355–358, 1980.

105. Meyers EF, Charles P: Prolonged adverse reactions to ketamine in children. *Anesthesiology* 49:39–40, 1978.

106. Aitkenhead AR, Willatts SM, Park GR, et al: Comparison of propofol and midazolam for sedation in critically ill patients. *Lancet* 11:704–709, 1989.

107. Harris CE, Grounds RM, Murray AM, et al: Propofol for long-term sedation in the intensive care unit. *Anaesthesia* 45:366–372, 1990.

108. Norreslet J, Wahlgreen C: Propofol infusion for sedation of children. *Crit Care Med* 18:890–892, 1990.

109. Farling PA, Johnston JR, Coppel DL: Propofol infusion for sedation of patients with head injury in intensive care. *Anaesthesia* 44:222–226, 1989.

110. Caravati EM, Bennett DL: Clonidine transdermal patch poisoning. *Ann Emerg Med* 17:175–176, 1988.

111. Sarnaik AP, Heidemann SM: Clonidine poisoning in children. *Crit Care Med* 18:618–620, 1990.

112. Fiser DH, Moss MM, Walker W: Critical care for clonidine poisoning in toddlers. *Crit Care Med* 18:1124–1128, 1990.

113. Anderson RJ, Hart GR, Crumpler CP, et al: Clonidine overdose: report of six cases and review of the literature. *Ann Emerg Med* 10:107–112, 1981.

114. Conner CS, Watanabe AS: Clonidine overdose: a review. *Am J Hosp Pharm* 36:906–911, 1979.

115. Hunyor SNB, Bradstock K, Somerville PJ, et al: Clonidine overdose. *Br Med J* 4:23, 1975.

116. Banner W, Lund ME, Clawson L: Failure of naloxone to reverse clonidine toxic effect. *Am J Dis Child* 137:1170–1171, 1983.

117. Mendoza JE, Medalie M: Clonidine poisoning with marked hypotension in a 2 year old child. *Clin Pediatr* 18:123–127, 1979.

118. Schieber RA, Kaufman ND: Use of tolazoline in massive clonidine poisoning. *Am J Dis Child* 135:77–78, 1981.

119. Yagupsky P, Gorodischer R: Massive clonidine ingestion with hypertension in a 9-month-old infant. *Pediatrics* 72:500–502, 1983.

120. Pai GS, Lipsitz DJ: Clonidine poisoning. *Pediatrics* 58:749–750, 1976.

121. Farsang C, Kunos G: Naloxone reverses the antihypertensive effect of clonidine. *Br J Pharmacol* 67:161–164, 1979.

122. Curtis MT, Lefer AM: Protective actions of naloxone in hemorrhagic shock. *Am J Physiol* 239:H415–H421, 1980.

123. Faden AI, Holaday JW: Opiate antagonists: a role in the treatment of hypovolemic shock. *Science* 205:317–318, 1979.

124. Holaday JW, Faden AI: Naloxone acts at central opiate receptors to reverse hypotension, hypothermia and hypoventilation in spinal shock. *Brain Res* 189:295–300, 1980.

125. Greenblatt DJ, Allen MD, Koch-Weser J: Accidental iron poisoning in childhood. *Clin Pediatr* 15:835–838, 1976.

126. Henretig FM, Karl SR, Weintraub WH: Severe iron poisoning treated with enteral and intravenous deferoxamine. *Ann Emerg Med* 12:305–309, 1983.

127. Krenzelok EP, Hoff JV: Accidental childhood iron poisoning: a problem of marketing and labeling. *Pediatrics* 63:591–596, 1979.

128. Reynolds LG, Kelin M: Iron poisoning—a preventable hazard of childhood. *S Afr Med J* 67:680–683, 1985.

129. Banner W, Tong TG: Iron poisoning. *Pediatr Clin North Am* 33:393–409, 1986.

130. Doolin EJ, Drueck C: Fatal iron intoxication in an adult. *J Trauma* 20:518–522, 1980.

131. Movassaghi N, Purugganan MD, Leikin S: Comparison of exchange transfusion and deferoxamine in the treatment of acute iron poisoning. *J Pediatr* 75:604–698, 1969.

132. Reissman KR, Coleman TJ: Acute intestinal iron intoxication. II. Metabolic, respiratory and circulatory effects of absorbed iron salts. *Blood* 10:45–51, 1955.

133. Tenenbein M, Israels SJ: Early coagulopathy in severe iron poisoning. *J Pediatr* 113:695–697, 1988.

134. Filpi RG, Majd M, LoPresti JM: Reversible gastric stricture following iron ingestion. *South Med J* 66:845–846, 1973.

135. Gandhi RK, Robarts FH: Hour-glass stricture of the stomach and pyloric stenosis due to ferrous sulfate poisoning. *Br J Surg* 49:613–617, 1962.

136. Einhorn AH: Iron poisoning. In Rudolph AM (ed): *Pediatrics*, ed 15. New York, Appleton-Century-Crofts, 1977, pp 790–793.

137. Anon: Iron. In Rumack BH (ed): *Poisindex*. Englewood, CO, Micromedex, 1980.

138. Czajka PA, Konrad JD, Duffy JP: Iron poisoning: an in vitro comparison of bicarbonate and phosphate lavage solution. *J Pediatr* 98:491–494, 1981.

139. Geffner ME, Opas LM: Phosphate poisoning complicating treatment for iron ingestion. *Am J Dis Child* 134:509–510, 1980.

140. Benjamin BI, Cortell S, Conrad ME: Bicarbonate-induced iron complexes and iron absorption: one effect of pancreatic secretions. *Gastroenterology* 53:389–396, 1967.

141. Koren G, Bentur Y, Strong D, et al: Acute changes in renal function associated with deferoxamine therapy. *Am J Dis Child* 143:1077–1080, 1989.

142. McGuigan MA, Lovejoy FH, Marino SK, et al: Qualitative deferoxamine color test for iron ingestion. *J Pediatr* 94:940–942, 1979.

143. Gordon GS, Ambruso DR, Robinson WA, Githens JH: Intranasal administration of deferoxamine to iron overloaded patients. *Am J Med Sci* 297:280–284, 1989.

144. Hedlund BE, Hallaway PE, Mahoney JR: High molecular weight forms of deferoxamine: novel therapeutic agents for treatment of iron-mediated tissue injury. *Adv Exp Med Biol* 264:235–246, 1990.

145. Mahoney JR, Hallaway PE, Hedlund BE, Ecton JW: Acute iron poisoning—rescue with macromolecular chelators. *J Clin Invest* 84:1362–1366, 1989.

146. Foxford R, Goldfrank L: Gastrotomy—a surgical approach to iron overdose. *Ann Emerg Med* 14:1223–1226, 1985.

147. Banner W, Vernon DD, Ward RM, et al: Continuous arteriovenous hemofiltration in experimental iron intoxication. *Crit Care Med* 17:1187–1190, 1989.

148. Sofer S, Tal A, Shahak E: Carbamate and organophosphate poisoning in early childhood. *Pediatr Emerg Care* 5:222–225, 1989.

149. Zwiener RJ, Ginsbury CM: Organophosphate and carbamate poisoning in infants and children. *Pediatrics* 81:121–126, 1988.

150. Kass R, Kochar G, Lippman M: Adult respiratory distress syndrome from organophosphate poisoning. *Am J Emerg Med* 9:32–33, 1991.

151. Joubert J, Joubert PH: Chorea and psychiatric changes in organophosphate poisoning. *S Afr Med J* 74:32–34, 1988.

152. Senanayake N, Karalliedde L: Neurotoxic effects of organophosphorus insecticides: an intermediate syndrome. *N Engl J Med* 316:761–763, 1987.

153. Karademir M, Erturk F, Kocak R: Two cases of organophosphate poisoning with development of intermediate syndrome. *Hum Exp Toxicol* 9:187–189, 1990.

154. Einhorn AH: Organophosphate insecticide poisoning. In Rudolph AM (ed): *Pediatrics*, ed 15. New York, Appleton-Century-Crofts, 1977, pp 793–795.

155. Mortensen ML: Management of acute childhood poisonings caused by selected insecticides and herbicides. *Pediatr Clin North Am* 33:421–425, 1986.

156. Farrar HC, Wells TG, Kearns GL: Use of continuous infusion of pralidoxime for treatment of organophosphate poisoning in children. *J Pediatr* 116:658–661, 1990.

157. Taylor P: Anticholinesterase agents. In Gilman AG, Goodman LS, Gilman A (eds): *The Pharmacologic Basis of Therapeutics*, ed 6. New York, Macmillan, 1980, pp 100–119, 1980.

158. Samani SM, Dube SN: Physostigmine—an overview as pretreatment drug for organophosphate intoxication. *Int J Clin Pharmacol Ther Toxicol* 27:367–387, 1989.

159. Besser R, Vogt T, Gutmann L: Pancuronium improves the neuromuscular transmission defect of human organophosphate intoxication. *Neurology* 40:1275–1277, 1990.

CHAPTER 65

Calcium and Calcium Antagonists in Shock and Ischemia

DIANA S. MALCOLM, Ph.D.

One of the primary characteristics of the shock syndrome in humans is a profound alteration of the physiologic regulation of the circulation, resulting in inadequate tissue oxygenation, anaerobic metabolism, organ failure, and death. Prolonged hemorrhage, cardiac failure, trauma, and sepsis are a few of the many recognized causes of shock. Septic shock develops in approximately 25% of the estimated 330,000 Gram-negative bacteremias that occur in the U.S. each year (1). Gram-negative sepsis is associated with an overall 50% mortality, even when treated under optimal situations (2). When further complicated by renal or respiratory failure, the mortality rate approaches 90 to 100% (3). Most of these patients die from progressive multiorgan failure, which is thought to result from the release of toxic substances from the infecting organisms (e.g., endotoxin), the release of secondary endogenous mediators, and altered metabolic status, resulting in progressive tissue ischemia.

Current clinical management of circulatory shock involves aggressive ventilatory support, fluid resuscitation, and pharmacotherapy directed at maintaining blood pressure and cardiac output. Despite these medical interventions and the availability of new and effective antibiotics, the mortality rate for septic shock has remained virtually unchanged (4). It is clear that new pharmacologic strategies, based on a better knowledge and understanding of the pathophysiologic mechanisms involved in shock, are necessary for more effective treatment. The purpose of this chapter is to review the laboratory and clinical evidence suggesting that calcium (Ca) blockers may be beneficial in the treatment of shock based on the hypothesis

that intracellular Ca overload plays an important part in the pathophysiology of ischemic injury in shock.

ROLE OF CALCIUM IN THE PATHOPHYSIOLOGY OF SHOCK

Calcium plays a critical role as a modulator and initiator of many essential cellular functions during physiologic or pathophysiologic conditions. Cellular responses to drugs, hormones, neurotransmitters, and other biologic messengers include the activation of specific receptors that in turn alter Ca channels or couple to second-messenger systems such as cyclic AMP and phosphatidylinositol. These major intracellular second messengers further modify biochemical events within the cell, in part through alteration of intracellular Ca availability. Recently, much attention has focused on the role of Ca in mediating or propagating the ischemic cell injury that occurs during shock. In order to better understand the possible mechanisms by which Ca may alter cellular function, it may be helpful to review the major steps involved in the regulation of cellular Ca homeostasis.

The vast majority of Ca in the circulation is bound to proteins such as albumin. However, it is the free (ionized) Ca^{2+} in equilibrium with the bound Ca, that provides the biologically functional Ca pool. In unstimulated cardiac and smooth muscle cells, free cytosolic Ca^{2+} concentrations range between 0.05 and 0.5 μmol, whereas Ca^{2+} concentrations in the extracellular milieu are approximately 1–5 μmol. Thus, the concentration gradient for free Ca^{2+} across the cell membrane is approximately 1 to 10,000 (intracellular to extracellular). The maintenance of this gradient is essential for cell viability since excessive increases in intracellular Ca can be destructive to the cell. The Ca gradient across the cell is maintained primarily by (*a*) the cell membrane, which is relatively impermeable to Ca; (*b*) Ca pumps within the membrane (CaATPase, Ca-sodium exchange); and (*c*) cellular organelles (sarco(endo)plasmic reticulum and mitochondria) that remove Ca from the cytosol. Many of these processes require a constant supply of energy.

In shock or other ischemic disorders, Ca homeostasis is disrupted, usually resulting in an abnormal accumulation of Ca within the cell (5–8). This accumulation of cytosolic Ca can be a consequence of either an increase in cell membrane Ca permeability and/or a decrease in activity of the cellular pumps or cellular organelles that sequester or remove Ca from the cell (e.g., as a result of ATP depletion). In septic shock, infecting agents may act directly on these Ca systems or indirectly, such as through the release of cytokines, to increase intracellular Ca levels, since endotoxin itself does not appear to alter calcium concentration.

An uncontrolled increase in cystolic Ca can disrupt a number of intracellular processes (9), which include excitation-contraction coupling, endocytosis and exocytosis, and enzyme activation. These processes may further exacerbate the hemodynamic and metabolic insufficiencies underlying the shock syndrome. For example, Ca-induced smooth muscle contraction in blood vessels (vasoconstriction) may produce or worsen ischemia by decreasing nutrient blood flow to tissues and cells. Among the intracellular mechanisms that may be involved, phospholipase activation (by Ca) can produce membrane damage and liberate free fatty acids (10). Furthermore, free fatty acid elevations can stimulate the production of free radicals and increase the production of platelet-activating factor and eicosanoids, including thromboxanes, prostacyclins, and leukotrienes (10). Some of these toxic products may cause additional cellular damage and a further disruption of Ca homeostasis. Increases in cytosolic Ca may also activate proteases, nucleases, and Ca-dependent ATPases and uncouple oxidative phosphorylation (11–13). Thus, although Ca is essential for cellular function, excessive increases in intracellular Ca may also damage the cell. It remains to be determined whether the alterations in Ca fluxes leading to intracellular Ca overload are a cause for the cellular metabolic derangements observed in shock or whether these changes are a result of other pathophysiologic processes occurring in shock.

RATIONALE FOR USING CALCIUM ANTAGONISTS IN SHOCK THERAPY

Figure 65.1 illustrates a proposed scheme of the pathophysiologic events occurring during sepsis that ultimately lead to the irreversible stages of septic shock (multiorgan failure). A similar scheme of events may occur during other forms of circulatory shock or ischemic disorders. Although it is unknown whether ischemia is a primary (or causative) effect or a secondary consequence of shock, it is known that prolonged ischemia leads to hemodynamic and metabolic derangements that are detrimental to the cell. These derangements include

decreased tissue oxygenation, decreased ATP levels, and accumulation of cellular metabolic products resulting in metabolic acidosis. As described above, an increase in cell membrane permeability can result in an influx of Ca into the cell, resulting in an intracellular Ca overload. Increased cytosolic Ca activates a host of intracellular processes that, if left unchecked, can lead to cellular destruction and eventual organ dysfunction and death. Thus, intracellular Ca accumulation or overload may be thought of as a common pathway for ischemic injury in shock. Based on the hypothesis that intracellular Ca overload is a mediator for cellular dysfunction in shock, it would be reasonable to assume that Ca-antagonists may prevent Ca accumulation within the cell and thus preserve cell/organ function and ultimately improve outcome.

A variety of pharmacological agents are currently available that may be useful in preventing intracellular Ca overload during shock. As a group, these drugs may be classified as Ca "antagonists." A Ca-antagonist may be loosely defined as a drug that alters the cellular action of Ca by inhibiting its entry and/or release or by interfering with one of its intracellular actions. Specifically, Ca-antagonists may be divided into at least three categories: (*a*) Ca-chelators (e.g., Ethylene Glycol-bis (β-amino-ethyl ether) N,N,N′,N′-tetraacetic acid (EGTA)), which lower circulating extracellular Ca levels and thus decrease Ca availability for entry into cells; (*b*) Ca channel blockers (e.g., verapamil, nifedipine, diltiazem), which block Ca entry into cells by interacting with Ca-specific channels (3); and (*c*) intracellular Ca-antagonists, which either inhibit sarcoplasmic reticular release of Ca (e.g., dantrolene) or inhibit intracellular Ca action (e.g., calmodulin antagonists).

A wide body of evidence supports the use of Ca-blockers in the treatment of myocardial ischemic disorders, and Ca-blockers are currently used for this purpose. Since tissue ischemia is also a hallmark of the shock syndrome, Ca-blockers may be useful in the treatment of shock. In addition, if intracellular Ca overload is important in the etiology of shock, Ca-blockers may afford additional protection. Since Ca blockers to date have not been tested clinically in the treatment of shock, this chapter focuses on the available laboratory data that support a role for Ca-blockers in the treatment of shock.

EFFECTS OF CALCIUM ANTAGONISTS IN ISCHEMIC DISORDERS

Ca-antagonists have been used extensively (and successfully) in the treatment of cardiac arrhythmias, myocardial ischemic syndromes, and systemic hypertension. In particular, extensive laboratory and clinical evidence has accumulated to suggest that Ca-antagonists may be useful in the treatment of myocardial infarction (14). In the ischemic heart, the Ca-antagonists verapamil and nifedipine have been shown to preserve high-energy phosphate compounds (ATP), improve cardiac function, improve myocardial perfusion, preserve normal metabolic activity, reduce infarct size, decrease oxygen demand, prevent intracellular Ca accumulation, and improve survival (15–20). Ca-blockers may afford myocardial protection from ischemia by (*a*) preventing Ca entry and cellular overload, (*b*) vasodilating coronary and systemic vessels, and/or (*c*) decreasing myocardial contraction and oxygen demands. In contrast, agents that increase Ca entry into the cell or

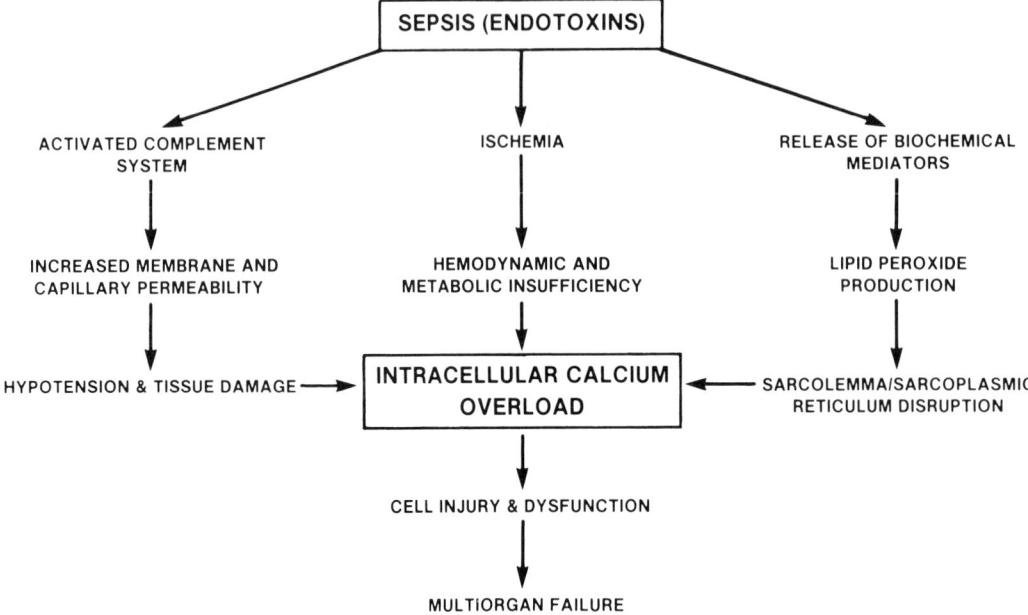

Figure 65.1. A proposed scheme of the pathophysiological events occurring during sepsis and leading to multiorgan failure (see text).

elevate extracellular Ca levels during ischemia have been shown to result in elevated myocardial muscle resting tensions and to exacerbate myocardial injury (6). Together, these findings support the hypothesis that elevated intracellular Ca levels contribute to myocardial cell necrosis during low perfusion states.

There is also evidence that Ca may be responsible for producing vasospasm and cellular dysfunction following cerebral ischemia. Although evidence to the contrary exists (21), Ca channel antagonists have been shown to improve cerebral tissue oxygenation, reduce cerebral vasospasm, and improve neurological recovery and survival in cats and rats following cerebral embolization (22, 23). Other research has shown that Ca channel antagonists also improve cerebral perfusion and neurological recovery following cardiac arrest (24–26).

Similar evidence is accumulating to suggest that Ca is a pathogenic mediator of cellular injury during ischemia in the kidney, liver, and skeletal muscle. In the kidney, verapamil treatment preserves inulin clearance and renal blood flow, protects against tubular necrosis, and prevents intracellular Ca accumulation following norepinephrine infusion (27, 28) and renal artery occlusion (29). Incubation of hepatocytes with Ca-free solutions has been shown to protect the cells against death caused by anoxia and hepatotoxins (8). Other studies show that elevated intracellular Ca levels can cause major ultrastructural damage to mitochondria and myofilaments within skeletal muscle (30, 31).

SPECIFIC EFFECTS OF CALCIUM ANTAGONISTS IN EXPERIMENTAL MODELS OF SHOCK

ENDOTOXIC AND SEPTIC SHOCK

As discussed in the preceding sections, Gram-negative bacteria are the most common cause of sepsis and septic shock,

and bacterial lipopolysaccharides (endotoxins) are considered to be primary factors in the development of the shock state (32). Like other shock syndromes, endotoxic shock is characterized by decreased organ perfusion leading to a decrease in cellular oxygen supply and nutrient delivery, with eventual cellular injury and death. Intracellular Ca overload has been postulated to be a common pathway for cellular injury and death in experimental endotoxic shock.

The success of Ca-blocker use in shock is dependent on (*a*) the presence of elevated intracellular Ca, which is associated with cellular dysfunction, and (*b*) the ability of Ca-blockers to prevent/reverse this increase in intracellular Ca, with a resultant improvement in cellular function and overall survival.

There are few published reports examining the effects of Ca-blockers on intracellular Ca regulation in endotoxic shock. The initial report from the laboratory of Lee and Lum (33) failed to show an increase in total tissue Ca in response to endotoxin administration. Moreover, they reported no change or a decrease in total tissue or mitochondrial Ca in various tissue organs of endotoxin-treated rats (33). In contrast, Sayeed and Maitra (34) reported a significant rise in cytosolic Ca in the livers of endotoxemic rats. Furthermore, Dudley, Maitra, and Sayeed (35) reported an increase in the fast exchangeable pool of intracellular Ca, but not in total tissue (skeletal muscle) Ca, in endotoxin-treated animals as compared with controls. Their findings emphasize the possibility that accumulations of Ca can occur in discrete intracellular compartments without the evidence of changes in total tissue calcium.

Since Lee and Lum (33) did not observe an increase in tissue Ca content, they did not determine the effects of Ca channel blockers on total Ca content in their study. They did report a dose-dependent reduction in mortality in endotoxemic animals treated with various Ca-blockers and concluded that this protection from mortality was probably not related to the prevention of Ca overload. In all published reports from Dr. Sayeed's laboratory, diltiazem pretreatment attenuated the endotoxin-induced rise in intracellular Ca in both liver and skeletal muscle. Furthermore, they reported that endotoxin inhibits the release of Ca from the endoplasmic reticulum when intracellular concentrations of Ca are high (34). They postulated that this attenuation of intracellular Ca mobilization may adversely affect cellular glucose production, which is Ca dependent. Importantly, diltiazem pretreatment restored intracellular Ca mobilization in the presence of endotoxin, suggesting that Ca-blockers may also improve the resultant carbohydrate dyshomeostasis seen in endotoxic shock.

A recent clinical study has shown that free intracellular Ca is elevated in lymphocytes from septic patients as compared with those from nonseptic critically ill patients or healthy human volunteers (36). Furthermore, circulating mononuclear cells obtained from septic patients presenting with multiorgan failure also demonstrated marked elevations in intracellular Ca levels (37). Further studies are needed to determine which tissues, cells, and organelles are affected by Ca overload and whether multiorgan failure is a result or cause of intracellular Ca overload. Finally, studies are needed to determine whether the benefit derived from Ca-blocker treatment is related to the reversal or prevention of Ca accumulation and subsequent improvement in organ function and survival.

On the other hand, a small but growing body of laboratory data suggests that Ca-blocker therapy is beneficial in the treatment of experimental shock. A metaanalysis of the data from prospective, randomized, controlled animals models of sepsis demonstrated that Ca-antagonist treatment afforded significant improvement in survival as compared with no treatment (38). Overall, treatment with a Ca-antagonist was associated with a survival rate 1.32 times that of the untreated groups ($P \leq 0.001$) (38). The most striking observation from laboratory animal studies is that in all (33, 39–42) but one reported case (43), survival was significantly improved. In the one study that did not demonstrate a benefit from Ca-blocker therapy, the animal number was too small for statistical significance (43), and although Ca-blocker therapy did not improve survival, it had no detrimental effects in the study. In several reported studies, Ca-blocker therapy more than doubled survival. Bosson et al (39) reported 7-day survival (which they consider permanent survival) to be 62% in treated dogs vs. 7% in control animals. Since these animals were given supportive measures including additional fluids throughout the experimental period (4 hr), as would be the case in a clinical setting, the encouraging findings from this study warrant further clinical study. Although it has been shown that pretreatment with Ca-blockers is more effective in improving survival than posttreatment (33), this does not necessarily suggest that Ca-blockers would be of limited value clinically. In these laboratory experiments, endotoxin was administered as a single lethal bolus; in contrast, the endotoxemia associated with clinical Gram-negative septicemia would ordinarily be expected to accumulate to a lethal level at a comparatively slow rate. Under the latter circumstances, Ca-blockers theoretically could be lifesaving.

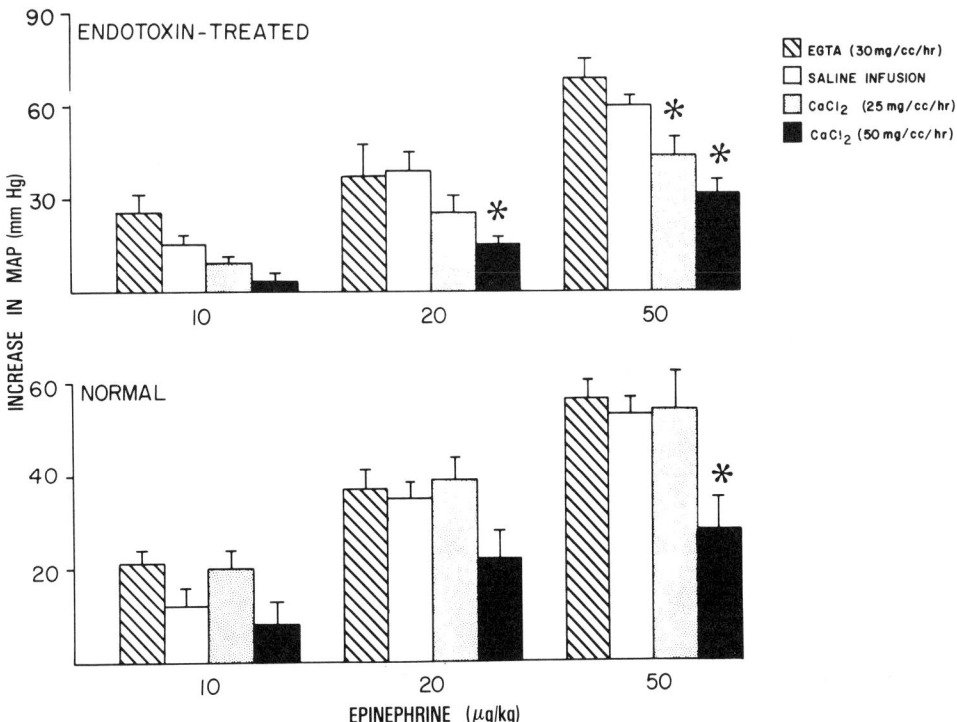

Figure 65.2. Effects of hypocalcemia and hypercalcemia on epinephrine-induced increases in mean arterial pressure (MAP) in normal and endotoxin-treated rats. Rats ($n = 8$) were rendered hypocalcemic (with EGTA infusion) or hypercalcemic (with $CaCl_2$ infusion) and then subjected to bolus injection of *Escherichia coli* endotoxin (5 mg/kg i.v.) or saline (normal group). Control rats were infused with saline (1 ml/hr i.v.). Sixty minutes postendotoxin or saline, rats were injected with incremental bolus doses of epinephrine (10, 20, 50 μg/kg i.v.) approximately 15 minutes apart. $CaCl_2$ infusions (50 mg/cc/hr) blunted epinephrine's pressor effects in normal and endotoxemic rats. EGTA infusions did not alter epinephrine's pressor effects. (* = $P < 0.05$.)

Other beneficial effects of Ca-blocker therapy during septic/endotoxic shock include improvements in mean arterial pressure (40, 41, 43), systemic vascular resistance (39, 44), cardiac output (43, 44), cardiac index (39), pulmonary artery pressure (39), left ventricular stroke volume (39), and organ blood flow (43). Ca-blocker therapy was also associated with a decrease in the incidence of disseminated intravascular coagulation (45) and the absence of intestinal mucosal injury following bacteremic shock (43). Metabolic indices were also improved. Not all of the reported salutary effects of Ca-blockers may be attributed to their Ca-blocking properties. It is likely that the known vasodilatory effects of Ca-blockers may have played an important role in the improved organ function and survival in some animals.

In addition to studies using Ca-antagonists, other reports suggest a significant role for Ca in the pathophysiology of shock. The author and co-workers were among the first to show that calcium chloride ($CaCl_2$) infusions (producing hypercalcemia) are detrimental in shock (38, 46, 47). $CaCl_2$ (50 mg/cc/hr i.v.) infusions elevated ionized circulating Ca levels by 100% and not only blunted epinephrine's pressor effects (Fig. 65.2) but also significantly increased mortality in endotoxemic rats (Fig. 65.3). In contrast, lowering circulating Ca levels by the intravenous administration of a chelator (EGTA) improved survival in endotoxic shock (Fig. 65.3) and did not impair epinephrine's pressor actions (Fig. 65.2) (47). Interestingly, the author and colleagues observed that verapamil injection (2.5 mg/kg i.v.) also produced a decrease in circulating ionized Ca^{2+} levels (40). Confirming the results of others (39), the authors were able to demonstrate that verapamil improved mean arterial pressure (Fig. 65.4) and increased 24-hour survival from 50% to 90% (40). Together, these findings suggest that lowering circulating Ca levels (with EGTA) or blocking its entry into cells (with verapamil) may protect cells from Ca overload and thus improve the shock state. Obviously, in a syndrome as complex as shock and with a class of drugs with several different modes of action, more studies are needed to determine the precise mechanism(s) involved in the protective effects of Ca antagonists in shock. To date, all laboratory findings strongly suggest that Ca-blocker therapy is beneficial in the treatment of shock, whether it results from endotoxemia or bacteremia. In light of the reported benefits of Ca-blockers on survival from septic/endotoxic shock studies, and the lack of reported detrimental effects associated with Ca-blocker use, clinical trials should be encouraged. It is possible that Ca-blockers may become promising adjunctive agents in the treatment of septic shock.

HEMORRHAGIC SHOCK

During the course of hemorrhagic shock, there is a significant degree of ischemic injury to many organs, including the heart, kidney, brain, and liver. Since Ca-antagonists have been shown to decrease ischemic damage and improve function in these organs, theoretically they should be of benefit in the treatment of hemorrhagic shock. Indeed, it has been shown by Hackel et al (48) that verapamil infusions in hemorrhaged dogs partially or completely prevented the development of ventricular subendocardial hemorrhage and necrosis and resulted in less intestinal mucosal hemorrhage. In these studies, verapamil-treated animals also had a significantly higher survival rate. Others have confirmed and extended these findings to demonstrate that verapamil treatment significantly improves mean arterial pressure and coronary blood flow, improves cardiac index, and decreases heart rate and total peripheral resistance during the course of hemorrhagic shock (15, 49, 50).

Although the majority of hemorrhagic shock studies employ verapamil, other Ca-blockers have been shown to be beneficial. Felodipine, a dihydropyridine Ca-antagonist, has been shown to restore renal and mesenteric blood flow (51) and to prevent renal failure (52) in dogs subjected to lethal hemorrhage. Pretreatment or posttreatment with felodipine was equally effective in improving survival and restoring mean arterial pressure in severely hemorrhaged rats (53). In addition

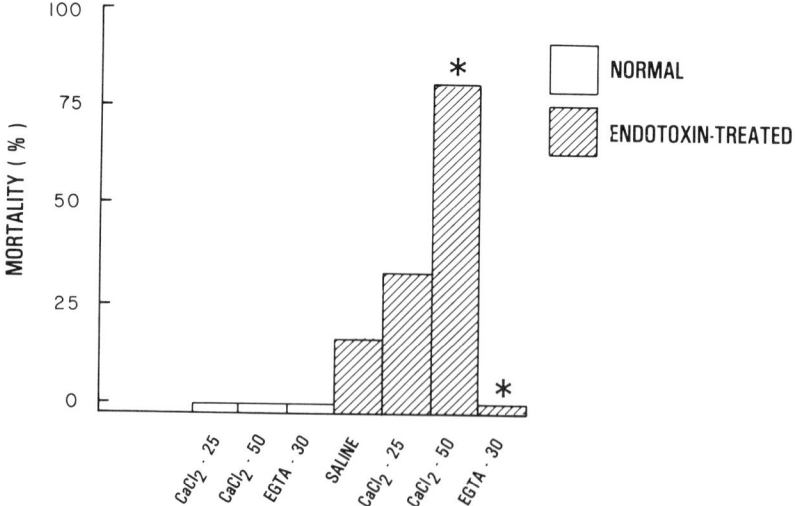

Figure 65.3. Effects of $CaCl_2$ and EGTA infusions on endotoxin mortality. Rats ($n = 8$) were infused with saline, $CaCl_2$, or EGTA and 30 minutes later injected with either saline (normals) or endotoxin (5 mg/kg i.v.). Animals were infused a total of 2 hours. Mortality was determined 24 hours postendotoxin injection. $CaCl_2$ infusions (50 mg/cc/hr) significantly increased endotoxin mortality, whereas EGTA infusions (30 mg/cc/hr) significantly decreased endotoxin mortality. (* = $P < 0.05$.)

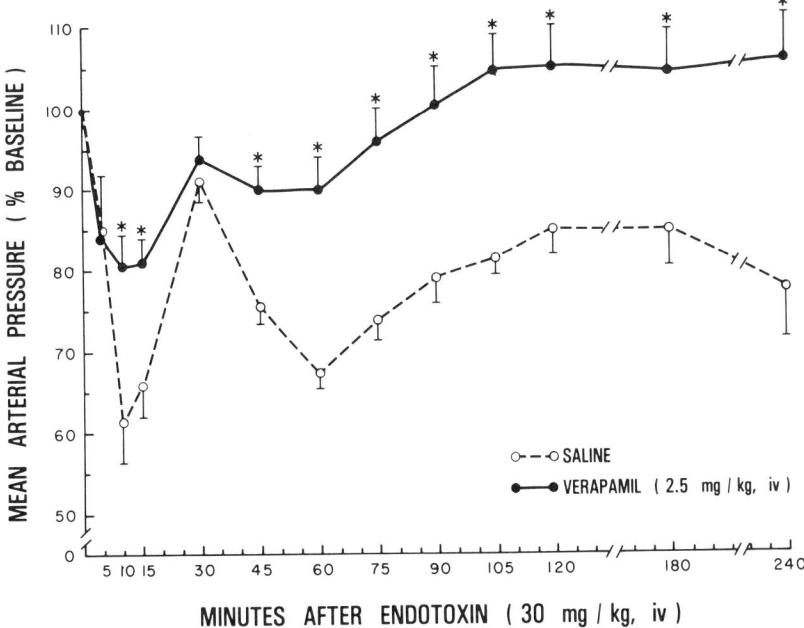

Figure 65.4. Effects of verapamil pretreatment on hemodynamic responses during endotoxic shock in rats. Verapamil pretreatment (2.5 mg/kg i.v., 15 minutes) significantly (* = $P < 0.05$) improved mean arterial pressure throughout the 4 hours postendotoxin (30 mg/kg i.v.) except at the 30-minute time point.

to improving survival, diltiazem has been shown to attenuate the hyperglycemic and tachycardic responses to hemorrhagic shock (54). Nitrendipine has also been reported to possess beneficial effects in hemorrhagic shock (55).

Not only have cardiovascular function, myocardial histology, and overall survival been shown to be improved by Ca-blockers, but it has also been documented that subcellular function is protected during the course of shock. Hess and Greenfield (56) have demonstrated a significant depression of Ca uptake by the sarcoplasmic reticulum and an uncoupling of Ca transport from ATP hydrolysis in the myocardium during hemorrhagic shock. In verapamil-treated animals, Ca uptake by the sarcoplasmic reticulum was not suppressed, and excitation-contraction remained tightly coupled. Although intracellular Ca levels were not measured in these studies, the observation that sarcoplasmic reticular Ca uptake was depressed suggests that intracellular Ca levels consequently were increased above normal in the untreated shocked animals. This finding would support the hypothesis that (a) intracellular Ca overload occurs during hemorrhagic shock and (b) that a defect in the sarcoplasmic reticulum may be a potential site or cause for the Ca overload. Thus, verapamil's beneficial effects in shock and ischemia may result from a stabilization of the sarcoplasmic reticulum with a subsequent decrease in intracellular Ca overload, resulting in improvement of myocardial function and overall survival (56).

In addition to stabilization of the sarcoplasmic reticulum, other mechanism(s) by which Ca-antagonists improve outcome in hemorrhagic shock may be involved. Some researchers have suggested that the beneficial effects of verapamil are not mediated by calcium channel blockade per se, but by unknown metabolic effects that preserve ATP (57). In addition, the ability of verapamil to mitigate myocardial and intestinal mucosal injury cannot be overlooked as a possible contributor

to the overall increase in survival observed in verapamil-treated animals. The prominent effects of verapamil and other Ca-antagonists on peripheral vascular smooth muscle may also play a significant role in improving shock outcome. Ca channel antagonists have a well-documented effect on Ca influx in vascular smooth muscle and are capable of directly producing peripheral and coronary artery vasodilation, reducing left ventricular afterload and improving cardiac output (56). Other researchers have shown that verapamil inhibits the development of portal hypertension and lowers circulating renin levels (suggesting improved renal perfusion) during the course of hemorrhagic shock (58).

SUMMARY

Ca plays a critical role as a modulator and initiator of many essential cellular functions during physiological or pathophysiological conditions. In shock and other ischemic disorders, Ca homeostasis is disrupted, usually resulting in an abnormal accumulation of Ca within the cell. Increased cytosolic Ca activates a host of intracellular processes that can lead to cellular destruction and eventual dysfunction and death. Based on the hypothesis that intracellular Ca overload is a mediator for cellular dysfunction in shock, the use of Ca channel blockers has been proposed to prevent Ca accumulation within the cell and thus preserve cell/organ function and ultimately improve outcome.

Ca channel blockers have been used extensively in the treatment of myocardial ischemic diseases. In the ischemic heart, Ca-blockers have been shown to prevent intracellular Ca accumulation, preserve normal metabolic activity, and improve cardiac function and survival. Similarly, Ca-blockers have been shown to have protective effects in ischemic brain, kidney, liver, and skeletal muscle.

Overwhelming evidence from laboratory studies suggests that Ca-blocker therapy is beneficial in the treatment of shock. The most striking observation is that Ca-blockers improve survival, in some cases even double survival, in shock. Other beneficial effects of Ca-blocker therapy include improvement in cardiovascular function and organ blood flow and prevention of ischemic tissue injury in septic shock. Conversely, infusion of CaCl has been shown to be detrimental in septic shock.

It remains to be determined whether intracellular Ca overload does indeed occur in the shock state and whether the benefit derived from Ca-blocker therapy is related to the reversal or prevention of Ca accumulation. It is likely that the known vasodilatory effects of Ca-blockers may have played an important role in improving organ function and survival in some animals. It also remains to be determined which Ca-blockers are the treatment of choice—preferably, a Ca-blocker with the least hypotensive effect.

To date, all laboratory findings strongly suggest that Ca-blocker therapy is beneficial in the treatment of shock, whether it results from endotoxemia, bacteremia, or hemorrhage. In light of the reported benefits of Ca-blocker therapy, their successful use in the treatment of ischemic diseases, and their well-documented clinical safety, clinical trials of Ca-blockers in the treatment of shock are warranted and long overdue. It is possible that, pending successful clinical testing, Ca-blockers may provide an important adjunctive strategy in the treatment of shock.

REFERENCES

1. Kreger BE, Craven DE, McCabe WR: Gram-negative bacteremia—re-evaluation of clinical features and treatment of 612 patients. *Am J Med* 68:344–355, 1980.
2. National Center of Health Statistics: Advance report, final mortality statistics. In *Monthly Vital Statistics Report* 33(3) (suppl), DHHS (PHS)84-1120, 1981.
3. Cohen CJ, Janis RA, Taylor DG, et al: Where do calcium antagonists act? In Opie LH (ed): *Calcium Antagonist and Cardiovascular Disease*. Raven Press, New York, pp 271–282, 1984.
4. Hale DJ, Robinson JA, Loeb HS, et al: Pathophysiology of endotoxin shock in man. In Proctor RA (ed): *Handbook of Endotoxin*, vol 4, *Clinical Aspects of Endotoxin Shock*. Elsevier Science Publishers, Amsterdam, pp 1–15, 1986.
5. Katz AM, Reuter H: Cellular calcium and cardiac cell death. *Am J Cardiol* 44:188-190, 1979.
6. Nayler WG, Poole-Wilson PA, Williams A: Hypoxia and calcium. *J Mol Cell Cardiol* 11:683–706, 1979.
7. Okuno F, Orrego H, Israel Y: Calcium requirements for anoxic liver injury. *Res Commun Chem Pathol Pharmacol* 39:437–444, 1983.
8. Schanne FAX, Kane AB, Young EE, et al: Calcium dependent toxic cell death: a final common pathway. *Science* 206:700–702, 1979.
9. Cheung JY, Bonventre JV, Malis CP, et al: Calcium and ischemic injury. *N Engl J Med* 314:1670–1676, 1986.
10. White BC, Winegar CD, Wilson RF, et al: Possible role of calcium blockers in cerebral resuscitation: a review of the literature and synthesis for future studies. *Crit Care Med* 11:202–207, 1983.
11. Carafoil E, Crampton M: Calcium ions and mitochondria. *Symp Soc Exp Biol* 30:89–115, 1976.
12. Lehninger AL: Mitochondria and calcium transport. *Biochem J* 119:129–138, 1970.
13. Villabobo A, Lehninger AL: Inhibition of oxidative phosphorylation in ascites tumor mitochondria and cells by intramitochondrial calcium. *J Biol Chem* 255:2457–2464, 1980.
14. Urthaler F: Review: role of calcium channel blockers in clinical medicine. *Am J Med Sci* 29:217–230, 1986.
15. Hess ML, Mahany TM, Greenfield LJ: Calcium channel blockers in shock. In Lefer AM, Schumer W (Eds): *Molecular and Cellular Aspects of Shock and Trauma*. Alan R. Liss, New York, pp 271–282, 1983.
16. Nayler WG, Ferrari R, Williams A: Protective effect of pretreatment with verapamil, nifedipine, and propranolol on mitochondrial function in the ischemic and reperfused myocardium. *Am J Cardiol* 46:242–248, 1980.
17. Reimer KA, Lowe JE, Jennings RB: Effect of the calcium antagonist verapamil on necrosis following temporary coronary artery occlusion in dogs. *Circulation* 55:581–587, 1977.
18. Sherman LG, Liang CS, Boden WE, et al: The effect of verapamil on mechanical performance of acutely ischemic and reperfused myocardium in the conscious dog. *Circ Res* 48:224–232, 1981.
19. Smith HJ, Singh BN, Nisbet HD, et al: Effects of verapamil on infarct size following experimental coronary occlusion. *Cardiovasc Res* 9:569–578, 1975.
20. Watts JA, Koch CD, Lanoue KF: Effects of calcium antagonist on energy metabolism: calcium and heart failure after ischemia. *Am J Physiol* 238:H909–H916, 1980.
21. Faden AI, Jacobs TP, Smith T: Evaluation of the calcium channel antagonist nimodipine in experimental spinal cord ischemia. *J Neurosurg* 60:796–799, 1984.
22. White BC, Winegar CD, Wilson RF, et al: Calcium blockers in cerebral resuscitation. *J Trauma* 23:788–793, 1983.
23. Wiernsperger N, Gypax P, Hofmann A: Calcium antagonist PY 108-068: demonstration of its efficacy in various types of experimental brain ischemia. *Stroke* 15:679–685, 1984.
24. Hoffmuster F, Kazda S, Krause HP: Influence of nimodipine on the postischemic changes of brain function. *Acta Neurol Scand* 60(suppl 72):58, 1979.
25. White BC, Gadzinski DS, Hoehner PJ, et al: Correction of canine cerebral cortical blood flow and vascular resistance after cardiac arrest using flunarizine, a calcium antagonist. *Ann Emerg Med* 11:118–126, 1982.
26. Winegar CD, Henderson O, White BC, et al: Early amelioration of neurologic deficit by lidoflazine after fifteen minutes of cardiopulmonary arrest in dogs. *Ann Neurol Med* 12:471–477, 1983.
27. Burke TJ, Arnold PE, Gordon JA, et al: Protective effect of intrarenal calcium membrane blockers before or after renal ischemia. *J Clin Invest* 74:1830–1841, 1984.
28. Malis DC, Cheung JY, Leaf A, et al: Effects of verapamil in models of ischemic acute renal failure in the rat. *Am J Physiol* 245:F735–F742, 1983.
29. Wait RB, White G, Davis JH: Beneficial effects of verapamil on postischemic renal failure. *Surgery* 94:276–282, 1983.
30. Duncan CJ, Smith JL: The effect of the ionophore A23187 on the ultrastructure and electrophysiological properties of frog skeletal muscle. *Cell Tissue Res* 173:193–209, 1976.
31. Publicover SJ, Duncan CJ, Smith JL: The use of A23187 to demonstrate the role of intracellular calcium in causing ultrastructural damage in mammalian muscle. *J Neuropathol Exp Neurol* 37:544–557, 1978.
32. McCabe WR: Gram-negative bacteremia. *Adv Intern Med* 19:135–158, 1974.
33. Lee HC, Lum BKB: Protective action of calcium entry blockers in endotoxin shock. *Circ Shock* 18:193–203, 1986.
34. Sayeed MM, Maitra SR: Effect of diltiazem on altered cellular calcium regulation during endotoxic shock. *Am J Physiol* 253:R549–R554, 1987.
35. Dudley CM, Maitra SR, Sayeed MM: Effect of diltiazem on cellular calcium alterations in skeletal muscle during endotoxic shock. *Prog Clin Biol Res* 264:373–378, 1988.
36. Zaloga GP, Washburn D, Black KW, Prielipp R: Human sepsis increases lymphocyte intracellular calcium. *Crit Care Med* 21:196–202, 1993.
37. Zaloga GP, Washburn D: Multiorgan failure is associated with elevated free intracellular calcium in human sepsis. *Chest* 94(suppl):6S, 1988.
38. Zaloga GP, Malcolm DS: Calcium in septic shock: a meta-analysis. In Neugebauer E, Holaday JW (eds): *Handbook on Mediators in Septic Shock*. CRC Press, Boca Raton, FL, pp 475–485, 1993.
39. Bosson S, Kuenzig M, Schwartz SI: Verapamil improves cardiac function and increases survival in canine *E. coli* endotoxin shock. *Circ Shock* 16:307–316, 1985.
40. Malcolm D, Zaloga G, Chernow B, et al: Calcium involvement in endotoxic shock: verapamil improves hemodynamics and survival in rats. *Circ Shock* 18:346, 1986.
41. Malcolm DS, Zaloga GP, Holaday JW: Calcium administration increases the mortality of endotoxic shock in rats. *Crit Care* 17:900–903, 1989.
42. Bosson S, Kuenzig M, Schwartz SI: Increased survival with calcium antagonists in antibiotic-treated bacteremia. *Circ Shock* 19:69–74, 1986.
43. Bosson S, Haglund U: Effects of nifedipine in feline septic shock. *Circ Shock* 19:125, 1986.
44. Griffin AJ, Goto M, Ow E, Sayeed M: Effect of diltiazem in the treatment of endotoxic shock in newborn puppies. *Circ Shock* 13:71A, 1984.
45. Lee HC, Hardman JM, Lum BKB: The effects of the calcium entry blockers nilvadipine and nitrendipine on endotoxin-induced disseminated intravascular coagulation. *Life Sci* 45:877–883, 1989.
46. Zaloga GP, Sager A, Black KW, Prielipp R: Low dose calcium administration increases mortality during septic peritonitis in rats. *Circ Shock* 37:226–229, 1992.
47. Zaloga GP, Willey S, Malcolm D, Chernow B, Holaday JW: Hypercalcemia attenuates blood pressure response to epinephrine. *J Pharmacol Exp Ther* 247:949–951, 1988.
48. Hackel DB, Mikat EM, Whalen G, et al: Treatment of hemorrhagic shock in dogs with verapamil. *Lab Invest* 41:356–359, 1979.
49. Hackel DB, Mikat EM, Whalen G: Effects of verapamil on heart and circulation in hemorrhagic shock in dogs. *Am J Physiol* 241:H12–H17, 1981.

50. Hess ML, Warner MF, Smith JM, et al: Improved myocardial hemodynamic and cellular function with calcium channel blockade (verapamil) during canine hemorrhagic shock. *Circ Shock* 10:119–130, 1983.

51. Sabouni M, Hodge K, Jandhyala BS: Restoration of renal and mesenteric hemodynamics by felodipine in a canine model of hemorrhagic shock. *Naunyn Schmiedebergs Arch Pharmacol* 337:465–470, 1988.

52. Chintala MS, Jandhyala BS: Renal failure in hemorrhagic shock in dogs: salutary effects of a calcium antagonist felodipine. *Naunyn Schmiedebergs Arch Pharmacol* 341:357–363, 1990.

53. Chintala MS, Jandhyala BS: Comparative evaluation of the effects of felodipine, hydralazine and naloxone on the survival rate of rats subjected to a "fixed volume" model of hemorrhagic shock. 32:219–229, 1990.

54. Maitra SR, Krikhely M, Dulchavsky SA, et al: Beneficial effects of diltiazem in hemorrhagic shock. *Circ Shock* 33:121–125, 1991.

55. Hock CE, Su JY, Lefer AM: Salutary effects of nitrenidine, a new calcium entry blocker in hemorrhagic shock. *Eur J Pharmacol* 97:37–46, 1984.

56. Hess ML, Greenfield LJ: Calcium entry blockers: potential applications in shock. *Adv Shock Res* 10:15–25, 1983.

57. Bourdillon PD, Poole-Wilson PA: The effects of verapamil, quiescence, and cardioplegia on calcium exchange and mechanical function in ischemic rabbit myocardium. *Circ Res* 50:360–368, 1982.

58. Whalen GF, Hackel DB, Mikat E: Prevention of portal hypertension and small bowel hemorrhage in dogs treated with verapamil during hemorrhagic shock. *Circ Shock* 70:399–404, 1980.

CHAPTER 66

Surfactant in Infant Respiratory Distress Syndrome and ARDS

RODOLFO I. GODINEZ, M.D., Ph.D.

MARYE H. GODINEZ, M.D.

RUSSELL C. RAPHAELY, M.D.

INTRODUCTION

Pulmonary surfactant has been characterized as a glycolipo-protein whose principal lipid component is phosphatidylcholine with palmitic acid esterified at both the 1 and 2 positions. Normal surfactant homeostasis leads to the maintenance of a functional residual capacity, at which ventilation-perfusion ratios are optimal; pulmonary compliance is high; and atelectasis is minimal. An absolute or relative absence of surfactant, or interference with its normal function, is associated with pulmonary dysfunction characterized by low functional residual capacity, low ventilation-perfusion, and abundant atelectasis.

The principal role attributed to surfactant consists of stabilization of the alveoli by its surface tension-lowering ability but has been postulated to include (*a*) the ability to "splint" the alveoli open at low internal alveolar diameters by forming a rigid monolayer; (*b*) preventing lung edema and transudation of fluid into alveoli; (*c*) aiding the removal of foreign particles from the airway; (*d*) assisting digestion of bacteria (1). Recently, immunologic functions have been attributed to pulmonary surfactant (2). The surfactant system would be that first exposed to pulmonary toxins, and it is possible that its ability to meet demands could be compromised in situations encountered in clinical medicine.

In this chapter we shall examine this fascinating substance in detail, and discuss its replacement therapies recently introduced into clinical use. The dysfunction, inactivation, and/ or lack of surfactant impacts on pathologic states commonly encountered in critical care.

THE SURFACTANT SYSTEM OF THE LUNG

COMPOSITION

Pulmonary surfactant, convincingly demonstrated by Pattle (3) and Clements (4) in the mid-1950s, is a mixture of lipids, specific apoproteins, and complex polysaccharides, that is best thought of as a functional system, even though we do not fully understand the role of all of its components. Phospholipids account for about 85 to 90% by weight of pulmonary surfactant, with proteins constituting around 5 to 10% (lesser amounts of neutral lipids and carbohydrates make up the balance). Of the phospholipids, phosphatidylcholine represents approximately 80%, 60% of which is dipalmitoylphosphatidylcholine or disaturated phosphatidylcholine. The next most abundant phospholipid is phosphatidylglycerol, an unusual acidic lipid primarily found in mitochondrial and bacterial membranes, but which represents 8 to 10% of surfactant lipids. The complete list of pulmonary surfactant lipids in normal lungs and in acute lung injury is given in Table 66.1

Surfactant proteins can be divided into two major groups, each representing approximately 2 to 4% of the total surfactant mass. The first group consists of surfactant apoprotein A (5), a highly glycosylated, collagen-like protein with molecular weights ranging from 26 to 36 kilodaltons (depending on

Table 66.1. Composition of Human Lung Surfactant (% Total Phospholipid)

Variable	Normal				ARDS		
Reference	*1*	*2*	*3*	*4*	*2*	*3*	*4*
Phosphatidylcholine	68.6	62.8	73.0	62.8	48.1	59.5	42.7
Phosphatidylethanolamine	8.4	4.8	2.6	4.8	18.7	4.3	27.9
Phosphatidylinositol	2.5	8.3	2.7	8.3	13.9	3.1	7.4
Phosphatidylglycerol	11.4	10.0	12.4	10.0	1.9	0.3	1.3
						(0–7.0)	
Sphingomyelin	2.1	7.4	3.7	7.4	14.2	17.5	15.9
Lysophosphatidylcholine	2.0	1.3	0.4	1.3	1	1.5	1.7
Phosphatidylserine	ND	4.5	3.3	ND	ND	13.0	ND

[1] Sadana T, Dhall K, Sanyal SN, et al: Isolation and chemical composition of surface-active material from human lung lavage. *Lipids* 23:551–558, 1988. Both sexes at autopsy, 4–6 observations.
[2] Pison U, Seeger S, Buchhorn R, et al. Surfactant abnormalities in patients with respiratory failure after multiple trauma. *Am Rev Respir Dis* 140:1033–1039, 1989. Both sexes volunteers, 10 observations.
[3] Hallman M, Spragg R, Harrell JH, et al. Evidence of lung surfactant abnormality in respiratory failure. *J Clin Invest* 70:673–683, 1982. Both sexes volunteers, 12 observations.
[4] Pison U, Obertacke U, Brand M, et al. Altered pulmonary surfactant in uncomplicated and septicemia-complicated courses of acute respiratory failure. *J Trauma* 30(1):19–26, 1990. Both sexes anesthetized patients for operation, 10 observations.

glycosylation) and lipophobic in nature. The second group is composed of two highly lipophilic, smaller proteins (molecular weights 4 to 18 kilodaltons), referred to as surfactant apoprotein B and surfactant apoprotein C. Both of these latter proteins will coextract with the lipids into organic solvents (6), a very important property that we will discuss later.

METABOLISM AND REGULATION

Over the last 25 years, much interest has been devoted to the study of pulmonary surfactant metabolism and the regulation of its synthesis and release. Evidence to date supports the thesis that synthesis of surfactant phospholipids and proteins takes place in the microsomal fraction (endoplasmic reticulum) of alveolar type II cells. They are then transported to the Golgi apparatus and packaged into the osmiophilic inclusion bodies (lamellar bodies) characteristic to the type II pneumocyte (7–9). Secretion of surfactant into the alveolar lumen occurs through the process of exocytosis, where the lamellar bodies fuse with the cell membrane, and their contents are extruded (10).

The control of surfactant synthesis and secretion is complex, involving multiple factors. It is beyond the scope of this chapter to cover this subject in depth, and the reader is directed to several excellent reviews and books on this subject (11–13). Suffice it to say that a variety of agents can positively influence surfactant secretion in adult subjects, among them mechanical factors (14, 15), adrenergic and cholinergic agonists (15, 16), and prostaglandins (15). Factors that negatively influence surfactant production or function will be addressed later.

Clearance of pulmonary surfactant takes place with an apparent half-life of around 20 hours and seems to primarily consist of recycling by type II cells (17), with a smaller contribution by alveolar macrophage degradation (18). Adrenergic agonists have been implicated in the control of surfactant clearance (19).

FUNCTION

The molecular characteristics of surfactants allow them to preferentially adsorb at a surface and to alter interfacial tension as their concentration varies. Pulmonary surfactant follows this principle in performing its physiologic role. The Young-Laplace equation for a sphere, or a bubble is

$$DP = 2T/r$$

where DP is the pressure drop across the bubble, r is the radius of the bubble, and T is the surface tension. This equation tells us that the pressure necessary to stabilize a bubble will vary inversely with its radius, unless the surface tension also varies directly with the radius (or area) of the bubble. In physiologic terms, as alveolar volume (area) decreases—as during exhalation—alveolar surface tension must also decrease in order to maintain stability and prevent collapse at physiologic transalveolar (transpleural) pressures. The converse principle is also true: greater transalveolar pressure will be needed to maintain alveolar volume in the absence of functional surfactant.

Pulmonary surfactant function is usually measured in vitro in a Langmuir-Wilhelmy balance, or with the pulsating bubble apparatus of Enhorning (20). For more details on these and other methods, as well as their advantages and disadvantages, see the review by Notter and Finkelstein (21).

Pulmonary surfactant is able to perform its function because of its composition. It is generally accepted that the principal surface-tension lowering activity arises from the unique abundance of dipalmitoylphosphatidylcholine, whose straight aliphatic chains and hydrophilic choline groups can readily form a stable monomolecular surface layer. It has become increasingly clear that the apoproteins of surfactant also play an important role. Surfactant apoprotein B and surfactant apoprotein C, the two small lipophilic proteins, appear to be essential if the optimal surface tension-lowering activity of surfactant (<5 mN/m)—both natural (5, 6), and exogenous (22)—is to be achieved. Surfactant apoprotein A probably is involved in the generation of tubular myelin, an alveolar form of surfactant associated with the formation of the surface film, and in the Ca^{2+}- and surfactant apoprotein B-dependent aggregation and adsorption of the phospholipids to the liquid surface (23). Surfactant apoprotein A may also be involved in the regulation of surfactant secretion and recycling (24, 25).

The most enigmatic component of surfactant is phosphatidylglycerol. Although it is found in relatively large amounts, and its increase in concentration closely parallels that of dipal-mitoylphosphatidylcholine during fetal maturation, its presence is not essential to surfactant function in terms of its surface tension-lowering activity, and it can be replaced by phosphatidylinositol without physiologic effect. Phosphatidylglycerol may have a regulatory role (26), may serve as a marker of acute lung injury, or it may simply be part of the process of secretion. It is of interest that phosphatidylglycerol release into bronchoalveolar lavage (BAL) is subject to β-adrenergic stimulation in an isolated perfused lung preparation although, under these conditions, its concentration does not parallel that of phosphatidylcholine (M. Godinez and R. Godinez, unpublished observation, 1992).

SURFACTANT DEFICIENCY STATES

In the absence of surfactant, surface forces will cause the collapse of alveoli at end-exhalation, unless the transalveolar pressure is increased in compensation. Even if the dysfunction is only partial (either deficient or partial inactivation), the equilibrium point at end-exhalation will occur at a lower bubble radius (alveolar volume, or functional residual capacity), thereby placing the lung at a mechanical disadvantage for the start of the next inspiration. Thus, the clinical manifestations of surfactant deficiency will be low lung volumes, decreased compliance, atelectasis, and altered ventilation-perfusion, leading to arterial hypoxemia. The two "respiratory distress syndromes"—infant and adult—have such a clinical presentation, and in both surfactant deficiency is implicated.

INFANT RESPIRATORY DISTRESS SYNDROME (IRDS)

Characteristically seen in premature infants, and associated with other conditions of the newborn such as meconium aspiration and infants of diabetic mothers, IRDS has generated enormous research activity at all levels since the association between altered surfactant homeostasis and IRDS was first described by Avery and Mead in 1959 (27). It is now well-accepted that in premature infants, IRDS is associated with an immaturity of the type II pneumocyte leading to surfactant deficiency and that maturation is under the control of, and can be induced by, glucocorticoids (28). Surfactant inactivation, rather than reduced production, is the likely mechanism of the functional deficiency of surfactant in meconium aspiration.

Functional tests for surfactant system maturation have been developed and are in common clinical use via evaluating amniotic fluid: the lecithin/sphingomyelin (L/S) ratio and the measurement of phosphatidylglycerol. Detailed descriptions of these tests may be found in any neonatology textbook and will not be repeated here.

ADULT RESPIRATORY DISTRESS SYNDROME (ARDS) OR ACUTE LUNG INJURY SYNDROME (ALIS)

ARDS is the pulmonary injury associated with a variety of acute pathologic conditions (sepsis, shock, multiple trauma, and interstitial pulmonary infections) that generate a systemic

or pulmonary inflammatory cascade. The many pathophysiologic similarities between IRDS and ARDS have led investigators to question whether a surfactant deficiency could be implicated in the clinical presentation of acute lung injury. Ashbaugh and coworkers (29) first reported increased minimum surface tension (>20 mN/m) when testing extracts from ARDS lungs. Ten years later, Petty (30) reported decreased lung volume and compliance in postmortem examination of lungs of a patient with ARDS. The BAL material from those lungs had normal lipid content but elevated protein content, and the minimum surface tension obtained was 20 mN/m (normal is <5 mN/m). Other investigators (31, 32) have also reported normal or increased phospholipid content of alveolar lining material from human ARDS lungs but abnormal composition consisting of decreased dipalmitoylphosphatidylcholine and phosphatidylglycerol, increased phosphatidylinositol, and higher-than-normal protein content. Pison and co-workers (33) found that decreased phosphatidylglycerol and increased phosphatidylinositol amounts in BAL were found as early as 6 hours after trauma and these levels normalized during recovery. In those patients who developed sepsis, percentage concentrations of alveolar phosphatidyslethanolamine increased, and phosphatidylcholine decreased. Liau et al (34) postulated that the low level of phosphatidylglycerol found in acute alveolar injury in dogs might be due to increased turnover of phosphatidylglycerol to diphosphatidylglycerol (DPG) (not detectable in lavage fluid), which might be used in repair of alveolar epithelial cells because they found a threefold increase in tissue levels during late recovery.

The role that translocated serum plasma proteins may have in the inactivation of surfactant in ARDS has been extensively investigated, since one of the hallmarks of acute lung injury is the accumulation of proteinaceous fluid in the alveoli as a result of altered capillary permeability (35–39). The evidence supports the concept that these proteins inactivate the surfactant already present in the alveolus. Another hallmark of acute inflammation in man as a consequence of trauma, burn injury, or infection is the increased concentrations of C-reactive protein. Li (39) found increased levels of C-reactive protein in BAL and demonstrated that the C-reactive protein bound to liposomes containing dipalmitoylphosphatidylcholine and phosphatidylglycerol. The result of this interaction was inhibition of the surface tension-lowering activity as measured with the Enhorning pulsating bubble apparatus. Furthermore, surfactant replacement (surfactant TA) was also inhibited by C-reactive protein in a dose-dependent manner.

One can envision a vicious cycle where surfactant inactivation, superimposed on type II pneumocyte dysfunction, increased capillary permeability with access of more protein and further inactivation would lead to the clinical manifestations of ARDS. An important finding in the works cited above is that plasma protein inactivation of surfactant can be blocked by increasing the concentration of surfactant, thereby restoring its biophysical properties; this result would have therapeutic implications.

Recent studies have focused on what role mediators of inflammation, particularly the cytokines, may play in the pathogenesis of the surfactant alterations seen in ARDS. Several studies have demonstrated an increase in serum cytokine levels, especially tumor necrosis factor (TNF) during acute lung injury. TNF appears to be the initiating point in the inflammatory cascade, and its importance in ARDS has been highlighted in several studies. Analysis of BAL fluid from patients with ARDS has shown high concentrations of TNF (40). The intratracheal (41) and intravenous (42) administration of TNF in experimental animals resulted in histologic and functional changes consistent with ARDS, and the exposure of a human pulmonary adenocarcinoma cell line to TNF resulted in decreased concentrations of surfactant apoprotein A, its messenger RNA, and messenger RNA for surfactant apoprotein B (43). More studies should be forthcoming on the specific effect of TNF and other inflammatory mediators on surfactant synthesis and secretion.

The administration of increased concentrations of oxygen in ARDS is almost universal and, although essential to maintain arterial oxygen content compatible with the preservation of aerobic bioenergetics, pulmonary oxygen toxicity probably compounds the original lung injury. The literature is somewhat equivocal on the subject of oxygen-mediated alterations of surfactant homeostasis. Young exposed male rats to 85% oxygen for 7 days and reported that an increase in number and size of type II cells was associated with substantial increases in surfactant disaturated phosphatidylcholine content in lung tissue (208%), lamellar body (450%), and lavage fractions (550%), compared to that in controls (44). However, studies of other authors, using various animal preparations and genders, have demonstrated decreased amounts of phospholipids and decreased synthesis of phosphatidylcholine (45–47). Time of exposure and FIO_2 appear to be factors in the determination of effects. Using male baboons, King et al (48) found that at 100% O_2 for 4 to 5 days, disaturated phosphatidylcholine levels decreased to 87% those of controls and the ratio of phosphatidylglycerol to phosphatidylinositol was 37% that of controls. Ventilation with 80% O_2 for 6 days resulted in smaller changes in disaturated phosphatidylcholine, but the ratio of the levels of phosphatidylglycerol to phosphatidylinositol remained the same. A progressive deterioration occurred despite reduction of the FIO_2 to 50% after 4.5 days of 100% O_2. These researchers concluded that the phosphatidylglycerol/ phosphatidylinositol ratio may be predictive of early oxygen-mediated lung injury. In addition, they found increased protein in the surfactant fraction that was not consistent with contamination with serum and cell protein. Further evidence of the profound effect of oxygen on surfactant metabolism was provided by Holm and co-workers (49), who exposed adult rabbits to 100% O_2 for 64 hours and found a 30% decrease in BAL phospholipid content and a threefold increase in protein levels. When the animals were returned to room air for 24 hours, BAL phospholipid levels declined 51%, and mean protein levels were up to eight times those of control values. It should be noted that these studies of oxygen toxicity were done on otherwise healthy animals, so that the combined effects of ARDS and one of its therapies (oxygen) on surfactant dynamics is not known. It is, however, safe to speculate that avoidance of toxic inspired oxygen concentrations would be beneficial in ARDS, if an alternative means could be employed to improve the low ventilation-perfusion ratios that dictate their use.

For further details on the subject of surfactant dysfunction in ARDS, including animal models of the acute lung injury, the following excellent reviews are suggested (11, 50–52).

SURFACTANT REPLACEMENT THERAPY

We have already alluded to the stimulation of research on lung metabolism that followed Avery and Mead's association of surfactant deficiency with IRDS. The natural extension of identifying a deficiency state is to attempt replacement of the missing natural substance (such as administering insulin in diabetes mellitus), and such has been the course with surfactant replacement therapy. Initial attempts at surfactant replacement involved the administration of nebulized sonicated phospholipids, mostly dipalmitoylphosphatidylcholine, to infants with IRDS, but the results were disappointing (53–55). Delivery of the replacement material was difficult, so dosages were not controlled. Furthermore there was not a complete understanding of the role of all the components of endogenous surfactant, especially the proteins. These early failures stimulated systematic investigation of composition and delivery systems and culminated in the first confirmed report of successful surfactant replacement therapy by Fujiwara's group in 1980 (56). Since then, surfactant replacement has become an accepted clinical therapy in IRDS and a promising experimental subject in ARDS. However, the search for the most perfect replacement is still underway. The remainder of this chapter will be devoted to an examination of the clinical and investigative use of exogenous surfactant preparations.

TYPES AND COMPOSITION

To date, at least seven types of exogenous surfactants have been used in clinical trials around the world. To minimize confusion and allow for rational comparison of results, Jobe and Ikegami (57) have proposed a useful classification scheme based on the origin of the material in question. "Natural" surfactants are those recovered from tissues or biologic fluids by lavage, filtration, or centrifugation, which is then subjected (except in the case of human amniotic fluid surfactant) to organic solvent lipid extraction. Lipophilic surfactant-associated proteins are present in these preparations. "Modified natural" surfactants are as above, with the subsequent addition or subtraction of components. "Artificial" surfactants are composed of materials synthesized in vitro and may contain substances not found in endogenous surfactant. Finally, "synthetic natural" surfactants are an in vitro reconstitution of natural surfactant with apoproteins obtained through recombinant DNA technology. All of the "recipes" detailed below fall under one of these types. At the present time, "synthetic natural" material is not available for clinical use.

NATURAL SURFACTANTS

Human Amniotic Fluid. Obtained by sucrose gradient centrifugation of amniotic fluid collected at the time of term-elective cesarean section, this material contains approximately 81% phospholipids, 9% neutral lipids, and 5% protein. The phospholipid composition is 63% phosphatidylcholine (40%

dipalmitoylphosphatidylcholine), 6% phosphatidylglycerol, and smaller amounts of phosphatidylinositol, phosphatidylethanolamine, and sphingomyelin. Cholesterol is the most abundant neutral lipid. All surfactant-associated proteins are present. The lypholized preparation is suspended in saline prior to use, with a recommended dose being approximately 60 mg phospholipid/kg (58).

Minced Porcine Lung.   Widely studied in Europe, this material (Curosurf, Chiesi Farmaceutici, Parma, Italy) is obtained from minced pork lung by saline extraction, differential centrifugation, and organic solvent extraction. The phospholipid fraction is isolated by chromatography and lypholized. The preparation thus obtained contains 99% phospholipids and 1% lipophilic protein. The final lipid composition is 80% phosphatidylcholine (46% dipalmitoylphosphatidylcholine), and smaller amounts of phosphatidylethanolamine, phosphatidylinositol, and sphingomyelin. Following suspension in saline, the recommended dose is 200 mg phospholipid/kg (59).

Calf Lung Lavage.   Neonatal calf lung surfactant extract (CLSE) or Infasurf (Forest Laboratories, NY) is in wide clinical use. Following saline lavage of calf lungs, the lipid fraction is concentrated by differential centrifugation, acetone precipitation, and organic extraction. The obtained material contains approximately 95% phospholipid, 4% neutral lipid (mainly cholesterol), and 1% lipophilic protein. The phospholipid composition is 79% phosphatidylcholine (80% dipalmitoylphosphatidylcholine), 6% phosphatidylglycerol, and 15% other polar lipids. A similar preparation, used extensively in Canada, is obtained from 6-month-old cows. The nitrogen-dried surfactants are suspended in saline prior to use and administered in a dose of 100 mg phospholipid/kg (60, 61).

MODIFIED NATURAL SURFACTANT

Fujiwara's original surfactant (56) consisted of material isolated from a saline extract of minced bovine lungs by centrifugation, acetone precipitation, and organic solvent extraction. Because of the dilution of surfactant lipids by structural lipids, supplementation with dipalmitoylphosphatidylcholine and phosphatidylglycerol was necessary to restore surface activity. In its present version, the extract is supplemented with dipalmitoylphosphatidylcholine, tripalmitin, and palmitate. The final composition is 88% phospholipid and 6% each of free fatty acids and triglyceride. Phosphatidylcholine represents 74% of the phospholipids while phosphatidylglycerol is 3%. Lipophilic proteins account for 3% of the dry weight. One preparation is stored as a lypholized powder (Surfactant TA) and dispersed in saline prior to administration. A second preparation, Survanta (Abbott Laboratories), is supplied as a refrigerated liquid dispersion. The recommended dose is 100 mg phospholipid/kg (62, 63).

ARTIFICIAL SURFACTANT

Two artificial preparations have been used with demonstrated clinical efficiency. The first one is a formulation of 70% dipalmitoylphosphatidylcholine and 30% phosphatidylglycerol (w/w) suspended in saline and is known as "artificial lung expanding compound" (ALEC). Recommended doses range from 50 to 100 mg phospholipid per treatment (64, 65).

The second preparation, Exosurf (Burroughs Wellcome), is composed of dipalmitoylphosphatidylcholine hexadecanol and the nonionic surfactant, tyloxapol, in the proportions of 13.5 : 1.5 : 1 w/w. The lyophilized mixture also contains 27.7% NaCl and is reconstituted with water prior to administration. The recommended dose is 67.5 mg dipalmitoylphosphatidylcholine/kg (66).

COMPARISON OF EXOGENOUS SURFACTANTS

The goal of the manufacturers has been to supply a product that would mimic the physicochemical properties of native surfactant and thus restore physiologic function. Only in the case of amniotic fluid extract, however, is native surfactant totally duplicated. Common to all of the other exogenous surfactant preparations is a preponderance of dipalmitoylphosphatidylcholine, with varying amounts of other substances either naturally occurring or man-made. Putting the differing lipid compositions aside, the major difference between the "natural" surfactant preparations and the artificial ones is the fact that the lung-derived formulations all contain varying amounts of surfactant apoprotein B and surfactant apoprotein C, while the artificial ones contain none. We have previously addressed the apparent role of surfactant-associated proteins in surfactant. In a recent publication (22), Hall and coworkers have systematically compared the biophysic properties and physiologic effects of CLSE, Survanta, and Exosurf, the three major products in clinical use. In oscillating bubble studies, Survanta and CLSE decreased surface tension to physiologic ranges, but Exosurf only achieved a minimum value of 29 mN/m. When surfactant apoprotein B and surfactant apoprotein C were added to Exosurf, the surface activity reached physiologic levels. An interesting finding was that tyloxapol alone (one of the components of Exosurf) had the same surface-active properties as those of the complete product. In studies with surfactant-depleted excised rat lungs, CLSE restored pressure-volume mechanics to 95% of the pre-depletion levels, while Survanta restored 50% and Exosurf only 10%. Addition of surfactant apoprotein B and surfactant apoprotein C brought Exosurf to 70% of control values. These authors conclude that the apoproteins are more effective than hexadecanol and tyloxapol in facilitating the ability of dipalmitoylphosphatidylcholine to lower surface tension in their model. The lower activity obtained with Survanta is ascribed to the presence of nonsurfactant lipids inherent to that formulation.

The conclusions which can be drawn from the study cited above and others (67–69) are that the apoproteins are essential if physiologic function is to be restored using exogenous surfactant. The fact that Exosurf is effective in the clinical setting can only lead to the conclusion that it either combines with endogenous apoproteins present in the alveoli, or that its dipalmitoylphosphatidylcholine is used as substrate through recycling for the production of new surfactant. Both these explanations are compatible with published observations on the effectiveness and time course of Exosurf therapy (70–73). A clinically important consequence of the apparent indirect action of Exosurf through combination with endogenous apoproteins or through recycling pathways, would be if this formulation is considered for use in the presence of protein inhibitor or type II cell dysfunction, as in ARDS.

Table 66.2. Recommended Dose of Surfactants in Clinical Use

Trade Name	Type	Source	Dose
Surfactant TA	Modified Natural	Minced bovine lung	100 mg phospholipid/kg body weight
Infrasurf	Natural	Calf lung lavage	100 mg phospholipid/kg body weight
Curosurf	Natural	Minced porcine lung	200 mg phospholipid/kg body weight
	Natural	Human amniotic fluid	60 mg phospholipid/kg body weight
ALEC	Artificial	DPPC:PG in saline	50–100 mg/treatment
HDL	Artificial	DPPC with high density lipoprotein	30 mg DPPC/dose
Exosurf	Artificial	DPPC, hexadecanol, tyloxapol	67.5 mg DPPC/kg body weight

METHODS OF ADMINISTRATION

Nearly all published studies on infants have used the Fujiwara method of endotracheal installation of liquid surfactant suspension through a small catheter advanced beyond the tip of the tracheal tube (56). The total dose is divided in quarters, and the infant's position is changed for each instillation to optimize distribution. Positive pressure ventilation, either manual or mechanical, is used between quarter doses. As decreased oxygenation often occurs during instillation, either cutaneous PO_2 or SPO_2 is monitored continuously and the FIO_2 increased as needed. Alternatively, a special tracheal tube adapter with a side port allows administration of the surfactant material without interruption of ventilation. This would seem to provide the advantage of minimizing any periods of hypoventilation and hypoxemia.

Lewis and coworkers (74) recently compared the effectiveness and efficiency of instillation or nebulization of Survanta in an adult rabbit lung injury model. A physiologic improvement ascribed to the therapy was seen in the nebulized surfactant group but not in the instilled group, even though the actual dose of surfactant deposited in the lungs by nebulization was 1/20th of the dose instilled. Of note is that a simple medication nebulizer was employed, and that foaming of the surfactant suspension was minimized by keeping the nebulizer on ice during the period of administration. It is tantalizing to speculate what effect using a more efficient nebulizer and employing ventilatory patterns that encourage aerosol deposition would have had on their results. Further studies, including clinical applications of this technique, should be forthcoming, especially in older patients with ARDS, where the amount of surfactant needed for the traditional instillation method would be prohibitive.

Essentially, all the clinical experience with surfactant replacement therapy has been obtained on neonates. Two treatment strategies have been used in study protocols: so-called "rescue" or therapeutic administration to infants manifesting the clinical syndrome of IRDS, or "prophylactic" administration at birth or soon thereafter, before IRDS is manifest. Similarly, doses of the various surfactant preparations, administered once or multiple times, have been established to obtain satisfactory results. Although this approach is practical in a patient population where risk factors are well-defined (gestational age, birth weight, antenatal lung maturation indices, etc), no such scheme will be possible in the case of ARDS. We would caution against the application of infant protocols and techniques to the more heterogeneous patient population with ARDS.

The recommended dose of surfactants in clinical use for IRDS is given in Table 66.2. In general, side effects of these agents are related to the method of administration—i.e., intratracheally—which may stimulate a vasovagal reflex causing bradycardia. Too rapid instillation of the substance may also stimulate the carina, inducing coughing. Use of appropriate monitoring, such as a pulse oximeter, will allow the physician to note the onset of bradycardia and/or decreased oxygen saturation and thus to slow the rate of instillation and/or treat the decreased heart rate with atropine. Because rapid changes in oxygenation and lung compliance may occur, ventilatory variables (tidal volume, end-tidal, or cutaneous carbon dioxide) should be closely monitored and the ventilatory parameters adjusted accordingly.

In its product literature, Exosurf Neonatal is reported to be associated with a 20 to 30% incidence of surfactant reflux after administration. If this event is observed, the tracheal tube should not be suctioned, but rather the inflating pressure on the ventilator may be increased 4 to 5 cm H_2O until the tube clears.

The danger of nosocomial sepsis is always a possibility and the need for sterility in dealing with the respiratory system is a maxim that should be continually reiterated.

SURFACTANT THERAPY IN IRDS

There are now more than 20 reports of controlled clinical trials with exogenous surfactant therapy in the neonatal age group, and more appear regularly. The results of these trials on thousands of infants are overwhelmingly positive. It is safe to say that this form of therapy has gained wide acceptance in the palliation of IRDS. We choose the term "palliation" purposefully, because we believe that exogenous surfactant should be viewed as a means of temporizing until endogenous production can attain levels compatible with life. The principal theoretical advantage of exogenous surfactant administration is its ability to minimize other supportive therapies (supplemental oxygen, continuous positive airway pressure, and mechanical ventilation) that may lead to lung injury and bronchopulmonary dysplasia. The variables measured in the trials of exogenous surfactant largely reflect the advantages mentioned above: lung mechanics (or the need for mechanical ventilation), PAO_2/FIO_2, incidence of parenchymal gas leaks, development of bronchopulmonary dysplasia (BPD), and overall survival. Other variables that may be related to IRDS and its conventional management (retinopathy of prematurity, intraventricular hemorrhage, patent ductus arteriosus, and even necrotizing enterocolitis) have also been studied.

As already mentioned, the results of these trials have been mostly positive. Although absolute numbers vary depending on the preparation used and the particular study, some general conclusions can be drawn: prophylaxis with natural surfactants in babies <30 weeks gestational age results in decreased incidence of IRDS, reduction in severity (as judged by O_2 ventilatory needs), and a decrease in the incidence of gas leaks. "Rescue" therapy had similar effects on established IRDS. Multiple doses were necessary for sustained effect. Mortality was reduced in some studies but was unchanged in others. Artificial surfactant (primarily Exosurf) did not reduce the incidence of IRDS when given prophylactically but had beneficial effects similar to those of the natural surfactants on the course and severity of established disease. The incidence of BPD with all preparations has been reported to be either reduced or unchanged, while the incidence of the associated conditions mentioned above remains unchanged. For a very complete description of surfactant therapy in IRDS the reader is referred to the excellent review by Yee and Scarpelli (75).

Very few adverse effects of exogenous surfactant administration in IRDS have been reported. Of note is the increased incidence of apnea seen with Exosurf but not reported with any other preparation (66). Whether the nonlipid components of this preparation are the causative agent is only speculation, and this phenomenon deserves further study.

A word of caution: the administration of exogenous surfactants should have the desired effect of reducing oxygen requirements and improving pulmonary mechanics, and these changes may occur rapidly. Changes in compliance could result in excessive tidal volumes being delivered to the infant if conventional time-cycled, pressure-limited ventilators are used. To safeguard against this problem, we feel it is essential that exhaled tidal volumes be carefully, if not continuously, monitored with a device capable of accurately measuring small volumes. Alternately, volume preset ventilatory modes may be considered, with reductions in the peak inflating pressure signaling the onset of surfactant action. A similar admonition is directed at supplemental oxygen administration, and frequent, if not continuous, monitoring of oxygenation should be practiced.

SURFACTANT THERAPY IN ARDS

As we have already noted, surfactant dysfunction is a prominent feature in the pathophysiology of ARDS. An absolute decrease, as well as an inactivation of surfactant by extrapulmonary proteins, leads to decreased surface activity in this condition. Most of our knowledge linking ARDS and surfactant dysfunction is fairly recent, and the understanding of the mechanisms implicated remains incomplete—unlike with IRDS. Also, unlike IRDS, the application of surfactant replacement therapy for ARDS has not been widely embraced. Only two reports are to be found in the literature describing attempts at surfactant replacement therapy in clinical settings (76, 77). This paucity of clinical application of a theoretically desirable therapy is somewhat disconcerting. A partial explanation may be that, unlike prematurity, animal models of ARDS look like ARDS but still are fully equivalent to the human disease. It is nonetheless encouraging to see that reports on laboratory investigations of surfactant replacement in animal models of ARDS are growing in number. Clinical trials are also underway, but no reports are yet available.

One of the pioneer studies of surfactant replacement in adult lung injury was done by Lachmann and coworkers (78)

using an in vivo lung lavage model with guinea pigs, although the argument could be made that the pathophysiology of this model mimics IRDS. Exogenous surfactant administration has shown positive effects in other models of lung injury caused by antilung serum (79), *N*-nitroso-*N*-methylurethane (74, 80), hyperoxia (81, 82), and *Pneumocystis carinii* pneumonia in immunocompromised rats (83).

FUTURE DIRECTIONS

Much work remains to be done before surfactant replacement therapy becomes as commonplace as other modalities employed in critical care. Exogenous surfactant administration in IRDS is well-accepted, but the search for the ideal formulation is not over. In the case of ARDS we are only starting to gather the necessary information that will lead to successful use of this therapy.

We believe that replacement therapy for surfactant deficiency states should not be the final answer but only a temporizing move, while ways to either prevent surfactant deficiencies or induce secretion of new surfactant are discovered. We have already seen this process occur in the case of prematurity, where induction of lung maturation in utero is an accepted practice. However, until prevention and induction are feasible, surfactant replacement will continue to decrease the morbidity and mortality associated with the dysfunction of the endogenous surface-active system of the lung.

REFERENCES

1. Hollingsworth M, Gilfillan AM: The pharmacology of lung surfactant secretion, *Pharmacol Rev* 36 (2):69–90, 1984.
2. Shimizu S, Vayuvegula B, Ellis M, et al: Regulation of immune functions by human surfactant. *Ann Allergy* 61:459–462, 1988.
3. Pattle RE: Properties, function and origin of the alveolar lining layer. *Nature* 175:1125–1126, 1955.
4. Clements JA: Surface tension of lung extracts. *Proc Soc Exp Biol Med* 95:170–172, 1957.
5. Possmayer F: Pulmonary perspective: a proposed nomenclature for pulmonary surfactant-associated proteins. *Am Rev Respir Dis* 138:990–998, 1988.
6. Whitsett JA, Ohning BL, Ross G, et al: Hydrophobic surfactant-associated protein in whole lung surfactant and its importance for biophysical activity in lung surfactant extracts used for replacement therapy. *Pediatr Res* 20:460–467, 1986.
7. Wright JR, Clements JA: Metabolism and turnover of lung surfactant. *Am Rev Respir Dis* 135:426–434, 1987.
8. Crecelius CA, Longmore WJ: Phosphatidic acid phosphatase activity in subcellular fractions derived from adult rat type II pneumocyte in primary culture. *Biochim Biophys Acta* 750:447–456, 1983.
9. Massaro GD, Massaro D: Granular pneumocytes. Electron microscopic radioautographic evidence of intracellular protein transport. *Am Rev Respir Dis* 105:927–931, 1972.
10. Ryan US, Ryan JW, Smith DS: Alveolar type II cells: studies on the mode of release of lamellar bodies. *Tissue Cell* 7:587–599, 1975.
11. Robertson B, van Golde LMG, Batenburg JJ (eds): *Pulmonary Surfactant*. Elsevier, Amsterdam, 1984.
12. Van Golde LMG, Batenburg JJ, Robertson B: The pulmonary surfactant system: biochemical aspects and functional significance. *Physiol Rev* 68:374–455, 1988.
13. Ballard PL: Hormonal regulation of pulmonary surfactant. *Endo Rev* 10:165–181, 1989.
14. Nicholas TE, Power JHT, Barr HA: Surfactant homeostasis in the rat lung during swimming exercise. *J Appl Physiol* 53:1521–1528, 1982.
15. Oyarzun MJ, Clements JA: Control of lung surfactant by ventilation, adrenergic mediators and prostaglandins in the rabbit. *Am Rev Respir Dis* 17:879–891, 1978.
16. Brown LAS, Longmore WJ: Adrenergic and cholinergic regulation of lung surfactant secretion in the isolated perfused rat lung and in the alveolar type II cell in culture. *J Biol Chem* 256:66–72, 1981.
17. Baritussio AG, Magoon MW, Goerke J, Clements JA: Precursor-product relationship between rabbit type II cell lamellar bodies and alveolar surface active material. Surfactant turnover time. *Biochim Biophys Acta* 666:382–393, 1981.
18. Jobe A, Kirkpatrick E, Gluck L: Labeling of phospholipids in the surfactant and subcellular fractions of rabbit lung. *J Biol Chem* 253:3810–3816, 1978.
19. Fisher AB, Dodia C, Chander A: Adrenergic mediators increase pulmonary retention of instilled phospholipids. *J Appl Physiol* 59:743–748, 1985.

20. Enhorning G: Pulsating bubble technique for evaluating pulmonary surfactant. *J Appl Physiol* 43:198–203, 1977.
21. Notter RH, Finkelstein JN: Pulmonary surfactant: an interdisciplinary approach. *J Appl Physiol* 57:1613–1624, 1984.
22. Hall SB, Venkitaraman AR, Whitsett JA, Holm BA, Notter RH: Importance of hydrophobic apoproteins as constituents of clinical exogenous surfactants. *Am Rev Respir Dis* 145:24–30, 1992.
23. Hagwood S, Benson BJ, Hamilton RL: Effects of a surfactant-associated protein and calcium ions on the structure and surface activity of lung surfactant lipids. *Biochemistry* 24:184–190, 1985.
24. Dobbs LG, Wright JR, Hagwood S, Gonzalez R, Venstrom K, Nellenbogen J: Pulmonary surfactant and its components inhibit secretion of phosphatidylcholine from cultured rat alveolar type II cells. *Proc Natl Acad Sci USA* 84:1010–1014, 1987.
25. Wright JR, Wager RE, Hagwood S, Dobbs L, Clements JA: Surfactant apoprotein Mr = 26,000–36,000 enhances uptake of liposomes by type II cells. *J Biol Chem* 262:2888–2894, 1987.
26. Gilfillan AM, Smart DA, Rooney SA: Phosphatidylglycerol stimulates cholinephosphate cytidylyltransferase activity and phosphatidylcholine synthesis in type II pneumocyte. *Biochim Biophys Acta* 835:141–146, 1985.
27. Avery ME, Mead J: Surface properties in relation to atelectasis and hyaline membrane disease. *Am J Dis Child* 97:517–523, 1959.
28. Farrell PM, Zachman RD: Induction of choline phosphotransferase and lecithin synthesis in the fetal lung by corticosteroids. *Science* 179:297–299, 1973.
29. Ashbaugh DG, Bigelow DB, Petty TL, Levine BE: Acute respiratory distress in adults. *Lancet* ii:319–323, 1967.
30. Petty TL, Reiss OK, Paul GW, Silvers GW, Elkins ND: Characteristics of pulmonary surfactant in adult respiratory distress syndrome associated with trauma and shock. *Am Rev Respir Dis* 115:531–536, 1977.
31. Von Wichert P, Kohl FV: Decreased dipalmitoyllecithin content found in lung specimens from patients with so-called shock-lung. *Eur Intensive Care Med* 3:27–30, 1977.
32. Hallman M, Spragg R, Harrell JH, Moser KM, Gluck L: Evidence of lung surfactant abnormality in respiratory failure. *J Clin Invest* 70:673–683, 1982.
33. Pison U, Obertacke U, Brand M, et al: Altered pulmonary surfactant in uncomplicated and septicemia-complicated courses of acute respiratory failure. *J Trauma* 30 (1):19–26, 1990.
34. Liau F, Redington Barret C, Loomis Bell AL, et al: Diphosphatidylglycerol in experimental acute alveolar injury in the dog. *J Lipid Res* 25:678–683, 1984.
35. Ikegami M, Jobe A, Jacobs H: A protein from airways of premature lambs that inhibits surfactant function. *J Appl Physiol* 57:1134–1142, 1984.
36. Fuchimukai T, Fujiwara T, Takahashi A, Enhorning G: Artificial pulmonary surfactant inhibited by proteins. *J Appl Physiol* 62:429–437, 1987.
37. Seeger W, Stohr G, Wolf HRD: Alteration of surfactant function due to protein leakage: special interaction with fibrin monomers. *J Appl Physiol* 58:326–328, 1985.
38. Holm BA, Notter RH: Effects of hemoglobin and cell membrane lipids on pulmonary surfactant activity. *J Appl Physiol* 63:1434–1442, 1987.
39. Li JJ, Sanders RL, McAdam KP, et al: Impact of C-reactive protein (CRP) on surfactant function. *J Trauma* 29:1690–1697, 1989.
40. Millar AB, Singer M, Meagher A, et al: Tumor necrosis factor in bronchopulmonary secretions of patients with adult respiratory distress syndrome. *Lancet* 712–714, Sept 23, 1989.
41. Fuchs HJ, Debs R, Patton JS, et al: The pattern of lung injury induced after pulmonary exposure to tumor necrosis factor-α depends on the route of administration. *Diagn Microbiol Infect Dis* 13:397–404, 1990.
42. Wheeler AP, Jesmock G, Brigham KL: Tumor necrosis factor's effects on lung mechanics, gas exchange, and airway reactivity in sheep. *J Appl Physiol* 68:2542–2549, 1990.
43. Wispe JR, Clark JC, Warner BB, et al: Tumor necrosis factor-alpha inhibits expression of pulmonary surfactant protein. *J Clin Invest* 86:1954–1960, 1990.
44. Young SL, Crapo JD, Kremers SA, Brumley GW: Pulmonary surfactant lipid production in oxygen-exposed rat lungs. *Lab Invest* 46:570–576, 1982.
45. Gross NJ, Smith DM: Impaired surfactant phospholipid metabolism in hyperoxic mouse lungs. *J Appl Physiol* 51:1198–1203, 1981.
46. Ward JA, Roberts RJ: Effect of hyperoxia on phosphatidylcholine synthesis, secretion, uptake and stability in newborn rabbit lung. *Biochim Biophys Acta* 796:42–50, 1984.
47. Holm BA, Matalon S, Finkelstein JN, Notter RH: Type II pneumocyte changes during hyperoxic lung injury and recovery. *J Appl Physiol* 65:2672–2678, 1988.
48. King RJ, Coalson JJ, Seidenfeld JJ, Anzueto AR, Smith DB, Peters JI: O₂ and pneumonia-induced lung injury. II. Properties of pulmonary surfactant. *J Appl Physiol* 67:357–365, 1989.
49. Holm BA, Notter RH, Siegle J, Matalon S: Pulmonary physiological and surfactant changes during injury and recovery from hyperoxia. *J Appl Physiol* 59:1402–1409, 1985.
50. Holm BA, Matalon S: Role of pulmonary surfactant in the development and treatment of adult respiratory distress syndrome. *Anesth Analg* 69:805–818, 1989.
51. Notter RH: Biophysical behavior of lung surfactant: implications for respiratory physiology and pathophysiology. *Semin Perinatol* 12:180–212, 1988.
52. Seeger W, Pison U, Buchhorn R, Obertacke U, Joka T: Surfactant abnormalities and adult respiratory failure. *Lung* 168 (suppl): 891–902, 1990.
53. Robillard E, Alaire Y, Dagenais-Perusse P, Baril E, Guilbeault A: Microaerosol administration of synthetic (β-γ-dipalmitoyl-α-lecithin) in the respiratory distress syndrome: a preliminary report. *Can Med Assoc J* 90:55–57, 1964.
54. Chu J, Clements JA, Cotton EK, Klaus MH, Sweet AY, Tooley WH: Neonatal pulmonary ischemis. *Pediatrics* 40 (suppl):709–782, 1967.
55. Ivey H, Roth S, Kattwinkel J: Nebulization of sonicated phospholipids (PL) for treatment of respiratory distress syndrome (RDS) of infancy (abst.). *Pediatr Res* 11:573, A1207, 1977.
56. Fujiwara T, Maeta H, Chida S, Morita T, Watabe Y, Abe T: Artificial surfactant therapy in hyaline-membrane disease. *Lancet* i:55–59, 1980.
57. Jobe A, Ikegami M: Surfactant for the treatment of respiratory distress syndrome. *Am Rev Respir Dis* 136:1256–1275, 1987.
58. Hallman M, Merrit TA, Schneider H, et al: Isolation of human surfactant from amniotic fluid and a pilot study of its efficacy in respiratory distress syndrome. *Pediatrics* 71:473–482, 1983.
59. Noack G, Berggren P, Curstedt T, et al: Severe neonatal respiratory distress syndrome treated with the isolated phospholipid fraction of natural surfactant. *Acta Pediatr Scand* 76:697–705, 1987.
60. Shapiro DL, Notter RH, Morin III FC, et al: Double-blind randomized trial of a calf lung surfactant extract administered at birth to very premature infants for prevention of respiratory distress syndrome. *Pediatrics* 76:593–599, 1985.
61. Enhorning G, Shennan A, Possmayer F, Dunn M, Chen CP, Milligan J: Prevention of neonatal respiratory distress syndrome by tracheal instillation of surfactant: A randomized clinical trial. *Pediatrics* 76:145–153, 1985.
62. Possmayer F: A proposed nomenclature for pulmonary surfactant-associated proteins. *Am Rev Respir Dis* 138:990–998, 1988.
63. Horbar JD, Soll RF, Sutherland JM: A multicenter randomized placebo-controlled trial of surfactant therapy for respiratory distress syndrome. *N Engl J Med* 320:959–965, 1989.
64. Ten Centre Study Group: Ten centre trial of artificial surfactant (artificial lung expanding compound) in very premature babies. *Br Med J* 294:961–966, 1987.
65. Morley CJ, Greenough A, Miller NG, et al: Randomized trial of artificial surfactant (ALEC) given at birth to babies from 23 to 34 weeks gestation. *Early Hum Dev* 17:476–478, 1988.
66. Exosurf pediatric sterile powder treatment IND protocol EXO-501. Burroughs Wellcome, Research Triangle Park, NC (BW Document THPR/89/0042) 1989.
67. Notter RH: Physical chemistry and physiological activity of pulmonary surfactant. In Shapiro DL, Notter RH (eds): *Surfactant Replacement Therapy.* Alan R Liss, New York, pp 19–70, 1989.
68. Holm BA, Venkitaraman AR, Enhorning G, Notter RH: Biophysical inhibition of synthetic lung surfactants. *Chem Phys Lipids* 52:243–250, 1990.
69. Holm BA, Notter RH: Surfactant therapy in adult respiratory distress syndrome and lung injury. In Shapiro DL, Notter RH (eds); *Surfactant Replacement Therapy.* Alan R Liss, New York, pp 273–304, 1989.
70. Durand DJ, Clyman RI, Heymann MA et al: Effects of a protein-free, synthetic surfactant on survival and pulmonary function in preterm lambs. *J Pediatr* 107:775–780, 1985.
71. Bose C, Corbet A, Bose G, et al: Improved outcome at 28 days of age for very low birth weight infants treated with a single dose of synthetic surfactant. *J Pediatr* 117:947–953, 1990.
72. Corbet A, Bucciarelli R, Goldman S, et al, the American Exosurf Pediatric Study Group: Decreased mortality rate among small premature infants treated at birth with a single dose of a synthetic surfactant: a multicenter controlled trial. *J Pediatr* 118:277–284, 1991.
73. Kendig J, Notter R, Cox C, et al: A comparison of surfactant as immediate prophylaxis and as rescue therapy in newborns of less than thirty weeks gestation. *N Engl J Med* 324:865–871, 1991.
74. Lewis J, Ikegamy M, Jobe A, Absolom D: Nebulized vs. instilled exogenous surfactant in an adult lung injury model. *J Appl Physiol* 71:1270–1276.
75. Yee WFH, Scarpelli EM: Surfactant replacement therapy. *Pediat Pulmonol* 11:65–80, 1991.
76. Richman PS, Spragg RG, Merritt TA, Robertson B, Curstedt T: Administration of porcine-lung surfactant to humans with ARDS: initial experience. *Am Rev Respir Dis* S135:A5, 1987.
77. Lachmann B: Surfactant therapy. *Resuscitation.* 18 Suppl:S37–49, 1989.
78. Lachmann B, Robertson V, Vogel J: In vivo lung lavage as an experimental model of the respiratory distress syndrome. *Acta Anesthesiol Scand* 24:231–236, 1980.
79. Lachmann B, Hallman M, Bergmann KC: Respiratory failure following antilung serum: study on mechanisms associated with surfactant system damage. *Exp Lung Res* 12:163–180, 1987.
80. Ryan SF, Liau DF, Bell AL, Hashim SA, Barret CR: Correlation of lung compliance and quantities of surfactant phospholipids after acute alveolar injury from N-nitroso-N-methylurethane in the dog. *Am Rev Respir Dis* 123:200–204, 1981.
81. Matalon S, Holm BA, Notter RH: Mitigation of pulmonary hyperoxic injury by administration of exogenous surfactant. *J Appl Physiol* 62:756–761, 1987.
82. Loewen GM, Holm BA, Milanowski I, Wild LM, Matalon S: Alveolar hyperoxic injury in rabbit receiving exogenous surfactant. *J Appl Physiol* 66:1087–1092, 1988.
83. Eijking EP, van Daal G-J, Tenbrinck R, et al: Effect of surfactant replacement on Pneumocystis carinii pneumonia in rats. *Intensive Care Med.* 17:475–478, 1991.

CHAPTER 67

Pharmacotherapy of Shock

EDMUND NEUGEBAUER, Ph.D
ALEX LECHLEUTHNER, M.D., Ph.D.
DIETER RIXEN, M.D.
STEFAN SAAD, M.D.

INTRODUCTION

The term "choc"—French for "push" or "impact"—was first published by the physician LeDran in 1743 (79) to describe the clinical status of patients following gunshot trauma. At that time it reflected the mistaken belief that the symptoms arose from fear or some other form of altered cerebral function. Not until the turn of the 19th century did one begin to understand the pathophysiology of this syndrome. In 1899 Crile initially realized that replacement of blood volume with intravenous fluid administration decreased mortality in experimental hemorrhagic shock (33). In the mid-20th century Wiggers (180) then introduced a new era of shock research in "the physiology of shock" followed by the advent of cardiopulmonary resuscitation by Liss in 1960 (84). From that time on, research in the wide field of medicine led to new aspects and insights into the pathophysiology and treatment of shock.

For most authors it is a sine qua non first to define a disease state (e.g., shock) before describing etiology, pathophysiology, diagnosis, and treatment. However, as demonstrated by history, definitions are a matter of change, depending on increasing knowledge and professional background of the scientists. It was Karl Popper in 1945 (122) who argued against strict definitions because they are always insufficient and incomplete. Instead he proposed to count several determinants of the state of the disease for description. This approach obviously has the advantage that new insights can be added without giving a new definition. Several commonly accepted determinants of shock are given in Table 67.1.

It is the aim of this chapter to present our current view on etiology, pathophysiology, and management of shock—with emphasis on pharmacotherapy—being aware that future investigations will be necessary to put the puzzle together.

PATHOPHYSIOLOGY OF SHOCK

CHANGES IN MACROCIRCULATION

Depending on cardiac output (CO) and the total systemic vascular resistance (SVR) in general, two hemodynamic states of shock can be distinguished: the hyperdynamic and hypodynamic state (88).

Hyperdynamic Shock State

Usually, shock develops with inadequate capillary perfusion by decreased CO following heart attack (cardiogenic shock) or blood/volume loss (hypovolemic shock). Early in septic shock, however, CO stays normal or increases because of an increased arteriovenous shunting. Therefore, the early phase of septic shock is characterized by only a slight decrease in blood pressure combined with normal or increased CO, tachycardia, and decreased SVR. The leading causes are most often bacteremia, endo-, or exotoxemia with inadequate mediator release or formation, followed by decrease of precapillary vascular tonus. The cerebral pyrogen reaction and the generalized sympathoadrenergic reaction stimulate the heart to an increased CO. The host counteracts to peripheral vasodilation as well as to a relative (and later on, an absolute) volume loss with a consecutive decrease in CO. This initial hyperdynamic state can progress to a subsequent hypodynamic state.

Hypodynamic Shock State

A decrease in CO leads to a decrease in blood pressure. The sympathoadrenergic response is initiated via aortic and carotid baroreceptors. Catecholamines and angiotensins are released. Heart rate, myocardial contractility, and SVR increase. Released or newly formed vasoactive substances lead to nonuniform effects in different vascular regions of various organs, depending on α- and β-receptor distribution.

Owing to α-adrenergic preference, the arterial vasculature of kidneys, skin, muscles, and splanchnics, as well as postcapillary venous regions, constricts. In the heart and brain, blood supply remains adequate, as α-receptors are scarce. This cardiovascular compensating mechanism prevents a further decrease in blood pressure and is known as "centralization."

CHANGES IN MICROCIRCULATION

Tissue perfusion not only relies on an adequate pressure gradient but also on the function of precapillary resistance, as well as the capacitative postcapillary venules. Furthermore, blood flow influences local perfusion (163): all shock states show a disturbance of the terminal vessels and aligning endothelial cells.

The terminal arterioles (precapillary resistance vessels) regulate the volume of flow into the capillary system. In shock, sympathoadrenergic stimulation leads to vasoconstriction of both precapillary and postcapillary vessels. As a result of precapillary constriction, the pressure gradient, the flow velocity, and the amount of capillary perfusion decrease (69). The spontaneous arteriolar vasomotion (48) is impaired, and capillary perfusion becomes irregular.

During further shock development, oxygen supply decreases, forcing the organism to generate energy by anaerobic glycolysis. Consequently, muscle, and liver cells especially, release lactate, followed by lactic acidosis. Disturbances in liver and renal function, with reduced lactate elimination, increase acidosis. Finally, intracellular acidosis inhibits the key enzymes of glycolysis, limiting this source of energy supply.

The decrease in oxygen supply, the shift to anaerobic glycolysis, and the consecutive acidosis alter the reaction of terminal resistance vessels in response to the continual sympathetic activities. The precapillary vessels dilate, while postcapillary vessels remain constricted (shock-specific vasomotion) (95).

Table 67.1. Commonly Accepted Determinants of Shock

Determinants of Shock
— Inadequate tissue perfusion
— Sustained loss of effective circulatory blood volume
— Breakdown of cellular metabolism and microcirculatory homeostasis
— Hypoperfusion of peripheral tissue that leads to a diminutive transcapillary exchange function
— Disproportion between oxygen delivery (VO₂) and oxygen demand (DO₂)

This situation results in an increase in blood flow to the capillary system, leading to a "pooling" effect in front of the venules. This volume shift again produces an additional hypovolemia in the macrocirculation. Additionally, the increased hydrostatic filtration pressure causes fluid loss into tissues. This extravasation is promoted by a mediator-induced increase in capillary permeability for larger molecules (e.g., proteins), which themselves can bind water (83). Thus, large molecular weight compounds also appear in the intraalveolar fluid, leading to pulmonary edema (capillary leak syndrome) (137). Local and systemic hematocrit, as well as blood viscosity, increases. This increase again adds to the reduced flow velocity. Erythrocytes aggregate and obstruct the capillary system. Additionally, leukocytes stick to the endothelium in shock, obstructing vessels, which leads to local ischemia (4). Circulatory shock finally exists when tissue perfusion is inadequate to maintain normal cellular functioning. These changes in microcirculation lead to the *circulus vitiosus of shock* (Fig. 67.1).

MEDIATOR RESPONSE IN CIRCULATORY SHOCK

Shock interferes with a complex system of feedback loops involving numerous regulatory systems. The catecholamines, the renin-angiotensin system, electrolytes, pituitary and adrenal hormones, eicosanoids, endorphins, neuropeptides, cytokines, and other mediators all influence normal homeostasis. Cells mainly responsible for mediator release/formation are macrophages/monocytes, neutrophils, platelets, endothelial cells, and mast cells (157). A prerequisite for developing adequate therapeutic interventions is the exact knowledge of mediator physiology and pathophysiology. Currently, we are far from having a clear-cut picture (58). Mediator release occurs at variable times throughout shock; many of them have positive homeostatic activities in shock states, others may contribute to the observed hemodynamic, pulmonary, and other abnormalities associated with circulatory shock.

Estimates of the current role of a single mediator or active substance as a "shock toxin" vary tremendously, depending on current shock paradigms, the state of shock progression (organ insufficiency), as well as the experimental conditions (model, species) studied (108). Table 67.2 gives an overview on currently described active substances as candidates for pathophysiologic reactions in shock. This list of mediators currently is comprised of more than 150 candidates. In order to evaluate which mediators are causally associated with the

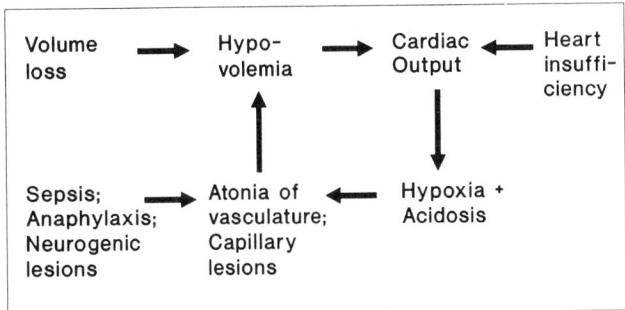

Figure 67.1. Schematic representation of the circulus vitiosus of shock.

Table 67.2. Active Substances as Candidates of Pathologic Reactions in Shock[a, b]

Classes of Chemical Substances	Active Substance (Single Compounds or Groups)	Specification or Examples of Active Substances
1. Biogenic amines	Histamine	
	Acetylcholine	
	Serotonin (5-HT)	
	Catecholamine	Epinephrine, norepinephrine, dopamine
2. Oligo- and polypeptides	Tyramine	
	Tachykinins	Substance P
	Bradykinins	Bradykinin, kallidine, prekallikrein, kininogen
	Peptide hormones	Neurotensin, somatostatin, vasoactive intestinal peptide (VIP), vasopressin, angiotensin, tPA, tPAI-1
	Endogenous opioids	Encephaline, β-endorphin
	Anaphylatoxins	C4a, C3a, C5a, C5b9
	Chemotactic factors	ECF-A, M-CSF, G-CSF, GM-CSF
	Endothelial cell factors	EDRF, (NO), endothelin
	Macrophage-derived factors	TNF, IL1- IL10, γ-interferon
3. Proteins	α-2-glycoprotein	
	Fibronectin	
	Chemotactic factors	Neutrophil chemotactic factor (NCF-A)
	Proteolytic enzymes	Hagemann factor (HFa), plasmine, chymase, tryptase, C1-esterase, arginine esterase, elastase, lactoferrin
	Acid hydrolases	β-Glucuronidase, arylsulphatase
4. Fatty acid derivatives	Prostaglandins	Prostaglandin E1, E2, D2, F_2-α
	Thromboxane	Thromboxane A2, B2
	Prostacyclin	Prostaglandin I2
	Leukotrienes	LTC4, LTD4, LTE4
	Arachidonic acid—metabolites	5-HETE, 5-HPETE
	Platelet-activating factors	PAF-acether and derivatives
5. Varia	Heparins	
	Nucleotides and nucleosides	ATP, inosine, cyclic nucleotides
	Ca—ions and Ionophores	Ca^{2+}, Calcium ionophore
	O_2—radicals	O_2^-, HO_2^-, H_2O_2, OH^-

[a] From Neugebauer E, Lorenz W, Maroske D, Barthlen W, Ennis M: The role of mediators in septic/endotoxic shock. A meta-analysis evaluating the current status of histamine. *Theor Surg* 2:1–28, 1987a.

[b] Active substances are defined as chemically identified compounds, mediating signals from cell to cell.

pathophysiology of shock, it is generally accepted to use the four classical Koch-Dale criteria as an initial approach (107):

1. *Presence in disease:* The circulating concentration of the active substance must be increased in the disease state.
2. *Absence in health:* The active substance must be absent or below pathologic values
3. *Eliciting disease by exogenous administration:* When administered alone, the substance must elicit some of the responses seen in shock.
4. *Blocking the effect by "antagonists" and preventing disease:* When the substance is inhibited in some way, the disease state must improve.

Unfortunately, much confusion exists owing to misinterpretation of published findings as to cause and effect. To increase empirical evidence for a causal relationship, several other types of association, mainly, bias in selection of patients or animal species/strains, measurement bias, the role of chance, and confounding bias, must be excluded. This goal can be achieved—thus coming to a more valid evaluation of the current status of single mediators in shock—by using the model of a decision tree as described by Neugebauer et al (104, 107) for all four Koch-Dale criteria.

In fulfilling all criteria, a causal relationship of a mediator in shock can be assumed, though not necessarily its relative

Table 67.3. Mediators with Proof of Causal Relationship to Shock[a]

Toxins	Endotoxins
Oligo- and polypeptides	Complement factors (C3a, C5a)
	Opioids (β-endorphin)
	Tumor necrosis factor (TNF), interleukins (IL1, IL6)
Fatty acid derivatives	Arachidonic acid metabolites (TXA_2, PGI_2, LTC4-E4)
	Platelet-activating factor (PAF)
Varia	Calcium

[a] From Holaday JW, Neugebauer E, Carr DB: Meta²—An analysis of meta-analyses of mediators in septic shock. In Neugebauer E, Holaday, JW (eds): *Handbook of Mediators in Septic Shock.* CRC Press, Boca Raton, FL, 1993, pp 523–534.

significance in the concert of mediators. For this, one has to apply further multicausal models, causal networks, or chaos research models, which will not be covered in this chapter (107). The list of mediators (Table 67.2) is reduced significantly when Koch-Dale criteria are applied. This leads to mediators listed in Table 67.3, for which today a causal relationship is more or less proven. Several therapeutic approaches have been developed to control inadequate mediator response. They will be described in a subsequent chapter.

METABOLIC RESPONSE IN CIRCULATORY SHOCK

In shock, glucagon and catecholamine secretion increase, with a subsequent shift in metabolism towards gluconeogenesis and triglyceride formation. Increased glucagon secretion causes hepatic glucose mobilization, resulting in hyperglycemia. Increased catecholamine secretion inhibits insulin release and reduces peripheral glucose uptake, contributing further to hyperglycemia. Despite the hyperglycemic state, the skeletal muscles—in need of energy—cannot utilize the circulating glucose because of the lack of relative insulin. Muscle proteolysis is initiated. Inhibition of pyruvate dehydrogenase activity makes skeletal muscles dependent on the oxygenation of branched-chain amino acids for energy, with an increase of alanine production (170). Alanine is then either expected in the kidney or utilized in the gluconeogenic process of the liver (153); further exacerbation of the hyperglycemia results. Increased alanine concentration also allows carbon fragments to enter the liver's tricarboxylic acid cycle, converting them to fatty acids via malonyl-CoA. Consequently, hypertriglyceridemia results, characteristically seen in septic patients. Unfortunately, malonyl-CoA additionally inhibits fatty acid oxidation and hepatic ketogenesis, which results in a decrease of ketone bodies available in sepsis for energy metabolism by skeletal muscle (154). Finally, sepsis also shifts metabolism toward an increase in hepatic protein synthesis, resulting in a production of "acute-phase proteins" (e.g., C-reactive protein, α-1-antitrypsin, and coeruloplasmine) (154).

TYPES OF CIRCULATORY SHOCK

The causes of shock can generally be attributed to alterations of one of the following four main hemodynamic parameters: quantity of blood volume; vascular tonus; cardiac performance and blood circulation. Thus, it is possible to divide circulatory shock into four major categories with different subgroups (Table 67.4), hypovolemic; distributive; cardiogenic; obstructive. Blood loss, accidental—or burn trauma, for instance—is a primary cause of volume reduction (hypovolemia). Bacterial factors, immunologic reactions, or neurovegetative discoordination lead to major microcirculatory changes in septic, anaphylactic, or neurogenic shock. Reduced cardiac performance (e.g. following heart attack) leads to cardiogenic shock, while circulatory arrest by obstruction to the outflow of blood from the heart (e.g., following pulmonary embolism,

Table 67.4. Main Classes of Circulatory Shock

1. Hypovolemic shock
Hemorrhagic/traumatic
Dehydrative
Burn
2. Distributive shock
Septic
Anaphylactic, anaphylactoid
Neurogenic
3. Cardiogenic shock
4. Obstructive shock
Pulmonary embolism
Cardiac tamponade
Pneumothorax

cardiac tamponade, or tension pneumothorax) leads to obstructive shock. Of course, a considerable overlap among shock states exists. Nevertheless, dividing "shock" into these four main categories is helpful for understanding the etiology and characteristics of the various shock states, as well as the different approaches to therapy.

HYPOVOLEMIC SHOCK

Hemorrhagic/Traumatic Shock

If hypovolemic shock is caused by acute blood loss, e.g., by gastrointestinal bleeding, aneurysm rupture, or traumatic vascular perforation, the term "hemorrhagic shock" is most appropriate. "Traumatic" or "hemorrhagic/traumatic shock" should be used if major tissue damage is associated.

The incidence of gastrointestinal bleedings in Germany totals up to 50 to 100/100,000 patients per year, with a mortality rate of more than 20% in ulcer bleedings (169). Taking into account data from Great Britain, the incidence of aortic aneurysm rupture is 5 : 100,000 per year, with a mortality of over 50% (70, 93). The incidence of traumatic vascular perforation is concomitant with civil or wartime situations, with mortality again correlating to injury localization and extension, as well as to the amount of blood loss. In the U.S., approximately 1700 traumatic injuries (respectively, 100 severe injuries) per 100,000 occur per year, leading to an annual mortality rate of 150,000 persons (28). It is the leading cause of death in people under 45 years of age.

Dehydrative Shock

Hypovolemia can also be caused by nonhemorrhagic conditions as, e.g., plasma or water/electrolyte loss (e.g., by diarrhea, vomiting, ileus, peritonitis, pancreatitis). In contrast to hemorrhagic shock, hemoconcentration occurs quickly, amplifying microthrombi development by blood flow reduction.

In shock following burn, massive volume loss and toxin release are dominant. The overall incidence of burn injuries is estimated as about 200 to 400/100,000 persons per year (135). Children and adults over 60 years are considered to be high-risk groups with high mortality rates (165).

DISTRIBUTIVE SHOCK

Septic Shock

At present, there is no unified definition available for "septic shock." The terms bacteremia, sepsis, septicemia, sepsis syndrome, and septic shock are used interchangeably in the literature. This imprecise terminology causes considerable confusion when used in comparative clinical investigations (16, 17). The definitions recently proposed by Bone (Table 67.5) should be provisionally accepted as working definitions.

Recent statistics estimate 400,000 cases of sepsis per year in the U.S. (97). About 5 cases of sepsis occur in 1000 in-hospital patients (119). In 20 to 40% of septic patients, septic shock develops. This statistic is accompanied by an increasing incidence of organ failure (73) and mortality (75). In the U.S., septic shock is estimated to cause 100,000 deaths annually (120).

Table 67.5. Proposed Delineation of Terminology (Bone (16), (17))

Term	Definition
Bacteremia	Positive blood culture
Septicemia	Old term, no longer to be used[a]
Sepsis	Clinical evidence of infection: tachypnea (respiration >20 breaths/min; if mechanically ventilated, minute ventilation >10 liters/min) Tachycardia (heart rate >90 beats/min) Hyperthermia or hypothermia (core or rectal temperature >101°F (38°C) or <96.1°F (35.5°C))
Sepsis syndrome[b]	Sepsis, plus evidence of altered organ perfusion (including one or more of the following): Acute changes in mental status Hypoxemia: PAO_2/FIO_2 <280 (without other pulmonary or cardiovascular disease at the cause) Increased lactate (more than upper limits of normal for the testing laboratory) Oliguria (documented urine output <0.5 ml/kg body weight for at least 1 hr (in patients with bladder catheter in place)
Septic shock	Sepsis syndrome with hypotension that is responsive to i.v. fluids or pharmacologic intervention (systemic BP < 90 mm Hg or decrease in mean arterial pressure by > 40 mm Hg from baseline in a hypertensive patient)
Refractory or nonresponsive septic shock	Sepsis syndrome with hypotension that lasts for >1 hr. These changes are not responsive to i.v. fluids (the equivalent of 500 ml of normal saline over 30 mins) or pharmacologic intervention (requiring vasopressors, e.g., dopamine >10 μg/kg × min).

[a] Sprung (160) suggests to define "septicemia" as "patients with bacteremia and sepsis."

[b] New suggested term is systemic inflammatory response syndrome (SIRS).

Although septic shock can also be triggered by fungi or viruses, statistics show that bacteria are most common, with *Escherichia coli, Klebsiella, Bacterioides, Pseudomonas,* and *Hemophilus* in decreasing frequency (114). Septic shock resulting from Gram-negative bacteria is caused by the release of lipopolysaccharide (endotoxin) from the bacterial wall, leading to a cascade of reactions in cell, immunologic, complement, coagulation, and mediator systems.

Septic shock is not a steady state but rather a dynamic process. In general, one can subdivide septic shock into an early hyperdynamic phase and a later hypodynamic phase (88).

A more specific division was given by Siegel et al (152) stressing the developmental aspect of septic shock. For demonstration, he chose a circle diagram with four physiologic states (A, B, C, and D states) representing increasing stages of severity. The prototype patient for any one of these four states could be described by specific physiologic patterns of multivariable means. Each of these prototype states was considered a grid point in a "multidimensional physiologic hyperspace." The multivariable physiologic state of an individual patient can be quantified by measuring his "distance" from each of the prototype points at a given moment in time.

Anaphylactic, Anaphylactoid Shock

Anaphylaxis is an IgE-mediated reaction to an antigen exposure. Anaphylactoid reactions manifest in a similar way, but are not IgE-mediated. In other words, the anaphylactic, in contrast to the anaphylactoid reaction, is an immunologic response. Data regarding the incidence and prevalence of anaphylaxis and the number of deaths owing to anaphylaxis are limited. Among the known cases, adverse reactions of antibiotics and contrast media are most common (14). The incidence of reactions to these substances is about 20 to 30%, with life-threatening reactions of about 0.1 to 0.5% (87).

The predominant pathophysiologic mechanism for anaphylactic or anaphylactoid shock is histamine release. Independent of its cause (either by immunologic IgE-response or nonimmunologic mechanism), histamine release response in clinical conditions shows a wide range of severity, from a single spot of erythema or a wheal up to severe hypotension, ventricular fibrillations, bronchospasm, or the death of a patient (85).

Neurogenic Shock

Neurogenic shock is mainly due to cerebral or spinal trauma. An estimate of the annual incidence of head injury requiring medical attention is 200/100,000 population (71). Approximately 8% of head-injured patients are comatose during the first days of postinjury and have a mortality of 30 to 50% (35). Reported spinal cord injury incidence rates range from 2.8 to 5/100,000 persons per year (52).

Neurogenic shock occurs when neurovegetative discoordination results in loss of sympathetic control to the heart and circulation by loss of vasomotor function. The loss of vasomotor responsiveness and autoregulation profoundly affects the pathologic process, with alteration of blood pressure also influencing the evolution of the lesion. In contrast to other shock states, "centralization" does not occur, leaving the heart and brain without blood flow. Hypotension by relative hypovolemia appears. Local changes occur in microcirculation, causing sludging of blood flow and resulting in a decrease in tissue oxygen tension. All of these changes combine to disrupt the microcirculation and to produce an ischemic insult to the brain or spinal cord.

CARDIOGENIC SHOCK

The principal cause for cardiogenic shock is a heart attack with at least 45% loss of muscle function (164), followed by arrhythmias, myogenic insufficiency, and acute heart compression (pericardial tamponade, pneumothorax, pulmonary emboli) (13). Hemodynamically, cardiogenic shock is an extreme form of left ventricular inefficiency with high left ventricular filling pressure and reduced CO. Sympathicoadrenergic reaction increases catecholamine levels, leading to increased positive inotropy and chronotropy but also to an increase of myocardial oxygen consumption. A low cardiac output, secondary to myocardial dysfunction and pump failure, is the terminal event of all irreversible forms of shock. The exact pathomechanism is unknown, but compromised coronary perfusion (significantly when BP is below 70 mm Hg), increased metabolic demand, a decline in the ratio of subendocardium to subepicardium perfused, and myocardial intestinal edema all play some role. Therapeutic interventions in cardiogenic shock are geared to increase cardiac output, restoring perfusion pressure and preserving myocardial tissue by limiting infarct size (61).

OBSTRUCTIVE SHOCK

In obstructive shock, failure of tissue perfusion results from vascular obstruction or mechanical impairment to the outflow of blood by the heart. The reasons for obstructive shock mainly include massive pulmonary embolism, cardiac tamponade, or tension pneumothorax.

It is estimated that venous thrombosis and pulmonary embolism are associated with 300,000 to 600,000 hospitalizations/year in the U.S. and that as many as 50,000 individuals die each year as a result of pulmonary embolism (116). The pulmonary vascular and cardiac effects of embolisms are a direct consequence of the degree of obstruction of the pulmonary vascular bed. Occlusion of pulmonary blood flow results in pulmonary hypertension and can reduce systemic pressure when occlusion is more than 50%. This form of obstructive shock differs from cardiac tamponade and tension pneumothorax in that both of these result from inadequate cardiac filling and output.

Cardiac tamponade can occur following trauma, spontaneous cardiac rupture, constrictive pericarditis, or malignant pericardial effusion. Cardiac tamponade results in any degree of cardiovascular instability from transient hypotension right up to cardiac arrest. In addition to manifestations of systemic hypoperfusion, the patient may have an increase in central venous pressure (CVP) or distended neck veins or a paradoxical pulse (94).

Pneumothorax is reported to be present in 15 to 50% of patients with blunt chest injuries and is almost invariably present with transpleural penetrating injuries (39). In addition to trauma, numerous diseases are associated with pneumothorax (e.g., asthma, chronic bronchitis, and emphysema). It may also occur spontaneously in the general population at a rate as high as 18/100,000 people (34). In tension pneumothorax, air accumulates progressively within the pleural cavity as the injury acts like a one-way valve letting air in but not out again. This activity leads to a shift of mediastinal structures to the opposite hemithorax, and compression of both the contralateral lung as well as the heart. This sequence in turn results in obstruction of blood return to the right side of the heart and reduction of cardiac output, unavoidably leading to an obstructive shock state.

SPECIFIC ORGAN FAILURES IN SHOCK

Since the final common pathway for all types of shock is inadequate cellular O_2 delivery, it is clear why shock can be the initiating factor for the development of multisystem organ dysfunction or failure as described in brief below.

THE BRAIN

Cerebral blood flow is protected by at least three different autoregulative mechanisms: (*a*) Inverse relationship to both arterial blood O_2 saturation and arterial PO_2-level, (*b*) direct relationship to arterial PCO_2 levels (123), and (*c*) autoregulation of perfusion by changes in perfusion pressure.

If mean arterial pressure decreases below 60 mm Hg or the A-VO_2 difference is more than 5 vol% and mixed venous PO_2 is below 30 torr (4 kPa) (76), however, cerebral perfusion also decreases. Reduction of cerebral blood flow can affect all levels of brain function. The most common clinical manifestation, however, is an acute disorder in mental state, varying from mild changes in acuity (altered mental status) to severe coma.

THE KIDNEYS

Renal blood flow is also protected by autoregulation. Unfortunately, renal perfusion decreases if arterial pressure falls below 60 mm Hg. This decrease results in oliguria or anuria. Although therapeutic increase of systemic blood pressure may be adequate, oliguria or anuria, respectively, may persist (143). Especially in septic shock, polyuric renal failure is common (45). At present, the pathogenesis of shock-related oliguria is unknown; preglomerular vasoconstriction persists, which influences the renin-angiotensin system, prostaglandin formation, and catecholamine release. Additionally, altered filtrate rediffusion through necrotic, damaged or obstructed tubuli may be responsible.

THE HEART

Cardiac failure manifests in reduced cardiac output, with consecutive tachycardia. With resulting coronary ischemia, rhythm disturbances, and systemic arterial hypotension, cardiac dysfunction becomes impaired. As the heart fails, left ventricular end-diastolic pressure increases, causing pulmonary edema and respiratory failure. In addition, although discussed controversially in the literature, specific polypeptides ("myocardial depressant factors") are considered to play a role in cardiac failure (2, 80, 120).

THE LUNGS

In studies of patients who develop multiple organ failure, pulmonary failure is often mentioned as the first event. Adult respiratory distress syndrome (ARDS) is the most severe and final stage of pulmonary failure. It was first described in 1967 (3) and was assumed to be shock-specific. Today, multiple pathogenetic factors are accepted as causes of ARDS (sepsis, mass transfusions, long-term ventilation, pancreatitis, oxygen intoxication, etc.). According to Royston (139), characteristics of this syndrome are:

—Respiratory failure requiring mechanical ventilation
—Bilateral diffuse infiltrates on the chest radiograph
—A low total respiratory system compliance
—Arterial hypoxemia refractory to increased inspired oxygen
—A low pulmonary artery occlusion pressure.

Morphologically, a vascular congestion, perivasal and/or interstitial edema, perivasal and alveolar bleeding, atelectasis, hyperplasia of alveolar cells, swelling of endothelial cells, then fibrin precipitation and later hyaline membranes are seen. Mortality is estimated at 60% (1, 9).

THE LIVER

In shock, α-adrenergic stimulation diverts up to 30% of the hepatic blood flow elsewhere as a compensating mechanism (23). This mechanism results in local hepatic hypoxia,

Table 67.6.   Basic (Level 1) Monitoring in ICU Patients with Shock

Parameter	Method	Frequency	Normal	Shock State	Dimension
Skin	Clinical assessment	D[a]	Dry pink	Cool, wet[b] livide, pale	-
Systolic blood pressure (BP)	Arterial line	C	>90	<90	mm Hg
Heart rate (HR)	ECG	C	<100	>100	min^{-1}
Central venous pressure (CVP)	Central venous line	D, h^{-1}	>5	<5	mm Hg
Urinary output	Urinary catheter	D, h^{-1}	>50	<50	ml h^{-1}
Mixed-venous oxygen sat. (SVO$_2$)	Central venous line	D[c], 4h^{-1}	>70	<70	%
Arterial oxygen saturation (SAO$_2$)	Pulsoximetry	C	>92	<92	%
Lactate	Lab analysis	D, 4h^{-1}			
Basic blood[d] parameters	Lab analysis	D, 4-8h^{-1}	<1.3	>1.3	mmol l^{-1}
	Lab analysis	D, different	-	-	-
End-tidal CO$_2$	Expiration airflow analysis	C	>32	<32[e] >42	%

[a] C, continuous; D, discontinuous; ECG, electrocardiographic monitor.
[b] In hyperdynamic shock state, skin is pink and warm.
[c] Continuously by fiberoptic catheter systems. (Data from Rasanen, et al (127)).
[d] For example, Hb, electrolytes, base-acid status, thrombocytes.
[e] Depending on setup of mechanical ventilator.

eventually leading to acidosis, increased lactate production, and liver malfunction. The phagocytic abilities of the liver's reticuloendothelial cells are affected, so that bacteria that would usually be filtered out are instead permitted to enter into the systemic circulation (32).

THE GASTROINTESTINAL TRACT

Changes in microcirculation also affect the gastrointestinal tract. Ischemic damage, especially of the mucosal layer, increases gut permeability by destruction of mucosal filter function (19, 37), leading to a "translocation" of bacteria and endotoxin from the gastrointestinal tract into the systemic circulation. As the reticuloendothelial system (RES) is reduced in its defense ability, elimination of such a large amount of endotoxin is impaired (130). The clinical picture of a septic reaction occurs. This "septic reaction" is not a consequence of classic septicemia, but rather a generalized inflammatory reaction towards, e.g., endotoxin. Also, stress-related stomach mucosal damage may be viewed as failure of the gastrointestinal tract. Superficial erosions progress in 6 hours; ulceration appears in as little as 2 days (140).

THE BLOOD

Early in shock, coagulation factors, fibrinogen, and the amount of platelets decrease (8). Because of endothelial cell damage, prostacyclin production—the most potent natural antiaggregating substance—is decreased. In addition, high catecholamine levels in response to shock further promote platelet aggregation. Also, neutrophil polymorphonuclear leukocytes sequestrate. Vasoactive substances from damaged platelets (100), as well as oxygen-free radicals and lysosomal enzymes from activated granulocytes (129), result in further damage to the vascular endothelial cells, leading to a circulus

vitiosus. In parallel to activated plasmatic coagulation, fibrinolysis is increased. Fibrin concentrations increase, and microthrombi develop. The activation of these pathways leads to consumption of coagulation factors and to disseminated intravascular coagulation (DIC) (128).

MANAGEMENT OF SHOCK

DIAGNOSIS OF SHOCK

Shock starts when oxygen delivery (DO$_2$) to the cells is inadequate to meet the metabolic demand (imbalance between O$_2$ demand and present O$_2$ delivery). Therefore, sufficient tissue perfusion and oxygenation are the major therapeutic goals in all types of circulatory shock (150). Although hypovolemia, absolute or relative, is common in all types of shock, early diagnosis remains a major problem. Which variables should be chosen, and when and how should they be measured? The more invasive the monitoring, the more data can be obtained. The increased use of invasive measures, however, is accompanied by an increase of complications (54). Invasive monitoring thus is only indicated if the benefits exceed the risk. In most cases in daily practice, a carefully obtained history, a precise clinical examination, and basic monitoring are sufficient to assess the cause and the initial status of a shock diagnosis.

BASIC (LEVEL 1) MONITORING AND PITFALLS IN INTERPRETATION

In the basic (level 1) monitored patient, a decreasing systolic blood pressure (BP), a decreased urinary output and an increased heart rate are the first easy-to-measure signs of shock in the ICU (Table 67.6). However, normal or high BP values, as well as sufficient urinary output, can also be noticed in patients with deep shock (41). In the critically ill patient, the frequently monitored central venous pressure (CVP) often gives only a poor reflection of left ventricular performance (47). Under low oxygen delivery ($\dot{D}O_2$) conditions (e.g., hemorrhagic, cardiogenic shock), blood flow decreases and leads to hypooxygenation of the tissue, despite the fact that the oxygen extraction mechanism is very efficient. Under other shock conditions (e.g., septic shock), several factors influence tissue oxygenation by decreasing oxygen extraction ($\dot{V}O_2$), despite a normal $\dot{D}O_2$. Microthrombi, vasoactive mediators, and alterations of endothelial cell function can impair $\dot{V}O_2$ (124). Disorders can, therefore, be noticed at the level of the microcirculation, as well as at the cellular level.

In healthy subjects, the extraction of O_2 ($\dot{V}O_2$) is independent of $\dot{D}O_2$. If $\dot{D}O_2$ decreases, $\dot{V}O_2$ increases and, at a certain point, the so-called "critical oxygen delivery" ($\dot{D}O_{2crit}$) (26, 63) (variable in different tissues), $\dot{V}O_2$ becomes $\dot{D}O_2$-dependent. In an early state of shock, a decreased $\dot{D}O_2$ can be estimated

Table 67.7. CO Interpretation according to SVO_2 and Lactate[a]

CO	SVO_2	Lactate	Probable Cause
High	High	Normal	Excessive blood flow
High	High	High	Septic shock ($\downarrow$ VO_2)
High	Low	Normal	$\uparrow$ VO_2
High	Low	High	Septic shock ($\uparrow$ VO_2)
Low	High	Normal	$\downarrow$ VO_2
Low	High	High	Septic shock ($\downarrow$ VO_2)
Low	Low	Normal	Low blood flow
Low	Low	High	Shock with low blood flow

[a] According to Vincent JL, de Boelpope C, Luypaert P: Association of amrinone with norepinephrine in endotoxic shock in dogs: an experimental study (abstr). *Crit Care Med* 16:402, 1988.

from a decreasing mixed venous O_2 saturation ($SVO_2 < 70\%$) (72) (see Table 67.8). However, it must be kept in mind that the correlation between SVO_2 and $\dot{D}O_2$ is hyperbolic, so that a decrease in the high saturation values reflects a high decrease of $\dot{D}O_2$ (132). A relevant increase of CO with any therapeutic manipulation in a deficit situation only leads to a slight increase in SVO_2, if $\dot{V}O_2$ is increasing in parallel (175). An increased CO with a high increase of SVO_2 ($>80\%$) only means an increase in arteriovenous shunting, not a better tissue oxygenation. Therefore, in progressive shock states, the SVO_2 became imprecise due to an inadequate $\dot{V}O_2$. Additional measurements of blood lactate (normal value about 1 mmol/liter) are necessary to estimate the level of anaerobic metabolism. However, also the interpretation of lactate levels may be difficult, because other parameters can influence them. The production of lactate is influenced by seizures, by decompensated diabetes, and by intoxications. The elimination of blood lactate is influenced by its mobilization in the liver. The relationship between cardiac output, SVO_2 and lactate levels, as well as possible explanations, is summarized in Table 67.7. Nevertheless, all of the above-mentioned basic monitoring measures are considered adequate in many shocked patients, and although they cannot predict outcome, they can be used intelligently to guide initial volume and vasoactive drug management.

ADVANCED (LEVEL 2) MONITORING AND PITFALLS IN INTERPRETATION

While volume depletion can be avoided by careful clinical examination in combination with continuous/discontinuous

Table 67.8. Advanced (Level 2) Monitoring in ICU Patients with Shock

Parameter	Calculation	Normal	Shock State	Optimal[a]	Dimension
Mean arterial pressure (MAP)	Direct measurement	80–100	<80	>84	mm Hg
Central venous pressure (CVP)	Direct measurement	1–9	<0 or >12	<5	mm Hg
Stroke index (SI)	CI/HR	30–50	<30	>48	ml/m²
Mean pulmonary arterial pressure (MPAP)	Direct measurement	11–15	>15	<15	mm Hg
Pulmonary arterial wedge pressure (PAWP)	Direct measurement	2–12	<0 or >18	>9.5	mm Hg
Cardiac index (CI)	Direct measurement	2.5–3.5	<2.5 or >3.5	>4.5	l/min/m²
Left ventricular stroke work index (LVSW)	SI*MAP*0.0144	44–68	<40	>55	gm*m/m²
Left cardiac work index (LCW)	CI*MAP*0.0144	3–4.6	<3	>5	kg*m/m²
Right ventricular stroke work index (RVSW)	SI*MPAP*0.0144	4–8	<4	>13	gm*m/m²
Right cardiac work index (RCW)	CI*MPAP*0.0144	0.4–0.6	<0.4	>1.1	kg*m/m²
Wedge-pressure (PCWP)	Direct measurement	10–12	<10	>12	mm Hg
Systemic vascular resistance index (SVRI)	79.92(MAP-CVP)/CI	900–1200 >1200	<900	<1450	dyn*sec/cm⁻⁵*m²
Pulmonary vascular resistance index (PVRI)	79.92(MPAP-WP)/CI	45–225	>226	<226	dyn*sec/cm⁻⁵*m²
Heart rate (HR)	Direct measurement	60–100	>100	<100	beats/min
Arterial-mixed venous O_2 content difference (C(a-v)O_2)	CaO₂-CvO₂	4–5.5	<4	<3.5	
O_2 consumption (VO₂)	C(a-v)O₂*CI*10	100–180	<100	>167	ml/min*m²
O_2 delivery (DO₂)	CaO₂*Ci*10	520–720	<520	>550	ml/min*m²
O_2 extraction rate (O₂ext)	CaO₂-CvO₂)*CaO₂	22–30	>30	<31	%

[a] Optimal values according to Shoemaker et al (146, 149).

Table 67.9. Circumstances that Can Lead to Misinterpretation of Haemodynamic Variables[a]

CVP	Different tonus in venous system
	High abdominal pressure
	Mechanical ventilation
	Tricuspidal valve insufficiency
	Ventricular positioning
PAP	Wrongly adjusted pressure adapter
	Misplacement (U-shaped back position)
	Tip partly occluded (e.g., blood clots)
PCWP	PEEP (142)
	Ventilation pressure (27)
	PAC-tip not in lung zone III (91, 101)
	Vasopressures
CO	Measurement not started end-expiratory
	Tricuspidal regurgitation (101)
	Intracardiac shunts (92)
	Low-output state (101)

[a] Directly measured pressures can be influenced by hydraulic problems in the measurement system.

Table 67.10. Future Alternatives to Pulmonary Artery Catheter

	References
Thoracic electrical bioimpedance	Bernstein (11), Sramek (161)
Doppler ultrasound	Moore and Haenel (99)
Mixed-venous oximetry	Waller et al (178)
Transcutaneous O_2 monitoring	Ruppel (141)

basic monitoring at "level 1" (BP, CVP, hemoglobin (HB), hematocrit (HC), pulse oximetry, and urinary output), these variables become less appropriate in other, more complex shock states, like septic shock, cardiogenic shock (low-output syndrome), or in mixed-shock situations. Especially in the development of septic shock, early parameters, like specific mediator monitoring, are not in daily clinical use, and the measurable variables, like fever or leukocyte counts, have a low discriminative power.

In this setting, the use of invasive pulmonary artery catheters (level 2 monitoring; see Table 67.8) offers the possibility of either intermittent (or, preferably, continuous) measurement of hemodynamic variables, which are a useful guide to wholebody O_2 delivery and utilization (31). However, the widespread use of pulmonary artery catheters (PAC) is not necessarily accompanied by a better outcome. Recently, it has been proposed that the population that really benefits from a PAC must be better defined by clinical trials (138). The incidence of complications in pulmonary artery catheterization ranges, depending on definition, from 0.4% (144) to 4% (155, 158) up to 12% (149). The pulmonary catheter delivers direct measures, as well as calculated hemodynamic variables (see Table 67.8). With this information, $\dot{V}O_2$ can be directly calculated via the Fick equation ($\dot{V}O_2 = CI \times C(a - v) O_2 \times 10$). Normal or high $\dot{V}O_2$ values, however, are not valid enough to exclude shock (172, 176) (see Table 67.7). With an increasing $\dot{V}O_2/\dot{D}O_2$ quotient, blood lactate levels also increase and reflect a serious shock state (102).

The administration of volume, vasoactive drugs, alterations in ventilation, and a diverse range of stimuli, including normal nursing procedures, can cause dramatic changes in mixed venous saturation and can thus lead to incorrect conclusions (Table 67.9). These changes, which reflect alterations in O_2 delivery and utilization, occur with such rapidity that they would be difficult to observe by using intermittent measurements or by monitoring only bulk flow. Moreover, continuous monitoring of mixed venous oxygenation allows a more accurate assessment of therapeutic interventions. The combination of continuous arteriovenous and mixed venous saturation measurements allows even closer monitoring of the delivery/utilization equation and has been shown to facilitate the adjustment of ventilation in the critically ill (127). Future alternatives

to a pulmonary artery catheter are listed in Table 67.10. Further evaluation, however, is necessary before advocating them as better alternatives.

In conclusion, the reasons for a change from level 1 to level 2 monitoring are always situations when level 1 parameters no longer reflect the clinical picture, which is worsening (e.g., cold wet skin, blue acra) or when therapeutic interventions lead to unexpected values (44).

ASSESSMENT OF OXYGENATION

Careful consideration of oxygenation is paramount to the therapy of shock. Hypoxia may occur at four different levels (5): (*a*) hypoxic hypoxia; (*b*) anemic hypoxia; (*c*) stagnant (low-flow) hypoxia; and (*d*) histiotoxic or cellular hypoxia.

Hypoxic hypoxia resulting in arterial hypoxemia is the form most readily identified. Pulmonary dysfunction as a result of ventilation-perfusion mismatching and frank pulmonary shunting is a common occurrence in the shocked patient. It may be the result of pulmonary edema, pulmonary infection, pulmonary embolism, or a functional disturbance secondary to vasoactive factors, and it is recognized by the measurement of arterial PO_2 and hemoglobin saturation.

Arterial O_2 content depends on the quantity of hemoglobin available to take up and to carry O_2 to the tissues, and *anemic hypoxia* may occur during or after blood loss. To avoid anemic hypoxia it has been recommended (61) that the hemoglobin concentration should be maintained above 10 g%, preferably by using fresh blood, and the arterial pH should be maintained between 7.26 and 7.36.

The *third form of hypoxia* is that associated with low cardiac output. Despite high PaO_2 and an adequate concentration of hemoglobin, hypoxia may result secondary to pump failure. Cardiac output is a major determinant of O_2 delivery; a small reduction in its value has important consequences for tissue metabolism.

In the final form of hypoxia in the shock syndrome (*histiotoxic or cellular hypoxia*) the O_2 consumption is reduced due to circulating "toxins" (e.g., cyanide, 2,3-dinitrophenol).

In conclusion, if hypoxia is diagnosed one must aim to maintain the HB > 10g%, the PaO_2 above 8 kPa, the hemoglobin saturation above 90%, and the cardiac index (CI) above 4.5 liters/min/m^2 (147).

THERAPY OF SHOCK

Regardless of the underlying etiology, the immediate end-points of therapy remain the same and depend upon the maintenance of an adequate delivery of substrate to respiratory tissues, with the prevention or reversal of anaerobic respiration (147, 148). Manipulation by altering blood flow, blood pressure, hemoglobin level, and hemoglobin saturation aim to optimize hemodynamics and improve outcome (61).

THERAPEUTIC GOALS

Shoemaker (146, 149) established a set of *therapeutic goals* to guide treatment. These goals include:

1. CI 50% greater than normal—4.5 liters/(min/m²);
2. O₂ delivery slightly greater than normal—600 ml/(min/m²);
3. O₂ consumption 30% greater than normal—170 ml/(min/m²);
4. Blood volume 500 ml in excess of norm—3.2 liters/m² for males and 2.8 liters/m² for females.

Using these "supranormal" values as guidelines, Shoemaker et al (149) have demonstrated a decrease in mortality in a prospective trial of critically ill postoperative patients. Table 67.11 summarizes the therapeutic goals in basic (level 1) monitored patients and the principles of therapy. *Thus, support of ventilation and initial therapy for hypotension are first-aid therapeutic procedures.* The consequence of failing to proceed aggressively can be irreversible organ failure, rather than full recovery.

MECHANICAL VENTILATION

Important signs to indicate the need for ventilatory support include cyanosis, severe tachhypnea or bradypnea, use of accessory muscles during breathing, and mental obtundation. In the absence of the full shock picture, intubation and mechanical ventilation should be instituted following assessment of gas exchange, work of breathing, and the ability to maintain a patent airway. Tissue availability of oxygen is dependent on oxygen delivery (DO₂), which is the product of cardiac output (in liters per minute) × arterial oxygen content (in vol%) × 10. Adequate oxygen delivery is affected by alterations of oxyhemoglobin dissociation, the presence of abnormal hemoglobins, binding of hemoglobin by carbon monoxide, microcirculatory blood flow changes and, at the cellular level, by blockade of oxidative phosphorylation (62, 74). The importance of maintaining O₂ delivery to tissues indicates that hemoglobin levels should be maintained at greater than 10 g% (or hematocrit 30 to 35%) in patients without a history of cardiac disease and above 11.5 g% if any cardiac disease is known (22). The PaO₂ should be above 70 mm Hg (9.3 kPa), while the saturation (pulse oximetry) should be at least 90%. SVO₂ data and blood lactate values should be interpreted together (133, 175; see also Table 67.7).

VOLUME REPLETION

Aggressive resuscitative measures for arterial hypotension should be undertaken whenever the systolic blood pressure is unacceptably low (e.g., less than 90 mm Hg) and there are signs of vital organ malfunction. The deficit of volume in the vascular bed is often underestimated, especially in septic shock. A slow capillary filling time, a reduced urinary output, or an increase in urinary osmolarity and a decreased natriuresis can reflect a volume deficit. Moreover, an early use of vasopressors can mask a volume deficit.

The objectives of intravenous fluid administration are twofold: to replace body fluid and to increase preload and cardiac output, which should increase O₂ delivery. Once hypovolemia as a cause of shock has been treated, it is possible to differentiate between two groups of patients: those with inadequate cardiac output (pump failure) and those with high cardiac output and impaired tissue perfusion owing to maldistribution of flow or diminished substrate utilization.

The choice of fluid for resuscitation remains a cause of considerable controversy (177). Appropriate cell-free solutions are crystalloids, colloids, hyperosmolar solutions, or a combination of them. As a result of the absence of a consensus view, it is not possible to be dogmatic about fluid replacement.

For many years, the colloid vs. crystalloid controversy focused on the formation of pulmonary edema. Numerous clinical studies comparing the effects of different types of intravenous solutions on the incidence as well as severity of respiratory complications have failed to convincingly demonstrate a clinically important difference between colloids and crystalloids. Discussion of the pros and cons are beyond the scope of this chapter.

Great interest has recently arisen in the use of hyperosmolar solutions. They have the advantage that small volumes of infused fluid can draw a large volume of intracellular water into the extracellular space. Some authors have achieved success in the treatment of refractory hypovolemic shock that has not responded to vigorous fluid replacement (36, 171). For immediate resuscitation of patients who have incurred multiple injuries, Holcroft et al (67) observed that the use of 7.5% NaCl/Dextran 70 solutions resulted in a better blood pressure response and in improved survival, compared with those obtained by using Ringer's solution. Other preliminary studies have emphasized the lack of complications associated with this type of hyperosmotic solution (90). In the treatment of burns, the role of hypertonic solutions have not been established, although early clinical results have been encouraging (98). In summary, hypertonic solutions currently represent an investigative form of therapy that must be further studied before they can be generally recommended.

Table 67.11. Therapeutic Goals in Basic (Level 1) Monitored Patients and Principles of Therapy

Parameter	Therapeutic Goal	Therapeutic Principles
Skin	Dry, warm, pink-colored	
Systolic blood pressure (BP)	> 90 mm Hg	Volume, inotropic agents α-receptor stimulation
Heart rate (HR)	< 100/min	Volume, antiarrhythmics, cardioversion
Central venous pressure (CVP)	> 5 mm Hg	Volume, α-receptor stimulation
Urinary output	> 50 ml/hr	Volume, salt, diuretics
Mixed venous oxygen saturation (SAO₂)	> 70%	Oxygen carriers, volume, inotropic agents
Arterial oxygen saturation (SAO₂)	> 90%	Oxygen carriers, oxygen insufflation, ventilatory support

Table 67.12.   Properties of Different Fluids for Volume Repletion in Shock

Fluid	Volume Effect[a] (Fluid:Blood)	Coagulation Abnormalities	Anaphylactoid Reactions	Half-Life
Colloids				
Hydroxyethyl 6% Starch	1.3:1	Possible	Rare	6–8 hr
Dextran 40	2:1	Possible	Possible[b]	6 hr
Gelatine	2:1	Rare	Rare	2–3 hr
Albumin 5%	1.3:1	Rare	Rare	5–6 hr
Crystalloids				
Ringer's solution	0.25:1	No	No	Minutes
Hypertonic solution	2:1	No	No[c]	Minutes
Blood products				
Fresh frozen plasma (FFP)	1:1	No/improved	Rare[d]	5–6 hr
Red blood cells (RBC)	1-1.5:1	No	Rare[d]	days

[a] According to Shippey et al (145) and Marini (91).
[b] Hapten pretreatment recommended.
[c] Hypernatremia, decreased intracellular volume, and hyperosmolarity are limiting factors in their use.
[d] Transfusion and infection risk have to be considered.

For the use of blood products, guidelines have been established in 1985, but they vary between medical institutions and in individual patients, particularly with the recent concern about transmissible illnesses (50) (see also separate chapter in this book). Table 67.12 summarizes common properties of different fluids for volume repletion.

In conclusion, the most important factor in the success of early volume repletion is the knowledge and experience of the nursing and medical staff, rather than the choice of fluid. Rapid and aggressive treatment is vital, and so an inexperienced team should be able to use either crystalloids or colloids with equal effectiveness (126). If the rate of administration is too slow, arterial hypotension or vasopressor use is unnecessarily prolonged; if too fast, the risk of pulmonary edema increases rapidly. At all times, the rate of fluid administration should be adjusted frequently, by using changes in BP, urine output, or evidence of emerging pulmonary edema as important clinical endpoints. Additional fluid administration is dictated by the clinical response to the initial fluid challenge (177) or by new information from hemodynamic monitoring.

INOTROPIC AGENTS AND VASODILATORS

Vasoactive drugs are the next line of pharmacologic defense in the treatment of shock. They may be required immediately to support blood pressure in the early stages of shock. When these agents cannot be discontinued following intravascular volume expansion, continued pharmacologic support is necessary. Two approaches can be used: enhancing CO through the use of inotropic agents or increasing systemic vascular resistance (SVR) through the use of vasopressors.

To use these drugs most efficiently, one has to consider that different shock states have different hemodynamic profiles (CO, PVR, SVR; see Table 67.13) and that many drugs have combined effects. A comparison of currently available agents of both groups is given in Table 67.14.

Catecholamines

After volume repletion, dopamine and dobutamine are the inotropic agents of first choice in the treatment of shock.

Table 67.13.   Characteristics of Hemodynamic Estimates in Different Types of Circulatory Shock

	Preload	CO[a]	PVR	SVR
Hemorrhagic	↓	↓	↑	↑
Anaphylactic	↓/↑	↓	↑↑	↓
Cardiogenic	↑	↓↓	↑	↑
Septic (hyperdynamic)	↓	↑	↑	↓↓
Septic (hypodynamic)	↓	↓	↑	↑

[a] CO, cardiac output; PVR, pulmonary vascular resistance; SVR, systemic vascular resistance.

Dopamine.   Dopamine is an endogenous precursor of norepinephrine and has multiple, dose-related effects. A low dose (0.5 to 3 μg/kg/min), β_2, and dopaminergic effects are evident, and enhanced blood flow to renal and splanchnic beds is prominent. Higher doses (5 to 10 μg/kg/min) have positive inotropic effects, while α-actions (vasoconstriction) are seen with infusion rates above 20 μg/kg/min.

Dobutamine.   Dobutamine is a synthetic congener of isoproterenol with primarily β_1 (cardiac)- but also β_2 (vasodilatory)-stimulating properties (decrease of PAOP), with only minor influence on renal and splanchnic areas. Dobutamine leads to a decrease in cardiac filling pressures and may, in contrast to dopamine, uncover insufficient volume load. These features make the use of dobutamine desirable, even in the presence of ischemic coronary disease, as long as heart rate is not unduly increased. In cardiac failure, a simultaneous infusion of low-dose dopamine (<5 mg/kg/min) enhances renal perfusion and urine output (134).

A dopamine- and dobutamine-resistant depression of the systemic blood pressure in an adequate volume state can be improved by the α-receptor agonist *norepinephrine*. Norepinephrine is a potent vasoconstrictor of renal and mesenteric vasculature. A combination with low-dose dobutamine (1 to 3 μg/kg/min) is often used to protect renal perfusion, although it has not been demonstrated in controlled trials that using this combination results in a decrease of acute renal failure. It must be emphasized that continuous monitoring of cardiac filling pressures, CO, O_2 delivery, and O_2 extraction is essential in order to assess these potentially hazardous pharmacologic interventions.

Table 67.14. Effects of Inotropic Agents and Vasodilators on Cardiac Output (CO) and Systemic Vascular Resistance (SVR)

Drug	Receptor Interaction	CO	SVR	Dose Range ($\mu g/kg/min$)
Epinephrine	$\alpha,\beta_1\ (\beta_2)$	↑↑	↑	0.02–0.5
Norepinephrine	α,β_1	0–↑	↑↑↑	0.05–0.5
Dopamine	$\beta_2,DR\ (\alpha)$	↑	↑	2–12
Dobutamine	β_1,β_2	↑↑	0–↑	2–12
Dopexamine	β_1,β_2,DR	↑↑	0–↑	0.9–5
Vasopressin	Angiotensin III[a]	0–↓	↑↑↑	5–20
Amrinone/enoximone	PDI	↑↑	↓↓	5–10
Nifedipine		0–↑	↓	0.5–10
Nitroglycerin		0–↑	↓	3–5
Nitroprusside		0–↑	↓	0.5–5
Prostacyclin	Other	↑	↓[b]	10–40[c]

[a] Specific receptor for angiotensin III in arteriolar muscle cells (Regoli et al (131)) and central stimulation (Doussout et al (40)).
[b] For a detailed discussion see Rademacher et al (125) and Bunting et al (24).
[c] In ng/KG/min.

Dopexamine. Dopexamine, a new synthetic catecholamine with β_1-, β_2-, and dopaminergic agonistic activities, was supposed to combine the advantages of dopamine and dobutamine. With low-dose dopexamine (up to 1.0 $\mu g/kg/min$), CO is enhanced by about 40% along with enhanced renal blood flow (25%) (82). In clinical use, the future role of dopexamine has to be evaluated (174).

Other Inotropic Agents

In shock states with high SVR and low catecholamine-refractory CO, byperidine *phosphodiesterase inhibitors (PDI; amrinone, Enoximone)* can enhance CO and reduce SVR (about 50%). This group of drugs acts as a nonreceptor-mediated inhibitor of the phosphodiesterase fraction III. While β-agonists enhance the synthesis of cAMP from ATP, the PDIs inhibit the degradation of cAMP to 5-adenosine-monophosphate (5-AMP) (89). In addition to these cardiac effects, they cause a decrease of calcium in the smooth vascular muscle cells, which leads to relaxation. This mechanism can explain the decrease of SVR that is observed with PDI. Their single use in septic state with low SVR is limited, and it can only be recommended in combination with vasopressors like norepinephrine (173). Intravenous amrinone is indicated as second-line, short-term therapy of severe refractory congestive heart failure. In severe trauma with impaired cardiac performance and high SVR, we have also experienced positive effects with this drug.

In severe, norepinephrine-resistant hypotension, as a last attempt, *angiotensin II* can be applied (167). In this and other bad prognostic shock states, blood pressure can be restored for a short time.

Another future alternative in situations with subsequent loss of cardiac sensitivity to β-adrenergic stimulation (receptor down-regulation) are *H_2-agonists.* Sarcolemmal H_2-receptors are not involved in the process of receptor down-regulation. Stimulation of H_2-receptors is characterized by a reduction of cardiac preload by H_2-receptor-mediated venodilatation, reduction of cardiac afterload by arteriolar dilation, and enhancement of cardiac contractility by direct inotropic action (H_2). Clinical studies from Baumann et al (6) have shown that administration of the H_2-receptor agonist *Impromidine* exerts beneficial effects in patients with severe catecholamine-insensitive heart failure. However, high costs of synthesis, the narrow therapeutic range, and the arrythmogenic potential of impromidine limit its introduction into broader clinical practice. Newer H_2 agonists, however, have been synthesized and await clinical testing (25).

Digoxin is seldom used in the initial therapy of shock but has long been used in the treatment of tachycardia and chronic congestive heart failure. In our hands, digoxin is used in patients with shock to treat tachycardia (arrhythmia absoluta); this application is under drug monitoring control.

Vasodilators

The rationale for the use of vasodilators, including nitroprusside nitrates, hydralazine, and prostacyclin, rests on the accepted theoretical consideration that the observed systemic hypotension is partly induced by arteriolar vasoconstriction with the opening up of many low-resistance arteriovenous shunts (30). The essential prerequisite for the use of vasodilators is normovolemia with adequate preload; otherwise, profound hypotension will ensue.

Nitroglycerin. Nitroglycerin is commonly employed to reduce excessive ventricular afterload and preload. Nitroglycerin is the drug of choice for acute ischemic myocardial pain and may be beneficial after resuscitation from cardiogenic shock once appropriate coronary perfusion pressure can be maintained (62). A cotreatment with ACE inhibitors can be useful, however, in severe shock. They force hypotension by blocking the production of angiotensin II (42). The use of vasodilators is limited by a concomitant fall of systemic blood pressure and an increase of renin levels, which leads to a reduced sodium urinary excretion (151).

CORTICOSTEROIDS

The justification for corticosteroid use in the treatment of shock is based on numerous in vitro and in vivo studies. Over the years, it has been demonstrated that pharmacologic doses given early contribute to preservation of the cardiac, hemodynamic (microcirculation), and cellular-metabolic function of organ systems (12, 56, 181). Current knowledge indicates that this protection is due to the inhibition of synthesis and release of a great number of inflammatory mediators (e.g., cytokines), as summarized by Neugebauer et al (112).

Although most experimental studies in hemorrhagic/traumatic shock, anaphylactic/anaphylactoid shock, neurogenic (CNS), and septic/endotoxic shock have repeatedly shown that survival can be improved when corticosteroids are given early (either before or early after the onset of shock) (110), there is good clinical evidence only in the prophylaxis of anaphylactoid shock (77), the treatment of CNS trauma (20a), and specific bacteremic/septic states such as *Pneumocystis carinii* pneumonia (20, 49), meningitis (53, 78, 117), and typhoid fever (64).

Clinical studies in *hemorrhagic/traumatic shock* up to now have shown a positive trend (111), but further randomized controlled trials with a more homogeneous study population (including trauma scores) are necessary before traumatic shock can be reliably accepted as a given indication for glucocorticoid treatment. Such a multicenter study is currently under way in Germany (Neugebauer, personal communication).

For the treatment of *sepsis and septic shock*, glucocorticoids are presently considered as being of no benefit, especially after the publication of two negative multicenter trials (15, 166). However, both studies have been strongly criticized (115, 109, 112, 156) because of the methodological drawbacks in study design and evaluation, as well as the neglect of basic pharmacokinetic principles. Moreover, a recent meta-analysis showed a positive effect on mortality of glucocorticoids in the subgroup of Gram-negative sepsis (81). This finding leads us to conclude that the "chapter" on steroid treatment for sepsis and septic shock is still open. A further study should be performed under therapeutic drug monitoring conditions (112).

APPROACHES TO "ANTIMEDIATOR" THERAPY IN SHOCK

General approaches to control or modulate inadequate mediator response as a result of an extensive triggering of the host defense mechanisms by exogenous stimuli and their endogenous products in shock are:

(1) Inhibition of cell activation (i.e., surgical therapy of septic focus);
(2) Inhibition of transcription, translation, or mediator synthesis;
(3) Inhibition of mediator release;
(4) Neutralization of circulating or tissue mediators, such as by specific antibodies or soluble receptors;
(5) Specific end-organ receptor blockade;
(6) Pharmacologic modulation of effector cell postreceptor responses (e.g., receptor down-regulation)
(7) Competitive inhibition of mediator-receptor interaction;
(8) Increased clearance of circulating mediators (e.g., plasmapheresis, dialysis).

INHIBITION OF EXOGENOUS CELL ACTIVATION

The early, reliable diagnosis of shock is the key to successful intervention at the level of cell activation. Management can be directed towards treating the specific initiating cause and thus may halt the downward spiral of events.

Space limitations do not allow a discussion of the different initial approaches in all types of shock. The possibilities in

sepsis syndrome may serve as an example since recent pharmacologic attempts were shown to be very encouraging (29). Once the sepsis syndrome has been diagnosed, intravenous antimicrobial therapy must be initiated—before culture results are available. A methodical search for the primary site of infection and, if possible, surgical therapy of the focus is the next essential step. After gaining knowledge about the infection's organism from culture specimens, the antibiotic regimen has to be changed to the appropriate drugs. Despite major advances with these conventional attempts to inhibit bacterial growth using antibiotics, mortality remains a significant problem.

Newer approaches by neutralization of endotoxin using immunotherapy have been shown to reduce mortality in patients with Gram-negative infections. This finding was demonstrated in two large, recent randomized trials using human monoclonal immunoglobulin (IgM) antibodies that binds to the lipid A domain of endotoxin (55, 182). For further discussion and for results of polyclonal immunoglobulin therapy, see references 18 and 46.

INHIBITION (MODULATION) OF ENDOGENOUS MEDIATOR RESPONSE

This subchapter aims to describe the current view on successful experimental and clinical therapeutic approaches against mediators shown to be causally involved in different types of circulatory shock (see Table 67.3).

Histamine.   For histamine, the oldest known shock mediator (104), the best evidence for its involvement in shock is available in anaphylactic/anaphylactoid shock data. For septic/endotoxic shock, results are still contradictory despite years of research (105, 106). In general, histamine can be blocked by inhibiting its synthesis via histidine-decarboxylase inhibitors (α-fluoromethylhistamine) (106), by inhibiting its release from mast cells (disodium chromoglycate), and by blockade of H_1- and H_2-receptors, using receptor antagonists.

Experimentally as well as clinically, the effect of H_1 and H_2 prophylaxis in anaphylactic/anaphylactoid shock is proven (86). For septic/endotoxic shock, recent experimental studies on animals show that a combination of H_1-receptor antagonism, combined with H_2 agonism, is therapeutically promising (136). Histamine synthesis inhibitors, however, have not been shown to reduce mortality (103).

Complement.   Complement system activation was studied in extensive experimental as well as clinical trials in various shock states (septic/endotoxic shock, anaphylactic/anaphylactoid shock, ARDS, trauma, burns, acute pancreatitis). Possibilities for inhibition are (*a*) prevention of cell activation by cause (removal of necrotic tissue, abscess drainage) or high-dose steroids and (*b*) complement inactivation by administration of antibodies toward factors of the alternative pathway (anti C5a-antibodies). A positive effect with anti C5a antibodies was only shown in endotoxic shock and bacterial septic shock in rats (159) and primates (59, 162). Although Stevens showed a significantly reduced mortality from 75% to 0% by antibody administration, no controlled clinical trial with anti C5a antibodies has yet been performed, possibly because a correlation between increased release of complement factors and complications such as ARDS is judged contradictory in different studies (7).

Opioids. Partial responsibility of endocrine opioid peptides for hypotension in septic shock was first shown by Holaday and Faden (65). This group and others could demonstrate an improvement of hemodynamics, cardiac output, cell integrity, and mortality with the opiate antagonist naloxone in different shock models (hemorrhagic shock, septic/endotoxic shock) and among different species. Although initial, prospective clinical studies were promising in septic shock (57, 121), subsequent randomized studies by Hughes (68) and DeMaria (38), using low doses of naloxone showed no improvement of hypotension and mortality. Answering open questions about dose and pharmacokinetics will be necessary before starting further clinical studies. An early, high-dose naloxone application in shock is most likely to be therapeutically beneficial.

Another promising development is application of thyrotropin-releasing hormone (TRH). TRH interacts with κ opiate receptors as well as with its own receptors in the CNS and periphery to eliminate the hypoperfusion without affecting analgesia (66). Currently, clinical studies in anaphylactic shock and spinal cord injury are being prepared.

Tumor Necrosis Factor (TNF). TNF, a cytokine, is mainly released by activated monocytes and macrophages. Given intravenously the whole spectrum of reaction to a Gram-negative septicemia can be simulated dose-related (96). TNF fulfills all 4 Koch-Dale criteria in different species. TNF can be inhibited by (*a*) inhibition of cell activation (e.g., neutralization of endotoxin by antibodies), (*b*) inhibition of synthesis (e.g., blocking transcription by glucocorticoids), and (*c*) binding TNF by specific anti-TNF antibodies. Mortality is reduced experimentally by anti-TNF antibodies in different rodents (rats, mice), rabbits, and monkeys given prophylactically (up to 2 hours prior to endotoxin or *Escherichia coli* shock) (168). A first clinical trial (43) showed no significant side effects to the antibody and an increase in MAP in patients with septic shock. Several multicenter trials are currently underway.

Interleukin 1 (IL-1). Interleukin 1 (IL-1) is another polypeptide hormone that shares many similarities with TNFα. Several lines of evidence implicate IL-1 in the development of sepsis. Many actions of IL-1 are regulated at the receptor level, and thus any agent that could bind to IL-1 receptors should be able to inhibit those actions. A naturally occurring IL-1 receptor antagonist (IL-1-ra) has been discovered and can be reproduced though recombinant technology. In several animal models of sepsis, administration of IL-1-ra improved hemodynamics, reduced severity of lactic acidemia, and markedly reduced mortality (118). Preliminary studies of the use of IL-1-ra in patients with sepsis were encouraging; a randomized multicenter trial is currently underway.

Arachidonic Acid Metabolites. In sepsis, polytrauma, and ARDS, activation of the classic cascade system (kallikrein-kinin, complement, coagulation, fibrinolysis) and further unspecific noxes leads to activation of membrane phospholipase and the subsequent production of free arachidonic acid. Metabolism via cyclooxygenase pathway leads to different prostaglandins and thromboxane A₂, eicosanoids with predominantly

vasoconstrictive effects (except prostacyclin), and platelet-activating effects. Metabolism via the lipooxygenase pathway leads to leukotriene formation, with an increase in vascular permeability. Pharmacologic approaches to influence these eicosanoid cascades are (*a*) inhibition of cell membrane activation by glucocorticoids and protease inhibitors, (*b*) inhibition of cyclooxygenase and/or lipooxygenase pathway by nonsteroidal antiinflammatory drugs (NSAIDs) (e.g., indomethacin, acetylsalicylicacid, antioxidants, or ibuprofen) or (*c*) selective inhibition (stimulation) of single products (TXA₂ synthesis inhibitors), (dazoxiben) or TXA₂ antagonists (e.g., ONO 3708).

An improvement in hemodynamics, catabolism, pulmonary function, autoaggregation and mortality because of NSAIDs in the early state of shock has been experimentally proven. To date, only four prospective studies exist (septic shock, surgical trauma, and sepsis), one of which demonstrates a reduction in mortality by ibuprofen in sepsis (10). A recent randomized multicenter trial in patients with severe sepsis by Haupt et al (60), however, was unable to detect significant differences in hemodynamic and respiratory values and mortality.

Platelet-Activating Factor (PAF). PAF is produced by neutrophils, eosinophils, monocytes/macrophages, platelets, and endothelial cells in shock (septic/endotoxic shock, trauma, ischemia). Several structurally different PAF receptor antagonists (BN 52021, CV 3988, WEB 2086, Kadsurenon, SRI 63-072, etc.) are able to block PAF effects, such as the increase of IL₁ and TNF production as well as the increased plasma proteases activity. Beneficial effects were demonstrated in experimental endotoxic shock models, such as the inhibition of mediator release (TNF, TXA₂, catecholamines), a reduction of late hypotension and of early pulmonary vascular resistance, the prevention of gastrointestinal bleeding and ulcer development, and a dose-dependent decrease of mortality (rats, mice, dogs, pigs). More clinical studies are still necessary (21).

Oxygen-Free Radicals. Oxygen radicals are part of the unspecific host defense; they are found basically in all cells under normal physiologic conditions. Cells usually prevent autodestruction by a series of endogenous antioxidants (enzymes) such as gluthation peroxidase (GSH), superoxide dismutase (SOD), and catalase. In pathologic situations such as ischemia and reperfusion, acute renal or liver insufficiency, pancreatitis, or ARDS, oxygen-free radicals are excessively produced. This overproduction can be blocked by inhibitors of production, such as allopurinol, mannitol, DMSO, folic acid, vitamin C and vitamin E, or by O₂ radical scavengers such as SOD, GSH, L-methionine, or desferrioxamine. Studies with experimental shock models (ARDS, endotoxin, ischemia, and hemorrhagic shock) demonstrate temporary improvement of several organ functions, such as for the lung, liver, and the kidneys. A critical analysis by Gerdin and Haglund (51) showed enormous species differences in various shock models. Until now, no clinical benefit in shock therapy has been demonstrated.

CONCLUSION

Increasing knowledge of the detailed pathophysiology of different types of shock has led to the development of

Table 67.15. Problems in Establishing a Therapeutic Benefit of Experimental Drugs under Clinical Trial Conditions of Shock[a]

(1) Lack of valid early diagnostic parameters to identify patient subgroups.

(2) Heterogenity of patients in etiology, severity, and duration of shock.

(3) Lack of statistical power to demonstrate a real existing benefit in subgroups (β-error).

(4) Failure to apply principles of clinical pharmacology (pharmacokinetics and pharmacodynamics).

[a] From Neugebauer E, Dietrich A, Lechleuthner A, Bouillon B, Eypasch E: Trends in circulatory shock: pharmacotherapy in shock syndromes: the neglected field of pharmacokinetics and pharmacodynamics. *Circ Shock* 36:312–320, 1992.

numerous drugs capable of blocking or even reversing the deleterious cycle of events. Analysis of the literature (see also previous chapter), however, reveals an obvious discrepancy between obtained experimental and clinical study results. Promising, even overwhelming, effects of therapeutic drugs in the laboratory often could not be verified in subsequent randomized clinical trials. In analyzing the clinical features of theoretically sound and experimentally attractive approaches, four categories of problems (outlined in Table 67.15) can be identified. A key difficulty in establishing a therapeutic benefit in clinical studies, apart from study design characteristics, is the lack of knowledge and application of principles of clinical pharmacokinetics and pharmacodynamics.

In shock states, the relationship between an administered fixed-dose regimen and the drug effect is strongly influenced by dynamic changes in absorption, distribution, metabolism, and elimination of the drug, all of which vary among individual patients. The usual standard dosage schedules of drugs tested in clinical trials accomplish little in some patients, cause serious toxicity in others, and are fully satisfactory in a few. Fixed dosages and schedules can be satisfactory only when a drug's therapeutic margin is very large, when its therapeutic "window" is large, and when its full therapeutic potential is not required. If a drug does not fulfill these prerequisites, drug testing trials, using fixed-dosage schedules, most often fail to show a significant therapeutic effects.

Better knowledge of the dose-effect relation of drugs, the factors that influence this relation, and the use of that knowledge in study designs may well clarify a series of current controversies about the efficacy of adjuvant drugs used in clinical shock research (113). The inclusion of therapeutic drug monitoring in clinical shock studies should be applied more frequently.

REFERENCES

1. Andreadis N, Petty TL: Adult respiratory distress syndrome. Problems and progress. *Am Rev Resp Dis* 132:1344–1346, 1985.
2. Archer LT: Myocardial dysfunction in endotoxin- and E. coli-induced shock: pathophysiological mechanisms. *Circ Shock* 15:261–280, 1985.
3. Ashbaugh DG, Bigelow DB, Petty TL: Acute respiratory distress in adults. *Lancet* ii:319–323, 1967.
4. Bagge U, Braide M: Microcirculatory effects of white blood cells in shock. *Prog Appl Microcirc* 7:43–47, 1985.
5. Barcroft J: On anoxaemia. *Lancet* ii:485, 1920.
6. Baumann G, Permanetter B, Wirtzfeld A: Possible value of H₂-receptor agonists for the treatment of catecholamine-intensive congestive heart failure. *Pharmacol Ther* 24:165–177, 1984.
7. Bengtsson A, Redl H, Heideman M, Schlag G: Complement in septic shock. In Neugebauer E, Holaday JW (eds): *Handbook for Mediators in Septic Shock.* CRP Press Inc., Boca Raton, FL, pp 231–257, 1993.
8. Bergentz S-E: On bleeding and clotting problems in post-traumatic states. *Crit Care Med* 4:41–45, 1976.
9. Bernard GR, Brigham KL: The adult respiratory distress syndrome. *Annu Rev Med* 36:195–205, 1985.
10. Bernard G, Reines HD, Metz CA, et al: Effects of a short course of ibuprofen in patients with severe sepsis. *AST* 138, 1988.
11. Bernstein DP: Continuous noninvasive real-time monitoring of stroke volume and cardiac output by thoracic electrical bioimpedance. *Crit Care Med* 14:898–901, 1986.
12. Bihari DJ, Tinker J: Steroids in intensive care. *Br J Hosp Med* 28:323–330, 1982.
13. Bleifeld W, Kupper W: Nosologie, Klinik und Therapie des kardiogenen Schocks. In Riecker G (ed): Springer, Berlin, pp 15–94, 1984.
14. Bochner BS, Lichtenstein LM: Anaphylaxis. *N Engl J Med* 324:1785–1790, 1991.
15. Bone RC, Fisher Jr CJ, Clemmer TP, Slotman GJ, Metz CA, Balk RA and the members of the study group: A controlled clinical trial of high-dose methylprednisolone in the treatment of severe sepsis and septic shock. *N Engl J Med* 317:653–658, 1987.
16. Bone RC: Let's agree on terminology. Definition of sepsis. *Crit Care Med* 19:973–976, 1991.
17. Bone RC: Sepsis, the sepsis syndrome, multi-organ failure: a plea for comparable definitions. *Ann Intern Med* 114:332–333, 1991b.
18. Bone RC: A critical evaluation of new agents for the treatment of sepsis. *JAMA* 266:1686–1691, 1991c.
19. Border JR, Hassett J, LaDuca J, et al: The gut origin septic states in blunt multiple trauma (ISS-40) in the ICU. *Ann Surg* 206:427–448, 1987.
20. Bozzette SA, Sattler FR, Clin J: A controlled trial of early adjunctive treatment with corticosteroids for *Pneumocystis carinii* pneumonia in the acquired immunodeficiency syndrome. *N Engl J Med* 323:1451–1457, 1990.
20a. Bracken MB, Shepard JM, Collins WF, et al: A randomized, controlled trial of methylprednisolone or naloxone in the treatment of acute spinal cord injury. *N Engl J Med* 322:1405–1411, 1990.
21. Braquet P, Paubert-Braquet M, Koltai H, Bourgain R, Bussolino F, Hosford D: Is there a case for PAF antagonists in the treatment of ischemic states? *Trends Pharmacol Sci* 10:23–30, 1989.
22. Bryan-Brown CW: Blood flow to organs: parameters for function and survival in critical illness. *Crit Care Med* 16:170–178, 1988.
23. Bulkley GB, Oshima A, Bailey RM: Pathophysiology of hepatic ischemia in cardiogenic shock. *Am J Surg* 151:87–97, 1986.
24. Bunting S, Gryglewski R, Moncada S, Vane JR: Arterial walls generate from prostaglandin endoperoxides a substance (prostaglandin X) which relaxes strips of mesenteric and coeliac arteries and inhibits platelet aggregation. *Prostaglandins* 12:897–913, 1976.
25. Buschauer A, Baumann G: Structure activity relationships of histamine H₂-agonists, a new class of positive inotropic drugs. In Timmerman H, Van der Goot H (eds): *New Perspectives in Histamine Research.* Birkhäuser Verlag, Basel, Agents & Actions (Suppl 33) pp 231–256, 1991.
26. Cain SM: Appearance of excess lactate in anesthetized dogs during anemic and hypoxic hypoxia. *Am J Physiol* 209:604–608, 1965.
27. Cengiz M, Crapo RO, Gardner RM: The effect of ventilation on the accuracy of pulmonary artery and wedge pressure measurements. *Crit Care Med* 7:502–507, 1983.
28. Champion HR, Copes WS, Sacco WJ, et al: The major trauma outcome study: establishing national norms for trauma care. *J Trauma* 30:1356–1365, 1990.
29. Cohen J, Glauser MP: Septic shock treatment. *Lancet* 338:736–739, 1991.
30. Cohn JN, Mathew JK, Franciosa JA: Chronic vasodilator therapy in the management of cardiac shock and intractable left ventricular failure. *Ann Intern Med* 81:777–781, 1974.
31. Connors Jr AF, McCaffree DR, Gray BA: Evaluation of right-heart catheterization in the critically ill patient without acute myocardial infarction. *N Engl J Med* 308:263–267, 1983.
32. Cowley RA, Hankins JR, Jones RT, Trump BF: Pathology and pathophysiology of the liver. In Cowley RA, Trump BF (eds): *Pathophysiology of Shock, Anoxia, and Ischemia.* Williams & Wilkins, Baltimore, pp 285–301, 1982.
33. Crile GW: *An Experimental Research into Surgical Shock.* JB Lippincott, Philadelphia, 1899.
34. Curtis P: Family practice grand rounds: spontaneous pneumothorax—a dilemma of management. *J Fam Pract* 6:367–373, 1978.
35. Dacey RG, Jane JA: Craniocerebral trauma. In Baker AB, Baker LH (eds): *Clinical Neurology.* Harper & Row, Philadelphia, 1984.
36. De Felippe J, Timouer J, Velasco IT, et al: Treatment of refractory hypovolaemic shock by 7.5% sodium chloride injections. *Lancet* ii:1002–1004, 1980.
37. Deitch EA, Winterton J, Li M, Berg R: The gut as a portal of entry for bacteremia. *Ann Surg* 205:681–692, 1987.
38. DeMaria A, Craven DE, Heffernan JJ, et al: Naloxone versus placebo in treatment of septic shock. *Lancet* i:1363–1365, 1985.
39. Dougall AM, Paul ME, Finely RJ, Holliday RL, Coles JC, Duff JH: Chest trauma: current morbidity and mortality. *J Trauma* 17:547–553, 1977.

40. Doursout M-F, Chelly JE, Hartley CJ, Szilagyi J, Montastruc JL, Buckley JP: Regional blood flows and cardiac function changes induced by angiotensin-II in conscious dogs. *J Pharmacol Exp Ther* 246:591–596, 1988.

41. Dries DJ, Waxman K: Adequate resuscitation of burn patients may not be measured by urine output and vital signs. *Crit Care Med* 19:327–329, 1991.

42. Errington ML, Rocha e Silva Jr M: On the role of vasopressin and angiotensin in the development of irreversible haemorrhagic shock. *J Physiol* (Lond) 242:119–141, 1974.

43. Exley AR, Cohen J, Buurman W, et al: Monoclonal antibody to TNF in severe septic shock. *Lancet* 335:1275–1276, 1990.

44. Expert Panel: The use of the pulmonary artery catheter. *Intensive Care Med* 17:1–8, 1991.

45. Fisher M: Non-oliguric renal failure. In *Intensive and Critical Care Medicine 1981–1985–1989*. Proceedings of the 4th World Congress on Intensive and Critical Care Medicine. King & Wirth, London, pp 314–316, 1985.

46. Fisher Jr CJ, Bellingan G: Immunotherapy of sepsis syndrome: a comparison of the available treatments. *Klin Wochenschr* 69 (Suppl XXVI):162–167, 1991.

47. Forrester JS, Diamond G, McHugh TG, Swan HJC: Filling pressures in the right and left side of the heart in acute myocardial infarction. *N Engl J Med* 285:190–193, 1971.

48. Funk W, Endrich B, Messmer K, Intaglietta M: Spontaneous arteriolar vasomotion as a determinant of peripheral vascular resistance. *Int J Microcirc Clin Exp* 2:11–25, 1983.

49. Gagnon S, Boota AM, Fisher MA, Baier H, Kirksey OW, Voie LL: Corticosteroids as adjunctive therapy for severe *Pneumocystis carinii* pneumonia in the acquired immuno-deficiency syndrome. *N Engl J Med* 323:1444–1450, 1990.

50. Gaudon AL, Tomasulo PS, Bergin JJ, et al: The Hospital Transfusion Committee Guidelines for Improving Practice. *JAMA* 253:540–543, 1985.

51. Gerdin B, Haglund U: Possible involvement of oxygen free radicals (OFR) in shock and shock related states. In Neugebauer E, Holaday JW (eds): *Handbook of Mediators in Septic Shock*. CRC Press, Inc., Boca Raton, FL, pp 457–473, 1993.

52. Gerhart KA: Spinal cord injury outcomes in a population-based sample. *J Trauma* 31:1529–1535, 1991.

53. Gigris NF, Farid R, Mikhail IA, Farray I, Sultan Y, Kilpatrich ME: Dexamethasone treatment for bacterial meningitis in children and adults. *Pediatr Infect Dis* 8:848–851, 1989.

54. Gore JH, Goldberg RJ, Spodick DH, Alpert JS, Dalen JE: A community wide assessment of the use of pulmonary artery catheters in patients with acute myocardial infarction. *Chest* 92:721–727, 1987.

55. Greenman RL, Schein RMH, Martin MA, et al: A controlled clinical trial of E-5 murine monoclonal IgM antibody to endotoxin in the treatment of gram(-) sepsis. *JAMA* 266:1097–1102, 1991.

56. Grimminger F, Seeger W: Regulation inflammatorischer Abläufe—Angriffspunkte und Grenzen steroidaler Antiphlogistika. *Med Welt* 41:951–964, 1990.

57. Groeger JA, Carton GC, Howland WS: Naloxone in septic shock. *Crit Care Med* 11:650–654, 1983.

58. Hack CE, Thijs LG: The orchestra of mediators in the pathogenesis of septic shock: a review. In Vincent JL (ed): *Update in Intensive Care and Emergency Medicine: Update 1991*. Springer Verlag, Berlin, pp 232–246, 1991.

59. Hangen DH, Stevens JH, Satoh PS, Hall EW, O'Hanley PT, Raffin TA: Complement levels in septic primates treated with anti-C5a antibodies. *J Surg Res* 46:195–199, 1989.

60. Haupt MT, Jastremski MS, Clemmer TP, et al: Effect of ibuprofen in patients with severe sepsis: a randomized, double blind, multicenter study. *Crit Care Med* 19:1339–1347, 1991.

61. Herkes RG, Bihari DJ: Management of shock. In Tinker J, Zapol WM (eds): *Care of the Critically Ill Patient*, ed 2. Springer-Verlag, Berlin, pp 259–284, 1991.

62. Higgins TL, Chernow B: *Pharmacotherapy of Circulatory Shock*. In Bone RC (ed): New Book Medical Publishers, 1987.

63. Hill EP, Willford DC, Moores WY, Bellamy R, Heydorn WH: Oxygen transport and oxygen consumption vs. cardiac output at different haematocrits. *Perfusion* 2:39–50, 1987.

64. Hoffman SL, Punjabi NH, Kumata S: Reduction of mortality in chloramphenicol treated severe typhoid fever by high-dose dexamethasone. *N Engl J Med* 310:82–88, 1984.

65. Holaday JW, Faden AI: Naloxone reversal of endotoxin hypotension suggests role of endorphins in shock. *Nature* 275:450–451, 1978.

66. Holaday JW, Long JB, Martinez-Arizala A, Chen H-S, Reynolds DG, Gurll N: Effects of TRH in circulatory shock and central nervous system ischemia. *Ann NY Acad Sci* 353:379–380, 1989.

67. Holcroft JW, Vassar MJ, Turner JE, Derlet RW, Kramer GC: 3% NaCl and 7.5% NaCl/Dextran 70 in the resuscitation of severely injured patients. *Ann Surg* 206:279–288, 1987.

68. Hughes GS Jr: Naloxone and methylprednisolone sodium succinate enhance sympathomedullary discharge in patients with septic shock. *Life Sci* 35:2319–2326, 1984.

69. Intaglietta M, Messmer K: Microangiodynamics, peripheral vascular resistance, and the normal microcirculation. *Int J Microcirc Clin Exp* 2:3–10, 1983.

70. Jenkins AM, Ruckley CV, Nolan B: Ruptured abdominal aortic aneurysm. *Br J Surg* 73:395–398, 1986.

71. Jennett B, Teasdale G (eds): *Management of Head Injuries*. FA Davis, Philadelphia, 1986.

72. Kandel G, Alberman A: Mixed venous oxygen saturation: its role in the assessment of the critically ill patient. *Arch Intern Med* 143:1400–1402, 1983.

73. Knaus WA, Draper EA, Wagner DP, Zimmerman JE: Prognosis in acute organ-system failure. *Ann Surg* 202:685–693, 1985.

74. Kox WJ, Christ F: Oxygen transport pattern in hemorrhagic and septic patients. In Vincent JL (eds): *Update in Intensive Care and Emergency Medicine: Update 1991*. Springer Verlag, Berlin, pp 113–119, 1991.

75. Kreger BE, Craven DE, McCabe WR: Gramnegative bacteremia. 4. Reevaluation of clinical features and treatment in 612 patients. *Am J Med* 68:344–355, 1980.

76. Lassen NA: Cerebral blood flow and oxygen consumption in man. *Physiol Rev* 39:183–238, 1959.

77. Lasser EC, Berry CC, Talner LB, Santini LC, Lang EV, et al: Pretreatment with corticosteroids to alleviate reactions to intravenous contrast material. *N Engl J Med* 317:845–849, 1987.

78. Lebel MH, Freij BJ, Syrogiannopoulos GA, et al: Dexamethasone therapy for bacterial meningitis: results of two double-blind, placebo-controlled trials. *N Engl J Med* 319:964–971, 1988.

79. LeDran, HF: *A Treatise, or Reflections Drawn from Practice on Gunshot Wounds* (translated). Clarke, London, 1743.

80. Lefer AM: Vascular mediators in ischemia and shock. In Cowley RA, Trump BF (eds): *Pathophysiology of Shock, Anoxia and Ischemia*. Williams & Wilkins, Baltimore, pp 165–181, 1981.

81. Lefering R, Neugebauer E, Saad S: Ist der Einsatz von Steroiden bei Sepsis sinnvoll? In: Gall, Beger NG, Ungeneur E. (eds): *Langenbecks Arch* (suppl): Chir. Forum 92 für experimentelle und klinische Forschung, Springer-Verlag, Berlin, pp 481–484, 1992.

82. Leier CV, Binkley PF, Carpenter J, Randolph PH, Unverferth DV: The cardiovascular pharmacology of dopexamine in patients with low output congestive heart failure. *Am J Cardiol* 62:94–99, 1988.

83. Lewis DH, Mellander S: Competitive effects of sympathetic control and tissue metabolites on resistance and capacitance vessels and capillary filtration in skeletal muscle. *Acta Physiol Scand* 56:162–188, 1962.

84. Liss HP: A history of resuscitation. *Ann Emerg Med* 15:65–72, 1986.

85. Lorenz W, Doenicke A, Schöning B, Ohmann C, Grote B, Neugebauer E: Definition and classification of the histamine release response to drugs in anaesthesia and surgery: studies in the conscious human subject. *Klin Wochenschr* 60:896–913, 1982.

86. Lorenz W, Dietz W, Ennis M, Stinner B, Doenicke A: Histamine in anaesthesia and surgery—a causality analysis. In Uvnäs B (ed): *Handbook of Exp. Pharmacology*, vol 97, *Histamine and Histamine Antagonists*, Springer, Berlin, pp 385–439, 1991.

87. Lorenz W, Ennis M, Doenicke A, Dick W: Perioperative uses of histamine antagonists. *J Clin Anesth* 2:345–360, 1990.

88. MacLean LD, Mulligan WG, McLean APH, Duff JH: Patterns of septic shock in man—a detailed study of 56 patients. *Ann Surg* 166:543–562, 1967.

89. Mancini D, LeJemtel TH, Sonnenblick EH: Intravenous use of amrinone for the treatment of the failing heart. *Am J Cardiol* 56:8B–15B, 1985.

90. Maningas PA, Mattox KL, Pepe PE, Jones RL, Feliciano DV, Burch JM: Hypertonic saline-dextran solutions for the prehospital management of traumatic hypotension. *Am J Surg* 157:528–534, 1989.

91. Marini JJ: Pulmonary artery occlusion pressure: clinical physiology, measurement and interpretation. *Am Rev Resp Dis* 128:319–325, 1983.

92. Marino PL: *The ICU Book*. Lea & Febiger, Philadelphia, 1991.

93. Marsch CH: Experience with abdominal aneurysms in a district general hospital. *Am R Coll Surg Engl* 62:294–299, 1980.

94. Marshall WG, Bell JL, Kouchoukos NT: Penetrating cardiac trauma. *J Trauma* 24:147–149, 1984.

95. Messmer K: Rheologische Grundlagen der Schocktherapie. *Internist* 23:445–449, 1982.

96. Michie HR, Wilmore DW: Sepsis, signals and surgical sequelae. *Arch Surg* 125:531–536, 1990.

97. MMWR (Morbidity and Mortality Weekly Report): Increase in national hospital discharge survey rates for septicemia—United States, 1979–1987. *JAMA* 263:937–938, 1990.

98. Monafo WW, Chuntrasakul C, Ayvazian VH: Hypertonic sodium solutions in the treatment of burn shock. *Am J Surg* 126:778–783, 1973.

99. Moore FA, Haenel JB: Alternatives to Swan-Ganz output monitoring. *Surg Clin North Am* 71:699–721, 1991.

100. Moulds RFW, Iwanov V, Young MJ: Vasoactive effects of platelet aggregates. *N Engl J Med* 311:198–199, 1984.

101. Nadeau S, Noble WH: Limitations of cardiac output measurement by thermodilution. *Can J Anesth* 33:780–784, 1986.

102. Nelson LD, Anderson HB, Garcia H: Clinical validation of a new metabolic monitor suitable for use in critically ill patients. *Crit Care Med* 15:951–959, 1987.

103. Neugebauer E, Beckurts T, Lorenz W, Maroske D, Merte H, Horeyseck G, Dietz W: Induced histidine decarboxylase in endotoxic shock: identification of the enzyme in rat liver and influence of its inhibitors on survival parameters. *Agents Actions* 18:23–29, 1986.

104. Neugebauer E, Lorenz W, Maroske D, Barthlen W, Ennis M: The role of mediators in septic/endotoxic shock. A meta-analysis evaluating the current status of histamine. *Theor Surg* 2:1–28, 1987(a).

105. Neugebauer E, Lorenz W, Maroske D, Barthlen W: Mediatoren beim septischen Schock; Strategien zu ihrer Sicherung und zur Einschätzung ihrer kausalen Bedeutung. *Chirug* 58:470–481, 1987b.

106. Neugebauer E, Lorenz W, Beckurts T, Maroske D, Merte H: Significance of histamine formation and release in the development of endotoxic shock: proof of current concepts by randomized controlled studies in rats. *Rev Infect Dis* 9:585–593, 1987c.

107. Neugebauer E, Lorenz W: Causality in circulatory shock: strategies for integrating mediators, mechanisms and therapies. *Prog Clin Biol Res* 264:295–305, 1988a.

108. Neugebauer E, Lorenz W, Schirren J, Dietrich A: Mediators in the pathogenesis of septic shock—State of the art. In Reinhart K, Eyrich K (eds): *Sepsis—An Interdisciplinary Challenge.* Springer, Berlin, pp 202–215, 1988b.

109. Neugebauer E, Schirren J, Lorenz W: High-dose steroids and sepsis (letter to the editor). *N Engl J Med* 318:514–516, 1988.

110. Neugebauer E, Bouillon B, Dietrich A, Lechleuthner A: Cortison: Standards und neue Tendenzen—Notfallindikation Schock. *Münch Med Wochenschr* 131:907–910, 1989.

111. Neugebauer E, Dietrich A, Bouillon B, Lorenz W, Lechleuthner A, Troidl H: Steroids in trauma patients—right or wrong? A qualitative meta-analysis of clinical studies. *Theor Surg* 5:44–53, 1990.

112. Neugebauer E, Dietrich A, Bouillon B, Lechleuthner A, Saad S: Glukokortikoide beim Polytrauma und bei Sepsis—Immer noch ein Thema? *Klin Wochenschr* 69(Suppl XXVI):211–223, 1991.

113. Neugebauer E, Dietrich A, Lechleuthner A, Bouillon B, Eypasch E: Trends in circulatory shock: pharmacotherapy in shock syndromes: the neglected field of pharmacokinetics and pharmacodynamics. *Circ Shock* in press, 1992.

114. Neuhof H, Lasch HG: Shock: Physiologie, Überwachung, Klinik, Therapie. In Bock HE, Gerok W, Hartmann F (eds): *Klinik der Gegenwart-Handbuch der praktischen Medizin,* Urban & Schwarzenberg, Baltimore, pp 939–1019, 1981.

115. Nicholson DP: Review of corticosteroid treatment in sepsis and septic shock: pro or con. *Crit Care Clin* 5:151–155, 1989.

116. NIHCCS (National Institute of Health Consensus Conference Statement): Prevention of venous thrombosis and pulmonary embolism. *JAMA* 256:744–749, 1986.

117. Odio CM, Faingezicht I, Paris M, et al: The beneficial effects of early dexamethasone administration in infants and children with bacterial meningitis. *N Engl J Med* 324:1525–1531, 1991.

118. Ohlson K, Björk P, Bergenfeldt M, Hageman R, Thompson RC: Interleukin-1 receptor anatagonist reduces mortality from endotoxin shock. *Nature* 348:550–552, 1990.

119. Parker MM, Parrillo JE: Septic shock: hemodynamics and pathogenesis. *JAMA* 250:3324–3327, 1983.

120. Parrillo JE: Septic shock in humans. Advances in the understanding of pathogenesis, cardiovascular dysfunction, and therapy. *Ann Intern Med* 113:227–242, 1990.

121. Peters WP, Johnson MW, Friedmann PA, Mitch WE: Pressor effect of naloxone in septic shock. *Lancet* i:529–539, 1981.

122. Popper KR: *The open society and its enemies. I. The spell of Plato. II. The high tide of prophecy: Hegel, Marx and the aftermath.* Routledge & Kegan Paul, London, 1945.

123. Prough DS, DeWitt DS: Cerebral protection. In Chernow B (ed): *The Pharmacologic Approach to the Critically Ill Patient.* Williams & Wilkins, Baltimore, pp 198–218, 1988.

124. Rackow EC, Astiz ME, Weil MH: Cellular oxygen metabolism during sepsis and shock: the relationship of oxygen consumption to oxygen delivery. *JAMA* 259:1989–1993, 1988.

125. Radermacher P, Santak B, Wüst HJ, Tarnow J, Falke KJ: Prostacyclin and right ventricular function in patients with pulmonary hypertension associated with ARDS. *Intensive Care Med* 16:227–232, 1990.

126. Raper RF, Fisher MMcD: Resuscitation in acute haemorrhage. *Anaesth Intensive Care* 12:212–216, 1984.

127. Rasanen J, Downes JB, Dehaven B: Titration of continuous positive airway pressure by real-time dual oxymetry. *Crit Care Med* 15:395–399, 1987.

128. Ratnoff OD: Disseminated intravascular coagulation. In Ratnoff OD, Forbes CD (eds): *Disorders of hemostasis.* Grune & Stratton, Orlando, FL, pp 289–319, 1984.

129. Redl H, Hammerschmidt DE, Schlag G: Augmentation by platelets of granulocyte aggregation in response to chemotaxins: studies utilizing an improved cell preparation technique. *Blood* 61:125–131, 1983.

130. Regel G, Dwenger A, Gratz KF, Nerlich ML, Sturm JA, Tscherne H: Humorale und zelluläre Veränderungen der unspezifischen Immunabwehr nach schwerem Trauma. *Unfallchirurg* 92:314–320, 1989.

131. Regoli D, Park WK, Rioux F: Pharmacology of angiotensin. *Pharmacol Rev* 26:69–123, 1974.

132. Reinhart K, Rudolph T, Bredle DL, Hannemann L, Cain SM: Comparison of central venous to mixed venous oxygen saturation during changes in oxygen supply/demand. *Chest* 95:1216–1221, 1989.

133. Reinhart K, Hannemann L, Kuss B: Optimal levels of O_2 delivery in the critically ill. *Intensive Care Med* 16:S149–S155, 1990.

134. Richard C, Ricome JL, Rimailho A, Bottineau G, Auzepy P: Combined hemodynamic effects of dopamine and dobutamine in cardiogenic shock. *Circulation* 67:620–626, 1983.

135. Rijn OJL, Grol MEC, Bouter M, Mulder S, Kester ADM: Incidence of medically treated burns in the Netherlands. *Burns* 17:357–362, 1991.

136. Rixen D, Lechleuthner A, Saad S, Buschauer A, Nagelschmidt M, Thoma S, Rink A, Neugebauer E: Beneficial effect of H2-agonism and H1-antagonism in rat endotoxic shock? (abstr.) *Circ Shock* 34:133, 1991.

137. Robin ED, Cary LC, Grenvik A, Glauser F, Gaudio R: Capillary leak syndrome with pulmonary edema. *Arch Intern Med* 130:66–71, 1972.

138. Robin ED: Death by pulmonary artery flow-directed catheter (editorial). *Chest* 92:727–731, 1987.

139. Royston D: Acute adult animal respiratory distress sydnrome: a sideways look at ARDS. *Br J Anaesth* 58:1207–1209, 1986.

140. Runciman WB, Skowronski GA: Pathophysiology of haemorrhagic shock. *Anaesth Intensive Care* 12:193–205, 1984.

141. Ruppel GL: *Manual of Pulmonary Function Testing,* ed 5. St. Louis, Mosby-Year Book, 1991.

142. Schmitt EA, Brantighan CO: Common artifacts of pulmonary artery and pulmonary artery wedge pressures: recognition and management. *J Clin Monit* 2:44–52, 1986.

143. Seybold D, Gessler U: Die Niere im Schock und Schockniere—Nosologie, Pathophysiologie, Klinik und Therapie. In Rieker G (ed): *Schock.* Springer, Berlin, pp 261–321, 1984.

144. Shah KB, Rao TK, Laughlin S: A review of pulmonary artery catheterization in 6245 patients. *Anesthesiology* 61:271–275, 1984.

145. Shippy CR, Appel PL, Shoemaker WC: Reliability of clinical monitoring to assess blood volume in critically ill patients. *Crit Care Med* 12:107–112, 1984.

146. Shoemaker WC, Bland RD, Appel PL: Therapy of critically ill postoperative patients based on outcome prediction and prospective clinical trials. *Surg Clin North Am* 65:811–833, 1985.

147. Shoemaker WC: Relation of oxygen transport patterns to the pathophysiology and therapy of shock states. *Crit Care Med* 13:230–243, 1987a.

148. Shoemaker WC: Circulatory mechanisms of shock and their mediators. *Crit Care Med* 15:787–794, 1987b.

149. Shoemaker WC, Appel PL, Kram HB, Waxman K, Lee TS: Prospective trial of supranormal values of survivors as therapeutic goals in high-risk surgical patients. *Chest* 94:1176–1186, 1988.

150. Shoemaker WC: Tissue perfusion and oxygenation: a primary problem in acute circulatory failure and shock states. *Crit Care Med* 19:595–596, 1991.

151. Shrier RW: Pathogenesis of sodium and water retention in high output and low output cardiac failure, nephrotic syndrome, cirrhosis and pregnancy. *N Engl J Med* 319:1065–1069, 1988.

152. Siegel JH, Cerra FB, Coleman B, et al: Physiological and metabolic correlations in human sepsis. *Surgery* 86:163–193, 1979.

153. Siegel JH, Vary TC: Sepsis, abnormal metabolic control and multiple organ failure syndrome. In Siegel JH (ed): *Trauma: Emergency Surgery and Critical Care.* Churchill Livingstone, Edinburgh, pp 411–502, 1987a.

154. Siegel JH: Physiologic and metabolic correlations in human septic shock. In *First Vienna Shock Forum,* Part A. *Pathophysiological Role of Mediators and Mediator Inhibitors in Shock.* Liss, New York, pp 439–457, 1987b.

155. Sise MJ, Hollingworth P, Brimm JE, Peters RM, Virgilio RW, Shackford SR: Complications of the flow-directed pulmonary artery catheter: a prospective analysis in 219 patients. *Crit Care Med* 9:315–318, 1981.

156. Sjölin J: High-dose corticosteroid therapy in human septic shock: Has the jury reached a correct verdict? *Circ Shock* 35:139–151, 1991.

157. Skarvan K: Mediatoren beim Trauma. *Med Welt* 45:525–532, 1989.

158. Slung HB, Scher KS: Complications of the Swan-Ganz catheter. *World J Surg* 8:76–81, 1984.

159. Smedegard G, Cui LX, Hugli TE: Endotoxin-induced shock in the rat. A role for C5a. *Am J Pathol* 135:489–497, 1989.

160. Sprung CL: Definitions of sepsis: Have we reached a consensus? *Crit Care Med* 19:849–851, 1991.

161. Sramek BB: Noninvasive Technique for Measurement of Cardiac Output by Means of Electrical Impedance. 5th International Conference of Electrical Bioimpedance. Tokyo, Japan, 1987.

162. Stevens JH, O'Hanley P, Shapiro JM, et al: Effects of anti-C5a antibodies on the adult respiratory distress syndrome in septic primates. *J Clin Invest* 77:1812–1816, 1986.

163. Sunder-Plassmann L, Messmer K: Funktionelle Veränderungen der Mikrozirkulation im Schock. In Ahnefeld FW, Bergmann H, Burri C, Dick W, Halmagyi M, Rügheimer E (eds): *Klinische Anästhesiologie und Intensivtherapie,* Bd V. Springer, Berlin, pp 76–86, 1974.

164. Swan HJC, Forrester JC, Diamond G, Chatterjee K, Parmeley WW: Hemodynamic spectrum of myocardial infarction and cardiogenic shock. *Circulation* 45:1097–1110, 1972.

165. Tejerina T, Reig A, Codina J, Safont J, Baena P, Mirabet V: An epidemiological study of burn patients hospitalized in Valencia, Spain, during 1989. *Burns* 18:15–18, 1992.

166. The Veterans Administration Systemic Sepsis Cooperative Study Group: Effect of high-dose glucocorticoid therapy on mortality in patients with clinical signs of systemic sepsis. *N Engl J Med* 317:659–665, 1987.

167. Thomas VL, Nielsen MS: Administration of angiotensin II in refractory septic shock. *Crit Care Med* 19:1084–1086, 1991.

168. Tracey KJ, Fong Y, Hesse DG, et al: Anti-cachectin/TNF antibodies prevent the fatal sequelae of experimental bacteremia in primates. *Nature* 330:662–664, 1987.

169. Troidl H, Vestweber KH, Kusche J, Bouillon B: Die Blutung beim peptischen Gastroduodenalulcus: Daten als Entscheidungshilfe für ein chirurgisches Therapiekonzept. *Der Chirurg* 57:372–380, 1986.

170. Vary TC, Siegel JH, Nakatani T, et al: Regulation of glucose metabolism by altered pyruvate dehydrogenase. *J Parenter Enteral Nutr* 10:351–355, 1986.

171. Velasco IT, Pontieri V, Rocha e Silva M, Lopes OU: Hyperosmotic NaCl and severe hemorrhagic shock. *Am J Physiol* 239:H664–H673, 1980.

172. Vincent JL, Dufaye P, Berré J, Leeman M, Degaute JP, Kahn RH: Serial lactate determinations during circulatory shock. *Crit Care Med* 11:449–451, 1983.

173. Vincent JL, de Boelpape C, Luypaert P: Association of amrinone with norepinephrine in endotoxic shock in dogs: an experimental study (abstr). *Crit Care Med* 16:402, 1988.

174. Vincent JL, Reuse C, Kahn RJ: Administration of dopexamine, a new adrenergic agent, in cardiorespiratory failure. *Chest* 96:1233–1236, 1989.

175. Vincent JL: O₂—demand, uptake and supply. *Intensive Care Med* 16(Suppl 2):S145–S148, 1990.

176. Vincent JL, Roman A, De Backer D, Kahn RJ: Oxygen uptake/supply dependency: effects of short term dobutamine infusion. *Am Rev Respir Dis* 142:2–7, 1990.

177. Vincent JL: The colloid-crystalloid controversy. *Klin Wochenschr* 69(Suppl XXVI):104–111, 1991.

178. Waller JL, Kaplan JA, Bauman DI, Cramer JM: Clinical evaluation of a new fiberoptic catheter oximeter during cardiac surgery. *Anesth Analg* 61:676–679, 1982.

179. West JB, Dollery CT, Naimark A: Distribution of blood flow in isolated lung; relation to vascular and alveolar pressures. *J Appl Physiol* 19:713–724, 1964.

180. Wiggers CI: *Physiology of Shock*. The Commonwealth Fund, New York, 1950.

181. Williams TJ, Yarwood H: Effect of glucocorticoids on microvascular permeability. *Am Rev Respir Dis* 141:539–543, 1988.

182. Ziegler EJ, Fisher CJ, Sprung CL: Treatment of gram negative bacteremia and septic shock with HA-1A human monoclonal antibody against endotoxin. *N Engl J Med* 324:429–436, 1991.

183. Holaday JW, Neugebauer E, Corr DB: Meta²—An analysis of meta-analysis of mediators in septic shock. In Neugebauer E, Holaday JW (eds): *Handbook of Mediators in Septic Shock*. CRC Press, Boca Raton, FL pp 523–534, 1993.

CHAPTER 68

Selective Digestive Decontamination in the Intensive Care Unit

JOHN D. LOCKREM, M.D.
JAMES K. STOLLER, M.D.

Infections continue to be the major cause of morbidity and mortality in critically ill patients despite the development of powerful and effective antibiotics and the institution of modern infection control techniques. A recent prospective study of 1304 patients from 16 intensive care units (ICUs) showed a 21.3% prevalence of acquired pneumonia, with a 38% mortality rate (1). As many as 90% of ICU patients may become infected after 1 week in the unit (2, 3). Approximately 275,000 cases of nosocomial pneumonia are estimated to occur in the United States each year, with a staggering economic impact (4).

Obviously, a successful strategy for preventing nosocomial infection rather than treating established infection would have enormous appeal and would be expected to reduce mortality, costs, and ICU length of stay. Interest in preventing nosocomial infection led to a trial of aerosolized polymyxin in the ICU of the Beth Israel Hospital in 1975 (5). Unfortunately, this early experience was disappointing and dampened enthusiasm for later approaches to antibiotic prophylaxis of ICU-associated pneumonias. In that study by Feeley, et al, aerosolized polymyxin E was administered specifically to prevent *Pseudomonas aeruginosa* pneumonia, which was associated with very high mortality (approximately 70%). Although aerosolized polymyxin E was effective in preventing pneumonia from *P. aeruginosa* (i.e., only one patient of the 292 study patients developed *Pseudomonas* pneumonia), pneumonia caused by other pathogens resistant to polymyxin developed, and the overall mortality rate from pneumonia increased. These results were ascribed to "emergence of resistance," but "superinfection" seems a

more apt description because all the microorganisms responsible for the pneumonias (*Proteus, Serratia, Pseudomonas maltophilia, Flavobacterium*) were intrinsically insensitive to polymyxin E.

As a result of this early experience and with a heightened respect for the risks of altering microbial ecology by prophylactic therapy, further investigation of antibiotic prophylaxis strategies was slowed, until interest was revived with studies of selective digestive decontamination. In an early selective digestive decontamination trial in multiple trauma patients begun in 1981 and reported in 1984 (6), Stoutenbeek et al demonstrated a reduction in respiratory tract infections from 59% to 8% (P < 0.0001) using a prophylactic selective digestive decontamination regimen. Unlike experience with aerosolized polymyxin, the goal of selective digestive decontamination is to suppress selectively aerobic Gram-negative bacilli in the gut, which most commonly cause nosocomial infections in the ICU.

PATHOGENESIS OF NOSOCOMIAL PNEUMONIA AND RATIONALE FOR SELECTIVE DIGESTIVE DECONTAMINATION

Infections may be classified as exogenous, caused by microorganisms from outside the patient, or endogenous, caused by microorganisms carried in the patient's oropharynx or gut. Endogenous infections in the ICU can be further classified as *primary*, caused by organisms colonizing the patient on admission to the hospital, or *secondary,* caused by organisms acquired during the hospital stay that are not part of the usual community flora. The pathogenesis of infection has been described (7) in three stages: (*a*) Acquisition of nosocomial (Gram-negative) bacteria and colonization of the digestive tract. Sources for the colonization are other patients and the hospital environment. (*b*) Colonization of other organs (e.g., skin, respiratory tract, urinary tract) by these same potentially pathologic microorganisms (PPM) without clinical signs of infection. (*c*) Development of clinically recognizable infection.

Recognizing that colonization with pathogens precedes infection, and that colonization may occur soon after hospitalization (8), selective digestive decontamination is a strategy that aims to block colonization with enteric Gram-negatives and yeast while selectively sparing endogenous organisms, mostly anaerobic flora. The endogenous flora help to control the overgrowth of aerobic bacteria (5), and these organisms have less pathogenic potential.

As originally described by Stoutenbeek et al, this strategy is accomplished by administering a mixture of antimicrobials in a sticky, water-soluble paste (Orabase, Squibb) to the oropharynx topically, and instilling a solution of the antibiotic mixture to the stomach, usually through a nasogastric tube. The originally described topical mixture consisted of *poly-myxin E, tobramycin,* and *amphotericin B* (PTA), 2% each, and was chosen for several very specific reasons: (*a*) the antibiotics are nonabsorbable and therefore achieve high concentrations in the gut lumen; (*b*) the antibiotics are bactericidal and do not require leukocyte activity to achieve effect; (*c*) the mixture does not alter endogenous anaerobic flora; and (*d*) the antibiotics are not inactivated by fecal contents. Additionally, polymyxin has been reported to act synergistically with tobramycin, especially against *Pseudomonas* sp (9).

The original regimen also included parenteral cefotaxime 50–100 mg/kg/day as an early part of the program in order to eradicate community pathogens such as pneumococcus, and to treat any established primary infection until the enteral elements had time to become effective. Cefotaxime was chosen for three reasons: (*a*) its wide spectrum of activity against "community" and "hospital" organisms; (*b*) high levels can be achieved in tracheal and bronchial secretions; and (*c*) it has a relatively low side effect profile (10). The three elements of selective digestive decontamination—oral, gastric, and intravenous antibiotics—are considered to work in concert to prevent the main sources of ICU-acquired pneumonia: exogenous pneumonias, from community microorganisms which threaten early after admission, and both primary and secondary endogenous pneumonias, which threaten later during hospitalization.

AVAILABLE STUDIES OF SELECTIVE DIGESTIVE DECONTAMINATION: REGIMENS USED

As summarized in Table 68.1, 25 trials of selective digestive decontamination currently are available and form the basis for current impressions about efficacy. As also reviewed elsewhere (9, 11), key aspects of these studies are summarized in this section. Since the original study by Stoutenbeek et al using a regimen of intravenous cefotaxime coupled with polymyxin, tobramycin, and amphotericin topically in the mouth and in suspension via nasogastric tube, several different regimens of selective digestive decontamination have been proposed. Deviations from the original regimen include deletion of the intravenous component, deletion of the oral antibiotic paste, and changes in the antibiotics administered to the oropharynx and stomach. Specifically, of the 25 available studies, eleven have employed the original regimen. Four trials deleted the topical oral antibiotics, and eight deleted systemic antibiotics altogether, while others (31, 32) substituted intravenous cephradine or trimethoprim for cefotaxime. In the four studies reported from the United States, nonavailability of topical tobramycin and amphotericin has required substitution of gentamicin for tobramycin/sulfamethoxazole and nystatin for amphotericin. Others have substituted a fluoroquinolone (e.g., norfloxacin) for the aminoglycoside.

The original rationale for including intravenous cefotaxime for the early phase of decontamination was to eradicate primary endogenous colonization and infection, and the first report by Stoutenbeek et al strengthened this impression by showing fewer acquired pneumonias in recipients of all three elements of selective digestive decontamination (topical oral, nasogastric, *and* intravenous cefotaxime) than in recipients of topical antibiotics only.

THE EFFICACY OF SELECTIVE DIGESTIVE DECONTAMINATION IN AVAILABLE TRIALS

Methodologic considerations regarding the design of selective digestive decontamination trials have been reviewed recently by van Saene et al (9) and Reidy et al (11). With these considerations in mind, the currently available literature shows a spectrum of study designs, summarized as follows:

1. Randomized clinical trials	13
Double-blind, placebo controlled	6
2. Consecutive (historical) controls	10
Crossover design	3
Observational cohort	1
3. Preliminary report one of which (22) appears to be a subset of a larger, subsequently fully reported study (28)	2

As summarized in Table 68.2, a variety of outcome measures have been examined. Twenty-three trials have examined rates of colonization as an outcome event, and 21 of these reported a significant reduction. In addition to diminishing colonization, long-term application of topical, nonabsorbable antibiotics has been found to eradicate oropharyngeal and gastric carriage of Enterobacteriaceae, Pseudomonadaceae, *Acinetobacter* spp, and yeasts. Finally, Brun-Buisson et al (17) successfully used selective digestive decontamination to interrupt an outbreak of infection by multi-resistant Enterobacteriaceae.

Acquired infection rates have been considered as outcomes in each of the 25 available studies and a significant reduction in the rate of acquired infection has been reported in 21 (84%). However, two of the most convincing studies, a 15-site multicenter trial reported by Gastinne, which found a decrease in Gram-negative pneumonias but not in total pneumonias or overall infections, and the study by Hammond, which found no efficacy at all in reducing infection, mortality, or antibiotic cost, have to be considered seriously in weighing

Table 68.1.   Design Elements of Available Controlled Trials of Selective Digestive Decontamination[a]

Center	N (Total)	Study Design[b]	Study Group[c]	Specified Exclusions[d]
Stoutenbeek (6)	122	Consec	Multiple trauma; > 5 days ICU	Prior antibiotics; existing infection
Unertl (12)	39	RCT	Neurologic injury; trauma; >4 days MV	Existing infection; WBC; ARDS
Wiesner (13)	30	Obs cohort	Liver transplant recipients	None
Ledingham (14)	324	Consec	Med/surg ICU	None
Kerver (15)	96	RCT	SICU >5 days on MV	None
Konrad (16)	165	Consec	SICU >4 days on MV	None
Brun-Buisson (17)	86	RCT	MICU stay >2 days; SAPS >2	Prior antibiotics; neutropenia
Ulrich (18)	100	RCT	Mixed ICU on MV; expected stay >5 days	None
Thulig (19)	200	Consec + X-over	TISS class III or IV; SICU >5 days MV >3 days	None
Aerdts (20)	56	RCT	MV >5 days	Pregnancy; age >16
Flaherty (21)	107	RCT	Cardiac surgery	None
Guillaume (22)	129	Consec + X-over	ICU stay >2 days	None
Cockerill (23)	150	RCT	Expected ICU LOS >3 days	Existing inf, antibiotic Rx for 24 hr
Tetteroo (24)	114	RCT	Esophageal resection	None
Sydow (25)	93	Consec	Mixed ICU >7 days; >4 days on MV	None
McClelland (26)	27	Consec	MV >5 days acute renal failure	None
Pugin (27)	52	RCT	SICU on MV >48 hrs	Transplant recipient
Godard (28)	131	Consec + X-over	All ICU patients	Postop patients, neutropenic
Hartenauer (29)	200	Consec + X-over	SICU ≥5 days, intubated within 3 days of study onset, TISS III or IV	None
Zobel (30)	50	RCT	PICU >4 days on MV	None
Fox (31)	24	Consec	Cardiac surg ICU; MV >4 days	None
Cerra (32)	46	RCT	SICU expected stay 7 days, hypermetabolic	MOF
Gastinne (39)	445	RCT multicenter	Ventilated ICU pts 15 ICU sites	GCS <4, neutropenia, overdose, SAPS >24, pregnancy, another clinical trial
Hammon[d] (40)	239	RCT	Ventilated ICU pts with expected intubation >48 hr	Expected ICU stay <5 days
Rocha (41)	101	RCT	Ventilated >3 days and stay in ICU >5 days	Suspected infection, neutropenia, antibiotics in prior 7 days

[a] As of February 1992. (Modified from van Saene, Stoutenbeek, and Stoller: Selective decontamination of the digestive tract (SDD) in the ICU: current status and future prospects. *Crit Care Med,* 20:691–703, 1992, with permission.)
[b] Consec = consecutive controls; Obs cohort = observational cohort; X-over = cross-over between different ICUs; RCT = randomized clinical trial.
[c] SICU = surgical ICU; MICU = medical ICU; MV = mechanical ventilation; SAPS = simplified acute physiological score; PICU = pediatric ICU. TISS = Therapeutic Intervention Scoring System.
[d] WBC = white blood cells; ARDS = adult respiratory distress syndrome; MOF = multiple organ failure; GCS = Glasgow coma scale.

existing evidence for efficacy. The other two reports showing no change in infection rates are the study by Fox et al (31), which, surprisingly, showed a reduction in ICU mortality rate in selective digestive decontamination recipients without a concomitant reduction in rates of colonization or acquired infection, and that by Brun-Buisson et al, in which no parenteral antibiotic was used and topical application of antibiotics in the oropharynx was replaced by rinsing with a solution of povidone-iodine. To the extent that rinsing the orophayngeal

cavity with chlorhexidine (in another study) (33) did not eradicate carriage of enteric Gram-negative bacteria and yeast in patients with radiation mucositis, it is possible that failure to reduce the rate of acquired infection in this study occurred because the topical antimicrobial did not decontaminate the oropharynx.

Mortality is an important outcome event, which has been considered in 16 trials, 7 of which have reported a decrease with selective digestive decontamination. Only 6 of the 16

Table 68.2. Outcome Measures and Results for Available Controlled Trials of Selective Digestive Decontamination[a]

Center	Types[b]	Efficacy Shown For[b]	Morbidity (%) Control/ SDD	Mortality (%) Control/SDD	Blinded Detection Specified
Stoutenbeek (6)	Col (T, R, Tr, U, W); Acq Inf; Resist; Antib use	Col; Acq Inf; Resist; Antib use	81/16[c]	-	No
Unertl (12)	Col (T, Tr); Acq Inf; Resist; Mort	Col; Acq Inf; Resist	70/21[c]	26/30	2 radiologists
Wiesner (13)	Col (T, R); Acq Inf	Col; Acq Inf	-/23	-/3	No
Ledingham (14)	Col (T, G, R, Tr, U); Acq Inf; Resist; Mort; Antib use	Col; Acq Inf; Resist; Mort; Antib use	24/10[c]	24/24 26/0[c] (trauma)	No
Kerver (15)	Col (T, R, Tr, U); Acq Inf; Resist; Mort; Antib use	Col; Acq Inf; Resist; Mort; Antib use	81/39[c]	32/39 17/4[c] (infection-related)	No
Konrad (16)	Col (T, R, Tr) Acq Inf; Resist	Col; Acq Inf	42/6[c]	22/30	No
Brun-Buisson (17)	Col (R); Acq Inf; Resist; Mort	Col with multiply resistant strain	33/32	10/8.5	No
Ulrich (18)	Col (T, R, Tr); Acq Inf; Resist; Mort (overall and infection-related)	Col; Acq Inf; Resist; Mort (overall and infection-related)	44/6[c]	54/31[c] 15/0[c] (infection-related)	No
Thulig (19)	Col (T, R, Tr); Acq Inf; Resist; Mort	Col; Acq Inf; Resist; Mort	46/10[c]	47/38 42/30	No
Aerdts (20)	Col (T, G, Tr) Acq Inf	Col; Acq Inf	69/6[c]	-	Radiologist
Flaherty (21)	Col (T, G; R); Acq Inf	Col (T, G); Acq Inf	27/12[c]	-	No
Guillaume (22)	Acq Inf; Mort; Time to onset of Acq Inf	Acq Inf; Mort; Time to onset of Acq Inf	21/3[c]	18/6[c]	No
Cockerill (23)	Col, Acq Inf, Mort, LOC, ventilator days, Therapeutic Antib use, Resist	Col, Acq Inf, Dur Vent	25.3%/ 13.3%	21%/14.6%	No
Tetteroo (24)	Col (N, T, G, R, Tr, U); Acq Inf; Mort; Resist; Antib use	Col; Acq Inf; Resist; Antib use	55/21[c]	3/5	No
Sydow (25)	Col; Acq Inf; Resist	Col; Acq Inf; Resist	75/7[c]	-	No
McClelland (26)	Col; Acq Inf; (Tr, U, W); Antib use	Col; Acq Inf; Antib use	83/33[c]	42/40	No
Pugin (27)	Col (Tr, G); Acq Inf Mort; Ox	Col; Acq Inf; Ox	78/16[c]	26/28	Yes
Godard (28)	Col (R); Total Acq Inf; Acq Inf/Pt; Mort	Col; Acq Inf/Pt	0.60/ 0.33[c,d]	18/12	Yes
Hartenauer (29)	Col (T, Tr, R, U); Acq Inf; Mort	Col; Acq Inf	10/45[c,e]	46/34	No
Zobel (30)	Col (T, Tr, G, U, R); Acq Inf; Mort	Col; Acq Inf	36/8	8/12	No
Fox (31)	Col; Acq Inf; Mort	Mort	NS (42/22)	67/17	No
Cerra (32)	Acq Inf, MOFS	Acq Inf	200%/88%[c]	48/52	Yes
Gastinne (39)	Mort, Acq Inf, Dur Vent, ICU LOS, Antib use	Gram-negative pneumonia	15%/12%	30%/34%	Yes
Hammond (40)	Mort, Acq Inf, ICU LOS, Hospital LOS, Antib use	None	34%/26%	21%/21%	Yes
Rocha (41)	Col, Acq Inf, Mort, Mort related to inf, cost, resist, LOS, Therapeutic Antib use	Col, Acq Inf, Mort, Mort related to inf, Therapeutic Antib Use	63%/26%	44%/21%	Yes

[a] As of February 1992. (Modified from van Saene, Stoutenbeek, and Stoller: Selective decontamination of the digestive tract (SDD) in the ICU: Current status and future prospects. *Crit Care Med* 20:691–703, 1992, with permission.)
[b] Col = colonization; Acq inf = acquired infection; Resist = resistance; Mort = mortality; Antib use = antibiotic use; N = nasal culture; T = throat (oropharynx) culture; G = gastric culture; R = rectal culture; Tr = tracheal culture; U = urine; Ox = oxygenation; W = wound culture; MOFS = multiple-organ failure syndrome; LOS = length of stay.
[c] $P < 0.0002$.
[d] Acquired infections per patient.
[e] For acquired bronchopulmonary infection.

have considered infection-specific (rather than crude overall) mortality rates in selective digestive decontamination recipients vs. controls (15, 17, 18, 24, 26, 41). This distinction may be important, because studies of selective disorder decontamination would not be expected to show a mortality advantage if most deaths were unrelated to the presence of infection. For example, in the study by Unertl et al, the most common cause of death in both the study and control groups was head trauma (12). The overall mortality rate was similar for both groups in the study by Kerver et al (15), but the rate of infection-related mortality was significantly lower in the selective digestive decontamination group. Still, the mortality results are not as consistent as the reduction in acquired infections, a finding that may challenge the notion that ICU patients die *of* rather than *with* infection. In support of this possibility, Gross and Antwerpen (34) demonstrated in a case-control study that "nosocomial infections appeared to favor a fatal outcome only in those whose condition was not terminal on admission."

Finally, emergence of resistance to Gram-negatives has not been reported in selective digestive decontamination studies to date, although surveillance has been limited to a maximum of 2½ years of follow-up (35). Ten of the 12 studies that specifically monitored resistance have reported no increase in resistant Gram-negative organisms with selective digestive decontamination, but emergence of resistant Gram-positive bacteria has been reported. In the study by Konrad et al (16) 20% of the *Staphylococcus aureus* isolates from the throat and upper airways were resistant to the cefotaxime used in the selective digestive decontamination arm, but the pneumonia rate in the selective digestive decontamination group (2 of 82 patients, 2.4%) was lower than in the control group (6 of 83 patients, 7%).

Seven of the nine studies that have measured antibiotic usage have reported a significant reduction in therapeutic antibiotic usage (Table 68.2).

EXPERIENCE WITH SELECTIVE DIGESTIVE DECONTAMINATION AT THE CLEVELAND CLINIC

In response to the weight of supportive literature, the authors' hospital recently has adopted selective digestive decontamination as standard therapy for eligible patients in the medical, surgical, and cardiovascular ICUs. This experience is reviewed briefly to report several practical details of using selective digestive decontamination.

Beginning in April 1991, selective digestive decontamination was initiated using a standard formulation as follows: (a) a sticky water-soluble paste (Orabase, Colgate-Hoyt, Canton, MA) to which is added by the pharmacy 2% each of polymyxin E and gentamicin, and nystatin, 100,000 units/g, to be applied to the buccal mucosa; and (b) a suspension to be placed down gastric tubes containing a mixture of polymixin E (10 mg/ml), gentamicin (8 mg/ml), and nystatin (200,000 units/ml). Gentamicin and nystatin were chosen because tobramycin and amphotericin B powders are not available in the U.S.A. A specific parenteral agent was not recommended, primarily because most of the patients involved had undergone surgery

and had already received perioperative prophylactic antibiotics; most of the remaining ICU patients were receiving antibiotics for documented or suspected infections.

Patients deemed eligible for the selective digestive decontamination program were mechanically ventilated and had been in the hospital for 48 hours. Intubation was expected to continue for at least 24 hours after ICU admission. Administration of selective disorder decontamination ended when the patient was extubated or was discharged from the ICU.

Compliance with the recommendations to administer selective digestive decontamination was generally high. Specifically, in the medical ICU, selective disorder decontamination use was monitored for 68 days beginning 6 months after initiating the selective digestive decontamination program. Of 731 total patient-days during this period, selective disorder decontamination eligibility occurred for 73% (531 patient-days), during which selective digestive decontamination was used in 83%. In the surgical ICU, 12 days were monitored, during which selective digestive decontamination eligibility occurred in 163 patient-days. Because of more rapid patient discharge from the surgical than the medical ICU, a smaller proportion of patient-days was eligible (33%), but the rate of compliance with selective digestive decontamination was similarly high (87%).

Impediments to complete compliance with selective digestive decontamination included the lack of a nasogastric tube in some patients with esophageal mucosal erosions, presence of a jejunal rather than a nasogastric feeding tube, gastrointestinal obstruction, oropharyngeal surgery, enterocutaneous fistulae, and failure to reorder selective digestive decontamination after reintubation for recurrent respiratory failure. Compliance was also more difficult among awake patients, who frequently complained about the unappealing taste and consistency (described by one patient as being "like tree bark"). To enhance palatability, the pharmacist suggested that the 15-g single-patient use jars should be kept at the bedside after use without refrigeration, which has reportedly improved the consistency. Furthermore, the taste has been improved by adding flavor extracts, including lemon and banana.

The cost to the pharmacy is $7.48 per 15-g jar of oral paste, and $23.89 per 30 ml of gastric suspension. The number of doses per jar varies by application technique, and the routine gastric dose is 10 ml per nasogastric tube every 6 hours. Assuming a 5-day duration of eligibility for selective disorder decontamination during which 2 jars of paste and 20 gastric doses are used, the cost per patient is $173.83. Future cost analyses must consider whether the aggregate cost of selective digestive decontamination is offset by the savings produced by reducing nosocomial infections and the associated costs of ICU care.

AREAS FOR FUTURE INVESTIGATION

Despite the extensive investigation to date, several issues regarding the efficacy and application of selective digestive decontamination remain unclear. Future studies should be designed to answer the specific questions that follow:

1. **What is the ideal selective digestsve decontamination regimen?** As mentioned previously and as summarized in Table 68.3, a wide variety of regimens has been collected

Table 68.3. Treatment Strategies in Available Controlled Trials of Selective Digestive Decontamination[a]

Center	Systemic Antibiotics[b]	SDD Regimen[b]	Specified Co-Maneuvers[b]
Stoutenbeek (6)	CFX	PTA;O+GI	Chest physiotherapy; vent circuit sterilized q1–3d
Unertl (12)	None	P Genta A; NA+O+GI	Steroids; handwashing; H_2 blockers + antacids; daily change of vent tubing; sterile suctioning q 6–8 hr
Wiesner (13)	CFX q 8h × 48 hr	P Genta Nyst; O+GI	Low bacterial diet
Ledingham (14)	CFX 4 days	PTA; O+GI	None
Kerver (15)	CFX 5–7 days	PTA; O+GI	Bladder irrigation; vent tube changed q 48 hr
Konrad (16)	CFX 3–4 days	PTA; O+GI	None
Brun-Buisson (17)	None	Neo Nal; GI	Oral povidone-iodine solution
Ulrich (18)	"Perioperative prophylaxis" + TMP >8 days	P Norf A; O+GI	None
Thulig (19)	CFX >4 days	PTA; O+GI	None
Aerdts (20)	CFX q 8h × 5 days	P Norf S; O+GI	None
Flaherty (21)	None	P Genta Nyst; O+GI	H_2-blockers or antacids; vs sucralfate without SDD in comparison group
Guillaume (22)	None	PT;GI	Oral povidone-iodine solution; GI ampho B to all patients
Cockerill (23)	CFX 3 days	P Genta Nyst; O+GI	None
Tetteroo (24)	CFX 4 days	PTA; O+GI	No H_2 blockers given; standard IV antibiotic prophylaxis in controls (Cefa + Met; 1 d)
Sydow (25)	CFX 4 days	PTA; O+GI	H_2 blockers; vent tube changed daily
McClelland (26)	CFX 4 days	PTA; O+GI	None
Pugin (27)	None	P Neo Vanc; O+GI	None
Godard (28)	None	T Col Ampho; GI	No sucralfate; antacid and/or H_2 blockers only; oral povidone and sodium carbonate rinse
Hartenauer (29)	CFX 4 days	PT Ampho; O+GI	Cimetidine and pirenzipine
Zobel (30)	CFX, duration NS	P Genta Ampho; O+GI	None
Fox (31)	Cephradine × 4 days	PTA; O + GI (oral solution—no paste)	No routine stress ulcer prophylaxis
Cerra (32)	None	Norf Nyst; GI	Nutritional support
Gastinne (39)	None	PTA; O & GI	None
Hammond (40)	CFX	PTA; O & GI	None
Rocha (41)	CFX	PTA; O & GI	Vent tubing Δ q 48 hr
Cockerill (23)	CFX	P, Genta, Nyst; O & GI	None

[a] As of February 1992. (Modified from van Saene, Stoutenbeek and Stoller: Selective decontamination of the digestive tract (SDD) in the ICU: Current status and future prospects. *Crit Care Med,* 20:691–703, 1992, with permission.)
[b] CFX = cefotaxime; TMP = trimethoprim; Cefa = cefamandole; Met = metronidazole; P = polymyxin; T = tobramycin; Genta = gentamicin; Neo = neomycin; Nal = nalidixic acid; Norf = norfloxacin; Ampho = amphotericin B; Nyst = nystatin; O = oropharyngeal decontamination; GI = gastrointestinal decontamination; NA = nasal decontamination; Vanc = vancomycin; Col = colistin; NS = not stated; A = amphotericin B; PTA, polymixin E tobramycin amphotericin B; PT, polymyxin E tobramycin.

under the heading "selective digestive decontamination", so variation in efficacy may relate to differing regimens. The largest experience has been accumulated with the original program of oral and gastric polymyxin, tobramycin, and amphotericin B, along with parenteral cefotaxime, but the comparative efficacy of other agents has not been examined critically. Future studies should be designed to compare results not only with control groups but also with groups receiving different regimens. In addition, the importance of the parenteral antibiotic should be confirmed, and the question about which intravenous agent is preferred should be resolved. Though Stoutenbeek et al chose cefotaxime because it spares anaerobic endogenous bacteria to prevent overgrowth by potentially pathologic microorganisms, this may not be the ideal parenteral agent for patients at risk for anaerobic and enterococcal infections, such as patients undergoing colon resections. Whether alternate parenteral agents reduce the effectiveness of selective digestive decontamination or encourage the development of resistant organisms is unknown at this time but is in need of further study.

2. Who will benefit from selective digestive decontamination? Among available trials, the patients treated with selective digestive decontamination vary greatly among series, which may also help to explain the differences in outcomes reported (Table 68.2). Future studies should be large enough to allow subgroup analysis, or be aimed at specific groups only to answer this question. Some trials have been quite specific, investigating only patients undergoing esophageal resection (24), liver transplantation (13), multiple trauma (6), or cardiac surgery (31), but more patients and more specific groups (such as those undergoing colonic resection, or those on broad-spectrum antibiotics for existing infections) should be examined.

Severity of illness using a method that predicts estimated hospital mortality early in the hospital course, such as APACHE II (36), APACHE III (37), or the Mortality Prediction Model (38) should be documented to help explain differences in outcome. For example, a difference in mortality is most likely to be demonstrable in the moderate severity range where the number of deaths is large enough to document a reduction by a specific intervention such as selective digestive decontamination. Examination of patients so ill as to be unlikely to survive no matter what is done, and of those who are expected to have extremely low mortality may yield information about colonization rates and cost of treatment, but may only confuse the issue of mortality.

Another area for investigation is the use of selective digestive decontamination preoperatively and postoperatively for those patients at risk for infectious complications, such as those undergoing pneumonectomy, or thoracoabdominal aortic aneurysm resections.

3. **What are the cost implications?** Trials specifically designed to clarify the impact of selective digestive decontamination on overall cost are necessary. The added cost of selective digestive decontamination administration must be balanced against possible reductions in acquired infections, antibiotic usage, length of stay, laboratory testing, necessity for additional medical consultations, nursing costs, ventilator days, and use of disposable equipment. A reduction in acquired infections should translate into savings to the patient, the hospital, and society, but this has not yet been established and should not be presumed.

CONCLUSION

The weight of evidence suggests that selective digestive decontamination is effective in preventing secondary colonization and acquired infection in critically ill patients. Ongoing debate surrounds its efficacy in reducing mortality and, to a lesser extent, its risk in selecting multiply resistant microorganisms. Further research is necessary to define the population most likely to benefit in terms of reduced morbidity, cost, and mortality before it can be recommended for routine use in all ICU patients.

REFERENCES

1. Langer M, Cigada M, Mandelli M, et al: Early onset pneumonia: multicenter study in intensive care units. *Intensive Care Med* 13:342–346, 1987.
2. Thorp JM, Richard WC, Telfer ABM: A survey of infection in an ICU. *Anesthesia* 34:643–650, 1979.
3. Northey D, Adess ML, Hartsuck JM, Rhoades ER: Microbial surveillance in a surgical ICU. *Surg Gynecol Obstet* 139:321–325, 1974.
4. Niederman MS: Strategies for the prevention of pneumonia. *Clin Chest Med* 8(3):543–556, 1987.
5. Feeley TW, du Moulin GC, Hedley-Whyte J, et al: Aerosol polymyxin and pneumonia in seriously ill patients. *N Engl J Med* 293:471–475, 1975.
6. Stoutenbeek CP, Stoutenbeek HKF, Miranda DR, et al: The effect of oropharyngeal decontamination using topical non-absorbable antibiotics on the incidence of nosocomial respiratory tract infections in multiple trauma patients. *J Trauma* 27:357–364, 1987.
7. Stoutenbeek CP, Van Saiene HK, Miranda DR, Zandstra DF: A new technique of infection prevention in the ICU by selective decontamination of the digestive tract. *Acta Anaesthesiol Belg* 3:209–221, 1983.
8. Hillman KM, Riordan T, O'Farrell SM, et al: Colonization of the gastric contents in critically ill patients. *Crit Care Med* 10:444–447, 1982.
9. van Saene HKF, Stoutenbeek CP, Stoller JK: Selective decontamination of the digestive tract (SDD) in the ICU: current status and future prospects. *Crit Care Med* 20:691–703, 1992.
10. Alcock SR: Use of short-term parenteral antibiotic as a supplement to SDD. In van Saene HKF, Stoutenbeek CP, Lawin P, McA Ledingham I (eds): *Infection Control by Selective Decontamination. Update in Intensive Care and Emergency Medicine*, vol. 7. Berlin-Heidelberg, Springer-Verlag, pp 102–108, 1989.
11. Reidy J, Ramsay G: Clinical trials of selective decontamination of the digestive tract: review. *Crit Care Med* 18:1449–1456, 1990.
12. Unertl K, Ruckdeschel G, Selbmann HK, et al: Prevention of colonisation and respiratory infections in long-term ventilated patients by local antimicrobial prophylaxis. *Intensive Care Med* 13:106–113, 1987.
13. Wiesner RH, Hermans PE, Rakela J, et al: Selective bowel decontamination to decrease Gram-negative aerobic bacterial and *Candida* colonization and prevent infection after orthotopic liver transplantation. *Transplantation* 45:570–574, 1988.
14. McA Ledingham I, Alcock SR, Eastaway AT, et al: Triple regimen of selective decontamination of the digestive tract, systemic cefotaxime, and microbiological surveillance for prevention of acquired infection in intensive care. *Lancet* 1:785–790, 1988.
15. Kerver AJH, Rommes JH, Mevissen-Verhage EAE, et al: Prevention of colonization and infection in critically ill patients: a prospective randomized study. *Crit Care Med* 16:1087–1093, 1988.
16. Konrad F, Schwalbe B, Heeg K, et al: Kolonisations-Pneumoniefrequenz und Resistenzentwicklung bei langzeitbeatmeten Intensivpatienten unter selektiver Dekontamination des Verdauungstraktes. *Anaesthesist* 38:99–109, 1989.
17. Brun-Buisson C, Legrand P, Rauss A, et al: Intestinal decontamination for control of nosocomial multiresistant Gram-negative bacilli. Study of an outbreak in an intensive care unit. *Ann Intern Med* 110:873–881, 1989.
18. Ulrich C, Harinck-de Weerd JE, Bakker NC, et al: Selective decontamination of the digestive tract with norfloxacin in the prevention of ICU-acquired infections: a prospective randomized study. *Intensive Care Med* 15:424–431, 1989.
19. Thulig B, Hartenauer U, Fegeler W, et al: Effektive Infektionskontrolle durch selektive Darmdekontamination (SDD) bei thoraxchirurgische Intensivpatienten. *Anaesthesist* 38:S352, 1988.
20. Aerdts SJ, Closever HA, van Dalen R, et al: Prevention of bacterial colonization of the respiratory tract and stomach of mechanically ventilated patients by a novel regimen of selective decontamination in combination with initial systemic cefotaxime. *J Antimicrob Chemother* 26(suppl A):59–76, 1990.
21. Flaherty J, Kabins SA, Weinstein RA: New approaches to the prevention of infection in intensive care unit patients. In van Saene HKF, Stoutenbeek CP, Lawin P, McA Ledingham I (eds): *Infection Control by Selective Decontamination. Update in Intensive Care and Emergency Medicine*, vol 7. Berlin-Heidelberg, Springer-Verlag, pp 184–188, 1989.
22. Guillaume C, Godard J, Bui-Xuan B, et al: Selective digestive tract decontamination (SDD) in a polyvalent intensive care unit (ICU). In: 29th ICAAC, Houston, Texas, USA, American Society of Microbiology, *Abstract* 325, 1989.
23. Cockerill FR, Muller SR, Anhalt JP, et al: Prevention of infection in critically ill patients by selective decontamination of the digestive tract. *Ann Intern Med* 117:545–553, 1992.
24. Tetteroo GWM, Wagenvoort JHT, Castelein A, et al: Selective decontamination to reduce Gram negative colonisation and infections after oesophageal resection. *Lancet* 335:704–707, 1990.
25. Sydow M, Burchardi H, Crozier TA, et al: Einfluss der selektiven Dekontamination auf nosokomiale Infektionen, Erregerspektrum und Antibioticaresistenz bei langzeitbeatmeten Intensivpatienten. *Anaesthesie Intensivtherapie Notfallmedizin* 25(6):416–423, 1990.
26. McClelland P, Murray AE, Williams PS, et al: Reducing sepsis in severe combined acute renal and respiratory failure by selective decontamination of the digestive tract. *Crit Care Med* 18:935–939, 1990.
27. Pugin J, Auckenthaler R, Lew D, Suter P: Oropharyngeal decontamination decreases incidence of ventilator-associated pneumonia. *JAMA* 265:2704–2710, 1991.
28. Godard J, Guillaume C, Reverdy ME, et al: Intestinal decontamination in a polyvalent ICU. *Intensive Care Med* 16:307–311, 1990.
29. Hartenauer U, Thulig B, Diemer W, et al: Effect of selective flora suppression on colonization, infection, and mortality in critically ill patients: a one-year, prospective consecutive study. *Crit Care Med* 19:463–473, 1991.
30. Zobel G, Kuttnig M, Grubhauer HM, et al: Reduction of colonization and infection rate during pediatric intensive care by selective decontamination of the digestive tract. *Crit Care Med* 19:1242–1246, 1991.
31. Fox MA, Peterson S, Fabri BM, et al: Selective decontamination of the digestive tract in cardiac surgical patients. *Crit Care Med* 19:1486–1490, 1991.
32. Cerra FB, Maddaus MA, Dunn DL, et al: Selective gut decontamination reduces nosocomial infections and length of stay but not mortality or organ failure in surgical ICU patients. *Arch Surg* 127:163–169, 1992.
33. Spijkervet FKL, van Saene HKF, Panders AK, et al: Effect of chlorhexidine rinsing on the oropharyngeal ecology in patients with head and neck cancer who have irradiation mucositis. *Oral Surg Oral Med Oral Pathol* 67:154–161, 1989.

34. Gross, PA, van Antwerpen C: Nosocomial infections and hospital deaths. A case-control study. *Am J Med* 75:658–662, 1983.

35. van Saene HKF, Stoutenbeek CP, Hart CA: Selective decontamination of the digestive tract (SDD) in ICU patients: a critical evaluation. *J Hosp Infect* 18:261–277, 1991.

36. Knaus WA, Draper EA, Wagner DP, Zimmerman JA: APACHE II: a severity of disease classification system. *Crit Care Med* 13:818–829, 1985.

37. Knaus WA, Wagner DP, Draper EA, et al: The APACHE III prognostic system: risk prediction of hospital mortality for critically ill hospitalized adults. *Chest* 100:1619–1636, 1991.

38. Lemeshow S, Teres D, Pastides H, et al: A method for predicting survival and mortality of ICU patients using objectively derived weights. *Crit Care Med* 13:519–525, 1985.

39. Gastinne H, Wolff M, Delatour F, et al: A controlled trial in intensive care units of selective decontamination of the digestive tract with nonabsorbable antibiotics. *N Engl J Med* 326:594–599, 1992.

40. Hammond J, Potgieter PD, Saunders GL, et al: Double-blind study of selective decontamination of the digestive tract in intensive care. *Lancet* 340:5–9, 1992.

41. Rocha LA, Martin MJ, Pita S, et al: Prevention of nosocomial infection in critically ill patients by selective decontamination of the digestive tract. *Intensive Care Med* 18:398–404, 1992.

CHAPTER 69

Drug Delivery Systems

JANE W. KWAN, B.S. PHARMACY, M.P.H.

Although increased emphasis has been observed in treating patients in alternative delivery settings, such as outpatient clinics or in patient homes, a growing percentage of hospital beds is dedicated to the critically ill. According to recent American Hospital Association statistics, approximately 8% of hospital beds are critical care beds (1). The expertise of the medical staff and the development of technology for use in the critical care environment has so raised the level of the quality of patient care that it has been said that American medical care in the critical care setting is the best in the world.

From the first recorded injection of drugs into the veins of living animals by Sir Christopher Wren in 1657, parenteral drug therapy has been so widely adopted and utilized in the U.S. that it is now estimated that 40% of all drugs administered in hospitals are given as injections, and more than 20,000,000 patients will receive intravenous therapy in hospitals this year.

The utilization of technology for the delivery of parenteral drugs, in general, has undergone a dramatic increase in the last 20 years. This increase is due to new developments in drug therapy, new methods for administering drugs, and the development of new computer technology. The technology of parenteral drug delivery systems has evolved to the point where drug therapy protocols are no longer dictated by the technical ability to deliver the drug, but rather drug therapy now dictates the development of infusion device technology.

The pressure of gravity has been used as the driving force for administration of intravenous solutions since the 17th century. The amount of pressure generated by gravity from a hanging i.v. is primarily dependent on the distance from the hanging

solution to the right atrium of the patient. In most cases the force of gravity is sufficient to overcome venous pressure. Under normal conditions, the venous system offers little resistance to fluid flow, approximately 10 to 30 mm Hg or less than 1 psi (1 psi = approximately 50 mm Hg). At a height of 36 inches, a hanging solution generates a pressure of approximately 65 mm Hg. Although this favorable pressure gradient exists, early studies demonstrated wide variations in the accuracy of gravity delivery, ranging from −63% to +50% (2, 3).

The typical method used for gravity delivery employed manual clamps and an in-line drip chamber through which drops of falling solution could be counted and regulated to achieve a specific delivery rate. A number of factors contribute to this variation in delivery accuracy. These factors include length and diameter of the administration set tubing and cannula; solution viscosity; drop size variations; changes in head height, i.e., the distance between the solution container and the patient; patient position; temperature; and backpressure due to changes in resistance to flow, e.g., patient blood pressure, clotting, or body position (4, 5). Additional factors include variations in size of drip-chamber orifice, plastic cold flow, clamp slippage, final filters, pressure changes in i.v. containers, rate of flow, temperature of the i.v. fluid, changes in needle position, and kinked tubing (6).

To improve delivery accuracy, mechanical devices, such as controllers and infusion pumps, were then developed. The primary difference between controllers and infusion pumps is that while controllers utilize gravity pressure to drive fluid delivery, infusion pumps generate positive pressure to overcome any in-line resistance to flow. Early controllers electronically counted drops, but such systems did not consistently achieve volumetric accuracy because of drop size variations. Today, special administration tubing sets have been developed for use with controllers to provide volumetric accuracy. The set contains an in-line chamber of a measured volume from which a precise volume is delivered.

When the pressure of gravity is insufficient to overcome in-line resistance, additional pressure, such as that provided by an infusion pump, is indicated. The occlusion pressure settings of infusion pumps range up to approximately 25 psi, although the recent trend is to reduce pressure settings, in the range of 8 to 10 psi. Minimizing pressure is a more critical clinical issue if vascular access is achieved by peripheral insertions, rather than by central venous catheters. Although there is no evidence indicating that the use of infusion pumps increases the incidence of infiltrations, the severity of infiltrations increases if undetected, particularly with high occlusion pressure settings on infusion pumps (7). Pumps today have also been developed that combine the functions of both a pump and a controller in a single device, allowing the user to select the operating mode.

CLASSIFICATION OF INFUSION PUMPS

Making an infusion pump selection decision requires an appropriate matching of the device to the clinical need. This decision requires a knowledge of the devices available on the market and what their capabilities are.

Infusion pumps can be classified in several ways. Mechanism of operation is one of the simplest methods of classification of infusion pumps. This classification scheme includes peristaltic systems, cassette systems, syringe pump systems, and elastomeric reservoir systems (8).

PERISTALTIC SYSTEMS

Peristaltic infusion pumps use a motor-driven mechanism to cause finger-like projections to squeeze the fluid-filled delivery tubing, thereby moving fluid toward the patient. Such systems may be either linear or rotary. In the linear system, tubing is massaged in a straight line (Fig. 69.1). In the rotary system, the tubing is coiled around a rotating cam that has projection points to press on the tubing (Fig. 69.2).

Some peristaltic pumps require the use of a special tubing set that has a flexible portion, e.g., made of silicone, that is "massaged" by the finger-like projections. An example of this peristaltic system is the Imed Gemini PC pump. Other peristaltic pumps have been designed to be used with standard tubing sets, at less cost than the dedicated type sets. The delivery accuracy of devices using the standard tubing sets is typically less than that of pumps using the specially designed sets. Examples of hospital-use peristaltic systems that use standard tubing sets are the Baxter Flo-Gard 6200 and the SIGMA 6000+.

CASSETTE SYSTEMS

Cassette systems use an administration set that contains an in-line chamber of a measured volume. The advantage of

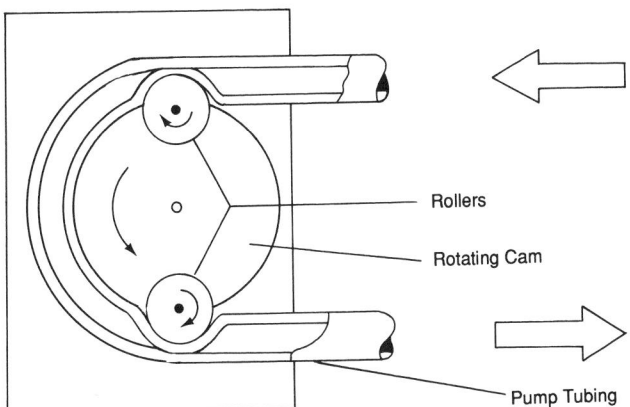

Figure 69.1. Rotary peristaltic mechanism.

the cassette system is its volumetric accuracy, while a potential disadvantage is the interruption of flow during the fill cycle, which is often dependent on the flow rate desired, e.g., a slow flow rate has a longer fill time than a high flow rate. A cassette system requires a fill cycle during which fluid moves into the chamber and a delivery cycle during which fluid is delivered out of the chamber (Fig. 69.3). An example of an infusion pump that uses the cassette type of mechanism is the Imed 980 infusion pump. Cassette sets are also more expensive than standard i.v. tubing. A safety feature of cassette tubing sets is that free flow is generally not possible even if a clamp is left open, a potential problem with standard i.v. tubing sets.

SYRINGE PUMPS

Syringe pumps have been developed that utilize both motor and nonmotor-driven mechanisms to move the syringe plunger and thereby cause fluid delivery. The movement may be continuous, as in spring mechanisms (Fig. 69.4), e.g., 3M AVI Medifuse and Healthtek Adfuse, or it may be intermittent, as in motor-driven lead screw mechanisms (Fig. 69.5), e.g., AutoSyringe AS20S. An innovative disposable syringe pump single-use system is the Prime CADI-120, a vacuum-driven syringe-style system. Another primary distinguishing feature between syringe pumps is the programmability of administration. Some syringe pumps are programmed to deliver a single dose, e.g., the entire contents of the syringe, so that the syringe must be replaced and the pump reprogrammed for delivery of each intermittent dose, e.g., Becton-Dickinson 360 Infuser or Rate Infuser II. Other programmable syringe pumps can deliver multiple doses from a single syringe, delivering a single dose over a defined time and repeating that delivery at a scheduled interval, e.g., Bard Harvard Mini-Infuser Model 400.

ELASTOMERIC RESERVOIR PUMPS

Currently available elastomeric reservoir pumps utilize the elastomeric pressure of a balloon-type reservoir to force fluid through a rate-controlling restrictor into the delivery pathway (Figs. 69.6 and 69.7). While elastomeric devices have primarily been used in the ambulatory setting (e.g., Baxter Infusor, Intermate, and Block Homepump), some have been used in acute care settings. The delivery accuracy of elastomeric

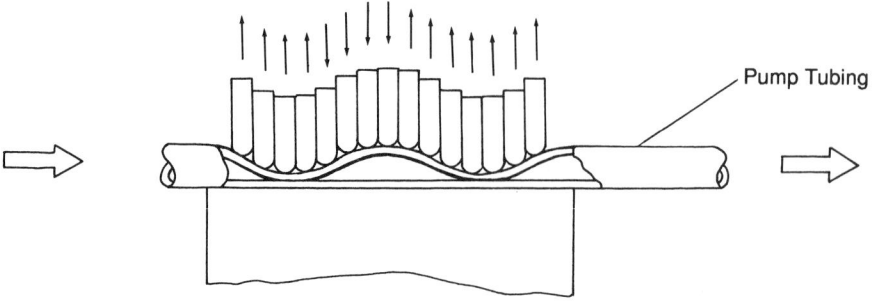

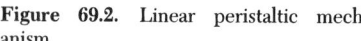
Figure 69.2. Linear peristaltic mechanism.

Pump Tubing

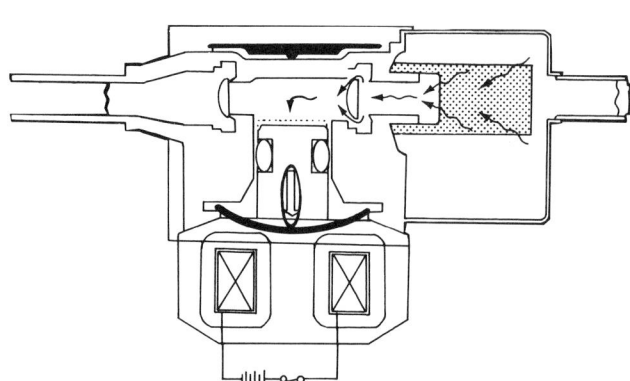

Figure 69.3. Piston cassette mechanism.

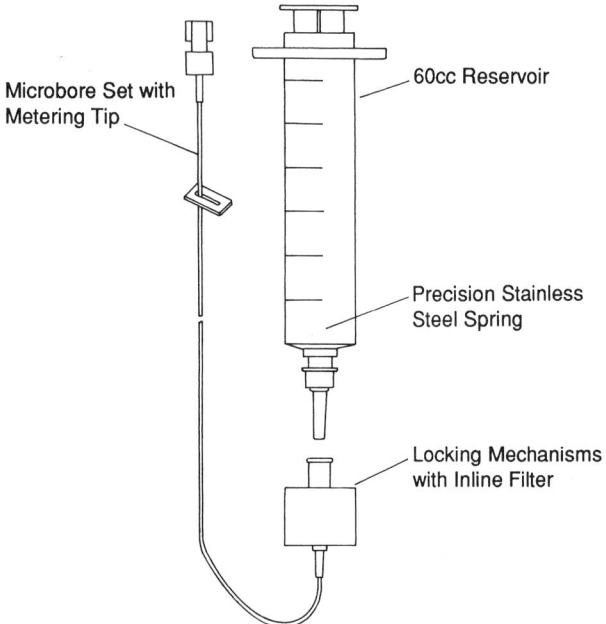

Microbore Set with
Metering Tip

60cc Reservoir

Precision Stainless
Steel Spring

Locking Mechanisms
with Inline Filter

Figure 69.4. Syringe spring mechanism Healthtek Adfuse.

devices (±10 to 15%) is more variable than that of electromechanical infusion pumps (±2 to 5%). This variability in flow rate is due to factors such as temperature and solution viscosity, which affect flow rate.

THERAPEUTIC CLASSIFICATION OF INFUSION PUMPS

The classification of infusion pumps by type of therapy is a useful classification, particularly when attempting to meet a particular delivery need. Typical therapeutic classifications for infusion pumps include total parenteral nutrition, antibiotics, pain management, chemotherapy, and hydration.

Total parenteral nutrition (TPN) is one of the earliest therapies for which the use of an infusion pump was designed and is often a part of the regimen for critically ill patients. Gravity is insufficient to deliver TPN solution with flow rate accuracy because of the viscosity of the high dextrose content solutions and the typically high flow rates required. Infusion pumps developed today for TPN delivery usually incorporate a flow-ramping capability to avoid hyper- or hypoglycemia at the start and end of infusion. A hospital type TPN infusion pump is the McGaw 522 Intelligent Pump. Ambulatory examples include the Abbott Provider Plus and the Pharmacia Deltec CADD TPN infusion pumps.

The delivery of parenteral antibiotics using an infusion pump may be accomplished in two ways: programming the delivery of a single dose at the time it is to be delivered or programming the delivery of multiple doses of a specified volume over a specified time period at a specified time interval. Most multiple-dose intermittent infusion pumps have a keep vein open (KVO) option to deliver a low flow rate of fluid between dose deliveries to maintain patency of vascular access.

Patient-controlled analgesia (PCA) is one of the fastest-growing methods of pain control today, both for the control of acute postoperative pain and for the chronic pain associated with cancer. PCA infusion pumps may be either worn externally for subcutaneous, intravenous, or epidural use, or may be implanted when an intrathecal delivery is required. Examples of hospital type PCA pumps that affix to an i.v. pole are the Harvard Bard PCA, the Abbott Lifecare PCA, and the IVAC PCA 310 Infuser. External ambulatory PCA pumps include the Abbott Pain Management Provider, the Bard Ambulatory PCA, and the Pharmacia Deltec CADD PCA.

PCA infusion pumps are designed to deliver PCA therapy, and are able to be programmed with the required delivery parameters (e.g., basal infusion rate, PCA dose, lockout interval, maximum dose limit). Retrieval of delivery history includes the number of attempts, injections, and the total dose received. This history is critical information when patients are being titrated to the lowest effective therapeutic dose. Using delivery history, the clinician is able to determine whether the prescribed regimen is effective in meeting patient needs or whether an adjustment must be made.

Most chemotherapy regimens for which infusion pumps have been used are for continuous infusions. Circadian administration, in which varying amounts of drug are delivered at different times of the day in order to take advantage of time-dependent physiologic responses, is a new programming feature that has been incorporated into infusion pumps, e.g., the Ivion Intelliject and Iflow Vivus. Chronotherapy, utilizing circadian administration, has recently been investigated in a number of chemotherapy protocols (9).

Continuous-infusion dobutamine for long-term management of congestive heart failure is a therapy that can be delivered in the home setting with ambulatory infusion pumps (10). Patients with prolonged hospitalizations who await a suitable donor for heart transplantation and could not be discontinued from dobutamine therapy were able to be discharged to home with ambulatory infusion pumps.

THE CRITICAL CARE SETTING

The critical care setting today is a multidisciplinary environment, in which the physician, nurse, and pharmacist work as a team in which each member has defined roles of responsibility. Pharmacists have begun to take more active roles in

the critical care area, and the development of critical care pharmacy satellites is increasingly being utilized to meet the pharmaceutical care needs of the critically ill patient (11).

Two emerging areas for pharmacy involvement with infusion pumps in the critical care area include the evaluation, selection, and provision of infusion devices and the provision of information concerning both the devices and the drugs being administered by them, e.g., drug dosing and incompatibilities with multiple drugs. Such activities are based on an application of the pharmacist's expertise and knowledge of drug therapy requirements to administration capabilities.

EVALUATION AND SELECTION

Selecting an infusion device requires a determination of the drug delivery requirements and the matching of the device to meet those requirements. The therapeutic application for which the device will be used, the delivery requirements of

Figure 69.5. Syringe lead screw mechanism.

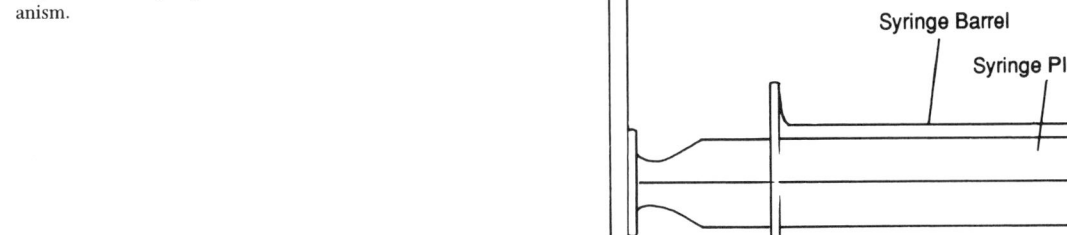
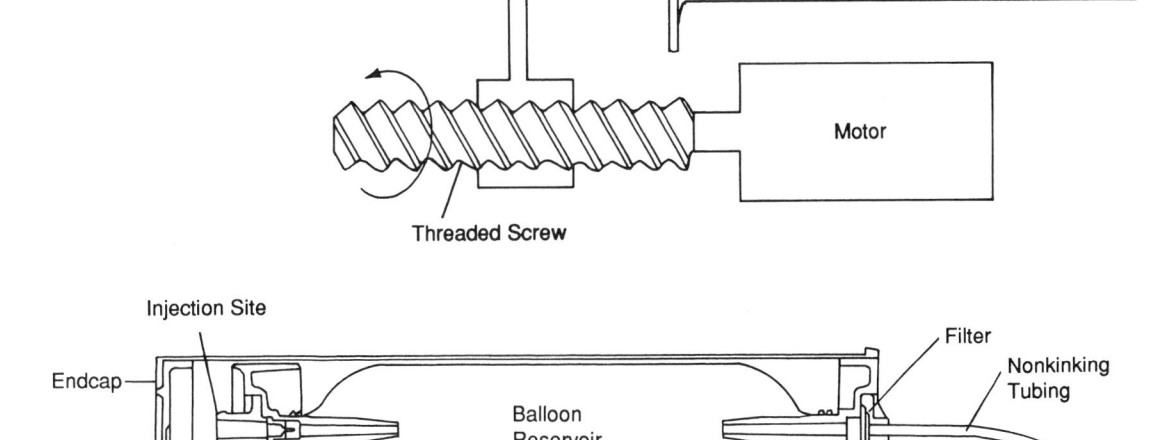

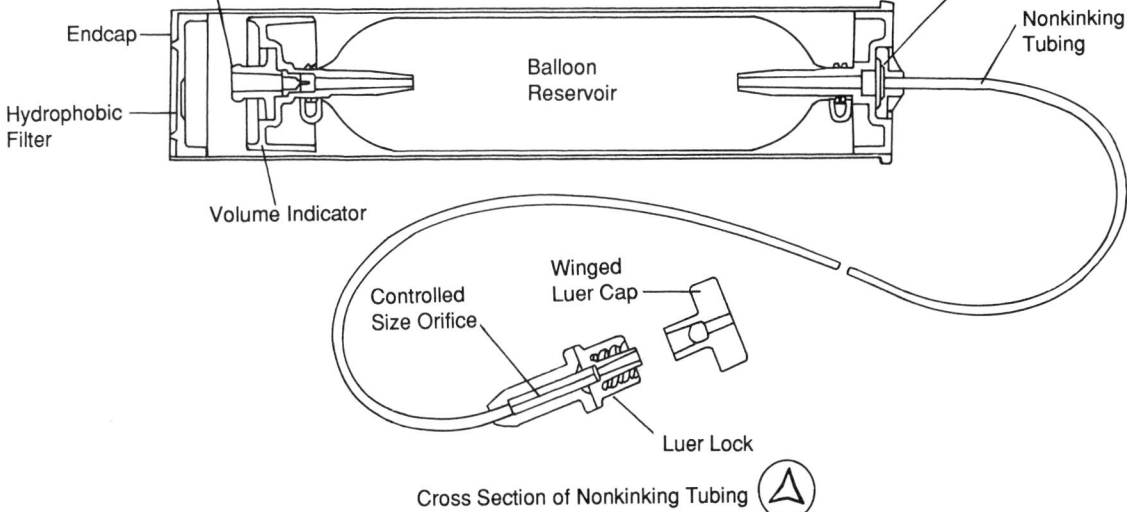

Figure 69.6. Elastomeric reservoir mechanism Baxter infusion.

that application, and the matching of those requirements to the infusion device will be the basic criteria on which a selection decision will be made. Although accuracy of delivery is the primary reason for using an electronic infusion device, there is no general agreement on specific criteria on which to base institutional selection decisions.

Selection criteria can be very narrow, focused on such factors as physical pump specifications, e.g., minimum/maximum flow rates and the presence of specific safety features, e.g., air-in-line alarms and both fluid-side and patient-side occlusions. Additional features to be considered include modes of delivery, size and weight dimensions, power source, service/maintenance requirements, reliability, and cost. Criteria can also reflect a broader scope, such as ease of use and multifunctionality. These broader factors are optimally evaluated with multidisciplinary input, i.e., from the various disciplines which will ultimately be responsible for pump operation and management.

Ease of use is of increased importance in selection decisions. Although staff in critical care areas utilize technology, perhaps to a greater degree than do staff in other areas of a hospital, a recent study indicated that inexperience with equipment and shortage of trained staff were the factors most often felt to contribute to preventable mishaps in an intensive therapy unit (12).

CRITICAL CARE APPLICATIONS

In critical care environments, infusion pumps, rather than controllers, are generally the drug delivery device of choice. While it has been estimated that 80 to 85% of fluid delivery needs are achievable by gravity infusion, the use of infusion pumps is clinically indicated for certain drugs. Many of these are drugs typically administered to the critically ill patient,

including sodium nitroprusside, oxytocin, dopamine, levarterenol, nitroglycerin infusion, streptokinase, urokinase, and antineoplastics (13, 14). Factors contributing to the need for infusion pumps include (*a*) the administration of drugs with a narrow therapeutic-toxic ratio—dobutamine, dopamine, isoproterenol, lidocaine, nitroglycerin, nitroprusside, procainamide, ritodrine, and vasopressin; (*b*) the need to deliver emergency drugs quickly and accurately, e.g., at very low or constant rates, without having to manually adjust drop rate; (*c*) the administration of a greater number of drugs to the critically ill patient than to the noncritical patient (15); and (*d*) the increased resistance to flow caused by these multiple i.v. lines.

While most studies seem to indicate that variations in actual delivery of fluid over short time intervals is not clinically significant, e.g., when drug half-life is more than 2 minutes, the effect of interruptions in flow continuity can result in variations in response to certain drugs with very short half-lives, e.g., nitroprusside with a half-life of 0.4 minutes (16–18). Such flow interruptions occur because of infusion pump mechanisms of action, e.g., cassette pump systems that require a fill cycle and a delivery cycle, syringe systems in which plunger movement is not continuous, or peristaltic systems in which there is a pause between peristaltic delivery movements.

The critically ill patient may have additional infusion considerations, for which infusion device technology offers advantages. These considerations include the need to titrate certain drugs, e.g., vasopressors and hypotensives; intraoperative administration of anesthetic drugs, where multiple changes in plasma concentration may be required to titrate the depth of anesthesia; fluid restriction requirements for many critically ill patients; the need to perform pharmacokinetic drug monitoring; blood and blood product transfusions; and the need

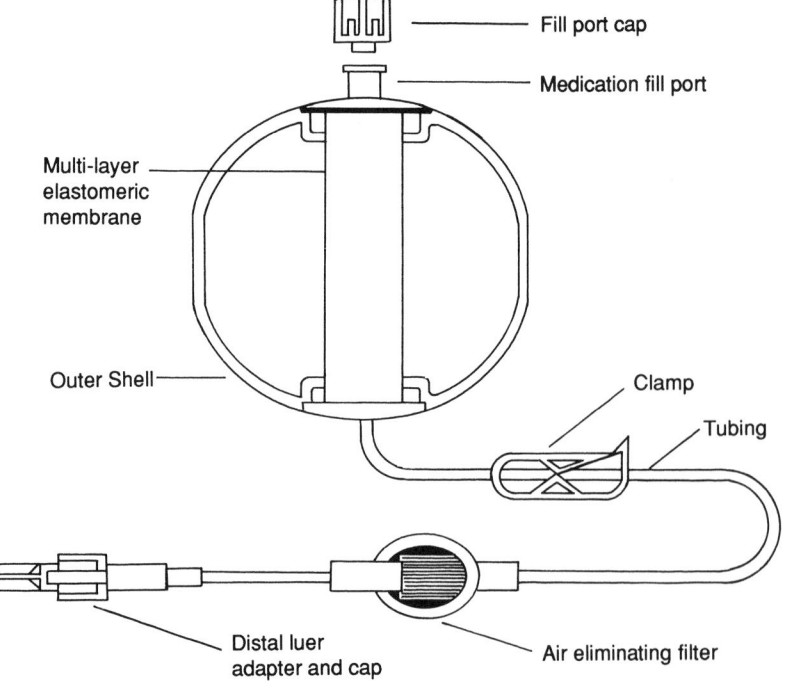

Figure 69.7.   Elastomeric reservoir mechanism Block Homepump.

to deliver certain drugs according to body weight dosing, e.g., nitroprusside, alfentanil, vecuronium, dobutamine, etc.

The titration of critical drugs is facilitated by new infusion pumps available today. The delivery of i.v. anesthetics by continuous-variable rate infusion, rather than via bolus injections, can also be titrated easily with infusion pumps (19). While older-model infusion pumps require stopping infusion to reprogram a change in flow rate, devices today can be programmed with a new flow rate without an interruption, and the new rate can be immediately implemented, e.g., Baxter AutoSyringe AS20GH2 and Medfusion 2010. Rapid infusions are facilitated by the ease of flow rate changes instead of relying on manual drop-count adjustments with a drip chamber. Minimizing volume for drug delivery in fluid-restricted patients is facilitated by using syringe pumps or by using multichannel infusion pumps that manifold together when one is using a single administration set.

Pharmacokinetic services are often provided by clinical pharmacy practitioners and are utilized in the appropriate dosing of aminoglycosides, vancomycin, theophylline, antiarrhythmics, and anticonvulsants (20). Such services result in improved quality of care through individualization of therapy, e.g., survival and time to response (21). A number of drug delivery device factors can influence the accuracy of pharmacokinetic monitoring, e.g., residual volume in administration tubing sets, mechanism of device operation, and device delivery accuracy of both volume and time (22, 23). Flow rate variability at very low flow rates (range of 1 ml/hr) to neonates has also been shown to have effects on pharmacologic responses, e.g., oscillations of transcutaneous PO_2 with low flow rate dopamine and of blood pressure with epinephrine infusions (24).

Several studies have been published demonstrating the ability of infusion pumps to deliver blood and blood products without damage. Although early infusion pumps, particularly peristaltic systems, caused a significant degree of hemolysis and were unsuitable for red blood cell delivery, many infusion pumps today can be used for delivery of blood components (25–27). The manufacturer of an infusion pump should be able to provide to potential users the results of blood delivery study testing. However, less expensive alternatives, e.g., pressure cuffs, can be used to facilitate the delivery of blood products.

The dosing of drugs by body weight requires a conversion from mass units of the desired dose to volume units for the desired flow rate. Many critical care drugs are dosed on a μg/kg/min or μg/kg/hr basis, and conversion tables have been developed to facilitate the accurate conversion of doses into a flow rate to be programmed into an infusion pump. Infusion pump programming for body weight dosing requires entering the appropriate drug concentration, e.g., in μg/ml or mg/ml the patient's body weight, e.g., in kilograms; and the desired dose. The infusion pump automatically delivers the appropriate infusion rate without a manual calculation and entry of the flow rate, minimizing the potential for calculation errors in critical situations. Examples of this type of infusion pump include the Baxter AutoSyringe AS20GH-2 and the Medfusion 2010 infusion pumps. Another novel approach to facilitate body weight dosing is that of drug-specific "smart labels" that affix magnetically to the face of an infusion pump (the Bard

Infus-O.R.) In order to achieve delivery accuracy, this system requires the use of a specific drug concentration and syringe size. Dose and body weight selections are made using a dial, and the appropriate flow rate is delivered.

Multichannel infusion pumps are available that can deliver from 2 to 10 solutions simultaneously or independently of the other. Many of these pumps have been targeted specifically for critical care areas, because of the large number of medications required in the typical critically ill patient. A knowledge of compatibility of combinations of critical care medications is critical information and is often provided by the manufacturer of multichannel infusion pumps to their users (28). The major advantages of the multichannel pump include improving patient safety by minimizing the amount of equipment at the patient bedside and reducing the inventory of infusion pumps required. Some multichannel devices can be programmed to deliver an automatic flush between incompatible medications administered sequentially and to program scheduled intermittent medications with a KVO in between. Examples of two-channel infusion pumps include the Baxter Flo-Gard 6300, the Imed Gemini PC-2, the AVI 840, and the Abbott Provider 6000; of a three-channel infusion pump, the MiniMed III; of four-channel infusion pumps, the Abbott Omniflow series, the Ivion Intelliject, and the IFlow Vivus 4000; of a 10-channel infusion pump, the Baxter Multiplex Series 100; and a modular system in which multiple pumps are stacked on each other on a single i.v. pole, the McGaw Horizon Modular Infusion System.

FUTURE TECHNOLOGY

An innovative concept in drug delivery technology that is still primarily in the research phase is that of using computerized feedback systems to monitor physiologic response and control drug delivery accordingly. Such systems may be either open loop or closed loop. In the open-loop system, physiologic response information is obtained externally to the delivery system. The information may be as simple as laboratory data that is interpreted by a clinician who then decides how to adjust delivery rate to achieve a change in physiologic response, or the information may have been obtained using a computerized pharmacokinetic model-driven system. In the closed-loop sytem, there is a direct connection between the physiologic monitoring system and the computer-controlled infusion pump for adjustment of drug infusion. When a well-defined relationship can be established between serum concentration and the desired effect and an algorithm derived for drug delivery, a feedback loop can be established, adjusting drug delivery to achieve the desired physiologic effect. If the feedback is accomplished automatically, i.e., via a physiologic sensor interfaced with a computer system that then adjusts drug delivery, a closed-loop system is achieved. The technological difficulty at this time lies in the development of the physiologic sensor to provide immediate data for a computer program. If drug delivery is adjusted based on physiologic data obtained from an external source, such as laboratory results or computerized pharmacokinetic models of predicted serum concentrations, and is then adjusted without a direct interface between physiologic sensor and drug delivery, the system is termed an open-loop system. The physiologic response data is obtained from a real-time biologic sensor; the desired effect is determined by a pharmacokinetic model; and a direct interface to the infusion system causes delivery of the desired flow rate to achieve the predicted response. The major obstacle to the development of such systems is the lack of a real-time biologic sensor to provide the direct data. The closed-loop system is theoretically of most benefit for drugs with a short duration of action or with complicated multicompartmental pharmacokinetic behavior that results in rapid changes of serum concentration. Several hospital type infusion pumps have a communications port built into the device, which can receive information to adjust drug delivery. Computer-assisted continuous-infusion devices have been developed to maintain constant drug levels of i.v. anesthetics, analgesics, and antihypertensives (29, 30). The only commercially available closed-loop infusion system currently on the market is the IVAC Titrator Sodium Nitroprusside Closed Loop Module—Model 10K for the delivery of nitroprusside to maintain arterial pressure after open heart surgery.

Bar code technology is increasingly being utilized in institutional settings. Such applications include documentation of drug administration to reduce chart documentation deficiencies (32), to control inventory (33), and for infusion pump management and programming. Systems such as the Abbott OmniFlow Therapist and the Block Verifuse utilize bar code technology to automate programming. These systems require a pharmacy-generated bar code label that contains administration information for the i.v. solution. The label is scanned using a wand or light pen, automatically programming the pump.

CONCLUSION

The integration of computer technology and infusion systems has revolutionized the patterns of American health care delivery. A high level of acute therapy to the severely ill patient can now be provided in alternative outpatient delivery settings, while an increasingly more sophisticated and technologically complex level of care is provided in the critical care setting. The use of infusion systems for the critically ill patient has improved patient outcomes, enhanced the effectiveness of i.v. therapy, decreased related morbidity and risk of complications, and saved staff time both in routine and emergency situations. Critical care therapy will no doubt continue to be enhanced with future innovations in infusion technology.

REFERENCES

1. *American Hospital Association Hospital Statistics:* American Hospital Association. 2:221, 1990.
2. Demoruelle JL, Harrison WL, Flora RE: Flow rate maintenance and output of intravenous fluid administration sets. *Am J Hosp Pharm* 32:177–185, 1975.
3. Kelly WN, Christensen LA: Selective patient criteria for the use of electronic infusion devices. *Am J IV Ther Clin Nutr* 10:18–28, 1983.
4. Flack FC, Whyte TD: Variations of drop size in disposable administration sets used for intravenous infusion. *J Clin Pathol* 28:510–512, 1975.
5. Merrick I, Merrick IM, Merrick TE: Comparison of drop size of intravenous administration sets. *Am J Hosp Pharm* 37:1346–1350, 1980.
6. Turco SJ, King RE: In *Remington's Pharmaceutical Sciences,* ed 17. Easton, PA, Mack Publishing, pp 1542–1551, 1985.
7. Phelps SJ, Helms RA: Risk factors affecting infiltration of peripheral venous lines in infants. *J Pediatr* 111:384–389, 1987.
8. Kwan JW: High-technology i.v. infusion devices. *Am J Hosp Pharm* 46(2):320–335, 1989.
9. Kwan JW: Chronotherapeutic applications in the oncology patient. *Highlights Antineoplastic Drugs* 7 (May/June):39–41, 1989.
10. Miller LW, Merkle EJ, Herrmann V: Outpatient dobutamine for end-stage congestive heart failure. *Crit Care Med* 18:S30–S33, 1990.
11. Dasta JF, Segal R, Cunningham A: National survey of critical-care pharmaceutical services. *Am J Hosp Pharm* 46:2308–2312, 1989.
12. Wright D, Mackenzie SJ, Buchan I, et al: Critical incidents in the intensive therapy unit. *Lancet* 338:676–678, 1991.
13. Robinson LA, Vanderveen TW: Pharmacy-based infusion pump program. *Am J Hosp Pharm* 34:697–705, 1977.
14. Kelly WN, Christensen LA: Selective patient criteria for the use of electronic infusion devices. *Am J IV Ther Clin Nutr* 10:18–28, 1983.
15. Dasta JF, Armstrong DK: Pharmacoeconomic impact of critically ill surgical patients. *Drug Intell Clin Pharm* 22:994–998, 1988.
16. Floyd RA: Effect of infusion pump fill-stroke flow interruptions on simulated serum concentrations of short half-life drugs. *Am J Hosp Pharm* 41:2399–2400, 1984.
17. Leff RD, True WR, Roberts RJ: A gravimetric technique for evaluating flow continuity from two infusion devices. *Am J Hosp Pharm* 44:1388–1391, 1987.
18. Mann HJ, Fuhs DW, Cerra FB: Effect of infusion pump fill-stroke flow interruption on response to sodium nitroprusside in surgical patients. *Clin Pharm* 7:214–219, 1988.
19. White PF: Clinical uses of intravenous anesthetic and analgesic infusions. *Anesth Analg* 68:161–171, 1989.
20. Ellinoy BR, Clarke JE, Wagers PW, Swinney RS: Comprehensive pharmaceutical service in a medical intensive care unit. *Am J Hosp Pharm* 41:2335–2342, 1984.
21. Bootman L, Wertheimer AI, Zaske D, et al: Individualizing gentamicin dosage regimens in burn patients with gram-negative septicemia: a cost benefit analysis. *J Pharm Sci* 68:267–272, 1979.
22. Nahata MC: Effect of i.v. drug delivery systems on pharmacokinetic monitoring. *Am J Hosp Pharm* 44:2538–2542, 1987.
23. Hurlbut JC, Thompson S, Reed MD: Influence of infusion pumps on the pharmacologic response to nitroprusside. *Crit Care Med* 19:98–101, 1991.
24. Stull JC, Erenberg A, Leff RD: Flow rate variability from electronic infusion devices. *Crit Care Med* 16:888–891, 1988.
25. Strayer AH, Henry DW, Erenberg A, et al: Administration of whole blood, packed red blood cells, and platelets using a multipurpose infusion pump. *Am J Hosp Pharm* 48:1970–1972, 1991.
26. Burch KJ, Phelps SJ, Constance TD: Effect of an infusion device on the integrity of whole blood and packed red blood cells. *Am J Hosp Pharm* 48:92–97, 1991.
27. Snyder EL, Rinder HM, Napychank P: In vitro and in vivo evaluation of platelet transfusions administered through an electromechanical infusion pump. *Am J Clin Pathol* 94:77–80, 1990.
28. Horrow JC, Digregoria GJ, Barbieri EJ, et al: Intravenous infusions of nitroprusside, dobutamine, and nitroglycerin are compatible. *Crit Care Med* 18:858–861, 1990.
29. Glass P, Jacobs J, Hawkins E, et al: Accuracy and efficacy of a pharmacokinetic model-driven device to infuse fentanyl for anesthesia during general surgery. *Anesthesiology* 69:A290, 1988.
30. McKinley S, Cade JF, Siganporia R, et al: Clinical evaluation of closed-loop control of blood pressure in seriously ill patients. *Crit Care Med* 19:166–170, 1991.
31. Bednarski P, Siclari F, Voigt A, et al: Use of a computerized closed-loop sodium nitroprusside titration system for antihypertensive treatment after open heart surgery. *Crit Care Med* 18:1061–1065, 1990.
32. Barry GA, Bass Jr GE, Eddlemon JK, et al: Bar code technology for documenting administration of large volume intravenous solutions. *Am J Hosp Pharm* 46:282–287, 1989.
33. Meyer GE, Brandell R, Smith JE, et al: Use of bar codes in inpatient drug distribution. *Am J Hosp Pharm* 48:953–966, 1991.

Index

Page numbers followed by *t* and *f* indicate tables and figures, respectively. Page numbers in boldface type indicate major discussions.